Veterinary
Pathology

Veterinary Pathology _____

THOMAS CARLYLE JONES,
B.S., D.V.M., D.Sc. (Hon.)

Professor of Comparative Pathology, New England Regional Primate Research Center, Harvard Medical School; Formerly: Director of Pathology, Angell Memorial Animal Hospital; Lt. Col. U.S. Army Veterinary Corps; Chief, Veterinary Pathology Section, Armed Forces Institute of Pathology.

RONALD DUNCAN HUNT,
B.S., D.V.M.

Professor of Comparative Pathology, Director, New England Regional Primate Research Center, Director Animal Research Center, Harvard Medical School.

FIFTH EDITION _____

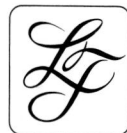

Lea & Febiger · *Philadelphia* · 1983

Lea & Febiger
600 Washington Square
Philadelphia, PA   19106
U.S.A.

Library of Congress Cataloging in Publication Data

Jones, Thomas Carlyle.
  Veterinary pathology.

  Rev. ed. of: Veterinary pathology / Hilton Atmore
Smith, Thomas Carlyle Jones, Ronald Duncan Hunt. 4th
ed. 1972.
  Bibliography: p.
  Includes index.
  1. Veterinary pathology.   I. Hunt, Ronald Duncan.
II. Smith, Hilton Atmore, 1895–1965.   Veterinary path-
ology.   III. Title.   [DNLM: 1. Pathology, Veterinary.
SF 769 J79va]
SF769.J65 1981   636.089′607   81-20820
ISBN 0-8121-0789-6   AACR2

Published in Great Britain by
Bailliere Tindall, London

PRINTED IN THE UNITED STATES OF AMERICA

Print No.   6   5   4   3   2   1

First Edition, 1957

Reprinted, 1958

Second Edition, 1961

Spanish Edition, 1962

Reprinted, 1963

Third Edition, 1966

Reprinted, 1968, 1970

Fourth Edition, 1972

Reprinted, 1974, 1976, 1977, 1978, 1979

Preface

In preparing this fifth edition, the authors have struggled to maintain the original objectives: a textbook of veterinary pathology useful to the veterinary student and a reference book that will be helpful to anyone interested in veterinary pathology. The emphasis continues to focus on anatomic pathology, including as much information on pathogenesis and molecular biology as space permits. In general pathology, recent research has yielded a large mass of data and evolved many new concepts of disease. The size of this book makes it necessary to condense all data and to select and compress theories ruthlessly. Some of these ideas will survive; we hope we have picked at least some of the survivors.

Every effort has been made to consider individual disease states by presenting a brief notation of their clinical features, followed by a succinct description of the gross, microscopic, ultrastructural, and biochemical lesions. Pathogenesis and etiology are also considered briefly and critically.

We hope that this book will stimulate and guide the student toward the further study of this fascinating field, still full of new things to discover. Pertinent references to current literature are provided and historical papers of value have been retained in the reference lists.

Our policy has been to be alert to new ideas based on well-documented data, to maintain a historical perspective, and to keep what is currently useful and likely to remain so. We make no claim to perfection and are always grateful to our colleagues who point out errors or make suggestions for improvement.

We have acknowledged contributions of photographs in the legends. Ideas are acknowledged by listing references. We are pleased to acknowledge the help of several individuals: Dorotha Anne Jones, for editorial assistance and typing; Dr. M. D. Daniel, for reading and commenting helpfully on Chapter 9; Dr. William Hadlow, for his continued interest and offers of photographs over the years; Professor Doctor Hansrudi Luginbühl, for his useful comments and advice; and Mrs. Barbara Luginbühl, for her secretarial assistance. We gratefully acknowledge the help of several members of the Primate Research Center staff: Virginia Werwath, Robin Saunders, Maureen Maguire, and Anne Marie Block, for extensive reference searches and typing of the manuscript; June Armstrong, for photo reproduction and preparation of graphic materials; and Sydney Fingold, for successful efforts to locate the more inaccessible references. We particularly thank Beverly Blake for her editorial assistance and the painstaking retrieval and organization of all original illustrations, which were required for this printing.

The support, encouragement, and patience of Mr. Christian C. F. Spahr, Jr. and his staff at Lea & Febiger are also gratefully acknowledged.

Southborough, Mass.

T.C. Jones
R.D. Hunt

Contents

CHAPTER

CHAPTER 1

Introduction, the Cell, Death of Cells and Tissues

Pathology is the study of the molecular, cellular, tissue or organismal response of the living body (animal or plant) when exposed to injurious agents or deprivations. Many of these injurious agents are chemical compounds, either inorganic or, more frequently, the product of living organisms, the most conspicuous of which are the disease-producing bacteria and viruses. Others consist of energy in such forms as heat and mechanical trauma applied to a harmful degree. While most pathologic conditions arise as a result of the exposure of body tissues to injurious substances, failure of access to various necessary materials such as proteins, minerals, vitamins, water and oxygen can have equally deleterious effects. Inherited factors also play an important role in pathology.

The key word in the definition of pathology is **response**, which represents a spectrum of reactions ranging from cell death to malignant transformation. When this response is deleterious to the individual, it is called disease.

The body is also subjected to many normal stimuli to which it responds in much the same, if not identical, fashions as it does to abnormal or deleterious stimuli. The inflammatory response accompanying menstruation in human beings is the same response that accompanies bacterial pneumonia; only the stimuli and the effect on the host vary. The processes of atrophy and necrosis in the normal disappearance of the thymus are not dissimilar from atrophy and necrosis resulting from an abnormal diminution of blood supply to an organ or part. Certain responses, such as death of a cell following anoxia, are passive, but most, such as inflammations, are active, and in most cases represent normal, life-saving defense reactions. When these reactions resolve or eliminate the insult, they may go unnoticed. When less perfect, clearly visible reactions follow, which may or may not resolve the insult. Thus, our defense reactions are good and bad, or better stated, well adapted and poorly adapted.

The vision a pathologist must develop is to recognize that all of these reactions are real, consistent, and recognizable. He must be aware of the advantages they serve the host as well as the disadvantages: both exist. Animals have not completely adapted to their environment, and as the environment is constantly changing, there is little chance they will.

To the extent that our limited knowledge permits any biologic science to be precise, pathology is that branch of medical studies which attempts to relate specific effects to definite causes. When, if ever, our understanding of the laws of pathology becomes perfect, then it will be possible to predict the effect of a disease-producing agent with just as much certainty as it is now possible to measure the force of gravity and predict the course of a falling body. Under what appear to be entirely comparable conditions, one animal survives an infection and one succumbs, one person develops a malignant neoplasm and another escapes. We pass these things off as biologic variations or differences in resistance and tell ourselves that such irregularities must be expected even in carefully conducted biologic experiments. But let no one suppose that each unexplained event is in reality without adequate and finite cause; it is only because of our incomplete information and knowledge of pertinent facts that we try to group such variable outcomes according to the laws of chance. Too much time has been wasted in considering pathology as a long list of separate observations upon diseased animals and tissues. The things that occur in health and disease are fully related to each other and are founded upon chemical and physical laws as constant as any in science.

The pathologist may approach the study of pathologic processes at any of several different levels. At the **population** level, the interaction of organisms to each other and to the environment under various adverse conditions may contribute to pathologic states. At the level of the **organism**, or individual, pathologic states are manifest by overt clinical signs (observable objectively) or by symptoms subjectively recognized by the human patient and are the result of interaction of changes in one or more organ systems. Specific pathologic changes in **organs** or **tissues** may be recognized by inspection of the gross specimen or by study of preparations under the light microscope. At the **cellular** level, some pathologic features may be recognized with the light microscope; others, involving intracellular organelles, may be visu-

alized only with the electron microscope. At the **molecular** level, the chemical reactions which underlie all pathologic processes may be studied, using the techniques of chemistry and to some extent electron microscopy. Study of pathologic changes at the molecular level is the latest approach to emerge and offers the most promise toward understanding the fundamental processes of pathology.

The careful anatomic study of gross and microscopic preparations (pathologic anatomy) has yielded a great deal of useful information about disease processes and still is valuable as a method of recognizing disease states. It is expected that the techniques and approaches of pathologic anatomy will continue to be useful in arriving at a diagnosis or for limiting the possible diagnoses and therefore are emphasized in this book. Skill and judgment in the use of these tools are not easily acquired but are currently necessary to the specialist in pathology. Deeper elucidation of pathologic problems, old and new, increasingly depend upon use of modern techniques, including those of electron microscopy and biochemistry.

We like to think of each injurious agent as causing a specific sort of injury and provoking a specific reaction on the part of the tissues and, in general, this is the case. The products of the tubercle bacillus, for instance, evoke a tissue response that is readily distinguishable from that resulting from the canine hepatitis virus. It is by virtue of these differences that it is possible to diagnose the type of disease to which the body is being subjected. On the other hand, if the young child falls and hurts his knee, or if he receives a spanking from his parent, the loud reaction is likely to be identical in both cases for the reason that a child of early age has only one way of expressing dissatisfaction, whatever its cause. Likewise, body cells and tissues have only a limited number of ways of reacting to a considerable variety of injurious agents. This is especially true in the central nervous system, where it is particularly difficult to decide from the type of reaction what the injurious agent may have been.

THE NORMAL CELL

Concepts concerning the structural and functional aspects of the cell have drastically changed due to the use of new techniques and instruments, particularly the electron microscope. This instrument makes it possible to clearly visualize many organelles whose existence within the cell heretofore were only speculative. It is now possible to demonstrate the structural basis for functions that biochemical techniques reveal at the molecular level. Many of these events underlie the processes that can ·be recognized as disease in the cell, tissue, or organism. Many structures, which are recognized as components of normal cells and whose function is at least partially understood, are most certainly involved in disease processes. However, relatively few of the morphologic changes at the ultrastructural level have been clearly established in relation to disease in the organism, although the list of ultramicroscopic lesions is growing rapidly. It is now important to understand the structural and functional components of the cell at the magnifications of the electron microscope in order to appreciate current research in pathology. In some particular disease problems this understanding is also necessary to arrive at a definitive diagnosis. A brief review of the current status of knowledge of the ultrastructure of cells is therefore considered pertinent in an introduction to pathology.

The **cell membrane** is not visible by the light microscope but has been presumed to surround the cytoplasm because of indirect indications: cytoplasm flows from the cell after it is pricked by a microdissection needle; cells shrink in hypertonic solution and swell in hypotonic solution; the cell is highly permeable to lipid-soluble substances and less permeable to ions—

suggesting that the cell membrane consists of lipid or lipoprotein. Ultra-thin sections of cells disclose that the limiting membrane has a remarkably constant structure, consisting of two electron-dense lines, each about 30Å thick, separated by a light line of about the same thickness. (Å or Au is the Ångström unit, equivalent to 0.0001 micron, and is named after the Swedish physicist, Anders J. Ångström [1814–1874].)

This trilaminar arrangement is remarkably similar in most animal cells and has been referred to by some as the "unit membrane." The two outer layers are currently believed to consist of protein, the intermediate layer of lipid. The membrane is not always smooth but may be evaginated to produce specialized structures such as **microvilli**, which increase absorptive surfaces on such cells as the epithelial cells lining intestinal villi. The brush border of some cells of the renal tubules is made up of similar microvilli. The cell membrane may also be invaginated into the cytoplasm, probably as a part of the process known as **pinocytosis**. This process results in the engulfing of a minute droplet of fluid from the interstitium. This fluid contains inorganic ions such as sodium, which in part are eliminated by a process that requires energy (the "sodium pump"). Although the cell membrane acts as a semipermeable membrane, permitting the passive transfer of substances varying in molecular size, chemical composition, and electrical charge, active regulatory mechanisms are necessary to maintain a cell in homeostasis. Active membrane transports called ion pumps depend on cellular production of large amounts of ATP supplied by mitochondrial and glycolytic phosphorylations. As we shall see, any disruption in these pumps will lead to cell death. Cells are not at equilibrium with their environment; sodium, calcium, and water must be moved from the cell and potassium and magnesium into the cell against the forces of Donnan equilibrium,

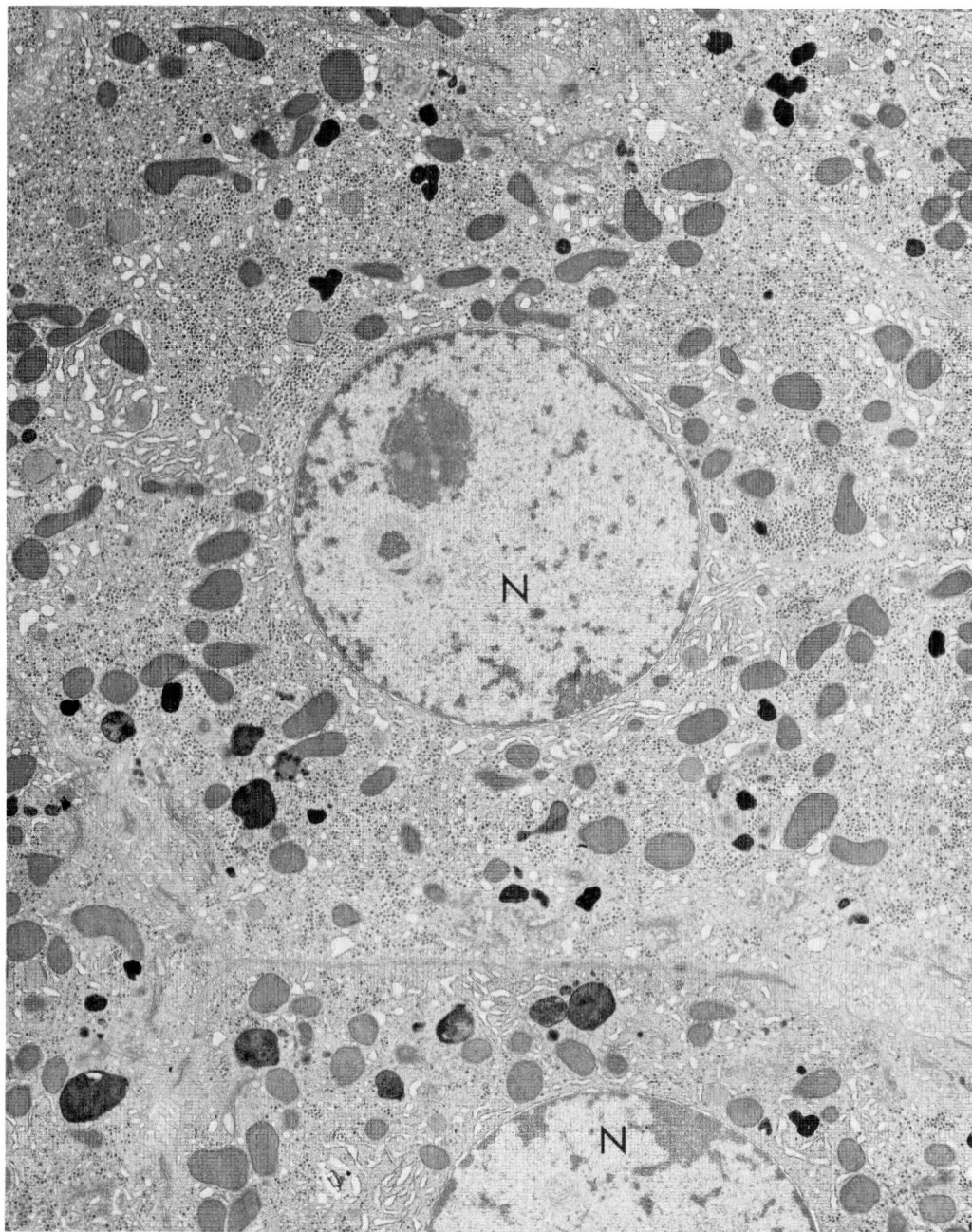

Fig. 1–1. The cell. Electron micrograph (× 10,350) of parts of three liver cells of an owl monkey (*Aotus trivirgatus*). Note: nucleus (N), mitochondria (membrane bound irregularly ovoid structures), lysosomes (electron dense bodies), glycogen (smallest dense granules), cell membranes (separating adjacent cells). (Courtesy of Dr. Norval W. King.)

exerted by the presence of negatively charged, nondiffusible intracellular macromolecules, chiefly protein.

Many modifications of the cell membrane structure occur in different situations, such as between adjoining cells or over free surfaces; these are interesting but will not be considered further here.

The **cytoplasm** of the normal cell, which under the light microscope appears to consist of eosinophilic, homogeneous to granular ground substance containing various inclusions and vesicles, contains an amazing array of organelles visible under the electron microscope. The number of each organelle varies with the type of cell and with its functional state. Among the most conspicuous are the **mitochondria**, which are discrete structures, visible with the light microscope, usually measuring 2 to 3 μ in length but often much longer. They vary in number, size, and shape, but usually appear as slender tubules with blind ends and are occasionally bent or folded. Often they are found in close proximity to structures which require energy, such as cardiac or skeletal muscle fibers or lipid globules. They were recognized in cells as early as 1850, but Benda, in 1898, was the first to use the term "mitochondrion." Each mitochondrion is outlined by an outer membrane, about 70 Å thick, separated by a clear space about 80 Å wide from a similar inner membrane. This inner membrane extends into the mitochondrion as lamellae, or tubular arrays called **cristae**. These cristae may be few in number, extending only a short distance into the matrix of the mitochondrion, or they may be numerous, closely packed, and bridge the width of the mitochondrion.

The more complex arrays of cristae appear to be associated with increased oxidative capacity. Differential centrifugation has been used to isolate mitochondria in quantities suitable for chemical analysis and to demonstrate that they are the principal sites of the oxidative reactions that make the energy in foodstuff available for cell metabolism. The necessary enzymes are situated for the most part in the membranes, presumably with spatial arrangements that permit the sequential events in the cytochrome chains linked to the Krebs cycle. Oxidative phosphorylation leads to the transfer of the energy released by oxidation to adenosine diphosphate (ADP) and its eventual storage in the form of adenosine triphosphate (ATP).

A complex system of membranes, which traverses the cytoplasm to form canaliculi, cisternae, vesicles, or parallel arrays, is known as the **endoplasmic reticulum** or **ergastoplasm**. Some of the membranes are smooth and are usually referred to as the **smooth-surfaced** or **agranular endoplasmic reticulum**. Others are studded with distinct granular bodies, **ribosomes**, and are therefore referred to as **rough-surfaced** or **granular endoplasmic reticulum**. This type has its greatest development in glandular cells which produce a secretion containing protein. However, synthesis of protein is known to be associated with ribosomes that may function adequately in the absence of endoplasmic reticulum. The endoplasmic reticulum appears to be necessary as a system of pathways that segregate the cell product, transport it to the Golgi region, store it temporarily, and later move it to the exterior of the cell.

The granular reticulum usually appears in electron micrographs as thin profiles of membranes that form flat saccular expanses, called **cisternae**, from a pair of membranes 300 to 600 Å apart. These membranes are continuous with one another at the end of their profile. These may be single, or more often, aggregated together and form intercommunicating tubules as well as cisternae. Vesicles may also be formed in isolated portions of the endoplasmic reticulum.

Smooth-surfaced (agranular) endoplasmic reticulum often appears to be continuous with the rough variety—differing only in the absence of ribosomes. This type of membrane is richest in cells of the endo-

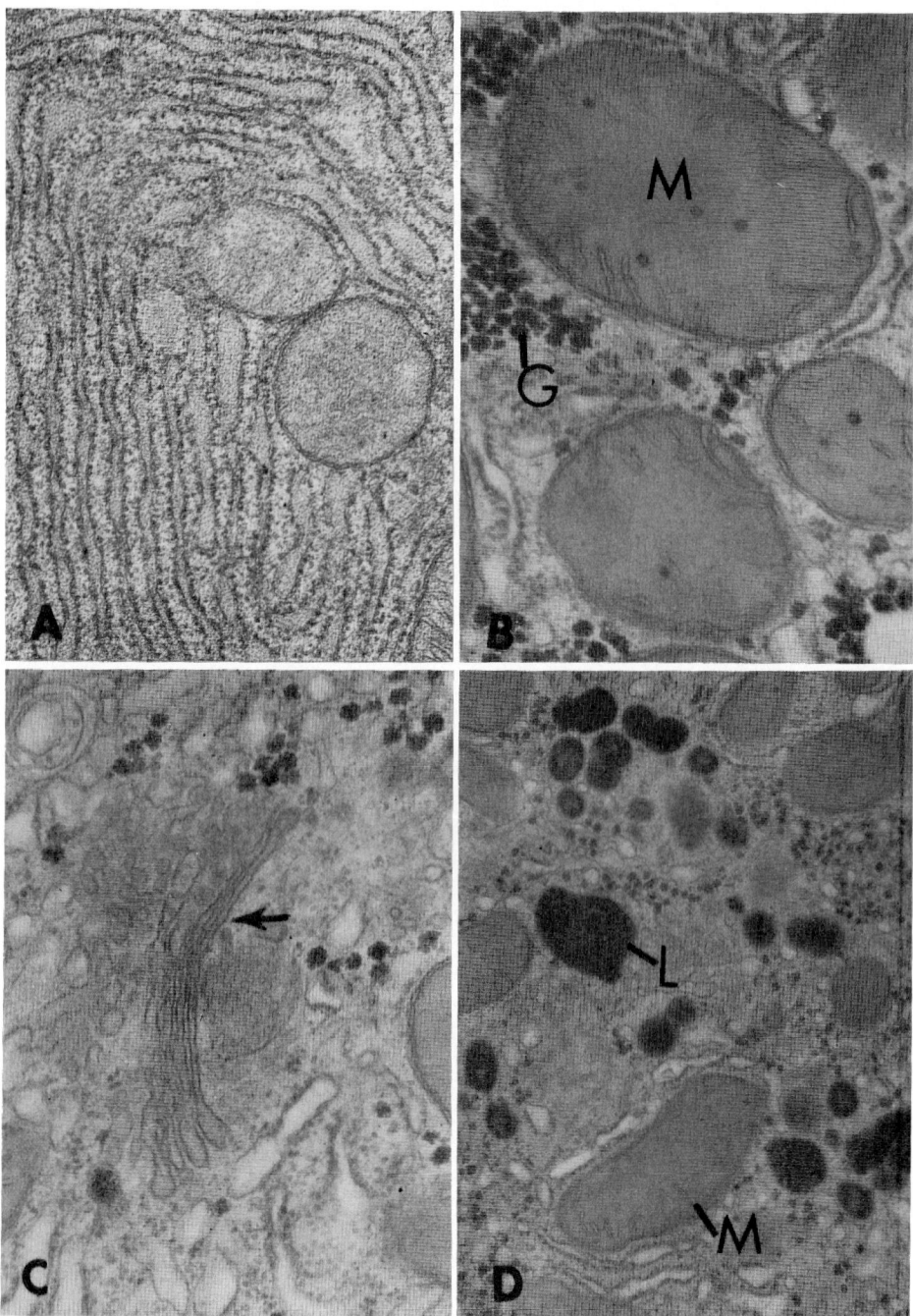

Fig. 1–2. Intracellular organelles in electron micrographs. *A*, Rough endoplasmic reticulum in a plasma cell (× 36,000). *B*, Mitochondria (M) and glycogen (G) (× 44,500). *C*, Golgi apparatus. Each preparation from owl monkeys (*Aotus trivirgatus*). *D*, Lysosomes (largest at L) and mitochondria (M) (× 22,900). (Courtesy of Dr. Norval W. King.)

crine glands, but may be caused to increase in liver cells by administration of certain drugs such as barbiturates. Thus, agranular reticulum is believed to be involved in the production of hormones, and it possibly has a role in detoxification.

The endoplasmic reticulum cannot be clearly visualized with the light microscope, but it was probably demonstrated many years ago in preparations of muscle cells impregnated with metal. Basic dyes stain structures in the cytoplasm which probably are cisternae, and these structures have been called basophilic bodies, Nissl substance, chromophilic substance, or ergastoplasm. The electron microscope was required to demonstrate the canalicular nature, reticular formation, and widespread occurrence of the endoplasmic reticulum.

The **Golgi complex**, or Golgi apparatus, was discovered by Golgi in 1898 in nerve cells that had been treated for a prolonged period in a solution of osmium tetroxide. Golgi called this structure the "internal reticular apparatus." Prolonged immersion in osmium tetroxide ("postosmication") is necessary to stain this structure, although it may be demonstrated by light microscopy following negative staining with toluidine blue. A long controversy over the actual existence of this structure, in part due to the failure to demonstrate it in living cells, was resolved by the use of the electron microscope. The complex is usually located near the nucleus and, in glandular cells, at the apical pole of the nucleus. Secreting granules are usually in close proximity.

In ultra-thin sections, the Golgi complex is made up of aggregations of closely packed, membrane-bound elements arranged parallel to one another and joined at their ends. These packets vary in length, are usually about 150 Å wide, and may be flat or curved. Clustered around the ends of these packets are many small vesicles, 400 to 800 Å in diameter. On the inner, or concave, surface of the complex, the cisternae

are often distended and contain secretory products. Secretory granules are usually adjacent and surrounded by a membrane apparently arising from the Golgi complex.

The functions of the Golgi complex are not entirely known, but it is believed that it assembles secretory products brought to it through the endoplasmic reticulum after synthesis by the ribosomes. Polysaccharides may be added by the Golgi complex to the protein brought to it. Lipid absorbed by cells of the small intestine may accumulate in the Golgi complex of intestinal epithelial cells, but the exact nature of the chemical events at this site is not known. It is possible that other functions may be found for this structure.

Lysosomes were originally found by differential centrifugation of tissue suspensions, and defined as membrane-bound particles containing one or more hydrolytic enzymes. Structures meeting this chemical definition are found with difficulty in electron micrographs by demonstrating, with cytochemical staining, the presence of acid phosphatase. Bodies containing this enzyme have diverse morphologic features in different tissues. The specific granules of neutrophils and eosinophils contain acid hydrolases and are therefore clearly lysosomes. Certain membrane-limited dense bodies, which are found in relation to the Golgi complex and in bile canaliculi in the liver, also meet the criteria for lysosomes. Morphologic criteria alone are not sufficient to identify lysosomes, hence much confusion will probably continue in connection with these structures within the cytoplasm of cells, except in cases in which electron microscopic and biochemical methods are used in concert.

The **centrioles** may be resolved with the light microscope as a pair of deeply stained short rods (sometimes called the diplosome). They are often adjacent to the nucleus in a zone known as the centrosome or cell center. Cytologists often refer to a line projected through the nucleus and the centrosome as the "cell axis." In some cells, the centrioles are surrounded by the Golgi complex; in others, they are located immediately beneath the cell membrane. One to forty pairs may occupy a single cell. The functions of the centrioles are not clear, but apparently include the organization of the cell, particularly during cell division. Their position, after they have replicated, at opposite poles of the nucleus during mitosis is significant in the movement of the chromosomes to opposite poles of the cytoplasm. The chromosomes are connected to dense bodies (satellites) adjacent to the centriole by means of the spindle fibers which in electron micrographs are seen to be **microtubules**. In ciliated cells, reduplicated centrioles form the "basal bodies," which give rise to the cilia and serve as their kinetic centers.

Structurally, the electron microscope reveals each centriole to consist of a hollow cylinder, 0.15 μ in diameter and up to 0.5 μ long. One end of this cylinder is open, the other closed. The pair is often arranged with each long axis perpendicular to the other. The wall of the cylinder is made up of nine evenly spaced, hollow fibrils or tubules, each in triplicate. In some cells, ill defined, often spherical bodies up to 700 Å in diameter are seen adjacent to the centriole. These pericentriolar structures are the satellites to which the "spindle fibers" are attached.

Electron micrographs of the **nucleus** confirm the presence of structures seen by light microscopy and resolve many details, but disclose few new organelles, in contrast to the rich lode found in the cytoplasm. The **nuclear envelope** consists of two membranes, each about 75 Å thick, separated by a space about 400 to 700 Å wide, the **perinuclear cisterna**. The outer membrane of the envelope is studded with ribosomes and often is continuous with endoplasmic reticulum of the cytoplasm. The nuclear envelope has its origin from these membranes. The inner and outer membranes of the nuclear envelope are diverted at intervals around circular structures called **nuclear pores**. These are not freely communicating fenestrations, but under high resolution appear to be closed by a characteristic membrane. These so-called pores may be the means of transfer of materials to and from the cytoplasm under enzymatic control. The perinuclear cisterna appears to be the means of exchange of most materials with the cytoplasm. Some cells have a third membrane on the inner surface of the nuclear envelope. This is a filamentous structure, moderately dense, about 300 Å thick, and is called the **fibrous lamina**. It appears to function as a supportive skeleton for the cell.

Most of the content of the nucleus is made up of basophilic material called **chromatin**. Its distribution and structure depends upon the type of cell, its functional state, and the fixation and staining procedures used. The most dense granular component forms masses of various sizes; it is called **heterochromatin** and is considered to be relatively inactive metabolically. One specific mass of chromatin, located adjacent to the nuclear envelope in cells of females, is the **sex chromatin**, representing the inactive X chromosome. The more loosely arranged chromatin granules make up the **euchromatin** and are considered to be in the metabolically active state. Both stain characteristically with Feulgen reagent, demonstrating the principal component to be deoxyribonucleic acid (DNA) (see Chapter 8).

The **nucleolus**, readily recognized with the light microscope, also has a characteristic ultrastructure. This organelle appears to have a key role in the synthesis of protein and metabolism of nucleic acids. It consists of a rounded mass of chromatin, usually eccentrically placed, basophilic, and staining specifically for ribonucleic acid (RNA). It disappears during mitosis, but in the interphase, the nucleus has two ultrastructural components. The **nucleolonema** appears as branching coarse strands that form a network. Under higher magnification these strands are seen to consist of a matrix in which are embedded dense granules resembling ribosomes. These granules are judged to be made up of ribonucleoprotein. The nucleolonema usually surrounds a spherical, apparently structureless component of the nucleolus, the **pars amorpha**.

The nucleus is not essential for the life of some cells, such as the mature erythrocyte and the epithelial cells in the interior of the lens, but it is necessary for the cell to divide or carry out complex metabolic activities. Present concepts make the DNA of the nucleus responsible for the character of the enzymes that control all functions of the cell and, by exact replication of the DNA and its distribution to daughter cells in the chromosomes, determine the characteristics of each cell generation. This is discussed further in Chapter 8.

Many **cell inclusions** are resolved in the cytoplasm in more detail with the electron microscope, although most have been recognized with the light microscope. These include secretory products, such as those found in anterior pituitary cells, pancreatic islets, and other endocrine cells. Similar inclusions are found in exocrine gland cells, such as in salivary, goblet, mucous, chief, pancreatic acinar, and Brunner's gland cells. Neurosecretory granules are another important cell inclusion. Pigments such as melanin and lipofuscin are included in this category, as are glycogen, lipid, and crystalline inclusions. These are described in detail in the appropriate chapters.

Cell Injury, Death, and Necrosis

Cellular death has been defined by Majno (1960) as a process during which the cell loses its integrity as a functional unit. A "point of no return" is visualized as a singular point beyond which damage to the cell is no longer reversible and the cell is dead. Death of tissue in the living body is known as necrosis. **Necrosis**, which will be discussed more fully later, includes the

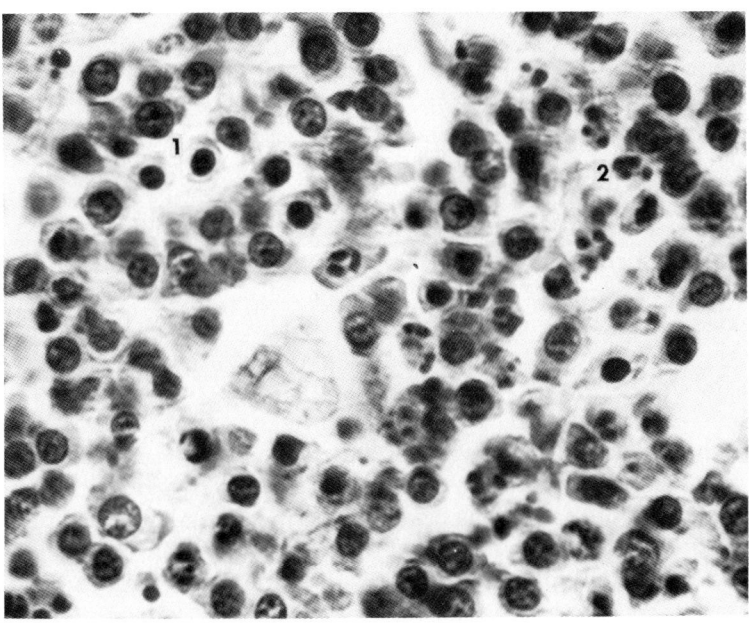

Fig. 1-3. Necrosis, evidenced by pyknosis and karyorrhexis of nuclei in neoplastic cells of a canine malignant lymphoma after treatment with nitrogen mustard. Pyknotic nuclei (*1*) are round, decreased in size and homogeneous; nuclei undergoing karyorrhexis (*2*) are fragmented into several pieces. (H & E, × 600.)

subsequent degeneration of a dead cell in the living body by hydrolytic reactions which convert the cell to a mass of debris or complete dissolution to simple inorganic compounds. In part, this decomposition results from the release of hydrolases from lysosomes, a process of self-digestion or **autolysis**. Dissolution of the cell is furthered by products of other cells, such as neutrophils, a process termed **heterolysis**. Heterolysis is an active event dependent on living tissues and therefore only occurs in the living body.

The term **necrobiosis** is used by some as a synonym for necrosis and by others to mean the death of cells at the end of their life span, as is natural in most healthy tissues.

Dissolution of cells not previously injured also follows death of the body. This also results from the process of autolysis, with no essential difference from autolysis of a dead cell in the living body. It is common to use the term autolysis as a strictly postmortem event, but this is not true. After death of the body, the term must be prefaced by the adjective **postmortem**. Products of putrefactive bacteria result in further decomposition after somatic death.

Thus, the changes in the dead cells and tissues are essentially the same whether they have died with the animal as a whole, which constitutes postmortem autolysis, or whether this particular group of cells died within the living animal, which by definition is necrosis. But, while the gross and microscopic appearances of dead cells remain the same regardless of which way they died, the significance to the pathologist is quite another matter. If it can be established that the observed changes occurred after the death of the patient, they have no connection with disease and are of no concern to the physician, pathologist, or biologist. But if the cells underwent necrosis, a process occurring within the living body which is obviously abnormal and unhealthy, this becomes something of great interest and concern in the study of

disease and to anyone undertaking to combat it. We propose first to describe the observable changes incident to death of cells and then to describe how necrosis can be distinguished from postmortem autolysis.

Since a fixative, such as a 10% solution of formalin, promptly puts a stop to lytic or other changes in body cells, it is customary in microscopic pathology to speak of a cell or tissue as living if its characteristics are those of cells that were living when placed in the fixative, and as dead if it shows any of the series of changes about to be discussed as occurring after death. These, if present, must have developed between the time of actual death of the cells and their fixation. As will be shown, it becomes a matter of prime importance for the pathologist to know whether he is dealing with "living" or "dead" cells and tissues.

The fact is that there is no way of saying exactly when the death of a cell occurred, but a minimum of six to twelve hours lapse between cell death and incontroversial recognition that the cell is dead by light microscopy. This is also influenced by the nature and severity of the injury and the cell type. These factors are also important in determining whether the injury will lead to cell death or reversible damage. For example, neurons and myocardial cells are more susceptible to anoxia than fibroblasts; renal tubular epithelium is more susceptible to mercuric ions than myocardium; hepatocytes are more susceptible to carbon tetrachloride than gastrointestinal epithelium; proximal convoluted tubular epithelium is more subject to injury than distal convoluted tubules. Cells with large amounts of hydrolytic enzymes, such as exocrine pancreas cells, undergo autolysis (ante- or postmortem) more rapidly than less active cells, such as fibroblasts.

CAUSES OF CELL INJURY AND DEATH

A wide number of environmental insults may lead to cell injury and death. These are dealt with in detail in subsequent chapters,

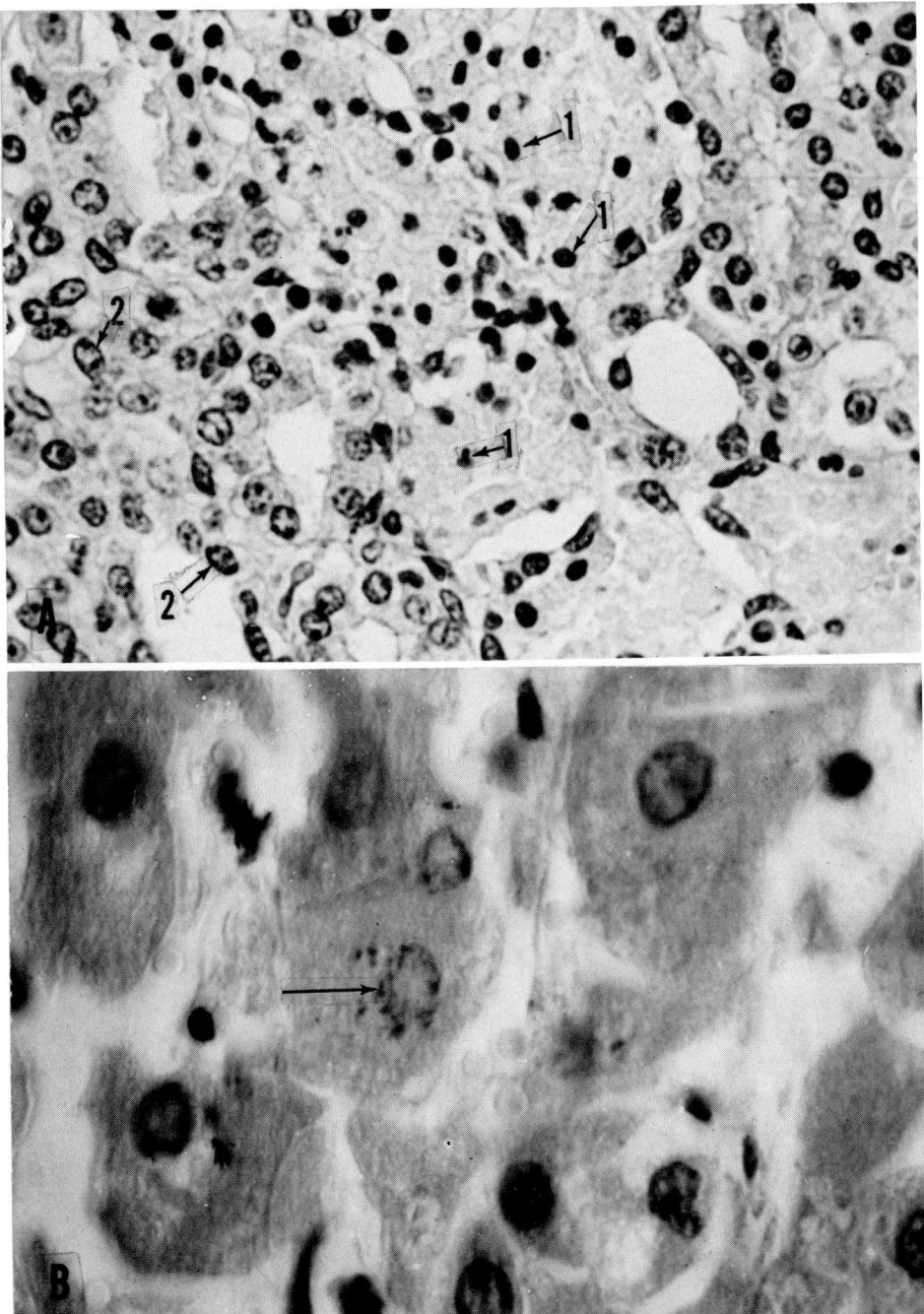

Fig. 1–4. *A*, Pyknosis. Small, round, densely staining nuclei (*1*) at the margin of an infarct in the kidney of a pig. Compare with the nuclei (2) of unaffected renal tubules. (× 490.) (Courtesy of Armed Forces Institute of Pathology.) Contributor: Lt. Col. F. D. Maurer. *B*, Karyorrhexis. Fragmentation of nuclear chromatin (arrow) in a liver cell of a dog. (× 800.) (Courtesy of Armed Forces Institute of Pathology.)

and the following represents generalizations.

Poisons

It is difficult to state exactly what is meant by the term poison. Included is the idea of a substance with a definite chemical structure, simple or complex, known or unknown, which produces injury when taken into or applied to the animal body. The injury may result from a number of mechanisms varying with the kind of poison, but many poisons produce injury either locally by direct contact or remotely when distributed in the blood. It is convenient to divide poisons into four classes according to their origin.

"**Chemical poisons**" are chemical preparations, usually articles of commerce such as drugs, insecticides, and a great variety of substances used in the industries. The insecticide, lead arsenate, is a good example; when ingested in a large amount and in somewhat concentrated form, it kills many of the cells with which it comes in contact, producing intestinal ulceration; taken in small amounts and suitably diluted over a period of time, it slowly destroys the delicate parenchymal cells of the liver, which it reaches by way of the blood. Strong acids and strong alkalies also belong in this group.

The toxins, or poisons of pathogenic microorganisms, are the principal means by which such organisms produce disease, necrosis of delicate parenchymatous cells often being a prominent feature. The necrophorus bacillus is outstanding for its ability to kill the tissues around it wherever it may localize. The blackleg organism kills the muscle tissue where it localizes.

Poisons produced by certain plants and animals cause cell death, either locally or in the cells of parenchymatous organs such as the liver and kidney. Even the common "chigger" (Trombicula sp.) causes necrosis of a zone around its tiny bite in susceptible humans. Hypersensitization may be a factor in this case. Slow death of hepatic or renal epithelium is a feature of many plant poisonings.

Toxins or **poisons produced by decomposition** processes in the body are well illustrated in the death of liver cells which follows severe burns in any part of the body. Absorbed toxic products from decomposing tissue at the site of the burn are considered responsible.

Viruses

Viruses and certain other intracellular parasites do not require toxins or poisons to injure cells, but rather interfere with cellular metabolism at the level of nucleic acid control. An infected cell cannot carry out life sustaining functions, such as protein synthesis and energy metabolism.

Lack of Proper Blood Supply

Not all tissues require the same amount of blood, but the minimum must be met or the tissue will die. The immediately critical requirement is that of oxygen. The arterial flow to a part can be partially or completely obstructed by lodged emboli and thrombosis within the artery, or by compression of the artery by ligatures, tourniquets (which should be temporarily released at intervals of 20 minutes), or the pressure of nearby tumors or abscesses. The blood vessels of the bowel are obstructed by twisting or compression of the mesentery in which they run, such as occurs in intestinal volvulus or intussusception. Ergotism (poisoning by ergot, the "smut" of grains and grasses) causes death of the extremities because its contractile effect on smooth muscle constricts the arteries until the more distal ones are obliterated. Poisoning by tall fescue grass (Festuca arundiacca) has a similar effect. Stagnation of the flow of blood in venous congestion is a factor in the necrosis of the central cells of the hepatic lobules whenever there is prolonged impairment of cardiac function (see toxic hepatitis).

Lack of Nerve Supply

It is still unsettled to what extent "trophic" nerve fibers are essential for proper nutrition of the tissues, but it is known that limbs and other parts suffer atrophy and necrosis of many cells when deprived of normal innervation. A good example is seen in "sweeney" of the horse. The animal, when put to heavy work without gradual conditioning, is prone to develop a sudden shoulder lameness, and in a very few days the supraspinatus or the infraspinatus muscle, or both, waste away until the skin lies almost in direct contact with the scapula. The collar puts undue pressure on the suprascapular nerve where it passes over the anterior edge of the scapula, impairing the continuity of many of its fibers. In the resultant paralyzed state of these muscles, many or most of their fibers disappear. In the case of some, the necrosis becomes complete; in others, the sarcoplasm is destroyed but the sarcolemma persists. These latter muscle fibers are capable of regeneration concurrently with the nerve fibers.

Pressure

Severe pressure suddenly applied would be classed as trauma, which is discussed next. Pressure necrosis is that which occurs as the result of long-continued, often relatively mild pressure. Spectacular examples are seen in bedsores (decubitus ulcers) and at the site of casts or bandages. An animal recumbent for some days, even though carefully bedded, will often suffer slow death of the skin and all soft tissues over the bony prominences of the body, such as the tuber coxae and the zygomatic arch. In spite of the best of nursing, the same unfortunate complications arise with even greater frequency in humans, for the reason that life commonly continues longer for the bed-fast human patient. Casts and bandages applied too tightly may be removed only to reveal an ulcerated and necrotic skin beneath. This is not to be confused with death of a whole limb which sometimes results from shutting off its circulation (lack of blood supply) by a tight cast or bandage. Slower in development but no less sure is the necrosis of parenchymal cells of soft organs as they yield to the continuous pressure of encroaching tumors or abscesses. In these cases, the necrosis proceeds so insidiously that few dead cells may be seen at any given moment, an example of necrosis detected by "absence of cell."

Mechanical and Thermal Injuries

Any number of forms of physical trauma can be severe enough to kill body cells in the area involved. This is readily believed by almost anyone whose thumb has accidentally borne the brunt of a hammer-blow intended for a nail. In addition to such purely mechanical injuries, heat and the various related forms of energy can have similar effects. The latter include light rays, ultraviolet rays, roentgen rays, radiations from radium and other radioactive substances, and electric current. All tend to coagulate protoplasm, thus killing the cells, and if sufficiently severe, to carbonize it.

The milder **burns** may not immediately kill even the epidermis but cause only erythema. They are known as burns of the **first degree**; however the epidermis usually desquamates a week later, as in the case of sunburns and mild burns by ultraviolet light. Burns of the **second degree** also produce a serous inflammatory exudate in the form of vesicles (blisters) between the epidermis and the dermis. **Third degree** burns kill the tissue outright to an appreciable depth.

Freezing kills cells directly by bursting their walls as well as by disarranging the colloidal suspensions of the protoplasm. However, extremities can suffer necrosis and gangrene without actually being frozen, for at near-freezing temperature the blood becomes a sludge and stops flowing, and the tissues die from lack of blood supply.

Nutritional Deficiencies and Excesses

Lack of essential nutrients will lead to death of cells by reducing available metabolites, or indirectly through such mechanisms as anoxia in severe iron deficiency anemia. Excesses of certain nutrients, such as vitamin A, calcium, or fluoride, may also lead to cell injury.

Immune Mechanism

Antigen-antibody reactions and cell-mediated immune responses may lead to cell injury. A variety of mechanisms may contribute, ranging from direct injury by a killer lymphocyte to indirect mechanisms dependent upon other chemicals or cells, such as neutrophils in the Arthus reaction.

EVENTS LEADING TO CELL DEATH

Despite the multiplicity of causes of cell injury, certain basic mechanisms and alterations appear to be operant following most insults. Only a few forms of cell injury have been studied in detail, and therefore generalizations to other situations may not be accurate. The effects of anoxia on the cell are the best understood, which provide the basis for this discussion, but similar mechanisms appear to be involved in exposure to infectious, chemical, and physical agents. Following injury a series of events unfold that ultimately lead to loss of integrity of cellular membranes and acute cellular swelling.

Acute Cellular Swelling. Swelling of cells is one of the earliest recognizable events following injury. If severe, it is recognizable at the light microscopic level and is known as **hydropic or vacuolar degeneration.** The cause of this phenomenon is a failure of the ionic pump mechanism. As stated earlier, cells are not at equilibrium with their environment, and an energy-dependent active process (ionic pump) is required to counteract the leaking of sodium and water into the cell and potassium from the cell through the permeable cell membrane. Any failure in the pump results in an influx of cations and water in an attempt to reach equilibrium with the environment, an event that ultimately leads to rupture of the cell.

In the case of hypoxia and some other injuries, mitochondrial function stops, curtailing the availability of ATP, without which the ionic pumps fail. Temporarily the anaerobic glycolytic pathway supplies ATP, but the release of lactic and other organic acids and the drop in cellular pH results in enzyme inhibition, especially of phosphofructokinase, further curtailing the production of ATP. Glycolysis results in a **decrease in glycogen,** which is one of the earliest recognizable events in all injury. The decrease in cellular pH causes clumping of nuclear chromatin and inactivation of nuclear RNA synthesis.

The decreased activity of the ionic pump is followed by an influx of sodium and calcium and a loss of potassium and magnesium. The increased water content results in dilation of the endoplasmic reticulum and swelling of the cell. Structures such as microvilli become distorted. The fall in ATP also results in decreased protein synthesis, further augmented by the loss of potassium. Mitochondrial membranes become more permeable and these organelles, in turn, swell. The change in mitochondrial membrane permeability results in leakage of enzymes into the cell sap and eventually through the altered cell membrane, into the extracellular space and subsequently the blood. Raised serum levels of these soluble enzymes provides a clinical diagnostic measurement to establish the existence of cell injury, and due to the uniqueness of isoenzymes, often identifies the affected organ.

Calcium also enters the cell and precipitates with phosphate on internal cell membranes. Calcium activates phospholipase, which leads to a loss of phospholipid from the cell membrane, resulting in further membrane dysfunction. The increase in cellular concentration of calcium ions may be of primary importance to the cell's passing the point of no return. It is at this stage that the damage has become irreversible and the cell has reached the point of no return or is dead. Lysosomes begin to swell and hydrolytic enzymes leak through their membranes, initiating the process of autolysis, leading to self-digestion, coagulation, and denaturation of cellular proteins. It has been postulated that cell death is the result of lysosomal enzyme release (suicide-bag hypothesis); however, most evidence indicates that this event follows cell death. Exceptions to this generalization include rupture of lysosomes in silicosis and gout.

Several other morphologic features are evident at about this time. Ribosomes disappear from the ER membranes, blebs and breaks appear in the cell membrane and membranes of internal organelles, nuclear chromatin loses its density, dense inclusions appear in the cytoplasm, and myelin figures may form. Myelin figures or inclusions result from release of hydrophilic phospholipids which form lamellar whorls of membranes resembling myelin.

As indicated, these events appear to be common to most forms of cell injury. A partial exception is direct damage to the cell membrane by physical, chemical, or immunologic injury. Here the loss of membrane integrity is immediate and cellular swelling more rapid, both occurring prior to a drop in ATP.

With initiation of autolysis, the cell enters the stage of necrosis, which is readily recognizable by light microscopic features and often gross changes.

Cloudy Swelling. Rudolph Virchow, in 1860, proposed the term, *"trübe schwellung"* (opaque swelling), to a describe a particular swelling characterized by an opaque cytoplasm due to protein accumulation. The translation of the term into English, "cloudy swellng," was approved by Virchow, but over the ensuing years, the term has been corrupted by application to

other changes, including acute cellular swelling. In the latter, the cells are actually less opaque due to water uptake. As the term no longer has precise meaning, it should be abandoned.

CHARACTERISTICS OF NECROTIC CELLS AND TISSUES

As indicated earlier, death of tissue is known as necrosis (noun), which includes the subsequent degeneration of the dead tissue. Dead tissue is called **necrotic** (adjective; e.g., necrotic tissue; necrotic myocardium). The active verb describing the process is **to necrotize** (syn. necrose), and agents leading to or causing the state of necrosis are called **necrotizing**.

Microscopic Appearance of Dead Tissue

(Note to the student: We frequently give the microscopic description before giving the gross characteristics. One reason for doing this is to impress upon you the fact that if the microscopic appearances are known, the gross picture can usually be deduced with considerable accuracy; the converse is not necessarily true. A part of the student's training should involve practice in these deductions.)

Changes in the Nucleus. Pyknosis. This is one of the common manifestations of the death of cells, although it must not be supposed that pyknosis will be seen in every dead cell. The pyknotic nucleus is **decreased in size** but **round**, more perfectly so than it was during life. The nucleus is **black** or nearly so when stained by ordinary stains, such as hematoxylin and eosin. This is because it is more acid in its reaction and attracts the basic hematoxylin; its nucleic acid is being set free. The pyknotic nucleus is **homogeneous**; it lacks the nucleolus, chromatin granules, and internal structure characteristic of most kinds of nuclei during life. Pyknosis is best seen in epithelial cells, leukocytes, and nerve cells. The elongated nuclei of connective tissue and muscle cells, of course, do not become round, but the loss of internal structure and the shrinking are conspicuous features of the dead smooth-muscle nucleus. Pyknosis is one of the earlier changes in point of time; ultimately the dead nucleus disappears altogether.

Karyorrhexis. Literally a breaking up of the nucleus, this term is used to designate the dead nucleus that is reduced to many tiny fragments, barely visible, and these may remain to mark the original position of the nucleus or they may be scattered over a considerable space. Karyorrhexis is seen occasionally and is a step in the development of caseous necrosis to be described later.

Karyolysis. This is dissolution of the nuclear material. When complete, the nucleus naturally is not seen, but the term is used to refer to the incomplete stages, when the nucleus appears as a hollow sphere, a ghost with only the nuclear membrane remaining.

A corollary process to karyolysis is **chromatolysis**. The stainable material of the nucleus, including the nucleolus, the chromosomes, and other visible structures, is known as **chromatin** because it gives the nucleus its color (blue by ordinary stains). In karyolysis, the chromatin is dissolved. The dissolved chromatin does not necessarily vanish but is in solution in the intracellular fluids of the vicinity, carrying its blue color with it. This accounts for a diffuse bluish discoloration in some unusual locations; for instance, if there is fibrin in the neighborhood, it will absorb the chromatin and become blue instead of its usual magenta.

Absence of the Nucleus. All of the preceding nuclear changes terminate in complete destruction of the nucleus. If the nucleus is absent, the cell is dead. The erythrocyte may be considered an exception, but it has lost, with its nucleus, its reproductive power and other characteristics of life.

Changes in the Cytoplasm. In some cases the cytoplasm may reveal relatively little change, but if changes in the nucleus indicate death, the cell should be considered dead. The following abnormalities of cytoplasm may be present.

Unusually Acidophilic Cytoplasm. The cytoplasm is acidophilic because its reaction is more basic than during life, hence it takes the acid stain, which is usually red (eosin). The cytoplasm, then, is a deeper red than usual. Cytoplasmic structure is obscured. This sign of death is prominent when the more delicate epithelial cells, such as those of renal tubules and liver, undergo the condition called coagulation necrosis, the nuclei being concomitantly pyknotic. The cytoplasm of dead polymorphonuclear neutrophils is also often conspicuously red-staining, as seen in pus. This acidophilia is believed to be largely the result of loss of nucleoproteins (ribonucleoprotein and deoxyribonucleoprotein), i.e., loss of basophilia, from the cytoplasm and nucleus, and an increase in positively charged reactive sites along polypeptide chains after denaturation.

Cytoplasmolysis. As the changes of death and necrosis progress, the cytoplasm tends to become less and less dense and ultimately disappears completely. It is possible for much of the cytoplasm to disappear while the cell remains alive, however, and therefore the decision whether the cell is living or dead under circumstances of partial lysis of cytoplasm should depend on the condition of the nucleus.

More Advanced Changes in the Cell as a Whole. *Loss of Cell Outline.* When the changes of necrosis are well advanced, it may be impossible to see the form and outline of the cells, although the material of which they are made is obviously still present. In applying this criterion, one must not be misled by failure to identify cell outlines, which are often indistinct in normal histology, such as those in stratified squamous epithelium and smooth muscle. The condition under consideration may be illustrated by the cells of an inflammatory exudate in which the nucleus, or remains of it, may still be visible, but the shape and nature of the cell are quite unde-

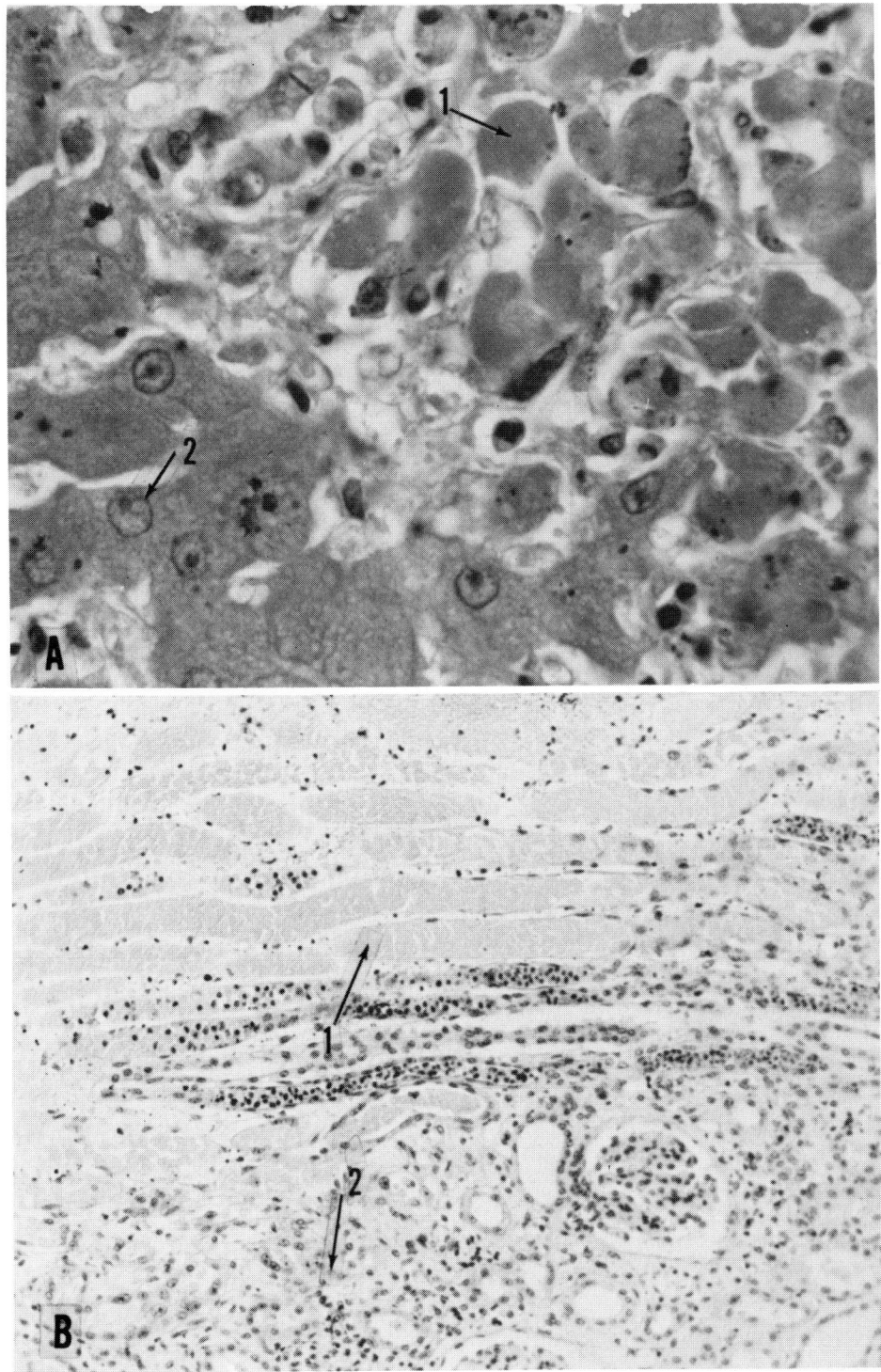

Fig. 1–5. *A*, Necrosis indicated by loss of nuclei (*1*) from liver cells of a dog. Compare with vesicular nuclei (*2*) containing nucleoli, in unaffected liver cells. (× 600.) Contributor: Dr. D. J. Carren. *B*, Necrosis, indicated by loss of differential staining in renal tubules (*1*) at the margin of an anemic infarct in the kidney of a pig. Normal renal tubules at (*2*). (× 125.) (Courtesy of Armed Forces Institute of Pathology.) Contributor: Lt. Col. F. D. Maurer.

terminable. Complete loss of cell outline is seen in caseous necrosis of a tubercle.

Loss of Differential Staining. Situations occur in which tissue can still be seen but the colors of nuclei and cytoplasm, as well as the colors characteristic of the different histologic tissues, cannot be distinguished. Chromatolysis has an important part in producing this condition. As an example, look at the mucosa of an intestine involved either in necrosis or postmortem autolysis. There is a stage in which the villi and glands are fairly well outlined, but not a single individual cell or structure can be identified. This represents both loss of differential staining and loss of cell outline.

Absence of Cell. If the cell cannot be found, it must be assumed to have died and autolyzed. Absence of cells that should be present has practical importance both within organs and tissues and on their surfaces. If the number of hepatic cells in a liver lobule, for instance, is less than we know to be normal, it can be concluded that the missing ones have died and have undergone autolysis and disappeared, one by one. On a surface such as the intestinal mucosa and the skin, when a cell dies there is commonly nothing to hold it in its place and it disappears through the process of **desquamation**, or sloughing. In the intestine such desquamated cells may often be seen mixed with fecal material and still showing rather satisfactory staining qualities. Those cells are dead by virtue of being desquamated if there is nothing else to show. If one sees the lining epithelium of a gland or duct, or the endothelium of a blood vessel free in the lumen, those cells must be considered dead even though they may stain rather well. Usually if they still stain well, the desquamation and death is a matter of postmortem autolysis and therefore of no significance, but if they come off during life they will never be reunited to their base and the process is one of necrosis. This is not an infrequent occurrence; the sloughing of the bronchial epithelium in bronchitis is an example, as well as the loss of acinar epithelium in mastitis.

Gross Characteristics of Dead Tissue

This subject will be discussed further under Differentiation between Necrosis and Postmortem Autolysis, but the following general characteristics may be pointed out:

Loss of Color. Dead tissue is regularly paler than living, except when it is well filled with blood, which makes it black. Hemolyzed blood is blackish-red, and if large amounts are present in the tissue, this will be the dominant color. Spotting with black and white usually has no other significance than this. Areas of necrosis are often conspicuous by their change in color.

Loss of Strength. Dead tissue has little strength, especially tensile strength. In lifting the intestine out of the cadaver at autopsy, a length of intestine, necrotic because of obstruction or infarction, or the whole intestine in case of advanced postmortem autolysis, may be too weak to support its own weight and it pulls apart as it is raised. The finger may be thrust with little resistance into a liver or lung that has undergone these changes.

Odors. Odors of putrefaction appear if the dead tissue was exposed to bacteria following gangrene or postmortem autolysis.

Necrosis. Such changes as caseation, liquefaction, and coagulation will be discussed under forms of necrosis, although most of them develop also during the process of postmortem autolysis. As an example, one sees brains which have been sent without preservation to the laboratory for examination for Negri bodies. In warm weather they sometimes arrive in a state of complete liquefaction.

DIFFERENTIATION BETWEEN NECROSIS AND POSTMORTEM AUTOLYSIS

Microscopic Appearances. The following considerations assist in deciding whether tissue died ante mortem or post mortem, that is, in distinguishing between necrosis and postmortem autolysis.

If one finds both living and dead tissue within the same microscopic section, it seems obvious that the dead part represents necrosis and not postmortem autolysis, but unfortunately things are not always so simple. Postmortem autolysis sometimes has a decidedly patchy distribution which is deceptive and justifies reliance on other criteria to decide between antemortem and postmortem death of tissue.

The erythrocytes within the blood vessels should be examined for sharpness of outline and for the degree to which they take the stain. Hemolysis of the blood cells in the blood stream, if present, took place after death, thus indicating a certain degree of postmortem autolysis of the whole specimen. Formalin-fixed erythrocytes stained with hematoxylin and eosin should stain a bright copper-red; with mercuric chloride fixation they are a rose-red. Alcohol fixation hemolyzes erythrocytes to empty circles, whatever stain is used. Erythrocytes separated by hemorrhage from the circulation and their source of oxygen undergo hemolysis within the living body. Hence they are not of value in determining the presence or absence of postmortem autolysis.

Necrotic tissue left in the body usually acts as an irritant, hence there should be at least a slight inflammatory zone of leukocytes and hyperemia in the living tissue that immediately surrounds the necrotic tissue.

Knowledge of the relative rate at which different tissues of the body tend to show the effects of postmortem autolysis may be of material assistance. The mucosa of the digestive tract undergoes these changes early because the usual autolysis is abetted by the action of the no longer inhibited digestive juices. Even earlier the lining of the gallbladder succumbs to autolysis intensified by the destructive action of bile. The medulla of the adrenal gland undergoes early postmortem liquefaction, so that it is not unusual to examine an otherwise rather well-preserved adrenal gland and find only a collapsed space where the medulla should be. The neurons are probably next to show the changes of postmortem autolysis; connective tissue is among the last to do so. In the kidney, autolysis proceeds more rapidly in proximal convoluted tubular epithelium than in distal convoluted tubular epithelium.

Gross Appearances. The problem is usually to decide at the start of an autopsy how long the animal has been dead. Autolysis and putrefaction are greatly inhibited by refrigerator temperature. At summer temperatures the postmortem deterioration that occurs in hours may almost equal the effect of as many days in the refrigerator. Sheep show serious postmortem changes very early because the insulating effect of the fleece prevents dissipation of the body heat, and the same is true of larger swine because of the insulating layer of fat. Postmortem changes proceed with unusual rapidity when the body temperature is very high at the time of death, as in heat stroke, and when it continues to rise even after death, as in tetanus, and when potentially putrefactive organisms are disseminated through the blood at the time of, or possibly before death (*Clostridium septicum*). An example of the latter phenomenon has at times resulted in a postmortem picture so startling as to be called "black disease," a name attributed to the almost universal blackish discoloration of congested, autolyzed tissues seen upon removal of the animal's skin. "Pulpy-kidney disease" has been described in sheep when autolytic and putrefactive softening have involved the kidneys especially. With or without more specific changes, such kidneys are severely congested and contain large numbers of clostridial organisms.

If the digestive tract of herbivorous animals is well filled with ingesta, fermentation and gas formation may, within a few hours, cause great distention of the digestive tract and consequently of the torso, and also press bloody foam out the nostrils and cause the rectal lining to protrude in a pseudo-prolapse. The distention due to

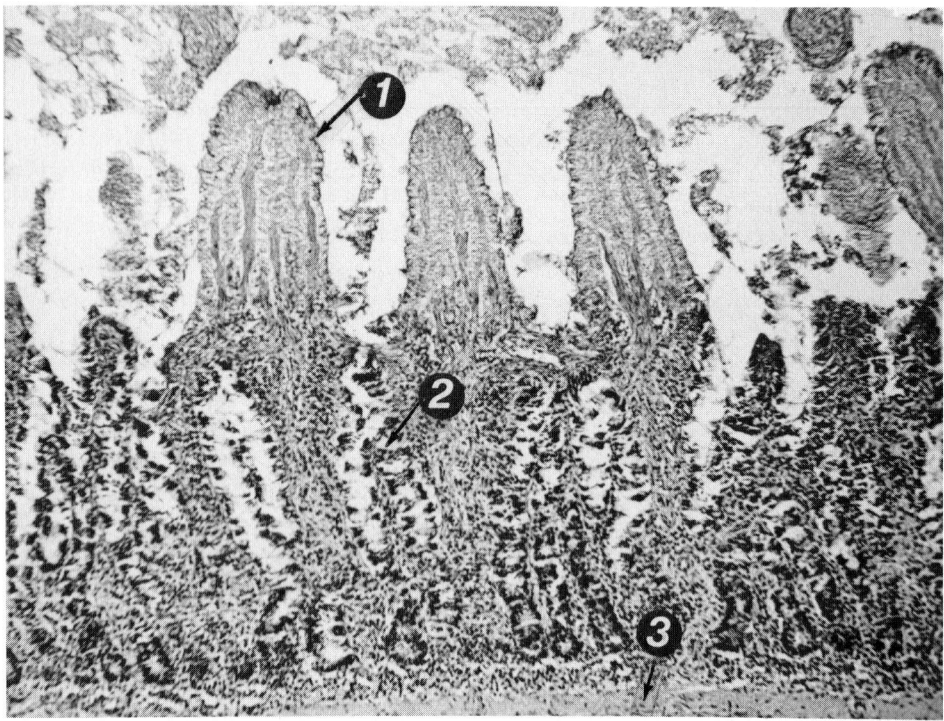

Fig. 1–6. Postmortem autolysis, small intestine of a dog. The villi (1) are denuded of epithelium which, however, is still present in the crypts (2). Muscularis mucosae at (3). (× 90.) (Courtesy of Armed Forces Institute of Pathology.) Contributor: Dr. R. O. Delano.

postmortem fermentation has to be distinguished from antemortem bloating (tympanites), a frequent cause of death in ruminants. Signs of anoxia usually accompany the bloating that occurred during life.

When postmortem changes are far advanced, the muscles are softened, pale red, watery, and resemble meat that has been cooked slightly. When postmortem autolysis is only moderately advanced, an important indication is **postmortem imbibition**. This is the result of the previously mentioned hemolysis of erythrocytes in the blood vessels. Their hemoglobin is released to go into solution in the blood plasma, and at the same time the walls of the blood vessels become more permeable to fluids as the result of postmortem autolysis. Consequently the red-tinged plasma leaks out into the surrounding tissues, or, as it is customarily expressed, is

"imbibed" by them. The result is a distinct dark red fringe along the course of each vessel, which is easily seen in white tissues such as the mesentery or omentum. "Imbibition of bile" is a similar leaking of bile through the autolyzed wall of the gallbladder to stain adjacent liver tissue a greenish hue to a varying depth, which is sharply delimited.

Further information is gained upon opening the heart. Ordinarily rigor mortis contracts the left ventricle strongly and empties it of blood. The right ventricle remains more or less filled with blood, and when this blood is hemolyzed a few hours postmortem, the lining of the ventricle assumes a lusterless but strong red color that does not wash off. If the left ventricle does contain blood and this is unclotted, it indicates that rigor mortis has not yet taken place, death being recent. However, after a lapse of 24 to 72 hours postmortem, depending upon temperature, the rigor has come and gone, allowing dark, hemolyzed blood from the disintegrating clot to run back into the ventricle. This latter indicates prolonged postmortem autolysis. If the left ventricle contains clotted blood, the body forces were too low at the time of death for rigor mortis to develop, as is often the case with lingering illness.

In the rumen, reticulum, and omasum of ruminants, an impressive sign of postmortem autolysis is desquamation of the epithelium. Within a surprisingly short time after death, this comparatively thick surface layer is completely displaced by the slightest touch.

The cause of postmortem autolysis is obvious and its importance to the pathologist is only that it be avoided if possible and that it be distinguished accurately from necrosis.

FORMS OF NECROSIS

Coagulation Necrosis

Coagulation necrosis results when denaturation of cellular protein proceeds to denaturation of hydrolytic enzymes as well, thus stopping the process of autolysis. Loss of water also favors denaturation without further decomposition. The tissue ultimately passes on to slow and imperceptible liquefaction through heterolysis. Coagulation necrosis is not seen in diseases in which large numbers of neutrophils are attracted to the dead tissues, owing to heterolysis.

Microscopic Appearance. Such tissue structures and cellular outlines as existed previously are still discernible. The nuclei are generally pyknotic but still readily visible. The cytoplasm is often strongly acidophilic.

Gross Appearance. The necrotic tissue is gray or white (unless filled with blood), firm, dense and often depressed as compared with surrounding living tissue.

Causes. Causes especially tending to produce this variety of necrosis include (1) local ischemia, as in infarcts, (2) the toxic products of certain bacteria, as in calf diphtheria, necrophorus enteritis, and other forms of necrobacillosis, (3) certain locally acting poisons, such as mercuric chloride, (4) the milder burns, whether produced by heat, electricity or roentgen rays, and (5) Zenker's necrosis of muscle.

Caseous Necrosis

Caseous necrosis occurs as part of the typical lesions of tuberculosis, syphilis (humans), ovine caseous lymphadenitis, and other granulomas. It results from a mixture of coagulated protein and lipid. Once the cause is removed, the caseous material is slowly liquefied and removed.

Microscopic Appearance. There is loss of cell outline and loss of differential staining. Cell walls and other histologic structures disappear, the tissue disintegrating to form a finely granular mass which has a purplish color (hematoxylin and eosin stain) resulting from the mixture of blue chromatin granules with red ones derived from the cytoplasm. Any pre-existing fibrillar structure will have disappeared.

Gross Appearance. The gross appearance is suggestive of "milk curds," or "cottage" cheese, hence the name, caseous. The necrotic tissue is dry but slightly greasy, firm but without any cohesive strength, so that it can be easily separated into granular fragments by a blunt instrument. The color is white, grayish, or yellowish.

Causes. Caseous necrosis is caused by the locally acting toxins of the specific microorganisms of the diseases already mentioned.

Liquefaction Necrosis

While most necrotic tissue slowly disappears by a process of insidious and imperceptible liquefaction, there are situations in which this change proceeds rapidly with accumulation of measurable amounts of fluid and without any noticeable precursor

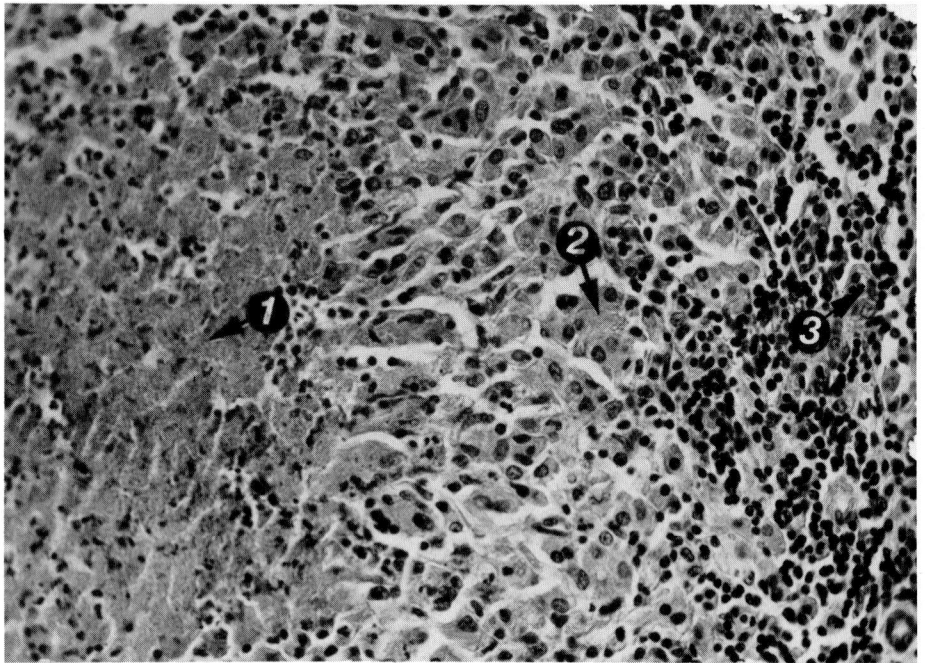

Fig. 1–7. Caseous necrosis *(1)* in the center of a tubercle in the lung of a monkey *(Macaca mulatta).* Epithelioid granulation tissue *(2)*, and lymphocytes *(3)* surround the caseous center. (× 260.) (Courtesy of Armed Forces Institute of Pathology.) Contributor: Army Veterinary School.

change in the dying cells. This process is known as liquefaction necrosis.

Occurrence. There are two principal situations in which noticeable liquefaction of dying tissue is encountered. The first is in the central nervous system; the second, in abscesses. Areas of liquefactive necrosis sometimes occur in tuberculous lungs, producing cavities of considerable size.

Microscopic Appearance. The necrotic area, be it large or small, appears as an empty space. The space not only is without any definitive lining, but its edges are frayed and irregular, and usually the cells on the edge may show some of the evidences of necrosis. A pink-staining proteinaceous precipitate may or may not remain from the liquid. The actual water is removed in the process of dehydration of the tissue preparatory to sectioning. In the case of an abscess, the liquid is represented by pus, which leaves a dehydrated residue of polymorphonuclear neutrophils, frag-

ments of destroyed tissue cells, fibrin, and nondescript debris.

Gross Appearance. This lesion is represented by a cavity, small or large, containing fluid which is usually cloudy. Assuming that the process is still in progress, the walls of the cavity are frayed and irregular and more or less softened. Such a fluid-filled space is not generally considered a cyst, since a true cyst involves the accumulation of fluid, usually a secretion, in a cavity that has a natural and permanent type of lining, usually epithelial. In liquefaction necrosis, the liquid usually is drained away by the lymphatics and the wall is merely the pre-existing tissue in the process of disintegration. In an abscess, the liquefaction is a minor aspect, the accumulation of inflammatory exudate being of transcendent importance.

Causes. The causes of liquefaction necrosis are included in those already given for necrosis in general. The reason that tissue liquefies in the brain and spinal cord almost as soon as it dies is considered to be the high content of lipids and the small amount of coagulable albumin present in these tissues. Also, an acid reaction of the tissue is essential. In the case of abscesses, the liquefaction of tissue is attributable to liquefying toxins (lysins), which have been demonstrated for most of the bacteria responsible. The leukocytes, which comprise most of the inflammatory exudate, also produce liquefying enzymes. The liquefaction of old pulmonary tubercles may be regarded as an end stage of the caseous necrosis which is typically encountered, since all necrotic tissue tends ultimately to disappear by a slow process of liquefaction. However, secondary pyogenic infection and lytic substances produced by the bacteria probably play an important part in liquefaction necrosis in these tubercles.

Necrosis of Fat

When adipose tissue undergoes necrosis, the fat is not infrequently decomposed, perhaps slowly, into its two constituent radicals, fatty acid and glycerin. The fatty acid then combines in various proportions with the metallic ions present, chiefly sodium, potassium, and calcium. The result is the formation of a soap within what was a fat cell, and the soap is not dissolved out, as fat is, by the fat solvents (xylene, etc.) used in the imbedding technique.

Microscopic Appearance. One sees the same adipose-connective-tissue cells as in the normal tissue, but the fat is replaced by a solid, opaque material, nearly homogeneous but sometimes pervaded by minute clear slits, marking the site of dissolved fatty-acid crystals. It takes a bluish or a pinkish tinge, depending on the presence of sodium or potassium respectively, or purple if calcium has been deposited. The nuclei tend to be pyknotic, but histologically are not of a type to show this change clearly.

Gross Appearance. Adipose tissue that has undergone this change loses its shiny and semitranslucent character to become opaque, whitish, and solid or slightly granular. It retains its previous position and extent indefinitely.

Causes. Two types of causative mechanism are recognized. The traditional **pancreatic necrosis of fat** occurs only in the abdominal cavity, and is the result of the fat-splitting action of pancreatic juice which has escaped from its proper ducts and channels because of some other lesion in the ductal system of the pancreas, such as invasion by a neoplasm. But the same type of change occurs outside the abdominal cavity due to pressure and mechanical trauma. It is known as **traumatic necrosis of fat** and is well exemplified in the subcutaneous and intermuscular fat in the sternal region of a cow which for some time has been in a position of sternal recumbency. Another form of fat necrosis also occurs in animals (most frequently in cattle) that is characterized by large masses or nodules of necrotic adipose tissue, particularly in the abdominal cavity or retroperitoneal tissue, in the absence of pancreatic disease. The resemblance to tumors has resulted in the synonym **lipomatosis.** If extensive, the lesions can lead to intestinal stenosis. Vitonec *et al.* (1975) have suggested that the disease is initiated by crystallization of fatty acids and their soaps when lipolysis exceeds the rate of fatty acid transport, thus differing from pancreatic or traumatic necrosis of fat. They compared the disease to sclerema neonatorum and adiponecrosis cutis neonatorum of human beings.

Significance. In the abdominal cavity, one searches for a pancreatic lesion, although the nonpancreatic type can be found here also.

Zenker's Necrosis

This condition, which is also known as **Zenker's degeneration,** occurs only in striated muscle. It is essentially a coagulation of proteins of the sarcoplasm.

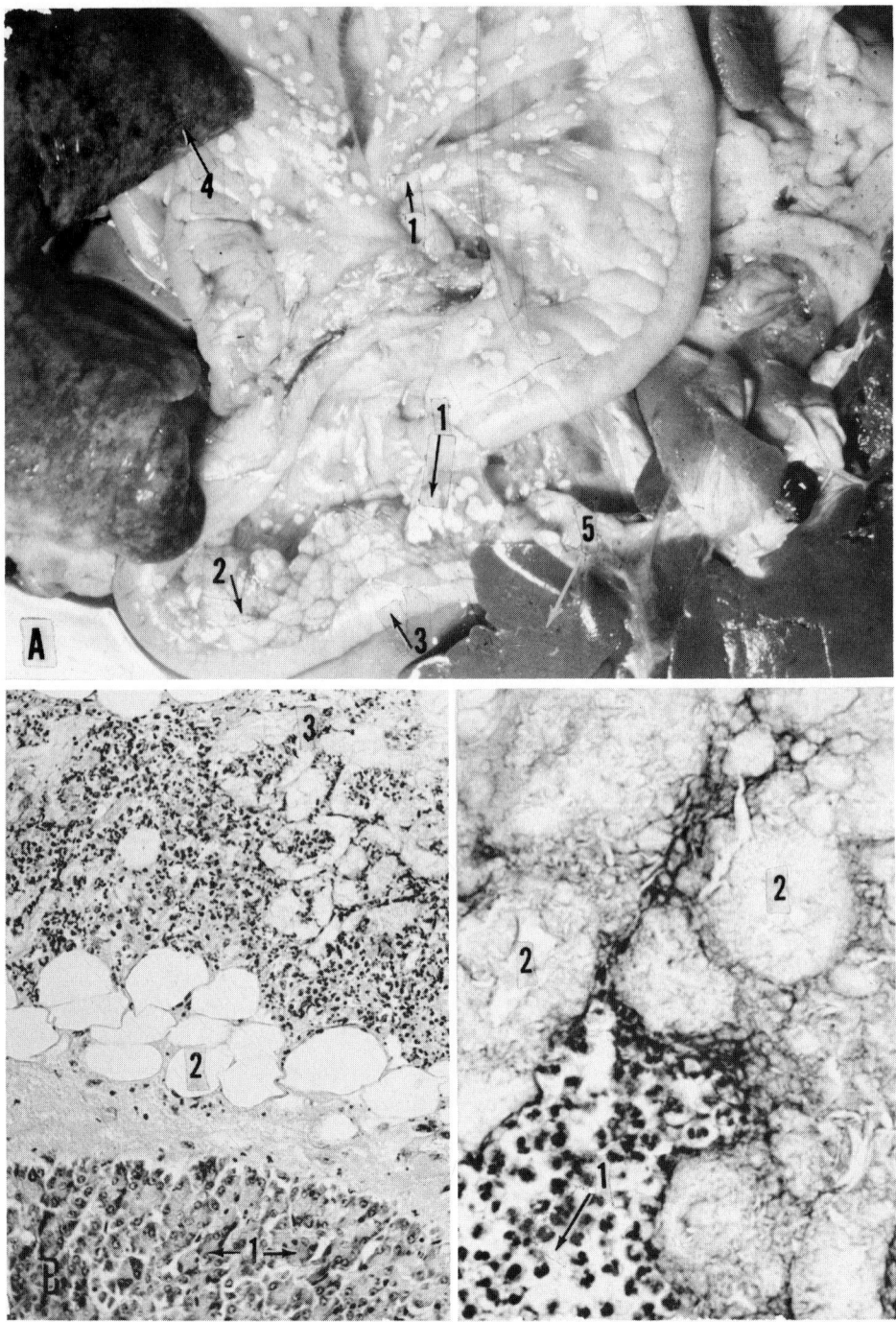

Fig. 1–8. Pancreatic necrosis of fat in the mesentery of a dog. *A*, Chalky appearing plaques (*1*), pancreas (*2*), duodenum (*3*), lung (*4*), and liver (*5*). *B*, Pancreas (*1*), normal fat cells (*2*) and necrotic fat (*3*) surrounded by leukocytes. (× 165.) *C*, Higher magnification of polymorphonuclear leukocytes (*1*) and necrotic (saponified) fat (*2*). (× 440.) (*B* and *C*, Courtesy of Armed Forces Institute of Pathology.) Contributor: Dr. Samuel Pollock.

Microscopic Appearance. The individual fibers are swollen, often greatly, and are homogeneous and hyaline in texture. The sarcoplasm is unusually acidophilic (red by ordinary stains), the myofibrils cannot be seen, and nuclei are small and dark.

Gross Appearance. If the involved area is large enough to be seen, the muscle is white or pale, rather shiny and somewhat swollen. The term **hyaline degeneration** has been used by some for this change in muscle, but will be reserved in this work for certain more specific lesions to be described later.

Causes. The causes are considered usually to be toxins of pathogenic microorganisms, since it occurs in connection with various systemic or local infections, but white-muscle diseases present a similar change.

The Outcome of Necrosis

Under exceptional circumstances, necrotic tissue may remain in the body for some time, but ultimately its disposal is accomplished along one of the following routes.

1. Liquefaction by autolysis and heterolysis and removal of the fluid by way of the blood and lymph. This is the usual termination when the number of dead cells in a given area at a given time is small, and larger masses may gradually follow the same course. As already stated, it is the rule in the central nervous system.

2. Liquefaction and formation of a cyst-like accumulation of fluid occurs occasionally, the fluid accumulating faster than it is drained away.

3. Liquefaction with abscess formation occurs when necrosis is part of the damage inflicted by pyogenic bacteria. It is accompanied by formation of a purulent exudate. The tendency is for abscesses to rupture, the pus making its way to the nearest free surface along a path of subsequently developing necrosis in the overlying tissue.

4. Encapsulation without liquefaction: When there is little moisture in the part, dead tissue may remain with little change, usually in the form of caseous or coagulative necrosis. It then acts as an irritant to surrounding living tissue and incites a cellular (leukocytic) inflammatory reaction around it. Before many days have passed, the reaction involves fibrosis and the formation of a fibrous capsule. Enclosed in this fibrous capsule, it may persist for a long time, doing the patient little or no harm. In addition to tubercles, dead helminth parasites within tissues are commonly encapsulated in this manner.

5. Desquamation or sloughing: If on an external or internal body surface, dead cells regularly lose their attachment to the underlying living tissue. Thin layers, such as an epithelial covering, are said to desquamate, that is, to come off in flat, scale-like fragments. Larger and deeper masses of tissue are said to "slough off." The desquamated epithelial cells are often seen clumped together in the lumen of glands, ducts, bronchi, renal tubules, or the intestine. The endothelial cells lining blood vessels behave similarly. Postmortem sloughing must be excluded.

6. Replacement by scar tissue ultimately follows as the terminal stage of abscesses, encapsulated areas, cystic cavities, infarcts, or diffuse loss of tissue such as occurs in the kidney and liver.

7. Calcification converts the dead tissue into a sandy mass. It is thus rendered inert and harmless, unless in such a location that the hard and irregular material interferes mechanically with movement or function of the nearby structures.

8. Gangrene supervenes when parts have become necrotic and exposed directly or indirectly to the external air and its saprophytic bacteria. This will presently be treated in detail.

9. Atrophy of the organ, tissue, or part is naturally an accompaniment of the necrosis and loss of any considerable number of cells.

10. Regeneration, the formation of new cells like those which were lost, is a fortu-

nate termination in some cases. The regenerated cells are produced by subdivision and multiplication of remaining cells that escaped or withstood the original necrotizing agent. This is seen commonly on epithelial surfaces, in the lining cells of pulmonary alveoli and bronchi, and in the parenchymatous cells of the liver and kidneys.

Cholesterol Clefts. Cholesterol clefts are encountered not infrequently as byproducts of necrosis. They are empty spaces left by crystals of cholesterol dissolved by the solvents used in preparation of the tissue. The crystals are readily recognized by their special shape, which is that of a flat, thin rhomboid plate with one corner cut out along lines parallel to the outer edges of the crystal. The dimensions of length and breadth commonly fall between 50 and 100

μ with a thickness of 5 to 10 μ. Since the crystal is dissolved in preparation of the tissue, what one sees in a microscopic section is the cleft-like empty space of approximately the same size and shape. Since the probability of this narrow slit being cut transversely is much greater than of its happening to lie in the plane of the section, one usually sees a narrow cleft perhaps 50 μ in length and bulging slightly at the middle. The crystals are anisotropic (birefringent) when seen in frozen sections.

The cholesterol is not usually seen grossly, but in large amounts, it is visible as a shiny, yellowish, granular, or flaky material.

Since the cholesterol that crystallizes in the tissues comes from the decomposed protoplasm of cells that have died, it is obvious that these clefts are found in re-

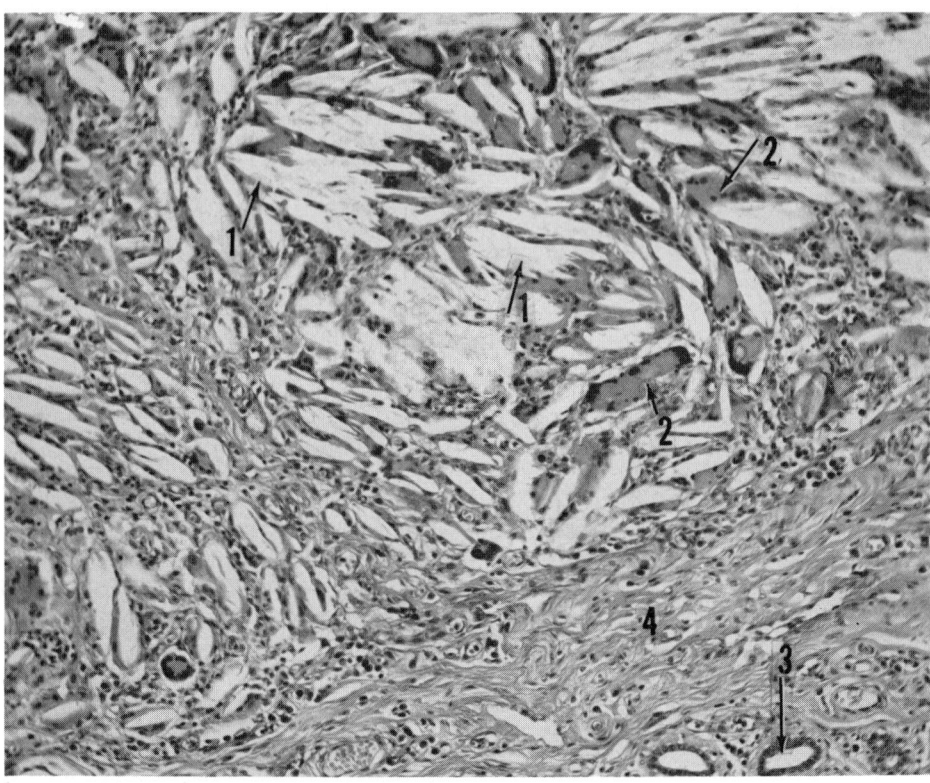

Fig. 1–9. Cholesterol clefts (*1*) at the site of old hemorrhage and necrosis in the mammary gland of a dog. Giant cells of foreign body type (*2*), mammary acini (*3*), connective tissue (*4*). (× 115.) (Courtesy of Armed Forces Institute of Pathology.) Contributor: Dr. W. H. Riser.

gions where there has been considerable necrosis of cells relatively rich in that substance. Such situations include the sites of old hemorrhages, old abscesses, atheromas, and sometimes dermoid and sebaceous cysts. Cholesterol also appears in the tissue of the liver and gallbladder when, for any reason, bile is entrapped there.

Gangrene

Moist gangrene is a condition in which necrotic tissue is invaded by saprophytic, and usually putrefactive, bacteria. Necrotic tissue accessible to air-borne bacteria regularly suffers such invasion; hence, we seldom speak of necrosis of limbs, ears, tails, lungs, intestines or udder, but rather of gangrene of those organs.

Microscopically, the condition is recognized as a mixture of coagulation and liquefaction necrosis in which large **bacilli** (rod-shaped bacteria) are demonstrated. They need not be numerous. By the ordinary hematoxylin-eosin stain, bacteria are bluish, but much less so than nuclei, and hazy in outline as compared with results achieved by the bacterial stains. Since many species of saprophytic bacteria are gas-formers, the gangrenous tissue may contain gas-bubbles, recognizable as empty spaces of various sizes, having no wall of their own, and tending to be spherical but subject to distortion by the pressure of adjoining histologic structures.

In moist gangrene, the affected part, be it a limb or an area of lung or intestine, is swollen, soft, pulpy, and usually dark or black in color. Depending on the kinds of bacteria present, it is likely to have a foul,

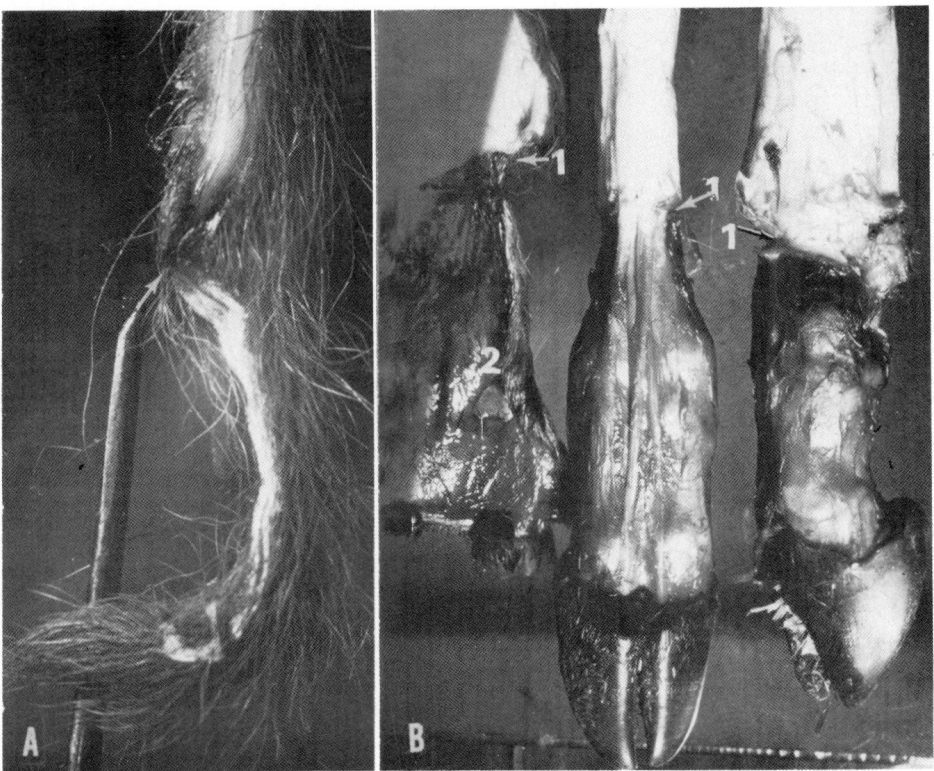

Fig. 1–10. *A*, Dry gangrene, ear (longitudinal section) of a calf (arrow) following ergot poisoning. *B*, Moist gangrene involving feet of same calf. Note sharp line of demarcation between black gangrenous and white living tissue (*1*); the skin, inside out, after removal (*2*).

putrefactive odor. During life, it is without body heat and insensible to touch or pain. This, the more frequent type, occurs in those tissues which are well-filled with blood at the time the necrosis begins.

Dry gangrene occurs in tissues that have a more limited content of blood and fluid, or in which the necrosis has developed slowly, with retardation of the natural circulation. Since dry tissue is not a favorable culture medium, the multiplication and spread of the bacteria is slow. The tissue becomes denatured or coagulated and the part becomes cool, shrivelled, leather-like, and discolored.

All areas of gangrene (moist and dry) are separated from the adjoining living tissue by **a line of demarcation**, which is readily seen grossly, either during life or after death, as a swollen, reddish or bluish zone of hyperemia and inflammation.

Causes. The causes of gangrene are the causes of necrosis plus the exposure to saprophytic bacteria. In the extremities, interference with the blood supply is the outstanding cause, as it is also in the intestine. In the lungs and udder, the toxic products of highly lethal bacteria are the usual causes. In the lungs, irritant medicines intended to be swallowed, but unskillfully allowed to pass down the trachea, set the stage for the growth of microorganisms, both pathogens and saprophytes.

Significance and Effect. The principal therapeutic efforts are usually directed toward stopping the spread of the gangrenous process, and this involves stopping the spread of cell death and necrosis, whatever the cause. Highly toxic substances are produced as steps in the decomposition of proteins in gangrenous tissue and elsewhere. These tend to be absorbed into the circulating blood of the adjacent living areas, with disastrous consequences to the patient. Indeed, in a weakened and moribund patient, we sometimes see **sapremia,** a condition in which the saprophytic bacteria, ordinarily growing only in dead organic matter, are able to survive in

the blood and be disseminated by it through the living body. For all of these considerations, amputation of a gangrenous extremity, even of the udder, is often necessary. In the case of the intestine, early surgical removal of the gangrenous portion with anastomosis of the healthy segments is the only hope for survival.

But nature does have her own remedy for gangrene in a patient with good resistance. The line of demarcation is an inflammatory zone of combat in which all of the body's protective devices, humoral and cellular, are drawn up in battle array to resist the entrance of harmful substances, living or otherwise, into the healthy tissues. Often these are successful, in which case separation of the dead tissue, even of bone, eventually causes the gangrenous extremity to drop off, and the stump slowly heals. In dry gangrene, this is the usual outcome, and the process may involve no startling changes in the general bodily health.

Gangrene of the uterus is possible on the basis of the definitions set forth. A gangrenous uterus, from its size and location, leads to a quickly fatal peritonitis by spread of the toxic products and pathogenic organisms. Superficial necrosis of the uterine lining, most often from irritant medicine, is possible, as it is with other mucous surfaces.

Gas Gangrene. Several species of anaerobic spore-forming bacteria, classified by Bergey (at this writing) in the genus *Clostridium,* have the faculty of growing both in dead organic matter and in living tissues. Hence they are both saprophytes and pathogens. They are able to kill animal tissue and then continue to multiply in it as saprophytes. They produce gas from constituents of the dead tissue, which appears as bubbles in the affected tissue. The group of diseases so produced are known as the gas gangrenes, including specifically malignant edema and blackleg in animals and nonspecific wound infections in humans. They constitute examples of gangrene and necrosis occurring without the previous action of some other necrotizing agent.

Infarction

Infarcts are localized areas of necrotic tissue resulting from sudden deprivation of their blood supply. The necrosis is coagulative in type, but the affected tissue eventually passes through the whole series of changes described for dead tissue, with ultimate complete disappearance. The area involved is ordinarily that supplied by a single "end-artery" whose flow has been arrested, and the boundaries are, therefore, sharply delimited.

As the tissue dies, its capillary network obviously dies with it, and there must be a line somewhere with dead capillaries on one side and living on the other. A certain amount of blood diffuses back from the living into the dead capillaries and these latter, being dead and without normal strength and resistance, permit escape of the blood into the surrounding necrotic tissue. Blood in the efferent veins doubtless flows back into the necrotic area in a similar way. Consequently, a recent infarct tends to fill with blood. Indeed it is this feature that gives the lesion its name, which is derived from the Latin *infarcire*, meaning to fill fully or to stuff.

Some infarcts, then, if seen before the stranded erythrocytes have undergone hemolysis (see Postmortem Autolysis) are filled with blood. These are called **hemorrhagic** or **red infarcts**. In other cases, the escaped blood never gets beyond a thin peripheral zone, leaving the bulk of the lesion with the pale color which is characteristic of necrosis. These are called **anemic** or **pale infarcts**. The existence of the two types has been explained by some as de-

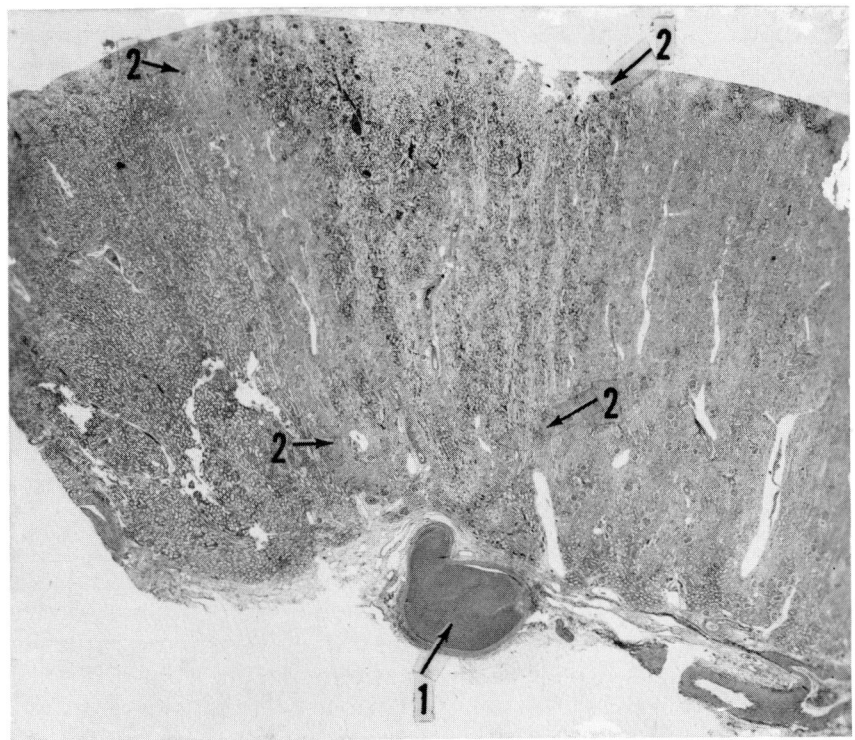

Fig. 1–11.   Infarct in the kidney of a pig infected experimentally with hog cholera virus. A thrombus is seen in an arciform artery (*1*), the margins of the infarct are indicated by arrows (*2*). (× 6.) (Courtesy of Armed Forces Institute of Pathology.) Contributor: Lt. Col. F. D. Maurer.

pending on the length of time that elapsed between formation of the infarcts and examinaton of the tissue, it having been theorized that all infarcts are hemorrhagic before the disappearance of the blood cells by autolytic processes, usually a matter of two to three days. Others believe that the amount of blood that escapes into the necrotic area is determined by the denseness or perviousness of the tissue in question. Certainly infarcts seen in the kidney, a dense and solid organ, are almost always anemic, and those in the pervious and lace-like tissue of the lung are invariably hemorrhagic.

Microscopic Appearance. The picture is that of coagulative necrosis, with or without the filling of the tissue spaces with blood, as just described. The shape of the necrotic area is that of the part supplied by the obstructed vessel below the point of obstruction. In sections of most organs, this is a triangular or wedged-shaped area, with its apex near the place of obstruction and its base at or just inside the organ's wall or capsule, which may have a sufficient blood supply of its own. Since necrotic tissue regularly constitutes an irritant to adjacent living tissues, an infarct has more or less of an inflammatory zone (hyperemia and leukocytes) surrounding it. Unfortunately for the diagnostician, this is sometimes slight. The smaller leukocytes must be carefully distinguished from the dark, angular fragments of nuclei of preexisting parenchymatous cells, which, in the peripheral zone of an infarct, may remain for some time in a state of karyorrhexis rather than disappearing promptly by karyolysis. Old infarcts are chiefly fibrous. In case a trifling amount of blood continues to flow, any structure having prior access to it may survive as a living oasis in the necrotic desert. Renal glomeruli, for instance, may persist indefinitely, although other microscopic components of the kidney have long since disappeared.

Gross Appearance. The red or white color has already been described. Hemorrhagic infarcts may protrude slightly above the surrounding tissues; the pale ones tend to be slightly depressed. Old infarcts are decidedly sunken on the surface. In all cases they are sharply demarcated. In the three-dimensional view, the triangular shape seen microscopically becomes pyramidal or conical; the affected area, as seen on the surface of the organ, is likely to be irregular. The pale infarct is a little denser and tougher than the surrounding tissue; the hemorrhagic one may be softer.

Cause. By definition (on which there is practically universal agreement), an infarct is an area of necrosis, and the cause of the necrosis is lack of proper blood supply. The cause of the lack of blood is ordinarily an obstruction in an artery or vein as a result of a lodged embolus.

Possibly there is some lack of precision in applying the name of infarct to areas which become filled with blood because of external pressure sufficient to prevent the venous outflow, but not sufficient to obstruct completely the stiffer-walled arteries. However, if the exit of blood is impossible, that which accumulates in a part soon becomes stagnant, no more oxygen or other nutrients can be brought in, and necrosis ensues. In this way, venous obstruction can be admitted as a cause, chiefly in the case of a strangulated intestine, and possibly in rare cases of occluding venous thrombi in other organs. It would seem proper, nevertheless, to insist on the demonstration of necrosis in any true infarct, since it is the death of the tissue, rather than the filling with blood, which is of principal significance to the patient.

Special Types and Diagnosis. Infarcts of the kidney are typically conical, with the apex usually near the corticomedullary junction and the path of the arcuate arteries. In dogs and pigs, an accompanying chronic valvular endocarditis is frequently demonstrable and may well be the source of the causative embolus. Infarcts of the kidney are rather frequent and typically anemic, may be multiple, and often heal, leaving only a narrow, fibrous scar.

Infarcts of the spleen are almost always hemorrhagic. Many shallow, subcapsular infarcts, difficult to distinguish from mere subcapsular hematomas, accompany hog cholera. Arterioles become obstructed due to swelling and hyperplasia of endothelial cells as an effect of the virus.

Infarcts of the myocardium, far rarer in animals than in man and usually of different etiology, are either red or gray at the time they are discovered.

Infarcts of the brain are usually anemic and quickly reach a state of liquefaction necrosis in accordance with the susceptibility of nervous tissue to that termination. The animal may survive, the infarcted area being represented by a sharp gap in the tissue. These are rare in animals.

Intestinal infarctions usually involve a considerable length of the bowel. They are always hemorrhagic, and large amounts of blood diffuse into the lumen through the necrotic tissue. They are ordinarily caused by strangulation of the bowel caught in a hernial sac or in a twisted loop of mesentery. In spite of the frequency of thrombosing injury to the anterior mesenteric artery by strongyle worms in the horse, emboli of sufficient importance to thwart the rather efficient system of arterial anastomosis are rare. Intestinal infarctions, unless promptly treated by surgical resection, undergo fatal gangrene through invasion of saprophytic bacteria from the intestinal lumen. Obstruction of the lumen of the bowel by some foreign body is frequent in the dog and produces the same hemorrhagic lesion if the obstruction is complete.

Infarcts can occur in the lung despite the only moderately effective circulation of the bronchial arteries as a secondary source of supply, but apparently only when that circulation is weakened by abnormally low blood pressure or some other interference. Emboli, single or multiple, brought in by way of the pulmonary artery are the usual cause. Because of the secondary bronchial circulation, as well as the extensive capillary network and the pervious nature of lung tissue, pulmonary infarcts are always hemorrhagic, the alveolar spaces being filled with blood.

In animals, infarction of the lung is not common. It is probable that some areas of lung, filled with blood in a lobular distribution, have been called infarcts without meeting the criterion of necrosis, and certainly without finding the embolus. It is not always easy to distinguish hemorrhagic infarction from simple hemorrhage or a localized hemorrhagic exudate.

True infarcts of the liver are almost nonexistent because both the portal vein and the hepatic artery supply large amounts of blood. If an infarct does occur, it is the result of obstruction of a branch of the hepatic artery apparently, for experimental obstruction of the portal vein has failed to have such an effect. Pseudo-infarcts, sometimes called Zahn's infarcts, have been reported, but these lack the essential feature of necrosis and are really areas of venous and sinusoidal engorgement on a multilobular scale. Except for this greater extent, such pseudo-infarcts might not look very different from the engorgement of sinusoids that accompanies central necrosis. A so-called infarct, in which the circumscribed area of affected hepatic tissue is whitened by degenerative changes and incipient necrosis, is stated to be characteristic of infection by *Clostridium hemolyticum bovis*.

Abraham, E. P.: Necrosis, calcification and autolysis. *In* General Pathology, 4th ed., edited by H. W. Florey. Philadelphia, W. B. Saunders Co., 1970.

Craig, J. M.: The etiology of liver necrosis in rats following administration of progesterone late in pregnancy. Lab. Invest., *19*:49–54, 1968.

de Duve, C.: The lysosome. Sci. Am., May, 64–72, 1963.

de Reulk, A. V. S., and Knight, J.: Ciba Foundation Symposium on Cellular Injury. Boston, Little Brown & Co., 1964.

Ericsson, J. L. E., and Biberfeld, P.: Studies on aldehyde fixation. Fixation rates and their relation to fine structure and some histochemical reactions in liver. Lab. Invest., 17:281–298, 1967.

Essner, E.: Endoplasmic reticulum and the origin of microbodies in fetal mouse liver. Lab. Invest., 17:71–87, 1967.

Farber, J. L., and El-Mofty, S. K.: The biochemical pathology of liver cell necrosis. Am. J. Pathol., 81:237–250, 1975.

Fawcett, D. W.: The Cell. Philadelphia, W. B. Saunders Co., 1966.

Harris, R. J. C. (ed.): The Interpretation of Ultrastructure. New York, Academic Press, 1962.

Herdson, P. B., Kaltenback, J. P., and Jennings, R. B.: Fine structural and biochemical changes in dog myocardium during autolysis. Am. J. Pathol., 57:539–557, 1969.

Hruban, Z., Slesers, A., and Orlando, R.: Structure of enzymes in vitro. Lab. Invest., 16:550–564, 1967.

Ito, T.: A pathological study on fat necrosis in swine. Jpn. J. Vet. Sci., 35:299–310, 1973.

Ito, T., Miura, S. Ohshima, K., and Numakunai, S.: Pathological studies of fat necrosis (lipomatosis) in cattle. Jpn. J. Vet. Sci., 30:141–150 & 3 plates, 1968.

Jennings, R. B., Gnoti, C. E., and Reiner, K. A.: Ischemic tissue injury. Am. J. Pathol., 81:179–198, 1975.

Jorgensen, F.: Electron microscopic studies of normal visceral epithelial cells. Lab. Invest., 17:225–242, 1967.

Kerr, J. R. F.: An electron-microscope study of liver cell necrosis due to heliotrine. J. Pathol., 97:557–562, 1969.

King, D. W., et al.: Cell death. I. The effect of injury on the proteins and deoxyribonucleic acid of Ehrlich tumor cells. II. The effect of injury on the enzymatic protein of Ehrlich tumor cells. III. The effect of injury on water and electrolytes of Ehrlich tumor cells. IV. The effects of injury on the entrance of vital dye in Ehrlich tumor cells. Am. J. Pathol., 35:369–381, 575–589, 835–849, 1067–1079, 1959.

Littefield, J. W., et al.: Studies on cytoplasmic ribonucleoprotein particles from the liver of the rat. J. Biol. Chem., 217:111–123, 1955.

Magee, P. N.: Toxic liver necrosis. Lab. Invest., 15:111–123, 1966.

Mahley, R. W., et al.: Lipid transport in liver. II. Electron microscopic and biochemical studies of alterations in lipoprotein transport induced by cortisone in the rabbit. Lab. Invest., 19:358–369, 1968.

Majno, G., LaGattuta, M., and Thompson, T. E.: Cellular death and necrosis: Chemical, physical and morphologic changes in rat liver. Virchows Arch. [Pathol. Anat.], 333:421–465, 1960.

Palade, G. E., and Porter, K. R.: Studies on the endoplasmic reticulum. I. Its identification in cells in situ. J. Exp. Med., 100:641–656, 1954.

Palade, G. E., and Siekovitz, P.: Pancreatic microsomes. An integrated morphological and biochemical study. J. Biophys. Biochem. Cytol., 2:671–691, 1956.

Panabokke, R. G.: An experimental study of fat necrosis. J. Pathol. Bact., 75:319–331, 1958.

Pearl, R.: The Biology of Death. Philadelphia, J. B. Lippincott Co., 1922.

Prichard, R. W.: Descriptions in pathology. Avoiding pathological descriptions. [Editorial, Amer. Med. Ass.] Arch. Pathol., 59:612–617, 1955. Reprinted Path. Vet., 3:169–177, 1966.

Ribelin, W. E., and DeEds, F.: Fat necrosis in man and animals. J. Am. Vet. Med. Assoc., 136:135–139, 1960.

Schlumberger, H. G.: Origins of cell concept in pathology. Arch. Pathol., 37:396–407, 1944.

Smuckler, E. A., and Trump, B. F.: Alterations in the structure and function of the rough surfaced endoplasmic reticulum during necrosis in vitro. Am. J. Pathol., 53:315–329, 1968.

Splitter, G. A., and McGavin, M. D.: Sequence and rate of postmortem autolysis in guinea pig liver. Am. J. Vet. Res., 35:1591–1596, 1974.

Tosteson, D. C.: Regulation of cell volume by sodium and potassium transplant. In The Cellular Function of Membrane Transport, edited by J. F. Hoffman. Englewood Cliffs, Prentice-Hall, 1964. pp. 3–22.

Trump, B. F., et al.: An electron microscopic study of mouse liver during necrosis in vivo (autolysis). Lab. Invest., 11:986–1016, 1962.

Trump, B. F., and Mergner, W. J.: Cell injury. In The Inflammatory Process, Vol. 1, edited by B. W. Zweifach, L. Grant, and R. T. McCluskey. New York, Academic Press, 1974. pp. 115–257.

Vitovec, J., Proks, C., and Valvoda, V.: Lipomatosis (fat necrosis) in cattle and pigs. J. Comp. Pathol., 85:53–59, 1975.

Vogt, M. T., and Farber, E.: On the molecular pathology of ischemic renal cell death. Reversible and irreversible cellular and mitochondrial alterations. Am. J. Pathol., 53:1–26, 1968.

Winborn, W. B., and Bockman, D. E.: Origin of lysosomes in parietal cells. Lab. Invest., 19:256–264, 1968.

CHAPTER 2

Cellular Infiltrations and Degenerations

A variety of endogenous substances may accumulate in normal or degenerating cells. Their presence is indicative of a metabolic abnormality in the affected cell, or at another site if the affected cell has merely passively acquired the substance. Such substances may or may not be harmful to the affected cell. Cell and tissue depositions of minerals and pigmented substances are treated separately in Chapter 3.

FATTY CHANGE

The intracellular accumulation of lipid (usually as neutral fat) occurs in the liver, kidney, and heart under various conditions, most of them pathologic. Since Virchow's time, efforts have been made to distinguish between physiologic and pathologic accumulations of fat in cells and to understand their significance to the function and survival of affected cells. Many terms have been developed over the years. Some may be considered synonyms; others, based upon concepts now considered invalid, should be abandoned. **Fatty metamorphosis, fatty deposition, intracellular lipid deposition** or **accumulation** are each considered synonymous with **fatty change**, the term currently considered most appropriate. The term **fat phanaerosis**, or **lipophanaerosis**, was based upon the invalid concept that fat was simply "unmasked" in affected cells, that is, the breakdown of lipoprotein membranes and complex lipids resulted in the visible droplets of lipid. This is now known to be not true. The term **fatty degeneration** was used to designate a presumed degenerative change which leads to necrosis of the cell and to distinguish it from **fatty infiltration**, an accumulation of fat that was readily reversible and did not lead to damage to the cell. It now appears that the criteria long considered to distinguish between the two are not supported by present evidence. We shall consider these terms to be less-preferred synonyms for fatty change.

Microscopic Appearance. In ordinary sections, fats and lipids appear in the cytoplasm as clear, unstained spherical spaces. This shape is due to the well-known fact that oil and water do not mix. The spaces are clear because they are empty, the fat having been dissolved by the solvents (alcohol, xylene, etc.) used in preparing the tissue for embedding in paraffin or celloidin. If it is desired that the lipids actually be retained, the sections must be cut on the freezing microtome. They can then be handled by techniques that involve a minimal use of fat solvents and be stained by special **fat stains**. Sudan III stains fats a yellowish-orange color; Sudan IV, also known as scarlet red or Scharlach red, gives

33

them a redder shade; osmic acid colors them black; Nile blue sulfate imparts a violet color, which is bluish in the case of fatty acids and reddish when neutral fats predominate. Certain techniques have been devised for the differential staining of true fats and lipids, but the distinction is somewhat more satisfactorily made by means of the polarizing microscope. True fats are isotropic, which means that the light coming through them vibrates in one plane. When viewed with the polarizing microscope, the analyzer can be turned so as to darken these completely. The common lipoidal substances are anisotropic, or birefringent, the light from them vibrating in two or more planes. As a result, these substances are not obliterated as the analyzer is turned. Under the polarizing microscope, little points of light in the form of a Maltese cross indicate the lipoid particles, which are especially likely to be esters of cholesterol.

In the liver, the fat appears as droplets in the cytoplasm of the epithelial cells. It is usually in the form of droplets so fine that a large number are contained within the cytoplasm of one cell, but at times there is a mixture of large and small droplets. Coalescence may lead to a single large vacuole displacing the cytoplasm and nucleus, leading to a cell resembling that of normal adipose tissue. The nucleus remains practically unchanged. Usually all parts of the liver are affected almost equally. Within the lobule, the distribution is likely to be zonal, as explained in the discussion of acute toxic hepatitis (Chap. 23). Most, if not all, droplets are true neutral fat.

In the kidney, lipids may be deposited in the epithelial cytoplasm of any of the tubules, but as a rule the proximal convoluted tubules or the ascending limbs of Henle's loops, located in the medullary rays, are involved almost exclusively. The droplets are small and indistinct and may easily be overlooked until a fat stain is made. In certain types of glomerular dis-

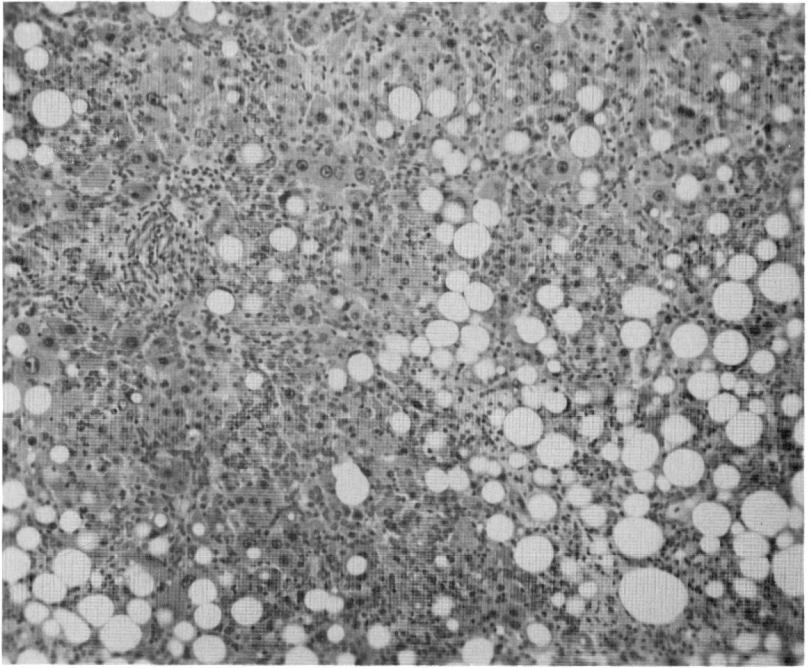

Fig. 2–1. Fatty change of the liver of a rat which received a diet deficient in choline and methionine. (H & E, × 115.)

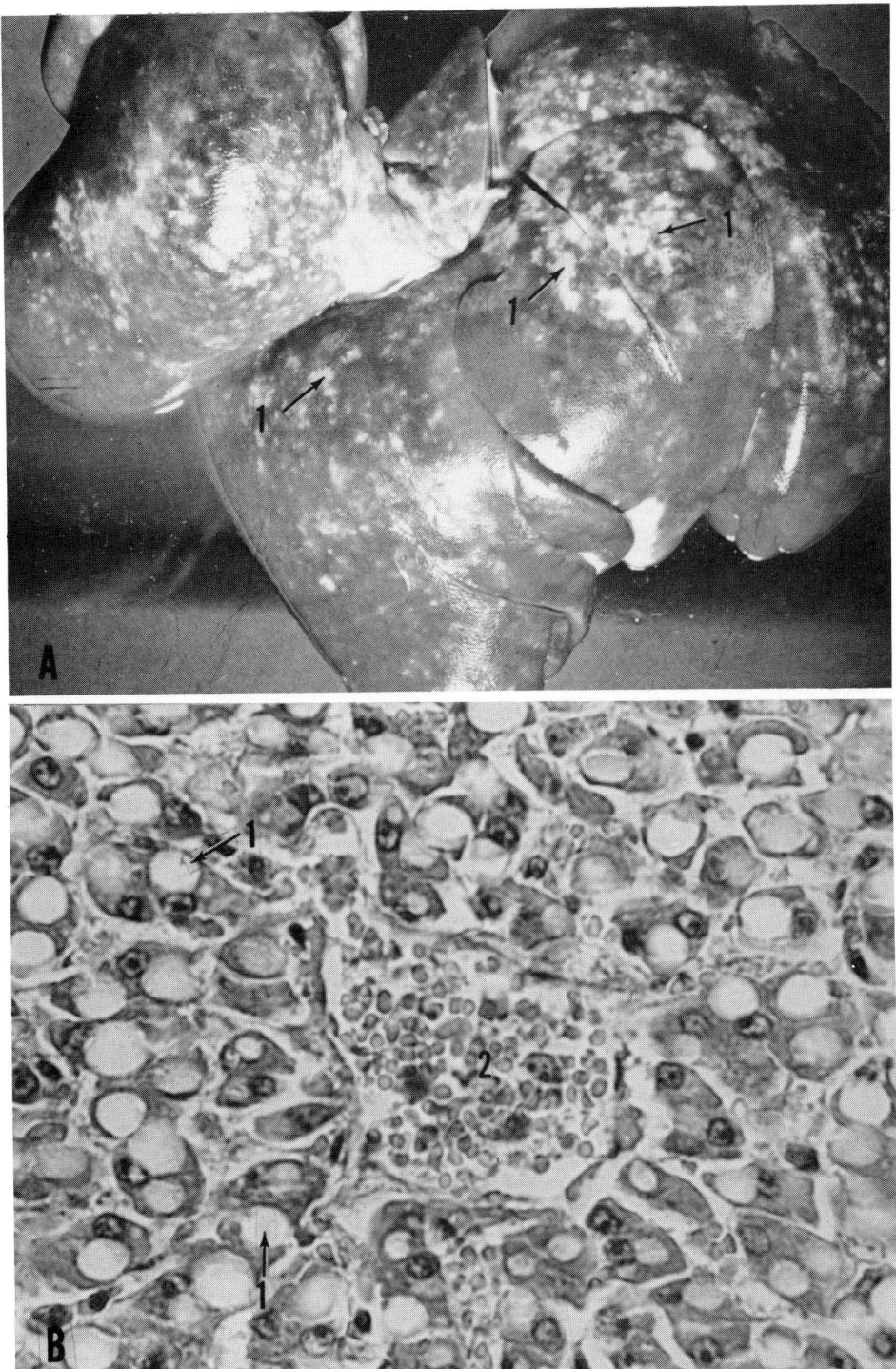

Fig. 2–2. Fatty change, liver of a dog given 200 ml of olive oil and cream six hours before (unexpected) death. *A*, Deposits of fat *(1)* are seen in all lobes. *B*, Fat droplets *(1)* in liver cells surrounding a central vein *(2)*. (Courtesy of Armed Forces Institute of Pathology.) Contributor: Dr. Melvin G. Rhoades.

ease, numerous fat droplets may be demonstrated by means of fat stains in the glomeruli, presumably in the epithelial cells. In cases in which the connective tissue surrounding Bowman's capsules has undergone inflammatory increase, fat stains may demonstrate fat droplets. Likewise, when the walls of arteries have suffered nephrosclerotic thickening, fat may often be stained in them. Rarely, fatty material has been stained in the lumens of the tubules toward the end of the excretory route.

In the heart, fat appears in fine droplets within the muscle cells. The affected cells are often grouped together in patches that alternate with unaffected areas. Fatty change in the heart is not easily detected without a suitable special stain. It has nothing to do with adipose cells, which occur normally in the coronary groove and which may extend a variable distance among the muscle bundles.

Lipids also occur in certain other cells and tissues, which will be mentioned in the discussion of causes.

Gross Appearance. Organs with intracellular fat accumulation are lighter in color and have a greasy cut surface. The color approaches that of normal adipose tissue; yellow, if carotenoids are dissolved in the fat, or white in species without carotenoids. Fat in the liver produces an enlargement of the organ which is limited by a tensely stretched capsule, a slight bulging of the cut surfaces when incised, and a less acute angle between its anterior and posterior surfaces where they join each other at the border of the organ. The liver is slightly or markedly lighter in color, approaching a tan or yellow which lacks the greenish tinge that goes with icterus. With rare exceptions, all parts of the liver are affected equally. The presence of fat lowers the specific gravity of the tissue; very fatty livers float in water. Extensive accumulations of lipids make the liver friable, that is, reduce its strength and toughness. It may be

possible to force the finger into the hepatic tissue with little resistance, and in being handled postmortem, a lobe may be fractured unavoidably. Summarizing, the fatty liver is recognized grossly by enlargement, light color, light weight, and friability.

Fat in the kidney may bring a slight irregularity in depth of color of the cut surface, but it is only detected with certainty when, as frequently happens in the dog, the ascending loops of Henle contain it. In such a case, medullary rays stand out as brilliant white streaks radially directed through the cortex but not reaching the capsule. Diffuse paleness of the renal tissue is seldom attributable to fatty changes.

In the heart, fatty degeneration cannot be judged accurately by gross examination.

Causes. Intracellular accumulation of lipid may occur in any of several situations that interfere with the transport or metabolism of fat, or in special instances, synthesis of protein. These mechanisms are best known in the liver. A short summary of the major means of transport and metabolism of fat by the liver follows: Fat is absorbed from the small intestine and transported by means of the plasma to the liver in **chylomicra**, tiny lipid particles consisting mostly of triglycerides, but also containing small amounts of protein and phospholipid. In the liver, triglycerides are hydrolyzed enzymatically to fatty acids. Protein is synthesized by the endoplasmic reticulum and combined with triglycerides to form several lipoprotein particles, which are released into the plasma (low density lipoproteins; very low density lipoproteins; high density lipoproteins). Under the influence of lipoprotein lipase, the lipids are deposited as fatty acids in adipose tissue. Mobilization of fat may return fatty acids to plasma and then to the liver. Also in the liver, esterification of fatty acids to triglyceride, phospholipid, or cholesterol ester may occur under enzymatic control.

Some of the mechanisms that may interfere with the transport and metabolism of lipid to result in fatty change are the following:

(1) **Excessive release of free fatty acids** from adipose tissue, resulting in delivery of increased amounts of these acids to the liver, heart, or kidney, which may not be able to utilize the increased free fatty acids, thence storing them as neutral fat. This is apparently the process involved in starvation.

(2) **Decreased utilization or oxidation of fatty acids** due to interference with cofactors essential to oxidation of long-chain fatty acids. Bacterial toxins (e.g., diphtheria toxin) are believed to produce their effect on fatty change in this manner.

(3) **Lipotrope deficiency** resulting in decreased phospholipid synthesis. Deficiency of methionine or choline decreases phospholipid synthesis, and their absence leads to esterification of diglycerides to triglycerides.

(4) **Fatty acids preferentially esterified to triglycerides.** This is believed to explain the fatty change in acute ethanol poisoning.

(5) **Failure of protein synthesis,** thus reducing the protein component available for the lipoprotein particles, which are the means of excretion of lipid from the liver. Examples may be found in experimental poisoning by ethionine, carbon tetrachloride, puromycin, or yellow phosphorus. Each of these cause dispersion of ribosomes from the endoplasmic reticulum, swelling of the endoplasmic reticulum, and accumulation of neutral fat in the cytoplasm. Dietary protein deficiency also leads to fatty change by interfering with the secretion of triglycerides.

Significance. Fatty change, the intracellular accumulation of lipids, is a process independent of other changes (e.g., necrosis), which results from one or more of the five mechanisms described previously (or others not described). These pathogenic mechanisms may be caused by many factors, such as toxins of poisonous plants (Chapter 16), or metabolic disorders (Chapter 17). In animals, aside from various poisonings, extensive fatty change is a constant feature of ketosis, toxemia of pregnant ewes, and diabetes mellitus.

Fatty change may be completely reversible or may lead to rupture and death of the cell. Although independent of necrosis, it may have the same causes, and often occurs in the same organ in association with necrosis. Interpretation of the significance of fatty change, once recognized in a specific case, requires consideration of all the possible causes and pathogenic mechanisms.

INTERSTITIAL OR STROMAL FATTY INFILTRATION

These terms currently are used to describe the deposition of lipids in the cytoplasm of adipose tissue cells found among the interstitial connective tissue cells throughout the animal body. If the amount of fat is excessive, obesity is used as a descriptive term. Adipose tissue cells may also replace muscle cells that atrophy for any reason.

EXTRACELLULAR ACCUMULATION OF LIPIDS

Lipid may occur outside of cells in some situations. Necrosis of cells may release lipids into extracellular spaces, where pooling may make them visible. Cholesterol is released from cells or pooled from lipoproteins in crystalline form ("clefts") as the result of hemorrhage. Fat may be seen in blood vessels also as emboli of adipose tissue or bone marrow. Fat droplets in renal tubular epithelium may be shed into the lumen to produce fatty casts.

FATTY DEGENERATION OF MYELIN

This is a condition in which myelin is destroyed with the production of stainable fat as a degeneration product. It will be treated in the study of the nervous system.

Abraham, E. P., and Robb-Smith, A. H. T.: Degenerative changes and some of their consequences. *In* General Pathology, 4th ed., edited by H. W. Florey. Philadelphia, W. B. Saunders Co., 1970.

Gordon, E. R., and Lough, J.: Ultrastructural and biochemical aspects during the regression of an ethanol-induced fatty liver. Lab. Invest., 26:154–162, 1972.

Isselbacher, K. J., and Greenberger, N. J.: Metabolic effects of alcohol on the liver. N. Engl. J. Med., 270:351–371, 1964.

Lombardi, B.: Considerations on the pathogenesis of fatty liver. Lab. Invest., 15:1–20, 1966.

Longnecker, D. S., Skinozuka, H., and Farber, E.: Molecular pathology of in vivo inhibition of protein synthesis. Am. J. Pathol., 52:891–915, 1968.

Kumar, V., Deo, M. G., and Ramalingaswami, V.: Mechanism of fatty liver in protein deficiency. An experimental study in the Rhesus monkey. Gastroenterology, 62:445–451, 1972.

Meldolesi, J., et al.: Cytoplasmic changes in rat liver after prolonged treatment with low doses of ethionine and adenine. An ultrastructural and biochemical study. Lab. Invest., 17:265–275, 1967.

————: Effects of carbon tetrachloride on the synthesis of liver endoplasmic reticulum membranes. Lab. Invest., 19:315–323, 1969.

Reynolds, E. S., and Yec, A. G.: Liver parenchymal cell injury. VI. Significance of early glucose-6-phosphate suppression and transient calcium influx following poisoning. Lab. Invest., 19:273–281, 1968.

Rubin, E., and Lieber, C. S.: The effects of ethanol on the liver. Int. Rev. Exp. Pathol., 11:177–232, 1972.

Schlunk, F. F., and Lombardi, B.: Liver liposomes. I. Isolation and chemical characterization. Lab. Invest., 17:30–38, 1967.

————: On the ethionine-induced fatty liver in male and female rats. Lab. Invest., 17:299–307, 1967.

GLYCOGEN AND GLYCOGEN STORAGE DISEASE

Since the visible changes in glycogenic infiltration are somewhat similar to those in lipidosis, it is convenient to consider the former at this point. Glycogen is sometimes picturesquely called animal starch, since its chemical formula resembles those of the true starches in being multiples of $C_6H_{10}O_5$. Carbohydrates of all kinds are

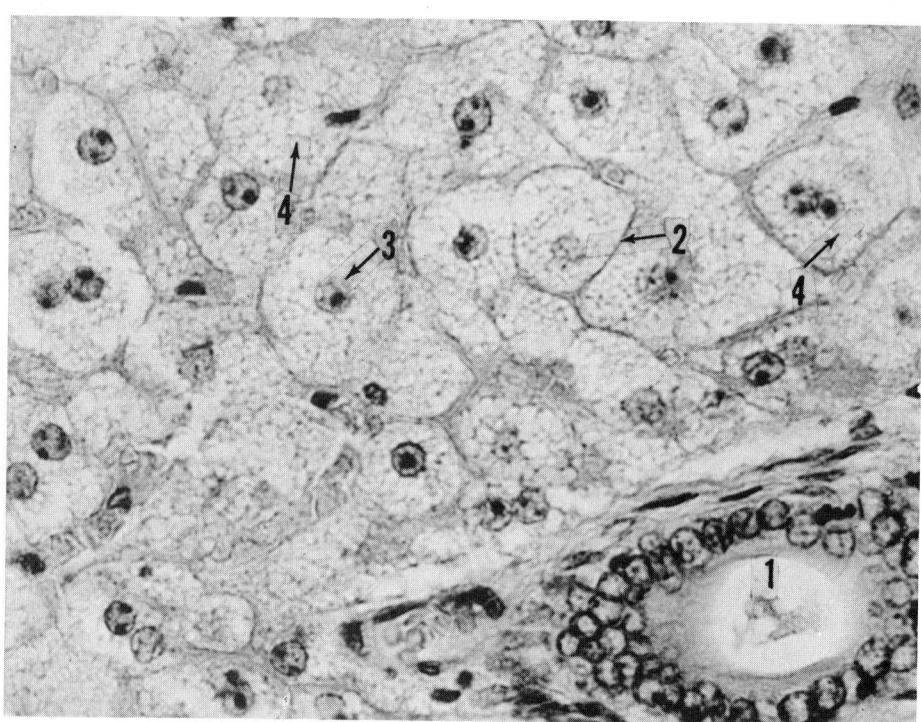

Fig. 2–3. Glycogen in liver cells of a dog. Glycogen is a normal finding in well nourished animals; it disappears rapidly in many diseased states. Bile duct (*1*), distinct walls of liver cells (*2*), centrally located nuclei (*3*) of hepatic cells, and fine droplets of glycogen (*4*), which fill the cytoplasm of these cells. (× 500.) (Courtesy of Armed Forces Institute of Pathology.) Contributor: Dr. Lester Barto.

normally carried in the blood as glucose (dextrose) to be stored as glycogen, chiefly in liver and muscle cells. Hence it is normal to find considerable amounts in these tissues.

Occurrence. Glycogen occurs pathologically in the cytoplasm of epithelial cells of the liver and kidneys, leukocytes, cardiac muscle, and less frequently, in smooth muscle, spleen, lymph nodes, and brain.

Microscopic Appearance. Whether the glycogen be normally or pathologically deposited, it is seen in the cytoplasm of cells as clear spaces or vacuoles. This is because glycogen, being soluble in water, is readily dissolved away in ordinary methods of tissue preparation. The empty spaces are not necessarily round nor do they always have sharp outlines, but they are clear. All of these facts help one to distinguish glycogenic infiltration from fatty change and from hydropic degeneration. Such

vacuoles in the epithelium of Henle's loops are almost surely due to glycogen.

The ultrastructural appearance of glycogen is characteristic (Fig. 2–4). The method of fixation influences the appearance of glycogen, but usually the electron microscope reveals its smallest unit as roughly isodiametric, slightly irregular particles, 150 to 300 Å in diameter. These, **beta particles,** usually coalesce to form aggregates called **alpha particles** or **rosettes.** The number of particles or rosettes vary greatly, as is to be expected, and may be present in such numbers to obscure most intracellular organelles.

The hepatic epithelium of well-nourished animals normally contains considerable glycogen, enough to give the cytoplasm a finely foamy appearance, varying with the amount and recentness of carbohydrate consumption.

Positive identification or differentiation

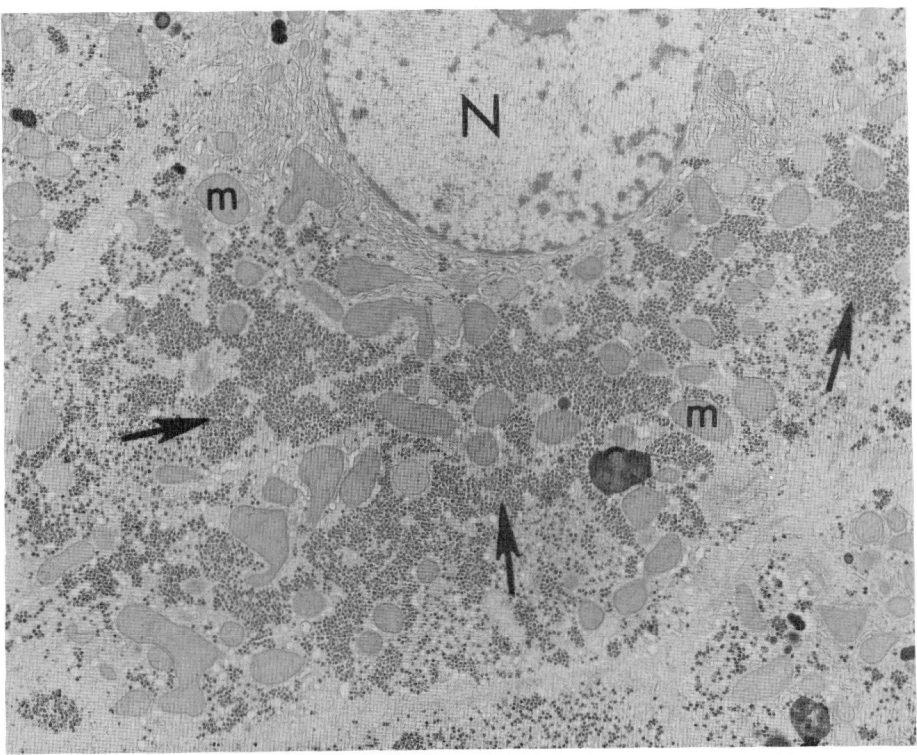

Fig. 2–4. Glycogen in a hepatocyte of an owl monkey (*Aotus trivirgatus*). Glycogen appears as numerous small electron dense granules (arrows). N, nucleus, m, mitochondria. (Courtesy of Dr. Norval W. King.)

depends upon special technique. The tissue is fixed in alcohol and alcoholic stains are used throughout, so that no water comes in contact with it. Best's carmine stain then colors the glycogen a bright pink.

Gross Appearance. Glycogen is not detected grossly.

Cause. The cause of glycogen infiltration in animals is almost always the result of hyperglycemia, as in diabetes mellitus. The fatty change so typical of diabetes mellitus may mark the presence of glycogen. In the kidney, glycogen infiltration of proximal convoluted tubule epithelium partially results from tubular reabsorption of excreted glucose.

Glycogen Storage Diseases

In people, several specific genetic defects in the enzymes involved in the metabolism and catabolism of glycogen result in the accumulation of glycogen in cells and are grouped as *glycogen storage diseases.* Ten different enzyme defects, leading to relatively distinct clinicopathologic entities, have been identified in man. At least two forms of glycogen storage disease have been recognized in animals.

Type II, or Pompe's disease, has been described in an apparently healthy cat (Sandstrom et al., 1969) and in three calves with muscular weakness (Edwards and Richards, 1979). The disease results from a deficiency of α-glucosidase, leading to glycogen storage in the brain, muscles, and liver. The glycogen is predominantly stored within membrane-bound bodies believed to be lysosomes. In other forms of glycogen storage disease, the glycogen is not membrane-bound.

Type III glycogen storage disease, or Cori's disease, has been reported in four female German Shepherd dogs (Rafiquzzaman, et al., 1976, Ceh, et al., 1976). This disorder results from a deficiency of the debranching enzyme, amylo-1, 6-glucosidase. Glycogen is stored diffusely throughout the cytoplasm of hepatocytes,

myocardium, skeletal muscle, smooth muscle, and nerve cells. At two months of age, the dogs developed dizziness, muscular weakness, and distended abdomen. At necropsy, the liver was grossly enlarged.

Significance. The glycogen is not in itself injurious, but its presence in these situations is indicative of other injury.

Ceh, L., Hauge, J. G., Svenkerud, R., and Strande, A.: Glycogenosis type III in the dog. Acta Vet. Scand., 17:210–222, 1976.

Edwards, J. R., and Richards, R. B.: Bovine generalized glycogenosis type II: a clinico-pathological study. Br. Vet. J., 135:338–348, 1979.

McAdams, A. J., Hug, G., and Bove, K. E.: Glycogen storage disease, types I to X: criteria for morphologic diagnosis. Hum. Pathol., 5:463–487, 1974.

Rafiquzzaman, M., Svenkerud, R., Strande, A., and Hauge, J. G.: Glycogenosis in the dog. Acta Vet. Scand., 17:196–209, 1976.

Sandstrom, B., Westman, J., and Ockerman, P. A.: Glycogenosis of the central nervous system in the cat. Acta Neuropathol., 14:194–200, 1969.

HYDROPIC DEGENERATION

Hydropic or vacuolar degeneration is a condition in which there is an increase in water, possibly in association with electrolytes or organic compounds within the cytoplasm of cells. The advanced stage of acute cellular swelling that accompanies most forms of cell death is an example of hydropic degeneration. Whether all forms of hydropic degeneration are synonymous with acute cellular swelling is not clear. Swollen, vacuolated cells are, however, encountered in many epithelial tissues, including the skin, liver, and kidney, in the apparent absence of death of cells. It may be acute cellular swelling before reaching the point of no return. An example that would appear to be an exception is osmotic nephrosis.

INTRACELLULAR ACCUMULATION OF PROTEIN

The accumulation of protein in cells leading to an increased cytoplasmic density or discrete eosinophilic droplets has been termed cloudy swelling, parenchymatous degeneration, albuminous degeneration, protein degeneration, and granular degeneration. Most of these terms are antiquated and have no particular meaning today. Some of these terms referred to acute cellular swelling, but most have no significance.

Hyaline droplets or protein droplets may occur in cells, especially in the kidney. Although previously called hyaline droplet degeneration, it is probably not a degenerative lesion but a nontoxic accumulation. The most common form of hyaline droplets occurs in the epithelium of the proximal convoluted tubule of the kidney. It results from leakage of protein through the glomerulus into the urine and subsequent reabsorption by pinocytosis. The pinocytotic vesicles fuse with lysosomes and the protein is digested. If accumulation exceeds the rate of digestion, microscopically visible droplets result. By light microscopy, these appear as round, highly eosinophilic droplets or granules of varying size, up to 10 μ in diameter. If the protein leakage is great, eosinophilic **albuminous casts** or **hyaline casts** are present in the tubular lumina.

HYALIN

Reference has just been made to hyaline droplet formation. The adjective "hyaline" is used to refer to any one of several substances that are white, glossy, solid, dense, and of smoothly homogeneous texture (*hyalos* Greek = glassy or glass-like). Substances described as hyalin (a noun) also occur as extracellular changes termed connective tissue hyalin and epithelial hyalin.

Connective-Tissue Hyalin

Connective-tissue hyalin is a substance formed in connective tissue and, since it represents a change that has taken place in that tissue, one may refer to the changed connective tissue as "hyaline connective tissue."

Occurrence. It occurs, therefore, in structures already formed wholly or partly of connective tissue. These include particularly (1) old scars, (2) the corpus albicans of the ovary, a physiologic scarring of the defunct corpus luteum, (3) the walls of arteriosclerotic blood vessels, and (4) other places where connective tissue has been chronically injured or deprived of nutrition.

Microscopic Appearance. The hyaline area is structureless and smoothly homogeneous under the microscope as well as to the naked eye. It is strongly acidophilic and stains a brilliant pink with the usual stains. When completely hyalinized, the connective tissue has no nuclei and no fibrils, but the boundaries of the hyaline area are indefinite, usually with a gradual transition through an outer zone, where nuclei are sparse, into the surrounding normal fibrous tissue.

Gross Appearance. The amount of hyaline material may be too small to be noticeable, but greater amounts are white, shiny, semitranslucent, and glassy, but uniformly solid and dense. Old scars are white, even in the skin of dark animals, partly because of the more or less hyaline connective tissue and partly because of the inability of the regenerated epithelium to develop pigmentation.

Causes. The fundamental cause is a lack of nutrition. Large scars are notorious for their poor blood supply. More immediate factors in its production are previous injury as well as advanced age of the individual or tissue. In many species, the placental villi become hyaline as the time of parturition approaches. Toxins or injurious substances carried in the circulating blood may be responsible for the change as it occurs in arteriosclerotic blood vessels, but this is obscure.

Significance. While not incompatible with the continued existence of the tissue involved, hyalinization is a degenerative process. The tissue functions less perfectly and connective tissue, so affected, has less than normal strength. It is also inelastic and inflexible, as may be observed in old scars. Once formed, it is relatively permanent. Hyalinization of a blood-vessel wall is by no means conducive to maintaining an even and normal blood pressure, and rupture of the vessel is to be feared.

Epithelial Hyalin

An obsolete synonym for epithelial hyalin is "colloid."

Occurrence. The occurrence of this change is usually limited to **corpora amylacea** (Latin for "starch-like bodies"), which may be found in (a) the prostate, most commonly of man, and (b) the lung. Also called corpora amylacea by neuro-pathologists are round, opaque bodies encountered in damaged areas of the white matter of the brain. They are 5 to 10 μ in diameter and more or less amphoteric (purplish) in their staining. They are considered to be the remains of astrocytes that have disappeared, usually following a stage of gliosis. The use of the term corpus amylaceum should be avoided for granules that are merely calcified, such as those often found in the mammary gland.

Microscopic Appearance. Corpora amylacea are rounded, homogeneous, or concentrically laminated bodies, staining pink, perhaps tinged zonally with blue, that lie within an alveolus of lung or prostate. They are not detected grossly.

Cause and Significance. Corpora amylacea received their name from the early belief that they were carbohydrate in nature, but it is now known that they are composed of protein. They are believed to result from pressure, dehydration, and a prolonged kneading action upon dead cells that have desquamated from the epithelial lining, held together probably by a little fibrin. Thus their presence indicates previous degeneration.

KERATOHYALIN

Keratin is another name for this substance, and the process of its formation may be called either keratinization or **cornification**. It may be normal or it may be pathologic because excessive in amount or abnormal in location. It is produced by the slow death of stratified squamous epithelial cells and is normal as the cornified layer, or stratum corneum, of the epidermis and certain other squamous epithelial structures.

Microscopic Appearance. In a state of complete cornification, this material appears as a solid, homogeneous, pink-staining mass or layer forming the superficial zone of stratified squamous epithelium. It blends gradually with the epithelium of the prickle-cell layer (stratum granulosum), becoming more and more cellular. In locations where it is constantly wet, it occasionally stains bluish.

Gross Appearance. It is that of a hard, colorless, more or less translucent, horny material. In the skin, it is likely to be accompanied by much wrinkling.

Occurrence, Causes, and Significance. Abnormal keratinization occurs in the following situations:

(1) In **calluses**, such as those that form on the human hand as the result of prolonged friction and pressure insufficient to cause blistering or erosion. Here it constitutes a physiologic and protective hypertrophy but becomes excessive. The same process may result from mild irritation by harness or saddle.

(2) **Corns** on the human foot are essentially similar to calluses, but they are more extensive and irritating because of location. **Corns in the horse's foot** start as a bruise, usually with underlying hemorrhage, and later involve excessive proliferation of the horn. Such lesions as these may also be viewed as excessive proliferative inflammations.

(3) In **warts,** which are focal papillary epithelial proliferations caused by a filterable virus. In addition to the total excess of epithelium, the cornified layer itself is excessive.

(4) In the bovine disease known as **specific hyperkeratosis** which is caused by poisoning by substances containing chlorinated naphthalenes.

(5) In the rare and unexplained disease

of man, cattle, and dogs called **ichthyosis,** in which horny scales appear all over the body (Figs. 18–3, 18–4).

(6) In **metaplasia** of some other kind of epithelium to stratified squamous epithelium. This occurs in urinary and other mucous membranes under the influence of avitaminosis-A, and in chemical irritation of the bronchial lining, where it may be a precancerous condition.

(7) In the "epithelial pearls" of **squamous-cell carcinoma**, in which the cornified layer finds itself the compressed core of an epithelial mass whose aberrant manner of growth has caused it to be "turned inside out."

Except in the last instance, excessive keratinization is caused by continued mild irritation of one kind or another.

While primarily a protective reaction, excessive keratohyalin can interfere with secretory and absorptive functions and can cause pain in a tissue under mechanical pressure. When the cause is removed, the excessive keratin disappears by desquamation.

AMYLOIDOSIS

In this disorder, various organs are infiltrated by a firm and solid extracellular substance called amyloid. While the name means starch-like, it is now known that amyloid is a protein that contains somewhat less than 5% carbohydrate.

Occurrence. Amyloidosis may affect any tissue and may be restricted to a single organ or be generalized. The spleen, liver, and kidneys are noteworthy as the sites of its earliest and most extensive formation. Lymph nodes and adrenal glands are also commonly involved. It is a slowly progressive disease which in the end may almost completely replace the affected organ or tissue.

In the spleen, the deposits either form between cells in the Malpighian corpuscles or along the sinuses. As the deposits enlarge in the Malpighian corpuscles, tiny nodules of white, firm material, which are visible grossly, impart a suggestion of a spleen sprinkled with sago or its more modern counterpart, tapioca grains, producing what is traditionally called a **sago spleen**.

In the liver, the deposits begin in the spaces of Dissé between the Kupffer cells and the hepatocytes, ultimately causing atrophy and necrosis of the hepatic parenchyma. Renal amyloidosis usually appears first in the glomeruli, although it may be restricted to the medulla, a finding common in cats. The glomerular deposits begin in the mesangium. In renal amyloidosis, amyloid fibrils may be detected in urinary sediment by electron microscopy. In most tissues, including the spleen, liver, and kidney, amyloid deposits favor the immediate vicinity, or the actual wall, of smaller blood vessels.

Microscopic Appearance. As already implied, amyloid is a dense and nearly homogeneous substance that replaces and obliterates pre-existing cells. The borders of the amyloid are relatively sharp, a fact which assists in distinguishing it from connective-tissue hyalin. With hematoxylin and eosin, this substance stains a slightly purplish pink. Reasonably specific staining reactions are obtained with Congo red, which stains amyloid orange and has an apple-green birefringence when viewed with polarized light. Although this is an excellent method of identification, it is not pathognomonic, especially if the tissues have been preserved with fixatives other than formalin. Thioflavin-T staining imparts fluorescence to amyloid with equal or greater specificity than Congo red birefringence. Toluidine blue staining of amyloid results in a reddish polarization color that is not affected by fixation. Although considerably less specific, cresyl violet stains amyloid a violet color.

Ultrastructurally, amyloid is composed of nonbranching fibers about 100 Å in diameter, which are composed of two twisted subfilaments about 40 Å in diame-

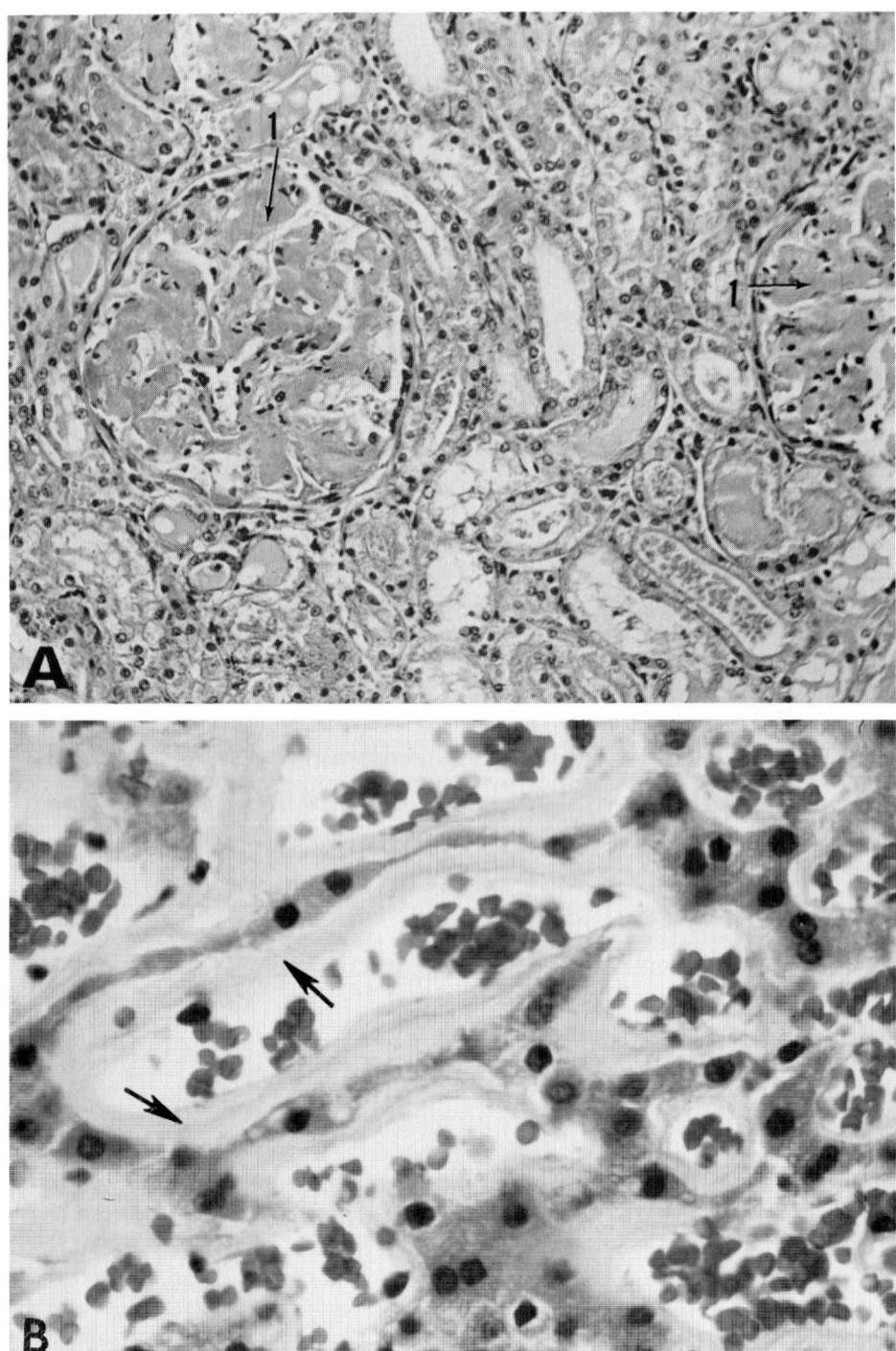

Fig. 2–5. *A*, Amyloidosis, kidney of a dog. Amyloid (*1*) is deposited in the glomerular tufts. (× 175.) (Courtesy of Armed Forces Institute of Pathology.) Contributor: Dr. C. L. Davis. *B*, Amyloidosis, liver of a monkey. Amyloid (arrows) is deposited in the space of Dissé between the hepatocytes and endothelial lining of the sinusoids. The hepatocytes are atrophic.

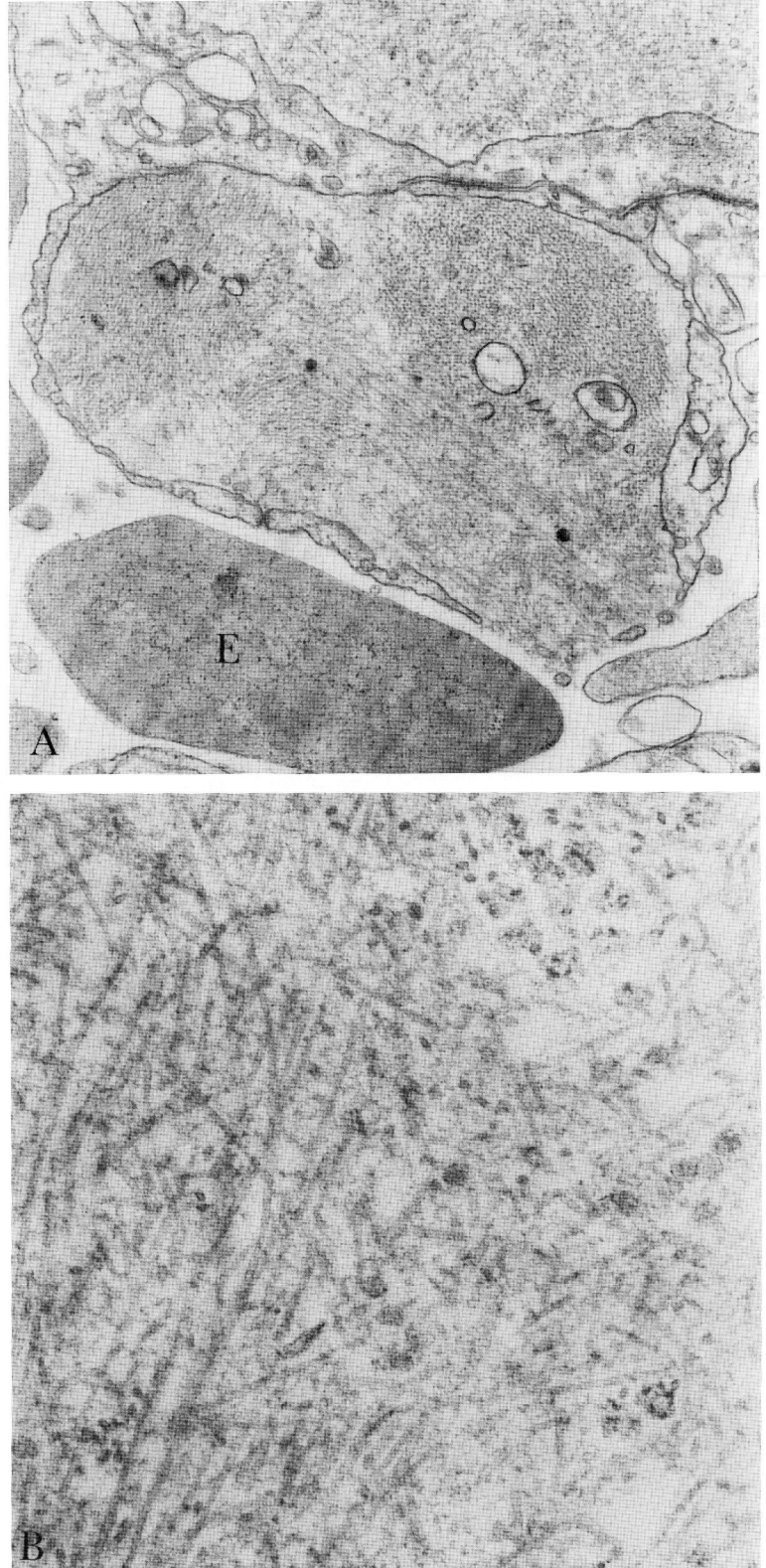

Fig. 2–6. Bovine renal amyloidosis. *A*, Electronmicrograph of subendothelial amyloid encircled by endothelial cytoplasm. E, erythrocyte. (Courtesy of Dr. E. Gruys and *Veterinary Pathology*.) *B*, Ultrastructure of amyloid fibrils in longitudinal and cross section. (Courtesy of Dr. E. Gruys.)

ter and separated by a 20 Å gap, which form a double helix of 1000 Å periodicity.

On fresh slices of tissue, the application of aqueous solutions of iodine, such as Lugol's, brings out the amyloid as a distinctly brown material. Following the iodine solution with dilute sulfuric acid changes the amyloid from brown to blue, which is possibly more conspicuous.

Gross Appearance. Small amounts of amyloid are not detected grossly. When accumulations are larger, this substance is white, opaque, and somewhat resembles lard but is firmer. The term lardosis (not lordosis) has been used as a synonym in some quarters. As a rule, organs other than the spleen show amyloidosis by a slight change in their general appearance rather than in the form of individual deposits. The liver, for instance, is larger, paler, and firmer than normal when extensively involved. Microscopic confirmation is essential.

Cause. Amyloidosis is classically divided into two major forms: primary and secondary. **Primary amyloidosis** occurs independently of any other disease. **Secondary amyloidosis** occurs in association with chronic diseases, especially long-standing infections such as tuberculosis and suppurative processes. It may also be associated with various neoplasms, especially lymphoma and multiple myeloma. It also occurs with frequency in horses that are used for the production of antibodies, and it can be induced experimentally by repeated injections of antigenic material, such as casein and certain drugs. Amyloidosis may also be associated with aging, and this is classified as **senile amyloidosis**. In human beings and mice, several types of **familial amyloidosis** are recognized, such as in familial Mediterranean fever. Whether the pathogenesis in these various forms of amyloidosis is different or the same is not known. Nor is it known whether, in fact, the protein deposits are of the same chemical composition in these various circumstances.

Amyloid is produced locally by reticuloendothelial cells, histiocytes, and plasma cells. It has been speculated that amyloid may also be transported by way of the blood and deposited at distant sites, but this is unproven. Teilum (1966) has postulated a two-phase cellular theory of local secretion. The first phase involves the proliferation and stimulation of pyroninophilic reticuloendothelial cells and plasma cells, resulting in elevated levels of γ-globulin in the plasma. In the second (amyloid) phase, the pyroninophilic cells are suppressed (or exhausted—by persistent stimulation or other means unknown) in their production of γ-globulin (which drops to lower levels in the plasma), and new generations of cells around blood vessels are recognized by material in their cytoplasm which is colored specifically by the periodic acid-Schiff (PAS) method. These PAS-positive cells are believed to produce amyloid in loco around blood vessels. The site of formation is in doubt, but amyloid fibrils have been identified in membrane-bound vesicles that resemble lysosomes. An associated increased rate of synthesis of α-, β-, and γ-globulins and the demonstration that purified amyloid proteins have in part a protein similar to the light chain of immunoglobulin suggests that amyloid may be a degradation product of immunoglobulin. Kisilevsky et al. (1976) suggest α_2-globulin as the most likely precursor.

Significance. Most examples are encountered at autopsy incidental to other diseases, such as those just mentioned. However, if death does not intervene from other causes, amyloidosis progresses to the point where vital functions are destroyed and it is fatal of itself. A cutaneous form of amyloidosis is described in horses (Chap. 18).

Barth, W. F., Gordon, J. K., and Willerson, J. T.: Amyloidosis induced in mice by *Escherichia coli* endotoxin. Science, *162*:694–695, 1968.

Benditt, E. P., and Eriksen, N.: Chemical characteristics of the substance of typical amyloidosis in monkeys. Acta Pathol. Microbiol. Scand., *80A* (Supp. 233):103–108, 1972.

————: Chemical similarity among amyloid substances associated with long standing inflammation. Lab. Invest., 26:615–625, 1972.

Berman, L., Stilmant, M., and Hayes, J. A.: Streptozotocin and renal amyloidosis in the Syrian hamster. Am. J. Pathol., 84:139–148, 1976.

Clark, L., and Seawright, A. A.: Generalized amyloidosis in seven cats. Path. Vet., 6:117–134, 1969.

Cohen, A. S.: Preliminary chemical analysis of purified amyloid fibrils. Lab. Invest., 15:66–83, 1966.

Cohen, A. S.: Amyloidosis. N. Engl. J. Med., 277:522–530, 1967.

Cooper, J. H.: Selective amyloid staining as a function of amyloid composition and structure. Histochemical analysis of the alkaline Congo red, standardized toluidine blue, and iodine methods. Lab. Invest., 31:232–238, 1974.

Cornelius, E. A.: Amyloidosis and renal papillary necrosis in male hybrid mice. Am. J. Pathol., 59:317–326, 1970.

Derosena, R., Koss, M. N., and Pirani, C. L.: Demonstration of amyloid fibrils in urinary sediment. N. Engl. J. Med., 293:1131–1133, 1975.

Gruys, E.: Ultrastructural and enzyme histochemical aspects of amyloidosis in the bovine renal medulla. Vet. Pathol., 12:94–110, 1975.

Gueft, B., and Ghidoni, J. J.: The site of formation and ultrastructure of amlyoid. Am. J. Pathol., 43:837–854, 1963.

Gueft, B., Kikkawa, Y., and Hirschl, S.: An electron-microscopic study of amyloidosis from different species. In Amyloidosis, edited by E. Mandema, L. Ruinen, J. H. Schalten, and A. S. Cohen. Amsterdam, Excerpta Med. Found., 1968.

Hadlow, W. J., and Reinhard, K. R.: Amyloidosis in the dog. Cornell Vet., 44:475–489, 1954.

Hass, G. M., Huntington, R., and Krumdieck, N.: Amyloid. Properties of amyloid deposits occurring in several species under diverse conditions. Arch. Pathol., 35:226–241, 1943.

Jakob, W.: Spontaneous amyloidosis of mammals. Vet. Pathol., 8:292–306, 1971.

Janigan, D. T.: Pathogenic mechanisms in protein-induced amyloidosis. Am. J. Pathol., 55:379–393, 1969.

Kisilevsky, R., Axelrad, M., Brunet, S., and Richards, M.: Effects of amyloid induction on plasma protein turnover, and its implication. Am. J. Pathol., 83:299–318, 1976.

Klatskin, G.: Non-specific green birefringence in Congo red-stained tissues. Am. J. Pathol., 56:1–14, 1969.

Murray, M., Rushton, A., and Selman, I.: Bovine renal amyloidosis: a clinico-pathological study. Vet. Rec., 90:210–216, 1972.

Nordstoga, K.: Amyloidosis in mink induced by repeated injections of endotoxin. Acta Pathol. Microbiol. Scand., 80A:159–168, 1972.

Rodgers, D. R.: Screening for amyloid with the thioflavin-T fluorescent method. Am. J. Clin. Pathol., 44:59–61, 1965.

Saeed, S. M., and Fine, G.: Thioflavin-T for amyloid detection. Am. J. Clin. Pathol., 47:588–593, 1967.

Schwartz, P., Wolfe, K. B., and Beuttas, J. T.: Spontaneous amyloidosis in mink. J. Comp. Pathol., 81:437–445 & 5 plates, 1971.

Shirahama, T., and Cohen, A. S.: Ultrastructural studies on renal peritubular amyloid experimentally induced in guinea pigs. I. General aspects. Lab. Invest., 19:122–131, 1968.

Shirahama, T., and Cohen, A. S.: Intralysosomal formation of amyloid fibrils. Am. J. Pathol., 81:101–116, 1975.

Slauson, D. O., Gribble, D. H., and Russell, S. W.: A clinicopathological study of renal amyloidosis in dogs. J. Comp. Pathol., 80:335–343, 1970.

Stünzi, H., Ehrensperger, F., Wild, P., and Leemann, W.: Systemic cutaneous and subcutaneous amyloidosis in the horse. Vet. Pathol., 12:405–414, 1975.

Teilum, G.: Amyloidosis: origin from fixed periodic acid-Schiff positive reticuloendothelial cells in loco and basic factors in pathogenesis. Lab. Invest., 15:98–110, 1966.

Trautwein, G.: Vergleichende Untersuchungen über das Amyloid und Paramyloid verschiedener Tierarten. I. Histomorphologie und färberische Eugenschaften des amyloids und paramyloids. Path. Vet., 2:297–327, 1965.

————: Vergleichende untersuchungen über das amyloid und Paramyloid verschiedener Tierarten. II. Histochemie des amyloids und Paramyloids. Path. Vet., 2:493–513, 1965.

Wolman, M.: Amyloid, its nature and molecular structure. Comparison of a new toluidine blue polarized light method with traditional procedures. Lab. Invest., 25:104–110, 1971.

Wolman, M., and Buber, J. J.: The cause of the green polarization color of amyloid stained with Congo red. Histochemie, 4:351–356, 1965.

Wright, J. R., Calkins, E., and Humphrey, R. L.: Potassium permanganate reaction in amyloidosis. A histologic method to assist in differentiating forms of this disease. Lab. Invest., 36:274–281, 1977.

Zòltowska, A., and Wrzolkowa, T.: Experimental amyloidosis in hamster. J. Pathol., 109:93–99, 1973.

Zucker-Franklin, D., and Franklin, E. C.: Intracellular localization of human amyloid by fluorescence and electron microscopy. Am. J. Pathol., 59:23–41, 1970.

PROTEINS, ALBUMINS, AND ALBUMINOUS FLUIDS

It is customary in pathology to refer to nonspecific protein substances by what is almost always their principal constituent, albumin. Pathologically or otherwise, these substances are encountered in the microscopic section in a variety of situations as precipitates from body fluids.

(1) The lumen of a blood vessel may be filled with a pink-staining, homogeneous

material. This is merely dehydrated plasma, with serum-albumin as its visible component, the cells having settled after death to some other part of the vessel.

(2) A similar precipitate is often seen in the renal tubules. In this case it is albumin (and other protein) precipitated and coagulated from the excreted urine, and the diagnosis is albuminuria or proteinuria. Sometimes the concentration may be so great that precipitation occurs during life, forming albuminous casts of the tubular lumens, which are recognizable in the voided urine. In sections of kidney, these are usually dense and deep-staining.

(3) Most of the various kinds of cysts are filled with albumin-containing fluid. The liquor folliculi, the "colloid" of the thyroid acini, and the salivary secretions are physiologic examples of similar fluids.

(4) In the case of serous inflammatory exudates or the transudate of edema, the only visible substance remaining is the precipitate of albumin and related proteins. These are seen, for example, filling the alveoli of the lung, as well as in tissue spaces anywhere.

Microscopic Appearance. Albumin precipitated as just outlined is usually smoothly homogeneous, although occasionally, with high magnification, it is in the form of uniformly fine granules. It stains a bright, clear pink by usual techniques. This purity of tint helps to distinguish albumin from amyloid and from fibrin, both of which have an appearance of opacity because they give impure hues based on a variety of wave-lengths.

Gross Appearance. All these substances look like a watery fluid unless, of course, the fluid is mixed with other substances, such as blood or pus.

FIBRIN

Fibrin is another proteinaceous substance, physiologic or pathologic, which the student must learn to recognize.

Occurrence. Fibrin is seen (1) wherever blood clots, as in internal hemorrhages, intravascular clots, be they antemortem (thrombi), or postmortem, (2) in the infrequent clotting of lymph, and (3) in fibrinous inflammatory exudates.

Microscopic Appearance. Fibrin stains' pink, but usually it is a "dirty" or smudgy pink. Ordinarily, it is in the form of minute, tangled fibrils readily visible with a magnification of 400 or 500 diameters (high, dry lens), but in some cases it forms a solid and practically homogeneous mass. One of the best examples of this is a fibrinous exudate in the pulmonary alveoli, which has to be distinguished from the albumin of a serous exudate, or inflammatory edema. If karyolysis has occurred in its vicinity, fibrin, sponge-like, absorbs the released chromatin, thereby becoming endowed with the blue color characteristic of nuclei.

Gross Appearance. Fibrin, as seen in clots from which the blood cells have been removed by washing, is a dull white, stringy material, the strands of which form a tangled mass. In fibrinous exudates, it is likely to be mixed with other exudative components, dead tissue, or fecal material (fibrinous enteritis), which modify its form and color.

Causes. The causes appear in the respective discussions of clotting and exudates.

Significance. Fibrin is formed by the coagulation of fibrinogen; hence its source is the blood, either directly or through the process of exudation. Fibrin is not innately a harmful substance; as an exudate upon a mucous or serous surface, it forms a valuable protective coating; by closing an opened blood vessel, it terminates the loss of blood which must otherwise be fatal. But in many situations, its ultimate effect is harmful if not disastrous. Clots, called thrombi, all too frequently develop within the vascular system, stopping the supply of blood to a certain part with the consequences portrayed under Necrosis. In the

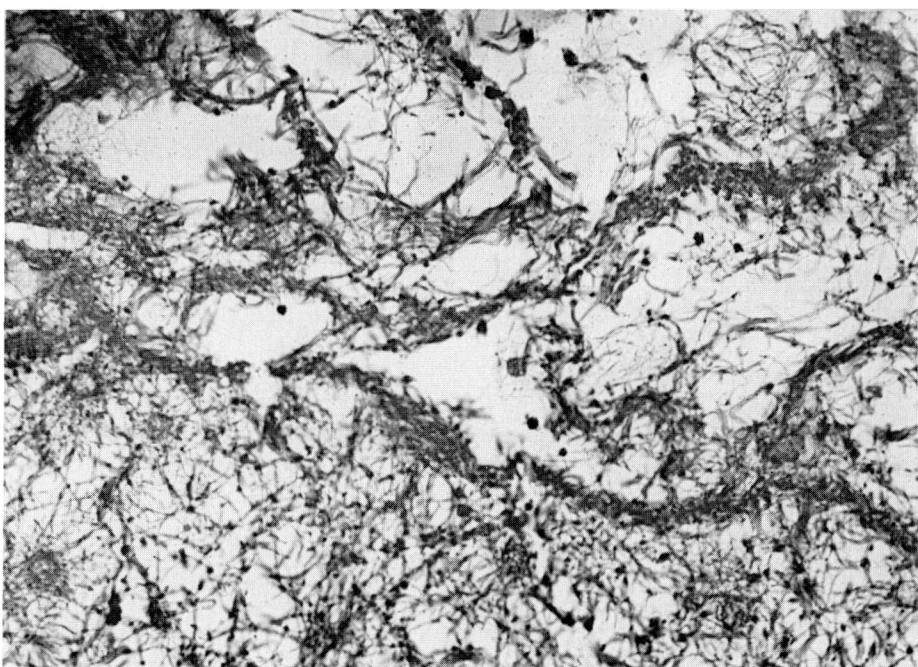

Fig. 2-7. Microscopic appearance of fibrin in a blood clot in the pulmonary vein of a dog. Note the thin interlacing fibrils.

pulmonary alveoli, it prevents the entrance of air. While covering and protecting a surface, it interferes more or less with the normal functioning of the surface cells.

As to the ultimate fate of fibrin, there are two possibilities. The fibrin may be completely liquefied by plasmin, or by the liquefying enzymes of leukocytes. On the other hand, the mere presence of fibrin appears to act as a stimulus for the proliferation of nearby fibroblasts, with the result that the latter grow into it, and in the course of some days, the fibrin has disappeared and fibrous connective tissue has taken its place, a process that is called **organization**. Thrombi are thus made permanent, as is also the solidification of the pulmonary alveoli. On surfaces that line potential cavities, such as the pleural and peritoneal cavities, there is the strong probability that the two apposed surfaces may be permanently tied together by fibrous **adhesions.** (See Fibrinous Inflammation.)

FIBRINOID DEGENERATION

Fibrinoid degeneration, or merely fibrinoid, is a currently popular name for small areas of nondescript material appearing in connective tissues in various locations. It is stained by the specific stains for fibrin and is strongly positive to the periodic-acid-Schiff reaction (PAS). In ordinary hematoxylin-eosin sections, it appears as a smudgy, pink material, always in connective tissue, with no distinct boundaries, not exactly necrotic but appearing to lack the numbers of nuclei that would be adequate for normal living tissue. Whether the material is homogenized fibrin from an inflammatory exudate or represents a degenerative change in the collagen or ground substance of connective tissue already present is in dispute. There is general agreement that the change is characteristic, and doubtless the result, of an antigen-antibody reaction going on locally in the connective tissue. It is therefore an outstanding feature of the "collagen diseases" of humans, such as rheumatic fever, periarteritis nodosa, and several others.

MUCUS AND MUCIN

Mucus (the corresponding adjective is "mucous") is a clear, glistening, water-like fluid, which is somewhat more viscid than water and which has lubricating properties that give a slimy, slippery impression. It consists of water plus a mucin, a compound containing a nucleoprotein. Due to the nucleic acid in the latter, mucins take the basic stain, which in usual techniques is blue (hematoxylin). (Note that the preceding protein substances have all taken some shade of red.) On the basis of their origin, two forms of mucin are recognized.

Epithelial Mucin. A product of epithelial cells, epithelial mucin occurs only upon mucous membranes, coming either from the mucous glands with which most mucous membranes are provided, or from those one-celled mucous glands called goblet cells.

A slight amount of mucus is normally secreted by most mucous membranes, especially those of the respiratory and digestive tracts. The "mucus of estrum," which is produced so copiously by the cervical glands at the estrual period, is a physiologic phenomenon. Excessive production on other occasions is a response to an irritant and will be treated in detail under Mucous Inflammation.

Connective-Tissue Mucin. Sometimes called **mucoid** to distinguish it from epithelial mucin, this is, potentially at least, one of the intercellular components of connective-tissue matrix. It is abundant in the connective tissue of the embryo and is responsible for the bluish staining of the embryonal type of connective tissue wherever found. Pathologically, it occurs in that reversion to embryonal connective tissue that we call mucoid degeneration.

Pseudomucin. This is a substance related to the true mucins but staining pink instead of blue. It is found in the cystic spaces of ovarian cystadenomas and cystadenocarcinomas.

MUCOID DEGENERATION

Equivalent to this condition are "myxomatous degeneration" and "mucoid atrophy of fat." "Serous atrophy of fat" is also practically synonymous, but owing, probably, to the formation of potassium soaps in the degenerating fat cells, there is a pinkish, rather than a bluish discoloration.

Occurrence. Mucoid degeneration occurs in tissues that normally contain at least small amounts of fibrous or adipose connective tissue. In this broad territory the more usual locations are (1) around the coronary groove of the heart and extending down between myocardial fibers, (2) in skeletal muscle, between its fibers and bundles, and (3) in the omentum and mesentery.

Microscopic Appearance. There is a proliferation of connective tissue of embryonal characteristics; its intercellular matrix has the bluish tinge of mucin; its scanty fibrils have a criss-cross arrangement; its hyperchromatic nuclei tend to be stellate, ovoid, or spherical. To some extent this connective tissue, which is moderate in amount, is added to the pre-existing elements, but such fibrillar or adipose connective tissue as may have been present tends to decrease in amount, to show pyknotic and prenecrotic changes, and to be replaced by the embryonal tissue.

Gross Appearance. An appreciable amount of mucoid degeneration produces an area where the tissue is translucent and watery underneath its shiny covering of serosa or other overlying membrane. When mingled with adipose tissue, as is usual, the whole process is obviously an area of degenerated, watery fat. One should watch for it, especially, in the coronary fat of the heart.

Causes. Certain sorts of blood-borne toxins may possibly play a part, but the principal causative role is to be attributed to lack of proper nutrition. Mucoid degeneration is the most conspicuous alteration accompanying ordinary starvation. Meat inspectors pay much attention to it as pointing to a state of malnutrition, which makes mere lack of fat and muscle a case calling for condemnation of the carcass. The condition can occur when the total amount of food is adequate, but when there is some serious shortcoming in its quality. It has been noted, for instance, in a lamb which was fed experimentally a diet containing no protein. It is an accompaniment of various wasting and cachectic diseases in their later stages. The possibility that local interference with nutrition may produce mucoid degeneration of a restricted area has to be considered.

Significance. Mucoid degeneration is important for what it indicates about general health. It has little effect upon function locally and is a change that is entirely reversible.

LYSOSOMAL STORAGE DISEASES, LEUKODYSTROPHIES AND LIPODYSTROPHIES

Lysosomal storage diseases are a group of inherited disorders in which lipid metabolites, most usually glycolipids and phospholipids (lipidoses), or mucopolysaccharides with or without lipids (mucopolysaccharidoses), accumulate in cells. The accumulations result from nearly complete or partial deficiencies of various catabolic lysosomal hydrolytic enzymes. Neurons are most often affected in the lipidoses, probably due to the high lipid content of the nervous system tissues. The mucopolysaccharidoses also involve neurons, but the liver, spleen, connective tissue, and other organs are also affected.

In several of the conditions, myelin metabolism is defective, leading to hypomyelinogenesis.

Over a score of lysosomal enzyme deficiency diseases have been recognized in human beings, but only a few have been described in animals. These are listed in Table 2–1.

GM$_1$ gangliosidosis has been described in Siamese cats (Baker et al., 1971; Handa and Yamakawa, 1971), a cat of unspecified breed (Blakemore, 1972), Friesian cattle (Donnelly et al., 1973), and a mixed breed dog (Read and Harrington, 1976). The disease is similar to the condition in man and results from an inherited deficiency of the lysosomal enzyme β-galactosidase. The trait is inherited as an autosomal recessive. The deficiency leads to accumulation of GM$_1$ ganglioside in neurons. In humans, there is also accumulation of a keratin sulfate-like mucopolysaccharide, and in addition to neurons, the liver, spleen, and kidney may be affected. Hepatocellular vacuolation and an unexplained aspermatogenesis is seen in affected cats. Neurons throughout the brain, spinal cord, ganglia, and retina are distended with finely granular, faintly basophilic material that displaces Nissl substance and nuclei. In frozen tissue reaction, the material is intensely PAS positive and stains faintly with fat-soluble dyes. Ultrastructurally, the stored material consists of spherical inclusions about 1 μm in diameter and composed of numerous concentric lamellae with an interlamellar periodicity of 500 to 600 mm.

Affected cats appear normal until two to three months of age, when discrete tremors of the head and pelvic limbs develop, which progress to generalized dysmetria and spastic quadriplegia at seven to eight months of age. At one year, there is an exaggerated acousticomotor response, impaired vision, and recurrent grand mal seizures. Friesian calves develop posterior incoordination, stiffness, and reluctance to move at about three months of age; this

Table 2–1.　Storage Diseases of Animals

Disease	Species	Reference
GM$_1$ gangliosidosis	Siamese cats	Baker et al., 1971
		Handa and Yamakawa, 1971
	Friesian cattle	Donnelly et al., 1972, 1973
	Dog	Read and Harrington, 1976
GM$_2$ gangliosidosis	German Shorthair Pointers	Karbe and Schiefer, 1967
		McGrath, et al., 1968
		Bernheimer and Karbe, 1970
	Yorkshire Swine	Read and Bridges, 1968
		Pierce et al., 1976
Sphingomyelin storage (Nieman-Pick disease)	Poodle dog	Bundza et al., 1979
	Cats	Chrisp et al., 1970
		Percy and Jortner, 1971
	FM Mice	Fredrickson et al., 1969
		Adachi et al., 1976
Globoid cell leukodystrophy (Krabbe's disease)	West Highland and Cairn Terriers	Fankhauser et al., 1963
		Fletcher et al., 1966, 1971
		Hirth and Nielsen, 1967
		Jortner and Jonas, 1968
		McGrath et al., 1969
	Cats	Johnson, 1970
	Dorset sheep	Pritchard et al., 1980
Glucocerebroside storage	Dogs	Hartley and Blakemore, 1973
	Sheep	Laws and Saal, 1968
	Swine	Sandison and Anderson, 1970
Mannosidosis	Angus cattle	Jolly, 1971, 1974
Neuronal glycoproteinosis (Lafora's disease) (Myoclonus epilepsy)	Basset Hounds Poodles	Holland, 1970
Metachromatic leukodystrophy	Mink	Brander and Palludan, 1965
	Cats	Hegreberg et al., 1971
Mucopolysaccharidosis	Domestic Short-Hair cat (Type I or Hurler's syndrome)	Cowell et al., 1976
		Jezyk et al., 1977
	Siamese cat (Type VI or Maroteaux-Lamy syndrome)	Haskins et al., 1979
	Cattle ("snorter" dwarfs)	Lorincz, 1964
		Hurst et al., 1975
Sudanophilic leukodystrophy	Jimpy mice	Torii et al., 1971
Ceroid lipofuscinosis	English Setter	Koppang, 1970
	Chihuahua	Rac and Giesecke, 1975
	Dachshund	Cummings and deLahunta, 1977

Table 2–1. Storage Diseases of Animals (Continued)

Disease	Species	Reference
	Siamese cat	Green and Little, 1974
	Cattle (Beefmaster)	Read and Bridges, 1969
	Sheep (South Hampshire)	Jolly and West, 1976
		Jolly et al., 1980
Chediak-Higashi disease	(See Chapter 22)	
Type II glycogen storage disease (Pompe's disease)	Cat	Sandstrom et al., 1969
	Cattle	Edwards and Richards, 1979
Type III glycogen storage disease (Cori's disease)	Dog	Rafiquzzaman et al., 1976
		Ceh et al., 1975

progresses to total incapacity and prostration between six and nine months of age.

GM₂ gangliosidosis (Tay-Sachs disease; amaurotic familial idiocy) results from a deficiency of one or more hexosaminidase enzymes (N-acetyl,β-hexosaminidase A), resulting in accumulation of a GM$_2$-ganglioside, a glycolipid. The human disease occurs in infantile and juvenile forms, with muscular weakness, amaurosis, mental retardation, and paralysis. A peculiar cherry-red spot occurs in the retina and optic atrophy often accompanies the blindness. The infantile form of the disease is more common among infants of Jewish descent and tends to be familial in incidence. The condition has been described in German Shorthair Pointers and Yorkshire swine, in which it is inherited as an autosomal recessive trait. Similar but less well-characterized conditions have been reported in English Setters, cattle, and cats. In affected dogs and swine, neurons in the brain, spinal cord, spinal ganglia, and retina have a foamy, vacuolated appearance. The material is PAS positive and stains with Sudan Black in frozen but not in paraffin sections. There is no demyelination. Ultrastructurally, the accumulations are membrane-bound laminated inclusions 0.6 to 1.0 μ in diameter. There is no involvement of visceral tissues, in contrast to the disease in human beings. Swine are

smaller than normal, and by three months of age, become incoordinated, which progresses to paralysis and eventual death. In dogs, incoordination is not clearly evident until about one year of age, although there are earlier signs of nervousness.

Sphingomyelin storage (Niemann-Pick disease) is a disorder of human beings resulting from the absence or reduction in sphingomyelinase, leading to accumulation of sphingomyelin, lysobisphosphatidic acid, and cholesterol in histiocytes. A similar disorder has been reported in FM mice, cats, and a Poodle dog, which is believed to be inherited as an autosomal recessive trait. There is vacuolation of neurons, hepatocytes, and reticuloendothelial cells of the liver, spleen, thymus, Peyer's patches, and lymph nodes. There is no demyelination. The stored material stains strongly with acid hematin and Nile Blue stains, and moderately with PAS and Luxol Fast Blue. Ultrastructurally, the inclusions are mixtures of loosely arranged membranes and electron-dense bodies. In mice, sphingomyelinase activity is described as normal, suggesting that the murine disease is analogous to one of the variants of Niemann-Pick disease of man. In the one example in a Poodle dog, sphingomyelinase was not demonstrable in the brain. In cats, enzyme determinations have not been reported. Clinically, in mice, cats,

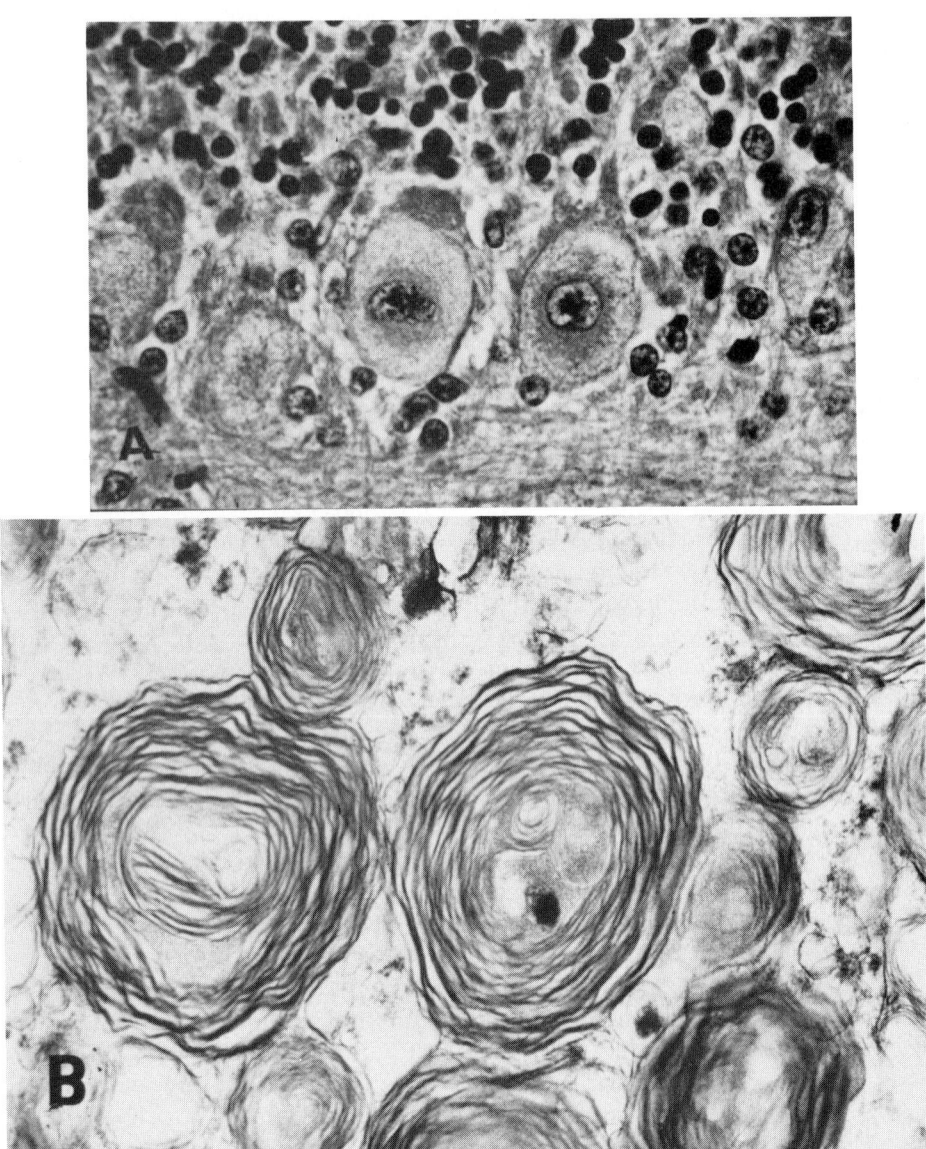

Fig. 2–8. GM₁ gangliosidosis in a cat. *A*, Glycoside-laden Purkinje cells. *B*, Ultrastructure of membranous inclusions in neuronal cytoplasm. (Courtesy of Dr. Henry J. Baker.)

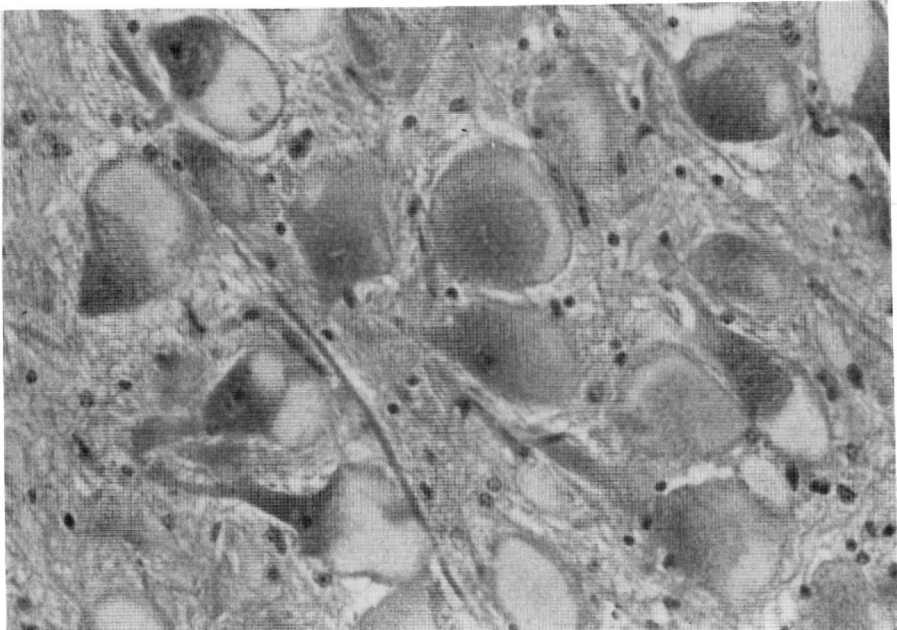

Fig. 2-9. Bovine GM$_1$ gangliosidosis. Swollen vacuolated neurons in the nucleus cuneatus of the medulla of a calf. (Courtesy of Dr. W. J. C. Donnelly.)

and the dog, there was a progressive ataxia, incoordination, hypermetria, and head tremor.

Globoid cell leukodystrophy (Krabbe's disease) results from a deficiency of the lysosomal enzyme, β-galactocerebrosidase. The disease was first described in human beings, but has since been documented in dogs (Cairn Terriers and West Highland White Terriers), Domestic Short-Hair cats, and polled Dorset sheep. It is inherited as a simple autosomal recessive trait. Galactocerebroside, which is localized in myelin sheaths, is synthesized and degraded by oligodendroglial cells. In the absence of the splitting enzyme, galactocerebroside accumulates in the large, macrophage-like cells known as globoid cells. There is resultant destruction of oligodendroglia, increased myelin breakdown, cessation of further myelination, and a paradoxic decrease in galactocerebroside production. In advanced examples, the white matter is soft and gray, and

peripheral nerves are larger and whiter than normal.

Microscopically, in the brain and spinal cord, there are bilaterally symmetric areas of demyelination accompanied by astrocytosis and large numbers of globoid cells, particularly surrounding blood vessels. There is also demyelination of peripheral nerves with swelling, fragmentation, and loss of axons and numerous globoid cells in the endoneurium. Globoid cells are large, foamy macrophages and Schwann cells with peripherally placed nuclei. The foamy cytoplasm is PAS-positive, nonsudanophilic, and nonmetachromatic. Electron microscopic studies of globoid cells have demonstrated two types of inclusions. One is straight or slightly curved and polygonal in cross section, and the other, small and round in cross section and twisted in profile.

The syndrome is characterized by progressive posterior paralysis with eventual forelimb paralysis. There may be tremors, ataxia, and impaired vision, ultimately leading to prostration, cachexia, and death.

Mannosidosis occurs in cattle and human beings as an inherited autosomal recessive trait. In cattle, it has been described in Angus and Murray Gray Calves in Australia, New Zealand, and recently in the United States. It was originally termed pseudolipidosis, but there is no storage of lipid. It is characterized by a deficiency of acid α-mannosidase leading to storage of mannose-rich oligosaccharides in lysosomes. Heterozygote individuals have α-mannosidase levels intermediate between normal cattle and those affected with the disease.

Pathologically, there is vacuolation of reticuloendothelial cells in the liver and lymph nodes, pancreatic exocrine cells, and neurons. The stored material stains with PAS, but easily washes out from tissue sections. Ultrastructurally, the vacuoles are membrane-bound and appear empty except for fragments of membranes and amorphous material.

Affected cattle are ataxic, incoordinated, have tremors, and fail to thrive, dying in the first year of life.

Neuronal glycoproteinosis (Lafora's disease; myoclonus epilepsy) is a rare disorder of human beings that has also been described in Basset Hounds and Poodles. It is characterized by accumulations of glycoproteins in neurons, but a specific enzyme defect has not been identified. The material is also not within lysosomes. In contrast to most other storage diseases, the inclusions do not result in a vacuolated cell, but rather in more discrete basophilic, PAS-positive cytoplasmic inclusions (Lafora bodies) in neurons and rarely in glial cells. They are located in the cell body as well as in dendrite processes, and in man (but not the dog), in myocardial fibers and liver cells. They are most frequent in Purkinje cells, cerebral cortex, motor nuclei, molecular layer of the cerebellum, and retina. These bodies are round, laminated,

basophilic in hematoxylin and eosin stains, and up to 32 μ in diameter. They are isotropic to polarized light and do not exhibit any autofluorescence. They are composed of a dense electron core surrounded by a fibrillar periphery without a limiting membrane. Histochemical and ultrastructural features of these bodies in dogs support the thesis that they consist of complex glycoprotein essentially similar to that reported in the human disease.

Clinically, the findings include somnolence, incoordination, convulsions, and progressive deterioration.

Glucocerebroside storage disease (Gaucher's disease) results from a deficiency of glucocerebrosidase (β-glucosidase), leading to accumulations of glucocerebroside [glycosyl (β-1,1) ceramide]. A single report (Hartley and Blakemore, 1973) describes a disease similar to the condition in man in an eight-month old Sydney Silky dog, and disorders resembling Gaucher's disease have been described in sheep (Laws and Saal, 1968) and a pig (Sandison and Anderson, 1970). The accumulated material results in large foamy cells (Gaucher cells), which are slightly eosinophilic and PAS-positive. The inclusions are membrane-bound aggregates of twisted, branching tubular structures, 40 to 60 nm in diameter and of indeterminate length. In the dog, Gaucher cells were observed in the hepatic sinusoids and in lymph nodes and tonsil. Neurons were also affected. The spleen was spared, in contrast to the disease in man. There is no demyelination. The dog was ataxic and hyperkinetic.

Metachromatic leukodystrophy (sulfatide lipidosis) is another metabolic defect of myelin metabolism, which is known as a familial disease of infants and has also been recognized in mink (Brander and Palludan, 1965) and cats (Hegreberg, et al., 1971). It results from a deficiency of arylsulfatase A. The features of the disease are degeneration of myelin sheaths, disorganization of myelin, and the presence of

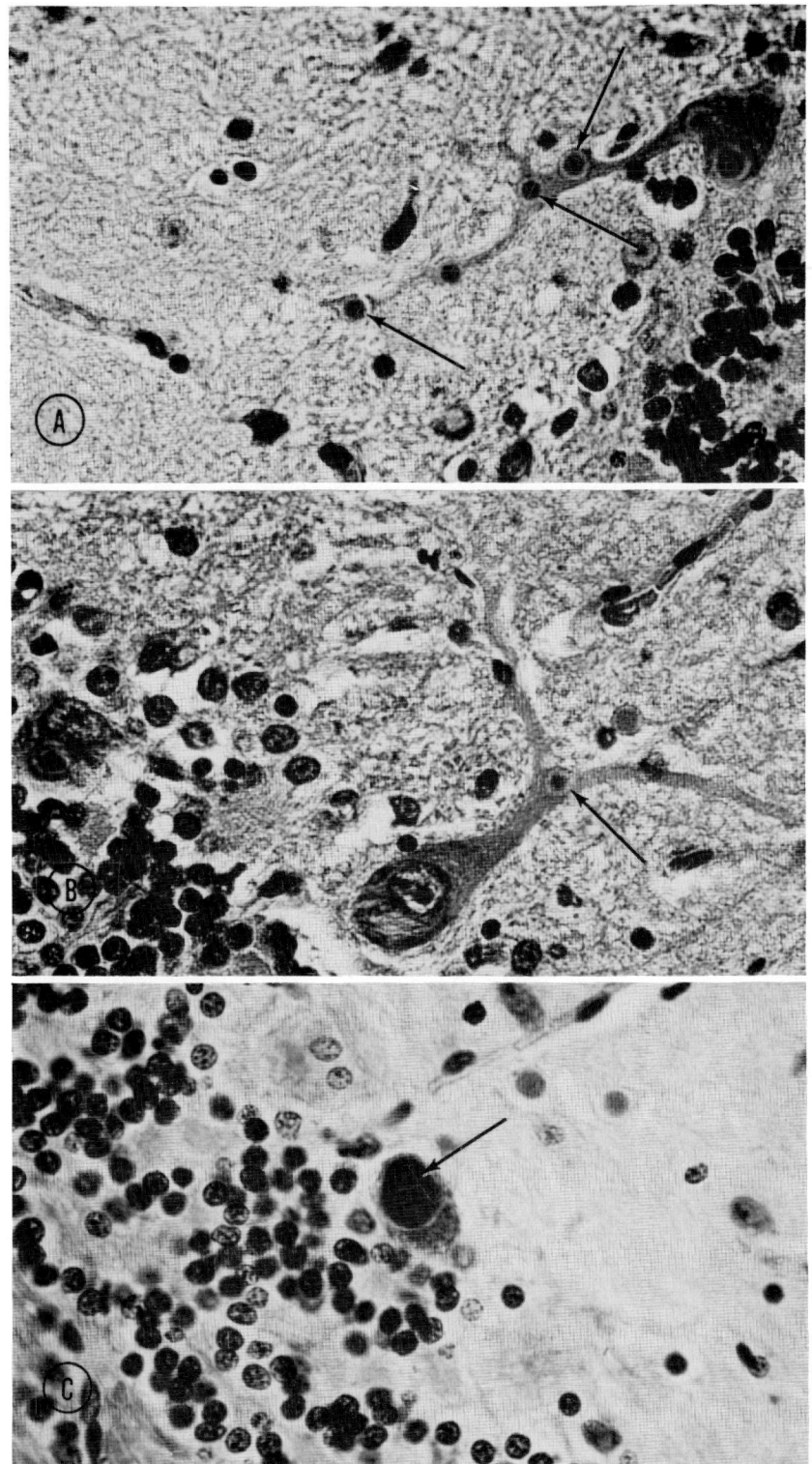

Fig. 2–10. Neuronal glycoproteinosis (Lafora's disease) in a dog. *A* and *B,* Purkinje cells containing discrete Lafora bodies. *C,* A single large Lafora body displacing nucleus of Purkinje cell. (Courtesy Dr. James M. Holland and *American Journal of Pathology.*)

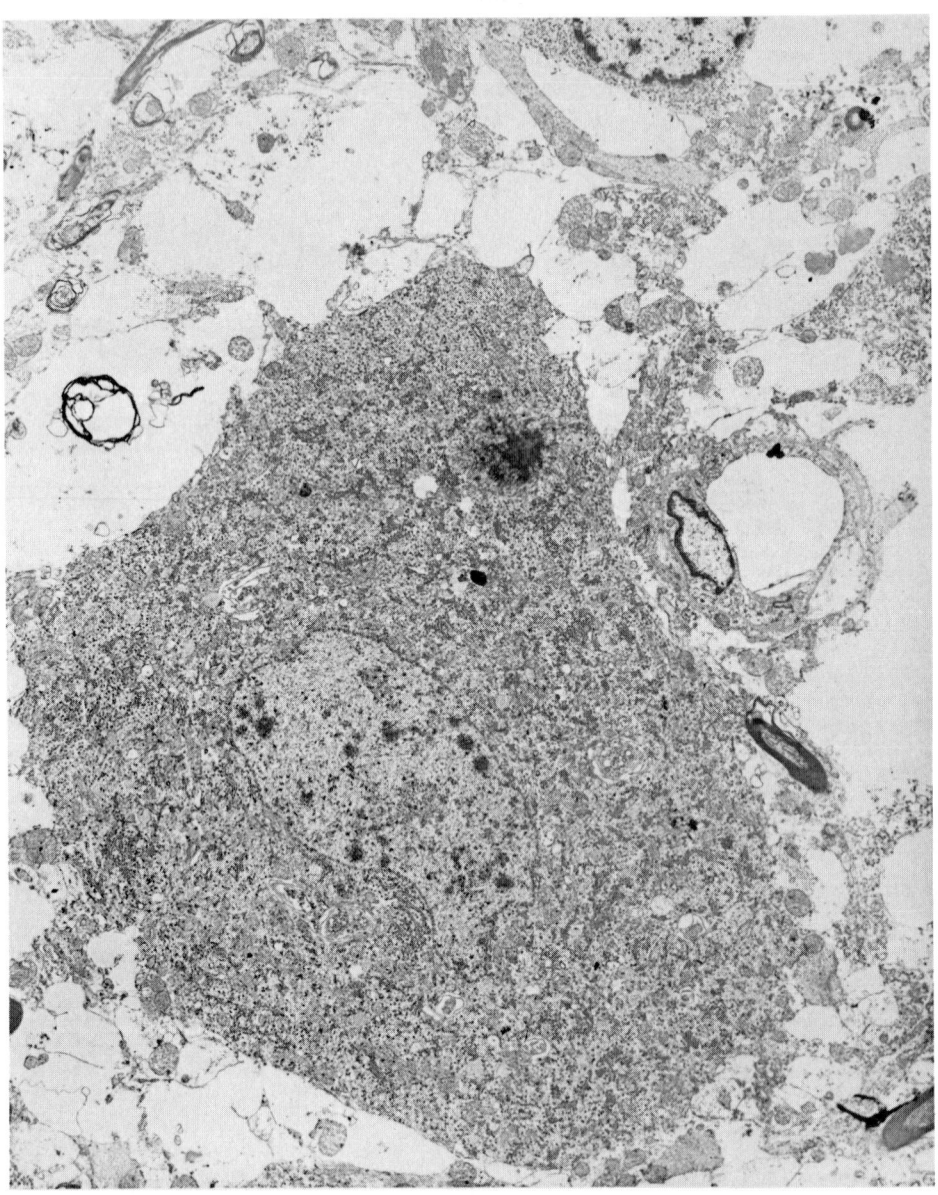

Fig. 2–11. Neuronal glycoproteinosis (Lafora's disease). A neuron with cytoplasmic inclusion or Lafora body. (Courtesy of Dr. W. C. Davis.)

metachromatic lipid material in macrophages in the brain, liver, kidney, white blood cells, and Schwann cells in peripheral nerves. The evidence points toward an autosomal, recessive mode of inheritance in the mink.

Mucopolysaccharidoses are a group of diseases resulting from deficiencies of one or more enzymes necessary for mucopolysaccharide catabolism. At least six different forms are recognized in human beings. Mucopolysaccharide-synthesizing cells, such a fibroblasts, endothelial cells, leukocytes, chondrocytes, and osteocytes, accumulate mucopolysaccharide in lysosomes, which results in a foamy appearance microscopically and eventual cellular dysfunction. Mucopolysaccharides also accumulate in lysosomes of other cell types, which take up but are incapable of catabolizing these substances. This involves most cell types, including hepatocytes, renal tubular epithelium, and reticuloendothelial cells. In addition, nerve cells cannot catabolize glycolipids, which accumulate in their cytoplasm. Mucopolysaccharides are water soluble, therefore lost with the usual methods of fixation and processing. If fixed in alcohol, they are stainable with alcian blue and are metachromatic with toluidine blue. Neuronal glycolipids can be demonstrated in frozen sections with alcian blue, PAS, or Sudan stains. They are also metachromatic with toluidine blue.

The mucopolysaccharidoses are inherited autosomal recessive diseases.

Mucopolysaccharidosis has been recognized in the Domestic Short Hair cat (Type I or Hurler's syndrome, due to deficiency of α-L-iduronidase), the Siamese cat (Type VI or Maroteaux-Lamy syndrome, due to deficiency of arylsulfatase B) and cattle (so called "snorter" dwarf cattle). The reported examples in animals are too few to generalize on the clinicopathologic findings, but the principal effect of dysfunction of mucopolysaccharide-synthesizing cells lies with skeletal deformities resulting from arrest of endochondrial bone growth. This leads to dwarfing, and facial and other abnormalities due to abnormally shaped bones. The cornea is opaque, and the liver and spleen are enlarged. In man, mental retardation occurs.

Sudanophilic leukodystrophy (neutral fat leukodystrophy) is characterized by dysmyelination, demyelination, and the accumulation of sudanophilic material in macrophages resulting from myelin breakdown in the brain. The disease is recognized in human beings, and an apparently analogous condition is seen in Jimpy mice (Torie et al., 1971). Mice develop tremors and generalized tonic seizures and usually die within 30 days of birth. There is almost total absence of myelin.

Ceroid lipofuscinosis (Batten's disease) is a disorder characterized by lysosomal accumulation of lipofuscin and ceroid in neurons and reticuloendothelial cells, especially in the spleen and lymph nodes. It is an autosomal recessive trait which is recognized in human beings and described in dogs (English Setter, Chihuahua, Dachshund), the Siamese cat, Beefmaster cattle, and South Hampshire sheep. Although the exact pathogenesis is not known, in dogs and man there is a marked reduction of p-phenylenediamine-mediated peroxidase. In English Setters, the disease has been called familial amaurotic idiocy and is characterized by progressive blindness, deafness, dullness, disorientation, ataxia, and muscular spasms commencing from 12 to 15 months of age. Sheep present similar clinical signs between 9 and 12 months of age. Both dogs and sheep rarely survive beyond the age of two years. Lipofuscin and ceroid pigments are discussed further in Chapter 3.

Chediak-Higashi disease is in part characterized by lysosomal accumulation of multilamellar bodies and lipofuscin pigment in multiple cell types. It is discussed in detail in Chapter 3.

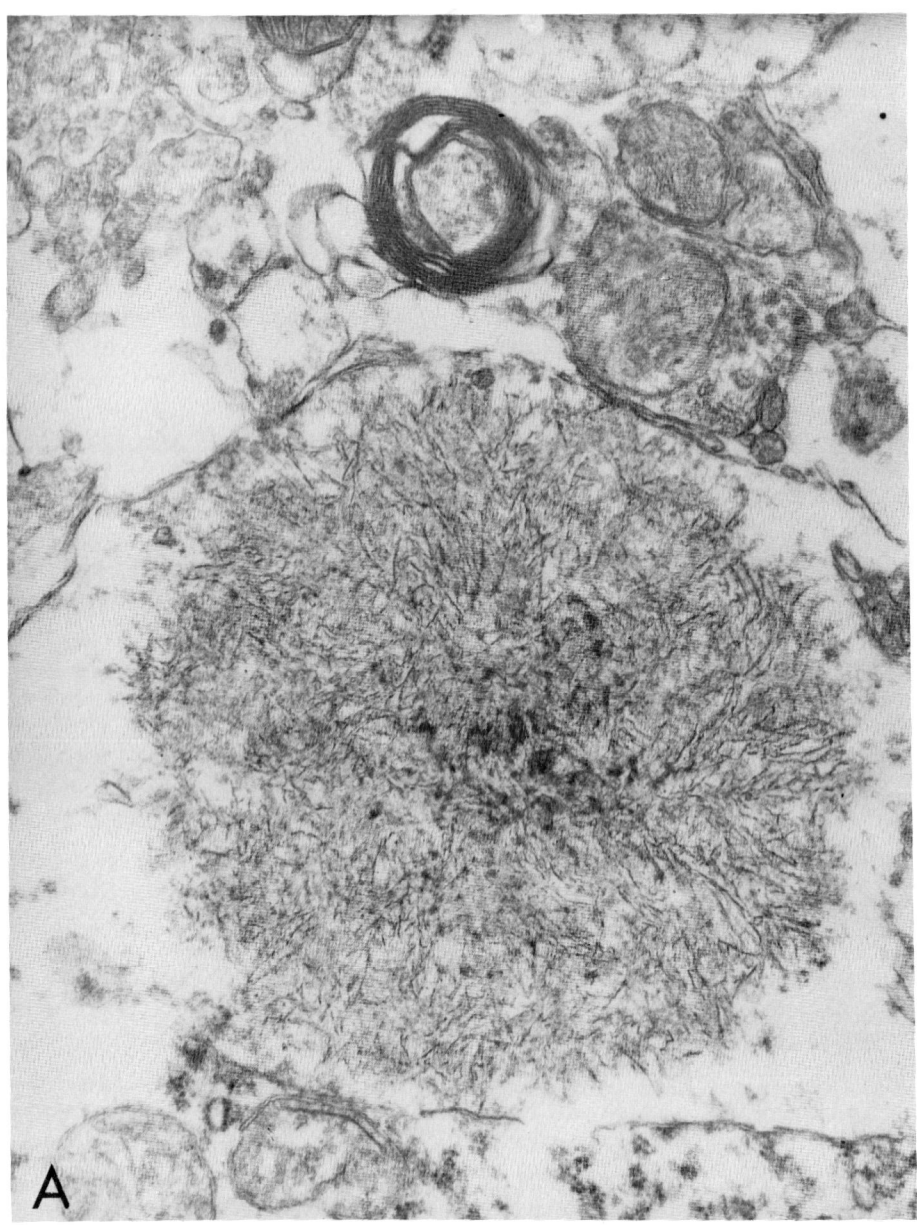

Fig. 2–12. Neuronal glycoproteinosis (Lafora's disease). *A*, Fibrillar form of inclusion. (Continued on facing page.)

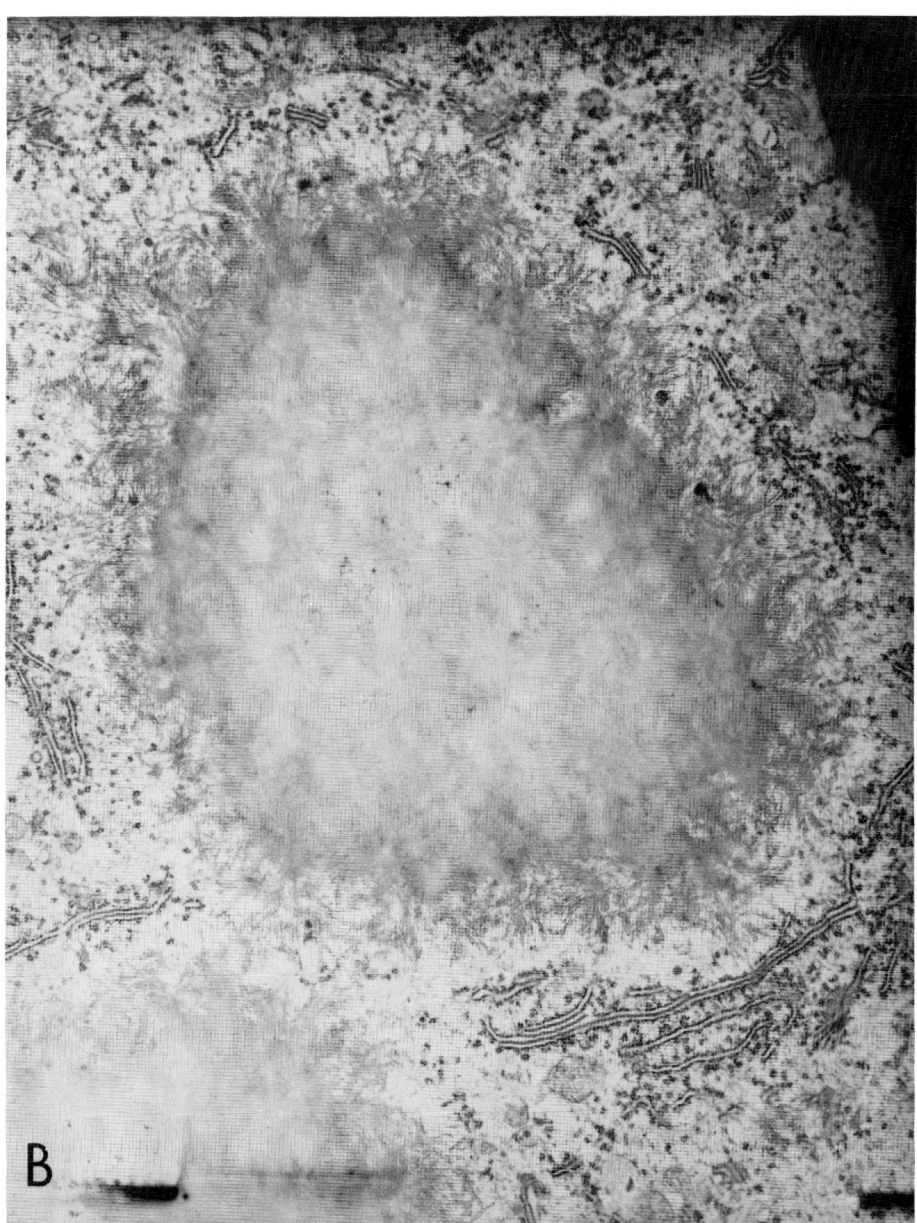

Fig. 2–12 (continued). *B*, Homogeneous form of inclusion. (Courtesy of Dr. W. C. Davis.)

Glycogen storage disease can result from deficiency of many different enzymes involved in glycogen catabolism. Only Pompe's disease (deficiency of α-glucosidase) is associated with storage in lysosomes. In the other forms, glycogen is freely dispersed throughout the cytoplasm. Glycogen storage disease is discussed in this chapter.

Other storage diseases, which have been described variably as leukodystrophies, lipodystrophies, lipidoses, and histiocytoses, have been reported in various species of animals, but the exact nature of the stored substance has not been identified. These may represent further examples of those disorders discussed previously or distinct diseases. The student is also referred to the section on disorders of myelin. At least another dozen lysosomal storage diseases in human beings have not been recognized in lower animals. Certain drugs, such as chloroquine, can cause neuronal and muscular lipodystrophy, and cytoplasmic vacuolation of cells may be seen in other conditions, which must be considered in differential diagnosis. An example is neuronal vacuolation in locoweed poisoning.

Adachi, M., Volk, B. W., and Schneck, L.: Animal model of human disease: Niemann-Pick disease type C. Am. J. Pathol., 85:229–231, 1976.

Anderson, H. A., and Palludan, B.: Leucodystrophy in mink. Acta Neuropathol., 11:347–360, 1968.

Baker, H.J., and Lindsey, J. R.: Animal model: Feline GM₁ gangliosidosis. Am. J. Pathol., 74:649–652, 1974.

Baker, H. J., Lindsey, J. R., McKhann, G. M., and Farrell, D. F.: Neuronal GM₁ gangliosidosis in a Siamese cat with β-galactosidase deficiency. Science, 174:838–839, 1971.

Bernheimer, H., and Karbe, E.: Morphologische und Neurochemische Untersuchungen van Zwei Formen der Amaurotischen Idiotie des Hundes. Nachweis einer GM₂ Gangliosidose. Acta Neuropathol. (Berl.), 16:243–261, 1970.

Bernheimer, H., and Seitelberger, F.: Uber das Verhalten der Ganglioside im Gehirn bei Zwei Fallen von Spatinfantiler Amaurotischer Idiotie. Wein Klin. Wochenschr., 80:163–164, 1968.

Blakemore, W. F.: GM₁ gangliosidosis in a cat. J. Comp. Pathol., 89:179–185, 1972.

Brander, N. R., and Palludan, B.: Leucoencephalopathy in mink. Acta Vet. Scand., 6:41–51, 1965.

Bundza, A., Lowden, J.A., and Charlton, K.M.: Nieman-Pick Disease in a Poodle Dog. Vet. Pathol., 16:530–538, 1979.

Ceh, L., Hauge, J. G., Svenkerud, R., and Strande, A.: Glycogenosis type III in the dog. Acta Vet. Scand., 17:210–222, 1976.

Chrisp, C. E., et al.: Lipid storage disease in a Siamese cat. J. Am. Vet. Med. Assoc., 156:616–622, 1970.

Christensen, E., and Palludan, B.: Late infantile familial metachromatic leucodystrophy in mink. Acta Neuropathol., 4:640–645, 1965.

Cork, L. C., et al.: GM₂ ganglioside lysosomal storage disease in cats with β-hexosaminidase deficiency. Science, 196:1014–1017, 1977.

Cowell, K. R., Jezyk, P. F., Haskins, M. E., and Patterson, D. F.: Mucopolysaccharidosis in a cat. J. Am. Vet. Med. Assoc., 169:334–339, 1976.

Cummings, J. F., and deLahunta, A.: An adult case of canine neuronal ceroid-lipofuscinosis. Acta Neuropathol. (Berlin), 39:43–51, 1977.

Donnelly, W. J. C., Hannan, J., Sheahan, B. J., and O'Connor, P. J.: Cerebrospinal lipidosis in Friesian calves. Vet. Rec., 91:225–226, 1972.

Donnelly, W. J., Sheahan, B. J., and Rogers, T. A.: GM₁ gangliosidosis in Friesian calves. J. Pathol., 111:173–179, 1973.

Dukes, T. W., Read, W. K., Bay, W. W., and Gleiser, C. A.: A drug-induced cerebrospinal lipodystrophy in the domestic chicken (Gassas domesticus). Can. J. Comp. Med., 35:208–211, 1971.

Fankhauser, R. H.: Degenerative, lipoidiotische Erkrankung des Zentralnervensystems bei zeve Hunden. Schweiz. Arch. Tierheilkd., 107:73–87, 1965.

Fankhauser, R. H., Luginbuhl, H., and Hartley, W. J.: Leukodystrophic vom Typhus Krabbe beim Hund. Schweiz. Arch. Tierheilkd., 105:198–207, 1963.

Farrell, D. F., et al.: Feline GM₁ gangliosidosis: biochemical and ultrastructural comparisons with the disease in man. J. Neuropathol. Exp. Neurol., 32:1–18, 1973.

Fredrickson, D. S., Sloan, H. R., and Hansen, C. T.: Lipid abnormalities in foam cell reticulosis of mice, an analogue of human sphingomyelin lipidosis. J. Lipid. Res., 10:288–293, 1969.

Fletcher, T. F., and Kurtz, H. J.: Animal model: globoid cell leukodystrophy. Am. J. Pathol., 66:375–378, 1972.

Fletcher, T. F., Kurtz, H. J., and Low, D. G.: Globoid cell leukodystrophy (Krabbe type) in the dog. J. Am. Vet. Med. Assoc., 149:165–172, 1966.

Fletcher, T. F., Kurtz, H. J., and Stadlan, E. M.: Experimental Wallerian degeneration in peripheral nerves of dogs with globoid leukodystrophy. J. Neuropathol. Exp. Neurol., 30:593–602, 1971.

Fletcher, T. F., Lee, D. G., and Hammer, R. F.: Ultrastructural features of globoid-cell leukodystrophy in the dog. Am. J. Vet. Res., 32:177–181, 1971.

Gleiser, C. A., et al.: Study of chloroquine toxicity and a drug-induced cerebrospinal lipodystrophy in swine. Am. J. Pathol., 53:27–45, 1968.

Green, P. D., and Little, P. B.: Neuronal ceroid-lipofuscin storage in Siamese cat. Can. J. Comp. Med., 38:207–212, 1974.

Hagen, L. O.: Lipid dystrophic changes in the central nervous system in dogs. Acta Pathol. Microbiol. Scand., *33*:22–35, 1953.

Handa, S., and Yamakawa, T.: Biochemical studies in cat and human gangliosidosis. J. Neurochem., *18*:1275–1280, 1971.

Hartley, W. J., and Blakemore, W. F.: Neurovisceral glucocerebroside storage (Gaucher's disease) in a dog. Vet. Pathol., *10*:191–201, 1973.

Haskins, M. E., et al.: Mucopolysaccharidosis in a Domestic Short-Haired cat—a disease distinct from that seen in the Siamese cat. J. Am. Vet. Med. Assoc., *175*:384–387, 1979.

Hegreberg, G. A., Norby, D. E., and Hamilton, M. J.: Lysosomal enzyme changes in an inherited dwarfism of cats. Fed. Proc., *33*:598, 1971.

Hegreberg, G. A., Thyline, H. C., and Francis, B. H.: Morphologic changes in feline leukodystrophy. Fed. Proc., *30*:341Abs, 1971.

Hirth, R. S., and Nielsen, S. W.: A familial canine globoid cell leukodystrophy ("Krabbe type"). J. Small Anim. Pract., *8*:569–575, 1967.

Holland, J. M., Davis, W. C., Prieur, D. J., and Collins, G. H.: Lafora's disease in the dog. A comparative study. Am. J. Pathol., *58*:509–530, 1970.

Howell, J. McC., and Palmer, A. C.: Globoid cell leucodystrophy in two dogs. J. Small Anim. Pract., *12*:633–642, 1971.

Hurst, R. E., Cezayirli, R. C., and Lorincz, A. E.: Nature of the glycosaminoglycanuria (mucopolysacchariduria) in brachycephalic "snorter" dwarf cattle. J. Comp. Pathol., *85*:481–486, 1975.

Jezyk, P. F., et al.: Mucopolysaccharidosis in a cat with arylsulfatase B deficiency: a model of Maroteaux-Lamy syndrome. Science, *198*:834–836, 1977.

Johnson, K. H.: Globoid leukodystrophy in the cat. J. Am. Vet. Med. Assoc., *157*:2057–2064, 1970.

Jolly, R. D.: The pathology of the central nervous system in pseudolipidosis of Angus calves. J. Pathol., *103*:113–121, 1971.

———: Animal model of human disease of mannosidosis of children, other inherited lysosomal storage diseases. Am. J. Pathol., *74*:211–214, 1974.

Jolly, R. D., and West, D. M.: Blindness in South Hampshire sheep: a neuronal ceroid-lipofuscinosis. NZ Vet. J., *24*:123, 1976.

Jolly, R. D., Janmaat, A., West, D. M., and Morrison, I.: Ovine ceroid-lipofuscinosis of Batten's disease. Neuropathol. Appl. Neurobiol., *6*:195–209, 1980.

Jortner, B. S., and Jonas, A. M.: The neuropathology of globoid-cell leucodystrophy in the dog. A report of two cases. Acta Neuropathol., *10*:171–182, 1968.

Karbe, E.: Gangliosidosis and other neuronal lipodystrophies with amaurosis in dogs. A comparative histopathological, histochemical, electron microscopical and biochemical study. Arch. Exp. Vet. Med., *25*:1–48, 1971.

Karbe, E.: Animal model of human disease: GM_2 gangliosidosis (amaurotic idiocies), types, I, II and III. Am. J. Pathol., *71*:151–154, 1973.

Karbe, E., and Schiefer, B.: Familial amaurotic idiocy in male German Shorthair Pointers. Pathol. Vet., *4*:223–232, 1967.

Koppang, N.: Neuronal ceroid-lipofuscinosis in English Setters. J. Small Anim. Pract., *10*:639, 1970.

Kosanke, S. D.: A study of the biochemical and morphological changes in GM_2-gangliosidosis of Yorkshire swine and the influence of chloroquine HCl upon these changes. Diss. Abstr. Int., *36B*:2101, 1975.

Kurtz, H. J., and Fletcher, T. F.: The peripheral neuropathy of canine globoid-cell leukodystrophy (Krabbe type). Acta Neuropathol., *16*:226–232, 1970.

Laws, L., and Saal, J. R.: Lipidosis of the hepatic reticulo-endothelial cells in a sheep. Austr. Vet. J., *44*:416–417, 1968.

Leav, I., Crocker, A. C., Petrak, M. L., and Jones, T. C.: A naturally occurring lipidosis in shell parakeets, *Melopsittacus undulatus*. Lab. Invest., *18*:433–437, 1968.

Leipold, H. W., Smith, J. E., Jolly, R. D., and Eldridge, F. E.: Mannosidosis of Angus calves. J. Am. Vet. Med. Assoc., *175*:457–459, 1979.

Lorincz, A. E.: Hurler's syndrome in man and snorter dwarfism in cattle. Clin. Orthop., *33*:104–118, 1964.

McGrath, J. T., Kelly, A. M., and Steinberg, S. A.: Cerebral lipidosis in the dog. J. Neuropathol. Exp. Neurol., *27*:141, 1968.

McGrath, J., Schutta, H., Yaseen, A., and Steinberg, S.: A morphologic and biochemical study of canine globoid leukodystrophy. J. Neuropathol. Exp. Neurol., *28*:171, 1969.

Patel, V., Koppang, N., Patel, B., and Zeman, W.: p-Phenylenediamine-mediated peroxidase deficiency in English Setters with neuronal ceroid-lipofuscinosis. Lab. Invest., *30*:366–368, 1974.

Percy, D. H., and Jortner, B. S.: Feline lipidosis. Light and electron microscopic studies. Arch. Pathol., *92*:136–144, 1971.

Pierce, K. R., Kosanke, S. D., Bay, W. W., and Bridges, C. H.: Animal model: porcine cerebrospinal lipodystrophy (GM_2 gangliosidosis). Am. J. Pathol., *83*:419–422, 1976.

Pritchard, D. H., Napthine, D. V., and Sinclair, A. J.: Globoid cell leucodystrophy in polled Dorset sheep. Vet. Pathol., *17*:399–405, 1980.

Rac, R., and Giesecke, C. T.: Lysosomal storage disease in Chihuahuas. Aust. Vet. J., *51*:403–404, 1975.

Rafiquzzaman, M., Svenkerud, R., Strande, A., and Hauge, J. G.: Glycogenesis in the Dog. Acta Vet. Scand., *17*:196–209, 1976.

Read, W. K., and Bridges, C. H.: Cerebrospinal lipodystrophy in swine. A new disease model in comparative pathology. Pathol. Vet., *5*:67–74, 1968.

———: Neuronal lipodystrophy. Occurrence in an inbred strain of cattle. Pathol. Vet., *6*:235–243, 1969.

Read, D. H., Harrington, D. D., Keenan, T.W., and Hinsman, E.J.: Neuronal-visceral GM_1 gangliosidosis in a dog with β-galactosidase deficiency. Science, *194*:442–445, 1976.

Ribelin, W. E., and Kintner, L. D.: Lipodystrophy of

the central nervous system in a dog. Cornell Vet., *46*:532–537, 1956.

Sakuragawa, N., et al.: Niemann-Pick disease experimental model: sphingomyelinase reduction induced by AY-9944. Science, *196*:317–319, 1977.

Sandison, A. J., and Anderson, L. J.: Histiocytosis in two pigs and a cow. Conditions resembling lipid storage disorders in man. J. Pathol., *100*:207–210, 1970.

Sandstrom, B., Westman, J., and Ockerman, P. A.: Glycogenosis of the central nervous system in the cat. Acta Neuropathol., *14*:194–200, 1969.

Sheahan, B. J., and Donnelly, W. J. C.: Enzyme histochemical and ultrastructural alterations in the brains of Friesian calves with GM_1 gangliosidosis. Acta Neuropathol., *30*:73–84, 1974.

Suzuki, Y., et al.: Studies in globoid leukodystrophy: enzymatic and lipid findings in the canine form. Exp. Neurol., *29*:65–75, 1970.

Torii, J., Adachi, M., and Volk, B. W.: Histochemical and ultrastructural studies of inherited leukodystrophy in mice. J. Neuropath. Exp. Neurol., *30*:278–289, 1971.

CHAPTER 3

Mineral Deposits, Pigments

This chapter is concerned with a discussion of pathologic deposits of minerals that are encountered in tissues upon gross or microscopic examination; general metabolism of minerals is treated elsewhere. Some mineral substances are detected because they are also pigments, i.e., they have an intrinsic color. Also included are pigments of organic origin, both endogenous and exogenous, which are encountered in tissues as normal components or as pathologic deposits.

PATHOLOGIC CALCIFICATION

By pathologic calcification is meant the deposition of calcium salts in tissues other than bone and teeth. The calcium is usually deposited as calcium phosphate and calcium carbonate, and may occur in the form of hydroxyapatite similar to that of normal bone. Often the salts are not chemically pure, but may be accompanied by other ions such as iron, which has led some to prefer the noncommittal term of **mineralization**.

Pathologic calcification may be divided into dystrophic calcification, metastatic calcification and calcinosis circumscripta. Calcinosis circumscripta is discussed separately under skin.

Dystrophic Calcification

Dystrophic calcification is the deposition of calcium salts in dead or degenerating tissues. It is not related to calcium content of blood, which normally is around 10 mg/100 ml. It may occur in practically any tissue or organ. While we refer ordinarily to the tissues of the patient, the term dystrophic calcification may be applied to the tissues of metazoan parasites that wander into various regions of the patient's body and perish there, as in trichinosis.

Microscopic Appearance. The calcium carbonate or phosphate is usually in irregular granules of microscopic size or a little larger. They usually take a characteristic purplish color from the basic hematoxylin stain, although occasionally, with minor variations in technique, the effect of eosin may predominate. The depth of color in the small particles encountered in microscopic sections depends on the thickness of the particle, and this often shows abrupt variation from point to point, as if the mineral were deposited in layers that decrease step by step toward the edge of the calcified granule. Everywhere the form and structure of the granule or clump of granules are entirely irregular and unpredictable, although they may be limited to the confines of a given histologic structure, such as the wall of a small artery.

Calcium salts can be demonstrated to greater advantage with special staining methods, such as the von-Kossa and alizarin-red-S techniques. However, certain calcium salts, such as calcium oxalate, do not stain with hematoxylin, nor do they react with the usual histochemical stains for calcium salts.

Gross Appearance. If freed from the surrounding tissue, the calcium particles would be white or gray, irregularly rounded, and often honeycombed. The material must be somewhat less dense than ordinary limestone, for small deposits often yield to the microtome knife with about an equal degree of fragmentation of the stone and the steel.

The most common way of detecting calcification grossly is to slice though the suspected area with a knife in search of a gritty sound and feeling. This is done routinely by meat inspectors examining for tuberculosis and other conditions in which calcification is a more or less constant feature.

Causes. The presence of dead or dying animal tissue is the fundamental cause of calcium deposition of this type. It is not related to an increased amount of calcium in the blood. What local factors initiate the precipitation of calcium are unknown, but is has been suggested that local alkalinity in dead tissue favors the precipitation. There is little evidence to support this hypothesis. Another suggestion is that fatty acids formed in necrotic tissue combine with calcium, forming soaps which are later replaced by phosphates and carbonates. No doubt this is important in fat necrosis, but again, there is little evidence to indicate this mechanism is involved in dystrophic calcification. Increased levels of alkaline phosphatase have been demonstrated within sites of dystrophic calcifica-

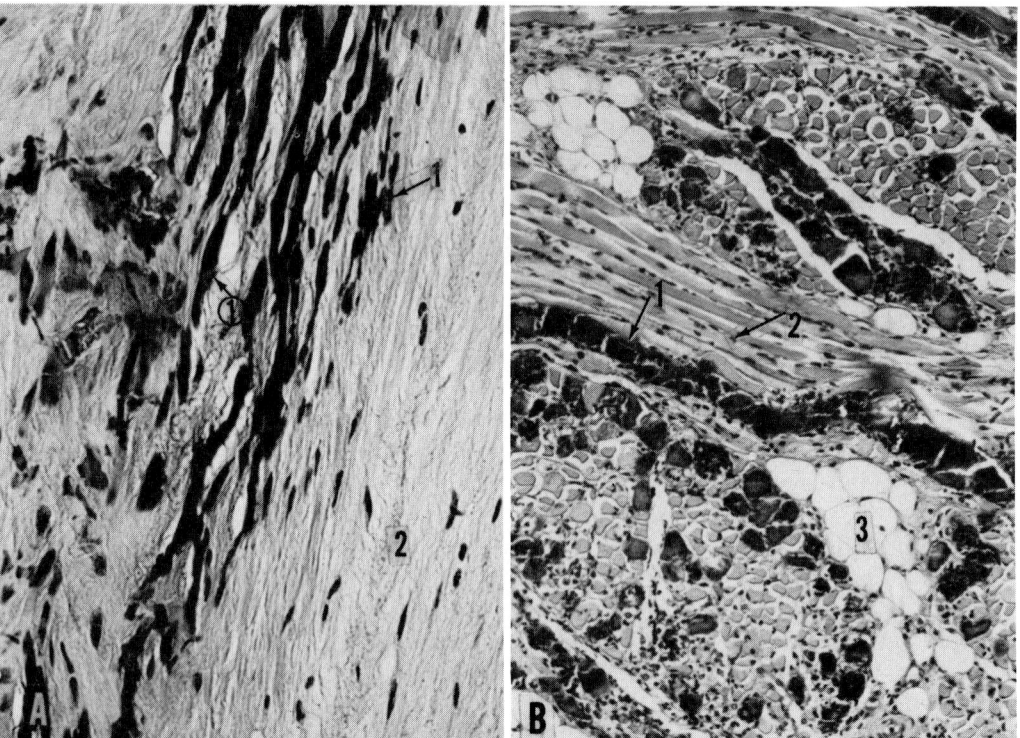

Fig. 3–1. Calcification. *A*, Deposits of calcium salts (*1*) in the myocardium of a cow. (× 300.) (Courtesy of Armed Forces Institute of Pathology.) Contributor: Dr. J. F. Ryff. *B*, Calcium deposition in skeletal muscles in the tongue of a foal possibly as a result of vitamin E deficiency. The calcium salt (*1*) replaces the sarcoplasm in many muscle bundles. A few unaffected bundles (*2*) remain. Normal fat cells (*3*) are present. (× 114.) (Courtesy of Armed Forces Institute of Pathology.) Contributor: Dr. W. O. Reed.

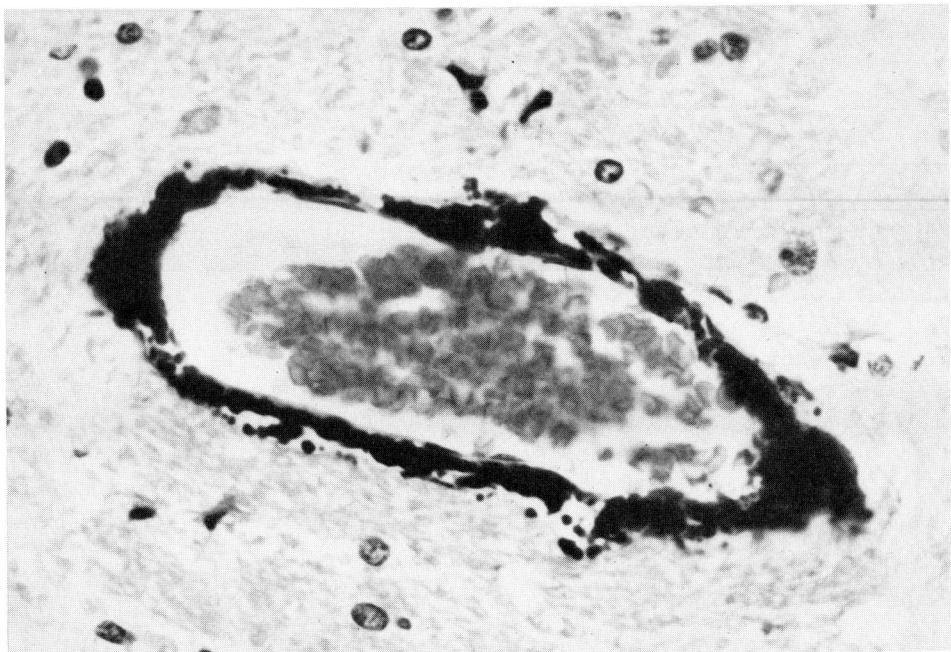

Fig. 3–2. Cerebrovascular siderosis, marmoset *(Saguinus oedipus).* Iron positive and calcium positive material in the wall of a cerebral arteriole. (Courtesy of New England Regional Primate Research Center, Harvard Medical School.)

tion, but it is not known whether this enzyme is involved in the deposition of calcium salts. Also, the enzyme cannot be demonstrated invariably.

Among the situations in which calcification is prone to develop are the caseous centers of tubercles (except avian) and caseous areas in some of the other granulomatous diseases, the rosettes and ensheathed colonies of actinomycosis and staphylococcic granuloma (botryomycosis), old thrombi, degenerating tumors and old areas of scarring, including the injured walls of atheromatous blood vessels. Also included are the remains, more or less encapsulated and scarred, of parasites such as trichinae, flukes, encysted tapeworm larvae, demodectic mites, and others, which have been unable to complete their life-cycles and have died within the tissues.

Significance. Calcium deposits are relatively permanent but are harmless unless, by virtue of their location, they interfere mechanically with some function or reduce the strength of a part. It will be recalled that calcification was listed as one of the ways by which the body disposes of dead tissue, since calcified material is functionally inert. Occasionally, calcification in certain locations may accompany and possibly be causally related to pathologic ossification.

Metastatic Calcification

Metastatic calcification is the precipitation of calcium salts as the result of a persistently high concentration of calcium in the blood. The tissues affected need not have been previously damaged. The staining qualities and gross appearance of the calcium salts do not differ from those described for dystrophic calcification.

Causes. Metastatic calcification can result from (1) primary hyperparathyroidism, but this condition is exceedingly rare, especially in animals; (2) renal failure, in which the excretion of phosphate is reduced, resulting in increased serum inorganic phosphate levels. Secondary hyperparathyroidism may develop in this situation which then accentuates calcium deposition. It becomes difficult to differentiate "dystrophic" from "metastatic" calcification under these circumstances, due to the presence of degenerating lesions of uremia. (3) Widespread calcification of the walls of arteries and other tissues can result from hypercalcemia produced by very large excesses of vitamin-D in the diet. In animals this may be encountered in livestock fed too enthusiastically with artificial vitamins. There is evidence that ultrastructural lesions precede renal calcification in

hypervitaminosis D in rats. By definition, one would have to reassess the use of the term metastatic if similar findings are encountered in other tissues and other forms of metastatic calcification.

Widespread calcification of tissues has been observed in several species (cattle, sheep, and goats) in different parts of the world. Evidence now indicates that certain plants containing the active principle of vitamin D (25-hydroxycholecalciferol) are responsible for these conditions. **Enzootic calcinosis** is the term applied in Germany, Austria, South Africa, and India. One plant, yellow oat (*Trisetum flavescens*), has been incriminated in Germany. A similar, if not identical, disease described in

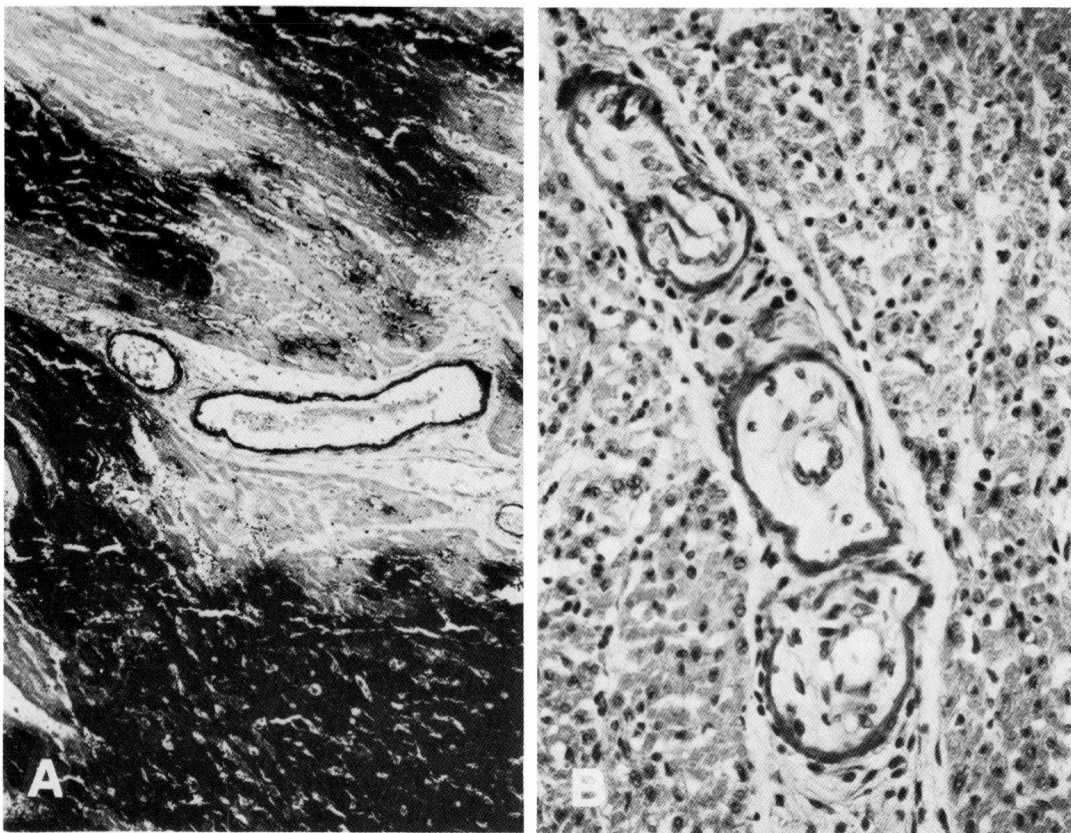

Fig. 3–3.   Calcinosis in young swine due to large doses of vitamin D₃. *A,* Mycocardium, severe calcification in muscle cells and elastica of arteries. Von Kossa stain. *B,* Myocardium of same piglet, calcium in elastica of small artery. (H & E stain.) (Courtesy of Prof. Dr. H. Luginbühl and Dr. H. Häni, with permission of the *Schweizer Archiv für Tierheilkunde.)*

Argentina and Brazil and designated **Enteque seco** has been reproduced experimentally by feeding a plant, *Solanum malacoxylon.* **Manchester wasting disease,** described in Jamaica, and **Naalehu disease,** reported from Hawaii, have similar features, and have recently been related to the consumption of *Solanum malacoxylon* (p. 978). Calcinosis with associated hypercalcemia has been identified in Florida in horses that have eaten leaves of a shrub, *Cestrum diurnam.*

The deposition of calcium salts is primary and most extensive in the elastica of the heart, aorta, and muscular arteries. Calcification also involves elastic fibers in the pulmonary parenchyma, trachea, bronchial cartilage, and heart valves. In severe cases in cattle and sheep, the flexor tendons of the forelimb are calcified, the bones are hard and dense, osteoarthritis is

seen in carpal and tarsal joints, and the inorganic phosphorus level in the blood is elevated. Calcification in the septa of the lungs may lead to ossification (Fig. 3–4).

In hyperadrenocorticism in the dog, calcification may occur in a variety of tissues, but especially in skin, lungs, and skeletal muscle. The mechanisms of this type of calcification are not understood.

PATHOLOGIC OSSIFICATION

Bone may be encountered in a variety of non-osseous tissues. Under most circumstances, it is abnormal and represents a form of metaplasia discussed in Chapter 4.

Occurrence. It is a feature of the normal ontogeny of the turkey that, as the bird approaches maturity, the tendons of its leg muscles turn to bone. In limited and variable degree, a similar change is not unknown in other species. **Ossification of the**

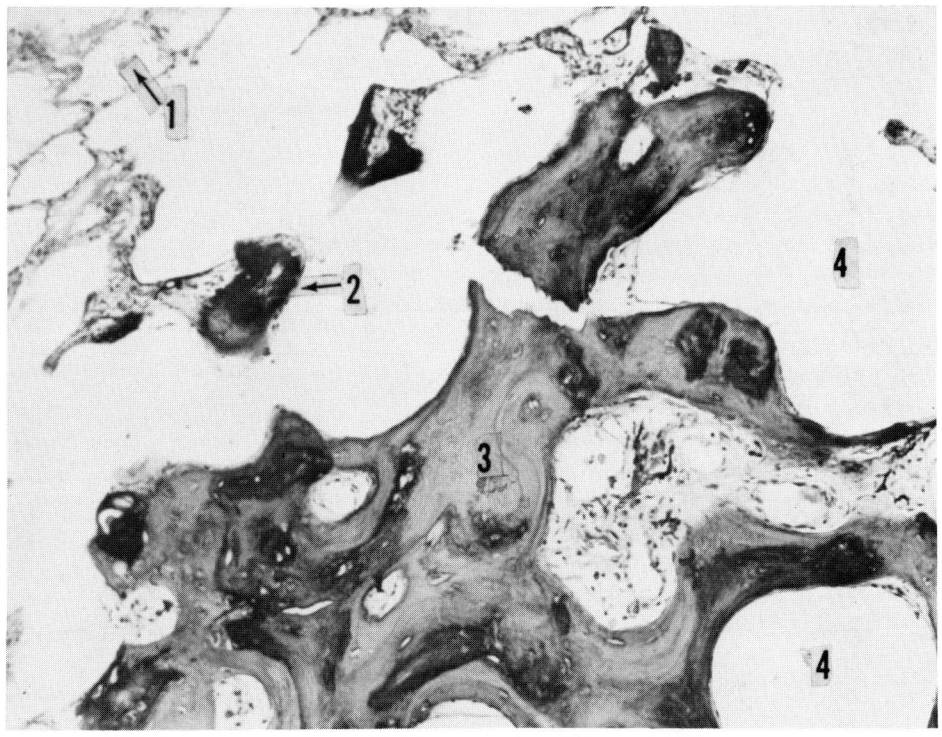

Fig. 3–4. Pathologic ossification of a bovine lung; seen in enzootic calcinosis. Alveoli (*1*), early calcification (*2*), and osteoid (*3*). Dilated alveolar spaces (*4*) are partially surrounded by bone. (× 250.) (Courtesy of Armed Forces Institute of Pathology.) Contributor: Dr. W. S. Bailey.

lateral cartilages of the horse's foot is an important cause of lameness. It occurs in the draft breeds, in older individuals, in those individuals that have had hard work on hard pavements, and in the forefeet, which bear the most weight. Rarely in old horses and old people there is partial ossification of tracheal or laryngeal cartilages, especially if these have been exposed to stresses or have had inflammatory processes nearby. Widespread formation of bony spicules in the interalveolar septa of the lung is not altogether rare. Hilton Smith in earlier editions reported dissecting a flat layer of bone measuring 3 by 4 cm from the wall of the renal pelvis of a bovine. He also encountered a flat plate of bone of larger size between the muscular layers of the abdominal wall of a pig. Both were in the vicinity of inflammatory processes. Injured muscle is prone to ossification, referred to as myositis ossificans.

Microscopic Appearance. Small bits of ossified tissue are best distinguished from mere calcification by means of the cells and lacunae that are found in the bone; calcified areas are acellular. Marrow may accompany the bony structures.

Causes. It appears that ossification is a response to prolonged irritation in older individuals in which there is an hereditary tendency in this direction. Heterotopic bone is also not infrequent at sites of dystrophic and metastatic calcification. Under these circumstances, fibroblasts differentiate to osteoblasts, which form osteoid, which calcifies to become bone in an identical manner to normal membranous bone formation.

Significance. The bony structures interfere mechanically with movement, and in the lung may well interfere with the exchange of oxygen.

de Barros, S., Pohlenz, J., and Santigo, C.: Zur Kalzinose beim Schaf. Dtsch. Tieraerztl. Wochenschr., 77:346–349, 1970.
Dämmrich, K., Dirksen, G. and Plank, P.: Ueber eine enzootische "Kalzinose" beim Rind. 3. Skelettveränderüngen. Dtsch. Tieraerztl. Wochenschr., 77:342–346, 1970.

Dirksen, G., et al.: Ueber eine enzootische "Kalzinose" beim Rind. 1. Klinische Beobactungen und Untersuchen. Dtsch. Tieraerztl. Wochenschr., 77:321–338, 1970.
Dirksen, G., Plank, P., Hänichen, T., and Spiess, A.: Ueber eine enzootische "Kalzinose" beim Rind. 5. Experimentelle Untersucherungen an Kaninchen mit selektiver Verfütterung von Knaufgras (*Dactylis glomerata*) Goldhafer (*Trisetum flavescens*) und einer Gräsergemisch. Dtsch. Tieraerztl. Wochenschr., 79:77–79, 1972.
Gill, B. S., Singh, M., and Chopra, A. K.: Enzootic calcinosis in sheep: clinical signs and pathology. Am. J. Vet. Res., 37:545–552, 1976.
Gilka, F., Corner, A. H., Sugden, E. A., and Friend, D. W.: Heterotopic calcification in swine. Vet. Pathol., 15:213–222, 1978.
Häni, H., Thomann, J., and Schäfer, H.: Zur Calcinose des Jungferkels. I. Beschreibung der Spontanfälle. Schweiz. Arch. Tierheilk., 117:9–18, 1975.
Häni, H., and Rossi, G. L.: Zur Calcinose des Jungferkels. II. Pathogenese. Schweiz. Arch. Tierheilk., 117:19–30, 1975.
Hänichen, T., Plank, P., and Dirksen, G.: Ueber eine enzootisch "Kalzinose" beim Rind. 2. Histomorphologische Befunde an den Weichgeweben. Dtsch. Tieraerztl. Wochenschr., 77:338–342, 1970.
Krook, L., et al.: Hypercalcemia and calcinosis in Florida horses; implication of the shrub *Cestrum diurnum*, as the causative agent. Cornell Vet., 64:26–56, 1975.
Pool, R. R., Williams, J. R., and Bulgin, M.: Disseminated calcinosis cutis in a dog. J. Am. Vet. Med. Assoc., 161:291–292, 1972.
Singh, G., Gill, B. S., and Randhawa, N. S.: Enzootic calcinosis in sheep: soil-plant-animal relationship. Am. J. Vet. Res., 37:553–556, 1976.
Tustin, R. C., et al.: Enzootic calcinosis of sheep in South Africa. J. S. Afr. Vet. Assoc., 44:383–395, 1973.
Weidmann, S. M.: Calcification of skeletal tissues. Int. Rev. Connect. Tissue Res., 1:339–377, 1963.

GOUT

Gout is a condition in which crystals of uric acid or urates are deposited in the tissues.

Occurrence. The disorder occurs in humans and in birds, but has not been clearly established in other species. Parts of the body involved are the articular and periarticular tissues, where the sharp crystals act as irritating foreign bodies, causing intense pain and acute inflammation. Attacks come and recede with poorly understood fluctuations in protein or purine metabolism.

In birds, two forms are found, the articular, like that just described, and the more frequent visceral form.

Most domestic animals have adequate amounts of the hepatic enzyme, **uricase**, which causes the relatively insoluble uric acid to be metabolized to the more soluble allantoin. This reduces the level of uric acid in the blood and limits its secretion in urine. Apes (Chimpanzees, Orangutans, and Gibbons) and certain South American primates (Squirrel monkey, Cebus, etc.) share with man the absence of hepatic uricase. Gout has not yet been reported in these species, however. One Old World monkey, the Rhesus, has adequate uricase, but it apparently has a less stable form.

The absence or inadequate amounts of uricase appear to be necessary for the occurrence of gout. Impaired renal excretion of uric acid may be associated with gout in birds. Normal circulating levels of polymorphonuclear leukocytes are necessary for inflammation to result from the presence of localized concentrations of urate crystals. The details of the molecular events in gout are still matters of dispute. It is proposed, however, that following deposition in tissues, urate crystals are phagocytized by leukocytes. The phagocytic vacuoles fuse with lysosomes, but rather then leading to digestion, the urate crystals damage the phagolysosome membrane, spilling hydrolytic enzymes into the cytoplasm, killing the cell, and freeing the urates, thus establishing a vicious cycle invoking an acute inflammatory response.

Microscopic Appearance. Inflammatory infiltrations, including many macrophages and foreign-body giant cells, in conjunc-

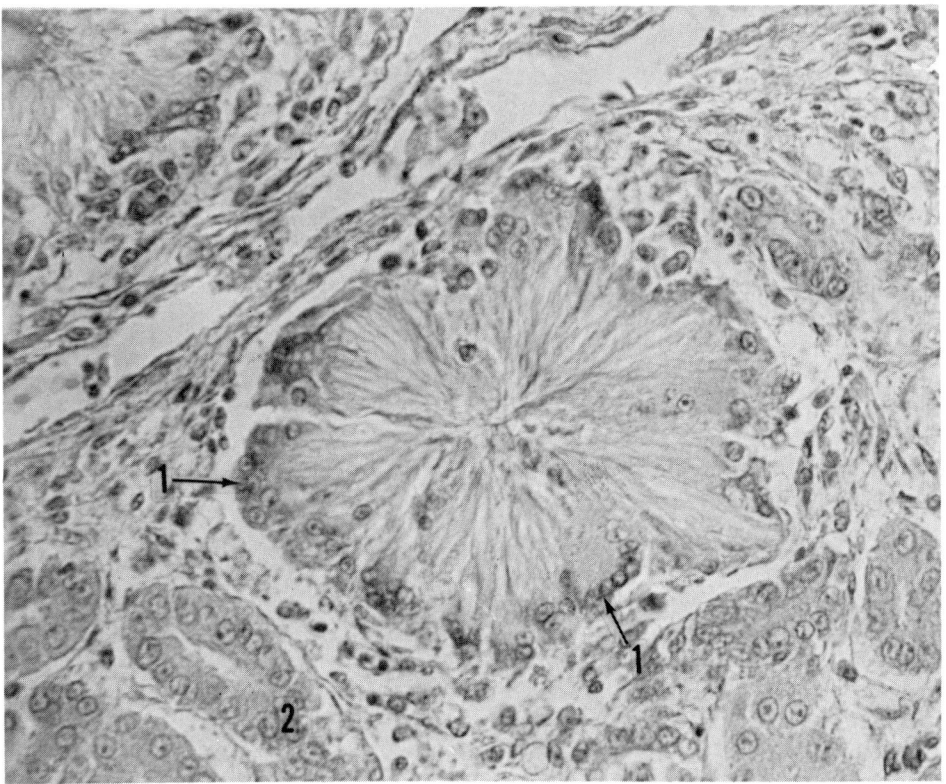

Fig. 3–5. Gout. Deposit of urate crystals in the kidney of a turkey. The urates are surrounded by multinucleated giant cells (*1*). Renal tubules (*2*). (× 425.) (Courtesy of Armed Forces Institute of Pathology.) Contributor: Dr. J. F. Olney.

tion with clusters of sharp acicular crystals, or spaces left after they dissolve, located in an articular surface, joint capsule, or adjacent tissues are indicative of articular gout. In the visceral gout of birds, various serous surfaces are covered with finely crystalline or almost amorphous material that does not stain.

Gross Appearance. Opportunities for necropsies of cases of this disease are rare except in birds, usually chickens or turkeys. The gross picture of the gouty joint is already obvious. The amount of precipitated material may be so great as to form grossly noticeable white, chalky masses in the tissues. Known as "tophi," these may occur in the subcutaneous tissues elsewhere than in the joints and may ulcerate, but without the severe pain that characterizes involvement of the joints.

In visceral gout, the serous surfaces in the body cavity and especially the outer surface of the pericardial sac are encrusted by a thin grayish layer having a metallic sheen. This appearance is diagnostic.

Causes. Uric acid and urates are decomposition products of nucleic acid metabolism. Just what happens is not clear, but it is known that in human patients, the concentration of uric acid in the blood is considerably increased (from 2.5 mg/100 ml to 4 mg/100 ml). The uric acid in the urine is low just before an attack, but becomes abnormally high as the attack develops. In birds, decrease in renal clearance of urates is associated with visceral gout.

In birds, the kidneys eliminate semisolid urates instead of urine and uric acid. In deficiency of vitamin A, the elimination of urates is severely impaired, one of the visible lesions being their accumulation in the ureteral ducts. Hence it is now customary to attribute visceral gout to this deficiency. However, the chemical aspects appear not to have been studied sufficiently, and there remains older experimental evidence linking this disorder to diets containing, if not too much protein, at least unusual kinds of protein.

Significance. The visceral gout of birds is seen only at necropsy. It is difficult to say whether any birds recover, but presumably recovery is possible with a suitable change in diet. Articular gout is stubbornly recurrent in afflicted humans and presumably so in the rare cases in animals.

Austic, R. E., and Cole, R. K.: Impaired renal clearance of uric acid in chickens having hyperuricemia and articular gout. Am. J. Physiol., 223:525–530, 1972.

Christen, P., et al.: Urate oxidase in primate phylogenesis. Europ. J. Biochem., 12:3–5, 1970.

Phelps, P., and McCarry, D. J., Jr.: Crystal-induced inflammation in canine joints. II. Importance of polymorphonuclear leukocytes. J. Exp. Med., 124:115–127, 1966.

Schlotthauer, C. E., and Bollman, J. L.: Spontaneous gout in turkeys. J. Am. Vet. Med. Assoc., 85:98–103, 1934.

Schlumberger, H. G.: Synovial gout in the parakeet. Lab. Invest., 8:1304–1318, 1959.

Shirahama, T., and Cohen, A. S.: Ultrastructural evidence for leakage of lysosomal contents after phagocytosis of monosodium urate crystals. Am. J. Pathol., 76:501–520, 1974.

Siller, W. G.: Avian nephritis and visceral gout. Lab. Invest., 8:1319–1357, 1959.

Spilberg, I.: Urate crystal arthritis in animals lacking Hageman factor. Arthritis Rheum., 17:143–148, 1974.

Wacker, W. E. C.: Man: sapient but gouty. N. Engl. J. Med., 283:151–152, 1970.

Weissmann, G., and Rita, G. A.: Molecular basis of gouty inflammation: Interaction of monosodium urate crystals with lysosomes and liposomes. Nature New Biol., 240:167–172, 1972.

PSEUDOGOUT

Lesions with clinical and radiologic features resembling articular gout have been described under this name. A more precise name, **chondrocalcinosis** has also been applied to this entity. A similar lesion has been described in a dog. In this case, a slowly enlarging radiopaque mass involved the joint of the fifth digit of one rear leg. The surgical specimen revealed a chalky-white mass attached to the joint capsule. Microscopically, the mass contained masses of crystalline material separated by islands of connective tissue and cartilage. The fine, needle-shaped crystals were identified as calcium pyrophosphate. The nature of the deposited material clearly

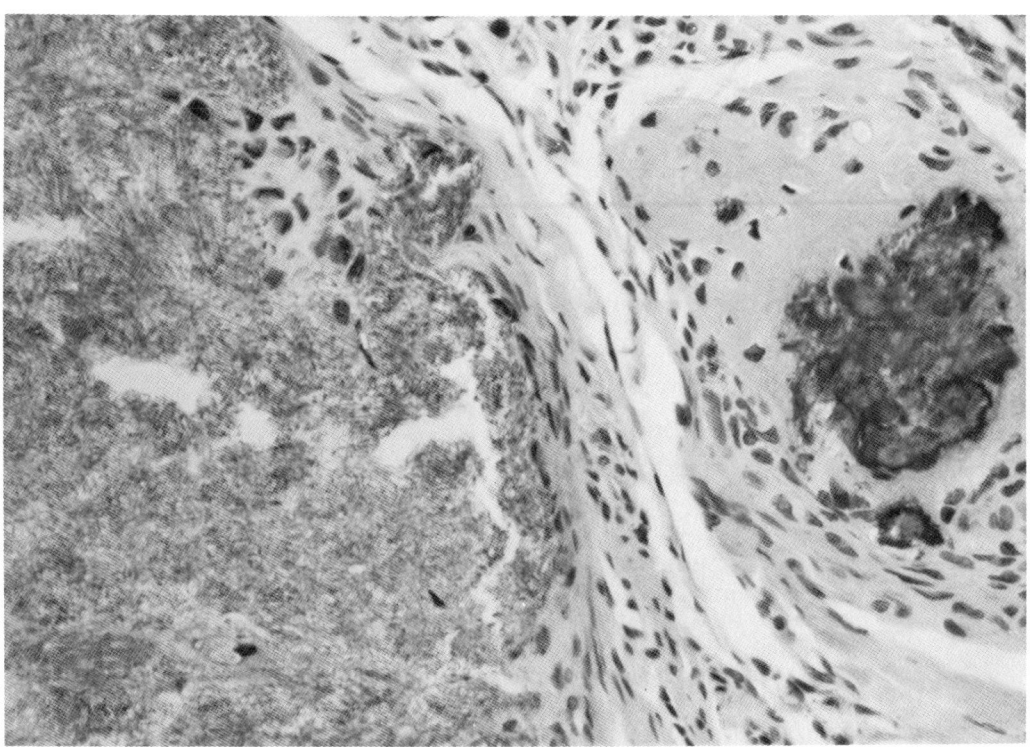

Fig. 3-6. Pseudogout. A mass of needle-shaped crystals and an island of cartilage in the skin of a dog. (Courtesy of Dr. J. P. Gibson.)

differentiates this lesion from gout, but the exact nature of this rare lesion has not been established.

Gibson, J. P., and Roenigk, W. J.: Pseudogout in a dog. J. Am. Vet. Med. Assoc., *161*:912–915, 1972.

PIGMENTS

There is nothing logical about considering together the diverse and unrelated substances customarily grouped as pigments except that, in surveying the various abnormalities that one may encounter in cellular pathology, it is convenient to have a look at all those substances that have color of their own instead of depending upon artificial staining to make them conspicuous.

A large number of pigments can be found in animal tissues. The ensuing discussion makes no attempt to cover all pigments, but rather is limited to those pigments that are encountered with frequency or are important components of animal diseases. For our purposes, pigments are classified as follows:

I. Exogenous pigments (those formed outside the body)
  A. Carbon
  B. Dusts
  C. Metals
  D. Tattoos
  E. Kaolin
  F. Carotenoids
II. Endogenous pigments (those formed inside the body)
  A. Phenolic pigments
     1. Melanin
  B. Hematogenous pigments
     1. Hemoglobins
     2. Hematins
     3. Parasitic pigments

Table 3–1.　Characteristics of Common Pigments as Seen in Tissue Sections

Pigment	Hematoxylin and Eosin	Polaroscopy	Iron Stains	Fat Stains	Acid Fast Stains	Other Distinguishing Characteristics
Carbon	Black	Isotropic	–	–	–	Resistant to all stains and bleaching agents and microincineration
Melanin	Yellow-brown to black	Isotropic	–	–	–	Reduce silver; bleached by $KMnO_4$; combusted by microincineration
Hemosiderin	Yellow-brown	Isotropic	+	–	–	Nonfluorescent
Acid hematins	Brown	Anisotropic	–	–	–	Removed by saturated alcoholic picric acid
Porphyrin	Usually not visible except in rodent Harderian gland	Slightly anisotropic	–	–	–	Fluorescent at 365 mμ
Bilirubin	Bright yellow	Anisotropic if crystalline	–	–	–	Gmelin's test positive; Nonfluorescent
Lipofuscins (wear and tear pigments and ceroid)	Yellow to brown	Isotropic	–	+	+	Fluorescent at 365 mμ

4. Hemosiderins
5. Bile pigments
6. Porphyrins (photosensitizing pigments)
C. Lipogenic pigments
   1. Tissue lipofuscins
   2. Ceroid
   3. Vitamin E deficiency pigment
D. Miscellaneous pigments
   1. Ochronosis pigment
   2. Dubin-Johnson pigment
   3. Cloisonné kidney

Carbon–Anthracosis

Anthracosis is the condition in which carbon particles are found as a black pigment in the tissues. Carbon is foremost among the exogenous pigments.

Occurrence. Carbon appears in the lungs and the lymph nodes that drain them and, rarely, in other organs when carried there in phagocytes. It is common in humans and animals that live in smoky cities, and as pointed out by Hilton Smith in the first edition of this text, universal among men and mules who work in coal mines. The mules have since left the mines, but black lungs still plague the miners.

Microscopic Appearance. Carbon appears as minute black granules either between cells or in their cytoplasm. In the lungs, it is in the alveolar walls and in the connective-tissue septa, usually within

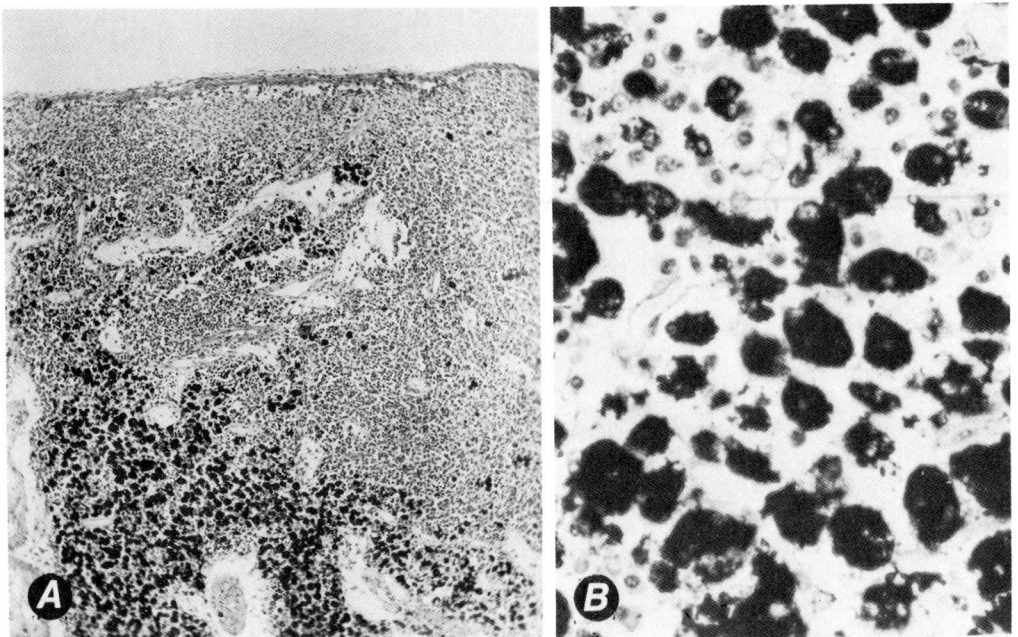

Fig. 3–7. Anthracosis, bronchial lymph node of an aged dog. *A*, Low power view (× 67), macrophages laden with carbon concentrated in the medulla. *B*, Higher power (× 594) of medulla—same lymph node. (Courtesy of Armed Forces Institute of Pathology.)

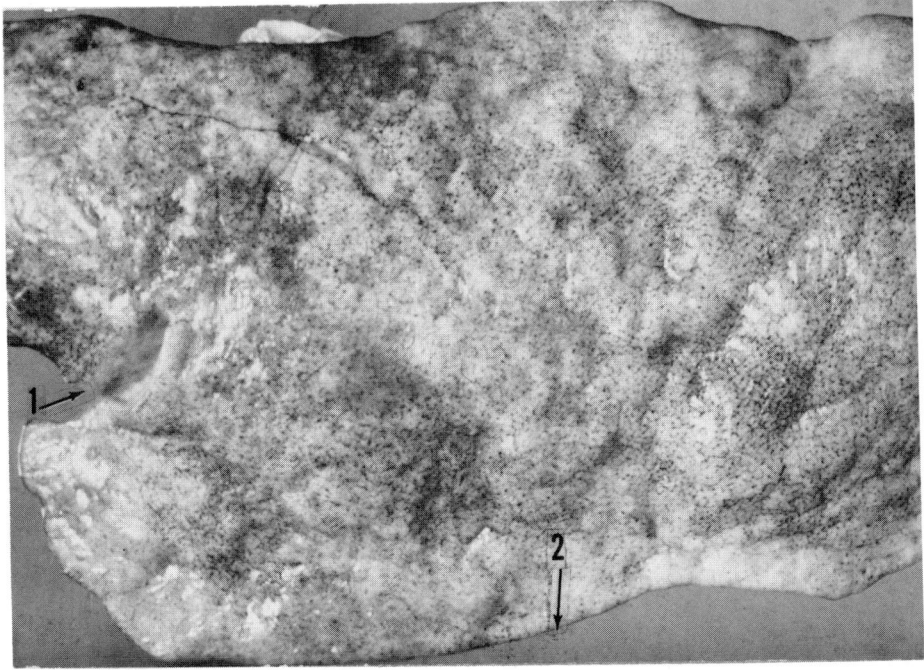

Fig. 3–8. Anthracosis, lung of a dog. Finely particulate collections of carbon are visible from the pleural surface. Cardiac notch (*1*) and ventral margin of lung (*2*).

macrophages. In the lymph nodes, it is chiefly between the lymphoid cells, but large mononuclear cells frequently phagocytize it and carry it elsewhere. Carbon can be distinguished from other pigments by its black color, and histochemically by its resistance to all solvents and bleaching agents.

Gross Appearance. Moderate or large amounts impart a mottling or speckling with black or gray to the lungs, the ventral portions of the lobes being affected more than the dorsal. Lymph nodes are likewise darkened. One must not confuse with anthracosis the black or brown color that almost invariably affects the medullary region of bovine lymph nodes. This discoloration is due to a soluble pigment presumed to come from recently hemolyzed blood. Since the pigment is soluble, it is not seen in microscopic preparations. Such lymph nodes do not reflect any form of ill health in the animal.

Causes and Significance. Anthracosis is due to repeated and continued inhalation of coal dust or smoke, which is the lot of thousands of human beings and animals living in cities. Men (and mules) working in coal mines are afflicted, so that the heavily blackened lung is called a miner's lung. Reasonable amounts of the pigment do little harm and cause no symptoms, but it remains in the tissues throughout life, and excessive amounts may cause slight fibrosis and are suspected of predisposing to pulmonary infections.

Dusts

When dust is inhaled, the organic particles are short-lived, owing to defensive mechanisms of the body. Several kinds of mineral dusts, however, leave visible particles in the pulmonary tissues. Collectively, dust retained in the lung is termed **pneumoconiosis**. Anthracosis is a specialized form of pneumoconiosis in which the dust particles are carbon. Several other mineral dusts are important causes of pneumoconiosis, some of which induce serious pulmonary disease.

Silicosis. **Silicon dioxide** is inhaled in rock quarries and mines or under any other conditions in which rock is being cut or sandblasted. Microscopically, silicon dioxide occurs in the tissues as fine, anisotropic crystals, which can only be visualized with polarized light. The crystals incite collagenous connective tissue proliferation, which takes the form of dense sclerotic nodules which may coalesce. The mechanism of action is through damage to lysosomes. Following phagocytosis and fusion with lysosomes, the lysosomal membrane is damaged through a hydrogen-bonding reaction between silicic acid and the membrane. Released lysosomal enzymes kill the phagocyte, freeing the silica particles, which are engulfed again to repeat the never-ending vicious cycle. A vascular or cellular inflammatory response does not occur. Grossly, the lungs are nodular and firm, and may be pigmented due to concomitant anthracosis.

Siderosis. **Iron dust** is inhaled chiefly as hematite or iron oxide from mines. The mineral does not incite fibrosis or an inflammatory reaction and is, therefore, of little significance. However, siderosis is often accompanied by silicosis. Microscopically, hematite and iron oxide appear as red crystals of varying size. They are anisotropic, appearing orange with polarized light, and iron can be specifically demonstrated with the Prussian blue reaction. The student should note that certain other iron salts and complexes may be black, blue, green, gray or brown, and not all react with the usual Prussian blue stain. In the gross specimen, hematite and iron oxide impart a brick red color to the lungs.

Asbestosis. Asbestos is widely used in the manufacture of fire-retardant insulating materials. Exposure to man or animals may result under many circumstances, but the most significant hazard to man occurs during manufacture or fabrication of products containing asbestos. Recognition of this hazard has led to changes in methods of manufacture of these products and restrictions in their use.

Under microscopic examination, asbestos occurs as fine, white anisotropic fibers and as asbestos bodies. Asbestos bodies are long beaded rods with rounded ends, which are yellow due to an iron coating that can be demonstrated with the Prussian blue reaction. Asbestos bodies are isotropic (dark under polarized light). Asbestos incites fibrous scarring of the pleura, around bronchioles and alveolar ducts, and within alveolar septae. Discrete nodules, as in silicosis, do not develop. Foreign body giant cells may form adjacent to the asbestos particles. In human beings, asbestosis has been associated with bronchogenic carcinoma and mesothelioma of the pleura and peritoneum. Grossly, the pleura is thickened and the lungs are firm.

Other Metals and Exogenous Pigments

Silver. The disorder known as **argyria** is of academic interest. Formerly certain infections were commonly treated with various organic silver compounds, of which argyrol is about the only present-day survivor. When large amounts were administered to human patients, silver was sometimes precipitated in the skin in amounts sufficient to impart to it a ghastly gray color. This was a permanent cosmetic injury of considerable importance to the victim. Obviously, the same would scarcely be true in animals.

Microscopically, silver occurs as an insoluble albuminate that is brown to black. It is deposited principally extracellularly between connective tissue fibers in the upper corium. Only a small amount may be found within macrophages. In some cases, deposits may also occur extracellularly in the liver and kidney. Silver does not produce injury nor incite a cellular reaction.

Lead. In chronic poisoning due to the prolonged ingestion or assimilation of small amounts of lead compounds, a blue-black discoloration is imparted to the gums. Of considerable diagnostic importance, it is most pronounced just above (or proximal to) the teeth, and is called the **lead line**. Chronic lead poisoning has occurred in animals as the result of eating pasturage contaminated by fumes and smoke from smelters, or drinking water similarly polluted. Ruminants and horses may ingest paint containing lead by chewing on painted wood surfaces. Puppies and children may chew on such surfaces or may eat pieces of paint scaled from old painted surfaces.

Bismuth. Occasionally in examining microscopic sections from the edge of a fistulous tract or sinus, such as might have been left by some penetrating foreign body, one sees a faint gray-black pigment in the form of minute granules in and between cells. Investigation reveals that this is a residue from a bismuth-containing paste or powder injected into the tract so that it could be visualized by roentgenologic examination, bismuth salts being opaque to x-rays. This and similar delicate pigments should be sought by low magnification with a strong light directed down upon the slide and reflected back into the microscope rather than by the usual light transmitted through the section.

Tattoos

A variety of pigments are used to produce tattoos. These include India ink, China ink, Bismark brown, cinnabar, and kurkuma. These pigments are inert and produce no tissue reaction. They are seen microscopically extracellularly between connective tissue fibers of the dermis and within macrophages.

Kaolin

Also known as China clay or Fuller's earth, kaolin is a kind of clay derived by disintegration of an aluminous material such as feldspar or mica. The essential mineral constituent is hydrated aluminum silicate (kaolinite), but the following elements may also be present: silicon (SiO_2), aluminum (Al_2O_3), iron (Fe_2O_3), titanium (TiO_2), calcium (CaO), magnesium (MgO), potassium (K_2O), sodium (Na_2O), manganese (MnO), copper (CuO), and sulfur (SO_3), with water, carbon, and organic matter.

Kaolin has been incriminated as a cause of pneumoconiosis (kaolinosis) in man and nonhuman primates, which leads to dense pulmonary scarring. It has also produced extensive subcutaneous granulomas in the pharyngeal and neck tissues of animals following overzealous administration of various kaolin containing products for gastrointestinal disease. The kaolin accidentally introduced into the subcutaneous tissue incites a striking influx of macrophages, producing dense nodules that displace adjacent tissues. The kaolin is visible as amorphous material and fine anisotropic crystals within macrophages.

Hartley, W. J., Mullins, J., and Lawson, B. M.: Nutritional siderosis in the bovine. NZ Vet. J., 7:99–105, 1959.

Heppleston, A. G.: Changes in the lungs of rabbits and ponies inhaling coal dust underground. J. Pathol., 67:349–359, 1954.

Higginson, J., Gerritsen, T., and Walker, A. R. P.: Siderosis in the Bantu of Southern Africa. Am. J. Pathol., 29:779–815, 1953.

Kilburn, K. H. (ed.): Pulmonary reactions to organic materials. NY Acad. Sci., 221: (entire volume).

Kleckner, M. S., Baggenstross, A. H., and Weir, J. F.: Iron-storage diseases. Am. J. Clin. Pathol., 25:915–931, 1955.

Lord, G. H., and Willson, J. E.: Foreign body granuloma in a Rhesus monkey. J. Am. Vet. Med. Assoc., 153:910–913, 1968.

Lynch, K. M., and McIver, F. A.: Pneumoconiosis from exposure to kaolin dust: kaolinosis. Am. J. Pathol., 30:1117–1127, 1954.

Selikoff, I. J.: Lung cancer and mesothelioma during prospective surveillance of 1249 asbestos workers, 1963–1974. Ann. N.Y. Acad. Sci., 271:448–456, 1976.

Selikoff, I. J., and Hammond, E. C.: Asbestos associated disease in United States shipyards. CA, 28:87–99, 1978.

Smith, B. L., Poole, W. S. H., and Martinovich, D.: Pneumoconiosis in the captive New Zealand Kiwi. Vet. Pathol., 10:94–101, 1973.

Suzuki, Y., and Churg, J.: Structure and development of the asbestos body. Am. J. Pathol., 55:79–107, 1969.

Taylor, F. A.: Pigment of anthracosis. Proc. Soc. Exp. Biol. Med., 48:70–72, 1941.

Taylor, K. E.: Ham discoloration due to iron injections. J. Am. Vet. Med. Assoc., 145:470–471, 1964.

Webster, I.: The ingestion of asbestos fibers. Environ. Health Perspect., 9:199–202, 1974.

Weller, W., and Ulmer, W. T.: Inhalation studies of coal-quartz dust mixture. Ann. NY Acad. Sci., 200:142–154, 1972.

Zaidi, S. H., Shanker, R., and Dogra, R. K. S.: Experimental infective pneumoconiosis: effect of asbestos dust and Candida albicans infection on lungs of Rhesus monkeys. Environ. Res., 6:274–286, 1973.

Carotenoid Pigments

The carotenoid pigments are fat-soluble pigments of plant origin. They include carotene-A, carotene-B (the precursor of vitamin A), and xanthophyll, all of which are greenish-yellow. They are classed as lipochrome pigments, which are not to be confused with the endogenous lipofuscin pigments.

Occurrence. Pigments of this group occur normally in the epithelial cells of the adrenal gland, lutein cells of the corpus luteum, epithelium of the testis and seminal vesicle, Kupffer cells of the liver, ganglion cells, the yolks of eggs, butter fat, and the adipose cells of animals, such as horses and Jersey and Guernsey cattle, which have a markedly yellow body fat. The amount of carotenoid pigments in tissues varies between species, owing to their relative efficiency in converting carotene-B to vitamin A and rejecting carotenoids in the ingesta that are not required for vitamin A synthesis. The efficiency for these two functions is low in such species as fowl, horses, cattle, humans, and nonhuman primates.

Pathologically, the same type of pigment occurs in small tumors known as xanthomas. These tumors are not true neoplasms, but appear to be a disorder of the reticuloendothelial system.

Lipochrome pigments are seen only grossly, since the material is soluble, and the color, diffuse and not pronounced.

Hepatic Carotenosis. Bovine livers sometimes appear a brilliant yellow, perhaps slightly reddish, but not with the greenish tinge that is characteristic of jaundice and retention of bile, nor with the pale yellow of fatty change. The pigment in this case is carotene, which in itself is harmless, but the affected livers also show toxic changes, consisting chiefly of focal or centrilobular necrosis and limited fatty change. These changes progress to varying degrees of portal cirrhosis and even almost complete replacement of the liver tissue by fibrous tissue; mild lymphocytic infiltrations are also present. Feeding such livers experimentally to rats produces similar toxic changes in the livers of the rats, but not accumulation of carotene. It is presumed that the carotene remains unconverted and unmetabolized because of the toxic injury to the liver cells, but this appears to be a peculiarity of the bovine species only. Investigators, working with material obtained at meat inspection, suspected some unknown toxic plant as the cause.

Livers filled with retained bile pigment in obstructive jaundice, in spite of their usual greenish tinge, may be confused with hepatic carotenosis. The two can be differentiated by extracting a sample of minced liver with ether and water. After thorough shaking, the lighter ether will rise to the top with the yellow color of the carotene, if this is present. The water below will be colored yellow by bilirubin, the pigment of icterus, if such is present. The fatty liver not only has a lighter yellow color but greater swelling if the condition is pronounced, and a lighter specific gravity, often being able to float on water.

Melanin

Passing to the **endogenous** group of pigments, the most important in the **autogenous** subgroup is melanin. Melanin is the pigment that gives color to the skin and hair and to the iris, and provides the black, reflection-proof inner coating of the eyeball.

While the complete chemistry of melanin is not known, it is considered to be formed from the amino acid, tyrosine, which, it will be recalled, differs from phenylalanine (β-phenyl, α-amino propionic acid) by having one hydroxy group attached to the phenyl group, and which therefore is also called hydroxyphenylalanine. Although the oxidative steps necessary to convert tyrosine to melanin are not known, the copper-containing enzyme, tyrosinase, is required. There also exists, by artificial production, the substance dihydroxyphenylalanine, which has one more hydroxy group attached to the phenyl ring. More will be said about this presently.

The mechanisms that control melanin formation are also poorly understood. It has been established in man and some animals that the pituitary produces two melanocyte stimulating factors; α-MSH and β-MSH. Although their function is not clear, they are believed to be important in man in the increased pigmentation seen in Addison's disease and in pregnancy. ACTH also has melanocyte stimulating potential, but to a significantly lesser degree than MSH. Hydrocortisone decreases MSH release from the pituitary.

Occurrence. Normal physiologic deposits of melanin include the following: In the epidermis of animals and humans, there is a small amount in light-colored individuals and more in darker ones. The melanin exists as minute brown or black granules in the cytoplasm of the epithelial cells, chiefly or entirely in the basal layer, the stratum germinativum. In black animals and Negroes, some of the pigment extends into cells of the intermediate layers. It is produced by specialized dendritic cells derived from the neural nest called melanoblasts, which transfer melanin by way of their processes to epithelial cells. The hairs partake of the same pigmentation to a degree somewhat proportional to that of the skin. In the hairs, the melanin is in the cortical substance, having been derived from the epithelium of the hair follicle. It is reported that the melanin granules are large in dark hairs, smaller in lighter hairs. Bay, brown, and even sorrel horses have a black skin, as do red and fawn cattle and red swine. In the dog and cat, this may not be the case, depending on the breed. In animals with white spots, both hair and skin are nonpigmented at these places. Gray horses owe their color to a mixture of white and black hairs over a black skin. White rabbits, white rats, white mice, and occasional individuals of any species are true **albinos**, having no pigment in hair, skin or elsewhere, except that the retina is not entirely devoid of pigment.

In some breeds of cattle, especially Jerseys, and in some breeds of dogs, such as Chows, the mucous membrane of the mouth shares the pigmentation of the adjacent skin. The same is true of hoofs—white hoof tissue growing from white skin—and this is largely true of horns.

Melanin gives color to the iris, and a thick, black zone of melanin is deposited in a layer of cells where the retina joins the choroid, which totally blackens the interior of the uveal space.

In some people and especially in sheep, melanin is found here and there in certain dendritic cells of the pia-arachnoid. In sheep this is common over the anterior part of the brain, but may be found even over the spinal cord. In some species, the substantia nigra of the brain is black because of melanin-containing nerve cells.

Melanin occurs pathologically, or at least abnormally, in the tumors known as melanomas, melanosis, acanthosis nigricans, such abnormalities of the human skin as freckles, hyperpigmentation of the skin associated with hyperadrenalism, and a rare, inherited disease in man (Dubin-Johnson syndrome) and mutant Corriedale sheep in which a hepatic excretionary defect results in accumulation of melanin pigment in hepatocytes.

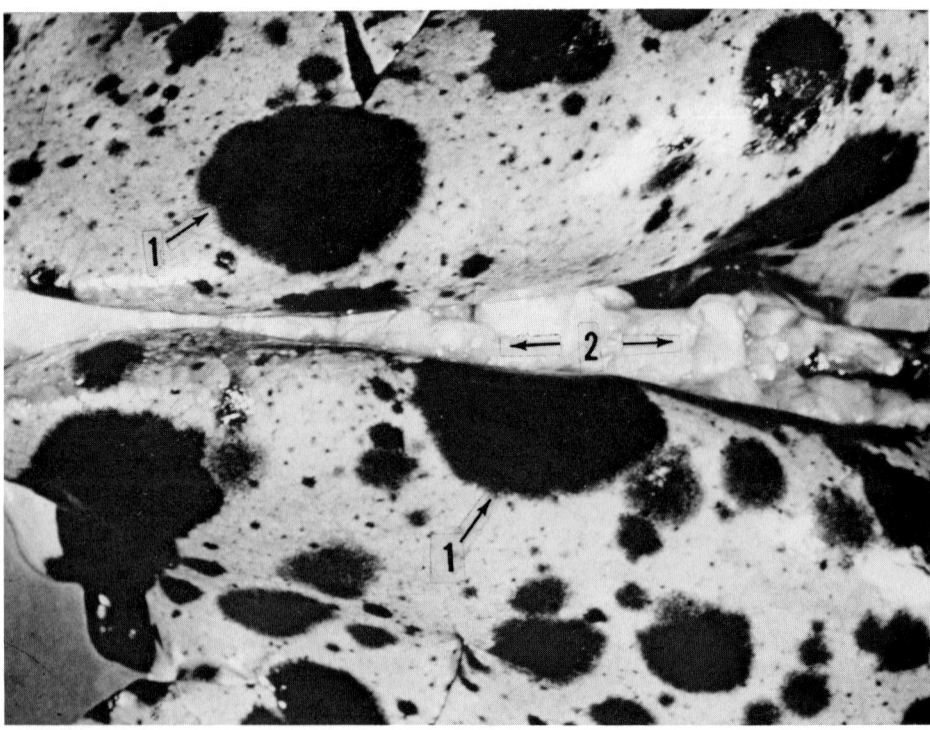

Fig. 3–9.   Melanosis, lung of sheep. Large deposits of melanin (*1*), mediastinum (*2*). (Courtesy of Dr. C. L. Davis.)

Melanosis is a deposition of melanin in various organs, especially the lungs and aorta, as rather spectacular black or brown spots of irregular shape and often a centimeter or more in greatest diameter. There is no change in the texture, consistency, or form of the tissue and no tendency toward neoplasia. The condition is most frequently encountered by meat inspectors, the animals being in normal health.

Albinism represents a pathologic absence of melanin. It is thought to result from an inability of the melanocyte to synthesize sufficient functionally active tyrosinase. Melanocytes are present in albinism and are structurally identical to normal melanocytes. Inability to form melanin occurs with the development of **achromotrichia** in copper deficiency in several animal species. As mentioned previously, copper is an essential component of tyrosinase. Focal depigmentation may occur in scars and radiation burns.

Microscopic Appearance. Melanin takes the form of minute, rounded granules of light or dark brown color located in the cytoplasm of cells. Ultrastructurally, the granules are extremely dense, ellipsoid, and measure 0.3 by 0.7 μ. In the skin, melanin lies in the cytoplasm of the basal and adjoining cells of the epidermis.

Certain investigators, using the "dopa reaction" and other special techniques, have shown that the melanin is produced in special cells just beneath the epithelium (or within it), which have long dendritic processes interspersed among the epithelial cells. These special cells are **melanoblasts** (or melanocytes). It is postulated that the pigment is transferred from them to the epithelial cells. Although in some other locations the presence of melanin may be attributable solely to dendritic cells of more or less similar morphology, it does not appear that all melanin formation can be accredited to cells of this type (for instance, in the substantia nigra), and it is difficult to reconcile this view with what one sees in day-to-day observations of skin sections. It is clear, however, that melanin does escape from its intracellular position, is seen extracellularly, is excreted in the urine in

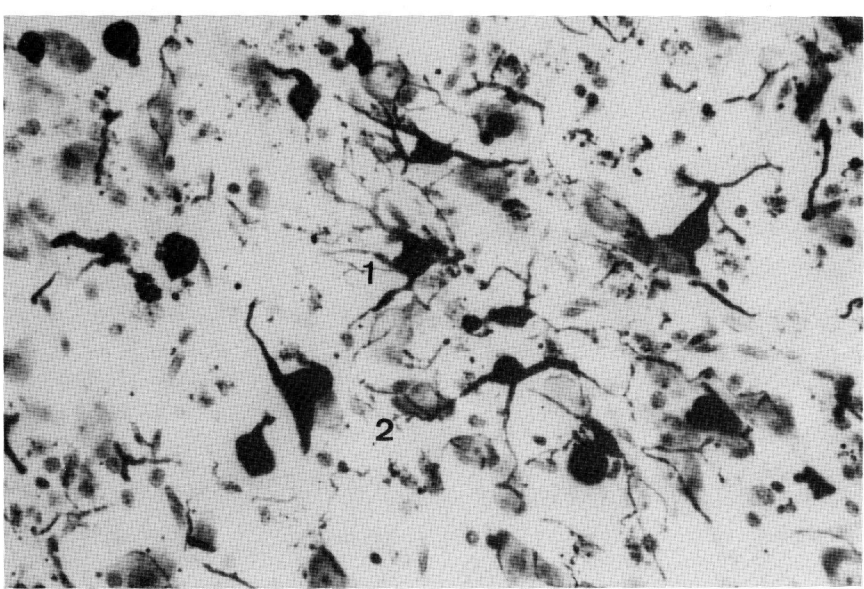

Fig. 3–10. Melanosis, thalamus of a goat. *(1)* Melanin-laden melanocytes with elongate processes; *(2)* melanophagic neurons. Luxol blue stain. (Courtesy of Dr. G. Bestetti, Prof. Dr. R. Fankhauser, and Prof. Dr. H. Luginbühl, Bern.)

cases of great overproduction (malignant melanomas), and is frequently phagocytized by ordinary reticuloendothelial macrophages. When laden with melanin, these phagocytes receive the special name of **melanophore** (or melanophage). The melanophores are often seen in the dermis beneath pigmented epithelium, and not infrequently migrate in great numbers to the regional lymph nodes, where they are recognized as large, round cells filled with pigment composed of finer granules than those of hemosiderin, with which melanin can be confused. The melanophore is not a producer of melanin, as can be shown by the **dopa reaction**.

The word "dopa" was coined from the key letters of dioxyphenylalanine, an older equivalent of dihydroxyphenylalanine, which received attention earlier in this section. If a section of fresh tissue is incubated with a suitable solution of this substance, the position of melanin-producing cells is indicated by a black granular precipitate. This is pigment formed by the action of the melanin-producing cells upon the dihydroxyphenylalanine. Such cells have the same action on (mono) hydroxyphenylalanine, which is tyrosine, as previously stated. The reaction is considered to be due to an enzyme, called dopa-oxydase (tyrosinase), existing in melanin-forming cells. The dopa reaction, then, is not a test for melanin, but for the power of producing melanin. Since it has to be performed upon frozen sections of unfixed or slightly fixed tissue, precise localization of the enzyme is not easy, but in general, dopaoxydase occurs where melanin occurs, except in the case of phagocytized and transported melanin. One may test for the actual presence of melanin granules by Fontana's silver solution, which turns such granules black.

Significance. Melanin itself is not harmful, although the melanomas, in which it is so conspicuously seen, are major threats to life. Melanosis is not harmful. In the skin, the amount of pigment increases with increased exposure to sunlight (or artificial ultraviolet rays), and it is considered to be of primary importance in protecting the tissues from sunburn. (See also Photosensitization.)

Fawcett, D. W.: An Atlas of Fine Structure. The Cell, Its Organelles and Inclusions. Philadelphia, W. B. Saunders, 1966.

Flatt, R. E., Nelson, L. R., and Middleton, C. C.: Melanotic lesions in the internal organs of miniature swine. Arch. Pathol., 93:71–75, 1972.

Gjesdal, F.: Investigations on the melanin granules with special consideration of the hair pigment. Acta Pathol. Microbiol. Scand., Suppl. 133:112, 1959.

Kaliner, G., Frese, K., Fatzer, R., and Fankhauser, R.: Thalamic melanosis in goats. Schweiz. Arch. Tierheilkd., 116:405–411, 1974.

Okum, M. R., Donnellan, B., Pearson, S. H., and Edelstein, L. M.: Melanin: A normal component of human eosinophils. Lab. Invest., 30:681–685, 1974.

Hematogenous Pigments

A variety of pigments are derivatives of hemoglobin metabolism. Certain are normal physiologic pigments, which may accumulate to excess, such as hemosiderin and bilirubin, and others are pathologic, such as methemoglobin and hematins formed by protozoan and metazoan parasites.

Hemoglobin

Hemoglobin, the normal pigment of erythrocytes, is in solution or in a colloidal state within those cells. Hemoglobin consists of a pigment, heme, plus the protein, globin. Heme is divisible into ferrous iron and a porphyrin (protoporphyrin III). The various porphyrins consist principally of four pyrrol rings with various hydrocarbon radicals attached to them. (Porphyrins will be discussed shortly.) The empirical formula of hemoglobin has been estimated to be approximately $C_{112}H_{1130}N_{214}S_2FeO_{245}$. It is noteworthy, however, that hemoglobin does not respond to the ordinary tests for iron compounds.

Hemoglobin imparts grossly to individual erythrocytes a straw-yellow color, which deepens to crimson red when a thick layer of erythrocytes is viewed in the fresh state. Hemoglobin ordinarily is not seen microscopically, however its presence is responsible for the eosinophilia of erythrocytes. Hemoglobin can be more specifically demonstrated by several histochemical techniques.

The gross tinctorial properties and chemistry of hemoglobin may be slightly altered under certain conditions, such as in some poisonings and due to postmortem changes. In normal hemoglobin, the iron is in the ferrous state and is either loosely oxygenated (it is not oxidized) and referred to as **oxyhemoglobin**, or has given up its oxygen store and referred to as **reduced hemoglobin**. The bright red of arterial blood is due to the presence of oxyhemoglobin; the dark red of venous blood is caused by reduced hemoglobin.

Methemoglobin is a true oxide of hemoglobin (ferric iron) and is dark red (often called chocolate brown), in contrast to bright red oxyhemoglobin. It is produced by poisonings with nitrites, chlorates, and some organic compounds. **Sulfhemoglobin** is a combination of reduced hemoglobin and inorganic sulfide and is a dark brown. It results from the action of nitrites and coal tar preparations (aniline, acetophenetidin, acetanilid) in the presence of excessive amounts of sulfur. A **sulfur methemoglobin** can form after death and cause a greenish discoloration to abdominal structures. **Carboxyhemoglobin,** which is a bright cherry-red, is the result of a combination of carbon monoxide with hemoglobin.

When erythrocytes undergo hemolysis, whether in the vessels after death, in an external or internal hemorrhage, or in a flask of blood withdrawn for some laboratory purpose, the anoxic hemoglobin slowly escapes and carries its dark red color to the surrounding fluids and tissues. Such discolored perivascular tissues after death represent postmortem imbibition. As stated previously, the color of hemoglobin is not seen microscopically.

Hematins

Hematins, or more properly **acid hematins,** are pigments formed by the action of acids on hemoglobin. They are not normal breakdown products. The most familiar of the acid hematins is **acid formalin hematin**, which is formed when acid aqueous solutions of formaldehyde act on blood-rich tissues. It appears in tissue sections as a dark brown, finely granular, anisotropic pigment that does not stain with iron stains. It may be seen both in vascular spaces and within (or on top of) various cellular elements. Acid formalin hematin is of no pathologic significance, but its presence can be annoying in that it must be differentiated from other pigments. It can be removed from tissue sections with saturated alcoholic picric acid. The use of neutral (pH 7.0) buffered formalin prevents its occurrence. A similar pigment may develop in extremely alkaline (above pH 8.0) formalin solutions. Other acid hematins that closely resemble acid formalin hematin can form from the action of acetic acid and hydrochloric acid. **Hydrochloric acid hematin** is often seen within and adjacent to gastric ulcers. It apparently forms from the action of gastric acid with hemoglobin.

Several parasitic diseases are associated with the deposition of hematin pigments in tissues. In **malaria**, hematins are present in parasitized erythrocytes and in the cytoplasm of reticuloendothelial cells in the spleen, lymph nodes, liver, and bone marrow. In each site, the pigment is yellow to dark brown and iron-negative. In erythrocytes, the pigment is anisotropic, whereas in reticuloendothelial cells, it is isotropic. The pigment is formed by the malarial parasites from the host's hemoglobin. Several species of trematodes produce pigments believed to be hematins. *Fascioloides magna* in the ruminant liver deposits a grossly visible pigment that accumulates adjacent to the parasite within macro-

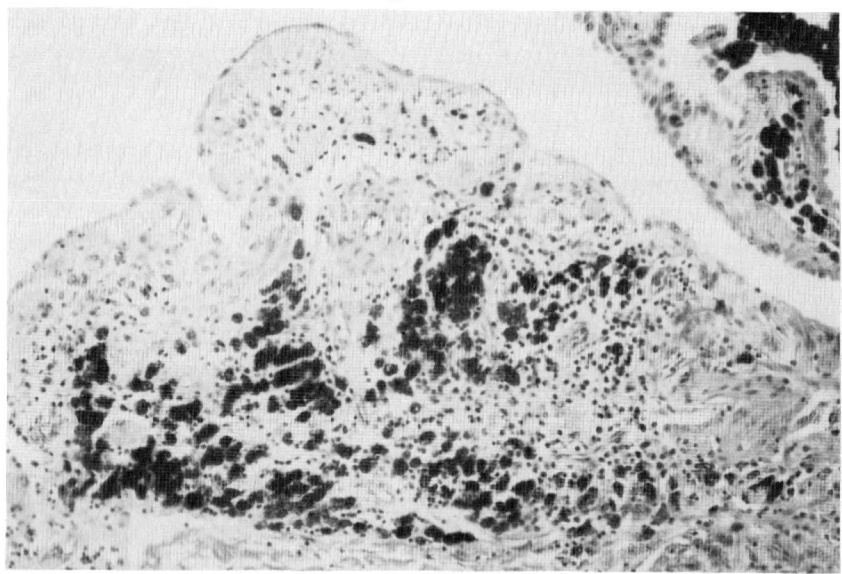

Fig. 3–11. *Pneumonyssus simicola* infestation of the lung of a rhesus monkey *(Macaca mulatta)*. Parasitic hematin pigments within macrophages adjacent to a bronchiole. (Courtesy of New England Regional Primate Research Center, Harvard Medical School.)

phages. Various species of *schistosomes* produce anisotropic, iron-negative hematins, which accumulate in macrophages of the liver, spleen, bone marrow, and lymph nodes.

Pneumonyssus simicola is associated with two pigments. One occurs as light brown to colorless, needle-like brightly anisotropic crystals, and the other, as finely granular brown to black granules that are variably anisotropic. Both pigments are believed to be derived from hemoglobin metabolized by the mite. In contrast to hematins, most of the pigment stains with the usual iron stains, although isolated crystals and granules may be negative.

Hemosiderin

Hemosiderin is a shiny, golden yellow or golden brown pigment derived from hemoglobin. It is usually seen within macrophages and does respond to the ordinary tests for iron; chemically, it is the same as ferritin.

Occurrence. It occurs principally in the red pulp of the spleen and in other places where there has been extensive disintegration of erythrocytes. Such places include the sites of old hemorrhages into the tissues, receding ovarian corpora hemorrhagica, and chronically congested lungs. Rarely, large amounts are seen within the epithelial cells of the liver, spleen, and kidneys, but these cases are discussed separately under the heading Hemochromatosis.

Microscopic Appearance. Hemosiderin commonly takes the form of glittering golden-colored spherules, 2 or 3 μ in diameter, packed into oval or rounded phagocytes. These macrophagic cells are commonly so full of pigment that the nucleus cannot be seen, but it is easy to surmise that the yellow, granular body is a cell because of its size, shape, and rounded outline. At times, the color tends more toward brown, and the arrangement in spherical granules is less evident. The presence of hemosiderin in the tissues is determined readily by an ordinary chemical test for its component iron, the **Prussian-blue reaction.** The application of a solution of potas-

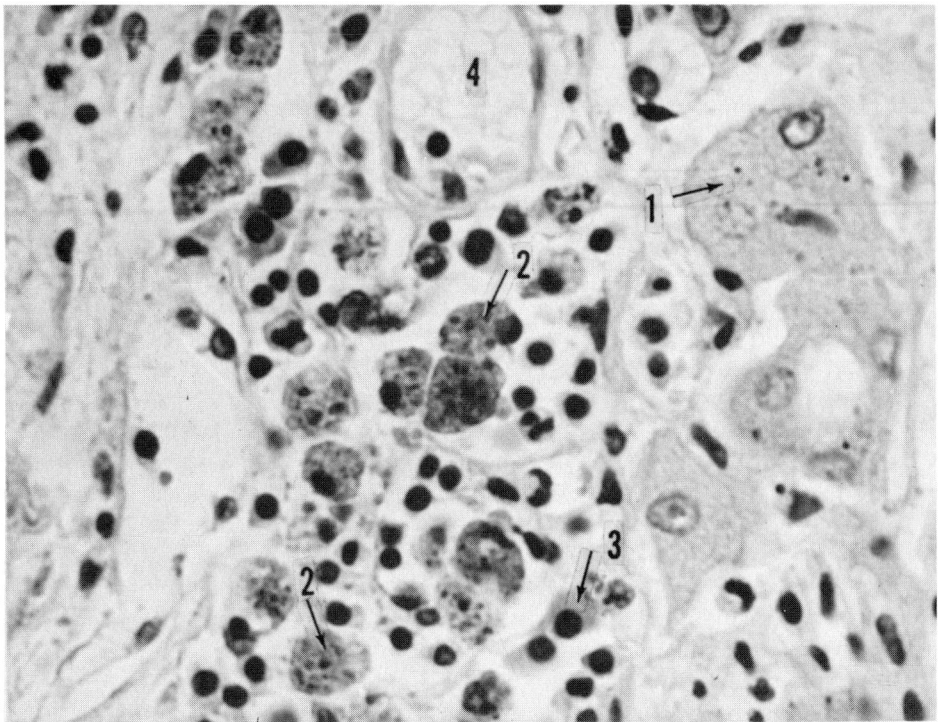

Fig. 3-12. Hemosiderin in portal area, liver of a dog. Liver cell (*1*) with distended bile canaliculus, macrophages (*2*) with engulfed granules of brown staining hemosiderin, plasma cells (*3*), and branch of portal vein (*4*). (× 650.) (Courtesy of Armed Forces Institute of Pathology.) Contributor: Dr. D. J. Carren.

sium ferrocyanide to the microscopic section following treatment with an acid turns hemosiderin a strong greenish blue, the potassium having been replaced by Fe to give ferric ferrocyanide, which, incidentally, is the common pigment of blue paints called Prussian blue. The same test can also be applied to fresh tissue, the whole area taking a diffuse bluish tinge if large amounts of hemosiderin are present.

Gross Appearance. Small amounts of hemosiderin are not detected grossly, but large accumulations impart a brownish color to the organ or tissue in which they occur.

Causes and Special Considerations. The cause of the formation of hemosiderin is the destruction, or hemolysis, of erythrocytes to an excessive degree. This happens locally when there has been hemorrhage into the tissues.

Hemosiderin accumulates in phagocytic cells of the spleen as the result of excessive hemolysis within the circulating blood, as in hemolytic anemia. It may also be deposited in the liver in both Kupffer cells and hepatocytes, and in the tubular lining cells and interstitium of the kidney.

Hemosiderin gathers in the spleen, lungs, and even other organs as the result of chronic passive congestion. Chronic congestion of the spleen is most likely to result from cirrhosis, along with congestion of the whole portal circulation.

Chronic passive congestion of the lungs is ordinarily due to disease of the heart, valvular insufficiency, or stenosis of the left side. Hence, when hemosiderin accumulates here, the macrophages of the lung, brilliant with their golden pigment and often lying conspicuously free in the alveolar lumens, are given the nickname of

heart-failure cells. Grossly, a brownish tinge is imparted to the lung tissue when the accumulation of hemosiderin is large. As a reaction to the constant pressure of the blood in the distended capillaries, there is a diffuse increase of connective tissue throughout the alveolar walls. This tends to make the whole lung leathery and somewhat hard, or as we say, indurated. On the basis of these two changes, it is common to refer to the condition as a whole as **brown induration** of the lungs.

Significance. The significance of hemosiderosis (the deposition of hemosiderin in the tissue) is merely that one of the foregoing disorders is present. The pigment in itself is not harmful, nor is it indestructible. In spite of the possibility that chronic passive congestion may be responsible for its presence in the spleen, large amounts almost always indicate hemolytic anemia. Such a spleen often also contains numerous giant cells of foreign-body type. Hemosiderosis is related to, but, we believe, separable from hemochromatosis.

Hemochromatosis

Hemochromatosis is a rare condition in human beings in which a pigment indistinguishable from hemosiderin is deposited in tremendous amounts in the cytoplasm of the epithelial cells of the liver and pancreas, as well as in kidneys, spleen, and various other organs in lesser amounts. It is accompanied by cirrhosis, apparently resulting from irritation by the pigment, by diabetes, probably causally related to the deposited pigment, although the islets are not destroyed, and by melanin pigmentation of the skin. On the basis of this triad of lesions, the name **bronzed diabetes** has been in common use clinically. The cause is thought to be an inborn metabolic defect. In view of the fact that the body normally limits its absorption of iron to its scanty needs and eliminates the element slowly or not at all, evidence suggests that the trouble may be in excessive absorption of that substance. It is agreed that this iron-containing pigment does not come from hemolysis; hence, it is not related to hemosiderosis. For this reason, the name, **cytosiderosis**, has been suggested.

In animals, the syndrome has not been reported, but in some instances, heavy deposition of what appears to be the same pigment is found in livers and kidneys. This is said to occur in equine infectious anemia, without the spleen being similarly involved. It also occurs in anemias due to deficiency of accessory hemoglobin-forming elements, copper and cobalt. Apparently, in those forms of anemia in which the hematopoietic tissue is active but unable to metabolize iron, iron accumulates in the tissues and is phagocytized in a form indistinguishable from hemosiderin. In all probability, increased amounts of iron are absorbed.

Zahawi (1957) has reported a condition in goats grazing the mountains of northern Iraq (inaccessible to other animals) in which 3.6% of 700 goats had brown or blackish kidneys due to heavy deposition of a hemosiderin-like pigment in the epithelium of the proximal convoluted tubules, sometimes with evidence of mild injury to the cells, apparently due to a deficiency of cobalt. Lesser amounts of this pigment were found in the Kupffer (rarely the epithelial) cells of the liver, and in reticuloendothelial cells of the spleen and lymph nodes. The testes suffered necrosis of much seminiferous epithelium and gave a Prussian-blue reaction. Other organs were normal. The goats were not clinically ill. The soil here contains as much as 4% copper and 30% iron, but is deficient in cobalt.

Hartley, W. J., Mullins, J., and Lawson, B. M.: Nutritional siderosis in the bovine. N. Z. Vet. J., 7:99–105, 1959.

Higginson, J., Gerritsen, T., and Walker, A. R. P.: Siderosis in the Bantu of Southern Africa. Am. J. Pathol., 29:779–815, 1953.

Kleckner, M. S., Baggenstross, A. H., and Weir, J. F.: Iron-storage diseases. Am. J. Clin. Pathol., 25:915–931, 1955.

Plummer, P. J. G.: Three cases of osteohaemo-chromatosis in cattle. Can. J. Comp. Med., 13:64–65, 1949.

Rimington, C.: Pigments of blood and bile. Lancet, 261:551–556, 1951.

———: Haems and porphyrins in health and disease. Acta Med. Scand., 143:161–196, 1952.

Sheldon, J. H.: Haemochromatosis. London, Oxford University Press, 1935.

Zahawi, S.: Symmetrical cortical siderosis of the kidney in goats. Am. J. Vet. Res., 18:861–867, 1957.

Bile Pigments

Since there is a normal destruction each day of an appreciable number of erythrocytes, a certain amount of hemoglobin is continually being metabolized. The iron and globin are reused by the body, and the porphyrin is changed to a soluble pigment, **bilirubin**, by reticuloendothelial cells in the bone marrow, spleen, and elsewhere. In the normal course of events, the bilirubin circulates in the blood until it reaches the liver, where it is excreted in the bile, being responsible for the color of the excreted product. It accumulates pathologically whenever and wherever the disintegration of erythrocytes becomes excessive. Its further history will be related shortly in connection with icterus.

Although bilirubin is a soluble substance ordinarily, there is occasionally encountered a yellowish pigment, especially at the site of old hemorrhages, which has long been called **hematoidin**. This is now believed to be the same as bilirubin, although it appears as a precipitate, presumably because the solution becomes locally or temporarily supersaturated. Neither bilirubin nor hematoidin are positive to the usual tests for iron. This, and the fact that it remains as angular, yellow crystals and is seldom phagocytized, are the principal features that distinguish hematoidin from hemosiderin, for both are formed under the same conditions and have the same significance.

Biliverdin is an intermediary product in the formation of bilirubin; it is of similar chemical structure, but it is green rather than yellow. Biliverdin is not ordinarily seen in tissue sections, but it is responsible in part for the blue-green discoloration of bruises.

In addition to their common presence at sites of hemorrhage, bile pigments are often seen in tissue sections under other circumstances. They may normally be observed in the bile ducts and gallbladder as bright orange–yellow, amorphous masses. In obstructive jaundice, bile pigments may be observed within bile canaliculi, Kupffer cells, hepatocytes, and occasionally in the epithelial cells of proximal convoluted tubules and portions of the loops of Henle in the kidney.

Hyperbilirubinemia (Icterus, Jaundice). The formation of bilirubin from the hemoglobin released from destroyed erythrocytes and its normal course to the liver have been referred to earlier; however, prior to considering icterus, it is well to examine these events more closely. In the breakdown of hemoglobin in the reticuloendothelial system, the cyclic structure of the iron-porphyrin compound (heme) is opened, and the iron is removed and reutilized by the body, as is the globin. The open-chained porphyrin is converted to a green pigment called **biliverdin**. Biliverdin is then reduced by biliverdin reductase to **bilirubin**, an orange-yellow pigment. Bound to albumin, bilirubin is then transported from the reticuloendothelial cell by way of the blood to the liver. In the hepatocyte, the pigment is separated from albumin and conjugated with glucuronic acid, and excreted in the bile as **bilirubin-diglucuronide**. The enzyme involved at this point is uridine diphosphoglucose glucuronyl transferase. The conjugated bilirubin in the intestine is reduced by bacteria to **urobilinogen** (mesobilirubinogen and stercobilinogen). Some urobilinogen is reabsorbed into the portal circulation and carried to the liver (enterohepatic circulation), where most of it is converted to a bilirubin-like compound and re-excreted into the bile. A small amount of the absorbed urobilinogen enters the general circulation and is excreted in the urine. The urobilinogen that is not reabsorbed from the intestine is oxidized in the lower intestine to **urobilin** and **stercobilin**, which are normal pigments of feces.

Three pigments in this scheme are of primary importance to the diagnosis of icterus: (1) bilirubin-diglucuronide, which is also called **conjugated bilirubin** or **direct-reacting bilirubin** (direct reaction to the Van den Bergh test) and cholebilirubin; (2) **nonconjugated bilirubin**, which is also called **indirect-reacting bilirubin** (indirect reaction to the Van den Bergh test), bilirubin, and hemobilirubin; and (3) urobilinogen.

Gross and Microscopic Appearance. Icterus is an important disorder clinically and postmortem in which bilirubin reaches such a high concentration in the circulating blood that the tissues of the whole body are tinged with yellow. Since yellow is a weaker color than red, one must look for it where the tissues normally are white or pale, such as the sclera of the eye, the omentum, and mesentery. In considering the color of adipose tissue as a basis for diagnosis, one must keep in mind the natural color of fat in the particular species and breed. The fat of horses, Jersey and Guernsey cattle, and certain nonhuman primates is normally yellow. Mucous membranes and other tissues normally reddish may display a yellowish tinge if the icterus is severe. Since the bilirubin is in solution and not sufficiently concentrated to form a visible precipitate upon dehydration, icterus is seen only *grossly*. However, when the amount of bile pigment (bilirubin) in the circulating blood is large, it is sometimes revealed in microscopic sections of the kidney by a brownish precipitate or bile-stained albumin in the lumens of the tubules and by a brownish tinge in the ordinarily pink-staining (hematoxylin and eosin) cytoplasm of the epithelial lining cells. If the icterus is of the obstructive type, microscopic sections of the liver may also reveal its presence by accumulations of bile pigment in the bile canaliculi and ducts.

Causes. Depending on the causative mechanism, icterus, or jaundice, is divided into three types: hemolytic, toxic, and obstructive.

Hemolytic jaundice is the result of excessive hemolysis of erythrocytes, ordinarily in the circulating blood. The more important diseased conditions in which this type of icterus is pronounced are piroplasmosis, anaplasmosis, leptospirosis (partially hemolytic), and equine infectious anemia. A similar destruction of erythrocytes occurs in infections by hemolytic streptococci, *Clostridium hemolyticum bovis,* and *Bacillus anthracis,* but in these cases other aspects of the disease usually overshadow the jaundice. Indeed, these bacterial infections may progress so rapidly that the patient does not survive the two or three days usually necessary for the development of icterus. Ricin, saponin, and possibly other plant poisons, potassium or sodium chlorate, pyrogallic acid, nitrobenzene, and lead (if chronically ingested) are hemolytic poisons that may or may not produce visible icterus. Most snake venoms owe much of their lethal potency to their hemolytic action, so that icterus is frequent after the lapse of a few days. Massive internal, usually intraperitoneal, hemorrhages result in icterus because of absorption of bilirubin from the disintegrating erythrocytes of the escaped blood. Icterus neonatorum is a form of hemolytic jaundice; it is discussed in connection with hemolytic anemia. Congenital hyperbilirubinemia, inherited as a single recessive gene in the Gunn rat, results in icterus and kernicterus. The basic enzyme defect is the virtual absence of uridine diphosphoglucose (UDP) glucuronyl transferase, which results in the accumulation of unconjugated bilirubin in the blood.

Toxic jaundice is caused by toxic substances acting upon the cells of the liver and producing hydropic degeneration, fatty change, and necrosis. Jaundice can result from these destructive changes in the liver in two ways. First, the hepatic cells may be damaged to such an extent that they cannot perform their excretory function. Hemobilirubin (unconjugated bilirubin) then remains in the blood, just as in hemolytic jaundice. Secondly, the swelling of the hepatic cells may be sufficient to block the bile canaliculi. The bile is excreted from the cell, but cannot pursue its course to the gallbladder and intestine. In this case, bilirubin-diglucuronide, or posthepatic bilirubin, accumulates in the liver, from whence it is reabsorbed into the blood. As a rule, both these processes go on simultaneously, so that both kinds of bilirubin accumulate in the blood.

The causes of this hepatic damage are, in general, those that cause acute toxic hepatitis. They include hepatic toxins developed in the course of certain infections and extraneous poisons. Outstanding in veterinary medicine are poisonings by lupines and vetches, by plants of the genus *Senecio* (ragwort, groundsel), the genus *Amsinckia* (tarweed), and others. Several inorganic poisons are capable of causing jaundice, but chronic copper poisoning is the one most often reported as actually being accompanied by icterus. Numerous infectious diseases are accompanied by severe hepatic injury, but leptospirosis is outstanding in its ability to produce toxic (as well as hemolytic) icterus.

Obstructive jaundice results from obstruction to the normal flow of bile. Retained anywhere in the biliary passageways, much of the bile is reabsorbed into the blood. (Some of it becomes dehydrated and is precipitated in the tissue as bile pigment.) The obstruction may be caused by (1) blocking of the bile canaliculi by swollen hepatic cells, (2) obstruction of the ducts, either inside or outside the liver by flukes, fimbriated tapeworms (*Thysanosoma actinioides*), or ascarids, (3) pressure on the intrahepatic ducts by the contracting fibrous tissue of biliary cirrhosis, (4) cholangitis, with swelling of the walls of the ducts, (5) gall stones, (6) pressure on any part of the ductal system by neoplasms, granulomas, or abscesses, or (7) pressure of inflammatory swelling on the slanting orifice of the bile duct as it enters the duodenum at the papilla duodeni in duodenitis. The acute angle at which the duct passes through the duodenal wall subjects it to easy closure by the compression of inflammatory swelling.

Diagnosis of Icterus. In mild cases, the clinical discoloration may not be unequivocal; therefore, laboratory tests are often employed to establish the diagnosis of jaundice with certainty. The **icterus index** is determined merely by comparing in a colorimeter the color of the blood serum with the yellow tint of a solution of potassium dichromate of standard strength. The **Van den Bergh reaction** depends on the addition of sulfanilic acid and sodium nitrite to the serum, and the change in color is a quantitative indication of the presence of bilirubin-diglucuronide. This is the **direct** Van den Bergh reaction. If alcohol is added to the mixture, hemobilirubin also reacts, constituting the **indirect** Van den Bergh reaction. Thus, hemolytic jaundice gives the indirect reaction and obstructive jaundice, the direct reaction, a valuable aid in differentiation. Toxic jaundice usually gives both direct and indirect reactions.

When the bile reaches the intestinal lumen, bacteria change it by chemical reduction into a substance called urobilinogen. Much of the urobilinogen is reabsorbed into the portal blood to be carried to the liver, which normally returns it to the bile, but when the hepatic cells have suffered the types of injury that accompany toxic hepatitis, the urobilinogen is imperfectly removed from the blood and remains to be excreted by the kidneys. Furthermore, the capacity of the liver to eliminate urobilinogen, as has also been pointed out with respect to bilirubin, is by no means unlimited. One can understand, then, that in hemolytic jaundice large amounts of urobilinogen are found in the feces and in the urine, for the amount of cholebilirubin originally excreted is maximal, contributing much urobilinogen to the feces, and the considerable excess above what the liver can decompose goes into the urine. In toxic jaundice, the amount in the urine is considerable, varying with the relative ability of the liver to excrete bilirubin and to decompose the resorbed urobilinogen. In obstructive jaundice, the amount of urobilinogen in the feces and in the urine is diminished, perhaps to zero. The actual test is usually made upon the urine, but the feces can also be tested.

It is also common practice to perform certain simple tests for bilirubin (bile) in the urine, the presence of which is called choluria. Since the kidneys are able to excrete bilirubin-diglucuronide but not hemobilirubin, it is obvious that the urine is acholuric in hemolytic icterus, but contains much bilirubin in obstructive jaundice. Because of its dual causative mechanism, toxic jaundice again falls between the two extremes, but some choluria is usually found.

Summarizing, we find that a high icterus index shows the presence of icterus. A positive direct Van den Bergh reaction indicates obstructive jaundice or, at least, the presence of bilirubin-diglucuronide, which may result from toxic jaundice as well as the obstructive type. A positive indirect Van den Bergh test shows the presence of hemobilirubin, which signifies either hemolytic jaundice or toxic jaundice with inability of the hepatic cells to function. With respect to urobilinogen in the urine, a certain amount is normal; smaller amounts or its absence indicate obstructive jaundice (no bile reaching the intestine); large amounts indicate hemolytic icterus with a normal degree of hepatic secretion or, in the absence of hemolytic disease, toxic jaundice with an impairment of the excretory function of the liver. With respect to the mere presence or absence of urinary

bilirubin, obstructive icterus is choluric, hemolytic icterus is acholuric.

Other laboratory tests are available for determining the degree of icterus, as well as general hepatic functions. Of course, if hemoglobinuria accompanies the icterus, it is practically safe to make a diagnosis of the hemolytic type.

Significance. From the foregoing, it becomes evident that jaundice is an important clue to any one of several different disorders. To profit by its existence, the diagnostician needs to have keen observation for its clinical appearance, access to the applicable laboratory tests, and a clear understanding of its pathogenic mechanisms. The bilirubin itself ordinarily is not a seriously harmful substance, although it may well be directly responsible for some subjective symptoms that humans feel, such as itching. It possibly contributes to the development of necrosis in the renal epithelium in the poorly understood "hepatorenal" syndrome. The most noteworthy harmful effect of bilirubin per se is seen in newborn animals and infants with kernicterus. In this disorder, most often associated with erythroblastosis fetalis, the hippocampus, basal nuclei, midbrain, medulla, and floor of the fourth ventricle are grossly yellow, and there is microscopic evidence of neuronal degeneration. Although the accumulation of bilirubin to high levels in blood and tissues does not appear particularly harmful in the adult human or animal, it does seriously affect the developing neonatal brain. One example in which kernicterus develops as a natural disease in animals is the congenital hyperbilirubinemia that is hereditary in the Gunn strain of rats. If the cause can be overcome, the accumulated bilirubin promptly disappears.

Arias, I. M.: Inheritable and congenital hyperbilirubinemia. Models for the study of drug metabolism. N. Engl. J. Med., 285:1416–1421, 1971.

Butcher, R. E., Vorhees, C. V., Kindt, C. W., and Keenan, W. J.: An experimental evaluation of phototherapy for hyperbilirubinemia in the Gunn rat. Am. J. Dis. Child., 123:575–578, 1972.

Campbell, C. B., et al.: The use of Rhesus monkeys to study biliary secretion with an intact enterohepatic circulation. Aust. N. Z. J. Med., 2:49–56, 1972.

Cornelius, C. E.: Dubin-Johnson syndrome. Comp. Pathol. Bull., 2:2, 1970.

Cornelius, C. E., and Arias, I. M.: Crigler-Najjar syndrome— animal model: hereditary nonhemolytic unconjugated hyperbilirubinemia in Gunn rats. Am. J. Pathol., 69:366–371, 1972.

Dowling, R. H., Mack, E., and Small, D. M.: Biliary lipid secretion and bile composition after acute and chronic interruption of the enterohepatic circulation in the Rhesus monkey. IV. Primate biliary physiology. J. Clin. Invest., 50:1917–1926, 1971.

Ford, E. J. H., and Gopinath, C.: The excretion of phylloerythrin and bilirubin by the horse. Res. Vet. Sci., 16:186–198, 1974.

Johnson, L., Sarmiento, F., and Blanc, W. A.: Kernicterus in rats with an inherited deficiency of glucuronyl transferase. Am. J. Dis. Child., 97:591–608, 1959.

Lester, R., and Schmid, R.: Bilirubin metabolism. N. Engl. J. Med., 270:779–786, 1964.

Quin, J. I.: The effect of surgical obstruction of the normal bile flow. Onderstepoort. J. Vet. Sci. Anim. Ind., 1:505–526, 1933.

Sawasaki, Y., Yamada, N., and Nakajima, H.: Studies on kernicterus. I. Gunn rat: An animal model of human kernicterus with marked cerebellar hypoplasia. Proc. Jpn. Acad., 49:840–845, 1973.

Schaffner, F., et al.: Mechanisms of cholestasis. VII. α-Naphthylisothiocyanate-induced jaundice. Lab. Invest., 28:321–331, 1973.

Schutta, H. S., and Johnson, L.: Electron microscopic observations on acute bilirubin encephalopathy in Gunn rats induced by sulfadimethoxine. Lab. Invest., 24:82–89, 1971.

Sherwood, L. M., and Parris, E. E.: Inheritable and congenital hyperbilirubinemia. N. Engl. J. Med., 285:1416–1421, 1971.

Shimada, K., Bricknell, K. S., and Finegold, S. M.: Deconjugation of bile acids by intestinal bacteria. Review of literature and additional studies. J. Infect. Dis., 119:273–281, 1969.

Snell, A. M.: Fundamentals in the diagnosis of jaundice. J. A. M. A., 138:274–279, 1948.

Yearly, R. A., and Grothaus, R. H.: The Gunn rat as an animal model in comparative medicine. Lab. Anim. Sci., 21:362–366, 1971.

Porphyrins, Photosensitizing Pigments: Photosensitization

Historically speaking, the condition known as photosensitization or, perhaps better, as photosensitizational dermatitis, has been recognized in farm animals for some time, especially but by no means exclusively in cattle and sheep. The clinical manifestations, appearing a number of hours after exposure to strong sunlight, include burning or itching sensations, erythema, and inflammatory edema, which is often extensive—in other words, the "rubor et tumor cum calore et dolore" that were recounted as the signs of inflammation nearly two thousand years ago. Often the inflammation is so severe that the skin is killed and the necrotic layer sloughs in a few days. These changes are strictly, and often sharply, limited to areas of the body surface that are in a position to receive the direct rays of strong light, and are unprotected by pigmentation of a dark skin or a thick coat of hair (or, of course, a blanket or a saddle). In cows the thinly haired and usually unpigmented teats, udder, and escutcheon are included. In sheep, the head and ears are the most vulnerable areas, and the edema is likely to be the most prominent inflammatory change, leading to the colloquial term **bighead**, or **geeldikkop**, which is a South African term meaning thick, yellow head. In New Zealand, an equivalent term is **facial eczema**. The ears in these sheep are so swollen that they bend downward; the face is deformed and the mandibular area is so distended and bulging with edematous fluid as to require differentiation from the noninflammatory "bottle-jaw" that is traditional in gastrointestinal helminthiasis. The cutaneous lesions usually heal after days or weeks, depending on the degree of severity, but shock and generally disturbed body functions have often been discernible at the beginning, and death is an occasional termination due to infection and gangrenous change in the raw, ulcerated areas where the skin is lost.

The lesion of photosensitization has nothing to do with sunburn, which is less severe. Photosensitization of the tissues is the result of the action of light upon some fluorescent pigment that has accumulated in them. A fluorescent pigment is one that

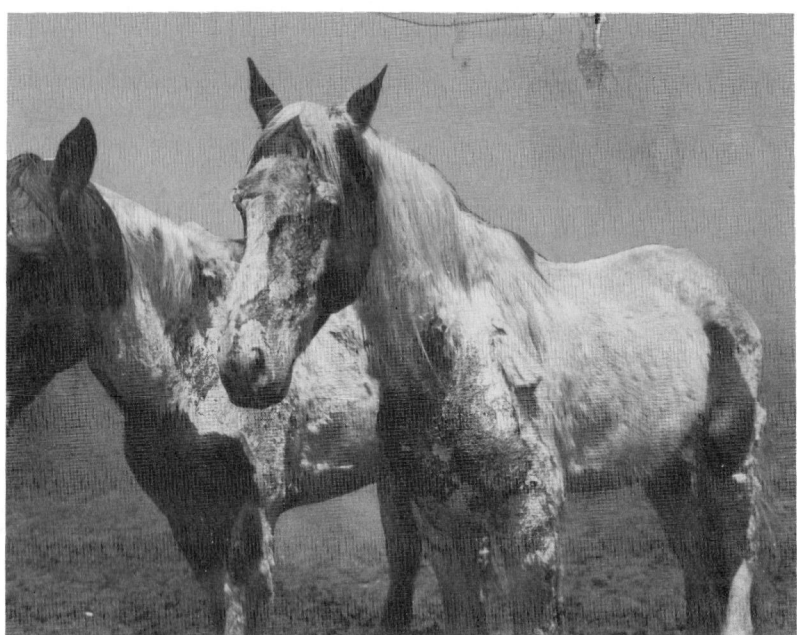

Fig. 3–13.   Photosensitization of skin of horses. Note that the lesions are in the white skin and not in the black areas of these spotted horses. From Bulletin 412 A Colorado State University, Poisonous and Injurious Plants in Colorado, 1950, by L. W. Durrell, Rue Jensen and Bruno Klinger. (Courtesy of Dr. Rue Jensen.)

accepts the incoming rays of light and transforms them into light of a longer wavelength (the process of fluorescence). Often the resulting color is red, since this is the color of the longest wavelength; doubtless some of the resulting energy is in the infrared portion of the spectrum. Experimentally, fluorescein, a dye noted for its fluorescent properties, can be injected into the blood and produce a certain photosensitization of the skin. In nature, the fluorescent, sensitizing pigments appear under three different and unrelated sets of circumstances, but the pigments, as far as they have been studied chemically, are relatives of hemoglobin and chlorophyll, being porphyrins or the related phylloerythrin, a degradation product of chlorophyll. Both chlorophyll and hemoglobin molecules have as their basic components four pyrrole radicals, tied together by methene groups (the basic structure of porphyrin). It is of philosophic interest that these, the principal pigments of the plant and animal kingdoms, are so nearly identical.

The three sets of circumstances which give rise to the presence of photosensitizing pigments in the tissues are **congenital porphyria**, in which there is a metabolic defect in porphyrin metabolism; **hepatotoxic photosentitization**, in which there is interference with the excretion of phylloerythrin; and **primary photosensitization,** in which preformed photosensitizing pigments are ingested, absorbed, and enter the general circulation. In none of these conditions is the pigment seen in usual microscopic preparations. In porphyria the pigment is grossly visible. In certain rodents (mice, rats, hamsters), the Harderian gland, an intraorbital lacrimal gland, normally secretes porphyrin, which accounts for the red or brown tears seen in these animals. The pigment can be seen in the Harderian gland microscopically as variably sized yellow to reddish granules.

Congenital Porphyria. Congenital porphyria has been described in cattle, swine, and cats as a metabolic defect in the synthesis of the normal heme pigment, ferroprotoporphyrin. The principal enzymatic defects in various types of porphyria in man and animals are still under study. One enzymatic defect in man and cattle is probably a partial deficiency of uroporphyrinogen III cosynthetase. This enzyme deficiency results in the overproduction of porphyrins of the type I series, which accumulate in the tissues (Romeo et al., 1970). The dominant forms of human hereditary porphyria (intermittent acute porphyria, hereditary coproporphyria, and variegate porphyria) appear to be based upon increased activity of hepatic δ-amino-levulinic acid synthetase (Meyer and Schmid, 1973). In cattle, the disease is believed to be inherited as a simple mendelian recessive, whereas in swine and cats, it is believed to be inherited as a dominant characteristic.

In cattle, the accumulation of porphyrins results in photosensitizational dermatitis when exposed to strong sunlight. Interestingly, photosensitizational dermatitis has not been reported in swine, even when white, or cats with congenital porphyria. The accumulation of porphyrins in dentine and bone gives rise to a red color, which has often gone by the misnomer, "osteohemochromatosis," or by the colorful term, "pink tooth." Affected bones and teeth elicit a strong reddish fluorescence with ultraviolet light, a useful aid to clinical and postmortem diagnosis. Because of increased excretion of porphyrin (porphyrinuria) in the urine, it is reddish brown, or at least tends to develop this color upon standing for a varying period from 10 minutes to 24 hours. This change must be differentiated from hemoglobinuria and myoglobinuria, and possibly from alkaptonuria (reported in man, one chimpanzee, and one orangutan). Fluorescence with ultraviolet light is one distinguishing feature. Discoloration of soft tissues due to the accumulation of porphy-

rin is less obvious, but may be encountered in the lungs or kidneys, which also fluoresce. Fluorescence can also be demonstrated in unstained tissue sections as well as in blood smears in which the erythrocytes fluoresce.

Except for its photosensitizing effect, this disorder is clinically harmless, as shown by Fourie (1953), who described an ox, imported to South Africa from Switzerland, which reached the ripe old age of 18 years while excreting 1.6 gm of porphyrin daily, and remaining in good health as long as he was stabled during the day. Exposed to sunlight, he promptly developed the usual lesions of photosensitization. At necropsy, the animal's teeth and bones were brown, and there was pigment in various internal organs.

Anemia has been reported in cattle and cats with porphyria, apparently resulting from inability to produce normal amounts of hemoglobin and a shortened life span of the erythrocyte.

Other forms of porphyria with varying clinical manifestations occur in humans. The interested student is referred to the chapter by Schmid (1966).

Clare, N. T., and Stephens, E. H.: Congenital porphyria in pigs. Nature, 153:252–253, 1944.

Cornelius, C. E., and Gronwall, R. R.: Congenital photosensitivity and hyperbilirubinemia in Southdown sheep in the United States. Am. J. Vet. Res., 29:291–295, 1968.

Flygers, V., and Levin, E. Y.: Animal model of human disease: Congenital erythropoietic porphyria. Am. J. Pathol., 87:269–272, 1977.

Fourie, P. J. J.: The occurrence of congenital porphyrinuria (pink tooth) in cattle in South Africa (Swaziland). Onderstepoort J. Vet. Sci., 7:535–566, 1936.

Fourie, P. J. J.: Does bovine congenital porphyrinuria (pink tooth) produce clinical disturbances in an animal which is protected against the sun? Onderstepoort J. Vet. Sci., 26:231–233, 1953.

Giddens, W. E., Labbe, R. F., Swango, L. J., and Padgett, G. A.: Feline congenital erythropoietic porphyria associated with severe anemia and renal disease. Am. J. Pathol., 80:367–386, 1975.

Glenn, B. L., Monlux, A. W., and Panciera, R. J.: A hepatogenous photosensitivity disease of cattle: I. Experimental production and clinical aspects of the disease. Pathol. Vet., 1:469–484, 1964.

Glenn, B. L., Panciera, R. J., and Monlux, A. W.: A

hepatogenous photosensitivity disease of cattle: II. Histopathology and pathogenesis of the hepatic lesions. Pathol. Vet., 2:49–57, 1965.

Glenn, B. L., Glenn, H. G., and Omtvedt, I. T.: Congenital porphyria in the domestic cat *(Felis catus)*: preliminary investigations on inheritance pattern. Am. J. Vet. Res., 29:1653–1657, 1968.

Glenn, B. L.: Feline porphyria. Comp. Pathol. Bull., 11 (No. 2), 1970.

Hancock, J.: Congenital photosensitivity in Southdown sheep. Proc. Ruakura NZ Farmers Conf. Week, 1949. Abstract, Vet. Bull. No. 3385:85, 1951.

Haydon, M.: Inherited congenital porphyria in calves. Can. Vet. J., 16:118–120, 1975.

Joergensen, S. K.: Congenital porphyria in pigs. Br. Vet. J., 115:160–175, 1959.

Johnson, L. W., and Schwartz, S.: Isotropic studies of erythrocyte survival in normal and porphyric cattle: Influence of light exposure, blood withdrawal and splenectomy. Am. J. Vet. Res., 31:2167–2178, 1970.

Kaneko, J. J.: Erythrokinetics and iron metabolism in bovine porphyria erythropoietica. Ann. NY Acad. Sci., 104:689–700, 1963.

Kaneko, J. J., Zinkl, J. G., and Keeton, K. S.: Erythrocyte porphyrin and erythrocyte survival in bovine erythropoietic porphyria. Am. J. Vet. Res., 32:1981–1986, 1971.

Meyer, U. A., and Schmid, R.: Hereditary hepatic porphyrias. Fed. Proc., 32:1649–1655, 1973.

Moore, W. E.: Metabolic acidosis in bovine erythropoietic porphyria during the neonatal period. Am. J. Vet. Res., 31:1561–1567, 1970.

Nestel, B. L.: Bovine congenital porphyria (pink tooth) with a note on five cases observed in Jamaica. Cornell Vet., 48:430–439, 1958.

Owen, L. N., Stevenson, D. E., and Keilin, J.: Abnormal pigmentation and fluorescence in canine teeth. Res. Vet. Sci., 3:139–146, 1962.

Rimington, C.: Some cases of congenital porphyrinuria in cattle: Chemical studies upon the living animals and post-mortem material. Onderstepoort J. Vet. Sci., 7:567–609, 1936.

Roe, D. A., Krook, L., and Wilkie, B. N.: Hepatic porphyria in weaning pigs. J. Invest. Dermatol., 54:53–64, 1970.

Romeo, G., Glenn, B. L., and Levin, E. Y.: Uroporphyrinogen III Cosynthetase in asymptomatic carriers of congenital erythropoietic porphyria. Biochem. Genet., 4:719–726, 1970.

Rudolph, W. G., and Kaneko, J. J.: Kinetics of erythroid bone marrow cells of normal and porphyric calves in vitro. Acta Haematol. (Basel), 45:330–335, 1971.

Schmid, R.: The porphyrias. In The Metabolic Basis of Inherited Disease, edited by J. B. Stanbury and J. B. Wyngaarden. 2nd ed. New York, McGraw-Hill Book Co., 1966.

Tobias, G.: Congenital porphyria in a cat. J. Am. Vet. Med. Assoc., 145:462–463, 1964.

Wass, W. M., and Hoyt, H. H.: Bovine congenital porphyria: studies on heredity; hematologic studies, including porphyrin analyses. Am. J. Vet. Res., 26:654–658, 1965.

Hepatogenous Photosensitization. The great majority of photosensitizations in animals are not of hemoglobinogenous origin, but are due to a derivative of the plant kingdom's counterpart of hemoglobin, namely chlorophyll. Furthermore, they depend upon toxic injury to the liver. When the chlorophyll of plants passes through the digestive process, one of the products is the pigment **phylloerythrin**. It differs from phylloporphyrin in having a ketone group attached to the sixth carbon atom, but for practical purposes can be classed with the porphyrins. Normally, this phylloerythrin, with its photosensitizing properties, is eliminated through the liver by the simple expedient of excreting it through the bile (where its brownish color joins that of bilirubin, that not-so-different derivative of the animal kingdom's hemoglobin). When the liver or its ductal system is injured in a way that interrupts this excretory function, the phylloerythrin, with its photosensitizing properties, reaches the skin by way of the circulating blood, and the results are the same as those from the presence of (hemoglobinogenous) porphyrin.

There is usually no specific morphologic pattern of liver injury, although the changes described for acute toxic hepatitis are usually in evidence. Often, but not invariably, toxic icterus is an easily recognized part of the general illness, and occasionally there are nervous disturbances and other signs of hepatic malfunction. In two forms of hepatogenous photosensitization, more specific hepatic lesions are seen. In "facial eczema" of sheep and alfalfa-associated photosensitization, there is a pericholangitis, which leads to occlusion of small bile ducts.

The causes of photosensitizing hepatitis are, in general, among those listed for acute toxic hepatitis, but it must be emphasized that only a small minority of toxic hepatic illnesses are accompanied by photosensitization. There may be several reasons for this, but the outstanding one is that the animal must be on a diet containing liberal amounts of chlorophyll (usually green pasture). Clare (1952), in his admirable monograph on photosensitization, listed the following agents as causing poisoning accompanied by photosensitization and by hepatic dysfunction and icterus: *Tribulus terrestris*, plants grown for forage in parts of South Africa, causing geeldikkop, also known as "thick yellow head," "thick ear," and geelsiekte; a mycotoxin from the fungus, *Pithomyces chartarum*, growing on perennial ryegrass and other pastures, causing facial eczema of sheep in New Zealand; *Lippia rehmanni*, a South African plant; *Lantana camara*, a verbena-like plant that occurs in the United States as well as in South Africa and Ceylon; sacahuiste (*Nolina texana*), found in western Texas; lechuguilla (*Agave lechugilla*), also a native of western Texas and nearby arid areas; second growth from stumps of the Brazilian tree called alecrim (*Holocalyx glaziovii*); panick grasses (*Panicum miliaceum et sp.*) in Australia and South Africa; leaves of the ngaio tree of New Zealand (*Myosporum laetum*), which affects horses as well as ruminants; the Australian grass *Brachiaria brizantha*; the American morenita (*Kochia scoparia*); *Tetradymia glabrata*, known as "coal-oil brush" in Utah and as "spring rabbit brush" in Nevada, and *Tetradymia canescens*, the "spineless horse-brush" of Utah; *Microcystis flos-aquae*, a blue-green alga that grows as a scum on lakes; the plant *Northecium ossifragum*, which causes the Norwegian disease of lambs called "alveld;" and *Kochia scoparia*, to which "black fever" is attributed. Other plants include the seeds of *Stryphnodendron obovatum*, *Erodium circutorium*, and Bermuda grass. A similar disorder is "yellowses," a disease of lambs in Scotland of uncertain cause.

Several of the above plants are discussed as to their general toxic aspects in Chapter 16. Some other plants, valuable as pasture or cured forage, have also been incriminated or suspected in outbreaks of photosensitizational dermatitis, among them some of the trefoils and bur clovers (*Medicago sp.*), Alsike or Swedish clover (*Trifolium hybridum*), as well as some plants of the cabbage family (rape, *Brassica rapa*, and kale, *Medicago denticulata*), not to mention the common perennial ryegrass, which forms so many of our winter pastures. Outbreaks of photosensitization occur at highly variable periods, often seasonal, and various explanations have been offered. Investigators in New Zealand have discovered that under certain conditions of growth, temperature, and humidity, fields producing these forages became heavily infested with a fungus known either as *Sporodesmium bakeri* or *Pithomyces chartarum*. The fungal growth, when first noticed, was so heavy that mowing machines were blackened by its dark spores. It was demonstrated in these cases that mycotoxin was really the toxic substance responsible for the photosensitization, rather than the plants themselves. A similar mechanism has been suggested for a photosensitizational dermatitis associated with Bermuda grass in the southern United States and also for a hepatogenous photosensitivity caused by feeding flood-damaged alfalfa. Further investigation is needed to determine to what extent an analogous situation may prevail with other plants. Numerous other plants have been suspected of causing photosensitization when eaten by livestock. A listing of these is included in the report by Aplin (1976).

In addition to these causes, there have occurred cases of photosensitization accompanied by toxic hepatic injury and icterus in cattle treated with phenanthridinium, a trypanocidal drug. Carbon tetrachloride poisoning, hepatic fascioliasis (liver flukes), and Rift Valley fever can also lead to hepatogenous photosensitization.

A hereditary defect in the hepatic phylloerythrin excretory mechanisms, which leads to photosensitivity, occurs in Southdown sheep. The disease, which is also associated with hyperbilirubinemia, has been described in New Zealand and the United States. No morphologic lesion is present in the liver. A second syndrome has been described in Corriedale sheep similar to the Dubin-Johnson syndrome in man, which is also associated with a failure to excrete phylloerythrin and with photosensitivity.

If further evidence is needed of the role of hepatic dysfunction in the production of photosensitization, it is furnished by the experimental work of Quin (1933), in which he produced photosensitization by ligation of the bile duct (obstructive jaundice) provided that fresh green plants were fed.

Allison, A. C., Magnus, I. A., and Young, M. R.: Role of lysosomes and of cell membranes in photosensitizaton. Nature, 209:874–878, 1966.

Aplin, T. E. H.: Plants in Australia Which When Eaten Produce Photosensitization in Livestock. South Perth Western Australia; Dept. Agr., 13 pp., 1976.

Arias, I., et al.: Black liver disease in Corriedale sheep: A new mutation affecting hepatic excretory function. J. Clin. Invest., 43:1249–1250, 1964.

Bailey, J. M., and Carbeck, R. B.: Porphyria hepatica with primary psychiatric manifestations. USAF Med. J., 9:1346–1350, 1958.

Betty, R. C., and Trikojus, V. M.: Hypericin and a non-fluorescent photosensitive pigment from St. John's Wort (Hypericum perforatum). Aust. J. Exp. Biol. Med. Sci., 21:175–182, 1943.

Blum, H. F.: Photodynamic Action and Diseases Caused by Light. New York, Reinhold Pub. Corp., 1941.

Brown, J. M. M.: Advances in "geeldikkop" (Tribulosis ovis) research. J. S. Afr. Vet. Med. Assoc., 30:97–111, 1959; 31:179–193, 1960.

———: Biochemical lesions in the pathogenesis of "geeldikkop" (Tribulosis ovis) and enzootic icterus in sheep in South Africa. Ann. NY Acad. Sci., 104:504–538, 1963.

Budiarso, I. T., Carlton, W. W., and Tuite, J. F.: Phototoxic syndrome induced in mice by rice cultures of Penicillium viridicatum and exposure to sunlight. Pathol. Vet., 7:531–546, 1970.

Camargo, W.: Photosensitization of cattle by Stryphnodendron obovatum. Biologico, 31:7–11, 1965.

Clare, N. T.: Photosensitivity in Diseases of Domestic Animals. Commonwealth Bureau Animal Health Revue Series, 3, 1952.

———: Photosensitized keratitis in young cattle following the use of phenothiazine as an anthelmintic. II. The metabolism of phenothiazine in ruminants. Aust. Vet. J., 23:340–344, 1947.

———: Photosensitization in animals. Adv. Vet. Sci., 2:182–211, 1955.

Collet, P., and Henry, E.: Photosensibilisation du dindon par le sarrazin. Bull. Soc. Sci. Vét., Lyon 54, 55:437–442, 1952–1953.

Cunningham, I. J., and Hopkirk, C. S. M.: Experimental poisoning of sheep by Ngaio (Myosporum laetum). NZ J. Sci. Tech. Sec. A, 26:333–339, 1945.

Egyed, M. N., Shlosberg, A., and Eilat, A.: The susceptibility of young chickens, ducks, and turkeys to the photosensitizing effect of Ammivisnaga seeds. Avian Dis., 19:830–833, 1975.

Ford, G. E.: Photosensitivity due to Erodium spp. Aust. Vet. J., 41:56, 1965.

Fowler, M. E., Berry, L. J., Bushnell, R., and Hinkley, H. S.: Sphenosciadium capitellatum (whiteheads) (Umbelliferae, Ed) toxicosis of cattle and horses. J. Am. Vet. Med. Assoc., 157:1187–1192, 1970.

Gordon, H. McL., and Green, R. J.: Phenothiazine photosensitization in sheep. Aust. Vet. J., 27:51–52, 1951.

Johnson, A. E.: Experimental photosensitization and toxicity in sheep produced by Tetradymia glabrata. Can. J. Comp. Med., 38:406–410, 1974.

Kellerman, T. S., et al.: Photosensitivity in South Africa. I. A comparative study of Asaemia axillaris (Thunb.) Harv. ex Jackson and Lasiospermum bipinnatum (Thunb.) Druce poisoning in sheep. Onderstepoort J. Vet. Res., 40:115–126, 1973.

Lora, R. P.: Fotosensibilización en ovinos merinos por consumo de Hypericum perforatum L. Bol. Zootec., Cordoba, 9:187–190, 1953.

Mathews, F. P.: Photosensitization and the photodynamic diseases of man and the lower animals. Arch. Pathol., 23:399–429, 1937.

McFarlane, D., Evans, J. V., and Reid, C. S. W.: Photosensitivity diseases in New Zealand. XIV. The pathogenesis of facial eczema. NZ J. Agric. Res., 2:194–200, 1959.

McGavin, M. D., Gronwall, R. R., Cornelius, C. E., and Mia, A. S.: Renal radial fibrosis in mutant Southdown sheep with congenital hyperbilirubinema. Am. J. Pathol., 67:601–612, 1972.

Mia, A. S., Gronwall, R. R., and Cornelius, C. E.: Bilirubin C turnover studies in normal and mutant Southdown sheep with congenital hyperbilirubinemia. Proc. Soc. Exp. Biol. Med., 133:955–959, 1970.

Mia, A. S., Cornelius, C. E., and Gronwall, R. R.: Increased bilirubin production from sources other than circulating erythrocytes in mutant Southdown sheep. Proc. Soc. Exp. Biol. Med., 136:227–230, 1971.

Mia, A. S., Gronwall, R. R., McGavin, M. D., and Cornelius, C. E.: Renal function defect in mutant Southdown sheep with congenital hyperbilirubinemia. Proc. Soc. Exp. Biol. Med., 137:1237–1241, 1971.

Mortimer, P. H.: The experimental intoxication of sheep with sporodesmin, a metabolic product of Pithomyces chartarum. III. Some changes in cellular components and coagulation properties of the blood, in serum proteins and in liver function. Res. Vet. Sci., 3:269–286, 1962.

Moses, C.: Photosensitivity as a cause of falsely positive cephalin-cholesterol flocculation tests. J. Lab. Clin. Med., 30:267–269, 1945.

Quin, J. I.: The effect of surgical obstruction of the normal bile flow. Onderstepoort J. Vet. Sci. Anim. Ind., 1:505–526, 1933.

Rimington, C.: Haems and porphyrins in health and disease. Acta Med. Scand., 143:161–196, 1952.

Rocha, E., and Silva, M.: En torno da etiologia da doença de fotosensibilização produzida pelo Holocalyx glaziovii. Biólogico. São Paulo, 9:187–194, 1943.

Shlosberg, A., Egyed, M. N., and Eilat, A.: The comparative photosensitizing properties of Ammi majus and Ammi visnaga in goslings. Avian Dis., 18:544–550, 1974.

Slater, T. F., and Riley, P. A.: Photosensitization and lysosomal damage. Nature, 209:151–154, 1965.

Synge, R. L. M., and White, E. P.: Photosensitivity diseases in New Zealand. XXIII. Isolation of sporodesmin, a substance causing lesions characteristic of facial eczema from Sporodesmium bakeri, Syd. NZ J. Agri. Res., 3:907–921, 1960.

Thornton, R. H., and Percival, J. C.: A hepatotoxin from Sporidesmium bakeri (Stemphylium botryosum) capable of producing facial eczema diseases in sheep. Nature, 183:63, 1959.

Tonder, E. M. van, Basson, P. A., and Rensburg, I. B. J. van: Geeldikkop: experimental induction by feeding the plant Tribulus terrestris L. (Zygophyllaceae). J. S. Afr. Vet. Assoc., 43:363–375, 1972.

Witzel, D. A., Dollahite, J. W., and Jones, L. P.: Photosensitization in sheep fed Ammi majus (Bishop's Weed) seed. Am. J. Vet. Res., 39:319–322, 1978.

Primary Photosensitization. There are several photosensitizational diseases in which neither hepatic injury, icterus, nor any form of porphyrinemia has been demonstrated. Two of these have long been known and have received considerable study, namely **fagopyrism**, poisoning by buckwheat (*Fagopyrum esculentum*), and **hypericism**, which is poisoning by *Hypericum perforatum* or closely related species. Common names for the *Hypericum* species include St. John's wort, goatweed, Tipton weed, amber, cammock, and Klamath weed. In both fagopyrism and hypericism, a red fluorescent pigment has been obtained from the plant itself and demonstrated in the blood. It appears that this pigment sensitizes the skin in the same way that phylloerythrin and certain other porphyrins do. The effective wavelengths of light in this process are near the middle of the visible spectrum, different from that which produces the hepatogenous type of photosensitization.

The commonly employed anthelmintic **phenothiazine** is also a cause of primary photosensitizational dermatitis. This drug is oxidized in the intestinal tract to phenothiazine sulfoxide, a photosensitive pigment which is usually metabolized by the liver. However, if it escapes the liver and enters the general circulation, dermatitis will develop upon exposure to sunlight. A damaged liver or the liver of young animals is less efficient in eliminating the sulfoxide. In addition to dermatitis, keratitis is a usual finding, owing to the excretion of phenothiazine sulfoxide in the tears and its entry into the aqueous humor. Photosensitization by this drug occurs most readily in swine, but cattle are also susceptible. Sheep are more resistant, apparently due to a greater efficiency of the sheep liver to reduce phenothiazine sulfoxide to phenothiazine sulfate.

A photosensitization of white chickens and ducks has been reported from Uruguay by Cassamagnaghi (1946) due to the seed of the umbelliferous plant, *Ammi visnaga*. Whether this is to be classed with fagopyrism and hypericism or with the hepatogenous photosensitizations has not been determined.

Summarizing, photosensitization as it is most frequently encountered in veterinary medicine involves a triad of hepatotoxic plants, fresh green feed in the diet, and exposure to direct sunlight. Exceptions exist (1) in the form of plants that supply a sensitizing pigment of their own, apparently involving no hepatic injury, (2) in certain animals that form porphyrins in their daily metabolism due to a hereditary metabolic defect, only sunlight being required to produce the characteristic dermatitis; and (3) certain drugs that have a direct photosensitizing effect.

Cassamagnaghi, A.: Accidentes de fotosensibilización de origen alimentico en los animales demésticos. An. Fac. de vet. Montevideo, 4:541–549, 1946.

Jha, G. J., and Iyer, P. K. R.: Pathology of photosensitization caused by experimental phenothiazine intoxication in cattle and sheep. Indian Vet. J., 43:1078–1084, 1966.

Kirksen, G., and Tammen, C.: Keratitis in young cattle resulting from photosensitization after prolonged medication. Dtsch. Tierarztl. Wochenschr., 71:545–548, 1964.

Kitsikis, A., Dimov, S., and Dubouch, P.: Study of the photosensitivity of *Papio anubis, Papio cynocephalus* and of their cross-mating. Electroencephalogr. Clin. Neurophysiol., 29:102, 1970.

Lapras, M., Mallein, R., and Touzin, J.: Photosensitization in a dog (chronic solar dermatitis). Study of the role of porphyrins. Rev. Med. Vet., 123:45–59, 1972.

Pace, N.: The etiology of hypericism, a photosensitivity produced by St. Johnswort. Am. J. Physiol., 136:650–656, 1942.

Serbanescu, T., and Balzamo, E.: The influence of thyrozine in photosensitive baboons, *Papio papio*. Electroencephalogr. Clin. Neurophysiol., 36:253–258, 1974.

Wender, S. H.: Action of photosensitizing agents isolated from buckwheat. Am. J. Vet. Res., 7:486–489, 1946.

Lipogenic Pigments

Lipogenic pigments constitute a group of colored substances derived mainly or partly from lipids. They are not the same as the lipochrome or carotenoid pigments. Numerous tissue pigments have been classified as lipogenic pigments, and the list of names designated to them is exhaustive, despite the fact that their individuality is not established.

Two pigments from the group are encountered with frequency or are of special pathologic significance. These are tissue lipofuscin and ceroid.

Lipofuscin

Synonyms include wear-and-tear pigment, the German abnutzen pigment, hemofuscin, pigment of brown atrophy, and lipochrome. The multiplicity of synonyms suggests the confusion that exists with respect to this pigment. The name lipofuscin (*lipo*, Greek for fat, and *fuscus*, Latin for dusky or dark) was introduced by Borst (1922). Lipofuscin in one view is believed to represent a homogeneous group of pigments that are derived from the oxidation of unsaturated tissue lipids or lipoproteins. Lipofuscin occurs in a variety of tissues and cell types, including the heart, skeletal muscle, liver, adrenal gland, neurons, thyroid, parathyroid, kidney, ovary, and testicle, and is referred to by the organ or tissue containing it, i.e., cardiac lipofuscin, hepatic lipofuscin. Lipofuscin is resistant to fat solvents and is sudanophilic (i.e., stains with fat stains), even after paraffin embedding procedures. It is usually acid-fast, but negative to iron stains.

Lipofuscin may occur in great quantity in organs undergoing cachectic or senile atrophy, imparting a brown color to them, constituting the pathologic entity known as **brown atrophy**. However, lipofuscin may be seen in tissues from animals that are not cachectic or aged, necessitating caution in interpreting its significance.

Neuronal lipofuscin has received particular attention because of a possible (however disputed) relation to aging in man and other species. It has been held that accumulation of lipofuscin in a neuron eventually interferes with its function and finally results in its destruction. This view is also contested, but it is established that in cases of one rare inherited disease, pigment does accummulate excessively and produces neurologic deficit and death. This disease, **neuronal ceroid-lipofuscinosis** was discussed in Chapter 2. The use of this name underlines the problem in distinguishing between ceroid and lipofuscin.

Microscopic Appearance. The pigment takes the form of minute yellowish or darker brown granules. In heart muscle cells, it is located chiefly near the poles of the nucleus; in skeletal muscle, it is found in any part of the fiber; and in most parenchymatous organs, such as the liver or adrenal gland, it is distributed throughout the cytoplasm. In neurons, lipofuscin granules are seen in the cytoplasm forming a diffuse halo around the nucleus, clustered at one side of the nucleus, or aggregated at one or both poles of the nucleus in a polar or bipolar configuration.

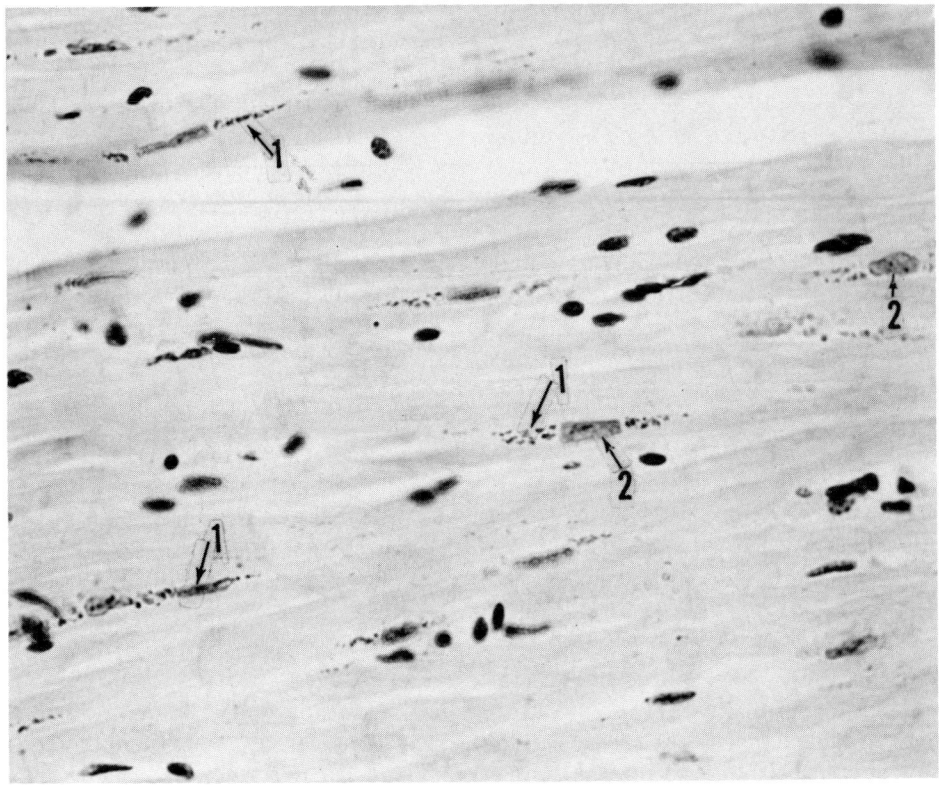

Fig. 3–14. Pigment of "brown atrophy" in a bovine heart. Granules of lipofuscin (*1*) in cardiac muscle cells at poles of nuclei (*2*). (× 440.) (Courtesy of Armed Forces Institute of Pathology.) Contributor: Barnes General Hospital.

Ultrastructure. Neuronal lipofuscin is osmiophilic, but also is demonstrable following potassium permanganate and potassium bichromate fixation. The forms of the granules, in order of frequency, are described by Hasan and Glees (1972) as follows: (1) homogeneous or uniformly electron-dense, (2) finely granular, (3) vacuolated, (4) lamellated or banded, (5) coarse granular, or (6) compound or heterogeneous (combinations of types). A single membrane has been demonstrated partially surrounding some of the granules. Electron-lucid areas, sometimes called vacuoles, are common, particularly in older animals, and may be visualized also by the freeze-etching technique. Aggregation of lipofuscin bodies is some-

times observed, resulting in larger granular masses.

Gross Appearance. If present in significant quantity, lipofuscin may impart a brownish tinge to cardiac and skeletal muscle.

Significance. The significance of lipofuscin cannot always be established, but it often points to some wasting disease, senility, or emaciation. The old dairy cows that display the pigment in their skeletal musculature are usually those that go to slaughter when their usefulness as milk-producers is at an end, the condition being found by the veterinary meat inspector. These animals are always more or less emaciated, and the brownish discoloration is one of the grounds for condemning them as cachectic. The relationship to ageing in various species has been discussed.

Unclassified Lipofuscins. A blackish pigment is frequently seen grossly and microscopically in bovine lymph nodes, chiefly but not exclusively in the thoracic, mesenteric, and supramammary nodes. Von Wyler (1952) has shown that it is limited to the medulla of the nodes, is minutely granular, intracellular (reticuloendothelial cells) or extracellular, and has histochemical properties and reactions that appear to place it with the "lipofuscins." While it increases with the age of the animal, being absent in calves, it can hardly be considered pathologic, since it is commonly encountered in perfectly healthy cattle at meat inspection.

Apparently limited to certain regions of Australia, a diffuse, blackish pigmentation of the livers of sheep has been called melanosis. Almost 100% of the sheep show the pigment, beginning a few weeks after being brought into the given area. There is a strong suspicion that it results from consumption, perhaps only at certain seasons, of foliage of the Mulga tree (*Acacia aneura*), a widely used forage for sheep in these semiarid areas, but limited experimentation has not confirmed this. Cattle, which consume the plant less often, develop the pigmentation occasionally. The livers may be slightly darkened or may reach a uniformly distributed dark gray. Microscopic examination shows that the pigment takes the form of minute granules, first in the cytoplasm of the hepatic cells, later in the Kupffer cells, also reaching the portal lymph nodes via macrophages or as free particles. The first particles seen in the cytoplasm of liver cells are yellow; later they become black (oxidation) and look like granules of melanin. Hans Winter (1961, 1963) has shown by extensive histochemical studies that the pigment is not melanin, but has the characteristics of "lipofuscin."

Ceroid

Ceroid was first described by Lillie (1941) as a pigment that developed in the liver of rats with experimentally-induced cirrhosis. It has since also been produced in the livers of cattle, horses, dogs, pigs, rats, and guinea pigs. Its development is

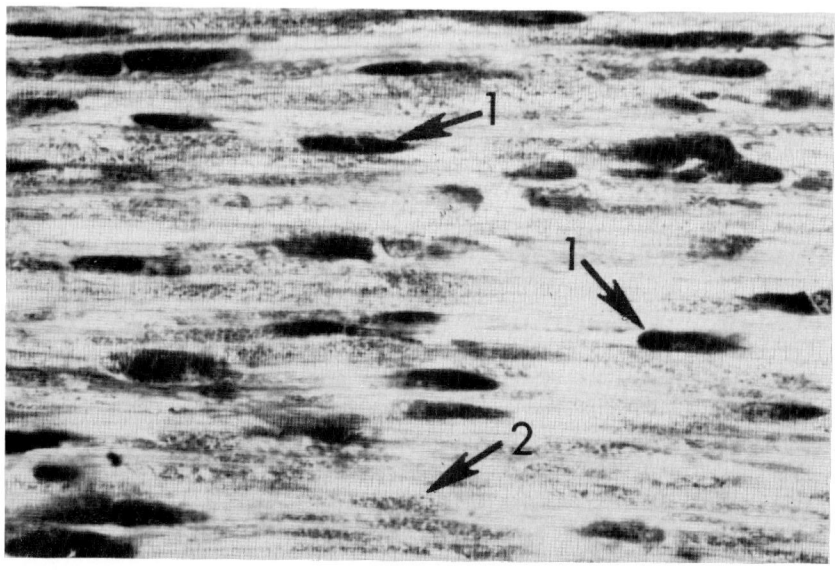

Fig. 3–15. Vitamin E deficiency pigment (ceroid). Large aggregates *(1)* and fine granules *(2)* of pigment in smooth muscle cells of the small intestine of a dog (PAS stain). (Courtesy of Dr. K. C. Hayes.)

related to choline deficiency, and like other lipofuscins, forms from unsaturated lipids. It occurs principally within macrophages but also within hepatocytes.

An essentially identical pigment occurs in **vitamin E deficiency** in a variety of animal species. This form of ceroid is not restricted to the liver, but also occurs within macrophages throughout the body, fat cells, cardiac muscle, smooth muscle of the spleen and intestine (so called "leiomyometaplasts"), and ganglion cells. Often the pigment is so abundant that it is visible grossly, giving rise to **yellow fat disease** or **brown dog gut**. **Microscopically**, both forms of ceroid are isotropic, granular to homogeneous, and yellow to brown. They are resistant to fat solvents and are sudanophilic even after paraffin embedding procedures. They are acid-fast and negative to iron stains. Ceroid is indistinguishable histochemically from lipofuscin. However, its occurrence under differing situations probably justifies, for the present, the continued use of this name.

Borst, M.: Pathologishe Histologie. Leipzig, Vogel, 1922.

Bourne, G. H.: Lipofuscin. Prog. Brain Res., 40:187–201, 1973.

Brizzee, K.R.: Ultrastructural studies on regional differences in lipofuscin accumulation in neuroglia of brain in nonhuman primates. Gerontologist, 14:36, 1974.

Casselman, W. G. B.: The in vitro preparation and histochemical properties of substances resembling ceroid. J. Exp. Med., 94:549–562, 1951.

Graham, C. E.: Distribution of lipofuscin in the squirrel monkey Saimiri sciurea. Histochem. J., 2:521–525, 1970.

Green, P. D., and Little, P. B.: Neuronal ceroid-lipofuscin storage in Siamese cats. Can. J. Comp. Med., 38:207–212, 1974.

Hasan, M., and Glees, P.: Electron microscopical appearance of neuronal lipofuscin using different preparative techniques including freeze-etching. Exp. Gerontol., 7:345–351, 1972.

Hasan, M., and Glees, P.: Genesis and possible dissolution of neuronal lipofuscin. Gerontologia, 18:217–236, 1972.

————: Lipofuscin in monkey lateral geniculate body—electron microscope study. Acta Anat. (Basel), 84:85–95, 1973.

Koppang, N.: Canine ceroid-lipofuscinosis—a model for human neuronal ceroid-lipofuscinosis and ageing. Mech. Ageing Dev., 2:421–445, 1973–1974.

Lee, C. S.: Histochemical studies of the ceroid pigments of rats and mice and its relation to necrosis. J. Natl. Cancer Inst., 11:339–349, 1950.

Lillie, R. D., Daft, F. S., and Sebrell, W. H., Jr.: Cirrhosis of the liver in rats on a deficient diet and the effect of alcohol. Public Health Rep., 56:1255–1258, 1941.

Mason, K. E., and Hartsough, G. R.: "Steatitis" or "yellow fat" in mink, and its relation to dietary fats and inadequacy of vitamin E. J. Am. Vet. Med. Assoc., 119:72–75, 1951.

Oliver, C., Essner, E., Zimring, A., and Haimes, H.: Age-related accumulation of ceroid-like pigment in mice with Chediak-Higashi syndrome. Am. J. Pathol., 84:225–238, 1976.

Schmidt, U.: Generalisierte Lipofuscinose bei einer Katze. Berl. Muench. Tieraerztl. Wochenschr., 87:70–73, 1974.

Sharma, S. P., and Manocha, S. L.: Lipofuscin formation in developing nervous system of squirrel monkeys consequent to maternal dietary protein deficiency during gestation. Mech. Ageing Dev., 6:1–14, 1977.

Trautwein, G. W.: The occurrence of acid-fast lipopigments in animals. Am. J. Vet. Res., 23:134–145, 1962.

von Wyler, R.: Über die pigmentierung der Rinderlymphknoten (Pigmentation of lymph nodes in cattle.) Acta Anat., 14:365–382, 1952.

Whitehair, C. K., Schaefer, A. E., and Elvehjem, C. A.: Nutritional deficiencies in mink with special reference to hemorrhagic gastroenteritis, "yellow fat" and anemia. J. Am. Vet. Med. Assoc., 115:54–58, 1949.

Winter, H.: An environmental lipofuscin pigmentation of livers. Studies on the pigmentation affecting the sheep and other animals in certain districts of Australia. University of Queensland, Papers by Faculty of Veterinary Science, 1:1–66, 1961.

Winter, H.: "Black kidneys" in cattle—a lipofuscinosis. J. Pathol. Bact., 86:253–258, 1963.

Miscellaneous Pigments

Ochronosis Pigment. Ochronosis is a feature of a rare hereditary disease of man known as alkaptonuria (urinary excretion of homogentisic acid) in which there is a deficiency of the enzyme homogentisic acid oxidase. Homogentisic acid is a product formed during the metabolism of phenylalanine and tyrosine. The urine in alkaptonuria turns dark upon standing, as the acid is oxidized to a melanin-like product. A pigment is also deposited within tissues, especially in the walls of blood vessels, cartilage, tendons, ligaments, and other dense collagenous connective tissues, endocrine glands, kidney, and lung.

The pigment is believed to be a polymer derived from homogentisic acid and has similarities to melanin. Microscopically, it is yellow to brown, isotropic, and iron-negative. A similar syndrome has been reported in a chimpanzee and an orangutan.

Dubin-Johnson Pigment. The Dubin-Johnson syndrome, or chronic idiopathic jaundice, was first described as a disease in man in 1954. The disorder, which is probably hereditary, is characterized by chronic icterus and an unidentified pigment in the liver cells. The pigment may be a lipofuscin but also shares many properties with melanin. An abnormality in the excretion of conjugated bilirubin is responsible for chronic icterus, but the mechanism of pigment formation is not known. Arias et al. (1964) described a similar disorder in Corriedale sheep. In addition to chronic icterus (also due to failure to excrete conjugated bilirubin) and hepatic pigmentation, photosensitivity occurred due to accumulation of phylloerythrin in serum. They suggested that the pigment was melanin and that the disorder appeared to be functionally identical with the Dubin-Johnson syndrome of man.

Cloisonné Kidney. First described by Al Zahawi (1957), in Cloisonné kidney a dark brown, iron-negative pigmentation occurs in the basement membranes of proximal convoluted tubules of the kidney, which imparts an appearance, in tissue section, reminiscent of enameled jewelry (Cloisonné). Al Zahawi described the condition in Angora goats. It has also been described by Light (1960) in castrated male Angora goats. Light did not see the condition in female or noncastrated male goats. The nature and significance of the condition is not known.

Arias, I., et al.: Black liver disease in Corriedale sheep: A new mutation affecting hepatic excretory function. J. Clin. Invest., 43:1249–1250, 1964.

Cornelius, C. E., Arias, I. M., and Osburn, B. I.: Hepatic pigmentation with photosensitivity: A syndrome in Corriedale sheep resembling Dubin-Johnson Syndrome in man. J. Am. Vet. Med. Assoc., 146:709–713, 1965.

Grossman, I. W., and Altman, N. H.: Caprine Cloisonné renal lesion. Arch. Pathol., 88:609–612, 1969.

Light, F. W.: Pigmented thickening of the basement membranes of the renal tubules of the goat ("Cloisonne kidney"). Lab. Invest., 9:228–238, 1950.

Zahawi, S.: Symmetrical cortical siderosis of the kidneys of goats. Am. J. Vet. Res., 18:861–867, 1957.

CHAPTER 4

Disturbances of Growth: Aplasia to Neoplasia

Disturbances of growth range from complete absence (aplasia) to uncontrolled proliferation (neoplasia). These two extremes always represent a pathologic state for which no known benefit can be ascribed, but many stages between the extremes occur under normal physiologic conditions or represent beneficial responses to various insults (although classified as disease). Thus, disturbances of growth are not unlike the responses discussed under inflammation (Chapter 6) or immune diseases (Chapter 7).

APLASIA (Agenesis)

Aplasia or agenesis is the complete failure of an organ or part to form during embryogenesis. Aplasia is also applied to the failure to form certain adult tissues that require continued replacement, as in aplastic anemia. Pathologically, the organ or part is missing. If the part is vital, fetal development may not proceed. Most examples in this category are not brought to the pathologist's attention owing to early abortion or resorption. Others may not be compatible with extrauterine life. As a result, most examples that are seen involve paired structures, such as the kidneys or gonads, or nonvital parts, such as a limb or the tail.

Causes. The causes of aplasia are generally not determined, but they may include inherited genetic defects such as taillessness in Manx cats or absence of the thymus in Nude mice. Various poisons may result in aplasia, such as thalidomide, which causes absence of limbs (amelia), and *Veratrum californicum*, which causes (among other abnormalities) absence of the palate and gross facial anomalies. Prenatal infections may also result in aplasia.

HYPOPLASIA

Hypoplasia is the failure of an organ or part to develop to its normal size. It differs from atrophy in that the atrophic organ has shrunk from a previously normal size, but the hypoplastic organ was never any larger. Obviously the disorder occurs during the period of growth, usually before birth, but also during postnatal growth. As with aplasia, the causes are usually obscure, but genetic defects (pituitary dwarfism), certain infectious agents (cerebellar hypoplasia), and certain poisons (thalidomide) can lead to hypoplasia.

ATROPHY

Atrophy is a shrinking, or wasting away, of an organ or tissue to less than its former, and less than its normal size. It may represent a normal physiologic event or a pathologic process. Atrophy can occur in two ways, although both may occur simultaneously in the same organ: (1) through a decrease in the number of constituent cells, necrosis having eliminated some of those normally present. Atrophy developing by this process is called **numerical atrophy**. The same result is attained (2) by a decrease in the size of each component cell, which constitutes **quantitative atrophy**. Most commonly, it is parenchymal rather than interstitial cells that undergo this change.

Atrophy may occur in any organ or tissue; it may involve the whole organ or a single cell.

Microscopic Appearance. Several microscopic features may indicate that atrophy has occurred. Cells of certain histologic types in an organ or tissue may be fewer than normal (numerical atrophy) or smaller than normal (quantitative atrophy). If an organ has a capsule, the wrinkled or undulating capsule may be the most obvious indication that the contents have atrophied. Attention may first be attracted by the fact that nonatrophied elements appear too large or too numerous. In the spleen, for example, the trabeculae may appear surprisingly large, with too many in a given microscopic field; in reality, they have come closer to each other because some of the intervening parenchyma has disappeared. For the same reason, the glomeruli of an atrophic kidney appear too numerous and too close together. Actually the change is in the numer of tubules; some have been destroyed, with a corresponding collapse of the remaining tissue to fill the unoccupied spaces. One should not be misled in this case by the kidney of a very young animal, which has many small, uniform glomeruli (renal corpuscles), while some of the tubules are not yet developed.

In atrophic muscle, the sarcoplasm grows narrower and disappears, leaving for a time the sarcolemma and endomysium, which bear a resemblance to fibrous tissue. In the liver, the hepatic cords may remain intact but become extremely narrow.

Gross Appearance. The organ or part is smaller than normal as determined by looking, by measuring, or by weighing. If a paired organ is the subject of scrutiny, it should always be compared with its fellow.

Causes. The causes of atrophy to some extent duplicate the causes of necrosis, which is not surprising since numerical atrophy involves previous necrosis. **Starvation and malnutrition** cause atrophy of almost the whole body, chiefly quantitative. In starvation the adipose tissue is consumed to produce the energy necessary to maintain life. As the fat becomes exhausted, the muscular and glandular tissues diminish, their protoplasm being catabolized and converted to the production of energy. Practically all organs suffer.

Lack of adequate blood supply brings deficiency of oxygen and quantitative atrophy of individual cells or numerical atrophy of the organ through necrosis of a certain percentage of the cells. For example, the stagnation of chronic passive congestion causes narrowing of the hepatic cords to half their former width and their ultimate disappearance.

Lack of proper innervation has already been noted as causing necrosis of muscle cells in "sweeney" of the horse's shoulder. In spite of what has been said about the necrosis, some of the muscle cells remain alive, undergoing only quantitative atrophy through loss of their sarcoplasm. It is these cells which regenerate most successfully when recovery supervenes.

Disuse atrophy represents a causative mechanism not encountered in the study of necrosis, but one of considerable importance with respect to atrophy. The wasting that occurs in an immobilized limb is a matter of common observation. It results from atrophy of both muscle and bone. Denervation atrophy obviously may also initiate disuse atrophy.

Prolonged **pressure** leads to atrophy, at first quantitative and later numerical with necrosis. This is striking when a neoplasm invades the liver, eventually replacing most of the hepatic tissue. As another illustration, it is possible to tell whether a horse has been working habitually by the slight depression of the healthy tissues where the collar or the saddle rests.

Certain **disturbances of endocrine glands** produce atrophy of structures dependent upon their secretions, as, for instance, atrophy of the testes in hypopituitarism. Prolonged **overwork** leads exceptionally to atrophy, as in the thyroid exhaustion following prolonged exophthalmic goiter.

Physiologic atrophy occurs under a variety of circumstances, the resorption of tadpole's tail in metamorphosis being a classic example. Similarly, the thymus practically disappears (involutes) as the individual advances beyond infancy. Other examples are involution of the uterus and mammary glands following pregnancy and lactation, respectively.

Classification of Atrophy. It is sometimes useful to divide atrophy into several classes depending on special accompanying features. **Simple atrophy** needs no explanation; the term is used when none of the other classifying adjectives apply. In **fatty atrophy**, the missing cells have been replaced by adipose tissue. This occurs, for instance, in physiologic atrophy of the thymus. In **fibrous atrophy,** sometimes called "fibroid" or "scirrhous" atrophy, proliferating fibrous tissue comes in as the pre-existing cells shrink and disappear. The proliferation of new connective tissue really constitutes a chronic inflammatory reaction. **Pigment atrophy** is that which is accompanied by deposition of pigment, namely the pigment of brown atrophy. **Mucoid atrophy of fat**, also known as **serous atrophy of fat**, has been discussed in connection with connective-tissue mucin and myxomatous degeneration.

Mechanisms. The mechanism of atrophy due to loss of cells involves cell death, autolysis, necrosis, and heterolysis, which have been discussed in Chapter 1. Reduction in the size of cells or qualitative atrophy, on the other hand, requires reduction in protoplasm without cell death. This is accomplished by isolating cellular components in membrane-bound vacuoles, called **autophagic vacuoles**, into which lysosomes discharge their contents, resulting in digestion of the cellular components. This process is known as **autophagy**. Cole et al. (1971) have shown that autophagic vacuoles form within five to ten minutes following occlusion of portal venous blood supply to a lobe of the liver, a process that leads to atrophy. What initiates autophagy is not known, but glucagon has been demonstrated to stimulate the process (Shelburne et al., 1973).

HYPERTROPHY

An increase in size of an organ or tissue to greater than its former and normal size is known as **organ hypertrophy**. It may result from an increase in the size of its constituent cells, which is called **cellular hypertrophy**, or an increase in the number of its constituent cells, which is called **hyperplasia**. Obviously, hyperplasia is restricted to organs and tissues in which the cells have retained the ability to undergo mitosis, a feature lost by many tissues. In general, hyperplasia is more effective in meeting increased functional demands than is hypertrophy.

Hypertrophy of most tissues and organs results from a combination of cellular hypertrophy and hyperplasia. Pure hypertrophy (without hyperplasia) occurs only in organs whose cells have generally lost the ability to undergo mitosis, for example, skeletal and cardiac muscle. However, even in muscle, limited cell division may accompany hypertrophy. Cellular hypertrophy results from the formation of new cytoplasm, including ribonucleic acid, protein, and mitochondria. Grossly, the organ is enlarged, and microscopically, the appearance is unchanged except the cells are larger, but this may be difficult to appreciate.

Classification. Two types of hypertrophy, not always clearly distinguishable from one another, are usually considered on the basis of their origin and probable cause. These are compensatory and hormonal hypertrophy.

Compensatory or Adaptive Hypertrophy. This enlargement may represent a physiologic or pathologic response. It is believed to result as a consequence of impaired function of a paired organ or part of an organ system. For example, loss of one kidney, for any reason, results in gradual enlargement of the remaining kidney, enabling it to compensate for the loss of function of the paired organ. Another example is found in the myocardium, which as a result of valvular deformities or hypertension, undergoes remarkable enlargement. Stenosis of the lumen of the pylorus of the stomach leads to hypertrophy of the gastric musculature; similar partial obstruction of the intestinal or urethral lumen leads to hypertrophy of the intestinal or bladder muscle, respectively. The enlargement of skeletal muscles as the result of repeated exercise is well known, and represents a physiologic compensatory hypertrophy.

Hormonal Hypertrophy. This most often is a physiologic phenomenon, but in some instances may be pathologic. The enlargement of the mammary gland at the approach of lactation involves hypertrophy, as well as hyperplasia (to be discussed), as does the great increase in size of the testes in birds and some mammals during the mating season.

Significance. Hypertrophy is a protective mechanism and a response to a need for increased function. Occasionally the enlarged organ may constitute a mechanical hindrance to some other function, as when enlargement of the heart muscle may distort the valves from their proper positions or cause the heart to fail due to inadequate blood supply. Note that, while the increase

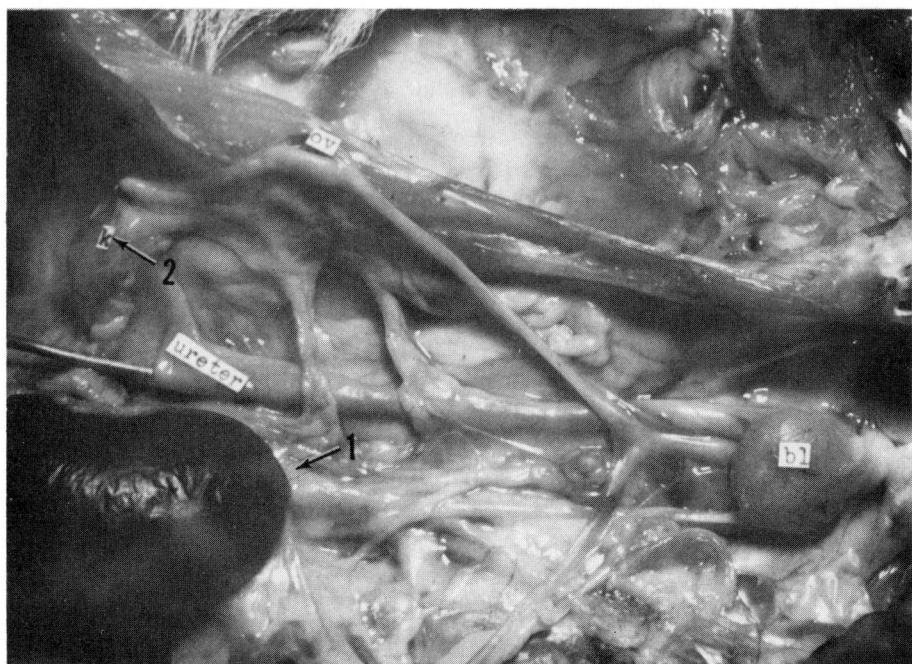

Fig. 4–1. Compensatory hypertrophy of right kidney *(1)*, resulting from congenital hypoplasia of left kidney *(k, 2)*. Left ovary *(ov)* and bladder *(bl)*. From a 5½-month-old female terrier which died of canine distemper.

in size occasioned by hypertrophy may be considerable, there are always definite limits to the maximum size attained. Once the stimulus for hypertrophy is withdrawn, the hypertrophic process regresses, although the hypertrophied organ rarely reverts to its previous size.

HYPERPLASIA

Hyperplasia is an absolute increase in number of cells, in response to functional demands or other stimuli, which leads to hypertrophy of the involved organ or tissue. Usually, only a single cell type in any given tissue is affected. As stated earlier,

hyperplasia is limited to cells capable of division. In certain organs the value of hyperplasia is negated by the inability to increase the number of functional units. For example, the number of pulmonary alveoli or renal nephrons cannot be increased, nor can those lost to disease be replaced, despite hypertrophy and hyperplasia of individual cells. This greatly limits its potential for increased function of these organs.

Gross and Microscopic Appearance. Gross and microscopic appearances vary with the tissue affected and the cause. Hyperplasia of a glandular organ usually

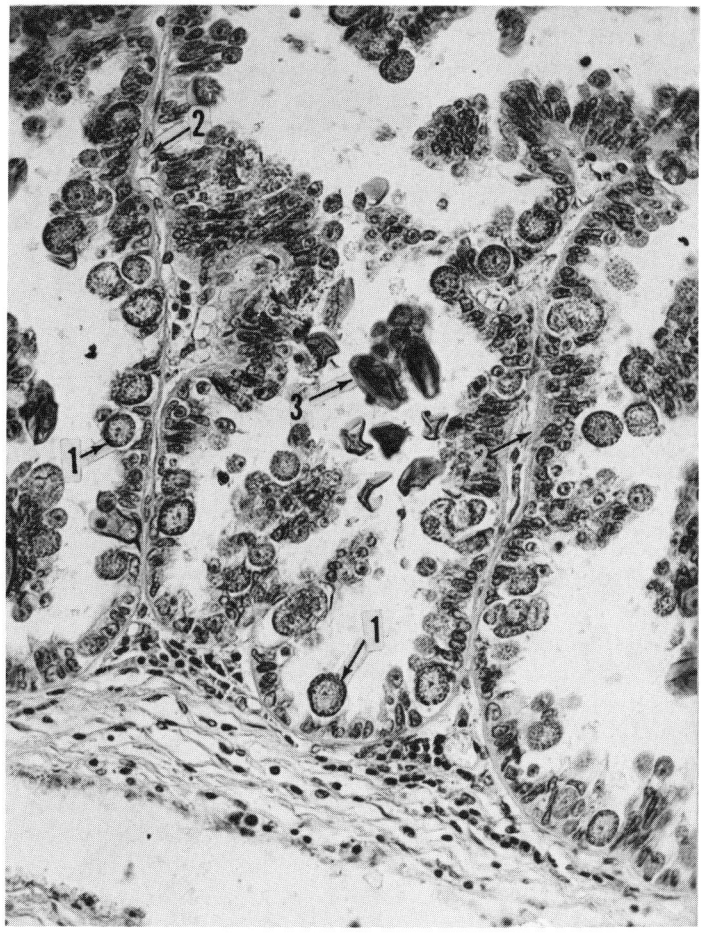

Fig. 4–2. Hyperplasia of intrahepatic biliary epithelium in liver of a rabbit infected with *Eimeria stiedae*. Gametocytes (*1*) and oocysts (*3*). Note the long fronds of hyperplastic epithelial cells supported by a delicate stroma (*2*). (× 250.) (Courtesy of Armed Forces Institute of Pathology.) Contributor: Dr. C. L. Davis.

involves an increase in height of the acinar epithelium and at the same time an increase in the number of its cells. Based on the same principle as the well-known fact that one can plant more hills of corn in a crooked row than a straight one, the contours of the acinar lining become crooked, wavy, and folded, often to the extent that papillary projections jut into the lumen. Indeed, the acinus may be more or less filled with reduplicated folding of an acinar lining that originally was in the form of a smoothly contoured circle. This is seen especially well in hyperplasia of the thyroid or prostate. In some instances, huge acini are formed at the expense of surrounding structures, as in **cystic glandular hyperplasia** of the endometrium or mammary gland. Hyperplastic conditions of the epidermis may take the form of increased thickness of the prickle-cell layer (stratum spinosum), which is known as **acanthosis**, or of the cornified layer, which is called **hyperkeratosis**. Hyperplasia, which accompanies many forms of chronic inflammation with its associated fibrosis, as in hepatic cirrhosis, may result in the formation of circumscribed, expanding nodules of proliferating cells. Hyperplastic cells usually have an increased nucleocytoplasmic ratio, although the number of cytoplasmic organelles may be increased. As expected, mitoses are more frequent.

Classification. As with hypertrophy, hyperplasia can be classified into two principal types, although multiple underlying stimuli may be operant in each.

Compensatory or Adaptive Hyperplasia. This may represent a physiologic or a pathologic response. Following surgical removal of a kidney or partial hepatectomy, there occurs a physiologic hyperplasia of the opposite kidney or remaining lobes of the liver. Pathologic destruction of one kidney will initiate the same physiologic hyperplasia. Similarly, loss of blood or reduced atmospheric oxygen tension leads to erythroid hyperplasia.

The term **regenerative hyperplasia** is sometimes applied in these circumstances.

Other pathologic stimuli initiate hyperplasia that is considered adaptive or compensatory, but the nature of the stimulus or true value of the response is usually unknown. Examples include lymphoid hyperplasia in response to infections (of clear value), hyperplasia of the bile duct epithelium in hepatic coccidiosis (uncertain value), epithelial or mesenchymal hyperplasia in pox viral infections, and epithelial hyperplasia associated with chronic irritation, as seen in corns.

Hormonal Hyperplasia. Hormonal hyperplasia may also be physiologic or pathologic. Hyperplasia of the mammary glands or uterus associated with puberty or pregnancy are physiologic events. In contrast, cystic glandular hyperplasia of either of these tissues associated with malfunction of the ovary is a pathologic event. The hyperplastic goiter of Graves' disease is another example of pathologic hormonal hyperplasia, as is iodine deficiency goiter.

Significance. In most respects, the significance of hyperplasia seems obvious. It sometimes appears to be but a short step from hyperplasia to the much more serious neoplasia. Still, there are comparatively few conditions in which there exists any strong evidence of hyperplasia leading to neoplasia. However, differentiation of many benign neoplasms and even some malignant neoplasms may be difficult. As with hypertrophy, hyperplasia terminates and regresses when the stimulus is withdrawn, but the organ may never revert to its original size.

METAPLASIA

Metaplasia is the substitution of one variety of adult, fully differentiated cells for another type of adult, fully differentiated cells. Metaplasia is a substitution and not a transformation. The new adult cell types are derived from reserve cells, which are pluripotential for differentiation. Metaplasia is usually considered a protective response, but the value is not always clear.

Occurrence. Metaplasia of columnar or cuboidal epithelium into stratified squamous epithelium, usually cornifying, occurs in the bronchi and bronchioles, in the gallbladder when irritated by gall stones, in the ducts of glands, and in the protruded parts of prolapsed organs such as the cervix. In deficiency of vitamin A, there is metaplasia of the epithelium in a variety of other locations, such as the lining of the renal pelvis.

Connective tissue undergoes metaplasia to cartilage or bone, and cartilage changes to bone in a variety of situations. In cattle, the formation of large numbers of bony spicules in thickened alveolar septa of the lung is not of exceptional rarity. Bony and cartilaginous metaplasia in adenocarcinomas and mixed tumors of the canine mammary gland is frequent and may be so extensive that the major part of the neoplasm consists of bone. The ossification of tendons and cartilage is a form of metaplasia which has already been described. Rarely, the scars of abdominal wounds develop bony layers.

Cause. The fundamental cause of metaplasia is a demand for a different kind of function, usually for protection against chronic irritation. The exact mechanisms are essentially unknown.

Significance. Metaplasia is almost always reversible, but it may precede neoplastic transformation. Most carcinomas of the human lung and cervix arise in metaplastic epithelium.

DYSPLASIA

Dysplasia (*dys* = disordered; *plassein* = to form) is disordered or abnormal devel-

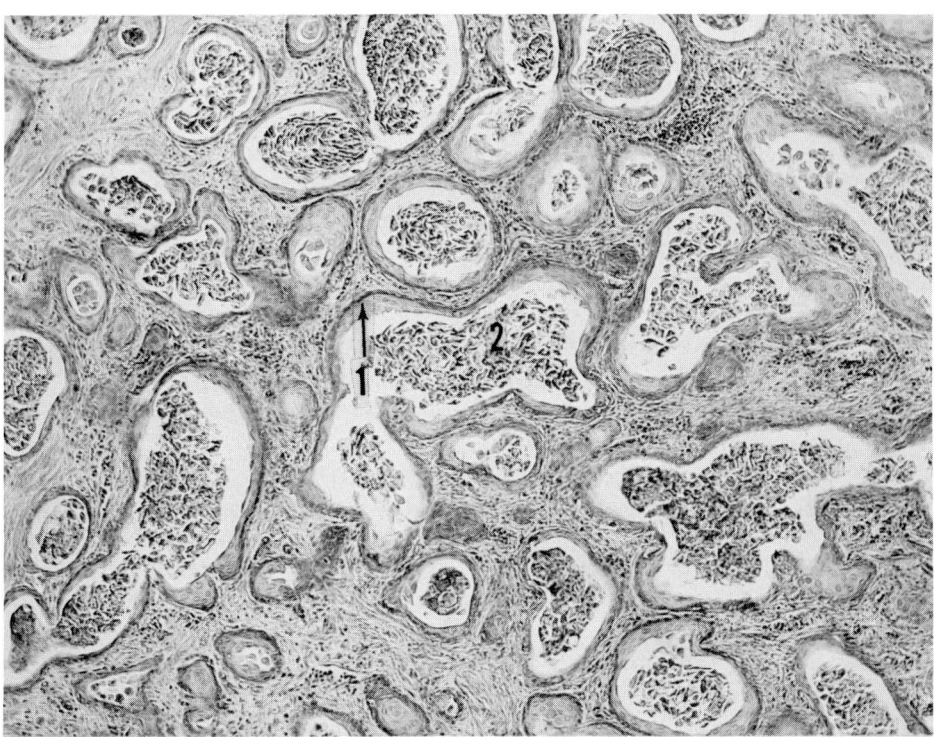

Fig. 4–3. Squamous metaplasia of prostate of a dog, resulting from estrogen production of a Sertoli cell tumor of the testis. Prostatic acini are lined with squamous epithelium (*1*) and filled with keratin debris (*2*). (× 70.) (Courtesy of Armed Forces Institute of Pathology.) Contributor: Dr. W. H. Riser.

opment of cells and tissues. It may occur in fetal or neonatal development, or in adult tissues that are continuously replaced. Dystrophia is sometimes used as a synonym, but this is incorrect (*trophe* = nourishment). Dystrophy represents a retrogressive change in a tissue after it has reached a stable adult state, as in nutritional muscular dystrophy.

Microscopic and Gross Appearances. Dysplasia occurring during development may or may not be reflected in a disordered microscopic appearance. In chondrodysplasia (chondrodystrophy) leading to abnormal endochondral bone growth and dwarfism, the cartilaginous growth plate is highly disorganized, whereas in hip dysplasia, the acetabulum is grossly misshapen, but microscopically not remarkable. In adult renewing tissues, dysplasia occurs predominantly in epithelia, especially the skin, mucous membranes, and mucosae of the gastrointestinal tract, cervix, and vagina. Here it is characterized microscopically by disruption of orientational relationships, variation in size and shape of cells (pleomorphism), hyperchromasia of nuclei, increase in nuclear to cytoplasmic ratio, and increased mitotic activity.

Cause. Dysplasia of development is probably caused by the same types of conditions as aplasia and hypoplasia. In adult renewing tissues, it is believed to result from chronic irritation and is considered reversible. It may, however, hallmark neoplastic transformation, an event well documented in dysplasia of metaplastic squamous epithelium of the human cervix. Dysplasia may be difficult to discern from anaplasia.

ANAPLASIA

Anaplasia is a reversion of cells to a more primitive and less differentiated type. Synonyms include dedifferentiation and undifferentiation. The cells lose structural and functional characteristics and morphologically resemble dysplastic tissue but

more so. There is great pleomorphism, with some cells becoming very large (giant) with hyperchromatic nuclei and an increased nuclear cytoplasmic ratio. Mitotic activity is increased, with many abnormal mitotic figures. Anaplasia is considered irreversible and a precursor of neoplasia. Anaplasia is also a feature of neoplastic tissue.

DEVELOPMENTAL ANOMALIES AND MALFORMATIONS

Developmental anomalies ordinarily originate before birth; indeed, in embryonic life, when the development of most body structures has its beginning. There are however exceptions. For example, if the epiphyseal cartilages of, let us say, the femur of a child or young animal suffer severe damage, as they may in chronic osteomyelitis, for instance, the bone grows no more and the individual has a shortened and deformed leg, a malformation.

Forms of Maldevelopment

The frequency of prenatal malformations is surprising; their wide variety is unbelievable. Most types have been given names, but these will be omitted here. Reflection on the various forms reveals that they depend upon one of several different errors in the developmental mechanism. Outstanding among these are:

Arrest of Development. This may occur in a certain part of the embryo, so that a certain structure is absent (aplasia) or too small (hypoplasia).

Failure of a Certain Embryonal or Fetal Structure to Disappear When it Normally Should. There are many examples of this, such as the persistence of the ductus arteriosus or the thyroglossal duct. Atresia ani is a rather common malformation that results from failure of the overlying skin to disappear from the anal opening.

Failure of Certain Openings, Grooves, and Fissures to Close Properly. Many of these are in the midline, such as cranioschisis and rachioschisis from lack of closure of the neural groove. Patent foramen ovale in the heart can be included here, as can persistent cloaca, in which the rectal and external genital openings are not separated.

Aberrant (Ectopic or Heterotopic) Structures. It is not highly extraordinary to find islands of pancreatic tissue in the wall of the stomach, or adrenal tissue in the kidney or pelvic tissues. Displacement of cutaneous and mucosal tissues into deeper areas is considered the proper explanation for the rather frequent appearance of dermoid cysts located near the exterior of the body, as well as for dentigerous cysts occurring in the head and neck, although just when such malformations become sufficiently complicated to be suspected of resulting from imperfect duplication is difficult to say.

Duplications. Each cell or group of cells of the early embryo is destined to produce, as it multiplies, a particular structure in the adult. If such a cell were to undergo division without any further specialization or differentiation toward a particular organ or tissue, it is obvious that two cells with identical potentialities would be produced, each destined to form identical body structures, of which there would be two instead of the usual one. If the cell doing this were the recently fertilized ovum, there would be two complete and identical individuals, or twins (of the identical or monozygotic variety).

The work of experimental embryologists indicates that a slightly different process occurs. The fertilized ovum normally divides into two blastomeres, or primitive daughter cells. In some simple animal species, these two blastomeres have been experimentally separated and each develops into a complete individual, an identical or uniovular twin. What must be almost complete separations of the two blastomeres has been accomplished by shaking or by inverting the ovum at this two-cell stage, with the resulting formation of double monsters, that is, twins like the

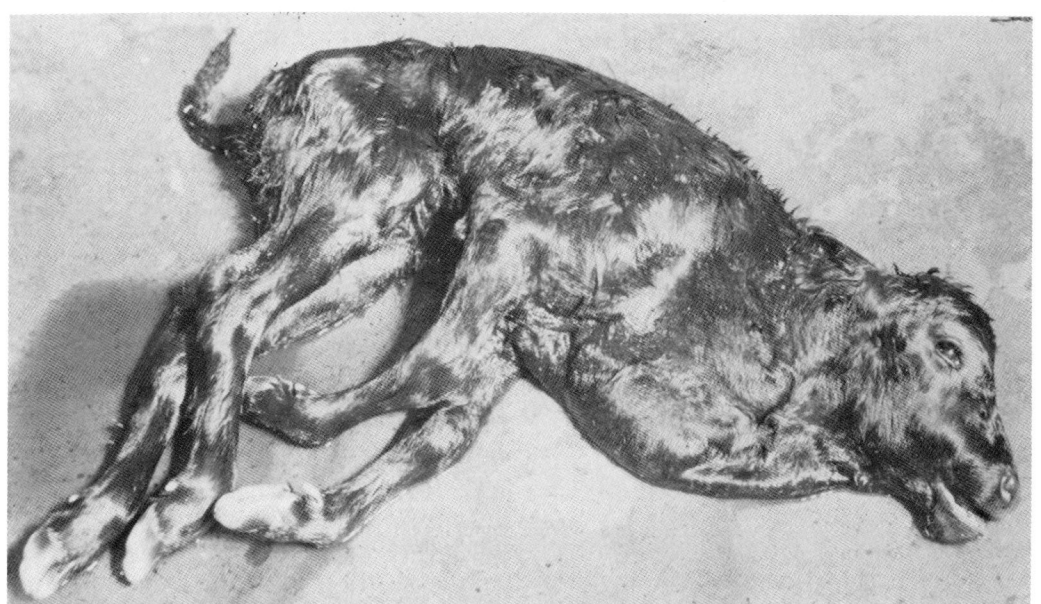

Fig. 4-4. *Ectopia cordis* in a newborn Angus calf, a full-term twin to a normal calf. The diaphragm was absent; abdominal viscera in the thorax; the heart in the subcutis of the neck. Some calves with this anomaly have lived several months or years.

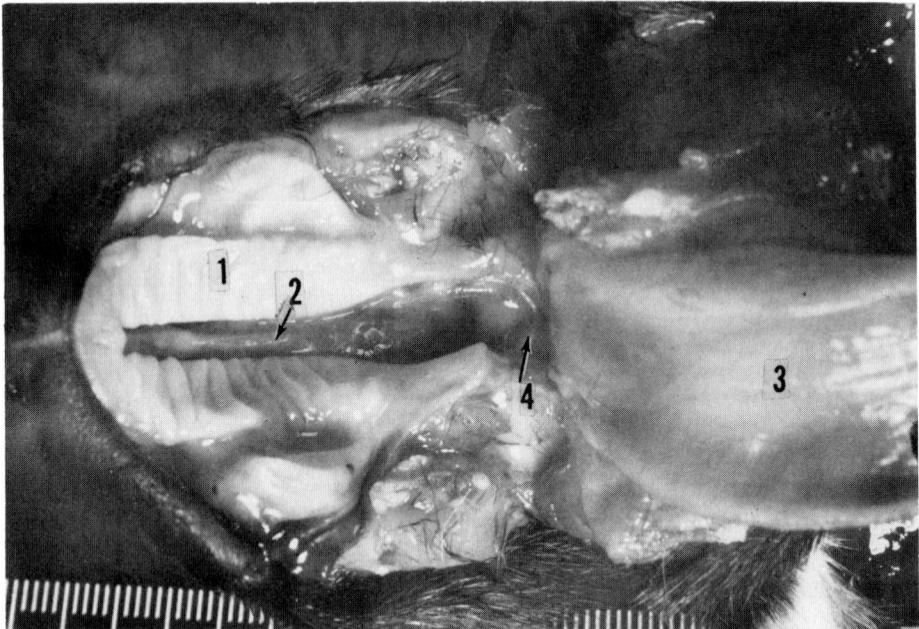

Fig. 4–5. Congenital anomaly. Cleft palate in a week-old bull dog. Hard palate (*1*), cleft (2) opening into nasal cavity, deflected tongue (3) and posterior nares (4).

Siamese twins, almost but not completely separated. In other experiments with certain amphibian species, monsters with two heads or anterior ends have been produced by constricting the developing embryo at a somewhat later stage (during gastrulation). This procedure involves not only the separation of groups of cells, but a division of the supply of certain chemical hormones called "organizers." These organizers have formed in the appropriate region of the embryo and are what supplies the necessary stimulus for the involved cells to differentiate into the particular types and structures needed—in this case, to form a head. If the plane of constriction is not exactly median, one of the heads is normal and the other is incomplete and imperfect in one way or another; usually it has only one eye. Double monsters and other radical malformations have also been produced by experimental embryologists in amphibian and similar lower animal species through such means as depriving the very early embryo of sufficient oxygen, by the application of minute amounts of certain toxic chemicals, or by lowering the temperature unduly.

There may be all degrees of duplication, such as two separate and perfect twins, two twins which are perfectly formed but joined together by more or less unduplicated tissue, such as belly to belly, back to back, or head to head. In such cases, the vital organs may or may not be duplicated. There may be duplication of almost any part of the animal's body: the muzzle, the head, the cephalothorax, the tail, the hind quarters, and others. There may be double pairs of fore or hind limbs; the latter are common.

As might be anticipated from the experimental results recorded above, the duplicated parts are not necessarily equal. Especially when the duplication is not a matter of right and left counterparts, the inequality is often such that one set of organs is more or less normal and perhaps functional, while the other recedes to a purely accessory status. We have seen a lamb that was born with two mouths, one in the normal place and one, considerably smaller, in the right subparotid region. The accessory mouth chewed when the main mouth chewed, secreted saliva, and had three rudimentary teeth, but it did not have an opening into the pharynx. The lamb was raised to well past a year of age (dying of an accident), and in the course of the animal's normal growth, the accessory mouth became relatively less and less prominent, since it grew but little.

Supernumerary parts, usually of minor nature, occur in some situations where the conception of duplication is less obvious but probably still applicable, for instance, in the case of supernumerary digits in man or animal. The extra digits are usually bilaterally symmetrical but practically always imperfect and purely accessory. Supernumerary breasts are described in the human female and male. Supernumerary (and rudimentary) teats are common in the cow. However, in the porcine and even the canine species, a somewhat variable number of pairs of mammae is considered normal. Likewise, the number of vertebrae and ribs is subject to certain normal variation in some species.

Inequality of duplicated parts attains its logical culmination when the accessory structure is no more than a shapeless mass, attached outside or inside the dominant individual and recognizable only as the microscope reveals its histologic components. Such a structure constitutes a teratoma. Since teratomas are likely sites for the development of malignant neoplasia, they are discussed in that connection.

Etiology

The causes of many congenital anomalies are essentially unknown; these are discussed in the appropriate chapters concerning organ systems. The important known causes of anomalies follow.

(1) Prenatal infection with a virus—for example, panleukopenia (cerebellar hypoplasia), Newcastle disease of chickens (ocular or auditory anomalies) Blattner and Williamson (1951), blue tongue of sheep and rickettsial infection. Most of these are associated with anomalies of the central nervous system.

(2) Intrauterine effects of poisons ingested by the mother—for example, the plant *Veratrum californicum*, thalidomide, selenium, molybdenum, trypan blue, and sodium salicylate.

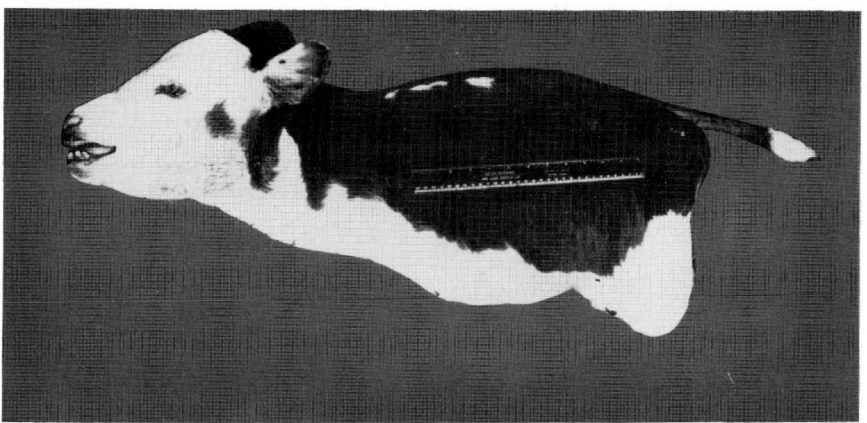

Fig. 4–6. Congenital anomaly, a calf born alive but without legs (amelia) lived three days without nourishment and was given euthanasia. A similar anomaly in pigs is reported by Hutt to be due to a single recessive gene.

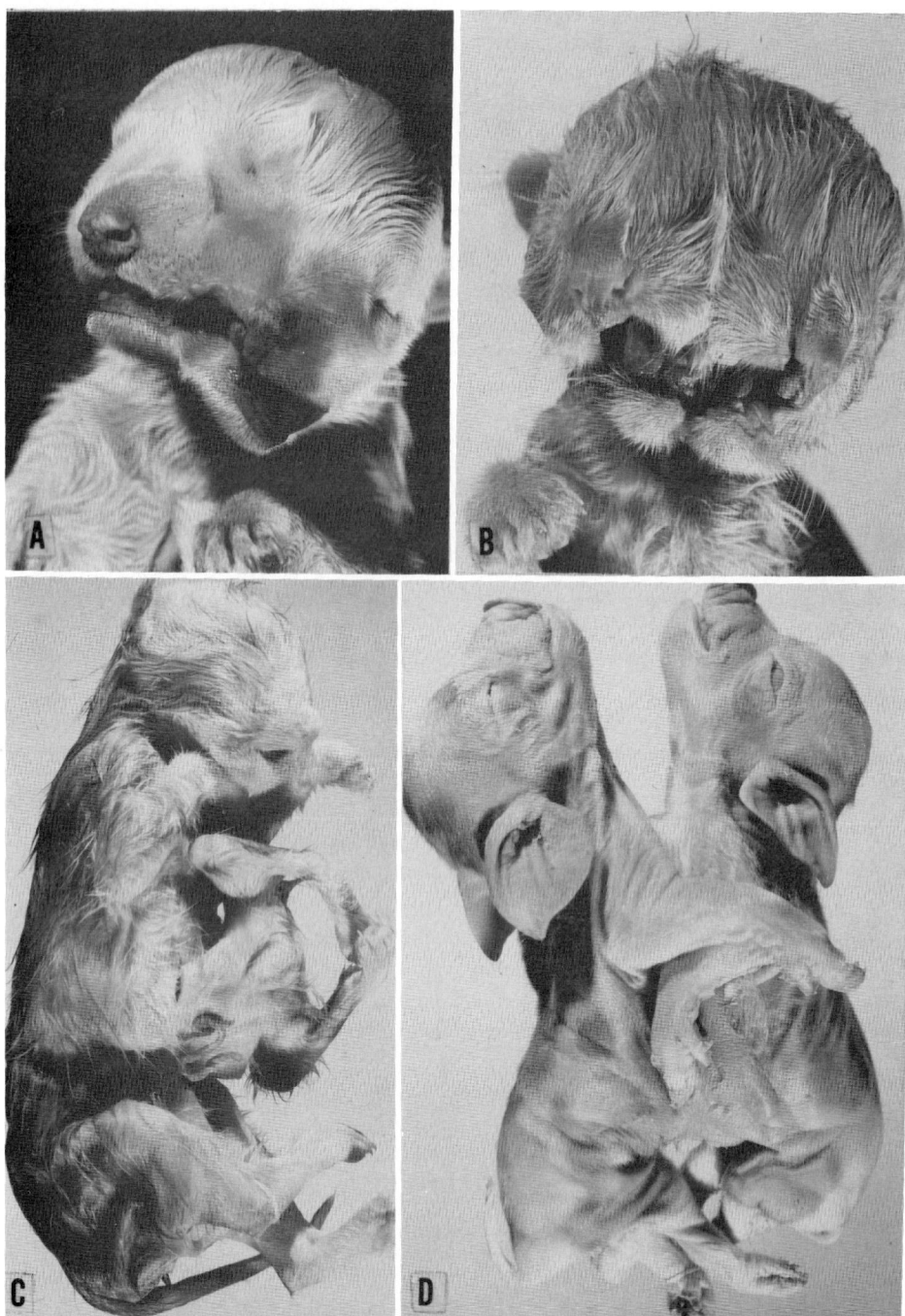

Fig. 4–7.   Congenital anomalies. *A*, Partial duplication of head (diprosopia) in a fox-terrier puppy which lived for two days. *B*, Diprosopia in a kitten. *C*, Twin kittens joined at the abdomen; one of them is only partially developed (heteradelphia). (Courtesy of Armed Forces Institute of Pathology.) Contributor: Major A. C. Girard. *D*, Twin pigs joined at the thorax (thoracopagus).

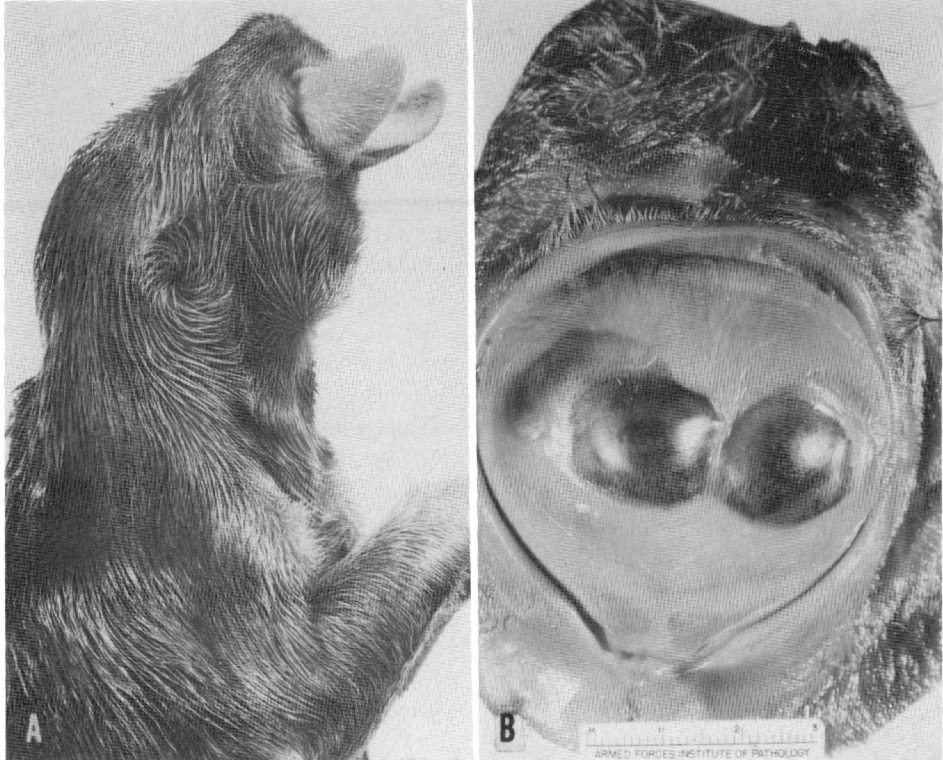

Fig. 4–8. Congenital anomalies. *A*, Absence of eyes (anophthalmia) and lower jaw in a newborn puppy. *B*, Partially fused eyes (synophthalmia or cyclopegia) in a newborn colt.

(3) Vitamin deficiencies—for example, vitamin A and folic acid.

(4) Experimentally, hyperthermia has induced congenital defects in many animals species, but its role in naturally occurring malformations is not known.

(5) Genetic factors—the recombination of mutant genes, inherited from one or (usually) both parents. These are discussed more fully in Chapter 8.

Baker, C. A., Hendrickx, A. G., and Cooper, R. W.: Spontaneous malformations in Squirrel monkey *(Saimiri sciureus)* fetuses with emphasis on cleft lip and palate. J. Med. Primatol., *6*:13–22, 1977.

Barron, C. N.: Ectopic Pancreas in the Dog. Acta Anat., *36*:344–352, 1959.

Berry, C.L., et al.: Non-mendelian developmental defects: animal models and implications for research into human disease. Bull. W.H.O., *55*:475–487, 1977.

Blattner, R. J., and Williamson, A. P.: Developmental abnormalities in the chick embryo following infection with Newcastle disease virus. Proc. Soc. Exp. Biol. Med., *77*:619–621, 1951.

Cole, S., Matter, A., and Karnovsky, M. J.: Autophagic vacuoles in experimental atrophy. Exp. Mol. Pathol., *14*:158–175, 1971.

Dennis, S. M., and Leipold, H. W.: Syndactylism in a neonatal lamb. Cornell Vet., *60*:23–27, 1970.

———: Aprosopia (facelessness) in lambs. Vet. Rec., *90*:365–367, 1972.

Goss, R. J.: Hypertrophy versus hyperplasia. Science, *153*:1615–1620, 1966.

Harris, H.: Cell growth and multiplication. *In* General Pathology, ed. by H. W. Florey. Philadelphia, W. B. Saunders Co., 1970.

Hughes, K. L., Haughey, K. G., and Hartley, W. J.: Spontaneous congenital developmental abnormalities observed at necropsy in a large survey of newly born dead lambs. Teratology, *5*:5–10, 1972.

Kalter, H., and Warkany, J.: Experimental production of congenital malformations in mammals by metabolic procedure. Physiol. Rev., *39*:69–115, 1959.

Landtman, B.: Relationship between maternal conditions during pregnancy and congenital malformations. Arch. Dis. Child., *23*:237–246, 1948.

Selby, L. A., Khalili, A., Stewart, R. W., Edmonds, L.

D., and Marienfeld, C. J.: Pathology and epidemiology of conjoined twinning in swine. Teratology, 8:1–9, 1973.

Shelburne, J. D., Arstila, A. V., and Trump, B. F.: Studies on cellular autophagocytosis. Cyclic AMP- and dibutyryl cyclic AMP-stimulated autophagy in rat liver. Am. J. Pathol., 72:521–540, 1973.

Thomson, R. G.: Congenital bronchial hypoplasia in calves. Path. Vet., 3:89–109, 1966.

NEOPLASIA

A neoplasm is a new growth of cells that (1) proliferate continuously without control, (2) bear a considerable resemblance to the healthy cells from which they arose, (3) have no orderly structural arrangement, (4) serve no useful function and (5) for the present, at least, have no clearly understood cause. There have been many definitions of neoplasm, but the above, changed but little from that offered by Mallory more than a generation ago, possibly comes as close as any to enlightening the novice on what the general public calls a "cancer." "Tumor" is a less precise but commonly used synonym, which originally meant a swelling, but now is reserved almost exclusively for enlargements of a neoplastic nature.

The "uncontrolled proliferation" and "no useful function" are the key points to any definition of neoplasia. For most of the processes discussed in previous chapters, the mechanisms controlling the reactions are more clearly understood, and although considered disease, represent reactions that serve a purpose, which is often life-saving, e.g., abscess, granuloma, hypertrophy, or hyperplasia.

General Characteristics

Manner of Growth. It is the **continuous proliferation**, the uncontrolled growth, that makes neoplasia the formidable and destructive process that it is. Rates of growth vary, and naturally the tumor of rapid growth is to be feared most. But there is also a difference in type of growth: neoplasms may grow by expansion or by invasion. In the tumor endowed with the power of invasive growth, the outermost cells multiply actively and unevenly and, as more room is required for the growing population, individual cells or small groups force themselves in amongst the cells and structures of the surrounding tissues. Since the invading tumor cells usually possess great vitality, they can endure more pressure and more successfully compete for oxygen and nutrient substances, with the result that the preexisting tissues are crowded out and disappear through necrosis of one cell after another.

Thus the tumor, able to grow by invasion, destroys whatever is in its path, even bone, and this continues until life itself is destroyed. The singular exception is cartilage, which is resistant to neoplastic invasion. Because of this great destructiveness, neoplasms of this nature are classed as **malignant**, while those that grow only expansively, much less dangerous to their host, are said to be **benign**. (Details of the differentiation between benign and malignant neoplasms are discussed on p. 122.)

One other feature of malignant neoplasms, which, indeed, is the *sine qua non* of malignancy, is the capacity for **metastasis**. Metastasis is the transport of tumor cells or tumor fragments from the primary neoplastic site to another location. Most often they are transported by way of lymphatics or veins. It is obvious that an invasive growth will sooner or later make its way into blood vessels and lymph vessels. As the neoplastic cells reach the lumen, they are in contact with the flowing stream, and it is not unusual for single cells or small groups of cells to be detached and carried away as emboli in the blood stream or lymph, as the case may be. They travel until their progress is stopped by lodgment in the fine meshes of the next lymph node or in small, terminal arterioles or capillaries. More often than not, lodgment occurs in the lungs, liver, spleen, or kidneys, whose capillary networks provide fine and extensive filters. The malignant neoplastic

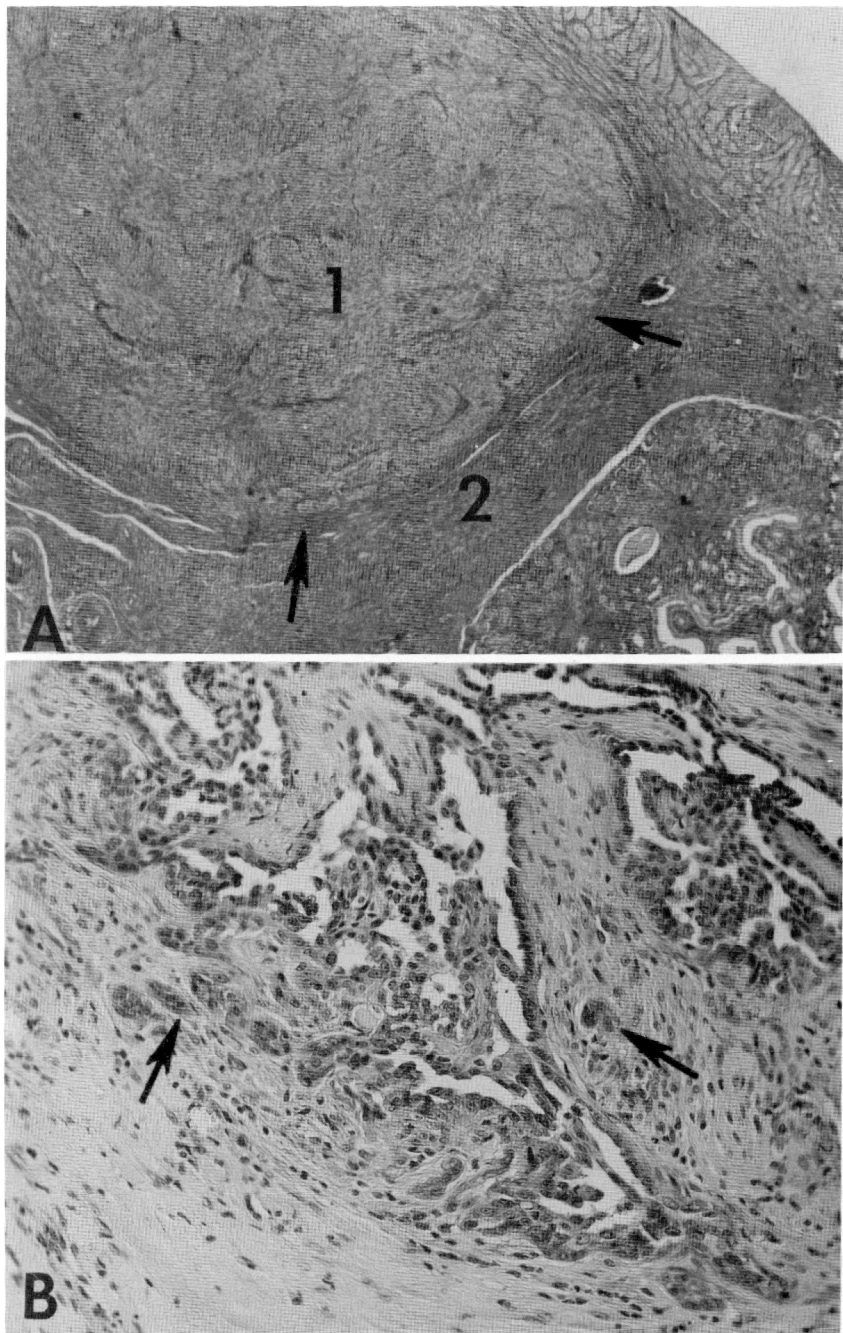

Fig. 4-9. Manner of growth of benign *vs* malignant neoplasms. *A*, Growth by expansion and compression of adjacent tissue. Note smooth junction (arrows) between the neoplasm (*1*) and normal tissue (*2*). From a leiomyoma of the canine uterus. *B*, Growth by invasion. Note extension of cells from the neoplasm into the stroma (arrows). From an adenocarcinoma of apocrine gland of the canine skin. (Courtesy of Armed Forces Institute of Pathology.)

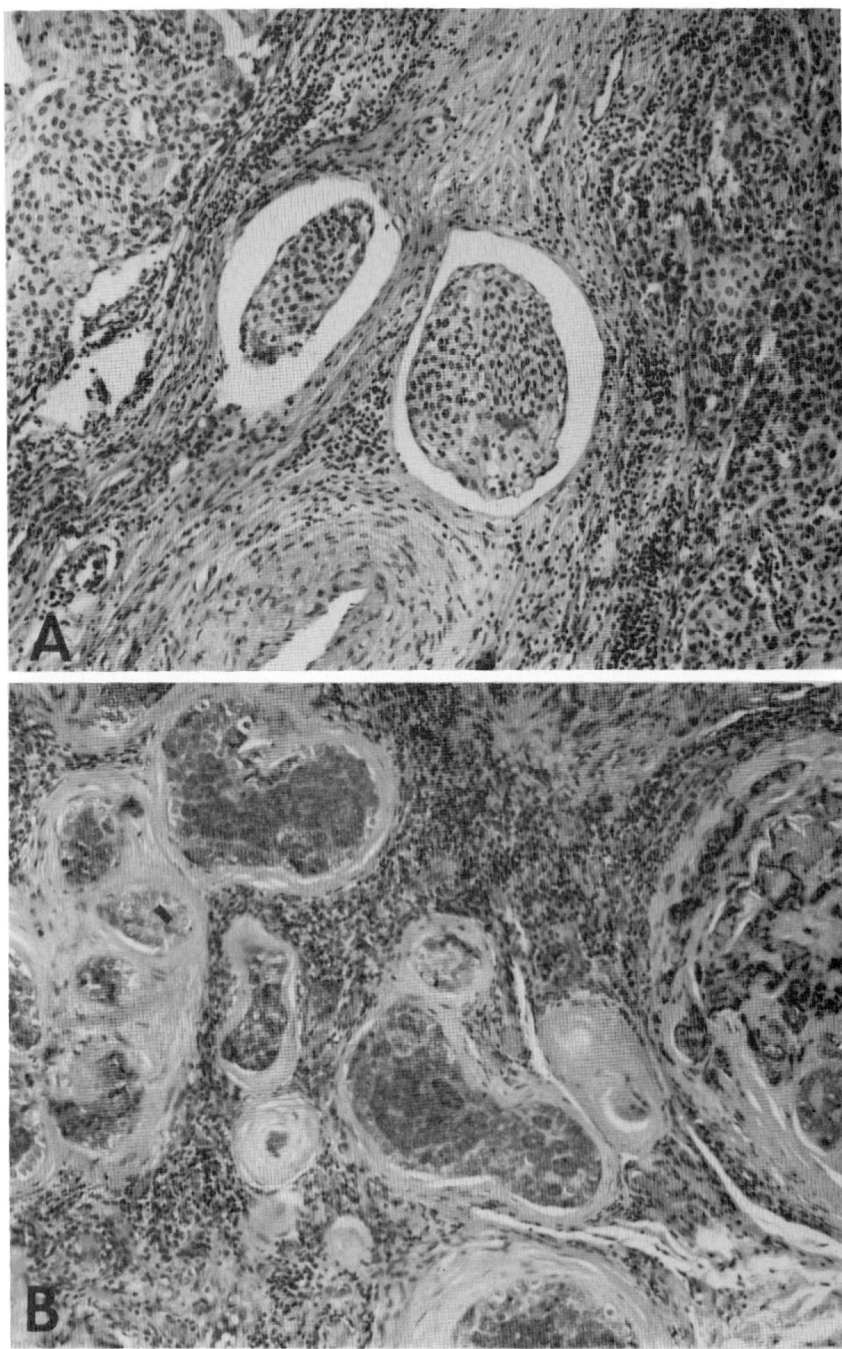

Fig. 4–10. Metastasis by way of lymphatics. *A*, Squamous cell carcinoma of the cervix in lymphatics. (Courtesy Harvard Medical School.) *B*, Tumor cells growing within sclerotic lymphatics adjacent to an adenocarcinoma of the canine mammary gland.

cells may die at their new location or multiply and continue their uncontrolled and disorderly growth at the point where they lodge, setting up a new colony, a **metastatic neoplasm**.

Malignant epithelial tumors (carcinomas) usually metastasize by way of lymphatics. Exceptions are carcinomas of the renal cells and hepatocytes, which are transported by veins. Sarcomas almost always metastasize by way of the blood. Malignant tumors may also disseminate by direct spread or detachment of fragments within coelomic cavities (e.g., peritoneal or pleural), bronchi, renal pelvis or ureter, cerebrospinal space, and other epithelial-lined cavities or structures. This form of metastasis is often referred to as **implantation**.

Normal tissues may enter the circulation and be carried as emboli to distant sites, but this usually is not referred to as metastasis. Examples include emboli of bone marrow following fractures, or trophoblasts from the placenta, a not infrequent occurrence in women and chinchillas. The trophoblast may continue to proliferate in its new location (usually the lung), resulting in a grossly visible, but nonneoplastic, nodule.

While malignant neoplasms have the sinister powers of both invasive and metastatic growth, the **benign neoplasm** is limited to the expansive type of growth. The tumor is able to grow outward, if on a body surface, or to exert expansive pressure against surrounding tissues, but the neoplastic and normal cells remain segregated along a fairly sharp line. Because of its inability to invade, the benign growth is not likely to penetrate a blood vessel, but if some of its cells do chance to be carried

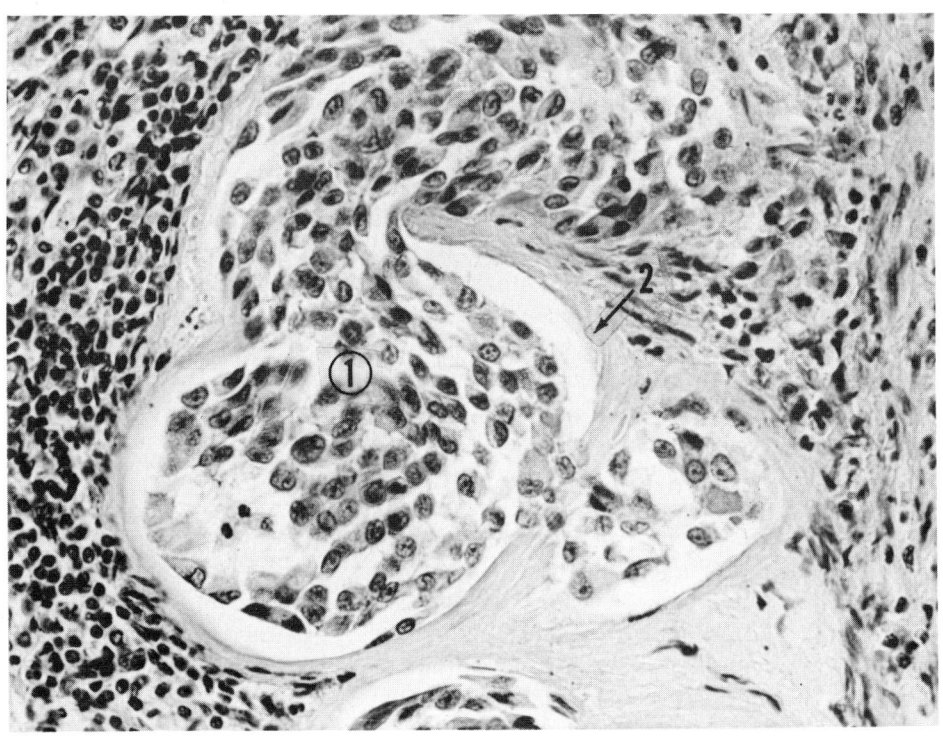

Fig. 4–11. Tumor embolus in a small splenic artery of a dog. The primary site of this undifferentiated carcinoma (1) was not determined. The artery wall is indicated at (2). An infarct resulted from this embolus. (× 350.) (Courtesy of Armed Forces Institute of Pathology.) Contributor: Dr. David E. Lawrence.

about by blood or lymph, they are usually not able to survive in a new location.

Microscopic Appearance. Neoplastic cells resemble cells from which they arose, providing the basis for our system of classification and nomenclature. The neoplastic cells are almost always of a single cell type. Rarely, however, a neoplasm may be composed of two or more types of neoplastic cells, as is the case with mixed tumors of the mammary gland (Figs. 4–14, 25–27). In proportion to their malignancy, tumor cells resemble less and less the histologic tissue from which they arose, even to the point that the tissue of origin cannot be guessed. This quality of not conforming to any histologic prototype in structure, arrangement and staining qualities is called **anaplasia**. Such cells are **anaplastic**, or undifferentiated. The **lack of orderly structural arrangement** will be appreciated by the student after a few tumors have been examined. He will find that, microscopically, the fibrous strands of a fibroblastic tumor run harum-scarum in all directions, and the epithelium of an epidermal tumor is surrounded by connective tissue stroma, whereas the opposite is the normal arrangement.

That the "nonconformist attitude" is not restricted to their physical appearance, but extends to their whole behavior and manner of living, is freely attested by their uncontrollably rapid rate and undisciplined manner of reproduction. It may be supposed that such cells are equally unorthodox in many of their metabolic processes; indeed, that there must be certain basic metabolic aberrations that permit them to flout so successfully what, for other cells, are basic laws. Chemists have found a few differences, the most important of which appears to be the much greater ability of neoplastic tissues to obtain energy by splitting glucose into lactic acid (called glycolysis). This apparently makes them more or less independent of an extensive supply of oxygen, which, to ordinary adult tissues, is essential.

Neoplastic cells lack contact inhibition of normal cells *in vivo* and *in vitro*, and are less tightly adherent to one another than normal cells. This is correlated with a decrease in calcium content in the neoplastic cell membranes and an increase in the negative charge on the cell surface, which might cause the cells to repel one another. The biochemical basis of invasiveness, however, remains unknown. To date, the only means of assessing the degree of malignancy, or indeed, of differentiating between malignant and benign neoplasms remains microscopic examination.

Function. Most neoplasms have no function at all. In general, the less differentiated the neoplasm is morphologically, the less its cells maintain differentiated biochemical functions. The neoplastic cells, however may retain to a greater or lesser degree their original roles. As an example, we see occasionally a tumor (adenoma) of the pancreatic islets. While its cells proliferate in a disorganized manner, they individually have an appearance similar to that of normal cells of the same kind. As islet cells should do, they secrete insulin, producing an excess of this substance with resultant hypoglycemia, which may be fatal. Certain interstitial-cell tumors of the testis have produced hypermasculinity and prostatic hyperplasia. Arrhenoblastomas of the ovary have brought masculinity to the female (human), as do also many adrenocortical tumors (man, bovines). The Sertoli-cell tumor of the dog's testis often has a marked feminizing effect. Adenomas of the thyroid may cause hyperthyroidism (toxic goiter). Several tumors of the hypophysis bring disorders of growth, depending on the particular hormone produced. Adenomas of the parathyroid cause decalcification of bones, hypercalcemia and even renal calculi, through their excessive secretion. Since none of these functions are useful, but often quite the contrary, the original definition of a neoplasm is not violated.

Neoplastic cells may also assume new functions. In man, some neoplasms that are not related to endocrine glands secrete hormones. For example, certain carcinomas of the lung secrete adrenocorticotropic hormone and antidiuretic hormone, and some adenocarcinomas of the colon secrete a substance with parathyroid-hormone activity. Comparable tumors have not been reported in animals. Functional abilities that are not detrimental are also evident in well-differentiated nonhormone-secreting neoplasms. For example, squamous cell carcinomas may produce keratin; osteosarcomas, bone; chondromas, cartilaginous matrix; adenocarcinomas, mucin; and hepatomas, bile.

The connective tissue and vascular stroma of neoplasms are derived from surrounding tissues and expand as the tumor grows, but are not themselves neoplastic, except in rare mixed tumors. The amount of stroma generally resembles that of the tissue of origin. It is usually more abundant in the more slowly growing neoplasms and minimal in rapidly growing neoplasms. Certain malignant epithelial tumors (carcinomas) stimulate connective tissue proliferation such that it may exceed the volume of neoplastic cells, a process referred to as a desmoplastic reaction. Neoplasms are subject to most of the pathologic processes of normal tissues, such as inflammation, necrosis, thrombosis, and infarction.

Gross Appearance. Gross appearances of neoplasms are seldom as informative as one would wish, but a few points will possibly be of assistance. The general conception of a neoplasm as an enlargement is ordinarily applicable, but there are exceptions. Some of the more malignant carcinomas and melanomas may never reach conspicuous size before they kill the patient through the effects of their metastases or by interfering with some vital function, such as the passage of food through the intestine. This remark refers to the primary, or original tumor. The metastatic tumors arising by transfer of cells from the primary are often called secondary tumors.

Cases are not rare in which the patient dies of a metastatic tumor without the primary tumor being discovered, even in a reasonably thorough autopsy. Such a primary neoplasm is referred to as an **occult** neoplasm. For instance, if a rather spherical, circumscribed tumor (these being gross characteristics of a metastatic rather than a primary growth) consisting of mucus-forming glandular epithelium (an adenocarcinoma) is found in the spleen, this is a metastatic tumor, because there is no mucus-forming glandular epithelium in the normal spleen. We must look for the primary tumor where such epithelium normally occurs, for instance, in the gastrointestinal mucosa. Adenocarcinomas of the intestine often consist of little more than a short stretch of annular thickening, and if there is no constriction of the lumen and no ulceration, it is quite possible for the inexperienced prosector to overlook such a tumor. A nicety of expression should be noted here: in this hypothetical case, the neoplasm is a tumor *of* the intestine but the growth in the spleen is not a tumor *of* the spleen; it is still an adenocarcinoma of the intestine, metastatic *in* the spleen. "Of" refers to the site of the primary tumor, always.

In contrast, some neoplasms may reach very large sizes. Before the days of surgical removal, instances were known in which human tumors weighed more than the patient. The same could occur in an animal if its life were conserved with equal care, but usually the daily struggle for food and with enemies terminates life at an earlier stage. Such tumors must obviously be of the benign variety; a malignant tumor would bring death before any such tremendous size was attained.

Tumors of any considerable size cause a bulging of the organ or part involved. This is especially noticeable in tumors arising in or just beneath the skin. Such protruding masses lead eventually to pressure necrosis of the overlying skin or mucous membrane with ulceration and bleeding.

Some malignant neoplasms (carcinomas) of the skin or mucous membranes ulcerate before they reach any noticeable gross proportions. In such cases, the ulcer may be the presenting sign. Benign epithelial tumors (papillomas) protrude in simple or complicated branching forms.

The cut cross-section usually reveals the tumor as a mass of foreign tissue of different color and consistency from that which surrounds it. The color is likely to be white or nearly so. Melanomas are typically black, although some are "amelanotic" and white. A few, such as the interstitial-cell tumor of the testis, are yellow. The consistency may be harder or softer than that of the surrounding tissue; one learns to recognize the tissue of lymphomas by its rather soft, homogeneous, white character. Incision not infrequently reveals hemorrhages, cysts, other special structures, and also areas of necrotic tissue.

Neoplastic tissue, bulging, ulcerated or otherwise, has to be distinguished from inflammatory granulomatous tissues, including those of actinomycosis, tuberculosis, and excessive granulation tissue of wound healing. Sometimes this can be done by the clinical history, the location, or the presence of abscesses, "sulfur granules," or other special structures. In most instances, the decision must await microscopic examination.

Classification of Neoplasms

The resemblance that tumor cells bear to the healthy cells from which they arose is the basis for our system or classification and nomenclature of neoplasms. Other systems of classification have been proposed, including an etiologic classification, but to date classification by histogenesis is the most satisfactory. There are many different kinds of neoplasms, corresponding to almost every type of cell recognized in histology. In addition, there are several tumors that are traceable, not to any tissue found in normal histology, but to a type of tissue occurring only at a certain stage of embryonal development.

Classification of neoplasms according to the different histologic types is of more than academic importance, for the various types differ greatly in their clinical course and effect on the patient, as well as in their responsiveness to various forms of treatment. Thus, it is the correlation of microscopic characteristics with clinical behavior that becomes the purpose of classification. Despite the generalities already described, certain tumors may be anaplastic or undifferentiated and behave relatively benignly, and some histologically benign tumors may be quick to metastasize.

Tumors are named for the cell or tissue of origin with an appropriate suffix to denote whether the neoplasm is benign or malignant. The suffix -oma, meaning tumor, is used for benign neoplasms of epithelial or mesenchymal origin. Thus a benign tumor of fibroblasts is a fibroma; of smooth muscle, a leiomyoma; of cartilage, a chondroma; and so forth. Epithelial neoplasms of glandular tissue are called adenomas, e.g., apocrine gland adenoma and mammary gland adenoma. Occasionally, adeno- is not included in the name, as in a benign neoplasm of hepatocytes called a hepatoma. For certain neoplasms, owing to convention or rules of etymology, -oma is not used, as for example, mast cell tumor or basal cell tumor.

If the neoplasm is malignant, the suffix -oma is preceded by the prefix carcin-, if the tumor is of epithelial origin, or sarc- if of mesenchymal origin. Thus, a malignant neoplasm of a glandular tissue is an adenocarcinoma; of fibroblasts, a fibrosarcoma. As with benign tumors, sometimes the carcin- or sarc- is eliminated and the word "malignant" substituted in the name, as with malignant melanoma or malignant lymphoma. A histologic classification of selected neoplasms is presented in Table 4–1.

Differentiation Between Benign and Malignant Neoplasms

From what has been said of the respective effects of benign and malignant neoplasms, it is obvious that one of the first

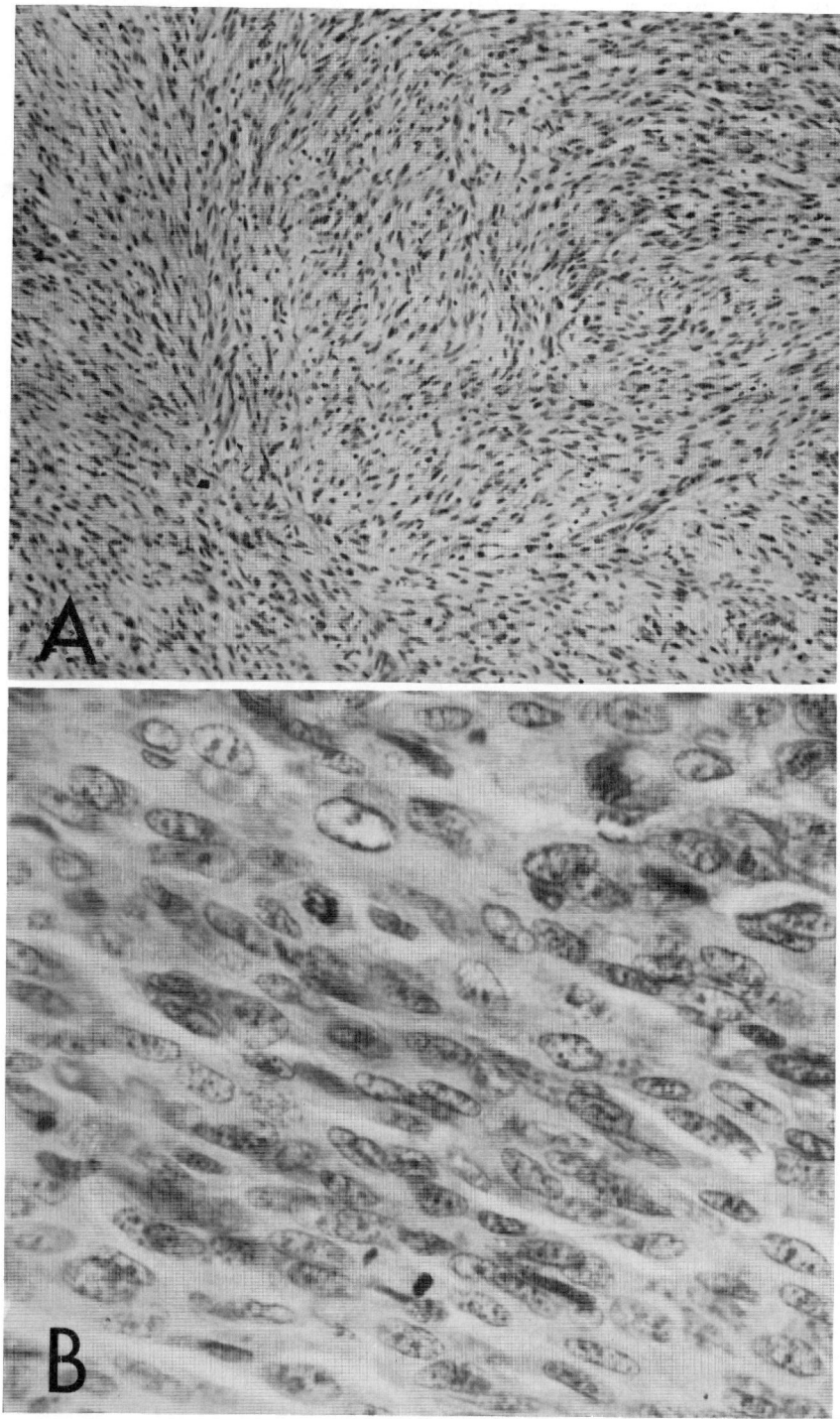

Fig. 4–12. Fibrosarcoma. The tissue and cells bear a resemblance to normal fibrous connective tissue. The pattern of growth, however, is disorganized, as evident in *A*, and the cells depicted in *B* are more plump and their nuclei more vesicular. (*B* Courtesy of Armed Forces Institute of Pathology.)

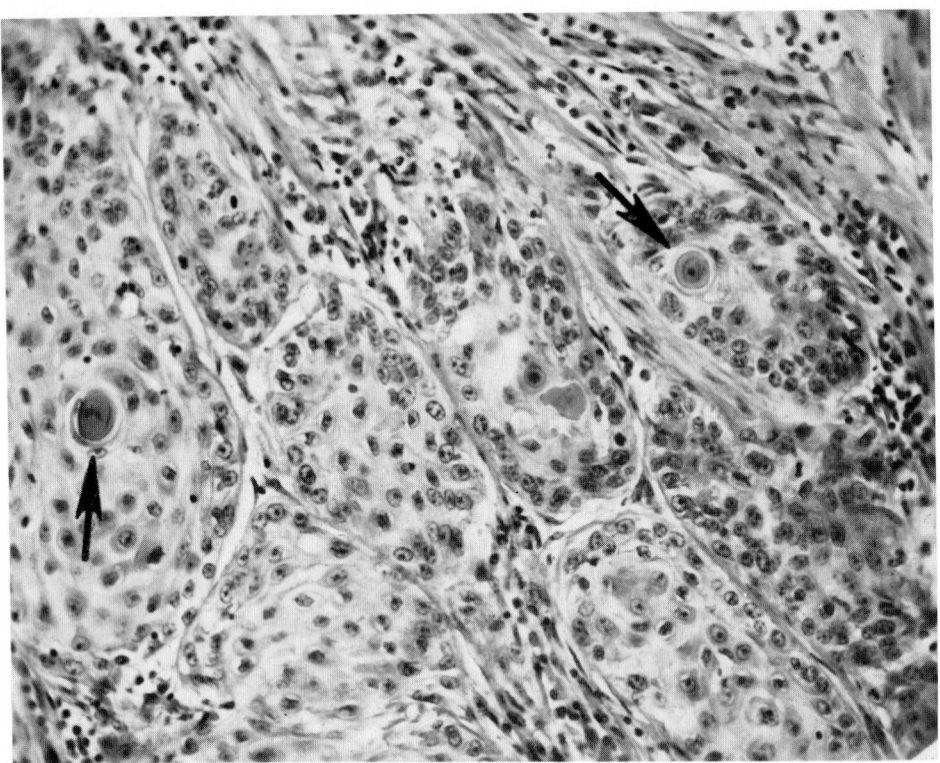

Fig. 4–13. Squamous cell carcinoma. The cells resemble normal squamous epithelium and mature from a basal layer through keratinization. Note keratin pearls (arrows). The pattern of growth, however, is disorganized. (Courtesy of Armed Forces Institute of Pathology.)

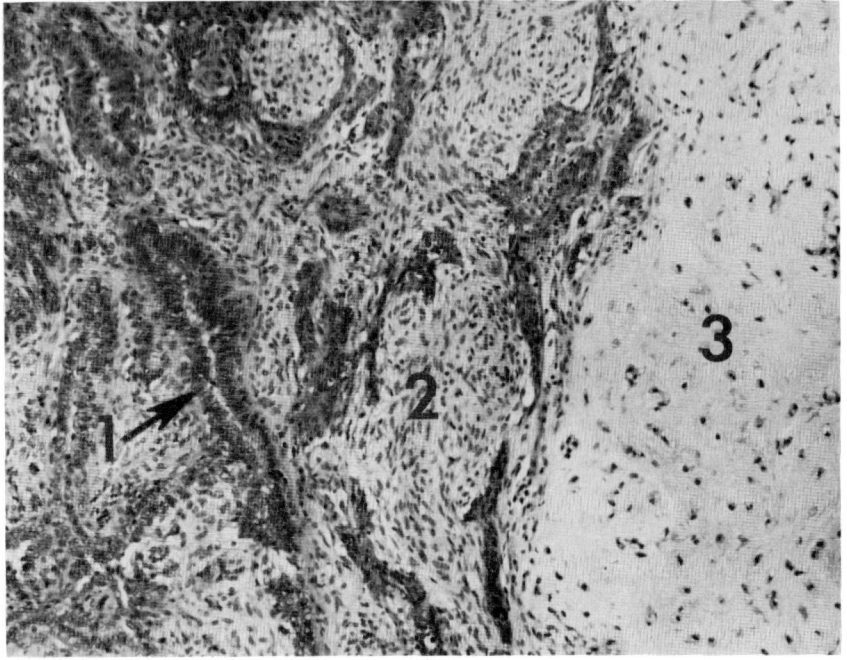

Fig. 4–14. Some neoplasms contain more than one type of neoplastic cell. In this mixed tumor of mammary gland from a dog, there are epithelial (1), myoepithelial (2) and cartilaginous components (3).

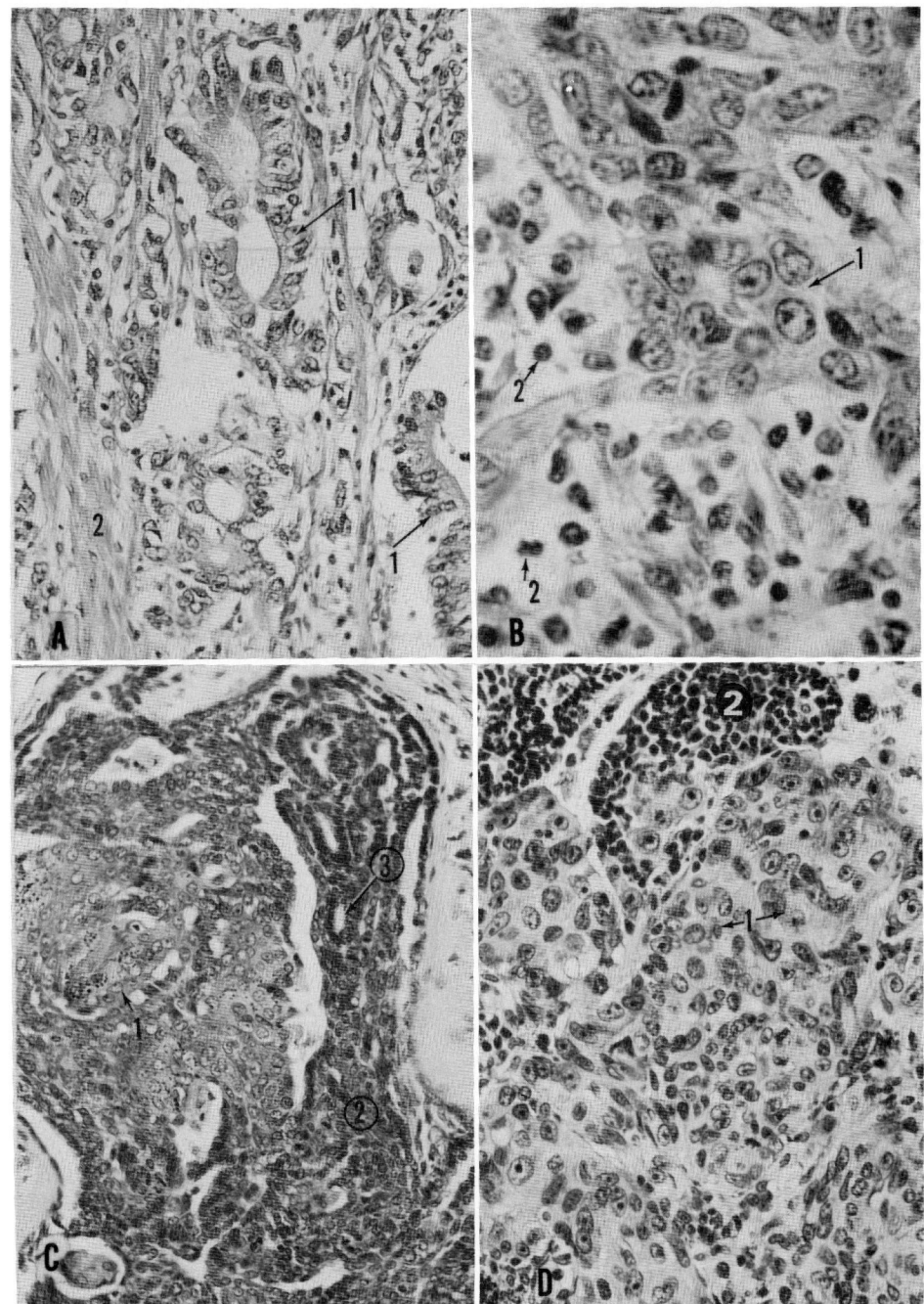

Fig. 4–15. Differences in the microscopic appearance of adenocarcinoma. *A*, Adenocarcinoma arising in the gastric mucosa and invading the stomach wall in an eight-year-old female Boston terrier. Neoplastic cells (*1*) form irregular acini as they invade the muscularis (*2*). Contributor: Dr. A. E. Rappoport. *B*, Undifferentiated cells (*1*) and lymphocytes (*2*) in an adenocarcinoma (× 750) in the mammary gland of a 25-year-old mare. Contributor: Dr. C. L. Davis. *C*, Squamous cells (*1*), solid nests (*2*) and acini (*3*) in an adenocanthoma of the mammary gland of a six-year-old female English setter. Contributor: Angell Memorial Animal Hospital. *D*, Solid nests of carcinoma cells (*1*) (medullary carcinoma) in a lymph node (*2*) metastasis of a primary adenocarcinoma of bile ducts of a 15-year-old beagle. (Courtesy of Armed Forces Institute of Pathology.) Contributor: Dr. D. N. Bader.

125

Table 4–1. Nomenclature of Selected Neoplasms

Tissue	Benign Tumor	Malignant Tumor
Connective Tissue		
Adult fibrous tissue	Fibroma	Fibrosarcoma
Embryonic fibrous tissue	Myxoma	Myxosarcoma
Cartilage	Chondroma	Chondrosarcoma
Bone	Osteoma	Osteosarcoma
Adipose tissue	Lipoma	Liposarcoma
Histiocytes	Histiocytoma	Malignant histiocytoma
Mast cells	Mast cell tumor	Malignant mast cell tumor
Endothelium		
Blood vessels	Hemangioma	Hemangioendothelioma (Hemangiosarcoma)
Lymph vessels	Lymphangioma	Lymphangiosarcoma
Muscle		
Smooth muscle	Leiomyoma	Leiomyosarcoma
Striated muscle	Rhabdomyoma	Rhabdomyosarcoma
Hematopoietic Tissue		
Erythroblasts	None	Erythroid leukemia
Myeloblasts	None	Myeloid leukemia
Lymphatic Tissue	None	Malignant lymphoma
Lymphoblasts		Lymphocytic (blastic) leukemia
Neural Tissue		
Glia	Glioma	Glioblastoma
Neurons	None	Neuroblastoma
Nerve sheath	Neurilemoma (Neurofibroma)	Neurogenic sarcoma (Neurofibrosarcoma)
Melanocytes	?	Malignant melanoma
Epithelium		
Squamous epithelium	Papilloma	Squamous cell carcinoma
Transitional epithelium	Papilloma	Transitional cell carcinoma
Glandular epithelium	Adenoma	Adenocarcinoma
Tumors Containing More Than One Neoplastic Cell Type		
Ovary	Teratoma	Malignant teratoma
Kidney	—	Embryonal nephroma
Mammary gland	—	Mixed mammary tumor
Salivary gland	—	Mixed tumor of salivary gland
Sweat gland	—	Mixed tumor of sweat gland

questions to be settled when neoplastic disease is encountered is that of whether the tumor is benign or malignant. Since this is commonly impossible by clinical examination alone, the task ordinarily falls to the pathologist.

It should be emphasized, however, that the benign and malignant classes are not set apart by an iron-clad boundary. Benignity is a relative quality, and certainly there are all degrees of malignancy. Still, it is possible in more than 90% of cases to predict the clinical behavior of a tumor from its histologic structure and other characteristics. (See Table 4–2.) The clinician will learn some things from the gross appearance of the tumor; the pathologist will determine more by applying the microscopic criteria of malignancy; but our most effective aid at times is a personal acquaintance with the characteristic life-history of each tumor entity. For instance, it is well known

Table 4–2. Comparison of Benign and Malignant Neoplasms

Characteristic	Benign	Malignant
Growth rate	Slow	Rapid
Growth limits	Circumscribed	Unrestricted
Mode of growth	Expansion	Invasion
Differentiation	Good	Anaplastic
Stroma	Usually abundant	Usually scant
Metastasis	None	Frequent
Recurrence	Rare	Frequent

that the usual carcinoma of the bovine orbit is prone to cause great destruction by direct invasion into surrounding tissues, but seldom metastasizes. This encourages the surgeon to hope for a complete cure in cases in which complete removal is possible. On the other hand, a similarly well-differentiated adenocarcinoma of the

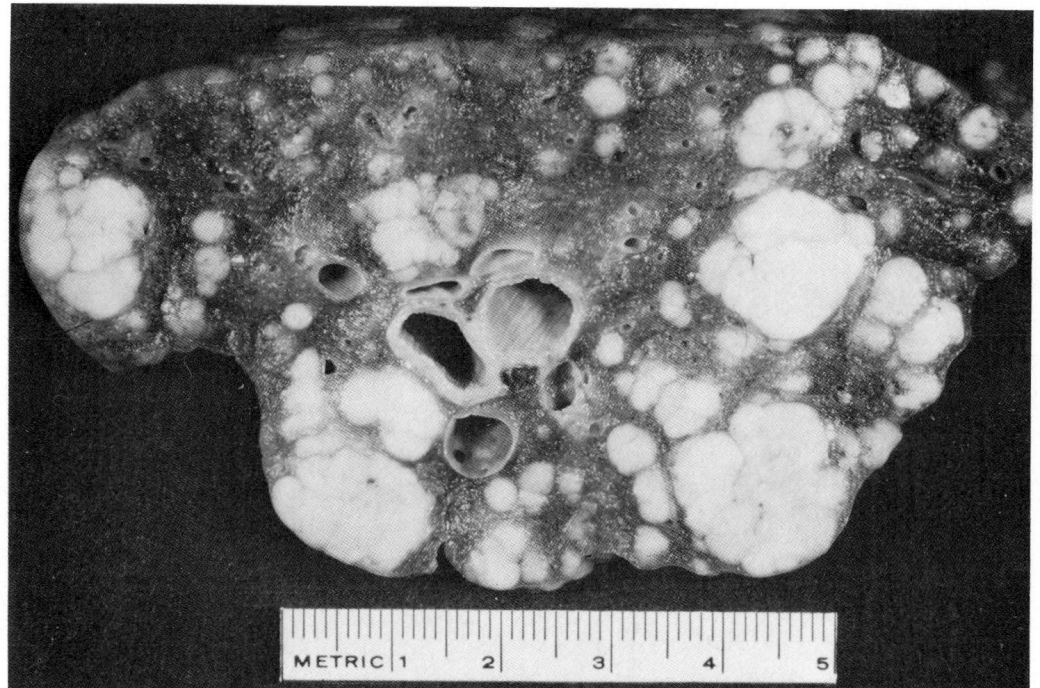

Fig. 4–16. Metastases in the lung from adenocarcinoma of the thyroid of an eight-year-old male Irish setter. Note that the single and confluent nodules are not all the same size. (Courtesy of Angell Memorial Animal Hospital.)

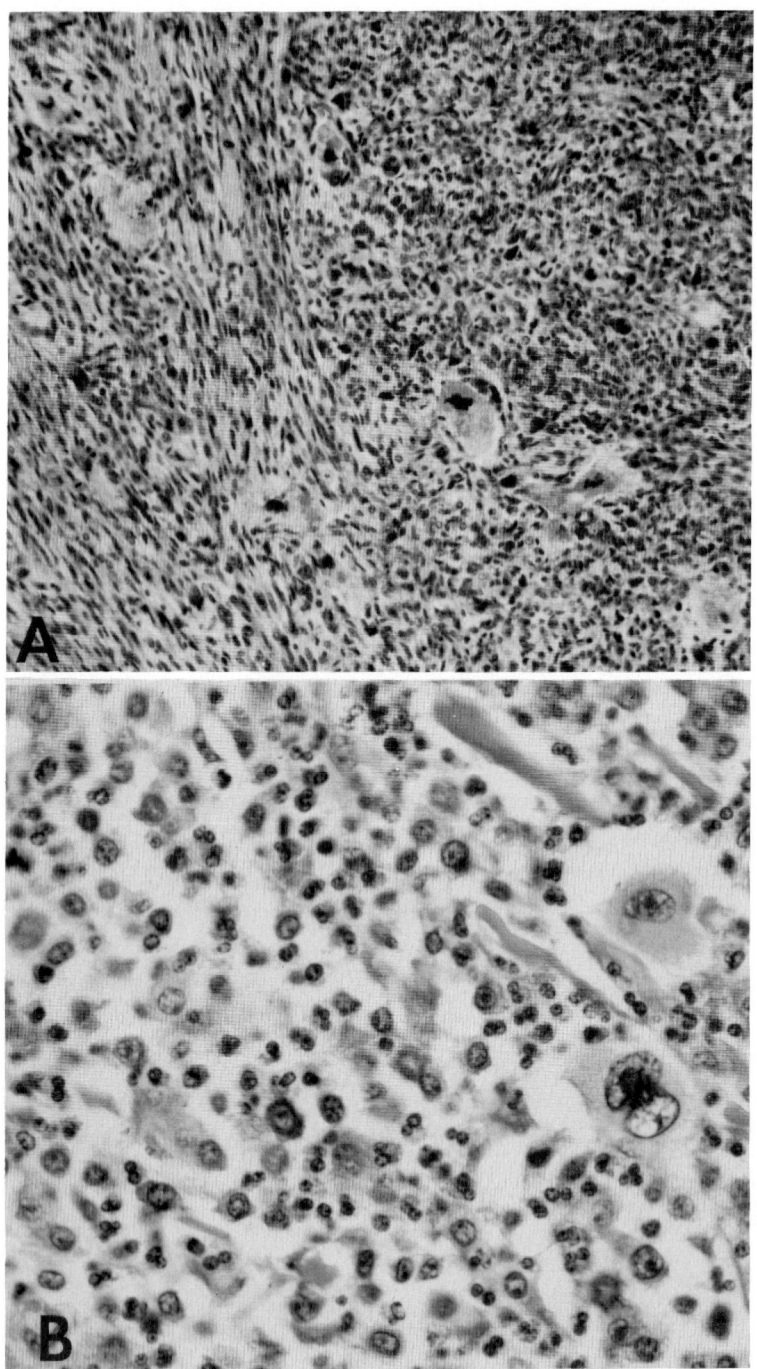

Fig. 4–17. Pleomorphism and tumor giant cells are often features of malignancy. *A*, Fibrosarcoma with disorderly pattern of growth and cellular pleomorphism. (Courtesy of Harvard Medical School.) *B*, Tumor giant cells in a canine mast cell tumor. (Courtesy of Armed Forces Institute of Pathology.)

canine mammary gland offers a much poorer prognosis. As another example, a seminoma in the dog has about the same histologic appearance as its human counterpart, but metastasis is much less likely than it is reputed to be in the human. Hopefully, more and better recorded observations on the outcome of tumors will bring a more accurate knowledge of many of them.

Microscopic Appearance. There are several accepted criteria to be considered in estimating the degree of malignancy of a neoplasm. The fundamental measure of malignancy is the **degree of anaplasia**, meaning the extent to which the neoplastic tissue diverges from the normal histologic pattern for the kind of tissue in question. Some tumors resemble the normal histology closely in the shape, size, and staining reactions of the cells and their nuclei, and are put together in a way that simulates closely the architecture of the parent tissue. These are usually benign. Proportionately as these characteristics deviate from the normal and as the neoplastic cells cease to resemble the normal or as they come to resemble the embryonal stages of such cells, so the degree of malignancy rises. Such growths are said to be anaplastic, or undifferentiated.

The **mode of growth** is of prime importance. If metastases are known to have occurred, the question of malignancy is obviously settled. If any extensive invasion can be demonstrated, the tumor is malignant. This criterion is useful especially in the early stages of epithelial tumors; if it can be shown that the neoplastic epithelial cells have infiltrated below the basement membrane, or the basal line where a theoretic basement membrane separates epithelium from connective tissue stroma, the tumor is malignant, a carcinoma. Some epithelial growths are characterized by extensive projections, with crowded folds and many subdivisions. These may project into the lumina of glands (prostate, mammary) or ducts, or into cystic structures, presenting a startling and bizarre appearance. If it can be shown that the epithelium always remains above the line corresponding to a basement membrane and does not infiltrate, the neoplasm is to be classed as benign. Indeed, the disorder may be only hyperplasia, as in the hyperplastic thyroid of cretinism.

The **degree of cellularity** is important in fibrous and similar neoplasms. Nuclei that are closely spaced, suggesting a large number of cells per unit of area, indicate malignancy.

If the **nuclei tend to be hyperchromatic**, taking a stronger nuclear stain (such as hematoxylin) than usual, they are thus more like embryonic cells, hence probably malignant. Nuclei of unusually large size are also significant.

Numerous mitotic figures (nuclei in some stage of mitosis) mean rapid growth, and the tumor is probably malignant. The kind of tumor is important here. Some characteristically show many mitoses; others do not, even though malignant.

Abnormal mitotic figures, such as division into three daughter nuclei instead of two, occur in some malignant tumors, and are significant if recognized.

Gross Appearance. These criteria afford some assistance in determining whether a tumor is benign or malignant. If it is growing on a surface and is pedunculated (attached only by a narrow neck), it is in all probability benign. Sessile tumors (relatively flat and having a broad base) are much more likely to be malignant. The rate of growth may also reflect degree of malignancy. Benign tumors generally grow slowly, and malignant tumors, rapidly. Ulceration is somewhat suggestive of malignancy, but may occur in either kind. Within the tissues, the tumor may have a distinct fibrous capsule. Such a tumor is probably benign. In the process of removal, the well-encapsulated, benign tumor may "shell out," like peas from the pod, leaving the smooth inner lining of the capsule. The physical examination should, of course, include careful examination for metastases in the regional lymph nodes and other accessible sites. Recurrence following surgical removal is much more frequent with malignant tumors than with benign tumors.

When tumors are encountered in such organs as lungs, liver, kidney, and spleen, the question arises whether they are **primary or metastatic**. The form of the growth is usually significant. Primary neoplasms are seldom regular in shape or smooth in outline. Metastatic growths, though obviously malignant, grow largely by expansion and produce a more or less spherical tumor. If more than one are present, one recalls the extreme improbability of several similar primary tumors developing in the same organ at the same time. If more than one organ is involved some, perhaps all, of the growths are metastatic.

General Characteristics of Mesenchymal and Epithelial Neoplasms

Mesenchymal Neoplasm. The major mesenchymal neoplasms are presented in Table 4–1. Further subdivisions and complete descriptions of each are presented in appropriate chapters. Benign mesenchymal tumors, almost without exception, closely resemble their tissue of origin in structure and functional products, and do not present major difficulties to diagnosis. Caution is required to differentiate nonneoplastic proliferations, such as granulation tissue from fibroma, or fibroma from leiomyoma, but gross and microscopic characteristics are usually adequate. The majority of malignant mesenchymal tumors (sarcomas) also resemble their tissue of origin, and do not present major diagnostic problems, but as to be expected, many lack morphologic individuality even to the point of making the differentiation of sarcoma from carcinoma difficult. In contrast to carcinomas, sarcomas display greater pleomorphism. Nuclei vary in size and shape, and multinucleated tumor giant cells are more frequent in sarcomas than in carcinomas. As discussed earlier, sar-

comas almost always metastasize by way of blood vessels.

Epithelial Neoplasms. Nomenclature of epithelial neoplasms is presented in Table 4–1. Specific neoplasms are described in chapters dealing with specific systems.

Benign neoplasms of epithelia are almost always well differentiated, and where present, well confined by basement membranes. Diagnosis is usually straightforward and obviously limited to the cell types present in the particular locale of the neoplasm. Malignant epithelial neoplasms (carcinomas) also usually resemble the parent tissue, but in some cases de-differentiation is so great as to preclude diagnosis. In these cases, special stains for cell products such as mucin, or ultrastructural examination for such characteristics as desmosomes may be helpful. Carcinomas usually metastasize by way of lymphatics, with the exception of carcinomas of the liver and kidney.

Causes of Neoplasms

Some specific causes of neoplasms have been identified, but the cause of most neoplasms is not known. Their elusive etiology is partly due to the fact that in most cases the cause is probably multifactorial. This is well exemplified by examining mammary adenocarcinoma in mice caused by virus, but different strains of mice vary in susceptibility, and under natural conditions, the virus rarely causes disease in male mice, while the incidence of cancer in female mice is greater in animals which have undergone one or more pregnancies. Thus, in addition to the virus, development of the mammary adenocarcinoma depends upon genotype, sex, and hormonal stimulation. Similar multifactorial correlations have been established for many neoplastic diseases.

Causally related factors that will be addressed include the following:
1. Fetal rests
2. Physical agents
   a. Chronic irritation
   b. Ionizing irradiation

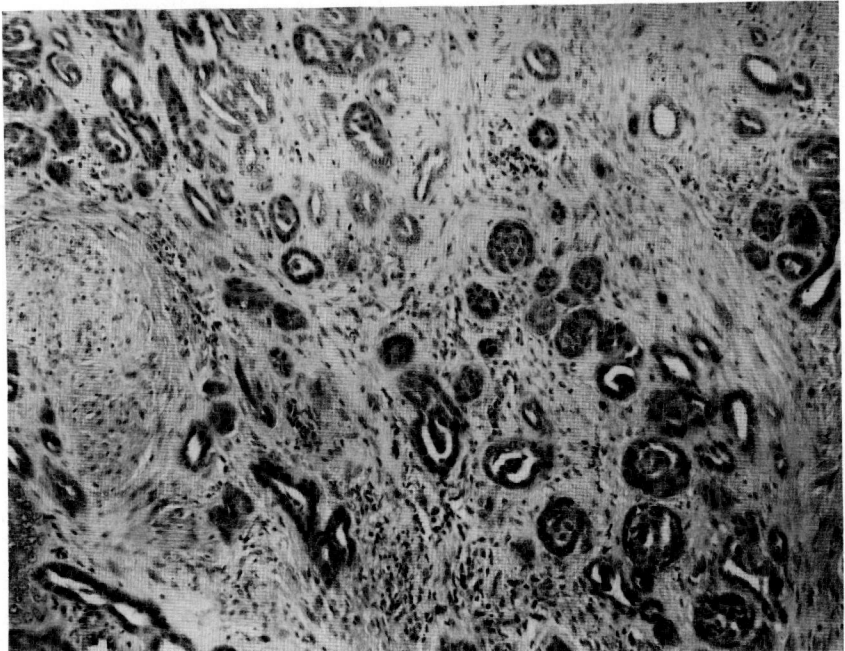

Fig. 4–18. Desmoplasia. Many epithelial neoplasms incite a proliferation of collagenous connective tissue. Such tumors are referred to as scirrhous. This is an example of a scirrhous adenocarcinoma of the canine mammary gland. Scirrhous adenocarcinomas are also seen in other locations, for example, the stomach and bovine uterus.

3. Chemical agents
4. Biologic agents
   a. Parasites
   b. Viruses
5. Hormones
6. Heredity
7. Age

Fetal Rests. Earlier students of neoplasia noticed that most neoplastic cells were remarkably similar in their microscopic appearance to their embryonal predecessors, and were inclined to view this feature in a causative light. They found, on rare occasions, neoplasms developing from islands of unmatured and undifferentiated tissues, or even what appeared to be tissues that should have formed one organ but were entrapped within another. The best example was the supposed inclusion within the kidney of tissue which, on the basis of similarity, should have been a part of the adrenal gland, the tumor being the well-known hypernephroma. From such

instances, fetal misplacements, fetal rests, and fetal inclusions were postulated to be the causes of neoplasms, **Cohnheim's theory of fetal residues.** A pronounced form of such misplacement of embryonal tissues is the teratoma, a slowly enlarging mass containing several histologic types of tissue. Such disorders of embryonal and fetal development do occur, areas of persistent embryonal tissue not being altogether rare in the young. The incidence of active neoplasia in such areas appears to be high, but it is by no means universal, and a direct causal relationship is no longer credited.

Physical Agents. Chronic Irritation. This came to occupy a prominent place in theories that were prevalent for many years, Virchow being one of its leading proponents. It was early observed that the incidence of squamous cell carcinoma was higher in scars resulting from severe burns, branding of cattle, and other injuries than in normal skin. What constituted the chronic irritation following apparently successful healing and the appearance of the neoplasm, or why the epithelium was different, was difficult to explain. It was observed that among the people of Khurdistan, India, carcinoma of the skin of the anterior abdominal wall is frequent, although almost unknown in other races and nationalities. These people have a custom of carrying a pot filled with live coals or hot stones resting on the anterior belly wall. A causative relationship seemed obvious, apparently in terms of heat and pressure, but it is difficult to rule out chemical carcinogens.

Similarly, the incidence of cutaneous neoplasms on the feet and legs appears to be much higher among bare-foot peoples than in the races whose feet are clad. At least such were the findings of Vos (1936), who reported 33.4% of all cutaneous carcinomas and 82.5% of malignant melanomas were on the feet or legs of Javanese natives, the corresponding figures in Holland being 0.7% and 22.5% respectively. Whether the feet and legs were exposed to any other irritant than physical trauma would be a matter for speculation.

No corresponding observations on animals have been compiled, but against the theory that ordinary mechanical injury, even though persistently repeated, causes neoplasia is the experience with millions of horses that have been used as draft animals. Injury and chronic ulcerated areas from pressure of the collar were unfortunately everyday occurrences in the days of horse-drawn implements and vehicles, but neoplasia at that site remained practically unknown.

The present tendency is to eliminate ordinary physical injury as a cause of neoplasia, but the same may not be said of certain other factors in the local environment.

Ionizing Irradiation. All forms of ionizing irradiation are carcinogenic. It is generally accepted that exposure to the ultraviolet rays of sunlight is responsible for the fact that as many as 90% of human cutaneous tumors occur on the unclothed parts of the body. The backs of the hands of many outdoor workers show areas of hyperkeratosis and hyperpigmentation which, in a certain number of instances, progress to carcinomas. Statistics show that such neoplasms are more frequent in the sun-drenched Southwest than in the more somber parts of the United States. Exposure to solar ultraviolet light causes a similar situation in cattle—ocular and periocular squamous cell carcinoma in white-faced Hereford cattle in the Southwest.

Human beings suffer from a rare disease, hereditarily recessive, called xeroderma pigmentosum (a pigmented, dry skin), in which owing to a great sensitivity to light, a dermatitis terminating in fatal carcinomatosis is inescapable before more than a few years of life have passed.

Ultraviolet rays have low penetrance, and neoplasms resulting from chronic exposure are limited to exposed surfaces. It is believed to cause its effects by molecular excitation of nucleic acid, leading to alteration and mutation of DNA.

Other forms of ionizing irradiation include gamma rays, x-rays, alpha particles, beta particles, and neutrons, all of which have been causally related to carcinogenesis. Roentgen rays (x-rays) are notorious for their carcinogenic effect when total exposure is excessive over an extended period of time, as in x-ray technicians, who, in the early history of roentgenology, worked without protective clothing or other safety devices. Ample experimental studies have confirmed these clinical observations. There is chronic dermatitis, then ulceration, and finally some of the ulcers develop into carcinomas, the whole process usually requiring several years.

Radium and thorium, when accidentally or experimentally introduced into the body, localize in the bone and produce chronic osteitis, in which osteosarcoma supervenes. The first knowledge of this fact came when it was found, as reported by

Martland (1931), that persons engaged in painting a radioactive preparation on watch dials to make them luminous, died of osteogenic sarcoma a few years later. Chronic or multiple exposures are much more apt to lead to neoplasia than a single exposure of the same magnitude. Although tumors of most types have been associated with irradiation, exposure to ionizing radiaton of high penetrating power is most often associated with various hematopoietic tumors (leukemias), and those of low penetrability, with tumors of the skin. The mechanism of carcinogenesis is believed to result from permanent aberrations in DNA. Another mechanism, however, is the activation of latent oncogenic viruses, which has been demonstrated in mice.

Chemical Carcinogens. The earliest evidence for chemical carcinogenesis was described in 1775 by Sir Percivall Pott. He observed that chimney-sweeps in London had a high incidence of carcinomas of the scrotum, which was almost unknown in other men. The carcinogenic nature of soot and gaseous products of combustion was unknown at that time, and the cause was explained as "chronic irritation." As tars and oils found more uses in our industrial age, the suspicion arose that neoplasms might result from contact with them. A number of persons attempted to demonstrate this experimentally. In 1915, two Japanese, Yamagiwa and Ichikawa, finally succeeded in producing cutaneous papillomas and carcinomas in the ears of rabbits after repeated applications of coal tar throughout a period of many months. Many similar experiments by various researchers brought out the fact that mice are readily susceptible to "tar cancer," rabbits somewhat less so, the other common laboratory animals being more refractory. Chemists naturally set out to discover the exact compounds or radicals that exert the carcinogenic effect. The first chemically pure hydrocarbons found to be carcinogenic were derivatives of 1:2-benzanthracene, such as 1:2:5:6-dibenzanthracene, the most powerful being 9:10-dimethyl-1:2-benzanthracene:

Another outstanding carcinogenic derivative is methylcholanthrene:

This substance has been directly synthesized and has also been prepared from cholic and desoxycholic acids of bile. This and the fact that desoxycholic acid itself has shown some carcinogenic effect have led to the suspicion that carcinogenic substances of similar composition may possibly be formed in animal tissues.

The list of chemical carcinogens has since expanded and includes a wide variety of diverse compounds, including polycyclic aromatic hydrocarbons, aromatic amines, alkylating agents, nitrosamines, natural products (see aflatoxins), azo dyes, and a multitude of others. Some of these act directly (direct-acting carcinogens or **proximal carcinogens**), such as alkylating agents, and others require enzymatic conversion within the body to an active form (**procarcinogens** or **distal carcinogens**), such as aromatic amines. They bind to nucleic acids, a process which may then lead to neoplastic transformation. There is usually a significant time lapse or latent period, often years, between exposure and the appearance of tumors. Carcinogenesis is dose-dependent, but once established, the continued presence of the carcinogen is not necessary, as it is with oncogenic viruses.

In general, chemical carcinogens produce carcinomas when applied externally to the epidermis, sarcomas when introduced into the connective tissues. However, the relative susceptibility or resistance of the various tissues is a factor, and under some circumstances, a carcinogenic substance causes neoplasia of a certain organ regardless of where or how it is introduced into the body. This is illustrated by the work of Orr (1943), who regularly produced carcinomas of the mammary glands of suitably susceptible mice by applying the carcinogen to the nasal mucosa. A few types of carcinogen appear to have a positive predilection for a particular organ or tissue, as, for instance, o-aminoazotoluene (used for dying leather) and other azo-compounds, which produce epithelial tumors of the liver when introduced in a variety of ways. On the other hand, the type of tumor produced sometimes appears to vary with the species of experimental animal, as in the work of Rigdon (1952), who produced cutaneous hemangiomas by the local application of methylcholanthrene to the skin of ducks, but obtained carcinomas when chickens were given the same treatment. All these differences probably depend on variations in susceptibility, which will be discussed shortly.

Biologic Agents. Parasites. As agents setting up irritation which may lead to neoplasia, parasites deserve some attention. Bilharziasis, better known as schistosomiasis *(Schistosoma hematobium)*, has been considered a cause of carcinoma of the human bladder, especially since the two conditions occur together and the incidence of carcinoma of the bladder is high in those populations (Egypt) which are heavily parasitized. The blood flukes produce considerable cystitis of a chronic nature, but they are not universally accepted as causing the neoplasms.

The small nematode *Gonglyonema (Spiroptera) neoplasticum*, which parasitizes the wall of the rat's stomach, occasions the development of carcinoma or a carcinoma-like proliferation of the gastric mucosa. The tumors were produced experimentally by Fibiger (1914) and what he considered pulmonary metastases occurred in some cases. More recently, some other plausible explanations have been offered for the pulmonary growths, causing some belief that the gastric tumors were really no more than inflammatory hyperplasia similar to that occurring in coccidiosis of the rabbit's gallbladder. There is also evidence that deficiency of vitamin A may have been an important factor in the production of these hyperplasias (Hitchcock and Bell, 1952).

Cysticercus fasciolaris, the cystic, or larval, stage of the tapeworm of the cat, *Taenia crassicolis (taeniaeformis)*, developing in the liver of rats, either naturally or experimentally, results in what some consider true sarcomatous proliferation of the connective tissue which surrounds the parasitic cysts (Bullock and Curtis, 1920; Dunning and Curtis, 1939, 1946).

In the dog, a nematode that is rather common in warm countries, *Spirocerca lupi,* invades the wall of the lower esophagus. One or more worms are often found at the center of spheroidal fibrous tumor, 1 or 2 cm. in diameter. These tumors, obviously resulting from the worm's presence, usually have the histologic structure of fibrosarcomas or osteosarcomas (metaplasia of fibrous tissue to bone). They commonly form a large mass extending into the mediastinal tissue and ulcerating on the esophageal surface. A number of them have been reported as metastasizing to the lungs (Seibold, et al., 1955) and other viscera. The evidence that the embedded worms have a causal relationship appears incontrovertible.

The occurrence of true neoplasia in connection with metazoan parasites is thus an apparent fact at present. If true carcinogenic effect is present we do not know whether it is physical or chemical.

Oncogenic Viruses. It has been known since 1908 that extracts of animal tumors, filtered to be free of cells and bacteria, were capable of inducing new tumors upon injection into a suitable host. The first such demonstration of a tumor-inducing (oncogenic) virus in avian leukosis was the work of Ellermann and Bang. Rous, in 1910, produced similar results with the fowl (Rous) sarcoma. These demonstrations of viral-associated neoplasms have been followed over the years by many others, as outlined in Table 4–3.

The evidence is overwhelming, therefore, that certain viruses can cause tumors in birds, invertebrates, and mammals. Incontrovertible proof is only lacking in man because of the difficulties and proscriptions in experimenting with the human species.

Oncogenic viruses may be either DNA- or RNA-containing viruses. Oncogenic RNA viruses are all classed as a single group called oncornaviruses or ret-

roviruses. Oncogenic DNA viruses include members of the *Herpesviruses, Poxviruses, Adenoviruses,* and *Papovaviruses.* With most oncogenic DNA viruses, infection of cells is followed either by production of new virions or a nonproductive infection in which the virus becomes masked, and which may lead to transformation to neoplasia. The viral DNA either becomes incorporated into the cell genome or exits as episomal DNA. In either case, it is passed on to all future generations of cells and must be continuously present. Experimentally purified viral DNA, in the absence of whole virus, is capable of causing neoplasia. Cells infected with RNA oncogenic viruses continuously produce viral particles after inducing neoplastic transformation, but without leading to cell lysis. These viral particles contain an enzyme, reverse transcriptase, which is capable of converting RNA into DNA, which then

Table 4–3. Some Viral-Induced Neoplasms

Year	Species	Type of Neoplasms	Author
1908	Chicken	Fowl leukosis	Ellermann and Bang
1910	Chicken	Fowl sarcoma	Rous
1920	Cow	Bovine papilloma	Magalhaes
1932	Dog	Oral papilloma	DeMonbreun and Goodpasture
1932	Rabbit	Fibroma	Shope
1933	Rabbit	Cutaneous papilloma	Shope
1933	Chicken	Lymphomatosis, myelomatosis	Furth
1936	Mouse	Mammary adenocarcinoma	Bittner
1938	Frog	Renal adenocarcinoma	Lucké
1943	Rabbit	Oral papilloma	Parsons and Kidd
1951	Horse	Cutaneous papilloma	Cook and Olson
1951	Mouse	Malignant lymphoma	Gross
1953	Mouse	Tumor of parotid gland	Gross
1953	Squirrel	Fibroma	Kilham, Herman, and Fisher
1954	Goat	Cutaneous papilloma	Moulton
1955	Deer	Fibroma	Shope et al.
1957	Mouse, hamster	Polyoma	Stewart and Eddy
1964	Cat	Malignant lymphoma	Jarrett et al.
1964	Rodents	Sarcoma	Harvey
1966	Mouse	Osteosarcoma	Finkel, Biskis, and Jinkins
1967	Guinea pig	Malignant lymphoma	Opler
1967	Mouse	Leukemia	Friend
1969	Simian primates	Malignant lymphoma	Melendez et al.
1969	Cat	Sarcoma	Snyder and Theilen
1971	Simian primates	Sarcoma	Theilen et al.

controls transformation. Oncogenic viruses and their respective neoplasms are discussed further in Chapter 9.

Hormones. Some investigators have been impressed by the similarity of the structural formulas of the carcinogenic hydrocarbons, such as benzanthracene and cholanthrene, to those of certain hormones produced in the body, particularly ovarian follicular estrogens, progesterone of the corpus luteum, testosterone of the testis, and the corticosterones of the adrenal gland, and have theorized that disordered metabolism of these hormones may result in their transformation into carcinogenic compounds. There is no real evidence that this happens, however, and the similarity of the formulas would appear to be no greater than that which exists between various carcinogenic and noncarcinogenic members of the anthracene or benzpyrene groups themselves.

The chemical relationship between the carcinogenic hydrocarbons and the bile acids has been mentioned. Here, again, any spontaneous transformation into carcinogenic substances remains hypothetical.

Limited experimentation has been reported on the production of neoplasms by the administration of massive doses of the estrogenic hormones. It appears that such hormones are able to induce hyperplastic and even neoplastic growth of the interstitial cells of the testes of mice. It has recently been shown in human beings that the administration of diethylstilbestrol during pregnancy is associated with an increased incidence of clear adenocarcinoma of the uterus in the children some 20 years later. There are reports of similar effects in other organs normally under hormonal control, such as the prostate.

Heredity. The vast amount of experimentation on this aspect of neoplasia, conducted chiefly in mice, has shown that whether one of the recognized carcinogens actually produces a tumor depends on the relative susceptibility of the individual.

The susceptibility or the lack of it is transmitted from one generation to the next. For instance, certain strains of mice are highly susceptible to carcinoma of the skin, but resistant to other types. Other strains have been bred which have a high susceptibility to mammary adenocarcinoma. Some families have a high resistance to all forms. These characteristics are thus to be considered hereditary, although neoplasms themselves are not inherited. Thus, it is inheritance of factors that control the susceptibility to various carcinogens which is the important point. This may be as simple as the inheritance of light skin color, predisposing to ultraviolet-light-induced skin cancer, or the susceptibility to a known oncogenic virus, but more often than not, the fundamental basis for decreased or increased susceptibility is not known. The high incidence of neoplasia in boxer dogs is an example of the latter. More will be said about the incidence of neoplasia in different species and breeds later.

Age. Most neoplasms occur with greater frequency in older animals. Whether this reflects an inherent change in cellular metabolism, the opportunity for a proper latent period, or an increased opportunity for exposure to carcinogens is not known. Most likely, all three factors are operant. Certain tumors, however, occur with greater frequency in young animals. Malignant lymphoma and canine histiocytoma, for example, tend to be diseases of young animals. In human beings, childhood cancers are predominantly of mesenchymal origin, whereas in adults, epithelial neoplasms predominate.

Tumor Immunity

Up to this point, from what has been discussed concerning both benign and malignant neoplasms, it would appear that the body lacks defense mechanisms against neoplasia. Once a neoplasm has been recognized, this is for all practical purposes true. Neoplasms, however, are immunogenic and do elicit a response in their hosts. The concept of immunologic surveillance has been advanced, which theorizes that an immune response destroys most cancer cells while in the early stage of tumor formation. There is little data, however, to support this theory. To the contrary, in animals and human beings with immunodeficiency disease (e.g., athymic nude mice), especially of cellular immunity, or in immunosuppressed animals and human beings, there is not a general increase in neoplasia except of the lymphoreticular system (i.e., the immune system itself). Schwartz's (1975) analysis proposes that this indicates a failure to terminate lymphoproliferation triggered by antigen, and not a failure of immunologic surveillance.

Experimentally, however, animals can be protected against neoplasia, and immunotherapy (bolstering the immune system) can lead to tumor regression, two observations providing hope for cancer control. The immunity is directed at new or uncovered antigens in or on tumor cells. These are termed tumor-associated antigens, tumor-specific antigens, tumor-regression antigens, or tumor-specific transplantation antigens, and are on the surface of tumor cells. Some tumors have antigens called oncofetal antigens, which are embryonic or fetal cell products reexpressed in tumor cells. A variety of new antigens are also present in and on viral-induced tumors unrelated to the above antigens. The antigens in tumors induced by chemical carcinogens are distinct for each tumor, even within the same animal and caused by the same chemical, whereas tumors induced by the same virus, even if of different histogenic origin, share tumor-associated antigens. The antigens induce both a humoral and a cellular immune response, but the latter is most effective in destroying cancer cells. Infiltrations with lymphocytes (presumably T cells) occur in and around many tumors, and statistical studies have shown longer sur-

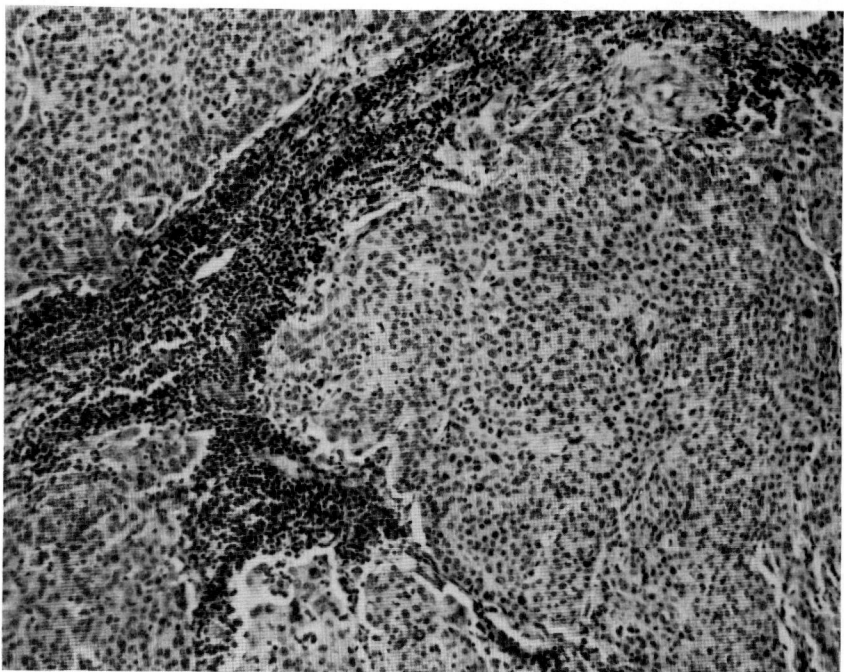

Fig. 4–19. Infiltration of lymphocytes within a squamous cell carcinoma. This may represent a cellular immune response.

vival time when these occur. Despite the immunogenicity of tumors, the defense mechanisms are incapable of stopping the progression of most neoplasms. This should not be surprising, as the immune system fails to afford protection to many chronic infectious diseases as well. Proposed explanations for this failure include the following: (1) all tumors do not bear foreign antigens, (2) the immune response is too weak, and (3) soluble blocking factors (antigen-antibody complexes) interfere with cellular immunity. Schwartz's (1975) analogy with pneumococcal pneumonia in man is appropriate: "It is the penicillin that cures the patient. The immune response protects against reinfection with pneumococci . . . ."

The Frequency of Neoplasms

A knowledge of "what kind of tumor occurs where and how often" not only satisfies a natural scientific curiosity, but is essential to studies of many sorts dealing with etiology and possible prevention. Unfortunately, precise information of this kind is not easy to obtain. Some of our best works on animal neoplasms have dealt with frequency of occurrence in a general way, without giving figures susceptible to precise tabulation and analysis. Certain variations in terminology and interpretation have been in vogue over the years and in some instances have rendered one author's report scarcely comparable with another's, not to mention the doubts that have existed in all minds concerning some of the more difficult classifications.

Although it is interesting to know which histologic types are found in a large series of neoplasms collected over the years at a clinic or hospital, this does not lead to data which are useful to study the frequency of particular tumors. In order to have information of value to determine rate of occurrence, the population from which the neoplasms came must be carefully and thoroughly defined. Only such data are of value in comparing trends under varying conditions. A few studies have been made of animals in which adequate laboratory identification of the neoplasms was combined with sound epidemiologic methods. Examples of studies which consider the epizootiologic aspects of neoplasia are found in the reports of Dorn, et al., 1966 and 1968; Anderson, et al., 1969 and Zaldivar, 1967. The kinds of tumors and their order of frequency in a specific organ or system are discussed further in appropriate chapters.

Neoplasia—General References

Anderson, L. J., and Sandison, A. T.: Tumours of connective tissues in cattle, sheep and pigs. J. Pathol., 98:253–263, 1969.

Anderson, L. J., Sandison, A. T., and Jarrett, W. F. H.: A British abattoir survey of tumours in cattle, sheep and pigs. Vet Rec., 84:547–551, 1969.

Andervont, H. B., and Dunn, T. B.: Occurrence of tumours in Wild House mice. J. Nat. Cancer Inst., 28:1153–1163, 1962.

Block, M. M., Opler, S. R., and Speer, F. D.: Microscopic structure of gastric carcinomas and their regional lymph nodes in relation to survival. Surg., Gynecol. Obstet., 98:725–734, 1954.

Bullock, F. D., and Curtis, M. R.: Experimental production of sarcoma of the liver of the rat. Proc. NY Pathol. Soc. N.S., 20:149–175, 1920.

Chapman, W. L., Jr., and Allen, J. R.: Multiple neoplasia in a Rhesus monkey, *Macaca mulatta*. Path. Vet., 5:342–352, 1968.

Chesterman, F. C., and Pomerance, A.: Spontaneous neoplasms in ferrets and polecats. J. Pathol. Bact., 89:529–533, 1965.

Davis, C. L., Leeper, R. B., and Shelton, J. E.: Neoplasms encountered in federally inspected establishments in Denver, Colorado. J. Am. Vet. Med. Assoc., 83:229–237, 1933.

Dorn, C. R., et al.: The prevalence of spontaneous neoplasms in a defined canine population. Am. J. Public Health. 56:254–265, 1966.

———: Survey of animal neoplasms in Alameda and Contra Costa Counties, California. I. Methodology and description of cases. J. Natl. Cancer. Inst., 40:295–305, 1968.

———: Survey of animal neoplasms in Alameda and Contra Costa Counties, California. II. Cancer morbidity in dogs and cats from Alameda County. J. Natl. Cancer Inst., 40:307–318, 1968.

Dunning, W. F., and Curtis, M. R.: Malignancy induced by *Cysticercus fasciolaris*: its independence of age of the host when infested. Am. J. Cancer, 37:312–328, 1939.

———: Multiple peritoneal sarcoma in rats from injection of washed ground, *Taenia* larvae. Cancer Res., 6:668–670, 1946.

Feldman, W. H.: Neoplasms of Domesticated Animals. Philadelphia, W. B. Saunders Co., 1932.

Fibiger, J.: Weitere Untersuchungen uber das Spiropteracarcinom der Ratte. Ztschr. Krebsforsch., 14:295–326, 1914.

Harvey, W. F., Dawson, E. K., and Innes, J. R. M.: Debatable tumors in human and animal pathology. Edinburgh M. J., 45:275–284, 1938; 46:256–266, 1939.

Hitchcock, C. R., and Bell, E. T.: Studies on the nematode parasite, Gonglyonema neoplasticum, and avitaminosis A in the forestomach of rats: comparison with Fibiger's results. J. Nat. Cancer Inst., 12:1345–1387, 1952.

Jackson, C.: Incidence and pathology of tumors of domesticated animals in South Africa. Onderstepoort. J. Vet. Sci., 6:3–460, 1936.

Kent, S. P.: Spontaneous and induced malignant neoplasms in monkeys. Ann. NY Acad. Sci., 85:819–827, 1960.

Kovacs, A. B., and Somogyvári, K.: (Incidence of tumours in domestic animals): Data from the Budapest Veterinary School for the past 50 years. Magy. Allatorv. Lap., 23:460–463, 1968, V.B., 39:2132, 1969.

Krook, L.: A statistical investigation of carcinoma in the dog. Acta Pathol. Microbiol. Scand., 45:407–422, 1954.

Lillie, R. D.: Histopathologic Technique. Philadelphia, Blakiston Co., 1947.

Loeb, W. F.: Leucyl aminopeptidase activity in canine neoplasia. Lab. Invest., 15:1118–1119, 1966.

Martland, H. S.: The occurrence of malignancy in radioactive persons. Am. J. Cancer, 15:2435–2516, 1931.

Mawdesley-Thomas, L. B.: Neoplasia in fish—a bibliography. J. Fish Biol., 1:187–207, 1969.

Meier, H., et al.: Epizootiology of cancer in animals. Ann. NY Acad. Sci., 108:617–1326, 1963.

Misdorp, W.: Tumors in newborn animals. Path. Vet., 2:328–343, 1965.

Monlux, A. W., Anderson, W. A., and Davis, C. L.: A survey of tumors occurring in cattle, sheep and swine. Am. J. Vet. Res., 17:646–677, 1956.

Mugera, G. M.: Canine and feline neoplasms in Kenya. Bull. Epizoot. Dis. Afr., 16:367–370, 1968; V.B., 39:2610, 1969.

Murray, M.: Neoplasms of domestic animals in East Africa. Br. Vet. J., 124:514–524, 1968.

Orr, J. W.: Mammary carcinoma in mice following the intranasal administration of methylcholanthrene. J. Pathol. Bact., 55:483–488, 1943.

Pamukcu, A. M.: An annotation on the occurrence of tumours in sheep. Br. Vet. J., 112:499–506, 1956.

Plummer, P. J. G.: A survey of six hundred and thirty-six tumours from domesticated animals. Can. J. Comp. Med., 20:239–251, 1956.

Pott, P.: Chirurgical observations relative to the cancer of the scrotum. London, 1775. Reprinted in Natl. Cancer Inst. Monograph, 10:7–13, 1963.

Ratcliffe, H. L.: Incidence and nature of tumors of captive wild animals and birds. Am. J. Cancer., 17:116–135, 1933.

Reyniers, J. A., and Sacksteder, M. R.: Tumorigenesis and the germfree chicken. Ann. NY Acad. Sci., 78:328–353, 1959.

Rigdon, R. H.: Tumors produced by methylcholanthrene in the duck. Arch. Pathol., 54:368–377, 1952.

Rous, P.: A transmissible avian neoplasm (sarcoma of the common fowl). J. Exp. Med., 12:697–705, 1910.

———: The virus tumors and the tumor problem. Am. J. Cancer, 28:233–272, 1936.

Schardein, J. L., Fitzgerald, J. E., and Kaump, D. H.: Spontaneous tumors in Holtzman source rats of various ages. Pathol. Vet., 5:238–252, 1968.

Schwartz, R. S.: Another look at immunologic surveillance. N. Engl. J. Med., 293:181–184, 1975.

Seibold, H. R., et al.: Observations on the possible relations of malignant esophageal tumors and Spirocerca lupi lesions in the dog. Am. J. Vet. Res., 16:5–14, 1955.

Vos, J. J. T.: Over huidkanker onder de inheemsche bevolking in Nederlandsch Oost-Indië. Geneesk. tijdschr. v. Nederl.-Indië. 75:283–294, 1935. [Skin cancer among the native population in the Dutch East Indies, Abst. Am. J. Cancer, 28:423–424, 1936.]

Webster, W. M.: Neoplasia in food animals with special reference to the high incidence in sheep. N. Z. Vet. J., 14:203–214, 1966.

Yamagiwa, K., and Ichikawa, K.: Experimentelle Studie über die Pathogenese der Epithelialgeschwulste. Mitt. Med. Fak. Tokio, 15:295–344, 1915.

Zaldivar, R.: Incidence of spontaneous neoplasms in beagles. J. Am. Vet. Med. Assoc., 151:1319–1321, 1967.

Viral-Induced Neoplasms

Bittner, J. J.: Some possible effects of nursing on the mammary gland tumor incidence in mice. Science, 84:162, 1936.

Cook, R. H., and Olson, C., Jr.: Experimental transmission of cutaneous papilloma of the horse. Am. J. Pathol., 27:1087–1097, 1951.

DeMonbreun, W. A., and Goodpasture, E. W.: Infectious oral papillomatosis of dogs. Am. J. Pathol., 8:43–56, 1932.

Dulbecco, R.: Viruses in carcinogenesis. Ann. Intern. Med., 70:1019–1029, 1969.

———: Cell transformation by viruses. Science, 166:962–968, 1969.

Ellermann, V., and Bang, O.: Experimentelle leukäemie bei Hühnern. Zentralbl. Bakt. 46:595–609, 1908.

Finkel, M. P., Biskis, B. O., and Jinkins, P. B.: Virus induction of osteosarcomas in mice. Science, 151:689–701, 1966.

Friend, C.: Cell-free transmission in adult Swiss mice of a disease having the character of a leukemia. J. Exp. Med., 105:307–318, 1967.

Furth, J.: Observations with a new transmissible strain of the Leucosis (leucemia) of fowls. J. Exp. Med., 53:243–267, 1931.

———: Lymphomatosis, myelomatosis and endothelioma of chickens caused by a filterable agent. 1. Transmission experiments. J. Exp. Med., 58:253–275, 1933.

Gross, L.: "Spontaneous" leukemia developing in C3H mice following inoculation, in infancy, with AK-leukemic extracts, or AK-embryos. Proc. Soc. Exp. Biol. Med., 76:27–32, 1951.

———: A filterable agent recovered from AK-leukemic extracts causing salivary gland carcinomas in C3H mice. Proc. Soc. Exp. Biol. Med., 83:414–421, 1953.

———: Viral etiology of "spontaneous" mouse leukemia: a review. Cancer Res., 18:371–381, 1958.

Habel, K.: Tumor viruses. Yale J. Biol. Med., 37:473–486, 1965.

Harvey, J. J.: An unidentified virus which causes the rapid production of tumours in mice. Nature, 204:1104–1105, 1964.

Huebner, R. J., and Todaro, G. G.: Oncogenes of RNA tumor viruses as determinants of cancer. Proc. Nat. Acad. Sci., 64:1087–1094, 1969.

Jarrett, W. F. H., et al.: Leukemia in the cat. Transmission experiments with leukemia (lymphosarcoma). Nature, 202:566–568, 1964.

Kilham, L., Herman, C. M., and Fisher, E. R.; Naturally occurring fibromas of Grey squirrels related to Shope's rabbit fibroma. Proc. Soc. Exp. Biol. Med., 82:298–301, 1953.

Lucké, B.: Carcinoma in the Leopard frog. Its probable causation by a virus. J. Exp. Med., 68:457–468, 1938.

Magalhaes, O.: Warts in cattle. Brazil-Med., 34:430, 1920.

Melendez, L. V., et al.: Herpesvirus Saimiri. II. Experimentally induced malignant lymphoma in primates. Lab. Anim. Care, 19:378–386, 1969.

Moulton, J. E.: Cutaneous papillomas on the udders of milk goats. North Am. Vet., 35:29–33, 1954.

Opler, S. R.: Observations on a new virus associated with guinea pig leukemia: preliminary note. J. Natl. Cancer Inst., 38:797–800, 1967.

Parsons, R. J., and Kidd, J. G.: Oral papillomatosis of rabbits. A virus disease. J. Exp. Med., 77:233–250, 1943.

Rous, P.: A transmissible avian neoplasm (sarcoma of the common fowl). J. Exp. Med., 12:697–705, 1910.

Shope, R. E.: Infectious papillomatosis of rabbits. J. Exp. Med., 58:607–624, 1933.

———: A transmissible tumor-like condition in rabbits. J. Exp. Med., 56:793–802, 1932.

———: An infectious fibroma of deer. Proc. Soc. Exp. Biol. Med., 88:533–535, 1955.

Snyder, S. P., and Theilen, G. H.: Transmissible feline fibrosarcoma. Nature, 221:1074–1075, 1969.

Stewart, S. E., et al.: The induction of neoplasms with a substance released from mouse tumors by tissue culture. Virology, 3:380–400, 1957.

Syverton, J. T.: Present status of studies on tumor-producing viruses. Natl. Cancer Inst. Mono. No. 4, 345–353, 1959.

Theilen, G. H., Gould, D., Fowler, M., and Dungworth, D. L.: C-type virus in tumor tissue of a Wooly monkey (*Lagothrix spp.*) with fibrosarcoma. J. Natl. Cancer Inst., 47:881–889, 1971.

CHAPTER 5

Disturbances of Circulation

Interference with circulation and therefore blood supply to vital organs may arise from a variety of mechanisms. The hemodynamic changes of concern in this chapter are thrombosis, hemorrhage, hyperemia, edema, and shock. Circulatory changes are also a principal manifestation of other entities, such as heart failure, primary vascular disease, and anemia, which are reviewed in other chapters, and changes in circulation are an integral component of the inflammatory process, which is discussed in the next chapter.

COAGULATION

When exposed to contact with injured cells, whether tissue cells, leukocytes, or even blood platelets, blood coagulates and forms a clot. The nonyielding and tenacious characteristics of the clot are due to a meshwork of fibrils of fibrin coupled with the adhesiveness of the platelets. The process of coagulation can be stated simply as the conversion of the plasma protein **fibrinogen** to **fibrin** by the action of an enzyme **thrombin**. This conversion is accelerated by the presence of **calcium ions** and a **heat labile accelerator**. The fibrin formed by this process, which is soluble, is subsequently converted to an insoluble polymerized fibrin by a specific globulin, **fibrin-stabilizing factor**. The production of thrombin for the conversion of fibrinogen to fibrin cannot be as simply stated. It is the result of a highly complex series of enzymatic events which lead to the conversion of **prothrombin** to thrombin.

In recent years a group of blood clotting factors have been identified. Although a Roman numeral terminology has been suggested by the International Committee on Blood Clotting Factors, these factors are also honored with numerous synonyms. The factors by both number and more important synonyms are:

Factor I —Fibrinogen

Factor II —Prothrombin

Factor III —Thromboplastin, Tissue thromboplastin

Factor IV —Calcium

Factor V —Proaccelerin, labile factor

Factor VII —Proconvertin, precursor of serum prothrombin conversion accelerator, Pro-SPCA

Factor VIII—Antihemophilic factor, Antihemophilic globulin Antihemophilic factor A

Factor IX —Christmas factor, Plasma thromboplastin component, PTC. Antihemophilic factor B

Factor X —Stuart-Prower factor

Factor XI —Plasma thromboplastin antecedent, PTA

Factor XII —Hageman factor

Factor XIII—Fibrin stabilizing factor

The participation of these factors in clot formation can be conveniently divided into an **intrinsic clotting mechanism** and an **extrinsic clotting mechanism**. The two mechanisms share certain factors but are initiated by different means. The factors concerned in each of these systems are as follows:

form, which in turn activates the Christmas factor (IX). The activation of Christmas factor requires the presence of calcium

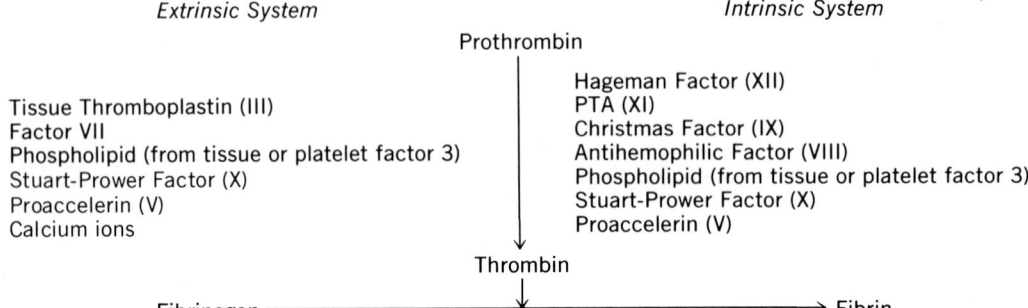

Extrinsic System

Prothrombin

Tissue Thromboplastin (III)
Factor VII
Phospholipid (from tissue or platelet factor 3)
Stuart-Prower Factor (X)
Proaccelerin (V)
Calcium ions

Intrinsic System

Hageman Factor (XII)
PTA (XI)
Christmas Factor (IX)
Antihemophilic Factor (VIII)
Phospholipid (from tissue or platelet factor 3)
Stuart-Prower Factor (X)
Proaccelerin (V)

Thrombin

Fibrinogen ⟶ Fibrin

Intrinsic Mechanism. The interaction of the clotting factors proceeds in an orderly sequential chain of reactions. The intrinsic mechanism, which is independent of tissue damage, is initiated by the activation of the Hageman factor (XII). In a test tube, contact with glass initiates this step. Blood collected into a tube lined with paraffin will not clot owing to the lack of a proper stimulus for the activation of the Hageman factor. It is not known what mechanism initiates this activation in vivo. Activated Hageman factor then converts thromboplastin antecedent (PTA : XI) to an activated

ions. Activated Christmas factor in the presence of calcium ions and phospholipid activates the antihemophilic factor (VIII), which in turn converts the Stuart factor (X) to an activated form. This conversion also requires calcium ions. Activated Stuart factor in the presence of phospholipid converts proaccelerin (V) to a prothrombin converting principle, which then converts prothrombin (II) to thrombin. This sequence of events can be illustrated after the "waterfall sequence" of Davie and Ratnoff (1964), or the "enzyme cascade" of MacFarlane (1964) as follows:

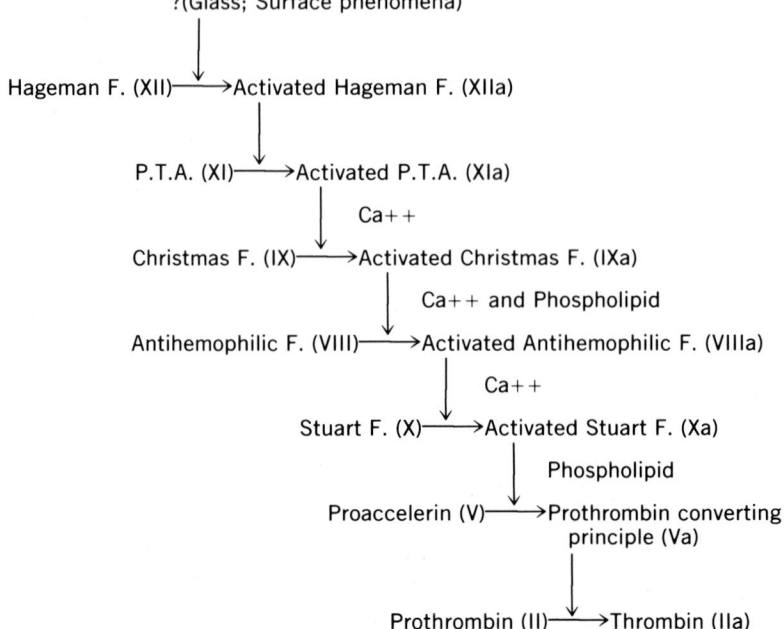

Extrinsic Mechanism. The extrinsic mechanism depends upon tissue injury and the release of tissue thromboplastin (III), which in the presence of calcium ions and factor VII activates the Stuart factor (X). The sequence of events then proceeds as in the intrinsic system as follows:

diphosphate (ADP) by injured endothelial cells. Experimentally, ADP has been shown to cause clumping of platelets. Certain prostaglandins also favor platelet aggregation, although others are inhibitory. Aspirin and other nonsteroid anti-inflammatory drugs inhibit the enzyme

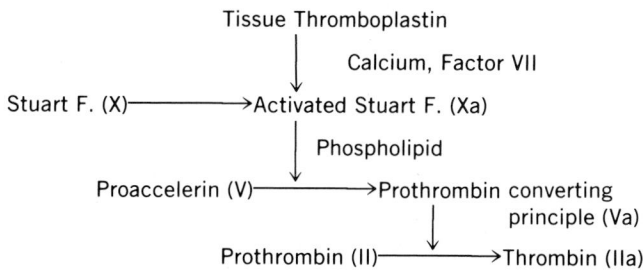

Thrombin formed by either mechanism converts fibrinogen to fibrin, as indicated at the beginning of this section. Illustrated, this proceeds as follows:

cyclooxygenase, which is necessary for prostaglandin synthesis. Platelets also contain serotonin and other factors that augment the inflammatory response.

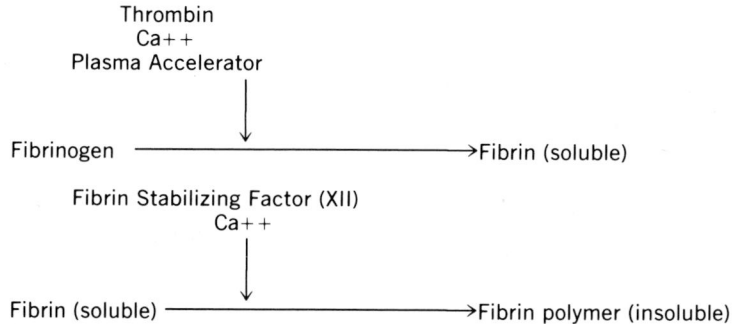

Noticeably absent from our discussion to this point is the **platelet**. Platelets contain fibrinogen, an antiheparin known as platelet factor r, calcium, and phospholipids, all of which favor coagulation. The principal role of platelets in hemostasis, however, is their ability to plug small rents in the vascular integrity. When a vessel wall is injured, platelets aggregate at the site of injury and adhere to the vessel wall and each other, forming a plug and a focus for the deposition of fibrin strands. The stimulus for this aggregation is unknown but it has been suggested that it may be the result of a release of adenosine

Prevention of Coagulation; Clot Dissolution. The prevention of coagulation is of equal importance to life as is clot formation. Blood must remain fluid to serve its multiplicity of vital functions. Although not entirely understood, several safeguards prevent coagulation. Normal plasma contains a potent **antithrombin substance**, which rapidly removes thrombin upon its formation. In addition, it is thought that an **antithromboplastin** exists. Though not normally present in plasma, **heparin** is an important inhibitor of coagulation. Heparin acts by forming an inactive complex with PTA (factor XI), preventing the activation of the Christmas factor (IX), and also by interfering with the activation of antihemophilic factor (VIII) and the formation of thrombin. The rate of blood flow, blood viscosity, the integrity of the lining endothelium, and the normal separation of formed elements from the vascular endothelium by plasma (laminar flow) are also important factors in maintaining the fluidity of blood. Alteration in these qualities predispose to coagulation and thrombosis.

In addition to factors that prevent clotting, a mechanism exists for clot **dissolution**. A fibrinolytic enzyme, **plasmin (fibrinolysin)**, is capable of dissolving clots. Plasmin is formed by the activation of a precursor, **plasminogen (profibrinolysin)**, which is normally present in plasma. Plasminogen activation is stimulated by a tissue activator, **fibrinolysokinase**, and also by **streptokinase** and **urokinase**.

Kinds of Blood Clots. Blood clots are of two kinds: (1) Clots formed in the flowing blood, which necessarily occur antemortem, and are called thrombi (singular, thrombus). The deposition of the clot in the flowing stream gives it certain identifying characteristics which will be described shortly. (2) Clots not formed in the flowing blood. These include clots formed in the vessels after death, called postmortem clots, and those formed outside of vessels as the result of hemorrhage. We naturally think of the latter as being formed to close the open vessel, but if the hemorrhage is so located that the blood flows into a body cavity or tissue spaces, the same clotting occurs there.

Abildgaard, C. F., Harrison, J., and Johnson, C. A.: Comparative study of blood coagulation in nonhuman primates. J. Appl. Physiol., *30*:400–405, 1971.

Baille, A. J., and Sim, A. K.: Activation of the fibrinolytic enzyme system in laboratory animals and in man. A comparative study. Thromb. Diath. Haemorrh., *25*:499–506, 1971.

Birndorf, N. I., Pearson, J. D., and Wredman, A.: Clotting system of monkeys. A comparison of coagulation factors and tests between cynomol-

gus monkeys *(Macaca irus)* and humans. Comp. Biochem. Physiol., *38*:157–160, 1971.

Braunwald, E.: Regulation of the circulation. N. Engl. J. Med., *290*:1124–1129, 1974.

Davie, E. W., and Ratnoff, O. D.: Waterfall sequence for intrinsic blood clotting. Science, *145*:1310–1312, 1964.

Deykin, D.: Emerging concepts of platelet function. N. Engl. J. Med., *290*:144–151, 1974.

Dooley, K. L., Zimmerman, H. E., Jr., and Mercer, H. D.: Effect of oxalic and malonic acids on the clotting mechanism of dogs. J. Am. Vet. Med. Assoc., *158*:346–348, 1971.

Droller, M. J.: Ultrastructure of the platelet release reaction in response to various aggregating agents and their inhibitors. Lab. Invest., *29*:595–606, 1973.

Gajewski, J., and Povar, M. L.: Blood coagulation values of sheep. Am. J. Vet. Res., *32*:405–409, 1971.

International Committee for the Nomenclature of Blood Clotting Factors: The nomenclature of blood clotting factors. J. A. M. A., *180*:733–735, 1962.

Kalowski, S., Howes, E. L., Jr., Margaretten, W., and McKay, D. G.: Effects of intravascular clotting on the activation of the complement system. The role of the platelet. Am. J. Pathol., *78*:525–536, 1975.

MacFarlane, R. G.: An enzyme cascade in the blood clotting mechanism, and its function as a biochemical amplifier. Nature, *202*:498–499, 1964.

Nageswara, G.: Plasma clotting of female Beagle dogs. Lab. Anim. Sci., *24*:757–762, 1974.

Rowsell, H. C.: The hemostatic mechanisms of mammals and birds in health and disease. Adv. Vet. Sci., *12*:337–410, 1968.

Singer, J. W.: The coagulation system of Rhesus monkeys, *Macaca mulatta*. Comp. Biochem. Physiol. [A], *40*:635–638, 1971.

Todd, M. E., McDevitt, E., and Goldsmith, E. I.: Blood-clotting mechanisms of nonhuman primates: choice of the baboon model to simulate man. J. Med. Primatol., *1*:132–141, 1972.

Ur, A.: The blood coagulation curve of some mammals. Res. Vet. Sci., *16*:204–207, 1974.

Weiss, H. J. (ed.): Platelets and their role in hemostasis. Ann. NY Acad. Sci., *201*, 1972.

Postmortem Clots

Except when death results from certain septicemias and anoxic conditions, the greater part of the blood is clotted in the venous system soon after life ceases. The arteries contract in rigor mortis so that little blood remains in them. Blood clots formed in this way, as well as those formed outside the vascular channels, whose nature is obvious, have to be distinguished from thrombi.

Microscopic Appearance. The visible components of these clots are the erythrocytes, leukocytes, fibrin, and precipitated proteins, chiefly albumin. In postmortem clots, these elements may be rather uniformly mixed, or the erythrocytes may have settled by force of gravity to the lowest parts of the vessel, to be overlain by leukocytes and the precipitated protein of the plasma. Laminations like those in thrombi, however, do not occur. A useful differential feature is the size of the fibrils of fibrin, which in this type of clot are uniformly fine, barely visible individually under the usual low-power magnification of 100 diameters.

Gross Appearance. The postmortem clot is dark red, smooth and shiny on the outside and molded to the vessel in which it is formed like jelly in its container, presents a uniform texture to the naked eye, and is entirely unattached to the vessel wall. Because of these characteristics, it is sometimes called a **currant-jelly clot**.

A **chicken-fat clot** results from settling and separation of the red cells from the fluid phase of the blood. This sedimentation is not different from that which occurs in a test tube. This type of postmortem clot is most likely to be found in the chambers of the heart and when postmortem clotting is delayed. Such a clot has the smooth and shiny surface of the currant-jelly, postmortem clot, but has the yellow color of plasma. It is not really attached to the vascular lining, but is commonly immobilized through being entangled in the cardiac valves and chordae tendineae.

Cause. The coagulation mechanisms discussed previously are responsible for postmortem clotting. The system is probably activated by the release of tissue thromboplastin generated from postmortem autolysis of endothelial cells, leukocytes, and erythrocytes, and also the activation of the intrinsic coagulation mechanism.

Significance. Postmortem clotting, like postmortem autolysis, requires only to be distinguished from antemortem changes of somewhat similar nature.

Antemortem Clots, Thrombosis

As previously stated, thrombi are clots formed in the flowing blood. This relatively slow process produces a clot of somewhat different qualities from those just described.

Microscopic Appearance. In addition to the components given for the postmortem clot, blood platelets, or thrombocytes, accumulate at the site of a thrombus and constitute a significant portion of this type of clot. The platelets tend to adhere strongly to each other, as well as to the vessel wall, forming somewhat amorphous, pink- or gray-staining masses which tend to alternate irregularly with layers or areas where fibrin and leukocytes, fibrin and erythrocytes, or fibrin alone predominate. Thus, a section through a thrombus tends to be irregularly laminated. If the section traverses the right part of the thrombus, its area of attachment can be seen. On the other hand, a section cut through the trailing end of an obturating thrombus may appear as a lonely island in the middle of the lumen of the vessel.

The fibrils of fibrin are relatively thick and heavy, a feature of prime importance in distinguishing the thrombus from a postmortem clot.

Gross Appearance. As seen at the necropsy table, a thrombus is friable and has a dull and irregularly roughened or somewhat stringy surface, in contrast to the shiny, currant-jelly aspect of the postmortem clot. The color is a mixture of red and gray, usually in irregular layers or laminations. On at least one side the thrombus will be found attached to the wall of the blood vessel. If the thrombus closes the lumen of the vessel entirely, it is an **occluding thrombus**. Rather frequently it occludes the lumen, except that there are one or several small openings which let a certain amount of blood pass through. This is a **canalized thrombus**. The canals come to be lined with endothelium continuous with that of the adjacent vessel wall.

Not too infrequently, the clotting process continues in the part of the thrombus which is distal to its area of attachment, without any further connection to the wall. The free end then trails downstream with the current and may attain surprising length. Such a thrombus is an **obturating thrombus**.

Causes. The causes of thrombosis are five. (1) Injury to the endothelial cells lining the vessel wall releases the thromboplastin and possibly adenosine diphosphate (ADP) to start the clotting process; it also causes the platelets to adhere to the area, which may be the very first step in thrombosis. The cause of the endothelial damage may be some local injury, such as phlebitis of infectious origin or external twisting, ligation, or contusion of the vessel. Repeated insertions of the hypodermic needle fall in this category, but fortunately, thrombosis following unskillful intravenous injections is less frequent than might be expected. Thrombosis inside the heart can occur just as readily as in the peripheral vessels and is relatively frequent. Endocarditis due to infection (*Streptococcus, Erysipelothrix*) is causative here. Injury by heartworms, *Dirofilaria immitis,* occasionally but not frequently is sufficient to have a similar effect.

(2) Roughness of the vessel lining, which sometimes remains after healing of some earlier injury, favors lodgment of platelets. If the platelets are slightly injured in this process, it is thought that they may release the necessary thromboplastin or ADP. Once started, it is easy to understand how the clotting process continues by virtue of thromboplastin derived from the disintegration of leukocytes enmeshed in the clot already formed.

(3) Slowing or stasis of the flow of blood theoretically may be considered as a secondary cause of thrombosis, but in reality it is of primary importance. Just as a log jam cannot hold in a swift river, so a thrombus forms with difficulty in a strongly moving stream. Aside from mechanical factors, the current of blood dissipates the thrombin downstream before it can exert its effect. Generalized slowing of the circulation occurs in connection with cardiac insufficiency, with its chronic passive congestion, hence thrombosis is to be feared in this condition. Localized venous congestion and stasis is the rule in extensive inflammations. This, along with vascular injury due to the infection usually present, accounts for the frequent thrombosis of vessels in extensive areas of inflammation, such as metritis.

(4) Disruption of the laminar flow of blood predisposes to thrombosis by allowing platelets and blood cells to contact the vascular endothelium. Normally these elements are separated from the vascular surface by a zone of plasma. Aneurysms, varices, lodged emboli, and extrinsic pressures all produce distortion, which results in a turbulence in the flow of blood.

(5) Changes in the composition of blood may also predispose to thrombosis. Thrombosis has been associated with an increase in the number and adhesiveness of platelets, which may follow surgical procedures, parturition, accidental trauma, and other conditions associated with extensive tissue damage. Thrombosis is frequent in human beings with polycythemia, which produces an increased viscosity of the blood. Increased secretion of catecholamines and epinephrine hasten coagulation and predispose to thrombosis.

Concepts concerning the mechanisms involved in coagulation and thrombosis are frequently changed, and many of the details are outside the scope of this text. The student is encouraged to read further, utilizing the references at the end of this section and following current literature.

Significance, Effects and Outcome. Thrombi in arteries completely or partially obstruct the flow of blood to the part supplied by the particular vessel. Depending on the local vascular anatomy, complete occlusion of the artery may be followed by necrosis, in accordance with principles already set forth, or a **collateral circulation** may fill the breach if the branches of nearby arteries anastomose with the terminal network of the occluded artery. If an area of necrosis results, it is called an infarct, as has already been explained.

Thrombosis, embolism, or any other disruption or impediment to arterial blood flow results in **ischemia** (Greek: to keep back blood) in the tissue supplied by the blood vessel. This lack of adequate blood leads to degenerative changes, which may reach necrosis. These effects were described in Chapter 1. Interruption of arterial blood flow to a specific tissue results in a sharply demarcated zone of necrosis in that tissue, corresponding to the distribution of the tributaries of the involved artery. This lesion is called an **infarct**.

In the horse, severe injury to the **anterior mesenteric artery** (rarely others) caused by invasion of larvae of *Strongylus vulgaris* and other worms is so common that every equine autopsy should include examination of this artery. Proliferative arteritis develops with more or less thrombosis or perhaps an aneurysm. Thrombi may so restrict the flow of blood to the small intestine that attacks of acute colicky indigestion become recurrent. This is the "thrombotic colic" described in clinical literature. In many of these cases, the artery returns to normal after the parasites leave, as shown by the much lower incidence of strongyle arteritis in late winter and spring than in the other half of the year.

Thrombosis of the **iliac arteries** is a cause of intermittent lameness of both hind legs in the horse. The obstruction is not complete; if it were, a fatal outcome would soon result, but the flow of blood is typically restricted to the extent that it is sufficient only for the resting animal. Upon vigorous exercise, agonizing and disabling pain arises due to anoxia of the involved muscles, only to disappear when the shortage of oxygen has been relieved by rest. Thrombosis in this location appears to be due also to the ravages of strongyle larvae, aberrant parasites in this case.

Thrombosis of coronary vessels due to atherosclerosis, so important in human medicine, is rare in domestic animals.

Despite all that may be said of thrombosis of arteries, the disorder, in general, occurs much more frequently in veins. This is because of the normally slower flow of blood and more easily produced stasis in veins. In humans bedridden from some other cause, thrombosis of the veins of the leg is prone to occur purely because of stagnation of the venous circulation and practical collapse of these almost empty veins. The same possibility in animals can be added to hypostatic congestion as another reason for frequently turning over a sick animal that is unable to do this for itself. Thrombosis and obstruction of veins tend to cause edema of the part drained because of retarded outflow of fluid.

Ever present in venous thrombosis, wherever it may be located, is the danger of fragments of the clot breaking off to be carried in the blood flow as emboli. These continue to float along until stopped at some bifurcation where the vascular lumens become too small to permit their passage. Venous thrombi may release emboli that pass through the heart and are stopped in the smaller vessels of the lungs or brain with fatal results.

Thrombi do not remain as such indefinitely. Many are slowly liquefied by plasmin and possibly by enzymes of leukocytes, the erythrocytes having disappeared by autolysis after two or three days. Others, unfortunately, undergo organization into fibrous connective tissue. Fibrin appears to be an especially fertile field for the multiplication of fibroblasts, which invade it from the surrounding fibrous tissue. The thrombus then becomes a permanent tissue.

The histopathologist needs to be alert in the recognition of such **old, organized**

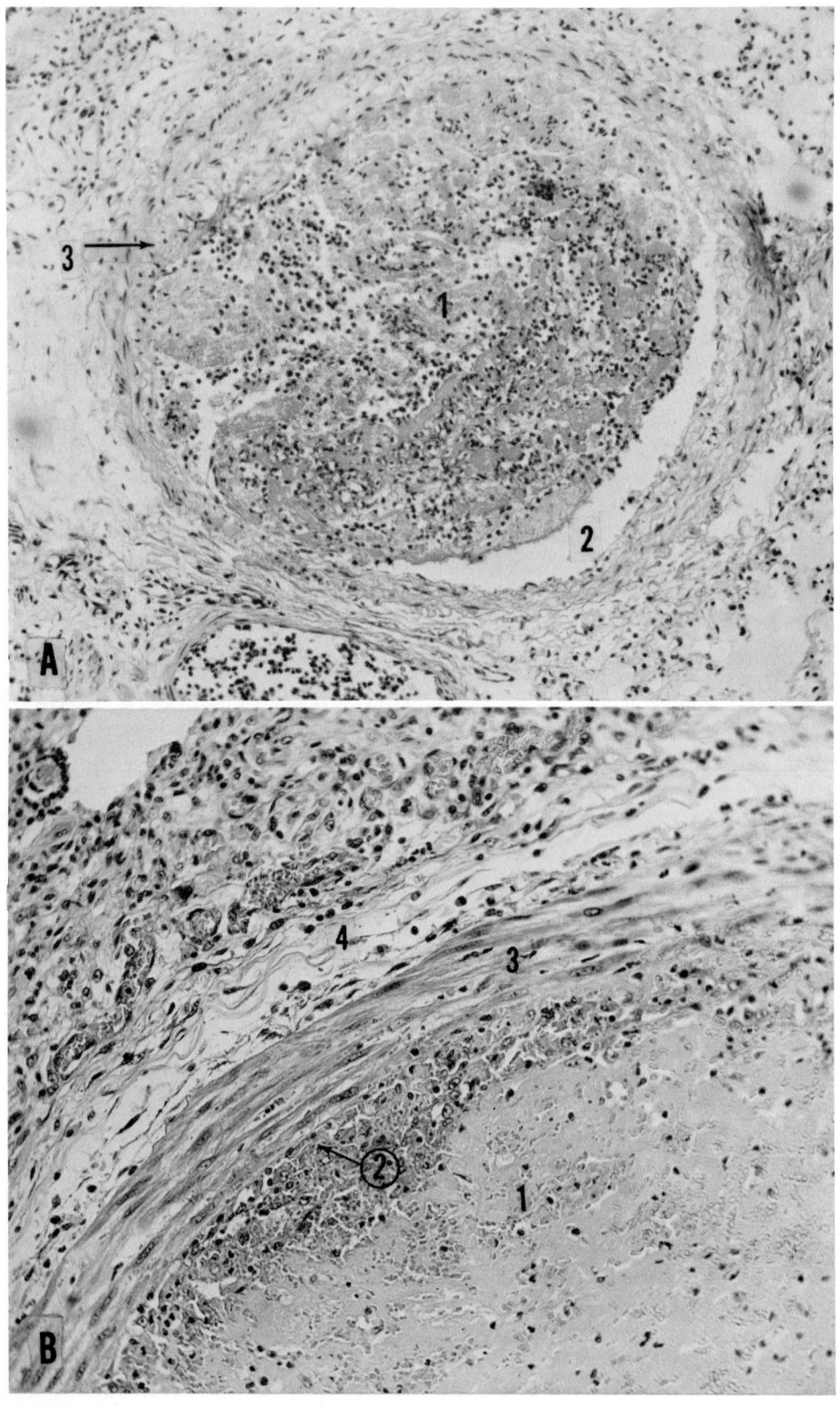

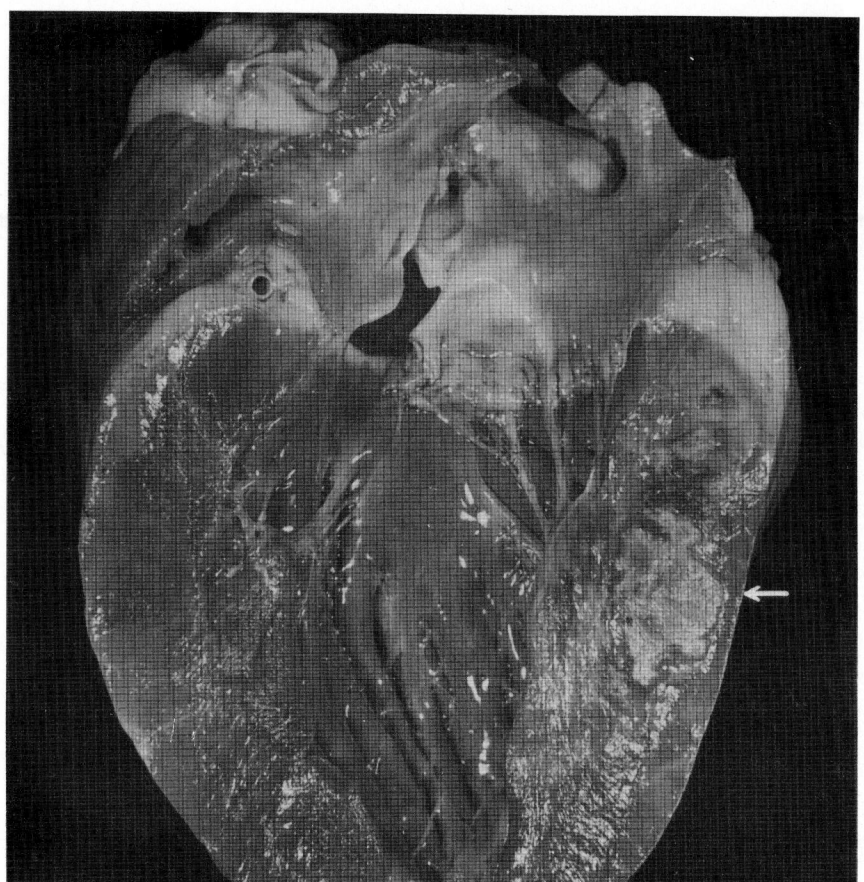

Fig. 5–2. Infarction of myocardium of left ventricle of heart of an eight-year-old male Airedale dog with malignant lymphoma. The infarction is believed to be the result of occlusion of a branch of the left coronary artery by tumor growth. (Courtesy of Angell Memorial Animal Hospital.)

Fig. 5–1. *A*, Thrombosis of branch of pulmonary artery, lung of a five-year-old Cocker Spaniel with pyometra. Thrombus (*1*), lumen of artery (*2*), attachment of thrombus to intima (*3*). (× 115.) (Courtesy of Armed Forces Institute of Pathology.) Contributor: Dr. Samuel Pollock.

B, Thrombosis of branch of pulmonary artery in an 11-year-old Scottish Terrier with chronic valvular endocarditis. Hyaline material in the thrombus (*1*), proliferation of endothelium (*2*), media of distended artery (*3*), and edema in the adventitia (*4*). (× 185.) (Courtesy of Armed Forces Institute of Pathology.) Contributor: Dr. Elihu Bond.

thrombi. The fibrous tissue is usually mature with no special features to make it conspicuous, except that it may take a circular arrangement. Usually, but not invariably, there are some remnants of the encircling smooth muscle. There may be some hemosiderin or hematoidin, the result of hemolysis of erythrocytes caught in the meshes of the developing clot. Occasionally, an irregular area of calcification may mark the site of decomposing fibrin and dead blood cells. Sometimes the whole mass is neatly encapsulated by an encircling fibrous wall. If the thrombus has been canalized, it may puzzle the inexperienced with one or more irregular blood passages that are much too large to be capillaries, but have no wall except a single endothelial layer, all buried in fibrous tissue.

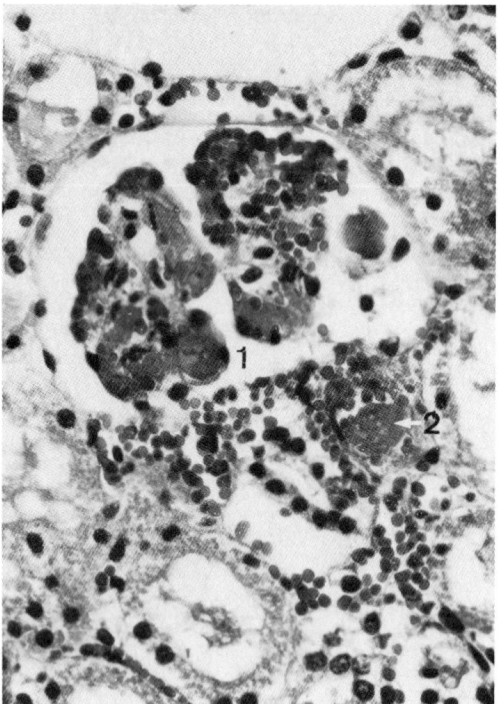

Fig. 5–3. Disseminated intravascular coagulation. Fibrinous emboli in capillaries (*1*) and afferent arteriole (2) of renal glomerulus of a pig with streptococcal sepsis. Streptococci were demonstrated by culture and by special stains in the emboli. (Courtesy of Prof. Dr. H. Luginbühl.)

Disseminated Intravascular Coagulation

An event posing a serious threat to life, recognized in man and with increasing frequency in animals, involves simultaneous coagulation within many vessels of the body. It has been associated with obstetric complications, malignant neoplastic disease, severe systemic infections, pregnancy, systemic lupus erythematosus, thrombotic microangiopathic hemolytic anemia, and granulomatous diseases. Species in which this condition has been recognized include dogs, swine, horses, rats, and Aleutian mink. The signs of bleeding are usually severe, with large confluent ecchymoses, prolonged bleeding from mucous membranes, surgical incisions, and venipuncture sites. Lesions have been described resembling those of the Shwartzman reaction, which may follow the repeated injection of bacterial endotoxin. In addition, the syndrome has been shown to follow injection of thrombin, thromboplastins and other procoagulant substances.

Bibbs, R. (ed.): Human Blood Coagulation, Haemostasis and Thrombosis. Philadelphia, F. A. Davis, 1972.

Deykin, D.: The clinical challenge of disseminated intravascular coagulation. N. Engl. J. Med., *283*:636–644, 1970.

Ganote, C. E., Seabra-Gomes, R., Nayler, W. G., and Jennings, R. B.: Irreversible myocardial injury in anoxic perfused rat hearts. Am. J. Pathol., *80*:419–450, 1975.

Garner, R., Chater, B. V., and Brown, D. L.: The role of complement in endotoxin shock and disseminated intravascular coagulation: experimental observations in the dog. Br. J. Haematol., *28*:393–401, 1974.

Genton, E., Gent, M., Hirsh, J., and Harker, L. A.: Platelet-inhibiting drugs in the prevention of clinical thrombotic disease. N. Engl. J. Med., *293*:1296–1300, 1975.

Gerrity, R. G., et al.: Endotoxin-induced vascular endothelial injury and repair. II. Focal injury, en face morphology, (^{3}H) thymidine uptake and circulating endothelial cells in the dog. Exp. Mol. Pathol., *24*:59–69, 1976.

Gunson, D. E., and Rooney, J. R.: Anaphylactoid purpura in a horse. Vet. Pathol., *14*:325–331, 1977.

Hawley, H. B., et al.: Disseminated intravascular coagulopathy during experimental pneumococcal sepsis: studies in normal and asplenic Rhesus monkeys. J. Med. Primatol., *6*:203–218, 1977.

Hoffman, R.: The disseminated intravascular coagulation syndrome (consumption coagulation) of domestic animals. *In* Fortschritte der Veterinärmedizin, No. 24, 100 pp. Tiergesundheitsdienst Bayern, Grub b. München, German Federal Republic, 1976.

Hoffstein, S., et al.: Cytochemical localization of lysoenzymal enzyme activity in normal and ischemic dog myocardium. Am. J. Pathol., 79:193–206, 1975.

Legendre, A. M., and Krehbiel, J. D.: Disseminated intravascular coagulation in a dog with hemothorax and hemangiosarcoma. J. Am. Vet. Med. Assoc., 171:1070–1071, 1977.

McKay, D. G., and Margaretten, W.: Disseminated intravascular coagulation in virus diseases. Arch. Intern. Med., 120:129, 1967.

Prathap, K.: Natural history of platelet rich mural thrombi in systemic arteries of hypercholesterolemic monkeys: light microscope and electron microscope observations. J. Pathol., 110:203–211, 1973.

Robboy, S. J., et al.: Pathology of disseminated intravascular coagulation (DIC). Human Pathol., 3:327–343, 1972.

Schiefer, B., and Searcy, G.: Disseminated intravascular coagulation and consumption coagulopathy. Can. Vet. J., 16:151–159, 1975.

Schoendorf, T. H., Rosenberg, M., and Beller, F. K.: Endotoxin-induced disseminated intravascular coagulation in nonpregnant rats. Am. J. Pathol., 65:51–58, 1971.

Selman, I. E., et al.: A respiratory syndrome in cattle resulting from thrombosis of the posterior vena cava. Vet. Rec., 94:459–466, 1974.

Spector, J. I., Lang, J. E., and Crosby, W. H.: Coagulation changes in baboons during acute experimental hemoglobinemia and dextran infusion. Am. J. Pathol., 78:469–476, 1975.

Thomson, G. W., McSherry, B. J., and Valli, V. E. O.: Endotoxin induced disseminate intravascular coagulation in cattle. Can. J. Comp. Med., 38:457–466, 1974.

EMBOLI AND EMBOLISM

Emboli are foreign bodies floating in the blood. Several kinds are recognized. Simple emboli, or **fibrinous emboli** (thromboemboli), are pieces of thrombi which have been broken loose by the force of the blood. In microscopic and gross appearance, they resemble thrombi. They are almost always found lodged at an arterial bifurcation or other place where the lumen of the artery becomes too small to permit their passage. The cause is obvious.

When an embolus of fibrin becomes arrested in a vessel, it usually brings with it a certain amount of thrombin, and the condi-

tions are met for the process of thrombosis to proceed. Hence, if the embolus itself does not entirely obstruct the flow of blood, the thrombus formed around it does so. Thus, the effect of the embolus is to produce obstruction with the same consequences as if it were a thrombus originally.

Fatty emboli are droplets of the patient's fat, which at normal body temperature has a consistency little beyond that of oil. Since oil and water do not mix readily, the fat remains as separate bodies in the circulating blood. While not detected grossly, they are readily seen microscopically if a fat stain is applied to the section in the usual way. Usually they fill the capillaries or arterioles, being lodged in them.

The cause of fat embolism is the sudden release of body fat from numbers of adipose cells. This may occur when a long bone is fractured with considerable splintering, and then subjected to movements that cause the jagged ends to jab into the marrow cavity repeatedly. (The animal must, of course, have passed the age when the cavity would contain red marrow.) Less easily, fatty embolism can occur from severe trauma of subcutaneous fat in obese individuals and occasionally from metabolic failure in diabetics.

Fat emboli in the heart, lung, or kidney have been known to result from the extreme fatty change of **deficiency hepatitis**, brought on by a deficiency of choline, methionine, or cystine. In these disorders, of experimental animals chiefly, the overloaded hepatic cells in the centers of the lobules sometimes rupture and discharge their accumulated fat, so that it coalesces into "fat cysts," whence the fat may find its way into the blood. (We must remember, of course, that many body fats are not far from their melting points at the temperature of the living body in a given species.) A similar situation has been known to occur in human alcoholics.

The emboli are usually numerous and are carried back to the heart and into the lungs, where they lodge as the blood passages divide and subdivide. Extensive fatty embolism is fatal through interference with the pulmonary circulation, and it constitutes a cause of unexpected death a short time subsequent to accidents of the nature just outlined. The condition occurs with some frequency in humans and probably is often overlooked in animals, fat stains being necessary to demonstrate it.

Gas emboli, usually air emboli, form as bubbles in the blood when there is a sudden and sufficient lowering of the ambient pressure. This occurs when aviators ascend rapidly to great heights, and possibly with more severity when construction workers emerge from underwater compartments in which the air pressure has been raised to several times that of normal atmospheric pressure. Such a compartment can be placed on the bottom of a river, and if the air pressure is greater than the water pressure, the water is forced out, permitting men to enter and work. These compartments are called by the French name, cais-

sons, and the disorder is called **caisson disease**. It is also known as the **bends**, because of the severe cramping pain that occurs when the individual is released from pressure. Since the blood has almost unhindered access to pulmonary alveolar air through walls that are quite pervious to gases, the air dissolves in the blood in proportion to the pressure, following ordinary laws of physics. The oxygen dissolved is readily utilized by the tissues, but the inert nitrogen, constituting four-fifths of the air, can only remain in solution, the blood being saturated for that particular pressure. If the pressure is suddenly reduced (by ascent of the worker from the caisson), there is nothing for the nitrogen to do but to bubble out. The gas bubbles are capable of stopping the flow in small capillaries and the condition is sometimes fatal. The remedy is to release the pressure slowly.

Rarely, air embolism may result from air being sucked into the venous circulation

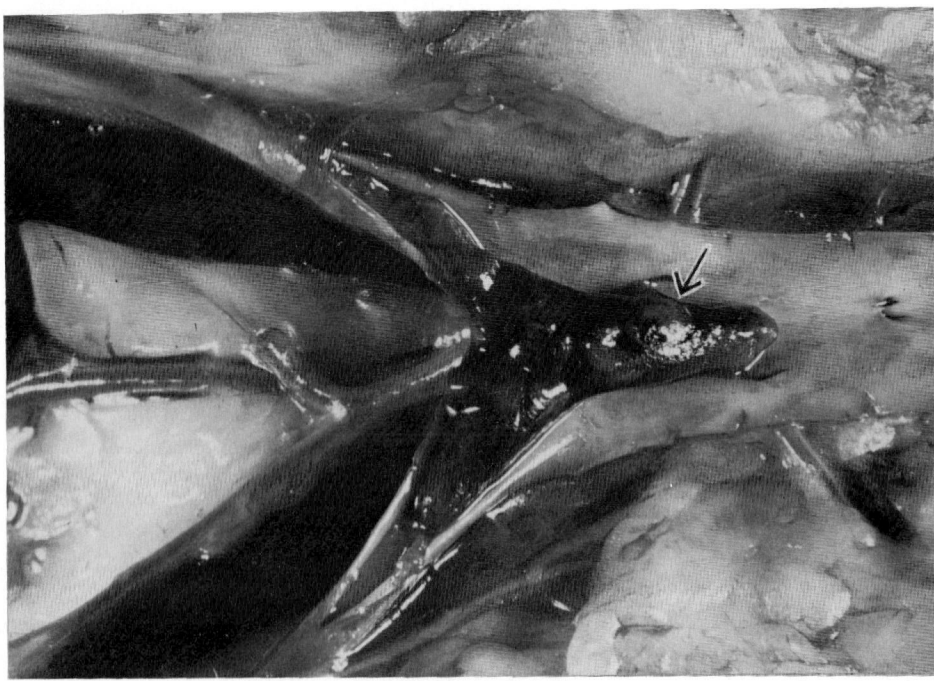

Fig. 5–4. Saddle embolus (arrow) at bifurcation of the aorta of an eight-year-old spayed female cat. This embolus presumably originated in the left atrium. (Courtesy of Angell Memorial Animal Hospital.)

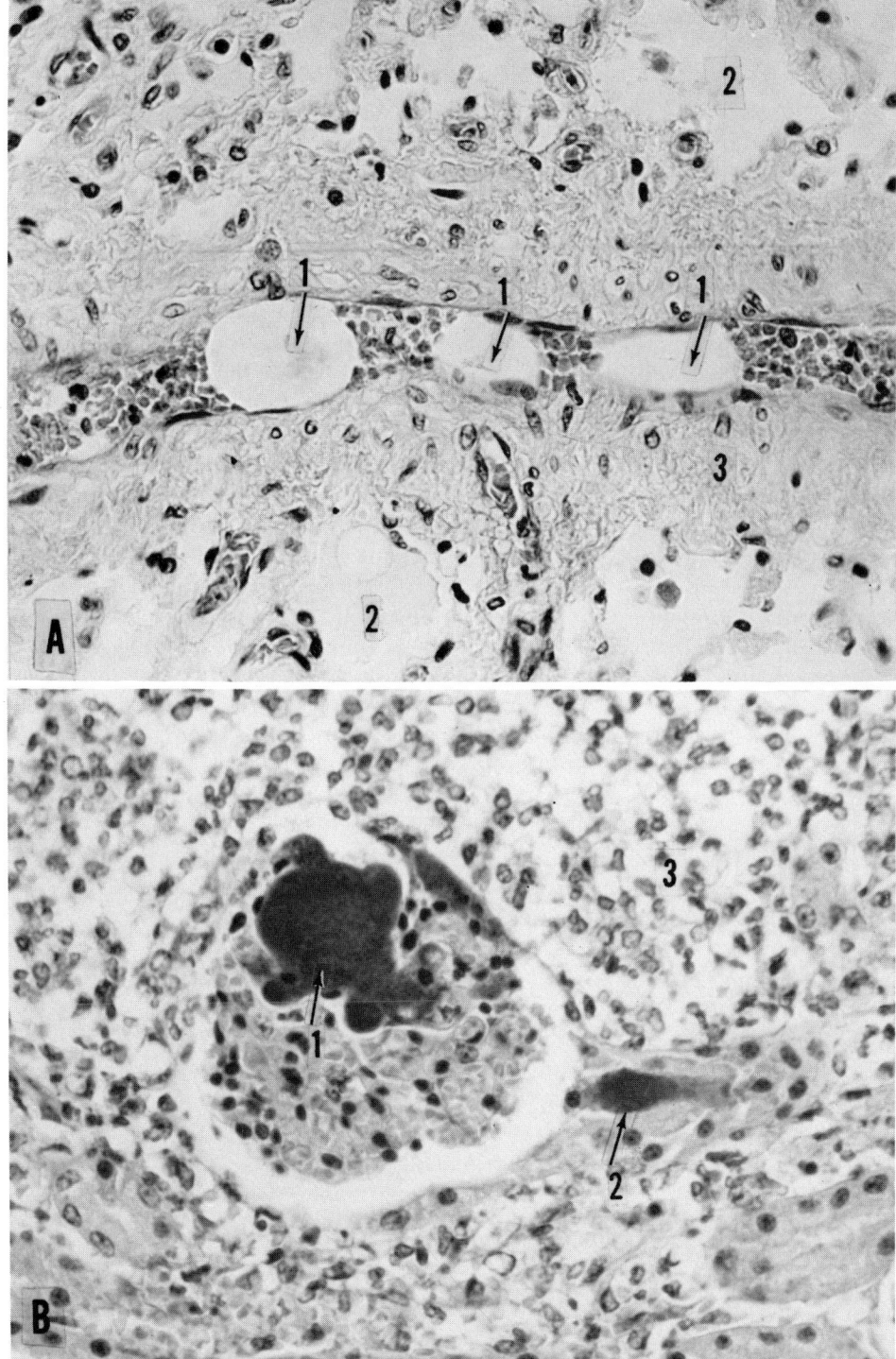

Fig. 5–5. *A*, Fatty emboli in a branch of the pulmonary artery of a dog hit and killed by an automobile. Globules of fat (*1*) expand the arterial wall and displace blood cells. Pulmonary alveoli (*2*) are present in the section. (× 395.) (Courtesy of Armed Forces Institute of Pathology.) Contributor: Dr. Elihu Bond.

B, Bacterial emboli in a renal glomerulus of a foal infected with *Shigella equuli*. A bacterial colony is seen in the glomerulus (*1*) and in the efferent tubule (*2*); leukocytes have accumulated around the glomerulus (*3*). (× 315). (Courtesy of Armed Forces Institute of Pathology.) Contributor: Army Veterinary Research Laboratory.

through large, gaping wounds so located that respiratory or other movements of the exposed fasciae and muscles can exert a pumping action. Less unusual is the pumping of air into surrounding tissues from such wounds, producing merely emphysema but not involving the blood.

The injection of air into the veins should be mentioned here. In some biologic laboratories, a routine method of killing experimental rabbits is to inject 10 ml of air into the ear vein. This causes almost instant death. However, a comparable lethal amount of air for a man or for most domestic animals would be much larger. The accidental inclusion of a little air in making an ordinary intravenous injection involves no danger.

Bacterial emboli are clumps of bacterial cells sometimes mechanically detached into the venous flow from heavily infected tissues. Such emboli are often stopped in capillaries, to which they are carried after leaving the heart. Interference with the circulation is insignificant, but such groups of bacteria usually multiply at the place where they lodge, and are much more likely to set up a new focus or center of infection than scattered, single cells would be. Such a transfer of infection is known as **metastasis**. While some organs are not a fertile field for the growth of certain species of bacteria, in general the frequency with which a given organ suffers from such metastases is proportional to two factors combined: the amount of blood flowing through it in a given time, and the extent of fine capillaries through which such blood is filtered. This means that liver, kidneys, and lungs are the most frequent recipients of metastatic infections.

Parasitic emboli include fragments of adult canine heartworms, *Dirofilaria immitis*, usually in the branches of the pulmonary artery, clumps of blood flukes, *Schistosoma sp.*, and possibly groups of agglutinated trypanosomes. Embolism of this kind is infrequent.

Emboli of **neoplastic cells** are occasion-

ally seen and must occur frequently, since it is by clumps of tumor cells carried in the blood that malignant neoplasms are able to colonize in new locations. The spot where a growing neoplasm breaks into a vein is frequently visible, and it is easy to understand how clumps of its cells or individual cells are broken off and carried away to lodge in a new location.

Spodogenous emboli are clumps of blood cells that have been agglutinated (glued together) by immunologic processes, such as the injection of incompatible types of blood. Also included in this classification are masses of precipitated protein that result from certain kinds of irritant chemicals injected into the blood. Chloral hydrate, commonly used as an anesthetic, is thought to produce such precipitation rarely, sometimes with death resulting.

Other types of emboli include red bone marrow emboli following fractures, amniotic fluid emboli, hepatic emboli following trauma to the liver, foreign bodies such as broken needles or hair introduced in venipuncture, and trophoblastic emboli, which occur in the chinchilla and in primates.

Jacobs, R. R., et al.: Fat embolism: A microscopic and ultrastructure evaluation of two animal models. Trauma, 13:980–993, 1973.
Naquet, R., et al.: Dynamics of air embolism in the monkey. Electroencephalogr. Clin. Neurophysiol., 34:788–789, 1973.
Tvedten, H. W., and Langham, R. F.: Trophoblastic emboli in a chinchilla. J. Am. Vet. Med. Assoc., 165:828–829, 1974.
Wingfield, W. E., and Corley, E. A.: Fatal air embolism associated with pneumourethography and pneumocystography in a dog. J. Am. Vet. Med. Assoc., 160:1616–1618, 1972.

FAILURE TO CLOT

Under certain conditions, there is partial or total interference with the normal clotting process. Such phenomena are of diagnostic interest to the pathologist studying postmortem material and of vital concern during life. The conditions in which the clotting power of the blood is seriously impaired include the following.

In **septicemic diseases**, the expected clotting in the vessels after death may not materialize. This is so much the rule in animals dead of anthrax that failure of the blood to clot is considered an important diagnostic sign. Anoxemia has been blamed for failure of the clotting mechanism, but this has not been proved.

Destructive lesions of the liver, such as occur in severe forms of acute and chronic hepatitis (cirrhosis) may result in failure of clotting due to deficiency of prothrombin, which is produced by the liver cells. We should be aware, however, of the great reserve capacity of the liver. The damage to hepatic cells must be severe and well-nigh universal if its effect is to be felt in impairment of this function. Fibrinogen, factor VII, the Stuart factor (factor X), and probably the Christmas factor (factor IX) are also synthesized by the liver.

Hypocalcemia theoretically can be included as a cause of failure to clot; however, it is unlikely that this mechanism is of importance in vivo. Calcium levels required to prolong coagulation time are well below those that would induce other clinical manifestations of hypocalcemia.

Deficiency of vitamin K (2-methyl-1, 4 naphthaquinone) can lower the amount of several clotting factors in the blood with resultant impairment of clotting. Vitamin K is required for the synthesis of prothrombin, Christmas factor (factor IX), Stuart factor (factor X), and factor VII. However, this deficiency is largely limited to the experimental laboratory, and is not likely to be encountered in animals fed any

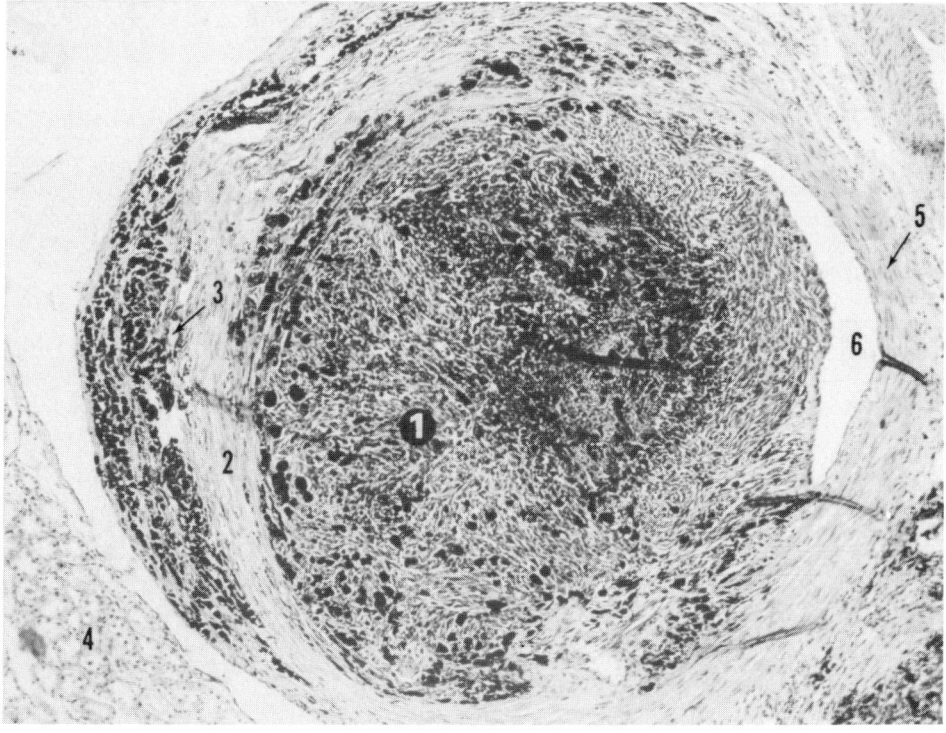

Fig. 5–6. Thrombosis of renal artery by implantation of a tumor embolus. The neoplasm was a malignant melanoma, primary in the oral mucosa of a nine-year-old dog. Tumor *(1)* attached to artery wall *(2)*, which has been penetrated by tumor cells *(3)*. Renal tubules *(4)*, uninvolved artery wall *(5)*, and lumen of the artery *(6)* (× 70.) (Courtesy of Armed Forces Institute of Pathology.) Contributor: Dr. F. L. Povar.

natural or ordinary diet, which usually contains ample vitamin K. Also, vitamin K is synthesized by bacterial action in the intestine.

Sweet-clover poisoning has resulted in uncontrollable and fatal hemorrhage in numerous bovine animals fed for several weeks or longer on sweet-clover hay *(Mellilotus alba et sp.)*. The active principle responsible for this action has been found to be *Dicumarol* (3,3'-methylenebis 4-hydroxycoumarin), also known as coumarin and dicoumarin. Dicumarol acts as an antagonist to vitamin K. (See Poisoning by Sweet Clover and Warfarin.)

Other poisons such as aspirin and cottonseed meal may cause the blood to fail to clot. The mechanisms involved are discussed in Chapter 16.

Thrombocytopenia or a diminished number of circulating platelets results in interference with clotting and hemorrhage. The disease occurs as a primary or idiopathic thrombocytopenia, in which case the cause is not known, and as secondary thrombocytopenia, resulting from certain poisonings, sensitivities, and other blood dyscrasias. Both forms are discussed in Chapter 22.

Hemophilia is an inherited defect of the coagulation mechanism. Several forms of the disease are known in man and animals, each affecting a specific coagulation factor. The types of hemophilia recognized at this writing in man and other animals are listed in Table 5–1, and are discussed in further detail in Chapter 22. Inherited coagulation defects which are known in man but not yet identified in animals include dysfibrinogenemia, prothrombin (factor II) deficiency, factor V deficiency (parahemophilia), factor XII deficiency (Hageman

Table 5–1. Inherited Bleeding Disorders

Disease	Defective Factor	Affected Species
Fibrinogen deficiency (hypofibrinogenemia, afibrinogenemia)	Factor I	Man, dogs, goats
Hypoproconvertinemia	Factor VII	Man, dogs
Classic hemophilia (hemophilia A)	Factor VIII	Man, dogs, horses, cats
Hemophilia B (Christmas disease)	Factor IX	Man, dogs
Stuart factor deficiency	Factor X	Man, dogs
Plasma thromboplastin antecedent (PTA) deficiency	Factor XI	Man, cattle, dogs
Von Willebrand's disease	Factor VIII, platelet adhesion, bleeding time	Man, swine, dogs
Thrombopathia (thrombasthenia, Glanzmann's disease)	Platelet function	Man, dogs, rats

trait), factor XIII (fibrin stabilizing factor) deficiency, and familial thrombocytopenia (Dodds, 1975).

Archer, R. K., and Bowden, R. S. T.: A case of true haemophilia in a Labrador dog. Vet. Rec., 71:560, 1959.

Bannerman, R. M., Edwards, J. A., and Kreimer-Birnbaum, M.: Investigation of potential animal models of thalassemia. Ann. NY Acad. Sci., 232:306–322, 1974.

Bowie, E. J. W., et al.: Tests of hemostasis in swine: normal values and values in pigs affected with von Willebrand's disease. Am. J. Vet. Res., 34:1405–1408, 1973.

Brinkhouse, K. M., Morrison, F. C., and Muhrer, M. E.: Comparative study of clotting defects in human, canine and porcine hemophilia. Fed. Proc., 11:409, 1952.

Brock, W. E., et al.: Canine hemophilia. Arch. Pathol., 76:464–469, 1963.

DeHeer, D. H., and Edgington, T. S.: Evidence for a B lymphocyte defect underlying the anti-A anti-erythrocyte autoantibody response of NZB mice. J. Immunol., 118:1858–1863, 1977.

Dodds, W. J.: Bleeding disorders. *In* Textbook of Veterinary Internal Medicine, Vol. 2, edited by S. J. Ettinger. Philadelphia, W. B. Saunders, 1975. pp. 1679–1698.

————: Canine factor X (Stuart-Prower factor) deficiency. J. Lab. Clin. Med., 82:560–566, 1973.

Field, R. A., Rickard, C. G., and Hutt, F. B.: Hemophilia in a family of dogs. Cornell Vet., 36:285–300, 1946.

Griggs, T. R., et al.: Von Willebrand factor: gene dosage relationships and transfusion response in bleeder swine—a new bioassay. Proc. Natl. Acad. Sci. USA, 71:2087–2090, 1974.

Hogan, A. G., Muhrer, M. E., and Bogart, R.: A hemophilia-like disease in swine. Proc. Soc. Exp. Biol. Med., 48:217–219, 1941.

Howell, J. McC., and Lambert, P. S.: A case of haemophilia A in a dog. Vet. Rec., 76:1103–1105, 1964.

Joshi, B. C., and Jain, N. C.: Detection of antiplatelet antibody in serum and on megakaryocytes of dogs with autoimmune thrombocytopenia. Am. J. Vet. Res., 37:681–685, 1976.

Kattlove, E. E., Shapiro, S. S., and Spivack, M.: Hereditary prothrombin deficiency. N. Engl. J. Med., 282:57–61, 1970.

Muhrer, M. E., et al.: Antihemophilic factor level in bleeder swine following infusions of plasma and serum. Am. J. Physiol., 208:508–510, 1965.

Mustard, J. F., et al.: Canine factor VII deficiency. Br. J. Haematol., 8:43–47, 1962.

Myers, L. J., Pierce, K. R., Gowing, G. M., and Leonpacher, R. J.: Pseudohemophilia in a dog. J. Am. Vet. Med. Assoc., 161:1028–1029, 1972.

Ratoff, O. D.: Hereditary defects in clotting mechanisms. Adv. Intern. Med., 9:107–179, 1958.

Rowsell, H. C., et al.: A disorder resembling hemophilia B (Christmas disease) in dogs. J. Am. Vet. Med. Assoc., 137:247–250, 1960.

Sanger, V. L., Mairs, R. E., and Trapp, A. L.: Hemophilia in a foal. J. Am. Vet. Med. Assoc., 144:259–264, 1964.

Spurling, N. W., Burton, L. K., Peacock, R., and Pilling, T.: Hereditary factor-VII deficiency in the Beagle. Br. J. Haematol., 23:59–67, 1972.

Spurling, N. W., Burton, L. K., and Pilling, T.: Canine factor-VII deficiency: Experience with a modified thrombotest method in distinguishing between the genotypes. Res. Vet. Sci., 16:228–239, 1974.

Storb, R., et al.: Canine hemophilia and hemopoietic grafting. Blood, 40:234–238, 1972.

Wurtzel, H. A., and Lawrence, W. C.: Canine hemophilia. Thromb. Diath. Haemorrh., 6:98–103, 1961.

HEMORRHAGE

Hemorrhage is the escape of blood from a vessel, whether it be to the outside of the body, into a body cavity, or into adjacent tissues. The ordinary rapid flow of blood through a break or cut in a vessel wall is called **hemorrhage by rhexis** (a bursting). Considerable amounts of blood may also be lost by a slow oozing of fluid and the escape of blood cells one by one through minute or imperceptible imperfections in the vessel walls. This is called **hemorrhage by diapedesis**.

Tiny hemorrhages that leave dots of blood not much larger than the point of a pin are called **petechiae** (singular, petechia). Somewhat larger hemorrhagic spots on a body surface or in the tissues are called **ecchymoses** (singular, ecchymosis). **Extravasations** refer to hemorrhages in the tissues spread over considerable areas.

When blood escapes into the tissues and produces a tumor-like enlargement, the mass usually goes by the name of **hematoma**, although **hematocyst** is more appropriate. A simple example is the common "blood blister," familiar to all who have aimed a hammer blow at a nail but somehow had it strike the thumb.

Causes. The causes of hemorrhage include any mechanical trauma cutting or breaking a blood vessel, necrosis or destruction of vessel wall, as by an ulcer or a spreading neoplasm, and rupture of a vessel weakened by aneurysm or atheroma. An **aneurysm** is a sharp bulging of the wall

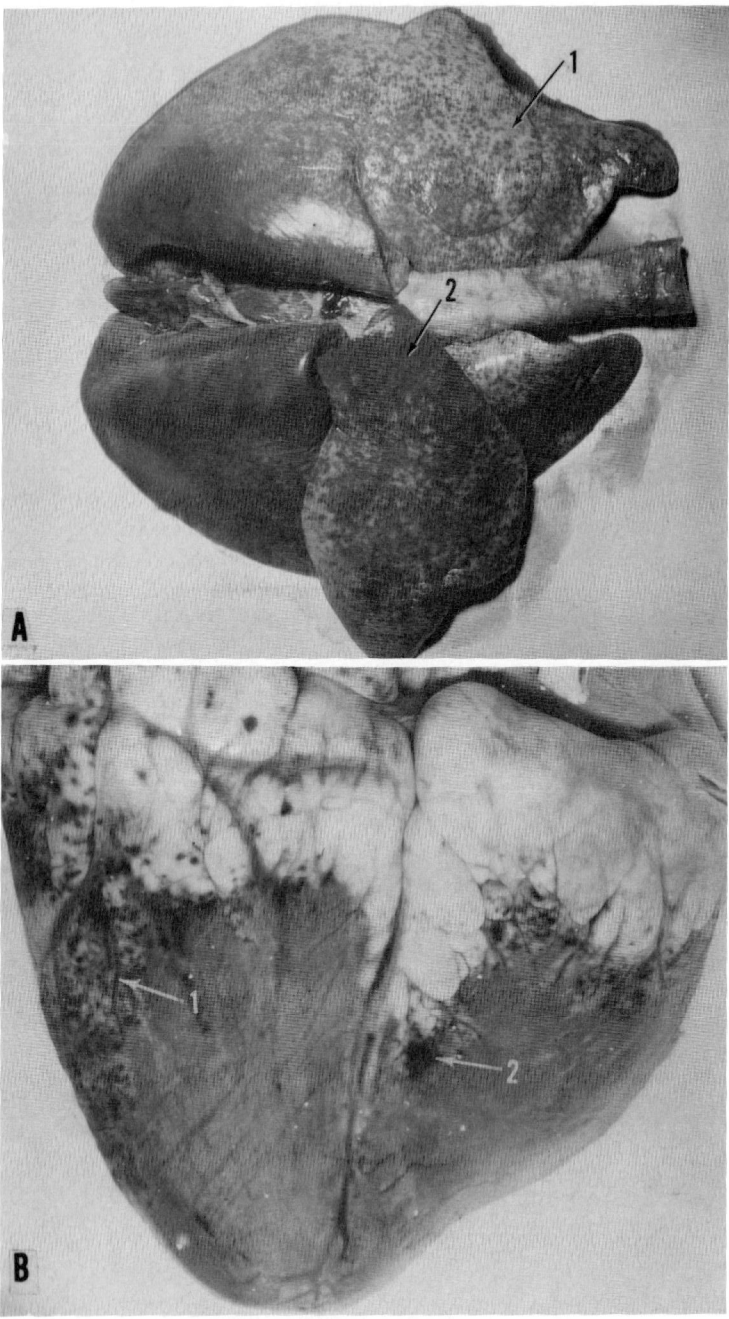

Fig. 5–7. Hemorrhage. *A*, Petechiae (*1*) and extravasations (*2*) of blood in the pleura of a dog dying of fulminant leptospirosis. *B*, Petechiae (*1*) and ecchymoses (*2*) in epicardium of the heart of a Hereford cow following intravenous injection of formalin solution.

of a blood vessel which occurs when the wall is weakened or partially destroyed. Aneurysms of the anterior mesenteric artery have been mentioned in connection with thrombosis. A **dissecting aneurysm** results from a special kind of rupture of the aorta or artery. As a result of trauma or disease (arteriosclerosis, lathyrism, aflatoxicosis), a weakened point in the wall yields to the pressure of blood, which ruptures the intima and forces its way along the vessel between layers of the media or even into the adventitia. The blood that "dissects" its way along the blood vessel may return at some distal point to the lumen, forming one or more new blood channels. Rupture through the adventitia of the aorta leads to massive, usually fatal hemorrhage. A rare but not unknown aneurysm may result from dead adult canine heartworms *(Dirofilaria immitis)* being forced into the pulmonary artery,

where they lodge as emboli. Their presence may result in aneurysmal dilatation and weakening of the arterial wall, which ruptures into a bronchus, leading to sudden death from exsanguination and suffocation.

Rupture of diseased (arteriosclerotic or atherosclerotic) blood vessels or of aneurysms is made more likely by the increase of blood pressure which goes with excitement or exercise. Aneurysms develop in the aorta of mutant *Blotchy* mice as a result of inherited cross-linking defects in collagen and elastica.

Toxic injury to capillary endothelium culminating in transient openings of punctiform size is chiefly responsible for petechiae and ecchymoses seen on serous and mucous membranes, as well as within the depths of the tissues. The causes of this toxic injury are several: toxins produced by septicemic infections, such as hog cholera,

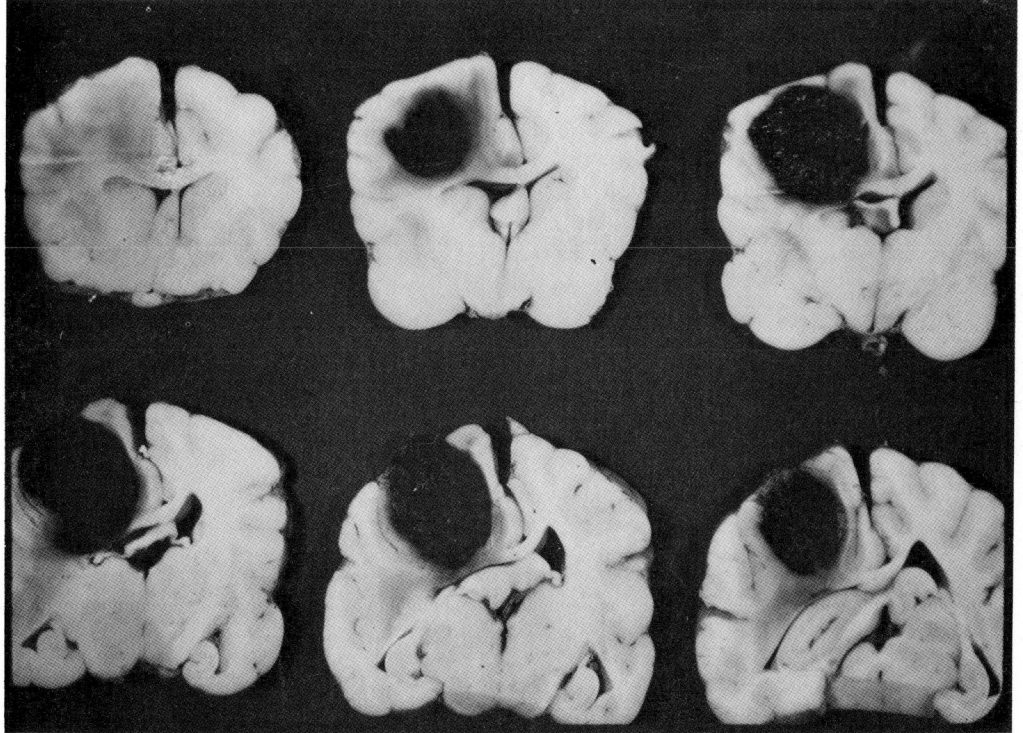

Fig. 5–8. Hemorrhage into brain as a complication of arteriosclerosis in a 12-year-old male Spitz dog. The brain has been sectioned at 1-cm intervals. (Courtesy of Angell Memorial Animal Hospital.)

pasteurellosis, anthrax, blackleg, and the probably allergic purpura hemorrhagica; certain plant poisonings, including bracken poisoning, and *Crotalaria* poisoning; various chemical poisonings, including arsenic; and certain digestive toxemias, especially enterotoxemia of sheep, in which the toxin of *Clostridium perfringens* is present.

Vitamin C deficiency, or **scurvy**, results in an increased capillary fragility leading to hemorrhage. Most animals synthesize adequate vitamin C and are not subject to deficiency. However, scurvy is frequently encountered in guinea pigs and nonhuman primates (monkeys and apes), which require an exogenous source of this vitamin.

Anoxia, whether it results from direct suffocation or from anemia or any other interference with adequate aeration of the blood, causes petechiae and ecchymoses. It may well be that many of the causes just listed are fundamentally an interference with oxidative processes.

Disorders of the clotting mechanism, such as that due to the action of dicoumarin and other substances listed under "Failure to Clot," can be considered secondary causes of hemorrhage once a slight weakness of the capillary wall develops. Whether such substances also injure the endothelial lining cells is unsettled.

Significance and Effect. In reviewing the results of hemorrhage, we have to consider the effects of the escaped blood, if it remains in the body cavities or tissues, and the effects of the loss of blood from the circulation. Blood that flows into the tissues or cavities of the body soon clots, and its subsequent history has been discussed under the heading of Clots. Its relation to icterus and to hemosiderin have been pointed out.

The location of hemorrhage is important

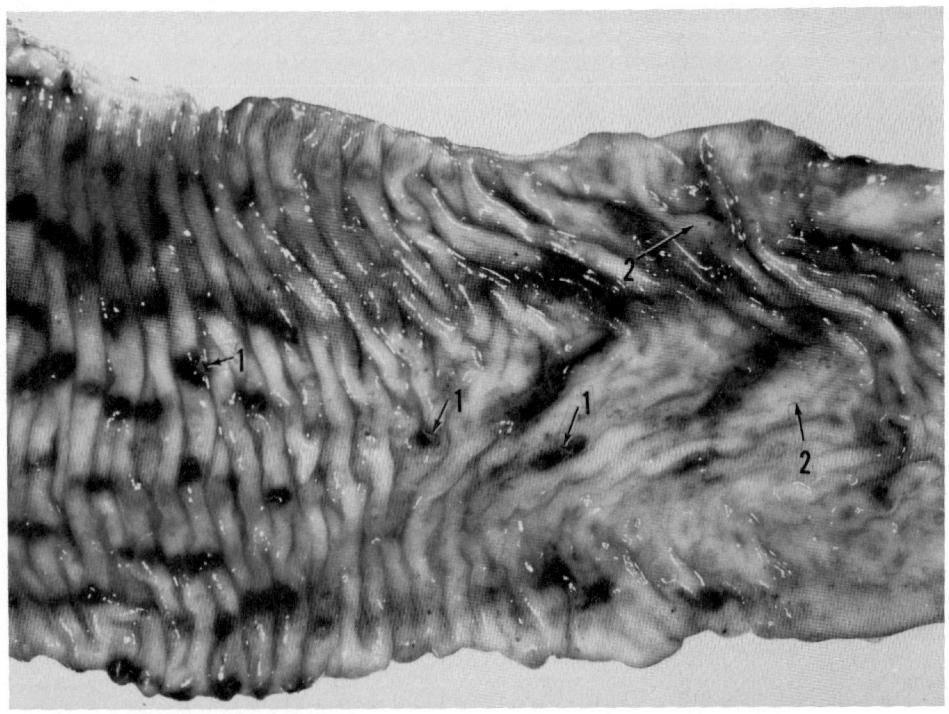

Fig. 5–9. Hemorrhages in the colon of a dog with rickettsiosis of "salmon poisoning." Ecchymoses (*1*) and petechiae (*2*). (Courtesy of Dr. Wm. J. Hadlow.)

to its significance. Hemorrhage into the brain may result in the loss of vital functions or permanent disability. Hemorrhage into the pericardial cavity may mechanically interfere with cardiac function. Hemorrhage into the trachea or bronchi may result in exsanguination or asphyxiation.

Loss of more than one-fourth or one-third of the total blood of the body will be fatal unless some of it is promptly replaced. Before this large amount is lost (25 or 30 pounds, or some 12 L in a 1000-pound horse), the arterial blood pressure drops markedly, which facilitates clotting and tends to reduce further loss, so that only the largest cuts or injuries result fatally.

Following loss of a considerable amount of blood, the volume of fluid is replaced within a hour or two by withdrawal from the intercellular spaces of the tissues, great thirst resulting. Leukocytes are replaced in one or two weeks; replenishment of the full number of erythrocytes is likely to require four to six weeks.

Chronic blood loss does not lead to the serious effects of massive bleeding. Rather, the continued loss of blood causes depletion of iron stores, resulting in iron-deficiency anemia.

Andrews, E. J., White, W. J., and Bullock, L. R.: Spontaneous aortic aneurysms in Blotchy mice. Am. J. Pathol., 78:199–210, 1975.
Ardran, G. M., Kemp, F. H., Hovell, G. J. R., and Woods, C. G.: Cephalohematoma in Squirrel monkeys. J. Am. Vet. Radiol. Soc., 18:70–75, 1977.

HYPEREMIA AND CONGESTION

Both these terms denote an excess of blood in the vessels of a given part. This can occur in either of two ways: too much blood being brought in by the arteries or too little being drained out by the veins. Some prefer the older term, congestion; some prefer to use the other. In either case, if too much blood is brought in by the arteries, the condition is said to be "active," if the blood simply remains because of impaired venous drainage, it is "passive." Some, therefore, speak of active and passive congestion; others, of active and passive hyperemia. A distinction is also made in that hyperemia, in itself, implies the active condition of too much arterial blood being brought in by dilated arterioles and capillaries, whereas congestion implies that the flow of blood, like the flow of vehicles on a busy street, is impeded because the elements next in front cannot move out fast enough. To make misunderstanding impossible, it is well to speak always of active hyperemia and passive congestion. However, on these pages, hyperemia will mean excessive arterial inflow, and congestion will signify interference with the venous exit. Synonymous with passive congestion is the term "venous congestion."

Active Hyperemia

This condition may occur in any organ or part of the body.

Microscopic Appearance. The capillaries are dilated and filled with blood. They also appear to be more numerous than before, simply because in the normal state some are empty and collapsed much of the time. Arteries and arterioles are also dilated, but this is seldom apparent after death because postmortem contraction of their musculature empties and closes their lumens.

Gross Appearance. To a greater or lesser extent, depending on its original color, the part takes on the bright red color of arterial blood. During life the part is also warmer than usual, and pulsating arteries may be felt which are not usually perceptible.

Causes. Active hyperemia is the first stage of inflammation, and the great majority of cases are of this nature. Heat locally applied, often as a therapeutic measure, promptly brings marked dilatation of the vessels. A person need only expose his bare skin in front of a fireplace to see it redden in a few moments. Increased physiologic activity leads to an increase of arterial blood, which supplies the oxygen and nutrients needed for the functions to be performed. This physiologic hyperemia is seen not only in muscles, but also in the stomach and intestines during digestion, and in the mammary gland at the start of lactation. On a somewhat different basis but still physiologic is the hyperemia, followed by congestion, which occurs in the decidual uterus at menstruation. Blushing is a transient hyperemia caused by a psychologic stimulus.

Significance and Effect. The significance and effect of active hyperemia are minor when it does not mark the onset of inflammation.

Passive Congestion

Passive congestion may occur in practically any part of the body, and it may be acute or chronic.

Microscopic Appearance. The capillaries and veins are dilated and full of blood; likewise, the sinusoidal blood spaces of the liver and spleen are filled with blood in cases in which these organs are involved. If the congestion is chronic, there is a slight or moderate increase of fibrous tissue in the walls of the veins, thickening and strengthening them, a sort of compensatory hypertrophy.

Acute passive congestion of the liver is frequently evidenced by sinusoidal capillaries and central veins that are conspicuously dilated but empty. This happens because, when a piece of liver is put in the fixative solution preparatory to microscopic sectioning, the blood oozes out into the solution, but the blood spaces retain their dilated shape. Also, the more central cells of the hepatic cords tend to disappear, leaving a central sea of blood, but this is discussed in the section on "Diseases of the Liver," as is the appearance of chronic congestion in this organ.

Gross Appearance. The congested part is slightly swollen and tends to have a bluish-red tinge. During life the temperature of the part may be discernibly lower than normal because new blood is not being brought in. After death, the bluish red darkens as postmortem hemolysis advances. Considerable amounts of blood can be squeezed from the cut surface. This is an important indication in such organs as the lungs and liver.

Causes. The most important cause, by far, of acute, generalized congestion is the diminished blood pressure that goes with a failing heart and vasodilation in the terminal stages of many infections and other diseases. The immediate cause of death is spoken of as generalized venous congestion or **congestive heart failure**. When this situation exists, at necropsy, one can see that the vena cava and large veins of the abdominal and thoracic cavities are large and dark, filled with blood which, quite likely, has clotted. The veins of the mesentery and intestinal walls are prominent and dark. The liver contains much blood, as do, probably, the lungs.

Chronic passive congestion of the lungs results from interference with the proper progress of the blood on the left side of the heart, in other words, from hindrance to its free and prompt movement from the pulmonary into the systemic circulation. Such interference occurs through either **insufficiency or stenosis of the mitral (left atrioventricular) valve**. Insufficiency results because of failure of the cusps of the valve to seat properly, which usually is the result of irregular thickening of their surfaces with inflammatory granulation tissue or fibrinous exudate. Or, the cusps may have become retracted through the shrinking of fibrous scars, so that they do not completely close the lumen. In either case when the ventricle contracts, some of the blood is forced backward through the leaky valve to impede the incoming flow from the pulmonary vein. Stenosis is a narrowing of the total size of the lumen. It results from the shrinking of fibrous scar tissue when the latter has developed around the base of the cusps. The effect again is to decrease the amount of blood that can pass the valve in a given time. All of these interfering derangements are the result of inflammation, valvular endocarditis, caused by infections, or by a congenital anomaly.

The aortic semilunar valve is subject to the same disorders as the mitral, although attacked less frequently. This does not directly affect the lungs but, in common with other valvular imperfections, leads to "compensatory" hypertrophy (really adaptive, as we have classified hypertrophy) of the left ventricle. This enlargement of the ventricle sometimes distorts the mitral valve to the extent that insufficiency develops, with the same pulmonary congestion.

Tricuspid (right atrioventricular) valvular disease is possibly more frequent in animals than mitral disease, and this valve is subject to the same insufficiency and stenosis. In this case, the blood is thrown back into the vena cava and its tributaries, the first appreciably expansible vascular channels being those of the liver. The result is **chronic passive congestion of the liver**. Chronic passive congestion of the liver may also be the result of severe obstruction of the flow of blood through the lungs, with retardation of the flow through the right side of the heart and backing up into the liver. Hypertrophy of the right ventricle is usually an accompaniment.

Cirrhosis makes it difficult for blood to get through the liver and causes chronic passive congestion of the portal venous system, including the spleen and intestines, usually with ascites.

Partial obstruction of any vein of considerable size leads to local congestion of its drainage area, unless collateral drainage is established. Such obstruction may be caused by thrombi or emboli, by stenosis as the result of fibrous scarring following phlebitis (as from repeated puncturing in intravenous administration of medicines) or by external pressure upon the vein from tumors or abscesses.

During the later stages of pregnancy, **pressure of the fetus** upon the femoral vein as it passes over the anterior border of the pubis causes chronic passive congestion (and consequent edema) of the hind leg. This occurs at least in the equine and bovine species, in which the single fetus reaches relatively large size and there is little opportunity for the tensions caused by the fetus to be shifted with changes in the mother's position. The same difficulty occurs in the human species, resulting in so-called **milk-leg**.

Gravity is the cause of **hypostatic congestion**. This is a congestion, often quite noticeable, of the organs and tissues on the

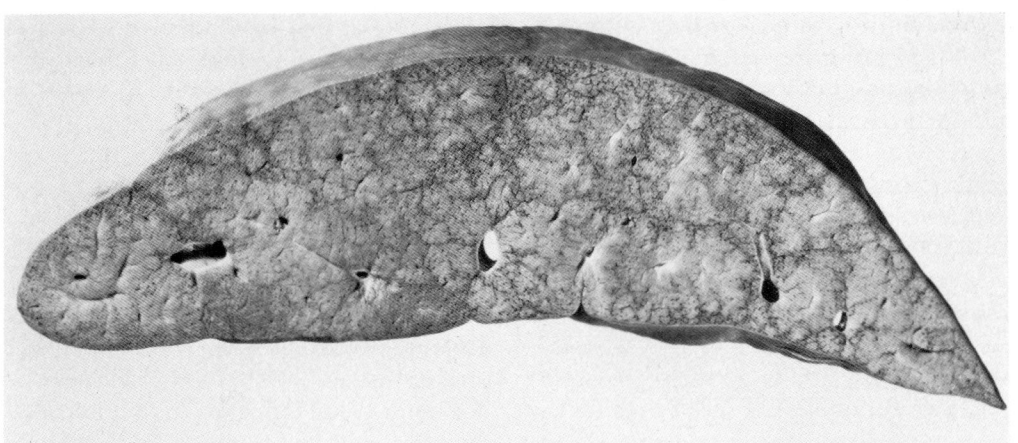

Fig. 5–10. Chronic passive congestion of the liver of an eight-month-old Hereford steer. The underlying lesions were large firm "vegetative" masses on the leaflets of the tricuspid valve. (Courtesy of Dr. W. J. Hadlow.)

lower side of a recumbent animal. Especially in large animals, there is a strong tendency for blood to gravitate to the lower side of the body. This may cause the death of an otherwise healthy horse confined for some hours in an unnatural position from which it cannot rise. The gravitational movement continues after death until clotting interferes, so that in many cadavers the condition is interpreted merely as a postmortem phenomenon. The prosector naturally takes this phenomenon into consideration in his interpretation of the gross lesions.

Significance and Effect. One of the effects of passive congestion is anoxia, since fresh blood cannot be brought in. Function is impaired; for instance, the congested udder does not secrete milk of normal quantity or quality; the congested intestine does not function properly. In delicate parenchymal cells, even necrosis may result. The slow movement of the current predisposes to thrombosis. Edema, which will be discussed presently, is a frequent result of either generalized or localized passive congestion.

The proliferation of connective tissue in chronic congestion has been mentioned. In the liver this thickens the walls of the central veins, almost nonexistent normally, and of the sinusoidal capillaries, the change being called **central cirrhosis**. Chronic passive congestion of the spleen is characterized by diffuse fibrosis of the red pulp, with hematoidin and hemosiderin conspicuous in amount.

Pulmonary chronic passive congestion produces the condition known as **brown induration of the lung**. The lung is indurated (hardened) because of fibrous thickening of the interalveolar septa, that is, of the capillary walls in them. This is visible microscopically and is detected grossly by a certain toughness and lack of resiliency. The brown color is due to hemosiderin. From the congested capillaries, there is a certain amount of hemorrhage by diapedesis into the alveoli. The pigment

released from the disintegrating erythrocytes is phagocytized as hemosiderin by reticuloendothelial cells, which remain to impart collectively their brownish color. Since chronic passive congestion of the lung is ordinarily the result of valvular heart disease, as just explained, the phagocytes filled with hemosiderin are called **heart-failure cells**.

EDEMA

Edema is a disorder characterized by an excessive accumulation of fluid (water) in the intercellular spaces, including the body cavities. Excessive fluid within the cells has already been defined as hydrops, or hydropic degeneration, and this definition will be respected here, in spite of a certain looseness in distinguishing between hydrops and edema which is occasionally encountered. The subject of edema has long been a confusing one, and many conflicting theories have been proposed concerning the mechanisms involved. Some of the confusion has come from a certain lack of consistency of ideas regarding edema and inflammation, so that in common medical parlance we formulate certain definitions but fail to abide by them.

May we begin by dispelling one or two fallacies that may have entered the student's mind from older sources, or from what may at first have seemed logical assumptions? (1) Edema is *not* caused by a heavy consumption of water. It is possible to fill an animal so full of water that serious disorders result, but edema is not one of them. (2) Edema is *not* caused by a heavy consumption of salt in the diet, notwithstanding the fact that depleting the patient's body of salts already accumulated in the tissues may be beneficial in causing greater elimination of water. (3) High blood pressure (ordinary arterial pressure) does *not* cause edema. This sometimes fatal disorder is all too common in human beings, but edema is not one of the signs.

Edema may be general or local. As the term is freely used, it may also be inflammatory or noninflammatory, but inflammatory edema, being a reaction to an irritant, is by definition an inflammation. (See Chapter 6.) Strict adherence to this concept in one's inner consciousness, if not in one's common phraseology, should considerably simplify the subject. In this discussion, edema means noninflammatory edema only.

Occurrence. Localized edema may occur in most organs and tissues, depending upon local causes. Generalized edema affects the body as a whole, but most of the fluid tends to accumulate, because of the force of gravity, in the lowest parts of the body, which are capable of stretching to make room for it. In quadrupeds, such places are along the ventral abdominal and chest wall and in and below the intermandibular space.

Microscopic Appearance. When tissue is edematous, the spaces between adjacent cells, fibrils, or other elemental structures are enlarged. During life they were, of course, filled with fluid; in the microscopic section there may or may not remain a faint, pink-staining residue of precipitated albumin, depending on the amount of albumin (and other protein) in the edema fluid. If the common technical procedure was followed of affixing the section to the glass slide with egg albumin, the beginner will need to guard against mistaking this fixative albumin, which becomes visible when slightly excessive, for the residue from an edema fluid. In case it is the fixative, the pink-staining albumin is visible outside the area of the section as well as in it.

Considerable judgment needs to be employed also in interpreting empty intercellular spaces. A certain but variable amount of space is left between cells by the shrinkage that occurs in the preparation of sections by the paraffin or similar techniques. These artificial spaces tend to be less numerous, less uniform in size, and less evenly distributed than the spaces that result from edema. Shrinkage follows natural lines of cleavage, which usually lie between one kind of tissue and another, although they do not separate epithelium from its connective-tissue base. A few erythrocytes, leukocytes, or fibrils of fibrin may be present, but any considerable number of the last two indicates inflammation.

Edema of the brain betrays itself first by distention of the perivascular (Fig. 5–11) and even the perineuronal spaces, but excessive shrinkage may be deceptive. The sulci are compressed and the convolutions flattened by pressure against the cranial wall, a situation more easily noticed grossly than microscopically. In edema of the lungs, the alveoli are filled with fluid. There is usually enough albuminous residue to render the condition noticeable microscopically.

Gross Appearance. The edematous part is swollen. Edematous swelling along the ventral belly wall is often of a thickness of several centimeters and rather sharply delimited, so that a conspicuous longitudinal ridge marks its boundaries along each side. The swelling commonly diffuses into the preputial region in males and fades out anteriorly in the sternal region. In other cases ("brisket-disease" of cattle), the swelling is most pronounced in the sternal region. Sometimes the edema is conspicuous externally only as a sagging protrusion of the submandibular tissues. This is especially true in sheep suffering from gastrointestinal parasitism, the condition called "bottle-jaw" among stockmen.

The swollen tissue has a firm and doughy consistency. It "pits on pressure," meaning that if the finger is pressed into the edematous tissue, the fluid is dispersed into nearby tissue spaces. When the finger is removed, the pit remains for a moment, since a certain interval of time is required for the fluid to filter back through the network of tissue cells and fibrils.

The cut surface, in well-marked cases, contains a pale yellowish fluid permeating the tissue strands. There may be slight clot-

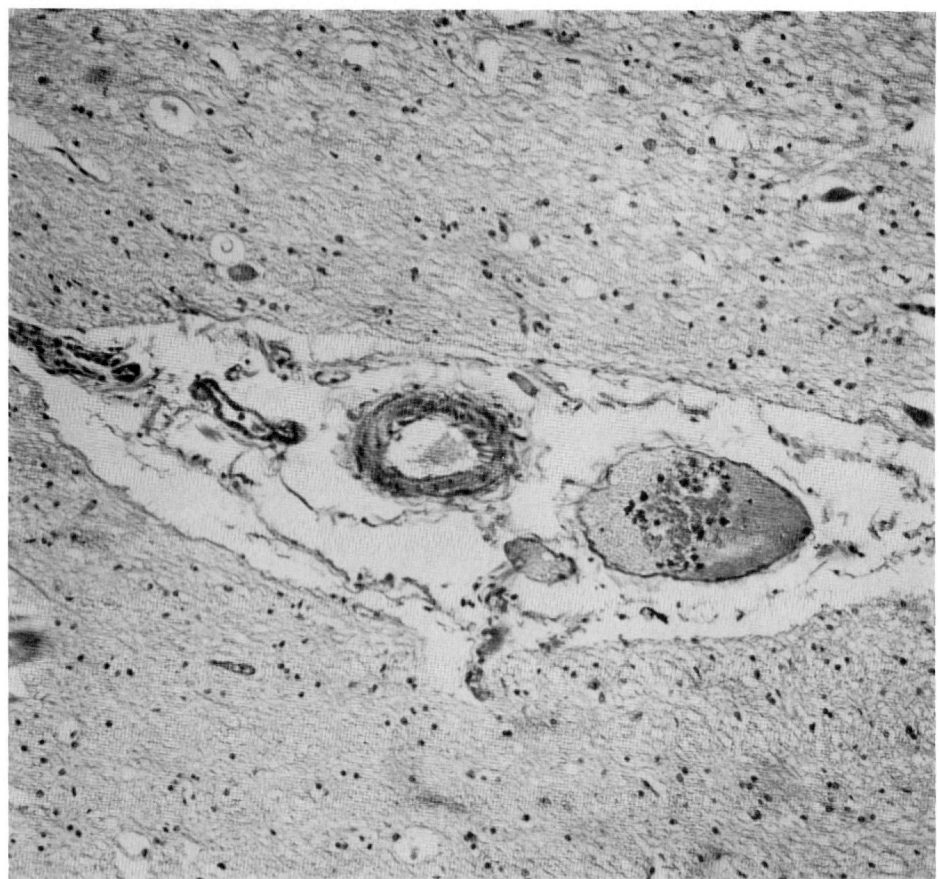

Fig. 5–11. Perivascular edema, brain of a horse. (H & E, × 200.)

ting, but usually the fluid drips from the cut surface; if pressure is applied, a much larger amount of fluid can be squeezed from the tissue.

During life the edematous part, if external, is cool as well as swollen. There is no redness and no sign of pain.

Edema of the lungs is best detected at autopsy by cutting through a lobe and squeezing the edges. If a watery fluid exudes, perhaps a little tinged with blood, the lung tissue being distended and of firm consistency, the condition is edema. If a definitely bloody fluid is pressed out, the lung is congested; if drops of pus appear, the condition is pneumonia. In edema of the peritoneal, pleural, or other serous cavities, the cavity is filled and often dis-

tended with a clear watery fluid. Edema of the brain is recognized less, perhaps, by the watery conditions of the tissue than by the flattening of the swollen gyri as they are pressed against the cranium.

The question of whether one is dealing with inflammatory or noninflammatory edema sometimes has to be answered by a study of all accompanying circumstances. The fluid of noninflammatory edema is called a **transudate**, because it is conceived as passing from the blood into the tissues purely as the result of deranged physiologic mechanisms. The fluid of inflammatory edema is called an **exudate**, being one of the types (serous) of exudates that characterize acute inflammation. If accessible for physical examination, a transudate can

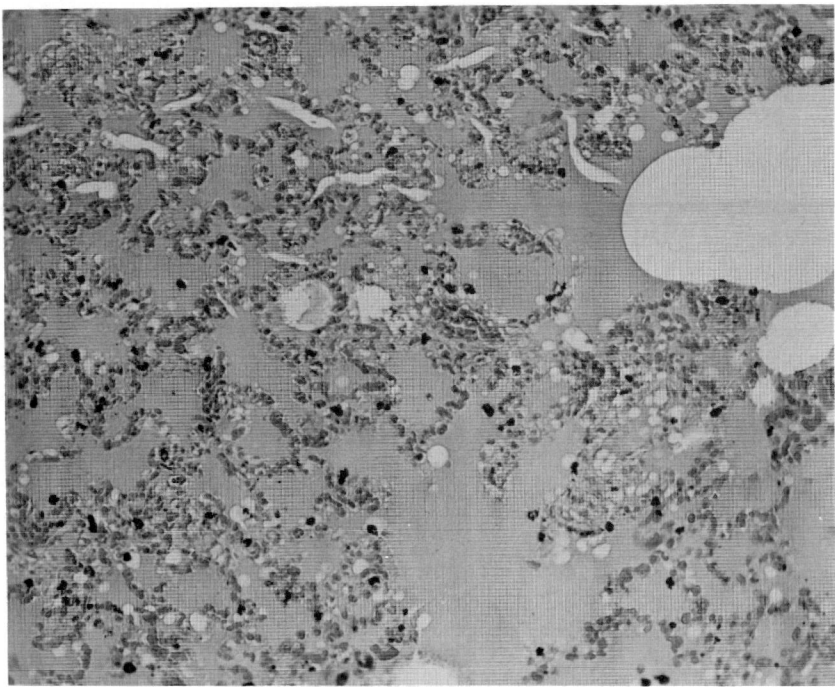

Fig. 5-12. Edema of the lung of a dog. Note homogeneous protein material fills alveoli. (H & E, × 170.) (Courtesy of Armed Forces Institute of Pathology.)

usually be differentiated from a serous exudate by the specific gravity. The specific gravity of a transudate is almost invariably less than 1.017, usually less than 1.015; that of serous exudate is ordinarily 1.017 or

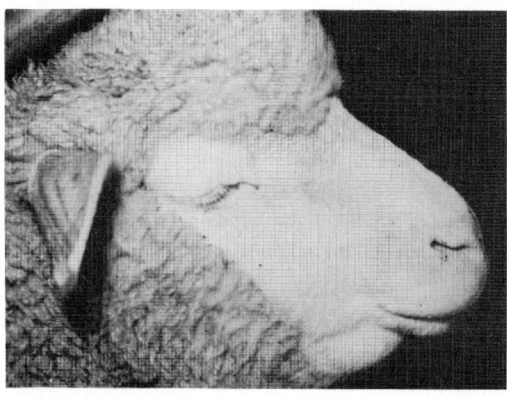

Fig. 5-13. Edema, subcutis, inframandibular region. Sheep with severe trichostrongylosis. Swollen tissue was doughy in consistency and pitted on digital pressure. (Courtesy of Dr. A. Tontis and Prof. Dr. H. Luginbühl.)

above. The difference is due to the much lower concentration of salts and colloids, especially albumin, in the transudate. Determinations of the total protein usually reveal less than 3% in the transudate of edema; it is likely to be considerably higher in an inflammatory exudate. As would be expected from these figures, the exudate leaves a heavier precipitate of protein, chiefly albumin, in the microscopic section, and inflammatory edema can usually be recognized on this basis. The exudate also contains an appreciable or even considerable number of leukocytes and often some fibrin; the transudate contains no more than traces of these, at most. Grossly, the exudate often includes some clotted fibrin, and there may be a frank fibrinous inflammation of some of the involved surfaces.

Causes. Physiologically, the blood enters a capillary with a hydrostatic pressure (blood pressure in the usual sense) of about

45 mm Hg. Since the walls of the capillaries are rather freely permeable to fluids and the smaller dissolved molecules, such as crystalloids, this pressure tends to expel those substances into the surrounding intercellular spaces. But this expulsive force is opposed by the (colloidal) osmotic pressure exerted by molecules that cannot pass through the capillary wall, chiefly the molecules of albumin and globulin, which together amount to about 6 gm/100 ml. This force has been computed in the human as 30 to 35 mm Hg, leaving an outward force of 10 to 15 mm Hg. Hence, at the arterial end of the capillary, much of the blood serum passes out into nearby intercellular spaces, where it is called lymph. As the blood current travels through the minute lumen of the capillary, its hydrostatic pressure is rapidly dissipated, declining to a figure between 11 and 16 mm Hg. By this time, the blood passing through the capillary has lost considerable water and has become a more concentrated solution, with a higher osmotic pressure than the 30 to 35 mm given for the arterial end. The fluid already in the tissues has an opposing osmotic pressure of its own, due to the substances dissolved in it. This osmotic attraction tends to draw the water out into the tissues. Toward the lower end of the capillary, this outward attraction is doubtless somewhat diminished because the incoming watery lymph has lowered its concentration of solutes. But this difference appears to be small and is usually disregarded. Conservatively disregarding both these extravascular changes in osmotic pressure, which would lessen the expellant force existing at the terminal end of the capillary, we still have at the venous end of the capillary some 11 to 16 mm of outward pressure opposed to 30 to 35 mm of inward osmotic pressure, a balance of 19 mm tending to draw fluid into the capillary. The result is a normal flow of fluid out of the capillary at its upper end and a return flow into the lumen at its venous end. Edema is the result of some interference with this normal flow.

Noninflammatory Edema. The fundamental disturbances operating to cause noninflammatory edema can be simplified to the following: decreased plasma colloid osmotic pressure, increased capillary blood pressure, obstruction of lymphatic drainage, and retention of sodium and water.

Decreased plasma colloid osmotic pressure is the result of hypoproteinemia. Loss of a large part of the albumin and globulin of the blood occurs in those forms of nephritis (or nephrosis) characterized by severe albuminuria. In the human species, at least, the loss of albumin is much greater than the loss of globulin, causing a "reversed albumin-globulin ratio" of 1 to 3 instead of the normal 3 to 1. In some domestic species (the bovine, especially), the proportion of albumin is normally much lower and the frequency of albuminuria much less; the precise value of the human analogy has not been adequately investigated. The preponderant loss of albumin is especially significant, for its molecules are small and more numerous than those of globulin, therefore exerting a dominant effect on the osmotic pressure. The above-described mechanisms, loss of protein and consequent loss of osmotic pressure, is the cause of the commonly encountered **renal edema**.

Serious deficiencies of blood protein also occur in starvation, protein deficiency, and cachexia, the amount assimilated from the diet being just too small to replenish losses. This situation is the cause of **nutritional edema** or **cachectic edema**.

Advanced liver disease, usually in the form of cirrhosis, can also lead to hypoproteinemia due to decreased synthesis of plasma proteins. The liver is the site of production of albumin, fibrinogen, and alpha and beta globulins.

Continued daily removal of blood protein can also deplete the available supply and produce hypoproteinemia. This occurs as a result of heavy infestation with bovine and ovine trichostrongyles and some other intestinal parasites, whose blood-sucking bites and possibly an anticoagulant toxin result in repeated minute hemorrhages in large numbers. This daily loss of blood with inadequate replacement accounts for the frequent cases of **parasitic edema**, as well as for the severe anemia.

Increased capillary blood pressure usually results from **venous stasis**. This name is given to passive congestion so severe that movement of the blood has all but stopped. Such a severe obstruction of the normal venous flow does two things to the veins and capillaries and the blood in them: it greatly increases the hydrostatic pressure in the veins and the venous ends of the capillaries, and it deprives the capillary endothelium, as well as the other tissue constituents of the area, of their normal supply of oxygen and quite possibly of other nutrients. This certainly does not improve the functional capacity of the capillary walls, and it is believed to weaken them to the point where they permit the passage of albumin and other large molecules. The effect of such a movement of molecules is to lower the osmotic pressure within the capillary and raise it in the surrounding tissue fluid. However, this **increased permeability** to large molecules becomes significant only in **inflammatory edema,** as is proved by the fact that the noninflammatory transudate contains such small amounts of protein.

The effects of (1) the increased intracapillary and venous hydrostatic pressure, (2) the lowered intracapillary osmotic pressure, and (3) the increased osmotic pressure in the intercellular fluid combine to neutralize the attractive forces (about 19 mm Hg) that draw fluid back into the capillary. The result is an increase of the fluid that stays in the intercellular spaces, and this constitutes edema.

Since the usual cause of venous stasis is impaired cardiac function, a weakened and worn-out heart, edema caused in this way is known as **cardiac edema**.

For practical purposes, the clinician or the pathologist may well ask himself which of the four kinds of edema—renal, nutritional, parasitic, or cardiac—is present in his patient. The first three exist by virtue of hypoproteinemia; the last results from impaired cardiac action and generalized venous stasis. The first steps to be taken in treatment depend on the answer to this question.

Obstruction to lymphatic drainage, which is similar to localized venous stasis, also results in edema. Examples of obstructed lymph drainage are seen in the case of lymph nodes invaded by neoplastic or granulomatous tissue so that the passage of lymph through them is blocked.

In some parts of the world, human lymph nodes become obstructed due to the adult filarial worm, *Filaria bancrofti,* whose microfilariae are mosquito-borne and found in the circulating blood. The area drained through such nodes becomes edematous. Lymph drainage may also be obstructed and cause edema in a rare condition known as **congenital hereditary lymphedema**, which results from the discontinuity or absence of lymph vessels. This condition has been described in children and young dogs.

A special case of obstructed lymph drainage is the accumulation of fluid in the meningeal spaces and ventricles of the brain, causing communicating and internal **hydrocephalus** respectively. Swelling or fibrous proliferations that would otherwise constitute insignificant anatomic derangements close the minute openings through which the lymph has to drain, resulting in continuous increase of fluid and pressure atrophy of the brain parenchyma.

A similar situation exists in the eye; obstruction of the lymph drainage causes increased fluid in the eyeball with destructive intraocular pressure and pressure

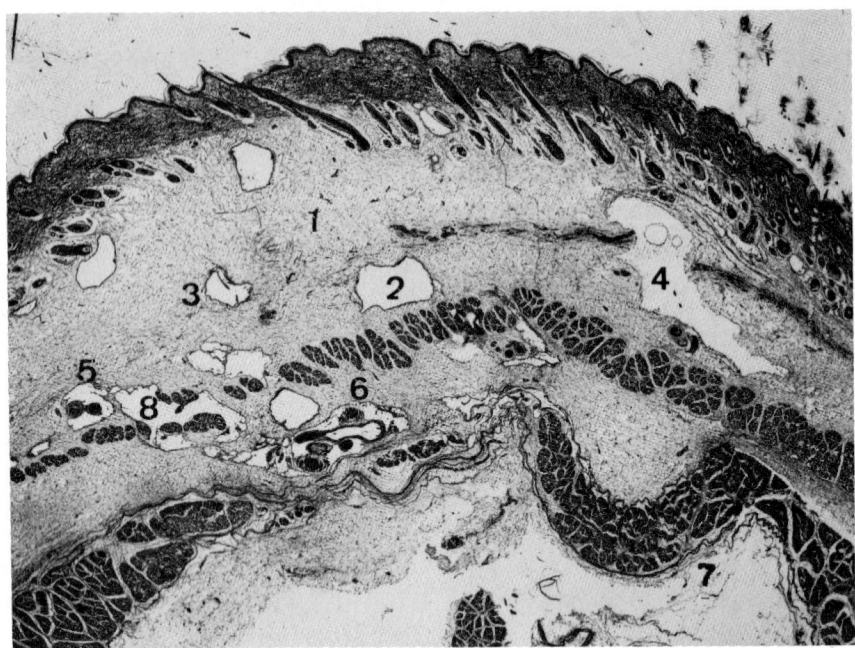

Fig. 5–14. Congenital hereditary lymphedema, one day old puppy. Section of skin of thorax. The subcutis (*1*) is thickened and contains edema of low protein content. Blood vessels are irregularly dilated (*2*), some vascular valves (*3*) appear ruptured, some lymph vessels surround thick-walled veins (*5*) or arteries (*6*). The panniculus muscle bundles are separated by edematous stroma (*7*) and by dilated lymph vessels (*8*). (Courtesy of Prof. Dr. H. Luginbühl and *Journal of Medical Genetics.*)

atrophy, a condition known as **glaucoma**. Edema within the optic papilla, known as **papilledema**, however, is due to increased intracranial fluid and intracranial pressure projected along the optic nerve within its meningeal covering.

Retention of sodium and water. As stated earlier, excess consumption of either salt or water by a normal individual does not cause edema. However, failure to excrete sodium in the urine resulting secondarily in water retention does lead to generalized edema. Reduced urinary excretion of sodium can occur in congestive heart failure and in nephrosis and nephritis. It is important to recall that these diseases also produce edema by other mechanisms as indicated earlier. Increased renal tubular reabsortion is believed to be the cause of renal retention of sodium. However, reduced glomerular filtration may also be important in these diseases.

Adrenal cortical hormones may also play a role in congestive heart failure and renal disease. These hormones (particularly aldosterone) cause retention of sodium and increased excretion of potassium. Edema is not infrequently encountered in patients receiving these steroids.

Significance and Effect. The fact already noted that edema is almost always of parasitic, nutritional, cardiac, or renal origin is of much practical significance to the diagnostician.

Edema fluid remaining for more than a few days tends to become organized with fibrous tissue, perhaps as a chronic inflammatory reaction, perhaps through clotting and subsequent organization. This fibrosis is marked in the edema due to lymphatic obstruction in human filariasis (*Filaria,* or *Wuchereria bancrofti*). The human limb becomes permanently and irregularly thickened to the point where it resembles an elephant's leg, causing the condition to be called **elephantiasis**. In spite of this fibrosing tendency, however, most edemas readily subside if the cause is removed. Surgical drainage, as of the edematous peritoneal cavity, helps but little, for with the cause unabated, the fluid soon returns.

Accumulation of fluid in the peritoneal cavity is called **ascites**; in the thorax, it is **hydrothorax**; in the pericardium, **hydropericardium**; in the scrotum, **hydrocele**. In most of these cases, the condition is an inflammatory edema or serous inflammation, but noninflammatory ascites is not rare. It may be a part of generalized edema, or it may result from stasis of the portal circulation caused, in most instances, by obstruction of the intrahepatic flow by the proliferated connective tissue of cirrhosis. Generalized subcutaneous edema is called **anasarca**. Noninflammatory hydropericardium occurs rarely in connection with myocardial venous stasis, but in animals, at least, practically all cases are inflammatory. **Hydrops amnii** is a noninflammatory edema of the amniotic sac.

Angioneurotic edema is a rare hereditary disease of human beings in which there is a deficiency of the inhibitor of the first components of complement (C1). This complement inhibitor helps to control the complement cascade (see Chapter 7), as well as to inhibit plasmin, kallikrein, and activated Hageman factor. In deficient individuals, it is believed that minimal trauma and tissue damage leads to edema through the generation of vascular permeability factors, which in normal individuals would be checked by the inhibitor (Frank et al., 1976).

Frank, M. M., Gelfand, J. A., and Atkinson, J. P.: Hereditary angioedema. The clinical syndrome and its management. Ann. Int. Med., *84*:580–593, 1976.

Ladds, P. W., Dennis, S. M., and Leipold, H. W.: Lethal congenital edema in Bulldog pups. J. Am. Vet. Med. Assoc., *159*:81–86, 1971.

Lieberman, A. H.: Current status of aldosterone in the etiology of edema. Arch. Intern. Med., *102*:990–997, 1958.

Luginbühl, H., et al.: Congenital hereditary lymphoedema in the dog. II. Pathological studies. J. Med. Genet., *4*:153–165, 1967.

Roberts, K. B.: Oedema. *In* General Pathology, 4th ed., edited by L. Florey. London, Lloyd-Luke Med. Books, Ltd., 1970. pp. 370–393.

SHOCK

Following immediately or within a few hours after severe traumatic injury to an extensive amount of tissue, or after a major operation, especially one involving considerable exposure and handling of the intestines, or as the result of severe pain of certain kinds, the baffling and often fatal disorder known as shock is likely to supervene. The sudden loss of a large amount of blood has practically the same effect, as does also the exudation of a large amount of serum a day or so after a widespread superficial burn.

The signs of shock may also be evoked experimentally in dogs or monkeys by administration of endotoxin or by withdrawal of sufficient amounts of blood to reduce the mean arterial pressure to about 40 mm Hg.

A patient suffering from shock is in the severest state of functional depression compatible with life, and life may cease at any moment. He is conscious but does not show it; humans can answer questions intelligently but do so only with slowness and reluctance. He feels cold and without strength; the body temperature is subnormal and the body surface has no warmth-giving circulation. The fundamental change is a tremendous fall in blood pressure; it is accompanied by the shallow and irregular respirations and the rapid but weak or even irregular pulse of a failing heart. In experimentally-induced shock, the syndrome may continue to progress to death after the hypotension has been maintained for a certain time, even after the blood volume has been restored.

Causes. In spite of extensive studies, all is not yet settled with respect to the etiologic mechanisms of shock. It seems clear that the volume of circulating blood is too small to fill the space in the vascular system, with the result that the heart has insufficient blood to fill its chambers. In the case of a sudden, severe hemorrhage, this is readily understood. Even the copious serous exudate that flows from a large burned area may conceivably reduce the volume of circulating blood sufficiently to produce the situation outlined, although one would suppose that a satisfied thirst would replenish the fluid of the blood as needed. But in the strictly typical cases of shock following operations or injuries, there is no loss of fluid to the exterior. In many instances there is edema of the lungs, and in the case of large muscular bruises, there is considerable exudation of serum into the bruised tissues (inflammatory edema). Some differences exist between species: in the dog, experimental shock usually results in hemorrhagic enterocolitis. In the baboon, the intestine is not so affected, but hemorrhage and edema occur in the lung. While the loss of some fluid can be explained in these ways, there are many examples of equally extensive edema without the syndrome of shock. It becomes apparent that the real reason for the lack of sufficient blood to fill the vascular channels is that the channels have stretched. To say it a little more precisely, each capillary has expanded until it holds more blood than formerly. This slight expansion becomes the more significant when we realize that it is normal in most, if not all, parts of the body for more than half of the capillaries to be closed at any given moment, especially if the organ or part is resting. The dilatation of capillaries, it may be said, is chiefly in the internal parts of the body, the abdominal area especially; these capillaries are found postmortem to be filled with the blood which should be passing through the heart.

While the type and degree of vasomotor innervation of capillaries is not positively known, there seems little doubt that the dilatation of the capillaries is a nervous phenomenon. The suddenness of the change as well as the circumstances under which it occurs would strongly indicate this. Another explanation has, however, had its advocates. This is that histamine or a histamine-like substance is liberated from injured tissues and that this substance both paralyzes the capillaries and increases their permeability. Following the theory further we see that the "increased permeability of the capillaries" is the same phenomenon that has already been explained in connection with inflammatory edema; increased permeability to large molecules, which escape into the intercellular fluid, raise its osmotic pressure and attract fluid into it. Experimentally, the injection of histamine has such an action, but there are several objections to attributing to it the condition we have defined as shock. Among the most practical of these are the following: in some of the causative situations, there is little destruction of tissue and little histamine produced; in many cases of shock, there is no edema; and it seems difficult to explain why a widely diffused substance in the blood would cause dilatation of capillaries in the splanchnic areas, but leave them constricted and empty in the peripheral parts of the body.

From the preceding paragraphs it should be obvious that shock is an entity that has multiple causes, but many of the causes act through similar mechanisms. Regardless of the original insult, shock is an inequality between blood volume and the capacity of the vascular system, which results from blood or fluid loss or vasodilation of neurogenic origin, and leads to a reduction of blood flow to the tissues. The latter causes anoxia, which may sustain and accentuate shock. Based on cause, shock can be classified as **hemorrhagic shock** (blood loss); **neurogenic shock** (trauma, pain, psychic); **traumatic (or surgical) shock** (probably neurogenic); **burn shock** (fluid loss); and **endotoxic (septic) shock** (from bacterial endotoxins).

Diagnosis. The diagnosis of shock is usually made clinically on the basis of the startling picture already outlined, but a reliably precise diagnosis often is not easy. It is probably for this reason that the exact limitations of the syndrome we call shock are open to doubt. On the one hand it must be distinguished from the fainting that results in some people from a sudden severe pain, such as may arise from a blow on the testicle or the periosteum. Fainting is a purely nervous reaction involving complete unconsciousness, but is of little more than momentary duration and is unaccompanied by the severe vascular disturbances characteristic of shock. Transient spells of complete unconsciousness are not unknown in animals, at least in the horse, but they appear to have causes other than nervous reflexes. It is doubtful that true fainting occurs in animals. At the other extreme, some have included with shock the premortal coma and near-coma which is often seen in fatal cases of many systemic diseases. If this usage were followed, the definition of shock would have to be broad, indeed.

The postmortem lesions of shock are described as severe congestion of the smaller vessels of the lungs, liver, and intestines especially, together with an ischemic state of the peripheral parts of the body. In the lungs, the congestion is accompanied not only by the presence of edema fluid in the alveoli, but also by appreciable hemorrhage into these spaces, a fact, which should differentiate the condition from pulmonary congestion and edema from cardiac causes, just as the absence of inflammatory cells should differentiate it from incipient pneumonia. The congestive state of the intestines may also be accompanied by edema and by hemorrhages. There may be small amounts of blood-tinged fluid in the peritoneal, pleural, or pericardial cavities. The spleen is empty and bloodless.

In patients that live a day or two, degenerative changes and necrosis may be found in the kidneys, liver, heart, adrenal cortex, lymph nodes, and spleen. With one or two exceptions, the lesions outlined here are similar to those of poisoning by alpha-naphthyl thiourea. However, the total absence of blood in the fluid in the lungs and elsewhere is an important differentiating feature. The kidneys are congested in the poisoned animals; the peripheral tissues are not strikingly bloodless. In both symptoms and lesions, points of marked similarity between shock and various other diseases could be named. But the essence of our concept of shock is that it is a reflex nervous phenomenon or something closely akin thereto, and not to be explained on the basis of any of the usual causes of disease, such as poisons, infections, or even trauma in its ordinary aspects. The lesions of the shock-like syndrome that follows severe hemorrhage naturally include little in the nature of congestion; all parts are ischemic. Another important differential feature is the fact that the intravenous administration of blood or isotonic solutions and serum substitutes is promptly beneficial following hemorrhage, but this is not true of shock.

The effects of shock are obvious. If death occurs, it is due largely to cerebral or myocardial ischemia.

Balis, J. U., Rappaport, E. S., Gerber, L., and Neville, W. E.: Development of lung lesions in endotoxin shock. Am. J. Pathol., 66:53a, 1972.

Balis, J. U., et al.: A primate model for prolonged endotoxin shock: blood-vascular reactions and effects of glucocorticoid treatment. Lab. Invest., 38:511–523, 1978.

Barton, R. W., Reynolds, D. G., and Swan, K. G.: Mesenteric circulatory responses to hemorrhagic shock in the baboon. Ann. Surg., 175:204–209, 1972.

Berman, I. R.: The lung lesion in shock. Adv. Exp. Med. Biol., 23:51–55, 1972.

Brungardt, J. M., Reynolds, D. G., and Swan, K. G.: Route of endotoxin delivery effects on canine mesenteric hemodynamics. Am. J. Physiol., 223:565–568, 1972.

Chang, J., and Hackel, D. B.: Comparative study of myocardial lesions in hemorrhagic shock. Lab. Invest., 28:641–647, 1973.

Coalson, J. J., et al.: Pathophysiologic responses of the subhuman primate in experimental septic shock. Lab. Invest., 32:561, 1975.

Herman, C. M., Moquin, R. B., and Horwitz, D. L.: Coagulation changes of hemorrhagic shock in baboons. Ann. Surg., 175:197–203, 1972.

Janson, P. M. C.: Study of lysosomal disruption during development of endotoxic shock in baboon. S. Afr. J. Surg., 12:81, 1974.

Margaretten, W., Howes, E. L., Jr., and McKay, D. G.: The effect of shock on the inflammatory response. Am. J. Pathol., *78*:159–170, 1975.

Pingleton, W. W., Coalson, J. J., and Guenter, C. A.: Significance of leukocytes in endotoxic shock. Exp. Mol. Pathol., *22*:183–194, 1975.

Rutherford, R. B., and Trow, R. S.: Pathophysiology of irreversible hemorrhagic shock in monkeys. J. Surg. Res., *14*:538–550, 1973.

Selkurt, E. E.: Physiological basis of circulatory shock. Status of investigative aspects of hemorrhagic shock. Fed. Proc., *29*:1832–1835, 1970.

Stickles, L. E., Jr.: Shock. Part 1: Basic origins and causes. Canine Pract., *2*:48–52, 1975.

Swan, K. G., and Reynolds, D. G.: Blood flow to the liver and spleen during endotoxin shock in the baboon. Surgery, *72*:388–394, 1972.

Vick, J. A., et al.: Treatment of hemorrhagic shock with a new vasodilator. Milit. Med., *138*:490–494, 1973.

CHAPTER 6

Inflammation

A pathologic phenomenon known and studied from ancient times, inflammation has long been defined as **the reaction of the tissues to an irritant**. Although, owing to its simplicity, this definition is difficult to surpass, two important characteristics that demand emphasis are omitted. First, inflammation is a dynamic process and not a state, and secondly, the process depends upon viable tissue. The definition proposed by Ebert (in Zweifach, *et al.*, 1965), though more cumbersome, is more complete: "Inflammation is a process which begins following sublethal injury to tissue and ends with complete healing." This definition also includes the end result of inflammation, i.e., healing, which is a part of the dynamic process and not a distinct entity unto itself. The basic meaning of the verb, "to inflame" is to "set fire to." Many who have suffered the agonies of a severe, acute inflammation in a tender spot will attest to the aptness of the name.

The clinical signs that characterize inflammation are, as stated by Celsus (30 BC–38 AD) in the first century A.D., and by every medical writer since that time, *rubor et tumor cum calore et dolore,* which, translated, means "redness and swelling with heat and pain." These signs and symptoms are known as the **cardinal signs** of inflammation. The redness is due to a great increase of blood in the inflamed part. The swelling comes from the increase of blood

and the additional presence of substances which, like sap from a tree, have exuded from the blood vessels into the surrounding tissues and are called exudates. The heat, objective but not subjective, also results from the increased flow of blood, carrying warmth to the periphery from the higher interior temperatures of the body. The pain is often attributed to increased pressure upon nerve endings, but it may well be that the irritating effects of toxic products are of greater significance, since the degree of pain that accompanies inflammations of apparently equal extent and severity may be highly variable. The Greek physician, Galen AD 130–200), later added loss of function as a fifth cardinal sign of inflammation. Pain-initiated reflex inhibition of muscle movements, mechanical swelling, and tissue destruction all contribute to loss of function.

Inflammation is both a beneficial phenomenon, when it leads to healing and a random series of events, seemingly without purpose, when it continues as a prolonged, unending process. It occurs in all the more complex forms of animal life. Without its protection, the animal races could not have survived their enemies, a fact which appears to have been first perceived by John Hunter (1728–1793) about 200 years ago. The body possesses potent defensive weapons of two quite different forms, its humoral antibodies and its reactive cells, chiefly the leukocytes. The effect of inflammation, with its hyperemic changes is to bring these defensive mechanisms into immediate contact with the irritant substance or the cells that have been injured by it. By this means the causative irritant, if still present, can often be destroyed or at least confined, which is the first prerequisite to recovery from the injury.

Although without inflammation survival is not possible, like other vital processes, inflammation may become aberrant and harmful. Diseases thought to be immunologic in origin, such as rheumatic fever, rheumatoid arthritis, glomerulonephritis, and disseminated lupus erythematosus, are associated with inflammatory reactions that provide no obvious benefit, but rather inflict harm upon the host.

NATURE AND KINDS OF IRRITANTS CAUSING INFLAMMATION

It may be advantageous to review here, before proceeding to a study of the inflammatory process itself, the **causes of inflammation**:

(1) **Pathogenic organisms** or, more precisely, the toxic and injurious substances produced by them. Included in this group are bacteria, viruses, fungi, protozoa and parasitic metazoa. More will be said later about the effects of each class.

(2) **Chemical poisons**, which are of endless variety. As explained under the heading of necrosis (which also is produced by many of them), poisons may act either upon the tissues with which they come in immediate contact or upon more distant cells, such as those of the liver, kidney and brain, which are often susceptible to highly diluted poisons in the blood. Some poisons, like cyanides and strychnine, kill without causing either inflammation or necrosis.

(3) **Mechanical and thermal injuries.** Prominent among these are burns by heat, electricity, light or other radiant energy.

Excessive cold, as well as blows and lacerations are also included.

(4) **Immune reactions.** An inflammatory reaction is associated with antigen-antibody interactions that occur under various circumstances. Included are delayed hypersensitivity, the Arthus reaction, the Shwartzman reaction, serum sickness, and certain autoimmune diseases.

Ryan, G. B., and Majno, G.: Acute inflammation: a review. Am. J. Pathol., 86:185–276, 1977.
Thomas, L.: Adaptive Aspects of Inflammation. Keynote address at Third Symposium, Int. Inflammation Club, Brook Lodge, Michigan, June 1–3, 1970.
Zweifach, B. W., Grant, L., and McClusky, R. I. (eds.): The Inflammatory Process. New York, Academic Press, 1965.

THE INFLAMMATORY PROCESS

Despite the simple manner in which inflammation has been defined, it is not a simple process, but rather a highly complex series of events, whether approached from its morphologic, physiologic, or biochemical characteristics. It is beyond our intentions to discuss each of these events in depth, but rather concentrate on morphologic changes and present the more accepted or plausible explanations for their development. The few pages devoted to inflammation in this chapter will hopefully provide a foundation upon which the student of pathology can build. The subject is classically covered with the completeness of current knowledge in *The Inflammatory Process*, second edition, edited by Zweifach, Grant, and McClusky, and in *Florey's General Pathology*. The inflammatory process, particularly when acute, is primarily a circulatory phenomenon involving changes in the amount and quality of blood reaching the affected area. These changes have already been alluded to in describing the cardinal signs of inflammation. Regardless of the nature of the injurious agent or the location of the insult, the basic character of the initial vascular response is remarkably similar. Only as inflammation progresses do features develop which depend upon the cause and allow for the morphologic classification of inflammation.

The Sequence of Vascular Events in Inflammation

The circulatory events of inflammation were determined with great nicety by Cohnheim (1839–1884) in 1867, and little has been added to our knowledge of the visual sequelae of the vascular events since his original description. The following sequence is based on Cohnheim's observations of the **vascular** changes.

Changes in the Blood Vessels. **Momentary constriction.** Immediately upon application of the irritant the vessels are constricted, apparently by a kind of stimulant action before the full effect of the irritant is felt. Because of its transitory character, this stage is of negligible importance.

Dilation of the vessels quickly supervenes, admitting more arterial blood and instituting the stage of hyperemia. This is believed to occur through relaxation of the arteriolar smooth muscle walls and of the precapillary sphincters. A noteworthy feature of the dilatation phenomenon is the startling increase in the number of capillaries visible in an inflamed area. This is due to the fact that unfilled capillaries, previously unseen, become distended and conspicuous. As far as acute inflammations are concerned, there is no actual proliferation. The cause of the dilation, which is predominantly restricted to arterioles and venules and not capillaries, is probably multiple, but as yet not completely understood. In part, the **axon reflex** or the so-called antidromic reflex is responsible for dilation at the site of injury and the associated dilation beyond the area of immediate injury. The vasomotor nerves are not necessary to the development of dilation or any other aspect of the inflammatory process. Of more importance in causing dilation, and of greater significance in altering vascular permeability, are the so-called **chemical mediators** of inflammation,

which will be discussed shortly. An increase in capillary and venule **blood pressure** is associated with the dilation of vessels.

Increased permeability of venules and capillaries develops more slowly, in connection with retardation of the flow, and permits the large molecules of blood protein and a few erythrocytes to leak through into the tissues. Leukocytes also pass through the walls with much greater ease than is normally the case. The exudative stage is thus instituted. Explanations for this increased permeability of the walls differ. Numerous theories have been advanced; some have since been disregarded and others are still in question. The effects of chemical mediators on the venule and capillary wall are probably the principal underlying factors in increasing permeability. An increase in local blood pressure and stretching of vessel walls also contribute to increased permeability. It is uncertain how these mechanisms actually affect the vessel wall and allow large molecules to escape. Undoubtedly the endothelial cells and/or their basement membranes are damaged. Most evidence suggests that materials pass between two adjacent endothelial cells and accumulate between the cell and the basement membrane, eventually leaving through "pores" or rents in the basement membrane. However, there is also evidence to indicate that materials may pass through the endothelial cell in pinocytotic vacuoles.

Changes in the Rate of Flow. **Acceleration of the rate of flow** naturally accompanies the preliminary dilatation of arterioles, but it soon gives way to **retardation of the vascular flow.** Loss of fluid from the blood, to be explained shortly, doubtless increases its viscosity, and a certain stickiness of the leukocytes also tends to slow its flow. These factors also account for the increased capillary hydrostatic pressure. The mere dilatation of capillaries and veins, following enlargement of the afferent arterioles, obviously provides space for a more lingering stream. Thus, retardation deepens into **stasis**, and passive congestion is established. This situation is much more favorable for the escape of molecular and cellular elements essential to the formation of an exudate.

Changes in the Blood Stream. **Distribution of the Erythrocytes.** Most of us are familiar with the appearance of a flooded river, in which floating debris is drawn to the center of the stream where the flow is fastest. In the normal blood stream, the majority of the erythrocytes are likewise found in the center of the flow, since this is in accordance with physical laws. But when the stream grows sluggish, the heavier solid elements cease to be drawn to the center and become more evenly distributed. This situation favors the escape of erythrocytes, and the same may well be true of the heavier molecules of globulin and albumin. And globulins are the bearers of the "humoral antibodies," which constitute specific defenses against the most outstanding of all irritants, the microorganisms of disease.

Margination of the Leukocytes (sometimes called "pavementing"). The white cells of the blood are naturally influenced by the same physical principles as those which govern the distribution of the erythrocytes, but leukocytes are motile individuals, masters, we can almost say, of their own destiny. As Hilton Smith wrote in an earlier edition: "And what is the behavior of the leukocytes in inflammation? Most of them are found along the walls of the vessels, that is, of the dilated capillaries. They appear to be searching and examining every inlet and bayou of the swollen and roughened capillary lining as if, like houseflies on a screen-door, they were looking for a way to get through. But let us say merely that they have developed some quality of adhesiveness toward the vessel wall, for we do not attribute intelligence to these cells. Or should we say that they are drawn toward the outside by some irresistible force, as a lover is drawn to his

lady fair? We also cannot exclude that injured endothelium, rather than leukocytes, may be the sticky surface. The adherence of nonmotile red blood cells and platelets suggests that the cells may not be acting like houseflies, but the vessel wall has become flypaper. However that may be, the leukocytes do stick and succeed in passing through the capillary walls, so that the surrounding tissue comes to be filled with them, where, it seems, lies their inevitable destiny." This metaphoric description gives a stimulating mental picture but pays scant heed to the complex processes, now uncovered by hard work, which mediate changes in the blood vessels and leukocytes. A summary list of these mediators of permeability and chemotaxis is presented in Table 6–1, and a discussion of them appears shortly.

Diapedesis (Emigration) of the Leukocytes. This process of passing into the adjacent tissue is known, by long-standing custom, as emigration or diapedesis of the

Table 6–1. Probable Mediators of Inflammation

(Endogenous Factors)	
From cells	
Histamine	
Serotonin (5-hydroxytryptamine)	
Slow reacting substance of anaphylaxis (SRS–A)	
Prostaglandins	
Cationic proteins	
Acid proteases	} From lysosomes
Neutral proteases	
Macrophage migration inhibiting factor (MIF)	
Chemotactic factors	} From lymphocytes
Skin reactive factors	
Lymph node permeability factor	
From plasma:	
Bradykinin	
Kallikrein	
Complement C3a, C5a, C567, C-kinin	
Fibrinopeptides	

leukocytes (diapedesis = Greek, "leaping through"). They do this by means of their power of ameboid movement. The migration evidently is not accomplished without difficulty for, when studied by means of intravital staining, they are seen to assume a surprising variety of bizarre forms and positions as they squirm through narrow crevices between the cells of the capillaries.

Whatever may be said of other phenomena of inflammation, this emigration of the leukocytes is not a matter of inert and inanimate particles moving in accordance with any law of physics. It is, rather, the action of living cells. The force that attracts them into the inflamed tissues is called **chemotaxis**, a chemical attraction. Chemotactic attraction and repulsion are by no means mythical; they have been demonstrated many times in the laboratory, using amebae or other kinds of protozoa as well as leukocytes in a fluid medium to which various attractive or repellant chemicals have been added at one end of the container.

The polymorphonuclear leukocytes apparently move along the endothelial surface until they reach a junction between two endothelial cells. They force pseudopodia through the intercellular cleft, squeeze through the endothelium, and migrate between the endothelial cells and basement membrane until they reach a point where they can escape through the basement membrane into the extracellular space. This point is often located where the basement membrane splits to enclose a pericyte. A second possibility is that neutrophils may digest the basement membrane with their own collagenase and thus escape its confines.

Lymphocytes do not stick to the endothelium or emigrate through the intercellular junctions of endothelium. Their emigration occurs later in the inflammatory process, and is currently believed to involve a route through the endothelial cells—not between them.

Of the many factors isolated and tested,

those that appear most important as chemotactic factors for neutrophils include soluble bacterial factors; a factor derived from complement (C3); and a complement-associated factor ($C\overline{567}a$). Separate factors have been isolated that are chemotactic to mononuclear cells. These include lysates from neutrophils, soluble bacterial factors, and serum-derived factors. Although each is clearly chemotactic *in vitro*, their precise role *in vivo* is not firmly established (see Ward, 1968).

Diapedesis of the Erythrocytes. Erythrocytes are not able to move through the endothelium by ameboid movement, but may escape through interepithelial cell gaps caused by migration of leukocytes, or through gaps or leaks produced in the endothelium by chemical mediators. Red blood cells do not stick to the capillary endothelium. The erythrocytes are not considered as having any effect on the inflammatory process. In some cases their number becomes great, leading to the designation of hemorrhagic inflammation.

Exudation of Serum. As would be expected, it is still easier for the fluid part of the blood to exude, or pass into, the tissues around the capillary than it is for cells to do so. As was shown in the study of edema, the retention or release of water from the blood vessels depends upon a balance of hydrostatic and osmotic pressures within and without the vessel. It seems safe to say that in inflamed tissue the causative agent has injured cells to the extent that many of their large and complex molecules have been broken into smaller ones and that these enter the intercellular lymph. Thus, the osmotic pressure of the extra-vascular tissue is increased. As indicated previously, the hydrostatic pressure at the venous end of the capillary is also increased. Both these factors tend to transfer fluid from the vessels into the tissues. The increased permeability of the venules and capillaries is sufficient to allow the largest molecules of protein to pass through, which was not the case in noninflammatory edema. These molecules also raise the extravascular osmotic pressure.

Thus, large amounts of fluid commonly exude into the inflamed area. Contrary to what we find in noninflammatory edema, the specific gravity of this exudate approaches that of the blood plasma itself, and all of the proteins of the plasma, including fibrinogen, appear in the exudate. This is a most beneficial situation. In the first place, the fluid greatly dilutes toxic substances formed within the body or introduced from without. In such conditions as bee-stings and snake-bites, this dilution process is of primary importance. An even more important benefit in infectious inflammations is the fact that this blood serum brings with it the globulins and antibodies, which bring to bear whatever humoral immunity the patient has against the infection in question.

From the fibrinogen of the exudate, fibrin forms. It is believed to afford a supporting framework on which leukocytes can better exercise their ameboid movement. It is difficult to point to the exact mechanism that places much fibrin in one inflammatory exudate and little in another, although the ultimate causes are reasonably well understood and will be discussed with fibrinous inflammation.

Cohnheim, J.: Lectures on General Pathology, Vol. I. Translated by A. B. McKee. London, New Syndenham Society, 1889.
Courtade, E. T., Tsuda, T., Thomas, C. R., and Dannenberg, A. M., Jr.: Capillary density in developing and healing tuberculous lesions produced by BCG in rabbits. Am. J. Pathol., 78:243–260, 1975.
Florey, H. W. (ed.): General Pathology. 4th ed. Philadelphia, W. B. Saunders, 1970.
Jones, D. B.: The morphology of acid mucosubstances in leukocytic sticking to endothelium in acute inflammation. Lab. Invest., 23:606–611, 1970.
Schwartz, L. W., and Osburn, B. I.: An ontogenic study of the acute inflammatory reaction in the fetal rhesus monkey. I. Cellular response to bacterial and nonbacterial irritants. Lab. Invest., 31:441–453, 1974.
Van Arman, C. G.: Brief review of mechanisms in chronic inflammation. Agents Actions, 6:104–106, 1976.
van Deurs, V., Ropke, C., and Westergaard, E.: Permeability properties of the postcapillary high-endothelial venules in lymph nodes of the mouse. Lab. Invest., 32:201–208, 1975.
Wallach, J. D.: The inflammatory response of Rainbow Trout. J. Am. Vet. Med. Assoc., 159:583–595, 1971.
Ward, P. A.: Chemotaxis of mononuclear cells. J. Exp. Med., 128:1201–1221, 1968.
———: Insubstantial leukotaxis. Lab. Clin. Med., 79:873–877, 1972.
———: Leukotaxis and leukotactic disorders. Am. J. Pathol., 77:520–538, 1974.
Zweifach, B. W., Grant, L., and McClusky, R. T.: The Inflammatory Process. 2nd ed. Academic Press, New York, 1974.

CHEMICAL MEDIATORS OF INFLAMMATION

Most of the preceding describes the early events of the inflammatory process. Why it happens and how it happens are questions for which we have few answers, although considerable progress has been made in recent years. Some answers were provided in the previous discussion, but only brief reference was made to the subject of chemical mediators. It is not our purpose to go far into the field of biochemistry, important though it is, but several chemical substances that participate in the inflammatory reaction must be mentioned. The constancy of the changes just outlined prompted the search for chemical mediators liberated regardless of the cause of the inflammatory reaction. Such studies are difficult at best, for discovering, and in particular, evaluating any given substance is a formidable task in the face of the multitude of events in the inflammatory reaction. Nevertheless, several substances have emerged that meet the requirements of chemical mediators constant to the inflammatory process.

Histamine. Histamine (β-imidazolyl-ethylamine) was one of the first chemicals associated with inflammatory reactions, and one of the few that is universally accepted as a chemical mediator. Histamine initiates the early vascular responses but only sustains them for 30 to 60 minutes. Histamine is then superseded by other mediators, which sustain the vascular reactions or induce what is called the delayed or prolonged vascular reaction. Histamine is widely distributed in tissues in the granules of **basophilic leukocytes** and **mast cells**. Following injury of most any nature, histamine is released from the granules, probably by enzymatic action, though details of release are still under investigation, as is its mode of action on the vessel.

Serotonin. The role of serotonin (5-hydroxytryptamine) in inflammation is less

least two factors, the **Hageman factor** (factor XII) and **plasminogen**. The activated forms of these factors, **plasmin** and **activated Hageman factor**, act upon serum **kallikreinogen** (prekallikrein) and convert it to an active enzyme, **kallikrein**. Kallikrein, which has weak inflammatory properties, in turn releases kinins from α_2-globulins known as kinogens. Schematically the events are as follows:

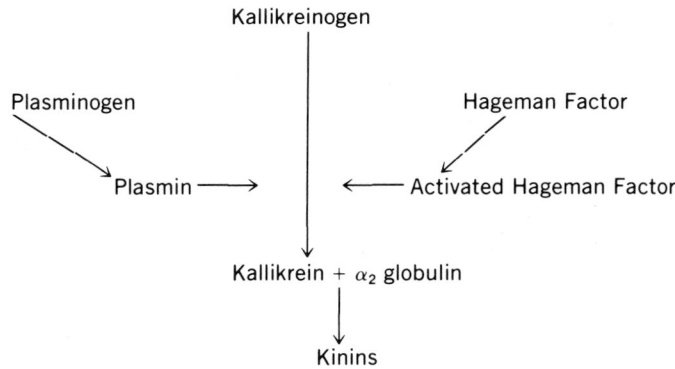

certain than that of histamine. It has vasoactive properties in most species, but vascular dilatation and increased permeability have only been clearly documented in the rat and mouse. In most all animals, serotonin is widely distributed in the enterochromaffin system, with its greatest concentration in the argentaffin cells of the gastrointestinal tract. It is also present in platelets and in the central nervous system. In the rat, mast cells also contain serotonin. Although experimentally serotonin can initiate the vascular phenomena of the inflammatory process, it probably is not of great significance.

Kinins. The kinins, **bradykinin** and **kallidin** are mediators that sustain the vascular reactions after the initial histamine response and cause pain associated with inflammation. Kinins are produced from normal serum precursors by the action of several enzymes in a sequence of events remarkably similar to the coagulation mechanism. In fact, the systems share at

In normal plasma, kallikrein is probably a group rather than a single enzyme, and the kinins in turn are probably several, though each would appear to be a closely related polypeptide.

Kinins are inactivated to inactive peptides by kinase.

Prostaglandins. These small, fatty-acid derivatives affect many biologic systems, including the inflammatory response, where they are believed to be of importance to the prolonged response and chemotaxis. PGE_1 and PGE_2 mediate increased vascular permeability, potentiate the effects of histamine and bradykinin in causing pain, and act as pyrogens causing fever. They are formed from fatty acids released from phospholipids during cell injury. Aspirin and certain other drugs inhibit prostaglandin synthesis through their action on cyclooxygenase.

Other Permeability Factors. Several other compounds affect vascular permeability, but their role in the inflammatory process or their nature is less certain than that of histamine and the kinins. A **globulin permeability factor** and a **lymph node permeability factor** have been studied in several species, but their exact nature and significance is not clear. *Hyaluronidase, lecithinases* and *nucleosides* have been suggested as permeability factors, but their role, if any, is uncertain. **Slow reactive substance of anaphylaxis (SRSA)**, an acid, sulfur-containing lipid that is released from immunologically sensitized cells, produces increased vascular permeability and contraction of smooth muscle. Several mediators are released during complement activation, as discussed elsewhere.

By virtue of their abilities to induce vasoconstriction and diminish vascular permeability, **epinephrine** and **norepinephrine** are well-established anti-inflammatory agents. Dopa and dopamine, two intermediaries in the formation of norepinephrine and epinephrine, are similarly anti-inflammatory. When absent, these compounds play a passive role in mediating the inflammatory response; therefore, degradation of these compounds is an important step in allowing the inflammatory process to develop. It is suggested that when tissues are damaged, the enzymes monamine oxidase, dopamine β-oxidase and dopa decarboxylase are activated to increase the formation and inactivation of epinephrine, norepinephrine, dopa, and dopamine.

Anti-inflammatory Effects of Glucocorticoids. Mention has been made elsewhere of the anti-inflammatory properties of epinephrine and its precursors, eosinophils, and other agents, but no endogenous or pharmacologic agent possesses anti-inflammatory properties as potent and effective as the glucocorticoids of the adrenal cortex. Indiscriminate "therapeutic" use of these compounds has more than once accentuated rather than cured disease. Corticoids suppress most aspects of the inflammatory process. They block increased vascular permeability, prevent exudation of inflammatory cells, impair intracellular destruction of bacteria, and impede the union of antigen and antibody. The mechanism of these actions is not clear, but probably multiple. One means may be through a stabilizing effect on the membranes of lysosomes and other intracellular granules, preventing the release of their contents.

Table 6-2.   Summary of Vascular Changes in Inflammation

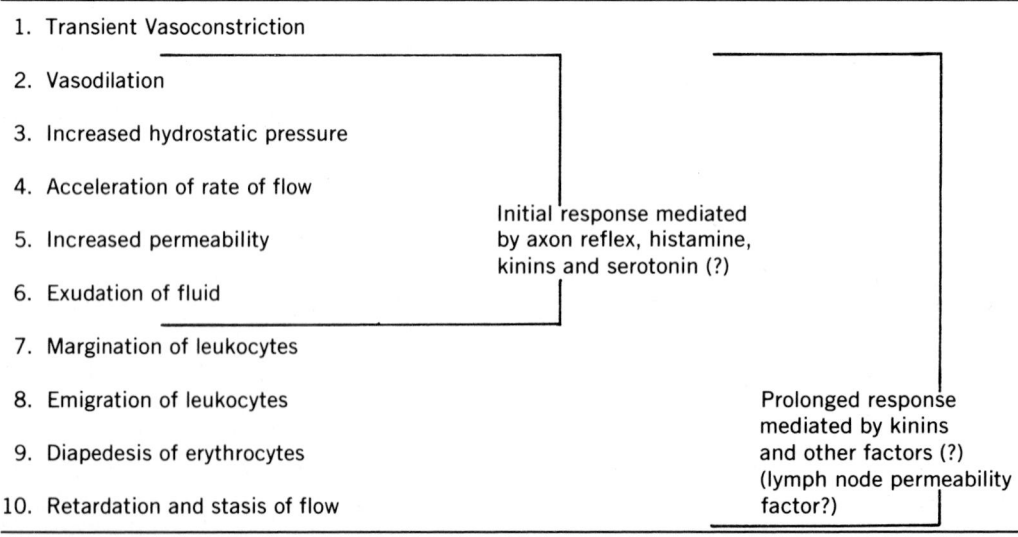

Aikawa, M., Schoenbechler, M. H., Barbaro, J. F., and Sadun, E. H.: Interaction of rabbit platelets and leukocytes in the release of histamine. Am. J. Pathol., 63:85–92, 1971.

Beaven, M. A.: Physiology in medicine: Histamine. N. Engl. J. Med., 294:30–36, 321–325, 1976.

Colman, R. W.: Formation of human plasma kinin. N. Engl. J. Med., 291:509–515, 1974.

Dickinson, J. O., and Huber, W. G.: Catabolism of orally administered histamine in sheep. Am. J. Vet. Res., 33:1789–1796, 1972.

Eggleston, P. A., and Eggleston, A. W.: Platelet and leukocyte aggregation associated with antigenic leukocyte histamine release. Lab. Invest., 31:421–424, 1974.

Eyre, P., and Lewis, A. J.: Production of kinins in bovine anaphylactic shock. Br. J. Pharmacol., 44:311–313, 1972.

Greaves, M. W.: Prostaglandins and Inflammation. *In* Prostaglandins: Physiological, Pharmacological and Pathological Aspects, edited by S. M. M. Karim. Baltimore, University Park Press, 1976, pp. 293–302.

Holroyde, M. C., and Eyre, P.: Immunologic release of histamine from bovine polymorphonuclear leukocytes. Am. J. Vet. Res., 36:1801–1802, 1975.

Onabanjo, A. C., and Maegraith, B. G.: Pathological lesions produced in the brain by kallikrein (kininogenase) in *Macaca mulatta* infected with *Plasmodium knowlesi*. Ann. Trop. Med. Parasitol., 64:237–242, 1970.

Ross, R., Glomset, J., Kariya, B., and Harker, L.: A platelet dependent serum factor that stimulates the proliferation of arterial smooth muscle cells in vitro. Proc. Nat. Acad. Sci., 71:1207–1210, 1974.

Rothwell, T. L. W., Prichards, R. K., and Love, R. J.: Studies on the role of histamine and 5-hydroxy-tryptamine in immunity against the nematode *Trichostrongylus colubriformis*. I. In vivo and in vitro effects of the amines. Int. Arch. Allergy, 46:1–13, 1974.

Seki, T., Miwa, I., Nakajima, T., and Erdos, E. G.: Plasma kallikrein-kinin system in non-mammalian blood: evolutionary aspects. Am. J. Physiol., 224:1425–1430, 1973.

Wahl, S. M., Arend, W. P., and Ross, R.: The effect of complement depletion on wound healing. Am. J. Pathol., 75:73–90, 1974.

Watters, J. W.: Effects of bradykinin and histamine on cerebral arteries of monkeys. Radiology, 98:299–303, 1971.

INFLAMMATION CLASSIFIED ACCORDING TO TYPE OF EXUDATE

Following the initial steps discussed up to this point, the inflammatory reaction may subside or continue, depending on the nature of the inciting stimulus. These stimuli, listed under causes, influence the reaction in different manners such that the course of the inflammatory process varies with the cause. What mediates this variance is unknown, but the chemical nature of the agent, the products of tissue necrosis, and in the case of bacteria, exotoxins and endotoxins, all probably participate. Morphologically, the process varies by the character of the exudate. While only a fluid, strictly speaking, can exude, the leukocytes and erythrocytes may leave the blood as part of the exudate. In this sense, exudates vary considerably, and it is desirable now to divide them, in spite of constant overlapping, into several types. Certain non-exudative mechanisms also enter into some forms of inflammation, which, it will be remembered, was defined as the reaction of the tissues to an irritant.

Serous Inflammation

Serous exudative inflammation is characterized by the exudation of blood serum, a clear, albuminous fluid. This is the form which is equivalent to **inflammatory edema**. A common method of more or less humanely killing small domestic or laboratory animals is to inject chloroform into the heart. This brings almost instantaneous death. If the injecting needle misses the heart and the chloroform is placed in the lungs, the animal commonly lives from one to two minutes. Examination of the lungs shows a red and slightly swollen area around the point of injection. Microscopically, the alveoli and the septa are filled with a uniformly pink-staining (hematoxylin and eosin) albuminous fluid. Almost any pathologist examining such a section will call the condition edema. By the definition of inflammation, it is obviously an inflammatory exudate.

Occurrence. This type of inflammation is especially frequent in serous cavities, doubtless because of the large areas of well-vascularized surfaces that line these cavities and the thinness of the surface mesothelium. Serous inflammation also occurs in the lungs, as the first stage in certain pneumonias, in response to various inhaled chemical irritants, and as the result of at least one irritant which is ingested and presumably eliminated through the lungs, namely, alpha-naphthyl-thiourea (the rat poison, ANTU). Blisters or vesicles, such as those that form in the skin after a bee-sting or a second-degree burn, or affect the mucosa in such diseases as aphthous fever, vesicular stomatitis, and vesicular exanthema, are examples of localized serous inflammation.

Microscopic Appearance. Microscopically, one sees a homogeneous, pink-staining precipitate like that already described under the topic of albumin; natural spaces are distended by it and artificial ones are created, as in the case of vesicles. With the precipitated fluid, there are usually a few scattered leukocytes of various kinds and traces of fibrin. The hyperemic and congested vessels are conspicuous.

Gross Appearance. A watery fluid fills the body cavities or tissue spaces; this differs little from the plasma of the blood. Neither is it easily distinguished from the fluid of true edema. The presence of small amounts of fibrin clinging to involved surfaces, or of a cloudiness caused by the presence of a few leukocytes, indicates an inflammatory origin. A red tinge, coming from small numbers of erythrocytes, also suggests but does not prove, that the fluid is an inflammatory exudate. The difference in the specific gravity of transudates and exudates has been mentioned. If the fluid is within vesicles, it is an exudate. In any case, hyperemia of surrounding tissues indicates that the fluid is of inflammatory origin.

Causes. This type of inflammation is usually caused by some moderately severe and often transient irritant. In the serous cavities, this is practically always an infection. Joint cavities constitute an exception in that a serous exudate, or excess of synovia, often results from the trauma of tears, sprains, and blows. In the peritoneal, pleural and pericardial cavities, colon organisms are frequently responsible, more rarely the actinobacillus and the virus of bovine encephalitis. In the spinal canal and cerebral cavity, an inflammatory increase of fluid accompanies most of the viral and bacterial infections which attack these nervous tissues, with a typical group of symptoms resulting from the increased intracranial pressure.

In the lungs, the usual cause is a bacterial or viral infection, which commonly goes on to produce the more severe purulent or fibrinous reactions some hours later. In fact, most pneumonias begin with a serous exudate, the so-called inflammatory edema. The bacterial causes include *Pasteurella multocida,* the bronchisepticus organism of dogs (formerly called *Brucella bronchisepticus*), possibly Hoffman's pseudodiphtheria bacillus (*Corynebacterium pseudodiphtheriticum*) and others; the viruses include that of psittacosis. The equine and porcine influenza and hog cholera viruses predispose to it, but it is difficult to say just what effects are due to the viruses and what to various bacteria that appear as secondary invaders. Various chemical irritants produce serous exudation in the lungs, chloroform already having been mentioned. Ordinarily they are chemicals that reach the lungs by inhalation and include many irritant gases. The inhalation of chloroform and even of ether tends to have the same effects, an unfavorable feature of their use as anesthetics. Similar to bee-stings, which have been mentioned, are the bites of many venomous creatures ranging from ants to serpents. The usual effect of a bite of the American rattlesnake (*Crotalus sp.*) is a tremendous local inflammatory edema, a serous exudate, even to the extent that the fluid passes through the overlying intact skin. Simple cutaneous abrasions, if of the right depth and severity, induce an exudate of this type. These are abrasions not quite deep enough to cause bleeding. An hour after the injury is inflicted, drops of yellowish fluid appear on the surface, where they dry and form a scab.

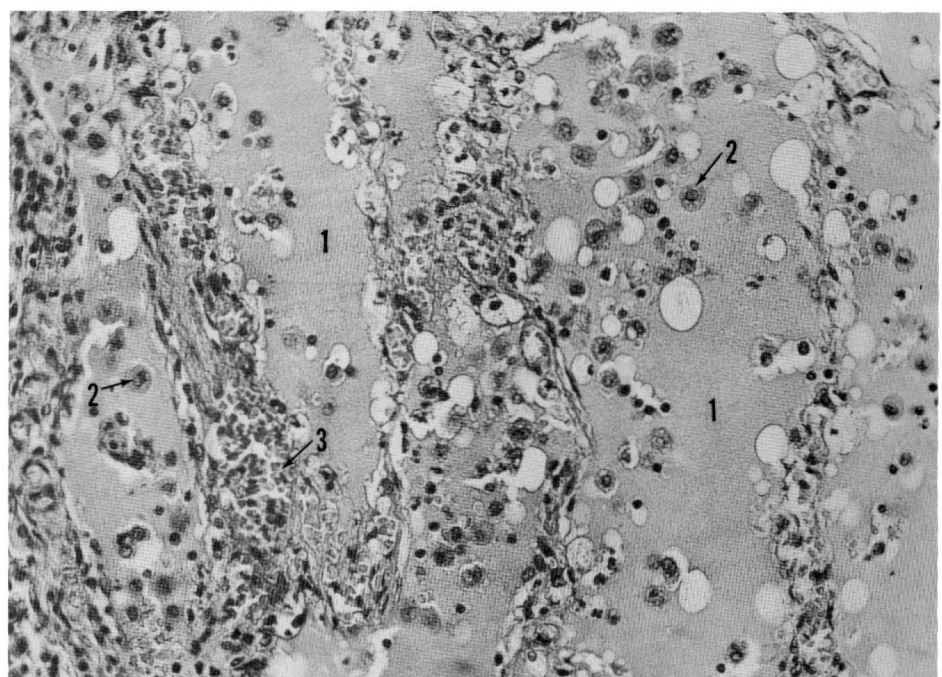

Fig. 6–1. Inflammatory edema of the lungs of an elephant with pulmonary tuberculosis. Albuminous fluid *(1)*, mononuclear cells *(2)*, and congested capillaries *(3)*. (× 300.) (Courtesy of Armed Forces Institute of Pathology.) Contributor: National Zoological Park.

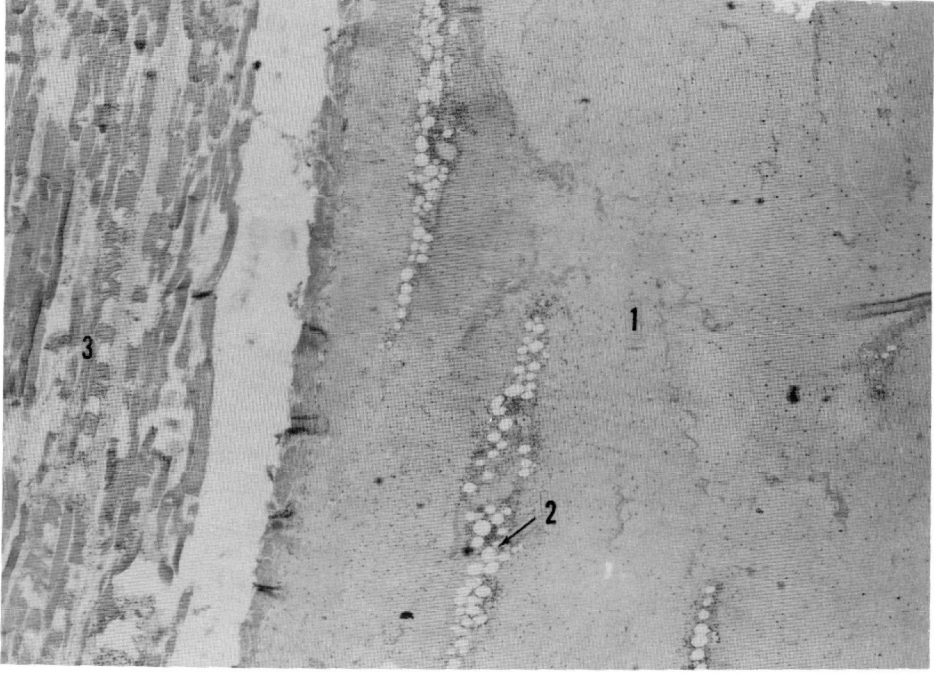

Fig. 6–2. Inflammatory edema in subcutaneous musculature of a horse with purpura hemorrhagica. Albuminous material *(1)* containing cells and fibrin; leukocytes accumulated around fat cells *(2)*, and skeletal muscle *(3)* with fibers separated by edema fluid. (Courtesy of Armed Forces Institute of Pathology.) Contributor: Army Veterinary Research Laboratory.

185

Significance and Effect. The first effect of serous exudation is to dilute any material with which it mixes. This is advantageous in case a toxin is present, because the most effective means of weakening the local effectiveness of a toxin is to dilute it a thousandfold. In case the host animal has antibodies to the toxin, the serous exudate is useful in bringing the toxin, in a diluted form, in contact with antibodies in the serum.

The pressure of exuded serum produces swelling of the part and interferes with its function, but any pain that is present usually must be attributed to other factors, judging from the sensations of persons who suffer from accumulations of noninflammatory fluids. Indeed, in pleuritis the severe pain disappears when the serous exudate arrives to lubricate and separate the hyperemic and severely irritated surfaces of visceral and parietal pleural membranes. Summarizing, it may be said that as long as an inflammation remains serous, it is comparatively mild. The fluid is promptly resorbed if the cause is overcome.

Fibrinous Inflammation

This type of inflammation is characterized by an exudate containing large amounts of fibrinogen, which clots, so that fibrin is the most conspicuous component, although the constituents of the other acute inflammatory exudates are present in some degree.

Occurrence. Fibrinous inflammation occurs chiefly on mucous and serous membranes, and is particularly frequent in the pericardial sac. The respiratory mucous membranes, from pharynx to lung alveoli, the pleura and peritoneum, synovial membranes, and the lower intestinal mucous membrane are also locations where this type of inflammation is prone to occur.

Microscopic Appearance. The dirty pink color and general appearance of fibrin have already been described. Microscopically, the fibrin is seen adherent to the surface

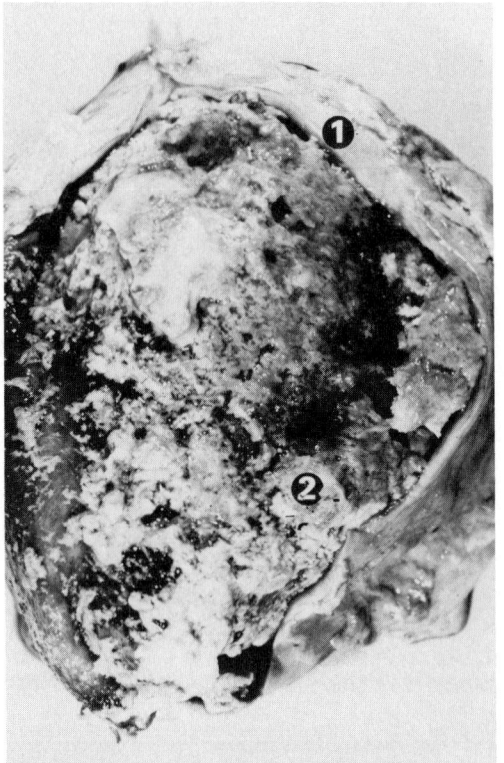

Fig. 6–3. Fibrinous exudate. Pericardium (*1*) and epicardium are covered by thick yellow fibrillar exudate with some hemorrhage (*2*). Young pig with streptococcal infection. (Courtesy of Prof. Dr. H. Luginbühl.)

that produced it, any detached fibrin seldom remaining as a part of the microscopic section. The fibrils may sometimes be traced into the epithelial or mesothelial cells of the parent surface. These latter, due to the toxic action of the irritant responsible for the fibrin, usually suffer necrosis. Coagulative necrosis is typical, but ultimately the cells pass through the various changes that are characteristic of dead tissue. With the fibrin, there are small but variable amounts of precipitated serum (protein), leukocytes, and even erythrocytes. The underlying living tissue is hyperemic. The amount of exudate may be minute or massive. Not infrequently, the exudate is formed in recurrent surges, or waves, so that one zone of exudate may be thin and lacelike, a second dense and deep-staining, and a third heavily sprinkled with leukocytes. In the pulmonary alveoli and less commonly in other places, the fibrin may be so densely packed as to form a solid, nonfibrillar mass. Since many leukocytes often accompany the fibrin and die in its vicinity, the already mentioned tendency of fibrin to suffer a blue-staining discoloration from karyolysis and chromatolysis is often pronounced, more so in one area than in another.

Gross Appearance. In the earliest stages, a dull and cloudy haze on a surface that should be smooth and shiny (serous membranes especially) is all that discloses the presence of a fibrinous exudate, but as the condition advances, a conspicuous covering of whitish fuzzy or stringy material develops. This may increase to a thickness of a centimeter with a shaggy outer surface, shreds of fibrin hanging here and there. The fibrin is sometimes reddened with blood, or it may be mingled with the fluid of a serous exudate, which may accompany the fibrinous variety. The layer of fibrin is at times dense and tough, and is then aptly called a **pseudomembrane** (false membrane), for it forms a white or yellowish sheet like a piece of thick paper.

Some fibrinous exudates form a layer that is readily loosened from the underlying parent tissue. Such a layer is called a croupous membrane, and the disorder is said to be **croupous inflammation**. The name comes from the "croup" of babies, an infection of the laryngeal and adjacent mucous membranes characterized by a detachable but voluminous and suffocating fibrinous exudate.

A **diphtheritic inflammation**, by contrast, is one in which the fibrinous exudate is so firmly attached to the underlying surface that is cannot be removed except by tearing off with it a superficial layer of bleeding tissue. This diphtheritic membrane is characteristic of human diphtheria, whence the name. Calf diphtheria

has an entirely different cause (the necrophorus organism), but the lesion is often much the same as that of human diphtheria.

Croupous exudates, perhaps more than the diphtheritic forms, are sometimes voluminous in amount and retain the shape of the structure in which they were molded, thus forming a **fibrinous cast**. Most astonishing fibrinous casts, several inches long and having the exact form of a bronchus and its branches, are sometimes coughed up by animals, commonly bovines, which may not appear very ill before or after the event. Hollow casts lining an intestine may be several feet in length. When voided with the feces, it may at first seem that the animal has passed a segment of its intestine. These are seen at least in horses and cattle.

Causes. Fibrinous inflammation usually arises in response to the attack of certain microorganisms. Prominent among these are the diphtheria bacillus, which attacks humans only, the necrophorus organism *Fusobacterium necrophorum (Sphaeropherus* or *Actinomyces necrophorus), Salmonella choleraesuis (Salmonella suipestifer),* which is thought to be the primary instigator of fibrinous enteritis in the pig, and the virus of avian laryngotracheitis. The viruses of feline infectious enteritis (panleukopenia), malignant catarrhal fever, and feline infectious peritonitis are somewhat less notable for the production of fibrinous exudates.

Many fibrinous exudates are mixed with the serous variety and are called serofibrinous; others are combined with purulent inflammation (to be described shortly), constituting a fibrinopurulent type. In these combined forms, we may list many causes of serous and purulent inflammations as causes of the fibrinous inflammations as well. This applies most frequently to the pyogenic organisms, to which the reaction is usually purulent.

In such cases, the part of the body involved appears to be an important factor in determining whether the exudate is fibrinous. It has been stated that fibrinous inflammation occurs chiefly on mucous and serous surfaces. This is so true that it seems proper to accord to the anatomic location a causative role. For example, any acute inflammation of the pericardium is almost sure to be fibrinous, serofibrinous, or fibrinopurulent. The same is likely to be true of inflammations of the pleura, peritoneum, and even the meninges.

Burns are at times followed by a fibrinous reaction, apparently without infection.

Significance and Effect. It is difficult to identify the exact mechanism responsible for the outpouring of fibrinogen. We are not aware of any other source than the usual clotting apparatus of the blood. Possibly hydrostatic and osmotic pressures are such that a large amount of blood plasma passes through the abnormally permeable capillaries (see vascular changes), deposits its fibrin, and then is reabsorbed.

As far as the inflamed area is concerned, the fibrin probably serves a number of useful purposes. We can believe that it prevents loss of blood (erythrocytes) through the dead and unprotected surface that usually underlies it (coagulative necrosis), and that it protects the underlying tissues from further irritation. Certainly a "sore throat" coated with a layer of exudate is less painful than it is after the coating has been removed. The strands of fibrin are believed by many to form a framework useful in supporting leukocytes as they migrate through the inflamed zone.

If the inflammation terminates with reasonable promptness, the underlying surface is regenerated and the fibrin is dissolved. On a free mucous surface, it may be sloughed, as in the case of the bronchial and intestinal casts previously mentioned. But on the serous surfaces and in the pulmonary alveoli, fibrin remaining for some days is likely to undergo **organization** by fibrous tissue in much the same way that a thrombus does. The fibroblasts build into the zone of fibrin by proliferation of those in the underlying tissue. Such fibrous tissue is permanent. It is especially unfortunate on serous surfaces, such as those of the pleura, pericardium, and peritoneum, for it tends to build across from one opposing surface to another, forming permanent **adhesions** that tie them together and prevent movement and function. Barring this contingency, the organized layer on a surface becomes, as the inflammation subsides, covered with mesothelial cells which form a surface similar to that which existed previously. If fibrin in the alveoli of the lung is organized, that portion of the lung is permanently converted into fibrous tissue, a process known as **carnification** (*carneus,* flesh).

Purulent Inflammation

Purulent inflammation and purulent exudates are characterized by pus. **Pus** is typically a liquid of creamy color and consistency, but it may be thin and almost watery, or inspissated and semisolid. Its creamy yellow color is changed to bluish or greenish if *Pseudomonas aeruginosa (Bacillus pyocyaneus)* is among the infecting bacteria. It carries a blackish discoloration if it comes from black hoofs of horses, the color reportedly being due to sulfides. The definitive characteristic of pus is the presence of numerous neutrophilic polymorphonuclear granulocytes. These "neutrophils," living or necrotic, together with necrotic cells of the preexisting tissue, more or less liquefied, and minor amounts of the other constituents of inflammatory exudates, including serum, constitute the ingredients of pus. When pus is present in major or minor degree, the inflammatory process is said to be purulent. (There is no such adjective as "pussy.")

The term suppurative inflammation or **suppuration** is a variant of the general term and implies that considerable amounts of pus are produced; usually it runs from a surface or fills cavities.

A **phlegmon**, or phlegmonous inflammation, is a condition in which appreciable amounts of pus are diffusely scat-

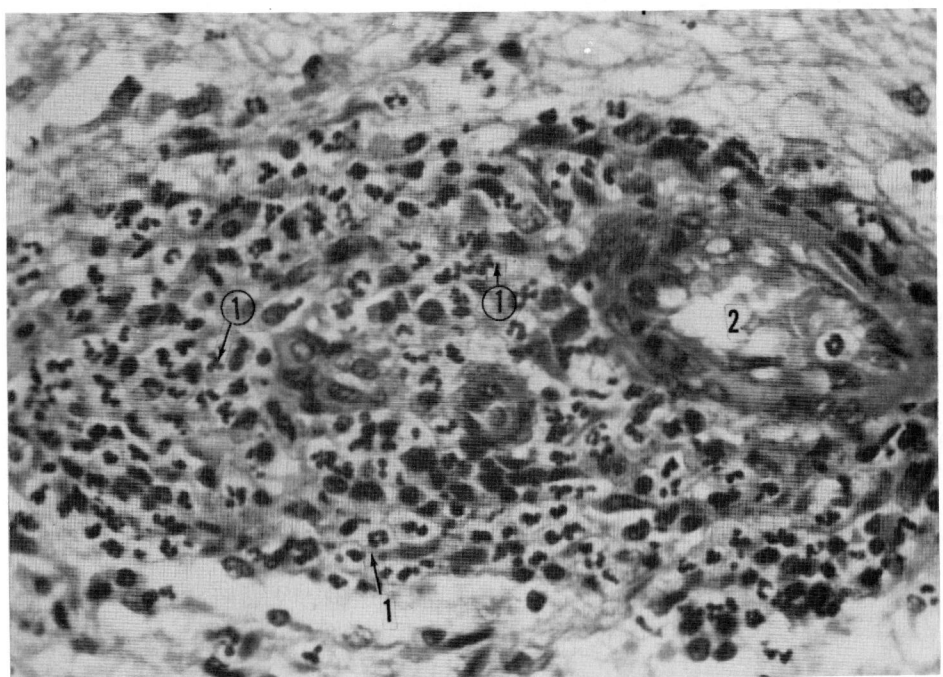

Fig. 6–4. Purulent inflammation. Polymorphonuclear neutrophilic leukocytes ("neutrophils" or "polymorphs") *(1)* adjacent to an artery *(2)* in the brain of a horse with generalized infection by *Streptococcus pyogenes*. Grossly visible abscesses were found elsewhere in the cerebrum. (× 600.) (Courtesy of Armed Forces Institute of Pathology.) Contributor: Army Veterinary Research Laboratory.

tered through a tissue, particularly the subcutis. **Cellulitis** is a more or less synonymous term. A phlegmon tends to spread indefinitely, in contrast to an abscess, in which the reaction and the causative infection are confined.

An **abscess** is defined as a circumscribed collection of pus. When well developed, it has a wall or capsule of fibrous tissue separating it from the surrounding tissue. In size, abscesses vary from microscopic to almost unlimited dimensions.

Microscopic Appearance. The appearance of considerable numbers of neutrophilic leukocytes in or on a tissue justifies a diagnosis of purulent inflammation. Usually these are seen in great numbers, but they do not need to be more numerous than accompanying lymphocytes for the purulent designation to be employed. It should be noted that lymphocytes, as well as plasma cells and macrophages, are present in varying numbers in many inflammatory reactions. Many of the neutrophils undergo necrosis and are recognized by their small size, dark and irregularly shaped nuclei, and acidophilic cytoplasm. In addition to hyperemia or congestion, a minor amount of fibrin, serum (as a pink-staining precipitate), and various other leukocytes, fixed, and wandering cells will be seen in conjunction with the neutrophils.

Gross Appearance. The purulent exudate consists of pus, the general appearance of which has been described as viscous, cream-colored fluid with possible variations extending from a watery consistency, such as results from some streptococcal infections, to a material that is practically a solid as the result of resorption of water. The red discoloration resulting from hemorrhage, the blue-green color coming from the pigment-forming pyocyaneus bacillus, and the black color from disintegrating hoof material have also been described. Pus may be seen exuding from an infected wound or mucous membrane. It may be confined within abscesses or the body cavities. Its presence in the pulmonary alveoli, a phase of pneumonia called gray hepatization, is demonstrated by incising the lung and pressing it out from the cut surfaces. The beginning student is familiar with it, if nowhere else, as the thick yellow and sometimes foul-smelling fluid which he expectorates or blows from his nose in the late stages of a "cold."

Causes. Purulent or suppurative inflammations are caused by **pyogenic bacteria**. The word pyogenic means "pus-forming." The principal members of this group of bacteria are the pyogenic bacilli, *Corynebacterium (Bacterium) pyogenes,* and its relatives, *C. renale* and *C. equi, Pseudomonas aeruginosa,* and rarely, *Escherichia (Bacillus) coli.* By pyogenic cocci we mean *Staphylococcus (Micrococcus) aureus* and its relatives, *Staph. albus* and *Staph. citreus,* the streptococci, and the human pathogens appearing as diplococci, *Streptococcus (Diplococcus) pneumoniae, Neisseria (Diplococcus) gonorrhoeae,* and *N. meningitidis.* The tubercle bacillus is a pus-former in the very earliest stages of infection, and tuberculous meningitis may be purulent simply because the patient dies before the usual type of tuberculous lesion becomes established. The reaction in several of the infectious granulomas tends to be purulent in the immediate vicinity of the invading organisms. Chief among these granulomas are actinomycosis, actinobacillosis, the form of staphylococcal granuloma formerly called botryomycosis, coccidioidomycosis, blastomycosis, glanders, and chronic tularemia.

There are a few other pathogens which, under certain circumstances of virulence and resistance, can be pyogenic, but the cocci and corynebacteria far outweigh all others in frequency, importance, and pyogenic potency. It is possible to produce a purulent lesion and abscesses by the direct injection into the tissues of various chemical irritants such as turpentine.

Significance and Effect. The liquefactive necrosis of tissue which is a feature of pus formation illustrates the fact that purulent inflammation is a prompt and violent reaction against irritant organisms. Along with the vigorous microphagic and other activities of the neutrophils, there is often effective production of humoral antibodies (immune bodies) as well as fever, all of which are potent defenses. These organisms also happen to be among the most vulnerable to available therapeutic agents.

Pus usually contains large numbers of the causative bacteria, living or dead, and the various toxic products of their metabolism. Confined pus is a source for absorption of toxic substances into the circulation, often with harmful results, including such visible changes as cellular swelling and necrosis of parenchymatous organs. **Toxemia** is the name given to such a state, meaning literally "toxins in the blood." Living organisms also find their entrance into the blood stream facilitated by confinement of the exudate containing them, so that some may be carried by the blood to new locations, where they colonize and multiply, a process called **metastasis**. For these reasons it is of the utmost importance that an abscess or other suppurative lesion have free drainage to the outside, surgical intervention sometimes being necessary.

Abscesses, however, may become sterile, the body defenses having killed all of the causative bacteria. The accumulated pus, with no way to escape, commonly remains for some time before being slowly liquefied and absorbed.

Hemorrhagic Inflammation

Hemorrhagic inflammation and hemorrhagic exudates are characterized by large numbers of erythrocytes which leave their normal channels by diapedesis to exude from a body surface or into nearby tissues. With them are any or all of the components of other types of exudates—serum, leukocytes and especially fibrin—so that the whole exudate bears some resemblance to clotted or unclotted blood.

Occurrence. While this type of inflammation occurs within the tissues in such diseases as blackleg, anthrax, pasteurellosis, and purpura hemorrhagica, it is especially prone to involve mucous surfaces. The lungs may also suffer this type of inflammation. Hemorrhagic gastritis and enteritis are among the commonest manifestations of this type of exudate.

Microscopic Appearance. With the components just listed, distinguishing hemorrhagic exudate from simple hemorrhage may be a problem. However, the various components of the blood are present in other than their normal proportions, and the constituents of exudates, such as fibrin, leukocytes, or both, are always more plentiful than in normal blood. Also, the exudate is diffuse in distribution, having come from an area, not from one or a few points, as would be the case with a simple hemorrhage.

Gross Appearance. Blood-colored material, sometimes fluid or semifluid, but usually clotted and of gelatinous consistency, appears on a surface or in tissue spaces. It is likely to be somewhat streaked or varying in color and consistency, revealing that the material is not pure clotted blood. The inflamed surface is deep red. It may be confused with the type of catarrhal inflammation in which the principal changes are severe hyperemia and loss of epithelium, but usually in the latter type, bloody fluid has not actually escaped from the tissue and the reddening of the surface is not quite so pronounced. Blood, whether as an exudate or as a hemorrhage, coming from any but the most posterior part of the gastrointestinal tract, colors the feces black. Coming from the lungs it is foamy from admixed air, but when it comes from the respiratory passages this is not the case.

Causes. The causes of hemorrhagic inflammation are microorganisms of high virulence and acute poisoning by certain chemicals when in contact in concentrated form with digestive or other mucous membranes, or when such substances are eliminated by way of mucous membranes, especially those of the lower bowel, bladder, or gallbladder. Among these substances are phenol, arsenic and phosphorus. The clotted exudate of laryngotracheitis of chickens has been mentioned as fibrinous. It is also hemorrhagic, with individual cases varying as to which type predominates. The pathogenic leptospirae and the virus of canine hepatitis are pathogens notable for causing hemorrhagic inflammation, doubtless the direct result of injury to vascular endothelium.

Significance and Effect. Hemorrhagic inflammation arises quickly and is all too likely to presage an early fatality, although in some instances it subsides with almost equal rapidity upon removal of the cause.

Catarrhal or Mucous Inflammation

The characteristic component of this type of inflammatory exudate is mucus, which comes from cells rather than from the blood. Mucus is produced by epithelial cells, either the mucous glands that open upon mucous membranes, or the one-celled mucous glands called goblet cells. For this reason, the occurrence of mucous or catarrhal inflammation is limited to mucous membranes. The number of goblet cells in a given mucous membrane can vary, increasing under proper stimuli, and it is possible for epithelia not normally equipped with them to develop mucus-secreting cells.

Microscopic Appearance. Commonly, the excessive mucus is readily visible as pale bluish or grayish strands of mucin clinging to the mucous membrane that produced it. The increased number of goblet cells may be conspicuously apparent. In many cases, however, another important feature is loss by necrosis and desquamation of much of the surface epithelium. Rather frequently this becomes the predominant feature of catarrhal inflammation, leaving the affected mucous membrane denuded of its epithelial covering, somewhat hyperemic, and containing slight or moderate infiltrations of lymphocytes. Thus, in spite of the fact that the fundamental idea of catarrh is a flowing, we come to speak of a catarrhal inflammation in which there is no flow of mucus. The hyperemia and the presence of reactive cells usually suffice to differentiate this condition from postmortem desquamation of the epithelium.

Gross Appearance. The predominantly mucous forms of catarrhal inflammation are recognized by the presence of the clear, slimy, mucin-containing fluid that has already been described as mucus. This is readily recognized on postmortem examination. During life it may even drip from the nostrils if the nasal mucosa is involved. Mucous colitis, a fairly common condition, can often be recognized clinically by opaque white shreds or patches of semidehydrated mucus adhering to the formed feces or mixed with the excrement if it is softer.

When the inflammation is characterized less by mucus than by hyperemia and loss of epithelium, the inflamed surface shows little but the red color of raw meat with slight swelling. Limited amounts of mucus or of fibrinous or purulent material may or may not be present. Not infrequently there is such an admixture of pus that the term mucopurulent is used. In mucous cholecystitis, the mucus may be seen imperfectly mixed with bile or it may not be discernible.

The increased flow of tears or of saliva that occurs when the respective regions of the body suffer suitable irritation is an entirely comparable reaction to mucous inflammation, although the secretions of the lachrymal and salivary glands differ from mucus.

Causes. The irritants that cause this type of inflammation are mild in character or of short duration. They include bacterial and viral infections of low virulence or in their early stages. A "cold" as seen most often in humans and poultry forms a good example, in its earlier stages, of catarrhal inflammation. Later the mucous exudate may become purulent.

Mildly or transiently irritating chemicals cause mucous inflammation. Inhaled formalin, chlorine, bromine, and chlorpicrin (tear gas) fall in this category, as do many antiseptics used in too great a concentration on delicate mucous membranes. There is considerable difference in what can be endured by the columnar epithelium of the cervix and uterus and by the squamous lining of the mouth.

Irritating foods in the digestive tract have the ability to set up catarrhal inflammation. In some cases it is difficult to say whether a case of transient catarrhal gastroenteritis is due directly to the food or to microorganisms in it, but mild forms are often caused by foods of improper quality for the species concerned or consumed excessively, or at a time when the nervous or other status of the digestive tract is not compatible with them (equine spasmodic colics, excessive horse meat in dogs). Along with the mild inflammation of the digestive mucosa, there is usually a transient diarrhea due to violent peristalsis and an increase of intraintestinal fluid, which can be viewed as a serous exudate.

The inhalation of ordinary dust, in considerable amounts, is sufficient to initiate a mucous reaction in the air passages.

Inhalation of substances containing foreign proteins to which the patient is hypersensitive causes copious mucous exudation in "hay fever" of humans.

Significance and Effect. The flow of mucus is protective in that it tends to wash away the irritating substance. If the cause is removed, the flow of mucus subsides and the lost epithelium is quickly restored by proliferation of a few cells that survive here and there. If the injurious agent continues to act, especially if it is a microorganism, the inflammation appears to lead to hypersensitivity and hyperactivity of mucous glands and a chronic catarrh, especially in the respiratory passages.

These five forms complete the list of acute exudative inflammations as they are usually classified. It is evident that a given case may represent a mixture of two or more types, and also that a reaction may change from a mild to a more severe form. Likewise, the severe forms may subside gradually, assuming a catarrhal character, not to mention chronic forms, which are yet to be considered. On the whole, however, the type of reaction encountered is likely to give a useful clue to the cause of the condition.

Lymphocytic Inflammation

Some inflammatory reactions are recognizable only by accumulations of lymphocytes in the tissues and a certain degree of hyperemia. We concur with a rather small group in placing these in a separate classification.

Occurrence. Lymphocytic inflammation occurs in (1) numerous infections of the central nervous system, (2) the islands of Glisson (portal spaces) of the liver, with or without hepatitis, (3) occasionally in mucous membranes, and (4) the kidney in such infections as subacute leptospirosis.

Microscopic Appearance. Lymphocytes gather singly or in clumps in the tissues, which otherwise may appear normal or only somewhat hyperemic. Frequently the lymphocytes form a more or less complete wreath around a blood vessel, from which they have doubtless emigrated. This is called **perivascular lymphocytic infiltration** or, in professional slang, "cuffing." It is especially common in the central nervous system. In the intestine, the lymphocytes are in the stroma (lamina propria) of the mucous membrane, where a certain number are considered normal.

Gross Appearance. When lymphocytic infiltration is the only evidence, the inflammation is not recognized grossly.

Causes. Chief among these are viral infections of the nervous system, in which perivascular lymphocytic infiltration is the typical and often the only visible expression of such infections as rabies, Aujeszky's disease, lymphocytic choriomeningitis, equine encephalomyelitis, and Teschen disease. Perivascular lymphocytic infiltration is not limited to viral diseases. Such infections as listeriosis and toxoplasmosis are characterized by the same lesion, but there are usually other signs also. The central nervous system is not the only location in which perivascular lymphocytic infiltration occurs, although it seems to have some peculiar predilection for this site. Possibly a partial explanation is that many of the viruses involved are of such generally limited virulence that they cannot injure other than the delicate nervous tissues and are not sufficiently destructive irritants to incite any of the more vigorous inflammatory reactions.

Toxic substances brought to the liver occasionally manifest themselves by lymphocytic infiltration, although ordinarily there are alterative (degenerative) changes in the parenchymal cells. Toxic and possibly some slightly virulent infectious agents acting over a period of time appear to be responsible for lymphocytic infiltration of the intestinal and other mucous membranes. Usually these inflammations reach the point where they can be classified as catarrhal or chronic proliferative.

Significance and Effect. The viral encephalitides usually terminate fatally. The microscopic diagnostician should remember that lymphocytes, perivascular or otherwise, are common at some distance from the center of disturbance in many inflammations of various types. These do not belong under the present classification.

Also, an inflammatory reaction of one of the more violent types may subside to the point where only a lymphocytic infiltration remains for a while. It should be kept in mind that the principal function of the lymphocytes is to mediate immunologic responses and their presence in tissues indicates such a response.

Granulomatous Inflammation

Prolonged (chronic) inflammation often has features described under the term granuloma and granulomatous response. This is based upon a misnomer ("granule" plus "oma," a tumor), but it is well ingrained into the literature. It must not be confused with **granulation tissue,** which will be described next.

A granuloma is a chronic inflammatory reaction principally consisting of closely packed collections of macrophages. They can be classified into two main types, **foreign body granulomas** and **hypersensitivity granulomas.** Foreign body granulomas form in response to agents which fail to evoke an immune response, such as silk sutures, splinters and oil. They consist of collections of macrophages, often in association with neutrophils surrounding the foreign object. The macrophages may fuse to form multinucleated giant cells, also known as **foreign body giant cells.** The nuclei in these cells are randomly distributed, in contrast to Langhans' type giant cells.

Hypersensitivity granulomas are the characteristic response to mycobacteria (tuberculosis), fungi, helminths and their

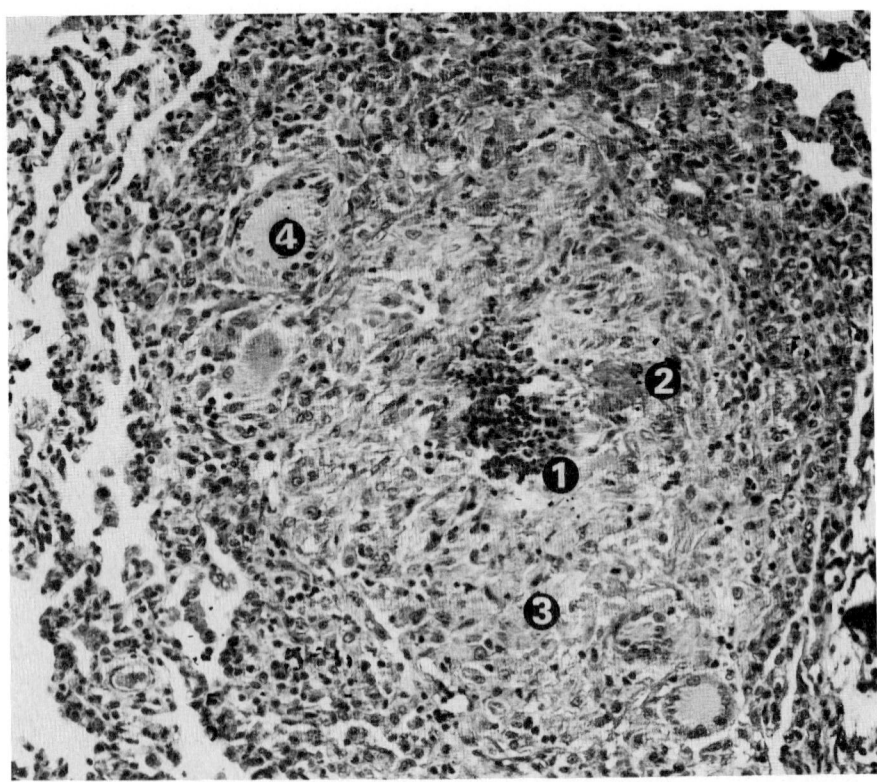

Fig. 6–5. Granulomatous inflammation. Tubercle in the lung of a rhesus monkey. In center of granuloma are neutrophils *(1)* and coagulation necrosis *(2)*. Macrophages *(3)* make up most of the lesion. Langhans' giant cell *(4)*. The periphery contains lymphocytes, plasma cells, monocytes, and few fibroblasts. (Courtesy of Prof. Dr. H. Luginbühl.)

ova, and many organisms that replicate intracellularly (e.g., *Brucella*). Histologically, they consist of focal collections of macrophages, many of which develop abundant eosinophilic cytoplasm and large pale nuclei, giving them an appearance not unlike some epithelial cells. This gave rise to the term **epithelioid cells,** which is still in use today. Fusion of macrophages to form multinucleated giant cells is also a feature of hypersensitivity granulomas, but the nuclei are usually arranged at the periphery of the cell with the cytoplasmic organelles in the center (Fig. 6–5). This type of giant cell is known as a **Langhans' type giant cell** and is typical of tuberculosis. Hypersensitivity granulomas are T-cell dependent, representing a form of delayed hypersensitivity. Why the reaction assumes the granulomatous feature in contrast to the usual delayed reaction is not known, but thought to result from the fact that the antigen is concentrated in an insoluble matrix. This is supported by the

fact that the tuberculin reaction, evoked by soluble protein derivatives of mycobacteria, is characterized by diffuse accumulations of mononuclear cells in contrast to the characteristic granuloma of tuberculosis.

Granulomas often become partially or completely surrounded by immature connective tissue which is infiltrated by lymphocytes. This granule may be sealed off by the connective tissue to eventually become a scar, or it may break down to expel its contents to incite further granulomas— in effect, fusing several granulomas together. Destruction of tissue may proceed simultaneously with these apparent efforts to contain the irritant and produce healing. These events lead to the characteristic histologic features that are called granulomatous inflammation.

Granulation Tissue

An important phenomenon in the process of inflammation is the formation of granulation tissue. This should not be con-

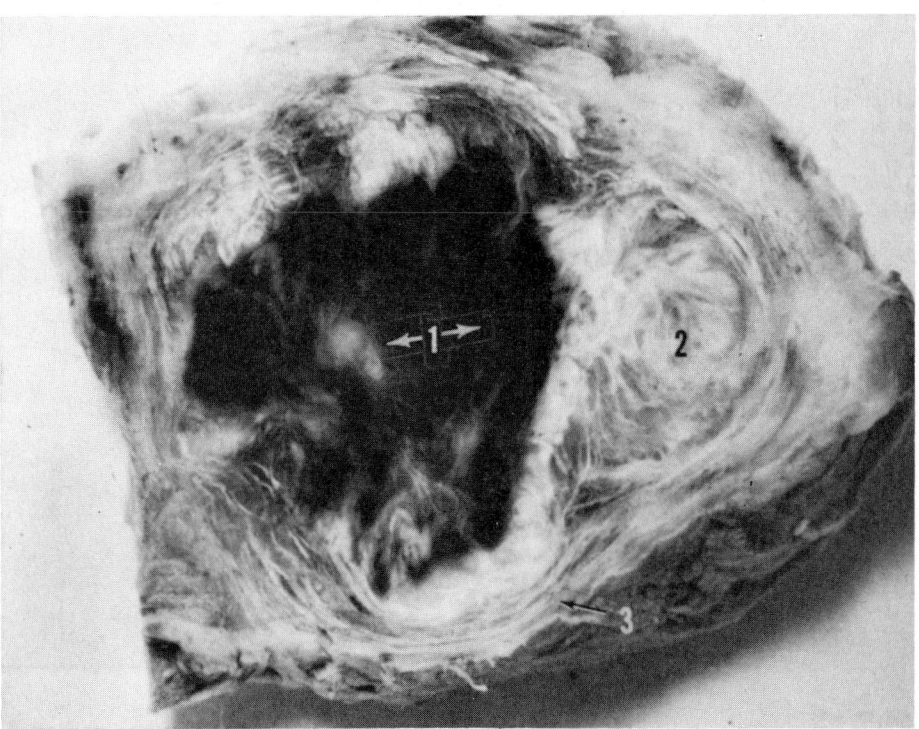

Fig. 6–6. Fibrous granulation tissue in a partially organized hematocyst in the abdominal wall of a horse. Old hemorrhage (*1*), fibrous connective tissue (*2*) forming a capsule (*3*).

fused with granulomatous inflammation described previously. The name comes from the gross appearance of this tissue. The surface, when seen with the naked eye, appears to bear many red "granules," which are actually the blunt ends of loops of new capillaries which are often perpendicular to the surface. Granulation tissue is most often encountered in large wounds that require filling in defects in connective tissue, and in the walls of sinus tracts leading to a foreign body.

Microscopic Appearance. Granulation tissue has a characteristic but sometimes confusing microscopic appearance. The fibroblasts, which are its principal component, are elongate fibrillar cells with plump, ovoid, hyperchromatic nuclei. Mitoses are frequent. These cells often form bundles or fasciculi, and these are rich in collagen in the deeper parts of the lesion. Many new capillaries with plump endothelial nuclei are present, and these vessels often run in parallel arrays perpendicular to the surface (Figs. 6–6 and 6–7). The zone nearest the surface often contains

neutrophils, erythrocytes, and cellular debris.

Gross Appearance. Granulation tissue on an exposed surface is apt to be ulcerated, red or bloody. The mass may bulge grotesquely above the surface. The surface is rough, granular under the scab due to the loops of new capillaries. The tissue in its deeper parts is apt to be white, tough, and hard, but less dense, edematous, and congested near the surface.

THE LEUKOCYTES IN INFLAMMATION

It is desirable to consider briefly the functions and capabilities of the various reactive cells in inflammatory processes.

Neutrophil Leukocytes

These cells, sometimes known as polymorphs, polymorphonuclear cells, and granulocytes, but for which the most popular designation is neutrophils, are the characteristic component of the purulent exudate and probably the most potent of the leukocytes in the inflammatory battle. The term **heterophil** is used to describe the

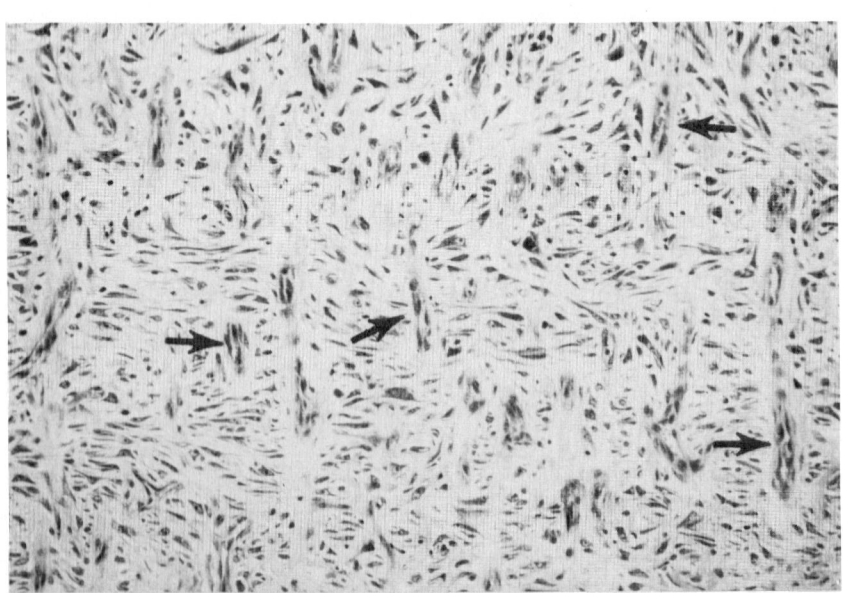

Fig. 6–7. Fibrous granulation tissue at the base of a healing ulcer of the rectum of a cow. The organization of new blood vessels (arrows) perpendicular to fibroblasts and collagen is typical and allows differentiation from fibroma. (Courtesy of Dr. C. L. Davis.)

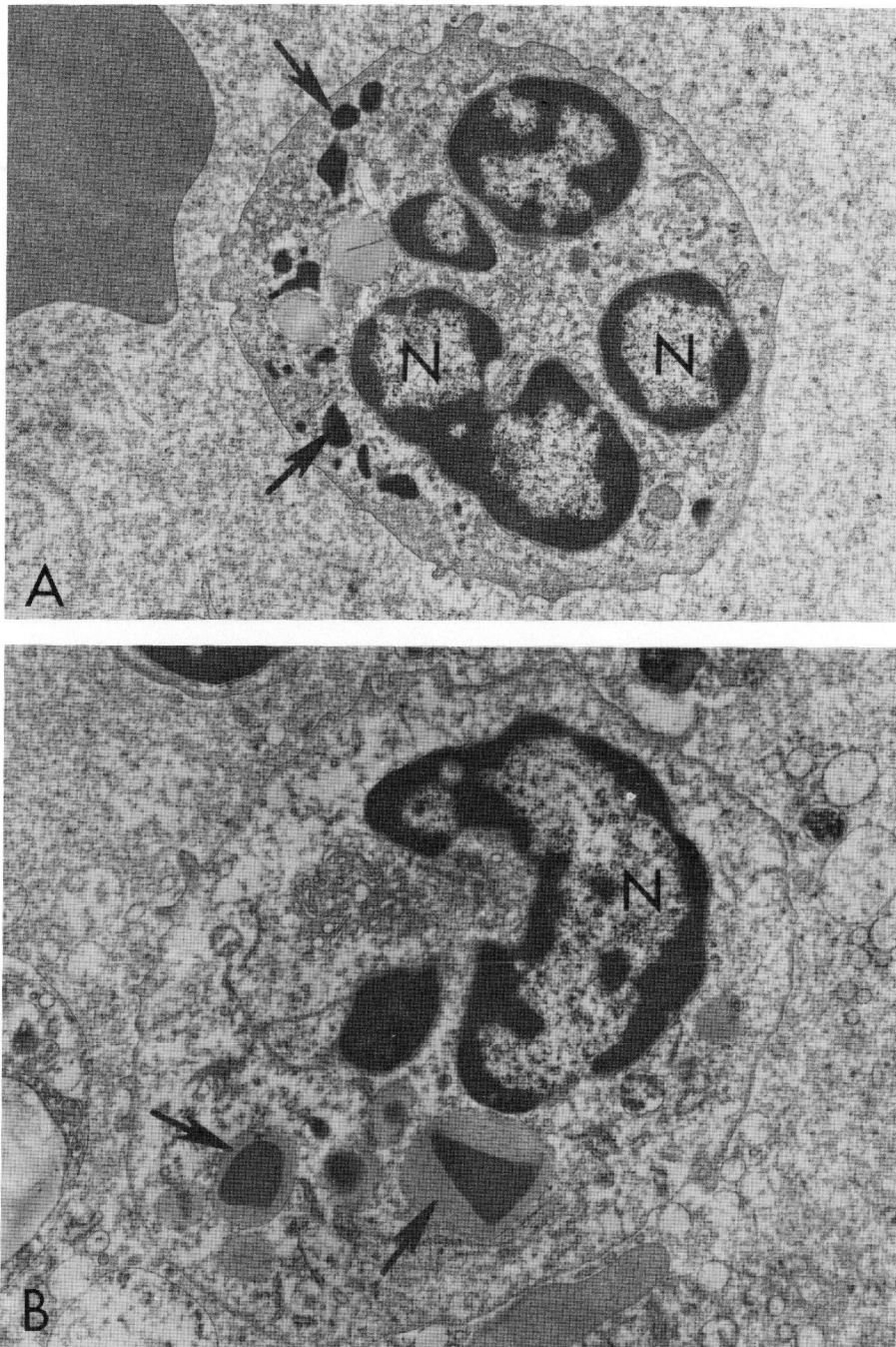

Fig. 6–8. Leukocytes in peripheral blood of a marmoset *(Saguinus nigricollis). A,* Neutrophil. The lobes of the nucleus *(N)* appear separate due to thin sectioning. The granules (arrows) resemble lysosomes. *B,* Eosinophil. The granules (arrows) contain dense crystalline bodies. (Courtesy of Dr. N. W. King, Jr.)

functional counterpart of the neutrophil in certain species such as the rabbit and guinea pig, in which the granules of the cells are eosinophilic. The less desirable term, pseudoeosinophil, has also been applied to the neutrophil of these species.

Formed in the bone marrow from primitive cells, the mature neutrophil, when released into the circulation, has a bizarre, multilobed nucleus and numerous cytoplasmic granules that resemble lysosomes. When observed by electron microscopy, the nuclear lobes often appear disconnected due to ultrathin sectioning. The chromatin is concentrated near the nuclear membrane. The granules are surrounded by a membrane, relatively uniform in size, round to elongate, and have a homogeneous, moderately electron-dense matrix. There is a paucity of organized cytoplasmic structures other than the granules. Mitochondria are generally few and little or no endoplasmic reticulum is present. A Golgi apparatus is usually evident. The granules contain a host of hydrolytic, oxidative, and proteolytic enzymes, as well as two antibacterial substances, **lysozyme** and **phagocytin**.

The half life of neutrophils is approximately six hours, requiring their continual replenishment both to the circulation and to inflammatory exudates, as neutrophils are end cells, incapable of division. It is not certain what constitutes the graveyard for dying neutrophils, but probably most leave the body to the outside world via the intestines, skin, and lungs.

The neutrophils leave the blood in large numbers in response to invasion and injury by pyogenic bacteria to enter the zone of inflammation, as explained in the description of purulent exudate. They reach the scene quickly, within a few hours, utilizing their marked ability of ameboid movement.

Their function of engulfing small particles is so readily observable that they are called the **microphages** of the body, a term coined by Metchnikoff in 1892. This phe-nomenon, known as **phagocytosis**, is probably the principal function of neutrophils. They may ingest foreign matter such as carbon, pigments, cellular debris, and most importantly, bacteria. To phagocytize bacteria, certain serum proteins called **opsonins** are required. Opsonins generally represent specific antibodies directed against the bacterium, although normal serum from nonimmunized or previously exposed individuals also contain proteins (which may in fact be specific antibodies) which coat bacteria and bind complement. Once engulfed, "digestible" materials are disposed of by "digestive" enzymes held by the neutrophil's granules. If perchance the material is "nondigestible," like a carbon particle, it is released upon the death of the short-lived neutrophil, to be engulfed by another neutrophil or possibly by a macrophage. Most bacteria are killed following phagocytosis, but not by usual enzymes such as proteases, for these living objects are resistant to most enzymes. Two substances, lysozyme and phagocytin, are held responsible for this ability.

Other functions ascribed to neutrophils include secretion of lytic substances to degrade dead bacteria and dead body cells, secretion of substances that augment the inflammatory reaction, secretion of chemotactic chemicals, and secretion of a pyrogen (fever-producing substance) to initiate and maintain fever.

The mechanisms involved in all aspects of phagocytosis continue to be studied in details that lie outside the scope of this book. The review by Stossel (1974) is recommended reading for one who wishes an overview of the subject.

As indicated, neutrophils, unlike some of the reactive cells, have no ability to multiply by mitosis or otherwise. Replacements for the large numbers killed on the inflammatory battleground have to come from their original source, the myeloid tissue in the red bone marrow. It is not surprising then that, as an acute suppurative inflammation develops, the number of neutrophils in the circulating blood is perceptibly, often markedly increased. Moderate increases in the numbers of these cells may also accompany certain toxemias, such as uremia, severe loss of blood, and pregnancy.

Practical use is made of this fact by determining the **total** and **differential white-cell counts** of the blood in the diagnosis of suspected pyogenic infections. The percentage of neutrophils among all leukocytes is increased in acute pyogenic infections in the human, dog, and horse from a normal of 60 to 70% up to 75 to 90%. In cattle, sheep, and swine, the normal of around 50% shows a similar tendency. The total leukocyte count of 6,000 to 10,000 per cubic millimeter in the human, with a somewhat higher normal in the domestic mammals, rises commonly to 12,000 to 15,000 and less often to 20,000, 30,000 or even higher in these infections, although in cattle the first 24 or 48 hours of an acute pyogenic process may actually be marked by a decrease. This inflammatory change is known as (neutrophilic) **leukocytosis**. It has to be distinguished from **leukemia**, a neoplastic increase in the numbers of one kind or another of white cells in the blood, sometimes to much higher levels. On the other hand, in some other infections, chiefly viral, there is a marked decrease in the white-cell count known as **leukopenia** or if the change is only in the neutrophils, as **neutropenia**.

Something can also be learned concerning the diagnosis and prognosis from the **Schilling count**. This consists in determining how many of the neutrophils are young ("juvenile," or "stab" from the German) cells. These should not exceed 6 per cent of the total white cells. If their number is higher, it indicates an active but possibly losing battle against a pyogenic invader, since larger numbers of juvenile forms appear only when production by the myeloblastic tissue is inadequate. A high neutrophil count consisting of mature types (horseshoe or multi-lobed nucleus) is a fa-

vorable sign. The term "shift to the left," based on a common way of writing the figures for the different types, is a frequent method of expressing an increase in the count of juvenile neutrophils.

Belcher, R. W., Carney, J. F., and Monahan, F. G.: An electron microscopic study of phagocytosis of *Candida albicans* by polymorphonuclear leukocytes. Lab. Invest., 29:620–627, 1973.

Boucek, M. M., and Snyderman, R.: Calcium influx requirement for human neutrophil chemotaxis: Inhibition by lanthanum chloride. Science, 193:905–907, 1976.

Boyne, R.: Observations on the alkaline phosphatase activity of leucocytes in adrenalectomised rats. Res. Vet. Sci., 14:234–238, 1973.

Brune, K., Schmid, L., Glatt, M., and Minder, B.: Correlation between antimicrobial activity and peroxidase content of leukocytes. Nature, 245:209–210, 1973.

Carlson, G. P., and Kaneko, J. J.: Intravascular granulocyte kinetics in developing calves. Am. J. Vet. Res., 36:421–425, 1975.

Guidry, A. J., Paape, M. J., and Miller, R. H.: In vitro procedure for measuring phagocytosis of blood neutrophils. Am. J. Vet. Res., 35:705–710, 1974.

Metchnikoff, E.: *Leçons sur la pathologie comparée de l'inflammation.* Paris, Masson, 1892.

Normann, S. J.: Kinetics of phagocytosis. III. Two colloid reactions, competitive inhibition, and degree of inhibition between similar and dissimilar foreign particles. Lab. Invest., 31:286–293, 1974.

Paape, M. J., Guidry, A. J., Kirk, S. T., and Bolt, D. J.: Measurement of phagocytosis of P-labeled *Staphylococcus aureus* by bovine leukocytes: Lysostaphin digestion and inhibitory effect of cream. Am. J. Vet. Res., 36:1737–1744, 1975.

Prasse, K. W., Kaeberie, M. L., and Ramsey, F. K.: Blood neutrophilic granulocyte kinetics in cats. Am. J. Vet. Res., 34:1021–1025, 1973.

Stossel, T. P.: Phagocytosis. N. Engl. J. Med. (I) 290:717–723, 1974; (II) 290:774–780, 1974; (III) 290:833–839, 1974.

Wetzel, B. K., Horn, R. G., and Spicer, S. S.: Fine structural studies on the development of heterophil, eosinophil, and basophil in rabbits. Lab. Invest., 16:349–382, 1967.

White, J. G., and Estensen, R. D.: Selective labilization of specific granules in polymorphonuclear leukocytes by phorbol myristate acetate. Am. J. Pathol., 75:45–60, 1974.

Eosinophil Leukocytes

The functions of the eosinophil leukocyte in the battle against disease have long been a matter of speculation and study, but still remain largely mysterious. It is well recognized that eosinophils are increased in numbers and must play an important part in allergic reactions such as asthma, the invasions by many (but not all) parasitic helminths and arthropods, and diseases of the skin.

The mature circulating eosinophil, produced in the bone marrow, varies in appearance between species. In most, the nucleus is slightly lobed but rarely to the extent of a mature neutrophil. As seen in man, dogs, and horses, the nucleus consists of two tear-drop lobes connected by a thin strand, whereas in the rat, the nucleus is usually an annular ring without distinct lobation. The cytoplasmic granules also vary in the different species, being unusually large in the horse, rod-like in the cat, ovoid in the sheep, cow, and pig, and round but variable in size in the dog. The ultrastructure of the eosinophil nucleus is similar to that of neutrophils, with condensation of chromatin at the periphery. The granules are membrane-bound structures with a moderately dense matrix in which is embedded a very dense structure of crystalline appearance. This crystalloid varies in shape from round (dog) to square (man) to rectangular (cat, rat). Other cytoplasmic organelles are not numerous; mitochondria are few and the endoplasmic reticulum is sparse. Eosinophils contain a complement of enzymes similar to those of the neutrophil, but lack detectable lysozyme and phagocytin. They have an unusually high concentration of peroxidase and contain histaminase.

Like neutrophils, eosinophils have a short life span (a few days) and are end-cells incapable of reproduction. Although the normal number in the circulating blood in most species is small, vast reserves are present in the marrow and in the walls of the intestines, lungs, skin, and vagina. Rapid changes can occur in the circulating number apparently from interchanges with the tissue pool. Adrenal cortical steroids induce a swift reduction or disappearance in eosinophils (eosinopenia) which accounts for the eosinopenia in shock or the "alarm" reaction. Experimen-

tal injection of histamine also induces eosinopenia.

As indicated, their function is obscure. They are motile and phagocytic and therefore presumed to play a role in engulfing and destroying particulate matter such as dead cells, bacteria, parasites, and very likely **antigen-antibody precipitates**. A most probable role of the eosinophil is as an antagonist to the inflammatory response. Recent evidence has shown that eosinophil extracts are antagonistic to histamine, serotonin, and bradykinin, all of which are mediators of the inflammatory response. This may also explain the close association of eosinophils to mast cells in tissues, which has led some to regard the eosinophil as a physiologic opposite of the mast cell. Eosinophils are also thought to play a role in the immune response, possibly accepting antigen or "information" from macrophages that have engulfed antigen.

In the tissues, eosinophils, with or without other leukocytes, congregate at the site of allergic reactions (lungs in asthma) and in the vicinity of animal parasites (intestinal worms, trichinae, and recent acute sarcosporidiosis). They have the ability to kill parasites that are coated with specific antibody. Eosinophils have receptors that bind them to antibody and then kill the parasite, presumably through a unique component of the eosinophil granule, the eosinophil major basic protein (MBP). MBP has been shown to kill parasites in vitro (David et al., 1980).

The reason for their presence in huge numbers in eosinophilic myositis has never been discovered. They are numerous in the sinuses of lymph nodes that drain other tissues containing eosinophils and also under other circumstances not understood. In the tissues and even on a glass slide, they are attracted by histamine, while they antagonize its action at the same time. This attraction is presumed to be the reason why they are drawn to the types of injury just mentioned, but it does not explain the selective attraction to these types of injury and not others.

Anderson, J. C.: A suggested role for colostral antibody in the eosinophil response of the piglet. Br. J. Exp. Pathol., 54:135–141, 1973.

Basten, A., Boyer, M. H., and Beeson, P. B.: Mechanism of eosinophil response of rats to *Trichinella spiralis.* J. Exp. Med., 131:1271–1287, 1970.

Basten, A., and Beeson, P. B.: Mechanism of eosinophilia. II. Role of the lymphocyte. J. Exp. Med., 131:1288–1305, 1970.

Cohen, S. G.: The eosinophil and eosinophilia. N. Engl. J. Med., 290:457–459, 1974.

David, J. R., et al.: Enhanced helminthotoxic capacity of eosinophils from patients with eosinophilia. N. Engl. J. Med., 303:1147–1152, 1980.

El-Hashimi, W.: Charcot-Leyden crystals. Formation from primate and lack of formation from nonprimate eosinophils. Am. J. Pathol., 65:311–324, 1971.

Hudson, G., Chin, K. N., and Maxwell, M. H.: Ultrastructure of simian eosinophils. J. Anat., 122:231–239, 1976.

Hung, K. S.: Electron microscopic observations on eosinophil leukocyte granules in dog blood. Anat. Rec., 174:165–174, 1972.

Morgan, J. E., and Beeson, P. B.: Experimental observations on the eosinopenia induced by acute infection. Br. J. Exp. Pathol., 52:214–220, 1971.

Olsson, I., Venge, P., Spitznagel, J. K., and Lehrer, R. I.: Arginine-rich cationic proteins of human eosinophil granules: Comparison of the constituents of eosinophilic and neutrophilic leukocytes. Lab. Invest., 36:493–500, 1977.

Parmley, R. T., and Spicer, S. S.: Cytochemical and ultrastructural identification of a small type granule in human late eosinophils. Lab. Invest., 30:557–567, 1974.

Spry, C. J. F.: Eosinophil structure and functions. Curr. Titles Immunol. Transplant Allerg., 4:81–84, 1976.

Walls, P. S., and Beeson, P. B.: Mechanism of eosinophilia. VIII. Importance of local cellular reactions in stimulating eosinophil production. Clin. Exp. Immunol., 12:111–119, 1972.

Basophil Leukocytes

Basophils are found in very low numbers in the circulating blood. They have a lobed nucleus and the cytoplasm contains deeply basophilic and metachromatic granules, which, like mast cells, contain histamine and heparin. Basophils and mast cells have similar functions but differ in origin. Basophils arise from precursors in the bone marrow, whereas mast cells are thought to arise from mesenchymal cells in connective tissue.

Both cell types function in hypersensitivity reactions moderated by IgE which, with antibody, binds to their surface, leading to release of histamine and heparin.

Hastie, R.: A study of the ultrastructure of human basophil leukocytes. Lab. Invest., 31:223–231, 1974.

Maxwell, M. H.: Comparison of heterophil and basophil ultrastructure in six species of domestic birds. J. Anat., 115:187–202, 1973.

Murata, F., and Spicer, S. S.: Ultrastructural comparison of basophilic leukocytes and mast cells in the guinea pig. Am. J. Anat., 139:335–352, 1974.

Yamada, Y., and Sonoda, M.: Basophils of ovine peripheral blood in electron microscopy. Jpn. J. Vet. Sci., 34:29–32, 1972.

Lymphocytes

The lymphocytes have received considerable discussion under the heading of Lymphocytic Inflammation. They appear in a great variety of acute and chronic inflammatory processes, but only in limited numbers. Probably because they have only limited powers of ameboid movement, they remain at some distance from the center of active acute inflammation. Frequently, many of them only succeed in getting just outside the blood vessel that brought them, constituting **perivascular lymphocytic infiltration**. They usually appear rather late in the course of an infection, some days after its beginning. They are not phagocytic.

Lymphocyte precursors are believed to be produced in the bone marrow, but depend for their development and eventual functions upon two primary lymphoid organs. These are clearly demonstrable in chickens and other birds as the **thymus** and **bursa of Fabricius**, a lymphocytic structure in the wall of the cloaca. In mammals, the latter anatomic structure has not been so clearly defined, but the bone marrow has been postulated as the **bursal equivalent.** The features of these two **primary lymphoid organs** (thymus and bursa) are: They appear early in embryonic life and proliferate in an antigen-free environment. Their cell populations of lymphocytes depend upon a stem-cell supply. Plasma cells and

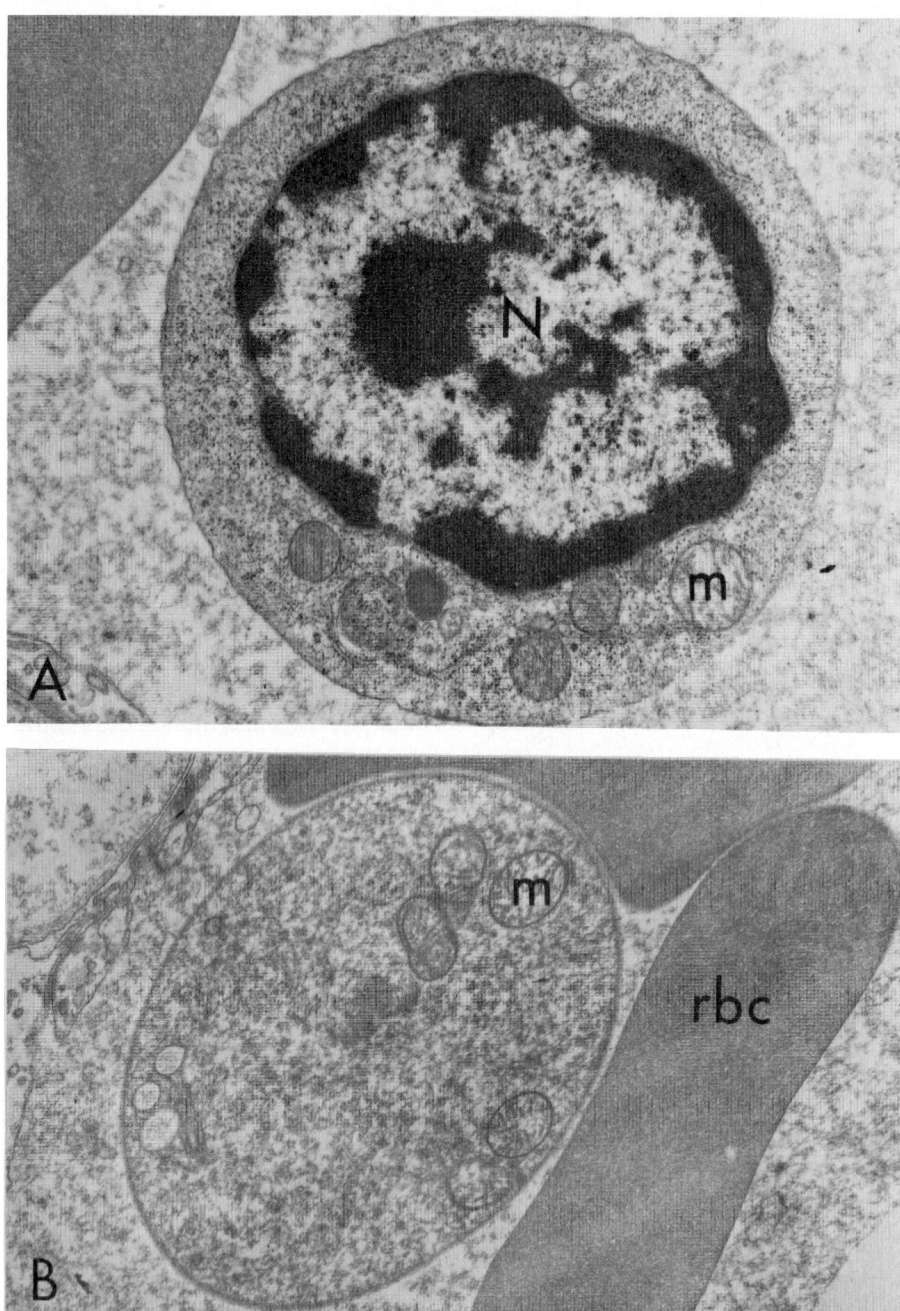

Fig. 6–9. *A*, Lymphocyte in peripheral blood of a marmoset *(Saguinus oedipus). N,* nucleus, *m,* mitochondria. *B*, Thrombocyte, *m,* mitochondria. (Courtesy of Dr. N. W. King, Jr.)

germinal centers are not seen in the normal, undamaged organ after antigenic stimulation. Removal of either organ (thymus or bursa) from the embryo before maturation of the lymphocytic system produces specific immunologic defects.

The **thymus** has been established (by neonatal thymectomy) to have the function of programming lymphocyte precursors, the **T lymphocytes**, giving them the capacity to induce **cell-mediated immunity**. This cell-mediated immunity is involved in: graft rejection; delayed hypersensitivity; graft-versus-host reactions; defense against intracellular organisms; and humoral response to certain antigens (such as red blood cells, demonstrated experimentally).

Animals and children who have no thymus, or a functionally deficient thymus, or have been neonatally thymectomized, are deficient in certain immunologic functions and manifest decreased immunity to infections, such as moniliasis and otherwise weakly pathogenic viruses. Naturally occurring immunologic deficiencies due to a thymic-deficient state are known in children (Di George's syndrome), nude mice, and Arabian foals.

Removal of the **bursa of Fabricius** of chickens by neonatal surgery, testosterone suppression, or irradiation by x-rays results in complete inhibition of production of antibodies and the absence of plasma cell precursors or **B lymphocytes**. As indicated, the functional equivalent of the bursa of Fabricius in birds has been postulated to exist in man and other mammals, but has not been clearly demonstrated anatomically. Removal of the sacculus rotundus, appendix, and Peyer's patches of the rabbit results in diminished antibody production. This has led to the theory that these organs of the rabbit may be functionally equivalent to the bursa of Fabricius.

The bursectomized chicken with severely diminished serum immunoglobulins, absence of plasma cells, but with cell-mediated immunity intact, appears to have its human equivalent in the Bruton type of agammaglobulinemia.

Thus, two functionally distinct but morphologically similar populations of lymphocytes exist in birds and mammals. Most circulating lymphocytes are T lymphocytes; B lymphocytes are largely restricted to lymphoid organs. T and B lymphocytes

Table 6–3. Summary of Characteristics of T and B Lymphocytes*

Characteristic	T-Lymphocytes	B-Lymphocytes
Origin:	Bone marrow	Bone marrow
Life span:	Months	Probably days or weeks
Recirculation pool:	Majority (60%)	Minority
Major localization:		
Lymph nodes:	Deep cortical, parafollicular	Subcapsular, medullary, germinal centers
Spleen:	Periarteriolar	Peripheral white pulp, red pulp
Peyer's patches:	Perifollicular	Central follicles
Phytohemagglutinin response:	Yes	No
Functions:		
Cell-mediated		
Immunity:	Yes	No (?)
Humoral immunity:		
Induction:	4+	4+
Antibody synthesis:	0	4+
Memory:	Yes	Yes

* After Craddock et al., 1971.

will be discussed further in Chapter 22, and their role in immunity in Chapter 7. See Table 6–3 for characteristics of these cells. A third class of lymphocytes exists; these do not have T or B cell markers. These lymphocytes bind and lyse antibody-coated cells. They are called *null cells* or *IgG labile cells* (see Chapter 7).

Lymphocytes are released via the major lymph channels to the blood stream, where they comprise a large percentage of the circulating leukocytes. Most are small cells containing a round nucleus and a narrow rim of cytoplasm. A smaller number of lymphocytes have larger nuclei with more prominent nucleoli and a greater amount of a more basophilic cytoplasm; these are called large lymphocytes. The cytoplasm of small lymphocytes contains only mitochondria and a few small vesicles, whereas large lymphocytes contain, in addition, a prominent Golgi apparatus and endoplasmic reticulum. Lymphocytes are not end cells; large lymphocytes are capable of division into small lymphocytes, and small lymphocytes, of differentiation to a large cell, which in turn is capable of division into small lymphocytes. Stimulation by such substances as phytohemagglutinin and antigens in previously immunized animals causes lymphocytes in blood or in vitro cultures to undergo mitosis and assume the appearance of lymphoblasts.

In contrast to granulocytes, which remain within the circulation until death or unless "called forth," lymphocytes do not normally remain in the blood stream continuously but recirculate from the blood back to the lymph. They enter lymphocytic follicles, lymph nodes, spleen, and other lymphoid organs such as Peyer's patches by passing across the walls of postcapillary venules. From the node or spleen, the lymphocytes then either directly re-enter the blood or travel via lymphatics to regain the blood circulation.

Plasma Cells

Plasma cells are not found in the blood, but are an important constituent of many inflammatory reactions. They are lymphocytes modified structurally for the production of gamma globulins. These cells are smoothly spherical or elliptical, with much more cytoplasm and therefore somewhat larger than a lymphocyte. The nucleus resembles that of a lymphocyte in being spherical and having a "clock-face" peripheral arrangement of chromatin granules. An important aid in recognition is the fact that the nucleus is almost always eccentrically placed in the cell. The cytoplasm appears homogeneous and as a rule, but not invariably, is a little more basophilic in its staining reaction than most cytoplasm, taking a nearly magenta shade of purplish red. Often the cytoplasm contains a distinct hyaline sphere called a **Russell body**. The electron microscopic features of the nucleus are not distinctive, however the cytoplasm, in addition to distinct Golgi bodies and mitochondria, is filled with an abundant amount of endoplasmic reticulum. Within the cisternae of the endoplasmic reticulum, homogeneous material (gamma globulin) is found which, as it increases in amount, dilates the cisterna and gives the Russell body its characteristic microscopic appearance.

Plasma cells do not undergo mitosis; they originate from lymphocytes. Once formed, they live a short life, about 12 hours. It is assumed that the plasma cell then dies, but it has not been proved that death is the fate; it is possible they change in morphology to remain in the tissues as "memory" cells for immunologic mechanisms.

The function of the plasma cell is the production of antibodies (immunoglobulins). Plasma cells produce all recognized types of humoral antibodies. The homogeneous material described above, which lies in the cisternae of the endoplasmic reticulum, represents accumulation of gamma-globulins produced by the cell.

Their occurrence seems to be influenced both by the type of injurious agent and the part of the body involved. With regard to the latter, the female reproductive tract is

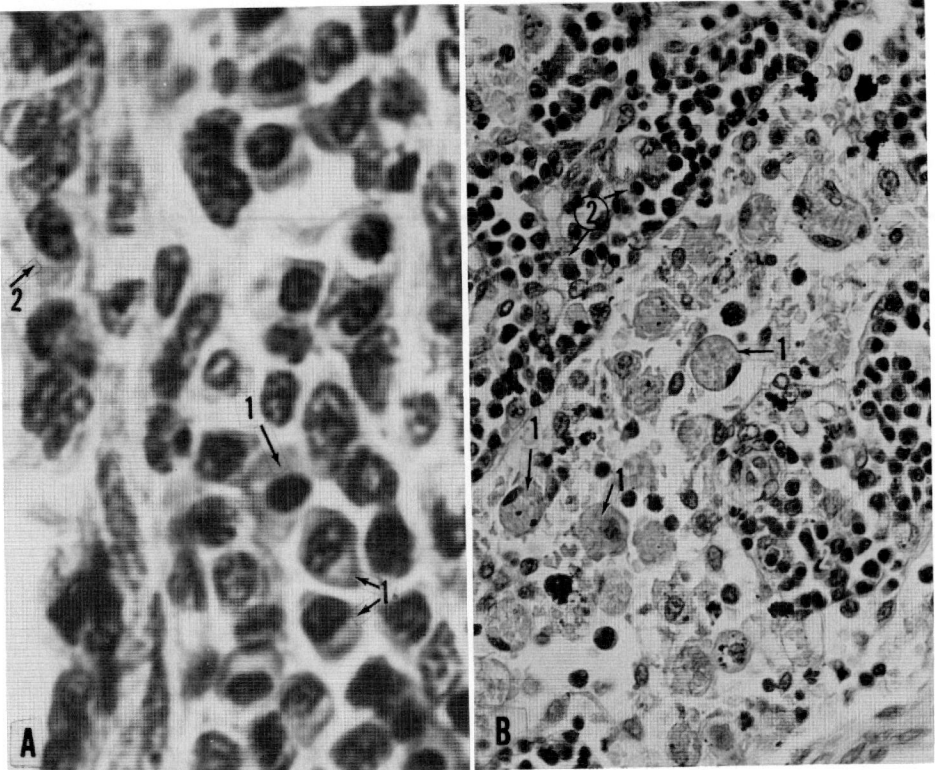

Fig. 6–10. *A*, Plasma cells in an intestinal villus of a dog. Plasma cells (*1*), intestinal epithelium (*2*). (× 1000.) (Courtesy of Armed Forces Institute of Pathology.) Contributor: Dr. Samuel Pollock. *B*, Erythrophagocytosis, lymph node of a dog with acute leptospirosis. Erythrocytes in macrophages (*1*), lymphocytes (*2*). (× 440.) (Courtesy of Armed Forces Institute of Pathology.) Contributor: Division of Veterinary Medicine, Walter Reed Army Institute of Research.

an outstanding location for plasma-cell reactions. Almost all inflammations here involve small or large numbers of plasma cells. They are also seen with some frequency in intestinal inflammations and in those of the male reproductive organs. The infections that bring them out are chronic in nature and include some of the granulomas. Plasma cells increase in the spleen and lymph nodes of rats affected with experimentally induced tumors.

Alexander, E. L., and Wetzel, B.: Human lymphocytes: similarity of B and T cell surface morphology. Science, *188*:732–734, 1975.

Craddock, C. G., Longmire, R., and McMillan, R.: Lymphocytes and the immune response. N. Engl. J. Med., (I) *285*:324–331, 1971; (II) *285*:378–384, 1971.

Eichberg, J. W., et al.: Thymus derived lymphocytes and bone marrow derived lymphocytes in nonhuman primates and effects of thymosin in vitro. Fed. Proc., *34*:966, 1975.

Friedenstein, A., and Goncharenko, I.: Morphological evidence of immunological relationships in the lymphoid tissue of rabbit appendix. Nature, *206*:1113–1115, 1965.

Helmreich, E., Kern, M., and Eisen, H. N.: The secretion of antibody by isolated lymph node cells. J. Biol. Chem., *236*:464, 1961.

Horsmanheimo, M.: Lymphocytic transformation and the Kveim test. Lancet, *1*:1120–1121, 1973.

Howard, J. C.: The life span and recirculation of marrow-derived small lymphocytes from the rat thoracic duct. J. Exp. Med., *135*:185–199, 1972.

Niblack, G. D., and Gengozian, N.: Identification of T and B lymphocytes in marmoset: A natural blood chimera. Fed. Proc., *34*:1013, 1975.

Sonoda, M.: Electron microscopy of lymphocytes in the peripheral blood of clinically healthy horses. Jpn. J. Vet. Sci., *33*:291–294, 1971.

Monocytes (reticuloendothelial cells)

The blood monocyte characteristically has an indented nucleus with condensation of the nucleoplasm near its membrane. The cytoplasm is similar in many ways to

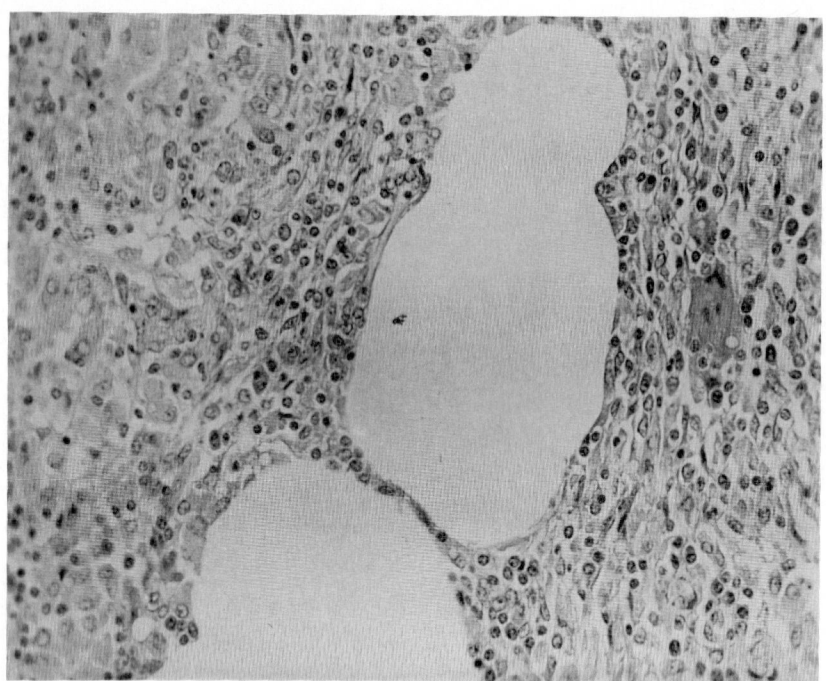

Fig. 6–11. Macrophages surrounding lipid foreign material (spaces) injected subcutaneously as an adjuvant in a tissue vaccine. Subcutis of a cow. (H & E, × 300.) (Courtesy of Armed Forces Institute of Pathology.) Contributor: Col. Fred. D. Maurer, V.C.

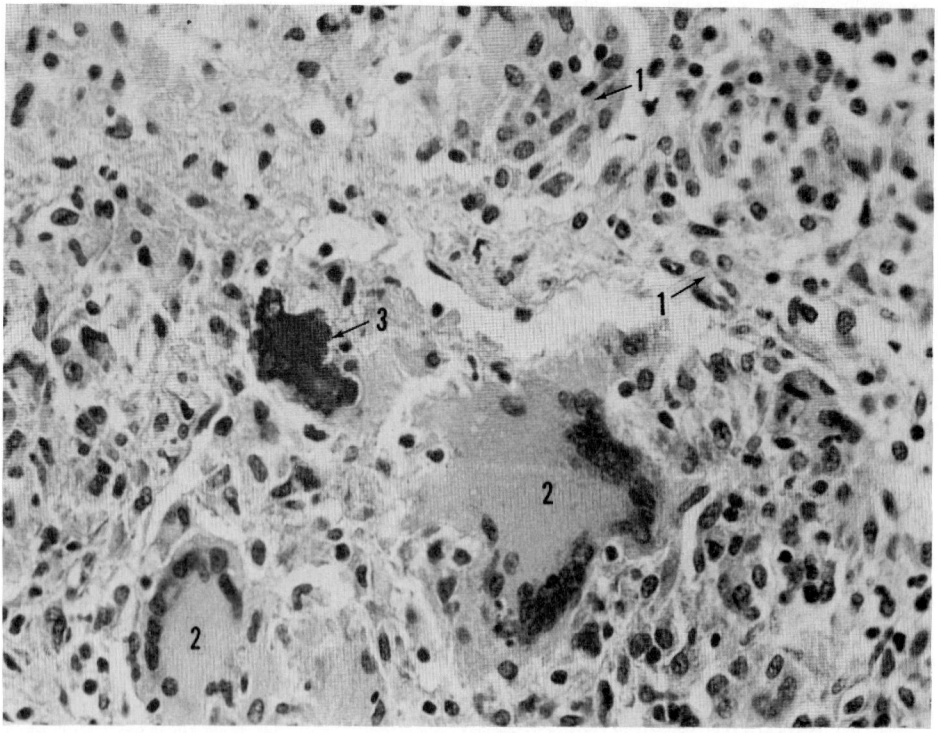

Fig. 6–12. Granulomatous inflammation in tuberculosis of an equine lung. Macrophages (*1*), Langhans' giant cells (*2*), and calcareous debris (*3*). (× 435.) (Courtesy of Armed Forces Institute of Pathology.) Contributor: Dr. J. R. M. Innes.

that of the lymphocyte, but is more abundant. It contains mitochondria, a well-formed Golgi apparatus, and rough and smooth endoplasmic reticulum which usually appears as "vesicles." Lysosomes or other "granules" are absent. The tissue macrophage has a similar structure to the monocyte, but also contains many membrane-bound granules. These granules are reminiscent of lysosomes and presumably contain a packet of enzymes, including lysozyme and acid-phosphatase.

Their functions include the phagocytosis of the microscopically larger particles, animate or inanimate, including the pathogenic bacteria responsible for their presence. This faculty gives them the name of **macrophages**, as contrasted with the mi-crophages, which are polymorphonuclear neutrophils. The macrophages frequently fuse together to form giant cells, which are able to phagocytize still larger particles, such as pathogenic yeast cells and fungi, of which the *Cryptococcus (Torula)* and the *Coccidioides* are among the largest. A **Langhans' giant cell** is of irregular shape and some 50 or 60 mμ in diameter. Its cytoplasm is fused into a homogeneous mass, but it has many spherical nuclei arranged in a more or less complete wreath just inside its hazy and indefinite periphery. A **foreign-body giant cell** is similar, except that its somewhat larger nuclei are piled up in a jumbled mass at the center of the cell.

Functions of the mononuclear cells other than phagocytosis are thought to include

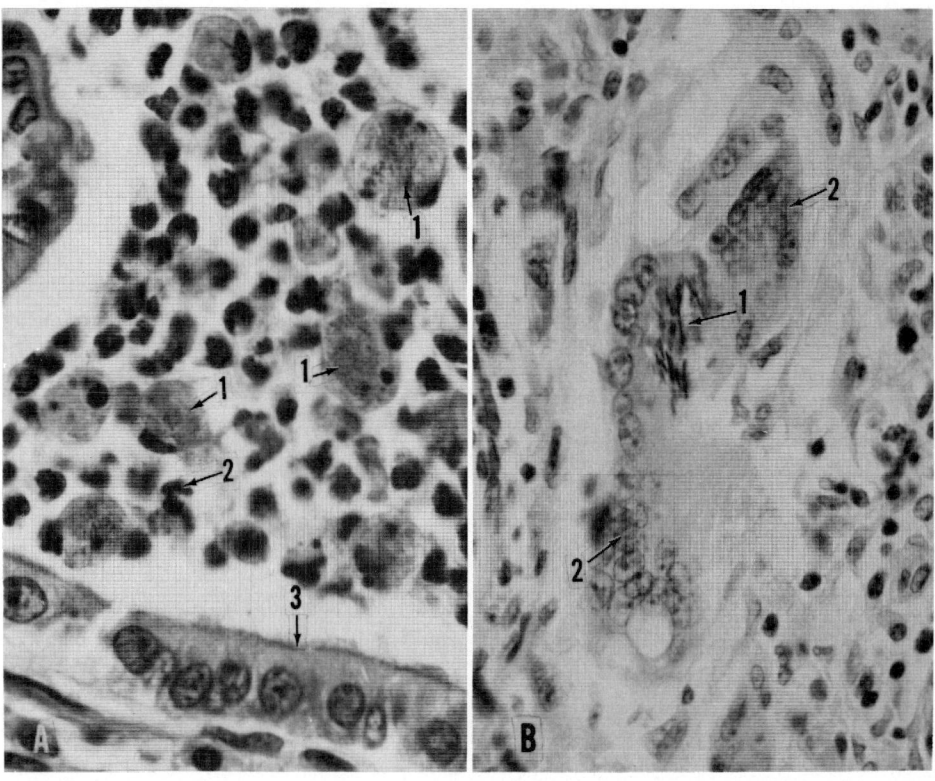

Fig. 6–13. *A*, Macrophages in a bronchiole of a foal infected with *Corynebacterium pyogenes*. Organisms in macrophages (*1*), neutrophils (*2*), bronchiolar epithelium (*3*) (× 1000) (Courtesy of Armed Forces Institute of Pathology.) Contributor: Army Veterinary School. *B*, Foreign body type giant cells in spermatic granuloma in a ram. Phagocytized spermatozoa (*1*), nuclei of giant cell (*2*). (× 648.) (Courtesy of Armed Forces Institute of Pathology.) Contributor: Dr. K. McEntee.

the secretion of various enzymes and neutralizing substances. They may also play a role in the immune processes by altering antigen or transferring antigen or "information" to an immunologically competent cell. Their function of providing a physical barrier in the form of a frequently wide zone of granulation tissue between the infected and healthy areas has been described in connection with granulomatous inflammation.

Adams, D. O.: The structure of mononuclear phagocytes differentiating in vivo. I. Sequential fine and histologic studies of the effect of *Bacillus Calmette-Guerin* (BCG). Am. J. Pathol., 76:17–48, 1974.

Adams, D. O.: The structure of mononuclear phagocytes differentiating *in vivo*. II. The effect of *Mycobacterium tuberculosis*. Am. J. Pathol., 80:101–116, 1975.

Adams, D. O.: The granulomatous inflammatory response. A review. Am. J. Pathol., 84:164–191, 1976.

Akpom, C. M., and Warren, K. S.: The inhibition of granuloma formation around *Schistosoma mansoni* eggs. Am. J. Pathol., 79:435–452, 1975.

Bhuyan, U. N., and Ramalingaswami, V.: Systemic macrophages mobilization and granulomatous response to BCG in the protein-deficient rabbit. Am. J. Pathol., 76:313–322, 1974.

Boros, D. L., and Warren, K. S.: The Bentonite granuloma. Characterization of a model system for infectious and foreign body granulomatous inflammation using soluble mycobacterial, histoplasma and schistosoma antigens. Immunology, 24:511–529, 1973.

Dannenberg, A. M., Jr.: Macrophages in inflammation and infection. N. Engl. J. Med., 293:489–493, 1975.

Leibovich, S. J., and Ross, R.: The role of the macrophage in wound repair. Am. J. Pathol., 78:71–100, 1975.

Nichols, B. A., and Bainton, D. F.: Differentiation of human monocytes in bone marrow and blood: Sequential formation of two granule populations. Lab. Invest., 29:27–40, 1973.

Papadimitriou, J. M., and Spector, W. G.: Origin, properties and fate of epithelioid cells. J. Pathol., 105:187–203, 1971.

Papadimitriou, J. M., Robertson, T. A., and Walters, M. N-I.: An analysis of the phagocytic potential of multinucleate giant cells. Am. J. Pathol., 78:343–358, 1975.

Polliack, A., and Gordon, S.: Scanning electron microscopy of murine macrophages: Surface characteristics during maturation, activation and phagocytosis. Lab. Invest., 33:469–477, 1975.

Ryan, G. B., and Spector, W. G.: Macrophage turnover in inflamed connective tissue. Proc. R. Soc. Lond. (Biol.), 175:269–292, 1970.

Seshadri, R. S., Brown, E. J., and Zipursky, A.: Leukemic reticuloendotheliosis: A failure of monocyte production. N. Engl. J. Med., 295:180–184, 1976.

Stanley, E. R., Hansen, G., Woodcock, J., and Metcalf, D.: Colony stimulating factor and the regulation of granulopoiesis and macrophage production. Fed. Proc., 34:2272–2278, 1975.

Tsuda, T., et al.: Mononuclear cell turnover in chronic inflammation. Am. J. Pathol., 83:255–268, 1976.

Unanue, E. R., and Benacerraf, B.: Immunologic events in experimental hypersensitivity granulomas. Am. J. Pathol., 71:349–364, 1973.

Unanue, E. R.: Secretory function of mononcuclear phagocytes. A review. Am. J. Pathol., 83:396–418, 1976.

Van Furth, R.: Origin and kinetics of monocytes and macrophages. Semin. Hematol.,7:125–141, 1970.

Van Furth, R., et al.: The mononuclear phagocyte system. A new classification of macrophages, monocytes. Bull WHO, 46:845–852, 1972.

Ward, P. A.: Chemotaxis of mononuclear cells. J. Exp. Med., 128:1201–1221, 1968.

Warren, K. S., Boros, D. L., Hang, L. M., and Mahmoud, A. A. F.: The *Schistosoma japonicum* egg granuloma. Am. J. Pathol., 80:279–294, 1975.

Mast Cells

Although mast cells are not usually looked upon as a cellular component of the inflammatory exudate, their probable relationship to the inflammatory process demands their consideration here. Mast cells arise from undifferentiated mesenchymal cells, and by mitosis from other mast cells. They are found in loose connective tissue throughout the body and in organs rich in connective tissue such as the mammary gland. Generally they are few in number in parenchymatous organs that contain little connective tissue, such as the kidney and liver. However, in certain species, even in these tissues they may be numerous. For example, the dog liver contains an appreciable number of mast cells. Neoplastic mast cells may circulate in the blood, as in the cat with mast cell tumor of the spleen.

Mast cells were named by Paul Ehrlich (1877), who noted that the cells were "stuffed" or overfed with metachromatic granules (*mast*, German, = well fed).

Mast cells vary in shape and size within and between species. The nucleus is round or oval and contains a prominent nu-

Table 6–4. Histochemical Determinations on Mast Cells*

Species	Heparin	Histamine	Serotonin 5-HTA	Chymotrypsin-like enzyme	Trypsin-like enzyme	Nonspecific esterase	Acid Phosphatase	β-Glucuron-idase	N-Acetyl-β-gluco-aminidase
Carp	±	–	–	–	–	–	–	–	–
Frog	+ to +++	–	–	–	–	++	+	+	++
Turtle	+ to ++	++	–	–	+++	–	–	–	–
Chicken	+ to ++	++	–	–	–	–	–	–	+++
Rat	+++	+++	+++	+++	++	+++	–	++	++
Monkey	+ to +++	+++	–	+	+++	++	++	++	+++
Man	++ to +++	++	–	+	+++	+	+	++	+++

+ to +++ = degree of positive reaction
± = equivocal reaction
– = negative reaction
 * = After Chiu and Lagunoff, 1972

5-HTA = 5-hydroxytryptamine

cleolus. The cytoplasm is distinctive, containing many spherical basophilic and metachromatic granules. The ultrastructure of the granule varies from finely granular to concentric lamellae of filaments presenting a whorled or scrolled pattern not dissimilar from the granules of the basophil. Mitochondria, Golgi, and endoplasmic reticulum are also found in the cytoplasm, although often obscured by the multitude of granules.

The granules contain, in addition to a variety of enzymes, heparin, histamine, and at least in the rat and mouse, serotonin. It is these compounds that relate the function of the mast cell to the inflammatory process. Each has been discussed earlier. Upon proper stimulation, which includes mechanical trauma, venoms, bacterial toxins, heat, cold, irradiation, etc., mast cells degranulate and release their vasoactive amines. Indeed, in an acute inflammatory response there is a reduction in stainable mast cells. The release of their contents is of prime importance in IgE hypersensitivity reactions, as mentioned under the discussion of basophils. In contrast, mast cells increase in number in chronic inflammatory processes.

The granules of mast cells from different species do not have the same histochemical content, suggesting that their function may also differ in various species. This is depicted in Table 6–4.

Of concern to the diagnostic pathologist is the neoplastic transformation of mast cells to produce the mast cell tumor. This is discussed in Chapter 18.

Benditt, E. P., and Lagunoff, D.: The mast cell. Its structure and function. Prog. Allergy., *8*:195–202, 1964.

Bloch, K. J., and Angevine, C.: Mast cells and mast cell sensitizing homocytotrophic antibodies. Rheumatology, 3:169–193, 1970.

Chiu, H., and Lagunoff, D.: Histochemical comparison of vertebrate mast cells. Histochem. J., 4:135–144, 1972.

Kessler, S., and Kuhn, C.: Scanning electron microscopy of mast cell degranulation. Lab. Invest., 32:71–77, 1975.

Ehrlich, P.: Beiträge zur Kenntniss der Anilinfärbungen und ihrer Verwendung in der mikroskopischen Tecknik. Arch. mikros. Anat., 13:263–277, 1877.

Komiyama, A., and Spicer, S. S.: Acid phosphatase demonstrated ultrastructurally in mast cell granules altered by pinocytosis. Lab. Invest., 32:485–491, 1975.

Murata, F., and Spicer, S. S.: Ultrastructural comparison of basophilic leukocytes and mast cells in the guinea pig. Am. J. Anat., *139*:335–352, 1974.

Padawer, J.: Phagocytosis of particulate substances by mast cells. Lab. Invest., 25:320–330, 1971.

Parmley, R. T., Spicer, S. S., and Wright, N. J.: The ultrastructural identification of tissue basophils and mast cells in Hodgkin's Disease. Lab. Invest., 32:469–475, 1975.

Spicer, S. S., Simson, J. A. U., and Farrington, J. E.: Mast cell phagocytosis of red blood cells. Am. J. Pathol., *80*:481–498, 1975.

Whur, P., and Gracie, M.: Histochemical comparison of mast cell and globule leucocyte granules in the rat. Experientia, 23:655–657, 1967.

THE DURATION OF INFLAMMATION

The duration of an illness is often identified by terms that indicate increasing length as **acute**, **subacute**, or **chronic**. These terms are also applied to the duration of inflammation.

Acute inflammation arises suddenly, often within a few hours, and progresses rather rapidly to recovery or death within a few days. The principal clinical features of such inflammation may be demonstrated by a simple experiment: Make a mild stroke injury on your arm by drawing something like the back corner edge of a ruler along the skin with moderate pressure. In a few minutes, a red, dull line appears along the course of the stroke, surrounded by a brighter red halo or flare. This is followed by swelling (wheal) of the dull red line. In addition to the redness and swelling, heat and pain are evident. These are the signs of inflammation.

The dull, red line is due to release of substances (particularly histamine) that cause dilation of small blood vessels. The flare is due to arteriolar dilation through axon reflex stimulation. The swelling (wheal) of the line of injury is due to release of substances that cause increased permeability of small blood vessels, and exudation of fluid, proteins, and sometimes cells. This last effect is the result of degranulation of mast cells, which releases histamine and other substances. This causes leakage of venules, producing the wheal at the site of the direct injury.

This type of acute inflammation is sometimes referred to as the **immediate transient response** to injury. More severe injury may result in an inflammatory response that is similar, but may reappear and last for hours. This is the **delayed prolonged response**. Examples of the causes of this type of injury include: sunburn (due to ultraviolet rays), mild heat, and some bacterial toxins. Some tissue extracts injected experimentally also cause this delayed response (pyrogen, an extract of rabbit leukocyte granules; also an extract of rabbit lymphocytes). An even more severe injury may result in an immediate response that persists for days or weeks. This is the **immediate prolonged response**. An example would be a severe burn. Leakage from capillaries and venules is immediate and severe. Damage to endothelium may result in thrombosis.

These experimental demonstrations of three facets of inflammation are not usually so clear-cut in nature, but sometimes may be evident. Usually they occur simultaneously.

Chronic inflammation may have some of the features of acute inflammation, but may be distinguished, not only by its longer duration, but by the nature of the exudation. Inflammation and repair tend to occur simultaneously, causing many types of cells to be present. All types of leukocytes, fibroblasts, and endothelial cells tend to be present. If the repair to connective tissue is extensive, the preponderant tissue will become granulation tissue.

Some types of irritants (tubercle bacilli, most pathogenic fungi, lipid) cause the predominant inflammatory cells to be macrophages, resulting in granulomatous inflammation. This also tends to be of long duration unless the immunologic and tissue defenses are totally adequate, in which case the irritant tends to be confined and walled off—encapsulated. Eventually this results in a dense scar.

The descriptive term **subacute** is sometimes used to indicate inflammation with duration between acute and chronic. It is not precise and cannot be described accurately in pathologic terms.

Wound healing is also of interest in connection with duration of inflammation. If a wound is made with a sharp instrument, is not contaminated with bacteria or foreign debris, and has its edges brought together promptly (and held there), the wound is apt to heal rather promptly, leaving little or no scar. This is called healing by **first intention**.

On the other hand, if the wound is accompanied by infection, hemorrhage, and other exudation into a gaping space and edges are not brought together, healing is delayed. Debris and infectious organisms must be neutralized, phagocytosed, and removed. Space filled by exudate is eventually replaced by granulation tissue, which finally contracts, pulling the edges of the wound together approximately but leaving a depressed scar and possibly contraction lines in the skin. This is healing by **second intention**.

HEALING AND REGENERATION

Healing is the process which, after an injurious agent has been overcome, restores the injured part as nearly as possible to its previous normal condition. The task commonly involves three phases: removal, repair, and regeneration.

Removal of the products of inflammation, such as exudates and dead cells, is usually accomplished by liquefaction, the fluid being readily absorbed into the lymph and blood. The fact that dead tissue tends to be liquefied by its own autolytic enzymes (autolysis) and by enzymes derived from inflammatory leukocytes (heterolysis) has already been reported. Several kinds of leukocytes are thought to produce substances aiding this process, as explained in immediately preceding pages. If the dead tissue is on a surface, the main mass desquamates or sloughs as soon as preliminary liquefaction has loosened its attachment. Everyone is familiar with a loosening of a scab, which is simply dried and hardened exudate.

Repair of damaged or disjoined parts is accomplished by proliferation of fibrous tissue, the building of a scar. Much more to be desired, however, is the healing by regeneration.

Regeneration is the process by which lost cells and tissues are replaced by others of the same kind. Some tissues regenerate readily; others do not, a situation that often determines what extent of recovery is possible from a given injury.

Epithelium can, in general, regenerate with considerable facility. That of the digestive, respiratory, and similar **mucous membranes**, of the lung alveoli following pneumonia, and of the endometrium after menstruation is readily replaced by multiplication of some few cells that remain, albeit in glands or ducts opening on the destroyed surfaces. Secretory epithelium of badly damaged **glands**, however, is commonly not replaced. This is true of the gastric glands, mammary gland, seminiferous tubules, and other glands. In the **liver**, the epithelial cells regenerate readily provided the framework of the lobule is intact; otherwise, there is often an unsuccessful attempt in the proliferation of large numbers of bile ducts. But these scarcely produce functioning hepatic tissue. In the **kidney**, individual cells of the tubular lining are replaced, but no new nephrons are formed. The **epidermis** readily regenerates from the edges of a wound, but accessory skin structures are not reproduced. Papillation and often pigmentation remain absent.

Muscle. Severed muscles are usually reunited by a fibrous scar that restores them to normal functional ability. Smooth and cardiac muscles never regenerate. A certain amount of regeneration sometimes occurs in voluntary striated muscle, with buds of muscle cells building out into the tissue of the fibrous union. Often these appear as multinucleated **giant-cells** which might be mistaken for foreign-body giant cells, since they have many nuclei and little sarcoplasm. If the sarcolemma remains intact, as in atrophy of a muscle, the sarcoplasm can be replaced.

Nerve. If a peripheral nerve is severed, the distal portion dies but is slowly regenerated by new growth from the proximal end. Rarely, perhaps, there is union of the proximal and the original distal ends. If a nerve cell body dies, the whole neuron dies and is not replaced, the peripheral process undergoing what is called **wallerian degeneration**. Sometimes, more or less perfect function is restored by training, e.g., for particular acts, by virtue of a new route being found to carry the impulse around the destroyed portion of the brain or cord. Neuroglia proliferate readily.

Blood. Restoration of blood has been treated under Hemorrhage.

Connective Tissue. It has already been seen that fibrous tissue proliferates readily, replacing its own kind or other tissues that are not able to regenerate. When young, it is areolar in arrangement, often rich in young capillaries. It becomes denser and less vascular with age, until finally old scars may be very dense and even hyaline, with a poor blood supply. (See Granulation Tissue.)

Cartilage and bone are regenerated first as fibrous tissue by multiplication of the undifferentiated connective-tissue cells of the perichondrium or periosteum, and, to a lesser extent, of the endosteum. In the healing of a fracture, the sequence is (1) hemorrhage, (2) clotting, the formation of fibrin, (3) organization of the fibrin by fibroblasts, as is prone to occur in fibrin anywhere, (4) calcification and ossification of the fibrous tissue into imperfect bone (the provisional callus), which is then slowly destroyed and replaced by more perfect bone (the true callus).

Tendons and ligaments regenerate slowly but perfectly as a rule.

Blood vessels are easily replaced by newly formed capillaries. These may become much larger than capillaries normally are, but a muscular coat (characteristic of arteries and veins) is seldom, if ever, developed.

Mesothelium of the serous surfaces is quickly regenerated.

FEVER

Fever has been occasionally noted as being a part of inflammation for centuries (Celsus, 30 BC–38 AD), and was for a long time thought to be disease itself. The first experiments designed to establish a relationship between inflammation and fever were carried out by Billroth and Frese, about 100 years ago, but the experiments were not conclusive (Atkins and Bodel, 1972). Currently, fever is distinguished from other hyperthermias (to be discussed later) on the basis of several characteristics: (1) The elevation in body temperature is generated by thermoregulation only, resulting from the action of exogenous or endogenous pyrogens on the preoptic anterior hypothalamic areas of the brain. (2) The increase in the thermopreferendum is evident, particularly at the outset of fever. Man and animals seek a warmer, more comfortable temperature during a "chill." (3) The higher temperature is maintained by a fully functional thermoregulatory system. The "set point" on the body "thermostat" is simply put at a higher temperature. (4) Antipyretic drugs, such as aspirin, can intervene in the febrile process to reduce the body temperature.

None of the foregoing criteria applies to the other hyperthermias.

Fever occurs in representative species of several phyla (Kluger, 1979). Live and dead bacteria have been used to produce fever in fishes, amphibians, reptiles, birds, and mammals. Antipyretic drugs have been shown to reduce the experimental fever in all of these species except amphibians. Studies to establish the effect of endogenous pyrogens (to be discussed) have not been completed on representative species of all of these phyla.

Newborn mammals (man, sheep, guinea pig) do not manifest fever in the presence of infections. Neonatal lambs and guinea pigs are refractory to bacterial pyrogens administered experimentally. Large doses of bacterial endotoxins, administered intravenously, will produce fever in the guinea pig, however. This apparent resistance to fever in the neonate is postulated to be due to immaturity of the mechanisms in the central nervous system or to an effect of circulating antipyretic substances. Such substances have been demonstrated in the blood of lambs and ewes close to the time of parturition (Cooper, et al, 1979).

The central system of temperature regulation is located in the preoptic anterior hypothalamus. Obliterative lesions at this site remove the ability to regulate body temperature.

The substances that cause fever (pyrogens) include a long list of exogenous materials, foremost of which is bacterial endotoxin. Circulating antigen-antibody complexes are also recognized as pyrogenic. The pyrogenic effect of prostaglandins has been described earlier.

The value of fever to the diseased host is still not clearly demonstrated, although some deleterious effects upon survival have been shown to occur experimentally when fever is abated by use of antipyretics. Philosophically, it seems that the ability to respond to infection by elevated temperature must have some beneficial effects. Otherwise, it would not have survived as a function in so many animal species.

Atkins, E., and Bodel, P.: Fever. N. Engl. J. Med., *286*:27–34, 1972.

Atkins, E., and Bodel, P.: Clinical fever: Its history, manifestations and pathogenesis. Fed. Proc., 38:57–63, 1979.

Bernheim, H. A., and Kluger, M. J.: Fever: effect of drug-induced antipyresis in survival. Science, 193:237–239, 1976.

Cranston, W. I.: Central mechanisms of fever. Fed. Proc., 38:49–51, 1979.

Cooper, K. E., Veale, W. L., Kasting, N., and Pittman, Q. J.: Ontogeny of fever. Fed. Proc., 38:35–38, 1979.

Dinarello, C. A.: Production of endogenous pyrogen. Fed. Proc., 38:52–56, 1979.

Greaves, M. W.: Prostaglandins and Inflammation. *In* Prostaglandins: Physiological, Pharmacological and Pathological Aspects, edited by S. M. M. Karim. Baltimore, University Park Press, 1976, pp. 293–302.

Kluger, M. J.: Phylogeny of fever. Fed. Proc., 38:30–34, 1979.

Pickering, G. W.: Fever. *In*, General Pathology, edited by H. W. Florey. 4th ed. London, Lloyd-Luke, Ltd., 1970, pp. 394–412.

Robinson, S. (ed.): Problems in temperature regulation and exercise. Fed. Proc., 32:1563–1622, 1973.

OTHER HYPERTHERMIAS

The body temperature is increased in several other conditions that do not conform to the definition of fever. Among those presently known are certain pathologic and pharmacologic states in man and animals, as follows: (1) **malignant hyperthermia** of man and swine; an inherited predisposition, triggered by certain drugs, with usually fatal hyperthermia; (2) **hypothalamic lesions**, natural or experimental, which destroy or disturb the temperature regulating center; (3) metabolic disease associated with **thyrotoxicosis** (hyperthyroidism) or with **pheochromocytoma** of the adrenal gland; (4) disturbance of **monoamine metabolism** in the central nervous system; (5) prolonged administration of **atropine**.

Hyperthermia of exercise is also recognized as a situation featuring elevated temperature. In this case, dissipation of heat is inadequate to dispose of heat generated by the exercise. Elevated temperature persists as long as the exercise continues. The physiologic mechanisms are not completely understood.

Heat Exhaustion (Heat Prostration, Heat Stroke)

Under certain conditions, animals are unable to eliminate sufficient heat to maintain body temperature at a level compatible with life. In the absence of adequate clinical study or a satisfactory history, the pathologist may have difficulty recognizing this syndrome and be at a loss for an adequate explanation of the animal's death. In those instances in which an adequate history is available, it is evident that the animal has been exposed to unusually high heat and humidity, a confined space, and some psychologic stress (fear, excitement). Often a dog will be bathed at a kennel, placed in a drying cage (or small cage) on a hot, humid day, then found dead an hour or two later. A common story is that the dog was left for a "short time" (usually, actually two or more hours) in the back of a station wagon while the owner is shopping, and the dog is very ill or dead when the shopping is finished. Other cases may involve shipping in a small, poorly ventilated crate or confinement in a truck, airplane, or railroad car in which the temperature and humidity become excessive. Swine may be affected when shipped in hot humid weather or during or after parturition under these conditions. Poorly conditioned horses may also succumb under these conditions. Any animal confined out in hot sun may be affected. Pet monkeys and cats are susceptible to this condition. Failure of a ventilating or cooling system may also be responsible for this syndrome.

The essential signs are high fever (106° to 110° F), which may be lowered by cold water or other cooling methods, severe hyperpnea and respiratory distress (dog), severe discomfort, congested mucosae, tachycardia, excitement, collapse, and sudden death. Fetuses in pregnant animals (swine) may die in utero and be delivered or retained to produce severe metritis.

Gross Appearance. Generalized hyperemia is most severe in the respiratory tract, especially in the lungs and tracheal and bronchial mucosae. Lungs may also be edematous and occasionally contain focal consolidations of bronchopneumonia. Other organs, such as heart, kidneys, meninges, lymph nodes, and muscles, may also be severely congested. Preexisting cardiac disease (e.g., dirofilariasis) or pulmonary disease (focal pneumonia) may accentuate the effect of heat and may contribute to the death of the animal. Unexpectedly extensive autolysis is often evident, particularly in dogs and swine.

Microscopic Appearance. The lesions are compatible with those seen grossly. The vasculature of the lungs is severely engorged and edema is evident in alveoli. Centrilobular necrosis, disassociation of hepatocytes, and congestion are often found in the liver. Subendocardial and subepicardial hemorrhages are found in the heart. Capillary congestion is evident in kidneys, meninges, lymph nodes, and other structures.

Diagnosis. The diagnosis of heat exhaustion depends upon consideration of several factors. The persistent high fever, distress, and sudden death of an animal that could have been exposed to high temperature and humidity should arouse suspicion. The gross hyperemia, especially of the respiratory system, unusually rapid autolysis, and absence of lesions of other specific infectious diseases are helpful factors in arriving at a diagnosis.

Busey, W. M., Coate, W. B., and Badger, D. W.: Histopathologic effects of nitrogen dioxide exposure and heat stress in cynomolgus monkeys. Toxicol. Appl. Pharmacol., 29:130, 1974.

Clowes, G. H. A., Jr., and O'Donnell, T. F., Jr.: Heat stroke. N. Engl. J. Med., 291:564–567, 1974.

Hickey, T. E., and Kelly, W. A.: Heatstroke in a colony of squirrel monkeys. J. Am. Vet. Med. Assoc., 161:700–703, 1972.

Krum, S. H., and Osborne, C. A.: Heatstroke in the dog: A polysystemic disorder. J. Am. Vet. Med. Assoc., 170:531–535, 1977.

Musacchia, X. J.: Fever and hyperthermia. Fed. Proc., 38:27–29, 1979.

Stitt, J. T.: Fever versus hyperthermia. Fed. Proc., 38:39–43, 1979.

Malignant Hyperthermia of Swine

This syndrome is also known as malignant hyperthermia syndome, malignant hyperpyrexia, porcine malignant hyperthermia, and acute stress syndrome in pigs.

Apparently similar to a familial syndrome of the same name in human patients, this disorder is triggered by certain anesthetic materials, particularly halothane and chloroform. It may also be the same as or similar to a disorder called acute stress syndrome in pigs, provoked by transport, exercise, and slaughtering. The syndrome is expressed by signs of tachypnea, hyperventilation, generalized muscular rigidity, blotchy cyanosis of skin, tachycardia, asystole, and death. Analyses of plasma reveal elevated levels of protein, electrolytes, creatinine phosphokinase, and serum aldolase. A study of biopsy specimens from skeletal muscle in vitro indicate an increased rate of depletion of adenosine triphosphate.

The trait has been found in specific families of swine of the following breeds: Landrace, Pietrain, Poland China, and Yorkshire.

Incomplete genetic evidence points toward dominant inheritance with variable penetrance. The possibility of involvement of two genes has not been excluded.

Microscopic Appearance. The microscopic and ultrastructural lesions apparently have not been described in detail, although skeletal muscles have been indicated to be "pale, soft, and exudative." Loss of striations and hyalinization of sarcoplasma has also been indicated. Involvement of other systems has not been reported.

Most attention has been given to the muscles, skeletal and cardiac, from the physiologic and biochemical viewpoint. One of the postulated mechanisms is that the triggering substance (halothane) may provoke the uncoupling of oxidative phosphorylation in susceptible pigs, reducing the capacity to synthesize adenosine triphosphate (ATP). A further postulate visualized sarcoplasmic Ca^{++} concentration to stimulate phosphorylase kinase, and indirectly, myosin ATPase. Elevated levels of cellular Ca^{++} may cause the uncoupling of oxidative phosphorylation; ATP is consumed; cellular levels of adenosine diphosphate (ADP) and inorganic phosphorus are increased. This stimulates glycolysis as mitochondria sequester Ca^{++}; oxygen consumption is increased, with an increase in temperature.

The mechanisms involved, particularly the nature of the provoking events, are not incontrovertibly understood. The reader is referred to the references and to current literature as this fascinating syndrome is studied further.

Allen, W. M., et al.: Experimentally induced acute stress syndrome in Pietrain pigs. Vet. Rec., 87:64–68, 1970.

Britt, B. A.: Etiology and pathophysiology of malignant hyperthermia. Fed. Proc., 38:44–48, 1979.

Campion, D. R., and Topel, D. G.: A review of the role of swine skeletal muscle in malignant hyperthermia. J. Anim. Sci., 41:779–786, 1975.

Eikelenboom, G., and Sybesma, W.: A possible mechanism for induction of porcine malignant hyperthermia syndrome. J. Anim. Sci., 38:504–596, 1974.

Hall, L. W., Trim, C. M., and Woolf, N.: Further studies of porcine malignant hyperthermia. Br. Med. J., 2:145–148, 1972.

Harrison, G. G., and Verburg, C.: Erythrocyte osmotic fragility in hyperthermia-susceptible swine. Br. J. Anaesth., 45:131–133, 1973.

Jones, E. W., et al.: Malignant hyperthermia of swine. Anesthesiology, 36:42–51, 1972.

STRESS

An animal learns that a certain thing or situation is harmless or dangerous, agreeable or disagreeable, and is content to approach it or avoid it without making any great effort to understand it. Fortunately for human progress, man is more curious and wishes to understand the various phenomena that he encounters. If this proves currently impossible, man has at least one last recourse: he gives the object or the phenomenon a name, and then he feels considerably more tranquil. Whole populations, indeed, are often content to talk glibly about a certain subject which they do not understand but for which they do have a name. Such names come and go and are widely used, often with a poor conception of what it is to which the name applies. Such a name is "stress." We are tempted to infer that "stress" is the cause of many poorly defined illnesses an animal (or person) may have.

Nearly a generation ago, Cannon (1929) pointed out that the observable signs and symptoms of fright, rage, or pain are entirely comparable to those that result from a suitable dose of epinephrine and are just what would be expected if a considerable amount of that substance were suddenly released into the circulation from the adrenal gland. If a cat is held at bay by a dog, the hair of the cat stands erect, its pupils dilate and its eyes bulge, its muscles are tense, its heart beats faster. Investigation shows that the level of blood sugar rises, making it immediately available for the production of energy, more blood flows into the musculature and less into the digestive organs, whose activities are held in relative abeyance. The bronchioles dilate, increasing the animal's capacity for rapid uptake of oxygen; the spleen empties its reserve erythrocytes into the circulation; even the clotting power of the blood is enhanced, as if in preparation for a wound. If the cat then decides to run, it is capable of extreme speed and unbelievably long jumps; its claws dig with unerring accuracy into the bark of an unfamiliar tree, up whose trunk it runs as if on level ground. This is the "alarm reaction" of Cannon.

Selye (1950) carried this idea further and has postulated an increase of various adrenal and pituitary hormones as one of the protective agencies operating against the "stress" of infections, cold, muscular fatigue, nervous strain, and even of heat and ionizing radiations. Following upon the epinephric reaction of Cannon, Selye theorized that increased adrenocortico-trophic hormone, ACTH, from the pituitary stimulated the adrenal cortex to greater release of various of its steroid hormones, which are sometimes known as "corticoids." The supply of all these hormones is held to be subject to exhaustion in the case of the prolonged "stress" of the disorders mentioned. The theory then goes on to propose that a number of stubborn and poorly understood diseases of man are due to an imbalance of the cortical hormones so produced. The basis for this theory was that the administration of certain of these cortical hormones (the mineralocorticoids) to experimental animals produced lesions similar to those found in many human diseases. Furthermore, these lesions are relieved or prevented by another group of cortical hormones (the glucocorticoids), of which cortisone is now a well-known example.

While adverse environmental stimuli are associated with certain diseases and lesions, such as gastric ulcers, colitis, hypertension, pneumonia, and general wasting, the causal relationships are not clear. Citing stress as a cause of disease should be considered most judiciously.

Selye, H.: The Physiology and Pathology of Exposure to Stress. Montreal, Acta, Inc., 1950.

Weiss, J. M.: Psychological factors in stress and disease. Sci. Am., 226:104–113, 1972.

CHAPTER 7

Immunopathology

Immunity or the resistance to disease is afforded by a highly complex interaction of mechanical, chemical, humoral, and cellular events and reactions which may act singly or more usually in concert, often associated with or as an integral and often necessary component of the inflammatory reaction (Chapter 6).

IMMUNE REACTIONS AND HYPERSENSITIVITY

In recent years, much attention has been directed to diseases resulting from reactions on the part of the immune system, which are grouped under the term hypersensitivity diseases, allergic diseases, or broadly under immunopathology. However, the specific hypersensitivity diseases, which are discussed later in this chapter, are not the usual outcome of immune reactions. The immune system affords each individual higher animal protection from invasion by other organisms, thus preserving individuality and preserving the species. Deficiencies in the immune system, such as hypogammaglobulinemia and thymic aplasia, which are on the opposite side of the coin from hypersensitivity, clearly reveal the importance of this system. The system, however, is far from perfect. It appears still to be in the process of evolving, as complete immunity to infectious disease is rarely achieved. Aside from natural or innate immunity, a significant time lag is required to produce protective levels of antibodies or call forth cellular immune responses, such that these systems do not afford the individual any protection from a highly virulent organism, as is clearly seen when the bacillus of anthrax invades a cow. Also, the hypersensitivity diseases point to the lack of perfection of the system. Although most all of the experimentally induced hypersensitivity diseases have naturally occurring analogs, these are not common, and some of the diseases are iatrogenic in origin. For example, the injection of large quantities of horse serum that can lead to serum sickness is clearly going to occur only at the hands of man. However, immune complex diseases leading to glomerulonephritis and other disorders in association with certain infections, such as lymphocytic choriomeningitis, do occur, and no benefit to the host is apparent, and autoimmune diseases (autoallergic), in which the immune system responds to the tissues of the host, are documented in several animal species, again with absolutely no recognizable advantage to the host.

NATURAL IMMUNITY

The most poorly understood but most perfect form of immunity is species variation in susceptibility to infectious diseases. Horses, swine, and cats are resistant to infection with the virus of canine distemper, which causes a serious disease in dogs. Feline panleukopenia virus affects felines, but not dogs, ruminants, or a number of other species. In addition to these absolute differences, relative degrees of resistance are seen with other infectious agents. *Bacillus anthracis* causes an acute fulminating fatal disease in cattle, whereas the disease is mild in dogs and horses, and chickens are entirely resistant. Within a species, certain breeds are more resistant than others, as exemplified by piroplasmosis in Zebu cattle *(Bos indicus)* vs domestic cattle *(Bos taurus)*. An excellent example is presented by the Epstein-Barr virus in human beings. It is believed to cause malignant lymphoma in some African children, has been shown to cause infectious mononucleosis in the United States, and yet most people become infected without evidence of disease. Similarly, many cats are exposed to feline leukemia virus, but only a few develop malignant lymphoma. The strain differences in disease incidence seen in laboratory mice is another dramatic example. Certain aspects of acquired immunity may be important in some of these differences, but most are genetically endowed. Age, sex, hormonal status, nutritional status, and environment also influence innate immunity. Only female mice which have had one or more pregnancies develop carcinoma of the mammary gland due to Bittner's virus, despite the fact that virgins and males are also infected. Rats deficient in iron are significantly more susceptible to salmonellosis than nondeficient rats. Young monkeys are susceptible to Rous sarcoma virus, but adults are resistant.

Aside from these imperfectly understood examples of resistance, other innate immune factors are recognized. A mechanical barrier is provided by the skin and mucous membranes, which prevents organisms from gaining entrance. Mucus entraps organisms and the action of cilia helps to sweep them away. Saliva, gastric acid and intestinal enzymes also afford protection. Tears and nasal and gastrointestinal secretions also contain the enzyme lysozyme, which is believed to be bactericidal, although its exact biologic function is not known.

Neutrophils and macrophages are capable of ingesting (phagocytosis) and digesting a variety of microorganisms in nonimmune (acquired immunity) hosts, although the process of phagocytosis is aided by acquired antibodies. The microbicidal mechanism is primarily the result of the generation of hydrogen peroxide and superoxide through myeloperoxidase in neutrophils and catalase in macrophages. Other molecules, such as cationic proteins and lactoferrin, which are also bactericidal, have been identified in neutrophils. Lysosomal hydrolytic enzymes do not kill bacteria, but act to digest and eliminate dead organisms. (However, many bacteria are not killed after phagocytosis; rather, bacterial products kill the phagocyte.)

Natural antibodies, which are identical to acquired antibodies, have been described as a component of natural immunity. Their existence, however, has been questioned. Many believe that they represent acquired antibodies resulting from specific but unrecorded stimuli. This seems a plausible explanation in view of the specific antibodies that man and animals have against infectious agents whose diseases go unrecognized (e.g., toxoplasmosis, histoplasmosis, canine hepatitis).

The cellular production of a protein, termed **interferon**, provides a defense mechanism against viruses and possibly other microbes. Interferon falls between innate immunity and acquired immunity, resembling the former in that it is nonspecific and without memory, but similar to acquired immunity in that its production depends upon infection with an invading organism(s). Although its production is also stimulated by certain bacterial, protozoan, and mycotic organisms, its activity appears to be most important in limiting viral diseases. Interferon is probably more important in limiting viral infections in nonimmune animals than are humoral antibodies.

It has long been recognized that an animal or tissue infected with a virus was resistant to infection with a second virus, a phenomenon labeled **viral interference**. It is now known that most viruses, upon infecting a cell, stimulate the production and release of a protein that prevents or interferes with the action of the same or another virus on new cells. Interferon is not virus-specific, but it is species- or host-specific. Its mode of action is not clear, but apparently it either hinders the formation of complete or infective virus or completely arrests viral replication. It has no effect on viral attachment or the entrance of virus into a cell or its release from a cell. It most likely interferes with synthesis of viral nucleic acid or viral proteins. Interferon is not in itself antiviral, but apparently it induces the cell to produce other proteins that inhibit viral replication by interfering with the synthesis of viral-coded, functional enzymes and structural coat proteins necessary for viral replication, such as viral RNA replicase, viral DNA polymerase, and thymidine kinase. Attempts have been made to use exogenous interferon or stimulate endogenous formation to treat viral diseases, but to date without significant success.

ACQUIRED IMMUNITY

Three features contrast innate or natural defenses with acquired immunity: (1) **acquired immunity requires prior stimulation to become active**, (2) **acquired immunity is highly specific**, and (3) **acquired immunity has memory**. Two principal mechanisms are included in acquired immunity: the production of humoral antibodies and cellular immunity (or delayed hypersensitivity).

Humoral Immunity

The adjective "humoral" is a vestige of the Hippocratic teachings. In the concept of the renowned Greek physician, the body contained four humors or fluids (blood, phlegm, black bile, and yellow bile), and diseases represented disorders of those humors (fluids). In modern medicine, humoral antibodies are the substances found in the body fluids (humors), chiefly the blood, which work against disease. Antibodies are formed in the body as the result of exposure to foreign substances, including inanimate chemicals as well as nonpathogenic and pathogenic microorganisms and their toxic products. Collectively, substances that stimulate the production of antibodies are known as antigens.

Antigens. Antigens, with few exceptions, are substances that are foreign to the host. The best antigens (the ones that induce the greatest antibody response) are high-molecular-weight proteins. Less complex polypeptides, polysaccharides, and nucleic acids may also be antigenic, but most simple chemicals cannot serve as antigens. However, if simple chemicals are conjugated to a protein, they can create a new recognizable antigenic site on that protein and induce antibodies to that reactive site which will also couple with the smaller molecule in the absence of its carrier protein. Such substances are called **haptens**.

Antibodies to antigens that are chemically similar may cross-react, a feature which may allow partial protection or immunity from similar microorganisms, and a feature which can obscure accurate diagnosis with serologic procedures. Most natural antigens have several antigenic determinants, each capable of stimulating an antibody against itself. Thus, for a given antigen there is a group of antibodies (not a single antibody), each with an affinity for the specific determinant of the antigen.

The antibody response to antigens can be greatly increased if presented in a substance that releases the antigens to the body slowly. Such substances are known as **adjuvants** and include oils, waxes, killed tubercle bacilli, alum, and aluminum hydroxide.

Antibodies. Antibodies are glycoproteins which, as indicated, react specifically with the antigenic determinant that induced their formation. They are part of the globulins of serum, and hence, they are collectively termed **immunoglobulins**. Five classes of immunoglobulins are recognized: IgG (7S), IgA, IgM (19S), IgD, and IgE. IgG accounts for the bulk of the immunoglobulins in serum. It is the principal antibody that combats microorganisms and also mediates many of the immediate type hypersensitivity reactions. IgM, the largest immunoglobulin, is the first antibody formed following antigen exposure. It functions as IgG. IgA is the major immunoglobulin in external secretions. It is produced locally by plasma cells in tissues, such as the mucosa of the gastrointestinal and respiratory tracts, and serves as a first line of defense. It also is believed to be important in local immediate hypersensitivity reactions, although IgE is the major antibody in such hypersensitivities. IgE, which is abundant in respiratory and intestinal mucosae, reacts with mast cells and basophils, which, with specific antigen, results in release of chemical mediators (histamine, serotonin). This action results in an inflammatory response permitting intravascular antibodies and leukocytes to gather at the site to combat the offending organism. However, if the antigenic stimulus is pollen or some other apparently harmless substance, the reaction serves no useful function and is considered an allergic response or disease. IgE is also important in providing protection against intestinal helminths. The function of IgD other than as an antigen receptor is not known. It is only present in trace amounts.

Antibodies may also be classed on the basis of function or in vitro properties. These include: (1) **antitoxins**, which chemically and quantitatively neutralize specific bacterial exotoxins (tetanus, diphtheria, botulism); (2) **agglutinins**, which agglutinate bacterial cells, sticking them together in such large masses that they spread to other areas of the body only with difficulty; (3) **precipitins**, which precipitate dissolved proteins, thus inhibiting their dissemination and chemical activity; (4) **lysins**, which lyse cells and gram-negative bacteria through activation of the complement

Table 7–1. Characteristics of Immunoglobulins

Immunoglobulin	Molecular Weight	Approx. Total % Immunoglobulin in Serum	Normal Functions
IgG	160,000	75%	Principal antiviral, antibacterial, and antitoxin
IgA	170,000	16%	Immunoglobulin of external secretions
IgM	900,000	7%	Initial antibody; functions as IgG
IgD	180,000	0.2%	Unknown
IgE	200,000	0.01%	Mediates vascular events of inflammation

sequence; and (5) **opsonins**, which facilitate and stimulate phagocytosis of bacterial cells (cocci and certain bacilli) by the microphages (neutrophils) or macrophages.

The mechanisms operant in such hypersensitivities as anaphylaxis, the Arthus phenomenon, or immune complex diseases are presented in the discussions of these entities. Many of these reactions fix (employ) complement, which is required for their ultimate success in combating invaders or eliciting hypersensitivity diseases. Such antibodies are referred to as **complement-fixing antibodies**. The reaction of an antibody with a microbial antigen does not necessarily imply destruction of the microbe. Antibodies that do destroy the agent are called **neutralizing antibodies**.

Following exposure to an antigen, there is a latent period of about four to six days before serum antibodies are detectable. The response peaks around 14 days after exposure and slowly declines after about 21 days. The principal component of this primary response is IgM. Upon second exposure, the latent period is shorter, the level of antibody is higher, it is maintained longer, and is predominantly IgG. This response is a function of the memory of the immune reaction, and is referred to as the **anamnestic response**. It is believed to result from an expanded population of lymphocytes specific to the antigen.

That antibodies are of cellular origin has been accepted for many years, but considerable confusion has existed about what cells are responsible for their formation, i.e., what cells are **immunologically competent**. Currently there are two recognized classes of immunologically competent cells: T lymphocytes and B lymphocytes. The exact manner in which lymphocytes effect their competence and their relationship to one another and to other cells is only partially understood. T lymphocytes are primarily responsible for cellular immunity, and B lymphocytes for the production of immunoglobulins.

Prior to recognition by a B lymphocyte, antigen is processed by the macrophages. Most of the antigen is catabolized by the macrophages, but some unaltered antigen is presented to B lymphocytes, which have specific receptor molecules on their plasma membrane. These receptors are immunoglobulin molecules, thought to be identical to those subsequently secreted by the interacting cell. Lymphocytes react by becoming a larger cell called a lymphoblast (immunoblast), which undergoes proliferation and differentiation into antibody-forming plasma cells, and presumably long-lived lymphocytes, which serve as memory cells. Although B lymphocytes can produce antibody in the absence of T cells, in most instances there is participation by T cells. These cells are called **helper T cells**, and although incapable of secreting antibody themselves, they are required to interact with B lymphocytes before the latter secrete antibodies. A counterpart of helper T cells also exists, a population of cells called **suppressor T cells**, which suppress both humoral and cellular immune responsiveness.

In the spleen and lymph nodes, B lymphocytes, which are of bone marrow origin (bursa of Fabricius in birds), are predominantly located in lymphocytic follicles around germinal centers. They account for about 15% of circulating lymphocytes. In contrast, in lymph nodes and spleen, T lymphocytes are located in interfollicular areas. They account for about 85% of circulating lymphocytes. B lymphocytes have specific receptors on their surfaces that are bound immunoglobulin molecules, thus providing a simple means of differentiating them from T cells. When antigen is presented to B cells, it is bound to the immunoglobulin receptors, which coalesce to form a single polar cap that is ingested by the cell. There follows a period of six to eight hours when the cell does not have surface receptors.

Morphologically, stimulation of the humoral immune system is characterized by development and enlargement of germinal centers in lymph nodes and spleen and the appearance of large numbers of plasma cells. Plasma cells also appear locally in mucosae, probably indicative of local IgA and possibly other immunoglobulin synthesis.

The mechanism by which a foreign protein induces the production of specific antibody has been the subject of extensive debate. Two theories have been set forth, and although to date both are hypothetic, they deserve brief consideration prior to our later discussion of hypersensitivity and autoimmunity. The **instructive theory** postulates that antigen, upon entering the body, comes into contact with immunologically competent cells and acts as a template to instruct the cell to produce a specific gamma globulin. This theory implies that any immunologically competent cell can be instructed to produce any specific antibody. This theory has been essentially discarded because (1) the template (antigen) would have to persist for the duration of the immunity, (2) it does not account for the anamnestic response, and (3) it does not allow an adequate explanation of the body's ability to recognize "self," or how an individual can be tricked into recognizing "nonself" as self.

Except under unusual circumstances, antibodies are not produced against one's own tissues. Yet, for a period of time, while the immune system is "immature," foreign proteins can be introduced which in later life will be recognized as self and not as foreign. This is well illustrated in freemartin cattle who share placental circulation, resulting in a transfer of cellular (and humoral) components. As adults, these dizygotic twins are chimerics which share blood groups and are immunologically tolerant of each other's tissues. Other experimentally induced forms of immunologic tolerance also support this phenomenon.

To explain recognition of self and nonself as well as to meet other objections to the instructive theory, Burnet advanced the **selective theory**, or clonal theory of antibody production. This theory proposes that clones of cells exist that have the inherent capacity to produce antibody upon stimulation by the proper antigen, and that this clone is stimulated to reproduce more cells with the same capacity. The theory indicates that, for every possible antigen (including self), a cell or clone of cells exists that has the genetically endowed ability to produce a specific antibody to that specific antigen, and that the antigen must find (select) the proper cell or cells with which to interact. To explain self-recognition and immunologic tolerance before birth, it is then theorized that body antigens of self interact with the proper cells, or clones, before birth, and before these cells have the ability to proliferate upon antigenic stimulus, and that this interaction results in the destruction of these clones.

Complement. The existence of the complement system has been recognized for several decades, but it is only within the past ten years that the complex nature of the system in normal immune mechanisms has been refined, and its roles in inflammation, phagocytosis, and many of the hypersensitivity diseases more clearly elucidated. The complement system amplifies both the protective functions of antibodies and hypersensitivity reactions. We will not attempt to describe the complexity of the system, but will rather point out a few important steps. For a detailed discussion, the student is referred to textbooks of immunology or the excellent review by Ruddy, Gigli, and Austen (1972).

There are nine components in the complement system. The interaction of all nine is required to lead to cell lysis or to a classic in vitro complement fixation reaction with red blood cells. The classic complement fixation reaction sequence is initiated with the interaction of antigen and antibody with complement, as depicted in Figure 7–1. Several active products are released during the sequence. AAC14 results in

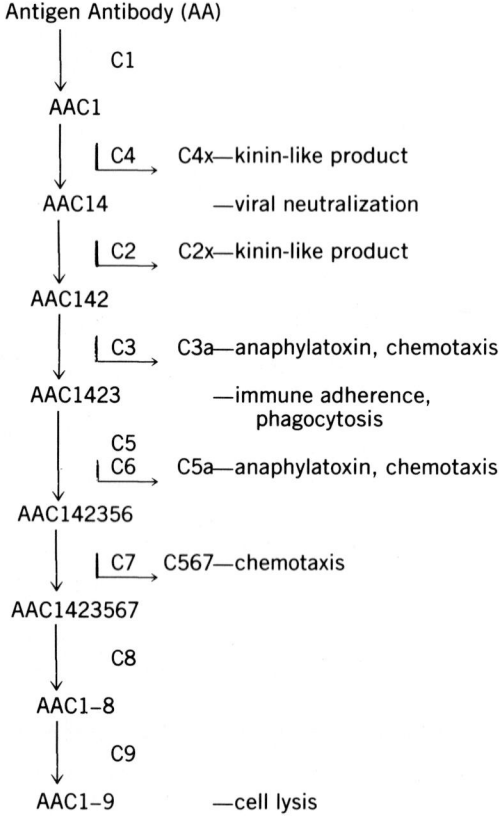

Antigen Antibody (AA)

↓ C1

AAC1

↓ | C4 → C4x—kinin-like product

AAC14   —viral neutralization

↓ | C2 → C2x—kinin-like product

AAC142

↓ | C3 → C3a—anaphylatoxin, chemotaxis

AAC1423   —immune adherence,
                           phagocytosis
       C5
     | C6 → C5a—anaphylatoxin, chemotaxis

AAC142356

↓ | C7 → C567—chemotaxis

AAC1423567

↓ C8

AAC1–8

↓ C9

AAC1–9   —cell lysis

Fig. 7–1. Complement system and active by-products.

viral neutralization. The interaction of C2 with AAC14 releases C3a, which has several biologic properties, including chemotaxis and that of an anaphylatoxin. The subsequent release of C5a aids in both of these reactions. AAC1423 causes immune adherence (opsonization) and enhances phagocytosis. Chemotaxis is also enhanced by the release of C567 after C7 is engaged in the sequence. AAC1423567 renders cells susceptible to lymphocytotoxicity. As indicated, cell lysis results at the final step, with the formation of C142356789. It is important to note that certain cells will be lysed (e.g., erythrocytes and gram-negative bacteria), but gram-positive bacteria are not susceptible to the lytic action of complement.

The complement sequence can also be activated in the absence of an antigen-antibody complex. This sequence is referred to as the **alternate pathway** for complement activation. In the alternate pathway, C3 is activated without triggering C1, C4, or C2. Initiators of this sequence include endotoxin and zymosan, which act with several serum proteins called properdins.

Cellular Immunity

The cellular immune response does not involve circulating antibodies and cannot be passively transferred with serum. It is, however, a form of acquired immunity, and like humoral immunity, it requires a stimulus, is highly specific, and has a memory. Cellular immunity accounts for the resistance and reaction associated with tuberculosis and the efficacy of the tuberculin reaction. Probably most organisms causing granulomatous diseases (Chapter 12) elicit a cellular immune response, including some of the simple bacteria (e.g., *Listeria sp.*, *Brucella sp.*), higher bacteria (e.g., *Mycobacterium sp.*), protozoa, and metazoan parasites. The cellular immune responses are also the major mechanisms of graft rejection, as well as the destruction (or attempted destruction) of endogenous neoplasms. The lesions of some viral diseases also result from cellular immune responses. The best example is lymphocytic choriomeningitis virus, which leads to the appearance of new (and foreign) membrane antigens on affected cells. In this disease the lymphocytic reaction can be prevented by suppressing the cellular immune response. In many other viral infections, the cytotoxic T-cell response to new membrane antigens is of key importance in combating the infection. The delayed hypersensitivity diseases are mediated through cellular immune mechanisms.

The details of the cellular immune response are less well understood than those operative in humoral immunity; however, it is clear that the thymus-derived lymphocytes (T lymphocytes) are the immunologically competent cells in this system. The latent period requires several days to two weeks to reach its peak. Upon second exposure, rather than an immediate response, the reaction begins slowly, peaking at 24 to 72 hours. The fact that cells must be brought to the antigen (rather than circulating antibodies) explains this delayed reaction. Antigen is first processed and presented to T cells by macrophages, analogous to the humoral immune system. Sensitized T cells in turn call forth additional macrophages, which accumulate at the reaction site. Macrophages are the principal cellular component of the inflammatory response of cellular immunity.

Microscopically, the delayed reaction is characterized by proliferation of large lymphocytes in the paracortical regions of lymph nodes. Some of these sensitized T cells enter the circulation and make contact with the stimulating antigen on first or second exposure. It is believed that contact occurs by chance, rather than by a specific chemotaxis. Upon recognition of the specific antigen(s), the T lymphocytes release substances called lymphokines, which attract monocytes (macrophages) from the blood stream. The sensitized lymphocytes may participate directly in destroying the antigen, especially in lysis of cells, but the macrophages called forth also elaborate cytotoxic materials as well as possess increased phagocytic ability. The macrophages, however, require activation by lymphokines. This is a specific reaction, but once activated, the macrophages are nonspecifically cytotoxic. If sensitized or activated T cells cause lysis of cells directly, they are called **killer cells, cytotoxic T cells,** or **cytolytic T cells.** These play a role in lysis of cells with new membrane antigens as occur in viral diseases, and on tumor cells. The destruction of the cell is believed to require intimate contact between the two, though a cytotoxic factor termed lymphotoxin may be released. Lymphokines also

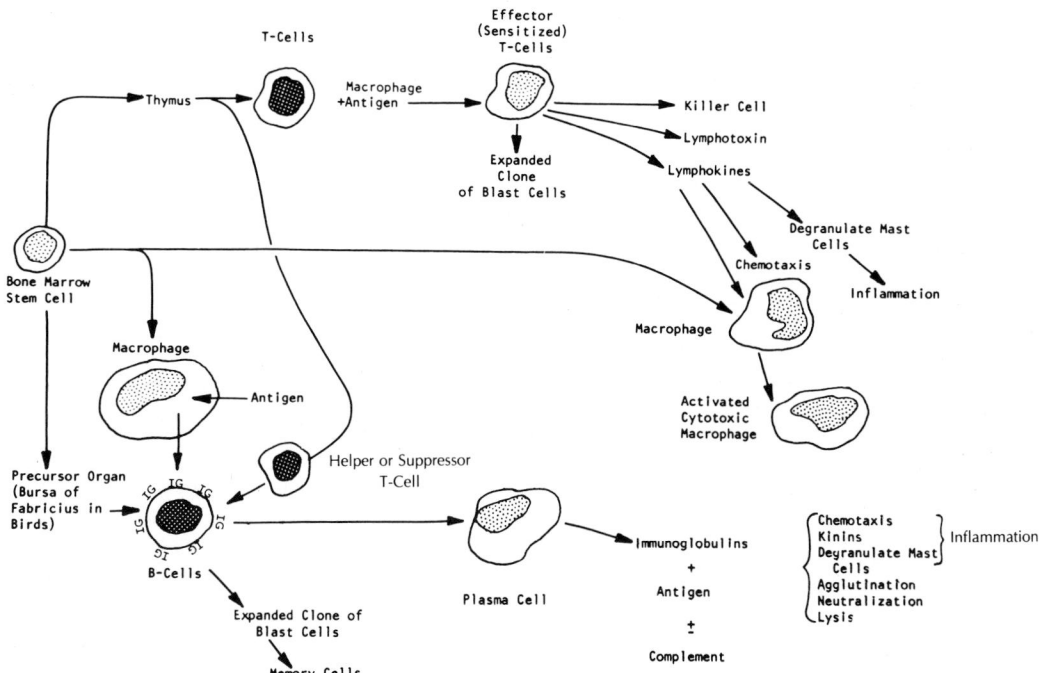

Fig. 7–2. Schematic representation of humoral and cellular immune systems and their interaction.

cause degranulation of mast cells and basophils, initiating the classic inflammatory results.

In certain of these reactions, most notably tuberculosis, macrophages differentiate into epithelioid cells, large polygonal cells with eosinophilic cytoplasm that, as the name implies, resemble epithelial cells. These cells apparently are not phagocytic. Their function is not known, but based on their numbers, must be important in some diseases. Fusion of macrophages results in the formation of multinucleated giant cells, which are conspicuous in many granulomatous diseases, but are not a feature of the cellular immune responses to tissue grafts and delayed hypersensitivity diseases. If elicited by the injection of tuberculin, this mononuclear cellular response is primarily perivenular and perivenous in distribution, but in granulomatous diseases this is not the case.

Neutrophils may be present in small numbers, but are not an essential component of delayed immunity. Complement also is not involved.

It is appropriate at this stage of our discussion to point out that humoral and cellular immunity work in concert. Although some reactions are purely humoral (lysis of foreign erythrocytes) and others apparently purely cellular (tuberculin reaction), both are often operative simultaneously.

In summary, cellular immunity mediated through T lymphocytes (1) regulates B cells as helper T cells or suppressor T cells, (2) provides resistance to certain bacteria, viruses, and other organisms, (3) is involved in transplantation and tumor immunity, and (4) is responsible for delayed hypersensitivity reactions.

We have seen that lysis of cells can be mediated through either antibody and complement, or cytotoxic T cells. There exists another class of lymphocytes which lack T or B cell markers and have thus been termed **null cells.** These cells loosely bind IgG and have therefore also been termed

IgG labile cells. They will bind to cells coated with IgG resulting in their lysis, a reaction described as **antibody-dependent cell cytotoxicity.**

The humoral and cellular immune systems and their interaction are depicted schematically in Figure 7–2.

IMMUNODEFICIENCIES

Genetic and congenitally acquired defects in the ability to form antibody or develop cell-mediated immunity have been recognized in human beings. Only a few have been identified in animals. Most often these deficiencies are associated with and indeed recognized by increased susceptibility to infection. Those with B cell or humoral defects are associated with infections by pyogenic organisms; those with T cell defects, with increased susceptibility to opportunistic organisms or organisms usually held in check as latent infections. The defect in several of these deficiencies, however, affects both systems. In several,

Table 7–2. Primary Immunodeficiency Disease

Probable Cell Defect	Disease
B	Agammaglobulinemia
B	Hypogammaglobulinemia
B	Selective immunoglobulin deficiency (dysgammaglobulinemia)
B	Transient hypogammaglobulinemia of infancy
T	Thymic aplasia (hypoplasia) (Di George syndrome, nude mouse)
T,B	Severe combined immunodeficiency
T,B	Partial immunodeficiency (Wiskott-Aldrich syndrome; Immunodeficiency with thrombocytopenia and eczema)
T,B	Immunodeficiency with ataxia telangiectasia
T,B	Immunodeficiency with dwarfism
T,B	Variable immunodeficiency Unclassified immunodeficiency; "acquired" hypogammaglobulinemia

there is an increased incidence of neoplastic diseases, suggesting the importance of immune surveillance in controlling transformed cells.

B Cell Deficiency. Agammaglobulinemia and Hypogammaglobulinemia. These diseases may result from **defective synthesis, increased catabolism,** or **excessive loss** of immunoglobulins. In human beings, defective synthesis occurs in several disorders, many of which are transmitted as genetic characteristics. In some, such as **X-linked agammaglobulinemia**, B cells are lacking in tissues and circulation, and the disorder manifests itself in early life. There is no detectable IgM, IgA, IgD, or IgE in serum, and IgG levels are less than 10% of normal. The transplacental transfer of maternal IgG affords protection of affected boys for the first few months of life. In contrast, a condition called **common, variable, unclassified immunodeficiency** ("acquired" hypogammaglobulinemia) may occur at any age, and be associated with either no B cells or normal or increased numbers of B cells. The B cells, however, fail to differentiate into immunoglobulin-secreting cells. Both sexes are affected. Other conditions exist in which one to several selective immunoglobulins are deficient (**dysgammaglobulinemia**), for example, IgA deficiency or IgG deficiency. Transient **hypogammaglobulinemia** of infancy is a rare condition in which there is an apparent delay in B cell maturation, and passively acquired IgG levels fall prior to synthesis by the infant.

Hypercatabolism of immunoglobulins leading to deficiency has been described in several forms in human beings but not in other animals. These include familial idiopathic hypercatabolic hypoproteinemia, Wiskott-Aldrich syndrome, and myotonic dystrophy.

Excessive loss of immunoglobulins (and other serum proteins) can occur in renal disease and gastrointestinal disease. Both glomerular and tubular damage can lead to losses, but intact immunoglobulin loss is greatest with glomerular disease. Gastrointestinal loss in man is associated with diseases that affect lymphatic drainage, such as lymphangiectasia, lymphatic fistulas, and Whipple's disease.

T Cell Deficiencies. Deficiencies of T cells generally result in more serious susceptibility to infection than B cell defects, owing to the needed cooperation of T cells for B cell function. In **severe combined immunodeficiency**, there are no T or B cells. The disease is also known as Swiss-type agammaglobulinemia, alymphocytosis, and thymic alymphoplasia. In man, the disease is hereditary and invariably fatal prior to two years of age, most often from viral infections. An essentially identical immunodeficiency has been described in horses of the Arabian breed by McGuire and associates (1974). It has not been seen in other breeds. As in man, there are no T or B cells; the foals cannot synthesize immunoglobulins and lack cell-mediated immunity. The disease is characterized by lack of immunoglobulins, lymphopenia, and death before four to five months of age. The most common secondary disease leading to death is pneumonia caused by viral, bacterial, fungal, or protozoal organisms. The important pathologic features focus on lymphoid organs. The thymus is aplastic or extremely hypoplastic, with only the epithelial components present. Lymph nodes contain few lymphocytes and totally lack follicles or germinal centers; there are no plasma cells. The spleen has a similar appearance. The disease is believed to be inherited as an autosomal recessive trait. An associated deficiency of adenosine deaminase has been found in human beings with severe combined immunodeficiency. Polmar et al. (1976) have provided evidence that indicates enzyme replacement therapy restores immunocompetence.

Congenital thymic aplasia or *Di George syndrome* results from a failure of normal embryogenesis of the thymus and parathyroid glands which are derived from the third and fourth pharyngeal clefts. In human beings, the disease is often associated with anomalies of the heart and major blood vessels and mental retardation. The thymus may be entirely aplastic or hypoplastic. In many children, T cell function improves with age, but if the cell-mediated immune response is severely impaired, death results from recurrent infections.

The **nude athymic mouse** has a counterpart of this disease in which there is complete aplasia of the thymus. The hairlessness is inherited as a recessive autosomal trait, which has nothing to do with thymic aplasia except that the latter is linked to this genetic trait. There are no T cells, but B cells with surface immunoglobulin receptors are present. Unless precautions are taken, the mice die within a few months of birth. Neonatally thymectomized mice are not as severely impaired, apparently due to migration of some T cells from the thymus prior to birth. A severe thymic hypoplasia has also been described in calves of the Black Danish breed by Brummerstedt et al. (1974). In these cattle the condition results from a genetic inability to absorb zinc.

Two strains of **dwarf mice** have a T cell defect: the **Snell-Bagg mouse** and the **Ames mouse**. After weaning, there is a progressive thymus atrophy and loss of T cell function, which can be prevented with growth hormone, prolonged nursing, or injections of mouse milk.

Other T Cell Deficiency States. Other deficiencies occur in human beings that have not been described in animals. In **immunodeficiency with ataxia telangiectasia** there is also a B cell deficiency. The patients have impaired T cell function and low levels or absent IgA and IgE. The syndrome **immunodeficiency with thrombocytoplasia and eczema (Wiskott-Aldrich syndrome)** is an X-linked recessive disorder with impaired T and B cell function.

Complement Deficiencies. Deficiencies in complement have been recognized in man, guinea pigs, mice, and rabbits. C3 and C5 deficiency in man has been associated with recurrent infections, but not in all patients. Deficiency of C4 in guinea pigs, C5 in mice, and C6 in rabbits has not been associated with increased incidence of infections. Apparently normal levels of C3 are sufficiently protective.

Viral Immunosuppression. This may follow infection with any of several viruses, particularly those that localize in lymphocytes and reticuloendothelial cells, such as the leukemia viruses. Immunosuppression may also accompany such diseases as canine distemper, hog cholera, and bovine virus diarrhea.

Immunosuppression may also result from certain nutrient deficiencies and exposure to toxic inorganic and organic chemicals. (See zinc, Chapter 17.)

HYPERSENSITIVITY REACTIONS AND DISEASES (Allergy-Atopy)

Hypersensitivity represents an accelerated or accentuated immune response to a degree that is often detrimental rather than beneficial. This is especially true when violent reactions, which may lead to death, develop in response to exposure to ordinarily innocuous substances. Allergic (allergy) or atopic (atopy) are synonyms.

Hypersensitivity reactions are classically divided into **immediate type** and **delayed type**. The immediate reactions include anaphylaxis (systemic anaphylaxis), acute allergic reactions (local anaphylaxis), cytotoxic hypersensitivity (cytotoxic anaphylaxis) and immune complex disease, which includes the Arthus reaction and serum sickness. Delayed reactions are classically illustrated by tuberculin sensitivity, transplant rejection, and contact dermatitis. Autoimmunity, a special form of hypersensitivity, is discussed separately.

Immediate Hypersensitivities

Anaphylaxis. Anaphylaxis can be experimentally demonstrated when an animal is given an intravenous injection of a protein such as albumin, blood serum of

Table 7–3. Hypersensitivity Diseases

	Classification	Principal Immunoglobulin	Manifestations	Mechanism of Damage
	Immediate Type			
I	a. Generalized anaphylaxis	IgE	Anaphylaxis	Mediators from reagin-sensitized cells
	b. Acute allergic reactions (localized anaphylaxis)	IgE	Urticaria, hives, asthma, GI allergy	Mediators from reagin-sensitized cells
II	Cytotoxic hypersensitivity (cytotoxic anaphylaxis)	IgG, IgM and Complement	Transfusion reactions, hemolytic anemia, thrombocytopenia	Complement
III	Arthus reaction or immune complex disease	IgG, IgM and Complement	Serum sickness, glomerulonephritis, vasculitis	Complement and polymorphonuclear leukocytes
	Delayed Type			
IV	Delayed hypersensitivity	NONE Sensitized T lymphocytes	Contact dermatitis: (drugs, poison ivy), tuberculosis, tuberculin reaction, graft rejection	Lymphokines from antigen-sensitized lymphocytes

another species of animal or, as first demonstrated by Portier and Richet in 1902, an extract of sea anemone. After a latent period of about ten days to two weeks, a second injection of the same substance is given in the same way. The dose and the material are such as would be harmless to a normal animal, but in this sensitized animal a violent and usually fatal reaction follows within a matter of minutes, a reaction known as anaphylaxis **(systemic anaphylaxis).**

Signs of Anaphylaxis. The signs of anaphylaxis vary between species, owing to variances in the target organ and relative sensitivities to the chemical mediators of the reaction. The fundamental reaction is constriction of smooth muscle. In the guinea pig, contraction of the smooth muscle of bronchioles is the outstanding effect, with dyspnea and partial or fatal suffocation. In the dog, contraction of venous passages, especially the hepatic veins, is the salient manifestation, with severe congestion of the liver and other splanchnic organs leading to hypotension or shock.

Horses, cats, and mice repond in a manner similar to guinea pigs. In cattle, cutaneous edema and dyspnea have been reported. In rats, the findings are those of increased vascular permeability and hemorrhage in the small intestine. In rabbits, constriction of pulmonary arteries and dilatation of the right heart occur. In contrast to other species, in rabbits, antigen-antibody complexes precipitate in pulmonary capillaries, accompanied by platelet and leukocyte clumps, which are primarily responsible for the pulmonary hypertension and death.

Pathologic findings are not dramatic in any species. Pulmonary edema, congestion and emphysema are characteristic of bronchiolar constriction. Splanchnic congestion and hemorrhage are seen in the rat and dog. The absence or reduction in number of mast cells (indicative of degranulation or disruption) is a usual feature, but often difficult to assess.

Anaphylaxis (and other immediate- but not delayed-type hypersensitivities) depends on circulating serum antibodies, which can be transferred to another individual. The combination of antibody with specific antigen results in the release of mediators of the reaction. Two types of interaction may lead to the release of mediators: (1) **cytotropic anaphylaxis,** and (2) **aggregate anaphylaxis.** A third reaction, which may lead to an anaphylactic type response, is considered separately under the heading Cytotoxic Hypersensitivity.

Cytotropic anaphylaxis is the usual mechanism of anaphylaxis. In cytotropic anaphylaxis, the antibodies (cytotropic antibodies) become fixed to receptors on target cells (e.g., mast cells and basophils). IgE antibodies are the most important class responsible for this form of hypersensitivity. The combination of antigen with the fixed antibody results in the release of mediators from the target cells. Complement is not necessary for this reaction. If passively transferred by the injection of cytotropic antibodies, a day or two is required before the antibodies become fixed and anaphylaxis can be induced.

In aggregate anaphylaxis, antigen and antibody combine in the serum, and this immune complex reacts with complement to release the polypeptides cleaved from C3 and C5 (C3a and C5a), once called anaphylatoxin. C3a and C5a cause the release of mediators from target cells, chiefly histamine from mast cells. Because fixation of antibodies is not required, anaphylaxis can be induced immediately after passive transfer of antibodies. Aggregate anaphylaxis is not the usual mechanism and requires large amounts of circulating antibody.

The mediators released from target cells, ultimately to cause constriction of smooth muscle, have been the subject of considerable investigation. The more important mediators include histamine, serotonin, bradykinin, slow reactive substance of anaphylaxis (SRS-A), and prostaglandins. Histamine, serotonin, and bradykinin are discussed in Chapter 6. SRS-A is a sub-

stance of unknown composition which was first isolated from guinea pigs with induced anaphylaxis. It acts on smooth muscle and causes bronchoconstriction. Prostaglandins have been identified in anaphylaxis and are known to cause contraction of smooth muscle. A substance termed eosinophil chemotactic factor of anaphylaxis (ECF-A) has been identified in anaphylaxis and in mast cells. The release of this substance is believed to attract eosinophils to sites of hypersensitivity reactions.

Acute Allergic Reactions. An acute allergic reaction called **local anaphylaxis** is a localized immediate hypersensitivity reaction. The reaction is often localized to the skin and, hence, it is often known also as **cutaneous anaphylaxis**. The reaction, however, need not be confined to the skin, as the nasal mucosa or lung is often the target organ. For many decades (if not centuries), it has been recognized that certain human beings, and occasionally animals, suffer from hypersensitivity to organic substances of great variety. If the offending substance is a particular food, the hypersensitivity is shown by digestive disturbances or cutaneous rashes (hives). If the object of the hypersensitivity is an inhaled substance, the result is either "hay fever," a seromucous inflammation of the upper air passages, asthma, a spasmodic and hypertropic narrowing of the bronchioles, or hypersensitivity pneumonitis. These allergic diseases are often called **atopy** or **atopic allergy**. These types of reaction require prior sensitization, although the offending substance and time of sensitization are often unknown and may be difficult to determine. The number and types of allergens (antigens) in these reactions are exhaustive, including pollens and other plant products, foods, molds, animal and bird dander, parasitic organisms, and parenterally injected substances, such as vaccines, antibiotics, and any other substance containing foreign proteins. The mechanism is believed to be the same as described for cytotropic anaphylaxis. The reaction depends upon the production of specific IgE antibody to the offending antigen. IgE becomes fixed to tissue mast cells, which release their contents upon subsequent attachment of antigen. Before identification, the IgE antibodies were referred to as *reagins,* a term still occasionally used.

In addition to fixed IgE antibodies, there are also circulating antibodies (predominantly IgG) specific for the antigen. These are also known as blocking antibodies, because they compete for the antigen, and if present in high enough levels, block the hypersensitivity reaction. Injection of repeated small doses of antigen (small enough to avoid systemic anaphylaxis) raises the level of blocking antibodies, a procedure used to immunize or desensitize individuals with atopic allergies, though often without great prophylactic value.

In man, localized anaphylaxis most often presents itself as hives, hay fever or asthma. In dogs the reaction is usually characterized by dermatitis regardless of route of entry of the antigen. Another example of this form of hypersensitivity is atypical interstitial pneumonia of cattle (hypersensitivity pneumonitis; pulmonary emphysema-adenomatous syndrome), a disease resembling farmer's lung of human beings.

Cytotoxic Hypersensitivity. Cytotoxic hypersensitivity or cytotoxic anaphylaxis is characterized by an antigen-antibody reaction on the surface of a cell which activates the complement system and results in cell lysis. This form of hypersensitivity is operant in transfusion reactions, erythroblastosis fetalis, autoimmune hemolytic anemia, certain forms of thrombocytopenia, and some viral anemias, such as equine infectious anemia. If the reaction does not fix complement, lysis does not occur, but the affected cells, if they are erythrocytes, agglutinate or are phagocytized by the reticuloendothelial system (erythrophagocytosis). Immune cytolysis may also be important in the lysis of cells altered by viruses and cancer cells (leukemia cells), both of which may bear foreign surface antigens.

Immune Complex Diseases. Immune complex diseases result from the interaction of antibody with soluble or fixed antigens and complement, leading to an inflammatory reaction. Immune complex disease includes the *Arthus reaction, serum sickness,* and *chronic immune complex disease.* The latter group constitutes the most important in animals. The offending antigen may be iatrogenically introduced foreign proteins, bacterial, parasitic, and viral proteins, autologous antigens, or unknown antigens.

The **Arthus reaction** is an expression of immediate hypersensitivity principally characterized by vasculitis. As with anaphylaxis, it depends upon circulating antibody. An experimentally initiated Arthus reaction consists of a focal area of inflammation and necrosis at the site of antigen injection in a previously sensitized animal. The injected antigen combines and precipitates with antibody and complement in vessel walls. The release of chemotactic complement components (C5a and C5b) attracts neutrophils, which infiltrate and surround the vessel. The participation of neutrophils is necessary for the necrosis, edema, hemorrhage, and thrombosis associated with the reaction. If neutrophil infiltration is blocked, the Arthus reaction does not develop. The exact manner in which neutrophils inflict their damage is not clear, but is related to release of lysosomal enzymes and activation of other processes of the acute inflammatory response.

Serum Sickness and Chronic Immune Complex Disease. Serum sickness is similar to the Arthus reaction in some respects, but classically it develops in individuals not previously sensitized to the responsible antigen. Instead, when a large amount of antigen such as horse serum is injected, some remains in circulation after the specific antibody response becomes evident, which is generally in 6 to 12 days. The resulting circulating antigen-antibody complex leads to the development of serum sickness. Although most of this complex is removed from circulation by the reticuloendothelial system, some is deposited in vessel walls along with complement. Released chemotactic factors from complement lead to an infiltration of neutrophils into the vessel wall, leading to a necrotizing vasculitis. Many vessels may be affected, but in particular lesions are seen in the major arteries, the endocardium and the renal glomeruli. This form of "immediate" hypersensitivity is referred to as acute serum sickness.

Chronic serum sickness is the result of the continuous (or repeated) exposure to antigen resulting in the formation of immune complexes in blood. This form is also known as **chronic immune complex disease**; it is important in the pathogenesis of many diseases of man and animals. The antigen may be an autoantigen, as in the autoimmune diseases, such as systemic lupus erythematosus (SLE) in man, autoimmune disease of New Zealand Black Mice, and SLE of dogs; viral antigens, as in lymphocytic choriomeningitis, equine infectious anemia, or Aleutian disease; or bacterial antigens, as seen in poststreptococcal glomerulonephritis of man. Although other lesions and other immune reactions may occur in some of these diseases (e.g., cytotropic hemolytic anemia in SLE dogs or delayed hypersensitivity in lymphocytic choriomeningitis), the most outstanding lesion results from the deposition of immune complexes as irregular, electron-dense granular deposits on the epithelial side of the basement membrane. These may or may not contain complement. The deposits ultimately lead to immune complex glomerulonephritis and chronic renal insufficiency. Deposition in vessel walls leads to vasculitis, as described for serum sickness and the Arthus reaction.

There are many forms of glomerular disease as well as vasculitis in which immunoglobulin, with or without complement, can be demonstrated by immunofluorescence, and which morphologically resemble known immune complex diseases. However, the antigens responsible for the formation of the complexes are usually unknown.

Delayed Hypersensitivity

Most of the features of delayed hypersensitivity were given in our discussion of **cell-mediated immunity** earlier in this chapter. The mechanisms and morphologic features are the same as those with the protective aspects of delayed immunity. In fact, it is a more difficult task to separate normal reaction from disease (although this philosophic question can be raised for any body reaction and can be argued *ad infinitum*). Delayed hypersensitivity is a component of the tuberculin reaction, tuberculosis, and probably most other granulomatous diseases, graft rejection, graft-versus-host reaction, the contact dermatitides, and some autoimmune diseases. The essential microscopic feature of most forms of delayed hypersensitivity is perivenular accumulation of mononuclear cells, which ultimately extend into adjacent tissues. As with immediate hypersensitivity reaction, the "allergens" are innumerable. Details of the histopathology of granulomatous diseases are found elsewhere (Chapter 6).

Transplant Rejection. Transplant rejection is characterized by a cellular reaction composed of small lymphocytes (T cells) and macrophages (attracted by mediators released from sensitized T cells). These cells, which surround and infiltrate the foreign tissue, are stimulated by histocompatibility antigens located on cell membranes of foreign tissues. Humoral antibodies are also elicited, but are not believed to play a major role in rejection.

Contact Dermatitis. This reaction is characterized by a slow onset (one, two, or up to ten days, depending on whether the exposure is primary or secondary) after exposure to a sensitizing antigen. The best known examples are poison ivy dermatitis in man and flea-bite dermatitis in dogs and cats. Histologically, the dermis is infiltrated with lymphocytes and macrophages. Hyperemia and edema of the dermis occur, and vesicles may form in the epidermis.

AUTOIMMUNITY

In the discussion of hypersensitivity, we saw how a normal process can become aberrant or over-reactive and become more harmful than the noxious stimuli initiating the reaction. Autoimmunity represents another aberrant reaction on the part of immunologic mechanisms that harm the host and for which no advantage can be found. As defined by Burnet (1969), autoimmunity is "a condition in which structural or functional damage is produced by the reaction of immunocytes or antibodies with normal components of the body." How can antibodies form against one's own tissues? What happens to self-recognition? Using Burnet's clonal theory of antibody formation, several conceivable mechanisms have been set forth to explain autoimmunity, however, the underlying cause in all cases is essentially unknown.

Anatomic Segregation of Antigen. If, during maturation of the immune system, a particular antigen is anatomically segregated or not formed until later in life, this antigen will not be recognized as self, as it will never have had the opportunity to inactivate immunologically competent clones capable of reacting to it. For all practical purposes, the antigen is foreign. This mechanism has been postulated for **Hashimoto's disease** of man and similar forms of **lymphocytic thyroiditis** in the dog. Spermatozoa and the lens of the eye are other examples of isolated antigens.

Alteration of Antigens. If tissues are altered so that new and foreign reactive antigenic sites are present, they will stimulate antibody formation. It is postulated that radiation-induced mutations, infections, and certain chemicals might produce antigenic alteration of tissue proteins.

Cross Reactions Between Antigens. If foreign antigens possess reactive sites in common with tissue proteins, the antibodies to the foreign antigen might react with tissue proteins. Rheumatic fever and glomerulonephritis in man may be the result of this type of cross reaction between tissue proteins and certain strains of streptococci.

Forbidden Clones. It has been postulated that autoimmunity might be caused by alteration of immunocytes with the appearance of new clones or a failure of the normal suppression mechanisms allowing clones to persist or reappear. These forbidden clones, as Burnet has called them, would then be capable of producing antibodies to tissue proteins. It is not known why new, forbidden, or abnormal clones appear, but it is believed that in certain individuals a genetic predisposition exists. Remember that the clonal selection theory of Burnet is itself hypothetic and not proven.

Whatever the mechanism, autoimmunity represents a failure to recognize self, and serious and often fatal diseases develop for which no satisfactory treatment exists.

Both humoral and cellular immunity contribute to autoimmune disease. Two humoral mechanisms may participate. In one, the antibody is directed against a specific fixed-tissue antigen restricted to a specific tissue. Examples include thyroiditis, encephalitis, and orchitis. In the second form, antibody reacts with antigen, forming immune complexes which are deposited in glomeruli or vessels, leading to disease at these sites. The process (but not the antigen) is essentially the same as described earlier for immune complex hypersensitivity diseases, and is appropriately termed **autologous immune complex disease**. There is also little tolerance to intracellular components, and their release is followed by the production of autoantibodies and/or immune T lymphocytes. This regularly follows tissue necrosis. However, the presence of such an autoimmune response does not imply disease leading to tissue injury, because antibody does not penetrate cell membranes.

Kinds of Autoimmune Diseases

In human beings, a variety of diseases are thought to be autoimmune in origin, whereas in animals the examples are fewer. The following are the more important of these.

Antiglomerular Basement Membrane Nephritis (Anti-GBM Nephritis, Goodpasture's Syndrome). This is a rare disease in which autoantibodies are made against glomerular basement membrane. In contrast to immune complex glomerulonephritis, the antibodies in this syndrome are deposited homogeneously along the basement membrane rather than as irregular deposits. The disease has been described in horses by Banks and Henson (1972). The condition can be induced experimentally by immunization with foreign GBM. Experimentally, interstitial nephritis can be induced by immunization with tubular basement membrane **(antitubular basement membrane nephritis)**. Spontaneous antitubular basement membrane nephritis is a rare disease of human beings and probably of animals.

Autoimmune Hemolytic Anemia. In this disease, antibodies are produced against an individual's own red blood cells, which accelerates their destruction by hemolysis and removal by the liver and spleen. Mice of the New Zealand Black (NZB) strain almost invariably develop autoimmune hemolytic anemia, as well as other immunologic lesions. It is also described in dogs (Miller et al., 1954; Lewis, 1974), and also in conjunction with other immunologic abnormalities. The anemia may be severe in dogs and is associated with hepatosplenomegaly and often with thrombocytopenia. Antibodies on red cells are demonstrable by the direct Coombs test.

Allergic Encephalomyelitis. This disease can be produced by the injection of central nervous system tissue from individuals of the same or other species. The responsible antigen is a protein of myelinated tissue. The lesions are those of vasculitis and destruction and demyelination of white matter, associated with infiltration of mononuclear cells. Humoral autoantibodies and sensitized T cells are demonstrable. Post-rabies vaccination encephalitis is an example of this disorder. Tissue culture vaccines, replacing rabbit-brain suspension vaccines, now preclude its development. The pathogenesis of demyelinating encephalitis associated with neurotropic viruses such as canine distemper also depend on an autoimmune response.

Lymphocytic Thyroiditis. One can experimentally induce lymphocytic thyroiditis by immunization with heterologous thyroglobulin. The disease is characterized as a chronic lymphocytic thyroiditis, with diffuse or focal infiltration of the thyroid gland with lymphocytes, and the appearance of lymphocytic follicles with germinal centers, macrophages, and plasma cells accompanying the infiltrate. Lymphocytes and plasma cells invade between thyroid epithelial cells, resulting in the destruction of the follicular epithelium and basement membrane, and ultimately in fibrosis as well as hyperplasia of the follicular epithelium. The disease occurs spontaneously in rats, dogs, an obese strain of chickens, and human beings, in whom it is known as Hashimoto's disease. In chickens, the disease results in hypothyroidism and obesity. In other species there is less severe hypothyroidism. Neonatal bursectomy, but not thymectomy, prevents or lessens the disease in chickens, indicating that the disorder is primarily the result of antithyroid antibodies. In other species, the pathogenesis has not been clarified but it is suspected that cell-mediated immunity may play an important role. Wick and Graf (1972) have described virus-like particles in degenerated thyroid epithelial cells in the obese strain of chicken, but not in normal White Leghorn chickens. The significance of these particles has not been determined.

In a closed colony of Beagle dogs, lymphocytic orchitis has been associated with lymphocytic thyroiditis. Both are presumed autoimmune in origin and in part genetically influenced.

Lupus Erythematosus (LE). This is a complex autoimmune disease of human beings and dogs. Antibodies are formed against a variety of tissue components, including DNA, RNA, and other nucleoproteins (all collectively called antinuclear antibodies), thyroglobulin, and erythrocyte membrane antigens. In man and dogs, diagnosis is established by the LE test. Upon incubation of blood or bone marrow, the breakdown of some cells releases DNA, which combines with serum anti-DNA antibodies, resulting in antigen-antibody aggregates that are engulfed by neutrophils as a large amorphous mass which pushes the nucleus to the side. These cells are called LE cells, and they are diagnostic.

The clinicopathologic picture is characterized by hemolytic anemia, thrombocytopenic purpura, leukopenia, fibrinoid degeneration of collagen, and arthritis. The antinuclear antibodies themselves cannot directly damage cells, as they cannot cross cell membranes. In the course of the normal turnover of cells, however, antinuclear antibodies form complexes with the released protein. These lead to autologous immune complex disease, which is of major importance to the pathogenesis of the disease leading to vasculitis (Arthus phenomenon) and immune complex glomerulonephritis. Renal failure is often the most serious concern in LE. The pathogenesis of the thrombocytopenia is not established. Antiplatelet antibodies have not been demonstrated. The cause of LE is not known. It has been suspected to be hereditary, but studies in dogs have not supported this hypothesis. Lewis et al. (1973) have presented evidence to suggest that a transmissible agent is associated with the canine disease. Beaucher et al. (1977) have speculated that the disease in man and dogs may be caused by a common environmental exposure, possibly an infectious agent.

New Zealand Black Mice Disease (NZB). This complex autoimmune disease of the NZB strain of mouse resembles lupus erythematosus. Autoantibodies form against red cell membranes and nuclear proteins. Mice develop hemolytic anemia and its associated clinicopathologic features, and autologous immune complex glomerulonephritis. A high incidence of malignant lymphoma and infection with C-type viruses has suggested an infectious syndrome. If a virus is incriminated as the cause in NZB mice, or in canine LE, what is currently considered an autoimmune disease may in fact be a conventional immune reaction to viral antigens.

Rheumatoid Arthritis. Human beings with rheumatoid arthritis and animals with comparable diseases have autoantibodies to gamma globulin, principally IgM and IgG. These antibodies are called rheumatoid factor, and are present in other disorders such as lupus erythematosus. The significance of rheumatoid factor to the pathogenesis of arthritis is not established, but in addition to its presence in serum, it is also demonstrated as an immune complex in synovial fluids.

Pemphigus Vulgaris. Pemphigus vulgaris is a disease characterized by bullae of the skin and mucous membranes leading to large ulcers. It results from the separation of epidermal cells from one another (acantholysis) due to degeneration of intercellular space substance and the loss of intercellular bridges. The disease occurs in man and has been described in dogs by Hurvitz and Feldman (1975). In the dog and man, autoantibodies directed against intercellular space substance are believed to play an important role in the pathogenesis of the disease. (See Chapter 18.)

Orchitis. Orchitis can be induced by immunization with spermatozoa or their antigens. The lesion is characterized by focal or diffuse infiltration of the testes, vas deferens, and epididymis with lymphocytes and lesser numbers of other mononuclear cells. Naturally occurring lymphocytic orchitis has been speculated to be of autoimmune origin. Fritz et al. (1976) have described the lesion in a closed colony of Beagle dogs in which there was also a high incidence of lymphocytic thyroiditis. Orchitis or epididymitis of infectious or other origin may be exacerbated by the release of spermatozoa to surrounding tissues.

Ophthalmitis. Immunization with lens protein, uveal antigen, and retinal antigens can induce ophthalmitis. The ensuing lesions are principally characterized by mononuclear infiltration of the uvea, often accompanied by multinucleated giant cells and granulomas. The role of autoantibodies in naturally occurring ophthalmitis is not clear, but circulating antibodies and cell-mediated immunity have been demonstrated in a high percentage of human beings with noninfectious uveitis.

Other Autoimmune Disorders. Autoimmune inflammation of other organs and tissues has been recognized in human beings and can be induced experimentally in laboratory animals. Examples include autoimmune insulitis leading to transient diabetes mellitus, autoimmune adrenalitis, myasthenia gravis, aplastic anemia, "idiopathic" neutropenia, thrombocytopenia, parathyroiditis, and pernicious anemia in man. Idiopathic polyneuritis (Coonhound paralysis; Guillain-Barré syndrome) of dogs has been speculated to be an autoimmune disease. Many organs and tissues share antigens, which may result in multiple organ disease following immunization with antigen from a single tissue. For example, the liver, kidney, duodenum, ileum, and colon have common antigens. This may explain the complexity of many autoimmune diseases.

Viruses and "Autoimmunity." Viral infections almost invariably elicit a humoral immune response, but in addition they may stimulate a cell-mediated immune response that is important to the pathogenesis of the lesions and to the resolution of the infection. This cell-mediated reaction, which has been variably termed a hypersensitivity reaction and an autoimmune response, is directed against viral-induced cell membrane antigens which are foreign to the host. These antigens are not viral capsid antigens, but new membrane antigens stimulated by the viral infection. It is important to note that humoral antibodies are also formed against these antigens. The reaction is aimed at the rejection of the virus-infected tissue by the host, a process essentially the same as transplant rejection. This, of course, results in the destruction of host tissues or organs, which may lead to resolution of the infection or, if extensive, death. In some examples, the suppression of cellular immunity prevents the reaction and the disease, suggesting that the responsible viral infection is essentially harmless.

This disease mechanism is best studied in lymphocytic choriomeningitis infection of mice. In this disease, if infection occurs in mice more than a few days old, an intense lymphocytic inflammatory response occurs in most all organs, which leads either to death, rejection of the infection, or a persistent infection. If infected in utero or at one day of age, an acute reaction does not follow, but a persistent infection is established. It was once thought the latter was an example of complete tolerance, but humoral and cell-mediated immune responses are elicited. A chronic disease results, with destruction of cells as well as the formation of virus-antibody immune complexes, leading to vasculitis and glomerulonephritis. Other viral infections in which similar mechanisms are important to their pathogenesis include lactic dehydrogenase infection of mice, Moloney sarcoma virus of mice, Aleutian disease of mink, equine infectious anemia, hog cholera, virus induced leukemias, and cytomegalovirus infection. With further study it will probably be demonstrated that most viral infections are associated with new membrane antigens and that certain unexplained autoimmune diseases are the result of viral infections.

Summarizing this account and earlier comments, viruses may induce several immunopathologic changes. These include (1) **depression of humoral and cellular immune response;** (2) **production of immune complexes and associated disease;** and (3) **stimulate new antigens on cell membranes, leading to cell destruction through either antibody and complement or cell-mediated immune responses.** Less well characterized is potentiation of immune response by certain viruses, such as lactic dehydrogenase virus and Venezuela equine encephalitis virus.

Allison, A. C., and Ferluga, J.: How lymphocytes kill tumor cells. N. Engl. J. Med., 295:165–167, 1976.

Atwal, O. S., Samagh, B. S., and Bhatnager, M. K.: A possible autoimmune parathyroiditis following ozone inhalation. II. A histopathologic, ultrastructural, and immunofluorescent study. Am. J. Pathol., 80:53–68, 1975.

Banks, K. L., and Henson, J. B.: Immunologically mediated glomerulonephritis of horses. II. Antiglomerular basement membrane antibody and other mechanisms in spontaneous disease. Lab. Invest., 26:708–716, 1972.

Barnhart, D. D., and Gengozian, N.: Actively induced thrombocytopenia in marmoset: possible autoimmune model. Clin. Exp. Immunol., 21:493–500, 1975.

Beaucher, W. N., Garman, R. H., and Condemi, J. J.: Familial lupus erythematosus: antibodies to DNA in household dogs. N. Engl. J. Med., 296:982–984, 1977.

Benacerraf, B., and Unanue, E. R.: Textbook of Immunology. Baltimore, London, Williams & Wilkins, 1979.

Bigazzi, P. E., and Rose, N. R.: Spontaneous autoimmune thyroiditis in animals as a model of human disease. Prog. Allergy, 19:245–274, 1975.

Bishop, D. W., Narbaitz, R., and Tessof, M.: Induced aspermatogenesis in adult guinea pigs injected with testicular antigen and adjuvant in neonatal stages. Dev. Biol., 3:444–485, 1961.

Boxer, L. A., Greensberg, M. S., Boxer, G. J., and

Stossel, T. P.: Autoimmune neutropenia. N. Engl. J. Med., 293:748–753, 1975.

Brand, A., Gilmour, D. G., and Goldstein, G.: Lymphocyte-differentiating hormone of bursa of Fabricius. Science, 193:319–321, 1976.

Brown, P. G., Glynn, L. E., and Holboro, E. J.: The pathogenesis of experimental allergic orchitis in guinea pigs. J. Pathol. Bact. (London), 86:505–520, 1963.

Brummerstedt, E. et al.: Lethal trait A46 in cattle. Nord. Vet. Med., 26:279, 1974.

Burnet, F. M.: Cellular Immunology. Melbourne, Melbourne University Press, 1969.

Burnet, F. M.: A reassessment of the forbidden clone hypothesis of autoimmune disease. Aust. J. Exp. Biol. Med. Sci., 50:1–9, 1972.

Collins-Williams, C., Chiu, A. W., and Varga, E. A.: The relationship of atopic disease and immunoglobulin levels with special reference to IgA deficiency. Clin. Allergy, 1:381–386, 1971.

Craddock, C. G., Longmire, R., and McMillan, R.: Lymphocytes and immune response. N. Engl. J. Med., 285:324–331, 378–384, 1971.

Craighead, J. E.: Virus induced insulitis in experimental animal models. Acta Endocrinol., 83 (Suppl. 205):123–128, 1976.

DeMartini, J. C.: Thymic hypoplasia and lymphopenia in a Siberian tiger. J. Am. Vet. Med. Assoc., 165:824–829, 1974.

Dieppe, P. A., Willoughby, D. A., Huskisson, E. C., and Arrigoni-Martelli, E.: Pertussis vaccine pleurisy: a model of delayed hypersensitivity. Agents Actions, 6:618–621, 1976.

Duncan, J. R., et al.: Persistent papillomatosis associated with immunodeficiency. Cornell Vet., 65:205–211, 1975.

Dvorak, A. M., Mihm, M. C., Jr., and Dvorak, H. F.: Morphology of delayed-type hypersensitivity reactions in man. II. Ultrastructural alterations affecting the microvasculature and the tissue mast cells. Lab. Invest., 34:179–191, 1976.

Egeberg, J., Junker, K., Kromann, H., and Nerup, J.: Autoimmune insulitis. Pathological findings in experimental animal models and juvenile diabetes mellitus. Acta Endocrinol., 83 (Suppl. 205):129–137, 1976.

Fritz, T. E., Lombard, L. S., Tyler, S. A., and Norris, W. P.: Pathology and familial incidence of orchitis and its relation to thyroiditis in a closed Beagle colony. Exp. Mol. Pathol., 24:142–158, 1976.

Fritz, T. E., Zeman, R. C., and Zelle, M. R.: Pathology and familial incidence of thyroiditis in a closed Beagle colony. Exp. Mol. Pathol., 12:14–30, 1970.

Gengozian, N., and McLaughlin, C. L.: Actively induced platelet bound IgG associated with thrombocytopenia in the marmoset. Fed. Proc., 36:379, 1979.

Goldgraber, M. B., and Kirsner, J. B.: Granulomatous lesions—an expression of a hypersensitive state. An experimental study. Arch. Pathol., 66:618–634, 1958.

Grossberg, S. E.: The interferons and their inducers: molecular and therapeutic considerations. N. Engl. J. Med., 287:13–19, 79–85, 122–127, 1972.

Hoffman, R., et al.: Suppression of erythroid-colony formation by lymphocytes from patients with aplastic anemia. N. Engl. J. Med., 296:10–13, 1977.

Hoschoian, J. C., Comini, E., and Andrada, J. A.: Experimental autoimmune adrenalities in the rat. J. Steroid Biochem., 7:481–489, 1976.

Howard, F. A., and Cronin, M. T. I.: Colostral transfer of anti-erythrocyte agglutinins from mare to foal. J. Am. Vet. Med. Assoc., 126:93–94, 1955.

Hurvitz, A. I., and Feldman, E.: A disease in dogs resembling human pemphigus vulgaris. J. Am. Vet. Med. Assoc., 166:585–590, 1975.

Izsof, Z.: Anafylaxia u ošípanych. [Anaphylaxis in pigs.] Čas československsk. Vet., 5:200–201, 1950.

Keuning, F. J., and Van der Slikke, L. B.: Role of immature plasma cells, lymphoblasts and lymphocytes in the formation of antibodies as established in tissue cultures. J. Lab. Clin. Med., 36:167–182, 1950.

Kolata, G. B.: Autoimmune diseases in animals: useful models for immunology. Science, 184:1360–1362, 1974.

Koller, L. D.: Immunosuppression produced by lead, cadmium and mercury. Am. J. Vet. Res., 34:1457–1458, 1973.

Korf, B. R., and Bloom, S. E.: Cytogenetic and immunologic studies in chickens with autoimmune thyroiditis. J. Hered., 65:219–222, 1974.

Krum, S. H., Cardinet, G. H., III, Anderson, B. C., and Holliday, T. A.: Polymyositis and polyarthritis associated with systemic lupus erythematosus in a dog. J. Am. Vet. Med. Assoc., 170:61–64, 1977.

Lane, F. C., and Unanue, E. R.: Requirement of thymus (T) lymphocytes for resistance to listeriosis. J. Exp. Med., 135:1104–1112, 1972.

Lennon, V. A., Lindstrom, J. M., and Seybold, M. E.: Experimental autoimmune myasthenia: a model of myasthenia gravis in rats and guinea pigs. J. Exp. Med., 141:1365–1375, 1975.

Lennon, V. A., Lindstrom, J. M., and Seybold, M. E.: Experimental autoimmune myasthenia gravis: cellular and humoral responses. Ann. N.Y. Acad. Sci., 274:283–299, 1976.

Lewis, R. M.: Spontaneous autoimmune diseases of domestic animals. In International Review of Experimental Pathology, Vol. 13. New York, Academic Press, 1974, pp. 55–82.

Lewis, R. M., et al.: Chronic allogeneic disease. I. Development of glomerulonephritis. J. Exp. Med., 128:653–679, 1968.

Lewis, R. M., and Borel, Y.: Canine rheumatoid arthritis. A case report. Arthritis Rheum., 14:67–72, 1971.

Lewis, R. M., and Hathaway, J. E.: Canine systemic lupus erythematosus presenting with symmetrical polyarthritis. Br. J. Small Anim. Pract., 8:273–284, 1967.

Lewis, R. M., Henry, W. B., Thornton, G. W., and Gilmore, C. E.: A syndrome of autoimmune hemolytic anemia and thrombocytopenia in dogs. Soc. Proc. J. Am. Vet. Med. Assoc., 1:140–163, 1963.

Lewis, R. M., and Schwartz, R. S.: Canine systemic lupus erythematosus. Genetic analysis of an established breeding colony. J. Exp. Med., 134:417–438, 1971.

Lewis, R. M., et al.: Canine systemic lupus erythematosus. Transmission of serologic abnormalities by cell-free filtrates. J. Clin. Invest., 52:1893–1907, 1973.

Lindstrom, J. M., Lennon, V. A., Seybold, M. E., and Whittingham, S.: Experimental autoimmune myasthenia gravis and myasthenia gravis: biochemical and immunochemical aspects. Ann. N.Y. Acad. Sci., 274:254–274, 1976.

Losos, G. J., Winter, A. J., and McEntee, K.: Induction of testicular degeneration in bulls by autoimmunization. Am. J. Vet. Res., 29:2295–2306, 1968.

Mansmann, R. A., Osburn, B. I., Wheat, J. D., and Frick, O.: Chicken hypersensitivity pneumonitis in horses. J. Am. Vet. Med. Assoc., 166:673–677, 1975.

Maplesden, D. C., Cote, J. F., and Mitchell, D.: Allergy in a horse. J. Am. Vet. Med. Assoc., 128:152, 1956.

McGuire, T. C., Banks, K. L., and Davis, W. C.: Alterations of the thymus and other lymphoid tissue in young horses with combined immunodeficiency. Am. J. Pathol., 84:39–54, 1976.

McGuire, T. C., Banks, K. L., Evans, D. R., and Poppie, M. J.: Agammaglobulinemia in a horse with evidence of functional T lymphocytes. Am. J. Vet. Res., 37:41–46, 1976.

McGuire, T. C., Banks, K. L., and Poppie, M. J.: Animal model of human disease: combined immunodeficiency (severe), Swiss-type agammaglobulinemia. Animal model: combined immunodeficiency in horses. Am. J. Pathol., 80:551–554, 1975.

McGuire, T. C., and Poppie, M. J.: Primary hypogammaglobulinemia and thymic hypoplasia in horses. Fed. Proc., 32:821, 1973.

McGuire, T. C., Poppie, M. J., and Banks, K. L.: Combined (B- and T-lymphocyte) immunodeficiency: A fatal genetic disease in Arabian foals. J. Am. Vet. Med. Assoc., 164:70–76, 1974.

McGuire, T. C., Poppie, M. J., and Banks, K. L.: Hypogammaglobulinemia predisposing to infection in foals. J. Am. Vet. Med. Assoc., 166:71–75, 1975.

Mellors, R. C., Siegel, M., and Pressman, D.: Histochemical demonstration of antibody localization in tissues. Lab. Invest., 4:69–89, 1955.

Miller, G., Swisher, S. N., and Young, L. E.: A case of autoimmune hemolytic disease in a dog. Clin. Res. Proc., 2:60–61, 1954.

Muscoplat, C. C., et al.: Lymphocyte subpopulations and immunodeficiency in calves with acute lymphocytic leukemia. Am. J. Vet. Res., 35:1571–1574, 1974.

Nevalainen, J., Fowlie, E., and Janigan, D. T.: Foreign serum-induced pancreatitis in mice. II. Secretory disturbances of acinar cells. Lab. Invest., 36:469–473, 1977.

Osburn, B. I.: Immune responsiveness of the fetus and neonate. J. Am. Vet. Med. Assoc., 163:801–803, 1973.

Parker, W.: Control of lymphocyte function. N. Engl. J. Med., 295:1180–1186, 1976.

Parsonson, I. M., Winter, A. J., and McEntee, K.: Allergic epididymo-orchitis in guinea pigs and bulls. Vet. Pathol., 8:333–351, 1971.

Patterson, R.: Ragweed allergy in the dog. J. Am. Vet. Med. Assoc., 135:178–180, 1959.

Patterson, R., Harris, K. E., Suszko, I. M., and Roberts, M.: Reagin mediated asthma in Rhesus monkeys and relation to bronchial cell histamine release and airway reactivity to carbocholine. J. Clin. Invest., 57:586–593, 1976.

Patterson, R., Zeiss, C. R., and Kelly, J. F.: Classification of hypersensitivity reactions. N. Engl. J. Med., 295:277–278, 1976.

Pelletier, M., and Montplaisir, S.: The nude mouse: a model of deficient T cell function. Methods Achiev. Exp. Pathol., 7:149–166, 1975.

Perryman, L. E., Hoover, E. A., and Yohn, D. S.: Immunologic reactivity to the cat: immunosuppression in experimental feline leukemia. J. Natl. Canc. Inst., 49:1357–1365, 1972.

Playfair, J. H. L.: Animal models of autoimmunity. In Current Titles in Immunology, Transplantation and Allergy, Vol. 1. London, Middlesex Hospital, Dept. of Immunology, 1974, pp. 1–3.

Polmar, S. H., et al.: Enzyme replacement for severe combined immunodeficiency disease. N. Engl. J. Med., 295:1337–1342, 1976.

Poppie, M. J., and McGuire, T. C.: Combined immunodeficiency in foals of Arabian breeding: evaluation of mode of inheritance and estimation of prevalence of affected foals and carrier mares and stallions. J. Am. Vet. Med. Assoc., 170:31–33, 1977.

Poskitt, T. R., Fortwengler, H. P., Jr., Bobrow, J. C., and Roth, G. J.: Naturally occurring immune-complex glomerulonephritis in monkeys (Macaca iris). Am. J. Pathol., 76:145–159, 1974.

Prieur, D. J., Olson, H. M., and Young, D. M.: Lysozyme deficiency—an inherited disorder of rabbits. Am. J. Pathol., 77:283–298, 1974.

Rabin, B. S., and Rogers, S.: Pathologic changes in the liver and kidney produced by immunization with intestinal antigens. Am. J. Pathol., 84:201–210, 1976.

Ruddy, S., Gigli, I., and Austen, K. F.: The complement system of man. N. Engl. J. Med., 287:489–495, 545–549, 592–596, 642–646, 1972.

Schultz, R. D., Scott, F. W., Duncan, J. R., and Gillespie, J. H.: Feline immunoglobulins. Infect. Immun., 9:391–393, 1974.

Schwartz, R. S.: Viruses and systemic lupus erythematosus. N. Engl. J. Med., 292:132–136, 1975.

Stevens, D. R., and Osburn, B. I.: Immune deficiency in a dog with distemper. J. Am. Vet. Med. Assoc., 168:493–498, 1976.

Stroble, C. P., and Glenn, M. W.: A fatal case of bovine anaphylaxis. J. Am. Vet. Med. Assoc., 126:227–232, 1955.

Strockbine, J. K.: Anaphylaxis and the ox warble. J. Am. Vet. Med. Assoc., 77:106–107, 1930.

Talal, N., and Steinberg, A. D.: The pathogenesis of autoimmunity in New Zealand Black mice. Curr. Top. Microbiol. Immunol., 64:79–103, 1974.

Thompson, D. B., Studdert, M. J., Beiharz, R. G., and Littlejohns, I. R.: Inheritance of a lethal immunodeficiency disease of Arabian foals. Aust. Vet. J., 51:109–113, 1975.

Tizard, I. R.: Macrophage-cytophilic antibodies and the function of macrophage-bound immuno-globulins. Bacteriol. Rev., 35:365–378, 1971.

Toyka, K. V., et al.: Study of humoral immune mechanisms by passive transfer to mice. N. Engl. J. Med., 296:126–131, 1977.

Tyrrell, D. A.: The role of interferon in the response to infection. Proc. Roy. Soc. Med., 62:13–14, 1969.

Waldman, T. A.: Disorders of immunoglobulin metabolism. N. Engl. J. Med., 281:1170–1177, 1969.

Weiden, P. L., et al.: Immune reactivity in dogs with spontaneous malignancy. J. Natl. Canc. Inst., 53:1049–1056, 1974.

Wells, P. W., Pass, D. A., and Eyre, P.: Acute systemic immediate hypersensitivity in pigs. Res. Vet. Sci., 16:347–350, 1974.

Wick, G.: Animal model of human disease: thyroiditis of chickens. Comp. Pathol. Bull., 8:3–4, 1976.

Wick, G., and Graf, J.: Electron microscopic studies in chickens of the obese strain with spontaneous hereditary autoimmune thyroiditis. Lab. Invest., 27:400–411, 1972.

Wick, G., Sundick, R. S., and Albine, B.: A review: the obese strain (OS) of chickens: an animal model with spontaneous autoimmune thyroiditis. Clin. Immunol. Immunopathol., 3:272–300, 1974.

Wilkie, B. N.: Hypersensitivity pneumonitis: experimental production in calves with antigens of Micropolyspora faeni. Can. J. Comp. Med., 40:221–227, 1976.

Williams, M. R., Maxwell, D. A. G., and Spooner, R. L.: Quantitative studies on bovine immunoglobulins, normal plasma levels of IgG_2, IgG_1, IgM and IgA. Res. Vet. Sci., 18:314–321, 1975.

Williamson, A. R.: Biosynthesis of antibodies. Nature, 231:359–362, 1971.

Wong, V. G., Green, W. R., McMaster, P. R., and Johnson, D. K.: Rhodopsin and autoimmune blindness in primates. Trans. Penn. Acad. Ophthalmol. Otolaryngol., 28:135–137, 1975.

Zweiten, M. J. van, Bhan, A. K., McCluskey, R. T., and Collins, A. B.: Studies on the pathogenesis of experimental antitubular basement membrane nephritis in the guinea pig. Am. J. Pathol., 83:531–541, 1976.

CHAPTER 8

Genetically Determined Disease; Cytogenetics

During recent years, many significant discoveries have been made in the field of genetics, particularly in application to genetically determined disease in humans. The fundamental nature of much of the new knowledge has inspired and challenged investigation in many disciplines; many of the new techniques are being used to explore disease problems. Although much of the work is being done in relation to human disease, most principles undoubtedly apply to animals. The search for models and the probe for underlying causes of genetically influenced disease in animals is challenging to the veterinary pathologist. It is now clear that genetic mechanisms are not only involved in transmitting characteristics from one generation to the next, but also are important in controlling the activities of cells in the body, particularly as they change from one cell generation to another.

The veterinary pathologist must understand the principles of genetics in order to judge the quality and significance of genetic evidence in the cause and pathogenesis of disease. He also needs to know enough about the field to communicate effectively with scientific colleagues who are geneticists. Complete discussion of this field is outside the scope of this book, but some of the principles will be recounted briefly, particularly those that now appear to be fundamental in disease processes.

The student is strongly advised to read further in the literature; some of the most pertinent information is found in the references listed at the end of this chapter. *Animal Genetics* by F. D. Hutt would be a delightful book with which to start. This book is precise and readable with Hutt's spritely style, and genetic principles are beautifully illustrated by examples in animals.

MENDELIAN GENETICS

The founder of genetics was undoubtedly the Austrian monk and teacher, Gregor Johann Mendel, whose careful studies of a few characteristics of garden peas led to the discovery of some basic principles that influence heredity in all living things. In **simple mendelian inheritance**, characteristics inherited from one generation by the next are controlled by unit characters called genes. Two of these units of inheritance occur in each of the cells of living creatures that reproduce sexually, one gene derived from each parent. In the gametes (ova, sperm) produced by the parents, these paired genes segregate from one another, each gamete acquiring half the number found in somatic cells. When two gametes unite at random to form a zygote, their genes recombine. By studying the

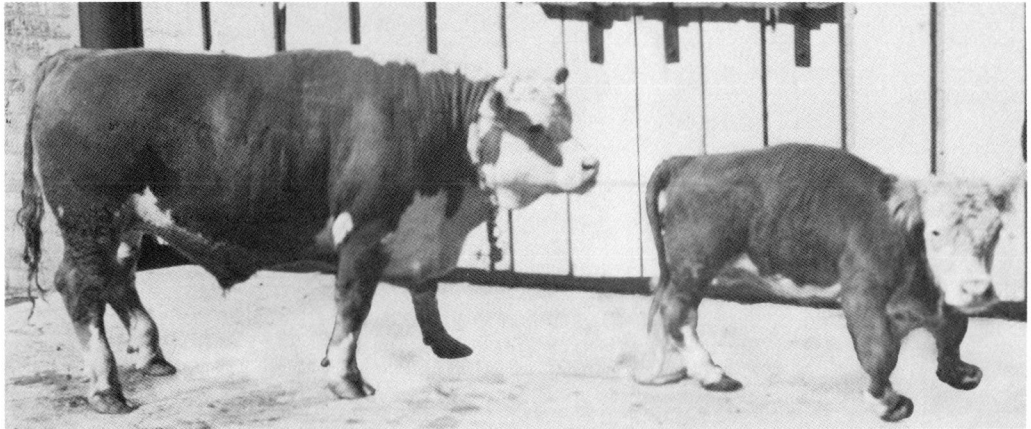

Fig. 8–1. Dwarfism 'C' in a Hereford calf. Note small size, large head, and distorted limbs in affected calf. Normal calf of same age and breed on left.

characteristics resulting from these recombinations, Mendel discovered the principle of **independent assortment**. It is now known, of course, that genes are carried in the chromosomes of cells and segregate independently if carried on different chromosomes, but if close together ("linked") on the same chromosome, they are more apt to remain together. Genes that occupy the same site **(locus)** on a chromosome can only be alternates for one another, and are called **alleles**. Genes located in the X or Y chromosome are called **sex-linked**, those in all other chromosomes are designated **autosomal**.

When the genes at one locus are the same from both parents (homozygous), only one characteristic controlled at this locus will be conveyed to the next generation, but when these genes are different (heterozygous), the sex cells (gametes) will contain alternate alleles in approximately equal numbers. In the heterozygous state, the characteristic manifest in the phenotype of the progeny may be controlled by only one gene, which in this case is considered **dominant**; the unexpressed gene is called **recessive**. In matings between heterozygotes, recombinations at random will result in homozygous dominant, heterozygous, and homozygous recessive zygotes in the approximate ratio of 1:2:1. Since the dominant gene will be expressed whenever present, the recessive gene will be expressed only when homozygous, thus giving a 3:1 ratio in the phenotype. This principle, reported by Mendel in 1865, is useful today in the study of genetically controlled disease conditions in man and animals.

The preceding paragraph illustrates the ratios that can be expected in progeny in animals heterozygous for a single gene that controls a hereditary defect. This is the simplest ratio that is useful as genetic evidence, but is only applicable to certain disease conditions, and only when all parents are heterozygous. Other ratios occur in progeny, depending upon the frequency of the controlling gene in the population.

Altman, P. L., and Dittmer, D. S. (ed.): Growth—including reproduction and morphological development. Table I, pp. 1–7. *In* Biological Handbook. Washington, D.C., Federation of American Society of Experimental Biology, 1962.

Emery, A. E. H.: Heredity, Disease and Man. Berkeley, University of California Press, 1968.

Grüneberg, H.: The Genetics of the Mouse. 3rd ed. The Hague, Bibliographia Genetica, 1963.

Hadorn, E.: Developmental Genetics and Lethal Factors. New York, John Wiley & Sons, 1961.

Hutt, F. B.: Inherited lethal characters in domestic animals. Cornell Vet., 24:1–25, 1934.

———: Genetic Resistance to Disease in Domestic Animals. Ithaca, Comstock Publishing Co., 1958.

————: Animal Genetics. New York, Ronald Press Co., 1964.

Innes, J. R. M., and Saunders, L. Z.: Comparative Neuropathology. New York, Academic Press, 1962.

Montague, F. A.: Genetic Mechanisms in Human Disease. Springfield, Charles C Thomas, 1961.

Pauling, L.: Molecular disease and evolution. Bull. N.Y. Acad. Med., 40:334–342, 1964.

Robinson, R.: Genetics of the domestic cat. Bibliographia Genetica, 18:271–362, 1959.

Srb, A. M., and Owen, R. D.: General Genetics. San Francisco, W. H. Freeman and Co., 1952.

DNA, RNA, AND THE GENETIC CODE

For a long time, nucleic acids have been known to occur in the nuclei of cells. A particular nucleic acid, deoxyribonucleic acid (DNA), is now believed to be the molecular substance with the characteristics needed to be genetic material—namely, it is self-replicating and it is able to control all chemical processes specific to the organism. In microbial systems, DNA has been shown to be the sole carrier of genetic information. Although perhaps best viewed as a theory at the present, strong evidence exists that DNA is the fundamental genetic material in all living things. The presumption of the truth of this hypothesis has led to great research efforts and many fundamental facts are emerging as a result.

Structure of DNA

The structure of the DNA molecule was first demonstrated in 1953 by Watson and Crick, whose findings (now amply confirmed) won them a Nobel Prize. The DNA molecule was shown by Watson and Crick to be made up of three types of "building blocks," viz., phosphate (which gives it acid properties), deoxyribose (a sugar), and four bases (two purines: adenine and guanine, and two pyrimidines: cytosine and thymine). The molecule consists of elongated chains in which the sugar and phosphate form a double helix around a central axis; these paired helical bands are linked together at regular intervals by pairs of bases (Fig. 8–2). These

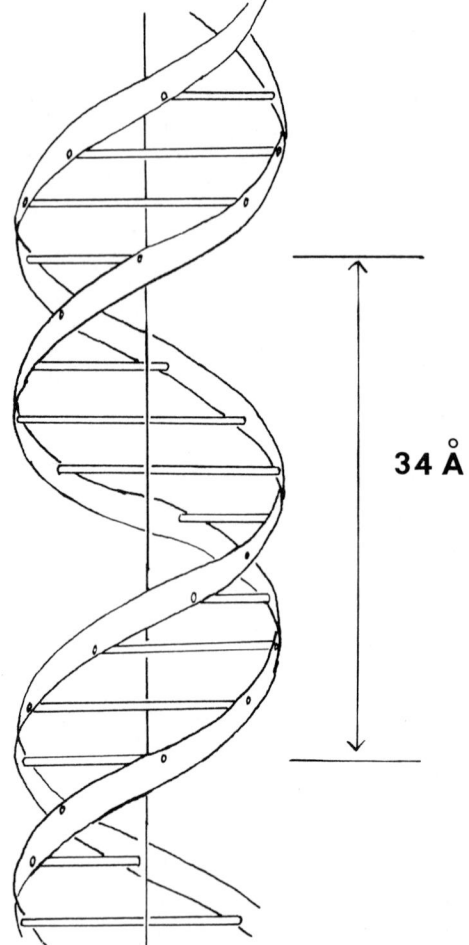

34 Å

Fig. 8–2. The deoxyribonucleic acid (DNA) model of Watson and Crick. The coiled double helix, made up of sugar (deoxyribose) and phosphate, form paired "backbones" which are held equal distances apart by base pairs (purines and pyrimidines) represented by the horizontal lines. (After Symonds, N. D., *Chromosomes in Medicine*, 1961, Wm. Heineman.)

bases are joined in specific ways: one purine is held to one pyrimidine by hydrogen bonds; i.e., adenine (A) is always paired with thymine (T), and guanine (G), with cytosine (C). Each single group, consisting of base pair, sugar, and phosphate, is sometime referred to as a **nucleotide**, and the DNA molecule, as a polynucleotide chain.

Replication of DNA is visualized by Watson and Crick as based upon the specific base-pairing of adenine-thymine and guanine-cytosine along the length of the molecule. As illustrated in Figure 8–3, this results in a pair of templates when the

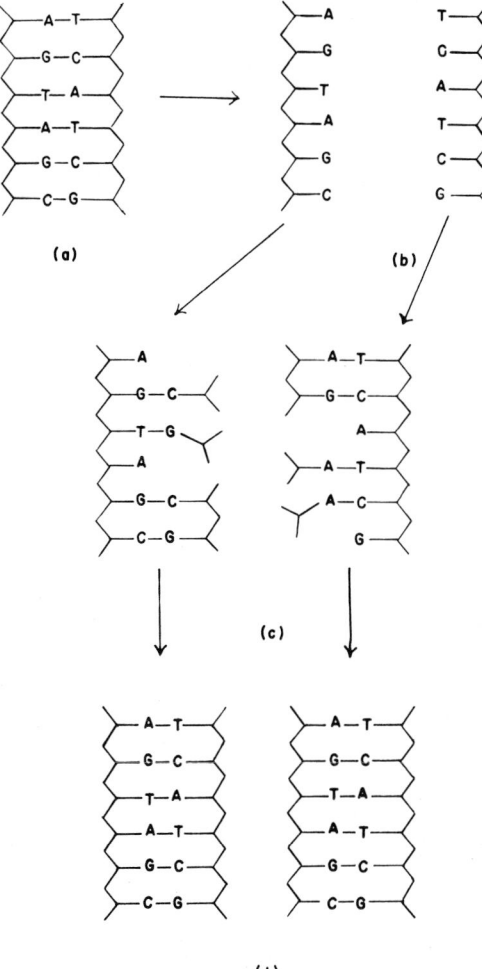

(a)

(b)

(c)

(d)

Fig. 8–3. Replications of DNA. In (a) the base pairs (adenine-thymine and guanine-cytosine) are represented by letters (A–T, G–C) separating the "backbone" of sugar-phosphate. In (b) the base pairs separate, leaving two single strands of DNA with bases in linear sequence. Enzymes and a source of energy cause binding of free bases with their sugar-phosphates to specific sites (c) resulting in two double strands of DNA (d) with exactly the same base sequence as the original (a). (After Symonds, *Chromosomes in Medicine*, 1961, Wm. Heineman.)

two chains of the DNA molecule separate. Bases, sugar, and phosphate that are free in the cell are combined, and the base pairs are joined at their specific sites to form a new polynucleotide chain. The specific sequential arrangement of the base-pairs along the molecule is therefore replicated as new double-stranded chains are formed, which exactly duplicate the parent DNA. This is an oversimplified explanation of a very complicated process, but outlines the basic concept which now seems to be amply confirmed.

The Control of Function by DNA

The synthesis of specific proteins is controlled by genetic factors, suggesting that at least some, if not all, of the genetic information carried by DNA concerns the sequence of amino acids in proteins. The sugar-phosphate part of the double helix is perfectly regular, but the sequence of the four base pairs along the length of the DNA molecule varies, and therefore must be the component which in some way determines the sequence of amino acids in proteins. The **genetic code** involves the specific means by which a sequence of nucleotides in the DNA molecule can, without ambiguity, determine the sequence of amino acids in a polypeptide chain (protein).

The view of Crick et al. (1957) of the coding problem involved the concept of nonoverlapping triplet codes. These are explained as follows: By designating each of the nucleotides by a letter, an arbitrary sequence along the chain may be designated as: AGTAGCTGC. If the code is a triple one, a sequence of three adjacent nucleotides is necessary to code for one amino acid. Assuming that AGC is such a sequence, and the code is nonoverlapping, then none of these three nucleotides, AGC, can be part of any adjacent triplet. The next triplet to the left, AGT, and the next to the right, TGC, would be codes for different amino acids. This triplet code therefore could be AGT AGC TGC; other combinations would be meaningless. It was shown by Crick et al. that it is theoretically possible to construct a number of codes of this type in which, of the 64 possible triplets, 20 could provide codes for individual amino acids. As 20 amino acids commonly make up proteins, these codes adequately satisfy the requirements of the coding problem.

The nucleotide triplet code for each amino acid has been demonstrated by experimental methods. Although specific for each amino acid, more than one code is effective for several of them. This is summarized succinctly by Jukes (1966).

The simplest explanation of protein synthesis, assuming that its specificity is determined by some such coding mechanism as just described, would be that it was assembled directly on the DNA. However, the site of protein synthesis has been shown experimentally to be in the cytoplasm of the cell; specifically in tiny particles called ribosomes, which contain a large quantity of **ribonucleic acid** (RNA). The molecule of RNA is similar to DNA, except that one of its bases, **thymine**, is replaced by a similar pyrimidine, **uracil**, and the sugar, deoxyribose, becomes ribose. It appears that RNA molecules are involved in the transfer of genetic information from the DNA of the nucleus to the cytoplasm; and within the ribosomes, act as templates for the synthesis of protein. This process as now visualized (Sutton, 1963) requires three types of RNA: **Messenger RNA** (mRNA, template RNA), which is unstable in most systems, and contains 1500 nucleotides; **ribosomal RNA**, which is stable, and contains 1650 and 3300 nucleotides; and **transfer RNA** (soluble RNA, sRNA, adapter RNA), which is stable and contains only 70 nucleotides. Twenty amino acids are necessarily present in the cell, plus 20 enzymes, each capable of attaching a specific amino acid to one of 20 specific **transfer RNA**'s. Each molecule of sRNA is believed to attach to its specific amino acid and, recognizing the sequence (code) of base pairs in

the **messenger RNA** in the ribosomes, attaches the amino acids in the proper sequence for the specific protein. After alignment in the proper order, condensation occurs between adjacent peptides to form the specific protein, which then separates from the sRNA, which in turn becomes available for further synthesis of protein.

The Gene and DNA

Each of the nonoverlapping regions of DNA, which contains a particular sequence of nucleotides and which indirectly controls the synthesis of one specific protein, can be called a gene. In this sense, it is a unit of function and can be subdivided into smaller units or **mutational sites**. The number of amino acids in a typical protein is in the order of 1000, and as three nucleotides are necessary to code for each amino acid, a gene contains about 3000 nucleotide pairs. A small organism, such as a virus, may contain sufficient DNA to include 100 genes of this size, while higher organisms may have enough DNA to provide as many as 1 million genes.

The student can visualize, by the use of the foregoing schemata, that a change or defect in one or more base pairs in DNA may lead to the formation of an abnormal protein or may preclude its production entirely. At the molecular level, such a change in base pairs is believed to be one underlying mechanism in **mutation.** Major errors can occur in DNA replication, sometimes involving chromosomal segments or whole chromosomes. These may have a significant effect upon the resultant phenotype. The recognition of abnormal phenotypes, in the language of the geneticist, represents pathologic diagnosis to the pathologist, and is the point of interest in much of this book.

The first disease clearly shown to be the result of genetic influences at the molecular level is sickle cell anemia of man. Pauling, et al., in 1949, found that the essential defect underlying the loss of erythrocytes involved the hemoglobin molecule. Amazing as it may seem, the concept of such genetic defects was thoroughly considered and expanded by Garrod in 1909. The introduction of biochemical techniques and philosophy into genetics resulted in development of an important modern area of research, sometimes called **molecular genetics.** Some genetic defects of man now recognized at the molecular level are phenylketonuria, alkaptonuria, cystinuria, cystinosis, glycinuria, galactosemia, and various glycogen storage diseases. For the most part, these defects are each controlled by a single recessive gene. The concept of the gene is still valid, but can now be considered in biochemical terms on the molecular level.

Studies with microbial organisms, particularly *Neurospora,* have disclosed that single enzymes control the synthesis of specific proteins, and each enzyme is determined by a specific gene. Organisms which are normally able to produce all of their nutritional needs from simple substances can be caused, by radiation-induced mutation, to lose the ability to synthesize one or more of these essential nutrients. Mutation of one gene results in the loss of one enzyme. These facts have led some (Pauling, 1949) to state that vitamin deficiency states are actually genetically determined diseases which are the result of the loss during evolution of the ability to synthesize the necessary vitamin. As an example, man and the guinea pig have each lost the ability to synthesize ascorbic acid, and therefore are subject to scurvy when this vitamin is absent from the diet. Most other animals still retain the capacity to synthesize ascorbic acid—presumably because they still have the gene that controls this function.

Jukes, Thomas H.: Molecules and Evolution. New York, Columbia University Press, 1966.

Kornberg, A.: Biologic synthesis of deoxyribonucleic acid. Science, *131*:1503–1508, 1960.

Pauling, L., Itano, H. A., Singer, S. J., and Wells, I. C.: Sickle cell anemia, a molecular disease. Science, *110*:543–548, 1949.

Sutton, H. E.: Genes and protein synthesis. *In* Second International Conference on Congenital Malformations, New York, International Medical Congress, Ltd., 1963.

Symonds, N. D.: DNA, Genes and Chromosomes. pp. 7–16. *In* Hamerton, J. L.: Chromosomes in Medicine. London, Wm. Heineman (Medical Books) Ltd., 1963.

Watson, J. D., and Crick, F. H. C.: Molecular structure of nucleic acids. A structure for deoxyribose nucleic acid. Nature, *171*:737–738, 1953.

Woese, C. R.: The Genetic Code: The Molecular Basis for Genetic Expression. New York, Harper & Row, 1967.

CHROMOSOMES

Shortly after the beginning of the 20th century, geneticists were enthusiastically testing the principles of Mendel in plants and animals. One of them (Sutton, 1902) observed that the multiplication and reduction-division of chromosomes in meiosis, preceding the formation of germ cells, could provide mechanisms for the segregation of genes, with recombinations occurring at fertilization in accord with mendelian principles. Thus, observations in genetics were combined with others in cytology to establish that genes are carried in chromosomes. This was the beginning of **cytogenetics.** The techniques of cytogenetics have long been used in the study of plants, but have only recently been shown to be applicable to animals. Phenomenal progress has been achieved in applying cytogenetic methods to the elucidation of human diseases in which abnormalities occur in the chromosomes. Only the beginning has been made in the study of chromosomes of other animals. However, enough has been learned to indicate that detectable abnormalities do occur in the chromosomes of animals, as well as man, and many of these abnormalities underlie the occurrence of genetically determined disease. Chromosomes are, therefore, of great interest to the veterinary pathologist.

Number and Morphology

Chromosomes are most readily studied at metaphase, at which time individual chromosomes are separately distinct and can be counted and studied morphologically. Appropriate techniques usually involve the culture of cells of the animal under study in order to obtain adequate numbers undergoing mitosis. Rapidly multiplying cells in tissue culture are treated with colchicine (or a related compound) in order to arrest many cells in the metaphase stage of mitosis. The cells are then expanded with hypotonic saline solution, forcing the chromosomes apart, permitting their fixation on a glass slide individually separated from one another. After proper staining, the chromosomes may be studied under the light microscope or, better, photographed. Photographic enlargements of the chromosomes (Fig. 8–4) are used to count their number, align them in homologous pairs in a systematic arrangements (called a karyotype) (Fig. 8–5) and to study their morphologic features. It is now possible to identify each individual chromosome and to locate some functional regions by means of specific staining techniques. Some of these demonstrate banded regions along the length of the chromosomes. The most common of these are called respectively, **Q bands** (from quinacrine), **G bands** (from Giemsa's stain), and **C bands** (constitutive heterochromatin). Two of these banding techniques are illustrated in Figure 8–6.

The number of chromosomes is characteristic for each species; each **somatic** cell in the body contains the same number of homologous pairs (diploid, **2n**), one derived from each parent. Following meiosis,

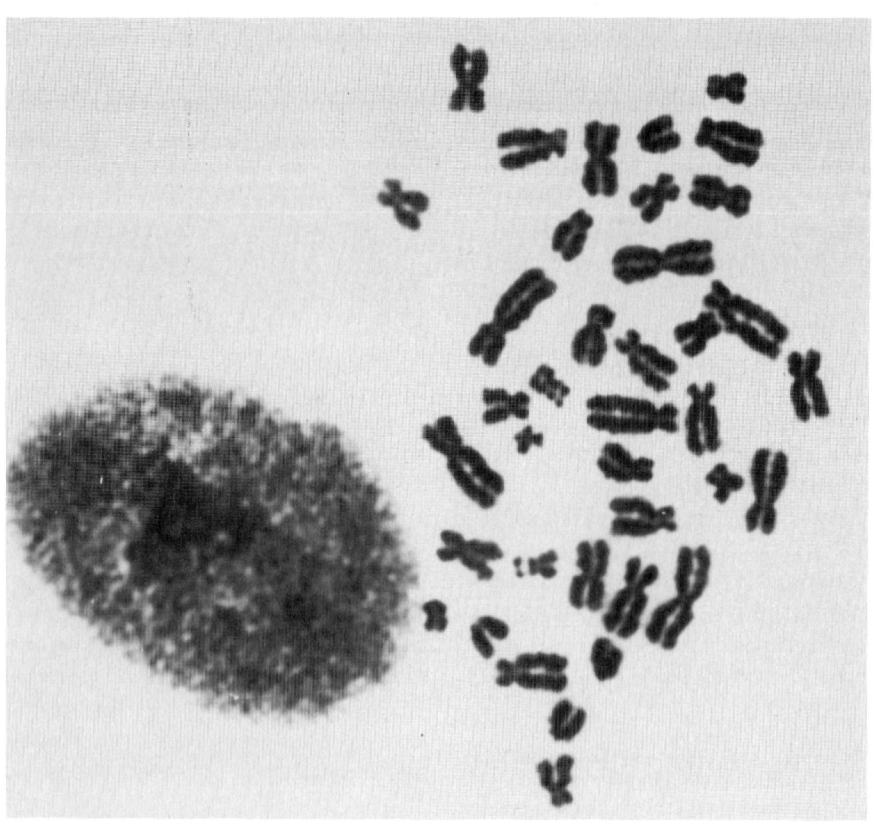

Fig. 8–4. Chromosomes of the cat *(Felis catus)* in metaphase. An interphase nucleus at the left. Smear prepared from cultures of lung treated with colchicine in vitro.

the germ cells each contain half the diploid number, therefore are haploid (**n**). Fertilization of the ovum restores the diploid number to the zygote. The determinors of sex are found in the **sex chromosomes**, which are individually distinguishable in most species. In most normal mammals, females have a pair of X chromosomes (XX), and males have one X and one much smaller Y chromosome (XY). In *Lepidoptera*, birds, reptiles, and some other animals, males are the homogametic sex, with two chromosomes (usually designated ZZ); females have one Z and a smaller chromosome designated W (ZW). Birds have many tiny chromosomes, called microchromosomes, which present difficulties in counting and tend to obscure the small W chromosome. Drones of honeybees are of particular interest because they have a haploid (**n**) number of chromosomes, all originating by parthenogenesis from unfertilized eggs.

The remaining chromosomes are called **autosomes**, which contain most of the genetic material. Genes that are carried in these chromosomes are called **autosomal**, in contrast to those carried on the X chromosome (the Y apparently determines only the male sex, does not carry other genes), which are called **sex-linked**. The pattern of inheritance differs between autosomal and sex-linked genes and lesions in the autosomal vs. the sex chromosomes have different effects, making their distinction important. Identification of the sex

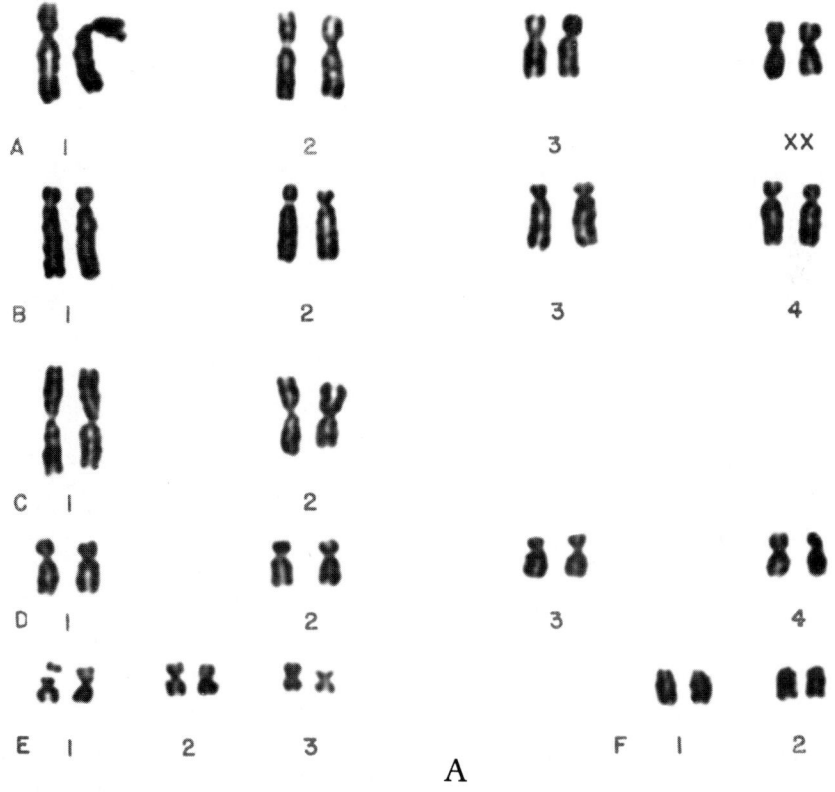

A

Fig. 8–5. Karyotype of the domestic cat, *Felis catus*, prepared according to the "San Juan System" (agreed upon by a group of scientists in San Juan, Puerto Rico, November, 1964). *A*, Female, from a cell cultured from the spleen. (Continued on page 248.)

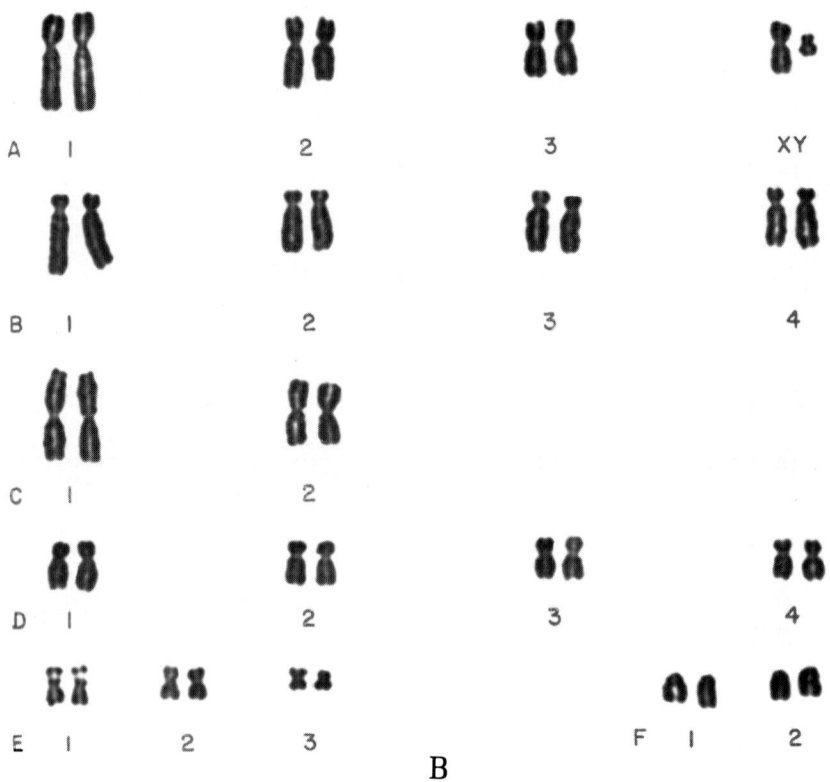

B

Fig. 8–5 (Cont'd).   B, Male cell, cultured from the kidney. Note that in this system the groups can be readily described, viz: Group A, large submetacentric chromosomes; Group B, large subtelocentrics; Group C, large metacentrics; Group D, small metacentrics or submetacentrics; Group E, small metacentrics (the first pair satellited); and Group F, small acrocentric chromosomes.

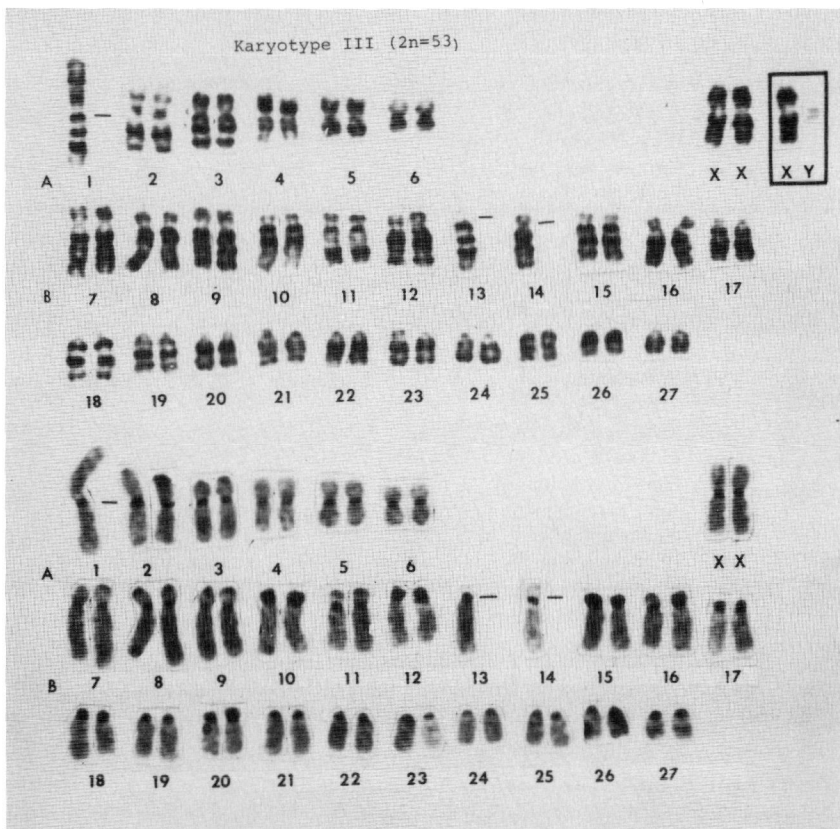

Fig. 8–6. Translocation of chromosomes by Robertsonian fusion, owl monkey *(Aotus).* Karyotype at top is prepared by the "G" method of banding. Note that large metacentric chromosome A1 is not paired and the long arm is identical to acrocentric chromosome B13, also not paired. Acrocentric chromosome B14, also single, has bands that identify it as the other arm of chromosome A1.

The lower karyotype is from the same owl monkey, but is prepared by the "C" banding method. The dense staining, usually at the centromere, indicates constitutive heterochromatin. (Courtesy of Dr. Nancy S. F. Ma, Harvard Medical School, New England Regional Primate Research Center.)

Table 8–1. Chromosomes of Some Common Species

Species		Chromosomes 2n	Sex Chromosomes	
Common Name	Scientific Name		Female	Male
Ass	Equus asinus	62	XX	XY
Mule	Equus mulus	63	XX	XY
Horse	Equus caballus	64	XX	XY
Przewalsky horse	Equus caballus przewalskii	66	XX	XY
Mrs. Hartmann's Mountain Zebra	Equus zebra hartmannae	32	XX	XY
Man	Homo sapiens	46	XX	XY
Mouse	Mus musculus	40	XX	XY
Dog	Canis familiaris	78	XX	XY
Cat	Felis catus	38	XX	XY
Rabbit	Oryctolagus cuniculus	44	XX	XY
Guinea pig	Cavia cobaya	64	XX	XY
Goat	Capra hircus	60	XX	XY
Sheep	Ovis aries	54	XX	XY
Cattle	Bos taurus	60	XX	XY
Zebu	Bos indicus	60	XX	XY
Pig	Sus scrofa	36/38	XX	XY
Fox	Vulpes fulva	38	XX	XY
Mink	Mustela vison	30	XX	XY
Parakeet	Melopsittacus undulatus	58	ZW	ZZ
Turkey	Meleagris gallopavo	81–82	ZW	ZZ
Duck	Anas platyrhyncha domestica	79–80	ZW	ZZ
Fowl	Gallus gallus	77–78	ZW	ZZ
Honey Bee	Apis mellifera	32 (16-drone)	ZW	ZZ

chromosomes may be facilitated by the use of autoradiography. Cultures of multiplying cells are exposed to tritiated thymidine that has been made radioactive. This substance is utilized by the replicating DNA, and can be identified later in the metaphase chromosomes by means of an autoradiograph, which is prepared from a photographic film placed over the cell preparation on the slide. After prolonged exposure, the film is developed in place over the chromosome spreads and the radioactivity is identified as blackened spots of silver grains. One or more of the sex chromosomes replicate out of phase with the autosomes and are heavily labelled by the radioactive thymidine.

The number of chromosomes currently believed to occur in several common species is indicated in Table 8–1. The correct number of human chromosomes was not settled until new techniques were introduced in 1958. Revisions in this table may be necessary as each species is studied more adequately with new techniques.

Benirschke, K., Brownhill, L. E., and Beath, M. M.: Somatic chromosomes of the horse, the donkey and their hybrids, the mule and the hinny. J. Reprod. Fertil., 4:319–326, 1962.

Benirschke, K., Low, R. J., Sullivan, M. M., and Carter, R. M.: Chromosome study of an alleged fertile mare mule. J. Hered., 55:31–38, 1964.

Borland, R.: The chromosomes of domestic sheep. J. Hered., 55:61–64, 1964.

Caspersson, T., Zech, L., and Johansson, C.: Differential binding of alkylating fluorochromes in human chromosomes. Exp. Cell Res., 61:315–319, 1970.

Chu, E. H. Y., and Bender, M. A.: Chromosome cytology and evolution in primates. Science, 133:1399–1405, 1961.

DeRobertis, E.: Advances in the ultrastructure of the nucleus and chromosomes. J. Nat. Cancer Inst. Mono. No. 14, May, 1964.

Eberle, P.: Comparative studies on sex chromosomes in different species. Genetica, 35:34–46, 1964.

Gustavsson, I.: The chromosomes of the dog. Hereditas, 51:187, 1964.

Hamerton, J. L. (ed.): Chromosomes in Medicine. London, Wm. Heinemann (Medical books) Ltd., 1961.

Hare, W. C. D., et al.: Cytogenetics in the dog and cat. J. Small Anim. Pract., 7:575–592, 1966.

Hsu, T. C., and Benirschke, K.: Atlas of Mammalian Chromosomes. Vol. 1–5. New York, Springer-Verlag, 1967–71.

Lehman, J. M., MacPherson, I., and Moorhead, P. S.: Karyotype of the Syrian hamster. J. Nat. Cancer Inst., 31:639–649, 1963.

Makino, S.: An Atlas of the Chromosome Numbers in Animals. Ames, Iowa State University Press, 1951.

Moore, W., Jr., and Lambert, P. D.: The chromosomes of the Beagle dog. J. Hered., 54:273–276, 1963.

Mukherjee, B. B., and Sinha, A. K.: Cytological evidence for random inactivation of X-chromosomes in a female mule complement. Proc. Nat. Acad. Sci., 51:252–254, 1964.

Rothfels, K., Aspden, M., and Mollison, M.: The W-chromosome of the budgerigar, Melopsittacus undulatus. Chromosoma, 14:459–467, 1963.

Stefos, K., and Arrighi, F. E.: Heterochromic nature of W chromosome in birds. Exp. Cell Res., 68:228–231, 1971.

Sutton, W. S.: The chromosomes in heredity. Biol. Bull., 4:231–251, 1902.

Wang, H. C., and Federoff, S.: Banding in human chromosomes treated with trypsin. Nature, 235:52–53, 1972.

Weitkamp, L. R., et al.: Inherited pericentric inversion of chromosome number two: a linkage study. Ann. Human Genet. (London), 33:53–59, 1969.

Wurster, D.H., and Benirschke, K.: Comparative cytogenetic studies in the order Carnivora. Chromosoma (Berl.), 24:336–382, 1968.

———: Indian Muntjac, Muntiacus muntjak: a deer with a low diploid chromosome number. Science, 168:1364–1366, 1970.

ABERRATIONS OF CHROMOSOMES

Surprisingly, abnormalities are not infrequent in chromosomes of animals, notwithstanding the admittedly preconceived idea that chromosomal material must be inviolate in order for the species to survive. A large variety of lesions occurs in chromosomes with alarming frequency, but subsequent death of the gamete or zygote has a species-cleansing effect, permitting only a few abnormal chromosomes to persist in the embryo through birth or into adult life. In spite of this "cleansing" mechanism, some chromosomal aberrations do persist and have a significant effect upon the adult phenotype. Several such abnormal chromosomes are known to underlie important disease syndromes in man, and an increasing number are being found in animals as the search is continued.

Aberrations in Number (Heteroploidy)

Possession of chromosome numbers (Table 8–1), other than the haploid (n) set in the gametes, or the diploid (2n) complement after fertilization, is called heteroploidy. If the abnormal number involves exact multiples of the haploid set, the resulting cells are called euploid and the condition euploidy or euploid heteroploidy. Examples of this condition have been found in mammalian embryos, particularly mice, although most of the affected animals die within the first days of embryonic life. The usual explanation for this abnormality is that the error occurs during meiosis, particularly in the ovum, and that distribution of the chromosome sets to the gametes is erroneous. For example, the polar body may fail to be extruded from the ovum, leaving the diploid set (2n) to be fertilized by a haploid sperm (n) resulting in a 3n (triploid) zygote. Various possibilities and their theoretic explanation are summarized by Russell (1962).

Aberrations in the number of chromosomes that do not involve exact multiples of the haploid (n) number are termed aneuploid heteroploidy. This may involve specific chromosomes in triple number (trisomy) or single number (monosomy), rather than the normal double dose. Errors of this type are more apt to persist into adulthood and result in significant abnormalities. Several of these are now known in man, involving either autosomes or sex chromosomes, and a few have been found in animals. These will be described later.

Duplications and deficiencies of a section of a chromosome may also occur, leaving the total number intact. Long known to occur in Drosophila and plants, these defects have now been observed in chromosomes of man and mouse. Deletion or duplication of a part of a chromosome may not necessarily be lethal, and may result in an abnormal phenotype. **Translocation** involves the rearrangement of genetic material of at least two nonhomologous chromosomes. This translocation may be reciprocal or nonreciprocal between the two chromosomes. If the zygote survives, and some (with this defect) do survive, genetic effects are usually evident in the resulting phenotype, and the translocations may be detected by cytologic study of the chromosomes.

Two more definitions are indicated before we consider some of the specific chromosomal abnormalities that have been discovered so far.

Mosaicism may refer to genes or to whole chromosomes, and usually means that more than one population of cells is present in the body, each population differing in some respect in their chromosomes or genes. Usual usage implies that the differing cell populations are inlaid by some error within the individual during its development. Chromosomal mosaicism, for example, could result from a defect (i.e., nondisjunction) in certain cells in the embryo, giving rise to two populations of cells, one with an extra X chromosome (XXY in a male), while the rest of the cells could be normal (XY).

Chimerism, in this context, implies mosaicism in which one cell type is acquired in utero from a twin. For example, Owen (1945) demonstrated that fraternal bovine twins, one male and one female, with placental anastomoses permitting exchange of hematopoietic cells during fetal life, could be shown later to have red blood cells of two types, one acquired in utero from its twin. Germ cells may also circulate in embryonic life and could give rise to germ cell chimerism.

Anomalies in Sex Chromosomes

In most mammals, male sex is determined by the presence of the Y chromosome, which is received by the zygote from the male parent. Somatic cells resulting from union of an X- and a Y-bearing gamete each contain one Y chromosome derived from the male and one X from the female parent (XY). The female zygote receives one X-bearing gamete from each parent, and therefore each somatic cell normally contains two X chromosomes (XX). Female cells during anaphase were

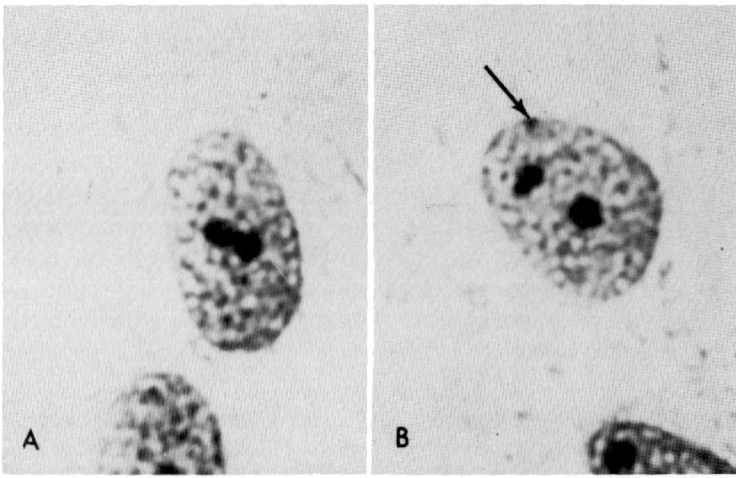

Fig. 8–7.   Sex chromatin in interphase nuclei. (H & E. × 1600.) *A*, Cell from buccal smear of normal male (XY) cat. Sex chromatin absent (negative). *B*, Nucleus from buccal smear of a tortoiseshell male cat (XXY). Barr Body (arrow) at nuclear membrane—one fewer than the number of X chromosomes in the cell.

discovered by Barr (in neurons of *Felis catus*) to differ from male cells in that a small heteropyknotic body was often demonstrable along the nuclear membrane in female cells only. This body (Fig. 8–7) is now called the Barr body or **sex chromatin**. According to the concept first proposed by Lyon (1962), this sex chromatin body consists of one of the X chromosomes, which is genetically inactivated. Presumably, inactivation of this X chromosome occurs early in embryonic life. This inactivated, heteropyknotic X chromosome could be either maternal or paternal in origin in different cells of the same animal. Apparently, only one X chromosome is needed in the activity of the cell, because if more X chromosomes are present in the cell, all but one will be inactivated and appear as sex chromatin. The number of sex chromatin bodies in a cell, therefore, will be one fewer than the number of X chromosomes present. An XX cell will contain one, an XXX cell, two, and an XXXX cell, three sex chromatin bodies. In the absence of sex chromatin, as in a male (XY) cell or an XO female cell, the cell is sometimes depicted as "sex chromatin negative." The sex chromatin is easily demonstrated with simple techniques and is therefore useful in studies of animals with heteroploidy involving the X chromosome.

Klinefelter's Syndrome. In the human subject, Klinefelter's syndrome is recognized in adolescence by small testes, and sometimes eunuchoid features, gynecomastia, low urinary excretion of 17-ketosteroids, and high excretion of gonadotropins. A slender, tall body build is most common, and frequently sexual hair is sparse. Many affected individuals are intellectually subnormal, and many later prove to be infertile. Most males with this syndrome are sex chromatin positive and therefore have more than one X chromosome in their somatic cells. The usual karyotypes are XXY, with most cells containing the extra X chromosome. The modal chromosome count is 47, one more

than the normal number. In some cases of this syndrome, some cells (10 to 50%) contain a different number of X chromosomes. Therefore, these are called XX/XXY mosaics. In come cases, XXYY, and in others, XXXY chromosomal configurations have been described. The cause of this abnormality is not known, but one theory ascribes it to nondisjunction of the X chromosome during gametogenesis. Nondisjunction may be further described as the failure of two chromosomes of a pair to migrate to opposite poles of the cells in meiosis. One gamete may receive both chromosomes and the next, none. The exact cause of this phenomenon is unknown.

The Tortoiseshell Male Cat. In the domestic cat, *Felis catus*, orange coat color and its alternative, black, are determined by genes within the X chromosome; therefore, they are sex-linked. The orange gene (O) is codominant with its allele for black (O$^+$), and both characteristics are expressed in the heterozygote. Modifying genes may result in a panoply of patterns and intensity of color, but the essential feature of the heterozygote is occurrence of both black and orange hair. The black hair may be diluted to blue and the orange hair to cream by the recessive gene for Maltese dilution (d), but the O/O$^+$ genotype still can be detected in the phenotype. This heterozygote is commonly called the tortoiseshell or "tortie." Cats in which the orange and black are mixed with white (due to a dominant gene, S, for piebald) are called "calico" or "tricolor."

Tortoiseshell cats are therefore heterozygous for two sex-linked alleles; therefore, they must have two X chromosomes and consequently must be females. Most tortoiseshells are females, but exceptional male torties sometimes occur. Most tortie males have been reported to be sterile, but a few were said to be fertile. Thuline and Norby (1961) demonstrated that blood cells of two tortoiseshell male cats contained one more than the normal

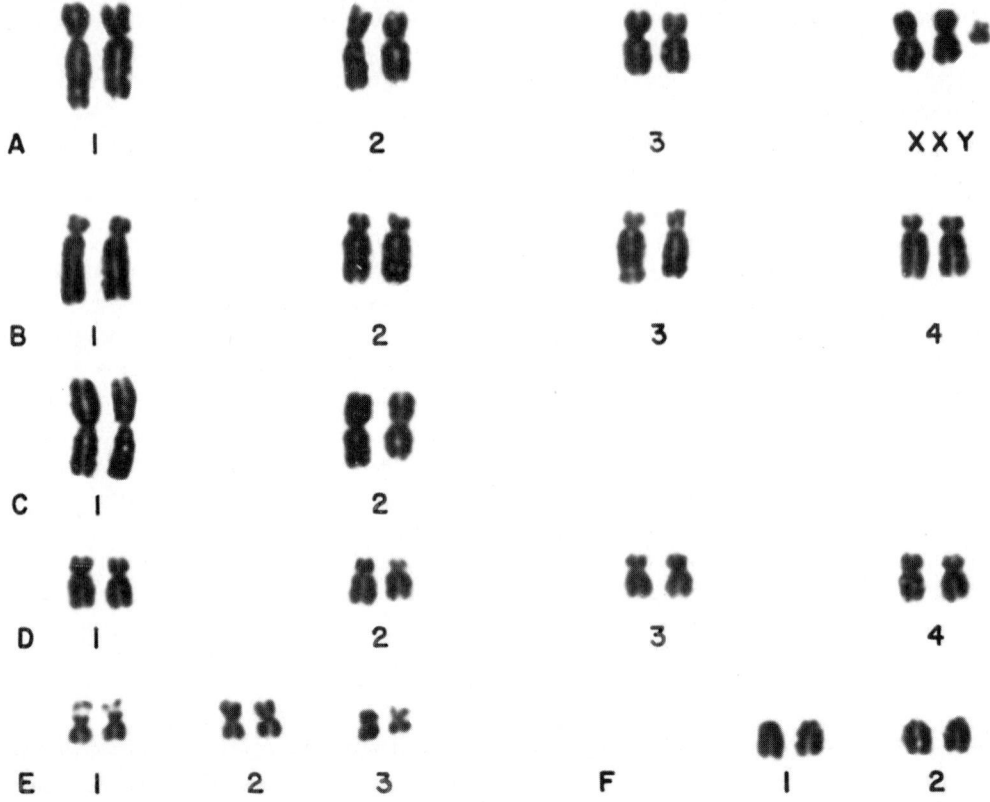

Fig. 8-8. Karyotype of a male tortoiseshell cat. Note the diploid (2n) number is 39 and the sex chromosomes are XXY.

number of chromosomes (2n—39). In our laboratory, we were able to identify the additional chromosome to be an X chromosome in two cats (Fig. 8-8). Further, in one case, XX/XY/XXY mosaicism was demonstrated. Both of these male cats had small testicles and lacked libido. A third male calico studied by Malouf and Benirschke (1967) had an XX/XY mosaic karyotype with a normal (2n—38) number of chromosomes. Chu, Thuline and Norby (1964) described triploid-diploid chimerism in a male tortoiseshell cat which was reportedly sterile, and whose testicles histologically contained Sertoli cells and spermatogonia, but no spermatids or spermatozoa. Cell cultures from the skin of the ear of this cat contained about 55% triploid cells (3n—57), with XXY sex chromosomes. Most of the remainder of the cells in these tissue cultures contained normal XX (2n—38) chromosomes. The two X chromosomes were believed to carry both alternative genes for yellow and black coat color; the Y chromosome was the male sex determinant. This syndrome in the cat appears to mimic Klinefelter's syndrome in man in many respects, and may provide a useful model for studies on its pathogenesis and etiology.

Anomalies of sex chromosomes similar to those described in Klinefelter's syndrome in man and in the tortoiseshell male cat have been reported in sheep (Bruere, Marshall and Ward, 1969), cattle (Rieck, Höhn and Herzog, 1969) and horses (Basrur, Kanagawa and Gilman, 1969).

Turner's Syndrome. A clinical syndrome in women described originally by Turner (1938) consisted of sexual infantilism, webbing of the neck, and cubitus valgus. Similar findings were reported by Ullrich (1930) in children, but sexual deficiency was not recognized in his patients. Oftentimes the syndrome is not recognized until puberty, when menstruation does not begin when expected. These patients are usually short in stature and of slightly lower than average intelligence. It is now known that most of the patients with this syndrome do not have sex chromatin in their somatic cells and have only 45 chromosomes, one less than the normal number of 46. The missing chromosome is the X; therefore, the karyotype can be designated as XO. The lack of this one X chromosome appears to underlie the clinical syndrome, but neither is the cause of the chromosomal abnormality known, nor is the mode of action of the missing X understood. Females of XO karyotype have been described in mice which were fertile and presumably otherwise normal, but this situation has not yet been uncovered in any other species. Gonadal dysgenesis associated with an XO karyotype has been described in mares (Hughes et al., 1975). The phenotype in these mares is unremarkable, except for sterility. Mice with XXY karyotype have also been reported, but no adequate comparison has been made with XXY individuals in man or cat (Russell, 1962).

Intersexes. An intersex or **gynandromorph** is defined as an animal or person with some ambiguity in genitalia or secondary sexual characteristics suggesting both male and female. **Hermaphroditism** includes those animals or persons with both male and female genitalia, external and internal. A **pseudohermaphrodite** has the external genitalia of one sex and the gonads of the opposite sex, the gonadal sex usually added as an adjective in its name. Thus, a male pseudohermaphrodite has female external genitalia and male gonads (testes). It is not unusual for both an ovary and testis, or a fused ovotestis, to be present in some intersexes.

Study of the chromosomes of such intersex animals has added new dimensions to the problem presented by such anomalies, and has led to new theories concerning the factors controlling determination of sexual characteristics. Intersexes have been described in many species, and increasing numbers are now being studied from the genetic and cytogenetic points of view. No completely consistent chromosomal pattern has yet emerged, but most affected animals appear to be chimeric as far as their sex chromosomes are concerned. This aspect has been reviewed in admirable detail in all species by Benirschke (1970).

Intersexuality has been studied at some length in swine (Basrur and Kanagawa, 1971; Melander et al., 1971; Bäckström and Henricson, 1971). In most cases, the affected pigs have an underdeveloped vulva, enlarged clitoris, and a scrotum, often containing one testis. Male accessory sex glands are often present internally, and a uterine body and two cornua may be found. An ovotestis is sometimes present at the anterior extremity of one or both uterine horns. The chromosome complement most often is normal female (38XX). Adult animals may behave sexually as either male or female. Inheritance has been postulated to be by means of a single recessive gene, but the data do not support this concept. In one study (Bäckström and Henricson, 1971), for example, a boar mated to eight sows produced 12 intersexes among 160 piglets. This frequency (0.075) of affected animals does not equal the expected frequency (0.25) from a homozygous recessive gene.

An intersex horse has been studied cytogenetically (Basrur, Kanagawa, and Podiachouk, 1970). In this animal, 64XX and 64XY chromosomal configurations were reported in gonadal tissue, and cells with XX, XY, XXY and XO karyotypes were found in other tissues.

Freemartinism. A problem of continued interest is the hypogonadism and sterility of female bovines which are carried in utero with a male twin. These particular heifers have been recognized for many years and are usually designated by a name of obscure origin: **freemartin**. The phenomenon of freemartinism is not thoroughly explained, but appears to be associated with several situations. First, the male and female cotwins share a common placental circulation in utero, which allows them to exchange hematopoietic and germ cells early in embryonic life. Second, the cells from one embryo establish themselves in the cotwin, producing chimerism, which can be demonstrated in sex chromosomes and erythrocyte antigens. The presence of XX cells in gonads and other tissues of male calves which are twins of females appears to reduce fertility, and the XY cells in the female cotwin is associated with sterility. However, in twin marmosets, germ cell chimerism is not associated with sterility; hence, a direct causal effect of the heterosexual germ cells is not established.

The earlier theory concerning the etiology of freemartinism induced the postulate that androgenic hormones produced by the testicles of the male twin had a deleterious effect upon the development of the female gonad. This theory still remains viable, although definitive evidence to support it has not yet been forthcoming.

Testicular Feminization. This anomaly affects the phenotypic expression of sexuality, is reported in human patients, and appears to have a counterpart in animals. The patient has female secondary sexual characteristics, including female external and internal genitalia, except for the presence of testes in place of ovaries. The karyotype in all cells is XY. This situation is explained on the basis of an inherited, single gene defect, which makes all tissues unresponsive to androgenic hormones, particularly testosterone. Thus, in spite of the presence of a functioning testis, male genitalia and secondary sex characteristics do not develop.

Ohno and Lyon (1970) have described a sex-linked genetic characteristic in mice which has these features of testicular feminization. These workers demonstrated that cells of mice homozygous for the defective gene are unable to respond to testosterone or dihydrotestosterone. This is demonstrated in renal tubular cells, in which alcohol dehydrogenase is produced in normal mice by stimulation with androgens, but no alcohol dehydrogenase is developed in mice homozygous for the defective gene. Similar cases have been described in sheep (Bruere, McDonald and Marshall, 1969) and cattle (Short, 1967).

Armstrong, C. N., and Marshall, A. J.: Intersexuality in Vertebrates Including Man. London, Academic Press, 1964.

Bäckström, L, and Henricson, B.: Intersexuality in the pig. Acta Vet. Scand., 12:257–273, 1971.

Basrur, P. K., Kanagawa, H., and Gilman, J. P. W.: An equine intersex with unilateral gonadal agenesis. Can. J. Comp. Med., 33:297–306, 1969.

Basrur, P. K., Kosaka, S., and Kanagawa, H.: Blood cell chimerism and freemartinism in heterosexual bovine quadruplets. J. Hered., 61:15–18, 1970.

Basrur, P. K., Kanagawa, H., and Podiachouk, L.: Further studies on the cell populations of an intersex horse. Can. J. Comp. Med., 34:294, 1970.

Basrur, P. K., and Kanagawa, H.: Sex anomalies in pigs. J. Reprod. Fertil., 26:369–371, 1971.

Benirschke, K.: Spontaneous chimerism in mammals. A critical review. Curr. Top. Pathol., 51:1–61, 1970.

Benirschke, K., and Brownhill, L. E.: Further observations on marrow chimerism in marmosets. Cytogenetics, 1:245–257, 1962.

Benirschke, K., et al.: Chromosome study of an alleged fertile mare mule. J. Hered., 55:31–38, 1964.

Biggers, J. D., and McFeely, R. A.: Intersexuality in domestic mammals. *In* Advances in Reproductive Physiology, ed. by A. McLaren. London, Logos Press, 1966.

Bruere, A. N.: Male sterility and an autosomal translocation in Romney sheep. Cytogenetics, 8:209–218, 1969.

Bruere, A. N., Marshall, R. B., and Ward, D. P. J.: Testicular hypoplasia and XXY sex chromosome complement in two rams: the ovine counterpart of Klinefelter's syndrome in man. J. Reprod. Fertil., 19:103–108, 1969.

Bruere, A. N., McDonald, M. F., and Marshall, R. B.: Cytogenetical analysis of an ovine male pseudohermaphrodite and the possible role of the Y chromosome in cryptorchidism of sheep. Cytogenetics, 8:148–157, 1969.

Cattanach, B. M.: XXY mice. Genet. Res., 2:156–160, 1961.

———: XO mice. Genet. Res., 3:487–490, 1962.

Carr, D. H.: Chromosome studies on abortuses and stillborn infants. Lancet, 2:603–606, 1963.

Chu, E. H. Y., Thuline, H. C., and Norby, D. E.: Triploid-diploid chimerism in a male tortoiseshell cat. Cytogenetics, 3:1–18, 1964.

Clendenin, T. M., and Benirschke, K.: Chromosome studies on spontaneous abortions. Lab. Invest., 12:1281–1292, 1963.

Clough, E., et al.: An XXY sex chromosome constitution in a dog with testicular hypoplasia and congenital heart disease. Cytogenetics, 9:71–77, 1970.

Dunn, H. O., McEntee, K., and Hansel, W.: Diploid-triploid chimerism in a bovine true hermaphrodite. Cytogenetics, 9:245–259, 1970.

Dunn, H. O., Vaughan, J. T., and McEntee, K.: Bilaterally cryptorchid stallion with female karyotype. Cornell Vet., 64:265–275, 1974.

Gerneke, W. H., and Coubrough, R. I.: Intersexuality in the horse. Onderstepoort J. Vet. Res., 37:211–215, 1970.

Hard, W. L.: The anatomy and cytogenetics of male pseudohermaphroditism in swine. Anat. Rec., 157:255–256, 1967.

Hughes, J. P., Kennedy, P. C., and Benirschke, K.: XO-gonadal dysgenesis in the mare (report of two cases). Equine Vet. J., 7:109–112, 1975.

Jones, T. C.: Anomalies of sex chromosomes in male tortoiseshell cats. In Comparative Mammalian Cytogenetics, ed. by K. Benirschke. Berlin-Heidelberg, Springer, 1969.

Kanagawa, H., and Basrur, P. K.: The leukocyte culture method in the diagnosis of freemartinism. Can. J. Comp. Med., 32:583–586, 1968.

Kosaka, S., et al.: Abnormal blood type and female type of chromosome in a male of heterosexual bovine twins. Jpn. J. Zootech. Sci., 40:238–242, 1969.

Krishnamurty, S., Macpherson, J. W., and King, G. J.: Intersexuality in Ontario swine. Can. J. Anim. Sci., 51:807–809, 1971.

Loughman, W. D., Frye, F. L., and Condon, T. B.: XY/XXY bone marrow mosaicism in three male tricolor cats. Am. J. Vet. Res., 31:307–314, 1970.

Lubs, H. A., and Ruddle, F. H.: Chromosomal abnormalities in the human population: estimation of rates based on New Haven newborn study. Science, 169:495–497, 1970.

Lyon, M. F.: Sex chromatin and gene action in the mammalian X chromosome. Am. J. Hum. Genet., 14:135–148, 1962.

Malouf, N., Benirschke, K., and Hoefnagel, D.: XX-XY chimerism in a tricolored male cat. Cytogenetics (Basel), 6:228–241, 1967.

McFeely, R. A., Hare, W. C. D., and Biggers, J. D.: Chromosome studies in 14 cases of intersex in domestic animals. Cytogenetics, 6:242–253, 1967.

McKusick, V. A.: On the X Chromosome of Man. Washington, D.C., Amer. Inst. Biol. Sci., 1964.

Melander, Y., Hanse, M. E. I., Holm, L., and Somley, B.: Seven swine intersexes with XX chromosome constitution. Hereditas, 69:51–58, 1971.

Miller, O. J.: The sex chromosome anomalies. Am. J. Obstet. Gynecol., 90:1078–1139, 1961.

Miyake, Y. I.: Cytogenetical studies on swine intersexes. Jpn. J. Vet. Res., 21:41–50, 1973.

Mukherjee, B. B., and Sinha, A. K.: Cytological evidence for random inactivation of X-chromosomes in a female mule complement. Proc. Nat. Acad. Sci., 51:252–254, 1964.

Owen, R. D.: Immunogenetic consequences of vascular anastomoses between bovine twins. Science, 102:400–401, 1945.

Payne, H. W., Willsworth, K., and DeGrott, A.: Aneuploidy in an infertile mare. J. Am. Vet. Med. Assoc., 153:1293–1299, 1968.

Rieck, G. W., Höhn, H., and Herzog, A.: Hypogonadismus, Intermittierender Kryptorchidismus und segmentäre Aplasia der Ductus Wolffii bei einem männlichen Rind mit XXY—Konstellation bsw. XXY/XX/XY—Gonosomen-Mosaik. Dtsch. Tierarztl. Wochenschr., 76:133–138, 1969.

Rigdon, R. H., and Mott, C.: Testis in the sterile hybrid duck. A histologic and histochemical study. Path. Vet., 2:553–565, 1965.

Russell, L. B.: Chromosome aberrations in experimental mammals. In Progress in Medical Genetics, Vol. II by A. G. Steinberg and A. G. Bearn. New York, Grune & Stratton, 1962.

Sampath Kumaran, J. D., and Iya, K. K.: Sex chromatin in bovines. Indian Vet. J., 42:377–383, 1965.

Short, R. V.: Reproduction. Ann. Rev. Physiol., 29:373–400, 1967.

Thuline, H. C., and Norby, D. E.: Spontaneous occurrence of chromosome abnormalities in cat. Science, 134:554–555, 1961.

Toyama, Y.: Sex chromosome mosaicisms in five swine intersexes. Jpn. J. Zootech. Sci., 45:551–557, 1974.

Anomalies in Autosomal Chromosomes

Autosomes would appear, at first examination, to be more frequently involved in defects than the sex chromosomes, simply because there are more of them. Clinical deviations related to abnormal sex chromosomes are, on the contrary, much more frequent in the human subject. The explanation may be that abnormal autosomes may be more apt to lead to death of the zygote, therefore leaving fewer abnormal living phenotypes. It does appear that lesions in autosomes do have a more serious effect on the individual than similar defects in sex chromosomes.

Trisomy. **Down's syndrome** or **mongolism** in children, although described over a hundred years ago (Down, 1866), is associated with one of two anomalies of autosomal chromosomes. Affected children are mentally retarded and have other physical features that characterize the syndrome. The cells of patients with this syndrome are usually aneuploid, with a chromosome number of 47. The extra chromosome is usually found to be one of the small acrocentric chromosomes defined as number 21. This trisomy was the first discovered, and apparently is the most frequent. Some children with Down's syndrome were subsequently found to have the normal number (2n—46) of chromosomes, but karyotype analysis revealed evidence of a translocation involving chromosome number 21.

Trisomy of a small acrocentric autosomal chromosome in a young female chimpanzee *(Pan troglodytes)* has been reported by McClure et al. (1969). This chimpanzee was born in the Yerkes Regional Primate Research Center from parents with normal karyotypes and phenotypes. The sire was 21 years old and the dam, 14, at the time of birth of the trisomic offspring. The dam had delivered a premature stillborn infant 28 months prior to this parturition. At birth, this chimp was in the low normal range of weight in comparison with other chimps born in this laboratory. She grew significantly slower than normal chimps. Several congenital anomalies were noted: bilateral partial syndactyly of the toes with clinodactyly, prominent epicanthus, hyperflexibility of the joints, and a short neck with excess skin folds. Several neurologic abnormalities were present, including absence of the Moro reflex, marked hypotonia, abnormal traction and suspension responses, and general inactivity. Several deficiencies in postural behavior were evident in comparison to other chimpanzees at the same age. Each of these features in this trisomic chimpanzee are similar to those observed in human infants with Down's syndrome. This raises interesting speculation about the possible homology of the small acrocentric chromosomes of man and chimpanzee.

Another defect of autosomes has been established as occurring repeatedly in man, and involves trisomy of chromosome 17 or 18. This defect has been associated with odd-shaped skull, low-set and malformed ears, micrognathia, webbing of the neck, probable mental retardation, and a congenital heart defect. A third autosomal abnormality, trisomy of the group 13–15 of large acrocentric chromosomes, has been found in children with multiple congenital anomalies such as harelip, cleft palate, and bilateral coloboma. Other abnormal chromosomes have been reported, but the above serve to illustrate aberrations in autosomes that result in viable but seriously altered phenotypes.

Malignant Disease and Chromosomes. In human cases of chronic granulocytic leukemia, cells have been found with a small isologous chromosome, presumably number 21, which has lost a quarter of its long arm. This "marker" chromosome is called the **Philadelphia or Ph[1] chromosome**, after the city in which it was first described (Nowell & Hungerford, 1961). The consistent occurrence of an extra and a marker chromosome in granulocytic leukemia of the mouse has been reported by Wald et al. (1963).

In cases of bovine lymphosarcoma (malignant lymphoma), interesting chromosomal alterations have been found. Basrur and associates (1964) described the occurrence of three large submetacentric chromosomes, resembling the X chromosome in this species, in a complement of 61 (2n) chromosomes (Fig. 8–9). In other cells cultured from the circulating blood of cattle affected with lymphosarcoma, Hare et al. (1964) have found several chromosomal abnormalities. Although some inconsistency between individuals was evident, in several cases modal chromosome numbers were heteroploid due to the presence of large extra telocentric and metacentric chromosomes and the loss of one X chromosome.

Dr. P. K. Basrur graciously permitted me to study karyotypes of cells cultured from five dogs with lymphosarcoma (malignant lymphoma). Two of the these were males; three, females. All had more than the nor-

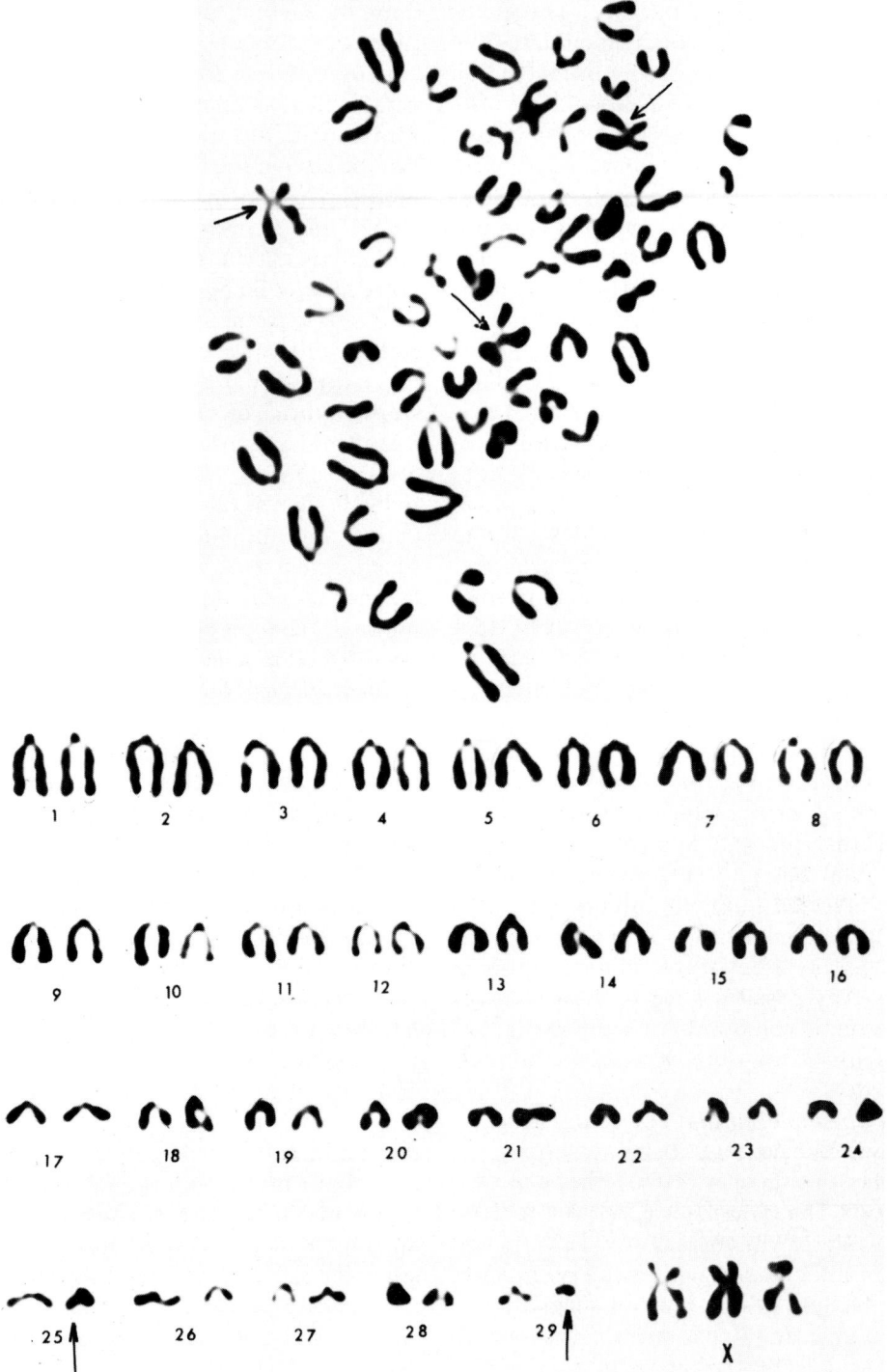

Fig. 8–9. Metaphase spread (top) and karyotype of a cell from a cow with malignant lymphoma (lymphosarcoma). Note the two large extra metacentric chromosomes and the total number (2n—61). (Courtesy of Dr. Parvathi K. Basrur, Ontario Veterinary College.)

mal number of metacentrics—two females with normal diploid complement (2n—78) had three (one more than normal) large submetacentric chromosomes, and one female with 2n—77 had two large and two smaller metacentric chromosomes. One male dog had a normal complement (2n—78), but an extra large metacentric chromosome was present. The second male dog with lymphosarcoma also had two large metacentrics and 2n—77. Further details may be found in the publication by Dr. Basrur (1966).

Malignant Lymphoma in Cats. This disease is accompanied by a panoply of chromosomal abnormalities in affected cells (Jones, 1969). Four groups of anomalies have been identified: (I) due to loss of a single chromosome in group E, resulting in a modal chromosome number of 37 (see normal karyotype, p. 247); (II) a single chromosome lost from group D, causing the modal number of chromosomes to be 37; (III) an additional acrocentric chromosome in group F, resulting in a total number of chromosomes of 39; (IV) additional chromosomes in groups C, D, E, and F, resulting in 2n numbers of 40 and 41. In a final category (V), no abnormalities were detected in the lymphomatous cells. This severe aneuploidy in malignant cells may be the effect of the feline lymphoma virus. Any possible effect of these changes in chromosome number on the malignant behavior of the cells is yet to be demonstrated.

Sterility in Hybrids. The mule, our best known hybrid, has been described as "without pride of ancestry or hope of posterity." The underlying reason for the mule's sterility is of much scientific interest and is still clouded with mystery. In spite of published descriptions of allegedly fertile mules, doubt has been expressed by Benirschke (1964) that reportedly fertile mules were actually mules. In his view, in fact, they may have been donkeys. Karyotype analysis now offers one approach to this problem, but is yet to be

done on such allegedly fertile mules. The domestic horse *(Equus caballus)* is now known to have a 2n number of 64 chromosomes; the ass *(Equus asinus)*, 62 chromosomes; and the mule, not unexpectedly, has the sum of the haploid number of each of his parents—namely, 63. Benirschke (1962) has demonstrated an intriguing panoply of chromosome numbers in many varieties of wild equines (Table 8–1). Variation in chromosome number and arrangement may provide an important mechanism that affects evolution. The sterile hybrid, on the other hand, presents a dead end in the development of new varieties or species. The cause of sterility in hybrids such as the mule is unknown. One of the possibilities is that unequal numbers of chromosomes are unable to pair off ("synapse") during that specific phase of meiosis. The problem has many aspects needing more adequate study.

Spontaneous Human Abortions. Studies by several investigators, particularly Benirschke (1963), Clendenin (1963), and Carr (1963) have uncovered chromosomal abnormalities in human aborted and stillborn fetuses. It appears likely that the chromosomal defects were causally related to the intrauterine death of these fetuses. Among the defects in the chromosomes of these abortuses or fetuses were the following: translocation on chromosome A (2n—46); trisomy of group E (pair 16) (2n—47); anencephaly, XO sex chromosomes (2n—45); triploidy and XXY sex chromosomes (2n—69); trisomy of group D (2n—47) and tetraploid cultures. It has been estimated that about one chromosomal abnormality occurs in 200 live births. These aberrations are much more frequent in aborted and stillborn fetuses; one estimate puts this frequency at about 30% of all spontaneously interrupted pregnancies (Benirschke, 1963).

The significance of finding defective chromosomes in these human patients is yet to be fully determined, but it appears that such defects may well contribute signficantly to the nonviable state of many human embryos.

The chromosomes of aborted animals of any species are yet to be studied. Such studies may prove to be quite revealing.

Basrur, P. K., Gilman, J. P. W., and McSherry, B. J.: Cytological observations on a bovine lymphosarcoma. Nature (Lond.), 201:368–371, 1964.
Basrur, P. K., and Gilman, J. P. W.: Chromosome studies in canine lymphosarcoma. Cornell Vet., 56:451–469, 1966.
Benirschke, K., Brownhill, L. E., and Beath, M. M.: Somatic chromosomes of the horse, the donkey, and their hybrids, the mule and the hinny. J. Reprod. Fertil., 4:319–326, 1962.
Benirschke, K.: Chromosomal studies on abortuses. Trans. New Eng. Obstet. Gyn. Soc., 17:171–183, 1963.
Benirschke, K., Low, R. J., Sullivan, M. M., and Carter, R. M.: Chromosome study of an alleged fertile mare mule. J. Hered., 55:31–38, 1964.
Benjamin, S. A., and Noronha, F.: Cytogenic studies in canine lymphosarcoma. Cornell Vet., 57:526–542, 1967.
Bruere, A. N., and Chapman, H. M.: Autosomal translocations in two exotic breeds of cattle in New Zealand. Vet. Rec., 92:615–618, 1973.
Carr, D. H.: Chromosome studies on abortuses and stillborn infants. Lancet, 2:603–606, 1963.
Clendenin, T. M., and Benirschke, K.: Chromosome studies on spontaneous abortions. Lab. Invest., 12:1281–1292, 1963.
Hare, W. C. D., et al.: Chromosomal studies in bovine lymphosarcoma. J. Nat. Cancer Inst., 33:105–118, 1964.
———: Cytogenetics in the dog and cat. J. Small Anim. Pract., 7:575–592, 1966.
Harvey, M. J. A.: An autosomal translocation in the Charolais breed of cattle. Vet. Rec., 89:110–111, 1971.
Jones, T. C.: Chromosomal analyses of feline lymphomas. Nat. Cancer Inst. Monograph No. 32, p. 95, 1969.
McClure, H. M., et al.: Autosomal trisomy in a chimpanzee: resemblance to Down's syndrome. Science, 165:1010–1012, 1969.
Miles, C. P., Moldavannu, G., Miller, D. G., and Moore, A.: Chromosome analysis of canine lymphosarcoma: two cases involving probable centric fusion. Am. J. Vet. Res., 31:783–790, 1970.
Nowell, P. C., and Hungerford, D. A.: Chromosome studies in human leukemia. II. Chronic granulocytic leukemia. J. Nat. Cancer Inst., 27:1013–1035, 1961.
Pollock, D.: A chromosome abnormality in Friesian cattle in Great Britain. Vet. Rec., 90:309–310, 1972.
Rich, M. A., Tsuchida, R., and Siegler, R.: Chromosome aberrations: their role in the etiology of murine leukemia. Science, 146:252–253, 1964.
Russell, L. B.: Chromosome aberrations in experimental mammals. In Progress in Medical Genetics. Vol. II, by A. G. Steinberg and A. G. Bearn. New York, Grune & Stratton, 1962.
Tsuchida, R., and Rich, M. A.: Chromosomal aberrations in viral leukemogenesis. I. Friend and Rauscher leukemia. J. Nat. Cancer Inst., 33:33–47, 1964.
Wald, N., et al.: The consistent occurrence of an extra and a marker chromosome in mouse granulocytic leukemia. Mamm. Cyto. Confer. Vergennes, Vermont, 1963.
Weber, W. T., Nowell, P. C., and Hare, W. C. D.: Chromosome studies of a transplanted and a primary canine venereal sarcoma. J. Nat. Cancer Inst., 35:537–547, 1965.

PATHOLOGIC STATES DETERMINED BY ONE OR MORE GENES

In conformity with our policy of considering pathologic entities in relation to their specific etiology when known, in the following section are described some entities that have been characterized adequately and for which convincing evidence of their genetic basis is available. The numbers of such diseases is increasing rapidly, and it is not possible to include all that should be so categorized. Some are listed in Tables 8–2 through 8–12; others may be found only in the references, or in the chapters directed toward the anatomic systems involved.

Lethal Genes

One should not be surprised, after consideration of even a few aspects of genetic mechanisms, to learn that some defective genes result in death of the zygote. This lethal effect may be expressed at any time after fertilization—in the embryo, fetus, newborn, or adult animal. Many other (sublethal) genes result in defects that lower vitality or produce other undesirable characteristics, but do not result in death. Most completely lethal genes are recessive and recognized only by their full expression in the homozygous animal. In most instances, one normal gene is sufficient to overcome the presence of the homologous abnormal gene.

An example to demonstrate present concepts concerning the pathogenesis of a characteristic controlled by a single lethal gene is found in hemophilia A, which occurs in nearly identical form in man and the dog. This gene is sex-linked—i.e., carried in the X chromosome. The female, with her two X chromosomes, can be either homozygous or heterozygous for this gene. The male, with only one X, can only be hemizygous. If his single X chromosome contains the abnormal gene, he will be affected with hemophilia. The affected male produces no factor VIII (antihemophilic globulin, AHG), which is needed to protect him against uncontrolled bleeding. The homozygous normal and the heterozygous female usually produce normal amounts of factor VIII, but in some instances (Graham et al., 1951), the heterozygote (carrier) produces somewhat reduced amounts of factor VIII. No matter which of several explanations now current for this phenomenon are most accurate, it can be seen that quantitative analysis of the specific protein or specific enzyme may provide a means of detecting the carrier heterozygote. This is a matter of potential importance in control of genetically determined diseases in animals.

One important and practical problem should be considered in the study of the effect of lethal or sublethal genes in animals. This involves what the pathologist would call specific pathologic diagnosis, and the geneticist, "identification of the phenotype." In some cases, simple clinical inspection may be adequate, but in most instances, careful study by chemical and pathologic methods is necessary. For example, clinically manifest cerebellar ataxia in young kittens may be found at necropsy to result from grossly recognizable hypoplasia of the cerebellum; from absence of Purkinje cells in the cerebellum; or from microscopically detectable encephalitic lesions in the cerebellum. These three lesions may each have different causes, only one, or none of them due to genetic factors. Much needs to be done in the elucidation of the character of the le-sions in animals as well as in underlying genetic mechanisms.

Mendelian ratios in progeny, study of pedigrees, test matings, coupled with adequate studies using clinical and pathologic techniques, are helpful in gaining presumptive evidence to decide whether a disease is merely congenital (acquired in utero and usually evident at birth) or whether it is also actually genetically controlled (i.e., inborn or inherited from the parents and the result of the recombination of genetic factors). Much more must be learned about the mechanisms involved at the molecular level before an adequate understanding is reached. The interactions of environmental factors (i.e., viruses, toxic chemicals, x-radiation, nutritional factors) must be more carefully studied to uncover all possible modes of action upon animal cells and particularly upon their genetic mechanisms (especially DNA and RNA).

Inherited Diseases

Evidence concerning the inherited nature of animal diseases is accumulating to the point that not enough space is available in this book to present the data adequately. A series of tables is included in this chapter to indicate the scope of this subject. In many cases, the disease entities are described in more detail in the chapters arranged by anatomic systems. In many cases, disease states that are probably hereditary are not described adequately or the genetic data is incomplete. This presents a challenge for the future. We also must make a clear distinction between congenital (present at birth) and hereditary (genetically determined) abnormalities.

Inherited Diseases of Two or More Anatomic Systems

Brandt, E. J., and Swank, R. T.: The Chediak-Higashi (Biege) mutation in two mouse strains. Am. J. Pathol., 82:573–588, 1976.

Ceh, L., Hauge, J. G., Svenkerud, R., and Strande, A.: Glycogenosis type III in the dog. Acta Vet. Scand., 17:210–222, 1976.

Erickson, R. P., Glueoksohn-Waelsch, S., and Cori, C. F.: Glucose-6-phosphatase deficiency caused by radiation-induced alleles at the albino locus in the mouse. Proc. Natl. Acad. Sci. U.S.A., 59:437–444, 1968.

Glenn, B. L., Glenn, H. G., and Omtvedt, I. T.: Congenital porphyria in the domestic cat (Felis catus): preliminary investigations on inheritance pattern. Am. J. Vet. Res., 29:1653–1657, 1968.

Giddens, W. E., Jr., Labbe, R. F., Swango, L. J., and Padgett, G. A.: Feline congenital erythropoietic porphyria associated with severe anemia and renal disease. Am. J. Pathol., 80:367–386, 1975.

Graham, J. B., Collins, D. L., and Brinkhous, K. M.: Assay of plasma antihemophilic activity in normal, heterozygous (hemophilia) and prothrombinogenic dogs. Proc. Soc. Exp. Biol. Med., 77:294, 1951.

Gross, S. R.: Animal models of glycogen storage conditions. West. J. Med., 123:194–201, 1975.

Hartley, W. J., and Blakemore, W. F.: Neurovisceral glucocerebroside storage (Gaucher's disease) in a dog. Vet. Pathol., 10:191–201, 1974.

Hocking, J. D., Jolly, R. D., and Batt, R. D.: Deficiency of alpha-mannosidase in Angus cattle. An inherited lysosomal storage disease. Biochem. J., 128:69–78, 1972.

Jolly, R. D., and Blakemore, W. F.: Inherited lysosomal storage disease: an essay in comparative medicine. Vet. Rec., 92:391–400, 1973.

Jolly, R. D., et al.: Identification of mannosidosis heterozygotes—factors affecting normal plasma alpha-mannosidase levels. NZ Vet. J., 22:155–162, 1974.

Jones, T.C.: Hereditary disease. In Pathology of Laboratory Animals, Vol. II, edited by K. Benirschke, F.M. Garner, and T.C. Jones. New York, Springer-Verlag, 1978, pp. 1981–2064.

Kaneko, J. J., and Mills, R.: Hematological and blood chemistry observations on neonatal normal and porphyric calves in early life. Cornell Vet., 60:52–60, 1970.

Keeling, M. E., McClure, H. M., and Kibler, R. F.: Alkaptonuria in an orangutan (Pongo pygmaeus). Am. J. Phys. Anthropol., 38:435–438, 1973.

Kramer, J. W., Davis, W. C., and Prieur, J.: The Chediak-Higashi syndrome of cats. Lab. Invest., 36:554–562, 1977.

Levin, E. Y., and Flyger, V.: Uroporphyrinogen III. Cosynthetase activity in the Fox squirrel (Sciurus niger). Science, 174:59–60, 1971.

Lyon, J. B., Jr., and Porter, J.: The relation of phosphorylase to glycogenolysis in skeletal muscle and heart of mice. J. Biol. Chem., 238:1–11, 1963.

Manktelow, W., and Hartley, W. J.: Generalized glycogen storage disease in sheep. J. Comp. Pathol., 85:139–145, 1975.

Mostafa, I. E.: A case of glycogenic cardiomegaly in a dog. Acta Vet. Scand., 11:197–208, 1970.

Padgett, G. A., Holland, J. M., Davis, W. C., and Henson, J. B.: The Chediak-Higashi syndrome: a comparative review. Curr. Top. Pathol., 51:175–194, 1970.

Phillips, N. C., Robinson, D., Winchester, B. G., and

Jolly, R. D.: Mannosidosis in Angus cattle. The enzymic defect. Biochem. J., 137:363–371, 1974.

Rafiquzzaman, M., Svenkerud, R., Strande, A., and Hauge, J. G.: Glycogenosis in the dog. Acta Vet. Scand., 17:196–209, 1976.

Renshaw, H. W., Davis, W. C., Funderberg, H. H., and Padgett, G. A.: Leukocyte dysfunction in the bovine homologue of the Chediak-Higashi syndrome of humans. Infect. Immun., 10:928–937, 1974.

Sandström, B., Westman, J., and Ockerman, P. A.: Glycogenosis of the central nervous system in the cat. Acta Neuropathol. (Berl.), 14:194–200, 1969.

Tobias, G.: Congenital porphyria in a cat. J. Am. Vet. Med. Assoc., 145:462–463, 1964.

Wass, W. M., and Hoyt, H. H.: Bovine congenital porphyria: Studies on heredity. Am. J. Vet. Res., 26:654–658, 1965.

Watkins, S. P., Jr., Binley, H., and Shulman, N. R.: Alkaptonuria in a chimpanzee. In Medical Primatology, 1970, edited by E. I. Goldsmith and J. Moor-Jankowski. Basel, S. Karger, 1971. pp. 297–298.

Whittem, J. H., and Walker, D.: "Neuronopathy" and "pseudolipidosis" in Aberdeen Angus calves. J. Pathol. Bacteriol., 74:281–288, 1957.

Windhorst, D. B., and Padgett, G. A.: The Chediak-Higashi syndrome and the homologous trait in animals. J. Invest. Dermatol., 60:529–537, 1973.

Inherited Diseases of Integument

Anderson, J. H., and Brown, R. E.: Cutaneous asthenia in a dog. J. Am. Vet. Med. Assoc., 173:742–743, 1978.

Edmonds, H. W., and Dolan, W. D.: Ichthyosis congenita fetalis, severe type (Harlequin fetus). Bull. Intern. Assoc. Med. Mus., 32:1–21, 1951.

Eldridge, F. E., and Atkeson, F. W.: Streaked hairlessness in Holstein-Friesian cattle. J. Hered., 44:265–271, 1953.

Green, M. C.: Chapter 8. In Biology of the Laboratory Mouse, edited by E. L. Green. New York, McGraw-Hill, 1964.

Halliwell, R. E. W., and Schwartzman, R. M.: Atopic disease in the dog. Vet. Rec., 89:209–214, 1971.

Hegreberg, G. A., Padgett, G. A., Gorham, J. R., and Henson, J. B.: Connective tissue disease of dogs and mink resembling Ehlers-Danlos syndrome of man. J. Hered., 60:249–254, 1969.

Hegreberg, G. A., Padgett, G. A., and Henson, J. B.: Connective tissue disease of dogs and mink resembling Ehlers-Danlos syndrome of man. III. Histopathologic changes of the skin. Arch. Pathol., 90:159–166, 1970.

Hjarre, A.: Vegetierende Dermatosen mit Reisenzellen-pneumonien bei Schwein. Dtsch. Tierarzl. Wochenschr., 60:105–110, 1953.

Hutt, F. B.: Inherited lethal characters in domestic animals. Cornell Vet., 24:1–25, 1934.

Hutt, F. B., and Frost, J. N.: Hereditary epithelial defects in Ayrshire cattle. J. Hered., 39:131–137, 1948.

Table 8–2.   Examples of Inherited Diseases of Two or More Anatomic Systems

Scientific and Common Names	Genetic Designation and Gene Symbol	Clinical and Pathologic Features; Species	References
Alkaptonuria	Unknown	Deficiency of homogentisic acid oxidase results in accumulation and excretion of homogentisic acid; urine turns brown to black on standing; ochronosis in human patients; rare event in chimpanzee and orangutan.	Watkins et al., 1971; Keeling, et al., 1973
Chediak-Higashi syndrome	A, r	Granules in cytoplasm of leukocytes and other cells; partial oculocutaneous albinism; increased susceptibility to infection; a bleeding tendency. Man, mice, cats, cattle, mink, a killer whale.	Brandt and Swank, 1976; Kramer et al., 1977; Padgett et al., 1970; Renshaw et al., 1974; Windhorst and Padgett, 1973
Glycogenoses (Glycogen storage diseases)	A, r	(1) Von Gierke's syndrome (man, mouse) results from deficiency of glucose-6-phosphatase, causing glycogen storage in liver, kidney, intestine.	Erickson et al., 1968; Gross, 1975
	A, r	(2) Pompe's disease—putative cases in dog (enzyme defect not demonstrated); hypertrophied heart, glycogen deposits in brain, liver, lungs, esophagus, kidneys.	Mostafa, 1970

	S, r	(3) Phosphorylase kinase deficiency in mice comparable to McArdle disease in man; temporary weakness and cramping of skeletal muscles following exercise; myoglobinuria.	Lyon and Porter, 1963; Gross, 1975
	Unknown	(4) Glycogen storage disease reported in sheep, dog, and cat; lesions described, but enzyme defect not yet identified.	Manktelow and Hartley, 1975; Sandström et al., 1969; Rafiquzzaman et al., 1976; Ceh et al., 1976
Mannosidosis (pseudolipidosis)	A, r	Associated with deficiency of lysosomal enzyme, α-mannosidase; ataxia, tremor of head, aggressive behavior, death usually in first year of life (cattle); similar disease in man.	Whittem and Walker, 1957; Hocking et al., 1972; Phillips et al., 1974; Jolly et al., 1974
Neurovisceral glucocerebrosidosis (Gaucher's disease)	A, r (?)	Cerebroside kerasin accumulates in reticuloendothelial cells; spleen, skin, bone and lung involved; reported in man and dog; enzyme deficiency: glucocerebrosidase	Jolly and Blakemore, 1973; Hartley and Blakemore, 1974
Porphyria (Erythropoietic porphyria)	A, D	Recognized in man, cattle, cats; porphyrins accumulate as brown, fluorescent pigment in bones and teeth; anemia and renal disease observed in cats; porphyrins in skin produce photosensitization in sunlight; apparently tolerated in Fox squirrel.	Glenn et al., 1968; Giddens et al., 1975; Kaneko and Mills, 1970; Levin and Flyger, 1971; Tobias, 1964; Wass and Hoyt, 1965

Table 8–3. Examples of Inherited Diseases of Integument

Scientific and Common Names	Genetic Designation and Gene Symbol	Clinical and Pathologic Features; Species	References
Atopy (Atopic disease)	Unknown	Recognized in dogs; pruritus, erythema, scaling of skin; occasionally purulent conjunctivitis; hypersensitivity to pollens exposed through respiratory route; IgE antibody produced; diagnosis by patch tests with ragweed pollen.	Halliwell and Schwartzman, 1971; Patterson, 1959; Rockey and Schwartzman, 1967; Schwartzman, 1965; Wittich, 1941
Atrichia (Hairlessness)	A, D	Gene is lethal in homozygous state in dogs; hairless animals are heterozygous for gene; homozygotes lack pinnae, may have stenotic esophagus; usually born dead. Several genes in mice, rats (*nude, rhino*, etc.); mink have similar effects.	Hutt, 1934; Green, 1934
Cutaneous asthenia; Dermatosparaxia; Fragility of skin; Ehlers-Danlos syndrome; Dermal asthenia	A, r	Disease known in cattle, dogs, cats, mink, and man; defect in collagen results in fragile skin that stretches and tears easily.	Anderson and Brown, 1978; Hegreberg et al., 1969, 1970; O'Hara et al., 1970; Patterson and Minor, 1977

Condition	Genetics	Description	References
Dermoid sinus; Epidermoid inclusion cyst	Unknown	Skin extends along midline of back deep down to vertebrae; cyst lined by stratified squamous epithelium with adnexa; recognized in Rhodesian Ridgeback dogs.	Stratton, 1964; Mann and Stratton, 1966
Epitheliogenesis imperfecta (Epithelial defects)	A, r (ep) "skinless"	Recognized in newborn calves (Ayrshire, Jersey, and Holstein breeds); absence of skin over patches of fetlocks and knees, sometimes over ears and muzzle; calves usually born alive.	Hutt and Frost, 1948; Hutt, 1964
Hairlessness, streaked	S, D "streaked hairlessness"	Vertical streaks of atrichia over the hips in heterozygous females; hemizygous males are presumed to die in utero. Recognized in Holstein-Friesian cattle.	Eldridge and Atkeson, 1953; Hutt, 1964
Ichthyosis fetalis ("Fish skin")	A, r	Similar lesions to Harlequin fetus in newborn infants; seen in newborn calves of Norwegian Red Poll cattle and probably other breeds; lesions of alopecia; scaly, fissured skin; hyperkeratosis and acanthosis; deep fissures in skin (Fig. 18–3).	Tuff and Gledish, 1949; Edmonds and Dolan, 1951; Julian, 1960
Vegetative dermatosis (Dermatosis vegetans)	A, r	Acanthosis and hyperkeratosis of skin; followed by microabscesses in dermal papillae and epidermis; lungs consolidated with macrophages and Langhans' giant cells; recognized in newborn piglets.	Hjarre, 1953; Jericho, 1974; Percy and Hulland, 1967, 1968, 1969

Table 8–4.   **Examples of Inherited Diseases of the Musculoskeletal System**

Scientific and Common Names	Genetic Designation and Gene Symbol	Clinical and Pathologic Features; Species	References
Achondroplasia (Bull-dog calves)	A, r	Fetus aborted 4th to 6th months of gestation; anasarca; phocomelia; prognathia, domed skull, protruding tongue; achondroplasia; Dexter breed heterozygous for gene; occurs also in other breeds of cattle.	Hutt, 1964; Stormont, 1958; Innes and Saunders, 1962
Acroteriasis congenita; Adactyly; Amputated	A, r	Known in Holstein-Friesian cattle; forelegs terminate at elbow, hindlegs at hocks; cleft palate; adentia; prognathism; distortion of maxillae; death near time of birth.	Stormont, 1958; Wiesner, 1960
Amelia, congenital Amputated	A, r	Piglets born alive with all limb appendages missing.	Hutt, 1964
Cartilaginous exostoses, multiple	Unknown	Cartilaginous masses on ribs, vertebral processes, long bones, usually at costochondral junctions or metaphyses. These exostoses consist of hyaline cartilage surrounding endochondral bone. Described in several breeds of dogs.	Banks and Bridges, 1956; Gee and Doige, 1970; Chester, 1971
Chondrodystrophy	A, r (cd)	Described in rabbits, resembles achondroplasia in this species; fetuses grossly fatter, more muscular; cartilages overgrown; shafts of long bones bowed and shortened.	Fox and Crary, 1971
Chondrodysplasia; Dwarfism; Dyschondroplasia	A, r (dan)	Described in Alaska Malamute; associated with hemolytic anemia; stunted growth evident about 3 months after birth; long bones shortened; end of bones and epiphyseal plates thickened; failure of ossification of cartilage in growth plate.	Fletch et al., 1973; Fletch and Pinkerton, 1972; Smart and Fletch, 1971; Subden et al., 1972

Dwarfism ("Snorter dwarfs")	A, r	Cattle involved, particularly Hereford and Angus breeds; calves are short in stature; fail to grow; bulging foreheads; malocclusion; nasal obstruction may cause dyspnea; severe mucopolysacchariduria reported in some cases.	Julian et al., 1959; Hutt, 1964; Hurst et al., 1975
Elbow dysplasia	Polygenic	Reported in many large breeds, more frequent in German Shepherd dogs; anconeal process not united; early osteoarthritis of elbow joints.	Corley et al., 1968; Ljunggren et al., 1966; Seer and Herov, 1969
Hip dysplasia; Acetabular dysplasia	Polygenic	Large breeds of dogs affected; more frequent in German Shepherds; acetabulum shallow; head of femur displaced; sometimes false joint formed; osteoarthritis.	Henricson and Olsen, 1959; Hutt, 1967, 1969; Seer and Hurov, 1969
Anury; Spina bifida; Brachyury; Taillessness	A, D (M) (Manx) (sb) rabbit	Manx breed of cat with varying degrees of anury, are heterozygous for M; homozygosity results in lethality; lesions include spina bifida, imperforate anus, rachischisis, sacral and coccygeal dysgenesis, and defects in lower spinal cord. Similar disease described in rabbits (sb) and cattle.	Crary et al., 1966; Howell and Siegel, 1963, 1966; James et al., 1969; Todd, 1961, 1964; Tomlinson, 1971; Leipold et al., 1974; Martin, 1971
Osteopetrosis	A, r (os) rabbit (op) mice	Described in man, mice (op), and rabbits (os); cortex of long bone severely thickened, may obliterate marrow; also occurs in two other mutant mice: grey-lethal (gl) and microphthalmic (mi).	Marks and Walker, 1969; Marks and Lane, 1976
Muscular dystrophy	A, r (dy) mice	Occurs in several species: mice (dy); mink, chickens, sheep, hamster, turkeys, and cattle; not identical but similar failure of muscles to develop.	Davidowitz et al., 1976; Pachter et al., 1976; Hegreberg et al., 1974; Julian and Asmundson, 1963; Harper and Parker, 1967; Hadlow, 1962; Homberger et al., 1963

Hutt, F. B.: Animal Genetics. New York, Ronald Press, 1964.

Jericho, K. W. F.: Dermatosis vegetans—giant cell pneumonitis in pigs: further observations and interpretations. Res. Vet. Sci., 16:176–181, 1974.

Julian, R. J.: Ichthyosis congenita in cattle. Vet. Med., 55:35–41, 1960.

Mann, G. E., and Stratton, J.: Dermoid sinus in the Ridgeback. J. Small Anim. Pract., 7:631–642, 1966.

O'Hara, P. J., Read, W. K., Romane, W. M., and Bridges, C. R.: A collagenous tissue dysplasia of calves. Lab. Invest., 23:307–314, 1970.

Patterson, R.: Ragweed allergy in the dog. J. Am. Vet. Med. Assoc., 135:178–180, 1959.

Patterson, D. F., and Minor, R. R.: Hereditary fragility and hyperextensibility of the skin of cats. A defect in collagen fibrillogenesis. Lab. Invest., 37:170–179, 1977.

Percy, D. H., and Hulland, T. J.: Dermatosis vegetans (vegetative dermatosis) in Canadian swine. Can. Vet. J., 8:3–9, 1967.

————: Evolution of multinucleate giant cells in dermatosis vegetans in swine. Pathol. Vet., 5:419–428, 1968.

————: The histopathological changes in the skin of pigs with dermatosis vegetans. Can. J. Comp. Med., 33:48–54, 1969.

Rockey, J. H., and Schwartzman, R. M.: Skin sensitizing antibodies: A comparative study of canine and human PK and PCA antibodies and a canine myeloma protein. J. Immunol., 98:1143–1151, 1967.

Schwartzman, R. M.: Atopy in the dog. In Comparative Physiology and Pathology of the Skin, edited by A. J. Rook and G. S. Walton. Oxford, Blackwell, 1965. pp. 557–559.

Stratton, J.: Dermoid sinus in the Rhodesian Ridgeback. Vet. Rec., 76:846–848, 1964.

Tuff, P., and Gledish, L. A.: Ichthyosis congenita hos Kalveren arvelig letal defekt. Nord. Vet. Med., 1:619–627, 1949.

Wittich, F. W.: Spontaneous allergy (atopy) in the lower animals. Seasonal hay fever (fall type) in a dog. J. Allergy, 12:247–251, 1941.

Inherited Diseases of Musculoskeletal System

Banks, W. C., and Bridges, C. H.: Multiple cartilaginous exostoses in a dog. J. Am. Vet. Med. Assoc., 129:131–135, 1956.

Chester, D. K.: Multiple cartilaginous exostoses in two generations of dogs. J. Am. Vet. Med. Assoc., 159:895–897, 1971.

Corley, E. A., Sutherland, T. M., and Carlson, W. D.: Genetic aspects of elbow dysplasia. J. Am. Vet. Med. Assoc., 153:543–547, 1968.

Crary, D. D., Fox, R. R., and Sawin, P. B.: Spina bifida in the rabbit. J. Hered., 57:236–243, 1966.

Davidowitz, J., Pachter, B. R., Philips, G., and Breinin, G. M.: Structural alterations of the junctional region in extraocular muscle of dystrophic mice. I. Modifications of sole-plate nuclei. Am. J. Pathol., 82:101–110, 1976.

Fletch, S. M., and Pinkerton, P. H.: An inherited anemia associated with hereditary chondrodysplasia in the Alaska Malamute. Can. Vet. J., 13:270–271, 1972.

Fletch, S. M., Smart, M. E., Pennock, P. W., and Subden, R. E.: Clinical and pathologic features of chondrodysplasia (dwarfism) in the Alaska Malamute. J. Am. Vet. Med. Assoc., 162:357–361, 1973.

Fox, R. R., and Crary, D. D.: A new recessive chondrodystrophy in the rabbit. Teratology, 4:245–246, 1971.

Gee, B. R., and Doige, C. E.: Multiple cartilaginous exostoses in a litter of dogs. J. Am. Vet. Med. Assoc., 156:53–59, 1970.

Hadlow, W. J.: Diseases of skeletal muscle. In Comparative Neuropathology, edited by J. R. M. Innes and L. Z. Saunders. New York, Academic Press, 1962. pp. 147–243.

Harper, J. A., and Parker, J. E.: Hereditary muscular dystrophy in the domestic turkey. J. Hered., 58:189–190, 1967.

Hegreberg, G. A., Camacho, A., and Gorham, J. R.: Histopathologic description of muscular dystrophy of mink. Arch. Pathol., 97:225–233, 1974.

Henricson, B., and Olson, S. E.: Hereditary acetabular dysplasia in the German Shepherd dog. J. Am. Vet. Med. Assoc., 135:207–210, 1959.

Homburger, F., et al.: Further morphologic and genetic studies on dystrophy-like primary myopathy of Syrian hamsters. Fed. Proc., 22:195–197, 1963.

Howell, J. M., and Siegel, P. B.: Phenotype variability of taillessness in Manx cats. J. Hered., 54:167–169, 1963.

————: Morphological effects of the Manx factor in cats. J. Hered., 57:100–104, 1966.

Hurst, R. E., Cezayirli, R. C., and Lorincz, A. E.: Nature of the glycosaminoglycanuria (mucopolysacchariduria) in brachycephalic "snorter" dwarf cattle. J. Comp. Pathol., 85:481–486, 1975.

Hutt, F. B.: Animal Genetics. New York, Ronald Press Co., 1964.

————: Genetic selection to reduce the incidence of hip dysplasia in dogs. J. Am. Vet. Med. Assoc., 151:1041–1048, 1967.

————: Developments in veterinary science. Advances in canine genetics, with special reference to hip dysplasia. Can. Vet. J., 10:307–311, 1969.

Innes, J. R. M., and Saunders, L. Z.: Comparative Neuropathology. New York, Academic Press, 1962.

James, C. C. M., Lassman, L. P., and Tomlinson, B. E.: Congenital anomalies of the lower spine and spinal cord in Manx cats. J. Pathol., 97:269–276, 1969.

Julian, L. M., Tyler, W. S., and Gregory, P. W.: The current status of bovine dwarfism. J. Am. Vet. Med. Assoc., 135:104–109, 1959.

Julian, L. M., and Asmundson, V. S.: Muscular dystrophy in the chicken. In Muscular Dystrophy, edited by G. H. Bourne and M. N. Golarz. New York, Hafner Publishing Co., 1963, pp. 457–498.

Leipold, H. W., Huston, K., Blauch, B., and Guffy, M.

M.: Congenital defects of the caudal vertebral column and spinal cord in Manx cats. J. Am. Vet. Med. Assoc., 164:520–523, 1974.

Ljunggren, G., Cawley, A. J., and Archibald, J.: The elbow dysplasias in the dog. J. Am. Vet. Med. Assoc., 148:887–891, 1966.

Marks, S. C., Jr., and Walker, D. G.: The role of the parafollicular cell of the thyroid gland in the pathogenesis of congenital osteopetrosis. Am. J. Anat., 126:299–314, 1969.

Marks, S. C., Jr., and Lane, P. W.: Osteopetrosis, a new recessive skeletal mutation on chromosome 12 of the mouse. J. Hered., 67:11–18, 1976.

Martin, A. H.: A congenital defect in the spinal cord of the Manx cat. Vet. Pathol., 8:232–238, 1971.

McGavin, M. D., and Baynes, I. D.: A congenital progressive ovine muscular dystrophy. Pathol. Vet., 6:513–524, 1969.

Pachter, B. R., Davidowitz, J., and Breinin, G. M.: Structural alterations of the junctional region in extraocular muscle of dystrophic mice. II. Hypertrophy of the neuromuscular junctional apparatus. Am. J. Pathol., 82:111–118, 1976.

Seer, G., and Hurov, L.: Elbow dysplasia in dogs with hip dysplasia. J. Am. Vet. Med. Assoc., 154:631–637, 1969.

Smart, M. E., and Fletch, S.: A hereditary skeletal growth defect in purebred Alaskan Malamutes. Can. Vet. J., 12:31–32, 1971.

Stormont, C.: Genetics and disease. Vet. Sci., 4:137–162, 1958.

Subden, R. E., Fletch, S. M., Smart, M. A., and Brown, R. G.: Genetics of the Alaskan Malamute chondrodysplasia syndrome. J. Hered., 63:149–152, 1972.

Todd, N. B.: The inheritance of taillessness in Manx cats. J. Hered., 52:228–232, 1961.

———: The Manx factor in domestic cats. J. Hered., 55:225–230, 1964.

Tomlinson, B. E.: Abnormalities of the lower spine and spinal cord in Manx cats. J. Clin. Pathol., 24:480, 1971.

Wiesner, E.: Die Erbschöden der landwertschaftlichen Nutztiere. Jena, Gustaf Fischer, 1960.

Inherited Diseases of Cardiovascular System

Dupont, J., et al.: Selection of three strains of rats with spontaneously different levels of blood pressure. Biomed (Express), 19:36–41, 1973.

Medoff, H. S., and Bongiovanni, A. M.: Age, sex and species variation on blood pressure in normal rats. Am. J. Physiol., 143:297–299, 1945.

Okamoto, K., and Aoki, K.: Development of a strain of spontaneously hypertensive rats. Jpn. Circ. J., 27:282–293, 1963.

Patterson, D. F.: Epidemiologic and genetic studies of congenital heart disease in the dog. Circ. Res., 23:171–202, 1968.

———: Canine congenital heart disease: Epidemiologic and etiologic hypotheses. J. Small Anim. Pract., 12:263–287, 1971.

Patterson, D. F., et al.: Hereditary patent ductus arteriosus and its sequelae in the dog. Circ. Res., 29:1–13, 1971.

Patterson, D. F.: Congenital defects of the cardiovascular system of dogs: studies in comparative cardiology. Adv. Vet. Sci. Comp. Med., 20:1–37, 1976.

Pyle, R. L., Patterson, D. F., and Chacko, S.: Genetics and pathology of discrete subaortic stenosis in the Newfoundland dog. Am. Heart J., 92:324–334, 1976.

Inherited Diseases of Hemic and Lymphatic System

Bannerman, R. M., Edwards, J. A., and Pinkerton, P. H.: Hereditary disorders of the red cell in animals. Prog. Hematol., 8:131–179, 1974.

Bannerman, R.M., and Edwards, J.A.: Hereditary anaemias in laboratory animals. Br. J. Haematol., 32:299–307, 1976.

Breukink, H. J., et al.: Congenital afibrinogenemia in goats. Zentralbl. Veterinärmed. [A], 19:661–676, 1972.

Brinkhous, K. M., Morrison, F. C., Jr., and Muhrer, M. E.: Comparative study of clotting defects in human, canine and porcine hemophilia. Fed. Proc., 11:409, 1952.

Brinkhous, K. M., and Graham, J. B.: Hemophilia in the female dog. Science, 111:723–724, 1959.

Chan, J. Y. S., et al.: von Willebrand disease "stimulating factor" in porcine plasma. Am. J. Physiol., 214:1219–1224, 1968.

Cornell, C. H., Cooper, R. G., Kahn, R. A., and Garb, S.: Platelet adhesiveness in normal and bleeder swine as measured in a Celite system. Am. J. Physiol., 216:1170–1175, 1969.

Cotter, S. M., Brenner, R. M., and Dodds, W. J.: Hemophilia A in three unrelated cats. J. Am. Vet. Med. Assoc., 172:166–168, 1978.

Dodds, W. J., Packham, M. A., Rowsell, H. C., and Mustard, J. F.: Factor VII survival and turnover in dogs. Am. J. Physiol., 213:36–42, 1967.

Dodds, W. J.: Canine von Willebrand's disease. J. Lab. Clin. Med., 76:713–721, 1970.

Dodds, W. J., and Kull, J. E.: Canine factor XI (plasma thromboplastin antecedent) deficiency. J. Lab. Clin. Med., 78:746–748, 1971.

Dodds, W. J.: Hereditary and acquired hemorrhagic disorders in animals. In Progress in Hemostasis and Thrombosis, Vol. II, edited by T. H. Spalt. New York, Grune and Stratton, 1974.

Edwards, J. A., and Bannerman, R. M.: Animal models of human disease—inherited hypochromic anemias of rodents. Comp. Pathol. Bull., 4:3–4, 1972.

Fass, D. N., Broackway, W. J., Owen, C. A., Jr., and Bowie, E. J. W.: Factor VIII (Willebrand) antigen and ristocetin-Willebrand factor in pigs with von Willebrand's disease. Thromb. Res., 8:319–327, 1976.

Field, R. A., Rickard, C. G., and Hutt, F. B.: Hemophilia in a family of dogs. Cornell Vet., 36:283–300, 1946.

Table 8–5.   Examples of Inherited Diseases of the Cardiovascular System

Scientific and Common Names	Genetic Designation and Gene Symbol	Clinical and Pathologic Features; Species	References
Patent ductus arteriosus	Polygenic	Principally studied in dogs; lesions vary in severity; fully patent ductus arteriosus results in left heart failure in about half of cases; small percentage develop pulmonary hypertension with right-to-left or bidirectional shunts.	Patterson et al., 1971; Patterson, 1968, 1971, 1976
Subaortic stenosis, discrete	Polygenic	Lesion occurs in dog, pig, cow, and man; best evidence for genetic determination is in dogs, especially Newfoundland breed; lesions found after 3 weeks of age range in severity from subclinical to well-developed subaortic ring causing death before sexual maturity.	Pyle, Patterson and Chacko, 1976
Hypertension	Polygenic	Spontaneous hypertension not dependent upon high salt diet; best studied in rats but probably occurs in many other species; increased blood pressure is a clinical sign; underlying disease is unknown; affects cardiovascular system and kidney especially.	Medoff and Bongiovanni, 1945; Okamoto and Aoki, 1963; Dupont et al., 1973

Fletch, S. M., Brueckner, P. J., and Pinkerton, P. H.: Hereditary hemolytic anemia and chondrodysplasia in the dog. Fed. Proc., 32:821, 1973.

Graham, J. B., Collins, D. L., and Brinkhous, K. M.: Assay of plasma antihemophilic activity in normal, heterozygous (hemophilia) and prothrombinopenic dogs. Proc. Soc. Exp. Biol. Med., 77:294, 1951.

Hogan, A. G., Muhrer, M. E., and Bogart, R.: A hemophilia-like disease in swine. Proc. Soc. Exp. Biol. Med., 48:217–219, 1941.

Hovig, T., et al.: Experimental hemostasis in normal dogs and dogs with congenital disorders of blood coagulation. Blood, 30:636–668, 1967.

Hutt, F. B., Rickard, C. G., and Field, R. A.: Sex-linked hemophilia in dogs. J. Hered., 39:2–9, 1948.

Kammerman, B., Gmür, J., and Stunzi, H.: Afibrogenämie beim Hund. Zentralbl. Veterinaermed., 18:192–194, 1971.

Kociba, G. J., et al.: Bovine plasma thromboplastin antecedent (factor XI) deficiency. J. Lab. Clin. Med., 74:37–39, 1969.

Leighton, R. L., and Suter, P. F.: Primary lymphedema of the hindlimb in the dog. J. Am. Vet. Med. Assoc., 175:369–374, 1979.

Luginbühl, H., Chacko, S. K., Patterson, D. F., and Medway, W.: Congenital hereditary lymphedema in the dog. 2. Pathological studies. J. Med. Genet., 4:153–165, 1967.

Lund, J. E., Padgett, G. A., and Gorham, J. R.: Additional evidence on the inheritance of cyclic neutropenia in the dog. J. Hered., 61:47–49, 1970.

Mustard, J. F., et al.: Canine factor VII deficiency. Br. J. Haematol., 8:43–47, 1962.

Patterson, D. L., Medway, W., Luginbühl, H., and Chacko, S.: Congenital hereditary lymphedema in the dog. I. Clinical and genetic studies. J. Med. Genet., 4:145–152, 1967.

Prasse, K. W., et al.: Pyruvate kinase deficiency anemia with terminal myelofibrosis and osteosclerosis in a Beagle. J. Am. Vet. Med. Assoc., 166:1170–1175, 1975.

Rowsell, H. C., et al.: A disorder resembling hemophilia B (Christmas disease) in dogs. J. Am. Vet. Med. Assoc., 137:247–250, 1960.

Standerfer, R. J., Templeton, J. W., and Black, J. A.: Anomalous pyruvate kinase deficiency in the Basenji dog. Am. J. Vet. Res., 35:1541–1544, 1974.

Windhorst, D. B., et al.: Intestinal malabsorption in the gray Collie syndrome. Fed. Proc., 26:260, 1967.

Cornelius, C. E., and Gronwall, R. R.: Congenital photosensitivity and hyperbilirubinemia in Southdown sheep in the United States. Am. J. Vet. Res., 29:291–295, 1968.

Cornelius, C. E.: Congenital hyperbilirubinemia, Gilbert's syndrome. Model No. 8. In Handbook: Animal Models of Human Disease. Armed Forces Institute of Pathology, Washington, D.C., 1972a.

Cornelius, C. E.: Congenital hyperbilirubinemia, Dubin-Johnson syndrome. Model No. 2. In Handbook: Animal Models of Human Disease. Armed Forces Institute of Pathology, Washington, D. C., 1972b.

Cornelius, C. E., and Arias, I. M.: Congenital hyperbilirubinemia, Crigler-Najjar syndrome. Model No. 26. In Handbook: Animal Models of Human Disease. Armed Forces Institute of Pathology, Washington, D. C., 1973.

Fox, R. R., and Crary, D. D.: Hereditary diaphragmatic hernia in the rabbit. Genetics and pathology. J. Hered., 64:333–336, 1973.

Hutt, F. B., and Lahunta, A. de: A lethal glossopharyngeal defect in the dog. J. Hered., 62:291–293, 1971.

Inherited Diseases of Urinary System

Bovee, K. C., Thier, S. O., Rea, C., and Segal, S.: Renal clearance of amino acids in canine cystinuria. Metabolism, 23:51–58, 1974.

Cordes, D. O., and Dodd, D. C.: Bilateral renal hypoplasia of the pig. Pathol. Vet., 2:37–48, 1965.

Cornelius, C. E., Bishop, J. A., and Schaffer, M. H.: A quantitative study of amino aciduria in Dachshunds with a history of cystine urolithiasis. Cornell Vet., 57:177–183, 1967.

Holtzapple, P. G., Rea, C., Bovee, K., and Segal, S.: Characteristics of cystine and lysine transport in renal and jejunal tissue from cystinuric dogs. Metabolism, 20:1016–1022, 1971.

Solomon, S.: Inherited renal cysts in rats. Science, 181:451–452, 1973.

Treacher, R. J.: Intestinal absorption of lysine in cystinuric dogs. J. Comp. Pathol., 75:309–322, 1965.

Tsan, M-F., et al.: Canine cystinuria: its urinary amino acid pattern and genetic analysis. Am. J. Vet. Res., 33:2455–2462, 1972a.

Tsan, M-F., Jones, T. C., and Wilson, T. H.: Canine cystinuria: intestinal and renal amino acid transport. Am. J. Vet. Res., 33:2463–2468, 1972b.

Inherited Diseases of Digestive System

Angus, K., and Young, G. B.: A note on the genetics of umbilical hernia. Vet. Rec., 90:245–247, 1972.

Cornelius, C. E., Arias, I. M., and Osburn, B. L.: Hepatic pigmentation with photosensitivity: A syndrome in Corriedale sheep resembling Dubin-Johnson syndrome in man. J. Am. Vet. Med. Assoc., 146:709–713, 1965.

Inherited Diseases of Genital System

Bardin, C. W., et al.: Pseudohermaphrodite rat: end organ insensitivity to testosterone. Science, 167:1136–1137, 1970.

Fox, R. R., and Crary, D. D.: Hypogonadia in the rabbit: genetic studies and morphology. J. Hered., 62:163–169, 1971.

Table 8–6.   Examples of Inherited Diseases of Hemic and Lymphatic Systems

Scientific and Common Names	Genetic Designation and Gene Symbol	Clinical and Pathologic Features; Species	References
Anemia, hemolytic	A, r (dan)	Intrinsic red blood cell defect found in dwarf Alaska Malamutes	Fletch et al., 1973
Anemia, stem cell		Anemia is associated with several mutant genes in mice; this group is usually macrocytic; some are associated with skeletal and other defects:	Bannerman et al., 1974; Edwards and Bannerman, 1972; Bannerman and Edwards, 1976
	A, r (W, W^u)	Dominant spotting, mouse, linkage group XVII	
	A, r (SL, SL^d)	Steel, mouse, linkage group IV	
	A, r (an)	Hertwigs anemia, mouse, linkage group VIII	
	A, r (dm)	Diminutive, mouse, linkage group V	
	A, D (Ts)	Tail short anemia, mouse, linkage group unknown	
Anemia, hypochromic	A, r (f)	Flex-tailed mouse, linkage group XIV, transitory anemia, siderocytes;	Bannerman and Edwards, 1976
	S, r (s/a)	Sex-linked anemia, mouse, associated with malabsorption of iron;	
	A, r (mk)	Microcytic anemia, mouse;	
	A, r (b)	Belgrade rat, severe anemia, often lethal;	
	A, r (hbd)	Hemoglobin deficit, mouse.	
Anemia, hemolytic (rodents)	A, r (sp)	Spherocytosis, deer mouse;	Bannerman and Edwards, 1976
	A, r (sph)	Spherocytosis, mouse, usually lethal;	
	A, r (ja)	Jaundice, mouse, intrinsic hemolysis, lethal;	
	A, r (ha)	Hemolytic, mouse, intrinsic red cell defect.	
Anemia, hemolytic	A, r	Basenji and Beagle dogs, associated with deficiency of pyruvic kinase.	Standerfer et al., 1974; Prasse et al., 1975
Cyclic neutropenia ("Gray collie syndrome")	A, r	Collie dogs associated with defect in coat color (gray collie); intermittent neutropenia results in decreased resistance to infection; intestinal malabsorption.	Lund et al., 1970; Windhorst et al., 1967

Disease	Genetics	Description	References
Hemophilia A; Factor VIII deficiency; Antihemophilia factor deficiency	S, r(h)	Several breeds of dogs involved; hemizygous males usually affected; homozygous females also exhibit hemophilia; deficiency of antihemophilic factor VIII results in failure of blood to clot; hemorrhages into joints, subcutis, and elsewhere may result in death; also reported in cats.	Hutt et al., 1948; Brinkhous and Graham, 1959; Field et al., 1946; Cotter et al., 1978; Brinkhous et al., 1952
Hemophilia B; Christmas disease	S, r	Deficiency of factor IX (plasma thromboplastin) results in hemorrhage.	Rowsell et al., 1960
Factor VII deficiency	A, r	Usually reported in Beagle dogs, mildly affected; require no treatment; homozygotes have about 1–4% of normal level of factor VII.	Mustard et al., 1962; Dodds et al., 1967; Hovig et al., 1967; Dodds, 1974
Factor X deficiency; Stuart-Prower factor deficiency	A, r	Described in family of Cocker Spaniel dogs; prolonged prothrombin time, Russell's viper venom time, and bleeding in newborn and young animals; less severe in adults—increased risk during surgery.	Dodds, 1974
Factor XI deficiency Plasma thromboplastin antecedent deficiency (PTA)	A, r	Described in cattle, dogs, and man; minor bleeding, except severe after surgery; low factor XI assay; prolonged partial thromboplastin and recalcification times; abnormal prothrombin consumption.	Kociba et al., 1969; Dodds and Kull, 1971
Factor XII; Hageman factor	A, r	Marine mammals, fowl, reptiles lack this factor; man and horse may occasionally be deficient; no effect on coagulation.	Dodds, 1974
Von Willebrand's disease	A, r	Swine and dogs reported to have disease resembling that in man; moderate to severe bleeding disorder, low factor VIII levels; prolonged bleeding times; reduced platelet retention.	Hogan et al., 1941; Chan et al., 1968; Cornell et al., 1969; Dodds, 1970; Fass et al., 1976
Afibrinogenemia; Hypofibrinogenemia	Unknown	Reported in dogs and goats; severe hemorrhagic diathesis in newborn; umbilical bleeding, subcutaneous bleeding, and mucosal hemorrhages; fibrinogen levels low to absent; decreased platelet retention and prolonged bleeding times.	Dodds, 1974; Kammerman et al., 1971; Breukink et al., 1972
Lymphedema, congenital, hereditary	A, D	Reported in dogs, man, swine, and cattle; obstruction of lymphatics at regional lymph nodes; distal lymphatics become distended; tissues edematous.	Patterson et al., 1967; Luginbühl et al., 1967; Leighton and Suter, 1979

Table 8–7. Examples of Inherited Diseases of the Digestive System

Scientific and Common Names	Genetic Designation and Gene Symbol	Clinical and Pathologic Features; Species	References
Diaphragmatic hernia	A, r (dh-1) (dh-2)	Hereditary form in the rabbit; diaphragmatic hernia occurs in many species but genetic data not available.	Fox and Crary, 1973
Umbilical hernia	A, D	Umbilical hernia reported in many species; genetic evidence in cattle indicates hereditary nature.	Angus and Young, 1972
Glossopharyngeal defect ("Bird tongue")	A, r	One report in dogs; genetic evidence adequate; tongue is narrow, edges curled upward; puppy unable to suckle and dies of starvation.	Hutt and Lahunta, 1971
Congenital hyperbilirubinemia; Gilbert's syndrome	A, r	Reported in Southdown sheep; hyperbilirubinemia with unconjugated bilirubin 50–60%; no jaundice; photosensitization due to retention of phylloerythrin from chlorophyl in green feed; death due to renal failure; liver fails to take up many organic anions such as bilirubin, phylloerythrin, sulfobromophthalein sodium, indocyanine green, rose bengal.	Cornelius and Gronwall, 1968; Cornelius, 1972a
Congenital hyperbilirubinemia; Dubin-Johnson-Sprinz-Nelson syndrome	A, r	Spontaneous disease in Corriedale sheep. Inherited excretory defect for organic anions results in accumulation of melanin pigment in liver cells. Photosensitivity results from retention of phylloerythrin; similar to Dubin-Johnson-Sprinz-Nelson syndrome in man.	Cornelius et al., 1965; Cornelius, 1972b
Congenital hyperbilirubinemia; Hereditary unconjugated hyperbilirubinemia of Gunn rats; Crigler-Najjar syndrome (man)	A, r	Acholuric jaundice in newborn infants (Crigler-Najjar syndrome) with kernicterus is similar to disease in Gunn strain of rats; both are caused by deficiency in hepatic uridine diphosphate (UDP) glucuronyl transferase activity.	Cornelius and Arias, 1973

Table 8–8. Examples of Inherited Diseases of Urinary System

Scientific and Common Names	Genetic Designation and Gene Symbol	Clinical and Pathologic Features; Species	References
Cystinuria; Cystine urolithiasis	A, r (sex-limited)	Reported in dogs and wolves. Cystine, an amino acid, secreted in increased amounts from kidneys; possibly defective transport mechanism involving renal tubules; precipitated cystine forms uroliths in bladder; may obstruct urethra. Similar disease in man.	Bovee et al., 1974; Cornelius et al., 1967; Holtzapple et al., 1971; Treacher, 1965; Tsan et al., 1972a,b
Polycystic disease, renal	A, r	Reported in dogs, cats, rats, man. Multiple cysts develop as animal matures, eventually displace renal tissue and interfere with function; cysts appear to arise from renal tubules.	Solomon, 1973
Renal hypoplasia, (bilateral) agenesis, dysgenesis	A, r	Reported in swine and many other species; kidneys in newborn animals much smaller than normal; unilateral hypoplasia and absence also occur.	Cordes and Dodd, 1965

Table 8–9.   Examples of Inherited Diseases of Genital System

Scientific and Common Names	Genetic Designation and Gene Symbol	Clinical and Pathologic Features; Species	References
Testicular feminization; Pseudohermaphroditism	S, r (Tfm)	Reported in women, mice, and rats; female phenotype (with vulva and vagina, but not ovaries or uterus); male gonads and male (XY) genotype; key tissues are insensitive to hormonal effects of testosterone; 20% of hemizygous (Tfm) mice develop seminomas in intraabdominal testes.	Lyon and Hawkes, 1970; Ohno, 1974; Bardin et al., 1970; Jones, 1978
Testicular hypoplasia	A, r	Reported in many breeds of cattle; genetic basis studied in Swedish Highland breed; one testicle smaller at birth; definitely hypoplastic at puberty. Spermatogenesis not complete.	Gledhill, 1973
Cryptorchidism	A, r	Genetic details not complete; more frequent in horses and dogs of several breeds; testicles fail to descend into scrotum; spermatogenesis arrested in intraabdominal location.	King, 1978
Hypogonadia	A, r (hg)	Described in rabbits; atrophy of ovaries or testes; aspermatogenesis or no ovogenesis.	Fox and Crary, 1971; Sawin and Crary, 1962

Table 8–10. Examples of Inherited Diseases of Endocrine System

Scientific and Common Names	Genetic Designation and Gene Symbol	Clinical and Pathologic Features; Species	References
Adrenal hyperplasia	A, r (ah)	Reported in rabbits; adrenals enlarged with extensive proliferation of zona fasciculata; medulla absent; many animals have "clubbed" feet; affected animals die shortly after birth.	Fox and Crary, 1972
Diabetes insipidus	A, r	Most studied in man, rats, mice, and dogs; pathologic defect in hypothalamo-neurohypophyseal system leads to decreased production of vasopressin, the antidiuretic hormone; severe polydypsia and polyuria may be controlled by administration of vasopressin.	Valtin et al., 1962; Sawyer et al., 1964; Moses and Miller, 1970; Silverstein et al., 1961
Diabetes mellitus	A, r (db) (mouse)	Several types of diabetes mellitus occur in man and many other species; some of these are hereditary; genetic data is most extensive on db mouse (diabetic and obese); see Chapter 26.	Hummel et al., 1966; Like et al., 1972; Mayer et al., 1951; Renold, 1968; Stearns and Bengs, 1977
Pituitary dwarfism; Nanosomia premordalis	A, SD (Dw)	Described in rabbits; homozygotes (Dw Dw) reduced in size; die shortly after birth; heterozygotes (Dw dw) survive; slightly reduced in size.	Greene et al., 1934; Greene, 1940; Sawin and Crary, 1964

Table 8–11. Examples of Inherited Diseases of Nervous System

Scientific and Common Names	Genetic Designation and Gene Symbol	Clinical and Pathologic Features; Species	References
Ataxia, hereditary	A, r (at) (ax)	Reported in cattle, cats, rabbits; must be differentiated from congenital viral infections; calves affected at 2–3 weeks of age ("jittery"); incoordination; leukodysplasia of cerebellum, midbrain, and medulla.	Saunders et al., 1952 a, b; O'Leary et al., 1962
Gangliosidosis, GM_1; Tay-Sachs disease	A, r	Reported in man, cattle, cats, swine; deficiency of β-galactosidase enzyme results in accumulation of GM_1 ganglioside in neurons; generalized neurologic disorder, fatal in all species.	Tay, 1881; Sachs, 1887; Baker et al., 1971; Handa and Yamakawa, 1971; Volk et al., 1972; Blakemore, 1972; Farrell et al., 1973; Donnelly et al., 1973
Gangliosidosis, GM_2	A, r	Reported in man, dog, cat; deficiency of β-hexosaminidase leads to storage of gangliosidase GM_2 in lysosomes in neurons; fatal, generalized neurologic disease.	Gambetti et al., 1970; Karbe, 1971; Cork et al., 1977

Globoid cell leukodystrophy	A, r	Reported in man, dogs, cats; reduced level of β-galactocerebrosidase causes accumulation of galactocerebroside in large phagocytes with foamy cytoplasm in white matter; globoid cells are characteristic of lesion.	Johnson, 1970; Boysen et al., 1974; Johnson et al., 1975
Neuronal abiotrophy	A, r	Reported in Swedish Lapland dogs; paralysis by 5 to 7 weeks of age; chromatolysis of neurons in cerebellum, spinal cord, and ganglia; axon and myelin degeneration in peripheral nerves; osteopenia of long bones.	Sandefeldt et al., 1973
Neuroaxonal dystrophy	A, r	Described in cats; signs of ataxia associated with abnormal dilute hair color; gross atrophy of cerebellar vermis; nerve cell processes undergo ballooning; electron-dense flocculent material, osmiophilic bodies, and filaments in axons.	Woodard et al., 1974
Spinal dysraphism; Syringomyelia	A, r	Described in Weimaraner dogs with a "hopping" gait, crouching stance, and abducted hindlegs; pathologic findings include anomalies of dorsal septum of spinal cord (absence of septum, rarefaction of septal and adjacent white matter); anomalies of central canal (hydromelia, syringomelia, duplication, absence); anomalies of central, dorsal, and ventral horns; anomalies of ventral median fissure.	Confer and Ward, 1972; McGrath, 1965

Table 8–12.   Examples of Inherited Diseases of Eye and Ear

Scientific and Common Names	Genetic Designation and Gene Symbol	Clinical and Pathologic Features; Species	References
Buphthalmos; Hydrophthalmos; Congenital or infantile glaucoma	A, r (?) (bu)	Reported in rabbits; increased intraocular pressure in one or both eyes; globe is enlarged; cornea may become bluish and ulcerated; occasional corneal rupture; interference with outflow from anterior chamber.	Auricchio and Wistrand, 1959; Harris et al., 1970
Cataract, hereditary; Posterior, subcapsular	A, r	Described in Miniature Schnauzers with posterior subcapsular or complete cataracts; cataracts in other breeds may be autosomal dominant.	Anderson and Schultz, 1958; Rubin et al., 1968
Cataract, hereditary, equatorial	A, r	Reported in Standard Poodles; opacities start at equator of lens, progress from young age to complete opacity.	Rubin and Flowers, 1972
Cataract, nuclear or cortical	A, r	Reported in Old English Sheepdogs; often associated with retinal detachment, not compared genetically with other types.	Koch, 1972
Collie ectasia syndrome; Scleral ectasia; Juxtapapillary staphyloma; Collie eye anomaly; Retinal detachment	A, r	Limited to Collies, manifestations vary; usually bilateral, chorioretinal dysplasia, excavation of optic disc (scleral coloboma), retinal detachment, intraocular hemorrhage.	Donovan and Wyman, 1965; Freeman et al., 1966; Roberts et al., 1965, 1966

Disease	Inheritance	Description	References
Hemeralopia (Day blindness)	A, r	Reported in Alaska Malamutes and Poodles; good vision in dim light but apparent blindness in bright light; also tested by scotopic-flicker fusion electroretinography.	Rubin et al., 1967
Hereditary deafness	A, r	Associated with white or partially white coat color; reported in cats, mink, dogs (White Boxer, Merle Collie); lesion is degeneration of organ of Corti.	Saunders, 1965; Adams, 1956; Bergsma and Brown, 1971; Bosher and Hallpike, 1965
Retinal dystrophy, Primary, type I; Progressive retinal atrophy; Photoreceptive abiotrophy; Retinitis pigmentosa	A, r	Reported in dogs: Gordon Setters, Irish Setters, Poodles, English Cocker Spaniels, Norwegian Elkhounds; progressive degeneration of neuroepithelium, migration of cells from pigment epithelium into peripheral retina.	Aguirre and Rubin, 1971a, 1971b, 1975; Barnett, 1969, 1970, 1976; Cogan and Kuwabara, 1965; Parry, 1953
Retinal dystrophy, type II; Central progressive retinal atrophy; Central retinal degeneration	A, r	Reported in several canine breeds: Labrador Retriever, Border Collie, Golden Retriever, English Springer Spaniel, Cardigan Welsh Corgi. Usually detected at 3- to 5-years of age; hypertrophy and migration of pigment epithelium in central fovea; rods and cones layer absent in affected area; abrupt change to normal retina in periphery.	Barnett, 1969; Parry, 1954

Gledhill, B. L.: Inherited disorders causing infertility in the bull. J. Am. Vet. Med. Assoc., 162:979–982, 1973.

Jones, T.C.: Hereditary disease. In Pathology of Laboratory Animals, edited by K. Benirschke, F.M. Garner, and T.C. Jones. New York, Springer Verlag, 1978. p. 1981–2064.

King, N. W.: The reproductive tract. In Pathology of Laboratory Animals, edited by K. Benirschke, F.M. Garner, and T.C. Jones. New York, Springer Verlag, 1978.

Lyon, M. F., and Hawkes, S. G.: X-linked gene for testicular feminization in the mouse. Nature, 227:1217–1219, 1970.

Ohno, S.: Animal model of human disease. Testicular feminization. Am. J. Pathol., 76:589–592, 1974.

Sawin, P. B., and Crary, D. D.: Inherited hypogonadia in the rabbit. Anat. Rec., 142:325, 1962.

Inherited Diseases of Endocrine System

Fox, R. R., and Crary, D. D.: A lethal recessive gene for adrenal hyperplasia in the rabbit. Teratology, 5:255, 1972 (abstract).

Greene, H. S. N., Hu, C. K., and Brown, W. H.: A lethal dwarf mutation in the rabbit with stigmata of endocrine abnormality. Science, 79:487–488, 1934.

Greene, H. S. N.: A dwarf mutation in the rabbit. J. Exp. Med., 71:839–856, 1940.

Hummel, K. P., Dickie, M. M., and Coleman, D. L.: Diabetes, a new mutant in the mouse. Science, 153:1127–1128, 1966.

Like, A. A., Lavine, R. L., Poffenbarger, P. L., and Chick, W. L.: Studies in the diabetic mutant mouse. VI. Evolution of glomerular lesions and associated proteinuria. Am. J. Pathol., 66:193–203, 1972.

Mayer, J., Bates, M. W., and Dickie, M. M.: Hereditary diseases in genetically obese mice. Science, 113:746–747, 1951.

Moses, A. M., and Miller, M.: Accumulation and release of pituitary vasopressin in rats heterozygous for hypothalamic diabetes insipidus. Endocrinology, 86:34–41, 1970.

Renold, A. E.: Spontaneous diabetes and/or obesity in laboratory rodents. In Advances in Metabolic Disorders, Vol. 3, edited by R. Levine and R. Luft. New York, Academic Press, 1968.

Sawin, P.B., and Crary, D.D.: Genetics of skeletal deformities in the domestic rabbit (Oryctolagus cuniculus). Clin. Orthopaed., 33:71–90, 1964.

Sawyer, W. H., Valtin, H., and Sokol, H. W.: Neurohypophyseal principles in rats with familial hypothalamic diabetes insipidus (Brattleboro strain). Endocrinology, 74:153–155, 1964.

Silverstein, E., Sokoloff, L., Mickelsten, O., and Jay, G. E.: Primary polydipsia and hydronephrosis in an inbred strain of mice. Am. J. Pathol., 38:148–158, 1961.

Stearns, S. B., and Bengs, C. A.: Structural and chemical alterations associated with hepatic glycogen metabolism in genetically diabetic (db) and in streptozotocin-induced diabetic mice. Lab. Invest., 37:180–187, 1977.

Valtin, H., Schroeder, H. A., Benirschke, K., and Sokol, H.: Familial hypothalamic diabetes insipidus in rats. Nature, 196:1109–1110, 1962.

Inherited Diseases of Nervous System

Baker, H. J., McKhann, G. M., and Farrell, D. F.: Neuronal GM1 gangliosidosis in a Siamese cat with β-galactosidase deficiency. Science, 174:838–839, 1971.

Blakemore, W. F.: GM1 gangliosidosis in a cat. J. Comp. Pathol., 82:179–185, 1972.

Boysen, B. G., Tryphonas, L., and Harries, N. W.: Globoid cell leukodystrophy in the Bluetick Hound dog. I. Clinical manifestations. Can. Vet. J., 15:303–308, 1974.

Confer, A. W., and Ward, B. C.: Spinal dysraphism: a congenital myodysplasia in the Weimaraner. J. Am. Vet. Med. Assoc., 160:1423–1426, 1972.

Cork, L. C., et al.: GM2 ganglioside lysosomal storage disease in cats with β-hexosaminidase deficiency. Science, 196:1014–1017, 1977.

Donnelly, W. J. C., Sheahan, B. J., and Kelly, M.: Betagalactosidase deficiency in GM1 gangliosidosis of Friesian calves. Res. Vet. Sci., 15:139–141, 1973.

Farrell, D. F., et al.: Feline GM1 gangliosidosis: biochemical and ultrastructural comparisons with the disease in man. J. Neuropathol. Exp. Neurol., 32:1–18, 1973.

Gambetti, L. A., Kelley, A. M., and Steinberg, S. A.: Biochemical studies in a canine gangliosidosis. J. Neuropathol. Exp. Neurol., 29:137–138, 1970.

Handa, S., and Yamakawa, T.: Biochemical studies in cat and human gangliosidosis. J. Neurochem., 18:1275–1280, 1971.

Johnson, G. R., Oliver, J. E., and Selcer, R.: Globoid cell leukodystrophy in a Beagle. J. Am. Vet. Med. Assoc., 167:380–384, 1975.

Johnson, K. H.: Globoid leukodystrophy in the cat. J. Am. Vet. Med. Assoc., 157:2057–2064, 1970.

Karbe, E.: (G-M2) Gangliosidosis and other neuronal lipodystrophies in amaurosis in the dog. A comparative histopathological, histochemical, electron microscope and biochemical study. Arch. Exp. Veterinaermed., 25:1–48, 1971.

McGrath, J. T.: Spinal dysraphism in the dog. Pathol. Vet., 2(Suppl 1):1–36, 1965.

O'Leary, J. L., et al.: Hereditary ataxia of rabbits: histopathologic alterations. Arch. Neurol., 6:123–137, 1962.

Sachs, B.: On arrested cerebral development with special reference to its cortical pathology. J. Nerv. Ment. Dis., 14:541, 1887.

Sandefeldt, E., et al.: Hereditary neuronal abiotrophy in the Swedish Lapland dog. Cornell Vet., 63(Suppl 3):1–71, 1973.

Saunders, L. Z., et al.: Hereditary congenital ataxia in Jersey calves. Cornell Vet., 42:559–591, 1952a.

Saunders, L. Z.: A checklist of hereditary and familial diseases of the central nervous system. Cornell Vet., 42:592, 1952b.

Tay, W.: Symmetrical changes in the region of the yellow spot in each eye of an infant. Trans. Ophthalmol. Soc. UK, 1:55, 1881.

Volk, B. W., Adachi, M., and Schneck, L.: The pathology of sphingolipidoses. Semin. Hematol., 9:317–348, 1972.

Woodard, J. C., Collins, G. H., and Hessler, J. R.: Feline hereditary neuroaxonal dystrophy. Am. J. Pathol., 74:551–556, 1974.

Inherited Diseases of the Eye and Ear

Adams, E. W.: Hereditary deafness in a family of Foxhounds. J. Am. Vet. Med. Assoc., 128:302–303, 1956.

Aguirre, G. D., and Rubin, L. F.: Progressive retinal atrophy (rod dysplasia) in the Norwegian Elkhound. J. Am. Vet. Med. Assoc., 158:208–217, 1971a.

———: The early diagnosis of rod dysplasia in the Norwegian Elkhound. J. Am. Vet. Med. Assoc., 159:429–433, 1971b.

———: Rod-cone dysplasia (progressive retinal atrophy) in Irish Setters. J. Am. Vet. Med. Assoc., 166:157–164, 1975.

Auricchio, G., and Wistrand, P.: The osmotic pressure in the aqueous humor of rabbits with congenital glaucoma. Acta Ophthalmol. 37:340–345, 1959.

Anderson, A. C., and Schultz, F. T.: Inherited (congenital) cataract in the dog. Am. J. Pathol., 34:965–975, 1958.

Barnett, K. C.: Primary retinal dystrophies in the dog. J. Am. Vet. Med. Assoc., 154:804–808, 1969.

———: Genetic anomalies of the posterior segment of the canine eye. Trans. Ophthalmol. Soc. UK, 89:301–318, 1970.

———: Comparative aspects of canine hereditary eye disease. Adv. Vet. Sci. Comp. Med., 20:39–67, 1976.

Bergsma, D. R., and Brown, K. S.: White fur, blue eyes and deafness in the domestic cat. J. Hered., 62:171–185, 1971.

Bosher, D. R., and Hallpike, F. R. S.: Observations on the histological features, development and pathogenesis of inner ear degeneration of the deaf white cat. Proc. Roy. Soc. Lond. [B], 162:147–170, 1965.

Cogan, D. G., and Kuwabara, T.: Photoreceptive abiotrophy of the retina in the Elkhound. Pathol. Vet., 2:101–128, 1965.

Donovan, E. F., and Wyman, M.: Ocular fundus anomaly in the collie. J. Am. Vet. Med. Assoc., 147:1465–1469, 1965.

Freeman, H. M., Donovan, R. H., and Schepens, C. L.: Retinal detachment, chorioretinal changes, and staphyloma in the collie. Arch. Ophthalmol., 76:412–421, 1966.

Harris, T. M., et al.: A comparison of corneal epithelium regeneration in normal and buphthalmic rabbits. Invest. Ophthalmol., 9:122–150, 1970.

Koch, S. A.: Cataracts in interrelated Old English Sheep dogs. J. Am. Vet. Med. Assoc., 160:299–301, 1972.

Parry, H. B.: Degeneration of the dog retina. II. Generalized progressive atrophy of hereditary origin. Br. J. Ophthalmol., 37:487–502, 1953.

———: Degeneration of the dog retina. VI. Central progressive atrophy with pigment epithelial dystrophy. Br. J. Ophthalmol., 38:653–668, 1954.

Roberts, S. R., Dellaporta, A., and Winter, F. C.: The Collie ectasia syndrome: Pathology of eyes of pups one to fourteen days of age. Am. J. Ophthalmol., 61:1468–1469, 1965.

———: The Collie ectasia syndrome: Pathology of eyes of young and adult dogs. Am. J. Ophthalmol., 62:728–752, 1966.

Rubin, L. F., Bourns, T. K. R., and Lord, L. H.: Hemeralopia in dogs: heredity of hermeralopia in Alaskan Malamutes. Am. J. Vet. Res., 28:355–357, 1967.

Rubin, L. F., Koch, S. A., and Huber, R. J.: Hereditary cataracts in Miniature Schnauzers. J. Am. Vet. Med. Assoc., 154:1456–1458, 1968.

Rubin, L. F., and Flowers, R. D.: Inherited cataract in a family of Standard Poodles. J. Am. Vet. Med. Assoc., 161:207–208, 1972.

Saunders, L. Z.: The histopathology of hereditary congenital deafness in white mink. Pathol. Vet., 2:256–263, 1965.

CHAPTER 9

Diseases Caused by Viruses

Viruses are now clearly identified as unique organisms that inhabit vertebrate, invertebrate, and plant hosts. The clear recognition that viruses are distinct organisms is found in Lwoff's (1957) definition: "Viruses are infectious, potentially pathogenic nucleoprotein entities possessing only one type of nucleic acid, which reproduce from their genetic material, are unable to grow and to undergo binary fission, and are devoid of metabolic enzymes." It is now known that viruses have many other unique characteristics, but this definition still serves its purpose.

Each virus must enter a living host cell in order to be reproduced, and the interactions between virus and host cell determine to a great extent whether the relationship is deleterious (pathogenic) or not (commensal). The effects produced by a specific virus upon the cells, tissues, and life of an animal are often quite specific, and the disease can be identified by the lesions seen by the light and electron microscope. Some viruses produce nonspecific or nonrecognizable effects upon their host's cells, and therefore must be detected by recovering the virus or identifying it immunologically (Chapter 7). In any case, it is always desirable to identify the virus involved in a specific infection but even this is not always adequate to establish a diagnosis. Some viruses are harbored by host cells and may be recovered under many circumstances, but have nothing to do with the disease under investigation. It is best to identify the specific viral agent in association with characteristic lesions that have been shown by experiment and experience to be the result of known viral agent.

CLASSSIFICATION AND NOMENCLATURE OF VIRUSES

In recent years, a significant body of information has been gathered concerning the biochemical, ultrastructural, and molecular characteristics of viruses. It is now possible to identify relationships between groups of viruses based upon these characteristics. Earlier, viruses were simply identified with the tissue, host, and disease from which they were recovered. Names for viruses and schemes for their classification are still evolving, but a system of nomenclature and classification has been started and tentatively accepted by an international body of virologists (Melnick, 1980; Fenner et al., 1974; Fenner, 1976). (See Tables 9–1 to 9–5.) This system will be utilized in this chapter to the extent possible. Note that similar viruses produce similar lesions and often have affinity for the same organ system.

The affinity (tropism) of viruses for specific tissues is one of the characteristics that have been used in grouping similar agents in the past. This feature varies, however, and many viruses infect numerous tissues,

Table 9–1. DNA-Containing* Viruses with Cubic Symmetry and Naked Nucleocapsid

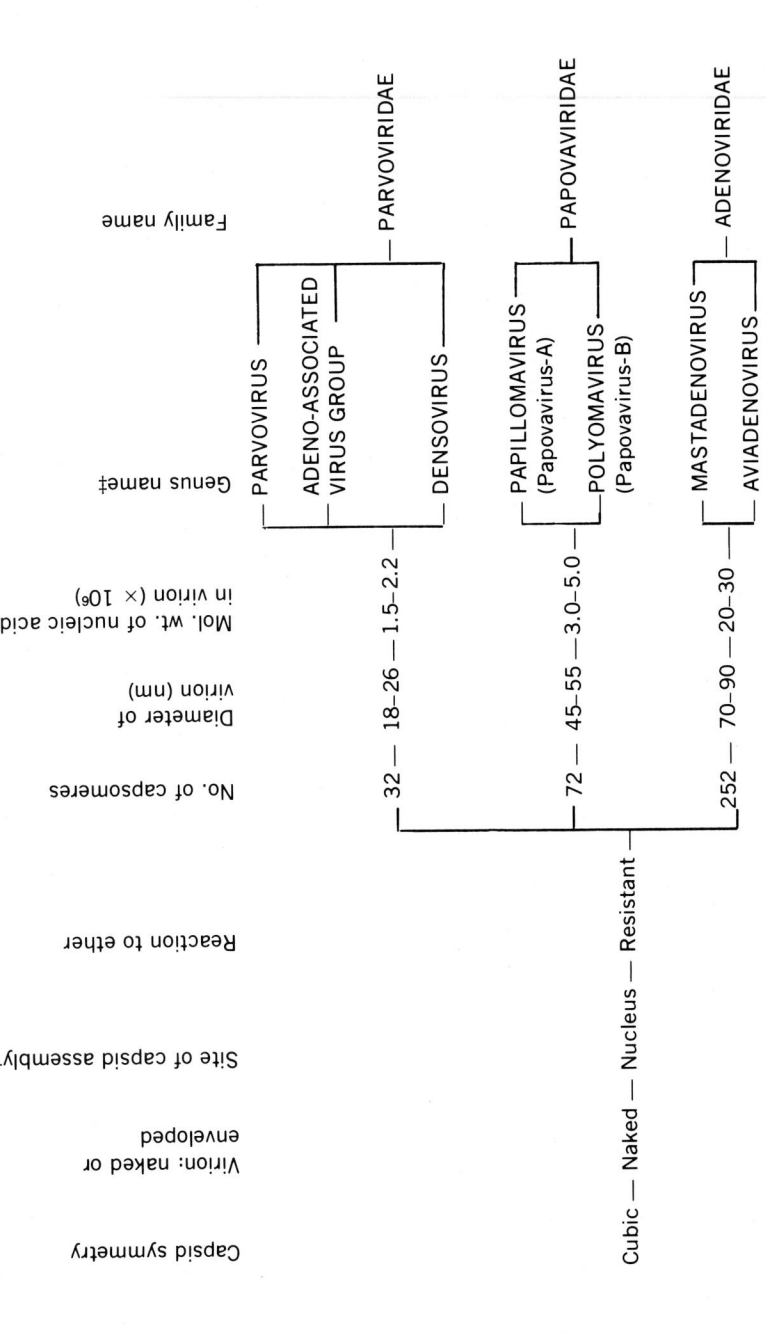

Capsid symmetry	Virion: naked or enveloped	Site of capsid assembly†	Reaction to ether	No. of capsomeres	Diameter of virion (nm)	Mol. wt. of nucleic acid in virion ($\times 10^6$)	Genus name‡	Family name
Cubic	Naked	Nucleus	Resistant	32	18–26	1.5–2.2	PARVOVIRUS / ADENO-ASSOCIATED VIRUS GROUP / DENSOVIRUS	PARVOVIRIDAE
				72	45–55	3.0–5.0	PAPILLOMAVIRUS (Papovavirus-A) / POLYOMAVIRUS (Papovavirus-B)	PAPOVAVIRIDAE
				252	70–90	20–30	MASTADENOVIRUS / AVIADENOVIRUS	ADENOVIRIDAE

* Among the DNA-containing viruses of vertebrates, all have double-stranded DNA except members of Parvoviridae, whose DNA is single-stranded within the virion.

† For the DNA-containing viruses whose capsid assembly takes place in the nucleus, a phase of replication occurs in the cytoplasm, as evidenced by the detection of viral messenger RNA associated with polyribosomes.

‡ Genus name, or group name if genus name is not yet assigned.

Courtesy of Dr. J. L. Melnick and Prog. Med. Virol. (Karger, Basel, 1980).

287

Table 9–2. DNA-Containing[a] Viruses with Envelopes or Complex Coats

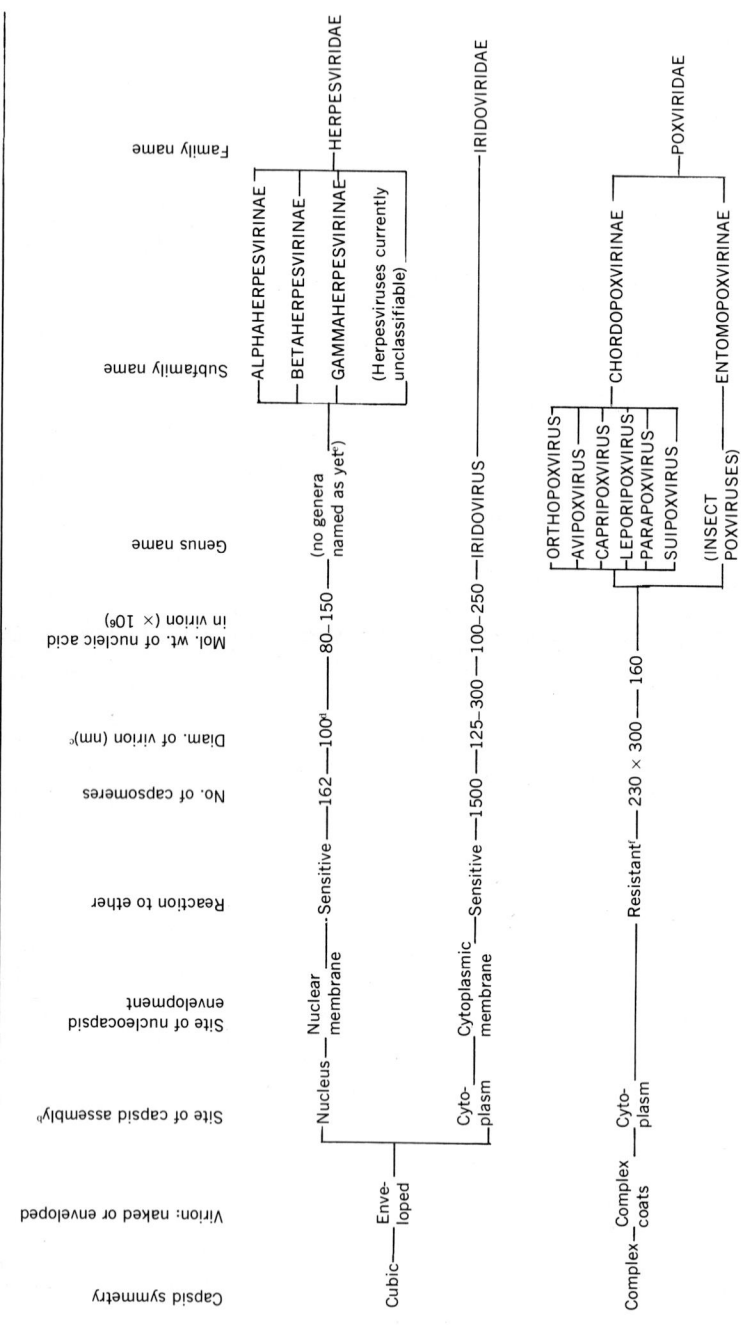

[a] Among the DNA-containing viruses of vertebrates, all have double-stranded DNA except members of Parvoviridae, whose DNA is single-stranded within the virion.
[b] For the DNA-containing viruses whose capsid assembly takes place in the nucleus, a phase of replication occurs in the cytoplasm, as evidenced by the detection of viral messenger RNA associated with polyribosomes.
[c] Diameter, or diameter × length.
[d] The naked virus is 100 mm in diameter; however, enveloped virions range up to 200 nm.
[e] In Herpesviridae, some genera have been set up provisionally, and two have been given English vernacular names (human cytomegalovirus group and murine cytomegalovirus group, within the subfamily Betaherpesvirinae).
[f] Members of the genera Orthopoxvirus and Avipoxvirus are ether-resistant, although other members of Poxviridae are sensitive to another lipid solvent, chloroform.
Courtesy of Dr. J. L. Melnick and Prog. Med. Virol. (Karger, Basel, 1980).

Table 9–3. RNA-Containing* Viruses with Cubic Capsid Symmetry

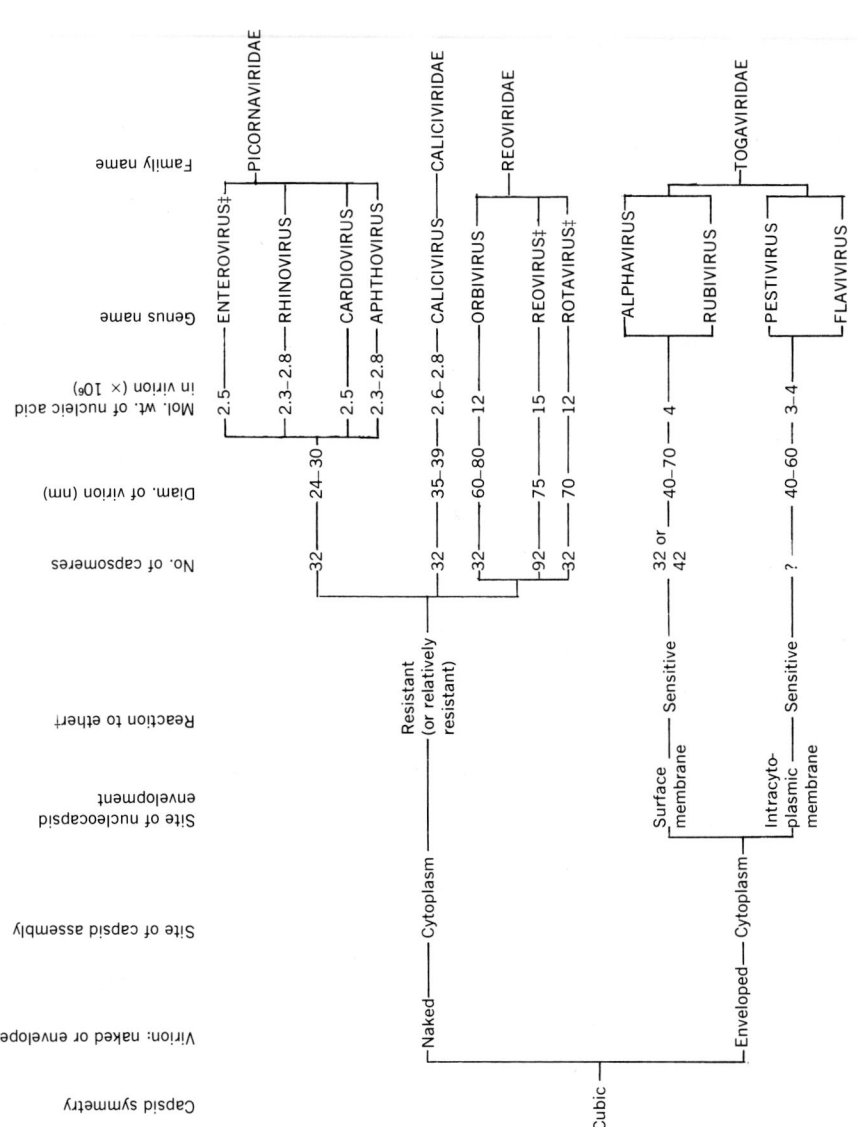

* Among the RNA-containing viruses of vertebrates, all have single-stranded RNA except members of Reoviridae, whose RNA is double-stranded.
† For most genera of Picornaviridae and Reoviridae, infectivity is resistant to treatment with lipid solvents; however, the orbiviruses are only partly resistant.
‡ Most of the RNA-containing viruses are sensitive to pH 3 treatment; exceptions are the enteroviruses, reoviruses and rotaviruses.
Courtesy of Dr. J. L. Melnick and Prog. Med. Virol. (Karger, Basel, 1980).

289

Table 9–4. RNA-Containing* Viruses with Helical Symmetry

Capsid symmetry	Virion: naked or enveloped	Site of capsid assembly	Site of nucleocapsid envelopment	Reaction to ether	Diam. of helix (nm)†	Diam. of virion (nm)‡	Mol. wt. of nucleic acid in virion (× 10⁶)	Genus name	Family name
Helical	Enveloped	Cytoplasm	Surface membrane	Sensitive	9–15	80–120	4–5	INFLUENZAVIRUS§	ORTHOMYXOVIRIDAE
					12–15	150–300	5–8	PNEUMOVIRUS	PARAMYXOVIRIDAE
					18	150–300	5–8	PARAMYXOVIRUS	
								MORBILLIVIRUS	
					18	60 × 180	3.5–4.6	VESICULOVIRUS	RHABDOVIRIDAE
								LYSSAVIRUS	
			Intracytoplasmic membrane	Sensitive	11–13	80–130	5–6	CORONAVIRUS	CORONAVIRIDAE
					8–9	100	6–7	BUNYAVIRUS	BUNYAVIRIDAE
								(Other genera)	

* Among the RNA-containing viruses of vertebrates, all have single-stranded RNA except members of Reoviridae, whose RNA is double-stranded.

† Diameter of ribonucleoprotein helix.

‡ Diameter, or diameter × length.

§ Influenza type C probably is a separate genus, but has not yet been so designated.

Courtesy of Dr. J. L. Melnick and Prog. Med. Virol. (Karger, Basel, 1980).

Table 9-5. RNA-Containing* Viruses with Architecture Unsymmmetric or Unknown

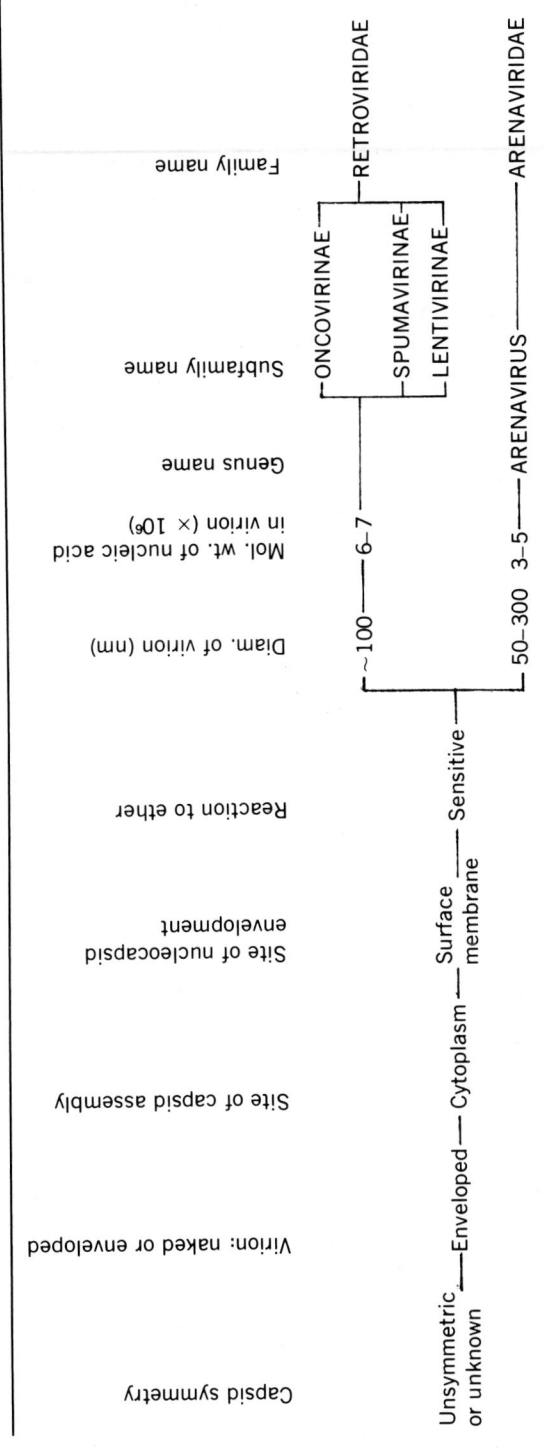

Capsid symmetry	Virion: naked or enveloped	Site of capsid assembly	Site of nucleocapsid envelopment	Reaction to ether	Diam. of virion (nm)	Mol. wt. of nucleic acid in virion ($\times 10^6$)	Genus name	Subfamily name	Family name
Unsymmetric or unknown	Enveloped	Cytoplasm	Surface membrane	Sensitive	~100	6–7		ONCOVIRINAE SPUMAVIRINAE LENTIVIRINAE	RETROVIRIDAE
					50–300	3–5	ARENAVIRUS		ARENAVIRIDAE

* Among the RNA-containing viruses of vertebrates, all have single-stranded RNA except members of Reoviridae, whose RNA is double-stranded. Courtesy of Dr. J. L. Melnick and Prog. Med. Virol. (Karger, Basel, 1980).

hence it is of limited value. **Neurotropic viruses**, for example, are those that have a predilection for cells of the nervous system. These include the viruses of rabies, equine encephalomyelitis, Teschen disease, poliomyelitis, mouse encephalomyelitis, and louping ill. Some viruses (pox, aphthous fever, vesicular stomatitis, xanthema, and warts) produce lesions principally in epithelium and are referred to as **epitheliotropic**. Viruses that attack the lung (swine, human, and equine influenza) are described as **pneumotropic**. Some of these characteristics are indicated in current names given viruses, such as *Adenovirus, Rhinovirus*, and *Enterovirus*.

Virologists have coined many names to identify individual viruses and groups of viruses. Some of these names have been "latinized" by adding a suffix. Virus groups with major similarities and some differences have been grouped into families and their name, by agreement, always ends in "-viridae." Closely similar viruses have been grouped into genera within each family; their names are italicized and end in "-virus." The origin and meaning of each of these coined words are taken up as each virus is considered.

ULTRASTRUCTURAL MORPHOLOGY OF VIRUSES

Each "virus-particle" **(virion)** has a central core of deoxyribonucleic acid (DNA) or ribonucleic acid (RNA) surrounded by a protein coat called the **capsid**. Morphologic units distinguishable within the capsid are called **capsomeres**. The nucleic acid core plus its capsid is referred to as the **nucleocapsid** (Fig. 9–1). The nucleocapsid may be surrounded by a lipoprotein **envelope (peplos)** or may lack this envelope ("naked"). This envelope is derived from nuclear or cytoplasmic membranes of the cell in which the virion is produced. The essential structure of the envelope is a phospholipid bilayer in which are embedded specific proteins. These phospholipids may be similar or identical to those of the

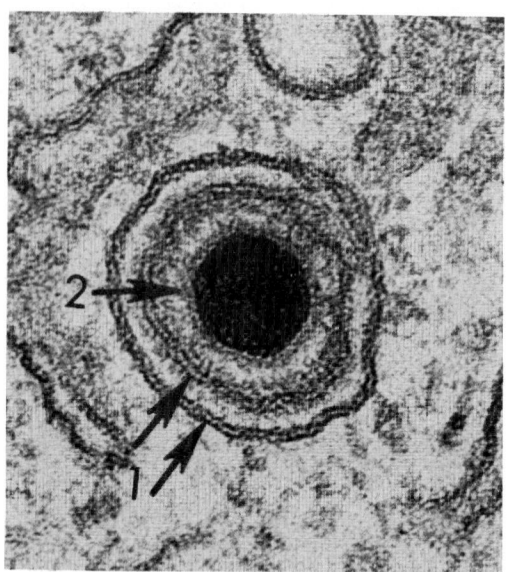

Fig. 9–1. Single virion of *Herpesvirus simplex* in tissue culture of rat cerebellum. Note envelopes *(1)* and capsid *(2)* surrounding the dense nucleoid. (× 220,000.) (Courtesy of Dr. J. E. Leestma and *Laboratory Investigation*.)

host cell. Radially-arranged structures, which may project from the outer surface of the envelope, are called **peplomers**. The envelope, therefore, is made up of an inner lipid layer, a protein coat, and peplomers as the outermost layer. Some virions may have more than one envelope.

The nucleocapsid of the virion contains the genome of the virus. The envelope contains the specificities that determine the viral antigenicity and interact with receptor sites on the cell membrane of the host cell to initiate infection.

Brown, F., and Hull, R.: Comparative virology of the small RNA viruses. J. Gen. Virol., 20:43–60, 1973.

Brown, F., and Tinsley, T. W. (eds.): Comparative virology (symposium). J. Gen. Virol., 20(suppl.):1–130, 1973.

Dalton, A. J., and Haguenau, F. (eds.): An Atlas of Ultrastructure of Animal Viruses and Bacteriophages. Vol. 5, Ultrastructure in Biological Systems. New York, Academic Press, 1973.

Fenner, F., et al.: The Biology of Animal Viruses. 2nd ed. New York, Academic Press, 1974.

Fenner, F.: Classification and Nomenclature of Viruses. (Second Report of the International Committee on Taxonomy of Viruses). Basel, S. Karger, 1976.

Horsvall, F. L., Jr., and Tamm, I. (eds.): Viral and Rickettsial Diseases of Man. 4th ed. Philadelphia, J. B. Lippincott, 1965.

Horzinek, M. C.: Comparative aspects of Togaviruses. J. Gen. Virol., 20:87–103, 1973.

Knudson, D. L.: Rhabdoviruses. J. Gen. Virol., 20:105–130, 1973.

Lwoff, A.: The concept of viruses. J. Gen. Microbiol., 17:239–253, 1957.

Maramorosch, K. (ed.): The Atlas of Insect and Plant Viruses. Vol. 8, Ultrastructure in Biological Sytems. New York, Academic Press, 1977.

Melnick, J. L.: Taxonomy of viruses, 1980. Prog. Med. Virol., 26:214–232, 1980.

Newman, J. F. E., Rowlands, D. J., and Brown, F.: A physico-chemical sub-grouping of the mammalian picornaviruses. J. Gen. Virol., 18:171–184, 1973.

Rueckert, R. R.: Picornaviral architecture. In Comparative Virology, edited by K. Maramorosch and E. Kurstak. New York, Academic Press, 1971.

Tinsely, T. W., and Longworth, J. F.: Parvoviruses. J. Gen. Virol., 20:71–75, 1973.

Wood, H. A.: Viruses with double stranded RNA genomes. J. Gen. Virol., 20:61–85, 1973.

POXVIRIDAE

Viruses classified in this family, Poxviridae, are responsible for infections in man, animals, birds, and insects. These viruses produce generalized disease with pustular (pock = pustule) lesions or benign tumors of the skin. The pox viruses are the largest animal viruses (Fenner et al., 1976), with complex, brick-shaped virions (300 × 240 × 100 mm) containing single linear molecules of double-stranded DNA, molecular weight 160 to 200 million daltons, and multiply and mature in the cytoplasm of host cells. The virions contain several enzymes including a transcriptase. The genera share a group antigen. In some (Parapoxvirus, Capripoxvirus, and swinepox virus), the virions are narrower than those of the others. Six genera have been named so far, but several viruses have not been classified. This is depicted in Table 9–6.

Diseases Caused by Orthopoxviruses

Smallpox (Variola)

This human disease is a highly contagious viral infection with a febrile onset, followed in a few days by characteristic cutaneous eruptions. Beginning as macules, these soon become papules, then vesicles, and finally, within about ten days, pustules, which undergo typical umbilication. The disease is observed in three clinical types: discrete, confluent, and hemorrhagic, in order of mounting mortality. A mild form of the disease, varioloid, is seen in persons who have been partially immunized by vaccination. A milder form of the disease, known as alastrim or variola minor, is caused by an immunologically indistinguishable but less virulent strain of virus. Except for a few small isolated endemic foci, smallpox no longer exists as a frank human disease.

The cutaneous lesion in smallpox begins as a circumscribed zone of congestion and lymphocytic infiltration in the dermal papillae underlying the affected epidermis. Epidermal cells swell, are isolated by extrusion of fluid between them, and eventually become necrotic. Before necrosis occurs, the epithelial cells contain eosinophilic cytoplasmic inclusions, **Guarnieri bodies**, composed of myriads of minute spherical granules, **Borrel** or **Paschen bodies**, believed to be the elementary visible form of the virus. As necrosis occurs in the affected epithelium, a clear vesicle forms and soon fills with neutrophils. This pustular lesion, which is from 2 to 4 mm in diameter, appears grossly to be both elevated above the surface and embedded in the skin. The contents of the pustule become desiccated, producing an umbilicated lesion; healing follows, and a deep, pitted scar is left. Hemorrhagic pneumonia and cutaneous and renal hemorrhages have been observed in fatal cases.

Vaccinia. Vaccinia is the virus used for immunization of man against smallpox. The origin of the virus is obscure. Classically, it was considered to have been derived from cowpox, but continuous passage over many years through man, laboratory animals, and tissue culture has resulted in the "creation" of a laboratory

Table 9-6. Pox Diseases Due to Poxviridae

	A. *Orthopoxvirus*	B. *Parapoxvirus*	C. *Capripoxvirus*	D. *Avipoxvirus*	E. *Leporipoxvirus*	G. **Unclassified*
Disease (species)	Variola (Smallpox)	Contagious ovine ecthyma (orf)	Sheep-pox	Fowlpox	Myxomatosis (rabbit)	Swinepox Horsepox
	Cowpox	Bovine papular stomatitis	Goatpox	Canarypox Sparrowpox Starlingpox	Fibroma (rabbit)	Molluscum contagiosum (man, chimp)
	Ectromelia Mousepox	Pseudocowpox (milker's nodules)	Lumpy skin disease (cattle)	Pigeonpox Robinpox	Fibroma (squirrel)	Yaba (monkey)
	Monkeypox Rabbitpox Buffalopox Raccoonpox Gerbilpox	Contagious ecthyma (chamois) Sealpox Camelpox		Turkeypox	Fibroma (hare)	Tana (man, monkey)
	Vaccinia					

* Genus *Entomopoxvirus*, viruses of insects, is not included in this table.
Ref: Fenner *et al.* 1974; Fenner, 1976

virus which, although infectious to a wide spectrum of animals, does not exist as a natural disease. Two major types of vaccinia occur, a dermatotropic strain and a neurotropic strain, properties developed by the method of propagating the virus in laboratory rabbits. The vaccinia virus, or closely related viruses, have been isolated from spontaneous diseases in several animal species, and certain of the pox diseases discussed in this section may not be distinct entities, but rather vaccinia infections. Vaccinia is known to be infectious for rabbits, mice, cattle, sheep, swine, monkeys, and man. The lesions produced in each of these species is similar to those described for smallpox.

Arita, I., and Henderson, D. A.: Smallpox and monkeypox in primates. Primates Med., 3:122–123, 1969.

Downie, A. W., and Dumbell, K. R.: Pox viruses. Ann. Rev. Microbiol., 10:237–252, 1956.

Fenner, F., and Burnet, F. M.: A short description of the pox-virus group (vaccinia and related viruses). Virology, 4:305–314, 1957.

Fenner, F.: The biological characters of several strains of vaccinia, cowpox, and rabbitpox viruses. Virology, 5:502–529, 1958.

Goodpasture, E. W., Woodruff, A. M., and Buddingh, G. J.: Vaccinial infection of the chorio-allantoic membrane of the chick embryo. Am. J. Pathol., 8:271–282, 1932.

Lillie, R. D.: Smallpox and vaccinia. Arch. Pathol., 10:241–291, 1930.

Joklik, W. K.: The poxviruses. Bacteriol. Rev., 30:33–66, 1966.

Lum, G. S., Soriano, F., Trejos, A., and Llerena, J.: Vaccinia epizootic in El Salvador. Am. J. Trop. Med. Hyg., 16:332–338, 1967.

Noble, J., Jr., and Rich, J. A.: Transmission of smallpox by contact and by aerosol routes in *Macaca irus*. Bull. WHO, 40:279–286, 1969.

Rhodes, A. J., and vanRooyen, C. E.: Textbook of Virology, 5th ed. Baltimore, Williams & Wilkins, 1968.

Wolman, M.: Pathologic findings in hemorrhagic smallpox (purpura variolosa): report of case with special reference to Feulgen's reaction in tissues. Am. J. Clin. Pathol., 21:1127–1138, 1951.

Woodroofe, G. M., and Fenner, F.: Serological relationships within the poxvirus group: an antigen common to all members of the group. Virology, 16:334–341, 1962.

Mousepox (Infectious Ectromelia)

The pox virus causing this disease is also classified in the genus *Orthopoxvirus* because of its immunologic affinities to others in the group (such as vaccinia and variola). Mousepox occurs in Europe and has, at times, been recognized in the United States. The disease may result in cutaneous or disseminated lesions. The clinical disease has been described as occurring in two forms: a rapidly fatal form, with few or no cutaneous lesions, and a chronic form characterized by ulceration of the skin, particularly the feet, tail, and snout. These are not dissimilar forms of the disease, but rather represent different stages in the pathogenesis of the infection. The infection begins with a primary lesion of the skin characterized by edema, ulceration, and ultimate scarring, which releases virus to the lymphatics and the blood, enabling it to localize and multiply in the liver and spleen. Virus is released from these organs, localizes in other viscera (salivary gland, lung, pancreas, lymph nodes, Peyer's patches, the small intestine, kidney, urinary bladder) and in the skin. The localization in the epidermis results in secondary skin lesions characterized by a generalized papular rash, which may progress to ulceration of the skin and gangrene of the extremities. If multiplication in the liver and spleen is exceptionally rapid, death may occur at this stage without premonitory clinical signs or a skin rash, except for the primary lesion, which may be small, absent, or overlooked. The lesions in this fulminating form of the disease are principally confined to the liver and spleen. In the liver, focal areas of necrosis are randomly distributed without any lobular pattern. The splenic lesions are also characterized by focal necrosis, which affects both the lymphoid follicles and the intervening reticuloendothelial tissue. Other visceral lesions may include focal necrosis of lymph nodes, Peyer's patches, mucosa of the small intestine, lung, kidney, urinary bladder, pancreas, and salivary gland. Eosinophilic, intracytoplasmic inclusion bodies may occur in all of these viscera. The primary and secondary skin lesions are characterized by spongiosis and ballooning degeneration of the epidermis, followed by necrosis and ulceration with a lymphocytic infiltration of the dermis. Eosinophilic intracytoplasmic inclusion bodies occur in the ballooned epithelial cells. During the stage of the secondary skin rash, conjunctivitis and blepharitis are frequent, and ulcers may occur on the tongue and buccal mucous membranes. Mortality ranges from 50 to 100%. If death does not occur in the stage of virus multiplication in the spleen and liver, recovery usually follows, unless the secondary cutaneous lesions are exceptionally severe or if gangrene occurs. In recovered mice, hairless scars may be present in the skin, and dense scars are usually present in the spleen.

The definitive diagnosis is based upon the demonstration of antihemagglutinins to vaccinia in the sera of convalescent mice, or cross-immunization of mice with the agents of vaccinia and mousepox, or viral isolation and identification.

Briody, B. A.: The natural history of mousepox. Viruses of Laboratory Rodents. Nat. Cancer Inst. Monogr., 20:105–116, 1966.

Dingle, J. H.: Infectious diseases of mice. In Snell, G. D.: Biology of the Laboratory Mouse. Philadelphia, Blakiston, 1941, Chap. 12, pp. 380–474.

Fenner, F.: Mousepox (infectious ectromelia of mice): A review. J. Immunol., 63:341–373, 1949.

————: The clinical features and pathogenesis of mouse pox (infectious ectromelia of mice). J. Pathol. Bact., 60:529–552, 1948.

Schell, K.: On the isolation of ectromelia virus from the brains of mice from a "normal" mouse colony. Lab. Anim. Care, 14:506–513, 1964.

Trentin, J. J.: An outbreak of mouse pox (infectious ectromelia) in the United States. I. Presumptive diagnosis. Science, 117:226–227, 1953.

Trentin, J. J., and Briody, B. A.: An outbreak of mouse pox (infectious ectromelia) in the United States. II. Definitive diagnosis. Science, 117:227–228, 1953.

Monkeypox

This specific infection of humans and nonhuman primates is of especial interest because of the close immunologic relation it bears to other members of this genus: *Orthopoxvirus*. The appearance of this virus in persons in one region of the Republic of Zaire, Africa, in a colony of *Macaca fascicularis* (crab-eating Macaque) in Copenhagen, Denmark, and in a large monkey colony in Pennsylvania caused much concern because of the difficulty of distinguishing it from the virus of variola (von Magnus et al., 1959; Prier et al., 1960; Marennikova et al., 1972; Cho and Wenner, 1973). The virus of monkeypox is clearly different from other viruses which may infect monkeys, such as Yaba and Tana pox viruses, which will be considered later in this text.

Signs. Clinical signs of monkeypox may be minimal prior to the appearance of cutaneous lesions, but in some animals edema of the face and eyelids may be conspicuous.

Lesions. The cutaneous lesions appear almost simultaneously and consist of multiple, discrete blanched papules about 1 to 4 mm in diameter, elevated or flattened on the skin surface. Many become umbilicated, with dark red-brown centers. A pustule filled with creamy grayish material may be expressed later from the lesion. Reddish-brown crusts cover the lesion, falling off in seven to ten days. These eruptions may be seen anywhere on the skin of the body and the oral, pharyngeal, or tracheal mucous membranes, but they are most common on the hands, feet, legs, and buttocks. In fatal cases, especially in infants, the lesions have a tendency to fill with hemorrhage.

In fatal cases, lesions may be found in some viscera. Foci of necrosis may occur in lymph nodes, spleen, and Peyer's patches. Petechiae and ecchymoses may rarely be found in skin, subcutis, peritoneum, omentum, gastrointestinal mucosae, and lungs.

The microscopic lesions are most striking in the skin. In early lesions, the epidermis undergoes localized acanthosis, with formation of broad, elongated rete ridges. Intracellular edema further increases the thickness of the epidermis. Coagulation necrosis precedes the formation of vesicles and later pustules in the epidermis. Often the necrosis affects specific layers of the epidermis. Intracytoplasmic inclusions are most numerous in epidermal cells at the margin of the necrotic or pustular lesion. These inclusions vary in size from 3 to 7 μ in diameter, and are irregular in shape, eosinophilic, and single or multiple. Similar inclusions within nuclei may be seen, but not in the same cells that contain cytoplasmic inclusions (Sauer et al., 1960)

Electron microscopic examination reveals characteristic pox virions, indistinguishable from others of this genus.

Arita, I., et al.: Outbreaks of monkeypox and serological surveys in nonhuman primates. Bull. WHO, 46:577–583, 1972.

Cho, C. T., and Wenner, H. A.: In vitro growth characteristics of monkeypox virus. Proc. Soc. Exp. Biol. Med., 139:916–920, 1972.

Cho, C. T., and Wenner, H. A.: Monkeypox virus. Bacteriol. Rev., 37:1–18, 1973.

Hall, R. D., Olsen, R. G., Pakes, S. P., and Yohn, D. S.: Differences in clinical and convalescent phase antibodies of Rhesus monkeys infected with monkeypox, Tanapox and Yaba. Infect. Immun., 7:539–546, 1973.

Heberling, R. L., and Kalter, S. S.: Induction, course, and transmissibility of monkeypox in baboon (*Papio cynocephalus*). J. Infect. Dis., 124:33–38, 1971.

Lourie, B., et al.: Human infection with monkey poxvirus. Laboratory investigations of six cases in West Africa. Bull. WHO, 46:633–639, 1972.

Magnus, P. von, Anderson, E. K., and Peterson, K. B.: A pox-like disease in cynomologous monkeys. Acta Path. Microbiol. Scand., 46:156–176, 1959.

Marennikova, S. S., Gurvish, E. B., and Shelukhina, E. M.: Comparison of the properties of five pox virus strains isolated from monkeys. Arch. Virol., 33:201–210, 1971.

Marennikova, S. S., et al.: Isolation and properties of the causal agent of a new variola-like disease (monkeypox) in man. Bull. WHO, 46:599–611, 1972.

Marennikova, S. S., Seluhina, E. M., Mal'ceva, N. N., and Ladnyj, I. D.: Poxviruses isolated from clinically ill and asymptomatically infected monkeys and a chimpanzee. Bull. WHO, 46:613–620, 1972.

Nicholas, A. H.: Poxvirus of primates. I. Growth of virus in vitro and comparison with other poxviruses. II. Immunology. J. Natl. Cancer Inst., 45:897–914, 1970.

Noble, J., Jr.: A study of New and Old World monkeys to determine the likelihood of a simian reservoir of smallpox. Bull. WHO, 42:509–514, 1970.

Prier, J. E., Sauer, R. M., Malsberger, R. G., and Sillaman, J. M.: Studies on a pox disease of monkeys. II. Isolation of the etiologic agent. Am. J. Vet. Res., 21:381–384, 1960.

Sauer, R. M., et al.: Studies on a pox disease of monkeys. I. Pathology. Am. J. Vet. Res., 21:377–380, 1960.

Cowpox

This disease in cattle is caused by a virus closely related to, but distinguishable from, vaccinia. The disease, which is not common, is mild, self-limiting, and its lesions are found only on the teats and udder. Microscopically the lesions resemble smallpox with vesiculation and cytoplasmic inclusions. The disease is spread by milking. Human infection may occur, with lesions usually limited to the hands. Experimental infection can be induced in rabbits, guinea pigs, mice, and monkeys. Cattle are also susceptible to vaccinia; infection usually resulting from exposure to a person recently vaccinated.

Downie, A. W., and Haddock, D. W.: A variant of cowpox virus. Lancet, May 24, 1049–1050, 1952.

Downie, A. W.: A study of the lesions produced experimentally by cowpox virus. J. Pathol. Bact., 48:361–378, 1939.

———: The immunological relationship of the virus of spontaneous cowpox to vaccinia virus. Br. J. Exp. Pathol., 20:158–176, 1939.

Hester, H. R., Boley, L. E., and Graham, R.: Studies on cowpox. I. An outbreak of natural cowpox and its relation to vaccinia. Cornell Vet., 31:360–378, 1941.

Maltseva, N. N., Akatova-Shelukhina, E. M., Yumasheva, M. A., and Marennikova, S. S.: The aetiology of epizootics of certain smallpox like infections in cattle and methods of differentiating vaccinia, cowpox and swine pox viruses. J. Hyg. Epidemiol. Microbiol. Immunol., 10:202–209, 1966.

Diseases Caused by Avipoxviruses

At least four antigenically related but distinguishable viruses are known to affect avian species. These are in general species-specific, but may infect hosts of other avian species. These pox diseases are known as **fowlpox** (avianpox, contagious epithelioma), **canarypox, pigeonpox, and turkeypox**. Much experimental work has been accomplished with these agents; hence, they are among the better known viruses. It was with the agent of fowlpox that Woodruff and Goodpasture (1930)

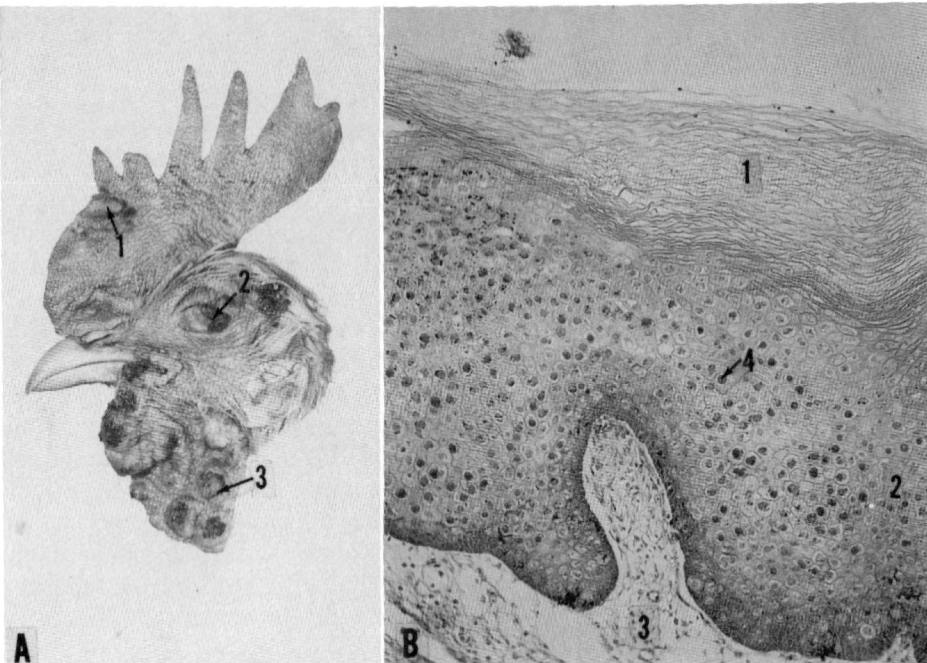

Fig. 9–2. *A.* Fowl pox. Lesions on comb *(1)*, eyelid *(2)*, and wattle *(3)* of a chicken. Contributor: Dr. C. L. Davis. *B*, Canary pox. Lesions (× 100), skin of the foot of a canary. Wide layer of keratin *(1)*, hyperplastic epidermis *(2)*, edema in dermis *(3)*, and Bollinger bodies *(4)*. (Courtesy of Armed Forces Institute of Pathology.) Contributor: Dr. J. Andrade dos Santos.

demonstrated that a single elementary (Borrel) body separated from the inclusion (Bollinger) body was capable of inducing typical infection. The spontaneous lesions in chickens occur in the skin of the head, particularly the comb and wattles, or in the mucosa of the mouth or nasal passages, where a diphtheritic membrane forms. Lesions on the feet, legs, and body are less common. A complete review of avianpox may be found in Biester and Schwarte (1965).

Biester, H. E., and Schwarte, L. H.: Diseases of Poultry, 4th ed. Ames, Iowa, Iowa State University Press, 1965.

Danks, W. B. C.: A histochemical study by microincineration of the inclusion body of fowl pox. Am. J. Pathol., *8*:711–716, 1932.

Giddens, W. E., Jr., et al.: Canary pox in sparrows and canaries *(Fringillidae)* and in weavers *(Polceidae)*. Pathology and host specificity of the virus. Vet. Pathol., *8*:260–280, 1971.

Goodpasture, E. W., Woodruff, A. M., and Buddingh, G. J.: Vaccinial infection of the chorio-allantoic membrane of the chick embryo. Am. J. Pathol., *8*:271–282, 1932.

Woodruff, C. E., and Goodpasture, E. W.: The infectivity of isolated inclusion bodies in fowl pox. Am. J. Pathol., *5*:1–9, 1929.

———: Relation of virus of fowl pox to specific cellular inclusions in the disease. Am. J. Pathol., *6*:713–720, 1930.

Woodruff, C. E.: Comparison of the lesions of fowl pox and vaccinia in the chick, with especial reference to the virus bodies. Am. J. Pathol., *6*:169–173, 1930.

Diseases Caused by Capripoxviruses

Three diseases result from infection by viruses of this genus, *Capripoxvirus:* **Sheep-pox, goatpox** and **lumpy skin disease**. Each virus usually is confined under natural conditions to one species, but human infection with goatpox has been reported (Sawhney, Singh and Malik, 1972). Many virus strains may be adapted from natural host species to others by repeated experimental passage (Sharma and Danda, 1972). As in other genera of pox viruses, the members of this genus are related by their immunologic characteristics.

Sheep-pox

Sheep-pox is prevalent in parts of North Africa, Asia, and Southern Europe, but is not known to occur in the United States. It is a serious disease with cutaneous lesions appearing in areas devoid of wool, such as the cheeks, lips, and nostrils. Hemorrhages are often an aftermath of vesicle formation, followed by pustule formation. Gelatinous edema of the subcutis may be observed in proximity to the epidermal lesions. The disease has a tendency to become generalized, resembling smallpox in this respect, and mortality rates may reach 50%.

The lesions in the epidermis are similar to those of other poxviruses, with localized acanthosis followed by vesiculation starting in the middle layers of epithelium. In addition, the edematous underlying dermis and subcutis contain many distinctive cells, called "cellules claveleuses" of Borrel or "sheep-pox cells." These cells, concentrated especially around blood vessels and between collagen bundles, have nuclei with marginated chromatin, nucleoli, and a large vacuole in the center of the nucleus. The cytoplasm of these cells varies in shape, some resembling monocytes, others resembling macrophages. Some cells are fusiform, with the appearance of fibroblasts. The cytoplasm of most of these cells contains eosinophilic inclusion bodies. These bodies, under the electron microscope, are sites of viral replication, with a granular matrix and round developing virions as well as some characteristic ovoid-shaped mature pox virions. These mature virus particles are also seen elsewhere in the cytoplasm. Similar lesions, of course, are seen in infected epithelial cells in the dermis (Murray, Martin and Koylu, 1973).

Severe necrotizing vasculitis involves dermal and subcutaneous blood vessels. This results in ischemic necrosis and intense infiltration by neutrophils in and around the affected blood vessels.

Goatpox

This disease exists in North Africa, the Middle East, parts of Europe and India. The virus is immunologically related but distinguishable from that of sheep-pox. It has been reported on rare occasions to infect men who are in close contact with goats (Sawhney, Singh and Malik, 1972). The disease has a somewhat longer incubation and is less severe than sheep-pox. The skin lesions are smaller in goatpox and are seldom hemorrhagic.

Bennett, S. C. J., Horgan, E. S., and Mensur, A. H.: The pox disease of sheep and goats. J. Comp. Pathol., 54:131–159, 1944.
Krishnan, E.: Pathogenesis of sheep-pox. Indian Vet. J., 45:297–302, 1968.
Likhachev, N. V., et al.: Some studies on the pathogenesis of sheep pox. Trudy Nauchno-Kontrol Inst. Vet. Preparatov., 12:9–12, 1964. Vet. Bull., 35:1736, 1965.
Murray, M., Martin, W. B., and Koylu, A.: Experimental sheep-pox: a histological and ultrastructural study. Res. Vet. Sci., 15:201–208, 1973.
Palgov, A. A.: Immunogenic properties of various sheep pox virus strains. Trudy Nauchno-Kontrol Inst. Vet. Preparatov., 12:32–45, 1964. Vet. Bull., 35:1735, 1965.
Plowright, W., MacLeod, W. G., and Ferris, R. D.: The pathogenesis of sheep-pox in the skin of sheep. J. Comp. Pathol., 69:400–413, 1959.
Sawhney, A. N., Singh, A. K., and Malik, B. S.: Goat-pox an anthropozoonosis. Indian J. Med. Res., 60:683–684, 1972.
Sen, D. C.: Immunobiological relationships of goat pox and sheep pox viruses. Indian J. Med. Res., 56:1153–1156, 1968.
Sen, K. C., and Datt, N. S.: Studies on goat pox virus. I. Host range pathogenicity. II. Serological reactions. Indian J. Vet. Sci., 38:388–393, and 394–398, 1968.
Sharma, S. N.: Studies on sheep and goat pox viruses. Summary of thesis, Agra Univ., 1966. Vet. Bull., 37:4682, 1967.
Sharma, S. N., and Dhanda, M. R.: Studies on sheep and goat pox viruses: pathogenicity. Indian J. Animal Health, 11:39–46, 1972.
Vigario, J. D., and Ferraz, F. P.: Study of sheep-pox virus synthesis by fluorescent antibody technique. Am. J. Vet. Res., 28:809–813, 1967.

Lumpy-Skin Disease

Lumpy-skin disease is a disease of cattle, restricted to Africa, caused by a poxvirus related to the viruses of sheep-pox and goatpox. It is thought to be transmitted by insect vectors. The disease is characterized by a generalized cutaneous eruption of round, firm nodules, varying from 0.5 to 5 cm in diameter. Nodules may also appear on oral, nasal and genital mucous membranes, and there is enlargement of the superficial lymph nodes. The mortality rate is generally low, but may approach 10%. Microscopically, the nodule is characterized by the inflammatory reaction in the dermis composed of edema, perivascular collections of lymphocytes, macrophages, plasma cells, and neutrophils, and proliferating fibroblasts. There is necrosis and vesicle formation in the overlying epidermis. Eosinophilic cytoplasmic inclusion bodies form in epithelial cells and macrophages. Necrosis of the entire nodule precedes healing which requires three to five weeks. Rabbits are experimentally susceptible to the virus.

The disease may be differentiated from a Herpesvirus infection (called Allerton virus), which is frequent in cattle in Kenya, by the microscopic lesions and by finding the characteristic pox virions in those lesions (Davies et al., 1971).

Ayre-Smith, R. A.: The symptoms and clinical diagnosis of lumpy-skin disease. Vet. Rec., 72:469–472, 1960.

Davies, F.G., Krauss, H., Lund, J., and Taylor, M.: The laboratory diagnosis of lumpy skin disease. Res. Vet. Sci., 12:123–127, 1971.

Munz, E. K., and Owen, N. C.: Electron microscopic studies on lumpy-skin disease virus type "neethling." Onderstepoort. J. Vet. Res., 33:3–8, 1966.

Weiss, K. E.: Lumpy skin disease. Virology Monographs, 3:109–131, 1968.

Diseases Caused by Leporipoxviruses

Infectious Myxomatosis of Rabbits

Infectious myxomatosis occurring spontaneously in South American rabbits was first described by Sanarelli in 1898. During the intervening years the malady has been observed in many other parts of the world, where it has decimated the wild rabbits and threatened the domesticated rabbit population. In *Oryctolagus sp.*, the disease is characterized by the appearance of firm, elevated nodules in the skin, particularly in the vicinity of the eyes, mouth, nose, ears, and genitalia. Purulent conjunctivitis is a rather constant feature. The disease runs a rapid, highly fatal course, with death occurring a week or two after onset of symptoms.

The etiologic agent is a poxvirus that can be readily transmitted to susceptible rabbits but not to other animals. Its relation to the virus of the Shope fibroma (p. 303) is indicated by the immunity of rabbits against myxomatosis after infection with the fibroma virus. The virus exists in a natural state in wild rabbits in South America *(Sylvilagus braziliani)* and California *(Sylvilagus bachmani)*, occurring as an enzootic disease characterized by local cutaneous swelling without systemic lesions or mortality. The disease is exceptionally rare in hares *(Lepus sp.)*, which are naturally resistant to the virus. In the European, or common laboratory rabbit *(Oryctolagus cuniculus)*, both wild and domestic, the virus produces a systemic disease with a mortality rate greater than 99%. In Australia and probably Europe, following the deliberate introduction of the virus into wild populations of *Oryctolagus cuniculus*, attenuated strains of myxoma virus have evolved which are less virulent and result in a disease with lower mortality rate. Also the extreme lethality of myxomatosis has resulted in the evolution of a population of rabbits in these geographic areas with genetic resistance to the disease. Mosquitoes and fleas serve as mechanical vectors for natural transmission of the virus.

Lesions. The lesions in the skin are described by Rivers as numerous elevated, round, or ovoid masses which sometimes cause the skin to appear purplish. Most of

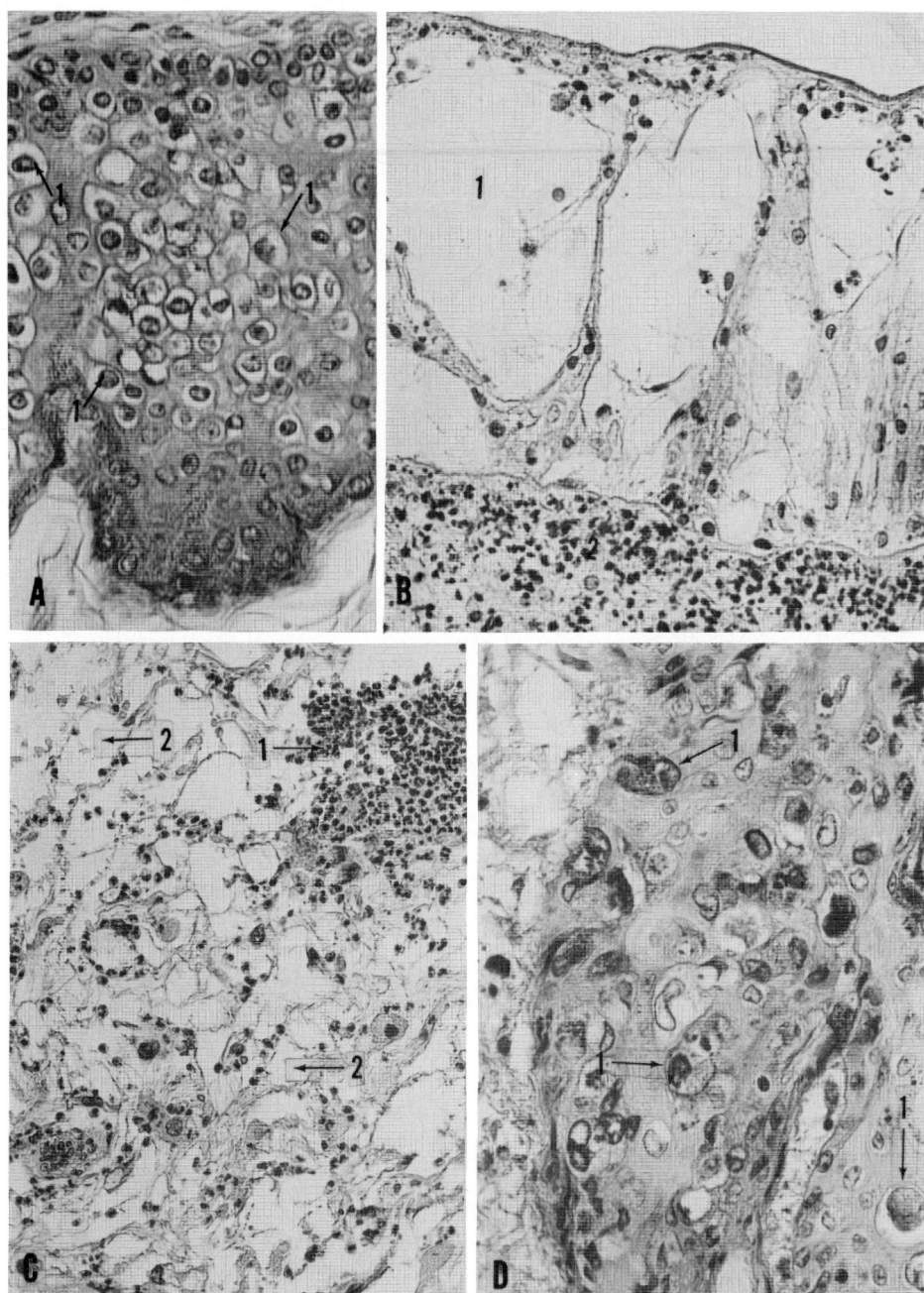

Fig. 9–3. Infectious myxomatosis of rabbits. *A,* Hyperplastic epidermis (× 365). Note large cells with vacuoles surrounding nuclei *(1). B,* Large vesicle *(1)* in epidermis in a later stage (× 395). *C,* Microabscess *(1)* and edematous spaces *(2)* in dermis (× 235). *D,* Giant, distorted nuclei *(1)* in the epidermis (× 395). (Courtesy of Armed Forces Institute of Pathology.) Contributor: Dr. J. Andrade dos Santos.

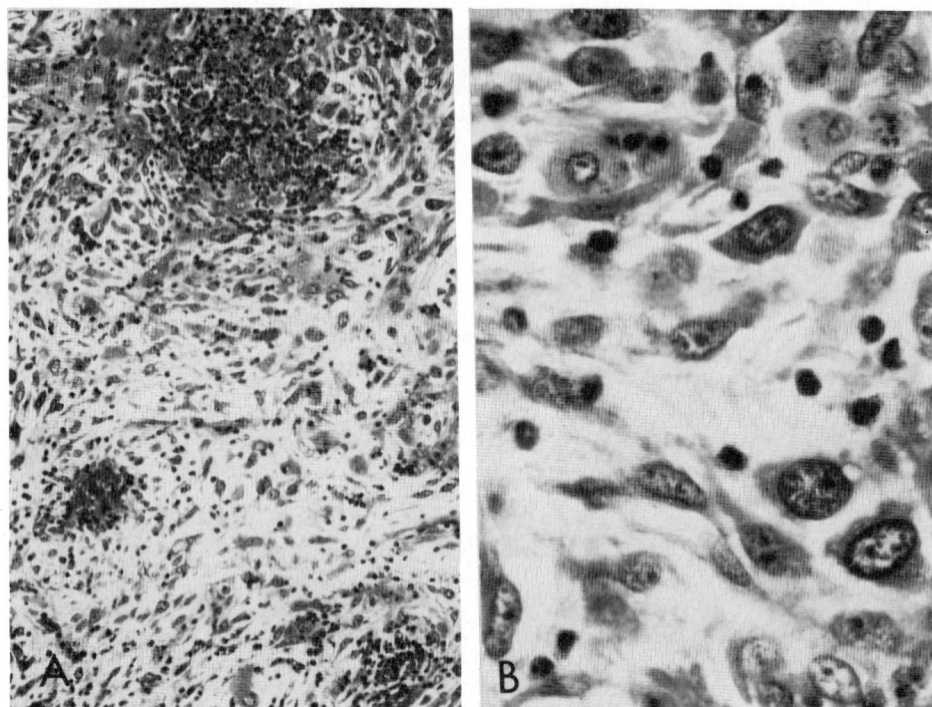

Fig. 9–4. Infectious myxomatosis, rabbit. *A*, Replacement of a lymph node by large "myxoma" cells. *B*, Higher magnification of "myxoma" cells in a lymph node. (Courtesy of Dr. F. Fenner.)

these nodules are firm and solid, but those near the genitalia may be edematous. Vesiculation of the epidermis over the lesions is evident grossly, and the vesicles are replaced by crusts, if the animal survives long enough. On cut section, the consistency of the cutaneous nodules is firm and tough, the epidermis is thickened or vesiculated, and the corium and subcutis contain gelatinous material interspersed with numerous blood vessels. The nodules are sometimes attached to the underlying musculature. The lymph nodes become enlarged, solid, and uniform in consistency.

Microscopically, the earliest change is increase in size and number of cells in the Malpighian layer, accompanied by the appearance of acidophilic granules, which increase in number and eventually fill the cytoplasm. Blue, rod-shaped bodies are sometimes seen among the acidophilic granules. The nuclei become swollen or vacuolated, and their chromatin is fragmented. The cells undergo dissolution to form vesicles in the epidermis, which subsequently coalesce into rather large bullae. In the underlying corium, large, stellate or polygonal cells appear along with much amorphous material, many neutrophils, and multinucleated cells. The nuclei of the stellate cells are swollen and contain some mitoses, and granules assumed to be ingested material are seen in the cytoplasm. These cells are often concentrated around blood vessels, and the endothelial cells of some vessels increase in number and size.

In the lymph nodes, hyperplasia of lymphoid cells occurs; the reticulum cells in the follicles increase in number and mix with a few neutrophils and eosinophils. The medulla is edematous, especially around vessels, and contains collections of neutrophils, eosinophils, mononuclear cells, and fibroblasts. Edema appears around small vessels and fibrin thrombi may be seen in the sinuses. Later many lymphocytes are lost, and overgrowth of reticuloendothelial cells interspersed with islands of neutrophils replaces most of the node. Later the reticulum may undergo cystic degeneration.

Diagnosis. Diagnosis is based on the clinical features, along with the gross and microscopic lesions, which are characteristic of the disease. Confirmation can be obtained by transmission of the disease to susceptible rabbits or virus isolation.

Fenner, F., and Ratcliffe, F. N.: Myxomatosis. Cambridge, Cambridge Univ. Press, 1965.

Fenner, F.: Myxomatosis. Br. Med. Bull., *15*:240–245, 1959.

Hurst, E. W.: Myxoma and the Shope fibroma. I. Histology of myxoma. Br. J. Exp. Pathol., *18*:1–15, 1937.

Rivers, T. M.: Observations on the pathological changes induced by virus myxomatosum (Sanarelli). J. Exp. Med., *51*:965–976, 1930.

Sanarelli, G.: Das myxomatogene virus; Beitrag zum Studium der Krankheitserreger ausserhalb des Sichtbaren. Zentralbl. Bakt., *23*:865–873, 1898.

Stewart, F. W.: The fundamental pathology of infectious myxomatosis. Am. J. Cancer *15*:2013–2028, 1931.

Shope Fibroma

Fibromas occurring naturally in the skin of wild cottontail rabbits *(Sylvilagus)* were described by Shope in 1932 and shown to be caused by a filtrable virus, classified as a poxvirus. These lesions are also transmitted experimentally to domestic rabbits *(Oryctolagus)*, and the agent was demonstrated to be related to that of infectious myxomatosis. The fibroma virus produces an effective immunity to subsequent infection by myxomatosis, although in other respects there is no resemblance between the two diseases.

Lesions. The lesions in the Shope fibroma are often multiple and are described as elevations of the skin by a fibrous mass; the overlying epidermis is thickened and sends bulbous, proliferating epithelium deep into the tumor. Large eosinophilic inclusions occur in the cytoplasm of the affected epidermal cells.

Viruses similar to the Shope fibroma virus have been reported to cause fibromas in brush rabbits *(Sylvilagus)* in California, fibromas in hares *(Lepus)* in Europe, and fibromas in gray squirrels in North America.

Cilli, V.: Aspetti Virologici del Fibroma di Shope e suoi Rapporti con il Mixoma di Sanarelli. G. Mal. Infet. Parassit., *10*:1017–1040, 1958.

Shope, R. E.: A transmissible tumor-like condition in rabbits. J. Exp. Med., *56*:793–802, 1932.

———: A filterable virus causing a tumor-like condition in rabbits and its relationship to virus myxomatosum. J. Exp. Med., *56*:803–833, 1932.

Diseases Caused by Parapoxviruses

Contagious Ovine Ecthyma

Synonyms for this disease are contagious pustular dermatitis, infectious labial dermatitis, "scabby mouth," "sore mouth," and "orf." Contagious ecthyma is an infectious poxvirus disease of sheep and goats in which vesicular or pustular lesions develop on the lips, oral mucous membranes, udder, and rarely, feet. It is also transmissible to man. The virus is immunologically related to the viruses of bovine papular stomatitis and pseudocowpox. The virus also appears to be related to the virus of ulcerative dermatosis of sheep. Mild transitory pustular lesions, particularly on the forearm, characterize the human disease, which has occurred after contact with infected sheep. Infection has been reproduced in sheep with material taken from such human lesions. The disease is known in the United States, Europe, and Australia. Screwworm *(Cochliomyia macellaria* and *Callitroga americana)* infestation of lesions is a serious complication of this disease in southern parts of the United States.

Lesions. The gross lesions appear as papules, vesicles, and then pustules, with necrosis and eventual sloughing of the affected areas. Microscopically, the lesions are sharply delimited, with the affected epidermis overlying a densely cellular dermis, richly vascular, and infiltrated with leukocytes and edema. The basal epidermal layer proliferates and appears to grow downward into the dermis. The superficial layers of the epidermis undergo degenerative changes consisting of vacuolation, ballooning degeneration, vesiculation, and pustule formation. In lambs, the disease may be more fulminant, and staphylococci are often present in the vesicles. Eosinophilic cytoplasmic inclusion bodies have been reported, but they are transitory and their specificity is not established.

Diagnosis. The diagnosis of contagious ecthyma is based on the characteristic lesions and isolation and identification of the virus. The disease must be differentiated from sheep-pox and ulcerative dermatosis. The virus is immunologically distinct from sheep-pox virus, and although related, separable from the virus of ulcerative dermatosis. The absence of inclusions in ecthyma is a point of histologic differentiation, as is also downgrowth of the basal layer of epidermis into the dermis, which does not occurr in sheep-pox or ulcerative dermatosis. The widespread cutaneous distribution of the lesions of sheep-pox and the preputial lesions of ulcerative dermatosis also aid in differential diagnosis.

Abdussalam, M.: Contagious pustular dermatitis. 2. Pathological histology. J. Comp. Pathol., 67:217–222, 1957.

———: Contagious pustular dermatitis. 3. Experimental infection (rabbits). J. Comp. Pathol., 67:305–319, 1957.

———: Contagious pustular dermatitis. 4. Immunological reactions. J. Comp. Pathol., 68:23–35, 1958.

Abdussalam, M., and Cosslett, V. E.: Contagious pustular dermatitis virus. 1. Studies on morphology. J. Comp. Pathol., 67:145–156, 1957.

Boughton, I. B., and Hardy, W. T.: Contagious ecthyma (sore mouth) of sheep and goats. J. Am. Vet. Med. Assoc., 85:150–178, 1934.

Park, V. M., Mackerras, I. M., Sutherland, A. K., and Simmons, G. C.: Transmission of contagious ecthyma from sheep to man. Med. J. Aust., 2:628–632, 1951.

Theiler, A.: Ecthyma Contagiosum of Sheep and Goats. Thirteenth and 14th Ann. Reports, Director, Vet. Ed. and Res., Union of South Africa, 1928, pp. 7–14.

Wheeler, C. E., and Cawley, E. P.: The microscopic picture of ecthyma contagiosum (orf) in sheep, rabbits, and men. Am. J. Pathol., 32:535–545, 1956.

Bovine Papular Stomatitis

A mild disease that causes lesions in and around the mouth of young cattle has been recognized from time to time in Europe and the United States. It does not cause serious illness, but in some respects simulates some features of certain important bovine diseases (aphthous fever, vesicular stomatitis, mucosal disease, and viral diarrhea). Several different names have been used to describe what may eventually prove to be a single disease entity: pseudoaphthous stomatitis, *stomatitis papulosa bovis specifica*, infectious ulcerative stomatitis, proliferative stomatitis, and esophagitis.

One viral agent has been isolated by Griesemer and Cole (1960), and the disease has been reproduced experimentally. This agent multiplies in tissue cultures of bovine kidney cells, but does not produce any cytopathogenic effect in these cultures. Guinea pigs, weanling mice, and chick embryos are apparently not susceptible. This virus may be the same as the infectious agent described by Olson and Palionis (1953) and Pritchard et al. (1958) because the diseases are similar, but exact comparisons have not been made. The virus has been shown to be closely related to paravaccinia (pseudocowpox virus) and to share antigenic properties with the virus of contagious ecthyma. The virus is infectious for man, producing erythematous papules on the hands and arms.

Signs. The disease affects young calves for the most part; clinical signs are mild and fever is not usually manifest, although viremia evidently occurs. The course of the disease is prolonged—usually several weeks.

Lesions. The lesions are found on the lips, muzzle, nostrils, gingivae, tongue, and oral mucosa generally, and in sacrificed

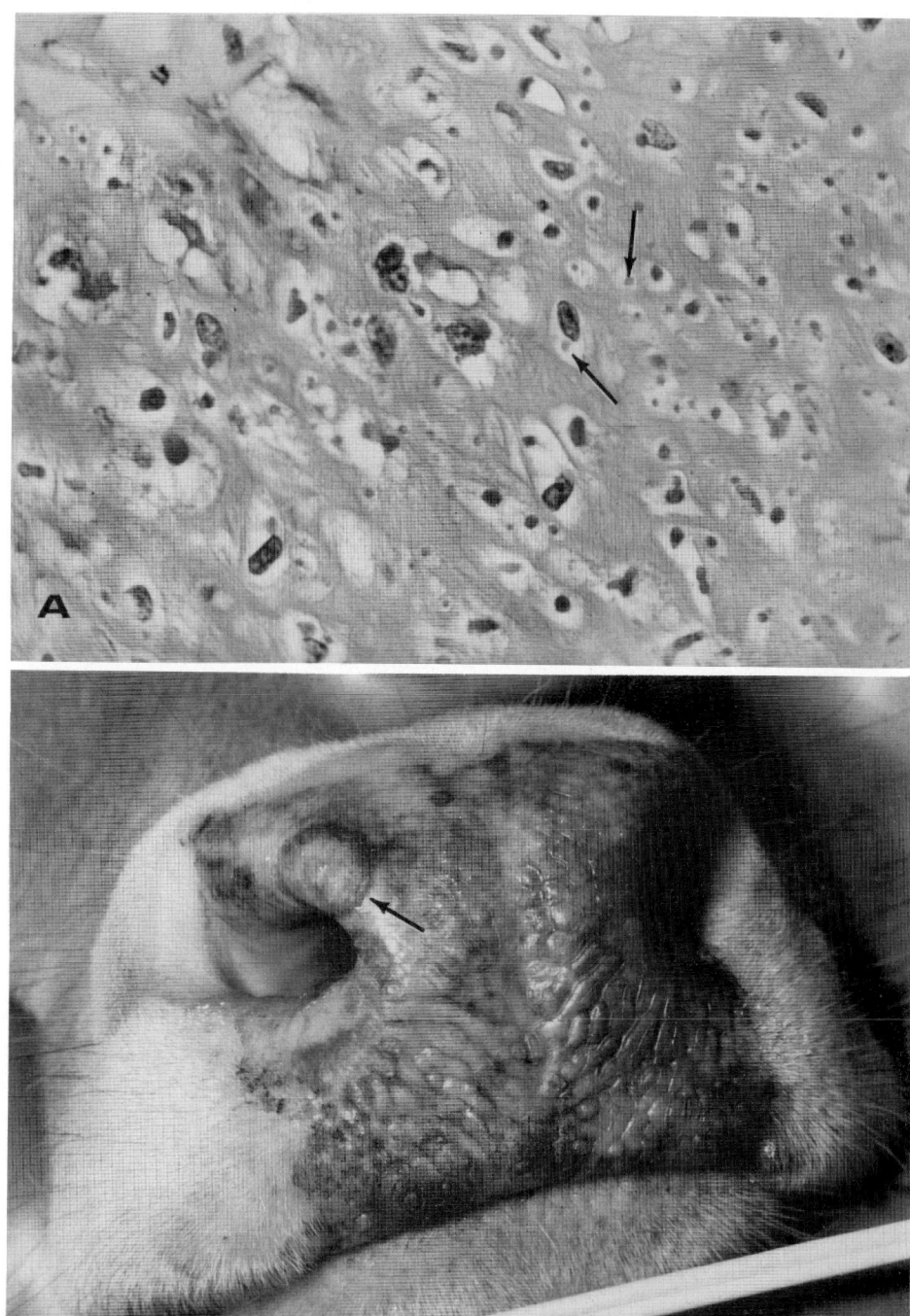

Fig. 9–5. Bovine papular stomatitis. *A*, Photomicrograph of epithelium containing eosinophilic inclusion bodies (arrows). *B*, Muzzle of a calf with an experimentally induced papular lesion of nostril (arrow). (Courtesy of Dr. Richard A. Griesemer, Ohio State University.)

305

animals, in the esophagus, rumen, reticulum and omasum. The earliest lesions are recognized grossly as small hyperemic foci 2 to 4 mm in diameter, often on the lower margin of the nostrils, occasionally on the palate or inner surface of the lips. In about a day, the center of these foci become elevated from the surface to form a low, convex, whitish papule. At this time, the epithelium, seen microscopically, is focally hyperplastic and contains focal areas of hydropic degeneration. These changes in the epithelium, up to 300 μ in diameter, are located for the most part in the superficial part of the **stratum spinosum**. Nuclei in these zones are often pyknotic and occasionally undergo karyorrhexis. As the disease progresses, the hydropic lesions move toward the surface, and the affected epithelial cells often contain spherical cytoplasmic inclusion bodies which are 10 μ or more in diameter, homogeneous, eosinophilic, and usually only one in a cell. Congestion of the adjacent lamina propria usually gives the papular lesion a reddish or pink hue at this time. As the lesions reach the surface, they become grossly roughened and may become infiltrated by neutrophils. The thickened epithelium may become eroded, leaving an elevated ulcer. Superficial erosion of the epithelium may appear in some instances rather than ulcers. These may become filled with pyogenic granulation tissue. Confluence of lesions often occurs. Healing is usually uneventful but prolonged.

Diagnosis. The diagnosis is usually based upon the mild clinical course, the gross and histologic appearance of the lesions, and the isolation and identification of the virus.

Buttner, D., et al.: The fine structure of the virions of contagious pustular dermatitis and bovine papular stomatitis. Arch. Ges. Virusforsch., *14*:657–673, 1964.

Carson, C. A., Kerr, K. M., and Grumbles, L. C.: Bovine papular stomatitis: experimental transmission from man. Am. J. Vet. Res., *29*:1783–1790, 1968.

Carson, C. A., and Kerr, K. M.: Bovine papular

stomatitis with apparent transmission to man. J. Am. Vet. Med. Assoc., *151*:183–187, 1967.

Griesemer, R. A., and Cole, C. R.: Bovine papular stomatitis. I. Recognition in the United States. J. Am. Vet. Med. Assoc., *137*:404–410, 1960.

———: Bovine papular stomatitis. II. The experimentally-produced disease. Am. J. Vet. Res., 22:473–481, 1961.

———: Bovine papillary stomatitis. III. Histopathology. Am. J. Vet. Res., 22:482–486, 1961.

Matthias, D., and Jakob, W.: Zur pathologischen Anatomie der Stomatitis papulosa infectiosa bovis. Mh. Vet. Med., *17*:265–274, 1962. VB *32*:4156, 1962.

Olson, C., Jr., and Palionis, T.: The transmission of proliferative stomatitis of cattle. J. Am. Vet. Med. Assoc., *123*:419–426, 1953.

Plowright, W., and Ferris, R. D.: Papular stomatitis of cattle in Kenya and Nigeria. Vet. Rec., *71*:718–722, 1959.

———: Papular stomatitis of cattle. II. Reproduction of the disease with culture-passaged virus. Vet. Rec., *71*:828–832, 1959.

Pritchard, W. R., Claflin, R. M., Gustafson, D. P., and Ristic, M.: An infectious ulcerative stomatitis of cattle. J. Am. Vet. Med. Assoc., *132*:273–278, 1958.

Pseudocowpox

The virus of pseudocowpox is called **paravaccinia** and is not related to vaccinia or cowpox. Paravaccinia virus is closely related to the viruses of contagious ovine ecthyma and bovine papular stomatitis. The lesions are limited to the teats and udders, appearing as red papules and vesicles. Microscopically there is proliferation of the subepithelial capillary network, vesicular degeneration of the epithelium and eosinophilic cytoplasmic inclusion bodies. Infection does not confer immunity. The disease is transmissible to man as "milkers' nodules," and oral lesions may develop in suckling calves.

Cheville, N. F., and Shey, D. J.: Pseudocowpox in dairy cattle. J. Am. Vet. Med. Assoc., *150*:855–861, 1967.

Duncan, A. G.: Milkers' nodules. Canad. Med. Assoc. J., *77*:339–342, 1957.

Friedman-Keen, A. E., Rowe, S. P., and Banfield, W. G.: Milkers' nodules. Isolation of poxvirus from a human case. Science, *140*:1335–1336, 1963.

Huck, R. A.: A paravaccinia virus isolated from cows' teats. Vet. Rec., *78*:503–504, 1966.

Laurence, B.: Cowpox in man and its relationship with milker's nodules. Lancet, *268*:764–766, 1955.

Liebermann, H.: Relationships between milker's nodules, udder pox, papular stomatitis and contagious ecthyma. Z. arztl. Fortbildung., *61*:447–448, 1967.

Nagington, J., Lauder, T. M., and Smith, J. S.: Bovine papular stomatitis, pseudocowpox and milker's nodules. Vet. Rec., *81*:306–313, 1967.

Nagington, J., Tee, G. H., and Smith, J. S.: Milker's nodule virus infection in Dorset and their similarity to orf. Nature, *208*:505–507, 1965.

Neal, E. J. E., and Calvert, H. T.: Milkers' nodules. Some observations on true and false cowpox apropos an outbreak in a closed community. Br. J. Derm., *79*:318–324, 1967.

Diseases Caused by Unclassified Poxviruses

Swinepox

This common disease in the Corn Belt of the United States principally affects young swine. The virus of swinepox is not related to that of vaccinia and is believed to be transmitted by the swine louse, *Haematopinus suis*, though a vector is not necessary for transmission. The incubation period is five to seven days, following which erythematous areas, then papules, 4 to 5 mm in diameter, appear. These lesions usually are limited to the underside of the body but may involve the skin generally. In the vesicular and pustular stages, the lesions often escape observation and are detected only when they have become umbilicated. Eosinophilic cytoplasmic inclusion bodies develop in epithelial cells. Swine are reported to be susceptible to vaccinia virus, and this is the most common and severe form of pox in swine in Europe. True swinepox also occurs in Europe.

Blakemore, F., and Abdussalam, M.: Morphology of the elementary bodies and cell inclusions in swine pox. J. Comp. Pathol., *66*:373–377, 1956.

Cheville, N. F.: The cytopathology of swine pox in the skin of swine. Am. J. Pathol., *49*:339–352, 1966.

Datt, N. S., and Orlans, E. S.: The immunological relationship of the vaccinia and pigpox viruses demonstrated by gel diffusion. Immunology, *1*:81–86, 1958.

Datt, N. S.: Comparative studies of pigpox and vaccinia viruses. II. Serological relationship. J. Comp. Pathol., *74*:70–80, 1964.

Kasza, L., and Griesemer, R. A.: Experimental swine pox. Am. J. Vet. Res., *23*:443–451, 1962.

McNutt, S. H., Murray, C., and Purwin, P.: Swine pox. J. Am. Vet. Med. Assoc., *74*:752–761, 1929.

Murray, C.: Swine pox. J. Am. Vet. Med. Assoc., *90*:326–330, 1937.

Nakamatsu, M., Gogo, M., and Morita, M.: Electron microscopy of the inclusion bodies in pigpox. Jap. J. Vet. Sci., *30*:289–297, 1968.

Molluscum Contagiosum

Molluscum contagiosum is a disease of man caused by a distinct poxvirus. The

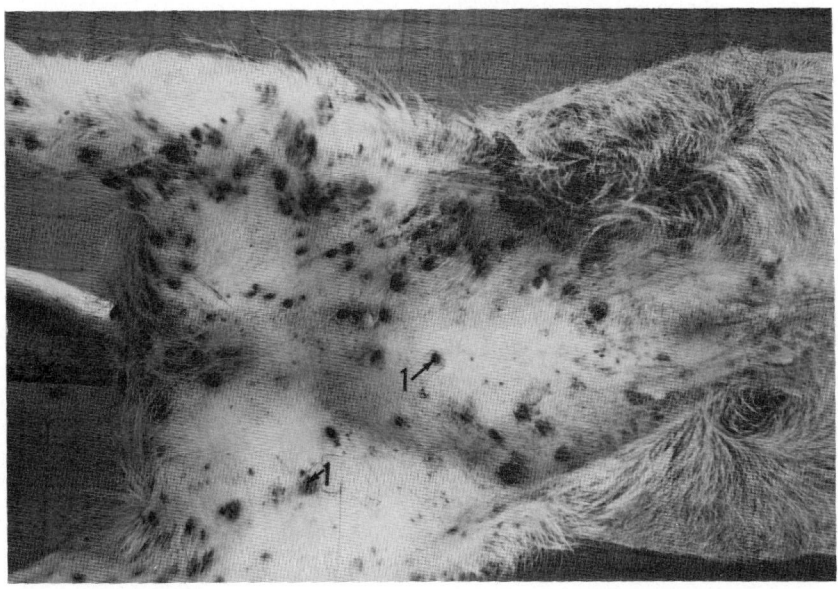

Fig. 9–6. Swine pox, abdomen of a pig. Note hemorrhagic appearance of pox lesions *(1)*.

lesions are characterized by epithelial hyperplasia and extremely large eosinophilic inclusion bodies, which enlarge to eventually occupy a whole cell. A disease histologically similar has been described in chimpanzees.

Douglas, J. D., et al.: Molluscum contagiosum in chimpanzees. J. Am. Vet. Med. Assoc., 151:901–904, 1967.
Goodpasture, W. E., and Woodruff, C. E.: Molluscum contagiosum. Am. J. Pathol., 7:1–9, 1931.

Ulcerative Dermatosis

Synonyms are infectious balanoposthitis, ulcerative vulvitis, lip and leg ulceration. Ulcerative dermatosis is a disease of sheep and goats characterized by an ulcerative dermatitis of the lips, legs, feet, prepuce, and vulva. The virus is a member of the poxvirus group and is immunologically related to the virus of contagious ovine ecthyma. The lesions are poorly studied but reportedly nonspecific in microscopic appearance, and lack the hyperplasia of epidermis seen in contagious ecthyma.

Flook, W. H.: An outbreak of venereal disease among sheep (ulcerative dermatosis). J. Comp. Pathol., 16:374–375, 1903.
McFadyean, J. A.: A contagious disease of the generative organ of sheep. J. Comp. Pathol., 16:375–376, 1903.
Roberts, R. S., and Bolton, J. F. A.: A venereal disease of sheep. Vet. Rec., 57:686–687, 1945.
Trueblood, M. S.: Relationship of ovine contagious ecthyma and ulcerative dermatosis. Cornell Vet., 56:521–526, 1966.
Tunnicliff, E. A.: Ulcerative dermatosis of sheep. Am. J. Vet. Res., 10:240–249, 1949.

Benign Epidermal Pox of Monkeys

Several pox diseases have been observed in captive primates in laboratories and zoos. Virus strains isolated from these outbreaks have been given various names and have been compared to one another to some extent. At this time it appears that these viruses are each related and produce a disease most closely resembling a "benign epidermal pox disease" described by Casey et al. (1967). The viruses in this group differ from that described as mon-

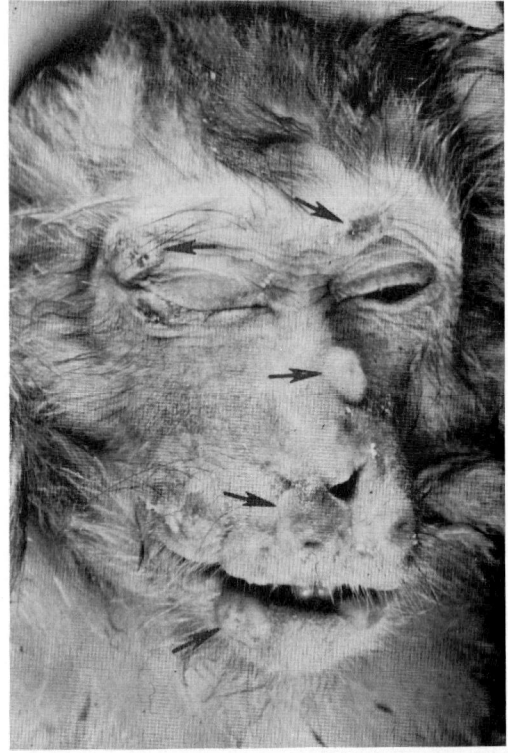

Fig. 9–7. Monkey pox. Numerous elevated pocks on the skin of the face of a macaque infected with "Oregon" monkey pox. (Courtesy of Dr. W. P. McNulty.)

keypox virus, a member of the genus *Orthopoxvirus*.

Yaba virus, a poxvirus which was first encountered in a laboratory colony of rhesus monkeys located in Yaba, Nigeria, has caused lesions in animal caretakers. This agent has been studied at length in the laboratory. Similar viruses have been encountered in outbreaks in colonies of monkeys in Oregon, Texas, and California. These strains have been referred to as the "Or Te Ca" pox viruses. Another virus, the Tana pox virus, was isolated (Downie et al., 1971) from people living along the Tana River in Kenya, Africa. Monkeys proved to be susceptible to this virus after experimental inoculation.

The disease and the lesions caused by this group of viruses are similar and may

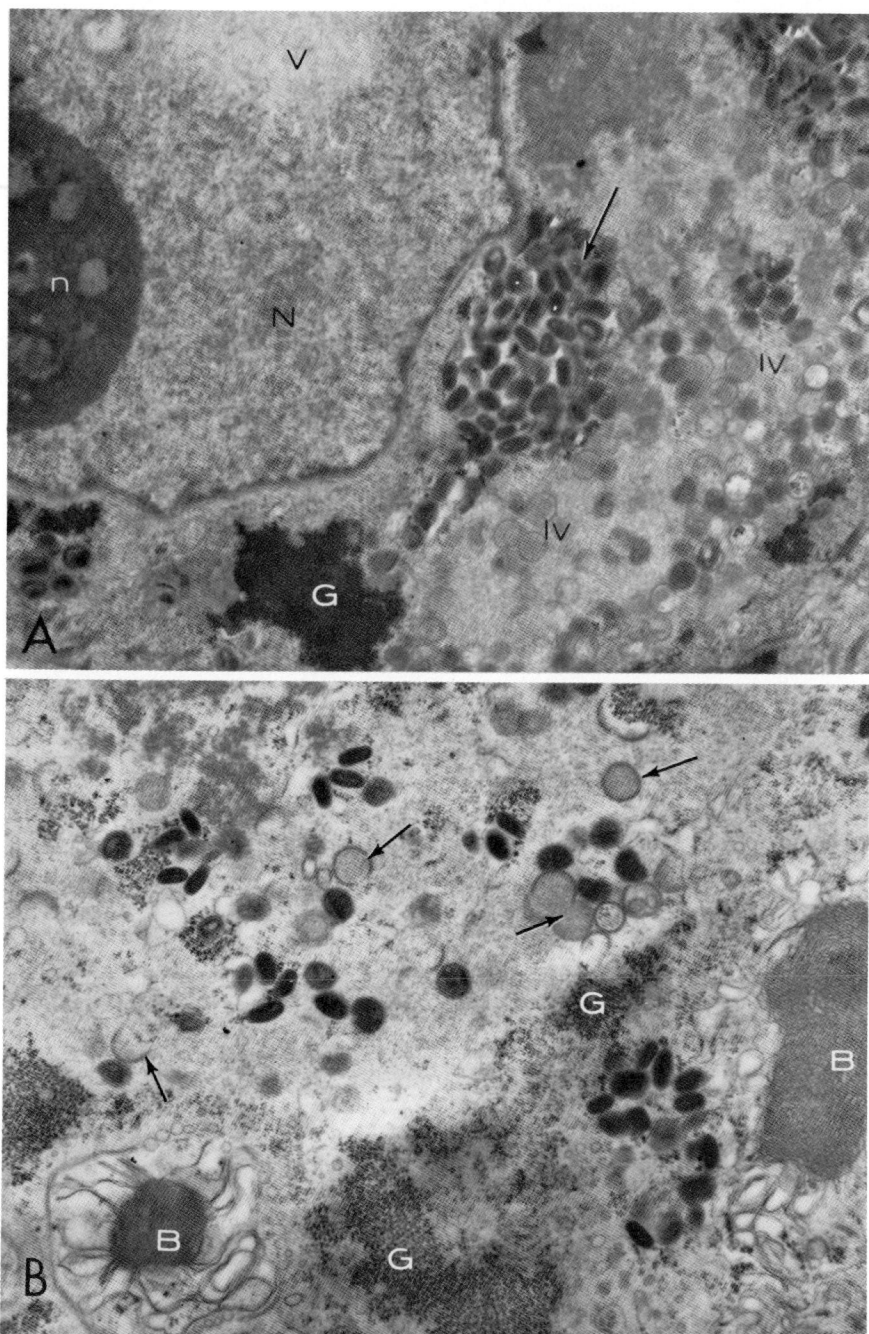

Fig. 9–8. Oregon monkey pox. *A*, Portion of an epithelial cell with nuclear vacuolization *(V)*; abundant mature viral particles (arrow) surrounded by immature particles *(IV)*. *G*, glycogen; *N*, nucleus; *n*, nucleolus (× 17,000). *B*, Immature viral particles (arrows) and dense crystalloid bodies *(B)*. *G*, glycogen (× 26,000). (Courtesy of Dr. W. P. McNulty.)

be considered together. The signs include brief febrile manifestations followed by the appearance of one or more solid masses in the epidermis, oral mucous membranes, or viscera. The lesions consist of proliferation of epithelial cells containing eosinophilic cytoplasmic inclusions. Necrosis of epidermis and inflammation in the dermis may follow, but vesicles are not usually formed. The disease usually runs a benign course.

Ambrus, J. L., Strandstrom, H. V., and Kawinski, W.: 'Spontaneous' occurrence of Yaba tumor in a monkey colony. Experimentia, 25:64–65, 1969.

Ambrus, J. L., and Strandstrom, H. V.: Susceptibility of Old World monkeys to Yaba virus. Nature (London), 211:876, 1966.

Behbehani, A. M., et al.: Yaba tumor virus. I. Studies on pathogenesis and immunity. Proc. Soc. Exp. Biol. Med., 129:556–561, 1968.

Casey, H. W., Woodruff, J. M., and Butcher, W. I.: Electron microscopy of a benign epidermal pox disease of rhesus monkeys. Am. J. Pathol., 51:431–446, 1967.

Cheville, N., et al.: Cytopathic changes in lesions of a pox disease in monkeys. Iowa State Univ. Vet., 30:77–81, 1968; Vet. Bull., 39:3328, 1969.

Crandell, R. A., Casey, H. W., and Brunlow, W. B.: Studies of a newly recognized poxvirus of monkeys. J. Infect. Dis., 119:80–88, 1969.

Downie, A. W., et al.: Tanapox: A new disease caused by a pox virus. Br. Med. J., 1:363–368, 1971.

Downie, A. W., and Espana, C.: Comparison of Tanapox virus and Yaba-like viruses causing epidemic disease in monkeys. J. Hyg. (Camb.), 70:23–33, 1972.

Downie, A. W., and Espana, C.: A comparative study of Tanapox and Yaba viruses. J. Gen. Virol., 19:37–49, 1973.

Gispen, R., Verlinde, J. D., and Zwart, P.: Histopathological and virological studies on monkeypox. Arch. Ges. Virusforsch., 21:205–216, 1967.

Grace, J. T., and Mirand, E. A.: Human susceptibility to a simian tumor virus. Ann. NY Acad. Sci., 108:1123–1128, 1963.

Grace, J. T., Jr., and Mirand, E. A.: Yaba virus infection in humans. Exp. Med. Surg., 23:213–216, 1965.

Hall, A. S., and McNulty, W. P., Jr.: A contagious pox disease in monkeys. J. Am. Vet. Med. Assoc., 151:833–838, 1967.

Kupper, J. L., Casey, H. W., and Johnson, D. K.: Experimental Yaba and benign epidermal monkey pox in Rhesus monkeys. Lab. Anim. Care, 20:979–988, 1970.

Luby, J. P.: Another zoonosis from monkeys—Tanapox. Ann. Intern. Med., 75:800–801, 1971.

McConnell, S., et al.: Monkeypox: experimental infection in chimpanzee (Pan satyrus) and immuniza-

tion with vaccinia virus. Am. J. Vet. Res., 29:1675–1680, 1968.

————: Protection of Rhesus monkeys against monkeypox by vaccinia virus immunization. Am. J. Vet. Res., 25:192–195, 1964.

McNulty, W. P., et al.: A pox disease in monkeys transmitted to man. Arch. Dermatol., 97:286–293, 1968.

Nivan, J. S. C., et al.: Subcutaneous growths in monkeys produced by poxvirus. J. Pathol. Bact., 81:1–14, 1961.

Olsen, R. G., and Yohn, D. S.: Immunodiffusion analysis of Yaba poxvirus structural and associated antigens. J. Virol., 5:212–220, 1970.

Peters, J. C.: An epizootic of monkey pox at Rotterdam Zoo. Int. Zoo Yearbook, 6:274–275, 1966.

Prier, J. E., et al.: Studies on a pox disease of monkeys. II. Isolation of the etiological agent. Am. J. Vet. Res., 21:381–384, 1960.

Rouhandeh, H., et al.: Properties of monkey pox virus. Arch. Ges. Virusforsch., 20:363–373, 1967.

Sauer, R. M., et al.: Studies on a pox disease of monkeys. I. Pathology. Am. J. Vet. Res., 21:377–380, 1960.

Tsuchiya, Y., and Rouhandeh, H.: Plaque formation by Yaba virus in cynomolgus monkey kidney cells. J. Natl. Cancer Inst., 47:219–222, 1971.

Tsuruhara, T.: Immature particle formation of Yaba poxvirus studied by electron microscopy. J. Natl. Cancer Inst., 47:549–554, 1971.

von Magnus, P., Anderson, E. K., Peterson, K. B.: A pox-like disease in cynomolgus monkeys. Acta Path. Microbiol. Scand., 46:156–176, 1959.

Wenner, H. A., et al.: Studies on pathogenesis of monkey pox. III. Histopathological lesions and sites of immunofluorescence. Arch. Ges. Virusforsch., 27:179–197, 1969.

Wenner, H. A., Macasaet, F. D., and Kamitsuka, P. S.: Monkey pox. I. Clinical, virologic and immunologic studies. Am. J. Epidemiol., 87:551–566, 1968.

Wenner, H. A., et al.: Studies on pathogenesis of monkey pox. II. Dose-response and virus dispersion. Arch. Ges. Virusforsch., 27:166–178, 1969.

Wolfe, L. G., Griesemer, R. A., and Farrell, R. L.: Experimental aerosol transmission of Yaba virus in monkeys. J. Natl. Cancer Inst., 41:1175–1195, 1968.

Yohn, D. S., Marmol, F. R., and Olsen, R. G.: Growth kinetics of Yaba tumor poxvirus after in vitro adaptation to Cercopithecus kidney cells. J. Virol., 5:205–211, 1970.

Rabbitpox

Outbreaks of pox have been described in rabbits caused by a virus indistinguishable from vaccinia. The disease may become generalized, with necrotizing lesions in the oral mucous membranes, lungs, liver, adrenal glands, testicles, and lymph nodes, in addition to cutaneous pocks. The skin lesions lack the vesicular character seen in most other poxvirus infections. Inclusion bodies have not been reported.

Christensen, L. R., Bond, E., and Matanic, B.: "Pockless" rabbit pox. Lab. Anim. Care, *17*:281–296, 1967.

Green, H. S. N.: Rabbit pox. I. Clinical manifestations and cause of the disease. II. Pathology of the epidemic disease. J. Exp. Med., *60*:427–440, 441–456, 1934.

Horsepox

Apparently an ancient disease of horses, horsepox is known in Europe but not in the United States. It is believed to be caused by an immunologically distinct virus, but the relationship of the horsepox virus to other poxviruses is not known. Lesions may occur on the lips, nose, oral mucosa, and genitalia. "Grease-heel," papular dermatitis and Uasin Gishu skin disease of the horse may represent other forms of horsepox.

Andrews, C., and Pereira, H. G.: Viruses of Vertebrates. 2nd ed. London, Bailliere, Tindal and Cassell, 1967.

Eby, C. H.: A note in the history of horse pox. J. Am. Vet. Med. Assoc., *132*:420–422, 1958.

Kaminjolo, J. S., Jr., and Winqvist, G.: Histopathology of skin lesions in Uasin Gishu skin disease of horses. J. Comp. Pathol., *85*:391–395, 1975.

McIntyre, R. W.: Virus papular dermatitis of the horse. Am. J. Vet. Res., *10*:229–232, 1949.

HERPETOVIRIDAE

This family contains at the moment only one genus, *Herpesvirus* (herpes = creeping), in which are grouped many viruses pathogenic for man and animals. Most of the *Herpesviruses* have been given species names based upon their usual host, but none of these names has been officially accepted at this time (1980). Table 9–5 presents a summary of the *Herpesviruses*, their hosts, species names, and the disease which they are considered to cause.

The nucleic acid of *Herpesviruses* is DNA and ultrastructurally the capsid is icosahedral in configuration surrounded by an envelope formed by the nuclear membrane of the host cell (Fig. 9–1). The virions are assembled in the nucleus, producing characteristic inclusions recognizable by the light microscope (Fig. 9–9). The envelope is acquired as the virion emerges by budding through the nuclear mem-

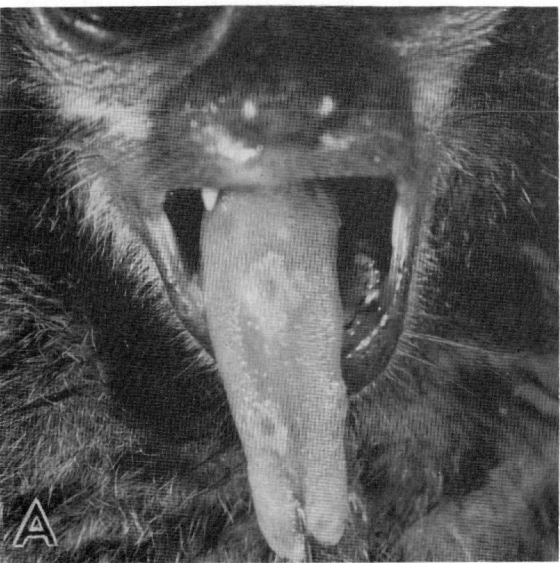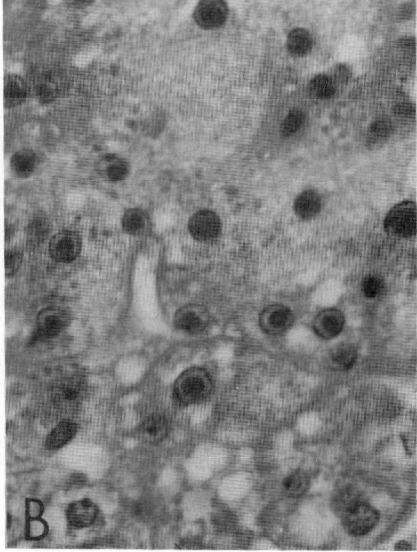

Fig. 9–9. *Herpesvirus simplex* infection of an owl monkey *(Aotus trivirgatus). A,* Ulcerative glossitis. *B,* Intranuclear inclusion bodies in hepatocytes. (Courtesy of New England Regional Primate Research Center, Harvard Medical School.)

brane. Each capsid contains 162 capsomeres enclosed within a lipoprotein envelope. Each virus produces a group-specific antibody, associated with the nucleocapsid and demonstrable by immunodiffusion. Several type-specific antigens are associated with the nucleocapsid and envelope.

The molecular characteristics of herpesviruses (Fenner et al., 1976) are summarized as follows: single linear molecule of double-stranded DNA, about 100 million daltons; icosahedral capsid 100 nm in diameter with 162 capsomeres, enclosed by an envelope 150 nm in diameter; multiplies in nucleus; matures by budding at nuclear

membrane. Group-specific antigens are associated with the nucleocapsid.

Fenner, F.: Classification and Nomenclature of Viruses. (Second Report of the International Committee on Taxonomy of Viruses.) Basel, S. Karger, 1976.

Diseases Caused by Herpesviruses

Herpesvirus Simplex Infection in Primates (Herpesvirus hominis)

Herpesvirus simplex infection is one of the oldest viral diseases known to man. The use of the word herpes in medicine can be traced as far back as Hippocrates, and descriptions clearly related to the disease

Table 9–7. Diseases Caused by Herpetoviridae (Genus: Herpesvirus)

Names of Viruses	Host(s)	Name of Disease
H. simplex, type 1	Human, marmosets, owl monkeys	Herpes simplex, oral, nasal rarely brain; generalized in marmoset
H. simplex, type 2	Human	Genital herpes
H. varicella-zoster	Human	Varicella and zoster
Epstein-Barr virus	Human	Infectious mononucleosis, probably Burkitt's lymphoma, and nasopharyngeal carcinoma
H. simiae, "B virus"	Nonhuman primates	Herpes B of nonhuman (Macaques esp.) primates; rarely affects humans
H. suis	Swine, cattle	Pseudorabies, Aujeszky's disease
H. canis	Canines	Canine herpes, upper respiratory tract
H. equi (Equine herpesvirus, type 1)	Equines	Equine rhinopneumonitis; equine viral abortion
H. spp	Bovines	Infectious bovine rhinotracheitis
H. felis	Felines	Infectious feline rhinotracheitis
H. bovis	Bovines	Malignant catarrhal fever
H. spp	Bovines	Herpesvirus mamillitis
Laryngotracheitis virus	Birds	Infectious laryngotracheitis
Marek's disease virus	Chickens	Avian lymphomatosis; Marek's disease
Lucké's virus	Frogs	Adenocarcinoma of kidney
H. saimiri	Squirrel monkey (Saimiri sciureus)	Carried by squirrel monkeys; experimentally produces malignant lymphoma in marmosets, rabbits, and owl monkeys
H. ateles	Spider monkey (Ateles spp.)	Carried by spider monkeys; experimentally produces malignant lymphoma in marmosets, rabbits, and owl monkeys
H. tamarinus	Squirrel monkeys, marmosets	Carried by squirrel monkeys; natural systemic disease in marmosets
Cytomegaloviruses	Specific for each disease	Many viruses, characteristic lesions in man, guinea pig, monkeys, swine

as now understood in man were published in the seventeenth century. Many early reports describe experimental transmission of *Herpesvirus simplex* to laboratory animals, such as rabbits, guinea pigs, mice, rats, and hamsters. *H. simplex* is an important spontaneous disease of owl monkeys (*Aotus trivirgatus*), a New World species, and gibbons (*Hylobates lar*), an anthropoid ape.

The Disease in Man. Man is the natural and reservoir host for *H. simplex*, assuming a role similar to the Rhesus monkey with *Herpesvirus B*, the Squirrel monkey with *Herpesvirus T*, and swine with *Herpesvirus suis*. Two antigenically different *H. simplex* viruses infect human beings. Type 1 usually affects the lips and oral mucosa; type 2 causes lesions on the genital mucosae of both sexes and is transmitted by coitus. Primary infection of type 1 virus occurs principally in young children, taking the form of an acute gingivostomatitis, which heals with no serious side effects. By adolescence or early adulthood, 90 to 95% of all individuals have become infected, as evidenced by the presence of serum neutralizing antibodies. Many people, despite the presence of serum neutralizing antibodies, suffer from periodic recurrence of secondary *H. simplex* infection for much of their lives, often with several episodes occurring each year. Recurrent lesions are believed to be the result of activation of a latent infection that persists in all infected individuals for life. A variety of stimuli have been associated with activation, including fever ("fever blister"), colds ("cold sore"), fatigue, menstruation, emotional distress, and certain foods.

Lesions. Recurrent lesions are characterized by small clusters of vesicles that rupture, leaving erosions or ulcers that heal in five to ten days. Hyperesthesia and neuralgia often precede the lesions and may persist for variable periods of time after healing. The mucocutaneous junction of the lip is the most frequent site, but the external nares, oral mucosa, conjunctiva, skin, esophagus, external genitalia, vagina, and cervix are not uncommon locations.

Microscopic features are ballooning degeneration, necrosis, intracellular edema, multinucleated giant cells, and intranuclear inclusion bodies. Virus is readily isolated during the course and up to three weeks after recovery. Interestingly, virus can be recovered from a proportion of the population (7 to 20%) in the absence of visible lesions.

H. simplex, type 1, infection in man is not always a benign disease. In neonates and young children, primary infection may lead to a fatal generalized disease affecting most organs and tissues, and in adults, fatal meningoencephalitis can develop. The lesions in both of these forms are characterized by focal necrosis and intranuclear inclusion bodies in the affected tissues. At present there is no satisfactory explanation for the occurrence of serious disease in the natural host for *H. simplex*. The finding, however, is not dissimilar from the effect of *H. suis* in its natural host, swine, or for *H. canis* in its probable natural host, the dog.

The Disease in Monkeys. In owl monkeys, *H. simplex* produces an epizootic disease with high morbidity and mortality rates. Following an incubation period of about seven days, there is a short clinical illness characterized by oral and labial ulceration, ulcerative dermatitis, conjunctivitis, anorexia, hyperesthesia, weakness and incoordination. Death is the usual outcome in two to three days. Lesions are widespread and identical both grossly and microscopically to those produced in this species by *Herpesvirus T*, except that encephalitis is frequent in *H. simplex* infection. The encephalitis is similar to *H. simplex* infection in man; the lesions are most extensive in the temporal lobes of the cerebral cortex, with extension in the frontal, parietal, and occipital lobes. Lesions may also occur in the thalamus and basal nuclei. The changes are principally characterized by widespread necrosis of neurons, with many neurons containing

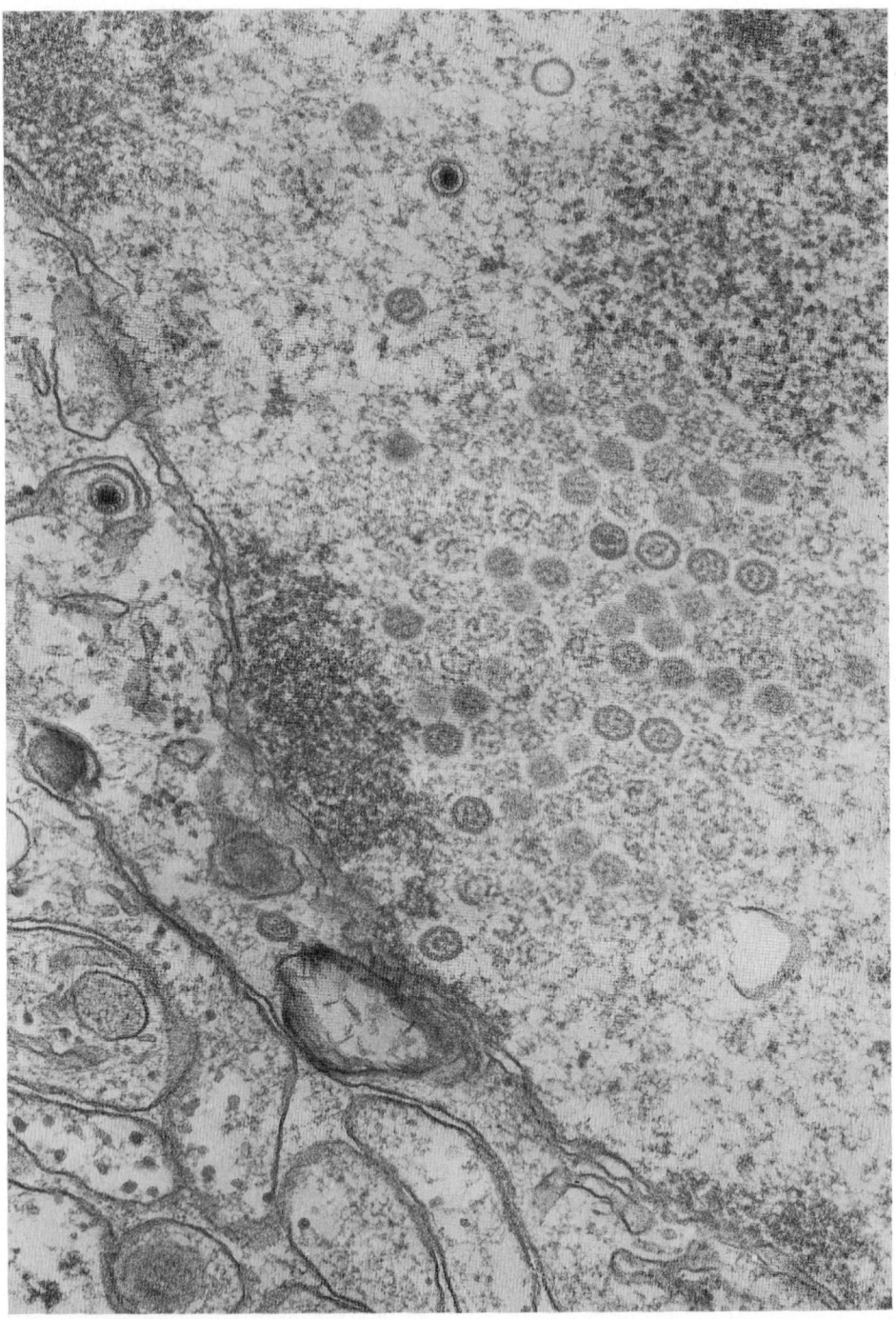

Fig. 9–10. Intranuclear inclusion body of *Herpesvirus simplex* in tissue culture. A crystalline array of viral particles lies within the nucleus (× 50,000). (Courtesy of Dr. J. E. Leestma and *Laboratory Investigation*.)

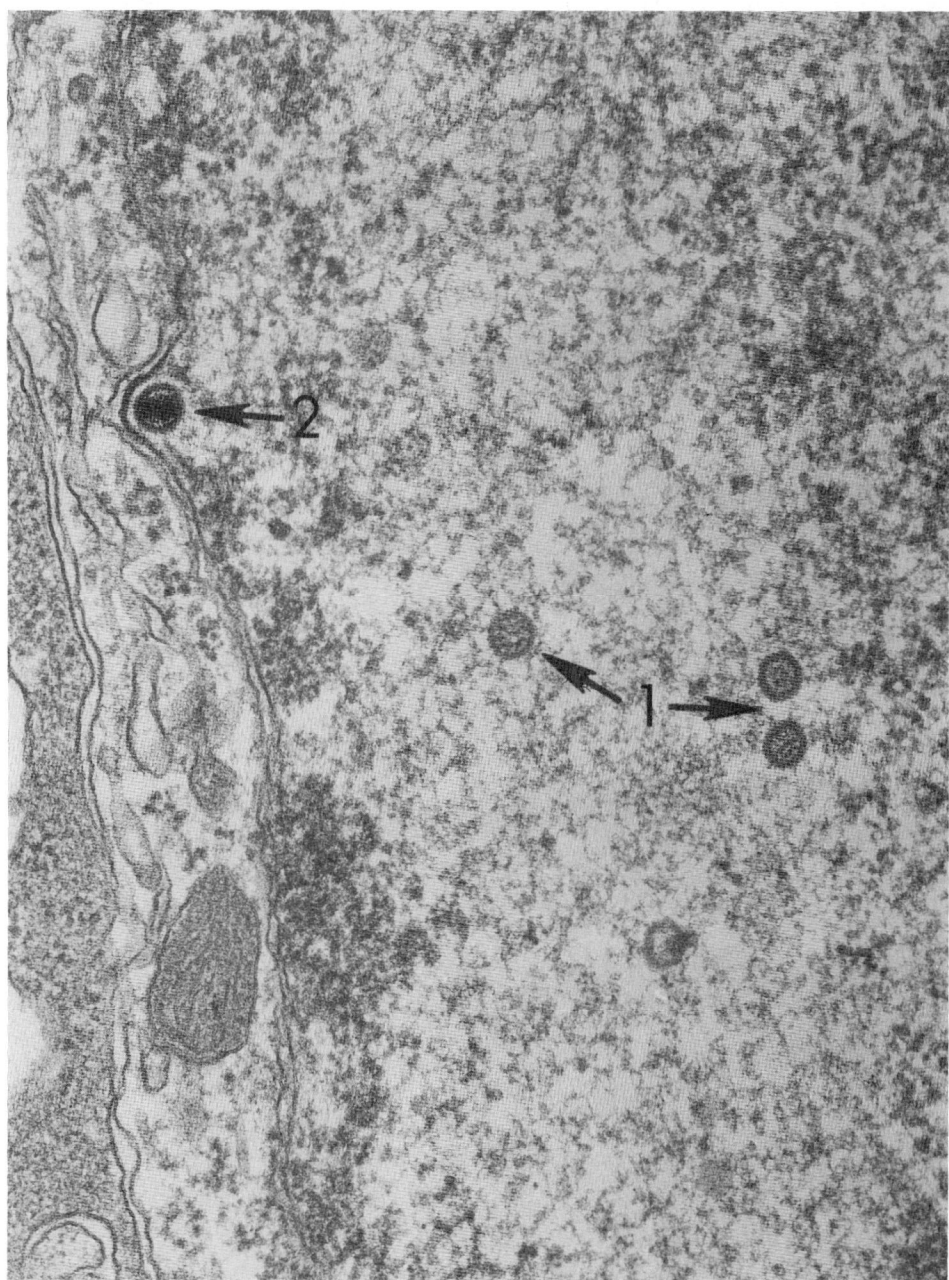

Fig. 9–11. *Herpesvirus simplex* infection in tissue culture of nervous tissue. Note un-enveloped viral particles in the nucleus *(1)*. A single virion *(2)* is approaching the bulging nuclear membrane, a stage preparatory to envelopment (× 40,000). (Courtesy of Dr. J. E. Leestma and *Laboratory Investigation*.)

intranuclear inclusion bodies. Gliosis and perivascular cuffing may or may not be prominent. *Herpesvirus simplex*, type 2, is the cause of ulcerative lesions on genital epithelium in both sexes and has been associated with squamous cell carcinomas of the cervix of women.

Diagnosis. A presumptive diagnosis of *H. simplex* infection in owl monkeys can be made on the basis of history and pathologic changes. However, generally the lesions cannot be distinguished from *Herpesvirus T* infection in this species; therefore, definitive diagnosis requires viral isolation and identification. In addition to the owl monkey, spontaneous *H. simplex* encephalitis has been reported in the gibbon, an anthropoid ape *(Hylobates lar)*, and marmosets *(Saguinus spp.)* have been shown to be experimentally susceptible to the virus. The virus may be isolated from blood, spleen, liver, adrenal glands and kidneys by co-cultivation with permissible cells, such as rabbit or owl monkey kidney cells.

Buddingh, G. J., Schrum, D. I., Lanier, J. C., and Guidry, D. J.: Studies of the natural history of Herpes simplex infections. Pediatrics, *11*:595–610, 1953.

Constantine, V. S., Francis, R. D., and Montes, L. F.: Association of recurrent Herpes simplex with neuralgia. J. Am. Med. Assoc., *205*:131–133, 1968.

Deinhardt, F., Holmes, A. W., Devine, J., and Deinhardt, J.: Marmosets as laboratory animals. IV. The microbiology of laboratory kept marmosets. Lab. Anim. Care, *17*:48–70, 1967.

Hunt, R. D., and Melendez, L. V.: Herpes virus infections of non-human primates: a review. Lab. Anim. Care, *19*:221–234, 1969.

Kaplan, A. S.: Herpes simplex and pseudorabies viruses. Virology Monographs 1969. New York, Springer-Verlag, pp. 1–115.

Katzin, D.S., Connor, J. D., Wilson, L. A., and Sexton, R. S.: Experimental Herpes simplex infection in the Owl monkey. Proc. Soc. Exp. Biol. Med., *125*:391–398, 1967.

Leestma, J. E., Bornstein, M. B., Sheppard, R. D., and Feldman, L. A.: Ultrastructural aspects of Herpes simplex virus infection in organized cultures of mammalian nervous tissue. Lab. Invest., *20*:70–78, 1969.

Leider, W., Magoffin, R. L., Lennette, E. H., and Leonards, L. N. R.: Herpes simplex virus encephalitis. Its possible association with reactivated latent infection. N. Engl. J. Med., *273*:341–347, 1965.

Melendez, L. V., Espana, C., Hunt, R. D., Daniel, M. D., and Garcia, F. G.: Natural Herpes simplex infection in Owl monkey *(Aotus trivirgatus)*. Lab. Anim. Care, *19*:38–45, 1969.

Miller, J. K., Hesser, F., and Tompkins, V. N.: Herpes simplex encephalitis. Ann. Int. Med., *64*:92–103, 1966.

Olson, L. C., Buescher, E. L., Artenstein, M. S., and Parkman, P. D.: Herpesvirus infections of the human central nervous system. N. Engl. J. Med., *277*:1271–1277, 1967.

Rhodes, A. J., and vanRooyen, C. E.: Textbook of Virology. Baltimore, Williams & Wilkins, 1962, pp. 136–146.

Smith, P. C., Yuill, T. M., Buchanan, R. D., Stanton, J. S., and Chaicumpa, V.: The gibbon *(Hylobates lar)*, a new primate host for *Herpesvirus hominis*. I. A natural epizootic in a laboratory colony. J. Infect. Dis., *120*:292–297, 1969.

Smith, P. C., Yuill, T. M., and Buchanan, R. D.: Natural and experimental infection of gibbons with Herpesvirus hominis. Ann. Prog. Report SEATO Med. Res. Lab. and SEATO Clinical Res. Cen., Bangkok, Thailand, pp. 258–261, 1958.

Szogi, S., and Berge, Th.: Generalized Herpes simplex in newborns. Acta Path. Microbiol. Scand., *66*:401–408, 1966.

Herpesvirus B Infection of Monkeys (Herpes-B, Herpesvirus simiae, B-virus)

The increasingly frequent use of monkeys of various species in medical research has stimulated interest in studies of the spontaneous diseases of these animals as a necessary corollary. In 1934, Sabin and Wright isolated a virus from the brain of a human patient who died following the bite of an apparently normal Rhesus monkey *(Macaca mulatta)*. The virus was shown subsequently to be carried by Old World monkeys of the genus *Macaca*, in which little or no disease is usually evident. Based on the presence of clinical disease, virus isolation, and/or serum neutralizing antibodies, the following species have been incriminated as natural reservoir hosts for the virus: *M. mulatta* (Rhesus); *M. fascicularis* (Cynomolgus, crab-eating Macaque); *M. fuscata* (Japanese Macaque) and *M. arctoides* (Stump-tail Macaque).

The Disease in Monkeys. The bulk of our knowledge of *Herpesvirus B* comes from studies with Rhesus monkeys. Following infection, clinical disease characterized by vesicles and ulcers, particularly on the dorsal surface of the tongue and on the mucocutaneous junction of the lip, may develop, but it is not known whether lesions invariably follow infection. In addition to the oral mucous membranes, vesicles and ulcers may also occur on the skin, and the virus may cause conjunctivitis. These lesions heal uneventfully in 7 to 14 days.

Microscopically, the lesions are characterized by ballooning degeneration and necrosis of epithelial cells and the presence of intranuclear inclusion bodies. Multinucleated epithelial cells containing intranuclear inclusion bodies are also usually present. Inclusion bodies may also be found in macrophages and in endothelial cells. During the course of clinical disease in the Rhesus and Cynomolgus monkey, visceral lesions may also develop. These are characterized by foci of necrosis in the liver, associated with intranuclear inclusion bodies. In the central nervous system neuronal necrosis and gliosis associated with minimal perivascular cuffing with lymphocytes may be found. Intranuclear inclusion bodies occur in glial cells and neurons. The lesions are most frequent in the nucleus and tract of the descending branches of the trigeminal nerve, between the roots of origin of the facial and auditory nerves, and at the roots of the trigeminal and facial nerves.

These natural lesions are intensified by the administration of cortisone and the intraspinal, intrathalamic, and intramuscular inoculation of inactivated poliomyelitis vaccine. These are procedures used in the testing of the safety of this vaccine. In monkeys in which the disease has been thus activated, a diffuse encephalomyelitis may occur and the architecture of the spinal cord may be destroyed at the site of the inoculation. Lymphocytic infiltration of the meninges and nerve roots, as well as neutrophils and focal demyelinization may be found in the lumbar region. Edema and necrosis occur, as well as diffuse glial infiltration in the medulla and pons, particularly at the midline, and perivascular lymphocytic infiltration is extensive. Diffuse necrosis may be seen in the floor of the fourth ventricle, and the inflammation may cause loss of ependymal cells and extend into the ventricle. Glial infiltrations are common in vestibular nuclei, medial longitudinal fasciculi, and nuclei of the spinal tracts of the fifth cranial nerve. Small glial foci may occur around the cerebral aqueduct, in the thalamus, putamen, caudate nucleus, and in the parietal and temporal cortex. The hippocampus, occipital cortex, amygdaloid, and hypothalamus are reportedly free of lesions in this accentuated form of the natural disease.

The infection spreads within a colony of monkeys by means of direct contact, fomites, and probably aerosols, until nearly 100% of the colony has become infected, as determined by the presence of serum neutralizing antibodies. Oral lesions are not encountered in every animal, which is explained in part by failure to observe them.

Once a monkey is infected with *Herpesvirus B*, it should probably be considered infected for life. Although recurrence of lesions, as in *Herpesvirus simplex* infection in man, has not been recognized (according to Dr. M. D. Daniel), the virus may be isolated from blood, urine, feces, and vaginal samples from animals without overt disease. Rhesus monkeys without demonstrable neutralizing antibodies, which were inoculated with *Herpesvirus B*, did not exhibit any sign of disease, but did develop high levels of neutralizing antibody and shed virus in oral, fecal, and corneal samples.

Herpesvirus B has not been demonstrated to produce spontaneous fatal disease in Rhesus monkeys, but in the Cynomolgus monkey the disease may be severe enough to lead to death.

The Disease in Man. The principal importance of *Herpesvirus B* is not its hazards to the reservoir hosts, but rather that the virus produces a fatal disease in man. Although the morbidity rate is low, of 18 cases reported, all but two have proved fatal. Most infections have followed a monkey bite. The disease is characterized clinically and pathologically by encephalomyelitis. Focal necrosis may occur in the liver, spleen, lymph nodes, and adrenal glands. Intranuclear inclusion bodies may be found in any affected tissue, but have not been demonstrated in all cases.

Diagnosis. A presumptive diagnosis can be made from the characteristic lesions. Due to the number of simian herpesviruses, definitive diagnosis requires isolation and identification of the virus. A rise in titer of serum neutralizing antibodies may support the diagnosis.

Davidson, W. L.: B virus infection in man. Ann. NY Acad. Sci., *85*:970–979, 1960.

Endo, M., et al.: Etude de Virus au Japan. Jap. J. Exp. Med., *30*:227–233, 385–392, 1960.

Gralla, E. J., Ciecura, S. J., and Delahunt, C. S.: Extended B-virus antibody determinations in a closed monkey colony. Lab. Anim. Care, *16*:510–514, 1966.

Hartley, E. G.: Naturally-occurring "B" virus infection in Cynomolgus monkeys. Vet. Rec., *76*:555–557, 1964.

Hull, R. N.: The Simian Viruses, Virology Monographs 2, New York, Springer-Verlag, 1968.

Hunt, R. D., and Melendez, L. V.: Herpes virus infections of non-human primates: a review. Lab. Anim. Care, *19*:221–234, 1969.

Keeble, S. A.: B virus infection in monkeys. Ann. NY Acad. Sci., *85*:960–969, 1960.

Keeble, S. A., Christofinis, G. J., and Wood, W.: Natural B-virus infection in Rhesus monkeys. J. Pathol. Bact., *76*:189–199, 1958.

Kirschstein, R. L., Van Hoosier, C. L., and Li, C. P.: Virus B-infection of the central nervous system of monkeys used for the poliomyelitis vaccine safety test. Am. J. Pathol., *38*:119–125, 1961.

Ruebner, B. H., et al.: Ultrastructure of *Herpesvirus simiae* (Herpes B virus). Exp. Mol. Pathol., *22*:317–325, 1975.

Sabin, A. B., and Wright, A. M.: Acute ascending myelitis following a monkey bite, with isolation of a virus capable of reproducing the disease. J. Exper. Med., *59*:115–136, 1934.

Sabin, A. B.: Studies on the B virus. I. The immunological identity of a virus isolated from a human case of ascending myelitis associated with visceral necrosis. Br. J. Exp. Pathol., *15*:248–269, 1934.

Shah, K. V., and Southwick, C. H.: Prevalence of antibodies to certain viruses in sera of free-living Rhesus and of captive monkeys. Indian J. Med. Res., *53*:488–500, 1965.

Herpesvirus T Infection of Monkeys (Herpesvirus M, Herpesvirus platyrrhinae I)

Herpesvirus T infection has many similarities to *Herpesvirus B* infection; however, the virus is distinct and the susceptible hosts are New World monkeys. *Herpesvirus T* is carried as a latent viral infection by the Squirrel monkey *(Saimiri sciureus)*. Based on evidence derived from circulating serum neutralizing antibodies, Cinnamon Ringtail monkeys *(Cebus albifrons)* and Spider monkeys *(Ateles spp.)* are also likely natural reservoir hosts. Although the morbidity rate is high, clinical disease is rarely seen in the reservoir host, and has only been documented in the Squirrel monkey where the lesions consist of vesicles and ulcers of the oral mucous membranes. The microscopic features are identical to *Herpesvirus B* infection in the Rhesus. Visceral lesions or changes in the central nervous systems are not known to occur. The disease in the reservoir hosts is not known to be fatal. Exacerbation of oral lesions is also not known to occur, but as with *Herpesvirus B* infection, the virus can be excreted in the absence of visible lesions. All available evidence suggests that latent infection remains for life.

Marmosets *(Saguinus spp.)* and Owl monkeys *(Aotus trivirgatus)* have a less fortunate relationship with *Herpesvirus T*. In these hosts, *Herpesvirus T* produces an epizootic disease of high morbidity and mortality rates. The clinical features, which develop following a 7- to 10-day incubation period, are characterized by anorexia, lassitude, oral and labial vesicles and ulcers, ulcerative dermatitis (especially of the face), and occasionally conjunctivitis. Hyperesthesia, as evidenced by intense scratching, may be the most obvious sign. After a course of two to three days, most animals become moribund and die.

Gross lesions consist of vesicles and/or ulcers of the skin, lips, oral cavity, esophagus, small intestine, cecum, and colon. Hemorrhage is present in most lymph nodes, the adrenal cortices and occasionally in the lung. Microscopically, variable sized foci of necrosis and intranuclear inclusion bodies are found in most organs and tissues of the body. Lesions are most frequent in the oral cavity, small and large intestine, liver, spleen, lymph nodes, adrenal cortex and various ganglia. Multinucleated giant cells are present in lesions of the oral cavity and skin. Encephalitis is not common, and when present, it is not extensive.

Diagnosis. In either the reservoir hosts or the fatally affected hosts, the characteristic lesions allow for a presumptive diagnosis. However, due to the occurrence of other herpesviruses in New World monkeys, the virus should be isolated and identified. In owl monkeys, the lesions of *Herpesvirus T* infection cannot be differentiated from those of *Herpesvirus simplex* infection.

Daniel, M. D., et al.: Isolation of Herpes-T virus from a spontaneous disease in Squirrel monkeys (*Saimiri sciureus*). Arch. Virusforsch., 22:324–331, 1967.

Holmes, A. W., Caldwell, R. G., Dedmon, R. E., and Deinhardt, F.: Isolation and characterization of a new Herpes virus. J. Immunol., 92:602–610, 1964.

Holmes, A. W., Devine, J. A., Nowakowski, E., and Deinhardt, F.: The epidemiology of a Herpes virus infection of New World monkeys. J. Immunol., 96:668–671, 1966.

Hunt, R. D., and Melendez, L. V.: Herpes virus infections of nonhuman primates: A review. Lab. Anim. Care, 19:221–234, 1969.

Hunt, R. D., and Melendez, L. V.: Spontaneous Herpes-T infection in the Owl monkey (*Aotus trivirgatus*). Path. Vet., 3:1–26, 1966.

King, N. W., Hunt, R. D., Daniel, M. D., and Melendez, L. V.: Overt Herpes-T infection in Squirrel monkeys (*Saimiri sciureus*). Lab. Anim. Care, 17:413–423, 1967.

Melendez, L. V., Hunt, R. D., Garcia, F. G., and Trum, B. F.: A latent Herpes-T infection in *Saimiri sciureus* (Squirrel monkey). *In* Some Recent Developments in Comparative Medicine, edited by R. N. T-W-Fiennes. pp. 393–397. London, Academic Press, 1966.

Additional Simian Herpesviruses

Several other herpesviruses that cause disease in nonhuman primates deserve brief mention. A fatal systemic infection has been described in African green or vervet monkeys (*Cercopithecus aethiops*), an Old World species. The agent, tentatively called the **Liverpool vervet monkey virus** was first isolated in England. The disease is characterized by the development of a generalized vesicular rash, which is followed by death in 24 to 48 hours. In addition to

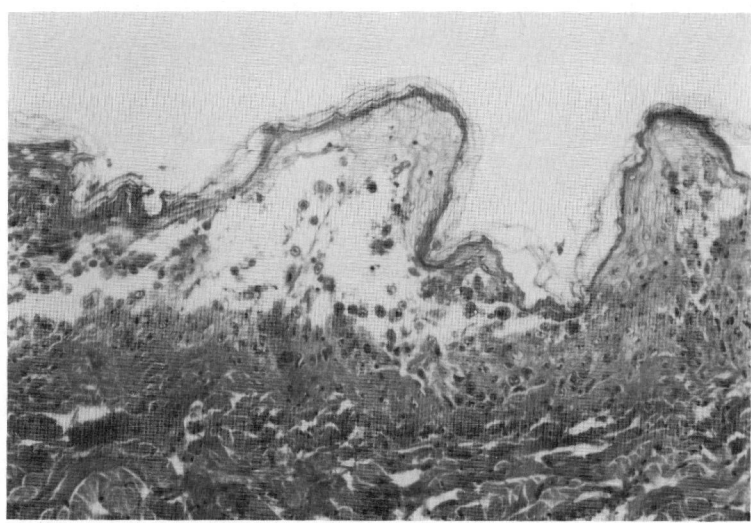

Fig. 9–12. Liverpool vervet monkey virus infection. Vesicular dermatitis of a vervet monkey (*Cercopithecus aethiops*). (Courtesy of Dr. E. Thorpe.)

epidermal vesicles, focal necrosis occurs in the lung, liver, and spleen. Intranuclear inclusion bodies are found in all affected tissues. Lesions have not been described in the oral cavity or central nervous system. The natural or reservoir host(s) for the virus is not known. A similar disease entity has been described in patas monkeys *(Erythrocebus patas)*. The causative agent is a herpesvirus and resembles the Liverpool vervet monkey virus but has not been completely classified.

An agent termed the **spider monkey herpesvirus** was isolated from a young spider monkey that died of a generalized infection with oral and labial erosions and ulcers. Further examples of spontaneous disease have not been reported.

Herpesvirus saimiri is carried in latent form by Squirrel monkeys *(Saimiri sciureus)*, but may be transmitted experimentally to Owl monkeys *(Aotus sp.)*, rabbits, or marmosets *(Saguinas sp.)*, producing malignant lymphoma in these animals. Another herpesvirus, *H. ateles*, is carried latently by spider monkeys *(Ateles sp.)* and also produces malignant lymphoma when inoculated into marmosets or owl monkeys. The malignant lymphoma caused by *H. saimiri* may result from contact between infected Squirrel monkeys and normal Owl monkeys.

Clarkson, M. J., Thorpe, E., and McCarthy, K.: A virus disease of captive vervet monkeys *(Cercopithecus aethiops)* caused by a new Herpesvirus. Arch. Virusforsch., 22:219–234, 1967.

Hull, R. N.: The Simian Viruses. Virology Monographs 2. New York, Springer-Verlag, 1968.

Hunt, R. D., and Melendez, L. V.: Herpes virus infections of non-human primates: A review. Lab. Anim. Care, 19:221–234, 1969.

Lennette, E. H.: Workshop on viral diseases which impede colonization of nonhuman primates. Nat'l Center for Primate Biology, Univ. of Calif. at Davis, May 22–24, 1968.

Malherbe, H., and Harwin, R.: Neurotropic virus in African monkeys. Lancet, 2:530, 1958.

Malherbe, H., Harwin, R., and Ulrich, M.: The cytopathic effects of Vervet monkey viruses. S. A. Med. J., 37:407–411, 1963.

Malherbe, H., and Strickland-Cholmley, M.: Virus from baboons. Lancet, 2:1300, 1969.

McCarthy, K., et al.: Exanthematous disease in Patas monkeys caused by a herpes virus. Lancet, 2:856–857, 1968.

Herpesvirus Canis Infection of Dogs

Herpesvirus canis was first isolated, characterized, and identified as the cause of a fatal systemic infection of neonatal puppies in 1965. From available evidence, it appears that dogs are the natural and reservoir hosts for this herpesvirus, in a manner analogous to *Herpesvirus simplex* in man, *Herpesvirus B* in monkeys, and *Herpesvirus suis* in swine. A high percentage of dogs become infected with the virus without history of associated illness, and the virus can be isolated from puppies and adult dogs in the absence of recognizable disease. Although adult dogs carry the virus as a latent infection, it has been shown to cause a mild tracheobronchitis. The occurrence of fatal infections in neonatal puppies appears to be analogous to the parallel condition of fatal *Herpesvirus simplex* in infants or fatal *Herpesvirus suis* in piglets. These are each an example of fatal disease in the same host which usually carries the virus as a latent infection.

Puppies are infected in utero or during birth by exposure to the virus in the vagina. The infection results in either stillbirth or an acute fatal disease in the first three weeks of life. After three to five weeks of age, infection is usually inapparent.

Lesions. The most striking gross pathologic change is hemorrhage, especially of the renal cortices and lungs, but the stomach, intestine, and adrenals may also contain hemorrhages. Serosanguineous fluid is usually present in the thoracic and abdominal cavities, and there is splenomegaly and enlargement of lymph nodes. Variably sized gray foci are often present in the lungs, kidneys, and liver.

Microscopically, the lesions in all tissues are characterized by focal necrosis and the presence of intranuclear inclusion bodies. These necrotizing lesions may be found in

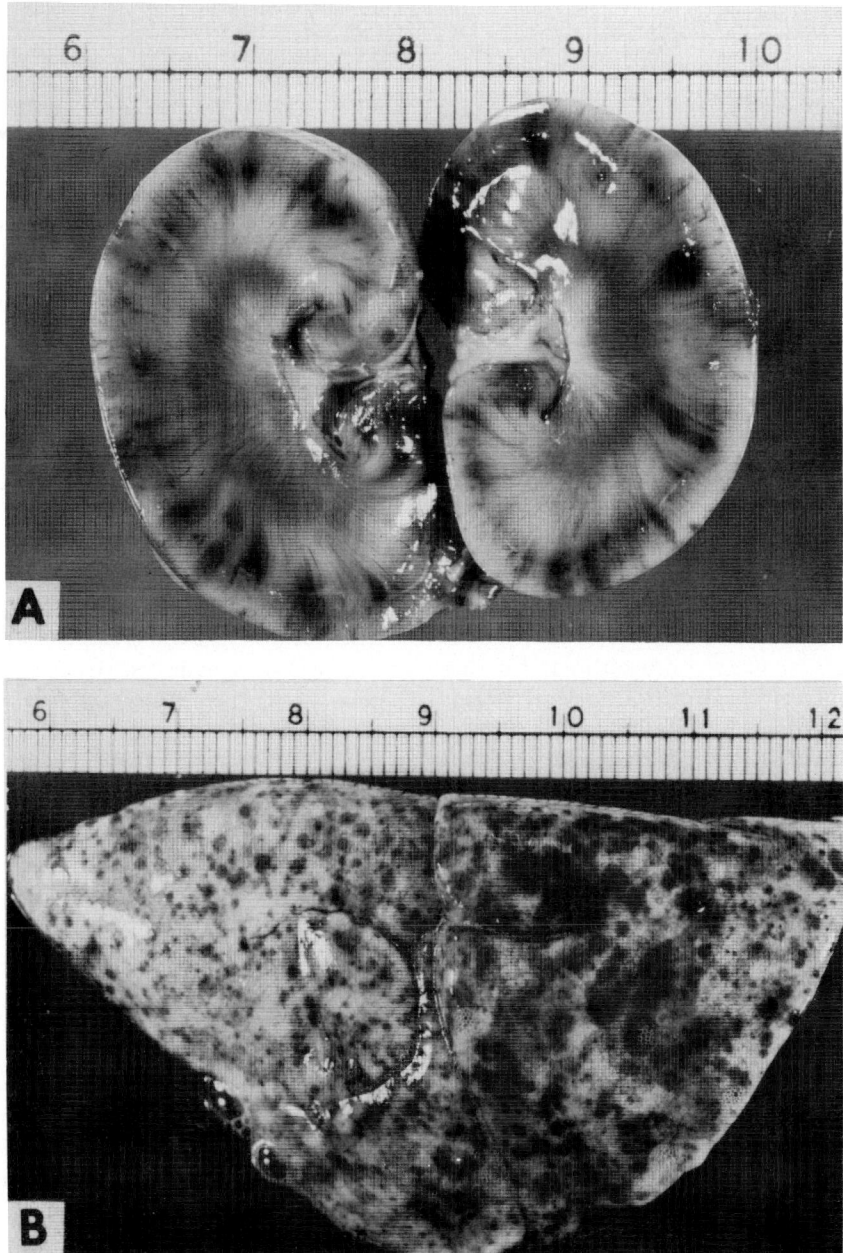

Fig. 9–13. *Herpesvirus canis* infection in a puppy. *A,* Hemorrhage and necrosis in renal cortex. *B,* Numerous petechiae, ecchymoses and suffusion in the lung. (Courtesy of Dr. T. J. Kakuk and *Laboratory Animal Care.*)

the lung, kidneys, liver, spleen, lymph nodes, adrenal, intestines, and brain. Usually the lesions are most extensive in the kidneys and lungs. The lesions in the central nervous system are those of a disseminated, nonsuppurative encephalomyelitis with focal malacia of the cerebral cortex, cerebellar cortex, basal ganglia, and gray columns of the spinal cord. Secondary lesions follow in the white matter. Infection in adult dogs is usually not associated with histopathologic changes, but the virus may produce a catarrhal tracheobronchitis with intranuclear inclusions in the lining epithelium. Inclusion bodies in both neonates and adults may be difficult to demonstrate unless an acid fixative such as Zenker's fluid has been employed.

Diagnosis. The characteristic necrotizing lesions and intranuclear inclusion bodies in neonatal or stillborn puppies allows for a presumptive diagnosis. Definitive diagnosis requires virus isolation and characterization. Dogs are natural hosts for this virus and subject to latent infection; therefore, virus isolation in the absence of characteristic histopathologic lesions must be interpreted with caution.

Carmichael, L. E., Strandberg, J. D., and Barnes, F. D.: Identification of a cytopathogenic agent infectious for puppies as a canine herpesvirus. Proc. Soc. Exp. Biol. Med., *120*:644–650, 1966.

Carmichael, L. E., Squire, R. A., and Krook, L.: Clinical and pathologic features of a fatal viral disease of newborn pups. Am. J. Vet. Res., *26*:803–814, 1965.

Cornwell, H. J. C., Wright, N. G., Campbell, R. S. F., and Roberts, R. J.: Neonatal disease in the dog associated with a Herpes-like virus. Vet. Rec., *79*:661–662, 1966.

Cornwell, H. J. C., and Wright, N. G.: Neonatal canine herpesvirus infection: a review of present knowledge. Vet. Rec., *84*:2–6, 1969.

Kakuk, T. J., et al.: Isolation of a canine herpesvirus from a dog with malignant lymphoma. Am. J. Vet. Res., *30*:1951–1960, 1969.

Kakuk, T. J., and Conner, G. H.: Experimental canine herpesvirus in the gnotobiotic dog. Lab. Anim. Care, *20*:69–79, 1970.

Karpas, A.: Experimental production of canine tracheobronchitis (kennel cough) with canine herpesvirus isolated from naturally infected dogs. Am. J. Vet. Res., *29*:1251–1257, 1968.

Karpas, A., et al.: Canine tracheobronchitis: isolation and characterization of the agent with experi-

mental reproduction of the disease. Proc. Soc. Exp. Biol. Med., *127*:45–52, 1968.

Lundgren, D. L., and Clapper, W. E.: Neutralization of canine herpesvirus by dog and human serums: a survey. Am. J. Vet. Res., *30*:479–482, 1969.

Percy, D. H., Olander, H. J., and Carmichael, L. E.: Encephalitis in the newborn pup due to a canine herpesvirus. Path. Vet., *5*:135–145, 1968.

Percy, D. H., et al.: Pathogenesis of canine herpesvirus encephalitis. Am. J. Vet. Res., *31*:145–156, 1970.

Spertzel, R. O., et al.: Recovery and characterization of a herpes-like virus from dog kidney cell cultures. Proc. Soc. Exp. Biol. Med., *120*:651–655, 1965.

Stewart, S. E., et al.: Herpes-like virus isolated from neonatal and fetal dogs. Science, *148*:1341–1343, 1965.

Wright, N. G., and Cornwell, H. J. C.: Experimental herpes virus infection in young puppies. Res. Vet. Sci., *9*:295–299, 1968.

Pseudorabies
(Infectious Bulbar Paralysis, Aujeszky's Disease, Mad Itch)

Pseudorabies, a disease to which many species are susceptible, is caused by a virus of the herpes group termed *Herpesvirus suis.* The disease was first described by Aujeszky (1902) in Hungary, but is now known to occur in many parts of the world, including the United States. Natural infection occurs in swine, cattle, dogs, cats, sheep, rats, and mink, but is of greatest importance in cattle, in which the disease is nearly always fatal. The infection is similar with respect to epizootiology, clinical signs, and pathologic changes to certain other herpesvirus infections, such as *Herpesvirus B* and *Herpesvirus simplex.*

Epizootiology and Signs. Swine and probably rats serve as the natural and reservoir hosts for *H. suis.* Swine are susceptible to infection, but adult animals rarely exhibit symptoms or die from the disease. In adult swine, a mild febrile, nonfatal disease may occur, but recovery is the rule. In piglets the infection is more severe, occurring as an acute illness which may lead to death in 24 to 48 hours without specific clinical signs. Piglets over four weeks of age may show signs of involvement of the central nervous system, usually as incoordination of the hind quarters, tremors,

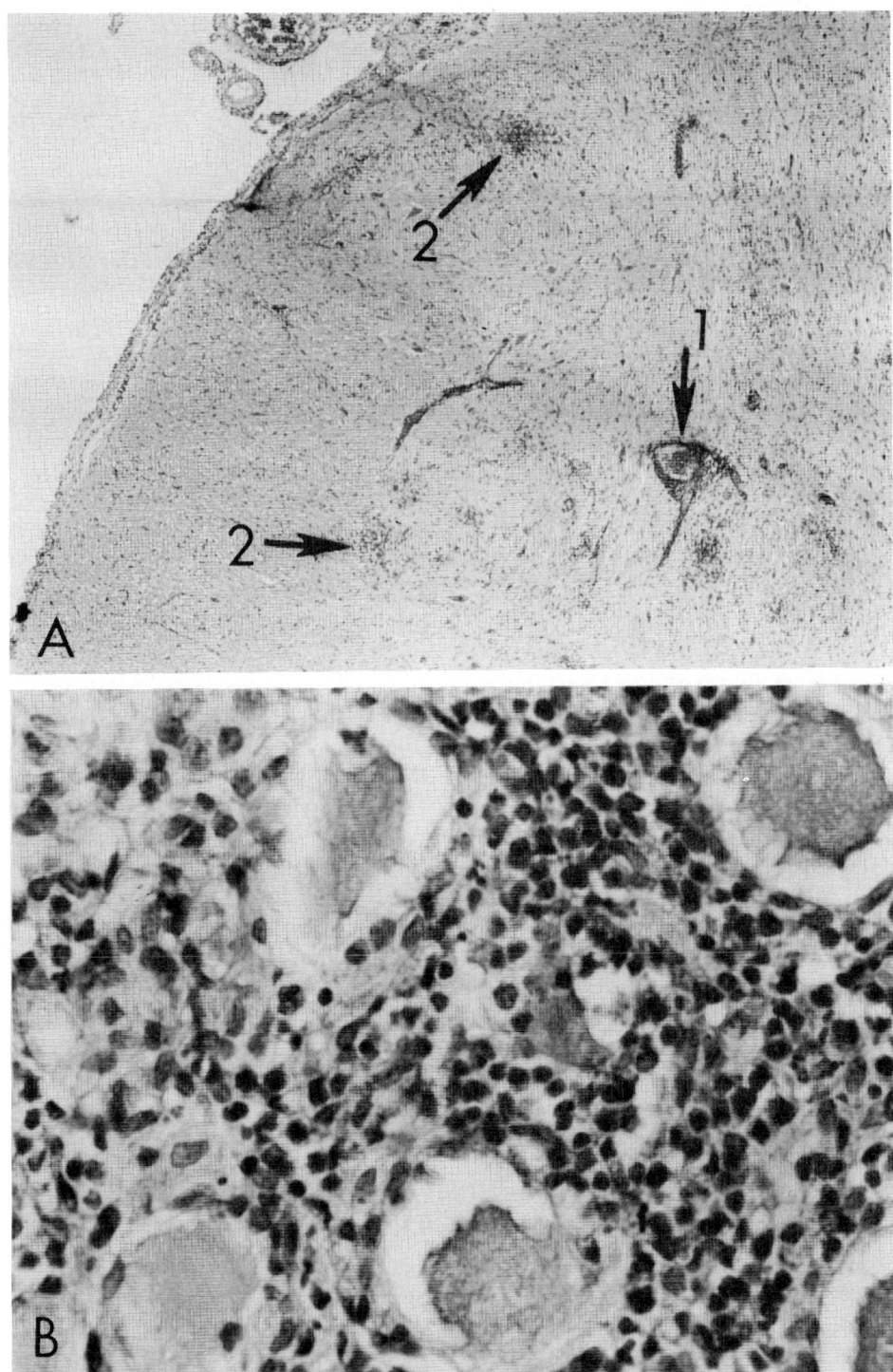

Fig. 9–14. Pseudorabies in a piglet. *A,* Encephalitis with perivascular cuffing *(1)* and glial nodules *(2). B,* Semilunar ganglioneuritis with ganglion cell necrosis, capsule cell proliferation and a pleomorphic cellular infiltrate. (Courtesy of Dr. H. J. Olander.)

convulsions, and eventual paralysis. Although not usual, older pigs may develop encephalitis and die of the infection. Intrauterine infection can occur, leading to abortion and stillbirth.

Young and adult swine may excrete the virus in the absence of clinical disease, a situation analogous to *Herpesvirus simplex* in man. This may represent activation of a latent infection. Swine with a subclinical infection, by nuzzling with their snout, may transmit the disease to cattle. Sheep are susceptible to experimental exposure to the virus by scarification of the skin, subcutaneous injection, and instillation into nasal passages, oral cavity, or conjunctival sac. The disease also occurs naturally among sheep housed with pigs, and it is transmitted by the nuzzling pigs in much the same manner that they convey the virus to cattle.

Intense itching develops in the skin of the bovine at the point of contact after about 50 hours. Frenzied scratching of this area by the animal causes ulceration of the skin, and secondary infection ensues. Paralysis may develop, and cattle may die rather suddenly with indications of bulbar involvement. Rabbits are particularly susceptible to artificial exposure to this disease; guinea pigs, somewhat less so. Monkeys are also readily infected by experimental means. The virus may be transmitted through the abraded skin simply by rubbing the nose of an infected rabbit against it.

Lesions. Following natural or experimental inoculation, *Herpesvirus suis* reaches the central nervous system by traveling up nerve fibers. Lesions occur in the nerve fibers, ganglia, and central nervous system in all species; their extent and distribution depending on the site of inoculation and duration of the illness. In general, central lesions are most extensive in the spinal ganglia, temporal cerebral cortex, and basal ganglia of the brain.

Local irritation and necrosis occur at the site of subcutaneous inoculation of rabbits and involve both fascia and musculature. The virus reaches the spinal ganglia, first affecting those on the side of the body where the inoculation was given. The lesions in the ganglia, which are believed to be the cause of the intense pruritus, consist of degeneration of neurons and proliferation of capsule cells and other glial cells. Intracranial inoculation of the rabbit is followed by lymphocytic proliferation in the meninges, proliferation of the subpial glia, and necrosis of superficially placed nerve cells. Intranuclear inclusions are observed in cells of all embryonic layers: nerve cells, glia, capillary endothelium, sarcolemmal cells, and Schwann cells. These inclusions, when stained by phloxine-methylene blue, reveal aggregations of coarse, pale pink granules or irregular, deeper pink granules. In the rabbit, death usually occurs as soon as the virus reaches the medulla and before microscopic lesions are visible at this site. Respiratory failure resulting from involvement of the medulla oblongata appears to be the cause of death. This may be true in other species as well.

In the guinea pig, the lesions are similar to those in the rabbit, although the guinea pig is somewhat more resistant to experimental infection. In the monkey, after intracerebral inoculation, degeneration and necrosis of cortical nerve cells are widespread, with intranuclear inclusions occurring in nerve and glial cells but not in mesodermal cells. No lesions are found in viscera.

In the bovine and ovine, the spontaneous disease resembles the experimental disease in the monkey. Moderate perivascular infiltration of lymphocytes and some foci of microglial proliferation are seen in the central nervous system, but most nerve cells are normal or exhibit only mild chromatolysis. A few inclusions are found.

In swine, the lesions in the central nervous system may be very mild or unrecognizable. There are vascular, perivascular, and interstitial lesions with slight nerve cell degeneration. Inclusion bodies are

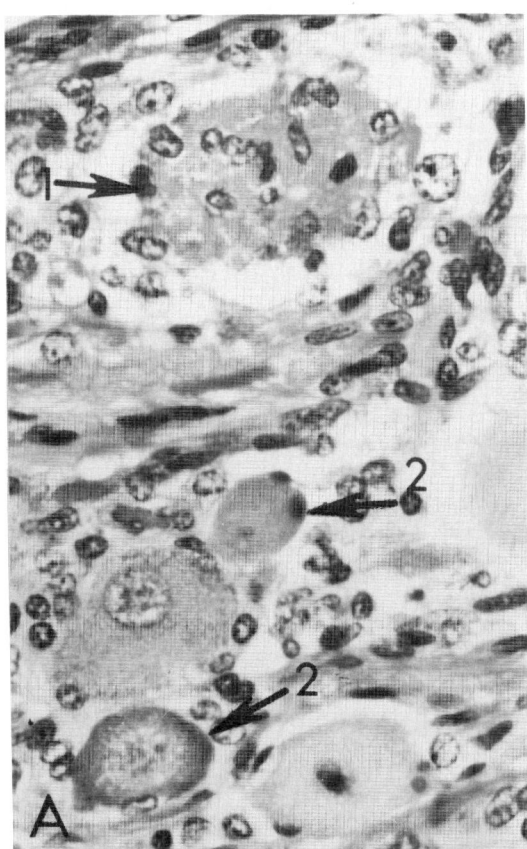 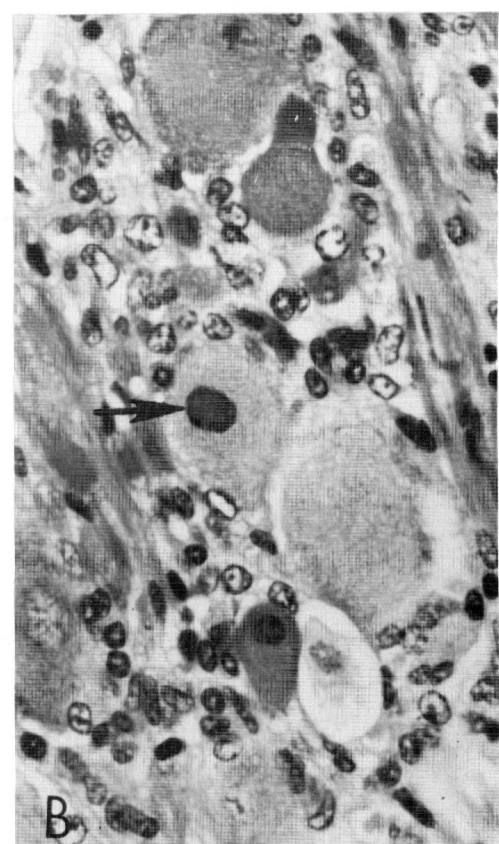

Fig. 9–15. Pseudorabies in a lamb. *A,* Dorsal root ganglioneuritis with a neuronophagic nodule *(1)* and neuron necrosis *(2). B,* A neuron containing an intranuclear inclusion body. (Courtesy of Dr. R. M. McCraken and Dr. C. Dow.)

present, but may be few in number. In addition to invasion of the nervous system, lesions are often present in other organs and tissues. Focal necrosis of pharyngeal mucosa, tonsils, lymph nodes, lungs, liver, and adrenal cortex associated with intranuclear inclusion bodies in both epithelial and mesenchymal cells are frequently encountered. Invasion of tissues outside the nervous system is unusual in other species, although adrenal cortical necrosis with inclusion bodies has been reported in experimental pseudorabies in sheep.

Diagnosis. Pseudorabies may be suspected in disease outbreaks in which animals die shortly after showing severe pruritus limited to a segment of the skin. Cattle or sheep in which the disease appears are almost always closely associated with swine or wild rats. The microscopic lesions in the skin and spinal ganglia are of some presumptive significance, but the final diagnosis of pseudorabies depends upon reproduction of the disease in experimental animals. This is most readily accomplished by the subcutaneous injection of rabbits with suspensions of nervous tissue from diseased animals. These rabbits will show intense, frenzied itching, with characteristic local inflammation of the skin. Death is due to respiratory failure, and the chief pathologic manifestations are necrotic changes in ganglion cells.

Aujeszky, A.: Über eine Neue Infektionskrankheit bei Haustiere. Zentralbl. f. Bakt., pt. 1, (Orig.), *32:*353–357, 1902.

Baskerville, A., and Lloyd, G.: Experimental infection of monkeys with *Herpesvirus suis* (Aujeszky's disease virus). J. Med. Microbiol., *10*:139–143, 1977.

Bergmann, B., and Becker, C.-H.: Studies on the pathomorphology and pathogenesis of Aujeszky's disease. I. Histopathology of the spinal ganglia, spinal nerve roots and spinal cord of guinea pigs after experimental infection. Path. Vet., *4*:97–119, 1967.

Boyse, E. A., et al.: The spread of a neurotropic strain of herpes virus into the cerebrospinal axis of rabbits. Br. J. Exp. Pathol., *37*:333–342, 1956.

Cernovsky, J.: Histopathology of the central nervous system in Aujeszky's disease. Veterinářství, *15*:176–178, 1965.

Corner, A. H.: Pathology of experimental Aujeszky's disease in piglets. Res. Vet. Sci., *6*:337–343, 1965.

Csontos, L., and Szeky, A.: Gross and microscopic lesions in the nasopharynx of pigs with Aujeszky's disease. Acta Vet. Hung., *16*:175–186, 1966.

Dow, C., and McFerran, J. B.: Experimental Aujeszky's disease in sheep. Am. J. Vet. Res., *25*:461–468, 1964.

———: The neuropathology of Aujeszky's disease in the pig. Res. Vet. Sci., *3*:436–442, 1962. VB 504–63.

———: The pathology of Aujeszky's disease in cattle. J. Comp. Pathol., *72*:337–347, 1962. VB 827–63.

———: Aujeszky's disease in the dog and cat. Vet. Rec., *75*:1099–1102, 1963. VB 1288–64.

———: Experimental studies on Aujeszky's disease in cattle. J. Comp. Pathol., *76*:379–385, 1966.

———: Experimental studies on Aujeszky's disease in sheep. Br. Vet. J., *122*:464–470, 1966.

Fraser, G., and Ramachandran, S. P.: Studies on the virus of Aujeszky's disease. I. Pathogenicity for rats and mice. J. Comp. Pathol., *79*:435–444, 1969.

Goto, H., Gorham, J. R., and Hagen, K. W.: Clinical observation of experimental pseudorabies in mink and ferrets. Jap. J. Vet. Sci., *30*:257–264, 1968.

Hanson, R. P.: The history of pseudorabies in the United States. J. Am. Vet. Med. Assoc., *124*:259–261, 1954.

Howarth, J. A., and DePaoli, A.: An enzootic of pseudorabies in swine in California. J. Am. Vet. Med. Assoc., *152*:1114–1118, 1968.

Huck, R. A., et al.: The isolation of Aujeszky's disease virus from dogs. Vet. Rec., *84*:232, 1969.

Hurst, E. W.: Studies on pseudorabies. I. Histology of the disease, with a note on the symptomatology. J. Exper. Med., *58*:415–433, 1933.

———: Studies on pseudorabies (infectious bulbar paralysis—mad itch). II. Routes of infection in the rabbit, with remarks on the relation of the virus to other viruses affecting the nervous system. J. Exp. Med., *59*:729–749, 1934.

Kaplan, A. S.: Herpes simplex and pseudorabies viruses. Virology Monographs, *5*:1–115, 1969.

Knosel, H.: Zur Histopathologie der Aujeszky's Chen Krankheit bei Hund und Katze. Zentbl. Vet. Med., *12B*:592–598, 1968.

———: Histopathology of Aujeszky's disease in pigs. Deutsch Tierarztl. Wschr., *72*:279–282, 1965.

Kojnok, J.: The role of carrier sows in the spreading of Aujeszky's virus carriership among fattening pigs. Acta Vet. Hung., *15*:282–295, 1965.

———: The role of pigs in the spreading of Aujeszky's disease among sheep and cattle. Acad. Sci. Hung., *12*:53–58, 1962.

Lucas, A., Metianu, T., and Atanasiu, P.: Maladie d'Aujeszky chez le chien en France. Annls. Inst. Pasteur, Paris, *110*:130–135, 1966.

Olander, H. J., et al.: Pathologic findings in swine affected with a virulent strain of Aujeszky's virus. Pathol. Vet., *3*:64–82, 1966.

Potgieter, L. N. D., Stair, E. L., Jr., Whitenack, D. L., and Morton, R. J.: Pseudorabies in swine in Oklahoma. J. Am. Vet. Med. Assoc., *170*:1413–1415, 1977.

Shahan, M. S., Knudson, R. L., Seibold, H. R., and Dale, C. N.: Aujeszky's disease (pseudorabies); a review with notes on two strains of the virus. North Am. Vet., *28*:440–449, 511–521, 1947.

Shope, R. E.: Experiments on the epidemiology of pseudorabies. I. Mode of transmission of the disease in swine and their possible role in its spread to cattle. J. Exp. Med., *62*:85–99, 1935.

———: Experiments on the epidemiology of pseudorabies. II. Prevalence of the disease among Middle Western swine and the possible role of rats in herd-to-herd infections. J. Exp. Med., *62*:101–117, 1935.

Infectious Bovine Rhinotracheitis
(Infectious Pustular Vulvovaginitis, Coital Exanthema, Vesicular Venereal Disease, Vesicular Vaginitis, Coital Vesicular Vaginitis or Coital Vesicular Exanthema)

First isolated in Colorado in association with a respiratory disease of cattle, the virus of infectious bovine rhinotracheitis (IBR) is now recognized as a herpesvirus of bovines of worldwide distribution. The virus can be carried by cattle as a latent infection and shed periodically in a manner believed to be similar to that seen with herpesviruses of other species such as man (*Herpesvirus simplex*), monkeys (*Herpesvirus-T* and *Herpsvirus-B*) and dogs (*H. canis*). In addition to causing an infectious upper respiratory disease, the virus has been demonstrated to cause conjunctivitis, encephalitis, mastitis, abortion, and systemic infection in calves. Each of these forms of the disease is generally (but not invariably) associated with the upper respiratory form of the disease. The virus of IBR has also been shown to be the cause of infectious pustular vulvovaginitis and balanoposthitis, which usually occurs in the absence of respiratory disease or the other forms of IBR. The respiratory, genital, and abortion forms are the most important and best studied of the manifestations of IBR.

Respiratory Form. Young cattle, assembled in large numbers as in feedlots, are most susceptible to the disease. The disease is highly infectious, with morbidity often approaching 100%. The symptoms begin with fever, anorexia, and a mucous nasal discharge, which later becomes mucopurulent and occasionally is tinged with blood. Respiratory distress is evidenced by dilated nostrils, mouth breathing, inspiratory dyspnea, and coughing. The course in most cases is about ten days, but in approximately 10% it may be prolonged. Chronically affected animals lose much flesh, and an estimated 3% die.

The gross lesions in cases of the rhinotracheitis form are usually limited to the nasal passages, paranasal sinuses, trachea, and bronchi. Thick mucopurulent exudate clings tenaciously to the congested, often edematous, nasal and turbinate mucosa. The lining of all paranasal sinuses is congested, glistens with excess mucus, and occasionally shows petechiae. The tracheal mucosa is similarly congested and covered with mucopurulent exudate. Severe edema in the wall of the trachea often extends into the walls of the major bronchi. In the trachea, the accumulation of edema between the mucosa and the cartilaginous rings may cause the wall to become as much as 2 cm thick, thereby decreasing the diameter of the lumen. Stenosis of the trachea contributes to the respiratory distress and may result in death from asphyxia or bronchopneumonia.

The microscopic lesions in calves experimentally infected with this virus have been described by Crandell, Cheatham, and Maurer (1959). The important lesions are concentrated in the mucosa of the upper respiratory tract, involving both stratified squamous and pseudostratified columnar epithelial cells. Twelve hours after infection, the cytoplasm of a few cells in the mucosa over the nasal septum, turbinates and nictitating membrane become pale and vacuolated, sometimes definitely granular or vesicular, with loss of cell outline. After 24 hours, similar lesions could be detected in the mucosa of the pharynx as well. By the end of 36 hours following inoculation, definite intranuclear inclusion bodies could be recognized in these cells (Fig. 9–16). Small irregular aggregates of pale acidophilic material first appeared among the nuclear chromatin and the chromatin became concentrated at the nuclear margins. The pink inclusion became more homogeneous as time elapsed, and eventually a distinct clear halo separated it from the marginated chromatin. The inclusions became more difficult to find after about 72 hours, but ulceration of nonspecific nature could be seen at this stage. The use of acid fixatives aids in the demonstration of the inclusion bodies.

During an outbreak of rhinotracheitis, the infection in very young calves may become generalized. The condition is acute and usually fatal, often with the absence of signs referable to the respiratory system. Pathologically, the lesions in this form of the disease consist of widespread focal necrosis. In both natural and experimental cases, focal necrosis has been observed in the respiratory epithelium, liver, kidney, spleen, lymph nodes, and the mucosa of the oral cavity, esophagus, and forestomachs. Intranuclear inclusion bodies have been described in each of these tissues.

Genital Form. Gillespie and co-workers (1957) discovered that IBR virus also causes another bovine disease with quite dissimilar manifestations. This disease, **infectious pustular vulvovaginitis**, has been known for many years, often under another name—such as, **coital exanthema, vesicular venereal disease, vesicular vaginitis, coital vesicular vaginitis,** or **coital vesicular exanthema**. It has been reported fre-

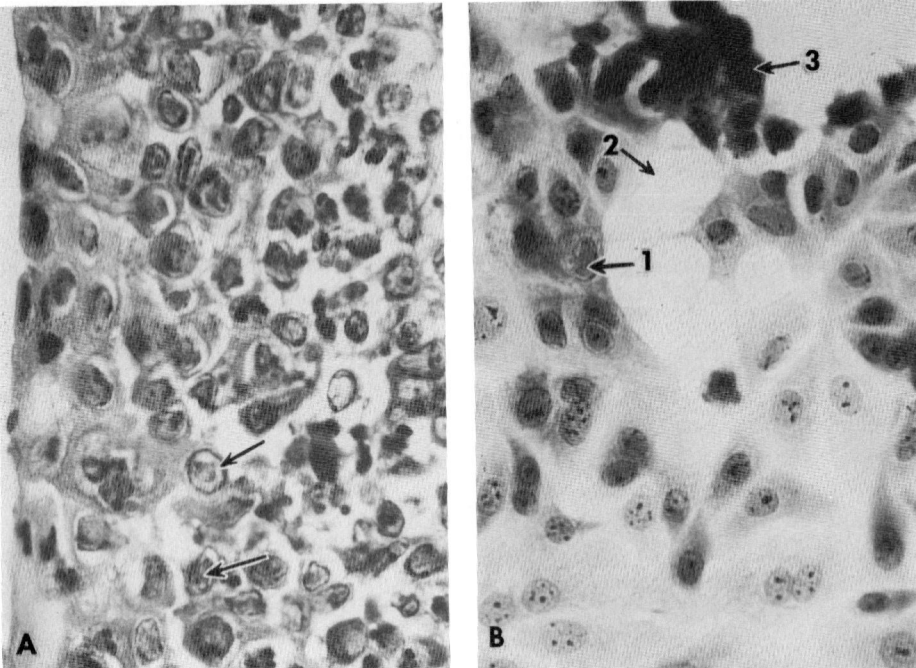

Fig. 9–16. Infectious bovine rhinotracheitis. *A,* Mucosa of nasal septum of a calf, 36 hours after infection. Intranuclear inclusions (arrows). (H & E, × 700.) *B,* Viral infected tissue culture of bovine renal cells. Effect of virus is indicated by *(1)* intranuclear inclusion bodies, and cytopathogenic effect evidenced by *(2)* vacuoles and *(3)* pyknotic nuclei. (H & E, × 390.) (Courtesy of Colonel Fred D. Maurer and Armed Forces Institute of Pathology.)

quently in Europe and occasionally in North America. This infection involves principally the female genital tract, as the name implies, but lesions may occur on male genitalia as well. The manifestations of this disease in the cow are described as appearing suddenly 24 to 72 hours following coitus with an infected bull. The mucosa of the vulva becomes reddened with dark red punctate foci, which shortly grow to form vesicles and pustules. These lesions are less than 0.1 to 5.0 mm in diameter and may be water-clear to yellowish-red in color. The pustules may form a yellowish membrane by coalescence. The membrane becomes detached shortly to reveal an underlying zone of ulceration. Some pain may be manifest during this stage, and the vulva may become obviously swollen. Affected bulls with similar lesions on the penis and prepuce, usually have a small amount of preputial exudate and may be left with some adhesions, although they usually recover completely in about two weeks. Some bulls have been reported to experience orchitis during the course of the disease, and there may be severe effects on reproductive efficiency. In the absence of secondary bacterial infection, the lesions usually heal in 10 to 14 days; however, repeated attacks may occur. It is not clearly established if repeated attacks always represent re-infection or possibly activation of a latent infection similar to recurrent *Herpesvirus simplex* infection in man. Cows and bulls can carry the virus in the absence of visible lesions. Microscopically, the lesions consist of foci of necrosis of the mucosal epithelium with an associated inflammatory reaction. Intranuclear inclusion bodies develop within epithelial cells.

Limited evidence suggests that the IBR

virus may cause a similar disease in sows and boars.

Abortion. The virus of IBR has recently been recognized as an important cause of abortion in cattle. The abortion generally follows the occurrence of the rhinotracheitis form of the disease or the use of modified live IBR vaccine. Two weeks to two months after the respiratory disease, or vaccination, up to 60% of a herd may abort. Although abortion may occur at any stage of pregnancy, it is most frequent in the third trimester. The critical period for exposure appears to be four and one-half to six and one-half months after conception. At the time of abortion, there is no recognizable clinical disease in the dam. Advanced postmortem autolysis is the most striking gross finding in the fetus, which is expelled 24 to 36 hours after intrauterine death. Microscopically characteristic lesions in the fetus consist of focal necrosis in the liver, lymph nodes, spleen, and kidney. Intranuclear inclusion bodies may be found in each of these tissues, but they may be difficult to demonstrate owing to the extensive autolysis. Nonspecific necrosis is seen in the placenta, which is believed to develop subsequent to fetal death.

The pattern of IBR abortion and the fetal lesions are remarkably similar to equine rhinopneumonitis abortion in mares. Both diseases are caused by herpes viruses.

Other Manifestations of IBR. Experimentally, IBR virus has caused mastitis characterized by focal necrosis and intranuclear inclusion bodies. The virus also causes conjunctivitis, which may occur in conjunction with or independently of the respiratory disease. Encephalitis caused by IBR virus has been reported in calves in Australia and the United States. The lesions are characterized by neuronal necrosis and intranuclear inclusion bodies in neurons. Perivascular cuffing with lymphocytes and a mononuclear meningeal infiltration is also seen. In view of the neurotropism exhibited by most members of the herpesvirus group, this finding is not surprising.

Diagnosis. A presumptive diagnosis of infectious bovine rhinotracheitis in any of its many forms can be based on characteristic clinical signs and the demonstration of necrotizing lesions containing intranuclear inclusion bodies. The diagnosis can be confirmed by isolation and characterization of the virus.

Abinanti, F. R., and Plumer, G. J.: The isolation of infectious bovine rhinotracheitis virus from cattle affected with conjunctivitis—observations on the experimental infection. Am. J. Vet. Res., 22:13–17, 1961.

Baker, J. A., McEntee, K., and Gillespie, J. H.: Effects of infectious bovine rhinotracheitis-infectious pustular vulvovaginitis (IBR-IPV) virus on newborn calves. Cornell Vet., 50:156–170, 1960.

Barenfus, B., et al.: Isolation of infectious bovine rhinotracheitis virus from calves with meningoencephalitis. J. Am. Vet. Med. Assoc., 143:725–728, 1963.

Cheatham, W. J., Crandell, R. A.: Occurrence of intranuclear inclusions in tissue culture infected with virus of infectious bovine rhinotracheitis. Proc. Soc. Exp. Biol. Med., 96:536–538, 1957.

Chow, T. L., Deem, A. W., and Jensen, R.: Infectious rhinotracheitis in cattle. II. Experimental reproduction. Proc. U. S. Livestock San. Assoc., 1955, pp. 151–167.

Chow, T. L., Palotay, J. L., and Deem, A. W.: Infectious rhinotracheitis in feedlot cattle III. An epizootiological study in a feedlot. J. Am. Vet. Med. Assoc., 128:348–351, 1956.

Chow, T. L., and Davis, R. W.: The susceptibility of mule deer to infectious bovine rhinotracheitis. Am. J. Vet. Res., 25:518–519, 1964.

Collier, J. R., Chow, T. L., Benjamin, M. M., and Deem, A. W.: The combined effect of infectious bovine rhinotracheitis virus and *Pasteurella hemolytica* on cattle. Am. J. Vet. Res., 21:195–198, 1960.

Corner, A. H., Greig, A. S., and Hill, D. P.: A histological study of the effects of the herpesvirus of infectious bovine rhinotracheitis in the lactating bovine mammary gland. Can. J. Comp. Med. Vet. Sci., 31:320–330, 1967.

Crandell, R. A., Cheatham, W. J., and Maurer, F. D.: Infectious bovine rhinotracheitis—the occurrence of intranuclear inclusion bodies in experimentally infected animals. Am. J. Vet. Res., 20:505–509, 1959.

French, E. L.: A specific virus encephalitis in calves: Isolation and characterization of the causal agent. Aust. Vet. J., 38:216–221, 1962.

———: Relationship between infectious bovine rhinotracheitis (IBR) virus and a virus isolated from calves with encephalitis. Aust. Vet. J., 38:555–556, 1962.

Gillespie, J. H., McEntee, K., Kendrick, J. W., and Wagner, W. C.: Comparison of infectious pustular vulvovaginitis agent with infectious bovine rhinotracheitis virus. Cornell Vet., 49:288–297, 1959.

Gillespie, J. H., Lee, K. M., and Baker, J. A.: Infectious bovine rhinotracheitis. Am. J. Vet. Res., *18*:530–535, 1957.

Griffin, T. P., Howells, W. V., Crandell, R. A., and Maurer, F. D.: Stability of the virus of infectious rhinotracheitis. Am. J. Vet. Res., *19*:990–992, 1958.

Hall, W. T. K., et al.: The pathogenesis of encephalitis caused by the infectious bovine rhinotracheitis virus. Aust. Vet. J., *42*:299–327, 1966.

Jensen, R., Griner, L. A., Chow, T. L., and Brown, W. W.: Infectious rhinotracheitis in feedlot cattle. I. Pathology and symptoms. Proc. U. S. Livestock San. A. (1955):189–199.

Kendrick, J. W. Gillespie, J. H., and McEntee, K.: Infectious pustular vulvovaginitis of cattle. Cornell Vet., *48*:458–495, 1958.

Kendrick, J. W., and Straub, O. C.: Infectious bovine rhinotracheitis infectious-pustular vulvovaginitis virus infection in pregnant cows. Am. J. Vet. Res., *28*:1269–1282, 1967.

Kennedy, P. C., and Richards, W. P. C.: The pathology of abortion caused by the virus of infectious bovine rhinotracheitis. Path. Vet., *1*:7–17, 1964.

Madin, S. H., York, C. J., and McKercher, D. J.: Isolation of the infectious bovine rhinotracheitis virus. Science, *124*:721–722, 1956.

McFeely, R. A., Merritt, A. M., and Stearly, E. L.: Abortion in a dairy herd vaccinated for infectious bovine rhinotracheitis. J. Am. Vet. Med. Assoc., *153*:657–661, 1968.

McKercher, D. G.: Infectious bovine rhinotracheitis. Adv. Vet. Sci., *5*:299–328, 1959.

McKercher, D. G., Moulton, J. E., and Jasper, D. E.: Virus and virus-like disease entities new to California. Proc. U. S. Livestock San. A. (1954).

McKercher, D. G., Moulton, J. E., Kendrick, J. W., and Saito, J.: Recent developments on upper respiratory disease of cattle. Proc. U. S. Livestock San A. (1955):151–167.

McKercher, D. G., Moulton, J. E., Madin, S. H., and Kendrick, J. W.: A newly recognized virus disease in cattle. Am. J. Vet. Res., *18*:246–256, 1957.

McKercher, D. G., Straub, O. C., Saito, J. K., and Woda, E. M.: Comparative studies of the etiological agents of infectious bovine rhinotracheitis and infectious pustular vulvovaginitis. Can. J. Comp. Med., *23*:320–328, 1959.

Miller, N. J.: Infectious necrotic rhinotracheitis of cattle. J. Am. Vet. Med. Assoc., *126*:463–467, 1955.

Mitchell, D., and Greig, A. S.: The incidence and significance of bovine herpesvirus (infectious bovine rhinotracheitis) antibodies in the sera of aborting cattle. Can. J. Comp. Med. Vet. Sci., *31*:234–238, 1967.

Molello, J. A., et al.: Placental pathology. V. Placental lesions of cattle experimentally infected with infectious bovine rhinotracheitis virus. Am. J. Vet. Res., *27*:907–915, 1966.

Owen, N. V., Chow, T. L., and Molello, J. A.: Bovine fetal lesions experimentally produced by infectious bovine rhinotracheitis virus. Am. J. Vet. Res., *25*:1617–1626, 1964.

Rosner, S. F.: Infectious bovine rhinotracheitis: Clinical review, immunity and control. J. Am. Vet. Med. Assoc., *153*:1631–1638, 1968.

Sattar, S. A., and Bohl, E. H.: Some studies of infectious bovine rhinotracheitis (IBR) virus infection in calves. Can. J. Comp. Med., *32*:587–592, 1968.

Saxegaard, F., and Onstad, O.: Isolation and identification of IBR IPV virus from cases of vaginitis and balanitis in swine and from healthy swine. Nord. Vet. Med., *19*:54–57, 1967.

Snowdon, W. A.: The IBR-IPV virus: reaction to infection and intermittent recovery of virus from experimentally infected cattle. Aust. Vet. J., *41*:135–142, 1965.

Schwarz, A. J. F., York, C. J., Zirhel, L. W., and Estela, L. A.: Modification of infectious bovine rhinotracheitis (IBR) virus in tissue culture and development of a vaccine. Proc. Soc. Exp. Biol. Med., *96*:453–458, 1957.

Van Kruiningen, H. J., and Bartholomew, R. C.: Infectious bovine rhinotracheitis diagnosed by lesions in a calf. J. Am. Vet. Med. Assoc., *144*:1008–1012, 1964.

Bovine Malignant Catarrh (Malignant Catarrhal Fever, Snotsiekte)

Malignant catarrh is an infectious disease of cattle in which the principal manifestations are catarrhal and mucopurulent inflammation of the eyes and nostrils, erosions in the oral mucosa, rapid emaciation, enlargement of lymph nodes, corneal opacity and nervous symptoms. The disease has a world-wide distribution, occurring in Europe, Africa, and the United States. There is good evidence to indicate that sheep are subject to an inapparent infection and act as carriers for the disease of cattle. In South and East Africa, a type of wild antelope (wildebeest) is believed to be a carrier. Rabbits are apparently the only laboratory animals that are experimentally susceptible. The disease usually appears only in cattle which are in contact with sheep or wildebeest. The cause is a virus that is classified as a member of the herpesvirus group.

Signs and Course. Experimental infection, after an incubation period of 14 to 60 days, is followed by high fever and catarrhal conjunctivitis and rhinitis, which are evidenced by mucopurulent discharge from the eyes and nose. This exudate characteristically streams from the eyes and nostrils, but soon dries and adheres. The eyes are sensitive to strong light; the cornea becomes opaque in the final stages.

There is rapidly developing emaciation. The skin of the muzzle is eroded and the nasal passages are obstructed by mucopurulent exudate. At the start of the fever, the inside of the mouth is merely congested, but in some cases erosions develop inside the cheeks and on the roof of the mouth that are reported to be grossly indistinguishable from the erosive oral lesions of rinderpest. Diarrhea is frequent and nervous manifestations are seen in the final stages. In mild forms of the disease, skin lesions may be observed. These consist of thickening and peeling, particularly of the skin of the neck, axillae, and perineum. The lymph nodes are swollen (an almost constant sign), and those that appear as small, subcutaneous nodules forming a chain along the jugular groove of the neck can be observed clinically.

Lesions. The principal gross lesions occur in the nostrils, respiratory tract, oral mucosa, eye, and lymph nodes, and less prominently in the intestinal tract. In the nostrils, sharply demarcated, irregularly shaped erosions of the mucosa are covered with a tenacious mucopurulent exudate. Microscopically, these lesions are seen to be the result of necrosis of the epithelium and intense lymphocyte infiltration of the underlying stroma. Cellular exudate may cover the surface of the eroded area. Lesions essentially similar develop in the oral and pharyngeal mucosae.

In the esophagus, rumen, reticulum and omasum, congestion, edema, and erosions have been described. In the abomasum, catarrhal inflammation of the mucosa develops occasionally and an increase of eosinophils in the submucosa has been reported. Erosions and ulcers may be present in the abomasum. The small and large intestines both show submucous hyperemia, edema, and an occasional nonspecific increase in eosinophils. Goblet cells are often increased in the small intestine, but croupous membranes are rare.

In the eye, congestion and edema are severe, particularly at the limbus; the lamina propria of the cornea is often edematous, the fibers being swollen and separated, and the corneal epithelium occasionally exhibits ballooning and vesicle formation. The iris stroma is usually congested and contains some inflammatory cells. Fibrinous exudate in the anterior and posterior chambers and occasionally posterior and anterior synechiae with leukocytic infiltration indicate iridocyclitis.

The liver and kidneys are often grossly enlarged and mottled. Grossly the renal cortex may contain gray to white foci which resemble infarcts. Microscopically, these lesions consist of collections of mononuclear cells. Similar infiltrates are found in the periportal tissues of the liver. The lymph nodes are swollen; sometimes entire nodes or areas seen on cut section are cherry pink and the cut surface often appears granular. The principal microscopic changes in these lymph nodes are reported to be dilatation of lymphatic channels and severe edema and proliferation of reticuloendothelial cells and lymphocytes. In the heart and skeletal muscles, perivascular infiltrations by lymphoid cells have been described. Foci of fatty infiltration may be found in the cardiac muscle fibers in some areas. The microscopic lesions of the skin resemble those of the oral cavity. The media and intima of arteries and arterioles in most tissues are infiltrated with lymphocytes, macrophages, plasma cells, and eosinophils. The endothelium may be swollen or hyperplastic.

In the brain, a "cooked" gross appearance and an odor resembling that of broth have been described, but the basis for these observations is not clear. Microscopic lesions that have been reported include edema and lymphocytic infiltration in the meninges, especially in the pia mater deep in the sulci. Perivascular edema and accumulation of lymphocytes, noted rather constantly, are particularly pronounced in the medulla, pons, olfactory bulb, corpus striatum, caudate nucleus and hippocampus, as well as in the cerebrum, cerebellum and spinal gray matter. Variable degenerative changes have been described in neurons, but are irregular in occurrence.

Although the condition is caused by a herpesvirus, the biologic behavior of this virus is unlike cytocidal herpesviruses, such as those of bovine viral rhinotracheitis, feline viral rhinotracheitis, or equine abortion. The behavior of the virus does, however, resemble lymphotropic herpesvirus, such as the Epstein-Barr virus or *H. saimiri*. As pointed out by Plowright (1968), Hunt and Billups (1979) and others: (1) no free virus is present in tissues of affected cattle, and virus cannot be recovered except by co-cultivation techniques; (2) the virus is associated with lymphocytes; (3) the virus induces classic herpetic CPE in vitro, but in affected cattle there is no herpetic necrosis, no inclusion body, or syncytial giant cell formation; (4) the disease is not considered contagious between cattle; (5) the incubation period is highly variable; and (6) the principal pathologic feature is lymphocytic proliferation and infiltration. Based upon the observations, these authors suggested that malignant catarrhal fever resembles malignant lymphoma or infectious mononucleosis of man.

Diagnosis. The diagnosis of malignant catarrh is often difficult. It may be differentiated from rinderpest by the greater infectivity and shorter course of rinderpest and its more pronounced gross intestinal lesions. The microscopic changes in the mucosae and lymph nodes are also of value in differentiating these two diseases. Considerably more study of malignant catarrh is needed, as are better methods for its recognition.

Berkman, R. N., Barner, R. D., Morrill, C. C., and Langham, R. F.: Bovine malignant catarrhal fever in Michigan. II. Pathology. Am. J. Vet. Res., 21:1015–1027, 1960.
Danskin, D., and Burdin, M. L.: Bovine petechial fever. Vet. Rec., 75:391–394, 1963. VB 3139–63.
Fourie, J. M., and Snyman, P. S.: Blouwildebeestoog. J. S. Afr. Vet. Med. Assoc., 13:43–47, 1942.
Hunt, R. D., and Billups, L. H.: Wildebeest-associated catarrhal fever in Africa: a neoplastic disease of cattle caused by an oncogenic Herpesvirus? Comp. Immun. Microbiol. Infect. Dis., 2:275–283, 1979.
Manjoer, M.: Renjakit Ingusan, a disease resembling malignant catarrhal fever in India. VB 2144, 1958.
Murray, R. B., and Blood, D. C.: An outbreak of bovine malignant catarrh in a dairy herd. I. Clinical and pathological observations. Can. Vet. J., 2:227–281, 1961. VB 32: 130, 1962.
Plowright, W.: The blood leukocytes in infectious malignant catarrh of the ox and rabbit. J. Comp. Pathol. Therap., 63:318–334, 1953.
———: Malignant catarrhal fever. J. Am. Vet. Med. Assoc., 152:795–804, 1968.
Stenius, P. I.: Bovine malignant catarrh. A statistical histopathological and experimental study. Bull. Inst. Path. Vet. College, Helsinki, 1952.

Equine Viral Rhinopneumonitis (Equine Virus Abortion)

A viral disease of the equine fetus, originally described in 1940 by Dimock et al., under the term "equine virus abortion," has since become well established as a cause of intrauterine death of near-term equine fetuses. It is a particular hazard in horse breeding establishments. In the same year, a filtrable virus was isolated by Jones and co-workers (1948) from young horses with a respiratory disease and was maintained for several years by serial passage through colts. This disease was responsible for a large number of deaths of horses in remount depots during World War II, usually from pneumonic complications. The disease was called equine influenza at the time, although no immunologic relationship could be demonstrated between this virus and that of swine or human influenza; furthermore, it has other characteristics quite different from those of the other influenza viruses. It is now recognized that the causative agent of rhinopneumonitis is a herpesvirus. Since the isolation of true influenza viruses from horses with respiratory diseases, the use of the term influenza should be restricted to those diseases alone. The appropriate term for equine herpesvirus infection is now accepted as equine viral rhinopneumonitis.

In 1954, Doll and co-workers adapted to hamsters and chick embryos the viruses isolated by Dimock and Jones, and demonstrated serologic and immunologic similarities between the two. They also showed that virus causing the respiratory disease of young horses could produce intrauterine death of near-term fetuses, in which the pathologic changes were characteristic of virus abortion. The lesions in fetuses dead of equine abortion and in animals with equine rhinopneumonitis also had distinct similarities, further evidence that the same etiologic agent was concerned. For this reason, equine viral abortion and equine rhinopneumonitis, although previously regarded as separate and distinct disease entities, can appropriately be considered together. The term equine viral rhinopneumonitis was first suggested by Doll for this disease complex, which is now recognized to occur worldwide. Since further study on this subject is needed, future developments may cause revision of present concepts of the nature of these diseases. German workers have described a similar disease of viral etiology, but the agent has not yet been compared with those encountered in the United States. Another disease which can now be separated, on the basis of its etiology and pathology, from the clinical "influenza" group, is equine viral arteritis, described by Doll et al.

Signs. Infection of the fetus with the agent of virus abortion has some characteristic features from which a presumptive diagnosis can often be made. The disease almost exclusively affects the fetus during the eighth to the eleventh months of pregnancy, the majority of abortions being in the ninth and tenth months. The fetus is expelled from the uterus promptly after death or, in some cases, before the heart beat stops, usually with no more difficulty than is experienced in normal parturition. Complications such as retained placenta, delayed involution and postparturient metritis are seldom encountered following abortion due to this viral agent. The mare usually recovers promptly, showing little more than a slight transitory fever. A storm of abortions may occur, as many as 90% of the pregnant mares in a band being affected, or the disease may be limited to only a small fraction of the susceptible mares.

In young horses from one to four years of age, the same virus produces a fever with abrupt onset about three days after intravenous or intranasal instillation of the virus. Slight congestion of nasal and conjunctival mucosae occurs, the animal is somewhat depressed, and a dry, hacking cough may develop; the fever usually subsides in two to four days and the animal recovers promptly. In complicated cases observed in natural outbreaks in large groups of horses, however, severe respiratory symptoms may appear, particularly when beta hemolytic streptococci are also involved. Death may result from pneumonia or, in a few cases, from purpura hemorrhagica or streptococcal septicemia. One late sequel is damage to the left recurrent laryngeal nerve, which produces paralysis of the vocal cords, causing characteristic sounds with each inspiration ("roaring").

Lesions. In the aborted fetus, the lesions are typically found in the lungs, liver, and lymph nodes, although some icteric discoloration, interlobular pulmonary edema, and excess peritoneal fluid are significant gross findings. The changes in the liver, which usually is congested, may be seen grossly as tiny gray subcapsular foci, usually from 2 to 5 mm in diameter, scattered throughout the lobules. Microscopically, these foci consist of sharply demarcated aggregations of necrotic liver cells. Liver cells surrounding the foci of necrosis often contain small eosinophilic intranuclear inclusions (Fig. 9–17). Enlargement of the nucleus or margination of the chromatin is seldom associated with these inclusions, which usually are quite small,

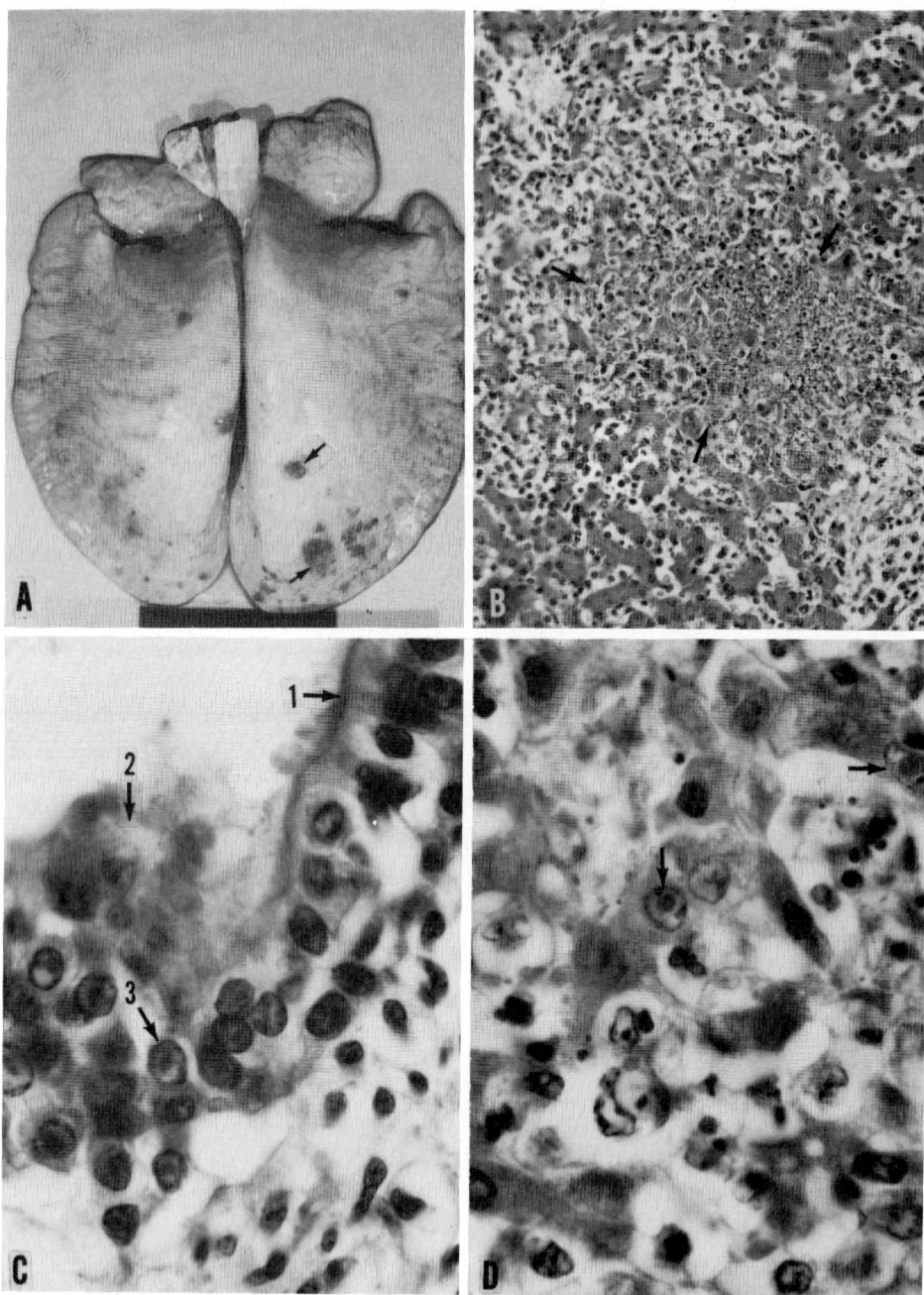

Fig. 9–17. Equine rhinopneumonitis. *A,* Hemorrhages in pleura, lung of an aborted fetus. *B,* Focal necrosis (arrows) in liver (× 145). *C,* Erosion and proliferation of bronchiolar epithelium (× 825). Bronchiolar epithelium *(1),* which is desquamated and hyperplastic at *(2)* and contains intranuclear inclusions *(3). D,* Intranuclear inclusions (arrows) in liver cells (× 825). (Courtesy of Armed Forces Institute of Pathology.) Contributor: Dr. Rufus Humphrey.

although large enough to replace most of the internal structure of the nucleus. In the lung, interlobular edema and excessive pleural fluid are constant gross lesions. The microscopic changes in the lung consist of cellular debris in the lumen of the bronchi and bronchioles, and partial or complete erosion of adjacent epithelium. In epithelial cells near the eroded areas, the nuclei contain eosinophilic inclusions like those in liver cells (Fig. 9–17). Similar intranuclear inclusions and foci of necrosis are found in the spleen and lymph nodes in many cases.

In the young adult animal, the lesions are often complicated by the effects of hemolytic streptococci and other bacteria which invade the respiratory system in association with the virus. Hemorrhagic or purulent bronchopneumonia is the most frequent finding in fatal cases, but disseminated abscesses or purpura hemorrhagica may also be found.

Diagnosis. Diagnosis of this infection in an aborted equine fetus is confirmed by the demonstration of characteristic lesions with intranuclear inclusions in the lung, liver, and other organs. Further confirmation may be accomplished by infection of suckling hamsters with suspensions of equine fetal tissues and demonstration of similar lesions in the liver of these animals; however, serial passage is usually necessary to adapt the virus to hamsters. Experimental intrauterine injection of mares in the ninth month of pregnancy almost invariably results in infection and abortion of the fetus, with characteristic lesions. Differential diagnosis of the respiratory form of rhinopneumonitis must include equine influenza and equine viral arteritis.

Three equine herpesviruses (equine herpesvirus types 2, 3 and equine cytomegalovirus), distinct from equine rhinopneumonitis virus, have recently been reported. Their pathogenicity has not been studied, but it necessitates caution in identifying herpesvirus isolates from horses. Recent reports have also associated a herpesvirus, believed to be distinct from equine rhino-pneumonitis virus, with vulvitis and balanitis in horses.

Dimock, W. W.: The diagnosis of virus abortion in mares. J. Am. Vet. Med. Assoc., 96:665–666, 1940.

Doll, E. R.: Intrauterine and intrafetal inoculations with equine abortion virus in pregnant mares. Cornell Vet., 43:112–121, 1953.

Doll, E. R., Richards, M. G., and Wallace, M. E.: Adaptation of the equine abortion virus to suckling Syrian hamsters. Cornell Vet., 43:551–558, 1953.

————: Cultivation of the equine influenza virus in suckling Syrian hamsters. Its similarity to the equine abortion virus. Cornell Vet., 44:133–138, 1954.

Doll, E. R., Wallace, M. E, and Richards, M. G.: Thermal, hematological, and serological responses of weanling horses following inoculation with equine abortion virus: its similarity to equine influenza. Cornell Vet., 44:181–190, 1954.

Doll, E. R., Bryans, J. T., McCollum, W. H., and Crowe, M. E. W.: Isolation of a filterable agent causing arteritis of horses and abortion by mares. Its differentiation from the equine abortion (influenza) virus. Cornell Vet., 47:3–41, 1957.

Girard, A., Greig, A. S., and Mitchell, D.: A virus associated with vulvitis and balanitis in the horse: a preliminary report. Can. J. Comp. Med., 32:603–604, 1968.

Hatziolas, B. C., and Reagan, R. L.: Neurotropism of equine influenza-abortion virus in infant experimental animals. Am. J. Vet. Res., 21:856–861, 1960.

Jeleff, W.: Beitrag zur fötalen Histopathologie des Virusaborts der Stute mit besonderer Berucksichtigung der Differentialdiagnose. Arch. Exp. Vet. Med., 11:906–920, 1959.

Jones, T. C., and Maurer, F. D.: Neutralization studies of the viruses of influenza A, influenza B and swine influenza with equine influenza convalescent serums. Am. J. Vet. Res., 3:179–182, 1942.

Jones, T. C., and Maurer, F. D.: The pathology of equine influenza. Am. J. Vet. Res., 4:15–31, 1943.

Jones, T. C., et al.: Transmission and immunization studies on equine influenza. Am. J. Vet. Res., 9:243–253, 1948.

Jones, T. C., Doll, E. R., and Bryans, J. T.: The lesions of equine viral arteritis. Cornell Vet., 47:52–68, 1957.

Karpas, A.: Characterization of a new herpes-like virus isolated from foal kidney. Ann. Inst. Pasteur. Paris, 110:688–696, 1966.

Matumoto, M., Ishizaki, R., and Shimizu, T.: Serologic survey of equine rhinopneumonitis virus infection among horses in various countries. Arch Ges. Virusforsch., 15:609–624, 1965.

McCollum, W. H., Doll, E. R., Wilson, J. C., and Johnson, C. B.: Isolation and propagation of equine rhinopneumonitis virus in primary monolayer kidney cell cultures of domestic animals. Cornell Vet., 52:164–173, 1962.

Pascoe, R. R., Spradbrow, P. B., and Bagust, T. J.: An equine genital infection resembling coital exanthema associated with a virus. Aust. Vet., 45:166–170, 1969.

Plummer, G., Bowling, C. P., and Goodheart, C. R.:

Comparison of four horse herpesviruses. J. Virol., 4:738–741, 1969.

Sályi, J.: Beitrag zur Pathohistologie des Virusabortus der Stuten. Arch. f. wissensch. u. prakt. Tierh., 77:244–253, 1941–42.

Straub, M.: Histology of catarrhal influenzal bronchitis and collapse of lung in mice infected with influenza virus. J. Pathol. Bact., 50:31–36, 1940.

Waldman, O., and Köbe, K.: Der seuchenhafte Husten (infektiose Bronchitis) des Pferdes. Zentralbl. f. Bakt., pt. 1, (Orig.) 133:49–59, 1934.

Westerfield, C., and Dimock, W. W.: The pathology of equine virus abortion. J. Am. Vet. Med. Assoc., 109:101–111, 1946.

Feline Viral Rhinotracheitis

The isolation and identification, by Crandell and Maurer (1958), of a virus clearly related to an upper respiratory disease of cats is of particular significance because the agent has been shown to be the cause of a widely disseminated disease of cats. Crandell and Maurer named this disease "feline viral rhinotracheitis," an apt designation that indicated its etiology as well as the species and anatomic structures affected. The virus has been characterized as a herpesvirus. The disease is manifest by sudden onset of sneezing and copious discharge of a mucous nasal exudate. This exudate may be seen clinging to the nostrils or on the forelegs as a result of the cat's efforts to clear its nose. Ulcerative glossitis frequently accompanies the respiratory signs. A transient fever occurs in the early stages. Young, recently weaned kittens are particularly susceptible, but the disease may affect cats of all ages. It is quite likely that this disease is responsible for much of the illness referred to as "coryza" which appears with such frequency in catteries and veterinary hospitals.

Lesions. The lesions are confined to the nasal cavities, tongue, pharynx, larynx, and trachea for the most part, only rarely involving the lungs. The virus attacks the respiratory and oral epithelium, resulting in necrosis of cells and, in early stages, the presence of intranuclear inclusions (Fig. 9–18). This change in the epithelium is followed by ulceration and leukocytic infiltration. The intranuclear inclusions can also be demonstrated in tissue cultures of the virus using feline kidney cells. The virus also produces giant cells and has a significant necrotizing effect upon the cells in the tissue culture.

Recent experimental evidence suggests that the virus may be an important cause of abortion and systemic disease of the neonate in a manner analogous to other herpesvirus infections such as *Herpesvirus simplex, H. canis,* and infectious bovine rhinotracheitis.

Crandell, R. A., and Despeaux, E. W.: Cytopathology of feline viral rhinotracheitis virus in cultures of feline renal cells. Proc. Soc. Exp. Biol. Med., 101:494–497, 1959.

Crandell, R. A., Ganaway, J. R., Niemann, W. H., and Maurer, F. D.: Comparative study of three isolates with the original feline viral rhinotracheitis. Am. J. Vet. Res., 21:504–506, 1960.

Crandell, R. A., and Madin, S. H.: Experimental studies on a new feline virus. Am. J. Vet. Res., 21:551–556, 1960.

Crandell, R. A., and Maurer, F. D.: Isolation of a feline virus associated with intranuclear inclusion bodies. Proc. Soc. Exp. Biol. Med., 97:487–490, 1958.

Crandell, R. A., et al.: Experimental feline viral rhinotracheitis. J. Am. Vet. Med. Assoc., 138:191–196, 1961.

Ditchfield, J., and Grinyer, I.: Feline rhinotracheitis virus: a feline herpesvirus. Virology, 26:504–506, 1965.

Hoover, E. A., Rokovsky, M. W., and Griesemer, R. A.: Experimental feline viral rhinotracheitis in the germfree cat. Am. J. Pathol., 58:269–282, 1970.

Karpas, A., and Routledge, J. K.: Feline herpes virus: isolations and experimental studies. Zbl. Vet. Med., 15:599–606, 1968.

Scott, F. W.: Evaluation of a feline viral rhinotracheitis-feline calicivirus disease vaccine. Am. J. Vet. Res., 38:229–234, 1977.

Walton, T. E., and Gillespie, J. H.: Feline viruses, VII. Immunity to the feline herpesvirus in kittens inoculated experimentally by the aerosol method. Cornell Vet., 60:232–239, 1970.

The Lucké Frog Kidney Carcinoma

Lucké described a carcinoma of the kidney, in 1934, as a frequent spontaneous tumor of the leopard frog (*Rana pipiens*) particularly in northern New England states. He later suggested that the disease was caused by a transmissible virus. Present evidence supports that the neoplasm is caused by a virus of the herpesvirus

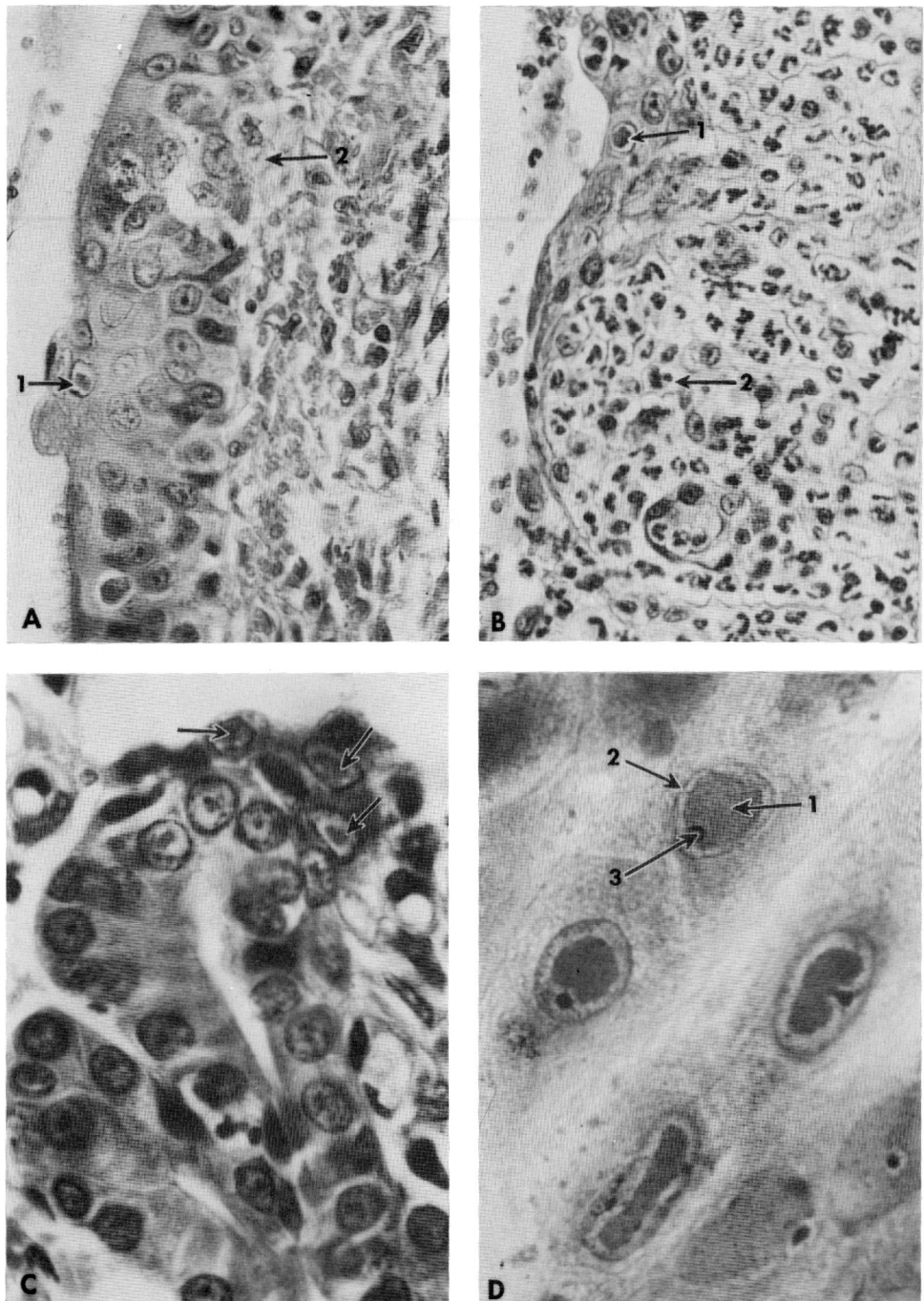

Fig. 9–18. Feline viral rhinotracheitis. *A,* Nasopharynx of cat infected with the virus. Intranuclear inclusion *(1)* and early necrosis *(2)* of the epithelium. (H & E, × 530.) B, Nasopharynx of cat, later stage of infection. Intranuclear inclusion *(1)* still present in mucosa and neutrophils *(2)* invading the necrotic epithelium. (H & E, × 530.) *C,* Intranuclear inclusions in nasal epithelium. (H & E, × 1190.) *D,* Intranuclear inclusion *(1)* in cells of feline kidney tissue culture. Marginated nuclear chromatin *(2)* and nucleolus *(3)*. (H & E, × 1100.) (Courtesy of Colonel Fred D. Maurer and Armed Forces Institute of Pathology.)

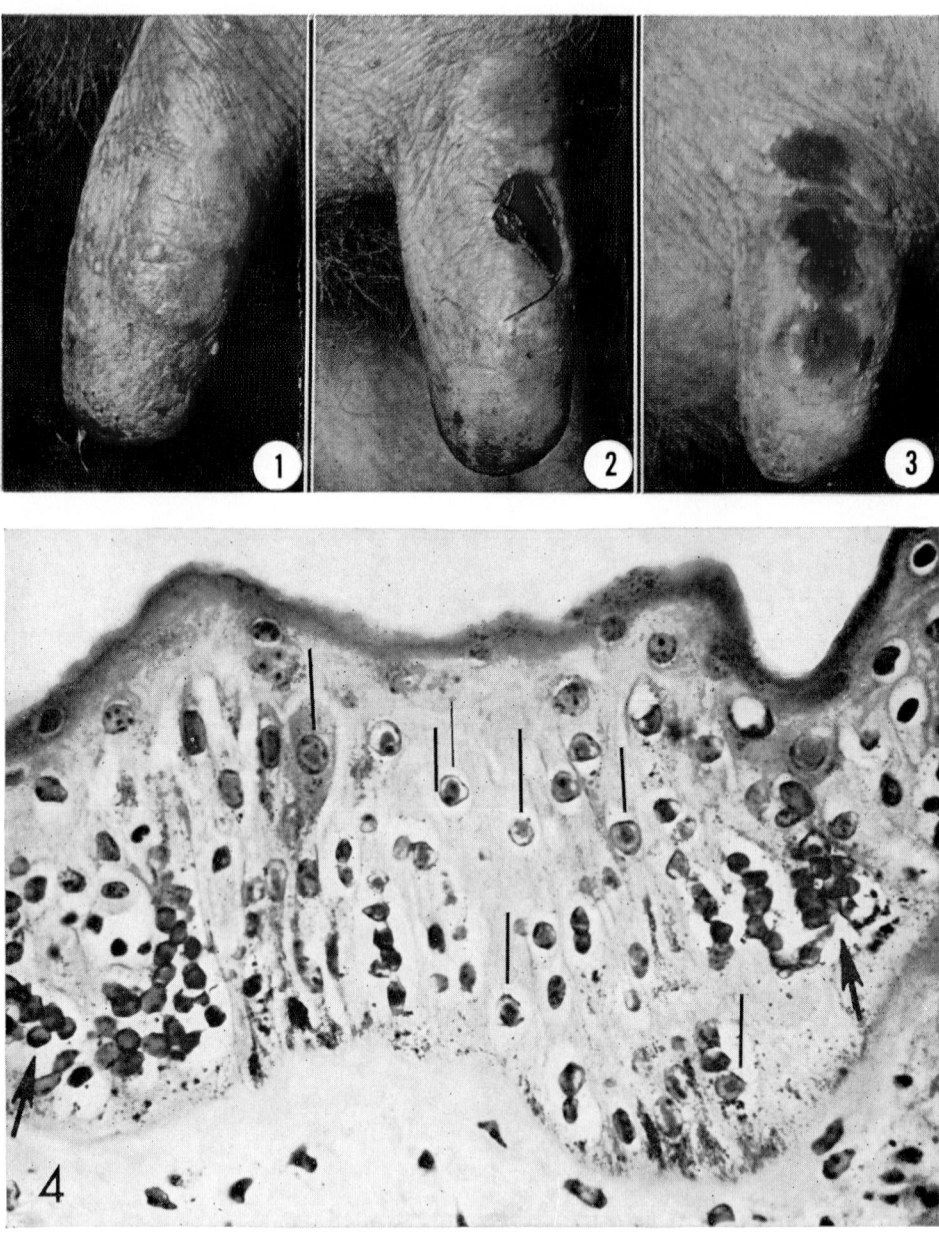

Fig. 9–19. Herpesvirus mamillitis. *(1)* Early raised plaque followed by *(2)* ulceration and *(3)* scab formation. *(4)* Epithelial cells of teat epithelium containing intranuclear inclusion bodies *(bars)*. Multinucleated cells are also evident (arrows). (Courtesy of Dr. W. B. Martin, Dr. I. M. Lauder, and *American Journal of Veterinary Research*.)

group. The tumors may occur in one or both kidneys as single or multiple white nodules. Microscopically, they appear as typical adenocarcinomas, with the unique exception that eosinophilic intranuclear inclusion bodies are often present.

Gross, L.: Oncogenic viruses. International Series of Monographs on Pure and Applied Biology, Vol. 11. New York, Pergamon Press, 1961.

Lucké, B.: A neoplastic disease of the kidney of the frog, *Rana pipiens*. Am. J. Cancer, 20:352–379, 1934.

———: Carcinoma in the Leopard frog. Its probable causation by a virus. J. Exp. Med., 68:457–468, 1938.

Bovine Ulcerative Mamillitis (Bovine Herpesvirus Mamillitis)

Although recognized earlier, a specific ulcerative disease of the bovine teat caused by a herpesvirus was first reported by Martin, Martin, and Lauder (1964). The virus, which is a distinct member of the herpesvirus group, is not distinguishable from the Allerton virus, a herpesvirus once thought to be associated with lumpy skin disease (now recognized as a poxvirus infection of cattle).

Lesions. The lesions of ulcerative mamillitis are usually confined to the teats, although lesions may spread to the skin of the udder. Beginning as local areas of erythema and edema, the lesions progress to vesicles which rupture, leaving scab-covered ulcers. Healing without visible scars generally occurs in 10 to 18 days, though lesions may persist up to three months. Microscopically, the features resemble other localized herpesvirus in-

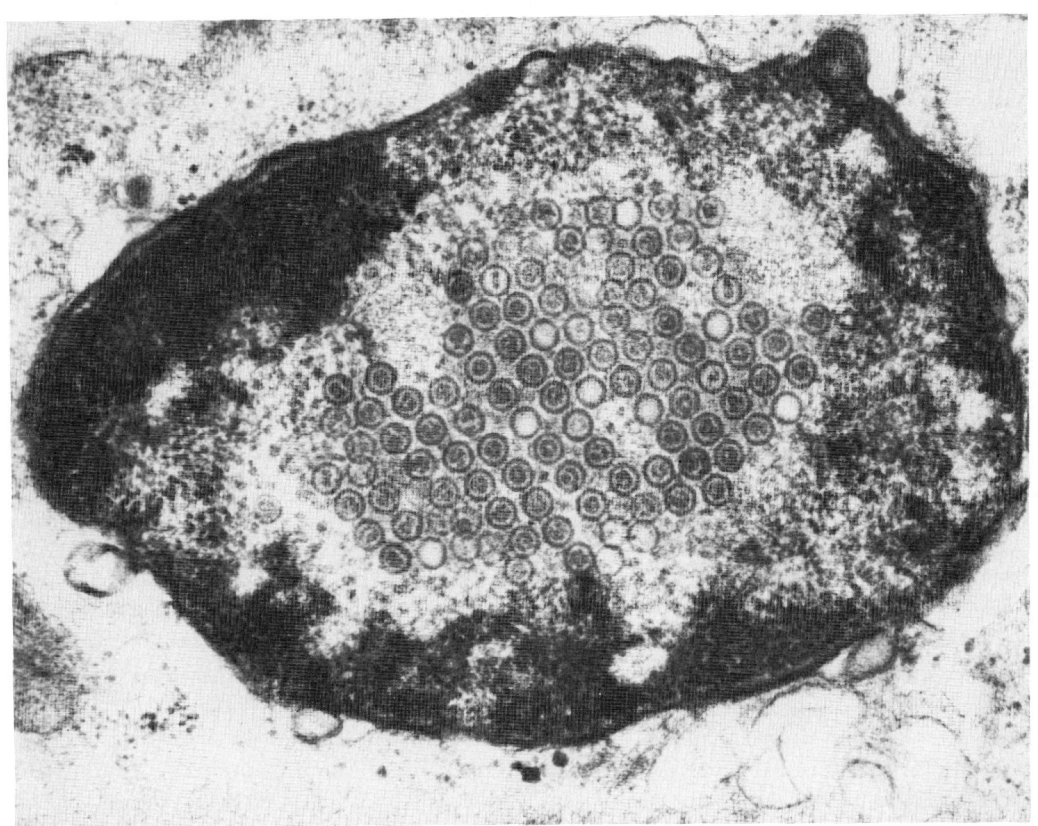

Fig. 9–20. Herpesvirus mamillitis. Numerous viral particles form an inclusion body in an epidermal cell (× 42,000). (Courtesy of Dr. W. B. Martin, Dr. I. M. Lauder, and *American Journal of Veterinary Research*.)

duced lesions (see *Herpesvirus simplex, B and T*). In the epidermis there is ballooning degeneration, intercellular edema, and necrosis leading to vesiculation. Multinucleated giant cells form within the epidermis. Intranuclear inclusion bodies are numerous in epithelial cells and giant cells. A cellular inflammatory response develops in the dermis.

Diagnosis. The disease must be differentiated from cowpox and pseudocowpox. Histologically, the presence of giant cells and intranuclear inclusion bodies differentiates herpesvirus infections from poxvirus infections, which are characterized by cytoplasmic inclusions. Viral isolation and identification allows a definitive diagnosis.

Martin, W. B., et al.: Pathogenesis of bovine mamillitis virus infection in cattle. Am. J. Vet. Res., 30:2151–2166, 1969.

———: Bovine ulcerative mamillitis caused by a herpesvirus. Vet. Rec., 78:494–497, 1966.

———: Characteristics of bovine mamillitis virus. J. Gen. Microbiol., 45:325–332, 1966.

Martin, W. B., Martin, B., and Lauder, I. M.: Ulceration of cows' teats caused by a virus. Vet. Rec., 76:15–16, 1964.

Rweyemamu, M. M., Johnson, R. H., and McCrea, M. R.: Bovine herpes mamillitis virus. III. Observations on experimental infection. Br. Vet. J., 124:317–323, 1968.

Rweyemamu, M. M., Johnson, R. H., and Tutt, J. B.: Some observations on herpes virus mamillitis of bovine animals. Vet. Rec., 79:810–811, 1966.

Rweyemamu, M. M., Osborne, A. D., and Johnson, R. H.: Observations on the histopathology of bovine herpes mamillitis. Res. Vet. Sci., 10:203–207, 1969.

Cytomegalic Inclusion Diseases

Cytomegalic inclusion diseases, which affect a variety of animal species including man, are caused by relatively host-specific viruses termed cytomegaloviruses, classified within the herpesvirus group. The viruses characteristically induce the formation of extremely large cells up to 40 μ in diameter, which bear large intranuclear inclusion bodies. Most of the cytomegaloviruses have a particular affinity for salivary glands. The infection is most often latent or subclinical, but under proper circum-

stances, overwhelming generalized and frequently fatal infection can develop. Specific cytomegaloviruses have been isolated from man, guinea pigs, mice, rats, African green monkeys *(Cercopithecus aethiops)*, swine (inclusion body rhinitis), ground squirrels, and horses. Although viruses have not been isolated, lesions compatible with cytomegalovirus infection have been seen in the Rhesus monkey *(Macaca mulatta)*, Cebus monkey, hamster, chimpanzee, gorilla, sheep, sand rat, and tarsier. As indicated, in most species the infection is of little concern, the principal importance lying in recognition and differential diagnosis. Therefore, we will only elaborate on three cytomegalic inclusion diseases to illustrate the host-virus relationships.

Cytomegalic Inclusion Disease in Man. Based on the presence of complement-fixing antibodies, cytomegalovirus infection is extremely common in man. Pathologically, the infection can be divided into two forms. In the **localized** form of the disease, inclusion-bearing megalocytes without associated tissue damage or inflammatory reaction are confined to the salivary gland. This is the most frequent expression of the disease in man and in various animal cytomegalovirus infections. **Generalized** cytomegalic inclusion disease, although less frequent, represents a serious and often fatal disorder. This form is most frequent in newborn children, who are believed to have become infected in utero. Less frequently it is seen in children beyond the neonatal period. Characteristic megalocytes and inclusion bodies may be found in the salivary glands, kidneys, liver, lungs, adrenals, thyroids, pancreas, thymus, and brain, often associated with necrosis and cellular infiltration. Often the child is subnormal in size. Surviving children may develop hydrocephalus, microcephaly, microphthalmia, and mental retardation. Generalized cytomegalic inclusion disease also occurs in adults, usually in association with neoplastic disease or immunosuppressive therapy.

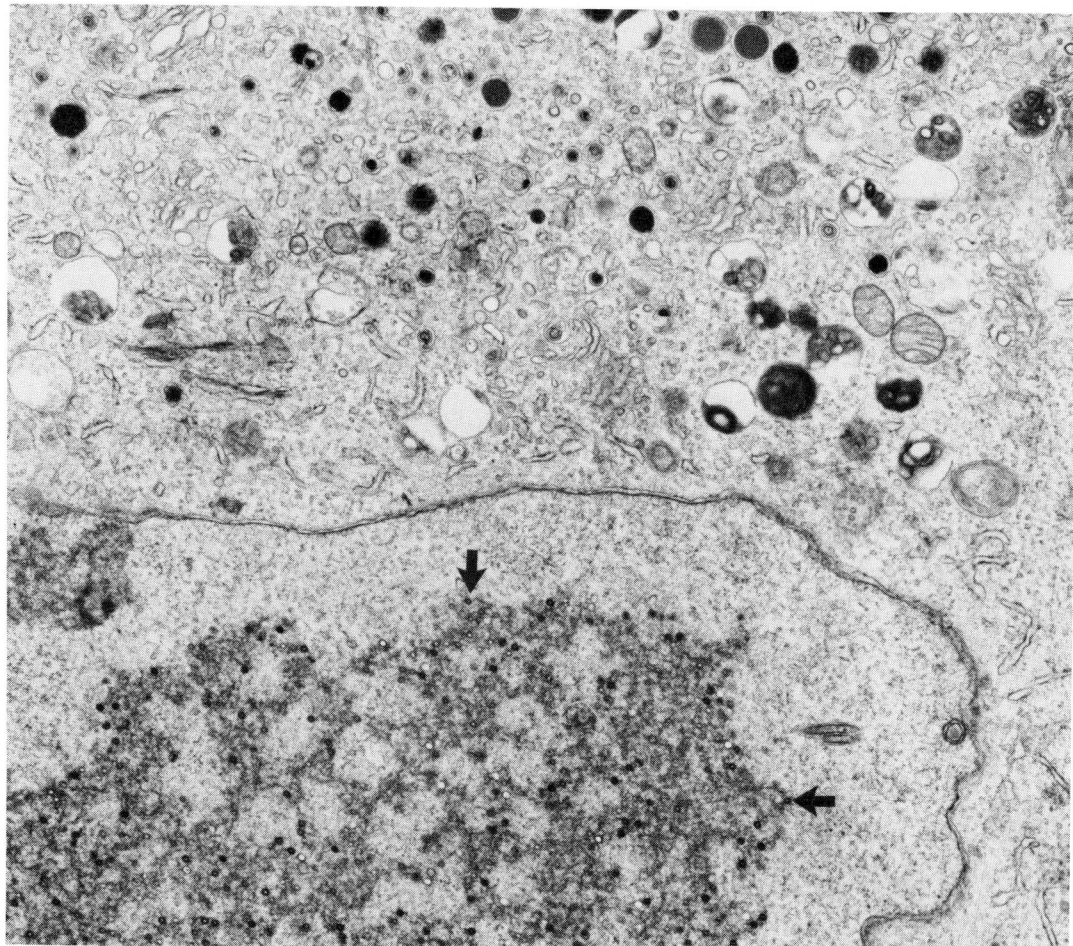

Fig. 9–21. Human cytomegalovirus in tissue culture of human fibroblast. The nucleus contains a large inclusion body consisting of virions, viral structural protein, and DNA (arrows). (Courtesy of Dr. N. W. King, Jr.)

Cytomegalic Inclusion Disease in Guinea Pigs. This spontaneous viral disease of guinea pigs has been the subject of considerable investigation. The disease, although not uncommon, is usually occult, and it is most frequently recognized by finding large eosinophilic or basophilic inclusion bodies in the nuclei of ducts of salivary glands. Experimental serial passage of the agent through young guinea pigs enhances its virulence until it can produce illness and even death. The infection is of interest in comparison with a cytomegalic inclusion disease of infants, in which the inclu-sion bodies are similar. The causative agents of the human and animal disease, however, are distinct.

The intranuclear inclusions in the guinea pig diseases are usually not accompanied by any specific necrosis or inflammatory changes. A salivary gland duct that otherwise appears normal may contain several enlarged epithelial nuclei, with margination of chromatin and a large central mass, which is either eosinophilic or slightly basophilic. The inclusion body has some resemblance to that of canine hepatitis.

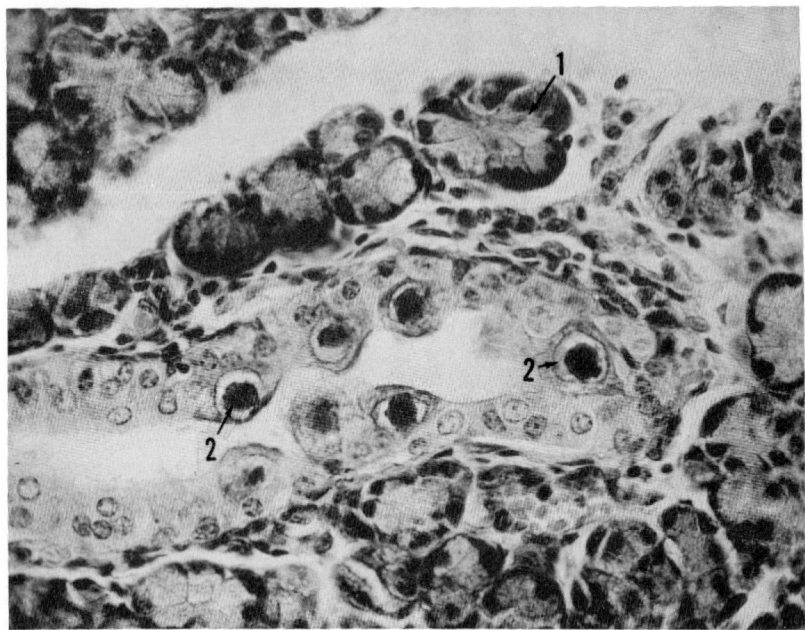

Fig. 9–22. Salivary gland virus disease in guinea pig (× 395). Salivary acinar epithelium *(1)*, intranuclear inclusions in epithelium of a duct *(2)*. (Courtesy of Armed Forces Institute of Pathology.) Contributor: Major C. N. Barron.

The virus may disseminate through the body of the guinea pig, particularly when its virulence is enhanced by serial passage, but apparently it localizes in the submaxillary salivary gland even when introduced into the subcutis. While the infection seldom causes much loss in colonies of laboratory animals, its presence makes the guinea pig unsuitable for research on other viruses whose lesions might be confused with those of the salivary gland virus.

Inclusion Body Rhinitis of Swine. Inclusion body rhinitis of swine is a cytomegalovirus disease first described in Great Britain in 1955. The disease, known to occur in Europe and the United States, principally affects two- to three-week-old piglets, producing a mild catarrhal to purulent rhinitis. Morbidity is high, but the disease has a low mortality rate, unless complicated by more serious secondary pathogens.

Microscopically, the picture is domi-nated by inclusion-bearing megalocytes in the glandular epithelium of the nasal cavity. Recovery is usually uneventful. In the experimentally induced disease, inclusion bodies are first seen ten days after infection, and are usually absent by 27 days. Inclusion bearing megalocytes have also been described in the kidney and salivary gland.

Black, P. H., Hartley, J. W., and Rowe, W. P.: Isolation of a cytomegalovirus from African green monkeys. Proc. Soc. Exp. Biol. Med., *112*:601–605, 1963.

Cole, R., and Kuttner, A. G.: A filterable virus present in the submaxillary glands of guinea pigs. J. Exp. Med., *44*:855–873, 1926.

Cowdry, E. V., and Scott, G. N.: Nuclear inclusions suggestive of virus action in the salivary glands of the monkey, *Cebus fatuellus*. Am. J. Pathol., *11*:647–658, 1935.

———: Nuclear inclusions in the kidneys of Macacus Rhesus monkeys. Am. J. Pathol., *11*:659–668, 1935.

Craighead, J. E., Hanshaw, J. B., and Carpenter, C. B.: Cytomegalovirus infection after renal allotrans-

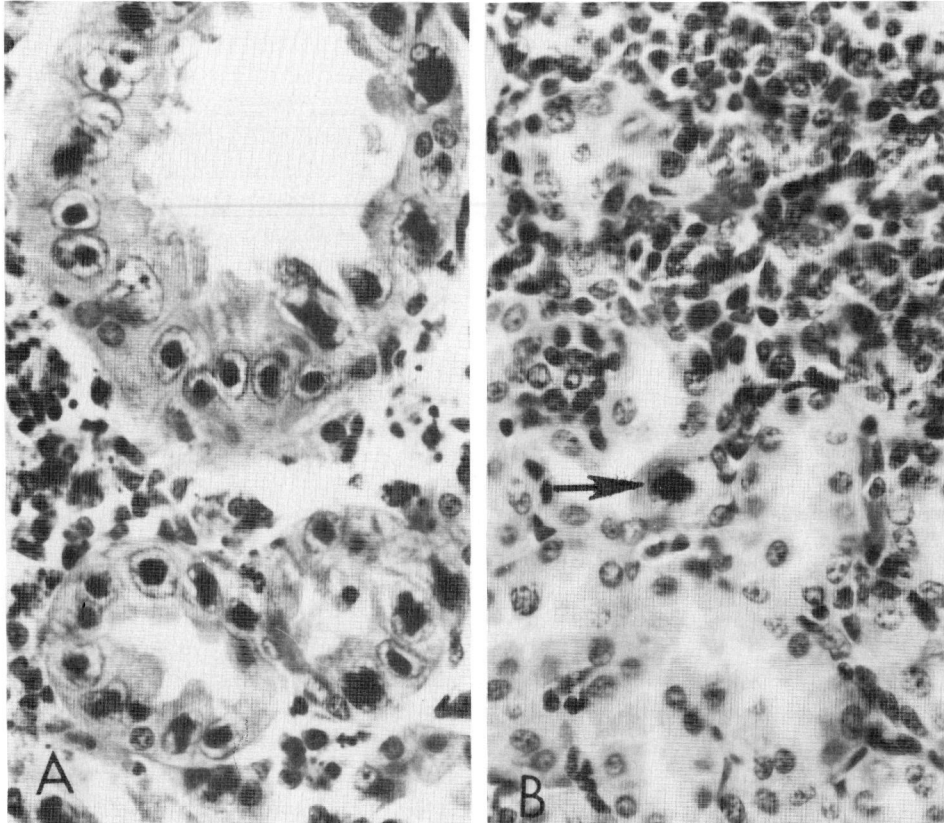

Fig. 9–23. Inclusion body rhinitis of swine. *A*, Numerous intranuclear inclusion bodies in nasal glands. (Courtesy of Dr. J. R. Duncan.) *B*, Intranuclear inclusion body (arrow) in renal tubular epithelial cell and lymphocytic nephritis. (Courtesy of Dr. D. F. Kelly.)

plantation. J. Am. Med. Assoc., *201*:725–728, 1967.

Diosi, P., Babusceac, L., and David, C.: Recovery of cytomegalovirus from the submaxillary glands of ground squirrels. Arch. Ges. Virusforsch., *20*:383–386, 1967.

Diosi, P., et al.: Incidence of cytomegalic infection in man. Pathologia et Microbiologia, *30*:453–468, 1967.

Done, T. C.: An "inclusion-body" rhinitis of pigs (preliminary report). Vet. Rec., *67*:525–527, 1955.

Duncan, J. R., Ramsey, F. K., and Switzer, W. P.: Electron microscopy of cytomegalic inclusion disease of swine (inclusion body rhinitis). Am. J. Vet. Res., *26*:939–947, 1965.

Duvall, C. P., et al.: Recovery of cytomegalovirus from adults with neoplastic disease. Ann. Int. Med., *64*:531–541, 1966.

Fetterman, G. H., et al.: Generalized cytomegalic inclusion disease of the newborn. Arch. Pathol., *86*:86–94, 1968.

Goodwin, R. F. W., and Whittleston, P.: Inclusion-body rhinitis of pigs: an experimental study of some factors that affect the incidence of inclusion bodies in the nasal mucosa. Res. Vet. Sci., *8*:346–352, 1967.

Hanshaw, J. B.: Cytomegalovirus complement-fixing antibody in microcephaly. N. Engl. J. Med., *275*:476–479. 1966.

Hanshaw, J. B.: Cytomegaloviruses. Virology Monographs, *3*:1–23, New York, Springer-Verlag, 1968.

Harding, J. D. J.: Inclusion body rhinitis of swine in Maryland. Am. J. Vet. Res., *19*:907–912, 1958.

Hsiung, G. D., et al.: Characterization of a cytomegalo-like virus isolated from spontaneously degenerated equine kidney cell culture. Proc. Soc. Exp. Biol. Med., *130*:80–84, 1969.

Hunt, R. D., Melendez, L. V., and King, N. W., Jr.: Cytomegalic inclusion disease in sand rats (*Psammomys obesus*): histopathologic evidence. Am. J. Vet. Res., *28*:1190–1193, 1967.

Johnson, K. P.: Mouse cytomegalovirus: placental infection. J. Infect. Dis., 120:445–450, 1969.

Kelly, D. F.: Pathology of extranasal lesions in experimental inclusion body rhinitis of pigs. Res. Vet. Sci., 8:472–478, 1967.

Kendall, O., et al.: Cytomegaloviruses as common adventitious contaminants in primary African green monkey kidney cell cultures. J. Nat. Cancer Inst., 42:489–496, 1969.

Kuttner, A. G.: Further studies concerning the filterable virus present in the submaxillary glands of guinea pigs. J. Exp. Med., 46:935–956, 1927.

Naeye, R. L.: Cytomegalic inclusion disease, the fetal disorder. Am. J. Clin. Pathol., 47:738–744, 1967.

Rabson, A. S., et al.: Isolation and growth of rat cytomegalovirus in vitro. Proc. Soc. Exp. Biol. Med., 131:923–927, 1969.

Rifkind, D.: Cytomegalovirus infection after renal transplantation. Arch. Intern. Med., 116:553–558, 1965.

Rinker, C. T., and McGraw, J. P.: Cytomegalic inclusion disease in childhood leukemia. Cancer, 20:36–39, 1967.

Smith, A. A., and McNulty, W. P., Jr.: Salivary gland inclusion disease in the tarsier. Lab. Anim. Care, 19:479–481, 1969.

Vogel, F. S., and Pinkerton, H.: Spontaneous salivary gland virus disease in chimpanzees. Arch. Pathol., 60:281–285, 1955.

Tsuchiya, Y., Isshiki, O., and Yamada, H.: Generalized cytomegalovirus infection in gorilla. Jap. J. Med. Sci. Biol., 23:71–73, 1970.

ADENOVIRIDAE

Many adenoviruses (adeno = gland), distinguished from one another by immunologic methods, have been isolated from mammals and birds. They are grouped together in the family Adenoviridae because of common ultrastructural features of the virion, chemical characteristics, and a common group antigen. Some of these viruses have the ability to transform cells in culture and to induce transplantable malignant tumors in newborn hamsters. These qualities make adenoviruses particularly useful in laboratory studies of viral actions. Some adenoviruses also produce disease in their definitive hosts in addition to their experimentally demonstrable oncogenic effects. Two genera are presently recognized: *Mastadenovirus* (masto = mammal), including viruses received from mammals, and *Aviadenovirus* (avi = bird), in which are grouped viruses isolated from avian species. Our attention in this text will be directed toward diseases produced in mammals by organisms classified in the genus *Mastadenovirus*.

All viruses in this family have a characteristic icosahedral structure in the virion, with fibers that project from each of the 12 vertices of the icosahedron. The icosahedral capsid contains 252 capsomeres, which also have an icosahedral array. The nucleic acid consists of a single linear molecule of double-stranded DNA. The virions have no envelope and are produced within the nucleus of the host cell, where a characteristic intranuclear inclusion is produced (Fenner et al., 1974). See Table 9–1.

The best studed adenoviruses include several serotypes isolated from human, simian, and avian hosts. Others have been recovered from many species, such as bovine, ovine, porcine, equine, murine, and canine types, which are currently identified by the species of origin and a number (for example, bovine adenovirus, type 3). Adenoviruses are often associated with respiratory disease, but in many instances, the causal relationship of the virus to a specific disease has not been well-established. A notable exception is the cause of infectious canine hepatitis, the first adenovirus to be studied.

Diseases Due to Mastadenoviruses

Infectious Canine Hepatitis (Hepatitis Contagiosa Canis, Canine Adenovirus Infection)

Although certain lesions of infectious canine hepatitis have been recognized for many years, its clinical features, its etiology, and its actual existence as a separate disease were not established until the classic report of Rubarth appeared in 1947. The disease has since been recognized in many parts of the world and it is now possible to differentiate it from other diseases such as canine distemper. Rubarth pointed out that fox encephalitis virus, shown by Green to be infective for dogs, undoubtedly was identical to the virus of canine hepatitis. This has since been confirmed.

Signs. Canine hepatitis principally affects young dogs. The infection is common, but most often it goes unnoticed or is inapparent. When clinical disease is evident, its course is rather variable but frequently peracute, with the first signs manifested only a few hours before death. More regularly, however, the illness is apparent for several days before death or recovery occurs. The disease starts with apathy, followed by anorexia and, in many cases, intense thirst. Severe, disfiguring subcutaneous edema of the head, neck, and ventral aspects of the trunk is a striking but rare manifestation. Vomiting and diarrhea, the latter with hemorrhage, are rather common symptoms, and abdominal pain is often expressed by moaning sounds. With onset, the temperature is elevated, but it may fall abruptly to subnormal levels as death approaches.

Signs referable to the central nervous system are uncommon and, when seen, take the form of clonic spasms of the extremities and neck, paralysis of the hind quarters, or in a rare case, extreme agitation. The mucous membranes usually appear anemic, sometimes slightly icteric, but rarely deeply jaundiced. Petechiae may occur on the anemic membranes, particularly those of the gingiva. Generally the tonsils are reddened and swollen, with the result that tonsillitis is often the initial diagnosis. Copious lacrimation with hyperemic conjunctivae is rather common. In an occasional animal, diffuse, opaque cloudiness in the cornea of one eye is associated with a decrease in the visual acuity of that eye, its extent depending on the severity of the lesion. This corneal cloudiness disappears spontaneously if the animal recovers. In the urine, albumin may be present in significant amounts, but usually that is its only abnormality. Other clinicopathologic findings include neutropenia and lymphopenia during the course, with a lymphocytosis during re-

covery; prolonged bleeding and coagulation times; and elevation of SGOT and SGPT.

Lesions. The virus of canine hepatitis has an obligate affinity for parenchymal and Kupffer cells of the liver and endothelial cells generally. Its lethal effect on cells of these types produces most of the lesions, both gross and microscopic, that can be attributed to the disease. Specific intranuclear inclusions, necrosis of cells, and in the case of endothelial cells, proliferation and increased vascular permeability with hemorrhage, are the pathologic evidence of this virus's affinity for these specific tissues. The only exceptions are seen in bone marrow and spleen, where intranuclear inclusions may be observed in cells which, although difficult to identify, are probably reticuloendothelial. In experimentally infected animals, it is possible to produce intranuclear inclusions in other tissues. For example, in animals injected via the cisterna magna with fox encephalitis virus, intranuclear inclusions develop in ependymal cells; in foxes inoculated by the testicular route, in interstitial cells; in dogs inoculated intraperitoneally, in the lining cells of the peritoneum. The gross appearance of the lesions is not diagnostic, for petechiae in any location are the most common manifestation. The liver and spleen are usually congested and somewhat enlarged, and the gallbladder wall is edematous and thickened.

The liver is enlarged and usually contains an increased amount of blood, which can be detected both grossly and microscopically. In addition to congestion of the major vessels, particularly the veins, the sinusoids exhibit lacunose dilatation that results in compression of adjacent parenchymal cells. This vascular dilatation of the sinusoids may be found in any part of the lobule. Characteristic are small, scattered focal areas of necrosis of parenchymal cells in which the distinctive staining properties of the cells are lost and their nuclei have often disappeared. Occasion-

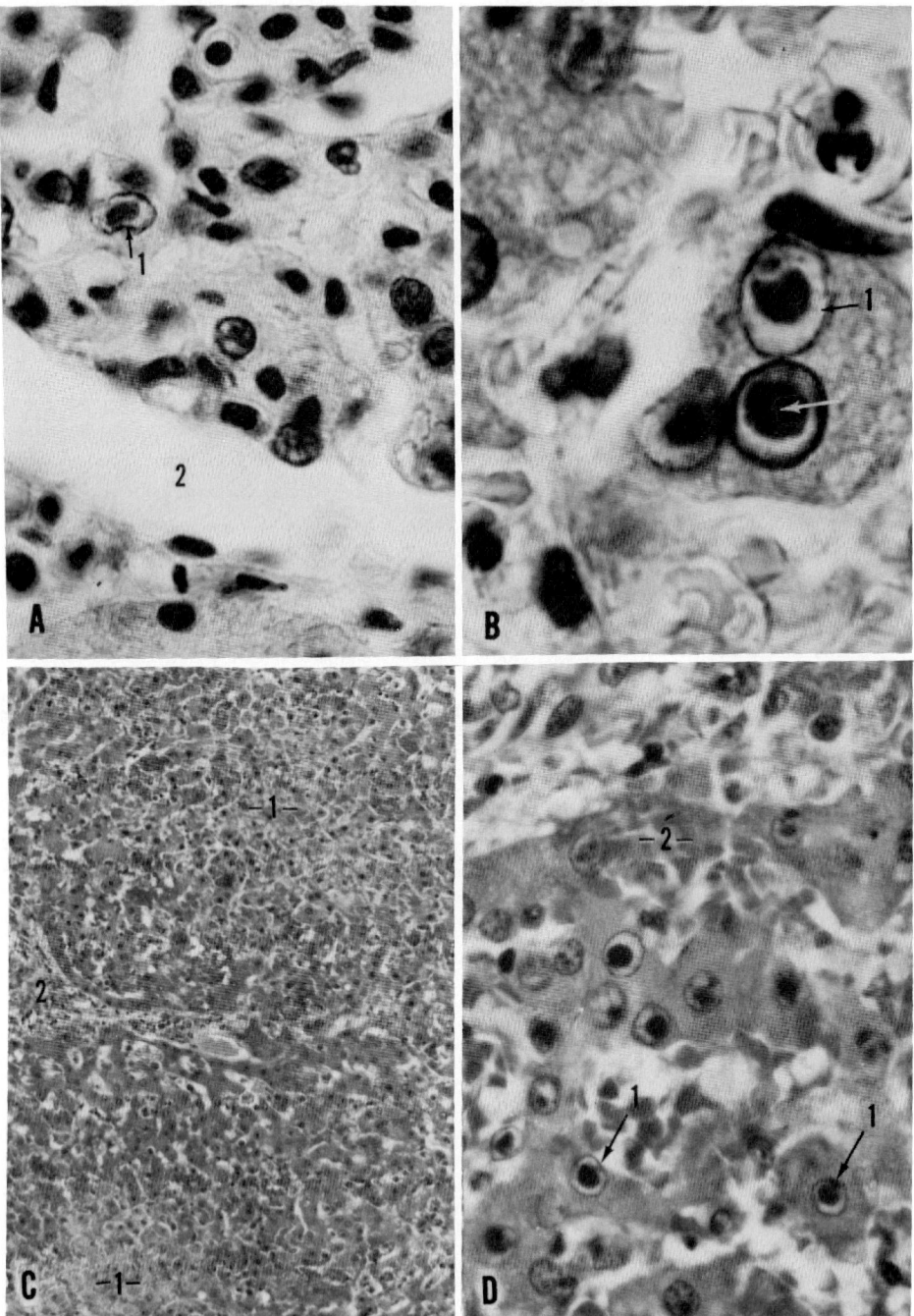

Fig. 9–24.   Infectious canine hepatitis. *A,* Intranuclear inclusion *(1)* in endothelial cell of glomerular tuft, Bowman's space *(2)* (× 1080). *B,* Intranuclear inclusion in hepatic cells (arrow) (× 1850). Note margination of nuclear chromatin *(1).* Contributor: Dr. N. Breslauer. *C,* Foci of necrosis *(1)* in liver (× 125). Portal area *(2). D,* Intranuclear inclusion *(1)* in liver cells (× 615). Note lacunose dilatation of sinusoids *(2).* (Courtesy of Armed Forces Institute of Pathology.) Contributor: Dr. W. J. Foster.

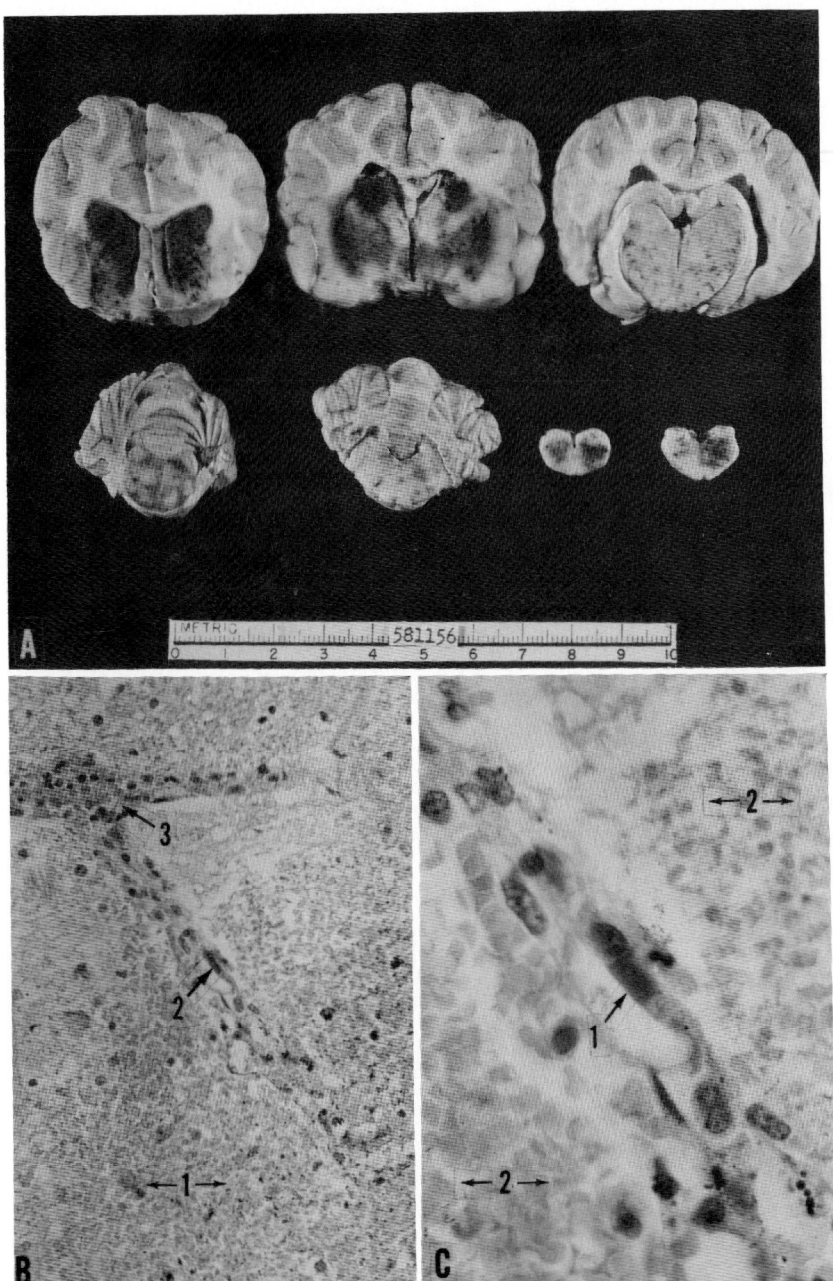

Fig. 9–25. Infectious canine hepatitis. Hemorrhages in the central nervous system. *A*, Bilaterally symmetrical hemorrhagic zones in the brain. *B*, One of the small hemorrhages (× 235) in the brain. Erythrocytes free in the brain parenchyma *(1)* originating in a ruptured capillary with an intranuclear inclusion *(2)* in an endothelial cell near the site of rupture. This vessel branches at *(3)*. *C*, Higher magnification of B (× 1100) with inclusion body *(1)* in the nucleus of an endothelial cell. There is adjacent hemorrhage *(2)*. (Courtesy of Armed Forces Institute of Pathology.) Contributor: Dr. D. L. Coffin.

ally, in the more advanced lesions, the outlines of the cells are no longer discernible. Intranuclear inclusion bodies are prominent, usually in partly degenerating cells adjacent to areas of necrosis. The nucleus is greatly enlarged, and its chromatin is displaced to its peripheral margin (margination of chromatin). The inclusion, which almost fills the nucleus, has a rather indistinct spherical outline and usually takes a somewhat basophilic tint in sections stained with hematoxylin and eosin. Except for a fine granularity, the inclusion body has little demonstrable internal structure. Similar inclusions may be found in the sinusoidal endothelial cells and the Kupffer cells. The enlargement and light yellowish brown color of the liver, seen grossly, may be caused by these lesions, but when congestion is paramount the liver is dark red. The capsule is often tense and the lobular design stands out distinctly.

In a high percentage of cases, the gallbladder wall is edematous, usually grayish, and thickened to as much as 5 mm. Sometimes hemorrhage and edema cause the gallbladder to appear reddish black. Fine precipitation of fibrinous exudate is frequently seen on the serosa of the gallbladder. The hepatic lymph nodes are often edematous and occasionally contain petechiae. Capillary rupture with intranuclear inclusions in endothelium can be demonstrated microscopically in liver and gallbladder.

The spleen is usually enlarged and contains an abnormal amount of blood. Infarcts are seldom seen. Intranuclear inclusions may be found without difficulty in cells presumed to be reticuloendothelial cells as well as in endothelial cells.

Lesions in the other visceral organs are inconstant and, when present, are related to changes in vascular endothelium. Petechiae surround small capillaries and intranuclear inclusions may be found in the endothelium of these vessels. Often near the site of hemorrhage, the number of endothelial cells on the inner surface of the vessels is increased. These changes can produce edema as well as hemorrhage, particularly in lymph nodes, mesentery, tonsils, and under serous surfaces.

In the kidney, intranuclear inclusions may be found microscopically in endothelial cells of the glomerular tufts. These inclusions are limited to one or two in each glomerulus and are rarely associated with any demonstrable lesion in nephrons. Occasionally intranuclear inclusions are present in epithelial cells of collecting tubules. Focal nonsuppurative interstitial nephritis has been described in dogs in the convalescent stages of experimental infectious canine hepatitis.

The lesions in the brain are directly related to the changes in capillary endothelium. The involved endothelial cells are increased in number, and some contain elongated intranuclear inclusions conforming to the shape of the enlarged nucleus, in which the chromatin is marginated. Many of the capillaries are surrounded by a small collar of hemorrhage. These hemorrhages may be particularly prominent in the thalamus, midbrain, pons, and medulla oblongata, with grossly demonstrable bilateral symmetry, or they may be diffusely distributed throughout the brain and, for the most part, microscopic. In a few instances, necrosis, loss of myelin, and occasional collections of glial cells are noted adjacent to affected vessels. These appear to be secondary to interference with circulation.

Carmichael (1964, 1965) has demonstrated that the ocular lesions that develop in dogs recovering from canine hepatitis are the result of an Arthus-type hypersensitivity reaction. Persistent virus within ocular tissues during the antibody response to the infection provides the proper prerequisites for an Arthus reaction. The principal lesion consists of iridocyclitis characterized by hyperemia, edema, and infiltration of plasma cells, neutrophils, and lymphocytes. The cornea is edematous

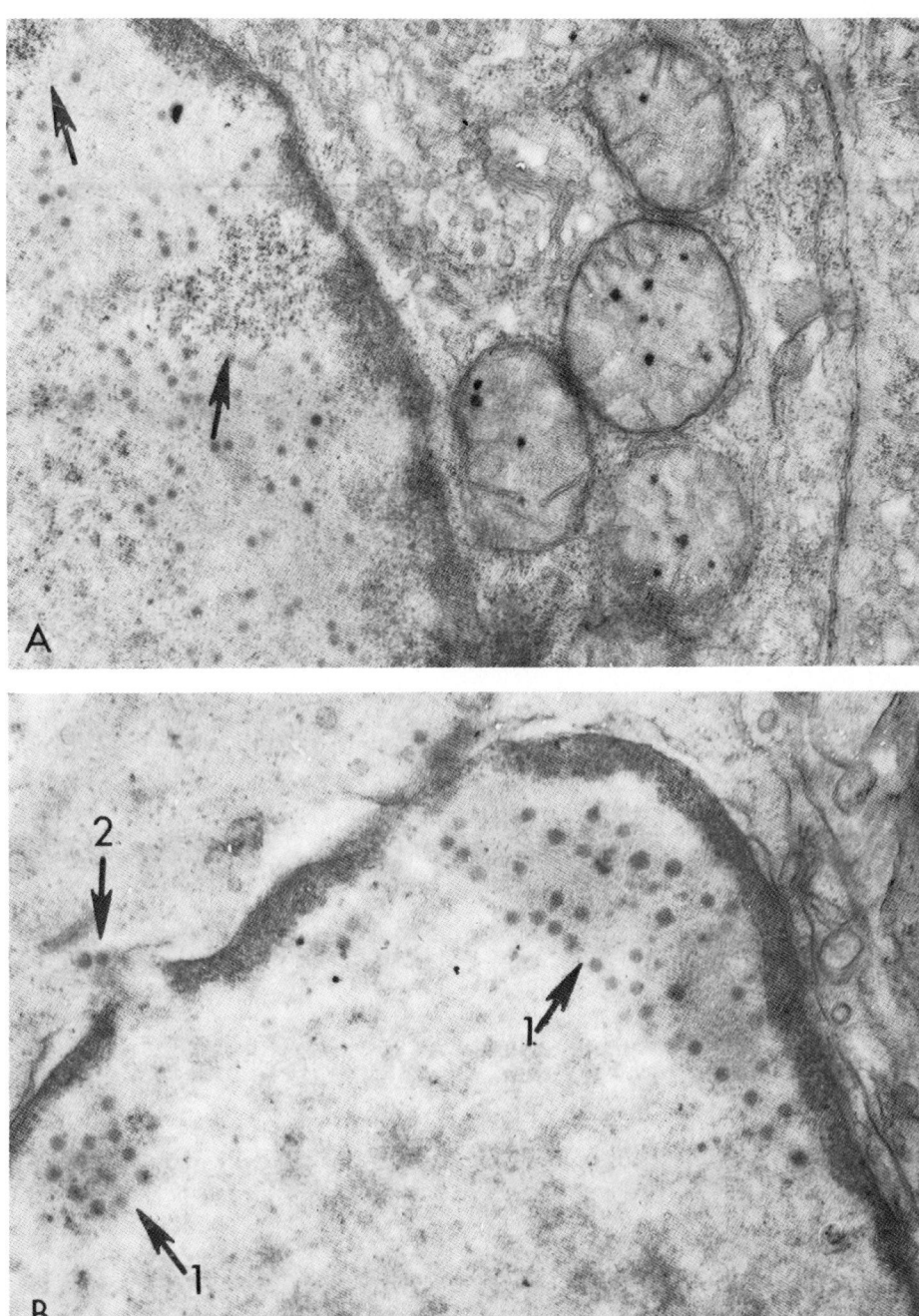

Fig. 9–26. Infectious canine hepatitis. *A,* Adenovirus particles (arrows) scattered throughout the nucleus of a hepatocyte (× 23,700). *B,* Virus particles in a hepatocyte nucleus associated with crystalline formations *(1).* Virus particles *(2)* are also escaping from the nucleus (× 30,000). (Courtesy of Dr. K. F. Givan and *Laboratory Investigation.*)

and infiltrated with neutrophils, lymphocytes, and macrophages. Inclusion bodies are not present, although during the acute stages of the disease (prior to the hypersensitivity reaction), they may be numerous in the ciliary body and iris.

Ultrastructural studies have demonstrated that the inclusion bodies of infectious canine hepatitis contain viral particles, but that the bulk of the inclusion body is composed of finely granular electron-dense material.

On the second and third days following experimental inoculation of the virus, virions are visible in electron micrographs of endothelial cells of renal glomeruli (Wright et al., 1973). Glomerular endothelial cells at this time are swollen, often occluding the capillary lumen; the cytoplasm contains vacuoles, and some cells are detached from the basement membrane. Some nuclei of these cells are pyknotic. Mesangial cells are often enlarged and contain small cytoplasmic vacuoles. Foot processes of epithelial cells are often fused; nuclei are often pyknotic, and the cytoplasm is swollen by intracellular edema, which disperses the mitochondria. Microvilli are partially lost, and the lumen of the tubule is often obliterated by the swollen cytoplasm or desquamated cellular debris.

Edema is evident around capillaries in the renal interstitium, and virions are present in nuclei of the endothelial cells.

Diagnosis. The diagnosis in the living animal is difficult because of the nonspecific nature of the symptoms. Microscopic demonstration of focal necrosis and intranuclear inclusions in surgically ablated tonsils or liver biopsy specimens is sufficient to confirm a presumptive clinical diagnosis. At necropsy, the diagnosis is not a problem. It is established by the demonstration of typical lesions associated with characteristic intranuclear inclusions. Fluorescent antibody techniques and viral isolation in tissue culture can be employed if necessary. This disease may occur in association with others, such as canine distemper or leptospirosis; hence, it may present a difficult but not insoluble diagnostic problem.

Appel, M., et al.: Pathogenicity of low-virulence strains of two canine adenovirus types. Am. J. Vet. Res., 34:543–551, 1973.

Appel, M., Carmichael, L. E., and Robson, D. S.: Canine adenovirus type 2—induced immunity to two canine adenoviruses in pups with maternal antibody. Am. J. Vet. Res., 36:1199–1202, 1975.

Carmichael, L. E.: The pathogenesis of ocular lesions of infectious canine hepatitis. Pathol. Vet., 1:73–95, 1964.

————: The pathogenesis of ocular lesions of infectious canine hepatitis. II. Experimental ocular hypersensitivity produced by the virus. Pathol. Vet., 2:344–359, 1965.

Coffin, D. L.: The pathology of so-called acute tonsilitis of dogs in relation to contagious canine hepatitis (Rubarth). J. Am. Vet. Med. Assoc., 112:355–362, 1948.

Coffin, D. L., and Cabasso, V. J.: The blood and urine findings in infectious canine hepatitis. Am. J. Vet. Res., 14:254–259, 1953.

Coffin, D. L., Coons, A. H., and Cabasso, V. J.: A histological study of infectious canine hepatitis by means of fluorescent antibody. J. Exp. Med., 98:13–20, 1953.

Correa, W. M.: Notas Preliminares sobré Hepatita a Virus dos Marrecos no Brasil. Rev. Fac. Med. Vet., Sao Paulo, 6:43–52, 1957.

Fenner, F., et al.: The Biology of Animal Viruses. 2nd ed. New York, Academic Press, 1974.

Fujimoto, Y.: Studies on infectious canine hepatitis. I. Histopathological studies on spontaneous cases. Jpn. J. Vet. Res., 5:51–70, 1957.

Garg, S. P., Moulton, J. E., and Sekhri, K. K.: Histochemical and electron microscopic studies of dog kidney cells in the early stages of infection with infectious canine heptitis virus. Am. J. Vet. Res., 28:725–730, 1967.

Givan, K. F., and Jezequel, A.-M.: Infectious canine hepatitis: a virologic and ultrastructural study. Lab. Invest., 20:36–45, 1969.

Green, R. G., and Dewey, E. T.: Fox encephalitis and canine distemper. Proc. Soc. Exp. Biol. Med., 27:129–130, 1929.

Green, R. G., Katter, M. S., Shillinger, J. E., and Hanson, K. B.: Epizoötic fox encephalitis. IV. The intranuclear inclusions. Am. J. Hyg., 18:462–481, 1933.

Green, R. G., and Shillinger, J. E.: Epizoötic fox encephalitis. VI. A description of the experimental infection in dogs. Am. J. Hyg., 19:362–391, 1934.

Hunt, R. D., et al.: A histochemical comparison of the inclusion bodies of canine distemper and infectious canine hepatitis. Am. J. Vet. Res., 24:1248–1255, 1963. VB 1343–64.

Innes, J. R. M.: Hepatitis contagiosa canis (Rubarth) in Great Britain. Vet. Rec., 61:173–175, 1949.

Kinjo, T., Yanagawa, R., and Fujimoto, Y.: Oncogenicity of infectious canine hepatitis virus in hamsters. Jpn. J. Vet. Res., 16:145–158, 1968.

Larin, N. M.: Epidemiological studies of canine virus hepatitis (Rubarth's Disease). Vet. Res., 70:295–297, 1958.

Lindblad, G., Branemark, P. I., and Lundstrom, J.: Capillary form and function in dogs with experimental *hepatitis contagiosa canis*: an intravital microvascular study. Acta Vet. Scand., 5:384–393, 1964.

Lindblad, G., and Bjorkman, N.: Ultra-structural alterations in sinusoidal endothelium of liver and bone marrow in dogs with experimental *hepatitis contagiosa canis*. Acta Pathol. Microbiol. Scand., 62:155–163, 1964.

Moulton, J. E., and Zee, Y. C.: Release of infectious canine hepatitis virus. Am. J. Vet. Res., 30:2051–2065, 1969.

Poppensiek, G. C., and Baker, J. A.: Persistence of virus in urine as factor in spread of infectious hepatitis in dogs. Proc. Soc. Exp. Biol. Med., 77:279–281, 1951.

Rubarth, S.: An acute virus disease with liver lesions in dogs (hepatitis contagiosa canis). A pathologico-anatomical and etiological investigation. Acta Path. Microbiol. Scand. (Suppl.), 69, 1947.

Sarma, P. S., et al.: Induction of tumors in hamsters with infectious canine hepatitis virus. Nature, 215:293–294, 1967.

Saunders, L. Z., Jubb, K. V., and Jones, L. D.: The intraocular lesions of hog cholera. J. Comp. Pathol., 68:375–379, 1958.

Seibold, H. R., and Green, J. E.: Virus-type inclusions in the epithelium of the canine renal medulla. J. Am. Vet. Med. Assoc., 125:385–386, 1954.

Wright, N. G.: Experimental infectious canine hepatitis. IV. Histological and immunofluorescence studies of the kidney. J. Comp. Pathol., 77:153–158, 1967.

Wright, N. G., et al.: Canine adenovirus respiratory disease: isolation of infectious canine hepatitis virus from natural cases and the experimental production of the disease. Vet. Rec., 90:411–416, 1972.

Wright, N. G., Thompson, H., Cornwell, H. J. C., and Morrison, W. I.: Ultrastructure of the kidney and urinary excretion of renal antigens in experimental canine adenovirus infection. Res. Vet. Sci., 14:376–380, 1973.

Bovine Adenoviral Infections

Bovine adenoviruses of several serotypes have been isolated from cattle in several parts of the U.S., Europe, Great Britain, Australia, and Japan. Some of them (Types 3 and 5) appear to be more pathogenic than others to young calves, producing disease concentrated in the respiratory and gastrointestinal tracts of these animals. The bovine adenoviruses have the biochemical and morphologic features of all of the Adenoviridae, but may be distinguished by the difference in serum-neutralizing antibodies induced by each type. Surveys of the presence of antibodies in the serum of cattle indicate that infection is widespread, and each infection may not result in overt disease.

Signs. The clinical signs are varied, as indicated by some of the descriptive colloquial names given to cases of this infection: pneumoenteritis of calves, respiratory tract disease, conjunctivitis, keratoconjunctivitis, febrile disease associated with rhinorrhea and diarrhea, and weak-calf syndrome. The disease is most often manifest in calves one to four weeks of age. Any beef or dairy breed may be affected. Signs of upper respiratory involvement, such as catarrhal rhinitis, sneezing, coughing, conjunctivitis, and lacrimal discharge associated with fever are often manifest. Tympanitis, colic, and diarrhea are frequent in most outbreaks. In the weak calf syndrome, edema and hemorrhage around joints result in lameness. Morbidity is usually low early in the course of an outbreak, but as many as 80% of all calves in a large herd may eventually exhibit signs of the disease. The mortality rate may be low.

Lesions. The lesions may be generalized or limited to the respiratory or gastrointestinal tracts. The characteristic gross lesions in the respiratory tract start in nasal passages as mucinous exudate, which eventually becomes mucopurulent. Diffuse congestion and hemorrhage in the lungs lead to consolidation of entire lobules in parts of the lung. Hemorrhage and edema are evident in the lymph nodes related to the respiratory tract, and petechiae and edema may be seen in the kidneys, adrenal cortex, myocardium, and wall of the intestine. Petechiae and edema are especially conspicuous around major joints in some outbreaks in which lameness is a frequent sign.

The microscopic lesions at the level of the light microscope characteristically involve endothelial cells, particularly of capillaries and small vessels, in which necrosis, edema, and hemorrhage are accompanied by characteristic intranuclear inclusions in endothelial cells. The inclusions vary in size, are usually basophilic in hematoxylin and eosin stains, and are surrounded by a clear zone that separates them from the nuclear membrane to which the chromatin is attracted ("marginated").

In experimental cases following intranasal and intratracheal instillation of virus, viral inclusions appear in respiratory epithelium and endothelial cells, particularly in bronchioles and alveolar septa. The bronchiolar epithelium may become multilayered and the lumen filled with cellular debris. Thickening of interalveolar septa is a common feature. Pulmonary lobules that are not consolidated may become atelectatic.

Ultrastructure examination of infected cells reveal most of the virions to be within the nucleus, a few in the cytoplasm. The virions appear round or hexagonal with an electron-dense core about 55 nm in diameter, surrounded by a dense capsid, giving an overall diameter of about 75 to 80 nm. Linear arrays of virions are common, and parallel membranes among them may give a crystalline appearance. The internal capsomeres and projecting fibers may be demonstrable at high magnification.

Bulmer, W. W., Tsai, K. S., and Little, P. B.: Adenovirus infection in two calves. J. Am. Vet. Med. Assoc., 166:233–238, 1975.

Cutlip, R. C., and McClurkin, A. W.: Lesions and pathogenesis of disease in young calves experimentally induced by a bovine adenovirus type 5 isolated from a calf with weak calf syndrome. Am. J. Vet. Res., 36:1095–1098, 1975.

Darbyshire, J. H., et al.: The pathogenesis and pathology of infection in calves with a strain of bovine adenovirus type 3. Res. Vet. Sci., 7:81–93, 1966.

Darbyshire, J. H.: Bovine adenoviruses. J. Am. Vet. Med. Assoc., 152:786–792, 1968.

———: Bovine adenoviruses. Prog. Exp. Tumor Res., 18:56–66, 1973.

Lehmkuhl, H. D., Smith, M. H., and Dierks, R. E.: A bovine adenovirus type 3: isolation, characterization, and experimental infection in calves. Arch. Virol., 48:39–46, 1975.

Mattson, D. E.: Adenovirus infection in cattle. J. Am. Vet. Med. Assoc., 163:894–896, 1973.

Mattson, D. E.: Naturally occurring infection of calves with a bovine adenovirus. Am. J. Vet. Res., 34:623–630, 1973.

Mohanty, S. B.: Comparative study of bovine adenoviruses. Am. J. Vet. Res., 32:1899–1905, 1971.

Phillip, J. I. H., and Sands, J. J.: The isolation of bovine adenovirus serotypes 4 and 7 in Britain. Res. Vet. Sci., 13:386–387, 1972.

Human Adenoviral Infections

The first human adenovirus was isolated from cultures of adenoidal tissue from infants (Rowe et al., 1953) and from military recruits with an acute respiratory illness (Hilleman and Werner, 1954). A large number of such adenoviruses have subsequently been isolated from human sources. It is evident that some of these viruses are responsible for respiratory disease, particularly in young people. Of even greater interest is the fact that many of these viruses produced undifferentiated neoplasms in newborn hamsters, starting at the site of inoculation (Merkow and Slifkin, 1973). Some types of adenovirus are oncogenic in the central nervous system of newborn Sprague-Dawley rats. Intracerebral inoculation of human adenovirus type 12 results in numerous medulloepitheliomatous tumors along the ventricular system in the brain and spinal cord of these rats.

Some adenoviruses have been associated with the occurrence of ileocecal intussusception in young children (Yunis et al., 1975).

Hilleman, M. R., and Werner, J. H.: Recovery of a new agent from patients with acute respiratory illness. Proc. Soc. Exp. Biol. Med., 85:183–188, 1954.

Merkow, L. P., and Slifkin, M. (eds.): Oncogenic adenoviruses. Prog. Exp. Tumor Res., 18:1–293, 1973.

Mukai, N., and Kobayashi, S.: Human adenovirus-induced medulloepitheliomatous neoplasms in Sprague-Dawley rats. Am. J. Pathol., 73:671–690, 1973.

Norrby, E.: Adenoviruses. In Comparative Virology, edited by K. Maramorosch and E. Kurstak. New York, Academic Press, 1971.

Rowe, W. P., et al.: Isolation of a cytopathogenic agent from human adenoids undergoing spontaneous degeneration in tissue culture. Proc. Soc. Exp. Biol. Med., *84*:570–573, 1953.

Yunis, E. J., Atchison, R. W., Michaels, R. H., and Decicco, F. A.: Adenovirus and ileocecal intussusception. Lab. Invest., *33*:347–351, 1975.

Murine Adenoviral Infections

A latent virus isolated by Hartley and Rowe (1960) from leukemic mice was shown to be a part of the Adenoviridae family. This agent is oncogenic in newborn hamsters, and under some conditions, it has a predilection for specific organs. Experimental infections may produce lesions concentrated in the central nervous system (Heck et al., 1972), or may result in severe necrotizing lesions in the adrenal cortex. This latter tissue affinity has evoked the idea that adenovirus infection might be an antecedent to adrenal cortical atrophy (Margolis et al., 1974; Hoenig et al., 1974).

Hartley, J. W., and Rowe, W. P.: A new mouse virus apparently related to the adenovirus group. Virology, *11*:645–647, 1960.

Heck, F. C., Jr., Sheldon, W. G., and Gleiser, C. A.: Pathogenesis of experimentally produced mouse adenovirus infection in mice. Am. J. Vet. Res., *33*:841–846, 1972.

Hoenig, E. M., Margolis, G., and Kilham, L.: Experimental adenovirus infection of the mouse adrenal gland II. Electron microscopic observations. Am. J. Pathol., *75*:375–394, 1974.

Margolis, G. Kilham, L., and Hoenig, E. M.: Experimental adenovirus infection of the mouse adrenal gland I. Light microscopic observations. Am. J. Pathol., *75*:363–374, 1974.

Equine Adenoviral Infection

Adenoviruses with specific serotype have been recovered from young foals with respiratory disease. Each of seven viral isolates from widely-dispersed outbreaks appear to be the same equine adenovirus (England et al., 1973). Certain Arabian foals are especially vulnerable due to an inherited immunodeficiency (McGuire and Poppie, 1973). The usual signs include sudden onset of fever with mucous to mucopurulent nasal discharge, cough, dyspnea, tachycardia, and increased respiratory rate, abnormal lung sounds, and in some instances, death.

Lesions. The lesions are usually confined to the respiratory tract, with mucopurulent rhinitis, tracheitis, and coniform, prune-colored consolidation of dependent portions of the lungs. Bronchiolar thickening results from proliferation of the lining epithelial cells and accumulation of leukocytes around the bronchiole. Necrosis of cells results in cellular debris partially or completely filling the lumen. Basophilic intranuclear inclusions are located in epithelial cells along the entire respiratory tract. These inclusions may also be found in association with focal necrosis in epithelial cells lining the renal pelvis, ureter, urinary bladder, and urethra; epithelial cells also affected include those of the conjunctiva, lacrimal glands, salivary glands, and the pancreas. Occasionally focal lesions may be found in the gastrointestinal tract.

Pulmonary consolidation is concentrated around affected bronchioles, with atelectasis, desquamation of alveolar lining cells, and thickening of the alveolar septa. Lymph nodes and splenic corpuscles are small, as is the thymus—features probably related to the inherited immunodeficiency.

The microscopic lesions are presumptively diagnostic, particularly if the typical virions may be demonstrated with the electron microscope. Isolation of the specific adenovirus is confirmatory in the presence of expected lesions.

Ardans, A. A., Pritchett, R. F., and Zee, Y. C.: Histologic, immunofluorescent, and electron microscopic studies of equine dermis cells infected with an equine adenovirus. Am. J. Vet. Res., *35*:431–436, 1974.

England, J. J., McChesney, A. E., and Chow, T. L.: Characterization of an equine adenovirus. Am. J. Vet. Res., *34*:1587–1590, 1973.

Johnston, K. G., and Hutchins, D. R.: Suspected adenovirus bronchitis in Arab foals. Aust. Vet. J., *43*:600–602, 1967.

McChesney, A. E., et al.: Adenoviral infection in suckling Arabian foals. Path. Vet., *7*:547–565, 1970.

McChesney, A. E., England, J. J., and Rich, L. J.: Adenoviral infection in foals. J. Am. Vet. Med. Assoc., *162*:545–549, 1973.

McChesney, A. E., et al.: Experimental transmission of equine adenovirus in Arabian and non-

Arabian foals. Am. J. Vet. Res., *35*:1015–1024, 1974.

McChesney, A. E., and England, J. J.: Adenoviral infection in foals. J. Am. Vet. Med. Assoc., *166*:83–85, 1975.

McGuire, T. C., and Poppie, M. J.: Hypogammaglobulinemia and thymic hypoplasia in horses: a primary combined immuno-deficiency disorder. Infect. Immun., *8*:272–277, 1973.

Studdert, M. J., Wilks, C. R., and Coggins, L.: Antigenic comparisons and serologic survey of equine adenoviruses. Am. J. Vet. Res., *35*:693–699, 1974.

Todd, J. D.: Comments on rhinoviruses and parainfluenza viruses of horses. J. Am. Vet. Med. Assoc., *155*:387–390, 1969.

Whitlock, R. H., Dellers, R. W., and Shively, J. N.: Adenoviral pneumonia in a foal. Cornell Vet., *65*:393–401, 1975.

Adenoviral Infections in Other Species

Swine. Most porcine adenoviruses are of low pathogenicity and can be isolated with some regularity from feces. Porcine adenovirus type 4, originally isolated from the brain of a ten-week-old pig with encephalitis, was subsequently shown to produce meningoencephalitis in gnotobiotic piglets following nasal or oral inoculation. At least four serotypes from swine are known at present.

Sheep. Adenoviruses have been identified in sheep in Scotland and Australia from animals suffering from respiratory disease. In one outbreak, lambs four to ten weeks of age were particularly affected; many were ill and several died. At least four serotypes have been identified as adenoviruses using gel diffusion tests to demonstrate the common antigen, and serum neutralization tests to differentiate the serotypes (McFerran et al., 1969; Sharp et al., 1974).

Monkeys. A large number of adenoviruses have been isolated from several monkey species, usually from tissue cultures of kidney or gastrointestinal cells. Many of these isolates have been shown to be oncogenic when inoculated into newborn hamsters, producing undifferentiated tumors in others, depending on the site of injection of the virus. At least one virus has been shown to be pathogenic in its natural host, illustrated by pancreatitis associated with infection in a Rhesus monkey (*Macaca mulatta*) (Chandler et al., 1974).

Chandler, F. W., Callaway, C. S., and Adams, S. R.: Pancreatitis associated with an adenovirus in a Rhesus monkey. Vet. Pathol., *11*:165–171, 1974.

Derbyshire, J. B., Clarke, M. C., and Collins, A. P.: Serological and pathogenicity studies with some unclassified porcine adenoviruses. J. Comp. Pathol., *85*:437–443, 1975.

Edington, N., Kasza, L., and Christofinis, G. L.: Meningoencephalitis in gnotobiotic pigs inoculated intranasally and orally with porcine adenovirus 4. Res. Vet. Sci., *13*:289–291, 1972.

Kasza, L.: Isolation of an adenovirus from the brain of a pig. Am. J. Vet. Res., *27*:751–758, 1966.

McFerran, J. B., Nelson, R., McCracken, J. M., and Ross, J. G.: Viruses isolated from sheep. Nature, *221*:194–195, 1969.

Merkow, L. P., and Slifkin, M.: Simian adenoviruses. Prog. Exp. Tumor Res., *18*:67–87, 1973.

Shadduck, J. A., Kasza, L., and Koestner, A.: Pathogenic properties of a porcine adenovirus. Lab. Invest., *16*:635, 1967.

Sharp, J. M., McFerran, J. B., and Rae, A.: A new adenovirus from sheep. Res. Vet. Sci., *17*:268–269, 1974.

IRIDOVIRIDAE

Viruses classified in the family Iridoviridae are grouped together on the basis of several common characteristics. Assembly of virions occurs in the cytoplasm of infected cells; a similar feature occurs in Poxviridae but not in other DNA viruses. The virus has complex structure with an outer icosahedral capsid, 190 nm in diameter, with about 1500 capsomeres. Most have no true envelope, except some invertebrate iridoviruses. The nucleic acid consists of a single linear molecule of double-stranded DNA, of 130 to 140 million daltons (Fenner et al., 1974).

Many of the viruses classified in this family reproduce in insects: *Tipula* iridescent virus, *Sericesthis* iridescent virus, *Chilo* iridescent virus, and *Aedes* iridescent virus. Vertebrate viruses include: Gecko virus, lymphocystic virus of fish, frog virus 3, and African swine fever virus (Hess, 1971).

African Swine Fever (Wart Hog Disease)

African swine fever was first recognized in domestic swine *(Sus scrofula)* taken to Africa by European settlers, who soon associated the disease with contact between domestic swine and wild wart hogs *(Phacochoerus africanus)*. For many years only an acute clinical form of the disease was known in domestic swine until about 1947, when imported swine, allowed free range in probable contact with wart hogs, developed a chronic form of the disease. This form of the disease made recognition more difficult and increased the chance of a carrier state in domesticated swine. The disease spread, in 1957, to Lisbon, Portugal, presumably from Angola by means of processed pork products, and by 1960 had spread to Spain. In 1971, a serious outbreak started in Cuba. Thus it is evident that African swine fever is no longer limited to Africa, and that expanded air travel from Africa may facilitate spread of the virus to other parts of the world.

Clinical Manifestations. A high fever characteristically precedes the appearance of other symptoms by several days. During this febrile period, affected swine may appear well and have a hearty appetite, then in their final 48 hours, they become depressed, weak, apathetic, cyanotic, develop cough and dyspnea, then die. With some strains of virus, vomiting and diarrhea may be observed.

As indicated, a more protracted course of the disease is now recognized, with recovery of some domesticated swine which may act as carriers of the virus. The wart hog has been proved to be a carrier, but no disease due to this virus has been recognized in this species.

Lesions. Changes grossly evident in African swine fever are similar in many respects to those of hog cholera, but are generally more severe. Lymph nodes, especially adrenal, hepatic, and gastric nodes, are usually diffusely hemorrhagic. Intralobular pulmonary edema is seen in about 40% of the swine that succumb; petechiae and ecchymoses are found in the pleura, pericardium, and peritoneum in most cases. Edema and congestion are frequent in the gallbladder and in the adjacent liver. Extensive perirenal, diffuse subcapsular, and pelvic hemorrhages are encountered in a few cases. Hemorrhages into the renal cortex, if found at all, are numerous. The spleen is engorged and swollen in about 10% of cases, while gastric ulceration is severe in about 20%. Catarrhal enteritis is commonly manifest. The stomachs of about 80% of the dead swine are full of feed, indicating the fulminant nature of the disease. Pneumonia is a rare complication.

The microscopic lesions in African swine fever have been studied critically and have been compared to those of hog cholera. The vascular lesions in African swine fever are similar to these of hog cholera, but result in more severe circulatory disturbances (edema, hemorrhages, infarction). Severe karyolysis of lymphocytes occurs in African swine fever in contrast to hog cholera, in which lymphopenia occurs, but no severe destruction of lymphocytes is found in sections. A particularly striking lesion in the African disease is found in the ellipsoids of the spleen, which become acellular and thus are clearly demonstrated in tissue sections (Fig. 9–27).

The lesions in natural cases of the chronic form of the disease have been described as consisting of pneumonia, fibrinous pericarditis, arthritis, and generalized enlargement of lymph nodes with hypoplasia of lymphocytic cells. Hypogammaglobulinemia accompanies these lesions. Pigs experimentally infected with virus of low virulence also exhibit pneumonia with some interstitial components, such as infiltration by lymphoid cells and thickening of alveolar walls, focal areas of consolidation with desquamation of alveolar lining cells, and localized zones of necrosis with organization around them. These lesions are equally evident in

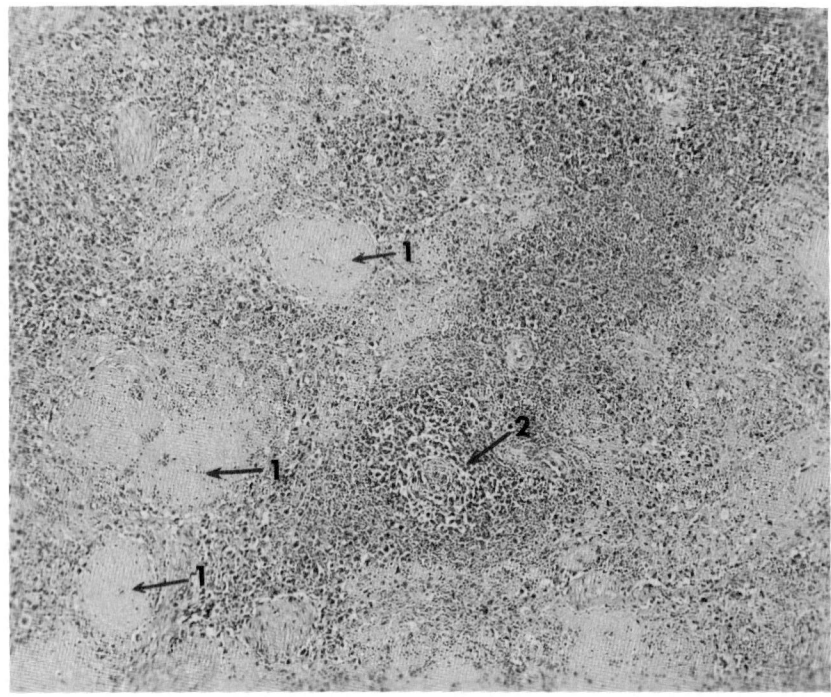

Fig. 9–27. Spleen of a pig with African swine fever. The splenic ellipsoids are enlarged and effaced by hyalin material (1). Lymphocytes (2) are for the most part necrotic or absent. (Courtesy of Colonel Fred D. Maurer and Armed Forces Institute of Pathology.)

animals which received several challenges of virus, including some given intratracheally. Aside from focal proliferation of lymphocytes and plasma cells in many parenchymatous organs, lesions in other systems also appear essentially nonspecific.

Diagnosis. The lesions and epizootiologic circumstances are helpful in acute cases of African swine fever. The prolonged cases and latent infections require the isolation and identification of the virus in appropriate tissue culture. Fluorescein-conjugated immune globulins have been used to identify viral antigens in tissues of affected swine with some degree of success.

Coggins, L.: African swine fever virus. Pathogenesis. Prog. Med. Virol., 18:48–63, 1974.

De Kock, G., Robbinson, E. M., and Keppel, J. J. G.: Swine fever in South Africa. Onderstepoort J. Vet. Sci. Anim. Ind., 14:31–93, 1940.

Detray, D. E.: African swine fever. Adv. Vet. Sci., 8:299–333, 1963.

Fenner, F., et al.: The Biology of Animal Viruses, 2nd edition. New York, Academic Press, 1974.

Greig, A.: Pathogenesis of African swine fever in pigs naturally exposed to the disease. J. Comp. Pathol., 82:73–79, 1972.

Hess, W. R.: African swine fever virus. Virol. Monogr., 9:1–33, 1971.

Heuschele, W. P., and Hess, W. R.: Diagnosis of African swine fever by immunofluorescence. Trop. Anim. Hlth. Prod., 5:181–186, 1973.

Konno, S., Taylor, W. D., and Dardiri, A. H.: Acute African swine fever. Proliferative phase in lymphoreticular tissue and the reticuloendothelial system. Cornell Vet., 61:71–84, 1971.

Konno, S., Taylor, W. D., Hess, W. R., and Heuschele, W. P.: Liver pathology in African swine fever. Cornell Vet., 61:125–150, 1971.

Malmquist, W. A., and Hay, D.: Hemadsorption and cytopathic effect produced by African swine fever virus in swine bone marrow and buffy coat cultures. Am. J. Vet. Res., 21:104–108, 1960.

Maurer, F. D., Griesemer, R. A., and Jones, T. C.: The pathology of African swine fever—a comparison with hog cholera. Am. J. Vet. Res., 19:517–539, 1958.

Montgomery, R. E.: On a form of swine fever occurring in British East Africa (Kenya Colony). J. Comp. Pathol. Therap., 34:159–191, 243–262, 1921.

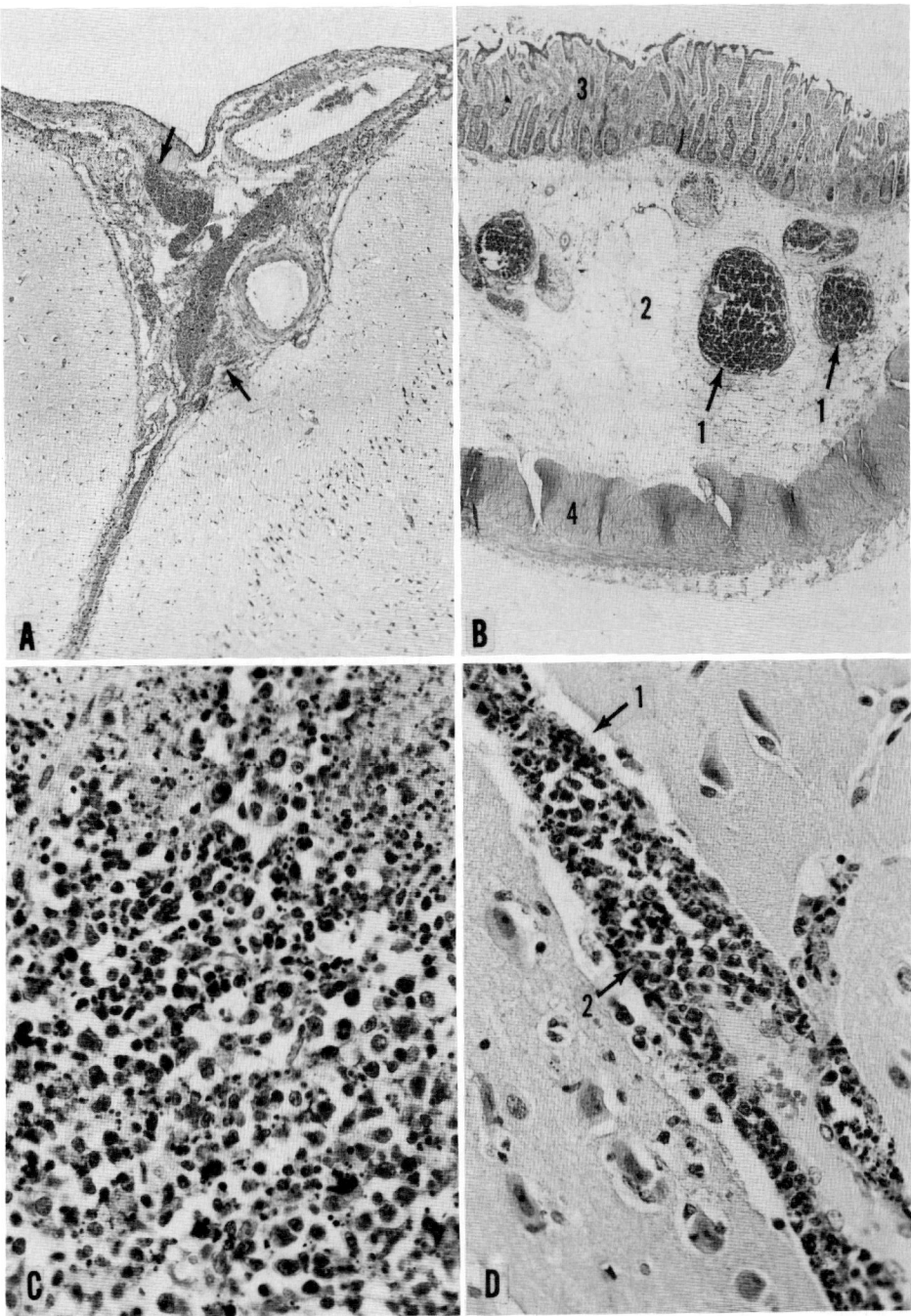

Fig. 9–28. African swine fever. *A,* Hemorrhages (arrows) in the pia mater (× 50). *B,* Congested submucosal veins *(1)*, edema in submucosa *(2)*, hemorrhage in mucosa *(3)* of the colon (× 26). The muscularis is indicated at *(4)*. *C,* Severe karyorrhexis involving lymphoid cells in a lymph node (× 395). *D,* A vein in the cerebral cortex (× 305). The Virchow-Robin space *(1)* is empty, but the wall of the vein *(2)* is infiltrated by lymphoid cells. (Courtesy of Lt. Col. F. D. Maurer.)

Moulton, J., and Coggins, L.: Comparison of lesions in acute and chronic African swine fever. Cornell Vet., 58:364–388, 1968.

Moulton, J. E., et al.: Pathologic features of chronic pneumonia in pigs with experimentally induced African swine fever. Am. J. Vet. Res., 36:27–32, 1975.

Pan, I. C., DeBoer, C. J., Hess, W. R., and Breese, S. S., Jr.: Purification of African swine fever virus. Fed. Proc., 30:354, 1971.

Pan, I. C., Trautman, R., DeBoer, C. J., and Hess, W. R.: African swine fever: hypergamma-globulinemia and the iodine agglutination test. Am. J. Vet. Res., 35:629–632, 1974.

Pan, I. C., Moulton, J. E., and Hess, W. R.: Immuno-fluorescent studies on chronic pneumonia in swine with experimentally induced African swine fever. Am. J. Vet. Res., 36:379–386, 1975.

PAPOVAVIRIDAE

It has long been recognized that the benign papillary lesions that originate on skin and mucosal surfaces are caused by viral infection and have morphologic and biologic features in common. In more recent years, it has also been shown that the viral agents from these lesions have many common morphologic and biochemical features. This has led to grouping these agents in the family Papovaviridae (a synthetic word; *pa* = papilloma, *po* = polyoma, *va* = vacuolating agent). This family is currently divided into two genera of viruses that differ in size but share many common structural and chemical properties: *Polyomavirus* and *Papillomavirus*.

Papovaviridae virions have icosahedral symmetry with 72 capsomeres and 420 structural subunits. Members of the genus *Polyomavirus* have virions with diameter of 45 nm and the molecular weight of their DNA is 3 million daltons. *Papillomavirus* virions are 55 nm in diameter and the molecular weight of the DNA is 5 million daltons. The base combinations of guanine + cytosine (G+C) also differ somewhat between these two genera. The virions are assembled in the nucleus and have no envelope.

The genus *Polyomavirus* (poly = many; oma = tumor) is made up of several viruses of considerable scientific interest because of their oncogenic and transforming effects

on cells in mammalian systems. Their pathogenicity in nature appears negligible. The specific viruses in this genus include SE polyoma virus of mice, K virus of rats, simian virus 40 (SV 40), rabbit vacuolating virus (plus others), and the viruses of multifocal leukoencephalopathy of man. The reader is referred to the list of references for additional information on these viruses.

The genus *Papillomavirus* contains the viral agents responsible for benign papillomatosis (warts, verrucae vulgaris) in man and other animals. The viruses in general appear to be specific for a single species. Some actually have narrow tissue specificities; for example, oral papillomatosis in rabbits and dogs is produced by viruses that differ from those which infect cutaneous surfaces. Most animal species which have been adequately studied are afflicted by their own variety of papillomatosis. The list of known susceptible species is added to from time to time.

Papillomatosis in Animals Due to Papillomavirus (Common Warts, Verrucae Vulgaris)

The common wart that adorns the finger of the small boy has its counterpart in nearly every animal species. In some animals, these warts are precise lesions that fastidiously refuse to grow anywhere but in a selected type of epithelium—in the mouth, for example. In others, massively huge and roughly keratinized warts indiscriminately involve large areas of the skin. Most warts are known from observation to be infectious by contact, and many have been shown by experiment to be transmissible with bacteria-free suspensions of macerated wart tissue. In cutaneous papillomas of the rabbit and goat, transformation of simple hyperplastic squamous epithelium to frankly malignant squamous cell carcinoma has been demonstrated. Thus it appears that papillomatoses represent infectious disease caused by viruses and characterized by benign hyperplasia of

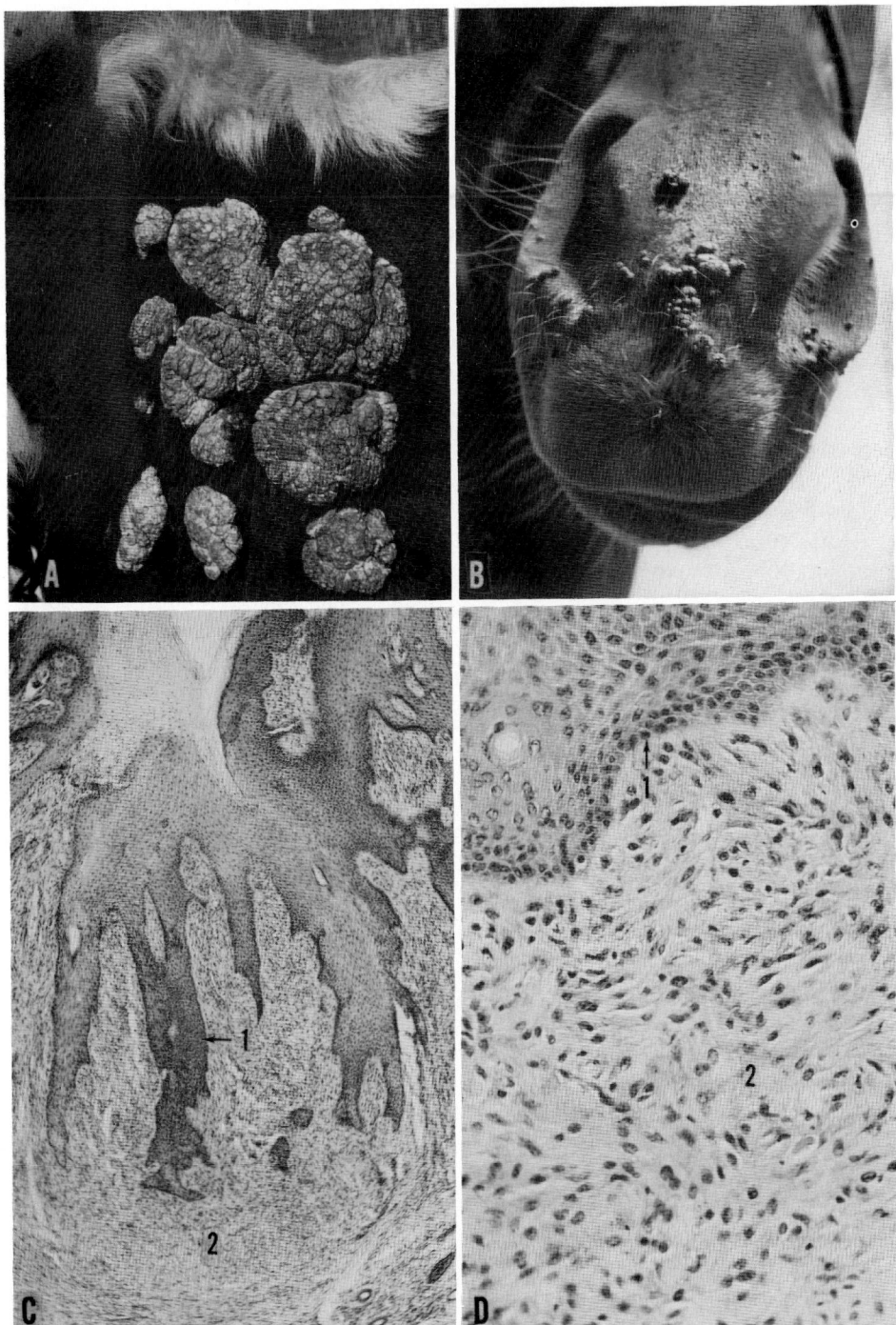

Fig. 9–29. *A,* Bovine papillomatosis (warts), neck of a Hereford steer. *B,* Equine papillomatosis, nose of a horse. Photographs courtesy of Dr. Carl Olson, Jr. *C,* Experimentally transmitted bovine papillomatosis (× 35) 41 days after inoculation. Note elongated growth of epidermis *(1)* and cellular dermis *(2)*. *D,* Higher magnification (× 210), with hyperplastic but sharply demarcated epidermis *(1)* and richly cellular dermis *(2)*. (Courtesy of Armed Forces Institute of Pathology.) Contributor: Dr. Carl Olson, Jr.

stroma and epithelium, which may, under certain circumstances, undergo malignant change. These viruses may therefore be considered among those which induce tumor formation.

Bovine Cutaneous Papillomatosis

In the bovine species, cutaneous papillomatosis is more frequent than in any other domestic animal. Its viral etiology seems to be well established. The disease is more common and severe in young animals; only partial immunity to reinfection develops, and neutralizing antibodies are not demonstrable in bovine serum. The disease is generally self-limiting and recovery without treatment is the usual course; but when lesions occur on the genitalia (see Fibropapillomas), they may interfere with reproduction.

An outbreak of papillomatosis described by Bagdonas and Olson (1953) involved 82 (74.5%) of a herd of 110 Hereford cattle in the course of 2½ years. The incubation period following intimate natural contact was 3½ to 4 months and the duration of disease was 1 to 5½ months, all animals recovering spontaneously. Papillomas were observed by these workers to be most frequent on the neck, chin, shoulder, and dewlap; less common on the ears, eyelids, throat, lips, and elsewhere. The site of the lesions depends to a great extent upon points of skin contact between affected and susceptible animals.

Lesions. The typical bovine wart appears grossly as a rough, cauliflower-like mass of varying size and irregular shape, elevated above the skin surface and attached by either a narrow stalk or a broad base. The lesions are first seen as numerous, closely spaced elevations of the skin, which are round and smooth but soon become rough and horny (Fig. 9–29).

Microscopically, the lesions are made up of greatly thickened epidermis, which is both acanthotic and hyperkeratotic, supported in elongated fronds by a core of hyperplastic dermis. In some lesions, par-

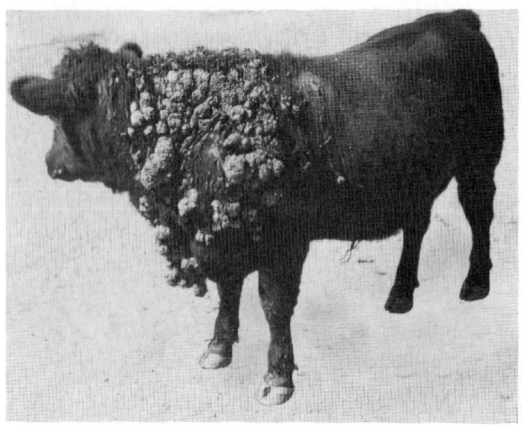

Fig. 9–30. Bovine cutaneous papillomatosis (warts). Aberdeen-Angus steer.

ticularly those induced experimentally by intradermal injection of the virus, overgrowth of the connective tissue elements of the dermis is a dominant feature. Thus the virus can induce proliferative growth in both epidermis and dermis. Electron microscopic and immunofluorescent studies indicate that the virus is present in the epithelial portion and the fibromatous portion of the papilloma. Epithelial cells of the stratum spinosum occasionally contain intranuclear eosinophilic, homogeneous structures, which may represent viral inclusion bodies.

Fibropapillomas of Bovine Genitalia

Certain papillary lesions of the penis of young bulls and vagina of cows have been shown to be transmissible, and McEntee (1950) has demonstrated that they are caused by the virus of cutaneous bovine papillomatosis. These fibropapillomas differ from ordinary warts not only in their location, but also in their structure, which is characterized by intense proliferation of connective tissue elements with only slight overgrowth of the overlying epithelium (Fig. 9–31). Interlacing bundles of large, spindle-shaped cells suggest fibroma or fibrosarcoma. Loss of epithelium and secondary infection may result in leukocytic

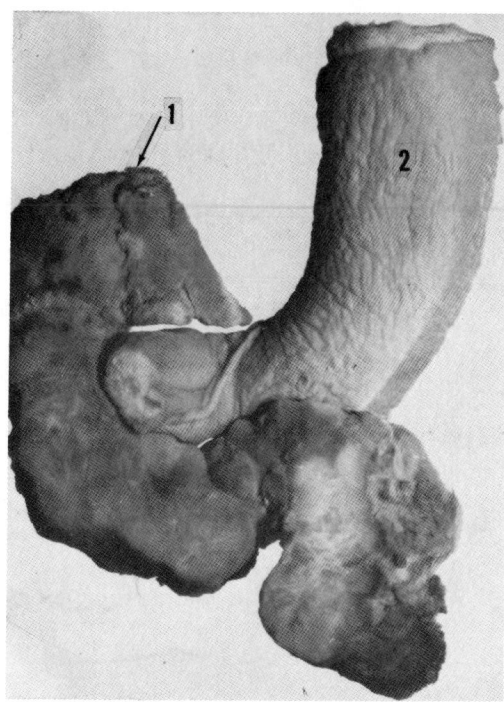

Fig. 9–31. Bovine fibropapillomatosis. Large roughly irregular mass *(1)* on the glans penis *(2)* of a bull.

infiltration and edema, which increase the cellularity of the lesion and add to the difficulties of interpretation by the uninitiated pathologist. This specific entity is readily recognized, however, by one familiar with its characteristics. The lesions in the genitalia often present surgical problems and may recur after excision, but they do not metastasize and are usually self-limiting.

Olson et al. (1959) have experimentally demonstrated that the bovine papilloma virus can induce fibromas and polyps of the bovine urinary bladder similar to the naturally occurring tumors associated with chronic enzootic hematuria. Olson and associates (1965) subsequently isolated a virus, resembling the bovine papilloma virus, from spontaneous urinary bladder tumors of cattle. Experimentally, the bovine papilloma virus has also been shown to induce fibromatous meningeal tumors in calves and hamsters, and fibromatous tumors in the skin of horses, hamsters, and mice.

Equine Sarcoid

The pathologic characteristics of this growth are presented in Chapter 18. The entity was first recognized by Jackson (1936) in South Africa, who found evidence suggesting that it was transferable from one part of the horse's body to another. He also thought that the abnormal proliferation was primarily epidermal, the underlying dermis later becoming affected and assuming a preponderant role. In these two respects he perceived a resemblance to the common warts (papillomas), which are known to have a viral origin.

Olson (1948) experimentally demonstrated what Jackson suspected, that the lesion can be transplanted from one cutaneous site to another in the same horse (autotransplantation). Later, Olson and Cook (1951) were able to produce a lesion resembling equine sarcoid by inoculating the horse's skin with material from bovine papillomas (warts), a unique crossing of species boundaries. Ragland and Spencer (1969) have confirmed these findings in ponies.

Equine Cutaneous Papillomatosis

Common warts are most frequent on the nose, muzzle, and lips of horses during their first and second years of life. These lesions are experimentally transmissible to horses by exposure of scarified skin to triturated suspensions of warts, before or after filtration through bacteria-retaining filters; calves, lambs, dogs, rabbits, and guinea pigs are not susceptible. Natural transmission between horses appears to occur through simple contact. The incubation period is two to three months; the duration of the lesions is about two months, spontaneous regression having occurred in all reported cases. Reinfection is rarely observed in animals which have recovered from the disease.

The papillomas of this equine disease are usually small, discrete, and attached by a narrow stalk, but in some cases they are very numerous and may be confluent. Small papillomas may appear as elongated, elevated nodules with a smooth surface, but larger ones have the rough surface characteristic of warts in other species.

Microscopically, hyperplastic, folded layers of squamous epithelium are supported by a thin core of connective tissue continuous with the dermis. Acanthosis and hyperkeratosis are prominent features in the affected epidermis. The outer layers of the acanthotic prickle cell layer exhibit so-called balloon degeneration, and aggregations of keratohyaline granules may be present in the cells. The lesions in general do not differ basically from those of papillomatosis in other species.

Canine Oral Papillomatosis

Infectious papillomas have been known for many years (McFadyean and Hobday, 1898) to occur in the oral cavity of young dogs. These lesions are transmissible by contact or through injection of bacteria-free suspensions of wart material, but will grow only on the oral mucosa. Skin and other epithelial surfaces are refractory to infection. Only dogs are susceptible; attempts to infect guinea pigs, rabbits, rats, mice, monkeys, and kittens have been unsuccessful. Although cutaneous warts do occur in dogs, apparently they are not caused by the same virus that induces the

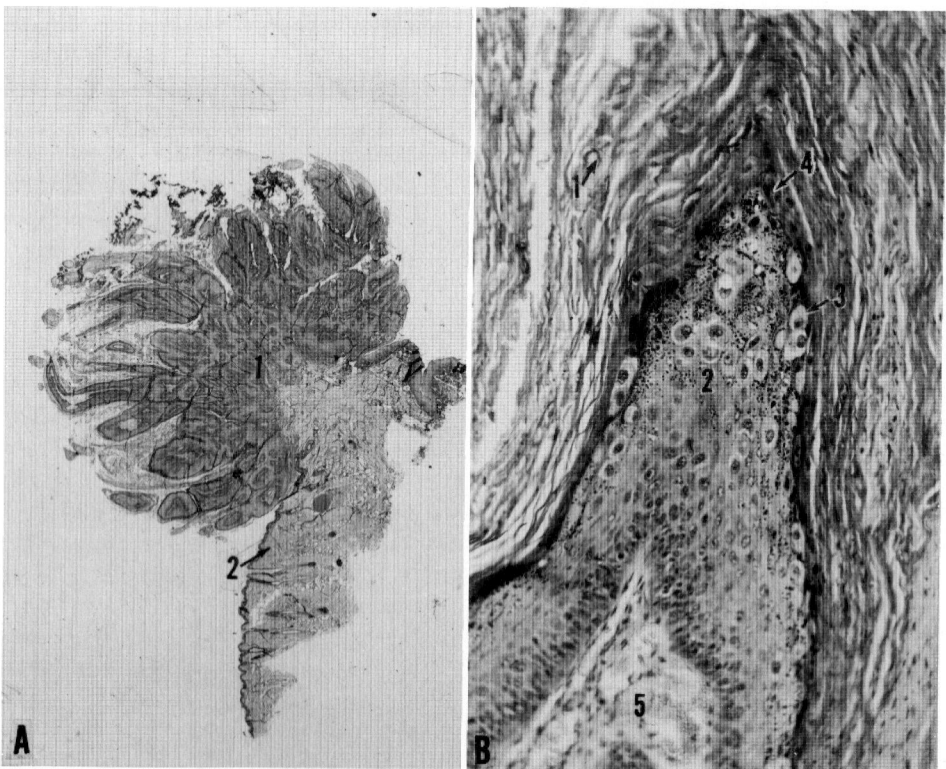

Fig. 9–32. Canine oral papillomatosis. *A*, A verrucous mass *(1)* arising from the junction of oral mucosa and skin *(2)* (× 7). *B*, Higher magnification (× 160). Note extensive layer of keratin *(1)*, long fronds of hyperplastic epidermis *(2)* containing some vacuoles *(3)* and eleidin granules *(4)* on a core of connective tissue stroma *(5)*. (Courtesy of Armed Forces Institute of Pathology.) Contributor: Dr. S. Pollock.

oral lesions. The duration of oral papillomas is usually from three to five months.

Lesions. The lesions may be single but more often are multiple, and in some dogs are so numerous as to interfere with mastication and deglutition. They occur anywhere on the oral mucosa, in the cheeks, tongue, palate, or pharynx, but do not extend below the epiglottis or into the esophagus. The papillomas are sharply delimited, single or confluent cauliflower-shaped masses with a roughened surface, elevated from the oral mucosa.

Microscopically, the earliest lesion is seen as a sharply circumscribed segment of hyperplastic epithelium in which mitotic figures are frequent. The prickle cell layer becomes progressively thicker as the lesion grows; some cells lose their intercellular bridges and there is beginning papillary formation. Hyperkeratosis becomes a prominent feature, and although cells of the malpighian layer remain normal in size, the squamous cells become larger, their cytoplasm vacuolated or filled with albuminous material. The nuclei of the squamous cells either become greatly enlarged, or, in the outer layers, shrunken and distorted. The superficial cells apparently drop out, leaving a meshwork in the thick keratin layer. In older lesions, a few cytoplasmic inclusions, 1 to 5 μ in diameter, may be seen just under the keratin layer. These are interpreted as keratohyaline masses. In some sections basophilic inclusions fill nuclei of epithelial cells. Viral particles have been demonstrated in epithelial nuclei and correlated with the development of the basophilic inclusions. The underlying corium is relatively unchanged, but it sends out long vascular fronds to support the finger-like projections of hyperplastic epithelium. A few plasma cells and lymphocytes may be seen in the stroma underlying old lesions.

Cutaneous Papillomatosis of Rabbits

An infectious papillomatosis of wild cottontail rabbits (*Sylvilagus*) was originally investigated by Shope (1933), hence is often referred to as the Shope papilloma. The warts in this disease are usually found in cases of natural infection involving the skin of the inner surface of the thighs, abdomen, or about the neck and shoulders. The lesions are black or gray, 0.5 to 1.0 cm in diameter and 1.0 to 1.5 cm in height, and are covered with a thick layer of keratin. They can be transmitted without difficulty from one cottontail rabbit to another by injecting or applying filtered or unfiltered wart suspensions to scarified skin. Evidence has been obtained to indicate that certain arthropods may transmit the virus of this disease. Although domestic rabbits (*Oryctolagus*) can be infected, the disease cannot be perpetuated in series in such breeds. However, once established in a domestic rabbit, the papillomas can persist for long periods, undergo malignant transformation, and kill the animal by metastasis. When these tumors become carcinomatous, they lose their pigment and differentiated characteristics, assume the features of squamous cell carcinoma, and can be transplanted to other domestic rabbits.

Oral Papillomatosis of Rabbits

Spontaneous papillomatosis of the oral cavity of domestic rabbits (*Oryctolagus*) has been described by Parson and Kidd (1943) and demonstrated to be the result of a virus infection. The viral agent is distinct from the Shope papilloma virus, which affects the epithelium of the skin but not the mouth. These spontaneous papillomas are small, discrete, gray-white nodules, either sessile or pedunculated. Usually multiple and sometimes numerous, they are almost always situated on the under-surface of the tongue, occasionally on the gums, and rarely on the floor of the mouth. The lesions are predominantly small, with a smooth dome-shaped surface, but occasionally are larger, sometimes attaining a diameter of 5 mm, with a rugose, cauliflower-like surface.

Microscopically, the lesions appear as discrete nodules of thickened, folded, hyperplastic epithelium, supported by sharply demarcated stroma which may form delicate papillae. In lesions of long standing, the prominent changes are seen in epithelial cells; those of the malpighian layer become large, coarsely vacuolated, and irregularly polyhedral in shape. The nuclei of all layers, particularly of the prickle cells, become enlarged, vesicular, and may contain eosinophilic or basophilic inclusion bodies. The inclusions contain viral particles. There is little tendency toward excessive keratinization of the affected epithelium; the outer layers merely appear denser and more eosinophilic in stained sections.

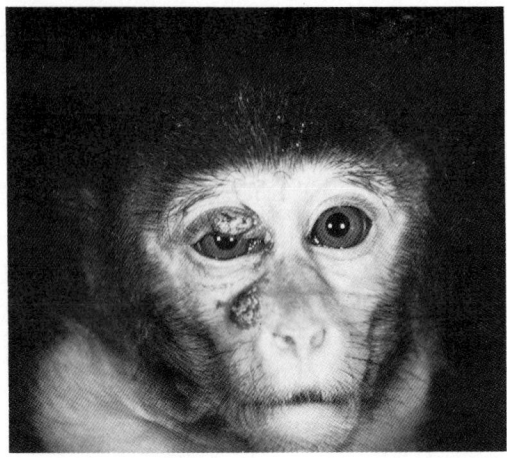

Fig. 9–33. Cutaneous papillomatosis of the face of a rhesus monkey *(Macaca mulatta)*. (Courtesy of New England Regional Primate Research Center, Harvard Medical School.)

Caprine Papillomatosis

Papillomatosis of goats may occur in either of two forms. Davis and Kemper (1936) described cutaneous warts on the head, face, shoulder, neck, and upper part of the forelimb, but not on the teats and udder, in one herd of Saanen goats. Moulton (1954) reported papillomatosis limited to the teats and udder in another herd of goats of the same breed. The outbreak described by Moulton was initiated by the introduction of an infected goat into the herd, with the strange result that 50 of 150 black goats were affected, while not one of the 50 white goats exhibited lesions. The disease in this herd was of long duration, papillomas persisting more than five months with little sign of regression. Some of them looked like cutaneous horns, reaching a length of 3 cm, and usually having a rod-like or conical, rather than a papillary, shape. Massive discoid tumors develop in some instances, with frank squamous cell carcinomas arising by dissociation and downgrowth of epithelium. Although there was no generalized metastasis, one of these squamous cell carcinomas metastasized to the supramammary lymph node. Of seven advanced lesions examined microscopically, four showed evidence of malignant transformation. Moulton was unable to cultivate the agent in chick embryos, and transmission to other goats was not attempted.

Papillomatosis of Monkeys

A papillomatous lesion of the skin of a brown Cebus monkey, described by Lucké, Ratcliffe, and Breedis (1950), was experimentally transmitted to another skin site on the same monkey and later to 11 of 13 other monkeys. Both Old and New World monkeys were included in the susceptible group. The incubation period was about two weeks; regression of the lesions occurred between the fourth and eighth months, and no evidence of malignancy was seen during a subsequent eight-month period of observation. This record adds another to the species of animals in which papillomatosis has been observed.

Bagdonas, V., and Olson, C., Jr.: Observations on the epizoötiology of cutaneous papillomatosis (warts) of cattle. J. Am. Vet. Med. Assoc., *122*:393–397, 1953.
———: Observations on immunity in cutaneous bovine papillomatosis. Am. J. Vet. Res., *15*:240–245, 1954.
Brobst, D. F., and Dulac, G. C.: Meningeal tumors induced in calves with the bovine cutaneous papilloma virus. Pathol. Vet., *6*:135–145, 1969.

Brobst, D. F., and Hinsman, E. J.: Electron microscopy of the bovine cutaneous papilloma. Pathol. Vet., 3:196–207, 1966.

Brobst, D. F., and Olson, C.: Histopathology of urinary bladder tumors induced by bovine cutaneous papilloma agent. Cancer Res., 25:12–19, 1965.

Cheville, N. F., and Olson, C. L.: Cytology of the canine oral papilloma. Am. J. Pathol., 45:848–872, 1964.

Cook, R. H., and Olson, C., Jr.: Experimental transmission of cutaneous papilloma of the horse. Am. J. Pathol., 27:1087–1097, 1951.

Dalmat, H. T.: Arthropod transmission of rabbit papillomatosis. J. Exp. Med., 108:9–20, 1958.

Davis, C. L., and Kemper, H. E.: Common warts (papillomata) in goats. J. Am. Vet. Med. Assoc., 88:175–179, 1936.

DeMonbreun, W. A., and Goodpasture, E. W.: Infectious oral papillomatosis of dogs. Am. J. Pathol., 8:43–56, 1932.

Fujimoto, Y., and Olson, C.: The fine structure of the bovine wart. Path. Vet., 3:659–684, 1966.

Gordon, D. W., and Olson, C.: Meningiomas and fibroblastic neoplasia in calves induced with the bovine papilloma virus. Cancer Res., 28:2423–2431, 1968.

Jackson, C.: The incidence and pathology of tumours of domesticated animals in South Africa. Onderstepoort J. Vet. Sci. Anim. Ind., 6:1–160, 1936.

Lucké, B., Ratcliffe, H., and Breedis, C.: Transmissible papilloma in monkeys. Fed. Proc., 9:337, 1950.

McEntee, K.: Transmissible fibropapillomas of the external genitalia of cattle. Rep. N. Y. State Veterinary College, Cornell Univ., Ithaca, N. Y., 1950–51, p. 28.

———: Fibropapillomas on the external genitalia of cattle. Cornell Vet., 40:304–312, 1950.

McFadyean, J., and Hobday, F.: Note on the experimental transmission of warts in the dog. J. Comp. Pathol. Ther., 11:341–344, 1898.

Moulton, J. E.: Cutaneous papillomas on the udders of milk goats. North Am. Vet., 35:29–33, 1954.

Olson, C., Jr.: Equine sarcoid; a cutaneous neoplasm. Am. J. Vet. Res., 9:333–341, 1948.

Olson, C., and Cook, R. H.: Cutaneous sarcoma-like lesions of the horse caused by the agent of bovine papilloma. Proc. Soc. Exp. Biol. Med., 77:281–284, 1951.

Olson, C., et al.: A urinary bladder tumor induced by a bovine cutaneous papilloma agent. Cancer Res., 19:779–782, 1959.

Olson, C., Pamukcu, A. M., and Brobst, D. F.: Papilloma-like virus from bovine urinary bladder tumors. Cancer Res., 25:840–849, 1965.

Parsons, R. J., and Kidd, J. G.: Oral papillomatosis of rabbits: a virus disease. J. Exp. Med., 77:233–250, 1943.

Penberthy, J.: Contagious warty tumors in dogs. J. Comp. Pathol. Ther., 11:363–365, 1898.

Ragland, W. L., and Spencer, G. R.: Attempts to relate bovine papilloma virus to the cause of equine sarcoid: Equidae inoculated intradermally with bovine papilloma virus. Am. J. Vet. Res., 30:743–752, 1969.

———: Attempts to relate bovine papilloma virus to the cause of equine sarcoid: immunity to bovine papilloma virus. Am. J. Vet. Res., 29:1363–1366, 1968.

Rdzok, E. J., Shipkowitz, N. L., and Richter, W. R.: Rabbit oral papillomatosis: ultrastructure of experimental infection. Cancer Res., 26:160–166, 1966.

Richter, W. R., Shipkowitz, N. L., and Rdzok, E. J.: Oral papillomatosis of the rabbit: an electron microscopic study. Lab. Invest., 13:430–438, 1964.

Robl, M. G., and Olson, C.: Oncogenic action of bovine papilloma virus in hamsters. Cancer Res., 28:1596–1604, 1968.

Rous, P., and Beard, J. W.: The progression to carcinoma of virus-induced rabbit papillomas (Shope). J. Exp. Med., 62:523–548, 1935.

Segre, D., Olson, C., Jr., and Hoerlein, A. B.: Neutralization of bovine papilloma virus with serums from cattle and horses with experimental papillomas. Am. J. Vet. Res., 16:517–520, 1955.

Shope, R. E.: Infectious papillomatosis of rabbits. J. Exp. Med., 58:607–624, 1933.

Tajima, M., Gordon, D. E., and Olson, C.: Electron microscopy of bovine papilloma and deer fibroma viruses. Am. J. Vet. Res., 29:1185–1194, 1968.

Voss, J. L.: Transmission of equine sarcoid. Am. J. Vet. Res., 30:183–191, 1969.

Watrach, A. M.: The ultrastructure of canine cutaneous papilloma. Cancer Res., 29:2079–2084, 1969.

Diseases Due to Polyomavirus

The virus first described by Sarah E. Stewart and Bernice E. Eddy of the National Institutes of Health serves to illustrate the complexities, contradictions and surprises encountered by investigators studying viruses in relation to neoplasms. The agent now called the S. E. (after Stewart and Eddy) polyoma virus was first encountered by Stewart in the course of an experiment to repeat the success of Gross, in 1951, in transmitting spontaneous lymphocytic leukemia of the mouse with cell-free extracts. To her surprise, mice (of the C$_3$H/Hen strain) inoculated with cell-free extracts of lymphomatous mouse tissue, did not acquire leukemia but, after eight to ten months, developed multiple tumors of the parotid salivary glands. Hybrid mice (C$_3$H$_f$ X AKR) inoculated with similar extracts, on the other hand, developed leukemia early in life. In further experiments with cell-free extracts of leukemic mouse tissues, pleomorphic tumors of salivary glands, kidneys, mammary gland, thymus, and adrenal gland appeared following inoculation of this cell-free material. Subsequently it was shown that the material contained a virus that could be cultivated in cultures of monkey kidney cells and mouse embryo tissues. Good evidence has been accumulated to establish this agent as a virus; much of this knowledge has been summarized by Eddy, 1960.

A few points are of interest concerning the pathologic effects of this virus. First, its presence results in intranuclear inclusion bodies in renal epithelium. Second, several host species are susceptible; for example, mice, Syrian hamsters, Chinese hamsters, rabbits, and rats. Third, a wide variety of neoplasms appear in these hosts following introduction of the polyoma virus. Some of these tumors are summarized by Stewart (1960) as follows:

1. pleomorphic tumors of salivary glands and mucous glands of head and neck
2. renal cortical tumors and renal sarcomas
3. epithelial thymomas
4. mammary adenocarcinomas and epidermoid carcinomas
5. bone tumors
6. mesotheliomas
7. subcutaneous sarcomas and hemangioendotheliomas
8. medullary adrenal carcinomas
9. other tumor types—thyroid adenocarcinoma and epidermoid carcinoma

Eddy, B. E.: The polyoma virus (B). Adv. Virus Res., 7:91–102, 1960.
————: Polyoma virus. Virology Monographs, 7:1–114, 1969.
Stewart, S. E.: The polyoma virus (A). Adv. Virus Res., 7:61–90, 1960.

PARVOVIRIDAE

The family Parvoviridae (parvo = small) is made up of unique DNA viruses that have a genome consisting of a single molecule of single-stranded DNA. Three genera make up this family: *Parvovirus* (la-

tent viruses H–1, H–3, RV, and X 14 of rodents; minute virus of mice; and tentatively, avian, porcine, and bovine parvoviruses, feline panleukopenia virus, hemorrhagic encephalopathy [rat] virus, mink enteritis virus, and canine parvovirus); *Densovirus* (viruses of insects); and one unnamed genus (which includes the satellite or adenovirus-associated viruses). Two other human viruses, the acute infectious gastroenteritis virus and hepatitis A virus, may also belong to the genus *Parvovirus*. The latent rat viruses cause severe disease when inoculated into newborn hamsters or rats, but do not appear to cause disease in adult rats. The "adenovirus-associated" viruses multiply only in the presence of "helper" adenovirus.

The Parvoviridae are the smallest viruses of vertebrates, and the measured diameter of the virion varies with different methods of staining and measurement. They are highly resistant to chemical and physical reagents, are not affected seriously by heat at 60° C for an hour, and are unaffected by ether, chloroform, or anionic detergents. Determination of the symmetry and number of capsomeres has been difficult and not completely resolved. They are polyhedral, but the exact number and arrangement appear not agreed upon at this time. The virions are not enveloped.

Some features of parvoviruses, which influence the nature, sites, and severity of lesions, are worth noting. Parvoviruses, particularly rat virus and feline panleukopenia virus, have an affinity for cells in mitosis—virions are assembled in these host cells in particular and lethal effects on these cells are extensive. The virus may become attached to red cells and pass through endothelial cells and placental barriers to establish fetal infection. The virus also attacks hepatic parenchymal cells, thus upsetting circulating hemostatic mechanisms, and thus may produce capillary hemorrhage by indirect effects. The rapidly dividing cells of the intestinal mucosa are favorite sites for infection and replication of parvoviruses, hence their principal effect is usually in the intestine. The affinity for the germinal epithelium of the developing cerebellum of the rat fetus or newborn cat and the ability of the virus to pass through the placenta underlies the production of cerebellar hypoplasia in the rat and cat.

Diseases Due to Parvoviruses

Feline Panleukopenia (Feline Distemper, Feline Enteritis, Agranulocytosis)

Feline panleukopenia is a highly contagious and usually fatal febrile disease of domestic cats, other *Felidae,* and mink. It is caused by a virus and is characterized clinically by severe panleukopenia, fever, and enteritis that results in extreme dehydration. Although the domestic house cat is the principal host, a variety of wild felines, mink, and raccoons are susceptible. The disease runs a rapid course. Its onset is marked by lassitude and abrupt elevation of temperature to 104 to 105° F. The fever is diphasic; it falls after about 24 hours and rises approximately 48 hours later. Severe leukopenia involving all of the granulocytic series (agranulocytosis) and all other leukocytes is a constant feature. Vomiting and intractable diarrhea also may be observed. Death frequently occurs shortly after the second peak of temperature.

Lesions. The gross lesions seen at necropsy usually consist of extreme dehydration and emaciation, with mucopurulent exudate on the nasal and lacrimal mucosae. The mucosa of the terminal part of the ileum is often covered with hemorrhagic exudate. The lymph nodes of the mesentery are edematous and somewhat enlarged. The bone marrow of the long bones often appears greasy, yellowish or white, and semifluid. The lack of hematopoietic marrow is obvious.

The principal microscopic lesions are found in the gastrointestinal tract and associated lymph nodes. The superficial layers of the mucosa in the small intestine are eroded, and the remaining epithelium has undergone proliferation. The crypts are dilated with mucus and lined with irregular, hyperplastic epithelial cells. Here inflammatory infiltration of the lamina propria occurs, but little change is seen in the submucosa. In some cases granular, eosinophilic intranuclear inclusions have been described in the lining epithelium remaining at the sites of erosion. These inclusions, when present, are helpful in diagnosis.

The changes in the lymph nodes are reported to be characteristic. Early in the disease the mesenteric lymph nodes are edematous and hyperemic and there is proliferation of reticuloendothelial cells. Erythrophagocytosis is seen in the center of the nodes, and intranuclear inclusions have been reported in a small percentage of monocytic cells.

As the disease progresses, the lymphoid cells become hyperplastic, and later, necrosis becomes evident. Marked hyperplasia of the secondary follicles may occur at some stages but appears to be transient, for it is not uniformly demonstrable post mortem. The changes in the spleen parallel those in the lymph nodes, except that the large secondary nodules are not so prominent. The bone marrow is specifically inhibited; the normal hematopoietic marrow is usually replaced by fatty marrow.

The studies by Rohovsky and Griesemer (1967) and Johnson et al. (1967) on experimental panleukopenia in germfree cats are of particular interest. Enteric lesions were not observed in germfree cats, but consistently developed in specific pathogen-free cats. The most significant findings in germfree cats were lymphocytic destruction, reticuloendothelial hyperplasia, severe thymic atrophy, and panleukopenia. Later studies indicate that viral infection is related to greater mitotic activity in intestinal epithelium of pathogen-free cats.

Diagnosis. A presumptive diagnosis usually can be based upon the symptoms

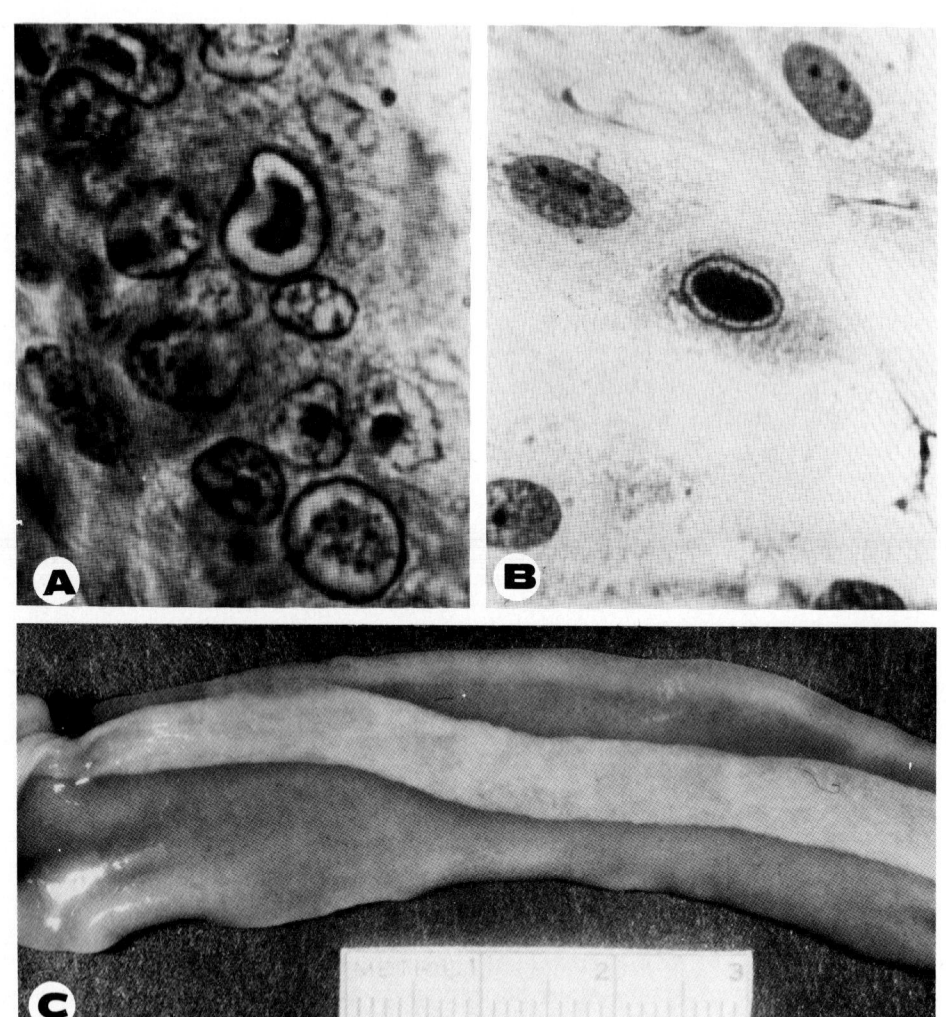

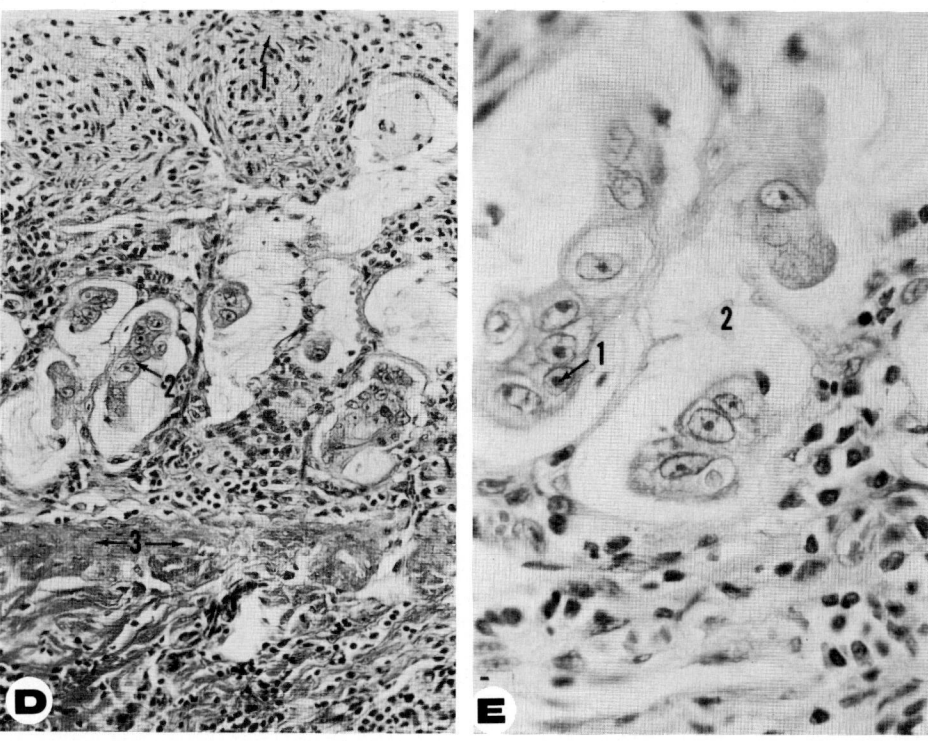

Fig. 9–34. *A*, Intranuclear inclusions of panleukopenia (infectious feline enteritis) virus. In intestinal epithelium of a cat five days following inoculation with the virus. *B*, Inclusion in culture of feline kidney cells five days after inoculation with virus. (Courtesy of Dr. John R. Gorham, Washington State University.) *C*, Fibrinous cast in the lumen of a seven-month-old male cat with panleukopenia. (Courtesy of Angell Memorial Animal Hospital.) *D*, Wall of a small intestine ($\times$ 210) of a cat. Loss of epithelium at tips of villi *(1)*, disorganization and proliferation of epithelial cells in crypts *(2)*. Note collection of mucus. *E*, Higher magnification ($\times$ 590) to show intranuclear inclusions *(1)* and collections of mucus *(2)*, muscularis mucosa *(3)*. (*D*, *E*, Courtesy of Armed Forces Institute of Pathology.) Contributor: Dr. J. T. Bryans.

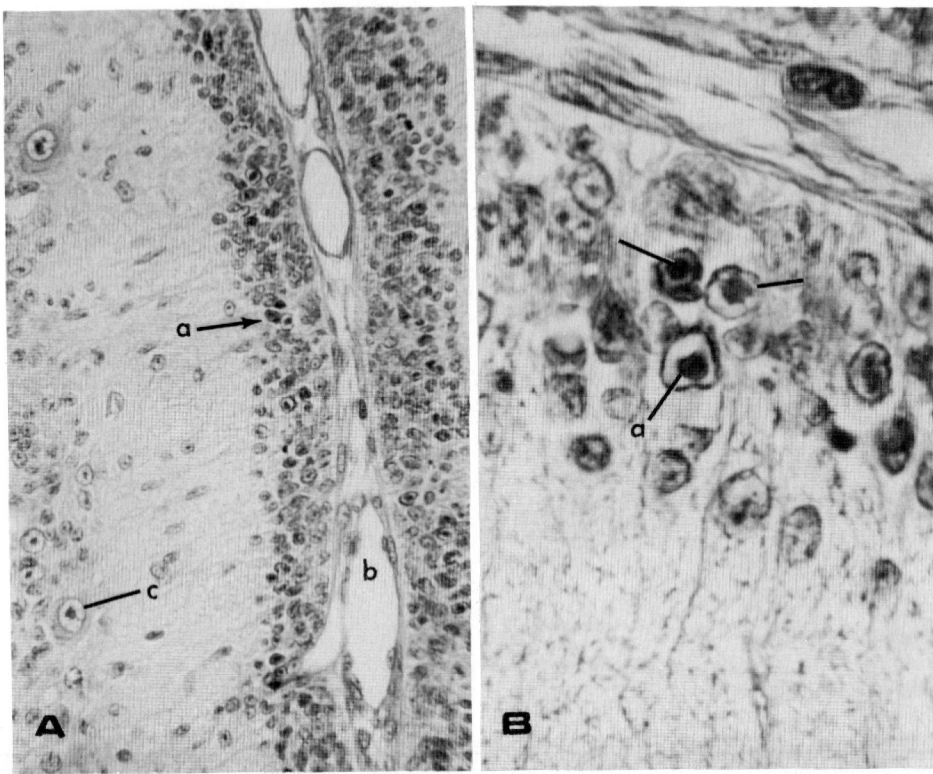

Fig. 9–35. Cerebellum of a 21-day old kitten which had received the panleukopenia virus at birth. *A*, Note intranuclear inclusions and necrotic cells in the cells of the germinal layer *(a)* adjacent to the vascular pia mater *(b)*, Purkinje cells at *(c)*. *B*, Higher magnification of *A*. Note intranuclear inclusions *(a)* and margination of chromatin in affected nuclei. (Courtesy of Dr. George Margolis, Dartmouth Medical School.)

and the agranulocytosis. Demonstration of intranuclear inclusions in the epithelial cells of the small intestine is helpful in postmortem diagnosis, but unfortunately they are not always present.

Panleukopenia and Cerebellar Hypoplasia. Kilham, Margolis, and Colby (1967) demonstrated that the virus of feline panleukopenia can produce cerebellar hypoplasia in kittens. The virus, when injected into the fetus or intravenously into a pregnant cat, invades cells of the external germinal layer of the fetal cerebellum, producing intranuclear inclusion bodies and necrosis, which leads to gross or microscopic "hypoplasia" of the cerebellum in the newborn kitten. Inclusion bodies may persist to the early neonatal period, but usually are not evident after birth. Virus, how-

ever, can be isolated from various tissues, especially the kidney, for several months. The virus has also been isolated from natural cases of cerebellar hypoplasia in kittens. Kilham (1966) had previously demonstrated that rat virus can induce cerebellar hypoplasia in kittens, rats, and hamsters. Although it appears that panleukopenia virus is an important cause of cerebellar hypoplasia in kittens, the relative importance of rat virus is undetermined. These studies are of great significance in that a viral etiology has been demonstrated for a disease accepted by many to represent a genetic abnormality.

Kilham's studies are also of interest because they demonstrated that feline panleukopenia virus could also induce cerebellar hypoplasia in ferrets, a species not considered susceptible to classic panleukopenia.

Bartholomew, T. T., and Gillespie, J. H.: Feline viruses. I. Characterization of four isolates and their effects on young kittens. Cornell Vet., 58:248–265, 1968.

Carlson, J. H., Scott, F. W., and Duncan, J. R.: Feline panleukopenia 1. Pathogenesis in germfree and specific pathogen free cats. Vet Pathol., 14:79–88, 1977.

Carlson, J. H., and Scott, F. W.: Feline panleukopenia. II. The relationship of intestinal mucosal cell proliferation rates to viral infection and development of lesions. Vet. Pathol., 14:173–181, 1977.

Csiza, C. K., de Lahunta, A., Scott, F. W., and Gillespie, J. H.: Pathogenesis of feline panleukopenia virus in susceptible newborn kittens. II. Pathology and immunofluorescence. Infect. Immun., 3:838–846, 1971.

Csiza, C. K., Scott, F. W., de Lahunta, A., and Gillespie, J. H.: Immune carrier state of feline panleukopenia virus-infected cats. Am. J. Vet. Res., 32:419–426, 1971.

————: Feline viruses. XIV. Transplacental infections in spontaneous panleukopenia of cats. Cornell Vet., 61:423–439, 1971.

————: Spontaneous feline ataxia. Cornell Vet., 62:300–322, 1972.

Farrell, R. K., Burger, D., Hartsough, G. R., and Gorham, J. R.: Relationship of mink virus enteritis virus and feline panleukopenia virus: rapid onset of mink virus enteritis virus protection after feline panleukopenia virus infection. Am. J. Vet. Res., 33:2351–2352, 1972.

Fowler, E. H., and Rohovsky, M. W.: Enzyme histochemistry of the small intestine in germfree and specific-pathogen-free cats inoculated with feline infectious enteritis (feline panleukopenia) virus. Am. J. Vet. Res., 31:2055–2060, 1970.

————: Enzyme histochemistry of lymphoid tissues in germfree cats inoculated with feline infectious enteritis (feline panleukopenia) virus. Am. J. Vet. Res., 31:2061–2069, 1970.

Gillespie, J. H.: Report of the panel of the colloquium on selected feline infectious disease. J. Am. Vet. Med. Assoc., 157:2043–2051, 1970.

Gillespie, J. H., and Scott, F. W.: Feline viral infections. Adv. Vet. Sci. Comp. Med., 17:163–200, 1973.

Hammon, W. D., and Enders, J. F.: A virus disease of cats principally characterized by aleucocytosis, enteric lesions and the presence of intranuclear inclusion bodies. J. Exp. Med., 69:327–351, 1939.

Herndon, R. M., Margolis, G., and Kilham, L.: The synaptic organization of the malformed cerebellum induced by perinatal infection with the feline panleukopenia virus (PL V). I. Elements forming the cerebellar glomeruli. II. The Purkinje cell and its afferents. J. Neuropathol. Exp. Neurol., 30:196–205, 1971.

Hersey, D. F., and Maurer, F. D.: Immunological relationship of selected feline viruses by complement fixation. Proc. Soc. Exp. Biol., 107:645–646, 1961.

Johnson, G. R., Koestner, A., and Rohovsky, M. W.: Experimental feline infectious enteritis in the germfree cat. Path. Vet., 4:275–288, 1967.

Johnson, R. H., Margolis, G., and Kilham, L.: Identity of feline ataxia virus with feline panleucopenia virus. Nature, Lond., 214:175–177, 1967.

Johnson, R. H.: Serologic procedures for the study of the feline panleukopenia. J. Am. Vet. Med. Assoc., 158:876–884, 1971.

Kilham, L., and Margolis, G.: Viral etiology of spontaneous ataxia of cats. Am. J. Pathol., 48:991–1011, 1966.

Kilham, L., Margolis, G., and Colby, E. D.: Congenital infections of cats and ferrets by feline panleukopenia virus manifested by cerebellar hypoplasia. Lab. Invest., 17:465–480, 1967.

————: Cerebellar ataxia and its congenital transmission in cats by feline panleukopenia virus. J. Am. Vet. Med. Assoc., 158:888–901, 1971.

Krunajevic, T.: Experimental virus enteritis in mink. Acta Vet. Scand., (Suppl.) 30:1–88, 1970.

Langheinrich, K. A., and Neilsen, S. W.: Histopathology of feline panleukopenia. J. Am. Vet. Med. Assoc., 158:863–872, 1971.

Larson, S., Flagstad, A., and Aalbaek, B.: Experimental feline panleucopenia in the conventional cat. Vet. Pathol., 13:216–240, 1976.

Lawrence, J. S., Syverton, J. T., Shaw, J. S., and Smith, F. P.: Infectious feline agranulocytosis. Am. J. Pathol., 16:333–354, 1940.

Lawrence, J. S., et al.: The virus of infectious feline agranulocytosis. II. Immunological relation to other viruses. J. Exp. Med., 77:57–64, 1943.

Lucas, A. M., and Riser, W. H.: Intranuclear inclusions in panleukopenia of cats. Am. J. Pathol., 21:435–465, 1945.

Percy, D. H., Scott, F. W., and Albert, D. M.: Retinal dysplasia due to feline panleukopenia virus infection. J. Am. Vet. Med. Assoc., 167:935–937, 1975.

Riser, W. H.: The histopathology of panleucopenia (agranulocytosis) in the domestic cat. Am. J. Vet. Res., 7:455–465, 1946.

Rohovsky, M. W., and Griesemer, R. A.: Experimental feline infectious enteritis in the germfree cat. Pathol. Vet., 4:391–410, 1967.

Scott, F. W., Csiza, C. K., and Gillespie, J. H.: Feline viruses. IV. Isolation and characterization of feline panleukopenia virus in tissue culture and comparison of cytopathogenicity with feline Picornavirus, Herpesvirus, and Reovirus. Cornell Vet., 60:165–183, 1970.

————: Feline viruses. V. Serum neutralization test for feline panleukopenia. Cornell Vet., 60:183–190, 1970.

————: Maternally derived immunity to feline panleukopenia. J. Am. Vet. Med. Assoc., 156:439–453, 1970.

Syverton, J. T., et al.: The virus of infectious feline agranulocytosis. I. Character of the virus: pathogenicity. J. Exp. Med., 77:41–56, 1943.

Canine Parvovirus Infection

Although a parvovirus (called "minute virus of canines") was isolated from normal dogs in 1970, it was not until 1978 that a parvovirus was associated with any disease of dogs. In 1978, an apparently new or heretofore unrecognized disease entity suddenly appeared in several parts of the world. Much remains to be learned of the ecology of the virus, but it is clear that the virus is related to that of feline panleukopenia. Canine parvovirus may represent a natural or laboratory mutant of feline panleukopenia virus.

Intestinal Form. The clinical and pathologic picture may occur in one of two forms, intestinal or cardiac. The intestinal form, which may occur in dogs of all ages but is most severe in young pups, is characterized by vomiting, diarrhea, and dehydration. There may be fever and leukopenia. Microscopically, there is a necro-

tizing enteritis of the small intestine reminiscent of feline panleukopenia, with dilated crypts and often regeneration of epithelium. Intranuclear inclusion bodies may be found in intestinal epithelial cells with the same low frequency as in cats with panleukopenia. These signs and lesions may occur in conjunction with the cardiac form.

Cardiac Form. The cardiac form is confined to puppies two to eight weeks of age. This form may exist with or without signs or lesions in the small intestine. Clinically, death may be sudden or follow a brief period of dyspnea and sometimes signs of enteritis. Microscopically, there are multiple foci of myocardial necrosis associated with a mononuclear cellular infiltrate. Fibrosis may be evident in dogs surviving

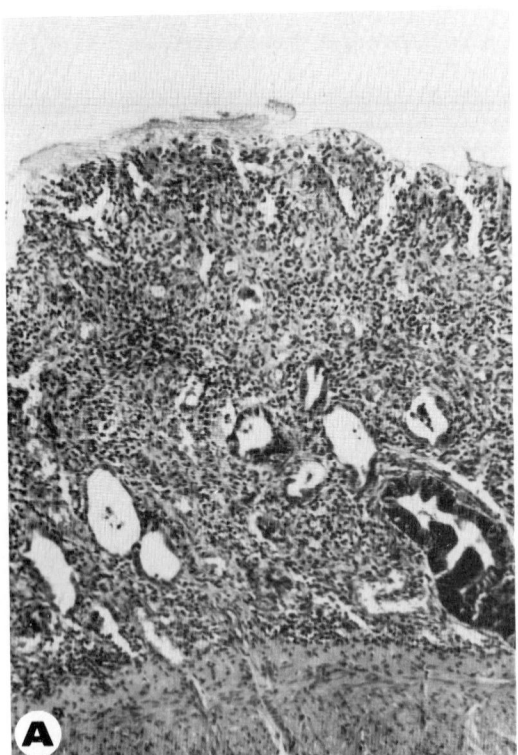
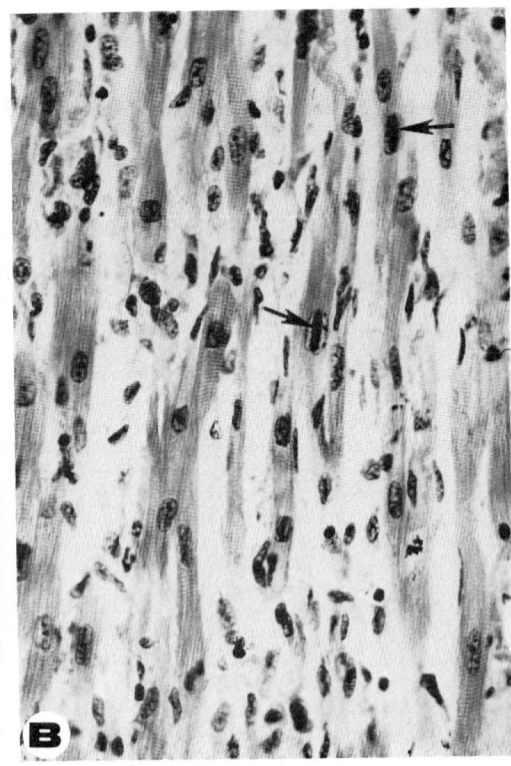

Fig. 9–36.   Canine parvovirus infection. *A*, Necrotizing enteritis, ileum. Note extensive necrosis and loss of epithelial cells lining villi and crypts resulting in collapse and fusion of villi. Scattered crypts are dilated and lined by hypertrophic, regenerating epithelial cells. *B*, Myocarditis, characterized by interstitial edema, sparse mononuclear inflammatory cell infiltration and basophilic intranuclear inclusion bodies in myofibers (arrows). (Courtesy, Dr. Norval W. King.)

an acute episode. Intranuclear inclusion bodies are present in myofibers.

Diagnosis. Diagnosis depends upon the lesions and isolation of the virus. The myocardial form is unique, but the intestinal form may be confused with other causes of enteritis, such as coronavirus infections. The latter is not usually milder clinically and is not associated with leukopenia nor significant necrosis of intestinal epithelium.

Appel, M. J. G., et al.: Status report: canine viral enteritis. J. Am. Vet. Med. Assoc., *173*:1516–1518, 1978.

Appel, M. J. G., et al.: Immunization against canine parvoviral infection. J. Am. Vet. Med. Assoc., *176*:448, 1980.

Carpenter, J. L., et al.: Intestinal and cardiopulmonary forms of parvovirus infection in a litter of pups. J. Am. Vet. Med. Assoc., *176*:1269–1273, 1980.

Hayes, M. A., et al.: Sudden death in young dogs with myocarditis caused by parvovirus. J. Am. Vet. Med. Assoc., *174*:1197–1203, 1979.

Robinson, W. F., et al.: Canine parvoviral myocarditis: a morphologic description of the natural disease. Vet. Pathol., *17*:282–293, 1980.

Bovine Parvovirus Infections

Bovine *Parvovirus* has been isolated from the intestinal tract of young calves afflicted with a severe but transitory diarrhea. It appears that each of several isolates are closely related and presumably the same agent. Bovine *Parvovirus* agglutinates human type O and guinea pig red blood cells; some strains agglutinate rat erythrocytes, but not red blood cells of any other species. Bovine strains are immunologically different from *Parvovirus* derived from any other species. The virions may be demonstrated in large numbers in nuclei of affected cells. They occur as fully developed dense capsids or as ring-like hexagonal empty capsids of the same size—20–22 nm in diameter.

Oral or intravenous administration of bovine *Parvovirus* to newborn calves results in mucoid to watery diarrhea 24 to 48 hours later. Intestinal cells at all levels of the digestive tract become infected, but those of the small intestine appear to be most clearly involved. Viremia persists for 4 to 6 days, but virus may be isolated from feces up to 11 days. The illness is usually transitory, but may be severe if complicated by other viral or bacterial infections. The diagnosis depends upon isolation and identification of the virus in cultures of bovine cells, or by demonstration of specific immunofluorescence or ultrastructurally typical virions in affected cells.

Abinanti, F. R., and Warfield, M. S.: Recovery of a hemadsorbing virus (Haden) from the gastrointestinal tract of calves. Virology, *14*:288–289, 1961.

Bates, R. C., Storz, J., and Reed, D. E.: Isolation and characterization of bovine parvoviruses. J. Infect. Dis., *126*:531–536, 1972.

Storz, J., Bates, R. C., Warren, G. S., and Howard, T. H.: Distribution of antibodies against bovine parvovirus 1 in cattle and other animal species. Am. J. Vet. Res., *33*:269–272, 1972.

Storz, J., and Bates, R. C.: Parvovirus infections in calves. J. Am. Vet. Med. Assoc., *163*:884–886, 1973.

Woods, G. T.: Bovine parvovirus 1, bovine syncytial virus, and bovine respiratory syncytial virus and their infections. Adv. Vet. Sci. Comp. Med., *18*:273–286, 1974.

Porcine Parvovirus Infection

Parvovirus is widespread in swine populations, judging by the demonstration of antibodies and recovery of strains of the agent. The principal effects of the virus appear to be upon reproduction, causing intrauterine deaths of fetuses. Abortion rarely occurs; infected swine fetuses undergo maceration or mummification, but are not usually expelled prematurely. Lesions of infected pig fetuses have not been described in detail, except to record the presence of virus in macerated or mummified fetuses. It may be possible that this virus, like other parvoviruses, becomes concentrated in embryonic tissues during the period of maximum growth rate.

Experimental infection of fetuses has been accomplished by injection of virus into the allantoic fluid, intravenously, intranasally, or orally, early in gestation. Some of the fetuses die in utero. Virus may be isolated from the live or dead fetuses, or viral antigen demonstrated by fluorescent antibody. In natural situations, increased frequency of serum-neutralizing antibodies to porcine parvovirus has been associated with decreased reproductive productivity in herds of swine.

Cartwright, S. F., Lucas, M., and Huck, R. A.: A small hemagglutinating porcine DNA virus. I. Isolation and properties. J. Comp. Pathol., *79*:371–377, 1969.
———: A small hemagglutinating porcine DNA virus. II. Biological and serological studies. J. Comp. Pathol., *81*:145–156, 1971.
Cutlip, R. C., and Mengeling, W. L.: Experimentally induced infection of neonatal swine with porcine parvovirus. Am. J. Vet. Res., *36*:1179–1182, 1975.
———: Pathogenesis of in utero infection: experimental infection of eight and ten-week-old porcine fetuses with porcine parvovirus. Am. J. Vet. Res., *36*:1751–1754, 1975.
Koestner, A., Kasga, L., Kindig, O., and Shattuck, J. A.: Ultrastructure alterations of tissue cultures infected with a pathogenic porcine adenovirus. Am. J. Pathol., *53*:651–665, 1968.
Lucas, M. H., Cartwright, S. F., and Wrathall, A. E.: Genital infection of pigs with porcine parvovirus. J. Comp. Pathol., *84*:347–350, 1974.
Mengeling, W. L.: Porcine parvovirus: frequency of naturally occurring transplacental infection and viral contamination of fetal porcine kidney cell cultures. Am. J. Vet. Res., *36*:41–44, 1975.
Mengeling, W. L., and Cutlip, R. C.: Pathogenesis of in utero infection: experimental infection of five-week-old porcine fetuses with porcine parvovirus. Am. J. Vet. Res., *36*:1173–1177, 1975.
———: Reproductive disease experimentally induced by exposing pregnant gilts to porcine parvovirus. Am. J. Vet. Res., *37*:1393–1400, 1976.
Mengeling, W. L., et al.: Fetal mummification associated with porcine parvovirus infection. J. Am. Vet. Med. Assoc., *166*:993–995, 1975.
Rodeffer, H. E., et al.: Reproductive failure in swine associated with maternal seroconversion for porcine parvovirus. J. Am. Vet. Med. Assoc., *166*:991–992, 1975.

Murine Parvovirus Infections

Parvovirus of rats and mice are of unusual interest because they have served as model systems for the study of the pathogenic effects of parvoviruses on different host cells and tissues. Rat parvovirus (rat virus) has been demonstrated by experimental inoculation of virus alone to produce a severe hemorrhagic encephalopathy in suckling rats. Similar effects may be produced in adult rats by combined injection of virus and administration of immunosuppressive doses of cyclophosphamide. In this system, the virus acts concurrently on the developing vascular tissue and upon other rapidly proliferating cells in the neonatal brain. The affinity of parvoviruses for cells in active mitosis is clearly evident. The dual effect upon endothelial and hepatic cells also serves to explain vascular hemorrhage and coagulation defects.

Baringer, J. R., and Nathanson, N.: Parvovirus hemorrhagic encephalopathy of rats. Electron microscopic observations of the vascular lesions. Lab. Invest., *27*:514–522, 1972.
Cole, G. A., Nathanson, N., and Rivet, H.: Viral hemorrhagic encephalopathy of rats. II. Pathogenesis of central nervous system lesions. Am. J. Epidemiol., *91*:339–348, 1970.
Lipton, H., Nathanson, N., and Hodous, J.: Enteric transmission of parvoviruses; pathogenesis of rat virus infection in adult rats. Am. J. Epidemiol., *96*:443–446, 1972.
Margolis, G., and Kilham, L.: Parvovirus infection, vascular endothelium, and hemorrhagic encephalopathy. Lab. Invest., *22*:478–488, 1970.
Nathanson, H., et al.: Viral hemorrhagic encephalopathy of rats. I. Isolation, identification, and properties of the HER strain of rat virus. Am. J. Epidemiol., *91*:328–338, 1970.

PICORNAVIRIDAE

A large number of viruses (Table 9–8) are grouped in the Family Picornaviridae (pico = small, rna = ribonucleic acid). These viruses are serologically distinct but similar in terms of their morphology and physical and chemical properties. They are responsible for a spectrum of illnesses in man and animals. At present only three genera are officially recognized although evidence has been presented (Fenner et al., 1974) to justify the establishment of three new groups: the encephalomyocarditis, Mengo, and ME viruses as a separate genus, *Cardiovirus* (cardio = heart); the foot and mouth disease (aphthous fever) virus as a new genus, *Aphthovirus*; and the equine rhinovirus as a new genus. These three new groups are proposed on the basis of differences in density in cesium chloride, base composition of RNA and

Table 9–8. Diseases Caused by Picornaviridae

Enterovirus	Rhinovirus (Aphthovirus)	Calicivirus
Poliomyelitis	Aphthous fever (foot and mouth disease)	Vesicular exanthema, swine
Coxsackie viruses	Rhinovirus, human, respiratory infection	Feline (picornavirus) calicivirus, respiratory infection
Encephalomyocarditis	Rhinovirus, bovine, respiratory infection	
Teschen disease	Rhinovirus, equine, respiratory infection	
Benign enzootic paresis of pigs		
Talfan disease		
Canadian viral encephalomyelitis		
Mouse (murine) encephalomyelitis		
Avian encephalomyelitis		
Bovine and porcine enterovirus infection		
Duck hepatitis		
Nodamura virus infection		

stability of virions at different pH values (Newman et al., 1973).

Viruses grouped in the Picornaviridae have an icosahedral capsid 20 to 40 nm in diameter and nonenveloped. The virions of genera *Enterovirus* and *Rhinovirus* are uniform, 20 to 30 nm in diameter. *Calicivirus* virions are slightly larger, 35 to 40 nm in diameter. The viral nucleic acid in the type species, *Poliovirus*, consists of a single linear molecule of single-stranded RNA with a molecular weight of 2.6 daltons. The RNA extraced from the virion is infectious, as is also the double-stranded form extracted from infected cells.

The electron microscope reveals picornaviruses to consist of small, spherical naked virions with a protein capsid encompassing a dense core of single-stranded RNA, 16 nm in diameter.

Diseases Caused by Enteroviruses

Poliomyelitis of Mice (Mouse Encephalomyelitis, Theiler's Disease)

A spontaneous disease of albino mice, characterized by progressive flaccid paralysis, particularly of the hind legs, was reported in 1934 by Theiler, who demonstrated its cause to be a filtrable virus. The disease is not transmissible to other laboratory animals. Although in nature few mice exhibit symptoms, large numbers with no apparent illness may carry the virus in the intestinal tract. The virus can be demonstrated by the intracranial inoculation of normal mice with bacteria-free suspensions of intestinal contents taken from carrier animals. The epizoötiologic characteristics, along with the selective distribution of the lesions in the central nervous system, are closely comparable with those of poliomyelitis in man. Theiler's virus is classified among the *Enteroviruses* and conforms to the biochemical and morphological characteristics of the genus. The virus usually inhabits the digestive tract and only rarely involves the central nervous system.

Lesions. Lesions of the murine disease are most constantly found in the substantia nigra, tegmentum, reticular formation, olivary nuclei, nuclei of the fifth and eighth nerves, red and dentate nuclei. Changes in the caudate nuclei are not often observed. The anterior horns of the spinal cord are severely involved after the onset of paralysis. The lesions consist not only of vascular and perivascular changes, but also of neuronal degeneration, necrosis, and neuronophagia. The virus not only causes destruction of neurons but also results in primary demyelination. This effect on myelinated fibers has been shown to be the result of immunologic response to the virus which can be negated by immunosuppression with cyclophosphamide or antiserum to mouse thymocytes (Dal Canto and Lipton, 1975; Lipton, 1975; Lipton and Dal Canto, 1976).

Diagnosis. The diagnosis can be established by demonstrating the lesions and isolation of the virus from infected animals. The virus can be identified by appropriate methods. Although apparently producing a disease analogous to human poliomyelitis, the virus is antigenically distinct from that of poliomyelitis.

Bodian, D., and Howe, H. A.: The significance of lesions in peripheral ganglia in chimpanzee and in human poliomyelitis. J. Exp. Med., 85:231–241, 1947.

Bodian, D.: Histopathological basis of clinical findings in poliomyelitis. Am. J. Med., 6:563–578, 1949.

Dal Canto, M. C., and Lipton, H. L.: Primary demyelination in Theiler's virus infection. An ultrastructural study. Lab. Invest., 33:626–637, 1975.

Daniels, J. B., Pappenheimer, A. M., and Richardson, S.: Observations on encephalomyelitis of mice, DA strain. J. Exp. Med., 96:517–530, 1952.

Lipton, H. L.: Theiler's virus infection in mice: an unusual biphasic disease process leading to demyelination. Infect. Immun., 11:1147–1155, 1975.

Lipton, H. L., and Dal Canto, M. C.: Theiler's virus-induced demyelination: Prevention by immunosuppression. Science, 192:62–64, 1976.

Olitsky, P. K.: Further studies of the agent in intestines of normal mice which induces encephalomyelitis. Proc. Soc. Exp. Biol. Med., 43:296–300, 1940.

————: A transmissible agent (Theiler's virus) in the intestines of normal mice. J. Exp. Med., 72:113–127, 1940.

Olitsky, P. K., and Schlesinger, R. W.: Histopathology of CNS of mice infected with virus of Theiler's disease (spontaneous encephalomyelitis). Proc. Soc. Exp. Biol. Med., 47:79–83, 1941.

Theiler, M.: Spontaneous encephalomyelitis of mice—a new virus disease. Science, 80:122, 1934.

————: Spontaneous encephalomyelitis of mice. J. Exp. Med., 65:705–719, 1937.

Theiler, M., and Gard, S.: Encephalomyelitis of mice. J. Exp. Med., 72:49–67, 1940.

————: Epidemiology of mouse encephalomyelitis. J. Exp. Med., 72:79–90, 1940.

Poliomyelitis in Primates

The virus responsible for poliomyelitis in man is the type species for the genus *Enterovirus*. The virus is a common, and apparently nonpathogenic, inhabitant of the digestive tract, and is also responsible for paralytic poliomyelitis of children and young adults. The virus, under natural conditions, may also be transmitted from human to nonhuman primates such as the chimpanzee *(Pan troglodytes* or *paniscus)*, gorilla *(Gorilla gorilla)*, orangutan *(Pongo pygmaeus).* and Rhesus monkey *(Macaca mulatta).* The virus may be carried in the intestines of these species and in some instances may cause paralytic poliomyelitis. The Rhesus *(Macaca mulatta)* and crab-eating Macaque monkey *(Macaca fascicularis)* have also been used extensively in testing the poliomyelitis vaccines, which have been so efficacious in reducing the frequency of paralytic poliomyelitis.

Allmond, B. W., Jr., Froeschle, J. E., and Guilloud, N. B.: Paralytic poliomyelitis in large laboratory primates. Virologic investigation and report on the use of oral poliomyelitis virus (OPV) vaccine. Am. J. Epidemiol., 85:229–239, 1967.

Guilloud, N. B., Allmond, B. W., Froeschle, J. E., and Fitz-Gerald, F. L.: Paralytic poliomyelitis in laboratory primates. J. Am. Vet. Med. Assoc., 155:1190–1193, 1969.

Douglas, J. D., Soike, K. F., and Raynor, J.: The incidence of poliovirus in chimpanzees *(Pan troglodytes).* Lab. Anim. Care, 20:265–268, 1970.

Graves, I. L., and Oppenheimer, J. R.: Human viruses in animals in West Benghal: An ecolo-analysis. Hum. Ecol., 3:105–130, 1975.

Viral Encephalomyocarditis

A disease characterized chiefly by myocarditis was first described by Helwig and Schmidt (1945) in certain nonhuman primates, namely, the gibbon and chimpanzee, from which a viral agent had been transferred to mice and other animals with the production of encephalomyelitis and myocarditis. The virus has since been iso-

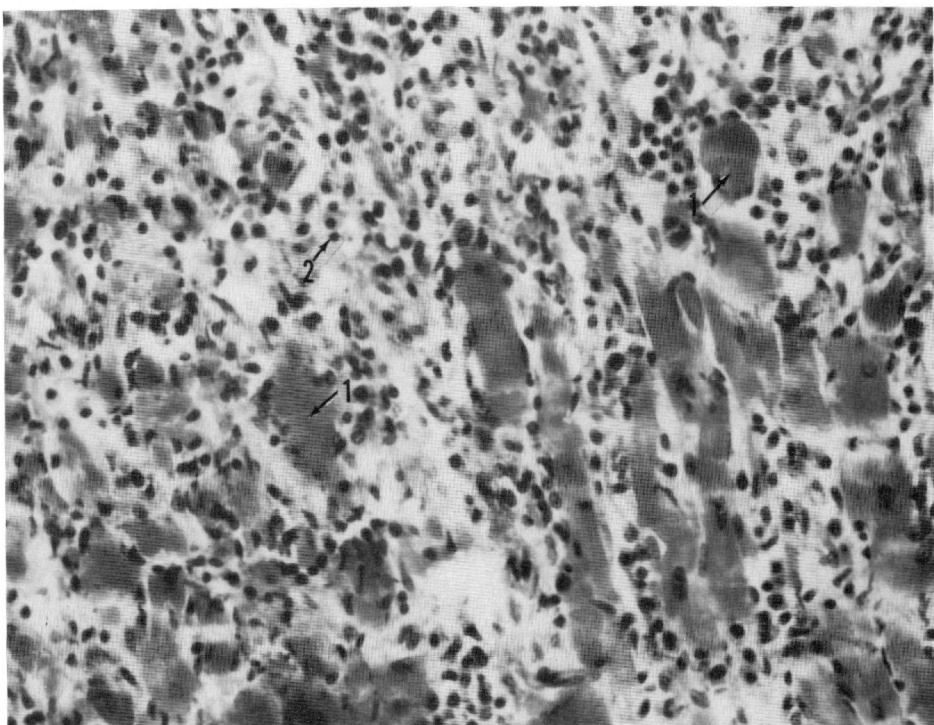

Fig. 9–37. Encephalomyocarditis, myocardium (× 350) of a gibbon. Fragmented myocardial fibers*(1)* are separated by intense infiltration of lymphocytes*(2)* and plasma cells. (Courtesy of Armed Forces Institute of Pathology.) Contributor: Lt. Col. F. C. Helwig.

lated from several animal species and associated with either encephalomyelitis, myocarditis, or both. As a spontaneous disease in animals, the disease is of greatest importance in nonhuman primates and swine, in which the virus produces a fatal myocarditis without encephalitis. The demonstration of neutralizing antibodies in human sera indicates that this agent might well be infectious for man. Wild rats probably serve as a reservoir for the virus.

The principal lesion of the disease is interstitial myocarditis. The heart usually is dilated and there is some slightly blood-tinged pericardial effusion. Occasionally bilateral hydrothorax and pulmonary edema are observed. The interstitial myocarditis seen microscopically is characterized by necrosis of myocardial fibers and rather intense infiltration with polymorphonuclear and mononuclear cells. The experimentally induced disease in mice usually results in encephalomyelitis as well as myocarditis. Hamsters and rats have been reported susceptible, with the resultant disease similar to that seen in mice. The virus is reported to induce myelitis in horses, and myocarditis in cattle. Rabbits and guinea pigs are somewhat refractory to experimental infection. Although microscopic calcification of muscle bundles has been described in guinea pigs in which attempts have been made to induce the infection, this change may not be due to the virus of encephalomyocarditis.

Craighead (1966, 1968) has obtained two variant strains of encephalomyocarditis virus through serial passage in either brain tissue (E-strain) or heart tissue (M-strain). In mice, the E strain is predominantly neurotropic, whereas the M strain principally affects the heart. In addition, the E strain produces necrosis of the acinar pancreas, parotid salivary gland, and lacrimal gland. In contrast, the M strain, which also affects the lacrimal gland, produces necrosis of the islets of Langerhans and diabetes mellitus. The experimental disease has evoked considerable interest.

Acland, H. M., and Littlejohns, I. R.: Encephalomyocarditis virus infection of pigs. 1. An outbreak in New South Wales. Austral. Vet. J., 51:409–415, 1975.

Burch, G. E., Tsui, C. Y., and Harb, J. M.: The early renal lesions of mice infected with encephalomyocarditis virus. Lab. Invest., 26:163–172, 1972.

Burch, G. E., Tsui, C. Y., and Harb, J. M.: Pancreatitis of mice infected with encephalomyocarditis virus. Path. Microbiol., 40:281–296, 1974.

Craighead, J. E.: Pathogenicity of the M and E variants of the encephalomyocarditis (EMC) virus. II. Lesions of the pancreas, parotid and lacrimal glands. Am. J. Pathol., 48:375–386, 1966.

———: Pathogenicity of the M and E variants of the encephalomyocarditis (EMC) virus. I. Myocardiotropic and neurotropic properties. Am. J. Pathol., 48:333–345, 1966.

Craighead, J. E., and McLane, M. F.: Diabetes mellitus: induction in mice by encephalomyocarditis virus. Science, 162:913–914, 1968.

Craighead, J. E., and Steinke, J.: Diabetes mellitus-like syndrome in mice infected with encephalomyocarditis virus. Am. J. Pathol., 63:119–129, 1971.

Craighead, J. E., Kanich, R. E., and Kessler, J. B.: Lesions of the islets of Langerhans in encephalomyocarditis virus-infected mice with diabetes mellitus-like disease. Am. J. Pathol., 74:287–300, 1974.

Farber, P. A., and Glascow, L. A.: Factors modifying host resistance to virus infection. II. Enhanced susceptibility of mice to encephalomyocarditis virus infection during pregnancy. Am. J. Pathol., 53:463–481, 1968.

Gainer, J. H.: Encephalomyocarditis virus infections in Florida, 1960–1966. J. Am. Vet. Med. Assoc., 151:421–425, 1967.

Gainer, J. H., Sandefur, J. R., and Bigler, W. J.: High mortality in a Florida swine herd infected with the encephalomyocarditis virus. An accompanying epizootiologic survey. Cornell Vet., 58:31–47, 1968.

Gainer, J. H.: Increased mortality in encephalomyocarditis virus-infected mice consuming cobalt sulfate: tissue concentrations of cobalt. Am. J. Vet. Res., 33:2067–2074, 1972.

Harb, J. M., Hiramoto, Y., and Burch, G. E.: Viral hepatitis in encephalomyocarditis virus-infected mice. Path. Microbiol., 40:65–78, 1974.

Hayashi, K., Boucher, D. W., and Notkins, A. L.: Virus induced diabetes mellitus. II. Relationship between beta cell damage and hyperglycemia in mice infected with encephalomyocarditis virus. Am. J. Pathol., 75:91–102, 1974.

Helwig, F. C., and Schmidt, E. C. H.: A filter passing agent producing interstitial myocarditis in anthropoid apes and small animals. Science, 102:31–33, 1945.

Littlejohns, I. R., and Acland, H. M.: Encephalomyocarditis virus infection of pigs. 2. Experimental disease. Austral. Vet. J., 51:416–422, 1975.

Roca-Garcia, M., and Sanmartin-Barberi, C.: The isolation of encephalomyocarditis virus from Aotus monkeys. Am. J. Trop. Med., 6:840–852, 1957.

Schmidt, E. C. H.: Virus myocarditis. Pathologic and experimental studies. Am. J. Pathol., 24:97–117, 1948.

Watt, D. A., and Spradbrow, P. B.: Experimental encephalomyocarditis virus infection of pigs. Austral. Vet. J., 50:316–319, 1974.

Encephalomyelitides of Swine

Certain viral agents have an affinity for the central nervous system of swine and cause diseases of some importance in the species. The virus of hog cholera, for example, may upon occasion attack the cells of the central nervous system. The lesions resulting from the presence of hog cholera virus may be distinguished with reasonable certainty by histologic methods utilizing that virus' affinity for the vasculature. Herpesvirus suis (pseudorabies) is highly neurotropic, producing encephalitis in piglets and other domestic animals. The lesions in pseudorabies are distinguished by the presence of intranuclear inclusion bodies. Japanese B encephalitis also affects pigs. Swine vesicular disease sometimes affects the central nervous system. Other viruses that have an even more selective affinity for the nervous system of swine have been recognized. The first of these is called Teschen disease, so named from the province of Czechoslovakia where the first outbreak was identified. Several outbreaks of porcine diseases with similar clinical features and histopathologic effects upon the central nervous system have been described subsequently from widely scattered parts of the world. These diseases have received various local names and

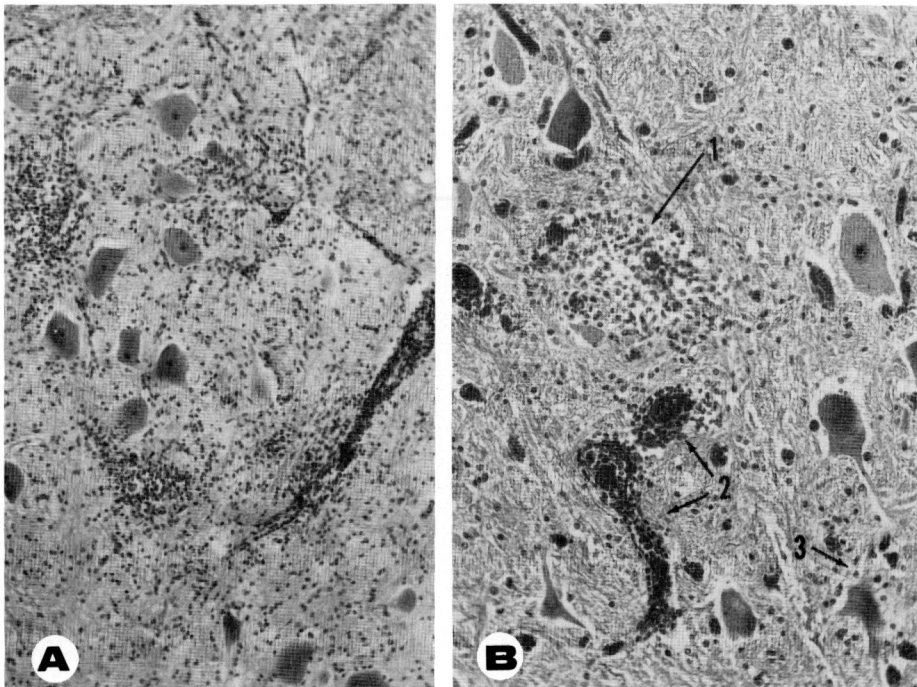

Fig. 9–38. *A*, Encephalomyelitis of swine ("benign enzootic paresis"). Ventral horn of spinal cord of a pig. (H & E, × 110.) (Courtesy of Dr. Aage Thordal-Christensen, Royal Veterinary and Agricultural College, Copenhagen.) *B*, Teschen disease. Ventral horn of spinal cord of a pig (× 160). Nodule of inflammatory cells *(1)*, perivascular "cuffing" by lymphocytes *(2)*, neuronophagia *(3)*. (Courtesy of Armed Forces Institute of Pathology.) Contributor: Dr. M. M. Kaplan.

have been studied with some intensity. Of particular importance is the development of evidence that similar viral agents, each now classified as an *Enterovirus*, are involved in these diseases. Each condition will be described briefly, comparisons made, and the present evidence outlined concerning their probable relationship to one another.

Teschen Disease. Teschen disease is also known as encephalomyelitis or poliomyelitis of swine, Bohemian pest, and meningo-encephalomyelitis suum. This disease occurs in many countries of central and western Europe, but is not clearly recognized in the Western Hemisphere. The causative virus is found in the central nervous system of infected pigs, at times in feces, transiently in the blood, and rarely in other tissues or excretions. The disease is limited to swine, and morbidity and mortality rates are both high in this species. Teschen disease is similar to poliomyelitis of man in that the virus may be isolated from the intestinal tract, and the ventral columns of gray matter in the spinal cord are rather constantly affected. However, in the porcine disease, the lesions in the cerebral cortex and cerebellum are much more extensive and indiscriminately located than in poliomyelitis. No immunologic relationship of the viruses of the two diseases has been demonstrated.

Pathogenesis. Following oral infection, the virus first invades and replicates in lymphatic tissue and epithelium of the colon, without leading to observable lesions in these tissues. Viremia follows, which allows spread of the virus to the central nervous system through the blood

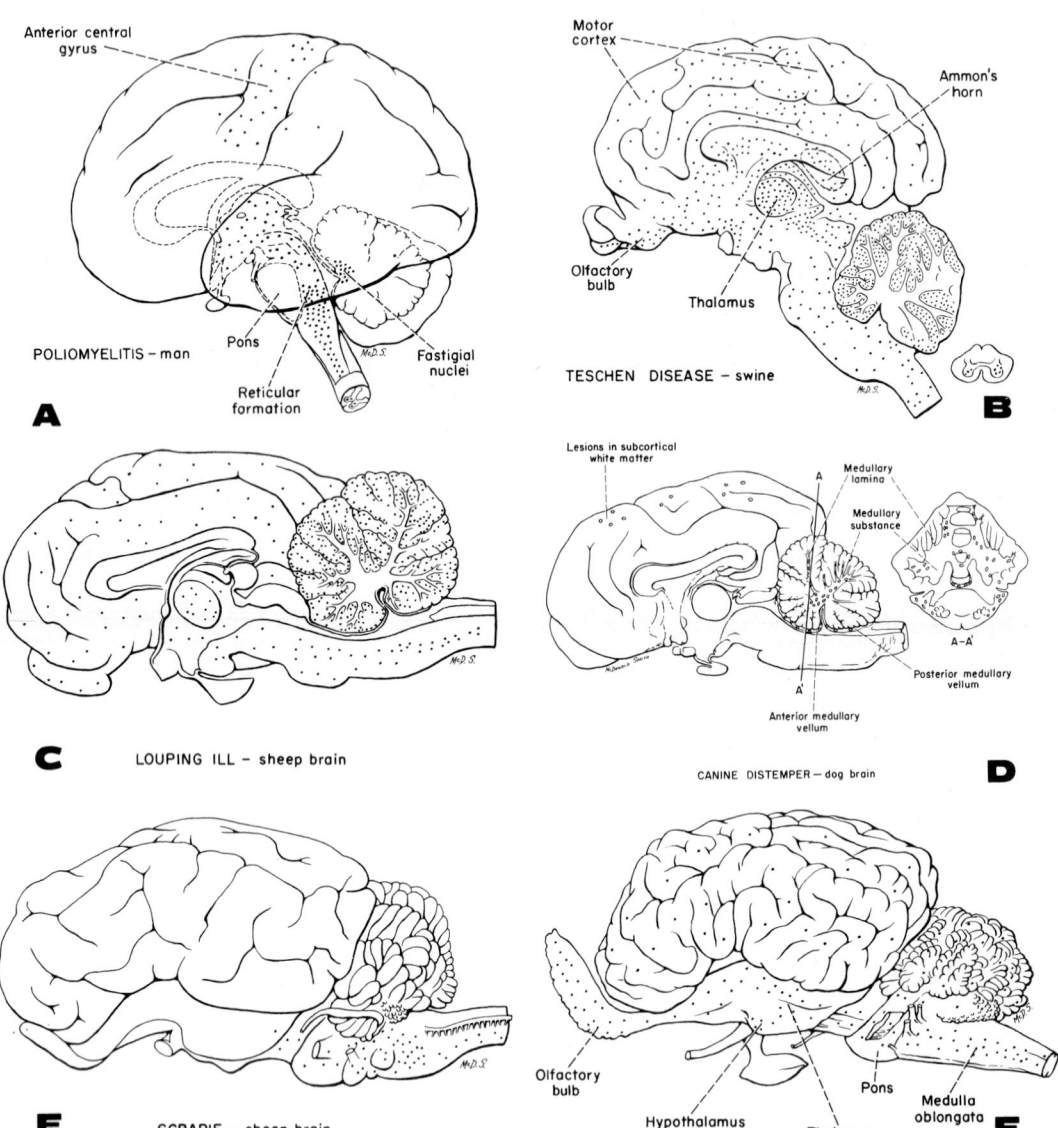

Fig. 9–39. Distribution of lesions in neurotropic viral diseases. *A*, Poliomyelitis in man. *B*, Porcine encephalomyelitis (Teschen disease), swine. *C*, "Louping ill," sheep. *D*, Canine distemper in the dog. *E*, "Scrapie," brain of a sheep. *F*, Equine encephalomyelitis, brain of a horse. (Courtesy of Armed Forces Institute of Pathology.)

stream. In the brain and spinal cord, the virus invades and replicates in neurons, glia, and capillary endothelial cells.

Signs. Following an incubation period of 10 to 20 days, the onset is usually accompanied by fever (104° to 105° F.), anorexia, lassitude, depression, and sometimes slight incoordination, particularly of the rear limbs. These symptoms are followed within a few hours or, at most, one to three days, by a stage of irritability and by stiffness of the extremities, and in severe cases, by tremors, nystagmus, violent clonic convulsions, prostration, and coma. Convulsions accompanied by loud squealing can be set off by a stimulus, such as a sudden noise. Stiffness and opisthotonus are the most persistent symptoms in some cases. A sudden drop in temperature followed by paralysis and death three or four days after onset is the usual course, although some animals die within 24 hours. Others survive but are left with a flaccid posterior paralysis. Usually, if held up on their feet, these swine will eat ravenously and can, in fact, be kept alive for long periods.

Swine of all ages are affected during epizootics, but once the disease is endemic, clinical disease is limited to newborn pigs and newly introduced pigs.

Lesions. No gross lesions specific for Teschen disease have been demonstrated in animals succumbing to this infection. Microscopic lesions are limited to the central nervous system. The virus attacks neurons of brain and cord, producing changes referable to the destruction of these nerve cells. The lesions have a specific distribution, a point that can be utilized to some extent in differential diagnosis. The spinal cord is constantly affected, the changes being principally limited to the ventral columns of the gray matter. The cerebellum also suffers rather intensely, with the Purkinje, molecular, and granular layers being involved in that order of decreasing severity. In some cases, the leptomeninges over the cerebellum are heavily infiltrated with lymphocytes. The thalamus also sustains considerable damage, and lesions of decreasing intensity occur in the basal nuclei, the base of the brain generally, olfactory bulbs, hippocampal gyrus, and the pons and medulla. The motor cortex, although more vulnerable than the rest of the cerebral cortex, is not a site of predilection.

In affected sites, multipolar nerve cells undergo degeneration of varying degree up to and including necrosis, accompanied by neuronophagia, inflammatory or glial nodules, occasional hemorrhage, and rather diffuse infiltration of leukocytes, predominantly lymphocytes. Rarely are neutrophils a part of the exudate in this disease. Accumulations of lymphocytes in the perivascular (Robin-Virchow) spaces are often seen. They are usually adjacent to lesions in the gray matter and may extend into the white matter; otherwise, the white matter is not involved.

Koestner (1966) demonstrated that the earliest lesion in neurons is detachment of ribosomes from endoplasmic reticulum, disappearance of ribosomal clusters followed by dilation of endoplasmic reticulum, and vesiculation (Fig. 9–40).

Diagnosis. The demonstration of typical microscopic lesions in the brain and spinal cord is sufficient for the presumptive diagnosis of Teschen disease. The preponderance of glial nodules, their distribution in the ventral columns of the spinal cord, the cerebral cortex and cerebellum, and the intense lymphocytic infiltration of the cerebellar leptomeninges are important to this decision. The definitive diagnosis requires that the virus be isolated and identified or that specific antibodies be demonstrable in increased quantities in the serum of recovered swine.

Benign Enzootic Paresis of Pigs (Poliomyelitis Suum). In 1959, Thordal-Christensen reported the results of studies on the clinical features, transmissibility, and pathologic anatomy of a disease of young swine first recognized in Denmark by Bendixen and Sjolte (1955). Some early cases were observed in pigs two to three

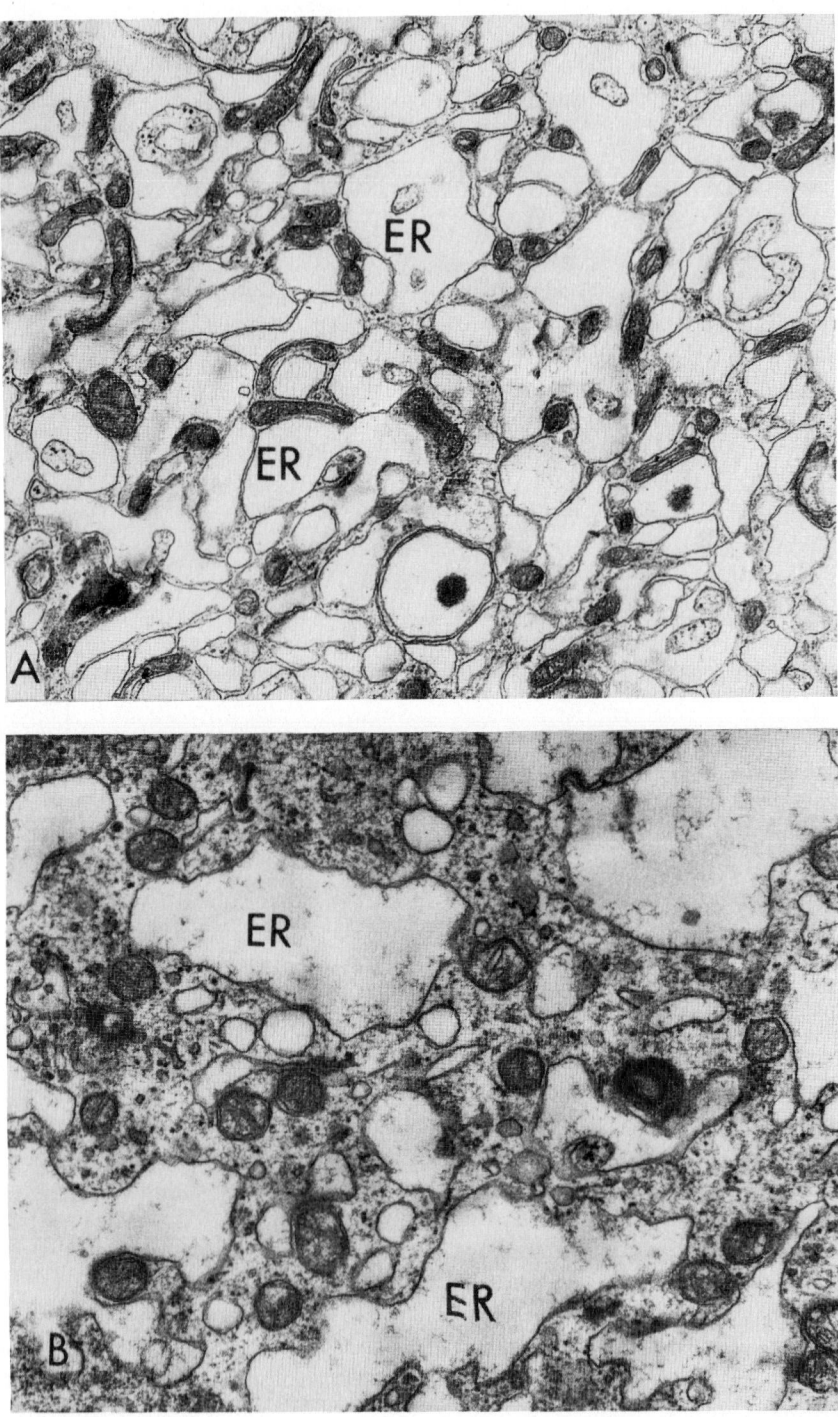

Fig. 9-40. Teschen disease of swine (porcine polioencephalomyelitis). *A,* Extensive vesiculation of neuronal endoplasmic reticulum cisternae (ER). (× 23,700.) *B,* Higher magnification of the dilated endoplasmic reticulum cisternae (ER). Mitochondria are compressed (× 35,000). (Courtesy of Dr. A. Koestner and *American Journal of Pathology*.)

months of age, but the most severe manifestations in natural cases involved unweaned piglets. The clinical signs were initiated by diminished control of the hind legs, ataxia, and "a weakened, hollow back." An elevated temperature was observed at this time. In many pigs, the nervous signs disappeared in a few days, but in others it became intensified until paresis of all four legs was apparent. Excitement, tremors, loss of equilibrium, and uncontrolled movements were manifest in many instances. Mortality rate was not usually high.

The microscopic lesions in this disease were essentially the same as for Teschen disease, but generally less intense and widespread. Aside from this quantitative difference, the lesions in enzootic paresis could not be distinguished from those of Teschen disease. Serum from pigs recovered from enzootic paresis will neutralize the virus of Teschen disease. It is apparent, therefore, that this disease described in Denmark is caused by a virus that is similar to the virus of Teschen disease, differing only in the severity of the disease that it causes.

Talfan Disease. In 1957, a disease of the nervous system of young swine was described from England. The clinical features, morbidity and mortality rates, microscopic lesions, and transmissibility closely resembled the Danish disease: enzootic paresis of swine. Later evidence indicated that enzootic paresis, Talfan, and Teschen disease are caused by closely related viruses, differing only in the virulence of the clinical manifestations.

Canadian Viral Encephalomyelitis (North American Encephalomyelitis). In 1960, Richards and Savan reported the occurrence of a transmissible viral encephalomyelitis in suckling pigs in Canada. The lesions, transmissibility, infectivity, morbidity and mortality rates were essentially the same as for Teschen disease. Convalescent serum from pigs recovered from Teschen disease would neutralize the virus of

this Canadian disease. These authors also presented evidence indicating that a similar disease has occurred in some swine herds in the United States. Koestner et al. (1962) confirmed this by demonstrating a similar viral encephalomyelitis in suckling pigs in Ohio. Therefore it appears that viral diseases essentially similar to, although less destructive than, Teschen disease occur in many parts of the world, including the Western Hemisphere.

Bendixen, H. C., and Sjolte, J. P.: Undersogelser Vedrørende Optrasden of Enzootish (Overførbar) Griselammelse (Poliomyelitis Suum) i Danmark. Nord. Vet. Med., 7:97–140, 1955.

Betts, A. O.: Porcine enteroviruses. *In* Diseases of Swine, 2nd ed., edited by H. W. Dunne. Ames, Iowa State Univ. Press, 1964.

Bück, G., and Guesnel, J. J.: Infectious paralysis of pigs (Teschen disease) in Madagascar. Bull. Epizoöt. Dis. Afr., 2:279–281, 1954.

Chaproniere, D. M., Done, J. T., and Andrewes, C. H.: Comparative serological studies on Talfan and Teschen diseases and similar conditions. Br. J. Exp. Pathol., 39:74–77, 1958.

Dobberstein, J.: Histopathologie des Zentralnervensystems bei der Poliomyelitis des Schweines. Ztschr. Infectionskr., 59:54–80, 1942.

Done, J. T.: The pathological differentiation of diseases of the central nervous system of the pig. (Proc. 75th Ann. Congr. B. V. A. Cambridge, 1957) Vet. Rec., 69:1341–1349, 1957.

Dunne, H. W.: Porcine enteroviruses. *In* Diseases of Swine, 4th ed., edited by H. W. Dunne and A. D. Leman. Ames, Iowa State Univ. Press, 1975.

Gardiner, M. R.: Polio-encephalomyelitis of pigs in Western Australia. Aust. Vet. J., 38:24–26, 1962. VB 2266–62.

Harding, J. D. J., Done, J. T., and Kershaw, G. F.: A transmissible polioencephalomyelitis of pigs (Talfan disease). Vet. Rec., 69:824–832, 1957.

Horstmann, D. M.: Experiments with Teschen disease (virus encephalomyelitis of swine). J. Immunol., 69:379–394, 1952.

Ishitani, B., et al.: Studies on a swine virus disease with nervous symptoms which occurred in the winter of this year. II. Histopathological observations. Jpn. J. Vet. Sci., 16:138–139, 1954.

Jones, T. C.: Encephalomyelitides. *In* Diseases of Swine, 4th ed., edited by H. W. Dunne and A. D. Leman. Ames, Iowa State Univ. Press, 1975.

Kaplan, M. M., and Meranze, D. R.: Porcine virus encephalomyelitis and its possible biological relationship to human poliomyelitis. Vet. Med., 43:330–341, 1948.

Kasza, L.: Swine polioencephalomyelitis viruses isolated from the brains and intestines of pigs. Am. J. Vet. Res., 26:131–137, 1965.

Kment, A.: Zur histopathologie des Zentralnervensystems bei der Teschener Schweinelähmung. Wien. Tierärztl. Wochenschr., 27:361–362, 1940.

Koestner, A., Kasza, L., and Holman, J. E.: Electron microscopic evaluation of the pathogenesis of porcine polioencephalomyelitis. Am. J. Pathol., 49:325–327, 1966.

Koestner, A., Long, J. F., and Kasza, L.: Occurrence of viral polioencephalomyelitis in suckling pigs in Ohio. J. Am. Vet. Med. Assoc., 140:811–814, 1962.

Long, J. F., Koestner, A., and Kasza, L.: Pericarditis and myocarditis in germfree and pathogen-free pigs experimentally infected with a porcine polioencephalomyelitis virus. Lab. Invest., 15:1128, 1966.

Long, J. F., Koestner, A., and Liss, L.: Experimental porcine polioencephalomyelitis in germfree pigs. A silver carbonate study of neuronal degeneration and glial response. Pathologia Vet., 4:186–198, 1967.

Manuelidis, E. E., Sprinz, H., and Horstmann, D. M.: Pathology of Teschen disease. Am. J. Pathol., 30:567–597, 1954.

Mayr, A., and Schwöbel, W.: Züchtung des Virus der ansteckenden Schweinelähmung (Teschener Krankheit) in der Gewebkulturen. Mh. prakt. Tierheilk., 8:49–51, 1956.

———: Die Züchtung des Virus der ansteckenden Schweinelähmung (Teschener Krankheit) in Nierengewebekulturen von Schwein and Charakterisierung des Kulturvirus. Zentbl. Bakt., Paras., Infekt. Hyg., 168:336–349, 1957.

Mills, J. H. L., and Nielsen, S. W.: Porcine polioencephalomyelitides. Adv. Vet. Sci., 12:33–104, 1968.

Richards, W. P. C., and Savan, M.: Viral encephalomyelitis of pigs. A preliminary report on the tranmissibility and pathology of a disease observed in Ontario. Cornell Vet., 50:132–155, 1960.

Sasahara, J., et al.: Studies of a swine virus disease with nervous symptoms which occurred in the winter of this year. I. Isolation of the virus. Jpn. J. Vet. Sci., 16:139, 1954.

Thordal-Christensen, A.: A Study of Benign Enzootic Paresis of Pigs in Denmark. Copenhagen, Carl FR. Mortensen, Ltd., 1959.

Treffny, L.: Massenerkrankungen von Schweinen in Teschner Land. Zverolekarsky Obzor., 23:235–236, 1930.

Watanabe, H., Pospisil, Z., Mensik, J.: Study on the pigs infected with virulent Teschen disease virus (KNM strain) with special reference to immunofluorescence. Jpn. J. Vet. Res., 19:87–102, 1971.

Swine Vesicular Disease

Any disease outbreak that affects cloven-hoofed animals and has clinical features of foot and mouth disease (aphthous fever) is bound to attract a great deal of attention. This was the case when in 1966, in Italy, a febrile disease of swine was recognized in association with vesicles on the mouth, snout, and feet. Lameness and ulcerations followed the early vesiculation (Nardelli et al., 1968). All these features are indistinguishable from the signs of foot and mouth disease. A distinctive *Enterovirus* has been identified in association with swine vesicular disease, making it possible to differentiate this infection from vesicular exanthema (calicivirus), aphthous fever *(Enterovirus* or *Aphthovirus)*, or vesicular stomatitis *(Vesiculovirus)*.

Swine vesicular disease now has been recognized in the United Kingdom, Hong Kong, Austria, France, Poland, and Italy. Some strains of the virus produce a disseminated encephalitis following natural or experimental exposure (Monlux et al., 1974, 1975). Also of interest is the close relationship, as determined by immunodiffusion tests, of the swine vesicular disease virus and Coxsackie B virus, a common pathogen to human beings. The swine virus also is suspected of infecting laboratory workers who have been in contact with it. It has been postulated (Brown, Talbot and Burrows, 1973) that the swine vesicular disease virus and Coxsackie B virus may have had the same antecedents. Coxsackie B virus has been associated with aseptic meningitis, encephalitis, myositis, orchitis, myocarditis, diarrhea, respiratory disease, and vesicular and papular rash in people. It also has been isolated from neonatal infants with a fulminating disease culminating in degenerative changes in many organs.

Lesions. Changes in the stratified epithelium are most evident in the skin of the coronary band of the hoof, the metatarsus and metacarpus, the snout, tongue, and tonsil. Coagulation necrosis in the malpighian layer results in vesiculation and sloughing, and is followed by regenerative pseudoepitheliomatous hyperplasia. Epithelial cells in renal pelvis, bladder, tonsillar crypts, ducts of pancreas, and salivary glands undergo degenerative changes, with formation of periodic acid-Schiff-positive material in individual cells

(Lenghaus and Mann, 1976). Some intradermal sweat glands undergo necrosis with subsequent collection of leukocytes. Nonspecific aggregations of leukocytes may be found in subepithelial stroma of the trachea, and in salivary glands.

Brown, F., Talbot, P., and Burrows, R.: Antigenic differences between isolates of swine vesicular disease virus and their relationship to Coxsackie B5 virus. Nature (London), 245:315–316, 1973.

Burrows, R., Greig, A., and Goodridge, D.: Swine vesicular disease. Res. Vet. Sci., 15:141–144, 1973.

Graves, J. H.: Serological relationship of swine vesicular disease virus and Coxsackie B virus. Nature (London), 245:314–315, 1973.

Lenghaus, C., and Mann, J. A.: General pathology of experimental swine vesicular disease. Vet. Pathol., 13:186–196, 1976.

Lenghaus, C., Mann, J. A., Done, J. T., and Bradley, R.: Neuropathology of experimental swine vesicular disease in pigs. Res. Vet. Sci., 21:19–27, 1976.

Monlux, W. S., Graves, J. H., and McKercher, P. D.: Brain and spinal cord lesions in pigs inoculated with swine vesicular disease virus (Hong Kong strain). Am. J. Vet. Res., 35:615–617, 1974.

Monlux, W. S., McKercher, P. D., and Graves, J. H.: Brain and spinal cord lesions in pigs inoculated with swine vesicular disease (UKG Strain) virus and coxsackievirus B5. Am. J. Vet. Res., 36:1745–1749, 1975.

Nardelli, L., et al.: A foot and mouth disease syndrome in pigs caused by an enterovirus. Nature (London), 219:1275–1276, 1968.

Diseases Caused by Rhinoviruses

The rhinoviruses are found in the upper respiratory tracts (*rhino* = nose) of man and animals. They, of course, conform to the overall characteristics of the family Picornaviridae and differ from the genus *Enterovirus* in a few respects. The rhinoviruses are acid-labile (pH 3) and have a buoyant density in cesium chloride of 1.38–1.43 g/cm^3. The virus of aphthous fever (foot and mouth disease) is currently placed in the genus *Rhinovirus*, but several differences in the virus have caused some (Newman et al., 1973) to propose that a separate genus, *Aphthovirus*, be created for this organism. Aphthous fever virus differs from other current rhinoviruses on the basis of density in cesium chloride (1.43 g/cm^3) and base composition of RNA.

Aphthous Fever (Foot and Mouth Disease, Epizoötic Aphtha)

Aphthous fever is an important and widespread disease caused by a virus with strong epitheliotropic features. The disease occurs naturally in cloven-hoofed animals, the most important of which are cattle, sheep, goats, and swine. It may also affect ruminants, such as deer, goats, and antelope, and under some conditions they act as reservoirs for the infection. Guinea pigs, suckling mice, birds, and carnivores are susceptible to experimental inoculation with the virus. Natural infection may occur in man, in whom the disease is usually mild and limited to acute fever associated with the appearance of vesicles on the hands, feet, and oral mucosae.

Although aphthous fever is prevalent in all of Europe, Africa, much of Asia, and in some countries of South America, the disease has been prevented from re-entering the United States since 1929, when a severe outbreak occurred in California. This and previous outbreaks were stamped out by stringent quarantine of infected areas and slaughter of exposed and infected animals. Important outbreaks have occurred in Mexico and Canada, but appear to have been controlled.

The virus occurs in seven principal antigenic types. These, in the international nomenclature, are designated as "A," "O" (Vallée and Carré) and "C" (Waldmann), SAT-1, SAT-2, SAT-3 (Galloway, Brooksby, and Henderson) (SA = South Africa), and Asia −1. Although the symptoms and lesions produced by each virus type are essentially similar, infection with one virus does not immunize against the others. In recent years numerous subtypes have been identified which are also antigenically distinct. These are designated by a subnumber, i.e., A_5.

As indicated earlier, this virus is presently included in the genus *Rhinovirus*, but it has been proposed that it be placed in a separate genus, *Aphthovirus*.

Pathogenesis. Features of particular significance in this disease are the extreme infectiousness of the virus and the ease with which it can be carried, not only by infected animals and their products, but mechanically by man and other animals. It may be transported on the shoes or clothing of human beings, in or on the bodies of migratory birds or animals, as well as in such products as raw hides, milk, bedding, and forage. Infection is presumed to occur per os, with primary aphthae developing on the lips or oral mucosae. The virus soon gains access to the blood stream and is widely disseminated through the body, producing secondary lesions in epithelial tissues. Only the greater severity and wider dissemination of the secondary lesions distinguish them from primary lesions. The virus can be isolated from the blood during the febrile stage and becomes concentrated in the fluid of epithelial vesicles when the temperature falls.

Signs. The signs are directly related to the lesions of the disease. Those in the oral mucosa produce excess salivation and make eating painful, thus causing the infected animal to refuse food and water. Smacking of the lips and tongue is characteristic. The epithelium of the dorsum of the tongue usually becomes eroded. Lesions of the feet may produce lameness. Aphthae may be detected around other parts of the body that are lightly haired, such as the skin of the udder, the vulva, and the conjunctiva.

In young animals (lambs and calves), acute gastroenteritis and myocarditis are common and the mortality rate is very high. In animal populations that have experienced exposure to the disease, the mortality rate is low, rarely more than 5% in adult animals, although certain virus strains can cause a mortality rate as high as 60%.

Lesions. On cattle, the distribution of the vesicular lesions is characteristic. The oral mucosa over the lips, dorsum of the tongue, and palate is most severely involved. Lesions occur in the skin near the coronary band adjacent to the interdigital space, and are also frequent in other areas in which the hair is sparse, such as the vulva, teats, and udder. The conjunctiva may be affected, as may be that part of the forestomach which is lined with squamous epithelium (rumen, reticulum, and omasum). Small epidermal vesicles may also occur in grossly normal skin of the brisket, abdomen, hock, carpus, and perineum. In addition to these specific vesicular lesions, punctate hemorrhages or diffuse edema of the mucosa may be observed in the abomasum and small intestine. The mucosa of the large intestine may be hyperemic and blue-red, and some animals may bear subpleural, subepithelial or subepicardial hemorrhages. These, however, are not considered primary lesions.

The specific lesions in their early stages are microscopic and are limited to the epithelium at the sites of predilection. The lesion starts with localized "balloon" degeneration of cells in the middle of the stratum spinosum of the epithelium. Here the intercellular prickles are lost; the epithelial cells become round and detached from one another; their cytoplasm takes an intensely eosinophilic stain, and their nuclei are pyknotic. Edema fluid containing bits of fibrin accumulates between and separates the cells. Neutrophils infiltrate the epithelium at this stage. Liquefaction necrosis and accumulation of serum and leukocytes produce vesicles roofed over by the compressed stratum corneum, lucidum, and granulosum, and extending down to the basal layer, which usually remains in place over the heavily congested dermis. These small vesicles **(aphthae)** coalesce to form bullae, which cause large areas of epithelium to be detached and easily shed or rubbed off. Loss of epithelium is most common on the dorsal surface of the anterior two-thirds of the bovine tongue, which is separated by a transverse notch from a dorsal eminence occupying the posterior third of the tongue. The entire epithelium over the anterior area may be lost, leaving a raw, red surface that oozes blood. The pain from this denuded area explains the severe anorexia which is often a sign. In addition to the virus, the vesicles contain necrotic epithelial cells, leukocytes, occasional erythrocytes and, in the late stages, bacteria. Small pleomorphic bodies have been described in lymphocytes and epithelial cells, but these have not been established as virus particles or specific "inclusions."

Lesions in the myocardium are most common in the fatal disease in very young calves or lambs, but also occur in pigs and young goats. The lesions observed in the wall and septum of the left ventricle, seldom in the atria, appear as small, grayish foci of irregular size, which may give the myocardium a somewhat striped appearance (so-called tiger heart). Microscopically, hyaline degeneration and necrosis of myocardial fibers are accompanied by an intense lymphocytic, occasionally neutrophilic, infiltration. The myocardial lesion is not strictly specific for infections with the virus of foot and mouth disease, but it is believed to be the one that most commonly causes death of newborn animals.

In the skeletal muscle, lesions similar to those in the myocardium may be observed. Sharply delimited areas of necrosis are seen grossly as gray foci of various sizes, and microscopically as necrosis of muscle bundles associated with rather intense leukocytic infiltration. A similar, but much more severe, acute myositis occurs in suckling mice experimentally inoculated with the virus. The susceptibility of the musculature of young mice is being utilized with increasing frequency in experimental study of the virus.

Diagnosis. In the differential diagnosis of aphthous fever (foot and mouth disease), it is necessary to consider all other so-called "vesicular diseases" such as vesicular exanthema, swine vesicular disease, and vesicular stomatitis. These cannot be differentiated with absolute certainty by their symptoms and lesions. It is necessary, therefore, to isolate and identify the virus or to demonstrate complement-fixing or virus-neutralizing antibodies in recovered cases. The agar gel diffusion reaction is also useful in detecting antigenic relationships. The immunofluorescent methods are used to detect viral antigen in cells (Mohanty and Cottral, 1970).

Capel-Edwards, M.: The susceptibility of small mammals to foot-and-mouth disease virus. Vet. Bull., *41*:815–823, 1971.

Daubney, R.: Foot and mouth diseases; the fixed virus types. J. Comp. Pathol. Ther., *47*:259–281, 1934.

Domanski, E., and Fitko, R.: Disturbances of the pituitary and other hormonal glands after foot and mouth disease. Proc. 16th Intern. Vet. Cong., Madrid. *2*:421–423, 1959.

Frenkel, H. S.: Histologic changes in explanted bovine epithelial tongue tissue infected with the virus of foot and mouth disease. Am. J. Vet. Res., *10*:142–145, 1949.

Gailiunas, P.: Microscopic skin lesions in cattle with foot-and-mouth disease. Arch. Ges. Virusforsch., *25*:188–200, 1968.

Gailiunas, P., Cottral, G. E., and Seibold, H. R.: Teat lesions in heifers experimentally infected with foot-and-mouth disease virus. Am. J. Vet. Res., *25*:1062–1069, 1964.

Galloway, I. A., Henderson, W. M., and Brooksby, J. B.: Strains of the virus of foot and mouth disease recovered from outbreaks in Mexico. Proc. Soc. Exp. Biol. Med., *69*:57–63, 1948.

Gillespie, J. H.: Propagation of Type C foot-and-mouth-disease virus in eggs and effects of the egg-cultivated virus on cattle. Cornell Vet., *45*:170–179, 1955.

McVicar, J. W., and Sutmoller, P.: Three variants of foot-and-mouth disease virus type O: cell culture characteristics and antigenic differences. Am. J. Vet. Res., *33*:1627–1634, 1972.

———: Three variants of foot-and-mouth disease virus type O: agar gel diffusion reactions. Am. J. Vet. Res., *33*:1635–1640, 1972.

Mohanty, G. C., and Cottral, G. E.: Immunofluorescent detection of foot-and-mouth disease virus in the esophageal-pharyngeal fluids of inoculated cattle. Am. J. Vet. Res., *31*:1187–1196, 1970.

Platt, H.: Observations on the pathology of experimental foot and mouth disease in adult guinea pigs. J. Pathol. Bact., *76*:119–131, 1958.

———: Phagocytic activity in squamous epithelium and its role in cellular susceptibility to foot-and-mouth disease. Nature, Lond., *190*:1075–1076, 1961. VB 104–62.

Seibold, H. R.: The histopathology of foot and mouth

disease in pregnant and lactating mice. Am. J. Vet. Res., 21:870–877, 1960.

Skinner, H. H.: Propagation of strains of foot and mouth disease virus in unweaned white mice. Proc. Roy. Soc. Med., 44:1041–1044, 1951.

Sutmoller, P., and McVicar, J. W.: Three variants of foot-and-mouth disease virus type O: Exposure of cattle. Am. J. Vet. Res., 33:1641–1648, 1972.

Terpstra, C.: Pathogenesis of foot-and-mouth disease in experimentally infected pigs. Bull. Off. Internat. Epizoot., 77:859–874, 1972.

Bovine Respiratory Infection and Rhinoviruses

The etiologic complexity of acute respiratory infection is no more clearly evident than in the bovine species. Respiratory disease in young cattle is common and often occurs in relation to transport of the animals. A large number of microorganisms have been recovered from cattle with upper respiratory infections, including the following viruses: infectious bovine rhinotracheitis-bovine herpesvirus, bovine viral diarrhea virus, parainfluenza-3, adenovirus, rhinovirus, syncytial viruses, other bovine herpesviruses, enteroviruses, and reoviruses. The confusing array of etiologic agents (some occur simultaneously) and clinical signs undoubtedly helped give origin to the designations bovine shipping fever complex, bovine respiratory tract disease, or bovine respiratory disease complex.

Rhinoviruses in man are generally associated with the common cold. Bovine rhinoviruses may be a factor in bovine upper respiratory disease, but are so often isolated in the company of other viruses and bacteria that their pathogenic properties may be questioned. Experimental infection with bovine rhinovirus in susceptible calves has resulted in some cases in fever, anemia, coughing, rhinitis, congestion in nasal turbinates and trachea, depression, and hyperpnea. Necropsy disclosed disseminated foci of atelectasis, interstitial lymphocytic infiltration, and some foci of pneumonic consolidation. Virus is recoverable from the upper respiratory tract. It may be concluded that bovine rhinovirus may produce a mild respiratory disease by itself. Other factors may be necessary to result in severe or fatal disease.

The diagnosis of rhinovirus infection depends upon isolation and identification of the virus or demonstration of an appropriate immunologic response.

Bögel, K.: Bovine rhinoviruses. J. Am. Vet. Med. Assoc., 152:780–783, 1968.

Mohanty, S. B., Lillie, M. G., Albert, T. F., and Sass, B.: Experimental exposure of calves to a bovine rhinovirus. Am. J. Vet. Res., 30:1105–1111, 1969.

Rosenquist, B. D., English, J. E., Johnson, D. W., and Loan, R. W.: Mixed viral etiology of a shipping fever epizootic in cattle. Am. J. Vet. Res., 31:989–994, 1970.

Rosenquist, B. D.: Rhinoviruses: isolation from cattle with acute respiratory disease. Am. J. Vet. Res., 32:685–688, 1971.

Rosenquist, B. D., and Dobson, A. W.: Multiple viral infection in calves with acute bovine respiratory tract disease. Am. J. Vet. Res., 35:363–365, 1974.

Diseases Due to Caliciviruses

Organisms classified in the genus *Calicivirus* are distinguished from other Picornaviridae by the cup-shaped structures on the surface of the virion (calici = cup). Also, polyacrylamide gel electrophoresis demonstrates that Caliciviruses have a single capsid protein with molecular weight of approximately 61,000 daltons. The virions are also slightly larger, 35 to 40 nm, than other Picornaviridae. Other chemical features also distinguish this genus (Bachrach and Hess, 1973). At present, three disease-producing caliciviruses have been identified: the virus of vesicular exanthema of swine, the San Miguel sea lion virus, and the feline calicivirus.

Vesicular Exanthema

Vesicular exanthema of swine is characterized by fever and vesicle formation in the epithelium of the snout, lips, nostrils, tongue, feet, and mammary glands. It was first described in 1935, by Traum, whose observations were made on garbage-fed swine in California. The occurrence of this disease in a geographic area from which aphthous fever had been eliminated only with great economic loss, and the similarity of the symptoms and lesions of the two diseases, magnified its importance. Actually, vesicular exanthema runs a mild, rapid course of about ten days and is almost never fatal. So that proper measures for control can be adopted, it is essential that it be differentiated from aphthous fever, vesicular stomatitis, and swine vesicular disease, which produce similar manifestations.

Vesicular exanthema has not been reported in swine in the United States since 1956, but epidemiologic evidence prompted Madin (1975) to postulate that the causative virus had its origin in some natural reservoir and was transmitted by feeding uncooked garbage to swine. This theory appears to be partially confirmed by the identification of the San Miguel sea lion virus from aborted sea lion fetuses on the island of San Miguel, California. This virus appears to be nearly identical to the calicivirus of vesicular exanthema. It seems likely that sea lion *(Zalophus c. californianus)* carcasses were fed to swine to cause the initial porcine infection, and that the disease was spread widely by uncooked pork scraps taken from railroad dining cars and fed to other swine.

Lesions. The lesions of vesicular exanthema appear 16 to 28 hours after experimental inoculation of vesicle fluid; they are slightly reddened areas at the sites of inoculation. Abrupt rise in temperature to as high as 107° F. is accompanied or followed shortly by the appearance of small vesicles filled with clear or straw-colored fluid. The vesicles occur in the epithelium of the snout, nose, lips, gums, tongue, between digits, around the coronary band, on the ball of the foot, or even in the dewclaws. They may develop on the udder and teats of nursing sows. Vesicles sometimes coalesce. Spontaneous rupture of all vesicles occurs after a few days and is soon followed by healing. The covering of eroded areas becomes brown and dry and gradually sloughs off. After seven to ten days, only slightly scarred areas are left at the sites of vesiculation. Ulceration and presumably secondary bacterial infections of lesions on the feet may cause a few of the heavier animals to remain lame for some time. The cutaneous lesions are believed to be morphologically indistinguishable from the intraepithelial lesions of foot and mouth disease, but systemic lesions are not seen in vesicular exanthema.

Diagnosis. The diagnosis of vesicular exanthema depends upon complement-fixation tests, animal inoculations or virus isolation and identification, which are necessary to distinguish it from foot-and-mouth disease, vesicular stomatitis, or swine vesicular disease.

Bachrach, H. I., and Hess, W. R.: Animal picornaviruses with a single species of capsid protein. Biochem. Biophys. Res. Commun., 55:141–149, 1973.

Bankowski, R. A., Keith, H. B., Stuart, E. E., and Kummer, M.: Recovery of the fourth immunological type of vesicular exanthema virus in California. J. Am. Vet. Med. Assoc., 125:383–384, 1954.

Crawford, A. B.: Experimental vesicular exanthema of swine. J. Am. Vet. Med. Assoc., 90:380–395, 1937.

Madin, S. H.: Vesicular exanthema. In Disease of Swine, 4th ed., edited by H. W. Dunne and A. D. Leman. Ames, Iowa State Univ. Press, 1975.

Madin, S. H., and Traum, J.: Experimental studies with vesicular exanthema of swine. Vet. Med., 48:395–400, 1953.

Sawyer, J. C.: Vesicular exanthema of swine and San Miguel sea lion virus. J. Am. Vet. Med. Assoc., 169:707–709, 1976.

Smith, A. W., and Akers, T. G.: Vesicular exanthema of swine. J. Am. Vet. Med. Assoc., 169:700–703, 1976.

Smith, A. W., Akers, T. G., Madin, S. H., and Vedros, N. A.: San Miguel sea lion virus isolation, preliminary characterization and relationship to vesicular exanthema of swine virus. Nature (London), 244:108–109, 1973.

Traum, J.: Vesicular exanthema of swine. J. Am. Vet. Med. Assoc., 88:316–334, 1936.

Feline Respiratory Disease Due to Calicivirus (Picornavirus Infection, Interstitial Pneumonia, Ulcerative Stomatitis, Feline Calicivirus Disease)

Many viruses have been isolated from cats during the course of respiratory diseases that are difficult to distinguish on the basis of clinical signs. Feline viral rhino-tracheitis, due to a feline *Herpesvirus,* appears to be the most frequent. Infection with organisms of the genera *Calicivirus* and *Reovirus* can also be distinguished by identifying the viral agent. Early references to feline picornavirus infection at this writing are referred to as feline *Calicivirus* infection, the current genus in the family Picornaviridae in which this virus is classified. These three viruses may be distinguished (Kahn and Gillespie, 1970) by their characteristic effects upon cultures of feline cells. *Herpesvirus* induces Cowdry type A inclusions in nuclei and the formation of multinucleated giant cells. Feline *Picornavirus (Calicivirus)* produces rapidly developing cytopathogenic effects on the culture cells without formation of inclusions or polykaryocytes; the cells become rounded with fibrillar processes and detach from the culture glass. Feline *Reovirus* infection of cultured cells causes slowly progressive cytopathic degeneration with formation of cytoplasmic viral inclusions.

Signs. Natural and experimental infection of susceptible cats result in fever (often biphasic), depression, anorexia, dyspnea or polypnea, pulmonary rales, and vesicles leading to ulcers of the nostrils, tongue, or hard palate. Sneezing may occur, but nasal or conjunctival discharge is not a significant feature (Kahn and Gillespie, 1971; Hoover and Kahn, 1975; Love, 1975).

Lesions. The effects of caliciviruses on the tissues vary with strains of differing virulence. The significant lesions include vesicles of the nostrils, tongue, oral mucosa, or hard palate. These vesicles are followed by further necrosis of cells in the epithelium, leaving sharply demarcated ulcers that heal slowly. Viral antigen may be demonstrated in cells at the margin of these ulcers by immunofluorescence technique (Holzinger and Kahn, 1970).

The lungs are affected by multifocal zones of interstitial pneumonia which start with interalveolar infiltration of cells, followed by adenomatous proliferation of al-veolar lining cells, with eventual shedding of these cells into the alveoli. These changes result in sharply demarcated, irregularly outlined gross lesions in the lungs. These are solid dark purple, often located near the periphery of the lung. Sharply demarcated bands of congestion in about a fifth of inoculated cats have been described (Holzinger and Kahn, 1970), but the underlying reason for this change has not been recognized. Ultrastructurally, virions may be seen in relation to smooth endoplasmic reticulum, often in vesicles (Love and Sabine, 1975). These may also be seen in crystalline arrays, along membranous cisternae, and in fine fibrillar material.

Diagnosis. Diagnosis is made by identification of the virus by isolation or immunologic means. The lesions may be helpful in distinguishing herpesvirus, and the initial effects of the virus, as mentioned previously, are helpful in distinguishing among *Herpesvirus, Calicivirus,* and *Reovirus* infections.

Flagstad, A.: Experimental picornavirus infection in cats. Acta Vet. Scand., *14*:501–510, 1973.

Holzinger, E. A., and Kahn, D. E.: Pathologic features of picornavirus infections in cats. Am. J. Vet. Res., *31*:1623–1630, 1970.

Hoover, E. A., and Kahn, D. E.: Lesions produced by feline picornaviruses of different virulence in pathogen-free cats. Vet. Pathol., *10*:307–322, 1973.

————: Experimentally induced feline calicivirus infection: clinical signs and lesions. J. Am. Vet. Med. Assoc., *166*:463–468, 1975.

Kahn, D. E., and Gillespie, J. H.: Feline viruses. X. Characterization of a newly-isolated picornavirus causing interstitial pneumonia and ulcerative stomatitis in the domestic cat. Cornell Vet., *60*:669–683, 1970.

Kahn, D. E., and Gillespie, J. H.: Feline viruses: pathogenesis of picornavirus infection in the cat. Am. J. Vet. Res., *32*:521–531, 1971.

Kahn, D. E., Hoover, E. A., and Bittle, J. L.: Induction of immunity to feline caliciviral disease. Infect. Immun., *11*:1003–1009, 1975.

Kahn, D. E., and Hoover, E. A.: Feline caliciviral disease: experimental immunoprophylaxis. Am. J. Vet. Res., *37*:279–284, 1976.

Love, D. N.: Pathogenicity of a strain of feline calicivirus for domestic kittens. Aust. Vet. J., *51*:541–546, 1975.

Love, D. N., and Sabine, M.: Electron microscopic observation of feline kidney cells infected with a feline calicivirus. Arch. Virol., *48*:213–228, 1975.

Povey, R. C., Wardley, R. C., and Jessen, H.: Feline picornavirus infection: the in vivo carrier state. Vet. Rec., *92*:224–229, 1973.

Studdert, M. J., Martin, M. C., and Peterson, J. E.: Viral diseases of the respiratory tract of cats: isolation and properties of viruses tentatively classified as picornaviruses. Am. J. Vet. Res., *31*:1723–1732, 1970.

REOVIRIDAE

The family of viruses called Reoviridae is presently made up of two accepted genera, *Reovirus* and *Orbivirus*, and another tentatively called *"Rotavirus."* The name Reoviridae is an acronym (R = respiratory, e = enteric, o = orphan), which gives a clue to the fact that many of these viruses were recovered from animals or people but not clearly associated with disease. Some have subsequently been shown to be pathogens. These viruses have a genome consisting of several separate pieces of double-stranded RNA, and they also share other properties: the virions are spherical, nonenveloped, contain a transcriptase, and are assembled in the cytoplasm of the host cells. Members of the *Reovirus* genus have a double capsid structure; *Orbivirus* has a single capsid structure. Orbiviruses multiply in vertebrates and arthropods; reoviruses multiply only in vertebrates.

Diseases Due to Reoviruses

The genus *Reovirus* contains three serotypes of mammalian origin that cross-react by immunofluorescence and complement-fixation tests, but can be distinguished by neutralization or hemagglutination-inhibition tests. Group-specific antigens have been demonstrated for mammalian and avian strains. Reoviruses of mammalian origin, in general, agglutinate human red blood cells.

The virions of *Reovirus* are spherical, 75 to 80 nm in diameter, with an outer capsid and a second inner one, sometimes called the core. Seven polypeptides have been identified in *Reovirus* virions, both in the inner and outer capsids. These proteins and other characteristics of the reoviruses have been studied in detail (Fenner et al., 1974). Characteristic intracytoplasmic inclusions are formed by reoviruses in host cells.

Early evidence for the pathogenic properties of reoviruses was unconvincing under natural or experimental conditions. More recent data indicate that specific reoviruses do have important pathogenic effects in calves (neonatal calf diarrhea), kittens (feline reovirus respiratory disease), and neonatal rodents. These are discussed briefly.

Fenner, F., et al.: The Biology of Animal Viruses, 2nd ed. New York, Academic Press, 1974.

Feline Respiratory Disease Associated With Reovirus

A *Reovirus*, isolated from the intestine of a kitten suspected to have died from feline panleukopenia, was identified by Scott et al. (1970) as a *Reovirus*, type 3; it produced conjunctivitis, lacrimation, and photophobia in susceptible kittens. Serum-neutralizing antibodies were demonstrated in 29% of cats tested in Ithaca, New York, indicating rather widespread distribution of the virus. The disease produced experimentally is mild, but the evidence suggests that *Reovirus* must be considered to be one of the viral genera which may affect cats.

Reovirus Infection in Other Species

Reoviruses have been isolated from many species of vertebrates, including man. A canine *Reovirus*, type 2, isolated from a puppy with upper respiratory disease (Binn et al., 1977), induced an antibody response indicating infection, but the disease has not yet been reproduced experimentally. Serotype 1 *Reovirus* has also been recovered from laboratory dogs (Massie and Shaw, 1966). This virus caused a brief febrile upper respiratory infection when injected into susceptible dogs. Type

3 *Reovirus* isolated from rats has been used to study intrauterine and neonatal infections in rats. Fetuses become infected but rarely exhibit any evidence of disease (Margolis and Kilham, 1973; Kilham and Margolis, 1973). Encephalitis may be induced by intracerebral injection of type 3 *Reovirus* in newborn mice. Swine harbor another *Reovirus*, type 1, which has low virulence in experimental infection (Baskerville et al., 1971). Five serotypes of avian reoviruses have been defined by neutralization tests; one has been associated with viral arthritis or tenosynovitis in poultry (Olson, 1978).

Baskerville, A., McFerran, J. B., and Conner, T.: The pathology of experimental infection of pigs with type 1 *Reovirus* of porcine origin. Res. Vet. Sci., *12*:172–174, 1971.

Binn, L. N., et al.: Recovery of *Reovirus*, type 2 from an immature dog with respiratory tract disease. Am. J. Vet. Res., *38*:927–929, 1977.

Csiza, C. K.: Characterization and serotyping of three feline *Reovirus* isolates. Infec. Immun., *9*:159–166, 1974.

Kilham, L., and Margolis, G.: Pathogenesis of intrauterine infection in rats due to *Reovirus*, type 3. I. Virologic studies. Lab. Invest., *28*:597–604, 1973.

Lamont, P. H.: Reoviruses. J. Am. Vet. Med. Assoc., *152*:807–813, 1968.

Margolis, G., Kilham, L., and Gonatas, N. K.: *Reovirus* type III encephalitis: observations of virus-cell interactions in neural tissues. I. Light microscopy studies. Lab. Invest., *24*:91–100, 1971.

Margolis, G., and Kilham, L.: Pathogenesis of intrauterine infections in rats due to *Reovirus* Type 3. II. Pathologic and fluorescent antibody studies. Lab. Invest., *28*:605–613, 1973.

Margolis, G., Kilham, L., and Baringer, J. R.: Identity of Cowdry type B inclusions and nuclear bodies: observations in reovirus encephalitis. Exp. Mol. Pathol., *23*:228–244, 1975.

Massie, E. L., and Shaw, E. O.: *Reovirus* Type I in laboratory dogs. Am. J. Vet. Res., *27*:783–787, 1966.

Olson, N. O.: Reovirus infections. *In* Diseases of Poultry, 7th ed., edited by M. S. Hofstad, et al. Ames, Iowa State Univ. Press, 1978.

Scott, F. W., Kahn, D. E., and Gillespie, J. H.: Feline viruses: isolation, characterization, and pathogenicity of a feline reovirus. Am. J. Vet. Res., *31*:11–20, 1970.

Walters, M. N.-I., et al.: Murine infection with *Reovirus*. III. Pathology of infection with types 1 and 2. Br. J. Exp. Pathol., *46*:200–212, 1965.

Diseases Due to Orbiviruses

The genus *Orbivirus* (orb = ring) contains viruses that multiply in arthropods as well as in vertebrates. In biologic behavior, therefore, these are arboviruses (arbo = arthropod-borne), a term that is no longer used in classification of viruses. Bluetongue virus is the type species. This virus has double-stranded RNA with a molecular weight of 15 million daltons, which occurs as ten separate pieces. The virion has an outer diffuse layer in which are found seven capsid polypeptides. The capsid is believed to be icosahedral, with 32 capsomeres, 8 to 11 nm in diameter. The inner core is about 55 nm in diameter. The virion is nonenveloped and contains a virus-specific transcriptase. The virions are assembled in the cytoplasm of host cells.

Bluetongue of Sheep (Catarrhal Fever of Sheep, "Soremuzzle")

This viral disease of sheep was first recognized in South Africa in 1902 and still remains a serious problem in that country. The first appearance of the disease outside South Africa was reported from Cyprus in 1949 (Gambles), but the virus was not identified in this or in a subsequent outbreak in Israel until 1952. Evidence that the disease had been introduced into the United States before 1951 is the report of Hardy and Price (1952), who observed a disease of sheep in Texas to which they applied the name "soremuzzle." They were unable to establish its cause and did not identify it with bluetongue. The following year McGowan (1953) reported a similar outbreak in California, and McKercher (1953) isolated the causative virus and demonstrated its identity with the agent of bluetongue, well known in South Africa.

The virus of bluetongue, now classified in the genus *Orbivirus*, has been shown in South Africa and the United States to be transmitted by biting insects of the genus *Culicoides*.

Cattle, goats, and deer are also susceptible to infection. In cattle, the infection is usually not apparent, although it may resemble the disease in sheep, only milder. Cattle may carry the virus for protracted periods of time, with sporadic viremia adequate for insect transmission. In Africa, the blesbok antelope is considered a reservoir host for the virus. In deer, the disease (and virus) is remarkably similar to **epizootic hemorrhagic disease** of deer.

Signs. High fever is the first sign (105° F.), associated with reddening of the nasal and oral mucosae with excessive salivation. A watery discharge from the nostrils later becomes mucous and may dry to form crusts. Edematous swellings arise in the lips, tongue, ears, face, and intermandibular space. Edema and cyanosis of the tongue are so striking that they have given the disease its name, even though they are not always present. Petechiae soon appear on the oral and nasal mucosae, where the epithelium apparently becomes thickened and is shed, leaving excoriations and bleeding points. With subsidence of the fever, flushing of the skin and feet appears; the coronets become warm and tender, and later the pink perioplic band turns red. Hemorrhage into the medullary canals of the growing horn at the junction of skin and hoof, according to Thomas and Neidtz (1947), leaves a "streaky zone" parallel to the periople. This irregular zone or line persists, but is moved away from the coronet with growth of the hoof, and its color gradually changes from bright red to brown because of the breakdown of hemoglobin in the exudate. The presence of this zone is of distinct value in identifying a previous attack of the disease. The changes in the hoof and adjacent skin are believed to be indications of an acute aseptic pododermatitis, as is laminitis in the equine.

The disease may terminate in severe emaciation, prostration, and muscular weakness (occasionally with torticollis) which may last three weeks or more, followed by pulmonary edema and death from pneumonia. In prolonged cases, a "break" in the growth of wool may cause the fleece to be shed.

The morbidity rate in mild outbreaks is usually abot 50% of a flock, with the mortality rate about 7%. In severe outbreaks, however, losses from death may reach 50%. Sheep of all ages are susceptible, but in the United States, adults seem to be affected more often than lambs.

Lesions. Although the gross manifestations of this disease apparently result from changes in the vascular system, the microscopic lesions of the vessels have not received adequate study. Severe engorgement is the most striking change in the vessels. Arteritis, characterized by endothelial hyperplasia and an infiltration of neutrophils and lymphocytes in the adeventitia, has been reported in the oral mucosa, brain, and placenta. Further study is needed, therefore, to establish the basic nature of the lesions in this disease. The changes around the mouth that characterize the disease clinically are most obvious at necropsy, and consist of hyperemia, edema, cyanosis, and multiple hemorrhages in the tongue and cheeks, with erosion and even ulceration of the epithelium. The cyanosis and edema of the lips and tongue, however, are not constant findings. Similar lesions may be present on the dental pad, hard palate, and gingivae.

The skin is hyperemic and the subcutis, particularly around the head and neck is edematous. Microscopic examination of the hoof and adjacent skin reveals intense hyperemia of the vascular corium, most concentrated at the tips of the dermal papillae, associated with edema and infiltration with neutrophils. The red "streak" or zone seen grossly in the wall of the hoof is the result of the accumulation of erythrocytes as well as neutrophils in the hollow medullary canals of the horny wall, which continue as channels from the dermal papillae.

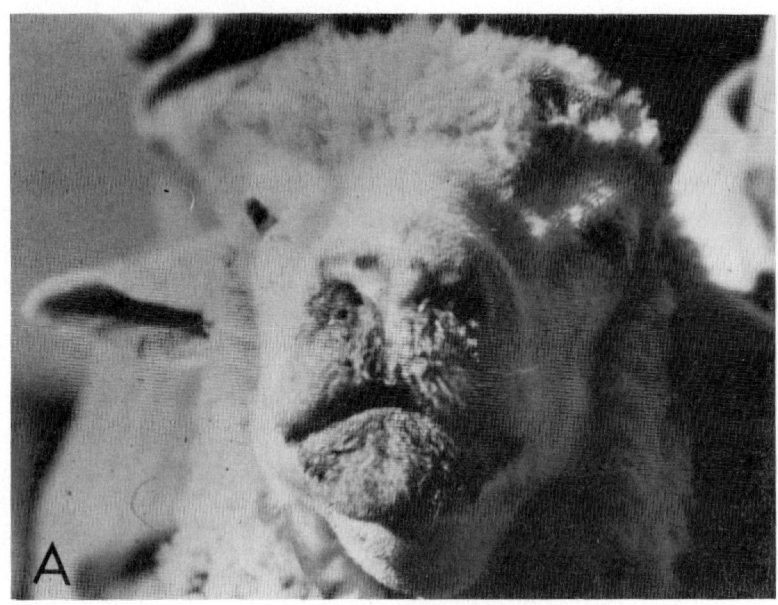

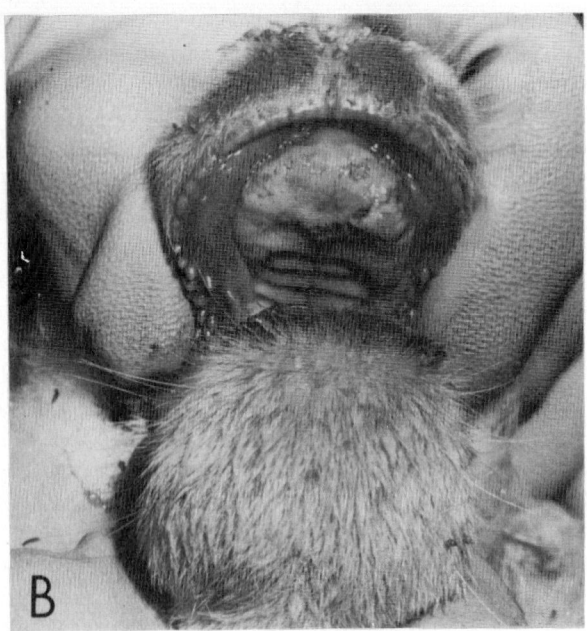

Fig. 9–41.   Bluetongue, sheep *(Orbivirus). A,* Edematous swelling of lips and nostrils. *B,* Ulcers of dental pad and swelling of lips and buccal mucosa. (Courtesy of Dr. J. G. Bowne and *Journal of the American Veterinary Medical Association.*)

At the periople, these channels may become dilated, although distal to the zone they are of capillary size.

The musculature usually contains foci of gross hemorrhage, which are associated with microscopic evidence of necrotic changes in muscle bundles. These changes have been described as hyalinization and loss of striations in the muscle bundles and pyknosis of sarcolemmal nuclei, followed by coagulation, irregular swelling and fragmentation of sarcoplasm. Proliferation of sarcolemmal nuclei and occasional calcific stippling of sarcoplasm have been reported. The pathogenesis of these changes is not clear, but it is possible that they are brought about by disturbance of the blood flow to the muscles.

In the digestive system, extravasations of blood from the mucosa of the abomasum and duodenum may be seen. The liver may have microscopic evidence of slight fatty change at the periphery of the lobules. The endocardium may be the site of extravasation of blood, and the pericardial sac may be distended with blood-tinged fluid. In the lungs, edema may be succeeded by pneumonia, which is not specific in character. In the spleen, slight congestion and enlargement are grossly apparent, and congestion, hemosiderosis, and some neutrophilic infiltration of the red pulp are visible microscopically.

Bluetongue vaccine prepared from modified live virus and administered to pregnant ewes has caused lesions in the central nervous system of their progeny. The critical period for exposure appears to be between the fourth and eighth weeks of gestation. Lambs may be stillborn, spastic, or most often, "dummies" which walk aimlessly, circle, bump into objects, are uncoordinated, and do not nurse unless helped. The congenital anomalies in the nervous system range from hydrocephalus to subcortical cysts in the cerebrum and cerebellum, with ex vacuo dilation of lateral ventricles. The studies of Young and Cordy (1964) have demonstrated that the

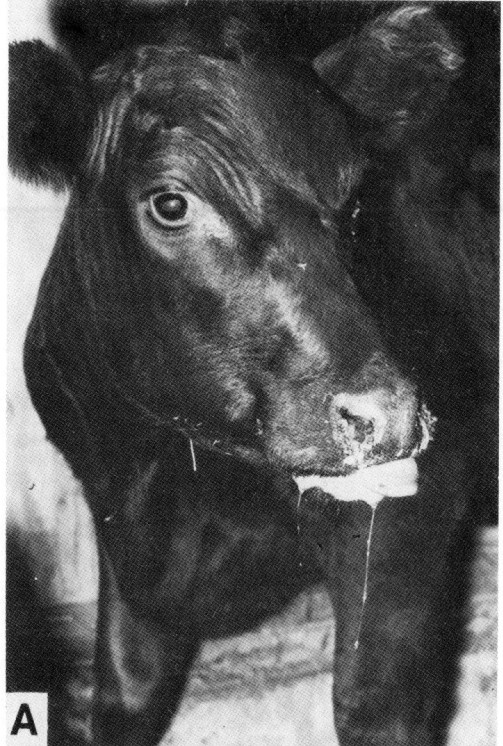

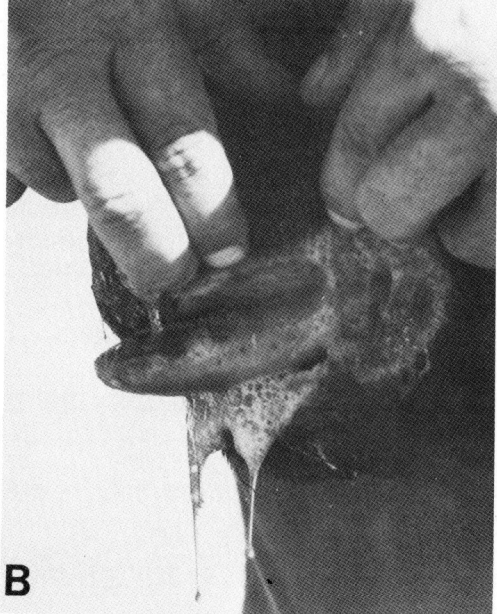

Fig. 9–42. Bluetongue, shorthorn heifer. *A,* The muzzle is dry and cracked and a mucopurulent exudate surrounds the nares. *B,* Erosions on the lateral surface of the tongue. (Courtesy of Dr. J. G. Bowne and *Journal of the American Veterinary Medical Association.*)

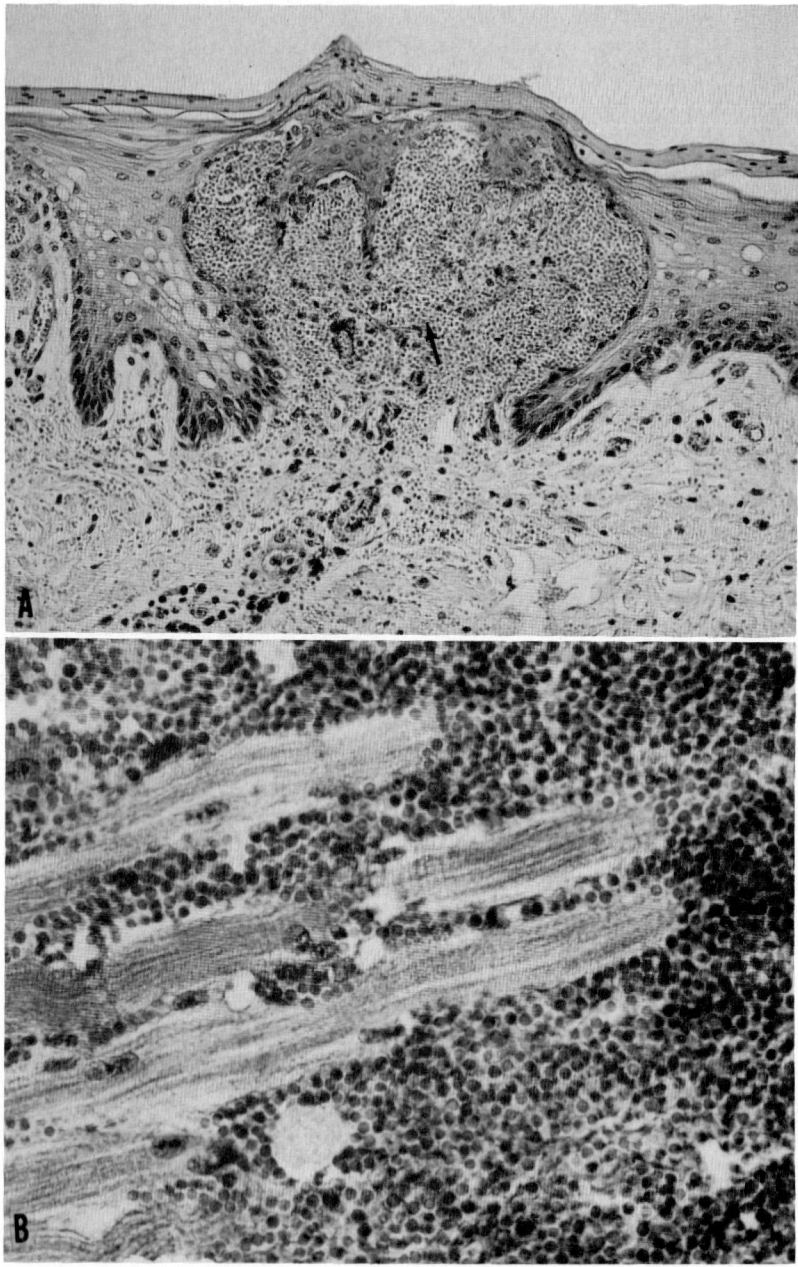

Fig. 9–43. Bluetongue. Hemorrhages in the tongue of a year-old ewe. *A,* Hemorrhage into a lingual papilla (arrow) (× 190). *B,* Severe hemorrhage isolating muscle bundles in the tongue (× 560). (Courtesy of Armed Forces Institute of Pathology.) Contributor: Dr. W. S. Monlux.

lesions are the result of an acute necrotizing meningoencephalitis. Although the clinical and gross findings of swayback (enzootic ataxia) may be similar, the two processes may be differentiated in that swayback is a dysmyelinating disease in which inflammatory changes do not occur.

Diagnosis. The clinical diagnosis may be made from the symptoms and gross lesions, but bluetongue must be differentiated from photosensitization, contagious ecthyma, foot-and-mouth disease, *Oestrus ovis* infestation, ulcerative dermatitis, and sheep-pox. In cattle, the disease must be differentiated from foot-and-mouth disease, rinderpest, vesicular stomatitis, infectious rhinotracheitis, mycotic stomatitis, and the bovine virus diarrhea-mucosal disease complex. At present, isolation and identification of the virus are necessary to confirm the diagnosis.

Anderson, C. K., and Jensen, R.: Pathologic changes in placentas of ewes inoculated with bluetongue virus. Am. J. Vet. Res., 30:987–999, 1969.

Becker, L. E., Narayan, O., and Johnson, R. T.: Comparative studies of viral infections of the developing forebrain. I. Pathogenesis of rat virus and bluetongue vaccine virus infections in neonatal hamsters. J. Neuropathol. Exp. Neurol., 33:519–529, 1974.

Bowne, J. G.: Bluetongue disease. Adv. Vet. Sci. Comp. Med., 15:1–46, 1971.

Bowne, J. G., Luedke, A. J., Jochim, M. M., and Metcalf, H. E.: Bluetongue disease in cattle. J. Am. Vet. Med. Assoc., 153:662–668, 1968.

De Kock, G., DuToit, R., and Neidtz, W. O.: Observations on blue tongue in cattle and sheep. Onderstepoort J. Vet. Sci. Anim. Ind., 8:129–181, 1937.

DuToit, R. M.: The transmission of blue tongue and horsesickness by Culicoides. Onderstepoort J. Vet. Sci. Anim. Ind., 19:7–16, 1944.

Gambles, R. M.: Blue tongue of sheep in Cyprus. J. Comp. Pathol. Ther., 59:176–190, 1949.

Griner, L. A., et al.: Bluetongue associated with abnormalities in newborn lambs. J. Am. Vet. Med. Assoc., 145:1013–1019, 1964.

Hardy, W. T., and Price, D. A.: Soremuzzle of sheep. J. Am. Vet. Med. Assoc., 120:23–25, 1952.

Hoff, G. L., Trainer, D. O., and Jochim, M. M.: Bluetongue virus and white-tailed deer in an enzootic area of Texas. J. Wildl. Dis., 10:158–163, 1974.

Hutcheon, D.: Malarial catarrhal fever of sheep. Vet. Rec., 14:629–633, 1902.

Luedke, A. J., Bowne, J. G., Jochim, M. M., and Doyle, C.: Clinical and pathological features of bluetongue in sheep. Am. J. Vet. Res., 25:963–970, 1964.

Luedke, A. J., Jochim, M. M., and Hones, R. H.: Bluetongue in cattle: effects of *Culicoides varipennis*-transmitted bluetongue virus on pregnant heifers and their calves. Am. J. Vet. Res., 38:1687–1695, 1977.

———: Bluetongue in cattle: effects of vector-transmitted bluetongue virus on calves previously infected in utero. Am. J. Vet. Res., 38:1697–1700, 1977.

McGowan, B.: An epidemic resembling soremuzzle or blue tongue in California sheep. Cornell Vet., 43:213–216, 1953.

McKercher, D. G., McGowan, B., Howarth, J. A., and Saito, J. K.: A preliminary report on the isolation and identification of the blue tongue virus from sheep in California. J. Am. Vet. Med. Assoc., 122:300–301, 1953.

Moulton, J. E.: Pathology of bluetongue of sheep. J. Am. Vet. Med. Assoc., 138:493–498, 1961.

Murray, J. O., and Trainer, D. O.: Blue-tongue virus in North American elk. J. Wildl. Dis., 6:144–148, 1970.

Nevill, E. M.: Cattle and Culicoides biting midges as possible overwintering hosts of bluetongue virus. Onderstepoort J. Vet. Res., 38:65–71, 1971.

Richards, W. P. C., and Cordy, D. R.: Bluetongue virus infection: pathologic responses of nervous systems in sheep and mice. Science, 156:530–531, 1967.

Shultz, G., and Delay, P. D.: Losses in newborn lambs associated with bluetongue vaccination of pregnant ewes. J. Am. Vet. Med. Assoc., 127:224–226, 1955.

Stair, E. L., Robinson, R. M., and Jones, P. L.: Spontaneous bluetongue in Texas white-tailed deer. Pathol. Vet., 5:164–173, 1968.

Thomas, F. C., and Miller, J.: A comparison of bluetongue virus and E. H. D. virus: electronmicroscopy and serology. Can. J. Comp. Med., 35:22–27, 1971.

Thomas, A. D., and Neidtz, W. O.: Further observations on the pathology of blue tongue in sheep. Onderstepoort J. Vet. Sci. Anim. Ind., 22:27–40, 1947.

Vosdingh, R. A., Trainer, D. O., and Easterday, B. C.: Experimental bluetongue disease in white-tailed deer. Can. J. Comp. Med. Vet. Sci., 32:382–387, 1968.

Young, S., and Cordy, D. R.: An ovine fetal encephalopathy caused by bluetongue vaccine virus. J. Neuropath. Exp. Neurol., 23:635–659, 1964.

Epizootic Hemorrhagic Disease of Deer

A serious, widely distributed disease of white-tailed deer (*Odocoileus virginianus*) was described in New Jersey by Shope et al. (1955), and demonstrated to be caused by a specific virus (Shope et al., 1960). The clinical signs of the disease include edema, especially around the head; rhinitis and glossitis, which may eventually produce ulcers; congestion and hemorrhage at the coronet of the hoof, which leads to transitory lameness. Experimentally infected animals exhibit severe fever and depression. The gross lesions consist of these hemorrhagic and necrotizing changes in skin and mucous membranes, edema which may be disseminated, and petechiae or ecchymoses in various serous membranes (peritoneum, pleura) as well as in muscles, joints, and viscera. Several species of wild ungulates appear to be susceptible.

These features in deer are indistinguishable from those produced by the bluetongue virus under natural or experimental conditions. The close similarity of the epizootic hemorrhagic fever virus to the bluetongue virus suggests that the two diseases may be the same. Some authorities consider them to be the same, but others point out that the viruses can be distinguished by serologic methods. The close relationship of the two diseases, coupled with the experimental infection of deer with bluetongue, suggests that they constitute one disease entity. It seems prudent, in light of the present evidence, to consider bluetongue and epizootic hemorrhagic disease of deer to be indistinguishable except by the serologic differences demonstrable in the two viruses.

Fletch, A. L., and Karstad, L. H.: Studies on the pathogenesis of experimental epizootic hemorrhagic disease of white-tailed deer. Can. J. Comp. Med., 35:224–229, 1970.

Fosber, S. A., Stauber, E. H., and Renshaw, H. W.: Isolation and characterization of epizootic hemorrhagic disease virus from white-tailed deer (Odocoileus virginianus) in eastern Washington. Am. J. Vet. Res., 38:361–364, 1971.

Griner, L. A., and Nelson, L. S.: Hemorrhagic disease in exotic ruminants in a zoo. J. Am. Vet. Med. Assoc., 157:600–603, 1970.

Hoff, G. L., and Trainer, D. O.: Experimental infection in North American elk with epizootic hemorrhagic disease virus. J. Wildl. Dis., 9:129–132, 1973.

———: Observations on bluetongue and epizootic hemorrhagic disease viruses in white-tailed deer.

I. Distribution of virus in the blood. II. Cross-challenge. J. Wildl. Dis., 10:25–31, 1974.

Karstad, L., Winter, A., and Trainer, D. O.: Pathology of epizootic hemorrhagic disease of deer. Am. J. Vet. Res., 22:227–235, 1961.

Prestwood, A. K., Kistner, T. P., Kellogg, F. E., and Hayes, F. A.: The 1971 outbreak of hemorrhagic disease among white-tailed deer of the southeastern United States. J. Wildl. Dis., 10:217–224, 1974.

Roughton, R. D.: An outbreak of a hemorrhagic disease in white-tailed deer in Kentucky. J. Wildl. Dis., 11:177–186, 1975.

Shope, R. E., MacNamara, L. G., and Margold, R.: Report on the deer mortality; epizootic hemorrhagic disease of deer. New Jersey Outdoors, 6:16–21, 1955.

———: A virus-induced epizootic hemorrhagic disease of the Virginia white-tailed deer (Odocoileus virginianus). J. Exp. Med., 111:155–170, 1960.

Stair, E. L., Robinson, R. M., and Jones, L. P.: Spontaneous bluetongue in Texas white-tailed deer. Path. Vet., 5:164–173, 1968.

Thomas, F. C., and Trainer, D. O.: Bluetongue virus in white-tailed deer. Am. J. Vet. Res., 31:271–278, 1970.

Thomas, F. C., and Miller, J.: A comparison of bluetongue virus and EHD virus: electromicroscopy and serology. Can. J. Comp. Med., 35:22–27, 1971.

Thomas, F. C., Willis, N., and Ruckerbauer, G.: Identification of viruses involved in the 1971 outbreak of hemorrhagic disease in southeastern United States white-tailed deer. J. Wild. Dis., 10:187–189, 1974.

Wilhelm, A. R., and Trainer, D. O.: A comparison of several viruses of epizootic hemorrhagic disease of deer. J. Inf. Dis., 117:48–54, 1967.

———: Hematological and virological studies of epizootic hemorrhagic disease of deer. Bull. Wildl. Dis. Assoc., 5:77–80, 89–94, 1969.

African Horse-Sickness

The apparently nonspecific name, African horse-sickness, applies to a specific and important disease of *Equidae* caused by a virus that is transmitted by several species of *Culicoides*. The disease was apparently present in South Africa when the first European settlers brought their horses and mules into that country in the 18th century, and has in recent years crossed the boundaries of several other countries—namely, Egypt, Israel, West Pakistan, Afghanistan, Cyprus, Iraq, Syria, Lebanon, Turkey, India, Iran, and Jordan. The entire problem has been adequately reviewed by Maurer and McCully (1963).

The etiologic agent is an *Orbivirus* similar to the bluetongue virus. Its host range includes horses, mules, donkeys, goats, dogs, and ferrets. The virions are icosahedral and measure 55 to 80 nm in diameter, depending on the method of preparation. Centrifugation in cesium chloride tends to remove the outer capsid layers, leaving the small capsid of 55 nm. The number of capsomeres has been reported to be 32 or 92. The virions contain double-stranded RNA and assembly occurs in the cytoplasm of host cells. The virus agglutinates red blood cells under appropriate conditions. The virus is infective for mice by intracerebral inoculation. Specific strains, which by passage via this route have become neurotropic for the mouse, are used extensively in the production of vaccine.

Signs. The clinical features of African horse-sickness usually are described as conforming to one of four types. The first is the least serious and is more often observed in partially immune animals, particularly donkeys. Mild fever, anorexia, dyspnea, and accelerated pulse rate may be all that is observed, followed by rapid recovery. The acute pulmonary form of the disease is recognized by an incubation period of three to five days, sudden onset of high fever (105–107° F.), and severe dyspnea due to pulmonary edema, often with frothy exudates in the nostrils. Sweating and coughing may occur, and death usually results within a few hours of onset of the pulmonary edema. This form has been described in dogs as well. A third clinical type of the disease is the subacute cardiac form, in which the incubation period and course are usually longer than in the pulmonary form. It is distinguished by the occurrence of edema of the head and neck, lips, eyelids, cheek, and tongue, and most characteristically, edematous bulging of the supraorbital fossa. Petechiae may appear on the ventral aspect of the tongue, abdominal pain and paralysis of the esophagus may be manifest, and death usually is due to cardiac failure and hypoxia. In a fourth, mixed form, a combination of pulmonary and cardiac lesions are found at necropsy.

Lesions. The lesions at necropsy usually can be correlated with the clinical form of the disease. The most striking changes are seen in the respiratory system. Hydrothorax usually accompanies the severe edema, which involves the subpleural and interlobular stroma and fills alveoli in many lobules. Frothy fluid usually fills the bronchi, trachea, and the rest of the upper respiratory tract. Fibrin and proteinaceous material are recognizable microscopically in the edematous tissues, and leukocytes may also be present. In some cases, these leukocytes may be present in sufficient numbers to suggest bronchopneumonia.

The cardiac lesions are also significant. Hydropericardium is usually present, along with petechiae and inflammatory edema in the epicardium. Disseminated foci of myocardial necrosis are seen microscopically, and are often accentuated by hemorrhages, which may be recognized grossly. Sometimes edema may involve the adventitia of arterioles, but otherwise, small blood vessels do not contain identifiable lesions.

Depletion of lymphocytes is usually evident in the spleen and lymph nodes; reticuloendothelial and plasma cells are usually increased in number, although the spleen is not usually enlarged. Some lymph nodes may be grossly hemorrhagic. The gastrointestinal tract may be involved. Edema around the pharynx may account for the presumed paralysis of the esophagus noted in some descriptions of the clinical features. Hemorrhage is common in the gastric mucosa. The liver is usually only congested. Hemorrhage and edema may be found in the kidneys, particularly involving the peripelvic fat.

Diagnosis. The diagnosis is usually made presumptively in enzootic regions from the clinical features and necropsy findings, but should be confirmed by recovery and identification of the virus. The method presently most suitable involves the intracerebral inoculation of mice and subsequent neutralization tests to determine the antigenic type.

Differentiation from equine viral arteritis should be considered because both diseases are characterized by edema and hemorrhage in the subcutis, heart, and lungs. The specific lesions in the musculature of arterioles in arteritis would be useful, but isolation and identification of the virus should also be undertaken. Infection by the virus of equine arteritis may be differentiated in the sera of affected horses by means of complement-fixation, serum-neutralization, and plaque reduction tests (McCollum et al., 1970). Specific immuno-fluorescence is also reported to be useful in detecting African horse-sickness virus in the spleen (Tessler, 1972).

Breese, S. S., Jr., Ozawa, Y., and Dardiri, A. H.: Electron microscopic characterization of African horse-sickness virus. J. Am. Vet. Med. Assoc., 155:391–400, 1969.

Henning, M. W.: Animal Diseases of South Africa, 3rd ed., Pretoria, Central News Agency, Ltd., 1956.

Howell, P. G: African horsesickness. FAO Agricult. Studies, 61:71–108, 1963.

Lecatsas, G., and Erasmus, B. J.: Electron microscopic study of the formation of African horse-sickness virus. Arch. Ges. Virusforsch., 22:442–450, 1967.

Maurer, F. D., and McCully, R. M.: African horsesickness—with emphasis on pathology. Am. J. Vet. Res., 24:235–266, 1963.

McCollum, W. H., Ozawa, Y., and Dardiri, A. H.: Serologic differentiation between African horse-sickness and equine arteritis. Am. J. Vet. Res., 31:1963–1966, 1970.

Piercy, S. E.: Some observations on African horse-sickness including an account of an outbreak amongst dogs. East African Agric. J., 17:1–3, 1951.

Reid, N. R.: African horse-sickness. Br. Vet. J., 118:137–142, 1961.

Tessler, J.: Detection of African horsesickness viral antigens in tissues by immunofluorescence. Can. J. Comp. Med., 36:167–169, 1972.

Wetzel, H., Nevill, E. M., and Erasmus, B. J.: Studies on the transmission of African horsesickness. Onderstepoort J. Vet. Res., 37:165–168, 1970.

Diseases Caused by Rotaviruses

The genus *Rotavirus* has been proposed to include Reoviridae that are antigenically related and infect the intestinal epithelium of infant calves, mice, children, lambs, and pigs. Members of this group have also been called "duoviruses." The virions of *Rotavirus* are 70 nm in diameter and morphologically resemble most closely those of *Orbivirus*. Direct immunofluorescence has been used to identify the agent in tissue cells and to demonstrate antigenic similarities among isolates from different species. The name of this genus was proposed by Flewett et al. (1974).

Neonatal Calf Diarrhea (Scours)

This serious disease of calves appears during the first seven days of life, affects most of the animals of the herd, and causes death of up to half of them. The principal

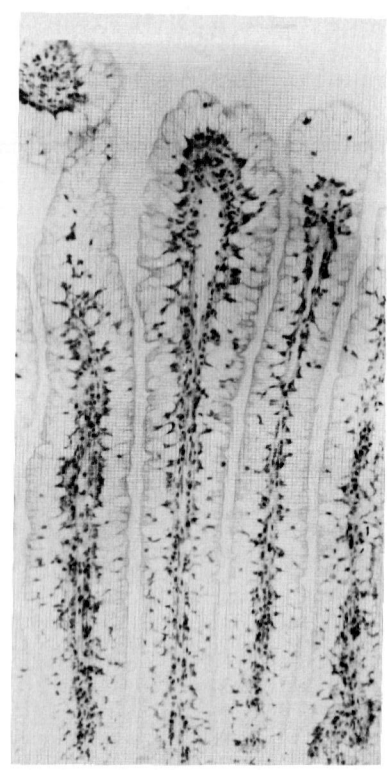

Fig. 9–44. Ileum of uninoculated control calf, 72 hours old. Villi are covered with tall columnar cells with nuclei at the base and the cytoplasm contains clear vacuoles. The lamina propria contains a lacteal and few other cells. (H & E) (Courtesy of Dr. C. A. Mebus and *Veterinary Pathology.*)

sign is the appearance of yellowish, watery feces, which soon leads to severe dehydration. This syndrome has been known for many years and has usually been attributed to enteric bacteria, such as *Escherichia coli*. Although multiple factors may well be involved and are not clearly understood, it seems likely that organisms such as the *Rotavirus* described by Mebus et al. (1971) may be the essential etiologic factor. Originally classified with the Reoviruses, this agent became the first of a group of similar viruses with common pathogenic features to be placed in the genus *Rotavirus* (Fletcher, et al., 1974).

Lesions. Mebus and colleagues demonstrated that the virus specifically attacks the epithelium of the small intestine of young calves. The virus replicates in intestinal epithelial cells near the tips of villi. Viral antigen is demonstrable in these cells by immunofluorescent techniques. Infected cells are desquamated and may be demonstrated in fecal preparations by this immunofluorescent technique. As epithelial cells are lost from the tips of villi, the desquamated cells are replaced by cuboidal, then by flattened squamous epithelial cells. Some villi may remain denuded for some time. The stroma of the villi becomes internally infiltrated with leukocytes.

Diagnosis. Diagnosis is greatly facilitated in clinical cases by the use of immunofluorescent staining of desquamated epithelial cells in fecal specimens. The technique has demonstrated that the

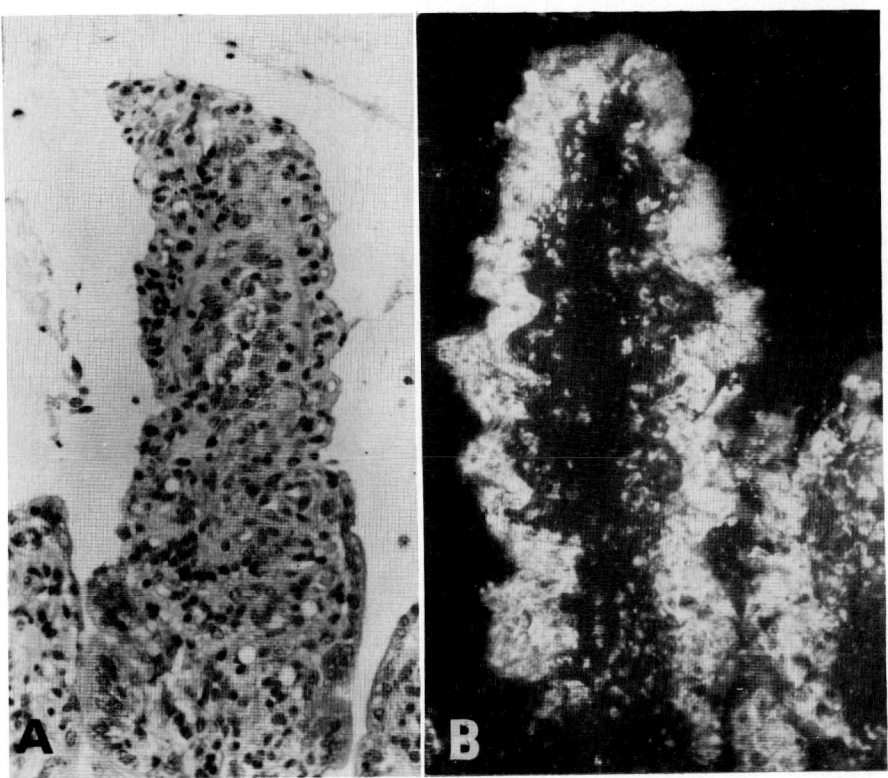

Fig. 9–45.   A villus of ileum of a calf infected with virus of neonatal calf enteritis (Rotavirus). *A*, From a calf killed 4.5 hours following onset of diarrhea. Epithelial cells are lost from the distal two-thirds of the villus. Cells are increased in the lamina propria. *B*, From a calf killed one-half hour after onset of diarrhea. Immunofluorescence demonstrates presence of viral antigen in epithelial cells of distal two-thirds of villus. (Courtesy of Dr. C. A. Mebus and *Veterinary Pathology*.)

Nebraska agent is widely distributed throughout the United States (White et al., 1970).

Bridger, J. C., and Woode, G. N.: Neonatal calf diarrhea: identification of the reovirus-like (rotavirus) agent in faeces by immunofluorescence and immune electron microscopy. Br. Vet. J., *131*:528–535, 1975.

Fernelius, A. L., et al.: Cell culture adaptation and propagation of a Reovirus-like agent of calf diarrhea from a field outbreak in Nebraska. Arch. Virusforsch., *37*:114–130, 1972.

Flewett, T. H., et al.: Relation between viruses from acute gastroenteritis of children and newborn calves. Lancet, 2:61–63, 1974.

Mebus, C. A., Underdahl, N. R., Rhodes, M. B., and Twiehaus, M. J.: Calf diarrhea (scours): reproduced with a virus from a field outbreak. Univ. Nebr. Res. Bull., *233*:1–16, 1969.

Mebus, C. A., Stair, E. L., Underdahl, N. R., and Twiehaus, M. J.: Pathology of neonatal calf diarrhea induced by a reo-like virus. Vet. Pathol., *8*:490–505, 1971.

Stair, E. L., Mebus, C. A., Twiehaus, M. J., and Underdahl, N. R.: Neonatal calf diarrhea: electron microscopy of intestines infected with a reovirus-like agent. Vet. Pathol., *10*:155–170, 1973.

White, R. G., Mebus, C. A., and Twiehaus, M. J.: Incidence of herds infected with a neonatal calf diarrhea virus. Vet. Med., *65*:487–489, 1970.

Epidemic Diarrheal Disease of Mice (Epizootic Diarrheal Disease of Mice, EDIM)

An enteric disease caused by a viral agent often presents a serious problem in colonies of laboratory mice, for it is hard to control and produces a very high mortality rate among suckling animals. Entire mouse colonies have been sacrificed in efforts to eliminate diseases.

Adult mice can become infected and eliminate the virus for varying periods of time in their feces; however, clinical disease does not occur.

The virus has been identified and classified in the genus *Rotavirus*. Virions have been visualized with the electron microscope (Adams and Kraft, 1963, 1967) in the cytoplasm of epithelial cells of small intestinal villi. The developing virions bud into swollen vesicles of endoplasmic reticulum to assume their mature, enveloped appearance. Dilated cysternae and accumulations of lipid increase in the cytoplasm, accompanied by aggregations of virions. These features give the epithelial cells, particularly near the tip of the villus, a vacuolated appearance under the light microscope. Infected cells may burst to shed their contents into the lumen, or may be desquamated totally.

The disease appears in suckling mice 10 to 15 days of age, but does not affect mice which have reached weaning age (22 days). Although the nursing females are ostensibly normal, their affected young appear somewhat shrunken or dehydrated, with dry whitish scales over the skin of the back and shoulder. Some mice have a cyanotic color, especially noticeable along the neck and between the shoulders. Diarrhea is evidenced by profuse soiling of the perineal region and tail with yellowish fecal material. Death often occurs soon after onset, but if mice survive more than two days, a tenacious somewhat darker material often stains the perianal region, and in such cases death may follow severe obstipation. In mild, uncomplicated cases, mice recover completely in two to five days, although the growth of some may be retarded.

The lesions, seen early in the infection, are concentrated in the epithelial cells of the small intestine, particularly near the tips of the villi. As indicated previously, the affected cells have vacuolated cytoplasm, associated with the presence of inclusions. Severely affected cells may rupture or be shed intact into the lumen (Adams and Kraft, 1967). The inclusion bodies, described originally by Pappenheimer and Enders (1947), are spherical, sharply outlined, 1 to 4 μ in diameter, and sometimes surrounded by a narrow clear halo. Laidlaw's acid fuchsin-phosphomolybdic acid-orange G stain reveals these inclusions to be intensely fuchsinophilic. They are eosinophilic with hematoxylin and eosin stain, and resemble the inclusion bodies of canine distemper.

Adams, W. R., and Kraft, L. M.: Epizootic diarrhea of infant mice: identification of the etiologic agent. Science, 141:359–360, 1963.

———: Electron-microscopic study of the intestinal epithelium of mice infected with the agent of epizootic diarrhea of infant mice (EDIM virus). Am. J. Pathol., 51:39–60, 1967.

Banfield, W. G., Kasnic, G., and Blackwell, J. H.: Further observations on the virus of epizootic diarrhea of infant mice. Virology, 36:411–421, 1968.

Cheever, F. S., and Mueller, J. H.: Epidemic diarrheal disease of suckling mice. I. Manifestations, epidemiology and attempts to transmit the disease. J. Exp. Med., 85:405–416, 1947.

———: Epidemic diarrheal disease of suckling mice. III. The effect of strain, litter and season on the incidence of the disease. J. Exp. Med., 88:309–316, 1948.

Kraft, L. M.: Two viruses causing diarrhea in infant mice. In The Problems of Laboratory Animal Disease, edited by R. J. C. Harris. New York, Academic Press, 1962, pp. 115–130.

———: Response of the mouse to the virus of epidemic diarrhea of infant mice. Neutralizing antibodies and carrier state. Lab. Anim. Care, 11:125–127, 1961.

Much, D. H., and Zajac, I.: Purification and characterization of epizootic diarrhea of infant mice virus. Infect. Immun., 6:1019–1024, 1972.

Pappenheimer, A. M., and Enders, J. F.: An epidemic diarrheal disease of suckling mice. II. Inclusions in the intestinal epithelial cells. J. Exp. Med., 85:417–422, 1947.

Pappenheimer, A. M., and Cheever, F. S.: Epidemic diarrheal disease of suckling mice. IV. Cytoplasmic inclusion bodies in intestinal epithelium in relation to the disease. J. Exp. Med., 88:317–324, 1948.

Rubinstein, D., Milne, R. G., Buckland, R., and Tyrell, D. A. J.: The growth of the virus of epidemic diarrhea of infant mice (EDIM) in organ cultures of intestinal epithelium. Br. J. Exp. Pathol., 52:442–445, 1971.

Wilsnack, R. E., Blackwell, J. H., and Parker, J. C.: Identification of an agent of epizootic diarrhea of infant mice by immunofluorescent and complement-fixation tests. Am. J. Vet. Res., 30:1195–1204, 1969.

Lethal Intestinal Disease of Infant Mice (LIVIM)

Lethal intestinal disease of infant mice is a viral infection of suckling mice characterized by diarrhea and a high mortality rate. Although similar to EDIM infection, the two diseases are caused by distinct viruses. LIVIM produces clinical disease in mice up to 16 to 20 days of age. As in EDIM, adults can become infected and shed the virus in the feces without clinical signs. Suckling mice develop diarrhea, do not suckle, become severely dehydrated and almost completely inactive. The mortality rate is high. Few gross changes occur. The stomach is empty, the small intestine often distended with gas, and unformed feces is present in the colon.

Microscopically, multinucleated epithelial cells are present in the villi of the small intestine. These and other cells slough, leaving ulcers. The villi decrease in size and number, resembling the atrophic villi of transmissible gastroenteritis of swine. Eosinophilic cytoplasmic inclusion bodies have been reported in the epithelial giant cells, but their specificity is not established.

Biggers, D. C., Kraft, L. M., and Sprinz, H.: Lethal intestinal virus infection of mice (LIVIM), an important new model for study of the response of the intesinal mucosa to injury. Am. J. Pathol., 45:413–422, 1964.

Kraft, L. M.: An apparently new lethal virus disease of infant mice. Science, 137:182–183, 1962.

Nonbacterial Gastroenteritis of Infants (*Rotavirus* Infection of Children, Neonatal Infantile Diarrhea)

A widespread and severe gastroenteritis of infants and children has been associated with a *Rotavirus*. This agent has been transmitted to a monkey (*Macaca nemestrina*) (Mitchell et al., 1977). The agent is similar to viruses identified in neonatal calf diarrhea, epizootic diarrhea of infant mice, porcine *Rotavirus* infection, and young lambs.

Flewett, T. H., et al.: Relation between viruses from acute gastroenteritis of children and newborn calves. Lancet, 2:61–63, 1974.

Holmes, I. H., Ruck, B. J., Bishop, R. F., and Davidson, G. P.: Infantile enteritis viruses: morphogenesis and morphology. J. Virol., 16:937–943, 1975.

Kapikian, A. Z., et al.; Reovirus-like agent in stools: association with infantile diarrhea and development of serologic tests. Science, 185:1049–1053, 1974.

———: New complement-fixation test for the human reovirus-like agent of infantile gastroenteritis. Lancet, 1:1056–1061, 1975.

Mebus, C. A., et al.: Diarrhea in gnotobiotic calves caused by the reovirus-like agent of human infantile gastroenteritis. Infect. Immun., *14*:471–474, 1976.

Mitchell, J. D., et al.: Transmission of rotavirus gastroenteritis from children to a monkey. Gut, *18*:156–160, 1977.

Torres-Medina, A., et al.: Diarrhea caused in gnotobiotic piglets by the reovirus-like agent of human infantile gastroenteritis. J. Infect. Dis., *133*:22–27, 1976.

Woode, G. N., et al.: Morphological and antigenic relationships between viruses (rotaviruses) from acute gastroenteritis of children, calves, piglets, mice and foals. Infect. Immun., *14*:804–810, 1976.

Porcine Rotaviral Enteritis

A syndrome of enteric disease is recognized clinically in piglets one to four weeks of age. The principal signs are diarrhea, anorexia, depression and occasional vomiting, with mortality rate from 7 to 20% of affected animals. This is often referred to as "milk scours," "white scours," or "three-week scours." One of the causative agents most likely to be involved in this clinical syndrome is a porcine rotavirus. This agent may be differentiated from the virus of transmissible gastroenteritis virus, porcine enterovirus, and enteropathogenic *Escherichia coli* (colibacillosis). Not only have rotaviruses been recovered from piglets during the course of enteric disease, but the agents have produced the disease in gnotobiotic pigs (Bohl et al., 1978; Hall et al., 1976; Chasey and Lucas, 1977).

Lesions. The virus has been demonstrated by immunofluorescent methods to replicate in epithelial cells near the tips of small-intestinal villi. These columnar cells undergo necrosis and are rapidly shed into the intesinal lumen. The changes may also be seen in other segments of the gastrointestinal tract.

The ultrastructurally demonstrable effects include severe distortion and loss of villi, accumulation of lipid droplets in the cytoplasm, formation of large vesicles in which virions may be seen, and mitochondria that are densely stained and vacuolated. Crystalline arrays of linear tubular components with dense viral particles may also be seen in some cells.

Diagnosis. The diagnosis may be established by identification of the rotavirus by isolation in tissue culture, or by direct demonstration of viral antigen in intestinal epithelial cells using immunofluorescence methods. The differentiation from the virus of transmissible gastroenteritis (a coronavirus) is particularly critical.

Bohl, E. H., et al.: Rotavirus as a cause of diarrhea in pigs. J. Am. Vet. Med. Assoc., *172*:458–463, 1978.

Chasey, D., and Lucas, M.: Detection of rotavirus in experimentally infected piglets. Res. Vet. Sci., *22*:124–125, 1977.

Hall, G. A., Bridger, J. C., Chandler, R. L., and Woode, G. N.: Gnotobiotic piglets experimentally infected with neonatal calf diarrhoea reovirus-like agent (rotavirus). Vet. Pathol., *13*:197–210, 1976.

Lecce, J. G., King, M. W., and Mock, R.: Reovirus-like agent associated with fatal diarrhea in neonatal pigs. Infect. Immun., *14*:816–825, 1976.

McNulty, M. S., et al.: A reovirus-like agent (rotavirus) associated with diarrhea in neonatal pigs. Vet. Microbiol., *1*:55–63, 1976.

Pearson, G. R., and McNulty, M. S.: Pathological changes in the small intestine of neonatal pigs infected with a pig reovirus-like agent (rotavirus). J. Comp. Pathol., *87*:363–375, 1977.

Saif, L. J., Bohl, E. H., Kohler, E. M., and Hughes, J. H.: Immune electron microscopy of transmissible gastroenteritis virus and *Rotavirus* (reovirus-like agent) of swine. Am. J. Vet. Res., *38*:13–20, 1977.

Theil, K. W., Bohl, E. H., and Agnes, A. G.: Cell culture propagation of porcine rotavirus (Reovirus-like agent). Am. J. Vet. Res., *38*:1765–1768, 1977.

Theil, K. W., et al.: Pathogenesis of porcine rotaviral infection in experimentally inoculated gnotobiotic pigs. Am. J. Vet. Res., *39*:213–220, 1978.

Woode, G. N., et al.: The isolation of reovirus-like agents (rotaviruses) from acute gastroenteritis of piglets. J. Med. Microbiol., *9*:203–209, 1976.

Rotaviral Infection in Other Species

Viruses of the genus *Rotavirus* appear to be widely distributed among mammals. In addition to the more extensively studied diseases in children, calves, piglets, and mice previously described, viral isolations have been reported from lambs (Snodgrass, et al., 1976; Snodgrass, Herring, and Gray, 1976; McNulty, et al., 1976); deer (Tzipori, Caple, and Butler, 1976) and foals (Flewett, Bryden, and Davies, 1975). It seems likely that these viruses may be found in many other species now that the appropriate techniques are available for their demonstration.

Flewett, T. H., Bryden, A. S., and Davies, H.: Virus diarrhea in foals and other animals. Vet. Rec., 96:477, 1975.

McNulty, M. S., et al.: Reovirus-like agent (Rotavirus) from lambs. Infect. Immun., 14:1332–1338, 1976.

Snodgrass, D. R., Smith, W., Gray, E. W., and Herring, J. A.: A rotavirus in lambs with diarrhea. Res. Vet. Sci., 20:113–114, 1976.

Snodgrass, D. R., Herring, J. A., and Gray, E. W.: Experimental rotavirus infection in lambs. J. Comp. Pathol., 86:637–642, 1976.

Tzipori, S., Caple, I. W., and Butler, R.: Isolation of a rotavirus from deer. Vet. Rec., 99:398, 1976.

TOGAVIRIDAE

The Togaviridae (toga = cloak) make up a large family of viruses which are distinguished by virions of characteristic morphology, consisting of a small nucleocapsid of cubic symmetry enclosed by an envelope of lipoprotein. The inner capsid is 20 to 40 nm in diameter; the lipoprotein envelope, 40 to 70 nm in diameter. The viral nucleic acid consists of single-stranded RNA of molecular weight of 4 million daltons. The virions are assembled in the cytoplasm of host cells; they mature and acquire their lipoprotein envelope by budding from cytoplasmic membranes (genus *Alphavirus*) or into intracytoplasmic membranes around vacuoles (genus *Flavivirus*). The purified RNA is infectious. Togaviridae are labile, readily inactivated by heat, acid, lipid solvent, and detergents.

The genus *Alphavirus* (A = alpha) is made up of those viruses formerly known as Group A arboviruses (ar = arthropod, bo = borne). These viruses have serologic cross-reactivity demonstrated by the hemagglutinin-inhibition tests. The arthropod vectors are mosquitoes, but some viruses may be transmitted congenitally by vertebrates. They may cause generalized infections with encephalitis in animals and man, but also result in inapparent infections in reptiles, birds, or mammals. The type species is the Sindbis virus. Other members of the genus are the equine encephalitis viruses—Eastern, Western, and Venezuelan, the Simliki Forest virus, Chikungunya virus, and 13 other named viruses.

The *Flavivirus* (flavi = yellow) genus is made up of the group formerly called the group B arboviruses. All cross-react serologically and are transmitted either by mosquitoes or ticks. The type species is the Dengue type 1 virus. Others include viruses of yellow fever, St. Louis encephalitis, West Nile, Dengue fever, Japanese encephalitis, Russian tick-borne encephalitis, Murray Valley encephalitis, and 27 other named viruses. Table 9–9 lists diseases caused by these viruses.

Table 9–9. Diseases Caused by Togaviridae

Alphavirus	Flavivirus	Pestivirus	Rubivirus
(Group A arboviruses)	(Group B arboviruses)	Hog cholera	Rubella (man)
Equine encephalomyelitis	Yellow fever	Bovine viral	
Western	Dengue type I	diarrhea-mucosal disease	
Eastern	St. Louis encephalitis	Equine arteritis	
Venezuelan	Japanese B encephalitis		
Semliki Forest virus	West Nile virus		
Chikungunya virus	Murray Valley encephalitis		
Sinbis virus	Russian tick-borne		
	encephalitis		
	Louping-ill virus		

Diseases Caused by Alphaviruses (Group A Arboviruses)

Equine Encephalomyelitis

A widespread disease of the central nervous system of horses was recognized in the United States as early as 1912 and was reported by Stange, who originally proposed the name "equine encephalomyelitis" (Anon., 1948). The disease was the cause of serious losses, particularly in the central part of the country, during the 1920s and 1930s. It was variously known as forage poisoning, cerebral spinal meningitis, staggers, Borna disease, botulism, and Kansas horse plague. During the summer of 1930, equine encephalomyelitis virus was isolated by Meyer, Haring, and Howitt (1931) from an affected horse. This important discovery was the forerunner of many significant advances in the understanding and control of viral encephalitis in many species, including man. The virus isolated by Meyer and colleagues is now known as the "Western" strain of equine encephalomyelitis virus, to distinguish it from an antigenically different virus isolated from horses in the eastern part of the United States, the "Eastern" strain (Ten Broeck and Merrill, 1933). A third strain of virus producing similar signs and lesions was isolated by Kubes and Rios (1939) from animals in Venezuela and is known as the "Venezuelan" strain. The Western strain occurs throughout most of the United States west of the Mississippi, but also has been recognized in several states along the Eastern Seaboard and in Central and South America. In contrast, the Eastern strain is principally limited to the Eastern Sea-

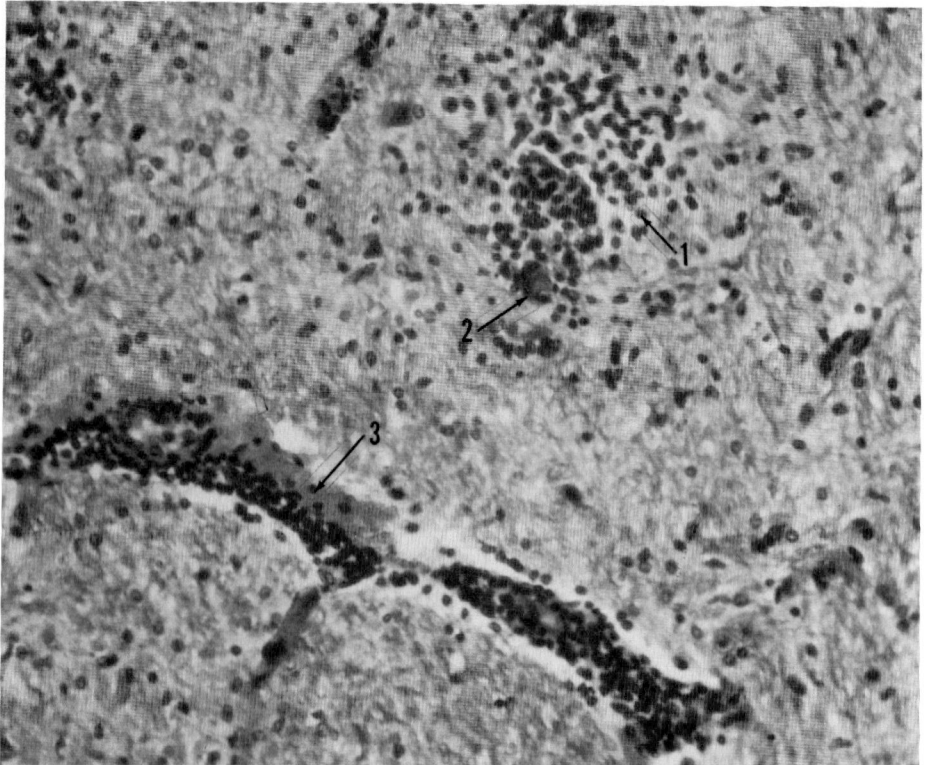

Fig. 9–46. Equine encephalomyelitis (Western strain), cerebrum of a horse (× 280). A nodule of lymphoid cells*(1)* adjacent to a neuron undergoing phagocytosis*(2)*. Lymphocytes*(3)* in the wall of a blood vessel and the Virchow–Robin space. (Courtesy of Armed Forces Institute of Pathology.) Contributor: Dr. L. T. Giltner.

board. The Venezuelan strain occurs in several South American countries, Panama, Trinidad, and Mexico. It also exists in Florida, and in 1971 a serious epizootic occurred in Mexico and Texas (Johnson and Martin, 1974).

The demonstration by Kelser, in 1933, that mosquitoes may serve as vectors of the virus of equine encephalomyelitis provided an explanation for many of its epizoötiologic features, and was followed by the discovery that the equine encephalomyelitis viruses are infective for large numbers of animals, including man.

Natural infection has been demonstrated in several species, such as calves (Pursell et al., 1976), pigs (Pursell et al., 1972), goats (Erickson et al., 1974), and dogs (Habluetzel et al., 1973). It has been proposed that wildlife (Bigler and McLean, 1973) serve as potential "sentinels" for detection of epidemic spread of the virus of the Venezuelan strain. Experimental infection of pregnant Rhesus monkeys *(Macaca mulatta)* with the Venezuelan virus results in congenital microencephaly, hydrocephalus, and cataracts in the fetuses (London et al., 1977).

It is now apparent that birds and reptiles serve as the main reservoirs for the virus, and that mosquitoes are the principal vectors. The prime vectors for the Western and Eastern strains are *Culex tarsalis* and *Culiseta melanura* respectively; however, other mosquitoes may also transmit the disease. *Aedes taeniorhynchus* is an important vector of the Venezuelan strain. The infection in most avian species is asymptomatic; however, in certain birds, such as the ring-neck pheasant, clinical disease with high mortality can occur. Owing to mosquito transmission, the disease is seasonal, with its greatest incidence in summer and fall, ending abruptly with the first killing frost.

Even though equine encephalomyelitis is an important disease in horses and man, infection of these species is rather incidental to the perpetuation of the virus, in that viremia generally is not adequate to infect mosquitoes. Since the signs and lesions caused by the three strains of virus are essentially the same, they will be considered together.

Signs. The signs, referable to derangement of the central nervous system, usually appear suddenly after an incubation period of one to three weeks. Affected animals lose awareness of their surroundings and wander about aimlessly, walk continuously in circles, are unresponsive to commands, and may collide with objects or crash through fences. High fever often occurs at the outset, but in some cases the body temperature has returned to normal by the time nervous symptoms appear. As the disease advances, stupor is evident and paralysis of various groups of muscles sets in. This flaccid paralysis increases rapidly, the animal lies down, is unable to regain its footing and soon succumbs. It is estimated that approximately 50% of horses infected with the Western strain of virus die; with the Eastern strain, this figure reaches 90%.

Lesions. No gross lesion can be considered characteristic of this disease. The viruses of equine encephalomyelitis attack neurons, hence the lesions are principally referable to damage of these cells. Affected neurons undergo various degenerative changes, culminating in necrosis. These changes are manifest by dissolution and loss of tigroid substance (tigrolysis) and chromatin (chromatolysis), fragmentation of the cell, and its removal by phagocytes (neuronophagia). This process attracts leukocytes and glial cells, which form small nodules around the injured neuron; such nodules may persist after all traces of the nerve cell are gone. The gray matter around affected neurons may also become edematous and diffusely infiltrated with lymphocytes, neutrophils, and small numbers of erythrocytes. Lymphocytes escaping from nearby arterioles are often trapped in the Virchow-Robin space to form a wide collar of densely packed cells around the blood vessel. This "perivascular cuffing" may extend into the white matter, where it is the only significant change. Perivascular cuffing is a striking microscopic finding, but it is not specific for equine encephalomyelitis; it occurs in numerous inflammatory lesions of the central nervous system.

Small intranuclear acidophilic inclusion bodies in neurons have been described by Hurst (1934) in Western equine encephalomyelitis of horses and laboratory animals, but because similar bodies have been demonstrated to occur in other viral diseases, it is doubted that they can be considered pathognomonic.

The distribution of the lesions in the central nervous system varies, depending somewhat on the strain of virus. With the Eastern strain, the gray masses are diffusely involved, the lesions are numerous, and neutrophils are often a prominent component of the exudate. The presence of these neutrophils appears to be the result of the severity of the infection and the short fatal course of the disease, thus is not absolutely diagnostic of the Eastern type. Infection with any strain of virus may result in lesions in the gray matter of the cerebral or cerebellar cortex, but they are most numerous in the olfactory bulbs, thalamus, hypothalamus, brain stem, and in both dorsal and ventral gray columns of the spinal cord. The gasserian and other ganglia may contain increased number of mononuclear cells.

In certain laboratory animals (rabbits, guinea pigs, mice) which have been experimentally infected, there is a tendency toward massive necrosis of certain olfactory centers (rhinencephalic cortex ventral to fissura rhinica and cornu Ammonis); however, other viruses may also affect these species in a like manner. A fatal encephalitis is produced by these viruses in man, with lesions comparable to those of the equine disease. Neutrophils are a much less prominent component of the exudate when the Western rather than the Eastern strain of virus is the etiologic agent involved. Western equine encephalomyelitis

in man produces widely disseminated lesions which are especially numerous in the putamen and caudate nuclei; fewer are found in the cerebral cortex and spinal cord.

Experimental infection of newborn mice with the virus of Eastern equine encephalomyelitis has been studied at the ultrastructural level by Murphy and Whitfield (1970). These investigators found that the initial changes were due to interstitial and perivascular edema, which resulted in extravascular space increasing throughout the infection. In neurons, cytoplasmic organelles were disorganized, with crenation, vacuolation, and breakdown of membranes. Virus nucleoids (28 nm in diameter) were formed in the cytoplasm of neurons and glial cells, but were not identified in endothelial cells. In the newborn mice infected with the Eastern strain, viral maturation occurred by budding of the nucleoids through plasma membranes. Complete virions were 55 nm in diameter and morphologically similar to other Togaviruses.

Diagnosis. A presumptive diagnosis may be made upon finding the microscopic lesions diffusely distributed through the gray matter of the central nervous system. A confirmed diagnosis can be made only on the basis of isolation and identification of the virus.

Specific identification of the Venezuelan strain of virus in tissues by use of fluorescence microscopy is a rapid and effective method (Erickson and Maré, 1975).

Albrecht, P.: Pathogenesis of neurotropic arbovirus infections. Curr. Top. Microbiol. Immunol., 43:44–91, 1968.
Anonymous: Editorial note. J. Am. Vet. Med. Assoc., 113:464, 1948.
Baker, A. B., and Noran, H. H.: Western variety of equine encephalitis in man. Arch. Neurol. Psychiatr., 47:565–587, 1942.
Bigler, W. J., and McLean, R. G.: Wildlife as sentinels for Venezuelan equine encephalomyelitis. J. Am. Vet. Med. Assoc., 163:657–661, 1973.
Chamberlain, R. W.: Vector relationships of the arthropod borne encephalitides in North America. Ann. NY Acad. Sci., 70:312–319, 1958.

Dill, G. S., Jr., Pederson, C. E., and Stookey, J. L.: A comparison of the tissue lesions produced in adult hamsters by two strains of avirulent Venezuelan equine encephalomyelitis virus. Am. J. Pathol., *72*:13–24, 1973.

Ehrenkranz, N. J., et al.: The natural occurrence of Venezuelan equine encephalitis in the United States. N. Engl. J. Med., *282*:298–302, 1970.

Erickson, G. A., Maré, C. J., Pearson, J. E., and Carbrey, E. A.: The goat as a sentinel for Venezuelan equine encephalomyelitis virus activity. Am. J. Vet. Res., *35*:1533–1536, 1974.

Erickson, G. A., and Maré, C. J.: Rapid diagnosis of Venezuelan equine encephalomyelitis by fluorescence microscopy. Am. J. Vet. Res., *36*:167–170, 1975.

Fothergill, L. D., Dingle, J. H., Farber, S., and Connerley, M. L.: Human encephalitis caused by virus of Eastern variety of equine encephalomyelitis. N. Engl. J. Med., *291*:411, 1938.

Gleiser, C. A., et al.: The comparative pathology of experimental Venezuelan equine encephalomyelitis infection in different animal hosts. J. Infect. Dis., *110*:80–97, 1962. VB 2271–62.

Gorelkin, L.: Venezuelan equine encephalomyelitis in an adult animal host: an electron microscopic study. Am. J. Pathol., *73*:425–442, 1973.

Gorelkin, L., and Jahrling, P. B.: Pancreatic involvement by Venezuelan equine encephalitis virus in the hamster. Am. J. Pathol., *75*:349–362, 1974.

Grayson, M. A., and Galindo, P.: Ecology of Venezuelan equine encephalitis virus in Panama. J. Am. Vet. Med. Assoc., *155*:2141–2145, 1969.

Habluetzel, J. E., Grimes, J. E., and Pigott, M. B., Jr.: Serologic evidence of naturally occurring Venezuelan equine encephalomyelitis virus infection in a dog. J. Am. Vet. Med. Assoc., *162*:461–462, 1973.

Haring, C. M., Howarth, J. A., and Meyer, K. F.: Infectious brain disease of horses and mules. North Am. Vet., *12*:29–36, 1931.

Hess, A. D., and Holden, P.: The natural history of the arthropod-borne encephalitides in the United States. Ann. NY Acad. Sci., *70*:294–311, 1958.

Hurst, E. W.: The histology of equine encephalomyelitis. J. Exp. Med., *59*:529–542, 1934.

Jahrling, P. B., and Scherer, W. F.: Histopathology and distribution of viral antigens in hamsters infected with virulent and benign Venezuelan encephalitis viruses. Am. J. Pathol., *72*:25–38, 1973.

Jennings, W. L., Allen, R. H., and Lewis, A. L.: Western equine encephalomyelitis in a Florida horse. Am. J. Trop. Med., *15*:96–97, 1966.

Johnson, K. M., and Martin, D. H.: Venezuelan equine encephalitis. Adv. Vet. Sci. Comp. Med., *18*:79–116, 1974.

Kelser, R. A.: Mosquitoes as vectors of the virus of equine encephalomyelitis. J. Am. Vet. Med. Assoc., *82*:767–771, 1933.

King, L. S.: Studies on Eastern encephalomyelitis; histopathology in the mouse. J. Exp. Med., *71*:107–112, 1940.

Kissling, R. E.: Host relationship of the arthropod-borne encephalitides. Ann. NY Acad. Sci., *70*:320–326, 1958.

Kubes, V., and Rios, F. A.: Causative agent of infectious equine encephalomyelitis in Venezuela. Science, *90*:20–21, 1939.

London, W. T., et al.: Congenital cerebral and ocular malformations induced in Rhesus monkeys by Venezuelan equine encephalitis virus. Teratology, *16*:285–296, 1977.

Meyer, K. F., Haring, C. M., and Howitt, B.: The etiology of epizoötic encephalomyelitis of horses in the San Joaquin Valley, 1930. Science, *74*:227–228, 1931.

Monlux, W. S., and Luedke, A. J.: Brain and spinal cord lesions in horses inoculated with Venezuelan equine encephalomyelitis virus (epidemic American and Trinidad strains). Am. J. Vet. Res., *34*:465–473, 1973.

Murphy, F. A., and Whitfield, S. G.: Eastern equine encephalitis virus infection: electron microscopic studies of mouse central nervous system. Exp. Mol. Pathol., *13*:131–146, 1970.

Peers, J. H.: Equine encephalomyelitis (Western) in man. Arch. Pathol., *34*:1050–1064, 1942.

Prior, M. G., and Agnew, R. M.: Antibody against Western equine encephalitis virus occurring in the serum of garter snakes (Colubridae: *Thamnophis*) in Saskatchewan. Can. J. Comp. Med., *35*:40–43, 1971.

Pursell, A. R., et al.: Naturally occurring and artificially induced Eastern encephalomyelitis in pigs. J. Am. Vet. Med. Assoc., *161*:1143–1147, 1972.

Pursell, A. R., Mitchell, F. E., and Seibold, H. R.: Naturally occurring and experimentally induced Eastern encephalomyelitis in calves. J. Am. Vet. Med. Assoc., *169*:1101–1103, 1976.

Roberts, E. D., Sanmartin, C., Payan, J., and Mackenzie, R. B.: Neuropathologic changes in 15 horses with naturally occurring Venezuelan equine encephalomyelitis. Am. J. Vet. Res., *31*:1223–1229, 1970.

Smart, D. L., Trainer, D. O., and Yuill, T. M.: Serologic evidence of Venezuelan equine encephalitis in some wild and domestic populations of southern Texas. J. Wildl. Dis., *11*:195–200, 1975.

Ten Broeck, C., and Merrill, M. H.: Serological differences between Eastern and Western equine encephalomyelitis virus. Proc. Soc. Exp. Biol. Med., *31*:217–220, 1933.

Weil, A., and Breslich, P. J.: Histopathology of the central nervous system in the North Dakota epidemic encephalitis. J. Neuropath. Exp. Neurol., *1*:49–58, 1942.

Diseases Caused by Flaviviruses

Japanese B Encephalitis

A viral encephalitis, primarily of man but to which cattle, swine, and horses are susceptible, has been described from the

Far East. The natural infection is most prevalent in Japan, but is known on Guam, Taiwan, Okinawa, and the Chinese mainland. The disease is insect-borne, transmitted by mosquitoes of the genus *Culex*. The demonstration of neutralizing and complement-fixing antibodies in cattle, swine, and horses with no history of frank disease has been used to establish the presence of inapparent infection. In swine, the virus is an important cause of abortion, stillbirth, and neonatal death. The sows are generally symptomless.

Lesions. In fatal infections in man, neuronophagic nodules are observed in all parts of the gray matter, with the thalamus, substantia nigra, nucleus basalis, and anterior horns of the spinal cord being most severely involved. In the spinal cord, the lesions tend to become confluent, whereas in the cerebral cortex and cerebellum, the lesions are generally discrete. The neuronophagic nodules indicate involvement of neurons.

In animals, including aborted and stillborn pigs, similar lesions are seen, particularly in the gray matter of the cerebral cortex and basal ganglia.

Diagnosis. Although the presence of typical lesions may suggest Japanese B encephalitis, they cannot with certainty be differentiated from those of louping ill, Teschen disease, or even equine encephalomyelitis. In order to make a definitive diagnosis, it is necessary to isolate the causative virus or demonstrate specific neutralizing antibody production following infection.

Burns, K. F.: Congenital Japanese B encephalitis of swine. Proc. Soc. Exp. Biol. N.Y., 75:621–625, 1950.
Burns, K. F., and Matumoto, M.: Japanese equine encephalomyelitis. J. Am. Vet. Med. Assoc., 115:112–115, 167–170, 1949.
————: Survey of animals for inapparent infection with the virus of Japanese B encephalitis. Am. J. Vet. Res., 10:146–149, 1949.
Haymaker, W., and Sabin, A. B.: Topographic distribution of lesions in the central nervous system in Japanese B encephalitis. Arch. Neurol. Psychiat., 57:673–692, 1947.

Webster, L. T.: Japanese B encephalitis virus; its differentiation from St. Louis encephalitis virus and relationship to louping-ill virus. J. Exp. Med., 67:609–618, 1938.
Zimmerman, H. M.: Pathology of Japanese B encephalitis. Am. J. Pathol., 22:965–991, 1946.

Ovine Encephalomyelitis (Louping III)

For many years, a disease of the nervous system has caused heavy losses among the sheep of Scotland, Northern Ireland, and England. Affected animals, usually lambs, exhibit a peculiar "louping" gait from which comes the common name for the disease. Pool, Brownlee, and Wilson (1930) isolated a virus from diseased lambs; the following year Hurst (1931) transmitted this agent to pigs, mice, and monkeys. The disease is not known to occur in the United States. The tick, *Ixodes ricinus*, transmits louping ill to sheep under natural conditions, which accounts for the seasonal occurrence of the disease. Natural fatal cases of the disease have been reported in horses (Timoney et al., 1976) and antibodies against louping ill have been detected in 10.9% of slaughtered horses in Ireland (Timoney, 1976). The disease has been described also as a mild nonfatal infection in laboratory workers.

Lesions. Louping ill virus produces lesions associated with the destruction of neurons diffusely distributed through the gray matter. Although these neuronal lesions are found throughout the cerebral cortex, they are most concentrated in the cerebellum, where loss of Purkinje cells and focal glial or inflammatory nodules are also observed. In the ventral horn of the spinal cord and medulla, motor neurons are often, but not consistently, affected. The lesions are similar in intensity and distribution to those of Teschen disease (porcine encephalomyelitis). The experimental lesions in sheep are similar to those that occur in the natural disease.

Louping ill has been experimentally transmitted to mice, pigs, and monkeys. In mice, it produces a uniformly fatal disease in which the principal change is diffuse encephalomyelitis, with neutrophilic infiltration and perivascular cuffing the prominent features. Necrosis in the hippocampus and granular layer of the cerebellum is also noted. In the monkey, symptoms of ataxia are produced and, while encephalomyelitis is less diffuse than in the mouse, the Purkinje cells in the cerebellum are largely destroyed and the anterior horn cells of the spinal cord are damaged. Cytoplasmic inclusion bodies in neurons have been described in mice and monkeys with experimental louping ill. They have not been found in the natural infection in sheep. In the pig, only the clinical manifestations of the experimental disease are known. They include hyperesthesia, tremors of the head and limbs, incoordination of movement, and inability to stand. Pigs usually recover from the experimental infection.

Diagnosis. A presumptive diagnosis can be made on the basis of the microscopic lesions in the brain and spinal cord, but definitive diagnosis depends upon isolation and identification of the virus.

Brownlee, A., and Wilson, D. R.: Studies in the histopathology of louping-ill. J. Comp. Pathol. Ther., *45*:67–92, 1932.

Doherty, P. C., and Reid, H. W.: Experimental louping-ill in sheep and lambs. II. Neuropathology. J. Comp. Pathol., *81*:331–336, 1971.

——: Louping-ill encephalomyelitis in the sheep. II. Distribution of virus and lesions in nervous tissue. J. Comp. Pathol., *81*:531–536, 1971.

Doherty, P. C., Reid, H. W., and Smith, W.: Louping-ill encephalomyelitis in the sheep. IV. Nature of the perivascular inflammatory reaction. J. Comp. Pathol., *81*:545–549, 1971.

Doherty, P. C., Smith, W., and Reid, H. W.: Louping-ill encephalomyelitis in the sheep. V. Histopathogenesis of the fatal disease. J. Comp. Pathol., *82*:337–344, 1972.

Doherty, P. C., Vantsis, J. T., and Hart, R.: Louping-ill encephalomyelitis in the sheep. VI. Infection of the 120 day foetus. J. Comp. Pathol., *82*:385–392, 1972.

Doherty, P. C., and Vantsis, J. T.: Louping-ill encephalomyelitis in the sheep. VII. Influence of immune status on neuropathology. J. Comp. Pathol., *83*:481–491, 1973.

Dow, C. and McFerran, J. B.: The neuropathology of experimental louping-ill in pigs. Res. Vet. Sci., *5*:32–38, 1964. VB 1342–64.

Findlay, G. M.: The transmission of louping-ill to monkeys. Br. J. Exp. Pathol., *13*:230–236, 1932.

Hurst, E. W.: Some observations on the pathogenesis of Eastern equine encephalomyelitis and louping-ill in young and old animals with special reference to routes of entry of the virus into the nervous system. J. Comp. Pathol. Ther., *60*:237–262, 1950.

——: The transmission of "louping-ill" to the mouse and the monkey: histology of the experimental disease. J. Comp. Pathol. Ther., *44*:231–244, 1931.

MacLeod, J., and Gordon, W. S.: Studies in louping-ill. II. Transmission by the sheep tick (Ixodes ricinus L.). J. Comp. Pathol. Ther., *45*:240–252, 1932.

Pool, W. A., Brownlee, A., and Wilson, D. R.: The etiology of "louping-ill." J. Comp. Pathol. Ther., *43*:253–290, 1930.

Reid, H. W., and Doherty, P. C.: Experimental louping-ill in sheep and lambs. I. Viraemia and the antibody response. J. Comp. Pathol., *81*:291–298, 1971.

Reid, H. W., and Doherty, P. C.: Louping-ill encephalomyelitis in the sheep. I. The relationship of viraemia and the antibody response to susceptibility. J. Comp. Pathol., *81*:521–529, 1971.

Timoney, P. I.: Louping ill: a serological survey of horses in Ireland. Vet. Rec., *98*:303, 1976.

Timoney, P. I., Donnelly, W. J. C., Clements, L. O., and Fenlon, M.: Encephalitis caused by louping ill virus in a group of horses in Ireland. Equine Vet. Res. J., *8*:113–117, 1976.

Wood, M.: Intranuclear inclusion bodies in the brain of guinea-pigs infected with louping ill virus with special reference to the effect of treatment with cyclophosphamide. Br. J. Exp. Pathol., *55*:56–63, 1974.

Diseases Caused by Pestiviruses

A tentative grouping of several important viral agents places a new genus, *Pestivirus*, in the family Togaviridae. This proposed group contains the viruses of hog cholera, bovine mucosal disease, equine arteritis, and simian hemorrhagic fever. Each of these viruses conforms to the physical and biochemical characteristics accepted for the family Togaviridae, which are defined as having an RNA genome, packed into a capsidal shell with icosahedral symmetry and surrounded by an envelope of lipoprotein (Horzinek, Maess, and Laufs, 1971). The virions of these viruses are 40 to 70 nm in diameter and contain isometric cores. Frequent deviations of the spherical shape of the virions are believed to be due to conformation of a loosely-fitting envelope. Immunologic similarities have been demonstrated between the viruses of hog cholera and bovine mucosal disease. It is possible that the taxonomic arrangement of these viruses may be changed in the future, but it seems advantageous to consider together diseases caused by these related viruses.

Horzinek, M., Maess, J., and Laufs, R.: Studies on the substructure of togaviruses, 11. Analysis of equine arteritis rubella, bovine viral diarrhea and hog cholera viruses. Arch. Virusforsch., *33*:307–318, 1971.

Spradbrow, P.: Arbovirus infections of domestic animals. Vet. Bull., *36*:55–61, 1966.

Hog Cholera (Swine Fever, Swine Plague)

Hog cholera is an acute, febrile, highly contagious, and frequently fatal disease of swine. First recognized as a separate entity by Salmon and Smith in 1885, its viral etiology was demonstrated by De Schweinitz and Dorset in 1903.

In 1962, a national program was instituted in the United States aimed at the eventual eradication of hog cholera. It was estimated at that time that four to five thousand herds of swine were suffering outbreaks of the disease each year. The program, conducted by state and federal officials and practicing veterinarians, was aimed at total eradication of the disease. Steps were taken to identify outbreaks of the disease, to prevent its spread by slaughter of infected and exposed animals, and to prevent movement of animals from any potentially infected area. The manufacture and use of all vaccines containing live or modified live virus was halted in 1969 because the vaccines were shown to be a source of new outbreaks. By 1974, the entire fifty states of the U.S. were declared to be free of hog cholera.

As the disease was restricted by these eradication measures, the florid, typical disease that had always been expected was rarely seen. Smoldering atypical cases of the disease were only identified as hog cholera following careful laboratory work involving infection of susceptible swine or identification of the virus by immunologic means.

All this may mean that current veterinary students in the United States will never encounter hog cholera as a disease problem, or may not recognize the disease should it appear. If the disease is now nonexistent in the U.S. and does not reappear, the following pages on hog cholera may not apply to the United States. However, it seems prudent to recount here the features of the disease should it reappear.

Signs. Following an incubation period of about three days after experimental exposure, or as many as seven days after field exposure, depression and a high fever (106° F.) are first manifest. These symptoms are accompanied by severe leukopenia, in which the total leukocyte count may be less than 4,000 mm^3 of blood. Although only a few animals in a herd may be infected initially, the disease spreads rapidly to all susceptible animals in contact with the disease. In addition to weakness and inappetence, nervous symptoms are commonly observed; these include lethargy, occasional convulsions, grinding of the teeth, and difficulty in locomotion. In swine with light skin, erythematous lesions appear, particularly on the skin of the abdomen, axillae, and inner surfaces of the legs. Most animals die less than ten days after the onset of symptoms; in a few that live longer, symptoms of intestinal and pulmonary involvement are more likely to be observed. In natural outbreaks, nearly 100% of susceptible animals in a herd may be expected to die. The disease in nature is limited to domestic and wild swine, but virus propagation can be accomplished experimentally in rabbits after modification of the virus by repeated alternate passage between swine and rabbits.

Infection with hog cholera virus of reduced virulence can result in a more protracted course which has been termed "chronic" hog cholera. Following an acute reaction and apparent remission, there is an exacerbation of the acute disease, result-

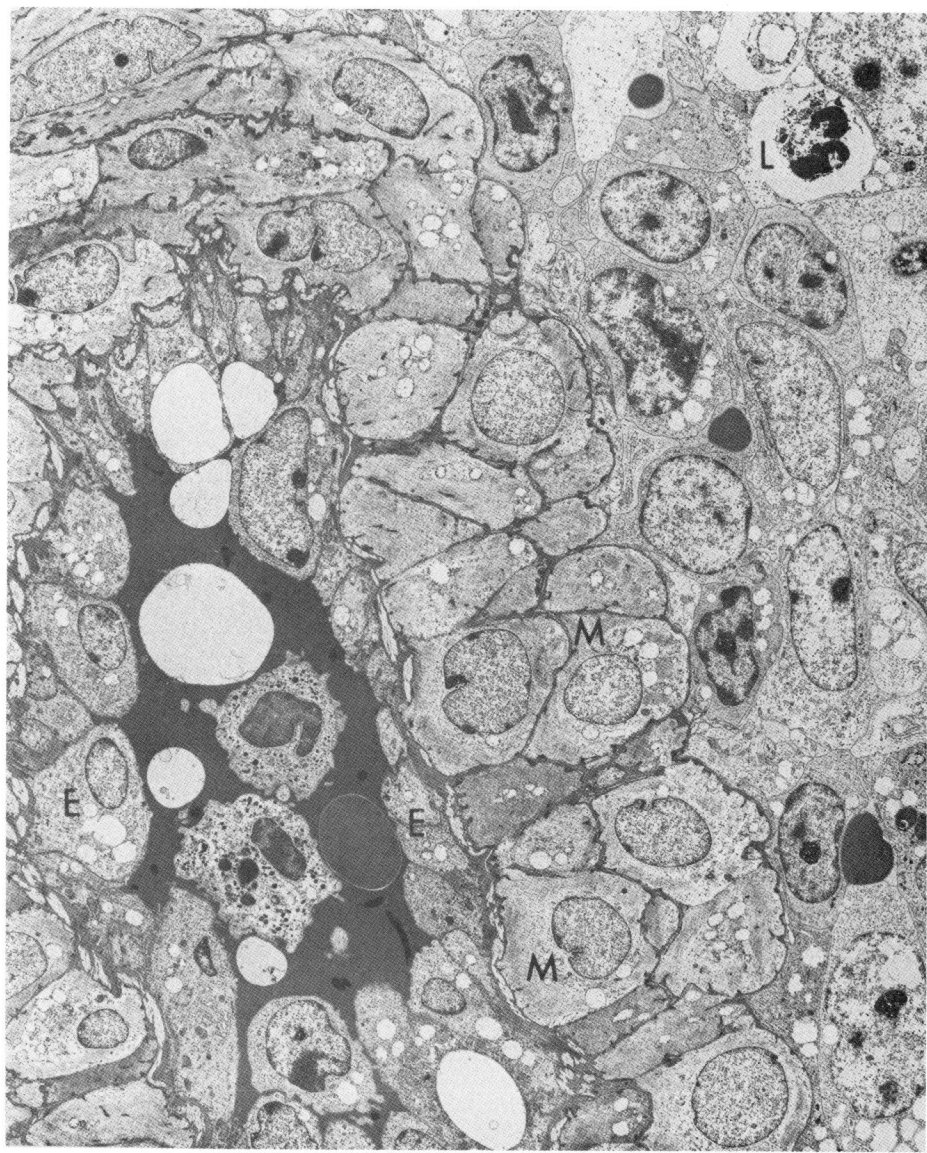

Fig. 9–47. Hog cholera. Swelling and degeneration of endothelial cells *(E)* and muscle cells *(M)* of a central arteriole of the spleen. A necrotic lymphocyte *(L)* is within a macrophage. (Courtesy Dr. N. F. Cheville and *Laboratory Investigation*.)

ing in death as late as 40 to 70 days after the initial signs of infection. These swine play an important role in the dissemination of hog cholera, because they excrete virus intermittently throughout the entire course of the infection. Swine vaccinated with live attenuated virus may also excrete virulent virus and serve as a source of infection to nonimmune swine.

A variety of fetal and neonatal abnormalities have been attributed to natural exposure to hog cholera virus or vaccination with modified live virus during pregnancy. The most critical period of exposure

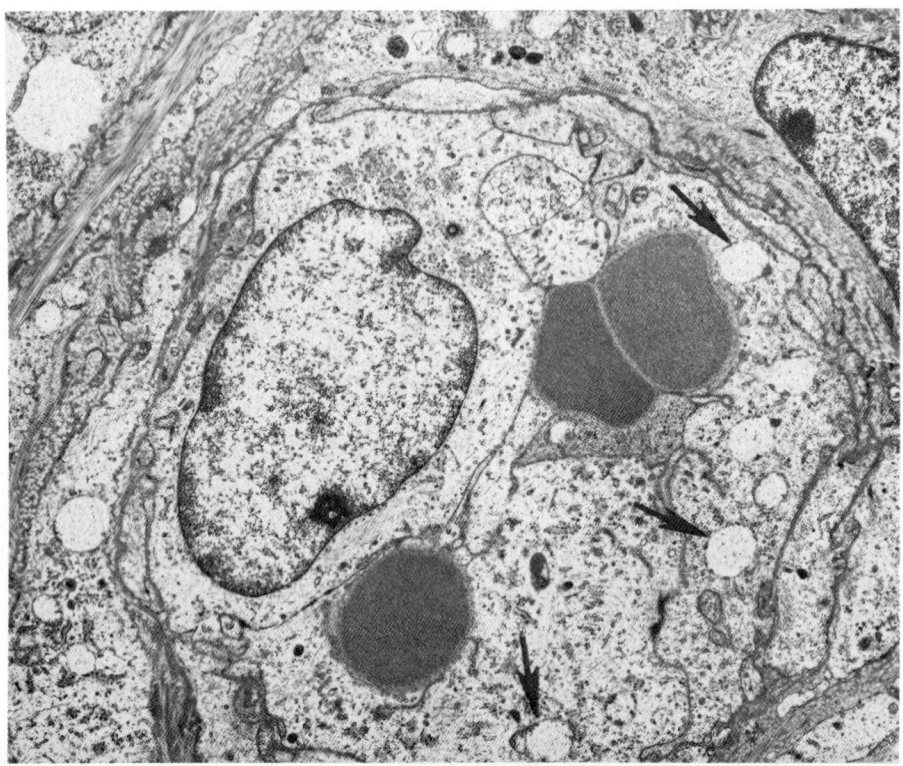

Fig. 9–48. Hog cholera. Swollen endothelial cells obliterating a capillary lumen. Mitochondria (arrows) are swollen and have lost their cristae. (Courtesy of Dr. N. F. Cheville.)

appears to be after 20 days gestation; however, earlier infection may result in embryonic death and adsorption. Abnormalities include mummification, anasarca, ascites, stillbirth, cerebellar hypoplasia, hypomyelinogenesis, congenital tremors, and neonatal death. Although the mechanism leading to these changes is not clear at present, virus crosses the placenta and invades fetal tissues, and can be demonstrated or isolated from the piglets. The immune status of the sow is not important to the development of fetal infection.

Lesions. The virus of hog cholera exerts a direct effect upon the vascular system, and the signs and lesions result from changes in the capillaries, precapillaries, arteries, and veins. For this reason, the gross lesions appear as areas of congestion, hemorrhage, or infarction, depending upon the organs involved and the severity

and duration of the vascular changes. In acute cases and in swine sacrificed early in the disease, gross lesions may be difficult to detect, but in cases of longer duration, they may be found in a wide variety of organs. According to Kernkamp (1939), gross lesions are seen in organs in the following order of frequency: kidney, lymph nodes, urinary bladder, skin (in white skinned animals), spleen, larynx, lungs, and large intestine. With less frequency, lesions are found in the heart, liver, small intestine, and stomach.

In the vascular system, the specific action of the virus is manifest grossly by petechiae and ecchymoses, but the nature of the lesions can be determined only by microscopic examination. The earliest and most pronounced lesions are found in the capillaries and precapillaries; some vessels are closed, others are dilated. The most

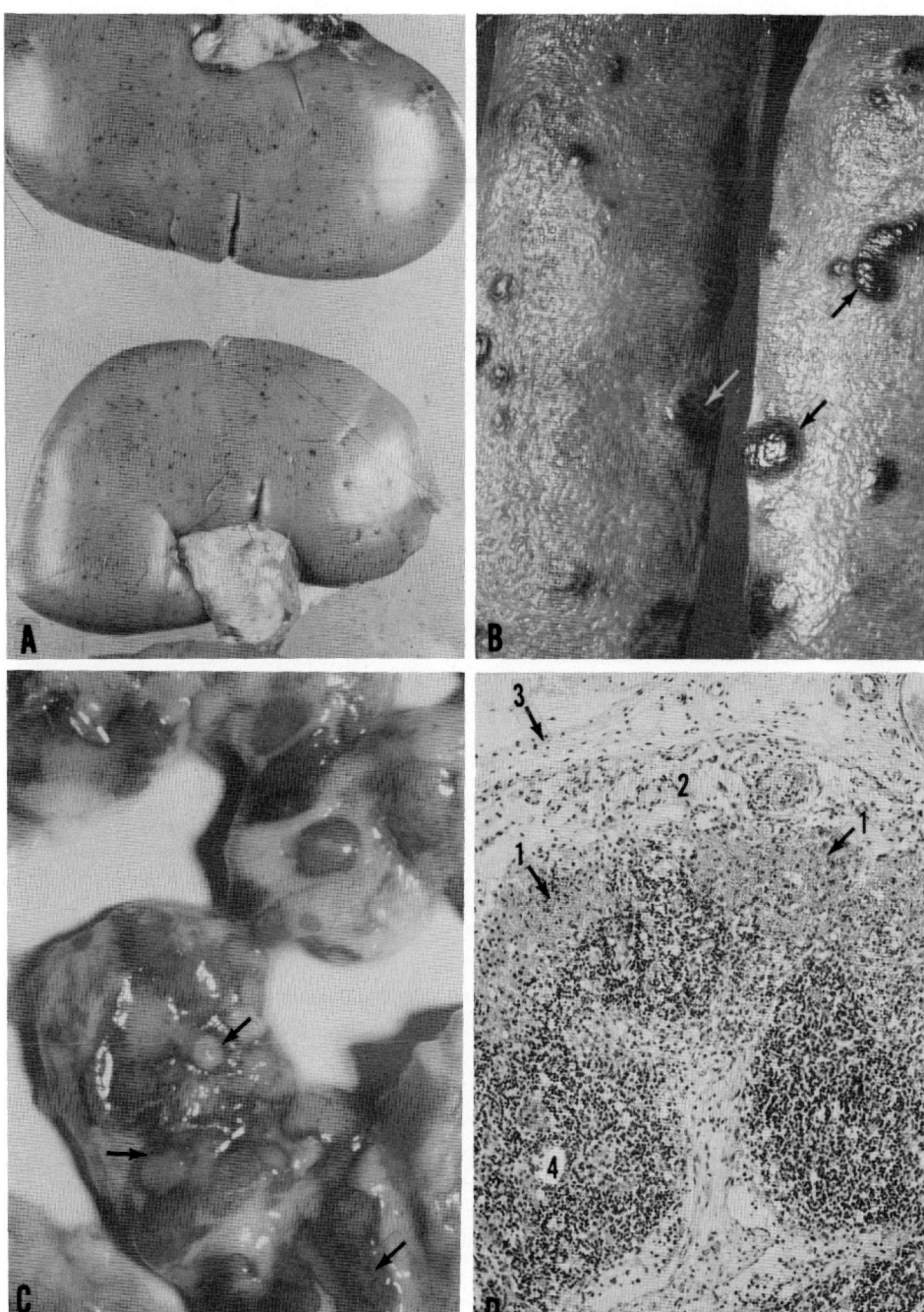

Fig. 9–49. Hog cholera. *A,* Petechiae in the kidney. *B,* Infarcts (arrows) in the spleen. *C,* Hemorrhages (arrows) in lymph nodes. *D,* Hemorrhages *(1)* in cell-poor substance of lymph node (× 90). Note that the subcapsular sinusoids *(2)* and capsule *(3)* are not involved. Lymphoid follicle at *(4).* (Courtesy of Armed Forces Institute of Pathology.)

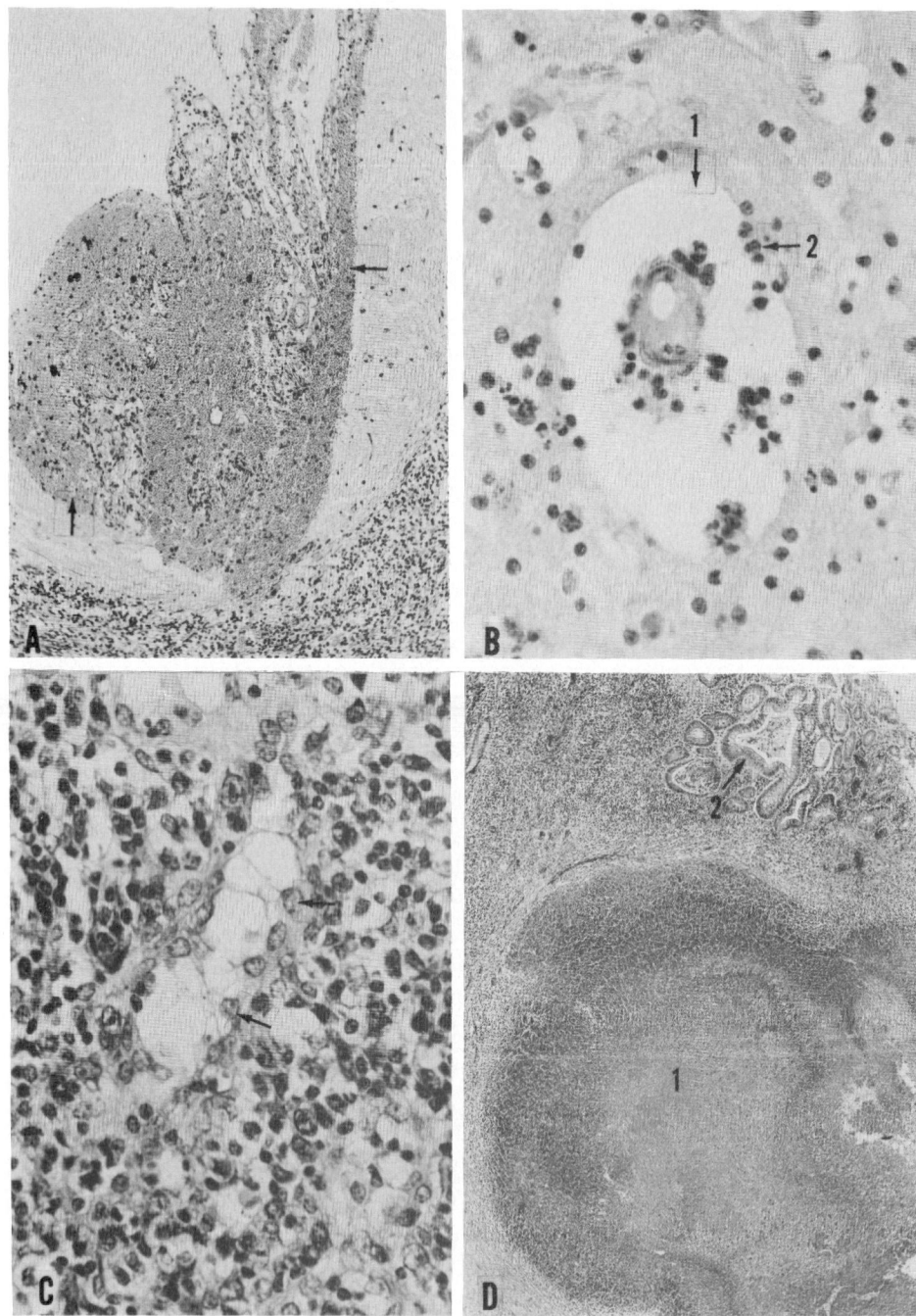

Fig. 9–50. Hog cholera. *A*, Hemorrhage (arrows) in the pia mater (× 75). *B*, Edematous distention *(1)* of Virchow-Robin space and aggregation of a few leukocytes *(2)* in the cerebrum (× 220). *C*, Proliferation of endothelial nuclei (arrows) in a lymph node (× 410). Contributor: Lt. Col. F. D. Maurer. *D*, Sharply demarcated zone of necrosis *(1)* in the colon (× 35). Epithelium is indicated at *(2)*. (Courtesy of Armed Forces Institute of Pathology.) Contributor: Lt. Col. F. D. Maurer.

constant change is swelling and proliferation of endothelial cells accompanied by a decrease in staining intensity. The endothelial nuclei are thus enlarged, increased in number, pale staining, and may pile up to occlude the lumen or be desquamated and lost. The capillary basement membrane is pale, eosinophilic, hyaline, and homogeneous, and these changes may extend to the collagen and reticulum fibers that surround the vessel. The capillary wall may become completely hyalinized, resulting in partial or complete occlusion (Fig. 9–50). Fat droplets may be seen in the capillary walls or in the surrounding area of necrosis. Thrombosis is rare in arterioles or smaller vessels. In small and medium-sized arteries, the lesions are similar to those in capillaries but are less frequent and more striking. In the larger of these arteries and in veins, swelling and proliferation of the endothelium are associated with separation and distention of fibers of the media and adventitia, perhaps by edema. The media and adventitia may be hyalinized, and occasionally necrosis is seen with an adventitial infiltrate of cells showing pyknosis and karyorrhexis. Thrombosis occasionally occurs in arteries involved in this manner. Similar lesions may be seen in veins but rarely in lymph vessels. Vascular changes are most severe in lymph nodes, spleen, and kidneys, and less severe in the nervous system, liver, intestine, skin, and other organs.

In the central nervous system, the lesions are related to the vasculature, and therefore may appear in any part of this system as early as six days after infection and before signs are observed. Aside from congestion of the vasculature, gross changes are not seen in the brain. The most striking microscopic lesion results from accumulation of lymphocytes in the perivascular (Virchow-Robin) spaces around arteries and veins (Fig. 9–50), and may be large enough to be detected in stained sections with very low magnification. This perivascular cuffing with lymphocytes, mononu-clear cells, plasma cells, and occasional eosinophils often outlines the vessel as it extends into the parenchyma from the pia-arachnoid. Neutrophils are not a part of the inflammatory exudate, but in severe cases, leukocytes may infiltrate the tissues surrounding the perivascular space. Hemorrhages may be observed around blood vessels, especially in the cerebellum and the spinal cord. Similarly, perivascular accumulations of mononuclear and red blood cells may be found in the choroid plexus. Conspicuously absent are thrombi, emboli, or patches of softening. Small nodules of proliferated microglia are present, particularly within white matter, but sometimes diffusely scattered through both white and gray matter. These small, sharply-outlined nodules are made up chiefly of microglial cells, but may include leukocytes. Such microglial nodules are rather subtle even in microscopic sections. Occasionally, Hortega cells containing many mitotic figures are seen in concentric arrangement around vessels. Of much less significance are the changes in the neurons which are neither specific nor common, but a few affected nerve cells may be noted adjacent to, or in areas of, glial proliferation. The large pyramidal cells are more likely to be damaged than are multipolar cells of the cortex and gray nuclei. Some Purkinje cells may be affected. In the involved neurons, the nucleus is swollen and located peripherally; its chromatin is fragmented and the nucleolus is absent. There may be tigrolysis of the cytoplasm, with vacuolation and loss of Nissl's granules. The cell membrane may be denticulated. Occasional neuronophagia and satellitosis are seen in the gray masses of the brain, cerebellum, and cord. There is no demyelination. Inclusion bodies resembling those described by Joest and Degen in Borna disease, and by Hurst in equine encephalomyelitis and poliomyelitis, are found in a few cases, but are not considered specific. These inclusions are intranuclear, round, homogeneous, acidophilic or occasionally basophilic, and several may be found in a single neuron.

In the spleen, infarction due to lesions in the arteries occurs in about 50% of the cases. Grossly, the infarcts are sharply outlined, red in color, irregular in shape, and elevated (Fig. 9–49); some are definitely wedge-shaped. Microscopically, degenerative changes in the wall of follicular or trabecular arteries are characterized by proliferation of endothelium, hyalinization, and necrosis in the media and adventitia with resultant thrombosis. Hemorrhagic infarction related to these vascular lesions is demonstrable as sharply demarcated areas of necrosis (Fig. 9–50).

Gross lesions are seen in one or more lymph nodes in more than 80% of animals that die of hog cholera. Even in nodes of the same animal, they vary from swelling and hyperemia with bright red, subcapsular hemorrhages outlining the periphery of the node, to dense, dark-colored hemorrhages obscuring the entire nodal architecture. In the milder lesions, the fresh hemorrhage is confined to the cell-poor substance, which in porcine lymph nodes lies just beneath the cortical and adjacent to the trabecular sinuses.* The cortical sinuses, even in hemorrhagic nodes, seldom contain red blood cells. Pronounced changes are usually observed in the capillaries, arterioles, and venules, particularly in the cell-poor substance. Swelling and proliferation of endothelial nuclei are striking, and are accompanied by occlusion of the lumen and duplication of the vessels. Diffuse accumulation of erythrocytes may obscure most of the histologic features of nodes that are severely involved.

In the skin, erythematous areas resulting from cyanosis are the most common gross lesions. They usually appear as areas of purplish discoloration, 1 to 15 cm in diameter, on the ventral surface of the abdomen

*The secondary follicles are located deep in the node near the trabeculae (Seifried and Cain, 1932). This is the reverse of the anatomic arrangement in most other species.

and the thorax, the medial surface of the thigh and leg, on the ears, on the medial surface of the forearm, in the skin of the perineum and snout. Edema and necrosis with sloughing are rare. The cyanotic changes usually can be readily detected in white-skinned swine, less easily in brown-skinned swine, and rarely in the black breeds. The typical changes in the vascular system also are responsible for these cutaneous lesions.

In the kidney, sharply demarcated petechiae, from 1 to 5 mm in diameter, are visible grossly just beneath the capsule and deep in the renal cortex. These petechiae give the kidney a characteristic appearance, which has been likened to that of a turkey egg (Fig. 9–49). Microscopically, hemorrhages are found in the interstitial stroma and in Bowman's spaces, and from the latter blood may flow into the convoluted tubules. These hemorrhages are related to the typical lesions in the vasculature.

The digestive system is most obviously affected in animals dying after a more prolonged course. Diffuse catarrhal inflammation may be seen, but is not specific for hog cholera. The characteristic lesion is a spherical ulcer in the mucosa, particularly of the colon. These ulcers are sharply circumscribed, single or multiple; they originate as small congested areas with adherent fecal material and develop into encrusted button-shaped foci ("button ulcers") a few millimeters in diameter. Cut section reveals a sharply demarcated zone of necrosis in the underlying mucosa and submucosa. This lesion develops following occlusion of a small artery by swelling and hydropic changes in its endothelium; thus the "button ulcer" is the result of infarction and evolves through the same sequence of events as the infarcts in the spleen.

Diagnosis. The diagnosis can usually be made on the basis of the clinical manifestations and gross and microscopic lesions. In the presence of fever without other symptoms, differentiation from acute systemic swine erysipelas may be a problem, but it can be solved by isolation of the organism of swine erysipelas from the blood stream. Acute arthritis, common in erysipelas, has specific diagnostic value because it does not occur in hog cholera. Teschen disease can be differentiated by the microscopic lesions found in the central nervous system. Confirmation of the diagnosis of hog cholera is accomplished by injection of blood or tissue filtrates from suspected swine into cholera-susceptible pigs, with controls receiving a large simultaneous dose of anticholera immune serum. The pigs receiving antiserum should remain well and the unprotected pigs sicken and die of hog cholera. This method obviously is suitable only for herd diagnosis. The virus can be isolated in tissue culture, but unfortunately most strains do not produce cytopathic effects. However, the presence of the virus can be demonstrated by the application of fluorescent antibody staining to infected cell cultures. This test has proven reliable and is replacing the older pig inoculation test. Fluorescent antibody staining can also be applied directly to tissue sections.

Baetz, A. L., Mengeling, W. L., and Booth, G. D.: Blood constituent changes associated with hog cholera virus infection of swine. Am. J. Vet. Res., 32:1479–1490, 1971.

Carbrey, E. A., et al.: Transmission of hog cholera by pregnant sows. J. Am. Vet. Med. Assoc., 149:23–30, 1966.

Cheville, N. F., and Mengeling, W. L.: The pathogenesis of chronic hog cholera (swine fever), histologic, immunofluorescent, and electron microscopic studies. Lab. Invest., 20:261–274, 1969.

Cheville, N. F., Mengeling, W. L., and Zinober, M. R.: Ultrastructural and immunofluorescent studies of glomerulonephritis in chronic hog cholera. Lab. Invest., 22:458–467, 1970.

De Schweinitz, E. A., and Dorset, M.: A form of hog cholera not caused by the hog cholera bacillus. Circular 41, U.S.D.A., BAI, Washington, D.C., September 28, 1903.

Dunne, H. W., and Clark, C. D.: Embryonic death, fetal mummification, stillbirth, and neonatal death in pigs of gilts vaccinated with attenuated live-virus hog cholera vaccine. Am. J. Vet. Res., 29:787–796, 1968.

Dunne, H. W., et al.: A study of an encephalitic strain of hog cholera virus. Am. J. Vet. Res., 13:277–289, 1952.

Dunne, H. W.: Hog cholera. In Diseases of Swine, 4th ed., edited by H. W. Dunne and A. D. Leman. Ames, Iowa State Univ. Press, 1975.

Dunne, H. W., Smith, E. M., and Runnells, R. A.: The relation of infarction to the formation of button ulcers in hog cholera infected pigs. Proc. Am. Vet. Med. Assoc., 1952, pp. 155–160.

Dunne, H. W., Reich, C. V., Hokanson, J. F., and Lindstrom, E. S.: Variations in the virus of hog cholera. A study of chronic cases. Proc. Am. Vet. Med. Assoc., 1955, pp. 148–153.

Emerson, J. L., and Delez, A. L.: Cerebrellar hypoplasia, hypomyelinogenesis, and congenital tremors of pigs, associated with prenatal hog cholera vaccination of sows. J. Am. Vet. Med. Assoc., 147:47–54, 1965.

Freeman, A.: All 50 states hog cholera free. J. Am. Vet. Med. Assoc., 165:158–162, 1974.

Helmboldt, C. F., and Jungherr, E. L.: Neuropathologic diagnosis of hog cholera. Am. J. Vet. Res., 11:41–49, 1950.

———: Further observations on the neuropathological diagnosis of hog cholera. Am. J. Vet. Res., 13:309–317, 1952.

Jefferies, J. C.: Hog cholera—where we are and what we must do. J. Am. Vet. Med. Assoc., 165:1004–1005, 1974.

Johnson, K. P., Ferguson, L. C., Byington, D. P., and Redman, D. R.: Multiple fetal malformations due to persistent viral infection. I. Abortion, intrauterine death, and gross abnormalities in fetal swine infected with hog cholera vaccine virus. Lab. Invest., 30:608–617, 1974.

Jones, R. K., and Doyle, L. P.: A study of encephalitis in swine in relation to hog cholera. Am. J. Vet. Res., 14:415–419, 1953.

Kernkamp, H. C. H.: Lesions of hog cholera: Their frequency of occurrence. J. Am. Vet. Med. Assoc., 95:159–166, 1939.

———: The blood picture in hog cholera. J. Am. Vet. Med. Assoc., 95:525–529, 1939.

Kresse, J. I., Stewart, W. C., Carbrey, E. A., and Snyder, M. L.: Swine buffy coat culture: an aid to the laboratory diagnosis of hog cholera. Am. J. Vet. Res., 36:141–144, 1975.

Lewis, P. A., and Shope, R. E.: The study of the cells of the blood as an aid to the diagnosis of hog cholera. J. Am. Vet. Med. Assoc., 74:145–152, 1929.

Loan, R. W., and Storm, M. M.: Propagation and transmission of hog cholera virus in nonporcine hosts. Am. J. Vet. Res., 29:807–811, 1968.

Mengeling, W. L., and Packer, R. A.: Pathogenesis of chronic hog cholera: host response. Am. J. Vet. Res., 30:409–417, 1969.

Mengeling, W. L., and Torrey, J. P.: Evaluation of the fluorescent antibody-cell culture test for hog cholera diagnosis. Am. J. Vet. Res., 28:1653–1659, 1967.

Peckham, J. C., Cole, J. R., Jr., and Pursell, A. R.: Fluorescent antibody and histopathologic procedures for hog cholera diagnosis. J. Am. Vet. Med. Assoc., 157:1204–1207, 1970.

Pirtle, E. C.: Hog cholera virus yields in swine kidney cells fused with beta-propiolactone-inactivated Sendai virus. Am. J. Vet. Res., 33:121–126, 1972.

Roehrer, H.: Histologische Untersuchungen bei Schweinepest. I. Lymphknotenveränderungen in akuten Fällen. Arch. f. Tierheilk., 62:345–372, 1930–31.

———: Histologische Untersuchungen bei Schweinepest. II. Veränderungen im Zentralnervensystem in akuten Fällen. Arch. Tierheilk., 62:439–462, 1930–31.

Salmon, D. E., and Smith, T.: Rep. Comm. Agr., Washington, D.C., 1885.

Saulmon, E. E.: Hog cholera eradication–dream or reality. J. Am. Vet. Med. Assoc., 163:1103–1105, 1973.

Saulmon, E. E.: Final phase of hog cholera eradication. J. Am. Vet. Med. Assoc., 164:304–306, 1974.

Seifried, O.: Histological studies on hog cholera. I Lesions in the central nervous system. J. Exp. Med., 53:277–289, 1931.

Seifried, O., and Cain, C. B.: Histological studies on hog cholera. II. Lesions of the vascular system. J. Exp. Med., 56:345–349, 1932.

———: Histological studies on hog cholera. III. Lesions in the various organs. J. Exp. Med., 56:351–362, 1932.

Solorzano, R. R., et al.: The diagnosis of hog cholera by a fluorescent antibody test. J. Am. Vet. Med. Assoc., 149:31–34, 1966.

Stewart, W. C., Carbrey, E. A., and Kresse, J. I.: Transplacental hog cholera infection in immune sows. Am. J. Vet. Res., 33:791–798, 1972.

———: Transplacental hog cholera infection in susceptible sows. Am. J. Vet Res., 34:637–640, 1973.

Stewart, W. C., et al.: Transmission of hog cholera virus by mosquitoes. Am. J. Vet. Res., 36:611–614, 1975.

Tidwell, Mac A., et al.: Transmission of hog cholera virus by horseflies (Tabanidae: Diptera). Am. J. Vet. Res., 33:615–622, 1972.

Bovine Viral Diarrhea—Mucosal Disease

A contagious disease of cattle in New York State was first described in 1946 by Olafson, McCallum and Fox, who demonstrated its viral etiology and termed the infection **virus diarrhea.** The disease was characterized by high morbidity and low (4 to 8%) mortality rates. Also in 1946, Childs described a disease of cattle in Canada similar to virus diarrhea, which was more severe and had a high mortality rate, although herd morbidity was low. In 1953, Ramsey and Chivers in Iowa described a syndrome nearly identical to that described by Childs, and named the syndrome **mucosal disease.** Pritchard et al., in

1954 and 1956, reported the occurrence of a disease in Indiana that closely resembled virus diarrhea in its clinical signs, morbidity, mortality, and gross and microscopic lesions. In the literature, this disease has become known as **Indiana virus diarrhea.** Diseases resembling virus diarrhea or mucosal disease have since been described in other parts of the United States and in Europe, Australia, and New Zealand.

At the outset, these two diseases appeared to differ in clinical and pathologic features and severity. As the disease has been studied further, these differences seemed less clear-cut. Serum from cattle recovering from both diseases neutralizes strains of both viruses in tissue culture systems (Gillespie et al., 1961). Although some

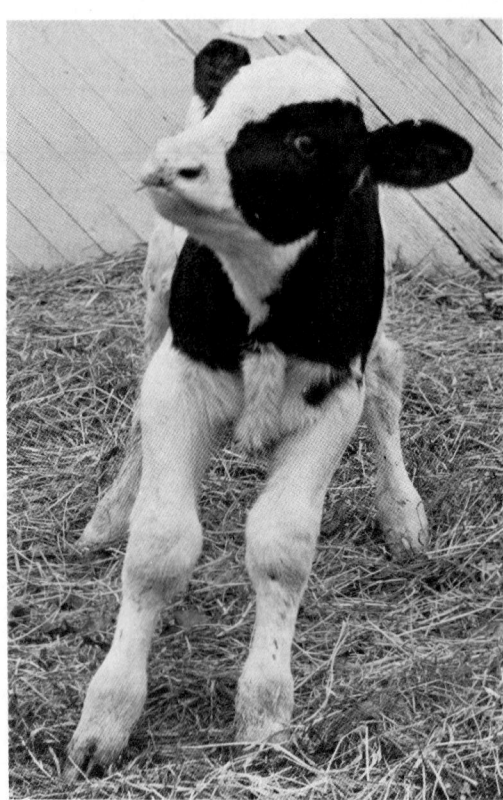

Fig. 9–51. Bovine viral diarrhea/mucosal disease. Cerebellar hypoplasia in a 3 day old Holstein calf. Virus was inoculated into the dam on the 150th day of pregnancy. Calf was blind and ataxic. (Courtesy of Dr. G. M. Ward and *Cornell Veterinarian.*)

differences in serotypes have been demonstrated (Fernelius et al., 1971), it now appears that the viral agents should be considered the same. A committee has recommended that the name **bovine viral
diarrhea-mucosal disease** should be
applied (Jensen et al., 1968). The virus has
infected pigs and causes intrauterine infection in sheep. The latter disease is described as Border disease.

Signs. The clinical signs include high
fever (105 to 108° F.), anorexia, depression,
and diarrhea, accompanied by excessive
salivation, with stringy mucus hanging
from the muzzle to the ground. Severe
leukopenia is observed rather constantly in
the early stages of the disease. Ulcers develop in the mouth, on the nose and muzzle of severely affected animals. Mucous or
mucopurulent nasal discharges are conspicuous in some animals; others cough
throughout the course of the disease. Disturbances in distribution of body heat may
be observed, with the ears, muzzle, and
extremities cold, and other parts of the
body very warm to the touch. The nasal
and oral mucosae are congested, varying
from pink to red. The conjunctiva may be
congested, but the eye is not otherwise involved. Dehydration and suspension of
milk secretion and rumination occur in severe infections, and the animals so affected
are weak and tend to be recumbent. Abortions, stillbirths, and mummified fetuses
are frequent following acute attacks, even
in animals that appear to be recovering.
Septic metritis following abortion may result in death. In the fetus, lesions similar to
those of the adult may be seen in the oral
cavity, esophagus, and abomasum. Calves

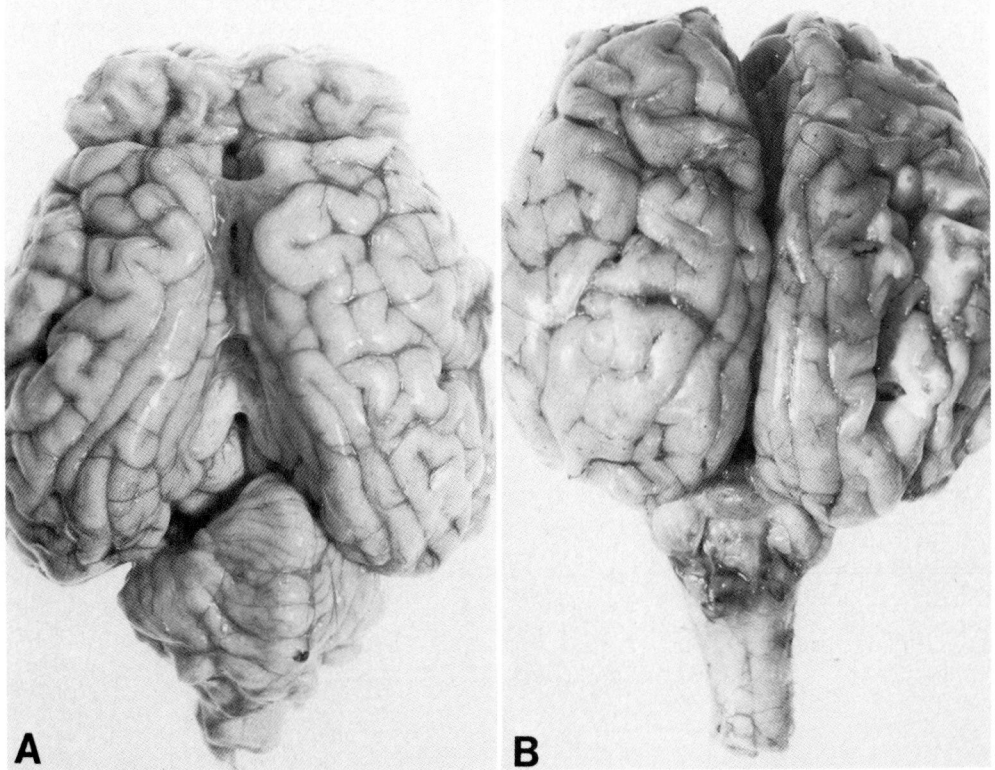

Fig. 9–52. Bovine viral diarrhea/mucosal disease. *A*, Brain of normal, uninoculated calf, one month old.
B, Brain of 33-day-old blind and ataxic calf. Severe hypoplasia of cerebellum. (Courtesy of Dr. G. M. Ward
and *Cornell Veterinarian*.)

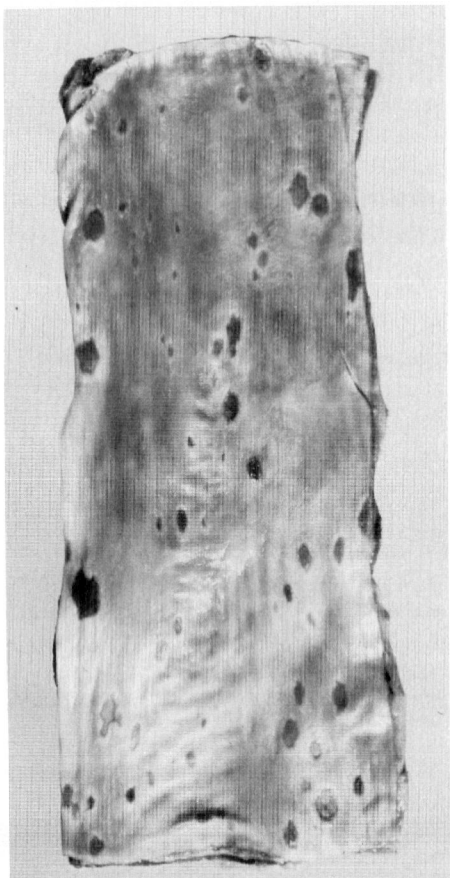

Fig. 9–53. Bovine viral diarrhea/mucosal disease. Esophageal ulcers in an Angus steer. (Courtesy of Dr. W. J. Hadlow.)

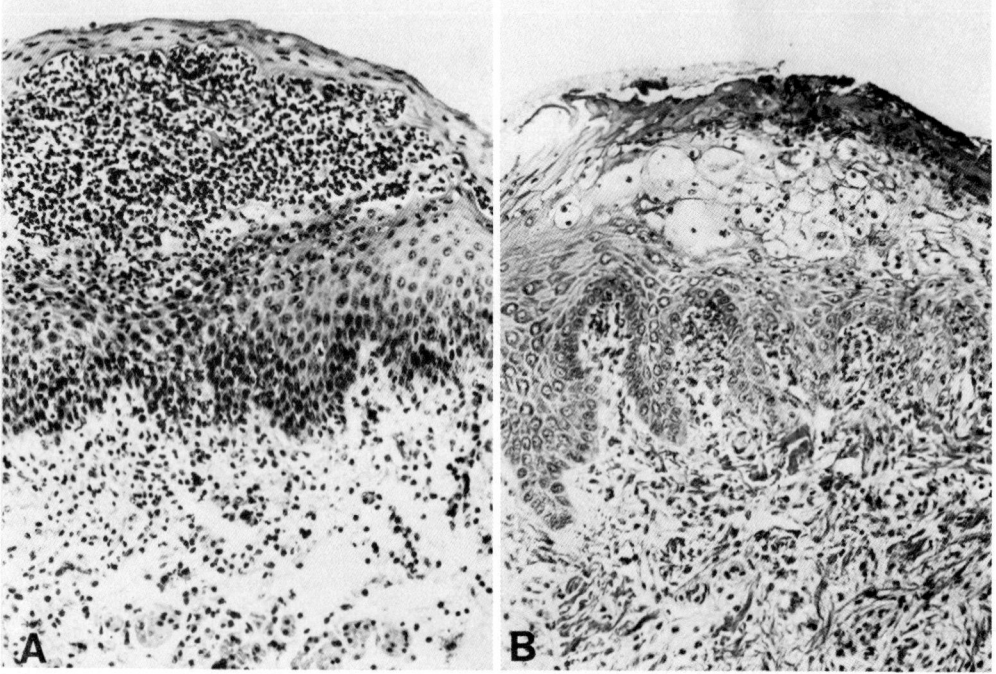

Fig. 9–54. Bovine viral diarrhea/mucosal disease. *A*, Esophagus of infected newborn calf. Necrosis of middle layers of epithelium with leukocytic infiltration. *B*, Buccal mucosa of an infected premature calf with necrosis of stratum germinativum of the epithelium. (Courtesy of Dr. G. M. Ward and *Cornell Veterinarian*.)

born alive may also exhibit signs and lesions of virus diarrhea. Congenital cerebellar hypoplasia, cataracts, retinal atrophy, microphthalmia, optic neuritis, and malformations of the choriocapillaries have been noted in calves born to naturally and experimentally infected dams. Observation of infected herds has shown that from 33 to 100% of the animals exhibit signs. The mortality rate is usually 4 to 8%.

Lesions. At necropsy, except for general dehydration and emaciation of the carcass, the principal gross lesions are found in the gastrointestinal tract. Sharply delimited, irregularly-shaped ulcers or erosions of the mucosa are found on the dental pad, palate, lateral surfaces of the tongue, and inside of the cheeks. Ulcers may also occur on the muzzle and at the external nares, although usually the nasal mucosae are merely reddened. On the mucous membrane of the pharynx, irregularly-shaped ulcers of varying size may be covered by a tenacious gray exudate. Necrotic lesions may be confined to the pharynx or may extend to the larynx. Some animals develop pneumonia.

In the esophagus, the entire mucous membrane may contain shallow erosions or ulcers with sharply delimited, irregular margins and a red base (Fig. 9–53). At times these lesions coalesce to form elongated ulcers or erosions, with necrotic material adhering to some.

The abomasal mucosa may be diffusely reddened or may contain petechiae and a few ulcers. Hemorrhages may be present in the leaves of the omasum. The mucosa of the small intestine is diffusely reddened, but prominent petechiae and ulcers are found only in the cecum. Hemorrhages have been observed in the vaginal mucosa, subcutis generally, and the epicardium.

Diagnosis. The resemblance of the lesions of virus diarrhea to the gastrointestinal lesions of rinderpest and the oral lesions of malignant catarrhal fever complicates the differential diagnosis. At present, cross-immunity and cross-serum neu-

tralization tests can be used to distinguish rinderpest from virus diarrhea. Malignant catarrh can be differentiated by its slower spread and the characteristic ocular, nasal, and brain lesions that it produces.

Archbald, L. F., et al.: Effects of intrauterine inoculation of bovine viral diarrhea-mucosal disease virus on uterine tubes and uterus of nonpregnant cows. Am. J. Vet. Res., *34*:1133–1138, 1973.

Baker, J. A., York, C. J., Gillespie, J. H., and Mitchell, G. B.: Virus diarrhea in cattle. Am. J. Vet. Res., *15*:525–531, 1954.

Bistner, S. I., Rubin, L. F., and Saunders, L. Z.: The ocular lesions of bovine viral diarrhea-mucosal disease. Pathol. Vet. *7*:275–286, 1970.

Braun, R. K., Osburn, B. I., and Kendrick, J. W.: Immunologic response of bovine fetus to bovine viral diarrhea virus. Am. J. Vet. Res., *34*:1127–1132, 1973.

Brown, T. T., et al.: Virus induced congenital anomalies of the bovine fetus. II. Histopathology of cerebellar degeneration (hypoplasia) induced by the virus of bovine viral diarrhea-mucosal disease. Cornell Vet., *63*:561–578, 1973.

———: Pathogenetic studies of infection of the bovine fetus with bovine viral diarrhea virus. I. Cerebellar atrophy. Vet. Pathol., *11*:486–505, 1974.

———: Pathogenetic studies of infection of the bovine fetus with bovine viral diarrhea virus. II. Ocular lesions. Vet. Pathol. *12*:394–404, 1975.

Carbrey, E. A., Stewart, W. C., Kresse, J. L., and Snyder, M. L.: Natural infection of pigs with bovine viral diarrhea virus and its differential diagnosis from hog cholera. J. Am. Vet. Med. Assoc., *169*:1217–1219, 1976.

Carlson, R. G., Pritchard, W. R., and Doyle, L. P.: The pathology of virus diarrhea of cattle in Indiana. Am. J. Vet. Res., *18*:560–568, 1957.

Casaro, A. P. E., Kendrick, J. W., and Kennedy, P. C.: Response of the bovine fetus to bovine viral diarrhea-mucosal disease virus. Am. J. Vet Res., *32*:1543–1562, 1971.

Childs, T.: X disease of cattle—Saskatchewan. Can. J. Comp. Med. Vet. Sci., *10*:316, 1970.

Fernelius, A. L., Lamber, G., and Booth, G. D.: Bovine viral diarrhea virus-host cell interactions: serotypes and their relationship to biotypes of cross neutralization. Am. J. Vet. Res. *32*:229–236, 1971.

Fernelius, A. L., et al.: Bovine diarrhea virus in swine: characteristics of virus recovered from naturally and experimentally infected swine. Can. J. Comp. Med., *37*:13–20, 1973.

———: Bovine viral diarrhea virus in swine, neutralizing antibody in naturally and experimentally infected swine. Can. J. Comp. Med., *37*:96–102, 1973.

Gillespie, J. H., Coggins, L., Thompson, J., and Baker, J. A.: Comparison of neutralization tests of strains of virus isolated from virus diarrhea and mucosal disease. Cornell Vet., *51*:155–159, 1961.

Gillespie, J. H., and Baker, J. A.: Studies on virus diarrhea. Cornell Vet., *49*:439–443, 1959.

Gillespie, J. H., Baker, J. A., and McEntee, K.: A cytopathogenic strain of virus diarrhea virus. Cornell Vet., *50*:73–79, 1960.

Gillespie, J. H., et al: The isolation of noncytopathic virus diarrhea virus from two aborted bovine fetuses. Cornell Vet., *57*: 564–571, 1967.

Gillespie, J. H.: Comments on bovine viral diarrhea-mucosal disease. J. Am. Vet. Med. Assoc., *152*:768–770, 1968.

Harkness, J. J., and Lamont, P. H.: Laboratory diagnosis of mucosal disease. Vet. Rec., *96*:17–18, 1975.

Hjerpe, C. A.: Atypical bovine virus diarrhea. J. Am. Vet. Med. Assoc., *144*:1278–1293, 1964.

Jensen, R., et al.: Report of Ad Hoc Committee on Terminology for the Symposium on Immunity to the Bovine Respiratory Disease Complex. J. Am. Vet. Med. Assoc., *152*:940, 1968.

Johnson, D. W., and Muscoplat, C. C.: Immunologic abnormalities in calves with chronic bovine viral diarrhea. Am. J. Vet. Res., *34*:1139–1142, 1973.

Kahrs, R. F., Scott, F. W., and de Lahunta, A.: Bovine viral diarrhea-mucosa disease, abortion and congenital cerebellar hypoplasia in a dairy herd. J. Am. Vet. Med. Assoc., *156*:851–857, 1970.

————: Congenital cerebellar hypoplasia and ocular defects in calves following bovine viral diarrhea-mucosal disease infection in pregnant cattle. J. Am. Vet. Med. Assoc., *156*:1443–1450, 1970.

Kendrick, J. W.: Bovine viral diarrhea-mucosal disease virus infection in pregnant cows. Am. J. Vet. Res., *32*:533–544, 1971.

Lambert, G., Fernelius, A. L., and Cheville, N. F.: Experimental bovine viral diarrhea in neonatal calves. J. Am. Vet. Med. Assoc., *154*:181–189, 1969.

Maess, J., and Reczko, E.: Electron optical studies of bovine viral diarrhea-mucosal disease virus. (BVDV). Arch. Virusforsch., *30*:39–46, 1970.

McCormack, P. E., St.-George-Grambauer, T. D., and Pulsford, N. F.: Mucosa type disease of cattle in South Australia. Aust. Vet. J., *35*:482–488, 1959.

Mills, J. H. L., Nielsen, S. W., and Luginbuhl, R. E.: Current status of bovine mucosal disease. J. Am. Vet. Med. Assoc., *146*:691–696, 1965.

Olafson, P., McCallum, A. D., and Fox, F. H.: An apparently new transmissible disease of cattle. Cornell Vet., *36*:205–213, 1946.

Olafson, P., and Rickard, C. G.: Further observations on the virus diarrhea (new transmissible disease) of cattle. Cornell Vet., *37*:104–106, 1947.

Pande, P. G., and Krishnamurthy, D.: Incidence and pathology of some recently recognized mucosal disease-like syndromes amongst cattle and buffaloes in India. Bull. Off. Int. Epiz., *55*:706–714, 1961. (VB 127–62.)

Peter, C. P., et al.: Cytopathologic changes of lymphatic tissues of cattle with the bovine virus diarrhea-mucosal disease complex. Am. J. Vet. Res., *29*:939–948, 1968.

Phillip, J. I. H., and Darbyshire, J. H.: Infection of pigs with bovine viral diarrhoea virus. J. Comp. Pathol., *82*:105–109, 1972.

Pritchard, W. R., Bunnell, D., Moses, H. E., and Doyle, L. P.: Virus diarrhea of cattle in Indiana. Ann. Rep. Purdue Agric. Exper. Sta., 1954.

Pritchard, W. R., Taylor, D. B., Moses, H. E., and Doyle, L. P.: A transmissible disease affecting the mucosae of cattle. J. Am. Vet. Med. Assoc., *128*:1–5, 1956.

Ramsey, F. K., and Chivers, W. H.: Mucosal disease of cattle. North Am. Vet., *34*:629–633, 1953.

Ramsey, F. K.: The pathology of a mucosal disease of cattle. Proc. Am. Vet. Med. Assoc., 1954, pp. 162–167.

Salisbury, R. M., et al.: A mucosal disease-like syndrome of cattle in New Zealand. Bull. Off. Int. Epiz., *56*:72–78, 1961. (VB 123–62.)

Schultz, L. E.: Pathologisch-Anatomische Befunde bei der Sogenannten "Mucosal Disease" (Schleimhautkrankheit) des Rindes. Dtsch. Tierärzt. Wochenschr., *66*:582–586, 1959.

Scott, F. W., Kahrs, R. K., and Parsonson, I. N.: A cytopathogenic strain of bovine viral diarrhea-mucosal disease virus. Cornell Vet., *62*:74–84, 1972.

Scott, F. W., et al.: Virus induced congenital anomalies of the bovine fetus. I. Cerebellar degeneration (hypoplasia), ocular lesions and fetal mummification following experimental infection with bovine viral diarrhea-mucosal disease virus. Cornell Vet., *63*:536–560, 1973.

Stewart, W.C., et al.: Bovine viral diarrhea infection in pigs. J. Am. Vet. Med. Assoc., *159*:1556–1563, 1972.

Taylor, D. O. N., Gustafson, D. P., and Claflin, R. M.: Properties of some viruses of the mucosal disease-virus diarrhea complex. Am. J. Vet. Res., *24*:143–149, 1963.

Tyler, D. E., and Ramsey, F. K.: Comparative pathologic, immunologic, and clinical responses produced by selected agents of the bovine mucosal disease-virus diarrhea complex. Am. J. Vet. Res., *26*:903–913, 1965.

Walker, R. V. L., and Olafson, P.: Failure of virus diarrhea of cattle to immunize against rinderpest. Cornell Vet., *37*:107–111, 1947.

Ward, G. M., et al.: A study of experimentally induced bovine viral diarrhea-mucosal disease in pregnant cows and their progeny. Cornell Vet., *59*:525–538, 1969.

Ward, G. M.: Bovine cerebellar hypoplasia apparently caused by BVD-MD virus. A case report. Cornell Vet., *59*:570–576, 1969.

————: Experimental infection of pregnant sheep with bovine viral diarrhea-mucosal disease virus. Cornell Vet., *61*:179–191, 1971.

————: Bovine viral diarrhea mucosal disease implicated in a calf with cerebellar hypoplasia and ocular disease. A case report. Cornell Vet., *61*:224–228, 1971.

Wheat, J. D., McKercher, D. G., and York, C. J.: Virus diarrhea in California. California Vet., *8*:26–28, 35, 1954.

Border Disease of Sheep (Fuzzy Lamb, Hairy-Shaker Lamb, Hypomyelinosis Congenita)

This congenital disease of lambs, named after the Welsh Border Country in which it was first recognized in 1959, has now been reported in Scotland, England, Ireland, United States, New Zealand, and Australia. Affected lambs are detected by their hairy coat at birth, severe tremors within a month, and poor growth and viability. Some are presumed to die in utero, although most are born alive. The disease has been transmitted to lambs in utero by injection of material from brains of affected lambs into the ewes during pregnancy. A viral agent is believed to be involved; serologic and experimental evidence points toward the virus of bovine mucosal disease-virus diarrhea as the causal agent. Affected ewes develop neutralizing antibodies against bovine mucosal disease virus and hog cholera—two immunologically related viruses.

Lesions. The gross lesions post mortem are not consistent. In a few lambs, the kidneys are slightly hyperplastic. In some the brain is small, the ventricles dilated, and the spinal cord narrow and unusually firm. Cystic lesions in the cerebral white matter are seen in some cases. The microscopic lesions in the brain and spinal cord consist of decreased production of myelin, increased number of cells, particularly glial cells, in the cerebral white matter, plus accumulation of lipid between the fascicles. Glial nuclei are increased in number, and in myelin stains, nerve fibers are twisted, distorted, and swollen, giving them a beaded appearance. Gitter cells are not usually conspicuous in spite of the apparent presence of lipid in the affected neuropile.

Barlow, R. M., and Dickinson, A. G.: On the pathology and histochemistry of the central nervous system in border disease of sheep. Res. Vet. Sci., 6:230–237, 1965.

Barlow, R. M., and Gardiner, A. C.: Experiments in border disease. I. Transmission, pathology and some serological aspects of the experimental disease. J. Comp. Pathol. Ther., 79:397–405, 1969.

Barlow, R. M., Gardiner, A. C., Storey, I. J., and Slater, J. S.: Experiments in border disease. II. Some aspects of the disease in the foetus. J. Comp. Pathol., 80:635–643, 1970.

Barlow, R. M.: Experiments in border disease. IV. Pathological changes in ewes. J. Comp. Pathol., 82:151–157, 1972.

Clarke, G. L., and Osburn, B. I.: Transmissible congenital demyelinating encephalopathy of lambs. Vet. Pathol., 15:68–82, 1978.

Dickinson, A. G., and Barlow, R. M.: The demonstration of the transmissibility of border disease of sheep. Vet. Rec., 81:114, 1967.

Durham, P. J. K., Forbes-Faulkner, J. C., and Poole, W. S. H.: Hairy shaker disease: preliminary studies on the nature of the agent, and the induced serological response. NZ Vet. J., 23:236–240, 1975.

Gard, G. P., Acland, H. M., and Plant, J. W.: A mucosal disease virus as a cause of abortion, hairy birth coat and unthriftiness in sheep. 2. Observations on lambs surviving for longer than seven days. Aust. Vet. J., 52:64–68, 1976.

Gardiner, A. C., and Barlow, R. M.: Experiments in border disease. III. Some epidemiological considerations with reference to the experimental disease. J. Comp. Pathol., 82:29–35, 1972.

Gardiner, A. C., Barlow, R. M., Rennie, J. C., and Keir, W. A.: Experiments in border disease. V. Preliminary investigations on the nature of the agent. J. Comp. Pathol., 82:159–161, 1972.

Hamilton, A., and Timoney, P. J.: B.V.D. virus and border disease. Vet. Rec., 91:468, 1972.

————: Bovine virus diarrhea/mucosal disease virus and border disease. Res. Vet. Sci., 15:265–267, 1973.

Huck, R. A.: Transmission of border disease in goats. Vet. Rec., 92:151, 1973.

Hughes, L. E., Kershaw, G. F., and Shaw, I. G.: "B" or border disease: an undescribed disease of sheep. Vet. Rec., 71:313–317, 1959.

Osburn, B. I., Clarke, G. L., Stewart, W. C., and Sawyer, M.: Border disease-like syndrome in lambs: antibodies to hog cholera and bovine viral diarrhea viruses. J. Am. Vet. Med. Assoc., 163:1165–1167, 1973.

Patterson, D. S. P., and Sweasey, D.: Hypocupraemia in experimental border disease. Vet. Rec., 93:484–485, 1973.

Patterson, D. S. P., et al.: Spinal cord lipids and myelin composition in border disease (*hypomyelinogenesis congenita*) of lambs. J. Neurochem., 24:513–522, 1975.

Plant, J. W., et al.: Immunological relationship between border disease, mucosal diseases and swine fever. Vet. Rec., 92:455, 1973.

Plant, J. W., Acland, H. M., and Gard, G. P.: A mucosal disease virus as a cause of abortion, hairy birth coat and unthriftiness in sheep. I. Infection of pregnant ewes and observations on aborted foetuses and lambs dying before one week of age. Aust. Vet. J., 52:57–63, 1976.

Porter, W. L., Lewis, K. H. C. and Manktelow, B. W.:
Hairy shaker disease of lambs. I. Acquired immunity, abortion and transmission via mucous
membranes. II. Further studies on acquired immunity, abortion and effects on foetal growth.
NZ Vet. J., 20:1–3, 4–7, 1972.
Richardson, C., Hebert, C. N., and Done, J. T.: Experimental border disease in sheep: dose-
response effect. Br. Vet. J., 132:202–208, 1976.
Storey, I. J., and Barlow, R. M.: Experiments in border
disease. VI. Lipid and enzyme histochemistry. J.
Comp. Pathol., 82:163–170, 1972.
Ward, G. M.: Experimental infection of pregnant
sheep with bovine viral diarrhea–mucosal disease virus. Cornell Vet., 61:179–185, 1971.
Winkler, C. E., Gibbons, D. F., and Shaw, I. G.:
Observations on the experimental transmissibility of border disease in sheep. Br. Vet. J.,
131:32–39, 1975.

Equine Viral Arteritis

An outbreak of an infectious disease of horses characterized by depression, edematous swelling of the limbs, intense pink or red discoloration of the conjunctiva, palpebral edema, abortion of pregnant mares, enteritis, and pneumonic complications, was described by Doll, Knappenberger and Bryans (1957). The filtrable agent that they isolated from the affected animals produces panleukopenia, abortion, and death in experimentally infected horses. The principal lesions of the disease, described by Jones, Doll and Bryans (1957), are based upon degenerative and inflammatory changes in the endothelium and media of small arteries. Some of the clinical features of equine viral arteritis are not unlike those described 50 or more years ago called equine influenza ("epizootic cellulitis" or "pink eye"), or more recently rhinopneumonitis. Early writers did not describe the microscopic lesions of epizootic cellulitis, nor did they identify the causative agent; thus, these important features cannot be compared with the lesions and virus of equine arteritis; however, equine rhinopneumonitis can be readily distinguished by its characteristic lesions and virus. The name **equine viral arteritis** proposed for this disease indicates both the nature of the etiologic agent and the basic lesions it produces.

Although this virus is not transmitted by arthropods, its morphologic, physical, and chemical characteristics justify its classification with the Togaviridae. The virion is assembled in the cytoplasm of infected cells and coated by budding into cytoplasmic vesicles. The virion is enveloped and about 58 nm in diameter. The nucleic acid consists of an infectious colinear molecule of single-stranded RNA, with a molecular weight of about 4 million daltons. Buoyant density of the RNA in Cs_2SO_4 is 1.65 g/ml (Van der Zeijst, Horzinek, and Moennig, 1975).

Lesions. The gross lesions in animals experimentally infected with the equine arteritis virus consist of congestion, edema, and petechiae in the conjunctiva, nasal mucosa, pharynx, larynx, and guttural pouches; edema of the subcutis of the legs and near sites of inoculation; hydrothorax and petechiae in the pleura; edema in the mediastinum, base of the heart, pericardium, and the interlobular pulmonary septa; edema and enlargement of the mediastinal lymph nodes; petechiae on the endocardium and epicardium; distention of the pericardial sac with fluid; and edema and petechiae in the mesentery, particularly along the course of the ileocecalcolic and anterior mesenteric arteries. In addition, the peritoneal cavity often contains an excessive amount of fluid, sometimes as much as 8 to 10 L; petechiae are frequent on the visceral as well as the parietal peritoneum and omentum; the mesenteric lymph nodes are large and edematous, some contain hemorrhages, and the wall of the small intestine, cecum and colon is often edematous and sometimes bloody in appearance. The distribution of edema in the intestine is characteristic; segments 1 to 3 feet long that are slightly to severely edematous alternate with segments of normal thickness. The mucosa over the edematous segments of intestine is rugose and the lumen is constricted. In the cecum,

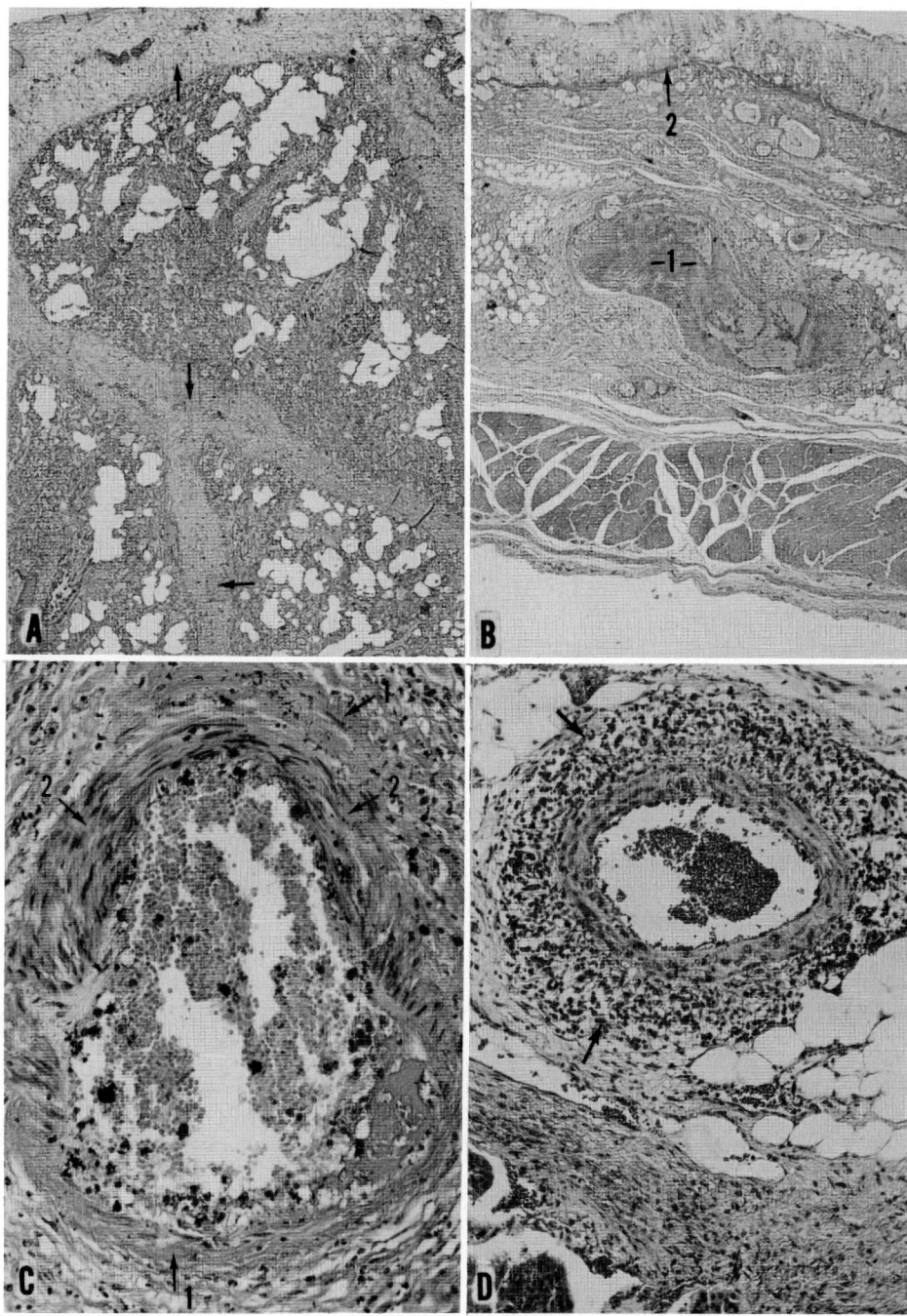

Fig. 9–55. Equine viral arteritis. *A*, Edema of the pleura and interlobular septa (arrows) (× 15). *B*, Thrombosis *(1)* of a submucosal artery in an infarcted segment of the small intestine. The muscularis mucosa *(2)* separates the necrotic mucosa and the congested, edematous submucosa. *C*, Early necrotizing lesion in the media of an artery in the submucosa of the cecum. Cellular debris and homogeneous eosinophilic material replaces the media *(2)*. *D*, An affected artery in the adrenal capsule. Note the intense infiltration of the adventitia by lymphocytes (arrows) and the concentric loss of cells of the media. (Courtesy of Armed Forces Institute of Pathology.) Contributor: Dr. E. R. Doll.

submucosal edema is often more severe at the apex than at the base or in other parts. Edema and petechiae may also be observed in the broad ligament and elsewhere. Hemorrhages into the adrenal cortex are frequent.

The microscopic lesions confirm the presence of widespread edema, vascular dilatation and, to a smaller extent, hemorrhages. Generally, the veins are fully distended with blood and the lymphatic vessels with lymph, but otherwise they are not affected. The small arteries throughout the body, however, show severe changes, especially in those tissues that exhibit gross lesions.

The most severe arterial lesions are usually seen in the submucosa of the cecum and colon. The earliest change is manifested by replacement of small parts of the arterial media by homogeneous eosinophilic material. This displaces the nuclei and cytoplasm of the muscular coat of the artery and is usually accompanied by edema and some cellular infiltration in the adventitia. In more advanced lesions, tiny areas of necrosis appear in the media, either as small foci involving a segment of the muscular coat or as more extensive, concentric zones of necrosis in the outer layers. This is accompanied by leukocytic infiltration into both the adventitia and the media. Scattered bits of nuclear chromatin are also in evidence in these areas.

Estes and Cheville (1970) have described the ultrastructure of the vascular lesions as predominantly endothelial cell damage characterized by dilation of cisternae, appearance of ribosome-like particles within cisternae of endoplasmic reticulum, and the presence of viral particles 58 nm in diameter within cytoplasmic vacuoles. Swelling of endothelial cells and platelet thrombi often obliterate capillary lumina. Edema appears to be the direct result of injury to capillaries. They suggested that degeneration of smooth muscle cells was a secondary lesion not associated with direct viral injury.

Diagnosis. The microscopic lesions of equine viral arteritis are characteristic enough to distinguish the disease from equine rhinopneumonitis, in which the characteristic lesions include foci of necrosis in lung, liver, and lymph nodes, with intranuclear inclusions.

The inflammatory lesions in the small arteries are observed in the adult horse in equine viral arteritis, but the necrotizing lesions and intranuclear inclusions of equine rhinopneumonitis are usually only found in the aborted fetus. The viruses of both diseases grow and produce cytopathogenic effects in monolayer cultures of renal cells of several species. This should permit more effective identification of the respective viruses to further confirm the specific diagnosis.

Bryans, J. T., Doll, E. R., Crowe, E. W., and McCollum, W. H.: The blood picture and thermal reaction in experimental, uncomplicated equine viral arteritis. Cornell Vet., 47:42–52, 1957.

Crawford, T. B., and Henson, J. B.: Viral arteritis of horses. Adv. Exp. Med. Biol., 22:175–183, 1972.

Doll, E. R., Bryans, J. T., McCollum, W. H., and Crowe, E. W.: Isolation of a filterable agent causing arteritis of horses and abortion by mares. Its differentiation from the equine abortion (influenza) virus. Cornell Vet., 47:3–41, 1957.

Doll, E. R., Knappenberger, R. E., and Bryans, J. T.: An outbreak of abortion caused by the virus of equine arteritis. Cornell Vet., 47:69–75, 1957.

Estes, P. C., and Cheville, N. F.: The ultrastructure of vascular lesions in equine viral arteritis. Am. J. Pathol., 58:235–253, 1970.

Jones, T. C., Doll, E. R., and Bryans, J. T.: The lesions of equine viral arteritis. Cornell Vet., 47:52–68, 1957.

McCollum, W. H., Doll, E. R., Wilson, J. C., and Johnson, C. B.: Propagation of equine arteritis virus in monolayer cultures of equine kidney. Am. J. Vet. Res., 22:731–735, 1961.

McCollum, W. H., Doll, E. R., Wilson, J. C., and Cheatham, J.: Isolation and propagation of equine arteritis virus in monolayer cell cultures of rabbit kidney. Cornell Vet., 52:452–458, 1962.

McCollum, W. H., Prickett, W. H., and Bryans, J. T.: Temporal distribution of equine arteritis virus in respiratory mucosa, tissues and body fluids of horses infected by inhalation. Res. Vet. Sci., 12:459–464, 1971.

Van der Zeijst, B. A. M., Horzinek, M. C., and Moennig, V.: The genome of equine arteritis virus. Virology, 68:418–425, 1975.

Wilson, J. C., Doll, E. R., McCollum, W. H., and Cheatham, J.: Propagation of equine arteritis virus previously adapted to cell cultures of equine kidney in monolayer cultures of hamster kidney. Cornell Vet., *52*:200–205, 1962.

Simian Hemorrhagic Fever

Simian hemorrhagic fever is a highly infectious disease of monkeys caused by a virus currently considered a member of the genus *Pestivirus*, family Togaviridae. The disease, which has only been reported in Old World primates of the genus *Macaca* (*M. mulatta, M. fascicularis, M. arctoides*), has occurred in primate colonies in Washington, D. C., California, England, and Russia. Clinical signs include rapid onset, fever, facial edema, cyanosis, anorexia, dehydration, epistaxis, melena, and cutaneous, subcutaneous, and retrobulbar hemorrhage. The course runs 10 to 15 days and the mortality rate is high.

Lesions. The gross and microscopic lesions are dominated by hemorrhage, which may be found in almost any organ or tissue, although most constantly in the skin, nasal mucosa, lung, gastrointestinal tract, perirenal tissues, renal capsule, adrenal gland, and periocular tissues. There is marked splenomegaly and necrosis of lymphocytic follicles of the spleen, lymph nodes, tonsils, and Peyer's patches. Thrombi are frequent in small veins and capillaries. Degenerative changes may occur in the liver, kidney, brain, and bone marrow, which are believed to be due to blood stasis and hypoxia.

Abilgaard, C., et al.: Simian hemorrhagic fever: Studies of coagulation and pathology. Am. J. Trop. Med. Hyg., 24:537–544, 1975.

Allen, A. M., et al.: Simian hemorrhagic fever. II. Studies in pathology. Am. J. Trop. Med., 17:413–421, 1968.

Giddens, W. E., Jr., et al.: The pathogenesis of simian hemorrhagic fever: hematologic and histopathologic studies. Lab. Invest., 32:424, 1975.

London, W. T.: Epizootiology, transmission and approach to prevention of fatal simian hemorrhagic fever in rhesus monkeys. Nature, 268:344–345, 1977.

Palmer, A. E., et al.: Simian hemorrhagic fever. I. Clinical and epizootiologic aspects of an outbreak among quarantine monkeys. Am. J. Trop. Med., 17:404–412, 1968.

Tauraso, N. M., et al.: Simian hemorrhagic fever. III. Isolation and characterization of a viral agent. Am. J. Trop. Med. Hyg., 17:422–431, 1968.

Tauraso, N. M., Kalter, S. S., Ratner, J. J., and Heberling, R. L.: Simian hemorrhagic fever. In Medical Primatology, edited by E. I. Goldsmith and J. Moor-Jankowski. Basel, S. Karger, 1971.

Trousdale, M. D., Trent, D. W., and Shelokov, A.: Simian hemorrhagic fever virus: a new togavirus (39111). Proc. Soc. Exp. Biol. Med., 150:707–711, 1975.

Wood, O., Tauraso, N., and Liebhaber, H.: Electron microscopic study of tissue cultures infected with simian haemorrhagic fever virus. J. Gen. Virol., 7:129–136, 1970.

Kyasanur Forest Disease

This disease, caused by a *Pestivirus*, is an infection of Old World monkeys (*M. radiata* and *Presbytis entellus*) and man, transmitted by a tick, *Haemophysalis spinigera*. Kyasanur Forest disease has not been described outside India. The hemorrhagic tendencies are generally more severe in simian hemorrhagic fever and marked splenomegaly and lymphocytic necrosis are not features of Kyasanur Forest disease. Nonsuppurative encephalomyelitis may occur in Kyasanur Forest disease. Mice are susceptible to Kyasanur Forest disease, but the virus of simian hemorrhagic fever does not kill mice, a point that can aid differentiation. Definitive diagnosis of either infection requires virus isolation and identification.

Goverdhan, M. K., et al.: Epizootiology of Kyasanur Forest disease in wild monkeys of Shimoga District, Mysore State (1957–1964). Indian J. Med. Res., 62:497–510, 1974.

Iyer, C. G. S., et al.: Kyasanur Forest disease. Part VII. Pathological findings in monkeys, Presbytis entellus and Macaca radiata, found dead in the forest. Indian J. Med. Res., 48:276–286, 1960.

Webb, H. E., and Burston, J.: Clinical and pathological observations with special reference to the nervous system in Macaca radiata infected with Kyasanur Forest disease virus. Trans. Royal Soc. Trop. Med. Hyg., 60:325–331, 1966.

Webb, H. E.: Kyasanur Forest disease virus infection in monkeys. Lab. Anim. Handb., 4:131–134, 1969.

Webb, H. E., and Chatterjea, J. B.: Clinico-pathological observations on monkeys infected with Kyasanur Forest disease virus, with special reference to the haemopoietic system. Br. J. Haemat., 8:401–413, 1962.

PARAMYXOVIRIDAE

Viruses classified in the family Paramyxoviridae (para = alongside, myxo = mucus) are enveloped viruses with RNA occurring as a single linear molecule with a molecular weight of about 7 million daltons. The nucleocapsid is tubular, with a diameter of about 18 nm and length of 1.0 nm. The nucleocapsid is enclosed within a lipoprotein envelope 150 nm or more in diameter. The viruses grouped in the genus *Paramyxovirus* all contain neuraminidase and agglutinate red blood cells. Viruses grouped in the genus *Morbillivirus*—canine distemper, rinderpest, and measles (Morbillus)—exhibit some cross-reactivity in serologic tests. Measles virus bears hemagglutinins but not neuraminidase. The viruses in the genus *Pneumovirus* (pneumo = lung) lack hemagglutinins and neuraminidase, but the virion and nucleocapsids are similar to all Paramyxoviridae. Table 9–10 lists these viruses.

Diseases Due to Paramyxoviruses

The genus *Paramyxovirus* currently contains the viruses that cause mumps in children, Newcastle disease in chickens, and parainfluenza viruses, which infect several species. This latter group is made up of serologically related viruses, which are conveniently and sensibly distinguished from one another by numbers.

Parainfluenza-1

Parainfluenza-1 viruses have been recovered from human beings, rats, mice, and swine. In children, this strain is incriminated, along with parainfluenza-2 and 3, in association with upper respiratory infection, "croup" of young children. The virus may be carried in upper respiratory passages by adults as well. Rats and mice are susceptible to this agent (also called Sendai virus), and may be infected from human carriers (Schels and Härtl, 1971). The virus, first described by Fukumi et al. (1954), may be carried as an inapparent infection or may be associated with epizootics of respiratory infection. (Zurcher et al., 1977; Burek et al., 1977).

Experimental infection by aerosol instillation of the virus intranasally into mice (Appell et al., 1971) results in rhinitis, tracheitis, broncheolitis, and bronchopneumonia. Hyperplasia of bronchiolar epithelium is accompanied by dense peribronchiolar infiltration by lymphocytes, followed by necrosis of bronchiolar epithelium and adjacent alveolar tissue. Resolution appears complete in nonfatal cases within about three weeks. Intracyto-

Table 9–10. Diseases Due to Paramyxoviridae

Paramyxovirus	Morbillivirus	Pneumovirus
Newcastle disease	Canine distemper	Pneumonia of mice
Mumps	Rinderpest	Respiratory-syncytial viruses
Parainfluenza-1 (human and murine)	Measles	
Parainfluenza-2 (human, simian, and avian)	Gastroenteritis of marmosets	
Parainfluenza-3 (human and bovine)		
Parainfluenza-4 (human)		
Other avian parainfluenza viruses		

plasmic inclusions are described in bronchial epithelium.

Natural cases in rats and mice may exhibit similar lesions with more extensive involvement of alveolar tissues. In rats, the peribronchiolar aggregations of lymphocytes tend to persist for months (Burek et al., 1977). In athymic, nude mice (Ward et al., 1976), the peribronchiolar lymphocytic response is much less conspicuous, not unexpected due to the immunologic deficit in nude mice. Hyperplasia of bronchiolar epithelial cells, phlebitis of venules, and squamous metaplasia of alveolar lining cells have been observed in these mice. Intranuclear inclusions, which contain crystalline arrays of virus typical of the paramyxoviruses, are seen rather than cytoplasmic inclusions noted in conventional mice.

Appell, L. H., Kovatch, R. M., Reddecliff, J. M., and Gerone, P. J.: Pathogenesis of Sendai virus infection in mice. Am. J. Vet. Res., *32*:1835–1841, 1971.
Burek, J. D., Zurcher, C., Van Nunen, M. C. J., and Hollander, C. F.: A naturally occurring epizootic caused by Sendai virus in breeding and aging rodent colonies. II. Infection in the rat. Lab. Anim. Sci., *27*:963–971, 1977.
Fukumi, H., Nishikawa, F., and Kitayama, T. A.: A pneumotropic virus from mice causing hemagglutination. Jpn. J. Med. Sci. Biol., *7*:345–363, 1954.
Parker, J. C., Tennant, R. W., Ward, T. G., and Rowe, W. P.: Enzootic Sendai virus infections in mouse breeder colonies within the United States. Science, *146*:936–938, 1964.
Parker, J. C., Tennant, R. W., and Ward, T. G.: Viruses of laboratory rodents. Nat. Cancer Inst. Monogr., *20*, 1966.
Schels, H., and Härtl, G.: Auftreten einer Parainfluenza-1 Virus (Sendai-Virus) Infektion in einer Versuchtstierzucht von Ratten. Zbl. Vet. Med., *18*:396–399, 1971.
Van der Veen, J., Poort, Y., and Bürchfield, D. J.: Experimental transmission of Sendai-virus infection in mice. Arch. Virusforsch., *31*:237–246, 1970.
Van Nunen, M. C. J., and Van der Veen, J.: Experimental infection with Sendai virus in mice. Arch. Virusforsch., *22*:388–397, 1967.
Ward, J. M., et al.: Naturally occurring Sendai virus infection of athymic nude mice. Vet. Pathol., *13*:36–46, 1976.
Zurcher, C., Burek, J. D., Van Nunen, M. C. J., and Meihuizen, S. P.: A naturally occurring epizootic caused by Sendai virus in breeding and aging rodent colonies. I. Infection in the mouse. Lab. Anim. Sci., *27*:955–962, 1977.

Parainfluenza-2

Parainfluenza-2 group contains isolates from human, canine, and simian sources (SV-41 and SV-5). Canine parainfluenza-2 virus (which resembles SV-5 closely) has been implicated in outbreaks of upper respiratory disease in dogs (Appel et al., 1970; Binn and Lazar, 1970; Black and Lee, 1970; Crandell et al., 1968; Cornwell et al., 1976). The natural disease is usually manifest by rhinitis, tracheitis, and bronchitis, with occasional bronchopneumonia. Experimental instillation of virus may result in bronchopneumonia. Multinucleated giant cells and cytoplasmic inclusions have been described in tissue cultures of the canine parainfluenza virus (Crandell et al., 1968).

Appel, M. J. G., and Percy, D. H.: SV 5-like parainfluenza virus in dogs. J. Am. Vet. Med. Assoc., *156*:1778–1781, 1970.
Binn, L. N., and Lazar, E. C.: Comments on epizootiology of parainfluenza SV5 in dogs. J. Am. Vet. Med. Assoc., *156*:1774–1777, 1970.
Bittle, J. L., and Emery, J. B.: The epizootiology of canine parainfluenza. J. Am. Vet. Med. Assoc., *156*:1771–1773, 1970.
Black, L. S., and Lee, K. M.: Infection of dogs and cats with a canine parainfluenza virus and the application of a conglutinating complement-absorption test on cat serums. Cornell Vet., *60*:120–134, 1970.
Crandell, R. A., Brumlow, W. B., and Davison, V. E.: Isolation of a parainfluenza virus from sentry dogs with upper respiratory disease. Am. J. Vet. Res., *29*:2141–2147, 1968.
Cornwell, H. J. C., et al.: Isolation of parainfluenza virus SV5 from dogs with respiratory disease. Vet. Rec., *98*:301–302, 1976.
Lazar, E. C., Swango, L. J., and Binn, L. N.: Serologic and infectivity studies of canine SV-5 virus. Proc. Soc. Exp. Biol. Med., *135*:173–176, 1970.

Parainfluenza-3

Parainfluenza-3 viruses have been recovered from respiratory disease in human, bovine, and ovine subjects. The structure of bovine parainfluenza-3 is indistinguishable from other paramyxoviruses. The virions, negatively stained, have a diameter ranging from 280 to 580 nm, and nucleocapsid diameter of 17 to 19 nm. Aggregates of nucleocapsid filaments

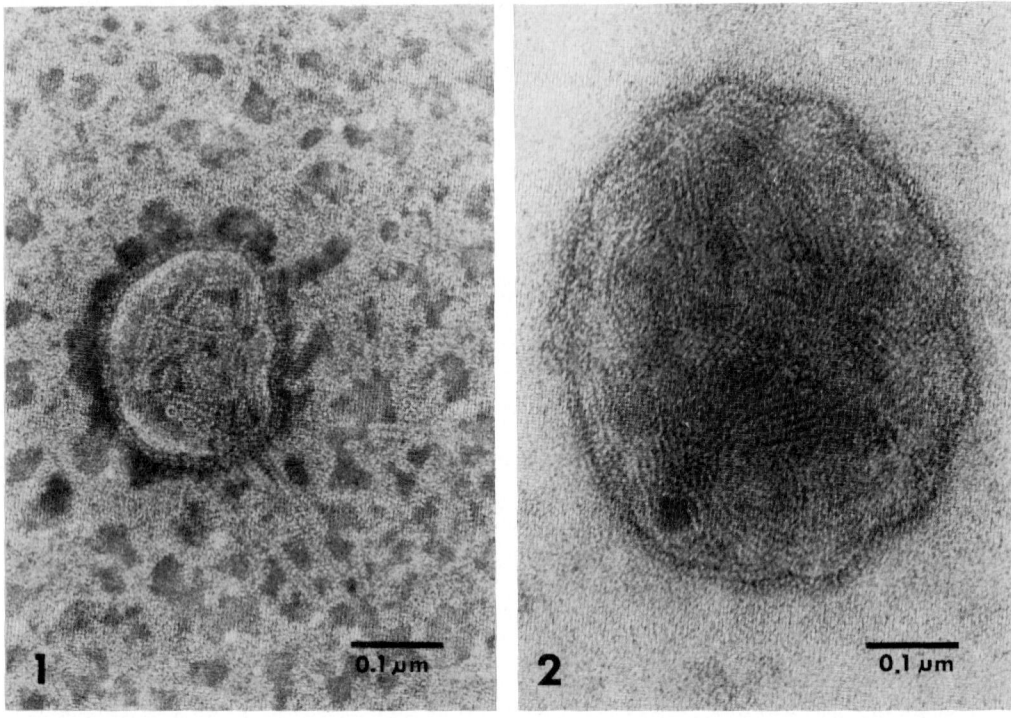

Fig. 9–56. Bovine parainfluenza-3 virus. *1* and *2*, Ultrastructure of virion containing filamentous nucleocapsids. (From McLean, A. M., and Doane, F. W.: The morphogenesis and cytopathology of bovine parainfluenza type 3 virus. J. Gen. Virol., *12*:271, 1971. Courtesy of Cambridge University Press.)

may be demonstrated in nuclei and cytoplasm of infected cells. The virions mature at the plasma membrane. In these structural features the virus resembles the measles group *(Morbillivirus)*, but antigenically it is more closely related to the other viruses classified in the genus *Paramyxovirus*. The agent produces typical cytopathic effects in cell cultures; hemadsorption is demonstrable with guinea pig erythrocytes, and hemagglutination is produced with guinea pig and human O-type red blood cells.

Parainfluenza-3 is clearly a pathogen as well. Human isolates are often associated with "croup" in young children; bovine strains are often recovered from upper respiratory disease ("shipping fever complex") and are pathogenic under experimental conditions. The virus is widespread among cattle, judging by the distribution of antibodies, and is likely one of the important pathogens in the shipping fever complex. The virus is often recovered in natural cases of respiratory disease in company with other viruses, such as infectious bovine rhinotracheitis, bovine enterovirus, streptococci, and *Corynebacterium* (Dunne et al., 1973).

Experimental infection of colostrum-deprived calves results in respiratory infection, with fever, dyspnea, coughing, rhinitis, and bronchopneumonia. The pulmonary lesions have a lobular distribution through the lungs, with concentration of lesions around bronchioles in many of them. Interstitial pneumonitis is a feature, with proliferation of septal cells and bronchiolar as well as alveolar epithelium. In early stages, syncytial giant cells are frequent in alveoli, and eosinophilic nuclear and cytoplasmic inclusions are present.

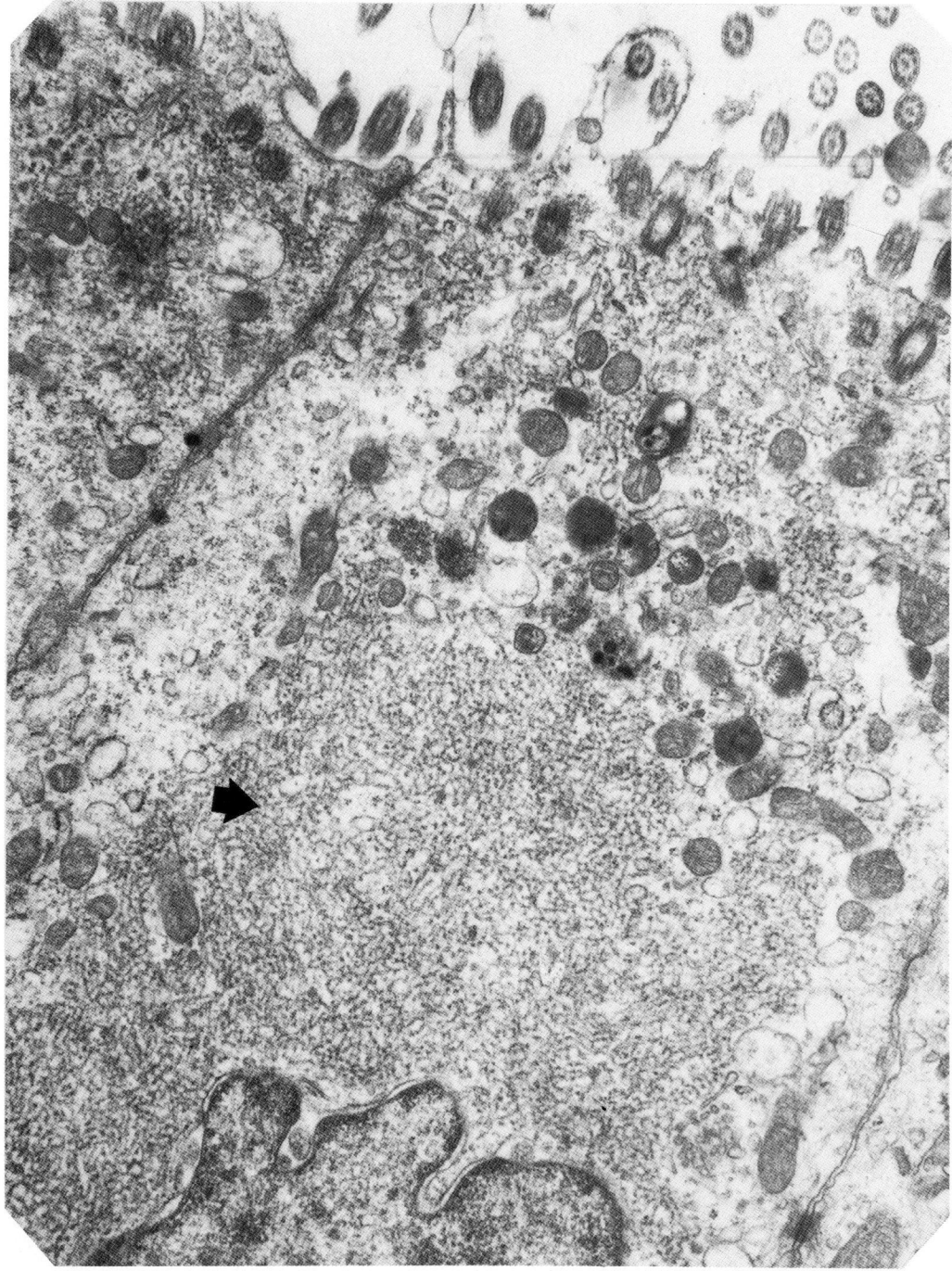

Fig. 9–57.   Bovine parainfluenza-3 virus. Infected bovine ciliated cell; aggregate of viral nucleocapsids, filamentous structures about 18 nm in diameter (arrow). (Courtesy of Dr. K–S. Tsai and *Infection and Immunity.*)

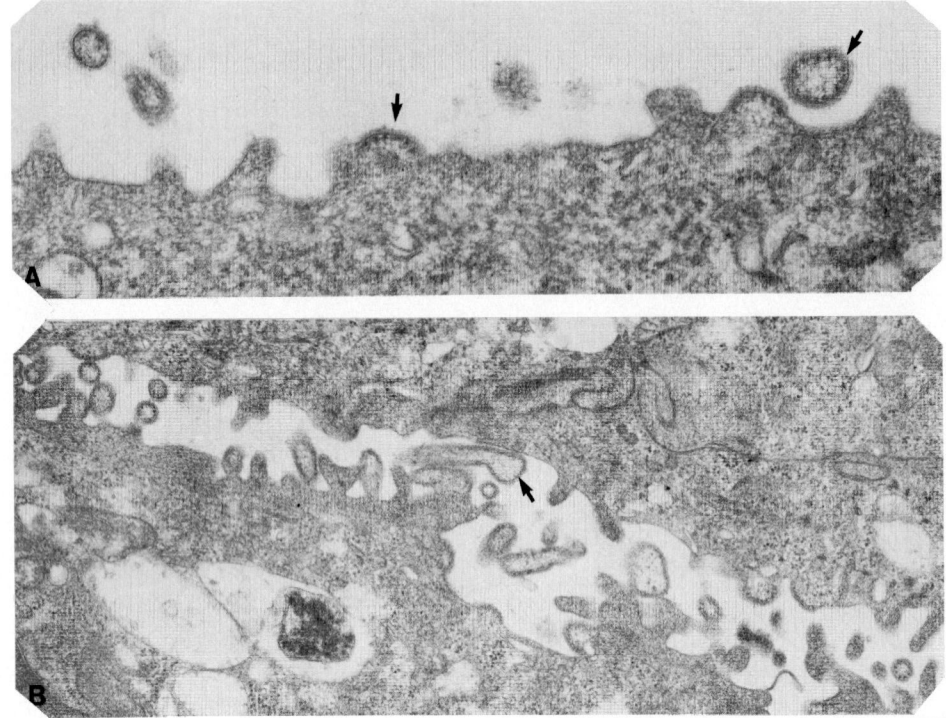

Fig. 9–58. Bovine parainfluenza-3 virus. Viral particles (arrows) and virus budding from cell membranes (arrows) in bovine cell from lining of small bronchiole. (Courtesy of Dr. K–S. Tsai and *Infection and Immunity.*)

These features may disappear as the disease progresses.

Parainfluenza-3 viruses have been isolated from domestic sheep and Rocky Mountain Bighorn sheep (Parks et al., 1972; Hore and Stevenson, 1969; Carter and Hunter, 1970). Their significance seems to be similar to that observed in cattle. Infection is widespread, and under certain conditions, disease may be produced.

Carter, M. E., and Hunter, R.: Isolation of parainfluenza type 3 virus from sheep in New Zealand. NZ Vet J., *18*:226–227, 1970.

Dawson, P. S., Darbyshire, J. H., and Lamont, P. H.: The inoculation of calves with parainfluenza 3 virus. Res. Vet. Sci., *6*:108–113, 1965.

Dunne, H. W., Ajinkya, S. M., Bubash, G. R., and Griel, L. C., Jr.: Parainfluenza-3 and bovine enteroviruses as possible important causative factors in bovine abortion. Am. J. Vet. Res., *34*:1121–1126, 1973.

Frank, G. H., and Marshall, R. G.: Parainfluenza-3 virus infection of cattle. J. Am. Vet. Med. Assoc., *163*:858–860, 1973.

Gale, C.: Role of parainfluenza-3 in cattle. J. Dairy Sci., *53*:621–625, 1970.

Hamdy, A. H.: Association of myxo-virus parainfluenza-3 with pneumoenteritis of calves: virus isolation. Am. J. Vet. Res., *27*:981–986, 1966.

Hore, D. E., and Stevenson, R. G.: Respiratory infection of lambs with an ovine strain parainfluenza type 3. Res. Vet. Sci., *10*:342–350, 1969.

McLean, A. M., and Doane, F. W.: The morphogenesis and cytopathology of bovine parainfluenza type 3 virus. J. Gen. Virol., *12*:271–279, 1971.

Omar, A. R., Jennings, A. R., and Betts, A. O.: The experimental disease produced in calves by the J121 strain of parainfluenza virus type 3. Res. Vet. Sci., *7*:379–388, 1966.

Parks, J. B., Post, G., Thorne, T., and Nash, P.: Parainfluenza-3 virus infection in Rocky Mountain bighorn sheep. J. Am. Vet. Med. Assoc., *161*:669–673, 1972.

Reisinger, R. C., Heddleston, K. I., and Manthei, C. A.: A myxovirus (SF-4) associated with shipping fever of cattle. J. Am. Vet. Med. Assoc., 135:147–152, 1959.

Stevenson, R. G., and Hore, D. E.: Comparative pathology of lambs and calves infected with parainfluenza virus type 3. J. Comp. Pathol., 80:613–618, 1970.

Swift, B. L., and Kennedy, P. C.: Experimentally induced infection of in utero bovine fetuses with bovine parainfluenza 3 virus. Am. J. Vet. Res., 33:57–63, 1972.

Swift, B. L.: Bovine parainfluenza-3 virus: experimental fetal disease. J. Am. Vet. Med. Assoc., 163:861–862, 1973.

Timoney, P. J.: Recovery of parainfluenza-3 virus from acute respiratory infection in calves. Irish Vet. J., 25:121–124, 1971.

Tsai, K. S., and Thomson, R. G.: Bovine parainfluenza type 3 virus infection; ultrastructural aspects of viral pathogenesis in the bovine respiratory tract. Infect. Immun., 11:783–803, 1975.

Woods, G. T., Sibinovic, K., and Marquis, G.: Experimental exposure of calves, lambs, and colostrum-deprived pigs to bovine myxovirus parainfluenza-3. Am. J. Vet. Res., 26:52–56, 1965.

Zygraich, N., Lobmann, M., and Huygelen, C.: Inoculation of hamsters with a temperature sensitive (ts) mutant of parainfluenza-3 virus. J. Hyg., 70:229–234, 1972.

Parainfluenza-4, 5

Parainfluenza-4 has so far been recovered only from human patients. Hsiung places several viruses of human and animal origin in a fifth group: Parainfluenza-5 (Hsuing, 1972). This writer places in this group simian virus five (SV-5), originally recovered from cell cultures from *Macaca mulatta* and *Macaca fascicularis*; virus SA from human nasal washings; DA virus— isolated from whole blood of a patient with infectious hepatitis; plus four other isolates from human patients.

Hsiung, G. D.: Parainfluenza-5 virus. Infection of man and animal. Prog. Med. Virol., 14:241–274, 1972.

Diseases Due to Morbilliviruses

The following relationships, based upon pathologic and immunologic similarities among the diseases of canine distemper, measles, and rinderpest, are now amply confirmed by the structural and biochemical similarities of the three viruses, which are now placed in the genus *Morbillivirus*. These viruses conform to the characteristics described for the family Paramyxoviridae.

A relationship between canine distemper and measles was first suggested by Pinkerton, Smiley, and Anderson (1945). Subsequently, an immunologic relationship was demonstrated between the viruses of canine distemper and measles and the viruses of canine distemper and rinderpest. The viruses of these three diseases and the pathologic processes are remarkably similar. As pointed out by Imagawa (1968), the main differences among measles, canine distemper, and rinderpest viruses are indicated by their natural hosts: measles virus causing natural disease in man and monkeys; canine distemper virus causing natural disease in *Canidae* (dog, wolf, fox), *Mustelidae* (weasel, ferret, mink), and *Procyonidae* (raccoon), and rinderpest virus causing natural disease in species of the order *Artiodactyla* (cattle, water buffalo, camel, goats, sheep).

That the three viruses are immunologically related is clearly demonstrated with cross-immunity studies. Measles virus will protect dogs against distemper. Distemper virus provides limited protection against measles. Rinderpest virus protects dogs against distemper, but distemper virus may or may not protect cattle against rinderpest. Measles virus can protect rabbits from rinderpest; however, cattle are not protected against rinderpest by measles virus. Also hyperimmune sera from natural hosts to each agent neutralizes heterologous virus to some degree. Pathologically, all three viruses produce multinucleated giant cells and both intranuclear and cytoplasmic eosinophilic inclusion bodies. A skin rash, common to measles, may also develop in distemper and rinderpest, and demyelinating encephalitis, which is common in distemper, is occasionally seen in measles and rarely in rinderpest. When adapted to experimental animals such as suckling mice, the pathologic processes induced by the three viruses become indistinguishable.

Canine Distemper

The common and serious disease of dogs known as canine distemper is caused by the virus originally described by Carré (1905), later studied extensively by Laidlaw and Duncan (1926), and now classified in the genus *Morbillivirus*. Bacterial organisms, particularly *Brucella bronchiseptica*, first isolated from fatal cases by Ferry (1911) and McGowan (1911), are now considered important secondary invaders, particularly in the presence of bronchopneumonia. The protean clinical manifestations of canine distemper have led to a great deal of confusion and difficulty, both in clinical diagnosis and experimental investigation of the disease. Many febrile diseases simulate certain features of canine distemper; in fact, only in recent years has clinical differentiation of such diseases as canine hepatitis, herpesvirus, parainfluenza, and leptospirosis been possible. Not only are dogs susceptible to the virus, but also other members of the family *Canidae* (wolves, coyotes), *Mustelidae* (ferrets, mink), *Viverridae* (Binturong), and *Procyonidae* (raccoon).

Signs. Exposure of susceptible dogs to the virus of Carré results in an acute fever, which appears after seven or eight days of incubation. Within 96 hours, the temperature usually drops rapidly to approximately normal levels, where it remains until the eleventh or twelfth day, when it climbs to a second peak. This diphasic fever curve is a characteristic feature of the disease. Coryza, purulent conjunctivitis, and bronchitis are manifest in varying degrees. Bronchopneumonia may occur. Very often, vesiculopustular lesions appear on the abdomen. In many cases, diarrhea leads to severe dehydration and emaciation. Nervous symptoms, characterized by chewing movements, excessive salivation, epileptiform seizures, and occasionally neuromuscular tics, are prominent in some outbreaks, having been observed in 50% of affected animals. Often neuro-logic signs are not manifest until after the respiratory signs have abated. Blindness and paralysis are less frequent nervous manifestations. Hyperkeratosis of the digital pads develops in some cases. Although the disease may occur in a mild, nonfatal form, most animals with severe nervous and enteric symptoms succumb to the infection.

Considerable confusion concerning the nervous manifestations of this disease has existed and much is still to be learned, particularly about the pathogenesis of the lesions. Variants of the virus have been suggested as the causative agents in infection of the central nervous system. That such variants occur, or that they are necessary to the production of the nervous symptoms, however, has never been established. Furthermore, evidence indicates that the virus of canine distemper can produce specific lesions of the central nervous system that develop in a high percentage of infected dogs even in the absence of clinically recognizable brain damage.

Lesions. In the respiratory system, purulent or catarrhal exudate may be found over the nasal and pharyngeal mucosae. In microscopic sections, characteristic cytoplasmic and intranuclear inclusion bodies often are seen in cells associated with the exudate. These inclusions are eosinophilic when stained by hematoxylin and eosin, and can be demonstrated distinctly by numerous other stains, particularly the Schorr S-3 stain. In the cytoplasm, they are round or ovoid and vary from 5 to 20 μ in diameter. They are usually homogeneous, sharply demarcated, and occasionally lie in vacuoles adjacent to the nucleus. The intranuclear inclusions, which are similar in appearance, cause only slight enlargement of the nucleus and little, if any, margination of the chromatin. The immunofluorescence technique may be used to demonstrate that these inclusions contain viral antigen.

In the lung, the lesions may be manifested by a purulent bronchopneumonia

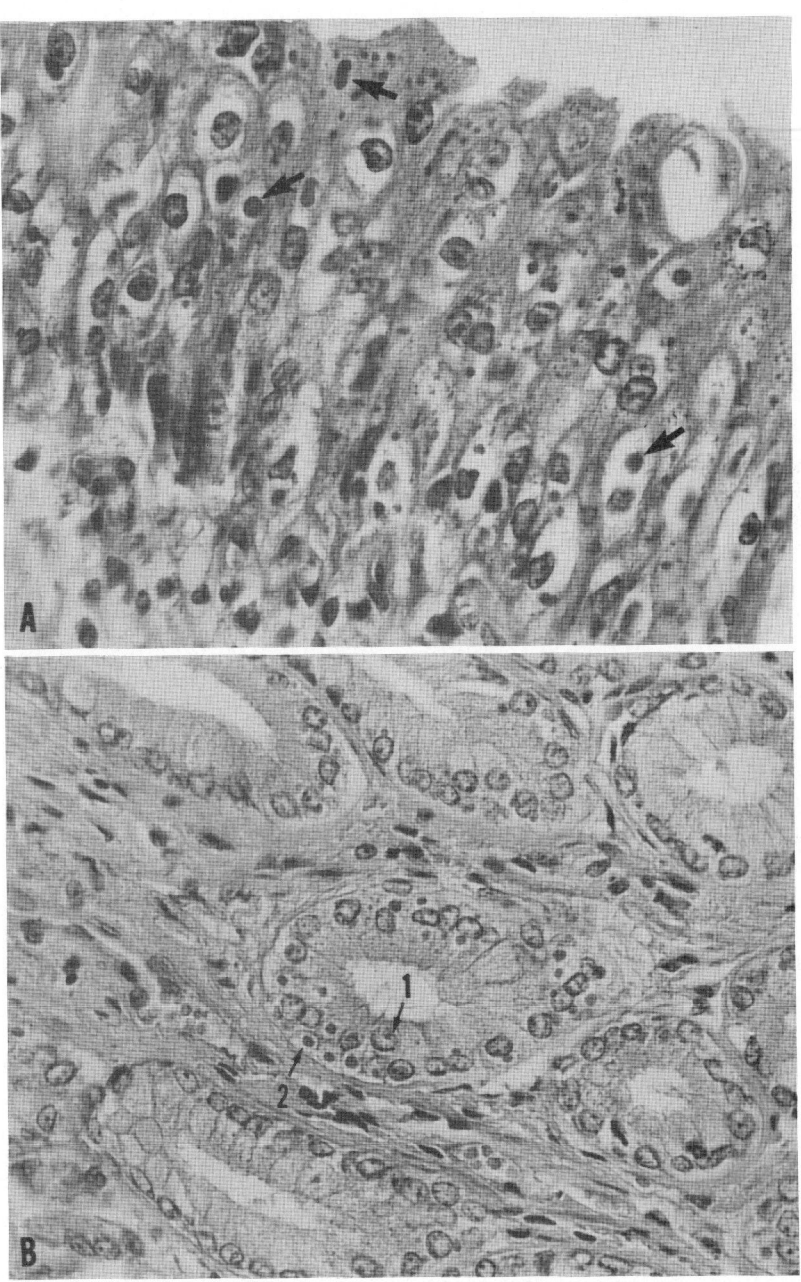

Fig. 9–59. Canine distemper. *A,* Inclusion bodies (arrows) in cytoplasm of epithelium of urinary bladder (× 525). Contributor: Dr. C. L. Davis. *B,* Intranuclear *(1)* and cytoplasmic *(2)* inclusion bodies in gastric epithelium (× 470). (Courtesy of Armed Forces Institute of Pathology.) Contributor: Dr. E. E. Ruebush.

in which bronchi and adjacent alveoli are filled with neutrophils, mucin, and tissue debris. In early stages, the exudate may contain some blood, neutrophils, and mononuclear cells. In other cases, collections of mononuclear cells lining alveolar walls or partially filling alveoli are the only evidence of infection. In some examples of this type, multinucleated giant cells form in the bronchial lining, alveolar septa, and free in alveoli. This form of giant cell pneumonia is similar to that associated with measles in man and monkeys. Cytoplasmic and less frequently intranuclear inclusions are found in these giant cells, in other mononuclear cells, and in cells of the bronchiolar and bronchial epithelium.

In the skin, particularly of the abdomen, a vesicular and pustular dermatitis may occur. The vesicles and pustules are confined to the malpighian layer of the epidermis, but some congestion of the underlying dermis is usual and lymphocytic infiltration is occasional. Nuclear or cytoplasmic inclusion bodies may be present within epithelial cells, especially those of sebaceous glands. On the foot-pads, extensive proliferation of the keratin layer of the epidermis results in a clinically recognizable lesion, which has given rise to the term "hard-pad disease." This lesion can develop in other diseases, for example, toxoplasmosis, and therefore is not specific for canine distemper.

The urinary epithelium, particularly of the renal pelvis and bladder, may contain congested vessels and microscopically demonstrable cytoplasmic or intranuclear inclusion bodies.

The stomach and intestines may contain large numbers of cytoplasmic and some intranuclear inclusions in the lining epithelium. Aside from these inclusions, few lesions are observed. In the large intestine, mucous exudate is often excessive; congestion and lymphocytic infiltration of the lamina propria may be demonstrable.

The spleen is often grossly enlarged and congested, and necrosis of lymphoid cells in the splenic follicles may be noted microscopically.

Of particular interest in the clinical diagnosis of distemper is the finding that cytoplasmic inclusions appear in some circulating neutrophils of affected dogs. The occurrence of these inclusions in leukocytes is good evidence that the virus is present, but their absence is of little value in determining the absence of the virus. Less frequently, similar inclusions are found in circulating lymphocytes. In some cases, inclusion bodies can be demonstrated in conjunctival epithelium.

Distemper does not induce significant lesions in the liver, although inclusions may be present in biliary epithelium. The presence of viral antigen in these inclusions is demonstrable with specific immunofluorescence technique.

In the central nervous system, the canine distemper virus has an affinity for the myelinated portions of the brain and spinal cord; thus, in contrast to such infections as equine encephalomyelitis, Teschen disease, and poliomyelitis, the neurons are not primarily affected. The distribution and nature of the lesions in canine distemper, therefore, differ from those in most other viral encephalitides. The lesions of canine distemper in the nervous system were at one time thought to be due to some other agent, and were often referred to as "McIntyre's encephalitis." The lesions can be detected only by microscopic study. They vary in intensity and scope, usually in direct relation to the severity and duration of the clinical disease. The structures most constantly affected are the cerebellar peduncles (brachium pontis, brachium conjunctivum, and restiform body), the anterior medullary velum, the myelinated tracts of the cerebellum, and the white columns of the spinal cord. The subcortical white matter of the cerebrum is usually spared. The lesions are characterized by rather sharply delimited areas of destruction, particularly in the myelinated tracts of the areas mentioned. Under the

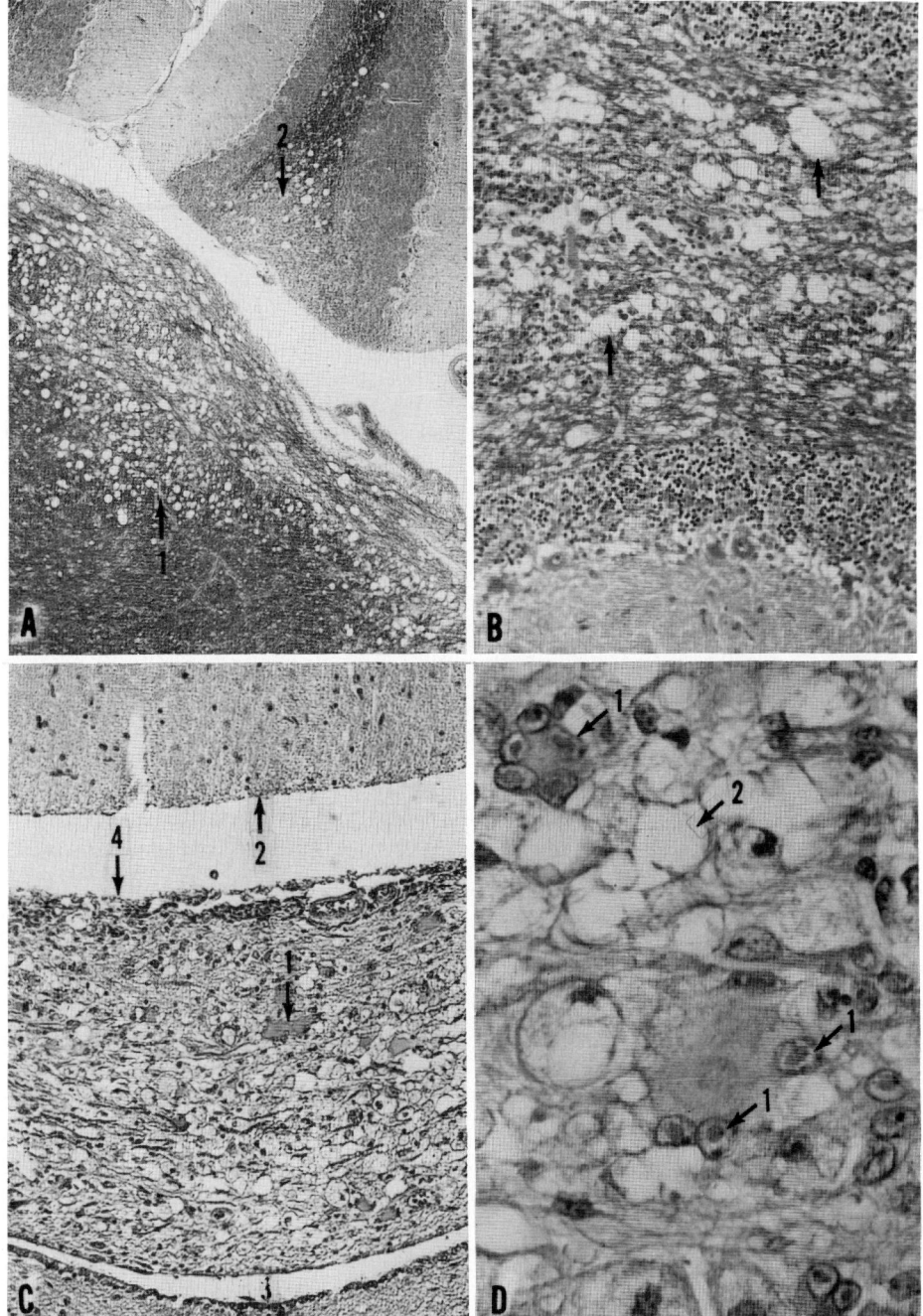

Fig. 9–60. Canine distemper. Lesions in the central nervous system. *A*, Status spongiosus in brachium pontis *(1)* and medullary part of folium *(2)* of cerebellum. Weil's stain (× 35). (Courtesy of Armed Forces Institute of Pathology.) Contributor: Dr. J. R. M. Innes. *B*, Spongy area in myelinated part of folium of cerebellum (× 150). (H & E stain.) Note large irregular vacuoles (arrows) and increased number of cells. Contributor: Dr. C. H. Beckman. *C*, Lesion in anterior medullary velum (× 100). (H & E stain.) "Gemistocytic" astrocytes *(1)*, cerebellar cortex *(2)*, fourth ventricle *(3)* and artifactually detached pia mater *(4)*. *D*, Higher magnification (× 600) of *C*. Intranuclear inclusions *(1)* in gemistocytes with fused cytoplasm. Large droplets of lipid (myelin) *(2)*. (Courtesy of Armed Forces Institute of Pathology.) Contributor: Dr. Elihu Bond.

low power of the microscope, especially in tissue stained by Weil's method, sharply delimited holes of irregular size give the affected tracts a "spongy" appearance (status spongiosa). Associated with this appearance are increased numbers of microglia and astrocytes and often collections of lymphocytes in the Virchow-Robin spaces around nearby vessels. Occasionally "gitter" cells are gathered around areas of necrosis in the white matter. Gemistocytic astrocytes or "gemistocytes" figure prominently in the exudate at many points. Intranuclear inclusions within "gemistocytes" and certain microglia are a characteristic feature of this lesion. In the cerebrum, the lesion is somewhat similar, but the most prominent microscopic feature is the apparent increase in the number of capillaries. This appearance may be due to proliferation of capillaries, or more likely, to distention and congestion of blood vessels and loss of surrounding parenchyma, causing the vasculature to appear more prominent. In many cases, lesions are limited to the cerebellar folia, the cerebellar peduncles, or the anterior medullary velum. In other cases, they are observed only in the anterior medullary velum, a delicate tract lying over the roof of the fourth ventricle.

Although overshadowed by the changes in the myelinated tracts, degenerative changes also develop in neurons, apparently resulting from both primary viral invasion and retrograde lesions secondary to axon damage. There is pyknosis, chromatolysis, gliosis, and neuronophagia. Rarely, cytoplasmic or nuclear inclusion bodies can be found in neurons. Neuronal necrosis may be present in the cerebral and cerebellar cortex, pontine and medullary nuclei, and spinal cord. In most cases, leptomeningitis, principally characterized by infiltrating lymphocytes, is present. Jubb, Saunders and Coates (1957) demonstrated that intraocular lesions occur in most cases of canine distemper. In the retina, there is congestion, edema, perivascular cuffing with lymphocytes, degeneration of ganglion cells, and gliosis. Neuritis of the optic nerve with demyelination and gliosis may also be present. Intranuclear inclusions are present in glia of the retina and optic nerve. The lesions lead to retinal atrophy of all layers. Swelling and proliferation of retinal pigment epithelium is also usually present.

According to one report (Crook and McNutt, 1959), inclusion bodies appeared in the bronchial epithelial cells as early as the fourth day after experimental intranasal infection of mink by means of aerosols. From the eighth to the thirty-second day, inclusions were numerous and large. Inclusions appeared a little later in reticuloendothelial cells of spleen, epithelium of intrahepatic bile ducts, bladder, renal pelvis, and intestine. Necrosis of lymphatic nodules of spleen, induced by pyknosis, and karyolysis of individual cells appeared almost simultaneously. Lesions in ferrets were similar.

Diagnosis. Postmortem diagnosis can be based upon a history of the typical clinical disease and the demonstration of characteristic lesions and cytoplasmic and intranuclear viral inclusions. Isolation of the virus is difficult but possible when susceptible puppies or ferrets are used. Some strains do not grow well in tissue culture. If adaptable to tissue culture, the cytopathic effects include the formation of giant cells and inclusion bodies. Positive identification of the virus should be accomplished by neutralization or cross-immunization studies. The disease can be differentiated from canine hepatitis by the predilection of the virus of the latter disease for parenchymal cells of the liver and endothelium, where it produces typical margination of chromatin and large, rather basophilic intranuclear inclusions. The postmortem diagnosis of canine distemper should not be made after examination of only one affected organ, but upon careful microscopic study of all organs, including the brain.

During life, clinical diagnosis can be confirmed by finding typical inclusion bodies in smears of cells of the respiratory epithelium or peripheral blood. Unfortunately, these inclusions are not present in all cases, hence their absence does not preclude the diagnosis of distemper. A fluorescence antibody technique recently introduced offers an excellent method for the demonstration of the virus in tissue smears and sections. In dogs, toxoplasmosis often occurs in association with canine distemper. Lesions of both diseases should be sought if evidence of either infection is apparent.

Adams, J. M., et al.: Old dog encephalitis and demyelinating diseases in man. Vet. Pathol., 12:220–226, 1975.

Appel, M. J. G.: Pathogenesis of canine distemper. Am. J. Vet. Res., 30:1167–1182, 1969.

Appel, M., and Robson, D. S.: A microneutralization test for canine distemper virus. Am. J. Vet. Res., 34:1459–1464, 1973.

Appel, M., Sheffy, B. E., Percy, D. H., and Gaskin, J. M.: Canine distemper virus in domesticated cats and pigs. Am. J. Vet. Res., 35:803–806, 1974.

Blanchard, G. L., Howard, D. R., Krehbiel, J. D., and Keller, W. F.: Amaurosis and associated electroretinographic alterations in canine distemper. J. Am. Vet. Med. Assoc., 163:976–978, 1973.

Broadhurst, J., MacLean, M. E., and Saurino, V.: Nasal inclusion bodies in dog distemper. Cornell Vet., 28:9–15,, 1938.

Burkhart, R. L., Poppensiek, G. C., and Zink, A.: A study of canine encephalitis, with special reference to clinical, bacteriological and postmortem findings. Vet. Med., 45:157–162, 1950.

Bussell, R. H., and Karson, D. T.: I. Canine distemper virus in ferret, dog, and bovine kidney cell cultures. II. Canine distemper virus in primary and continuous cell lines of human and monkey origin. Arch. Ges. Virusforsch., 17:163–182 and 183–202, 1965.

Cabasso, V. J.: Canine distemper and hardpad disease. Vet. Med., 47:417–423, 1952.

Cabasso, V. J., Stebbins, M. R., and Cox, H. R.: Experimental canine distemper encephalitis and immunization of puppies against it. Cornell Vet., 44:153–167, 1954.

Carré, H.: Sur la maladie des jeunes chiens. Compt. Rend. Acad. d. Sc., 140:689–690, 1905.

Cello, R. M., Moulton, J. E., and McFarland, S.: The occurrence of inclusion bodies in the circulating neutrophils of dogs with canine distemper. Cornell Vet., 49:127–146, 1959.

Coffin, D. L. and Liu, Chien: Studies on canine distemper infection by smears of fluorescein-labeled antibody. Virology, 3:132–145, 1947.

Confer, A. W., Kahn, D. E., Koestner, A., and Krakowka, S.: Biological properties of a canine distemper virus isolate associated with demyelinating encephalomyelitis. Infect. Immun., 11:835–844, 1975.

————: Comparison of canine distemper viral strains: an electron microscopic study. Am. J. Vet. Res., 36:741–748, 1975.

Cornwell, H. J. C., Campbell, R. S. F., Vantsis, J. T., and Penny, W.: Studies in experimental canine distemper. I. Clinico-pathological findings. J. Comp. Pathol., 75:3–17, 1965.

Cornwell, H. J. C., Laird, H. M., and Wright, N. G.: Ultrastructural features of canine distemper virus infection in a dog kidney cell line. J. Gen. Virol., 12:281–292, 1971.

Cornwell, H. J. C., Vantsis, J. T., Campbell, R. S. F., and Penny, W.: Studies in experimental canine distemper. II. Virology, inclusion body studies and haematology. J. Comp. Pathol. Ther., 75:19–34, 1965.

Crook, E., and McNutt, S. H.: Experimental distemper in mink and ferrets. II. Appearance and significance of histopathological changes. Am. J. Vet. Res., 20:378–383, 1959.

De Monbreun, W. A.: Histopathology of natural and experimental canine distemper. Am. J. Pathol., 13:187–212, 1937.

Fairchild, G. A., Steinberg, S. A., and Cohen, D.: The fluorescent antibody test as a diagnostic test for canine distemper in naturally infected dogs. Cornell Vet., 61:214–223, 1971.

Ferry, N. S.: Etiology of canine distemper. J. Infect. Dis., 8:399–420, 1911.

Fischer, K.: Einschlusskörperchen bei Hunden mit Staupé Enzephalitis und Anderen Erkrankungen des Zentralnervensystems. Pathol. Vet., 2:380–410, 1965.

Gibson, J. P., Griesemer, R. A., and Koestner, A.: Experimental distemper in the gnotobiotic dog. Path. Vet., 2:1–19, 1965.

Gillespie, J. H.: Some research contributions on canine distemper. J. Am. Vet. Med. Assoc., 132:534–537, 1958.

Greene, R. G., and Evans, C. A.: A comparative study of distemper inclusions. Am. J. Hyg., 29:73–87, 1939.

Hartley, W. J.: A post-vaccinal inclusion body encephalitis in dogs. Vet. Pathol., 11:301–312, 1975.

Hoff, G. L., Bigler, W. J., Proctor, S. J., and Stallings, L. P.: Epizootic of canine distemper virus infection among urban raccoons and gray foxes. J. Wildl. Dis., 10:423–428, 1974.

Hsiung, G. D., and Swack, N. S.: Myxovirus and pseudomyxovirus groups. *In* Pathology of Simian Primates, edited by R. N. T–W Fiennes. Part II. Basel, S. Karger, 1972. pp. 537–571.

Hurst, E. W., Cooke, B. T., and Melvin, P.: Nervous distemper in dogs. A pathological and experimental study with some references to demyelinating diseases in general. Aust. J. Exp. Biol. Med. Sci., 21:115–126, 1943.

Imagawa, D. T.: Relationships among measles, canine distemper and rinderpest viruses. Prog. Med. Virol., 10:160–193, 1968.

Jubb, K. B., Saunders, L. Z., and Coates, H. V.: The intraocular lesions of canine distemper. J. Comp. Pathol. Ther., 67:21–29, 1957.

King, L. S.: Disseminated encephalomyelitis of the dog. Arch. Pathol., 28:151–162, 1939.

Koestner, A., and Long, J. F.: Ultrastructure of canine distemper virus in explant tissue culture of canine cerebellum. Lab. Invest., 23:196–201, 1970.

Koprowski, H., et al.: A study of canine encephalitis. Am. J. Hyg., 51:63–75, 1950.

Krakowka, S., McCullough, B., Koestner, A., and Olsen, R.: Myelin-specific autoantibodies associated with central nervous system demyelination in canine distemper virus infection. Infect. Immun., 8:819–827, 1973.

Krakowka, S., Confer, A., and Koestner, A.: Evidence for transplacental transmission of canine distemper virus: two case reports. Am. J. Vet. Res., 35:1251–1254, 1974.

Krakowka, S., Hoover, E. A., Koestner, A., and Ketring, K.: Experimental and naturally occurring transplacental transmission of canine distemper virus. Am. J. Vet. Res., 38:919–922, 1977.

Kriesel, H. R.: A comparative study of the manifestations and histopathology of canine distemper and experimental fox encephalitis infection in dogs. Cornell Vet., 28:324–330, 1938.

Laidlaw, P. P., and Dunkin, G. W.: Studies in dog distemper: III. The nature of the virus. J. Comp. Pathol. Ther., 39:222–230, 1926.

Lentz, O.: Über spezifische Veränderungen an den Ganglienzellen wut—und staupekranker Tiere. Ein Beitrag zu unseren Kenntnissen über die Bedeutung und Entstehung der Negrischen Körperchen. Ztschr. Hyg. Infectionskr., 62:63–94, 1908–1909.

Lincoln, S. D., Gorham, J. R., Ott, R. L., and Hegreberg, G. A.: Etiologic studies of old dog encephalitis. I. Demonstration of canine distemper viral antigen in the brain in two cases. Vet. Pathol., 8:1–8, 1971.

Lincoln, S. D., Gorham, J. R., Davis, W. C., and Ott, R. L.: Studies of old dog encephalitis. Vet. Pathol., 10:124–129, 1973.

MacIntyre, A. B., Trevan, D. J., and Montgomerie, R. F.: Observations on canine encephalitis. Vet. Rec., 60:635–648, 1948.

Mangi, R. J., et al.: A canine distemper model of virus-induced anergy. J. Infect. Dis., 133:556–563, 1976.

McCullough, B., Krakowka, S., and Koestner, A.: Experimental canine distemper virus-induced lymphoid depletion. Am. J. Pathol., 74:155–170, 1974.

———: Experimental canine distemper virus-induced demyelination. Lab. Invest., 31:216–222, 1974.

McGowan, J. P.: Some observations on a laboratory epidemic principally among dogs and cats, in which the animals affected presented the symptoms of the disease called distemper. J. Pathol. Bact., 15:372–426, 1911.

Padmanaban, V. D., and Menon, U. K.: Electron micrographic studies on canine distemper virus. Indian Vet. J., 49:348–350, 1972.

Page, W. G., and Green, R. G.: An improved diagnostic stain for distemper inclusions. Cornell Vet., 32:265–268, 1942.

Perdrau, J. R., and Pugh, L. P.: The pathology of disseminated encephalomyelitis of the dog (the "nervous form of canine distemper"). J. Pathol. Bact., 33:79–91, 1930.

Pinkerton, H., Smiley, W. L., and Anderson, W. A. D.: Giant cell pneumonia with inclusions. A lesion common to Hecht's disease, distemper and measles. Am. J. Pathol., 21:1–23, 1945.

Poste, G.: Electron microscopic study of nuclear and nucleolar changes in cells infected with canine distemper virus (CDV). Archiv. ges. Virusforsch., 37:183–190, 1972.

Ribelin, W. E.: The incidence of distemper in canine encephalitis cases. Am. J. Vet. Res., 14:96–104, 1953.

Richter, W. R., and Moize, S. M.: Ultrastructural nature of canine distemper inclusions in the urinary bladder. Pathol. Vet., 7:346–352, 1970.

Tajima, M., Itabashi, M., and Motohashi, T.: Light and electron microscopic studies of lymph node of mink exposed to canine distemper virus. Am. J. Vet. Res., 32:913–924, 1971.

Warren, J.: The relationships of the viruses of measles, canine distemper and rinderpest. Adv. Virus Res., 7:27–60, 1960.

Watson, A. D. J., and Wright, R. G.: The ultrastructure of inclusions in blood cells of dogs with distemper. J. Comp. Pathol., 84:417–427, 1974.

———: Ultrastructure of cytoplasmic inclusions in circulating lymphocytes in canine distemper. Res. Vet. Sci., 17:188–192, 1974.

Whittem, J. H., and Blood, D. C.: Canine encephalitis, pathological and clinical observations. Aust. Vet. J., 26:73–83, 1950.

Wisnicky, W., and Wipf, L.: Significance of inclusion bodies of distemper. Am. J. Vet. Res., 3:285–288, 1942.

Wisniewski, H. C., Raine, S., and Kay, W. J.: Observations on viral demyelinating encephalomyelitis canine distemper. Lab. Invest., 26:589–599, 1972.

Wright, N. G., Cornwell, H. J. C., and Thompson, H.: Canine distemper: current concepts in laboratory and clinical diagnosis. Vet. Rec., 94:86–92, 1974.

Rinderpest (Cattle Plague)

Rinderpest has been a serious disease of cattle from antiquity, and is today the foremost cause of death in cattle in Africa and Asia. Fortunately it is not present in the Western Hemisphere or in Europe. The mortality in cattle varies from 25 to 90%, depending on the strains of virus involved and the resistance of the animals. The incubation period is from six to nine days after infection by contact, but only two or three days following experimental injection of the virus. In addition to cattle, sheep, swine, goats, deer, camels, and buffalo are susceptible to natural or artificial infection with rinderpest virus. The virus is immunologically and pathologically related to the viruses of canine distemper and measles. The virus is currently classified in the genus *Morbillivirus* and family Paramyxoviridae.

Signs. The onset of illness is indicated by a sharp rise in temperature to 104 to 105° F., accompanied by restlessness, dryness of the muzzle, and constipation. Within a day or two, nasal and lacrimal discharges appear. Other manifestations are photophobia, depression, excessive thirst, starry coat, retarded rumination, anorexia, leukopenia, and excessive salivation. A maculopapular rash may develop on those parts of the body where the hair is fine. The fever usually reaches its peak on the third to the fifth day, but drops abruptly with the onset of diarrhea, even though other symptoms are intensified. Lesions in the oral mucosa may appear by the second or third day of fever, but usually do not become conspicuous until after the onset of diarrhea. As the diarrhea increases in severity, it is accompanied by abdominal pain, accelerated respiration, occasional cough, severe dehydration and emaciation, which are followed by prostration, subnormal temperature, and death, usually after a course of 6 to 12 days.

Lesions. The rinderpest virus has a particular affinity for lymphoid tissue and for epithelial tissues of the gastrointestinal tract, in which it produces severe and characteristic effects.

In lymphoid tissue, the virus causes necrosis of lymphocytes, which is striking in microscopic sections of lymph nodes, spleen, and Peyer's patches. The destruction of lymphocytes is first evidenced by a fragmentation of nuclei in the germinal centers, and in a short time most of the mature lymphocytes disappear. The lymph follicles are involved to various degrees, depending upon the severity and stage of

the disease in which they are examined. Multinucleated giant cells containing eosinophilic cytoplasmic inclusion bodies are often present. Rarely, intranuclear inclusions are seen in these cells. Edema and congestion of capillaries are also seen microscopically, but only the edema can be detected grossly. The destruction of lymphoid cells leaves a fibrillar, somewhat eosinophilic and acellular matrix in place of the lymphoid follicles. The matrix may be surrounded by lymphocytes, plasma cells, nuclear debris and macrophages. Although these changes in lymphoid tissue are essentially the same in lymph nodes and in the Peyer's patches, grossly they are seen to better advantage in the latter, which may be darkened with hemorrhage and slough out, leaving deep craters in the intestinal wall.

The replication of viral nucleoprotein and the pathogenic effects on lymphocytic cells which precede the necrosis have been studied by Tajima and Ushijima (1971). These authors demonstrated, in experimentally-infected cattle, that the inclusion bodies seen with the light microscope are made up of aggregations of strands of nucleocapsids. These viral structures appear as tubules in longitudinal section, circular in cross-section, and have characteristic cross-striations that indicate their helical structure. These nucleocapsids are seen in the nucleus of reticuloendothelial cells, displacing the nuclear chromatin toward the nuclear membrane. Aggregations of these structures in the nucleus or cytoplasm result in the inclusion bodies, which may be seen with the light microscope. The nucleocapsids are assembled at the plasma membrane and, by budding outward, result in the formation of the mature virion, enveloped by the plasma membrane. Aside from intercellular edema, disorganization of cristae of mitochondria, and displacement of cell organelles by masses of viral nucleocapsids, few ultrastructural effects of the virus are seen. Lymphocytes usually contain only a few nucleocapsids, but undergo necrosis extensively, probably indicating increased sensitivity of these cells to the virus.

In the experimental disease in the rabbit, this affinity for lymphocytes is particularly well demonstrated in the Peyer's patches, in the sacculus rotundus, and appendix, where rather characteristic lesions, grossly chalk-white, stand out individually in contrast to the adjacent flesh-colored tissues. When viewed from the serous surface, these collections of lymphoid follicles have the appearance of white hexagonal tile separated by dark cement.

In the digestive system of cattle, the rinderpest virus produces typical lesions in the epithelium, varying with the anatomic features of the parts of the digestive tract affected. Application of the virus to the oral mucosa does not readily produce infection, which suggests that the virus is carried to the oral mucosa by the blood stream. In the squamous epithelium of the oral cavity, the first evidence of the presence of the virus is necrosis of a few epithelial cells in the deep layers of the stratum malpighii. These affected cells have pyknotic and fragmented nuclei and irregular, eosinophilic cytoplasm; they appear shrunken and are separated from the adjoining epithelium by a clear space. As these necrotic areas increase in size and extend toward the surface, the cornified layer above them becomes elevated and causes them to appear grossly as tiny, grayish-white, slightly raised puncta. Multinucleated giant cells form in the stratum spinosum. Eosinophilic cytoplasmic inclusion bodies form in the mucosal epithelial cells and giant cells. Intranuclear inclusion bodies are reportedly rarely seen. Vesicles are not formed in this disease. The foci of necrosis in the epithelium usually remain discrete for a time, but later coalesce to form large areas of erosion. Since the basal layer of the squamous epithelium is rarely penetrated, ulcers seldom form. The erosions are shallow, with a red, raw-appearing floor, bounded by essentially normal epitheli-

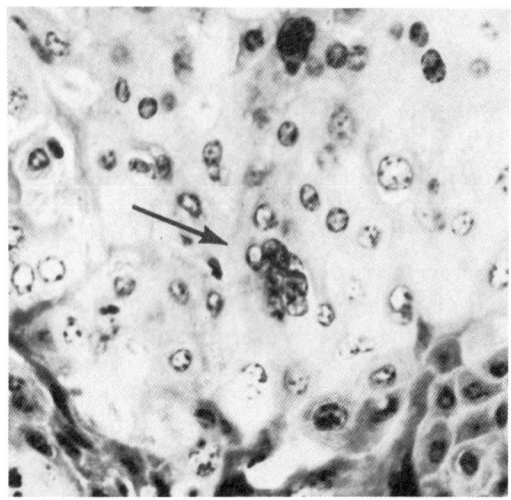

Fig. 9-61. Rinderpest. A multinucleated giant cell in the lingual mucosa. A small intranuclear inclusion body is evident. (Courtesy of Dr. W. Plowright.)

um, which provides a sharply demarcated margin. The lesions in the oral mucosa have a selective distribution: the inside of the lower lip, the adjacent gum, the cheeks near the commissures, and the ventral surface of the free portion of the tongue. In severe cases, they may extend from these sites to the hard palate and pharynx, and in fulminant cases to all the mucous surfaces of the tongue with the singular exception of the anterior seven-eighths of its dorsal surface. The esophageal lesions, particularly those of its upper third, are similar to those in the mouth and pharynx, but usually less severe. The rumen, reticulum, and omasum rarely exhibit any lesions, although in a few instances small eroded foci are found in the omasal leaves.

The abomasum is one of the most common sites of the lesions of rinderpest. They are most severe and consistent in the pyloric region, where necrotic foci of microscopic size in the epithelium are accompanied by capillary congestion and hemorrhage in the underlying lamina propria. This results in the gross appearance of irregularly outlined, superficial streaks of color, ranging from bright red to dark brown. The lesions tend to follow the edges of the broad plicae as streaks extending into the fundus, but becoming more numerous and diffuse in the flattened portion of the pylorus. Edema may be extensive in the submucosa of plicae, involving an entire fold and causing it to appear grossly thickened and gelatinous on cross section. As necrosis of the epithelium progresses, the infected areas become slate colored and the epithelium sloughs away, leaving sharply outlined irregular erosions with a red, raw floor oozing blood. In cases of relatively longer standing, black clotted blood may partially or completely fill these pits in the mucosa. Often the most tenacious portion of the clot is at the periphery of the erosion and clings to the edges, leaving the center open. Deep ulceration occasionally occurs, with microscopic evidence of penetration of the muscularis mucosae. In fatal cases, the lumen of the abomasum is usually empty, except for blood-tinged mucous material.

In the small intestine, severe lesions are less common than in the mouth, abomasum or large intestine, but streaks of hemorrhage and, less frequently, erosions along the crest of the folds of mucous membrane may be found, particularly in the initial part of the duodenum and terminal ileum. Peyer's patches are exceptionally vulnerable, and even in the presence of relatively normal adjacent mucous membrane, the lymphoid tissue may become so necrotic that patches slough out, leaving deep, raw craters in the intestinal wall.

The large intestine, as a rule, is more seriously damaged than the small intestine, with prominent lesions around the ileocecal valve, at the cecocolic junction, and in the rectum. In the cecum, lesions may be confined to the region of the ileocecal valve. In well-developed cases of rinderpest, the crest of the folds of mucous membrane throughout the cecum are bright red because of the numerous petechiae. These may be interpreted as diffuse hemorrhages unless examined closely under a good light, when they are seen to be sharply demarcated spots, 0.5 to 1.0 mm in diameter, immediately beneath the most superficial layer of cells. In early lesions, the petechiae are bright red, but they become darker and tend to coalesce as the lesion ages. Microscopic examination reveals that most of the spots that grossly appear to be hemorrhages are, in fact, greatly distended capillaries, packed with erythrocytes, in the lamina propria. Streaks of congestion along the folds of mucosa produce a characteristic "barred" or "zebra-striped" appearance. As the disease progresses and the mucosa becomes eroded, diffuse congestion and bleeding from the raw surfaces may occur over large areas. When the intestine is opened, the mucosa is diffusely red and the lumen contains dark, partially clotted blood.

At the cecocolic junction, there is a segment of intestine about 4 inches long in which the wall is normally thickened and the mucosal rugae, which are broader than in either the cecum or colon, are arranged both transversely and longitudinally. This transverse arrangement is in contrast to that in the colon, where the rugae are longitudinal. Histologically, in this area, numerous tiny infundibula are formed by invaginations of epithelium through the muscularis mucosa. In the submucosa, these form goblet-shaped structures with collections of lymphocytes and sometimes lymphoid follicles along their base. These histologic characteristics influence both the gross and microscopic lesions that occur in this segment of the intestine. Since the virus invades both the epithelium and the lymphoid cells, the lesions are accentuated. Necrosis of the lymphoid tissues and closure of the orifice at the neck of the infundibula result in isolation of necrotic tissue in the submucosa. This attracts some leukocytic infiltrate which contributes to the thickening of the wall. Erosion of epithelium, particularly at the opening of the infundibula, gives rise to small raw pits deeper than those elsewhere in the intestine. Congestion is likely to be greater in this segment and the increased thickness of the wall is partly the result of edema in the submucosa and muscularis.

The changes in the colon and rectum vary in intensity from a few longitudinal streaks of congestion along the crest of the folds of the mucosa to erosions of the mucosal epithelium, which may be so extensive that only small islands of intact mucous membrane remain. The lumen is filled with dark, partially coagulated blood, which has oozed from the raw surfaces. The characteristic streaks of congestion and hemorrhage are more frequent and striking in the rectum than in the colon.

The liver is affected only secondarily in rinderpest, with chronic passive congestion resulting from cardiac and pulmonary complications as the usual lesion. In the gallbladder, however, the lesions appear to be related specifically to the virus; they are similar to those in the lower part of the intestinal tract, varying from scattered petechiae to diffuse blotches of hemorrhage with occasional free bleeding into the lumen.

In the respiratory system, the epithelium is susceptible to the virus. Petechiae may appear on the turbinates, and erosions as well as petechiae may occur in the larynx if the oral mucosa is severely involved. In the trachea, streaks of hemorrhage in the mucosa are almost invariably found in the cases with well-developed lesions elsewhere. Most common are longitudinal streaks of rusty hemorrhage in the anterior third of the trachea, but the erosions usually associated with congestion and hemorrhage are rare. The lungs seem to be involved only secondarily. In animals killed early in the course of illness or which die after two or three days of illness, the lungs usually appear grossly normal. In longstanding cases in which diarrhea, dehydration, emaciation, and prolonged recumbence with labored respiration have been symptoms, necropsy may reveal both inter-

lobular and alveolar emphysema accompanied by congestion and hemorrhage of varying degree and occasionally by small areas of consolidation. Microscopically, there is no evidence of cellular damage directly attributable to the virus, but interlobular and interalveolar as well as alveolar emphysema may be observed. Vascular congestion can usually be explained on the basis of hypostasis.

The lesions of the heart also appear to be secondary, and are seen only in cases of prolonged duration. The most nearly constant finding is subendocardial hemorrhage over the papillary muscles of the left ventricle; seldom is the right ventricle involved. The myocardium is frequently flaccid and bears streaks of light color, but microscopic examination rarely discloses significant changes.

In the urinary system, there may be evidence of edema around the renal pelvis and occasional desquamation of pelvic epithelium. The nephrons are affected in only a few instances, usually in cases of long duration. In the urinary bladder, the epithelium may be desquamated and the underlying stroma infiltrated with erythrocytes. The infiltrates are seen grossly as thin red blotches, measuring as much as 2 mm in diameter, with irregular and fading edges. Sometimes they become confluent.

Lesions in the skin, though not frequent, may be seen as a maculopapular rash over the sparsely haired portions of the body, the vulva, and prepuce. Microscopically, they resemble those of the oral mucosa.

Diagnosis. The clinical, gross, and microscopic features of the disease are adequate for a presumptive diagnosis, which should, however, be confirmed by serologic methods, particularly in geographic areas in which the disease is not enzoötic. Confirmation of the diagnosis should be accomplished by a challenge of immune and normal control animals with splenic suspensions from animals believed to have died of rinderpest. A serum virus neutralization test on cattle can also be

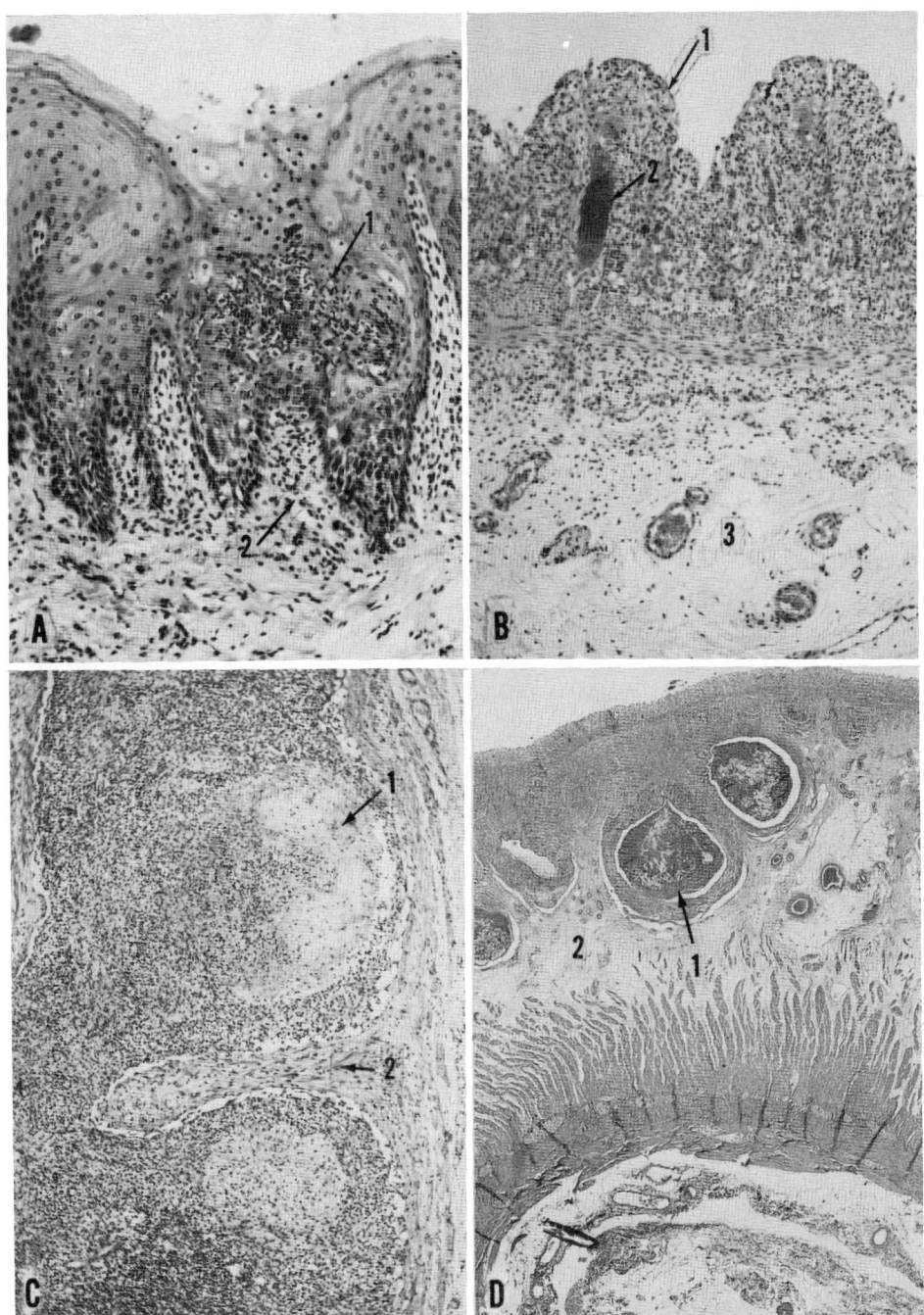

Fig. 9–62. Rinderpest. *A*, Early necrotizing lesion *(1)* in the epithelium of the tongue of a cow. Some edema and leukocytic infiltration *(2)* of the underlying stroma. *B*, Erosion of the epithelium *(1)*, congestion of the capillaries *(2)* in lamina propria of the mucosa, and edema *(3)* of the submucosa of the cecum (× 75). *C*, Necrosis of lymphoid cells *(1)*, leaving only fibrillar and nuclear debris in lymphoid follicles. A cortical trabeculus *(2)* extends from the capsule of this lymph node (× 48). *D*, Lesion (× 15) at ceco-colic junction. Infundibuli filled with necrotic debris *(1)*, edema in submucosa *(2)*, which separates the bundles of the inner muscularis. (Courtesy of Armed Forces Institute of Pathology.) Contributor: Lt. Col. F. D. Maurer.

done, but it is costly and requires adequate isolation facilities and virus titration controls. The virus can be isolated and identified in tissue culture, where its cytopathic effect includes the formation of multinucleated cells and intranuclear and cytoplasmic inclusion bodies.

Differential diagnosis must include other acute gastroenteric infections such as viral diarrhea-mucosal disease and malignant catarrhal fever.

Imagawa, D. T.: Relationships among measles, canine distemper and rinderpest viruses. Progr. Med. Virol., *10*:160–193, 1968.

Maurer, F. D., Jones, T. C., Easterday, B., and De Tray, D.: The pathology of rinderpest. Proc. Am. Vet. Med. Assoc., 1955. pp. 201–211, 1955.

Plowright, W.: Rinderpest virus. Virology Monogr., *3*:25–110, 1968.

Scott, G. R.: Rinderpest. Adv. Vet. Sci., *9*:113–224, 1964.

Tajima, M., and Ushijima, T.: The pathogenesis of rinderpest in the lymph nodes of cattle. Light and electron microscopic studies. Am. J. Pathol., *62*:221–236, 1971.

Yamanouchi, K., et al.: Pathogenesis of rinderpest virus infection in rabbits. I. Clinical signs, immune response, histological changes, and virus growth patterns. Infect. Immun., *9*:199–205, 1974.

————: Pathogenesis of rinderpest virus infection in rabbits. II. Effect of rinderpest virus on the immune functions of rabbits. Infect. Immun., *9*:206–211, 1974.

Measles (Rubeola, Monkey Intranuclear Inclusion Agent, *Morbillus*)

Measles is a highly infectious exanthematous viral disease of man, principally children. The virus and its pathologic effects are closely related to canine distemper and rinderpest. In addition to the characteristic exanthematous rash, measles infection in man may result in primary giant cell pneumonia and encephalomyelitis. Secondary bronchopneumonia is an important complication. Microscopically, the rash is characterized by vesiculation and necrosis of epithelial cells with an associated inflammatory response in the dermis. Epithelial cells may contain intranuclear inclusion bodies, and multinucleated giant cells are often present. The most characteristic pathologic feature is the Warthin-Finkeldey lymphoid giant cell, which is found in lymph nodes, spleen, Peyer's patches, appendix, and tonsils. These cells contain up to 100 small, deeply basophilic nuclei which only rarely bear inclusions. Primary pneumonia is also characterized by giant cells, but here the cells have fewer, more leptochromatic nuclei, and both intranuclear and cytoplasmic eosinophilic inclusion bodies are often present. In measles encephalomyelitis, there is congestion, hemorrhage, perivascular cuffing, and demyelination.

The virus of measles is currently grouped with the viruses of canine distemper and rinderpest in the genus *Morbillivirus* and family Paramyxoviridae. The viruses in this genus are morphologically similar and share many common antigens, demonstrable by neutralization, neutralization-enhancement, complement-fixation, immunofluorescence, immunodiffusion, hemolysis-inhibition and hemagglutination-inhibition tests (Orvell and Norrby, 1974). The nucleocapsid components of these three viruses cannot be distinguished from one another by immunologic means. Each nucleocapsid has an elongated, tubular structure with cross-striations indicating a helical configuration. The virions are assembled at the plasma membrane by budding to form roughly spherical virions.

Measles is also known to be infectious for several species of monkeys, including Rhesus *(Macaca mulatta)*, Cynomolgus *(M. fascicularis)*, Taiwan macaque *(M. cyclopis)*, baboons *(Papio spp.)*, African green *(Ceropithecus aethiops)*, Colobus monkeys *(Colobus guereza)*, squirrel monkeys *(Saimiri sciureus)*, and marmosets *(Saguinus* and *Callithrix sp.)*. Although measles is rare in their native habitats, few Rhesus monkeys escape infection once they are brought into captivity. Clinical disease is rarely recorded, either because it is mild or initial infection occurred enroute to the laboratory. However, monkeys may exhibit conjunctivitis and an exanthematous rash which lasts for three to four days. The disease is rarely if ever fatal. In newly imported animals dying of other causes, or killed in the course of experimentation, visceral lesions resulting from measles infection are encountered with some frequency, even in the absence of a rash. Most often these are characterized by giant cell pneumonia with intranuclear and cytoplasmic inclusion bodies within giant cells and respiratory epithelial cells. Lymphoid giant cells are less frequent than in human measles, but may be present.

In marmosets, measles may be more serious. Epizootics with high mortality rates have occurred (Levy and Mirkovic, 1971; Fraser et al., 1978), apparently the result of variant viruses with greater virulence.

In addition to pneumonia, marmosets develop gastritis and enterocolitis. There is thinning and sloughing of surface epithelium. Large syncytial cells are present near the eroded surface of mucosa and within the crypts. These large cells often contain eosinophilic intranuclear inclusions. Crypts are often dilated and contain neutrophils. Foci of necrosis, multinucleated giant cells, and inclusion bodies may also be present in the liver, kidney, uterus, pancreas, and salivary gland.

Certain strains of measles virus have been associated with a chronic, usually fatal, disease of the central nervous system, most often affecting young children. This disease has been named **subacute sclerosing panencephalitis.** Experimentally-induced disease has been described in macaques and studied in hamsters and mice. One variant has been attributed as the cause of hydrocephalus in experimentally-infected suckling hamsters (Haspell and Rapp, 1975).

Diagnosis. Presumptive diagnosis can be established on the basis of the characteristic lesions. Definitive diagnosis requires viral isolation and identification.

Albrecht, P., and Schumacher, H. P.: Markers for measles virus. I. Physical properties. Arch. ges Virusforsch., 36:23–35, 1972.

Albrecht, P., et al.: Subacute sclerosing panencephalitis: experimental infection in primates. Science, 195:64–66, 1977.

Albrecht, P., et al.: Fatal measles infection in marmosets: pathogenesis and prophylaxis. Inf. Immun., 27:969–978, 1980.

Barringer, J. R., and Griffith, J. F.: Experimental measles virus encephalitis. A light, phase, fluorescence, and electron microscopic study. Lab. Invest., 23:335–346, 1970.

Breitfeld, V., et al.: Fatal measles infection in children with leukemia. Lab. Invest., 28:279–291, 1973.

Byington, D. P., and Johnson, K. P.: Subacute sclerosing panencephalitis virus in immunosuppressed adult hamsters. Lab. Invest., 32:91–97, 1975.

Covell, W. P.: The occurrence of intranuclear inclusions in monkeys unaccompanied by specific signs of disease. Am. J. Pathol. 8:151–158, 1932.

Fankhauser, R., Freudiger, U., Vandevelde, M., and Fatzer, R.: Purkinjezellatrophie nach Masernvirus Vakzinierung beim Hund. Schweiz. Arch. Neurol. Neurochir. Psychiatr., 112:353–363, 1973.

Fraser, C. E. O., et al.: A paramyxovirus causing fatal gastroenterocolitis in marmoset monkeys. Prim. Med., 10:261–270, 1978.

Hall, W. C., Kovatch, R. M., Herman, P. H., and Fox, J. G.: Pathology of measles in Rhesus monkeys. Vet. Pathol., 8:307–319, 1971.

Haspell, M. V., and Rapp, F.: Measles virus: an unwanted variant causing hydrocephalus. Science, 187:450–451, 1975.

Herndon, R. M., Rena-Descalzi, L., Griffin, D. E., and Coyle, P. K.: Age dependence of viral expression: electron microscopic and immunoperoxidase studies of measles virus replication in mice. Lab. Invest., 33:544–553, 1975.

Imagawa, D. T.: Relationships among measles, canine distemper and rinderpest viruses. Prog. Med. Virol., 10:160–193, 1968.

Kamahora, J.: Experimental pathology of measles in monkeys. Jpn. J. Med. Sci. Biol., 18:51, 1965.

Kamahora, J., and Nii, S.: Pathological and immunological studies of monkeys infected with measles virus. Arch. Ges. Virusforsch., 16:161–167, 1965.

Levy, B. M., and Mirkovic, R. R.: An epizootic of measles in a marmoset colony. Lab. Anim. Sci., 21:33–39, 1971.

Manning, P. J., Banks, K. L., and Lehner, N. D. M.: Naturally occurring giant cell pneumonia in the Rhesus monkey (Macaca mulatta). J. Am. Vet. Med. Assoc., 153:899–904, 1968.

Meyer, H. M., Jr., Brooks, B. E., Douglas, R. D., and Rogers, N. G.: Ecology of measles in monkeys. Am. J. Dis. Child., 103:307–313, 1962.

Nishikawa, F., Sugiyama, T., Takasaka, M., and Honjo, S.: Epidemiology of myxo-paramyxovirus infections among cynomolgus monkeys imported for laboratory use. Jpn. J. Med. Sci. Biol., 27:249–262, 1974.

O'Brien, T. C., Albrecht, P., Tauraso, N. M., and

Burns, G. R.: Properties of a measles-virus neuropathic for rhesus monkeys. Arch. ges. Virusforsch., 39:228–239, 1972.

Ono, K., Iwa, N., Kato, S., and Konobe, T.: Demonstration of viral antigen in giant cells formed in monkeys experimentally infected with measles virus. Biken J., 13:329–337, 1970.

Örvell, C., and Norrby, E.: Further studies on the immunologic relationships among measles, distemper, and rinderpest viruses. J. Immunol., 113:1850–1858, 1974.

Phillips, I. R., Colman, G., and Clarke, M.: Measles in monkeys. Vet. Rec., 97:436, 1975.

Potkay, S., Ganaway, J. R., Rogers, N. G., and Kinard, R.: An epizootic of measles in a colony of Rhesus monkeys (Macaca mulatta). Am. J. Vet. Res., 27:331–334, 1966.

Raine, C. S., Feldman, L. A., Sheppard, R. D., and Bornstein, M. B.: Subacute sclerosing panencephalitis virus in cultures of organized central nervous tissue. Lab. Invest., 28:627–640, 1973.

Raine, C. S., et al.: Subacute sclerosing panencephalitis virus: Observations on a neuroadapted and non-neuroadapted strain in organotypic central nervous system cultures. Lab. Invest., 31:42–53, 1974.

Raine, C. S., Byington, D. P., and Johnson, K. P.: Subacute sclerosing panencephalitis in the hamster: ultrastructure of the acute disease in newborns and weanlings. Lab. Invest., 33:108–116, 1975.

Remfry, J.: Measles epizootic with five deaths in newly imported rhesus monkeys (Macaca mulatta). Lab. Anim., 10:49–57, 1976.

Ruckle-Enders, G.: Comparative studies of monkey and human measles-virus strains. Am. J. Dis. Child., 103:297–307, 1962.

Rustigian, R., Winston, S. H., Bellanti, J. A., and Clark, L. A.: Neutralizing antibody and lymphocyte mediated, colony forming inhibition responses to measles infection in Cercopithecus aethiops monkeys. J. Infect. Dis., 132:511–519, 1975.

Scott, G. B. D., and Keymer, I. F.: The pathology of measles in Abyssinian colobus monkeys (Colobus guereza): a description of an outbreak. J. Pathol., 117:229–233, 1975.

Sergiev, P. G., Ryazantseva, N. E., and Shroit, I. G.: The dynamics of pathological processes in experimental measles in monkeys. Acta Virol., 4:265–273, 1960.

Shishido, A., and Yamanouchi, K.: Encephalomyelitis induced by paramyxovirus in non-human primates with a special reference to possible viral etiology of multiple sclerosis. Neurology (Minneap.), 26:83–84, 1976.

Soto, P. J., Jr., and Deauville, G. A.: Spontaneous simian giant cell pneumonia with coexistent B virus infection. Am. J. Vet. Res., 25:793–805, 1964.

Taniguchi, T., Kamahora, J., Kato, S., and Hagiwara, K.: Pathology in monkeys experimentally infected with measles virus. Med. J. Osaka University, 5:367–379, 1954.

Ueda, S., Otsuka, T., and Okuno, Y.: Experimental

subacute sclerosing panencephalitis (SSPE) in a monkey by subcutaneous inoculation with a defective SSPE virus. Biken J., 18:179–181, 1975.

Yamanouchi, K., et al.: Giant cell formation in lymphoid tissues of monkeys inoculated with various strains of measles virus. Jpn. J. Med. Sci. Biol., 23:131–145, 1970.

ORTHOMYXOVIRIDAE

Now grouped together in this family are the "true" influenza viruses, currently classified in one genus: *Influenzavirus*. The genome of this family consists of seven separate pieces of single-stranded RNA, with a total molecular weight of 5 million daltons. The tubular nucleocapsid is about 6 to 9 nm in diameter and makes up the type-specific antigen (Type A, B, or C). The lipoprotein envelope is 80 to 120 nm in diameter, and contains the strain-specific antigens (hemagglutinin and neuraminidase). The virion contains a transcriptase and matures by budding from the plasma membrane. Multiplication occurs in the nucleus and cytoplasm of infected cells.

The peplomers which project from the surface of the virion are well-defined in electron micrographs. Two glycoprotein peplomers have been identified: the hemagglutin and the neuraminidase. Upon initial isolation, some strains have a filamentous form, but produce the roughly spherical virions with conspicuous peplomers on the surface as they become adapted to cell culture systems. The name, Orthomyxovirus, was developed from the action of early strains upon mucus (ortho = correct, true; myxo = mucus).

Diseases Due to Influenza Viruses

Influenza viruses have been studied at great length and are still of intense interest, not only because they have such a worldwide distribution and spread so rapidly among the human population, but they also infect many species of animals. Passage through cells of different species appears to be one of the means for these viruses to alter their antigenicity. The nomenclature used to identify different isolates of influenza is quite involved but outside the scope of this book. Of interest in our context is the fact that three types of influenza—A, B, and C—are identified on the basis of the antigenic characteristics of the nucleocapsids. Type A viruses have been recovered from many species of animals and birds and are distinguishable on the basis of their antigens associated with the lipoprotein envelope. Types B and C viruses appear to be limited to human hosts. One genus, *Influenzavirus,* has been officially adopted so far.

One of the serious features of human influenza A viruses is that a new antigenic variant appears about once each decade. A major segment of the population has no immunity to the new variant, resulting in a major pandemic. This change in antigenicity may be due to a mutagenic event involving the virus, or to genetic recombination from two viruses replicating in the same animal cells, resulting in a new hybrid that has a selective advantage. This concept assumes that this hybridization takes place in a susceptible animal population, an assumption that is increasingly supported by the evidence. Human influenza A has been demonstrated in a broadening number of animal species: chickens, ducks, turkeys, horses, cats, dogs, monkeys, and swine.

Anschutz, W., Scholtissek, C., and Rott, P.: Genetic relationship between different influenza strains. Med. Microbiol. Immunol., *158*:26–31, 1972.

Berendt, R. F.: Simian model for the evaluation of immunity to influenza. Infect. Immun., *9*:101–105, 1974.

Boudreault, A., Pavilanis, V., Lussier, G., and Di Franco, E.: Lesions observed in monkeys following intracerebral inoculation of live influenza virus. Symp. Ser. Immunobiol. Standard, *20*:158–163, 1973.

Downie, J. C., and Laver, W. G.: Isolation of a type A influenza virus from an Australian pelagic bird. Virology, *51*:259–269, 1973.

Easterday, B. C., and Couch, R. B.: Animal influenza: its significance in human infection. J. Infect. Dis., *131*:602–612, 1975.

Laver, W. G., and Webster, R. G.: Studies on the origin of pandemic influenza. III. Evidence implicating duck and equine influenza viruses as possible progenitors of the Hong Kong strain of human influenza. Virology, *51*:383–391, 1973.

London, W. T., Fuccillo, D. A., Sever, J. L., and Kent, S. G.: Influenza virus as a teratogen in rhesus monkeys. Nature, *225*:483–484, 1975.

Lussier, G., Boudreault, A., Pavilanis, V., and DiFranco, E.: Lesions of the central nervous system induced in non-human primates by live influenza viruses. Can. J. Comp. Med., *38*:398–405, 1974.

Marois, P., Boudreault, A., and DiFranco, E.: Response of ferrets and monkeys to intranasal infection with human, equine and avian influenza viruses. Can. J. Comp. Med., *35*:71–76, 1971.

Miyoshi, K., et al.: Influenza virus encephalitis in squirrel monkeys receiving immunosuppressive therapy. J. Immunol., *106*:1119–1121, 1971.

Narayan, O., et al.: Pathogenesis of lethal influenza virus infection in turkeys. J. Comp. Pathol., *82*:129–137, 1972.

Narayan, O.: Pathogenesis of lethal influenza virus infection in turkeys. II. Central nervous system phase of infection. J. Comp. Pathol., *82*:139–146, 1972.

Nikitin, T., Cohen, D., Todd, J. D., and Lief, F. S.: Epidemiological studies of A/Hong Kong: 68 virus infection in dogs. Bull. WHO, *47*:471–479, 1972.

O'Brien, T. C., and Tauraso, N. M.: Antibodies to type A influenza viruses in sera from nonhuman primates. Arch. ges. Virusforsch., *40*:359–365, 1973.

Paniker, C. K. J., and Nair, C. M. G.: Experimental infection of animals with influenzavirus types A and B. Bull. WHO, *47*:461–463, 1972.

Paniker, C. K. J., and Nair, C. M. G.: Infection with A2 Hong Kong influenza virus in domestic cats. Bull. WHO, *43*:859–862, 1970.

Sereda, V. N.: Aetiology of influenza of domestic animals. Acta Virologica, *18*:222–228, 1974.

Sever, J. L.: Virus infections and malformations. Fed. Proc., *30*:114–117, 1971.

Shortridge, K. F., Belyavin, G., and Bidwell, D. E.: The occurrence of human influenza virus antibodies in the sera of certain wild species of animal. Brief report. Arch. ges. Virusforsch., *32*:286–290, 1970.

Styk, B., et al.: Experimental infection of horses with A-equi 2/Miami/1/63 and human A2/Hong Kong/1/68 influenza viruses. III. Immunodiffusion study of the antibody response. Acta Virol. Prague, *14*:35–46, 1970.

Todd, J. D., and Cohen, D.: Studies of influenza in dogs. I. Susceptibility of dogs to natural and experimental infection with human A2 and B strains of influenza virus. Am. J. Epidemiol., *87*:426–439, 1968.

Tumova, B., and Schild, G. C.: Antigenic relationships between type A influenzaviruses of human, porcine, equine and avian origin. Bull. WHO, *47*:453–460, 1972.

Webster, R. G.: On the origin of pandemic influenza viruses. Curr. Top. Microbiol. Immunol., *59*:75–105, 1972.

WHO Expert Committee on Influenza: A revised system of nomenclature for influenza viruses. Bull. WHO, *45*:119–124, 1972.

Equine Influenza

The term influenza has been in use for centuries to describe respiratory diseases of man and animals, often being used as a catch-all diagnosis for diseases of uncertain cause. Influenza should be restricted to those specific diseases caused by agents classified within the orthomyxoviridae, genus *Influenzavirus*. Specific disease-associated influenza viruses have been isolated from man, swine, equines, and birds. Equine influenza virus was first isolated and identified in 1958 in Czechoslovakia (A/Equi 1 serotype). A second serotype (A/Equi 2) was isolated in 1963 in Miami. Both serotypes are of worldwide distribution, and cause similar syndromes which are highly infectious, spreading rapidly.

Signs. Clinical signs include nasal discharge, cough, dyspnea, fever, depression, and reluctance to move. The illness lasts two to seven days. The disease is rarely if ever fatal in adult horses, but death is reported in young foals. Secondary bacterial infection may complicate the disease in both adult and young animals.

Lesions. The lesions of equine influenza have been studied histologically in a few instances. As summarized by Gerber (1970), erosions of mucosae have been noted in the nose, pharynx, larynx, and trachea. In the lung, the lesions have been described as peribronchitis, bronchitis with hyaline membranes in alveoli, periarteritis, and bronchopneumonia.

Diagnosis. Positive diagnosis depends on demonstrating serum-neutralizing antibodies or isolation and identification of the virus. The clinical disease must be differentiated from other respiratory diseases. Equine rhinopneumonitis may resemble influenza, but as a respiratory disease it is principally an infection of young horses. Differentiating features of equine viral arteritis include edema of the limbs, colic, diarrhea, conjunctivitis, and photophobia. Viral arteritis is also associated with abortion during the course or in early convalescence. Rhinovirus and parainfluenza virus infections of horses produce respiratory illnesses which are indistinguishable from influenza except by identification of the specific virus involved.

Blaskovic, D.: Experimental infection of horses with equine influenza viruses. *In* Proceedings of Second International Conference of Equine Infectious Diseases, Paris, 1969, edited by J. T. Bryans and H. Gerber, Basel, S. Karger, 1970. pp. 111–117.

Frerchs, G. N., Burrows, R., and Frerchs, C. C.: Serological response of horses and laboratory animals to equine influenza vaccines. *In* Equine Infectious Diseases III, edited by J. T. Bryans and H. Gerber. Basel, S. Karger, 1973. pp. 503–509.

Gerber, H.: Clinical features, sequelae and epidemiology of equine influenza. *In* Proceedings of Second International Conference of Equine Infectious Disease, Paris, 1969, edited by J. T. Bryans and H. Gerber. Basel, S. Karger, 1970. pp. 63–80.

Hofer, B., et al.: An investigation of the etiology of viral respiratory disease in a remount depot. *In* Equine Infectious Diseases III, edited by J. T. Bryans and H. Gerber. Basel, S. Karger, 1973.

Hoyle, L.: The influenza viruses. Virology Monographs, *4*:1–375, 1968.

Martone, F., Palomba, E., Bonaduce, D., and Simone, L. De.: Influenza in horses due to myxovirus influenza A/equi-2. Characteristics of six strains isolated in Naples in 1971. Clinica Vet., *97*:345–353, 1974.

McQueen, J. L., Steele, J. H., and Robinson, R. Q.: Influenza in animals. Adv. Vet. Sci., *12*:285–336, 1968.

Powell, D. G., et al.: The outbreak of equine influenza in England April/May, 1973. Vet. Rec., *94*:282–287, 1974.

Rose, M. A., Round, M. C., and Beveridge, W. I. B.: Influenza in horses and donkeys in Britain, 1969. Vet. Rec., *86*:768–769, 1970.

Rouse, B. T., and Ditchfield, W. J. B.: The response of ponies to Myxovirus influenzae A-equi-2. III. The protective effect of serum and nasal antibody against experimental challenge. Res. Vet. Sci., *11*:503–507, 1970.

Rouse, B. T.: Equine influenza immunization—the role of nasal antibody—a review. Aust. Vet. J., *47*:146–148, 1971.

Sibalin, M., Jaksch, W., Pötsch, F., and Bürki, F.: Zwei Ausbrüche equiner Influenza des Typs A₂ in Österreich. Wien. Tierarz. Monat., *58*:421–427, 1971.

Sinvinova, O., et al.: Isolation of a virus causing respiratory disease in horses. Acta Virol., *2*:52–61, 1958.

Styk, B., et al.: Experimental infection of horses with A-equi 2/Miami/1/63 and human A₂/Hong Kong/1/68 influenza viruses. III. Immunodiffusion study of the antibody response. Acta Virol., *14*:35–46, 1970.

Todd, J. D., Lief, F. S., and Cohen, D.: Experimental infection of ponies with the Hong Kong variant of human influenza virus. Am. J. Epidemiol., 92:330–336, 1970.

Waddell, G. H., Teigland, M. B., and Sigel, M. M.: A new influenza virus associated with equine respiratory disease. J. Am. Vet. Med. Assoc., 143:587–590, 1963.

Swine Influenza

Swine influenza is an infectious respiratory disease of swine caused by a virus in the genus *Influenzavirus,* family Orthomyxoviridae, acting in synergy with a gram-negative bacterial organism, *Hemophilus influenzae suis.* The swine influenza virus is closely related to the viruses of human influenza type A; in fact, its transmission to laboratory animals (mice, ferrets) by Shope was the opening step to extensive work with similar viruses to which man is susceptible. Shope was also the first to postulate that swine influenza resulted from the infection of swine by the virus responsible for the 1918 pandemic of influenza. This view has been reinforced somewhat by the recent appearance of swine influenza A in the human population, fortunately not in pandemic form. It now seems likely that several species (man, swine, horse, chicken, turkey) are susceptible to influenza A, and that some could be vehicles for infection, transmission, and modification of virus strains. In addition, Shope demonstrated that the swine lungworm can act as intermediate host and reservoir for the swine influenza virus during interenzoötic periods. The virus is introduced into susceptible pigs by lungworm larvae; infection is provoked by the presence of *H. influenzae suis;* then the disease can spread to other pigs in the herd by direct contact. Swine, ferrets, and mice are susceptible to the experimental disease. There is some experimental evidence to indicate that two- to three-week old swine undergo severe pneumonia when inoculated with swine influenza virus during the migration of *Ascaris suum* larvae through the lungs.

Signs. The disease principally affects young pigs; after an incubation period of 24 to 48 hours, they exhibit fever, rhinitis, cough, and inappetence. These symptoms usually abate after three to five days, but in some cases transitory fever may recur within three weeks. Dyspnea associated with severe pulmonary involvement is observed in some cases, and death occurs following severe pneumonia. The mortality rate is usually not high (around 1%), but in some outbreaks may assume serious proportions. The morbidity rate may approach 100%.

Lesions. The specific lesions of swine influenza are restricted to the trachea, bronchi, bronchioles, alveolar ducts, and alveoli. The gross evidence of pathologic changes in these structures consists in part of mucopurulent exudate, which lies over the tracheal and bronchial mucosae and fills smaller branches of the bronchi. Plugging of these bronchi and bronchioles results in sharply demarcated, prune-colored areas of atelectasis. Consolidation of lung parenchyma occurs around the bronchi, starting adjacent to their finer branches. Experimental intranasal exposure of swine to the virus alone results in atelectasis restricted to the pendant portions of the lung, especially in the cardiac, apical, and intermediate lobes. The addition of *H. influenzae suis* to the inoculum produces more extensive pulmonary involvement: atelectasis extends to include the pendant portions of the diaphragmatic lobes, and peribronchial consolidation of the upper portions of all lobes occurs. Mucopurulent exudate in the bronchial system is also more extensive. Frank pneumonic consolidation and fibrinous pleuritis develop in affected animals exposed concurrently to unfavorable conditions, such as cold wet weather and shipping.

The microscopic changes that follow the intranasal instillation of swine influenza virus in mice, described by Dubin (1945), appear to parallel those that occur in swine. In mice, the virus produces necrosis of the lining cells of alveoli and bronchi and, to a smaller extent, those of the lower part of the trachea. Because of the loss of nuclei and hyalinization of cytoplasm of the epithelial cells, this necrotic process often appears as a hyaline membrane. Proliferation of the epithelial cells accompanies these necrotic changes and persists after they have disappeared. In the bronchi and bronchioles, the growth of epithelium progresses to such a remarkable degree that it fills the adjacent alveoli. These intra-alveolar plugs of epithelial cells begin to degenerate about the fourteenth day and some alveoli are reopened. The epithelium of the bronchi and bronchioles is restored during the third week of convalescence. The pneumonia is featured by necrosis of alveolar walls with formation of hyaline membranes lining the alveolar sacs, accompanied by congestion, focal hemorrhages, severe perivascular and intralobular edema, and infiltration with inflammatory leukocytes, principally mononuclear cells. Areas of collapse of lung parenchyma appear as early as the second day as a result of obstruction of bronchi by pus, mucus, and desquamated cells. These areas of atelectasis may become heavily infiltrated with leukocytes. Peribronchiolar alveoli are often consolidated as the result of infiltration of mononuclear cells or the ingrowth of respiratory epithelium. Consolidated alveoli are restored to a functional state by necrosis and phagocytic removal of the cells with which they are filled.

Diagnosis. The symptoms and gross and microscopic lesions provide a basis for the presumptive diagnosis of swine influenza. Definitive diagnosis depends upon demonstration of significant elevation of virus-neutralizing or antihemagglutinin antibodies in the sera of swine during the course of an infection, or upon isolation and identification of the swine influenza virus, type A.

Dubin, I. N.: A pathological study of mice infected with the virus of swine influenza. Am. J. Pathol., 21:1121–1134, 1945.

Easterday, B. C.: Influenza virus infection of the suckling pig. Acta Vet. Brno., 40:33–42, 1971.

Harkness, J. W., Schild, G. C., Lamont, P. H., and Brand, C. M.: Studies on relationships between human and porcine influenza. I. Serological evidence of infection in swine in Great Britain with an influenza A virus antigenically like human Hong Kong/68 virus. Bull. WHO, 46:721–728, 1972.

Hoyle, L.: The influenza viruses. Virology Monographs, 4:1–375. New York, Springer–Verlag, 1968.

Kundin, W. D.: Hong Kong A-2 influenza virus infection among swine during human epidemic in Taiwan. Nature, 228:857, 1970.

Kundin, W. D., and Easterday, B. C.: Hong Kong influenza infection in swine: experimental and field observation. Bull. WHO, 47:489–491, 1972.

Mensik, J., Valick, L., and Pospisil, Z.: Pathogenesis of swine influenza infection produced experimentally in suckling piglets. Multiplication of virus in the respiratory tract of suckling piglets in the presence of colostrum derived specific antibody in their blood stream. Zbl. Vet. Med. B, 18:665–678, 1971.

Pereira, H. G.: Swine influenza. Nature, 261:10, 1976.

Pirtle, E. C.: Incidence of antibody to swine influenza virus in Iowa breeder and butcher pigs correlated with signs of influenza-like illness. Am. J. Vet. Res., 34:83–86, 1973.

Popovici, V., et al.: Infection of pigs with an influenza virus related to the A2/Hong Kong/1/68 strain. Acta Virol., 16:363, 1972.

Renshaw, H. W.: Influence of antibody-mediated immune suppression on clinical, viral, and immune responses to swine influenza infection. Am. J. Vet. Res., 36:5–14, 1975.

Schnurrenberger, P. R., Woods, G. T., and Martin, R. J.: Serologic evidence of human infection with swine influenza virus. Am. Rev. Respir. Dis., 102:356–361, 1970.

Shope, R. E.: The etiology of swine influenza. Science, 73:214–215, 1931.

———: The swine lungworm as a reservoir and intermediate host for swine influenza virus. I. The presence of swine influenza virus in healthy and susceptible pigs. J. Exp. Med., 74:41–47, 1941.

———: Swine influenza. Experimental transmission and pathology. J. Exp. Med., 54:349–359, 1931.

———: The swine lungworm as a reservoir and intermediate host for swine influenza virus. II. The transmission of swine influenza virus by the swine lungworm. J. Exp. Med. 74:49–68, 1941.

———: The swine lungworm as a reservoir and intermediate host for swine influenza virus. III. Factors influencing transmission of the virus and the provocation of influenza. J. Exp. Med., 77:111–126, 1943.

———: The swine lungworm as a reservoir and intermediate host for swine influenza virus. IV. The demonstration of masked swine influenza virus in lungworm larva and swine under natural conditions. J. Exp. Med., 77:127–138, 1943.

Shortridge, K. F., et al.: Persistence of Hong Kong influenza virus variants in pigs. Science, 196: 1454–1455, 1977.

Smith, T. F., et al.: Isolation of swine influenza virus from autopsy lung tissue of man. N. Engl. J. Med., *294*:708–710, 1976.

Straub, M.: The microscopical changes in the lungs of mice infected with influenza virus. J. Pathol. Bact., *45*:75–78, 1937.

———: The histology of catarrhal influenza bronchitis and collapse of the lung in mice infected with influenza virus. J. Pathol. Bact., *50*:31–36, 1940.

Styk, B., et al.: Antibody against Hong Kong influenza viruses in pigs. Acta Virol., *15*:211–219, 1971.

Underdahl, N. R.: The effect of *Ascaris suum* migration on the severity of swine influenza. J. Am. Vet. Med. Assoc., *133*:380–383, 1958.

Urman, H. K., Underdahl, N. R., and Young, G. A.: Comparative histopathology of experimental swine influenza and virus pneumonia of pigs in disease-free swine. Am. J. Vet. Res., *19*:913–917, 1958.

RHABDOVIRIDAE

In the family Rhabdoviridae (rhabdo = rod) are grouped several viruses currently divided into two genera, *Vesiculovirus* and *Lyssavirus*. These viruses have bullet-shaped virions measuring 70 by 175 nm. The virus is enveloped and contains a single-stranded RNA with molecular weight of about 4 million daltons. The virions have been further described as rigid but fragile cylinders with one hemispherical (rounded) end and one flattened end,

Table 9–11. Diseases Caused by Rhabdoviridae

Vesiculovirus	Lyssavirus
Vesicular stomatitis virus	Rabies virus
Bovine ephemeral fever virus (cattle, sheep, Diptera)	Lagos bat virus
Hemorrhagic septicema virus (trout)	Nigerian shrew virus
Cocal virus (birds)	Kern Canyon virus (bats)
Flanders-Hart-Park virus (birds and Diptera)	
Mt. Elgon bat virus (bats and Diptera)	
Sigma virus (Drosophila)	
Potato yellow dwarf virus (plants)	
Lettuce necrotic yellow virus (plants)	

which usually buds off last. The lipoprotein envelope contains conspicuous peplomers which contain glycoprotein. Within the lipoprotein envelope is a membrane that contains the M protein (29,000 daltons). The nucleocapsid consists of a continuous strand, 5 nm wide, with a helical structure and repeating subunits. The virion contains a transcriptase. Table 9–11 lists these viruses.

Diseases Due to Vesiculoviruses

Two viruses that cause disease in mammals are currently classified in the genus *Vesiculovirus*, namely, the viruses of vesicular stomatitis and bovine ephemeral fever.

Vesicular Stomatitis

The virus of vesicular stomatitis may naturally affect swine, cattle, horses, and man, producing a disease which has close similarities to aphthous fever (foot and mouth disease) and vesicular exanthema. Vesicular stomatitis is present only in the warm months of the year, appearing in the late spring and disappearing with the coming of freezing weather. It is most common in cattle and horses, but severe outbreaks have been reported in swine in serum-producing biologic plants. Insect vectors are believed to represent the principal means of transmission.

Evidence has been developed (Donaldson, 1970) to indicate that bats (*Myotus lucifugus lucifugus*) are susceptible to the virus of vesicular stomatitis, and that the virus may be transmitted by mosquitoes (*Aedes aegypti*) to mice under experimental conditions. Bats could therefore serve as hosts for the virus, maintaining it in the ecology and spreading it by their own movements. The virus may be transmitted by phlebotomine sandflies (Tesh et al., 1972).

Under experimental conditions, the virus produces encephalitis in mice, horses, cattle, and sheep (Miyoshi, Harter and Hsu, 1971; Frank et al., 1945).

Lesions. The lesions of vesicular stomatitis are usually described as vesicular, but Seibold and Sharp (1960) disagree with this concept as a consequence of their study of experimentally infected bovine tongues. These investigators found the basic histologic alterations to be (1) intercellular edema in the middle of the malpighian layer, resulting in a filigree appearance, but not usually vesiculation; (2) necrosis of epithelial cells in the middle of the malpighian layer and usually sparing the basal layer; and (3) inflammatory cellular infiltration by heterophils and monocytes into the necrotic zones of epithelium. In some lesions, the intraepithelial edema becomes abundant enough to result in a vesicle, but this occurs in less than 30% of the experimental lesions. This observation is in agreement with several field experiences in which vesiculation was rarely observed clinically.

Nonvesiculated lesions terminate by dehydration of the superficial layers of epithelium—edema fluid apparently escaping through vertical cracks in the *stratum corneum.* Lesions with large vesicles or bullae usually lose the overlying epithelial layers, leaving a thin layer of basal cells over the congested dermis. These eroded lesions therefore have the characteristic red, raw appearance. Healing proceeds by regrowth of the epithelium from the remaining basal cells.

The ultrastructural features of the lesions of vesicular stomatitis (Proctor and Sherman, 1975) confirm the occurrence of intercellular edema and necrosis of superficial epithelial cells (keratinocytes). Virions bud from the plasma membrane and are seen in intracellular vesicles. Replication of desmosomes is a prominent feature at opposing cell membranes, and numerous free desmosomes accumulate in the cytoplasm. This phenomenon appears to be the result of endocytosis of the desmosomes after breaks occur in the related plasma membrane. Enlarging intracellular vesicles eventually isolate epithelial cells, especially keratinocytes, which undergo necrosis.

Diagnosis. The lesions of vesicular stomatitis are essentially similar in distribution, location, and microscopic appearance to those of aphthous fever and vesicular exanthema. The lesions of these three diseases cannot be definitively distinguished on morphologic grounds in spite of the less conspicuous vesiculation evident in vesicular stomatitis. Vesicular stomatitis, unlike aphthous fever, rarely causes myocarditis and is almost never fatal. The virus may be seen in ultramicroscopic sections or isolated for identification in tissue culture systems.

Brooksby, J. B.: Vesicular stomatitis and foot-and-mouth disease differentiation by complement-fixation. Proc. Soc. Exp. Biol. Med., 67:254–258, 1948.

Chow, T. L., Hansen, R. R., and McNutt, S. H.: Pathology of vesicular stomatitis in cattle. Proc. Am. Vet. Med. Assoc., 1951, pp. 119–124.

Chow, T. L., and McNutt, S. H.: Pathological changes of experimental vesicular stomatitis of swine. Am. J. Vet. Res., 14:420–424, 1953.

Donaldson, A. I.: Bats as possible maintenance hosts for vesicular stomatitis virus. Am. J. Epidemiol., 92:132–136, 1970.

Dal Canto, M. C., Rabinowitz, S. G., and Johnson, T. C.: An ultrastructural study of central nervous system disease produced by wild-type and temperature-sensitive mutants of vesicular stomatitis virus. Lab. Invest., 35:185–196, 1976.

———: In vivo assembly and maturation of vesicular stomatitis virus. Lab. Invest., 35:515–524, 1976.

Fields, B. N., and Hawkins, K.: Human infection with the virus of vesicular stomatitis during an epizootic. N. Engl. J. Med., 277:989–994, 1967.

Frank, A. H., Appleby, A., and Seibold, H. R.: Experimental intracerebral infection of horses, cattle and sheep with the virus of vesicular stomatitis. Am. J. Vet. Res., 6:28–38, 1945.

Miyoshi, K., Harter, D. H., and Hsu, K. C.: Neuropathological and immunofluorescence studies of experimental vesicular stomatitis virus encephalitis in mice. J. Neuropathol. Exp. Neurol., 30:266–277, 1971.

Proctor, S. J., and Sherman, K. C.: Ultrastructural changes in bovine lingual epithelium infected with vesicular stomatitis virus. Vet. Pathol., 12:362–377, 1975.

Ribelin, W. E.: The cytopathogenesis of vesicular stomatitis virus infection in cattle. Am. J. Vet. Res., 19:66–73, 1958.

Seibold, H. R. and Sharp, J. B., Jr.: A revised concept of the pathologic changes of the tongue in cattle with vesicular stomatitis. Am. J. Vet. Res., *21*:35–51, 1960.

Shahan, M. S., Frank, A. H., and Mott, L. O.: Studies on vesicular stomatitis with special reference to a virus of swine origin. J. Am. Vet. Med. Assoc., *108*:5–19, 1946.

Srihongse, S.: Vesicular stomatitis virus infection in Panamanian primates and other vertebrates. Am. J. Epidemiol., *90*:69–76, 1969.

Sudia, W. D., Fields, B. N., and Calisher, C. H.: The isolation of vesicular stomatitis virus (Indian strain) and other viruses from mosquitoes in New Mexico, 1965. Am. J. Epidemiol., *86*:598–602, 1967.

Tesh, R. B., Chaniotis, B. N., and Johnson, K. M.: Vesicular stomatitis virus (Indiana serotype): transmission by phlebotomine sandflies. Science, *175*:1477–1479, 1972.

Tesh, R. B., Peralta, P. H., and Johnson, K. M.: Ecologic studies of vesicular stomatitis virus. I. Prevalence of infection among animals and humans living in an area of endemic VSV activity. Am. J. Epidemiol., *90*:225–261, 1969.

Bovine Ephemeral Fever
(Bovine Epizootic Fever,
Three-day Sickness,
Stiff Sickness)

This subtle disease was apparently known in Africa as early as 1867, but its exact nature was obscure until 1967, when Westhuizen first isolated and identified the etiologic agent. The viral agent was identified as having features similar to those of vesicular stomatitis and rabies, and is currently classified as a *Vesiculovirus* (family Rhabdoviridae). The natural disease is recognized by the transitory fever, inappetence, hyperpnea or dyspnea of short duration, mucous to purulent nasal discharge, shivering, and a shifting lameness. In some cases, rumination may cease for a few days and ruminal stasis, diarrhea, or constipation may occur. Occasional posterior paralysis has been described. Many animals become ill but few die from the disease.

Bovine ephemeral fever has been reported from Africa, Asia, and Australia. Epizootiologic features, such as seasonal appearance of the disease, failure of transmission by contact, apparent spread by leaps over long distances, and the tendency for outbreaks to occur during seasons of heavy rainfall, indicate that the virus is probably transmitted by biting insects. Experiments with stable flies and mosquitoes indicate that they are probably not responsible for transmission of this virus. *Culicoides* species are suspected to be the vectors in Australia, but confirming evidence is lacking.

Lesions. Gross lesions reported in natural and experimental cases include generalized vascular engorgement, edematous lymph nodes, congestion of abomasal mucosa, hydropericardium, hydrothorax, rhinitis, tracheitis, and pulmonary emphysema. Tendovaginitis, fasciculitis, and cellulitis and focal necrosis of muscle have also been described. Petechiae may be seen in epineurium of peripheral nerves.

Lesions noted with the light microscope appear to be limited to venules and capillaries, particularly in muscles, tendon sheaths, synovial membranes, fascia, and skin. Endothelial cells may be hyperplastic, and the vessels surrounded by edema and leukocytic infiltration. Some vessel walls are necrotic; others, thrombosed. Hemosiderosis of spleen and lymph nodes has also been associated with the disease.

Diagnosis. Diagnosis may be confirmed by isolation and identification of the virus, or by identifying viral antigens in tissues of affected animals by specific immunofluorescent techniques.

Basson, P. A., Pienaar, J. G., and van der Westhuizen, B.: The pathology of ephemeral fever: a study of the experimental disease in cattle. J. S. Afr. Vet. Med. Assoc., *40*:385–393, 395 & 397, 1969.

Burgess, G. W.: Bovine ephemeral fever: a review. Vet. Bull., *41*:887–895, 1971.

Doherty, R. L., Standfast, H. A., and Clark, I. A.: Adaptation to mice of the causative virus of ephemeral fever of cattle from an epizootic in Queensland, 1968. Aust. J. Sci., *31*:365–366, 1969.

Doherty, R. L., Carley, J. G., Dyce, A. L., and Snowdon, W. A.: Virus strains isolated from arthropods during an epizootic of bovine ephemeral fever. Aust. Vet. J., *48*:81–86, 1972.

Heuschele, W. P.: Bovine ephemeral fever. I. Characteristics of the causative virus. Arch. ges. Virusforsch., *30*:195–202, 1970.

Holmes, I. H., and Doherty, R. L.: Morphology and development of bovine ephemeral fever virus. J. Virol., *5*:91–96, 1970.

Ito, Y., Tanka, Y., Inaba, Y., and Omori, T.: Electron microscopic observations of bovine epizootic fever virus. Natl. Inst. Anim. Hlth. Qt., Tokyo, 9:35–44, 1969.

Lecatsas, G.: The structure of bovine ephemeral fever virus. J. S. Afr. Vet. Med. Assoc., 40:230, 1969.

Lecatsas, G.: Further observations on the ultrastructure of ephemeral fever virus. Onderstepoort J. Vet. Res., 37:145–146, 1970

Matumoto, M., et al.: Behavior of bovine ephemeral fever virus in laboratory animals and cell cultures. Jpn. J. Microbiol., 14:413–421, 1970.

Murphy, F. A., Taylor, W. P., Mims, C. A., and Whitfield, S. G.: Bovine ephemeral fever virus in cell culture and mice. Archiv. Ges. Virusforsch., 38:234–249, 1972.

Parsonson, I. M., and Snowdon, W. A.: Ephemeral fever virus. I. Excretion in semen of infected bulls and attempts to infect female cattle by the intrauterine inoculation of virus. II. Experimental infection of pregnant cattle. Aust. Vet. J., 50:329–334, 335–337, 1974.

Snowdon, W. A.: Bovine ephemeral fever: the reaction of cattle to different strains of ephemeral fever virus and the antigenic comparison of two strains of virus. Aust. Vet. J., 46:258–266, 1970.

Theodoridis, A.: Fluorescent antibody studies on ephemeral fever virus. Onderstepoort J. Vet. Res., 36:187–190, 1969.

Theodoridis, A., and Lecatsas, G.: Variation in morphology of ephemeral fever virus. Onderstepoort J. Vet. Res., 40:139–142, 1973.

Tzipori, S., and Spradbrow, P. B.: Development and behaviour of a strain of bovine ephemeral fever virus with unusual host range. J. Comp. Pathol., 84:1–8, 1974.

Tzipori, S.: The susceptibility of young calves and newborn to bovine ephemeral fever virus. Aust. Vet. J., 51:254–255, 1975.

van der Westhuizen, B.: Studies on bovine ephemeral fever. I. Isolation and preliminary characterization of a virus from natural and experimentally produced cases of bovine ephemeral fever. Onderstepoort J. Vet. Res., 34:29–40, 1967.

Young, J. S.: Ephemeral fever and congenital deformities in calves. Aust. Vet. J., 45:574–576, 1969.

Diseases Due to Lyssaviruses

At least four viruses are now grouped in the genus *Lyssavirus,* based upon ultrastructural morphology of the virion and certain immunologic affinities. Each of these viruses have a rod or bullet-shaped virion, characteristic of the family Rhabdoviridae, and may be distinguished from other members of the family (such as vesicular stomatitis virus) by means of complement-fixation and neutralization tests. These viruses include the well-established virus of **rabies,** the **Lagos Bat** virus, the **Mokola** (Ib An 27377) **virus,** and the **Kotonkan** virus.

The Lagos Bat virus was first isolated from frugivorous bats *(Eidolon helvum)* in Nigeria (Boulger and Porterfield, 1958). It was subsequently shown to kill three-day-old mice by intracerebral inoculation, but not by the intraperitoneal route. This virus does not kill guinea pigs, rabbits, or one species of African monkey *(Cerocebus torquatus).*

The Mokola virus was originally isolated from the brains of shrews *(Crocidura spp.)* collected in Nigeria and subsequently from the brains of children succumbing to a neurologic disorder. The virus is pathogenic for mice, and neutralizing antibodies have been demonstrated in cattle, sheep, goats, swine, and birds in Nigeria. More recent studies indicate that both the Lagos bat and Mokola viruses produce fatal disease in dogs and monkeys *(M. mulatta)* when inoculated intracerebrally (Tignor et al., 1973; Percy et al., 1973).

A fourth *Lyssavirus,* Kotonkan virus, was recovered from the brains of *Culicoides.* Reactions to the complement-fixation and fluorescent antibody tests are similar to those of the Mokola virus, but not the same if the neutralization test is used. Neutralizing antibodies to this virus have been demonstrated in the sera of man, cattle, rodents, insectivores, sheep, and horses (Shope et al., 1970; Kemp et al., 1972; Tignor et al., 1973; Kemp et al., 1973).

Rabies (Hydrophobia, Lyssa, Rage, Tollwut)

Rabies is a viral encephalitis to which almost all mammals, including man, are susceptible. The virus is usually present in the saliva of infected animals and is transmitted by their bite; therefore, the disease is most common in carnivores such as dogs, wolves, and foxes. As a rule, rabies in man results from the bite of a rabid dog, wolf, fox, or skunk. These animals also transmit the disease to cattle, horses, and sheep, which, however, seldom spread it

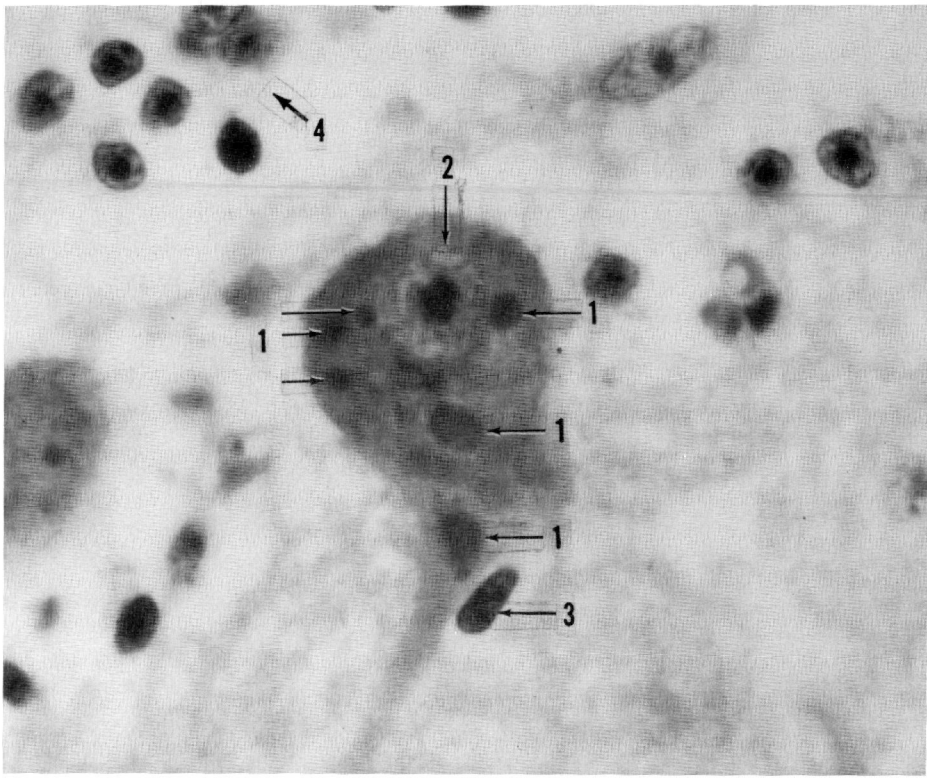

Fig. 9–63. Rabies, cerebellum of a cow (×1350). An unusual number of Negri bodies *(1)* are present in a Purkinje cell. Nucleus of the Purkinje cell*(2)*, nucleus of a microglial cell*(3)*, and cells of a granular layer*(4)*. Schleifstein modification of the Wilhite stain. (Courtesy of Armed Forces Institute of Pathology.) Contributor: Lt. Col. F. D. Maurer.

further. Insectivorous and frugivorous bats have in recent years been shown to harbor the virus, often without clinical signs of disease. These animals may have an important role in the dissemination of the virus and its survival in nature during interepizootic periods. In some parts of the world, vampire bats are important in the spread of the disease to other animals and man. A specific paralytic rabies in cattle, **derriengue,** transmitted by vampire bats, is an important problem in parts of Central and South America (Martell et al., 1974). Bats are the only animals that can become infected with, and excrete, rabies virus without developing clinical disease leading to death. In domestic animals, rabies is most frequent in cattle, dogs, and cats.

Wildlife rabies is most prevalent in skunks, foxes, raccoons, and bats.

Pathogenesis. The initial interactions between the rabies virus and cells in a tissue culture system have been studied by Iwasaki, Wiktor, and Koprowski (1973). These investigators found that within five minutes of the time a suspension of virus was added to the culture, virions were aligned perpendicular to the plasma membrane and engulfed within pinocytic vesicles and intracytoplasmic vacuoles. One hour later, virions were fused (by the "flat" end) to cell membranes, and release of the internal structures (nucleocapsids, etc.) of the virions into the cell was evident. Specific antibodies appeared in infected cells by four hours following inoculation. This specific antigen, demonstrated by fluorescent antibody, was present in most cells, and persisted for at least 96 hours. Budding of newly-formed virions started within six hours of initial exposure and reached a maximum within 24 hours. This period corresponded to the time of maximum recovery of virus from the cultures. After this 24 hours, increased numbers of virions and matrices were evident in the cytoplasm of infected cells, continuing to increase for at least 72 hours. Starting at 48 hours, focal degeneration of cells was evident in relation to the accumulating virions. Accumulation of dense bodies, fibrillar viral structures forming circumscribed matrices, and degenerated cell organelles become conspicuous features.

The transit of infectious virus particles from an inoculation site to the central nervous system has been studied in detail by Murphy et al. (1973) with three *Lyssaviruses*, by following them through the tissues by means of fluorescence, tissue titration of virus, and electron microscopy. Virus injected into muscle first enters and replicates in muscle cells, then virions are shed into extracellular spaces. Then neuromuscular and neurotendinal spindles nearby are involved. Peripheral nerves later become infected—apparently only axons support production of progeny virus and viral nucleocapsids. The infection extends progressively to dorsal root ganglia of ipsilateral segments of the lumbar spinal cord. Accumulation of large amounts of viral antigen in spinal cord prompts the conclusion that the virus reaches the synaptic junctions of the spinal cord by way of the peripheral nerve axioplasm, and replication occurs especially in the spinal cord.

Replication of virus becomes intense in most neuronal cells in the central nervous system, and eventually spreads centrifugally to involve neuronal cells throughout the body (Murphy et al., 1973). In experimental situations, virus reaches sites such as taste buds in the mouth and olfactory cells in the nose, where replication is intense—increasing chances for the spread of virus in saliva or nasal secretions.

Signs. Following the bite of a rabid animal, or penetration of the virus through the skin by some other means, the incubation period varies from a few days to several months. The clinical symptoms usually appear in one of two forms: the "dumb" and the "furious." In the dumb form of rabies, the animal falls into a stupor and has the peculiar staring expression associated with paralysis of the muscles of mastication. In the "furious" form, the animal goes into rages, biting and slashing at any moving object or even inanimate objects, such as sticks and trees. The furious champing of the jaws is accompanied by excessive salivation; the saliva streams from the mouth or is churned into foam which may adhere to the lips and face. A radical change in temperament occurs; wild animals that normally shun man will venture into the open and attack human subjects. The rabid dog, fox, or wolf tends particularly to attack a moving person or animal. Paralysis may follow either the "furious" or "dumb" stage of the disease. Death occurs within ten days of the first symptoms.

Although the view was long held that rabies infection always ended fatally, evidence has accumulated to indicate that this is not true. By using modern techniques to demonstrate viral infection, it has been demonstrated that some animals and people recover from rabies infection, and some clinically inapparent infections do occur (Bell, et al., 1972; Baer and Olson, 1972; Doege and Northrop, 1974; Fekadu, 1975).

Lesions. The lesions of rabies are microscopic, limited to the central nervous system, and extremely variable in extent. They may be subtle and indiscernible except for early necrosis of neurons with specific cytoplasmic inclusion bodies in the affected nerve cells. In some cases, diffuse encephalitis is demonstrated by perivascular cuffing, neuronophagic nodules, and other indications of destruction of neurons throughout the brain. These changes tend to be particularly prominent in the brain stem, the hippocampus, and the gasserian ganglia. According to Lapi, Davis, and Anderson (1952), specific lesions develop earlier and more constantly in the gasserian ganglia than elsewhere in the nervous system, and may be present even before specific inclusion bodies can be demonstrated. These lesions consist of focal proliferation of the capsule cells surrounding the ganglion cells, mild infiltration of lymphocytes and plasma cells, and encroachment of proliferating glial cells upon the neurons. These collections of proliferating glial cells replacing neurons are known as

Babes nodules. They may be seen in association with inclusion bodies in the cytoplasm of nearby ganglion cells.

In 1903, spherical cytoplasmic inclusion bodies with specific tinctorial characteristics were described by Negri in neurons of dogs, cats, and rabbits experimentally infected with rabies virus. These inclusion bodies have subsequently been called **Negri bodies,** and are accepted as specific indications of infection with rabies virus. This wide acceptance of Negri bodies as proof of rabies has developed in spite of a prolonged controversy regarding the exact nature of these inclusions. Negri's idea that they were protozoan is not generally held today. Electron microscopic observations indicate that Negri bodies

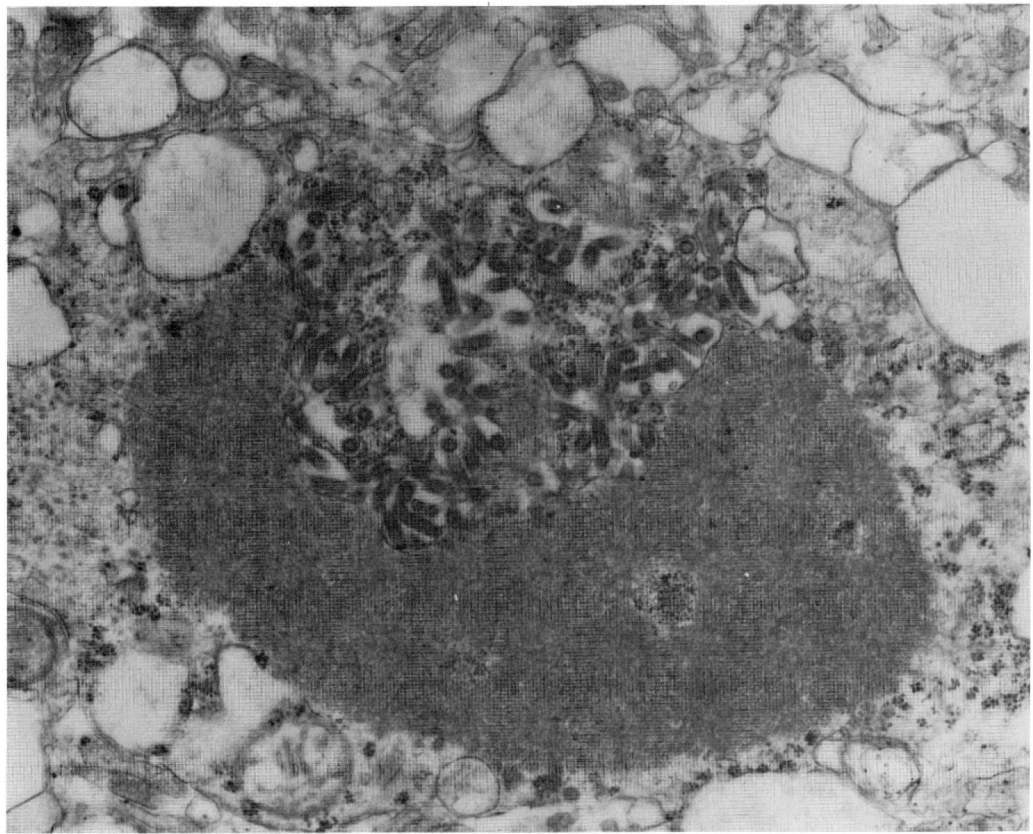

Fig. 9–64. Rabies, hippocampus, fox. A neuronal inclusion containing bullet-shaped and rod-shaped virus particles. (× 30,000.) (Courtesy of Dr. R. E. Dierks and *American Journal of Pathology.* Electronmicrograph taken by Dr. F. A. Murphy.)

represent well-defined electron-dense masses, which may or may not contain or be associated with rabies virions. The nature and significance of the matrix is not understood, but may represent a necessary component for viral replication or a reaction on the part of the infected neuron. Negri bodies are not always present in rabies, and certain strains of rabies virus do not produce inclusion bodies, indicating that Negri bodies are not necessary for viral replication. Negri bodies are always intracytoplasmic; in the rabid dog they are found most readily in the hippocampus, but in cattle they are more numerous in the Purkinje cells of the cerebellum. It is possible for all neurons, even those of the ganglia, to contain these inclusions. Negri bodies have a distinct limiting membrane and may be encircled by a narrow, clear halo. In tissue sections, they usually measure from 2 to 8 μ in diameter. One or several may be present in an affected nerve cell. These inclusions may be entirely within the cell body or they may occur in dendrites, where they are likely to be elongated, conforming to the shape of these processes. A granular, slightly basophilic internal structure can be demonstrated in preparations with Mann's stain.

The staining characteristics of the Negri body are of considerable interest. The hematoxylin and eosin method does not differentiate Negri bodies well. They become only a slightly darker shade of the color of the surrounding cytoplasm, but the clear halo may serve to delimit them. The Schleifstein modification of the Wilhite stain is particularly successful with tissue fixed in Zenker's solution. When stained by this method, Negri bodies are bright magenta, contrasting with the purplish cytoplasm of the neuron; red blood cells are somewhat yellowish or copper colored. The Williams modification of the van Gieson's stain gives a similar effect. In impression smears, Seller's stain is effective; the inclusion body is bright red or magenta against the pale blue background of the neuronal cytoplasm. Mann's and Giemsa's stains are also useful, particularly in impression smears. No matter which stain is used, it is important that the person who examines material to confirm the diagnosis be thoroughly familiar with the characteristics of the stain and the appearance of Negri bodies. The final recognition of Negri bodies should not be left to the novice.

Moulton (1954), who has studied the histochemical characteristics of the Negri body, has found that it gives positive reactions to stains for protein, arginine, tyrosine, and alpha-amino acids. The inner granules are positive for desoxyribonucleic acid and organic iron. The periodic acid-Schiff reaction is inconclusive. Negative reactions are obtained in tests for ribonucleic acid, glycogen, hyaluronic acid, mucopolysaccharides, ascorbic acid, neutral fats, phospholipids, cholesterol, inorganic iron, calcium, alkaline phosphatase, dehydrogenase, and cytochrome oxidase.

When the virus centrifugally invades the salivary gland, degenerative changes leading to necrosis may be encountered in the acinar epithelium, principally affecting mucogenic cells of the mandibular salivary gland. Virus can readily be demonstrated by fluorescent antibody techniques and electron microscopy within these cells. A moderate infiltration of lymphocytes and plasma cells accompanies the degenerative changes.

Diagnosis. The diagnosis of rabies can be based upon the symptoms if they are typical, but should be confirmed by laboratory examination. Demonstration of typical Negri bodies is considered diagnostic; however, the brains of as many as 30% of infected animals may not contain demonstrable Negri bodies. In cases in which Negri bodies cannot be demonstrated, animal (mouse) inoculations should be done.

Mice of all ages are susceptible to rabies virus, but newborn mice under three days of age are most sensitive. Following intracerebral inoculation, newborn mice usually succumb within 14 days, but should be examined daily for at least four weeks before the test is considered negative. The virus is demonstrated in the brains of mice that die by finding Negri bodies, by a neutralization test in other mice, or preferably, by the fluorescent antibody identification of the virus. Rabies virus may also be isolated by injecting suspected brain suspensions into tissue cultures using BHK–21 cell lines. Positive results can be obtained in 24 hours, and the virus identified by the fluorescent antibody method.

The fluorescent antibody technique is useful in specific identification of rabies inclusion bodies. In this method, specific antirabic serum is conjugated with a fluorescent dye and used to treat suspected impressions or other cell preparations. The Negri body absorbs the labeled antibody in the antirabic serum, which clings to and identifies the Negri body as it fluoresces typically under ultraviolet light. With suitable controls, this method is quite specific in identification of antigens of rabies virus, even when Negri bodies cannot be demonstrated by conventional staining techniques.

In those animals in which rabies is suspected but cannot be demonstrated, an attempt should be made to determine the cause of death or cause of encephalitis. Diseases to consider are canine hepatitis, toxoplasmosis, distemper in dogs, *Oestrus ovis* infestation in sheep, and listeriosis in sheep and cattle. The brain, spinal cord, or meninges may also be involved by diseases of unknown etiology. Differentiation of canine hepatitis and canine distemper are of considerable importance, since inclusion bodies may occur in both of these diseases. Both are also much more common in dogs than is rabies. In canine hepatitis involving the brain, intranuclear inclusions are found in endothelial cells in association with rupture of capillary walls and microscopic hemorrhages. The inclusions of canine distemper are most readily demonstrable in glial cells, particularly in the nuclei of gemistocytic astrocytes and microglia. Fluorescence antibody techniques show that distemper inclusions occur in neurons, but they are less readily demonstrable with other methods. Cytoplasmic inclusions are less frequently found in the brain in canine distemper.

Groups of tiny spherical bodies without a definite limiting membrane are encountered in the cytoplasm of neurons of nonrabid animals. Since at one time they were thought to be associated with rabies, they were given the name "Lyssa bodies." It now seems clear that they are not specific for rabies. They have been described in the dog, cat, skunk, fox, and laboratory white mouse. Although they can be easily confused with Negri bodies, they lack an internal structure, are more acidophilic, and are highly refractile. In the brains of normal cats, other cytoplasmic inclusions with tinctorial characteristics essentially the same as those of Negri bodies have been described. These feline inclusions cannot be differentiated morphologically from Negri bodies; therefore, it may be necessary to resort to animal inoculation or fluorescent antibody techniques when rabies is suspected in the cat.

Arko, R. J., Schneider, L. G., and Baer, G. M.: Nonfatal canine rabies. Am. J. Vet. Res., 34:937–938, 1973.
Baer, G. M., and Olson, H. R.: Recovery of pigs from rabies. J. Am. Vet. Med. Assoc., 160:1127–1128, 1972.
Baer, G. M., and Cleary, W. F.: A model in mice for the pathogenesis and treatment of rabies. J. Infect. Dis., 125:520–527, 1972.
Beauregard, M., Boulanger, P., and Webster, W. A.: The use of fluorescent antibody staining in the diagnosis of rabies. Can. J. Comp. Med., 29:141–147, 1965.
Behymer, D. E., et al.: Observations on the pathogenesis of rabies: experimental infection with a virus of coyote origin. J. Wildl. Dis., 10:197–203, 1974.
Bell, J. F., Gonzalez, M. A., Diaz, A. M., and Moore, G. J.: Nonfatal rabies in dogs: experimental studies and results of a survey. Am. J. Vet. Res., 32:2049–2058, 1971.
Bell, J. F., Sancho, M. I., Diaz, A. M., and Moore, G. J.: Nonfatal rabies in a enzootic area: results of a

survey and evaluation of techniques. Am. J. Epidemiol., 95:190–198, 1972.

Boulger, L. R., and Porterfield, J. S.: Isolation of a virus from Nigerian fruit bats. Trans. Roy. Soc. Trop. Med. Hyg., 52:421–424, 1958.

Boulger, L. R.: Natural rabies in a laboratory monkey. Lancet, 1:941–943, 1966.

Burns, K. F., Shelton, D. F., and Grogan, E. W.: Bat rabies: experimental host transmission studies. Ann. NY Acad. Sci., 70:452–466, 1958.

Constantine, D. G., Emmons, R. W., and Woodie, J. D.: Rabies virus in nasal mucosa of naturally infected bats. Science, 175:1255–1256, 1972.

Covell, W. P., and Danks, W. B. C.: Studies on the nature of the Negri body. Am. J. Pathol., 8:557–571, 1932.

Debbie, J. G., and Trimarchi, C. V.: Pantropism of rabies virus in free-ranging rabid red fox, Vulpes fulva. J. Wildl. Dis., 6:500–506, 1970.

Debbie, J. G.: Rabies. Prog. Med. Virol., 18:241–256, 1974.

Dierks, R. E., Murphy, F. A., and Harrison, A. K.: Extraneural rabies virus infection. Virus development in fox salivary gland. Am. J. Pathol., 54:251–273, 1969.

Doege, T. C., and Northrop, R. L.: Evidence for inapparent rabies infection. Lancet, 2:826–829, 1974.

du Plessis, J. L.: The topographical distribution of Negri bodies in the brain. J. S. Afr. Vet. Med. Assoc., 36:203–207, 1965.

Enright, J. B.: Bats and their relation to rabies. Ann. Rev. Microbiol., 10:369–392, 1956.

Fekadu, M.: Asymptomatic non-fatal canine rabies. Lancet, 1:569, 1975.

Fischman, H. R.: Fluorescent antibody staining of rabies-infected tissues embedded in paraffin. Am. J. Vet. Res., 30:1213–1221, 1969.

Fischman, H. R., and Schaeffer, M.: Pathogenesis of experimental rabies as revealed by immunofluorescence. Ann. NY Acad. Sci., 177:78–97, 1971.

Fischman, H. R., and Strandberg, J. D.: Inapparent rabies virus infection of the central nervous system. J. Am. Vet. Med. Assoc., 163:1050–1055, 1973.

Goodpasture, E. W.: Studies of rabies with reference to neural transmission of virus in rabbits and structure and significance of Negri bodies. Am. J. Pathol., 1:547–582, 1925.

Herzog, E.: Histologic diagnosis of rabies. Arch. Pathol., 39:279–280, 1945.

Hottle, G. A., et al.: Electron microscopy of rabies inclusion (Negri) bodies. Proc. Soc. Exp. Biol., NY, 77:721–723, 1951.

Iwasaki, Y., Wiktor, T. J., and Koprowski, H.: Early events of rabies virus replication in tissue cultures: an electron microscopic study. Lab. Invest., 28:142–148, 1973.

Iwasaki, Y., and Clark, H. F.: Cell to cell transmission of virus in the central nervous system. II. Experimental rabies in mouse. Lab. Invest., 33:391–399, 1975.

————: Rabies virus infection in mouse neuroblastoma cells. Lab. Invest., 36:578–584, 1977.

Jenson, A. B., et al.: A comparative light and electron microscopic study of rabies and Hart Park virus encephalitis. Expl. Molec. Pathol., 7:1–10, 1967.

Kemp, G. E., et al.: Mokola virus. Further studies on IbAn27377, a new rabies-related etiologic agent of zoonosis in Nigeria. Am. J. Trop. Med. Hyg., 21:356–359, 1972.

————: Kotonkan, a new rhabdovirus related to Mokola virus of the rabies serogroup. Am. J. Epidemiol., 98:43–49, 1973.

Lapi, A., Davis, C. L., and Anderson, W. A.: The gasserian ganglion in animals dead of rabies. J. Am. Vet. Med. Assoc., 120:379–384, 1952.

Larghi, O. P., and Jimenez, E.: Methods for accelerating the fluorescent-antibody test for rabies diagnosis. Appl. Microbiol., 21:611–613, 1971.

Martell, D., Montes, F. C., and Alcocer, B. R.: Transplacental transmission of bovine rabies after natural infection. J. Infect. Dis., 127:291–293, 1973.

Martell, M. A., et al.: Experimental bovine paralytic rabies—"derriengue." Vet. Rec., 95:527–530, 1974.

Matsumoto, S.: Electron microscope studies of rabies virus in mouse brain. J. Cell. Biol., 19:565–591, 1963.

McQueen, J. L.: Rabies diagnosis. Special application of fluorescent antibody techniques. Proc. 63rd Meet. U.S. Livestock Sanit. Assn. San Francisco. 1959. pp. 356–373.

Mitchell, F. E., and Monlux, W. S.: Diagnosis and incidence of rabies in a selected group of domestic cats. Am. J. Vet. Res., 23:435–442, 1962.

Moulton, J. E.: A histochemical study of the Negri bodies of rabies. Am. J. Pathol., 30:533–543, 1954.

Murphy, F. A., Bauer, S. P., Harrison, A. K., and Winn, W. C., Jr.: Comparative pathogenesis of rabies and rabies-like viruses: viral infection and transit from inoculation site to the central nervous system. Lab. Invest., 28:361–376, 1973.

Murphy, F. A., Harrison, A. K., Winn, W. C., and Bauer, S. P.: Comparative pathogenesis of rabies and rabies-like viruses: infection of the central nervous system and centrifugal spread of virus to peripheral tissues. Lab. Invest., 29:1–16, 1973.

Negri, A.: Beitrag zum Studium der Aetiologie der Tollwuth. Ztschr. Hyg. Infektionskr., 43:507–528, 1903.

Ninomiya, S.: Histopathologic studies on salivary glands of rabid dogs with special reference to parotid and mandibular glands. Appendix: on cervical lymph nodes. Gumma J. Med. Sci. Japan, 4:117–127, 1955.

Percy, D. H., Bhatt, P. N., Tignor, G. H., and Shope, R. E.: Experimental infection of dogs and monkeys with two rabies serogroup viruses, Lagos Bat and Mokola (IbAn 27377). Gross pathologic and histopathologic changes. Vet. Pathol., 10:534–549, 1973.

Richardson, J. H., and Humphrey, G. L.: Rabies in imported nonhuman primates. Lab. Anim. Sci., 21:1082–1083, 1972.

Schindler, R.: Studies on the pathogenesis of rabies. Bull. WHO, 25:119–126, 1961. V.B. 1091–62.

Shope, R. E., et al.: Two African viruses serologically

and morphologically related to rabies virus. J. Virol., 6:690–692, 1970.

Szlochta, H. L., and Habel, R. E.: Inclusions resembling Negri bodies in the brains of nonrabid cats. Cornell Vet., 43:207–212, 1953.

Thompson, S. W., et al.: The protein nature of the matrices of Negri bodies. Am. J. Vet. Res., 21:636–643, 1960.

Tierkel, E. S.: Rabies. Adv. Vet. Sci., 5:183–226, 1959.

Tignor, G. H., Shope, R. E., Bhatt, P. N., and Percy, D. H.: Experimental infection of dogs and monkeys with two rabies serogroup viruses, Lagos bat and Mokalo (IbAn27377): clinical, serologic, virologic, and fluorescent antibody studies. J. Infect. Dis., 128:471–478, 1973.

Vernon, S. K., Neurath, A. R., and Rubin, B. A.: Electron microscopic studies on the structure of rabies virus. J. Ultrastruct. Res., 41:29–42, 1972.

von Mickwitz, C. V.: Einschlusskorperchen in den Ganglienzellen des Ammonshornes und des Thalamus von Hausund Zookatzen. Path. Vet., 3:569–587, 1966.

Webster, L. T.: Rabies. New York, The Macmillan Co., 1942.

Winkler, W. G., Baker, E. F., Jr., and Hopkins, C. C.: An outbreak of non-bite transmitted rabies in a laboratory animal colony. Am. J. Epidemiol., 95:267–277, 1972.

Zlotnik, I., and Grant, D. P.: The relationship between immunity and the pathology of the CNS of mice infected with the CVS strain of rabies. Br. J. Exp. Pathol., 54:534–552, 1973.

RETROVIRIDAE

The family Retroviridae, formerly called the group Leukovirus, contains several RNA viruses, tentatively grouped into three subfamilies. The family has the following characteristics: The virion contains a virus-specified RNA-dependent DNA polymerase and other enzymes; the genome consists of a linear molecular of single-stranded RNA with molecular weight of 10 to 12 million daltons; the RNA consists of three or four linked pieces which may be associated with a tubular nucleocapsid, and the nucleocapsid is enclosed within a capsid of cubic symmetry, enclosed in an envelope. This envelope bears type-specific antigens. The virion, about 100 nm in diameter, also carries species-specific antigens, such as murine

Table 9–12. Diseases Caused by Retroviridae (Leukovirus)

Oncovirinae (RNA Tumor Viruses)	Spumavirinae (Foamy viruses, inapparent infections)	Lentivirinae (Visna and related agents)

Type C oncovirus group
 Murine sarcoma/leukemia
  viruses
 Feline sarcoma/leukemia viruses
 Baboon endogenous type C
  viruses
 Bovine type C oncovirus
 Porcine type C oncovirus
 Rat type C oncovirus
 Feline type C oncovirus
 Wooley monkey and gibbon
  sarcoma/leukemia virus
 Owl monkey type C virus
 Avian type C viruses
   Chicken leukemia/sarcoma
 virus
   Avian reticuloendotheliosis virus
 Reptilian type C virus
Type B oncovirus group
 Mouse mammary tumor virus
 Guinea pig mammary tumor
  virus
	Bovine syncytial virus
	Feline syncytial virus
	Hamster syncytial virus
	Human foamy virus
	Simian foamy virus
	 (9 serotypes)
		Ovine progressive pneumonia
		 (visna/maedi)
		Ovine pulmonary adenomatosis
		 (jaagsiekte)
		Equine infectious anemia

or feline types, and also antigens which are interspecies-specific (e.g., avian or rodent) (Fenner et al., 1974).

No generic name has been assigned by the International Committee on Taxonomy of Viruses to any of the groups of viruses currently included in the Retroviridae. Three subfamilies have been designated however: Oncovirinae, Spumavirinae and Lentivirinae (Table 9–12).

Fenner, F., et al.: The Biology of Animal Viruses, 2nd ed. New York, Academic Press, 1974.

Diseases Caused by Lentivirinae

Four viruses have been tentatively grouped in the subfamily Lentivirinae. These are the viruses of visna, maedi, progressive pneumonia, and equine infectious anemia. These viruses have the general characteristics of "slow" viruses, which produce diseases with a prolonged but predictable incubation period lasting months to years; progressive lesions are caused by the virus during its incubation period and the clinical course is protracted with serious disease or death (Sigurdsson, 1954). Other "slow" viruses have been identified, but are as yet unclassified. These include scrapie of sheep, mink encephalopathy, kuru, and Creutzfeldt-Jakob disease of man.

Visna and maedi, which are variants of the same agent, have several physical and chemical similarities to the oncogenic RNA viruses. Their virions have similar ultrastructural morphologic features; they develop similarly in cells and the number and general pattern of their viral proteins appear to be related. They both contain single-stranded RNA and a RNA-directed DNA polymerase. Visna appears to interfere with replication of murine leukemia and sarcoma virus in cell cultures but, although molecular hybridization indicates that visna and maedi viruses share common nucleic acid sequences, they do not anneal similarly with Rauscher murine leukemia or mouse mammary tumor virus,

indicating the nucleic acids of visna and maedi are not closely related to the two rodent tumor viruses (Harter et al., 1973; Takemoto et al., 1973).

Visna/Maedi (Ovine Progressive Pneumonia, Chronic Viral Encephalomyelitis of Sheep)

A chronic viral encephalomyelitis of sheep was first reported in Iceland by Sigurdsson, Thormar, and Palsson in 1935. The name visna, an Icelandic word for shrinkage or wasting, was applied to indicate one clinical feature of the paralyzed sheep. A chronic progressive pneumonia in sheep was recognized in 1939 by Gislason (Guadnadottir, 1974) and named "maedi," an Icelandic word meaning dyspnea. It is now believed that visna and maedi are caused by the same virus. A disease similar to maedi, described in the Netherlands and named **zwoegerziekte,** is also caused by the same virus. The same or a similar virus appears to be involved in the progressive pneumonia (Marsh, 1923) described in sheep in Montana (Kennedy et al., 1968). This viral infection, with its incubation period of two to three years and its progressive nature, is a prototype of the "slow" viral infections.

Lesions. Although, when originally encountered, the virus appeared to affect either the lungs or the central nervous system, it now seems evident that both systems may be affected in the same animal. The lesions in the central nervous system consist of zones of demyelination with destruction of paraventricular white matter in the cerebellum and cerebrum. Similar lesions have a focal distribution in the spinal cord. The demyelinated zones are surrounded by gliosis and lymphocytic infiltration. The meninges of both brain and spinal cord are usually infiltrated by lymphocytes and other mononuclear cells.

The lesions in the central nervous system result in severely increased numbers of cells in the cerebrospinal fluid (pleocytosis). This is of value in distinguishing the

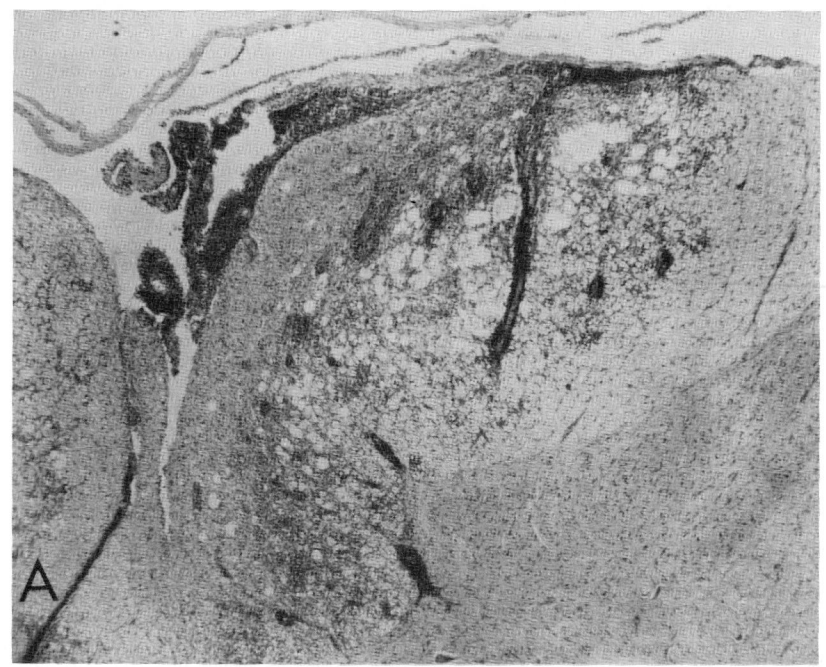

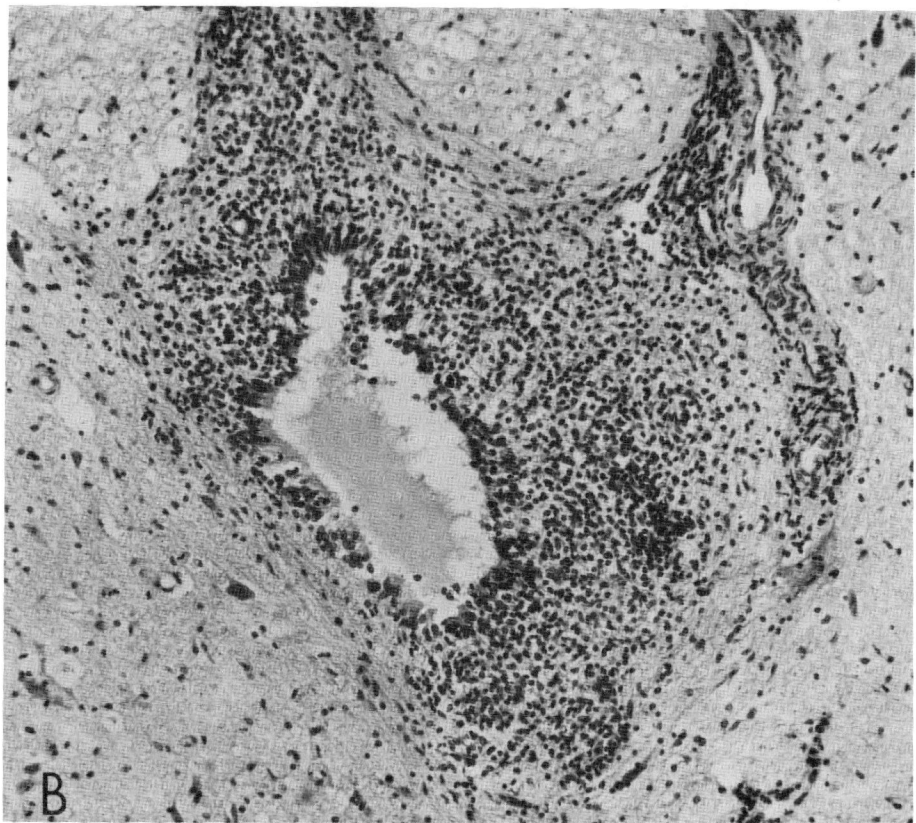

Fig. 9–65. Visna. *A*, Leptomeningeal infiltrate, perivascular cuffing, and microcavitation of lumbar spinal cord. *B*, Cellular infiltration surrounding central canal of cervical spinal cord. (Courtesy of Dr. Páll A. Pálsson.)

467

clinical disease from scrapie, which does not result in pleocytosis.

Gross Lesions. The gross lesions of the pulmonary form of this infection (maedi) are quite characteristic. The lungs do not collapse fully when the thorax is opened. They have a dense, rubbery consistency, but do not appear consolidated. All lobes have a uniform grayish yellow to grayish blue color and are of uniform consistency. This feature contrasts markedly with the sharp differences between normal and consolidated areas in lungs with usual acute pneumonia. The lungs are distended, appear large, and actually weigh two to five times as much as normal adult sheep lungs (which weigh 300 to 500 g). The cut surface is dry and exudate cannot be expressed, except possibly some mucus from the large bronchi.

Microscopic Lesions. The microscopic lesions reveal that the loss of elasticity and compressibility as well as the grayish color are due to a great increase in thickness of the alveolar walls. This thickening may be so great that the alveolar spaces are obliterated. The thickening is caused by proliferation and infiltration of reticuloendothelial or mesenchymal cells which invade the septa everywhere. As is the case in many types of reticuloendothelial proliferation, the cells vary from large round mononuclear forms, some of which appear to be macrophages, to short fibroblastic cells. Hyperemia of the interalveolar capillaries is a feature in early stages. The smooth muscle of the alveolar ducts (terminal bronchioles) is hyperplastic. Lymph nodules occur along the course of the bronchi and bronchioles. Alveolar lining cells in alveoli near the bronchi tend to become swollen and cuboidal in shape. A few large mononuclear cells contain one or more peculiar cytoplasmic inclusions, 1 to 3 μ in diameter, which take a soft bluish gray color by Giemsa's stain. These are probably specific for the disease.

The bronchial and mediastinal lymph nodes are enlarged because of lymphocytic hyperplasia and inflammatory proliferation. Localized chronic adhesive pleuritis occurs in a few cases. Aside from a few scattered aggregations of lymphocytes occasionally found in the liver, no visceral lesion is found outside the thorax.

Boer, G. F. de: Zwoegerziekte virus, the causative agent for progressive interstitial pneumonia (maedi) and meningo-leucoencephalitis (visna) in sheep. Res. Vet. Sci., *18*:15–25, 1975.

Coward, J. E., Harter, D. H., and Morgan, C.: Electron microscopic observations of visna virus-infected cell cultures. Virology, *40*:1030–1038, 1970.

Georgsson, G., et al.: The ultrastructure of early visna lesions. Acta Neuropathol., *37*:127–135, 1977.

Gudnadottir, M.: Visna-maedi in sheep. Prog. Med. Virol., *18*:336–349, 1974.

Haase, A. T.: The slow infection caused by visna virus. Curr. Top. Microbiol. Immunol., *72*:101–156, 1975.

Haase, A. T., Traynor, B. L., and Ventura, P. E.: Infectivity of visna virus DNA. Virology, *70*:65–79, 1976.

Haase, A. T., et al.: Slow persistent infection caused by visna virus: role of host restriction. Science, *195*:195–176, 1977.

Harter, D. H., et al.: The relationship of visna, maedi and RNA tumor viruses as studied by molecular hybridization. Virology, *52*:287–291, 1973.

Harter, D. H., and Coward, J. E.: Sheep progressive pneumonia viruses: "slow" cytolytic agents with tumor virus properties: a review. Tex. Rep. Biol. Med., *32*:649–664, 1974.

Kennedy, R. C., Eklund, C. M., Lopez, C., and Hadlow, W. J.: Isolation of a virus from the lungs of Montana sheep affected with progressive pneumonia. Virology, *35*:483–484, 1968.

Lin, F. H., and Thormar, H.: Substructures and polypeptides of visna virus. J. Virol., *14*:782–790, 1974.

Lycke, E., and Svennerholm, B.: Tumor incidence in visna virus inoculated mice. Experientia, *32*:514–515, 1976.

Macintyre, E. H., Wintersgill, C. J., and Thormar, H.: Morphological transformation of human astrocytes by visna virus with complete virus production. Nature New Biol., *237*:111–113, 1972.

Macintyre, E. H., Wintersgill, C. J., and Vatter, A. E.: A modification in the response of human astrocytes to visna virus. Am. J. Vet. Res., *35*:1161–1163, 1974.

Marsh, H.: Progressive pneumonia in sheep. J. Am. Vet. Med. Assoc., *62*:458–473, 1923.

Mehta, P. D., and Thormar, H.: Comparative studies of visna and maedi viruses as antigens. Infect. Immun., *11*:829–834, 1975.

Narayan, O., Silverstein, A. M., Price, D., and Johnson, R. T.: Visna virus infection of American lambs. Science, *183*:1202–1203, 1974.

Narayan, O., Griffin, D. E., and Chase, J.: Antigenic shift of visna virus in persistently infected sheep. Science, *197*:376–378, 1977.

Nathanson, N., et al.: Pathogenesis of visna. II. Effect of immunosuppression upon early central nervous system lesions. Lab. Invest., 35:441–451, 1976.

Nobel, T. A., Neumann, F., and Klopfer, U.: Pathological changes in lungs of imported sheep with special reference to maedi. Refuah Veterinarith., 30:19–23, 1973.

Oldstone, M. B. A., Lampert, P. W., Lee, S., and Dixon, F. J.: Pathogenesis of the slow disease of the central nervous system associated with WM 1504 E virus. Am. J. Pathol., 88:193–212, 1977.

Palsson, P. A., Georgsson, G., Petursson, G., and Nathanson, N.: Experimental visna in Icelandic lambs. Acta Vet. Scand., 18:122–128, 1977.

Panitch, H., et al.: Pathogenesis of visna. III. Immune responses to central nervous system antigens in experimental allergic encephalomyelitis and visna. Lab. Invest., 35:452–460, 1976.

Petursson, G., et al.: Pathogenesis of visna. I. Sequential virologic, serologic and pathologic studies. Lab. Invest., 35:402–412, 1976.

Ressang, A. A., Stam, F. C., and DeBoer, G. F.: A meningo-leucoencephalomyelitis resembling visna in Dutch Zwoeger sheep. Pathol. Vet., 3:401–411, 1966.

Schlom, J., Harter, D. H., Burny, A., and Spiegelman, S.: DNA polymerase activities in virions of visna virus, a causative agent of a "slow" neurological disease. Proc. Natl. Acad. Sci. USA, 68:182–186, 1971.

Sigurdsson, B.: Maedi, a slow progressive pneumonia of sheep: an epizootiological and pathological study. Br. Vet. J., 110:255–270, 1954.

Sigurdsson, B., Grimsson, H., and Palsson, P. A.: Maedi, a chronic progressive infection of sheeps' lungs. J. Infect. Dis., 90:233–241, 1952.

Sigurdsson, B., and Palsson, P. A.: Visna of sheep. A slow demyelinating infection. Br. J. Exp. Pathol., 39:519–528, 1958.

Sigurdsson, B., Thormar, H., and Palsson, P. A.: Cultivation of visna virus in tissue culture. Arch. ges. Virusforsch., 10:368–381, 1960.

Sigurdsson, B.: Observations on three slow infections of sheep, with general remarks on infections which develop slowly and some of their special characteristics. Br. Vet. J., 110:341–354, 1954.

Sigurdsson, B., Palsson, P. A., and Grimsson, H.: Visna, a demyelinating transmissible disease of sheep. J. Neuropathol. Exp. Neurol., 16:389–403, 1957.

Sigurdsson, B., Palsson, P. A., and van Bogaert, L.: Pathology of visna (transmissible demyelinating disease of sheep in Iceland). Acta Neuropath., 1:343–362, 1962.

Takemoto, K. K., Aoki, T., Garon, C., and Sturm, M. M.: Comparative studies on visna, progressive pneumonia, and Rous sarcoma viruses by electron microscopy. J. Natl. Cancer Inst., 50:543–547, 1973.

Thormar, H.: Physical, chemical, and biological properties of visna virus and its relationship to other animal viruses. Natl. Inst. of Neurological Diseases and Blindness Monograph No. 2:335–340, 1965.

Jaagsiekte (Ovine Pulmonary Adenomatous, Pulmonary Carcinoma of Sheep)

Derived from Afrikaans words meaning "drive" (jaagt) and "sickness," jaagsiekte is the South African name of a neoplastic disease, of older sheep, which may first reveal its existence by dyspneic and anoxic symptoms following the stress of strenuous exertion such as a long drive. The disease runs a progressive afebrile course of several months or longer. It has many points of similarity to Marsh's ovine progressive pneumonia, but one difference is the considerable catarrhal nasal discharge which is characteristic of jaagsiekte. Besides South Africa, the malady occurs in Europe, England, Iceland, Israel, and Peru.

It is well established that jaagsiekte is transmissible to susceptible sheep by contact, aerosol, and intratracheal or intrapulmonary injection of affected lung tissue from sheep with the disease. A herpesvirus has been isolated (MacKay, 1969; Smith and MacKay, 1969) from tissue culture of macrophages from sheep with pulmonary adenomatosis. The etiologic significance of this virus has not been proved. In ultrastructural, thin sections studied with the electron microscope, rare particles were observed which have the morphologic features of "C" particles, characteristic of RNA tumor viruses (Perk, Hod, and Nobel, 1971). These particles were rare, approximately 100 mμ in diameter, located within cisternae of the granular endoplasmic reticulum and budding from the membranes of cisternae. Intracytoplasmic clusters of structures that resemble the naked form of murine type-A particles were seen. Virus particles budding from cell surfaces were also seen. Alveolar macrophages in affected sheep also contained many mycoplasmas (see Chapter 10), whose significance has not been established.

Biochemical evidence has been added to the morphologic data supporting the presence of an RNA tumor virus in lungs of sheep with pulmonary adenomatosis (Perk et al., 1974). The tumorous lungs contained particles with a reverse transcriptase and a 60–70 sRNA. Extracts of these lung tumors were observed by electron microscopy to contain type C virus particles characteristic of rodent RNA tumor viruses.

Martin et al. (1976) reproduced the disease by the combined endobronchial injection of herpesvirus and the RNA reverse transcriptase virus. The RNA virus alone also produced small lesions, but less extensive than in sheep which received both agents.

Thus it appears that the exact nature of the causative agent or agents in jaagsiekte have not been established incontrovertibly. We have placed our discussion of this disease at this position in the text in spite of the controversies surrounding the etiologic agent.

Lesions. The lesions of jaagsiekte commence as a number of separate foci, from which they spread throughout the lung. They consist of accumulations of large mononuclear cells which are possibly derived both from the blood in the hyperemic capillaries and by proliferation and hypertrophy of alveolar lining cells to cuboidal or columnar cells. Papillary projections may extend from alveolar septa into the alveoli. The result is a pronounced thickening of the alveolar walls and their interstices, and partial obliteration of the alveolar spaces by tissue resembling an adenoma. Lymphocytes accompany the reticuloendothelial cells, but proliferated fibroblasts appear to be practically absent until the later stages, when fibrosis is extensive. A certain number of mononuclear cells and lymphocytes spill over, as it were, into the alveoli and, accompanied by a few neutrophils, appear as an exudate in some of the

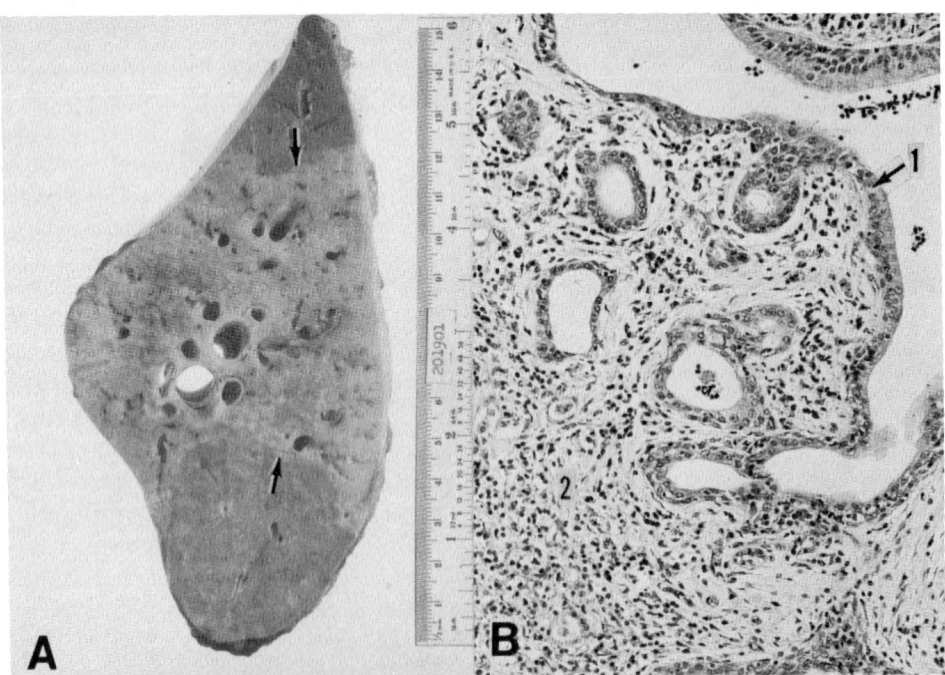

Fig. 9–66. *A,* Ovine progressive pneumonia. Lung of a sheep. Note solid area of consolidation (arrows) in center of lung. *B,* The same lung as *A* (× 130). Note hyperplasia of epithelium of bronchioles*(1)* and alveolar ducts, and intense inflammation and fibrosis that obliterate the alveoli*(2).* Contributor: Dr. Hadleigh Marsh. (Courtesy of Armed Forces Institute of Pathology.)

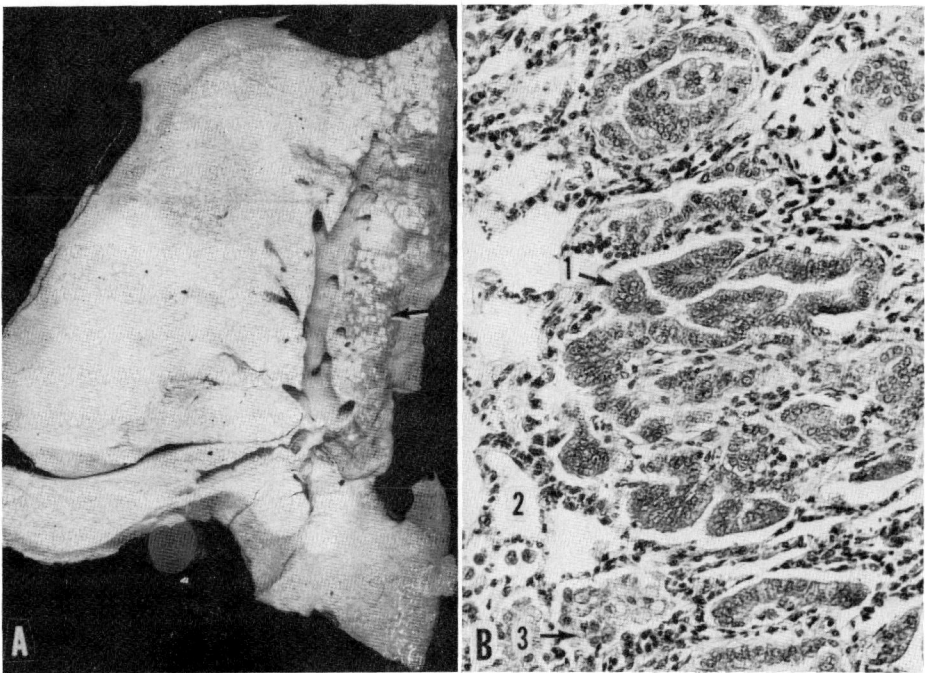

Fig. 9–67. *A,* Pulmonary adenomatosis (jaagsiekte). Lung of a sheep. Note nodules (arrow) of gray consolidation in some areas, diffuse solid zones in others. Contributor: Col. M. W Hale. *B,* Pulmonary adenomatosis in a sheep lung (× 195). Note columnar cells *(1)* which fill alveoli. Some alveoli are intact *(2),* others filled with macrophages *(3).* Contributor: Dr. T. F. Shirlaw. (Courtesy of Armed Forces Institute of Pathology.)

bronchi. There is, however, never any exudate comparable to that seen in the acute exudative pneumonias. The peribronchiolar lymph nodules are also hyperplastic and markedly enlarged, as is true in Marsh's progressive pneumonia and other chronic inflammations of the lungs. Metastatic lesions consisting of adenomatous foci in bronchial and mediastinal lymph nodes comparable to those seen in the lung have been reported by numerous authors. Less frequently the metastases are associated with a desmoplastic reaction similar to that encountered in certain carcinomas. A few reports have described extra-thoracic metastases to sites such as muscle and kidney. The proliferative nature of the pulmonary lesion coupled with metastases is strong evidence that jaagsiekte is neoplastic and malignant.

Diagnosis. The differentiation of jaagsiekte from maedi takes into consideration the distribution of lesions, focal in the former, uniformly diffuse in the latter, the tendency for the intraseptal proliferation to include young fibroblastic forms in maedi, the much greater tendency toward "adenomatosis" in jaagsiekte, and the occurrence of cellular inclusions in maedi. Differentiation from Marsh's ovine progressive pneumonia is on much less certain grounds. Ordinarily there is much less "adenomatosis" in the disease described by Marsh than there is in jaagsiekte, although Cowdry and Marsh (1927) suspected that they might be identical; present evidence indicates that they are not the same disease, but both may be present in the same animal.

Chauhan, H. V. S., and Singh, C. M.: Studies on the pathology of pulmonary adenomatosis complex of sheep and goats. II. Viral pneumonitis (a typical pneumonia). Indian J. Anim. Sci., *41*:272–276, 1971.

Cowdry, E. V., and Marsh, H.: Comparative pathology of South African jaagziekte and Montana progressive pneumonia of sheep. J. Exper. Med., 45:571–586, 1927.

Cuba-Caparo, A.: Adenomatosis Pulmonar de los Ovinos en el Peru. Bull. Off. Int. Epiz., 56:840–849, 1961.

Cuba-Caparo, A., De La Vega, E., and Copaira, M.: Pulmonary adenomatosis of sheep, metastasizing bronchiolar tumors. Am. J. Vet. Res., 22:673–682, 1961.

Damodaran, S.: Ovine pulmonary adenomatosis (jaagziekte). Indian Vet. J., 37:127–138, 1960. Abstr. Vet. Bull., No. 2895, 1960.

de Kock, G.: The transformation of the lining of the pulmonary alveoli with special reference to adenomatosis in the lungs (jaagziekte) of sheep. Am. J. Vet. Res., 19:261–269, 1958.

Dualde Perez, C.: Studies of ovine pulmonary adenomatosis in Spain. Proc. 17th World Vet. Congr. Hanover, 1:347–355, 1963.

Duran-Reynals, F., et al.: The pulmonary adenomatosis complex in sheep. Ann. NY Acad. Sci., 70:726–742, 1958.

Enchev, S.: Pulmonary adenomatosis of sheep in Bulgaria. I. Epidemiology, symptoms and pathology. II. Metastasis in pulmonary lymph nodes. Abstr. Vet. Bull. No. 1992, 1962.

Enchev, S., Tomov, T., and Ivanov, I.: (Pulmonary adenomatosis of sheep in Bulgaria.) Izv. Inst. Pat. Zhivotni, Sofia, 6:365–367, 1958. Abstr. Vet. Bull. No. 2621, 1959.

Hod, I., Perk, K., Nobel, T. A., and Klopfer, U.: Lung carcinoma of sheep (jaagsiekte). III. Lymph node, blood, and immunoglobulin. J. Natl. Cancer Inst., 48:487–507, 1972.

Kharole, M. U., and Kalra, D. S.: Cases of sheep pulmonary adenomatosis (jaagsiekte) from Haryana and Rajasthan, histopathological evidence. HAU J. Res. Hissar, 3:226–226b, 1973.

MacKay, J. M. K.: Tissue culture studies of sheep pulmonary adenomatosis (jaagsiekte). J. Comp. Pathol., 79:141–146, 1969.

Malmquist, W. A., Krauss, H. H., Moulton, J. E., and Wandera, J. G.: Morphologic study of virus-infected lung cell cultures from sheep pulmonary adenomatosis. Lab. Invest., 26:528–533, 1972.

Mandon, A.: La jaagsiekte de l'afrique du sud. Rec. méd. vet. exotique, 8:25–32, 1935.

Markson, L. M., and Terlecki, S.: The experimental transmission of ovine pulmonary adenomatosis. Pathol. Vet., 1:269–288, 1964.

Martin, W. B., et al.: Experimental production of sheep pulmonary adenomatosis (jaagsiekte). Nature, 264:183–184, 1976.

Mitchell, D. T.: Investigations into jaagsiekte or chronic catarrhal-pneumonia of sheep. Union of So. Africa, Dept. Agric., Rep. of Dir. of Vet. Research, 1915, 3 and 4, 585–614.

Nisbet, D. I., MacKay, J. M. K., Smith, W., and Gray, E. W.: Ultrastructure of sheep pulmonary adenomatosis. (jaagsiekte). J. Pathol., 103:157–162, 1971.

Nobel, T. A., Neumann, F., and Klopfer, U.: Histological patterns of the metastases in pulmonary adenomatosis of sheep (jaagsiekte). J. Comp. Pathol., 79:537–540, 1969.

Nobel, T. A., Klopfer, U., Neumann, F., and Trainin, Z.: Clinicopathological investigations in sheep pulmonary adenomatosis. (jaagsiekte). Zentbl. Vet. Med., 18B:9–14, 1971.

Nobel, T. A.: Pulmonary adenomatosis (jaagsiekte) in sheep with special reference to its occurrence in Israel. Refuah Vet., 15:67–73 (In Hebrew) and 101 (In Engl.), 1958.

Perk, K., Hod, I., and Nobel, T. A.: Pulmonary adenomatosis of sheep (jaagsiekte). I. Ultrastructure of the tumor. J. Natl. Cancer Inst., 46:525–537, 1971.

Perk, K., Hod, I., Nobel, T. A., and Klopfer, U.: Some pathogenetic aspects of ovine pulmonary carcinoma (jaagsiekte). Refuah Veterinarith. 29:15–19, 1972.

Perk, K., Hod, I., Presentey, B., and Nobel, T. A.: Lung carcinoma of sheep (jaagsiekte). II. Histogenesis of the tumor. J. Natl. Cancer Inst., 47:197–205, 1971.

Perk, K., Michalides, R., Spiegelman, S., and Schlom, J.: Biochemical and morphologic evidence for the presence of an RNA tumor virus in pulmonary carcinoma of sheep (jaagsiekte). J. Natl. Cancer Inst., 53:131–135, 1974.

Shirlaw, J. F.: Studies on jaagsiekte in Kenya. Bull. Epiz. Dis. Afr., 7:287–302, 1959. Abstr. Vet. Bull., No. 2896, 1960.

Sigurdsson, B.: Adenomatosis of sheep lungs. Experimental transmission. Arch. ges. Virusforsch., 8:51–58, 1958.

Smith, W., and Mackay, J. M. K.: Morphological observations on a virus associated with sheep pulmonary adenomatosis (jaagsiekte). J. Comp. Pathol., 79:421–424, 1969.

Stevenson, R. G.: Respiratory diseases of sheep. Vet. Bull., 39:747–759, 1969.

Tustin, R. C., and Geyer, S. M.: Transmission of ovine jaagsiekte using neoplastic cells grown in tissue culture. J. S. Afr. Vet. Med. Assoc., 42:181–182, 1971.

Wandera, J. G.: Sheep pulmonary adenomatosis (jaagsiekte). Adv. Vet. Sci. Comp. Med., 15:251–283, 1971.

Wandera, J. G., and Krauss, H.: The ultrastructure of sheep pulmonary adenomatosis. Zentbl. Vet. Med., 18A:325–334, 1971.

Wandera, J. G.: Experimental transmission of sheep pulmonary adenomatosis (jaagsiekte). Vet. Rec., 83:478–482, 1968.

Equine Infectious Anemia (Swamp Fever)

Infectious anemia of equines, a viral disease with worldwide distribution, is not only an important economic problem, but also a model useful for the study of mechanisms involved in prolonged persistence of the virus in the host and its pathogenic effects. Once the virus gains access to a susceptible animal, it can be demonstrated in the circulating blood as long as the animal lives. The infection may be almost subclinical, or it may be acute with febrile manifestations and a rapidly fatal outcome. Infected horses have lived as long as 18 years with few signs, yet, at any time, minute amounts of their blood injected into normal horses will induce acute fatal infectious anemia. Little demonstrable immunity results from this infection. Horses that apparently have recovered from the acute disease may suddenly exhibit severe symptoms and die after exposure to some deleterious influence (hard work, for example, or injection of an additional though minute amount of infectious anemia virus). It would seem that host and parasite, under some conditions, maintain a delicate balance. Equines (horses, mules, asses) are the only species susceptible to natural or experimental exposure.

The virus is transmitted by the bite of a mosquito *(Anopheles psorophora* or *Culex pipiens quinquefasciatus),* biting fly *(Stomoxys calcitrans, Tabanus fuscicostatus),* or by the transfer of a minute amount of blood from an infected horse to a normal one by the use of unsterilized hypodermic needles, tattoo needles, curry-combs or items of equipment, such as harness, bit, or saddle. The disease is not spread by ordinary contact.

The virus of equine infectious anemia was demonstrated to be filterable in 1904 (Vallée and Carré, 1904) and the clinical disease had been described in 1843 (Henson and McGuire, 1974), but significant progress in understanding the virus and its pathogenesis has begun only in recent years. The virus was cultivated in vitro for the first time by Kobayashi in 1961, in tissue culture of horse bone marrow and horse leukocytes. Complement-fixation by the virus was demonstrated by Kono and Kobayashi in 1966. Following these events, significant progress has been made toward understanding the virus and detecting infected horses (Henson and McGuire, 1974).

The virus is currently classified in the family Retroviridae, subfamily Lentivirinae, genus not named. Its nucleic acid is RNA and the virions bear an RNA-dependent DNA polymerase (reverse transcriptase). The virus is ether-sensitive but resistant to trypsin. It has an average buoyant density of 1.15 gm/ml in cesium chloride (CeCl). The virions are approximately 90 to 140 nm in diameter, and may be covered with a single limiting membrane. The dense nucleocapsid is 40 to 63 nm in diameter. The virus does not agglutinate red blood cells, has a group-specific antigen, and bears surface antigens, which vary to some extent.

Antigens in the virus of equine infectious anemia have been demonstrated by complement-fixation, complement-fixation-inhibition, precipitin, and immunofluorescence techniques. Humoral antibody response is not quantitatively deficient in infected animals; thus, loss of antibody response cannot be accepted in explanation of the life-long persistence of the virus in the equine host. An agar-gel immunodiffusion test, developed by Coggins, has proved effective in detecting antibodies and the presence of virus in horses (Coggins and Norcross, 1970; Coggins et al., 1972).

Clinical Manifestations. For purposes of description, the **clinical disease** is usually divided into three types: acute, subacute, and chronic. Cases of the disease, however, often fall partially in two or more of these groups, and in the various stages may pass through all three. The pathologic manifestations within each clinical type are similar to those in the other two; nonetheless, this classification is convenient, and even though it is arbitrary, it will be followed in the discussion of clinical and pathologic features.

Acute equine infectious anemia is characterized by rapid onset of high fever (to 108° F.) following an incubation period of one to three weeks. The fever is accompanied by extreme weakness, excessive thirst, inappetence, depression, edema of lower abdomen, and sublingual or nasal hemorrhages. Such an attack leads to death in less than a month or is followed by survival, with the disease assuming the subacute or chronic form. Anemia is not a prominent feature at the onset, but there is a gradual reduction in circulating red blood cells, the normal count of 8 million dropping to about 4 million in most cases.

In the subacute form, the disease is manifested by relapsing fever and recurrence of other symptoms at irregular intervals. The symptoms during these exacerbations are similar to those of the acute type, but generally less severe. The attacks may increase in severity, with gradual weight loss, debility, edema of dependent parts, and unsteady gait becoming increasingly evident. Death may supervene during any of these recurrent attacks. Pallor of mucous membranes usually indicates the loss of circulating erythrocytes, which may fall as low as 1.5 million/cu mm, and as a rule, the sedimentation rate is greatly increased. Accentuation of symptoms may be brought about by hard work, starvation, "blood letting," or other unfavorable factors.

The chronic form of the disease may develop after the animal has passed through an acute infection, or it may occur in the absence of an obvious attack. Experimental injection of minute amounts of the virus often results in chronic infectious anemia. Some animals appear to be in good health except for transient febrile manifestations at intervals of a month or two. Others remain thin in spite of a good diet, occasionally show edema under the thorax and abdomen, and may become weak or incoordinate. The red cell count is usually 2 to 3 million/cu mm below normal, but evidence of severe anemia is seldom observed.

Pathogenesis. The anemia that appears intermittently in this disease seems to be due principally to destruction of red blood cells by an immunologically-mediated mechanism. Erythrocytes of infected horses are coated with antiviral antibodies and complement 3 (McGuire, Henson, and Quist, 1969a, b). This binding to the cell surface results in increased osmotic fragility, shortened half life, and erythrophagocytosis. Plasma hemoglobin increases and serum haptoglobin levels decrease in infected animals. These findings point toward hemolysis as most important in genesis of the anemia. Another, probably less important, factor is depression of the bone marrow during acute episodes, as indicated by a decrease in both plasma iron turnover and utilization of radioactive iron.

Renal glomeruli are affected in horses with active disease. The glomeruli have thickened basement membranes and mesangium, cells are increased in numbers, and neutrophils are present. Equine immunoglobulin (IgG) and complement 3 (C3) can be demonstrated in the mesangium and on basement membranes (Banks et al., 1972). It appears that this glomerulitis is the result of deposition of virus-antibody complexes that have been demonstrated in the peripheral circulation. The immunologic factors involved in lesions in other organs have not been studied adequately, but it appears likely that immunologic factors may also be involved in the induction of lesions in other organs such as the liver.

Lesions. The nature of the lesions found upon necropsy of horses dead of infectious anemia or sacrificed during its course depends to a great extent upon the clinical type of the disease and the duration of the illness. In other words, an animal that dies during an attack following several exacerbations characteristic of the chronic form of the disease will exhibit different tissue changes than one that dies following a single acute attack. It is convenient, therefore, to describe the lesions in relation to the clinical type of the disease.

General. Acute Type. Icterus, edema, and hemorrhage are the principal gross findings at necropsy. Edema is most prominent

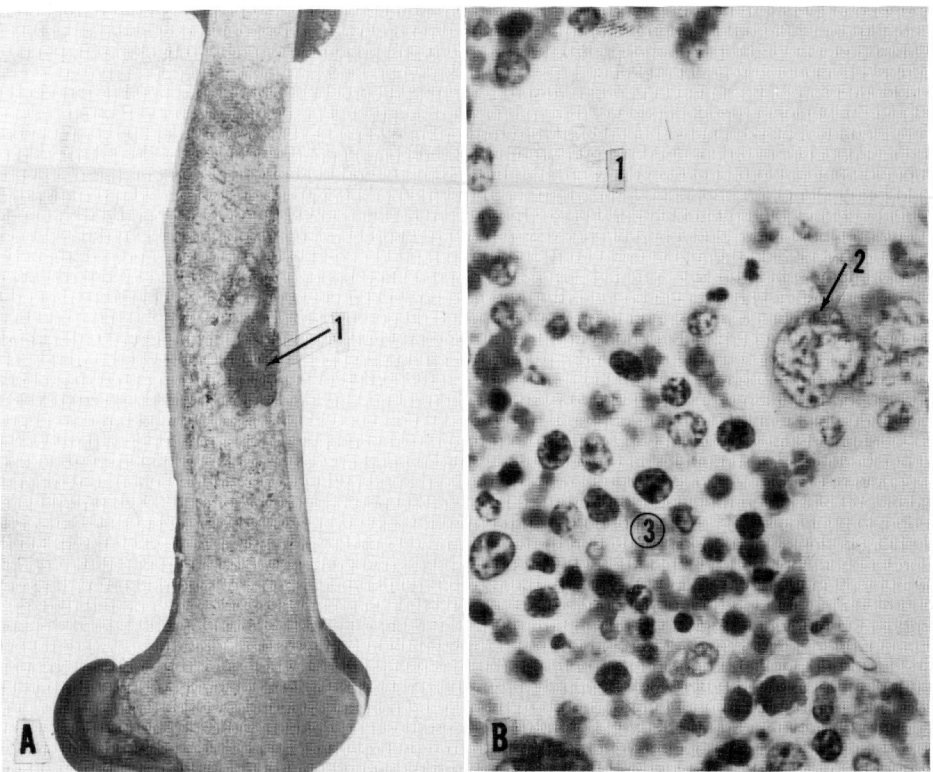

Fig. 9–68. Equine infectious anemia. *A*, Femur of an adult horse suffering from the chronic type of the disease. Hematopoietic marrow *(1)* in the center of the shaft, which at this age is normally made up entirely of fat. *B*, Hematopoietic marrow (× 1000) replacing fatty marrow of the femur. Fat cells *(1)* are infiltrated by hematopoietic cells, including megakaryocytes *(2)* and myeloid cells *(3)*. (Courtesy of Armed Forces Institute of Pathology.) Contributor: Army Veterinary Research Laboratory.

in the subcutis of the ventral wall of the abdomen, at the base of the heart, and in the perirenal and sublumbar fat. The hemorrhages are petechial or, less frequently, ecchymotic, and are found in the edematous areas or in serous membranes, particularly the pleura and peritoneum. Swelling of the parenchymatous organs is frequent and will be more fully described in connection with each system.

SUBACUTE TYPE. Edema and hemorrhages may be features, but they are likely to be less conspicuous than anemia, swelling and pigmentation of the liver, enlargement of the spleen, lymph nodes, and kidneys, and hyperplasia of the bone marrow.

CHRONIC TYPE. Hypertrophy of the spleen and bone marrow may be the only pathologic changes in a sacrificed animal.

Heart. ACUTE TYPE. The heart is usually enlarged, with the ventricles increased in size, and the myocardium, pale and flabby. Hemorrhages and edema occur in the epicardium and pericardium and the pericardial sac may contain excessive amounts of clear or sanguineous fluid. Microscopically, edema and hemorrhages are found, along with some lymphocytic infiltration of the adventitia of myocardial vessels.

SUBACUTE TYPE. In the myocardium, some muscle bundles have microscopically visible hyaline degeneration associated with varying degrees of leukocytic infiltration.

The majority of the infiltrating cells are lymphocytes, which tend to concentrate around blood vessels.

CHRONIC TYPE. Little of specific significance can be found.

Liver. ACUTE TYPE. The liver may be grossly enlarged, red to dark brown, and occasionally exhibits hemorrhages. Microscopic examination usually reveals edema and lymphocytic infiltration of Glisson's capsule, congestion and dilatation of sinusoids, swelling of Kupffer cells (some containing hemosiderin), macrophages containing hemosiderin in the sinusoids, and sometimes loss of liver cells at the center of lobules.

SUBACUTE TYPE. The liver is usually enlarged, dark brown, firm, and on its cut surface, the lobular markings are more distinct than on that of the normal organ. The distended central veins and the adjacent sinusoids may be evident grossly as dark brown or red puncta in a meshwork of dark brown lines. The microscopic changes are often striking, although not every section of the liver will be affected equally. The central veins are congested with blood; the sinusoids show lacunose dilatation and are filled with lymphocytes, plasma cells, macrophages containing hemosiderin or erythrocytes, and reticuloendothelial cells. The reticuloendothelial cells often form small nodules of cells within the sinusoids and occasionally in portal areas. The Kupffer cells are enlarged and often filled with hemosiderin. Stains for iron clearly demonstrate this hemosiderosis in affected livers. Liver cells are often compressed by the enlargement of sinusoids, contain some pigment, and may be reduced in number. Glisson's capsule usually contains many lymphocytes, plasma cells, and some histiocytes. Myeloid cells have been described in these portal areas by some observers in cases of prolonged duration, but megakaryocytes have not been seen.

CHRONIC TYPE. The lesions are not constant or as striking as in the subacute type, although the same microscopic changes may be seen in lesser degree. The gross appearance of the liver is not distinctive.

Spleen. ACUTE TYPE. The spleen is nearly twice normal size. The capsule is tense and may bear petechiae. The cut surface is turgid, cherry or dark red, and somewhat granular, with little liquid component. Hemorrhagic infarcts have been reported, but are inconstant. The splenic follicles may be less prominent and more widely separated than usual. Microscopically, the red pulp is increased in volume and very cellular, although in some sections severe congestion or hemorrhagic infarction of the splenic sinusoids obscures other details. This increase in volume of the red pulp, which widens the distance between the trabeculae and the splenic corpuscles, is due to infiltration of the cords of Bilroth with mononuclear cells. These cells are individually discrete and have irregular, somewhat eosinophilic cytoplasm and round, hyperchromic nuclei. They are monotonously uniform in size and shape and often occur in aggregations around sinusoids. These cells are believed to arise in the reticuloendothelium and to be immature lymphoid cells. Myeloid cells, megakaryocytes, and erythroblasts are seldom found. Eosinophils (normal in the equine spleen) are still present, but hemosiderin (common in the equine spleen) is reduced in amount.

SUBACUTE AND CHRONIC TYPES. The spleen may be the only visceral organ in which gross or microscopic evidence of this smouldering viral infection can be seen. The spleen is enlarged; its cut surface is light red or reddish brown, somewhat turgid and does not exude fluid. The trabeculae are usually widely separated, as are the splenic corpuscles which are enlarged and clearly visible in some gross specimens. In older affected horses, the enlarged, soft, nonfibrous organ has more nearly the appearance of the spleen of colts under one year of age. Microscopic evidence of reticuloendothelial hyperplasia in the cords of Bilroth, similar to that described for the acute form, is the basis for its gross appearance. Hemosiderin is usually present in macrophages, but is not increased in amount.

Lymph Nodes. ACUTE TYPE. The changes in lymph nodes, which may be enlarged, mimic those described in the spleen. If death occurs early, there is atrophy and necrosis of lymphocytes. If more prolonged, the lesions are proliferative, characterized by replacement of the normal cytoarchitecture by diffuse sheets of mononuclear cells considered to be reticuloendothelial cells or immature lymphocytes. There may be cellular infiltration of the trabeculae, capsule, and perinodal fat.

SUBACUTE AND CHRONIC TYPES. The proliferative response with replacement of normal structures by reticuloendothelial and lymphoid cells is generally more pronounced than in the acute type.

Bone Marrow. ACUTE TYPE. The normally fatty marrow usually contains red or yellowish red areas which, upon microscopic examination, are seen to be areas of active hematopoietic marrow.

SUBACUTE TYPE. The centers of long bones contain large areas of red, somewhat edematous, and occasionally hemorrhagic-appearing marrow.

CHRONIC TYPE. The marrow of the long bones, even in aged horses, is predominantly red rather than fatty. This hyperplasia of the hematopoietic marrow is more obvious in the gross specimen than in microscopic sections, since this effect is quantitative. The microscopic picture is one of hematopoietic marrow with myeloid and erythroid elements in approximately normal proportion. It is obvious from these findings that hematopoiesis is not depressed but rather stimulated, probably as the result of destruction of erythrocytes. Large numbers of reticuloendothelial and lymphoid cells are interposed between the erythroid and myeloid elements.

Kidney. ACUTE TYPE. The kidneys are usually involved in the edema that affects the perirenal tissues, particularly in the region of the pelvis. Intense infiltration of immature lymphoid cells into the interstitial stroma of both cortex and medulla is especially prominent around blood vessels and occasionally around glomeruli. This lymphoid infiltration takes on a nodular distribution in some cases. There is generally an increased cellularity to the mesangium of the glomeruli. Immunoglobulins and complement have been demonstrated with immunofluorescent techniques.

SUBACUTE AND CHRONIC TYPES. The lymphoid cells may be present in smaller numbers.

Other Organs. ACUTE TYPE. It is possible for all organs and tissues of the body to show evidence of the reticuloendothelial hyperplasia described in spleen, lymph nodes, liver, and kidney, but this change is not constant nor particularly distinctive. In the adrenal gland, lymphoid cell masses may separate parenchymal cells in much the same manner as in the liver. Endothelial cells of the adrenal have been reported to contain hemosiderin.

SUBACUTE AND CHRONIC TYPES. No distinctive alterations are found in other organs.

Hematologic Changes. The anemia is characteristically normocytic and normochromic. Reticulocytosis or other evidence of increased erythropoiesis is not evident. The anemia appears to result from a combination of hemolysis, erythrophagocytosis, and a decreased production of erythrocytes. The response of the bone marrow has received little attention; although usually described as hyperplastic, there is little evidence of increased erythropoiesis. To the contrary, studies of Obara and Nakajima (1961) and McGuire et al. (1969) indicate both a decrease in erythrocyte lifespan and production. Following an immediate lymphopenia, the disease is characterized by lymphocytosis and the appearance of iron-laden monocytes or siderocytes in the peripheral blood. Thrombocytopenia is a usual finding. Serum levels of gamma globulin are usually increased in the acute stages, and the Coombs' test is reportedly positive.

Diagnosis. A presumptive diagnosis can be made in the living animal during acute exacerbations of the disease or by recognizing characteristic gross and microscopic lesions at necropsy. Definitive diagnosis, however, depends upon specific identification of the virus in the affected animal or following its isolation in horse leukocyte cultures. The gel-diffusion test is particularly useful in detecting humoral antibodies in the serum of infected horses. The presence of these antibodies is consistently associated with virus, hence is a useful method to detect the virus. Fluorescein-labeled immunoglobulins are useful to demonstrate viral antigens in infected tissues.

Banks, K. L.: Monocyte activation in horses persistently infected with equine infectious anemia virus. Infect. Immun., *12*:1219–1221, 1975.

Banks, K. L., Henson, J. B., and McGuire, T. C.: Immunologically mediated glomerulitis of horses. I. Pathogenesis in persistent infection by equine infectious anemia virus. Lab. Invest., *26*:701–707, 1972.

Breaud, T. P., Steelman, C. D., Roth, E. E., and Adams, W. V., Jr.: Apparent propagation of the equine infectious anemia virus in a mosquito (*Culex pipiens quinquefasciatus* Say) ovarian cell line. Am. J. Vet. Res., *37*:1069–1070, 1976.

Burns, S. J.: Equine infectious anemia: Plasma clearance times of passively transferred antibody in foals. J. Am. Vet. Med. Assoc., *164*:64–65, 1974.

Carrier, S. P., Boulanger, P., and Bannister, G. L.: Equine infectious anemia: sensitivity of the agar-gel immunodiffusion test, and the direct and the indirect complement-fixation tests for the detection of antibodies in equine serum. Can. J. Comp. Med., *37*:171–176, 1973.

Coggins, L., and Norcross, N. L.: Immunodiffusion reaction in equine infectious anemia. Cornell Vet., *60*:330–335, 1970.

Coggins, L., Norcross, N. L., and Nusbaum, S. R.: Diagnosis of equine infectious anemia by immunodiffusion test. Am. J. Vet. Res., *33*:11–18, 1972.

Coggins, L.: Mechanism of viral persistence in equine infectious anemia. Cornell Vet., *65*:143–151, 1975.

Coggins, L., and Auchnie, J. A.: Control of equine infectious anemia in horses in Hong Kong. J. Am. Vet. Med. Assoc., *170*:1299–1301, 1977.

Crawford, T. B., McGuire, T. C., and Henson, J. B.: Detection of equine infectious anemia virus in vitro by immunofluorescence. Arch. Virusforschung, *34*:332–339, 1971.

Hawkins, J. A., et al.: Role of horse fly (*Tabanus fuscicostatus* Hine) and stable fly (*Stomoxys calcitrans* L.) in transmission of equine infectious anemia to ponies in Louisiana. Am. J. Vet. Res., *34*:1583–1586, 1973.

———: Transmission of equine infectious anemia virus by *Tabanus fuscicostatus*. J. Am. Vet. Med. Assoc., *168*:63–64, 1976.

Henson, J. B., and McGuire, T. C.: Immunopathology of equine infectious anemia. Am. J. Clin. Pathol., *56*:306–314, 1971.

Henson, J. B., McGuire, T. C., and Gorham, J. R.: The detection of precipitating antibodies in equine infectious anemia and partial purification of the antigen. Arch. Ges. Virusforschung, *35*:385–391, 1971.

Henson, J. B., and McGuire, T. C.: Equine infectious anemia. Prog. Med. Virol., *18*:143–159, 1974.

Hjärre, A.: Die Leberveränderungen bei der Infektiösen Anämie des Pferdes. Münch. Tierärztl. Wochenschr., *87*:26–31, 1936.

Ishitani, R.: Equine infectious anemia. Natl. Inst. Anim. Health Q. (Tokyo), *10*(Suppl.):1–28, 1970.

Ito, Y.: Morphogenesis of equine infectious anaemia virus. Acta Virol. (Praha), *18*:352–354, 1974.

Johnson, A. W.: Equine infectious anemia: the literature 1966–1975. Vet. Bull., *46*:559–574, 1976.

Kemen, M. J., Jr., and Coggins, L.: Equine infectious anemia: transmission from infected mares to foals. J. Am. Vet. Med. Assoc., *161*:496–499, 1972.

Kobayashi, K.: Studies on the cultivation of equine infectious anemia *in vitro*. II. Propagation of the virus in horse bone marrow culture. Virus, *11*:189–201, 1961.

———: Studies on the cultivation of equine infectious anemia virus *in vitro*. III. Propagation of the virus in leukocyte cultures. Virus, *11*:249–256, 1961.

Kobayashi, K., and Kono, Y.: Propagation and titration of equine infectious anemia virus in horse leukocyte culture. Natl. Inst. Anim. Health Quart., *7*:8–20, 1967.

Konno, S., and Yamamoto, H.: Pathology of equine infectious anemia. Proposed classification of pathologic types of disease. Cornell Vet., *60*:393–449, 1970.

Kono, Y., Kobayashi, K., and Fukunaga, Y.: Immunization of horses against equine infectious anemia (EIA) with an attenuated EIA virus. Natl. Inst. Anim. Health Q. (Tokyo), *10*:113–122, 1970.

Kono, Y., and Kobayashi, K.: Complement-fixation test of equine infectious anemia. I. Specificity of the test. Natl. Inst. Anim. Health Q. (Tokyo), *6*:194–203, 1966.

Matheka, H. D., Coggins, L., Shively, J. N., and Norcross, N. L.: Purification and characterization of equine infectious anemia virus. Arch. Virol., *51*:107–114, 1976.

McGuire, T. C., Henson, J. B., and Quist, S. E.: Viral-induced hemolysis in equine infectious anemia. Am. J. Vet. Res., *30*:2091–2097, 1969.

———: Impaired bone marrow response in equine infectious anemia. Am. J. Vet. Res., *30*:2099–2113, 1969.

McGuire, T. C., Henson, J. B., and Keown, G. H.: Equine infectious anaemia: the role of Heinz bodies in the pathogenesis of anaemia. Res. Vet. Sci., *11*:354–357, 1970.

McGuire, T. C., Perryman, L. E., and Henson, J. B.: Immunoglobulin composition of the hypergammaglobulinemia of equine infectious anemia. Fed. Proc., *29*:435, 1970.

McGuire, T. C., Crawford, T. B., and Henson, J. B.: Immunofluorescent localization of equine infectious anemia virus in tissue. Am. J. Pathol., *62*:283–294, 1971.

McGuire, T. C., and Crawford, T. B.: Demonstration of circulating infectious virus-antibody complexes in equine infectious anemia. Fed. Proc., *31*:635, 1972.

———: Induction of a cell membrane antigen by equine infectious anemia virus. Am. J. Vet. Res., *39*:385–386, 1978.

Moore, R. W., Redmond, H. E., Katada, M., and Wallace, M.: Growth of the equine infectious anemia virus in a continuous-passage horse leukocyte culture. Am. J. Vet. Res., *31*:1569–1575, 1970.

Nakajima, H., Tanaka, S., and Ushimi, C.: Physicochemical studies of equine infectious anemia virus. IV. Determination of the nucleic acid type in the virus. Arch. Ges Virusforsch., *31*:273–280, 1970.

Nakajima, H., Yoshino, T., and Ushimi, C.: Equine infectious anemia virus from infected horse serum. Infect. Immun., *10*:667–668, 1974.

Obara, J., and Nakajima, H.: Kinetics of iron metabolism in equine infectious anemia. Jpn. J. Vet. Sci., *23*:247–252, 1961.

———: Lifespan of ^{51}Cr-labeled erythrocytes in equine infectious anemia. Jpn. J. Vet. Sci., *23*:207–209, 1961.

Perryman, L. E., McGuire, T. C., Banks, K. L., and Henson, J. B.: Decreased C3 levels in a chronic virus infection: equine infectious anemia. J. Immun., *106*:1074–1078, 1971.

Siegler, R., Lane, I., Moran, S., and Leavitt, P.: Anemia virus as a distinct component of the murine leukemia-sarcoma complex of viruses. Cancer Res., *33*:1858–1861, 1973.

Squire, R. A.: Equine infectious anemia: a model of immunoproliferative disease. Blood, *32*:157–169, 1968.

Stein, C. D., Osteen, O. L., Mott, L. O., and Shahan, M. S.: Experimental transmission of equine infectious anemia by contact and body secretions and excretions. Vet. Med., *39*:46–52, 1944.

Umphenour, N. W., Kemen, M. J., and Coggins, L.: Equine infectious anemia: a retrospective study of an epizootic. J. Am. Vet. Med. Assoc., *164*:66–69, 1974.

Ushimi, C., Nakajima, H., and Tanaka, S.: Demonstration of equine infectious anemia viral antigen by immunofluorescence. Natl. Inst. Anim. Health Q. (Tokyo), *10*:90–91, 1970.

Vallée, H., and Carré, H.: Nature infectieuse de l'anémie du cheval. CR Acad. Sci., *139*:331–333, 1904.

Yoshino, T., Yamamoto, H., and Okaniwa, A.: Fine structure of basophilic round cells of the spleen and lymph node in equine infectious anemia.

Natl. Inst. Anim. Health Q. (Tokyo), *10*:11–25, 1970.

Yoshino, T., and Yamamoto, H.: Electron microscopy of small lymphoid cells in the chronic type of equine infectious anaemia. Natl. Inst. Anim. Health Q. (Tokyo), *11*:21–40, 1971.

Yamamoto, H., Yoshino, T., Nakajima, H., and Ishitani, R.: Relationship between histopathological and serological findings in field cases of equine infectious anemia. Natl. Inst. Anim. Health Q., *12*:193–200, 1972.

Diseases Due to Oncovirinae

The Oncovirinae or RNA tumor viruses include a large number that have been associated with tumors of animals (Table 9–12). The type C oncovirus group is of particular interest, but we shall describe only those diseases produced by the feline leukemia virus.

Feline Leukemia Virus

Transmission of feline malignant lymphoma was first demonstrated by Jarrett et al. (1964a) by inoculation of newborn kittens with a suspension from lymphomatous feline lymph nodes. C-type particles (oncornavirus) were demonstrated to be part of the original inoculum (Jarrett et al., 1964b). The existence and identity of the virus, named "feline leukemia virus" by Jarrett, has been amply confirmed, and the virus is currently classified as one of the Retroviridae family, subfamily Oncovirinae (Table 9–12). This agent and others identified subsequently have evoked intense scientific interest. The virus may be transmitted by direct contact, and viral infection is associated with numerous pathologic states.

The feline leukemia virus is associated with, and the apparent cause of, the following disorders:

1. Malignant lymphoma, which may appear in several forms with solid tumors variously distributed (thymic, multicentric, or alimentary). Malignant lymphocytic cells may reach the circulation in the presence

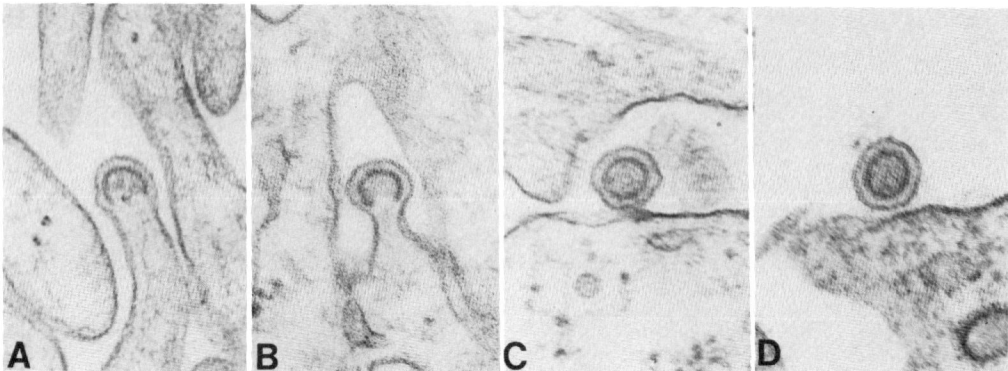

Fig. 9–69. Development of virions of *Retroviridae* (C-type particles). Progressive stages in the development of the virion on a cytoplasmic membrane are seen in A through D. (Courtesy of Dr. Norval W. King, Jr. and *Proceedings of National Academy of Science.*)

or absence of solid tumors.

2. Lymphocytic leukemia.

3. Anemia, in the presence or absence of malignant lymphoma, but associated with the presence of the virus. This anemia may be hemolytic in type, the red blood cells macrocytic and normochromic, with anisocytosis, reticulocytosis, and normoblasts in the circulation and increased erythropoiesis in bone marrow, spleen, and liver (extramedullary hematopoiesis). The anemia may also be manifest by no normoblastic response, depletion of bone marrow of erythroblasts, no extramedullary hematopoiesis, and normocytic and normochromic erythrocytes. About 50% of cats with malignant lymphoma also have anemia, which is not due to replacement of bone marrow with malignant cells. In some instances in the presence of virus, a transient, hemolytic anemia develops and is followed by the appearance of malignant lymphoma.

4. Glomerulonephritis is increased in frequency in cats infected with the feline leukemia virus. This appears to involve an immunologic mechanism.

5. Immunosuppression is one of the effects of the virus. This is manifest by atrophy of the thymus, depletion of thymic-derived (T) lymphocytes, and increased susceptibility to intercurrent infections. In some circumstances, a significant immune response to the virus follows infection and leads to resistance to malignant lymphoma.

Diagnosis. The presence of the virus may be demonstrated by electron microscopic photographs of replicating C-type particles (Figs. 9–69 to 9–71). A fluorescent antibody test is used to detect antigen in leukocytes in blood smears (Hardy et al., 1973). A third method is to isolate the virus in feline cell cultures from the plasma or oral swabs of cats. The pathologic manifestations of malignant lymphoma, leukemia, and anemia are described elsewhere.

Brian, D. A., Thomason, A. R., Rottman, F. M., and Velicer, L. F.: Properties of feline leukemia virus. III. Analysis of the RNA. J. Virol., 16:535–545, 1975.

Essex, M., Cotter, S. M., and Carpenter, J. L.: Feline virus-induced tumors and the immune response: recent developments. Am. J. Vet. Res., 34:809–812, 1973.

Hardy, W. D., Jr., et al.: Feline leukemia virus: occurrence of viral antigen in the tissues of cats with

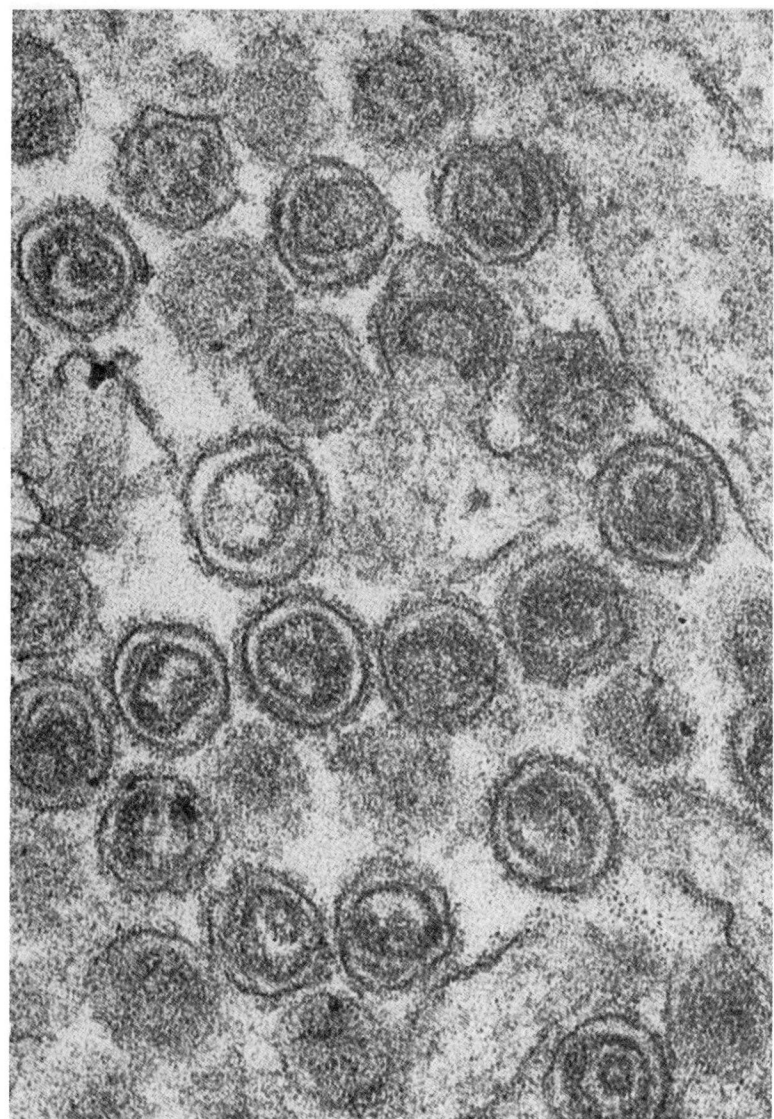

Fig. 9–70. Feline malignant lymphoma virus. Intracellular mature C-type viral particles (approximately ×
150,000). (Courtesy of Dr. G. H. Theilen.)

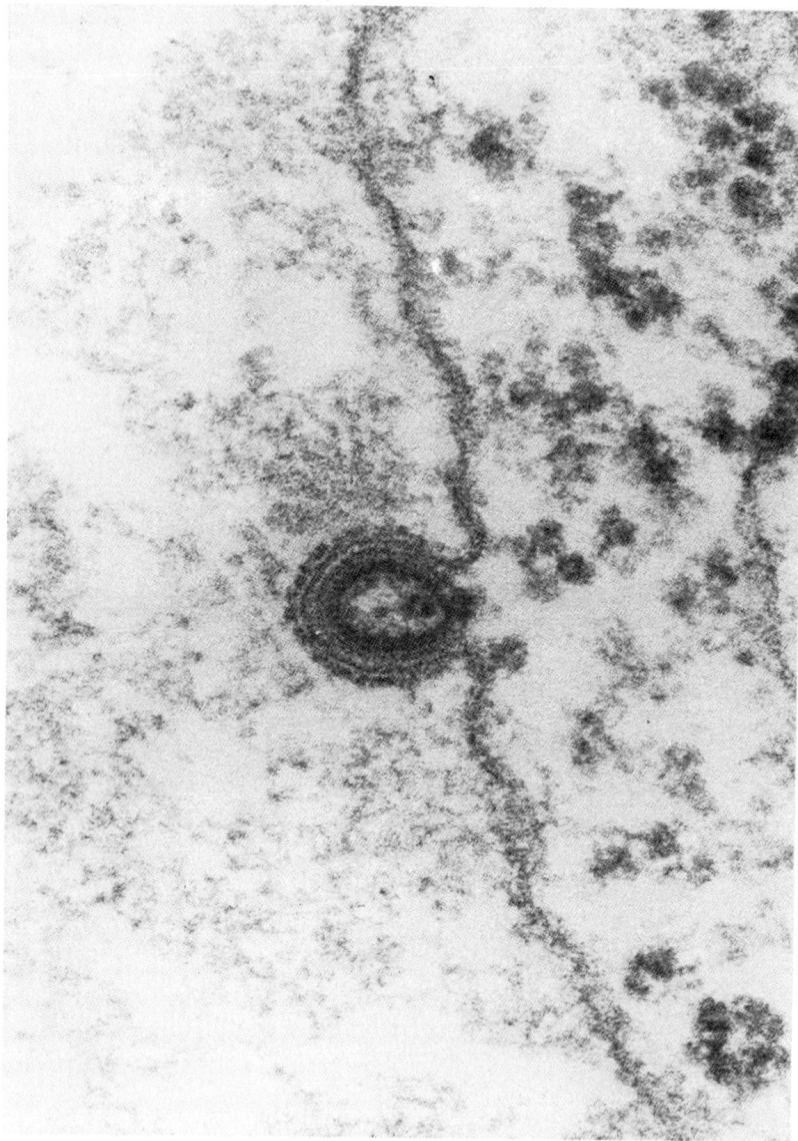

Fig. 9–71. Feline malignant lymphoma virus. Advanced stage of the budding process of the C-type virus from the cytoplasmic membrane of a lymphocyte (approximately × 200,000). (Courtesy of Dr. G. H. Theilen.)

lymphosarcoma and other diseases. Science, 166:1019–1021, 1969.

———: Horizontal transmission of feline leukemia virus. Nature, 244:266–269, 1973.

Hinshaw, V. S., and Blank, H.: Isolation of feline leukemia virus from clinical specimens. Am. J. Vet. Res., 38:55–57, 1977.

Jarrett, W. F. H., et al.: Transmission experiments with leukemia. Nature, 202:566–567, 1964a.

Jarrett, W. F. H., Crawford, E. M., Marten, W. B., and Davie, F.: A virus-like particle associated with leukaemia. Nature, 202:567–568, 1964b.

Jarrett, W. F. H., et al.: Horizontal transmission of leukaemia virus and leukaemia in the cat. J. Natl. Cancer Inst., 51:833–841, 1973.

Jarrett, O.: Natural history of feline leukaemia virus. J. Small Anim. Pract., 16:409–413, 1975.

Kawakami, T. G., et al.: C-type viral particles in plasma of cats with feline leukemia. Science, 158:1049–1050, 1967.

Mackey, L. J., Jarrett, W. F. H., Jarrett, O., and Laird, H. M.: An experimental study of virus leukemia in cats. J. Natl. Cancer Inst., 48:1663–1670, 1972.

Povey, C.: Viral diseases of cats: current concepts. Vet. Rec., 98:293–299, 1976.

Sarma, P. S., et al.: Differential host range of viruses of feline leukemia-sarcoma complex. Virology, 64:438–446, 1975.

Sliski, A. H., Essex, M., Meyer, C., and Todaro, G.: Feline oncornavirus-associated cell membrane antigen: expression in transformed nonproducer mink cells. Science, 196:1336–1339, 1977.

Mammary-Tumor Milk Virus

It has been known for many years that the offspring of hybrid mice produced by pairs from two inbred strains have an increased incidence of certain mammary tumors if their mothers are descendants of strains in which the incidence of mammary tumors is high. Bittner demonstrated in 1936 that a factor in the milk of the mice from the affected strains is responsible for the production of these tumors, even though they do not appear until the offspring mature. The frequency of tumors could be sharply reduced in mice with the same genetic background by putting them to nurse on foster mothers that did not carry the factor. The mammary-tumor milk agent is known to be a virus. The virus, which is transmitted in milk, infects infant mice when nursing, whether or not the mother has mammary cancer, as infected mice may be "latently" infected and excrete virus in the absence of disease. Newly infected mice may similarly transmit the virus to their offspring without developing mammary tumors. Once infected, development of mammary tumors requires a genetic susceptibility and appropriate hormone influence, which is usually provided by pregnancy.

Not all mammary tumors in mice are related to this virus, for several transplantable tumors have been recognized in mice which are free of the milk agent. The murine mammary tumor associated with the milk agent is of much interest in experimental oncology, as it provides a link in the chain of evidence pointing toward the viral etiology of neoplasia.

Bentvelzen, P., and Hilgers, J.: Murine mammary tumor virus. In Viral Oncology, edited by G. Klein. New York, Raven Press, 1980. pp. 311–355.

Gross, L.: Oncogenic viruses. International Series of Monographs on Pure and Applied Biology, Vol. 11. New York, Pergamon Press, 1961.

Gross, L.: Oncogenic Viruses, 2nd edition. New York, Pergamon Press, 1970. pp. 238–280.

ARENAVIRIDAE

The family Arenaviridae contains several viruses that usually infect rodents but may spread to man or other animals. The virions are spherical or pleomorphic, measuring 50 to 300 nm in diameter. The particles contain a variable number of electron-dense granules, 20 to 25 nm in diameter, which have a sandy appearance, giving the group its name (arenosus = sandy). A dense, lipid, double layer membrane surrounds the virion, which contains a core made up of particles similar to ribosomes. The virion proteins include two glycopeptides and two polypeptides. The genome consists of a single-stranded RNA in several segments differing in molecular weight. Virions are readily inactivated by acid, heat, radiation, or lipid solvent. Their buoyant density in sucrose is 1.17 to 1.18 g/cm^3. Replication occurs in the cytoplasm of host cells. Transmission occurs by means of contaminated food, water, air, or inoculation. This group of

Table 9–13.   Diseases Due to Arenaviridae (Genus: Arenavirus)

Lymphocytic choriomeningitis virus
Lassa virus
Tacaribe complex:
  Amapori virus
  Juniri virus
  Latino virus
  Machupo virus
  Parana virus
  Pichinde virus
  Tacaribe virus
  Tamiami virus

viruses causes several important hemorrhagic fevers of man (Lassa, Machupo, and Juniri viruses—Table 9–13). The family at present contains one genus, *Arenavirus;* the type species is the lymphocytic choriomeningitis virus.

Diseases Due to Arenavirus

Arenaviruses are associated with several diseases, including lymphocytic choriomeningitis, Bolivian hemorrhagic fever, and Lassa fever.

Lymphocytic Choriomeningitis

Lymphocytic chloriomeningitis is a viral disease to which man and many animals are susceptible. House mice and, to a smaller degree, other animals may harbor the virus without showing signs, except in the rare case in which fatal paralytic meningoencephalitis develops. The virus has been demonstrated in laboratory and house mice, monkeys, dogs, guinea pigs, roaches, ticks, and man. Experimental infection has also been produced in most of these species, but in rabbits, young chickens, hamsters, and horses, few symptoms follow experimental exposure, although these animals may harbor the virus for several days.

The disease not only is capable of invalidating experimental results, it is also a hazard to laboratory workers, for it is believed that man may become infected through the intact skin and conjunctiva or by inhalation or ingestion of the virus. Blood sucking insects, such as mosquitoes and ticks, may also transmit the disease. The course in man is usually two or three weeks and fortunately is rarely fatal.

Colonies of laboratory mice are likely to harbor the virus of lymphocytic choriomeningitis unless special precautions have been taken. Intrauterine transmission is the principal means of spread within a colony, although virus is also shed in urine and feces. Most mice, therefore, are either infected at birth or early in the neonatal period, and they carry the virus throughout their lives. Circulating antibody does not develop when the infection occurs in utero or in the neonatal period. Only about 20% of these mice, however, show signs of infection, and less than 2% die of the disease. Usually only young mice exhibit symptoms of the spontaneous infection: drowsiness, emaciation, and roughened fur. Affected animals often sit alone in a corner, moving reluctantly, and then slowly and stiffly. Paralysis, tremors, and spastic convulsions, which characterize the experimental disease, are not seen in the spontaneous infections.

The experimental disease may be induced in normal mice by intracerebral injection of virus-containing material, and in mice harboring the virus, by intracerebral introduction of sterile inoculum, such as broth. Either method will result in symptoms and lesions indistinguishable from those of the spontaneous disease in 3 to 13 days. General malaise, roughened fur, and the tendency to sit quietly alone are apparent in the experimentally infected mouse. When lifted by its tail, rapid leg motions are followed by tremors and convulsions. If released during such a convulsion, the mouse may fall with the hind legs stiffly stretched out, the tail rigid, and the back humped. It may drag itself around by the

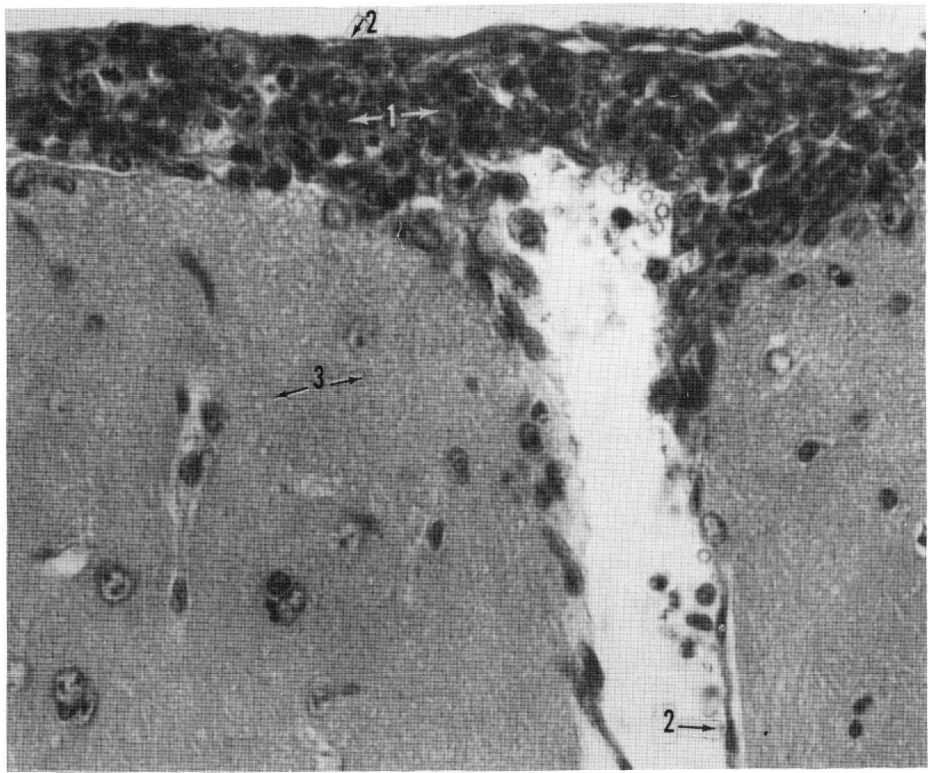

Fig. 9–72. Lymphocytic choriomeningitis, cerebrum of a mouse (× 865). Lymphocytes *(1)* infiltrate and elevate the pia *(2)*. Cerebral cortex *(3)*. (Courtesy of Armed Forces Institute of Pathology.) Contributor: Army Medical School.

front legs with the rear limbs extended. Death usually follows in two or three days.

Lesions. Gross lesions in mice and in other species are rather meager and not especially characteristic; they include serous pleural exudation, fatty changes in the liver, and enlargement of the spleen. Microscopically, lymphocytic infiltration of the meninges is characteristic, being most severe in the experimentally induced disease. The changes are most pronounced in the pia-arachnoid at the base of the brain, in the choroid plexus, and sometimes in perivascular spaces of submeningeal and subependymal vessels. Lymphocytic infiltration may also be detected in other organs, such as liver and lungs, usually concentrated around small blood vessels.

Similar lesions dominate the microscopic picture in other species affected with the disease.

Pathogenesis. Immunologic competency of the host is important in determining whether the virus will be tolerated, producing no disease, or whether severe lesions will result, ending fatally. In tolerantly infected female mice, the virus replicates in the placenta, and in vitro, it infects embryos, which become carriers without lesions. This same situation may be produced in offspring by inoculating pregnant mice with virus between 0 to 11 days following mating (Cole et al., 1971). Tolerant infection may also be produced by inoculating newborn mice with the lymphocytic choriomeningitis virus. Adult mice, inoculated intracerebrally, develop severe meningitis and succumb in a few days. This lethal disease is completely avoided by giving the adult mice an immunosuppressant (cyclophosphamide) on the third day of infection. Lesions in meninges and cerebellum (necrosis of granular cells) may develop as rats or mice carrying the infection reach a certain age. The phenomenon also appears to be mediated by immune mechanisms.

At one time it was believed that no circulating antibody was present in tolerantly infected mice with circulating virus, but it has been shown that antibody is present in the form of antigen-antibody complexes. These complexes are believed responsible for an immune-mediated glomerulonephritis that appears later in the life of these animals.

Early in experimental infection, the presence of viral antigen may be demonstrated by immunofluorescence in choroid plexus, ependymal epithelium, and arachnoid cells of the meninges. With the electron microscope, virions may be demonstrated enmeshed in the microvillus border and budding from the plasma membranes of cells of the choroid and ependyma.

Retinopathy has also been described in intracerebrally inoculated newborn rats. The virus is first demonstrable by immunofluorescence in the optic nerve, then the inner nuclear layer of the retina, the pigment epithelium, and all the layers of the retina. This results in destruction of the retina with little inflammatory infiltration (Monjan et al., 1972). Behavioral alterations have also been attributed to infection with the lymphocytic choriomeningitis virus (Hotchin and Seegal, 1977).

Cerebellar hypoplasia may also be produced in neonatal rats with this virus. This has been used to study this immune-mediated lesion of the cerebellum (Del Cerro et al., 1975).

Cole, G. A., Gilden, D. H., Monjan, A. A., and Nathanson, N.: Lymphocytic choriomeningitis virus: pathogenesis of acute central nervous system disease. Fed. Proc., *30*:1831–1841, 1971.

Dalldorf, G.: Lymphocytic choriomeningitis of dogs. Cornell Vet., *33*:347–350, 1943.

del Cerro, M., Nathanson, N., and Monjan, A. A.: Pathogenesis of cerebellar hypoplasia produced by lymphocytic choriomeningitis virus infection of neonatal rats. II. An ultrastructural study of the immune-mediated pathology. Lab. Invest., *33*:608–617, 1975.

Hirsch, M. S., Moellering, R. C., Jr., Pope, H. G., and Poskanzer, D. C.: Lymphocytic-choriomeningitis-virus infection traced to a pet hamster. N. Engl. J. Med., *291*:610–612, 1974.

Hotchin, J.: The contamination of laboratory animals with lymphocytic choriomeningitis virus. Am. J. Pathol., *64*:747–769, 1971.

Hotchin, J., et al.: Lymphocytic choriomeningitis in a hamster colony causes infection of hospital personnel. Science, *185*:1173–1174, 1974.

Hotchin, J., and Seegal, R.: Virus-induced behavioral alteration of mice. Science, *196*:671–674, 1977.

Lillie, R. D., and Armstrong, C.: Pathology of lymphocytic choriomeningitis in mice. Arch. Pathol., *40*:141–152, 1945.

Mims, C. A.: Effect on the fetus of maternal infection with lymphocytic choriomeningitis (LCM) virus. J. Infect. Dis., *120*:582–597, 1969.

———: Immunofluorescence study of the carrier state and mechanism of vertical transmission in lymphocytic choriomeningitis infection in mice. J. Pathol. Bact., *91*:395–402, 1966.

Monjan, A. A., Silverstein, A. M., and Cole, G. A.: Lymphocytic choriomeningitis virus-induced retinopathy in newborn rats. Invest. Ophthalmol., *11*:850–856, 1972.

Oldstone, M. B., and Dixon, F. J.: Pathogenesis of chronic disease associated with persistent lymphocytic choriomeningitis viral infection. II. Relationship of the antilymphocytic choriomeningitis immune response to tissue injury in chronic lymphocytic choriomeningitis disease. J. Exp. Med., *131*:1–19, 1970.

Skinner, H. H., and Knight, E. H.: Natural routes for post-natal transmission of murine lymphocytic choriomeningitis. Lab. Anim., *7*:171–184, 1973.

———: Factors influencing pre-natal infection of mice with lymphocytic choriomeningitis virus. Arch. Ges. Virusforsch., *46*:1–10, 1974.

Smadel, J. E., and Wall, M. J.: Identification of the virus lymphocytic choriomeningitis. J. Bact., *41*:421–430, 1941.

Traub, E.: An epidemic in a mouse colony due to lymphocytic choriomeningitis. J. Exp. Med., *63*:533–546, 1936.

Walker, D. H., Murphy, F. A., Whitfield, S. G., and Bauer, S. P.: Lymphocytic choriomeningitis: ultrastructural pathology. Exp. Mol. Pathol., *23*:245–265, 1975.

Bolivian Hemorrhagic Fever

This is a disease of man principally, but several species are susceptible, including rhesus monkeys *(Macaca mulatta)*. This disease occurs in South America, particularly Bolivia and Argentina, and is caused by an *Arenavirus*. Several viral strains of the Tacaribe complex, particularly the Machupo virus, are involved. It must be differentiated from **simian hemorrhagic fever,** a disease of Old World monkeys, caused by a *Pestivirus*, family Togaviridae.

This disease is manifest in rhesus monkeys experimentally exposed to the virus by skin rash, lymphadenopathy, splenomegaly, and hemorrhages, especially from nostrils. Death may occur within two weeks, depending on the dose of virus administered. The gross findings in these animals with an acute clinical course may be summarized as follows: splenomegaly, edema of meninges, hydropericardium, enlarged friable liver, enlarged lymph nodes, and hemorrhages in heart, brain, and nares. The lesions seen with the light microscope include: disseminated necrosis of liver cells with acidophilic inclusions (Councilman bodies) in hepatocytes and Kupffer cells; necrosis of intestinal epithelium, particularly at tips of villi, but often involving cells in the crypts as well; and necrosis of the adrenal cortex and some lymph nodes.

Animals that succumb after a course of more than 18 days usually are found to have nonsuppurative meningitis, necrosis of lymphocytes in lymph nodes, focal degeneration of myocardium with hemorrhages, hypoplasia of lymphocytes and reticuloendothelial cells in some nodes, and depletion of lymphocytes in others.

Eddy, G. A., Scott, S. K., Wagner, F. S., and Brand, O. M.: Pathogenesis of Machupo virus infection in primates. Bull. WHO, *52*:516–521, 1975.

McLeod, C. G., Jr., Stookey, J. L., Eddy, G. A., and Scott, S. K.: Pathology of chronic Bolivian hemorrhagic fever in the rhesus monkey. Am. J. Pathol., *84*:211–224, 1976.

Terrell, T. G., Stookey, J. L., Eddy, G. A., and Kastelli, M. D.: Pathology of Bolivian hemorrhagic fever in the rhesus monkey. Am. J. Pathol., *73*:477–494, 1973.

Lassa Fever

Lassa fever was first recognized as a new disease of human beings in 1969 in the course of an outbreak on the Jos plateau of Nigeria, West Africa. The disease may be subclinical, but florid cases occur, with death in some instances within four weeks. Guinea pigs and squirrel monkeys *(Saimiri sciureus)* have been experimentally infected with the virus, an *Arenavirus*, resulting in a severe viremia and fatal outcome. Transfer of virus to African multimammate rats *(Mastomys natalensis)* resulted in persistent viremia at high titer, but no obvious illness in these animals. This species is believed to provide one reservoir for the virus in nature.

The experimental infection in squirrel monkeys results in high viral titers and lesions in many organs at death. These lesions may be summarized as necrosis of lymphocytes in the spleen, necrosis of renal tubular epithelium, myocarditis, arteritis, and disseminated necrosis of hepatocytes. In animals with a survival time of 28 days or longer, choriomeningitis may be evident. The infection and its effects on the hosts are similar to that seen in the type species: lymphocytic choriomeningitis viral infection.

Buckley, S. M., and Casals, J.: Lassa fever, a new virus disease of man from West Africa. III. Isolation and characterization of the virus. Am. J. Trop. Med. Hyg., *19*:680–691, 1970.

Frame, J. D., Baldwin, J. M., Gocke, D. J., and Troup, J. M.: Lassa fever, a new virus disease of man from West Africa. I. Clinical description and pathological findings. Am. J. Trop. Med. Hyg., *19*:670–676, 1970.

Walker, D. H., Wulff, H., Lange, J. V., and Murphy, F. A.: Comparative pathology of Lassa virus infection in monkeys, guinea-pigs, and *Mastomys natalensis*. Bull. WHO, *52*:523–534, 1975.

Walker, D. H., Wulff, H., and Murphy, F. A.: Experimental Lassa virus infection in the squirrel monkey. Am. J. Pathol., *80*:261–278, 1975.

CORONAVIRIDAE

The virions of this family of viruses are pleomorphic enveloped particles averaging about 100 nm in diameter. Unique club-shaped peplomers, about 15–20 nm long, project from the envelope, giving the appearance of a crown in negatively stained electron micrographs (*corona* = crown). The genome consists of one molecule of single-stranded RNA with molecular weight of nine million daltons. The particles multiply in the cytoplasm of host cells and mature by budding through cytoplasmic reticulum.

Avian infectious bronchitis virus, the type species for the single genus, *Coronavirus,* is quite distinct immunologically. Several of the coronaviruses of mammals cross-react serologically. Some viruses of the group agglutinate the red blood cells of other species, e.g., human coronavirus and hemagglutinating encephalitis virus of piglets.

Coronaviruses are sensitive to ether but are clearly not related to any known myxo- or paramyxovirus. Their RNA codes for six or seven polypeptides, four of which are glycoproteins. Buoyant density of the virions in sucrose is 1.17 to 1.19 g/cm^3. Neuraminidase is not present. The virions mature by budding into cytoplasmic vesicles. Coronaviruses have been associated with the common cold and gastroenteritis in humans, and are known to be causative agents in several animal diseases.

Diseases Due to Coronavirus

A list of coronaviruses appears in Table 9–14. The name of each of these viruses identifies the disease with which it is associated.

Transmissible Gastroenteritis of Swine

First described by Doyle and Hutchings (1946), transmissible gastroenteritis of swine is a highly contagious viral disease of swine, especially young pigs. It now is established that the causative agent is a *Coronavirus* that meets the morphologic, physical, and chemical characteristics of this genus. This virus may be distinguished from another porcine coronavirus, the hemagglutinating encephalomyelitis virus of piglets, which agglutinates and hemabsorbs, in vitro, the red blood cells of chicks, hamsters, and rats. The transmissible gastroenteritis virus lacks these properties and also can be distinguished by the viral neutralization test.

Signs. In pigs under ten days of age, the disease is characterized by acute diarrhea, vomition, excessive thirst, weight loss, and dehydration, which lead to death in two to five days. Morbidity and mortality rates may approach 100%. In older piglets and adults, clinical signs may not be apparent or there may be profuse diarrhea, vomition, depression, and failure to gain or maintain weight. The morbidity rate in older swine may also approach 100%, but mortality rate is low.

Lesions. In pigs dying of transmissible gastroenteritis, few gross findings are evident. The carcass is dehydrated and curdled milk is usually present in the stomach. The mucosa of the stomach and small intestine is congested and often contains petechiae. Microscopically, there is marked atrophy of the villi of the small intestine. Villous length is reduced several

Table 9–14. Diseases Due to Coronaviridae (Genus: Coronavirus)

Avian infectious bronchitis virus	Calf neonatal diarrhea coronavirus
Human coronavirus	Murine hepatitis virus
Porcine transmissible gastroenteritis virus	Porcine hemagglutinating encephalitis virus
Rat coronavirus	Rat sialodacryoadenitis virus
Turkey bluecomb disease virus	Feline infectious peritonitis virus

fold and they are lined with flattened to cuboidal epithelial cells rather than the normal columnar cells. The brush border of the epithelium is irregularly absent, the cytoplasm vacuolated, and the nuclei small and often pyknotic. The lamina propria is infiltrated with mononuclear cells and neutrophils, but inflammatory exudation is not a striking feature. Thake (1968) has demonstrated that the villous atrophy is the combined effect of viral-induced villous cell destruction and improper maturation of cells as they advance from the crypts to the villi. Focal necrosis of the gastric mucosa has been described. In most cases there is evidence of nephrosis. Hydropic and hyalin droplet degeneration are present in the epithelium of proximal convoluted tubules and proteinaceous casts may be numerous. Okinawa and Maeda (1966) have described reticuloendothelial hyperplasia and loss of lymphocytes in lymph nodes and spleens of experimentally infected pigs.

Studies with the electron microscope reveal virions of the transmissible gastroenteritis virus within microcanaliculi, a network of cytoplasmic tubules of plasmalemma origin that is believed to be involved in the uptake of macromolecules of colostrum during the first days of life (Wagner et al., 1973). It is postulated that the virions are taken into cells through these microcanaliculi, which are present for only a few days after birth. This would possibly explain the increased susceptibility of newborn animals. Newly replicated virions appear to mature by budding into cytoplasmic vacuoles surrounded by plasma membranes. As virus particles accumulate in the cell, the cell ruptures to release the virus. The cell is disrupted and desquamated at this point.

Diagnosis. Presumptive diagnosis can be made by the clinical signs supported by finding the histopathologic lesions in the small intestine.

The virus of transmissible gastroenteritis may be identified by specific immunofluorescence or by neutralization in tissue culture systems. It may be distinguished from the hemagglutinating encephalomyelitis virus by its lack of hemagglutination of erythrocytes in vitro.

Ackerman, L. J., Morehouse, L. G., and Olson, L. D.: Transmissible gastroenteritis in three-week-old pigs: study of anemia and iron absorption. Am. J. Vet. Res., 33:115–120, 1972.

Bay, W. W., Doyle, L. P., and Hutchings, L. M.: The pathology and symptomatology of transmissible gastroenteritis. Am. J. Vet. Res., 12:215–218, 1951.

Butler, D. G., Gall, D. G., Kelly, M. H., and Hamilton, J. R.: Transmissible gastroenteritis. Mechanisms responsible for diarrhea in an acute viral enteritis in piglets. J. Clin. Invest., 53:1335–1342, 1974.

Derbyshire, J. B., Jessett, D. M., and Newman, G.: An experimental epidemiological study of porcine transmissible gastroenteritis. J. Comp. Pathol., 79:445–452, 1969.

Doyle, L. P., and Hutchings, L. M.: A transmissible gastroenteritis in pigs. J. Am. Vet. Med. Assoc., 108:257–259, 1946.

Ferris, D. H.: Epizootiologic features of transmissible swine gastroenteritis. J. Am. Vet. Med. Assoc., 159:184–194, 1971.

Frederick, G. T., and Bohl, E. H.: Local and systemic cell-mediated immunity against transmissible gastroenteritis, an intestinal viral infection of swine. J. Immunol., 116:1000–1004, 1976.

Hooper, B. E., and Haelterman, E. O.: Lesions of the gastrointestinal tract of pigs infected with transmissible gastroenteritis. Can. J. Comp. Med., 33:29–36, 1969.

Lucas, M. H., and Napthine, P.: Fluorescent antibody technique in the study of three porcine viruses: transmissible gastroenteritis virus, vomiting and wasting disease virus and the parvovirus 59E/63. J. Comp. Pathol., 81:111–117, 1971.

McClurkin, A. W., and Norman, J. O.: Studies on transmissible gastroenteritis of swine. II. Selected characteristics of a cytopathogenic virus common to five isolates from transmissible gastroenteritis. Can. J. Comp. Med. Vet. Sci., 30:190–198, 1966.

McClurkin, A. W., Stark, S. L., and Norman, J. O.: Transmissible gastroenteritis (TGE) of swine: the possible role of dogs in the epizootiology of TGE. Can. J. Comp. Med., 34:347–349, 1970.

Mengeling, W. L.: Porcine coronaviruses: co-infection of cell cultures with transmissible gastroenteritis virus and hemagglutinating encephalomyelitis virus. Am. J. Vet. Res., 34:779–783, 1973.

Mishra, N. K., and Ryan, W. L.: Ribonucleic acid synthesis in porcine cell cultures infected with transmissible gastroenteritis virus. Am. J. Vet. Res., 34:185–188, 1973.

Moon, H. W., Norman, J. O., and Lambert, G.: Age dependent resistance to transmissible gastroenteritis of swine (TGE). I. Clinical signs and some mucosal dimensions in small intestine. Can. J. Comp. Med., 37:157–166, 1973.

Moon, H. W., et al.: Age-dependent resistance to transmissible gastroenteritis of swine. III. Effects of epithelial cell kinetics on coronavirus production and on atrophy of intestinal villi. Vet. Pathol., 12:434–445, 1975.

Morin, M., Morehouse, L. G., Solorzano, R. F., and Olson, L. D.: Transmissible gastroenteritis in feeder swine: clinical immunofluorescence and histopathological observations. Can. J. Comp. Med., 37:239–248, 1973.

Morin, M., and Morehouse, L. G.: Transmissible gastroenteritis in feeder pigs: observations on the jejunal epithelium of normal feeder pigs and feeder pigs infected with TGE virus. Can. J. Comp. Med., 38:227–235, 1974.

Morin, M., Morehouse, L. G., Solorzano, R. F., and Olson, L. D.: Transmissible gastroenteritis in feeder swine: role of feeder swine in the epizootiologic features. Am. J. Vet. Res., 35:251–255, 1974.

Okinawa, A., and Maeda, M.: Histopathology of transmissible gastroenteritis in experimentally infected newborn piglets. I. Lesions in the digestive tract. Nat. Inst. Anim. Health Q. (Tokyo), 5:190–201, 1965.

———: Histopathology of transmissible gastroenteritis in experimentally infected newborn piglets. II. Lesions in organs other than digestive tract and pathologic features of TGE. Nat. Inst. Anim. Health Q. (Tokyo), 6:64–72, 1966.

Olson, L. D.: Induction of transmissible gastroenteritis in feeder swine. Am. J. Vet. Res., 32:411–417, 1971.

Olson, D. P., Waxler, G. L., and Roberts, A. W.: Small intestinal lesions of transmissible gastroenteritis in gnotobiotic pigs: A scanning electron microscopic study. Am. J. Vet. Res., 34:1239–1245, 1973.

Pensaert, M., Haelterman, E. O., and Burnstein, T.: Transmissible gastroenteritis of swine: virus-intestinal cell interactions. I. Immunofluorescence, histopathology and virus production in the small intestine through the course of infection. Arch. Ges. Virusforsch., 31:321–334, 1970.

Pensaert, M., Haelterman, E. O., and Hinsman, E. J.: Transmissible gastroenteritis of swine: virus-intestinal cell interactions. II. Electron microscopy of the epithelium in isolated jejunal loops. Arch. Ges. Virusforsch., 31:335–351, 1970.

Phillip, J. I. H., Cartwright, S. F., and Scott, A. C.: The size and morphology of T. G. E. and vomiting and wasting disease viruses of pigs. Vet. Rec., 88:311–312, 1971.

Reynolds, D. J., Garwes, D. J., and Gaskell, C. J.: Detection of transmissible gastroenteritis virus neutralizing antibody in cats. Arch. Virol., 55:77–86, 1977.

Roberts, A. W., Trapp, A. L., and Carter, G. R.: Laboratory diagnosis of transmissible gastroenteritis by immunofluorescence. Vet. Med. Small Anim. Clin., 68:612–614, 1973.

Saif, L. J., Bohl, E. H., Kohler, E. M., and Hughes, J. H.: Immune electron microscopy of transmissible gastroenteritis virus and *Rotavirus* (reovirus-like agent) of swine. Am. J. Vet. Res.,38:13–20, 1977.

Sprino, P. J., Morilla, A., and Ristic, M.: Intestinal immune response of feeder pigs to infection with transmissible gastroenteritis virus. Am. J. Vet. Res., 37:171–176, 1976.

Stone, S. S., Stark, S. L., and Phillips, M.: Transmissible gastroenteritis virus in neonatal pigs: intestinal transfer of colostral immunoglobulins containing specific antibodies. Am. J. Vet. Res., 35:339–345, 1974.

Thake, D. C.: Jejunal epithelium in transmissible gastroenteritis of swine. Am. J. Pathol., 53:149–168, 1968.

Thake, D. C., Moon, H. W., and Lambert, G.: Epithelial cell dynamics in transmissible gastroenteritis of neonatal pigs. Vet. Pathol., 10:330–341, 1973.

Thorsen, J., and Djurickovic, S.: Experimental immunization of sows with inactivated transmissible gastroenteritis (TGE) virus. Can. J. Comp. Med., 35:99–102, 1971.

Trapp, A. L., Sanger, V. L., and Stalnaker, E.: Lesions of the small intestinal mucosa in transmissible gastroenteritis-infected germfree pigs. Am. J. Vet. Res., 27:1695–1702, 1966.

Underdahl, N. R., et al.: Isolation of transmissible gastroenteritis virus from lungs of market-weight swine. Am. J. Vet. Res., 35:1209–1216, 1974.

Underdahl, N. R., Mebus, C. A., and Torres-Medina, A.: Recovery of transmissible gastroenteritis virus from chronically infected experimental pigs. Am. J. Vet. Res., 36:1473–1476, 1975.

Wagner, J. E., Beamer, P. D., and Ristic, M.: Electron microscopy of intestinal epithelial cells of piglets infected with a transmissible gastroenteritis virus. Can. J. Comp. Med., 37:177–188, 1973.

Waxler, G. L.: Lesions of transmissible gastroenteritis in the pig as determined by scanning electron microscopy. Am. J. Vet. Res. 33:1323–1328, 1972.

Porcine Coronaviral Encephalomyelitis

Two clinical entities in neonatal swine, both due to coronaviruses, have been described. The first disease, manifest by encephalomyelitis, was reported by Alexander et al. (1959) in Canada. The etiologic agent was called "hemagglutinating encephalomyelitis virus." The second clinical entity, reported from England, was named after its clinical features: "vomiting and wasting disease of piglets" (Cartwright et al., 1969). The causative agent of this disease proved to be a virus similar or identical to the hemagglutinating encephalomyelitis virus. Thus it appears that similar viruses may produce different clinical pictures under differing conditions.

Signs. Baby pigs usually manifest the first signs of the disease four to seven days following birth, with anorexia, lethargy, vomiting, and constipation, soon followed by signs of involvement of the central nervous system. These signs include: hyperesthesia (squealing and paddling movements in response to a sudden noise), stilted gait, and progressive posterior paralysis. In advanced stages, the pigs lie prostrate, are dyspneic, blind, and show nystagmus and coma. The vomiting and wasting disease also starts within a few days following birth with vomiting and retching, inappetence, and excessive thirst (with impaired ability to drink). They fail to gain weight, become emaciated, and usually die within a week or two. A few surviving animals fail to grow normally.

Lesions. Lesions in the central nervous system are, in essence, a nonsuppurative encephalomyelitis with glial nodules, diffuse gliosis, and perivascular aggregations of lymphocytes. This is characteristic of the experimental disease also. Experimental infection by nasal instillation results in focal and diffuse interstitial and peribronchiolar pneumonia.

Diagnosis. Diagnosis is based presumptively upon the clinical signs and the lesions, but must be confirmed by identification of the virus. The virus grows well in primary pig kidney cell cultures in appropriate medium and causes multinucleated syncytia to appear one or two days after inoculation. The virus may be identified by serum neutralization tests in pig kidney cultures or by hemagglutination-inhibition tests with convalescent serum. Other immunologic tests, such as immunofluorescence tests on cells in culture, agar-gel immunodiffusion, and hemadsorption plaque assay tests may be used. Not only must the infectious agent be distinguished from other coronaviruses, but

also from the Teschen disease group of enteroviruses.

Alexander, T. J. L., Richards, W. P. C., and Roe, C. K.: An encephalomyelitis of suckling pigs in Ontario. Can. J. Comp. Med., 23:316–319, 1959.

Appel, M., Greig, A. S., and Corner, A. H.: Encephalomyelitis of swine caused by a hemagglutinating virus. IV. Transmission studies. Res. Vet. Sci., 6:482–489, 1965.

Cartwright, S. F., et al.: Vomiting and wasting disease of piglets. Vet. Rec., 84:175–176, 1969.

Cutlip, R. C., and Mengeling, W. L.: Lesions induced by hemagglutinating encephalomyelitis virus strain 67N in pigs. Am. J. Vet. Res., 33:2003–2009, 1972.

Greig, A. S., et al.: A hemagglutinating virus producing encephalomyelitis in baby pigs. Can. J. Comp. Med. Vet. Sci., 26:49–56, 1962.

Greig, A. S.: Hemagglutinating encephalomyelitis virus infection. *In* Diseases of Swine, 4th ed., edited by H. W. Dunne and A. D. Lemon. Iowa State Univ. Press, Ames, 1975, Chap. 17, pp. 385–390.

Mengeling, W. L., and Cutlip, R. C.: Experimentally induced infection of newborn pigs with hemagglutinating encephalomyelitis virus strain 67N. Am. J. Vet. Res., 33:953–956, 1972.

Mengeling, W. L., and Coria, M. F.: Buoyant density of hemagglutinating encephalomyelitis virus of swine. Comparison with avian infectious bronchitis virus. Am. J. Vet. Res., 33:1359–1363, 1972.

Mengeling, W. L.: Porcine coronaviruses: coinfection of cell cultures with transmissible gastroenteritis virus and hemagglutinating encephalomyelitis virus. Am. J. Vet. Res., 34:779–783, 1973.

Mitchell, D.: Encephalomyelitis of swine caused by a hemagglutinating virus. I. Case histories. Res. Vet. Sci., 4:506–510, 1963.

Phillips, J. I. H., Cartwright, S. F., and Scott, A. C.: The size and morphology of T.G.E. and vomiting and wasting disease viruses of pigs. Vet. Rec., 88:311–312, 1971.

Richards, W. P. C., and Savan, M.: Viral encephalomyelitis of pigs. A preliminary report on the transmissibility and pathology of a disease observed in Ontario. Cornell Vet., 50:132–155, 1960.

Feline Infectious Peritonitis

For several years, evidence has indicated that feline infectious peritonitis is caused by a virus, namely, the disease is readily transmitted by means of peritoneal fluid filtered through a membrane of average pore diameter of 100 nm; bacteria, chlamydia, and mycoplasma have not been recovered, and viral particles have been demonstrated in tissues of experimentally

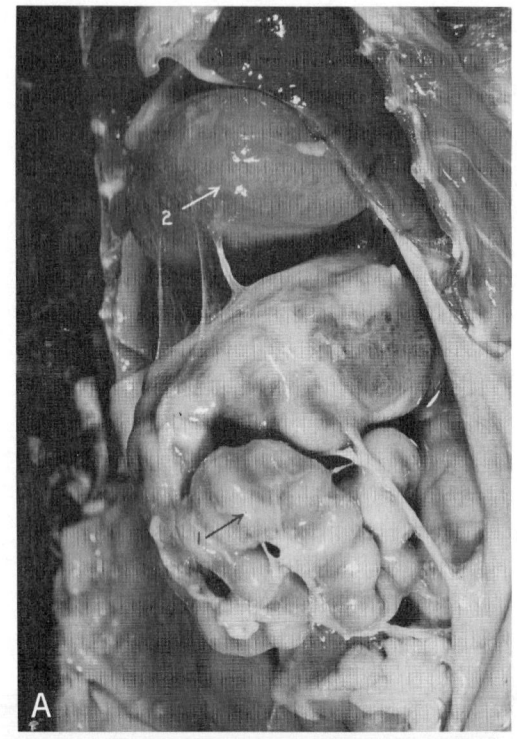

Fig. 9–73. Infectious feline peritonitis. *A,* Organizing fibrinous peritonitis in a four-year-old female cat. The exudate binds the intestines together *(1)* and covers and compresses the liver *(2). B,* Chronic organizing peritonitis in a 15-year-old female cat. Cloudy fluid *(1)* distends the abdomen, the parietal peritoneum is thick and tough *(2),* the mesentery *(3)* is short and thick, and the liver *(4)* is compressed and distorted in shape by the exudate covering its capsule. *C,* Another view of the liver in *B,* with thick, tough fibrous exudate on the capsule, compressing and distorting the liver. (Courtesy of Angell Memorial Animal Hospital.)

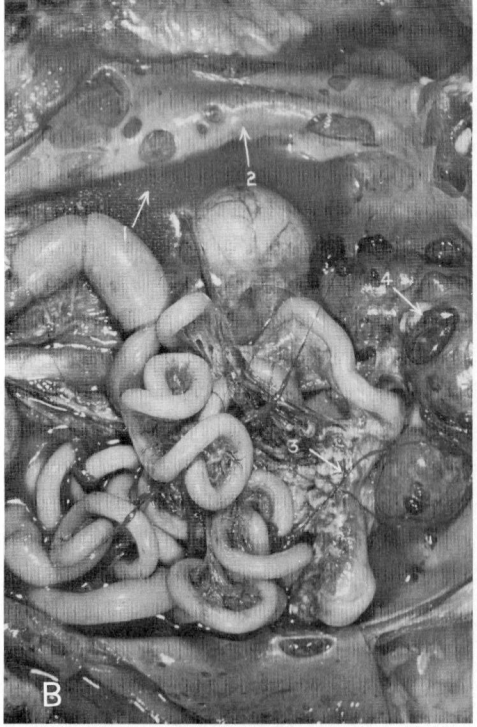

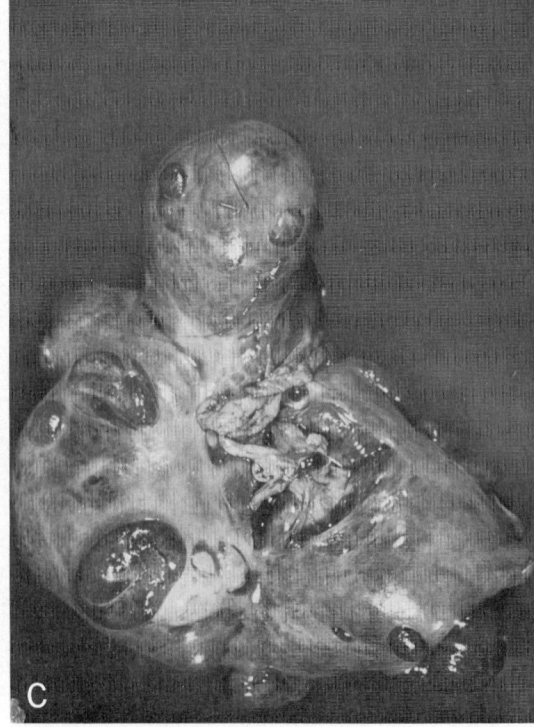

infected kittens. Cultivation of the organism has been difficult, and progress toward its taxonomic classification has been slow. It is now known (Pedersen, 1976) that this agent is heat-sensitive, ether-labile, relatively resistant to phenol, and inactivated by room temperature within 24 hours. The virus is also inactivated by viricidal concentrations of chlorhexidine and benzalkonium chloride.

The virions are 70 to 75 nm in diameter, with a central, roughly doughnut-shaped nucleoid 50 to 55 nm in diameter. The virions are enveloped with spike-shaped peplomers projecting from the envelope. Viral antigens are demonstrable by immunofluorescent methods. The virus is tentatively classified in the genus *Coronavirus*.

Signs. The disease, which is most frequent in young cats, is characterized by persistent fever, anorexia, depression, weight loss, and ascites leading to gradual abdominal enlargement. Other signs may include vomiting, diarrhea, and dyspnea. The disease is invariably fatal, following a course of two weeks to two months.

Lesions. The abdominal cavity contains excessive fluid, often up to 1 L. The fluid is yellow, viscid, and transparent, though it may contain flakes of fibrin. A gray-white granular exudate is present over all serosal surfaces, being especially thick over the liver and spleen. A similar fibrinous exudate extends into the scrotum and may also be present in the thoracic cavity. Small, discrete white foci of necrosis are often present throughout the liver. In protracted cases, organization of fibrinous exudate can result in severe distortion of abdominal viscera. Microscopically, the peritonitis, or pleuritis, is a classic fibrinous inflammation consisting of a layer of fibrin of varied thickness containing cellular debris overlying a zone of neutrophils, lymphocytes, and macrophages. Fibroplasia and proliferation of capillaries may accompany the exudate in protracted cases. The inflammatory process may extend beneath the serosa into any of the affected tissues. The focal

hepatic necrosis is accompanied by an inflammatory reaction. Similar necrotic foci may be found microscopically in the spleen, kidneys, pancreas, lymph nodes, and muscular layers of the gastrointestinal tract. While not usual, purulent and mononuclear meningitis may be seen.

The peritoneal exudate contains large amounts of immunoglobulin, principally IgG; hypergammaglobulinemia is also a feature of the natural disease. Granulomatous lesions, which appear to be part of this syndrome but have not been established by the demonstration of the virus in the lesions, have been described in tissues other than the peritoneum. These include meninges, eye, and spinal cord.

Diagnosis. The clinical signs are usually sufficient for diagnosis of the disease in the living animal. The gross and microscopic features are not duplicated by other forms of peritonitis. Specific immunofluorescence may be demonstrated in tissues of cats infected with the virus.

Doherty, M. J.: Ocular manifestations of feline infectious peritonitis. J. Am. Vet. Med. Assoc., *159*:417–424, 1971.

Gouffaux, M., Pastoret, P. P., Henroteaux, M., and Massip, A.: Feline infectious peritonitis, proteins of plasma and ascitic fluid. Vet. Pathol., *12*:335–348, 1975.

Hardy, W. D., Jr., and Hurvitz, A. I.: Feline infectious peritonitis: experimental studies. J. Am. Vet. Med. Assoc., *158*:994–1002, 1971.

Holzworth, J.: Some important disorders of cats. Cornell Vet., *53*:157–160, 1963.

Krum, S., Johnson, K., and Wilson, J.: Hydrocephalus associated with the noneffusive form of feline infectious peritonitis. J. Am. Vet. Med. Assoc., *167*:746–748, 1975.

Legendre, A. M., and Whitenack, D. L.: Feline infectious peritonitis with spinal cord involvement in two cats. J. Am. Vet. Med. Assoc., *167*:931–932, 1975.

Montali, R. J., and Strandberg, J. D.: Extraperitoneal lesions in feline infectious peritonitis. Vet. Pathol., *9*:109–121, 1972.

Osterhaus, A. D., Horzinek, M. C., and Ellens, D. J.: Untersuchungen zur Ätiologie der Felinen Infektiösen Peritonitis. Berl. Munch. Tierärztl. Wochenschr., *89*:135–137, 1976.

Pedersen, N. C.: Morphologic and physical characteristics of feline infectious peritonitis virus and its growth in autochthonous peritoneal cell cultures. Am. J. Vet. Res., *37*:567–572, 1976.

Pedersen, N. C.: Serologic studies of naturally occurring feline infectious peritonitis. Am. J. Vet. Res., 37:1449–1454, 1976.

Potkay, S., Bacher, J. D., and Pitts, T. W.: Feline infectious peritonitis in a closed breeding colony. Lab. Anim. Sci., 24:279–289, 1974.

Robison, R. L., Holzworth, J., and Gilmore, C. E.: Naturally occurring feline infectious peritonitis: signs and clinical diagnosis. J. Am. Vet. Med. Assoc., 158:981–986, 1971.

Slauson, D. O., and Finn, J. P.: Meningoencephalitis and panophthalmitis in feline infectious peritonitis. J. Am. Vet. Med. Assoc., 160:729–734, 1972.

Ward, B. C., and Pederson, N.: Infectious peritonitis in cats. J. Am. Vet. Med. Assoc.,154:26–35, 1969.

Ward, J. M., Munn, R. J., Gribble, D. H., and Dungworth, D. L.: An observation of feline infectious peritonitis. Vet. Rec., 83:416–417, 1968.

Ward, J. M.: Morphogenesis of a virus in cats with experimental feline infectious peritonitis. Virology, 41:191–194, 1970.

Ward, J. M., Gribble, D. H., and Dungworth, D. L.: Feline infectious peritonitis: experimental evidence for its multiphasic nature. Am. J. Vet. Res., 35:1271–1275, 1974.

Watson, A. D. J., Huxtable, C. R. R., and Bennett, A. M.: Feline infectious peritonitis. Aust. Vet. J., 50:393–397, 1974.

Wolfe, L. G., and Griesemer, R. A.: Feline infectious peritonitis. Pathol. Vet., 3:255–270, 1966.

Zook, B. C., King, N. W., Robison, R. L., and McCombs, H. L.: Ultrastructural evidence for the viral etiology of feline infectious peritonitis. Pathol. Vet., 5:91–95, 1968.

Rat Coronavirus Infection

A newly-isolated *Coronavirus* has been recovered from the lungs of wild and laboratory-reared rats (Parker et al., 1970). This virus is similar to other members of the *Coronavirus* genus, but may be distinguished by means of neutralization tests. The virus is clearly related to but not the same agent that causes sialodacryoadenitis in rats (Bhatt et al., 1972). The rat coronavirus grows well in cultures of rat kidney cells, producing a characteristic cytopathic effect (necrosis and polykaryocytic cells) as well as a complement-fixing antigen. Original isolations were made from pooled lung tissue of rats which were inoculated into weanling, disease-free rats, and subsequently put into primary rat kidney cultures. Intranasal instillation of suspensions of the rat coronavirus into newborn rats results in respiratory disease leading to death by the sixth to the twelfth day. Rats older than 48 hours have much greater resistance but do develop respiratory disease, and some die. Rats infected when older than 21 days exhibit no outward signs of illness.

The principal lesions in the lungs of experimentally infected rats are hyperemia, diffuse interstitial pneumonitis with mononuclear cells, and focal atelectasis. Compensatory emphysema may be seen in some lungs, and severe bronchopneumonia sometimes occurs, presumably due to secondary bacterial infection.

Bhatt, P. N., Percy, D. H., and Jonas, A. M.: Characterization of the virus of sialodacryoadenitis of rats: a member of the coronavirus group. J. Infect. Dis., 126:123–130, 1972.

Parker, J. C., Cross, S. S., and Rowe, W. P.: Rat coronavirus (RVC): a prevalent, naturally occurring pneumotropic virus of rats. Arch. Ges. Virusforsch., 31:293–302, 1970.

Sialodacryoadenitis of Rats

This synthetic term (sialo = saliva; dacryo = lacrimal; adenitis = inflammation of gland) is used to identify a specific inflammation of salivary and lacrimal glands of rats. The causative agent is a virus classified in the genus *Coronavirus*. The disease was first described by Innes and Stanton (1961) in rats housed in two different laboratories. A large number of rats are affected, but few die from the disease.

Signs. The neck of affected rats is swollen with the head sunk into the neck, giving the rats the short, "hunched head and neck appearance of guinea pigs." The thickening is due to the enlarged submaxillary glands, with surrounding edematous tissues. Gross edema may be seen at necropsy involving the intermandibular space to the base of the neck. The submaxillary glands grossly appear swollen, tense, edematous, and congested.

Lesions. The histologic appearance of the submaxillary salivary gland and the nearby harderian gland is characteristic of acute inflammation affecting all parts of each gland. The lobules are separated from one another by edematous and fibrinous exudate plus infiltration by neutrophils, lymphocytes, histiocytes, and connective tissue cells. Hemorrhage is not conspicuous. Mast cells are present only in small numbers. The parenchyma of the gland is very much altered due to distortion and loss of acinar and ductal cells, with intense infiltration by inflammatory cells and edema. Loss of cells appears to progress by involving a few at a time with no massive necrosis. No specific cytologic features occur in the disease, distinguishing it from the greatly enlarged nuclei and inclusions that occur in cytomegalovirus infection.

In some instances, squamous metaplasia of duct epithelium occludes the lumen and results in changes in the gland due to obstruction. Keratinization of these squamous cells is not a feature, however. The harderian gland may manifest similar lesions; the appearance of red tears on the cheek due to porphyrins in the lacrimal secretion may indicate involvement of this gland.

Bhatt, P. N., Percy, D. H., and Jonas, A. M.: Characterization of the virus of sialodacryoadenitis of rats: a member of the coronavirus group. J. Infect. Dis., *126*:123–130, 1972.

Innes, J. R. M., and Stanton, M. F.: Acute disease of the submaxillary and harderian glands (sialodacryoadenitis) of rats with cytomegaly and no inclusion bodies. Am. J. Pathol., *38*:455–468, 1961.

Jacoby, R. O., Bhatt, P. N., and Jonas, A. M.: Pathogenesis of sialodacryoadenitis in gnotobiotic rats. Vet. Pathol., *12*:196–209, 1975.

Jonas, A. M., et al.: Sialodacryoadenitis in the rat. A light and electron microscopic study. Arch. Pathol., *88*:613–622, 1969.

Coronaviral Calf Diarrhea

Many organisms—bacteria, fungi, mycoplasma, chlamydia, or viruses—have been implicated in diseases of young calves in which the principal clinical manifestation is diarrhea. Among the viruses listed in this category are bovine viral diarrhea/mucosal disease, infectious bovine rhinotracheitis virus, adenovirus, enterovirus, calf pneumonia/enteritis virus, and rotavirus. To this list must be added a coronavirus, first reported by Stair et al. (1972) as causing a diarrheal disease of young calves. This organism conforms morphologically, physically, and chemically to other members of the genus *Coronavirus.*

Lesions. The virus has an affinity for the epithelial cells of the villi of the small intestine. Replication of the virus in these cells is accompanied by loss of epithelium and blunting of the villi. In the colon, surface epithelial cells are also attacked, with loss of surface cells and cystic dilatation and accumulation of cellular debris in underlying crypts.

Diagnosis. The virus can be demonstrated by suitable immunofluorescent techniques in affected cells in the small and large intestine and in affected reactive lymph nodes of the mesentery. Virus can also be demonstrated specifically in intestinal epithelial cells shed into the intestinal lumen. Diagnosis depends upon confirmed identification of the etiologic agent.

Mebus, C. A., Stair, E. L., Rhodes, M. B., and Twiehaus, M. J.: Neonatal calf diarrhea: propagation, attenuation, and characteristics of a coronavirus-like agent. Am. J. Vet. Res., *34*:145–150, 1973.

———: Pathology of neonatal calf diarrhea induced by a coronavirus-like agent. Vet. Pathol., *10*:45–64, 1973.

Mebus, C. A., Newman, L. E., and Stair, E. L., Jr.: Scanning electron, light, and immunofluorescent microscopy of intestine of gnotobiotic calf infected with calf diarrheal coronavirus. Am. J. Vet. Res., *36*:1719–1726, 1975.

Sharpee, R. L., Mebus, C. A., and Bass, E. P.: Characterization of a calf diarrheal *Coronavirus.* Am. J. Vet. Res., *37*:1031–1041, 1976.

Stair, E. L., Rhodes, M. B., White, R. G., and Mebus, C. A.: Neonatal calf diarrhea: purification and electron microscopy of a coronavirus-like agent. Am. J. Vet. Res., *33*:1147–1156, 1972.

Murine Hepatitis

A murine virus originally isolated by Cheever et al. (1949) in connection with disseminated encephalomyelitis, and subsequently as a closely related strain from cases of hepatitis (Gledhill et al., 1951), is now recognized as the mouse hepatitis virus, a *Coronavirus*. This virus has a tendency to be latent in laboratory mouse colonies, but may produce disease under favorable conditions. In one instance, its pathogenic properties were accentuated when combined with a protozoan parasite of low pathogenicity: *Eperythrozoon coccoides*. It may be more virulent also in concert with mouse leukemia virus in the same host. It is, therefore, of importance to research involving mice.

Lesions. The lesions involve hepatic cells which become necrotic in focal zones throughout the liver. Kupffer cells also may become infected. Many types of cells may be infected, and lymphocytes are massively destroyed in spleen and lymph nodes by the virus. Encephalomyelitis may be seen, especially with certain strains of the virus.

Diagnosis. Diagnosis is confirmed by identification of the virus in the presence of compatible lesions.

Cheever, F. S., Daniels, J. B., Pappenheimer, A. M., and Bailey, O. T.: A murine virus (JHM) causing disseminated encephalomyelitis with extensive destruction of myelin. I. Isolation and biologic properties of the virus. J. Exp. Med., *90*:181–194, 1949.
Gledhill, A. W., and Andrewes, C. H.: A hepatitis virus of mice. Br. J. Exp. Pathol., *32*:559–568, 1951.
Gledhill, A. W., Dick, G. W. A., and Andrewes, C. H.: Production of hepatitis in mice by the combined action of two filterable agents. Lancet, *2*:509–511, 1952.

Other Coronaviral Diseases

Coronaviruses have been demonstrated in human beings in association with upper respiratory infections. Several strains of virus have been isolated from people with "colds," and it appears that as many as 15% of human "colds" may be due to coronaviruses (McIntosh, 1974). In a few instances, bronchitis and pneumonia have resulted from infection with these viruses.

The type species of the coronaviruses is the avian infectious bronchitis virus, the cause of this acute respiratory disease of chickens. This virus is widespread among poultry flocks, and several strains have been isolated. The original description of avian infectious bronchitis was published by Schalk and Hawn (1931), and the agent was first grown in embryonated hen's eggs by Beaudette and Hudson (1937).

A *Coronavirus* has been isolated from military dogs during the course of an outbreak of diarrhea, and has been shown to produce nonlethal intestinal disease in neonatal dogs (Keenan et al., 1976). The causative agent of bluecomb disease of turkeys (coronaviral enteritis of turkeys) has also been shown to be a *Coronavirus* (Pomeroy, 1978). It seems likely that viruses of this genus will eventually be recovered from most vertebrate species.

Beaudette, F. R., and Hudson, C. B.: Cultivation of the virus of infectious bronchitis. J. Am. Vet. Med. Assoc., *90*:51–60, 1937.
Estola, T.: Coronaviruses, a new group of animal RNA viruses. Avian Dis., *14*:330–336, 1970.
Keenan, K. P., Jervis, H. R., Marchwicki, R. H., and Binn, L. N.: Intestinal infection of neonatal dogs with canine coronavirus 1–71: Studies by virologic, histologic, histochemical, and immunofluorescent techniques. Am. J. Vet. Res., *37*:247–256, 1976.
McIntosh, K.: Coronavirus: a comparative review. Curr. Top. Microbiol. Immunol., *63*:85–129, 1974.
Pomeroy, B. S.: Coronaviral enteritis of turkeys. *In* Diseases of Poultry, 7th ed., edited by M. S. Hofstad, et al. Ames, Iowa State Univ. Press, 1978, pp. 633–640.
Schalk, A. F., and Hawn, M. C.: An apparently new respiratory disease of baby chicks. J. Am. Vet. Med. Assoc., *78*:413–422, 1931.

BUNYAVIRIDAE

This family of viruses derives its name from Bunyamwera, a place in Uganda, Africa, where the type species (Bunyamwera virus) was isolated. One genus has been named, *Bunyavirus*, and contains at least 84 named viruses, which are subdivided into ten serologically related groups. Most of the viruses are transmitted by mosquitoes, some by ticks. Transovarial transmission is known in some of them. Additional possible members of the family Bunyaviridae include at least 48 viruses, and at least two unnamed genera. Among these is the as yet unassigned virus of Rift Valley fever, which will be discussed on following pages.

The principal features of the family Bunyaviridae follow. The virions are spherical and enveloped, 90 to 100 nm in diameter. The envelope contains at least one virus-specified glycopeptide. The internal ribonucleoprotein occurs in long strands 2 to 2.5 nm wide. The genome consists of a single-stranded RNA in three pieces, with molecular weights of about 4, 2, and 0.8×10^6 daltons and total molecular weight of 6 to 7×10^6 daltons. The virions develop in the cytoplasm of host cells and mature by budding into smooth-surfaced membranes in or adjacent to the Golgi region.

Rift Valley Fever

Rift Valley fever is an acute viral disease which, in nature, principally affects sheep and cattle, causing heavy mortality rates in young lambs and calves and abortion in pregnant ewes and cows. Human beings may contract the infection during the course of an epizootic among domestic animals or by handling the virus in the laboratory. Sometimes human cases of an influenzal type may provide the first indication of the existence of an epizootic of Rift Valley fever. Montgomery in 1912 was the first to report the disease as an acute and highly fatal infection of lambs, and Stordy published similar observations the year following. Both reports were from Kenya, where the disease occurred on farms in the Rift Valley, a geologic depression that starts in Iran, continues through North and Central Africa, and ends in eastern Transvaal. Like many other newly reported diseases of unknown etiology, this one was named for the location where it was first observed, and not until 1931 was it established as a distinct entity by Daubney, Hudson and Garnham (1931), who were the first to demonstrate that it could be transmitted to susceptible animals. Rift Valley fever has a wide distribution in Africa, but has not been recognized in domestic animals outside of that continent.

Although the virus may be transmitted to susceptible animals by inoculation of infected blood or serum, in nature it is usually transmitted by arthropod vectors. The culicine mosquitoes, particularly *Eretmapodites chrysogaster*, have been shown experimentally to be capable of transmitting the disease. Experimental transmission of the virus to goats, mice, rats, wild rodents, and golden hamsters, as well as to its natural hosts, has been successful. The African buffalo, ferrets, and monkeys, both New World and Old World, are susceptible, although some species of primates appear to have resistance. Cats merely exhibit transitory febrile symptoms, and dogs, guinea pigs, rabbits, mongooses, hedgehogs, tortoises, frogs, and birds are refractory to artificial infection. Man is particularly susceptible and can easily become infected.

Signs. After an extremely short incubation period, from 20 to 72 hours after infection, the course in young lambs is brief. They may be disinclined to move, refuse to eat, exhibit some form of abdominal pain, and shortly thereafter become recumbent and unable to rise. Death may occur within 24 hours. It is not unusual for lambs to die before symptoms are observed. In adult sheep also, the disease often is not recognized; the infected animal is found dead without having displayed any indication of illness. Vomiting may be observed as the only symptom, but pregnant ewes usually abort in the course of the illness or during convalescence. In cattle, the disease may appear as a storm of abortions; the symptoms also are frequently indefinite, being manifest by a brief febrile period with inappetence, profuse salivation, diarrhea, abdominal pain, roughened hair coat, and cessation of lactation. The mortality rate in cattle is not high, but erosions of the buccal mucosae, necrosis of the skin of the udder or scrotum, laminitis, and coronitis may occur.

In man, the initial symptoms, after an incubation period of four to six days, are malaise, nausea, hyperthermia, epigastric pain, and a sensation of fullness over the region of the liver. There is usually complete anorexia, followed by rigors, violent headache, characteristic flushing of the face, injection of the conjunctiva, photophobia, aching pains in the back and joints, vertigo, and sometimes epistaxis. The disease in man is rarely fatal and immunity follows recovery, but serious sequelae such as thrombophlebitis, retinopathy, and retinal detachment have been reported.

Lesions. The disagreement in the literature concerning the characteristic gross and microscopic changes in Rift Valley fever indicate the need for further study. Varying manifestations in the susceptible species also create problems. According to Schultz (1951) and others, the most constant and characteristic lesions are found in the liver. In sheep, the organ is grossly enlarged, its surface is mottled gray to grayish red or purple, and bears numerous gray to white subcapsular, opaque foci. Microscopically, these foci are seen as areas of necrosis involving parenchymal cells near the central veins. The affected liver cells have swollen, eosinophilic, hyaline

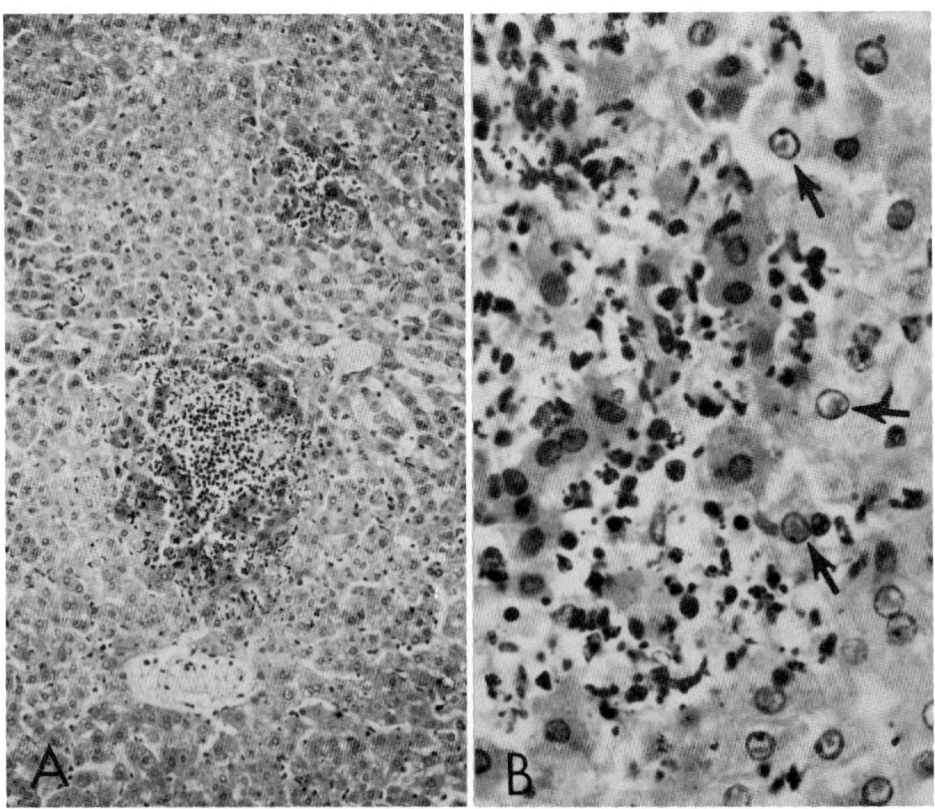

Fig. 9–74. Rift Valley fever, experimental infection in a hamster. *A*, Focal hepatic necrosis accompanied by purulent inflammation. *B*, Higher magnification illustrating small eosinophilic intranuclear inclusion bodies (arrows) in hepatocytes.

cytoplasm, and pyknotic or fragmented nuclei, their appearance suggesting the Councilman bodies of yellow fever. Findlay (1933) has described intranuclear inclusions, but their specificity is in doubt. They have also been seen in experimental animals, but inclusion bodies do not form in tissue culture. The studies of McGavran and Easterday (1963) suggest that the inclusion bodies present a degenerative change, in that they were not formed of viral particles. The frequent "paracentral" location of the liver lesion is suggestive of the changes associated with anoxia. In lambs, the liver usually is gray to reddish brown, but sometimes ochre yellow, and the distribution of the gray necrotic lesions is likely to be more diffuse than in adult sheep.

The gallbladder wall may be thickened by edema and contain subserosal hemorrhages, particularly near its attachment to the liver.

The visible mucosae are usually cyanotic and the vessels of the skin and subcutis are injected, particularly over the head and neck. The mammary gland may be grossly purple in color, but no mastitis is present. Hemorrhages may occur in the subcutis of the axillae and the medial and lower aspects of the limbs.

Hemorrhages may also be seen in the peritoneum of the gastrointestinal tract and diaphragm, as well as under the pleura, pericardium, endocardium, and in the myocardium. Similar hemorrhages may occur in the submucosa and muscularis of the gastrointestinal tract, in the pancreas, kidney, adrenal, lung, thymus, and lymph nodes (especially those of the mesentery). The lymph nodes are enlarged, appear moist and reddened, and the mesenteric and periportal nodes may contain numerous hemorrhages. Necrotic foci among lymphoid cells, with infiltration of neutrophils, vascular congestion, and edema, may be detected microscopically.

Ulceration of the intestinal mucosa may be seen in the terminal portion of the ileum, the cecum, and the initial part of the colon. Hemorrhagic lesions in some cases involve the entire gastrointestinal tract, but possibly are due to secondary factors.

The lungs are invariably hyperemic and edematous, often with subpleural and diffuse hemorrhages. Consolidation, particularly in the apical and cardiac lobes, may be fibrinous in character. In addition to bearing hemorrhages, the kidneys are usually slightly enlarged and show histologic evidence of nephrosis (swelling and loss of cell outline in tubular epithelium, albuminous casts in convoluted and collecting tubules, hemosiderin in tubular epithelium, congestion).

The spleen is usually enlarged and exhibits subcapsular petechiae. The malpighian bodies are indistinct because of reduction of lymphocytes. In the red pulp, hemorrhages with adjoining masses of pyknotic and fragmented nuclei may be seen, and sometimes collections of neutrophils.

Diagnosis. Rift Valley fever should be suspected in outbreaks of highly fatal disease affecting both lambs and calves, especially if persons associated with the sick animals or who handle infective materials display mild febrile symptoms. In addition, the occurrence of abortion in adult animals and the presence of the gross and microscopic lesions, particularly those of the liver, are believed to permit a presumptive diagnosis. Neutralization of infective blood by immune serum, using mice as test animals, confirms the diagnosis. A serum neutralization test with mice may also be employed.

Alexander, R. A.: Rift Valley fever in the Union. J. S. Afr. Vet. Med. Assoc., 22:105–111, 1951.

Daubney, R., Hudson, J. R., and Garnham, P. C.: Enzootic hepatitis or Rift Valley fever. An undescribed virus disease of sheep, cattle and man from East Africa. J. Pathol. Bact., 34:545–579, 1931.

Davies, F. G., Clausen, B., and Lund, L. J.: The pathogenicity of Rift Valley fever virus for the baboon. Trans. R. Soc. Trop. Med. Hyg., 66:363–365, 1972.

Easterday, B. C.: Rift Valley fever. Adv. Vet. Sci., 10:65–127, 1965.

Easterday, B. C., McGavran, M. H., Rooney, J. R., and Murphy, L. C.: The pathogenesis of Rift Valley fever in lambs. Am. J. Vet. Res., 23:470–479, 1962.

Findlay, G. M.: Rift Valley fever or enzoötic hepatitis. Tr. R. Soc. Trop. Med. Hyg., 25:229–265, 1932.

———: Cytological changes in the liver in Rift Valley fever with special reference to the nuclear inclusions. Br. J. Exp. Pathol., 14:207–219, 1933.

Findlay, G. M., and Howard, E. M.: The susceptibility of rats to Rift Valley fever in relation to age. Ann. Trop. Med., 46:33–37, 1952.

Mackenzie, R. D., Findlay, G. M., and Stern, R. O.: Studies on neurotropic Rift Valley fever virus: the susceptibility of rodents. Br. J. Exp. Pathol., 17:352–361, 1936.

McGavran, M. H., and Easterday, B. C.: Rift Valley fever virus hepatitis. Light and electron microscopic studies in the mouse. Am. J. Pathol., 42:587–607, 1963.

McIntosh, B. M., Dickinson, D. B., and dos Santos, I.: Rift Valley fever. 3. Viraemia in cattle and sheep. 4. The susceptibility of mice and hamsters in relation to transmission of virus by mosquitoes. J. S. Afr. Vet. Assoc., 44:167–169, 1973.

Sabin, A. B., and Blumberg, R. W.: Human infection with Rift Valley fever virus and immunity twelve years after single attack. Proc. Soc. Exp. Biol. Med., 64:385–389, 1947.

Schultz, K. C. A.: The pathology of Rift Valley fever or enzoötic hepatitis in South Africa. J. S. Afr. Vet. Med. Assoc., 22:113–120, 1951.

Schwentker, F. F., and Rivers, T. M.: Rift Valley fever in man. Report of a fatal laboratory infection complicated by thrombophlebitis. J. Exp. Med., 59:305–313, 1934.

Smithburn, K. C., Haddow, A. J., and Gillett, J. D.: Rift Valley fever: isolation of the virus from wild mosquitoes. Br. J. Exp. Pathol., 29:107–121, 1948.

DISEASES DUE TO UNCLASSIFIED VIRUSES

Most viruses of interest as disease-producing agents of vertebrates have been at least tentatively classified in a family as proscribed by the International Committee on Taxonomy of Viruses. A few remain, however, which are not well enough understood to place in any accepted taxon. These include the agents that cause hepatitis B and C of man, Borna disease of horses, and the "unconventional viruses" which are responsible for the **spongiform encephalopathies** of animals and man (Table 9–15). These unconventional viruses differ from all others in many important biologic, physical, and chemical fea-

Table 9–15.   Diseases Due to Unclassified Viruses

Spongiform encephalopathies:
  Scrapie (sheep and goats)
  Transmissible mink encephalopathy
  Kuru (man)
  Creutzfeldt-Jakob disease (man)
Aleutian disease (mink)
Borna disease (horse)
Marburg virus disease (man)
Hepatitis B and C (man)

tures: they are resistant to formaldehyde, beta-propiolactone, EDTA (ethylene-diamine-tetra-acetate), proteases (trypsin, pepsin), nucleases (ribonucleases A and III, dioxyribonuclease I), heat (to 80° C.; they are incompletely inactivated at 100° C.), ultraviolet radiation (at 2540 Å), ionizing radiation (x-rays), and ultrasonic energy. They have an atypical ultraviolet action spectrum—2370 Å causes six times the inactivation produced by 2540 Å. The viruses are not visible as recognizable virions by electron microscopy. No viral proteins have been demonstrated.

The unique biologic characteristics of these unconventional viruses may also be listed: the incubation period is long (months to years or decades); no significant inflammatory response is elicited in affected tissues; the lesions are progressive and essentially always terminate in death; the tissue changes are characteristically degenerative (widespread neuronal degeneration, amyloid, astrocytic gliosis); no inclusion bodies are found; interferon is not produced, and interference with the production of interferon by other viruses is not demonstrated; there is no sensitivity to interferon; no interference has been demonstrated with conventional viruses (at least 30 of them); infectious nucleic acid is not demonstrable; no viral antigenicity has been found; immunosuppression or immunopotentiation does not alter the incubation period, course, or duration of the disease; immune B cell and T cell functions are intact; no cytopathic effect on infected cells is demonstrable in vitro; and individual animals vary in their susceptibility to high doses of the agent.

This group of unconventional viruses has some resemblance to viroids, which are known as causative agents of certain plant diseases, such as the potato spindle tuber disease, chrysanthemum stunt, and citrus exocortis. These infectious units are believed to be composed only of nucleic acid, and they resemble the agent of scrapie in some features, leading to the postulation that scrapie virus is a viroid (Diener, 1974). However, evidence consisting of failure to extract scrapie virus from infected mouse brain using a phenol-extraction method suggests that scrapie virus may not be a viroid (Ward et al., 1974).

The unconventional viruses of scrapie, mink encephalopathy, kuru, and Creutzfeldt-Jakob disease do have some characteristics in common with conventional viruses (Gajdusek, 1977). These properties are: they are filterable to 25 nm average pore diameter (scrapie, mink encephalopathy) or 100 nm (kuru, Creutzfeldt-Jakob virus); all individuals in most species succumb to high lethal doses of virus; the viruses replicate in the brain, reaching titers of 10^8 to 10^{12}/g of brain; the viruses replicate first in the spleen and other reticuloendothelial cells, later in the brain; the viruses have a shortened incubation period following "adaptation" to a new host; most have a specific host range; in some species (sheep and mice), susceptibility is under genetic control; strains of virus vary in virulence and pathogenicity; clonal selection of strains from "wild stock" is possible, and slow-growing strain of scrapie virus will interfere with replication of a fast-growing strain in mice.

Kuru

Kuru is the name applied to a neurologic disease that afflicted certain primitive people of New Guinea. These people had a common language and observed ritualistic cannibalism of near relatives. The occurrence of kuru in families led to the assumption that the disease was hereditary. After a description of the lesions of kuru was published, Hadlow (1959) drew attention to the unique similarities of the lesions of kuru to those of scrapie, and pointed out that failures to transmit the disease to animals may have resulted from lack of anticipation of the prolonged incubation period. Hadlow's perception was correct; the first successful transmission of kuru was to a chimpanzee after an incubation period of many months (Gajdusek and Gibbs, 1971). Subsequently, the disease has been transmitted to Old and New World monkeys, mink, and ferrets (Gajdusek, 1977).

Creutzfeldt-Jakob Disease

This is a rare, presenile dementia of human patients which is found worldwide and sometimes has a familial pattern. Using the experience gained with kuru, an infectious agent has been transmitted from human patients to chimpanzees, Old and New World monkeys, and cats. This success has enlarged the possibilities of gaining better understanding of the cause and nature of this disease, and has stimulated the search for viruses in other human neuropathies, such as multiple sclerosis, Alzheimer's disease, Parkinson's disease, and many others.

"Scrapie" of Sheep (Ovine Spongiform Encephalopathy)

"Scrapie" is the colloquial name of a disease of sheep and, rarely, goats, derived from the principal clinical manifestation, which is almost continuous scraping of the skin against any reasonably stationary object as a result of the intense pruritus the animal suffers. The disease has been known in Scotland for at least two centuries, but has spread to Canada and the United States only in recent years. Present evidence indicates that the etiologic agent is a filtrable agent that can be experimentally transmitted by intracerebral passage of suspensions of medulla and spinal cord of affected animals.

The disease has a prolonged incubation period, as much as one-and-one-half to five years in nature and four to six months following intracerebral inoculation. The course of the disease is from two to twelve months. However, both the incubation period and course vary with the genotype of the sheep. Although certain individuals are resistant, the nature of the resistance is unknown. Mice, which are susceptible to experimental infection, are a useful laboratory animal. Many points remain obscure, and further study of this interesting disease is needed. The disease called "rida" in Iceland is probably the same as scrapie.

Scrapie is the prototype of the so called "slow" viral diseases of animals and man, with its prolonged course and progressive, serious lesions. It is also the first of the spongiform encephalopathies of man or animals shown to be transmissible (Cuillé and Chelle, 1936). It has been postulated (Gajdusek, 1977) that the infectious agent of scrapie of sheep has in various ways been transmitted to man to produce the spongiform encephalopathies known as kuru, Creutzfeldt–Jakob disease, and familial Alzheimer's disease. It also appears that transmissible mink encephalopathy is caused by an agent the same as, or similar to, the virus of scrapie. Supporting this concept is the transmission of a comparable disease from infected sheep to mink.

Signs. The signs, which appear in adult sheep, are usually characterized at the outset by restlessness and a startled look, the eyes having a fixed and wild expression. The pupils are dilated. The sheep may hold its head down and wag it as if hunting a fly. Its movements are aimless, and stiffness of the forelegs results in a trotting gait, a characteristic that gives the disease its German name, *Trabberkrankheit.* The animal usually grinds its teeth. Twitching, at first confined to the lips, soon involves the muscles of the shoulders and thighs as well. The

voice may be altered. If startled, the animal may fall in an epileptiform seizure of rather brief duration. The skin irritation apparently starts in the lumbar region, then may involve the rest of the body surface. The intense pruritus causes the sheep to rub against objects rather continuously until the wool coat is almost completely lost. Scratching the back of an affected animal will cause it to grind its teeth and show a characteristic rapid twitching of the lips. Incoordination may be followed by paralysis and inability to stand, and finally the animal dies.

Lesions. No characteristic gross lesion is found in this disease, the specific tissue alterations being limited to microscopic changes in the medulla oblongata, pons, midbrain, and spinal cord. The most striking and diagnostic lesion is the presence of large vacuoles in the cytoplasm of neurons, associated with rather diffuse astrogliosis and occasional accumulation of lymphocytes in the Virchow-Robin spaces. These lesions are most numerous in nuclei of the medulla, and are not found in the cerebral cortex or cerebellum. Sections taken just anterior to the calamus scriptorius are most likely to contain affected cells, therefore these should be selected for microscopic examination aimed at establishing the diagnosis. The nuclear masses in the medulla most frequently involved are the reticular formation and the medial vestibular and lateral cuneate nuclei. Vacuolated neurons are found less frequently in the hypoglossal nuclei, the inferior olive, and the gray columns of the spinal cord. In experimentally transmitted cases, the lesions tend to be more widespread. The possibility that vacuolization of nerve cells might be an artifact has been considered, and some controversy has existed on this point. It does appear, however, that the altered neurons containing vacuoles represent one quite constant microscopic alteration recognizable in this disease. In some cases, PAS-positive plaques are found in the molecular and granular layers of the cerebellum. Neutral fat can sometimes be demonstrated in the white matter, but otherwise demyelination is not obvious. The exact distribution of the tissue changes and the correlation between them and the symptoms are yet to be established. In the experimental disease in sheep, goats, and mice, in addition to the changes described there is widespread status spongiosus. Lesions in muscles have been reported in some studies, but the possibility exists that these changes are the result of a concurrent disease.

Ultrastructural studies have in general confirmed the presence of membrane-bound vesicles in affected neurons and their processes. Some disagreement persists concerning the presence of viral particles. Some workers describe viral particle budding from intracytoplasmic membranes, others report tubular structures suggesting nucleocapsids of naked nucleic acid, and still others contend that only membranous alterations can be detected. At this juncture, the infective agent appears not to have been visualized with certainty.

Diagnosis. The diagnosis is based upon the clinical symptoms and is confirmed by histologic examination of the brain and spinal cord, with particular emphasis on the medulla oblongata, pons, and midbrain. Especial study should be given sections from that area of medulla immediately cranial to the calamus scriptorius.

Adams, D. H., and Field, E. J.: The infective process in scrapie. Lancet, 2:714–716, 1968.

Alter, M., Frank, Y., Doyne, H., and Webster, D. D.: Creutzfeldt-Jakob disease after eating ovine brains? N. Engl. J. Med., 292:927, 1975.

Barnett, K. C., and Palmer, A. C.: Retinopathy in sheep affected with natural scrapie. Res. Vet. Sci., 12:383–385, 1971.

Beck, E., and Daniel, P. M.: Neuropathological studies in primates suffering from experimental kuru or Creutzfeldt-Jakob disease. Adv. Neurol., 10:341–346, 1975.

Beck, E., et al.: Experimental kuru in the spider monkey: histopathological and ultrastructural studies of the brain during early stages of incubation. Brain, 98:595–620, 1975.

Bertrand, I., Carré, H., and Lucam, F.: La tremblante du mouton. Rec. Méd. Vet., 113:586–603, 1937.

———: La tremblante du mouton. Rec. Méd. Vet., 113:540–561, 1937.

Bignami, A., and Parry, H. B.: Electron microscopic studies of the brain of sheep with natural scrapie. I. The fine structure of neuronal vacuolation. Brain, 95:319–326, 1972.

———: Electron microscopic studies of the brain of sheep with natural scrapie. II. The small nerve processes in neuronal degeneration. Brain, 95:487–499, 1973.

Brownell, B., Campbell, M. J., and Greenham, L. W.: The experimental transmission of Creutzfeldt-Jakob disease. J. Neuropathol. Exp. Neurol., 35:98, 1976.

Brownlee, A.: Histopathological studies of scrapie, an obscure disease of sheep. Br. Vet. J., 96:254–259, 1940.

Bruce, M. E., and Fraser, H.: Amyloid plaques in the brains of mice infected with scrapie: morphological variation and staining properties. Neuropathol. Appl. Neurobiol., 1:189–202, 1975.

Chandler, R. L.: Encephalopathy in mice produced by inoculation with scrapie brain material. Lancet, 1:1378, 1961.

Chandler, R. L.: Observations on the ultrastructure of the spinal cord, spleen and lymph nodes of mice inoculated with scrapie. Res. Vet. Sci., 10:292–293, 1969.

Cho, H. J., et al.: Virus-like particles from both control and scrapie-affected mouse brain. Nature, 267:459–460, 1976.

Cuillé, J., and Chelle, P. L.: La maladie dite tremblante du mouton est-elle inoculable? C. R. Acad. Sci., 203:1552–1554, 1936.

Dickinson, A. G.: Scrapie. Nature, 252:179–180, 1974.

Dickinson, A. G., Stamp, J. T., Renwick, C. C., and Rennie, J. C.: Some factors controlling the incidence of scrapie in Cheviot sheep injected with a Cheviot-passaged scrapie agent. J. Comp. Pathol., 78:313–321, 1968.

Dickinson, A. G., Fraser, H., and Outram, G. W.: Scrapie incubation time can exceed natural lifespan. Nature, 256:732–733, 1975.

Diener, T. O.: Is the scrapie agent a viroid? Nature (New Biol), 235:218–219, 1972.

Diener, T. O.: Viroids: the smallest known agents of infectious disease. Annu. Rev. Microbiol., 28:23–39, 1974.

Espana, C., et al.: Transmission of Creutzfeldt-Jakob disease to the stumptail macaque *(Macaca arctoides)*. Proc. Soc. Exp. Biol. Med., 149:723–724, 1975.

Field, E., and Shenton, B. K.: Rapid diagnosis of scrapie in the mouse. Nature, 240:104–106, 1972.

———: Rapid immunological method for diagnosis of natural scrapie in sheep. Nature, 244:96–97, 1973.

———: A rapid immunologic test for scrapie in sheep. Am. J. Vet. Res., 35:393–395, 1974.

Fuccillo, D. A., Kurent, J. E., and Sever, J. L.: Slow virus diseases. Annu. Rev. Microbiol., 28:231–264, 1974.

Gajdusek, D. C.: Slow-virus infections of the nervous system. N. Engl. J. Med., 276:392–400, 1967.

————: Unconventional viruses and the origin and disappearance of kuru. Science, 197:943–960, 1977.

Gajdusek, D. C., and Gibbs, C. J.: Transmission of two subacute spongiform encephalopathies of man (kuru and Creutzfeldt-Jakob disease) to New World monkeys. Nature, 230:588–591, 1971.

————: Transmission of kuru from man to rhesus monkey (Macaca mulatta) 8½ years after inoculation. Nature, 240:351, 1972.

————: Subacute and chronic diseases caused by atypical infections with unconventional viruses in aberrant hosts. Perspect. Virol., 8:279–311, 1973.

Gajdusek, D. C., Gibbs, C. J., Jr., and Alpers, M. (eds.): Slow, latent, and temperate virus infections. Nat. Inst. Neurological Diseases and Blindness Monographs, No. 2, 1965.

Gibbons, R. A., and Hunter, G. D.: Nature of the scrapie agent. Nature (Lond.), 215:1041–1043, 1967.

Gibbs, C. J., Jr., and Gajdusek, D. C.: Transmission of scrapie to the cynomolgus monkey (Macaca fascicularis). Nature, 236:73–74, 1972.

————: Experimental subacute spongiform virus encephalopathies in primates and other laboratory animals. Science, 182:67–68, 1973.

Griffith, J. S.: Self-replication and scrapie. Nature, 215:1043–1044, 1967.

Hadlow, W. J.: Scrapie and kuru. Lancet, 2:289–290, 1959.

————: The pathology of experimental scrapie in the dairy goat. Res. Vet. Sci., 2:289–314, 1961. VB 549–562.

Haig, D. A., and Clarke, M. C.: Multiplication of the scrapie agent. Nature, 234:106–107, 1971.

Hanson, R. P., et al.: Susceptibility of mink to sheep scrapie. Science, 172:859–861, 1971.

Harcourt, R. A., and Anderson, M. A.: Naturally-occurring scrapie in goats. Vet. Rec., 94:504, 1974.

Herzberg, L., et al.: Creutzfeldt-Jakob disease: hypothesis for high incidence in Libyan Jews in Israel. Science, 186:848, 1974.

Holman, H. H., and Pattison, I. H.: Further evidence on the significance of vacuolated nerve cells in the medulla oblongata of sheep affected with scrapie. J. Comp. Pathol. Ther., 53:231–236, 1940–1943.

Hotchin, J., and Buckley, R.: Latent form of scrapie virus: a new factor in slow-virus disease. Science, 196:668–671, 1977.

Hunter, G. D.: Scrapie. Prog. Med. Virol., 18:289–306, 1974.

Hunter, G. D., Collis, S. C., Millson, G. C., and Kimberlin, R. H.: Search for scrapie-specific RNA and attempts to detect an infectious DNA or RNA. J. Gen. Virol., 32:157–162, 1976.

Lamar, C. H., Gustafson, D. P., Krasovich, M., and Hinsman, E. J.: Ultrastructural studies of spleen, brains, and brain cell cultures of mice with scrapie. Vet. Pathol., 11:13–19, 1974.

Lampert, P., Hooks, J., Gibbs, C. J., Jr., and Gajdusek, D. C.: Altered plasma membranes in experimental scrapie. Acta Neuropathol., 19:81–93, 1971.

Leader, R. W., and Hurvitz, A. I.: Interspecies patterns of slow virus diseases. Annu. Rev. Med., 23:191–200, 1972.

Manuelidis, E. E.: Transmission of Creutzfeldt-Jakob disease from man to the guinea pig. Science, 190:571–572, 1975.

Manuelidis, E. E., et al.: Experimental Creutzfeldt-Jacob disease transmitted via the eye with infected cornea. N. Engl. J. Med., 296:1334–1336, 1977.

Marsh, R. F.: Slow virus diseases of the central nervous system. Adv. Vet. Sci. Comp. Med., 18:155–178, 1974.

Marsh, R. F., and Kimberlin, R. H.: Comparison of scrapie and transmissible mink encephalopathy in hamster. II. Clinical signs, pathology and pathogenesis. J. Infect. Dis., 131:104–110, 1975.

Masters, C. L., et al.: Experimental kuru in the gibbon and sooty mangabey and Creutzfeldt-Jakob disease in the pigtailed macaque. With a summary of the host range of the subacute spongiform virus encephalopathies. J. Med. Primatol., 5:205–209, 1976.

Morris, J. A., and Gajdusek, D. C.: Encephalopathy in mice following inoculation of scrapie sheep brain. Nature (London), 197:1084–1086, 1963.

Mould, D. L., and Smith, W.: The causal agent of scrapie. I. Extraction of the agent from infected sheep tissue. II. From infected goat tissue. J. Comp. Pathol., 72:97–105 and 106–112, 1962.

Narang, H. K.: Virus-like particles in natural scrapie of the sheep. Res. Vet. Sci., 14:108–110, 1973.

————: An electron microscopic study of natural scrapie sheep brain: further observations on virus-like particles and paramyxovirus-like tubules. Acta Neuropathol. (Berl.), 28:317–329, 1974.

Narang, H. K., Shenton, B., Giorgi, P. P., and Field, E. J.: Scrapie agent and neurones. Nature, 240:106–107, 1972.

Palmer, A. C.: Studies in scrapie. Vet. Rec., 69:1318–1328, 1957.

Pattison, I. H., and Jebbett, J. N.: Histopathological similarities between scrapie and cuprizone toxicity in mice. Nature, 230:115–117, 1971.

————: Clinical and histological recovery from the scrapie-like spongiform encephalopathy produced in mice by feeding them with cuprizone. J. Pathol., 109:245–250, 1973.

Pattison, I. H., and Jones, K. M.: The possible nature of the transmissible agent of scrapie. Vet. Rec., 80:2–9, 1967.

Pattison, I. H., Gordon, W. S., and Millson, G. C.: Experimental production of scrapie in goats. J. Comp. Pathol., 69:300–312, 1959.

Perry, H. B.: Scrapie: A transmissible hereditary disease of sheep. Nature (Lond.), 185:441–443, 1960.

Peterson, D. A., et al.: Transmission of kuru and Creutzfeldt-Jakob disease to marmoset monkeys. Intervirology, 2:14–19, 1973/1974.

Schulman, S., Vick, N. A., Blank, N. K., and Fernandez, C.: Transmission of Jakob-Creutzfeldt disease from man to rhesus monkey. J. Neuropathol. Exp. Neurol., 35:117, 1976.

Stockman, S.: Contribution to the study of the disease known as scrapie. J. Comp. Pathol. Ther., 39:42–59, 1926.

Ward, R. L., Porter, D. D., and Stevens, J. G.: Nature of the scrapie agent: evidence against a viroid. J. Virol., 14:1099–1103, 1974.

Wilson, D. R., Anderson, R. D., and Smith, W.: Studies in scrapie. J. Comp. Pathol. Ther., 60:267–282, 1950.

Wright, P. A. L.: The histopathology of the spinal cord in scrapie disease of sheep. J. Comp. Pathol., 70:70–83, 1960.

Zlotnik, I.: The histopathology of the brain stem of sheep affected with experimental scrapie. J. Comp. Pathol., 68:428–438, 1958.

———: The histopathology of the brain of goats affected with scrapie. J. Comp. Pathol., 71:440–448, 1961.

Zlotnik, I., et al.: Further observations on experimental transmission of Creutzfeldt-Jakob disease from man to squirrel and spider monkeys. Neuropathol. Appl. Neurobiol., 2:125–130, 1976.

Mink Encephalopathy

Mink encephalopathy is a transmissible disease of mink that was originally described in Wisconsin, later in Idaho, Ontario, Canada, and East Germany. Although the transmissible agent has not been isolated, it is filterable and unusually resistant to heat, ether, and formaldehyde, similar to the scrapie virus. The incubation period in the experimentally transmitted disease in mink is five to ten months. Ferrets and nonhuman primates can be experimentally infected.

The clinical signs are characterized by slowly progressive locomotor incoordination, excitability, late somnolence, and occasionally convulsions. Death follows a course of three to eight weeks. Lesions are restricted to the central nervous system, where widespread neuronal degeneration and marked astrogliosis are found in the cerebrum, cerebellum, and brainstem. The gray matter may have a spongy appearance. Neurons, especially in the cerebellar peduncles, may contain cytoplasmic vacuoles similar to those seen in scrapie.

Burger, D., and Hartsough, G. R.: Encephalopathy of mink. II. Experimental and natural transmission. J. Infect. Dis., 115:393–399, 1965.

———: Transmissible encephalopathy of mink. Nat. Inst. Neurol. Dis. and Blindness Monograph No. 2: 297–305, 1965.

Eckroade, R. J., Zu Rhein, G. M., Marsh, R. F., and Hanson, R. P.: Transmissible mink encephalopathy: Experimental transmission to the squirrel monkey. Science, 169:1088–1090, 1970.

Grabow, J. D., et al.: Transmissible mink encephalopathy agent in squirrel monkeys. Serial electroencephalographic, clinical and pathologic studies. Neurology (Minneap.), 23:820–832, 1973.

Hartsough, G. R., and Burger, D.: Encephalopathy of mink. I. Epizoologic and clinical observations. J. Infect. Dis., 115:387–392, 1965.

Hartung, J., Zimmermann, H., and Johannsen, U.: Infektiöse Enzephalopathie beim Nerz. 1. Mitteilung: Klinisch-epizootiologische und experimentelle Untersuchungen. Mh. Vet. Med., 25:385–388, 1970.

Johannsen U., and Hartung, J.: Infektiöse Enzephalopathie beim Nerz. 2. Mitteilung: Pathologisch-morphologische Untersuchungen. Mh. Vet. Med., 25:389–395, 1970.

Marsh, R. F., et al.: A preliminary report on the experimental host range of the transmissible mink encephalopathy agent. J. Infect. Dis., 120:713–719, 1969.

Marsh, R. F., Miller, J. M., and Hanson, R. P.: Transmissible mink encephalopathy: studies on the peripheral lymphocyte. Infect. Immun., 7:352–355, 1973.

Marsh, R. F., and Hanson, R. P.: Transmissible mink encephalopathy: Infectivity of corneal epithelium. Science, 187:656, 1975.

Marsh, R. F., Sipe, J. C., Morse, S. S., and Hanson, R. P.: Transmissible mink encephalopathy. Reduced spongiform degeneration in aged mink of the Chediak-Higashi genotype. Lab. Invest., 34:381–386, 1976.

ZuRhein, G. M., Eckroade, R., and Marsh, R. F.: Experimental transmissible mink encephalopathy (TME) in mink, monkey, and hamster. Electron microscopic studies. J. Neuropathol. Exp. Neurol., 30:124, 1971.

Borna Disease

A viral encephalitis principally affecting horses, which occurs in Europe but not in the Western Hemisphere, derives its name from Borna, in Saxony (Germany), where a severe outbreak was first described. In Bavaria, however, the disease is known as *Kopfkrankheit*. Although caused by a different virus, the lesions are similar in type and distribution to those in western equine encephalomyelitis. Acidophilic intranuclear inclusion bodies (**Joest bodies**) are found in neurons, particularly in the hippocampus, and are considered by some to be quite specific. Definite diagnosis, however, is based upon demonstration of the virus or viral antibodies. Natural infection with the virus also occurs in sheep. Rabbits, which are easily infected, are useful as experimental subjects.

In contrast to other equine viral encephalitides, an insect vector is not needed for transmission and the disease is not seasonal.

The causative agent has been established as a virus, but its exact taxonomic position among viruses has not been established. It has been compared to "slow viruses" because of the long incubation period and progressive nature of the disease. With the electron microscope, crystalline arrays have been described, as well as some clusters of filaments. The identity of these structures in relation to the virus has not been established. The large granular inclusions seen in Borna disease have not been proved to be associated with the virus.

Anzil, A. P., and Blinzinger, K.: Electron microscopic studies of rabbit central and peripheral nervous system in experimental Borna disease. Acta Neuropathol. (Berl.), 22:305–318, 1972.

Anzil, A. P., Blinzinger, K., and Mayr, A.: Persistent Borna virus infection in adult hamsters. Arch. Ges. Virusforsch., 40:52–57, 1973.

Blinzinger, K., and Anzil, A. P.: Large granular nuclear bodies (karyosphaeridia) in experimental Borna virus infection. J. Comp. Pathol., 83:589–596, 1973.

Cohrs, P.: Das Nervensystem. In Lehrbuch der Speziellen Pathologischen Anatomie der Haustiere, 3rd ed., edited by K. Nieberle and P. Cohrs. Jena, Fischer, 1949, pp. 455–456.

Joest, E., and Degen, K.: Über eigentümliche Kerneinschlüsse der Ganglienzellen bei der enzootische Gehirn-Rückenmarksentzündung der Pferde. Z. Infectionkr., 6:348–356, 1909.

Ludwig, H., Becht, H., and Groh, L.: Borna disease (BD), a slow virus infection. Biological properties of the virus. Med. Microbiol. Immunol. (Berl.), 158:275–289, 1973.

Nicolau, S., and Galloway, I. A.: L-Encephalo-Myélite Enzootique Expérimentale (Maladie de Borna). Ann. Inst. Pasteur, 44:457–523 and 673–696, 1930.

Seifried, O., and Spatz, H.: Die Ausbreitung der encephalitischen Reaktion bei der Bornaschen Krankheit der Pferde und deren Beziehungen zu die Encephalitis epidemica, der Heine-Medinschen Krankheit und der Lyssa des Menschen. Z. Neurol. Psychiat., 124:317–382, 1930.

Aleutian Disease of Mink

A few years ago breeders of mink found that unusual colors in mink fur could bring a premium in the market place. This led to the selection of animals with any of several mutant genes which in the homozygous state could result in a coat color different from the wild type. One of the first of these unusual coats was a blue color, due to a single recessive gene, which came to be called "Aleutian." After animals with this color became reasonably numerous, a serious disease appeared among them—hence the name "Aleutian disease." It is now known that other types of mink are also susceptible, but most natural cases occur in Aleutian or sapphire mink (the latter are homozygous for the Aleutian gene [a] and for another mutant gene [p] as well). The disease is more rapidly progressive in mink homozygous for the Aleutian gene than in non-Aleutian type mink, in which the disease is more protracted, lasting several months or years. The increased susceptibility of mink homozygous for the Aleutian gene is believed to be explained in part in that all such mink have an inherited anomaly of granule-producing cells designated the Chediak-Higashi syndrome.

Hartsough is credited by Helmboldt and Jungherr (1958) with first recognizing the disease in 1946, and one of the first reports was by Hartsough and Gorham (1956). The disease is known in all parts of the world in which mink are raised.

The etiologic agent is a virus with buoyant density in CeCl of 1.37 to 1.38; virions are about 23 nm in diameter, and some have a ring structure. It has been suggested that the virus should be considered a member of the Parvovirus genus, but its nucleic acid has not yet been clearly identified, hence it is presently considered as unclassified (Chesebro, et al., 1975). This situation may soon change as methods to purify the virus are developed.

The virus is transmitted by contact and is present in saliva and urine. "Vertical" transmission also occurs through the placenta to the fetus. Viremia usually persists throughout the course of the disease.

Signs. The disease is manifest in affected mink by lethargy, anorexia, cachexia, and occasionally with fever, which may reach 107° F. Blood often exudes from the mouth and sometimes from the anus. Young kits tend to die within a few days after signs of illness are seen, but most adults live for several weeks. Some may survive for many months, but among animals which show signs, 90% or more can be expected to die.

There is a progressive thrombocytopenia and anemia. The anemia is believed to result from hemorrhage associated with defective hemostasis and depression of erythropoiesis secondary to uremia. The thrombocytopenia has been shown to result from episodic intravascular coagulation with removal of fibrinogen and platelets from the circulation. Intravascular coagulation with deposition of incompletely polymerized fibrin in glomeruli is believed to play an important role in the pathogenesis of glomerular lesions in Aleutian disease, although the glomerulonephritis may represent a form of immune-complex disease.

Of particular interest is the severe hypergammaglobulinemia, first reported by Henson et al. (1961) and subsequently confirmed by others. The changes in the serum proteins are the result of elevation in the gamma globulin fraction, due to increase in the 7 S components of euglobulin. In normal pastel or Aleutian mink, gamma globulin constitutes 15 to 20% of the serum proteins. In mink affected with Aleutian disease, the gamma globulin may constitute as much as 65% of the serum proteins. The highest levels of gamma globulin are found in those cases with the most widespread accumulation of plasma cells in the tissues, a point to be described later.

Lesions. The lesions of Aleutian disease are characterized chiefly by disseminated focal accumulations of plasma cells in several organs; hyaline and inflammatory changes in the walls of small arteries; dilatation and proliferation of intrahepatic bile ducts; focal or diffuse interstitial fibrosis of the kidneys, glomerulonephritis, hemorrhages and focal encephalomalacia with nonsuppurative leptomeningitis. The large number of plasma cells in the tissues is a consistent feature of the disease and is undoubtedly the source of the excessive gamma globulins found in the serum. Obel (1959) considered these plasma cells to be neoplastic but it must be realized that these cells appear quite well differentiated and do not usually compress, invade and displace normal tissue as decisively as frankly neoplastic cells can be seen to do. According to Helmboldt and Jungherr (1958), the lesions, consisting largely of plasma cells and lymphocytes, were found in a series of 40 cases in the following organs: liver (85 per cent), brain (80 per cent), kidney (60 per cent) and lung (48 per cent). Arteritis was noted in small arteries in about 28 per cent of their cases. These lesions were characterized by hyalin changes in the media, infiltration of media and adventitia by lymphoid cells and eventual occlusion of the lumen with hyalin. These changes are indistinguishable from those of periarteritis nodosa. In severely diseased mink, plasma cell infiltration and arteritis may be found in any organ or tissue. The kidneys not only contain arterial lesions and accumulations of lymphocytes and plasma cells, but focal or diffuse fibrosis of the interstitial tissues may be evident. Glomerular tufts may be thickened due to deposition of a hyalin PAS-positive material, and some convoluted tubules may be distended with protein. Leader (1963), and Henson and co-workers (1967, 1968) have described the pathogenesis and ultrastructural features of the renal lesions.

The gross lesions conform to those one would expect to result from the microscopic lesions in arteries. Small (3 mm.) ulcers are often found in the mouth, particularly on the gums and buccal mucosa and may be covered with a diphtheritic membrane. The kidneys are often three times normal size, pale orange to yellow color, frequently mottled with white punctate areas. Stellar hemorrhages may be seen in the renal capsule which is not usually adherent to the underlying cortex. The liver may be enlarged as much as twice normal size and have a mahogany color. The spleen is enlarged from twice to five times its normal size but otherwise not remarkable grossly. The lungs may contain patches of red color which are visible on the surface and extend deeply into the parenchyma. In a few cases, the colon may contain free blood and in others, the tissues may be obviously anemic.

The pathogenesis of Aleutian disease has received considerable attention in recent years. An immunologic basis for lesions in arterioles and glomeruli seems likely from the following evidence: Immune complexes consisting of viral antigen, immunoglobulin (IgG), and complement (C3) are deposited in glomerular capillary walls and mesangium, presumably associated with the high level of circulating IgG and probably immune complexes. The lesions in arterioles in mink infected with the virus may be completely suppressed by the administration of an immunosuppressive drug, cyclophosphamide (Cheema et al., 1972). The presence of very high complement-fixing titers to viral antigen in infected mink indicates that the elevated circulating level of immunoglobulin (IgG) is probably the result of stimulation of plasma cells by viral antigens.

The occurrence of lymphoreticular proliferation, simulating lymphoma or Hodgkin's disease in children, is mimicked in Aleutian mink infected with the Aleutian disease virus. These mink, which are homozygous for the Chediak-Higashi syndrome, therefore simulate the human disease in several respects (Hadlow et al., 1972).

Diagnosis. The diagnosis of Aleutian disease can be made with certainty from the histologic lesions which are distinguishable from infection with avian tubercle bacilli (granulomas containing acid-fast bacilli), canine distemper (cytoplasmic and intranuclear inclusion bodies), and steatitis (inflammation and ceroid pigment in adipose tissues). The hypergammaglobulinemia is also useful to confirm presumptive diagnosis based upon clinical signs.

Basrur, P. K., Gray, D. P., and Karstad, L.: Aleutian disease (plasmacytosis) of mink. III. Propagation of the virus in mink tissue cultures. Can. J. Comp. Med. Vet. Sci., 27:301–306, 1963.
Bazeley, P. L.: The nature of Aleutian disease in mink. I. Two forms of hypergammaglobulinemia as related to method of disease transmission and type of lesion. J. Infect. Dis., 134:252–270, 1976.
Chapman, I., and Jimenez, F. A.: Aleutian-mink disease in man. N. Engl. J. Med., 269:1171–1174, 1963.
Cheema, A., Henson, J. B., and Gorham, J. R.: Aleutian disease of mink. Prevention of lesions by immunosuppression. Am. J. Pathol. 66:543–556, 1972.
Chesebro, B., Bloom, M., Hadlow, W., and Race, R.: Purification and ultrastructure of Aleutian disease virus of mink. Nature, 254:456–457, 1975.
Cho. H. J., and Ingram, D. G.: Pathogenesis of Aleutian disease of mink: nature of the antiglobulin reaction and elution of antibody from erythrocytes and glomeruli of infected mink. Infect. Immun., 8:264–271, 1973.
Drommer, W., and Trautwein, G.: Pathogenesis of Aleutian disease in the mink. VII. Chronic hepatitis with proliferation of bile ducts. Vet. Pathol., 12:77–93, 1975.
Eklund, C. M., et al.: Aleutian disease of mink: properties of the etiologic agent and the host responses. J. Infect. Dis., 118:510–526, 1968.
Gorham, J. R., Leader, R. W., and Henson, J. B.: Neutralizing ability of hypergammaglobulinemia serum on the Aleutian disease virus of mink. Fed. Proc., 22:265, 1963.
Goudas, P., Karstad, L., and Tabel, H.: Ultraviolet inactivation of the infective agent of Aleutian disease of mink. Can. J. Comp. Med., 34:118–121, 1970.
Hadlow, W. J., Race, R. E., and Jackson, T. A.: Lymphoreticular proliferative disease in mink homozygous for the Aleutian gene. J. Natl. Cancer Inst., 49:1455–1457, 1972.
Hartsough, G. R., and Gorham, J. R.: Aleutian disease in mink. Nat. Fur News, 28:10–11, 38, 1956.
Helmboldt, C. F., and Jungherr, E. L.: The pathology of Aleutian disease in mink. Am. J. Vet. Res., 19:212–222, 1958.

Henson, J. B., Leader, R. W., Gorham, J. R., and Padgett, G. A.: The sequential development of lesions in spontaneous Aleutian disease of mink. Pathol. Vet., *3*:289–314, 1966.

———: The sequential development of ultrastructural lesions in the glomeruli of mink with experimental Aleutian disease. Lab. Invest., *19*:153–162, 1968.

Henson, J. B., Gorham, J. R., and Tanaka, Y.: Renal glomerular ultrastructure in mink affected by Aleutian disease. Lab. Invest., *17*:123–139, 1967.

Henson, J. B., Leader, R. W., and Gorham, J. R.: Hypergammaglobulinemia in mink. Proc. Soc. Exp. Biol. Med., *107*:919–920, 1961.

Henson, J. B., Gorham, J. R., Leader, R. W., and Wagner, B. M.: Experimental hypergammaglobulinemia in mink. J. Exp. Med., *116*:357–364, 1962.

Johnson, M. I., Henson, J. B., and Gorham, J. R.: The influence of genotype on the development of glomerular lesions in mink with Aleutian disease virus. Am. J. Pathol., *81*:321–336, 1975.

Karstad, L.: Aleutian disease. A slowly progressive viral infection of mink. Curr. Top. Microbiol. Immunol., *40*:9–21, 1967.

Karstad, L., and Pridham, T. J.: Aleutian disease of mink. 1. Evidence of its viral etiology. Can. J. Comp. Med. Vet. Sci., *26*:97–102, 1962.

Kenyon, A. J., Trautwein, G., and Helmboldt, C. F.: Characterization of blood serum proteins from mink with Aleutian disease. Am. J. Vet. Res., *24*:168–173, 1963.

Kenyon, A. J., Helmboldt, C. F., and Nielsen, S. W.: Experimental transmission of Aleutian disease with urine. Am. J. Vet. Res., *24*:1066–1067, 1963.

Kenyon, A. J., and Helmboldt, C. F.: Solubility and electrophoretic characterizations of globulins from mink with Aleutian disease. Am. J. Vet. Res., *25*:1535–1541, 1964.

Leader, R. W., Wagner, B. M., Henson, J. B., and Gorham, J. R.: Structural and histochemical observations of liver and kidney in Aleutian disease of mink. Am. J. Pathol., *43*:33–53, 1963.

McGuire, T. C., Crawford, T. B., Henson, J. B., and Gorham, J. R.: Aleutian disease of mink: detection of large quantities of complement-fixing antibody to viral antigen. J. Immunol., *107*:1481–1482, 1971.

McKay, D. G., Phillips, L. L., Kaplan, H., and Henson, J. B.: Chronic intravascular coagulation in Aleutian disease of mink. Am. J. Pathol., *50*:899–916, 1967.

Obel, A-L.: Studies on a disease in mink with systemic proliferation of the plasma cells. Am. J. Vet. Res., *20*:384–393, 1959.

Padgett, G. A., Gorham, J. R., and Henson, J. B.: Epizootiologic studies of Aleutian disease. I. Transplacental transmission of the virus. J. Infect. Dis., *117*:35–38, 1967.

Pan, I. C., Tsai, K. S., and Karstad, L.: Glomerulonephritis in Aleutian disease of mink: histological and immunofluorescence studies. J. Pathol., *101*:119–127, 1970.

Pan, I. C., Tsai, K. S., Grinyer, I., and Karstad, L.: Glomerulonephritis in Aleutian disease of mink:

ultrastructural studies. J. Pathol., *102*:33–40, 1970.

Porter, D. D., Larsen, A. E., and Porter, H. G.: The pathogenesis of Aleutian disease of mink. III. Immune complex arteritis. Am. J. Pathol., *71*:331–344, 1973.

Porter, D. D., and Larsen, A. E.: Aleutian disease of mink. Prog. Med. Virol., *18*:32–47, 1974.

Sung, J. H., and Okada, K.: Neuronal inclusions in Aleutian mink: a light and electron microscopic study. J. Neuropathol. Exp. Neurol., *28*:160–161, 1969.

Trautwein, G. W. and Helmboldt, C. F.: Aleutian disease of mink. 1. Experimental transmission of the disease. Am. J. Vet. Res., *23*:1280–1288, 1962.

Wagner, B. M.: Aleutian disease of mink. Arthritis Rheum., *6*:386–391, 1963.

Marburg Virus Disease (Vervet Monkey Disease)

First described in 1967 in Marburg and Frankfurt, Germany, and Belgrade, Yugoslavia, Marburg virus disease is principally of importance as an infection of man contracted from Vervet monkeys (African green monkey; *Cercopithecus aethiops*). Of thirty cases reported in 1967, seven were fatal. The majority of cases occurred in laboratory workers in contact with monkey tissues; four occurred in hospital personnel caring for the patients. Following an incubation period of five to seven days, the clinical course was characterized by fever, headache, backache, prostration, vomiting, diarrhea, and an exanthematous rash. The rash later became hemorrhagic, and bleeding developed in the lungs and gastrointestinal tract. Pathologic findings were dominated by widespread focal necrosis, especially of the liver, lymphatic tissues, kidney, pancreas, adrenal glands, and skin. Nonsuppurative encephalitis with glial nodules and hemorrhage was also present.

The agent, although apparently a virus, has not at present been fully characterized or classified. However, the isolate, as well as human patient tissues, were highly virulent for Vervet monkeys and also for rhesus monkeys (*Macaca mulatta*), squirrel monkeys (*Saimiri sciureus*), guinea pigs, and hamsters. The disease, which is uniformly fatal, mimics the picture seen in man. In guinea pigs and hamsters, intracyto-plasmic granules believed to represent the infective agent are found in hepatocytes and epithelial cells of the kidney and lung. Infected animals excrete infectious material and all tissues are infective. The disease has developed in uninoculated monkeys housed with experimentally infected animals.

The virus has been observed with the electron microscope to consist of tubular structures which may become numerous in infected cells. These tubules measure about 55 nm in diameter, containing an electron-lucent axial channel measuring about 20 nm in diameter. These filaments often become closely-packed in parallel arrays, forming an inclusion visible by the light microscope (Murphy et al., 1971).

Bechtelsheimer, H., Jacob, H., and Solcher, H.: Zur Neuropathologie der Dursch Grune Meerkatzen (Cercopithecus aethiops) Ubertragenen Infektionskrankheiten in Marburg. Dtsche. Med. Wochenschr., 93:602–604, 1968.

————: The neuropathology of an infectious disease transmitted by African green monkeys (Cercopithecus aethiops). Germ. Med. Mth., 14:10–12, 1969.

Bowen, E. T. W., et al.: Vervet monkey disease: studies on some physical and chemical properties of the causative agent. Br. J. Exp. Pathol., 50:400–407, 1969.

Gedigk, P., Bechtelsheimer, H., and Korb, G.: Die pathologische Anatomie der "Marburg-Virus"—Krankheit (sog. "Marburger Affenkrankheit"). Dtsch. Med. Wochenschr., 93:590–601, 1968.

Hofmann, H., and Kunz, C.: Ein mauspathogener Stamm des "Marburg-Virus" (Rhabdovirus simiae). Arch. Ges. Virusforsch., 32:244–248, 1970.

Kalter, S. S., Ratner, J. J., and Heberling, R. L.: Antibodies in primates to the Marburg virus. Proc. Soc. Exp. Biol. Med., 130:10–12, 1969.

Kissling, R. E., Robinson, R. Q., Murphy, F. A., and Whitfield, S. G.: Agent of disease contracted from green monkeys. Science, 160:888–890, 1968.

Korb, G., Bechtelsheimer, H., and Gedigk, P.: Die Wichtigsten Histologischen Befunde Bei der Marburg Virus Krankheit. Jahrgang, 19:1089–1096, 1968.

Maass, G., Haas, R., and Oehlert, W.: Experimental infections of monkeys with the causative agent of the Frankfurt-Marburg syndrome (FMS). Lab. Anim. Handb., 4:155–165, 1969.

Martini, G. A.: Marburg virus disease. Postgrad. Med. J., 49:542–546, 1973.

————: Marburg agent disease: in man. Trans. R. Soc. Trop. Med. Hyg., 63:295–302, 1969.

Monath, T. P.: Lassa fever and Marburg virus disease. WHO Chron., 28:212–219 1974.

Murphy, F. A., et al.: Marburg virus infection in monkeys: ultrastructural studies. Lab. Invest., 24:279–291, 1971.

Murphy, F. A., Simpson, D. I. H., and Whitfield, S. G.: Marburg virus infection in monkeys. Ultrastructural studies. Med. Chir. Dig., 1:325–332, 1972.

Saenz, A. C.: Disease in laboratory personnel associated with vervet monkeys. I. A general report on the outbreak. Primates Med., 3:129–134, 1969.

Siegert, R., Shu, H. L., and Slenczka, W.: Isolierung und Identifizierung des "Marburg-virus." Dtsch. Med. Wochenschr., 93:604–612, 1968.

Simpson, D. I. H.: Vervet monkey disease: transmission to the hamster. Br. J. Exp. Pathol., 50:389–392, 1969.

Simpson, D. I. H., Zlotnik, I., and Rutter, D. A.: Vervet monkey disease. Experimental infection of guinea pigs and monkeys with the causative agent. Br. J. Exp. Pathol., 49:458–464, 1968.

Simpson, D. I. H.: Marburg virus disease: experimental infection of monkeys. Lab. Anim. Handb., 4:149–154, 1969.

————: Marburg agent disease: in monkeys. Trans. R. Soc. Trop. Med. Hyg., 63:303–309, 1969.

Zlotnik, I., Simpson, D. I. H., and Howard, D. M. R.: Structure of the vervet-monkey disease agent. Lancet, 2:26–28, 1968.

Zlotnik, I.: Marburg agent disease: pathology. Trans. R. Soc. Trop. Med. Hyg., 63:310–327, 1969.

Zlotnik, I., and Simpson, D. I. H.: The pathology of experimental vervet monkey disease in hamsters. Br. J. Exp. Pathol., 50:393–399, 1969.

CHAPTER 10

Diseases Caused by Mycoplasmatales, Rickettsiales and Spirochaetales

In this chapter, consideration is given to diseases caused by infectious organisms that are not clearly defined as viruses (Chapter 9), simple bacteria (Chapter 11), higher bacteria, fungi (Chapter 12), or protozoa (Chapter 13). Organisms classified in the Orders Mycoplasmatales, Rickettsiales, and Spirochaetales each have distinctive characteristics that determine their pathogenicity, hence it is appropriate to consider them together. Pathogens in each order will be discussed briefly, followed by more detailed consideration of each disease produced by pathogenic species.

The relationships of the organisms to be considered and their current classification are depicted in Table 10–1.

MYCOPLASMOSIS

The infectious agent involved in contagious bovine pleuropneumonia was first recognized by Nocard and Roux (1898) who were able to demonstrate the tiny organisms from infected bovine lungs by culturing them in celloidin bags implanted in the peritoneal cavity of rabbits. The organisms were seen undergoing brownian motion under the light microscope, and were later proved to cause the disease in susceptible cattle. This organism is now called *Myco-*

plasma mycoides (or *M. mycoides mycoides*), and it is the type species of the genus *Mycoplasma.*

Organisms of this genus are now considered to be the smallest free-living microbes that can be passed through bacteria-retaining filters. They grow on agar media without living cells, forming small, microscopically visible, disc-shaped colonies with a dark, thicker center and lighter colored periphery. The electron microscope reveals the organisms to be pleomorphic, with no definite cell wall. This feature has caused the order of Mycoplasmatales to be placed in a special category—Class IV, Mollicutes (meaning soft skin). The organisms form elongated branching shapes in which may be seen ovoid to round structures, which give the filaments a beaded appearance. These are sometimes called "elementary bodies," representing a reproductive stage of the organism.

Mycoplasma may be saprophytic, as is *M. laidlawii (Acholeplasma laidlawii)*, originally isolated from sewage.

For many years the awkward name "pleuropneumonia-like-organism" or "PPLO" was applied to all *Mycoplasma* other than the causative agent of bovine pleuropneumonia. Fortunately, specific

Table 10–1.   Classification of Organisms

Order:	Mycoplasmatales
Family:	Mycoplasmataceae
Genus:	*Mycoplasma*
Order:	Spirochaetales
Family:	Spirochaetaceae
Genera:	*Leptospira*
	Treponema
	Borrelia
	Spirochaeta
Order:	Rickettsiales
Family:	Rickettsiaceae
Genera:	*Rickettsia*
	Rochalimaea
	Coxiella
	Cowdria
	Erhlichia
	Neorickettsia
Family:	Bartonellaceae
Genera:	*Bartonella*
	Grahamella
Family:	Anaplasmataceae
Genera:	*Anaplasma*
	Paraanaplasma
	Aegyptianella
	Haemobartonella
	Eperythrozoon
Order:	Chlamydiales
Family:	Chlamydiaceae
Genus:	*Chlamydia*

names are now available for most identifiable organisms in this genus. PPLO still remains in the older literature and may emerge to confound the newcomer.

Identification of species of organisms within the genus *Mycoplasma* is based on several characteristics, including type of growth on specific media (appearance of colonies, turbidity in liquid media, hemolysis by some species, pH in glucose broth), microscopic morphology, pathogenicity in animals, and using specific antiserum, the growth inhibition test (using paper disc), complement-fixation test, agar gel precipitation, or agglutination tests. Details of these tests may be found in Hayflick (1969) and Maramorosch (1973).

Organisms now classified as Mycoplasmatales have been associated with true viruses that grow in colonies of *Mycoplasma*. The first viral strains isolated in this category, called Mycoplasmatales viruses, contain DNA as their nucleic acid, and their growth may be inhibited by specific antiserum. The role of these viruses in animal disease has not been established at the time this is written (Maramorosch, 1973).

Several species of *Mycoplasma* have been isolated from animals, and the number recovered from human beings is increasing. Unfortunately, not all species of named organisms have been compared with one another, hence interrelationships of organisms within the genus are essentially unknown. Some organisms that produce very small colonies on agar have been isolated from man and animals. These organisms, called T-mycoplasma (T is for "tiny"), seem to fit in the Family Mycoplasmataceae, but some believe they should be placed in a separate genus. One of the distinctive features of these T-mycoplasms (also called *Ureaplasma*) is their need for urea in the growth medium.

One point of interest is the occurrence of tiny pleomorphic forms in the cycle of certain bacteria, so-called **L-forms** or **L-phase**. The L-phase organisms were first recognized by Dr. Kleineberger-Nobel in 1935 in cultures of *Streptobacillus moniliformis*. She coined the term L-form after the Lister Institute where her discovery was made. It is currently believed that these L-forms do not represent a transitional stage between bacteria and mycoplasma. Therefore, the term L-phase of bacteria is more appropriate.

Freundt, E. A.: Present status of the medical importance of mycoplasmas. Pathol. Microbiol., 40:155–187, 1974.

Hayflick, L. (ed.): The Myoplasmatales and the L-Phase of Bacteria. New York, Appleton-Century-Crofts, 1969.

Hill, L. R.: Prospective for mycoplasma classification using multivariate analysis methods. Med. Microbiol. Immunol., 157:101–112, 1972.

Maramorosch, K. (ed.): Mycoplasma and mycoplasma-like agents of human, animal, and plant diseases. Ann. NY Acad. Sci., 225:5–532, 1973.

Neimark, H. C.: Division of mycoplasmas into subgroups. J. Gen. Microbiol., 63:249–263, 1971.

Bovine Pleuropneumonia

This infectious disease of cattle is caused by a specific organism, currently called *Mycoplasma mycoides* (Novak, 1929). Some of the synonyms for this organism are: "pleuropneumonia organism," *Asterococcus mycoides* (Borrell, 1910), *Coccobacillus mycoides peripneumoniae* (Martiznovski, 1911), *Micromyces peripneumoniae bovis contagiosae* (Frosch, 1923), *Mycoplasma peripneumoniae* (Novak, 1929), *Astromyces peripneumoniae bovis* (Wroblewski, 1931), and *Borrelomyces peripneumoniae* (Turner, Campbell and Dick, 1935).

A similar pleuropneumonia in goats is caused by an organism now classified as *Mycoplasma mycoides* var. *capri*.

The disease has been known as a specific entity for over 200 years. In the nineteenth century it spread from Europe to many parts of the world, including the United States. It was eliminated from this country before 1892 by an intensive campaign involving slaughter and quarantine of infected and exposed animals, and fortunately it has not reappeared. About 1854, the disease was introduced from Holland into South Africa, where it spread rapidly, causing the death of over 100,000 cattle in a two-year period. It has remained an extremely important disease in Africa, second only to rinderpest as an economic problem. At present, the disease is distributed over much of the world with the exception of the western hemisphere. A feature that adds to the difficulty of controlling the spread of pleuropneumonia is that it may exist in a symptomless form in some animals which, nonetheless, are carriers.

The disease affects cattle primarily, although buffalo, goats, and sheep apparently are susceptible to artificial infection. Mice, rabbits, guinea pigs, horses, camels, and swine are not susceptible.

Signs. In the typical case, after a prolonged and variable incubation period, the animal exhibits pneumonia, which clinically is indistinguishable from that of nonspecific etiology. In the acute stage, a dry and painful cough, which later becomes moist, is followed by labored respiration with grunting, halting expiration.

Table 10–2. Diseases Due to Mycoplasmas

Disease	Genus and Species
Bovine pleuropneumonia	*Mycoplasma mycoides* v. *mycoides*
Other bovine mycoplasmoses:	
Mastitis	*M. agalactiae* v. *bovis*
Seminal vesiculitis and epididymitis	*M. bovigenitalium*
Infectious bovine keratoconjunctivitis	*M. bovoculi*
Enzootic pneumonia of calves	*M. bovirhinis, M. dispar,* T-mycoplasma, *Ureaplasma* sp.
Contagious caprine pleuropneumonia	*M. mycoides* v. *capri*
Contagious agalactia of goats and sheep	*M. agalactiae*
Other mycoplasmoses in goats and sheep:	
pneumonia	*M. ovipneumoniae, M. arginini*
arthritis, pleuritis and pericarditis	*Mycoplasma* sp.
keratoconjunctivitis	*Mycoplasma* sp.
Murine chronic respiratory disease	*M. pulmonis*
Murine mycoplasmal arthritis	*M. arthritidis*
Mycoplasmal arthritis and polyserositis in swine	*M. hyosynoviae, M. hyorhinis*
Enzootic mycoplasmal pneumonia of swine	*M. hyopneumoniae, M. hyorhinis*

When the lungs are extensively involved, respiratory distress is exhibited by dyspnea so severe that the animal stands with its elbows turned out. In the later stages, there may be mucopurulent discharge from the nose and sometimes edematous infiltration of the lower thorax. Weakness and emaciation usually become apparent, and swelling of the joints (polyarthritis) is sometimes seen in young calves. The organism may invade the placenta and fetus, resulting in abortion.

Lesions. In the typical case of pleuropneumonia, the lesions of the lung are characteristic. They usually are limited to one lung, occasionally are bilateral, but never symmetrically involve contralateral lungs. The pleural cavity over the affected lung usually contains an excess of pleural fluid, which may be blood-stained and include strands of fibrin; as a rule, the pleura is adherent to the thoracic wall at some points. The parenchyma does not collapse when the thorax is opened but remains firm and raised above the relatively normal adjacent lung tissue. The cut surface has a marbled appearance, with red and grayish areas of parenchyma separated by thick yellowish interlobular septa. The presence of unequally distended lymph spaces often imparts a "beaded" appearance to these septa. In cases of long standing, zones of necrosis within groups of lobules tend to become sequestrated from the adjacent lung and surrounded by a dense layer of connective tissue. Within these sequestra, which often are large, the original configuration of lung parenchyma may be retained for a time. Eventually abscesses may form in the encapsulated tissue, and their rupture may cause an acute exacerbation of the symptoms, or the entire sequestrum may be converted to scar tissue.

The outstanding histologic characteristic of the lung is the separation of the lobules into distinct compartments by the heavily thickened interlobular septa, in which there is not only edema but organization as well. The lobules contain areas in which the alveoli are patent, although they are completely consolidated in many others. A particularly intense infiltration of round cells, chiefly lymphocytes and plasma cells, is seen around blood vessels and bronchi. Similar focal collections of leukocytes are found within the interlobular septa.

The lesions in other organs are not specific for this disease, but the liver may be infiltrated by round cells in the hepatic triads, with necrosis of individual liver cells near central veins. These necrotic liver cells are acidophilic, have dark pyknotic nuclei, and are believed by some to be the result of gradual anoxia. In the spleen, the germinal centers may be enlarged, mature lymphocytes decreased in number, plasma cells increased, and red blood cells and blood pigment present in excessive amounts.

Diagnosis. The diagnosis may be established by the history, the clinical symptoms, the gross and microscopic lesions, and recovery of the organism. A complement fixation test can also be used to establish the nature of the infection in acute cases, but it is less significant in long-standing cases because the complement-fixing antibody gradually decreases in titer.

Cottew, G. S., and Leach, R. H.: Mycoplasmas of cattle, sheep and goats. *In* The Mycoplasmatales and the L-Phase of Bacteria, edited by L. Hayflick. New York, Appleton-Century-Crofts, 1969. pp. 527–570.

Daubney, R.: Contagious bovine pleuropneumonia. Note on experimental reproduction and infection by contact. J. Comp. Pathol. Ther., *48*:83–96, 1935.

Johnston, L. A. Y., and Simmons, G. C.: Bovine pneumonias in Queensland with particular reference to the diagnosis of contagious bovine pleuropneumonia. Aust. Vet. J., *39*:290–294, 1963. VB 823–64.

Masiga, W. N., Windsor, R. S., and Read, W. C. S.: A new mode of spread of contagious bovine pleuropneumonia. Vet. Rec., *90*:247–248, 1972.

Mettam, R. W. M.: Contagious pleuropneumonia of goats in East Africa. Pan African Agri. Vet. Conf., Bul. 8E, 1929.

Nocard, E., and Roux, E. R.: Le Microbe de la péripneumonia. Ann. Inst. Pasteur (Paris), *12*:240–262, 1898.

Oghiso, Y., et al.: Pathological studies on bovine pneumonia in special references to isolation of mycoplasmas. Jpn. J. Vet. Sci., 38:15–24, 1976.

Piercy, D. W.: Synovitis induced by intra-articular inoculation of inactivated *Mycoplasma mycoides* in calves. J. Comp. Pathol., 80:549–558, 1970.

Piercy, D. W. T., and Bingley, J. B.: Fibrinous synovitis in calves inoculated with killed *Mycoplasma mycoides*. Elevated plasma fibrinogen concentration and increased permeability of the synovium. J. Comp. Pathol., 82:279–290, 1972.

Piercy, D. W. T.: Reaction to killed *Mycoplasma mycoides* in joints in specifically sensitized calves. J. Comp. Pathol., 82:291–294, 1972.

Thomas, C. L., and Hidalgo, R. J.: Comparison of three methods of differentiating bovine mycoplasma. Am. J. Vet. Res., 39:519–522, 1978.

Windsor, R. S., Masiga, W. N., and Boarer, C. D. H.: A single comparative intradermal test for the diagnosis of contagious bovine pleuropneumonia. Res. Vet. Sci., 17:5–23, 1974.

Other Bovine Mycoplasmoses

Several distinct species of *Mycoplasma* have been recovered from bovine animals and some of these organisms have been shown to be pathogens. Efforts to classify the *Mycoplasma* based on careful and thorough study of each isolate have established several distinct, named species. Synonymous names are frequent and in many instances the organisms associated with disease are not specifically identified in the literature. More than one serotype may be involved in infecting the same organ system, complicating the clear relationship of organism to disease.

Bovine Mastitis

One form of mastitis in bovine animals is caused by *Mycoplasma agalactiae v. bovis* (*M. bovimastitidis, M. bovi-agalactiae,* or *M. bovis*). The organism was originally recovered in pure culture from the mammary gland of a cow affected with severe mastitis. The characteristic disease was produced in normal cows by instilling cultures of this organism (Hale et al., 1962).

Lesions. The lesions involve mammary acini, interlobular ducts, and interstitial stroma. At the outset, all acini in the lobule become filled with purulent exudate. The interlobular ducts may also become filled with neutrophils, and the epithelium becomes hyperplastic. As the disease progresses, the ductal epithelium undergoes squamous metaplasia, and some ducts and acini are filled with lipogranulomatous exudate. The interstitial stroma is initially edematous and infiltrated by lymphocytes and plasma cells, but eventually undergoes fibrosis. Eosinophils are a frequent component of the exudate, both in natural and experimental infections.

Bovine Genital Infections

Mycoplasma bovimastitidis has also been isolated from the genital tract of cows (Edward et al., 1947), and by experimental inoculation, has caused purulent **endometritis, salpingitis,** and localized **peritonitis** in pregnant heifers (Hartman et al., 1964; Hirth and Nielsen, 1966). This organism may be responsible for some cases of sterility or low fertility in bovine animals.

Lesions. The lesions in experimentally infected cows were not evident grossly, and were limited to the uterus, oviducts, and related peritoneum. The endometrium was at first edematous, then infiltrated with lymphocytes and plasma cells. Neutrophils soon were evident in the lumen. The lymphocytic inflammation often extended to the serosal surface of the uterus and oviducts. In long-standing lesions, collections of lymphocytes and sometimes eosinophils were noted in the stroma surrounding uterine glands.

Diagnosis depends upon recognizing the lesions histologically and isolating and identifying the causative *Mycoplasma.*

Injection of cultured *M. agalactiae v. bovis* into the amniotic sac of pregnant heifers resulted in necrotizing, purulent placentitis followed by death and expulsion of the fetus (Stalheim and Proctor, 1976). The organism has also been isolated from joint fluid of cattle with naturally-acquired arthritis.

Seminal vesiculitis and **epididymitis** in bulls may be the result of infection by *Mycoplasma bovigenitalium.* Experimental infection has resulted in inflammatory disease in these and other parts of the genital tract of the bull. *M. bovigenitalium* has been isolated from joints affected with acute **arthritis,** and it has been suggested that it is the cause of **bovine granular vulvovaginitis.** The organism has been recovered from this disease, and has caused the disease when instilled into the vagina of normal cows. The gross lesions of bovine granular vulvovaginitis consist of mucopurulent discharge and the appearance of tiny granular elevations of the vulvar and vaginal epithelium. Microscopically, these elevated nodules consist of aggregations of lymphocytes that elevate and thin the overlying epithelium. The epithelium sometimes is necrotic, and the stroma is edematous and infiltrated by eosinophils.

Infectious Bovine Keratoconjunctivitis

This disease is associated with *Mycoplasma bovoculi* (or *M. oculi*). This organism, isolated and named by Langford and Leach (1973), appears to be an important etiologic factor in some cases. (See Chapter 28.)

Enzootic Pneumonia of Calves

Mycoplasma have been associated with what has been called enzootic pneumonia of calves, usually accompanied by bacteria and sometimes by viruses; in some instances, the mycoplasma appear to be pathogenic. *Mycoplasma bovirhinis* has been recovered from the nose and lungs of cattle with respiratory disease, from the udder of cows with mastitis, and from the lungs of bovine animals with pneumoenteritis. The disease in each instance has rarely been reproduced experimentally with *M. bovirhinis,* which presumably rapidly loses virulence in culture (Cottew and Leach, 1969). *Mycoplasma dispar,* and T-mycoplasma have been associated with pulmonary lesions (Gourlay, Mackenzie and Cooper, 1970). In other studies, *M. dispar, Ureaplasma spp.* have been isolated from pneumonic lungs and shown to be pathogenic upon experimental exposure to

calves (Pirie and Allen, 1975). Thus it appears that some mycoplasma (in addition to *M. mycoides var. mycoides*) may produce a type of pneumonia in calves.

Lesions. The lesions are usually limited to a few lobules in apical or cardiac lobes and result in consolidation of small groups of lobules, sharply demarcated from adjacent ones. Microscopically, the lesions are centered around bronchioles, with purulent exudate and debris in the lumen and nodules of lymphocytes distorting the bronchial wall. This is consistent with the fact that mycoplasma grow on epithelial surfaces of the respiratory tract. This type of bronchiolitis is reminiscent of the lesions of murine chronic respiratory disease.

Al-Aubaidi, J. M., McEntee, K., Lein, D. H., and Roberts, S. J.: Bovine seminal vesiculitis and epididymitis caused by *Mycoplasma bovigenitalium.* Cornell Vet., 62:581–596, 1972.

Afshar, A.: Genital diseases of cattle associated with mycoplasma. Vet. Bull., 37:879–884, 1967.

Bennett, R. H., Carroll, E. J., and Jasper, D. E.: Skin-sensitivity reactions in calves inoculated with *Mycoplasma bovis* antigens: humoral and cell-mediated responses. Am. J. Vet. Res., 38:1721–1730, 1977.

Bennett, R. H., and Jasper, D. E.: Immunosuppression of humoral and cell-mediated responses in calves associated with inoculation of *Mycoplasma bovis.* Am. J. Vet. Res., 38:1731–1738, 1977.

Blom, J., Erno, H., and Birch-Andersen, A.: Mycoplasmosis: experimental seminal vesiculitis. Electron microscopy of infected tissue. Acta Pathol. Microbiol. Scand., 81B:176–178, 1973.

Clyde, W. A., Jr.: Mycoplasma species identification based upon growth inhibition by specific antisera. J. Immunol., 92:958–965, 1964.

Cottew, G. S., and Leach, R. H.: Mycoplasmas of cattle, sheep and goats. *In* The Mycoplasmatales and the L-Phase of Baceria, edited by L. Hayflick, New York, Appleton-Century-Crofts, 1969, pp. 527–570.

Edward, D. C., Hancock, J. L., and Hignett, S. L.: Isolation of a Pleuropneumonia-like Organism from the Bovine Genital Tract. Vet. Rec., 59:329–330, 1947.

Erno, H., and Blom, E.: Mycoplasmosis: experimental and spontaneous infections of the genital tract of bulls. Acta Vet. Scand., 13:161–174, 1972.

———: Mycoplasmosis: experimental seminal vesiculitis. Demonstration of locally occurring antibody. Acta Vet. Scand., 14:332–334, 1973.

Erno, H.: Bovine mycoplasmas: Identification of 100 strains isolated from semen of bulls. Acta Vet. Scand., 16:321–323, 1975.

Gois, M., Kuksa, F., and Franz, J.: Isolation of *Mycoplasma bovigenitalium* from the semen of a boar. Vet. Rec., 93:47–48, 1973.

Gourlay, R. N.: Significance of *Mycoplasma* infections in cattle. J. Am. Vet. Med. Assoc., 163:905–908, 1973.

Gourlay, R. N., and Leach, R. H.: A new mycoplasma species isolated from pneumonic lungs of calves (*Mycoplasma dispar* sp. nov.). J. Med. Microbiol., 3:111–123, 1970.

Gourlay, R. N., Mackenzie, A., and Cooper, J. E.: Studies of the microbiology and pathology of pneumonic lungs of calves. J. Comp. Pathol., 80:575–584, 1970.

Gourlay, R. N., and Thomas, L. H.: The experimental production of pneumonia in calves by the endobronchial inoculation of T-mycoplasmas. J. Comp. Pathol., 80:585–594, 1970.

Hale, H. H., Helmboldt, C. F., Plastridge, W. N., and Stula, E. F.: Bovine mastitis caused by a *Mycoplasma* species. Cornell Vet., 52:582–591, 1962.

Hartman, H. A., Tourtellotte, M. E., Nielsen, S. W., and Plastridge, W. N.: Experimental bovine uterine mycoplasmosis. Res. Vet. Sci., 5:303–310, 1964.

Hirth, R. S., and Nielsen, S. W.: Experimental pathology of bovine salpingitis due to mycoplasma insemination. Lab. Invest., 15:1132–1133, 1966.

Hirth, R. S., Nielsen, S. W., and Tourtellotte, M. E.: Characterization and comparative genital tract pathogenicity of bovine mycoplasmas. Infect. Immun., 2:101–104, 1970.

Hirth, R. S., Tourtellotte, M. E., and Nielsen, S. W.: Cytopathic effects and ultrastructure of *Mycoplasma agalactiae var. bovis* (Donetta strain). Infect. Immun., 2:105–111, 1970.

Hjerpe, C. A., and Knight, H. D.: Polyarthritis and synovitis associated with *Mycoplasma bovimastitidis* in feedlot cattle. J. Am. Vet. Med. Assoc., 160:1414–1418, 1972.

Howard, C. J., Anderson, J. C., Gourlay, R. N., and Taylor-Robinson, D.: Production of mastitis in mice with human and bovine ureaplasmas (T-mycoplasmas). J. Med. Microbiol., 8:523–529, 1975.

Jasper, D. E., Al-Aubaidi, J. M., and Fabricant, J.: Epidemiologic observations on mycoplasma mastitis. Cornell Vet., 64:407–415, 1974.

Karbe, E., Nielsen, S. W., and Helmboldt, C. F.: Pathology of experimental mycoplasma mastitis in the cow. Zentbl. Vet. Med., 14B:7–31, 1967.

Langford, E. V.: Mycoplasma infections in the bovine genital tract. Can. Vet. J., 15:300–301, 1974.

Langford, E. V., and Leach, R. H.: Characterization of mycoplasma isolated from infectious bovine keratoconjunctivitis: *M. bovoculi* sp. nov. Can. J. Microbiol., 19:1435–1444, 1973.

Langford, E. V., Ruhke, H. L., and Onoviran, O.: *Mycoplasma canadense*, a new bovine species. Int. J. Systematic Bacteriol., 26:212–219, 1976.

Leach, R. H.: Further studies on classification of bovine strains of Mycoplasmatales, with proposals for new species. *Acholeplasma modicum* and *Mycoplasma alkalescens*. J. Gen. Microbiol., 75:135–153, 1973.

Nicolet, J., and Buttiker, W.: Isolation of *M. bovoculi* from eye lesions of cattle in the Ivory Coast. Vet. Rec., 95:442–443, 1974.

Parsonson, I. M., Al-Aubaidi, J. M., and McEntee, K.: *Mycoplasma bovigenitalium*: experimental induction of genital disease in bulls. Cornell Vet., 64:240–264, 1974.

Pirie, H. M., and Allan, E. M.: Mycoplasmas and cuffing pneumonia in a group of calves. Vet. Rec., 97:345–349, 1975.

Rovozzo, G. C., Luginbuhl, R. E., and Helmboldt, C. F.: A *Mycoplasma* from a bovine causing cytopathogenic effects in calf kidney tissue culture. Cornell Vet., 53:560–566, 1963.

Ruhnke, H. L., and van Dreumel, A. A.: The isolation of T-mycoplasma from pneumonic lungs of a calf. Can. J. Comp. Med., 36:317–318, 1972.

Shimizu, T., Nosaka, D., and Nakamura, N.: An enzootic of calf pneumonia associated with *Mycoplasma bovirhinis*. Jap. J. Vet. Sci., 35:535–537, 1973.

Singh, U. M., Doig, P. A., and Ruhnke, H. L.: Mycoplasma arthritis in calves. Can. Vet. J., 12:183–185, 1971.

Stalheim, O. H. V., and Proctor, S. J.: Experimentally induced bovine abortion with *Mycoplasma agalactiae* subsp. *bovis*. Am. J. Vet. Res., 37:879–884, 1976.

Contagious Caprine Pleuropneumonia

This respiratory disease of goats, caused by a myocoplasma, is an important economic problem in large parts of the world. It occurs in some African countries, the Soviet Union, Turkey, Greece, Iran, Syria, Spain, Afghanistan, the Arabian Peninsula, China, Burma, India, Mongolia, and South America. The causative organism, *Mycoplasma mycoides var capri* is difficult to maintain in culture, but has been clearly identified by careful studies.

Although the disease is not a widespread problem in the United States, several strains of *Mycoplasma* have been recovered from goats in this country, including in at least one instance, *Mycoplasma mycoides var capri* (Jonas and Barber, 1969, Barber and Yedloutschnig, 1970).

Signs. The signs usually seen include fever, nasal discharge, accelerated respiration, and depression. Incubation periods have been recorded as 8 to 28 days for the natural infection and 3 to 24 days for the experimentally induced disease. The mortality rate is high, often reaching 100% in an outbreak.

Lesions. The pulmonary lesions resemble those of bovine pleuropneumonia, except that sequestration of lung tissue is rare. In the peracute form, the lungs are uniformly consolidated with fibrinopurulent exudate on the pleura. In the less fulminant form, the pulmonary lobules have a variegated appearance. Edema is extensive in the interlobular septa and under the pleura. Fibrinous exudate covers the pleura.

Barber, T. L., and Yedloutschnig, R. J.: Mycoplasma infections of goats. Cornell Vet., *60*:297–308, 1970.
Cottew, G. S., and Leach, R. H.: Mycoplasmas of cattle, sheep and goats. *In* The Mycoplasmatales and the L-Phase of Bacteria, edited by L. Hayflick. New York, Appleton-Century-Crofts, 1969. pp. 527–570.
Jonas, A. M., and Barber, T. L.: *Mycoplasma mycoides var capri* isolated from a goat in Connecticut. J. Infect. Dis., *119*:126–129, 1969.

Contagious Agalactia of Goats and Sheep

This disease has been known for about a century in many countries where goats and sheep are important sources of milk and meat for human consumption. Contagious agalactia has been reported to occur in Romania, Yugoslavia, Switzerland, many Mediteranean countries, Sudan, Iran, the Soviet Union, Pakistan, and India. The disease causes considerable economic loss, principally from lowered milk production. Goats appear to be more susceptible in nature, but sheep are infected readily by experimental methods. The causative organism, *Mycoplasma agalactiae,* was first isolated by Bridré and Donatien (1923).

Experimental infection with *M. agalactiae* results in bacteremia, followed by excretion of organisms in milk within six days (Watson et al., 1968). Mammary infection persists for months, and the organisms may be isolated from blood, milk, or joint fluid.

Signs. The signs appear first at lambing time as mastitis in the lactating females. The milk may become greenish-yellow,

and the solids tend to sediment. Lameness frequently appears, particularly in males. Keratoconjunctivitis is also occasionally evident.

Mycoplasma agalactiae has been associated with **granular vulvovaginitis** of goats in India (Singh, Rajya, and Mohanty, 1974). The lesions consist of multiple tiny nodules of lymphocytes and plasma cells in the lamina propria and muscularis of the vagina and vulva. These aggregations of lymphocytes are visible grossly as tiny translucent granules that elevate the mucosa. This appearance led to the descriptive term, granular vulvovaginitis.

Bridré, J., and Donatien, A.: Le Microbe de l'agalaxie contagieuse et sa culture in vitro. C. R. Acad. Sci. (Paris), *177*:841–843, 1923.
Singh, H., Rajya, B. S., and Mohanty, G. C.: Granular vulvovaginitis (GVV) in goats associated with *Mycoplasma agalactiae.* Cornell Vet., *64*:435–442, 1974.
Singh, N., Rajya, B. S., and Mohanty, G. C.: Pathology of *Mycoplasma agalactiae* induced granular vulvovaginitis (GVV) in goats. Cornell Vet., *65*:363–373, 1975.
Turner, A. W.: Pleuropneumonia group of diseases. *In* Infectious Diseases of Animals, edited by Stableforth, A. W. and Galloway, L. A. Vol. 2, Butterworth, London, 1959. pp. 437–480.
Watson, W. A., Cottew, G. S., Erdag, O., and Arisoy, F.: The investigation of the pathogenicity of *Mycoplasma* organisms isolated from sheep and goats in Turkey. J. Comp. Pathol., *78*:283–291, 1968.

Other Mycoplasmoses in Goats and Sheep

Aside from the two *Mycoplasma,* *M. mycoides var capri* and *M. agalactiae,* which are important pathogens of goats and sheep in many parts of the world, several *Mycoplasma* have been isolated from diseased tissues in the United States. In some instances, evidence is convincing that the organisms recovered caused the disease. In others, it appears that *Mycoplasma* may be carried by essentially healthy sheep and goats.

Mycoplasma recovered from pneumonic ovine lungs caused septicemia and arthritis in susceptible lambs (Boidin et al., 1958). *M. ovipneumoniae,* isolated from pneumonic lungs of sheep in Australia and the United States, produced an interstitial pneumonia upon experimental inoculation of young lambs (St. George and Carmichael, 1975). In this disease, thickening of alveolar septae, proliferation of alveolar lining cells, hyperplasia of bronchiolar epithelium, and atelectasis have been described. A fatal disease in goats with fibrinopurulent arthritis, fibrinous pleuritis, pericarditis, and lymphadenopathy has been associated with *Mycoplasma* (Cordy et al., 1955). Keratoconjunctivitis of prolonged duration has also been associated with *Mycoplasma* (McCauley et al., 1971).

Mycoplasma arginini has been isolated from pneumonic lungs of wild big-horn sheep *(Ovis canadensis)* and domestic goats (Al-Aubaidi et al., 1972).

Al-Aubaidi, J. M., Taylor, W. D., Bubash, G. R., and Dardiri, A. H.: Identification and characterization of *Mycoplasma arginini* from bighorn sheep *(Ovis canadensis)* and goats. Am. J. Vet. Res., 33:87–90, 1972.

Alley, M. R., Quinlan, J. R., and Clarke, J. K.: The prevalence of *Mycoplasma ovipneumoniae* and *Mycoplasma arginini* in the respiratory tract of sheep. NZ Vet. J., 23:137–142, 1975.

Barile, M. F., Guidice, R. A. Del., and Tully, J. G.: Isolation and characterization of *Mycoplasma conjunctivae sp* from sheep and goats with keratoconjunctivitis. Infect. Immun., 5:70–76, 1972.

Boidin, A. G., Cordy, D. R., and Adler, H. E.: A pleuropneumonia-like organism and a virus in ovine pneumonia in California. Cornell Vet., 48:410–430, 1958.

Cordy, D. R., Adler, H. E., and Yamamoto, R.: A pathogenic pleuropneumonia like organism from goats. Cornell Vet., 45:50–68, 1955.

Cottew, G. S.: Characterization of mycoplasmas isolated from sheep with pneumonia. Aust. Vet. J., 47:591–596, 1971.

Cottew, G. S., and Leach, R. H.: Mycoplasmas of cattle, sheep and goats. *In* The Mycoplasmatales and the L-Phase of Bacteria, edited by L. Hayflick. New York, Appleton-Century-Crofts, 1969. pp. 527–570.

Cottew, G. S., and Lloyd, L. C.: An outbreak of pleurisy and pneumonia in goats in Australia attributed to a mycoplasma species. J. Comp. Pathol., 75:368–374, 1965.

Hamdy, A. H., Pounden, W. D., and Ferguson, L. C.: Microbial agents associated with pneumonia in slaughtered lambs. Am. J. Vet. Res., 20:87–90, 1959.

Krauss, H., and Wandera, J. G.: Isolation and properties of *Mycoplasma* from the respiratory tract of sheep with jaagsiekte in Kenya. J. Comp. Pathol., 80:389–397, 1970.

Langford, E. V.: Mycoplasma and associated bacteria isolated from ovine pink-eye. Can. J. Comp. Med., 35:18–21, 1971.

McCauley, E. H., Surman, P. G., and Anderson, D. R.: Isolation of *Mycoplasma* from goats during an epizootic of keratoconjunctivitis. Am. J. Vet. Res., 32:861–870, 1971.

McGowan, B., Moulton, J. E., and Shultz, G.: Pneumonia in California lambs. J. Am. Vet. Med. Assoc., 131:318–323, 1957.

St. George, T. D., Sullivan, N. D., Love, J. A., and Horsfall, N.: Experimental transmission of pneumonia in sheep with mycoplasma isolated from pneumonia sheep lung. Aust. Vet. J., 47:282–283, 1971.

St. George, T. D., and Carmichael, L. E.: Isolation of *Mycoplasma ovipneumoniae* from sheep with chronic pneumonia. Vet. Rec., 97:205–206, 1975.

Murine Chronic Respiratory Disease (Chronic Murine Pneumonia, Epizootic Bronchiectasis of Rats, Infectious Catarrh of Rats, Rodent Pulmonary Mycoplasmosis)

For many years, chronic infection of the respiratory system of laboratory rats has been an important disease problem. Evidence now available indicates that *Mycoplasma pulmonis* is the cause of a specific syndrome that involves the nasal passages, nasal sinuses, middle ear, larynx, trachea, bronchi, and lungs. Rats are most commonly affected, but mice may be infected experimentally and by contact with infected rats. The evidence that *Mycoplasma pulmonis* is the causative agent may be summarized as follows: (1) the organism may be isolated from natural cases, identified in culture, transferred to disease-free rats, in which the typical lesions result, and recovered from these lesions; (2) the organisms can be specifically identified in association with the lesions by means of fluorescence antibody; (3) the organisms may be demonstrated in large numbers on the surface of epithelial cells in the lesions by means of the electron microscope; (4) no putative virus has been shown to cause the disease and no known virus has been demonstrated in the experimentally induced lesions.

Mycoplasma pulmonis was first isolated by Kleineberger and Steabben (1937). The pathogenicity of the organism has been convincingly demonstrated by Kohn and Kirk (1969), Lindsay et al. (1971), and others.

Signs. Some rats may be severely affected but display few indications. Others may exhibit purulent rhinitis with nasal and ocular discharge, coughing, sneezing, and snuffling. Involvement of the inner ear often results in loss of equilibrium, twisting, and rotary movements. A rat held up by the tail will characteristically undergo rapid twisting or twirling motions. In the late stages, infected rats may exhibit polypnea, humped posture, inactivity, roughened hair coat, and loss of weight. Usually death occurs sporadically, and often lesions are detected only by postmortem examination following sacrifice.

Lesions. Purulent exudate in the nasal cavities, middle, and internal ear may be recognized grossly, but in some instances can be detected only by aspiration of material with a capillary pipette. Similar exudate may be present in the trachea and bronchi. The subepithelial stroma of the entire upper respiratory tract is infiltrated by lymphocytes and plasma cells.

The lungs often have a gross gray color and characteristically have a cobblestone appearance on the surface due to the dilated and thick-walled bronchi. In early lesions, the walls of bronchi are thick due to collections of lymphocytes and plasma cells. In long-standing cases, the bronchi become dilated and often contain pus. This bronchiectasis is often the dominant and characteristic feature. Squamous metaplasia of the bronchial epithelium is a frequent finding. Atelectasis often occurs, and some alveoli may be involved.

The electron microscope reveals large numbers of mycoplasma organisms on the surface of epithelial cells in intimate contact with the villi. Some organisms may be seen in membrane-bound vacuoles within these cells. Lymphocytes and plasma cells predominate in the tissue exudate involving the bronchial wall.

Diagnosis. The microscopic lesions are characteristic and adequate for presumptive diagnosis of murine mycoplasmosis. Confirmation may be accomplished (1) by cultural isolation of *Mycoplasma pulmonis* from bronchial, tracheal, or nasal exudate, (2) by demonstration of mycoplasma antigens in tissue sections of lung, using immunofluorescence, (3) by transmission of the disease to germ-free rats or mice, or (4) by demonstration of mycoplasma in electronmicrographs of the lesions.

Cassell, G. H., Lindsey, J. R., and Baker, H. J.: Immune response of pathogen-free mice inoculated intranasally with *Mycoplasma pulmonis*. J. Immunol., *112*:124–136, 1974.

Clyde, W. A.: Mycoplasma species identification based upon growth inhibition by specific antisera. J. Immunol., *92*:958–965, 1964.

Coleman, E. J., Zbijewska, J. R., and Smith, N. L.: Hematologic values in chronic murine pneumonia. Lab. Anim. Sci., *21*:721–726, 1971.

Ebbesen, P.: Chronic respiratory disease in BALB/c mice. I. Pathology and relation to other murine lung infections. Am. J. Pathol., *53*:219–233, 1968.

Ebbesen, P.: Chronic respiratory disease in BALB/c mice. II. Characteristics of the disease. Am. J. Pathol., *53*:235–243, 1968.

Ganaway, J. R., Allen, A. M., Moore, T. D., and Bohner, H. J.: Natural infection of germ-free rats with *Mycoplasma pulmonis*. J. Infect. Dis., *127*:529–537, 1973.

Gay, F. W., Maguire, M. E., and Baskerville, A.: Etiology of chronic pneumonia in rats and a study of the experimental disease in mice. Infect. Immun., *6*:83–91, 1972.

Giddens, W. E., Jr., Whitehair, C. K., and Carter, G. R.: Morphologic and microbiologic features of trachea and lungs in germ-free, defined-flora, conventional, and chronic respiratory disease-affected rats. Am. J. Vet. Res., *32*:115–130, 1971.

————: Morphologic and microbiologic features of nasal cavity and middle ear in germ-free, defined-flora, conventional, and chronic respiratory disease-affected rats. Am. J. Vet. Res., *32*:99–114, 1971.

Halliwell, W. H., McClune, E. L., and Olson, L. D.: *Mycoplasma pulmonis*-induced otitis media in gnotobiotic mice. Lab. Anim. Sci., *24*:57–61, 1974.

Jersey, G. C., Whitehair, C. K., and Carter, G. R.: *Mycoplasma pulmonis* as the primary cause of chronic respiratory disease in rats. J. Am. Vet. Med. Assoc., *163*:599–604, 1973.

Juhr, N. C.: Studies on chronic murine pneumonia. Pathogenesis of *Mycoplasma pulmonis* infection in the rat. Z. Versuchstierkd., *13*:217–223, 1971.

Kappel, H. K., Nelson, J. B., and Weisbroth, S. H.: Development of a screening technic to monitor a Mycoplasma-free Blu:(LE) Long-Evans rat colony. Lab. Anim. Sci., 24:768–772, 1974.

Kleineberger, E., and Steabben, D. B.: On a pleuropneumonia-like organism in lung tissue of rats, with notes on the clinical and pathologic features of the underlying condition. J. Hyg. (Camb.), 37:143–153, 1937.

————: On the association of the pleuropneumonia-like organism L₃ with bronchiectatic lesions in rats. J. Hyg. (Camb.), 40:223–227, 1940.

Kohn, D. F., and Kirk, B. E.: Pathogenicity of Mycoplasma pulmonis in laboratory rats. Lab. Anim. Care., 19:321–330, 1969.

Kohn, D. F.: Sequential pathogenicity of Mycoplasma pulmonis in laboratory rats. Lab. Anim. Sci., 21:849–855, 1972.

————: Bronchiectasis in rats infected with Mycoplasma pulmonis—an electron microscopy study. Lab. Anim. Sci., 21:856–861, 1972.

Lemcke, R. M.: Association of PPLO infection and antibody response in rats and mice. J. Hyg. (Camb.), 59:401–412, 1961.

Lindsey, J. R., et al.: Murine chronic respiratory disease. Significance as a research complication and experimental production with Mycoplasma pulmonis. Am. J. Pathol., 64:675–717, 1971.

Organick, A. B., and Lutsky, I. I.: Mycoplasma pulmonis infection in gnotobiotic and conventional mice: aspects of pathogenicity including microbial enumeration and studies of tracheal involvement. Lab. Anim. Sci., 26:419–429, 1976.

Overcash, R. G., Lindsey, J. R., Cassell, G. H., and Baker, H. J.: Enhancement of natural and experimental respiratory mycoplasmosis in rats by hexamethylphosphoramide. Am. J. Pathol., 82:171–190, 1976.

Taylor-Robinson, D., et al.: Fetal wastage as a consequence of Mycoplasma pulmonis infection in mice. J. Reprod. Fertil., 42:483–490, 1975.

Thomson, C., and Hill, A.: The direct inoculation of Mycoplasma pulmonis into rat lungs. J. Comp. Pathol., 82:81–85, 1972.

Tvedten, H. W., Whitehair, C. K., and Langham, R. F.: Influence of vitamins A and E on gnotobiotic and conventionally maintained rats exposed to Mycoplasma pulmonis. J. Am. Vet. Med. Assoc., 163:605–612, 1973.

Murine Mycoplasmal Arthritis

Arthritis is a reasonably frequent occurrence in laboratory rats and mice. In many instances this disease is associated with the presence of *Mycoplasma arthritidis*, a rather ubiquitous organism. The organism has been recovered from infected joints, heart blood, abscesses, a transmissible sarcoma, and submaxillary glands of rats. It is also pathogenic for mice but most other laboratory animals are refractory to infec-

tion. The joints of the limbs are most frequently involved. Usually only a single joint is involved, but occasionally two or more are affected. The joints are swollen, hot, tender, and fixed, as in acute arthritis in any species. After a time, proliferation of synovia and accumulation of fluid in the joint is accompanied by the appearance of purulent and lymphocytic inflammation in the adjacent tissues. Other organisms may also cause arthritis in these species; among them are *Streptococci* and *Streptobacillus moniliformis*. Arthritis has been produced in mice by injection of *Mycoplasma pulmonis* (Barden and Tully, 1969).

Barden, J. A., and Tully, J. G.: Experimental arthritis in mice with Mycoplasma pulmonis. J. Bacteriol., 100:5–10, 1969.

Findlay, G. M., Mackenzie, R. D., MacCallum, F. O., and Klieneberger, E.: The aetiology of polyarthritis in the rat. Lancet, 11:7–10, 1939.

Freundt, E. A.: Arthritis caused by Streptobacillus moniliformis and pleuropneumonia-like organisms in small rodents. Lab. Invest., 8:1358–1375, 1959.

Hannan, P. C. T., and Hughes, B. O.: Reproducible polyarthritis in rats caused by Mycoplasma arthritidis. Ann. Rheum. Dis., 30:316–321, 1971.

Harwick, H. J., Kalmanson, G. M., Fox, M. A., and Guze, L. B.: Mycoplasmal arthritis of the mouse: Development of cellular hypersensitivity to normal synovial tissue. Proc. Soc. Exp. Biol. Med., 144:561–563, 1973.

Hill, A., and Dagnall, G. J. R.: Experimental polyarthritis in rats produced by Mycoplasma arthritidis. J. Comp. Pathol., 85:45–52, 1975.

Sokoloff, L.: Osteoarthritis in laboratory animals. Lab. Invest., 8:1209–1217, 1959.

Stewart, D. D., and Buck, G. E.: The occurrence of Mycoplasma arthritidis in the throat and middle ear of rats with chronic respiratory disease. Lab. Anim. Sci., 25:769–773, 1975.

Mycoplasmal Arthritis and Polyserositis in Swine

Inflammatory lesions in the pericardium, pleura, peritoneum, and joints are often recognized in young swine. The etiologic factors are often unknown, but one common cause is *Mycoplasma hyorhinis*. McNutt et al. (1945) were the first to recover an infectious agent, distinguishable from *Erysipelothrix rhusiopathiae*, from young pigs by inoculating developing chick embryos. Material from infected

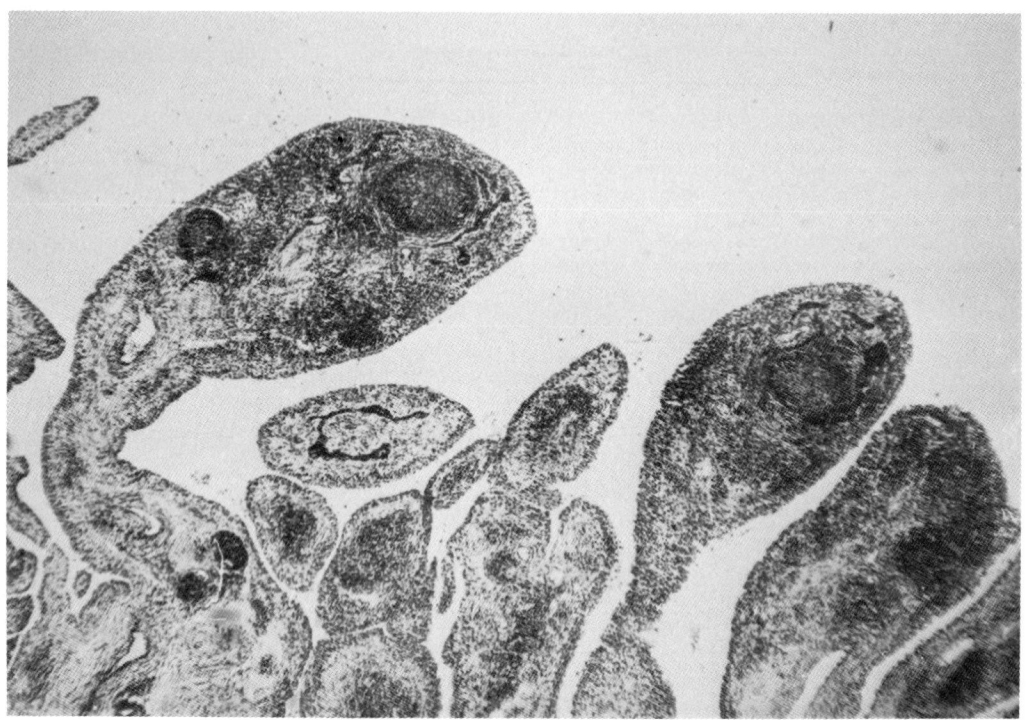

Fig. 10–1. *Mycoplasma hyorhinis* arthritis. Villous hypertrophy of synovial membrane in an affected pig. Focal collections of lymphocytes are present within the thickened villi. (Courtesy of Dr. J. R. Duncan and *American Journal of Veterinary Research.*)

chick embryos, when injected into young pigs, caused pleuritis, pericarditis, peritonitis, and arthritis in the pigs. Switzer, in 1953, demonstrated a similar agent from the nasal passages of swine with atrophic rhinitis, and observed that it formed intracellular organisms in chick embryos. These organisms were subsequently classified in the pleuropneumonia group (Carter and McKay, 1953) and named *Mycoplasma hyorhinis* by Switzer (1955). This organism now appears to be most frequently involved in polyserositis of young pigs in nature, and will result in disease following experimental inoculation.

M. hyorhinis will also cause severe acute arthritis in young pigs when inoculated intravenously or intraperitoneally (Barden and Decker, 1971; Barden et al., 1973; Barthel et al., 1972; Decker and Barden,

1975; Duncan and Ross, 1973; Ennis et al., 1971; and Ross et al., 1973).

Lesions. The lesions of the experimental disease are described in detail by Roberts et al. (1963). The pericarditis, pleuritis, and peritonitis (collectively sometimes spoken of as "polyserositis") is rather characteristic; each serous surface is affected in essentially the same way. Within six days following intraperitoneal instillation of organisms, fibrinopurulent exudate may be seen grossly on serous surfaces. This exudate becomes more extensive at ten days following inoculation, but wanes by the thirtieth day. The peritoneum and pleura are severely involved, the pericardium much less so in the experimental disease. The full-blown lesion consists of fibrinopurulent exudate on the serous surface, with swelling and disorganization of the serosal lining cells. Underlying these cells are lym-

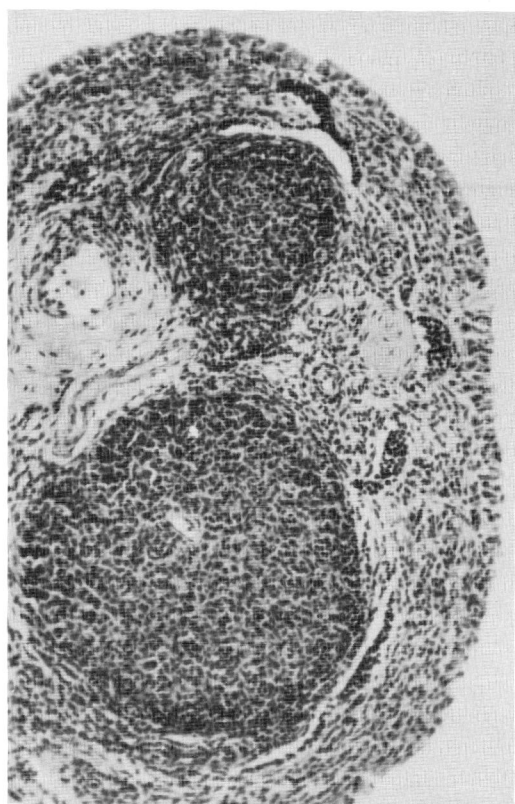

Fig. 10-2. *Mycoplasma hyorhinis* arthritis. Lymphocytic nodule in hypertrophic synovial villus. (Courtesy of Dr. J. R. Duncan and *American Journal of Veterinary Research.*)

phocytes, macrophages, and plasma cells. Hyperemia and vascularization are features during this stage. As the disease runs its course, after 15 to 30 days, the fibrinous exudate may organize, particularly over the pleura and peritoneal surfaces. This results in adhesions, which may persist for a long time. In an occasional case, severe exudation in the pericardial sac may lead to organizing epicarditis, which eventually interferes with cardiac function. The lymphocytic exudate sometimes extends into the subpleural alveoli and Glisson's capsule of the liver, but otherwise does not affect parenchymatous organs. The tunica vaginalis may be affected by extension from the peritoneum. In some cases, lym-phocytic leptomeningitis may be demonstrable.

The most frequent cause of mycoplasmal arthritis under natural conditions is *Mycoplasma hyosynoviae* (synonym: *M. suidaniae*). Swine weighing 75 to 100 pounds are most commonly affected with acute arthritis. The organisms are commonly carried on nasal and pharyngeal mucosae (Switzer and Ross, 1975).

One or more joints may become involved in this infection, with swelling, congestion and pain resulting in lameness. In the least severely affected joints and early in the course of the disease, the joint capsule may be slightly hyperemic and the synovial fluid excessive in volume. In more severely affected joints, the synovial fluid becomes yellow or turbid and may contain strands of fibrin. Neutrophils are numerous in such synovial fluid. The synovial membranes may become edematous, hyperemic, and yellowish in color. The membranes contain large numbers of lymphocytes and macrophages. The villi are edematous, redundant, and hyperemic. Nodules of lymphocytes sometimes form. In young swine, disorganization may be seen in the columns of cartilage in the epiphyseal plate. The cartilage columns lose their straight orderly arrangement and are distorted and irregular, with congested vascular spaces between them. Fibrous thickening of the joint capsule may result in partial or complete ankylosis of the affected joint.

Mycoplasma hyoarthrinosa and *Mycoplasma granularum* are two mycoplasmas distinct from *Mycoplasma hyorhinis* which have been reported to induce polyarthritis in swine. These two organisms have not been clearly differentiated at this time from *M. hyosynoviae.*

Diagnosis. The diagnosis of mycoplasma infections is based upon the gross and microscopic lesions and the demonstration of the organisms by cultural methods, immunofluorescence, or electron microscopy.

The "fibrinous-serosa-joint inflammation" of young pigs, called **Glässer's disease**, is pathologically nearly identical to *M. hyorhinis* infection, but Hjärre and Wramby (1942) associated Glässer's disease with swine influenza and infection with *Hemophilus influenzae suis*. Based on recent evidence it now seems reasonably certain that *H. influenzae suis* and *M. hyorhinis* are distinct causes of polyserositis and arthritis in swine. Hjärre reserves the eponym Glässer's disease for the disease caused by *H. influenzae suis*, and distinguishes it from mycoplasmosis in that purulent meningitis is found in 80% of spontaneous cases of Glässer's disease, whereas purulent meningitis is not a feature of mycoplasma infection. However, as noted previously, meningitis may develop in *M. hyorhinis* infection. For accurate differentiation, attempts should be made to culture both organisms.

Barden, J. A., and Decker, J. L.: *Mycoplasma hyorhinis* swine arthritis. 1. Clinical and microbiologic features. Arthritis Rheum., *14*:193–201, 1971.

Barden, J. A., Decker, J. L., Dalgard, D. W., and Aptekar, R. G.: *Mycoplasma hyorhinis* swine arthritis. III. Modified disease in Piney Woods swine. Infect. Immun., *8*:887–890, 1973.

Barthel, C. H., Duncan, J. R., and Ross, R. F.: Lactic dehydrogenase activity in plasma and synovial fluid of normal and *Mycoplasma hyorhinis*-infected swine. Am. J. Vet. Res., *32*:2011–2020, 1971.

Barthel, C. H., Duncan, J. R., and Ross, R. F.: Histologic and histochemical characterization of synovial membrane from normal and *Mycoplasma hyorhinis*-infected swine. Am. J. Vet. Res., *33*:2501–2510, 1972.

Carter, G. R., and McKay, K. A.: A pleuropneumonia-like organism associated with infectious atrophic rhinitis of swine. Can. J. Comp. Med., *17*:413–416, 1953.

Cordy, D. R., Adler, H. E., and Yamamoto, R.: A pathogenic pleuropneumonia-like organism from goats. Cornell Vet., *45*:50–68, 1955.

Cordy, D. R., Adler, H. E., and Berg, J.: The pathogenicity for swine of a pleuropneumonia-like organism from goats. Cornell Vet., *48*:25–30, 1958.

Davenport, P. G., Shortridge, E. H., and Voyle, B.: Polyserositis in pigs caused by infection with mycoplasma. NZ Vet. J., *18*:165–167, 1971.

Decker, J. L., and Barden, J. A.: *Mycoplasma hyorhinis* arthritis of swine: A model for rheumatoid arthritis. Rheumatology, *6*:338–345, 1975.

Duncan, J. R., and Ross, R. F.: Fine structure of the synovial membrane in *Mycoplasma hyorhinis* arthritis in swine. Am. J. Pathol., *57*:171–186, 1969.

Duncan, J. R., and Ross, R. F.: Experimentally induced *Mycoplasma hyorhinis* arthritis of swine: pathologic response to 26th post-inoculation week. Am. J. Vet. Res., *34*:363–366, 1973.

Ennis, R. S., et al.: *Mycoplasma hyorhinis* swine arthritis. II. Morphologic features. Arthritis Rheum., *14*:202–211, 1971.

Glässer, K., Hupka, E., and Wetzel, R.: Die Krankheiten des Schweines. 5th ed., Hanover, M. and H. Schaper Verlag, 1950.

Hjärre, A.: Enzootic virus pneumonia and Glässer's disease of swine. Adv. Vet. Sci., *4*:235–263, 1958.

Hjärre, A., and Wramby, G.: On Fibrinös Serosaledinflammation (Glässer) Hos Svin. Skand. vet.-tidskr, *32*:257–289, 1942.

King, S. J.: Porcine polyserositis and arthritis—with particular reference to mycoplasmosis and Glasser's disease. Aust. Vet. J., *44*:227–230, 1968.

Lecce, J. G.: Porcine polyserositis with arthritis isolation of a fastidious pleuropneumonia-like organism and *Hemophilus influenzae suis*. Ann. NY Acad. Sci., *79*:670–676, 1960.

McNutt, S. H., Leith, T. S., and Underbjerg, G. K.: An active agent isolated from hogs affected with arthritis. Am. J. Vet. Res., *6*:247–251, 1945.

Meyling, A., and Friss, N. F., Serological identification of a new porcine myocoplasma species, *M. flocculare*. Acta Vet. Scand., *13*:287–289, 1972.

Moore, R. W., Redmond, H. E., and Livingston, C. W., Jr.: Pathologic and serologic characteristics of a mycoplasma causing arthritis in swine. Am. J. Vet. Res., *27*:1649–1656, 1966.

Neil, D. H., et al.: Glasser's disease of swine produced by the intratracheal inoculation of Haemophilus suis. Can. J. Comp. Med., *33*:187–193, 1969.

Potgieter, L. N. D., and Ross, R. F.: Identification of *Mycoplasma hyorhinis* and *Mycoplasma hyosynoviae* by immunofluorescence. Am. J. Vet. Res., *33*:91–98, 1972.

Potgieter, L. N. D., and Ross, R. F.: Demonstration of *Mycoplasma hyorhinis* and *Mycoplasma hyosynoviae* in lesions of experimentally infected swine by immunofluorescence. Am. J. Vet. Res., *33*:99–105, 1972.

Roberts, D. H., Johnson, C. T., and Tew, N. C.: The isolation of *Mycoplasma hyosynoviae* from an outbreak of porcine arthritis. Vet. Rec., *90*:307–309, 1972.

Roberts, E. D., Switzer, W. P., and Ramsey, F. K.: Pathology of the visceral organs of swine inoculated with *Mycoplasma hyorhinis*. Am. J. Vet. Res., *24*:9–18, 1963.

———: The pathology of *Mycoplasma hyorhinis* arthritis produced experimentally in swine. Am. J. Vet. Res., *24*:19–31, 1963.

Robinson, F. R., Moore, R. W., and Bridges, C. H.: Pathogenesis of *Mycoplasma hyoarthrinosa* infection in swine. Am. J. Vet. Res., *28*:483–496, 1967.

Ross, R. F., Dale, S. E., and Duncan, J. R.: Experimentally induced *Mycoplasma hyorhinis* arthritis of swine: immune response to 26th post-inoculation week. Am. J. Vet. Res., *34*:367–372, 1973.

Ross, R. F., Switzer, W. P., and Duncan, J. R.: Experimental production of *Mycoplasma hyosynoviae* arthritis in swine. Am. J. Vet. Res., 32:1743–1750, 1971

Ross, R. F., and Spear, M. L.: Role of the sow as a reservoir of infection for *Mycoplasma hyosynoviae*. Am. J. Vet. Res., 34:373–378, 1973.

Switzer, W. P.: Mycoplasmosis. *In* Diseases of Swine, edited by H. W. Dunne. 2nd ed. Ames, Iowa State Univ. Press, 1964, pp. 498–507.

———: Studies on infectious atrophic rhinitis of swine. I. Isolation of a filterable agent from the nasal cavity of swine with atrophic rhinitis. J. Am. Vet. Med. Assoc., 123:45–47, 1953.

———: Studies on infectious atrophic rhinitis. IV. Characterization of a pleuropneumonia-like organism isolated from the nasal cavities of swine. Am. J. Vet. Res., 16:540–544, 1955.

Switzer, W. P., and Ross, R. F.: Mycoplasmal diseases. *In* Diseases of Swine, edited by H. W. Dunne and A. D. Leman, 4th ed. Ames, Iowa State University Press, 1975, pp. 741–764.

Enzootic Mycoplasmal Pneumonia of Swine

The etiology of this widespread pulmonary disease of swine has been in question until recently, although the disease, "virus pig pneumonia" or "enzootic pneumonia of swine," has been recognized for many years (Schofield, 1956). On the basis of experimental infection of young gnotobiotic pigs with pure cultures of *Mycoplasma*, demonstration of the organisms in association with the lesions ultrastructurally and by immunofluorescence, and recovery of *Mycoplasma* from affected lungs, it appears that these organisms are the principal if not sole cause of this pneumonia of swine. The organism *M. hyopneumoniae* (synonym: *M. suipneumoniae*) is the principal organism involved, although in some cases *M. hyorhinis* is recovered.

Signs. The clinical signs are limited to a prolonged course with poor weight gain, chronic cough, and high morbidity and low mortality rates.

Lesions. The gross lesions are seen principally in the apical and cardiac lobes of the lung, with lobular consolidations and atelectasis, enlarged peribronchial lymph nodes, and sometimes serofibrinous pleuritis, peritonitis, and pericarditis. These latter findings are similar to those seen in mycoplasmal polyserositis and arthritis in swine.

The microscopic lesions include peribronchial and peribronchiolar accumulations of lymphocytes and plasma cells in large numbers, with some cellular and mucous exudate in the lumen. Mucous-secreting cells in the bronchiolar and bronchial epithelium are hyperplastic and produce excess mucus. Neutrophils, lymphocytes, and macrophages accumulate between alveoli, and in some instances fill the alveoli. In some cases, lymphocytic encephalitis may be found.

Ultrastructure. Ultrastructural studies (Livingston et al., 1972; Baskerville and Wright, 1973) reveal that the mycoplasma are in the lumen of bronchi and bronchioles, applied to the surface of epithelial cells, and occasionally enclosed by invagination of the cell membrane near the ciliated border. Organisms are not usually found in alveoli, although purulent and lymphocytic exudate may be conspicuous at this site. Hyperplasia of type II pneumocytes is frequent (Baskerville, 1972). The pathogenic mechanisms are obscure, although it appears that excessive mucous secretion and partial bronchiolar occlusion may cause the exudate in alveoli. The organisms on the surface of the bronchial and bronchiolar epithelium may inhibit ciliary activity and stimulate secretion of mucus. The organisms are also thought to produce peroxide, which may affect cells lining airways and alveoli.

Diagnosis. The diagnosis may be established by finding characteristic microscopic lesions and the demonstration of mycoplasma on the bronchial or bronchiolar surface epithelium with electronmicroscopic preparations or by immunofluorescence (Potgieter and Ross, 1972).

Baskerville, A.: Development of the early lesions in experimental enzootic pneumonia of pigs: an ultrastructural and histological study. Res. Vet. Sci., 13:570–578, 1972.

Baskerville, A., and Wright, C. L.: Ultrastructural changes in experimental enzootic pneumonia of pigs. Res. Vet. Sci., 14:155–160, 1973.

Furlong, S. L., and Turner, A. J.: Isolation of *Mycoplasma hyopneumoniae* and its association with pneumonia of pigs in Australia. Aust. Vet. J., *51*: 28–31, 1975.

Gois, M., Pospisil, Z., Cerny, M., and Mrva, V.: Production of pneumonia after intranasal inoculation of gnotobiotic piglets with three strains of *Mycoplasma hyorhinis*. J. Comp. Pathol., *81*:401–409, 1971.

Goodwin, R. F. W., Pomeroy, A. P., and Whittlestone, P.: Production of enzootic pneumonia in pigs with a mycoplasma. Vet. Rec., *77*:1247–1249, 1965.

Goodwin, R. F. W.: Experiments on the transmissibility of enzootic pneumonia of pigs. Res. Vet. Sci., *13*:257–261, 1972.

Hjärre, A.: Enzootic virus pneumonia and Glasser's disease of swine. Adv. Vet. Sci., *4*:235–263, 1958.

Huhn, R. G.: Enzootic pneumonia of pigs: a review of the literature. Vet Bull., *40*:249–257, 1970.

Lam, K. M., and Switzer, W. P.: Mycoplasmal pneumonia of swine: Development of an indirect hemagglutination test. Am. J. Vet. Res., *32*:1731–1736, 1971.

Lam, K. M., and Switzer, W. P.: Mycoplasmal pneumonia of swine: active and passive immunizations. Am. J. Vet. Res., *32*:1737–1742, 1971.

Lam, K. M., and Switzer, W. P.: Mycoplasmal pneumonia of swine: serologic response in pigs. Am. J. Vet. Res., *33*:1329–1332, 1972.

L'Ecuyer, C., and Boulanger, P.: Enzootic pneumonia of pigs: identification of a causative *Mycoplasma* in infected pigs and in cultures by immunofluorescent staining. Can. J. Comp. Med., *34*:38–46, 1970.

Livingston, C. W., Stari, E. L., Underdahl, N. R., and Mebus, C. A.: Pathogenesis of mycoplasmal pneumonia in swine. Am. J. Vet. Res., *33*:2249–2258, 1972.

Maré, C. J., and Switzer, W. P.: Mycoplasma hyopneumoniae. A causative agent of virus pig pneumonia. Vet Med. Small Anim. Clin., *60*:841–846, 1965.

———: Virus pneumonia of pigs: drug and ether sensitivity of a causative agent. Am. J. Vet. Res., *27*:1671–1675, 1966.

———: Virus pneumonia of pigs: filtration and visualization of a causative agent. Am. J. Vet. Res., *27*:1677–1685, 1966.

———: Virus pneumonia of pigs: Propagation and characterization of a causative agent. Am. J. Vet. Res., *27*:1687–1693, 1966.

Marley, J., Spradbrow, P. B., and Watt, D. A.: The isolation of mycoplasmas from porcine pneumonias. Aus. Vet. J., *47*:375–378, 1971.

Potgieter, L. N. D., and Ross, R. F.: Demonstration of *Mycoplasma hyorhinis* and *Mycoplasma hyosynoviae* in lesions of experimentally infected swine by immunofluorescence. Am. J. Vet. Res., *33*:99–106, 1972.

Roberts, D. H.: Experimental infection of pigs with *Mycoplasma hyopneumoniae (suipneumoniae)*. Br. Vet. J., *130*:68–74, 1974.

Schofield, F. W.: Virus pneumonia-like (VPP) lesions in the lungs of Canadian swine. Can. J. Comp. Med., *20*:252–266, 1956.

Switzer, W. P.: Mycoplasmal pneumonia of swine. J. Am. Vet. Med. Assoc., *160*:653–654, 1972.

Switzer, W. P., and Ross, R. F.: Mycoplasmal diseases. *In* Diseases of Swine, edited by H. W. Dunne and A. D. Leman. 4th ed. Ames, Iowa State Univ. Press, 1975. pp. 741–764.

Terpstar, J. E., Akkermans, J. P. W. M., and Pomper, W.: A mycoplasma as a cause of enzootic pneumonia of a swine. Neth. J. Vet. Sci., *2*:5–11, 1969.

Mycoplasmosis in Other Species

Man and Other Primates. Several species of *Mycoplasma* may be recovered from the oral, respiratory, and genital mucosae of man and several other primate species. In only a few instances are these organisms clearly associated with any disease process. *Mycoplasma pneumoniae* (Eaton's agent) is clearly associated with many cases of **primary atypical pneumonia**. This respiratory disease is especially prevalent among young adults closely associated with one another, as are recruits in a military camp. The urogenital tract may be colonized by *Ureaplasma urealyticum* (T-mycoplasma) and sometimes associated with "nongonococcal" urethritis. An etiologic role for *Mycoplasma* in human rheumatoid arthritis has been suspected, but the evidence for such a role at this time is controversial.

Mycoplasma species recovered from human beings, for which no pathogenic effect has been demonstrated, include several organisms that have also been found on mucosae of some nonhuman primates. These organisms include the following species (with known hosts in parentheses): *Mycoplasma orale*, type 1 (*Pongo pygmaeus*—orangutan); *M. orale*, type 2 (*Cercopithecus aethiops*—African green monkey, *Macaca mulatta*—Rhesus monkey, *Pan troglodytes*— chimpanzee, and *Pongo pygmaeus*); *M. orale*, type 3 (*Cercopitheus aethiops* and *Pongo pygmaeus*); *M. hominis* (*C. aethiops, M. mulatta*, and *Pan troglodytes*); *M. fermentans* (*C. aethiops*); *M. salivarium* (*C. aethiops, M. mulatta, Gorilla*

gorilla, *Pan troglodytes*, and *Pongo pyg-maeus*); and *Mycoplasma primatum (C. aethiops)* (Barile, 1973; Madden, et al., 1970 a and b; Hutchison, et al., 1970; Hill, 1977).

Marmosets are susceptible (Mutanda and Ufson, 1977) to experimental inoculation of *Mycoplasma pneumoniae*, but Rhesus monkeys *(Macaca mulatta)* are somewhat resistant (Friedlaender et al., 1976). *Ureaplasma* (T-mycoplasma) have been recovered from genital mucosae of chimpanzees, and are thought to be related to infertility (Brown et al., 1976; Swenson and O'Leary, 1977). Similar organisms have been found in the oropharynx and genital tract of marmosets *(Callithix jacchus)* (Furr et al., 1976), and in the genital tract of Talapoin monkeys *(Miopithecus talapoin)* in association with reproductive failure (Kundsin et al., 1975).

It was suggested that arthritis in a Rhesus monkey *(Macaca mulatta)* was due to mycoplasma on the basis of complement-fixation tests, but organisms were not recovered (Obeck et al., 1976).

Guinea Pigs. Organisms identified as *Mycoplasma caviae, Mycoplasma sp.*, and *Acholeplasma sp.* have been isolated from conventional and "specific pathogen-free" guinea pigs. These organisms maintain themselves in the nasal cavity and vagina, but no disease has been associated with them (Hill, 1971, Stalheim and Matthews, 1975).

Dogs. *Mycoplasma* have been recovered repeatedly from conjunctiva, respiratory system, and genital tracts of dogs. The organisms that are the most frequent inhabitants of dogs, and therefore called "canine species" of *Mycoplasma*, are *Mycoplasma spumans, M. canis, M. maculosum, M. edwardii, M. cynos, M. molare*, and *M. gateae*. The last species is also isolated frequently from cats. Some organisms have been recovered from lesions, such as in pneumonic lungs, and may have an etiologic relationship to the disease. Viruses (such as adenoviruses) and bacteria are often present as well, and reproduction of the disease with *Mycoplasma* often fails. The pathogenic significance of mycoplasma in dogs therefore remains equivocal at this time (Armstrong et al., 1972; Rosendal, 1972, 1973a, b, 1974, 1975; Binn et al., 1968).

Cats. At least three *Mycoplasma* species and one *Acholeplasma* species have been recovered from sick and normal cats with some frequency. Tan and Miles (1974) recovered 407 strains from 236 sick cats in New Zealand. Table 10–3 shows some species isolated with the frequency indicated.

Although association with severe conjunctivitis appears established in many cases in which *Mycoplasma felis* was isolated, in many instances an etiologic relationship has not been clearly established. *M. felis* has occasionally been associated with upper respiratory diseases in which viruses and *Chlamydia* have also been recognized. Commensal or synergistic rela-

Table 10–3. Mycoplasma Recovered from Cats

Genus/Species	Organisms recovered from		
	Sick Cats %	Sick Cats sacrificed %	Well Cats %
M. felis	29.7	38.0	4.4
M. arginini	16.5	9.2	6.7
M. gateae	46.2	43.1	62.2
A. laidlawii	0.5	0	22.2

tionships have been suspected among these organisms, but not proved.

Mycoplasmoses in Man and Other Primates

Barile, M. F.: Mycoplasmal flora of simians. J. Infect. Dis., 127:S17–S20, 1973.
Brown, W. J., Jacobs, N. F., Jr., Arum, E. S., and Arko, R. J.: T-strain mycoplasma in the chimpanzee. Lab. Anim. Sci., 26:81–83, 1976.
Freundt, E. A.: Present status of the medical importance of Mycoplasmas. Pathol. Microbiol., 40:155–187, 1974.
Friedlaender, R. P., et al.: Experimental production of respiratory tract infection with *Mycoplasma pneumoniae* in Rhesus monkeys. J. Infect. Dis., 133:343–346, 1976.
Furr, P. M., Taylor-Robinson, D., and Hetherington, C. M.: The occurrence of ureaplasmas in marmosets. Lab. Anim., 10:393–398, 1976.
Hill, A.: The isolation of mycoplasmas from nonhuman primates. Vet. Rec., 101:117, 1977.
Hutchison, V. E., Pinkerton, M. E., and Kalter, S. S.: Incidence of mycoplasma in nonhuman primates. Lab. Anim. Care, 20:914–922, 1970.
Kundsin, R. B., et al.: T-strain mycoplasmas and reproductive failure in monkeys. Lab. Anim. Sci., 25:221–224, 1975.
Madden, D. L., et al.: The isolation and identification of mycoplasma from *Macaca mulatta*. Lab. Anim. Care, 20:467–470, 1970a.
————: The isolation and identification of mycoplasma from *Cercopithecus aethiops*. Lab. Anim. Care, 20:471–473, 1970b.
————: *Mycoplasma moatsii*, a new species isolated from recently imported grivet monkeys (*Cercopithecus aethiops*). Intl. J. Syst. Bact., 24:459–464, 1974.
Mutanda, L. N., and Ufson, M. A.: Experimental *Mycoplasma pneumoniae* infection of marmosets. Lab. Anim. Sci., 27:119, 1977.
Obeck, D. K., Toft, J. D., II, and Dupuy, H. J.: Severe polyarthritis in a rhesus monkey: suggested mycoplasma etiology. Lab. Anim. Sci., 26:613–618, 1976.
Swensen, C. E., and O'Leary, W. M.: Genital ureaplasmas in nonhuman primates. J. Med. Primatol., 6:344–348, 1977.

Mycoplasmoses in Guinea Pigs

Hill, A.: *Mycoplasma caviae*, a new species. J. Gen. Microbiol., 65:109–113, 1971.
Stalheim, O. H. V., and Matthews, P. J.: Mycoplasmosis in specific-pathogen-free and conventional guinea pigs. Lab. Anim. Sci., 25:70–73, 1975.

Mycoplasmoses in Dogs

Armstrong, D., et al.: Canine pneumonia associated with mycoplasma infection. Am. J. Vet. Res., 33:1471–1478, 1972.

Binn, L. N., et al.: Upper respiratory disease in military dogs: bacterial, mycoplasma and viral studies. Am. J. Vet. Res., 29:1809–1815, 1968.
Rosendal, S.: Mycoplasmas as a possible cause of enzootic pneumonia in dogs. Acta Vet. Scand., 13:137–139, 1972.
————: *Mycoplasma molare*, a new canine mycoplasma species. Int. J. Syst. Bact., 23:49–54, 1973a.
————: Canine mycoplasmas 1: cultivation from conjunctivae, respiratory and genital tracts. Acta Pathol. Microbiol. Scand., 81B:441–445, 1973b.
————: *Mycoplasma cynos*, a new canine *Mycoplasma* species. Int. J. Syst. Bact., 23:125–130, 1974.
————: Canine mycoplasmas. I. Cultural and biochemical studies of type and reference strains. II. Serological studies of type and reference strains, with a proposal for the new species, *Mycoplasma opalescens*. Acta Pathol. Microbiol. Scand., 83B:457–462, 463–470, 1975.

Mycoplasmoses in Cats

Campbell, L. H., Snyder, S. B., Reed, C., and Fox, J. G.: *Mycoplasma felis*-associated conjunctivitis in cats. J. Am. Vet. Med. Assoc., 163:991–995, 1973.
Tan, R. J. S., and Miles, J. A. R.: Characterization of mycoplasmas isolated from cats with conjunctivitis. NZ Vet. J., 21:27–32, 1973.
————: Incidence and significance of mycoplasmas in sick cats. Res. Vet. Sci., 16:27–34, 1974.

RICKETTSIAL DISEASES

Microorganisms classified in the Family Rickettsiaceae (order: Rickettsiales) include several causative agents of disease in man and animals. The organisms are minute obligate parasites which are found in the cytoplasm of tissue cells but not in erythrocytes. The organisms are frequently transmitted from one vertebrate species to another by arthropod vectors. Six pathogenic genera are presently included in this family: *Rickettsia*, *Rochalimaea*, *Coxiella*, *Cowdria*, *Ehrlichia*, and *Neorickettsia*. See Table 10–4.

The genus *Rickettsia* contains six species that are pathogenic for man and animals, and are transmitted by arthropod vectors. One organism, *Rochalimaea quintana* (formerly *Rickettsia quintana*), the cause of Trench fever, has been placed in a separate genus because of its ability to grow on media devoid of living cells (Bergey, 1974). The diseases caused by these organisms generally have severe febrile manifesta-

Table 10–4.   Diseases Due to Rickettsiaceae

Genus and Species	Vectors	Hosts*	Disease
Rickettsia prowazekii	Lice (Pediculus humanus)	Man (guinea pig)	Typhus fever
R. typhi	Rat louse (Polyplax spinosus) Rat flea (Xenopsylla cheopis) Human flea (Pulex irritans) Human louse (Pediculus humanus)	Man, rats, and mice	Murine typhus of man
R. rickettsii	Ticks (Dermacentor andersoni, D. variabilis, Haemaphysalis leporis palustris, Amblyomma americanum)	Man, squirrels, rabbits, mice	Rocky Mountain spotted fever
R. conori	Dog ticks (Rhipicephalus sanguineus and others)	Man, rodents (guinea pig)	Boutonneuse fever
R. tsutsugamushi	Trombiculid mites (Leptotrombidium akamushi, etc.)	Man, Rhesus, gibbon, (guinea pig, hamster, moles, rats, gerbils, mice)	Tsutsugamushi fever (scrub typhus)
R. akari	Mites (Allodermanyssus sanguineus)	Man, mice and other rodents (guinea pigs)	Rickettsial pox
Rochalimaea quintana	Lice (Pediculus humanus)	Man (rhesus)	Trench fever
Neorickettsia helminthoeca	Fluke (Nanophyetus salmincola)	Dogs, foxes, bears	Salmon disease of dogs and foxes (canine neorickettsiosis)
Coxiella burnetii	Ticks (many species—also aerosol transmission)	Man, cattle, sheep, goats, birds (rabbits, guinea pigs, hamsters, mice)	Q fever
Cowdria ruminatum	Ticks (Amblyomma sp.)	Cattle	"Heartwater"
Ehrlichia bovis (Rickettsia bovis)	Ticks (Rhipicephalus sp., Hyalomma sp.)	Cattle, wild ruminants	Bovine ehrlichiosis ("mild disease of cattle")
E. ovina (Rickettsia ovis)	Ticks (Rhipicephalus bursa, Hyalomma sp.)	Sheep	Ovine ehrlichiosis ("mild disease of sheep")
E. canis (Rickettsia canis)	Ticks (Rhipicephalus sanguineus)	Dogs	Canine ehrlichiosis
Ehrlichia sp.	Ticks (?)	Horses	Equine ehrlichiosis

* Experimentally susceptible host in parentheses ( )

tions and may terminate fatally. The agent causes severe disease in the arthropod vectors, and in some instances the natural disease in animals is severe and fatal. In some (typhus fever, trench fever), man is the only host, although other species are susceptible to experimental inoculation. The essential features of the rickettsioses are summarized in Table 10–4.

Weiss, E., and Moulder, J. W.: Rochalimaea. In Bergey's Manual of Determinative Bacteriology, 8th ed., edited by R. E. Buchanan and N. E. Gibbons. Baltimore, Williams & Wilkins, 1974, pp. 890–891.

Q Fever

A febrile disease of slaughterhouse workers was originally described in Australia by Derrick (1937), who named the disease "Q" fever (Q for query, i.e., of questionable or unknown etiology). The disease occurs in widely scattered parts of the world, including the United States and Europe. The infectious agent, now classified with the rickettsial organisms and called *Coxiella burnetii (Rickettsia burnetii, R. diaporica),* is harbored by cattle, sheep, and probably other species, and can be transmitted by ticks *(Dermacentor andersoni, D. occidentalis, Rhipicephalus sanguineus, Otobius megnini,* and others). Man may acquire the infection by contact with freshly slaughtered infected cattle or by consuming raw milk or butter in which the organisms are present. The organisms can be passed through filters that retain most bacteria, but they are demonstrable in tissues stained by Giemsa or Macchiavello methods, where they appear as minute pleomorphic organisms in the form of lanceolate rods, 0.05 μ in width and 0.5 μ long, as bipolar forms about 1.0 μ in length, or as diplobacillary forms which attain a length of 1.5 μ. Clusters of these organisms appear in the cytoplasm of tissue cells and occasionally are seen extracellularly. *Coxiella burnetii* are poorly stained by ordinary bacterial methods, thus conforming to the characteristics of other rickettsiae.

Lesions. Organisms have been recovered from cows that exhibited no signs of infection, and postmortem examination of such animals has disclosed few, if any, specific lesions. It is necessary to study the tissues of experimentally infected guinea pigs for information concerning the lesions of Q fever. According to Lillie (1942), the lesions in guinea pigs are characterized by focal perivascular exudation of lymphoid cells, less often monocytes and fibroblasts, and "vascular endotheliosis," particularly in the myocardium, lungs, alveolar tissue generally, adrenals, renal cortex and medulla, and epididymis. In the lungs, small foci made up of collections of epithelioid cells are seen in alveoli, and some lymphocytes and other mononuclear cells are located in the interalveolar stroma.

In later stages of the disease, small nodules of epithelioid cells are found in the spleen, liver, and vertebral marrow; less often in the heart, mediastinal and mesenteric fat, pancreas, kidney, adrenal, bladder mucosa, testicle, and brain. These small granulomas often contain large, multinucleated giant cells, which may replace the entire nodule. Serous exudate is common in alveolar tissues of the renal pelvis and rare in the epididymis.

In mice inoculated intranasally or intraperitoneally, Perrin and Bengston (1942) have shown that nodular or patchy granulomatous lesions develop in the spleen, liver, kidneys, and adrenals. Nodular and patchy areas of aplasia and necrosis also occur in the bone marrow. Proliferative changes in the lung and exudation of mononuclear cells are also observed in mice inoculated intranasally.

Diagnosis. Recognition of infection in cattle depends upon the isolation and identification of organisms, usually by inoculation of guinea pigs. Neutralization tests using convalescent serum to protect guinea pigs are of value in differential diagnosis. A complement-fixation test is also employed.

Behymer, D. E., et al.: Q fever *(Coxiella burnetii)* investigations in dairy cattle: persistence of antibodies after vaccination. Am. J. Vet. Res., 36:781–784, 1975.

Biberstein, E. L., et al.: A survey of Q fever *(Coxiella burnetii)* in California dairy cows. Am. J. Vet. Res., 35:1577–1582, 1974.

Curet, L. B., and Paust, J. C.: Transmission of Q fever from experimental sheep to laboratory personnel. Am. J. Obstet. Gynecol., 114:566–568, 1972.

Davis, G. E., Cox, H. R., Parker, R. R., and Dyer, R. E.: A filter-passing infectious agent isolated from ticks. I. Isolation from *Dermacentor andersoni,* reactions in animals and filtration experiments. II. Transmission by *Dermacentor andersoni.* III. Description of the organism and cultivation experiments. IV. Human infection. Pub. Health Rep., 53:2259–2282, 1938.

Derrick, E. H.: "Q" fever, a new fever entity: clinical features, diagnosis and laboratory investigation. Med. J. Aust., 2:281–299, 1937.

Enright, J. B., et al.: Q fever antibodies in birds. J. Wildl. Dis., 7:14–21, 1971.

————: The behavior of Q fever rickettsiae isolated from wild animals in northern California. J. Wildl. Dis., 7:83–90, 1971.

Heggers, J. P., Billups, L. H., Hinrichs, D. J., and Mallavia, L. P.: Pathophysiologic features of Q fever-infected guinea pigs. Am. J. Vet. Res., 36:1047–1052, 1975.

Lillie, R. D.: Pathologic histology in guinea pigs following intraperitoneal inoculation with the virus of "Q" fever. Pub. Health Rep.,57:296–306, 1942.

Parker, R. R., Bell, E. J., and Stoerner, H. G.: "Q" fever—a brief survey of the problem. J. Am. Vet. Med. Assoc., 114:55–60, 124–130, 1939.

Perrin, T. L., and Bengston, I. A.: The histopathology of experimental "Q" fever in mice. Pub. Health Rep., 57:790–798, 1942.

Randhawa, A. S., Dieterich, W. H., Jolleu, W. B., and Hunter, C. C.: Coxiellosis in pound cats. Feline Pract., 4:37–38, 1974.

Salmon Disease of Dogs and Foxes ("Salmon Poisoning," Canine Neorickettsiosis)

A febrile, often fatal, disease of dogs and foxes has been known for some time to be associated with a diet that includes salmon, trout, and other fish. The disease is related to infection by a small intestinal fluke, *Troglotrema (Nanophyetus) salmincola*, whose encysted metacercariae are carried in fish of the family Salmonidae, which thus serve as intermediate hosts. Earlier observations indicate that a rickettsial organism is the probable etiologic agent of the disease, the fluke acting only as a reservoir for the infection. This complex biologic pattern in host-parasite relationship is of unusual interest. The disease is not spread by contact, but can be produced by feeding the dog or fox fish infected with metacercariae of *Troglotrema salmincola*. It can be transmitted by intraperitoneal injection of blood of an infected dog, suspensions of washed flukes from infected dogs, or metacercariae from fish.

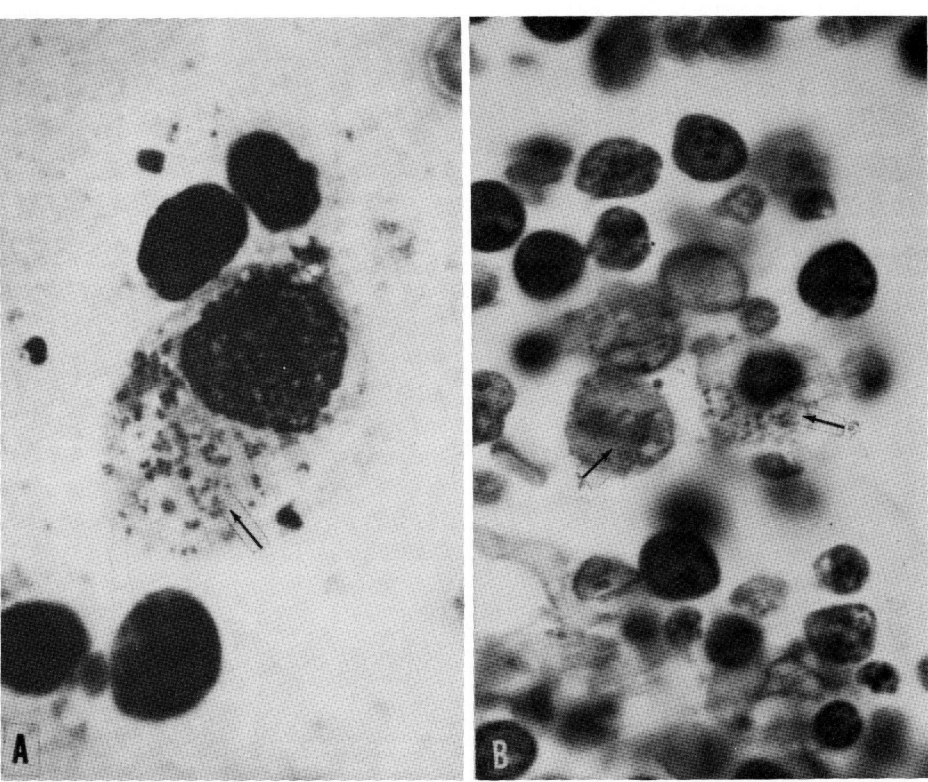

Fig. 10–3. "Salmon Disease" in a dog. *A*, Smear from a mesenteric lymph node. (Giemsa stain, × 1500.) *B*, Tissue section from another lymph node. (Giemsa stain, × 500.) Arrows indicate organism, *Neorickettsia helmintheca.* (Courtesy of Dr. Wm. J. Hadlow.)

Signs. The signs usually appear about five days after the ingestion of infected fish, starting as a fever, which continues four to eight days. Anorexia is a characteristic feature, and is accompanied by depression, weakness, and weight loss. Vomiting and diarrhea, with scant, yellowish, watery, or occasionally bloody and mucoid feces, accompanied by tenesmus, are prominent manifestations. Occasionally, a serous nasal discharge is observed, and a tenacious conjunctival exudate may collect at the inner canthus of the eye.

Lesions. According to Cordy and Gorham (1950), lymphoid tissues suffer particularly in this disease; the visceral nodes of the abdomen may be enlarged to six times normal size (Fig. 23–17), with the somatic lymph nodes somewhat less severely affected. These enlarged nodes are usually yellowish with prominent white follicles in their cortex. Some edema may surround them, and occasionally an opaque grayish fluid can be expressed from a nodule. The tonsils, which are enlarged and yellowish with prominent follicles and occasional petechiae, may be everted from the fossae. The spleen is often enlarged. The splenic follicles are prominent in foxes but unrecognizable in dogs. The lymphoid tissue of the intestinal tract is especially hyperplastic (Fig. 23–17). The intestinal contents may include free blood, especially in animals in which flukes have damaged the intestinal mucosa. Petechiae usually are seen in the intestinal mucosa, particularly over the enlarged lymphoid follicles. Bleeding from small ulcers may be noted in the pylorus. Intussusception of the small intestine is not uncommon. Although the liver often appears grossly normal, rupture is a possibility, with hemoperitoneum as the usual consequence. Hemorrhages have been observed in the gallbladder and the urinary bladder. The lungs usually are studded with many bright or dark red subpleural hemorrhagic puncta, 5 to 20 mm in diameter.

The microscopic findings, prominent in the lymph nodes, are dominated by hyperplasia of reticuloendothelial elements and depletion of small lymphocytes. Foci of necrosis are frequent and many include hemorrhages. Elementary bodies of *Neorickettsia* in reticuloendothelial cells, both in sinuses and parenchyma, are demonstrated by Giemsa or Macchiavello's stain. The thymus in younger dogs is the site of prominent changes, including depletion of small lymphocytes, proliferation of reticuloendothelial cells, increase in neutrophils, and the presence of small islands of necrosis throughout the gland. In the intestine, flukes may be demonstrated deep in the intestinal villi and occasionally in duodenal glands. There is surprisingly little tissue reaction to these flukes, aside from a few foci of neutrophils and slight increase in lymphoid and plasma cells in the lamina propria. Small hemorrhages in the intestinal mucosa or submucosa may be seen, although not necessarily in relation to the flukes.

According to Hadlow (1957), the brain contains microscopic lesions in 91% of fatal cases. These changes consist of: "(a) slight to moderate accumulation of mononuclear cells in the leptomeninges, most intense over the cerebellum, (b) cellular exudative and proliferative changes in sheaths of small and medium-sized intracerebral blood vessels; and (c) focal collections of glial, mesenchymal cells, or both." The intracerebral lesions, less intense than those of the meninges, occur in the cerebral cortex, brain stem, and cerebellum. Similar lesions may occur in the neurohypophysis. Aside from the hemorrhages, which are recognized grossly, microscopic changes in other viscera are minimal and believed to be nonspecific.

Diagnosis. Of particular significance in the diagnosis of this disease are the small intracytoplasmic "elementary" bodies in reticuloendothelial cells in lymphoid tissue and occasionally in large mononuclear cells of liver, lungs, and blood. These bodies are coccoid or coccobacillary in shape and uniformly about 0.3 μ in diameter. With Giemsa's stain, these bodies are purple; with Macchiavello's stain, red or blue; with Levaditi's method, black or dark brown; with hematoxylin and eosin, pale bluish violet. They are gram-negative. In some cells, they form nearly solid "plaques" filling the cytoplasm. In some smears, they are found free, apparently released from ruptured cells. They have not been observed in epithelium, endothelium, fibroblasts or muscle cells.

The organisms have been propagated in tissue cultures and may be demonstrated by specific immunofluorescence (Brown et al., 1972; Kitao et al., 1973).

An unnamed rickettsial organism has been demonstrated in black bears (Ursus americana) infected with Troglotrema salmincola; this organism differs serologically and by immunofluorescence from Neorickettsia helminthoeca, and produces a slightly different disease in dogs. This disease has been called "Elokomin fluke fever" (after the Elokomin River in Washington) (Farrell et al., 1973; Sakawa et al., 1973; and Kitao et al., 1973). Another agent, Rickettsia sennetsu, is believed to be the cause of Hyuga or Kagami fever, and was isolated from human patients in Kyushu, Japan. The human disease follows consumption of raw bora fish (Mugil cephalus), and it appears that an endoparasite of the fish may be the vector host (Kitao et al., 1973).

Brown, J. L., Huxsoll, D. L., Ristic, M., and Hildebrandt, P. K.: In vitro cultivation of Neorickettsia helminthoeca, the causative agent of salmon poisoning disease. Am. J. Vet. Res., 33:1695–1706, 1972.

Cordy, D. R., and Gorham, J. R.: The pathology and etiology of salmon disease in the dog and fox. Am. J. Pathol., 26:617–637, 1950.

Farrell, R. K., Leader, R. W., and Johnston, S. D.: Differentiation of salmon poisoning disease and Elokomin fluke fever: studies with the black bear (Ursus americanus). Am. J. Vet. Res., 34:919–922, 1973.

Frank, D. W., McGuire, T. C., Gorham, J. R., and Farrell, R. K.: Lymphoreticular lesions of canine neorickettsiosis. J. Infect. Dis., 129:163–171, 1974.

Hadlow, W. J.: Neuropathology of experimental salmon poisoning of dogs. Am. J. Vet. Res., 18:898–908, 1957.

Karr, S. L., and Wong, M. M.: Experimental infection of monkeys with Nanophyetus salmincola. J. Parasitol., 60:358, 1974.

Kitao, T., Farrell, R. K., and Fukuda, T.: Differentiation of salmon poisoning disease and Elokomin fluke fever: Fluorescent antibody studies with Rickettsia sennetsu. Am. J. Vet. Res., 34:927–928, 1973.

Philip, C. B., Hadlow, W. J., and Hughes, L. E.: Neorickettsia helmintheca, a new rickettsia-like disease agent of dogs in western United States transmitted by a helminth. Proc. 6th Internat. Cong. Microbiol. (Rome), 4:70–82, 1953.

Sakawa, H., Farrell, R. K., and Mori, M.: Differentiation of salmon poisoning disease and Elokomin fluke fever: Complement fixation. Am. J. Vet. Res., 34:923–926, 1973.

Weiseth, P. R., Farrell, R. K., and Johnston, S. D.: Prevalence of Nanophyetus salmincola in ocean-caught salmon. J. Am. Vet. Med. Assoc., 165:849–850, 1974.

"Heartwater" of Cattle, Sheep and Goats

The name of this disease, which is rather important on the African continent, is derived from its characteristic lesion: hydropericardium. The causative agent, Cowdria (formerly Rickettsia) ruminantium, is an intracellular parasite transmitted by ticks (genus Amblyomma). It is currently differentiated from the Rickettsia, which may be transmitted through the egg to succeeding generations of ticks. C. ruminantium may be carried through metamorphosis of larva to nymph or nymph to adult, but not through the egg. The organism is a tiny rod-shaped, often diplococcoid organism, which can be demonstrated with Giemsa's stain in endothelial cells of the jugular vein, vena cava, renal glomerular capillaries, and cerebral gray matter. It is gram-negative, cannot be cultivated on artificial media, and is not demonstrable in the circulating blood.

The organisms seen with the electron microscope are quite pleomorphic, in coccoid, ovoid, filamentous, irregular, horseshoe, and polygonal shapes, measuring roughly 0.49 μ to 2.7 μ in diameter. Each organism is enclosed within a two-unit membrane and contains a structure made up of electron-dense granules ("cytoplasm") and less dense fibrillar material ("nucleoid"). The organisms are found in the cytoplasm of cells and, in the mature form at least, are bound by a cell membrane that separates them from cytoplasmic organelles. The organisms multiply by binary fission and apparently by multiple budding as well (du Plessis, 1970, 1975; Pienaar, 1970).

The clinical manifestations are high fever and nervous manifestations, death resulting from systemic infection—often with distention of the pericardial sac by serous exudate.

du Plessis, J. L.: Pathogenesis of heartwater: I. *Cowdria ruminantium* in the lymph nodes of domestic ruminants. Onderstepoort. J. Vet. Res.,37:89–95, 1970.

————: Electron microscopy of *Cowdria ruminantium* infected reticulo-endothelial cells of the mammalian host. Onderstepoort. J. Vet. Res., 42:1–13, 1975.

Haig, D. A.: Tickborne rickettsioses in South Africa. Adv. Vet. Sci., 2:307–325, 1955.

Henning, M. W.: Animal Diseases of South Africa, 3rd ed., Pretoria, Central News Agency, Ltd., 1956.

Pienaar, J. G., et al.: Studies on the pathology of heartwater *(Cowdria Rickettsia) ruminantium* Cowdry, 1926. I. Neuropathological changes. Onderstepoort J. Vet. Res., 33:115–138, 1966.

Pienaar, J. G.: Electron microscopy of *Cowdria (Rickettsia) ruminantium* (Cowdry, 1926) in the endothelial cells of the vertebrate host. Onderstepoort. J. Vet. Res., 37:67–78, 1970.

Canine Ehrlichiosis (Canine Rickettsiosis, Tropical Canine Pancytopenia)

Caused by *Ehrlichia canis*, canine ehrlichiosis is principally of importance in Africa and India, although it also exists in the United States, Southeast Asia, the Virgin Islands, Puerto Rico, and Florida. The disease is transmitted by the tick, *Rhipicephalus sanguineus*. The organism multiplies in reticuloendothelial cells, lymphocytes, and monocytes, and can be visualized in stained smears of peripheral blood or tissue impressions, although often with difficulty. The life cycle of the parasite is not yet completely understood, but three intracellular forms can be recognized. Initial bodies are small (1 to 2 μ) spherical structures, which are believed to develop into larger bodies described as mulberry bodies or morulae, composed of multiple subunits. The morula is thought to dissociate to small granules called elementary bodies. The disease is usually mild, except in young puppies or when complicated by another disease, such as infection with *Babesia canis*.

Signs. Ewing (1965, 1969) describes the clinical signs as recurrent fever, serous nasal discharge, photophobia, vomiting, splenomegaly, and signs of central nervous system derangement. Epistaxis, emaciation, and edema of the limbs may also be observed (Hildebrandt et al., 1973). Pancytopenia and hypergammaglobulinemia, with increased levels of gamma globulin and glycoglobulin in the serum, are clinical features observed late in the disease (Burghen et al., 1971).

Lesions. The lesions encountered grossly consist of hemorrhages in the mucosae of the gastrointestinal and urogenital tracts and kidney, edematous or hemorrhagic enlargement of most lymph nodes, and edema of the limbs. Many animals are emaciated at the time of death, and epistaxis may be evident at this time. Rarely, icterus is observed (Hildebrandt et al., 1973).

The microscopic lesions consist of widespread perivascular accumulations of lymphoreticular and plasma cells, particularly in the meninges, kidneys, liver, and lymphopoietic tissues. The bone marrow is usually hypoplastic. Degeneration and acute necrosis is common in the center of lobules of the liver, presumably the result of anemia. In the central nervous system, hemorrhages and plasma cell accumulations occur in the meninges, and occasionally lymphocytic and plasma cell infiltrations are present in the brain parenchyma. These lesions have been interpreted as immunoproliferative manifestations (Hildebrandt et al., 1973).

Diagnosis. The diagnosis may be confirmed by identifying the organisms in sections of tissues in fatal cases. Serologic identification of specific antibodies may be accomplished by an indirect immunofluorescence test (Ristic et al., 1972). The organisms in tissues may also be identified by using the electron microscope.

Amyx, H. L., and Huxsoll, D. L.: Red and gray foxes—potential reservoir hosts for *Ehrlichia canis*. J. Wildl. Dis., 9:47–50, 1973.

Buhles, W. C., Jr., Huxsoll, D. L., and Ristic, M.: Tropical canine pancytopenia: Clinical, hematologic, and serologic response of dogs to *Ehrlichia canis* infection, tetracycline therapy, and challenge inoculation. J. Infect. Dis., 130:357–367, 1974.

Burghen, G. A., et al.: Development of hypergammaglobulinemia in tropical canine pancytopenia. Am. J. Vet. Res., 32:749–756, 1971.

Carter, G. B., Seamer, J., and Snape, T.: Diagnosis of tropical canine pancytopaenia (*Ehrlichia canis* infection) by immunofluorescence. Res. Vet. Sci., 12:318–322, 1971.

Ewing, S. A.: Canine ehrlichiosis. Adv. Vet. Sci., 13:331–353, 1969.

Ewing, S. A., and Buckner, R. G.: Manifestations of babesiosis, ehrlichiosis, and combined infections in the dog. Am. J. Vet. Res., 26:815–828, 1965.

Ewing, S. A., Roberson, W. R., Buckner, R. G., and Hayat, C. S.: A new strain of *Ehrlichia canis*. J. Am. Vet. Med. Assoc., 159:1771–1774, 1971.

Groves, M. G., Dennis, G. L., Amyx, H. L., and Huxsoll, D. L.: Transmission of *Ehrlichia canis* to dogs by ticks *(Rhipicephalus sanguineus)*. Am. J. Vet. Res., 36:937–940, 1975.

Hildebrandt, P. K., et al.: Pathology of canine ehrlichiosis (tropical canine pancytopenia). Am. J. Vet. Res., 34:1309–1320, 1973.

Huxsoll, D. L., et al.: *Ehrlichia canis*—the causative agent of a haemorrhagic disease of dogs. Vet. Rec., 85:587, 1969.

———: Laboratory studies of tropical canine pancytopenia. Exp. Parasitol., 31:53–59, 1972.

Immelman, A., and Button, C.: *Ehrlichia canis* infection (tropical canine pancytopenia or canine rickettsiosis). J. S. Afr. Vet. Assoc., 44:241–245, 1973.

Leeflang, P., and Perie, N. M.: A comparative study of the pathogenicities of Old and New World strains of *Ehrlichia canis*. Trop. Anim. Health Prod., 4:107–108, 1972.

Nims, R. M., et al.: Epizootiology of tropical canine pancytopenia in Southeast Asia. J. Am. Vet. Med. Assoc., 158:53–63, 1971.

Nyindo, M. B. A., Ristic, M., Huxsoll, D. L., and Smith, A. R.: Tropical canine pancytopenia: in vitro cultivation of the causative agent-*Ehrlichia canis*. Am. J. Vet. Res., 32:1651–1658, 1971.

Ristic, M., et al.: Serological diagnosis of tropical canine pancytopenia by indirect immunofluorescence. Infect. Immun., 6:226–231, 1972.

Seamer, J., and Snape, T.: *Ehrlichia canis* and tropical canine pancytopaenia. Res. Vet. Sci., 13:307–314, 1972.

Simpson, C. F.: Structure of *Ehrilichia canis* in blood monocytes of a dog. Am. J. Vet. Res., 33:2451–2454, 1972.

Simpson, C. F.: Relationship of *Ehrlichia canis*-infected mononuclear cells to blood vessels of lungs. Infect. Immun., 10:590–596, 1974.

Smith, R. D., Ristic, M., Huxsoll, D. L., and Baylor, R. A.: Platelet kinetics in canine ehrlichiosis: evidence for increased platelet destruction as the cause of thrombocytopenia. Infec. Immun., 11:1216–1221, 1975.

Smith, R. D., et al.: Development of *Ehrlichia canis*, causative agent of canine ehrlichiosis, in the tick *Rhipicephalus sanguineus* and its differentiation from a symbiotic rickettsia. Am. J. Vet. Res., 37:119–126, 1976.

———: Isolation in Illinois of a foreign strain of *Ehrlichia canis*, the causative agent of canine ehrlichiosis (tropical canine pancytopenia). J. Am. Vet. Med. Assoc., 166:172–174, 1975.

Stephenson, E. H., and Osterman, J. V.: Canine peritoneal macrophages: cultivation and infection with *Ehrlichia canis*. Am. J. Vet. Res., 38:1815–1819, 1977.

Walker, J. S., et al.: Clinical and clinicopathologic findings in tropical canine pancytopenia. J. Am. Vet. Med. Assoc., 157:43–55, 1970.

Ovine and Bovine Ehrlichiosis ("Tick-Borne Fever," "Mild Disease of Sheep")

Febrile disease of a mild, nonfatal nature has been associated with tick infestation in both sheep and cattle. Experimentally, a febrile disease may be transmitted between sheep and cattle. In Great Britain, the Netherlands, and Finland, a rickettsial organism called *Ehrlichia phagocytophilia* (*Rickettsia phagocytophilia*, *Cytoecetes phagocytophilia*, or *Cytoecetes bovis*) has been identified as the causative agent. Goats are also believed to be susceptible, and the organism has also been isolated from wild deer in Great Britain. The vector in Europe is believed to be the tick, *Ixodes ricinus*.

On the African continent, similar organisms isolated from sheep and cattle, and named respectively, *Ehrlichia ovina* and *Ehrlichia bovis*, have been associated with febrile illness in these animals. Transmission between sheep and cattle is possible, and the organisms have not been clearly differentiated at this time. Ticks of the genus *Hyalomma* have been identified as vectors of the bovine disease; other ticks, especially *Rhipicephalus bursa*, are thought to transmit the disease among sheep.

The identification of the organisms is crucial to specific diagnosis. Many reports of clinical studies in the literature fail to record this essential information. Further studies are needed to clarify the specific nature of these disease entities.

Buchanan, R. E., and Gibbons, N. E.: Bergey's Manual of Determinative Bacteriology. 8th ed. Baltimore, Williams & Wilkins, 1974, pp. 894–895.

Foster, W. N. M., and Cameron, A. E.: Thrombocytopenia in sheep associated with experimental tick-borne fever infection. J. Comp. Pathol., 78:251–254, 1968.

Foster, W. N. M., Foggie, A., and Hisbet, D. I.: Haemorrhagic enteritis in sheep experimentally infected with tick-borne fever. J. Comp. Pathol., 78:255–258, 1968.

Gordon, W. S., Brownlee, A., Wilson, D. R., and MacLeod, J.: Tick-borne fever. J. Comp. Pathol., 45:301–312, 1932.

Hudson, J. R.: The recognition of tick-borne fever as a disease of cattle. Br. Vet. J., 106:3–17, 1950.

Equine Ehrlichiosis

This infrequent disease has been described in horses in the foothills of the Sacramento Valley in California and has been studied experimentally (Gribble, 1969; Stannard et al., 1969).

The disease may be transmitted experimentally with blood-containing organisms. Sheep, goats, and dogs develop a mild experimental disease. Cattle do not appear to be susceptible. Ticks are suspected but not yet proved to be carriers in nature.

Signs. The clinical features include fever, anorexia, depression, edema of the legs, and ataxia. Clinical laboratory findings include leukopenia. thrombocytopenia, elevated plasma icterus index, decreased packed cell volume, and lymphopenia. The organisms appear as granular bodies in the cytoplasm of neutrophils and eosinophils.

Lesions. The experimentally-induced lesions in horses and donkeys are seen grossly as petechiae, ecchymoses, and edema in muscles, fascia, and subcutis. Icterus is frequent and orchitis common. The microscopic lesions consist of arteritis and phlebitis, particularly in muscles and fascia, but also in kidneys, heart, brain, and lungs. The blood vessels undergo necrosis as well as swelling of endothelium and smooth muscle cells. This is accompanied by accumulation of lymphocytes, plasma cells, and occasionally neutrophils.

Diagnosis. The diagnosis, based upon clinical findings, may be confirmed by the demonstration of organisms in neutrophils or eosinophils. They stain characteristically blue with Giemsa's or Wright-Leishman's stain and are gram-positive. The organisms are spherical, single or multiple, and vary in size from 200 mμ to 5 μ in diameter. The pleomorphic organisms, with two peripheral membranes, may be demonstrated with the electron microscope.

Gribble, D. H.: Equine ehrlichiosis. J. Am. Vet. Med. Assoc., 155:462–469, 1969.

Lewis, G. E., Jr., Huxsoll, D. L., Ristic, M., and Johnson, A. J.: Experimentally induced infection of dogs, cats, and nonhuman primates with *Ehrlichia equi* etiologic agent of equine ehrlichiosis. Am. J. Vet. Res., 36:85–88, 1975.

Sells, D. M. et al.: Ultrastructural observations on *Ehrlichia equi* organisms in equine granulocytes. Infect. Immun., 13:273–280, 1976.

Stannard, A. A., Gribble, D. H., and Smith, R. S.: Equine ehrlichiosis: A disease with similarities to tick-borne fever and bovine petechiae fever. Vet. Rec., 84:149–150, 1969.

Bovine Petechial Fever (Ondiri Disease)

An infrequent disease, reported only from Kenya and Tanzania, bovine petechial fever resembles equine ehrlichiosis in clinical signs and gross lesions. The causative agent, named by Tyzzer in 1938, is *Cytoecetes ondiri*, a member of the family Rickettsiaceae. The organisms are demonstrable in neutrophils of infected cattle as irregular spheroid bodies or morulae. The infection is often confined to particular paddocks or woodlots, and is suspected, but not proven to be carried by an arthropod vector.

Cooper, J. E.: Attempted transmission of the Ondiri disease (bovine petechial fever) agent to laboratory rodents. Res. Vet. Sci., 15:130–133, 1973.

Danks, W. B. C.: (First description of bovine petechial fever). Annu. Report Agri. Dept., p. 375, Kenya, 1933.

Davies, F. G., Odegaard, O. A., and Cooper, J. E.: The morphology of the causal agent of bovine petechial fever (Ondiri disease). J. Comp. Pathol., 82:241–246, 1972.

Dawe, P. S., Ohder, H., Wegener, J., and Bruce, W.: Some observations on bovine petechial fever (Ondiri disease) passaged in sheep. Bull. Epizoot. Dis. Afr., 18:361–368, 1970.

Jaffery, M. S., and Mwangota, A. U.: Hyperacute bovine petechial fever. Vet. Rec., 95:212–213, 1974.

Snodgrass, D. R.: Pathogenesis of bovine petechial fever. Latent infections, immunity, and tissue distribution of Cytoecetes ondiri. J. Comp. Pathol., 85:523–530, 1975.

Snodgrass, D. R., Karstad, L. H., and Cooper, J. E.: The role of wild ruminants in the epidemiology of bovine petechial fever. J. Hyg., 74:245–250, 1975.

Walker, A. R., Cooper, J. E., and Snodgrass, D. R.: Investigations into the epidemiology of bovine petechial fever in Kenya and the potential of trombiculid mites as vectors. Trop. Anim. Health Prod., 6:193–198, 1974.

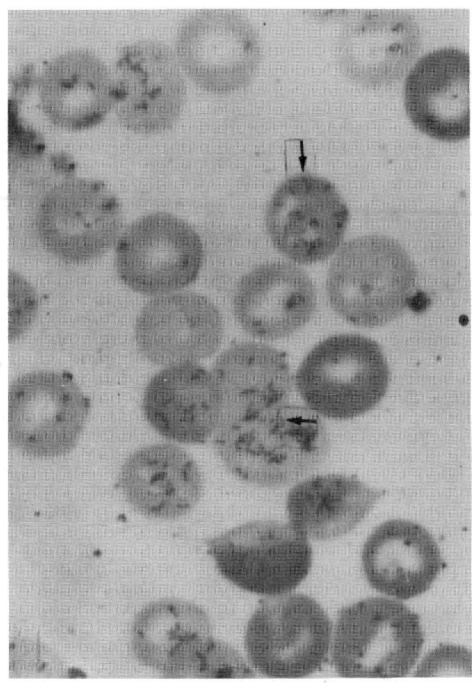

Fig. 10–4. *Bartonella* (arrows) in human blood. (× 1650.)

DISEASES DUE TO BARTONELLACEAE

In this category will be considered diseases caused by organisms presently classified in the Family *Bartonellaceae*. (See Table 10–5). These small, markedly pleomorphic organisms are found in erythrocytes of several species. The organisms take Giemsa's stain intensely, but are only lightly stained with aniline dyes. They are gram-negative. They are distinguished from protozoa by the absence of recognizable cytoplasm around their nucleus.

Two genera currently make up this family: *Bartonella,* and *Grahamella;* each of them contains parasitic species. *Bartonella bacilliformis,* the only species now recognized in this first genus, is the cause of a disease syndrome of man called Oroya fever, verruga peruviana, or Carrion's disease. This organism parasitizes the erythrocytes, reticuloendothelial system and

Table 10–5. Diseases Due to Bartonellaceae

Organism	Vectors	Hosts	Disease
Bartonella bacilliformis	*Phlebotomus sp.*	Man	Human bartonellosis (Oroya fever, *Verruga peruviana*)
Grahamella talpae	Unknown	Moles *(Talpa sp.)*	Erythrocytes parasitized
G. peromysci	Unknown	Deer, mice *(Peromyscus leucopus novaboracensis)*	Erythrocytes parasitized

vascular endothelium, occurring in the form of tiny polymorphous cocci and rods. Human bartonellosis is of considerable importance in South America, particularly in Peru and Colombia, but also occurs in Central America. It is transmitted by several species of *Phlebotomus*.

The second genus in this Family, *Grahamella*, consists of rod- to club-shaped organisms, 0.1 to 1.0 μ in size, which occur in the erythrocytes of several hosts. Two species, *Grahamella talpae*, a parasite of voles, and *Grahamella peromysci*, a parasite of deer mice, are currently recognized. These organisms stain light blue with Giemsa's stain; the club-shaped ends of the organism are usually a darker blue.

DISEASES DUE TO ANAPLASMATACEAE

In the present scheme of classification, this Family, Anaplasmataceae (Order Rickettsiales), now contains organisms grouped in five genera (8th edition, *Bergey's Manual* of *Determinative Bacteriology*). These genera are *Anaplasma, Paranaplasma, Aegyptianella, Haemobartonella,* and *Eperythrozoon.* These organisms are obligate parasites, found on or within erythrocytes or free in the plasma of wild and domestic vertebrates. Stained with Giemsa's stain, the organisms appear as rod-shaped, spherical, coccoid, or ring-shaped bodies, reddish-violet, and 0.2 to 0.4 μm in diameter. Each organism is enclosed in a membrane with an internal structure that resembles rickettsiae (Fig. 10–3). The organisms may occur in short chains or irregular groups within erythrocytes or in plasma. They are gram-negative, not acid-fast, multiply by binary fission, and are transmitted by arthropods. Anemia is the usual clinical feature manifest in infected animals.

Anaplasmosis

The organisms responsible for the disease, anaplasmosis, are presently grouped into a single genus, *Anaplasma*. Three species are of pathogenic importance: *Anaplasma m. marginale, A. marginale centrale,* and *A. ovis* (Table 10–6). With Romanowsky-type stains, such as Giemsa's, these organisms appear as dense, bluish-purple, homogeneous round structures within erythrocytes near the margin or in the center of the cell. With the electron microscope, these structures are separated from the cytoplasm of the erythrocyte by a membrane that encloses one to eight subunits, or initial bodies, which are the parasitic bacteria. The organisms are each 0.3 to 0.4 μm in diameter, and enclose electron-lucid plasma in which are embedded electron-dense aggregates of fine granular material (Fig. 10–5).

Another genus, *Paranaplasma*, currently contains two species: *P. caudatum* and *P. discoides*. These organisms are found in cattle infected with *Anaplasma marginale* (Kreier and Ristic, 1963), and may be distinguished by their infectivity for cattle, but not for deer or sheep, and by their distinctive morphology. By electron microscopy and fluorescent antibody stain, *P. caudatum* is seen to have a distinctive body and an appendage which may resemble a tail, loop, or ring connecting two organisms into a dumbbell shape. *Paranaplasma discoides* may be distinguished in water-lysed erythrocytes, using phase microscopy, as ovoid, disc-shaped structures with a dense mass at each pole. The pathogenic effect of these two organisms is not clearly established.

Anaplasma marginale, which parasitizes the red cells of cattle, causes an important disease of world-wide distribution. The disease is unusual in that infection results in overt disease only in adult animals; most young calves undergo an inapparent infection unless splenectomized prior to exposure. Fever of short duration is manifest in adult cattle but may be undetected or overshadowed by the later findings. Anemia is the essential effect produced by the organism and is manifest by weakness, pallor of mucosae, accelerated respiration, jaun-

Table 10–6. Diseases Due to Anaplasmataceae

Organism	Vectors	Hosts	Disease
Anaplasma marginale, marginale	Ticks, horseflies	Cattle, zebu, water buffalo, bison, deer, elk, camel, blesbuck, and duiker	Severe anaplasmosis
A. marginale, centrale	Ticks, horseflies	Cattle	Mild anaplasmosis
A. ovis	Ticks, horseflies	Sheep and goats	Mild to severe anaplasmosis
Paranaplasma caudatum	Probably ticks and horseflies	Cattle	Mixed infection with *A. marginale*
P. discoides	Probably ticks and horseflies	Cattle	Mixed infection with *A. marginale*
Aegyptianella pullorum (*A. granulosa, A. granulosa penetrans, Babesia pullorum, Balouria anserina, B. gallinarum, Spirochaeta granulosa penetrans*)	Ticks (*Argas persicus*)	Chickens, geese, ducks, turkeys, guinea fowl, pigeons, quail, ostrich	Aegyptianellosis
Haemobartonella muris (*Bartonella muris*)	Rat louse (*Polyplax spinulosa*)	Albino mouse, albino rat, some wild mice, hamster	Anemia only following splenectomy
H. felis (*Eperythrozoon felis*)	Unknown	Domestic cat	Hemobartonellosis
H. canis (*Bartonella canis*)	Unknown	Domestic dog	Anemia only following splenectomy
Eperythrozoon coccoides (*Gyromorpha musculi*)	Mouse louse (*Polyplax serrata*)	Albino and wild mice, albino rats, rabbits, and hamsters	Eperythrozoonosis
E. ovis	Horsefly, other arthropods	Sheep, goats, deer	Anemia
E. suis	Unknown	Swine	"Icteroanemia"
E. parvum	Pig louse (*Haematopinus suis*)	Swine	Anemia following splenectomy
E. wenyonii (*Haemobartonella wenyonii*)	Unknown	Cattle	Anemia following splenectomy

dice, decreased red cell count and hemoglobin, occasionally muscular trembling, depression, anorexia, and excessive salivation. Anemia results from increased destruction of parasitized erythrocytes by the reticuloendothelial system and not by hemolysis, therefore, hemoglobinuria is not seen. Autoimmunity has been suggested as a cause of the erythrocyte destruction, but this has not been confirmed. Death occurs in many cases, but recovery is not infrequent, the recovered animals remaining carriers of the infection for some time.

The organism, *Anaplasma marginale*, is a tiny spherical body, 0.3 to 0.8 μm in diame-

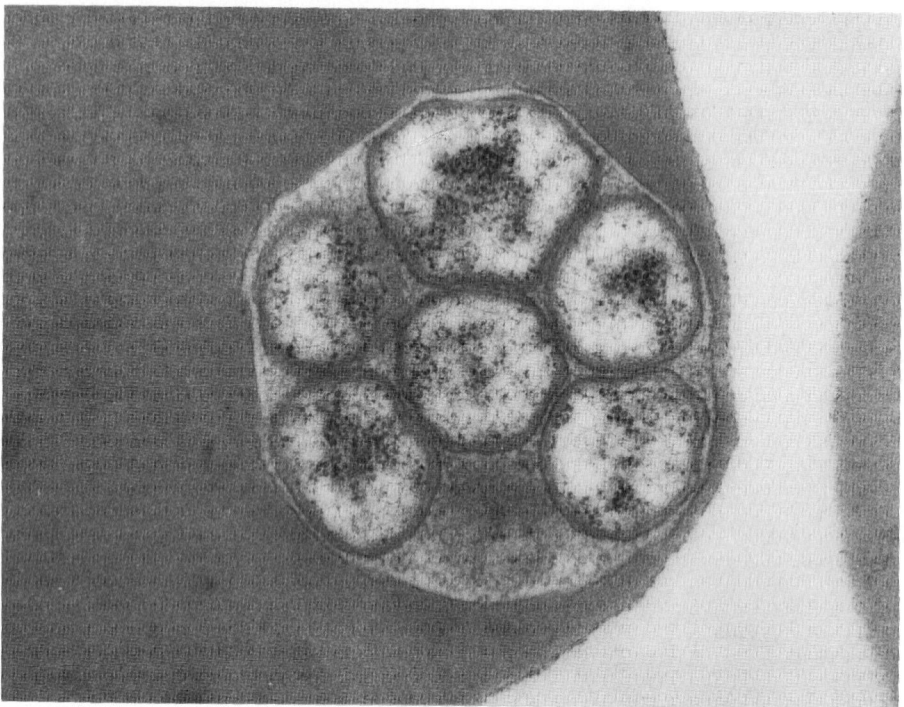

Fig. 10–5. *Anaplasma marginale.* An anaplasma body (marginal body) containing six subunits (initial bodies.) (× 60,000.) (Courtesy of Dr. C. T. Simpson and *American Journal of Veterinary Research.*)

ter, which is found within the cytoplasm of erythrocytes near the periphery of the cell. It is best demonstrated in blood smears with Giemsa stain. Studies by Ristic and Watrach (1963) with the electron microscope and with fluorescent antibody indicate that four developmental stages of *Anaplasma* are recognizable in infected erythrocytes. These stages are (a) early stage, consisting of **initial bodies**—the infective form, (b) mixed population with marginal and initial bodies, (c) vigorous growth and transfer, and (d) massive multiplication with a predominance of marginal bodies. According to these workers, after penetration of the erythrocytic cell membrane by initial bodies, the organisms reproduce by binary fission and pass through the four stages of development, then are transferred to other mature erythrocytes by direct contact between cells. Simpson and co-workers (1967) described

the initial body as spherical and surrounded by a double membrane. The marginal body contains up to six subunits (initial bodies) and is surrounded by a single membrane.

Microfibrillar structures between erythrocytes appear to facilitate exchange of organisms. A fluorescence technique using acridine orange has been shown to be useful by Gainer (1961) in identifying *Anaplasma,* as has the fluorescence antibody technique described by Ristic and Watrach (1963). The infection can be transmitted to a normal animal by carrying over a minute amount of blood. This can occur by the use of improperly sterilized bleeding needles, or by dehorning or castration without prior aseptic precautions, but usually in nature is spread by bites of ticks (*Boöphilus annulatus,* and others), biting flies (*Tabanus sp.*), and less often by mosquitoes (*Psorophora sp.*). Ticks are the most important vectors because they can carry the organisms for long periods of time. The transfer in utero between bovine mother and fetus has also been reported. The presence of carriers has long posed a problem in the control of the disease. The detection of such carriers is rarely possible by examination of blood smears, but a complement-fixation test can be used to detect carriers.

Lesions. The gross postmortem findings in fatal cases are those of severe anemia, with pallor of the tissues and occasionally with icterus. The spleen is usually greatly enlarged, with reddish-brown pulp and enlarged splenic follicles. The liver is enlarged, has rounded edges, and is yellowish in cases with icterus. The gallbladder is usually distended with dark grumous bile. Petechiae in the pericardium may be encountered, and catarrhal inflammation may be evident in the gastrointestinal tract. The microscopic findings indicate severe demands upon the hematopoietic system, with hyperplasia of the bone marrow and extramedullary hematopoiesis in the spleen and other organs. *Anaplasma* can be demonstrated with difficulty in erythrocytes in tissue sections.

The number of organisms demonstrable in smears of peripheral blood is highly variable. Prior to the onset of anemia, the majority of erythrocytes may harbor organisms, but with their sudden removal from the circulation, their numbers decrease. Immature erythrocytes (reticulocytes) that enter the circulation in response to the anemia are, for reasons poorly understood, resistant to the parasites.

Whether *Anaplasma centrale* warrants consideration as a separate species is doubtful; it may be a variant of *A. marginale*. It produces a mild infection in cattle, and has been employed to immunize cattle to *A. marginale*. *A. centrale* usually localizes near the center of the red blood cell.

Anaplasma ovis is infectious for sheep and goats. Cattle are not susceptible. The disease is mild, only rarely resulting in clinical signs of anemia.

Diagnosis. The diagnosis is based upon the clinical signs and demonstration of *Anaplasma* in erythrocytes. The complement-fixation test can be used for the detection of clinically silent carriers.

Amerault, T. E., Mazzola, V., and Roby, T. O.: Gram-staining characteristics of *Anaplasma marginale*. Am. J. Vet. Res., 34:552–555, 1973.

Buening, G. M.: Hypolipoidemia and hypergammaglobulinemia associated with experimentally induced anaplasmosis in calves. Am. J. Vet. Res., 35:371–374, 1974.

Carson, C. A., Sells, D. M., and Ristic, M.: Cell-mediated immune response to virulent and attenuated *Anaplasma marginale* administered to cattle in live and inactivated forms. Am. J. Vet. Res., 38:173–179, 1977.

————: Cell-mediated immunity related to challenge exposure of cattle inoculated with virulent and attenuated strains of *Anaplasma marginale*. Am. Vet. J. Res., 38:1167–1172, 1977.

Christensen, J. F., and Howarth, J. A.: Anaplasmosis transmission by Dermacentor occidentalis taken from cattle in Santa Barbara County, California. Am. J. Vet. Res., 27:1473–1475, 1966.

Cox, F. R., and Dimopoullos, G. T.: Demonstration of an autoantibody associated with anaplasmosis. Am. J. Vet. Res., 33:73–76, 1972.

Cox, H. U., Hart, L. T., and Dimopoullos, G. T.: Adenosine triphosphatase activity associated with bovine erythrocyte membranes during infection with *Anaplasma marginale*. Am. J. Vet. Res., 35:773–779, 1974.

Espana, C., Espana, E. M., and Gonzalez, D.: *Anaplasma marginale*. I. Studies with phase contrast and electron microscopy. Am. J. Vet. Res., 20:795–805, 1959.

Fowler, D., and Swift, B. L.: Abortion in cows inoculated with *Anaplasma marginale*. Theriogenology, 4:59–67, 1975.

Franklin, T. E., and Redmond, H. E.: Observations on the morphology of *Anaplasma marginale* with reference to projections or tails. Am. J. Vet. Res., 19:252–253, 1958.

Gainer, J. H.: Demonstration of *Anaplasma marginale* with the fluorescent dye, acridine orange, comparisons with the complement-fixation test and Wright's stain. Am. J. Vet. Res., 22:882–886, 1961.

Gates, D. W., and Roby, T. O.: The status of the complement-fixation test for the diagnosis of anaplasmosis in 1955. Ann. NY Acad. Sci., 64:31–39, 1956.

Jones, E. W., Kleiwer, I. O., Norman, B. B., and Brock, W. E.: *Anaplasma marginale* infection in young and aged cattle. Am. J. Vet. Res., 29:535–544, 1968.

Jones, E. W., Norman, B. B., Kliewer, I. O., and Brock, W. E.: *Anaplasma marginale* infection in splenectomized calves. Am. J. Vet. Res., 29:523–533, 1968.

Keeton, K. S., and Jain, N. C.: Scanning electron microscopic studies of *Paranaplasma sp.* in erythrocytes of a cow. J. Parasitol., 59:331–336, 1973.

Kreier, J. P., and Ristic, M.: Anaplasmosis XII. The growth and survival in deer and sheep of the parasites present in the blood of calves infected with the Oregon strain of *Anaplasma marginale*. Am. J. Vet. Res., 24:697–702, 1963.

Kreier, J. P., Ristic, M., and Schroeder, W.: Anaplasmosis, XVI. The pathogenesis of anemia produced by infection with anaplasma. Am. J. Vet. Res., 25:343–352, 1964.

Kuttler, K. L.: Clinical and hematologic comparison of *Anaplasma marginale* and *Anaplasma centrale* infections in cattle. Am. J. Vet. Res., 27:941–946, 1966.

Lotze, J. C., and Yiengst, M. J.: Mechanical transmission of bovine anaplasmosis by the horsefly, *Tabanus sulcifrons* (Macquart). Am. J. Vet. Res., 2:323–326, 1941.

———: Studies on the nature of anaplasma. Am. J. Vet. Res., 3:312–320, 1942.

Morris, H., and Ristic, M.: Serum opsonins in anaplasmosis and their in vitro effect on erythrophagocytosis. Ztschr. Tropenmed. Parasitol., 21:191–197, 1970.

Morris, H., Ristic, M., and Lykins, J.: Characterization of opsonins eluted from erythrocytes of cattle infected with *Anaplasma marginale*. Am. J. Vet. Res., 32:1221–1228, 1971.

Piercy, P. L.: Transmission of anaplasmosis. Ann. NY Acad. Sci., 64:40–48, 1956.

Ristic, M., and Watrach, A. M.: Studies in anaplasmosis. II. Electron microscopy of *Anaplasma marginale* in deer. Am. J. Vet. Res., 22:109–116, 1961.

———: Anaplasmosis. VI. Studies and a hypothesis concerning the cycle of development of the causative agent. Am. J. Vet. Res., 24:267–277, 1963.

Roby, T. O., et al.: Immunity in bovine anaplasmosis after elimination of *Anaplasma marginale* infections with imidocarb. Am. J. Vet. Res., 35:993–995, 1974.

Ryff, J. F., Weibel, J. L., and Thomas, G. M.: Relationship of ovine to bovine anaplasmosis. Cornell Vet., 54:407–414, 1964.

Schmidt, H.: Manifestations and diagnosis of anaplasmosis. Ann. NY Acad. Sci., 64:27–30, 1956.

Schroeder, W. F., and Ristic, M.: Anaplasmosis. XVII. The relation of autoimmune processes to anemia. Am. J. Vet. Res., 26:239–245, 1965.

Simpson, C. F.: Morphologic alterations of *Anaplasma marginale* in calves after treatment with oxytetracycline. Am. J. Vet. Res., 36:1443–1446, 1975.

Simpson, C. F., Kling, J.M., and Love, J. N.: Morphologic and histochemical nature of *Anaplasma marginale*. Am. J. Vet. Res., 28:1055–1065, 1967.

Smith, J. E., McCants, M., and Jones, E. W.: Erythrocyte enzyme activity during experimental anaplasmosis. Int. J. Biochem., 3:345–350, 1973.

Summers, W. A., and Padgett, F.: Electron microscopy of negatively stained *Anaplasma marginale* Theiler, 1910. Am. J. Vet. Res., 31:1679–1686, 1970.

Trueblood, M. S., Swift, B. L., and Bear, P. D.: Bovine fetal response to *Anaplasma marginale*. Am. J. Vet. Res., 32:1089–1090, 1971.

Young, M. F., Kuttler, K. L., and Adams, L. G.: Experimentally induced anaplasmosis in neonatal isohemolytic anemia-recovered calves. Am. J. Vet. Res., 38:1745–1747, 1977.

Haemobartonellosis

Organisms of the genus *Haemobartonella* are currently classified in the family Anaplasmataceae (Table 10–6). The organisms are obligate parasites, found within shallow or deep indentations of the cell wall of red blood cells. The organisms occur as cocci or chains of coccoid organisms, in pairs or in groups, in indentations of the surface of erythrocytes. They stain well with Giemsa's stain but poorly with many other aniline dyes. They are not acid-fast, are gram-negative, and have a limiting membrane but not a cell wall or nucleus (Fig. 10–6). Growth of *Haemobartonella* is inhibited by arsenicals and tetracyclines but not by penicillin or streptomycin. They have not been cultivated outside the host.

Only three species have been accepted as valid (Bergey's Manual of Determinative Bacteriology, 8th Edition). These are *Haemobartonella muris*, *H. felis*, and *H. canis*. Several other species have been identified in various hosts and await validation as distinctive species. These include: *H. peromyscii* var *maniculata*, from the gray-backed deer mouse; *H. microtii*, the vole; *H. tyzzeri*, the guinea pig; *H. bovis*, cattle; *H. sturmanii*, buffalo; *H. peromyscii*, the deer mouse; *H. blarinae*, the short-tailed shrew; and *H. sciuri*, the gray squirrel. Haemobartonella infections of erythrocytes have also been reported in an owl monkey (*Aotus*), rhesus monkeys (*Macaca mulatta*), and squirrel monkeys (*Saimiri sciureus*). In most species, with the exception of the cat, the disease is mild or without clinical signs until the host is splenectomized. Removal of the spleen is followed by anemia in most infected animals.

Aikawa, M., and Nussenzweig, R.: Fine structure of *Haemobartonella sp.* in the squirrel monkey. J. Parasitol., 58:628–630, 1972.

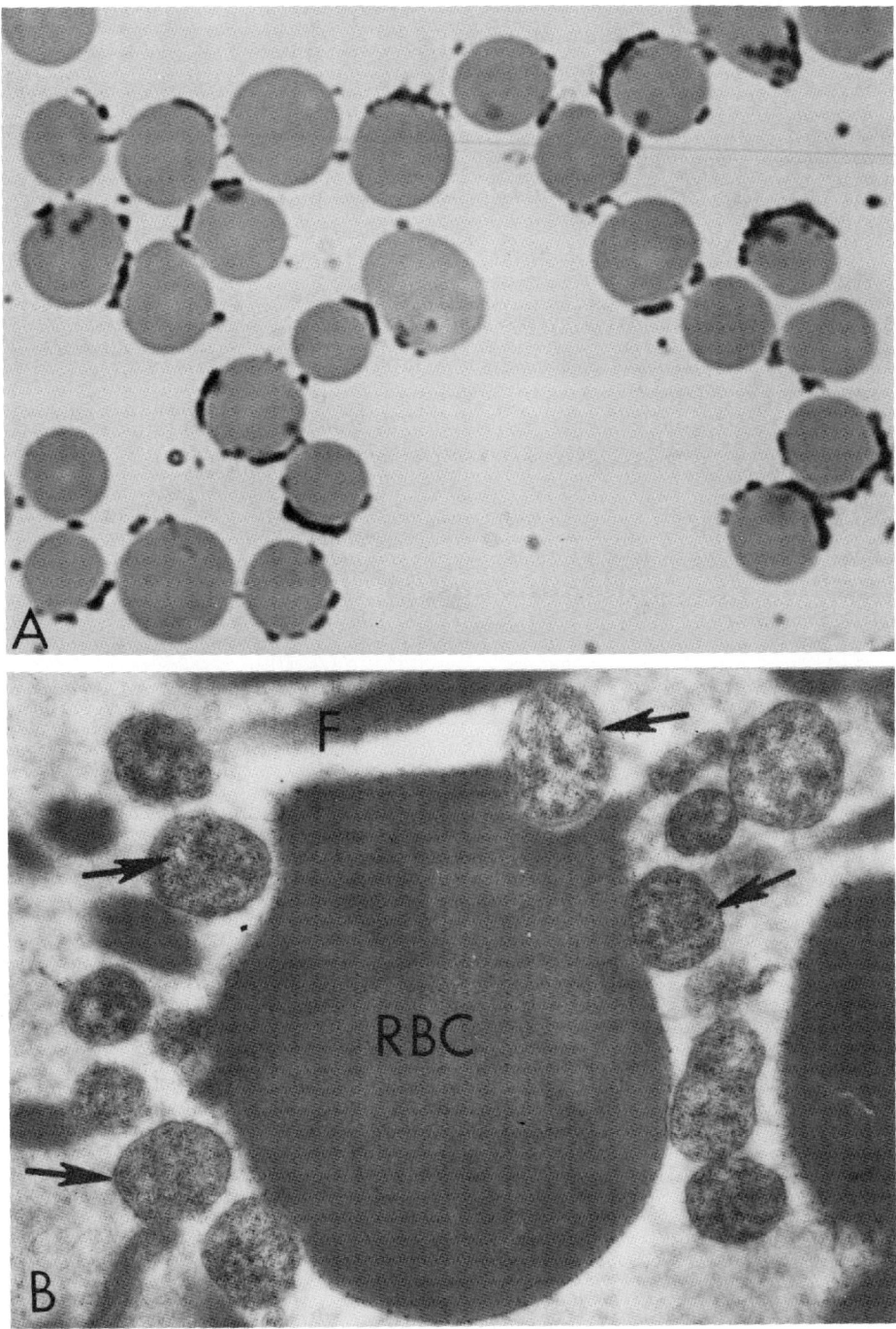

Fig. 10–6. *Haemobartonella bovis. A,* Organisms on periphery and surface of erythrocytes (RBC) from a splenectomized calf. *B,* Coccoid and rod-shaped organisms (arrows) on an erythrocyte. (× 40,000.) *F,* fibrin. (Courtesy of Dr. C. F. Simpson and *American Journal of Veterinary Research.*)

Baker, H. J., Cassell, G. H., and Lindsey, J. R.: Research complications due to *Haemobartonella* and *Eperythrozoon* infections in experimental animals. Am. J. Pathol., 64:625–652, 1971.

Benjamin, M. M., and Lumb, W. V.: *Haemobartonella canis* infection in a dog. J. Am. Vet. Med. Assoc., 135:388–390, 1959.

Carr, D. T., and Essex, H. E.: Bartonellosis: a cause of severe anemia in splenectomized dogs. Proc. Soc. Exp. Biol. Med., 57:44–45, 1944.

Ingle, R. T.: *Bartonella* Infection in a dog. North Am. Vet., 27:501–502, 1946.

Lotze, J. C., and Bowman, G. W.: The occurrence of *Bartonella* in cases of anaplasmosis and in apparently normal cattle. Proc. Helminth. Soc., Washington, D. C., 9:71–72, 1942.

Love, J. N., and McEwen, E. G.: Hypoglycemia associated with haemobartonella-like infection in splenectomized calves. Am. J. Vet. Res., 33:2087–2090, 1972.

Maede, Y., and Sonoda, M.: Studies of the feline haemobartonellosis. III. Scanning electron microscopy of *Haemobartonella felis*. Jpn. J. Vet. Sci., 37:209–211, 1975.

McKeen, A. E., Ziegler, R. F., and Giles, R. C.: Scanning and transmission electron microscopy of *Haemobartonella canis* and *Eperythrozoon ovis*. Am. J. Vet. Res., 34:1196–1201, 1973.

Mulhern, C. R.: A note on two blood parasites of cattle, (*Spirochaeta theileri* and *Bartonella bovis*), recorded for the first time in Australia. Aust. Vet., 22:118–119, 1946.

Peters, W., Molyneux, D. H., and Howells, R. E.: *Eperythrozoon* and *Haemobartonella* in monkeys. Ann. Trop. Med. Parasitol., 68:47–50, 1974.

Pryor, W. H., and Bradbury, R. P.: *Haemobartonella canis* infection in research dogs. Lab. Anim. Sci., 25:566–569, 1975.

Simpson, C. F., and Love, J. N.: Fine structure of *Haemobartonella bovis* in blood and liver of splenectomized calves. Am. J. Vet. Res., 31:225–231, 1970.

Small, E., and Ristic, M.: Morphologic features of *Haemobartonella felis*. Am. J. Vet. Res., 28:845–851, 1967.

Tanaka, H., et al.: Fine structure of *Haemobartonella muris* as compared with *Eperythrozoon coccoides* and *Mycoplasma pulmonis*. J. Bact., 90:1735–1749, 1965.

Tyzzer, E. E.: "Interference" in mixed infections of *Bartonella* and *Eperythrozoon* in mice. Am. J. Pathol., 17:141–153, 1941.

————: A comparative study of *Grahamellae*, *Haemobartonellae* and *Eperythrozoa* in small mammals. Proc. Am. Philos. Soc., 85:359–398, 1942.

Venable, J. H., and Equing, S. A.: Fine structure of *Hemobartonella canis* (Rickettsiales: Bartonellacea) and its relation to the host erythrocyte. J. Parasitol., 54:259–268, 1968.

Weinman, D.: On the cause of the anemia in *Bartonella* infection of rats. J. Infect. Dis., 63:1–9, 1938.

Feline Infectious Anemia (Feline Haemobartonellosis)

The studies of Flint and co-workers (1959) have done much to clarify the clinical and etiologic aspects of this disease, which is now recognized with increasing frequency in the domestic cat. Most of the available evidence points toward the parasite of erythrocytes, *Haemobartonella felis*, as the etiologic agent. This organism is seen as coccoid, ring, or rod-shaped bodies on the erythrocytes of affected cats. These are best seen in blood smears stained with Giemsa's or Wright's stain (Fig. 10–7). The natural mode of transmission is not known, but the disease has been reproduced following the injection of 0.5 ml of feline blood containing parasitized erythrocytes. In contrast to the situation in rodents and dogs, in which splenectomy is necessary to cause overt disease, cats are naturally susceptible to this disease and fatal illness often results.

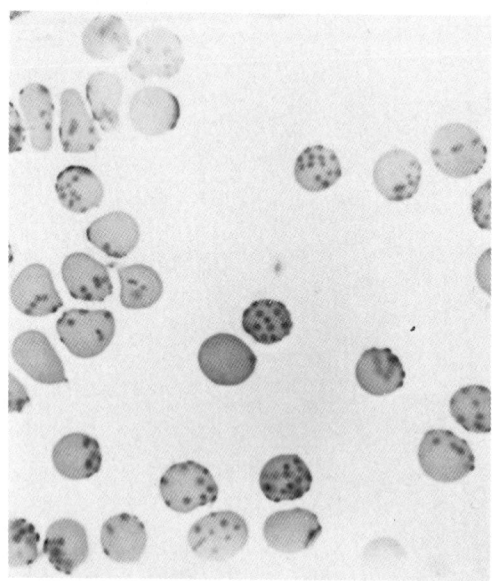

Fig. 10–7. *Haemobartonella felis* on the erythrocytes of cat with feline infectious anemia. (Giemsa stain, × 1200.) (Photograph by Dr. Rue Jensen, contributed by Dr. Jean C. Flint, Colorado State University.)

In its earliest stages, feline infectious anemia (haemobartonellosis) is manifest by fever, anorexia, depression, and macrocytic, hemolytic anemia. The anemia is evidenced by pale, occasionally icteric, mucous membranes, weakness, and a characteristic blood picture in which the hemoglobin and packed cell volumes are severely decreased. The hemoglobin levels usually decrease from a normal of 11 g/100 ml of blood to as low as 1.5 g in severe cases. Levels of 6.0 g/100 ml of blood or lower are usually considered typical of this disease. Macrocytosis and anisocytosis are usually prominent features, and in early stages, nucleated erythrocytes are present in large numbers. Reticulocytes are also increased in number, and some of them may contain the organisms, *Haemobartonella felis*. These organisms are not readily demonstrable in all stages of the disease which complicates the diagnostic problem in many cases.

The leukocyte count in the acute stage is usually elevated, a point of diagnostic significance in eliminating panleukopenia, but as the disease progresses, the leukocyte count gradually falls. After a prolonged illness, leukopenia may be severe and abnormal "reticuloendothelial cells" may appear in the peripheral circulation.

Severely affected animals may die with evidences of a severe hemolytic anemia, others may recover, with or without treatment, and still others will undergo relapses and eventually die following a prolonged illness.

Lesions. The lesions in fatal cases have not been adequately documented, and the cases of prolonged duration present some particularly challenging problems in the postmortem recognition of fatal cases, and in understanding the pathogenesis of the disease. The postmortem findings in cats which die following an acute episode are usually quite characteristic. Icterus is a feature in some acute cases. The spleen is enlarged many times, and its cut surface is dark, firm, and bulges when cut. Microscopically, this appearance is due to congestion and extramedullary hematopoiesis. Hemoglobin may stain the urine in the bladder and hemorrhages may be present, particularly on serous surfaces. Fatty infiltration may be evident in pale yellowish color of the liver and central or paracentral necrosis may also be seen in microscopic sections of this organ. These changes are believed to be secondary to the anemia. The bone marrow is usually solidly red in the long bones and contains large numbers of hematopoietic cells in approximately normal proportions. The lymph nodes are usually grossly enlarged and moist in all parts of the body, and microscopic sections reveal that the enlargement is due to reactive hyperplasia.

The lesions found at necropsy of animals which die after the prolonged illness, described previously, are often subtle and at this point not clearly understood. The reactive hyperplasia of lymph nodes seen in the acutely fatal case, is also a feature of the illness of longer duration, and the spleen may be large but not as hyperplastic. Icterus is rarely evident, and the bone marrow is hyperplastic. Ulceration of intestinal mucosae may be present, and sometimes hemorrhage may follow this ulceration. (See color plate II.)

Demaree, R. S., Jr., and Messmith, W. B.: Ultrastructure of *Haemobartonella felis* from a naturally infected cat. Am. J. Vet. Res., *33*:1303–1308, 1972.

Flint, J. C., and Moss, L. C.: Infectious anemia in cats. J. Am. Vet. Med. Assoc., *122*::45–48, 1953.

Flint, J. C., Roepke, M. H., and Jensen, R.: Feline infectious anemia. I. Clinical aspects. Am. J. Vet. Res., *19*:165–168, 1958.

———: Feline infectious anemia. II. Experimental cases. Am. J. Vet. Res., 20:33–40, 1959.

Hatakka, M.: Haemobartonellosis in the domestic cat. Acta Vet. Scand., *13*:323–331, 1972.

Jain, N. C., and Keeton, K. S.: Scanning electron microscopic features of *Haemobartonella felis*. Am. J. Vet. Res., 34:697–700, 1973.

Maede, Y., and Hata, R.: Studies on feline haemobartonellosis. II. The mechanism of anemia produced by infection with *Haemobartonella felis*. Jpn. J. Vet. Sci., 37:49–54, 1975.

Maede, Y., and Sonoda, M.: Studies of the feline haemobartonellosis. III. Scanning electron microscopy of *Haemobartonella felis*. Jpn. J. Vet. Sci., 37:209–211, 1975.

Small, E., and Ristic, M.: Morphologic features of *Haemobartonella felis*. Am. J. Vet. Res., 28:845–851, 1967.

Eperythrozoonosis

Increasing numbers of parasites that attack red blood cells have been discovered in animals. Organisms grouped in the genus *Eperythrozoon* are among the latest of these to be recognized. This genus is presently grouped in the family Anaplasmataceae; the organisms are similar to *Haemobartonella* and are often distinguished with difficulty. The principal features differentiating *Haemobartonella* from *Eperythrozoon* are that eperythrozoa occur both in the erythrocytes of the host and in the plasma, whereas *Haemobartonella* rarely are found free in the plasma, and are seldom in ring forms, which are frequent in *Eperythrozoon*. Five species of *Eperythrozoon* are currently accepted as valid (Table 10–6) (Kreier and Ristic, 1974). Each organism can be clearly distinguished by its specific immunologic effects upon the host, hence it is of practical importance to identify clearly the causative agent in each of these infections of erythrocytes.

Eperythrozoon are seen in blood smears stained by Giemsa's method as tiny pleomorphic structures within the erythrocytes, lying on their surface or free in the plasma. The organisms are delicate pale purple to pinkish purple, and predominantly in ring-shapes 0.5 to 1.0 μ in diameter or occasionally slightly larger. Triangular, ovoid, rod, dumbbell, and tennis-racket shapes may be seen. One to a dozen organisms may be present in a single red blood cell, and large numbers are uniformly distributed through the plasma. Organisms are much more numerous in blood smears taken at the height of infection.

The mode of transmission is not clearly established for all species of *Eperythrozoon*, but arthropods are generally suspected. *Eperythrozoon coccoides*, which infects mice, is transmitted by a louse, *Polyplax serrata*. Biting flies have been tentatively incriminated as vectors in other hosts. Experimental infection is greatly facilitated by the use of splenectomized animals.

Signs. The clinical manifestations of eperythrozoonosis are best known and quite similar in sheep and swine. In both species, evidence of infection may appear spontaneously, particularly in young animals exposed to other deleterious influences, such as helminthic parasitism, or may be brought forth by splenectomy of animals already harboring the infection. The natural disease in swine has been called "ictero-anemia," and has similarities to anaplasmosis of herbivora. It is, of course, distinguished with difficulty from anaplasmosis when sheep are involved. The symptoms start with fever (104 to 107° F.), which appears six to ten days following exposure or splenectomy of animals with latent infection. This is accompanied by gradually increasing depression and weakness. The total red blood cell count drops precipitously to 1 to 2 million per cubic millimeter, hemoglobin is decreased to 2 to 4 g/100 ml, and the packed red cell volume goes down to 4 to 7%. The icteric index is elevated to 18 to 25, and the sedimentation rate is greatly accelerated, reaching 75 mm/minute in some cases. The white cell count is usually not changed, although leukocytosis occurs in a few cases. Death may occur in an acute episode, as described, but animals recover more frequently and then are prone to have repeated recrudescences.

Lesions. The gross lesions are compatible with the hemolytic anemia resulting from the effect of *Eperythrozoon* upon the red blood cells. Icterus is a prominent feature, the blood is thin and watery, the liver is yellowish brown and the gallbladder contains thick gelatinous bile. Hydropericardium and ascites are present in some cases and the heart is pale and flabby. Petechiae may be seen in the mucosa of the urinary bladder. The bone marrow is predominantly red rather than fatty.

Microscopic changes are seen in the bone marrow, which is hyperplastic, and the liver, which is rich in hemosiderin, shows some fatty change and central or paracentral necrosis of liver lobules. The latter is presumed to be an effect of anoxia. The organisms are difficult to demonstrate in tissue sections.

Diagnosis. Eperythrozoonosis must be differentiated from anaplasmosis, haemobartonellosis, babesiosis, and other hemolytic anemias. The differentiation is most readily made by the precise identification of the causative organisms in the erythrocytes.

Adams, E. W., et al.: Eperythrozoonosis in a herd of purebred Landrace pigs. J. Am. Vet. Med. Assoc., *135*:226–228, 1959.

Glasgow, L. A., Murrer, A. T., and Lombardi, P. S.: *Eperythrozoon coccoides.* II. Effect on interferon production and role of humoral antibody in host resistance. Infect. Immun., *9*:266–272, 1974.

Keeton, K. S., and Jain, N. C.: *Eperythrozoon wenyoni*: a scanning electron microscope study. J. Parasitol., *59*:867–873, 1973.

Kreier, J. P., and Ristic, M.: Morphologic, antigenic, and pathogenic characteristics of *Eperythrozoon ovis* and *Eperythrozoon wenyonii.* Am. J. Vet. Res., *24*:488–500, 1963.

Kreier, J. P., and Ristic, M.: Genus V, *Eperythrozoon,* Schilling, 1928, 1854. *In* Bergey's Manual of Determinative Bacteriology, 8th ed., edited by R. E. Buchanan and N. E. Gibbons, Baltimore, Williams and Wilkins Co., 1974.

Neitz, W. O.: *Eperythrozoonosis* in sheep. Onderstepoort J. Vet. Sci. Ind., *9*:9–30, 1937.

Smith, A. R., and Rahn, T.: An indirect hemagglutination test for the diagnosis of *Eperythrozoon suis* infection in swine. Am. J. Vet. Res., *36*:1319–1322, 1975.

Splitter, E. J.: *Eperythrozoon suis,* the etiologic agent of ictero-anemia or an anaplasmosis-like disease in swine. Am. J. Vet. Res., *11*:324–330, 1950.

Splitter, E. J., and Williamson, R. L.: Eperythrozoonosis in swine. A preliminary report. J. Am. Vet. Med. Assoc., *116*:360–364, 1950.

Sutton, R. H., and Jolly, R. D.: Experimental *Eperythrozoon ovis* infection of sheep. NZ Vet. J., *21*:160–166, 1973.

DISEASES DUE TO CHLAMYDIACEAE

The organisms previously placed together as the psittacosis-lymphogranuloma-trachoma group are currently classified in a separate order, Chlamydiales; a single family, Chlamydiaceae, and one genus, *Chlamydia* (Bergey's Manual of Determinative Bacteriology, edition 8, 1974). The name of this genus, *Chlamydia,* supplants several now considered obsolete: *Miyagawanella* (Brumpt, 1938); *Bedsonia* (Meyer, 1953); *Prowazekia* (Coles, 1953), and *Rakeia* (Levaditi, Roger, and Destombes, 1964). Two species are presently accepted as valid: *Chlamydia psittaci* and *Chlamydia trachomatis.*

Chlamydia are minute bacterial organisms that propagate only within host cells of vertebrates, including man, other mammals and birds. The organisms are nonmotile, spherical, and have three developmental stages: the elementary body, the initial body, and the intermediate body. The **elementary body** is a spherule measuring 0.2 to 0.4 μm in diameter; it is electron-dense and contains a nucleus and many ribosomes surrounded by a multilaminated wall. This elementary body is the infectious form of the organism; it is taken into host cells by phagocytosis. The **initial body** is a larger spherule, 0.8 to 1.5 μm in diameter, with a thin wall containing nuclear fibrils and ribosomal structures. The initial body is the vegetative form, which divides by fission within the host cell. The **intermediate body** is a transitional stage between the initial and elementary bodies.

After phagocytosis by a host cell, elementary bodies enlarge to become initial bodies, which divide by fission within a cytoplasmic vesicle formed by invagination of the host's cell wall. Daughter cells of the initial bodies continue to divide, then develop laminated walls and a dense nuclear mass (intermediate form), then decrease in size to become the infectious elementary bodies. Rupture of the cytoplasmic vesicle and cell wall releases the elementary bodies, which may infect other host cells.

The cells walls of *Chlamydia* are gram-

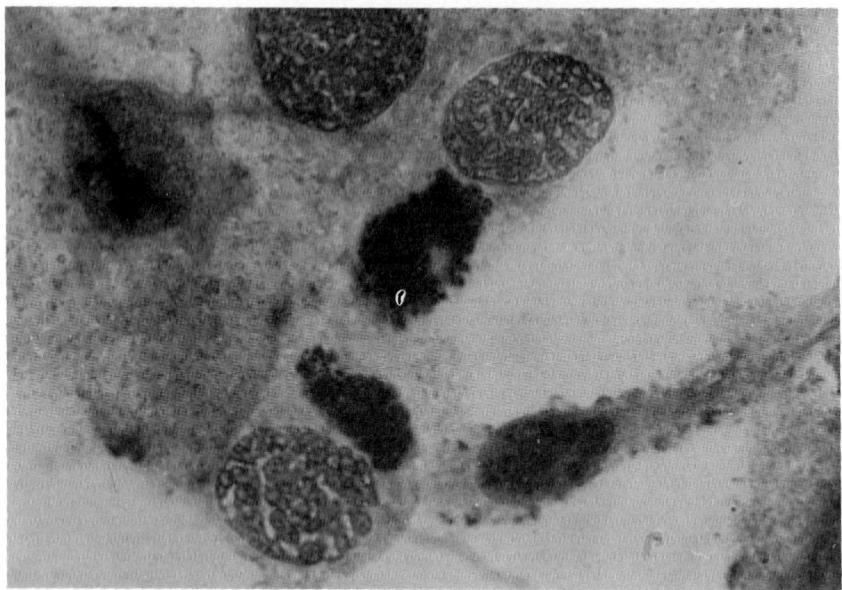

Fig. 10–8. Chlamydial inclusions 60 hours after infection in vitro with the agent of ovine abortion. (Courtesy of Dr. J. Storz.)

negative, similar chemically to gram-negative bacteria. The intracellular organisms may be stained with Giemsa's, Machiavello's, Gimenez's, or Castenada's methods. They may also be demonstrated in unstained preparations (wet mounts) of infected cells with a phase-contrast optical system. They have characteristic features under the electron microscope.

Chlamydia depend upon host cells for energy and do not grow outside such cells. They can catabolize glucose, pyruvic acid, or glutamic acid and produce carbon dioxide. Multiplication is inhibited by tetracyclines, penicillin, and 5-fluorouracil. An antigenically similar 100° C-stable lipoglycoprotein may be demonstrated in all members of this genus.

Chlamydia trachomatis may be differentiated from *C. psittaci* by its less compact colonies in host cells and the tendency of organisms to be distributed throughout the cytoplasm; by the production of iodine-staining compounds in the intracytoplasmic vesicles; and by the inhibition of growth of organisms in the yolk sac of chicken embryos with the use of sodium sulfadiazine. Strains of these two organisms are now believed to be involved in most infections of birds, man, and other mammals (Page, 1974).

Certain organisms have been so poorly characterized that it is not possible to ascertain whether they should be classified as *Chlamydia. Colesiota conjunctivae (Rickettsiae conjunctivae, Ricolesia bovis; R. conjunctivae bovis)* has been found in association with conjunctivitis of sheep, goats, and cattle in South Africa. Apparently this organism is not the cause of keratoconjunctivitis in cattle in the United States. Conjunctivitis and keratoconjunctivitis in chickens in South Africa is caused by another organism, *Colesiota conjunctivagalli (Ricolesia conjunctivae). Ricolesia lestoquardii (Rickettsia conjunctivae-suis)* causes conjunctivitis and keratitis in swine.

Brumpt, E.: *Rickettsia intracellulaire stomacale (Rickettsia culicis* N. Sp.) de *Culex fatigans.* Ann. Parasitol., *16*:153–158, 1938.

Coles, J. D. W.: Classification of rickettsiae pathogenic to vertebrates. Ann. NY Acad. Sci., 56:457–483, 1953.

Harshbarger, J. C., Chang, S. C., and Otto, S. V.: Chlamydia (with phages), Mycoplasmas and Rickettsia in Chesapeake Bay bivalves. Science, 196:666–668, 1977.

Jones, H., Rake, G., and Stearns, B.: Studies on lymphogranuloma venereum. III. The action of the sulfonamides on the agent of lymphogranuloma venereum. J. Infect. Dis., 76:55–69, 1945.

Levaditi, J. C., Roger, F., and Destombes, P.: Tentative de classification des Chlamydiaceae (Rake, 1955) tenante compte de leurs affinités tissulaires et du leur épidemiologie. Ann. Inst. Pasteur (Paris), 107:656–662, 1964.

Matsumoto, A., and Manire, G. P.: Electron microscopic observations on the fine structure of cell walls of Chlamydia psittaci. J. Bact., 104:1332–1337, 1970.

Meyer, K. F.: Psittacosis group. Ann. NY Acad. Sci., 56:545–556, 1953.

Page, L. A.: Revision of the family Chlamydiaceae Rake (Rickettsiales): Unification of the psittacosis-lymphogranuloma venereum-trachoma group of organisms in the genus Chlamydia Jones, Rake and Stearns, 1945. Int. J. Systemat. Bacteriol., 16:223–252, 1966.

Page, L. A.: Order II. Chlamydiales Storz and Page, 1971. In Bergey's Manual of Determinative Bacteriology, 8th ed., edited by R. E. Buchanan and N. E. Gibbons. Baltimore, Williams & Wilkins, 1974.

Pienaar, J. G., and Schutte, A. P.: Occurrence and pathology of chlamydiosis in domestic and laboratory animals.: a review. Onderstepoort J. Vet. Res., 42:77–89, 1975.

Tamura, A., Matsumoto, A., Manire, G. P., and Higashi, N.: Electron microscopic observations on the structure of the envelopes of mature elementary bodies and developmental reticulate forms of Chlamydia psittaci. J. Bact., 105:355–360, 1971.

Psittacosis (Ornithosis, Parrot Fever)

A febrile pulmonary disease of man, believed since the latter half of the nineteenth century to be contracted from sick parrots ("parrot fever"), is caused by an infectious agent harbored not only by parrots, but also by a wide variety of other birds. Psittacine birds (family Psittacidae), including parrots, parakeets, cockatoos, macaws, cockatiels and masked love birds, were the first in which the infection was demonstrated, both in an inapparent form and with obvious signs of illness. Several birds, including finches, canaries, and rice birds, acquire the infection by contact with parrots and transport the disease to man. Pigeons, ducks, fulmars, sea gulls, chickens, and turkeys are naturally infected and serve as reservoirs for human infection. Probably the distribution of the agent of psittacosis will eventually be found to be much wider and to include many more hosts than presently recognized.

The causative agent of psittacosis is presently referred to as Chlamydia psittaci. Its biologic and morphologic features are discussed in the preceding section.

Signs. The disease in man is manifest by sudden onset of a febrile illness with upper respiratory involvement, usually accompanied by pneumonia or pneumonitis and severe debility. Although the disease is not usually fatal, deaths occur with alarming frequency in some outbreaks. Antibiotic therapy has reduced the death rate dramatically.

In birds, psittacosis may appear as a fulminant, highly fatal disease or as a smouldering, inapparent infection demonstrable only by laboratory study or the appearance of the disease in human contacts. Infection in birds does not produce characteristic clinical manifestations; hence necropsy and laboratory examination are necessary for definitive diagnosis. Infected parrots or parakeets are sleepy, listless, and refuse to eat. Their wings droop and their feathers can be pulled out easily. After two or three weeks of illness, greenish and occasionally blood-tinged feces stain the feathers around the cloaca. The mortality rate is likely to be higher in parrots than in parakeets, but losses, particularly among young birds, may be great in both species.

Lesions. Psittacine birds that die of the disease or are sacrificed while they have definite symptoms are emaciated, and have many maculae, 2 to 4 mm in diameter, on the skin over the body and legs. The nares may be plugged with mucopurulent exudate. Fibrinous or fibrinopurulent exudates are found over the pericardial sac, peritoneum, pleura, or air sacs. The liver is enlarged, its edges are rounded, and it is yellowish, with mottling or patchy discoloration in shades of green or brown. In some cases it may be studded with petechiae and small yellowish foci of necrosis. The spleen is rather constantly enlarged, dark blood red, and occasionally has yellowish necrotic foci on its surface. The kidneys may be swollen, pale, and friable. The lungs are affected only rarely and the changes are limited to a few small areas of consolidation.

In parrots, parakeets, and other psittacine birds with latent infection, the spleen may be greatly enlarged, but no other gross lesions are apparent.

The microscopic changes in tissues in acute symptomatic psittacosis are associated with the presence of the organism in various tissue cells. The spleen is moderately to intensely infiltrated by mononuclear cells containing organisms, and its hemosiderin content is often increased. Hyperplasia of the reticuloendothelial cells is commonly observed. The liver often contains focal lesions involving isolated islands of parenchymal cells that undergo necrosis and replacement by a mass of hyaline amorphous material. Fibrin and lymphocytes may be noted on the liver capsule, and the portal areas are rich in lymphocytes and plasma cells. The tubular epithelium of the kidney may be packed with large numbers of LCL bodies; these are minute, spherical basophilic bodies, discovered by Levinthal, Coles, and Lillie. Destruction of this epithelium is followed by interstitial accumulation of epithelioid and lymphocytic cells. In the lungs, a few alveoli may contain seruous exudate, but frank pneumonic consolidation is rare. The superficial mucosa of the intestine is usually eroded, and the underlying lamina propria and submucosa are infiltrated with lymphocytes and plasma cells.

Diagnosis. The clinical manifestations and gross features at necropsy are generally insufficient for definite diagnosis. Necropsies must be performed by aseptic methods with adequate protection for the prosector,

and especial care must be taken to prevent desiccation and subsequent scattering of any infective material. Histologic study of smears or sections of peritoneal or pericardial lesions, liver or spleen stained by the Macchiavello, Castañeda or Giemsa method will disclose intracellular organisms in most acute cases. Intracranial or intraperitoneal injection of mice with tissue suspensions from birds suspected of having the infection in a symptomless form usually causes death in four or five days, and organisms are demonstrable in the mouse tissues. In some instances, at least one blind passage is required to establish the agent in mice. The organism also grows well in embryonated eggs and tissue culture.

The complement-fixation test is of value in the detection of antibodies in birds that have latent infections or are convalescent.

Beasley, J. N., Davis, D. E., and Grumbles, L. C.: Preliminary studies on the histopathology of experimental ornithosis in turkeys. Am. J. Vet. Res., *20*:341–349, 1959.

Beasley, J. N., Watkins, J. R., and Bridges, C. H.: Experimental ornithosis in calves. Am. J. Vet. Res., *23*:1192–1199, 1962.

Bland, J. C. W., and Canti, R. G.: The growth and development of psittacosis virus in tissue cultures. J. Pathol. Bact., *40*:231–241, 1935.

Durfee, P. T., Pullen, M. M., Currier, R. W., II, and Parker, R. L.: Human psittacosis associated with commercial processing of turkeys. J. Am. Vet. Med. Assoc., *167*:804–808, 1975.

Lillie, R. D.: The pathology of psittacosis in animals and the distribution of *Rickettsia psittaci* in the tissues of man and animals. Nat. Inst. Health Bull. 161, pp. 47–66, 1933.

Meyer, K. F.: Ornithosis and psittacosis. *In* Diseases of Poultry, 3rd ed., edited by H. E. Biester and L. H. Schwarte. Ames, Iowa State College Press, 1952. pp. 569–618.

Pierce, K. R., Moore, R. W., Carroll, L. H., and Bridges, C. H.: Experimental ornithosis in ewes. Am. J. Vet. Res., *24*:1176–1188, 1963.

Todd, W. J., and Storz, J.: Ultrastructural cytochemical evidence for the activation of lysosomes in the cytocidal effect of *Chlamydia psittaci.* Infect. Immun., *12*:638–646, 1975.

Tomlinson, T. H., Jr.: An outbreak of psittacosis at the National Zoological Park, Washington, D. C. Pub. Health Rep., *56*:1073–1081, 1941.

Wachendorfer, J. G.: Epidemiology and control of psittacosis. J. Am. Vet. Med. Assoc., *162*:298–303, 1973.

Sporadic Bovine Encephalomyelitis

A disease of young calves and, less frequently, older cattle, described by McNutt in Iowa, has now been reported in several states—Idaho, South Dakota, California, Oklahoma, and Texas—as well as Australia, Europe, and Japan. It probably is more widespread than published reports indicate. The disease is caused by an infectious agent currently designated as *Chlamydia psittaci (C. pecoris)*.

Organisms identified as *Chlamydia psittaci* have been recovered from several different disease syndromes of cattle, including enteritis of calves, latent intestinal infection of cattle, pneumonia, polyarthritis, placental infection, and epizootic abortion. These syndromes are taken up on following pages as they were described originally as distinct, separate diseases. It is well to keep in mind that as strains of the organisms are studied more extensively, it may become apparent that only one causative organism is involved, even though many different organ systems are affected. If this proves to be true, the disease should be identified as psittacosis or chlamydiosis, which may have varying clinical and pathologic manifestations.

Signs. The onset is sudden, with fever (105° to 107° F.), anorexia, depression, decreased activity, excessive salivation with drooling, and nasal discharge. Dyspnea with a cough is observed in about half the cases, but diarrhea, either mild or severe, is more common. Within a few days, calves have difficulty in walking, exhibiting stiffness and knuckling in the fetlock joints. They move aimlessly in circles, stagger, and fall with the head extended in opisthotonos. In the final stages, the limbs appear weak or paralyzed; death occurs in five to seven days in most cases, rarely being delayed for as long as a month.

Although calves are most susceptible, the report of Menges et al. (1953) indicates that adult cattle are also subject to the infection. These authors reported 21 herds totalling 1,774 cattle of all ages, of which 269 (15%) exhibited symptoms and 75 (28% of those affected) died from the disease. Among 892 calves in these herds, however, 224 (25%) contracted the disease and 64 (29% of those affected) died. Outbreaks of sporadic bovine encephalomyelitis usually follow introduction of new animals into a herd.

Lesions. The most constant gross lesion in fatal cases is serofibrinous peritonitis. Excessive amounts of clear yellow peritoneal fluid are present in early cases; in more prolonged cases, adhesive strands of fibrin form an exudate over the omentum, liver, and spleen. The spleen is sometimes enlarged. A similar fibrinous exudate lies over the pleura and pericardium in about half the fatal cases. A patchy lobular pneumonia may be seen in a few instances. The brain and spinal cord usually appear edematous and their vasculature is congested.

The microscopic lesions consist of fibrinous peritonitis, pleuritis, pericarditis, and perisplenitis, with addition of severe, diffuse meningoencephalomyelitis. The entire brain and spinal cord are involved in an intense inflammatory reaction, the meninges at the base of the brain being particularly affected. Proliferation of vascular endothelium and infiltration of the vessel walls with mononuclear and occasionally polymorphonuclear cells may be observed. Severe damage to neurons, both in brain and cord, has been described, and is believed by some to be secondary to the severe vascular lesions. Minute elementary bodies are demonstrable in mononuclear cells in the serosal exudates and in the brain or spinal cord. These bodies occur singly or in small clusters in the cytoplasm of these cells. They vary in size, but usually are less than a micron in diameter. They stain a pink-red with Macchiavello's stain.

In guinea pigs, a fatal disease may be experimentally induced with this agent, the organisms being demonstrable in the guinea pig tissues. Chick embryos are also susceptible; the embryos are killed in five to seven days, after adaptation of the agent.

Diagnosis. The gross and microscopic lesions are characteristic although not diagnostic of sporadic bovine encephalomyelitis. Demonstration of the typical elementary bodies is helpful. Transmission of this disease to the guinea pig with subsequent demonstration of the elementary bodies is confirmatory. All clinical and pathologic data must be carefully evaluated to eliminate rabies, "shipping fever," listeriosis, and malignant catarrhal fever.

Littlejohns, I. R., Harris, A. N. A., and Harding, W. B.: Sporadic bovine encephalomyelitis. Aust. Vet. J., 37:53, 1961. (VB 3956–61).
McNutt, S. H.: A preliminary report of an infectious encephalomyelitis of cattle. Vet. Med., 35:228–231, 1940.
McNutt, S. H., and Waller, E. F.: Sporadic bovine encephalomyelitis (Buss disease). Cornell Vet., 30:437–448, 1940.
Menges, R. W., Harshfield, G. S., and Wenner, H. A.: Sporadic bovine encephalomyelitis. Studies on pathogenesis and etiology of the disease. J. Am. Vet. Med. Assoc., 122:294–299, 1953.
Omori, T., Ishii, S., and Matumoto, M.: Miyagawanellosis of cattle in Japan. Am. J. Vet. Res., 21:564–573, 1960.
Price, D. A., and Hardy, W. T.: Sporadic bovine encephalomyelitis—isolation and antibiotic susceptibility of a Texas strain. J. Am. Vet. Med. Assoc., 128:308–310, 1956.
Tustin, R. C., Maré, J., and van Heerden, A.: A disease of calves resembling sporadic bovine encephalomyelitis. J. S. Afr. Vet. Med. Assoc., 32:117–123, 1961. (VB 129–62.)
Wenner, H. A., Harshfield, G. S., Chang, T. W., and Menges, R. W.: Sporadic bovine encephalomyelitis. II. Studies on the etiology of the disease. Isolation of nine strains of an infectious agent from naturally infected cattle. Am. J. Hyg., 57:15–29, 1953.
Wenner, H. A., Menges, R. W., and Carter, J.: Sporadic bovine encephalomyelitis. A serologic survey of cattle in the midwestern United States. Cornell Vet., 45:68–77, 1955.

Polyarthritis of Calves

In essentially analogous circumstances as described under polyarthritis of sheep, a variety of infectious organisms are capable of inducing polyarthritis in calves. *Mycoplasma mycoides* infection and vaccination can cause polyarthritis, and unidentified *Mycoplasma sp.* have been isolated from

polyarthritis by Moulton (1953) and Simmons and Johnson (1963). *Erysipelas insidiosa* and a variety of other bacteria (*Salmonella, Pasteurella,* diplococci, streptococci, staphylococci) often following umbilical infection, are also known to cause polyarthritis. Studies by Storz and colleagues (1966) indicate that polyarthritis in calves can result from infection by *Chlamydia psittaci.* The organism has been isolated from field cases of polyarthritis and induced arthritis following experimental inoculation. The infection as described by Storz et al. principally affected calves one to three weeks of age, and was characterized by involvement of practically all joints of the limbs, as well as vertebral and mandibular articulations. The joints were swollen and the synovial tissues edematous and thickened. The synovial fluid of the joints and tendon sheaths was increased in volume, turbid, yellow-gray, and contained numerous flakes of fibrin. Large plaques of fibrin often adhered to the synovial tissue and filled the pouches of the joint cavities. Cellular elements of the synovial fluid were increased in number and elementary bodies could be demonstrated in monocytic cells and synovial cells in smears stained with Giemsa.

Chlamydia frequently inhabit the digestive tracts of bovine animals. Usually the infection remains inapparent in adult cattle, but in young calves, the organisms cause enteritis and may reach the blood to be carried to the joints. Under experimental conditions, the organisms produce severe enteritis in newborn calves, but in adult cattle, the carrier state is more apt to result (Page et al., 1973; Smith et al., 1973; Doughri et al., 1973, 1974; Eugster and Storz, 1971).

Doughri, A. M., Altera, K. P., and Storz, J.: Host cell range of chlamydial infection in the neonatal bovine gut. J. Comp. Pathol., 83:107–114, 1973.
Doughri, A. M., Altera, K. P., Storz, J., and Eugster, A. K.: Ultrastructural changes in the *Chlamydia*-infected ileal mucosa of newborn calves. Vet. Pathol., 10:114–123, 1973.

Doughri, A. M., Young, S., and Storz, J.: Pathologic changes in intestinal chlamydial infection of newborn calves. Am. J. Vet. Res., 35:939–944, 1974.

Eugster, A. K., Joyce, B. K., and Storz, J.: Immunofluorescence studies on the pathogenesis of intestinal chlamydial infections in calves. Infect. Immun., 2:351–359, 1970.

Eugster, A. K., and Storz, J.: Effect of colostral antibodies on the pathogenesis of intestinal chlamydial infections in calves. Am. J. Vet. Res., 32:711–718, 1971.

Eugster, A. K., and Storz, J.: Pathogenetic events in intestinal chlamydial infections leading to polyarthritis in calves. J. Infect. Dis., 123:41–50, 1971.

Hughes, K. L., Edwards, M. J., Hartley, W. J., and Murphy, S.: Polyarthritis in calves caused by *Mycoplasma sp.* Vet. Rec., 78:276–281, 1966.

Moulton, J. E., Rhode, E. R., and Wheat, J. D.: Erysipelatous arthritis in calves. J. Am. Vet. Med. Assoc., 123:335–340, 1953.

Page, L. A., Matthews, P. J., and Smith, P. C.: Natural intestinal infection with *Chlamydia psittaci* in a closed bovine herd: serologic changes, incidence of shedding, antibiotic treatment of herd, and biologic characteristics of the chlamydiae. Am. J. Vet. Res., 34:611–614, 1973.

Simmons, G. C., and Johnston, L. A. Y.: Arthritis in calves caused by *Mycoplasma sp.* Aust. Vet. J., 39:11–14, 1963.

Smith, P. C., Cutlip, R. C., and Page, L. A.: Pathogenicity of a strain of *Chlamydia psittaci* of bovine intestinal origin for neonatal calves. Am. J. Vet. Res., 34:615–619, 1973.

Storz, J., Smart, R. A., Marriott, M. E., and Davis, R. V.: Polyarthritis of calves: isolation of psittacosis agents from affected joints. Am. J. Vet. Res., 27:633–641, 1966.

Storz, J., Shupe, J. L., Smart, R. A., and Thornley, R. W.: Polyarthritis of calves: experimental induction by a psittacosis agent. Am. J. Vet. Res., 27:987–995, 1966.

Epizootic Bovine Abortion

First described in California in 1956 by Howarth, epizootic bovine abortion represents an important cause of abortion in cattle in the United States and Europe. It is caused by *Chlamydia psittaci*; however, the natural mode of transmission is uncertain. The studies of Reed et al. (1975) indicate that at least one strain of *Chlamydia psittaci* may inhabit the intestinal tract of cattle and can produce the lesions of epizootic bovine abortion. This intestinal strain is also antigenically similar to *Chlamydia* recovered from cases of epizootic bovine abortion. *Chlamydia psittaci* is also known to be associated with bovine urogenital infections, and may result in venereal transmission (Storz et al., 1968, 1976). The disease has many similarities to enzootic abortion of ewes. Pregnant cattle are susceptible to experimental infection with the ovine agent, and pregnant sheep are susceptible to experimental infection with the bovine agent; however, the exact relationship of the two agents and disease requires further study.

Epizootic bovine abortion is principally a disease of the fetus, causing abortion, stillbirth, or birth of weak calves which die within a few days. No clinical evidence of disease is seen in the cow either before or after abortion. Abortions usually occur between the seventh and ninth months of gestation, but earlier abortion may occur. The abortion rate may exceed 75% of the pregnant animals in a herd.

Lesions. The pathologic features have been described in detail by Kennedy et al. (1960) and Kwapien et al. (1970). Gross findings in the fetus include subcutaneous edema, pleural and peritoneal effusion, generalized enlargement of lymph nodes, splenomegaly, petechiae on the oral mucous membranes, larynx, trachea, and conjunctivae, small gray foci in the myocardium and kidneys, and most characteristically a swollen, friable, coarsely nodular liver.

Microscopically, the basic histologic change is described as a granulomatous inflammatory process that may involve any or all body organs, but in particular the liver, meninges, brain, kidney, heart, and skin. Individual lesions consist of focal necrosis and collections of macrophages, epithelioid cells, lymphocytes and neutrophils. Lesions in lymph nodes may contain Langhans type giant cells. Marked reticuloendothelial hyperplasia accounts for the gross lymphadenopathy and splenomegaly.

The placenta in natural abortion has been described as edematous but of little diagnostic value. In the experimental disease, necroses of cotyledons, edema, accumulation of fibrinopurulent exudate, and a leathery tough consistency have been described.

Diagnosis. The clinical, gross, and microscopic findings should allow presumptive diagnosis, which can be supported by demonstrating cytoplasmic elementary bodies in impression smears of placenta or fetal organs stained by Macchiavello, Giemsa or Gimenez techniques. Definitive diagnosis requires isolation and identification of the infectious agent.

Bassan, Y., and Ayalon, N.: Abortion of dairy cows inoculated with epizootic bovine abortion agent (Chlamydia). Am. J. Vet. Res., *32*:703–710, 1971.

Howarth, J. A., Moulton, J. E., and Brazier, L. M.: Epizootic bovine abortion characterized by fetal hepatopathy. J. Am. Vet. Med. Assoc., *128*:441–449, 1956.

Kennedy, P. C., Olander, H. J., and Howarth, J. A.: Pathology of epizootic bovine abortion. Cornell Vet., *50*:417–429, 1960.

Kwapien, R. P., et al.: Pathologic changes of placentas from heifers with experimentally induced epizootic bovine abortion. Am. J. Vet. Res., *31*:999–1015, 1970.

McKercher, D. G.: Cause and prevention of epizootic bovine abortion. J. Am. Vet. Med. Assoc., *154*:1192–1196, 1969.

McKercher, D. G., Wada, E. M., Robinson, E. A., and Howarth, J. A.: Epizootiologic and immunologic studies of epizootic bovine abortion. Cornell Vet., *56*:433–450, 1966.

McKercher, D. G., et al.: Vaccination against epizootic bovine *(Chlamydial)* abortion. J. Am. Vet. Med. Assoc., *163*:889–890, 1973.

Page, L. A., and Smith, P. C.: Placentitis and abortion in cattle inoculated with chlamydiae isolated from aborted human placental tissue. Proc. Soc. Exp. Biol. Med., *146*:269–275, 1974.

Reed, D. E., et al.: Comparison of antigenic structure and pathogenicity of bovine intestinal *Chlamydia* isolate with an agent of epizootic bovine abortion. Am. J. Vet. Res., *36*:1141–1144, 1975.

Storz, J.: Comparative studies on EBA and EAE, abortion diseases of cattle and sheep resulting from infection with psittacosis agents. *In* Abortion Diseases of Livestock, edited by L. C. Faulkner. Springfield, Charles C Thomas, 1968.

Storz, J., McKercher, D. G., Howarth, J. A., and Straub, O. C.: The isolation of a viral agent from epizootic bovine abortion. J. Am. Vet. Med. Assoc., *137*:509–514, 1960.

Storz, J., Call, J. W., Jones, R. W., and Miner, M. L.: Epizootic bovine abortion in the Intermountain Region. Some recent clinical, epidemiologic and pathologic findings. Cornell Vet., *57*:21–37, 1967.

Storz, J., Carroll, E. J., Ball, L., and Faulkner, L. C.: Isolation of a psittacosis agent *(Chlamydia)* from

semen and epididymis of bulls with seminal vesiculitis syndrome. Am. J. Vet. Res., *29*:549–555, 1968.

Storz, J. et al.: Urogenital infection and seminal excretion after inoculation of bulls and rams with Chlamydiae. Am. J. Vet. Res., *37*:517–520, 1976.

Enzootic Abortion of Ewes

First reported in 1950 by Stamp in Scotland, enzootic abortion of ewes has since been recognized in Europe and the United States. The disease is caused by *Chlamydia psittaci;* closely related to the causative agent of epizootic bovine abortion. Abortion usually occurs in the last month of gestation, but earlier abortion, stillbirth, and birth of weak lambs may occur. Fetal membranes are ofen retained, which results in clinical disease in the ewe; otherwise, specific signs of infection are not seen in the ewe. Placentitis is the major lesion. Cotyledons are gray to dark red and the periplacentome is thickened, opaque yellow-pink, and covered with a flaky, clay-colored exudate. The uterine surface of the chorion is of tough, granular consistency, pink-yellow, and covered with a flaky, yellowish exudate. Microscopically there is focal necrosis, edema, vasculitis, and a mononuclear cell infiltration. Cytoplasmic elementary bodies can be demonstrated in tissue sections or smears stained by the Giemsa, Macchiavello or Gimenez techniques. Lesions in the lamb are not striking. They resemble those of epizootic bovine abortion, but of lesser degree.

Diagnosis. Diagnosis is based on clinical and pathologic findings supported by demonstration of elementary bodies or isolation of the infectious agent.

Djurov, A.: Die pathohistologishen Veränderungen der Feten beim enzootischen Virusabort der Schafe. Zentralbl. Veterinaermed. [B], *19*:578–587, 1972.

Krauss, H., Wandera, J. G., and Lauerman, L. H., Jr.: Isolation and identification of *Chlamydia* in Kenya sheep and serologic survey. Am. J. Vet. Res., *32*:1433–1438, 1971.

Novilla, M. N., and Jensen, R.: Placental pathology of experimentally induced enzootic abortion in ewes. Am. J. Vet. Res., *31*:1983–2000, 1970.

Parker, H. D., Hawkins, W. W., Jr., and Brenner, E.: Epizootiologic studies of ovine virus abortion. Am. J. Vet. Res., 27:869–877, 1966.

Parker, H. D.: A virus of ovine abortion—isolation from sheep in the United States and characterization of the agent. Am. J. Vet. Res., 21:243–250, 1960.

Pavlov, N., and Vesselivova, A.: Morphology of the natural infection in lambs with the virus of lamb abortion. Zentbl. Vet. Med., 12B:517–526, 1965.

Stamp, J. T., McEwen, A. D., Watt, J. A. A., and Nisbet, D. I.: Enzootic abortion in ewes. I. Transmission of the disease. Vet. Rec., 62:251–254, 1950.

Storz, J.: Comparative studies on EBA and EAE, abortion diseases of cattle and sheep resulting from infection with psittacosis agent. In Abortion Diseases of Livestock, edited by L. C. Faulkner. Springfield, Charles C Thomas, 1968.

Studdert, M. J.: Bedsonia abortion of sheep. II. Pathology and pathogenesis with observations on the normal ovine placenta. Res. Vet. Sci., 9:57–64, 1968.

Studdert, M. J., and McKercher, D. G.: Bedsonia abortion of sheep. I. Aetiological studies. Res. Vet. Sci., 9:48–56, 1968.

Studdert, M. J., and Kennedy, P. C.: Enzootic abortion of ewes. Nature (Lond.), 203:1088–1089, 1964.

Tunnicliff, E. A.: Ovine virus abortion. J. Am. Vet. Med. Assoc., 136:132–134, 1960.

Chlamydial Pneumonia of Cattle and Sheep

Organisms of the genus *Chlamydia* have been isolated from naturally-occurring cases of **enzootic pneumonia** of cattle, sheep, and goats. Cultures of these organisms on chicken yolk-sac preparations inoculated intratracheally in these species have also produced the disease. The relationship of these respiratory organisms to the *Chlamydia* that have been incriminated in sporadic bovine encephalomyelitis, polyarthritis of cattle or sheep, epizootic bovine abortion, or enzootic abortion of ewes is not at all clear. It appears that the organisms are all of the same species (*Chlamydia psittaci*), but may differ in some minor antigens or in pathogenicity. As was mentioned in the discussion of sporadic bovine encephalomyelitis, each of the "syndromes" described in the literature may be differing clinical and pathologic aspects of the same etiologic complex. The answer lies in more thorough comparisons of the strains of *Chlamydia* involved.

Cattle have been experimentally susceptible to ovine pneumonia isolates, and sheep, to the bovine isolates. Enzootic pneumonia which is principally, but not exclusively, of importance in young animals, is clinically nonspecific, characterized by fever, nasal discharge, cough, dyspnea, and depression.

Lesions. Lesions, which are comparable in cattle and sheep, are most often restricted to the anterior lobes of the lung. Microscopically the lesions are dominated by an extensive infiltration of lymphocytes, macrophages, and plasma cells, particularly in the bronchiolar mucosa and surrounding bronchioles and blood vessels, but also within alveolar septae. The exudate often has a follicular arrangement, and compresses bronchioles and alveoli. Bronchioles and alveoli contain macrophages and variable numbers of neutrophils, but purulent exudate is lacking unless secondary bacterial invaders initiate a more characteristic picture of bronchopneumonia, as is often the case. There is proliferation and epithelialization of alveolar lining cells, which contributes to alveolar consolidation.

Diagnosis. As in other infections caused by *Chamydia psittaci*, elementary bodies are more easily demonstrated in tissue impressions than tissue sections. Positive diagnosis requires isolation of the causative organism. It is essential that this infection be distinguished from the "enzootic pneumonia" caused by *Mycoplasma*. The lymphocytic aggregations around the bronchial tree are characteristic of the microscopic lesions of mycoplasmosis. The organisms also may be differentiated by their morphology and cultural characteristics.

Carter, G. R., and Rowsell, H. C.: Studies on pneumonia of cattle. II. An enzootic pneumonia of calves in Canada. J. Am. Vet. Med. Assoc., 132:187–190, 1958.

Dungworth, D. L., and Cordy, D. R.: The pathogenesis of ovine pneumonia. II. Isolation of virus from faeces: comparison of pneumonia caused by faecal, enzootic abortion and pneumonitis viruses. J. Comp. Pathol. Ther., 72:71–79, 1962.

———: The pathogenesis of ovine pneumonia. I. Isolation of a virus of the PL group. J. Comp. Pathol. Ther., 72:49–70, 1962.

Ide, P. R.: The etiology of enzootic pneumonia of calves. Can. Vet. J., 11:194–202, 1970.

Matumoto, M., et al.: Studies on the disease of cattle caused by a psittacosis-lymphogranuloma group virus (Miyagawanella). VI. Bovine pneumonia caused by this virus. Jpn. J. Exp. Med., 25:23–34, 1955.

McKercher, D. G.: A virus possibly related to the psittacosis-lymphogranuloma-pneumonitis group causing a pneumonia in sheep. Science, 115:543–544, 1952.

Omar, A. R.: The aetiology and pathology of pneumonia in calves. Vet. Bull., 36:259–273, 1966.

Palotay, J. L., and Christensen, M. S.: Bovine respiratory infections. I. Psittacosis-lymphogranuloma venereum group of viruses as etiological agents. J. Am. Vet. Med. Assoc., 134:222–230, 1959.

Phillip, J. I. H., et al.: Pathogenesis and pathology in calves of infection by Bedsonia alone and by Bedsonia and reovirus together. J. Comp. Pathol., 78:89–99, 1968.

Storz, J.: Psittacosis-lymphogranuloma agents in bovine pneumonia. J. Am. Vet. Med. Assoc., 152:814–819, 1968.

Polyarthritis of Sheep

One form of so-called "stiff-lamb-disease" is not the result of lesions in the muscles, but in the joints. Various organisms have been incriminated from time to time, including *Erysipelothrix rhusiopathiae (insidiosa)* and *Mycoplasma*. A specific and rather widespread cause of arthritis appears to be *Chlamydia psittaci* (Fig. 10–9), which can be isolated from joints, feces, cerebrospinal fluid, urine, blood, and viscera. Affected lambs are detected by a characteristic lameness involving one or more joints. Some lambs are depressed, with a high fever (106° F.), others lose weight and are slow to recover. Some animals appear to recover completely, but others remain permanently lame.

Lesions. The lesions in early stages consist for the most part of serofibrinous or fibrinous synovitis, occasionally with edema around the affected joint and greenish-gray masses of material in the articular spaces. Microscopically, affected synovial membranes are edematous; lining cells are swollen, often disorganized, detached, and covered with fibropurulent debris. The subsynovial connective tissue contains granulomatous accumulations of mononuclear cells. In most examples, large numbers of elementary bodies can be demonstrated in smears or sections of synovia or joint fluid stained with Giemsa's or Macchiavello's stain; however, arthritis may persist in the absence of demonstrable organisms.

Diagnosis. The diagnosis can be made by isolation of the infective agent in chick embryos, tissue culture, or guinea pigs, and demonstration of elementary bodies in association with characteristic lesions.

Cutlip, R. C.: Electron microscopy of cell cultures infected with a chlamydial agent causing polyarthritis of lambs. Infect. Immun., 1:499–502, 1970.

Cutlip, R. C., and Ramsey, F. K.: Ovine chlamydial polyarthritis: Sequential development of articular lesions in lambs after intraarticular exposure. Am. J. Vet. Res., 34:71–76, 1973.

Hopkins, J. B., Stephenson, E. H., Storz, J., and Pierson, R. E.: Conjunctivitis associated with chlamydial polyarthritis in lambs. J. Am. Vet. Med. Assoc., 163:1157–1160, 1973.

Mendlowski, B., and Segre, D.: Polyarthritis in sheep. I. Description of the disease and experimental transmission. Am. J. Vet. Res., 21:68–73, 1960.

Mendlowski, B., Kraybill, W. H., and Segre, D.: Polyarthritis in sheep. II. Characteristics of the causative virus. Am. J. Vet. Res., 21:74–80, 1960.

Norton, W. L., and Storz, J.: Observations on sheep with polyarthritis produced by an agent of the psittacosis-lymphogranuloma venereum trachoma group. Arthritis Rheum., 10:1–12, 1967.

Shupe, J. L., and Storz, J.: Pathologic study of psittacosis-lymphogranuloma polyarthritis of lambs. Am. J. Vet. Res., 25:943–951, 1964.

Stevenson, R. G., and Robinson, G.: The pathology of pneumonia in young lambs inoculated with Bedsonia. Res. Vet. Sci., 11:469–474, 1970.

Storz, J., et al.: Polyarthritis of lambs induced experimentally by a psittacosis agent. J. Infect. Dis., 115:9–18, 1965.

Storz, J., Shupe, J. L., James, L. F., and Smart, R. A.: Polyarthritis of sheep in the Intermountain Region caused by a psittacosis-lymphogranuloma agent. Am. J. Vet. Res., 24:1201–1206, 1963.

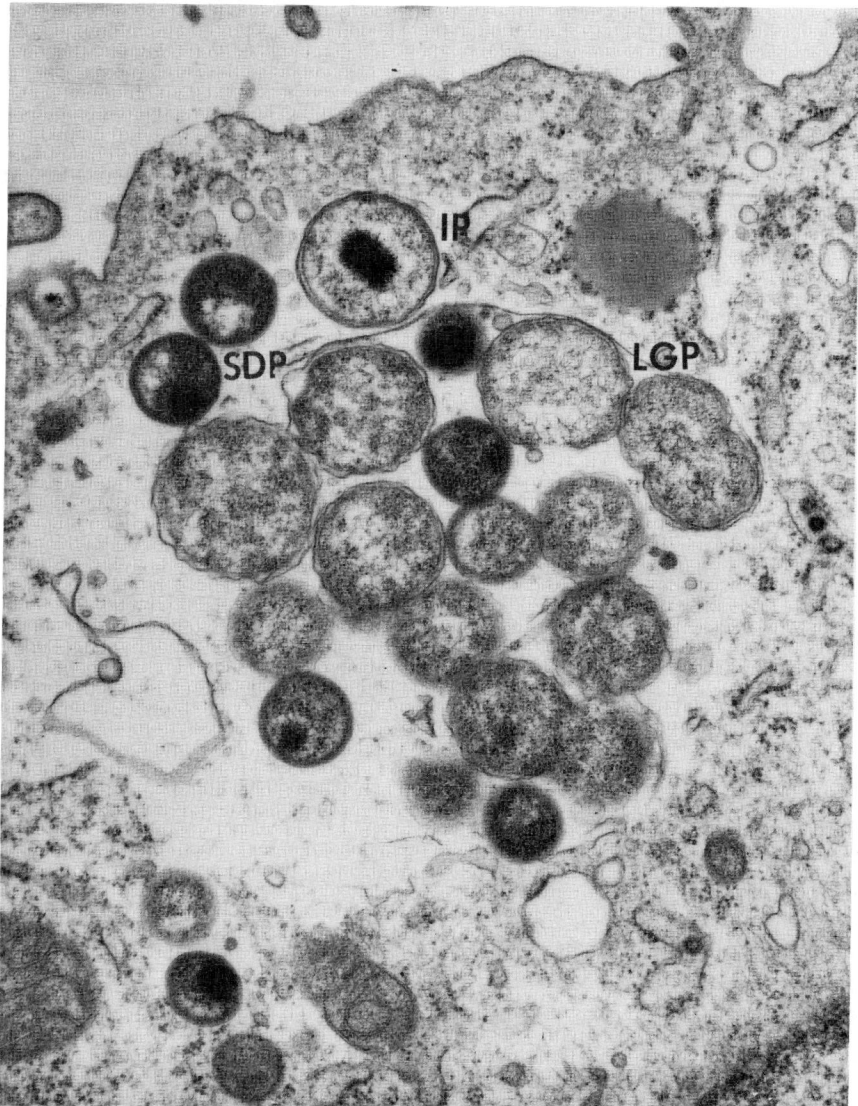

Fig. 10-9. Electron micrograph of a chlamydial inclusion of the agent of polyarthritis of lambs in tissue culture. There are several stages of development recognizable: small dense particles *(SDP)*, intermediate particles *(IP)*, and large granular particles *(LGP)*, some of which are dividing. (Courtesy of Dr. Randall C. Cutlip and *Infection and Immunity.*)

Feline Pneumonitis

Feline pneumonitis, a chlamydial infection of domesticated cats, is a problem in catteries and in experimental laboratories where cats are congregated. The disease starts as an acute upper respiratory infection, with sneezing and catarrh; later symptoms are nasal and conjunctival mucous discharges, transitory fever, and some inappetence. The disease runs a course of about two weeks and terminates fatally in a small percentage of cases. It may be adapted to mice by serial passage of infected material inoculated intranasally. A feature of value in the recognition of the disease is the presence of elementary bodies of the organism, which can be demonstrated most readily in the lung tissues of experimentally infected mice and occasionally in feline tissues.

Lesions. Aside from catarrhal inflammatory changes in the upper respiratory passages, the principal lesions are usually found in the lungs. Sharply demarcated patches of what appears to be consolidation may be seen in the various lobes. These patches are usually light reddish brown to gray or even prune-colored, contrasting sharply with the light pink lung tissue.

Microscopic examination reveals that these affected areas are distributed around terminal bronchioles and consist principally of alveolar collapse rather than consolidation, although in some areas inflammatory cells, lymphoid and polymorphonuclear, fill the alveoli. Of diagnostic significance is the presence of elementary bodies, which usually appear in loose aggregates in the cytoplasm of epithelial and mononuclear cells. These bodies are tiny spherical structures, approximately .5 μ in diameter. In smears, they stain selectively with Macchiavello's stain, appearing brightly eosinophilic and usually coccoid. In some instances, the elementary bodies coalesce into a plaque, forming a solid eosinophilic body which distends the cytoplasm of epithelial and occasionally of leukocytic cells. These organisms are currently considered to be a strain of *Chlamydia psittaci.* Older names include *Chlamydia felis* and *Miyagawanella felis.*

Schachter, Ostler and Meyer (1969) have described a case of acute keratoconjunctivitis in man caused by the feline pneumonitis agent.

Baker, J. A.: A virus causing pneumonia in cats and producing elementary bodies. J. Exp. Med., 79:159–172, 1944.

Hoover, E. A., Kahn, D. E., and Langloss, J. M.: Experimentally induced feline chlamydial infection (feline pneumonitis). Am. J. Vet. Res., 39:541–547, 1978.

Mitzel, J. R., and Strating, A.: Vaccination against feline pneumonitis. Am. J. Vet. Res., 38:1361–1363, 1977.

Schachter, J., Ostler, H. B., and Meyer, K. R.: Human infection with the agent of feline pneumonitis. Lancet, May 31:1063–1065, 1969.

Other Chlamydial Infections

Inclusion Conjunctivitis of Guinea Pigs. This natural disease was first described by Murray (1964) as a mild, self-limiting conjunctivitis of young guinea pigs. The inclusions in impressions of conjunctival epithelium are similar to those found in human inclusion blennorrhea (conjunctivitis). The causative organism in guinea pigs has the characteristics of *Chlamydia psittaci,* rather than those of *Chlamydia trachomatis,* the agent in the human disease. The genital tract of guinea pigs may be infected with organisms isolated from conjunctiva, then cultivated on chick embryo yolk-sacs. This experimental disease resembles lymphogranuloma-venereum and trachoma of the human patient to some extent (Mount et al., 1972, 1973; Howard et al., 1976; Reed et al., 1977; and Robinson, 1969).

Enzootic Pneumonia in Rabbits. This disease, not uncommon in young rabbits, is considered, with good reason, to be caused by *Pasteurella multocida.* In a few instances, Flatt and Dungworth (1971) were able to recover *Chlamydia* from occult lesions in lungs of apparently healthy young rabbits. The significance of this infection in pulmonary disease of rabbits appears yet to be established.

Chlamydial Polyarthritis in Foals. In one case, described by McChesney et al. (1974), *Chlamydia* were cultured from joint exudate from a young foal with spontaneous polyarthritis. This disease appears to be much less frequent in foals than in lambs or calves.

Chlamydial Infection in Dogs. Although chlamydial antibody titers have been demonstrated in as many as 50% of dogs in some surveys, clinical disease is reported much less frequently in this species. Dogs are susceptible to experimental infection, however (Young et al., 1972). A *Chlamydial* agent recovered from a case of ovine polyarthritis produced disease in five of six dogs when inoculated intraperitoneally or intravenously. The principal lesions were focal necrosis of the liver, lymphocytic and reticuloendothelial hyperplasia in spleen and lymph nodes, acute leptomeningitis, and polyarthritis.

Chlamydial Infections in Muskrats and Snowshoe Hares. Strains of *Chlamydia* were isolated from dead muskrats *(Ondatra zibethicus)* and snowshoe hares *(Lepus americanus)* during an outbreak in Saskatchewan, Canada in 1961 (Spalatin et al., 1966). Experimental infection in these species was reproduced with these cultures of *Chlamydia* (Iversen, et al., 1970).

Follicular Conjunctivitis of Sheep. A specific ocular disease of sheep is known in Australia as contagious conjunctivo-keratitis, pink eye, snow blindness, or heather blindness. This has been compared to trachoma of man by Cooper (1974). *Chlamydia* isolated from affected sheep have been propagated in yolk-sac cultures and subsequently used to reproduce the disease in susceptible sheep (Cooper, 1974). *Chlamydia* have also been isolated from the conjunctival sac of sheep suffering from a similar disease, follicular conjunctivitis, in the United States (Storz et al., 1967).

Chlamydial Infections of Nonhuman Primates. Natural infection of two crab-eating Macaques *(Macaca fascicularis)* with *Chlamydia* has been reported by Morita et al. (1971). Taiwan Rock Macaques *(Macaca cyclopis)* are susceptible to experimental infection with *Chlamydia trachomatis*, originally isolated from human trachoma. Owl monkeys *(Aotus sp.)* are even more susceptible to trachoma infection and have been used extensively in research on this disease (Fraser and Bell, 1971, Fraser et al., 1975; Fraser, 1976). *Chlamydia trachomatis*, isolated from a human patient with nongonococcal urethritis, produced urethritis and persist-ent infection after instillation into the urethra of male Baboons (DiGiacomo et al., 1975).

Cooper, B. S.: Transmission of chlamydia-like agent isolated from contagious conjunctivo-keratitis of sheep. NZ Vet. J., 22:181–184, 1974.

DiGiacomo, R. F., Gale, J. L., Wang, S. P., and Kiviat, M. D.: Chlamydial infection of male baboon urethra. Br. J. Vener. Dis., 51:310–313, 1975.

Flatt, R. E., and Dungworth, D. L.: Enzootic pneumonia in rabbits: naturally occurring lesions in lungs of apparently healthy young rabbits. Am. J. Vet. Res., 32:621–626, 1971.

——: Enzootic pneumonia in rabbits: microbiology and comparison with lesions experimentally produced by *Pasteurella multocida* and a chlamydial organism. Am. J. Vet. Res., 32:627–637, 1971.

Fraser, C. E. O., and Bell, S. D.: Experimental trachoma in owl monkeys and Taiwan monkeys. *In* Medical Primatology, 1970, edited by E. I. Goldsmith, and J. Moor-Jankowski. Basel, S. Karger, 1971. pp. 783–791.

Fraser, C. E. O., McComb, D. E., Murray, E. S., and MacDonald, A. B.: Immunity to chlamydial infections of eye. Arch. Ophthalmol., 94:518–521, 1975.

Fraser, C. E. O.: The owl monkey *(Aotus trivirgatus)* as an animal model in trachoma research. Lab. Anim. Sci., 26:1138–1141, 1976.

Howard, L. V., O'Leary, M. P., and Nichols, R. L.: Animal model studies of genital chlamydial infections. Immunity to re-infection with guinea pig inclusion conjunctivitis agent in the urethra and eye of male guinea pigs. Br. J. Vener. Dis., 52:261–265, 1976.

Iversen, J. O., et al.: The susceptibility of muskrats and snowshoe hares to experimental infection with a chlamydial agent. Can. J. Comp. Med., 34:80–89, 1970.

McChesney, A. E., Becerra, V., and England, J. J.: Chlamydial polyarthritis in a foal. J. Am. Vet. Med., Assoc., 165:259–261, 1974.

Morita, M., Yoshizawa, S., and Inaba, Y.: Spontaneous cases of a disease of cynomolgus monkeys *(Macaca irus)* probably caused by the psittacosis-lymphogranuloma-trachoma group *(Chlamydia)*. Jpn. J. Vet. Sci., 33:261–270, 1971.

Mount, D. T., Bigazzi, P. E., and Barron, A. L.: Infection of genital tract and transmission of ocular infection to newborns by the agent of guinea pig inclusion conjunctivitis. Infect. Immun., 5:921–926, 1972.

——: Experimental genital infection of male guinea pigs with the agent of guinea pig inclusion conjunctivitis and transmission to females. Infect. Immun., 8:925–930, 1973.

Murray, E. S.: Guinea pig inclusion conjunctivitis virus. I. Isolation and identification as a member of the psittacosis-lymphogranuloma-trachoma group. J. Infect. Dis., 114:1–12, 1964.

Reed, C., Campbell, L. H., and Soave, O. A.: Limited survey of genital infection by guinea pig inclusion conjunctivitis agent. Am. J. Vet. Res., *38*:1383–1387, 1977.

Robinson, G. W.: A naturally occurring latent bedsonia infection in guinea-pigs. Br. Vet. J., *125*:23–25, 1969.

Spalatin, J., et al.: Agents of psittacosis-lymphogranuloma venereum group, isolated from muskrats and snowshoe hares in Saskatchewan. Can. J. Comp. Med., *30*:260–264, 1966.

Storz, J., Pierson, R. E., Marriott, M. E., and Chow, T. L.: Isolation of psittacosis agents from follicular conjunctivitis of sheep. Proc. Soc. Exp. Biol. Med., *125*:857–860, 1967.

Young, S., Storz, J., and Maierhofer, C. A.: Pathologic features of experimentally induced chlamydial infection in dogs. Am. J. Vet. Res., *33*:377–383, 1972.

DISEASES DUE TO SPIROCHAETACEAE

These bacterial organisms, commonly called spirochetes, are currently grouped in one order, Spirochaetales, containing a single family, Spirochaetaceae. This family is made up of five genera, three of which contain pathogenic species (Table 10–7). These organisms are slender, helically coiled, single-celled bacteria measuring 3 to 500 μ in length. They are flexuous, may occur in chains held together by an outer envelope, and may assume the shape of a planar wave. They multiply by transverse fission. They are motile, do not form endospores, and are best observed with phase-contrast or dark-field microscopy. These bacteria may be free-living, com-

Table 10–7.   Genera of Spirochaetaceae

I. *Spirochaeta*. Five species free-living in water, sewage; none are pathogenic.

II. *Cristispira*. Many organisms found in marine and fresh water species of bivalve and univalve mollusks; none known to be pathogenic.

III. *Treponema*. Four pathogenic and seven nonpathogenic species are recognized (see Table 10–9).

IV. *Borrelia*. Nineteen species recognized, exact relationships yet to be determined (see Table 10–10).

V. *Leptospira*. One species recognized; many serotypes identified and named; cause leptospirosis in man and animals (see Table 10–8).

mensal, or parasitic. Specific species are causes of important diseases of man (syphilis, yaws, pinta, relapsing fever, leptospirosis) and animals (spirochetosis, leptospirosis, and borreliosis).

Leptospirosis

The nomenclature of organisms in the genus *Leptospira* is presently in a state of flux, due to insufficient accepted taxonomic data with which different isolates may be compared to one another (Turner, 1974). It has been customary to identify isolates of *Leptospira* from man and animals by serotypes, based upon response of the organisms to the agglutination reaction and cross-agglutinin absorption tests, using antisera prepared in rabbits. Until the taxonomic indecision is resolved, it appears most useful to refer to these organisms by the serotype designation. Only one species is recognized presently: *Leptospira interrogans*. All other pathogenic strains are referred to as serotypes (such as *canicola*, *icterohemorrhagiae*, and *pomona*). Pathogenic *Leptospira* serotypes are not limited to a single host species (Table 10–8).

Organisms in the genus *Leptospira* conform to the general characteristics of the family Spirochaetaceae and have some specific features. The spiral organisms are single, flexuous, and helical, with bent, hooked, or curved ends. Their dimensions are 6–20 μm or more in length by 0.1 μm in diameter. They are motile by means of axial filaments (axistyle), but have no external flagellae. They are best visualized by darkfield microscopy as well as the electron microscope. They may be stained with some silver-impregnation methods, but are not differently stained by aniline dyes.

The electron microscope reveals that the organisms consist of a cellular body wound on an axistyle with an external sheath surrounding both elements (Figure 10–10). The cell body, approximately circular in transverse section, contains nuclear material, cytoplasm, and a limiting cell membrane. The axistyle is a single structure,

Table 10–8. Diseases Due to Leptospira (Leptospira interrogans)

Serotype	Host Species (isolated from)	Disease
icterohemorrhagiae	man, rat, dog, cattle	Weil's disease (man)
		Leptospirosis (dogs)
canicola	dogs, man, cattle	Leptospirosis (dogs)
		Canicola fever (man)
		Hemoglobinuria (cattle)
pomona	swine, cattle, sheep,	Abortion, stillbirths (swine)
	man, horses, sea lions	Abortion, mastitis (cattle)
		Swineherd's disease (man)
		Abortion, stillbirths (sheep)
		Periodic ophthalmia (horses)
grippotyphosa (bovis)	cattle, swine	Stillbirths (swine)
		Infectious hemoglobinuria (cattle)
		Reproductive failure (cattle)
hardjo	man, cattle	Infertility, abortion, mastitis (cattle)
patoc	cattle	Leptospirosis (cattle)
hebdomadis	man, cattle	Leptospirosis (cattle)
sejore	man, cattle	Leptospirosis
saxkoebing	man, cattle	Leptospirosis
kennewicki	cattle	Leptospirosis
illini	cattle	Leptospirosis (low pathogenicity)
australis A	man, cattle	Leptospirosis (man, cattle)
autumnalis	man, cattle	Leptospirosis (man, cattle)
ballum	man, cattle	Leptospirosis (man, cattle)
bataviae	man, cattle	Leptospirosis (man, cattle)
copenhageni	man, cattle	Leptospirosis (man, cattle)
tarassovi	man, cattle	Leptospirosis (man, cattle)

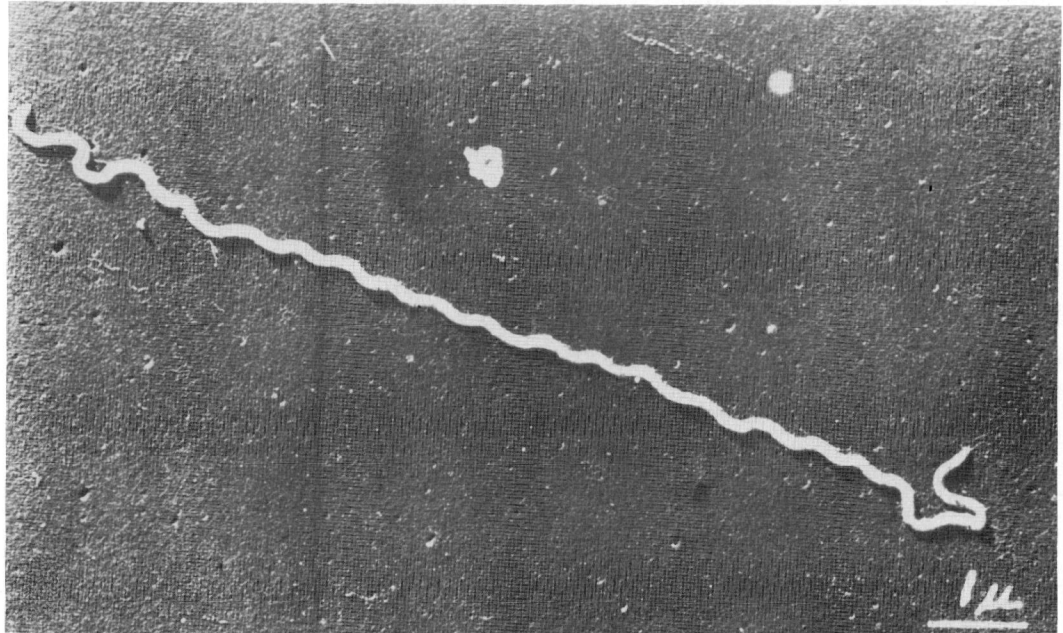

Fig. 10–10. Electron photomicrograph of *Leptospira canicola*. (Courtesy of Division of Veterinary Medicine, Walter Reed Army Institute of Research.)

consisting of two filaments, each of which is inserted near one terminal end of the organism. The free ends are near the middle of the organism.

Leptospira are aerobic and may be cultivated on media containing inorganic salts, buffered with phosphates. Some media containing serum enhance the growth of certain serotypes.

Some of the more prevalent serotypes are listed in Table 10–8.

Turner, L. H.: Genus V. Leptospira, Noguchi, 1917. *In* Bergey's Manual of Determinative Bacteriology, eighth ed., edited by R. E. Buchanan and N. E. Gibbons. Baltimore, Williams & Wilkins, 1974.

Canine Leptospirosis

Leptospira interrogans, serotype *canicola* is the common organism that infects dogs, but serotype *icterohemorrhagiae* occurs in a small percentage of cases of leptospiral infection in this species. Large numbers of dogs have been shown to have demonstrable antibodies to leptospirae in their serum; the incidence of significant antibody titer has reached 40% in some surveys. The clinical disease in dogs is also extremely common. The canine disease may appear as an acute febrile disease with icterus, dehydration, vomiting, bloody diarrhea, accelerated red blood cell sedimentation, albuminuria, severe debility, and often fatal outcome. However, some animals recover from this acute disease only to succumb to uremia from the nephritis that follows localization of leptospirae in the kidneys. In some cases, the acute icteric phase may not occur or may be inapparent, the uremic manifestations being the first indications of illness to be recognized. Dogs affected in this manner exhibit dehydration, loss of weight, weakness, vomiting (often bloody in character), diarrhea, and "uremic" breath.

Lesions. For convenience, the lesions in these "acute" and "subacute" phases of the disease will be described separately.

Acute Phase. In dogs dying during the "acute" or septicemic stage of the disease, the lesions are dominated by severe dehydration and icterus, with many petechiae on the pleura, peritoneum, and nasal and oral mucosae. The liver usually exhibits characteristic microscopic changes, although few may be recognized grossly. The most striking lesion is in the liver cells, which shrink and become disassociated from one another, breaking up the normal columns of liver cells into individually discrete cells. This individualization of liver cells (Fig. 10–11) is not limited solely to leptospirosis, but is particularly striking in this disease. The affected liver cells often have coarsely granular, eosinophilic cytoplasm and small hyperchromic nuclei. Regeneration of liver parenchyma may at times be evidenced by binucleate cells, large hyperchromic nuclei, and mitotic figures. Foci of necrosis of liver parenchyma may be found, but stainable lipoid material is seldom present. Bile retention is indicated by plugging of bile canaliculi, but larger bile ducts usually are empty. Kupffer cells contain large amounts of hemosiderin, and portal vessels are usually congested. Characteristic leptospirae may be demonstrated with appropriate silver impregnation technique. These organisms are seen in sinusoids and within liver cells as slender, tightly coiled, spiral organisms with hook-shaped ends (Fig. 10–12).

The changes in the kidney during this acute stage, except for grossly visible petechiae, may be somewhat subtle, but are definite and recognizable upon careful microscopic examination. The glomeruli may show little change, but convoluted tubules are usually severely altered. The epithelial cells of the convoluted tubules in particular areas are swollen, coarsely granular, and deeply eosinophilic, or vacuolated and partially or completely desquamated into the lumen. In some tubules, only the bare basement membrane of the tubule is left. In others, the lumen is filled with eosinophilic epithelial cytoplasmic debris, in which are some nuclei and occasional erythrocytes. Some

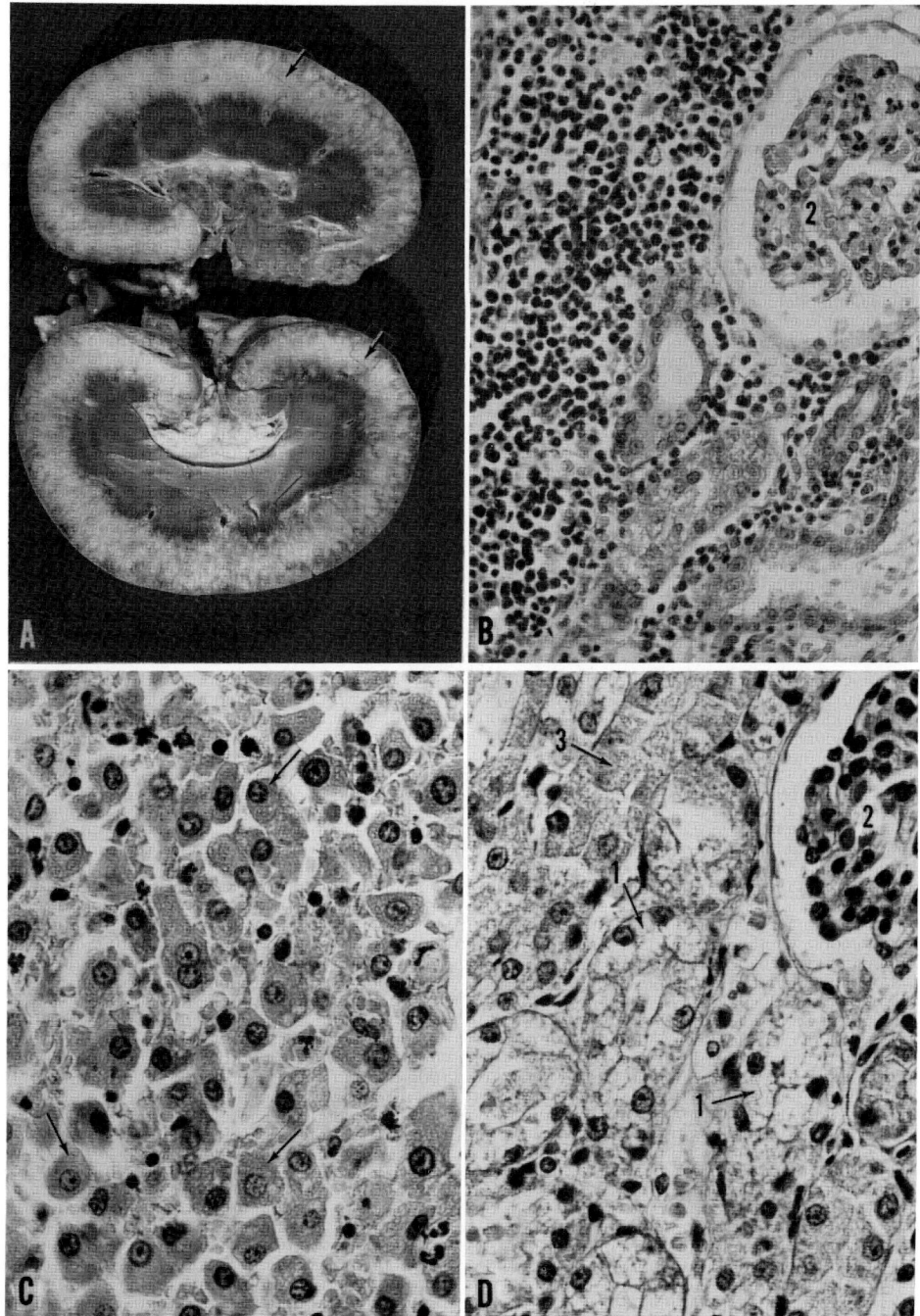

Fig. 10–11. Leptospirosis in the dog. *A,* Kidney of a dog with active infection following a subacute course. Note gray masses (arrows) replacing cortex. Contributor: Dr. C. L. Davis. *B,* Accumulation of lymphoid cells *(1)* in renal cortex in subacute case (× 260). Note glomerulus is spared. Contributor: USAF Hospital, Lackland Air Force Base. *C,* The liver in acute leptospirosis (× 490). Note dissociation of liver cells (arrows), which disrupts liver cell columns. *D,* The kidney in acute leptospirosis (× 490). Same dog as *C.* Note vacuoles in cytoplasm of some convoluted tubules *(1).* The glomerulus *(2)* and other convoluted tubules *(3)* are not affected. (Courtesy of Armed Forces Institute of Pathology.) Contributor: Division of Veterinary Medicine, Walter Reed Army Institute of Research.

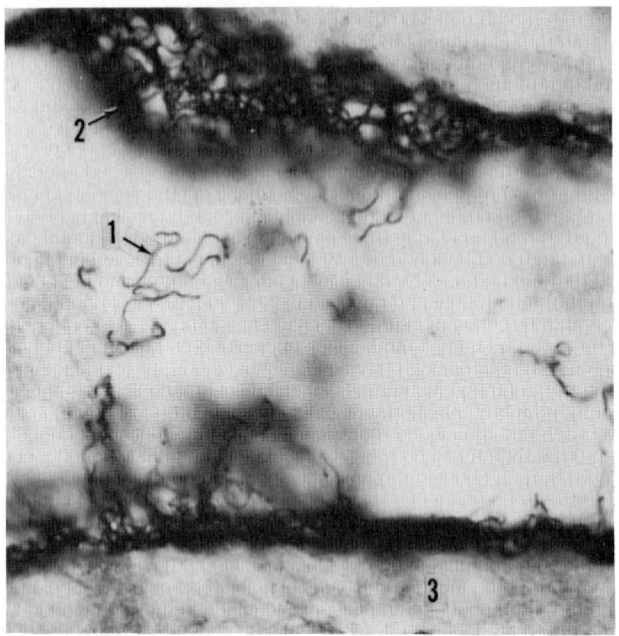

Fig. 10–12. Leptospirosis. Leptospira (× 1670) in the lumen *(1)* and in the epithelium *(2 and 3)* of a convoluted tubule, kidney of a dog with subacute infection. (Courtesy of Armed Forces Institute of Pathology.) Contributor: U. S. Army Veterinary Research Laboratory.

tubules may contain regenerating epithelium, as indicated by mitoses, hyperchromatic nuclei, and cells that coalesce to appear as multinucleated giant cells. Leptospirae are demonstrable singly or in small groups in affected tubules by use of silver impregnation techniques. Affected tubules are usually surrounded by lymphocytes, plasma cells, and occasional erythrocytes, which diffusely infiltrate the interstitial stroma.

Lymph nodes and spleen are usually grossly enlarged and may contain areas of edema and hemorrhage. Microscopically, there is a paucity of mature lymphocytes and an apparent increase in reticular cells. Erythrocytes are often present in the medullary sinuses, either free or in macrophages. Diffuse hemorrhages are common in the fundic portion of the gastric mucosa, and may be associated with necrosis, neutrophilic infiltration, and desquamation of the mucosa. Hemorrhages also may be seen in the submucosa and less frequently in the muscularis. The intestine may contain small petechiae in the serosa and mucosa, but these are not so severe as

those in the stomach, nor are the hemorrhages associated with necrosis.

Hemorrhages and areas of edema may be seen in other organs, such as myocardium, submucosa and muscularis of the urinary bladder, adrenal gland, pancreas, gallbladder, and lung. In the lung, gross hemorrhages on the pleural surface may be particularly striking, the entire surface being covered with tiny spherical hemorrhages or larger ones a few millimeters in diameter.

Subacute Phase. Animals that live through or escape the "acute" septicemic form of the disease, only to die from uremia due to renal involvement, may manifest a subacute course. At necropsy of such animals, dehydration, emaciation, and a strong "uremic" odor are observed, but icterus and hemorrhages are unusual. The renal lesions are most significant; those in other viscera are inconstant or related only to uremia. The kidneys are grossly enlarged, the surface usually is smooth, the capsule is tense and white or grayish, sometimes with hemorrhages showing through from the parenchyma. The renal parenchyma cuts with only slightly increased resistance, but the cut surface is moist and turgid, bulging away from the capsule. Petechiae may be seen anywhere on the cut surface, but the most striking changes usually are located at the corticomedullary junction. Here grayish masses of firm, turgid tissue replace the normal renal parenchyma. This gray tissue may form a wide band on the inner margin of the cortex or may obliterate most of the cortex. In animals sacrificed during recovery, these lesions may be focal in pattern.

The microscopic appearance of these lesions is characteristic. Convoluted tubules undergoing degenerative changes are surrounded or replaced by large dense masses of cells, including lymphocytes, plasma cells, macrophages, occasional neutrophils, and sometimes small nests of erythrocytes. Although convoluted tubules are severely affected, glomeruli are often spared or involved only secondarily. Except in cases treated with antibiotics, silver preparations demonstrate leptospirae in the lumen of tubules or in the cytoplasm of the tubular epithelium. The organisms occur singly or in tangled nests (Fig. 10–12).

Lesions resulting from uremia are found elsewhere in the body. They include severe gastric hemorrhages with microscopic deposits of calcium in the gastric mucosa and calcareous deposits in the walls of the aorta and large arteries (Fig. 21–12).

Bloom, F.: Histopathology of canine leptospirosis. Cornell Vet., *31*:266–268, 1941.

Carlos, E. R., et al.: Leptospirosis in the Philippines: canine studies. Am. J. Vet., Res., *32*:1451–1454, 1971.

Coffin, D. L., and Maestrone, G.: Detection of leptospires by fluorescent antibody. Am. J. Vet. Res., *23*:159–164, 1962.

Jones, T. C., Roby, T. O., Davis, C. L., and Maurer, F. D.: Control of leptospirosis in war dogs. Am. J. Vet. Res., *6*:120–128, 1945.

Meyer, K. F., Stewart-Anderson, B., and Eddie, B.: Canine leptospirosis in the United States. J. Am. Vet. Med. Assoc., *95*:710–729, 1939.

Monlux, W. S.: III. Clinical pathology of canine leptospirosis. Cornell Vet., *38*:109–121, 1948.

————: Pathology of canine leptospirosis. Cornell Vet., *38*:199–208, 1948.

Morton, H. E., and Anderson, T. F.: Morphology of *Leptospira icterohemorrhagiae* and *L. canicola* as revealed by the electron microscope. J. Bact., *45*:143–146, 1943.

Moulton, J. E., and Howarth, J. A.: The demonstration of *Leptospira canicola* in hamster kidneys by means of fluorescent antibody. Cornell Vet., *57*:523–532, 1957.

Bovine Leptospirosis

Leptospiral organisms have been recovered from, or demonstrated in, tissues of cattle which were manifesting a wide gamut of clinical symptoms: mastitis, fever, icterus, emaciation, hemoglobinuria, abortion, occasional anemia, transient leukopenia, and death, particularly involving young animals. The variety of clinical signs that may occur in bovine leptospirosis not only indicates the need for laboratory tests to establish the diagnosis, but also emphasizes the importance of maintaining a critical attitude regarding all evidence pointing toward the infection. It now appears, however, that leptospirae are well established as an agent of disease in the bovine species. The principal serotype found in the United States is *pomona*, but other serotypes also infect this species (Table 10–8).

Lesions. The disease in cattle in many respects parallels its counterpart in dogs. It may occur in an **acute septicemic form** or as a **chronic nephritic type** of disease. The latter is rarely fatal. The lesions in these two bovine types are similar to those observed in dogs. In the acute case, icterus, a swollen yellowish liver and petechiae are the principal gross findings, as in the dog. Hemolytic anemia, which is not a feature of the canine disease, accounts for hemoglobinuria and partially contributes to the icterus and hepatic lesions. Microscopic changes include portal hepatic lymphocytic infiltration, with splenic hemosiderosis in some outbreaks and severe centrilobular necrosis of the liver in others. In certain outbreaks in Israel with organisms of the *grippotyphosa* serotype, leptospirosis took a protracted clinical course. The microscopic lesions included hepatic cell dissociation, cholangitis, and congestion and hemosiderosis of the spleen. In the kidneys, swelling and disorganization of convoluted tubular epithelium were associated with bile pigment and hemoglobin in the lumen.

Animals that survive the systemic disease have grayish to white focal lesions in the kidney parenchyma. These foci are usually discrete and scattered through the cortex, not concentrated at the corticomedullary junction, as is often the case in dogs. Microscopically, the principal lesions are based upon changes in the tubular epithelium. The epithelial cells and affected tubules have granular, swollen, or vacuolated cytoplasm, sometimes associated with fragmentation of the cytoplasm and detachment of the cells. These affected tubles are surrounded by dense masses of leukocytes, chiefly lymphocytes and plasma cells. In some cases, syncytial giant cells of the Langhans' type have been described. Leptospirae are usually, but not constantly, demonstrable in sections impregnated with silver, located within affected tubular epithelium or in the lumen of the tubule.

Leptospiral abortion, which usually occurs in the latter half of pregnancy, is not associated with specific lesions in the placenta or fetus.

Amatredo, A.: Bovine leptospirosis. Vet. Bull., 43:875–891, 1975.

Baker, J. A., and Little, R. B.: Leptospirosis in cattle. J. Exp. Med., 88:295–307, 1948.

Birch-Anderson, A., Hougen, K. H., and Borg-Peterson, C.: Electron microscopy of Leptospira. I. Leptospira strain pomona. Acta Pathol. Microbiol. Scand. (B), 81:665–676, 1973.

Burdin, M. L.: Renal histopathology of Leptospira grippotyphosa in farm animals in Kenya. Res. Vet. Sci., 4:423–430, 1963.

Cordy, D. R., and Jasper, D. E.: The pathology of an acute hemolytic anemia of cattle in California associated with leptospira. J. Am. Vet. Med. Assoc., 120:175–178, 1952.

Ellis, W. A., and Michna, S. W.: Experimental leptospiral abortion in cattle. Vet. Rec., 94:255, 1974.

Hadlow, W. J., and Stoenmer, H. G.: Histopathologic findings in cows naturally infected with Leptospira pomona. Am. J. Vet. Res., 16:45–56, 1955.

Hanson, L. E.: Immunologic problems in bovine leptospirosis. J. Am. Vet. Med. Assoc., 163:919–920, 1973.

Imbabi, S. E., Sleight, S. D., Conner, G. H., and Schmidt, D. A.: Experimental leptospirosis: Leptospira canicola infection in calves. Am. J. Vet. Res., 28:413–419, 1967.

Killinger, A. H., et al.: Immunity to leptospirosis: Renal changes in vaccinated cattle given challenge inoculum. Am. J. Vet. Res., 37:93–94, 1976.

Langham, R. F., Morse, E. V., and Morter, R. L.: Pathology of experimental ovine leptospirosis. Leptospira pomona infections. J. Infect. Dis., 103:285–290, 1958.

Miller, N. F., and Wilson, R. B.: Electron microscopic study of the relationship of Leptospira pomona to the renal tubules of the hamster during acute and chronic leptospirosis. Am. J. Vet. Res., 28:225–235, 1967.

Morsi, H. M., Shibley, G. P., and Strother, H. L.: Renal leptospirosis: challenge exposure of vaccinated and nonvaccinated cattle to Leptospira icterohaemorrhagiae and Leptospira canicola. Am. J. Vet. Res., 34:175–179, 1973.

Murphy, J. C., and Jensen, R.: Experimental pathogenesis of leptospiral abortion in cattle. Am. J. Vet. Res., 30:703–713, 1969.

Reinhard, K. R., Tierney, W. F., and Roberts, S. J.: A study of two enzootic occurrences of bovine leptospirosis. Cornell Vet., 40:148–164, 1950.

Reinhard, K. R.: A clinical pathologic study of experimental leptospirosis of calves. Am. J. Vet. Res., 12:282–291, 1951.

Reinhard, K. R., and Hadlow, W. J.: Experimental bovine leptospirosis—pathological, hematological, bacteriological and serological studies. Proc. Am. Vet. Med. Assoc., pp. 205–216, 1954.

Porcine Leptospirosis

Swine are susceptible to several serotypes of Leptospira. In the United States serotype pomona appears to be the most important organism. The disease has not been studied as extensively in swine as it has in dogs and cattle, but it is recognized that infection with leptospirae may occur as a subclinical infection or be associated with acute hepatitis and icterus, subacute or chronic nephritis, and reproductive disorders characterized by abortion, stillbirth, and the birth of weak piglets which may die.

The gross and microscopic manifestations of leptospirosis in swine have not been adequately studied. Renal lesions have been described that mimic those in cattle. There is tubular degeneration and an intense focal lymphocytic infiltration. Leptospirae are demonstrable in the lumens and epithelium of the tubules and in the nodules of lymphocytic infiltration. In the pig, like most other susceptible species, leptospirae localize in the kidneys and are shed in the urine for protracted periods of time.

Stillborn pigs and aborted fetuses, which are expelled mainly in the last third of gestation, are often macerated, precluding accurate examination. The most characteristic lesion in abortuses and stillborns is focal necrosis of the liver, without significant cellular infiltration. Organisms can generally be isolated, but may be difficult to demonstrate in tissues.

Chaudhary, R. K., Fish, N. A., and Barnum, D. A.: Experimental infection with *L. pomona* in normal and immune piglets. Can. Vet. J., *7*:106–112, 1966.

Fennestead, K. L., and Borg-Petersen, C.: Experimental leptospirosis in pregnant sows. J. Infect. Dis., *116*:57–66, 1966.

Gochenour, W. S., Jr., Johnson, R. V., Yager, R. H., and Gochenour, W. S.: Porcine leptospirosis. Am. J. Vet. Res., *13*:158–160, 1952.

Gsell, O.: Leptospirosis Pomona, die Schweinehüterkrankheit. Schweiz. Med. Wochenschr., *76*:237–241, 1946.

Hanson, L. E., Reynolds, H. A., and Evans, L. V.: Leptospirosis in swine caused by serotype *grippotyphosa*. Am. J. Vet. Res., *32*:855–860, 1971.

Langham, R. F., Morse, E. V., and Morter, R. L.: Experimental leptospirosis. V. *Leptospira pomona* infection in swine. Am. J. Vet. Res., *19*:395–400, 1958.

Michna, S. W., and Campbell, R. S. F.: Leptospirosis in pigs: Epidemiology, microbiology and pathology. Vet. Rec., *84*:135–138, 1969.

Morsi, H. M., Shibley, G. P., and Strother, H. L.: Antibody response of swine to *Leptospira canicola* and *Leptospira iceterohaemorrhagiae*. Am. J. Vet. Res., *34*:1253–1256, 1973.

Shibley, G. P., Morsi, H. M., Strother, H. L., and Clark, M.: Renal leptospirosis: exposure of vaccinnated and nonvaccinated swine to *Leptospira icterohaemorrhagiae* and *Leptospira canicola*. Am. J. Vet. Res., *34*:1171–1174, 1973.

Sleight, S. D., Langham, R. F., and Morter, R. L.: Experimental leptospirosis: the early pathogenesis of *Leptospira pomona* infection in young swine. J. Infect. Dis., *106*:262–269, 1960.

Leptospirosis in Other Species

Serologic evidence indicates that leptospirosis is a relatively common infection in horses. Bryans (1955) demonstrated agglutinins for serotypes *icterohemorrhagiae, pomona,* or *canicola* in 30% of 512 mature horses. More recent studies indicate approximately the same frequency of elevated antibody titers among horses in California and Northeast United States (Smith et al., 1976; Verma et al., 1977). In horses inoculated with serotype *pomona,* Bryans observed a mild transient disease characterized by fever, hemolytic anemia, and icterus. In contrast to other species, leptospirae were not present in the urine of experimentally infected horses. The relationship of leptospirosis to periodic ophthalmia in horses is discussed in Chapter 28.

Both Old and New World nonhuman primates are experimentally susceptible to leptospirosis, but the natural disease has not been described in New World species and appears to be infrequent in Old World species. Cats are susceptible to several serotypes of leptospira, but infection has not been associated with clinical or pathologic changes. Disease resembling acute leptospirosis in cattle has been reported in sheep naturally infected with *Leptospira. Leptospira interrogans,* serotype *pomona,* has been associated with illness, abortions, and stillbirths among California sea lions (Vedros et al., 1971; Smith et al., 1974).

Arean, V. M.: The pathologic anatomy and pathogenesis of fatal human leptospirosis (Weil's disease). Am. J. Pathol., *40*:393–423, 1962.

Bohl, E. H., Powers, T. E., and Ferguson, L. C.: Abortion in swine associated with leptospirosis. J. Am. Vet. Med. Assoc., *124*:262–264, 1954.

Breese, S. S., Jr., Gochenour, W. S., Jr., and Yager, R. H.: Electron microscopy of leptospiral strains. Proc. Soc. Exp. Biol. Med., *80*:185–188, 1952.

Bryans, J. T.: Studies on equine leptospirosis. Cornell Vet., *45*:16–50, 1955.

Carlos, E. R., et al.: Leptospirosis in the Philippines: feline studies. Am. J. Vet. Res., *32*:1455–1456, 1971.

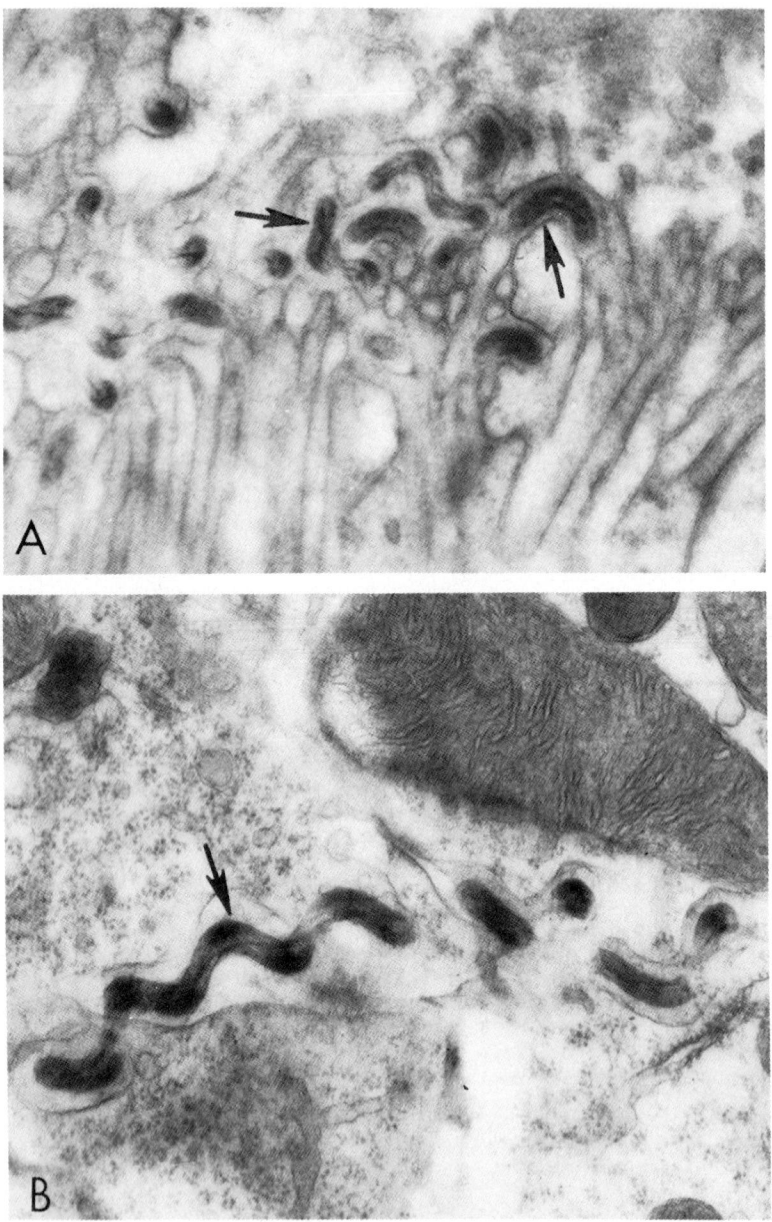

Fig. 10–13.   Leptospirosis. *A*, *Leptospira pomona* closely associated with microvilli of a proximal convoluted tubule cell in the kidney of a hamster. *B*, *Leptospira pomona* within a proximal tubule cell in the kidney of a hamster. (Courtesy of Dr. N. G. Miller and *American Journal of Veterinary Research*.)

Decker, M. J., Freeman, M. J., and Morter, R. L.: Evaluation of mechanisms of leptospiral hemolytic anemia. Am. J. Vet. Res., *31*:873–878, 1970.

De Freitas, D. C., et al.: Notas sobre Leptospirose Equina (in Brazil). Arq. Inst. Biol. (Sao Paulo), *27*:93–96, 1960. VB 1788–62.

Donham, K. J., and Crawford, R. P.: Effects of fluorescein isothiocyanate labeling on staining characteristics of a fluorescent antibody conjugate for the diagnosis of leptospirosis. Am. J. Vet. Res., *34*:267–271, 1973.

Famatiga, E. G.: Leptospirosis in Philippine monkeys. Southeast Asian J. Trop. Med., *4*:316–318, 1973.

Fear, F. A., et al.: A leptospirosis outbreak in a baboon *(Papio sp.)* colony. Lab. Anim. Care, *18*:22–28, 1968.

Gochenour, W. S., Jr., Gleiser, C. A., and Ward, M. K.: Laboratory diagnosis of leptospirosis. Ann. NY Acad. Sci., *70*:421–426, 1958.

Hartley, W. J.: Ovine leptospirosis. Aust. Vet. J., *28*:169–170, 1952.

Heusser, H.: Die periodische Augenentzündung, eine Leptospirose? Schweiz. Arch. Tierheilk., *90*:287–312, 1948.

Jacusiel, F.: Problem of leptospirosis in Israel. Refuah Vet., *6*:121–124, 1949.

Lucke, V. M., and Crowther, S. T.: The incidence of leptospiral agglutination titres in the domestic cat. Vet. Rec., *77*:647–648, 1965.

Marshall, R. B.: Ultrastructural changes in renal tubules of sheep following experimental infection with *Leptospira interrogans* serotype *pomona*. J. Med. Microbiol., *7*:505–508, 1974.

Michna, S. W., and Campbell, R. S. F.: Leptospirosis in wild animals. J. Comp. Pathol., *80*:101–106, 1970.

Minette, H. P.: Leptospirosis in primates other than man. Am. J. Trop. Med. Hyg., *15*:190–198, 1966.

Minette, H. P., and Shaffer, M. F.: Experimental leptospirosis in monkeys. Am. J. Trop. Med. Hyg., *17*:202–212, 1968.

Nervig, R. M., Ellinghausen, H.C., Jr., and Cardella, M. A.: Growth, virulence, and immunogenicity of *Leptospira interrogans* serotype *szwajizak*. Am. J. Vet. Res., *38*:1421–1424, 1977.

Roberts, S. J.: Sequelae of leptospirosis in horses on a small farm. J. Am. Vet. Med. Assoc., *133*:189–194, 1958.

Roth, E. E.: Leptospirosis in wildlife in the United States. Proc. Am. Vet. Med. Assoc., pp. 211–218, 1964.

Shive, R. J., et al.: Leptospirosis in Barbary apes *(Macaca sylvana)*. J. Am. Vet. Med. Assoc., *155*:1176–1178, 1969.

Smith, A. W., Brown, R. J., Skilling, D. E., and DeLong, R. L.: *Leptospira pomona* and reproductive failure in California sea lions. J. Am. Vet. Med. Assoc., *165*:996–999, 1974.

Smith, B. P., and Armstrong, J. M.: Fatal hemolytic anemia attributed to leptospirosis in lambs. J. Am. Vet. Med. Assoc., *167*:739–741, 1975.

Smith, R. E., Williams, I. A., and Kingsbury, E. T.: Serologic evidence of equine leptospirosis in the Northeast United States. Cornell Vet., *66*:105–109, 1976.

Smith, R. E., Reynolds, I. M., and Sakai, T.: Experimental leptospirosis in pregnant ewes. III. Pathologic features. Cornell Vet., *50*:115–122, 1960.

Stalheim, O. H. V.: Leptospirosis diagnosis by immunofluorescence: Improved procedure for antigen preparation. Am. J. Vet. Res., *32*:2107–2110, 1971.

Vedros, N. A., et al.: Leptospirosis epizootic among California sea lions. Science, *172*:1250–1251, 1971.

Verma, B. B., Biberstein, E. L., and Meyer, M. E.: Serologic survey of leptospiral antibodies in horses in California. Am. J. Vet. Res., *38*:1443–1444, 1977.

Watson, A. D. J., and Wannan, J. S.: The incidence of leptospiral agglutinins in domestic cats in Sydney. Aust. Vet. J., *49*:545, 1973.

Yager, R. H., Gochenour, W. S., Jr., and Wetmore, P. W.: Recurrent iridocyclitis (periodic ophthalmia) of horses. I. Agglutination and lysis of leptospiras by serums deriving from horses affected with recurrent iridocyclitis. J. Am. Vet. Med. Assoc., *117*:207–209, 1950.

Treponemal Infections

Spirochaetal organisms of the genus *Treponema* are responsible for several natural diseases of man and a few diseases of animals (Table 10–9). Animals are susceptible to several of the human pathogens following experimental exposure.

Swine Dysentery (Porcine Ulcerative Spirochaetosis)

Piglets 8 to 14 weeks of age appear to be most susceptible to this disease, first described by Doyle (1944). The disease appears to be highly infectious by the rapidity of its spread through a herd. The principal manifestation is severe diarrhea with copious amounts of mucus, blood, and fibrinous exudate in the feces. One serious effect is a failure of affected piglets to grow.

The etiology has been in controversy for many years. *Vibrio coli* was initially found in great numbers in affected colons, but its ability to cause the disease by itself has been equivocal. Suspensions of affected colonic mucosa cause the disease rather consistently when administered orally to gnotobiotic (germ-free) or conventional

Table 10–9. Diseases Due to *Treponema*

Organism	Disease and Host
Treponema pallidum	Syphilis in human beings; rabbits susceptible to experimental exposure; hamsters and guinea pigs resistant
T. pertenue	Yaws of human beings; rabbits and hamsters susceptible; guinea pigs refractory
T. carateum	Pinta or Carate in human beings; chimpanzees susceptible; rabbits, hamsters, and guinea pigs resistant
T. paraluis-cuniculi	Venereal spirochaetosis of rabbits (rabbit spirochaetosis); latent infection can be produced in mice, guinea pigs, and hamsters
T. phagedenis, macrodentium, refringens, denticola, orale, scoliodontum, and *vincentii*	Nonpathogenic species; cultivatable
T. hyodysenteriae	Presumptive name of organism associated with swine dysentery

pigs. A large spirochaete (tentative name: *Treponema hyodysenteriae*) has been demonstrated in large numbers in the colon of affected swine. The disease may be experimentally produced by administration of pure cultures of *T. hyodysenteriae* to conventional, but not to gnotobiotic piglets. In combination with pure cultures of an enteric anaerobe *Bacteroides vulgatus,* however, *T. hyodysenteriae* produces characteristic signs and lesions in gnotobiotic piglets. The disease is more severe when another anaerobe, *Fusobacterium necrophorum,* is added to the mixture. Thus it appears that a combination of organisms is necessary to cause this disease.

Lesions. The lesions are restricted to the colon, cecum, and rectum, but are most constant and severe in the spiral colon. The affected mucosa is folded and rugose, covered with a fibrinous mucinous exudate with foci of hemorrhage and eventually ulcers. Microscopically, the mucosa is particularly involved; initially it is thickened, then the superficial cells become necrotic and are sloughed. The fibrinous mucous exudate becomes conspicuous on the surface. Mucus lost from the goblet cells fills the crypts. The lamina propria becomes distended with leukocytes as epithelial cells are lost. Crypts and epithelial cells contain many spirochaetes. Other organisms, including *Vibrio coli* may exist in large numbers in the lumen of the crypts and among tissue debris in the lumen.

Diagnosis. The diagnosis is established by the nature of the lesions and by demonstrating the spirochaetes in the colonic mucosa, using silver stains, immunofluorescent techniques or electron microscopy.

Akkermans, J. P. W. M., and Pomper, W.: Aetiology and diagnosis of swine dysentery. Tijdschr. Diergeneeskd., *98*:649–654, 1973.

Blandford, T. B., Bygrave, A. C., Harding, J. D. J., and Little, T. W. A.: Suspected porcine ulcerative spirochaetosis in England. Vet. Rec., *90*:15, 1972.

Doyle, L. P.: A vibrio associated with swine dysentery. Am. J. Vet. Res., *15*:3–5, 1944.

———: Enteritis in swine. Cornell Vet., *35*:103–109, 1945.

———: Etiology of swine dysentery. Am. J. Vet. Res., *9*:50–51, 1948.

Hamdy, A. H., and Glenn, M. W.: Transmission of swine dysentery with *Treponema hyodysenteriae* and *Vibrio coli.* Am. J. Vet. Res., *35*:791–798, 1974.

Harcourt, R. A.: Porcine ulcerative spirochaetosis. Vet. Rec., *92*:647–648, 1973.

Harris, D. L., and Glock, R. D.: Swine dysentery. J. Am. Vet. Med. Assoc., *160*:561–565, 1972.

Harris, D. L., Glock, R. D., Christensen, C. R., and Kinyon, J. M.: Swine dysentery. I. Inoculation of pigs with *Treponema hyodysenteriae* (new species) and reproduction of the disease. Vet. Med. Small Anim. Clin., *67*:61–64, 1972.

Harris, D. L., Kinyon, J. M., Mullin, M. T., and Glock, R. D.: Isolation and propagation of spirochetes from the colon of swine dysentery affected pigs. Can. J. Comp. Med., *36*:74–76, 1972.

Harris, D. L., et al.: Swine dysentery: Studies of gnotobiotic pigs inoculated with *Treponema hyodysenteriae, Bacteroides vulgatus,* and *Fusobacterium necrophorum.* J. Am. Vet. Med. Assoc., 172:468–471, 1978.

Hughes, R., Olander, H. J., Gallina, A. M., and Morrow, M. E.: Swine dysentery. Induction and characterization in isolated colonic loops. Vet. Pathol., 9:22–37, 1972.

Hughes, R., Olander, H. J., and Williams, C. B.: Swine dysentery: Pathogenicity of *Treponema hyodysenteriae.* Am. J. Vet. Res., 36:971–978, 1975.

Hughes, R., Olander, H. J., Kanitz, D. L., and Quershi, S.: A study of swine dysentery by immunofluorescence and histology. Vet. Pathol., 14:490–507, 1977.

Hunter, D., and Clark, A.: The direct fluorescent antibody test for the detection of *Treponema hyodysenteriae* in pigs. Res. Vet. Sci., 19:98–99, 1975.

Kennedy, G. A., Strafuss, A. C., and Schoneweis, D. A.: Scanning electron microscopic observations on swine dysentery. J. Am. Vet. Med. Assoc., 163:53–55, 1973.

Kennedy, G. A., and Strafuss, A. C.: Scanning electron microscopy of the lesions of swine dysentery. Am. J. Vet. Res., 37:395–401, 1976.

Liven, E., and Saxegaard, F.: The isolation of a *Treponema hyodysenteriae*-like organism associated with swine dysentery in Norway. Acta Vet. Scand., 16:324–326, 1975.

Meyer, R. C., Simon, J., and Byerly, C. S.: The etiology of swine dysentery. I. Oral inoculation of germ-free swine with *Treponema hyodysenteriae* and *Vibrio coli.* Vet. Pathol., 11:515–526, 1974.

———: The etiology of swine dysentery. II. Effect of known microbial flora, weaning and diet on disease production in gnotobiotic and conventional swine. Vet. Pathol., 11:527–534, 1974.

Morales, G. A., Gianella, H., and Beltran, L. E.: Swine dysentery associated with *Treponema hyodysenteriae*-like organisms in Colombia. Trop. Anim. Health Prod., 7:211–212, 1975.

Wilcock, B. P., and Olander, H. J.: Studies on the pathogenesis of swine dysentery. I. Characterization of the lesions in colons and colonic segments inoculated with pure cultures or colonic contents containing *Treponema hyodysenteriae.* Vet. Pathol., 16:450–465, 1979.

Venereal Spirochaetosis of Rabbits (Treponematosis of Rabbits, Rabbit Syphilis, Cuniculosis, Vent Disease)

A natural disease of domesticated rabbits, caused by *Treponema paraluis-cuniculi (T. cuniculi)*, should be distinguished from the infection produced experimentally in rabbits by injection of *Treponema pallidum* from lesions of human syphilis. The rabbit spirochaetosis is readily transmitted by coitus and may spread rapidly through a breeding colony of rabbits (Small and Newman, 1972).

Lesions. Initial lesions may be observed on the skin of the face, nostrils, ears, prepuce, and perineum, consisting of tiny, slightly raised, erythematous, hyperkeratotic lesions, occasionally with tiny vesicles. These vesicles contain treponemes, which are demonstrable by dark-field examination. These early lesions of the skin tend to regress in a few months.

Lesions on the penis and adjacent prepuce consist of lymphocytes, heterophils, and macrophages lying under the squamous epithelium. Injection of organisms into the testes results in replacement of testicular tubules by lymphocytic masses with large numbers of macrophages and plasma cells. Lymph nodes contain many nests of epithelioid cells, which replace much of the lymphocytic tissue.

Diagnosis. The diagnosis may be established by the demonstration of treponemes in darkfield preparations. The organisms are difficult to demonstrate in tissue sections with silver stains. Serologic tests useful in detecting infection in a colony include the use of a fluorescent treponemal antigen and a rapid plasma reagin card test (Small and Newman, 1972).

Bayon, H.: A new species of *Treponema* found in the genital sores of rabbits. Br. Med. J., 2:1159, 1913.

Hougen, K. H., Birch-Andersen, A., and Jensen, H. J. S.: Electron microscopy of *Treponema cuniculi.* Acta Pathol. Microbiol. Scand. (B), 1:15–26, 1973.

Noguchi, H.: Venereal spirochaetosis in American rabbits. J. Exp. Med., 35:391–408, 1922.

Small, J. D., and Newman, B.: Venereal spirochetosis of rabbits (rabbit syphilis) due to *Treponema cuniculi*: a clinical, serological, and histopathological study. Lab. Anim. Sci., 22:77–89, 1972.

Smith, J. L., and Pesetsky, B. R.: The current status of *Treponema cuniculi*: Review of the literature. Br. J. Vener. Dis., 43:117–127, 1967.

Warthin, A. S., Buffington, E., and Wanstrom, R. C.: A study of rabbit spirochaetosis. J. Infect. Dis., 32:315–332, 1923.

Borreliosis

Spirochaetal organisms of the genus *Borrelia* have been identified in epidemic and

Table 10–10.   Diseases Due to *Borrelia*

Organism	Vector	Geographic Distribution	Disease
Borrelia anserina	*Argus persicus, A. reflexus, A. miniatus*, others	Worldwide	Avian borreliosis, borreliosis or spirochaetosis of birds
B. recurrentis	*Pediculus humanus* (body louse)	Potentially cosmopolitan	Human epidemic relapsing fever (louse-borne fever)
B. hispanica	*Ornithodorus erraticus*	Middle East; Mediterranean	Human endemic relapsing fever, (tick-borne fever)
B. hermsii	*O. hermsi*	North America	"
B. duttonii	*O. moubata*	Africa	"
B. parkeri	*O. parkeri*	North America	"
B. venezuelensis	*O. rudis*	South America	"
B. mazzottii	*O. talaje*	Mexico and Guatemala	"
B. persica	*O. tholozani*	Central Asia Middle East	"
B. turicatae	*O. turicata*	North and South America	"
B. latyschewii	*O. tartakovskyi*	Central Asia	"
B. caucasica	*O. verrucosus*	Caucasus	"
B. braziliensis	*O. braziliensis*	Brazil	"
B. dugesii	*Ornithodoros dugesi*	Mexico	Human endemic (tick-borne) relapsing fever
B. graingeri	*O. graingeri*	East Africa	"
B. crocidurae	*O. erraticus, sonrai*	Africa, Near East, Central Asia	Mildly pathogenic for man
B. harveyi	unknown	Africa	Mildly pathogenic for man, monkeys, mice, rats
B. tillae	*O. zumpti*	South Africa	Borreliosis in rats, mice, monkeys
B. theileri	*Rhipicephalus decoloratus, R. evertsi, Boophilus micropus*	South Africa Australia	Borreliosis of cattle and horses

endemic relapsing fever in man, avian spirochaetosis, and many lice and ticks (Table 10–10). Several isolates, recovered from ticks in widely scattered parts of the world, have been assigned species names which future studies may prove to be unwarranted. Until these organisms can be compared, their taxonomic relationships remain unsettled.

Louse-Borne Relapsing Fever (Epidemic Relapsing Fever)

This human disease, caused by *Borrelia recurrentis*, has been reproduced in Grivet monkeys *(Cercopithecus aethiops)*. This organism causes a clinical course and pathologic lesions similar to those of the human disease.

Signs. Initially, fever, inactivity, and leukocytosis are associated with spirochaetes circulating in the blood. After the initial infection, lasting four to seven days, the signs subside, but relapses then follow after four to six days of remission. Convalescence may last up to 22 days; death may occur during the first episode, but it is more likely during the second or third remission. (Judge et al., 1974a, 1974c).

Lesions. The lesions in Grivet monkeys are similar to those in man, with severe purulent myocarditis, focal necrosis, and leukocytic infiltration in spleen and liver. Infarcts in the spleen are also frequent. Spirochaetal organisms may be seen in the lesions of each organ (Judge et al., 1974b).

Avian Borreliosis or Spirochaetosis

This is a disease of poultry with worldwide distribution. It is described in detail by Gross (1978).

Felsenfeld, O.: *Borrelia.* Meth. Microbiol., *8*:75–94, 1973.

Felsenfeld, O., and Wolf, R. J.: Immunology of borreliosis in nonhuman primates. Fed. Proc., *34*:1656–1660, 1975.

Gross, W.B.: Spriochaetosis. *In* Diseases of Poultry, 7th ed., edited by M. S. Hofstad et al. Ames, Iowa State Univ. Press, 1978. pp. 330–334.

Judge, D. M., LaCroix, J. T., and Perine, P. L.: Experimental louse-borne relapsing fever in the grivet monkey, *Cercopithecus aethiops.* I. Clinical course. Am. J. Trop. Med. Hyg., *23*:957–961, 1974a.

————: Experimental louse-borne relapsing fever in the grivet monkey, *Cercopithecus aethiops.* II. Pathology. Am. J. Trop. Med. Hyg., *23*:962–968, 1974b.

————: Experimental louse-borne relapsing fever in the grivet monkey, *Cercopithecus aethiops.* III. Crisis following therapy. Am. J. Trop. Med. Hyg., *23*:969–973, 1974c.

Other Spirochaetal Infections

Spirochaetal organisms have been seen in the large intestine of man and nonhuman primates (Takeuchi et al., 1971; Takeuchi and Zeller, 1972) in close association with the microvilli of the brush border. The organisms are associated with loss of microvilli and are seen in contact with the plasma membrane but apparently do not result in any changes within the intestinal cell membrane. At present these organisms are difficult to study, and their pathogenic significance is not clear. Further study of these organisms and their effects on intestinal epithelial cells is needed.

Takeuchi, A., Sprinz, H., and Sohn, A.: Intestinal spirochetosis in the monkey and man. Lab. Invest., *24*:450, 1971.

Takeuchi, A., and Zeller, J. A.: Ultrastructural identification of spirochetes and flagellated microbes at brush border of large intestinal epithelium of the Rhesus monkey. Infect. Immun., *6*:1008–1018, 1972.

CHAPTER 11

Diseases Due to Simple Bacteria

The microorganisms that once were classified as simple bacteria (order Eubacteriales) are ubiquitous in nature, and include many pathogenic species. It is convenient to consider the diseases caused by such pathogens together, even though the organisms are undeniably heterogeneous, because the diseases that they cause have some similarities. Among them are some of the diseases first shown to be caused by specific bacteria, and consequently used for studies that established basic principles of etiology and immunology. While data concerning the causative organisms of many of the diseases are plentiful, little has been recorded in regard to the pathogenesis and the nature of the specific lesions. While these earlier investigations had their place in the development of bacteriology as an important science, it is no longer enough to isolate an organism and, using it, to reproduce a disease in another animal. The disease itself must be precisely identified and the relation of the suspected etiologic agent to the specific disease must be clearly established. The need for thoroughness is emphasized by the doubts that now exist concerning the actual role of some organisms that for years had been considered the sole cause of specific diseases. The challenge to the pathologist is clear. It is for him to investigate the conditions under which these diseases occur and the precise effects of the pathogen on the host. Even some of the first of these diseases to be recognized, anthrax, for example, could be restudied with profit in the light of present day knowledge and with modern techniques.

In this chapter, the student will note that infections caused by simple bacteria commonly are fulminant and overwhelming, although more prolonged or even smoldering infections may occur. The tissue reactions are often serous, fibrinous, or hemorrhagic in severe infections of short duration, with purulent and granulomatous changes appearing in those of increasingly longer duration. In many fulminant diseases, the recognizable morphologic changes are subtle and easily overlooked, necessitating careful observation and good pathologic technique.

Reclassification of bacteria and changes of genus and species names by taxonomists often present a dilemma to those of us who are interested in the diseases caused by specific organisms. This reordering is usually, but not always, the result of new knowledge of the characteristics of bacteria, leading to new concepts about their relationships to one another. Changes in names of pathogenic organisms are often based upon perceptions that have no relation to the disease. One problem follows due to the practice of naming diseases after the name of the organism—for example, vibriosis after *Vibrio*. The name of this genus was recently changed to *Campylobacterium,* hence the introduction of a new term for the disease: "campylobacteriosis." If it were not for the fact that the causal relation of specific organisms to infectious disease is important, our resistance to this exercise would be greater and our protests more vehement! We shall try to provide the older terms along with the most contemporary to encourage historical perspectives of the development and refinement of knowledge about bacterial diseases.

Bruner, D. W., and Gillespie, J. H.: Hagan's Infectious Diseases of Domestic Animals. 6th ed. Ithaca, Cornell Univ. Press, 1973.
Buchanan, R. E., and Gibbons, N. E.: Bergey's Manual of Determinative Bacteriology. 8th ed. Baltimore, Williams & Wilkins, 1974.
Dunne, H. W., and Leman, A. D. (eds.): Diseases of Swine. 4th ed. Ames, Iowa State Univ. Press, 1975.
Hofstad, M. S., et al. (eds.): Diseases of Poultry. 7th ed. Ames, Iowa State Univ. Press, 1978.

ANTHRAX

Anthrax is not only of current significance as an infection of animals and man, but also of historical interest, for it was investigated intensively by the founders of bacteriology. Robert Koch, in 1876, was the first to isolate the causative organism in pure culture and to reproduce the disease with the culture. Pasteur, Rous, and Chamberland, in 1881, demonstrated active immunization with attenuated anthrax cultures in the famous experiment at Pouilly-le-Fort. Their dramatic demonstration of the immunizing properties of attenuated cultures of anthrax bacilli, before a special French Commission, has been hailed for years as a significant milestone in the history of bacteriology.

Anthrax is principally a disease of herbivorous animals, but it may affect a wide variety of species, including man. Sheep and cattle are most susceptible; horses and mules are slightly more resistant to natural infection. Swine are even more resistant, as are dogs, cats, and other species, although anthrax does occur in these animals. In the more susceptible species (sheep, cattle, horses), the disease is usually seen as a fulminant septicemia. In the more resistant animals (swine), the disease may be localized and confined to the regional lymph nodes, particularly those of the cervical region. Man usually acquires anthrax from contact with infected animals or animal products (hides, wool, shaving brushes made from infected hog bristles), the disease being manifest as a localized, persistent cutaneous pustule, malignant carbuncle, or as a systemic, pulmonary, often fatal disease, **wool-sorters' disease.**

The causative organism, *Bacillus anthracis,* is a relatively large, encapsulated, rod-shaped bacillus, which produces spores. It grows well under aerobic conditions and is gram-positive. In smears from the tissues, it often appears as chains of square-ended rods, but spores are not formed until there has been exposure to air. Giemsa's stain should reveal red capsules on a minority of the organisms. It is the only pathogenic member of a large group of closely related aerobic bacilli. The organism grows in soil and organic material, hence a region in which infection has flourished may be rendered potentially hazardous for many years after the disease has apparently been eliminated. On the other hand, infected animal products are the chief source of virulent organisms. Aside from carcasses of animals dead of the disease, animal wastes and such products as wool, bristles, and hides from abattoirs have been implicated in many infections. Inadequately sterilized fertilizer and bone meal may harbor virulent anthrax bacilli. Infection can apparently follow ingestion or inhalation of spores or vegetative forms of the organism. It has also been produced by experimental inoculation through various routes.

Signs. The signs of anthrax are variable and may be overlooked in cases of short duration, death being the first indication of the presence of disease. In those instances in which symptoms have been ob-

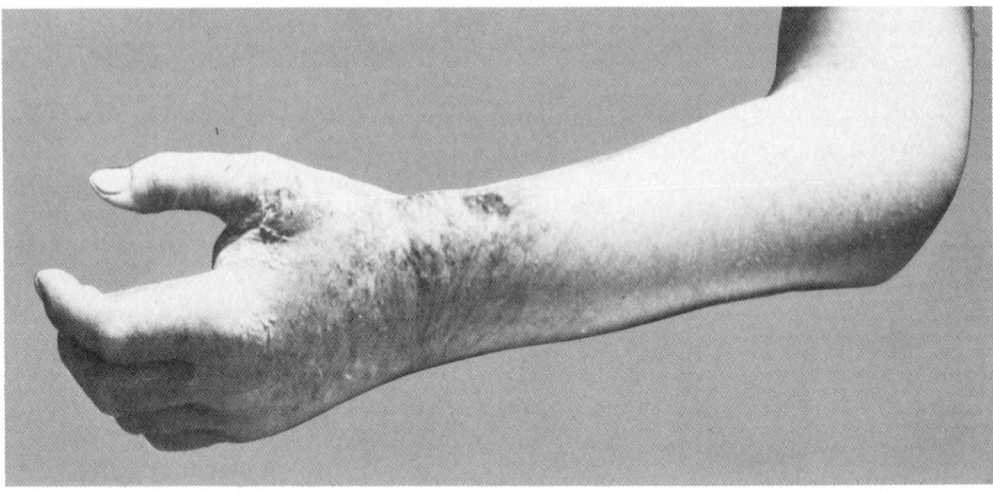

Fig. 11–1. Cutaneous anthrax in man. This man and his wife skinned a cow recently dead of anthrax. The carcas was fed to hogs, which soon exhibited "quinsey." *Bacillus anthracis* was isolated in pure culture from the lesion illustrated, from the swine, and the cow. The wife escaped infection. (Courtesy of Dr. Hubert Schmidt.)

served, anthrax is recognized as a febrile disease with manifestations of depression, weakness, bloody discharges from body orifices, cyanosis, dyspnea, and occasional edematous subcutaneous swellings. Most animals so affected die within a few hours or a day. Swine which have fed upon the carcasses of diseased sheep or cattle may exhibit nothing more than local infection of the pharynx, with enlargement of the cervical lymph nodes. The cutaneous form, malignant carbuncle of man, ordinarily is not recognized in animals.

Lesions. The gross lesions in fatal cases of the disseminated form of anthrax include edematous and hemorrhagic changes in any part of the body, particularly in serous membranes. The spleen is greatly enlarged and engorged with dark, unclotted blood. Lymph nodes are usually swollen, edematous, and occasionally hemorrhagic. Lesions in other organs are inconstant, although hemorrhages and swelling may occur in the intestinal tract, liver, and kidneys. In localized infections in swine, edema, and hemorrhages are seen in the pharynx and cervical lymph nodes. In cases of longer standing, the lymph nodes become enlarged and solid, with yellowish foci surrounded by fibrous connective tissue.

The microscopic findings in generalized cases are dominated by the presence of large numbers of anthrax bacilli in the blood and most other tissues. These large rod-shaped organisms can be demonstrated in smears or tissue sections, but they cannot be distinguished from saprophytic bacilli without culturing them and determining their pathogenicity in laboratory animals. In the spleen, the architecture is obscured by the presence of large numbers of erythrocytes. The lymphoid follicles are not discernible; only the trabeculae remain as tiny islands in a sea of red cells and nuclear débris, which floods the splenic sinuses and the cords of Bilroth. Bacilli are readily demonstrated in sections of the spleen with Gram's stain (Fig. 11–2).

A cytolytic toxin is a product of anthrax bacilli. This toxin has been shown experimentally in the rat to have a direct effect upon endothelial cells in pulmonary capillaries and venules. Within a few minutes following exposure to the toxin, ultrastructural studies reveal the formation of "blis-

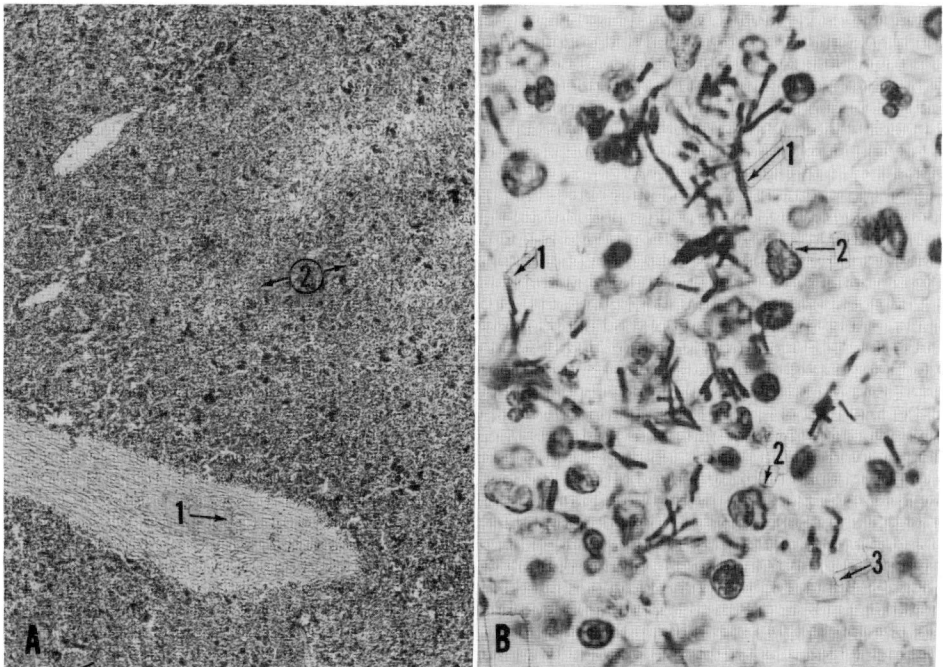

Fig. 11-2. *A*, Anthrax. Spleen in a fatal bovine case (H & E, × 62). Lymphoid elements are obscured and trabeculae *(1)* are widely separated by the massive hemorrhage *(2)*. *B*, Spleen of a guinea pig which was experimentally infected with anthrax from a bovine (× 1500). Gram's stain of a tissue section. Note gram-positive bacilli *(1)*, lymphoid cells *(2)*, and erythrocytes *(3)*. (Courtesy of Armed Forces Institute of Pathology.) Contributor: Dr. C. L. Davis.

ters" by the accumulation of plasma under the cell membrane of the endothelial cells. This injury to the endothelium leads to leakage of plasma and the formation of thrombi at this site. These localized effects are believed to be the direct cause of the pulmonary edema. This localized injury to endothelial cells, rather than generalized diffuse intravascular coagulation, such as occurs in shock or the Shwartzman reaction, is believed to be the pathogenetic mechanism involved in acute pulmonary anthrax (Dalldorf et al., 1969).

Localized infection in lymph nodes of swine result in foci of necrosis surrounded by a layer of granulation tissue. Giant cells usually are not present.

Diagnosis. Presumptive diagnoses are made largely upon the basis of the history (few premonitory symptoms, with sudden death of several animals in a herd) and the characteristic gross lesions found at necropsy. The diagnosis is confirmed by demonstration of *Bacillus anthracis* in large numbers in blood and tissues of animals dead of the disease. It is important that the organisms be identified and differentiated from saprophytes upon the basis of pathogenicity as well as morphologic and cultural characteristics. Inoculation of organisms, usually intraperitoneally, kills a mouse in 12 to 24 hours, a guinea pig in 24 to 36 hours. Organisms are readily seen in and cultured from the tissues of such inoculated animals.

Beall, F. A., and Dalldorf, F. G.: The pathogenesis of the lethal effect of anthrax toxin in the rat. J. Infect. Dis., *116*:377–389, 1966.

Dalldorf, F. G., et al.: Transcellular permeability and thrombosis of capillaries in anthrax toxemia. Lab. Invest., *21*:42–51, 1969.

Dalldorf, F. G., Kaufmann, A. F., and Brachman, P. S.: Wool-sorters' disease. An experimental model. Arch. Pathol., 92:418–426, 1971.

Fried, B. M.: The infection of rabbits with the anthrax bacillus by way of the trachea. Arch. Pathol., 10:213–223, 1930.

Fox, M. D., et al.: Anthrax in Louisiana, 1971: epizootiologic study. J. Am. Vet. Med. Assoc., 163:446–451, 1973.

———: An epizootiologic study of anthrax in Falls County, Texas. J. Am. Vet. Med. Assoc., 170:327–333, 1977.

Gleiser, C. A.: Pathology of anthrax infection in animal hosts. Fed. Proc., 26:1518–1521, 1967.

Plotkin, S. A., et al.: An epidemic of inhalation anthrax, the first in the twentieth century. I. Clinical features. Am. J. Med., 29:992–999, 1960.

Ross, J. M.: On the histopathology of experimental anthrax in the guinea pig. Br. J. Exp. Pathol., 36:336–342, 1955.

Smith, H., and Stoner, H. B.: Anthrax toxic complex. Fed. Proc., 26:1554–1558, 1967.

Stiles, G. W.: Isolation of the *Bacillus anthracis* from spinose ear ticks *Ornithodorus Megnini*. Am. J. Vet. Res., 5:318–319, 1944.

Van Ness, G. B.: Ecology of anthrax. Science, 172:1303–1307, 1971.

Other Infections Due to Bacillus

Bacillus anthracis has for many years been considered the only pathogenic member of the genus *Bacillus* (endospore-forming, gram-positive, aerobic or facultative anaerobic rod-shaped organisms). It appears that one other member of this large group of organisms is also pathogenic under certain conditions. *Bacillus cereus (B. anthracoides, B. pseudoanthracis)* has been associated with food poisoning in human beings, and with abortion or perinatal mortality in sheep and cattle. These events have been experimentally reproduced by intravenous inoculation of pregnant sheep and cattle. Organisms in pure culture have been recovered from affected fetuses.

Smith, I. D., and Frost, A. J.: The pathogenicity to pregnant ewes of an organism of the genus *Bacillus*. Aust. Vet. J., 44:17–19, 1968.

Smith, I. D.: Ovine perinatal mortality associated with *Bacillus cereus*. Res. Vet. Sci., 13:499–501, 1972.

Wohlgemuth, K., Bicknell, E. J., and Kirkbride, C. A.: Abortion in cattle associated with *Bacillus cereus*. J. Am. Vet. Med. Assoc., 161:1688–1690, 1972.

Wohlgemuth, K., Kirkbride, C. A., Bicknell, E. J., and Ellis, R. P.: Pathogenicity of *Bacillus cereus* for pregnant ewes and heifers. J. Am. Vet. Med. Assoc., 161:1691–1695, 1972.

CLOSTRIDIAL INFECTIONS

Organisms of the genus *Clostridium* are sporulating, anaerobic bacteria of rather large size, usually about 0.8 μ in width and 3 to 8 μ in length. Most members of the

Table 11–1. Pathogenic Clostridiae

Species		Disease
Cl. chauvoei		Blackleg
Cl. septicum		Malignant edema, braxy
Cl. hemolyticum		Bovine bacillary hemoglobinuria
Cl. novyi		Black disease
Cl. perfringens		
Type A	Gas gangrene and enteritis in man	
B	Lamb dysentery	
C	Struck	
D	Enterotoxemia	
E	Enterotoxemia	
Cl. sordelli		Wound infections
Cl. carnis		Wound infections
Cl. histolyticum		Wound infections
Cl. botulinum		Botulism (see Table 11–2)
Cl. tetani		Tetanus

genus are nonpathogenic and are commonly found in soil and intestinal tracts of man and animals. Several members of the group are responsible for a number of important diseases of man and animals. Some of these will be described briefly. Pathogenic members of the genus are listed in Table 11–1.

Blackleg

The causative agent of blackleg, *Clostridium chauvoei* (*C. feseri, Bacillus chauvoei,* bacillus of symptomatic anthrax), produces an acute, highly fatal disease of cattle and occasionally of other species, such as sheep, goats, and swine. The infection appears sporadically in certain areas where the organisms live in the soil. In some instances, the disease has appeared in cattle which have access to a newly excavated pond. It is postulated that disturbing the soil in some way exposes the bacteria or causes them to become pathogenic (Barnes et al., 1975). It runs an acute, usually fatal course, and affected animals are often found dead though signs of illness have not been observed.

Lesions. The lesions consist of crepitant swellings in the musculature, particularly of the extremities, which produce a stiff characteristic extension of the limbs a short time after death. Affected muscles incised at necropsy are dark brown or dark red, streaked with black. Some areas appear moist and upon pressure yield dark, gas-filled exudate. Other groups of muscles are dry and sponge-like, with numerous gas bubbles. A peculiar sweetish odor may be noticed. The subcutaneous tissues overlying affected muscles are usually yellowish,

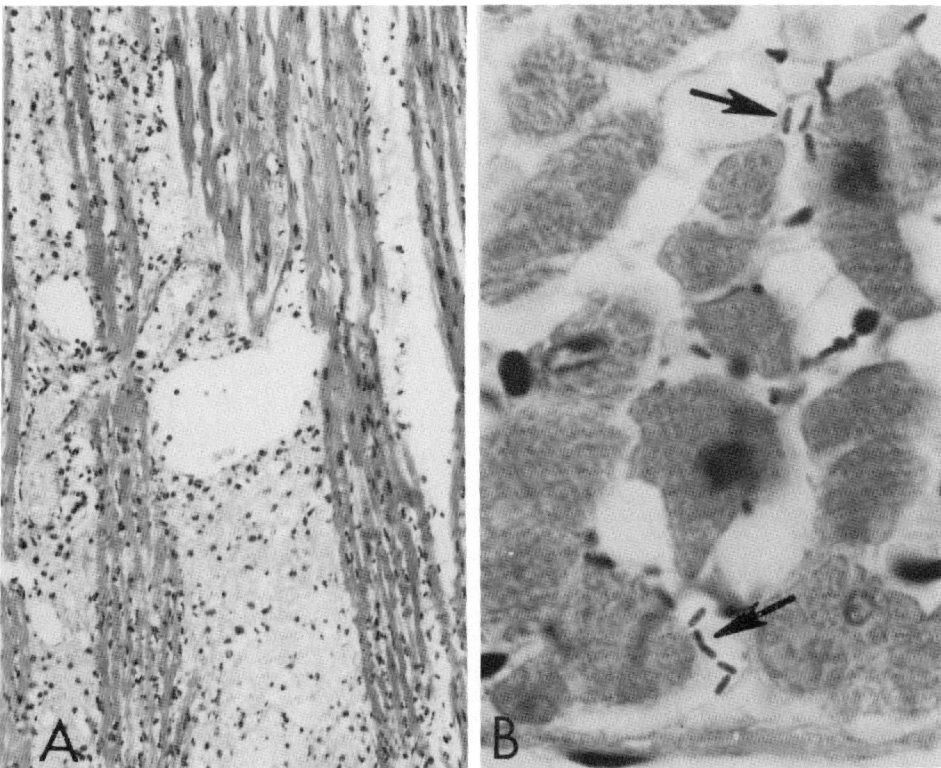

Fig. 11–3. Blackleg, bovine muscle. *A,* Fragmented myofibers are separated by edema, cellular infiltration, and gas bubbles. *B,* The large causative bacilli (arrows) demonstrated with Giemsa stain. (Courtesy of Dr. C. L. Davis.)

gelatinous, blood-tinged, and contain gas bubbles. Similar lesions are frequently demonstrated in the heart, rarely in tongue (could be confused here with "woody tongue"), or even as diffuse hemorrhagic lesions in the lung.

Microscopically, the essential lesions are found in the skeletal musculature. Gas bubbles in the fixed tissues are indicated by spherical spaces separating muscle bundles and fascia. There are irregular areas of necrosis and collections of neutrophils and lymphocytes along the muscle septa. Edema is infrequent. Gram-positive organisms are demonstrable in the sections, appearing singly or in small, irregular clumps.

The pathogenesis of the disease is not understood. It does not appear to result from wound infection. The disease is most frequent in young animals (six months to two years of age) on a good plane of nutrition.

Diagnosis. The diagnosis may be confirmed by the characteristic gross lesions, and by demonstration of fairly numerous single or possibly paired bacilli with rounded ends and occasional spores near, but not at the end, of the cell. As is typical of the clostridia, the spore is of somewhat greater diameter than the bacillus in which it forms. The organism grows only under strict anaerobic conditions. Fluorescein-labeled antiserum is useful in specifically identifying organisms in tissues or smears.

Bovine Bacillary Hemoglobinuria

A disease apparently first described in California in 1916 by K. F. Meyer, it occurs principally in sharply delimited geographic areas in the western and southern United States, but has been reported in Wisconsin and New Zealand. It is characterized by sudden onset of hemoglobinuria, high fever, collapse, and death within a day or two.

Lesions. At necropsy, affected cattle have large areas of infarction in their livers as the most constant lesion, although hemor-

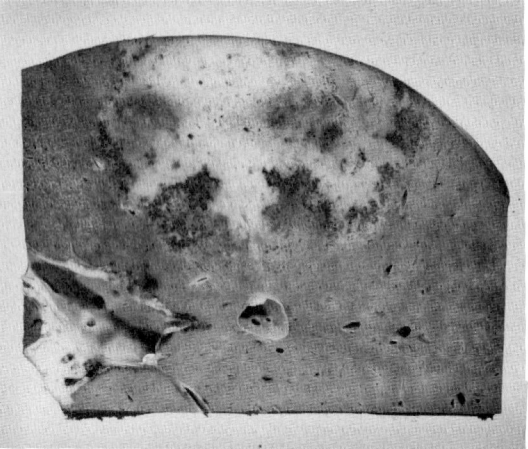

Fig. 11–4. Bovine bacillary hemoglobinuria. Necrotic lesion in liver of a two-year-old Holstein heifer. (Courtesy of Dr. W. J. Hadlow.)

rhages and hematuria are also prominent. Vawter and Records (1926) isolated *Clostridium hemolyticum* (*Clostridium hemolyticus bovis*) from early cases and were able to produce fatalities, but not characteristic lesions in cattle. The disease has been observed to spread with certain cattle imported into Montana, and its occurrence has been more frequent in regions in which *Fasciola hepatica* (liver fluke) is prevalent.

Many aspects of the pathogenesis of this disease remain to be explained, but available evidence suggests that following ingestion of *Cl. hemolyticum*, the bacteria localize in the liver and remain latent until an anaerobic environment is created by hepatic injury. Migration of liver flukes is believed to represent an important mode of initiating hepatic damage with resultant activation of the organism. Exotoxins produced by *Cl. hemolyticum* contribute to further hepatic damage with the production of the characteristic "infarct." Venous thrombi, which are usually present in the liver, enhance the development of the lesion, but are not believed to initiate the process. Olander et al. (1966) described activation of the disease by liver biopsy and have reproduced the disease in rabbits.

Diagnosis. Diagnosis is based on the pathologic findings (hepatic infarct, hemoglobinuria) and isolation of *Cl. hemolyticum.* The disease must be differentiated from many other situations in the bovine which are accompanied by hemoglobinuria. According to Van Ness and Erickson (1964), *Cl. hemolyticum* finds favorable growth conditions in marshy land in which the water supply is alkaline (pH 8.0 or higher) and rich in organic matter.

Malignant Edema

Originally isolated by Pasteur, who called it *"Vibrion septique,"* *Clostridium septicum* is another ubiquitous organism that grows in soil but may produce infection in animals. Malignant edema is seen as a sequel of wounds such as those incurred in shearing or docking, or in parturition attended by unskilled persons who ignore aseptic precautions. It is most frequent in horses, sheep, and cattle, is rare in dogs and cats, but has been reported in antelopes (Gallagher, 1972).

The disease is characterized by a febrile course of short duration with hot, painful swelling at sites of infection. These swollen areas later become even more edematous, but less painful and cooler. At necropsy, the involved tissues are edematous, frequently hemorrhagic, and contain some gas bubbles. Septicemia often occurs, with hemorrhages distributed throughout the body. The lungs are congested and edematous. Serous, blood-tinged effusion from the peritoneum may also be observed. *Clostridium septicum* is readily demonstrable in the affected tissues.

Braxy

Braxy (bradsot) is an acute infection of sheep caused by *Clostridium septicum* characterized by hemorrhagic abomasitis. The disease is principally of importance in Scotland and Scandinavia. The infection mainly affects young sheep and usually occurs during the winter months. Death is sudden, with few or no clinical signs. The wall of the abomasum is thickened, edematous, and hemorrhagic. Similar lesions may be encountered in the small intestine. The large causative bacilli can be seen in tissue section and are readily isolated from the lesions.

Black Disease

Also known as infectious necrotic hepatitis, black disease is an acute fatal infection of sheep and rarely cattle, caused by *Clostridium novyi. (Cl. oedematiens).* The organism is widely distributed in soil as three strains (A, B, C), and is a frequent inhabitant of the intestinal tract of sheep. The type B organism is the most frequent strain in black disease.

Black disease was first reported in Australia, but subseqently has been recognized in New Zealand, United States, United Kingdom, Europe, Turkey, India and Mali in Africa (Bagadi, 1974). Similarities with the pathogenesis, etiology and lesions of bovine bacillary hemoglobinuria are obvious. A similar disease has also been described in a horse (Dumaresq, 1939). In a high percentage of animals in enzootic areas, *Cl. novyi* pass through the intestinal wall and lodge in the liver, where they remain as a latent infection. An anaerobic environment produced by the migration of liver flukes (*Fasciola hepatica, Dicrocoelium dendriticum*) activates the bacteria, which release exotoxins, further contributing to hepatic necrosis and producing fatal toxemia. Death may result without premonitory signs. Pathologic changes include characteristic multiple foci of necrosis in the liver, petechiae on the epicardium and endocardium, and hydropericardium. Subcutaneous venous congestion causes a dark discoloration of the pelt, which resulted in the name black disease.

Diagnosis is based on pathologic findings and isolation of *Cl. novyi.* The organisms may be demonstrated with fluorescent antibody technique in smears or sections of the liver, but since the organisms are normal inhabitants at this site and proliferate rapidly after death from any cause, the clinical manifestations and gross and microscopic lesions must also be considered in establishing a diagnosis.

Gas Gangrene

Gas gangrene, the human counterpart of malignant edema, is a wound infection caused by *Clostridium spp*. Improved treatment of wounds, particularly war wounds, has greatly reduced the frequency of this infection. In addition to malignant edema, clostridial wound infections in animals include the species *Cl. perfringens, Cl. novyi, Cl. sordelli, Cl. feseri, Cl. histolyticum,* and *Cl. carnis.*

Tetanus

Tetanus, or "lockjaw," occurs in man and animals. It has become far less frequent than in the past because of more effective treatment of wounds and widespread use of tetanus toxoid. The causative organism, *Clostridium tetani,* is a normal inhabitant of the intestinal tract of herbivorous animals and grows well in humus-rich soil. It is a gram-positive, sporulating, anaerobic, rod-shaped bacillus. Tetanus is usually a sequel of wounds, often insignificant ones such as nail-pricks, or those produced by castration, docking, shearing, or even during parturition. The anaerobic environment of certain wounds allows germination of the spores, multiplication of the organism, and release of exotoxin. The exotoxin is not histolytic and probably does not contribute to local tissue destruction. The toxin is a neurotoxin, which becomes fixed to the gray matter of the central nervous system, where it diminishes or abolishes synaptic inhibition.

The disease is characterized by prolonged spasmodic contractions of muscles, with extension of limbs, stiffness, and immobilization. The muscles of mastication are often affected, immobilizing the jaws. The entire musculature is eventually involved and death follows. Diagnosis is based on clinical signs and a history of trauma; however, a wound is often not demonstrable, and if present the bacilli are difficult to demonstrate. Specific lesions have not been described.

Enterotoxemia

Cl. perfringens Type D. Recognized in fattening lambs and less regularly in adult sheep, this disease is characterized by brief nervous symptoms and sudden death. Decreasing the total amount of food or changing from a high concentration of grains with little roughage to a ration consisting almost entirely of hay or similar material appears to be an effective preventive measure. Lambs are usually found dead, but if an observer is present, he may detect a period of one-half to a few hours during which opisthotonos progresses into premortal coma. In a few cases, convulsions take the place of coma and death is still more prompt. Occasionally, animals show a desire to push the forehead against a solid wall, which is the characteristic attitude of "blind staggers" as seen in many forms of indigestion in various species. Some investigators have found these acute symptoms to be preceded by a day or more of anorexia and diarrhea or mucus-covered feces, at least in some individuals.

Lesions. Postmortem lesions that have attracted most attention are petechial or ecchymotic hemorrhages beneath the epicardial and endocardial surfaces, the serous surfaces of the intestines, in abdominal muscles, in the diaphragm, and in the thymus. Hydropericardium is usually noted. In addition to distortion of other values in the blood chemistry, there is pronounced glycosuria. Also noted by some observers are distention of the rumen, reticulum, the abomasum, and the lower intestines by ingesta and gas. Mild catarrhal gastroenteritis is sometimes visible. A distended gallbladder frequently provides further evidence of digestive malfunction. In addition, there is often a tendency toward the development of "pulpy kidney." Neurologic signs are explained (at least in part) by lesions of the nervous system, which consist of bilaterally symmetrical focal malacia of the basal ganglia, substantia nigra, and thalamus, and demyelination in the internal capsule, subcortical white matter, and cerebellar peduncles.

The ultrastructural changes in experimental disease (Morgan and Kelley, 1974) consist of periaxonal and intramyelinic edema in cerebellar white matter and swelling of axon terminals and dendrites in gray matter adjacent to lateral ventricles. Swelling of mitochondria is also an early feature. Occlusion of capillaries by aggregated platelets, accompanied by petechiae in relation to the malacia, suggests that changes in vascular endothelium may be the primary effect of the toxin. This concept is supported by evidence that the capillaries in affected parts of the brain leak conspicuously within 20 minutes following administration of *Cl. perfringens* type D toxin (Morgan, Kelley, and Buxton, 1975).

It has been demonstrated by Bennetts (1932) and confirmed by others that the intestinal contents of these lambs contain large numbers of clostridial organisms and significant amounts of the thermolabile toxin of *Clostridium perfringens,* type D (synonyms: *Cl. welchii,* type D; *Cl. ovitoxicus*). This toxin is promptly fatal to lambs and laboratory animals when injected parenterally, but under ordinary circumstances, quite harmless when given by mouth. There is nothing remarkable about the presence of *Cl. perfringens* organisms in the digestive tract; in fact, it would be unusual if these and other soil-borne clostridia were absent. The toxin must be significant, especially since its injection appears to reproduce the characteristic disease, but it has been demonstrated in the intestine of healthy lambs as well, and just why it is absorbed into the circulation in some individuals and not in others has never been fully explained. Experimentally, it has produced the disease when introduced into a lamb's alimentary tract

previously injured or at least functionally impaired by such procedures as partially paralyzing the bowel with opium and belladonna, distending it with an excessive amount of milk, or irritating it with a heavy feeding of corn meal. Ligation of the jejunum has produced terminal symptomatology apparently identical with that which accompanies death from enterotoxemia.

From the evidence available, which is extensive, it appears that this disease is initiated as the result of excessive quantities of a concentrated diet, culminating in the absorption of the fatal but normally unabsorbed toxin of *Cl. perfringens,* type D. The effectiveness of active immunizing agents against this organism is debated and difficult to determine because of the unpredictability of naturally occurring cases. It is not contended that the organism is a tissue pathogen in the ordinary sense (but see "pulpy kidney disease," Chapt. 24).

Enterotoxemia caused by *Cl. perfringens* type D has also been reported in calves and goats. The clinical and pathologic findings are comparable to those in lambs.

In addition to classic *type D* enterotoxemia, *Cl. perfringens* **types A, B, C and E** cause enterotoxemias in animals.

***Cl. perfringens* Type A.** Type A enterotoxemia has been reported in lambs and calves as an acute syndrome of short course and high mortality, characterized by intense icterus and hemolytic anemia with hemoglobinuria. Lesions include icterus, anemia, excess pericardial fluid, dark kidneys, and an enlarged, friable liver.

***Cl. perfringens* Type B.** Type B enterotoxemia, better known as "lamb dysentery," is of principal importance in lambs less than two weeks of age. Death may occur without premonitory signs, but usually the lambs are reluctant to suckle, lying down, and exhibiting signs of pain. The feces become semifluid, brownish, and contain blood. The characteristic lesion is hemorrhagic enteritis, often with ulceration. Petechiae and ecchymoses are common on serous membranes of the epicardium and endocardium and the pericardial cavity contains excess fluid. An essentially identical type B enterotoxemia occurs in calves, which is largely restricted to the first ten days of life and characterized by severe hemorrhagic enteritis. Type B enterotoxemia has also been reported in foals during the first two days of life; lesions are again characterized by hemorrhagic enteritis with ulceration.

Cl. perfringens Type C. Two distinct forms of type C enterotoxemia have been described. The first form of type C enterotoxemia to be described was called **struck**, a disease of adult sheep in Britain. It occurs most commonly during the winter and early spring months. Clinical signs usually are not noted. The lesions are hemorrhagic enteritis with ulceration of the mucosa particularly of the jejunum and duodenum. A striking feature is peritonitis with a large volume of clear yellow fluid in the peritoneal cavity.

In the United States, a form of type C enterotoxemia known as **enterotoxic hemorrhagic enteritis** occurs in calves and lambs in the first few days of life. Clinically there is diarrhea, but as with other forms of enterotoxemia, death often occurs in the absence of noted signs. The lesions, as described by Griner and co-workers (1953), are similar in both species, and are characterized by hemorrhagic enteritis with ulceration. Hemorrhages are frequent beneath the epicardium, in the thymus and elsewhere. In both species, bacteria identified as *Clostridium perfringens (welchii)*, type C, were numerous in the bowel contents. The evidence that this organism was responsible was that, in the case of the calves, the disease was reproduced by feeding a pure culture together with cornmeal and milk (a concentrated and irritant food for a newly born calf). In the case of the lambs, susceptible animals were protected by an antiserum against this organ-

ism. The condition is to be regarded as an enterotoxemia rather than a mere enteritis because bacteria-free filtrates of the intestinal contents were promptly lethal when injected into mice, the toxic substance being inactivated by heat, as is characteristic of bacterial exotoxins.

Type C enterotoxemia also occurs in suckling piglets, usually during the first week of life. Most affected pigs die within 12 to 48 hours after onset of clinical signs, which include depression, dehydration, and diarrhea that is often bloody. The pathologic changes, which have been described in detail by Hogh (1969), are dominated by a hemorrhagic or necrotizing enteritis principally affecting the jejunum. There is hemorrhagic lymphadenitis of draining lymph nodes, serosanguineous fluid in the peritoneal, pleural, and pericardial cavities, and hemorrhage in the epicardium, endocardium, and kidneys.

Cl. perfringens Type E. Type E *Clostridium perfringens* have been found in calves and lambs, but the status of the disease with respect to frequency or importance is not known. Available data do not suggest that the disease is of significance.

Botulism

Clostridium botulinum, another member of this group of anaerobic sporulating pathogens, is responsible for an extremely serious food intoxication, **botulism**. This disease is important in man, resulting from consumption of inadequately sterilized canned food in which the organisms have produced their powerful neurotoxin. Wild ducks that feed upon the muddy contaminated bottoms of shallow ponds or lakes may contract the disease, and losses in some instances have been great. Botulism also occurs in chickens fed spoiled canned foods (beans, etc.), and in that species it causes a peculiar torticollis, aptly named "limber neck." Nutritionally deficient cattle which have fed upon animal carcasses have acquired botulism from the bits of

Table 11–2.   Botulism in Animals and Man

Type	Principal Victims	Commonest Vehicles	Greatest Frequency
A	Man, chicken	Canned vegetables, fruits, meat, and fish	Western United States
B	Man, horse	Meat, usually pork; silage and forage	Eastern United States, Europe
Ca	Wild birds	Fly larvae, rotting vegetation	North and South America, South Africa, Australia
Cb	Cattle, sheep, horse, mink	Silage, carrion	Australia, Europe, North America
D	Cattle	Carrion	South Africa
E	Man, mink	Fish and marine animal foods	United States, Canada, Japan, Northern Europe
F	Man	Liver paste	Denmark

decaying meat clinging to the bones. No specific lesions are known.

Clostridium botulinum produces several antigenically distinguishable toxins, each requiring a specific antitoxin. These toxins have different host ranges and are usually found in specific food products or environments. Table 11–2, adapted from Scholtens and Coohon (1964), summarizes some of these relationships.

Although immunologically distinct, the pharmacologic effects of the toxins are identical. They do not act on the central nervous system, but rather on the peripheral nervous system at the myoneural junction. Their paralytic effect is apparently mediated through the prevention of the release of acetylcholine. How the release of acetylcholine is inhibited is not known.

Bagadi, H. O.: Infectious necrotic hepatitis (black disease) of sheep. Vet. Bull., *44*:385–388, 1974.

Bagadi, H. O., and Sewell, M. M. H.: Influence of postmortem autolysis on the diagnosis of infectious necrotic hepatitis (black disease). Res. Vet. Sci., *17*:320–322, 1974.

Baldwin, E. M., Jr., Frederick, L. D., and Ray, J. D.: The control of ovine enterotoxemia by the use of *Clostridium perfringens* type D bacteria. Am. J. Vet. Res., *9*:296–303, 1948.

Barnes, D. M., Bergeland, M. E., and Higbee, J.M.: Selected blackleg outbreaks and their relation to soil excavation. Can. Vet. J., *16*:257–259, 1975.

Bennetts, H. W.: Infectious enterotoxemia of sheep in Western Australia. Bull. Commonwealth of Australia, Council for Sci. Indust. Rsch., 57, 1932.

Bergeland, M. E.: Pathogenesis and immunity of *Clostridium perfringens* type C enteritis in swine. J. Am. Vet. Med. Assoc., *160*:568–571, 1972.

Britton, J. W., and Cameron, H. S.: So-called enterotoxemia in lambs in California. Cornell Vet., *34*:19–29, 1944.

———: Experimental reproduction of so-called enterotoxemia. Cornell Vet., *35*:1–8, 1945.

Bullen, J. J.: Enterotoxemia of sheep: *Clostridium welchii*, Type D, in the alimentary tract of normal animals. J. Pathol. Bact., *64*:201–206, 1952.

Clapp, H. W., and Graham, W. R.: An experience with *Clostridium perfringens* in Cesarean derived barrier sustained mice. Lab. Anim. Care, *20*:1081–1086, 1970.

Crowe, D. T., Jr., and Kowalski, J. J.: Clostridial cellulitis with localized gas formation in a dog. J. Am. Vet. Med. Assoc., *169*:1094–1096, 1976.

DiGiacomo, R. F., and Missakian, E. A.: Tetanus in a free-ranging colony of *Macaca mulatta:* a clinical and epizootiologic study. Lab. Anim. Sci., 22:378–383, 1972.

Dodd, S.: The aetiology of black disease. J. Comp. Pathol., 34:1–26, 1921.

Dumaresq, J. A.: A case of black disease in the horse. Aust. Vet. J., 15:53–57, 1939.

Durand, M., Loquerie, R., and Haschick, S.: (An outbreak of blackleg caused by *Clostridium welchii.*) Arch. Inst. Pasteur, Tunis, 39:73–81, 1962. VB 116–63.

Edgar, G.: On the occurrence of black disease bacilli in the livers of normal sheep, with some observations on the causation of the disease. Aust. Vet. J., 4:133–141, 1928.

Eklund, M. W., Poysky, F. T., Meyers, J. A., and Pelroy, G. A.: Interspecies conversion of *Clostridium botulinum* type C to *Clostridium novyi* type A by bacteriophage. Science, 186:456–458, 1974.

Ellender, R. D., Jr., Hidalgo, R. J., and Grumbles, L. C.: Characterization of five clostridial pathogens by gas-liquid chromatography. Am. J. Vet. Res., 31:1863–1866, 1970.

Fjølstad, M.: The effects of *Clostridium botulinum* toxin type C given orally to goats. Acta Vet. Scand., 14:69–80, 1973.

Gallagher, J.: Malignant oedema in antelopes. Vet. Rec., 90:367–369, 1972.

Gardner, D. E.: Pathology of *Clostridium welchii* type D enterotoxaemia. I. Biochemical and haematological alterations in lambs. J. Comp. Pathol., 83:499–507, 1973.

———: Pathology of *Clostridium welchii* type D enterotoxaemia. II. Structural and ultrastructural alterations in the tissues of lambs and mice. J. Comp. Pathol., 83:509–524, 1973.

———: Pathology of *Clostridium welchii* type D enterotoxaemia. III. Basis of the hyperglycaemic response. J. Comp. Pathol., 83:525–529, 1973.

Genigeorgis, C.: Public health importance of *Clostridium perfringens.* J. Am. Vet. Med. Assoc., 167:821–827, 1975.

Gitteo, M.: Botulism in mink: an outbreak caused by type-C toxin. Vet. Rec., 71:868–871, 1959.

Goldman, P. M., Andrews, E. J., and Lang, C. M.: A preliminary evaluation of *Clostridium sp.* in the etiology of hamster enteritis. Lab. Anim. Sci., 22:721–724, 1972.

Griesemer, R. A., and Krill, W. R.: Enterotoxemia of beef calves—30 years' observation. J. Am. Vet. Med. Assoc., 140:154–158, 1962.

Griner, L. A., and Bracken, F. K.: *Clostridium perfringens* (type C) in acute hemorrhagic enteritis of calves. J. Am. Vet. Med. Assoc., 122:99–102, 1953.

Griner, L. A., and Carlson, W. D.: Enterotoxemia of sheep. I. Effects of *Clostridium perfringens* type D toxin on the brains of sheep and mice. II. Distribution of I[131] radioiodinated serum albumin in brains of *Clostridium perfringens* type D intoxicated lambs. III. *Clostridium perfringens* type D antitoxin titers of normal, nonvaccinated lambs. Am. J. Vet. Res., 22:429–442, 443–446, 447–448, 1961.

Griner, L. A., and Johnson, H. W.: *Clostridium perfringens* (type C) in hemorrhagic enterotoxemia of lambs. J. Am. Vet. Med. Assoc., 125:125–127, 1954.

Harrison, S. G., and Borland, E. D.: Deaths in ferrets *(Mustela putorius)* due to *Clostridium botulinum* type C. Vet. Rec., 91:576–577, 1973.

Harshfield, G. S., Cross, F., and Hoerlein, A. B.: Further studies on overeating (enterotoxemia) of feedlot lambs. Am. J. Vet. Res., 3:86–91, 1942.

Hauschild, A. H. W., Niilo, L., and Dorward, W. J.: I. Enteropathogenic factors of food-poisoning *Clostridium perfringens* type A. II. Response of ligated intestinal loops in lambs to an enteropathogenic factor of *Clostridium perfringens* type A. Can. J. Microbiol., 16:331–338, 1970.

Hauschild, A. H. W., Walcroft, M. J., and Campbell, W.: Emesis and diarrhea induced by enterotoxin of *Clostridium perfringens* type-A in monkeys. Can. J. Microbiol., 17:1141–1143, 1971.

Helmy, N.: Experimental clostridial infection in dogs. Tijdschr. Diergeneeskd., 83:1089–1096, 1958.

Herd, R. P., and Riches, W. R.: An outbreak of tetanus in cattle. Aust. Vet. J., 40:356–357, 1964.

Hogh, P.: Necrotizing infectious enteritis in piglets, caused by *Clostridium perfringens* type C. I. Biochemical and toxigenic properties of the Clostridium. Acta Vet. Scand., 8:26–38, 1967.

———: Necrotizing infectious enteritis in piglets, caused by *Clostridium perfringens* type C. II. Incidence and clinical features. Acta Vet. Scand., 8:301–323, 1967.

———: Necrotizing infectious enteritis in piglets, caused by *Clostridium perfringens* type C. III. Pathologic changes. Acta Vet. Scand., 10:57–83, 1969.

Jamieson, S.: Studies in black disease. 1. The occurrence of the disease in sheep in the north of Scotland. Vet. Rec., 60:11–14, 1948.

———: The identification of *Clostridium oedematiens* and an experimental investigation of its role in the pathogenesis of infectious necrotic hepatitis ("black disease") of sheep. J. Pathol. Bact., 61:389–402, 1949.

Jansen, B. C.: The toxic antigenic factors produced by *Clostridium botulinum* types C and D. Onderstepoort J. Vet. Res., 38:93–98, 1971.

Jasmin, A. M.: Enzyme activity in *Clostridium hemolyticum* toxin. Am. J. Vet. Res., 8:289–293, 1947.

Kalmbach, E. R.: Western duck sickness: a form of botulism. U.S.D.A. Tech. Bull. 411, 1934.

Kao, I., Drachman, D. B., and Price, D. L.: Botulinum toxin: mechanism of presynaptic blockade. Science, 193:1256–1258, 1976.

Katitch,, R. V.: Conceptions modernes sur la pathogénie des enterotoxémies du mouton. Bull. Off. Int. Epiz., 56:929–934, 1961.

Keast, J. C., and McBarron, E. J.: A case of bovine enterotoxaemia. Aust. Vet. J., 30:305–306, 1954.

Macrae, D. R., Murray, E. G., and Grant, J. G.: Entero-toxaemia in young suckled calves. Vet. Rec., 55:203–204, 1943.

Marsh, H., and Tunnicliff, E. A.: Enterotoxemia in feedlot lambs in connection with an outbreak of coccidiosis. J. Am. Vet. Med. Assoc., *104*:13–14, 1944.

Marshall, S. C.: The isolation of *Clostridium hemolyticum* from cattle in New Zealand. NZ Vet. J., 7:115–119, 1959.

McDonel, J. L., and Duncan, C. L.: Histopathological effect of *Clostridium perfringens* enterotoxin in the rabbit ileum. Infect. Immun., *12*:1214–1218, 1976.

McDonel, J. L., Chang, L. W., Pounds, J. G., and Duncan, C. L.: The effects of *Clostridium perfringens* enterotoxin on rat and rabbit ileum: an electron microscopic study. Lab. Invest., *39*:210–218, 1978.

Meyer, K. F.: Studies to diagnose a fatal disease of cattle in the mountainous regions of California. J. Am. Vet. Med. Assoc., *48*:552–565, 1916.

Moon, H. W., and Bergeland, M. E.: *Clostridium perfringens* type C enterotoxemia of the newborn pig. Can. Vet. J., *6*:159–161, 1965.

Morgan, K. T., and Kelly, B. G.: Ultrastructural study of brain lesions produced in mice by the administration of *Clostridium welchii* type D toxin. J. Comp. Pathol., *84*:181–191, 1974.

Morgan, K. T., Kelly, B. G., and Buxton, D.: Vascular leakage produced in the brains of mice by *Clostridium welchii* type D toxin. J. Comp. Pathol., *85*:461–466, 1975.

Muth, O. H.: Control of pulpy kidney disease (entero-toxemia) of lambs. J. Am. Vet. Med. Assoc., *104*:144–147, 1944.

Muth, O. H., and Morrill, D. R.: Control of enterotoxemia (pulpy kidney disease) in lambs by the use of alum precipitated toxoid. Am. J. Vet. Res., 7:355–357, 1946.

Niilo, L., Hauschild, A. H. W., and Dorward, W. J.: Immunization of sheep against experimental *Clostridium perfringens* type A enteritis. Can. J. Microbiol., *17*:391–395, 1971.

Niilo, L.: Mechanism of action of the enteropathogenic factor of *Clostridium perfringens* type A. Infect. Immun., 3:100–106, 1971.

Niilo, L., Moffatt, R. E., and Avery, R. J.: Bovine "enterotoxemia." II. Experimental reproduction of the disease. Can. Vet. J., 4:288–298, 1963.

Olander, H. J., Hughes, J. P., and Biberstein, E. L.: Bacillary haemoglobinuria: induction by liver biopsy in naturally and experimentally injected animals. Pathologia Vet., 3:421–450, 1966.

Pamukcu, A. M.: Hemorrhagic encephalomyelitis due to botulism in cattle in Turkey. Zentralbl. Veterinärmed., 1:707–722, 1954.

Plaisier, A. J.: Enterotoxaemia in piglets caused by *Clostridium perfringens* type C. Tijdschr. Diergeneeskd., *96*:324–340, 1971.

Quinlivan, T. D., and Wedderburn, J. F.: Bacillary haemoglobinuria in cattle in New Zealand. NZ Vet. J., 7:113–115, 1959.

Quortrup, E. R., and Sudheimer, R. L.: Detection of botulinus toxin in the blood stream of wild ducks. J. Am. Vet. Med. Assoc., *102*:264–266, 1943.

Ramsay, W. R.: An outbreak of tetanus-like disease in cattle. Aust. Vet. J., *49*:188–189, 1973.

Rastas, V. P., Myers, G. H., and Lesar, S.: Bacillary hemoglobinuria in Wisconsin cattle. J. Am. Vet. Med. Assoc., *164*:1203–1204, 1974.

Records, E., and Vawter, L. R.: Bacillary hemoglobinuria of cattle and sheep. Bull. No. 173, Univ. of Nevada, June, 1945.

Roberts, T. A., Keymer, I. F., Borland, E. D., and Smith, G. R.: Botulism in birds and mammals in Great Britain. Vet. Rec., *91*:11–12, 1972.

Roberts, R. S., Guven, S., and Worrall, E. E.: *Clostridium oedematiens* in the livers of healthy sheep. Vet. Rec., *86*:628–629, 1970.

Safford, J. W., and Smith, L. deS.: A study of the epizootiology of bacillary hemoglobinuria. Proc. 91st Ann. Meet. Am. Vet. Med. Assoc., 1954. pp. 159–161.

Schofield, F. W.: Enterotoxemia (sudden death) in calves due to *Clostridium welchii*. J. Am. Vet. Med. Assoc., *126*:192–194, 1955.

Scholtens, R. G., and Coohon, D. R.: Botulism in animals and man, with special reference to type E, *Clostridium botulinum*. Sci. Proc. AVMA, 224–230, 1964.

Shreeve, J. E., and Edwin, E. E.: Thiaminase-producing strains of *Cl. sporogenes* associated with outbreaks of cerebrocortical necrosis. Vet. Rec., *94*:330, 1974.

Sinclair, K. B.: Black disease—a review. Br. Vet. J., *112*:196–200, 1956.

Smith, L. D.: The control of bacillary hemoglobinuria. Proc. 60th Ann. Meet. U. S. Livestock San. Assoc., Chicago, 1956, pp. 135–138. VB 1716–1958.

———: Clostridial diseases of animals. Adv. Vet. Sci., 3:463–524, 1957.

Smith, L., Davis, J. W., and Libke, K. G.: Experimentally induced botulism in weanling pigs. Am. J. Vet. Res., *32*:1327–1330, 1971.

Van Kampen, K. R., and Kennedy, P. C.: Experimental bacillary hemoglobinuria. II. Pathogenesis of the hepatic lesion in the rabbit. Pathologia Vet., 6:59–75, 1969.

———: Experimental bacillary hemoglobinuria: intrahepatic detection of spores of *Clostridium haemolyticum* by immunofluorescence in the rabbit. Am. J. Vet. Res., *29*:2173–2177, 1968.

Van Ness, G. B., and Erickson, K.: Ecology of bacillary hemoglobinuria. J. Am. Vet. Med. Assoc., *144*:492–496, 1964.

Vawter, L. R., and Records, E.: Recent studies on ictero-hemoglobinuria of cattle. J. Am. Vet. Med. Assoc., *68*:494–513, 1926.

Wanasinghe, D. D.: An outbreak of enterotoxaemia due to *Clostridium welchii* type D in goats. Ceylon Vet. J., *21*:62–65, 1973.

Wright, G. P.: The neurotoxins of *Clostridium botulinum* and *Clostridium tetani*. Pharmacol. Rev., 7:413–465, 1955.

STREPTOCOCCAL INFECTIONS

Certain of the gram-positive spherical organisms that occur in chains and are classified in the genus *Streptococcus* are pathogenic for man and animals. The frequency of these infections has decreased greatly during the past few years because

Table 11–3. Streptococcal Infections

Lancefield Group	Organism	Disease
A	S. pyogenes	Scarlet fever in man, various pyogenic infections, and occasionally a cause of bovine mastitis
B	S. agalactiae	Bovine mastitis
C	S. equi	Strangles
	S. zooepidemicus	Various pyogenic infections
	S. dysgalactiae	Bovine mastitis
	S. equisimilis	Respiratory infection in man
	S. genitalium	Equine genital infection and abortion
D	S. faecalis	Usually not pathogenic
E	S. uberis	Bovine mastitis
	Streptococcus spp.	Cervical lymphadenitis in swine
F thru O	Streptococcus spp.	Various species in these groups have been isolated from infections of the respiratory and genital mucous membranes of man and animals, and in bovine mastitis

of the widespread use of antibiotics. Some are still seen from time to time and will be discussed briefly. Some of the more important pathogenic streptococci are listed in Table 11–3, subdivided according to Lancefield's serologic groups and their associated diseases.

Strangles (Adenitis Equorum)

Strangles is an infectious respiratory disease of young horses characterized by sudden onset of fever and upper respiratory catarrh, followed by acute swelling and later by abscess formation in the submaxillary, parapharyngeal, and other lymph nodes. A beta-hemolytic streptococcus, *Streptococcus equi,* is constantly present in pure culture in the abscesses and is generally conceded to be the cause of the disease. Strangles may occur in connection with, and be accentuated by, outbreaks of equine rhinopneumonitis, but the work of Bazeley (1943) indicates that *Streptococcus equi* alone can produce the disease. Experimentally, new, rapidly growing cultures of these streptococci have been shown to produce the disease, while older cultures are avirulent.

The symptoms are characteristic, although they vary strikingly in severity. The edematous swelling of the pharyngeal regions may produce inspiratory dyspnea, which gives the impression that the animal is strangling. The submaxillary lymph nodes become enlarged, hot, and soon form abscesses which yield large quantities of creamy yellowish pus when they rupture spontaneously or are incised. In uncomplicated cases, recovery usually follows drainage of the abscess, but in some the infection spreads to other lymph nodes or reaches the general circulation. In such cases, abscesses may form in any organ but are more frequent in the lungs, kidneys, liver, and spleen, and less commonly in the brain. Fatal outcome may be expected in overwhelming infections or in those instances in which abscesses form in a critical organ.

Lesions. Organisms that penetrate the respiratory mucosa cause acute inflammation in the adjoining structures, particularly the lymph nodes, where abscesses form. In some cases, abscesses of microscopic size have been demonstrated in parapharyngeal lymph nodes by one of us (Jones) within 24 hours of the first evidence of fever. Such abscesses may become encapsulated or, more commonly, rupture into the oral or pharyngeal cavities or

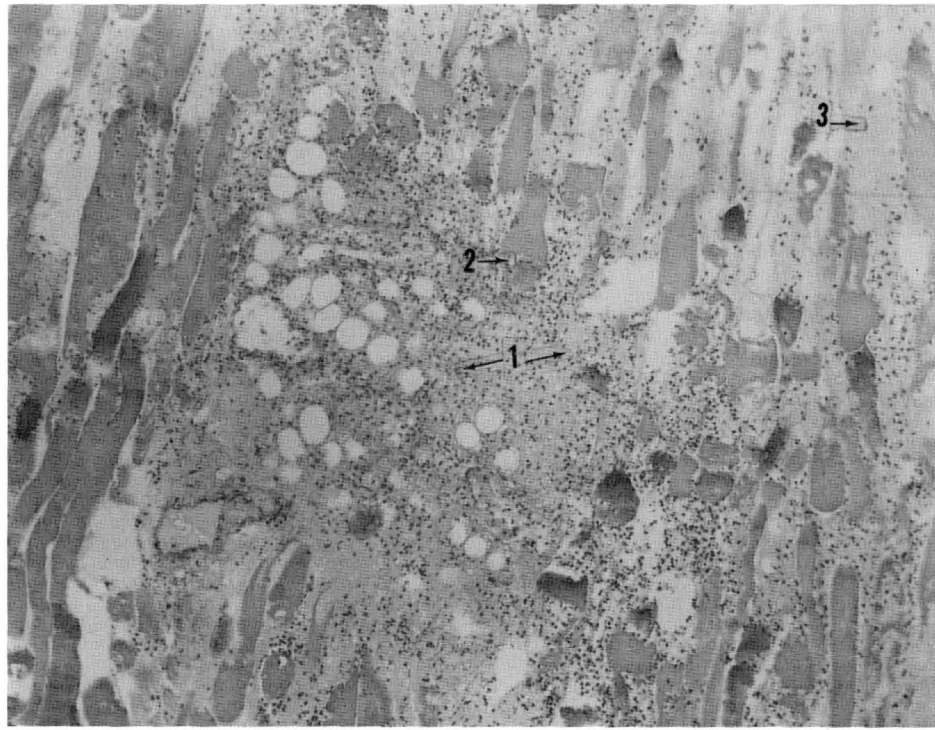

Fig. 11–5. Inflammatory edema in panniculus muscle of a horse with purpura hemorrhagica following respiratory infection with *Streptococcus pyogenes* (× 100). Septic emboli were found in adjacent tissues. Note cellular and albuminous exudate *(1)*, fragmented muscle bundles *(2)*, and loss of muscle fiber *(3)*. (Courtesy of Armed Forces Institute of Pathology.) Contributor: Army Veterinary Research Laboratory.

through the skin of the intermandibular region. Catarrhal or purulent rhinitis, in addition to lymphadenitis, is an invariable feature in fetal cases. Metastatic abscesses occur in the lung (sometimes with cavitation), liver, kidney, spleen, and occasionally the brain. Septicemia is sometimes observed, with abscesses few or absent.

Abscesses in the retropharyngeal lymph nodes may drain into the guttural pouches, leading to empyema of these structures (Knight et al., 1975).

Purpura hemorrhagica may be a complication of strangles, and in such cases, large subcutaneous areas of edema and hemorrhage are associated with septic emboli in blood vessels of the tissues involved.

Diagnosis. The clinical history, the presence of characteristic gross lesions, and the demonstration of *Streptococcus equi* in abscesses are sufficient to establish the diagnosis at necropsy. Demonstration and identification of the organisms in submaxillary or other abscesses will confirm the clinical diagnosis in living animals.

Streptococcal Mastitis

Bovine mastitis is widespread, particularly in dairy herds, and constitutes an important economic problem. Gram-positive coccoid organisms, occurring in short or long chains (streptococci), are commonly associated with inflammation of the bovine mammary gland and are generally regarded as important in the etiology. Other factors, such as trauma and exposure to cold, may be influential in the production of the lesions, but *Streptococcus agalactiae* is an obligate parasite of the mammary gland, and the mastitis produced by *Strep-tococcus agalactiae* represents a specific contagious disease of cattle. Other strep-tococci which do not require the mammary gland for survival are also important as causes of mastitis, but the associated diseases are not solely dependent upon the presence of the bacterium as is the case with *Streptococcus agalactiae*. These include *Streptococcus uberis, Streptococcus dysgalactiae, Streptococcus fecalis, Strep-tococcus zooepidemicus,* and members of Lancefield groups G and L. In a few instances, streptococci of human origin (*Streptococcus pyogenes*) may be involved in outbreaks of bovine mastitis and contribute to concomitant epidemics of "septic sore throat" in persons who drink the milk. Bovine mastitis is described more fully in Chapter 25.

Genital Infections

Streptococcus genitalium is encountered in the cervix and uterus of mares, where it is believed to contribute to inflammation that may result in sterility. The organisms in the genital tract are usually accompanied by catarrhal inflammation, which sometimes is followed by purulent exudation. When conception does occur in infected mares, the fetus is usually aborted during the early months of pregnancy. The lesions in aborted fetuses are not distinctive, even though *Streptococcus genitalium* may be present throughout their tissues.

Cervical Lymphadenitis of Swine

Abscesses (jowl abscess) are not infrequent in the cervical lymph nodes of swine. Streptococci of Lancefield group E are the most commonly isolated organisms; however, other bacterial species, including group C streptococci, *Corynebacterium pyogenes, Pasteurella multocida,* and *Staphylococcus aureus* have also been recovered from abscesses of cervical lymph nodes.

The disease may be transmitted to susceptible swine by instilling virulent cultures into the nasal or oral cavities. Transmission to other swine by direct contact has been demonstrated, and some swine may recover from the disease but still harbor the streptococci in the nasal or oral cavities and be a source of contagion. Hematogenous spread of the organisms occurs occasionally, leading to abscesses in other parts of the body, or to streptococcal endocarditis or meningitis. Immunization is now possible through use of a preparation made from a mutant, less virulent strain of group E streptococci.

Streptococcal Infections of Guinea Pigs

Streptococcal infections of Lancefield's type C are not infrequently encountered in enzootic infections of guinea pigs. Abscesses occur in the lymph nodes of the head and neck, and may lead to generalized dissemination of the organisms to pleura, lungs, peritoneum, pericardium, or lymph nodes generally. The organism most frequently isolated is usually designated *Streptococcus zooepidemicus, S. pyogenes animalis,* or simply serologic group C streptococci.

The lesions in the localized form are usually described as abscesses of lymph nodes, filled with cream-colored pus, sometimes reaching large size. The reaction in pleural and peritoneal surfaces is usually fibrinopurulent, with thromboses and necrotic zones in infarcted lungs. The disease may be differentiated from pneumococcal infection by identification of the organisms.

Neonatal Streptococcal Infections

Streptococcal infections are a particular hazard of the neonatal period in man and most domestic animals, particularly foals, calves, lambs, and pigs. Infection is usually thought to gain entrance by way of the umbilicus, but there is little evidence to substantiate this portal of entry. The infection most often results in suppurative polyarthritis ("joint-ill") and meningitis, but localization in the valvular endocardium, kidneys, and choroid of the eye are not infrequent, especially in lambs. Despite the virulence of streptococci in neonates, the strains usually isolated from neonates are not pathogenic for adult animals.

Wound and Other Infections

Local purulent inflammation may follow infection of wounds by streptococci and this may spread to distant organs. The tissue reaction is basically purulent, although encapsulation of abscesses may occur, giving the lesion a more granulomatous appearance as healing takes place. A necrotizing dermatitis due to streptococci of Lancefield's group G has been described in laboratory mice (Stewart et al., 1975). Group A streptococci have been shown to induce osteomyelitis and arthritis in swine following experimental inoculation (Wood et al., 1971). Rabbits have also been shown to be susceptible to group E streptococci (Cutlip and Shuman, 1971). Group G streptococci have been recovered from abscesses in cervical lymph nodes and skin of the feet and legs of cats housed in a laboratory (Goldman and Moore, 1973).

Pneumococcal Infections in Animals

Pneumococci are occasionally associated with infections in man and laboratory animals (nonhuman primates, guinea pigs, rats, and mice). The organisms, named *Streptococcus pneumoniae (Micrococcus* or *Diplococcus pneumoniae)* are coccoid and appear in pairs or short chains. They have no Lancefield group antigen; they are encapsulated with a distinct polysaccharide capsule. About 80 types have been identified, based on the antigenic component of the polysaccharide capsule.

Pulmonary and extrapulmonary lesions due to *S. pneumoniae* have been described by Parker, Russell, and DePaoli (1977) in laboratory colonies of guinea pigs. The lesions are commonly seen in pericardium, pleura, or peritoneum, but also affect the pregnant uterus. Less frequently, abscesses may be seen in many organs.

Streptococcus pneumoniae is often carried in the upper nasal passages of man and nonhuman primates, and has been encountered in meningitis, panophthalmitis, peritonitis, and septicemia in *Macaca mulatta, M. fascicularis,* and chimpanzees. Many laboratory primates are susceptible to experimental infection.

Pneumococcal septicemia has also been described in calves (McCrea, 1971).

Armstrong, C. H., and Payne, J. B.: Bacteria recovered from swine affected with cervical lymphadenitis (jowl abscess). Am. J. Vet. Res., 30:1607–1612, 1969.

Armstrong, C. H., Boehm, P. N., and Ellis, R. P.: Experimental transmission of streptococcic lymphadenitis (jowl abscess) of swine. Am. J. Vet. Res., 31:823–829, 1970.

Bazeley, P. L.: Studies with equine streptococci. 5. Some relations between virulence of *Streptococcus equi* and immune response in the host. Aust. Vet. J., 19:62–85, 1943.

Blakemore, E., Elliott, S. D., and Hart-Mercer, J.: Studies on suppurative polyarthritis (joint-ill) in lambs. J. Pathol. Bact., 52:57–82, 1941.

Cobb, L. M., Hepworth, P. L., and Heywood, R.: Pneumococcal leptomeningitis in cynomolgus monkeys *(Macaca fascicularis)*. Vet. Rec., 99:84, 1976.

Collier, J. R., and Noel, J.: Streptococcic lymphadenitis of swine: a contagious disease. Am. J. Vet. Res., 32:1501–1506, 1971.

————: Streptococcic lymphadenitis of swine: an immune carrier of *Streptococcus suis.* Am. J. Vet. Res., 32:1507–1510, 1971.

————: Streptococcal lymphadenitis of swine: prolonged carrier state and bacterial dynamics in the induction of disease. Am. J. Vet. Res., 35:799–802, 1974.

Collier, J. R., Shaffer, H. D., and Shultz, M.: Evaluation of a vaccine for control of streptococcic lymphadenitis of swine. J. Am. Vet. Med. Assoc., 169:697–699, 1976.

Cutlip, R. C., and Shuman, R. D.: Susceptibility of rabbits to infection with Lancefield's group E streptococci. Cornell Vet., 61:607–616, 1971.

Elliot, S. D., Alexander, T. J. L., and Thomas, J. H.: Streptococcal infection in young pigs. II. Epidemiology and experimental production of the disease. J. Hyg. Camb., 64:213–220, 1966.

Field, H. I., Butain, D., and Done, J. T.: Studies on piglet mortality. I. Streptococcal meningitis and arthritis. Vet. Rec., 66:453–455, 1954.

Fox, J. G., and Soave, O. A.: Pneumococcic meningoencephalitis in a rhesus monkey. J. Am. Vet. Med. Assoc., 159:1595–1597, 1971.

Gibbons, W. J.: The histopathology of mastitis. Cornell Vet., 28:240–249, 1938.

Goldman, P. M., and Moore, T. D.: Spontaneous Lancefield group G streptococcal infection in a random source cat colony. Lab. Anim. Sci., 23:565–566, 1973.

Gosser, H. S., and Olson, L. D.: Chronologic development of streptococcic lymphadenitis in swine. Am. J. Vet. Res., 34:77–82, 1973.

Gunning, O. V.: Joint-ill in foals (pyosepticemia). Vet. J., 103:47–67, 104–111, 129–148, 1947.

Herman, P. H., and Fox, J. G.: Panophthalmitis associated with diplococcic septicemia in a rhesus monkey. J. Am. Vet. Med. Assoc., 159:560–562, 1971.

Isaki, L. S., Bairey, M. H., and Van Patten, L. K.: Response of vaccinated swine to group E streptococcus exposure. Cornell Vet., 63:579–588, 1973.

Jones, F. S.: The streptococci of equines. J. Exp. Med., 30:159–178, 1919.

Jones, J. E. T.: The experimental production of streptococcal endocarditis in the pig. J. Pathol., 99:307–318, 1969.

Kaufmann, A. F., and Quist, K. D.: Pneumococcal meningitis and peritonitis in rhesus monkeys. J. Am. Vet. Med. Assoc., 155:1158, 1969.

Keeling, M. E., and McClure, H. M.: Pneumococcal meningitis and fatal enterobiasis in a chimpanzee. Lab. Anim. Sci., 24:92–95, 1974.

Knight, A. P., Voss, J. L., McChesney, A. E., and Bigbee, H. G.: Experimentally induced *Streptococcus equi* infection in horses with resultant guttural pouch empyema. Vet. Med. Small Anim. Clin., 70:1194–1195, 1198–1199, 1975.

Kunstyr, I., and Matthiesen, T.: Two forms of streptococcal infection (serologic group C) in guinea pigs. Z. Versuchstierkd., 15:348–357, 1973.

McCrea, C. T.: Pneumococcal septicaemia in calves. Vet. Rec., 88:518–519, 1971.

McDonald, T. J., and McDonald, J. S.: Streptococci isolated from bovine intramammary infections. Am. J. Vet. Res., 37:377–381, 1976.

Miller, W. T., and Johnson, H. W.: Differential staining of sections of unpreserved bovine udder tissue affected with mastitis. U.S.D.A., Washington, D. C., Circular No. 514, 1939.

Mitchell, C. A., and Plummer, P. J. G.: Septic arthritis caused by *Streptococcus equi*. Can. J. Comp. Med., 6:24–25, 1942.

Morrill, C. C.: A histopathological study of the bovine udder. Cornell Vet., 28:196–210, 1938.

Murphy, J. M.: The relationship of teat mucous membrane topography to age, breed, and incidence of udder infection in cows. Cornell Vet., 35:41–47, 1945.

Parker, G. A., Russell, R. J., and De Paoli, A.: Extrapulmonary lesions of *Streptococcus pneumoniae* infection in guinea pigs. Vet. Pathol., 14:332–337, 1977.

Riley, M. G. I., Morehouse, L. G., and Olson, L. D.: Distribution of group E streptococcus in head and neck regions of swine. Am. J. Vet. Res., 34:1163–1166, 1973.

———: Detection of tonsillar and nasal colonization of group E streptococcus in swine. Am. J. Vet. Res., 34:1167–1170, 1973.

Schmitz, J. A., Olson, L. D., Schueler, R. L., and Gosser, H. S.: Isolation of group E streptococcus from the blood of swine with streptococcic lymphadenitis. Am. J. Vet. Res., 33:449–452, 1972.

Schmitz, J. A., and Olson, L. D.: Susceptibility of swine of various ages to streptococcic lymphadenitis. Am. J. Vet. Res., 33:1995–2002, 1972.

———: Transmission of streptococcic lymphadenitis by carrier swine. Am. J. Vet. Res., 34:189–190, 1973.

Schueler, R. L., Morehouse, L. G., and Olson, L. D.: Intravenous exposure of swine to group E streptococci: clinical signs, hemic and lymphatic distribution of streptococci, and resistance to subsequent exposure. Am. J. Vet. Res., 33:1797–1800, 1972.

Schueler, R. L., Morehouse, L. G., and Olson, L. D.: Intravenous exposure of swine to group E streptococci: Articular and cardiac lesions associated with experimentally induced septicemic infection of swine with group E streptococci. Am. J. Vet. Res., 33:1801–1812, 1972.

Shuman, R. D., and Wessman, G. E.: Swine abscesses caused by Lancefield's group E streptococci. XII. Specificity of serological tests for their detection with relation to non-groupable beta hemolytic streptococci. Cornell Vet., 64:178–200, 1974.

Stewart, D. D., Buck, G. E., McConnell, E. E., and Amster, R. L.: An epizootic of necrotic dermatitis in laboratory mice caused by Lancefield group G streptococci. Lab. Anim. Sci., 25:296–302, 1975.

Taranta, A., et al.: Experimental streptococcal infections in nonhuman primates. *In* Medical Primatology 1970, edited by E. I. Goldsmith and J. Moor-Jankowski. Basel, S. Karger, 1971. pp. 748–760.

Wessman, G. E., and Shuman, R. D.: Swine abscesses caused by Lancefield's group E streptococci. XI. Application of the hemagglutination test to demonstrate a correlation between the antigens of group E and *Streptococcus uberis*, and their relation to antibodies induced by unknown organisms. Cornell Vet., 63:618–629, 1973.

Windsor, R. S., and Elliott, S. D.: Streptococcal infection in young pigs. IV. An outbreak of streptococcal meningitis in weaned pigs. J. Hyg. (Camb), 75:69–78, 1975.

Wood, R. L., Cutlip, R. C., and Shuman, R. D.: Osteomyelitis and arthritis induced in swine by Lancefield's group A streptococci (*Streptococcus pyogenes*). Cornell Vet., 61:457–470, 1971.

STAPHYLOCOCCAL INFECTIONS

Coccoid bacterial organisms, which are gram-positive and occur in packets, are classified in the genus *Staphylococcus*. Occasionally they are pathogenic for man and animals. These organisms are widespread in nature and frequent inhabitants of the normal skin. It is not surprising, therefore, that staphylococci commonly infect wounds and are present in cutaneous abscesses, boils, and furuncles. Staphylococci are frequent inhabitants in both veterinary and human hospitals, and represent a serious threat to surgical, debilitated, and diseased patients. Many strains (particularly hospital strains) are resistant to a variety of antibiotics and present formidable therapeutic problems. Some strains produce toxins that cause gastroenteritis ("food poisoning") in man following consumption of contaminated food in which the bacteria have been allowed to grow (Fey, 1978).

Granulomatous Staphylococcal Mastitis

Occurring with moderate rarity, and reported from Europe, the United States, and Australia, this bovine disease has gone under the etiologically incorrect name of "actinomycotic mastitis." The pathologic and etiologic characteristics are also those of the granulomatous disease that has been known as "botryomycosis." Since the older writers mention botryomycosis as occurring in the udders of mares, we presume it is correct to say that mares are subject to this form of mastitis, although there appear to be no reports of it in recent times. Lesions identical to those described in the mammary gland (botryomycosis) may be encountered in other animal species and in a variety of tissues, including the skin, skeletal muscle, and uterus.

One or more quarters of the udder are hard and moderately enlarged, but neither hot nor painful, the onset being insidious

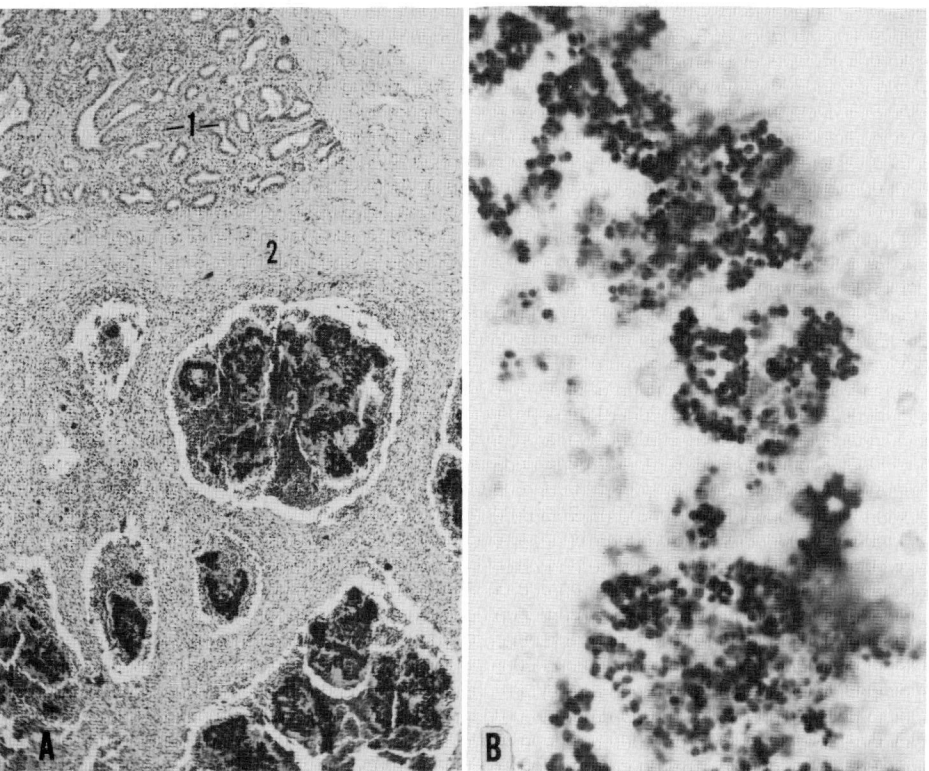

Fig. 11–6. Granulomatous staphylococcal mastitis, udder of a cow. *A,* Mammary lobules *(1)* are separated by dense bands of connective tissue *(2)* from the colonies of staphylococci *(3)* which are surrounded by a narrow zone of pus (× 48). *B,* Part of a bacterial colony stained by Gram's method (× 1000). Note spherical staphylococci. (Courtesy of Dr. E. A. Benbrook.)

and unperceived. The flow of milk is negligible or nonexistent, but the general health of the animals has generally been unimpaired.

Microscopic study reveals that each interlobular septum, normally so thin as to be almost imperceptible, has proliferated until it forms a distinct fibrous capsule. The average diameter of these roughly spherical lobules is about a centimeter, and the whole affected area, which may be the entire quarter, is composed of these circular compartments packed together. Inside each fibrous capsule is a zone of reticuloendothelial granulation tissue entirely comparable to that of actinomycosis and actinobacillosis. Within the granulation tissue there are one or, as a rule, several minute abscesses, or masses of polymorphonuclear neutrophils. Within each focus of purulent exudate, there are brilliant, red-staining (hematoxylin and eosin) "rosettes," which also closely simulate the rosettes of actinomycosis and actinobacillosis, showing however less tendency to form "clubs" at the periphery. The Gram stain shows these rosettes to be packed with cocci, although the organisms often have died out in the center, the oldest part of the colony (Fig. 11–6).

Grossly, the outlines of the lobular capsules are readily seen on the cut surface, and a droplet of pus may ooze from each barely visible abscess. The rosettes are seldom sufficiently firm that they can be felt with the fingers, as they usually can in actinomycosis.

Cultural studies of the causative cocci have shown that they differ in no significant manner from *Staphylococcus aureus*. Various theories have been proposed as to why this staphylococcus should produce a chronic granulomatous reaction so different from the acute serofibrinopurulent form, which is the rule. It is believed that a delicately close balance between pathogenicity of the invader and the resistance of the host may well be involved.

Diagnosis should be practically certain from the gross examination of the tissue, but histopathologic examination with demonstration of the organism leaves no room for doubt. Cultural or direct microscopic examination of the milk reveals only *Staphylococcus aureus*, with no evidence of its granulomatous propensities.

Other Staphylococcal Infections

The ubiquitous distribution of staphylococci on cutaneous surfaces and in the environment should cause one to be skeptical of their pathogenic significance in lesions of exposed surfaces. However, under some circumstances, these organisms do cause disease. In one example, staphylococcal dermatitis in young mink may have resulted from abrasions of the skin by their mothers' teeth (Crandell et al., 1971). Purulent inflammation in the dermis was associated with ulceration of the epidermis in this instance.

Lesions similar to those seen in granulomatous staphylococcal mastitis were described in mice (strain: C57 BL/6 Bd) maintained under "specific-pathogen-free" conditions (Shults et al., 1973). Several tissues were infected, with colonies of staphylococci surrounded by a zone of neutrophils, which in turn were contained by bands of fibrous connective tissue. In some cases, pieces of hair, acting as foreign bodies, appeared to form the nidus for the infection. Dermatitis attributed to staphylococci has also been described in Mongolian gerbils (*Meriones unguiculatus*) (Peckman et al., 1974).

Vesicular lesions have been described in the skin of guinea pigs inoculated with material containing *Staphylococcus aureus* (Tessler, 1973).

Albiston, H. E.: Actinomycosis of the mammary gland of cows in Victoria. Aust. Vet. J., 6:2–22, 1930.

Anderson, J. C.: Experimental staphylococcal mastitis in the mouse: the effect of inoculating different strains into separate glands of the same mouse. J. Comp. Pathol., 84:103–111, 1974.

Brown, R. W.: Intramammary infections produced by various strains of *Staphylococcus epidermidis* and *Micrococcus*. Cornell Vet., 63:630–645, 1973.

Chandler, R. L.: Ultrastructural pathology of mastitis in the mouse. A study of experimental staphylococcal and streptococcal infections. Br. J. Exp. Pathol., *51*:639–645, 1970.

Crandell, R. A., Huttenhauer, G. A., and Casey, H. W.: Staphylococcic dermatitis in mink. J. Am. Vet. Med. Assoc., *159*:638–639, 1971.

Dennis, S. M.: Perinatal staphylococcal infections of sheep. Vet. Rec., *79*:38–40, 1966.

Derbyshire, J. B.: The pathology of experimental staphylococcal mastitis in the goat. J. Comp. Pathol. Ther., *68*:449–454, 1958.

Fey, H.: Staphylokokken-Enterotoxine in Lebensmitteln und deren Nachweis. Chem. Rundshau, *31*:6–9, 1978.

Morrill, C. C.: A histopathological study of the bovine udder. Cornell Vet., *28*:196–210, 1938.

Pattison, I. H.: Histological examination of the teats of goats affected with streptococcal mastitis. J. Comp. Pathol. Ther., *62*:1–5, 1952.

Peckham, J. C., et al.: Staphylococcal dermatitis in Mongolian gerbils. Lab. Anim. Sci., *24*:43–47, 1974.

Schalm, O. W., Lasmanis, J., and Jain, N. C.: Conversion of chronic staphylococcal mastitis to acute gangrenous mastitis after neutropenia in blood and bone marrow produced by an equine antibovine leukocyte serum. Am. J. Vet. Res., *37*:885–890, 1976.

Shults, F. S., Estes, P. C., Franklin, J. A., and Richter, C. B.: Staphylococcal botryomycosis in a specific pathogen-free mouse colony. Lab. Anim. Sci., *23*:36–42, 1973.

Smith, H.: Two cases of actinomycotic mastitis. J. Am. Vet. Med. Assoc., *84*:635–644, 1934.

Sorenson, G. H.: *Micrococcus indolicus.* Some biochemical properties, and the demonstration of six antigenically different types. Acta Vet. Scand., *14*:301–326, 1973.

Spencer, G. R., and McNutt, S. H.: Pathogenesis of bovine mastitis. Am. J. Vet. Res., *11*:188–198, 1950.

Tessler, J.: Vesicular lesions produced in guinea pigs by a *Staphylococcus aureus* strain. Can. J. Comp. Med., *37*:323–324, 1973.

Thawley, D. G., Marshall, R. B., Cullinane, L., and Markham, J.: Atypical staphylococcal mastitis in a dairy herd. J. Am. Vet. Med. Assoc., *171*:425–428, 1977.

VIBRIOSIS (Campylobacterosis)

For many years, bacteria classified in the genus *Vibrio* have been considered causative agents in diseases of cattle, sheep, and man. Taxonomists have now decided that some of the *Vibrio* organisms should be classified among spiral and curved bacteria (Spirillaceae) and called *Campylobacter* (campylo = curved) (Buchanan and Gibbons, 1974). *Campylobacter fetus* is the current name proposed for *Vibrio fetus, Spirillum fetus,* or *Vibrio fetus* var *venerealis,* and the organism is responsible for abortion and infertility in cattle. This organism is transmitted by coitus and does not multiply in the intestinal tract.

Campylobacter fetus subspecies *intestinalis (Vibrio fetus* var *intestinalis)* is believed responsible for abortion in sheep (occasionally, in cattle) and human infection. The organism is found in the intestinal tract and gallbladder of man and animals.

Campylobacter fetus subspecies *jejuni (Vibrio jejuni, V. hepaticus,* possibly *Vibrio coli, Campylobacter jejuni,* or *Campylobacter coli)* is found in the intestine of aborted ovine fetuses and in the intestine of normal cattle, swine, sheep, goats, chickens, turkeys, and wild birds. It has been identified also in human enteritis (food poisoning).

Campylobacter sputorum (Vibrio sputorum) is apparently nonpathogenic, since it is found in the genital tracts of normal male and female cattle and sheep and in semen, preputial, and vaginal mucus of normal animals.

Organisms that currently remain in the genus *Vibrio* include *Vibrio cholerae,* the cause of human cholera (which is pathogenic experimentally for dogs, guinea pigs, and infant rabbits); *Vibrio parahaemolyticus,* found in sea food, which may produce acute enteritis in human beings; and *Vibrio aquillarum* and *V. fischeri,* which are found in sea water, diseased fish, and marine animals.

In cattle, transmission of vibriosis is entirely venereal, either by coitus or in the course of artificial insemination. The infection in cattle is principally characterized by temporary infertility and prolonged estrus cycles. The cow is infected during breeding, and although fertilization and implantation are normal, *Campylobacter fetus* soon kills the embryo and incites endometritis. Neither the death of the embryo nor the endometritis are manifest by clinical signs. Endometritis may prevent conception at succeeding estrus periods, but most cattle will conceive prior to resolution of the disease. Recovered cows are usually resistant to reinfection. Rarely, *Campylobacter fetus* will cause late abortion. The infection in the bull does not induce lesions or sterility. Bulls usually recover spontaneously, but certain bulls and cows can carry the organism for protracted periods of time. Passive transfer of infection by the bull is considered unlikely, because growth of organisms on the penis or within the prepuce is necessary in order for numbers of organisms to be adequate to cause infection in the cow (Clark et al., 1975).

In contrast to cattle, vibriosis in sheep is not a venereal disease. The oral route is believed to be the principal means of transmission. The infection is characterized by late abortion, stillbirth, or birth of weak lambs which usually die soon after birth. Following abortion, certain ewes may carry the organism.

Lesions. The lesions of vibriosis in cattle are subtle. In experimentally induced disease, Estes and coworkers (1966) described the lesions as a subacute, diffuse mucopurulent endometritis. The uterine glands contain neutrophils, lymphocytes, eosinophils, and sloughed epithelium. The uterine mucosa is infiltrated with lymphocytes, plasma cells, neutrophils, and eosinophils, especially beneath the surface epithelium, and around uterine glands and blood vessels.

In sheep, the placenta is intensely invaded, becomes necrotic and detached, and the fetus is aborted. Autolytic changes in natural cases usually preclude adequate pathologic study of the fetus and placenta. Studies of experimentally induced vibriosis in sheep by Jensen, Miller, and Molello (1961) have provided the following concepts of the pathogenesis of the disease: Maternal bacteremia with *Campylobacter fetus* is followed by localization of the organisms in the hilar zone of the placentomes; arteriolitis results in the vessels in the septa, capillary walls become necrotic, and some are thrombosed; *Campylobacter fetus* penetrate from the maternal blood through capillaries or arterioles to gain access to the hematomas formed between the chorion and the septa; the bacteria proliferate in the hematoma and stimulate accumulation of leukocytes in the hematoma and septa. At this point, the organisms gain access to the epithelial cells of the chorion by active penetration or by phagocytosis. These cells become engorged with organisms. From these infected chorionic epithelial cells (or from the hematoma), organisms gain access to the adjacent chorionic capillaries whose cells become engorged with bacteria and some lumens are occluded. From this point the organisms have free access to the fetal circulation. Edema of the chorionic villi is conspicuous at this time and desquamation between septa and villi results in separation. The fetus dies, presumably as the result of bacteremia and possibly toxemia, but also possibly by hypoxia resulting from separation of maternal and fetal placenta. The fetus and placenta decompose rapidly, sometimes become macerated, and are expelled to contaminate the environment. Vulvitis and vaginitis often follow. As indicated, lesions of diagnostic significance are generally absent in the fetus, but in about 10% of the aborted fetuses, lesions are present in the liver, which aid diagnosis. These consist of focal necrotizing hepatitis, which is observable grossly as tan to gray foci 1 mm to 2 cm in diameter.

Osborne and Smibert (1964) have suggested that vibrionic abortion may be the result of a hypersensitivity to *Campylobacter fetus* toxin, rather than an infectious process. Their experimental studies clearly demonstrated allergic phenomena, but whether this explains natural abortion will require further investigation. Experimental exposure of pregnant cows to *Campylobacter fetus* subspecies *intestinalis* results in generalized infection and death of the fetus, presumably due to its lack of immune competence (Osburn and Hoskins, 1970).

Diagnosis. The diagnosis in sheep is usually based upon clinical signs and gross lesions, usually confined to the uterus, its contents, vagina, and vulva. The uterine wall is edematous, the placentomes swollen, soft, and pale. Purulent exudate and blood may accumulate between the chorion and endometrium in interplacentomal areas of the uterus. Smears of the placenta usually reveal typical organisms in large numbers. Confirmation by culture and identification of the organisms is advisable.

In cattle, the clinical signs should cause suspicion of vibriosis, but confirmation is necessary to differentiate from trichomoniasis. If the abortus is viable, the organism can be cultured. However, this is not usual, hence culture of cervicovaginal mucus should be attempted. The agglutination test employed on cervical mucus is also of value, but the specific fluorescence antibody test appears to be most reliable and less time-consuming (Andrews and Frank, 1974). Culture can also be employed on preputial scrapings for diagnosis of infection in the bull. Infected bulls can also be identified by test-mating to disease-free heifers.

Andrews, P.J., and Frank, F. W.: Comparison of four diagnostic tests for detection of bovine genital vibriosis. J. Am. Vet. Med. Assoc., *165*:695–697, 1974.

Ardrey, W. B., Armstrong, P., Meinershagen, W. A., and Frank, F. W.: Diagnosis of ovine vibriosis and enzootic abortion of ewes by immunofluorescence technique. Am. J. Vet. Res., *33*:2535–2538, 1972.

Blachman, U., Goss, S. J., and Pickett, M.J.: Experimental cholera in the chinchilla. J. Infect. Dis., *129*:376–384, 1974.

Boncyk, L. H., Brack, M., and Kalter, S. S.: Hemorrhagic-necrotic enteritis in a baboon (*Papio cynocephalus*) due to *Vibrio fetus*. Lab. Anim. Sci., *22*:734–738, 1972.

Bryner, J. H., Estes, P. C., Foley, J. W., and O'Berry, P. A.: Infectivity of three *Vibrio fetus* biotypes for gallbladder and intestines of cattle, sheep, rabbits, guinea pigs, and mice. Am. J. Vet. Res., *32*:465–470, 1971.

Bryner, J. H., O'Berry, P. A., Estes, P. C., and Foley, J. W.: Studies of vibrios from gallbladder of market sheep and cattle. Am. J. Vet. Res., *33*:1439–1444, 1972.

Buchanan, R. E., and Gibbons, N. E.: *Bergey's Manual of Determinative Bacteriology*, 8th ed. Baltimore, Williams & Wilkins, 1974.

Clark, B. L., Dufty, J. H., Monsborough, M. J., and Parsonson, I. M.: Studies on venereal transmission of *Campylobacter fetus* by immunized bulls. Aust. Vet. J., *51*:531–532, 1975.

Corbeil, L. B., Corbeil, R. R., and Winter, A. J.: Bovine venereal vibriosis: activity of inflammatory cells in protective immunity. Am. J. Vet. Res., *36*:403–406, 1975.

Corbeil, L. B., et al.: Bovine venereal vibriosis: ultrastructure of endometrial inflammatory lesions. Lab. Invest., *33*:187–192, 1975.

Dobson, A. W., Bierschwal, C. J., Jr., and McDougle, H. C.: Induced estrus as an aid in detection of bovine genital vibriosis by means of the virgin heifer test. J. Am. Vet. Med. Assoc., *156*:1584–1588, 1970.

Dozsa, L., Mitchell, R. G., and Olson, N. O.: Histologic changes of the uterine mucosa following the duration of *Vibrio* infection and the subsequent development of immunity. Am. J. Vet. Res., *23*:769–776, 1962.

Eden, A. N.: Perinatal mortality caused by *Vibrio fetus*. J. Pediatr., *68*:297–304, 1966.

Estes, P. C., Bryner, J. H., and O'Berry, P. A.: Histopathology of bovine vibriosis and the effects of vibrio fetus extracts on the female genital tract. Cornell Vet., *56*:610–622, 1966.

Faulkner, L. C.: Abortion Diseases of Livestock. Springfield, Charles C Thomas, 1968.

Felsenfeld, O., Gyr, K., and Wolf, R. H.: Malnutrition and susceptibility to infection with *Vibrio cholerae* in vervet monkeys (*Cercopithecus aethiops*). 1. Induction of protein, B-vitamin complex and calorie malnutrition. J. Med. Primatol., *5*:186–194, 1976.

Ghosh, H. K.: The pathogenesis of experimental cholera. J. Med. Microbiol., *3*:427–440, 1970.

Hacking, M. A., and Budd, J.: Vibrio infection in tropical fish in a freshwater aquarium. J. Wildl. Dis., *7*:273–280, 1971.

Kendrick, J. W., Williams, J., Crenshaw, G. L., and Vestal, T. J.: Fertility and immune reaction of heifers vaccinated with the adjuvanted *Vibrio fetus* vaccine. J. Am. Vet. Med. Assoc., *158*:1531–1535, 1971.

Keusch, G. T., Grady, G. F., Deschner, E. E., and Weinstein, L.: Biochemical effects of cholera enterotoxin. III. Intestinal protein synthesis in the infant rabbit. Lab. Invest., *28*:593–596, 1973.

Jensen, R., Miller, V. A., and Molello, J. A.: Placental pathology of sheep with vibriosis. Am. J. Vet. Res., *22*:169–185, 1961.

Lowrie, D. B., and Pearce, J. H.: The placental localization of *Vibrio fetus*. J. Med. Microbiol., *3*:607–614, 1970.

McCarthy, D. H., Stevenson, J. P., and Roberts, M. S.: Vibriosis in rainbow trout. J. Wildl. Dis., *10*:2–7, 1974.

Moon, H. W., Cutlip, R. C., Amtower, W. C., and Matthews, P. J.: Intraepithelial vibrio associated with acute typhlitis of young rabbits. Vet. Path., *11*:313–326, 1974.

DISEASES DUE TO SIMPLE BACTERIA

Morse, E. V.: *Vibrio parahaemolyticus*: a cause of foodborne illness. J. Am. Vet. Med. Assoc., *169*:1236,
1976.

Osborne, J. C., and Smibert, R. M.: Vibrio fetus toxin.
I. Hypersensitivity and abortifacient action. Cornell Vet., *54*:561–572, 1964.

Osborne, J. C.: Pathologic responses in animals after
vibrio toxin shock. Am. J. Vet. Res.,
26:1056–1067, 1965.

Osburn, B. I., and Hoskins, R. K.: Experimentally
induced *Vibrio fetus* var. *intestinalis* infection in
pregnant cows. Am. J. Vet. Res., *31*:1733–1741,
1970.

————: Infection with *Vibrio fetus* in the immunologically immature fetal calf. J. Infect. Dis., *123*:32–40,
1971.

Redman, D. R., Trapp, A. L., Hamdy, A. H., and Bell,
D. S.: Ovine vibriosis in Ohio. J. Am. Vet. Med.
Assoc., *143*:1094–1095, 1963.

Samuelson, J. D., and Winter, A. J.: Bovine vibriosis:
the nature of the carrier state in the bull. J. Infect.
Dis., *116*:518–592, 1966.

Shires, G. M. H., and Kramer, T. T.: Filtration of
bovine cervicovaginal mucus for diagnosis of
vibriosis, using the fluorescent antibody test. J.
Am. Vet. Med. Assoc., *164*:398–401, 1974.

Schutte, A. P., McConnell, E. E., and Bosman, P. P.:
Vibrionic abortion in ewes in South Africa: preliminary report. J. S. Afr. Vet. Med. Assoc.,
42:223–226, 1971.

Wilkie, B. N., and Winter, A. J.: Location of *Vibrio
fetus* var. *venerealis* within the endometrium of
the cow. Infect. Immun., *3*:854–856, 1971.

————: Bovine vibriosis: the distribution and specificity of antibodies induced by vaccination and
infection and the immunofluorescent localization
of organism in infected heifers. Can. J. Comp.
Med., *35*:301–312, 1971.

Williams, C. E., et al.: Ovine campylobacterosis: Preliminary studies of the efficacy of the in vitro
serum bactericidal test as an assay for the potency
of *Campylobacter (Vibrio) fetus* subsp *intestinalis*
bacterins. Am. J. Vet. Res., *37*:409–415, 1976.

Swine erysipelas is an important disease
in many parts of the world. Not only does
the causative organism produce infections
in swine, but also in a wide variety of other
species, including birds (turkeys, chickens, geese, ducks, pigeons, parrots, and
quail, and many other wild species),
sheep, fish, and porpoises. It is responsible for **erysipeloid** of man, particularly of
persons who work in slaughterhouses and
fish markets. The cutaneous lesions of
erysipeloid are usually local, but may
explode into a fulminant disease, with

widespread exanthematous or bullous lesions on the hands, face, or body.

The causative organism, *Erysipelothrix
rhusiopathiae (E. insidiosa)*, is small,
pleomorphic, and rod-shaped, either
straight or curved. It is gram-positive and
may have a beaded appearance. The organism forms tiny colonies on ordinary agar
media. It survives for long periods in decaying flesh and in water, and is resistant
to such preservative processes as salting,
smoking, and pickling. A rapid and economical method for isolating and identifying *E. rhusiopathiae*, using triple sugar iron
agar, has been described (Vickers and
Bierer, 1958).

In swine, the disease presents diverse
manifestations that often make its clinical
recognition difficult. It may appear as an
acute febrile disease with high mortality
rate, death occurring before any specific
lesions can be detected. In less severe infections, appearance of rhomboid-shaped
areas of intense erythema in the skin are
characteristic and have suggested the
common name, "diamond-skin disease,"
frequently applied to this entity. These
erythematous lesions may progress to necrosis, with large patches of epidermis
sloughing as healing occurs. Another frequent clinical manifestation results from
localization of organisms in the joints. Arthritis in one or more joints is manifested
by sudden onset of painful hot swelling,
particularly of the carpal or tarsal articulations. Vegetative endocarditis is a common
sequel and may result in sudden death.
Hypersensitivity appears to play an important role in this disease, but evidence is still
accumulating on this point. Lesions closely
resembling the arthritic disease have been
produced in swine, lambs, and rabbits by
direct instillation of cell-free materials from
cultures of *E. rhusiopathiae* (Ajmal, 1971;
Piercy, 1971; White and Puls, 1969).

Lesions. In acute septicemic cases of
swine erysipelas, nonspecific lesions such
as hemorrhages may occur in serous surfaces and elsewhere. Specific lesions of

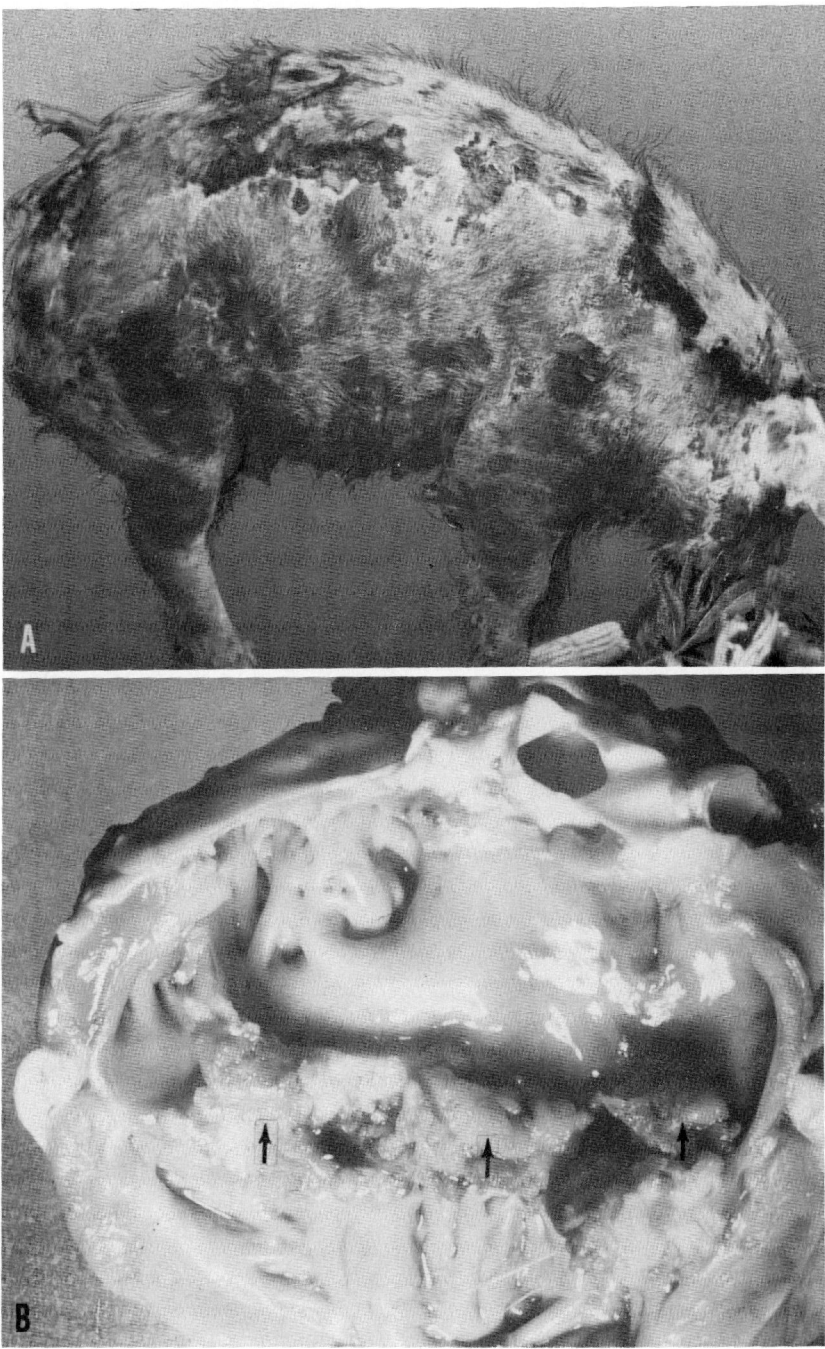

Fig. 11–7. Swine erysipelas. *A*, Sloughing of large areas of skin. *B*, Valvular endocarditis affecting the left atrioventricular (bicuspid or mitral) valve (arrows).

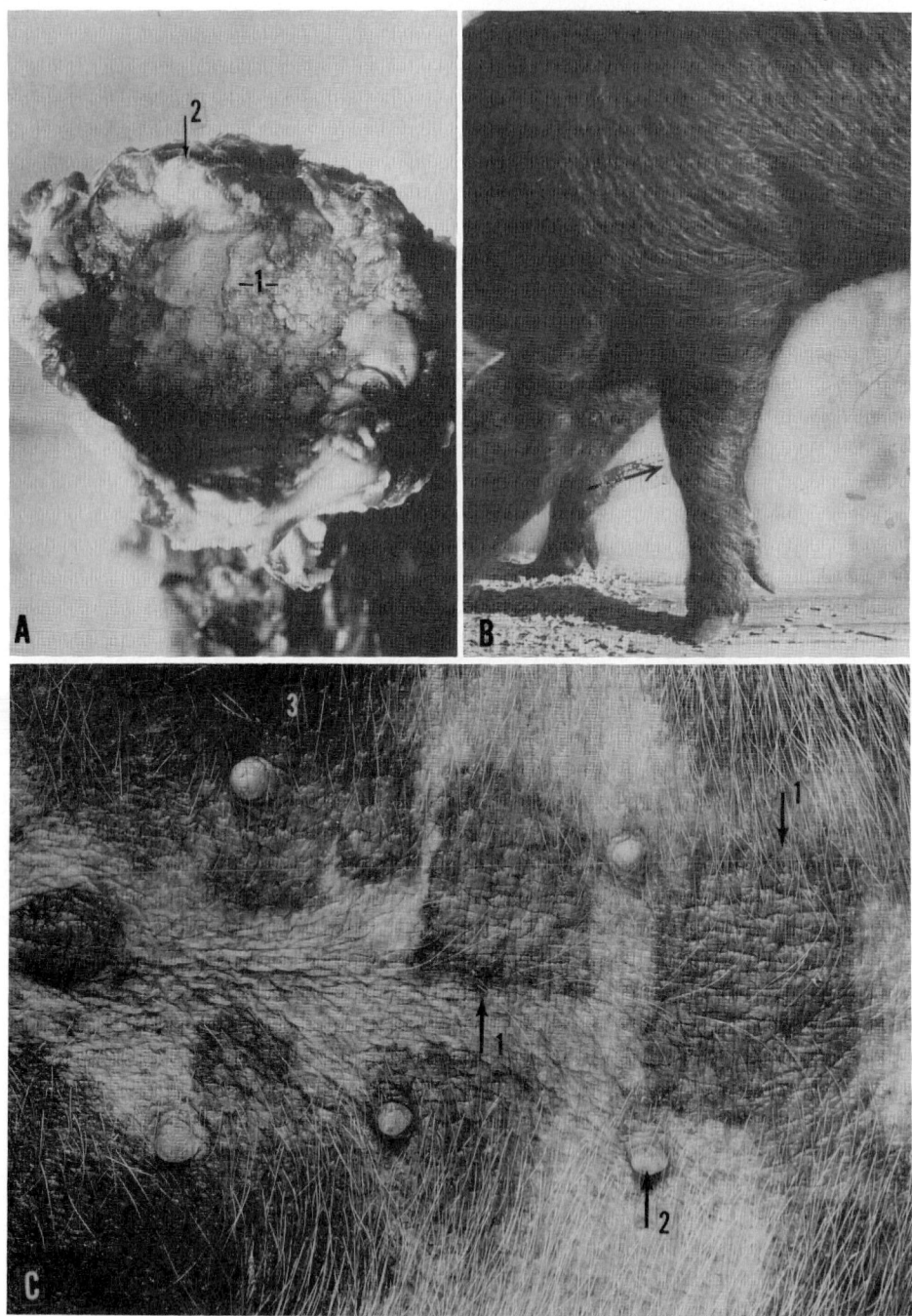

Fig. 11–8. Swine erysipelas. *A*, Arthritis, with roughened synovial surface *(1)* and thick joint capsule *(2)*. *B*, Acute arthritis with enlargement of the joint (arrow). *C*, Rhomboid areas of congestion in the skin ("diamond skin disease"). Note sharp margin *(1)* of the lesion. Normal teat *(2)* and pigmented skin *(3)*. (Courtesy of Armed Forces Institute of Pathology.) Contributor: Bureau of Animal Industry, U. S. Department of Agriculture.

diagnostic significance develop as the disease progresses. The distinguishing lesions of the less florid disease are found in the skin, synovial membranes, and endocardium. The cutaneous lesions, which are most common on the abdomen but may occur anywhere on the skin, vary in size but are almost always of diamond, rhomboid, or rectangular shape, sharply demarcated from the adjacent normal skin. At first they are bright red, but later they become purplish and eventually a dark bluish color. Necrosis in older lesions accounts for darkening of the skin; the overlying epidermis dries and eventually peels off. Forcible removal of scabs from an incompletely healed lesion uncovers a raw, bleeding surface. The reason for the shape of the skin lesions is not thoroughly understood, although the lesions themselves are believed to result from bacterial thrombosis of small cutaneous vessels. More thorough studies of the morphologic changes in the skin are definitely needed.

In affected joints, lesions of more chronic nature may be recognized grossly. The joint capsule is obviously enlarged, thickened, and distended with excessive fluid, and the articular surfaces are roughened. Rugose thickening of the joint capsule is particularly evident at the margins of the articular surfaces. Microscopically, the joint capsule is seen to be infiltrated with lymphoid cells, occasional nests of neutrophils are present, and the synovial lining is prominent and often thrown up into folds. Cell detritus and leukocytes may be found free in the lumen of the joint capsule.

Lesions in the heart are usually the consequence of subacute bacterial endocarditis. Most prominent are the large, irregularly coarse masses on the leaves of the mitral (bicuspid) valve or, less often, on the pulmonary valves. These nodular masses project into the lumen of the left ventricle and at times almost occlude it. The material adheres rather tenaciously to the valve leaflets, but it can be broken loose. Hypertrophy of the affected ventricle occurs in cases of long standing. Microscopically, the thickened valves are covered with fibrinous exudates made up of zones of organization, necrosis, leukocytes, and colonies of *Erysipelothrix*. The organisms can be more readily demonstrated by the use of a tissue Gram's stain.

Diagnosis. Typical symptoms and lesions are usually sufficient for diagnosis, but recovery and identification of the organism is necessary in acute septicemic cases and advisable in others.

Ajmal, M.: Experimental *Erysipelothrix* arthritis. Parts I. and II. Res. Vet. Sci., *12*:403–411, 412–419, 1971.

Chineme, C. N., Slaughter, L. J., and Highley, S. W.: Cardiovascular lesions associated with erysipelas in a sheep. J. Am. Vet. Med. Assoc., *162*:278–279, 1973.

Drew, R. A.: Erysipelothrix arthritis in pigs as a comparative model for rheumatoid arthritis. Proc. R. Soc. Med., *65*:994–998, 1972.

Drommer, W., Schulz, L-Cl., and Pohlenz, J.: Experimental infection of erysipelas in the pig. Disturbance of permeability and malacia in the central nervous system. Pathol. Vet., *7*:455–473, 1970.

Ehrlich, J. C.: *Erysipelothrix rhusiopathiae* infection in man. Arch. Int. Med., *78*:565–577, 1946.

Geissinger, H. D.: Acute and chronic *Erysipelothrix rhusiopathiae* infection in white mice. J. Comp. Pathol., *78*:79–88, 1968.

Harrington, R., Jr., and Ellis, E. M.: Salmonella and erysipelothrix infection in swine: a laboratory summary. Am. J. Vet. Res., *36*:1379–1380, 1975.

Hirsch, D. C., Boorman, G. A., and Jang, S. S.: Erysipelas in a black and red tamarin. J. Am. Vet. Med. Assoc., *167*:646–647, 1975.

Hubrig, T., and Kielstein, P.: Untersuchungen zur Rotlaufallergie. (Allergy in Swine Erysipelas.) Zbl. Vet. Med., *8*:869–895, 1961. VB 662–62.

Klauder, J. V.: *Erysipelothrix rhusiopathiae* infection in swine and in human beings. Arch. Dermat. Syph., *50*:151–159, 1944.

Marcato, P. S.: Histopathology of renal lesions in acute swine erysipelas. Acta Med. Vet. (Napoli), *9*:1–19, (I.e.f.g.) 1963. VB 1204–64.

Morita, M., Nozaki, C., Shibuga, S., and Okamoto, M.: Histopathology of muscle in experimental acute swine erysipelas. Jpn. J. Vet. Sci., *35*:261–267, 1973.

O'Brien, J. J., Baskerville, A., and McCracken, A.: Chronic rheumatoid arthritis in pigs associated with *Erysipelothrix* infection. Ir. Vet. J., *27*:21–25, 1973.

Papp, E., and Sikes, D.: Electrophoretic distribution of protein in the serum of swine with rheumatoid-like arthritis. Am. J. Vet. Res., *25*:1112–1119, 1964.

Piercy, D. W. T.: Synovitis induced by killed *Erysipelothrix rhusiopathiae*. Extended reaction in passively immunized lambs. J. Comp. Pathol., *81*:557–562, 1971.

Rebhun, W. C.: *Erysipelothrix insidiosa* septicemia in neonatal calves. Vet. Med. Small Anim. Clin., *71*:684–686, 1976.

Rosenwald, A. S., and Dickinson, E. M.: Swine erysipelas in turkeys. Cornell Vet., *29*:61–67, 1939.

Sakuma, S., Doi, K., and Okaniwa, A.: Pathology of experimental *Erysipelothrix insidiosa* infection in rats. Natl. Inst. Anim. Health Q. (Tokyo), *13*:80–90, 1973.

Sakuma, S., Doi, K., Okawa, H., and Okaniwa, A.: Vascular and perivascular lesions in experimental *Erysipelothrix insidiosa* infection in rats. Natl. Inst. Anim. Health Q. (Tokyo), *13*:203–210, 1973.

———: Articular lesions in experimental *Erysipelothrix insidiosa* infection in rats. Natl. Inst. Anim. Health Q. (Tokyo), *15*:86–93, 1975.

Seibold, H. R., and Neal, J. E.: Erysipelothrix septicemia in the porpoise. J.Am. Vet. Med. Assoc., *128*:537–539, 1956.

Sikes, D., Neher, G. M., and Doyle, L. P.: Studies on arthritis in swine. I. Experimental erysipelas and chronic arthritis in swine. Am. J. Vet. Res., *16*:349–366, 1955.

———: Swine erysipelas I. A discussion of experimentally induced disease. J. Am. Vet. Med. Assoc., *128*:277–281, 1956.

Sikes, D. E., et al.: Electrophoretic and serologic changes of blood serum of arthritic (rheumatoid) dogs infected with *Erysipelothrix insidiosa*. Am. J. Vet. Res., *32*:1083–1087, 1971.

Shuman, R. D., Wood, R. L., and Monlux, W. S.: Sensitization by *Erysipelothrix rhusiopathiae* (insidiosa) with relation to arthritis in pigs. I, II, III, IV. Cornell Vet., *55*:378–386, 387–396, 397–411, 444–453, 1966.

Simpson, C. F., Wood, F. G., and Young, F.: Cutaneous lesions in a porpoise with erysipelas. J. Am. Vet. Med. Assoc., *133*:558–560, 1958.

Sokoloff, L.: Comparative pathology of arthritis and rheumatism. Recent developments. Sci. Proc. AVMA, 1964. pp. 231–238.

Timoney, J. F., Jr., and Berman, D. T.: Erysipelothrix arthritis in swine: serum-synovial fluid gradients for antibody and serum proteins in normal and arthritic joints. II. Bacteriologic and immunopathologic aspects. Am. J. Vet. Res., *31*:1405–1409, 1411–1421, 1970.

Timoney, J. F., Jr.: Erysipelas arthritis in swine: concentrations of complement and third component of complement in synovia. Am. J. Vet. Res., *37*:5–8, 1976.

———: Erysipelas arthritis in swine: lysosomal enzyme levels in synovial fluids. Am. J. Vet. Res., *37*:295–298, 1976.

Tontis, A., et al.: Zur chronischer Rotlauf-Polyarthritis beim Lamm. Dtsch. Tierarzl. Wochenschr., *84*:113–116, 1977.

Vickers, C. L., and Bierer, B. W.: Triple sugar iron agar as an aid in the diagnosis of erysipelas. J. Am. Vet. Med. Assoc., *133*:543–544, 1958.

Wallach, J. D.: Erysipelas in two captive Diana monkeys. J. Am. Vet. Med. Assoc., *171*:979–980, 1977.

Wellmann, G., Thal, E., and Gravell, I.: chronic *Erysipelothrix rhusiopathiae* infection in laboratory rats. I. Attempts to produce chronic erysipelas by the injection of killed organisms. J. Comp. Pathol., *75*:267–273, 1965.

———: Chronic *Erysipelothrix rhusiopathiae* infection in laboratory rats. II. Influence of vaccination on the development of the disease. J. Comp. Pathol., *75*:275–279, 1965.

White, T. G., and Puls, J. L.: Induction of experimental chronic arthritis in rabbits by cell-free fragments of *Erysipelothrix*. J. Bact., *98*:403–406, 1969.

White, T. G., Puls, J. L., and Mirikitani, F. K.: Rabbit arthritis induced by cell-free extracts of *Erysipelothrix*. Infect. Immun., *3*:715–722, 1971.

Wood, R. L., and Packer, R. A.: Isolation of *Erysipelothrix rhusiopathiae* from soil and manure of swine-raising premises. Am. J. Vet. Res., *33*:1611–1620, 1972.

Wood, R. L.: Survival of *Erysipelothrix rhusiopathiae* in soil under various environmental conditions. Cornell Vet., *63*:390–410, 1973.

———: Isolation of pathogenic *Erysipelothrix rhusiopathiae* from feces of apparently healthy swine. Am. J. Vet. Res., *35*:41–43, 1974.

INFECTIONS DUE TO HAEMOPHILUS ORGANISMS

Haemophilus influenzae is an important secondary agent in human influenza. It also is a primary agent as a cause of upper respiratory infections and pneumonia, and is the commonest cause of purulent meningitis in infants and children. *H. influenzae* has also been associated with polyarthritis in man.

Along with the swine influenza virus, *Haemophilus (H. influenza suis) suis* plays an essential role in the pathogenesis of swine influenza. Swine influenza is discussed in Chapt. 9. *H. influenza suis* also produces a polyserositis and polyarthritis in swine which is known as Glässer's disease. The syndrome closely resembles that induced by mycoplasma infection in swine, and is discussed in Chapt. 10. *Haemophilus parahemolyticus* has been isolated with consistency from a porcine pleuropneumonia by investigators in Switzerland, Canada, and Great Britain (Hani et al., 1973; Schiefer and Greenfield, 1974; Little, 1970; Little et al., 1971). In Western Canada, lesions suggesting an adenovirus infection have been described (Schiefer et al., 1974) suggesting that an adenovirus may have an etiologic role.

Lesions. The lesions include fibrinous pleuritis, pulmonary vascular thromboses, and necrotizing pneumonia. Hani et al. (1973) point out that the early lesions in the preacute disease resemble those of endotoxin shock. These changes are alveolar and interlobular edema, dilatation of lymph vessels, congestion, hemorrhage, and intravascular fibrinous thrombosis. This view was supported by the production, in swine, of bilateral renal cortical necrosis (typical of the generalized Shwartzman reaction) by intravenous injection of sterile suspensions of pneumonic lung.

Infectious embolic meningoencephalitis was recognized and described in cattle by Griner, Jensen, and Brown (1956). An outbreak of a similar disease occurred in feedlot cattle in California in 1958. Kennedy and associates (1960) described this disease, isolated an unusual bacterial organism, and reproduced the disease by intravenous inoculation to calves with cultures of this organism. The organism, currently named *Haemophilus somnus*, has been recovered from many similarly affected cattle in Western United States and Canada (Van Dreumel, Curtis and Ruhnke, 1970; Dukes, 1971). This organism has also been associated with sporadic bovine abortion (Van Dreumel and Kierstead, 1975). Clinical signs are often not observed, but may include fever, opisthotonus, ataxia, weakness, blindness, paralysis, and death. Less acute disease is characterized by signs referable to the respiratory tract or polyarthritis.

Lesions. Grossly, the most characteristic lesions are single or multiple hemorrhagic foci in the brain. Any part of the brain may be affected. Petechiae and ecchymoses may be present in any viscus, lymph nodes are often enlarged, and serofibrinous laryngitis, tracheitis, polyarthritis, pleuritis, pericarditis, and peritonitis are frequent

findings. Microscopically, the basic and characteristic lesion of the disease is vasculitis, with thrombosis and septic infarction. Vasculitis is most frequent in the brain, but may be generalized. The lesions in the respiratory tract, joints, and body cavities are nonspecific. Diagnosis depends upon the clinical signs, lesions, and isolation of the causative agent, which is a gram-negative coccobacillus with cultural characteristics of *Haemophilus somnus.*

An acute septicemia of lambs caused by *Haemophilus agni* has been described by Kennedy et al. (1958). Clinical signs include fever, depression and reluctance to move, but since the course is usually less than 12 hours, affected animals are often found dead without premonitory signs.

Lesions. Gross changes are dominated by multiple hemorrhages throughout the body, including skeletal muscle where they are reported to be of diagnostic value. Focal necrosis of the liver and splenomegaly are almost constant findings. Fibrinopurulent arthritis, choroiditis, and basilar meningitis may develop in the rare lamb surviving 24 hours or more. Microscopically identifiable generalized bacterial embolism and vasculitis account for the gross findings. All tissues may be involved, but particularly the liver and skeletal muscle. Definitive diagnosis requires isolation and identification of *H. agni.*

In horses, a condition known as contagious equine metritis is caused by a bacillus tentatively classified as *Haemophilus equigenitalis* (see Chapter 25).

Bailie, W. E., Anthony, H. D., and Weide, K. D.: Infectious thromboembolic meningoencephalitis (sleeper syndrome) in feedlot cattle. J. Am. Vet. Med. Assoc., *148*:162–166, 1966.

Crandell, R. A., Smith, A. R., and Kissil, M.: Colonization and transmission of *Haemophilus somnus* in cattle. Am. J. Vet. Res., *38*:1749–1751, 1977.

Dukes, T. W.: The ocular lesions in thromboembolic meningoencephalitis (TEME) of cattle. Can. Vet. J., *12*:180–182, 1971.

Griner, L. A., Jensen, R., and Brown, W. W.: Infectious embolic meningoencephalitis in cattle. J. Am. Vet. Med. Assoc., *129*:417–421, 1956.

Hani, H., König, H., Nicolet, J., and Scholl, E.: Zur Haemophilus-Pleuropneumonie beim Schwein. V. Pathomorphologie. Schweiz. Arch. Tierheilkd., *115*:191–203, 1973.

———: Zur Haemophilus-Pleuropneumonie beim Schwein. VI. Pathogenese. Schweiz. Arch. Tierheilkd., *115*:205–212, 1973.

Kennedy, P. C., Frazier, L. M., Theiler, G. H., and Biberstein, E. L.: A septicemic disease of lambs caused by *Hemophilus agni* (new species). Am. J. Vet. Res., *19*:645–654, 1958.

Kennedy, P. C., et al.: Infectious meningo-encephalitis in cattle, caused by a haemophilus-like organism. Am. J. Vet. Res., *21*:403–409, 1960.

Little, T. W. A.: Haemophilus infection in pigs. Vet. Rec., *87*:399–402, 1970.

Little, T. W. A., and Harding, J. D. J.: The comparative pathogenicity of two porcine haemophilus species. Vet. Rec., *88*:540–545, 1971.

Panciera, R. J., Dahlgren, R. R., and Rinker, H. B.: Observations on septicemia of cattle caused by a *Haemophilus*-like organism. Path. Vet., *5*:212–226, 1968.

Schiefer, B., et al.: Porcine *Hemophilus parahemolyticus* pneumonia in Saskatchewan. I. Natural occurrence and findings. Can. J. Comp. Med., *38*:99–104, 1974.

Schiefer, B., and Greenfield, J.: Porcine *Hemophilus parahemolyticus* pneumonia in Saskatchewan. II. Bacteriological and experimental studies. Can. J. Comp. Med., *38*:105–110, 1974.

Van Dreumel, A. A., Curtis, R. A., and Ruhnke, H. L.: Infectious thromboembolic meningoencephalitis in Ontario feedlot cattle. Can. Vet. J., *11*:125–130, 1970.

Van Dreumel, A. A., and Kierstead, M.: Abortion associated with *Hemophilus somnus* infection in a bovine fetus. Can. Vet. J., *16*:367–370, 1975.

COLIBACILLOSIS

Shortly after birth, the intestinal tract of most, if not all, animals becomes colonized by certain bacteria—a symbiotic and usually favorable relationship. One of the most important of these organisms is a gram-negative rod-shaped bacterium, *Escherichia coli*. Under certain conditions involving changes in the host or the bacterium, these usually harmless organisms may become severely pathogenic. Much study of the resulting disease in animals and man has led to concepts involving several pathogenetic mechanisms that lead to distinctive forms of colibacillosis. It is useful to consider this disease syndrome from the pathogenetic viewpoint, making it possible to understand the varied clinical and pathologic manifestations which in the past have appeared to be the manifestations of several diseases (Moon, 1974; Fey, 1972).

Enterotoxic Colibacillosis. (Enteric colibacillosis, enteric *E. coli* infection, *E. coli* diarrhea, cholera-like *E. coli* infection, travelers' diarrhea.) This form is most common naturally in young piglets, calves, and lambs, but also occurs in babies and adult human beings. It may be reproduced in several species. The pathogenic *Escherichia coli* adhere to the mucosa and proliferate in the lumen of the small intestine, producing a potent enterotoxin, which stimulates excessive secretion of fluid from the intestinal mucosa. This loss of fluid causes the principal sign (diarrhea) and often leads to dehydration and death in the young. This secretion of fluid occurs from the intestinal epithelial cells located in the crypts of the small intestine. This effect and fluids produced appear to be similar in infection with both *E. coli* and *Vibrio cholerae*. The fluids (Moon, 1974) are generally alkaline, isotonic in comparison to serum, low in protein and ions of calcium and magnesium, and high in sodium and carbonate (Moon et al., 1971). The lesions are minimal in the intestinal epithelium, even in experimental cases. The goblet cells discharge their contents, but no other significant changes are noted by light or electron microscopy.

Enterotoxemic Colibacillosis. (Enteric-toxemic colibacillosis of calves, edema disease of swine.) In this form of *E. coli* infection, the organisms grow in the small intestine, producing toxin that is absorbed and acts elsewhere. This toxin is different from enterotoxin, and is considered to be a neurotoxin (edema disease principle), which acts as an antigen, leading to vascular response to hypersensitivity. In swine, this form is manifest by edema in gastric, colonic, palpebral, subcutaneous, and central nervous tissues (see also edema disease, Chap. 23). This noninflammatory edema results from vascular damage, which leads to hypertension and later vasculitis, with hyaline necrosis of arterial and arteriolar walls. Some strains of *E. coli* produce both the edema disease principle and the enterotoxin, resulting in both the enterotoxic and enterotoxemic forms of the disease simultaneously.

Local Invasive Colibacillosis. This form of colibacillosis occurs naturally in man and has been reproduced experimentally in laboratory animals. So far this form has not been recognized as a natural occurrence in animals. The organisms have the ability to penetrate and destroy the intestinal epithelial cells. The ability of these particular strains of *E. coli* to invade epithelial cells, particularly those of the colon, is similar to that shown by *Shigella*. The signs and lesions that result are dysentery, fever, and multiple foci of ulcerative enteritis.

Septicemic Colibacillosis. (Colisepticemic form.) In this form of the disease, the organisms invade the host (possibly through the oral cavity, respiratory system, pharynx, or umbilicus) and produce an **endotoxin** that apparently causes the lesions. Unless the enterotoxic form occurs simultaneously, the bacteria do not reach the small intestine. Thus diarrhea or intestinal lesions do not occur. This form is most dramatic and best described in young calves (Fey, 1972). Calves that are deficient in immunoglobulin (usually as a result of failure to receive colostrum) are most susceptible.

The signs and lesions are typical of bacterial arthritis, polyserositis, meningitis, ophthalmitis, and pyelonephritis, with bacterial emboli and necrotizing, purulent, or fibrinous exudation.

Thus, different strains of *Escherichia coli* have the ability, under certain conditions of the host, to produce pathologic manifestations involving at least four pathogenetic mechanisms. It appears likely that concepts will change or details will deepen with respect to this problem, since many investigators are currently conducting research on it.

Botes, H. J. W.: Fatal enterobacterial septicaemia in lambs. J. S. Afr. Vet. Med. Assoc., 37:17–25, 1966.

Christie, B. R., and Waxler, G. L.: Experimental colibacillosis in gnotobiotic baby pigs. I. Microbiological and clinical aspects. II. Pathology. Can. J. Comp. Med., 37:261–270, 271–280, 1973.

Clugston, R. E., and Nielsen, N. O.: Experimental edema disease of swine (*E. coli* enterotoxemia). I. Detection and preparation of an active principle. Can. J. Comp. Med., 38:22–28, 1974.

Clugston, R. E., Nielsen, N. O., and Roe, W. E.: Experimental edema disease of swine (*E. coli* enterotoxemia). II. The development of hypertension after the intravenous administration of edema disease principle. Can. J. Comp. Med., 38:29–33, 1974.

Clugston, R. E., Nielson, N. O., and Smith, D. L. T.: Experimental edema disease of swine (*E. coli* enterotoxemia). III. Pathology and pathogenesis. Can. J. Comp. Med., 38:34–43, 1974.

Dam, A.: Experimental infection of newborn piglets and weanling pigs with haemolytic *E. coli*, strain A₁, serotype 0149:K91:H10. Acta Vet. Scand., 12:293–296, 1971.

Drees, D. T., and Waxler, G. L.: Enteric colibacillosis in gnotobiotic swine. I. A fluorescence microscopic study. II. An electron microscopic study. Am. J. Vet. Res., 31:1147–1157, 1159–1171, 1970.

Du Pont, H. L., et al.: Pathogenesis of *Escherichia coli* diarrhea. N. Engl. J. Med., 285:1–9, 1971.

Fey, H.: Colibacillosis in Calves. Bern, Hans Huber, 1972.

Fox, M. W., and Haynes, E.: Neonatal colibacillosis in the dog. J. Small Anim. Pract., 7:599–603, 1966.

Gangarosa, E. J., and Merson, M. H.: Epidemiologic assessment of the relevance of the so-called enteropathogenic serogroups of *Escherichia coli* in diarrhea. N. Engl. J. Med., 296:1210–1213, 1977.

Gay, C. C.: *Escherichia coli* and neonatal disease of calves. Bact. Rev., 29:75–101, 1965.

Ginder, D. R.: Urinary tract infection and pyelonephritis due to *Escherichia coli* in dogs infected with canine adenovirus. J. Infect. Dis., 129:715–719, 1974.

Guerrant, R. L., et al.: Effect of *Escherichia coli* on fluid transport across canine small bowel: mechanism and time-course with enterotoxin and whole bacterial cells. J. Clin. Invest., 52:1707–1714, 1973.

Gyles, C. L., and Barnum, D. A.: A heatlabile enterotoxin from strains of *Escherichia coli* enteropathogenic for pigs. J. Infect. Dis., 120:419–426, 1969.

Hornich, M., et al.: Enteric *Escherichia coli* infections. Morphological findings in the intestinal mucosa of healthy and diseased piglets. Vet. Path., 10:484–500, 1973.

Johannsen, U.: Pathology and pathogenesis of spontaneous coli enterotoxaemia and the experimental coli endotoxin syndrome in pigs. VII. Pathology of the mesenteric nodes. Arch. Exp. Veterinaermed., 28:455–475, 1974.

Jones, J. E. T., and Smith, H. W.: Histological studies on weaned pigs suffering from diarrhea and oedema disease produced by oral inoculation of *Escherichia coli.* J. Pathol., *97*:168–172, 1969.

Kohler, E. M.: Pathogenesis of neonatal enteric colibacillosis of pigs. J. Am. Vet. Med. Assoc., *160*:574–581, 1972.

Kurtz, H. J., and Short, E. C., Jr.: Pathogenesis of edema disease in swine: Pathologic effects of hemolysin, autolysate, and endotoxin of *Escherichia coli* (0141). Am. J. Vet. Res., *37*:15–24, 1976.

Logan, E.F., and Penhale, W.J.: Studies on the immunity of the calf to colibacillosis. V. The experimental reproduction of enteric colibacillosis. Vet. Rec., *91*:419–423, 1972.

McClure, H. M., Strozier, L. M., and Keeling, M. E.: Enteropathogenic *Escherichia coli* infection in anthropoid apes. J. Am. Vet. Med. Assoc., *161*:687–689, 1972.

Meyer, R. C., Saxena, S. P., and Rhoades, H. E.: Polyserositis induced by *Escherichia coli* in gnotobiotic swine. Infect. Immun., *3*:41–44, 1971.

Meyer, R. C., and Simon, J.: Generalized infection of gnotobiotic piglets with *E. coli* of feline origin. Am. J. Pathol., *63*:57–64, 1971.

———: Experimental peracute colibacillosis. Gastrointestinal lesions in gnotobiotic piglets. Vet. Pathol., *9*:360–367, 1972.

Miniats, O. P., and Gyles, C. L.: The significance of proliferation and enterotoxin production by *Escherichia coli* in the intestine of gnotobiotic pigs. Can. J. Comp. Med., *36*:150–159, 1972.

Monteverde, J. J., and Garbers, G. V.: Enterobacterial infections in horses. I. *Escherichia coli* 023 H16 in fatal septicaemia and polyarthritis. Revta Med. Vet. B. Aires, *45*:263–270, 273–279, 1964.

Moon, H. W., Nielsen, N. O., and Kramer, T. T.: Experimental enteric colibacillosis of the newborn pig: histopathology of the small intestine and changes in plasma electrolytes. Am. J. Vet. Res., *31*:103–112, 1970.

Moon, H. W., Whipp, S. C., and Baetz, A. L.: Comparative effects of enterotoxins from *Escherichia coli* and *Vibrio cholerae* on rabbit and swine small intestine. Lab. Invest., *25*:133–140, 1971.

Moon, H. W.: Pathogenesis of enteric diseases caused by *Escherichia coli.* Adv. Vet. Sci. Comp. Med., *18*:179–211, 1974.

Moon, H. W., Whipp, S. C., and Skartvedt, S. M.: Etiologic diagnosis of diarrheal diseases of calves: frequency and methods for detecting enterotoxin and K99 antigen production by *Escherichia coli.* Am. J. Vet. Res., *37*:1025–1029, 1976.

Musa, B. E., et al.: Physiologic and pathologic changes in calves given *Escherichia coli* endotoxin or *Pasteurella multocida.* Am. J. Vet. Res., *33*:911–916, 1972.

Nielson, N. O., Moon, H. W., and Roe, W. E.: Enteric colibacillosis in swine. J. Am. Vet. Med. Assoc., *153*:1590–1606, 1968.

Pearson, G. R., McNulty, M. S., and Logan, E. F.: Pathological changes in the small intestine of neonatal calves with enteric colibacillosis. Vet. Pathol., *15*:91–101, 1978.

Rutter, J. M., and Anderson, J. C.: Experimental neonatal diarrhoea associated with an enteropathogenic strain of *Escherichia coli* in piglets. Vet. Rec., *88*:520–521, 1971.

Schiff, L. J., et al.: Enteropathogenic *Escherichia coli* infections: increasing awareness of a problem in laboratory animals. Lab. Anim. Sci., *22*:705–708, 1972.

Shreeve, B. J., and Thomlinson, J. R.: Hypersensitivity in young piglets: its relation to the pathogenesis of *Escherichia coli* disease. J. Med. Microbiol., *3*:377–385, 1970.

———: *Escherichia coli* disease in the piglet. A pathological and bacteriological investigation. Br. Vet. J., *126*:444–451, 1970.

———: Hypersensitivity of young piglets to *Escherichia coli* endotoxin. J. Med. Microbiol., *4*:307–318, 1971.

Sojka, W. J.: Enteric diseases in new-born piglets, calves and lambs due to *Escherichia coli* infection. Vet. Bull., *41*:509–522, 1971.

Spradbrow, P. V., and Cole, A. M.: The production of calf pneumonia with *Escherichia coli* and a bovine picornavirus. J. Comp. Pathol., *81*:551–555, 1971.

Staley, T. E., Jones, E. W., and Corely, L. D.: Attachment and penetration of *Escherichia coli* into intestinal epithelium of the ileum in newborn pigs. Am. J. Pathol., *56*:371–392, 1969.

Staley, T. E., Jones, E. W., Corely, L. D., and Anderson, I. L.: Intestinal permeability to *Escherichia coli* in the foal. Am. J. Vet. Res., *31*:1481–1483, 1970.

Stevens, J. B., Gyles, C. L., and Barnum, D. A.: Production of diarrhea in pigs in response to *Escherichia coli* enterotoxin. Am. J. Vet. Res., *33*:2511–2526, 1972.

Tennant, B., Harrold, D., and Reina-Guerra, M.: Physiologic and metabolic factors in the pathogenesis of neonatal enteric infections in calves. J. Am. Vet. Med. Assoc., *161*:993–1007, 1972.

Waxler, G. L., and Britt, A. L.: Polyserositis and arthritis due to *Escherichia coli* in gnotobiotic pigs. Can. J. Comp. Med., *36*:226–233, 1972.

Wray, C., and Thomlinson, J. R.: The effects of *Escherichia coli* endotoxin in calves. Res. Vet. Sci., *13*:546–553, 1972.

———: Anaphylactic shock to *Escherichia coli* endotoxin in calves. Res. Vet. Sci., *13*:563–569, 1972.

———: Lesions and bacteriological findings in colibacillosis of calves. Br. Vet. J., *130*:189–199, 1974.

———: Factors influencing occurrence of colibacillosis in calves. Vet. Rec., *96*:52–56, 1975.

INFECTIONS DUE TO KLEBSIELLA

Klebsiella pneumoniae (Friedlander's bacillus) is another normal inhabitant of the gastrointestinal tract that has a pathogenic potential. Under conditions which presently are poorly understood, *Klebsiella* may be a causative factor in pneumonia or septicemia in man or animals. Nonhuman primates are particularly susceptible to these organisms.

Fox, J. G., and Rohovsky, M. W.: Meningitis caused by *Klebsiella spp* in two rhesus monkeys. J. Am. Vet. Med. Assoc., 167:634–636, 1975.

———: Klebsiella in monkeys. J. Am. Vet. Med. Assoc., 168:276, 1976.

Giles, R. C., Jr., Hildebrandt, P. K., and Tate, C.: *Klebsiella* air sacculitis in the owl monkey (*Aotus trivirgatus*). Lab. Anim. Sci., 24:610–616, 1974.

Kageruka, P., Mortelmans, J., and Vercruysse, J.: *Klebsiella pneumoniae* infections in monkeys. Acta Zool. Pathol. Antverp., 52:83–88, 1971.

Schmidt, R. E., and Butler, T. M.: Klebsiella-enterobacter infections in chimpanzees. Lab. Anim. Sci., 21:946–949, 1972.

Walker, R. I., and Chesbro, W.: *Klebsiella pneumoniae* and *Staphylococcus aureus* infections in mice: differences in uremia and ammoniagenesis. Infect. Immun., 12:571–575, 1975.

Wyand, D. S., and Hayden, D. W.: Klebseilla infection in muskrats. J. Am. Vet. Med. Assoc., 163:589–592, 1973.

INFECTIONS DUE TO CORYNEBACTERIUM

Bacterial organisms classified in the genus *Corynebacterium* are involved in a wide variety of lesions in many domestic and wild animals, as well as in man. The best known organism in this genus is *Corynebacterium diphtheriae*, the causative agent of human diphtheria. Other members of this group are often referred to collectively as "diphtheroid bacteria." The lesions produced by various species of *Corynebacterium* show much variety: the tissue reaction to some is essentially suppurative, as it is to many of the simpler bacteria; the reactions to others is granulomatous. Because of these variations in pathologic characteristics, it is rather difficult to place these infections in a single group, but since the bacteriologic classification in current use includes this genus within the order Eubacteriales, all infections with *Corynebacterium* will be discussed together.

The bacteria making up this genus are gram-positive, nonacid-fast, and occasionally "beaded" in stained sections. They grow slowly on ordinary media, some species producing hemolysis on blood agar. Artificial inoculation of laboratory animals usually gives rise to purulent reactive lesions. *Corynebacterium* has some similarities to organisms in the genera *Mycobacterium* and *Nocardia*, including a common cell wall antigen, which may be responsible for complement-fixing antibodies to paratuberculosis (Johne's disease) in cattle infected with *Corynebacterium renale* (Buchanan and Gibbons, 1974; Gilmour and Goudswaard, 1972).

Corynebacterium pyogenes is a common and important organism in pyogenic processes in cattle, swine, sheep, and goats. In cattle, the organisms are found in abscesses, many of which are heavily encapsulated, and in necrotic and suppurative pneumonias. They have also been isolated from the suppurative arthritis and umbilical infections in calves, and from purulent metritis and mastitis in cows. In swine, the "diphtheroid" organisms produce diseases resembling those of cattle; infection often follows farrowing and arthritis is a common manifestation. In sheep and goats, purulent pneumonias and abscesses in the upper respiratory tract have been described.

Corynebacterium renale is commonly associated with "bacillary" pyelonephritis of cattle, in which chronic purulent cystitis and urethritis accompany the inflammatory changes in the ureters and renal pelvis. Horses and sheep may become infected, but dogs rarely. *Corynebacterium suis* has been associated with a similar cystitis and pyelonephritis in swine.

Corynebacterium ulcerans is a strain that appears to be intermediate between *C. diphtheriae* and *C. pseudotuberculosis* and has been recovered from the nasopharynx of persons with upper respiratory infection (Buchanan and Gibbons, 1974). It appears to be the causative agent in infection of bite wounds and pulmonary abscesses in nonhuman primates (*Macaca mulatta*, *M. fascicularis*, and *Presbytis entellus*) (May, 1972). The organism has also been isolated

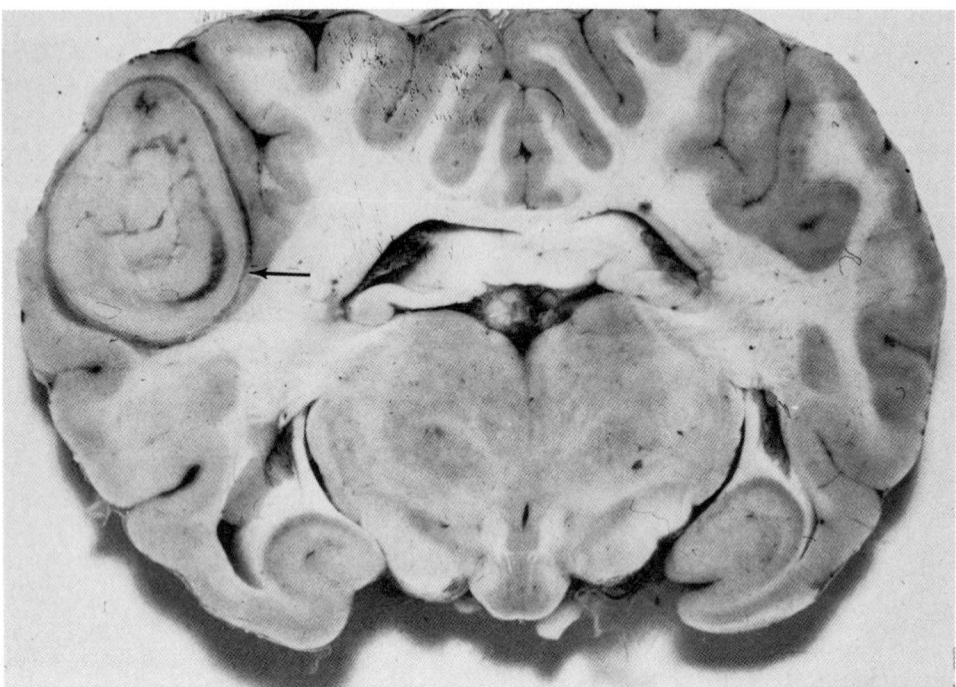

Fig. 11–9. Abscess in the cerebral cortex of a three-year-old male deer. *Corynebacterium pseudotuber-culosis* was recovered in pure culture from the abscess.

from cases of mastitis in dairy cattle and a bonnet macaque *(Macaca radiata)* (Fox and Frost, 1974).

Corynebacterium pseudotuberculosis (C. ovis, Preiz-Nocard baccilus) is the cause of ulcerative lymphangitis of horses and caseous lymphadenitis or pseudotuberculosis of sheep and goats. The lesions in the latter have some distinctive features, hence will be described in more detail.

Corynebacterium kutscheri (C. pseudotuberculosis murium) is the cause of pseudotuberculosis in mice and rats. The lesions consist of disseminated caseopurulent foci, particularly in the lungs, lymph nodes, liver, and kidneys (see also *Yersinia pseudotuberculosis).*

Corynebacterium equi is involved in a specific pneumonia of foals and has been isolated from arthritic joints in lambs and from granulomatous lesions in swine. In foals, the infection may be limited to the lungs, with lobular distribution of lesions,

or it may be systemic, with abscess formation in many viscera. The microscopic lesion is often characterized by the large numbers of macrophages in the exudate. These cells usually contain demonstrable bacteria in large numbers.

Ovine Caseous Lymphadenitis (Pseudotuberculosis of Sheep and Goats)

Caseous lymphadenitis often occurs as an inapparent infection in sheep and goats, but occasionally it causes overt disease and sometimes death. Signs are rarely recorded, although superficial lymph nodes may become abscessed and lesions in the lungs may produce respiratory distress. The entity is most likely to be encountered as an incidental finding in slaughtered animals. The causative organism is *Corynebacterium pseudotuberculosis (Corynebacterium ovis),* a gram-positive diphtheroid bacillus, but the mode of infection is unknown.

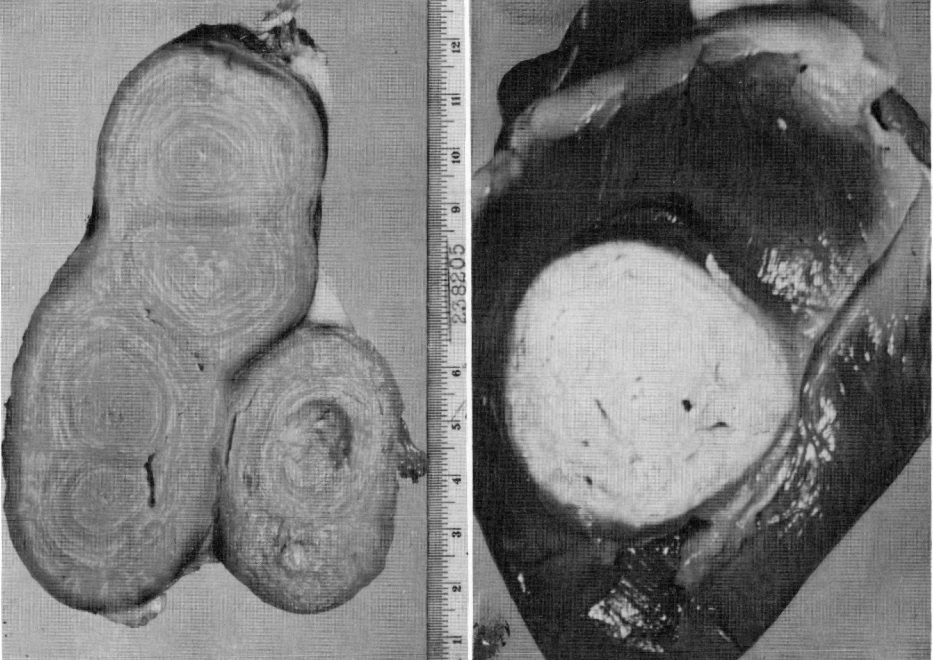

Fig. 11–10. Caseous lymphadenitis. *A,* Thoracic lymph nodes of a sheep. Note concentric laminations. (Courtesy of Armed Forces Institute of Pathology.) Contributor: Dr. C. L. Davis. *B,* A lesion in the myocardium of a sheep. (Courtesy of Dr. C. L. Davis.)

Lesions. The lesions are found in the lungs and lymph nodes, particularly the prescapular, prefemoral, and mediastinal nodes, and less often in the kidney and other viscera. Microscopic evidence indicates that the lesion starts as a small nidus of epithelioid cells, but is soon overtaken by caseation necrosis, which becomes the predominant feature. The central caseous mass is soon surrounded by a thin layer of epithelioid cells admixed with lymphocytes, to which an external reinforcing layer of fibrous connective tissue is added. As the lesion grows, the epithelioid and fibrous reactive layers undergo necrosis, the epithelioid layer dying earlier. While the fibrous layer still remains visible, new reactive layers form outside it and successively become necrotic. The result is a spherical, onion-like, concentrically laminated mass which may reach a diameter of several centimeters. Calcification may occur, but giant cells are not seen.

The gross appearance of lymph nodes is characteristic, the entire node being greatly enlarged and almost replaced by a single globoid lesion. In cross section it is concentrically laminated, layers of fibrous capsule alternating with caseous, friable material that may be greenish and occasionally gritty. In the lungs, the lesions may resemble an abscess, with a central, semifluid mass of yellowish or greenish pus.

Diagnosis. The gross and microscopic features, if typical, are practically diagnostic. Identification of the causative organism depends upon demonstrating its diphtheroid morphology and accepted cultural characteristics. Pathogenicity tests are commonly unfruitful.

Biberstein, E. L., Knight, H. D., and Jang, S.: Two biotypes of *Corynebacterium pseudotuberculosis.* Vet. Rec., 89:691–692, 1972.
Buchanan, R. E., and Gibbons, N. E.: Bergey's Manual of Determinative Bacteriology, 8th ed. Baltimore, Williams & Wilkins, 1974.

Cameron, C. M., and Purdom, M. R.: Immunological and chemical characteristics of *Corynebacterium pseudotuberculosis* cell walls and protoplasm. Onderstepoort J. Vet. Res., *38*:83–92, 1971.

Chattopadhyay, S. K., Pachalag, S. V., Banerjee, S., and Bandyopadhyay, M. C.: Pathological and bacteriological studies of lung abscess in sheep. Ind. J. Anim. Health, *13*:53–55, 1974.

Cimprich, R. E., and Rooney, J. R.: *Corynebacterium equi* enteritis in foals. Vet. Pathol., *14*:95–102, 1977.

Feldman, W. H., Moses, H. E., and Karlson, A. G.: *Corynebacterium equi* as a possible cause of tuberculous-like lesions of swine. Cornell Vet., *30*:465–481, 1940.

Foss, J. O.: Identification of *Corynebacterium renalis* from the kidney and bladder of a horse. J. Am. Vet. Med. Assoc., *104*:27, 1944.

Fox, J. G., and Frost, W. W.: *Corynebacterium ulcerans* mastitis in a bonnet macaque *(Macaca radiata)*. Lab. Anim. Sci., *24*:820–822, 1974.

Giddens, W. E., Jr., Keahey, K. K., Carter, G. R., and Whitehair, C. K.: Pneumonia in rats due to infection with *Corynebacterium kutscheri*. Pathol. Vet., *5*:227–237, 1968.

Gilmour, N. J. L., and Goudswaard, J.: *Corynebacterium renale* as a cause of reactions to the complement fixation test for Johne's disease. J. Comp. Pathol., *82*:333–336, 1972.

Hard, G. C.: Examination by electron microscopy of the interaction between peritoneal phagocytes and *Corynebacterium ovis*. J. Med. Microbiol., *5*:483–491, 1972.

Hartigan, P. J., Griffin, J. F. T., and Nunn, W. R.: Some observations on *Corynebacterium pyogenes* infection of the bovine uterus. Theriogenology, *1*:153–167, 1974.

Hinton, M.: Bovine abortion associated with *Corynebacterium pyogenes*. Vet. Bull., *42*:753–756, 1972.

Hinton, M.: *Corynebacterium pyogenes* and bovine abortion. J. Hyg. (Camb), *72*:365–368, 1974.

Hiramune, T., Inui, S., Murase, N., and Yanagawa, R.: Virulence of three types of *Corynebacterium renale* in cows. Am. J. Vet. Res., *32*:237–242, 1971.

Hughes, J. P., Biberstein, E. L., and Richards, W. P. C.: Two cases of generalized *Corynebacterium pseudotuberculosis* infection in mares. Cornell Vet., *52*:51–62, 1962.

Hull, F. E., and Taylor, E. L.: Abscess affecting the central nervous system of sheep. Am. J. Vet. Res., *2*:356–357, 1941.

Marsh, H.: *Corynebacterium ovis* associated with arthritis in lambs. Am. J. Vet. Res., *8*:294–298, 1947.

May, B. D.: *Corynebacterium ulcerans* infections in monkeys. Lab. Anim. Sci., *22*:509–513, 1972.

McAllister, H. A., and Keahey, K. K.: Infection of a hedgehog *(Erinaceus albiventris)* by *Corynebacterium pseudotuberculosis*. Vet. Rec., *89*:280, 1971.

Percy, D. H., Ruhnke, H. L., and Soltys, M. A.: A case of infectious cystitis and pyelonephritis of swine caused by *Corynebacterium suis*. Can. Vet. J., *7*:291–292, 1966.

Platt, H.: Septicaemia in the foal. A review of 61 cases. Br. Vet. J., *129*:221–229, 1973.

Scheckmeister, I. L.: Pseudotuberculosis in experimental animals. Science, *123*:463–464, 1956.

Schiefer, B., Pantekoek, J. F. C. A., and Moffatt, R. E.: The pathology of bovine abortion due to *Corynebacterium pyogenes*. Can. Vet. J., *15*:322–326, 1974.

Smith, R. E., Reynolds, I. M., Clark, G. W., and Milbury, J. A.: Fetoplacental effects of *Corynebacterium pyogenes* in sheep. Cornell Vet., *61*:573–590, 1971.

Soltys, M. A.: *Corynebacterium suis* associated with a specific cystitis and pyelonephritis in pigs. J. Path. Bact., *81*:441–446, 1961.

Van Pelt, R. W.: Infectious arthritis in cattle caused by *Corynebacterium pyogenes*. J. Am. Vet. Med. Assoc., *156*:457–465, 1970.

BRUCELLOSIS

The discovery and identification of three species of bacteria, now grouped in the genus *Brucella*, were important steps in the development of knowledge concerning the complex disease of man and animals now known as **brucellosis**. *Brucella melitensis*, the first to be recognized, was isolated in 1887 from the spleen of patients dead of "Mediterranean" or "gastric fever" (later "Malta fever") by David Bruce, whose name is identified with the organism and the disease. It was several years later (1905) before the infection was traced to the milk goat, which even today is the most common source of the organism, although it also has been isolated from the milk of infected cattle and from aborted fetuses of sheep.

A second step, in 1897, was the isolation and identification of *Brucella abortus* from aborted bovine fetuses and fetal membranes by the Danish veterinarian, Frederick Bang. The infection of cattle caused by that organism has since been known as "Bang's disease" or "Bang's abortion disease." Eventually it was proved that the causative organism was ubiquitous, natural infections occurring not only in cattle, but in man, horses, fowl, sheep, dogs, deer, and bison. One important source of infection for man is cow's milk, although contact with aborted bovine fetuses or slaughtered cattle has also produced the disease. The characteristic undulating or

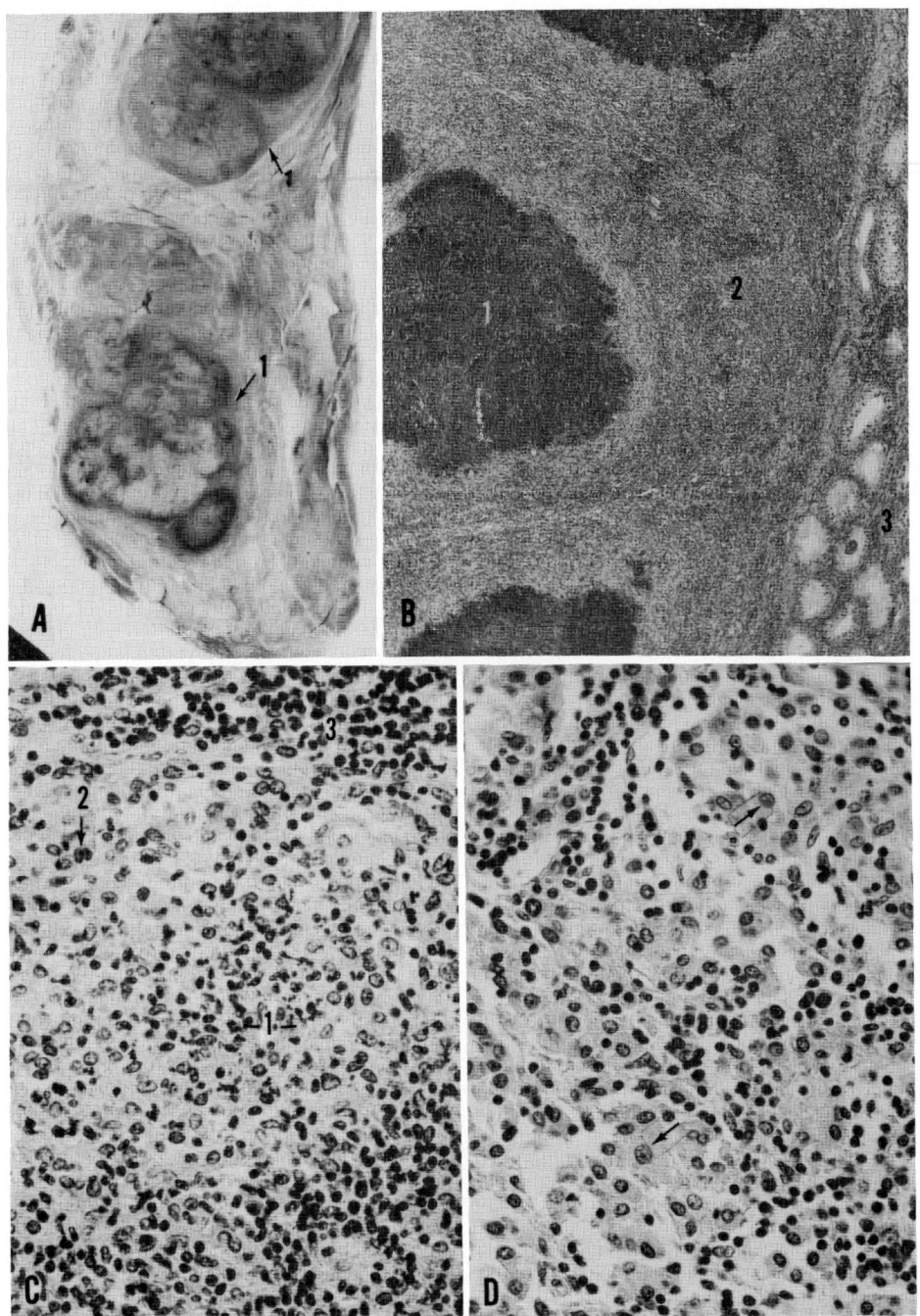

Fig. 11–11. Brucellosis. *A*, Granulomatous lesions *(1)* in the seminal vesicle of a bull. Contributor: Bureau of Animal Industry, U. S. Department of Agriculture. *B*, Necrotic foci *(1)* surrounded by epithelioid granulation tissue *(2)*, displacing seminiferous tubules *(3)* of swine testicle. Contributor: Dr. H. C. H. Kernkamp. *C*, Experimental brucellosis, lung of guinea pig (× 300). Necrotic center *(1)* surrounded by epithelioid cells *(2)* and lymphocytes *(3)*. *D*, Another field of *C* (× 300). Epithelioid cells (arrows) mixed with lymphocytes. (Courtesy of Armed Forces Institute of Pathology.) Contributor: Dr. J. Victor.

recurrent fever often observed in the human disease has given rise to the name "undulant fever."

The third organism to be included in the genus *Brucella* was originally identified by Traum in 1914 in aborted swine fetuses. This organism, *Brucella suis*, also infects man and, in addition, has been isolated from naturally infected horses, cattle, fowl, and dogs. The disease in man, usually acquired from contact with swine, differs little from brucellosis caused by *Brucella abortus*, except that it tends to be more severe and persistent.

The three species of the genus *Brucella* (*melitensis, abortus*, and *suis*) are similar in morphologic and other characteristics but can be differentiated by bacteriologic methods. Some bacteriologists, however, contend that each of these is but a strain of the same species. For our purposes, members of the genus *Brucella* may be described as small, gram-negative bacillary organisms varying from 0.4 to 3.0 μ in length and 0.4 to 0.8 μ in width, with coccoid forms outnumbering rod forms under some cultural conditions. *Brucella abortus* differs from *Br. suis* and *Br. melitensis* in one particular cultural characteristic: it requires reduced oxygen tension for initial cultivation on artificial media, although after several passages it will grow under ordinary atmospheric conditions. Of importance to the laboratory study of these organisms is the high susceptibility of the guinea pig to artificial infection. In that rodent, it produces a septicemic disease with multiple lesions grossly resembling those of tuberculosis.

Two other species are included in the genus *Brucella: Brucella ovis*, which causes chronic epididymitis in rams, and *Brucella canis*, which causes abortion in dogs.

Signs. Each of the five species of brucella has an affinity for the male and female reproductive organs, and the clinical signs are referable to these systems, most often presenting as abortion or epididymitis and orchitis. However, the organisms may localize in other organs and tissues, such as mammary gland, lymph nodes, joints, bone, and cartilage, resulting in diverse clinical signs. Bovine brucellosis, which is usually spread by contact with infective uterine discharges, is principally characterized by abortion between the seventh and eighth months of gestation. Although once a major cause of abortion, bovine brucellosis is no longer a significant cause of bovine abortion in the United States, owing to the use of strain 19 vaccine and testing programs. In bulls, the principal clinical sign is sterility. Swelling of the scrotum may be observed, but clinical signs of orchitis usually are not obvious. Strain 19 vaccine is pathogenic for bulls, producing identical lesions to natural infection.

Brucellosis in swine, which is usually transmitted by coitus, causes abortion between the second and third months of gestation. Orchitis occurs in infected boars. Skeletal localization appears to be more frequent in swine than in other species.

Brucella melitensis infection in sheep and goats is associated with late abortion. It is not an important infection in the United States. *Brucella ovis* is principally associated with epididymitis in rams, though reportedly invasion of the pregnant uterus occurs, which can result in abortion. *Brucella canis* infection in dogs causes abortion between 45 and 55 days of gestation, and epididymitis and orchitis.

Lesions. The lesions of brucellosis in animals are as protean as the clinical manifestations. The tendency of the organisms to circulate throughout the body in the blood at one stage and to localize in certain organs at a later stage is typical, but differs between species. It is difficult to generalize about the anatomic manifestations of brucellosis, but since the basic tissue response appears to be the same in all lesions, it will be described before the gross manifestations are discussed.

When living *Brucella* organisms localize in tissues, they attract phagocytic cells.

After they are engulfed, they grow and multiply in the cytoplasm of these cells, hence, the predominant manifestation is the accumulation of epithelioid cells. Thus an early lesion in a nonsensitized animal appears microscopically as a tiny nodule of epithelioid cells surrounded by a narrow zone of lymphocytes. As the disease progresses and the host becomes sensitized to the organisms, caseous necrosis occurs in the center of larger lesions and fibrous tissue is laid down at the periphery. Necrosis of cells attracts neutrophils and lymphocytes, which may become important elements of the tissue reaction. Frank abscesses are rarely formed, for the tissue reaction is not purulent. In some instances inflammation is diffuse; epithelioid cells, lymphocytes, and neutrophils make up the exudate, and nodules or frank granulomas seldom form.

The gross lesions are often subtle and rarely diagnostic. They have been described most clearly in organs that exhibit clinically recognizable manifestations. For example, the bovine placenta is believed to show specific changes when infected with *Brucella abortus*. In early placental lesions, the fetal cotyledons are dull and granular in appearance, and the intercotyledonary chorion is edematous. Microscopically, many organisms may be demonstrated in chorionic epithelial cells. More advanced lesions appear as yellowish granular necrotic areas on the surface of the fetal cotyledons; the rest of the chorion is opaque and thickened, with a leathery consistency. A sticky, brownish, odorless exudate, that resembles soft caramel candy may adhere to the chorion. The aborted fetus is edematous, with serosanguineous fluid in the body cavities. Fetal bronchopneumonia is nearly always present, characterized principally by a mononuclear cell infiltrate with lesser numbers of neutrophils.

The bovine mammary gland and the supramammary lymph nodes are common sites of localization of *Brucella abortus*, and induration may be the result. Microscopically, diffuse inflammation has been demonstrated, with lymphocytes and neutrophils predominating and collections of epithelioid cells and occasional Langhans' giant cells present in some areas. The epididymis and testicle of the bull occasionally exhibit lesions due to localization of *Br. abortus*. The scrotum becomes enlarged and indurated, features that can be detected in the living animal. The thickened tunica vaginalis usually surrounds large areas of thick fibrous connective tissue, which may compress or replace the testicle or epididymis. In rare instances, necrosis of the contents of the sac formed by the tunica may result in suppuration, rupture, and discharge of the contents. *Br. abortus* can usually be recovered in pure culture from the affected scrotal contents.

In swine, *Brucella suis* most frequently produces lesions in the uterus, but it may also localize in other organs. The infected uterine mucosa usually bears tiny white to yellowish nodules, which may reach a diameter of 5 mm. These nodules are firm and sometimes contain a central caseous mass. Similar lesions may occur in the spleen, liver, kidney, lymph nodes, and bone. Large abscesses, also attributed to this organism, have been described in the spleen, subcutis, thorax, and tendon sheaths of swine. Similar inflammatory processes have been noted in the epididymis, testicle, and seminal vesicles of the boar. Generalized infections have reportedly produced granulomatous lesions diffusely distributed throughout the viscera.

In rams, *Brucella ovis* infection characteristically involves the tail of the epididymis. The lesions begin as perivascular edema and lymphocytic infiltration, with subsequent hyperplasia and degeneration of the tubular epithelium and intertubular fibrosis. Escape of spermatozoa from damaged tubules incites a granulomatous response, which accounts for the major alteration of the epididymis. Primary lesions do not occur in the testicle; however, stasis results in secondary testicular degeneration. Fetal lambs experimentally infected with *Brucella ovis* develop inflammatory changes in the lung, liver, lymph nodes, spleen, and kidneys. The nature of the lesions varies from reticuloendothelial hyperplasia to well-formed nodules of reticuloendothelial cells, lymphocytes, and plasma cells. Necrosis and a cellular infiltration occur in the placenta.

Brucella canis infection in the bitch is accompanied by uterine and placental lesions analogous to bovine brucellosis. Bronchopneumonia is seen in aborted pups. Lesions described in a spontaneous outbreak in a laboratory colony of dogs included hyperplasia and plasmacytosis of lymph nodes, orchitis, epididymitis, prostatitis, and hyaline thickening of glomerular tufts (Gleiser et al., 1971). One clinical case of *B. canis* infection in a human patient has been reported in association with an infected dog in the household (Swenson et al., 1972).

In horses, *Brucella bovis* has been isolated from persistent necrotizing and purulent lesions involving the ligamentum nuchae. These lesions may occur near the occipital attachment of the ligamentum nuchae; at this site, the age-old name "poll evil" indicates some of its clinical characteristics. In the region of the thoracic attachment of the ligamentum nuchae, similar necrotizing and purulent lesions have led to its being called "fistulous withers." Other organisms, such as *Spheropherus necrophorus*, have also been recovered from such lesions, but *Brucella* appear to be the important pathogens.

Brucella abortus infection is occasionally reported in dogs. The lesions, attributed to infection, include arthritis, orchitis, epididymitis, and abortion.

Brucella neotomae, a species recovered from wood rats (*Neotoma lepida*) and ticks from them, appears to be rare and appar-

ently of little significance to public or animal health (Meyer, 1974).

Diagnosis. The precise diagnosis of brucellosis is often difficult, either in man or animals. The agglutination test and skin sensitivity (brucellin) tests are used, but neither is infallible. Isolation of the organism in cases with suggestive symptoms and lesions is generally necessary for definitive diagnosis. An antiglobulin test (Coombs) has been considered helpful, although nonspecific, in studying brucellosis in vaccinated herds (Beh and Lascelles, 1974). The direct fluorescent antibody test has been used to specifically identify *Br. abortus* in aborted bovine tissue. The organisms appear in clumps due to their localization in epithelioid cells (Cobel, 1973).

Anderson, W. A., and Davis, C. L.: Nodular splenitis in swine associated with brucellosis. J. Am. Vet. Med. Assoc., *131*:141–145, 1957.

Angus, R. D., Brown, G. M., and Gue, C. S., Jr.: Avian brucellosis: a case report of natural transmission from cattle. Am. J. Vet. Res., *32*:1609–1612, 1971.

Beh, K. J., and Lascelles, A. K.: The use of the antiglobulin test in the diagnosis of bovine brucellosis. Res. Vet. Sci., *14*:239–244, 1974.

Biberstein, E. L., McGowan, B., Olander, H., and Kennedy, P. C.: Epididymitis in rams. Study on pathogenesis. Cornell Vet., *54*:27–41, 1964.

Bicknell, S. R., Bell, R. A., and Richards, P. A.: *Brucella abortus* in the bitch. Vet. Rec., *99*:85–86, 1976.

Brown, I. W., Forbus, W. D., and Kerby, G. P.: The reaction of the reticulo-endothelial system in experimental and naturally acquired brucellosis of swine. Am. J. Pathol., *21*:205–232, 1945.

Brown, G. M., Pietz, D. E., and Price, D. A.: Studies on the transmission of *Brucella ovis* infection in rams. Cornell Vet., *63*:29–40, 1973.

Carmichael, L. E.: Canine abortion caused by *Brucella canis*. J. Am. Vet. Med. Assoc., *152*:605–616, 1968.

Clegg, F. G., and Rorrison, J. M.: Brucella abortus infection in the dog: a case of polyarthritis. Res. Vet. Sci., *9*:183–185, 1968.

Cobel, M. J.: The direct fluorescent antibody test for detection of *Brucella abortus* in bovine abortion material. J. Hyg. (Camb), *71*:123–129, 1973.

Cuba-Caparo, A., and Myers, D. M.: Pathogenesis of epididymitis caused by *Brucella ovis* in laboratory animals. Am. J. Vet. Res., *34*:1077–1086, 1973.

Denny, H. R.: Brucellosis in the horse. Vet. Rec., *90*:86–91, 1972.

Deyoe, B. L.: Histopathologic changes in male swine with experimental brucellosis. Am. J. Vet. Res., *29*:1215–1220, 1968.

Deyoe, B. L.: Immunology and public health significance of swine brucellosis. J. Am. Vet. Med. Assoc., *160*:640–642, 1972.

Delez, A. L., Hutchings, L. M., and Donham, C. R.: Studies in brucellosis in swine. VI. Clinical and histological features of intracutaneous reactions to fractions of *Brucella suis*. Am. J. Vet. Res., *8*:225–234, 1947.

Feldman, W. H., and Olson, C.: Spondylitis of swine associated with bacteria of the brucella group. Arch. Pathol., *16*:195–210, 1933.

Fredrickson, L. E., and Barton, C. E.: A serologic survey for canine brucellosis in a metropolitan area. J. Am. Vet. Med. Assoc., *165*:987–989, 1974.

George, L. W., and Carmichael, L. E.: A plate agglutination test for the rapid diagnosis of canine brucellosis. Am. J. Vet. Res., *35*:905–910, 1974.

Gleiser, C. A., Sheldon, W. G., Van Hoosier, G. L., and Hill, W. A.: Pathologic changes in dogs infected with a brucella organism. Lab. Anim. Sci., *21*:540–545, 1971.

Hamilton, P. K.: The bone marrow in brucellosis. Am. J. Clin. Pathol., *24*:580–587, 1954.

Harris, A. M., et al.: Enzootic *Brucella canis*—an occult disease in a research canine colony. Lab. Anim. Sci., *24*:796–799, 1974.

Henderson, R. A., Hoerlein, B. F., Kramer, T. T., and Meyer, M. E.: Discospondylitis in three dogs infected with *Brucella canis*. J. Am. Vet. Med. Assoc., *165*:451–455, 1974.

Hill, W. A., van Hoosier, G. L., Jr., and McCormick, N.: Enzootic abortion in a canine production colony. I. Epizootiology, clinical features, and control procedures. Lab. Anim. Care, *20*:205–208, 1970.

Hofstad, M. S.: The changes produced by *Brucella abortus* in the milk and udder of cows infected with Bang's disease. Cornell Vet., *32*:289–294, 1942.

Huddleson, F. I.: Brucellosis in Man and Animals. New York, The Commonwealth Fund, 1939.

Jacob, Kl.: Das bruzellöse Granulom. Path. Vet., *1*:41–63, 1964.

Jones, L. M., et al.: Taxonomic position in the genus *Brucella* of the causative agents of canine abortion. J. Bact., *95*:625–630, 1968.

Jones, L. M., and Berman, D. T.: Antibody response, delayed hypersensitivity, and immunity in guinea pigs induced by smooth and rough strains of *Brucella abortus*. J. Infect. Dis., *124*:47–57, 1971.

Kennedy, P. C., Frazier, L. M., and McGowan, B.: Epididymitis in rams: pathology and bacteriology. Cornell Vet., *53*:303–319, 1963.

Kernkamp, H. C., Roepke, M. H., and Jasper, D. E.: Orchitis in swine due to *Brucella suis*. J. Am. Vet. Med. Assoc., *108*:215–221, 1946.

Langenegger, J., and Szedhy, A. M.: (Brucellosis of domestic equidae: isolation of *Brucella abortus* from bursitis of the withers in Brazil.) Arq. Inst. Biol. Anim. Rio de J., *4*:49–63, 1963. VB 1193–64.

McCaughey, W. J., and Purcell, D. A.: Brucellosis in bulls. Vet. Rec., *91*:336–337, 1973.

McCormick, N., Hill, W. A., Van Hoosier, G. L., Jr., and Wende, R.: Enzootic abortion in a canine

production colony. II. Characteristics of the associated organism, evidence for its classification as *Brucella canis*, and antibody studies on exposed humans. Lab. Anim. Care, *20*:205–208, 1970.

McErlean, B. A.: Undulating fever, posterior paresis and arthritis in a dog apparently due to brucellosis. Vet. Rec., *79*:567–569, 1966.

Meinershagen, W. A., Frank, F. W., and Waldhalm, D. G.: *Brucella ovis* as a cause of abortion in ewes. Am. J. Vet. Res., *35*:723–724, 1974.

Meyer, M. E.: Advances in research on brucellosis, 1957–1972. Adv. Vet. Sci. Comp. Med., *18*:231–250, 1974.

Moore, J. A., and Kakuk, T. J.: Male dogs naturally infected with *Brucella canis*. J. Am. Vet. Med. Assoc., *155*:1352–1358, 1969.

Osburn, B. I.: The relation of fetal age to the character of lesions in fetal lambs infected with *Brucella ovis*. Path. Vet., *5*:395–406, 1968.

Osburn, B. I., and Kennedy, P. C.: Pathologic and immunologic responses of the fetal lamb to *Brucella ovis*. Path. Vet., *3*:110–136, 1966.

Peery, T. M., and Belter, L. F.: Brucellosis and heart disease. II. Fatal brucellosis. A review of the literature and report of new cases. Am. J. Pathol., *36*:673–697, 1960. VB 3516–60.

Percy, D. H., Egwu, I. N., and Jonas, A. M.: Experimental *Brucella canis* infection in the monkey (*Macaca arctoides*). Can. J. Comp. Med., *36*:221–225, 1972.

Pickerill, P. A., and Carmichael, L. E.: Canine brucellosis: control programs in commercial kennels and effect on reproduction. J. Am. Vet. Med. Assoc., *160*:1607–1615, 1972.

Prichard, W. D., Hagen, K. W., Gorham, J. R., and Stiles, F. C., Jr.: An epizootic of brucellosis in mink. J. Am. Vet. Med. Assoc., *159*:635–637, 1971.

Swenson, R. M., Carmichael, L. E., and Cundy, K. R.: Human infection with *Brucella canis*. Ann. Intern. Med., *76*:435–438, 1972.

Van Hoosier, G. L., Jr., McCormick, N., and Hill, W. A.: Enzootic abortion in a canine production colony. III. Bacteremia, antibody response, and mercaptoethanol sensitivity in agglutinins in naturally infected dogs. Lab. Anim. Care, *20*:964–968, 1970.

Whiting, R. D., White, B. M., and Stiles, F. C., Jr.: An epizootic of *Brucella melitensis* infection in Texas. J. Am. Vet. Med. Assoc., *157*:1860–1863, 1970.

INFECTIONS DUE TO BORDETELLA

The genus *Bordetella*, gram-negative, aerobic rods, contains two pathogenic species: *B. pertussis* and *B. bronchiseptica*. *Bordetella pertussis* is associated with respiratory infection ("whooping cough") in children. *Bordetella bronchiseptica* has many synonyms: *Bacillus bronchicanis*, *Bacillus bronchisepticus*, *Bacterium bron-*

chisepticus, Alcaligenes bronchisepticus, and *Hemophilus bronchisepticus. Bordetella bronchiseptica* has been recovered from the respiratory tract of many species and has been associated with some viral infections, such as canine distemper. Under some conditions, this organism may be the sole infectious cause of respiratory disease.

This organism has been associated with upper respiratory disease and bronchopneumonia in puppies, foals, cats, monkeys, rabbits, and guinea pigs. It was the apparent cause of pneumonia, otitis media, and meningitis in "lesser bushbabies" *(Galago senegalensis)* (Kohn and Haines, 1977). It has also been incriminated in experimentally induced pneumonia in germ-free piglets (Meyer and Beamer, 1973). The organism has also been identified in cases of atrophic rhinitis in swine. See Chapter 20.

The diagnosis is usually decided on the basis of recovery and identification of the organisms in association with specific lesions.

Fisk, S. K., and Soave, O. A.: *Bordetella bronchiseptica* in laboratory cats from central California. Lab. Anim. Sci., 23:33–35, 1973.

Harris, D. L., and Switzer, W. P.: Immunization of pigs against *Bordetella bronchiseptica* infection by parenteral vaccination. Am. J. Vet. Res., 33:1975–1984, 1972.

Holt, L. B.: The pathology and immunology of *Bordetella pertussis* infection. J. Med. Microbiol., 5:407–424, 1973.

Kohn, D. F., and Haines, D. E.: *Bordetella bronchiseptica* infection in the lesser bushbaby *(Galago senegalensis).* Lab. Anim. Sci., 27:279–280, 1977.

Mather, E. C., et al.: *Bordetella bronchiseptica* associated with infertility in a mare. J. Am. Vet. Med. Assoc., 163:76, 1973.

Meyer, R. C., and Beamer, P. D.: *Bordetella bronchiseptica* infections in germ-free swine: an experimental pneumonia. Vet. Pathol., 10:550–556, 1973.

Saxegaard, F., Teige, J., Jr., and Fjellheim, P.: Equine bronchopneumonia caused by *Bordetella bronchiseptica.* A case report. Acta Vet. Scand., 12:114–115, 1971.

Snyder, S. B., Fisk, S. K., Fox, J. G., and Soave, O. A.: Respiratory tract disease associated with *Bordetella bronchiseptica* infection in cats. J. Am. Vet. Med. Assoc., 163:293–294, 1973.

Stanbridge, T. N., and Preston, N. W.: Experimental pertussis infection in the marmoset: type specificity of active immunity. J. Hyg. (Lond), 72:213–228, 1974.

Thompson, H., McCandlish, I. A. P., and Wright, N. G.: Experimental respiratory disease in dogs due to *Bordetella bronchiseptica.* Res. Vet. Sci., 20:16–23, 1976.

TULAREMIA

The history of tularemia begins in 1910, with the isolation of a bacterial organism from lesions of a "plague-like disease" of ground squirrels by McCoy. He named the organism *Bacterium tularense* after Tulare County, California, in which the first infected ground squirrels had been found. The organism was subsequently designated *Pasteurella tularensis* and more recently *Francisella tularensis.* Accidental infection of laboratory workers with this organism was soon to follow, and eventually the natural occurrence of the human disease was established. A human disease in Utah, for several years popularly known as "deer-fly fever," was later identified as tularemia. Localized cutaneous ulceration and lymphadenitis followed the bite of a

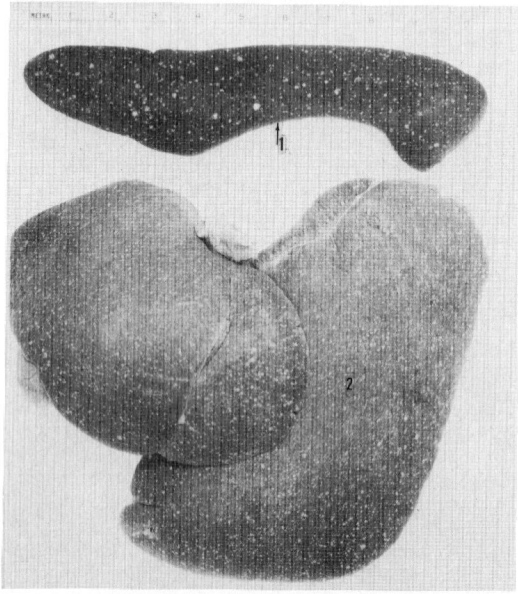

Fig. 11–12. Tularemia, spleen *(1)* and liver *(2)* of a ground hog *(Marmota flaviventer).* Note uniform distribution of tiny white foci. (Courtesy of Armed Forces Institute of Pathology.) Contributor: Dr. E. Francis.

blood-sucking fly, *Chrysops discalis*, which is probably responsible for spread of the disease among wild animals. A more important source of human infection was established by Francis (1925), who demonstrated tularemia organisms in the livers of wild rabbits collected from a market in Washington, D.C. (Fig. 11–13). "Rabbit-fever," well known among men in the rabbit market, also proved to be tularemia, a form of the disease that still is the most common.

"Conjunctivitis tularensis" in persons who have dressed wild jack rabbits is also recognized as a form of tularemia. The disease in all its forms is limited to laboratory workers or to persons who handle wild rabbits or wild rodents, and is now known to be distributed over practically the entire United States. Although wild rabbits and rodents are the common reservoir of infection, tularemia has been recognized in dogs. Most mammals are undoubtedly susceptible, and in the laboratory the guinea pig is readily infected. A naturally-acquired infection in a pet squirrel monkey *(Saimiri sciureus)* was attributed to exposure to wild-caught animals in the pet shop (Emmons et al., 1970).

Lesions. In man, the first sign of tularemia usually is a small cutaneous indurated swelling at the site of an insect bite or on the fingers or hands following the dressing of wild rabbits. Hot, painful swelling, occasionally with suppuration, soon extends to the regional lymph nodes; the cutaneous lesion may ulcerate; other lymph nodes and the abdominal viscera may become involved. Widespread involvement of lymph nodes and viscera generally results in death.

In rabbits and ground squirrels, the disease is usually recognized by the discovery of multiple chalky focal lesions scattered through the liver, spleen, and lymph nodes. These vary from pinpoint size to

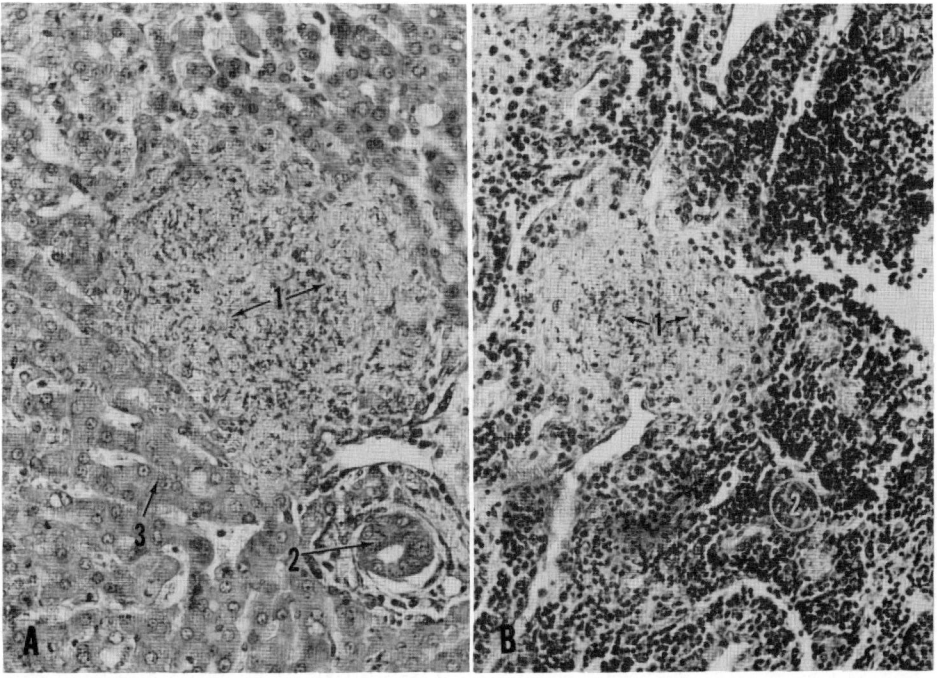

Fig. 11–13. Tularemia. *A*, Liver of a rabbit (× 120). Note necrotic focus *(1)* near portal area containing bile duct *(2)*. Intact liver columns *(3)*. *B*, Lymph node (× 210) of a rabbit. Necrotic lesions *(1)* displacing lymphoid cells *(2)*. (Courtesy of Armed Forces Institute of Pathology.) Contributor: Dr. W. J. Hadlow.

large, irregularly shaped foci several millimeters in diameter.

Microscopically, a central mass of caseous necrosis is surrounded by a zone of lymphocytes, mixed with a few neutrophils and macrophages. Early lesions may have a purulent core, but it is soon replaced by necrotic tissue debris. Thrombosis of small blood vessels is frequent and areas of necrosis may coalesce. The causative organisms, being gram-negative, are difficult to demonstrate in tissue sections, but are present in large numbers, particularly in phagocytes at the margin of lesions.

Diagnosis. The diagnosis can be made upon the basis of the gross and microscopic lesions, the isolation of the causative organisms, or specific identification with fluorescence antibody techniques. Increased agglutination-antibody titer is of value in nonfatal human cases. Tularemia must be differentiated from other diseases that produce similar lesions in the liver. These include Tyzzer's disease, salmonellosis, listeriosis, toxoplasmosis, and mousepox.

Coffee, W. M., and Miller, J.: Acute canine tularemia. J. Am. Vet. Med. Assoc., 102:210–212, 1943.

Emmons, R. W., Woodie, J. D., Taylor, M. S., and Nygaard, G. S.: Tularemia in a pet squirrel monkey *(Saimiri sciureus)*. Lab. Anim. Care, 20:1149–1153, 1970.

Francis, E.: Tularemia. J. Am. Med. Assoc., 84:1243–1250, 1925.

Goodpasture, E. W., and House, S. J.: The pathologic anatomy of tularemia in man. Am. J. Pathol., 4:213–226, 1928.

Gratzl, E.: Spontane Tularämie bei Hunden. Wein. Tierärztl. Mschr., 47:489–499, 1960. VB 1379–61.

Johnson, H. N.: Natural occurrence of tularemia in dogs used as a source of canine distemper virus. J. Lab. Clin. Med., 29:906–915, 1944.

Moe, J. A., et al.: Pathogenesis of tularemia in immune and nonimmune rats. Am. J. Vet. Res., 36:1505–1510, 1975.

Quin, A. H., Jr.: Tularemia, a disease transmissible from animal to man. North. Am. Vet., 6:36–38, 1925.

Schricker, R. L., Eigelsbach, H. T., Mitten, J. Q., and Hall, W. C.: Pathogenesis of tularemia in monkeys aerogenically exposed to *Francisella tularensis* 425. Infect. Immun., 5:734–744, 1972.

Tulis, J. J., Eigelsbach, H. T., and Kerpsack, R. W.: Host-parasite relationship in monkeys administered live tularemia vaccine. Am. J. Pathol., 58:329–336, 1970.

INFECTIONS DUE TO PSEUDOMONAS ORGANISMS

Organisms currently classified in the genus *Pseudomonas* are responsible for at least three diseases of animals, glanders *(Pseudomonas mallei)*, melioidosis *(P. pseudomallei)*, and purulent infections *(P. aeruginosa)*.

Glanders

An age-old respiratory disease of equines and man, glanders is now rare in the United States but still common in some parts of Asia. The respiratory mucosae and lungs are most frequently affected, but disseminated lesions may occur. Nasal involvement is indicated by a copious and persistent nasal discharge, which is first catarrhal, later purulent. Ulceration often occurs in the nasal mucosa, and chronic cough may indicate pulmonary infection. Cutaneous involvement ("farcy") produces indolent ulcers in the skin, with thickening of the superficial lymphatics, sometimes leading to abscesses in superficial lymph nodes.

The causative organism *Pseudomonas mallei (Malleomyces mallei, Loefferella mallei, Pfeiferella mallei, Bacillus mallei, Actinobacillus mallei)* is a short, rod-shaped organism with rounded ends. It is gram-negative, nonsporulating, aerobic, and an obligate parasite. Infection is passed from one animal to another through inhalation of nasal exudates or possibly by ingestion of contaminated food or water. Man appears to have rather good resistance, but when infection does take place, the outcome is usually fatal. Guinea pigs, dogs, rabbits, and cats are susceptible to the disease, and guinea pigs are most adaptable to laboratory investigation. Intraperitoneal injection of infected material into male guinea pigs (Strauss test) will result in acute purulent orchitis in three or four

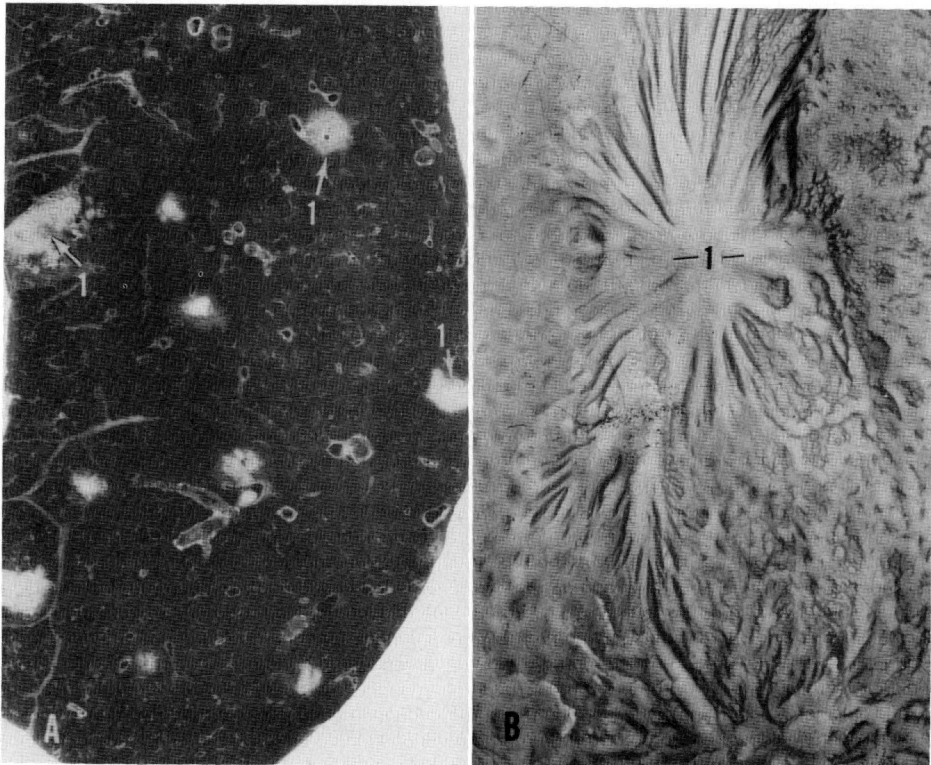

Fig. 11–14. Glanders. *A*, Sharply demarcated consolidated lesions *(1)* in the lung of a horse. (Courtesy of Armed Forces Institute of Pathology.) Contributor: Capt. R. A. Kelser, *B*, Scar *(1)* in the nasal mucous membrane of a horse. (Courtesy of School of Veterinary Medicine, Texas A&M University.)

days, and the organisms can be isolated in pure culture from the testicular lesions.

Lesions. The nasal lesions of glanders appear as erosive, deep ulcerations of the mucosa, particularly over the septum. After a prolonged course, the ulcers heal, leaving star-shaped scars. The pulmonary lesions are usually discrete granulomatous nodules resembling tubercles, but occasionally they coalesce. In a few cases, the disease is manifested as acute purulent bronchopneumonia. The granulomas usually have a caseous necrotic center surrounded by epithelioid cells, a few giant cells, and some lymphocytes. Granulomas occasionally occur in the liver, spleen, or other viscera.

The skin lesions, most frequent on the legs, appear as persistent ulcers connected by tortuous, indurated, thick-walled lymphatics. Superficial lymph nodes often become involved, suppurating and discharging thick tenacious pus. Healing occurs slowly with scarring, and the healed areas may break down, leaving persistent indolent ulcers.

Diagnosis. Clinical diagnosis is usually confirmed by means of the intradermal mallein test, which has been an effective means for detecting asymptomatic infections and making control of the disease possible. Diagnosis at necropsy is based upon the presence of typical lesions and the demonstration of *P. mallei* by cultural methods or guinea pig inoculation.

Buchanan, R. E., and Gibbons, N. E.: Bergey's Manual of Determinative Bacteriology, 8th ed. Baltimore, Williams & Wilkins, 1974.

Mendelson, R. W.: Glanders. US Armed Forces Med. J., *1*:781–784, 1950.

Melioidosis

An organism which is in some ways similar to the causative agent of glanders is *Pseudomonas pseudomallei (Malleomyces, pseudomallei, Loefferella mallei, Flavobacterium pseudomallei, Bacilli whitmori, Loefferella whitmori, Pfeiferella whitmori)*. However, the causative agents of glanders and melioidosis can be distinguished from one another by their morphology and biochemical characteristics. Although infection may be latent, melioidosis is frequently a fatal disease of man, nonhuman primates, rabbits, guinea pigs, goats, swine, dogs, horses, and cattle. It is most important in Laos, Thailand, and Ceylon, but has also been reported in Malaysia and Australia. The disease has come to recent attention in the United States following importation of infected nonhuman primates (stumptailed macaque, *Macaca arctoides*; pigtailed macaque, *M. nemestrina*; and chimpanzee, *Pan troglodytes*). Military dogs serving in the war in Vietnam were also occasionally reported to be infected.

Lesions. According to Omar (1963), the lesions are characterized by the formation of granulomatous nodules with a caseous center, which in some cases become purulent. The solid, granulomatous nature of the nodules distinguishes them from frank abscesses. The organisms are found in colonies in the nodules' caseous center, surrounded by layers of granulation tissue, which give the gross appearance a laminated character. Giant cells are seldom seen, but purulent reaction, particularly in confluent nodules, is not infrequent.

In young swine, the lungs are most frequently affected by bronchopneumonia, and the intrathoracic lymph nodes are edematous or contain granulomas. In adult swine, nodules are more apt to be seen involving lungs, thoracic lymph nodes, liver, spleen, and less often, other lymph nodes.

Affected goats usually are emaciated, have a head tilt, and terminally are comatose. The lesions are usually more widely distributed than in swine, and the nodules smaller. Ulcers may be found in the mucosa of the nasal septum and trachea; nodules and consolidated areas occur in the lungs, and multiple nodules are evident in the respiratory lymph nodes, spleen, and liver. A few nodules may be found in the heart, wall of the cecum, bladder wall, and mesentery. Nodules are also described in the lungs of affected horses, 2 to 3 mm in diameter, with a yellowish caseous center. The lungs may be edematous and consolidated; peritoneal effusion is evident, and occasionally purulent pyelitis may be associated with the presence of the organism.

Diagnosis. The diagnosis is dependent upon demonstration of the causative organism, *Pseudomonas pseudomallei* in characteristic lesions and their isolation and identification.

Butler, T. M., Schmidt, R. E., and Wiley, G. L.: Melioidosis in a chimpanzee. Am. J. Vet. Res., *32*:1109–1117, 1971.

Fournier, J.: La Mélioidose et le B. De Whitmore Controverses Épidémiologiques et Taxonomiques. Bull. Soc. Path. Exot., *58*:753–765, 1965.

Kaufmann, A. F., et al.: Melioidosis in imported non-human primates. J. Wildl. Dis., *6*:211–219, 1970.

Ketterer, P. J., Donald, B., and Rogers, R. J.: Bovine melioidosis in south-eastern Queensland. Aust. Vet. J., *51*:395–398, 1975.

Moe, J. B., Stedham, M. A., and Jennings, P. B.: Canine melioidosis. Clinical observation in three military dogs in Vietnam. Am. J. Trop. Med. Hyg., *21*:351–355, 1972.

Nguyen-Ba-Luong: La melioidose porcine au Viet-Nam. Bull. Off. Int. Epiz., *56*:964–976, 1964.

Omar, A. R., Cheah Kok Kheong, and Mahendranathan, T.: Observations on porcine melioidosis in Malaya. Br. Vet. J., *118*:421–429, 1962. VB 416–63.

Omar, A. R.: Pathology of melioidosis in pigs, goats and a horse. J. Comp. Pathol., *73*:359–372, 1963.

Retnasabapathy, A., and Joseph, P. G.: A case of melioidosis in a macaque monkey. Vet. Rec., *79*:72–73, 1966.

Rogers, R. J., and Andersen, D. J.: Intrauterine infection of a pig by *Pseudomonas pseudomallei*. Aust. Vet. J., *46*:292, 1970.

Stedham, M. A.: Melioidosis in dogs in Vietnam. J. Am. Vet. Med. Assoc., *158*:1948–1950, 1971.

Strauss, J. M., et al.: Melioidosis with spontaneous

remission of osteomyelitis in a macaque (*Macaca nemestrina*). J. Am. Vet. Med. Assoc., *155*:1169–1175, 1969.

Thonn, S., et al.: Note sur une Epizootie de Mélioidose Porcine au Cambodge. (Outbreak of melioidosis in pigs in Cambodia.) Rev. Elevage., *13*:175–179, 1960. VB 1004–61.

Pseudomonas Aeruginosa

Pseudomonas aeruginosa (Bacterium aeruginosum, B. aerugineum, Micrococcus pyocyaneus, Bacillus aeruginosus, B. pyocyaneus, Pseudomonas pyocyanea, Bacterium pyocyaneum, or *Pseudomonas polycolor)* is associated with the production of blue-green pigments and sporadic infection of plants, animals, and man. It has been associated with "leaf spot" of tobacco *(P. polycolor)* and a disease in grasshoppers. Usually, infections in man or animals are associated with some debilitating condition, such as severe burns, extensive surgical operations, and the use of broad-spectrum antibiotics, corticosteroids, or antimetabolites. Nearly all domestic and laboratory animals have been reported to be sporadically infected, and in some (mink, chinchilla), severe epizootics have occurred.

The organism is a small, gram-negative, rod-shaped organism, 1.5 to 3 μ in length and 0.3 to 0.6 μ wide. It is actively motile, with one to three polar flagellae, and does not produce spores. It is not acid-fast, some strains may be encapsulated, and it may occur singly, in pairs, or in short chains. Most, but not all, strains produce characteristic blue-green pigment in tissues and in cultures. The pigments are complex and include pyocyanin and fluorescent pigments. Other substances with antibiotic and bacteriocidal properties have been recovered from the organisms. Their pathogenic properties appear to be due to extracellular toxins, including protease and lecithinase, produced by the organisms.

Lesions. The lesions in acute fulminant cases are described as vasculitis with infiltration by large numbers of bacteria in the walls, but not in the lumen of arteries and veins. Hemorrhages, necrosis, and edema of surrounding tissues are often seen microscopically. More prolonged generalized infection results in the formation of abscesses in any tissue or organ.

Bucher, G. E., and Stephens, J.M.: A disease of grasshoppers caused by the bacterium *Pseudomonas aeruginosa* (Schroeter) Migula. Can. J. Microbiol., *3*:611–625, 1957.

Cross, M. R., Cooper, J. E., and Needham, J. R.: Observations on a post-operative septicaemia in experimental dogs with particular reference to *Pseudomonas aeruginosa.* J. Comp. Pathol., *85*:445–451, 1975.

Dominguez, J., Crasem, D., and Soave, O.: A case of pseudomonas osteomyelitis in a rabbit. Lab. Anim. Sci., *25*:506, 1975.

Ediger, R. D., Rabstein, M. M., and Olson, L. D.: Circling in mice caused by *Pseudomonas aeruginosa.* Lab. Anim. Sci., *21*:845–848, 1972.

Luis, P. I., and Soltys, M. A.: *Pseudomonas aeruginosa.* Vet. Bull., *41*:169–177, 1971.

Olson, L. D., and Ediger, R. D.: Histopathologic study of the heads of circling mice infected with *Pseudomonas aeruginosa.* Lab. Anim. Sci., *22*:522–527, 1972.

CHROMOBACTERIOSIS

Chromobacterium violaceum (Chromobacterium janthinum, C. manilae, C. laurentium) is a motile, rod-shaped, gram-negative bacterium which, in appropriate culture media, produces a violet colored pigment, violacein. This identifying pigment is soluble in ethanol, but not in chloroform or water. It is an aerobic or facultative anaerobic bacterium that grows well in water and soil in tropical and subtropical climates, and upon occasion has infected man and animals. Infections have been reported from southern United States, Malaya, Philippines, and Thailand.

In addition to man, fatal infections have been reported in swine, cattle, buffalo, nonhuman primates (gibbons, macaques, a guenon) and a Malaysian Sun bear. The disease is usually manifest as an acute septicemia with few premonitory signs and death in a day or two. In swine, a few cases with prolonged duration have been observed.

Lesions. The lesions are seen as large, circumscribed foci of necrosis in liver, spleen, lungs, kidneys, and adrenal glands. Organisms can usually be recovered from all of these organs and the blood in fatal cases. The microscopic appearance of the lesions is usually one of sharply circumscribed foci of necrosis with little or no inflammatory reaction. In cases with prolonged duration, some encapsulation of the necrotic tissue may be evident.

Diagnosis. The diagnosis may be suspected from the nature of the lesions and confirmed by recovery of the organisms in culture.

Audebaud, F., et al.: Isolement d'un *Chromobacterium violaceum* á partir de lesions hepatiques observées chez un singe *Cercopithecus cephus* étude et pouvoir pathogéne. Ann. Inst. Pasteur, 87:413–417, 1954.
Groves, M. G., et al.: Natural infections of gibbons with a bacterium producing violet pigment (*Chromobacterium violaceum*). J. Infect. Dis., 120:605–610, 1969.
Johnsen, D. O., Pulliam, J. D., and Tanticharoenyos, P.: *Chromobacterium* septicemia in the gibbon. J. Infect. Dis., 122:563, 1970.
Johnson, W. M., DiSalvo, A. F., and Steuer, R. R.: Fatal *Chromobacterium violaceum* septicemia. Am. J. Clin. Pathol., 56:400–406, 1971.
Joseph, P. G., et al.: *Chromobacterium violaceum* infection in animals. Kajian Vet., 3:55–66, 1971.
McClure, H. M., and Chang, J.: *Chromobacterium violaceum* infection in a non-human primate (*Macaca assamensis*). Lab. Anim. Sci., 26:807–810, 1976.
Sipple, W. L., Medina, G., and Atwood, M. B.: Outbreaks of disease in animals associated with *Chromobacterium violaceum*. I. The disease in swine. J. Am. Vet. Med. Assoc., 124:467–471, 1954.
Sneath, P. H. A.: A study of the bacterial genus *Chromobacterium*. Iowa State J. Sci., 34:243–500, 1960.
Wooley, P. G.: *Bacillus violaceus manilae* (a pathogenic organism). Bull. Johns Hopkins Hosp., 16:89–93, 1905.

SALMONELLOSIS

The genus *Salmonella* is made up of many species of antigenically related bacterial organisms which are gram-negative, rod-shaped, 0.4 to 0.6 μ wide and 1 to 3 μ long. They do not form spores, are usually motile, and in culture regularly ferment glucose but not lactose. All the known species are pathogenic for man, animals, or both. The taxonomic classification of *Salmonella* is based upon the identification by serologic methods of the antigens in the cell wall (O antigens, from the German, ohne Hauch) and flagellae (H antigens, from German, Hauch). This system has led to the identification of more than 1200 serotypes, most of which have been given species names. Rather than deal with this mind-boggling mass of data we chose to list in Table 11–4 some of the common *Salmonella* that have been associated with disease in man and animals.

Certain of these cause specific diseases and are host specific, such as *S. abortus-equi* in equine abortion, and *S. typhi* in human typhoid fever. Other serotypes are not host specific, producing disease, usually gastroenteritis or septicemia, in several hosts. For example *S. typhimurium* produces gastroenteritis, occasionally leading to septicemia, in cattle, horses, rodents, swine, and man. These organisms are often secondary invaders in virus diseases, such as hog cholera, but are believed to contribute greatly to losses from death. Overcrowding, transport and exposure to cold also increase susceptibility to salmonella. The infections are most frequent and of greatest concern in young animals. Recovered animals may become carriers and shed salmonella in their feces, representing a serious obstacle to control of the infection.

Salmonella, often originating in birds or mammals, are responsible for a specific "food poisoning" in man. These organisms produce a toxin that causes severe gastroenteritis, with nausea, vomiting, cramps, and diarrhea, which characteristically appears 18 to 24 hours following ingestion of contaminated food. Fatalities are uncommon, but explosive outbreaks can be alarming and involve large numbers of people.

Lesions. The lesions of salmonellosis or "paratyphoid fever" in animals are those of enterocolitis and septicemia. The stomach and proximal small intestine are usually spared, with enteritis commencing in the

Table 11–4. Salmonellosis

Organism	Hosts	Disease
S. cholerae-suis	Swine	Enteritis, septicemia
S. typhi (*Bacterium typhi,* *Eberthella typhi*)	Man	Typhoid fever
S. paratyphi-A	Man	Paratyphoid-A
S. schottmuelleri (*Bacterium paratyphi-B,* *B. schottmuelleri*)	Man, rarely animals	Enteric fever, paratyphoid-B
S. typhimurium	Rodents, many other animals and man	Gastroenteritis, septicemia, "food poisoning"
S. enteritidis	Man and other species	Enteritis
S. gallinarum	Poultry	Enteritis, septicemia, fowl typhoid
S. give	Cattle	Enteritis
S. pullorum	Chicks	Enteritis, septicemia, "pullorum disease"
S. abortus-equi	Horses	Abortion
S. dublin	Cattle, swine, sheep	Abortion, enteritis, septicemia, osteomyelitis, meningitis
S. anatum	Ducks, monkeys	Enteritis, septicemia

ileum and extending through the colon. The mucosa is hyperemic to frankly hemorrhagic, thickened, often covered with a red, yellow, or gray exudate, and may contain distinct ulcers. Microscopically in the mucosa there is hemorrhage, edema, necrosis, and leukocytic infiltration principally composed of macrophages. Lesions in other organs are less consistent. Although not pathognomonic, more specific lesions are found in the liver. These include small foci of necrosis and the so-called "paratyphoid nodules" ("typhoid" nodules in typhoid fever of man). The latter consist of small aggregations of reticuloendothelial cells (histiocytes, macrophages), which may occur in association with or independent of hepatic necrosis. The Kupffer cells become prominent and the sinusoids may contain numerous leukocytes.

Reticuloendothelial hyperplasia is present in lymph nodes and the spleen, which may cause enlargement of these tissues. Hemorrhage and necrosis is common in mesenteric lymph nodes. In septicemic cases there are, invariably, petechiae or ecchymoses on the pleura, peritoneum, endocardium, kidney, and meninges.

In the septicemic form, microscopic examination reveals fibrinoid necrosis of vessel walls and hyaline material deposited in glomerular capillaries and minor vessels of the dermis. This material is believed to be the result of thrombosis with fibrin and densely packed erythrocytes (Nordstoga, 1974). This situation has been compared to the generalized Shwartzman reaction (Chapter 7) by Nordstoga (1970), and has been reproduced in swine by the intravenous injection of killed *Salmonella cholerasuis*, which was repeated 24 and 48 hours later. This procedure resulted in disseminated vascular thromboses and bilateral cortical necrosis of the kidneys characteristic of the generalized Shwartzman reaction.

Villous atrophy has been described in the ileum of pigs infected with *Salmonella cholera-suis* (Arbuckle, 1975). An experimental pneumonia due to the same organism has also been reported (Baskerville and Dow, 1973).

Of especial interest is the study by Innes, Wilson and Ross (1956) of an epizootic disease associated with *Salmonella enteritidis* infection in hamsters. This highly fatal disease was reproduced experimentally in other hamsters with *Salmonella* recovered from spontaneous cases; the organisms were then demonstrated in the induced disease. The lesions included erosion of intestinal epithelium and necrosis of intestinal lymphoid nodules with characteristic focal necrosis in liver and spleen. Of particular interest, however, was the occurrence of phlebothrombosis in the pulmonary veins, with few or no pneumonic changes, but occasionally accompanied by septic emboli in the renal glomeruli.

Rectal stricture in swine has been observed (Wilcock and Olander, 1977a) to follow prolonged ulcerative proctitis associated with the infection due to *Salmonella typhimurium*. The strictures result from annular fibrous thickening of the submucosa and muscularis at a point 2 to 5 cm anterior to the anus. Partial or complete obstruction of the rectum occurs with subsequent distention of the rectum, colon, and abdomen with stunting of growth and emaciation. This syndrome has been reproduced experimentally by infecting pigs with *Salmonella typhimurium* (Wilcock and Olander, 1977b).

Abortion in mares caused by *S. abortus-equi* is no longer a common disease in the United States. Characteristically, most abortions caused by this agent occur between the sixth and ninth months of gestation. The placenta is edematous and contains focal hemorrhage and necrosis. There is usually edema and hemorrhage of the fetus, but specific lesions are lacking. Infected foals born at term are weak and die within a few days, often with suppurative polyarthritis.

Diagnosis. Salmonellosis can be suspected on the basis of gross and histopathologic findings; however, the le-

sions are not specific, and isolation of the causative agent in association with lesions is necessary for confirmation. An immunofluorescence technique for identification of *Salmonella* in tissues has been developed (Harrington and Ellis, 1972).

Altman, R., Gorman, J. C., Bernhardt, L. L., and Goldfield, M.: Turtle-associated salmonellosis. II. The relationship of pet turtles to salmonellosis in children in New Jersey. Am. J. Epidemiol., 95:518–520, 1972.

Arbuckle, J. B. R.: Villous atrophy in pigs infected with *Salmonella cholerae-suis*. Res. Vet. Sci., 18:322–324, 1975.

Armstrong, W. H.: Occurrence of *Salmonella typhimurium* infection in muskrats. Cornell Vet., 32:87–89, 1942.

Aserkoff, B., Schroeder, S. A., and Brachman, P. S.: Salmonellosis in the United States—a five year review. Am. J. Epidemiol., 92:13–24, 1970.

Baskerville, A., and Dow, C.: Pathology of experimental pneumonia in pigs produced by *Salmonella cholerae suis*. J. Comp. Pathol., 83:207–215, 1973.

Bruner, D. W., and Morgan, A. B.: Salmonella infection of domestic animals. Cornell Vet., 39:53–63, 1949.

Buchanan, R. E., and Gibbons, N. E.: Bergey's Manual of Determinative Bacteriology, 8th ed. Baltimore, Williams & Wilkins, 1974.

Carter, P. B., and Collins, F. M.: The route of enteric infection in normal mice. J. Exp. Med., 139:1189–1203, 1974.

Cordy,. D. R., and Davis, R. W.: An outbreak of salmonellosis in horses and mules. J. Am. Vet. Med. Assoc., 108:20–24, 1946.

Good, R. C., May, B. D., and Kawatomari, T.: Enteric pathogens in monkeys. J. Bact., 97:1048–1055, 1969.

Gorham, J. R., Cordy, D. R., and Quortrup, E. R.: Salmonella infections in mink and ferrets. Am. J. Vet. Res., 10:183–192, 1949.

Harbourne, J. F., Randall, C. J., Luery, K. W., and Wallace, J. G.: *Salmonella paratyphi B* infection in dairy cows: Part 1. Vet. Rec., 91:112–114, 1972.

Harrington, R. Jr., and Ellis, E. M.: Immunofluorescence technique for detection of *Salmonella* in tissues of swine. Am. J. Vet. Res., 33:445–447, 1972.

Hinton, M. H.: *Salmonella dublin* abortion in cattle. Vet. Rec., 93:162, 1973.

Hornick, R. B., et al.: Typhoid fever: pathogenesis and immunologic control. N. Engl. J. Med., 283:686–691, 1970.

Innes, J. R. M., Wilson, C., and Ross, M. A.: Epizoötic *Salmonella enteritidis* infection causing septic pulmonary phlebothrombosis in hamsters. J. Infect. Dis., 98:133–141, 1956.

Kent, T. H., Formal, S. B., and Labrec, E. H.: Salmonella gastroenteritis in rhesus monkeys. Arch. Pathol., 82:272–279, 1966.

Meinershagen, W. A., Waldhalm, D. G., and Frank, F. W.: *Salmonella dublin* as a cause of diarrhea and abortion in ewes. Am. J. Vet. Res., 31:1769–1771, 1970.

Nordstoga, K.: Porcine salmonellosis. I. Gross and microscopic changes in experimentally infected animals. Acta Vet. Scand., 11:361–369, 1970.

Nordstoga, K., and Fjolstad, M.: Porcine salmonellosis. II. Production of the generalized Shwartzman reaction by intravenous injections of disintegrated cells of Salmonella cholerae-suis. Acta Vet. Scand., 11:370–379, 1970.

———: Porcine salmonellosis. III. Production of fibrinous colitis by intravenous injections of a mixture of viable cells of Salmonella cholerae-suis and disintegrated cells of the same agent or hemolytic Escherichia coli. Acta Vet. Scand., 11:380–389, 1970.

Nordstoga, K.: Porcine salmonellosis: a counterpart to the generalized Shwartzman reaction. Origin of hyaline material precipitated in minute vessels. Acta Pathol. Microbiol. Scand., 82A:690–702, 1974.

O'Connor, P. J., Rogers, P. A. M., Collins, J. D., and McErlean, B. A.: On the association between salmonellosis and the occurrence of osteomyelitis and terminal dry gangrene in calves. Vet. Rec., 91:459–460, 1972.

Peterson, K. J., and Coon, R. E.: Salmonella typhimurium infection in dairy cows. J. Am. Vet. Med. Assoc., 151:344–350, 1967.

Rout, W. R., Formal, S. B., Dammin, G. J., and Giannella, R. A.: Pathophysiology of Salmonella diarrhea in the rhesus monkey: intestinal transport, morphological and bacteriological studies. Gastroenterology, 67:59–70, 1974.

Seghetti, L.: Observations regarding Salmonella choleraesuis (var. kunzendorf) septicemia in swine. J. Am. Vet. Med. Assoc., 109:134–137, 1946.

Smith, H. W., and Jones, J. E. T.: Observations on experimental oral infection with Salmonella dublin in calves and Salmonella choleraesuis in pigs. J. Pathol. Bact., 93:141–156, 1967.

Takeuchi, A., and Sprinz, H.: Electronmicroscope studies of experimental salmonella infection in the preconditioned guinea pig. II. Response of the intestinal mucosa to the invasion by Salmonella typhimurium. Am. J. Pathol., 51:137–161, 1967.

Tutt, J. B., and Hoare, D. I. B.: Disease associated with S. typhimurium in cattle. Vet. Rec., 95:334–337, 1974.

Wenkoff, M. S.: Salmonella typhimurium septicemia in foals. Can. Vet. J., 14:284–287, 1973.

Wilcock, B. P., and Olander, H. J.: The pathogenesis of porcine rectal stricture. I. The naturally occurring disease and its association with salmonellosis. Vet. Pathol., 14:36–42, 1977a.

———: The pathogenesis of porcine rectal stricture. II. Experimental salmonellosis and ischemic proctitis. Vet. Pathol., 14:43–55, 1977b.

ACTINOBACILLOSIS

Infections by *Actinobacillus equuli* and *Actinobacillus lignieresi* will be considered.

Actinobacillus Equuli

A specific infection of equines appearing during the neonatal period is caused by *Actinobacillus equuli (Shigella equuli, S. equirulis, S. viscosa)*. The organism, a tiny rod-shaped bacterium, that is gram-negative and nonsporulating, may be distinguished by its cultural and antigenic characteristics. It has been recovered in numerous instances from newborn foals, the disease being contracted in utero, at parturition, or during the first days after birth. Most infected foals die within the first three days of life, sometimes within 18 hours, but others may survive for a month or longer. Occasionally adult horses are affected. The organisms have been isolated from involved joints, fetal membranes, viscera (especially kidneys), umbilical cord or heart blood, and occasionally from infected verminous lesions in mesenteric arteries. *Actinobacillus equuli* is the most common cause of **pyosepticemia neonatorum**, "joint-ill," "navel ill," or "septicemia of foals."

The disease must be suspected in newborn foals which are weak, unable to stand to nurse, have swollen, hot, and painful joints, fever, and depression, or which die suddenly within a few days of birth.

Lesions. Lesions may be difficult to discern in foals which die shortly after birth with a fulminant, septicemic infection, but if the foal survives a few days, gross lesions may become recognizable. Infected joints are enlarged and contain excessive amounts of synovial fluid admixed with sanguineous or purulent exudate. The most characteristic gross changes are observed in the kidney, in which tiny gray foci, approximately equal in size, are uniformly distributed throughout the cortex. The renal medulla may contain hemorrhages, but it is remarkably free from the gray foci, which are demonstrable microscopically as tiny abscesses. These abscesses result from a shower of bacterial emboli that lodge in the capillaries, particularly in the glomerular tufts. Similar abscesses may occur in other organs, but much less frequently than in the kidney.

Actinobacillus equuli has been reported infrequently as the cause of infection in swine. The disease is described as septicemic, affecting young pigs usually, but occasionally adults. In one case, the organism was isolated from a vegetative lesion on the endocardium in a 10-day-old piglet. The organism is reportedly carried in the nasopharynx of horses, which may be a source of infection for foals and swine.

Diagnosis. Diagnosis can be confirmed by isolation of the organisms or by demonstration of typical gross and microscopic lesions in which the bacteria are present.

Baker, J. P.: An outbreak of neonatal deaths in foals due to *Actinobacillus equuli.* Vet. Rec., 90:630–632, 1972.

Dimock, W. W., Edwards, P. R., and Bullard, J. F.: *Bacterium viscosum equi:* a factor in joint-ill and septicemia in young foals. J. Am. Vet. Med. Assoc., 73:163–172, 1928.

Edwards, P. R.: Studies on *Shigella equirulis.* Kentucky Agr. Exper. Sta. Bull. No. 320, 1931.

Edwards, P. R., and Taylor, E. L.: *Shigella equirulis* infection in a sow. Cornell Vet., 31:392–393, 1941.

Webb, R. F., Cockram, F. A., and Pryde, L.: The isolation of *Actinobacillus equuli* from equine abortion. Aust. Vet. J., 52:100–101, 1976.

Werdin, R. E., Hurtgen, J. P., Bates, F. Y., and Borgwardt, F. C.: Porcine abortion caused by *Actinobacillus equuli.* J. Am. Vet. Med. Assoc., 169:704–706, 1976.

Windsor, R. S.: *Actinobacillus equuli* infection in a litter of pigs and a review of previous reports on similar infections. Vet. Rec., 92:178–180, 1973.

Actinobacillus Lignieresi

Infection with *Actinobacillus lignieresi* (named for J. Ligniéres) produces signs and gross lesions that resemble those of actinomycosis, but differ in several respects. This organism may infect the jaw of cattle, but with far greater frequency it invades the tongue ("woody tongue"), lymph nodes of the head, neck, and thorax, less often the lung, and rarely other organs.

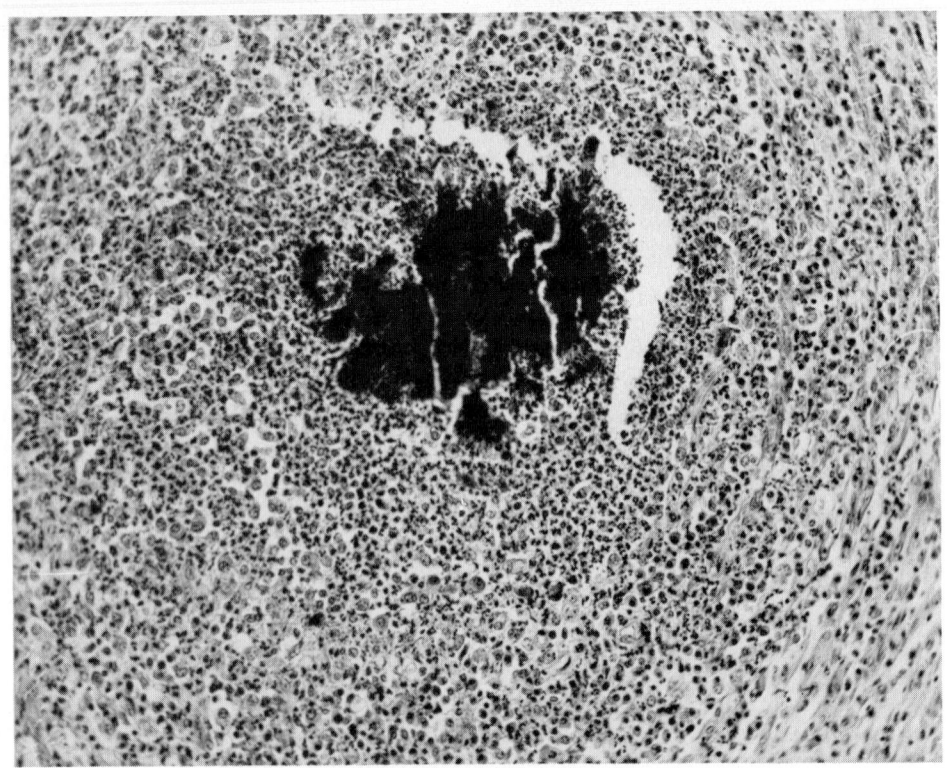

Fig. 11–15. Actinobacillosis, lung of a cow (× 160). Colony of *Actinobacillus lignieresi* in the center of a tiny abscess. (Courtesy of Armed Forces Institute of Pathology.) Contributor: Dr. C. L. Davis.

This infection in cattle is therefore much more frequent in soft tissues than in bones—a point of differentiation from actinomycosis. In the rare instances in which actinobacillosis occurs in sheep, it affects the soft tissues and lymph nodes related to the mouth and pharynx. Generalized infections have been described in man and experimentally inoculated guinea pigs. Localized soft tissue infection has been reported in dogs.

Lesions. Microscopically, the lesions closely resemble actinomycosis, with discrete colonies of organisms surrounded by radiating clubs, suspended in pus, and encapsulated with rather dense connective tissue. The colonies tend to be much smaller, the radiating clubs longer and more slender, and the purulent exudate more abundant than in actinomycosis. Gram's stain of smears or sections reveals gram-negative, rod-shaped organisms in the center of the colonies, but they may be difficult to detect because of the acidophilic staining of the background.

In the tongue, where the abscesses are usually small, diffuse proliferation of connective tissue sometimes causes such great enlargement that the stiff, partially immobile tongue protrudes from the mouth. This is the so-called woody tongue of cattle. In lymph nodes, the usual change consists of the formation of an abscess, one to several centimeters in diameter, filled with thick, smooth, shiny pus that has marked cohesive but slight adhesive properties. In the lungs and other tissues, the abscesses are usually much smaller.

Diagnosis. In tissue sections, gram-negative material in the center of the colonies suffices to distinguish actinobacillosis from actinomycosis, nocardiosis and staphylococcus infections ("botryomycosis"). Demonstration of rosettes and the absence of gram-positive organisms in fresh preparations also establish the diagnosis in bovine material. Culture and identification of the organisms may be used to confirm the diagnosis.

Campbell, S. G., Whitlock, R. W., Timoney, J. F., and Underwood, A. M.: An unusual epizootic of actinobacillosis in dairy heifers. J. Am. Vet. Med. Assoc., *166*:604–606, 1975.
Chladek, D. W., and Ruth, G. R.: Isolation of *Actinobacillus lignieresi* from an epidural abscess in a horse with progressive paralysis. J. Am. Vet. Med. Assoc., *168*:64–66, 1976.
Cutlip, R. C., Amtower, W. C., and Zinober, M. R.: Septic embolic actinobacillosis of swine: a case report and laboratory reproduction of the disease. Am. J. Vet. Res., *33*:1621–1626, 1972.
Kim, B. H., Phillips, J. E., and Atherton, J. G.: *Actinobacillus suis* in the horse. Vet. Rec., *98*:239, 1976.
Mair, N. S., et al.: *Actinobacillus suis* infection in pigs: a report of four outbreaks and two sporadic cases. J. Comp. Pathol., *84*:113–119, 1974.
Moon, H. W., Barnes, D. M., and Higbee, J. M.: Septic embolic actinobacillosis. A report of 2 cases in New World monkeys. Pathol. Vet., *6*:481–486, 1969.
Osbaldiston, G. W.: Enteric actinobacillosis in calves. Cornell Vet., *62*:364–371, 1972.
van Tonder, E. M., and Bolton, T. F. W.: The isolation of *Actinobacillus seminis* from bovine semen: a preliminary report. J. S. Afr. Vet. Med. Assoc., *41*:287–288, 1970.

BACILLARY DYSENTERY
(Shigellosis)

Primates are the only hosts which are naturally susceptible to infection with dysentery bacilli. The disease is well known in man and has been described in a variety of nonhuman primate species. It represents a disease of particular importance and frequency in Old World monkeys. *Shigella flexneri* is the most prevalent pathogen, but *Sh. sonnei*, and *Sh. dysenteriae* also occur with frequency. The strains of these shigellae species are infectious to man, but they are not the strains that produce severe dysentery in man, and fortunately, transmission from monkey to man is rare. The infection is readily transmissible between monkeys and often occurs as an epizootic. Control is hampered by infectious carriers which shed the bacilli in the absence of clinical disease.

Clinically, the dysentery varies from mild diarrhea to severe watery or mucoid diarrhea mixed with blood. Animals become dehydrated and rapidly lose condition. The pathologic changes are varied, nonspecific, and usually confined to the colon. The colonic mucosa is swollen and granular, with patchy or diffuse hemorrhage. Ulceration may or may not be present. The intestinal lumen contains varied quantities of mucus and blood. Other findings may include serosal petechiae, hyperemia of the mesentery, and enlarged and hemorrhagic mesenteric lymph nodes.

Lesions. Microscopically, the colitis is characterized by hyperemia, edema, hemorrhage, necrosis, and desquamation of the mucosal epithelium. Large numbers of neutrophils and macrophages infiltrate the mucosa. The submucosa is usually edematous and hyperemic, but only rarely is there necrosis or cellular exudation. In electron micrographs, the organisms may be seen within the intestinal epithelial cells, either free in the cytoplasm or surrounded by a membrane. It is by means of this ability to penetrate epithelial cells that *Shigella* exert their pathogenic effects.

Diagnosis. Diagnosis requires isolation and identification of the causative organism.

Arya, S. C., Vergheses, A., Agarwal, D.S., and Pal, S. C.: Shigellosis in rhesus monkeys in quarantine. Lab. Anim., 7:101–109, 1973.

Cooper, J. E., and Needham, J. R.: An outbreak of shigellosis in laboratory marmosets and tamarins (family: Callithricidae). J. Hyg., 76:415–424, 1976.

Formal, S. B., et al.: Fluorescent-antibody and histological study of vaccinated and control monkeys challenged with Shigella flexneri. J. Bact., 91:2368–2376, 1966.

Formal, S. B., Gemski, P. Jr., and Giannella, R. A.: Mechanisms of Shigella pathogenesis. Am. J. Clin. Nutr., 25:1427–1432, 1972.

Lapin, B. A., and Yakoovleva, L. A.: Comparative Pathology in Monkeys. Springfield, Charles C Thomas, 1963.

Lemen, R., Lemen, S., Morrish, R., and Tooley, W.: Marasmus and shigellosis in two infant gorillas. J. Med. Primatol., 3:365–369, 1974.

Levine, M. M., Dupont, H. L., and Formal, S. B.: Pathogenesis of Shigella dysenteriae 1 (Shiga) dysentery. J. Infect. Dis., 127:261–270, 1973.

Mannheimer, H. S., and Rubin, L. D.: An epizootic of shigellosis in a monkey colony. J. Am. Vet. Med. Assoc., 155:1181–1185, 1969.

Mulder, J. B.: Shigellosis in nonhuman primates. A review. Lab. Anim. Sci., 21:734–738, 1971.

Ogawa, H.: Experimental approach in studies on pathogenesis of bacillary dysentery—with special references to the invasion of bacilli into intestinal mucosa. Acta Pathol. Jpn., 20:261–277, 1970.

Rout, W. R., Formal, S. B., Giannella, R. A., and Dammin, G. J.: Pathophysiology of Shigella diarrhea in rhesus monkey: intestinal transport, morphological and bacteriological studies. Gastroenterology, 68:270–278, 1975.

Takasaka, M., et al.: Experimental infection with Shigella sonnei in cynomolgus monkeys (Macaca irus). Jpn. J. Med. Sci. Biol., 22:389–393, 1969.

———: Bacillary dysentery in cynomolgus monkeys following the administration with Shigella flexneri 2A by the anal route. Jpn. J. Med. Sci. Biol., 24:379–385, 1971.

Takeuchi, A., Formal, S. B., and Sprinz, H.: Experimental acute colitis in the rhesus monkey following peroral infection with Shigella flexneri: an electron microscopic study. Am. J. Pathol., 52:503–529, 1968.

Takeuchi, A., Sprinz, H., La Brec, E. H., and Formal, S. B.: Experimental bacillary dysentery—an electron microscopic study of the response of the intestinal mucosa to bacterial invasion. Am. J. Pathol., 47:1011–1044, 1965.

Takeuchi, A., Jervis, H. R., and Formal, S. B.: Animal model of human disease: monkey shigellosis or dysentery. Am. J. Pathol., 81:251–254, 1975.

Weil, J. D., Ward, M. K., and Spertzel, R. O.: Incidence of Shigella in conditioned rhesus monkeys (Macaca mulatta). Lab. Anim. Sci., 21:434–437, 1971.

PASTEURELLOSIS

Among the gram-negative facultatively anaerobic rod-shaped bacteria is a group of organisms placed in the genus *Pasteurella* (after Louis Pasteur, who described the type species, *Pasteurella multocida* and demonstrated it to be the cause of fowl cholera). At present, two groups of organisms have been removed from *Pasteurella* by the taxonomists and placed in two new genera, *Yersinia* and *Francisella*. Both of these contain pathogenic organisms that cause disease and are described elsewhere. At one time, on the basis of host-species specificity, many *Pasteurella* were given names identifying them with the usual mammalian host. These names (such as *Pasteurella bovicida, bubalseptica, equiseptica, gallinae, lepiseptica, oviseptica*) are no longer used because they are believed to represent strains of *P. multocida* (the "umbrella species").

Pasteurella multocida (P. cholerae-

gallinarum, P. bollingeri, P. septica, Bacterium multocidum, B. bipolare multocidum or Bacillus bipolaris septicus) is one of four species now left in the genus Pasteurella. **Pasteurellosis** is the overall designation of infections in mammalian species caused by Pasteurella. P. multocida is associated with several clinical entities, such as hemorrhagic septicemia and shipping fever of cattle, fowl cholera, swine plague, "snuffles," pneumonia, and septicemia in rabbits, and pneumonia and hemorrhagic septicemia in sheep. It is unlikely that P. multocida is the sole cause of disease in any of the preceding clinical syndromes. It may be only a secondary invader following debilitating conditions or infections with viruses, mycoplasma, or chlamydia.

Pasteurella haemolytica has been found commonly in enzootic pneumonia of sheep, a septicemia of lambs, sometimes in association with P. multocida in pneumonia in cattle, and as a disease of fowls resembling fowl cholera. It has also been isolated from cases of meningitis and arthritis in calves and mastitis in cows and ewes.

Pasteurella pneumotropica occasionally causes enzootic pneumonic diseases of mice, rabbits, and other laboratory animals. It may occur in the nasopharynx of man and dogs. It occasionally is isolated from wound infections in human patients.

Pasteurella ureae, the fourth member of this genus, occurs infrequently in the noses of healthy people but may be associated with ozena and other nasal infections.

Lesions. The gross lesions in fatal cases of pasteurellosis are diverse and hardly specific. In cattle, losses following shipping (shipping fever, shipping pneumonia) are usually the result of pneumonia, consolidation of the lung being most frequent in the apical portions, less often extending to the diaphragmatic lobes. Interlobular edema may be present but seldom prominent, nor are hemorrhages outstanding in the bovine disease. Pneumonic pasteurellosis is usually associated with Pasteurella haemolytica. Organisms are reportedly numerous in the pneumonic areas of the lung.

Widespread petechiae are the principal findings in "hemorrhagic septicemia" of cattle, which is believed to be caused by Pasteurella multocida. In rabbits, upper respiratory symptoms ("snuffles") may be followed by pleuritis and pneumonia or by acutely fatal septicemia, in which the blood teems with Pasteurella. Petechiae on the pericardium and serous surfaces are often the only lesions evident grossly.

Fowl cholera most commonly affects chickens, but ducks, swans, turkeys, geese and other birds are susceptible. The disease is usually an overwhelming, fulminant bacteremia in these species. Pathologic changes observed at necropsy may be limited to a few petechiae on the heart and pericardium, swelling of the spleen, and slight congestion of the upper part of the digestive tract. Swine may be infected with Pasteurella as a complication or sequel of hog cholera or swine influenza. Pneumonic lesions are commonly found at necropsy of swine.

Biberstein and Kennedy (1959) have described a septicemic disease of lambs associated with the presence of Pasteurella haemolytica. This is apparently similar to the disease described by Stamp (1955) in Scotland. The important gross lesions in fatal cases were hemorrhages on serosal surfaces, with congestion and edema in lungs and lymph nodes. Bacterial colonies, rarely associated with much inflammation, were demonstrated microscopically in the lungs, liver, spleen, and adrenal cortex. These colonies were often in capillaries and were considered to be characteristic of the disease.

Backmoro, D. K., and Casillo, S.: Experimental investigation of uterine infections of mice due to Pasteurella pneumotropica. J. Comp. Pathol., 82:471–475, 1972.

Bagadi, H. O., and Razig, S. E.: Caprine mastitis caused by Pasteurella mastitidis (P. haemolytica). Vet. Rec., 99:13, 1976.

Benjamin, S. A., and Lang, C. M.: Acute pasteurellosis in owl monkeys (Aotus trivirgatus). Lab. Anim. Sci., 21:258–262, 1971.

Biberstein, E. L., and Kennedy, P. C.: Systemic pasteurellosis in lambs. Am. J. Vet. Res., 20:94–101, 1959.

Carter, G. R.: Pasteurella infections as sequelae to respiratory viral infections. J. Am. Vet. Med. Assoc., 163:863–864, 1973.

———: Pasteurellosis: *Pasteurellosis multocida* and *Pasteurella hemolytica*. Adv. Vet. Sci., 11:321–379, 1967.

Ericson, C., and Juhlin, I.: A case of *Pasteurella multocida* infection after a cat bite. Acta Path. Microbiol. Scand., 46:47–50, 1951.

Flatt, R. E., and Dungworth, D. L.: Enzootic pneumonia in rabbits: microbiology and comparison with lesions experimentally produced by *Pasteurella multocida* and a chlamydial organism. Am. J. Vet. Res., 32:627–638, 1971.

Fox, R. R., Norberg, R. F., and Meyers, D. D.: The relationship of *Pasteurella multocida* to otitis media in the domestic rabbit (*Oryctolagus cuniculus*). Lab. Anim. Sci., 21:45–48, 1971.

Gilmour, N. J. L., Thompson, D. A., and Fraser, J.: The recovery of *Pasteurella haemolytica* from the tonsils of adult sheep. Res. Vet. Sci., 17:413–414, 1974.

Grey, C. L., and Thomson, R. G.: *Pasteurella haemolytica* in the tracheal air of calves. Can. J. Comp. Med., 35:121–128, 1971.

Hagen, K. W.: Enzootic pasteurellosis in domestic rabbits. I. Pathology and bacteriology. J. Am. Vet. Med. Assoc., 133:77–80, 1958.

Harris, G.: An outbreak of pasteurellosis in lambs. Vet. Rec., 94:84–85, 1974.

McAllister, H. A., and Carter, G. R.: An aerogenic *Pasteurella*-like organism recovered from swine. Am. J. Vet. Res., 35:917–922, 1974.

Moore, T. D., Allen, A. M., and Ganaway, J. R.: Latent *Pasteurella pneumotropica* infection of the intestine of gnotobiotic and barrier-held rats. Lab. Anim. Sci., 23:657–661, 1973.

O'Sullivan, B. M., Bauer, J. J., and Stranger, R. S.: Bovine mastitis caused by *Pasteurella multocida*. Aust. Vet. J., 47:576, 1971.

Pass, D. A., and Thomson, R. G.: Wide distribution of *Pasteurella haemolytica* type 1 over the nasal mucosa of cattle. Can. J. Comp. Med., 35:181–186, 1971.

Rogers, R. J., and Elder, J. K.: Purulent leptomeningitis in a dog associated with an aerogenic *Pasteurella multocida*. Aust. Vet. J., 43:81–82, 1967.

Savage, N. L., and Sheldon, W. G.: Torticollis in mice due to *Pasteurella multocida* infection. Can. J. Comp. Med., 35:267–268, 1971.

Schaaf, van der, A., Mullink, J. W. M. A., Nikkels, R. J., and Goudswaard, J.: *Pasteurella pneumotropica* as a causal microorganism of multiple subcutaneous abscesses in a colony of Wistar rats. Z. Versuchstierkd., 12:356–362, 1970.

Smith, I. M., Betts, A. O., Watt, R. G., and Hayward, A. H. S.: Experimental infections with *Pasteurella septica* (serogroup A) and an adeno or enterovirus in gnotobiotic piglets. J. Comp. Pathol., 83:1–12, 1973.

Snyder, S. B., Fox, J. G., and Soave, O. A.: Subclinical otitis media associated with *Pasteurella multocida*

infections in New Zealand white rabbits (*Oryctolagus cuniculus*). Lab. Anim. Sci., 23:270–272, 1973.

Stamp, J. T., Watt, J. A. A., and Tomlinson, J. R.: *Pasteurella hemolytica* septicemia in lambs. J. Comp. Pathol., 65:183–196, 1955.

Thigpen, J. E., Gupta, B. N., and Feldman, D. B.: *Pasteurella multocida* infection in the opossum (*Didelphis virginiana*). Lab. Anim. Sci., 24:922–923, 1974.

Thomson, R. G., Benson, M. L., and Savan, M.: Pneumonic pasteurellosis of cattle: Microbiology and immunology. Can. J. Comp. Med., 33:194–206, 1969.

Ward, G. M.: Development of a *Pasteurella*-free rabbit colony. Lab. Anim. Sci., 23:671–674, 1973.

Watson, W. T., Goldsboro, J. A., Williams, F. P., and Sueur, R.: Experimental respiratory infection with *Pasteurella multocida* and *Bordetella bronchiseptica* in rabbits. Lab. Anim. Sci., 25:459–464, 1975.

YERSINIOSIS

Three species of bacteria now make up the genus *Yersinia: Yersinia pestis, Y. pseudotuberculosis,* and *Y. enterocolitica. Yersinia pestis (Pasteurella pestis)* is the cause of bubonic plague in man, rats, ground squirrels, and other rodents, and is transmitted generally by the rat flea. *Y. pseudotuberculosis* and *Y. enterocolitica* produce enteric and systemic diseases which are similar but not identical. Unfortunately, both diseases have been described as "pseudotuberculosis," largely because of the gross appearance of the visceral lesions. We suggest that the term "yersiniosis" be used for these two infections. This may reduce the confusion slightly (see *Corynebacterium* infections, p. 607). Perhaps our taxonomist friends will not change the genus name before these words appear in print.

Yersinia pseudotuberculosis infection principally causes disease in rodents and birds, but has been reported in many other species, including man, rabbits, mice, deer, cats, swine, monkeys, sheep, goats, chinchillas, mink, horses, and many exotic mammals. The infection may occur as a fatal acute septicemia with few specific gross lesions, or more often, as a chronic infection that results in discrete white or gray nodules in the liver, spleen, lymph nodes, and lung. Enteric lesions may also occur, similar to those described for *Y. enterocolitica*.

Microscopic lesions of *Y. pseudotuberculosis* consist of a necrotic core of pus and bacteria surrounded by a zone of macrophages. Epithelioid cells may be present in lesions of prolonged duration, and a fibrous capsule may be formed. Giant cells are absent. In the intestine, especially the lower ileum, the necrotic lesions containing colonies of organisms often include the mucosa to the level of muscularis mucosa.

Yersinia enterocolitica, a similar organism distinguishable from *Y. pseudotuberculosis*, seems to have a smaller host range; at least, so far it has been reported in fewer species (man, nonhuman primates, dogs, chinchillas, pigs, horses, and cows). In man and nonhuman primates, it produces an enteric infection, usually limited to intestines and mesenteric lymph nodes, but it may become generalized in some instances and result in visceral lesions. Ulcers in Peyer's patches in the lower ileum have been described, as well as focal necrosis in liver, spleen, and lymph nodes. Colonies of organisms are seen under the light microscope in the necrotic zones, which in turn are surrounded by neutrophils and macrophages.

Bronson, R. T., May, B. D., and Ruebner, B. H.: An outbreak of infection by *Yersinia pseudotuberculosis* in nonhuman primates. Am. J. Pathol., 69:289–308, 1972.

Cappucci, D. T., Jr., et al.: Caprine mastitis associated with *Yersinia pseudotuberculosis*. J. Am. Vet. Med. Assoc., 173:1589–1590, 1978.

Carter, P. B.: Animal model of human disease: *Yersinia enteritis*. Animal model: oral *Yersinia enterocolitica* infection of mice. Am. J. Pathol., 81:703–706, 1976.

Dsikidse, von E. K., Pekerman, S. M., Gorislawets, J. J., and Baloewa, E. J.: Pseudotuberkulose bei roten Meerkatzen *(Erythrocebus patas patas)*. Z. Versuchstierkd., 14:147–153, 1972.

Feldman, W. H., and Karlson, A. G.: Pseudotuberculosis. *In* Diseases Transmitted from Animals to Man, 5th ed., edited by T. G. Hull. Springfield, Charles C Thomas, 1963, pp. 605–623.

Hirai, K., et al.: *Yersinia pseudotuberculosis* infection occurred spontaneously in a group of patas monkeys *(Erythrocebus patas)*. Jpn. J. Vet. Sci., 36:351–355, 1974.

Hubbert, W. T.: *Yersiniosis* in mammals and birds in the U.S. Am. J. Trop. Med. Hyg., 21:458–463, 1972.

Krogstad, O.: *Yersinia enterocolitica* infection in goats. A serological and bacteriological investigation. Acta Vet. Scand., 15:597–608, 1974.

Langford, E. V.: *Pasteurella pseudotuberculosis* associated with abortion and pneumonia in the bovine. Can. Vet. J., 10:208–211, 1969.

———: *Pasteurella pseudotuberculosis* infections in western Canada. Can. Vet. J., 13:85–87, 1972.

———: *Yersinia enterocolitica* isolated from animals in the Fraser Valley of British Columbia. Can. Vet. J., 13:109–113, 1972.

Leader, R. W., and Baker, G. A.: A report of two cases of *Pasteurella pseudotuberculosis* infection in the chinchilla. Cornell Vet., 44:262–267, 1954.

Mair, N. S., White, G. D., Schubert, F. K., and Harbourne, J. F.: *Yersinia enterocolitica* infection in the bushbaby (Galago). Vet. Rec., 86:69–71, 1970.

Mair, N. S., and Ziffo, G. S.: Isolation of *Y. pseudotuberculosis* from a foal. Vet. Rec., 94:152–153, 1974.

Mair, N. S., et al.: *Pasteurella pseudotuberculosis* infection in the cat: two cases. Vet. Rec., 81:461–462, 1967.

McClure, H. M., Weaver, R. E., and Kaufmann, A. F.: Pseudotuberculosis in nonhuman primates: infection with organisms of the *Yersinia enterocolitica* group. Lab. Anim. Sci., 21:376–382, 1971.

Messerli, J.: *Yersinia pseudotuberculosis*, Erreger einer Mastitis beim Rind. Zentralbl. Bakteriol [Orig. A], 222:280–282, 1972.

Mortelmans, J., and Kageruka, P.: *Pasteurella pseudotuberculosis* infections in monkeys. Lab. Anim. Handb., 4:95–98, 1969.

Nilehn, B., Sjostrom, B., Damgaard, K., and Kindmark, C.: *Yersinia enterocolitica* in patients with symptoms of infectious disease. Acta Pathol. Microbiol. Scand., 74:101–113, 1968.

Nilehn, B.: Studies on *Yersinia enterocolitica*, with special reference to bacterial diagnosis and occurrence in human enteric disease. Acta Pathol. Microbiol. Scand. Suppl., 206:1–48, 1969.

Obwolo, M. J.: A review of yersiniosis *(Yersinia pseudotuberculosis* infection). Vet. Bull., 46:167–171, 1976.

Otsuki, K., et al.: Isolation of *Yersinia enterocolitica* from monkeys and deer. Jpn. J. Vet. Sci., 35:447–448, 1973.

Robinson, M.: *Pasteurella pseudotuberculosis* infection in the cat. Vet. Rec., 91:676–677, 1972.

Tsubokura, M., Otsuki, K., and Itagaki, K.: Studies on *Yersinia enterocolitica*. I. Isolation from swine. Jpn. J. Vet. Sci., 35:419–424, 1973.

Weber, J., Finlayson, N. B., and Mark, J. B. D.: Mesenteric lymphadenitis and terminal ileitis due to *Yersinia pseudotuberculosis*. N. Engl. J. Med., 283:172–174, 1970.

LISTERIOSIS

A small, rod-shaped, gram-positive bacterial organism, *Listeria* (formerly *Lis-*

terella) monocytogenes, has been found in association with a number of diseases of man and animals and is undoubtedly the principal cause of some of them. Pure cultures of the organism have been obtained from human patients with meningitis, chickens with lesions of myocardial necrosis, rabbits with mononucleosis, and certain rodents (gerbil) with liver lesions. The most important infection of lower animals occurs in cattle, sheep, and goats in the form of encephalomyelitis (Listerella or Listeria encephalitis or "circling disease"). The organism has been recovered in cases of abortion in man, cattle, sheep, and goats, as well as from the central nervous system of young swine which died with nervous manifestations. A systemic or septicemic form of listeriosis has been described in man, calves, lambs, swine, dogs, cats, rodents, and birds. *Listeria* has also been found incidentally in bovine mesenteric lymph nodes.

It is obvious that the clinical manifestations of listeriosis are diverse, since they include abortion in man, cattle, sheep, and goats, and meningeal or encephalitic infection in man, cattle, sheep, goats, and swine, and systemic (septicemic) infection in man, cattle, sheep, swine, dogs, cats, and rodents. Involvement of the central nervous system, considered most characteristic of the disease in ruminants, is manifested by abnormal posturing of the animal's head and neck and its walking aimlessly in a circle ("circling"). The conditions under which infection is likely to occur are poorly understood, although evidence points to certain feeding practices as predisposing to the disease.

Lesions. The lesions are best approached by considering listeriosis in these forms: encephalitis, septicemia, and abortion.

Encephalitis. The lesions in the central nervous system can be recognized only by microscopic examination and are confined to the brain stem, particularly the medulla oblongata and spinal cord. The primary lesion is a circumscribed collection of mononuclear cells, with or without neutrophils, in close proximity to blood vessels. Diffuse cellular infiltration and frank microabscesses may occur, but there is relatively little tissue necrosis. Nerve cells can be destroyed, but the lesions are not restricted to gray matter. In some cases, the gasserian ganglia are involved. The organisms, being gram-positive, can be demonstrated in tissue sections without difficulty with appropriate stains. They are found in the center of the lesions in the medulla oblongata or spinal cord. Intense meningeal infiltration of lymphoid cells is a characteristic accompaniment.

Visceral lesions similar to those described below in septicemic listeriosis may be encountered in both cattle and sheep with listeric encephalitis.

Septicemia. Generalized listeriosis is most frequent in newborn and infants. The most characteristic lesion in this form is focal necrosis of the liver, and less frequently of the spleen, lymph nodes, lungs, adrenal glands, myocardium, gastrointestinal tract, and brain. Microscopically, the lesions consist of focal areas of necrosis infiltrated with mononuclear cells and some neutrophils. The organisms are easily demonstrated with appropriately stained tissue sections.

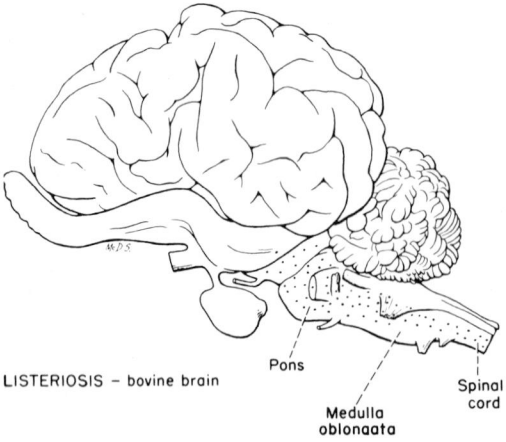

LISTERIOSIS – bovine brain

Pons

Spinal cord

Medulla oblongata

Fig. 11–16. Listeriosis, bovine brain. Localization of lesions indicated by dots in pons, medulla and spinal cord. Compare with Fig. 9–39.

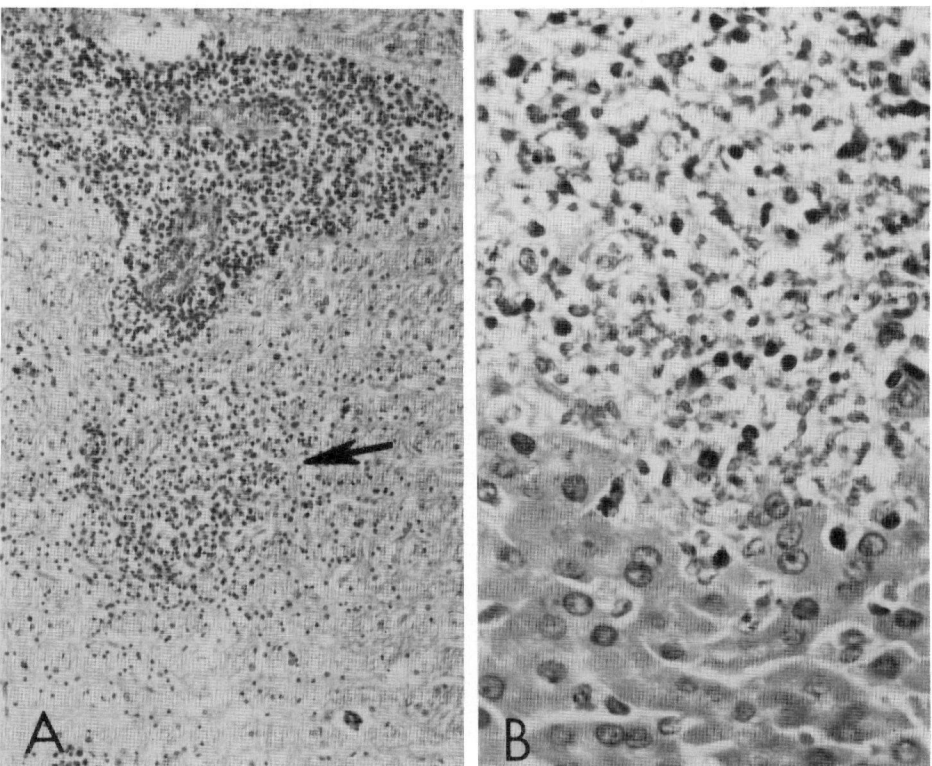

Fig. 11–17. Listeriosis. *A*, Brain of a cow. Note perivascular cuffing and a "microabscess" (arrow). Courtesy of Dr. C. L. Davis. *B*, Liver of a rat. There is focal necrosis with a moderate infiltration of neutrophils. (Courtesy of Animal Research Center, Harvard Medical School.)

Abortion. Listeric abortion in animals is principally of importance in cattle and sheep. Abortion usually occurs in the last quarter of gestation without signs of infection in the dam. The fetus dies in utero and may be severely autolyzed when finally expelled. If not obscured by autolysis, focal hepatic necrosis containing stainable organisms in the fetal liver is the principal lesion of diagnostic value.

Pathogenesis. Listeria have the ability to penetrate epithelial cells (conjunctiva, urinary bladder, and intestine), where they multiply, destroy the cells, and then are released to be phagocytized. Transport by macrophages is thought to result in a septicemic phase in some cases (Rácz, Tenner, and Mérö, 1972). Evidence points toward the centripetal movement of organisms within branches of the trigeminal nerve,

eventually to reach the medulla oblongata. Bacteria appear to move along fiber tracts, but also within axons (Borman et al., 1960; Charlton and Garcia, 1977). In experimentally-infected ewes in the latter half of gestation, *Listeria* were believed to penetrate the placenta and reach the fetal liver. Here multiplication occurred, resulting in the death of the fetus (Smith et al., 1970).

Diagnosis. The diagnosis of listeric encephalitis can be confirmed in suspicious cases by demonstration of the typical microscopic lesions, which include the combination of (1) microabscesses, diffuse purulent inflammation or glial nodules, (2) perivascular accumulation of lymphocytes, (3) lymphocytic leptomeningitis, and the gram-positive organisms associated with these lesions. Although the lesions in listeric septicemia and abortion are less specific than in listeric encephalitis, demonstration of the organisms within the necrotic lesions allows presumptive diagnosis. Confirmation can be made by isolation of the organisms in appropriate culture media inoculated with suspensions of tissue.

Attleberger, M. H., and Seibold, H. R.: Listeria infection of bovine mesenteric lymph nodes. J. Am. Vet. Med. Assoc., 128:202–204, 1956.

Biester, H. E., and Schwarte, L. H.: Listerella infection in swine. J. Am. Vet. Med. Assoc., 96:339–342, 1940.

Borman, G., Olson, C., and Segre, D.: The trigeminal and facial nerves as pathways for infection of sheep with Listeria monocytogenes. Am. J. Vet. Res., 21:993–1000, 1960.

Busch, L. A.: Human listeriosis in the United States 1967–1969. J. Infect. Dis., 123:328–331, 1971.

Busch, R. H., Barnes, D. M., and Sautter, J. H.: Pathogenesis and pathologic changes of experimentally induced listeriosis in newborn pigs. Am. J. Vet. Res., 32:1313–1320, 1971.

Charlton, K. M., and Garcia, M. M.: Spontaneous listeric encephalitis and neuritis in sheep. Light microscopic studies. Vet. Pathol., 14:297–313, 1977.

Charlton, K. M.: Spontaneous listeric encephalitis in sheep. Electron microscopic studies. Vet. Pathol., 14:429–434, 1977.

Cordy, D. R., and Osebold, J. W.: The neuropathogenesis of Listeria encephalomyelitis in sheep and mice. J. Infect. Dis., 104:164–173, 1959.

Decker, R. A., Roger, J. J., and Lesar, S.: Listeriosis in a young cat. J. Am. Vet. Med. Assoc., 168:1025, 1976.

Gray, M. L., and Killinger, A. H.: Listeria monocytogenes and listeric infections. Bact. Rev., 30:309–382, 1966.

Harcourt, R. A.: Listeria monocytogenes in a piglet. Vet. Rec., 78:735, 1966.

Jakob, W.: Further experiments on the pathogenesis of cerebral listeriosis in sheep. I. Pathological changes caused by freshly-isolated strains. Arch. Exp. Veterinaermed., 20:367–381, 1966.

Kidd, A. R. M., and Terlecki, S.: Visceral and cerebral listeriosis in a lamb. Vet. Rec., 78:453–454, 1966.

Killinger, A. H., and Mansfield, M. E.: Epizootiology of listeric infection in sheep. J. Am. Vet. Med. Assoc., 157:1318–1324, 1970.

King, L. S.: Primary encephalomyelitis in goats associated with listerella infection. Am. J. Pathol., 16:467–478, 1940.

Ladds, P. W., Dennis, S. M., and Njoku, C. O.: Pathology of listeric infection in domestic animals. Vet. Bull., 44:67–74, 1974.

Macleod, N. S. M., Watt, J. A., and Harris, J. C.: Listeria monocytogenes type 5 as a cause of abortion in sheep. Vet.Rec., 95:365–367, 1974.

McCallum, R. E., and Sword, C. P.: Mechanisms of pathogenesis in Listeria monocytogenes infection. IV. Hepatic carbohydrate metabolism and function in experimental listeriosis. Infect. Immun., 1:183–189, 1970.

———: Mechanisms of pathogenesis in Listeria monocytogenes infection. V. Early imbalance in host energy metabolism during experimental listeriosis. VI. Oxidative phosphorylation in mouse liver mitochondria during experimental listeriosis. Infect. Immun., 5:863–871, 872–878, 1972.

McClure, H. M., and Strozier, L. M.: Perinatal listeric septicemia in a Celebese black ape. J. Am. Vet. Med. Assoc., 167:637–638, 1975.

Miller, J. K., and Burns, J.: Histopathology of Listeria monocytogenes after oral feeding to mice. Appl. Microbiol., 19:772–775, 1970.

Moore, R. M., and Zehmer, R. B.: Listeriosis in the United States. J. Infect. Dis., 127:610–611, 1973.

Njoku, C. O., Dennis, S. M., and Cooper, R. F.: Listeric abortion studies in sheep. I. Maternofetal changes. Cornell Vet., 62:608–627, 1972.

Njoku, C. O., and Dennis, S. M.: Listeric abortion studies in sheep. II. Feto-placental changes. Cornell Vet., 63:171–172, 1973.

———: Listeric abortion studies in sheep. IV. Histopathologic comparison of natural and experimental infection. Cornell Vet., 63:211–219, 1973.

Njoku, C. O., Dennis, S. M., and Noonday, J. L.: Listeric abortion studies in sheep. III. Fetoplacental-myometrial interaction. Cornell Vet., 63:193–210, 1973.

Olafson, P.: Listerella encephalitis (circling disease) of sheep, cattle, and goats. Cornell Vet., 30:141–150, 1940.

Pulst, H.: Listeriosis in a foal. Mh. Veterinaermed., 19:742–744, 1964.

Rácz, R., Tenner, K., and Mérö, E.: Experimental listeria cystitis. I. A light microscope study in guinea-pigs, with special regard to the facultative intracellular parasitism of Listeria monocytogenes. Virchows Arch. [Cell Pathol.], 8:96–105, 1971.

———: Experimental listeria enteritis. I. An electron microscopic study of the epithelial phase in experimental listeria infection. Lab. Invest., 26:694–700, 1972.

Rittenbach, P., and Martin, J.: Experimental listeriosis in domestic and experimental animals. VIII. Experimental listerial abortion in ewes. Arch. Exp. Veterinaermed., 19:681–730, 1965.

Smith, R. E., Reynolds, I. M., Clark, G. W., and Millbury, J. A.: Experimental ovine listeriosis. IV. Pathogenesis of fetal infection. Cornell Vet., 60:450–462, 1970.

Smith, R. E., Reynolds, I. M., and Bennett, R. A.: Listeria monocytogenes and abortion in a cow. J. Am. Vet. Med. Assoc., 126:106–110, 1955.

Smith, R. E., Reynolds, I. M., and Clark, G. W.: Experimental ovine listeriosis. I. Inoculation of pregnant ewes. Cornell Vet., 58:169–179, 1968.

Young, S.: Listeriosis in cattle and sheep. In Abortion Diseases of Livestock, edited by L. C. Faulkner. Springfield, Charles C Thomas, 1968. pp. 95–107.

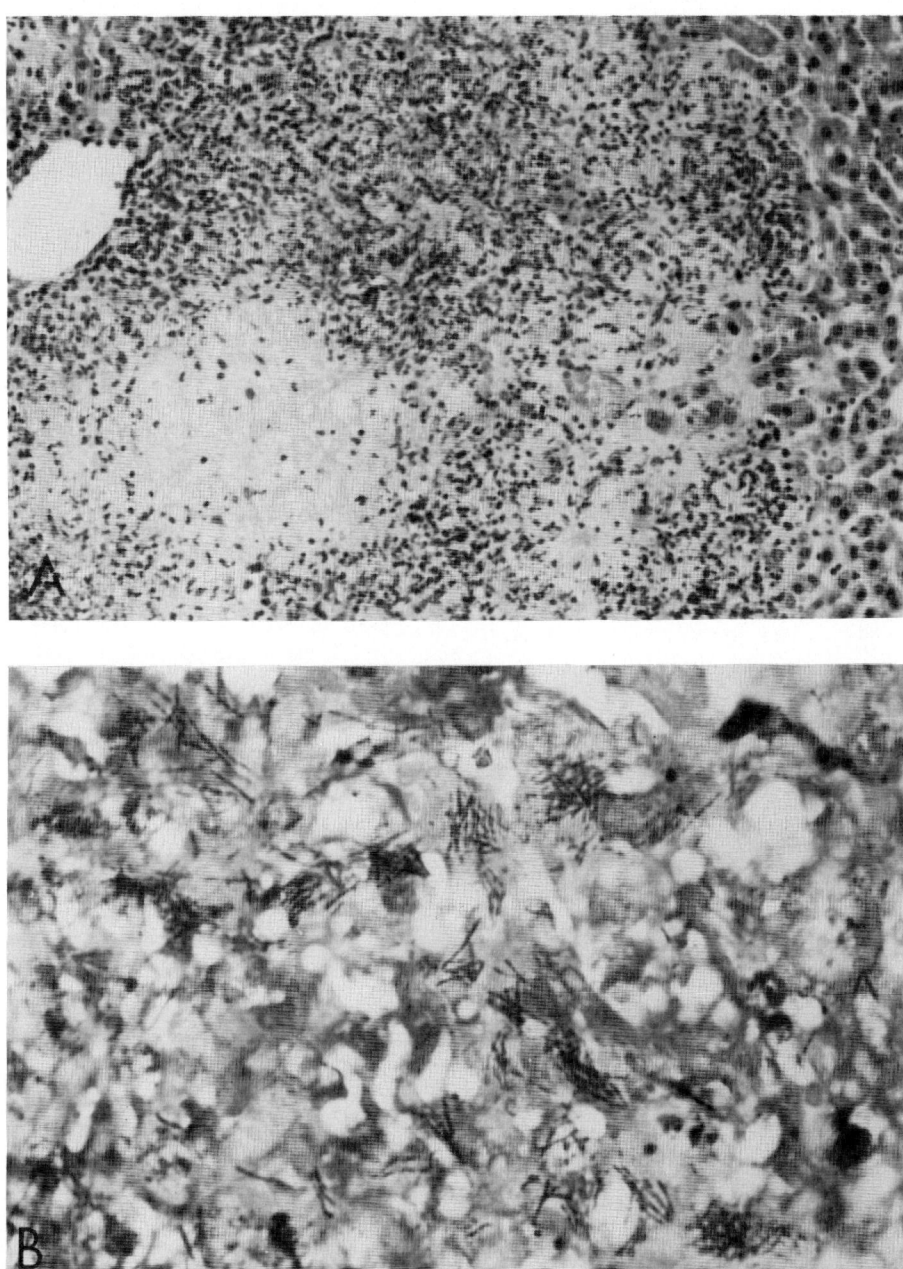

Fig. 11-18.   Tyzzer's disease in a mouse. *A*, Focal hepatic necrosis surrounded by a zone of inflammatory cells. *B*, Filamentous *Bacillus piliformis* in the cytoplasm of hepatocytes (Gomori's methenamine silver stain). (Courtesy of Dr. C. L. Davis.)

TYZZER'S DISEASE

Tyzzer's disease was originally described as an infection of mice caused by *Bacillus piliformis,* a gram-negative, curved rod 10 to 40 μ long and 0.5 μ or less wide (Tyzzer, 1917). The organism is an obligate intracellular parasite which has only been cultivated in tissue culture. *B. piliformis* appears to live as a saprophyte in many mouse colonies, producing disease under adverse environmental conditions and other forms of stress.

Lesions. The gross lesions consist of circular gray-white foci 1 to 2 mm in diameter on the capsular and cut surfaces of the liver. Microscopically, these foci consist of focal areas of hepatic necrosis surrounded by a zone of neutrophils and a lesser number of lymphocytes and macrophages. Numerous organisms are present around the necrotic foci in the inflammatory zone and in intact hepatocytes. They usually cannot be seen in hematoxylin and eosin stained tissue sections, but are clearly evident in sections stained by the Giemsa, Gomori's methenamine silver, and methylene blue techniques. Organisms are also found in intestinal epithelial cells, occasionally resulting in necrotizing enteritis. The mesenteric lymph nodes may contain small abscesses.

Tyzzer's disease has been demonstrated with increasing frequency in recent years as a disease of several species, including rats, gerbils, rabbits, monkeys, muskrats, dogs, cats, hamsters, and horse foals.

Allen, A. M., et al.: Tyzzer's disease syndrome in laboratory rabbits. Am. J. Pathol., *46*:859–882, 1965.

Carlton, W. W., and Olander, H. J.: Tyzzer's disease in a dog. J. Am. Vet. Med. Assoc., *168*:602–604, 1976.

Carter, G. R., Whitenack, D. L., and Julius, L. A.: Natural Tyzzer's disease in mongolian gerbils *(Meriones unguiculatus).* Lab. Anim. Care, *19*:648, 651, 1969.

Cutlip, R. C., Amtower, W. C., Reall, C. W., and Matthews, P. J.: An epizootic of Tyzzer's disease in rabbits. Lab. Anim. Sci., *21*:356–361, 1971.

Fujiwara, K., et al.: Pathogenic and antigenic properties of the Tyzzer's organisms from feline and hamster cases. Jpn. J. Exp. Med., *44*:365–372, 1974.

———: Tyzzer's disease in mice: pathologic studies on experimentally infected animals. Jpn. J. Exp. Med., *33*:181–194, 1963.

Ganaway, J. R., Allen, A. M., and Moore, T. D.: Tyzzer's disease. Am. J. Pathol., *64*:717–732, 1971.

———: Tyzzer's disease of rabbits: isolation and propagation of *Bacillus piliformis* (Tyzzer) in embryonated eggs. Infect. Immun., *3*:429–437, 1971.

Goto, N., et al.: Fine structure of the Tyzzer's organism in the feline liver. Jpn. J. Exp. Med., *44*:373–378, 1974.

Hall, W. C., and Van Kruiningen, H. J.: Tyzzer's disease in a horse. J. Am. Vet. Med. Assoc., *164*:1187–1189, 1974.

Harrington, D. D.: Naturally-occurring Tyzzer's disease *(Bacillus piliformis* infection) in horse foals. Vet. Rec., *96*:59–63, 1975.

———: *Bacillus piliformis* infection (Tyzzer's disease) in two foals. J. Am. Vet. Med. Assoc., *168*:58–59, 1976.

Jonas, A. M., Percy, D. H., and Craft, J.: Tyzzer's disease in the rat. Its possible relationship with megaloileitis. Arch. Pathol., *90*:516–528, 1970.

Karstad, L., Lusis, P., and Wright, D.: Tyzzer's disease in muskrats. J. Wildl. Dis., *7*:96–99, 1971.

Kovatch, R. M., and Zebarth, G.: Naturally occurring Tyzzer's disease in a cat. J. Am. Vet. Med. Assoc., *162*:136–138. 1973.

Kubokawa, K., et al.: Two cases of feline Tyzzer's disease. Jpn. J. Exp. Med., *43*:413–421, 1973.

McLeod, C. G., Stookey, J. L., Harrington, D. G., and White, J. D.: Intestinal Tyzzer's disease and spirochetosis in a guinea pig. Vet. Pathol., *14*:229–235, 1977.

Onodera, T., and Fujiwara, K.: Naso-encephalopathy in suckling mice inoculated intranasally with the Tyzzer's organism. Jpn. J. Exp. Med., *43*:509–522, 1973.

Poonacha, K. B., and Smith, H. L.: Naturally occurring Tyzzer's disease as a complication of distemper and mycotic pneumonia in a dog. J. Am. Vet. Med. Assoc., *169*:419–420, 1976.

Port, C. D., Richter, W. R., and Moize, S. M.: An ultrastructural study of Tyzzer's disease in the Mongolian gerbil *(Meriones unguiculatus).* Lab. Invest., *25*:81–87, 1971.

———: Tyzzer's disease in the gerbil *(Meriones unguiculatus).* Lab. Anim. Care, *20*:109–111, 1970.

Pulley, L. T., and Shively, J. N.: Tyzzer's disease in a foal. Light and electron-microscopic observations. Vet. Pathol., *11*:203–211, 1974.

Saunders, L. Z.: Tyzzer's disease. J. Nat. Cancer Inst., *20*:893–897, 1958.

Stedham, M. A., and Bucci, T. J.: Spontaneous Tyzzer's disease in a rat. Lab. Anim. Care, *20*:743–748, 1970.

Takasaki, Y., Oghiso, Y., Sato, K., and Fujiwara, K.: Tyzzer's disease in hamsters. Jpn. J. Exp. Med., *44*:267–270, 1974.

Tyzzer, E. E.: A fatal disease of the Japanese waltzing mouse caused by spore-bearing bacillus *(Bacillus piliformis,* N. Sp.). J. Med. Res., *38*:307–338, 1917.

White, D. J., and Waldron, M. M.: Naturally-occurring Tyzzer's disease in the gerbil. Vet. Rec., *85*:111–114, 1969.

Whitwell, K. E.: Four cases of Tyzzer's disease in foals in England. Equine Vet. J., 8:118–122, 1976.

INFECTIONS DUE TO MORAXELLA

Gram-negative cocci and coccobacilli are currently grouped in the family Neisseriaceae and contain four genera, three of which are of interest because of their pathogenicity (Neisseria, Branhamella, and Moraxella contain pathogenic species); organisms in the Genus Acinetobacter are saprophytic. Moraxella bovis is associated with infectious **bovine keratoconjunctivitis** ("pink eye") and is believed to be at least one of the causes of this disease. Subconjunctival or intracorneal inoculation of cattle with pure cultures results in severe keratoconjunctivitis that simulates the natural disease. Sunlight or ultraviolet light are also required. Bovine rhinotracheitis virus will also produce severe keratoconjunctivitis under these experimental conditions.

The clinical features of this bovine disease are summarized as: acute onset of photophobia, excessive lacrimation, purulent blepharitis, ulceration with peripheral vascularization of the cornea, and iridospasm.

Generalized and localized infections of piglets with a Moraxella sp. have been described in Denmark (Larsen, Billie, and Nielsen, 1973).

Hughes, D. E., et al.: Effects of vaccination with a Moraxella bovis bacterin on the subsequent development of signs of corneal disease and infection with M. bovis in calves under natural environmental conditions. Am. J. Vet. Res., 37:1291–1295, 1976.

Larsen, J. L., Billie, N., and Nielsen, N. C.: Occurrence and possible role of Moraxella species in pigs. Acta Pathol. Microbiol. Scand., 81B:181–186, 1973.

Nayar, P. S. G., and Saunders, J. R.: Infectious bovine keratoconjunctivitis. I. Experimental production. Can. J. Comp. Med., 39:22–31, 1975.

————: Infectious bovine keratoconjunctivitis. II. Antibodies in lacrimal secretions of cattle naturally or experimentally infected with Moraxella bovis. Can. J. Comp. Med., 39:32–40, 1975.

Pedersen, K. B.: Moraxella bovis isolated from cattle with infectious keratoconjunctivitis. Acta Pathol. Microbiol. Scand., 78B:429–434, 1970.

Pugh, G. W., Jr., Hughes, D. E., and McDonald, T. J.: Bovine infectious keratoconjunctivitis: serological aspects of Moraxella bovis infection. Can. J. Comp. Med., 35:161–166, 1971.

Pugh, G. W., Jr., and Hughes, D. E.: Bovine infectious keratoconjunctivitis: carrier state of Moraxella bovis and the development of preventive measures against disease. J. Am. Vet. Med. Assoc., 167:310–313, 1975.

Pugh, G. W., Jr., Hughes, D. E., Schulz, V. D., and Graham, C. K.: Experimentally induced infectious bovine keratoconjunctivitis: resistance of vaccinated cattle to homologous and heterologous strains of Moraxella bovis. Am. J. Vet. Res., 37:57–60, 1976.

Pugh, G. W., et al.: Infectious bovine keratoconjunctivitis: comparison of a fluorescent antibody technique and cultural isolation for the detection of Moraxella bovis in eye secretions. Am. J. Vet. Res., 38:1349–1352, 1977.

INFECTIONS DUE TO NEISSERIA

Gram-negative cocci, in the genus Neisseria (family Neisseriaceae) are principally human pathogens, but some cause infection in animals. Neisseria gonorrhoeae ("gonococcus") is the cause of the human venereal disease, gonorrhea. The chimpanzee is susceptible to experimental exposure to this organism. Neisseria meningitidis ("meningococcus") is the cause of some cases of meningitis in human patients.

Neisseria ovis, tentatively classified in this genus, has been recovered from the conjunctival sac of sheep with keratoconjunctivitis or with clinically normal cornea and conjunctiva. Pure cultures of this organism, injected into the cornea, only rarely produce any significant disease in sheep. The role of this organism as a sole pathogen for sheep remains in question.

Brown, W. J., Lucas, C. T., and Kuhn, U. S. G.: Gonorrhea in the chimpanzee: infection with laboratory-passed gonococci and by natural transmission. Br. J. Vener. Dis., 48:177–179, 1972.

Buchanan, R. E., and Gibbons, N. E.: In Bergey's Manual of Determinative Bacteriology, 8th ed. Baltimore, Williams & Wilkins Co., 1974.

Spradbrow, P.: Experimental infection of the ovine cornea with Neisseria ovis. Vet. Rec., 88:615–616, 1971.

CHAPTER 12

Diseases Caused by Higher Bacteria and Fungi

The diseases to be described in this chapter have been grouped together not only for the reason that their causative agents are related, but also because the reactions these agents provoke in their hosts have certain striking similarities. Many of these diseases are characterized by the formation of epithelioid granulation tissue and thus may be conveniently classified as the "infectious granulomas." Included in this group are:

Actinomycosis	Cryptococcosis
Nocardiosis	Histoplasmosis
Dermatophilus	Epizootic
infection	lymphangitis
Necrobacillosis	Phycomycoses
Tuberculosis	Sporotrichosis
Paratuberculosis	Candidiasis
Leprosy	Geotrichosis
Aspergillosis	Lobomycosis
Blastomycosis	Paecilomycoses
Coccidioidomycosis	Phaeohypho-
Adiaspiromycosis	mycosis
Nasal granuloma of	Dermatomycoses
cattle	Prototheocosis
Maduramycosis	Mycotoxicoses

The superficial mycoses (dermatophytoses, tinea, ringworm) also have a different reaction pattern, influenced more perhaps by the cutaneous habitat of the organism than by its intrinsic properties.

The term **mycetoma** is applied in man and animals to those mycotic infections that are localized in the subcutis but may also affect adjacent bone (maduramycosis, rhinosporidiosis). **Systemic mycoses** may be localized, but more often they affect several organ systems or may be widely disseminated (blastomycosis, cryptococcosis, histoplasmosis). Although possibly redundant, it is nonetheless pertinent to point out that the more closely organisms are related biologically, the more nearly identical will be the tissue reactions of their parasitized hosts. The infectious granulomas are of particular importance to the pathologist, because his techniques are especially valuable in arriving at their precise diagnosis.

Baker, R. D. et al. (ed).: International symposium on opportunistic fungus infections. Lab. Invest., 11:1017–1241, 1962.

Connole, M. D., and Johnston, L. A Y.: A review of animal mycoses in Australia. Vet. Bull., 37:145–153, 1967.

Emmons, C. W., Binford, C. H., Utz, J. P., and Kwon-Chung, K. J.: Medical Mycology. 3rd ed. Philadelphia, Lea & Febiger, 1977.

Kaplan, W.: Epidemiology of the principal systemic mycoses of man and lower animals and the ecology of their etiologic agents. J. Am. Vet. Med. Assoc., 163:1043–1047, 1973.

Kelley, D. C., and Mosier, J. E.: Public health aspects of mycotic diseases. J. Am. Vet. Med. Assoc., 171:1168–1170, 1977.

McGinnis, M. R., and Hilger, A. E.: A key to the genera of medically important fungi. Mycopathologia, 45:269–283, 1971.

Metzger, J. F., Kase, A., and Smith, C. W.: Identification of pathogenic fungi in surgical and autopsy specimens by immunofluorescence. Mycopathologia, 17:335–344, 1962. VB 467–63.

Saunders, L. Z.: Fungous diseases. *In* Diseases Transmitted from Animals to Man, edited by T. G. Hull. Springfield, Charles C Thomas, 1955, Chap. 23.

———: Systemic fungous infections in animals. Cornell Vet., 38:213–238, 1948.

Swartz, J. H., Medrek, T. F., and Robboy, S. J.: A new stain for systemic fungi in tissue. Am. J. Clin. Pathol., 57:27–29, 1972.

ACTINOMYCOSIS

Actinomycosis is the result of infection by organisms classified in the genus *Actinomyces*. The classic disease occurs in cattle, but many species may be infected under natural conditions. The currently recognized organisms, their hosts, and the diseases they cause are summarized in Table 12–1. The name of this disease has often been applied erroneously to somewhat similar infections, such as actinobacillosis and nocardiosis, which are caused by different etiologic agents. The most frequent and obvious manifestation of actinomycosis in cattle is the hard, irregular enlargement that results from infection of the mandible or, less often, the maxilla, and gives the disease its common name, "lumpy jaw." Similar infection of the mandible has been observed in wild ruminants such as elk. In dogs, actinomycosis usually affects soft tissues and may become generalized. In man, the cheek, mouth, skin of the chest, appendix, and intestine are the usual sites of involvement. Actinomycotic infection of the porcine mammary glands is not uncommon, and the organisms also have been identified in association with *Brucella abortus* in equine "fistulous withers."

Lesions. The organisms grow in tenacious colonies of microscopic size, located in tiny purulent centers surrounded by dense granulation tissue, which displaces the nearby normal tissues. When the organisms penetrate bone, it becomes enlarged and honeycombed as a result of destructive rarefaction and regenerative proliferation. The cut surface of the lesion usually is white and glistening from the dense connective tissue in which the small abscesses are embedded. Occasional sinus

Table 12–1. Actinomycosis

Organism	Host Species	Disease or Anatomic Systems Affected
Actinomyces bovis	Cattle, swine, horses, elk, man (experimentally: mice, hamsters)	Mandible, soft tissues, or generalized
A. israelii	Man, cattle (occasionally) (experimentally: hamsters, mice, rabbits)	Soft tissues, may be generalized
A. suis	Swine	Mammary gland
A. eriksonii	Man	Abscesses, subcutis, or lung
A. odontolyticus	Man	Oral cavity—associated with dentinal caries
A. viscosus	Man, hamster (experimentally: rats, mice)	Associated with periodontal disease
A. naeslundii	Man (experimentally: rats, mice)	Associated with periodontal disease in rats, caries in man
A. humiferus	Soil	Not pathogenic

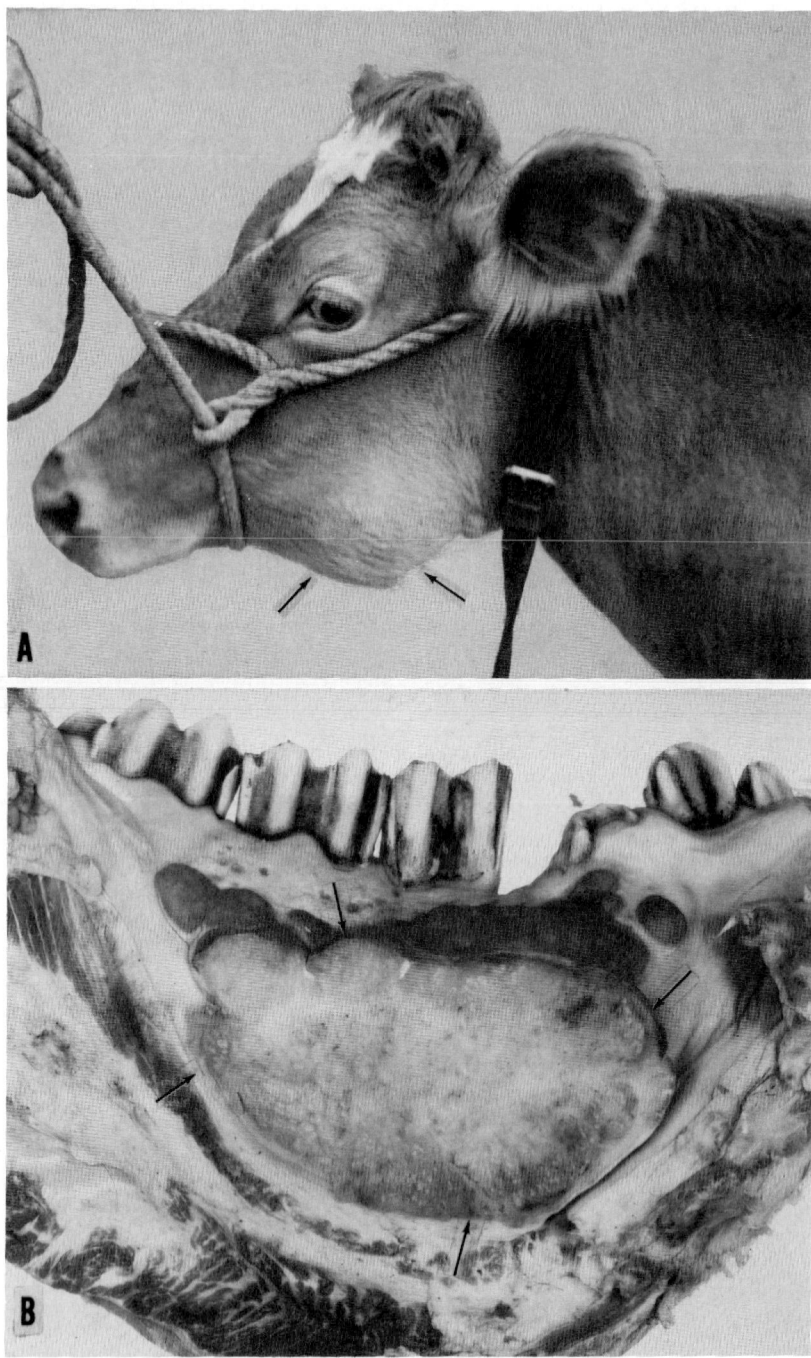

Fig. 12–1. Actinomycosis. *A,* Lesions in mandible of a Guernsey cow. Case from clinic of College of Veterinary Medicine, Iowa State University. *B,* Gross specimen from mandible of a similar case. (Courtesy of Armed Forces Institute of Pathology.) Contributor: Major Lytle, V.C.

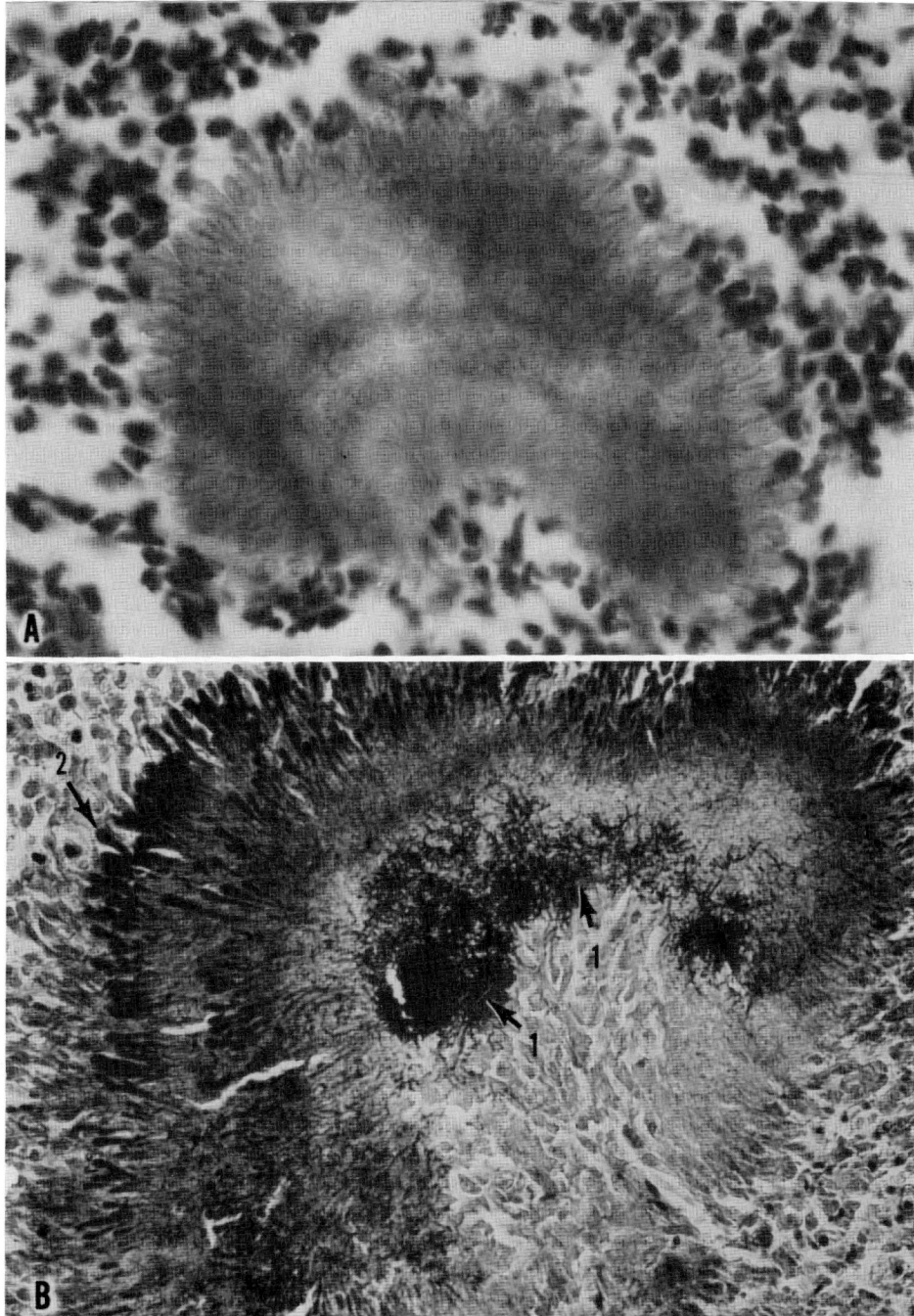

Fig. 12–2. Actinomycosis. *A,* Colony of *Actinomyces bovis* (× 500), in a tissue section stained with hematoxylin and eosin. Contributor: Major Lytle, V.C. *B,* A similar colony of *Actinomyces bovis* (× 500) in a tissue section stained by Gram's method. Note tangled, branching, gram-positive organisms in the center (*1*) surrounded by zones of radiating club-shaped structures (*2*). (Courtesy of Armed Forces Institute of Pathology.) Contributor: Dr. H. R. Seibold.

tracts may be demonstrated, with drainage through the skin or into the oral cavity. Expression of the yellowish pus from the abscesses yields tiny, hard masses called "sulfur granules," because of their gross consistency and yellowish color. Microscopically, these masses may appear as rosettes, and although early investigators considered them the "ray fungus," they are now known to be merely separate colonies of actinomyces organisms growing in characteristic fashion. In sections stained with hematoxylin and eosin, a colony appears as an eosinophilic, irregularly-shaped mass, 20 microns or more in diameter, surrounded by a zone of radially arranged projections with rounded ends, their shape suggesting Indian clubs or baseball bats. These radiating clubs are usually coarse, 3 to 10 μ in diameter and 10 to 30 μ in length, and brightly eosinophilic. Although their exact nature is not understood, it appears likely that they are a product of the cells of the host, rather than of the infecting organism.

The central part of the colony can be demonstrated by Gram's stain to be made up of a tangled mass of gram-positive, rod-shaped, or long filamentous organisms, which are often beaded and occasionally branched. Beyond the radiating clubs there is usually a zone of neutrophils, surrounded by an outer area of large mononuclear (epithelioid) cells with abundant, often foamy, cytoplasm. Giant cells of the Langhans' type and lymphocytes are occasionally found in this region. The dense, moderately vascular connective tissue that separates the many abscesses from one another usually encapsulates the entire lesion.

The colonies of actinomyces may become calcified in cases of long standing, in which event they assume a gritty texture as blue-staining granules of calcium salts replace the organisms.

Diagnosis. The characteristic lesions can be identified positively by using Gram's stain on sections of fixed tissue to differ-

entiate the gram-positive organisms at the center of the colonies. Organisms can also be demonstrated in smears of fresh, unfixed material stained by Gram's method. Successful cultures must be maintained under reduced oxygen tension, but they are seldom essential for diagnosis. The rosettes with the shiny, refractile, radiating clubs can be demonstrated in wet preparations of fresh pus compressed under a coverglass and examined with reduced illumination.

Differential diagnosis must include other granulomatous infections, but in particular actinobacillosis, nocardiosis, and staphylococcosis (botryomycosis). The morphology of the bacterial colonies, and individual organisms and their staining reactions, which differ in each of these infections, allow ready differentiation.

Al-Doory, Y.: A bibliography of actinomycosis. Mycopathologia, 44:1–88, 1971.

Altman, N. H., and Small, J. D.: Actinomycosis in a primate confirmed by fluorescent antibody technics in formalin fixed tissues. Lab. Anim. Sci., 23:696–700, 1973.

Ayers, K. M., and DePaoli, A.: Actinomycosis of the testes and spermatic cord in a dog. Vet. Pathol., 14:287–288, 1977.

Bestetti, G.: Morphology of the "sulphur granules" (Drusen) in some actinomycotic infections. A light and electron microscopic study. Vet. Pathol., 15:506–518, 1978.

Brown, J. R., and von Lichtenberg, F.: Experimental actinomycosis in mice. Arch. Pathol., 90:391–402, 1970.

Chastain, C. B., et al.: Actinomycotic peritonitis in a dog. J. Am. Vet. Med. Assoc., 168:499–501, 1976.

Coleman, M., and Georg, L. K.: Comparative pathogenicity of Actinomyces naeslundii and Actinomyces israelii. Appl. Microbiol., 18:427–432, 1969.

Davenport, A. A., Carter, G. R., and Patterson, M. J.: Identification of Actinomyces viscosus from canine infections. J. Clin. Microbiol., 1:75–78, 1975.

Georg, L. K., Brown, J. M., Baker, H. J., and Cassell, G. H.: Actinomyces viscosus as an agent of actinomycosis in the dog. Am. J. Vet. Res., 33:1457–1470, 1972.

Ginsberg, A., and Little, A. C. W.: Actinomycosis in dogs. J. Path. Bact., 60:563–572, 1948.

Martin, H. M.: Actinomycosis of the dog and cat. Univ. of Pennsylvania Bull. Veterinary Extension Quarterly, No. 87:15–19, June 16, 1942.

Menges, R. W., Larsh, H. W., and Habermann, R. T.: Canine actinomycosis. J. Am. Vet. Med. Assoc., 122:73–78, 1953.

Pine, L. and Overman, J. R.: Determination of the structure and composition of the "sulphur granules" of *Actinomyces bovis*. J. Gen. Microbiol., 32:209–223, 1963. VB 4260–63.

Robboy, S. J., and Vickery, A. L.: Tinctorial and morphologic properties distinguishing actinomycosis and nocardiosis. N. Engl. J. Med., 282:593–596, 1970.

Ryff, J. F.: Encephalitis in a deer due to *Actinomyces bovis*. J. Am. Vet. Med. Assoc., 122:78–80, 1953.

Sautter, J. H., Rowsell, H. C., and Hohn, R. B.: Actinomycosis and actinobacillosis in dogs. North Am. Vet., 34:341–346, 1953.

Shahan, M. S., and Davis, C. L.: The diagnosis of actinomycosis and actinobacillosis. Am. J. Vet. Res., 3:321–328, 1942.

Swerczek, T. W., Schiefer, B., and Nielsen, S. W.: Canine actinomycosis. Zentbl. Vet. Med., 15B:955–970, 1968.

NOCARDIOSIS

Infections with aerobic, gram-positive, filamentous organisms, which under some conditions have "acid-fast" staining properties, occur in man and animals, particularly dogs. The organisms have been known under several names (*Actinomyces asteroides, Cladothrix asteroides, Actinomyces gypsoides*), but at present are grouped in the genus *Nocardia* (*Nocardia asteroides*), from which comes the name nocardiosis. The lesions and organisms are sufficiently unlike those of actinomycosis to permit their differentiation.

Lesions. In dogs, infection of the lungs and pleura or skin is most common, although systemic infection can occur and the organisms may localize in peritoneal and pleural cavities, in the brain, or in any visceral organ. The lesions are seen microscopically as tangled, indistinct colonies of organisms surrounded by necrotic cellular debris, purulent exudate, and granulation tissue. The colonies are not surrounded by radiating clubs. The organisms can usually be demonstrated in the tissues as gram-positive, branching filaments, which are acid-fast when appropriately stained. Cultural identification of the organism is necessary to establish the diagnosis, although presumptive diagnoses can be made from tissue sections.

Nocardiosis is less frequent in other species, but is a sporadic cause of bovine mastitis and pneumonia in monkeys. The lesions in these or other species are similar to those described in the dog. The organism recovered from dogs and nonhuman primates has sometimes been identified as *Nocardia caviae*, a species closely related to *N. asteroides*.

Nocardia farcinica (which may be identical to *Nocardia asteroides*) is reportedly the cause of a disease of cattle known as **bovine farcy**. The infection is not known in the United States, but has been described in the Sudan, the Far East, and Latin America. The disease occurs as a chronic suppurative granulomatous inflammation of the skin, lymphatics, and draining lymph nodes, usually confined to the limbs. In fatal infections, there is metastasis to the lungs, liver, spleen, and internal lymph nodes.

Infection of the bovine fetus and placenta with resulting abortion has been associated with nocardiosis.

Awad, F. I. and Karib, A. A.: Studies on bovine farcy (nocardiosis) among cattle in the Sudan. Zentralbl. Veterinaermed., 5:265–272, 1958.

Bakerspigel, A.: An unusual strain of *Nocardia* isolated from an infected cat. Can. J. Microbiol., 19:1361–1365, 1973.

Bohl, E. H., et al.: Nocardiosis in the dog. J. Am. Vet. Med. Assoc., 122:81–85, 1953.

Boncyk, L. H., McCullough, B., Grotts, D. D., and Kalter, S. S.: Localized nocardiosis due to *Nocardia caviae* in a baboon (*Papio cynocephalus*). Lab. Anim. Sci., 25:88–91, 1975.

Brown, A. R., and Osborne, A. D.: A case of canine nocardiosis. Vet. Rec., 74:371–373, 1962. VB 2568–62.

Cuttino, J. T., and McCabe, A. M.: Pure granulomatous nocardiosis: a new fungus disease distinguished by intracellular parasitism. Am. J. Pathol., 25:1–47, 1949.

Ginsberg, A., and Little, A. C. W.: Actinomycosis in dogs. J. Pathol. Bact., 60:563–572, 1948.

Jonas, A. M., and Wyand, D. S.: Pulmonary nocardiosis in the rhesus monkey. Importance of differentiation from tuberculosis. Pathol. Vet., 3:588–600, 1966.

Kinch, D. A.: A rapidly fatal infection caused by *Nocardia caviae* in a dog. J. Pathol. Bact., 95:540–546, 1968.

Mahajan, V. M., et al.: Experimental pulmonary nocardiosis in monkeys. Sabouraudia, 15:47–50, 1977.

McClure, H. M., Chang, J., Kaplan, W., and Brown, J. M.: Pulmonary nocardiosis in an orangutan. J. Am. Vet. Med. Assoc., *169*:943–945, 1976.

Mitten, R. W.: Vertebral oesteomyelitis in the dog due to Nocardia-like organisms. J. Small Anim. Pract., *15*:563–570, 1974.

Mostafa, I. E.: Bovine nocardiosis (cattle farcy). A review. Vet. Bull., *36*:189–193, 1966.

Pier, A. C.: Nocardiosis in animals. Proc. 66th Ann. Meet. U. S. Livestock Sanit. Assn. Washington, 1962, pp. 409–415, 1963. VB 3872–63.

Pier, A. C., and Fichtner, R. E.: Serologic typing of *Nocardia asteroides* by immunodiffusion. Am. Rev. Respir. Dis., *103*:698–707, 1971.

Pier, A. C., Gray, D. M., and Fossatti, M. J.: *Nocardia asteroides*—a newly recognized pathogen of the mastitis complex. Am. J. Vet. Res. *19*:319–331, 1958.

Ridell, M.: Taxonomic study of *Nocardia farcinica* using serological and physiological characters. Int. J. Systematic Bacteriol., *25*:124–132, 1975.

Rodriguez, I. G.: Aportacion al Estudio de las Nocardiosis del Caballo. Una Enzootia de *Nocardiosis Equina*. Bol. Inf. Cons. Col. Vet. Esp., *8*:747–757, 1961. VB 1416–62.

Smith, I. M., and Hayward, A. H. S.: *Nocardia caviae* and *Nocardia asteroides*: comparative bacteriological and mouse pathogenicity studies. J. Comp. Pathol., *81*:79–87, 1971.

Swerczek, T. W., Trutwein, G., and Nielsen, S. W.: Canine nocardiosis. Zentralbl. Veterinaermed., *15B*:971–978, 1968.

Thordal-Christensen, A., and Clifford, D. H.: Actinomycosis (nocardiosis) in a dog. Am. J. Vet. Res., *14*:298–306, 1953.

Wohlgemuth, K., Knudtson, W., Bicknell, E. J., and Kirkbride, C. A.: Bovine abortion associated with *Nocardia asteroides*. J. Am. Vet. Med. Assoc., *161*:273–288, 1972.

DERMATOPHILUS INFECTION
(Cutaneous Streptothricosis)

Infection by the actinomycete *Dermatophilus congolensis* has been termed mycotic dermatitis, cutaneous streptothricosis, lumpy wool, strawberry foot rot, cutaneous actinomycosis, and other terms that contain erroneous implications regarding the nature of the causal agent. Dermatophilus infection (the preferred designation) has been described in cattle, sheep, goats, deer, horses, dogs, monkeys, cats, fowl, raccoons, lizards, cottontail rabbits, polar bears, and man. Rabbits, mice, and guinea pigs have been experimentally infected. In each of these species with the exception of man, the gross and histopathologic changes are similar.

Lesions. The infection is limited to the skin, producing raised, alopecic, and sometimes papillomatous lesions covered by thick keratinaceous incrustations. The lesions may be well circumscribed or confluent and may affect the skin of any portion of the body. In some instances, the organisms may reach lymph nodes resulting in a granulomatous response.

The microscopic features are unique and best understood by explaining the pathogenesis of the infection. The organism invades and multiplies within the epidermis as branching filaments, which divide in a characteristic multidimensional fashion, giving rise to multiple rows of coccoid organisms. They do not invade the dermis, but induce an extensive purulent exudate beneath the epidermis, separating it from the dermis. The invaded epidermis cornifies and a new epidermis forms under the exudate, which in turn is invaded by hyphae at the periphery of the lesion. A second inflammatory exudate separates the new epidermis from the dermis, and a third epithelium is generated. The process is repeated, resulting in a thick scab composed of alternate strata of cornified epidermis and exudate. The organisms can usually be seen in hematoxylin and eosin stained tissue sections, and are clearly seen as gram-positive filaments or chains of cocci in sections stained with the Gram's technique.

The disease is transmitted by the coccoid forms, which result from the multidimensional division of the hyphae. This stage, known as a zoospore, is motile and released when the scabs are exposed to moisture. Transmission can be direct or indirect through contaminated water or grasses. Insect transmission, which has been demonstrated with flies and ticks, is believed to be a principal means of spreading zoospores.

Diagnosis. Diagnosis can usually be made from the morphology of the exudate and demonstration of the organisms. If necessary, the organism can be cultured.

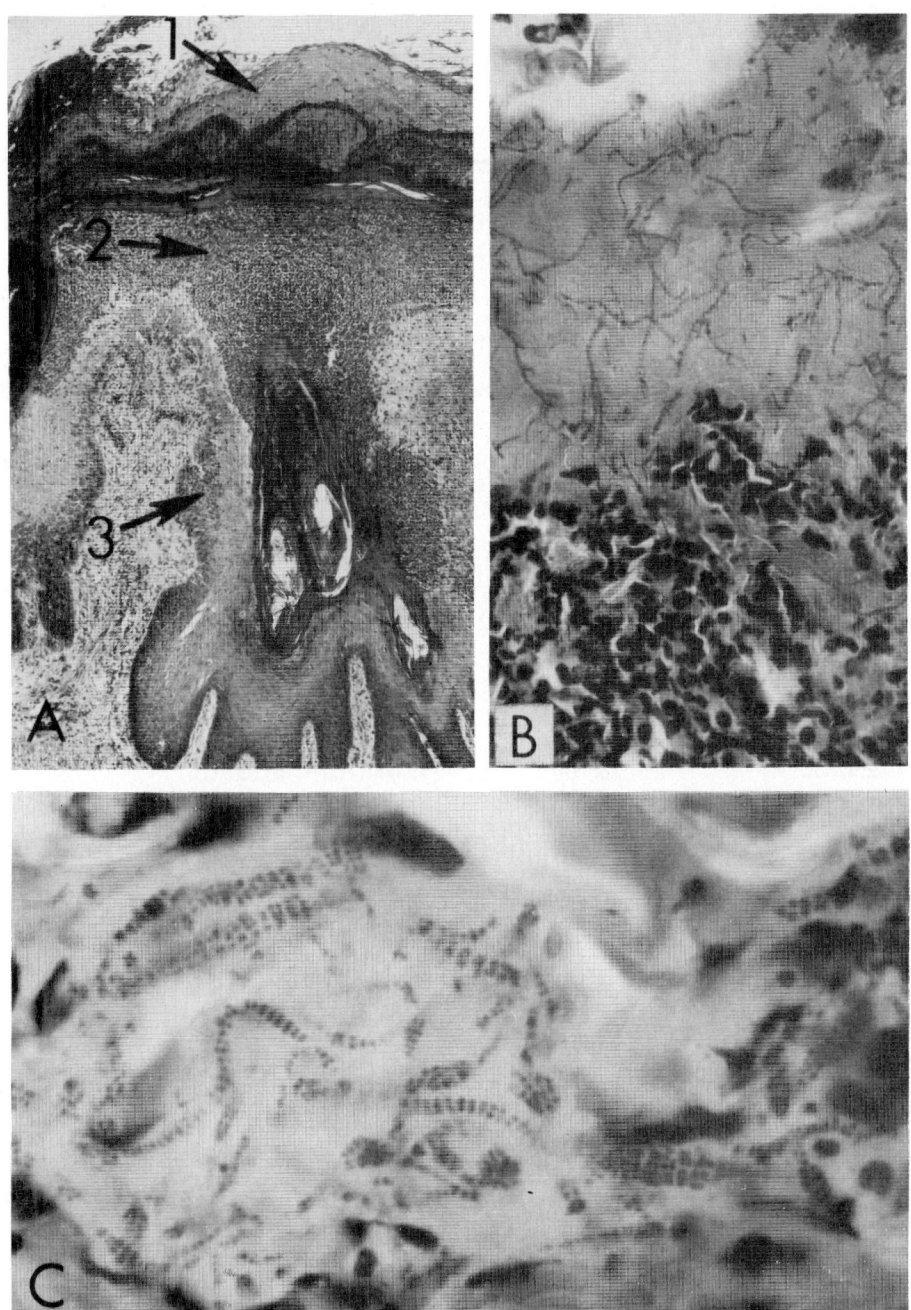

Fig. 12–3. Dermatophilus infection, skin, owl monkey (*Aotus trivirgatus*). *A,* Characteristic lamination of cornified epithelium (*1*), purulent exudate (*2*), and regenerating epithelium (*3*). *B,* Mycelia in cornified epithelium. *C,* Characteristic multidimensional division of *Dermatophilus congolensis*. (Courtesy Dr. N. W. King, Jr.)

Abu-Samra, M. T., Imbabi, S. E., and Mahgoub, S. el.: Experimental infection of domesticated animals and the fowl with *Dermatophilus congolensis.* (Vet Bull *46*:5055, 1976) J. Comp. Pathol., *86*:157–172, 1976.

Bentinck-Smith, J., Fox, F. H., and Baker, D. W.: Equine dermatitis (cutaneous streptothricosis) infection with dermatophilus in the U.S. Cornell Vet., *51*:334–349, 1961.

Bridges, C. H., and Romane, W. M.: Cutaneous streptothricosis in cattle. J. Am. Vet. Med. Assoc., *138*:153–157, 1961.

Chastain, C. B., et al.: Dermatophilosis in two dogs. J. Am. Vet. Med. Assoc., *169*:1079–1080, 1976.

Fox, J. G., et al.: Dermatophilosis (cutaneous streptothricosis) in owl monkeys. J. Am. Vet. Med. Assoc., *163*:642–644, 1973.

Gordon, M. A.: The genus *Dermatophilus.* J. Bact., *88*:509–522, 1964.

Jenkinson, D. M.: The skin surface: An environment of *Dermatophilus congolensis. In* Dermatophilus Infection in Animals and Man, edited by D. H. Lloyd and K. C. Sellers. New York, Academic Press, 1976, pp. 146–161.

Jones, R. T.: Subcutaneous infection with *Dermatophilus congolensis* in a cat. J. Comp. Pathol., *86*:415–421, 1976.

Kaplan, W.: Dermatophilosis in primates. *In* Dermatophilus Infection in Animals and Man, edited by D. H., Lloyd and K. C. Sellers. New York, Academic Press, 1976, pp. 128–140.

Kelley, D. C., and Bida, S. A.: Epidemiological survey of streptothricosis (kirchi) in northern Nigeria. Bull. Epizoot. Dis. Afr., *18*:325–328, 1970.

King, N. W., et al.: Cutaneous streptothricosis (dermatophiliasis) in owl monkeys. Lab. Anim. Sci., *21*:67–74, 1971.

Kistner, T. P., Shotts, E. B., Jr., and Greene, E. W.: Naturally occurring cutaneous streptothricosis in a white tailed deer. Path. Vet., *7*:1–6, 1970.

LeRiche, P. D.: The transmission of dermatophilosis (mycotic dermatitis) in sheep. Aust. Vet. J., *44*:64–67, 1968.

McClure, H. M., Kaplan, W., Bonner, W. B., and Keeling, M. E.: Dermatophilosis in owl monkeys. Sabouraudia, *9*:185–190, 1971.

Migaki, G.: Dermatophilosis in a titi monkey (*Callicebus moloch*). Am. J. Vet. Res., *37*:1225–1226, 1976.

Montali, R. J., Smith, E. E., Davenport, M., and Bush, M.: Dermatophilosis in Australian bearded lizards. J. Am. Vet. Med. Assoc., *167*:553–556, 1975.

Newman, M. S., Cook, R. W., Appelhof, W. K., and Kitchen, H.: Dermatophilosis in two polar bears. J. Am. Vet. Med. Assoc., *167*:561–564, 1975.

Oduye, O. O.: Effects of various induced local environmental conditions and histopathological studies in experimental *Dermatophilus congolensis* infection on the bovine skin. Res. Vet. Sci., *19*:245–252, 1975.

Richard, J. L., Pier, A. C., and Cysewski, S. J.: Experimentally induced canine dermatophilosis. Am. J. Vet. Res., *34*:797–799, 1973.

Richard, J. L., and Pier, A. C.: Transmission of *Dermatophilus congolensis* by *Stomoxys calcitrans* and *Musca domestica.* Am. J. Vet. Res., *27*:419–423, 1966.

Roberts, D. S.: *Dermatophilus* infection. Vet. Bull., *37*:513–521, 1967.

———: The histopathology of epidermal infection with the actinomycete, *Dermatophilus congolensis.* J. Pathol. Bact., *90*:213–216, 1965.

Salkin, I. F., Gordon, M. A., and Stone, W. B.: Dual infection of a white-tailed deer by *Dermatophilus congolensis* and *Alternaria alternata.* J. Am. Vet. Med. Assoc., *167*:571–573, 1975.

Salkin, I. F., Gordon, M. A., and Stone, W. B.: Dermatophilosis among wild raccoons in New York State. J. Am. Vet. Med. Assoc., *169*:949–951, 1976.

Searcy, G. P., and Hulland, T. J.: Dermatophilus dermatitis (streptothricosis) in Ontario. I. Clinical observations. II. Laboratory findings. Can. Vet. J., *9*:7–15 & 16–21, 1968.

Shotts, E. B., and Kistner, T. P.: Naturally occurring cutaneous streptothricosis in a cottontail rabbit. J. Am. Vet. Med. Assoc., *157*:667–670, 1970.

Smith, C. F., and Cordes, D. O.: Dermatitis caused by *Dermatophilus congolensis* infection in polar bears (*Thalacotos maritimus*). Br. Vet. J., *128*:336–371, 1972.

Stannard, A. A., and Jang, S. S.: Dermatophilosis in a lamb. J. Am. Vet. Med. Assoc., *163*:1161–1164, 1973.

NECROBACILLOSIS

Several necrotizing disease processes involving herbivorous animals have been associated with the presence of a certain anaerobic, nonsporulating, gram-negative, filamentous organism, currently named *Spherophorus necrophorus (Fusiformis necrophorus, Fusobacterium necrophorum).* There is little doubt that this organism can be recovered from animal lesions, but there is serious question that it is the sole, or even the primary, cause of disease. Since these lesions are encountered with some frequency, it appears advisable to describe them briefly and express the hope that future research will contribute to a better understanding.

In horses, a severe necrotizing disease of the feet appears in animals which are forced to remain for long periods in deep, manure- and urine-soaked mud. This "gangrenous dermatitis" usually starts at the heel or in the deep structures of the frog, and results in irregular areas of

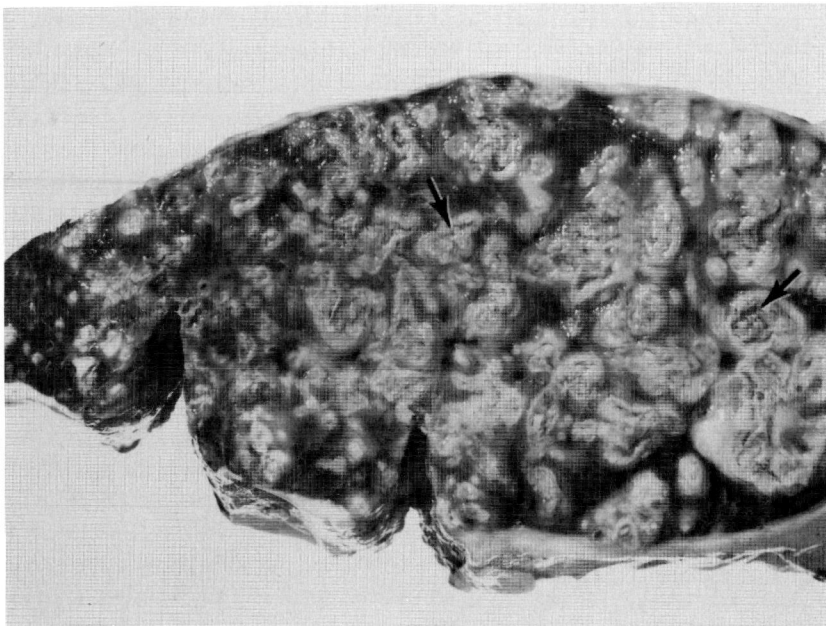

Fig. 12–4. Necrobacillosis. Irregularly shaped necrotic and encapsulated lesions (arrows) in a bovine spleen. (Courtesy of Dr. Wm. J. Hadlow.)

sharply demarcated necrosis involving large amounts of tissue. It often produces serious disability.

In cattle, necrophorus organisms are found in the elevated, tenacious, necrotic plaques of the larynx, pharynx, and trachea, commonly referred to as "calf diphtheria." They also have been demonstrated in bovine cases which terminated fatally in pneumonia. Large, sharply delimited foci of necrosis also occur in the liver and spleen of adult cattle, particularly those which are heavily fed. The hepatic lesions are associated with ulcerations of the rumen and are discussed further in Chapter 23. In the Sudan, the disease in cattle has been reported to involve the subcutis, lymph vessels, and nodes, with occasional spread to internal organs, or in some cases the internal organs are infected without apparent lesions in the subcutis. (See "bovine farcy.") Foot rot of cattle (infectious pododermatitis) is invariably associated with *Spherophorus necrophorus.*

Synergistic effects in bovine foot rot have been demonstrated using two organisms, *Spherophorus necrophorus* and *Bacterioides melaninogenicus,* to infect the interdigital skin of normal cattle (Berg and Loan, 1975). Typical lesions were induced and the organisms were recovered from the affected tissues.

Ulcerative, necrotizing stomatitis and enteritis in swine have been questionably attributed to *Spherophorus necrophorus,* as has a disfiguring type of rhinitis ("bull-nose"). The similarity of the external appearance of the nose of affected swine is some evidence that this latter entity might have been confused in the past with atrophic rhinitis.

In sheep, the necrophorus organism is associated with an obligate parasite, *Fusiformis nodosus,* and possibly a third organism, *Spirochaeta penortha,* in ovine foot rot. Foot abscess and "lip-and-leg ulceration" have also been ascribed to necrophorus infection. However, it is doubtful that this organism is the cause of these diseases in sheep.

Berg, J. N., and Loan, R. W.: *Fusobacterium nec-rophorum* and *Bacteroides melaninogenicus* as etiologic agents of foot-rot in cattle. Am. J. Vet. Res., *36*:1115–1122, 1975.

Britton, J. W.: An unusual infection in a foal. Cornell Vet., *37*:391–393, 1947.

Cross, R. F.: Influence of environmental factors on transmission of ovine contagious foot rot. J. Am. Vet. Med. Assoc., *173*:1567–1568, 1978.

Egerton, J. R., and Roberts, D. S.: Vaccination against ovine foot-rot. J. Comp. Pathol., *81*:179–185, 1971.

Egerton, J. R., and Merritt, G. C.: Serology of foot-rot: antibodies against *Fusiformis nodosus* in normal affected, vaccinated and passively immunized sheep. Aust. Vet. J., *49*:139–145, 1973.

Egerton, J. R., Roberts, D. S., and Parsonson, I. M.: The aetiology and pathogenesis of ovine foot-rot. I. A histological study of the bacterial invasion. J. Comp. Pathol., *79*:207–215, 1969.

Jensen, R., Flint, J. C., and Griner, L. A.: Experimental hepatic necrobacillosis in beef cattle. Am. J. Vet. Res., *15*:5–14, 1954.

Mackey, D. R.: Calf diphtheria. J. Am. Vet. Med. Assoc., *152*:822–823, 1968.

Marsh, H.: Necrobacillosis of the rumen in young lambs. J. Am. Vet. Med. Assoc., *104*:23–25, 1944.

Roberts, D. S., and Egerton, J. R.: The aetiology and pathogenesis of ovine foot-rot. II. The pathogenic association of *Fusiformis nodosus* and *F. nec-rophorus*. J. Comp. Pathol., *79*:217–227, 1969.

Simon, P. C., and Stovell, P. L.: Isolation of *Sphaerophorus necrophorus* from bovine hepatic abscesses in British Columbia. Can. J. Comp. Med., *35*:103–106, 1971.

———: Diseases of animals associated with *Sphaerophorus necrophorus*: characteristics of the organism. Vet. Bull., *39*:311–315, 1969.

Stewart, D. J.: An electron microscopic study of *Fusiformis nodosus*. Res. Vet. Sci., *14*:132–134, 1973.

Warner, J. F., Fales, W. H., Sutherland, R. C., and Teresa, G. W.: Endotoxin from *Fusobacterium nec-rophorum* of bovine hepatic abscess origin. Am. J. Vet. Res., *36*:1015–1025, 1975.

TUBERCULOSIS

Tuberculosis remains one of the most prevalent and devastating diseases of man and animals in spite of great strides made in its control and treatment. Although susceptibility to infection varies among species, tuberculosis occurs in all species of domestic animals and birds and in most wild animals, but presents a particularly serious problem in cattle, swine, domestic birds, and captive subhuman primates. Throughout most of the world, the bovine disease is widespread, but in the United States, Denmark and some other countries, its incidence has been greatly reduced by tuberculin testing and elimination of infected animals. In these countries, the control of bovine tuberculosis has dramatically reduced the prevalence of infection of the bovine type in man and animals.

The causative agents are acid-fast bacilli classified in the genus *Mycobacterium*. Three principal species cause tuberculosis, i.e., human, bovine, and avian organisms presently classified as *M. tuberculosis, M. bovis,* and *M. avium* respectively (Wayne et al., 1969). These organisms produce similar lesions, closely resemble one another morphologically, being small acid-fast bacillary forms, but vary in cultural characteristics, antigenic composition, and pathogenicity to various species (Table 12–2).

Susceptibility to Tuberculosis. Most vertebrates are susceptible to infection with tubercle bacilli *(Mycobacterium tuberculosis, M. bovis* and *M. avium)* under laboratory conditions. This susceptibility varies in degree in different species, and affects the frequency of the disease. The intensity and frequency of exposure to the organisms are also important factors in the prevalence of tuberculosis. Only in a few kinds of animals is the disease maintained in enzootic or epizootic numbers within the species. These include man, cattle, buffalo, voles, and fowl. For example, swine are often infected but appear to obtain the infection from cattle, fowl, or man. Monkeys become infected from exposure to infected people. In most other infections with tubercle bacilli, the organisms are not confined to one host species.

Among the species most susceptible to tuberculosis (Francis, 1958; Dannenberg, 1978) is a group made up of Old World monkeys (macaques, especially), guinea pigs, rabbits, and primitive people who have not been exposed to the organisms. Monkeys are exposed when captured and placed in contact with infected people. Guinea pigs and rabbits are not usually

Table 12–2. Mycobacterial Infections

Organism	Hosts	Disease
Mycobacterium tuberculosis (tubercle bacillus)	Man, cattle, dogs, nonhuman primates (experimentally: guinea pigs, hamsters)	Tuberculosis
M. bovis (bovine tubercle bacillus)	Cattle, man, swine, occasionally nonhuman primates, dogs, cats, parrots (experimentally: rabbits, guinea pigs, calves, hamsters, mice)	Tuberculosis
M. avium (avian tubercle bacillus)	Fowl, birds, local lesions in swine; occasionally primates, including man; rarely catttle, sheep [experimentally: rabbits, mice, guinea pigs (local lesions)]	Avian tuberculosis
M. ulcerans	Man (experimentally: mice, rats)	Ulceration of skin
M. microti (vole bacillus)	Vole (experimentally: guinea pigs, rabbits, calves)	Tuberculosis
M. marinarum	Fish, man	Acid-fast infection of fish, "swimming pool granuloma" in man
M. scrofulaceum	Children, swine	Cervical lymphadenitis
M. intracellulare (Battey bacillus)	Man; rarely swine, opossum	Chronic pulmonary disease, occasionally systemic disease
M. vaccae	Cattle (rare)	Mammary gland, skin lesions
M. fortuitum	Cattle, man, frog (experimentally: guinea pigs, rabbits, mice)	Local abscesses, occasionally pulmonary disease, mastitis, nodular infection of frog *(Gia)*
M. paratuberculosis	Cattle, sheep (experimentally: goats)	Paratuberculosis, Johne's disease
M. leprae (leprosy bacillus)	Man, armadillo (experimentally: armadillo)	Leprosy, Hansen's disease
M. lepraemurium (rat leprosy bacillus)	Rats	Granulomatous "nodular" disease of skin and lymph nodes; "rat leprosy"
Mycobacterium sp	Buffalo (India), frogs (South America), cats (Australia)	Nodular skin disease

infected in nature, but are very susceptible to experimental exposure.

The next most susceptible group of animals includes bovidae (cattle, sheep, goats, buffaloes), elephants, camels, swine, and modern man. Many other wild species become infected under zoo conditions.

A third group of animals with a somewhat lesser degree of susceptibility includes fowl, horses, asses, and mules.

Species with lowest susceptibility to tuberculosis include dogs, cats, mink, ferrets, hamsters, rats, and mice. Natural infection is rare in these species, and large numbers of organisms are required to produce experimental infection.

Atypical mycobacteria, culturally distinct from the three classical tubercle bacilli, have become increasingly important as causes of tuberculosis in man (Table 12–2).

Lesions. The characteristic microscopic lesion is the tubercle, starting as a cluster of neutrophils surrounding the invading bacilli, but replaced in a few hours by a whorl of macrophages (epithelioid, endothelioid, reticuloendothelial cells), which usually represents the earliest stage

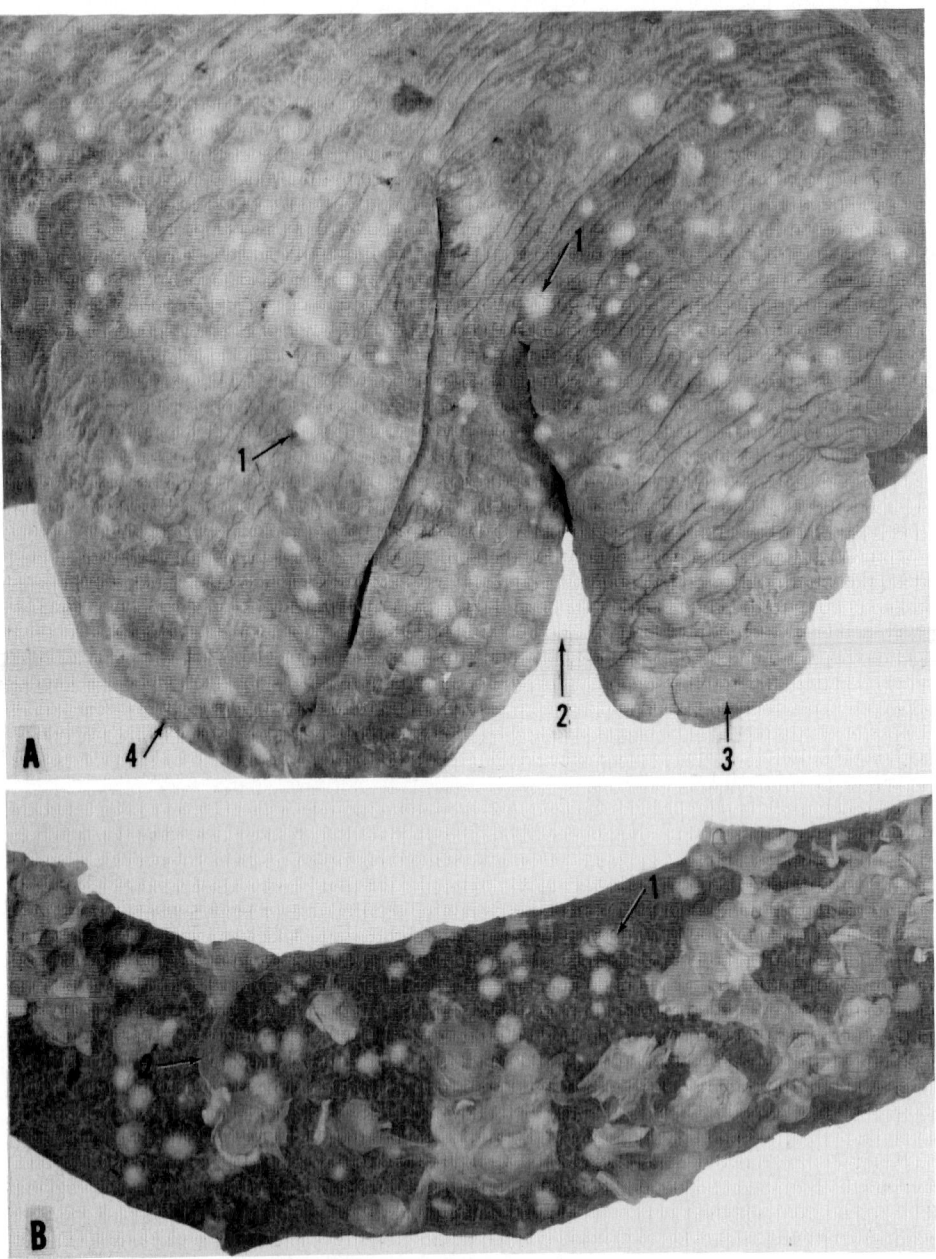

Fig. 12–5. Tuberculosis in swine. *A,* Lung. Sharply demarcated nodules (*1*) elevating the pleura. Cardiac notch (*2*), apical lobe (*3*), and inferior border (*4*) of the lung. *B,* Nodules in the spleen (*1*), adhesions of mesentery (*2*). (Courtesy of Armed Forces Institute of Pathology.) Contributor: Dr. B. A. Walter.

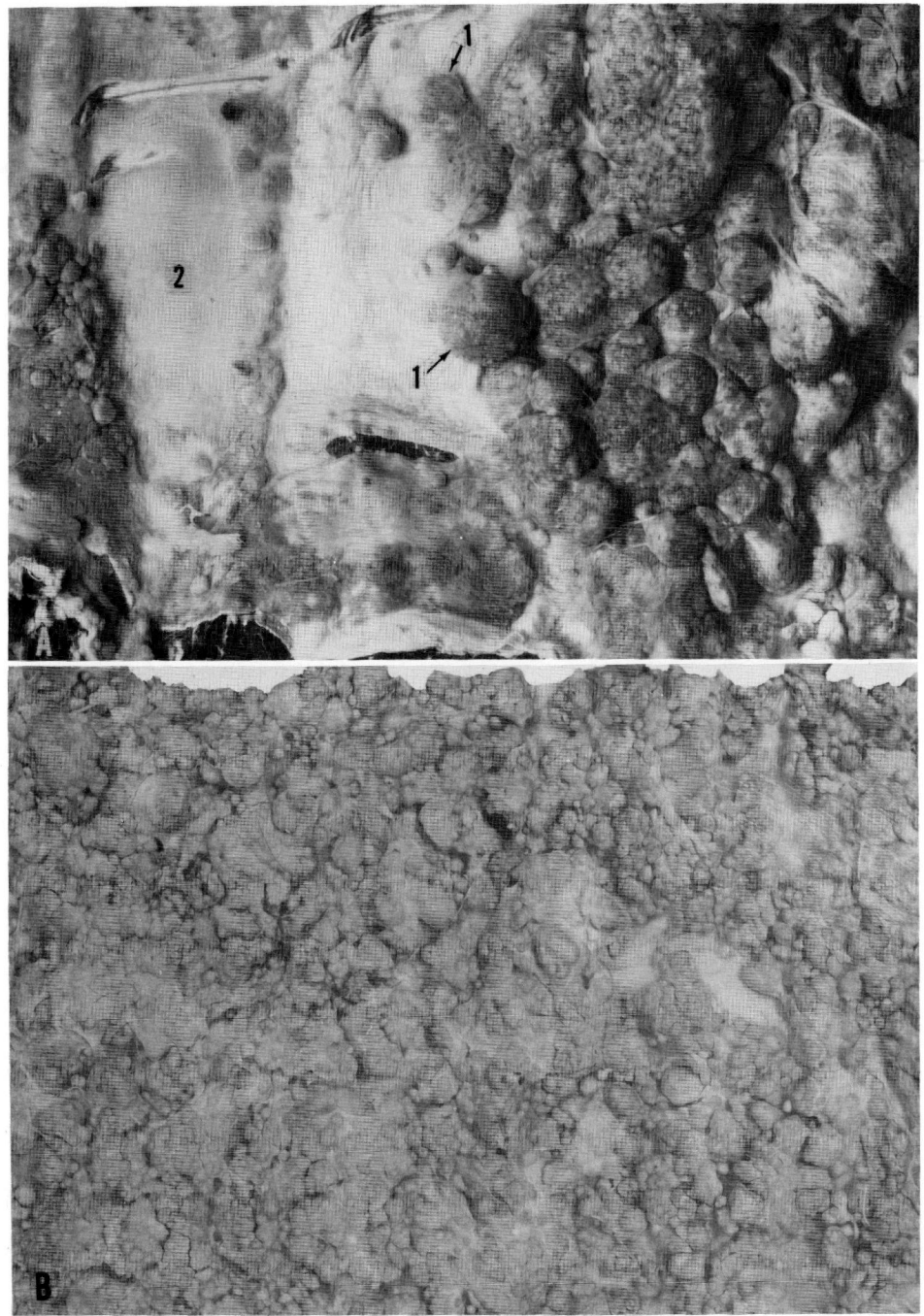

Fig. 12–6. Bovine tuberculosis. *A,* Involvement of pleura by coarse nodules (*1*). Inner surface of rib (2). Contributor: Major Lytle, V.C., U.S. Army. *B,* Tuberculous involvement of the omentum of a cow. (Courtesy of Armed Forces Institute of Pathology.) Contributor: Station Veterinarian, U.S. Army, Fort Bayard, N.M.

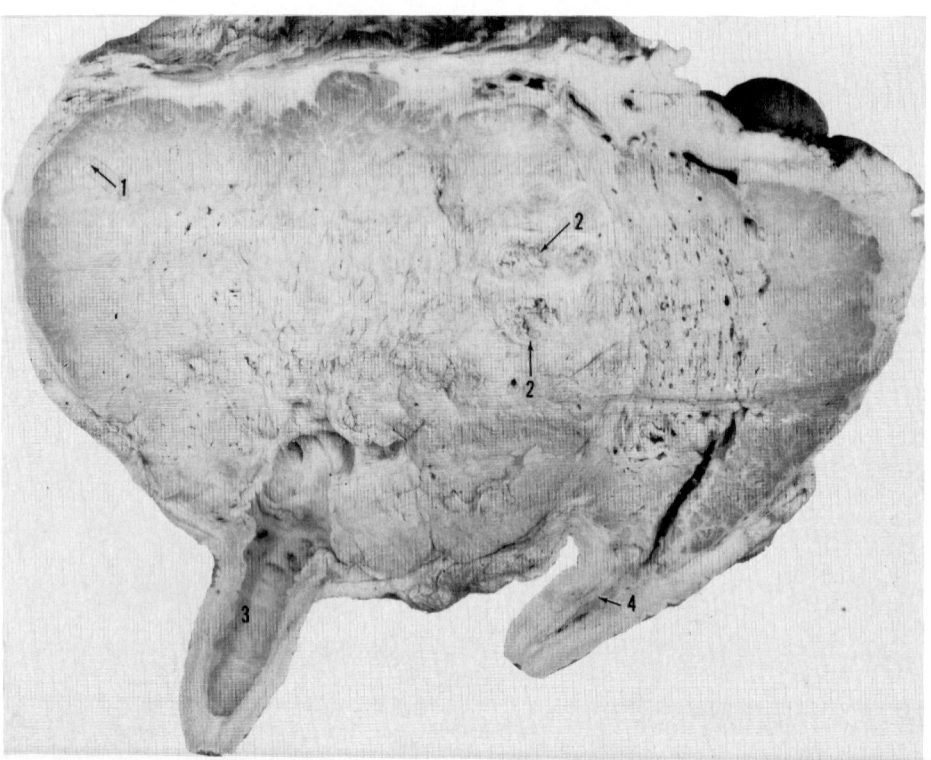

Fig. 12–7. Tuberculous mastitis, udder of a cow. Tiny discrete tubercles are seen at *(1)*, confluent lesions with central necrosis at *(2)*, normal teat canal *(3)*, partially obstructed canal *(4)*. (Courtesy of Armed Forces Institute of Pathology.) Contributor: Major Lytle, V.C., U.S. Army.

encountered. The epithelioid cells encircle and engulf the bacteria, but do not inhibit the growth of the lesion. As the tubercle bacilli multiply and produce toxic substances, the adjacent cells undergo caseous necrosis, and more epithelioid granulation tissue is laid down around the caseous center. The cells making up the granulation tissue have abundant, foamy, pale, acidophilic cytoplasm, and round, often eccentrically placed, nuclei. These cells may coalesce to form Langhans' giant cells, which are syncytial cells as much as 50 μ in diameter, with huge irregular masses of pale acidophilic cytoplasm and a number of round nuclei arranged in the form of a wreath or crescent at the periphery. The cell wall may be so indistinct that the cytoplasm appears to blend with adjacent tissues (Figs. 12–9, 12–10).

Langhans' giant cells may contain droplets of lipid and tubercle bacilli, the latter being demonstrable with acid-fast stains. Tubercle bacilli in varying numbers can also be demonstrated in the cytoplasm of epithelioid cells and in the caseous necrotic debris. The granulation tissue is usually surrounded by a zone of lymphocytes, arranged diffusely, in clumps, or near blood vessels. As the lesion ages, it becomes encapsulated by connective tissue of varying thickness. Calcification may occur in the caseous center of the tubercle, except in avian tuberculosis, where it is practically unknown.

A simple tubercle is usually between 1 mm and 2 cm in diameter, but larger conglomerate tubercles may be formed by the growth and coalescence of one or more adjacent single tubercles. Although they may

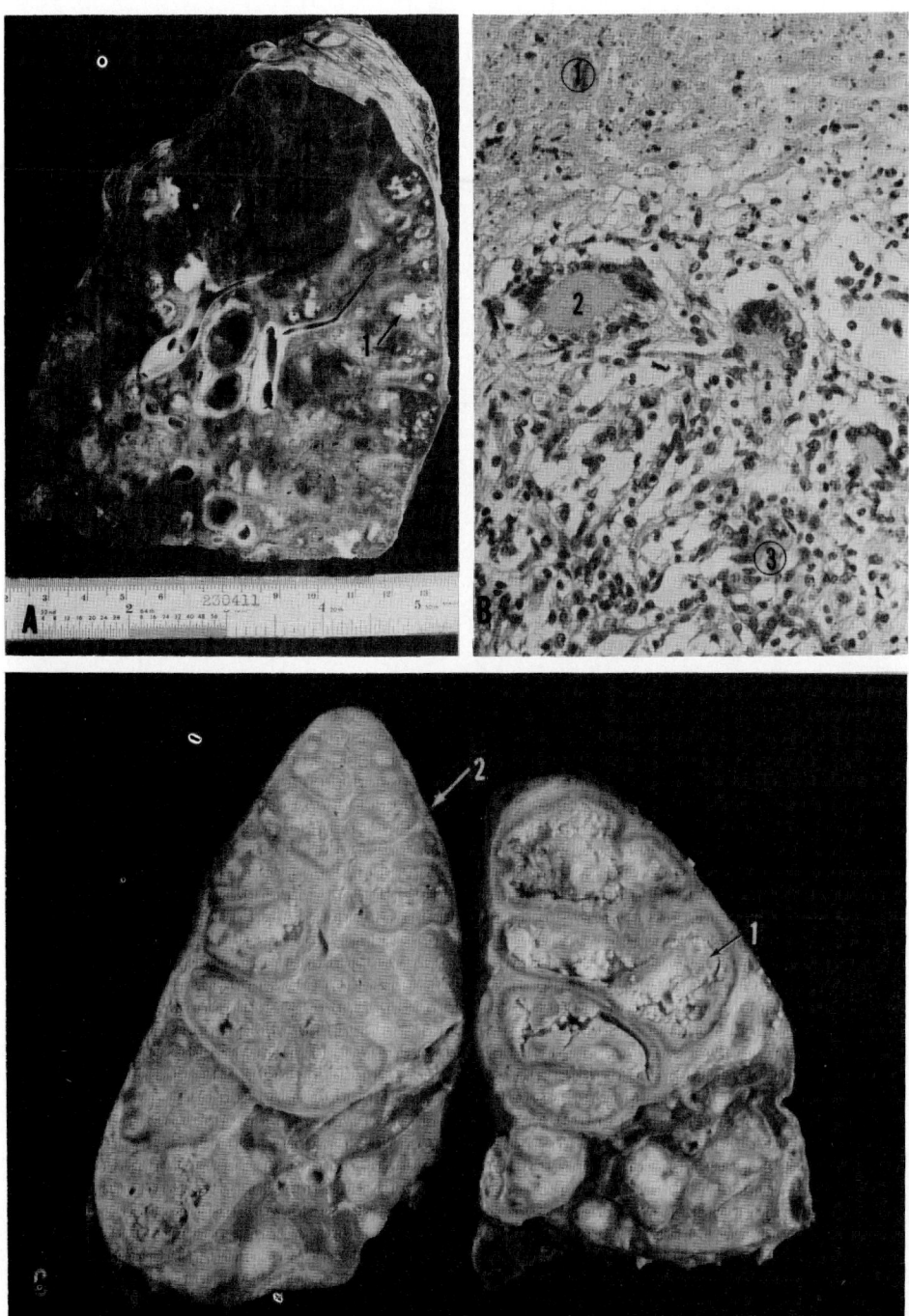

Fig. 12–8. *A*, Lobular pneumonia of tuberculosis. lung of a tapir. The white foci (*1*) represent pus in consolidated lobules, contrasting with less consolidated lung (*2*). Contributor: National Zoological Park. *B*, Margin of a tubercle in a bovine lung (× 260). Caseous necrosis (*1*), Langhans' giant cell (*2*), and epithelioid cells (*3*). *C*, Consolidated apical lobes of a bovine lung. Same as Case *B*. Note caseous areas (*1*) and thickening of pleura (*2*) and interlobular septa. (Courtesy of Armed Forces Institute of Pathology.) Contributor: Dr. Wm. H. Feldman.

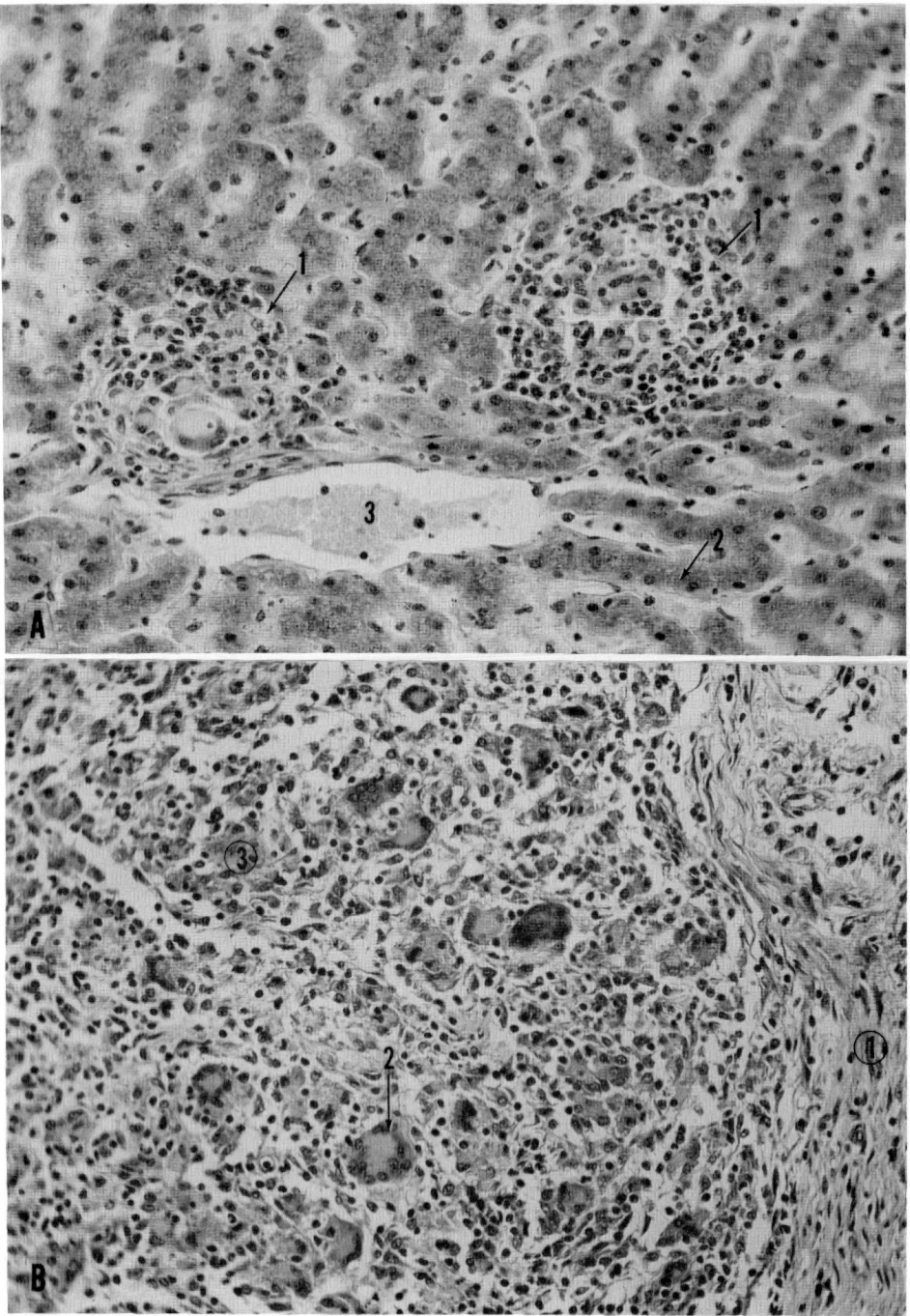

Fig. 12–9. Tuberculosis in a horse. *A*, Early tubercles in the liver (*1*) (× 260). Liver cell columns (*2*), central vein (*3*). *B*, Margin of a well-developed tubercle in the liver (× 260). The lesion is encapsulated (*1*) and contains many Langhans' giant cells (*2*) and epithelioid cells (*3*). (Courtesy of Armed Forces Institute of Pathology.) Contributor: Dr. J. R. M. Innes.

attain almost any shape and size, the structural relations still persist. If the bacteria in the lesion are eventually overcome, the tubercle will be reduced to a small mass of fibrous or hyaline scar tissue. This is recognized as a healed tubercle. If healing does not take place, secondary infection with other organisms may occur, to be followed by suppuration or by liquefaction necrosis that produces cavitation.

Infection with tubercle bacilli does not always result in the formation of typical tubercles. This is particularly true of meningeal tuberculosis, a rapidly fatal infection in which the pathologic changes consist of a scanty fibrinous or fibrinopurulent exudate on the surface of the pia mater and only a scattering of epithelioid cells in the meninges. Tissue reaction of a similar diffuse type may occur in overwhelming infections in sensitized animals.

The gross appearance of a tubercle, whether deep in soft tissue like liver and lungs, or bulging from a mucous or serous surface, is usually that of a firm or hard, white, gray, or yellow nodule. On cut section, its yellowish, caseous, necrotic center is dry and solid in contrast to the pus in an abscess. Calcification is common in many animals, and in sectioning a tubercle, a gritty sensation and grating sound indicate the presence of calcareous material.

Occasionally a tubercle breaks into a blood vessel, or by other means the blood is seeded with large numbers of tubercle bacilli, which lodge in capillaries of the parenchyma of visceral organs, where they give rise to myriad tubercles, 2 to 3 mm in diameter, all of the same age and size. Because these lesions suggested a sprinkling of millet seeds to early observers, they gave the name **miliary tuberculosis** to infection of this rapidly fatal type.

Lesions in Different Species. Although the general features of tuberculosis are evident in lesions from most species, certain differences in tissue reaction are more or less specific. In the **bovine,** calcification is often prominent, particularly in lymph

nodes. Disseminated tubercles over the pleural and peritoneal surfaces are also fairly common. The appearance of these individual tubercles, usually from 0.5 to 1.0 cm in diameter, gives this manifestation a common descriptive name—pearl disease. Of particular interest are certain bovine skin lesions which, though histologically indistinguishable from those of typical tuberculosis, are not caused by infection with tubercle bacilli. Acid-fast bacilli that apparently do not cause systemic disease produce these tuberculoid lesions. The organisms *(M. vaccae)* can be shown by bacteriologic methods to differ from the usual tubercle bacilli, but they do produce sensitivity to bovine tuberculin, a point of considerable practical importance.

In the **horse,** the lesions of tuberculosis are usually of chronic, proliferative character, and rarely exhibit caseation or calcification. Alimentary infection is the usual form, with possible extension elsewhere (Fig. 12–9). In **birds** also, calcification is seldom observed. The lesions of tuberculosis of the avian type in swine appear as multiple encapsulated foci, a few millimeters in diameter, scattered throughout the lymph nodes, particularly those of the head and cervical region. In **dogs,** pulmonary lesions rarely calcify, nor is caseation a prominent feature; diffuse infiltration of epithelioid cells usually predominates, but Langhans' giant cells are rare.

In **nonhuman primates,** the disease is usually pulmonary and may run a fulminating course; miliary lesions are frequent, caseation is often prominent, and calcification is rare. Langhans' giant cells may be numerous or absent. A Siamese **cat** infected with the avian-type organism was found to have granulomatous, calcified lesions in lymph nodes and diffuse consolidation of the lungs with epithelioid cells, in which no giant cells, caseous necrosis, nor calcification were present.

Infection by Mycobacterium avium in Monkeys. An enteric infection with acid-fast organisms long recognized in nonhu-

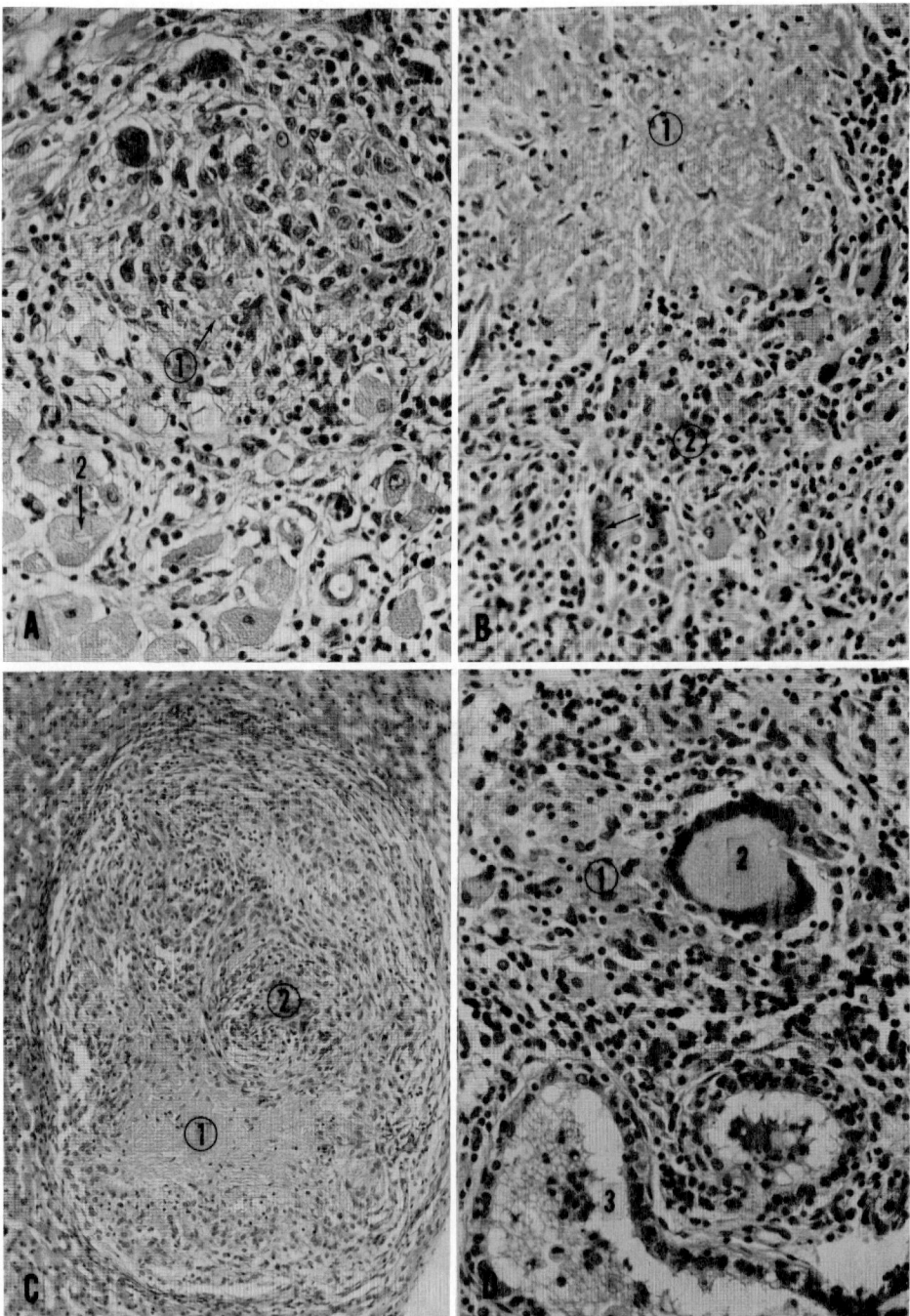

Fig. 12–10. Tuberculous lesions in different species. *A*, Tuberculous myocarditis in a pig (× 260). Note epithelioid cells (*1*) displacing myocardial fibers (*2*). Contributor: Dr. C. L. Davis. *B*, Tubercle in the spleen of a pig (× 260). Caseous necrosis (*1*), epithelioid cells (*2*), and giant cells (*3*). Contributor: Dr. C. L. Davis. *C*, Confluent tubercles in the liver of a dog (× 100). Note caseous necrosis (*1*) and epithelioid cells (*2*). Giant cells are absent. Contributor: Dr. R. B. Oppenheimer. *D*, Tuberculous mastitis in a cow (× 260). Note epithelioid cells (*1*), Langhans' giant cell (*2*), and mammary acinus (*3*). (Courtesy of Armed Forces Institute of Pathology.) Contributor: Dr. Wm. H. Feldman.

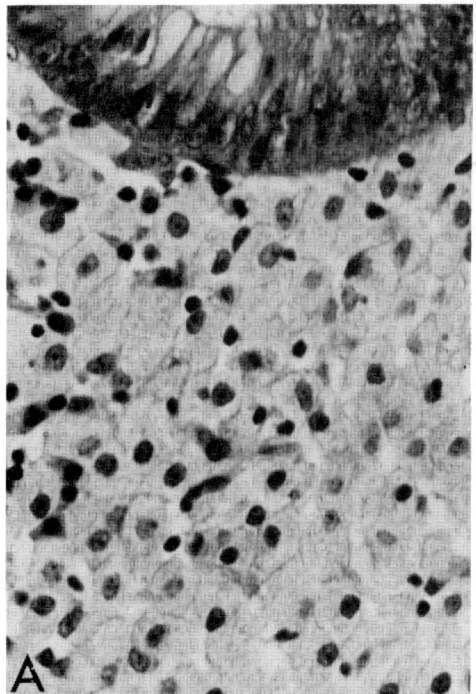

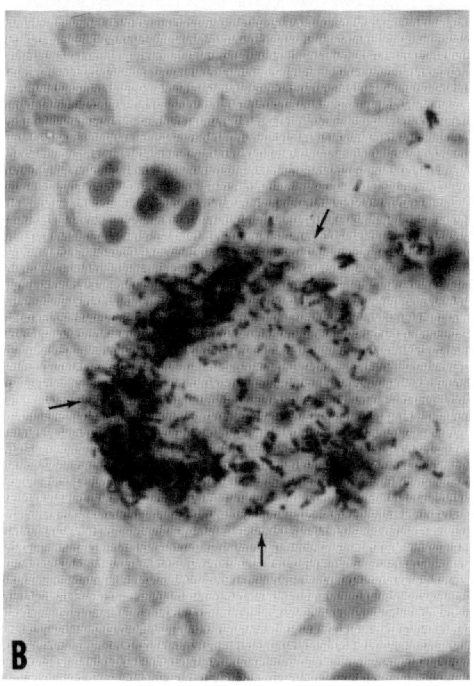

Fig. 12–11. Avian tuberculosis in a monkey. *A*, Large macrophages (epithelioid cells) in the lamina propria of the small intestine. *B*, A single macrophage (arrows) filled with tubercle bacilli (acid-fast stain). *B*, Contributed by Dr. C. L. Davis.

man primates is now known to be caused by the avian tubercle bacillus. The disease has been seen particularly in Old World monkeys, especially macaques. The clinical signs include persistent diarrhea and gradual emaciation. The lesions are found in the small intestines, ileum especially, but may also involve the cecum and colon. The principal gross lesions include rugose thickened mucosa and submucosa. Histologic preparations reveal the lamina propria and submucosa of the affected intestine to be filled and distended by macrophages (epithelioid cells). The cytoplasm of these cells is seen by appropriate stains to be packed with acid-fast organisms. Calcification, caseous necrosis or fibrosis are seldom seen, but an occasional Langhans' type giant cell may be evident. Sometimes the lesions extend to the mesenteric lymph nodes, visceral organs, or even subcutis.

In many respects the gross and microscopic findings resemble those of paratuberculosis. Isolation and identification of the organisms is necessary to distinguish this specific infection in nonhuman primates.

Pathogenesis. Inhalation of tubercle bacilli commonly precedes the formation of a primary lesion in the lung, usually in one of the diaphragmatic lobes. If the infection is overcome, this lesion may heal, leaving only a dense hyaline scar. This process, however, sensitizes the animal to products of tubercle bacilli, causing the tissues to respond much more violently to subsequent exposures. If the primary lesion does not heal, the infection may travel via the lymphatic channels along the respiratory tree toward the tracheal and bronchial lymph nodes. Secondary tubercles developing along the course of these lymphatics, which lie adjacent to the bronchial epithelium, may protrude into the bronchi, rupture, and discharge virulent bacilli into the lumen, thus permitting infection of terminal alveoli and resulting in tuberculous pneumonia. It is also possible for bacilli that are discharged into the respiratory passages to be coughed up and then swallowed, thus infecting the digestive system secondarily. Organisms may also gain access to the blood by rupture of veins or through lymphatics, and thus be carried to any part of the body. Infection of the digestive tract in children in all probability results from ingestion of infected milk, meat or other food. In any species, circumscribed lesions develop in the mucosa or submucosa and the organisms may spread by way of the lymphatics to lymph nodes and thence to other tissues. Spread to bone, spleen, kidneys, genitalia and mammary glands from intestinal lesions is not uncommon. Skin lesions may develop as a consequence of systemic dissemination or by direct contact when tubercle bacilli presumably gain access through abraded skin.

On the cellular level, the pathogenic events may be followed from the first entrance of tubercle bacilli to the lung or other tissue. These initial infecting bacilli are ingested by macrophages (epithelioid cells), which vary in enzyme content and microbicidal ability. If these factors are adequate, the bacilli are destroyed by microbicidal activity and then lysed by enzymes in the macrophage. If not destroyed, the tubercle bacilli grow and are released by necrosis of the macrophage, phagocytized by other macrophages, or transported elsewhere by macrophages. Usually, if the organisms are not destroyed, the center of the lesion becomes caseous due to the accumulation of necrotic macrophages. Liquefaction necrosis results in extracellular growth of tubercle bacilli, with accumulation of large numbers of organisms.

Blood-borne or tissue macrocytes, destined to become macrophages, arrive at the site of the lesion in an ineffectual state and must be "activated" locally to function. This is accomplished under the stimulation provided by the bacilli, their products, and the lymphokines produced by T-lymphocytes. This process is accelerated by the state of delayed hypersensitivity.

Hypersensitivity in Tuberculosis. Cellular hypersensitivity (delayed hypersensitivity) and cellular immunity play an important role in the pathogenesis of tuberculosis and account for (1) the striking difference between the reaction of an animal previously exposed to tuberculosis versus an animal which has never been infected, and (2) the effectiveness of tuberculin testing.

In previously exposed or vaccinated animals, the cellular reaction around tubercle bacilli develops within a few days, whereas in an unexposed individual, tubercle bacilli may remain at the site of inoculation and proliferate without inciting a response for as long as a week. Exposure to mycobacterial proteins results in hypersensitivity, which is expressed in the response of macrophages and lymphocytes which, when re-exposed or continuously exposed, are stimulated to proliferate and emigrate from the blood stream and accumulate at the site of tubercle bacilli or their extracts. Cellular hypersensitivity requires about 10 to 14 days to develop following natural infection. An increased capacity of macrophages to destroy tubercle bacilli is associated with the development of hypersensitivity. The latter cellular immunity, which is closely linked with hypersensitivity but which probably depends on mycobacterial lipids and polysaccharides, is mainly nonimmunologic in nature because it shows little specificity to tubercle bacilli, the "immune" macrophages having increased ability to destroy a variety of infectious agents. In contrast, cellular hypersensitivity is relatively specific to tuberculin. The net effect of calling forth "immune" macrophages is beneficial in overcoming infection and preventing its spread. However, if the mycobacterial products responsible for hypersensitivity are present in high concentrations, they cause necrosis of "sensitized" macrophages, which contributes to caseous necrosis of the reactive nodules of macrophages and lymphocytes. Obviously, circulatory phenomena and toxic products derived from the dying cells also contribute to necrosis. Delayed hypersensitivity is also held responsible, at least in part, for the liquefaction of the caseous foci, which provides an ideal locale for proliferation of tubercle bacilli separated from the host's defense reaction.

Thus hypersensitivity provides (1) a means of diagnosis (tuberculin), (2) the principal mechanism of combatting and resolving tuberculosis, and (3) a detrimental effect by killing macrophages (epithelioid cells). Hypersensitivity is described further in Chapter 7.

Diagnosis. The diagnosis of tuberculosis in the living animal may be based upon roentgenographic findings, the tuberculin test, and demonstration of the organisms in exudates or excretions. Several tests are being developed to identify immunologic features of tubercle bacilli, but are not yet established or in widespread use. These include a specific lymphocyte immunostimulation test, an indirect fluorescent antibody test, a bentonite flocculation test, and a soluble antigen fluorescence antibody test (Affronti et al., 1973; Condoulis et al., 1974; Fife et al., 1970).

In tissues obtained surgically or at necropsy, demonstration of acid-fast organisms within typical tubercles is sufficient to establish the diagnosis, although bacteriologic isolation of the organism is necessary to establish its type. Acid-fast bacteria *(Mycobacteria)* appear to infect many different species, hence it is important that in each instance organisms be recovered in culture for careful identification.

Ando, M., and Dannenberg, A. M., Jr.: Macrophage accumulation, division, maturation, and digestive and microbicidal capacities in tuberculous lesions. IV. Macrophage turnover, lysosomal enzymes and division in healing lesions. Lab. Invest., *27*:446–472, 1972.

Affronti, L. F., Fife, E. H., and Grow, L.: Serodiagnostic test for tuberculosis. Am. Rev. Respir. Dis., *107*:822–825, 1973.
Barton, M. D., and Acland, H. M.: *Mycobacterium avium* serotype 2 infection in a sheep. Aust. Vet. J., *49*:212–213, 1973.
Bone, J. F., and Soave, O. A.: Experimental tuberculosis in owl monkeys *(Aotus trivirgatus)*. Lab. Anim. Care, *20*:946–948, 1970.
Boughton, E.: Tuberculosis caused by *Mycobacterium avium*. Vet. Bull., *39*:457–465, 1969.
Brooks, O. H.: Observations on outbreaks of Battey type mycobacteriosis in pigs raised on deep litter. Aust. Vet. J., *47*:424–427, 1971.
Builbride, P. D. L., et al.: Tuberculosis in the free-living African (Cape) buffalo *(Syncerus caffer caffer,* Sparrman). J. Comp. Pathol., *73*:337–348, 1963. VB 811–64.
Capucci, D. T., Oshea, J. L., and Smith, G. D.: Epidemiologic account of tuberculosis transmitted from man to monkey. Am. Rev. Respir. Dis., *106*:819–823, 1972.
Cassidy, D. R., Morehouse, L. G., and McDaniel, H. A.: *Mycobacterium avium* infection in cattle: a case series. Am. J. Vet. Res., *29*:405–410, 1968.
Cheville, N. F., and Richards, W. D.: The influence of thymic and bursal lymphoid systems in avian tuberculosis. Am. J. Pathol., *64*:97–122, 1971.
Clarkson, M. J., and Smith, M. W.: An outbreak of tuberculosis in experimental monkeys caused by the bovine organism. Trans. R. Soc. Trop. Med. Hyg., *63*:24, 1969.
Condoulis, W. V., Soltysik, L. M., and Baram, P.: The in vitro assay of tuberculin hypersensitivity in *Macaca mulatta*. J. Med. Primatol., *3*:251–258, 1974.
Dannenberg, A. M., Jr.: Pathogenesis of pulmonary tuberculosis in man and animals: Protection of personnel against tuberculosis. In Mycobacterial Infections in Zoo Animals, edited by R. J. Montali. Washington, D. C., Smithsonian Institution Press, 1978.
Dannenberg, A. M.: Cellular hypersensitivity and cellular immunity in the pathogenesis of tuberculosis: specificity, systemic and local nature, and associated macrophage enzymes. Bact. Rev., *32*:85–102, 1968.
Englert, H. K. and Nassal, J.: Untersuchungen über das pathologisch-histologische Bild der durch die 3 Typen des Tuberkulose-erregers hervogerufenen Veränderungen beim Rind. Rindertuberk. u. Brucellose., *10*:21–27, 1961. VB 2048–61.
Feldman, W. H.: Histology of experimental tuberculosis in different species. Arch. Pathol., *11*:896–913, 1931.
———: Spontaneous tuberculous infections in dogs. J. Am. Vet. Med. Assoc., *85*:653–663, 1934.
Feldman, W. H., and Fitch, C. P.: Histologic features of the intradermic reactions to tuberculin in cattle. Arch. Pathol., *22*:495–509, 1936.
Feldman, W. H.: Avian Tuberculosis Infections. Baltimore, Williams & Wilkins Co., 1938.
Fife, E. H., Jr., Kruse, R. H., Toussaint, A. J., and Staab, E. V.: Serodiagnosis of simian tuber-

culosis by soluble antigen fluorescent antibody (Safa) tests. Lab. Anim. Care, *20*:969–978, 1970.

Fox, J. G., et al.: Tuberculosis spondylitis and Pott's paraplegia in a Rhesus monkey *(Macaca mulatta)*. Lab. Anim. Sci., *24*:335–339, 1974.

Francis, J.: Tuberculosis in Animals and Man. A Study in Comparative Pathology. London, Cassell and Co., Ltd., 1958.

Hime, J. M., Keymer, I. F., Boughton, E., and Birn, K. J.: Tuberculosis in a red deer *(Cervus elaphus)* due to an atypical mycobacterium. Vet. Rec., *88*:616–617, 1971.

Hix, J. A., Jones, T. C., and Karlson, A. G.: Avian tubercle bacillus infection in a cat. J. Am. Vet. Med. Assoc., *138*:641–647, 1961.

Innes, J. R. M.: The pathology and pathogenesis of tuberculosis in domesticated animals compared with man. Br. Vet. J., *96*:42–50, 96–105, 391–407, 1940.

———: Tuberculosis in the horse. Br. Vet. J., *105*:373–383, 1949.

Johnson, D. C., et al.: An epizootic of bovine tuberculosis in Georgia. J. Am. Vet. Med. Assoc., *167*:833–837, 1975.

Jorgensen, J. B., Haarbo, K., Dam, A., and Engbaek, H. C.: An enzootic of pulmonary tuberculosis in pigs caused by *M. avium*. I. Epidemiological and pathological studies. Acta Vet. Scand., *13*:56–67, 1972.

Kaufmann, A. F., Moulthrop, J. I., and Moore, R. M.: A perspective of simian tuberculosis in the United States—1972. J. Med. Primatol., *4*:278–286, 1972.

Karlson, A. G., Seibold, H. R., and Wolf, R. H.: *Mycobacterium abscessus* infection in owl monkey *(Aotus trivirgatus)*. Pathol. Vet., *7*:448–454, 1970.

Karlson, A. G., and Thoen, C. O.: *Mycobacterium avium* in tuberculous adenitis of swine. Am. J. Vet. Res., *32*:1257–1261, 1971.

Lau, D. T., Fuller, J. M., and Sumner, P. E.: Tuberculosis in a pig-tailed macaque. J. Am. Vet. Med. Assoc., *161*:696–699, 1972.

Leathers, C. W., and Hamm, T. E., Jr.: Naturally occurring tuberculosis in a Squirrel monkey and a Cebus monkey. J. Am. Vet. Med. Assoc., *169*:909–911, 1976.

Lesslie, I. W., and Davies, D. R. T.: Tuberculosis in a horse caused by the avian type tubercle bacillus. Vet. Rec., *70*:82–84, 1958.

Lindsey, J. R., and Melby, E. C., Jr.: Naturally occurring primary cutaneous tuberculosis in the rhesus monkey. Lab. Anim. Care, *16*:369–385, 1966.

Machotka, S. V., Chapple, F. E. III., and Stookey, J. L.: Cerebral tuberculosis in a rhesus monkey. J. Am. Vet. Med. Assoc., *167*:648–650, 1975.

McGavin, M. D., Mallmann, V. H., Mallmann, W. L., and Morrill, C. C.: Pathological changes in calves injected intradermally with *Mycobacterium intracellulare* serotype Davis and *M. avium* serotype 2. Vet. Pathol., *14*:56–66, 1977.

McLaughlin, A. R., and Moyle, A. I.: An epizootic of bovine tuberculosis. J. Am. Vet. Med. Assoc., *164*:396–397, 1974.

Miller, C. E., and Kinard, R.: A case of generalized

bone tuberculosis in a rhesus monkey. Lab. Anim. Care, *14*:264–267, 1964.

Mitchell, M. D., et al.: Swine tuberculosis in South Dakota. J. Am. Vet. Med. Assoc., *167*:152–153, 1975.

Montali, R. J. (ed.): Mycobacterial Infections of Zoo Animals. Washington, D. C., Smithsonian Institution Press, 1978.

Moore, T. D., Allen, A. M., Ganaway, J. R., and Sevy, C. E.: A fatal infection in the opossum due to *Mycobacterium intracellulare*. J. Infect. Dis., *123*:569–578, 1971.

Moreland, A. F.: Tuberculosis in New World primates. Lab. Anim. Care, *20*:262–264, 1970.

Nielsen, S. W., and Spratling, F. R.: Tuberculous spondylitis in a horse. Br. Vet. J., *124*:503–508, 1968.

Olson, G. A., and Woodard, J. C.: Miliary tuberculosis in a reticulated python. J. Am. Vet. Med. Assoc., *164*:733–735, 1974.

Pinto, M. R. M., Jainudeen, M. R., and Panabokke, R. G.: Tuberculosis in a domesticated Asiatic elephant *Elephus maximus*. Vet. Rec., *93*:662–664, 1973.

Renner, M., and Bartholomew, W. R.: Mycobacteriologic data from two outbreaks of bovine tuberculosis in nonhuman primates. Am. Rev. Respir. Dis., *109*:11–16, 1974.

Richardson, A.: The experimental production of mastitis in sheep by *Mycobacterium smegmatis* and *Mycobacterium fortuitum*. Cornell Vet., *61*:640–646, 1971.

Sesline, D. H., et al.: *Mycobacterium avium* infection in three rhesus monkeys. J. Am. Vet. Med. Assoc., *167*:639–645, 1975.

Smith, A. W., and Wolochow, H.: Comparison of old tuberculin and purified protein derivative in *Macaca mulatta*. Lab. Anim. Sci., *23*:373–376, 1973.

Smith, E. K., and Ruebner, B. H.: Granulomatous enteritis and amyloidosis associated with *Mycobacterium avium* in *Macaca nemestrina*. Fed. Proc., *29*:284, 1970.

Smith, E. K., et al.: Avian tuberculosis in monkeys, a unique mycobacterial infection. Am. Rev. Respir. Dis., *107*:469–471, 1973.

Smithwick, R. W., and David, H. L.: Acridine orange as a fluorescent counterstain with the auramine acid fast stain. Tubercle, *52*:226–231, 1971.

Snider, W. R.: Tuberculosis in canine and feline populations. Review of the literature. Am. Rev. Respir. Dis., *104*:877–887, 1971.

Snider, W. R., et al.: Tuberculosis in canine and feline populations. Study of high risk populations in Pennsylvania 1966–1968. Am. Rev. Respir. Dis., *104*:866–876, 1972.

Snyder, S., Peace, T., Soave, O., and Lund, J.: Tuberculosis in an owl monkey *(Aotus trivirgatus)*. J. Am. Vet. Med. Assoc., *157*:712–713, 1970.

Snyder, S. B., and Fox, J. G.: Tuberculin testing in rhesus monkeys *(Macaca mulatta)*: a comparative study using experimentally sensitized animals. Lab. Anim. Sci., *23*:515–521, 1973.

Stamp, J. T.: Tuberculosis of the bovine udder. J. Comp. Pathol. Ther., *53*:220–230, 1943.

Thoen, C. O., et al.: *Mycobacterium bovis* infection in baboons *(Papio papio).* Arch. Pathol., *101*:291–293, 1977.

——: Experimentally induced *Mycobacterium avium* serotype 8 infection in swine. Am. J. Vet. Res., *37*:177–182, 1976.

Thoen, C. O., Himes, E. M., Weaver, D. E., and Spangler, G. W.: Tuberculosis in brood sows and pigs slaughtered in Iowa. Am. J. Vet. Res., *37*:775–778, 1976.

Unanue, E. R.: Secretory functions of mononuclear phagocytes. Am. J. Pathol., *83*:396–417, 1976.

Wayne, L. G., Runyon, E. H., and Kubica, G. P.: Mycobacteria: a guide to nomenclatural usage. Am. Rev. Resp. Dis., *100*:732–734, 1969.

Youmans, G. P.: Relation between delayed hypersensitivity and immunity in tuberculosis. Am. Rev. Respir. Dis., *111*:109–114, 1975.

PARATUBERCULOSIS (Johne's Disease)

Paratuberculosis is a specific infection with an acid-fast organism, *Mycobacterium paratuberculosis,* which is known to affect cattle, sheep and goats, and is suspected of causing disease in swine and horses. It is a wasting illness with a prolonged course, during which intractable diarrhea results in dehydration, emaciation, and eventually death. The disease is of worldwide distribution and constitutes an important economic problem in cattle, but is less frequently encountered in other species. Many laboratory animals are resistant; however, infection has been established in rabbits, mice, rats, hamsters, guinea pigs, and moles. Successful transmission in both laboratory animals and ruminants usually requires exposure at an early age. Swine, horses, and chickens have also been shown to be susceptible to oral and intravenous inoculation of *Mycobacterium paratuberculosis.*

Infection in cattle and sheep does not always lead to clinical disease, however; even in the absence of recognizable infection, the organism is shed in the feces, providing a source of infection for young animals. Although lesions are usually restricted to the intestinal tract and lymph nodes, the organism can infect the uterus, which may lead to congenital infection and abortion.

Lesions. The terminal part of the ileum is the most common site of the specific lesions, which also occur in the remainder of the small and large intestines and the mesenteric lymph nodes. Microscopic sections reveal the lamina propria of the mucosa to be closely packed with large, discrete epithelioid cells that have abundant foamy cytoplasm and are frequently multinucleated. These cells also infiltrate and

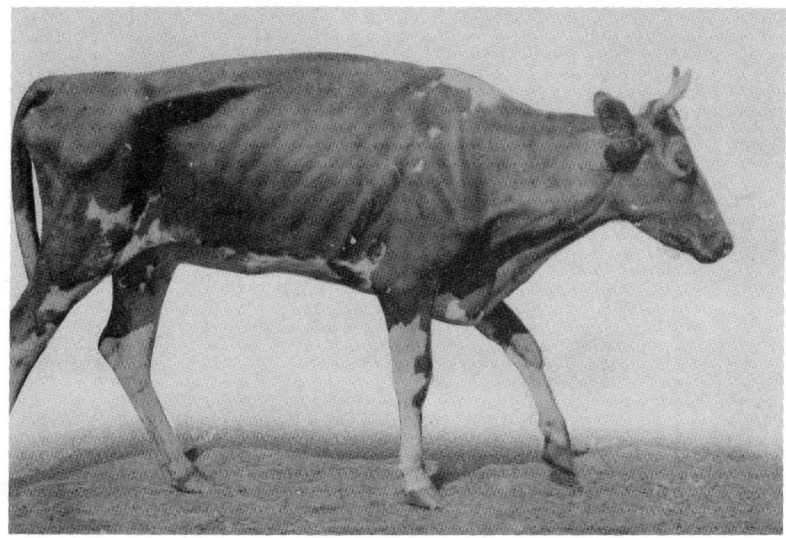

Fig. 12–12. Paratuberculosis. Emaciation and dehydration are significant features in this affected cow.

thicken the submucosa, but leave the muscularis mucosae and the muscularis intact. Nests of these same epithelioid cells may be found in mesenteric lymph nodes, but seldom elsewhere. In impression smears or sections through these lesions, Ziehl-Neelsen's stain demonstrates quantities of acid-fast, rod-shaped organisms crowding the cytoplasm of the epithelioid cells.

Secondary changes in the intestinal mucosa in paratuberculosis include edema, which results from local interference with circulation, nests of neutrophils, and increased numbers of eosinophils, the latter perhaps explainable on the basis of helminthic parasitism. Of importance is the absence of caseous necrosis, nodule formation, calcification, and increased vascularization. In contrast to cattle, nodule formation with necrosis and calcification has been described in sheep and goats.

The gross appearance is directly related to the microscopic changes. The affected intestinal wall is thickened, sometimes edematous, and its mucosal surface bears many broad, closely placed, transverse folds, or rugae. These rugae result from thickening of villi and give the surface a corrugated appearance, which does not disappear when the intestinal wall is stretched (Fig. 12–13).

Although lesions are usually confined to the intestines and lymph nodes, generalized infection has been described in both naturally and experimentally infected cattle, sheep, and goats, with lesions in the liver, spleen, lungs, kidneys, uterus, placenta, and nonmesenteric lymph nodes.

Diagnosis. The gross lesions in the intestine are highly suggestive, but confirmation of the diagnosis depends on the demonstration of epithelioid cells containing acid-fast bacilli in huge numbers in smears or sections of mucosa or submucosa. In about 60% of affected cattle, the lesions and organisms extend into the colon and rectum, which makes it possible to diagnose the disease in the living animal by microscopic examination of mucosal scrapings collected per rectum.

The diffuse nature of the lesions, their confinement to the intestinal mucosa and mesenteric lymph nodes, and the presence of myriads of acid-fast bacilli serve to dif-

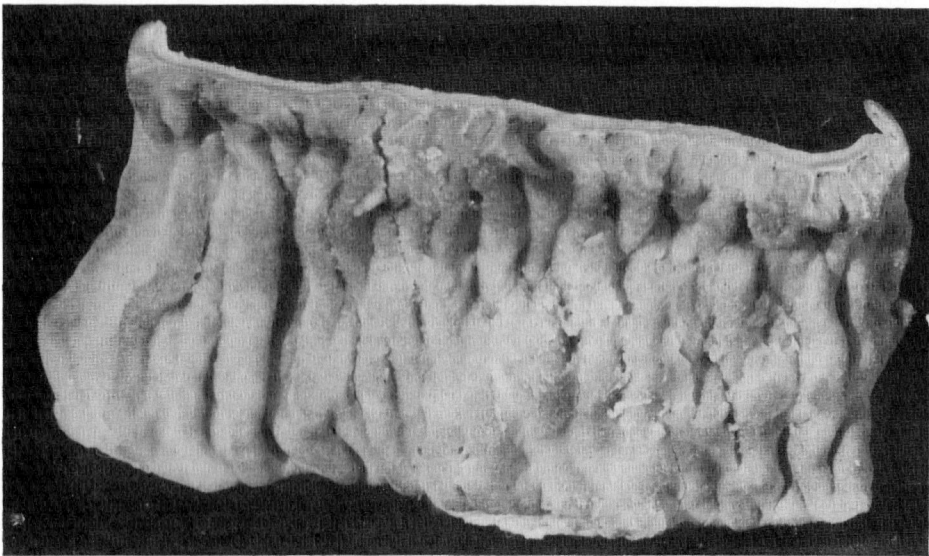

Fig. 12–13. Paratuberculosis (Johne's Disease), small intestine of a cow. Note thick, rugose mucosa. (Courtesy of Armed Forces Institute of Pathology.) Contributor: Dr. Edward Records.

ferentiate paratuberculosis from tuberculosis, in which nodule formation, fibrosis, abscess formation, necrosis, calcification, and but few acid-fast bacilli are characteristic. In sheep and goats, lesions with caseation and calcification require greater caution in differentiating tuberculosis; however, the diffuse distribution of the lesions of paratuberculosis usually allows this distinction.

Avian tubercle bacilli produce similar lesions in nonhuman primates. Culture and identification of the organisms is essential in this and all other infections with acid-fast organisms.

The intradermal johnin test and the complement-fixation test are aids to clinical diagnosis, but neither is completely satisfactory.

Aalund, O., Hoerlein, A. B., and Adler, H. C.: The migration test on circulating bovine leukocytes and its possible application in the diagnosis of Johne's disease. Acta Vet. Scand., 11:331–334, 1970.

Boever, W. J., and Peters, D.: Paratuberculosis in two herds of exotic sheep. J. Am. Vet. Med. Assoc., 165:822–823, 1974.

Buergelt, C. D., et al.: Lymphocyte transformation: an aid in the diagnosis of paratuberculosis. Am. J. Vet. Res., 38:1709–1715, 1977.

Buergelt, C. D., Hall, C., McEntee, K., and Duncan, J. R.: Pathological evaluation of paratuberculosis in naturally infected cattle. Vet. Pathol., 15:196–207, 1978.

Doyle, T. M.: Foetal infection in Johne's disease. Vet. Rec., 70:238, 1958.

Gilmour, N. J. L.: Recent research on Johne's disease. Vet. Rec., 77:1322–1326, 1965.

Goudswaard, J., and Terporten-Pastoors, W. W. M.: Johne's disease in goats; comparison of serological tests. Neth. J. Vet. Sci., 4:93–112, 1972.

Goudswaard, J., Gilmour, N. J. L., Dijkstra, R. G., and Van Beek, J. J.: Diagnosis of Johne's disease in cattle: a comparison of five serological tests under field conditions. Vet. Rec., 89:461–462, 1976.

Hallman, E. T., and Witter, J. F.: Some observations on the pathology of Johne's disease. J. Am. Vet. Med. Assoc., 83:159–187, 1933.

Harding, H. P.: Experimental infection with *Mycobacterium johnei*. 2. Histopathology of infection in experimental goats. J. Comp. Pathol., 67:37–52, 1957.

———: The histopathology of *Mycobacterium johnei* infection in small laboratory animals. J. Pathol. Bact., 78:157–169, 1959.

Hatakeyama, H., et al.: An outbreak of Johne's disease among sheep in Japan. Nat. Int. Anim. Hlth. Quart. Tokyo, 3:21–31, 1963. (In Engl.)

Hole, N. H.: Johne's disease. Adv. Vet. Sci., 4:341–387, 1958.

Howarth, J. A.: Paratuberculous enteritis in sheep. Cornell Vet., 27:223–234, 1937.

Johne, H. A., and Frothingham, L.: Ein eigenthümlicher Fall von Tuberculose beim Rind. Deutsch. Zeit Thiermed verg. Pathol., 21:438–454, 1895.

Kim, J. C. S., Sanger, V. L., and Whitenack, D. L.: Ultrastructural studies of bovine paratuberculosis (Johne's disease). Vet. Med. Small Anim. Clin., 71:78–83, 1976.

Kopecky, K. E.: Distribution of bovine paratuberculosis in the U. S. J. Am. Vet. Med. Assoc., 162:787–788, 1973.

———: Distribution of paratuberculosis in Wisconsin by soil regions. J. Am. Vet. Med. Assoc., 170:320–324, 1977.

Kopecky, K. E., Larsen, A. B., and Merkal, R. S.: Uterine infection in bovine paratuberculosis. Am. J. Vet. Res., 28:1043–1045, 1967.

Kluge, J. P., Monlux, W. S., Kopecky, K. E., and Lehmann, R. P.: Experimental paratuberculosis in sheep after oral, intratracheal, or intravenous inoculation: lesions and demonstration of etiologic agent. Am. J. Vet. Res., 29:953–962, 1968.

Larsen, A. B., Moon, H. W., and Merkal, R. S.: Susceptibility of swine to *Mycobacterium paratuberculosis*. Am. J. Vet. Res., 32:589–595, 1971.

———: Susceptibility of horses to *Mycobacterium paratuberculosis*. Am. J. Vet. Res., 33:2185–2189, 1972.

Larsen, A. B., and Moon, H. W.: Experimental *Mycobacterium paratuberculosis* infection in chickens. Am. J. Vet. Res., 33:1231–1236, 1972.

Larsen, A. B., Miller, J. M., and Kopecky, K. E.: Susceptibility of the Mongolian gerbil (*Meriones unguiculatus*) to *Mycobacterium paratuberculosis*. Am. J. Vet. Res., 37:1113–1114, 1976.

Larsen, A. B., and Kopecky, K. E.: *Mycobacterium paratuberculosis* in reproductive organs and semen of bulls. Am. J. Vet. Res., 31:255–258, 1970.

———: Studies on the intravenous administration of johnin to diagnose Johne's disease. Am. J. Vet. Res., 26:673–675, 1965.

Larsen, A. B., Vardaman, T. H., and Merkal, R. S.: An extended study of a herd of cattle naturally infected with Johne's disease. I. The significance of the intradermal johnin test. Am. J. Vet. Res., 24:91–93, 1963.

Lominski, I., Cameron, J., and Roberts, G. B. S.: Experimental Johne's disease in mice. J. Pathol. Bact., 71:211–221, 1956.

Majeed, S., and Goudswaard, J.: Aortic lesions in goats infected with *Mycobacterium johnei*. J. Comp. Pathol., 81:571–576, 1971.

Merkal, R. S.: Laboratory diagnosis of bovine paratuberculosis. J. Am. Vet. Med. Assoc., 163:1100–1102, 1973.

Merkal, R. S., Richard, J. L., Thurston, J. R., and Ness, R. D.: Effect of methotrexate on rabbits infected with *Mycobacterium paratuberculosis* or *Dermatophilus congolensis*. Am. J. Vet. Res., 33:401–407, 1972.

Merkal, R. S., Larsen, A. B., and Booth, G. D.: Analysis of the effects of inapparent bovine paratuberculosis. Am. J. Vet. Res., 36:837–838, 1975.

Merkal, R. S., Kopecky, K. E., Monlux, W. S., and Quinn, L. Y.: Experimental paratuberculosis in sheep after oral, intratracheal, or intravenous inoculation: serologic and intradermal tests. Am. J. Vet. Res., 29:963–969, 1968.

Merkal, R. S., Kopecky, K. E., Larsen, A. B., and Ness, R. D.: Immunologic mechanisms in bovine paratuberculosis. Am. J. Vet. Res., 31:475–486, 1970.

M'Fadyean, J.: Histology of the lesions of Johne's disease. J. Comp. Pathol. Ther., 31:73–87, 1918.

Minett, F. C.: The diagnosis of Johne's disease by cultural methods. J. Pathol. Bact., 54:209–219, 1942.

Nakamatsu, M., Fujimoto, Y., and Satoh, H.: The pathological study of paratuberculosis in goats, centered around the formation of remote lesions. Jpn. J. Vet. Res., 16:103–120, 1969.

O'Brien, J. J., Baskerville, A., and McClelland, T. G.: Johne's disease in sheep in Northern Ireland. Br. Vet. J., 128:359–365, 1972.

Omar, A. R., Lim, S. Y., and Retnasabapathy, A.: Placentitis and abortion in a cow probably caused by Mycobacterium johnei. Kajian Vet. Singapore, 1:39–43, 1967.

Patterson, D. S. P., and Allen, W. M.: Chronic mycobacterial enteritis in ruminants as a model of Crohn's disease. Proc. R. Soc. Med., 65:46–49, 1972.

Pearson, J. K. L., and McClelland, T. G.: Uterine infection and congenital Johne's disease in cattle. Vet. Rec., 67:615–616, 1955.

Rajya, B. S., and Singh, C. M.: Studies on the pathology of Johne's disease in sheep. III. Pathologic changes in sheep with naturally occurring infections. Am. J. Vet. Res., 22:189–203, 1961.

Rankin, J. D.: The experimental production of Johne's disease in laboratory rabbits. J. Pathol. Bact., 75:363–366, 1958.

————: The present knowledge of Johne's disease. Vet. Rec., 70:693–697, 1958.

Simon, J. and Brewer, R. L.: Investigation of Johne's disease in three cattle herds. J. Am. Vet. Med. Assoc., 143:263–266, 1963.

Taylor, A. W.: Experimental Johne's disease in cattle. J. Comp. Pathol., 63:355–367, 1953.

van Ulsen, F. W.: Paratuberkulose bij een dwergezel (Equus asinus form dom.) Tijdschr. Diergeneeskd., 95:446–448, 1970.

LEPROSY IN THE ARMADILLO

The nine-banded armadillo (*Dasypus novemcinctus*, Linn) has recently been reported to develop disseminated (lepromatous) leprosy following experimental injection of leprosy bacilli (*Mycobacterium leprae*) from human patients (Storrs, 1971;

Kirchheimer and Storrs, 1971). This finding, now amply confirmed, has stimulated needed research on this age-old but yet poorly understood human disease. Much remains to be learned if leprosy is to be thoroughly understood and the most effective means to treat and control the disease are to become available.

Not only is the armadillo fully susceptible to experimental infection with leprosy bacilli, but also is naturally infected with *M. leprae* in certain parts of southern Louisiana (Walsh et al., 1975). In these natural cases, large numbers of acid-fast bacilli are demonstrable in many organs, including skin, lymph nodes, spleen, and liver. As in the disease in man, the organisms do not grow in laboratory media, but multiply profusely in armadillo tissues. This provides a needed source of organisms for study. Natural leprosy has also been reported in the chimpanzee (Donham and Leininger, 1977; Leininger et al., 1978).

Balentine, J. D., Chang, S. C., and Issar, S. L.: Infection of armadillos with *Mycobacteriumn leprae*. Arch. Pathol. Lab. Med., 100:175–181, 1976.

Convit, J., and Pinardi, M. E.: Leprosy: confirmation in the armadillo. Science, 184:1191–1192, 1974.

Donham, K. J., and Leininger, J. R.: Spontaneous leprosy-like disease in a chimpanzee. J. Infect. Dis., 136:132–136, 1977.

Kirchheimer, W. F., and Storrs, E. E.: Attempts to establish the armadillo (*Dasypus novemcinctus*, Linn) as a model for the study of leprosy. 1. Report of lepromatous leprosy in an experimentally infected armadillo. Int. J. Lepr., 39:692–701, 1971.

Leininger, J. R., Donham, K. J., and Rubino, M. J.: Leprosy in a chimpanzee. Pathology of the disease and characterization of the organism. Vet. Pathol., 15:339–346, 1978.

Meyers, W. M., Kavernes, S., and Binford, C. H.: Comparison of reactions to human and armadillo lepromins in leprosy patients. Int. J. Lepr., 43:218, 1975.

Storrs, E. E.: The nine-banded armadillo: A model for leprosy and other biomedical research. Int. J. Lepr., 39: 702–703, 1971.

Storrs, E. E., Walsh, G. P., Burchfield, H. P., and Binford, C. H.: Leprosy in the armadillo: new model for biomedical research. Science, 183:851–852, 1974.

Walsh, G. P., et al.: Leprosy-like disease occurring naturally in armadillos. J. Reticuloendothel. Soc., 18:347–351, 1975.

LEPROSY OF BUFFALOES
(Lepra Bubalorum)

A disease of water buffaloes (carabao) characterized by persistent cutaneous and subcutaneous nodules on the legs and lower parts of the abdomen and thorax occurs in Java and other East Indian countries. It is of particular interest because of the similarity of its histologic features to those of human leprosy. Apparently the disease is uncommon and ordinarily does not result in death or serious disability. The causative organism, although demonstrable in tissue, has not been cultured successfully. A similar but even less frequent disease (Lepra bovinum) has been described in cattle in the East Indies.

Lesions. The cutaneous nodules result from accumulation of large numbers of epithelioid cells in the dermis. Microscopically, these individually discrete cells are seen to have greatly distended, foamy, often vacuolated cytoplasm in which numerous acid-fast bacilli are demonstrable. The large vacuoles are believed to be the result of lipid production by the bacilli and are identical to those in the large "lepra cells" of human leprosy. Giant cells of Langhans' type may be seen, but caseation necrosis and calcification do not occur. The gross appearance of the lesion is not distinctive. A solid, uniform nodule, with a diameter as great as 4 to 5 cm, may be firmly attached to the dermis and elevate the epidermis.

Diagnosis. In countries where the disease occurs, the diagnosis can be made on the basis of the collections of "lepra cells" in the dermis, these cells being laden with acid-fast bacilli.

Lobel, L. W. M.: Lepra bubalorum. Int. J. Lepr., 4:79–96, 1936.

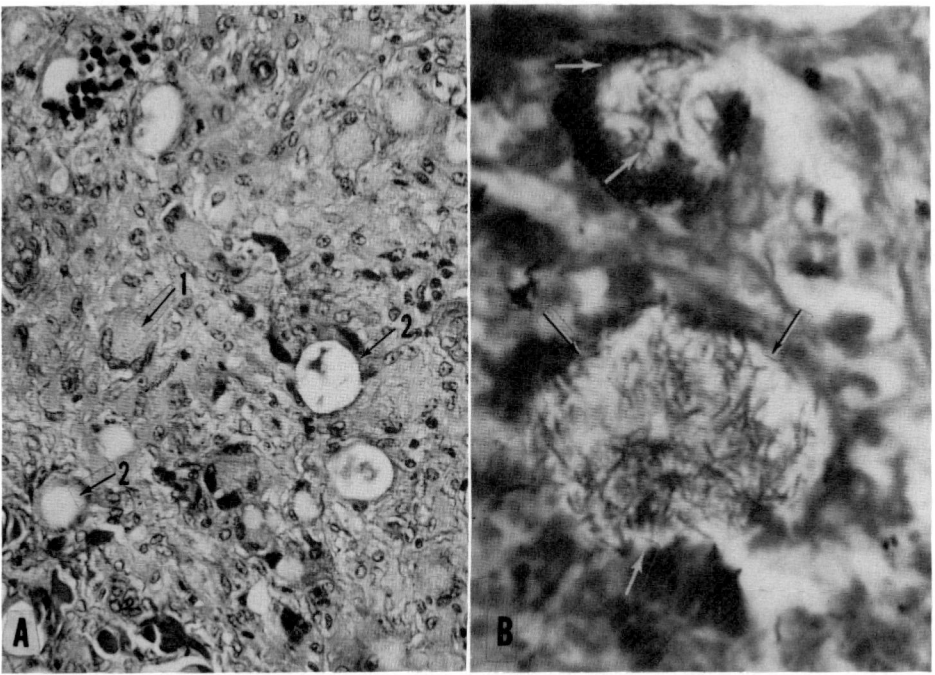

Fig. 12–14. Leprosy of buffaloes. *A*, A section of a dermal nodule (× 300). Giant cells (*1*) and large macrophages, many containing large "globules" (*2*). *B*, Higher magnification (× 1250) of a section stained for acid-fast bacilli. The "globules" (arrows) are filled with acid-fast organisms. (Courtesy of Armed Forces Institute of Pathology.) Contributor: Dr. K. W. Wade.

MURINE LEPROSY

Murine leprosy, a spontaneous disease of rats and mice that closely resembles human leprosy, was first described in 1902 by Stefansky. This disease has been studied extensively during the intervening years in attempts to gain information applicable to its human counterpart. The murine infection has been propagated by transfer of tissue suspensions containing the acid-fast bacilli, but the organisms have not been successfully cultivated outside the body of living animals. Progressive disease has been established in mice and rats, and nonprogressive infection has been produced in rabbits and monkeys, but not in guinea pigs. The causative organism is now considered to be *Mycobacterium lepraemurium*, which can be differentiated by appropriate means from *Mycobacterium leprae*, the human leprosy bacillus.

Lesions. The lesions in murine leprosy are the result of aggregations of cells packed with bacilli, diffusely infiltrating the dermis, subcutis, and all viscera except the kidney, or forming nodules in these tissues. These enlarged cells with foamy cytoplasm laden with acid-fast bacilli are called "lepra cells." They usually are derived from the reticuloendothelial system, but occasionally from epithelial cells of the epidermis, testicular tubules, or epididymis. Some lepra cells contain such excessive numbers of bacilli and such quantities of lipid that they form vacuolated globi, identical with those that occur in human or bovine leprosy (Fig. 12–14).

Although murine leprosy occurs as a spontaneous disease in laboratory rodents, it is of particular importance as a symbiont which can be studied to gain information applicable to human leprosy.

Granulomas resembling the nodular lesions of leprosy have been described in frogs, but their significance and relationship to leprosy have not been established.

Closs, O., and Haugen, O. A.: Experimental murine leprosy. 3. Early local reaction to *Mycobacterium lepraemurium* in C311 and C57/BL mice. Acta Pathol. Microbiol. Scand. A, *83*:51–58, 1975.
Fite, G. L.: Leprosy: The pathology of experimental rat leprosy. U. S. Nat. Health Bull. No. 173, pp. 45–76, U. S. Pub. Health Service, Washington, D. C., 1940.
Krakower, C., and Gonzales, L. M.: Mouse leprosy. Arch. Pathol., *30*:308–329, 1940.
Lowe, J.: Rat leprosy, a critical review of the literature. Int. J. Lepr., *5*:311–328, 463–482, 1937.
Machicao, N., and La Placa, E.: Lepra-like gram-ulomas in frogs. Lab. Invest., *3*:219–227, 1954.
Pinkerton, H., and Sellards, A. W.: Histological and cytological studies of murine leprosy. Am. J. Pathol., *14*:435–442, 1938.
Sellards, A. W., and Pinkerton, H.: The behavior of murine and human leprosy in foreign hosts. Am. J. Pathol., *14*:421–434, 1938.
Stefansky, W. K.: Eine lepraähnliche Erkrankung der Haut und der Lymphdrüsen bei Wanderraten. Zentralbl. Bakteriol., Orig. (pt. 1), *33*:481–487, 1903.

FELINE LEPROSY

Leprosy of the domestic cat (*Felis catus*) was first described in New Zealand (Bowman et al., 1962) as a nontuberculous granulomatous disease involving the dermis and subcutis. The disease has at this writing been reported in Australia, Great Britain, Netherlands, United States, and Canada. The causative agent has been identified as identical to *Mycobacterium lepraemurium* (Leiker and Poelma, 1974).

Lesions. The lesions usually appear as single or multiple nodules involving the skin and subcutis in almost any part of the body. The epidermis is occasionally ulcerated. The microscopic appearance is characteristic with large numbers of macrophages (epithelioid cells) replacing the dermis or subcutis. These cells are often large with foamy cytoplasm. Langhans' type giant cells are infrequent; caseous necrosis, calcification, or fibrosis are not usually seen. Appropriate stains reveal the epithelioid cells to be filled with acid-fast bacilli. These organisms fail to grow on any presently available media.

Brown, L. R., May, C. D., and Williams, S. E.: A non-tuberculous granuloma in cats. N. Z. Vet. J., *10*:7–9, 1962.

Lawrence, W. E., and Wickham, N.: Cat leprosy: infection by a bacillus resembling *Mycobacterium lepraemurium*. Aust. Vet. J., *39*:390–393, 1963.

Leiker, D. L., and Poelma, F. G.: On the etiology of cat leprosy. Int. J. Lepr., *42*:312–315, 1974.

Poelma, F. G., and Leiker, D. L.: Cat leprosy in the Netherlands. Int. J. Lepr., *42*:307–311, 1974.

Robinson, M.: Skin granuloma of cats associated with acid-fast bacilli. J. Small Anim. Pract., *16*:563–567, 1975.

Scheifer, B., Gee, B. R., and Ward, G. E.: A disease resembling feline leprosy in Western Canada. J. Am. Vet. Med. Assoc., *165*:1085–1087, 1974.

Wilkinson, G. T. A.: A non-tuberculous granuloma of the cat associated with an acid-fast bacillus. Vet. Rec., *76*:777–778, 833–834, 1964.

ASPERGILLOSIS

Infection with mycotic organisms of the genus *Aspergillus*, particularly *A. fumigatus*, is most prevalent in birds but may occur in mammals. The organisms are extremely common in nature, occurring on foodstuffs and plants as a white, fluffy mold. Young chicks and turkey poults are believed to become infected from contaminated bedding, usually while they are in the brooder stage of growth, hence the term "brooder pneumonia." Captive penguins, especially the King or Emperor varieties in zoölogical gardens, are particularly susceptible to aspergillosis. Horses, cats, dogs, rabbits, and rarely sheep and cattle have been reported to be infected. Infection of the guttural pouch in horses results in a clinical syndrome manifest by recurrent epistaxis and visual and locomotor disturbances. The infectious granulomata may spread from the guttural pouch to the nasal cavity and, via the optic nerves, to the optic chiasma and cerebrum.

In man, the body openings, especially the external ear, are more frequently involved than the lungs. The skin has also been suggested as the portal of entry in

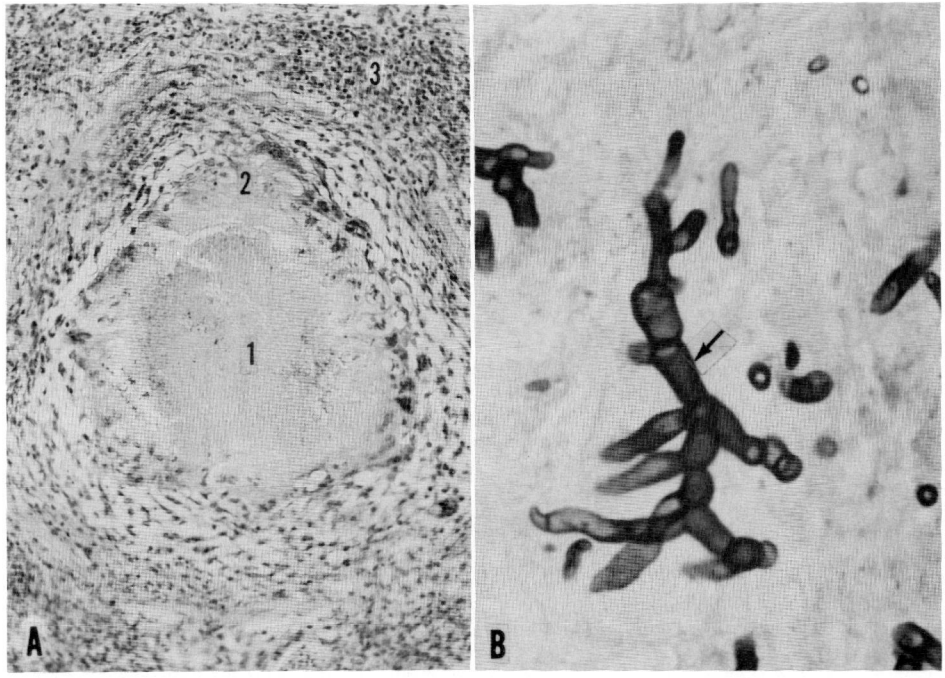

Fig. 12–15. Aspergillosis. *A,* Granuloma in lung of a chick (× 185). Necrotic center *(1)* of the granuloma is surrounded by giant cells *(2)* and lymphocytes *(3)* in connective tissue. *B,* Gridley fungus stain of a section (× 840) to demonstrate the septate, branching fungus. (Courtesy of Armed Forces Institute of Pathology.) Contributor: Dr. C. L. Davis.

human cases following immunosuppression. *Aspergillus fumigatus,* is the most important cause of mycotic placentitis and abortion in cattle, and has been reported in swine. Debilitating conditions and prolonged antibiotic therapy predispose to infection in both man and animals.

Lesions. The disease in birds may take several forms: (1) a diffuse pneumonic form, (2) a nodular pulmonary form, or (3) a diffuse infection of the air sacs. Aspergillosis in the first two forms may also occur in mammals. Gross examination of the lungs may disclose areas of consolidation, either diffuse or nodular, and thickening of the walls of air sacs (in birds) with a white moldy growth on the surface. The infection may become generalized or may be limited to one organ. Spherical nodules suggesting tuberculosis may be seen in the lungs and occasionally in other viscera.

Microscopically, the nodular lesions consist of a central core of caseation necrosis in which the organisms are found, surrounded by a wide zone of epithelioid granulation tissue. Giant cells of the foreign body type may be present, as well as lymphocytes and fibroblasts. The organisms in these granulomas appear as short, slender, septate, branching filaments, 3 or 4 μ wide and about 8 μ long. The organisms are poorly stained with hematoxylin and eosin, but stains for glycogen (PAS, Bauer's, Gridley's fungus) differentiate the mycelia by coloring the cell wall intensely. Short mycelia may appear to be almost spherical, but true spores are not found. On surfaces exposed to air, such as those of air sacs and the lining of external orifices and trachea, the organisms may produce long aerial mycelia bearing conidiophores, which project into the lumen. The mycelial

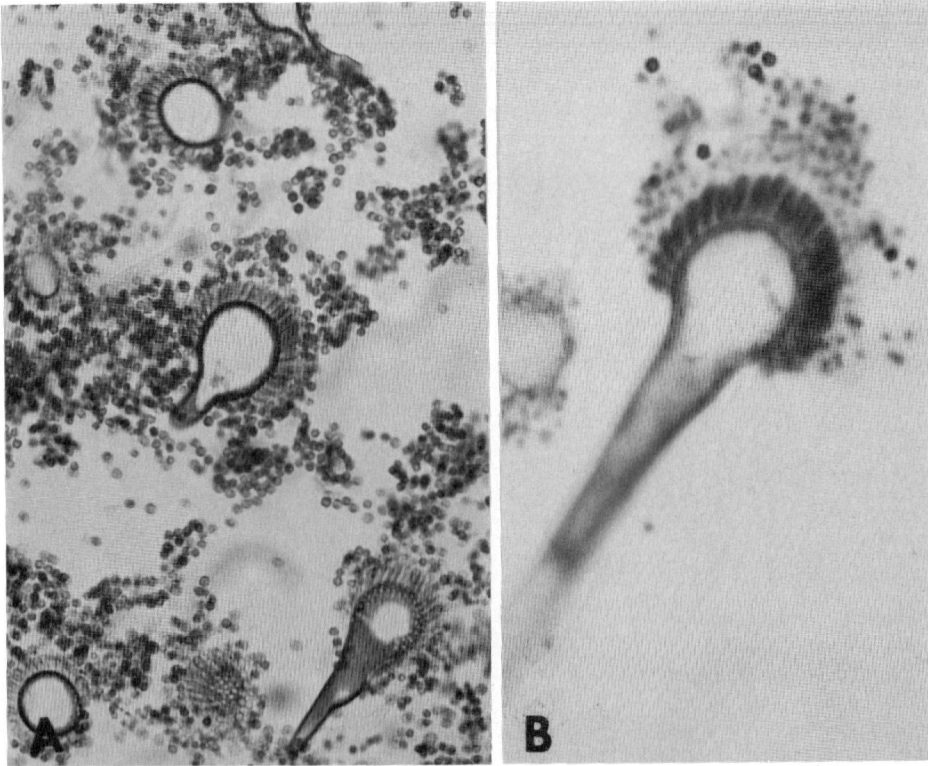

Fig. 12–16. Aspergillosis, lung of a chicken. *A,* Conidiophores of *Aspergillus fumigatus.* These sporulating structures only form in the presence of a high oxygen tension. *B,* Higher magnification of a conidiophore.

growth in these sites is like that in cultures on artificial media. In cattle, club formation surrounding the fungi is sometimes seen similar to that in actinomycosis and certain other mycotic infections.

Diagnosis. The diagnosis can be confirmed by demonstrating the characteristic organisms with their slender, dichotomously branching septate hyphae, in tissue sections, or recovering them in cultures from typical lesions.

Ainsworth, G. C., and Rewell, R. E.: The incidence of aspergillosis in captive wild birds. J. Comp. Pathol. Ther., 59:213–224, 1949.

Austwick, P. K. C.: The presence of *Aspergillus fumigatus* in the lungs of dairy cattle. Lab. Invest., 11:1065–1072, 1962.

Davis, C. L., and Schaefer, W. B.: Cutaneous aspergillosis in a cow. J. Am. Vet. Med. Assoc., 141:1339–1343, 1962. VB 1497–63.

Eggert, M. J., and Romberg, P. F.: Pulmonary aspergillosis in a calf. J. Am. Vet. Med. Assoc., 137:595–596, 1960.

Griffin, R. M.: Pulmonary aspergillosis in the calf. Vet. Rec., 84:109–111, 1969.

Hatziolos, B. C., Sass, B., Albert, T. F., and Stevenson, M. C.: Ocular changes in a horse with gutturomycosis. J. Am. Vet. Med. Assoc., 167:51–54, 1975.

Hill, M. W. M., Whiteman, C. E., Benjamin, M., and Ball, L.: Pathogenesis of experimental bovine mycotic placentitis produced by *Aspergillus fumigatus*. Vet. Pathol., 8:175–192, 1971.

Lingard, D. R., Gosser, H. S., and Monfort, T. N.: Acute epistaxis associated with guttural pouch mycosis in two horses. J. Am. Vet. Med. Assoc., 164:1038–1041, 1974.

Mason, R. W.: Porcine mycotic abortion caused by *Aspergillus fumigatus*. Aust. Vet. J., 47:18–19, 1971.

Merkow, L. P., et al.: The pathogenesis of experimental pulmonary aspergillosis. An ultrastructural study of alveolar macrophages after phagocytosis of *A. flavous* spores *in vivo*. Am. J. Pathol., 62:57–74, 1971.

Mohler, J. R., and Buckley, J. S.: Pulmonary mycosis of birds—with report of a case in a flamingo. U.S.D.A. Circular 58, Washington, D.C., 1904.

Patton, N. M.: Cutaneous and pulmonary aspergillosis in rabbits. Lab. Anim. Sci., 25:347–350, 1975.

Pier, A. C., Cysewski, S. J., and Richard, J. L.: Mycotic abortion in ewes produced by *Aspergillus fumigatus*: intravascular and intrauterine inoculation. Am. J. Vet. Res., 33:349–356, 1972.

Prystowsky, S. D., et al.: Invasive aspergillosis. N. Engl. J. Med., 295:655–658, 1976.

Purnell, D. M.: Enhancement of tissue invasion in murine aspergillosis by systemic administration of suspensions of killed *Corynebacterium parvum*. Am. J. Pathol., 83:547–556, 1976.

Smith, G. R.: Experimental aspergillosis in mice: aspects of resistance. J. Hyg., 70:741–754, 1972.

Tan Kheng Khoo, Kenji Sugai, and Tan Kim Leong: Disseminated aspergillosis. Case report and review of the world literature. Am. J. Clin. Pathol., 45:697–703, 1966.

Weber, A., and Rudolph, R.: Mycotic rhinitis in two dogs caused by *Aspergillus fumigatus*. Zentralbl. Veterinaermed. B, 19:503–510, 1972.

Whiteman, C. E., Benjamin, M. M., Ball, L., and Hill, M. W. M.: Bovine aspergillosis produced by the inoculation of conidiospores of *Aspergillus fumigatus* into a mesenteric or jugular vein. Vet. Pathol., 9:408–425, 1972.

Wood, G. L., et al.: Disseminated aspergillosis in a dog. J. Am. Vet. Med. Assoc., 172:704–707, 1978.

BLASTOMYCOSIS (North American Blastomycosis, Gilchrist's Disease)

Blastomycosis is an infectious disease of man and animals caused by a fungus, *Blastomyces dermatitidis* (*Zymonema dermatitidis, Gilchristia dermatitidis*). In man, the disease occurs as a cutaneous mycosis or as a pulmonary infection which may precede fatal dissemination. The disease has been reported in dogs (pulmonary, disseminated), horses (mammary gland), and cats (cutaneous, pulmonary). The disease is infrequent in most animals, but when it does occur in the dog, it is usually severe, often fatal. Pulmonary infection is most common in dogs, but dissemination of the organisms may result in involvement of any system. Although the frequency and distribution of the disease in animals are not accurately known, it appears to be most frequent in the Missouri Valley of the United States.

South American blastomycosis is of interest in contrast with North American blastomycosis, which is considered in greater detail. The South American disease is caused by *Paracoccidioides braziliensis*, an organism that also affects man and animals, but which can be differentiated in tissues by its manner of budding. This organism reproduces in tissues by multiple budding, in contrast to the single bud that grows out from the cell wall of each

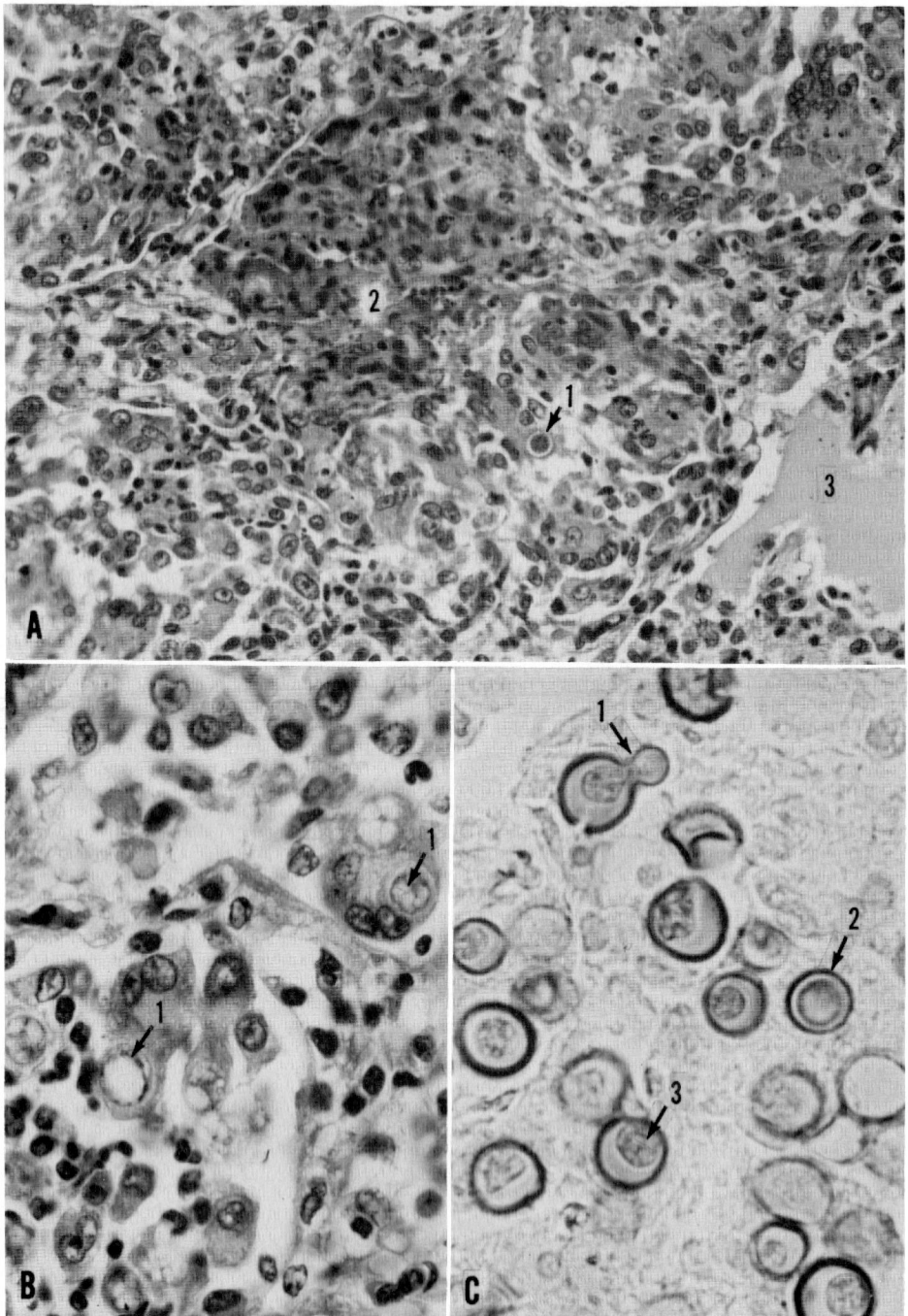

Fig. 12–17. Blastomycosis in canine lung. *A, Blastomyces dermatitidis (1)* surrounded by large masses of epithelioid cells (2), alveolus (3) (× 210). Contributor: Dr. W. H. Riser. *B,* Numerous organisms (1) in macrophages in alveoli in a fulminant case (× 660). Contributor: Dr. J. R. Rooney II. *C,* Higher magnification (× 1050) of a section stained with Gridley's fungus stain. Note budding (1), thick walls (2), and the internal structure of the organisms (3). (Courtesy of Armed Forces Institute of Pathology.) Contributor: Dr. C. G. Loosli.

spherule of *Blastomyces dermatitidis* (Fig. 12–17).

Lesions. In the human skin, intraepithelial abscesses with epithelioid reaction in the dermis and subcutis, ulceration, and slow healing of the epidermis are described. In the lungs of dogs, circumscribed gray nodules of solidification may be seen in some cases, and diffuse consolidation of the lung, with the cut surfaces yielding purulent exudate, in others. Microscopically, the pulmonary lesion is characterized by intensive infiltration by epithelioid cells, in which foci of neutrophils and diffusely distributed lymphocytes may be found. Caseation necrosis may occur, and although some fibroblasts are recognizable, there is little tendency toward encapsulation of the lesions. Multinucleated giant cells of the foreign body type may be seen, but Langhans' giant cells are rare. Calcification is infrequent.

The causative organisms are found in the lesions, free, or in macrophages, as spherical, yeast-like cells, 8 to 20 μ in diameter, with double-contoured walls. In hematoxylin and eosin-stained sections, the organisms usually are seen as a central granular mass surrounded by a refractile, double-contoured unstained zone which is bounded by a thin outer wall. An occasional cell may be seen extruding a daughter cell (budding). Stains for bound glycogen (PAS, Bauer's, Gomori's methenamine silver, Gridley's fungus) will stain the outer wall of the organism selectively, differentiating it more clearly from the surrounding tissue.

The lesions may be limited to the lungs, but dissemination with abscess formation has been described in the subcutis, spleen, kidneys, lymph nodes, liver, brain, bones, adrenal glands, eye and intestines.

Diagnosis. Microscopic examination of affected tissues is necessary to establish the diagnosis. The organisms can be demonstrated readily in typical lesions and can be stained differentially with glycogen stains (PAS, Bauer's, Gridley's fungus). They are

larger than *Histoplasma capsulatum*, smaller than *Coccidioides immitis* (a fungus that contains endospores and does not reproduce by budding), and they do not have the wide, mucicarmine-staining capsule of *Cryptococcus neoformans*. The tissue reactions in histoplasmosis and cryptococcosis are also unlike that of blastomycosis. Cultural identification of the organisms is of value, but it is more important that any fungus recovered in culture also be demonstrated in characteristic lesions.

Alden, C. L., and Mohan, R.: Ocular blastomycosis in a cat. J. Am. Vet. Med. Assoc., *164*:527–528, 1974.

Benbrook, E. A., Bryant, J. B., and Saunders, L. Z.: Blastomycosis in the horse. J. Am. Vet. Med. Assoc., *112*:475–478, 1948.

Easton, K. L.: Cutaneous North American blastomycosis in a Siamese cat. Can. Vet. J., 2:350–351, 1961.

Furcolow, M. L., Busey, J. F., Menges, R. W., and Chick, E. W.: Prevalence and incidence studies of human and canine blastomycosis. II. Yearly incidence studies in three selected states, 1967–1970. Am. J. Epidemiol., *92*:121–131, 1970.

Furcolow, M. L., Smith, C. D., and Turner, C.: Supportive evidence by field testing and laboratory experiment for a new hypothesis of the ecology and pathogenicity of canine blastomycosis. Sabouraudia, *12*:22–32, 1974.

Johnson, W. D., and Lang, C. M.: Paracoccidioidomycosis (South American blastomycosis) in a squirrel monkey *(Saimiri sciureus)*. Vet. Pathol., *14*:368–371, 1977.

Kurtz, H. J., and Sharpnack, S.: *Blastomyces dermatitidis* meningoencephalitis in a dog. Path. Vet., *6*:375–377, 1969.

Lacroix, L. J., Riser, W. H., and Karlson, A. G.: Blastomycosis in the dog. North Am. Vet., *28*:603–606, 1947.

Landay, M. E., Mitten, J., and Millar, J.: Disseminated blastomycosis in hamsters. II. Effect of sex on susceptibility. Mycopathol. Mycol. Appl., *42*:73, 1970.

Marx, M. B., Jones, M. B., Kimberlin, D. S., and Furcolow, M. L.: Survey of histoplasmin and blastomycin test reactors among thoroughbred horses in central Kentucky. Am. J. Vet. Res., *33*:1701–1705, 1972.

Saunders, L. Z.: Cutaneous blastomycosis in the dog. North Am. Vet., *29*:650–652, 1948.

Seibold, H. R.: Systemic blastomycosis in dogs. North Am. Vet., *27*:162–168, 1946.

Sheldon, W. G.: Pulmonary blastomycosis in a cat. Lab. Anim. Care, *16*:280–285, 1966.

Shull, R. M., Hayden, D. W., and Johnston, G. R.: Urogenital blastomycosis in a dog. J. Am. Vet. Med. Assoc., *171*:730–735, 1977.

Soltys, M. A., and Sumner-Smith, G.: Systemic mycoses in dogs and cats. Can. Vet. J., *12*:191–199, 1971.

Trevino, G. S.: Canine blastomycosis with ocular involvement. Path. Vet., *3*:652–658, 1966.

Turner, C., Smith, C. D., and Furcolow, M. L.: Frequency of isolation of *Histoplasma capsulatum* and *Blastomyces dermatitidis* from dogs in Kentucky. Am. J. Vet. Res., *33*:137–141, 1972.

Williamson, W. M., Lombard, L. S., and Getty, R. E.: North American blastomycosis in a Northern Sea lion. J. Am. Vet. Med. Assoc., *135*:513–514, 1959.

Wilson, R. W., Van Dreumel, A. A., and Henry, J. N. R.: Urogenital and ocular lesions in canine blastomycosis. Vet. Pathol., *10*:1–11, 1973.

COCCIDIOIDOMYCOSIS
(Coccidioidal Granuloma)

Coccidioidomycosis has been recognized as a human disease since 1892, when the first case was reported by Posada from Argentina. It is most prevalent in the arid regions of southwestern United States, but isolated cases have been seen worldwide. Coccidioidomycosis was first recognized as a spontaneous infection of animals by Giltner, who reported a bovine case in 1918. It is now known to occur in a wide variety of wild and domesticated animals, including wild deer, Bengal tigers, mice, pocket mice, grasshopper mice, Kangaroo rats, pack rats, ground squirrels, gorillas, monkeys, dogs, sheep, and cattle. The disease has also been reported in a horse (Zontine, 1958). In man, the disease may occur as an acute, febrile, upper respiratory infection with a short, favorable course (so-called Valley fever) or as a progressive, intractable disease with disseminated lesions and fatal outcome. In animals, the disease usually assumes the chronic progressive form, although an inapparent pulmonary infection has been recognized in cattle.

The causative organism, *Coccidioides immitis (Oidium coccidioides)*, may live in the soil, and inhalation of spores from this source will initiate the disease in either man or animals. Direct transmission from one animal host to another apparently does not occur, although certain rodents have been suspected of being reservoirs of infection. The organisms grow well in cultures, producing aerial mycelia which form a small, fluffy-white, spherical colony. In tissues, however, mycelial structures are not observed, the fungus taking the form of spherules 5 to 50 μ in diameter with double-contoured walls. Reproduction in tissues is by endosporulation, hence endospores may be found in some of the larger spherules.

Signs are absent in many cases, particularly in cattle, and the first indications of infection are lesions of pulmonary lymph nodes found in apparently healthy animals at the time of slaughter. Generalized infections run a slow course; the signs are nonspecific and may include emaciation, inappetence, low-grade fever and occasional cough.

Lesions. The gross lesions of coccidioidomycosis resemble those of tuberculosis in many respects. They may appear as discrete or confluent granulomas, with or without suppuration or calcification. In cattle, the lesions often are limited to small nodules in the lungs and, more frequently, to nodules or diffuse enlargements of bronchial or mediastinal lymph nodes. Large or small purulent foci may be surrounded by a wide band of granulation tissue and a fibrous capsule. Incision of an affected lymph node may permit the expression of thick yellowish pus. In the disseminated form of the disease, as in the dog, grayish nodules of various sizes may be found in the lungs, lymph nodes, liver, spleen, meninges, eye, bone marrow, and other organs. The nodules are usually irregular in size and shape and may or may not exude material when put under pressure. At times a close relation to the larger blood vessels may be demonstrated. In some species (dog, monkeys), lesions may be disseminated throughout the skeletal system. Ocular involvement may also occur as the presenting lesion.

The microscopic appearance is characteristic, but varies to some extent in relation to the developmental stage of the fungus which predominates in the lesion. The largest spherules, often filled with endo-

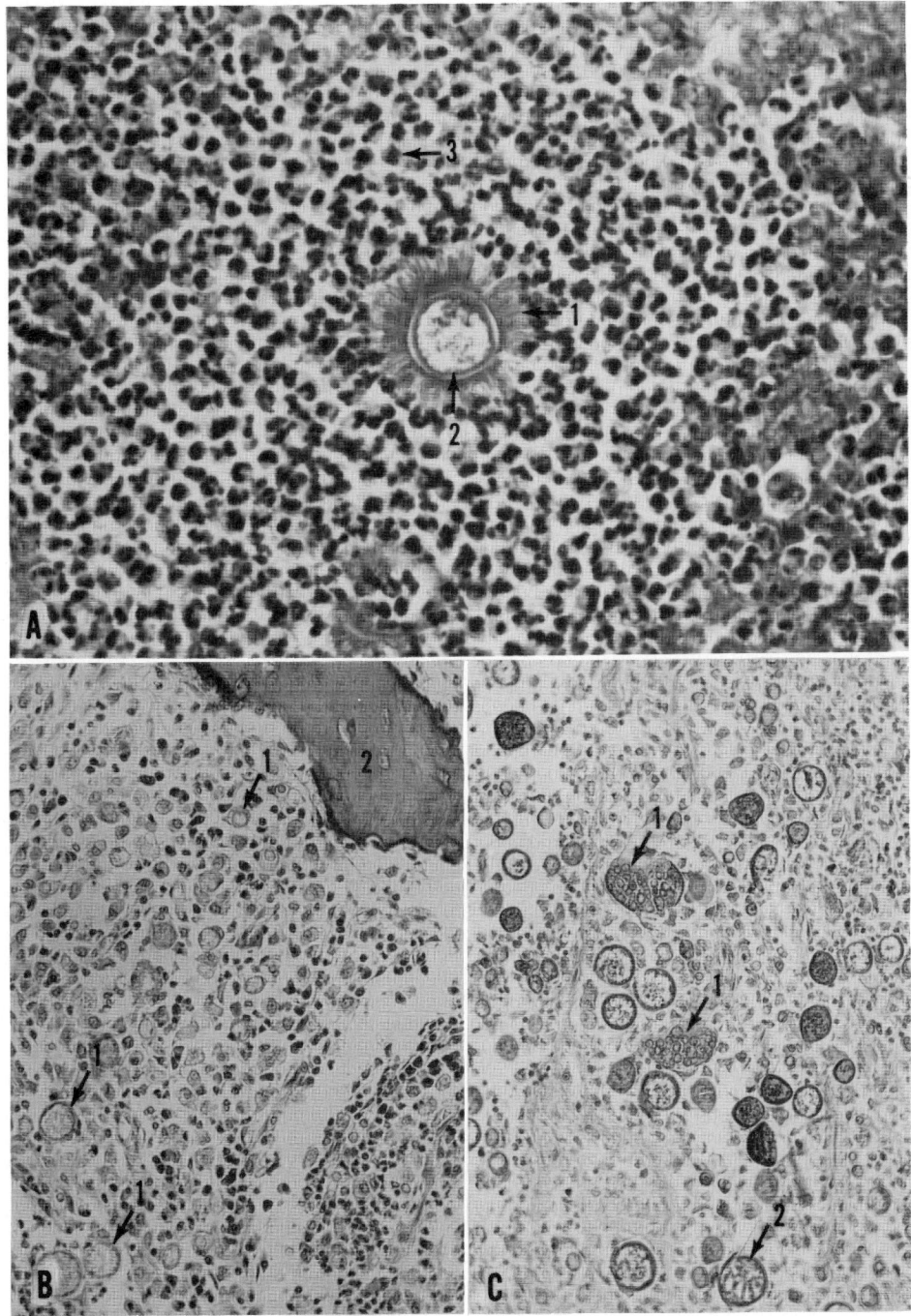

Fig. 12–18. Coccidioidomycosis. *A,* Lesions in a mediastinal lymph node of a cow (× 100). Note radiating club-shaped structures (*1*) around the thick-walled organism (*2*), which lies in a pool of neutrophils (*3*). Contributor: Dr. H. R. Seibold. *B,* Lesion in bone marrow of a dog (× 185). Organisms (*1*) of various sizes in macrophages which replace the normal marrow. Bone trabecula (*2*). *C,* Another section of *B* stained with Gridley's fungus stain (× 235). Large organisms (*1*) filled with endospores which are just starting to develop in smaller organisms (*2*). (Courtesy of Armed Forces Institute of Pathology.) Contributor: Dr. H. A. Smith.

spores, are usually surrounded by a wide zone of epithelioid cells, admixed with a few neutrophils and some lymphocytes. In cattle, these large spherules may be surrounded by a corona of radiating club-shaped structures (Fig. 12–18), somewhat resembling the "rosette" around a colony of *Actinomyces bovis*. When the wall of a large spherule ruptures, releasing its endospores, the tissue reaction becomes rich in neutrophils and lymphocytes, with fewer epithelioid cells. As these endospores mature, leukocytes and epithelioid cells tend to predominate in the inflammatory exudate. As organisms in all stages may occur in a single lesion, mixed tissue reactions are common. The organisms within the cytoplasm of Langhans' giant cells are clearly seen in sections stained with hematoxylin and eosin, but stains for bound glycogen (PAS, Gridley's fungus, Bauer's) will demonstrate the double-contoured wall selectively. In the liver, spleen, and lung, the lesions are usually spherical and sharply circumscribed and obviously are expanding to displace normal tissues; in lymph nodes and bone marrow, the feature of circumscription is usually lost. In the meninges, spherical nodules of microscopic size, containing one or two organisms in a mantle of epithelioid cells, may appear in the pia-arachnoid.

Diagnosis. Microscopic demonstration of the organisms in characteristic lesions usually establishes the diagnosis. When organisms are few, special stains (PAS, Gridley's fungus, Bauer's) are helpful in revealing them. The size of the largest spherules (up to 50 μ), the presence of endospores and absence of budding serve to distinguish *Coccidioides immitis* from *Blastomyces dermatitidis* or *Cryptococcus neoformans*. The spherules of *Emmonsia parva* may be similar in appearance and even larger in size, but they do not contain endospores.

Ashburn, L. L., and Emmons, C. W.: Spontaneous coccidioidal granuloma in the lungs of wild rodents. Arch. Pathol., 34:791–800, 1942.
Breznock, A. W., Henrickson, R. V., Silverman, S., and Schwartz, L. W.: Coccidioidomycosis in a rhesus monkey. J. Am. Vet. Med. Assoc., 167:657–661, 1975.
Cieplak, W., and Merbs, C. F.: Coccidioidomycosis in an Arizona chimpanzee colony. Am. J. Phys. Anthrop., 47:123, 1977.
Crane, C. S.: Equine coccidioidomycosis. Vet. Med., 57:1073–1074, 1962. VB 1503–63.
Davis, C. L., Stiles, G. W., Jr., and McGregor, A. N.: Pulmonary coccidioidal granuloma; a new site of infection in cattle. J. Am. Vet. Med. Assoc., 91:209–215, 1937.
Emmons, C. W.: Coccidioidomycosis. Mycologia, 34:452–463, 1942.
Farness, O. J.: Coccidioidal infection in a dog. J. Am. Vet. Med. Assoc., 97:263–264, 1940.
Forbus, W. D., and Bestebreurtje, A. M.: Coccidioidomycosis: a study of 95 cases of the disseminated type with special reference to the pathogenesis of the disease. Mil. Surgeon, 99:653–719, 1946.
Giltner, L. T.: Occurrence of coccidioidal granuloma (oidiomycosis) in cattle. J. Agric. Res., 14:533–542, 1918.
Henrickson, R. V., and Biberstein, E. L.: Coccidioidomycosis accompanying hepatic disease in two Bengal tigers. J. Am. Vet. Med. Assoc., 161:674–677, 1972.
Hugenholtz, P. G. et al.: Experimental coccidioidomycosis in dogs. Am. J. Vet. Res., 19:433–439, 1958.
Maddy, K. T.: Disseminated coccidioidomycosis of the dog. J. Am. Vet. Med. Assoc., 132:483–489, 1958.
McKenney, F. D., Traum, J., and Bonestell, A. E.: Acute coccidiomycosis in a mountain gorilla (*Gorilla beringeri*) with anatomical notes. J. Am. Vet. Med. Assoc., 104:136–140, 1944.
Pappagianis, D., Vanderlip, J., and May, B.: Coccidioidomycosis naturally acquired by a monkey, *Cerocebus atys*, in Davis, California. Sabouraudia, 11:52–55, 1973.
Pryor, W. H., Jr., Huizenga, C. G., Splitter, G. A., and Harwell, J. F., Jr.: *Coccidioides immitis* encephalitis in two dogs. J. Am. Vet. Med. Assoc., 161:1108–1112, 1972.
Rapley, W. A., and Long, J. R.: Coccidioidomycosis in a baboon recently imported from California. Can. Vet. J., 15:39–41, 1974.
Reed, R. E., Hoge, R. S., and Trautman, R. J.: Coccidioidomycosis in two cats. J. Am. Vet. Med. Assoc., 143:953–956, 1963.
Rehkemper, J. A.: Coccidioidomycosis in the horse. A pathologic study. Cornell Vet., 49:198–211, 1959.
Shively, J. N., and Whiteman, C. E.: Ocular lesions in disseminated coccidioidomycosis in 2 dogs. Pathol. Vet., 7:1–6, 1970.
Smith, H. A.: Coccidioidomycosis in animals. Am. J. Pathol., 24:223–233, 1948.
Stiles, G. W., and Davis, C. L.: Coccidioidal granuloma (coccidioidomycosis). Its incidence in man and animals and its diagnosis in animals. J. Am. Med. Assoc., 119:765–769, 1942.
Zontine, W. J.: Coccidioidomycosis in the horse, a case report. J. Am. Vet. Med. Assoc., 132:490–492, 1958.

ADIASPIROMYCOSIS (Haplomycosis)

A mycotic organism with wide geographic distribution, originally called *Haplosporangium parvum*, and most recently named *Emmonsia parva*, has been reported to produce infection in many wild animals, such as ground squirrels, pocket mice, white-footed mice, Kangaroo rats, pine squirrels, muskrats, beavers, rock and cottontail rabbits, mink, martins, skunks, weasels, wood rats, a fox, and raccoons. These organisms have also been found in the lungs of a dog and a goat, each succumbing to another disease (nephritis and poisoning respectively). Both of us have

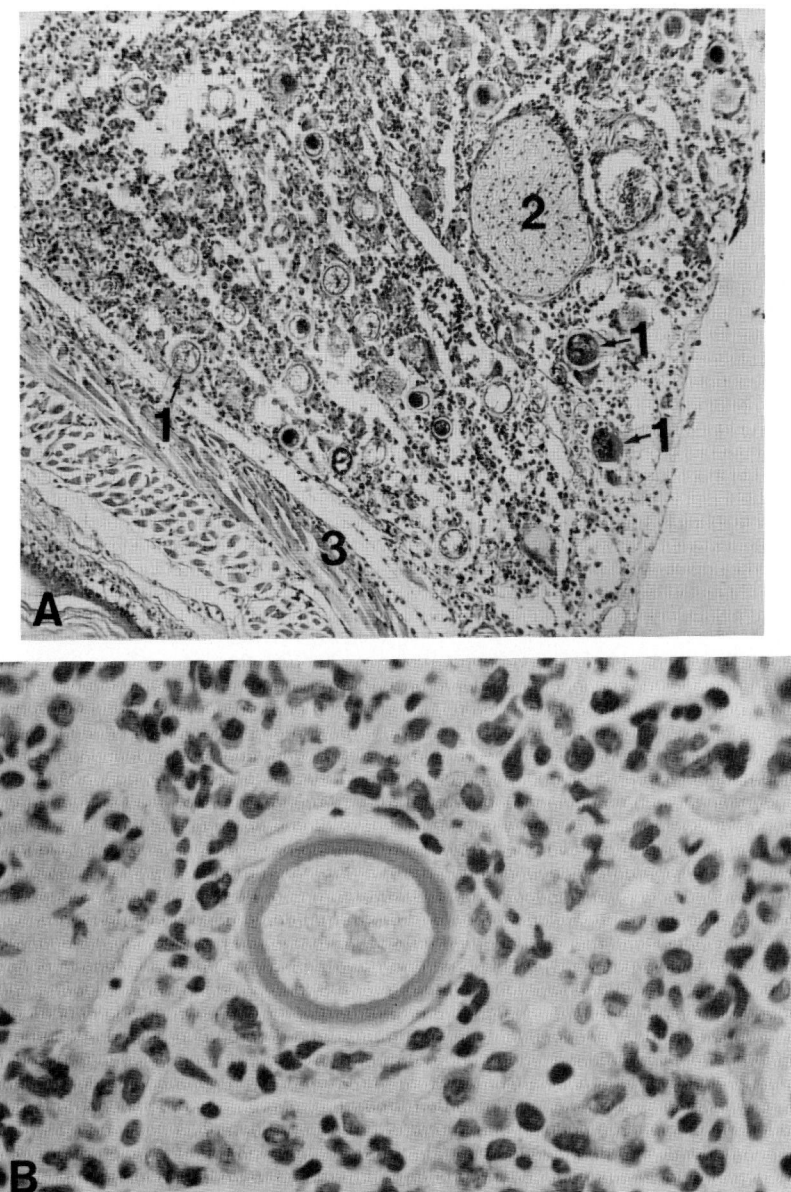

Fig. 12–19.   Adiaspiromycosis. *A,* Organism (*1*) without endospores in mediastinum of a mouse. Nerve (*2*), esophagus (*3*). (Preparation courtesy of Dr. R. T. Haberman.) *B,* A single spherule in the lung of an armadillo. Note thick wall and absence of endospores. (Courtesy of Animal Research Center, Harvard Medical School.)

observed organisms with the morphology of *E. parva* in sections of lungs of nine-banded armadillos. The name for the disease produced by this organism was proposed by Emmons (1948). Although skin sensitivity of cattle to products of growth of *Haplosporangium* (haplosporangin) has been demonstrated, and gross contamination of barnyard soils is known, natural infection of domesticated animals has not been recognized. However, it is altogether possible that domestic animals may become infected if conditions are suitable.

Emmons and Jellison (1960) have pointed out that the organism described above was improperly classified and have accepted its classification by Ciferri and Montemartini (1959) in a new genus as *Emmonsia parva*. Emmons and Jellison also suggest that a parasitic form of this genus be called *Emmonsia crescens* (n.sp.). The large spherule formed in tissues by *E. crescens*, which grows in size but does not form endospores, is called an *adiaspore* by these authors. Further, they suggest that the disease be called *adiaspiromycosis*, indicating a mycosis in which no multiplication or dissemination of the organism occurs beyond its original site of implantation.

Although *Emmonsia parva* may occur naturally in the same animals that harbor *Coccidioides immitis* (p. 672), these two organisms apparently are only distantly related and can be differentiated both in tissues and in culture. *Emmonsia parva* is uninucleate, does not produce progressive disease in rodents, reproduces in culture by means of sporangioles rather than arthrospores, and does not produce endospores in tissues. The lesions observed in spontaneous infections with this organism are usually limited to the lungs, which suggests inhalation of the organisms. In the tissues of the host, the organisms grow from rather minute forms to large (up to 270 μ) spherical structures with thick, double-contoured walls. Endospores are not formed in tissues; in fact, no reproduction of organisms takes place in tissues, hence

the disease is not progressive and the extent of involvement is related to the number of organisms inhaled. In spite of the very large size of some of the spherules of *Emmonsia*, only a mild tissue reaction is evoked in the host. Epithelioid cells and occasional giant cells are seen engulfing the organisms (Fig. 12–19). Mild lymphocytic infiltration may be present, but neutrophils are few and usually are adjacent to smaller spherules, which appear to be increasing in size.

Ashburn, L. L., and Emmons, C. W.: Experimental Haplosporangium infection. Arch. Pathol., *39*:3–8, 1945.

Cano, R. J., and Taylor, J. J.: Experimental adiaspiromycosis in rabbits: host response to *Chrysosporium parvum* and *C. parvum var. crescens* antigens. Sabouraudia, *12*:54–63, 1974.

Ciferri, R., and Montemartini, A.: Taxonomy of *Haplosporangium parvum*. Mycopath. Mycol. Appl., *10*:303–316, 1959.

Emmons, C. W.: Coccidioidomycosis and haplomycosis. Proc. Fourth Internat. Cong. Trop. Med. Malaria, *2*:1278–1286, Washington, D. C., 1948.

Emmons, C. W., and Ashburn, L. L.: The isolation of *Haplosporangium parvum* (n. sp.) and *Coccidioides immitis* from wild rodents. Their relationship to coccidioidomycosis. Pub. Health Rep., *57*:1715–1727, 1942.

Emmons, C. W., and Jellison, W. L.: *Emmonsia crescens sp. n.* and adiaspiromycosis (haplomycosis) in mammals. Ann. NY Acad. Sci., *89*:91–101, 1960.

Koller, L. D., Patton, N. M., and Whitsett, D. K.: Adiaspiromycosis in the lungs of a dog. J. Am. Vet. Med. Assoc., *169*:1316–1317, 1976.

Koller, L. D., and Helfer, D. H.: Adiaspiromycosis in the lungs of a goat. J. Am. Vet. Med. Assoc., *173*:80–81, 1978.

Menges, R. W., and Habermann, R. T.: Isolation of *Haplosporangium parvum* from soil and results of experimental inoculations. Am. J. Hyg., *60*:106–116, 1954.

Otcenasek, M., Krivanec, K., and Slais, J.: *Emmonsia parva* as causal agent of adiaspiromycosis in a fox. Sabouraudia, *13*:52–57, 1975.

NASAL GRANULOMA OF CATTLE

Polypoid or sessile masses in the nasal cavity of cattle have occasionally been reported from some parts of the country. This so-called nasal granuloma appears to be a definite clinical entity. Although its etiology is not clearly established, there is evidence that fungi may be involved, and it is

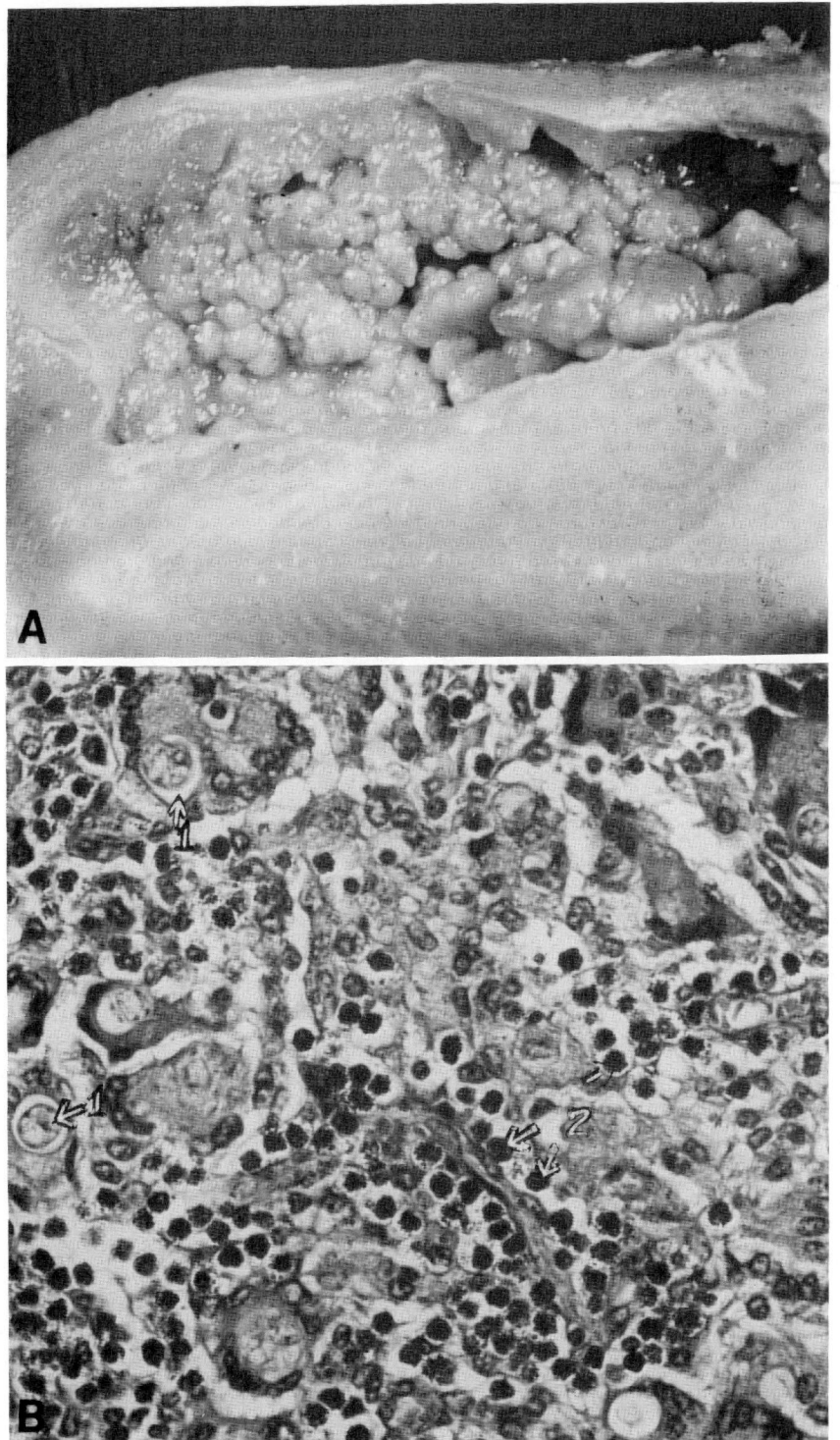

Fig. 12–20. Nasal granuloma of cattle. *A*, Polypoid masses on nasal septum. (Courtesy of Dr. C. L. Davis.) *B*, Section of a nasal granuloma (H & E, × 400.) Note fungal organisms (*1*) and eosinophils (*2*).

possible that more than one causative agent may be concerned. There is little to suggest a relation between nasal granuloma in cattle in the United States and rhinosporidiosis, although such a possibility must be admitted. Spherical organisms, undoubtedly fungal, were described in histologic sections of nasal granulomas, and cultures of *Helminthosporum* were recovered from these lesions by Davis and Shorten (1936), but the disease was not reproduced experimentally. Comparisons of the infection with haplomycosis and coccidioidomycosis have been made, but no conclusions reached.

Lesions. The lesions are confined to the external nares and appear as nodules that project from any part of the nasal mucosa into the nasal cavity (Fig. 12–20). The resulting partial obstruction may be accentuated by accumulation over the nodules of mucous and purulent exudates, which also stream from the external nostrils. The nodules have a glistening surface and are grayish yellow to red on cut section. Microscopically, the lesions underlying the elevated and often ulcerated nasal epithelium consist of granulation tissue, in which epithelioid and foreign-body giant cells predominate. Lymphocytes and eosinophils may make up a large part of some lesions. Spherical bodies, with thick walls and indistinct contents suggesting a fungus, are often seen within epithelioid and giant cells. In some reported cases, these organisms have not been found, although the possibility remains that they were present in parts of the lesion not examined microscopically.

Bridges (1960) has reviewed the problem of bovine nasal granuloma, has studied material from previously reported cases, and published three cases from central Texas. He was able to demonstrate both pigmented and nonpigmented hyphae and chlamydospores in the lesions, and by comparing their morphologic features, he determined that these organisms were a species of *Helminthosporum*. This organism

has been isolated from cases of maduramycosis, suggesting that nasal granuloma is merely a form of this latter disease. It is apparent that the Texas lesion is somewhat different from that of rhinosporidiosis as it is known in South America, and also differs from the bovine nasal granuloma of cattle in India, in which a fluke, *Schistosoma nasalis*, is demonstrable.

Bridges, C. H.: Maduramycosis of bovine nasal mucosa (nasal granuloma of cattle) Cornell Vet., 50:469–484, 1960.
Creech, G. T., and Miller, F. W.: Nasal granuloma in cattle. Vet. Med., 28:279–284, 1933.
Davis, C. L., and Shorten, H. L.: Nasal swelling in a bovine. J. Am. Vet. Med., Assoc., 89:91–96, 1936.
Dikmans, G.: Nasal granuloma in cattle in Louisiana. North Am. Vet., 15:20–24, 1934.
Roberts, E. D., McDaniel, H. A., and Carbrey, E. A.: Maduramycosis of the bovine nasal mucosa. J. Am. Vet. Med. Assoc., 142:42–68, 1963.
Robinson, V. B.: Nasal granuloma. Am. J. Vet. Res., 12:85–89, 1951.

MADURAMYCOSIS (Maduramycotic Mycetoma, Madura Foot)

An age-old disease of barefooted people ("Madura foot") was originally named after an area in which the disease was first described (Madura, India). Many different organisms have been recovered from such cases and may well have etiologic significance. The clinical disease in human patients has been divided into "eumycetomas," caused by *Eumycetes* or true fungi; "actinomycetomas," caused by organisms of the genera *Actinomyces, Nocardia, Actinomadura,* and *Streptomyces;* "botryomycosis," caused by *Staphylococci, Actinobacillus lignieresi, Escherichia coli, Proteus sp, Pseudomonas aeruginosa,* and nonhemolytic streptococci. In this section, only those lesions in animals caused by true fungi will be considered.

In tissues, the causative organisms currently grouped under this term form definite colonies or "grains" which are composed of cohesive masses of large segmented mycelial filaments with well-defined walls, chlamydospores, or other spores and, in most cases, pigment (Fig.

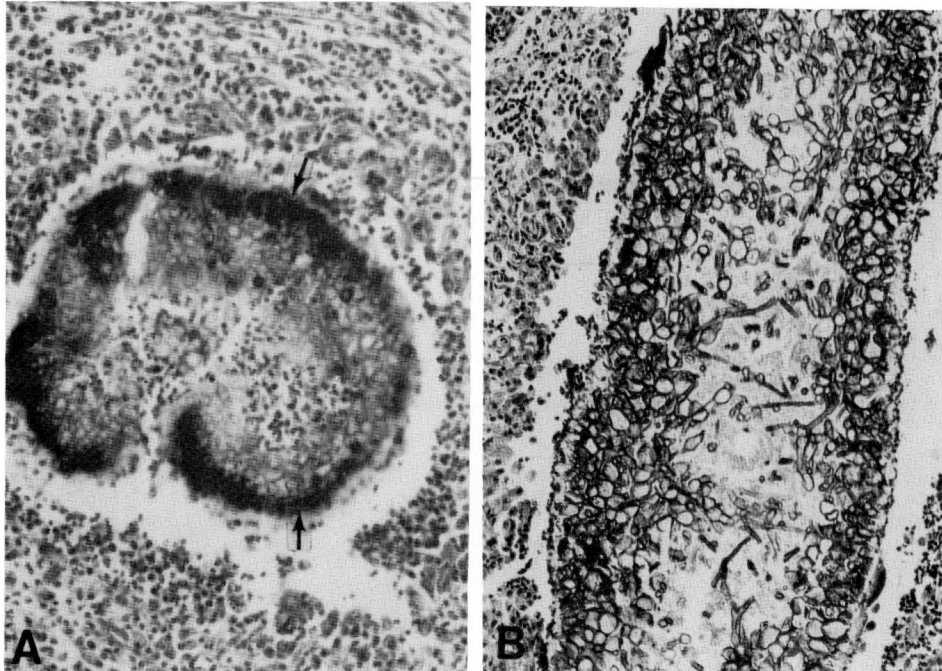

Fig. 12–21. Maduramycosis. *A*, Nasal granuloma in a horse (× 224). Note pigment in tenacious colony. (Courtesy of Armed Forces Institute of Pathology.) Contributor: Dr. Leon Z. Saunders. *B*, Granuloma of one year's duraction in the foot of a dog (× 130). *Curvularia geniculata* was isolated from the lesion. Note colony of organisms without pigment.

12–21). Fungi that do not produce pigment are involved in "white-grained maduramycosis." Colonies that contain pigment are visible to the unaided eye as "black grains," suggesting tiny bits of coal.

Among the fungal organisms that have been identified from lesions characteristic of maduramycosis are the following: *Allescheria boydii*, *Curvularia geniculata*, and *Brachycladium spiciferum*. Only the latter two have been recovered and identified in cultures.

Lesions. The lesions of maduramycosis are distinguished by the presence of discrete black or brown colonies of fungi, which appear grossly as tiny black or brown flecks ("grains") 1 to 3 mm wide, embedded in a large mass of granulation tissue. These colonies are tenaciously discrete and can be expressed by pressure from the narrow zone of pus that surrounds them. The lesions in animals are most fre-

quent on the extremities, but may involve the nasal mucosa, peritoneum, or skin at any site. The coiled glands of the foot pad of dogs appear to be sites of predilection. These mycotic granulomas may become quite large and are generally resistant to any treatment short of surgical excision.

The microscopic appearance is distinctive. Colonies of the fungi are seen as brown, irregularly spherical bodies embedded within a pocket of neutrophils. These purulent centers are separated by abundant amounts of granulation tissue richly infiltrated with macrophages, plasma cells, and lymphocytes. The organisms in the fungal colony cling together tenaciously and form an outer coronal zone made up of coarse, irregular, often swollen hyphae and thick-walled chlamydospores. The center of the colony is usually less dense and contains many branching, septate hyphae. The hyphae are of irregular length, but rarely more than 10 μ in width. The chlamydospores have thicker walls, are usually spherical, and may attain a diameter of 25 μ or more. The periodic-acid Schiff (PAS), Bauer's and Gridley's fungus stains are particularly useful in demonstrating the morphology of the fungi in tissue sections (Fig. 12–21).

Diagnosis. The diagnosis may be made by demonstration of typical fungal colonies in characteristic granulomas. Organisms should be cultured in order to establish the identity of the causative agent.

Bridges, C. H.: Maduromycotic mycetomas in animals. *Curvularia geniculata* as an etiological agent. Am. J. Pathol., *33*:411–427, 1957.

Bridges, C. H., and Beasley, J. N.: Maduromycotic mycetomas in animals—*Brachycladium spiciferum,* Bainier as an etiologic agent. J. Am. Vet. Med. Assoc., *137*:192–201, 1960.

Brodey, R. S., et al.: Mycetoma in a dog. J. Am. Vet. Med. Assoc., *151*:442–451, 1967.

Emmons, C. W., Binford, C. H., Utz, J. P., and Kwon-Chung, K. J.: Medical Mycology, 3rd ed. Philadelphia, Lea & Febiger, 1977.

Schauffler, A. F.: Maduromycotic mycetoma in an aged mare. J. Am. Vet. Med. Assoc., *160*:998–1000, 1972.

Seibold, H. R.: Mycetoma in a dog. J. Am. Vet. Med. Assoc., *127*:444–445, 1955.

CRYPTOCOCCOSIS (Torulosis, European Blastomycosis)

Cryptococcosis is being recognized with increasing frequency in many animal species and is well known in man. The causative organism, *Cryptococcus neoformans* (*Cryptococcus hominis,* or *Torula histolytica*), is a yeast-like fungus which may live in a nonparasitic state in nature. The organisms are found in soil, manure, and dust, from which sources both animals and man may be infected. Direct transmission of the disease between animals or from animals to man has not been demonstrated. In man, and in some animals as well, the organism has an affinity for the cerebrospinal meninges, but it may attack the respiratory system, the mammary gland, or several systems of the body.

Cryptococcosis has been reported in cattle, swine, horses, cats, dogs, marmoset (*Saguinus sp.*), rhesus (*Macaca mulatta*),

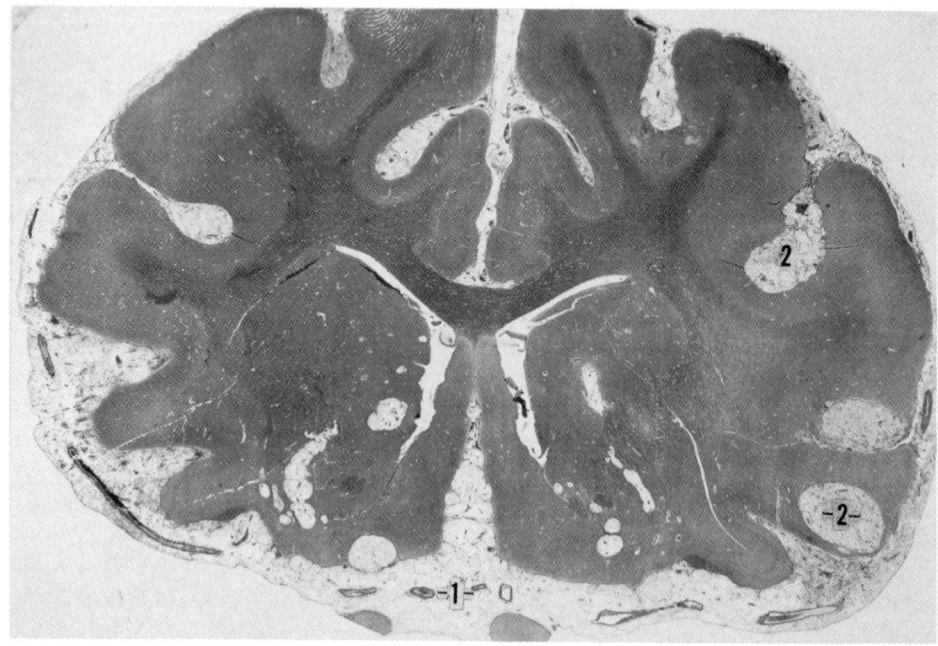

Fig. 12–22. Cryptococcosis, brain of a cat. Large masses of organisms in leptomeninges (*1*) give them an edematous appearance and result in distention of depths of sulci (*2*). (Courtesy of Armed Forces Institute of Pathology.) Contributor: Dr. John Mills.

Taiwan *(M. cyclopis),* and patas monkeys *(Erythrocebus patas),* and the cheetah. The manifestations of cryptococcosis depend upon the organs or systems involved; therefore, no constant clinical syndrome can be described. In cats, nasal obstructions resembling neoplasms have been associated with pulmonary infection, and subsequently the meninges have been involved. In horses also, the upper nasal cavity appears to be a site of predilection for the initial lesions. Outbreaks of intractable mastitis have been reported in dairy cattle, but though the supramammary lymph nodes were involved, dissemination throughout the body was the exception. Not infrequently, in many species, the presenting sign is enlargement of lymph nodes.

Lesions. The gross lesions are not diagnostic. In the lungs, peritoneum, nasal mucosae, and similar structures, they appear as granulomatous nodules, sometimes with ulceration of the contiguous mucous membranes. Affected lymph nodes are enlarged, apparently from edema, and the cut surfaces have a definitely mucinous quality. The involved meninges are thickened with translucent material grossly resembling edema. In the mammary gland, diffuse or patchy induration may be observed.

While the gross changes are inconclusive, the microscopic findings are diagnostic. The organisms occur in tissues as ovoid or spherical, thick-walled, yeast-like bodies which occasionally show single budding and are surrounded by a wide gelatinous capsule (Fig. 12–23). The cell inside the capsule is usually 5 to 20 μ in diameter; the capsule increases the overall diameter to a maximum of 30 μ. In sections stained with hematoxylin and eosin, the cell wall and sometimes its contents are visible, but the capsule remains unstained. This capsule stains selectively by the mucicarmine technique and the periodic acid-Schiff (PAS) method for glycogen.

In most situations, the organisms grow and multiply rapidly, forming a cystic space occupied by myriads of organisms, whose mucoid capsules account for the glistening appearance and slimy consistency encountered grossly. This is a prominent feature in the brain, the organisms growing in the pia mater over the surface and deep into the cerebral convolutions, where they form cystic areas and displace the brain parenchyma. Cystic lesions may occur in lungs, adrenal glands, lymph nodes, and mammary glands. In such sites, the tissue reaction of the host is difficult to detect, although occasional macrophages with engulfed organisms may be found. In some sites, the organisms are less numerous and the tissue reaction much more profound. In lesions of this type, which may be adjacent to a cystic lesion, numerous endothelial cells with an admixture of lymphocytes are partially or completely surrounded by connective tissue. This granulomatous reaction is particularly prominent in some cases of cryptococcal mastitis, but has also been observed in lesions in the brain, lung, and other organs.

The lesions tend to depend upon the growth stage of the organisms. Shadomey and Lurie (1971), in experimental studies with mice, demonstrated that essentially no tissue reaction is evoked by large cryptococcal organisms with wide capsules. Hyphal fragments and small round or oval organisms produce severe granulomata with central necrosis and microabscesses. As the organism increases in size, the tissue reaction tends to be less severe.

Diagnosis. The diagnosis is readily made from characteristic microscopic lesions, in which the organisms can be demonstrated and identified culturally or morphologically. The wide mucoid capsule, which selectively absorbs the mucicarmine stain, differentiates *Cryptococcus neoformans* in tissue from *Blastomyces dermatitidis.* The budding of *Cryptococcus neoformans,* as well as its smaller size and capsule, serves to distinguish it from *Coccidioides immitis,*

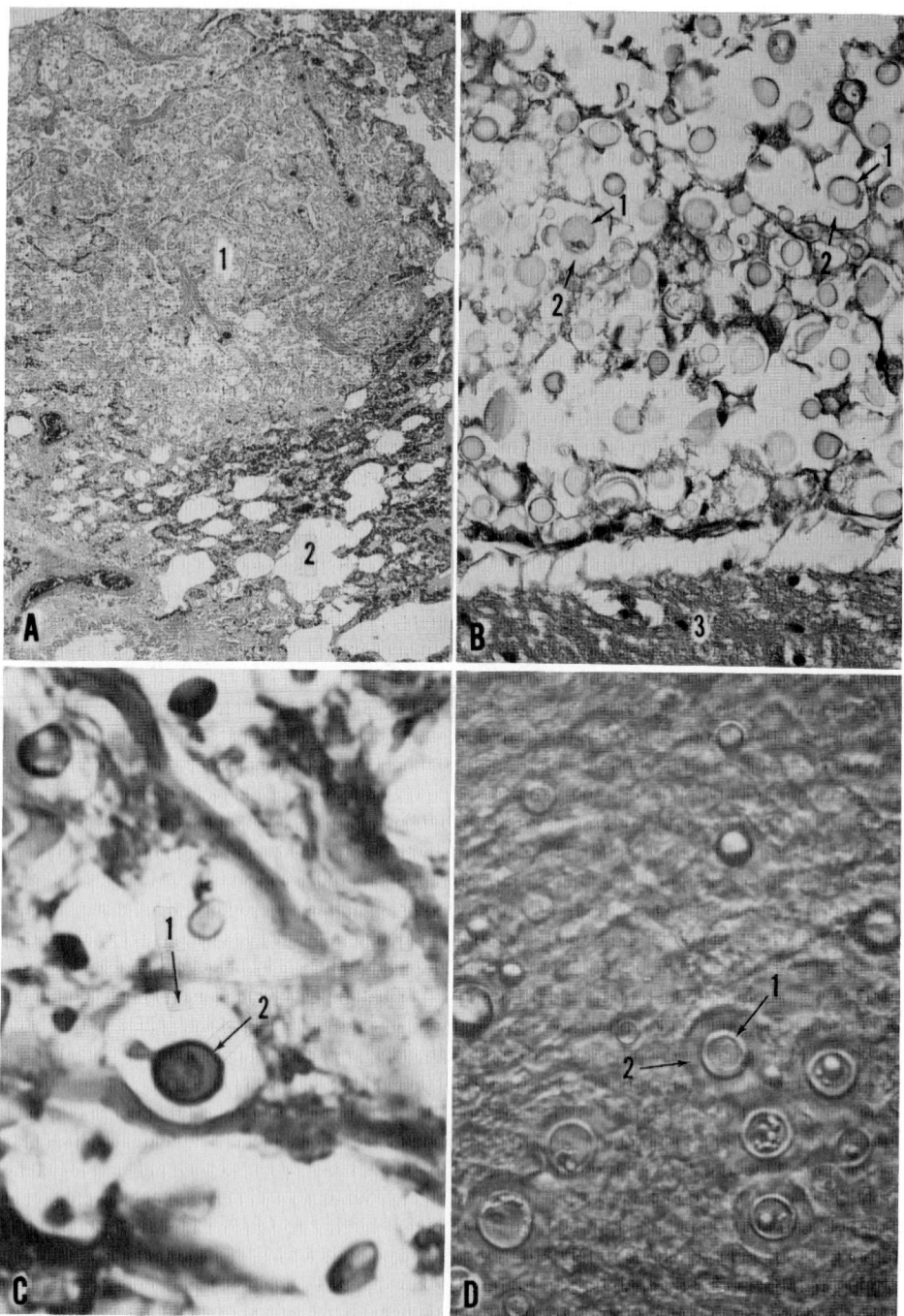

Fig. 12–23.   Cryptococcosis. *A,* Lung of a cat (× 48). Consolidated area (*1*) filling and compressing alveoli (*2*). *B,* Organisms in pia mater of a cat (× 300). Note spherical organisms (*1*) surrounded by a wide, clear capsule (*2*). Cerebral cortex (*3*). Contributor: Dr. John Mills. *C,* Organisms in cat lung (× 1045), same case as *A.* Note wide unstained capsule (*1*) surrounding a budding organism (*2*). (Courtesy of Armed Forces Institute of Pathology.) Contributor: Dr. Jean Holzworth. *D,* Unstained smear preparation viewed with phase contrast. Cell body (*1*) and capsule (*2*) (× 925).

which produces endospores and is not encapsulated.

Al-Doory, Y.: Bibliography of cryptococcosis. Mycopathol. Mycol. Appl., *45*:1–60, 1971.

Barron, C. N.: Cryptococcosis in animals. J. Am. Vet. Med. Assoc., *127*:125–132, 1955.

Dickson, J., and Meyer, E. P.: Cryptococcosis in horses in Western Australia. Aust. Vet. J., *46*:558, 1970.

Erwin, C. F. P., and Rac, R.: Cryptococcosis infection in a horse. Aust. Vet. J., *33*:97–98, 1957. Vet. Bull. 390, 1958.

Frothinghan, L.: A tumor-like lesion in the lung of a horse caused by a blastomyces (*Torula*). J. Med. Res., *8*:31–42, 1902.

Garner, F. M., Ford, D. F., and Ross, M. A.: Systemic cryptococcosis in 2 monkeys. J. Am. Vet. Med. Assoc., *155*:1163–1168, 1969.

Gelatt, K. N., McGill, L. D., and Perman, V.: Ocular and systemic cryptococcosis in a dog. J. Am. Vet. Med. Assoc., *162*:370–375, 1973.

Herin, V. and Dormal, R.: (Cerebral *Cryptococcus neoformans* infection in a horse in the Congo.) Ann. Soc. belge Med. trop., *42*:865–970, 1962. VB 3099–63.

Holzworth, J.: Cryptococcosis in a cat. Cornell Vet., *42*:12–15, 1952.

Holzworth, J., and Coffin, D. L.: Cryptococcosis in the cat. Cornell Vet., *43*:546–550, 1953.

Howell, J. McC., and Allan, D.: A case of cryptococcosis in the cat. J. Comp. Pathol., *74*:415–418, 1964.

Innes, J. R. M., Seibold, H. R., and Arentzen, W. P.: The pathology of bovine mastitis caused by *Cryptococcus neoformans*. Am. J. Vet. Res., *13*:469–475, 1952.

Johnston, L. A. Y., and Lavers, D. W.: Cryptococcal meningitis in a cat in North Queensland. Aust. Vet. J., *39*:306–307, 1963. VB 828–64.

Kavit, A. Y.: Cryptococcic arthritis in a Cocker Spaniel. J. Am. Vet. Med. Assoc., *133*:386–389, 1958.

Krogh, P., Basse, A., Hesselholt, M., and Bach, A.: Equine cryptococcosis: a case of rhinitis caused by *Cryptococcus neoformans* serotype A. Sabouraudia, *12*:272–278, 1974.

Littman, M. L., and Zimmerman, L. E.: Cryptococcosis (Torulosis, or European Blastomycosis). New York, Grune & Stratton, 1956.

Olander, H. J., Reed, H., and Pier, A. C.: Feline cryptococcosis. J. Am. Vet. Med. Assoc., *142*:138–143, 1963.

Roberts, E. D., et al.: Feline cryptococcosis. Iowa State Univ. Vet., *26*:30–33, 1963–64.

Rubin, L. F., and Craig, P. H.: Intraocular cryptococcosis in a dog. J. Am. Vet. Med. Assoc., *147*:27–32, 1965.

Scott, E. A., Duncan, J. R., and McCormack, J. E.: Cryptococcosis involving the postorbital area and frontal sinus in a horse. J. Am. Vet. Med. Assoc., *165*:626–627, 1974.

Seibold, H. R., Roberts, C. S., and Jordan, E. M.: Cryptococcosis in a dog. J. Am. Vet. Med. Assoc., *122*:213–215, 1953.

Shadomey, H. J., and Lurie, H. I.: Histopathological observations in experimental cryptococcosis caused by a hypha-producing strain of *Cryptococcus neoformans* (Coward strain). Sabouraudia, *9*:6–9, 1971.

Simon, J., Nichols, R. E., and Morse, E. V.: An outbreak of bovine cryptococcosis. J. Am. Vet. Med. Assoc., *122*:31–35, 1953.

Sly, D. L., London, W. T., Palmer, A. E., and Rice, J. M.: Disseminated cryptococcosis in a Patas monkey (*Erythrocebus patas*). Lab. Anim. Sci., *27*:694–699, 1977.

Smith, D. L. T., Fisher, J. B., and Barnum, D. A.: Generalized *Cryptococcus neoformans* infection in a dog. Can. Med. Assoc. J., *72*:18–20, 1955.

Sutmöller, P., and Poelma, F. G.: *Cryptococcus neoformans* infection (torulosis) of goats in the Leeward Islands Region. W. Ind. Med. J., *6*:225–228, 1957.

Takos, M. J., and Elton, N. W.: Spontaneous cryptococcosis of marmoset monkeys in Panama. Arch. Pathol., *55*:403–407, 1953.

Trautwein, B. and Nielsen, S. W.: Cryptococcosis in 2 cats, a dog and a mink. J. Am. Vet. Med. Assoc., *140*:437–442, 1962.

Wagner, J. L., Pick, J. R., and Kirgman, M. R.: *Cryptococcus neoformans* infection in a dog. J. Am. Vet. Med. Assoc., *153*:945–949, 1968.

Weidman, F. D., and Ratcliffe, H. J.: Cryptococcosis in a cheetah at the Philadelphia Zoo. Arch. Pathol., *18*:362–369, 1934.

Weitzman, I., Bonaparte, P., Guevin, V., and Crist, M.: Cryptococcosis in a field mouse. Sabouraudia, *11*:77–79, 1973.

HISTOPLASMOSIS

Histoplasmosis is an infectious, but not contagious, mycotic disease of man and lower animals. The causative organism, *Histoplasma capsulatum,* grows readily in culture media and soil as a white to brown mold that bears spores of two types: spherical, minutely spiny **microconidia,** 3 to 4 μ in diameter, and spherical, or rarely clavate, **macroconidia,** 8 to 12 μ in diameter, with evenly spaced finger-like projections over the surface. The parasitic phase in the mammalian host develops from either of these conidia into a yeast-like form.

Although for many years the disease in man was believed to occur only as a rare, consistently fatal, disseminated infection, it is now known that an acute nonfatal form is much more prevalent both in man and lower animals. The disease is not spread by direct contact between hosts, but it may appear in animals and man sharing the same environment. So-called epidemics of histoplasmosis are thus related to an environmental source of infection rather than to spread of contagion from host to host. Both the benign inapparent and the fatal disseminated forms of the disease occur in a wide variety of animals, including dogs, cats, cattle, horses, guinea pigs, bats, rats, mice, woodchucks, skunks, opossums, foxes, and raccoons. Cattle and monkeys (*Macaca mulatta* and *M. fascicularis*) have been used to produce diagnostic serum.

It has been reported from many parts of the United States, South and Central America, and less frequently other parts of the world, but apparently histoplasmosis is most common in certain regions of the United States, specifically those bordering the Missouri, Ohio and Mississippi Rivers. This impression may be misleading and merely reflect the more thorough studies that have been conducted in these areas. It is highly probable that most cases of his-

toplasmosis both animal and human, are neither recognized nor reported.

The benign form of the disease in animals is seldom recognized unless pulmonary lesions are present or organisms are recovered at necropsy, although in some instances x-ray examination has revealed lesions in subjects with histoplasmin sensitivity. Benign histoplasmosis in man may become apparent as an acute febrile pneumonitis with weight loss and adenopathy, or by roentgenologic evidence of dense, sometimes calcified "coin lesions" in the lungs, usually associated with histoplasmin sensitivity. The fatal disseminated form in animals, observed most frequently in dogs, usually runs a prolonged course with progressive loss of weight, lymphadenopathy, diarrhea, weakness, anemia, hepatomegaly, and ascites. Although histoplasmosis is difficult to recognize in the living animal, it has been diagnosed from the signs and course

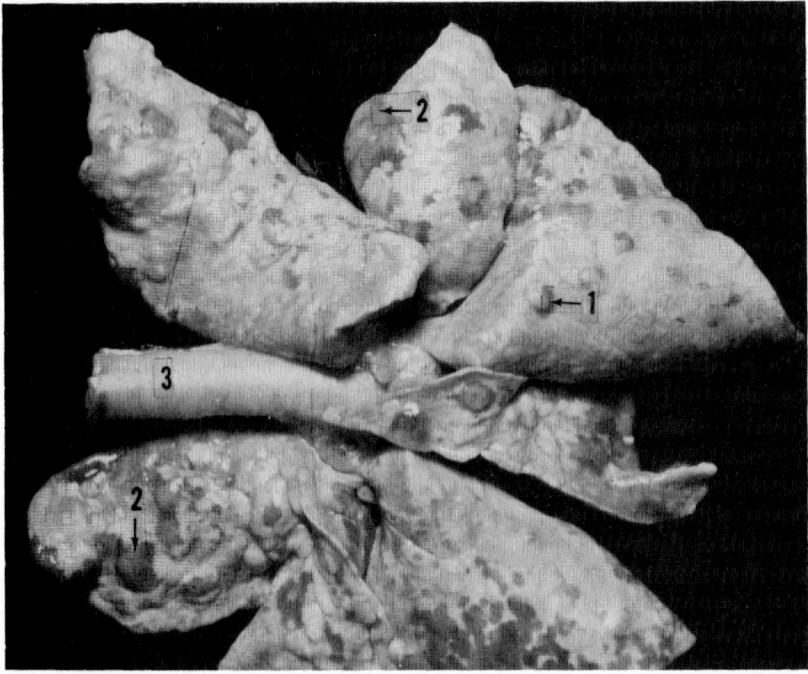

Fig. 12-24. Histoplasmosis. Nodules (*1*) in the lung of a dog. Consolidated lobules (*2*). Trachea (*3*). (Courtesy of Armed Forces Institute of Pathology.) Contributor: Dr. Karl S. Harmon.

and confirmed by demonstration of organisms in the circulating blood.

Lesions. The dominant feature of the tissue changes in histoplasmosis is the extensive proliferation of reticuloendothelial cells (macrophages, endothelioid, epithelioid cells), many of which contain yeast forms of the causative organism, either a few or so many that the cytoplasm is distended and tremendously enlarged. It is the proliferation of reticuloendothelial cells that causes displacement of normal tissues, interference with function, and gross enlargement of organs. The disease has been more adequately studied in the dog, hence the following remarks on the lesions apply especially to the dog.

The lungs in the benign form may have only a few discrete, well-encapsulated nodules or islands of epithelioid cells, some of which may contain demonstrable organisms. With recovery, these lesions regress to fibrocalcareous nodules that remain in the lung for years. In the disseminated form, the alveoli and interstitial stroma may be flooded with lymphocytes, plasma cells, and epithelioid cells, many containing organisms. The yeast-like bodies, which are always located in the cytoplasm, are irregularly egg-shaped and measure from 2 by 3 μ to 3 by 4 μ. In sections stained with hematoxylin and eosin, a central, spherical, usually basophilic body is surrounded by an unstained zone, which in turn is encircled by a thin cell wall. This may give the impression of a capsule around the central body, but the organism has no true capsule; the clear halo is actually within the cell wall. By the periodic acid-Schiff (PAS), Bauer's or Gridley's fungus method, the wall is stained selectively, leaving its contents unstained, thus the organism appears as an empty red ring. These stains are particularly useful in visualizing organisms when only a few are present and in differentiating them from other phagocytized particles, especially tissue debris.

The lymph nodes in the disseminated disease are tremendously enlarged by the proliferation of reticuloendothelial cells. Grossly, the nodes are firm and uniform in appearance, not unlike those of malignant lymphoma. The reticuloendothelial proliferation in severely affected nodes may obliterate the normal nodal architecture. Necrosis, purulent inflammation, and calcification are seldom observed, nor are multinucleated giant cells common. The predominant cell is mononuclear with tremendously expanded cytoplasm, often packed with organisms. Lymphocytes and plasma cells may be present in smaller numbers.

The spleen is enlarged to several times its normal size, light gray, and firm as the result of the reticuloendothelial proliferation, which masks much of the splenic architecture.

The liver is also enlarged, firm, and light gray because of the diffuse interlobular and intralobular proliferation of reticuloendothelial cells. These cells displace liver parenchyma and thus obviously interfere with liver function. As elsewhere, there is little tendency for encapsulation of the lesions in the disseminated form. Lymphocytes and plasma cells may be present in varying numbers.

The intestine, when involved, has a thickened rugose or nodular mucosal surface, and its wall is thickened by reticuloendothelial proliferation in the lamina propria and submucosa. Ulceration is unusual. The lymph nodules and adjacent lymph nodes are greatly enlarged, their architecture distorted by the characteristic large macrophages laden with organisms. The ileocecal junction and the adjacent lymph nodes are often severely affected.

The adrenal glands may be largely replaced by macrophages filled with organisms. This is particularly striking in fatal cases, but less so in affected animals sacrificed before the terminal stages of the disease.

Other organs, including skin, pancreas,

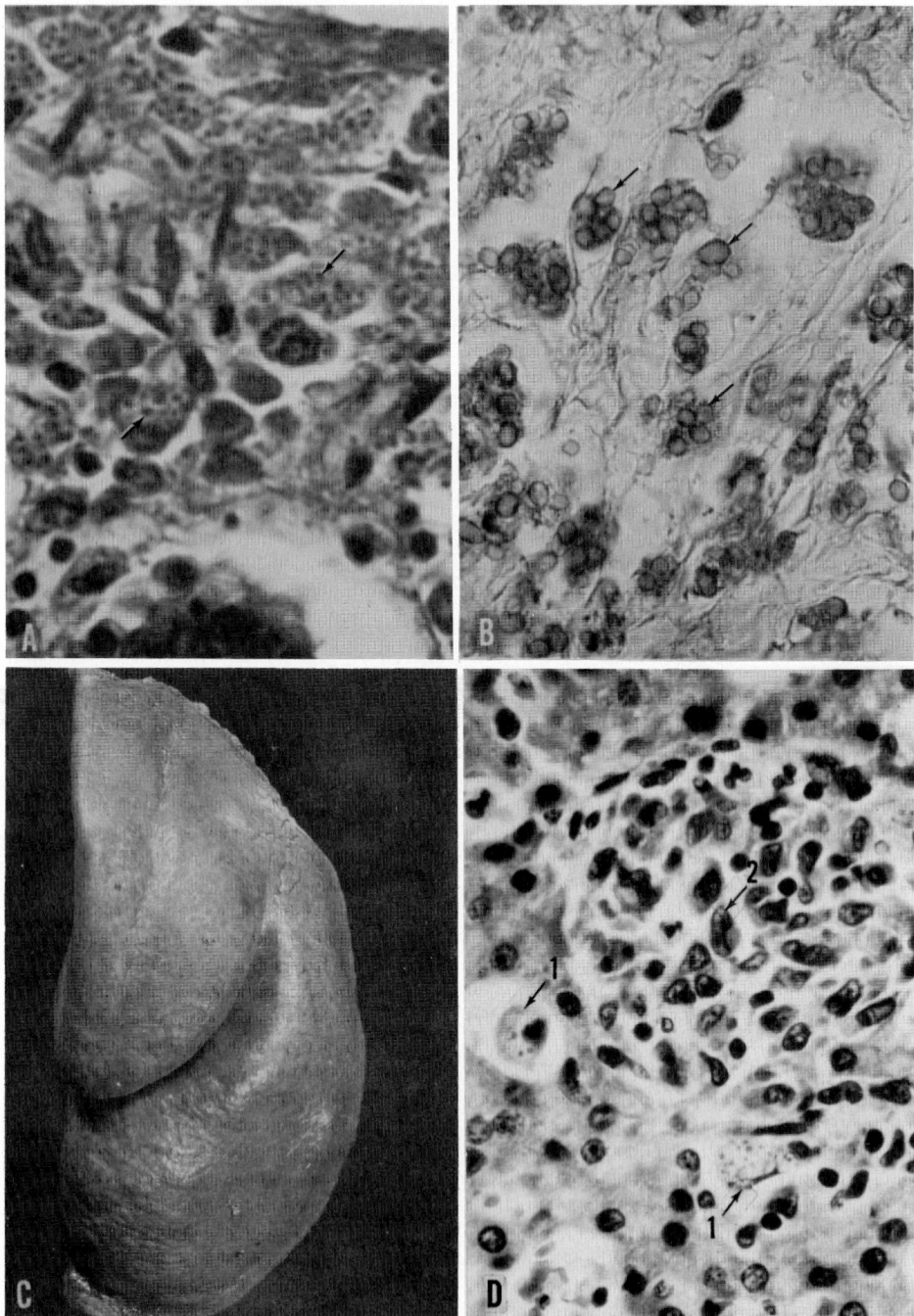

Fig. 12–25. Histoplasmosis. *A*, Macrophages (arrows) laden with *Histoplasma capsulatum* in submucosa of the ileum (× 1000) of a dog. Contributor: Dr. R. F. Birge. *B*, Organisms (arrows) stained by Gridley's fungus stain. The cell wall is stained red, causing the organisms to look larger than in *A*, although the magnification is the same (× 1000). *C*, Enlarged gray liver of a dog. Same as Case *B*. Contributor: Dr. Karl S. Harmon. *D*, Lesion in the liver (× 630) of a dog. Note macrophages laden with organisms (*1*) and reticuloendothelial cells (*2*). (Courtesy of Armed Forces Institute of Pathology). Contributor: Dr. H. R. Seibold.

heart, genitalia, and kidneys, are usually less severely affected, but may be involved by the characteristic reticuloendothelial proliferation.

Diagnosis. In the living animal, the diagnosis can be established by demonstration of typical reticuloendothelial proliferation and organisms in tissues at biopsy (tonsils, lymph node, liver). In some cases macrophages containing *H. capsulatum* can be demonstrated in smears of the circulating blood. Microscopic examination of tissue sections usually permits definitive diagnosis, but in some cases identification of the organisms in cultures is advisable. The organism of epizootic lymphangitis (*Histoplasma farciminosum*) cannot be differentiated in tissue sections, hence, cultures are necessary to distinguish these two infections. However, the different geographic distribution and the anatomic location of the two diseases usually eliminate difficulty. Some malignant neoplasms (malignant lymphoma, reticulum cell sarcoma), in which tissue necrosis and phagocytosis of cell debris have occurred, may have gross and microscopic features erroneously suggesting histoplasmosis, but can be distinguished by the absence of unequivocal organisms. Stains for bound glycogen (PAS, Bauer's, Gridley's fungus) are helpful in differential staining of the organisms. Differentiation of other mycotic organisms is not difficult in tissue sections, because *Blastomyces dermatitidis* is larger and exhibits budding, *Coccidioides immitis* is larger and forms endospores, and *Cryptococcus neoformans* is larger, has a wide mucoid capsule, and undergoes prominent budding.

Ackerman, N., Cornelius, L. M., and Halliwell, W.: Respiratory distress associated with histoplasma-induced tracheobronchial lymphadenopathy in dogs. J. Am. Vet. Med. Assoc., *163*:963–967, 1973.

Bauman, D. S., and Chick, E. W.: Experimental histoplasmosis in rhesus monkeys. Infectious dose and extrapulmonary dissemination determination. Chest, *63*:254–258, 1973.

————: Acute cavitary histoplasmosis in rhesus monkeys: influence of immunological status. Infect. Immun., *8*:245–248, 1973.

Birge, R. F., and Riser, W. H.: Canine histoplasmosis. North Am. Vet., *26*:281–287, 1945.

Cordy, D. R.: Histoplasmosis in a dog. Cornell Vet., *39*:339–343, 1949.

Correa, W. M., and Pacheco, A. C.: Naturally occurring histoplasmosis in guinea pigs. Can. J. Comp. Med. Vet. Sci., *31*:203–206, 1967.

Del Favero, J. E., and Farrell, R. L.: Experimental histoplasmosis in gnotobiotic dogs. Am. J. Vet. Res., *27*:60–66, 1966.

De Monbreun, W. A.: The dog as a natural host for *Histoplasma capsulatum.* Am. J. Trop. Med., *19*:565–588, 1939.

Dumont, A., and Robert, A.: Electron microscopic study of phagocytosis of *Histoplasma capsulatum* by hamster peritoneal macrophages. Lab. Invest., *23*:278–286, 1970.

Emmons, C. W.: Histoplasmosis. Bull. NY Acad. Med., *31*:627–638, 1955.

Emmons, C. W., and Ashburn, L. L.: Histoplasmosis in wild rats. Pub. Health Rep., *63*:1416–1422, 1948.

Farrell, R. L., and Cole, C. R.: Experimental canine histoplasmosis with acute fatal and chronic recovered courses. Am. J. Pathol., *53*:425–445, 1968.

Harmon, K. S.: Histoplasmosis in dogs. J. Am. Vet. Med. Assoc., *108*:60–62, 1948.

Kaplan, W., Kaufman, L., and McClure, H. M.: Pathogenesis and immunological aspects of experimental histoplasmosis in the cynomolgus monkey (*Macaca fascicularis*). Infect. Immun., *5*:847–926, 1972.

Lamas da Silva, J. M., Barbosa, M., and Hipolito, O.: (*Histoplasma capsulatum* infection in a dog in Brazil.) Arq. Esc. Vet. Minas Gerais., *13*:101–106, 1962.

Menges, R. W., Habermann, R. T., Selby, L. A., and Behlow, R. F.: *Histoplasma capsulatum* isolated from a calf and a pig. Vet. Med., *57*:1067–1070, 1962. VB 1909–63.

Menges, R. W., et al.: Ecologic studies of histoplasmosis. Am. J. Epidemiol., *85*:108–119, 1967.

Panciera, R. J.: Histoplasmic (*Histoplasma capsulatum*) infection in a horse. Cornell Vet., *59*:306–312, 1969.

Rowley, D. A., Habermann, R. A., and Emmons, C. W.: Histoplasmosis: pathologic study of fifty cats and fifty dogs from Loudon County, Virginia. J. Infect. Dis., *95*:98–108, 1954.

Seibold, H. R.: Histoplasmosis in a dog. J. Am. Vet. Med. Assoc., *109*:209–211, 1946.

Selby, L. A., Menges, R. W., and Habermann, R. T.: Survey for blastomycosis and histoplasmosis among stray dogs in Arkansas. Am. J. Vet. Res., *28*:345–349, 1967.

Sharbaugh, R. J., DiSalvo, A. F., Goodman, N. L., and Reddick, R. A.: Serologic aspects of experimental histoplasmosis in cattle. J. Infect. Dis., *127*:186–189, 1973.

Tomlinson, W. J., and Grocott, R. G.: Canine histoplasmosis. A pathologic study of the three reported cases and the first case found in the Canal Zone. Am. J. Clin. Pathol., *15*:501–507, 1945.

Wilson, T. M., Kierstead, M., and Long, J. R.: Histoplasmosis in a Harp seal. J. Am. Vet. Med. Assoc., *165*:815–816, 1974.

EPIZOOTIC LYMPHANGITIS

Epizootic lymphangitis is a disease of the skin and superficial lymphatics of horses, caused by a mycotic organism currently known as *Histoplasma farciminosum* (*Cryptococcus farciminosus, Blastomyces farciminosus, Saccharomyces farciminosus, Endomyces farciminosa, Saccharomyces equi*, or *Zyomonema farciminosum*). This organism is yeast-shaped in tissue but forms mycelia in cultures, in many respects resembling *Histoplasma capsulatum*. The disease probably no longer occurs in the United States, but still is common in some other countries, notably China, India, Egypt, and Sudan. The clinical features are those of chronic indurative ulceration of the skin, especially of the limbs, with thickening of the superficial lymphatics, enlargement of regional lymph nodes, formation of abscesses and discharge of purulent material, followed by the development of new indolent ulcers. Less frequently, infection may occur as conjunctivitis or nasolacrimal infection, and rarely becomes generalized, involving internal viscera.

The mode of transmission is not established. Direct contact does not appear important unless infective material is conveyed to previously injured skin. Experimentally, flies (*Musca* and *Stomoxys*) have been shown capable of transmitting the infection.

With the exception of rabbits, most laboratory animals are refractory to infection.

Lesions. Sections of the cutaneous lesions reveal granulomatous tissue reactions with a predominance of large macrophages, their cytoplasm distended with oval organisms, each about 2.0 by 3.0 μ, and enveloped by a thin capsule. The central mass of the fungus is demonstrable in sections stained with hematoxylin and eosin; the peripheral capsule remains un-

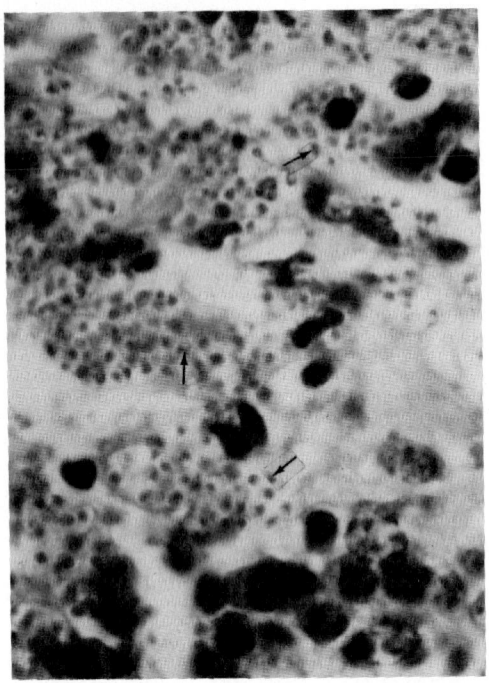

Fig. 12–26. Epizootic lymphangitis, skin of a mule (× 1200). Large number of *Histoplasma farciminosum* (arrows) are seen in macrophages. (Courtesy of Armed Forces Institute of Pathology.) Contributor: Ninth Medical Service Detachment Laboratory, U.S. Army.

stained. Stains for bound glycogen (PAS, Bauer's and Gridley's fungus stain) identify the capsule selectively, staining it red and leaving the central body unstained. The organisms are very similar to *Histoplasma capsulatum* in tissues; in fact, their appearance suggests that the two organisms should be carefully compared. Mycelial forms of *H. farciminosum* have been described in tissues but are usually absent.

Diagnosis. The diagnosis of epizootic lymphangitis can be confirmed by the demonstration of typical organisms in characteristic lesions, in tissue sections, cultures or stained smears of exudate.

Fawi, M. T.: *Histoplasma farciminosum*, the aetiological agent of equine cryptococcal pneumonia. Sabouraudia, *9*:123–125, 1971.

Fouad, K., Saleh, M. S., Sokkar, S., and Shouman, M. T.: Studies on lachrymal histoplasmosis in donkeys in Egypt. Zentralbl. Veterinaermed. B, 20:584–593, 1973.

Khater, A. R., Iskander, M., and Mostafa, A.: A histomorphological study of cutaneous lesions in equine histoplasmosis (epizootic lymphangitis). J. Egypt Vet. Med. Assoc., 28:165–174, 1968.

Singh, T.: Studies on epizootic lymphangitis. I. Modes of infection and transmission of equine histoplasmosis *(Epizootic lymphangitis)*. Indian J. Vet. Sci., 35:102–110, 1965.

Singh, T., and Varmani, B. M. L.: Studies on epizootic lymphangitis. A note on pathogenicity of *Histoplasma farciminosum* (Rivolta) for laboratory animals. Indian J. Vet. Sci., 36:164–167, 1966.

———: Some observations on experimental infection with *Histoplasma farciminosum* (Rivolta) and the morphology of the organism. Indian J. Vet. Sci., 37:47–57, 1967.

THE PHYCOMYCOSES

The term "phycomycosis" was introduced by Emmons et al. to provide a convenient name for mycoses caused by fungi placed in the class Phycomycetes. This class, Phycomycetes, is no longer recognized as valid by taxonomists, but the term is useful to apply to certain mycoses in which no culture has been obtained but the fungus in sections conform to certain morphologic criteria. The phycomycoses in this context currently include: **mucormycosis, entomophthoramycosis, oomycosis, rhinosporidiosis,** and **trichomycetosis** (see Table 12–3). A large number of fungi are involved and knowledge of their pathogenicity for animals is incomplete; therefore, only a few will be considered in this text.

Mucormycosis

This disease category includes infections by several fungi, classified in the order Mucorales. The fungi grow in tissues as coarse, nonseptate, branching filamentous organisms which result in infectious granulomas. Many species, including man, may be infected. Lesions are found on body surfaces and lymph nodes, and sometimes may be disseminated. Placentitis in bovine animals is a particular infection with these organisms and will be considered further. The specific species identified so far as pathogens are listed in Table 12–3.

Lesions. The gross lesions of mucormycosis are rather nonspecific. Ulcers with

Table 12–3. The Phycomycoses

Disease	Mycotic Organisms	Hosts
Mucormycosis	*Absidia corymbifera (Mucor corymbifera, Lichtheimia corymbifera)*	Cattle, man
	Mucor spp.	Cattle (abortion)
	Cunninghamella spp.	Man
	Mortierella wolfii	Man, cattle
	Rhizopus cohnii	Young pigs, man, cattle (abortion)
	Rhizopus microsporus	Suckling pigs
Entomophthoramycosis .	*Basidiobolus haptosporus*	Man
	Basidiobolus ranarum	Horse
	Entomophthora coronata (Conidiobolus coronatus)	Horse, chimpanzee, man, insects (rhinomycosis)
Oomycosis	*Saprolegnia ferax*	Fish
	Hyphomyces destruens	Horse (hyphomycosis destruens)
	Coelomomyces spp.	Mosquito larvae
Rhinosporidiosis (Chytoidiomycetes)	*Rhinosporidium seeberi*	Horse, man, dog, cattle, ducks, geese
Trichomycetosis	Class Zygomycotina (4 orders)	Arthropods

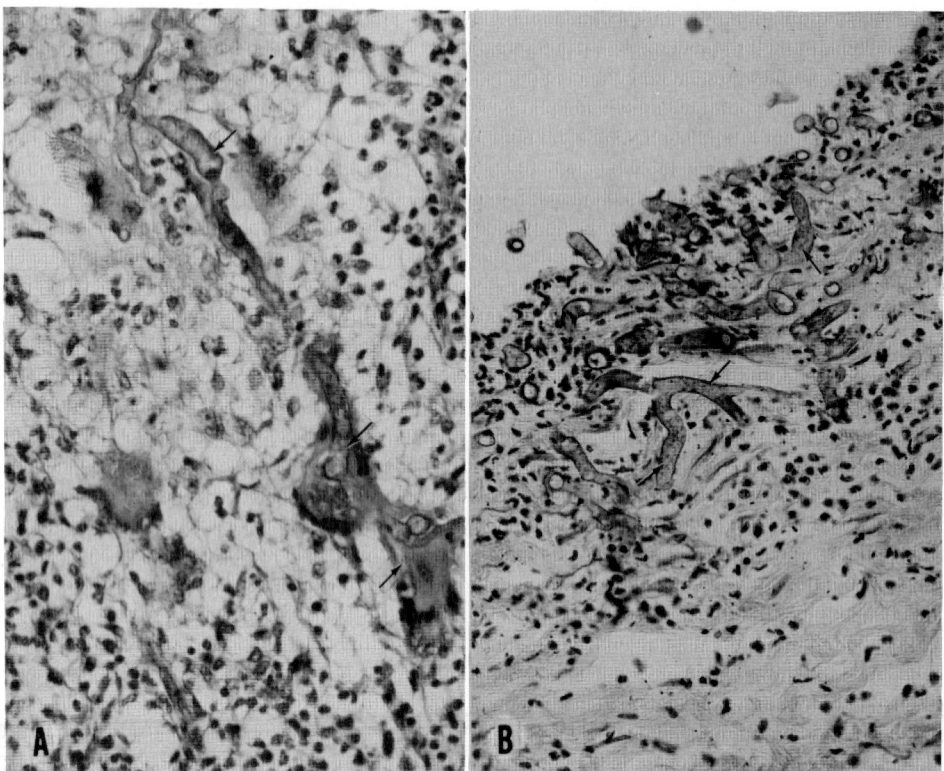

Fig. 12–27. Mucormycosis. *A*, Bovine mesenteric lymph node (× 310). Note long mycelium (arrows) in a large giant cell. (Courtesy of Dr. C. L. Davis.) *B*, Organisms (arrows) in the depths of an ulcer in the stomach of a dog (× 130). (Courtesy of Armed Forces Institute of Pathology.) Contributor: Dr. M. A. Troy.

raised edges may occur in the stomach; affected lymph nodes in cattle may be enlarged and replaced by yellowish granulomas with caseous or calcareous foci within them. Similar caseous lesions may be seen in any affected organ.

Microscopically, epithelioid granulation tissue with varying degrees of necrosis and calcification replaces normal tissues. Lymphocytic infiltration may be intense, and giant cells are often present. In cattle, particularly in the mesenteric lymph nodes, eosinophils are often conspicuous. The organisms appear in giant cells or necrotic zones as irregular, coarse hyphae, which are often branched but rarely septate. The organisms are readily demonstrable with hematoxylin and eosin stains, but are more distinctly outlined by the periodic acid-Schiff (PAS) reaction. There can be little

doubt that this organism grows in tissue and that host cells react specifically to its presence.

Diagnosis. Specific diagnosis should be based upon demonstration of characteristic organisms in typical granulomatous lesions. Isolation of organisms from the lesions is necessary for their further identification and study, but histologic demonstration of the fungus within tissues that are obviously reacting to its presence is critical in establishing the causal relationship in an individual lesion. Identification of the organism recovered from cultures is not decisive, because these fungi grow free in nature and can easily contaminate cultures taken under many circumstances.

Angus, K. W., Renwick, C. C., and Robinson, G. W.: Segmental necrosis of the ileum in a lamb associated with a phycomycete. Vet. Rec., *88*:654–656, 1971.

Christiansen, M.: Mucormykose beim Schwein. I. Mittelung. Virchows Arch. [Pathol. Anat.], *273*:829–858, 1929.

Davis, C. L., Anderson, W. A., and McCrory, B. R.: Mucormycosis in food-producing animals. J. Am. Vet. Med. Assoc., *126*:261–267, 1955.

Dawson, C. O.: Phycomycoses in animals in the tropics. Ann. Soc. Belg. Med. Trop., *52*:357–364, 1972.

Fragner, P., Vitovec, J., Vladik, P., and Proks, C.: Liver disease in hog caused by *Rhizopus cohnii*. Mycopathologia, *49*:249–254, 1973.

Gisler, D. B., and Pitcock, J. A.: Intestinal mucormycosis in the monkey *(Macaca mulatta)*. Am. J. Vet. Res., *23*:365–366, 1962.

Gitter, M., and Austwick, P. K. C.: Mucormycosis and moniliasis in a litter of suckling pigs. Vet. Rec., *71*:6–11, 1959.

Gleiser, C. A.: Mucormycosis in animals. J. Am. Vet. Med. Assoc., *123*:441–445, 1953.

Gregory, J. E., Golden, A., and Haymaker, W.: Mucormycosis of the central nervous system. Bull. Johns Hopkins Hosp., *73*:405–419, 1953.

Hessler, J. R., et al.: Mucormycosis in a rhesus monkey. J. Am. Vet. Med. Assoc., *151*:909–913, 1967.

Knudtson, W. U., Bergeland, M. E., and Kirkbride, C. A.: Bovine fetal cerebral absidiomycosis. Sabouraudia, *13*:299–302, 1975.

Martin, J. E., et al.: Rhino-orbital phycomycosis in a rhesus monkey. J. Am. Vet. Med. Assoc., *155*:1253–1257, 1969.

Pohlenz, J., Ehrensperger, F., and Breer, C.: Spontane Todesfälle infolge Mukormykose des Vormagens beim Rind. Schweiz. Arch. Tierheilkd., *115*:161–168, 1973.

Rapp, J. P., and McGrath, J. T.: Mycotic encephalitis in weanling rats. Lab. Anim. Sci., *25*:477–480, 1975.

Shirley, A. G. H.: Two cases of phycomycotic ulceration in sheep. Vet. Rec., *77*:675–677, 1965.

Symeonidis, A., and Emmons, C. W.: Granulomatous growth induced in mice by *Absidia corymbifera*. Arch. Pathol., *60*:251–258, 1955.

Bovine Mycotic Placentitis (Mycotic Abortion)

Premature expulsion of the bovine fetus upon occasion has been demonstrated to be associated with an infection of the placenta by one of several species of molds. The demonstration of granulomatous lesions in relation to the presence of fungi in the placenta may be accepted as good evidence that these organisms cause infection that may result in abortion ("mycotic abortion"). A better name is mycotic placentitis, because the placenta is principally involved even though the fetus may also be infected.

Twenty-four species of fungi have been isolated from cases of mycotic placentitis, but it appears that *Aspergillus fumigatus* is the most frequent pathogen—it has been recovered in 60% of the reported cases. *Absidia ramosa*, *Absidia corymbifera*, and *Rhizopus* and *Mucor spp.* have also been recovered with some frequency. Other species are rarely reported, and some doubt may remain as to the pathogenic significance of some of them. Infection is generally believed to result from dissemination of organisms via the circulation rather than by direct infection of the genital tract. One of the facts that support this belief is that the disease has been reproduced experimentally by the intravenous injection of fungal spores.

Lesions. The lesions of mycotic placentitis are found in the placenta of the aborted bovine fetus, but the affected dam rarely exhibits any signs or lesions that could characterize the disease. Affected placentae are described as having enlarged, thickened cotyledons that retain much of the maternal placenta, are thickened at the margins, and necrotic in the center. The intracaruncular zones may have a thickened, leathery appearance. Hemorrhage and hyperemia are reported to be prominent in histologic sections of early lesions and are accompanied by neutrophilic and eosinophilic leukocytes. Necrosis tends to separate the maternal and fetal layers of the placenta, and the organisms are demonstrable in this zone by appropriate staining techniques (Gridley's, Bauer's, PAS). The organisms are also recoverable from these lesions with suitable culture media. Although thick, encrusted, corrugated lesions have been seen in bovine fetuses from which fungi (*Aspergillus fumigatus*, particularly) were isolated, the histologic nature of the cutaneous lesions have not been determined. The organisms may be recovered from the stomach of aborted bovine fetuses, but no lesions have been described in the stomach.

Experimental intravenous inoculation of 5 million spores of *Mortierella wolfii* into pregnant cows resulted in focal mycotic pneumonia, placentitis, and death within four days. Smaller doses of spores led to nonfatal pneumonia in cattle (Cordes et al., 1972). *Aspergillus fumigatus* and *A. ramosa* appear to be less virulent under these experimental conditions. In experimental bovine infections with *Aspergillus fumigatus* (Hillman and McEntee, 1969), organisms were demonstrated in necrotic zones in the placenta and endometrium and in association with edema, necrosis, and neutrophil infiltration of the walls of arteries in the chorioallantois.

Equine Mycotic Placentitis (Mycotic Abortion)

It is of interest to record that lesions have been found by Mahaffey and Adam (1964) in the placentae of Thoroughbred mares, indicating that fungi may also be a cause of abortion in the equine species. These workers have demonstrated fungal organisms histologically in lesions in equine placentae and have isolated organisms identified as *Aspergillus* and *Mucor species*. Further studies will be required to determine the significance of these infections in *Equidae*.

Cysewski and Pier (1968) have experimentally induced mycotic abortion in ewes with intravenous inoculation of spores of *Aspergillus fumigatus*. The role of fungi in spontaneous abortion of ewes has not been established.

Ainsworth, G. C., and Austwick, P. K. C.: Fungal Diseases of Animals. Rev. Series 6, 1959. Commonwealth Agric. Bureaux, Farnham Royal, Bucks, England.

Bridges, C. H.: Mycotic diseases in mammalian reproduction. *In* Comparative Aspects of Reproductive Failure, edited by K. Benirschke. New York, Springer-Verlag, 1967.

Carter, M. E., Cordes, D. O., di Menna, M. E., and Hunter, R.: Fungi isolated from bovine mycotic abortion and pneumonia with special reference to *Mortierella wolfii*. Res. Vet. Sci., 14:201–206, 1973.

Cordes, D. O., Carter, M. E., and di Menna, M. E.: Mycotic pneumonia and placentitis caused by *Mortierella wolfii*. II. Pathology of experimental infection of cattle. Vet. Pathol., 9:190–201, 1972.

Cordes, D. O., di Menna, M. E., and Carter, M. E.: Mycotic pneumonia and placentitis caused by *Mortierella wolfii*. I. Experimental infections in cattle and sheep. Vet. Pathol., 9:131–141, 1972.

Counter, D. E.: An outbreak of mycotic abortion apparently due to mould-infected sugar beet pulp. Vet. Rec., 93:425, 1973.

Cysewski, S. J., and Pier, A. C.: Mycotic abortion in ewes produced by *Aspergillus fumigatus*: pathologic changes. Am. J. Vet. Res., 29:1135–1151, 1968.

di Menna, M. E., Carter, M. E., and Cordes, D. O.: The identification of *Mortierella wolfii* isolated from cases of abortion and pneumonia in cattle and a search for its infection source. Res. Vet. Sci., 13:439–442, 1972.

Hillman, R. B.: Bovine mycotic placentitis in New York State. Cornell Vet., 59:269–288, 1969.

Hillman, R. B., and McEntee, K.: Experimental studies on bovine mycotic placentitis. Cornell Vet., 59:289–302, 1969.

Mahaffey, L. W., and Adam, N. M.: Abortions associated with mycotic lesions of the placenta in mares. J. Am. Vet. Med. Assoc., 144:24–32, 1964.

White, L. O., and Smith, H.: Placental localisation of *Aspergillus fumigatus* in bovine mycotic abortion: enhancement of spore germination in vitro by foetal tissue extracts. J. Med. Microbiol., 7:27–34, 1974.

Wohlgemuth, K., and Knudtson, W.: Bovine abortion associated with *Candida tropicalis*. J. Am. Vet. Med. Assoc., 162:460–461, 1973.

Entomophthoramycosis

Fungal organisms in the family Entomophthoraceae have been identified as the cause of infectious granulomas in the skin and mucous membranes (nasal, oral) of several species. *Entomophthora coronata* has been identified in such lesions in several horses (Bridges et al., 1962; Chauhan et al., 1973). A single case of rhinophycomycosis has been described in a wild chimpanzee (Roy and Cameron, 1972). An infection in the skin of a horse due to *Basidiobolus ranarum* has been described (Van Overeem, 1925).

Bridges, C. H., Romane, W. M., and Emmons, C. W.: Phycomycosis of horses caused by *Entomophthora coronata*. J. Am. Vet. Med. Assoc., 140:673–677, 1962.

Chauhan, H. V. S., et al.: A fatal cutaneous granuloma due to *Entomophthora coronata* in a mare. Vet. Rec., 92:425–427, 1973.

Roy, A. D., and Cameron, H. M.: *Rhinophycomycosis entomophthorae* occurring in a chimpanzee in the wild in East Africa. Am. J. Trop. Med. Hyg., 21:234–237, 1972.

Van Overeem, C.: Beitrage zur Pilzflora von Nieder-
ländisch Indien. 10. Ueber ein merkwürdiges
Vorkommen von *Basidiobolus ranarum* Eidom.
Bull. Jardin Bot., 7:423–431, 1925.

Oomycosis

Diseases caused by fungi classified in
the class Oomycetes have been grouped as
the oomycoses. *Saprolegnia ferax* is considered to be the cause of a common mycosis
of fish. *Coelomomyces spp.* are mycotic
pathogens of mosquito larvae. Also presently included in this class, Oomycetes, is
Hyphomyces destruens, the cause of
hyphomycosis destruens ("leeches," bursatti), a dermal mycosis of horses known
for nearly a hundred years. This organism
has recently been classified (Austwick and
Copland, 1974) as a member of the class
Oomycetes, order Peronosporales. Its isolation and culture were first reported by
Bridges and Emmons in 1961. The disease
is manifest by massive infectious granulomas in the subcutis, particularly of the
legs. The greatly thickened subcutis contains necrotic foci, which may lead through
fistulous tracts to ulcers in the skin. Spread
sometimes occurs to the regional lymph
nodes, but usually remains localized for a
long time.

Austwick, P. K. C., and Copland, J. W.: Swamp
cancer. Nature, 250:84, 1974.
Bridges, C. H., and Emmons, C. W.: A phycomycosis
of horses caused by *Hyphomyces destruens.* J. Am.
Vet. Med. Assoc., 138:579–589, 1961.
Connole, M. D.: Equine phycomycosis. Aust. Vet. J.,
49:214–215, 1973.
Hutchins, D. R., and Johnston, K. G.: Phycomycosis
in the horse. Aust. Vet. J., 48:269–278, 1972.
Murray, D. R., Ladds, P. W., Johnson, R. H., and Pott,
B. W.: Metastatic phycomycosis in a horse. J. Am.
Vet. Med. Assoc., 172:834–836, 1978.

Rhinosporidiosis

Infection of the nasal mucosae with a
fungus, *Rhinosporidium seeberi,* is known in
man, horses, cattle, dogs, and aquatic
birds (ducks and geese). It is common in
man in India and is reported infrequently
in North and South America.

In animals, as in man, the organism invades the subepithelial stroma of the nasal

mucosa, where it induces chronic inflammation and often results in polyp formation. The polyps are single or multiple, irregular in size and shape, and may become
large enough to occlude the nasal passages.
In the horse in the Americas, the nasal
polyps are reportedly limited in extent,
amenable to surgery, and probably self-
limited in duration.

Microscopic examination of the polyps
discloses a stroma filled with spherical
organisms (Fig. 12–28) with a thick,
double-contoured wall. These spherules
vary in size, depending upon their stage of
development, the largest (sporangium)
measuring nearly 300 μ and the smallest
(spore) about 2.0 μ in diameter. The round
daughter cells, or endospores, formed
within the sporangium are released by rupture of the cell wall at the so-called pore,
where it is thinnest. In the spore form, the
organisms gain access to the tissues, where
they continue their life cycle, developing
into sporangia containing innumerable
endospores. The fragmented cell walls
from mature organisms appear to excite the
most intense tissue reaction, which in
places may encapsulate the organism with
dense connective tissue. The growing, living organisms attract inflammatory infiltration consisting principally of lymphocytes with few epithelioid cells.

Ainsworth, G. C., and Austwick, P. K. C.: Fungal
Diseases of Animals. Rhinosporidiosis. Review
Series No. 6, Commonwealth Bureau of Animal
Health. Common. Agric. Bureaux, Farnham
Royal, Bucks, England 44–45, 1959.
Davidson, W. R., and Nettles, V. F.: Rhinosporidiosis
in a wood duck. J. Am. Vet. Med. Assoc.,
171:989–990, 1978.
Fain, A., and Herin, V.: Two cases of nasal rhino-
sporidiosis in a wild goose and a wild duck.
Mycopathol. Mycol. Appl., 8:54–61, 1967.
Jungerman, P. F., and Schwartzman, R. M.: Rhino-
sporidiosis. In Veterinary Medical Mycology.
Philadelphia, Lea & Febiger, 1972, pp. 40–47.
Myers, D. D., Simon, J., and Case, M. T.: Rhino-
sporidiosis in a horse. J. Am. Vet. Med. Assoc.,
145:345–347, 1964.
Smith, H. A., and Frankson, M. C.: Rhinosporidiosis
in a Texas horse. Southwest Vet., 15:22–24, 1961.
Stuart, B. P., and O'Malley, N.: Rhinosporidiosis in a
dog. J. Am. Vet. Med. Assoc., 167:941–942, 1975.

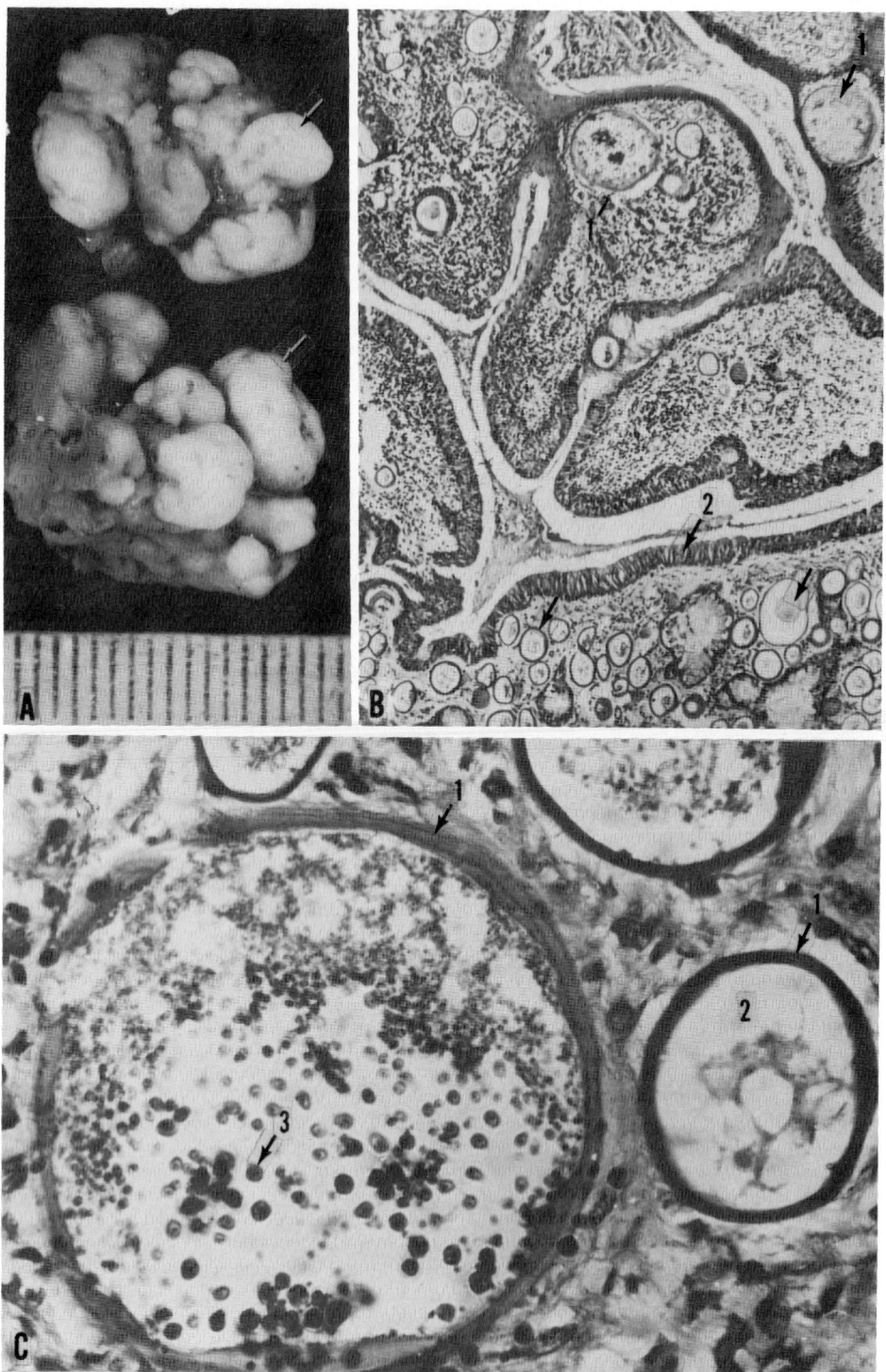

Fig. 12–28. Rhinosporidiosis. *A*, Polypoid masses from nasal mucosa of a horse. *B*, Section (× 100) of one of the polyps. *Rhinosporidium seeberi* containing endospore (*1*) or as empty cysts, elevating the mucous membrane (*2*). *C*, The organism (× 600); note thick wall (*1*), empty organisms (*2*), and others containing small and large (*3*) endospores. (Courtesy of Armed Forces Institute of Pathology.) Contributor: Col. M. W. Hale.

Weller, C. V., and Riker, A. D.: *Rhinosporidium seeberi:* pathological histology and report of the third case from the United States. Am. J. Pathol., 6:721–732, 1930.

Zschokke, E.: Ein rhinosporidium beim Pferd. Schweitz. Arch. Tierheilkd., 55:641–650, 1913.

SPOROTRICHOSIS

Sporotrichosis is a fungous disease that occurs both in man and animals, the horse being the most frequently affected lower animal. The causative organism, *Sporotrichum schenkii*, grows as a mold with aerial mycelia in culture, but is restricted to irregular club- or cigar-shaped forms in tissues. Chronic peritonitis and orchitis can be produced experimentally in male rats, mice, and hamsters by the intraperitoneal injection of material containing *S. schenkii*. In experimentally induced lesions, the organisms are much more numerous and more easily seen and identified. The disease runs a slow, obstinate course and does not become generalized.

Lesions. The lesions of sporotrichosis occur in the skin and cutaneous lymphatics, particularly over the legs, thorax, and abdomen. Spherical nodules, from 1 to 4 cm in diameter, are formed in the dermis and subcutis along the course of cutaneous lymphatics, which are thickened and pursue a tortuous course between the nodules. Occasionally, the nodules ulcerate, yield small amounts of thick, creamy pus, and then heal very slowly. Microscopic sections of the nodules reveal a purulent center surrounded by a wide band of epithelioid granulation tissue containing giant cells and lymphocytes. The lesion is usually surrounded by a dense connective-tissue capsule. The organisms in the lesion are not demonstrable with ordinary hematoxylin and eosin stains, but are stained by the periodic acid-Schiff (PAS) method or by modifications of this technique, such as the Gridley's fungus stain. The bound glycogen in the capsule of the organism makes it possible to visualize it in tissue sections. Demonstration of the organisms in sections, cultures, or laboratory animals is necessary to distinguish sporotrichosis from the cutaneous form of glanders (farcy), which is clinically similar.

Barbee, W. C., Ewert, A., and Davidson, E. M.: Animal model of human disease: sporotrichosis. Am. J. Pathol., 86:281–284, 1977.

Davis, H. H., and Worthington, E. W.: Equine sporotrichosis. J. Am. Vet. Med. Assoc., 145:692–693, 1964.

Jones, T. C., and Maurer, F. D.: Sporotrichosis in horses. Bul. U. S. Army Med. Dept. No. 74:63–73, 1944.

Kaplan, W., and Ochoa, A. G.: Application of the fluorescent antibody technique to the rapid diagnosis of sporotrichosis. J. Lab. Clin. Med., 62:835–841, 1963. VB 1251–64.

Kier, A. B., Mann, P. C., and Wagner, J. E.: Disseminated sporotrichosis in a cat. J. Am. Vet. Med. Assoc., 175:202–204, 1979.

CANDIDIASIS (Moniliasis, Thrush)

Candidiasis, caused by species of the fungus *Candida* (most usually *Candida albicans),* is principally a superficial mycosis of mucous membranes. It is encountered most frequently in avian species, affecting the mouth, esophagus, crop, and proventriculus. Superficial infection of oral mucous membranes is also the most common form of candidiasis in mammals, where it has been seen in man, cats, cattle, swine, and nonhuman primates. Systemic candidiasis, though rare, has been described in man, mice, and calves. Infection may also involve the skin of man and animals, and in man, *Candida sp.* may cause bronchitis, pneumonia, and vulvovaginitis. It has been reported as a cause of bovine mastitis and abortion. Candidiasis is most common in young animals, debilitated patients, and as a complication of protracted antibiotic therapy.

Lesions. The gross lesions in the superficial form of candidiasis are characterized by a white pseudomembrane overlying the skin or mucous membranes. Microscopically, the membrane is composed of masses of entangled pseudohyphae and budding yeast-like organisms 3 to 4 μ in diameter, which invade the epithelium, but rarely beyond the basal layer. The organisms can be difficult to discern in hematoxylin and eosin stained tissue sections, but are clearly demonstrated with the periodic acid-Schiff, Gridley and Gomori methenamine silver techniques. A leukocytic infiltration predominantly composed of neutrophils and lymphocytes accumulated beneath the epidermis. Lesions in systemic candidiasis, which may involve various internal organs but in particular the kidneys, are characterized by necrosis and suppuration. Rarely is a granulomatous reaction encountered.

The yeast form of *Candida albicans* has been demonstrated to be significantly more pathogenic under experimental conditions than the mycelial form. It has also been suggested that infection with candidiasis may give rise to a false tuberculin test under some conditions (Wikse et al., 1970).

Diagnosis. Diagnosis depends upon demonstration of the organisms in characteristic lesions.

Budtz-Jorgensen, E.: Immune-response to *C. albicans* in monkeys with experimental candidiasis in palate. Scand. J. Dent. Res., *81*:360–371, 1973.

Goetz, M. E., and Taylor, D. O. N.: A naturally occurring outbreak of *Candida tropicalis* infection in a laboratory mouse colony. Am. J. Pathol., *50*:361–369, 1967.

Goldstein, E., et al.: Studies on the pathogenesis of experimental *Candida guilliermondii* infection in mice. J. Infect. Dis. *115*:293–302, 1965.

Kaufmann, A. F., and Quist, K. D.: Thrush in a rhesus monkey: report of a case. Lab. Anim. Care, *19*:526–527, 1969.

Kral, F., and Uscavage, J. P.: Cutaneous candidiasis in a dog. J. Am. Vet. Med. Assoc., *136*:612–615, 1960.

McCullough, B., Moore, J., and Kuntz, R. E.: Multifocal candidiasis in a capuchin monkey (*Cebus apella*). J. Med. Primatol., *6*:186–191, 1977.

Mills, J. H. L., and Hirth, R. S.: Systemic candidiasis in calves on prolonged antibiotic therapy. J. Am. Vet. Med. Assoc., *150*:862–870, 1967.

Patterson, D. R., et al.: *Candida albicans* infections associated with antibiotic and corticosteroid therapy in spider monkeys. J. Am. Vet. Med. Assoc., *164*:721–722, 1974.

Ray, T. L., and Wuepper, K. D.: Experimental cutaneous candidiasis in rodents. J. Invest. Dermatol., *66*:29–33, 1976.

Reynolds, I. M., Miner, P. W., and Smith, R. E.: Cutaneous candidiasis in swine. J. Am. Vet. Med. Assoc., *152*:182–186, 1968.

Schmidt, R. E., and Butler, T. M.: Esophageal candidiasis in a chimpanzee. J. Am. Vet. Med. Assoc., *157*:722–723, 1970.

Simonetti, N., and Strippoli, V.: Pathogenicity of the Y form as compared to M form in experimentally induced *Candida albicans* infections. Mycopathologia, *51*:19–28, 1973.

Wikse, S. E., Fox, J. G., and Kovatch, R. M.: Candidiasis in simian primates. Lab. Anim. Care, *20*:957–963, 1970.

GEOTRICHOSIS

Geotrichosis is a rare mycosis of man and animals caused by *Geotrichum candidum*, a fungus common on fruits, vegetables, and dairy products. It has been described as causing mastitis and abortion in cattle, lymphadenitis in swine, and a systemic infection in a dog. In man, geotrichosis has been described as a chronic bronchitis, stomatitis, enteritis, conjunctivitis, dermatitis, and disseminated mycosis.

Lesions. The lesions, described by Lincoln and Adcock (1968) in a dog, consisted of necrotizing pneumonia, lymphadenitis, nephritis, adrenalitis, and mycocarditis; well-defined granulomas in the liver, spleen, bone marrow, and brain; and a mononuclear choroiditis of the eye. Organisms were associated with each of these lesions, occurring as intra- and extracellular round to ovoid yeast-like cells, 3 to 7 μ in diameter. Branching, septate hyphae and chains of round yeast-like cells resembling pseudohyphae of *Candida albicans* were also present.

Diagnosis. Diagnosis requires demonstration of the organism in tissue section and differentiation from *Candida albicans*. Isolation of the organism is necessary for positive identification, but cannot be relied upon as the sole means of diagnosis owing to the ubiquitous presence of *Geotrichum spp.* in nature.

Cutaneous geotrichosis has been reported by Spanoghie, Devos and Vianene (1976) in aged red flamingoes (*Phoenicopterus ruber*) kept for 16 years in a zoo in Brussels, Belgium. Lesions on the webs and legs of these birds contained organisms, demonstrated by culture and histologic sections. The infection was transmitted to chickens and mice. Pathogenesis was believed to be the result of aging and trauma to the feet of the flamingoes.

Lincoln, S. D., and Adcock, J. L.: Disseminated geotrichosis in a dog. Path. Vet., 5:282–289, 1968.

Spanoghie, L., Devos, A., and Vianene, N.: Cutaneous geotrichosis in the red flamingo *(Phoenicopterus ruber)*. Sabouraudia, 14:37–42, 1976.

LOBOMYCOSIS
(Lobo's Disease, Keloidal Blastomycosis)

Lobo's disease, or keloidal blastomycosis, is a chronic granulomatous infection of the human skin caused by a fungus, *Loboa loboi*. The first description of the disease in an animal species was in an Atlantic bottlenose dolphin *(Tursiops truncatus)* by Migaki and associates (1971). Prior to this report the infection had been reported only in man, where the occurrence is restricted to Brazil, Surinam, and Costa Rica. The dolphin was from Florida waters. A second, confirmatory case, with presumptive evidence of other cases in dolphins in Florida waters, has been published (Caldwell et al., 1975).

Lesions. The lesions, which are localized in the skin without visceral involvement, are characterized by dense collections of histiocytes and multinucleated giant cells with little proliferation of fibrous connective tissue. Small collections of neutrophils are usually present. The causative organisms are principally located within histiocytes and giant cells, appearing as round to oval yeast-like bodies 5 to 10 μ in diameter, containing a faintly basophilic central body 1 to 2 μ in diameter. They are often arranged in branching chains connected by short, thick tubes. They are best demonstrated with stains for carbohydrates (PAS, Gridley).

Diagnosis depends on demonstrating the characteristic organisms in tissue sections; the fungus has not been successfully cultured.

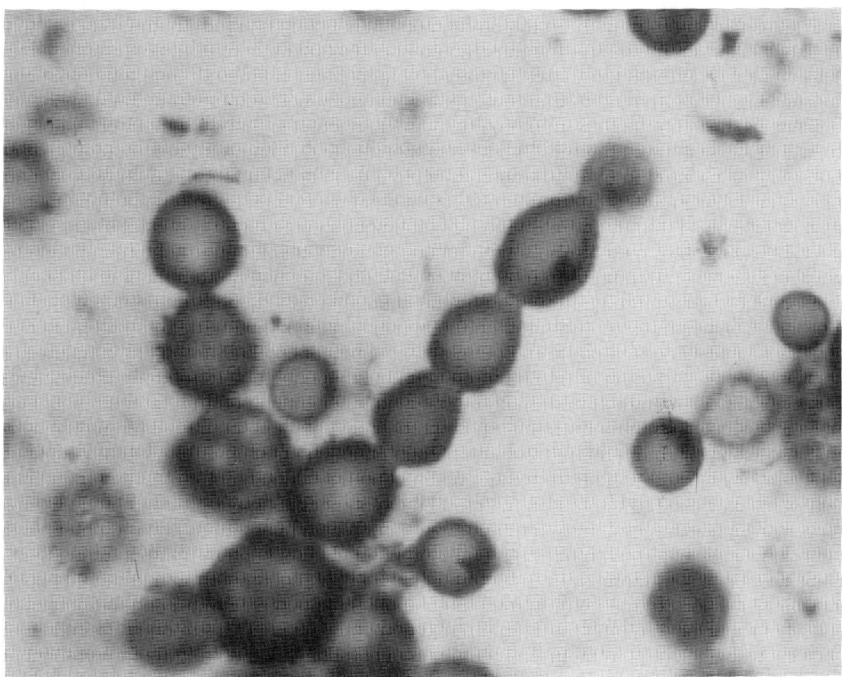

Fig. 12–29. Lobomycosis, Atlantic bottlenose dolphin. A branching chain of the fungus *Loboa loboi*. (Courtesy of Dr. G. Migaki.)

Caldwell, D. K., et al.: Lobomycosis as a disease of the Atlantic bottle-nosed dolphin *(Tursiops truncatus)* (Montagu, 1821). Am. J. Trop. Med. Hyg., *24*:105–114, 1975.

Migaki, G., Valerio, M. G., Irvine, B., and Garner, F. M.: Lobo's disease in an Atlantic bottlenose dolphin. J. Am. Vet. Med. Assoc., *159*:578–582, 1971.

Woodard, J. C.: Electron microscopic study of lobomycosis *(Loboa loboi).* Lab. Invest., *27*:606–612, 1972.

PAECILOMYCOSIS

Although usually considered a non-pathogenic species and common laboratory contaminant, *Paecilomyces variota* has been identified in a few cases as infecting man or animals. The organisms resemble *Penicillium* species under the light microscope, but do not produce greenish blue colonies and differ in the shapes of their conidia and colonies. Localized cutaneous and disseminated infections have been reported in dogs, a horse with equine infectious anemia, a human patient with endocarditis following cardiac surgery, and pulmonary infection in a Giant Aldabra tortoise.

Lesions. The lesions are usually granulomatous and may be disseminated throughout the body, involving lungs, liver, bone, bone marrow, brain, and other tissues.

Jang, S. S., Biberstein, E. L., Slauson, D. P., and Suter, P. F.: Paecilomycosis in a dog. J. Am. Vet. Med. Assoc., *159*:1775–1779, 1971.

Patnaik, A. K., et al.: Paecilomycosis in a dog. J. Am. Vet. Med. Assoc., *161*:806–813, 1972.

Uys, C. J., Don, P. A., Schrire, W., and Barnard, C. N.: Endocarditis following cardiac surgery due to the fungus *Paecilomyces.* S. Afr. Med. J., *37*:1280–1296, 1963.

van den Hoven, E., and McKenzie, R. A.: Suspected paecilomycosis in a dog. Aust. Vet. J., *50*:368–369, 1974.

PHAEOHYPHOMYCOSIS
(Phaeomycotic Granuloma)

This term has been applied to a group of mycotic infections, subcutaneous or systemic, caused by fungi that grow in the hosts' tissues with dark-walled (dematiacious) septate mycelia. Some questions have been raised about the appropriateness of this terminology, and it should be differentiated from "phaeomycotic cyst," which is applied to a type of mycotic subcutaneous infection in man caused by *Phialophora spinifera, Ph. gougeroti,* and other organisms. A similar disease caused by a pigmented fungus has been described in frogs *(Rana pipiens)* and called "chromomycosis" (Rush, Anver and Beneke, 1974).

The disease, infrequently described under the name phaeohyphomycosis in animals (horse and cat), has been associated with the fungus *Drechslera spicifera.* The lesions usually consist of purulent centers surrounded by wide zones of epithelioid granulomatous tissue.

Hill, J. R., Migaki, G., and Phemister, R. D.: Phaeomycotic granuloma in a cat. Vet. Pathol., *15*:559–561, 1978.

Kaplan, W., et al.: Equine phaeohyphomycosis caused by *Drechslera spicifera.* Can. Vet. J., *16*:205–208, 1975.

Muller, G. H., Kaplan, W., Ajello, L., and Padhye, A. A.: Phaeohyphomycosis caused by *Drechslera spicifera* in a cat. J. Am. Vet. Med. Assoc., *166*:150–154, 1975.

Rush, H. G., Anver, M. R., and Beneke, E. S.: Systemic chromomycosis in *Rana pipiens.* Lab. Anim. Sci., *24*:646–655, 1974.

DERMATOMYCOSES (Trichophytosis, Ringworm, Favus, Tinea, Superficial Mycoses, Dermatophytosis)

Dermatomycoses are those infections of the skin and its adnexae caused by the dermatophytic fungi (dermatophytes). These fungi comprise many species that inhabit the skin of man or animals and produce lesions under certain conditions. Not only may animals serve as reservoirs for human infection, but man may transmit his infection to animals. The dermatomycoses are characterized by growth of organisms upon or within the hairs, in the stratum corneum of the epidermis in the hair follicles, or the nails. The infection does not disseminate to deeper structures of the body.

The generally accepted mycologic classification of the dermatophytes proposed by Emmons (1934) on the basis of their morphologic characteristics in cultures separates these fungi into three genera (*Trichophyton, Microsporum,* and *Epidermophyton*), which include all species pathogenic for man and animals. Practically all of the human pathogens in this group also produce lesions in animals. Unfortunately, the fungi that cause particular lesions in animals have not always been adequately identified, and several fungi can cause lesions that are clinically indistinguishable. Therefore, precise association of specific agents with characteristic lesions is not always possible. The plethora of synonyms and duplication of names are also confusing to the student. Table 12–4 condenses essential information concerning some identified fungi of this group with their current names and the lesions with which they may be associated. The

student is referred to the papers of Georg and associates (1954, 1957) relative to the clinical and mycologic differentiation of the dermatomycoses.

In man, superficial mycoses are often classified by the anatomic site of the lesions as well as their clinical appearance. Several different fungi may be involved in one clinical entity. Animals are often the source of these organisms, hence some reference to these human entities is of interest. **Tinea pedis,** "athlete's foot" or ringworm of the feet, is associated with *Epidermophyton floccosum,* various species of *Trichophyton,* and rarely, species of *Microsporum* or *Candida albicans.* **Tinea unguium,** ringworm of the nails (onychomycosis) is usually caused by *Trichophyton rubrum* or *T. mentagrophytes.* **Tinea cruris,** ringworm of the groin or "jock itch," results from infection with *Epidermophyton*

Table 12–4. Dermatomycoses

Dermatophyte	Disease	Hosts Commonly Affected
Genus *Trichophyton* (Malmsten, 1845)		
T. mentagrophytes	Ringworm, tinea barbae	Mice, rats, muskrats, chinchillas, cattle, man, horses, sheep, dogs, cats, swine, goats, rabbits, monkey, guinea pigs
T. rubrum	Ringworm, tinea barbae	Man, dogs, foxes, primates, mice, squirrels, muskrats, etc.
T. tonsurans	Tinea capitis	Man
T. schoenleini	Tinea favosa	Man, cats, mice, rats, rabbits
T. concentricum	Tinea imbricata, tropical ringworm	Man
T. violaceum	Tinea imbricata	Man
T. verrucosum	Tinea favosa, ringworm	Cattle, man, horses, dogs, sheep
T. megnini	Tinea favosa	Man
T. gallinae	Favus, tinea favosa	Chickens, turkeys, man
T. equinum	Ringworm, tinea barbae	Children, horses
T. quinkeanum	Ringworm	Man, horses
Genus *Microsporum* (Gruby, 1843)		
M. canis	Sporadic ringworm	Dogs, cats, man, sheep, monkeys, calves, gibbons
M. audouini	Epidemic ringworm of scalp	Children, dogs, monkeys
M. gypseum	Sporadic ringworm of scalp, favus	Man, dogs, cats, horses
M. nanum	Ringworm	Swine
M. distortum	Ringworm	Monkeys, dogs
Genus *Epidermophyton* (Sabouraud, 1910)		
E. floccosum	Tinea pedis ("athlete's foot")	Man

floccosum and species of *Trichophyton.* **Tinea corporis, tinea circinata,** ringworm of the body, is caused by various species of *Trichophyton* and *Microsporum,* involves the glabrous (smooth and hairless) skin, and results in either simple scaling or deep granulomas. **Tinea imbricata,** scaly ringworm, is a disease of the tropics and apparently caused by a single fungus, *Trichophyton concentricum.* **Tinea barbae,** "barber's itch," or ringworm of the beard, is caused by various species of *Trichophyton* and *Microsporum.* The lesions may be superficial or deep, and infection is often contracted from animals, particularly cattle.

Tinea capitis, ringworm of the scalp and hair, is most common in children but may affect adults. The causative organisms, various species of *Trichophyton* and *Microsporum,* may be acquired by contact with infected animals or children. *Microsporum audouini* is most commonly involved, but *M. canis* and *M. gypseum* produce deeper, more severe lesions.

Trichophyton tonsurans also is known to produce widespread fungous infections of the scalp. **Tinea favosa,** favus or honeycomb ringworm, is also a chronic dermatophytosis caused by *Trichophyton schoenleini, T. violaceum,* or *Microsporum gypseum.* It is usually limited to the scalp and is characterized by yellowish, cup-shaped crusts (scutula) that have a peculiar "mousey" odor. The disease may produce scarring or permanent alopecia, and may spread to the glabrous skin and nails.

Lesions. The lesions of dermatomycosis are limited to the hairs, nails, epidermis and dermis. The fungi grow within or upon the surface of the stratum corneum or the hairs. Growth of the fungi often binds hairs together or causes them to shed, depending upon the fungus and host. Dry, scaly, or powdery crusts may form, or the hair may be bound together in a **scutulum,** which leaves a red, sometimes raw and bleeding surface when it is removed. The lesions are often circumscribed and may

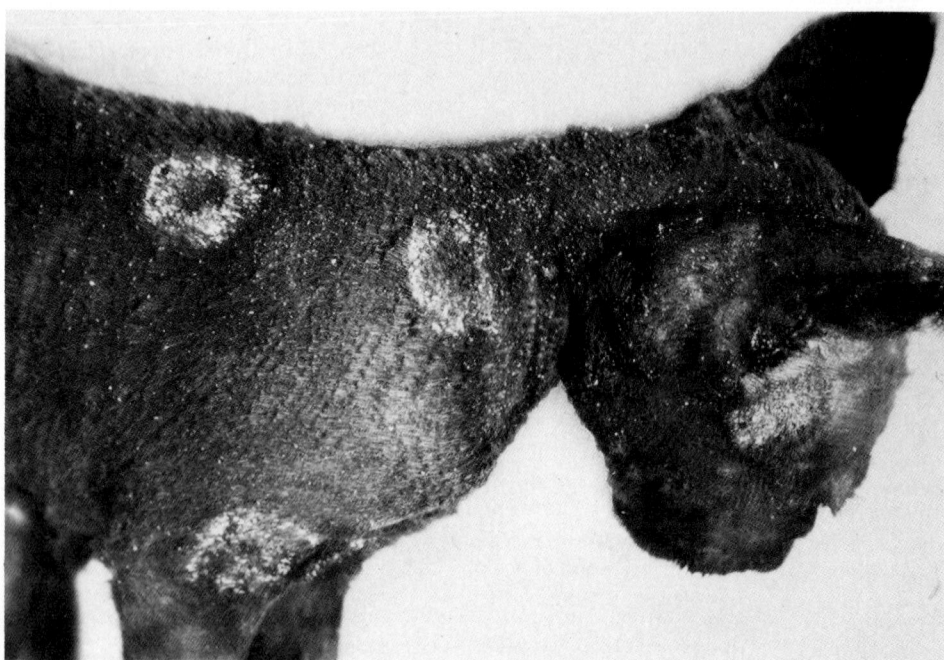

Fig. 12–30. Dermatomycosis ("ringworm") due to *Microsporum canis,* in a kitten. (Courtesy of Angell Memorial Animal Hospital.)

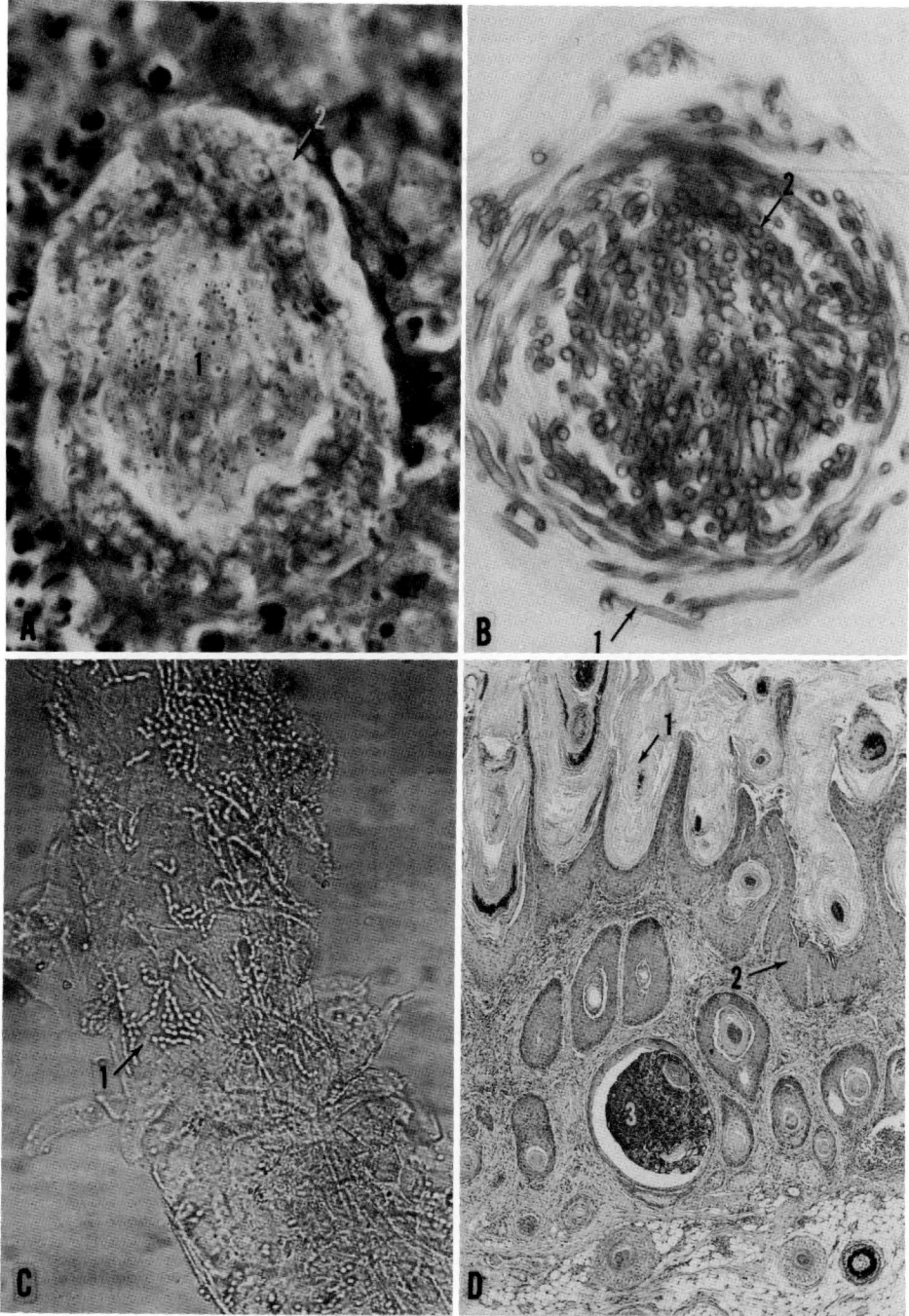

Fig. 12–31. Dermatomycosis. *A,* Hair follicle (× 730) in the skin of a monkey. Hematoxylin and eosin stain. Organisms are indistinctly seen in hair (*1*) and surrounding it (*2*). *B,* Replicate section of *A,* (× 730) stained with Gridley's fungus stain. Note hyphae of fungi in longitudinal (*1*) and cross section (*2*). *C,* A fresh preparation of hair, showing fungi on surface (*1*) of the hair. *D,* Skin of monkey (× 35). Same case as *A* and *B.* Note severe hyperkeratosis (*1*), acanthosis (*2*), and abscess in one hair follicle (*3*). (Courtesy of Armed Forces Institute of Pathology.) Contributor: Dr. Mervin G. Rhoades.

involve any part of the skin surface. The name "ringworm" is suggested by the circinate lesions that sometimes result from the outward growth of the organisms from the healing areas in the center.

The microscopic appearance of the lesions is subtle and easily overlooked in routine sections. Thickening of the stratum corneum may be all that can be seen in sections stained with hematoxylin and eosin, but special methods, such as Bauer's stain, the periodic acid-Schiff (PAS) reaction, and the Gridley's fungus stain often make it possible to recognize the fungi in tissue sections. Hypertrophy of the epidermis occurs in severe cases, accompanied by congestion and lymphocytic infiltration of the underlying dermis. In deeper infections in which the hair follicles are involved, severe destruction of the follicle with much resulting inflammation in the dermis may be seen. Organisms also can be identified in hairs and skin scrapings cleared with a concentrated aqueous solution of sodium or potassium hydroxide and examined under the microscope, using decreased illumination.

Diagnosis. The clinical recognition of some of the superficial mycoses is facilitated by the use of filtered ultraviolet light (Wood's light) to examine the lesions in a darkened room. Some species, particularly of *Microsporum*, exhibit fluoresence under the ultraviolet light, making it possible to recognize mild infections. In dogs and cats, *Microsporum canis* is the commonest cause of ringworm, but *Trichophyton mentagrophytes* and *Microsporum gypseum* are recovered occasionally by suitable cultural methods. Cattle and horses are more apt to be infected with *Trichophyton mentagrophytes.*

Abu-Samra, M. T., Imbabi, S. E., and Mähgoub, E. S.: *Microsporum canis* infection in calves. Sabouraudia, 13:154–156, 1975.

Ajello, L.: A taxonomic review of the dermatophytes and related species. Sabouraudia, 6:147–159, 1968.

Bagnall, B. G., and Grunberg, W.: Generalized *Trichophyton mentagrophytes* ringworm in capuchin monkeys *(Cebus nigrivitatus).* Br. J. Dermatol., 87:565–570, 1972.

Baker, H. J., Bradford, L. G., and Montes, L. F.: Dermatophytosis due to *Microsporum canis* in a rhesus monkey. J. Am. Vet. Med. Assoc., 159:1607–1611, 1971.

Banks, K. L., and Clarkson, T. B.: Naturally occurring dermatomycosis in the rabbit. J. Am. Vet. Med. Assoc., 151:926–929, 1967.

Cadigan, C., Jr., and Chaicumpa, V.: Infections among Thai gibbons and humans caused by atypical *Microsporum canis.* Lab. Anim. Sci., 23:226–231, 1973.

Connole, M. D.: A review of dermatomycoses of animals in Australia. Aust. Vet. J., 39:130–134, 1963. VB 3871–63.

Emmons, C. W.: Dermatophytes. Natural grouping based upon the form of the spores and accessory organs. Arch. Dermat. Syph., 30:337–362, 1934.

Emmons, C. W., Binford, C. H., Utz, J. P., and Kwan-Chung, K. J.: Medical Mycology, 3rd ed. Philadelphia, Lea & Febiger, 1977.

Errington, P. L.: Observations on a fungus skin disease of Iowa muskrats. Am. J. Vet. Res., 3:195–201, 1942.

Fowle, L. P., and Georg, L. K.: Suppurative ringworm contracted from cattle. Arch. Derm. Syph., 56:780–793, 1947.

Fuentes, C. A., Bosch, Z. E., and Boudet, C. C.: Occurrence of *Trichophyton mentagrophytes* and *Microsporum gypseum* on hairs of healthy cats. J. Invest. Dermat., 23:311–313, 1954.

Fuentes, C. A., and Aboulafia, R.: *Trichophyton mentagrophytes* from apparently healthy guinea pigs. Arch. Dermat. Syph., 71:478–480, 1955.

Georg, L. K.: The diagnosis of ringworm in animals. Vet. Med., 49:157–166, 1954.

Georg, L. K., Kaplan, W., and Canap, L. B.: Equine ringworm with special reference to *Trichophyton equinum.* Am. J. Vet. Res., 18:798–810, 1957.

Ginther, O. J.: Clinical aspects of *Microsporum nanum* infection in swine. J. Am. Vet. Med. Assoc., 146:945–953, 1965.

Grappel, S. F., Bishop, C. T., and Blank, F.: Immunology of dermatophytes and dermatophytosis. Bacteriol. Rev., 38:222–250, 1974.

Hoerlein, A. B.: Studies on animal dermatomycoses. I. Clinical studies. Cornell Vet., 35:287–298, 1945.

———: Studies on animal dermatomycoses. II. Cultural studies. Cornell Vet., 35:299–307, 1945.

Kaplan, W., Hopping, J. L., Jr., and Georg, L. K.: Ringworm in horses caused by the dermatophyte, *Microsporum gypseum.* J. Am. Vet. Med. Assoc., 131:329–332, 1957.

Kushida, T., and Watanabe, S.: Canine ringworm caused by *Trichophyton rubrum:* probable transmission from man to animal. Sabouraudia, 13:30–32, 1975.

Leeper, A. W. D.: Experimental bovine *Trichophyton verrucosum* infection. Preliminary clinical, immunological and histological observations in primarily infected and reinoculated cattle. Res. Vet. Sci., 13:105–115, 1972.

Menges, R. W., and Georg, L. K.: An epizoötic of ringworm among guinea pigs caused by

Trichophyton mentagrophytes. J. Am. Vet. Med. Assoc., *128*:395–398, 1956.

Parrish, H. J., and Craddock, S.: A ringworm epizoötic in mice. Br. J. Exp. Pathol., *12*:209–212, 1931.

Pascoe, R. R., and Connole, M. D.: Dermatomycosis due to *Microsporum gypseum* in horses. Aust. Vet. J., *50*:380–383, 1974.

Scott, D. B.: An outbreak of ringworm in Karakul sheep caused by a physiological variant of *Trichophyton verrucosum* Bodin. Onderstepoort J. Vet. Res., *42*:49–52, 1975.

Vries, G. A. de, and Jitta, C. R. J.: An epizootic in horses in the Netherlands caused by *Trichophyton equinum* var. *equinum*. Sabouraudia, *11*:137–139, 1973.

Young, C.: *Trichophyton mentagrophytes* infection of the Djungatian hamster *(Phodopus sungorus)*. Vet. Rec., *94*:287–289, 1974.

PROTOTHECOSIS

Colorless algae of the genus *Prototheca*, though usually saprophytic, have been reported to cause disease in man and animals. Although the infection appears to be rare, *Prototheca spp.* have been associated with cutaneous granulomas in man, dogs, and deer, generalized infection in dogs, mastitis in cattle, and granulomatous lymphadenitis in man, deer, and cattle. In tissue section, *Prototheca spp.* appear as round to oval organisms 3 to 20 μ in greatest diameter, with a refractile wall, granular cytoplasm, and a single nucleus. Reproduction occurs by endosporulation, which gives rise to single organisms containing several daughter cells (endospores). The cell wall stains poorly in hematoxylin and eosin stained tissue sections, but is strongly positive to stains for carbohydrate (PAS, Gridley's, Bauer's, G.M.S.). Tissue reaction may be minimal or the organism may incite granulomatous inflammation characterized by central necrosis surrounded by macrophages, epithelioid cells, lymphocytes, and foreign-body and Langhans' type giant cells.

Chlorellosis. In a single case in a lamb, Cordy (1973) described an infection due to algae differing from *Prototheca* by their production of bright green pigment. The production of this pigment, presumably chlorophyl, serves to differentiate the genus *Chlorella* from *Prototheca*. The exact relationship of these organisms as patho-

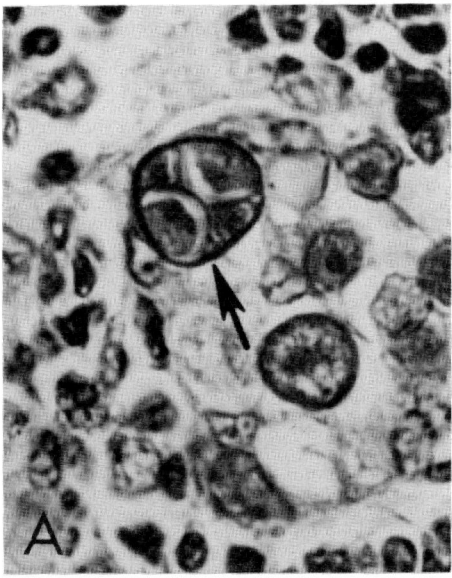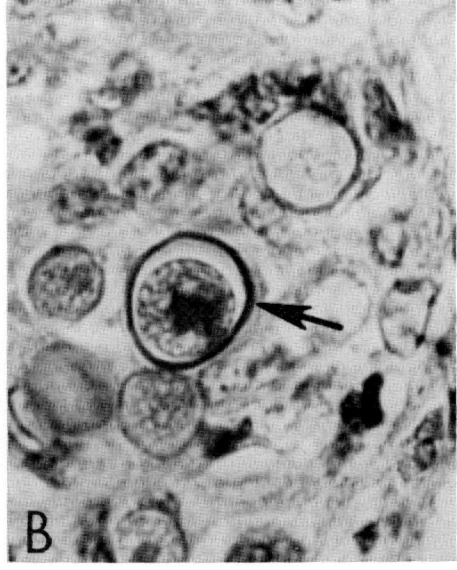

Fig. 12–32. Protothecosis, bovine lymph node. *A*, Several organisms, one composed of four daughter cells within a single cell wall (arrow), Mayer's mucicarmine stain. *B*, Single organisms have distinct cell walls (arrow) and one or more nuclei, Mayer's mucicarmine stain. (Courtesy of Dr. G. Migaki and *Pathologia Veterinaria*.)

gens is yet to be determined. The disease in the lamb was discovered at necropsy by the presence of bright green necrotic lesions in the liver and hepatic lymph nodes. Necrotic lesions were scattered at random throughout the liver, with organisms concentrated near the periphery of the necrotic material. Some fatty change was evident in liver cells, but little inflammatory reaction surrounded the necrosis. Necrosis and accumulation of organisms was apparent in the periphery of hepatic lymph nodes, and the afferent lymphatics were occluded with algae and exudate. Efforts to transmit the infection to other lambs were unsuccessful.

Diagnosis. Diagnosis requires demonstration of the organism in tissue section. Positive identification of the organism requires isolation on artificial medium, but isolation in the absence of demonstrating tissue invasion should be viewed with caution.

Buyukmihci, N., Rubin, L. F., and DePaoli, A.: Prototothecosis with ocular involvement in a dog. J. Am. Vet. Med. Assoc., *167*:158–161, 1975.

Carlton, W. W., and Austin, L.: Ocular prototothecosis in a dog. Vet. Pathol., *10*:274–280, 1973.

Cordy, D. R.: Chlorellosis in a lamb. Vet. Pathol., *10*:171–176, 1973.

Davies, R. R., Spencer, H., and Wakelin, P. V.: A case of human protothecosis. Trans. R. Soc. Trop. Med. Hyg., *58*:448–451, 1964.

Frank, N., Ferguson, L. C., Cross, R. F., and Redman, D. R.: Prototheca, a cause of bovine mastitis. Am. J. Vet. Res., *30*:1785–1794, 1969.

Migaki, G., Garner, F. M., and Imes, G. D., Jr.: Bovine protothecosis. A report of three cases. Path. Vet., *6*:444–453, 1969.

Povey, R. C., Austwick, P. K. C., Pearson, H., and Smith, K. C.: A case of prothothecosis in a dog. Path. Vet., *6*:396–402, 1969.

Rogers, R. J.: Protothecal lymphadenitis in an ox. Aust. Vet. J., *50*:281–282, 1974.

Sudman, S. M., Majka, J. A., and Kaplan, W.: Primary mucocutaneous protothecosis in a dog. J. Am. Vet. Med. Assoc., *163*:1372–1374, 1973.

van Kruiningen, H. J.: Protothecal enterocolitis in a dog. J. Am. Vet. Med. Assoc., *157*:56–63, 1970.

van Kruiningen, H. J., Garner, F. N., and Schiefer, B.: Protothecosis in a dog. Path. Vet., *6*:348–354, 1969.

MYCOTOXICOSES (Moldy Feeds)

The term "mold" is a rather indefinite designation for practically any of the hundreds of species of filamentous fungi. The word is seldom applied to pathogenic fungi, practically all molds being saprophytes. Following the usual concept that a pathogen grows and multiplies in the tissues, we have discussed fungi having that ability in connection with the specific infectious disease produced by each. There remain to be considered a large number of instances in which illness or death is more or less clearly attributable to the ingestion of molds or their products in or on the animal's feed. Collectively, these are grouped as mycotoxicoses. Diseases resulting from mycotoxins have been recognized for centuries, ergotism having been described in the Middle Ages and used medicinally for several hundred years. Other conditions were associated with molds earlier this century, such as stachybotryotoxicosis of horses in the U.S.S.R. in the 1940s, and facial eczema in sheep in New Zealand in the 1950s. With the recognition of aflatoxicosis in the 1960s, interest in mycotoxins expanded rapidly, and many new and old diseases were recognized as being caused by toxic metabolites of molds. The search for other mycotoxins has resulted in the laboratory identification of additional mycotoxins, many of which have not yet been associated with naturally occurring disease, although such an association is to be expected.

There are no common clinical or pathologic features to mycotoxicoses. Many are hepatotoxic, but their effects are varied ranging from neoplasia to neurologic dysfunction. Some of the more important and better studied mycotoxicoses are listed in Table 12–5. More detailed discussions of certain of these follow.

Austwick, P.K.C.: Mycotoxins. Br. Med. Bull., *31*:222–229, 1975.

Bacon, C.W., Porter, J.K., and Robbins, J.D.: Toxicity and occurrence of Balansia on grasses from toxic fescue pastures. Appl. Microbiol., *29*:553–556, 1975.

Crump, M.H.: Slaframine (slobber factor) toxicosis. J. Am. Vet. Med. Assoc., *163*:1300–1302, 1973.

di Menna, M.E., and Mortimer, P.H.: Experimental myrotheciotoxicosis in sheep and calves. NZ Vet. J., *19*:246–248, 1972.

Greenway, J.A., and Puls, R.: Fusariotoxicosis from barley in British Columbia. I. Natural occurrence and diagnosis. Can. J. Comp. Med., 40:12–15, 1976.

Hayes, A.W., Neville, J.A., and Hollingsworth, E.B.: Acute toxicity of rubratosin B in dogs. Toxicol. Appl. Pharmacol., 25:606–616, 1973.

Lillihoj, E.B.: Feed sources and conditions conducive to production of aflatoxin, *Ochratosin, Fusarium* toxins, and zearalenone. J. Am. Vet. Med. Assoc., 163:1281–1284, 1973.

Martinovich, D., Mortimer, P.H., and di Menna, M.E.: Similarities between so-called Kikuyu poisoning of cattle and two experimental mycotoxicoses. NZ Vet. J., 20:57–58, 1972.

Martinovich, D., and Smith, B.: Kikuyu poisoning of cattle. I. Clinical and pathological findings. NZ Vet. J., 21:55–63, 1973.

Newberne, P.M.: Mycotoxins: toxicity, carcinogenicity, and the influence of various nutritional conditions. Environ. Health Perspect., 9:1–32, 1974.

Pier, A.C.: An overview of the mycotoxicoses of domestic animals. J. Am. Vet. Med. Assoc., 163:1259–1261, 1973.

Purchase, I.F.H. (ed.): Mycotoxins. Amsterdam, Elsevier Scientific Publishing Company, 1974.

Shreeve, B.J., and Patterson, D.S.P.: Mycotoxicosis. Vet. Rec., 97:279–280, 1975.

Smalley, E.G.: T-2 toxin. J. Am. Vet. Med. Assoc., 163:1278–1280, 1973.

Smith, B., and Martinovich, D.: Kikuyu poisoning of cattle. 2. Epizootiological aspects. NZ Vet. J., 21:85–89, 1973.

Wilson, B.J., and Harbison, R.D.: Rubratoxins. J. Am. Vet. Med. Assoc., 163:1274–1275, 1973.

Wilson, B.J., Yang, D.T.C., and Boyd, M.R.: Toxicity of mould-damaged sweet potatoes (*Ipomoea batatas*). Nature, 227:521–522, 1970.

Wogan, G.N., Edwards, G.S., and Newberne, P.M.: Acute and chronic toxicity of rubratoxin B[1]. Toxicol. Appl. Pharmacol., 19:712–720, 1971.

Ergot

Most of the agricultural "small grains" and many different grasses are parasitized by the ascomycetic fungus, *Claviceps purpurea*. Each sclerotium of the fungus is a hard, black, elongated body that destroys and replaces a grain or seed of the maturing plant, being usually somewhat larger than the neighboring grains. These sclerotia constitute the substance known as ergot, which is used as a drug and whose poisonous properties have long been familiar. As late as the early nineteenth century, human beings were not infrequently poisoned by contaminated flour. In animals, including birds, poisoning may occur through the feeding of contaminated grain, but in her-

bivora, it results more frequently from the use of hay or straw containing a considerable proportion of parasitized plants.

In general, the action of ergot is to stimulate smooth muscle. This action upon the uterine musculature is responsible for its use as an oxytocic. Long-continued contraction of the vascular musculature is the principal basis for its poisonous effects. The usual manifestation of chronic poisoning by ergot, which is known as ergotism, consists of dry gangrene of the limbs, tail, and ears, so that after several weeks of ingestion of small amounts the most distal parts of the extremities may drop off (see Chapter 1). The early stages are characterized by lameness, irregular gait, and evidence of pain in the feet, the posterior extremities being chiefly affected. Palpation of the parts involved shows them to be cold and insensitive. These signs may begin as early as a week after the first consumption of contaminated material. Occasionally, the gangrene has been moist instead of dry, at least in the feet and phalanges. As would be expected, there is usually a clear line of demarcation and an inflammatory zone just proximal to it. In birds, the comb, tongue and beak become gangrenous. Less noticeable signs based upon involvement of the gastrointestinal musculature may precede or accompany those arising in the extremities. They include indigestion, colic, vomiting, and either diarrhea or constipation. Pregnant animals often abort. There is decreased milk production (agalactia), which may be the only sign in swine.

The above-described signs mark the usual "gangrenous form." In the rare "spasmodic form" (convulsive form, nervous form), there are tonic contractions of the flexors of the limbs, trembling of the muscles, opisthotonos, tetanic spasms of the whole body, convulsions, delirium, and death. This type of reaction is presumed to be related to failing blood supply in the central nervous system.

The postmortem lesions are obvious in the gangrenous cases. In addition, conges-

Table 12–5. Mycotoxicoses

Disease	Fungus	Toxin	Species (exp.)*	Major Pathologic Feature	Principal Plant	Geographic Location
Gangrenous ergotism	*Claviceps purpurea*	Ergotamine, other alkaloids (lysergic acid derivatives)	Cattle, horses, pigs, man (all suscep.) / Swine	Gangrene / Agalactia	Grains, grasses	Worldwide
Convulsive or nervous ergotism	*Claviceps paspali, C. purpurea*	Ergotamine, other alkaloids (lysergic acid derivatives)	All	Unknown	Dallis grass	Worldwide
Aflatoxicosis	*Aspergillus flavus*	Aflatoxins	Poultry, dogs, swine, cattle, man (sheep, cat, guinea pig, monkey, rat), trout	Toxic hepatitis, cirrhosis, hepatic adenomas and adenocarcinomas	Groundnut meal, cereals	Worldwide
Facial eczema	*Pithomyces chartarum*	Sporodesmin	Sheep, cattle	Toxic hepatitis, cirrhosis, photosensitization	Pasture plants	New Zealand, Australia, South Africa, Texas
Slobbers	*Rhizoctonia leguminicola*	Slaframine (converted to acetylcholine-like compound)	Cattle	Salivation	Red clover	Midwestern U.S.
Lupinosis	*Phomopsis leptostromiformis*	Unknown	Sheep, horses, cattle, swine, (goat, dog, rabbit, mouse)	Toxic hepatitis, cirrhosis	Lupines	Europe, New Zealand, Australia, South Africa, Montana
Porcine vulvovaginitis	*Fusarium roseum*	Zearalenone (estrogenic)	Swine (guinea pigs, rabbits)	Hyperplasia of uterus, vagina, mammary gland	Corn, barely, wheat	Worldwide
Ill-defined (diarrhea, tremors, convulsions)	*Penicillium cyclopium*	Cyclopiazonic acid	Sheep, horses, cattle, (rats)	Toxic hepatitis	Many foods	England
Ill-defined	*Penicillium rubrum*	Rubratoxins	Swine, cattle, (dogs, guinea pigs, mice, rabbits, cats)	Hepatic necrosis	Corn, other foods	United States (probably worldwide)

Disease	Fungi	Toxin	Species affected[*]	Effects	Substrate	Geographic distribution
Stachybotryotoxicosis	Stachybotrys alternans, S. chartarum	Stachybotryotoxin (satratoxin)	Horses, man, (cattle, sheep, swine, guinea pigs, mice, poultry)	Hemorrhagic necrosis and ulceration of mouth, stomach, intestine; leukopenia	Hays	U.S.S.R., Eastern Europe
Alimentary toxic aleukia	Fusarium poae, F. sporotrichioides	Unknown	Man	Dermatitis, stomatitis, leukopenia, lymphoid necrosis	Grains	U.S.S.R.
Unknown	Fusarium, Cephalosporium, Myrothecium, Trichothecium, Trichoderma	Trichothecenes	(Mice, rats, calves, swine, cats)	(Dermatitis, gastroenteritis; hemorrhages, radiomimetic effect)	Corn, barley, rice (many plants)	Worldwide
Cardiac beriberi (Shoshin-Kakke)	Penicillium citreoviride	Citreoviridin	Man	Cardiac distress, neurologic signs (Tremors, convulsions paralysis)	Rice	Japan
Hepatic necrosis	Penicillium islandicum	Luteoskyrin cyclochlorotine	Man, chicks (Mice, rabbits)	Toxic hepatitis (Toxic hepatitis, cirrhosis, hepatocarcinoma)	Rice	Japan
"Atypical interstitial pneumonia" of cattle	Fusarium solani, F. frimbriata	4-Ipomeanol	Cattle	Pulmonary edema, alveolar cell proliferation, hyaline membranes (Toxic hepatitis)	Sweet potatoes	U.S.A.
Mold nephrosis of swine; bovine abortion(?)	Aspergillus ochraceus, Penicillium viridicatum	Other toxins Ochratoxins, citrinin	(Sheep, cattle, mice) Swine Cattle (Rats, mice, dogs)	Toxic nephrosis Abortion (Toxic hepatitis, toxic nephrosis, fetal death & resorption)	Maize, wheat, barley, oats, alfalfa (others)	Denmark, Ireland, Wisconsin
Unknown	Aspergillus versicolor	Sterigmatocystin	Man (rats, monkey)	Hepatic & renal necrosis, cirrhosis hepatoma	Decaying animal and vegetable products	Worldwide
Moldy corn poisoning, equine encephalomalacia	Unknown (Fusarium moniliforme?)	Unknown	Horses	Encephalomalacia	Corn	Worldwide
Neurotoxicosis	Penicillium patulum	Patulin	Cattle	Unknown	Malted barley, wheat	Europe, U.S.A., Japan
Kikuyu poisoning	Myrothecium verrucaria, M. roridum	Trichothecenes(?)	Cattle, sheep	Ulcerative rumenitis, reticulitis, omasitis	Kikuyu grass (Pennisetum clandestinum)	New Zealand
Fescue foot	Balansia spp.?	Probably a mycotoxicosis, but not proved (see Fescue grass, Chapter 16).				

* Experimentally susceptible species in parentheses.

tion and occasionally hemorrhage are described in the visceral organs.

Another related fungu$, *Claviceps paspali,* produces different effects on animals and is therefore considered separately.

Anderson, J.F., and Werdin, R.E.: Ergotism manifested as agalactia and gangrene in sows. J. Am. Vet. Med. Assoc., *170:*1089–1091, 1977.

Burfening, P.J.: Ergotism. J. Am. Vet. Med. Assoc., *163:*1288–1290, 1973.

Dillon, B.E.: Acute ergot poisoning in cattle. J. Am. Vet. Med. Assoc., *126:*136, 1955.

Dollahite, J.W.: Ergotism produced by feeding *Claviceps cinera* growing on Tobosagrass (*Hilaria mutica*) and Galletagrass (*Hilaria jamesii*). SW Vet., *16:*295–296, 1963.

Greatorex, J.C., and Mantle, P.G.: Effect of rye ergot on the pregnant sheep. J. Reprod. Fertil., *37:*33–41, 1974.

Lumb, J.W.: Ergotism of cattle in Kansas. J. Am. Vet. Med. Assoc., *81:*812–816, 1932.

Mantle, P.G., and Gunner, D.E.: Abortions associated with ergotised pastures. Vet. Rec., *77:*885–886, 1965.

Woods, A.J., Jones, J.B., and Mantle, P.G.: An outbreak of gangrenous ergotism in cattle. Vet. Res., *78:*742–749, 1966.

Dallis Grass Poisoning (Claviceps Paspali)

A so-called ergot, *Claviceps paspali,* grows upon Dallis grass (*Paspalum dilatatum*), a pasture plant of the southern United States, and produces what is known as Dallis-grass poisoning (**paspalum staggers**). This ergot (sclerotium), like the seed it replaces, is much smaller than that of *Claviceps purpurea* and often of a brownish color. Symptoms of Dallis-grass poisoning appear after cattle have had access to parasitized seedheads of the grass for a few or several days. They are essentially nervous in character and manifest as (1) nervous hyperirritability, excitability, and even belligerency, and (2) muscular incoordination. The latter is worse when the cow or horse is excited and results in frequent falling and eventual inability to stand. Many animals recover with a change in feed. Gross lesions are minimal and microscopic studies appear to have been neglected. However, some have attributed certain forms of dermatitis to this fungus.

A symptomatically similar disease has occurred in certain years among cattle on the "bunch grass" ranges of the northern Rocky Mountain regions (Columbia basin of the state of Washington), and an ergot on the grass has been suspected. Neurologic sequelae have also been associated with Bermuda-grass and rye grass, but the cause or relation to a mycotoxin has not been established. *Penicillium spp.* and *Aspergillus spp.* are also known to produce neurotoxins that cause tremors and other neurologic signs in domestic and experimental animals. (The term ergotism, as commonly understood, applies only to the disease caused by *C. purpurea. C. paspali* is not associated with gangrene.)

Cysewski, S.J.: Paspalum staggers and Tremorgen intoxication in animals. J. Am. Vet. Med. Assoc., *163:*1291–1292, 1973.

Perek, M.: *Claviceps paspali* in pasture as a cause of poisoning in cattle in Israel. Refuah Vet., *12:*106–110, 1955.

———: Ergot and ergot-like fungi as the cause of vesicular dermatitis (sod disease) in chickens. J. Am. Vet. Med. Assoc., *132:*529–533, 1958.

Simms, B.T.: Dallis grass poisoning. Auburn Veterinarian, Summer, 1945.

Tatrishvili, P.S.: (Pathology of experimental *Claviceps paspali* poisoning in livestock.) Trud. Vesesoyuz Inst. Eksp. Vet., *20:*226–237, 1957. Abstr. Vet. Bull. No. 3383, 1958.

Aflatoxins (Mycotoxin, Aflatoxicosis, Groundnut Poisoning, Toxin of Aspergillus spp.)

Historically, mycotoxins have been suggested as a cause of morbidity in animals since 1901 (Buckley, and MacCallum, 1901), but the existence of aflatoxin appears to have been first indicated by the natural occurrence of an animal disease following much the same pattern that led to the discovery of dicoumarin. Seibold and Bailey (1952) described an epizootic toxic hepatitis ("hepatitis X") in dogs, which was later demonstrated by Newberne, Bailey, and Seibold (1955) to be the result of feeding commercial dog foods that contained contaminated peanut meal. The presence of mycotoxins in moldy feedstuff was further supported by the report of

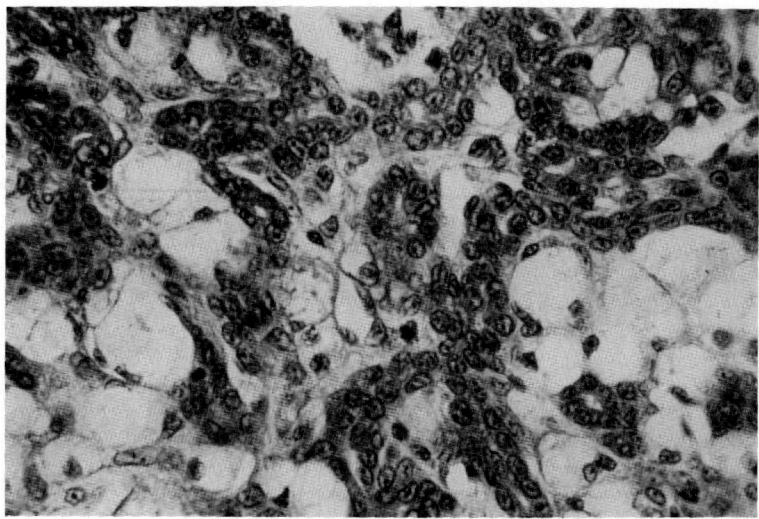

Fig. 12–33. Poisoning due to aflatoxin. Liver of rat, proliferation of bile ducts and vacuoles in hepatocytes. (Courtesy of Dr. Paul M. Newberne.)

Burnside et al. (1957) of a disease of cattle and swine; toxin-producing strains of molds were isolated from the suspected feeds and subsequently used to induce a toxic disease in animals. The chemical isolation of aflatoxins was first achieved (DeJongh et al., 1962) in the course of searching for the toxic principle in groundnut meal known to be poisonous for turkeys (Blount, 1961; DeJongh et al., 1962). It now appears that all domestic species thus far tested and fish are susceptible to poisoning by aflatoxins; furthermore, aflatoxins are suspected as etiologic agents of liver disease in man. The literature on the subject is now voluminous.

Currently, ten aflatoxin fractions have been isolated and differentiated from one another by their fluorescence, R_F values on thin-layer chromatography, and structural identification and synthesis. These toxins are produced by the growth in cereal grains, nuts, and seed products of certain molds of the *Aspergillus flavus* group and *Penicillium puberulum*.

Signs. The clinical signs in acute cases in dogs appear in 2 to 14 days (average five days) and consist of anorexia, icterus, bile-stained urine, prostration, occasional blood in feces, vomition (sometimes bloody), epistaxis, and rarely convulsions. Chronic cases after one to two months may exhibit icterus, ascites, loss of weight, occasional edema of the legs, elevated blood urea nitrogen (BUN), and prolonged clearance time for Bromsulphalein; fever is rarely observed. The signs in other species are similar when recognized, and for the most part are related to the interference with liver function. The susceptibility to aflatoxin B_1 as measured by LD_{50} has been determined experimentally to vary among different species. The following animals are listed in approximate order of decreasing susceptibility: duckling, rabbit, turkey, chicken, neonatal rat, cat, pig, dog, trout, guinea pig, rhesus monkey, adult rat, cattle, and sheep. However, the strain of animal and its nutritional status can have a profound effect on the response.

The clinical pathologic features of aflatoxin poisoning have been most clearly demonstrated in experimentally poisoned swine (Gumbmann and Williams, 1969; Cysewski et al., 1968; and Sisk, Carlton, and Curtin, 1968). Biochemical changes

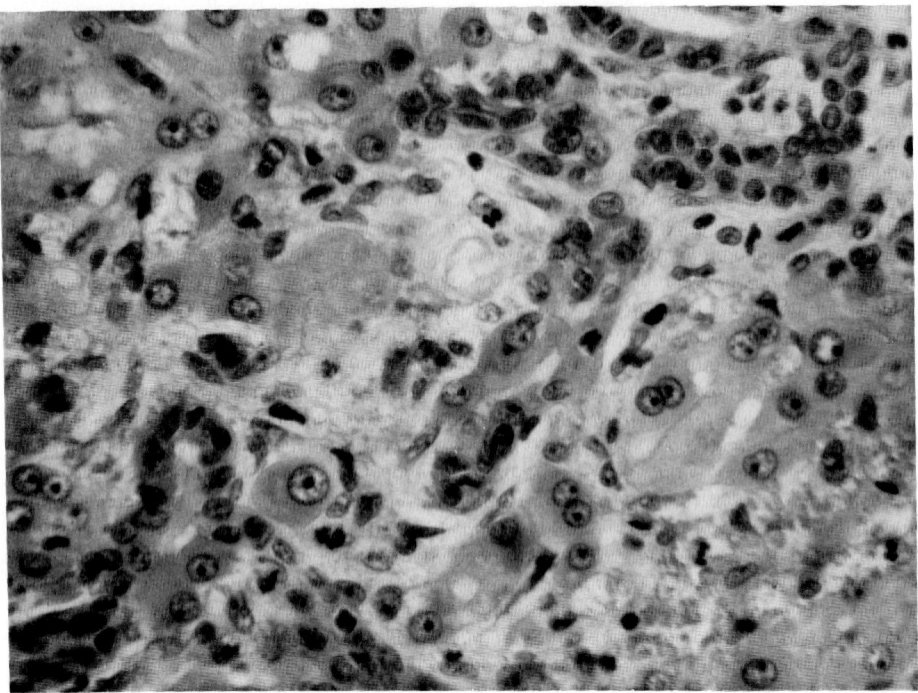

Fig. 12–34. Poisoning due to aflatoxin. Liver of dog. Proliferation of bile ducts, disorganization of hepatocytes. (Courtesy of Dr. Paul M. Newberne.)

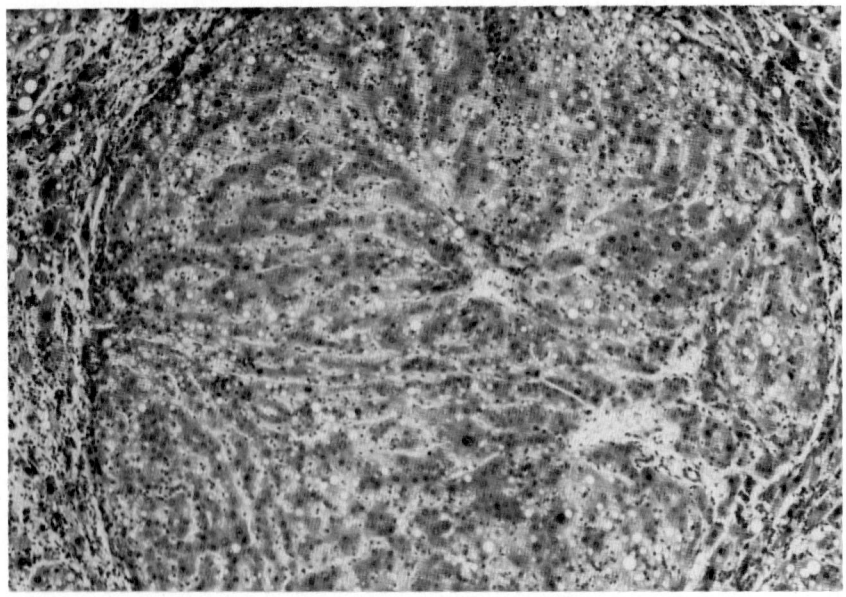

Fig. 12–35. Poisoning by aflatoxin. Hepatoma of rat. (Courtesy of Dr. Paul M. Newberne.)

depend upon hepatic injury, and their time of occurrence is related to the dose administered. Doses adequate to produce death within 72 hours will result in detectable liver damage within three hours and several alterations in liver function within six hours. The serum levels of glutamic oxaloacetic transaminase (GOT), ornithine carbamyl transferase (OCT), alkaline phosphatase (APase), and isocitric dehydrogenase (IDH) are markedly elevated. These enzymes are concomitantly lost from the damaged liver. Expectedly, the serum levels of the following are reduced: albumin, albumin-globulin ratio, nonprotein nitrogen (NPN), urea nitrogen (UN) and adenine nucleotides (AN). Leukocyte counts and prothrombin times are usually elevated within 24 hours of such a lethal poisoning. Chromatographic demonstration of metabolites of aflatoxins in urine plus clinical pathologic or histologic demonstration of liver damage are considered adequate for definitive diagnosis.

Lesions. The principal lesions occur in the liver and may be classified as toxic hepatitis. Natural cases usually result from repeated ingestion of toxin, and therefore the hepatic lesions are seen in various stages, but it should be pointed out that lesions are not necessarily specific. Single nonlethal or lethal doses have been given to many different animals under experimental conditions, revealing variation in response among different species (Newberne and Butler, 1969). One of the most constant responses to aflatoxin B_1 is proliferation of small bile ductules at the periphery of hepatic lobules. This appears in all species tested so far. Changes in hepatocytes (vacuolization, fatty change, loss of parenchyma, pyknosis) leading to necrosis are usually localized in one part of the hepatic lobule, depending on the species. These effects are **periportal** in ducklings, cats, adult rats, turkey, chickens, and rhesus monkeys; **midzonal** in rabbits, and **centrilobular** in pigs, dogs, guinea pigs, and cattle. Diffuse necroses are seen in neonatal rats and trout, with hemorrhage a conspicuous feature in the latter.

Edema of the gallbladder has been noted frequently in the dog and pig.

Nodular regeneration of hepatic lobules

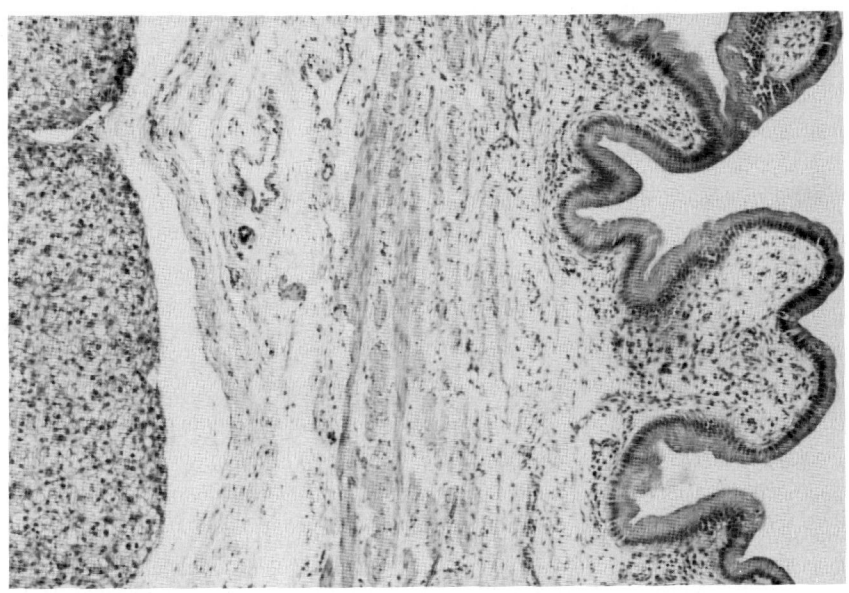

Fig. 12-36. Poisoning due to aflatoxin. Edema of the gallbladder of a dog. (Courtesy of Dr. Paul M. Newberne.)

has been observed in the duckling, pig, trout, guinea pig, turkey, chicken, and rhesus monkey. Fibrosis or cirrhosis has been reported in the duckling, pig, guinea pig, turkey, chicken, rhesus monkey, and cow, but occurrence of true cirrhosis is still under debate. Occlusive lesions in hepatic venules have also been reported in cattle.

The carcinogenic activity of aflatoxin is well established, although the exact conditions under which neoplasia develops are not completely understood. Hepatomas, hepatic cell carcinomas and cholangiocarcinomas have been produced by feeding aflatoxin to ducklings, guinea pigs, turkeys, chickens, trout, swine, rats, monkeys, and one sheep.

Adamson, R.H., Correa, P., and Dalgard, D.W.: Brief communication: occurrence of a primary liver carcinoma in a rhesus monkey fed aflatoxin $B_1^{1,2}$. J. Nat. Cancer Inst., 50:549–553, 1973.

Blount, W.P.: Turkey "X" disease. J. Br. Turkey Fed., 9:52, 1961.

Buckley, S.S., and MacCallum, W.G.: Acute haemorrhagic encephalitis prevalent among horses in Maryland. Am. Vet. Rev., 25:99–102, 1901.

Burnside, J.E., et al.: A disease of swine and cattle caused by eating mouldy corn. II. Experimental production with pure cultures of mould. Am. J. Vet. Res., 18:817–824, 1957.

Butler, W.H., and Barnes, J.M.: Carcinoma of the glandular stomach in rats given diets containing aflatoxin. Nature, Lond., 209:90, 1966.

Carnaghan, R.B.A., Lewis, G., Patterson, D.S.P., and Allcroft, R.: Biochemical and pathological aspects of groundnut poisoning in chickens. Path. Vet., 3:601–615, 1966.

Cysewski, S.J., et al.: Clinical pathologic features of acute aflatoxicosis in swine. Am. J. Vet. Res., 29:1577–1590, 1968.

DeJongh, H., et al.: Investigation of the factor in groundnut meal responsible for "turkey X disease." Biochem. Biophys. Acta, 65:548–551, 1962.

Ellis, J., and DiPaolo, J.A.: Aflatoxin B_1 induction of malformations. Arch. Pathol., 83:53–57, 1967.

Gagné, W.E., Dungworth, D.L., and Moulton, J.E.: Pathologic effects of aflatoxin in pigs. Path. Vet., 5:370–384, 1968.

Gumbmann, M.R., and Williams, S.N.: Biochemical effects of aflatoxin in pigs. Toxic. Appl. Pharmacol., 15:393–404, 1969.

Harding, J.D.J., et al.: Experimental groundnut poisoning in pigs. Res. Vet. Sci., 4:217–229, 1963.

Hodges, F.A., et al.: Mycotoxins: aflatoxin isolated from Penicillium puberulum. Science, 145:1439, 1964.

Kraybill, H.F.: The toxicology and epidemiology of mycotoxins. Trop. Geogr. Med., 21:1–18, 1969.

Krishnamachari, K.A.V.R., Bhat, R.V., Nagarajan, V., and Tilak, T.B.G.: Hepatitis due to aflatoxicosis. An outbreak in western India. Lancet, 1:1061–1063, 1975.

Legator, M.S.: Mutagenic effects of aflatoxin. J. Am. Vet. Med. Assoc., 155:2080–2083, 1969.

Madhavan, T.V., Tulpule, P.G., and Gopalan, C.: Aflatoxin-induced hepatic fibrosis in rhesus monkeys. Pathological features. Arch. Pathol., 79:466–469, 1965.

McGavin, M.D., and Knake, R.: Hepatic midzonal necrosis in a pig fed aflatoxin and horse fed moldy hay. Vet. Pathol., 14:182–187, 1977.

Newberne, J.W., Bailey, W.S., and Seibold, H.R.: Notes on a recent outbreak and experimental reproduction of hepatitis X in dogs. J. Am. Vet. Med. Assoc., 127:59–62, 1955.

Newberne, P.M., Carlton, W.W., and Wogan, G.N.: Hepatomas in rats and hepatorenal injury in ducklings fed peanut meal or Aspergillus flavus extract. Path. Vet., 1:105–132, 1964.

Newberne, P.M., et al.: Histopathologic lesions in ducklings caused by Aspergillus flavus cultures, culture extracts and crystalline aflatoxins. Toxic. Appl. Pharmacol., 6:542–556, 1964.

Newberne, P.M., Russo, R., and Wogan, G.N.: Acute toxicity of aflatoxin B_1 in the dog. Path. Vet., 3:331–340, 1966.

Newberne, P.M., Harrington, D.H., and Wogan, G.N.: Effects of cirrhosis and other liver insults on induction of liver tumors by aflatoxin in rats. Lab. Invest., 15:962–969, 1966.

Newberne, P.M., Rogers, A.E., and Wogan, G.N.: Hepatorenal lesions in rats fed a low lipotrope diet exposed to aflatoxin. J. Nutr., 94:331–343, 1968.

Newberne, P.M., and Rogers, A.E.: Carcinoma, thymidine uptake, and mitosis in the liver of rats exposed to aflatoxin. NZ Med. J., 67:8–17, 1968.

Newberne, P.M., and Wogan, G.N.: Sequential morphologic changes in aflatoxin B_1 carcinogenesis in the rat. Cancer Res., 28:770–781, 1968.

Newberne, P.M., and Butler, W.H.: Acute and chronic effects of aflatoxin on the liver of domestic and laboratory animals: a review. Cancer Res., 29:236–250, 1969.

Rogers, A.E., and Newberne, P.M.: The effects of aflatoxin B_1 and dimethylsulfoxide on thymidine-3H uptake and mitosis in rat liver. Cancer Res., 27:855–864, 1967.

Seibold, H.R., and Bailey, W.S.: An epizootic of hepatitis in the dog. J. Am. Vet. Med. Assoc., 121:201–206, 1952.

Serck-Hanssen, A.: Aflatoxin-induced fatal hepatitis? A case report from Uganda. Arch. Environ. Health., 20:729–731, 1970.

Sisk, D.B., Carlton, W.W., and Curtin, T.M.: Experimental aflatoxicosis in young swine. Am. J. Vet. Res., 29:1591–1602, 1968.

Sporn, M.B., Dingman, C.W., Phelps, H.L., and Wogan, G.N.: Alfatoxin B: binding to DNA in vitro and alterations of RNA metabolism in vivo. Science, 151:1539–1541, 1966.

Svoboda, D., Grady, H.J., and Higginson, J.: Aflatoxin B_1 injury in rat and monkey liver. Am. J. Pathol., 49:1023–1051, 1966.

Tulpule, P.G., Madhavan, T.V., and Gopalan, C.: Effect of feeding aflatoxin to young monkeys. Lancet, *1*:962–963, 1964.

Wilson, B. J., Teer, P.A., Barney, G.H., and Blood, F.R.: Relationship of aflatoxin to epizootics of toxic hepatitis among animals in southern U.S. Am. J. Vet. Res., *28*:1217–1230, 1967.

Wogan, G.N., and Newberne, P.M.: Dose-response characteristics of aflatoxin B$_1$ carcinogenesis in the rat. Cancer Res., *27*:2370–2376, 1967.

Wragg, J.B., Ross, V.C., and Legator, M.S.: Effect of aflatoxin B$_1$ on the deoxyribonucleic acid polymerase of *Escherichia coli*. Proc. Soc. Exp. Biol. Med., *125*:1052–1055, 1967.

Lupinosis

Lupinosis or European lupinosis was recognized as distinctive from other forms of lupine poisoning in the nineteenth century. Early workers suggested that the plant poisoning characterized by neurologic signs was due to a specific alkaloid, but that lupinosis was the result of a hepatotoxic factor possibly related to a fungus. Despite these early observations, confusion between the two syndromes continued until well into the twentieth century. It is now recognized that lupinosis is caused by a mycotoxin produced by the fungus *Phomopsis leptostromiformis* which may grow on sweet and bitter lupines. Lupinosis occurs in Europe, New Zealand, Australia, South Africa, and a single report (Marsh et al., 1916) suggests it has occurred in Montana.

Field outbreaks of lupinosis are restricted mainly to sheep, owing to greater use of lupines as a forage crop for sheep; however, the disease is reported in cattle, horses, and pigs. Experimentally, goats, dogs, rabbits, and mice are susceptible. Clinically, there is anorexia, icterus, and death within a few days to two weeks after exposure. Serum glutamic oxaloacetic transaminase, lactic dehydrogenase, alkaline phosphatase, and bilirubin are elevated in the serum. Pathologically, there is pronounced icterus, and the liver is enlarged, yellow, and friable.

Lesions. The hepatic lesions are initially characterized by focal necrosis, principally in the central and midzonal regions. The lesions progress to scarring, characterized by interlinking radiating bands of connective tissue connecting central and periportal regions, resulting in distortion of the normal lobular pattern. There is hyperplasia of bile ductules and Kupffer cells.

Gardiner, M.R.: Lupinosis—an iron storage disease of sheep. Aust. Vet. J., *37*:135–140, 1961.

———: Recent advances in lupinosis research—a progress report. J. Dep. Agric. West Aust., *5*:890–897, 1964.

———: Mineral metabolism in sheep lupinosis. I. Iron and cobalt. J. Comp. Pathol., *75*:397–408, 1965.

———: The pathology of lupinosis of sheep, gross and histopathology. Pathol. Vet., *2*:417–445, 1965.

———: Mineral metabolism in sheep lupinosis. II. Copper. J. Comp. Pathol., *76*:107–120, 1966.

———: Fungus-induced toxicity in lupinosis. Br. Vet. J., *122*:508–516, 1966a.

———: Lupinosis. Adv. Vet. Sci., *11*:85–138, 1967.

Gardiner, M.R., and Parr, W.H.: Pathogenesis of acute lupinosis in sheep. J. Comp. Pathol., *77*:51–62, 1967.

Gardiner, M.R., and Petterson, D.S.: Pathogenesis of mouse lupinosis induced by a fungus (*Cytospora spp.*) growing on dead lupins. J. Comp. Pathol., *82*:5–13, 1972.

Marasas, W.F.O.: *Phomopsis leptostromiformis.* In Mycotoxins, ed. by I. F. H. Purchase. Amsterdam, Elsevier Scientific Publishing Company, 1974.

Marsh, C.D., Clawson, A.B., and Marsh, H.: Lupines as poisonous plants. U. S. D. A. Bull., *405*:1, 1916.

Papadimitriou, J.M., Bradshaw, R.D., Petterson, D.S., and Gardiner, M.R.: Histological, histochemical and biochemical study of the effect of the toxin of lupinosis on murine liver. J. Pathol., *112*:45–53, 1974.

Papadimitriou, J.M., Walter, M.N.-I., Petterson, D.S., and Gardiner, M.R.: Hepatic ultrastructural changes in murine lupinosis. J. Pathol., *111*:221–228, 1973.

Facial Eczema

Facial eczema is one of the earlier-recognized diseases caused by a mycotoxin. First described in sheep in New Zealand, cattle are also affected; it is also recognized in Australia and South Africa, and is suspected to occur in the United States. It results from the mycotoxin **sporodesmin,** produced by the fungus *Pithomyces chartarum,* which is a saprophyte on certain pastures. It is most often associated with ryegrass, and the disease is most frequent in the fall.

Lesions. The toxin is principally a hepatotoxin, and the outstanding lesion from which the disease gets its name is the result of hepatotoxic photosensitization due to circulating phylloerythrin. Cholangiohepatitis, characterized by necrosis of biliary epithelium, fibrosis, and ductular hyperplasia, is the outstanding hepatic lesion. Focal hepatic necrosis and regenerative hyperplasia may be seen. Extrahepatic bile ducts are enlarged and edematous, as is the wall of the gallbladder. Hemorrhage in the wall of the gallbladder and urinary bladder are common.

A phototoxic syndrome, characterized by ophthalmitis and dermatitis, has been produced in mice by Budiarso et al. (1972), and McCracken et al. (1974), with *Penicillium viridicatum*, the mold associated with nephrosis in swine.

Budiarso, I.T., Carlton, W.W., and Tuite, J.F.: Phototoxic syndrome induced in mice by rice cultures of *Penicillium viridicatum* and exposure to sunlight. Pathol. Vet., 7:531–546, 1970.

Dodd, D.C.: The pathology of facial eczema. Symposium on Facial Eczema Research. Proc. New Zealand Soc. Anim. Prod., 19th Annual Conf., 48–52, 1959.

McCracken, M.D., Carlton, W.W., and Tuite, J.: *Penicillium viridicatum* mycotoxicosis in the rat. I. Ocular lesions. II. Scrotal lesions. III. Hepatic and gastric lesions. Food Cosmet. Toxicol., *12*:70–88, 89–98, 99–105, 1974.

Mortimer, P.H., and Taylor, A.: The experimental intoxication of sheep with sporodesmin, a metabolic product of *Pithomyces chartarum*. I. Clinical observations and findings at postmortem examination. Res. Vet. Sci., *3*:147–171, 1962.

Richard, J.L.: Mycotoxin photosensitivity. J. Am. Vet. Med. Assoc., *163*:1298–1300, 1973.

Synge, R.L.M., and White, E.P.: Sporodesmin: a substance from *Sporodesmium bakeri* causing lesions characteristic of facial eczema. Chem. Indust., *49*:1546–1547, 1959.

Ochratoxicosis (Mold Nephropathy of Swine)

A peculiar nephropathy of swine in Denmark was recognized and associated with feeding moldy grains by Larson in 1928. A similar disease has been seen in Ireland. Horses are suspected also to have suffered the same mycotoxicosis. Krogh and associates (1978) identified *Penicillium viridicatum* as the fungus most likely to be

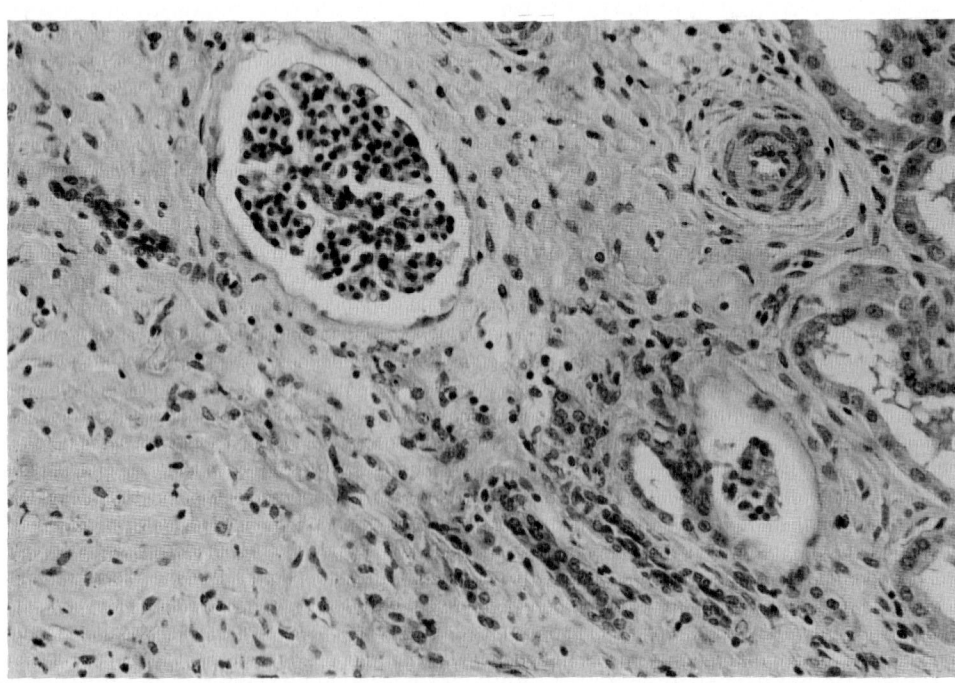

Fig. 12–37. Mycotoxic porcine nephropathy due to ochratoxin. Extensive cortical fibrosis represents the advanced stage of the disease. (Courtesy of Dr. P. Krogh.)

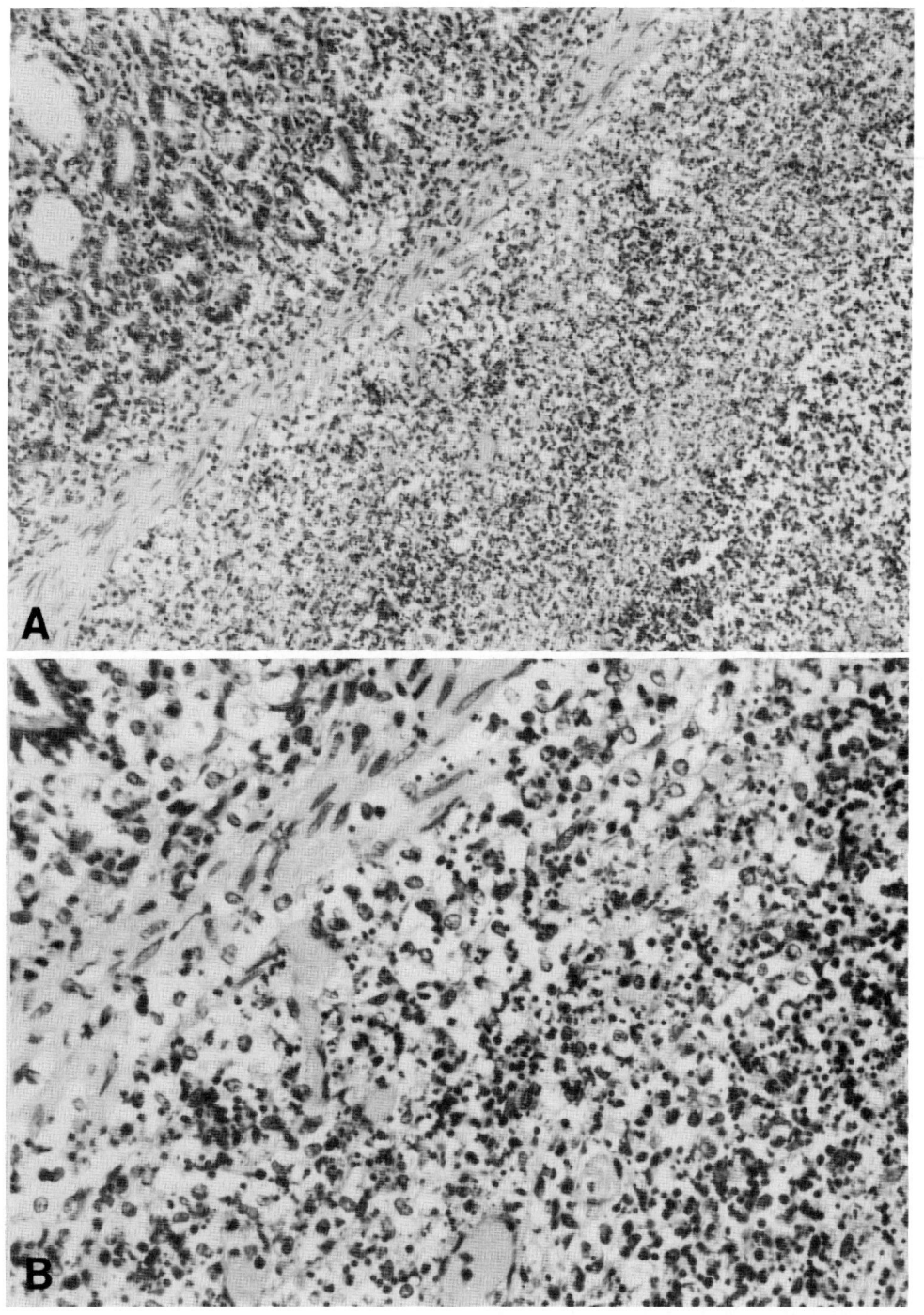

Fig. 12–38. Experimental ochratoxin A poisoning. *A,* Necrosis of submucosal lymphoid tissue in colon of a Beagle dog. *B,* High magnification of submucosal lymphoid necrosis. (Courtesy of Drs. W. W. Carlton and G. M. Szczech.)

causally related to the disease and demonstrated its nephrotoxicity. Although *P. viridicatum* was shown to produce oxalate, the nephropathy did not resemble oxalate nephrosis, nor did oxalates reproduce the disease. Two mycotoxins, ochratoxin A and citrinin, have been identified in *P. viridicatum*, and both have been shown to be nephrotoxic in swine as well as in rats, mice, and dogs. Ochratoxin A is believed to be the mycotoxin of principal importance. This mycotoxin is also produced by *Aspergillus ochratus,* from which it was actually first isolated.

The outstanding clinical signs of value are polydipsia, polyuria, and dehydration. There is increased urinary excretion of leucine aminopeptides, glucose, and protein, and serum creatine and urea nitrogen are elevated. Growth rate is significantly retarded.

Lesions. Pathologically, the lesions are restricted to the kidney. Grossly, the kidneys are enlarged, gray-yellow, and firmer than normal. Ochratoxin in swine is specifically toxic to the proximal convoluted tubule. Microscopically, the epithelial cells lose their brush border and become shorter than usual, with enlarged vesicular nuclei. Later, there is pyknosis and necrosis of the cells, which may slough to the lumen. The tubular basement membranes become greatly thickened. Secondarily, there is peritubular fibrosis, which becomes progressively more extensive until most of the kidney, including the glomeruli, are sclerotic. These lesions have been reproduced in swine experimentally poisoned. The report of Szczech et al. (1973) also described necrotizing gastroenteritis as a feature of experimental ochratoxicosis in swine, similar to that seen in other species experimentally exposed.

Experimentally, ochratoxin is also nephrotoxic in dogs, rats, chicks, and trout. The effect is principally on the proximal convoluted tubule, but degeneration of the distal tubule has also been described. In contrast to swine, lesions develop in other tissues in these species. These include fatty change and focal necrosis of the liver; focal erosive and ulcerative enteritis and colitis; and proctitis and necrosis of lymphoid tissues. Carlton et al. (1973) have experimentally induced a disease characterized by marked perirenal edema and renal necrosis by feeding swine a strain of *P. viridicatum* that did not produce citrinin or ochratoxin. The significance of this finding was not understood.

Ochratoxin is suspected to be a cause of abortion in cattle fed moldy hay. Fetal death and resorption have been produced in rats. Ochratoxin is also suspected to cause a fatal chronic nephropathy of human beings in the Balkans (Krogh et al., 1977).

Applegate, K.L. and Chipley, J.R.: Ochratoxins. Adv. Appl. Microbiol., *16:*97–109, 1973.

Buckley, H.G.: Fungal nephrotoxicity in swine. Irish Vet. J., *25:*194–196, 1971.

Carlton, W.W., and Tuite, J.: Nephropathy and edema syndrome induced in miniature swine by corn cultures of *Penicillium viridicatum.* Pathol. Vet., *7:*68–80, 1970.

Carlton, W.W., Tuite, J., and Caldwell, R.: *Penicillium viridicatum* toxins and mold nephrosis. J. Am. Vet. Med. Assoc., *163:*1295–1297, 1973.

Friis, P., Hasselager, E., and Krogh, P.: Isolation of citrinin and oxalic acid from *Penicillium viridicatum* West and their nephrotoxicity in rats and pigs. Acta Pathol. Microbiol. Scand., *77:*559–560, 1969.

Kitchen, D.N., Carlton, W.W., and Hinsman, E.J.: Ochratoxin A and citrinin induced nephrosis in Beagle dogs. III. Terminal renal ultrastructural alterations. Vet. Pathol., *14:*392–406, 1977.

Kitchen, D.N., Carlton, W.W., and Tuite, J.: Ochratoxin A and citrinin induced nephrosis in Beagle dogs. I. Clinical and clinicopathological features. Vet. Pathol., *14:*154–172, 1977.

Krogh, P.: Causal association of mycotoxic nephropathy. Acta Pathol. Microbiol. Scand. Suppl., *269:*1–28, 1978.

Krogh, P., Hald, B., Pleština, R., and Čeović, S.: Balkan (endemic) nephropathy and foodborne ochratoxin A: Preliminary results of a survey of foodstuffs. Acta Pathol. Microbiol. Scand. (B), *85:*238–240, 1977.

Krogh, P., et al.: Experimental porcine nephropathy. Changes of renal function and structure induced by ochratoxin A-contaminated feed. Acta Pathol. Microbiol. Scand. 32 (Suppl. 246) 22 pp., 1974.

Larsen, S.: On chronic degeneration of the kidneys caused by mouldy rye (in Danish). Maanedsskr Dyrl., *40:*259–284, 289, 300, 1928.

Munro, I.C., et al.: Toxicologic changes in rats fed graded dietary levels of ochratoxin A. Toxicol. Appl. Pharmacol., 28:180–188, 1974.

Rafiquzzaman, M.: Experimental *Penicillim viridicatum* toxicosis in rats. Acta Vet. Scand. Suppl., 47, 36 pp, 1974.

Still, P.E., Macklin, A.W., Ribelin, W.E., and Smalley, E.B.: Relationship of ochratoxin A to foetal death in laboratory and domestic animals. Nature, 234:563–564, 1971.

Szczech, G.M., Carlton, W.W., and Hinsman, E.J.: Ochratoxicosis in Beagle dogs. III. Terminal renal ultrastructural alterations. Vet. Pathol., 11:385–406, 1974.

Szczech, G.M., Carlton, W.W., and Tuite, J.: Ochratoxicosis in Beagle dogs. I. Clinical and clinicopathological features. Vet. Pathol., 10:135–154, 1973.

————: Ochratoxicosis in Beagle dogs. II. Pathology. Vet Pathol., 10:219–231, 1973.

Szczech, G.M., Carlton, W.W., Tuite, J., and Caldwell, R.: Ochratoxin A in swine. Vet Pathol., 10:347–364, 1973.

Estrogenic Mycotoxicosis

Species of *Fusarium*, which infect various grains, produce a mycotoxin known as zearalenone, which has estrogenic activity. A disease of sows has been recognized which results from consumption of *F. roseum*-infected barley and maize in the United States, Canada, Australia, Ireland, and Europe. The toxicosis simulates estrus, resulting in enlarged vulvae, mammary glands, and nipples, and occasionally prolapse of the vagina. Sows are infertile and may demonstrate nymphomania or pseudopregnancy. The ovaries are atrophic, and the uterus and cervix are grossly enlarged.

Lesions. Microscopically, there is ovarian follicular atresia, and edema and cellular proliferation of all layers of the uterus and ductular proliferation in the mammary glands. Focal squamous metaplasia may be seen in the tubular reproductive organs and mammary ducts. Stillbirths, small litters, and neonatal mortality may also result. Miller et al. (1973) also described incoordination of the hindlimbs in pigs born to exposed sows. In males, signs of feminization include testicular atrophy, swelling of the prepuce, and enlargement of the mammary gland.

Zearalenone toxicity is suspected to be responsible for similar occurrences and reduced fertility in cattle. Swine, rats, mice, guinea pigs, rabbits, and poultry are experimentally susceptible.

Bristol, F.M., and Djurickovic, S.: Hyperestrogenism in female swine as the result of feeding mouldy corn. Can. Vet. J., 12:132–135, 1971.

Chang, K., Kurtz, H.J., and Mirocha, C.J.: Effects of the mycotoxin zearalenone on swine reproduction. Am. J. Vet. Res., 40:1260–1267, 1979.

Kurtz, H.J., et al.: Histologic changes in the genital tracts of swine fed estrogenic mycotoxin. Am. J. Vet. Res., 30:551–556, 1969.

McErlean, B.A.: Vulvovaginitis of swine. Vet. Rec., 64:539–540, 1952.

McNutt, S.H., Purevin, P., and Murray, C.: Vulvovaginitis in swine. J. Am. Vet. Med. Assoc., 73:484–492, 1929.

Miller, J.K., Hacking, A., Harrison, J., and Gross, V.J.: Stillbirths, neonatal mortality and small litters in pigs associated with the ingestion of *Fusarium* toxin by pregnant sows. Vet. Rec., 93:555–559, 1973.

Mirocha, C.J., and Christensen, C.M.: Oestrogenic mycotoxins synthesized by *Fusarium. In* Mycotoxins, edited by I. F. H. Purchase. Amsterdam, Elsevier, 1974, pp. 129–148.

Rensburg, I.B.J. van, Marasas, W.F.O., and Kellerman, T.S.: Experimental *Phomopsis leptostromiformis* mycotoxicosis of pigs. J. S. Afr. Vet. Assoc., 46:197–204, 1975.

Roine, K., Korpinen, E.L., and Kallela, K.: Mycotoxicosis as a probable cause of infertility in dairy cows. Nord. Vet. Med., 23:628–633, 1971.

Sharma, V.D., Wilson, R.F., and Williams, L.E.: Reproductive performance of female swine fed corn naturally molded or inoculated with *Fusarium roseum*, Ohio isolates B and C. J. Anim. Sci., 38:598–602, 1974.

Moldy Corn Poisoning

As evident from Table 12–5, many different mycotoxin-producing molds may contaminate corn, and therefore the term "moldy corn poisoning" may encompass a number of distinctly different syndromes. The term is also used somewhat loosely to include toxicities due to other mold-infected grain, such as barley or oats. In horses, moldy corn poisoning usually refers to a leukoencephalomalacia. In most other species, the diseases are most often characterized by damage to the liver.

Equine leukoencephalomalacia associated with the feeding of moldy corn has been recognized in the United States and other parts of the world since the nineteenth century. The experimental work of Schwarte, Biester and Murray (1937) clearly established the causative status of moldy corn. The specific mold or mycotoxin has not been identified. *Fusarium moniliforme* has been associated with a recent occurrence in Egypt and South Africa; however most attempts to reproduce the disease have failed.

Affected horses are drowsy, tend to circle and stagger, and develop paralysis. The lesions, which are often grossly visible, consist of softening and liquefactive necrosis, chiefly of the white matter of the cerebrum. There is edema and congestion, but little cellular inflammatory reaction.

As indicated, moldy corn is most often associated with liver disease in other species. An example is the experience described by Sippel, Burnside and Atwood (1953) in cattle and swine. The principal lesions in these animals, when acutely affected, were variously located petechiae, ecchymoses, and massive hemorrhages, together with acute toxic hepatitis and toxic tubular nephrosis. These animals died after an illness of one or two days characterized by great weakness, staggering, and early jaundice. In cases of long duration, the hemorrhages were minimal, and the toxic changes in liver and kidneys, of increasing extent and importance. Centrilobular necrosis was sometimes so severe that it led to replacement of almost the whole lobule with blood, as is the case with gossypol poisoning. The kidneys, in addition to hydropic degeneration and necrosis of the cortical tubules and fatty change in the medullary rays, showed generalized dilation of the tubules and atrophy of the glomeruli. This disease was reproducible by the artificial feeding of the moldy corn, but not by cultures of any of the molds isolated. However, Sippel produced similar lesions by feeding cultures of *Aspergillus glaucus* and *A. clavatus* to calves, and *Penicillium regulosum* to mice. As is evident from Table 12–5, rubratoxin is the most likely mycotoxin to have been involved in this example. *Aspergillus flavus*, the producer of aflatoxin, may also contaminate corn.

Albright, J.L., et al.: Moldy corn toxicosis in cattle. J. Am. Vet. Med. Assoc., 144:1013–1019, 1964.

Bailey, W.S., and Groth, A.H., Jr.: The relationship of hepatitis-X of dogs and moldy corn poisoning of swine. J. Am. Vet. Med. Assoc., 134:514–516, 1959.

DoRego Chaves, L.: Doença de sintomatologia nervosa causada por intoxicaçã pelo milho. Rev. Milit. Remonta Vet., 10:199–215, 1950.

Hori, M., et al.: A fungus isolated from malt root feed causing mass death in cows. J. Jpn. Vet. Med. Assoc., 7:56–63, 1954. (In Japanese.) Abstr. Vet. Bull. 2533, 1955 *(Penicillium urticariae)*.

Lapcevic, E., Pribicevic, S., and Kozic, L.: (Poisoning in horses with the wheat rust fungus, *Puccinia graminis*.) Vet. Glasn., 7:268–271, 1953. (In Croat.; German summary.)

Muhrer, M.E., and Gentry, R.F.: A hemorrhagic factor in mouldy lespedeza hay *(Lespedeza stipulacea)*. Exper. Sta. Res. Bull. 429, Univ. Missouri, Columbia, 1948.

Schwarte, L.H., Biester, H.E., and Murray, C.: A disease of horses caused by feeding moldy corn. J. Am. Vet. Med. Assoc., 90:76–85, 1937.

Sippel, W.L., Burnside, J.E., and Atwood, M.B.: A disease of swine and cattle caused by eating moldy corn. Proc. Am. Vet. Med. Assoc., 1953, pp. 174–181.

Wilson, B.J., and Maronpot, R.R.: Causative fungus agent of leucoencephalomalacia in equine animals. Vet. Rec., 88:484–486, 1971.

CHAPTER 13

Diseases Due to Protozoa

In man's scheme of classification of the animal kingdom, unicellular animals are grouped in one phylum: Protozoa. In a current classification (Kudo, 1966), Protozoa are divided into two subphyla: Plasmodroma and Ciliophora. Subphylum Plasmodroma is arranged in four classes:

Class 1. Mastigophora—protozoa with one or more flagella; three types of nutrition (**holophytic**—synthesizing simple carbohydrates from carbon dioxide and water by chlorophyll contained in chloroplasts; **holozoic**—involving capture, ingestion, digestion, and assimilation of organic materials and excretion of waste products; **saprozoic**—utilizing simple dissolved organic or inorganic compounds requiring no enzymes or special organelles); free-living and parasitic; parasitic genera include: *Trypanosoma, Leishmania, Giardia, Trichomonas, Histomonas,* and *Hexamita.*

Class 2. Sarcodina—protozoa with thin pellicle; form pseudopodia; free-living and parasitic; parasitic genera in the order Amoebida include: *Hartmanella, Acanthamoeba, Endamoeba, Entamoeba, Endolimax,* and *Iodamoeba.*

Class 3. Sporozoa—without locomotor organs; produce spores at end of life cycle; all parasitic. Sporozoa is a complex class that includes a large number of parasitic organisms within two principal orders, several families, and multiple genera. The order *Coccidia* includes the genera *Eimeria, Isospora, Klosiella, Toxoplasma, Besnoitia, Hammondia, Cystoisospora, Sarcocystis, Frenkelia, Cryptosporidia,* and *Tyzzeria.* The order *Hemosporidia* includes the genera *Babesia, Plasmodia, Theileria, Cytauxzoon, Hemoproteus, Leucocytozoon,* and *Hepatazoon.*

Class 4. Cnidosporidia—formerly grouped with the Sporozoa; have unique spores with one to six polar filaments; one or more sporoplasms; parasites of bees, silkworms, and fishes; two genera of interest: *Nosema* and *Encephalitozoon.*

The subphylum Ciliophora contains protozoa with cilia, cirri, or other compound ciliary structures for locomotion; two kinds of nuclei—a macronucleus and micronucleus; holozoic and saprozoic nutrition; majority are free living, few are parasitic. Of two classes, Suctoria and Ciliata, only the latter contains a parasitic genus of interest in this text: *Balantidium.*

In this chapter, the effects of protozoa upon various animal hosts are described and the life cycles of some of the parasitic protozoa are outlined, with emphasis on those features that influence pathogenesis. In some instances, the effects upon the host have been rather clearly demonstrated and the tissue changes are well known; in others, practically nothing is known. The poorly understood protozoan diseases of animals, therefore, present many challenges to the research-minded veterinary pathologist.

Belding, D.L.: Textbook of Clinical Parasitology, 2nd ed. New York, Appleton Century-Crofts, 1952.

Cole, C.R., et al.: Some protozoan diseases of man and animals: anaplasmosis, babesiosis and toxoplasmosis. Ann. NY Acad. Sci., 64:25–277, 1956.

Hammond, D.M., and Long, P.L. (eds.): The Coccidia. Eimeria, Isospora, Toxoplasma, and Related Genera. Baltimore, University Park Press, 1973.

Henning, M.W.: Animal Diseases in South Africa, 3rd ed. Pretoria, Central News Agency, 1957.

Kudo, R.R.: Protozoology, 5th ed. Springfield, Charles C Thomas, 1966.

Levine, N.D.: Protozoan Parasites of Domestic Animals and Man. Minneapolis, Burgess Pub. Co., 1961.

Soulsby, E.J.L.: Helminths, Arthropods and Protozoa of Domesticated Animals (Mönnig), 6th ed. Philadelphia, Lea & Febiger, 1968.

Weinman, D., and Ristic, M.: Infectious Blood Diseases of Man and Animals. Diseases Caused by Protista. Vol. II. The Pathogens, the Infections and the Consequences. New York and London [Vol. 2], Academic Press, 1968.

COCCIDIOSIS

Coccidiosis is the name applied to the disease produced by protozoa of genera of the order Coccidia.

Clinically, "**coccidiosis**" is applied to the diseases produced by the genera *Eimeria* and *Isospora*. The order Coccidia, however, includes many additional parasitic organisms, but the diseases associated with these are generally named after the appropriate genera, e.g., toxoplasmosis, sarcosporidiosis. Most of the protozoa within the latter group were once thought to have only a tissue phase to their life cycles; however, it is now recognized that these also have an enteric cycle. Thus, the enteric phases of *Toxoplasma*, *Sarcosporidia*, *Besnoitia*, and other organisms would also be included under the disease classification of coccidiosis. Many coccidia affect animals and birds, the tissues attacked depending upon the rather obligate preferences of each parasite. Coccidiosis is especially common in cattle, sheep, and poultry, and represents a disease of major economic importance. A few of the important coccidial parasites of animals are listed in Table 13–1.

Life Cycle. The life cycles of coccidia are similar and must be understood in order to visualize their effects upon the host. The oöcysts are thick-walled, usually ovoid forms of the organism which resist drying and provide the means of transfer of infection from one host to another. The oöcysts of each species are distinctive morphologically, but have essentially similar features. Within the genus *Eimeria*, each fully-matured oöcyst contains four sporocysts, each sporocyst bearing two sporozoites, a total of eight sporozoites to each oöcyst. Oöcysts of *Isospora* contain two sporocysts, each with four sporozoites; thus the total number of sporozoites is also eight. Each oöcyst has at one pole a tiny pore, the **micropyle,** which is sealed by a substance which, like the rest of the wall, is resistant to drying as well as to many chemical substances. When oöcysts are ingested and reach the small intestine, the trypsinkinase of the pancreatic juice digests the seal of the micropyle, and through this opening the tiny sporozoites, now vigorously motile, escape from the oöcyst.

In hepatic coccidiosis of the rabbit, the sporozoites reach the intrahepatic bile ducts through the portal veins or lymphatics, not by way of the common bile duct. Intestinal infection is believed to take place by direct invasion of the intestinal epithelium. Each sporozoite enters a single epithelial cell, where it undergoes asexual development known as **schizogony.** The sporozoite gradually increases in size and complexity, becoming first a trophozoite and finally a **schizont,** which literally fills the cytoplasm of the host cell, displacing the nucleus to one pole. Each mature schizont contains many elongated spores, similar morphologically to sporozoites, but known as **merozoites.** The schizont ruptures its own and the host's cell wall, liberating the merozoites, which infect other epithelial cells and continue this asexual life cycle.

Table 13–1. Examples of Tissue Localization of Coccidia

Host	Coccidia	Tissues Affected
Chicken	*Eimeria tenella*	Ceca
Chicken	*Eimeria necatrix*	Small intestine, ceca
Chicken	*Eimeria brunetti*	Small intestine, ceca
Chicken	*Eimeria acervulina*	Small intestine, ceca
Dog, cat	*Isospora bigemina,* *I. canis,* and *I. felis*	Intestine
Dog, cat	*Eimeria canis* and *E. felis*	Intestine
Rabbit	*Eimeria stiedae*	Intrahepatic bile ducts
Rabbit	*Eimeria magna*	Intestine
Rabbit	*Eimeria neoleporis*	Cecum
Cattle	*Eimeria bovis*	Intestine
Cattle	*Eimeria zuernii*	Intestine
Sheep	*Eimeria ninakohlyakimovae*	Intestine
Sheep, goats	*Eimeria arloingi (ovina)*	Small intestine
Sheep, goats	*Eimeria parva*	Intestine
Sheep, goats	*Eimeria intricata*	Intestine
Swine	*Eimeria scrofae*	Intestine
Swine	*Isospora suis*	Intestine
Swine	*Eimeria scabra*	Intestine
Geese	*Eimeria truncata*	Renal tubules
Equidae	*Eimeria leuckarti*	Small intestine
Equidae	*Klossiella equi*	Renal tubules
Mice	*Klossiella muris*	Renal tubules
Mice	*Eimeria falciformis*	Intestine
Rats	*Eimeria nieschulzi*	Small intestine
Rats	*Eimeria separata*	Cecum and colon
Rats	*Hepatozoon muris*	Schizogony—liver Gametocytes—leukocytes
Man	*Isospora hominis*	Intestine
Frogs	*Isospora lieberkuhni*	Renal tubules
Guinea pigs	*Klossiella cobayae*	Renal tubules
Turkey	*Eimeria adenoides*	Small intestine, ceca
Turkey	*Eimeria meleagrimitis*	Small intestine

At a certain stage, some of the merozoites enter into the sexual phase of the life cycle, known as **gametogenesis.** Each of these predestined merozoites develops within an individual host epithelial cell, into a female form, **macrogamete,** or its male counterpart, a microgametocyte, which eventually ruptures to release a large number of tiny motile **microgametes.** One of the microgametes unites with a single macrogamete, which, upon being so fertilized, soon becomes an oöcyst. Further development within the oöcyst, known as **sporogony,** requires oxygen and certain other conditions which are met outside the body of the host. When the oöcysts are taken in with food or water by a new host, the life cycle is repeated.

This cycle, which is usually enteric, is depicted in Figure 13–1 and is consistent for all species of *Eimeria*. Other members of the order Coccidia have a similar enteric cycle, but in addition have an asexual tissue phase (extraintestinal phase), most often in an intermediate host, although certain animals may host both the enteric and tissue cycles. The tissue cycle has two stages, an acute infection characterized by cellular necrosis, and a chronic infection characterized by more or less dormant or

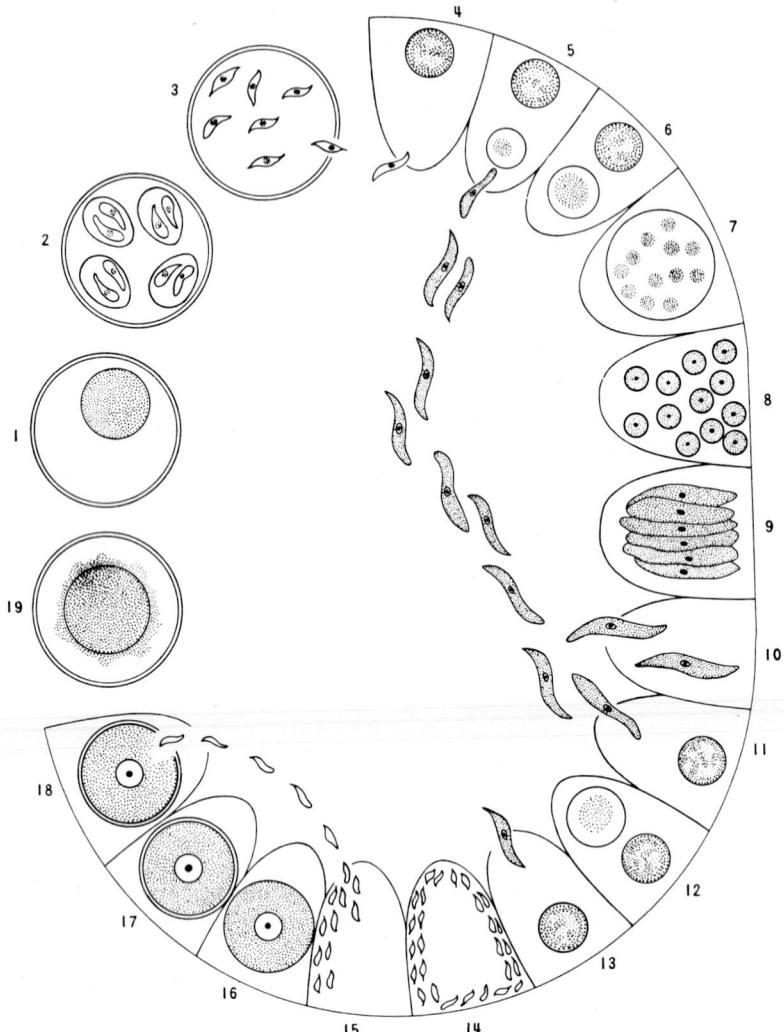

Fig. 13–1. Life cycle of *Eimeria* (diagrammatic). (*1*) Oöcyst, (*2*) sporulated oöcyst, (*3*) liberation of sporozoites, (*4*) sporozoites entering epithelial cells, (*5–11*) schizogony: formation of schizonts and merozoites, (*12*) sporogony: formation of macrogametocyte, (*13–15*) sporogony: formation of microgametocytes, (*16–17*) development of macrogametocyte, (*18*) fertilization, (*19*) formation of oöcyst.

latent collections of organisms. Following ingestion of oöcysts and the release of sporozoites, individual organisms, termed **tachyzoites,** invade beyond the gastrointestinal tract and enter cells of other viscera. The tissue specificity varies with organism: *Toxoplasma* invade most cell types; *Hammondia,* lymphoid cells; *Sarcocystis,* hepatocytes; *Frenkelia,* hepatocytes and Kupffer cells. The organisms multiply by internal budding (**endodyogeny)** producing a group of tachyzoites (analogous to a schizont and erroneously called a pseudocyst) which eventually destroys the cell; the tachyzoites then infect another cell, repeating the cycle. This phase of acute infection may go unnoticed or be associated with extensive tissue necrosis, as in acute toxoplasmosis.

The chronic phase is characterized by

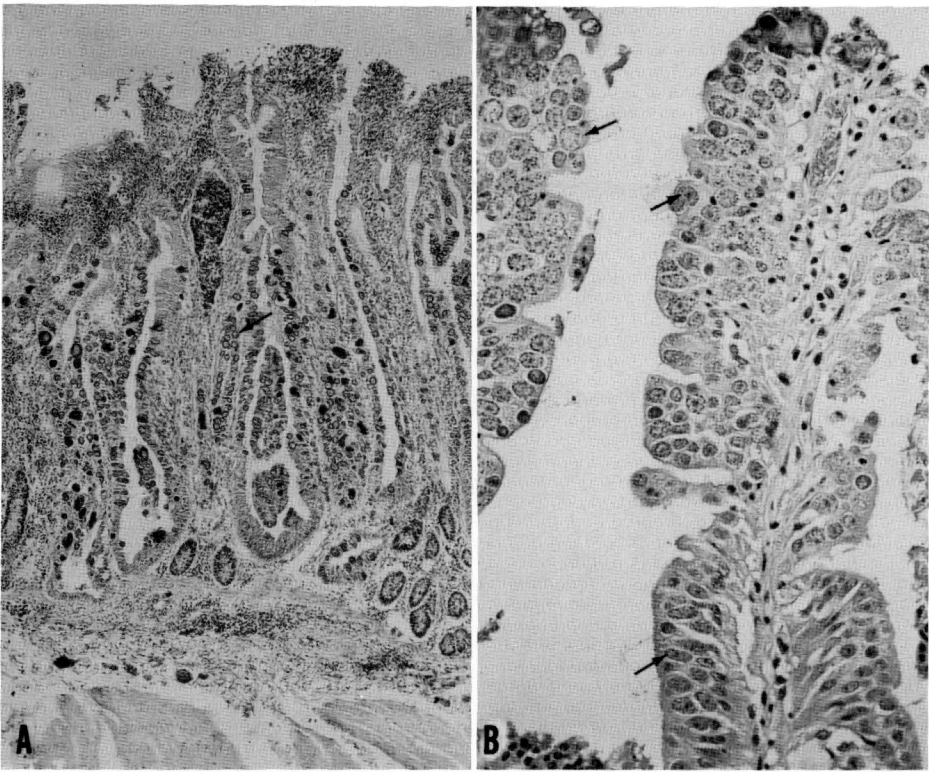

Fig. 13–2. Intestinal coccidiosis. *A*, Small intestine of a goat (× 50). Note elongated crypts and villi lined with hyperplastic, tall columnar epithelial cells containing coccidia (arrow). Contributor: Dr. L. Z. Saunders. *B*, Small intestine of a mink (× 260). Many coccidia (arrows) in epithelial cells. (Courtesy of Armed Forces Institute of Pathology.) Contributor: Dr. C. L. Davis.

formation of cysts containing individual organisms called **bradyzoites,** which slowly multiply by endodyogeny. The cysts localize in specific sites, again peculiar to each organism: *Sarcocystis* and *Hammondia* in skeletal and cardiac muscle; *Frenkelia* in brain and spinal cord, *Besnoitia* in fibroblasts; and *Toxoplasma* in many cell types.

Completion of the cycle depends on the carnivorous habits of the final hosts, in which the sexual cycle occurs in the intestinal epithelium. This newer knowledge has resulted in multiple names for certain coccidia (formerly considered single organisms). For example, *Isospora bigemina* of dogs and cats is now recognized as the sexual stage for species of *Toxoplasma, Sarcosporidia, Hammondia,* and *Besnoitia.*

Examples of these cycles are depicted in Fig. 13–3.

Clinical Manifestations. Coccidiosis affects the living host in many ways, depending upon the tissue preference of the particular parasite involved and the number of oöcysts in the initial infection. Most of these parasites attack the mucosa of the intestinal tract; therefore symptoms are predominantly enteric. Sudden onset of bloody diarrhea with fever, followed by dehydration, emaciation, and occasionally death, are the expected manifestations, but more frequently, little or no evidence of infection is observed in the living animal. Hepatic coccidiosis in rabbits is rarely accompanied by diarrhea, and young animals may die suddenly without showing any obvious signs of disease, although

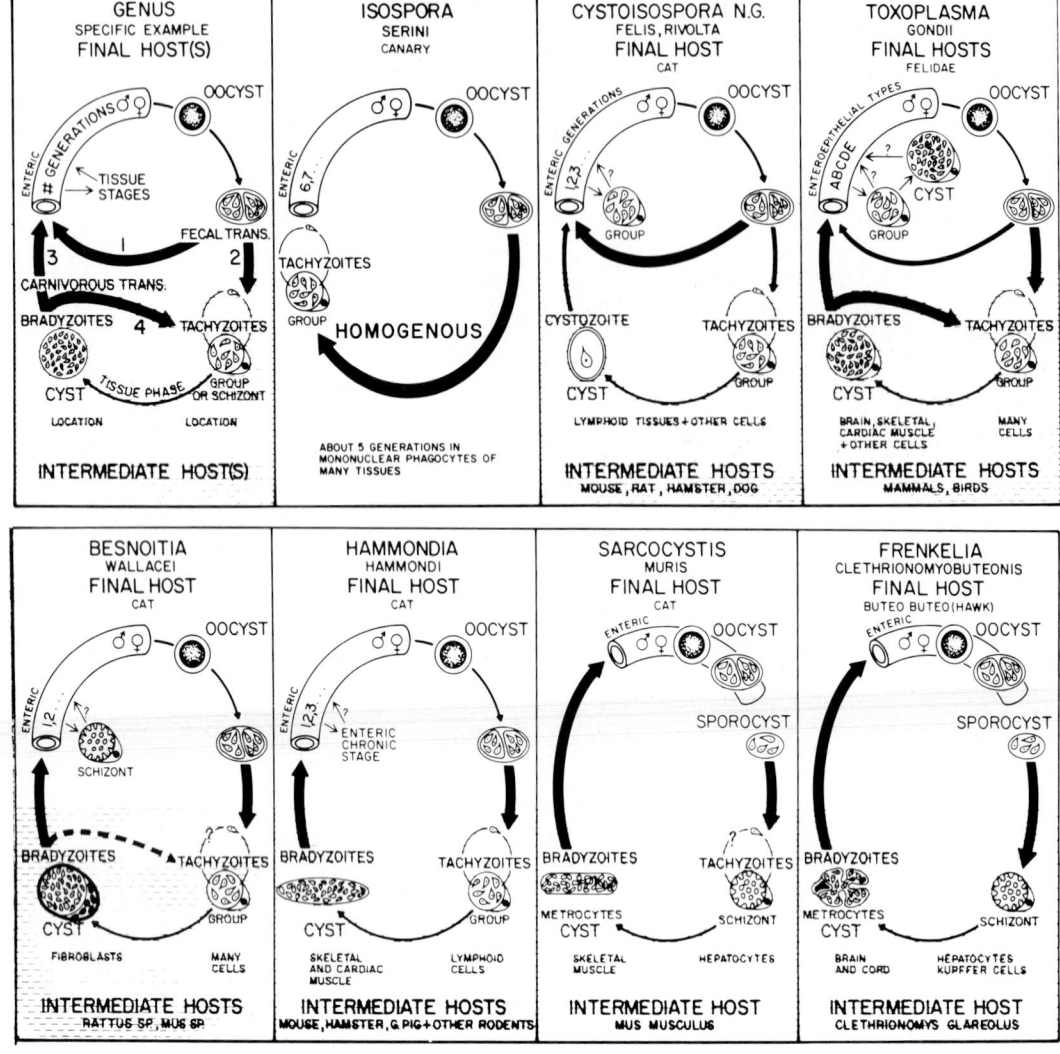

Fig. 13–3. The several types of cycles of *Isospora* and Coccidia other than *Eimeria*. The first panel depicts the several pathways by four arrows: *1*, oöcyst to same host (homogenous, fecal); *2*, oöcysts to intermediate host (heterogenous, fecal); *3*, cyst to final host (heterogenous, carnivorous); and *4*, cyst to intermediate host (homogenous, carnivorous). In the other panels, the heavy arrows indicate the most important route of transmission for the various parasites (Courtesy of Dr. J. K. Frenkel and *Journal of Parasitology*, 63:611, 1977).

jaundice and emaciation may be recognized in older animals.

Lesions. Coccidia are obligate intracellular parasites whose development within the cytoplasm of epithelial cells results in the death of each cell that is parasitized. The total effect on the host depends upon (1) the magnitude of the initial infecting dose of oöcysts, which determines the number of cells invaded at the outset by sporozoites, and (2) the spread of infection during schizogony, which is affected to a great extent by immunity acquired by the host. As increasing numbers of organisms enter the sexual phase (gametogenesis), infection of new cells by merozoites diminishes and the disease gradually abates.

When many cells of the intestinal

epithelium are parasitized at one time, the denuded mucosa may bleed freely, and intense inflammation involves the lamina propria and sometimes the submucosa. As large numbers of epithelial cells are destroyed, the remaining epithelium is stimulated to replace that which was lost. This eventually causes hyperplasia of the intestinal epithelium, which is cast into long papillary fronds as replacement of epithelial cells exceeds their loss. In lesions exhibiting this hyperplasia, coccidia in various stages of gametogenesis are most numerous. This is in contrast to the erosive, hemorrhagic stages, in which organisms in various stages of schizogony are most common.

Hepatic coccidiosis in the rabbit, due to *Eimeria stiedae,* affects the intrahepatic biliary epithelium in somewhat the same manner that other species of coccidia affect the intestinal epithelium. The destruction of biliary epithelium dominates the picture in early lesions, but in those animals in which the course is somewhat longer, proliferation of this epithelium becomes the predominant feature. The bile ducts become enormously enlarged by proliferation of epithelium, which is thrown up into papillary folds simulating adenomatous hyperplasia. These greatly enlarged segments of the bile ducts displace the adjacent liver parenchyma and appear grossly as irregularly shaped grayish areas, which are seen as depressions in the surface of the capsule (Fig. 4–2).

The gross lesions of intestinal coccidiosis may be envisaged from the foregoing account to appear as intensely congested, eroded, and bleeding areas of certain segments of the small intestine, sometimes alternating with, or replaced by, areas in which the mucosa is opaque and thickened.

Diagnosis. The clinical diagnosis is usually based upon the presence of oöcysts in fecal specimens, associated with sudden onset of typical bloody diarrhea. The microscopic lesions at necropsy are charac-teristic and are confirmed by demonstrating the organisms in tissue sections.

Barker, I. K., and Remmler, O.: The endogenous development of *Eimeria leuckarti* in ponies. J. Parasitol., *58*:112–122, 1972.

Biester, H. E., and Murray, C.: Studies in infectious enteritis of swine. VIII. *Isospora suis* (N. Sp.) in swine. J. Am. Vet. Med. Assoc., *85*:207–219, 1934.

Davis, C.L., Chow, T.L., and Gorham, J.R.: Hepatic coccidiosis in mink. Vet. Med., *48*:371–373, 1953.

Davis, L.R., and Bowman, G.W.: The endogenous development of *Eimeria zurnii*, a pathogenic coccidium of cattle. Am. J. Vet. Res., *18*:569–574, 1957.

Dubey, J.P.: Experimental *Isospora canis* and *Isospora felis* infection in mice, cats, and dogs. J. Protozool., *22*:416–417, 1975.

Gräfner, G., Graubmann, H.-D., and Dobbriner, W.: Hepatic coccidiosis in mink caused by a new species, *Eimeria hiepei*. Mh. Vet. Med., *22*:696–700, 1967. V.B. *38*:2638, 1968.

Hammond, D.M., Davis, L.R., and Bowman, G.W.: Experimental infections with *Eimeria bovis* in calves. Am. J. Vet. Res., *5*:303–311, 1944.

Hitchcock, D.J.: The life of *Isospora felis* in the kitten. J. Parasitol., *41*:383–397, 1955.

Klesius, P.H., Kramer, T.T., and Frandsen, J.C.: *Eimeria stiedai*: delayed hypersensitivity response in rabbit coccidiosis. Exp. Parasitol., *39*:59–68, 1976.

Lee, C.D.: The pathology of coccidiosis in the dog. J. Am. Vet. Med. Assoc., *85*:760–781, 1934.

Lepp, D.L., and Todd, K.S., Jr.: Life cycle of *Isospora canis* Nemeseri, 1959 in the dog. J. Protozool., *21*:199–206, 1974.

Levine, N.D., and Ivens, V.: Isospora species in the dog. J. Parasitol., *51*:859–864, 1965.

Levine, P.P.: A new coccidium pathogenic for chickens, *Eimeria brunetti*, N. Sp. (Protozoa: Eimeriidae). Cornell Vet., *32*:430–439, 1942.

———: Subclinical coccidial infection in chickens. Cornell Vet., *30*:127–132, 1940.

Lotze, J.C.: The pathogenicity of the coccidian parasite *Eimeria arloingi* in domestic sheep. Cornell Vet., *42*:510–517, 1952.

Pout, D.D.: Review article: Coccidiosis of sheep. Vet. Bull., *39*:609–618, 1969.

Pout, D.D.: Coccidiosis of lambs. III. The reaction of the small intestinal mucosa to experimental infections with *E. arloingi* "B" and *E. crandallis*. IV. The clinical response to infection of *E. arloingi* "B" and *E. crandallis* in laboratory-reared lambs. Br. Vet. J., *130*:45–53, 54–61, 1974.

Ruiz, A.V.: On the natural history of coccidial infections in range and feeder cattle. Zentralbl. Veterinaermed., *20B*:594–602, 1973.

Scholtyseck, E.: (Electron microscopy of schizogony in *Eimeria perforans* and *E. (stiedae)*. Z. Parasitkde., *26*:50–62, 1965. V.B. *36*:515, 1966.

Sharma Deorani, V.P.: Histopathological studies in natural infection of goat coccidiosis. Indian Vet. J., *43*:122–127, 1966.

Sivadas, C.G., Rajan, A., and Nair, M.K.: Studies on pathology of coccidiosis in goats. Indian Vet. J., 42:474–479, 1965.

Smetana, H.: Coccidiosis of the liver in rabbits. I. Experimental study on the excystation of oocysts of *Eimeria stiedae*. Arch. Pathol., 15:175–192, 1933.

———: Coccidiosis of the liver in rabbits. II. Experimental study on the mode of infection of the liver by sporozoites of *Eimeria stiedae*. Arch. Pathol., 15:330–339, 1933.

———: Coccidiosis of the liver in rabbits. III. Experimental study of the histogenesis of coccidiosis of the liver. Arch. Pathol., 15:516–536, 1933.

Spindler, L.A.: Investigations on coccidia of sheep and goats. Am. J. Vet. Res., 26:1068–1070, 1965.

Stockdale, P.H.G., and Niilo, L.: Production of bovine coccidiosis with *Eimeria zuernii*. Can. Vet. J., 17:35–37, 1976.

Vetterling, J.M.: Endogenous cycle of the swine coccidium *Eimeria debliecki* Douwes, 1921. J. Protozool., 13:290–300, 1966.

———: Prevalence of coccidia in swine from six localities in the United States. Cornell Vet., 56:155–166, 1966.

TOXOPLASMOSIS

Toxoplasma gondii, a small crescentic protozoön parasite, was first described in 1908, in material from a small rodent, the gondi, by Nicolle and Manceaux (1908) but its widespread distribution in the animal kingdom was not generally recognized until more than 20 years later. The organisms were rediscovered by Sabin and Olitsky in 1935 in the brains of guinea pigs that were being used to propagate encephalitis viruses. Shortly thereafter the incrimination of *Toxoplasma* as the cause of a diffuse encephalitis and chorioretinitis in a 31-day old infant by Wolfe, Cowan and Paige (1939) stimulated great interest in toxoplasmosis.

Life Cycle. Studies of Work and Hutchinson (1969) demonstrated an infective cyst in feces of cats experimentally infected with toxoplasma from mouse tissues. This cyst was identified by Frenkel, Dubey and Miller (1969) as an oöcyst, typical of the genus *Isospora*, and associated with schizonts, micro-, and macrogametocytes in the intestinal epithelium. These findings clarified a previously elusive life cycle and led the way to understanding the life cycle of other poorly understood organisms, such as sarcosporidia. The life cycle of *Toxoplasma* (Fig. 13–3) recognizes the cat as the final host. The organism undergoes schizogeny in the cat's intestine to produce oöcytes, which are resistant to environmental influences and are infective after sporogeny. The sporulated oöcysts can survive long periods and remain infective for intermediate hosts, which may develop either acute or chronic infection, characterized respectively by formation of groups of tachyzoites or cysts of bradyzoites in a variety of tissues. Most mammals and birds as well as cats may serve as intermediate hosts. Infection of intermediate hosts and cats may follow exposure to cat feces or materials contaminated by cat feces (soil, sand boxes, etc.), or consumption of or exposure to infected tissues containing tachyzoites or bradyzoites. Congenital transmission may also occur in intermediate hosts during the acute phase by invasion of tachyzoites across the placenta.

The sexual stages in the intestinal tract have been observed so far only in cats, but the disease caused by the asexual parasites (tachyzoites and bradyzoites) is known to occur in man and nearly all wild and domesticated mammals and birds.

Clinical Manifestations. The intestinal infection in felines is not associated with clinical signs or pathologic lesions of any consequence; therefore the disease, toxoplasmosis, usually refers to the results of the tissue phase in intermediate or final hosts.

Most infections with *Toxoplasma* go unrecognized. The incidence of infection approaches 75% in some populations of animals and human beings. As the organisms can infect a variety of cell types, a wide diversity of manifestations have been attributed to toxoplasmosis, making it difficult to ascribe limits to the clinical signs. The organisms apparently can also persist in tissue for long periods, producing lesions and signs only under certain as yet incompletely understood circumstances.

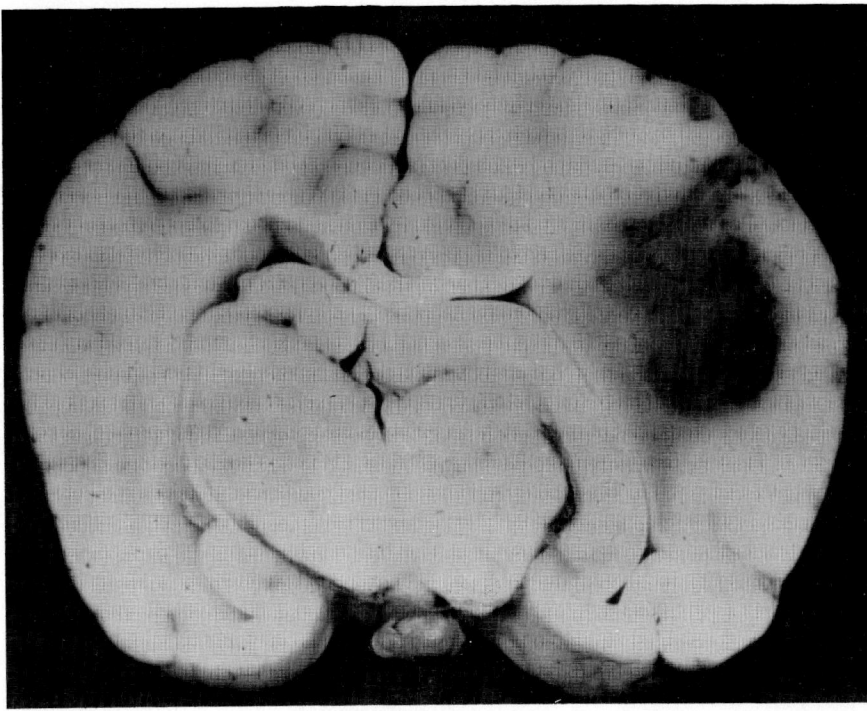

Fig. 13–4. Toxoplasmosis. Necrotic and hemorrhagic lesion in the left cerebral hemisphere of a four-year-old poodle. Myriads of *Toxoplasma gondii* were demonstrated in microscopic sections of this lesion. (Courtesy of Angell Memorial Animal Hospital.)

Immunosuppression can lead to reactivation, and in some instances, it appears that the concomitant presence of a virus or other deleterious influence makes it possible for *Toxoplasma* to produce clinical signs and fatal infections. The organisms most often affect the brain, myocardium, lymph nodes, lungs, intestinal muscularis, pancreas, liver, uterus, and placenta; hence symptoms of toxoplasmosis may be referable to involvement of any one or more of these organs. In man, toxoplasmosis is recognized most frequently as a congenitally acquired infection of the newborn, manifested by encephalitis, chorioretinitis, microencephaly, macroencephaly, cerebral calcifications, convulsive disorders, and mental retardation. In adults, chorioretinitis, lymphadenopathy, myocarditis, pneumonia, and meningoencephalitis have been associated with *Toxoplasma*.

Characteristics of Toxoplasma. *Toxoplasma gondii* is believed to be the single species of this parasite that infects all varieties of animals and man. The organism is readily maintained in the laboratory by cultivation in the peritoneal cavity of the mouse or in tissue cultures. In these situations, the organism is crescentic or arc-shaped, with one end rounded and the other pointed. It measures 2 to 4 μ in width and 4 to 7 μ in length. It has a nucleus, most clearly demonstrated with Giemsa's stain, located near one pole of the cell. Its cytoplasm may contain chromatin and glycogen granules, but there is neither demonstrable centrosome nor kinetoplast (see trypanosomiasis). Electron microscope studies indicate that there is a truncated cone, "conoid," at the anterior end with several homogeneous fibrils called "toxonemes" extending from it toward the

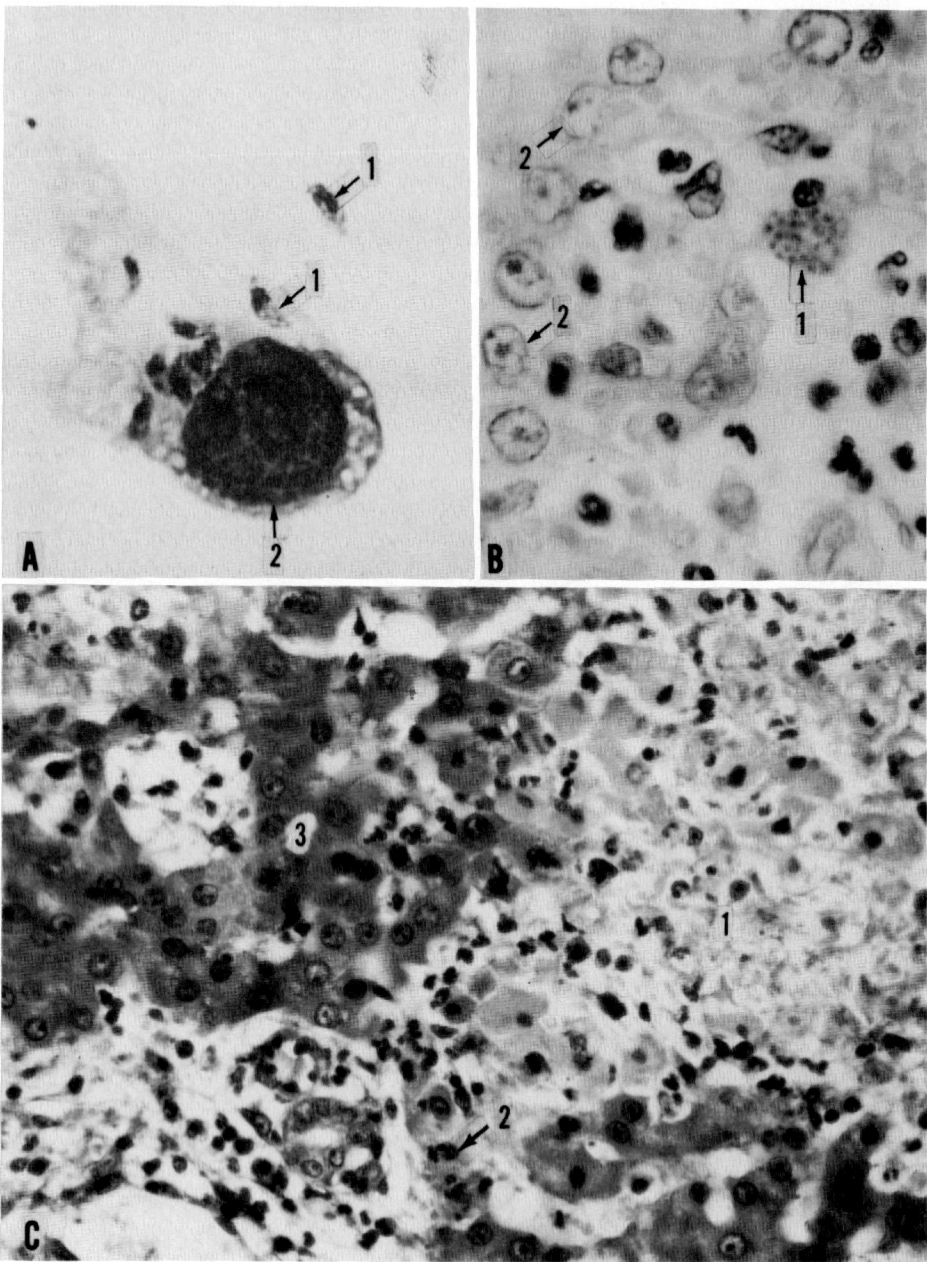

Fig. 13–5. Toxoplasmosis. *A,* Tachyzoites of *Toxoplasma gondii (1)* in mouse peritoneum, most organisms in macrophage *(2).* Contributor: Dr. W. B. Dublin. *B,* Tachyzoites of *Toxoplasma gondii (1)* in lung of a cat. Note proliferation and cuboidal shape *(2)* of cells lining alveoli. Contributor: Dr. M. Zimmerman. *C,* Sharply demarcated necrotic lesion *(1)* in liver of a dog (× 500). Necrotic *(2)* and viable *(3)* liver cells are present. (Courtesy of Armed Forces Institute of Pathology.) Contributor: Angell Memorial Animal Hospital.

blunter end of the cell. The organisms are frequently found in parallel pairs, indicating that reproduction occurs by longitudinal division. These organisms, heretofore considered as the only form of *Toxoplasma*, now appear to be tachyzoites, which have the ability to multiply in animal tissues and form collections of organisms which under certain conditions (especially in the brain) may become encysted collections of bradyzoites.

In tissue sections, tachyzoites of *Toxoplasma* may be crescentic, but also occur in rounded and ovoid form. Presumably because of shrinkage in fixation, the organisms usually appear smaller in sections than in smears, about 2 μ wide and 4 μ long. They are most frequently found in the cytoplasm of cells, but may be free. A large number of the organisms may be encountered in a single cell or may be contained by a thin, poorly defined membrane, which is believed to be the remnant of the wall of a host cell by some, a product of the parasite by others. Chronic infection is characterized by larger cysts filled with bradyzoites, which represent a resting stage of the parasite, because they are often seen in the absence of reaction in the adjacent host tissues, and they are apparently more resistant to deleterious influences in this stage.

Electron photomicrographs and histochemical studies indicate that the cyst wall is actually formed by the organisms, thus the term "pseudocyst" is not valid.

Lesions. From experimental evidence, infection with *Toxoplasma* is believed to result first in parasitemia, then in localiza-

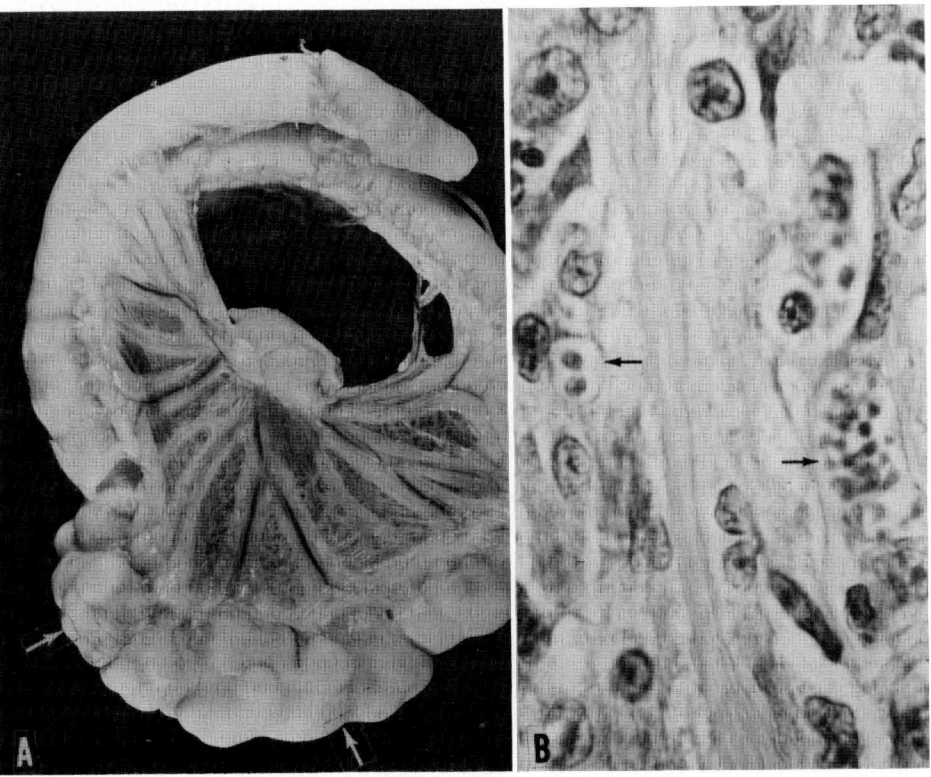

Fig. 13-6. Toxoplasmosis. *A,* Nodular granulomatous lesion in the intestinal muscularis of a cat. *B,* Involved muscularis of intestine ($\times$ 1283). Tachyzoites of *Toxoplasma gondii* in small and large groups within smooth muscle cells (arrows). (Courtesy of Armed Forces Institute of Pathology.) Contributor: Dr. Leo L. Lieberman.

tion and multiplication of the organisms in various tissues. This localization may be followed by active lesions in the affected tissue or, for unknown reasons, by encystment of the *Toxoplasma*, in which form they remain viable for a long time. This occult infection is most likely to occur in the brain, where living organisms have been found several years following infection: after two years in dogs and rats and three years in pigeons. *Toxoplasma* bradyzoites may therefore be demonstrable in microscopic sections of animal tissues in which the injury to the host may be intense, minimal, or nonrecognizable. The judgment of the pathologist may be severely tested in deciding just what influence, if any, *Toxoplasma* may have in a particular case. However, in active toxoplasmosis, the microscopic findings in a particular organ are reasonably characteristic, hence will be considered under each organ.

In the **brain,** active infection is indicated by diffuse nonsuppurative infiltration of brain parenchyma, particularly adjacent to the meninges, which may be similarly infiltrated. Lymphocytic cells accumulate within the Robin-Virchow spaces and are scattered through the parenchyma. Vacuoles may occur in the white matter. *Toxoplasma* tachyzoites may be found scattered singly or in pairs through the parenchyma or in aggregations containing up to 50 organisms. Necrotizing lesions have been observed in the basilar arteries in the cat, but their relationship to toxoplasmosis is not clearly established.

The **liver** in frank toxoplasmosis contains large, sharply delimited, microscopic-sized areas of coagulation necrosis involving any part of the hepatic lobules. The necrotic areas, containing eosinophilic material and cell debris, are surrounded by apparently normal hepatic cells with little or no cellular reaction. Tachyzoites may be found within liver or Kupffer cells, in cysts containing a large number of organisms, or singly or in pairs scattered sparsely in both

the necrotic and viable tissues. Organisms may be few in number even when severe necrosis is present.

The **lung** has rather striking changes, particularly in cats, although other species may develop similar lesions. The changes are particularly evident in the alveolar walls, whose lining becomes cuboidal or columnar and rich in cells, suggesting in this respect the appearance of fetal lung (so-called "fetalization" of lung). This feature also has superficial resemblances to pulmonary adenomatosis. The alveoli are filled with large mononuclear cells and leukocytes with aggregations of *Toxoplasma* in the cells lining the alveoli. These lesions have a nodular distribution throughout the lung, appearing grossly as small, gray, tumor-like masses scattered throughout one or all lobes. Foci of alveolar wall necrosis may accompany this change or may be the only lesion evident.

The **lymph nodes,** particularly those contiguous to affected parenchymal organs, are commonly involved in active cases. They are usually enlarged to several times their normal size, are firm in consistency and densely congested. Extensive coagulation necrosis is seen microscopically, usually in sharply demarcated but irregular zones with slight leukocytic infiltration around the margins. Tachyzoites may be found adjacent to these necrotic areas, particularly in endothelial cells of veins, but may be within the cytoplasm of monocytic cells or free in the tissues.

Ulcers in the **intestine,** presumably resulting from necrosis of submucosal lymph nodules, have been described in toxoplasmosis. Upon occasion, *Toxoplasma* invade the muscularis of the intestine, where a chronic necrotizing lesion followed by production of granulation tissue results in large, grossly detectable granulomatous nodules, which may replace the wall and impinge upon the lumen. The organisms are clearly demonstrable in small and large groups in the muscularis and the granulation tissue.

The **pancreas** may be a site of localization in toxoplasmosis, and here the acute necrotizing lesions arouse intense lymphocytic infiltration, edema, and swelling.

The **eye** may be infected in human adults, and ocular infection has been reported in animals. The lesion is one of granulomatous chorioretinitis in which *Toxoplasma* are demonstrable.

The **myocardium** is frequently invaded by *Toxoplasma,* which may be present in large or small groups within the cytoplasm of cardiac muscle cells. In some instances, severe lymphocytic inflammation is evoked; in others, the organisms are present with little associated inflammation.

Placental invasion leads to focal necrosis, often accompanied by calcification. Tachyzoites are found free and within trophoblasts. Abortion may follow with or without invasion of the fetus. This usually follows acute infection of the pregnant animal, but abortion may also follow reactivation of chronic infection. In the infected fetus, lesions are most common in the brain. Placental transmission may also cause stillbirth and neonatal death.

Diagnosis. The diagnosis of toxoplasmosis in the living animal is presently more of a problem than at necropsy. The complement fixation, neutralization, hemagglutination, Sabin-Feldman dye, and latex agglutination tests are valuable tests to demonstrate antibodies, but due to the high percentage of serologic positivity, demonstration of antibody cannot distinguish between current and past infection. Detection of circulating antigen or isolation of organisms by mouse inoculation or other means permit recognition of active infection. At necropsy, the demonstration of *Toxoplasma* in tissue sections in characteristic lesions should be supported by isolation of the organisms whenever possible. In tissue sections, the microscopic appearance of *Sarcocystis*, leishmanial forms of *Trypanosoma cruzi, Besnoitia besnoitia, Hammondia hammondi,* and sporozoites of Coccidia must be differentiated from *Toxoplasma.* The size (about twice as large) and definite cyst wall around *Sarcocystis* are reliable points of differentiation. The leishmanial forms of *Trypanosoma cruzi* may be distinguished by their centrosome and

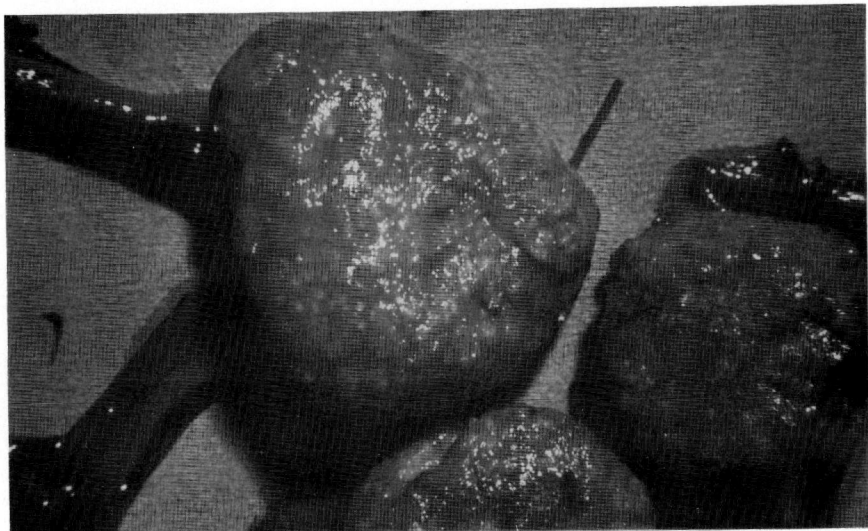

Fig. 13–7. Bovine toxoplasmosis. Multiple foci of necrosis in the placental cotyledons. (Courtesy of Dr. W. A. Watson.)

kinetoplast, which can be seen in some of the organisms. *Besnoitia* may be distinguished by the giant nuclei in the well-developed wall of the cyst, in which the small organisms are found.

Tissue stages of *Hammondia* are more difficult to differentiate, but the facts that intermediate hosts are limited to rodents, in which groups of tachyzoites are limited to lymphoid cells, and that cysts are limited to striated muscle are helpful. The application of the fluorescent antibody test to tissue sections or smears provides a useful method to more specifically identify *Toxoplasma*.

Hammondia hammondi (Frenkel and Dubey, 1975) is an organism which is similar to *Toxoplasma* and classified in the same family. It has a two-host cycle, with sexual reproduction in the intestine of cats (*Isospora bigemina*). Various rodents serve as intermediate hosts. Tachyzoites proliferate in lymphoid cells and cysts of bradyzoites are limited to skeletal and cardiac muscle. Dogs have been shown to be experimentally susceptible intermediate hosts, but the role of *Hammondia* in clinical or pathologic disease has not been determined.

Archer, J.F., Beverley, J.K.A., Watson, W.A., and Hunter, D.: Further field studies on the fluorescent antibody test in the diagnosis of ovine abortion due to toxoplasmosis. Vet. Rec., 88:178–180, 1971.

Averill, D.R., Jr., and deLahunta, A.: Toxoplasmosis of the canine nervous system. Clinicopathologic findings in four cases. J. Am. Vet. Med. Assoc., 159:1134–1141, 1971.

Beverley, J.K.A., Watson, W.A., and Payne, J.M.: The pathology of the placenta in ovine abortion due to toxoplasmosis. Vet. Rec., 88:124–128, 1971.

Beverley, J.K.A., Watson, W.A., and Spence, J.B.: The pathology of the foetus in ovine abortion due to toxoplasmosis. Vet. Rec., 88:174–178, 1971.

Capen, C.C., and Cole, C.R.: Pulmonary lesions in dogs with experimental and naturally occurring toxoplasmosis. Path. Vet., 3:40–63, 1966.

Chessum, B.S.: Reactivation of toxoplasma oocyst production in the cat by infection with *Isospora felis*. Br. Vet. J., 128:33–36, 1972.

Crowley, J.P.: Abortion and prenatal mortality in sheep associated with toxoplamosis. Irish J. Agric. Res., 3:159–164, 1964.

Dubey, J.P.: Experimental *Hammondia hammondi* infection in dogs. Br. Vet. J., 131:741–743, 1975.

Dubey, J.P., and Frenkel, J.K.: Cyst-induced toxoplasmosis in cats. J. Protozool., 19:155–177, 1972.

———: Immunity to feline toxoplasmosis: modification by administration of corticosteroids. Vet. Pathol., 11:350–379, 1974.

Dubey, J.P., Miller, N.L., and Frenkel, J.K.: The *Toxoplasma gondii* oocyst from cat feces. J. Exp. Med., 132:636–662, 1970.

Feldman, H.A.: Toxoplasmosis: an overview. Bull. N.Y. Acad. Med., 50:110–127, 1974.

Ferguson, D.J.P., Hutchison, W.M., Dunachie, J.F., and Siim, J.C.: Ultrastructural study of early stages of asexual multiplication and microgametogony of *Toxoplasma gondii* in the small intestine of the cat. Acta Pathol. Microbiol. Scand., 82B:167–181, 1974.

Frenkel, J.K.: Ocular lesions in hamsters with chronic *Toxoplasma and Besnoitia* infection. Am. J. Ophthalmol., 39:203–225, 1955.

———: Host, strain and treatment variation as factors in pathogenesis of toxoplasmosis. Am. J. Trop. Med. Hyg., 2:390–415, 1953.

Frenkel, J.K.: Toxoplasmosis: parasite life cycle, pathology and immunology. *In* The Coccidia, edited by D. M. Hammond and P. L. Long. Baltimore, University Park Press, 1973, pp. 343–410.

Frenkel, J.K., and Dubey, J.P.: Toxoplasmosis and its prevention in cats and man. J. Infect. Dis., 126:664–673, 1972.

———: *Hammondia hammondi*: a new coccidium of cats producing cysts in muscle of other mammals. Science, 189:222–224, 1975.

Frenkel, J.K., Dubey, J.P., and Miller, N.L.: *Toxoplasma gondii*: fecal forms separated from eggs of the nematode *Toxocara cati*. Science, 164:432–433, 1969.

———: *Toxoplasma gondii* in cats: fecal stages identified as coccidian oocysts. Science, 167:893–896, 1970.

Garnham, P.C.C., Baker, J.R., and Bird, R.G.: Fine structure of cystic form of *Toxoplasma gondii*. Br. Med. J., 83:83–84, 1962. VB 1462–62.

Gavin, M.A., Wanks, T., and Jacobs, L.: Electron microscopic studies of reproducing and interkinetic *Toxoplasma*. J. Protozool., 9:222–234, 1962.

Ghorbani, M., and Hafizi, A.: Assessment of the latex agglutination slide test for detection of toxoplasmic infection. Trop. Geogr. Med., 26:91–93, 1974.

Gustafson, P.V., Agar, H.D., and Cramer, D.I.: An electron microscope study of "*Toxoplasma*." Am. J. Trop. Med. Hyg., 3:1008–1022, 1954.

Hartley, W.J.: Some investigations into the epidemiology of ovine toxoplasmosis. N.Z. Vet. J., 14:106–117, 1966.

Hartley, W.J., and Kater, J.C.: The pathology of toxoplasma infection in the pregnant ewe. Res. Vet. Sci., 4:326–332, 1963. VB 2333–63.

Hartley, W.J., Lindsay, A.B., and MacKinnon, M.M.: Toxoplasma meningioencephalomyelitis and myositis in a dog. N.Z. Vet. J., 6:124–127, 1958.

Hartley, W.J., and Moyle, G.: Observation on an outbreak of ovine congenital toxoplasmosis. Aust. Vet. J., 44:105–107, 1968.

Hutchison, W.M., Dunachie, J.F., Siim, J. Chr., and Work, K.: Coccidian-like nature of *Toxoplasma gondii*. Br. Med. J., 1:142–144, 1970.

Katsube, Y., et al.: Studies of toxoplasmosis. I. Isolation of toxoplasma from muscles of humans, dogs and cats. Jpn. J. Med. Sci. Biol., *20*:413–419, 1967.

Koestner, A., and Cole, C.R.: Neuropathology of canine toxoplasmosis. Am. J. Vet. Res., *21*:813–830, 1960.

———: Neuropathology of porcine toxoplasmosis. Cornell Vet., *50*:362–384, 1960.

Meier, H., Holzworth, J., and Griffiths, R.C.: Toxoplasmosis in the cat, 14 cases. J. Am. Vet. Med. Assoc., *131*:395–414, 1957.

Mocsari, E., and Szemeredi, G.: Diagnostical value of the complement fixation test and the fluorescent antibody method in the laboratory diagnosis of toxoplasmosis. Acta Vet. Hung., *19*:21–27, 1969.

Moller, T., and Nielsen, S.W.: Toxoplasmosis in distemper-susceptible carnivora. Path. Vet., *1*:189–203, 1964.

Munday, B.L.: Transmission of *Toxoplasma* infection from chronically infected ewes to their lambs. Br. Vet. J., *128*:71–72, 1972.

Nakabayashi, T., et al.: Studies on the detection of *Toxoplasma gondii* with mouse inoculation method and fluorescent antibody technic in slaughtered pigs. Trop. Med. Nagasaki, *11*:16–26, 1969.

Nicolle, C., and Manceaux, L.: Sur une infection à corps de Leishman (ou organismes voisins) du gondi. Compt. Rend. Acad. d. Sc., *147*:763–766, 1908.

Olafson, P., and Monlux, W.S.: *Toxoplasma* infection in animals. Cornell Vet., *32*:176–190, 1942.

Piper, R.C., Cole, C.R., and Shadduck, J.A.: Natural and experimental ocular toxoplasmosis in animals. Am. J. Ophthalmol., *69*:662–668, 1970.

Pridham, T.J., and Belcher, J.: Toxoplasmosis in mink. Can. J. Comp. Med., *22*:99–106, 1958.

Raizman, R.E., and Neva, F.A.: Detection of circulating antigen in acute experimental infections with *Toxoplasma gondii*. J. Infect. Dis., *132*:44–48, 1975.

Riemann, H.P., et al.: Equine toxoplasmosis: a survey for antibodies to *Toxoplasma gondii* in horses. Am. J. Vet. Res., *36*:1797–1800, 1975.

Saxen, E., and Saxen, L.: The histological diagnosis of glandular toxoplasmosis. Lab. Invest., *8*:386–394, 1959.

Sheffield, H.G., and Melton, M.L.: *Toxoplasma gondii:* transmission through feces in absence of *Toxocara cati* eggs. Science, 164:431–432, 1969.

———: *Toxoplasma gondii:* The oocyst, sporozoite, and infection of cultured cells. Science, *167*:892–893, 1970.

Siim, J.C., Hutchison, W.M., and Work, K.: Transmission of *Toxoplasma gondii*. Further studies on the morphology of the cystic form in cat faeces. Acta Path. Microbiol. Scand., *77*:756–757, 1969.

Smith, C.: Staining of *Toxoplasma* in histological sections. Br. J. Ophthalmol., *37*:504–505, 1953.

Tisseur, H., et al.: Histological diagnosis of toxoplasmosis in animals. Recl. Med. Vet., *142*:15–23, 1966.

Vainisi, S.J., and Campbell, L.H.: Ocular toxoplasmosis in cats. J. Am. Vet. Med. Assoc., *154*:141–152, 1969.

Wanko, T., Jacobs, L., and Gavin, M.A.: Electron microscope study of toxoplasma cysts in mouse brain. J. Protozool., *9*:235–242, 1962.

Watson, W.A., and Beverley, J.K.A.: Ovine abortion due to experimental toxoplasmosis. Vet. Rec., *88*:42–45, 1971.

———: Epizootics of toxoplasmosis causing ovine abortion. Vet. Rec., *88*:120–124, 1971.

Werner, H., and Egger, I.: Latent toxoplasma infection of the uterus and its importance for pregnancy. II. Influence on the course of pregnancy in mice. Zentbl. Bakt. Parsit. I., *208*:122–135, 1968. V.B. *39*:1059, 1969.

Werner, H., Janitschke, K., and Köhler, H.: Über Beobachtungen an Marmoset-Affen *Saguinus (Oedipomidas) oedipus* nach oral und intraperitonealer Infektion mit verschiedenen zystenbildunden Toxoplasma—Stämmen unterschiedlicher Virulenz. Zentbl. Bakt. Parsit. I., *209*:553–569, 1969. V.B. *39*:4568, 1969.

Wildführ, W.: Elektronenmikroskopische Untersuchungen zur Morphologie und Reproduction von *Toxoplasma gondii*. Zentbl. Bakt. Parsit., *200*:525–547, 1966. V. B. *36*:4707, 1966.

Wilson, S.G., et al.: Toxoplasmosis in pigs. An experimental study of oral infection and infection through the skin. Vet. Rec., *81*:313–317, 1967.

Work, K.: Toxoplasmosis with special reference to transmission and life cycle of *Toxoplasma gondii*. Acta Pathol. Microbiol. Scand., Suppl. 221, 51 pp., 1972.

Work, K., and Hutchison, W.M.: The new cyst of *Toxoplasma gondii*. Acta Pathol. Microbiol. Scand., *77*:414–424, 1969.

SARCOSPORIDIOSIS

Tiny tubular cysts filled with crescentic bodies have been recognized for over a century as extremely common within skeletal and cardiac muscle fibers of aquatic birds and most mammals, particularly herbivora. They were first described by Miescher in 1843 in the musculature of a house mouse and were later called "Miescher's bodies, sacs, or tubules." Their classification, life cycle, source of infection, and significance were, however, a complete mystery until Rommel et al. (1972), Heydorn and Rommel (1972), Fayer and Johnson (1974), and Ruiz and Frenkel (1976) demonstrated that the parasitic cysts in muscle represent intermediate stages of intestinal coccidia, and that the life cycle is similar to that of *Toxoplasma* (Fig. 13–8). They are currently classified as Protozoa in the class Sporozoa, family Sarcocystinae. Only a few sarcosporidia have been

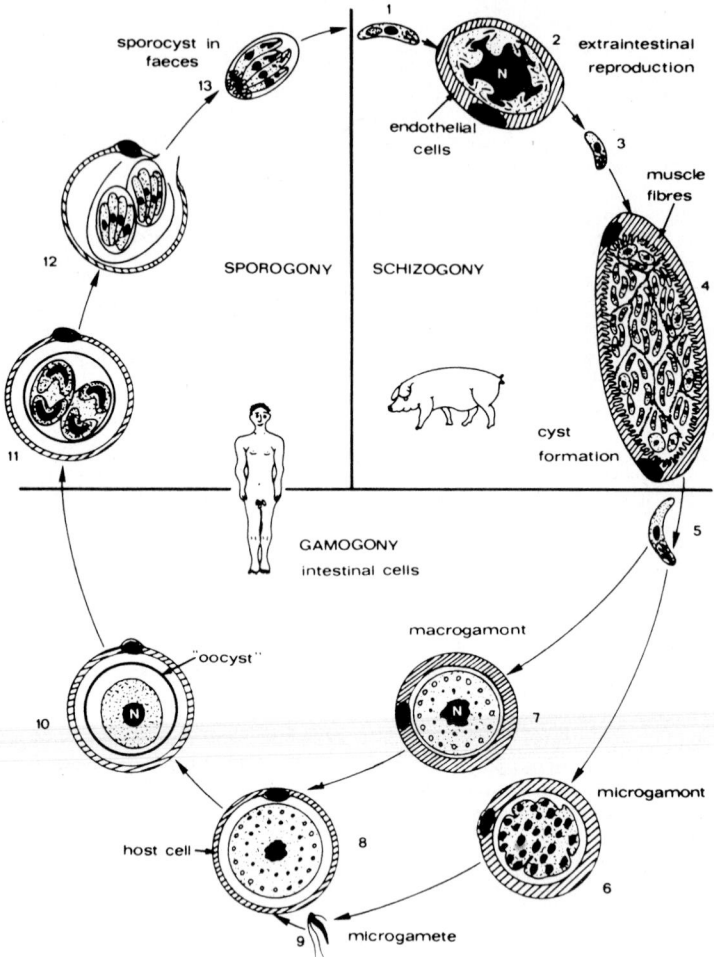

Fig. 13–8. Diagrammatic representation of the life cycle of *Sarcocystis suihominis*. (Courtesy of Dr. J. K. Frenkel and *Zeitschrift für Parasitenkunde*.)

studied in any detail and correlated with specific intestinal coccidia.

Over the years, numerous species names of uncertain validity have been applied to members of the genus *Sarcocystis*. These include such examples as *Sarcocystis tenella* (sheep); *S. blanchardi* and *S. fusiformis* (cattle); *S. miescheriana* (swine); and *S. bertrami* (horses). Of special interest is another type found in the tongue, esophagus, and occasionally other muscles of sheep. This type, called *Balbiania gigantea*, forms quite large, grossly visible, multinucleated saccules containing a fibrillar network within which myriads of crescentic spores are

found. This is apparently a variant of the species called *S. tenella*.

In light of present knowledge, all these names should be abandoned. It is now known that *Sarcosporidia*, like *Toxoplasma*, have a two-host life cycle: a sexual cycle in definitive hosts characterized by gamogony and sporogony; and an asexual cycle in muscle cells of intermediate hosts characterized by merogony.

Life Cycle. Using *Sarcocystis muris* (the type species) as an example (see Fig. 13–3), the intermediate hosts, mice, become infected following ingestion of sporulated oocysts. Sporozoites first multiply in the

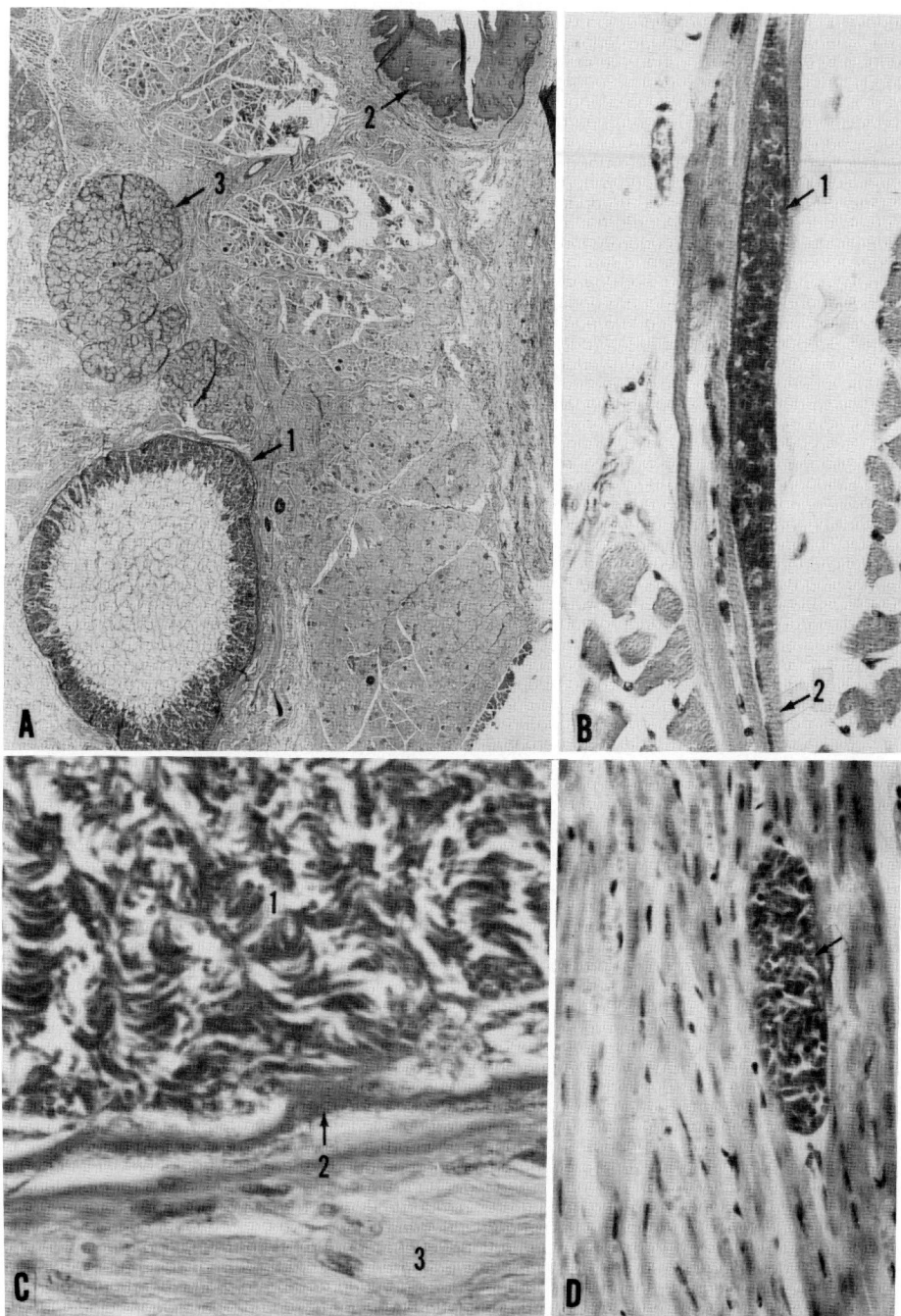

Fig. 13–9. Sarcosporidiosis. *A, Balbiania gigantea (1)* in the tongue of a sheep (× 15); lingual epithelium *(2)*, and lingual salivary glands *(3)*. *B, Sarcocystis blanchardi (1)* in the tongue of a cow (× 330). Note the muscle bundle *(2)* contains the organism. *C,* Higher magnification of organisms in *A* (× 650). Note spores *(1)*, cyst wall *(2)*, and muscle fibers *(3)*. (Courtesy of Armed Forces Institute of Pathology.) Contributor: Dr. C. L. Davis. *D, Sarcocystis blanchardi* in the myocardium of a cow (× 330).

liver, forming schizonts of tachyzoites, which subsequently invade skeletal muscle, first as metrocytes and then as large numbers of bradyzoites forming the typical sarcocystis cyst. The cycle is completed when the final host, cats, ingest muscle containing bradyzoites. The life cycle of *S. suihominis* is depicted in Figure 13–8.

The final hosts for many species of *Sarcocystis* have not been identified. Both cats and dogs have been identified as final hosts for bovine, ovine, porcine, and equine sarcosporidia. The intestinal stage in dogs and cats was formerly called *Isospora bigemina*. Human beings are hosts for the sexual stages of sarcosporidia of bovines and swine. The intestinal stage in man was previously called *Isospora hominis*. Based on the two hosts involved in the life cycles of sarcosporidia, new nomenclature has been proposed. Table 13–2 lists the nomenclature presented by Dubey (1976) and Frenkel et al. (1979).

The sarcocysts within muscle fibers are variable in size but usually become slightly wider than a muscle fiber and several times longer than their width. The wall of the cyst appears clear or hyaline and may have a diagonally laminated structure. There are often tiny strands or septae extending from the wall, which divide the cyst into tiny subcompartments in which the bradyzoites lie. The bradyzoites are strongly basophilic and elliptical or banana-shaped, each measuring about 4 by 8 μ. There is often degeneration in the centers of larger sarcocysts.

Lesions. The pathogenicity of *Sarcocystis* is also unsettled, although the organisms may be numerous in cardiac and skeletal muscles throughout the body. The sarcocysts are not encountered in smooth muscle cells or in any tissues of the body other than skeletal and cardiac muscle.

In most examples in which the parasites are encountered, the sarcolemma is displaced but no inflammatory reaction is evident. In some heavily parasitized bovine hearts, Jones has noted that Purkinje fibers (specialized muscle fibers) have also contained numerous sarcocysts, but whether their presence had any effect

Table 13–2. Nomenclature of Some Sarcocystis Species

Sarcocystis Species	Intermediate Host (muscle sporocyst stage)	Final Host (intestinal stage)	Former Names
S. bovifelis	Bovine	Cat	S. fusiformis
S. bovicanis	Bovine	Dog	S. blanchardi
S. bovihominis			S. hirsuta
	Bovine	Man, Monkey	(Isospora bigemina, I. hominis)
S. ovifelis	Sheep	Cat	S. tenella
			Balbiania gigantea
S. ovicanis	Sheep	Dog	(Isospora bigemina)
S. suicanis	Pig	Dog	S. miescheriana
S. suihominis	Pig	Man	(Isospora bigemina, I. hominis)
S. equicanis	Horse	Dog	S. bertrami
S. muris	Mouse	Cat	

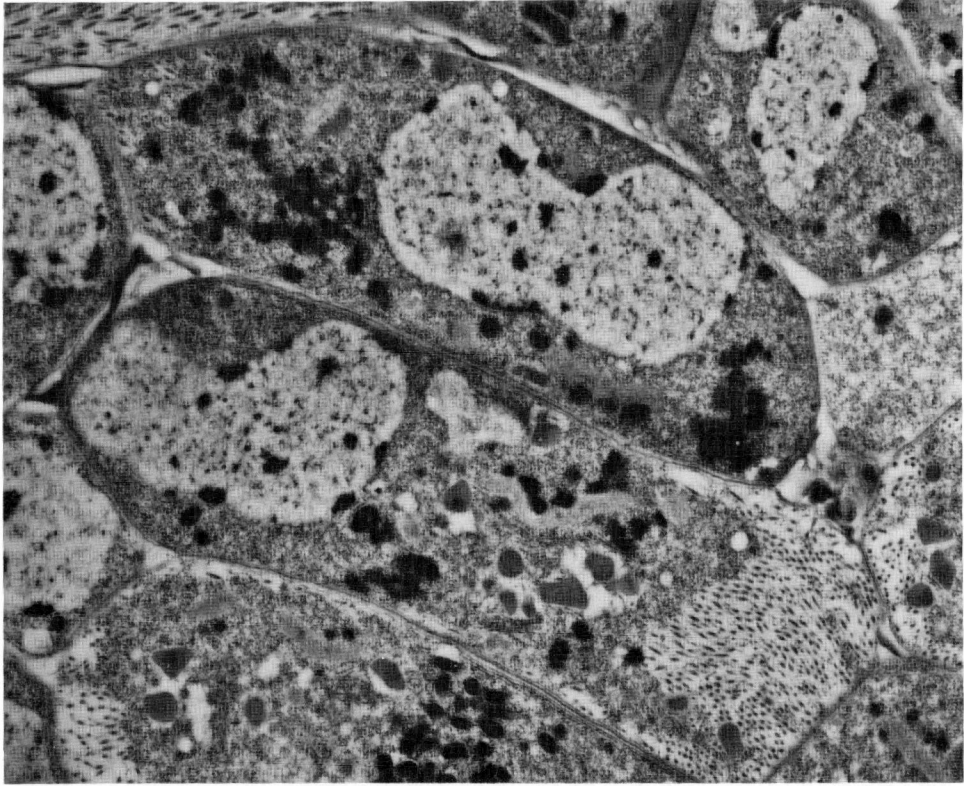

Fig. 13-10. *Sarcocystis fusiformis.* Electron micrograph (× 18,000). (Courtesy of Dr. Charles F. Simpson and *The Journal of Parasitology.*)

upon the conduction system remains unknown.

Occasionally, myositis and muscle necrosis are encountered in association with sarcosporidiosis, but cause and effect is difficult to ascertain. It is currently believed that rupture of sarcocysts stimulates an inflammatory reaction, which may be granulomatous in nature.

Certain cases of **eosinophilic myositis** in the bovine have been attributed to sarcosporidiosis, but this interpretation is felt to be based upon insufficient evidence. Although *Sarcocystis* may be present in moderate numbers in muscles affected with eosinophilic myositis, it is rare that the lesions and parasites can be topographically related and no changes are evident in the organisms. The more valid conclusion is that eosinophilic myositis of unknown etiology may occur in skeletal muscle already affected with sarcosporidiosis.

Overwhelming infection leading to clinical signs and death has been reported in calves (Frelier et al., 1977, 1979; Schmitz and Wolf, 1977).

Members of the genus *Frenkelia* are protozoa similar to sarcosporidia and classified in the same family. Sexual reproduction in the final host (various predatory birds) occurs in intestinal epithelium. Upon ingestion of sporulated oöcysts (sporocyst) by intermediate hosts, the organisms undergo schizogony in hepatocytes and Kupffer's cells, and subsequently form extremely large, multilobulated cysts filled with bradyzoites in the central nervous system (Fig. 13–11). They were previously termed M-organisms or *Toxoplasma microti*. The cysts have been observed in

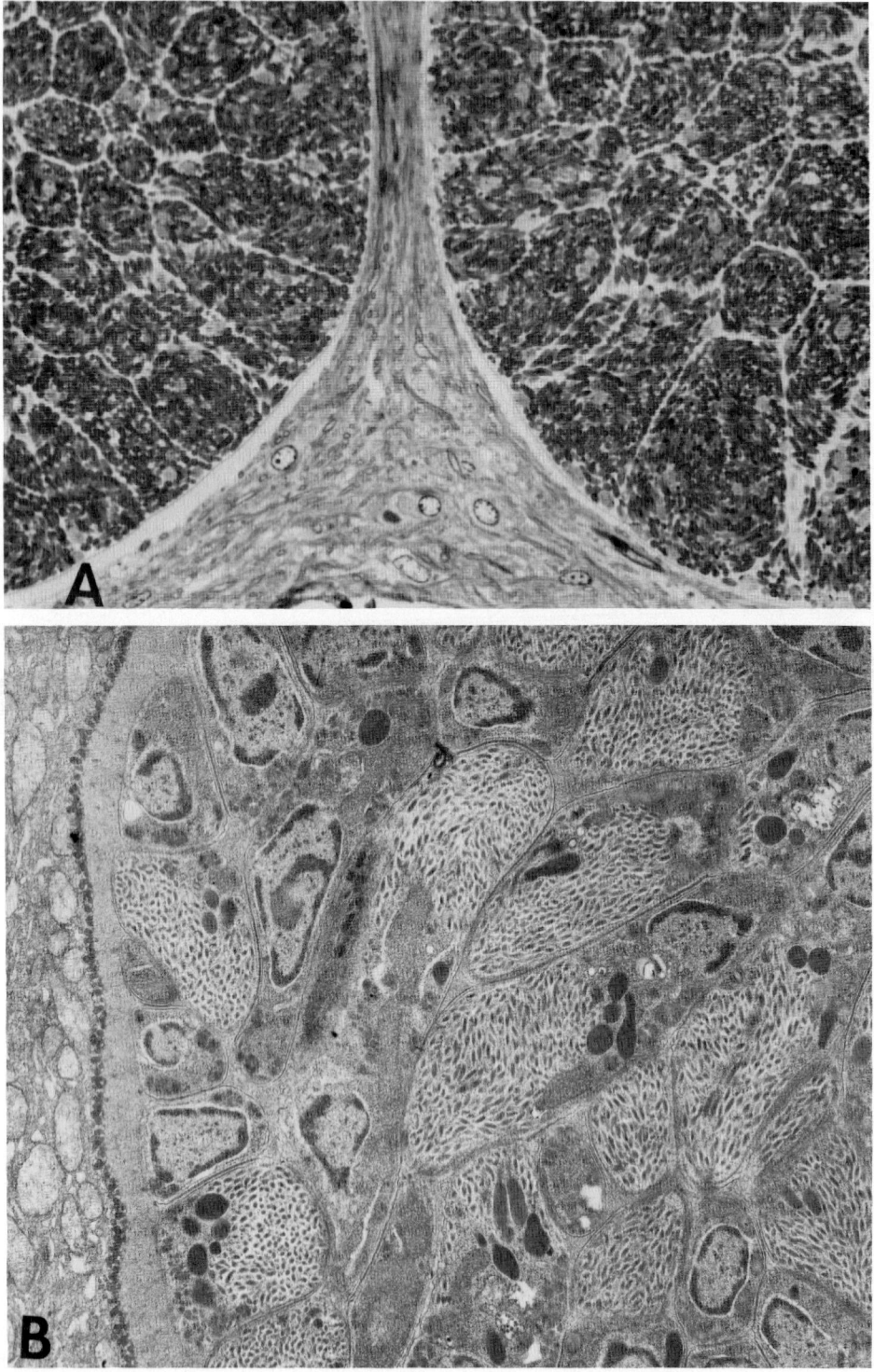

Fig. 13–11. *Frenkelia* sp. in the brain of a rat. *A*, Metrocyst containing numerous crescent-shaped bradyzoites separated by fine interlacing septae. (Courtesy of Dr. N. W. King, Jr. and *Veterinary Pathology.*) *B.* Ultrastructure of bradyzoites of *Frenkelia.* (Courtesy of Dr. N. W. King, Jr.)

voles, meadow mice *(Microtus sp.),* lemmings, muskrats, and rats. Usually there is no reaction to their presence, but granulomatous type inflammation is occasionally encountered, presumably after rupture of a cyst. Degeneration in the center of the cysts is not unusual.

Diagnosis. The diagnosis of sarcosporidiosis depends upon identification of sarcocysts, usually in tissue sections. *Sarcocystis* has often been confused with *Toxoplasma,* an error which should not occur because the spores are nearly twice as large (4 by 8 μ) and, in contrast to *Toxoplasma,* enclosed within a thick cyst wall. The eccentric nucleus of *Toxoplasma* is not demonstrable in *Sarcocystis.* The cysts of *Besnoitia* may be distinguished by their thick wall and location—squamous epithelium, blood vessel walls, connective tissue; they are not usually found in striated muscle cells.

Biocca, E.: Class toxoplasmatea. Critical review and proposal of the new name *Frenkelia gen. n.* for M-organism. Parasitologia, 10:89–98, 1968.

Dubey, J.P.: A review of sarcocystis of domestic animals and of other coccidia of cats and dogs. J. Am. Vet. Med. Assoc., 169:1061–1078, 1976.

Fayer, R.: Sarcocystis: Development in cultured avian and mammalian cells. Science, 168:1104–1105, 1970.

Fayer, R.: Development of *Sarcocystis fusiformis* in the small intestine of a dog. J. Parasitol., 60:660–665, 1974.

Fayer, R., and Johnson, A.J.: Development of *Sarcocystis fusiformis* in calves infected with sporocysts from dogs. J. Parasitol., 59:1135–1137, 1973.

———: *Sarcocystis fusiformis:* development of cysts in calves infected with sporocysts from dogs. Proc. Helminth. Soc. Washington, 41:105–108, 1974.

Ford, G.E.: Prey-predator transmission in the epizootiology of ovine sarcosporidiosis. Aust. Vet. J., 50:38–39, 1974.

Frelier, P., Mayhew, I.G., Fayer, R., and Lunde, M.N.: Sarcocystosis: a clinical outbreak in dairy calves. Science, 195:1341–1342, 1977.

Frelier, P.F., Mayhew, I.G., and Pollock, R.: Bovine sarcocystosis: pathologic features of naturally occurring infection with *Sarcocystis cruzi.* Am. J. Vet. Res., 40:651–657, 1979.

Hayden, D.W., King, N.W., Jr., and Murthy, A.S.K.: Spontaneous *Frenkelia* infection in a laboratory-reared rat. Vet. Pathol., 13:337–342, 1976.

Heydorn, A.-O., and Rommel, M.: Beitrage zum Lebenszyklus der Sarkosporidien. II. Hund und Katze als Ubertrager der Sarkosporidien des

Rindes. Berl. Munch. Tieraerztl. Wochenschr., 85:121–123, 1972.

Markus, M.B., Killick-Kendrick, R., and Garnham, P.C.C.: The coccidial nature and life cycle of Sarcocystis. J. Trop. Med. Hyg., 77:248–259, 1974.

Miescher, F.: Ueber Eigenthümliche Schläuche in den Muskeln einer Hausmaus. Ber. ü. d. Verhandl. Naturforsch. Gesellsch. Basel, 5:198–203, 1843.

Munday, B.L., and Corbould, A.: The possible role of the dog in the epidemiology of ovine sarcosporidiosis. Br. Vet. J., 130:9–11, 1974.

Rommel, M., and Heydorn, A.-O.: Beitrage zum Lebenszyklus der Sarkosporidien. III. *Isospora hominis* (Railliet and Lucet, 1891) Wenyon, 1923, eine Dauerform der Sarkosporidien des Rindes und des Schweins. Berl. Munch. Tieraerztl. Wochenschr., 85:143–145, 1972.

Rommel, M., Heydorn, A.-O., and Gruber, F.: Beitrage zum Lebenszyklus der Sarkosporidien. I. Die Sporozyste von *S. tenella* in den Fazes der Katze. Berl. Munch. Tieraerztl. Wochenschr., 85:101–105, 1972.

Ruiz, A., and Frenkel, J.K.: Recognition of cyclic transmission of *Sarcocystis muris* by cats. J. Infect. Dis., 133:409–418, 1976.

Rzepczyk, C.M.: Evidence of a rat-snake life cycle for Sarcocystis. Int. J. Parasitol., 4:447–449, 1974.

Sahasrabudhe, V.K., and Shah, H.L.: The occurrence of *Sarcocystis sp.* in the dog. J. Protozool., 13:531, 1966.

Schmitz, J.A., and Wolf, W.W.: Spontaneous fatal sarcocystosis in a calf. Vet. Pathol., 14:527–531, 1977.

Simpson, C.F.: Electron microscopy of *Sarcocystis fusiformis.* J. Parasitol., 52:607–613, 1966.

BESNOITIOSIS

A chronic debilitating and occasionally fatal disease with cutaneous and systemic manifestations in cattle and horses has been described from South Africa and called besnoitiosis after the cyst-forming protozoa, *Besnoitia besnoiti.*

Earlier names for the organism, *Globidium besnoiti,* and the disease, "globidiosis," appear to have been based on erroneous data and therefore should be abandoned. Similar organisms have been found in the blue wildebeest *(Connochaetes taurinus),* impala *(Aepyceros melampus),* and a kudu *(Tragelaphus strepsiceros)* in the Transvaal of South Africa (McCully et al., 1966). Rabbits are susceptible to experimental infection, develop cutaneous lesions similar to those of cattle, and therefore serve as a good experimental model (Bigalke et al., 1967).

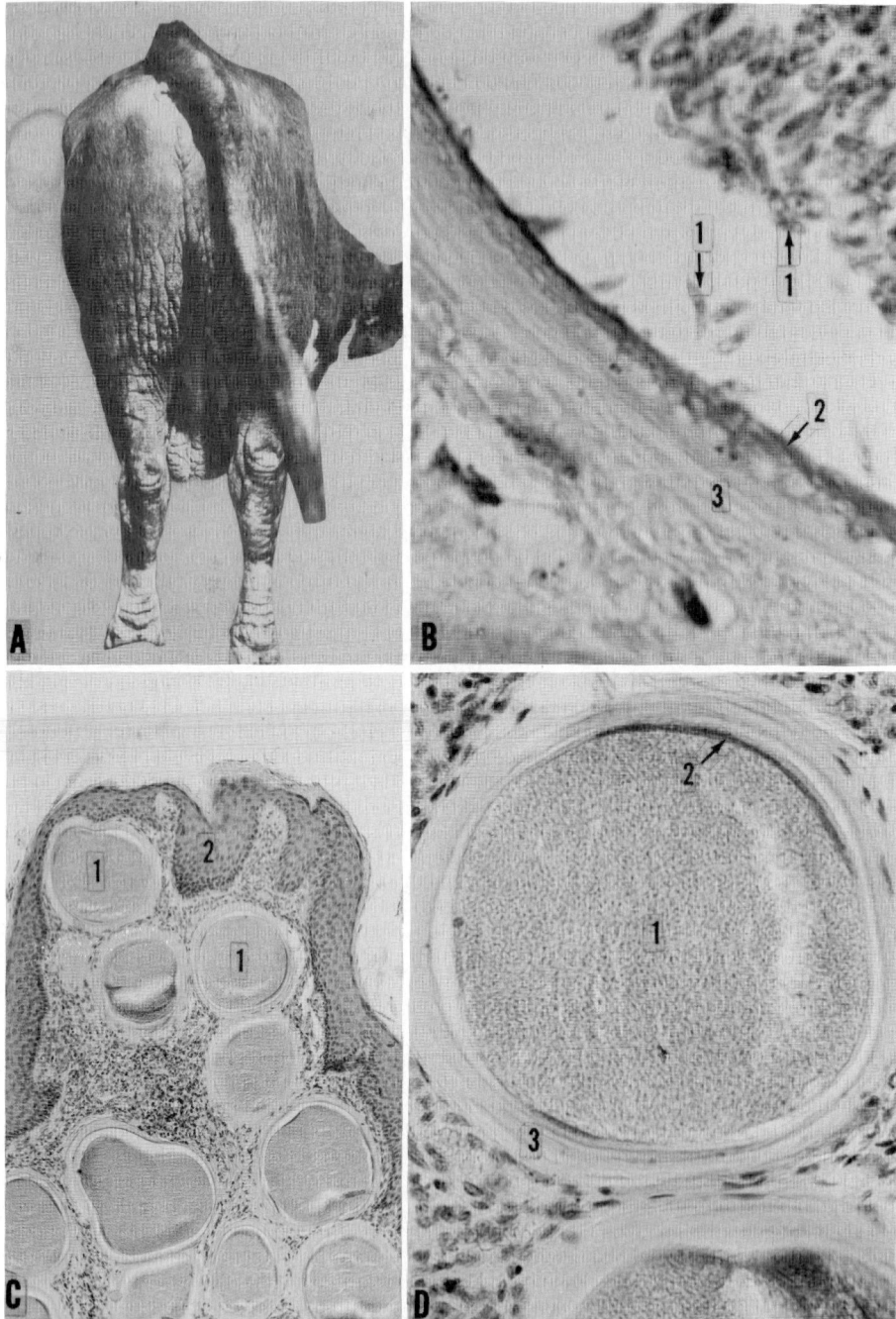

Fig. 13–12. Besnoitiosis. *A,* Thickened rugose skin of thigh, legs, and scrotum of Hereford bull in South Africa. *B,* High magnification (× 1300) of the wall of a cyst containing spores *(1),* acellular wall *(2)* and a dense fibrous capsule *(3).* From the dermis of a burro. Contributor: Col. J. H. Rust, III. *C,* Section of skin of the bull shown in *A* (× 75). Note cysts *(1)* in dermis, covered by acanthotic epidermis *(2). D,* Higher magnification (× 330) of *C.* Cyst filled with spores *(1),* large nucleus flattened against cyst wall *(2),* and fibrous component of the wall *(3).* (Courtesy of Armed Forces Institute of Pathology.) Contributor: Dr. Wm. S. Monlux.

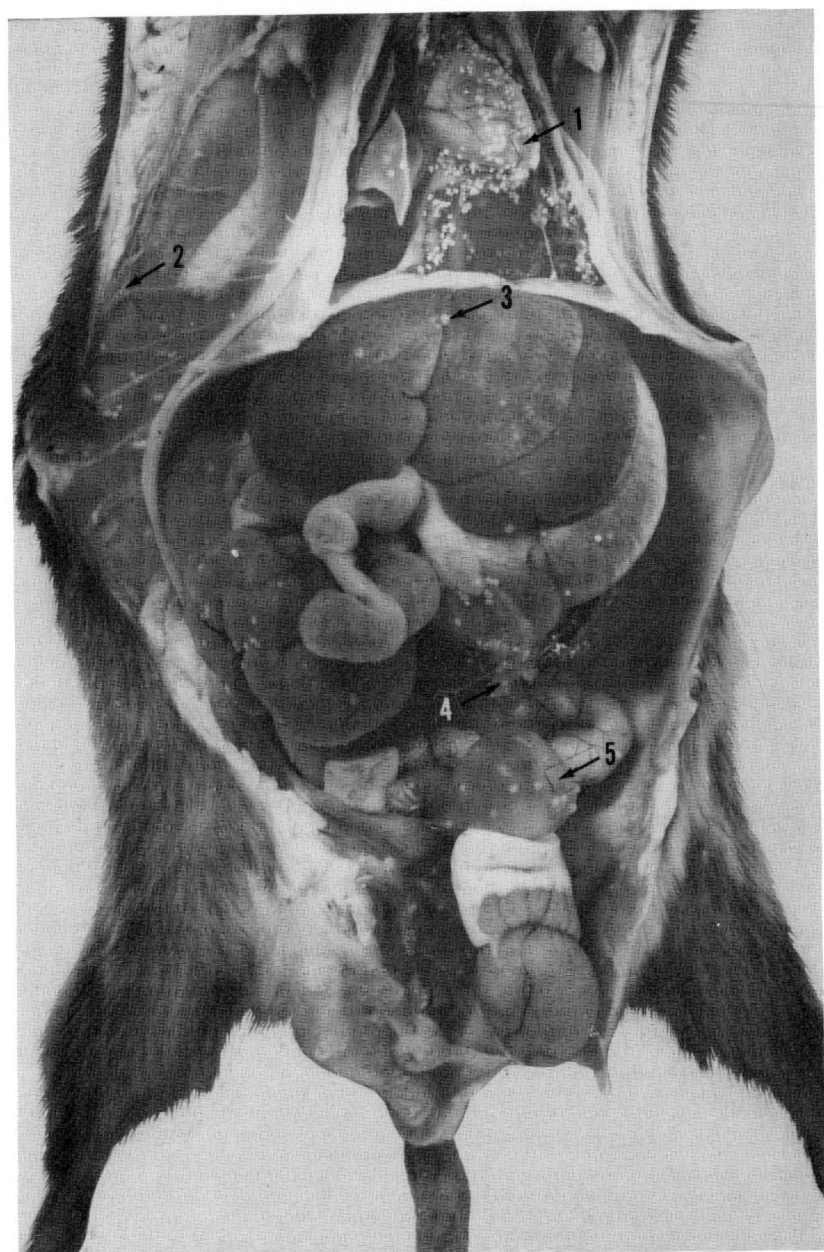

Fig. 13–13. *Besnoitia jellisoni* in pleura and pericardium*(1)*, subcutis*(2)*, serosa of the liver*(3)*, mesentery *(4)*, and urinary bladder*(5)* of a deer mouse*(Peromyscus sp.)*. Photograph courtesy of Dr. W. J. Hadlow.

Natural infection has also been described in reindeer and caribou in Alaska (B. tarandi), white footed mice in Idaho, Kangaroo rats in Utah (B. jellisoni), lizards in Panama (B. darlingi), and several other species. Similar organisms have been described in so called "Bangkok hemorrhagic disease" of chickens. Although minor differences have been detected in these Besnoitia, it is not known whether they actually represent different species.

Life Cycle. Besnoitia are classified in the family Sarcocystinae, subfamily Toxoplasmatinae, as is the genus *Toxoplasma* and the genus *Hammondia*. It has a two-host life cycle (Fig. 13–12), with sexual reproduction occurring in the intestinal tract of the final host, leading to production of oöcysts. Upon ingestion of oöcysts by intermediate hosts, the organisms invade many cell types, producing small groups of tachyzoites indistinguishable from *Toxoplasma*. This acute infection usually goes unrecognized. Tachyzoites subsequently invade fibroblasts and produce large cysts filled with bradyzoites, the infectious stage for the final host. The cysts are very large, often up to 2 mm in diameter, and hence may be visible to the unaided eye.

The organisms in cattle, horses, and burros are encountered most frequently in the cyst form, at which stage they have an unmistakable appearance. The cysts are smoothly spherical in well-fixed tissues, 0.1 to 0.5 mm in diameter, and are surrounded by a dense, uniformly eosinophilic wall which is homogeneous or concentrically laminated and appears to come from host tissue. Inside this wall are one or more giant ovoid nuclei which become compressed against the periphery by the enlarging mass of spores within. These giant nuclei are surrounded by a narrow band of cytoplasm which encircles the inner wall and sends one or more narrow dividing septa across the cyst. The inner contents are made up of many tiny crescentic spores, which in size and morphology are similar to *Toxoplasma*.

Lesions. The lesions in cattle and horses are closely related to the organisms, which may not only localize in the skin but may spread to all parts of the body. The cutaneous lesions are usually seen grossly as thickened, rugose, partially hairless areas of skin, particularly on legs, thighs, and scrotum. The microscopic picture is dominated by the large spherical cysts, which may occur in deeper areas and are frequently seen in the walls of small blood vessels. Invasion of the scrotum, epididymis, and testis, as well as upper gastrointestinal tract, is common and may be accompanied by a severe granulomatous tissue reaction, particularly when numerous spores are released into the tissue. In contrast, the mature cysts with their wide, hyaline wall are usually surrounded by little other inflammatory tissue reaction.

The lesions in antelopes appear to be limited to the presence of the cysts in the cardiovascular system. The intima of veins, such as the jugular and peripheral veins of limbs, is the site of predilection for the cysts, although some may be found in the muscularis or adventitia. In the impala, cysts are found especially in the walls of subcutaneous lymphatics. Some organisms may be found in the endocardium (McCully et al., 1966).

Diagnosis. The diagnosis is based upon demonstration of the organisms in tissue sections.

Bigalke, R.D., and Naude, T.W.: The diagnostic value of cysts in the scleral conjunctiva in bovine besnoitiosis. J. S. Afr. Vet. Med. Assoc., 33:21–27, 1962.

Bigalke, R.D., et al.: The relationship between *Besnoitia* of antelopes and *Besnoitia besnoiti* (Marotel, 1912) of cattle. Bull. Off. Int. Epizootol., 66:903–905, 1966.

———: Studies on the relationship between *Besnoitia* of blue wildebeest and impala, and *Besnoitia besnoiti* of cattle. Onderstepoort J. Vet. Res., 34:7–28, 1967.

Binninger, C.E., and McGuire, T.C.: Atypical globidiosis in a lamb. J. Am. Vet. Med. Assoc., 151:606–608, 1967.

Bwangamoi, O.: Besnoitiosis and other skin diseases of cattle (*Bos indicus*) in Uganda. Am. J. Vet. Res., 29:737–743, 1968.

Campbell, J.G.: Bangkok haemorrhagic disease of chickens: an unusual condition associated with an organism of uncertain taxonomy. J. Pathol. Bact., *68*:423–429, 1954.

Frenkel, J.K.: Ocular lesions in hamsters with chronic *Toxoplasma* and *Besnoitia* infection. Am. J. Ophthalmol., *39*:203–255, 1955.

————: *Besnoitia wallacei* of cats and rodents: with a reclassification of other cyst-forming isosporid coccidia. J. Parasitol., *63*:611–628, 1977.

Hadwen, S.: Cyst-forming protozoa in reindeer and caribou, and a sarcosporidian parasite of the seal (*Phoca richardi*). J. Am. Vet. Med. Assoc., *61*:374–382, 1922.

Jellison, W.L.: On the nomenclature of *Besnoitia besnoiti*, a protozoan parasite. Ann. N. Y. Acad. Sci., *64*:268–270, 1956.

Jellison, W.L., Fullerton, W.J., and Parker, H.: Transmission of the protozoan *Besnoitia jellisoni* by ingestion. Ann. N. Y. Acad. Sci., *64*:271–274, 1956.

McCully, R.M., et al.: Observations on besnoitia cysts in the cardiovascular system of some wild antelopes and domestic cattle. Onderstepoort J. Vet. Res., *33*:245–275, 1966.

Neuman, M.: An outbreak of besnoitiosis in cattle. Refuah Vet., *19*:106–110, 1962.

Pols, J.W.: The artificial transmission of *Globidium besnoiti* Marotel, 1912, to cattle and rabbits. J. S. Afr. Vet. Med. Assoc., *25*:37–44, 1954.

————: Studies on bovine besnoitiosis with special reference to the aetiology. Onderstepoort J. Vet. Res., *28*:265–356, 1960. VB 1426–61.

————: Preliminary notes on the behavior of *Globidium besnoiti* Marotel, 1912, in the rabbit. J. S. Afr. Vet. Med. Assoc., *25*:45–47, 1954.

Schulz, K.C.A.: A report on naturally acquired besnoitiosis in bovines with special reference to its pathology. J. S. Afr. Vet. Med. Assoc., *31*:21–35, 1960. VB 1427–61.

Terrell, T.G., and Stookey, J.L.: *Besnoitia bennetti* in two Mexican burros. Vet. Pathol., *10*:177–184, 1973.

Wallace, G.D., and Frenkel, J.K.: Besnoitia species (Protozoa, Sporozoa, Toxoplasmatidae): recognition of cyclic transmission by cats. Science, *188*:369–371, 1975.

KLOSSIELLA

These coccidia localize in the convoluted tubules of the kidney. Among these parasites are: *Klossiella equi*, in horses, zebras, and asses (*Equidae*); *Eimeria truncata* in the goose; and *Klossiella cobayae* in the guinea pig. *Klossiella* has also been described in the kidneys of mice and rats. Schizogony occurs in endothelial cells and epithelium of Bowman's capsule, releasing merozoites which infect tubular epithelial cells, where gametogenesis occurs. Oöcytes are shed in the urine. Although these organisms destroy some renal epithelium, their total effect appears slight. Usually there are no clinical signs; the parasites are usually found incidentally at necropsy.

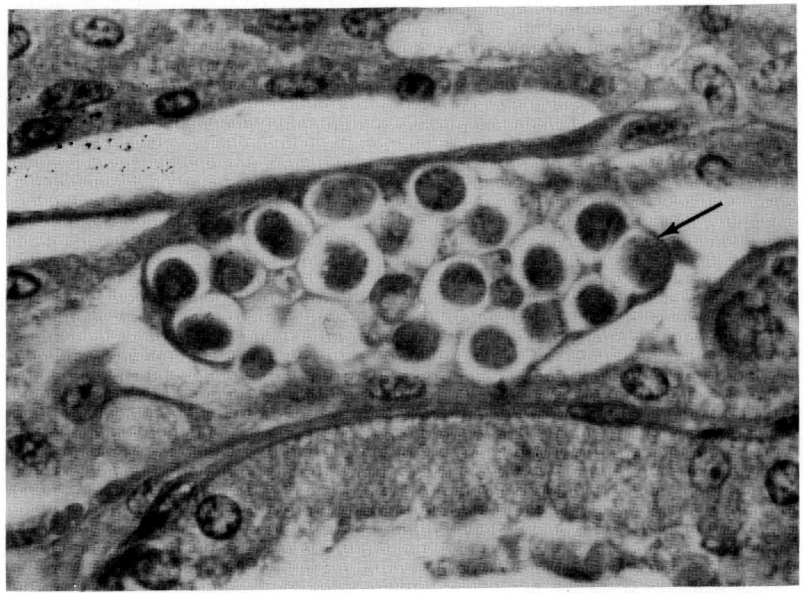

Fig. 13–14. *Klossiella equi* in convoluted renal tubules of a zebra. Specimen courtesy of Dr. M. J. Eggert.

Beemer, A.M., Kuttin, E.S., and Birnbaum, S.C.: Occurrence of *Klossiella* N. sp. in rats. Refuah Vet., 29:61–65, 1972.

Cossel, L.: Nierenbefunde beim Meerschweinchen bei Klossiellen-Infektion (*Klossiella cobayae*). (Zur Kenntnis der speziellen Pathologie der Versuchstiere). Schweiz. allgem. Pathol. Bakteriol., 21:62–73, 1958.

Hartman, H.A.: The protozoan parasite, *Klossiella equi*, in the Mexican burro. Am. J. Vet. Res., 22:1126–1129, 1961.

Meshorer, A.: Interstitial nephritis in the spiny mouse (*Acomys cahirinus*) associated with *Klossiella sp.* infection. Lab. Anim., 4:227–232, 1970.

Mullin, S.W., and Colley, F.C.: *Eimeria and Klossia spp.* (Protozoa: Sporozoa) from wild mammals in Borneo. J. Protozool., 19:406–408, 1972.

Pierce, L.: Klossiella infection of the guinea pig. J. Exp. Med., 23:431–442, 1916.

Seibold, H.R., and Thorsen, R.E.: *Klossiella equi*, N. sp. (Protozoa-Klossielidae) from the kidney of an American jack. J. Parasitol., 41:285–288, 1955.

Seidelin, H.: *Klossiella sp.* in the kidney of a guinea pig. Ann. Trop. Med. Parasitol., 8:553–564, 1941.

Smith, T., and Johnson, H.P.: On a coccidium (*Klossiella muris*, gen. et. spec. Nov) parasitic in the renal epithelium of the mouse. J. Exp. Med., 6:303–316, 1902.

Vetterling, J.M., and Thompson, D.E.: *Klossiella equi* Baumann, 1946 (Sporozoa: Eucoccidia: Adeleina) from equids. J. Parasitol., 58:589–594, 1972.

Winter, H., and Watt, D.: *Klossiella hydromyos n. sp.* from the kidneys of an Australian water rat (*Hydromys chrysogaster*). Vet. Pathol., 8:222–231, 1971.

CRYPTOSPORIDIOSIS

Members of the genus *Cryptosporidium* parasitize intestinal epithelium of a variety of animal species, including cattle, swine, sheep, rabbits, mice, guinea pigs, monkeys, birds, and snakes. Cryptosporidia are classified as coccidia, but differ from most other members in that all stages are extremely small and difficult to distinguish in usual tissue preparations. Ultrastructural studies or the use of thin tissue sections allows differentiation of trophozoites,

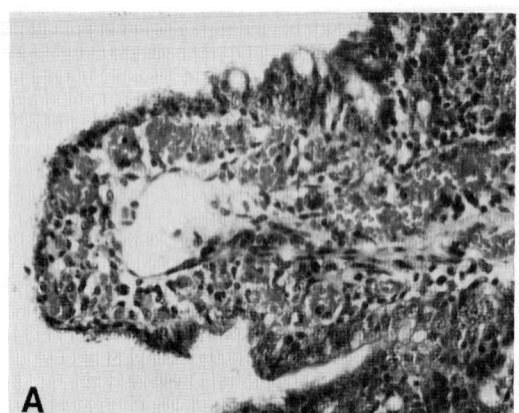

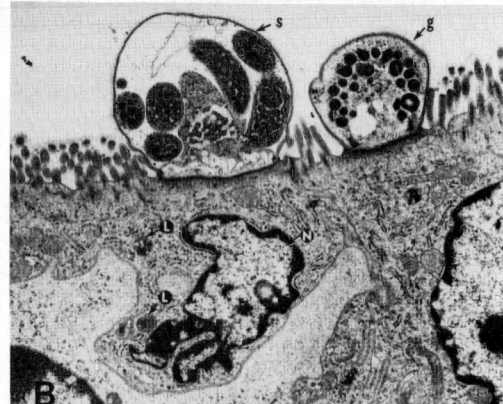

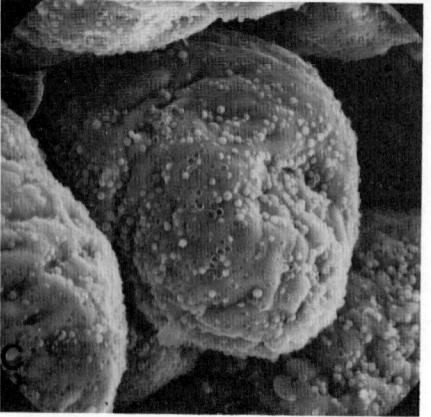

Fig. 13–15. Cryptosporidiosis in calves. *A,* Atrophic intestinal villus with numerous, barely discernible cryptosporidia adherent to the surface. *B,* Schizont (s) and gamete (g) in brush border of intestinal epithelium. *C,* Scanning electron micrograph of atrophic villus. Many cryptosporidia (white nodules) adherent to surface. Black circles are craters left when parasites leave surface or are rinsed off. (Courtesy of Dr. Harley W. Moon and *Journal of the American Veterinary Medical Association.*)

schizonts containing merozoites, macro- and microgametocytes, and oöcysts, all of which are under 3 μ in diameter. The organisms are fragile, and if fixation is not immediate, the infection is apt not to be recognized. Oöcysts are not easily demonstrable in fecal specimens, complicating diagnosis.

In tissue sections of small intestine or colon, the small, basophilic organisms are found embedded in microvilli of intestinal epithelial cells or just inside the cell membrane near the apical surface. Lesions may be minimal. Infected cells may be slightly more eosinophilic than normal, but extensive necrosis is not a feature of infection. There may be villous atrophy and cellular infiltration of the lamina propria with lymphocytes and plasma cells and lesser numbers of neutrophils and eosinophils. Clinical signs are usually inapparent, but chronic diarrhea has been associated with cryptosporidiosis, especially in young animals.

Diagnosis depends on demonstration of the organisms. The use of the Giemsa stain and thin sections is helpful.

Barker, I.K., and Carbonell, P.L.: *Cryptosporidium agni* sp. n. from lambs, and *Cryptosporidium bovis* sp. n. from a calf, with observations on the oocyst. Z. Parasitenkd., *44*:289–298, 1974.

Cockrell, B.Y., Valerio, M., and Garner, F.M.: Cryptosporidiosis in the intestines of rhesus monkeys (*Macaca mulatta*). Lab. Anim. Sci., *24*:881–887, 1974.

Fletcher, O.J., Munnell, J.F., and Page, R.K.: Cryptosporidiosis of the bursa of Fabricius of chickens. Avian Dis., *19*:630–639, 1975.

Kennedy, G.A., Kreitner, G.L., and Strafuss, A.C.: Cryptosporidiosis in three pigs. J. Am. Vet. Med. Assoc., *170*:348–350, 1977.

Meuten, D.J., Kruiningen, H.J. van, and Lein, D.H.: Cryptosporidiosis in a calf. J. Am. Vet. Med. Assoc., *165*:914–917, 1974.

Panciera, R.J., Thomassen, R.W., and Garner, F.M.: Cryptosporidial infection in a calf. Vet. Pathol., *8*:479–484, 1971.

Pohlenz, J., Moon, H.W., Cheville, N.F., and Bemrick, W.J.: Cryptosporidiosis as a probable factor in neonatal diarrhea of calves. J. Am. Vet. Med. Assoc., *172*:452–457, 1978.

Schmitz, J.A., and Smith, D.H.: Cryptosporidium infection in a calf. J. Am. Vet. Med. Assoc., *167*:731–732, 1975.

ENCEPHALITOZOONOSIS
(Nosematosis)

Encephalitozoon cuniculi, a minute organism presently classified with the Protozoa, is best known as a cause of encephalitis and nephritis of rabbits, but it may also infect laboratory rats, mice, guinea pigs, and monkeys, and has been reported in cats, dogs, and human beings. Infection in all susceptible species is often subclinical.

Life Cycle. Findings by Nelson (1962) and Lainson et al. (1964) indicate that this organism at one point in its life cycle develops a capsule and extrudes a polar filament. Organisms maintained by intraperitoneal inoculation of mice also have a developmental cycle and fine structure typical of protozoa classified as Microsporidia, particularly in the family Nosematidae. It has consequently been suggested that the organism be named *Nosema cuniculi* and the disease, "nosematosis." However, further studies with the life cycles of these organisms indicate that the species from mammals differs significantly from those that infect invertebrates and therefore should not be included in the genus, *Nosema.* The name *Encephalitozoon cuniculi* therefore appears to be valid for the mammalian parasite.

Of interest is the association of organisms of the family Nosematidae with diseases of bees, silkworms, and other invertebrate species. *Nosema apis* is the cause of destructive "nosema-disease" of honey bees, *Apis mellifica.* The organisms infect the midgut wall and malpighian tubules of the adult bees, especially the workers, although drones and queens are susceptible (Kudo, 1966).

Nosema bombycis may infect most cells of the silkworm, *Bombyx mori,* in any stage of development (embryo, larva, pupa, adult). Numerous tiny brownish-black foci are scattered over the body of the silkworm, giving rise to such names as "pebrine" and "Fleckenkrankheit." The organisms invade and multiply in the ova, infecting larvae before hatching, and often causing their death before pupation. Several other species of *Nosema* have been identified as parasites of mosquitoes, tapeworms, and beetles (Kudo, 1966).

Encephalitozoon cuniculi has been isolated from rabbit brain and cultivated on monolayer cell cultures from rabbit choroid plexus by Shadduck (1969). The development of this method of pure culture in vitro of this organism will undoubtedly facilitate its study.

Subclinical infections and encephalitis in man have also been associated with this organism (Matsubayashi et al., 1959). The possibility of transplacental passage of this organism was proposed by Innes, et al. (1962), and more recently demonstrated by Hunt et al. (1972).

Lesions. The lesions associated with infection are most characteristic in rabbits. The usual experience is to find the lesions and the organisms incidentally in histologic sections from rabbits which have shown no recognizable signs of infection, although in rare cases paralysis and death have been attributed to the parasite. In the brain, focal lesions are chiefly in the cerebral cortex, but may occur anywhere. Microscopic-sized granulomas made up of epithelioid cells surrounding a tiny necrotic center are the common finding in these occult infections. Larger areas of necrosis may be seen in fatal cases, and perivascular lymphocytic cuffing may be prominent. The organisms are demonstrable in the necrotic centers of the granulomas, usually appearing singly as

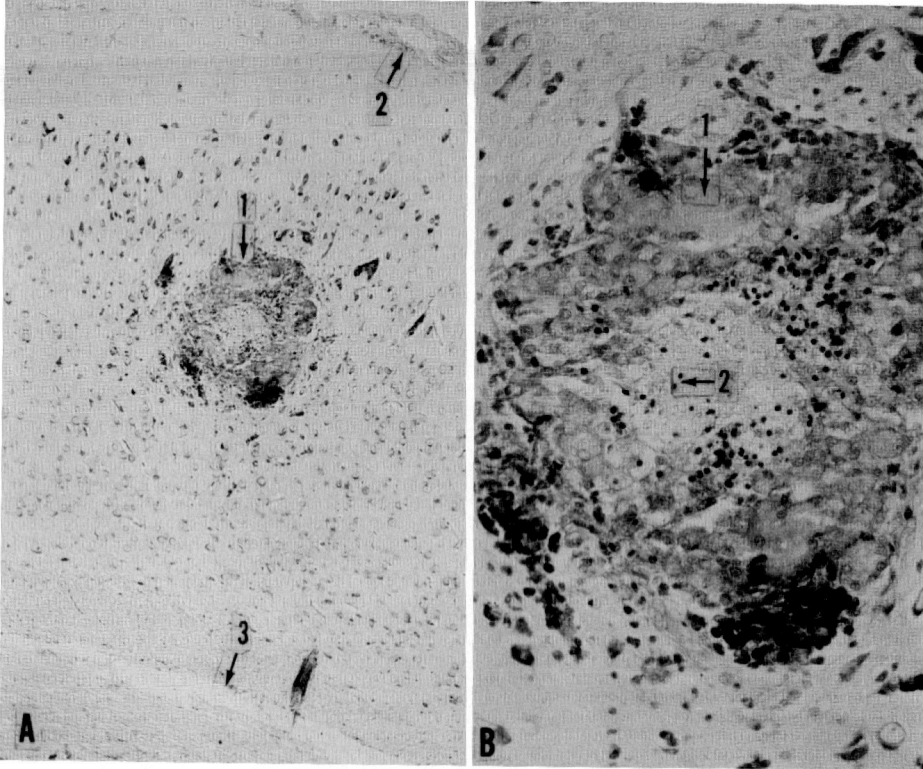

Fig. 13–16. Encephalitozoon infection, brain of a rabbit. *A*, Low power (× 45) to show granuloma *(1)* in the cerebral cortex. Pia mater *(2)* and ependyma *(3)* of lateral ventricle. *B*, Higher magnification of granuloma. Large, foamy macrophages *(1)* surrounding necrotic center containing organisms *(2)*. (Courtesy of Armed Forces Institute of Pathology.) Contributor: U. S. Army Environmental Health Laboratory.

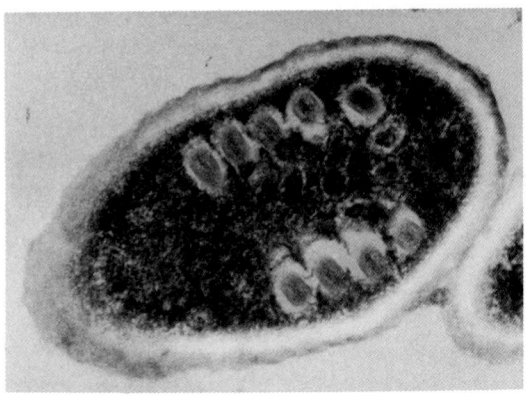

Fig. 13–17. *Encephalitozoon cuniculi* (× 36,800). Note cross section of polar filament. (Courtesy of Dr. J. A. Shadduck, Ohio State University, and *Science.*)

short, plump, rod-shaped bodies with rounded ends, measuring about 1 by 2 μ. They are stained intensely by silver impregnation methods (Warthin-Starry), accept Giemsa's stain, are acid-fast and gram-

positive, but are usually not visible in sections stained with hematoxylin and eosin.

Encephalitozoon cuniculi is also a cause of chronic nephritis characterized by lymphocytic infiltration, granulomas, and small focal scars. The organisms may be found in association with the lesions and in tubular epithelium. Myocarditis and vasculitis have also been attributed to encephalitozoonosis. The organism is apparently capable of infecting a variety of cell types and in time will undoubtedly be associated with lesions in other organs, but it clearly has a predilection for the brain and kidney.

Diagnosis. Diagnosis depends upon demonstrating the organisms in tissue section, isolation in tissue culture, or mouse inoculation. In the mouse peritoneum, the organism may be demonstrated to extrude its polar filament and be actively motile. Electron micrographs reveal the polar filament when it is coiled within the body of the parasite and enveloped by membranes.

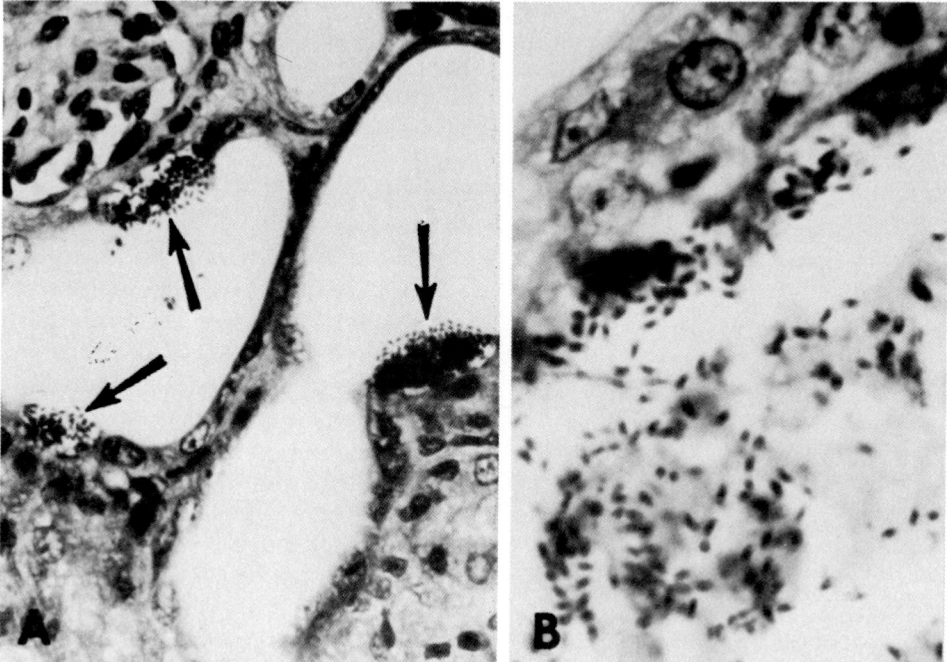

Fig. 13–18. Encephalitozoonosis, rabbit. *A, Encephalitozoon (Nosema) cuniculi* (arrows) within renal tubular epithelial cells. *B,* Organisms being extruded from epithelial cells and free within tubular lumen.

Occasionally it may be seen in longitudinal array (Fig. 13–17). The spores are about 2 microns long and also contain a laminated structure known as the polaroplast. Serologic tests have also been developed.

Anver, M.R., King, N.W., and Hunt, R.D.: Congenital encephalitozoonosis in a squirrel monkey (Saimiri sciureus). Vet. Pathol., 9:475–480, 1972.

Basson, P.A., et al.: Nosematosis: report of a canine case in the republic of South Africa. J. S. Afr. Vet. Med. Assoc., 37:3–9, 1966.

Buyukmihci, N., Bellhorn, R.W., Hunziker, J., and Clinton, J.: Encephalitozoon (Nosema) infection of the cornea in a cat. J. Am. Vet. Med. Assoc., 171:355–357, 1977.

Connor, D.H., Strano, A.J., and Neafie, R.C.: Nosema—a recently recognized pathogen of man. Lab. Invest., 30:371, 1974.

Cox, J.C., Walden, N.B., and Nairn, R.C.: Presumptive diagnosis of Nosema cuniculi in rabbits by immunofluorescence. Res. Vet. Sci., 13:595–597, 1972.

Flatt, R.E., and Jackson, S.J.: Renal nosematosis in young rabbits. Pathol. Vet., 7:492–497, 1970.

Hunt, R.D., King, N.W., Jr., and Foster, H.L.: Encephalitozoonosis: evidence for vertical transmission. J. Infect. Dis., 126:212–214, 1972.

Innes, J.R.M., Zeman, W., Frenkel, J.K., and Borner, G.: Occult, endemic encephalitozoonosis of the central nervous system of mice. J. Neuropathol. Exp. Neurol., 21:519–533, 1962.

Koller, L.D.: Spontaneous Nosema cuniculi infection in laboratory rabbits. J. Am. Vet. Med. Assoc., 155:1108–1114, 1969.

Kudo, R.R.: Protozoology, 5th ed. Springfield, Charles C Thomas, 1966.

Lainson, R., Garnham, P.C.C., Killick-Kendrick, R., and Bird, R.G.: Nosematosis, a microsporidial infection of rodents and other animals, including man. Br. Med. J., 2:470–472, 1964.

Matsubayashi, H., et al.: A case of encephalitozoon-like body infection in man. Arch. Pathol., 67:181–187, 1959.

Nelson, J.B.: An intracellular parasite resembling a microsporidian associated with ascites in Swiss mice. Proc. Soc. Exp. Biol. Med., 109:714–717, 1962.

Nordstoga, K., and Westbye, K.: Polyarteritis nodosa associated with nosematosis in blue foxes. Acta Pathol. Microbiol. Scand., 84A:291–296, 1976.

Pakes, S.P., Shadduck, J.A., and Cali, A.: Fine structure of Encephalitozoon cuniculi from rabbits, mice, and hamsters. J. Protozool., 22:481–488, 1975.

Perrin, T.L.: Toxoplasma and Encephalitozoon in spontaneous and in experimental infections of animals. Arch. Pathol., 36:568–578, 1943.

Petri, M., and Schiodt, T.: On the ultrastructure of Nosema cuniculi in the cells of the Yoshida rat ascites sarcoma. Acta Pathol. Microbiol. Scand., 66:437–446, 1966.

Plowright, W.: An encephalitis-nephritis syndrome in dog probably due to congenital Encephalitozoon infection. J. Comp. Pathol, Therap., 62:83–92, 1952.

Rensburg, I.B.J. van, and Plessis, J.L. du: Nosematosis in a cat: a case report. J. S. Afr. Vet. Med. Assoc., 42:327–331, 1971.

Shadduck, J.A.: Nosema cuniculi: in vitro isolation. Science, 166:516–517, 1969.

Weiser, J.: Nosema muris, n. sp. a new microsporidian parasite of the white mouse (Mus musculus. L.). J. Protozool., 12:78–83, 1965.

Wosu, N.J., et al.: Diagnosis of encephalitozoonosis in experimentally infected rabbits by intradermal and immuno-fluorescence tests. Lab. Anim. Sci., 27:210–216, 1977.

AMEBIASIS

Parasitic protozoa classified within the Class Sarcodina—those with pseudopodia—are best known as pathogens of man, but also of nonhuman primates and less frequently other animals. These organisms usually inhabit the intestinal tract and may be present in the absence of recognizable effects. However, under some circumstances, severe dysentery may result from their presence. The ameba may ulcerate and invade the intestinal wall, and possibly migrate to the liver or brain, resulting in "amebic" abscesses.

(The student will note that the diphthong (oe) is used in the names of some of these protozoa but, in the United States, is dropped in referring to the disease or organisms generally. Another point of possible confusion lies in the names of amebae of the genera Entamoeba and Endamoeba. At one time these organisms were considered in one genus; currently, they are separated. Entamoeba includes pathogens of man and other mammals; Endamoeba are generally found in lower invertebrates.)

The most important pathogen in this group appears to be Entamoeba histolytica, the cause of amebic dysentery in man, chimpanzee, rhesus monkey, dog, cat, rat, and pig. The pathogenetic mechanisms of this organism are not fully understood although it requires bacteria to survive in the intestinal tract and lives in many cases without causing overt disease. Fully 10%

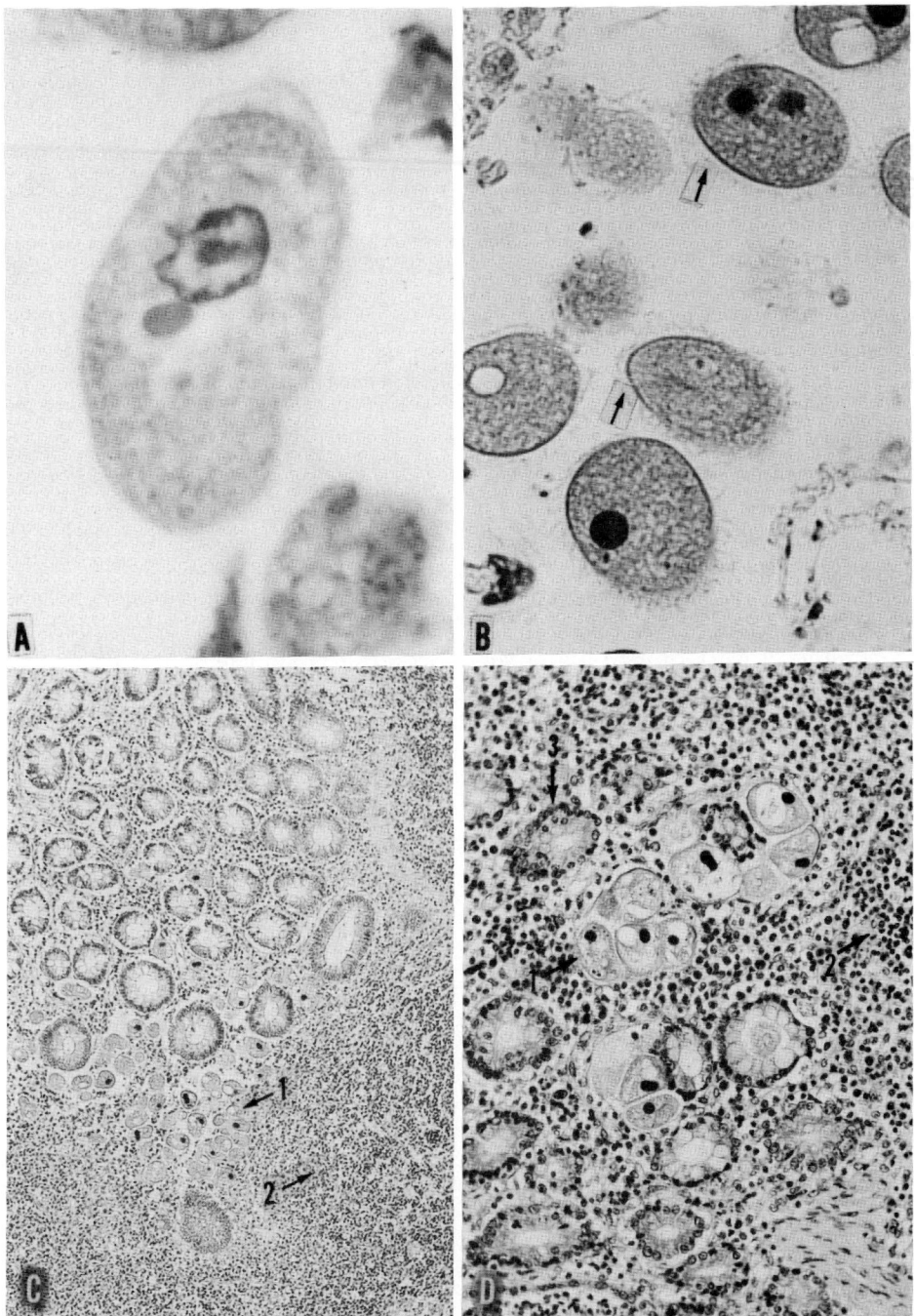

Fig. 13–19. *A, Entamoeba histolytica* (× 1750) in experimental amebiasis in a kitten. Contributor: Dr. H. E. Melleney. *B, Balantidium coli* (× 600) from colon of an orangutan. Note cilia (arrows). *C, Balantidium coli (1)* deep in the mucosa of the colon of an orangutan (× 75). Note lymphocytes *(2)*. Contributor: National Zoological Park. *D, Balantidium coli* (× 185) in mucosa of ileum of a pig *(1)*, lymphocytes *(2)*, and intestinal epithelium *(3)*. (Courtesy of Armed Forces Institute of Pathology.) Contributor: Lt. Col. F. D. Maurer.

of normal people studied in some surveys (Soulsby, 1968) are shown to be asymptomatic carriers. The organism may be transmitted between hosts by contamination of food or water by food handlers who are carriers, by means of cysts borne by flies or cockroaches, or by consumption of contaminated water, in which amebic cysts may survive for long periods.

Lesions. Once infection is established, reproduction is by binary fission, and under appropriate but unknown circumstances, trophozoites invade and undermine the mucosa, leading to variously sized ulcers. The trophozoites may be found deep in the wall of the colon, usually associated with a flask-shaped ulcer of the mucosa. The parasite is presumed to secrete a lytic enzyme under some as yet undetermined circumstances. Ulcerative colitis may lead to amebic abscesses in the liver or brain, at least in man, chimpanzees, and rhesus monkeys. One significant property of *E. histolytica* is its tendency to phagocytize erythrocytes.

The trophozoites of amebae are recognized in tissue sections as irregularly spherical organisms without cilia but often having pseudopodia. They have a distinct or indistinct nucleus, depending upon the species, and their abundant cytoplasm is often vacuolated and may contain phagocytized erythrocytes or tissue debris. Their over-all size is variable, as they range from 10 to 60 μ in diameter. They may be seen in intestinal crypts, in necrotic foci in the submucosa, or at the margins of sharply demarcated ulcers.

Diagnosis. The diagnosis may be made tentatively by identifying trophozoites of *E. histolytica* in the feces in the presence of dysentery, and confirmed by demonstrating the organisms in ulcers or abscesses.

Brandt, H., and Tamayo, R.P.: Pathology of human amebiasis. Hum. Pathol., *1*:351–385, 1970.
Burrows, R.B., and Lillis, W.G.: Intestinal protozoan infection in dogs. J. Am. Vet. Med. Assoc., *150*:880–883, 1967.

Jordan, H.E.: Amebiasis *(Entamoeba histolytica)* in the dog. Vet. Med. Small Anim. Clin., *62*:61–64, 1967.
Miller, M.J., and Bray, R.S.: *Entamoeba histolytica* infections in the chimpanzee *(Pan satyrus)*. J. Parasitol., *52*:386–388, 1966.
Mortelmans, J., Vercruysse, J., and Kageruka, P.: Three pathogenic intestinal protozoa of anthropoid apes: *Entamoeba histolytica, Balantidium coli* and *Troglodytella abrassarti. In* Proceedings of Third International Congress of Primatology, Vol. 2, edited by J. Biegert and W. Leutenegger. Basel, S. Karger, 1971, pp. 187–191.
Rees, C.W.: Pathogenesis of intestinal amoebiasis in kittens. Arch. Pathol., *7*:1–26, 1929.
Sebesteny, A.: Pathogenicity of intestinal flagellates in mice. Lab. Anim., *3*:71–77, 1969.
Soulsby, E.J.L.: Helminths, Arthropods and Protozoa of Domesticated Animal, 6th ed. Philadelphia, Lea & Febiger, 1968.

GIARDIASIS

Protozoa of the genus *Giardia* are pyriform in shape and bilaterally symmetrical. The anterior end is rounded and the posterior is elongated, nearly pointed. The convex ventral surface bears a large sucking disc. Each organism has four pair of flagella. These organisms are common inhabitants of the small intestine and colon of man and animals.

Although the pathogenicity of these organisms has been disputed, infection with *Giardia* is associated with dysentery, especially in young animals and children. The organisms localize in the small intestine on the surface of epithelial cells. Cellular infiltration of the lamina propria accompanies the presence of the organisms, but the lesions and the clinical signs are usually minimal.

Several species of *Giardia* and their hosts have been identified: *Giardia lamblia* (man), *G. canis* (dog), *G. cati* (cat), *G. chinchillae* (chinchilla), and *G. bovis* (cattle).

Burrows, R.B., and Lillis, W.G.: Intestinal protozoan infections in dogs. J. Am. Vet. Med. Assoc., *150*:880–883, 1967.
Kudo, R.R.: Protozoology, 5th ed. Springfield, Charles C Thomas, 1966.
Soulsby, E.J.L.: Helminths, Arthropods and Protozoa of Domesticated Animals, 6th ed. Philadelphia, Lea & Febiger, 1968.

PNEUMOCYSTOSIS

A protozoan organism of uncertain taxonomic classification, *Pneumocystis carinii* is known to inhabit the pulmonary alveoli of man and animals, and under certain conditions, causes severe disruption of respiratory function. *Pneumocystis* pneumonia has been recognized in man, dogs, horses, swine, goats, and monkeys, and the organisms have been identified in the lungs of many additional species in the absence of clinical disease. Human beings and animals suffering from disorders of the lymphoreticular system or immune mechanisms (e.g., agammaglobulinemia), or who undergo adrenocorticosteroid therapy, may develop the disease. It is also associated with malignant lymphoma and other diseases of the bone marrow. Similar

activation of latent infection has been reported in rats treated with cortisone acetate (Frenkel, Good and Shultz, 1966). Although the organisms in the various hosts are morphologically indistinguishable, some evidence indicates that each may be specific for the respective species. Failure to infect hamsters and rabbits with rat strains, and the absence of common complement-fixing antigens in human and rat strains, supports this concept of species specificity. Infection with other organisms, particularly *Corynebacterium kutscheri* and *Aspergillus sp.*, may complicate the disease in rats.

The organisms are located in alveoli adjacent to the surface of alveolar lining cells, and may become numerous enough to entirely fill some alveoli. Alveolar lining cells may become enlarged, but inflammatory

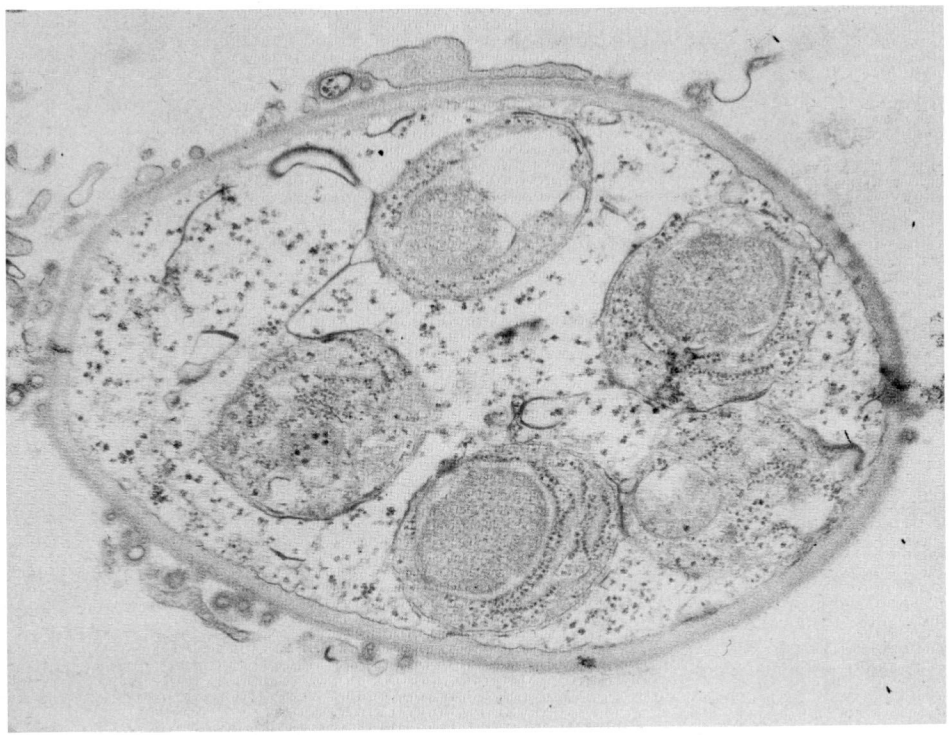

Fig. 13–20. *Pneumocystis carinii*, from the lung of a rat following treatment with cortisone acetate. Electron micrograph (× 25,000) of thick-walled organism with five intracystic bodies. (Courtesy of Drs. Earl G. Barton, Jr., Wallace G. Campbell, Jr. and *The American Journal of Pathology*.)

response to the organisms is usually minimal. The organisms may be seen with the light microscope as spherical cysts about 4.5 μ in diameter, sometimes slightly wrinkled, cup-shaped or crescentic. Some cysts contain intracystic bodies about 1 μ in diameter; as many as eight of these bodies have been identified within a single cyst. Gomori's methenamine silver stain and the PAS stain are useful in delineating these organisms.

Electron micrographs reveal thick- and thin-walled organisms containing intracystic bodies. The thin-walled organisms have been interpreted to be trophozoites. The thick-walled organisms contain one to eight intracystic bodies, which are limited by a pellicle, which is continuous with membranous structures in the cytoplasm of the cyst (Fig. 13–20). The completely developed intracystic body contains rough endoplasmic reticulum, a single mitochondrion, vacuoles, and a nucleus containing a nucleolus. These bodies apparently escape from the cyst through defects in the cyst wall and grow to be trophozoites as large as 5 μ in diameter, and contain particles resembling glycogen and lipid. Since liposomes, dense bodies, Golgi apparatus, and cytosomes are not present, it is believed that these organisms do not utilize phagocytic processes, and may metabolize substances of low molecular weight obtained from adjacent cells or intra-alveolar fluid (Barton and Campbell, 1969).

Barton, E.G., and Campbell, W.G., Jr.: *Pneumocystis carinii* in lungs of rats treated with cortisone acetate. Ultrastructural observations relating to the life cycle. Am. J. Pathol., *54*:209–236, 1969.

Chandler, F.W., McClure, H.M., Campbell, W.G., Jr., and Watts, J.C.: Pulmonary pneumocystosis in nonhuman primates. Arch. Pathol. Lab. Med., *100*:163–167, 1976.

Copland, J.W.: Canine pneumonia caused by *Pneumocystis carinii*. Aust. Vet. J., *50*:515–518, 1974.

Farrow, B.R.H., Watson, A.D.J., Hartley, W.J. and Huxtable, C.R.R.: Pneumocystis pneumonia in the dog. J. Comp. Pathol., *82*:447–453, 1972.

Frenkel, J.K., Good, J.T., and Shultz, J.A.: Latent pneumocystis infections of rats, relapse, and chemotherapy. Lab. Invest., *15*:1559–1577, 1966.

Seibold, H.R., and Munnell, J.F.: *Pneumocystis carinii* in a pig. Vet. Pathol., *14*:89–91, 1977.

Shively, J.N., et al.: *Pneumocystis carinii* pneumonia in two foals. J. Am. Vet. Med. Assoc., *162*:648–652, 1973.

Shively, J.N., Moe, K.K., and Dellers, R.W.: Fine structure of spontaneous *Pneumocystis carinii* pulmonary infection in foals. Cornell Vet., *64*:72–88, 1974.

HARTMANNELLOSIS— ACANTHAMEBIASIS

Certain protozoa in the class Sarcodina, order Amoebida, have been incriminated as pathogenic in certain tissues of man and animals. These have been identified as belonging to one of two closely related and similar genera: *Hartmannella* or *Acanthamoeba*. A species name has not been applied, but at the moment the genus *Hartmannella* is favored, and the disease is called hartmannellosis. Spontaneous cases of meningoencephalitis in man (Butt, 1966) have been attributed to this organism, as has a case of gangrenous bronchopneumonia in a bull (McConnell, Garner and Kirk, 1968).

Lesions. A case of disseminated acanthamebiasis in a dog has been described by Ayers et al. (1972). The central nervous system lesions are characterized by a hemorrhagic purulent and necrotizing inflammation. An amebic meningoencephalitis caused by an ameboflagellate of the genus *Naegleria* is recognized in human beings and has been experimentally reproduced in mice and monkeys.

Diagnosis. The organisms are reportedly cultivatable without difficulty, but also may be identified in tissue sections. They are usually present in large numbers in the lesion and are seen in two forms, with some intermediate types. In Ziegler's hematoxylin-eosin stain (Ziegler, 1944), the large form is about 9 to 12 μ in diameter, acidophilic, with a thin wall and one (occasionally two) central basophilic body, the karyosome. This karyosome serves to differentiate *Entamoeba histolytica* which

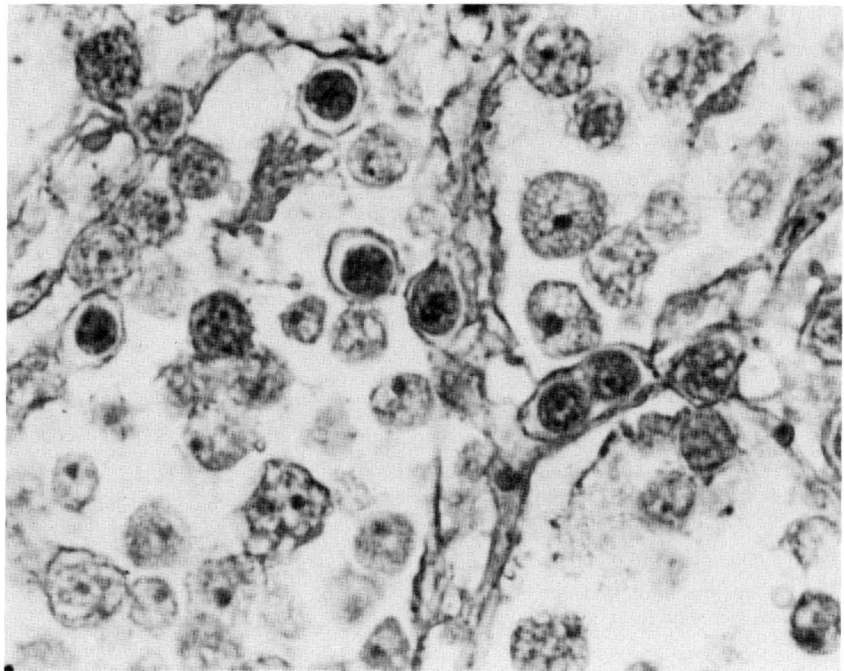

Fig. 13–21. *Hartmannella sp.* from a bovine lung (× 900). Note trophozoite and cyst forms. (Courtesy of Col. F. N. Garner, V.C., Armed Forces Institute of Pathology.)

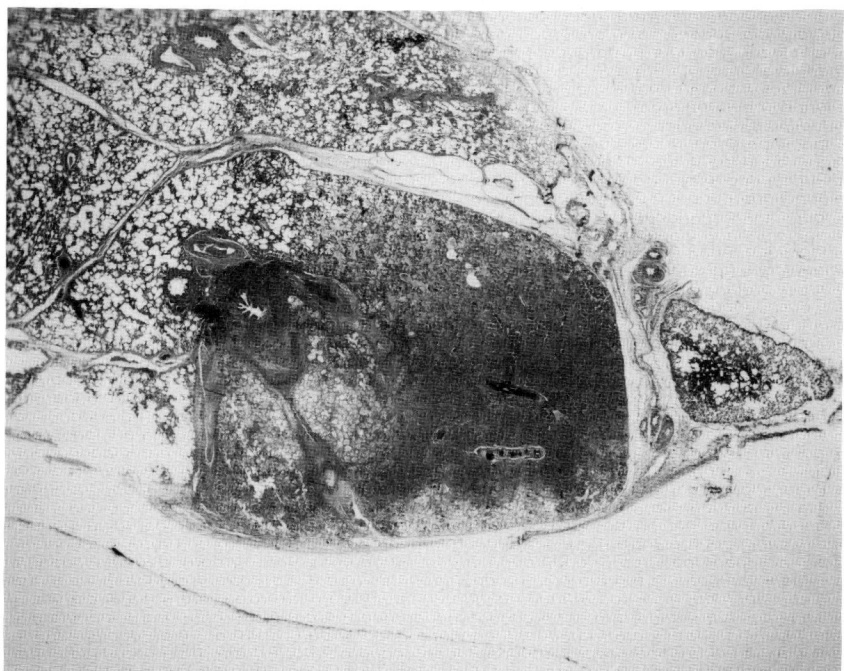

Fig. 13–22. Pneumonia, lung of a bull due to *Hartmannella sp.* (Courtesy of Col. F. N. Garner, V.C., Armed Forces Institute of Pathology.)

does not have one. This form, considered the trophozoite, has a moderate affinity for Gomori's methenamine silver stain, and periodic acid Schiff (PAS) reaction, and is blue to amphophylic with Giemsa's stain. The second form of *Hartmannella* is somewhat smaller (9 to 10 μ in diameter), more uniform in size, and has a membranous capsule which is often separated from the central body by a clear halo. These cystic forms are more basophilic in sections stained with hematoxylin and eosin. The PAS reaction is strongly positive, and the organisms are quite argentophilic in Gomori's methenamine silver stain.

The diagnosis may be established by recovering and identifying the organisms in association with necrotizing lesions. The organisms may be identified in microscopic sections by their presence in typical lesions and their characteristic morphology and staining properties.

Ayers, K.M., Billups, L.H., and Garner, F.M.: Acanthamoebiasis in a dog. Vet. Pathol., 9:221–226, 1972.

Butt, C.G.: Primary amebic meningoencephalitis. N. Engl. J. Med., 274:1473–1476, 1966.

Culbertson, C.G., Smith, J.W., Cohen, H.K., and Minner, J.R.: Experimental infection of mice and monkeys by *Acanthamoeba*. Am. J. Pathol., 35:185–197, 1959.

Martinez, A.J., Nelson, E.C., and Duma, R.J.: Primary amebic meningoencephalitis, *Naegleria* meningoencephalitis. CNS protozoal infection. Am. J. Pathol., 73:545–548, 1973.

McConnell, E.E., Garner, F.M., and Kirk, J.H.: Hartmannellosis in a bull. Pathol. Vet., 5:1–6, 1968.

Ziegler, E.E.: Hematoxylin-eosin tissue stain, an improved and uniform technique. Arch. Pathol., 37:68–69, 1944.

TRICHOMONIASIS

Protozoa in the class Mastigophora include a family, Trichomonadidae, of flagellated organisms, some of which are pathogenic. Two genera are of special interest: *Tritrichomonas* (with three anterior flagella) and *Trichomonas* (with four anterior flagella). Organisms of the genus *Giardia* were discussed previously.

Tritrichomonas foetus is the cause of **bovine trichomoniasis,** an important genital infection in cattle. The organism is transmitted by coitus and results in vaginitis in the female and balanitis in the male. Infection of the uterus or placenta may result in endometritis or placentitis, which terminates in early abortion and sometimes in sterility. Pyometra may result from uterine infection when the cervix is closed and the uterus fills with fluid teeming with trichomonads.

The diagnosis is established by demonstrating *Tritrichomonas foetus* in vaginal, uterine, or preputial exudates in association with a herd history of decreased fertility, abortions, vaginitis, metritis, and balanitis. Direct microscopic examination may not be adequate if numbers of trichomonads are small, as is often the case in bulls. Culture of the organisms is more accurate. Test matings are also effective in diagnosing infected bulls.

Tritrichomonas suis is found in the digestive and upper respiratory tracts of swine, but its pathogenicity is not completely established. *Trichomonas gallinae* is the etiologic agent in **avian trichomoniasis,** a serious inflammation of the upper gastrointestinal tract of pigeons, turkeys, chickens, and wild birds. *Trichomonas vaginalis* is found in the vagina, urethra, and prostate of women and men. It may be carried without producing signs, especially in men, but also may result in vaginitis or urethritis. It is transmitted by coitus. *Tritrichomonas fecalis (T. equi)* is a common organism of the intestinal flora of normal horses. It has been blamed as a cause of gastroenteritis, but there is no good evidence in support of this supposition. Other species of trichomonads have been suspected in cases of gastrointestinal infection (Bennett and Franco, 1969) but it is difficult to prove that these organisms are pathogenic in the digestive tract where they may thrive in the absence of disease.

Bennett, S.P., and Franco, D.A.: Equine protozoan diarrhea (equine intestinal trichomoniasis) at Trinidad racetracks. J. Am. Vet. Assoc., 154:58–60, 1969.

Clark, B.L., White, M.B., and Banfield, J.C.: Diagnosis of *Trichomonas foetus* infection in bulls. Aust. Vet. J., 47:181–183, 1971.

Damron, G.W.: Gastrointestinal trichomonads in horses: occurrence and identification. Am. J. Vet. Res., 37:25–28, 1976.

Soulsby, E.J.L.: Helminths, Arthropods and Protozoa of Domesticated Animals (Mönnig), 6th ed. Philadelphia, Lea & Febiger, 1968.

Todorovic, R., and McNutt, S.H.: Diagnosis of *Trichomonas foetus* infection in bulls. Am. J. Vet. Res., 28:1581–1590, 1967.

BALANTIDIASIS

The only member of the ciliated Protozoa, the Infusoria, which is of pathogenic significance (and this is questionable) is *Balantidium coli (B. suis)*. This comparatively large, single-celled organism is a natural inhabitant of the digestive tract of swine, man, and sometimes other vertebrates, usually living in the lumen or between the villi and causing no recognizable effect on the host. Under some imperfectly understood circumstances, *Balantidium coli* will invade the intestinal mucosa, penetrating into the submucosa, localizing particularly in lymphoid nodules. Occasionally, it may reach the genital tract. This tissue penetration results in varying degrees of acute inflammation in the vicinity and may result in some manifestations of enteric disease. Since its pathogenicity is questioned and most certainly limited, *Balantidium coli* is of interest to the pathologist as an organism that might be present with frank pathogens, but should not be mistakenly considered the cause of every disease with which it is associated (Fig. 13–19B,C,D).

Hatziolos, B.C.: Balantidium in bovine respiratory tract. Delt. Hellen. Kten. Hetair., 24:8–18, 1973.

Savchenko, V.F., and Karput, I.M.: Pathology and histology of Balantidium infection in pigs. Uchen. Zap. Vitebsk. Vet. Inst., 22:22–26, 1970.

TRYPANOSOMIASIS

Trypanosomiasis is often thought of as an exotic disease that occurs only in tropical Africa, India, and other far-off places. It is true that this disease is most serious in man and animals in certain regions of the world, but trypanosomes are distributed throughout all parts of the globe, often producing no recognizable disease in the host in which they reside. The disease in man with many names, such as **African sleeping sickness, tsetse fly disease, maladie du sommeil, Schlaffkrankheit,** and **doenca do sono,** has influenced the course of history, particularly in Africa, by denying people the use of certain lands and causing them to go to war over those areas relatively free of the disease. The disease in domesticated livestock has also played a similar historical role. Although urbanization and control measures have reduced the frequency of the disease, it still remains a serious problem in some areas of Africa and South America.

Life Cycle. These protozoa are flagellated, motile parasites that frequent the blood of many vertebrate and invertebrate hosts and localize in tissues, sometimes in a nonflagellated form. Trypanosomes have certain common anatomic features such as: an ovoid or rounded body in the nonflagellate stage, and a slender elongate body when it becomes flagellated; the flagellum arises from the dot-shaped blepharoplast and extends to or projects from the anterior pole of the organism; an undulating membrane extends along the border of the organism, with the flagellum forming its margin; a spherical or rod-shaped structure, the parabasal body, together with the blepharoplast, makes up the kinetoplast. A relatively large round or ovoid nucleus containing a more deeply staining karyosome is usually located near the middle of the body.

Trypanosomes multiply by longitudinal fission, but the exact details of their division are unknown. They may be cultivated in noncellular media, tissue cultures, or chick embryos, but are commonly maintained by experimental infection of laboratory animals. The life cycle in nature involves both vertebrate and invertebrate hosts, the latter acting as vectors of the

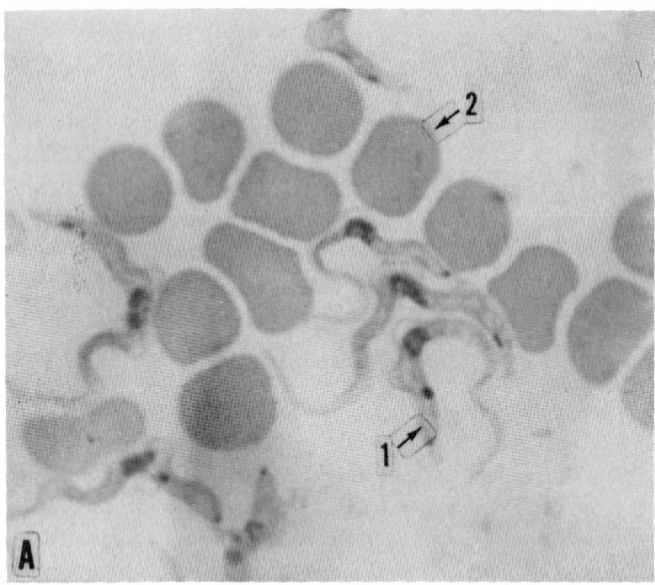

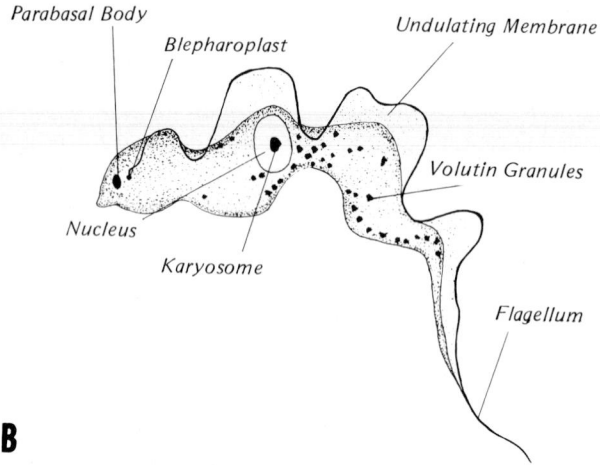

Fig. 13–23. Trypanosomiasis. *A, Trypanosoma equiperdum (1)* in the blood of a rat. Erythrocyte *(2)*. (Courtesy of Armed Forces Institute of Pathology.) Contributor: Dr. Kent Davis. *B*, Diagram of the morphology of a trypanosome.

infection. Mechanical transmission of trypanosomes may be accomplished by certain biting flies (*Tabanus, Stomoxys*), but definite cyclic development occurs in the body of the true invertebrate hosts (*Glossina, Triatoma*). In these hosts, the trypanosomes multiply in various forms in the digestive tract, and eventually migrate as infective forms to the salivary glands, in preparation for infection of a new vertebrate host.

Trypanosomes usually can be identified by their morphologic features, such as size, shape, position, arrangement, and development of the organelles, but no completely satisfactory classification scheme has yet been devised. Most species of trypanosomes do not produce serious effects upon their host, but a few are important pathogens (Table 13–3).

Pathogenesis. The pathogenesis of trypanosomiasis in man or animals is not

Table 13–3. Important Trypanosomes of Man and Animals

Species	Definitive Host	Intermediate Hosts (Vectors)	Geographic Distribution	Disease
T. lewisi	Rats	Fleas—several species	Cosmopolitan	None
T. theileri	Cattle	Tabanid flies	Cosmopolitan	None
T. melophagium	Sheep	Louse fly *(Melophagus ovinus)*	Temperate zones	None
T. theodori	Horses	Louse fly *(Lipoptena caprina)*	Palestine, Syria	None
T. cruzi	Man, armadillo, cat, opossum, dog	"Kissing bug" *(Triatoma sp.)*	S. America	Chagas' disease South American trypanosomiasis
T. evansi	Horse, mule, ass, cattle, buffalo	Horse flies *(Tabanidae* and *Stomoxys)*	Africa, Asia, S. America, Far East	Surra
T. equiperdum	Horse, ass	Trans. by coitus	Cosmopolitan	Dourine
T. vivax (uniforme)	Cattle, sheep, horse, goat, camel	Tsetse fly *(Glossina sp.)*	Central and S. America, Martinique, Guadaloupe, Mauritius and Africa	Souma
T. caprae	Horse, sheep, cattle	Tsetse fly	Tanzania Nyasaland	Trypanosomiasis
T. congolense, dimorphon	Cattle, horse, goat, sheep, ass, pig, dog, camel	Tsetse fly	Tropical Africa	Trypanosomiasis
T. simiae	Monkey, pig, horse, sheep	Tsetse fly	East Africa	Trypanosomiasis
T. brucei	Man, domestic and wild mammals, except goats	Tsetse fly	Tropical Africa	Nagana
T. rhodesiense	Man, antelope	Tsetse fly	East Africa	Acute "sleeping sickness"
T. gambiense	Man, antelope	Tsetse fly	Tropical Africa	Chronic "sleeping sickness"

thoroughly understood. The mechanisms that induce disease or cause death are essentially unknown. According to Weinman (1968), death cannot be explained on the basis of terminal hypoglycemia, anoxia, acidosis, or elevated potassium levels in the plasma. Some hepatic dysfunction is indicated by elevated serum levels of glutamic oxaloacetic and glutamic pyruvic transaminase. Anemia may be severe enough to cause death, but its pathogenesis is not settled. Erythrophago-cytosis may play a role, but there is gathering evidence that the anemia is immunologically mediated. Hypersensitivity to trypanosomal antigens may explain some acute deaths, through such reactions as anaphylaxis. Immune-mediated mechanisms may also contribute to the lesions of more chronically infected animals, leading to the extensive mononuclear tissue infiltrates and immune-complex glomerulonephritis. Except for *Trypanosoma cruzi*, the organisms do not invade tissue cells and therefore do not produce effects by direct destruction of cells. No specific tissue response has been recognized, although reticuloendothelial proliferation has been described in spleen and liver.

Specific Infections. *Dourine.* A disease of Equidae, dourine has a cosmopolitan distribution but is now rare in the United States. In contrast to other trypanosomiases, the causative agent, *Trypanosoma equiperdum*, is transmitted by coitus, rarely by biting flies. The disease is manifest by edematous lesions in the genital tract and ventral body wall, persistent ulcerous plaques in the genitalia and skin, and occasionally by anemia, incoordination, and paralysis. The causative trypanosome is demonstrable in the lesions, particularly those of the genitalia. The lesions are those of a mononuclear or granulomatous inflammation. Rabbits and deer mice are experimentally susceptible.

Nagana. (Tsetse Fly Disease). Nagana is most commonly used as a collective term for African trypanosomiasis of domesticated animals, particularly those infections caused by *Trypanosoma brucei* (Bruce, 1894), *T. congolense* (Broden, 1904), and *T. vivax* (Ziemann, 1905). The local term "Souma" is sometimes applied to infection with *T. vivax*. A large number and variety of wild animals may serve as reservoirs of infection, apparently with impunity to themselves. Nagana occurs in all domesticated animals in tropical Africa, resulting in acute or chronic manifestations with irregular fever, anemia, emaciation, subcutaneous edema, weakness, conjunctivitis, photophobia, lacrimation, and neurologic signs of tremor, hyperexcitability, incoordination, paresis, dullness, and coma. Death may occur following an acute illness or after a prolonged course, during which gradual wasting is a dominant feature. Postmortem examination usually discloses severe emaciation with edematous changes in all fatty tissues. The lymph nodes are swollen, edematous, occasionally with hemorrhage in the medulla; the liver is enlarged and congested. The spleen is either enlarged, normal, or atrophic with prominent malpighian corpuscles. Hemorrhages are common, particularly in subendocardial and epicardial locations. Pericardial fluid may be excessive. Congestion and hemorrhage may be a prominent feature in the gastrointestinal tract. Trypanosomes are found in blood and other body fluids as well as free in tissues, where they incite an inflammatory reaction, predominantly mononuclear. Mononuclear inflammation may occur in virtually every body tissue, including skeletal muscle, myocardium, brain, spinal cord, and meninges, eye, liver, adrenal gland, uterus and skin. Lymph nodes and spleen are hyperplastic. Erythrophagocytosis may be conspicuous throughout the reticuloendothelial system.

Surra. The important trypanosomiasis of Asia occurs principally in Equidae, but dogs, elephants, and ruminants may be infected, and wild ruminants can act as reservoirs. Camels are also susceptible, and guinea pigs can be experimentally infected. The causative organism, *Trypanosoma evansi* (Evans, 1880), is transmitted mechanically by the bite of horse flies (*Tabanus, Stomoxys*). The disease is recognized most frequently in a severe form with paroxysms of intermittent fever associated with trypanosomes in the blood; gradual emaciation in spite of good appetite; serous nasal discharge; patchy alopecia; petechiae and ecchymoses of visible mucosae; weakness and incoordination; edema of the limbs, lower abdomen, and thorax; icterus; progressive anemia, and fatal termination.

Mal de Caderas. This trypanosomiasis of tropical and subtropical South America, which affects Equidae in particular, is caused by *Trypanosoma equinum* (Voges, 1901). The disease is an acute infection similar to surra.

Murrina de Caderas (Derrengadera de caderas). This occurs in Central America and is caused by *Trypanosoma hippicum,*

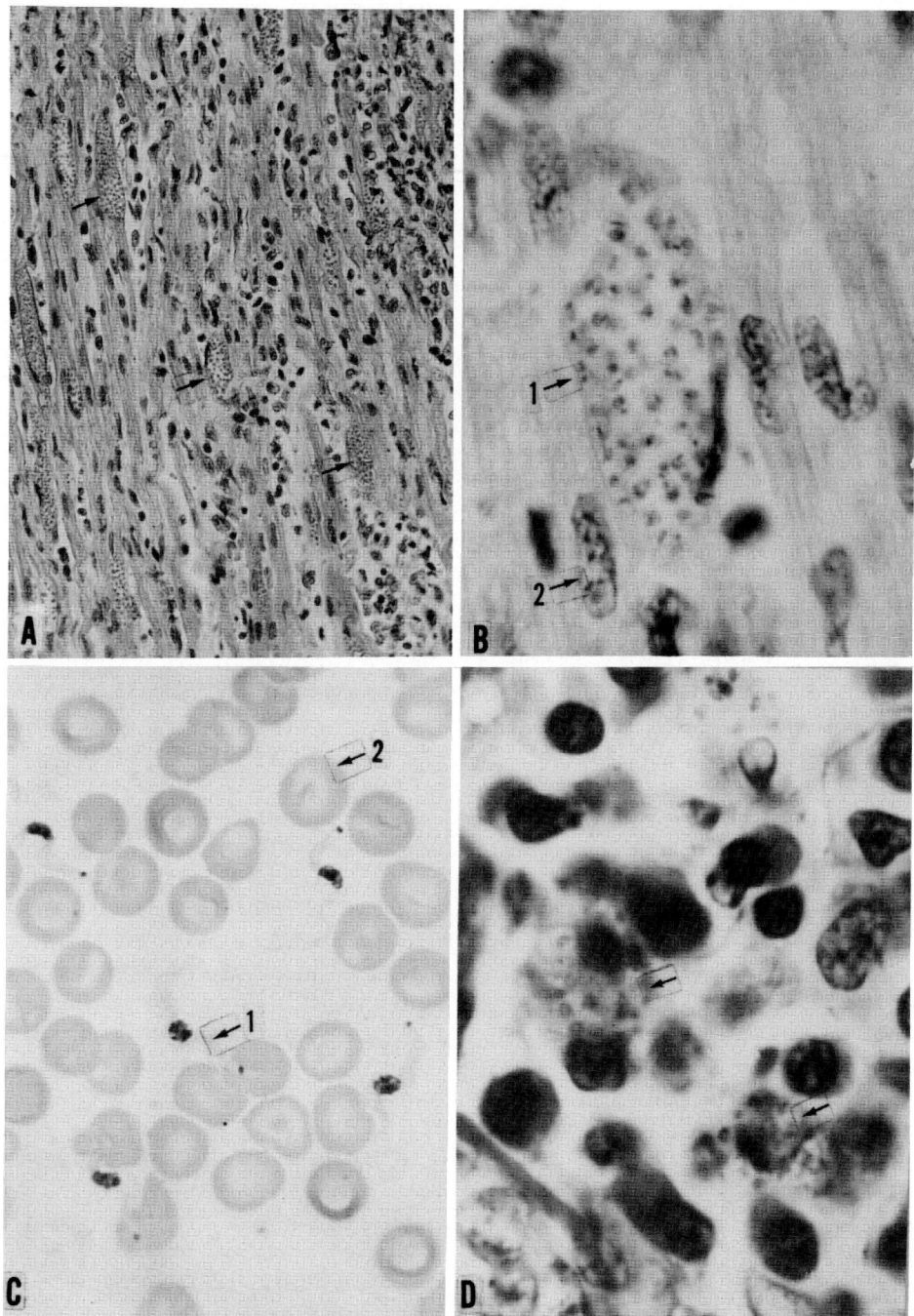

Fig. 13–24. *A, Trypanosoma cruzi* (arrows) (× 240) in the myocardium of a dog. *B,* Higher magnification (× 1240) showing leishmanial forms of *Tr. cruzi* in the cytoplasm *(1)* of a cardiac muscle bundle. One nucleus of a cardiac muscle cell is indicated by *(2).* Contributor: Dr. Francisco Laranja. *C, Tr. cruzi (1)* in the blood of a rat. Erythrocytes *(2).* Contributor: Lt. Col. F. D. Maurer. *D.* Leishmaniasis, lymph node of dog (× 1780); organisms (arrows) are in cytoplasm of macrophages. (Courtesy of Armed Forces Institute of Pathology.) Contributor: Dr. W. S. Bailey.

first described by Darling in 1910. Horses and mules are particularly susceptible; cattle act as reservoirs of infection. The disease is essentially similar to surra, although a more prolonged course is described, with weakness, emaciation, anemia, ecchymoses, edema, splenomegaly and paralysis being important features.

Chagas' Disease (American Trypanosomiasis). *Trypanosoma cruzi* was shown in 1909 by Chagas to be the cause of human trypanosomiasis in South America. The vectors were also proved by Chagas to be reduviid or "kissing" bugs (*Triatoma*). Dogs, cats, armadillos, monkeys, and small wild animals harbor the infection and are believed to be subject to a disease similar to the human infection. *Trypanosoma cruzi* is of particular interest because it assumes the typical trypanosomal form in the blood and tissues of mammals, in cultures, and in the intestine and rectum of insects, but it also occurs in leishmanial forms in both mammalian cells and tissue cultures, and develops transitional forms, typical of *Leptomonas* and *Crithidia*, intracellularly in mammals, in cultures, and in intestines of insects. Thus, this trypanosome appears to be closely related to *Leishmania*; in fact, it demonstrates a relationship between the two genera. One classification (Weinman, 1968) places *Trypanosoma cruzi* in a new genus, *Schizotrypanum*. It is further suggested that South American trypanosomiasis is no longer a specific name because a new trypanosome, *Trypanosoma rangelis*, has been found to affect man in the Americas.

Clinical Manifestations. The clinical manifestations are significantly related to damage in the brain and myocardium, although in some species (man, mouse, dog), edema may be a prominent feature. These edematous swellings occur in the subcutaneous fasciae and muscles and elevate the skin. Congestive heart failure with ascites and passive congestion of liver and spleen may also occur. Nervous manifesta-

tions point toward brain involvement, and cardiac collapse follows infection of the myocardium.

Lesions. The lesions result in part from the growth and activity of *T. cruzi* in the blood, but are most influenced by its intracellular activities. The initial lesion, seen in man following the bite of a reduviid bug, is a hard, red, painful edematous mass occurring at the site of the bite. This soon subsides as the organisms spread. The lymph nodes may become enlarged, edematous, and show intense histiocytic proliferation, and occasionally may contain microabscesses. Giant cells may form and contain leishmanial forms of *T. cruzi*. The heart is particularly affected. Myocardial fibers are penetrated by the organism, which proliferates, filling and destroying muscle cells and resulting in severe myocarditis. The heart becomes enlarged, the myocardium mottled with yellow, and the pericardial sac distended with fluid. Large cystic collections of leishmanial forms are demonstrable microscopically in cardiac muscle cells. The experimental disease in mice often results in myocarditis, particularly in the right ventricle. The right ventricle becomes distended and the ventricular wall thin. Passive congestion of liver and spleen is an expected result.

Skeletal and smooth muscles may also be invaded by this organism. In man, infection of smooth muscle of esophagus and colon may result in megaesophagus and megacolon. This finding has not been reported in animals.

In the brain, *T. cruzi* produces edema and congestion, particularly in the meninges, with some perivascular lymphocytic infiltration. Nodules of mononuclear and glial cells may occur throughout the brain. Within these areas the leishmanial forms of the trypanosomes are found in the cytoplasm of cells and free in the tissue. Destruction of neurons may lead to chronic neurologic sequelae.

The testicle may be severely invaded by

T. cruzi; the germinal cells become laden with organisms, and intense lymphocytic infiltration occurs in the interstitial stroma.

Diagnosis. The diagnosis depends upon demonstration of *T. cruzi* in blood or tissues of infected animals.

Chagas, C.: Ueber eine neue Trypanosomiasis des Menschen. Mem. Inst. Oswaldo Cruz (Rio de Janeiro), *1*:159–218, 1909.

Fernandez, D.B., Rico, F., and Dumag, P.U.: Observations on an outbreak of surra among cattle. Philipp. J. Anim. Ind., *21*:221–224, 1965. V.B. 37:517, 1967.

Fiennes, R.N.T.W., Jones, E.R., and Laws, S.G.: The course and pathology of *Trypanosoma congolense* (Broden) disease of cattle. J. Comp. Pathol. Ther., *56*:1–27, 1946.

Hoare, C.A.: Evolutionary trends in mammalian trypanosomes. Adv. Parasitol., *5*:47–91, 1967. V.B. 39:2852, 1969.

——: The classification of mammalian trypanosomes. Ergebn. Mikrobiol. Immunitatsforsch., *39*:49–57, 1966. V.B. 36:3868, 1966.

——: Nagana. Trans. R. Soc. Trop. Med. Hyg., *64*:531–532, 1971.

——: **The Trypanosomes of Mammals. A Zoological Monograph. Oxford and Edinburgh, Blackwell, 1972.**

Ikede, B.O.: Ocular lesions in sheep infected with *Trypanosoma brucei.* J. Comp. Pathol., *84*:203–213, 1974.

Ikede, B.O., and Losos, G.J.: Pathological changes in cattle infected with *Trypanosoma brucei.* Vet. Pathol., *9*:272–277, 1972.

——: Pathology of the disease in sheep produced experimentally by *Trypanosoma brucei.* Vet. Pathol., *9*:278–289, 1972.

——: Spontaneous canine trypanosomiasis caused by *T. brucei*: meningoenceophalomyelitis with extra-vascular localization by trypanosomes in the brain. Bull. Epizoot. Dis. Afr., *20*:221–228, 1972.

——: Pathogenesis of *Trypanosoma brucei* infection in sheep. I. Clinical signs. II. Cerebro-spinal fluid changes. III. Hypophysial and other endocrine lesions. J. Comp. Pathol., *85*:23–31, 33–36, 37–44, 1975.

Isoun, T.T.: The histopathology of experimental disease produced in mice infected with *Trypanosoma vivax.* Acta Trop., *32*:267–272, 1975.

Johnson, C.M.: Cardiac changes in dogs experimentally infected with *Trypanosoma cruzi.* Am. J. Trop. Med., *18*:197–206, 1938.

Kaliner, G.: *Trypanosoma congolense.* II. Histopathologic findings in experimentally infected cattle. Exp. Parasitol., *36*:20–26, 1974.

Killick-Kendrick, R.: The diagnosis of trypanosomiasis of livestock; a review of current techniques. Vet. Bull., *38*:191–197, 1968.

Kobayashi, A., Tizard, I.R., and Woo, P.T.K.: **Studies on the anemia in experimental African trypanosomiasis. II. The pathogenesis of the** anemia in calves infected with *Trypanosoma congolense.* Am. J. Trop. Med. Hyg., *25*:401–406, 1976.

Koberle, F.: Chagas' disease and Chagas' syndromes: The pathology of American trypanosomiasis. *In* Advances in Parasitology, Vol. 6, edited by B. Dawes. New York, Academic Press, 1968, pp. 63–116.

Kumar, R., Kline, I.K., and Abelmann, W.H.: Experimental *Trypanosoma cruzi* myocarditis. Relative effects upon the right and left ventricles. Am. J. Pathol., *57*:31–48, 1969.

Leach, T.M.: African trypanosomiases. Adv. Vet. Sci. Comp. Med., *17*:119–162, 1973.

Losos, G.J., and Ikede, B.O.: Review of pathology of diseases in domestic and laboratory animals caused by *Trypanosoma congolense, T. vivax, T. brucei, T. rhodesiense* and *T. gambiense.* Vet. Path. Suppl. ad 9, 1972.

Lumsden, W.H.R.: Pathobiology of trypanosomiasis. *In* Pathology of Parasitic Diseases. Lafayette, Ind., Purdue University Studies, 1971, pp. 1–14.

MacKenzie, P.K.I., and Cruickshank, J.G.: Phagocytosis of erythrocytes and leucocytes in sheep infected with *Trypanosoma congolense* (Broden 1904). Res. Vet. Sci., *15*:256–262, 1973.

Marsden, P.D., and Hagstrom, J.W.C.: Trypanosoma cruzi in the saliva of Beagle puppies. Trans. R. Soc. Trop. Med. Hyg., *60*:189–191, 1966.

McCully, R.M., and Neitz, W.O.: Clinicopathological study on experimental *Trypanosoma brucei* infections in horses. II. Histopathological findings in the nervous system and other organs of treated **and untreated horses reacting to Nagana. Onderstepoort J. Vet. Res., *38*:141–176, 1971.**

Mortelmans, J., and Neetens, A.: Ocular lesions in experimental *Trypanosoma brucei* infection in cats (and dogs). Acta Zool. Path. Antverp., *62*:149–172, 1975.

Moulton, J.E., Coleman, J.L., and Gee, M.K.: Pathogenesis of *Trypanosoma equiperdum* in rabbits. Am. J. Vet. Res., *36*:357–366, 1975.

Moulton, J.E., Coleman, J.L., and Thompson, P.S.: Pathogenesis of *Trypanosoma equiperdum* in deer mice (*Peromyscus maniculatus*). Am. J. Vet. Res., *35*:961–976, 1974.

Moulton, J.E., and Krauss, H.H.: Ultrastructure of *Trypanosoma theileri* in bovine spleen culture. Cornell Vet., *62*:124–137, 1972.

Moulton, J.E., and Sollod, A.E.: Clinical, serologic, and pathologic changes in calves with experimentally induced *Trypanosoma brucei* infection. Am. J. Vet. Res., *37*:791–802, 1976.

Nagle, R.B., et al.: Experimental infections with African trypanosomes: VI. Glomerulonephritis involving the alternate pathway of complement activation. Am. J. Trop. Med. Hyg., *23*:15–26, 1974.

Naylor, D.C.: The haematology and histopathology of *Trypanosoma congolense* infection in cattle. I. Introduction and histopathology. Trop. Anim. Health Prod., *3*:95–100, 1971.

Ormerod, W.E.: Taxonomy of the sleeping sickness trypanosomes. J. Parasitol., *53*:824–830, 1967. V.B. 38:535, 1968.

Packchanian, A.: Studies on *Trypanosoma gambiense* infection in various species of experimental animals. Tex. Rep. Biol. Med., 22:707–715, 1964.

Pavlov, P., and Christoforov, L.: The pathogenicity of *Trypanosoma equiperdum*. Proc. 1st Int. Congr. Parasit. Roma, 1:323–324, 1966. V.B. 37:2050, 1967.

Rees, J.M., and Clarkson, M.J.: Serum proteins in trypanosomiasis of sheep. Trans. R. Soc. Trop. Med. Hyg., 61:14, 1967. V.B. 37:2536, 1967.

Soltys, M.A., and Woo, P.: Multiplication of *Trypanosoma brucei* and *Trypanosoma congolense* in vertebrate hosts. Trans. R. Soc. Trop. Med. Hyg., 63:490–494, 1969.

Srivastava, R.V.N., Malhotra, M.N., and Iyer, P.K.R.: Pathology of experimental *Trypanosoma evansi* infection in dogs. Indian J. Anim. Sci., 39:307–314, 1969.

Weinman, D.: The human trypanosomiases. Chapter 17. *In* Infectious Blood Diseases of Man and Animals, edited by D. Weinman, and M. Ristic. New York, Academic Press, 1968.

LEISHMANIASIS

Infections of man and animals with protozoan organisms of the genus *Leishmania* have various local names but can be grouped together on the basis of their common characteristics. Three species are recognized as important pathogens: *Leishmania donovani*, the cause of visceral leishmaniasis, kala azar, or dum dum fever; *L. tropica*, the agent of cutaneous leishmaniasis, Oriental sore, or Delhi sore; and *L. braziliensis*, which causes the entity called mucocutaneous or American leishmaniasis, espundia, or several other names. The organisms are classified in the family Trypanosomidae, which includes five parasitic genera: *Trypanosoma* (vertebrate and invertebrate hosts), *Leishmania* (vertebrates and invertebrates), *Leptomonas*, *Crithidia*, and *Herpetomonas* (parasites of invertebrate hosts).

Leishmania occur in vertebrate hosts in the leishmanial form, which is a small, ovoid protozoan about 1 to 2 μ wide by 2 to 4.5 μ long, with neither flagellum nor undulating membrane. In Romanovsky-stained preparations, it has pale blue cytoplasm containing, near the posterior end, a reddish nucleus with a deeper staining central karyosome. Tangential and anterior to the nucleus is a deep violet, rod-shaped body, the kinetoplast, which contains the parabasal body and the dot-shaped blepharoplast. In its invertebrate host (sandflies) or in cultures, the organisms assume shapes varying from the leishmanial to the leptomonad form, the latter being slender and spindle-shaped, from 14 to 20 μ in length and 1.5 to 4 μ in width. This form is motile by means of a flagellum that arises from the blepharoplast and projects from the anterior pole of the organism.

Life Cycle. *Leishmania* reproduce in the vertebrate host by longitudinal binary fission, but the complete life cycle and maintenance of virulence depend upon an intermediate host or vector. Many species of sandflies (*Phlebotomus*) are involved in the transmission of *Leishmania* and are necessary for their perpetuation, but certain flies, such as *Stomoxys calcitrans*, may mechanically transmit the infection.

Clinical Manifestations. **Visceral leishmaniasis,** or kala azar (*L. donovani*), occurs naturally in man, dogs, cats, squirrels, cattle, horses, and sheep, but many laboratory animals, especially hamsters and dogs, are susceptible to experimental infection. The disease has a wide geographic distribution, but is most prevalent in countries bordering the Mediterranean, large areas of Africa, India, and China. It also occurs in Argentina, Colombia, Brazil, and Venezuela in South America, but cases reported in the United States originated elsewhere. Visceral leishmaniasis in animals usually is observed as a chronic debilitating disease with periods of fever and gradual weight loss, with anemia appearing in the terminal stages. A history of persistent cutaneous ulcers that heal slowly may sometimes be obtained. In the United States, the disease should be suspected in animals imported from areas where the disease is known to occur.

Cutaneous leishmaniasis (*L. tropica*) occurs principally in those Southern European and North African countries bordering the Mediterranean. The reservoirs for human infections are various wild rodents,

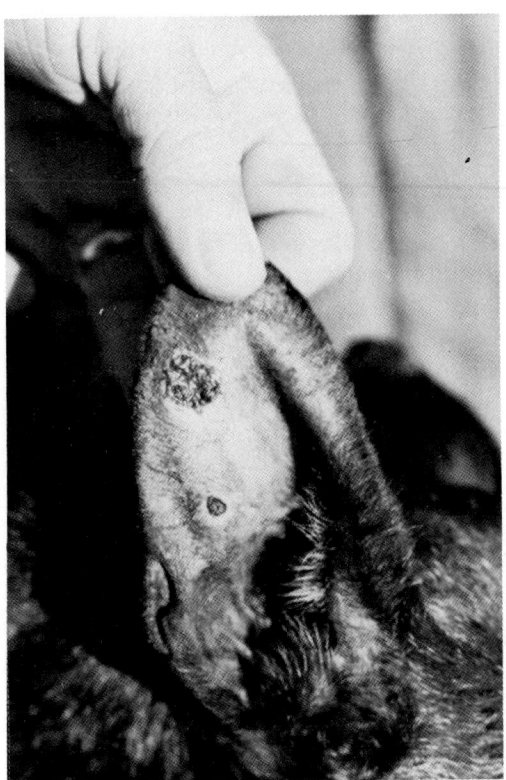

Fig. 13–25. Cutaneous leishmaniasis. Elevated ulcerated lesions in skin of the ear of a dog. (Courtesy of Dr. A. Herrer and *American Journal of Tropical Medicine and Hygiene.*)

although dogs, mice, guinea pigs, and monkeys are susceptible to experimental infection.

American or **mucocutaneous leishmaniasis** *(L. braziliensis)* occurs in Mexico and Central America, is particularly prevalent in Brazil, Venezuela, Colombia, and Peru, but is unknown in Chile. Animals are not frequently found infected in nature, although ground squirrels, dogs, cats, and monkeys are susceptible.

Lesions. The organisms of visceral leishmaniasis stimulate the production of large numbers of huge macrophages with cytoplasm filled with leishmanial forms. The lymph nodes and spleen are particularly involved by reticuloendothelial hyperplasia, although the liver, bone marrow, kidney, and less often, other viscera

and skin may be infected. The gross findings at necropsy, therefore, consist of severe emaciation; enlarged lymph nodes, spleen and liver; sometimes pallor of mucosae and serous surfaces; soft red bone marrow; and ulcers in the intestine. *Leishmania donovani* are found in histologic preparations of any of these organs, occurring in the cytoplasm of the enlarged macrophages. The lymph nodes may show moderate fibrosis as well as reticuloendothelial hyperplasia. Macrophages also replace large areas in the spleen and infiltrate portal zones in the liver. The bone marrow may be hyperplastic or replaced largely with macrophages filled with *Leishmania* (see Fig. 13–24D).

In cutaneous and mucocutaneous leishmaniasis, the dermis becomes filled with large numbers of macrophages, lymphocytes, plasma cells, and rarely, eosinophils. Numerous parasites are present within the macrophages. The lesions progress to well-defined, deep ulcers.

Diagnosis. Other diseases that also cause proliferation of reticuloendothelium present the most problems in differential diagnosis. These include histoplasmosis, toxoplasmosis (some cases), salmon disease, blastomycosis, and epizootic lymphangitis. Final determination must be based upon demonstration and identification of the causative organisms in tissue sections, smears or cultures. Tissues taken by biopsy are most useful to demonstrate the organisms in a living animal or human patient.

Galati, P.: Reperto di Trombosi Multipla in cane con Leishmoniosi Viscerale. (Multiple thrombosis in a dog with visceral leishmaniasis) Atti. Soc. ital. Sci. Vet., *12*:508–512, 1958. VB 3789–59.

Herrer, A., and Christensen, H.A.: Natural cutaneous leishmaniasis among dogs in Panama. Am. J. Trop. Med. Hyg., *25*:59–63, 1976.

McConnell, E.E., Chaffee, E.F., Cashell, I.G., and Garner, F.M.: Visceral leishmaniasis with ocular involvement in a dog. J. Am. Vet. Med. Assoc., *156*:197–203, 1970.

Rioux, J-A., Golvan, Y-J., and Houin, R.: Mixed *Hepatozoon canis* and *Leishmania canis* infection in a dog in the Sete Area, France. Annls. Parasit. Hum. Comp., *39*:131–135, 1964. V.B. 1302, 1965.

Stauber, L.A.: Experimental leishmaniasis in the chinchilla. J. Parasitol. (abstract), 39:11, 1953.

Thorson, R.E., Bailey, W.S., Hoerlein, B.F., and Seibold, H.R.: A report of a case of imported visceral leishmaniasis of a dog in the United States. Am. J. Trop. Med. Hyg., 4:18–22, 1955.

Wolf, R.E.: Immune response to *Leishmania tropica* in *Macaca mulatta*. J. Parasitol., 62:209–214, 1976.

MALARIA

Malaria has been recognized as an important disease of man in most recorded history and is still one of the most important infectious diseases in spite of great strides toward its eradication. The disease is thought of as especially prevalent in tropical and subtropical regions, but is not unknown in temperate parts of the globe. It is especially deleterious to young children, often combining with hookworm, tuberculosis, and other diseases to debilitate and kill. The name of the malady, *malaria*, comes from the Italian words *mala* (bad) and *aria* (air), in reference to the "miasmic vapors" which were believed to come from swamps.

One of the causative parasites was discovered by a French Army physician, Laveran, who in 1880 found what are now considered to be microgametocytes, probably of the organism now called *Plas-*

modium falciparum. It was not until after the turn of the century that Sir Ronald Ross (1910) demonstrated mosquitoes to be the "miasmas" arising from swamps to spread the disease.

The causative protozoa, classified among the sporozoa, are currently all members of the genus *Plasmodium*, which includes many pathogenic species. Man, birds, and nonhuman primates are now known to be the vertebrate hosts for these organisms. Of particular interest is the discovery (Eyles, Coatney and Getz, 1960) that man is susceptible to certain of the simian plasmodia. Thus, simian malarias not only may serve as models for human malaria, but also may be a source for human infection (Manwell, 1968). Simian malaria is also encountered in monkeys imported into laboratories, where it may interfere with the experimental data garnered from these animals. Thus, malaria is now viewed as a group of diseases caused by different species of *Plasmodium*.

Life Cycle. The life cycles of *Plasmodium*, as far as currently known, are quite similar. Two hosts are required: (1) vertebrates (man, other mammals, birds, and reptiles), in which schizogony takes place in erythrocytes and other cells; and (2) invertebrate blood-sucking insects (mosquitoes). The cycle is started when a female mosquito penetrates the skin of the vertebrate host, introducing sporozoites into the peripheral circulation. After a few days of exoerythrocytic development in endothelial cells or hepatocytes, the parasites enter red blood cells. Here they are called **schizonts.** Initially these schizonts appear as small rings that grow and divide to develop into many (24 or more) **merozoites,** tiny nucleated bodies which are released into the plasma as the cell disintegrates. These merozoites may be phagocytized by leukocytes or infect other red blood cells. This repeated schizogony, progressing geometrically, results in the paroxysmal recurrence of the signs of fever and anemia. Some of the merozoites develop into

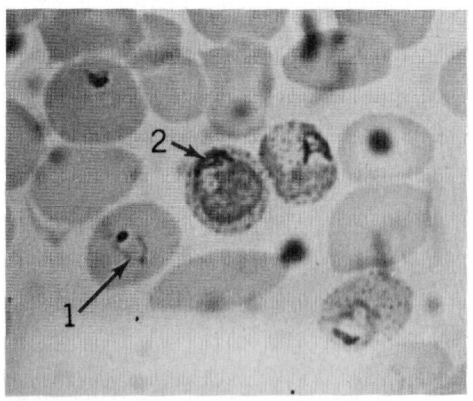

Fig. 13–26. Malaria in a cynomolgus monkey (*Macaca fascicularis*). Schizonts *(1)* and gametocytes *(2)* of *Plasmodium cynomolgi* are present in erythrocytes. (Courtesy of New England Regional Primate Research Center, Harvard Medical School.)

gametocytes, and remain in the blood as macro- and microgametocytes until ingested by a mosquito or eliminated by phagocytosis as their life span is completed. The organisms incompletely catabolize hemoglobin, leaving a brownish pigment, hemozoin, easily visible on stained smears.

The macro- and microgametocytes ingested by female mosquitoes (the males do not ingest blood) undergo further development in the stomach of the mosquito— the macrogametocyte becomes one macrogamete and the microgametocyte becomes 4 to 8 microgametes. Fusion of gametes results in a motile zygote called oökinete, which enters the gastric mucosa of the mosquito and becomes an oöcyst, which lies in the stroma adjacent to the gastric epithelium. Repeated nuclear divisions result in the formation of many sporozoites, which are set free by rupture into the hemolymph, permitting migration to the salivary glands of the mosquito. From this site, the sporozoites are available to infect a new vertebrate host when the female mosquito takes her blood meal.

The life cycle of *Plasmodium* closely resembles that of Coccidia, in that an asexual stage (schizogony), passed in the tissue of the vertebrate host, is continued by a sexual stage with sporozoite formation. The differences are that Coccidia have a form that is spent outside any host (oöcyst) and the sexual stages develop in the vertebrate host; the sexual stages in *Plasmodium* occur in the alimentary tract of a blood-sucking arthropod, and no form occurs that can survive outside the body of a host.

Clinical Manifestations. The signs in malaria are related to the numbers of parasites in the blood, and appear 5 to 14 or more days following infection; the incubation period depends to some extent upon the exoerythrocytic period of the parasites. Bouts of chills and fever appear at intervals roughly comparable to the periods of reproduction of the malaria parasite. The terms tertian (third) and quartan (fourth)

apply to the usual interval between paroxysms. After a 48-hour cycle, as is the case in *Plasmodium vivax* and *P. falciparum* infection, the signs reappear on the third day *(tertian)*. In the case of *quartan* malaria, the cycle of the parasite (*P. malariae*) is about 76 hours, and the signs reappear each fourth day. Malaria due to *P. falciparum* may also have a cycle less than 48 hours (*subtertian*) due to presence of two broods of parasites. These features are covered in Table 13–4. Relapses often occur in human malaria, sometimes after long intervals, thus providing a carrier state. This state also appears to occur in other animals.

Lesions. The pathologic effects of malaria vary to some extent with the organism involved, but are similar in most vertebrate hosts. The destruction of parasitized erythrocytes results in hemolysis and anemia, to which most of the clinical and pathologic findings can be ascribed. Splenomegaly is rather constant and rupture may occur. Hepatomegaly usually occurs, and the liver has a dark color due to the presence of malaria pigment (hemazoin) in Kupffer cells. Hemorrhages in the brain may be associated with blood vessels occluded by parasitized red blood cells and thrombi.

The hemolysis in malaria is the result of alteration of erythrocyte membranes by the parasites. Immunohemolytic anemia has been postulated, but such mechanisms do not seem to be important to the pathogenesis of the anemia. However, immune complex glomerulonephritis may accompany acute and chronic infection.

Diagnosis. The diagnosis of malaria is usually established by demonstrating the organisms in erythrocytes in thin or thick smears stained with Giemsa's or Wright-Giemsa's stain.

Abilgaard, C., Harrison, J., DeNardo, S., Spangler, W., and Gribble, D.: Simian *Plasmodium knowlesi* malaria: studies of coagulation and pathology. Am. J. Trop. Med. Hyg., 24:764–768, 1975.

Coatney, G.R.: Simian malarias in man: facts, implications, and predictions. Am. J. Trop. Med. Hyg., 17:147–155, 1968.

Table 13–4. Malarias

Organism	Vertebrate Hosts	Disease	Geographic Distribution
Plasmodium falciparum	Man	Malignant tertian, falciparum, or subtertian malaria	Widely distributed in tropics, some in subtropics
P. malariae	Man, chimpanzee	Quartan malaria	Philippine Islands, India
P. ovale	Man	Mild tertian malaria	Africa, Philippines and India
P. vivax	Man, chimpanzee (experimental)	Benign tertian or vivax malaria	Tropical, subtropical, some temperate regions, South and North America, England, Sweden, Argentina, Australia, Natal
P. knowlesi	*Macaca fascicularis* (crab-eater macaque) *M. cyclopis* (Taiwan macaque) Man (experimental) *M. nemestrina* *Presbytis melalophus*	Simian malaria	Malaya, Philippines
P. gallinaceum	Domestic fowl (other birds suscept. exper.)	Avian malaria	India
P. relictum	Penguins, sparrows, many birds	Avian malaria	U.S.A. (zoos)
P. brazilianum	*Cebus apella* (capuchin), *Alouatta seniculus,* *A. fusca* (howler monkeys), *Cacajao calvus* (uakari), *Chiropotes chiropotes* (saki), *Ateles paniscus p.,* *A. paniscus chamek* (spider monkey), *Lagothrix lagotricha,* *L. cana* (woolly monkeys), *Brachyteles arachnoides* (woolly spider monkey), *Callicebus torquatus* (titi), *Saimiri sciureus* (squirrel monkey), occasionally man	Simian malaria (quartan type)	South and Central America
P. simium	*Alouatta fusca, Brachyteles arachnoides,* occasionally man	Simian malaria (benign-tertian type)	Brazil

Table 13–4.   Malarias (Cont'd)

Organism	Vertebrate Hosts	Disease	Geographic Distribution

P. cynomolgi	*Macaca fascicularis,*
	  M. nemestrina
	  (pig-tailed macaque),
	M. cyclopis
	  (Taiwan macaque),
	M. radiata (bonnet mon-
	  key),
	Cynopithecus niger,
	  Presbytis sp.
		Simian malaria	Philippines, Taiwan,
			  Malaya, Java, Ceylon,
			  India, Cambodia,
			  Pakistan

P. coatneyi	*Macaca fascicularis*	Simian malaria	Philippines, Malaya

P. inui	*Macaca fascicularis,*
	  M. mulatta (rhesus),
	M. radiata,
	M. nemestrina,
	M. cyclopis,
	Cynopithecus
	  niger, Presbytis sp.
		Simian malaria	Indochina, Philippines,
			  tropical Asia

P. fieldi	*M. nemestrina* *M. fascicularis*	Simian malaria	Malaya
P. fragile	*M. radiata, M. sinica*	Simian malaria	Ceylon
P. simiovale	*M. sinica*	Simian malaria	Ceylon
P. pitheci	*Pongo pigmaeus* (orangutan)	Simian malaria	Borneo
P. youngi	*Hylobates lar* (gibbon)	Simian malaria	Malaya
P. jefferyi	*Hylobates lar*	Simian malaria	Malaya
P. eylesi	*Hylobates lar*	Simian malaria	Malaya
P. hylobates	*Hylobates lar*	Simian malaria	Java
P. gonderi	*Cerocebus galeritus,* *C. aterrimus,* *C. atys, Mandrillus* *leucophaeus*	Simian malaria	West Africa
P. reichenowi	*Gorilla gorilla* (gorilla), *Pan troglodytes* (chimpanzee)	Simian malaria	West and Central Africa
P. rhodhaini	*Pan troglodytes*	Simian malaria	West and Central Africa
P. schwetzi	*Gorilla gorilla* *Pan troglodytes*	Simian malaria	West and Central Africa

Hepatocystes
  (Plasmodium)
  kochi
  (Hepatocystes
  simiae)
	Cercopithecus sp
	Papio sp, etc.
		Simian malaria
		Hepatocystis
			Africa

Collins, W.E.: Primate malarias. Adv. Vet. Sci. Comp. Med., *18*:1–23, 1974.

Conrad, M.E.: Pathophysiology of malaria. Hematologic observations in human and animal studies. Ann. Intern. Med., *70*:134–141, 1969.

Contacos, P.G., and Collins, W.E.: *Plasmodium malariae:* transmission from monkey to man by mosquito bite. Science, *165*:918–919, 1969.

Eyles, D.E., Coatney, G.R., and Getz, M.E.: Vivax type malaria parasite of macaques transmissible to man. Science, *131*:1812–1813, 1960.

Garnham, P.C.C.: Malaria in mammals excluding man. Adv. Parasitol., *5*:139–204, 1967.

Held, J.R.: Primate malaria. Ann. NY Acad. Sci., *162*:587–593, 1969.

Hutt, M.S.R., Davies, D.R., and Voller, A.: Malarial infections in *Aotus trivirgatus* with special reference to renal pathology. II. *P. falciparum* and mixed malaria infections. Br. J. Exp. Pathol., *56*:429–438, 1975.

Laveran, C.L.A.: Nature parasitaire des accidents de l'impaludisme; Description d'un nouveau parasite trouvé dans le sang des malades atteintes de fievre palustre. Paris, Bailliere, 1881.

Manwell, R.D.: Malaria. *In* Infectious Blood Diseases of Man and Animals, Vol. II, edited by D. Weinman and M. Ristic. New York, Academic Press, 1968, pp. 25–95.

Miller, L.H.: Distribution of mature trophozoites and schizonts of *Plasmodium falciparum* in the organs of *Aotus trivigatus,* the night monkey. Am. J. Trop. Med. Hyg., *18*:860–865, 1969.

Rigdon, R.H.: Hemoglobinuria (blackwater fever) in monkeys. A consideration of the disease in man. Am. J. Pathol., *25*:195–209, 1949.

Ross, R.: The Prevention of Malaria. London, Murray, 1910.

Schmidt, L.H.: Infections with *Plasmodium falciparum* and *Plasmodium vivax* in the owl monkey: model systems for basic biological and chemotherapeutic studies. Trans. R. Soc. Trop. Med. Hyg., *67*:446–474, 1973.

Voller, A.: Immunopathology of malaria. Bull. WHO, *50*:177–186, 1974.

Voller, A., Davies, D.R., and Hutt, M.S.R.: Quartan malarial infections in *Aotus trivirgatus* with special reference to renal pathology. Br. J. Exp. Pathol., *54*:457–468, 1973.

Young, M.D., Baerg, D.C., and Rossan, R.N.: Parasitological review: experimental monkey hosts for human plasmodia. Exp. Parasitol., *38*:136–152, 1975.

HEPATOCYSTES

Hepatocystes (or *Hepatocystis*) *kochi* is a protozoan organism until recently named *Plasmodium kochi,* which is parasitic in many species of nonhuman primates. The organism is found in primates in the genera. *Cercopithecus, Papio, Hylobates,* and *Macaca.* Other species, such as leaf-nosed bats (*Hipposideros armiger armiger*) and red-bellied tree squirrels (*Callosciurus sciurus*), have been reported to be infected. One vector is reported to be *Culicoides adersi.*

One distinguishing feature of this parasite is its production of grossly visible cysts in the liver of vertebrate hosts. This cyst, called a **merocyst,** starts by invasion of a single hepatic cell by a merozoite, which grows within the hepatocyte, causing it to undergo hypertrophy as the parasite grows. Continued growth of the organism eventually results in a many-celled structure as large as 2 mm in diameter with a central, fluid-filled space. The outer wall is occupied by myriads of tiny **merozoites,** which are released when the cyst ruptures. These merozoites then parasitize erythrocytes, producing ring forms and eventually

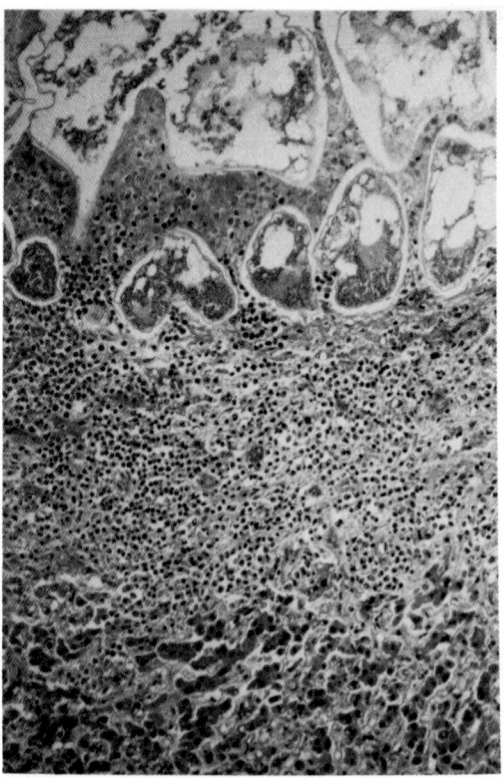

Fig. 13–27. *Hepatocystis kochi,* liver of a baboon. The section includes part of the cyst (top), a zone of reaction, and liver cells (bottom).

gametocytes. Gametogony is believed to take place in the invertebrate host, *Culicoides adersi.*

This merocyst initially destroys a single hepatic cell and displaces others as the organism grows. Varying degrees of tissue reaction result, presumably depending upon immunologic factors. The host may react by surrounding the cyst with epithelioid granulation tissue and multinucleated giant cells, finally with fibrous connective tissue. Recently ruptured cysts may be surrounded by hemorrhage. A fibrous scar eventually results.

Desowitz, R.S.: Observations on Hepatocystis of white-cheeked gibbon (*Hylobates concolor*). J. Parasitol., *56:*444–446, 1970.

Garnham, P.C.C.: Exoerythrocytic schizogony in *Plasmodium kochi*, Laveran. A preliminary note. Trans. Roy. Soc. Trop. Med. Hyg., *40:*719–722, 1947.

————: The developmental cycle of *Hepatocystes (Plasmodium) kochi* in the monkey host. Trans. Roy. Soc. Trop. Med. Hyg., *41:*601–616, 1948.

Manwell, R.D., and Kuntz, R.E.: Hepatocystis in Formosan mammals with a description of a new species. J. Protozool., *13:*670–672, 1966.

Shiroishi, T., Davis, J., and Warren, M.: *Hepatocystis* in white-cheeked gibbon, *Hylobates concolor.* J. Parasitol., *54:*168, 1968.

Vickers, J.H.: *Hepatocystis kochi* in Cercopithecus monkeys. J. Am. Vet. Med. Assoc., *149:*906–908, 1966.

Warren, McW., Shiroishi, T., and Davis, J.: A hepatocystis-like parasite of the gibbon. Trans. Roy. Soc. Trop. Med. Hyg., *62:*4, 1968.

HEPATOZOON INFECTIONS

Organisms of the genus *Hepatozoon* are placed in the class Sporozoa of the Protozoa and contain several pathogenic species. Schizogony occurs in endothelial cells of the liver and gametocytes may be found in erythrocytes or leukocytes of the vertebrate host, depending upon the species of the protozoa. Sporogony occurs in bloodsucking arthropods.

Life Cycle. Hepatozoon canis infects dogs, cats, hyenas and jackals in the Middle East, North Africa, Italy and the Far East. The developmental cycle of the organism involves the brown dog tick, *Rhipicephalus sanguineus,* which, when infected, carries

sporocysts in its body cavity. Ingestion of the infected vector tick by the vertebrate host results in release of **sporozoites,** which penetrate the intestinal wall to reach the spleen, liver, lungs, lymph nodes, myocardium, and bone marrow by way of the blood stream. The parasites enter tissue cells to become **schizonts,** reproducing several generations in these cells. Eventually, **merozoites** are produced, which parasitize erythrocytes or leukocytes and become **gametocytes,** or **gamonts.** These gametocytes become differentiated into macro- and microgametocytes in the body of the vector tick, and sexual union results in a motile zygote, the **oökinete.** This oökinete migrates to the hemocoel of the tick, where it grows to a large oöcyst, 100 μ in diameter, in which large numbers of sporozoites are formed within sporocysts. The sporozoites are released from the oöcyst after the tick is ingested by the vertebrate host.

Clinical Manifestations. Most often, the parasites are encountered as incidental findings in the absence of clinical signs or tissue reaction. However, infection may lead to signs of fever, anemia, splenomegaly, progressive emaciation, and sometimes paralysis. Death may occur four to eight weeks following outset of clinical signs.

Lesions. The lesions are those of anemia and focal necrotizing granulomas in affected tissues.

Diagnosis. The diagnosis is based on demonstration of the organisms—gametocytes in leukocytes in blood smears, or schizonts in biopsy or necropsy specimens of liver, spleen, bone marrow, or other tissue. Intercurrent disease apparently accentuates the pathogenicity of hepatozoon (McCully et al., 1975).

Several other organisms of this genus are known to infect vertebrates; some of them are: *Hepatozoon cuniculi* (host: rabbit in Europe); *H. muris* (brown rat, *Rattus norvegicus,* or black rat, *Rattus rattus;* the vector is the rat mite, *Echinolaelaps echid-*

minus); *H. procyonis* (raccoon); *Hepatozoon sp.* (impala in South Africa); *H. musculi* (white mouse in England).

Basson, P.A., et al.: Observations on a Hepatozoon-like parasite in the impala. J. S. Afr. Vet. Med. Assoc., *38*:12–14, 1967. V.B. 37:4651, 1967.

Klopfer, U., Nobel, T.A., and Neumann, F.: Hepatozoon-like parasite (schizonts) in the myocardium of the domestic cat. Vet. Pathol., *10*:185–190, 1973.

McCully, R.M., et al.: Observations on naturally acquired hepatozoonosis of wild carnivores and dogs in the Republic of South Africa. Onderstepoort J. Vet. Res., 42:117–133, 1975.

Schneider, C.R.: *Hepatozoon procyonis* Richards, 1961, in a Panamanian raccoon, *Procyon cancrivorus panamensis* (Goldman). Rev. Biol. Trop., *15*:123–135, 1968.

Soulsby, E.J.L.: Helminths, Arthropods and Protozoa of Domesticated Animals (Mönnig), 6th ed., Philadelphia, Lea & Febiger, 1968.

BABESIOSIS (Piroplasmosis, Tick Fever, "Red Water")

Organisms of the genus *Babesia*, Protozoa of the order Sporozoa, parasitize the erythrocytes of a wide variety of vertebrate hosts, multiplying in the erythrocytes by means of binary fission, giving rise to two or four daughter individuals. Ticks act as intermediate host-vectors in which the parasites reproduce, sometimes penetrating the egg to infect the young tick. Bovine babesiosis (piroplasmosis, Texas, or tick fever) was the first infection of any kind to be shown to be transmitted by an arthropod vector (Smith and Kilborne, 1893); this was a major scientific achievement and milestone in the conquest of disease. Of the 71 species in the genus *Babesia*, only a few affect domestic animals. *Babesia spp.* have been considered to be relatively host-specific, but recently cross-species infections have been recognized. Dogs, cattle, horses, sheep, swine, human beings, and nonhuman primates are susceptible to one or more separate species of *Babesia*, but the general features of the disease are similar in all hosts.

The clinical manifestations of babesiosis are so capriciously variable that they are of little help in diagnosis. The signs common to most cases include fever, malaise, listlessness, anorexia, and anemia. Icterus, hemoglobinuria, and ascites may appear during late stages and progressive debility terminates in death. Infection in young animals is usually mild and affords future protection.

Babesia are found in the circulating erythrocytes of mammals as pyriform or ovoid bodies, usually in pairs, the larger of which measure 4 to 5 μ by 2 to 3 μ (*B. bigemina*), and the smaller, 1.5 μ by 0.4 μ (*B. divergens*). They are readily distinguished from *Plasmodium spp.* by the absence of hemoglobin-derived pigment. *Babesia spp.* completely catabolize hemoglobin, whereas *Plasmodium spp.* retain a brownish pigment, hemozoin. They are particularly well demonstrated by Romanovsky-type stains. The important pathogens of domestic animals are listed in Table 13–5. Several other species of *Babesia* are apparently tolerated by animals with little ill effect; these can be found in the listing of Levine (1971).

Bovine Babesiosis (Texas Fever, Tick Fever, Piroplasmosis). This disease of cattle is of historical interest because it has now been virtually eliminated from the southern United States, where it was once prevalent. Its eradication was accomplished by elimination of the tick vector, *Boöphilus annulatus*. Babesiosis is still present in many other parts of the world.

Lesions. The gross lesions of the bovine disease are of interest. Necropsy of the emaciated carcasses of animals dead of the disease discloses the blood to be thin and watery and the plasma is red-tinged. The subcutaneous, subserous, and intramuscular connective tissue is edematous and yellow, and the fat is similarly affected. Gastroenteritis is indicated by swelling and patchy reddening of the abomasal and intestinal mucosa. Icteric discoloration is clearly recognizable in all viscera. The spleen is constantly enlarged four to five times normal size, and its parenchyma is soft and dark red. The splenic corpuscles are usually prominent. The liver is en-

Table 13–5. Babesia Infections

Organism	Animals Affected	Geographic Distribution	Tick Vectors
B. bigemina	Cattle, zebu, water buffalo, deer	Central and South America, Africa, Australia, Southern Europe	*Boophilus annulatus,* *B. microplus,* *B. australis,* *B. calcaratus,* *B. decoloratus,* *Rhipicephalus evertsi,* *Rh. bursa,* *Rh. appendiculatus,* *Haemaphysalis punctata*
B. bovis	Cattle, roe deer, stag	Southern Europe, Africa, Asia	*Ixodes ricinus,* *I. persulcatus,* *Boophilus calcaratus,* *Rhipicephalus bursa*
B. argentina	Cattle	Central and South America, Australia	*Boophilus miroplus*
B. divergens	Cattle	Northern Europe	*Ixodes ricinus,* *Dermacentor reticulatus*
B. major	Cattle	Europe, Africa	*Haemophysalis punctata*
B. canis	Dog, wolf, jackal	Asia, Africa, Southern Europe, United States, Central and South America, Soviet Union	*Rhipicephalus sanguineus,* *Dermacentor reticulatus,* *D. marginatus,* *Haemophysalis leachi,* *Hyalomma plumbeum*
B. gibsoni	Dog, wolf, fox, jackal	India, Ceylon, China, Turkestan, North Africa, United States	*Haemaphysalis bispinosa,* *Rhipicephalus sanguineus*
B. equi	Horse, mule, donkey, zebra	Asia, Africa, United States, Europe, South America, Soviet Union	*Dermacentor reticulatus,* *D. marginatus,* *Rhipicephalus bursa,* *Rh. sanguineus,* *Rh. evertsi,* *Hyalomma excavatum,* *Hy. plumbeum,* *Hy. dromedarii*
B. caballi	Horse, donkey, mule	Southern Europe, Asia, Soviet Union, Africa, Panama, United States	*Dermacentor marginatus,* *D. silvarum,* *D. nitens,* *Hyalomma excavatum,* *Hy. dromedarii,* *Hy. scupense,* *Rhipicephalus bursa,* *Rh. sanguineus,* *Dermacentor reticulatus*
B. motasi	Sheep, goats	Southern Europe, Middle East, Soviet Union, Asia, Africa	*D. silvarum,* *Haemaphysalis punctata,* *Rhipicephalus bursa*
B. ovis	Sheep, goats	Tropics, Southern Europe, Soviet Union	*Rh. bursa*
B. trautmanni	Pig, wart hog, bush pig	Southern Europe, Soviet Union, Congo, Tanzania	*Rh. turanicus,* *Rh. sanguineus,* *Boophilus decoloratus,* *Dermacentor reticulatus*
B. felis	Domestic cat, wildcat, lion, leopard, puma, American lynx	Sudan, South Africa, U. S. (Zoos)	*Unknown*

larged and yellow-brown, with the gallbladder distended with dark green bile. The lungs are slightly edematous and the urinary bladder usually contains red-colored urine.

The microscopic findings are characteristic of severe hemolytic anemia. *Babesia* may be demonstrable in large numbers in capillaries in the brain and optic choroid, even though they cannot be found elsewhere. The organisms in these sites are described as being both free in the lumen and in packed erythrocytes.

Equine Babesiosis (Piroplasmosis). Recently recognized for the first time in the United States, this disease is arousing some concern. Two species of *Babesia* are responsible for the disease in equine hosts but are not infective for other mammals. This genus-specificity is characteristic of these hemoprotozoan parasites. *Babesia caballi* affects horses, mules, and donkeys, as does *B. equi,* which has also been found in zebras. *B. caballi* may be distinguished by their appearance in erythrocytes, where they occur as paired pyriform bodies, 2.5 × 4.0 μ in maximum dimensions, with their pointed ends meeting at an acute angle. *B. equi* may be distinguished by their occurrence in erythrocytes in groups of four with pointed ends meeting to form a Maltese cross. The trophozoites are smaller (seldom exceeding 2.0 μ in length) and more pleomorphic, with round, oval, and ring forms. Groups of four are common because of their tendency to divide into four daughter trophozoites. *B. equi* is considered to be more pathogenic than *B. caballi.*

Clinical Manifestations. The clinical signs are variable and are related for the most part to the destruction of erythrocytes: fever, anemia, icterus, weakness, and occasionally hemoglobinuria and subcutaneous edema around the head. Respiratory signs may result from the anemia and be intensified by pneumonia.

Lesions. The findings at post mortem also indicate destruction of erythrocytes and the secondary effects of anemia. Eryth-

rophagocytosis and hyperplasia of hematopoietic tissues in spleen, bone marrow, and liver may be evident, plus centrilobular necrosis in the liver as a consequence of anoxia. Excessive fluid in peritoneal, pericardial, and pleural sacs may be a feature.

Canine Babesiosis. This disease is distributed worldwide, and two causative organisms have been identified: *B. canis* in the Western Hemisphere, Africa, Europe, parts of Asia and the Soviet Union; *B. gibsoni* in India, Ceylon, China, Turkestan, North Africa and recently in the United States (Anderson et al., 1979). Considering the ubiquitous distribution of the vector brown dog tick, *Rhipicephalus sanguineus,* the disease should be anticipated to occur in any part of the Western Hemisphere. Natural infection with *B. canis* (and other *Babesia*) has been demonstrated in splenectomized men. Experimental splenectomy of rhesus monkeys has been shown to render them susceptible to the disease.

Clinical Manifestations. The signs in the early acute case start with high fever, which may undergo remission and exacerbation, enlarged spleen, ataxia, bilateral chemosis and anemia, often with fewer than 3 million erythrocytes/cu mm of blood. Organisms may be demonstrated in large numbers in circulating erythrocytes at this time. As the disease progresses, fever abates, anemia continues, icterus appears, and conjugated as well as unconjugated bilirubin is excreted in the urine. The excretion of conjugated bilirubin indicates injury to the liver, as well as hemolysis in severe, prolonged cases. Injury to the kidney is indicated by anuria and elevated urea nitrogen in blood, proteinuria, plus cellular and granular casts in urine. Damage to the liver is indicated by elevated glutamic pyruvic transaminase in serum and by prolonged clearance time for sulfobromophthalein (Bromsulphalein). Alkaline phosphatase levels in serum may also be elevated.

Brown (cited by Malherbe, 1956) has

noticed involvement of masseter muscle in dogs with babesiosis. This results in inability to open the mouth and in manifestations of severe pain if the jaw is forcibly opened. The outcome of this muscular involvement is not reported, but the clinical similarity to so-called "eosinophilic myositis" of dogs is noteworthy.

Lesions. The trophozoites of *Babesia canis* are usually numerous in erythrocytes in the early stages, but may become difficult to find later, although the anemia persists. It has been suggested that an immunologic basis for the anemia may be present in the later stages. On occasion, dogs may harbor organisms for months without manifesting severe disease (Ewing, 1965).

The lesions are related to the anemia and possibly to the occlusion of small blood vessels by heavily parasitized, clumped erythrocytes. Thrombosis of ophthalmic veins have been reported and may explain the severe chemosis noted in many cases (Basson and Pienaar, 1965). Large numbers of organisms in clumps of erythrocytes have been seen in capillaries in the brain, and in some instances frank thrombosis is evident. These tend to be distributed in the brain in a bilaterally symmetrical manner, producing grossly visible hemorrhages. Hypoxia, due to the anemia, also appears to be a possible factor in the induction of lesions, particularly in the brain and liver. Similar vascular lesions appear to be the basis for focal edema and necrosis of skeletal muscle, liver, spleen, and lymph nodes.

Human Babesiosis. Human babesiosis was first reported in 1957 (Skrabalo) in a patient in Yugoslavia affected with *Babesia bovis.* Additional reports have followed from various parts of the globe, most examples occurring on Nantucket Island, Massachusetts, due to infection with *B. microti*, a babesiosis of mice and rodents. *B. divergens* has also been identified in a human patient. The disease is especially severe in splenectomized patients.

Diagnosis. The diagnosis is confirmed by identification of *Babesia* in blood smears, but all clinical manifestations must be judiciously weighed because of their variety and the occurrence of non-pathogenic *Babesia* in animals which may be ill from other causes. The organisms may be identified by their morphology and their stimulation of specific antibodies in the serum of infected animals. These antibodies may be detected by hemagglutination, complement fixation, fluorescent antibody and agglutination tests.

Allen, P.C., Frerichs, W.M., and Holbrook, A.A.: Experimental acute *Babesia caballi* infection. I. Red blood cell dynamics. Exp. Parasitol., *37*:67–77, 1975.

Anderson, J.F., et al.: Canine *Babesia* new to North America. Science, *204*:1431–1432, 1979.

Basson, P.A., and Pienaar, J.G.: Canine babesiosis: a report on the pathology of three cases with special reference to the "cerebral" form. J. S. Afr. Vet. Med. Assoc., *36*:333–341, 1965.

Bishop, J.P., and Adams, L.G.: Combination thin and thick blood films for the detection of *Babesia* parasitemia. Am. J. Vet. Res., *34*:1213–1214, 1973.

Brocklesby, D.W., Sellwood, S.A., Harradine, D.L., and Young, E.R.: *Babesia major* in Britain: blood-induced infections in splenectomized and intact calves. Int. J. Parasitol., *3*:671–680, 1973.

Brown, J.M.M., cited by Malherbe, W.D.: The manifestations and diagnosis of *Babesia* infections. Ann. NY Acad. Sci., *64*:128–146, 1956.

Callow, L.L., and Johnston, L.A.Y.: *Babesia spp.* in the brains of clinically normal cattle and their detection by a brain smear technique. Aust. Vet. J., *39*:25–31, 1963.

Curnow, J.A., and Curnow, B.A.: An indirect haemagglutination test for the diagnosis of *Babesia argentina* infection in cattle. Aust. Vet. J., *43*:286–290, 1967.

Dammin, G.J.: Babesiosis. *In* Seminars in Infectious Disease. Vol. I., edited by L. Weinstein and B. Fields. New York, Stratton Intercontinental Medical Book Corp., 1978.

Dennig, H.K.: Influence of splenectomy on latent piroplasmosis in horses. Berl. Muench. Tierarztl. Wochenschr., *78*:204–209, 1965.

Dorner, J.L.: A hematologic study of babesiosis of the dog. Am. J. Vet. Clin. Pathol., *1*:67–75, 1967.

Ewing, S.A.: Observations on leukocytic inclusion bodies from dogs infected with *Babesia canis*. J. Am. Vet. Med. Assoc., *143*:503–506, 1963.

———: Observations on the persistence and recurrence of *Babesia canis* infection in dogs. Vet. Med. Small Clin., *60*:741–744, 1965.

———: Method of reproduction of *Babesia canis* in erythrocytes. Am. J. Vet. Res., *26*:727–733, 1965.

———: Evaluation of methods used to detect *Babesia*

canis infections in dogs. Cornell Vet., *56*:211–220, 1966.

Fitzpatrick, J.E.P., et al.: Human case of piroplasmosis (babesiosis). Nature, *217*:861–862, 1968.

Garnham, P.C.C., et al.: Human babesiosis in Ireland: further observations and the medical significance of this infection. Br. Med. J., *2*:768–770, 1969.

Garnham, P.C.C., and Voller, A.: Experimental studies on *Babesia divergens* in rhesus monkeys with special reference to its diagnosis by serological methods. Acta Prot. Warszwa, *3*:183–187, 1965.

Hirsh, D.C., et al.: An epizootic of babesiosis in dogs used for medical research. Lab. Anim. Care, *19*:205–208, 1969.

Levine, N.D.: Taxonomy of the piroplasms. Trans. Am. Microsc. Soc., *90*:2–33, 1971.

Maegraith, B., Gilles, H.M., and Devakul, K.: Pathological processes in *Babesia canis* infections. G. Tropenmed. Parasit., *8*:485–514, 1957. V.B. 369–59.

Mahoney, D.F.: Circulating antigens in cattle infected with *Babesia bigemina* or *B. argentina*. Nature (Lond.), *211*:422, 1966.

Malherbe, W.D.: The manifestations and diagnosis of *Babesia* infections. Ann. NY Acad. Sci., *64*:128–146, 1956.

———: Clinico-pathological studies of *Babesia canis* infection in dogs. I. The influence of the infection on Bromsulphalein retention in the blood. J. S. Afr. Vet. Med. Assoc., *36*:25–30, 1965.

———: Clinico-pathological studies of *Babesia canis* infection in dogs. II. The influence of the infection on plasma transaminase activity. III. The influence of the infection on plasma alkaline phosphatase activity. J. S. Afr. Vet. Med. Assoc., *36*:173–178, 179–182, 1965.

———: Clinico-pathological studies of *Babesia canis* infection in dogs. V. The influence of the infection on kidney function. J. S. Afr. Vet. Med. Assoc., *37*:261–264, 1966.

Maurer, F.D.: Equine piroplasmosis—another emerging disease. J. Am. Vet. Med. Assoc., *141*:699–702, 1962.

Neitz, W.O.: Classification, transmission and biology of piroplasms of domestic animals. Ann. NY Acad. Sci., *64*:56–111, 1956.

Popovic, N.A., and Ristic, M.: Diagnosis of canine babesiasis by a gel precipitation test. Am. J. Vet. Res., *31*:2201–2204, 1970.

Riek, R. F.: Babesiosis. *In* Infectious Blood Diseases of Man and Animals, Vol. 2, edited by D. Wienman and M. Ristic. New York, Academic Press, 1968, pp. 219–268.

Rogers, R.J.: Observations on the pathology of *Babesia argentina* infections in cattle. Aust. Vet. J., *47*:242–247, 1971.

Ruebush, T.K.,II, et al.: Human babesiosis on Nantucket Island. Clinical features. Ann. Intern. Med., *86*:6–9, 1977.

Scholtens, R.G., Braff, E.K., Healy, G.R., and Gleason, N.: A case of babesiosis in man in the United States. Am. J. Trop. Med. Hyg., *17*:810–813, 1968.

Schroeder, W.F., Cox, H.W., and Ristic, M.: Anaemia, parasitaemia, erythrophagocytosis, and haemagglutinins in *Babesia rodhaini* infection. Ann. Trop. Med. Parasitol., *60*:31–38, 1966.

Seneviratna, P.: The pathology of *Babesia gibsoni* (Patton, 1910) infection in the dog. Ceylon Vet. J., *13*:107–110, 1965.

———: Studies of *Babesia gibsoni* infections of dogs in Ceylon. Ceylon Vet. J., *13*:1–6, 1965.

Shortt, H.E.: Human infections with *Babesia*. Trans. R. Soc. Trop. Med. Hyg., *69*:519–521, 1975.

Sibinovic, S., Sibinovic, K.H., and Ristic, M.: Equine babesiosis: diagnosis by bentonite agglutination and passive hemagglutination tests. Am. J. Vet. Res., *30*:691–695, 1969.

Simpson, C.F.: Electron microscopic comparison of *Babesia spp.* and hepatic changes in ponies and mice. Am. J. Vet. Res., *31*:1763–1768, 1970.

Simpson, C.F., Kirkham, W.W., and Kling, J.M.: Comparative morphologic features of *Babesia caballi* and *Babesia equi*. Am. J. Vet. Res., *28*:1693–1697, 1967.

Sippel, W.L., et al.: Equine piroplasmosis in the United States. J. Am. Vet. Med. Assoc., *141*:694–698, 1962.

Skrabalo, Z., and Deanovic, A.: Piroplasmosis in man. Report on a case. Doc. Med. Geogr. Trop., *9*:11–16, 1957.

Smith, T., and Kilborne, F.L.: Investigations into the nature, causation and prevention of Texas or Southern cattle fever. U. S. Dept. Agric. Bur. Anim. Ind. Bull. No. 1, 1893.

Todorivic, R.A.: Bovine babesiasis: its diagnosis and control. Am. J. Vet. Res., *35*:1045–1052, 1974.

———: Serological diagnosis of babesiosis: a review. Trop. Anim. Health. Prod., *7*:1–14, 1975.

Western, K.A., et al.: Babesiosis in a Massachusetts resident. N. Engl. J. Med., *283*:854–856, 1970.

Wright, I.G.: An electron microscopic study of intravascular agglutination in the cerebral cortex due to *Babesia argentina* infection. Int. J. Parasitol., *2*:209–215, 1972.

THEILERIASIS

Protozoan parasites of the genus *Theileria*, like *Babesia*, are found in the erythrocytes but reproduce by schizogony in lymphocytes or histiocytes, and are classified in the family Theileriidae. Two related genera are *Gonderi*, whose members reproduce by schizogony in lymphocytes and by fission in erythrocytes, and *Cytauxzoön*, which multiply by schizogony in histiocytic cells and by fission in erythrocytes. Table 13–6 indicates the important pathogenic *Theileria*.

Table 13-6. Theileriases

Organism	Animals Affected	Geographic Distribution	Tick Vector
Theileria parva	Cattle, African buffalo, Indian water buffalo	Africa	*Rhipicephalus appendiculatus*
Th. annulata	Cattle, zebu, water buffalo	North Africa, Middle & Far East, Southern Europe, Soviet Union	*Hyalomma detritum, H. dromedarii, H. excavatum, H. turanicum, H. savignyi, H. plumbeum, H. scupense*
Th. mutans	Cattle, deer	Africa, Asia, Australia, Soviet Union, United States, England	*Rhipicephalus appendiculatus, Rh. evertsi, Haemaphysalis bispinosa, H. punctata*
Th. hirci	Sheep, goats	North & East Africa, Iraq, Turkey, Soviet Union, Greece	*Rhipicephalus bursa* (?)
Th. ovis	Sheep, goats	Africa, Asia, India, Soviet Union, Europe	*Rhipicephalus bursa, Rh. evertsi, Dermacentor sylvarum, Haemaphysalis sulcata, Ornithodorous lahorensis*
Th. lawrencei	Cattle, buffalo	Africa	*Rhipicephalus appendiculatus*
Th. cervi	White tailed deer	United States	Unknown

Theileria parva, the cause of East Coast fever, a disease of cattle of much importance in Africa, is transmitted by several species of ticks, most of them in the genus *Rhipicephalus* and *Hyalomma.* Schizogony occurs in the cytoplasm of lymphocytes and histiocytes in peripheral blood or in lymph nodes, spleen, liver, and other organs. The schizonts, which are up to 12 μ in diameter, contain numerous nuclei, and are called **Koch's bodies** after their discoverer, are considered characteristic of the disease. Upon disruption, the process may be repeated in other lymphocytes, or the organisms may enter red blood cells as tiny rod-, comma-, or ring-shaped bodies, somewhat smaller than *Babesia,* which do not undergo further division.

Unlike babesiosis, recovery from East Coast fever not only results in solid immunity, but the organisms disappear from the body and hence are not in position to cause relapses or result in a carrier state.

Clinical Manifestations. The clinical manifestations start with fever, which appears about 15 days following exposure by the bite of infected ticks. Several days after *Theileria* becomes demonstrable in the blood, the appetite is gradually lost, rumination ceases, and milk secretion decreases. The superficial lymph nodes become noticeably enlarged, the muzzle dry, the hair coat rough, and salivation as well as lacrimation becomes excessive. Respiratory distress may follow pulmonary edema, and death may result from asphyxia. In some cases, death follows gradual emaciation, delirium, and coma. When signs relevant to central nervous system are present, the disease has been termed "**turning disease**." In all forms of theileriasis, anemia of varying severity may occur, which has been postulated to be of immune origin. There is generally leukopenia.

Lesions. The most constant lesions found at necropsy consist of generalized enlargement of lymph nodes, pulmonary edema and emphysema, and subcutaneous and intramuscular edema. The spleen is of normal size. Excessive pericardial and pleural fluid may be present, and the liver is generally enlarged, yellowish, and frequently mottled. White foci of various sizes may be seen in the renal cortex. The meninges may be congested and focal hemorrhage present in the brain.

The principal microscopic finding is proliferation of lymphocytic cells in lymph nodes, spleen, Peyer's patches, and elsewhere. Blood vessels, including cerebral vessels, may be filled with parasitized lymphocytes, which apparently impede blood flow, leading to focal infarction.

Koch's bodies may be found in tissue sections of many organs.

Infection with other species of *Theileria* is usually mild. *Th. annulata* is the cause of tropical theileriasis in cattle, which is similar to East Coast fever. *Th. mutans* is widely distributed, but of little pathologic importance. *Th. hirci* and *Th. ovis* also rarely cause clinical disease in sheep. *Th. lawrencei* causes what is called **Buffalo disease** or **Corridor disease** which, if severe, resembles East Coast fever.

Gonderia bovis is an organism similar to *Theileria* but lacks an erythrocytic stage. Infection, if severe, is similar to theileriasis.

Cytauxzoonosis, caused by a species of *Cytauxzoon* within the family Theileriidae, is an infection thought to have been limited to various wild ungulates in Africa. However, a disease pathologically similar has been reported in domestic cats in the

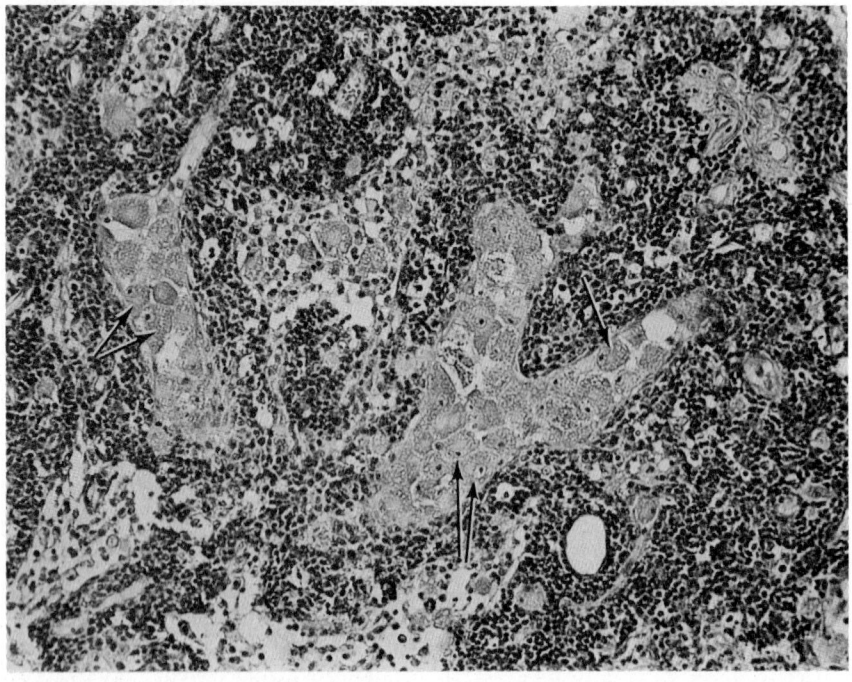

Fig. 13–28. Feline *Cytauxzoon* infected cells (arrows) in veins and sinuses of a mesenteric lymph node of a cat. Typically, nuclei of infected cells are not distinct and the cytoplasm appears foamy. (Courtesy of Dr. Ann Kier.)

United States (Wagner, 1976). *Cytauxzoon* undergoes schizogony in histiocytes and reticuloendothelial cells, with subsequent development of small organisms which may or may not divide in erythrocytes. The infection in cats was fatal and characterized by large numbers of schizonts in vascular endothelium of the liver, lung, spleen, and lymph nodes.

Diagnosis. The diagnosis of theileriasis depends upon demonstration of the organisms in erythrocytes and in lymphocytes (Koch's bodies). Babesiosis is the most important disease from which it must be differentiated. Various tests for circulating antibodies have also been used with success.

Barnett, S.F.: Theileriasis. *In* Infectious Blood Diseases of Man and Animals, edited by D. Wienman and M. Ristic. New York, Academic Press, 1968, pp. 269–328.

Burridge, M.J.: Application of the indirect fluorescent antibody test in experimental East Coast fever (*Theileria parva* infection of cattle). Res. Vet. Sci., 12:338–341, 1971.

Burridge, M.J., and Kimber, C.D.: The indirect fluorescent antibody test for experimental East Coast fever (*Theileria parva* infection of cattle). Evaluation of a cell culture schizont antigen. Res. Vet. Sci., 13:451–455, 1972.

Hooshmand-Rad, P.: The pathogenesis of anaemia in *Theileria annulata* infection. Res. Vet. Sci., 20:324–329, 1976.

Hooshmand-Rad, P., and Hawa, N.J.: Malignant theileriosis of sheep and goats. Trop. Anim. Health Prod., 5:97–102, 1973.

Jarett, W.F.H., and Brocklesby, D.W.: Preliminary electron microscopic studies on East Coat fever. Parasitol., 55:13, 1965.

————: A preliminary electron microscopic study of East Coast fever (*Theileria parva* infection). J. Protozool., 13:301–310, 1966.

Krier, J.P., Ristic, M., and Watrach, A.M.: *Theileria sp.* in a deer in the United States. Am. J. Vet. Res., 23:657–663, 1962.

Matson, B.A.: Theileriosis due to *Theileria parva, T. lawrencei* and *T. mutans.* Bibliography 1897–1966. Weybridge: Commonwealth Bureau of Animal Health, pp. 44, 1967.

McCully, R.M., Keep, M.E., and Basson, P.A.: Cytauxzoonosis in a giraffe [*Giraffa camelopardalis* (Linnaeus, 1758)] in Zululand. Onderstepoort J. Vet. Res., 37:7–9, 1970.

Rensburg, I.B.J. van: Bovine cerebral theileriosis: a report of five cases with splenic infarction. J. S. Afr. Vet. Assoc., 47:137–141, 1976.

Splitter, E.J.: *Theileria mutans* associated with bovine anaplasmosis. J. Am. Vet. Med. Assoc., 117:134–135, 1950.

Steck, W.: Histologic studies on East Coast fever. South Africa, Onderstepoort, 13th & 14th Reports, Part 1, 1928, pp. 243–282.

Wagner, J.E.: A fatal cytauxzoonosis-like disease in cats. J. Am. Vet. Med. Assoc., 168:585–588, 1976.

Wilde, J.K.H.: East Coast fever. Adv. Vet. Sci., 11:207–259, 1967.

CHAPTER 14

Diseases Caused by Parasitic Helminths and Arthropods

Metazoan parasites comprise a large and diverse group of organisms of considerable importance to veterinary medicine throughout the world. In the United States, many parasitisms of animals have been well controlled, and most of those affecting human beings have been reduced to a minimum. In many countries, however, metazoan parasites remain among the most frequent and important causes of disease, for example, schistosomiasis in man. In addition to being primary causes of disease, metazoan parasites may also serve as vectors for other infectious organisms. This is especially true of arthropods, which serve as vectors for many viruses as well as protozoan and metazoan parasites.

PARASITIC HELMINTHS

Parasitic helminths, or worms, are important incitants of disease in all species of animals. Although these parasites in many instances produce little serious damage to the host, they are never beneficial and in some instances can produce severe and even fatal disease. The effect of various helminths upon animal hosts is given chief consideration in this chapter. Life cycles, host range, immunity, and infectivity are discussed only in so far as they influence the lesions resulting from parasitism. The reader is referred to standard texts and the selected references at the ends of these topics for more detailed information on the many other important aspects of helminthic parasitism (helminthiasis).

The parasitic helminths to be considered in this chapter are classified by the International Code of Zoological Nomenclature in three phyla, as follows:

Phylum Platyhelminthes, including the **trematodes** or **flukes,** and the **cestodes** or **tapeworms;**

Phylum Nemathelminthes, including the **nematodes** or **roundworms,** which infect a wide variety of hosts including animals, man, and plants; and

Phylum Acanthocephala, including the **thorny-headed worms,** a few of which are important parasites of animals.

Effects of Helminthic Parasites Upon the Host

Helminthic parasites produce deleterious effects upon their hosts in a wide variety of ways. These can be outlined as follows:

1. Mechanically interfere with function
   a. Obstruct blood or lymph channels
      (1) Right ventricle and pulmo-

nary artery—*Dirofilaria immitis* (dog)

(2) Carotid arteries—*Elaeophora schneideri* (sheep)

(3) Lymphatic channels—*Dracunculus insignis* (dog)

(4) Mesenteric arteries—*Strongylus vulgaris* (horse)

(5) Aorta—*Spirocerca lupi* (dog); *Strongylus vulgaris* (horse)

(6) Vena cava—*Schistosoma bovis; S. hematobium*

b. Obstruct ducts or tracts

(1) Bile duct—liver flukes, ascarids, fringed tapeworms

(2) Esophagus—*Spirocerca lupi* (dog)

(3) Intestinal lumen—ascarids, tapeworms

(4) Respiratory tract—*Filaroides osleri, Metastrongylus apri*

(5) Urinary tract—*Dioctophyma renale*

c. Attach to or utilize functional tissue

(1) Stomach mucosa—*Trichostrongylus axei* (sheep, cattle), *Draschia megastoma* (horses)

(2) Small intestine—hookworms

(3) Cecum and large intestine—strongyles (horses), cecal worms (turkeys, dogs)

d. Act as foreign bodies, with resultant tissue reactions displacing normal structures

(1) Schistosome ova (flukes)

(2) Dead larvae of many nematodes—*Toxocara canis, Dirofilaria immitis*

2. Invade and displace cells and tissues, producing necrosis and loss of function

a. Skin—hookworm larvae, *Habronema* larvae, *Rhabditis sp., Onchocerca* larvae, *Elaeophora schneideri* larvae, *Stephanofilaria stilesi*

b. Liver—giant liver flukes, kidney worm larvae, cysticercus, echinococcus and coenurus cysts, ascarid larvae, *Capillaria hepatica* (rat, man)

c. Intestinal wall—nodular worms (*Esophagostomum sp.*), larvae of strongyles (horses)

d. Brain and spinal cord—coenurus, echinococcus, filaria, other helminth larvae

e. Lung—lungworms, ascarid larvae, hookworms

f. Musculature—trichinae, cysticerci

3. Devour blood and thereby cause anemia:

a. Hookworms (dogs, cattle)

b. Stomach worms (cattle and sheep)

4. Utilize food needed by the host:

a. Tapeworms

b. Ascarids

5. Induce or predispose to neoplasia:

a. Esophagus—*Spirocerca lupi* (dog)

b. Liver—*Cysticercus fasciolaris* (rat)

c. Urinary bladder—*Schistosoma hematobium* (man)

6. Introduce bacterial or other infection into tissues of the host:

a. Lungs—lungworms, ascarid larvae

b. Intestinal wall—hookworms, nodule worms, salmon flukes (dog)

c. Cecum—cecal worms (histomonads of turkeys)

d. Perirenal tissues—*Stephanurus dentatus*

7. Devour tissues of host:

a. Ascarids

b. Stomach worms

8. Secrete toxic products (hemolysins, histolysins, anticoagulants):

a. Hookworms, nodule worms

b. Stomach worms

c. Strongyles

Identification of Helminths in Tissues

The discovery of one or more fragments of a helminth in histologic sections of tissue presents a challenge to the pathologist. In order to evaluate fully the significance of such a finding, he must know the potentialities of the parasite; whence it came; where it was going when trapped by the fixative; and what its total effect upon the host might be. The identification of the parasite is therefore critical. Complete, well-preserved specimens should be secured for referral to a parasitologist whenever possible. However, presumptive identification of the parasite can often be made from fragments of the organism in tissues, or it may be possible to tease parasites in recognizable form from fixed gross tissues. Although far from complete, the information concerning the appearance of helminths in tissue sections is now sufficient to permit the recognition of many species.

In determining the identity of a parasite in tissues, several factors may be utilized to narrow the field of consideration: the host and its usual parasites, the anatomic location of the parasite, the nature of the tissue reaction, and, most important, the morphologic features of the parasite itself. Helminths must also be differentiated from arthropods and pentastomids, which may be encountered in tissue sections. (These organisms are discussed at the end of this chapter.) Identification of these major groups of parasitic metazoa by morphologic features is aided by the following key, based on Chitwood and Lichtenfels, 1972.

1.
   A. Internal organs embedded in parenchymatous matrix; body usually flattened dorsoventrally ....Platyhelmintha 2
   B. Internal organs suspended or free in body cavity; body usually not flattened 3
2.
   A. Segmented, attached by scolex, contain calcareous corpuscles, lack digestive tract, muscle layers separated ....Cestoda

   B. Leaf-shaped, attached by suckers, lack calcareous corpuscles, have digestive tract ..Trematoda
3.
   A. Somatic musculature not striated (smooth), attached to body wall throughout length 4
   B. Somatic musculature striated, attached to body wall only at ends 6
4.
   A. Hypodermis thicker than muscular layer, contains lacunar channels, digestive system absent .... Acanthocephala
   B. Hypodermis thinner than muscular layer, with no lacunar channels, digestive system present, but may be rudimentary 5
5.
   A. Cuticle usually with areoles; lateral hypodermal chords absent; ventral nerve chord usually prominent; digestive system rudimentary ....Nematomorpha
   B. Cuticle may be smooth, striated, or annulated, but areoles absent; hypodermal chords present; digestive system well developed .. ..Nematoda
6.
   A. Chitinous exoskeleton may be segmented, with jointed appendages ....Arthropoda
   B. Pseudosegmented, if present, pseudopodia not jointed ....Pentastomida

Nematodes have an external cuticle supported by a thin membrane, the hypodermis, within which is a muscular wall surrounding the body cavity. They have an alimentary canal and the sexes are separate. All of these features can be detected in cross sections of the adults and, in some cases, of the larvae. Further, the midsomatic muscular wall of the nematodes has some distinguishing features. The muscle cells are arranged longitudinally in a single layer just within the hypodermis and, in cross section of helminths of most species, are seen to be divided into four groups by cords of cells (chords) of the hypodermis, which project toward the center. Thus, one dorsal, one ventral, and two lateral chords are formed by the hypodermis. These cells in many species are also distinctive, varying in size and number. Nematodes are said to have a **polymyarian** somatic musculature *(Ascaris, Filaria,* and *Dracunculus)* when numerous long slender muscle cells, which run lengthwise along the body wall, protrude into the body cavity and are divided into four longitudinal units by dorsal, ventral, and lateral chords made up of a single row of cells (Fig. 14–6). Those nematodes with closely packed, somewhat flattened muscle cells in units containing three or four cells are classified as **meromyarian,** and include such genera as *Enterobius, Ancylostoma,* and *Necator.* In a third group of nematodes, the muscle cells, although closely packed, are not divided by chords, the body cavity being completely surrounded by longitudinally running muscle cells. This group is classified as **holomyarian** and includes the genus *Trichuris.*

The eggs or larvae can be used as a guide in the identification of some adult parasites in tissues. Sections are often made through the ovary or uterus of adult worms, in which numerous ova or larvae are present. The size, shape, and shell of many ova are distinctive for the species; for example, the ovoid egg with double-contoured shell of *Strongylus,* the single polar eminence of ova of *Oxyuris,* and the double polar eminence of ova of *Capillaria* (Fig. 14–21). Some nematodes are viviparous, the ova embryonating and hatching in the uterus, the larvae escaping as free forms *(Dirofilaria);* others are ovoviviparous and produce ova which are embryonated, but the larvae are still within the egg shell when they are expelled from the parasite *(Spirocerca).*

Trematodes and cestodes generally can be differentiated from nematodes in tissue sections. They are flat dorsoventrally and they do not have a body cavity, although some of the larval forms may be suspended in a bladder (see cysticerci). Most of them are hermaphroditic, hence male and female sex organs can often be seen in tissue sections of a single parasite. The anatomic site in which cestodes and trematodes are found, the nature of the tissue reaction they evoke, and their structural form are often guides to the tentative identification of these parasites in tissues. Familiarity with their life cycle, host range, and morphology is thus an asset to the pathologist.

The cestodes possess a specialized structure, the scolex, which can often be detected in larval forms as well as in adult in tissue sections. The scolex may bear two or more elongated suctorial grooves, or may have cup-shaped sucking discs, and a proboscis. In some species, the proboscis is armed with characteristic hooklets (Fig. 14–29). An external cuticle surrounding a germinal layer from which scolices or brood capsules containing scolices may arise also serves to identify cestodes in tissue sections. The body of cestodes is almost always segmented. The outer longitudinal muscles are separated from the inner circular muscles by parenchyma within which are suspended calcareous corpuscles. Cestodes lack a digestive tract.

In contrast to cestodes, trematodes are leaf-shaped and nonsegmented. They contain a digestive tract, lack calcareous corpuscles, and the longitudinal and circular muscle layers are close to one another. Their cuticle is usually thinner than that of cestodes. The eggs of trematodes are also distinctive. They are usually pigmented, operculated, and birefringent (anisotropic). The presence of some trematodes in the body may be determined by the identification of the ova of the parasite, even though the adult is not found. This is of particular value in schistosomiasis, in which many ova are carried by the blood stream to various organs, where they become embedded in small granulomas. Some of the filarid worms are seldom seen in adult form in the tissues, but their larval forms are sufficient for diagnosis.

Immunity to Parasites

Parasites elicit humoral antibodies and cellular hypersensitivity (delayed immunity) responses, and both are probably involved in the expulsion of adult and larval stages of parasites. Most evidence suggests that the delayed immune response mediated by T-cells is the most important of the two. Delayed or cellular hypersensitivity has been demonstrated specifically in the course of infections by several parasites, namely, *Trichinella spiralis*, *Trichostrongylus colubriformis*, *Ancylostomum caninum*, *Nippostrongylus brasiliensis*, *Ascaris suum*, *Schistosoma mansoni*, *Fasciola hepatica*, and *Hymenolepis nana*. The mechanism of expulsion is not fully elucidated. Although direct interaction between antibody or memory T-cells and the offending parasite may lead to expulsion through the various means discussed in Chapter 7, the immune induction of a nonspecific inflammatory response is believed to be the principal mechanism.

Belding, D.L.: Textbook of Clinical Parasitology, 3rd ed. New York, Appleton-Century-Crofts, Inc., 1965.

Benbrook, E.A.: Outline of Parasites Reported for Domesticated Animals in North America, 6th ed. ·Ames, Iowa State Univ. Press, 1963.

Chitwood, M., and Lichtenfels, J.R.: Identification of parasitic metazoa in tissue sections. Exp. Parasitol., 32:407–519, 1972.

Flynn, R.J.: Parasites of Laboratory Animals. Ames, Iowa State Univ. Press, 1973.

Georgi, J.R.: Parasitology for Veterinarians. 2nd ed. Philadelphia, W. B. Saunders, 1974.

Griffiths, H.J.: A Handbook of Veterinary Parasitology: Domestic Animals of North America. Minneapolis, Univ. of Minnesota Press, 1978.

Herms, W.B.: Medical Entomology, 6th ed. New York, The Macmillan Co., 1969.

Jarrett, W.F.H., Miller, H.R.P., and Murray, M.: The relationship between mast cells and globule leucocytes in parasitic infections. Vet. Rec., 80:505–506, 1967.

Kelly, J.D.: Mechanisms of immunity to intestinal helminths. Aust. Vet. J., 49:91–97, 1973.

Lapage, G.: Veterinary Parasitology. 2nd ed. Springfield, Charles C Thomas, 1968.

Larsh, J.E., Jr., and Race, G.J.: Allergic inflammation as a hypothesis for the expulsion of worms from tissues: a review. Exp. Parasitol., 37:251–266, 1975.

Larsh, J.E., Jr.: Delayed (cellular) hypersensitivity in parasitic infections. Am. J. Trop. Med. Hyg., 16:735–745, 1967.

Larsh, J.E., Jr., and Weatherly, N.F.: Cell-mediated immunity in certain parasitic infections. Curr. Top. Microbiol. Immunol., 67:113–137, 1974.

————: Cell-mediated immunity against certain parasitic worms. Adv. Parasitol., 13:183–222, 1975.

Lichtenfels, J.R.: Helminths of domestic equids. Proc. Helminthol. Soc. Wash., 42:1–92, 1975.

Ogilvie, B.M., and Jones, V.E.: *Nippostrongylus brasiliensis*: a review of immunity and the host/ parasite relationship in the rat. Exp. Parasitol., 29:138–177, 1971.

Poynter, D.: Some tissue reactions to the nematode parasites of animals. Adv. Parasitol., 4:321–383, 1966.

Sloss, M.W., and Kemp, R.L.: Veterinary Clinical Parasitology. 5th ed. Ames, Iowa State Univ. Press, 1978.

Soulsby, E.J.L.: Helminths, Arthropods and Protozoa of Domesticated Animals, 6th ed. Philadelphia, Lea & Febiger, 1968.

Whitlock, J.H.: Diagnosis of Veterinary Parasitisms. Philadelphia, Lea & Febiger, 1960.

Whur, P.: Relationship of globule leucocytes to gastrointestinal nematodes in the sheep, and *Nippostrongylus brasiliensis* and *Hymenolepis nana* infections in rats. J. Comp. Pathol., 76:57–65, 1966.

Ascariasis (Common Roundworm Infection, Ascarid Worm Infection)

Ascarids (phylum: Nemathelminthes; family: Ascaridae) are extremely common roundworms whose adult forms are found in abundance in the gastrointestinal tracts of birds and mammals throughout the world. Ascarids occur not only in great numbers but in many varieties, most of them being host-specific. Certain ascarids that are morphologically indistinguishable, such as those that infect man and swine, are host-specific and rarely develop to maturity in other than the true host.

The adults are usually large robust worms found in the small intestine, the cecal worms of chickens being an exception. The eggs are thick-shelled and unsegmented when laid, and a period of incubation and two molts within the shell are required before the embryo becomes infective. The eggs are resistant to desiccation, low temperatures and many chemical agents. Young animals are particularly susceptible to infection with ascarids; many adults lose their ascarid parasites spontaneously.

A few representative species are listed in Table 14–1 by the names currently preferred.

In the evolutionary extension of their range of final hosts to include birds and terrestrial and aquatic mammals, the life cycles of the ascarids and the migratory behavior of their larvae have been modified in many ways. The larvae or eggs of some species are ingested by an intermediate host (insect larvae, amphibia, rodents, or insectivora), in whose tissues they usually remain and develop to second stage larvae, until they gain access to the definitive host. This phenomenon has been demonstrated in several ascarids of veterinary importance, namely, *Ascaris columnaris (Baylisascaris columnaris)*, *Toxocara canis*, *Toxocara cati*, and *Toxascaris leonina*. Other helminths of this group do not utilize an intermediate host (none require it); the embryonated eggs are ingested by the host, the infective larvae

Table 14–1. Representative Species of Ascaridae

Species of Ascarid	Definitive Hosts
Ascaris lumbricoides (suum)	Man, swine (var. *suis*)
Toxocara canis	Dog, man (rarely)
Toxocara cati	Cat, dog, wildcat, lion, leopard, man (rarely)
Toxascaris leonina	Dog, cat, lion, tiger, fox
Neoascaris vitulorum	Cattle
Parascaris equorum	Horse
Ascaridia galli	Chickens, turkeys

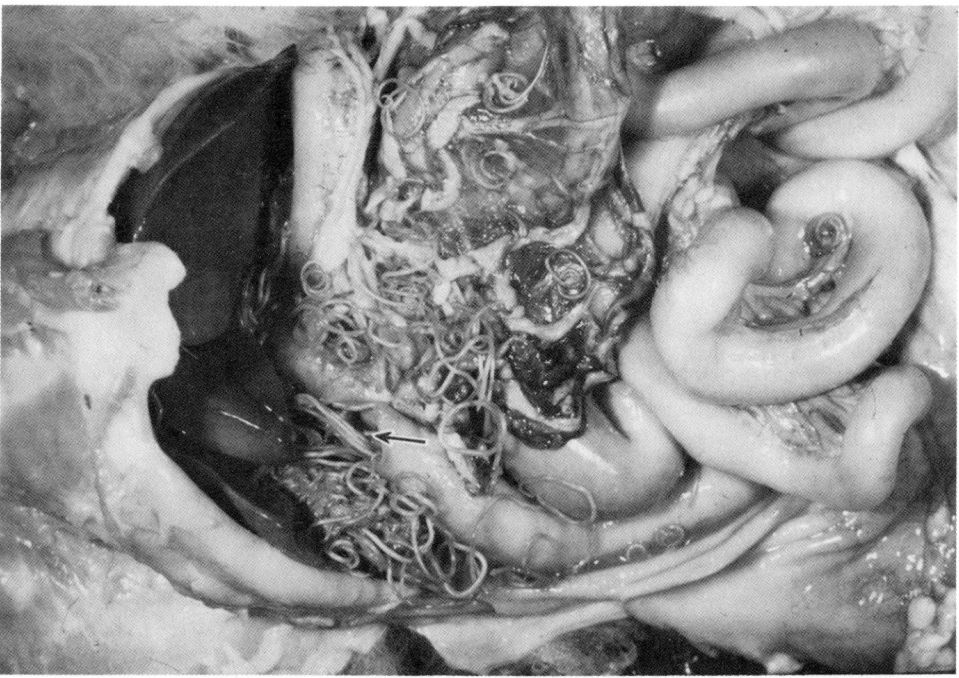

Fig. 14–1. Ascariasis. Unusually severe infection of a seven-week-old Collie puppy with *Toxocara canis*, resulted in rupture of duodenum (arrow) and death. (Photo courtesy of Angell Memorial Animal Hospital.)

escape from the egg and invade the host tissues, and then development to the adult form is completed at the end of their migration through the tissues. The lesions produced are determined by the migratory patterns the specific larvae follow, which are of three principal types.

(1) Infective larvae penetrate the intestinal wall, pass through the liver to the lungs, break through the alveoli, gain entrance to the bronchi, ascend the trachea, are swallowed, and then develop into adults in the intestinal lumen. This "tracheal migration" of larvae is characteristic of *Ascaris lumbricoides* (man), *A. lumbricoides* var. *suis* (swine), *Parascaris equorum* (horses), and *Toxocara canis* (dogs).

(2) Larvae migrate not only through the liver and lungs, but also through the somatic tissues, sometimes causing prenatal infection of the fetus. This has been demonstrated with *Toxocara canis* (dogs), *Toxocara cati* (cats), and *Neoascaris vitulorum* (cattle). Neonatal infection may result from transmammary passage of as-

carid larvae. Prenatal and transmammary neonatal infection does not require exposure of the pregnant or lactating animal to infection with resultant migration, but may follow activation of larvae localized in various tissues from previous exposure.

(3) Larvae penetrate the wall of the intestine, where they develop without involving other somatic or visceral tissues; then return to the intestinal lumen to become adults. This pattern is followed by *Toxascaris leonina.*

The migratory pattern also varies with the source of infection. For example, tissue migration follows exposure of cats to infectious eggs of *T. cati,* but in cats exposed to infectious larvae within an intermediate host, the parasites develop in the wall of the intestine, similarly to *Toxascaris leonina,* and do not migrate.

The age of the host also affects larval migration. In young puppies exposed to *T. canis,* most larvae migrate through lungs to mature to adulthood in the intestine; whereas in older dogs, most larvae localize in tissues as second-stage larvae

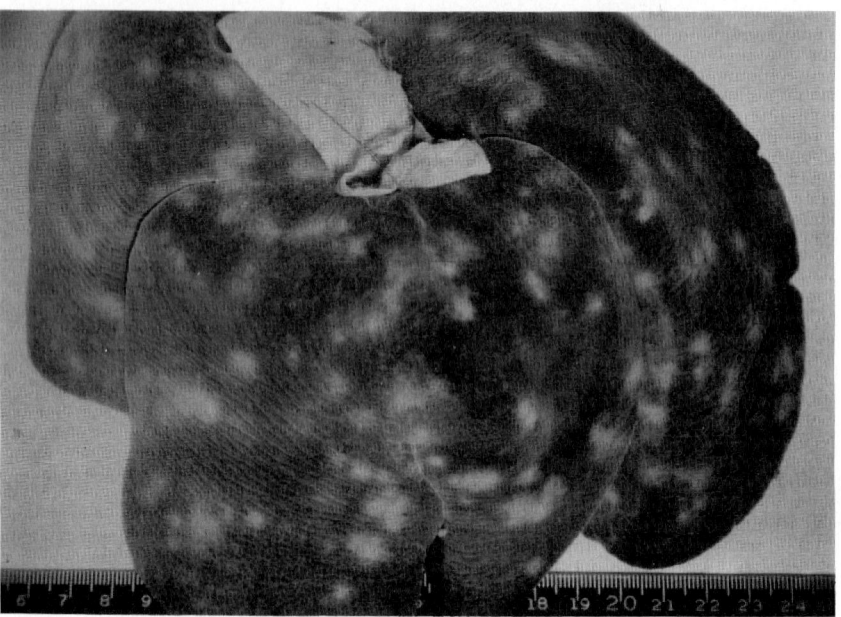

Fig. 14–2.   Ascariasis, liver of a young pig. Gray, fibrous areas are caused by migration of ascaris larvae.

and fail to produce patent infections. Whether this is a phenomenon of age or acquired immunity has not been determined.

It is readily apparent that ascarid larvae can penetrate various tissues of the host, where they may remain for some time and produce tissue damage. While the intestinal wall, the liver, and the lungs are the common routes for larval migration, any tissue of the body could be invaded. The interval between ingestion of infective forms and the appearance of eggs in the feces of the final host is called the **prepatent period.** Obviously this is a period during which the host can sustain serious damage from the migration and development of larvae in the tissues. The prepatent period for different species of worms varies; it may be relatively long, for example, 60 or more days for *A. lumbricoides.*

Lesions. Adult ascarids ordinarily live free in the lumen of the small intestine. They feed on the intestinal contents, occasionally abrade the mucosa and, by a swimming movement, maintain their position in the tract in spite of peristaltic action. Their motility may be enhanced by several factors, among which are increased temperature (fever in the host) and starvation. On the other hand, they may be unable to maintain their position against the exaggerated peristalsis that occurs in diarrhea or after purging, and be swept out of the intestine. When their motility increases, it is not uncommon for ascarids to move into the stomach or the hepatic or pancreatic ducts. In the bile ducts, they may produce obstruction, with icterus a prominent manifestation. Jaundice of this origin is a fairly common reason for condemnation of hog carcasses inspected in abattoirs. Adult ascarids remaining in their usual location may become so numerous as to cause obstruction of the intestinal lumen, which may be

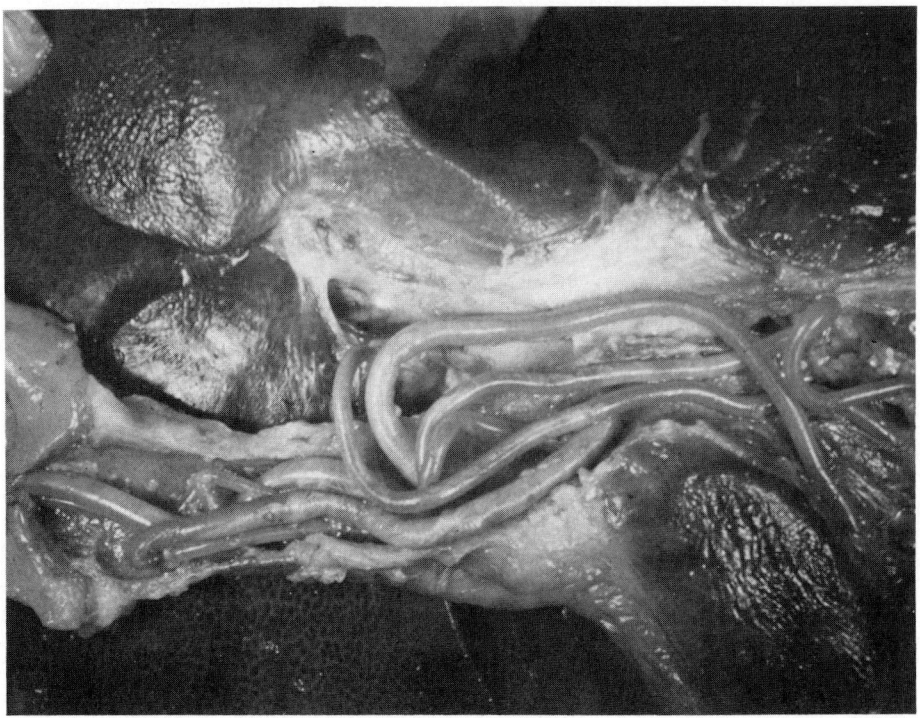

Fig. 14-3. *Ascaris lumbricoides, var. suis* in bile ducts of a pig. (Courtesy of Dr. C. L. Davis.)

fatal, particularly in young animals. On occasion, penetration of the intestinal wall has produced peritonitis in the host. Inanition in the host and retardation of growth of the young animal are the most common effects produced by ascarids, for they deprive the host of food and interfere with its digestive processes.

The lesions produced by the infective larvae during their migration and development in the tissues of the host range from minimal to severe. As the larvae migrate, tissues along the route are damaged and reparative processes become part of the pathologic picture. Larvae that penetrate the intestinal mucosa may carry bacteria into the tissues. In the liver, heavy infection with larvae often produces rather intense inflammation, with edema, neutrophils, eosinophils and lymphocytes as components of the inflammatory reaction. Larvae may be identified in a central mass of characteristic caseous necrosis surrounded by epithelioid cells, eosinophils, lymphocytes, and neutrophils. The portal areas are most severely involved, but subsequent fibrosis may obliterate entire lobules. However, in the average case seen at necropsy, tissue changes are negligible. In swine, a diffuse, subcapsular fibrosis is believed to mark the sites of previous larval invasion of the liver. Larval migration through the lungs sets up an inflammatory reaction that may result in mild to severe respiratory involvement, and which usually heals with few residual lesions. Hemorrhages occur as the larvae break out of the pulmonary capillaries to enter the alveoli, and in heavy infection loss of bronchiolar epithelium and infiltration of leukocytes may be additional features.

Ascarid larvae may wander throughout the body and produce granulomatous nodules in many sites. They are most commonly encountered in the kidney, but may localize in any tissue, including the liver, lung, myocardium, brain, eye, and lymph nodes.

Although adult ascarids are relatively host-specific, larvae are less so and may migrate within the tissues of many different species. The name **visceral larval migrans** has been given to the syndrome caused by ascarid larvae migration in abnormal hosts. It is especially important in young children, where it is usually caused by *Toxocara canis*, but it can occur in almost any species by any of the migratory ascarids (see also cerebrospinal nematodiasis).

Diagnosis. Clinical diagnosis of ascariasis is established by demonstration of ova or adults in the feces and the correlation of these findings with the clinical symptoms. During the prepatent period, ova will not be found in the feces, although immature forms may be present in the tissues or intestinal lumen. Ascarid larvae may be identified in tissue sections and their relationship to lesions clearly demonstrated. Serologic tests are useful to diagnose visceral larval migrans, which may mimic many granulomatoses and occasionally neoplastic diseases. Eosinophilia usually accompanies larval migrans. Occlusion of hepatic ducts by adult ascarids may occur, and is usually recognized at necropsy.

Barron, C.N., and Saunders, L.Z.: Visceral larva migrans in the dog. Pathol. Vet., 3:315–330, 1966.

Dubey, J.P.: *Toxocara cati* and other intestinal parasites of cats. Vet. Rec., 79:506–508, 1966.

Fernando, S.T., et al.: Precipitin reactions in monkeys (*Macaca sinica*) experimentally infected with *Toxocara canis* and in children with visceral larva migrans syndrome. J. Comp. Pathol., 80:407–414, 1970.

Fernando, S.T., Vasudevan, B., Jegatheeswaran, T., and Sooriyamoorthi, T.: The nature of resistance of immune puppies to superinfection with *Toxocara canis*: evidence that immunity affects second- but not fourth-stage larvae. Parasitology, 66:415–422, 1973.

Fitzgerald, P.R., and Mansfield, M.E.: Visceral larva migrans (*Toxocara canis*) in calves. Am. J. Vet. Res., 31:561–566, 1970.

Greve, J.H.: Age resistance to *Toxocara canis* in ascarid-free dogs. Am. J. Vet. Res., 32:1185–1192, 1971.

Hayden, D.W., and Van Kruiningen, H.J.: Experimentally induced canine toxocariasis: laboratory examinations and pathologic changes, with emphasis on the gastrointestinal tract. Am. J. Vet. Res., *36*:1605–1614, 1975.

Koutz, F.R., Groves, H.F., and Scothorn, M.W.: The prenatal migration of *Toxocara canis* larvae and their relationship to infection in pregnant bitches and in pups. Am. J. Vet. Res., *27*:789–795, 1966.

Matoff, K., and Komandarey, S.: Comparative studies on the migration of the larvae of *Toxascaris leonina* and *Toxascaris transfuga*. Z. Parasitenkd., *25*:538–555, 1965.

Mitchell, J.R.: Detection of *Toxocara canis* antibodies with the fluorescent antibody technique. Proc. Soc. Exp. Biol. N.Y., *117*:267–270, 1964.

Moncol, D.J., and Batte, E.F.: Peripheral blood eosinophilia in porcine ascariasis. Cornell Vet., *57*:96–107, 1967.

Morrow, D.A.: Pneumonia in cattle due to migrating *Ascaris lumbricoides* larvae. J. Am. Vet. Med. Assoc., *153*:184–189, 1968.

Mossalam, I., Hosney, Z., and Atallah, O.A.: Larva migrans of *Toxocara cati* in visceral organs of experimental animals. Acta Vet. Acad. Sci. Hung., *21*:405–412, 1971.

Okoshi, S., and Usui, M.: Experimental studies on *Toxascaris leonina*. VI. Experimental infection of mice, chickens and earthworms with *Toxascaris leonina*, *Toxocara canis* and *Toxocara cati*. Jpn. J. Vet. Sci., *30*:151–166, 1968.

Olson, L.J.: Ocular toxocariasis in mice: distribution of larvae and lesions. Int. J. Parasitol., *6*:247–251, 1976.

Rubin, L.F., and Saunders, L.Z.: Intraocular larva migrans in dogs. Pathol. Vet., *2*:566–573, 1965.

Schwartz, B.: Experimental infection of pigs with *Ascaris suum*. Am. J. Vet. Res., *20*:7–13, 1959.

Scothorn, M.W., Koutz, F.R., and Groves, H.F.: Prenatal *Toxocara canis* infection in pups. J. Am. Vet. Med. Assoc., *146*:45–48, 1965.

Shalkop, W.T., et al.: Report on investigations of icterus in swine. North Am. Vet., *34*:257–262, 1953.

Swerczek, T.W., Nielsen, S.W., and Helmboldt, C.F.: Transmammary passage of *Toxocara cati* in the cat. Am. J. Vet. Res., *32*:89–92, 1971.

Tomimura, T., Yokota, M., and Takiguchi, H.: Experimental visceral larva migrans in monkeys. I. Clinical, hematological, biochemical and gross pathological observations of monkeys inoculated with embryonated eggs of the dog ascarid, *Toxocara canis*. Jpn. J. Vet. Sci., *38*:533–538, 1976.

Ueckert, B.: Larva migrans, a review. Southwestern Vet., *15*:223–230, 1962.

Wilder, H.C.: Nematode endophthalmitis. Tr. Amer. Acad. Ophthalmol., (Oct):99–108, 1950.

Wiseman, R.A.: Toxocariasis in man and animals. Vet. Rec., *84*:214–216, 1969.

Ancylostomiasis (Hookworm Disease)

Hookworms (family: Ancylostomidae) are important parasites of mammals and in some parts of the world produce widespread disease in man. These parasites are cosmopolitan in distribution, although limited to certain areas by environmental conditions such as moisture and temperature. One or more species of hookworm occur in every domestic mammal, with the singular exception of the horse. Hookworms as a group have several characteristics that influence their pathological effects and therefore merit brief mention: (1) they have well-developed buccal cavities containing tooth-like structures, and all suck blood from the host; (2) adults normally inhabit the small intestine; eggs are passed in the feces, hatch under suitable conditions into rhabditiform larvae, which after two molts become filariform and may infect another host by penetration of the skin or through ingestion; (3) infective larvae that penetrate the skin or that are ingested migrate to the lungs and gain access to the intestine via the tracheal route; (4) some larvae may be carried by the blood to other tissues, where they usually die, but may also lead to persistent infection with third-stage larvae residing within muscle fibers; (5) although most hookworm species are host-specific, many can penetrate the epidermis of aberrant hosts, producing a specific dermatitis **(creeping eruption)**; (6) during migration or reactivation of persistent infection, larvae may pass through the placenta and infect the fetus, where further development is arrested until after birth; (7) larvae

Table 14–2. Important Hookworms and Their Hosts

Hookworm	Definitive Host
Ancylostoma duodenale	Man
Necator americanus	Man, monkeys
Ancylostoma caninum	Dog, cat
Ancylostoma braziliense	Dog, cat
Uncinaria stenocephala	Dog, fox
Bunostomum phlebotomum	Cattle
Bunostomum trigonocephalum	Sheep, goats
Globecephalus urosubulatus	Swine

of at least one species (*Ancylostoma caninum*) appear in the milk to infect suckling young. A few important hookworms are listed under the names currently in use in Table 14–2.

Clinical Manifestations. Signs produced in the host by hookworms depend upon the effect of both the adults and the infective larvae. The third stage (infective) larvae penetrate the intact skin, producing ancylostome dermatitis in the natural host (in man, "ground itch," "coolie's itch" or "water itch"). In aberrant hosts, e.g., *Ancylostoma braziliense* in man, infective larvae penetrate the epidermis and migrate for short distances in the dermis, producing indurated reddish papules from which linear serpiginous tunnels, 1 to 2 mm in diameter, extend for a few centimeters. This lesion is known as creeping eruption. In their natural host, the infective larvae, after penetrating the skin, invade the lungs. The usual symptoms are cough, and in severe cases, pneumonia.

The adult hookworms, which attach themselves to the mucosa of the small intestine, may produce symptoms of anemia (usually microcytic, hypochromic) in the host. These include pallor of the mucosae, hypoproteinemia, weakness, diarrhea, and progressive emaciation, with cardiac failure and death resulting in some cases.

Lesions. Infective larvae may excite severe dermatitis during their migration through the skin of sensitized animals. The tissue reaction is usually limited to the vicinity of the migratory path of the larvae and is not distinctive, although lymphocytes, eosinophils, and macrophages predominate in the exudate that infiltrates the dermis. These larvae may also breach the placenta and cause prenatal infection in the young. The most severe effects of the larval invasion are seen in the lung. As the larvae break into the alveoli from the pulmonary capillaries, hemorrhage occurs, and in heavy infections may be severe. Leukocytic infiltra-

tion follows, sometimes of such severity as to amount to lobular pneumonia. Secondary bacterial infection is believed to contribute to this lesion in many instances. Fibrosis of affected lung parenchyma is a common sequel. From the alveoli, the larvae invade the bronchial tree, are coughed up, and then swallowed to reach the small intestine of the host.

The adult hookworms have buccal tooth-like structures and a powerful esophagus, which permits them to draw bits of intestinal mucosa into their buccal cavity. In addition, they secrete an anticoagulant and inhibit platelet aggregation, which promotes the sucking of blood at a rapid rate; in some instances, intact erythrocytes are passed through the digestive tracts of the parasite. Worms may change position, leaving a lesion denuded of epithelium, from which blood continues to flow and through which bacteria can enter the tissues. The destructive effect upon the mucosa gives rise to enteritis, and the loss of blood, to anemia. It is now believed that in most instances the anemia of hookworm disease is entirely attributable to loss of blood. Anemia may be severe, the erythrocyte content of the blood dropping to 25% of normal in some cases. The blood loss usually results in hyperplasia of the hematopoietic elements of the bone marrow, which may be accompanied by myeloid metaplasia in the spleen. There is blunting and fusion of intestinal villi and inflammation and fibrosis of the lamina propria, which leads to defective nutrient absorption.

Diagnosis. The diagnosis can be confirmed clinically by demonstration of hookworm ova in the feces. At necropsy, adult worms may be found attached to the mucosa of the small intestine. Larvae may be demonstrable microscopically in tissue sections, but this is a matter of chance.

Baker, K.P., and Grimes, T.D.: Cutaneous lesions in dogs associated with hookworm infestation. Vet. Rec., *87*:376–379, 1970.

Buelke, D.L.: Hookworm dermatitis. J. Am. Vet. Med. Assoc., *158:*735–739, 1971.

Lee, K.T., Little, M.D., and Beaver, P.C.: Intracellular (muscle-fiber) habitat of *Ancylostoma caninum* in some mammalian hosts. J. Parasitol., *61:*589–598, 1975.

Migasena, S., Gilles, H.M., and Maegraith, B.G.: Studies in *Ancylostoma caninum* infection in dogs. I. Absorption from the small intestine of amino-acids, carbohydrates and fat. Ann. Trop. Med. Parasitol., *66:*107–128, 1972.

———: Studies in *Ancylostoma caninum* infection in dogs. II. Anatomical changes in the gastrointestinal tract. Ann. Trop. Med. Parasitol., *66:*203–207, 1972.

Miller, T.A.: Blood loss during hookworm infection, determined by erythrocyte labeling with radioactive chromium. I. Infection of dogs with normal and with x-irradiated *Ancylostoma caninum.* J. Parasitol., *52:*844–855, 1966.

———: Blood loss during hookworm infection, determined by erythrocyte labeling with radioactive [51]chromium. II. Pathogenesis of *Ancylostoma braziliense* infection in dogs and cats. J. Parasitol., *52:*856–865, 1966.

Orihel, T.C.: *Necator americanus* infection in primates. J. Parasitol., *57:*117–121, 1971.

Pacenovsky, J., and Brezanska, M.: Penetration of *Bunostomum phlebotomum* larvae into the body of cattle. Vet. Med. Praha., *13:*277–383, 1968. V.B. *39:*2583, 1969.

Soulsby, E.J.L., Venn, J.A.J., and Green, K.N.: Hookworm disease in British cattle. Vet. Rec., *67:*1124–1125, 1955.

Spellman, G.G., Jr., and Nossel, H.L.: Anticoagulant activity of dog hookworm. Am. J. Physiol., *220:*922–927, 1971.

Stone, W.M., and Girardeau, M.: Transmammary passage of *Ancylostoma caninum* larvae in dogs. J. Parasitol., *54:*426–429, 1968.

Trichostrongylosis

The superfamily Trichostrongyloidea includes several helminths that are important parasites of cattle and sheep. Trichostrongyles of a number of species may infect the hosts simultaneously, producing severe damage which is manifested by anemia, cachexia, diarrhea, debility, and sometimes death (particularly in lambs and calves). For this reason, trichostrongylosis may be considered an entity, although the parasitic genera involved in the clinical syndrome may differ in individual cases.

Helminths of the superfamily Trichostrongyloidea are small, slender worms in which the buccal cavity is absent or rudimentary, without leaf crowns, and usually toothless; their spicules are usually long and filiform or short and stout with protuberances. Their life cycle is direct; ellipsoidal ova pass to the ground in the feces of the host, hatch into filariform larvae, develop through larval stages in the soil, and produce infection in a new host when they are ingested with fresh grass. There is no migratory stage and the adults are found in the abomasum or small intestine, where they molt to the fourth stage. See Table 14–3.

Table 14–3. Representative Species of Trichostrongyloidea

Parasite	Location of Adult	Host(s)
Haemonchus contortus	Abomasum	Sheep (cattle)
H. placei	Abomasum	Cattle (sheep)
Ostertagia ostertagi	Abomasum	Cattle
O. circumcincta	Abomasum	Sheep
Trichostronglyus axei	Abomasum, small intestine, stomach	Cattle
T. colubriformis	Small intestine	Equine, swine, cattle, sheep
Cooperia punctata	Small intestine	Cattle (sheep)
C. curticei	Small intestine	Sheep
Nematodirus filicollis	Small intestine	Cattle, sheep
N. spathiger	Small intestine	Sheep
Hyostrongylus rubidus	Stomach	Swine

Haemonchus contortus and the similar *H. placei* ("barber-pole worm," "twisted stomach worm," or "common stomach worm") are the largest of the group. Infective third-stage larvae, after they are ingested, reach the abomasum, molt to the fourth stage, and attach themselves to the mucosa. After feeding on the host's blood for about 18 days, they reach sexual maturity. Eggs appear in the feces of the host 19 to 21 days after ingestion of the filiform larvae. The adult worms live free in the lumen but feed by piercing the mucosa with their pharyngeal lancets to suck blood. Not only do they rob the host of large quantities of blood, but they leave lacerations on the mucosa which predispose to gastritis. Haemonchosis is the most important of the trichostrongylid infections, and may result in significant herd or flock mortality rates.

The small trichostrongyles include helminths of the genera *Ostertagia* (*O. ostertagi*, the brown stomach worm), *Trichostrongylus* (*T. axei*—hairlike stomach worm, *T. colubriformis*), *Cooperia* (*C. punctata*) and *Nematodirus* (*N. filicollis*, *N. spathiger*, *N. battus*). Each of these genera includes several species besides those mentioned. The life cycle of these worms is similar to that of *Haemonchus contortus*, except that their embryonated eggs are highly resistant to drying and may accumulate on the ground during the dry season, then produce overwhelming infections when all larvae hatch at the same time, as the rainy season starts. These parasites also differ from *Haemonchus* in that they penetrate the tissues of the host. The infective larvae of *Trichostrongylus axei* burrow into the mucosa of the abomasum or stomach. Larvae of *Ostertagia* also penetrate the mucosa of the abomasum, but burrow deeper, remain longer, and generally cause more damage to the gastric wall. The parasites develop to maturity in small nodules; the adults may emerge completely or may be seen partially projecting from the nodules in the

mucosa. Other species of *Trichostrongylus*, *Cooperia* and *Nematodirus* invade the mucosa of the small intestine, and produce superficial erosions and sloughing of the mucosa, which may result in protein loss (hypoproteinemia), diarrhea, gastroenteritis, and death, especially in young animals. Microscopically, the mucosa is atrophic and infiltrated with an admixture of inflammatory cells.

Clinical Manifestations. The signs of trichostrongylosis are most severe in young or malnourished animals and may appear rather suddenly after rains that have broken a dry season. Anemia is the most outstanding symptom in acute infections, due to *Haemonchus*; lambs, in particular, may die from loss of blood without warning. In more prolonged infections, anemia is associated with edematous swellings under the jaw and sometimes the ventral abdomen (see p. 164). The body fat is replaced by gelatinous tissue (see mucoid degeneration, p. 50), hence emaciation is seldom apparent. Affected animals grow progressively weaker, their gait becomes staggering; death follows after prolonged illness. In cases in which the small trichostrongyles predominate, diarrhea with thin, fetid, black-colored feces may be noted in addition to anemia and cachexia.

Lesions. Necropsy findings in haemonchosis are dominated by the severe anemia in acute cases, the mucous membranes as well as the viscera appearing extremely pale or chalk-white, the blood, thin and watery. In cases of longer standing, anemia is also in evidence, but edematous swellings in the subcutis under the jaw and abdomen may be seen as well. Excessive amounts of fluid are usually present in the thoracic, pericardial, and peritoneal cavities. The body fat undergoes mucoid degeneration and becomes highly edematous. The liver is light brown and friable, and contains areas of fatty change. The abomasum may contain large numbers of worms, which remain actively motile as long as the body is warm. Shallow ulcers or many small red bite marks may be present in the mucosa as a result of the feeding habits of *Haemonchus contortus*. Small, round nodules, 1 to 2 mm in diameter, in the abomasal mucosa mark the points at which parasites of the *Ostertagia* and *Trichostrongylus* species have penetrated the walls. Trichostrongylid nodules are characterized by inflammatory cell infiltration and fibrosis surrounding the larvae. Catarrhal or hemorrhagic abomasitis, gastritis, or enteritis are found, depending upon the location of the parasite. Focal hemorrhage is encountered in intestinal trichostrongylosis, where invasion of larvae usually does not cause inflammatory nodules. Villus atrophy of varying degrees also occurs in intestinal trichostrongylosis.

Diagnosis. Although demonstration of ova in the feces will identify some infections, fatal trichostrongylosis can occur during the prepatent period. For this reason, when herd problems are encountered, it may be necessary to sacrifice an animal or two to establish the presence of this disease conclusively. The finding of helminths in large numbers in the abomasum and small intestine of animals which have been anemic and the demonstration of characteristic gross changes at necropsy are considered sufficient for diagnosis in most situations. Worms of the genera *Trichostrongylus*, *Ostertagia*, and *Cooperia* are so small that some usually competent veterinarians miss finding them even in fatal cases. Washings from which the coarser ingesta have been removed by a sieve should be examined with a hand lens or dissecting microscope. The parasites are also subject to autolysis and may be missed if necropsy is delayed.

Stomach Worms of Other Species

Hyostrongylus rubidus, a parasite similar to *Haemonchus sp.*, is common in swine but ordinarily of little significance. It has

been reported occasionally to produce ulcerations or diphtheric gastritis in which the mucosa is covered with a yellowish membrane or tenacious mucous exudate. The mucosa becomes thickened, hyperemic, and infiltrated with large numbers of lymphocytes. In areas of erosion or ulceration, neutrophils, eosinophils, and fibrin are part of the exudate. Larvae and adults lie in dilated gastric glands, which may be observed grossly as small nodules or cysts. Their lining undergoes mucoid metaplasia. The life cycle is direct.

Species of *Physaloptera* (order Spuroidea) parasitize the stomach and duodenum of cats, dogs, rodents, monkeys, and other animals. Infection follows ingestion of an intermediate host, which includes cockroaches, crickets, and beetles. The adults attach to the mucosa and suck blood, and leave small erosions and ulcers when they change positions. Hyperplasia of the gastric mucosa may lead to nodular projections resembling tumors.

Gnathostoma spinigerum is a gastric parasite of dogs, cats, and occasionally other species, including swine and man. Two intermediate hosts are required, a cyclops and fresh water fish. Larvae encysted in fish are released and migrate through the liver and other viscera, eventually penetrating the wall of the stomach where the adults reside in thick-walled cysts.

Barker, I.K.: Intestinal pathology associated with *Trichostrongylus colubriformis* infection in sheep: histology. Parasitology, 70:165–171, 1975.
———: A study of the pathogenesis of *Trichostrongylus colubriformis* infection in lambs with observations on the contribution of gastrointestinal plasma loss. Int. J. Parasitol., 3:743–757, 1973.
———: Scanning electron microscopy of the duodenal mucosa of lambs infected with *Trichostrongylus colubriformis*. Parasitology, 67:307–314, 1973.
———: Relationship of abnormal mucosal microtopography with distribution of *Trichostrongylus colubriformis* in the small intestines of lambs. Int. J. Parasitol., 4:153–163, 1974.
———: Location and distribution of *Trichostrongylus colubriformis* in the small intestine of sheep during the prepatent period, and the development of villus atrophy. J. Comp. Pathol., 85:417–426, 1975.

Baskerville, A., and Ross, J.G.: Observations on experimental and field infections of pigs with *Hyostrongylus rubidus*. Br. Vet. J., *126*:538–542, 1970.

Becklund, W.W., and Walker, M.L.: Nematodirus of domestic sheep, *Ovis aries*, in the United States with a key to the species. J. Parasitol., *53*:777–781, 1967.

Coop, R.L., Angus, K.W., and Mapes, C.J.: The effect of large doses of *Nematodirus battus* on the histology and biochemistry of the small intestine of lambs. Int. J. Parasitol., *3*:349–361, 1973.

Daengsvang, S.: Infectivity of *Gnathostoma spinigerum* larvae in primates. J. Parasitol., *57*:476–478, 1971.

Dodd, D.C.: Hyostrongylosis and gastric ulceration in the pig. NZ Vet. J., *8*:100–103, 1960.

Durham, P.J.K., and Elliott, D.C.: Experimental *Ostertagia* infection of sheep: pathology following a single high dose of larvae. NZ Vet. J., *23*:193–196, 1975.

Gardiner, M.R.: Pathological changes and vitamin B$_{12}$ metabolism in sheep parasitised by *Haemonchus contortus*, *Ostertagia* spp. and *Trichostrongylus colubriformis*. J. Helminthol., *40*:63–67, 1966.

Hotson, I.K.: Ostertagiosis in cattle. Aust. Vet. J., *43*:383–388, 1967.

Jennings, F.W., et al.: Experimental *Ostertagia ostertagi* infections in calves: studies with abomasal cannulas. Am. J. Vet. Res., *27*:1249–1257, 1966.

Kates, K.C., and Turner, J.H.: Observations on the life cycle of *Nematodirus spathiger*, a nematode parasitic in the intestine of sheep and other ruminants. Am. J. Vet. Res., *16*:105–115, 1955.

Kendall, S.B., Thurley, D.C., and Peirce, M.A.: The biology of *Hyostrongylus rubidus*. I. Primary infection in young pigs. J. Comp. Pathol., *79*:87–95, 1969.

Martin, W.B., Thomas, B.A.C., and Urquhart, G.M.: Chronic diarrhea in housed cattle due to atypical parasitic gastritis. Vet. Rec., *69*:736–739, 1957.

Nicholson, T.B., and Gordon, J.G.: An outbreak of helminthiasis associated with *Hyostrongylus rubidus*. Vet. Rec., *71*:133, 1959.

Osborne, J.C., Batte, E.G., and Bell, R.R.: The pathology following single infections of *Ostertagia ostertagi* in calves. Cornell Vet., *50*:223–224, 1960.

Ritchie, D.S., Anderson, N., and Armour, J.: The pathology of lesions seen in bovine ostertagiasis. Proc. 1st Int. Congr. Parasit. Roma, *2*:851–852, 1966.

Ritchie, J.D.S., et al.: Experimental *Ostertagia ostertagi* infections in calves: parasitology and pathogenesis of a single infection. Am. J. Vet. Res., *27*:659–667, 1966.

Ross, J.G., and Todd, J.R.: Biochemical, serological and haematological changes associated with infections of calves with the nematode parasite, *Ostertagia ostertagi*. Br. Vet. J., *121*:55–64, 1965.

Ross, J.G., and Dow, C.: The course and development of the abomasal lesion in calves experimentally infected with the nematode parasite *Ostertagia ostertagi*. Br. Vet. J., *121*:228–233, 1965.

Ross J.G., Purcell, A., Dow, C., and Todd, J.R.: Experimental infections of calves with *Trichostrongylus axei*: observations on lethal infections. Res. Vet. Sci., *9*:314–318, 1968.

Rowlands, D.ap.T., and Probert, A.J.: Some pathological changes in young lambs experimentally infected with *Nematodirus battus*. Res. Vet. Sci., *13*:323–329, 1972.

Sharma, K.M.L.: Studies on total serum proteins and serum proteins in calves experimentally infected with *Ostertagia ostertagi*. Indian J. Anim. Hlth., *7*:93–96, 1968. V.B. *39*:1184, 1969.

Stockdale, P.H.G.: The pathogenesis of *Hyostrongylus rubidus* in growing pigs. Br. Vet. J., *130*:366–373, 1974.

Stockdale, P.H.G., Ashton, G.K., Howes, M.A., and Ewert, E.: Hyostrongylosis in Ontario. Can. Vet. J., *14*:265–268, 1973.

Oesophagostomiasis (Nodule Worm Disease)

An important parasitic disease is produced in cattle, sheep, and goats in many parts of the world by the nodule worms, *Oesophagostomum radiatium*, *Oe. columbianum*, and other species. Similar species also infect swine (*O. dentatum*) and nonhuman primates. The parasite is a small slender nematode that has a direct life cycle. Adults in the large intestinal lumen produce ova that pass out in the feces, and after a period outside the host, develop into infective larvae. These larvae, upon ingestion by another host, penetrate the intestinal mucosa, become encysted, molt in the submucosa, and eventually return to the lumen, where they reach maturity. Percutaneous infection has been demonstrated experimentally, but is not considered of importance to natural transmission.

Clinical Manifestations. Signs are most often observed in young animals; profuse diarrhea is the most constant sign, and apparently is more intense when the larvae are returning from the submucosa to the intestinal lumen. Heavy infections of long standing usually result in chronic diarrhea, anemia, emaciation, cachexia, prostration, and death. Even though symptoms are mild, lesions may be found at postmortem inspection.

Lesions. The exudation of mucus and inflammatory cells from the intestinal mucosa of the host is believed to be the response to irritation caused by substances secreted by the adult parasite, perhaps from its cephalic or esophageal glands. It is thought that this exudate is the chief source of food for the worms, for they are not blood suckers, neither do they attach themselves to the mucosa or cause obstruction of the lumen. Although the mechanism is not understood, the adult parasites do cause intestinal hemorrhage, which may lead to anemia.

The larvae, on the other hand, produce severe and striking lesions (Fig. 14–4). They penetrate the mucosa at any point from the pylorus to the anus in order to reach the deeper parts of the submucosa, where they encyst and undergo a molt. Some may encyst in the lamina propria on the superficial face of the muscularis mucosae, but most of them are found in the submucosa on the deeper side of the muscularis mucosae. Larvae are capable of migrating into the peritoneal cavity and encysting in walled-off granulomas on the surface of various abdominal viscera. In initial infections, the larvae shed a striated skin and return to the intestinal lumen as fourth-stage larvae in five or six days, having produced only transitory inflammation in the mucosa and submucosa, but their ecdysis leads to small ulcers and intestinal bleeding. Some fourth-stage larvae of *O. columbianum* have been demonstrated to undergo a second intestinal invasion, where further development is usually arrested. In contrast, local tissue sensitivity develops in animals repeatedly exposed to these parasites, and the subsequent entry of larvae into the submucosa evokes an intense tissue reaction. Large numbers of eosinophils, lymphocytes, macrophages, and foreign body giant cells surround the larvae and infiltrate the adjacent submucosa and mucosa. The center of these lesions becomes

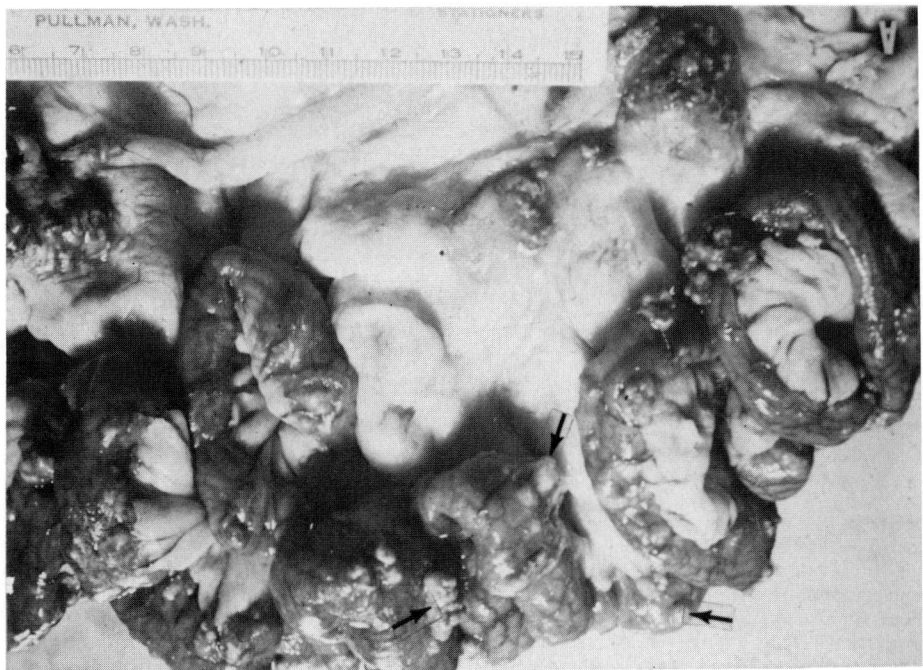

Fig. 14–4. Oesophagostomiasis, small intestine of a sheep. Subserosal nodules are indicated by arrows. (Courtesy of Dr. C. L. Davis.)

caseated, often calcified, and is surrounded by a dense capsule, which preserves the nodular character of the lesions. A few larvae survive and escape by wandering through the muscularis, but most of them die without finding their way back to the lumen.

The nodules may become infected and enlarged and displace the muscularis to serve as a nidus for local or generalized peritonitis, but usually they remain as calcified, encapsulated nodules. These lesions give the intestine a nodular appearance as they thicken the wall and project from the serosal surface. When present in large numbers, these nodules sometimes interfere with peristalsis and intestinal absorption.

Diagnosis. Clinical diagnosis may be made by finding eggs or fourth-stage larvae in fecal specimens. At necropsy, the lesions are recognized by their characteristic gross and microscopic features, for which the popular term, nodule disease, is an especially graphic summation.

Andrews, J.S., and Maldonado, J.F.: Intestinal pathology in experimental bovine esophagostomiasis. Am. J. Vet. Res., 3:17–27, 1942.

Berger, H., and Ribelin, W.E.: Pathology of the swine nodular worm, Oesophagostomum dentatum in rabbits. J. Parasitol., 55:1099–1101, 1969.

Bremner, K.C.: Pathogenetic factors in experimental bovine oesophagostomosis. V. Intestinal bleeding as cause of anemia. Exp. Parasitol., 27:236–245, 1970.

Bremner, K.C., and Fridemanis, R.: Oesophagostomum radiatum in calves: intestinal hemorrhage associated with larval emergence. Exp. Parasitol., 36:424–429, 1974.

Bremner, K.C., and Keith, R.K.: Oesophagostomum radiatum: adult nematodes and intestinal hemorrhage. Exp. Parasitol., 28:416–419, 1970.

Dash, K.M.: The life cycle of Oesophagostomum columbianum (Curtice, 1890) in sheep. Int. J. Parasitol., 3:843–851, 1973.

Dobson, C.: Globule leucocytes, mucin and mucin cells in relation to Oesophagostomum columbianum infections in sheep. Aust. J. Sci., 28:434, 1966.

————: Pathological changes associated with Oesophagostomum columbianum infestations in sheep: haematological observations on control worm-free and experimentally infected sheep. Aust. J. Agric. Res., 18:523–538, 1967.

Elek, P., and Durie, P.H.: The histopathology of the reactions of calves to experimental infection with the nodular worm, Oesophagostomum radiatum (Rudolphi, 1803). II. Reaction of the susceptible host to infection with a single dose of larvae. Aust. J. Agric. Res., 18:549–559, 1967.

Gerber, H.M.: Percutaneous infestation of calves and lambs with Oesophagostomum spp. J. S. Afr. Vet. Assoc., 46:273–275, 1975.

Hass, D.K., Brown, L.J., and Young, R., Jr.: Infectivity of Oesophagostomum dentatum larvae in swine. Am. J. Vet. Res., 33:2527–2534, 1972.

McCracken, R.M., and Ross, J.G.: The histopathology of Oesophagostomum dentatum infections in pigs. J. Comp. Pathol., 80:619–623, 1970.

Skelton, G.C., and Griffiths, H.J.: Oesophagostomum columbianum: experimental infection in lambs. Effects of different types of exposure in the intestinal lesions. Pathol. Vet., 4:413–434, 1967.

Dirofilariasis (Canine Filariasis, Heart Worm Disease)

Animals and human beings are subject to infection with a number of filarial (*Filarioidea*) parasites. A selected list is presented in Table 14–4. The "heart worm," *Dirofilaria immitis*, is one of the more important filarial parasites which is not uncommon, particularly in the southern and eastern coastal regions of the United States. Dogs, cats, foxes, wolves, muskrats, and rarely other species, such as horses, sea lions, and human beings, have been reported to be infected. *Dirofilaria repens* is a subcutaneous parasite of dogs, cats, and rarely man in Europe and the Far East. Adult worms of a closely related species, *Dirofilaria tenuis*, have been reported in the subcutis of raccoons (*Procyon lotor*) in Florida and Louisiana (Orihel and Beaver, 1965). This species has also been found in the subcutis of man, as has *Dirofilaria conjunctivae*.

The adult worms are slender, almost thread-like, filarial parasites. Males, 12 to 30 cm long, and females 25 to 31 cm long, are found in the right ventricle of the heart, less often in the right auricle or the pulmonary arteries. The males and females copulate in these sites; the viviparous female releases highly motile microfilariae, which circulate with the blood. These microfilariae are taken up from the cutaneous

Table 14–4. Filarial Parasites of Animals

Filarial Parasite	Definitive Host	Adult Location	Intermediate Host
Parafilaria multipapillosa	Equidae	Skin	*Haematobia atripalpis*
Setaria cervi	Bovidae	Abdominal cavity	Mosquitoes
S. digitata	Bovidae	Abdominal cavity	Mosquitoes
S. marshalli	Bovidae	Abdominal cavity	Mosquitoes
S. equina	Equidae	Abdominal cavity	Mosquitoes
Stephanofilaria stilesi	Bovidae	Skin	*Lyperosia titillans* *Haematobia irritans*
St. assamensis	Bovidae	Skin	*Musca conducens*
Loa loa	Man	Eye, skin	*Chrysops spp.*
Loa papionis	Nonhuman primates	Subcutis	*Chrysops spp.*
Dirofilaria immitis	Canidae, Felidae	Right ventricle	Mosquitoes
D. repens	Canidae, Felidae	Subcutis	Mosquitoes
D. tenuis	Procyonidae	Subcutis	Mosquitoes
D. corynodes	Monkeys	Subcutis	Mosquitoes
Dipetalonema reconditum	Canidae	Subcutis	Mosquitoes
D. perstans	Man, apes	Thoracic and abcominal cavities	Ceratopogonids
D. dracunculoides	Canidae	Peritoneum	*Hippobosca longipennis*
D. gracile	Monkeys	Abdominal cavity	Mosquitoes
Elaeophora schneideri	Bovidae, Cervidae	Subcutis	Tabanidae
Brugia malayi	Man, apes, monkeys	Lymphatics	Mosquitoes
B. pahangi	Canidae, Felidae	Lymphatics	Mosquitoes
B. patei	Canidae, Felidae	Lymphatics	Mosquitoes
Wuchereria bancrofti	Man	Lymphatics	Mosquitoes
Onchocerca cervicalis	Equidae	Ligamentum nuchae	Ceratopogonids
O. reticulata	Equidae	Subcutaneous connective tissue	Ceratopogonids
O. gibsoni	Bovidae	Subcutaneous connective tissue	Ceratopogonids
O. lienalis	Bovidae	Subcutis	Simuliidae
O. gutterosa	Bovidae	Ligamentum nuchae	Simuliidae
O. volvulus	Man	Subcutaneous connective tissue	Simuliidae
Dracunculus medinensis	Man, horse, dog, monkey	Subcutis	Copepods
D. insignis	Canidae	Subcutis	Copepods
Dioctophyma renale	Swine, dog, man	Kidney	*Cambarincola chirocephala* *Ameirus melas*
Wehrdikmansia cervipedis	Cervidae	Skin	Simuliidae

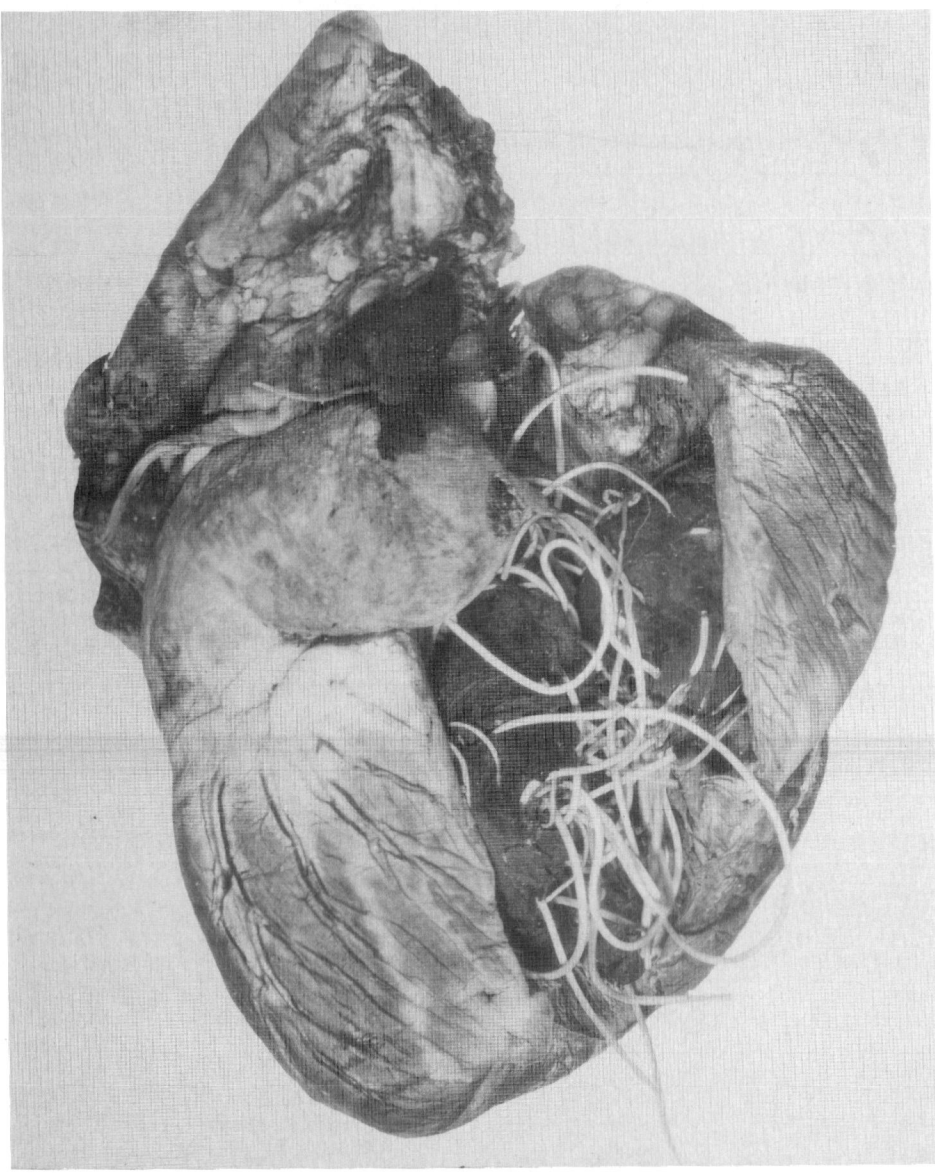

Fig. 14–5. Dirofilariasis. Many adult *Dirofilaria immitis* in right ventricle (opened) of a dog. (Courtesy of Armed Forces Institute of Pathology.) Contributor: Col. Wm. P. Hill, V.C.

circulation by certain biting insects (mosquitoes), in whose bodies they undergo stages of development. The infective filariae then gain access to the tissues of a new host through the bite of the intermediate host. These filarial larvae undergo further development in muscles, sub-cutaneous, and adipose tissues of the new host. When they reach a length of about 5 cm, they enter veins and are carried to the right heart. The cycle is complete when adult filariae start reproduction in the right ventricle of the host.

Clinical Manifestations. The disease in its earliest stages may give rise to few signs, but severely affected animals will

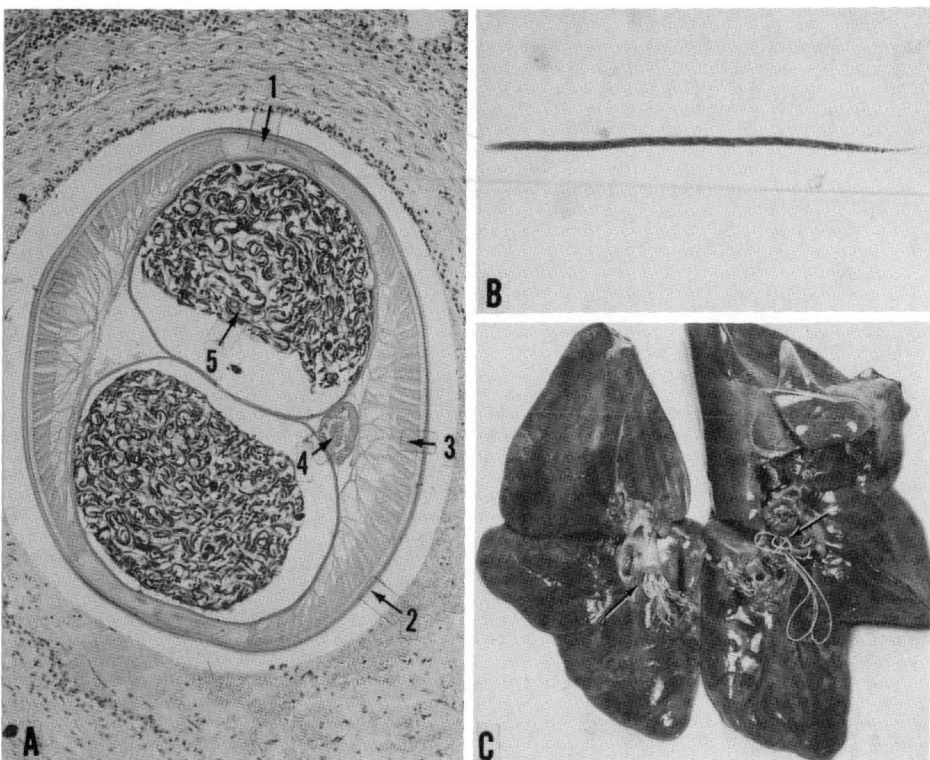

Fig. 14–6. Dirofilariasis. *A,* Adult female *Dirofilaria immitis* in a branch of the pulmonary artery of a dog. Note lateral chord cells *(1),* continuous with the hypodermis which lies just under the cuticula *(2).* The musculature of the worm *(3),* its digestive tube *(4)* and uterus filled with microfilariae *(5)* are clearly seen. (Courtesy of Armed Forces Institute of Pathology.) Contributor: Army Veterinary Research Laboratory. *B,* A single microfilaria of *Dirofilaria immitis* in a fixed specimen from peripheral blood. *C, D. immitis* filling the pulmonary arteries (arrows).

exhibit shortness of breath, weakness, cardiac enlargement, hepatomegaly, ascites, occasionally hypertrophic pulmonary osteoarthropathy (p. 1180) and may die with failure of the right heart. In a few instances, fatal outcome may be the result of pulmonary embolism by adult *Dirofilaria,* which die and are swept into the smaller branches of the pulmonary artery. In one case, we have observed dead worms lodged in the pulmonary artery, resulting in a thrombus and aneurysm in the branch of this artery supplying the diaphragmatic lobe. Subsequent rupture of the aneurysm into the adjacent bronchus resulted in severe hemoptysis and exsanguination in a few minutes.

Lesions. The principal effects of *Dirofilaria immitis* are produced by the adult worms, which interfere with circulation through the right heart. It is assumed that mechanical interference applied over rather long periods produces compensatory hypertrophy and enlargement of the right ventricle; insufficiency of the right heart results in passive congestion of the lungs, liver, and spleen, as well as ascites. Occasional adults die and are transported through the pulmonary artery to the lungs where they produce pulmonary embolism. This complication is relatively infrequent, except in dogs treated with certain filaricidal drugs.

Changes in the pulmonary arterial sys-

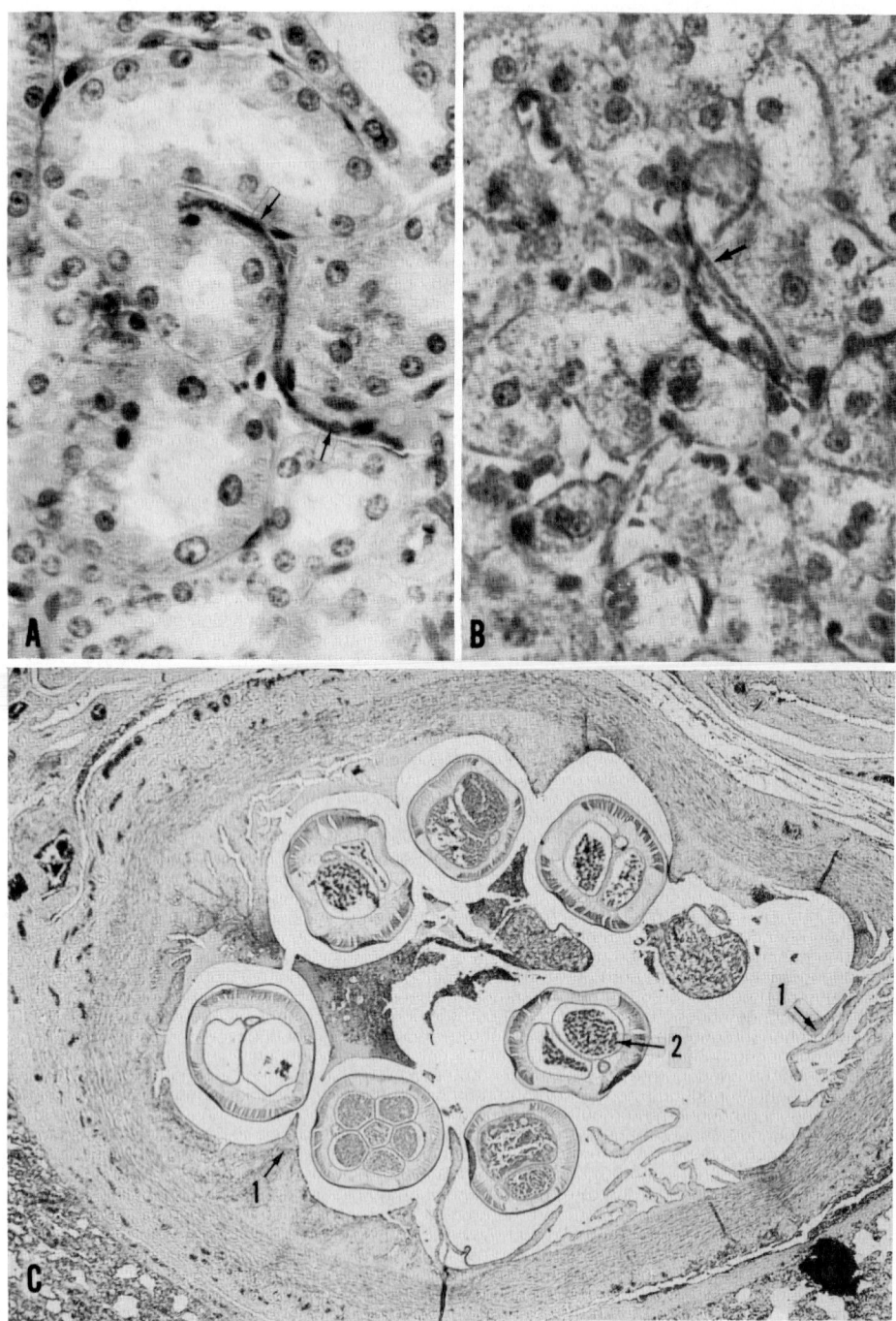

Fig. 14–7. Dirofilariasis. *A*, Microfilaria (arrows) in a capillary in the renal cortex (× 300). *B*, Microfilaria (arrow) in sinusoid of liver (× 515). *C*, Adult *Dirofilaria immitis* in the pulmonary artery (× 30). Note villous proliferation of intima *(1)* and microfilaria *(2)* in uterus of a female worm. (Courtesy of Armed Forces Institute of Pathology.) Contributor: Army Veterinary Research Laboratory.

tem of infected dogs have been described (Adcock, 1961, Porter, 1951). They include the formation of longitudinally arranged rows of villous projections of the intima into the lumen (Fig. 14–7) of the pulmonary arteries, with diffuse thickening of the subintima; severe endothelial proliferation in small pulmonary arterioles, sometimes with almost complete obliteration of the lumen; and medial hypertrophy of certain of the larger pulmonary arterioles.

In heavy infestations, *D. immitis* may occupy the vena cava, resulting in phlebosclerosis of the vena cava and hepatic veins. Rarely, adult parasites are found in the left side of the heart, aorta, or peripheral arteries, and occasionally outside the vascular tree in such locations as the peritoneal cavity, eye, or ventricles of the brain.

The microfilariae that circulate freely with the blood appear to produce little tissue damage, for they are found rather frequently in tissue sections, usually in the absence of a demonstrable inflammatory or other tissue reaction. Some microfilariae die, however, and a small granuloma usually forms around them. Such tiny granulomas have been seen in the interstitial stroma of the kidney in infected dogs. Interstitial nephritis and cystitis have been observed in dogs infected with *Dirofilaria,* but the causal relationship of the parasite to these lesions has not been established.

Diagnosis. Presumptive clinical diagnosis can be based upon the symptoms.

Adult worms can be visualized as radiolucencies using angiocardiography, a technique of value to assess extent of damage and effect of treatment. Diagnosis is confirmed by demonstration of microfilariae in peripheral blood; however, absence of circulating microfilariae does not preclude infection. Microfilariae can be identified by direct microscopic examination of fresh whole blood smears, serum extruded from clotted blood, filtrates of blood, or centrifugal sediment from a blood sample in which the red cells have been "laked" by addition of water or other nonphysiologic solution. The microfilariae are actively motile in fresh blood and measure 307 to 322 μ in length and 5 to 6 μ in width. The anterior end of the microfilaria is bluntly rounded and devoid of nuclei near the tip. Postmortem diagnosis can be made by finding adult filariae in the right ventricle or by demonstration of microfilariae in capillaries in tissue sections.

Newton and Wright (1956) have identified two kinds of microfilariae in the blood of dogs in the United States. One type is the larval stage of *Dirofilaria immitis;* the other, *Dipetalonema reconditum,* a relatively innocuous parasite whose adult forms are found in the subcutis and which is transmitted by fleas. The differentiation of the microfilariae of these two worms is often of practical importance. According to these authors, the microfilariae of these two filarial species can be differentiated by their average size and morphology after

Table 14–5. Comparison of *Dirofilaria immitis* and *Dipetalonema reconditum*

Dirofilaria immitis	*Dipetalonema reconditum*
Microfilaria:	*Microfilaria:*
Length: 307–322 μ	Length: 269–283 μ
Width: 6.7–7.1 μ	Width: 4.3–4.8 μ
Tails: mostly straight	Tails: curved, "button-hook"
Develop in mosquitoes *(Anopheles quadrimaculatus)*	Develop in fleas *(Ctenocephalus canis)*
Adults:	*Adults:*
Found in right ventricle and pulmonary artery	Found in subcutis

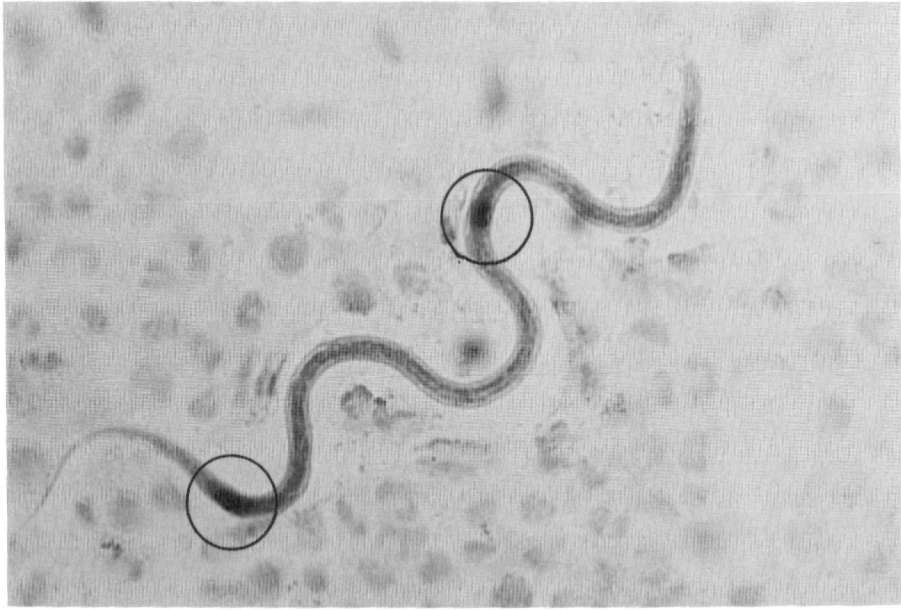

Fig. 14–8. Microfilaria of *Dirofilaria immitis* stained for the demonstration of acid phosphatase activity. Two distinct bands of activity at the excretory and anal pores (circles) allow accurate differentiation from microfilariae of *Dipetalonema reconditum* in which acid phosphatase activity is uniformly distributed. The background is stained with methyl green. (Courtesy of New England Regional Primate Research Center, Harvard Medical School.)

they are prepared by suitable means. About 1 ml of whole blood containing microfilaria is dropped into 10 ml of 1% formalin solution, which is shaken, centrifuged, and the supernatant decanted. A few drops of 1:1000 methylene blue solution are added to the sediment, which is then placed on a slide, a cover slip placed over it, and examined under a microscope. An ocular micrometer is used to make measurements of several microfilariae. If only a few microfilariae are present, a greater concentration may be obtained by allowing 5 to 15 ml of blood to clot and collecting the extruded serum, into which the microfilariae tend to migrate.

The comparison of these two parasites given in Table 14–5 may be helpful.

Chalifoux and Hunt (1971) have demonstrated that the two species of microfilariae can be accurately differentiated on the basis of localization of acid phosphatase activity in the parasites. In microfilariae of *Dirofilaria immitis*, acid phosphatase activity is limited to narrow bands at the excretory and anal pores, whereas in microfilariae of *Dipetalonema reconditum*, the enzyme activity is uniformly distributed throughout the parasite (Fig. 14–8). The technique has also been used to differentiate *Brugia malayi* from *Brugia pahangi*, two filarial parasites of man.

Abbott, P.K.: Feline dirofilariasis in Papua. Aust. Vet. J., 42:247–249, 1966.

Adcock, J.L.: Pulmonary arterial lesions in canine dirofilariasis. Am. J. Vet. Res., 22:655–662, 1961.

Beaver, P.C., and Orihel, T.C.: Human infection with filariae of animals in the United States. Am. J. Trop. Med. Hyg., 14:1010–1029, 1965.

Bemrick, W.J., Buchli, B.L., and Griffiths, H.J.: Development of *Dirofilaria immitis* in *Anopheles quadrimaculatus* after exposure of the microfilariae to a freezing temperature. J. Parasitol., 51:954–957, 1965.

Chalifoux, L., and Hunt, R.D.: Histochemical differentiation of *Dirofilaria immitis* and *Dipetalonema reconditum*. J. Am. Vet. Med. Assoc., 158:601–605, 1971.

Forrester, D.J., Jackson, R.F., Miller, J. F., and Townsend, B.C.: Heartworms in captive

California sea lions. J. Am. Vet. Med. Assoc., *163*:568–570, 1973.

Griffiths, H.J., Schlotthauer, J.C., and Gehrman, F.W.: Feline dirofilariasis. J. Am. Vet. Med. Assoc., *140*:61, 1962.

Gulber, D.J.: A comparative study of the distribution, incidence and periodicity of the canine filarial worms *Dirofilaria immitis* Leidy and *Dipetalonema reconditum* Grassi in Hawaii. J. Med. Entomol., *3*:159–167, 1966.

Hirth, R.S., and Nielsen, S.W.: Vascular lesions of *Dirofilaria immitis* in the red fox. J. Am. Vet. Med. Assoc., *149*:915–919, 1966.

Jackson, R.F., von Lichtenberg, F., and Otto, G.F.: Occurrence of adult heartworms in the venae cavae of dogs. J. Am. Vet. Med. Assoc., *141*:117–121, 1962.

Klein, J.B., and Stoddard, E.D.: *Dirofilaria immitis* recovered from a horse. J. Am. Vet. Med. Assoc., *171*:354–355, 1977.

Kotani, T., et al.: Pathological studies on the ectopic migration of *Dirofilaria immitis* in the brain of dogs. Jpn. J. Vet. Sci., *37*:141–154, 1975.

Lavers, D.W., Spratt, D.M., and Thomas, C.: *Dirofilaria immitis* from the eye of a dog. Aust. Vet. J., *45*:284–286, 1969.

Lindsey, J.R.: Identification of canine microfilariae. J. Am. Vet. Med. Assoc., *146*:1106–1114, 1965.

Live, I., and Stubbs, E.L.: The diagnosis of filariasis in the dog. J. Am. Vet. Med. Assoc., *92*:686–690, 1938.

Ludlam, K. W., Jachowski, L.A., Jr., and Otto, G.F.: Potential vectors of *Dirofilaria immitis*. J. Am. Vet. Med. Assoc., *157*:1354–1359, 1970.

Mantovani, A., and Jackson, R.F.: Transplacental transmission of microfilariae of *Dirofilaria immitis* in the dog. J. Parasitol., *52*:116, 1966.

Montgomery, C.A., Redington, B.C., Jervis, H.R., and Hockmeyer, W.T.: Histochemical differentiation of *Brugia malayi* and *Brugia pahangi*. Fed. Proc., *33*:592, 1974.

Newton, W.L., and Wright, W.H.: The occurrence of a dog filariid other than *Dirofilaria immitis* in the United States. J. Parasitol., *42*:246–258, 1956.

———: A reevaluation of the canine filariasis problem in the United States. Vet. Med., *52*:75–78, 1957.

Nishimura, T., Kondo, K., and Shoho, C.: Human infection with a subcutaneous *Dirofilaria immitis*. Biken J., *7*:1–8, 1964.

Orihel, T.C., and Beaver, P.C.: Morphology and relationship of *Dirofilaria tenuis* and *Dirofilaria conjunctivae*. Am. J. Trop. Med. Hyg., *14*:1030–1043, 1965.

Porter, W.B.: Chronic *Cor Pulmonale* in dogs with *Dirofilaria immitis* (heart-worms) infestations. Trans. Assoc. Am. Physicians, *64*:328–334, 1951.

Rothstein, H., and Brown, M.L.: Vital staining and differentiation of microfilaria. [*D. immitis* and *Dipetalonema*.] Am. J. Vet. Res., *21*:1090–1094, 1960.

Schnelle, G.B., Roby, T.O., Young, R.M., and Jones, T.C.: Canine filariasis. North Am. Vet., *26*:155–164, 1945.

Schnelle, G.B., and Jones, T.C.: *Dirofilaria immitis* in the eye and in an interdigital cyst. J. Am. Vet. Med. Assoc., *107*:14–15, 1945.

Slonka, G.F., Castleman, W., and Krum, S.: Adult heartworms in arteries and veins of a dog. J. Am. Vet. Med. Assoc., *170*:717–719, 1977.

Sonoda, M., and Kobayashi, K.: Electron microscopic studies on the morphology of microfilariae of *Dirofilaria immitis*. I. Observations of the whole body. Jpn. J. Vet. Res., *13*:67–70, 1965. V.B. *36*:3565, 1966.

Stackhouse, L.L., and Clough, E.: Clinical report: five cases of feline dirofilariasis. Vet. Med. Small Anim. Clin., *67*:1309–1310, 1972.

Taguchi, M., Takehara, B., and Uriu, I.: Aberrant *Dirofilaria immitis* in the lateral ventricle of the brain in a dog. J. Jpn. Vet. Med. Assoc., *12*:430–432, 1959. (Engl. summary.) VB *30*:1499, 1960.

Tashjian, R.J., et al.: Angiocardiography in canine heartworm disease. Am. J. Vet. Res., *31*:415–436, 1970.

Tulloch, G.S., et al.: Prepatent clinical, pathologic, and serologic changes in dogs infected with *Dirofilaria immitis* and treated with diethylcarbamazine. Am. J. Vet. Res., *31*:437–448, 1970.

von Lichtenberg, F., Jackson, R.F., and Otto, G.F.: Hepatic lesions in dogs with dirofilariasis. J. Am. Vet. Med. Assoc., *141*:121–128, 1962.

Williams, J.F., Williams, C.S.F., Signs, M., and Hokama, L.: Evaluation of a polycarbonate filter for the detection of microfilaremia in dogs in Central Michigan. J. Am. Vet. Med. Assoc., *170*:714–716, 1977.

Winter, H.: The pathology of canine dirofilariasis. Am. J. Vet. Res., *20*:366–371, 1959.

Dracunculosis

Parasitism by the "guinea-worm" is usually considered to occur only in tropical or subtropical countries, but this is not wholly correct because the disease does occur in North America. The North American guinea-worm, *Dracunculus insignis* (Leidy, 1858), has been reported to parasitize the subcutis of the dog, mink, otter, raccoon, and skunk in states as widely separated as New Hampshire, Missouri, Texas, and New York. The raccoon appears to be the most favorable host in North America.

The adult female is a slender (0.3 to 0.5 cm in width), thread-shaped worm about 20 to 28 cm long, resembling the true "guinea-worm," *D. medinensis* (serpentworm, dragon-worm, medina-worm), which parasitizes man and other hosts in the Orient. The adult female of *D. medinensis* may be differentiated by its length, 60 to 70 cm. The adult female of *D. insignis*, intertwined among the connective tissues of the subcutis, usually on one of the legs, deposits her living larvae through a small orifice in the skin at the apex of the small nodule formed by the parasite. The larvae are extruded when the lesion is in contact with water, apparently facilitating access to their intermediate host, a cyclops. The larvae become infective in these crustaceans and reach the next definitive host when it drinks the water in which the crustaceans live. The infective larvae are released from the intermediate host in the intestine of the adult host. The larvae then presumably migrate through the tissues, become mature, and eventually reach the subcutis.

These parasites are more annoying than serious, but may be removed with some difficulty by pulling them through the opening in the skin or by careful surgical dissection. Upon occasion, the larvae may be demonstrated in the circulating blood. Here they may be distinguished from the microfilaria of *Dirofilaria immitis* and *Dipetalonema reconditum* by their characteristic long tapering tail.

Benbrook, E.A.: The occurrence of the guinea worm, *Dracunculus medinensis*, in a dog and a mink with a review of this parasitism. J. Am. Vet. Med. Assoc., 96:260–263, 1940.

Beverley-Burton, M., and Crichton, V.F.J.: Attempted experimental cross infections with mammalian guinea-worms, *Dracunculus spp.* (Nematoda: Dracunculoidea). Am. J. Trop. Med. Hyg., 25:704–708, 1976.

Chandler, A.C.: The guinea-worm, *Dracunculus insignis* (Leidy, 1858). A common parasite of raccoons in east Texas. Am. J. Trop. Med., 22:153–157, 1942.

Cheatum, E.L., and Cook, A.H.: On the occurrence of the North American guinea-worm in mink, otter, raccoon, and skunk in New York State. Cornell Vet., 38:421–423, 1948.

Crichton, V.F.J., and Beverley-Burton, M.: Observations on the seasonal prevalence, pathology and transmission of *Dracunculus insignis* (Nematoda: Dracunculoidea) in the raccoon (*Procyon lotor* (L)) in Ontario. J. Wldlf. Dis., 13:273–280, 1977.

Elder, C.: Dracunculiasis in a Missouri dog. J. Am. Vet. Med. Assoc., 124:390–391, 1954.

Georgi, J.R.: Parasitology for Veterinarians. 2nd ed. Philadelphia, W. B. Saunders, 1974.

Johnson, G.C.: *Dracunculus insignis* in a dog. J. Am. Vet. Med. Assoc., 165:533, 1974.

Lapage, G.: Veterinary Parasitology. 2nd ed. Springfield, Charles C Thomas, 1968.

Schwabe, C.W., Meier, H., and Bent, C.F.: A case of dracontiasis in a New England dog. J. Parasitol., 42:651, 1956.

Tirgari, M., and Radhakrishnan, C.V.: A case of *Dracunculus medinensis* in a dog. Vet. Rec., 96:43–44, 1975.

Turk, R.D.: Guinea-worm (*Dracunculus insignis*, Leidy 1858) infection in a dog. J. Am. Vet. Med. Assoc., 117:215–216, 1950.

Equine Strongylidosis

Strongyles, or sclerostome worms of the family Strongylidae, are responsible for an equine disease with protean manifestations, conveniently designated **strongylidosis**. The adult forms of the parasites are found for the most part in the lumen or attached to the wall of the cecum and large colon of Equidae (horses, asses, mules, zebras). The life cycle of this group of helminths is direct, since it involves no intermediate host, but many of the larvae migrate through the tissues, each producing rather distinctive lesions. The "large" strongyles are slender worms, about 1 to 2 inches in length, which occur as one of three species: *Strongylus vulgaris*, *S. edentatus*, and *S. equinus*. The "small" strongyles, which seldom exceed 12 mm in length, are much more numerous (about 36 species of the genera *Triodontophorus*, *Craterostomum*, *Oestophagodontus*, *Trichonema*, *Poteriostomum*, and *Gyalocephalus* are known), but they are less injurious to the host, since they neither attach themselves to the intestinal mucosa nor ingest blood, as do the larger varieties. These smaller worms, however, contribute to the parasitic burden of the host, for they may be present in very large numbers, not only in the cecum and large colon, but also in the small intestine.

The disease known as **mal seco** in Argentina has been shown (Segal, 1959) to be equine strongylidosis.

Clinical Manifestations. Signs are varied and depend upon the severity of the infection caused by the adult worms and the anatomic localization of the larval forms.

General debility, weakness, emaciation, and anemia can result from the presence of numerous large strongyles in the cecum and colon. The larvae of *Strongylus vulgaris* often give rise to lesions in the mesenteric arteries, resulting in intestinal infarction manifested by severe abdominal pain. The larvae may also produce thrombi in the aorta or iliac arteries, which may partially occlude these vessels, causing serious weakness in one or both rear limbs—this symptom is accentuated by exercise. The migration of larvae through the intestinal wall and subperitoneal fat does not provoke obvious symptoms, even though numerous larval forms may be seen in these tissues at necropsy.

Specific Strongyles. **Strongylus vulgaris,** the common or double-toothed strongyle, is found in the cecum, usually attached to the mucosa. The males are about 16 mm in length, the female approximately 24 mm, and as a rule, the worms are red from ingested blood. The life cycle is direct; eggs pass in the feces and first-stage larvae hatch out, eventually developing to second-stage and finally to third-stage infective larvae. Following ingestion, third-stage larvae penetrate the wall of the intestine, molt in the submucosa, and penetrate terminal branches of intestinal arteries. This migration results in small hemorrhages throughout the wall of the intestine and an infiltration of lymphocytes, neutrophils, and eosinophils. There is similar inflammation and thrombosis of submucosal arteries, which contain fourth-stage larvae. The parasites migrate up the lumen of mesenteric arteries to reach the anterior mesenteric artery at one of its major branches by three or four weeks after infection, where they remain for three or more months. Here they are responsible for striking arterial lesions, particularly in the anterior mesenteric artery, and less frequently in the aorta, iliac, renal, and other arteries.

The strongyle larvae burrow into the intimal stroma of the artery and evoke proliferation of intima and endothelium, sometimes associated with hemorrhage and necrosis. Fibrin and cellular debris accumulate over the roughened intimal areas, extend out into the lumen, and occasionally cause occlusion. In reasonably long-standing cases, the wall of the artery becomes greatly thickened by the proliferation of both intimal and adventitial fibrous tissue. Collections of lymphocytes often gather in the thickened wall of the artery. This is the most common lesion and is appropriately regarded as **verminous arteritis.** In a less common lesion, the arterial wall becomes both thickened and sacculated, forming a dilated segment with a relatively smooth lining. This is properly considered a **verminous aneurysm.** Rupture of such aneurysms is almost unknown, although in some encountered at necropsy the wall is extremely thin at certain points.

The worms are found in the lumen of the affected artery, firmly attached to the intima and associated with varying degrees of inflammation. In some cases, only a few parasites are seen in an arterial lesion, in others, as many as 50 may be found. The worms may also be found at times in emboli or thrombi that arise from those arterial lesions. Fifth-stage larvae have been found in association with lesions in the spinal cord of a pony, and similar spinal lesions, without the parasite, have been reported in the horse (Pohlenz, et al., 1965). Upon maturing to young adults, parasites return to the intestine by way of lumens of arteries, again inducing local hemorrhage and inflammation.

Strongylus equinus, the triple-toothed strongyle, sclerostome, or bloodworm, is found in its adult form in the cecum and rarely in the colon of equines. It is usually attached to the mucosa and engorged with blood. The male is about 35 mm long; the female, up to 55 mm. The life cycle of *S. equinus* is known to be direct, but the migratory path of the immature worm has not been fully traced. The third-stage lar-

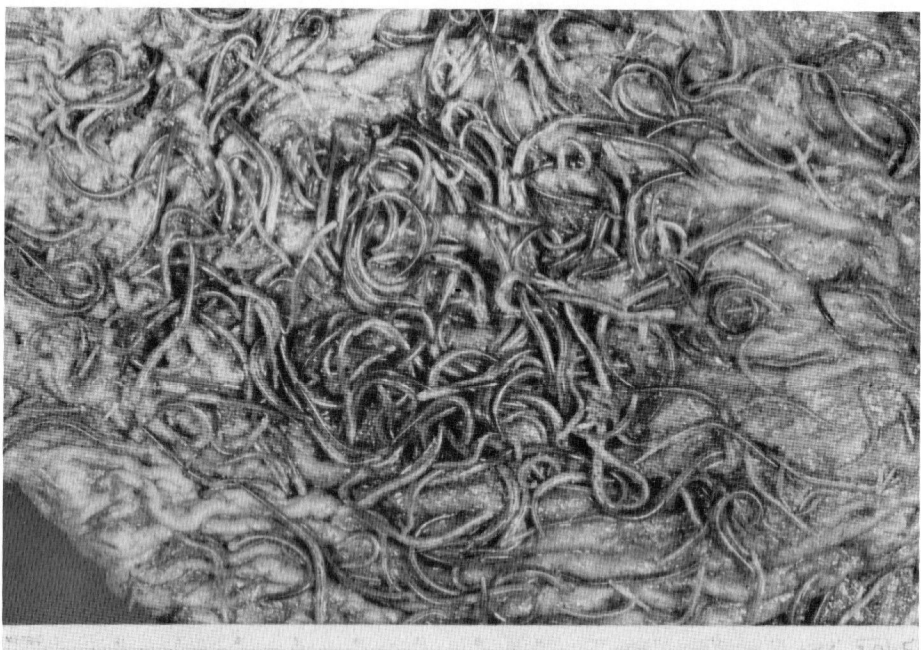

Fig. 14–9. Equine strongylidosis. Adult *Strongylus equinus* in the cecum of a two-year-old gelding. (Courtesy of Dr. C. R. Cole, Ohio State University.)

vae that have been ingested are believed to penetrate the intestine, producing small inflammatory nodules in which they develop to fourth-stage larvae. After about 11 days the larvae migrate through the peritoneal cavity to the liver, where they remain for six to seven weeks. The exact route to the liver has not been established, but is probably by way of portal veins. They then return to the peritoneal cavity and enter the pancreas. When they develop to young adults, it is presumed that they migrate directly to the lumen of the intestine, but their route has not been determined.

Strongylus edentatus, the toothless strongyle, occurs in adult form in the cecum and colon of equines, usually attached to the mucosa. The males are about 28 mm long; the females as much as 44 mm. The life cycle is direct; infective third-stage larvae penetrate the wall of the intestine and reach the liver by way of portal veins.

The larvae develop to fourth-stage larvae, which migrate within the liver, producing necrosis and inflammation. Larvae are believed to leave the liver within hepatic ligaments, making their way to the colon within the mesentery. In the wall of the colon, the larvae develop to young adults and then enter the lumen.

S. edentatus infection is associated with striking nodules in the small and large intestines, which have been termed **haemonomelasma ilei** by Cohrs (1954). The subserous masses are about 3 mm high, 5 mm wide, and one to several centimeters long. These lesions, when fresh, are bright red from recent hemorrhage; later they turn to shades of yellow and brown as the blood cells disintegrate to release blood pigment, which remains as hematoidin or hemosiderin.

Microscopically, these subserosal lesions are made up of edema, connective tissue, free red blood cells, leukocytes, macrophages, blood pigment, and in some sections, a central fragment of caseous necrotic debris. It is difficult to find larvae in the subserosal lesions, but occasionally a tract can be followed through the muscularis into the submucosa. Occasionally, the offending larvae may be cut in cross section in histologic preparations. These lesions, in spite of their florid appearance, seem to have little effect upon the host; hence their proper evaluation is of importance.

Larvae of any of the migrating strongyles may occasionally be encountered in aberrant locations, such as the lung or brain. The small strongyles also have direct life cycles and are believed to develop in small nodules in the wall of the large intestine similar to *Oesophagostomum* species.

Another member of the family Strongylidae which closely resembles equine strongyles as well as *Oesophagostomum sp.*, is *Chabertia ovina*, which inhabits the colon of sheep, goats, cattle, and wild ruminants. The males of the species measure up to 14 mm long; females, as much as 20 mm. They have a large buccal capsule on the anterior end which they use to attach to the mucosa of the colon. They draw in a piece of mucosal epithelium, digest it with their esophageal secretions, and may ingest blood. Hemorrhages and loss of blood to the parasite may terminate in anemia and death to the host. The life cycle is comparable to species of *Oesophagostomum* with a histotropic phase in the small intestine, but *Chabertia* do not cause nodules to form. A deleterious effect upon the growth of wool has also been ascribed to this parasite.

Diagnosis. Quantitative determinations of the strongyle ova in the feces are used to estimate the parasitic burden in the living animal. This is necessary because these parasites are so common that a few ova in a fecal specimen have no diagnostic significance. The diagnosis of equine strongylidosis must be based upon mature evaluation of all symptoms and ova counts.

Verminous arteritis and lesions due to migration of the parasite are usually recognized at necropsy.

Blackwell, N.J.: Colitis in equines associated with strongyle larvae. Vet. Rec., 93:401–402, 1973.

Cohrs, P.: Lehrbuch der Speziellen Pathologischen Anatomie der Haustiere 3rd ed. Jena, Fisher, p. 299, 1954.

Duncan, J.L., and Pirie, H.M.: The life cycle of *Strongylus vulgaris* in the horse. Res. Vet. Sci., 13:374–379, 1972.

————: The pathogenesis of single experimental infections with *Strongylus vulgaris* in foals. Res. Vet. Sci., 18:82–93, 1975.

Foster, A.O., and Clark, H.C.: Verminous aneurysm in equines of Panama. Am. J. Trop. Med., 17:85–99, 1937.

Herd, R.P.: The parasitic life cycle of *Chabertia ovina* (Fabricius, 1788) in sheep. Int. J. Parasitol., 1:189–199, 1971.

Herd, R.P., and Arundel, J.H.: Life cycle, pathogenicity and immunogenicity of *Chabertia ovina*. Vet. Rec., 84:487–488, 1969.

Little, P.B., Lwin, U.S., and Fretz, P.: Verminous encephalitis of horses: experimental induction with *Strongylus vulgaris* larvae. Am. J. Vet. Res., 35:1501–1510, 1974.

Ogbourne, C. P.: Studies of the epidemiology of *Strongylus vulgaris* infection of the horse. Int. J. Parasitol., 5:423–426, 1975.

Pohlenz, J., Schulze, D., and Eckert, J.: (Spinal infection with *Strongylus vulgaris* in a pony.) Dtsch. Tieaerztl. Wochenschr., 72:510–511, 1965. V.B. 36:1472, 1966.

Ross, J.G., and Todd, J.R.: The pathogenicity of *Chabertia ovina* in calves. Vet. Rec., 83:682–683, 1968.

Segal, M.: "Mal seco," enfermedad de equinos, contribución al conocimiento de su etiopatogenia, observaciones y experiencia en Junin de los Andes (Nequen) Rev. Vet. Milit. Buenos Aires, 7:3–10, 66–68, 70–74, 106, 108–116, 1959. VB 752–60.

Spirocercosis

Infection with the spiruroid worm, *Spirocerca lupi* (*Spirocerca sanguinolenta*, *Spiroptera sanguinolenta*, *Filaria sanguinolenta*, esophageal worm) is particularly common in certain of the southern United States, but it has also been reported from many parts of the world. The adult worms, which are usually bright red, have been found coiled in nodules in the wall of the esophagus, aorta, stomach and other organs of the dog, fox, wolf, and cat. The males measure 30 to 54 mm long; the females, 54 to 80 mm. The eggs are thick-walled, about 37 by 15 μ in maximum dimensions, and contain larvae when deposited.

Life Cycle. The life cycle of this helminth is complex. The embryonated eggs are passed in the feces and do not hatch until ingested by certain coprophagous beetles. In these intermediate hosts, the larvae develop into the infective (third) stage, then encyst. If eaten by an abnormal host (paratenic host), such as a frog, snake, lizard, or any one of many birds and mammals, the larvae burrow into the mesentery, where they remain in a viable state for some time. If infected beetles or other transport hosts are eaten by one of the final hosts (dog, fox, wolf, cat), the larvae penetrate the stomach wall, and by following the course of the arteries, migrating through adventitia and media, they reach the wall of the aorta and localize in the adventitia, usually of the upper thoracic portion. The parasites reach the aorta one to two weeks after ingestion and develop there for about 90 days, when they migrate to the adjacent esophagus and burrow into its wall, where they develop to adults in cystic nodules. Patent infection is established 50 to 70 days later, with the eggs reaching the esophageal lumen through a small opening in the nodule. Rarely, the adults localize in an abnormal location, such as the wall of the stomach or lungs.

Clinical Manifestations. Signs may be absent in mild infections, or persistent vomiting may be caused by esophageal obstruction. Sudden death from hemorrhage from aortic lesions has been reported.

Lesions. The principal lesions in this disease are produced by the adult worms as a result of their localization in the adventitia of the aorta and the submucosa of the esophagus. The worms become the center of a tumor-like nodule in the aortic wall, which may initiate the formation of aneurysm, with possible rupture and fatal hemorrhage. In microscopic sections of active lesions in the aorta, worms may be found in areas of the adventitia and media where normal tissue is destroyed and replaced by leukocytes and debris. Sometimes the worms are seen burrowing into the media, with necrotic tracts leading to the intima. The intimal stroma undergoes considerable proliferation. In most instances, however, the worm eventually departs from the aortic media or adventitia for the esophagus, leaving a lesion in the wall in the aorta. It is not uncommon to observe well-developed worm-containing nodules in the esophagus of the same animal in which there is evidence of previous localization of the aorta. On the intimal surface, these lesions appear as roughened, slightly elevated plaques of various sizes or as depressed aneurysmal scars.

The esophageal lesions are most common near its terminus, usually a few centimeters from the cardia of the stomach. Grossly, one or several nodules are seen on the luminal surface elevating the epithelium a centimeter or more. One or several worms may be embedded in each nodule, with parts of the worms protruding from a small orifice. Cross section of one of the nodules usually reveals a thick fibrous wall partially covered by epithelium, enclosing a cavity containing worms and yellowish pus. Microscopically, the worms form the center for a mass of neutrophils, surrounded by a thick wall of connective tissue infiltrated with macrophages, lymphocytes, and plasma cells. Strangely, eosinophils are usually absent. The adult worms have a thick cuticle surrounding a meromyarian muscle wall, interrupted by a double row of very large specialized muscle cells arranged along each side of the body cavity. Ova within the gravid uterus are flattened and ovoid, and are embryonated before they are discharged through the genital pore.

Seibold et al. (1955) have described a "deformative ossifying spondylitis" in the

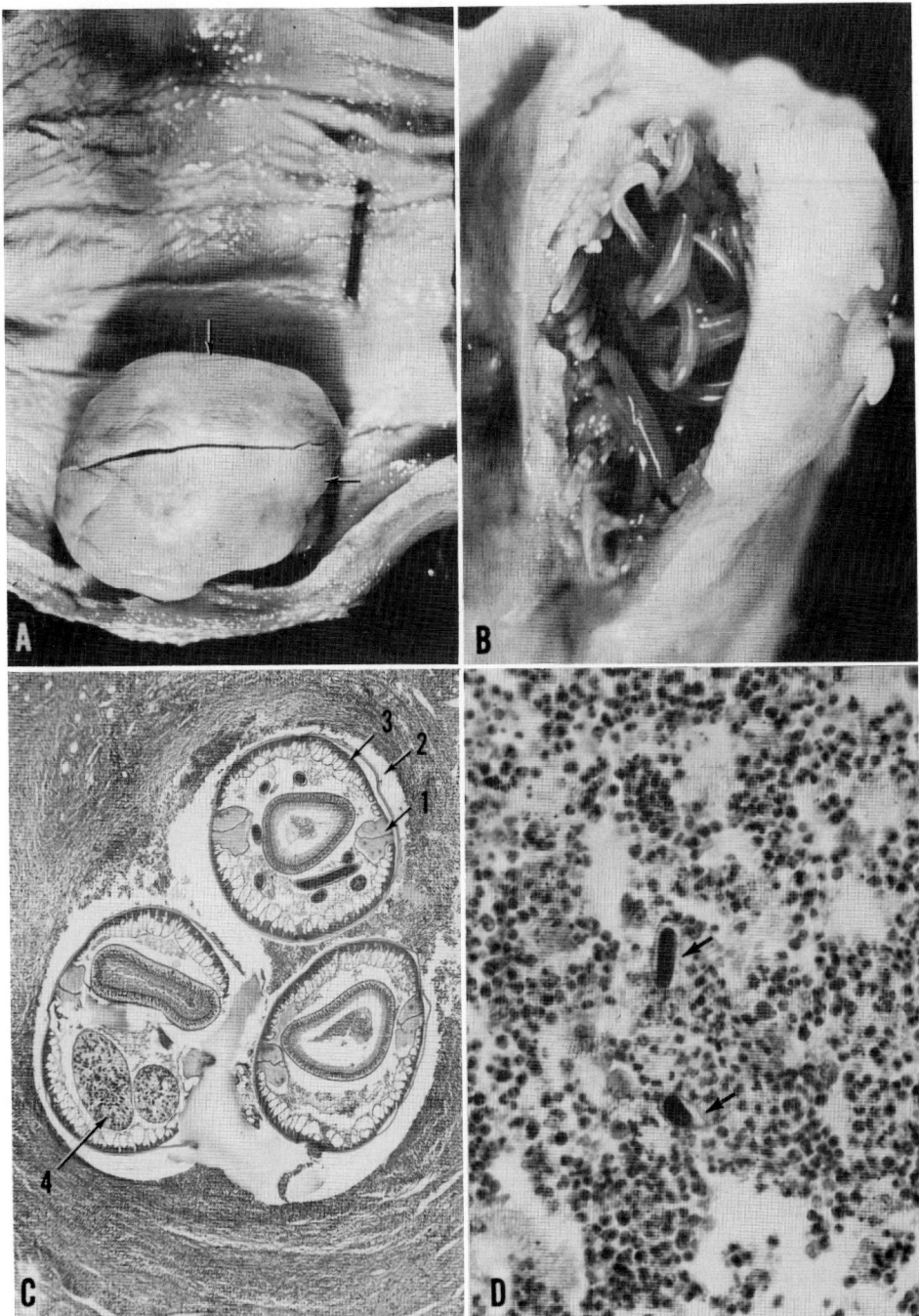

Fig. 14–10.   Spirocercosis. *A,* Nodule (arrows) in thoracic esophagus of a dog. *B,* A nodule opened to show the coiled nematodes within. Photographs courtesy of Major C. N. Barron. *C,* Section through a nodule (× 48) containing adult worms. Note lateral chord cells *(1),* cuticula *(2),* muscle cells *(3),* and uterus filled with ova *(4).* Contributor: Major C. N. Barron. *D,* Ova of *Spirocerca lupi* (× 300) surrounded by pus in an esophageal nodule. (Courtesy of Armed Forces Institute of Pathology.) Contributor: Major C. N. Barron.

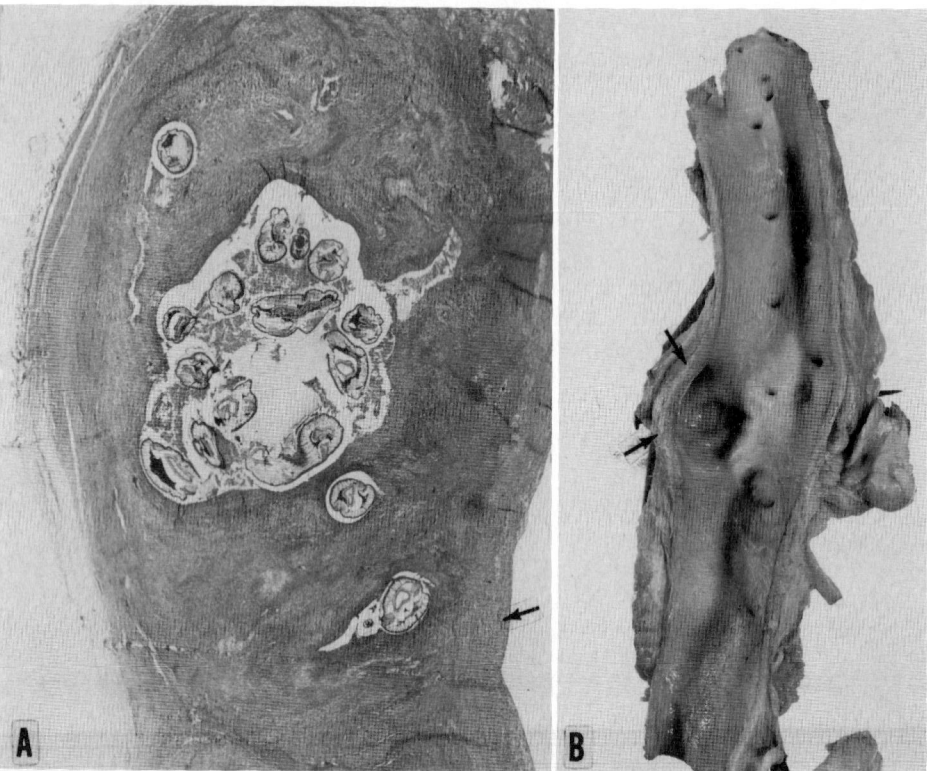

Fig. 14–11. Spirocercosis. *A*, Section of aorta (× 12) with a large worm-filled nodule in the adventitia. The intima is indicated by an arrow. Contributor: Dr. H. R. Seibold. *B*, A large sacculate lesion (arrows) in the aorta resulting from spirocercosis. (Courtesy of Armed Forces Institute of Pathology.) Contributor: Major C. N. Barron.

thoracic vertebrae of the host, which they believe is related to the migration and encystment of *Spirocerca lupi*. This lesion is characterized by irregular coarse exostoses of the ventral surfaces of the bodies of certain thoracic vertebrae. These writers also described osteosarcomas or fibrosarcomas originating in the wall of the esophagus in intimate relation to the lesions of *Spirocerca lupi*. While it has not been established that the parasite is the cause of the neoplasms, the close association suggests such a relationship. Additional significance to this relationship has been provided by the work of Ribelin and Bailey (1958). Also described by Seibold et al. was the frequent manifestation of hypertrophic pulmonary osteoarthropathy in dogs with large esophageal tumors, some of which had metastasized to the lungs and other viscera.

Diagnosis. Infection with *Spirocerca lupi* in the living animal can be confirmed by the identification of embryonated ova in the feces. Postmortem diagnosis is easily made by demonstration of characteristic lesions in the aorta, esophagus, or ventral face of thoracic vertebrae in association with the adult parasites.

Anantaraman, M., and Se, K.: Experimental spirocercosis in dogs with larvae from a paratenic host, *Calotes versicolor*, the common garden lizard in Madras. J. Parasitol., *52*:911–912, 1966.

Bannor, T.T.: Canine spirocercosis—cause of fatal haemorrhage in an Alsatian dog. Vet. Rec., *98*:302, 1976.

Bwangamoi, O.: Spirocercosis in Uganda and its association with fibrosarcoma in a dog. J. Small Anim. Pract., *8*:395–398, 1967.

Chhabra, R.C., and Singh, K.S.: Life history of *Spirocerca lupi*: route of migration of histotropic juveniles in dog. Indian J. Anim. Sci., *42*:540–547, 1972.

Chowdhury, N., and Pande, B.P.: The development of the infective larvae of the canine oesophageal tumour worm *Spirocerca lupi* in rabbits and its histopathology. Z. Parasitenkd., *32*:1–10, 1969.

Dixon, K.G., and McCue, J.F.: Further observations on the epidemiology of *Spirocerca lupi* in the southern United States. J. Parasitol., *53*:1074–1075, 1967.

Murray, M.: Incidence and pathology of *Spirocerca lupi* in Kenya. J. Comp. Pathol., *78*:401–405, 1968.

Murray, M., Campbell, H., and Jarrett, W.H.F.: *Spirocerca lupi* in a cheetah. E. Afr. Wildl. J., *2*:164, 1964.

Rajan, A., and Mohiyuddeen, S.: Incidence of spirocercosis in some uncommon sites. Kerala J. Vet. Sci., 5:139–142, 1974.

Ressang, A.A., and Hong, L.Y.: The occurrence of *Spirocerca lupi* in the Indonesian dog and its relation to neoplasm formation. Commun. Vet. Bogor, 7:9–17 (Ind.), 1963.

Ribelin, W.E., and Bailey, W.S.: Esophageal sarcomas associated with *Spirocerca lupi* infection in the dog. Cancer, 2:1242–1246, 1958.

Seibold, H.R., et al.: Observations on the possible relation of malignant esophageal tumors and *Spirocerca lupi* lesions in the dog. Am. J. Vet. Res., 16:5–14, 1955.

Cerebrospinal Nematodiasis (Neurofilariasis, Setariasis)

Certain nematodes have selective affinity for the central nervous system, and several may accidentally wander into the brain or spinal cord, resulting in paralytic diseases. For many years, obscure neuroparalytic symptoms of unknown cause have been observed seasonally in animals in the Far East, particularly in Japan, Korea, India, and Ceylon. In sheep and goats, such a clinical entity has been known as "lumbar paralysis," while a similar disease in horses has been called "kumri" (Hindustani for "weakness of the loin"). The observations of Innes (1953) have done much to characterize these diseases pathologically and to explain both their symptomatology and etiology. Most of the studies in the Far East have been conducted by Japanese workers (Innes, 1951). The presence of nematodes in the central nervous system in animals with obscure paralytic signs has also been reported in sheep in New York State by Kennedy et al. (1952) and in moose in Minnesota by Fenstermacher (1934). Tiner (1953) observed death of mice, squirrels, and guinea pigs preceded by nervous symptoms that developed after exposure to infective larvae of certain *Ascaris* species, especially ascarids from raccoons.

Setaria digitata, a natural parasite of the bovine, has been incriminated as one of the more important causes of parasitic encephalitis in sheep, goats, and horses in the Far East. *Pneumostrongylus tenuis* (*Elaphostrongylus, Odocoileostrongylus, Parelophostrongylus*, and *Neurofilaria cornellensis*), described by Kennedy and Whitlock (1952) as a normal parasite of white-tailed deer (*Odocoileus virginianus*), has been demonstrated to invade the brain of deer, sheep, goats, moose, elk, and other cervids. The adults normally reside in the subdural space, with larvae passing by way of the blood stream to the lungs, where they are coughed up and pass to the outside through the gastrointestinal wall. The parasite requires a snail as an intermediate host.

Angiostrongylus cantonensis, a parasite of rats, normally migrates through the brain as part of its life cycle in rats, and has been recognized as a cause of eosinophilic meningoencephalitis in man. Various species of ascarids are occasionally encountered in the brain, and *Ascaris columnaris* is an important cause of cerebral nematodiasis in rabbits, groundhogs, and squirrels.

Micronema deletrix, which is apparently a saphrophytic nematode, has been recognized as a cause of encephalitis in horses in the United States and Egypt, as well as a cause of nasal granulomas in horses. Larvae of *Strongylus vulgaris* are one of the more important causes of verminous encephalitis in horses in the United States. *Meningioma peruzzi* and *Dipetalonema perstans* have been found in the brain of monkeys. The latter species,

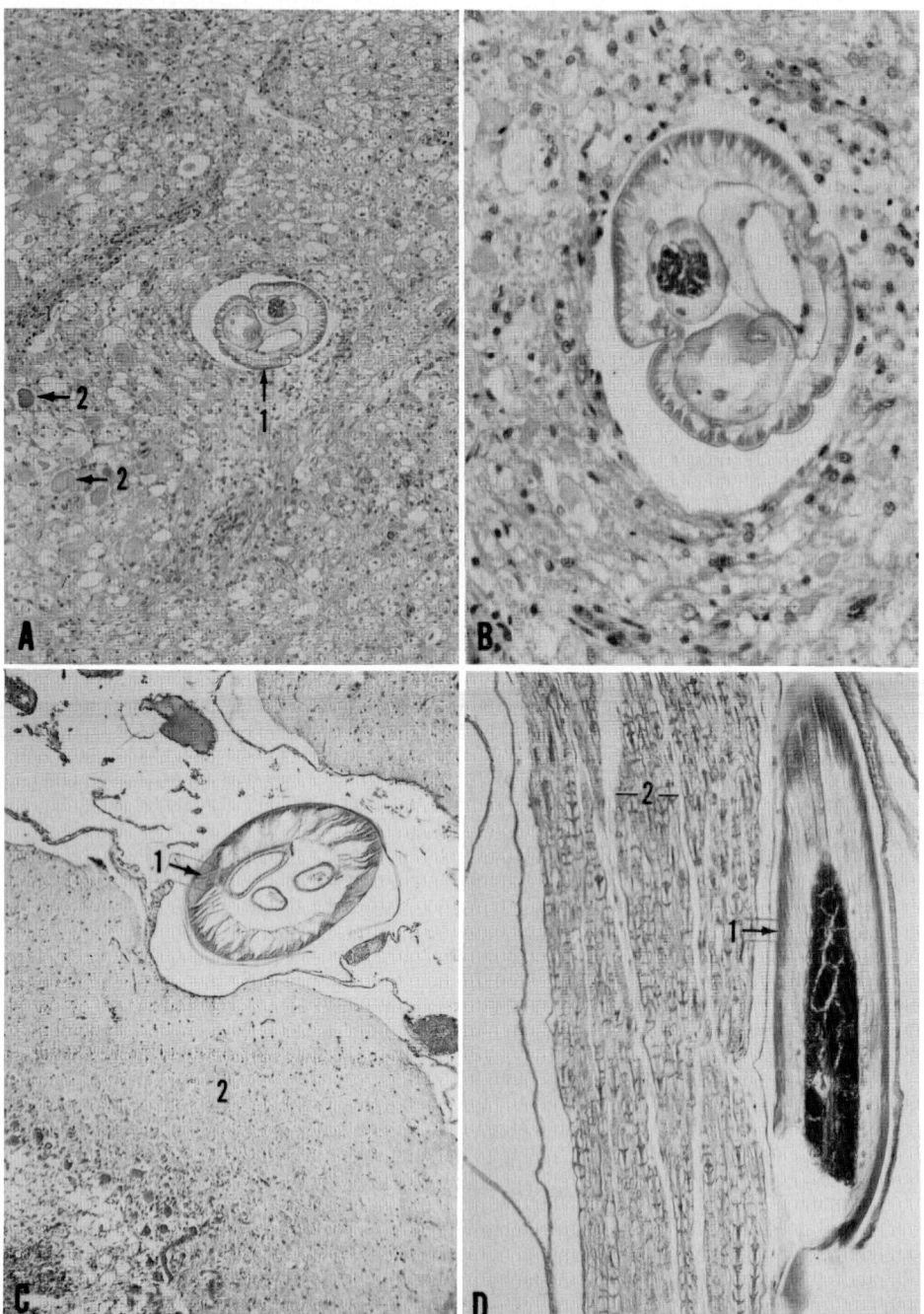

Fig. 14–12. Cerebrospinal nematodiasis. *A,* Nematode *(1)* in the spinal cord (× 77) of a sheep. Note swollen axones *(2). B,* Higher magnification (× 215) to show the parasite in greater detail. Contributor: Dr. Peter Olafson. *C,* Nematode *(1)* in the pia mater (× 53) of a horse. Cerebellar cortex *(2). D,* Another larva *(1)* in the longitudinal section (× 100) in a spinal nerve *(2)* from the same horse as *C.* (Courtesy of Armed Forces Institute of Pathology.) Contributor: 406th Medical General Laboratory.

as well as *Wuchereria bancrofti* and *Loa loa*, may invade the brain of human beings.

Similar diseases due to unidentified helminths have been described in a variety of domestic and wild animals. *Guretia paralysans* is a filarid that resides in spinal veins of cats and may be responsible for paralysis.

Tiner (1953, 1954) observed signs of central nervous system dysfunction and death of rodents and rabbits after exposure to infective larvae of certain ascarids. *Baylisascaris (Ascaris) procyonis* larvae from raccoons and *B. (Ascaris) columnaris* from skunks led to death as early as ten days after exposure.

Larvae of ascarids from carnivore final hosts, such as procyonids (raccoons) or mustelids (badgers, fishers, martens, skunks), may be responsible for outbreaks of cerebrospinal ascariasis that have occurred in rabbits (Dade et al., 1975; Nettles et al., 1975), groundhogs, and zoo rodents (see Kelly and Innes, 1966; Schueler, 1973). Such infected intermediate hosts in natural environments would be among the most available prey as food for final hosts.

Clinical Manifestations. Manifestations of cerebrospinal nematodiasis are extremely varied, as might be expected from the lesions to be described. Mildly affected animals may show only motor weakness, incoordination, or slight loss of balance. Animals with severe lesions may exhibit paresis of one or all limbs, the hind legs being most frequently and severely affected. The onset may be dramatically sudden in some cases, more insidious in others; death may intervene within a few days, or recovery may follow, with or without residual nervous manifestations, such as drooping of eyelid or ear, weakness, or impaired gait.

Lesions. Grossly visible lesions are unusual, except in those infrequent instances in which hemorrhage occurs in the primary malacic focus caused by the migration of the parasites. Meticulous microscopic study of the brain and spinal cord is usually necessary to uncover the areas affected. The primary foci may be single or multiple, and occur in any part of the central nervous system, although the spinal cord and thalamus appear to be favored sites. The lesions are usually asymmetrical, each appearing as a solitary, raggedly bound focus of cavitation, rarely containing hemorrhage. Under low magnification, these foci appear as cracks, crevices, or spongy areas, and in some, tracts leading from the nearby meninges can be detected. Under higher magnification, it will be seen that nervous tissue is partially or completely lost in the center of the affected zone. Around this, axis cylinders in cross section appear as large, irregularly shaped, rounded bodies, which are stained darkly eosinophilic in hematoxylin and eosin preparations and are heavily impregnated when the Bodian method is employed. Longitudinal sections of these axis cylinders show that they are irregularly enlarged, tortuous, and fragmented.

Axons similarly affected are seen in ascending and descending tracts extending above and below the primary malacic locus. Axonal damage is associated with swelling and distortion of myelin sheaths, and in long-standing cases, with glial proliferation. The secondary (wallerian) degeneration is no different from that observed as a frequent consequence of injuries to the central nervous system. The degenerative lesion in nerve fiber tracts may lead to the primary lesion if sufficient numbers of serial sections are prepared and examined.

Cellular infiltration composed of lymphocytes, neutrophils, or occasionally eosinophils is frequently observed in the pia mater near the primary malacic foci. These cells may also be seen in irregular nests in the pia arachnoid, in subdural and epidural locations, and sometimes extending along the spinal nerve roots. Perivascular lymphocytic cuffing may be prominent adjacent to primary malacic foci.

The offending helminths will be seen in

tissue sections only fortuitously, unless a diligent search of serial sections through characteristic lesions is made. It is assumed that migratory larvae not only can invade nervous tissue, but can also wander out again. In some cases it is possible to demonstrate the parasites only by filtration of the spinal fluid, although evidence of their invasion of nervous tissue may be readily found.

Diagnosis. Definitive diagnosis can be made only after meticulous microscopic examination of the central nervous system. Typical lesions must be found, and some should contain the causative nematodes. Clinical diagnosis is made in geographic regions in which the disease is enzoötic, but at present can be based only upon presumptive evidence.

Alden, C., Woodson, F., Mohan, R., and Miller, S.: Cerebrospinal nematodiasis in sheep. J. Am. Vet. Med. Assoc., 166:784–786, 1975.

Anderson, R.C.: Neurological disease in moose infected experimentally with *Pneumostrongylus tenuis* from white-tailed deer. Pathol. Vet., 1:289–322, 1964.

———: The development of *Pneumonstrongylus tenuis* in the central nervous system of white-tailed deer. Pathol. Vet., 2:360–379, 1965.

———: The pathogenesis and transmission of neurotropic and accidental nematode parasites of the central nervous system of mammals and birds. Helminth. Abstr., 37:191–210, 1968.

Anderson, R.C., et al.: Further experimental studies of *Pneumonstrongylus tenuis* in cervids. Can. J. Zool., 44:851–861, 1966.

Anderson, R.C., and Strelive, U.R.: The transmission of *Pneumonstrongylus tenuis* to guinea pigs. Can. J. Zool., 44:533–540, 1966.

———: Experimental cerebrospinal nematodiasis (*Pneumonstrongylus tenuis*) in sheep. Can. J. Zool., 44:889–894, 1966.

———: The penetration of *Pneumonstrongylus tenuis* into the tissues of white-tailed deer. Can. J. Zool., 45:285–289, 1967.

———: The effect of *Pneumonstrongylus tenuis* (Nematoda: Metastrongyloidea) on kids. Can. J. Comp. Med., 33:280–286, 1969.

Beautyman, W., and Woolf, A.L.: An ascaris larva in the brain in association with acute anterior poliomyelitis. J. Pathol. Bact., 63:635–647, 1951.

Church, E.M., Wyand, D.S., and Lein, D.H.: Experimentally induced cerebrospinal nematodiasis in rabbits (*Oryctolagus cuniculus*). Am. J. Vet. Res., 36:331–335, 1975.

Dade, A.W., Williams, J.F., Whitenack, D.L., and Williams, C.S.F.: An epizootic of cerebral nematodiasis in rabbits due to *Ascaris columnaris*. Lab. Anim. Sci., 25:65–69, 1975.

Fenstermacher, R.: Further studies of diseases affecting moose. Univ. Minnesota Agric. Exper. Sta. Bull. 308, 1934.

Ferris, D.H., Levine, N.D., and Beamer, P.D.: *Micronema deletrix* in equine brain. Am. J. Vet. Res., 33:33–38, 1972.

Innes, J.R.M.: Necrotizing encephalomyelitis (or encephalomyelomalacia) of unknown aetiology in goats in Ceylon with similarities to setariasis of sheep, horses and goats in Japan. (Including a brief review of nervous diseases of goats.) Br. Vet. J., 107:187–203, 1951.

Innes, J.R.M., and Shoho, C.: Cerebrospinal nematodiasis. Focal encephalomyelomalacia of animals caused by nematodes (*Setaria digitata*). A disease which may occur in man. Arch. Neurol. Psychiat., 70:325–349, 1953.

Innes, J.R.M., and Pillai, C.P.: Kumri—so-called lumbar paralysis—of horses in Ceylon (India and Burma), and its identification with cerebrospinal nematodiasis. Br. Vet. J., 111:223–235, 1955.

Kelly, W.R., and Innes, J.R.M.: Cerebrospinal nematodiasis with focal encephalomalacia as a cause of paralysis of beavers (*Castor canadensis*) in the Dublin Zoological Gardens. Br. Vet. J., 122:285–287, 1966.

Kennedy, P.C., Whitlock, J.H., and Roberts, S.J.: Neurofilariosis, a paralytic disease of sheep. I. Introduction, symptomatology, pathology. Cornell Vet., 42:118–124, 1952.

Kurtz, H.J., Loken, K., and Schlotthauer, J.C.: Histopathologic studies on cerebrospinal nematodiasis of moose in Minnesota naturally infected with *Pneumonstrongylus tenuis*. Am. J. Vet. Res., 27:548–557, 1966.

Little, P.B.: Cerebrospinal nematodiasis of Equidae. J. Am. Vet. Med. Assoc., 160:1407–1413, 1972.

Loken, K.I., et al.: *Pneumonstrongylus tenuis* in Minnesota moose (*Alces alces*). Bull Wildl. Dis. Assn., 1:7, 1965.

Nettles, V.F., Davidson, W.R., Fisk, S.K., and Jacobson, H.A.: An epizootic of cerebrospinal nematodiasis in cottontail rabbits. J. Am. Vet. Med. Assoc., 167:600–602, 1975.

Orihel, T.C., and Esslinger, J.H.: *Meningonema peruzzii* gen. et sp. n. (Nematoda: Filarioidea) from the central nervous system of African monkeys. J. Parasitol., 59:437–441, 1973.

Richter, C.B., and Kradel, D.C.: Cerebrospinal nematodosis in Pennsylvania groundhogs (*Marmota monax*). Am. J. Vet. Res., 25:1230–1235, 1964.

Rubin, H.L., and Woodard, J.C.: Equine infection with *Micronema deletrix*. J. Am. Vet. Med. Assoc., 165:256–258, 1974.

Schueler, R.L.: Cerebral nematodiasis in a red squirrel. J. Wldlf. Dis., 9:58–60, 1973.

Shoho, C., and Tanaka, T.: Further observations on cerebrospinal nematodosis in animals. II. The problems of reinfection of nematodes and clinically-silent cases. Br. Vet. J., 111:102–111, 1955.

Smith, H.J., and Archibald, R.McG.: Moose infected

with the common cervine parasite, *Elaphostrongylus tenuis*. Can. Vet. J., *8*:173–177, 1967.

Sprent, J.F.A.: On the invasion of the central nervous system by nematodes. I. The incidence and pathological significance of nematodes in the central nervous system. Parasitology, *45*:31–40, 1955.

———: On the invasion of the central nervous system by nematodes. II. Invasion of the nervous system by ascariasis. Parasitology, *45*:41–55, 1955.

Swanstrom, O.G., Rising, J.L., and Carlton, W.W.: Spinal nematodosis in a horse. J. Am. Vet. Med. Assoc., *155*:748–753, 1969.

Swerczek, T.W., and Helmboldt, C.F.: Cerebrospinal nematodiasis in groundhogs (*Marmota monax*). J. Am. Vet. Med. Assoc., *157*:671–674, 1970.

Tiner, J.D.: The migration, distribution in the brain and growth of ascarid larvae in rodents. J. Infect. Dis., *92*:105–113, 1953.

———: Fatalities in rodents caused by larval *Ascaris* in the central nervous system. J. Mammol., *34*:153–167, 1953.

———: The fraction of *Peromyscus leucopus* fatalities caused by raccoon ascarid larvae. J. Mammal., *35*:589–592, 1954.

Whitlock, J.H.: *Elaphostrongylus*, the proper designation of *Neurofilaria*. Cornell Vet., *49*:3–27, 1959.

Wilder, H.C.: Nematode endophthalmitis. Tr. Am. Acad. Ophthalmol., (Oct):99–108, 1950.

Trichinosis (Trichiniasis, Trichinelliasis)

Although animals are seldom observed to be seriously affected by trichinosis, they are the source of infection for man, in whom the disease may be debilitating or fatal. The causative agent is a tiny, slender nematode that spends its adult life in the mucosa of the small intestine of a wide variety of animals, including man, domestic and wild swine, rats, bears, dogs, and cats. The female is 3 to 4 mm in length and the male about half as long. The females are viviparous, producing larvae which are the principal excitants of symptoms and lesions, because they burrow through tissues and encyst in striated muscles. The causative parasite, *Trichinella spiralis*, is classified among the Nematoda under the family Trichinellidae and is the chief pathogen in this family. Based on crossbreeding experiments, it has recently been demonstrated that there are several other species of *Trichinella;* however, the parasites are morphologically identical.

Life Cycle. Completion of the life cycle of *Trichinella spiralis* depends upon consumption by the host of raw or undercooked flesh containing encysted larvae. Pork products provide the principal source of infections for man. The infective larvae are released from the ingested muscle by the action of digestive juices; then, in rapid succession, undergo four molts and mature into adults. After copulation the male dies, but the female burrows into the lamina propria of the intestinal villi and deposits large numbers of larvae in the lymphatic spaces. Some larvae may escape into the intestinal lumen, but most of them are carried to the blood stream and reach the musculature. The larvae invade the muscle bundles, where they encyst and remain throughout the life of the host. Further development of the parasite follows upon ingestion of the infected muscle by another host. The fetuses of rats, mice, and rabbits may become infected *in utero* under experimental conditions (Hartmannova and Chroust, 1969).

Clinical Manifestations. The symptoms and signs of trichinosis, rarely observed in animals, are varied and often nonspecific in man. Even in man, small numbers of trichina larvae undoubtedly can reach the muscle without provoking detectable symptoms, but in large numbers they produce muscular pain, nausea, vomiting, diarrhea, fever, edema of the face, increased respiratory rate, and urticarial skin manifestations. Invasion of cardiac muscle by the larvae may result in feeble or dicrotic pulse, muffled heart sounds, systolic murmur, or palpitation. When larvae invade the central nervous system, a plethora of signs may appear, including disorientation, apathy, stupor, delirium, paralysis, and coma. The most significant clinical laboratory evidence of the infection is in the blood cell count. Leukocytosis with eosinophilia, which in extreme cases may reach 90%, is characteristic. Although fluctuating within wide limits, the circulating eosinophilia may persist for months or even years. Identification of adult trichinae in the stools, or demonstration of larvae in

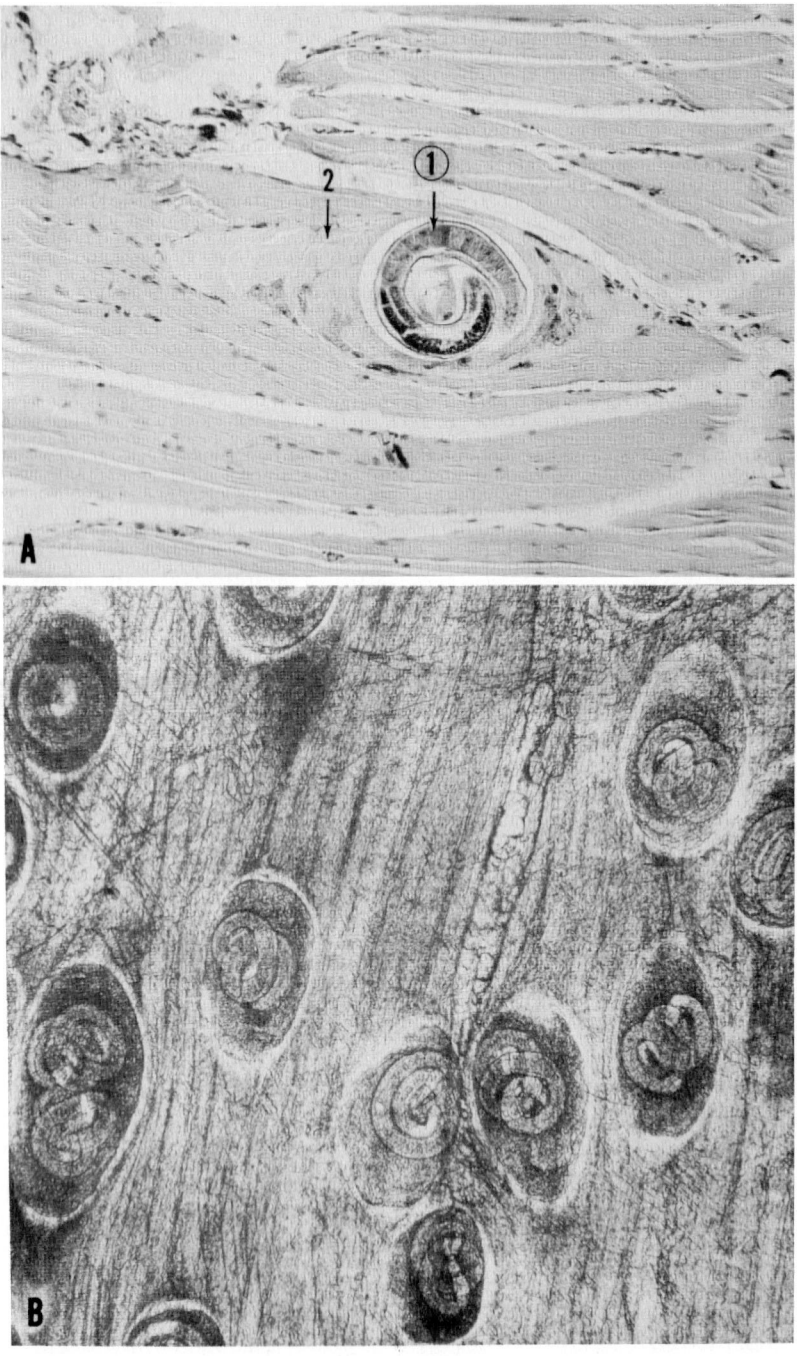

Fig. 14–13.   Trichinosis. *A, Trichinella spiralis* larva *(1)* encysted in a skeletal muscle bundle of a rat. Note capsule *(2)* around nematode (× 80). (Courtesy of Armed Forces Institute of Pathology.) Contributor: Dr. J. C. Swartz. *B,* Crush preparation of skeletal muscle containing *Trichinella spiralis* larvae.

biopsy specimens of muscle, is decisive in confirming the clinical diagnosis of trichinosis.

Lesions. Except for transitory catarrhal enteritis provoked by the activities of the adults, the lesions of trichinosis are confined to the skeletal and, to a much smaller extent, the cardiac musculature, and are the result of invasion and encystment of the larvae. In man, the muscles most frequently and heavily parasitized are the diaphragmatic, intercostal, masseteric, laryngeal, lingual, and ocular. The heart muscle may be invaded by young larvae during the time that they are being liberated in the intestinal villi, but encysted larvae are rarely found in cardiac muscle. The larvae penetrate the skeletal muscle bundles, most frequently near the tendinous portion, eliciting some inflammatory reaction in the adjacent stroma. This inflammation, which is evidenced by the presence of edema, neutrophils, lymphocytes, and eosinophils, soon subsides as each larva becomes encased in a muscle bundle. The sarcoplasm is replaced at the site of invasion by the encapsulated worm, and adjacent parts of the muscle bundle may undergo some degenerative changes. The sarcolemma is distorted by the parasite; the nuclei are increased in size and number; the sarcoplasm may be granular and its cross striations lost. Droplets of fatty material collect in the sarcolemma near the poles of the cyst containing the parasite. Often after a period of time calcium salts are deposited, first in the thick hyaline capsule around the parasite, now dead or dying, and later in the parasite itself. Fully calcified lesions, appearing as short chalk-colored streaks in skeletal muscle, can occasionally be detected by examination with the naked eye.

Diagnosis. Histologic demonstration of the trichina larvae in the muscles of animals is sufficient to establish the nature of the parasitism, but not enough to prove that the larvae were the cause of any clinical symptoms. This is a somewhat academic problem in animals, although of more importance in man. Trichina larvae can be demonstrated by digestion of muscle and collection of the parasites in the Baermann apparatus.

A European meat inspection practice utilizes bits of fresh skeletal muscle (usually the diaphragm) which are compressed between two heavy glass plates and examined under low magnification, a practice originally advocated by Virchow and practiced since 1866. Larvae are readily recognized in these preparations, but in mild infections this method may not disclose any larvae. Routine histologic sections will also reveal the encysted larvae coiled within a hyaline membrane inside a muscle bundle (Fig. 14–13).

Cypess, R.H., Lubiniecki, A., DeSeau, V., and Siebert, J.R.: Observations on trichinosis in the Rhesus monkey. J. Med. Primatol., *6*:23–32, 1977.

Geller, E.H., and Zaiman, H.: Incidence of infection with *Trichinella spiralis* in dogs. J. Am. Vet. Med. Assoc., *147*:253–254, 1965.

Georgi, J.R.: Parasitology for Veterinarians. 2nd ed. Philadelphia, W. B. Saunders, 1974.

Hartmannova, B., and Chroust, K.: Congenital trichinellosis. Acta Univ. Agric. Fac. Vet. Brno., *37*:93–103, 1968. VB *39*:1198, 1969.

Holzworth, J., and Georgi, J.R.: Trichinosis in a cat. J. Am. Vet. Med. Assoc., *165*:186–191, 1974.

Hörning, B.: Short report concerning *Trichinella* in Switzerland (1975–1976). Wiadom. Parazytol., *24*:123–124, 1978.

Hunt, G.R.: *Trichinella spiralis* in dogs and cats. Parasitology, *53*:659, 1967.

Lin, T-M., and Olson, L.J.: Pathophysiology of reinfection with *Trichinella spiralis* in guinea pigs during the intestinal phase. J. Parasitol., *56*:529–539, 1970.

Ogbourne, C.P.: Epidemiological studies on horses infected with nematodes of the family Trichonematidae (Witenberg, 1925). Int. J. Parasitol., *5*:667–672, 1975.

Pullen, M.M., Seymour, M.R., and Zimmermann, W.J.: Trichinosis in sows slaughtered at a Kentucky abattoir. J. Am. Vet. Med. Assoc., *171*:1171–1172, 1977.

Sadun, E.H., Anderson, R.I., and Williams, J.S.: Fluorescent antibody test for the serological diagnosis of trichinosis. Exp. Parasitol., *12*:423–433, 1962. VB 2041–63.

Shaikenov, B., Tazieva, Z.Ch., and Hörning, B.: The etiology of sylvatic trichinellosis in Switzerland. Acta Tropica, *34*:327–330, 1977.

Steele, J.H., and Arambulo, P.V., III.: Trichinosis. A world problem with extensive sylvatic reservoirs. Int. J. Zoon., *2*:55–75, 1975.

Strafuss, A.C., and Zimmermann, W.J.: Hematologic changes and clinical signs of trichinosis in pigs. Am. J. Vet. Res., 28:833–838, 1967.

Sulzer, A.J.: Indirect fluorescent antibody tests for parasitic diseases. I. Preparation of a stable antigen from larvae of *Trichinella spiralis*. J. Parasitol., 51:717–721, 1965.

Pulmonary Nematodiasis (Lungworm Disease, Dictyocauliasis, Dictyocaulosis, Metastrongylidosis, Verminous Pneumonia)

Certain thread-like worms are distinguished by their parasitic habitat: the respiratory passages (trachea, bronchi, alveoli) of numerous domesticated and wild animals. These lungworms often produce disease which may lead to death, but surprisingly often they live in the lungs with little apparent effect upon the host. Usually each host has its specific lungworm, but a few related animals (deer and sheep, sheep and cattle) may share the same parasite.

Life Cycle. The life cycle of each worm in this group is essentially similar to that of the others, differing only in detail. The adults live embedded in the mucosa of the trachea or in the lumen of the trachea, bronchi, or bronchioles. Copulation occurs here, and eggs are laid in these sites. They are either coughed up and swallowed, the larvae developing in the digestive tract, or more commonly, remain in the alveoli until they have undergone embryonation. The larvae that hatch in the alveoli are coughed up, swallowed, and eliminated with the feces.

Dictyocaulus species have a direct life cycle with the larvae hatching in the lung or gastrointestinal tract. Infective third stage larvae are ingested and penetrate the intestinal mucosa and migrate to mesenteric lymph nodes where they develop to fourth stage larvae. The fourth stage larvae reach the lungs by way of lymphatics and pulmonary arteries to enter the pulmonary alveoli and ultimately bronchioles and bronchi where they reach sexual maturity.

Capillaria spp. have a life cycle similar to

Dictyocaulus, however, the infective larvae develop within the egg which does not hatch until ingested. *Filaroides spp.* also have direct life cycles, but the larvae do not require a period of development before reaching the infective stage; first stage larvae in fresh feces are infectious.

All other lungworms have indirect life cycles. *Protostrongylus* requires snails; *Muellerius, Crenosoma*, and *Aelurostrongylus* require snails or slugs; *Metastrongylus* requires earthworms.

Angiostrongylus cantonensis, which requires mollusca as intermediate hosts, passes part of its life cycle in the brain before reaching pulmonary arteries in the lung. Aberrant infection in human beings can lead to an eosinophilic meningoencephalitis which may be fatal. Man is exposed to infection through ingesting intermediate hosts which include prawns and crabs, or produce contaminated by excreta from slugs, another intermediate host. Dogs, rabbits, monkeys, calves and pigs have been shown to be experimentally susceptible in which the parasite also localizes in the brain. *A. vasorum* does not migrate through the brain. It requires slugs and snails as intermediate hosts. *Crenosoma vulpis* reaches the lungs via the portal circulation, liver and hepatic vein. Heavy infestation may result in hepatic necrosis.

Clinical Manifestations. The signs of lungworm disease may be barely recognizable or so severe that death results. Severe infection is limited almost exclusively to young animals. The presence of a few lungworms usually causes only a hacking cough. Heavy infections, however, may result in labored respiration, anorexia, diarrhea, and stunted growth. Occasionally, death may follow pulmonary consolidation caused by secondary bacterial infection of occluded bronchioles and alveoli.

Lesions. As the infective larvae break through the capillary and alveolar walls, they cause some hemorrhage into the lu-

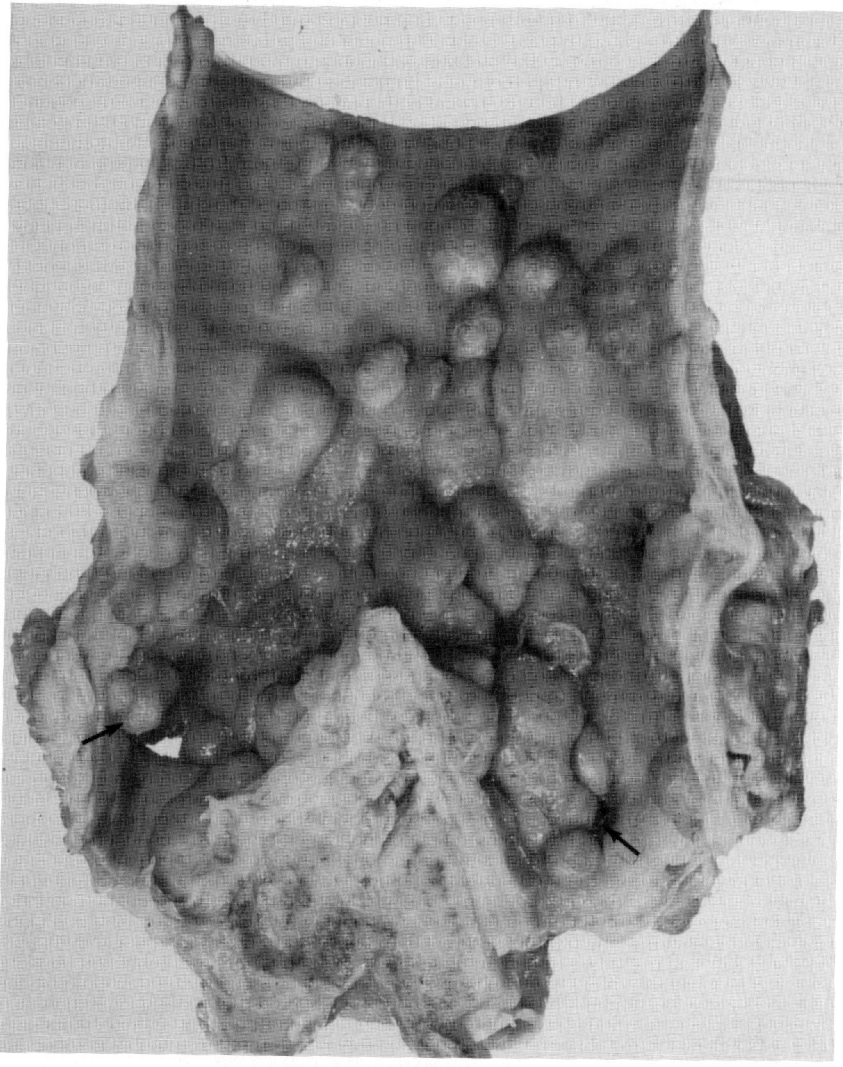

Fig. 14–14. Pulmonary nematodiasis. Nodules containing adult *Filaroides osleri* in the tracheal mucosa near the bifurcation. Note that the nodules produce partial stenosis of the lumen of the bronchi (arrows). (Courtesy of Armed Forces Institute of Pathology.) Contributor: Dr. F. D. Gentry.

mens of alveoli. This hemorrhage and the reparative process that follows may result in consolidation of alveoli, but usually this is transitory and involves only a fraction of the lung. In animals sensitized by previous exposure, the inflammatory reaction to infective larvae is more intense. Entire lobules may become filled with leukocytes, among which eosinophils predominate. As the lungworms grow to maturity, they move toward the alveolar ducts from the alveoli, establishing their adult abode in the bronchioles or bronchi. Their presence in this part of the respiratory tract produces some irritation which attracts leukocytes and an excessive amount of mucus. This exudate often occludes the bronchioles and leads to atelectasis or consolidation of the related alveoli. Most lungworm adults, feeding head down

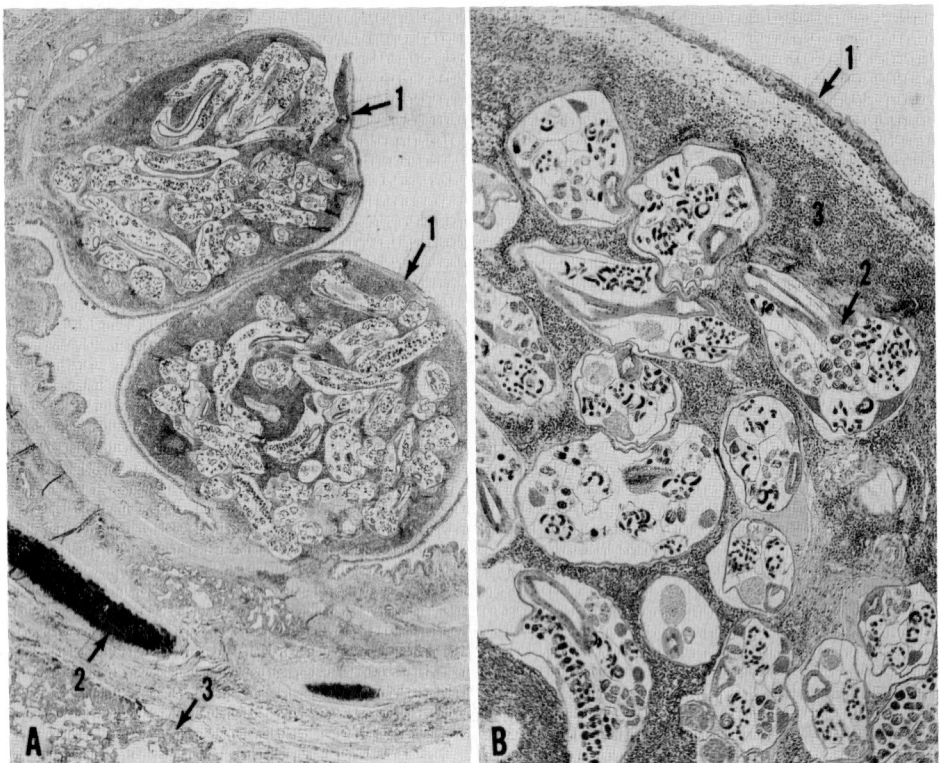

Fig. 14–15. Pulmonary nematodiasis. *A*, Two nodules filled with adult *Filaroides osleri* in the bronchial mucosa of a dog (× 13). The epithelium *(1)* is elevated. Bronchial cartilage *(2)* and lung parenchyma *(3)*. *B*, Enlarged view (× 50) of one of the nodules in *A*. Bronchial epithelium *(1)*, adult worms containing larvae *(2)*, lymphocytic inflammatory reaction *(3)*. (Courtesy of Armed Forces Institute of Pathology.) Contributor: Dr. F. D. Gentry.

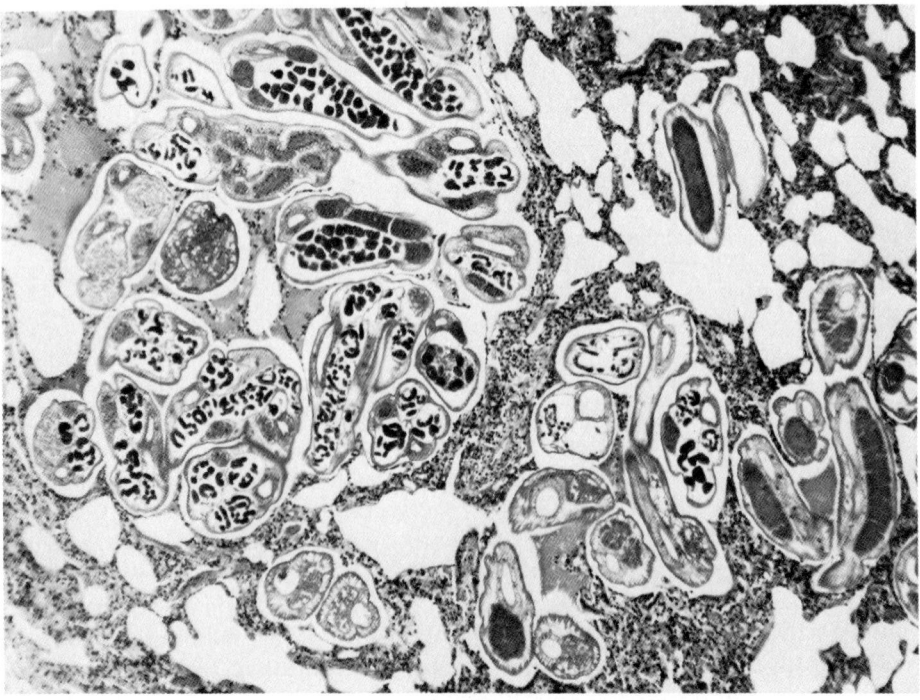

Fig. 14–16. Pulmonary nematodiasis. *Filaroides cebus* within pulmonary alveoli of a squirrel monkey.

upon mucus and cellular detritus in the bronchial tree, deposit ova which lodge in the alveoli, where they embryonate to become larvae. These embryonating ova act as foreign bodies, provoking inflammation that results in consolidation of viable lung. Secondary bacterial infection may intervene at any time, with purulent pneumonia the usual sequel. Emphysema is common in unconsolidated parts of the lungs.

The lesions produced by certain other lungworms differ in important respects from these described. The adults of the dog lungworm, *Filaroides osleri*, for example, are found in granulomatous nodules

in the mucosa of the trachea or bronchi, occasionally in sufficient numbers to occlude the respiratory passage and produce death from asphyxia, or rarely rupture of a nodule and subsequent pneumothorax. The life cycle and mode of infection of this parasite are unknown. *F. milksi* and *F. hirthi* incite similar granulomatous nodules in the lung, which can be seen grossly beneath the pleura. *Muellerius* in sheep reside in alveoli, rather than the bronchial tree, and incite a granulomatous response. The cat lungworm, *Aelurostrongylus abstrusus*, has been the subject of some dispute. The habitat of the adults is in small branches of

Table 14–6. Common Lungworms

Hosts	Parasite	Site of Adult Parasite
Cattle, deer, mouse, reindeer, pig	*Dictyocaulus viviparus* (cattle lungworm)	Trachea, bronchi
Cat	*Aelurostrongylus abstrusus* (cat lungworm)	Right ventricle, pulmonary artery
Deer, sheep, goat, cattle, other ruminants	*Dictyocaulus filaria* (thread lungworm, sheep lungworm),	Bronchioles
	Protostrongylus rufescens,	Bronchioles
	Protostrongylus brevispiculum	Bronchioles
Dog	*Filaroides osleri*	Mucosa of trachea and bronchi
Dog	*F. milksi*	Bronchi, bronchioles, alveoli
Dog	*F. hirthi*	Bronchi, bronchioles, alveoli
Mink	*F. martis*	Peribronchial connective tissue
Monkeys	*F. cebus*	Bronchioles, alveoli
Fox, dog, wolf, cat	*Capillaria aerophila* (fox lungworm)	Trachea, bronchi, bronchioles
Horse, donkey, tapir	*Dictyocaulus arnfieldi* (horse lungworm)	Bronchi and bronchioles
Sheep, goats	*Muellerius capillaris (minutissimus)* (hair lungworm),	Alveoli
	Cystocaulus ocreatus	Alveoli
Swine	*Metastrongylus apri (elongatus),*	Trachea, bronchi, bronchioles
	M. pudendotectus,	Trachea, bronchi, bronchioles
	M. salmi	Trachea, bronchi, bronchioles
Rabbits (wild)	*Protostrongylus boughtoni* (rabbit lungworm)	Bronchi, bronchioles
Foxes, dogs, cats	*Crenosoma vulpis*	Bronchi, trachea
Skunks	*Crenosoma canadensis*	Bronchi, bronchioles
Cat, leopard, tiger	*Bronchostrongylus subcrenatus*	
Dog, fox	*Angiostrongylus vasorum*	Pulmonary artery
Rat, fox	*Angiostrongylus cantonensis*	Pulmonary artery
Mink	*Perostrongylus pridhami*	Bronchioles, alveolar ducts

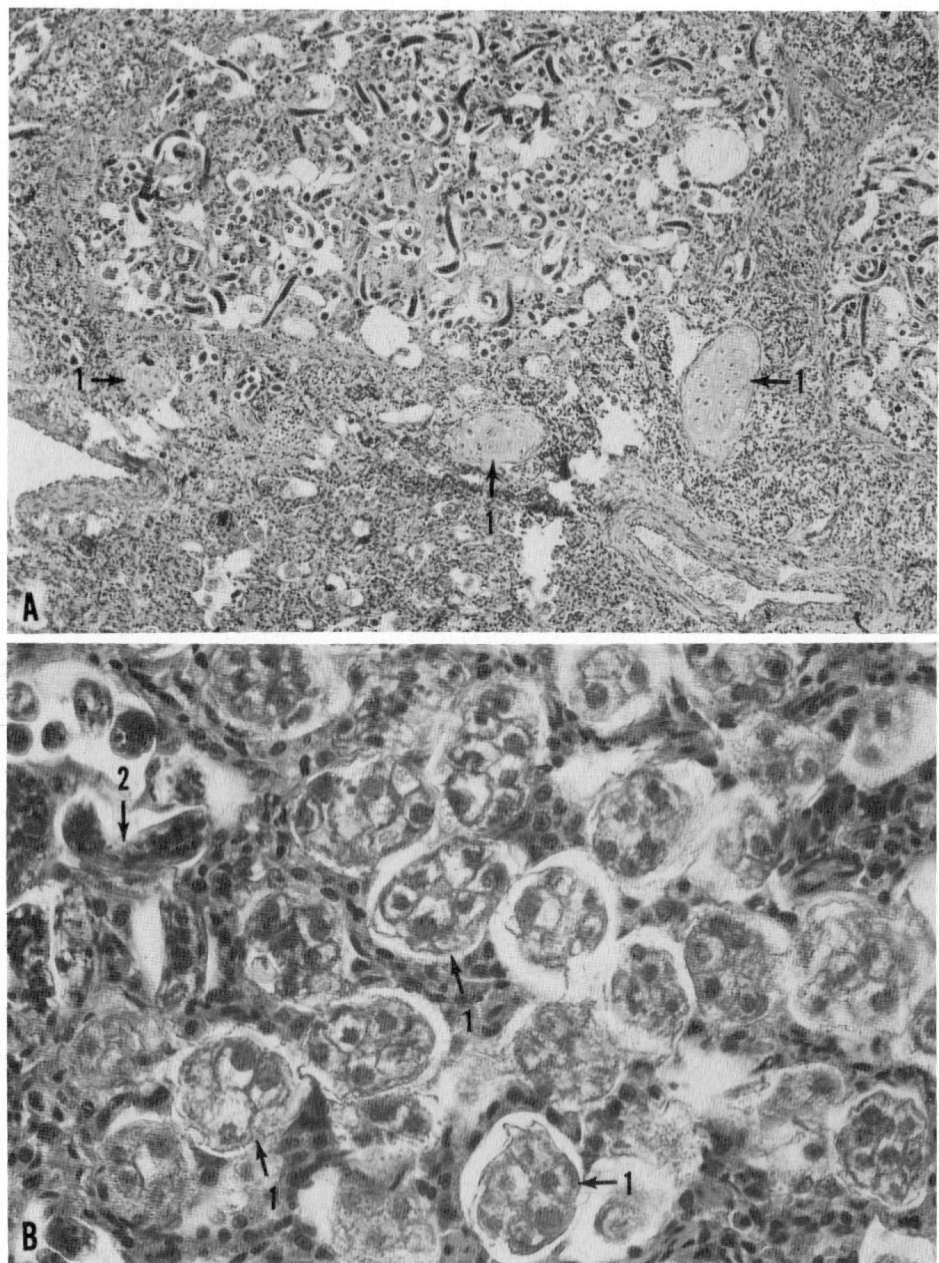

Fig. 14–17. Pulmonary nematodiasis. *Aelurostrongylus abstrusus* in the lung of a cat. *A,* Larvae filling a small bronchus outlined by its cartilage *(1)* (× 83). *B,* Another area in the same lung with embryonating ova *(1)* in alveoli and larvae in alveolar duct *(2)* (× 385). (Courtesy of Armed Forces Institute of Pathology.) Contributor: Dr. W. S. Bailey.

the pulmonary arteries or the right ventricle, where they produce ova that break through capillary walls into alveoli. Larvae developing from the ova move into alveolar ducts and bronchioles, are coughed up and swallowed, to pass out with the feces. These ova and larvae may cause interstitial pneumonia with considerable loss of air space in sharply circumscribed parts of the lung, but apparently only very heavy parasitism results in death of the host. The larvae that reach the outside must, according to present opinion, be ingested by certain molluscs (snails and slugs) in order to continue their life cycle. A dissenting opinion indicates that mice may act as the first intermediate host. Transport hosts, such as frogs, toads, lizards, snakes, and birds, may ingest the molluscs containing the third-stage infective larvae. The final host, the cat, becomes infected by eating a transport host or the true intermediate host.

Evidence has accumulated to associate infection by *Aelurostrongylus abstrusus* and *Toxocara cati* with characteristic lesions in the wall of branches of the pulmonary artery (Fig. 21–17) of cats. The lesion consists of hyperplasia of the media and fibrosis of the intima, which nearly obliterates the lumen. The effect of this change is to produce a sharply-demarcated stenosis of the artery, which decreases the blood supply to varying-sized segments of the lung. The exact mechanism that causes this lesion is not understood, but the effect is clearly demonstrable by experimental infection with either of these parasites (Hamilton, 1966; Jonas et al., 1970).

Diagnosis. The diagnosis of lungworm disease can be suspected from the signs and confirmed by identifying lungworm

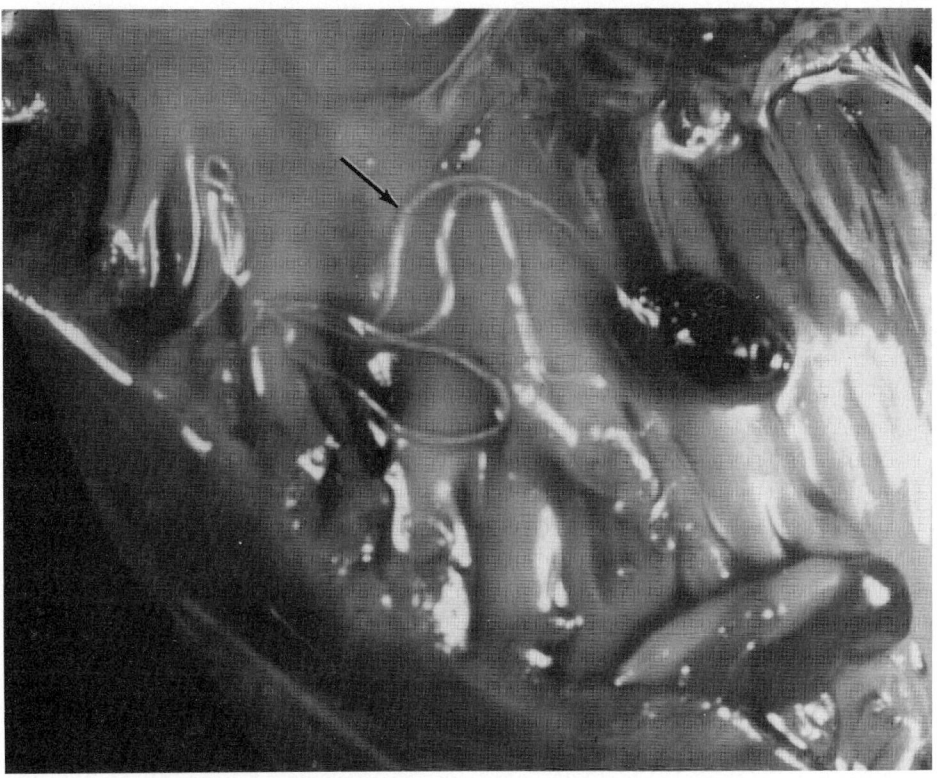

Fig. 14–18. *Aelurostrongylus abstrusus* (adults) in right ventricle of a four-year-old male tabby and white cat. (Courtesy of Angell Memorial Animal Hospital.)

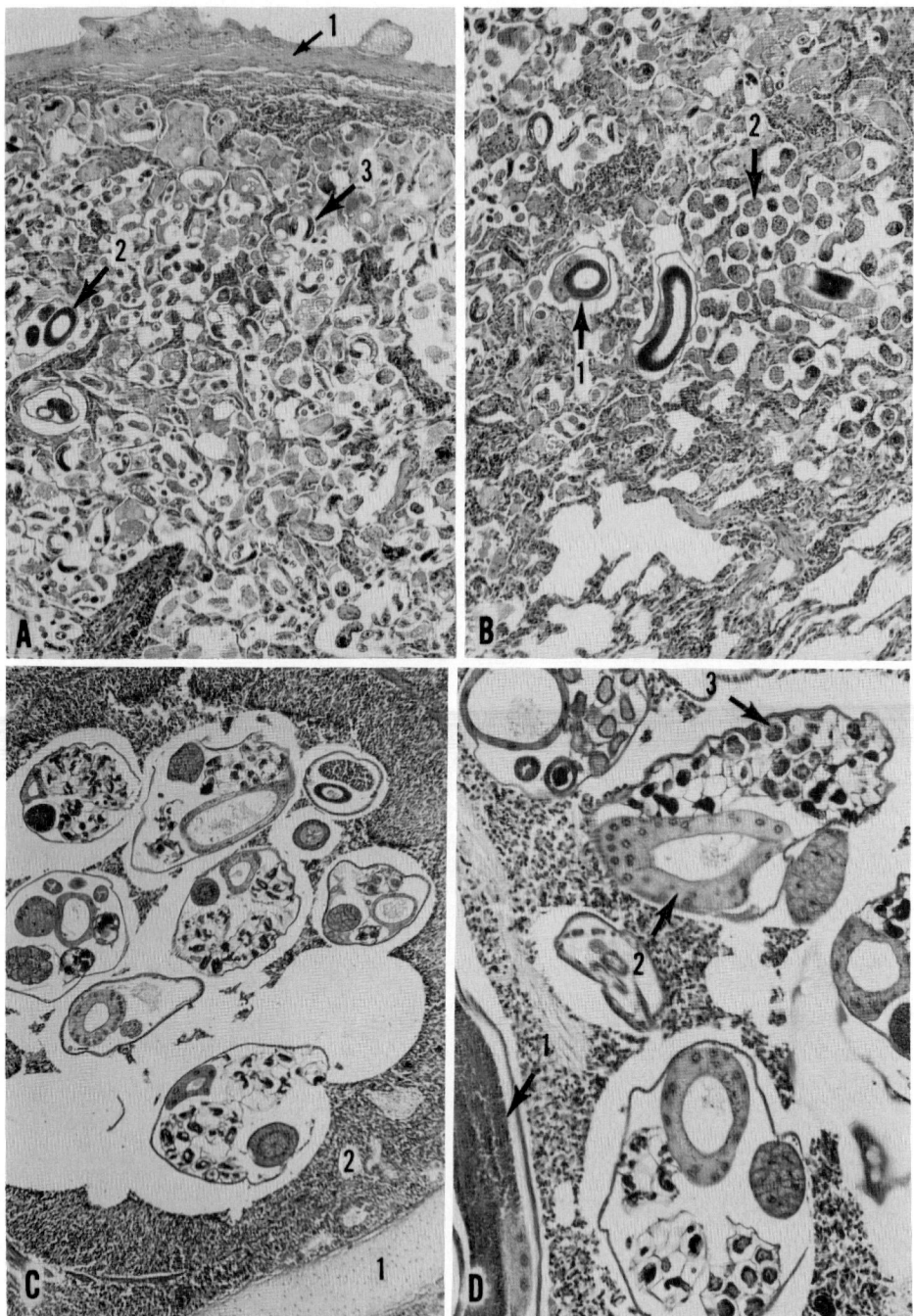

Fig. 14–19.   Pulmonary nematodiasis. *A, Muellerius minutissimus* in the lung (× 45) of a bighorn sheep
(*Ovis canadensis*). Note the pleura *(1)*, young adult worms *(2)* and larvae *(3)*. *B,* Higher magnification of *A*
(× 70), showing young adult larvae *(1)* and embryonating ova *(2)*. Most alveoli are consolidated.
Contributor: Dr. C. L. Davis. *C, Metastrongylus apri* in a bronchus of a pig (× 62). Bronchial cartilage *(1)*
and inflammatory exudate in the mucosa *(2)*. *D,* Slightly higher magnification (× 75) of *C,* showing adult
worms in longitudinal *(1)* and cross section. The intestinal tube *(2)* and ovary *(3)* can be recognized.
Contributor: Dr. R. J. Byrne. (*A, D,* Courtesy of Armed Forces Institute of Pathology.)

larvae in the feces of the living animal. Demonstration of adult lungworms in the bronchi or bronchioles and ova and larvae in the lung parenchyma at necropsy is often necessary to establish the nature of a herd infection. Careful examination with the naked eye and use of the hand lens are advisable, especially when searching for the smaller lungworms, and histopathologic examination is recommended.

Alicata, J.E.: Present status of *Angiostrongylus cantonensis* infection in man and animals in the tropics. J. Trop. Med. Hyg., 72:53–63, 1969.

Beresford-Jones, W.P.: Observations on *Muellerius capillaris* (Muller, 1889), Cameron 1927. II. Experimental infection of mice, guinea-pigs, and rabbits with third stage larvae. Res. Vet. Sci., 7:287–291, 1966.

Burrows, C.F., O'Brien, J.A., and Biery, D.N.: Pneumothorax due to *Filaroides osleri* infestation in the dog. J. Small Anim. Pract., 13:613–618, 1972.

Cameron, T.W.M.: Observations on the life history of *Aelurostrongylus abstrusus* (Railliet) the lungworm of the cat. J. Helminthol., 5:55–66, 1927.

Dodd, K.: *Angiostrongylus vasorum* (Baillet, 1866) infestation in a Greyhound kennel. Vet. Rec., 92:195–197, 1973.

Dorrington, J.E.: Preliminary report on the transmission of *Filaroides osleri* (Cobbold, 1879) in dogs. J. S. Afr. Vet. Med. Assoc., 36:389, 1965, VB 36:3563, 1966.

———: *Filaroides osleri*: (Cobbold, 1879) infestation in the dog. J. S. Afr. Vet. Med. Assoc., 38:91, 1967. VB 38:1942, 1968.

———: Studies on *Filaroides osleri* infestation in dogs. Onderstepoort. J. Vet. Res., 35:225–285, 1968. VB 39:1684, 1969.

Dubey, J.P., Beverley, J.K.A., and Crane, W.A.J.: Lung changes and *Aelurostrongylus abstrusus* infestation in English cats. Vet. Rec., 83:191–194, 1968.

Georgi, J.R., Georgi, M.E., Fahnestock, G.R., and Theodorides, V.J.: Transmission and control of *Filaroides hirthi* lungworm infection in dogs. Am. J. Vet. Res., 40:829–831, 1979.

Hamilton, J.M.: The number of *Aelurostrongylus abstrusus* larvae required to produce pulmonary disease in the cat. J. Comp. Pathol., 77:343–346, 1967.

———: Parenteral infection of the cat by larvae of *Aelurostrongylus abstrusus*. J. Helminthol., 43:31–34, 1969.

———: Experimental lungworm disease of the cat. Association of the condition with lesions of the pulmonary arteries. J. Comp. Pathol., 76:147–157, 1966.

Hamilton, J.M., and McCaw, A.W.: I. The role of the mouse in the life cycle of *Aelurostrongylus abstrusus*. II. An investigation into the longevity of first stage larvae of *Aelurostrongylus abstrusus*. J. Helminthol., 41:309–312 , 313–320, 1967.

Heyneman, D., and Lim, B-L.: *Angiostrongylus cantonensis*: proof of direct transmission with its epidemiological implications. Science, 158:1057–1058, 1967.

Hirth, R.S.: *Filaroides hirthi* infection in Beagle dogs used for research. Bull. SPEP, 5:11–17, 1977,

Hirth, R.S., and Hottendorf, G.H.: Lesions produced by a new lungworm in Beagle dogs. Vet. Pathol., 10:385–407, 1973.

Hobmaier, M.: Newer aspects of the lungworm (*Crenosoma*) in foxes. Am. J. Vet. Res., 2:352–354, 1941.

Jarrett, W.F.H., McIntyre, W.I.M., and Urquhart, G.M.: The pathology of experimental bovine parasitic bronchitis. J. Pathol. Bact., 73:183–193, 1957.

Jindrak, K.: The pathology of radicular involvement in angiostrongylosis as observed in experimentally infected calves and pigs. Virchows. Arch. Path. Anat., 345:228–237, 1968.

Jindrak, K., and Alicata, J.E.: Comparative pathology in experimental infection of pigs and calves with larvae of *Angiostrongylus cantonensis*. J. Comp. Pathol., 78:371–382, 1968.

———:Experimentally induced *Angiostrongylus cantonensis* infection in dogs. Am. J. Vet. Res., 31:449–456, 1970.

John, D.T., and Martinez, A.J.: Eosinophilic meningoencephalitis in mice infected with *Angiostrongylus cantonensis*. Am. J. Pathol., 80:345–348, 1975.

Jonas, A.M., Swerczek, T.W., and Downing, S.E.: Vaso-occlusive pulmonary hypertension. A feline model system. Lab. Invest., 22:502, 1970.

Jubb, K.V.: The lesions caused by *Filaroides milksi* in a dog. Cornell Vet., 50:319–325, 1960.

Michel, J.F., and MacKenzie, A.: Duration of the acquired resistance of calves to infection with *Dictyocaulus viviparus*. Res. Vet. Sci., 6:344–395, 1965.

Mills, J.H.L., and Nielsen, S.W.: Canine *Filaroides osleri* and *Filaroides milksi* infection. J. Am. Vet. Med. Assoc., 149:56–63, 1966.

Poynter, D., and Selway, S.: Diseases caused by lungworms. Vet. Bull., 36:539–554, 1966.

Rose, J.H.: Lungworms of the domestic pig and sheep. Adv. Parasitol., 11:559–599, 1973.

Rosen, L., Ash, L.R., and Wallace, G.D.: Life history of the canine lungworm *Angiostrongylus vasorum* (Baillet). Am. J. Vet. Res., 31:131–143, 1970.

Shoho, C.: Observations on rats and rabbits infected with *Angiostrongylus cantonensis* (Chen). Br. Vet. J., 122:251–258, 1966.

Simpson, C.F., et al.: Pathological changes associated with *Dictyocaulus viviparus* (Block) infection in calves. Am. J. Res., 18:747–755, 1957.

Stockdale, P.H.G.: Pulmonary lesions in mink with a mixed infection of *Filaroides martis* and *Perostrongylus pridhami*. Can. J. Zool., 48:757–759, 1970.

———: The pathogenesis of the lesions elicited by *Aelurostrongylus abstrusus* during its prepatent period. Pathol. Vet., 7:102–115, 1970.

Stockdale, P.H.G., and Hulland, T.J.: The patho-
genesis, route of migration, and development of
Crenosoma vulpis in the dog. Pathol. Vet., 7:28–
42, 1970.
Subramaniam, T., D'Souza, B.A., and Victor, D.A.:
Broncho-pneumonia in baby pigs due to *Metastrongylus apri*. Indian Vet. J., 44:121–127, 1967.
Taffs, L.F.: Lungworm infection in swine. Vet. Rec.,
80:554, 1967.
Tangchai, P., Nye, S.W., and Beaver, P.C.:
Eosinophilic meningoencephalitis caused by
angiostrongyliasis in Thailand. Am. J. Trop.
Med. Hyg., 16:454–461, 1967.
Wilson, G.I.: Investigations on the pathogenicity and
immunology of *Dictyocaulus filaria* in sheep and
goats. Diss. Abstr., 26:5612–5613, 1966. VB
37:619, 1967.

RENAL DIOCTOPHYMOSIS

The giant kidney worm *Dioctophyma renale (Eustrongylus gigas, Ascaris renalis)* is
an uncommon parasite of the dog and
mink, and rarely of other animals and man.
The adult worms are found in the renal
pelvis, occasionally in the intestinal lumen
and the peritoneal cavity. The right kidney
is more frequently affected than the left.
The female is a surprisingly large, cylindrical, reddish nematode, 20 to 100 cm in
length. The male is smaller, 14 to 40 cm
long. The life cycle of *D. renale* has not
been resolved. Although unconfirmed,
Woodhead (1950) has reported that gravid
females deposit ova in the renal pelvis,
which pass out with the urine and hatch
when swallowed by an annelid worm,
Cambarinocola chirocephala. This worm is
parasitic to crayfish, and the first stage
larvae of *D. renale* encyst in the crayfish.
This intermediate host is eaten by a bull-
head fish, *Ameirus melas*. The parasitic larvae pass through the third into the fourth
stage and encyst in the liver and mesentery. Mink, and presumably dogs, become
infected with *D. renale* by eating the fish.
Apparently, other species of fish may also
carry the infective larvae. The clinical
diagnosis is confirmed by the presence of
the brownish yellow ova, with their thick,
pitted shells and bipolar caps, in the urine.

The adult worms with their habitat in the
renal pelvis produce hydronephrosis,

which eventually destroys all the functional kidney. The contralateral kidney
undergoes compensatory hypertrophy in
the usual case, but bilateral renal involvement is obviously fatal.

Cooperrider, D.E., Robinson, V.B., and Staton, L.B.:
Dioctophyma renale in a dog. J. Am. Vet. Med.
Assoc., 124:381–383, 1954.
de Alencar, R.A., Jr.: Renal dioctophymosis in a dog.
Biologico., 32:34–36, 1966. VB 36:4403, 1966.
Eubanks, J.W., and Pick, J.R.: *Dioctophyma renale* infection in a dog. J. Am. Vet. Med. Assoc.,
143:164–169, 1963.
Hallberg, C.W.: *Dioctophyma renale* (Goetze, 1782). A
study of the migration routes to the kidneys of
mammals and resultant pathology. Am. Mi-
croscop. Soc., 72:351–363, 1953.
McLeod, J.A.: *Dioctophyma renale* infections in Man-
itoba. Can. J. Zool., 45:505–508, 1967.
McNeil, C.W.: Pathological changes in the kidney of
mink due to infection with *Dioctophyma renale*
(Goetze, 1782), the giant kidney worm of mammals. Am. Microscop. Soc., 67:257–261, 1948.
Osborne, C.A., et al.: *Dioctophyma renale* in the dog. J.
Am. Vet. Med. Assoc., 155:605–620, 1969.
Woodhead, A.E.: Life history cycle of the giant kidney
worm, *Dioctophyma renale* (Nematoda), of man
and many other mammals. Am. Microscop. Soc.,
69:21–46, 1950.

Habronemiasis

The stomach worms of horses are of three
species: *Habronema muscae, H. majus (H.
microstoma),* and *Draschia megastoma (Habronema megastoma).* The adult nematodes
are small and slender and are found in
nodules in the submucosa of the stomach.
Severe infections may interfere with gastric function, but a few parasites rarely
have any significant clinical effect. The life
cycle of each of these three parasites is similar in that eggs and larvae passed in the
feces are ingested by larvae (maggots) of
the housefly (*Musca domestica*), or in the
case of *H. majus,* by the larvae of the stable
fly. The larvae undergo further development in the pupae of the fly and migrate as
infective larvae into the proboscis of the
adult flies. The infective larvae are believed
to be deposited on the lips of horses and
eventually swallowed, to develop into
adults in the stomach. The occurrence of
the helminth larvae in lesions of the skin
suggests that they may gain access to the

host through the epidermis and migrate to the stomach.

According to de Jesus (1963), *H. muscae* is associated with diffuse gastritis; *H. microstoma,* with gastric ulcers, and *H. megastoma,* with granulomatous gastritis.

Cutaneous habronemiasis (summer sores), a persistent disease of the skin of equines, results from the activity of larvae of stomach worms, especially *Draschia megastoma.* The larvae are deposited on the skin by the housefly, which is attracted to some pre-existing ulceration or wound in the skin. Lesions are particularly common in the skin of the pectoral region, between the forelegs. The larvae penetrate deeply into the dermis and elicit granulomatous tissue in which eosinophils are conspicuous. The skin loses its hair and becomes encrusted by serous exudate, which oozes from the surface. It is believed by some that these particular larvae, which can be expressed by deep scrapings with pressure from the cutaneous lesions, do not complete the life cycle of the parasite, therefore, they do not reach the stomach. This lesion is not uncommon in horses during the summer months, but its true nature is often not suspected until larvae expressed from the lesion are identified by microscopic examination.

de Jesus, Z.: Observations on habronemiasis in horses. Philipp. J. Vet. Med., *2:*133–152, 1963. VB 35:3901, 1965.

Dikmans, G.: Skin lesions of domestic animals in the United States due to nematode infestation. Cornell Vet., *38:*3–23, 1948.

Lewis, J.C., and Seddon, H.R.: Habronemic conjunctivitis. J. Comp. Pathol. Ther., *31:*87–94, 1918.

Strongyloidosis

Nematodes of the family Strongyloididae occur both as parasites of the intestinal tract of man and animals and as free-living nonparasitic worms. Common parasitic species and their hosts are: *Strongyloides westeri* (equines), *S. stercoralis* (man), *S. ransomi* (swine), *S. papillosus* (cattle), *S. ratti* (rats), *S. simiae; S. fülleborni, S. cebus* (monkeys), *S. tumefaciens* (cats), and *S. canis* (dogs).

Life Cycle. The parasitic female is a filariform nematode about 2.0 mm long, which burrows into the lamina propria of the intestinal mucosa, where it deposits embryonated ova. The presence of these worms in the intestinal mucosa may result in diarrhea, which in most animals is of short duration, with the infection abating and providing immunity to reinfection. In some species, however, severe persistent enteric symptoms occur, occasionally terminating in death. The embryonated ova passed in the feces are not always recognized because hatching occurs promptly, and the larvae often escape detection by the methods of examination commonly employed. After leaving the host, free-living rhabditiform larvae may develop into infective larvae or pass through one or more free-living generations. Larvae gain access to a new host by penetrating the skin and entering the venous circulation, in which they are carried to the lungs. The larvae break into the alveoli and gain the bronchi, then are coughed up and swallowed to reach the intestine, where they develop into adults. Transmammary and prenatal infection has been demonstrated for some species of *Strongyloides* in the absence of intestinal parasitism, a situation similar to that of some species of ascarids. These routes are believed to be of major importance in swine infected with *S. ransomi.* The adult worm may occasionally be encountered in microscopic sections of the intestinal mucosa, taken routinely at necropsy. The adult worms burrow into the intestinal mucosa, localizing in the lamina propria, but rarely penetrating below the muscularis mucosae.

Lesions. The presence of these worms causes a local tissue reaction with infiltration of neutrophils, lymphocytes, eosinophils, and epithelioid cells (granulomas). Heavy parasitism may lead to extensive pulmonary and intestinal hemorrhage. Peritonitis may be the result of secondary

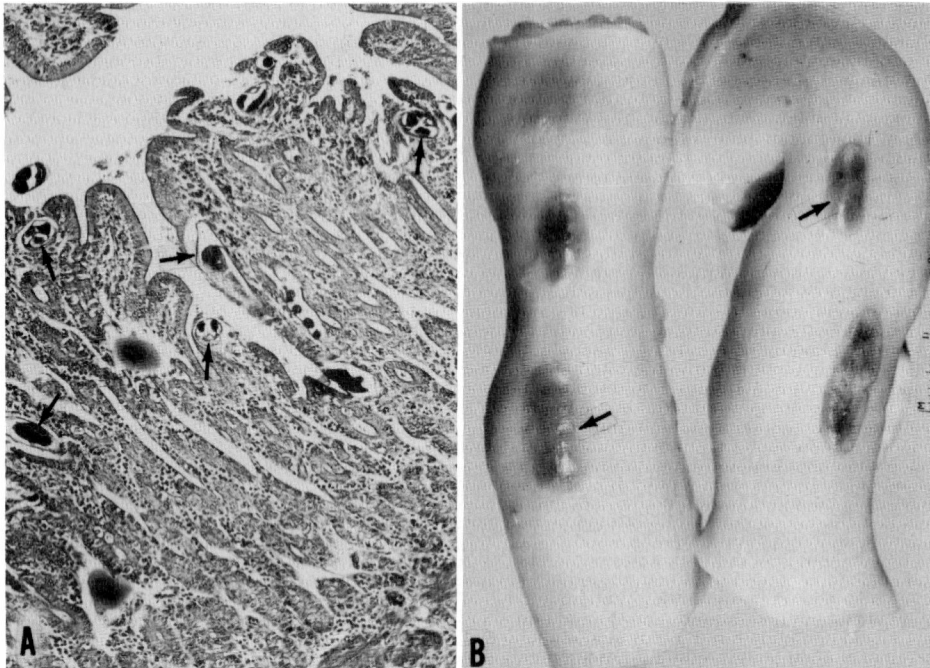

Fig. 14–20. *A,* Strongyloidosis *(Strongyloides westeri),* small intestine of a colt (× 75). Numerous small immature worms (arrows) burrowing in mucosa. Contributor: Dr. L. Z. Saunders. *B,* Strongyloidosis. Subserous lesions, "haemomelasma ilei," caused by migrating strongyle larvae (arrows) in ileum of horse. (Courtesy of Armed Forces Institute of Pathology.) Contributor: Lt. Col. T. C. Jones.

infection following penetration of the intestinal wall. Hyperinfection as the result of completion of the reproductive cycle within one host has been reported. In this situation, the larvae hatch in the lower intestine, then are believed either to penetrate the intestinal wall or to enter the vascular system directly, then undergo molts within the one host, producing a superabundance of adult worms in the intestine. In this manner, severe infection can occur even though the original number of infecting larvae is not large. It is generally believed that severe and fatal strongyloidosis is likely to occur only in man or animals debilitated from faulty nutrition or other factors.

Diagnosis. Diagnosis of strongyloidosis presents some problems because the usual flotation methods are not satisfactory to demonstrate the larvae, which embryonate and escape from the ova while still in the hosts' intestinal tract. The Baermann apparatus may be used to concentrate the larvae and they can be found in scrapings of the intestinal wall, but less readily in histologic sections.

Drudge, J.H., and Lyons, E.T.: Equine parasites, problems and control. Pract. Vet., *49:*5–7, 9, 1978.

Greer, G.J., Bello, T.R., and Amborski, G.F.: Experimental infection of *Strongyloides westeri* in parasite-free ponies. J. Parasitol., *60:*466–472, 1974.

Lyons, E.T., Drudge, J.H., and Tolliver, S.C.: On the life cycle of *Strongyloides westeri* in the equine. J. Parasitol., *59:*780–787, 1973.

Moncol, D.J.: Supplement to the life history of *Strongyloides ransomi* Schwartz and Alicata, 1930 (Nematoda: Strongyloididae) of pigs. Proc. Helminthol. Soc. Wash., *42:*86–92, 1975.

Moncol, D.J., and Batte, E.G.: Transcolostral infection of newborn pigs with *Strongyloides ransomi.* Vet. Med. Small Anim. Clin., *61:*583–586, 1966.

Pfeiffer, H., and Supperer, R.: Studies on the genus Strongyloides. VII. Prenatal infection in pigs.

Wien. Tieraerztl. Mschr., 53:90–94, 1966. VB 36:3144, 1966.

Stewart, T.B., Stone, W.M., and Marti, O.G.: Strongyloides ransomi: Prenatal and transmammary infection of pigs of sequential litters from dams experimentally exposed as weanlings. Am. J. Vet. Res., 37:541–544, 1976.

Stone, W.M., and Simpson, C.F.: Larval distribution and histopathology of experimental Strongyloides ransomi infection in young swine. Can. J. Comp. Med., 31:197–202, 1967. VB 38:1483, 1968.

Supperer, R.: Studies on the genus Strongyloides. VI. Prenatal infestation in pigs. Berl. Muench. Tierarztl. Wochenschr., 78:108–110, 1965. VB 35:4294, 1965.

Turner, J.H., and Shalkop, W.T.: Larval migration and accompanying pathological changes in experimental ovine strongyloidiasis. J. Parasitol., 44:28–38, 1958.

Pinworms

Several members of the family Oxyuridae are parasitic in animals and human beings. These include *Enterobius vermicularis* (man), *E. anthropopitheci* (apes and monkeys), *Oxyuris equi* (equines), *Skrjabinema ovis* (sheep and goats), *Passalurus ambigus* (rabbits), *Syphacia obvelata* (rodents), and *Aspicularis tetraptera* (mice).

Life Cycle. The life cycle is direct. Fertilized adult females lay singly operculated eggs in clusters in the perianal region. The eggs reach the infectious stage within a few hours, and are either licked off by a new host or fall off and are subsequently ingested. The larvae are released in the intestine and mature to adults which reside in the cecum or colon. Fertilized females migrate to the lower rectum and anus to deposit their eggs.

Lesions. Pinworms are relatively innocuous parasites and are rarely associated with serious disease. The activities of the female worm result in pruritus, and heavy infestation is thought to cause ulcerative colitis. The adult worms do not attach themselves to the mucosa, but in ulcerative colitis they and larvae may migrate into the mucosa. Whether the association with ulcerative colitis and tissue invasion is coincidental or caused by other factors is not established.

Diagnosis. Diagnosis of pinworm infestation is usually made by recognizing adult worms at the anus or eggs recovered from the perianal area. Cellophane or similar clear, sticky tape is useful to recover the eggs.

Drudge, J.H., and Lyons, E.T.: Equine parasites, problems and control. Pract. Vet., 49:5–7, 9, 1978.

Georgi, J.R.: Parasitology for Veterinarians. 2nd ed. Philadelphia, W. B. Saunders, 1974.

Kuntz, R.E., and Myers, B.J.: Parasites of South American primates. Int. Zoo Yearbook, 12:61–68, 1972.

Lapage, G.: Veterinary Parasitology. 2nd ed. Springfield, Charles C Thomas, 1968.

Lichtenfels, J.R.: Helminths of domestic equids. Proc. Helminthol. Soc. Wash., 42:1–92, 1975.

Moore, G., and Myers, B.J.: Parasites of non-human primates. In Annual Proceedings Am. Assoc. Zoo Vet., Washington, D.C., 1974, pp. 79–86.

Schmidt, R.E., and Prine, J.R.: Severe enterobiasis in a chimpanzee. Pathol. Vet., 7:56–59, 1970.

Slocombe, J.O.D., and McCraw, B.M.: Gastrointestinal nematodes in horses in Ontario. Can. Vet. J., 14:101–105, 1973.

Sloss, M.W., and Kemp, R.L.: Veterinary Clinical Parasitology. 5th ed. Ames, Iowa State Univ. Press, 1978.

Capillariasis

A parasite of mice, rats, dogs, beavers, muskrats, hares, peccaries, and monkeys, *Capillaria hepatica (Hepaticola hepaticola),* may sometimes accidentally infect man. The adult worm is a slender nematode related to whipworms (*Trichuris sp.*) but without the broader posterior extremity. The adults live in the liver parenchyma, where ova and excreta accumulate, causing tissue destruction leading to fibrosis. The life cycle is continued only if the infected liver is eaten by a new host, in which the ova are released but do not hatch. Ova passed with the feces of this second host embryonate on the ground to reach the infectious stage. Ova ingested by a third host contain larvae that penetrate the intestinal wall, eventually reaching the liver. The disease is not uncommon in wild rodents, but is rarely encountered in laboratory animals. The carnivorous habits of its hosts obviously are necessary to the perpetuation of *Capillaria hepatica.*

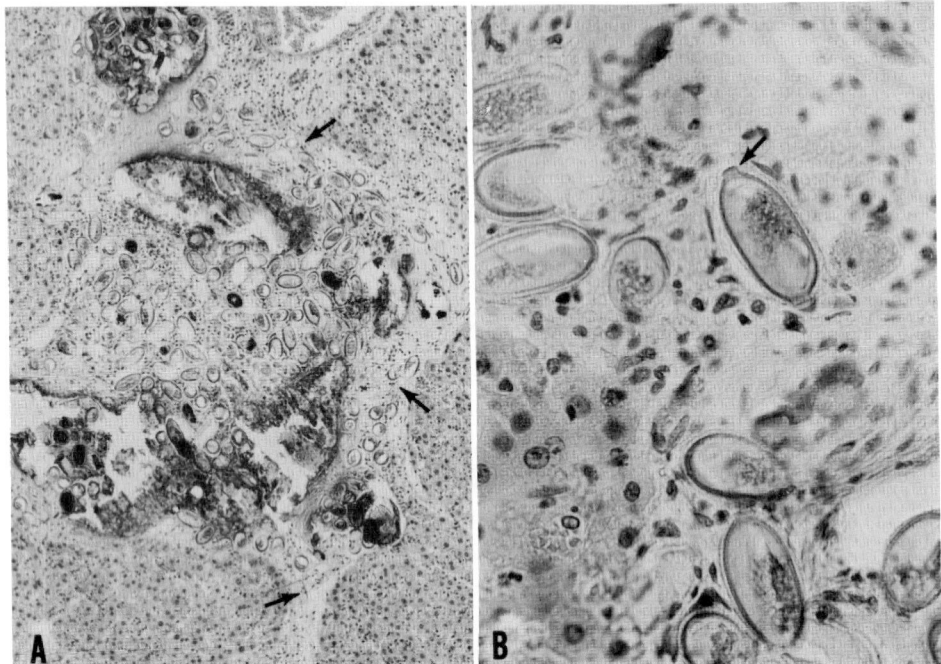

Fig. 14–21. *Capillaria hepatica* infection in the liver of a rat. *A*, Accumulation of ova in portal areas (arrows) with resultant fibrosis (× 76). *B*, Higher magnification (× 440), note ova with polar eminence (arrow) at each end, characteristic of the genus.

Capillaria feliscati and C. plica. These slender worms are about 30 to 60 mm long, and are found in the urinary bladder and occasionally the renal pelvis. *C. feliscati* has been reported from cats and *C. plica* from dogs, cats, and foxes. It is possible that these helminths are identical. The worms produce little effect on the urinary tract. Their presence may be detected by microscopic demonstration of ova in the urine.

Capillaria aerophila is a related species that infects the lung. In rats, a parasite within this same family, *Trichosomoides crassicauda,* inhabits the urinary bladder with no apparent ill effects.

Schmidt, R.E., and Prine, J.R.: Severe enterobiasis in a Chimpanzee. Pathol. Vet., 7:56–59, 1970.
Waddell, A.H.: *Capillaria feliscati* in the bladder of cats in Australia. Aust. Vet. J., 43:297, 1967.
———: Further observations on *Capillaria feliscati* infections in the cat. Aust. Vet. J., 44:33–34, 1968.

Weisbroth, S.H.: Diagnosis of *Trichosomoides crassicauda* in laboratory rats. BLU:LETTER (Blue Spruce Farms, Inc., Altamont, NY), 2:2–3, 1970.
Weisbroth, S.H., and Scher, S.: *Trichosomoides crassicauda* infection of a commercial rat breeding colony. I. Observations on the life cycle and propagation. Lab. Anim. Sci., 21:54–61, 1971.

Trichuriasis

The so-called **whipworms** include members of the Trichuridae, which were named to indicate that one part of their body is thick, the rest thin—resembling the shape of a whip. Interestingly, the name *Trichuris* means "hair-tail" and resulted from failure to observe that the posterior portion of the worm is thickest. "Hair-head" (*Trichocephalus*) is presumably more correct, but *Trichuris* has priority. Several species are of interest: *Trichuris ovis* is found in the cecum of cattle, sheep, goats, and many wild ruminants; *T. suis* inhabits the cecum of the

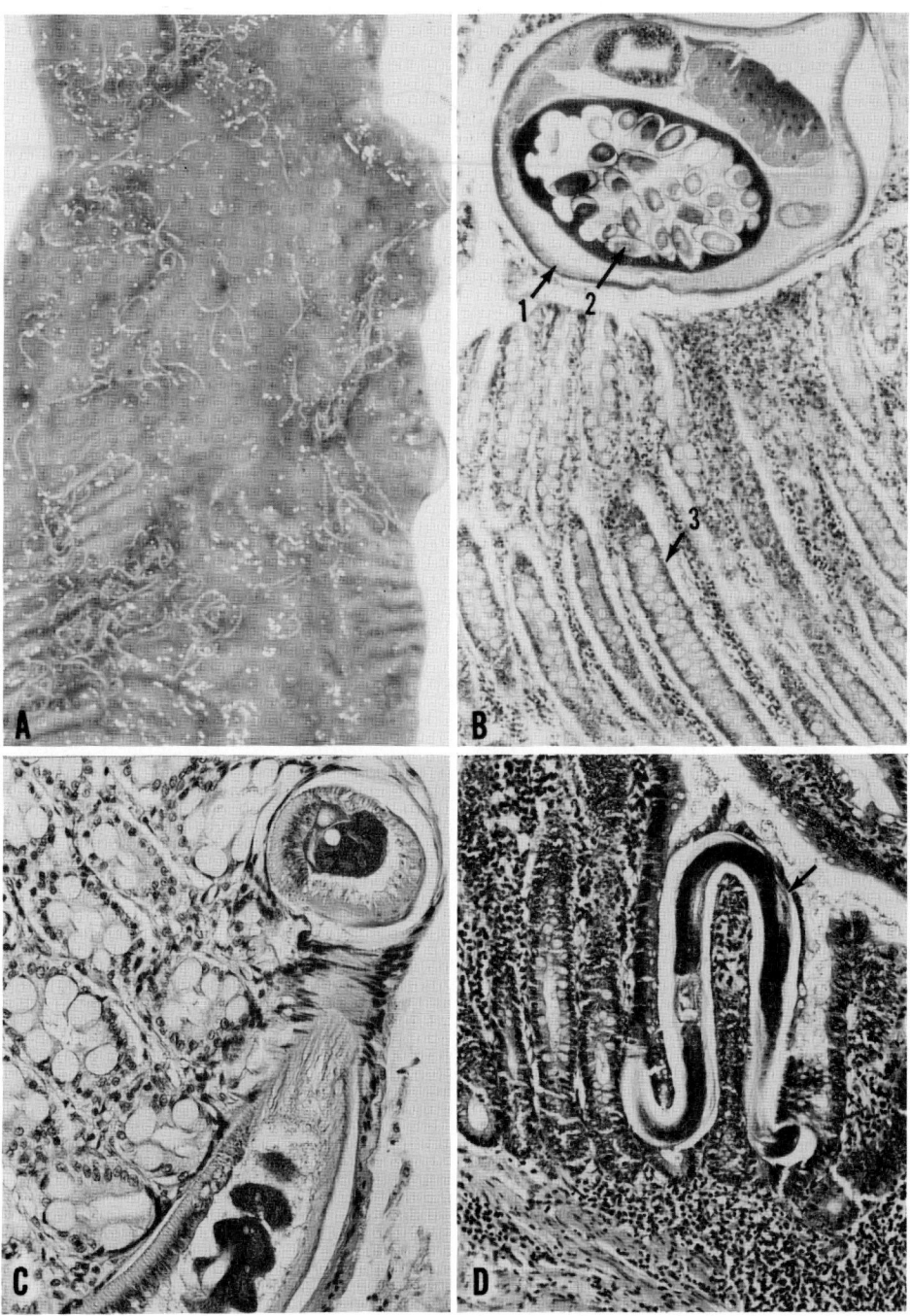

Fig. 14–22.   *A,* Trichuriasis, colon of a dog. Contributor: Army Veterinary School. *B, Trichuris vulpis* in the mucosa of the colon of a dog (× 100). Note muscular layer in wall *(1)* and ova in uterus *(2)* of the worm. Lymphocytic infiltration of the lamina propria separates the epithelial components *(3). C,* Another segment of *Tr. vulpis* (× 200) embedded in the mucosa of the colon. Contributor: Army Veterinary School. *D,* Strongyloidosis, small intestine of a spider monkey. Note the worm (arrow) buried in the mucosa. Contributor: Dr. C. N. Woolsey. *(A, B, D,* Courtesy of Armed Forces Institute of Pathology.)

domestic and wild pig and wild boar. It is similar if not identical morphologically to *T. trichiura,* which is parasitic in man and other primates. The dog may be infected experimentally with this parasite. Other species include *T. globulosa,* which inhabits the cecum of camels, sheep, goats and other ruminants, particularly in South Africa and *T. vulpis,* which infects foxes and dogs. Recently, *T. suis* has been shown to be capable of infecting man.

The parasites are oviparous. Infective eggs are ingested and hatch in the intestine, liberating larvae that penetrate the mucosa of the cecum and colon. After a period of about two weeks, the posterior portion protrudes into the intestinal lumen while the filamentous head remains embedded in the mucosa.

Although light to moderate infections produce little detectable effects, heavy parasitic loads may lead to catarrhal, hemorrhagic, or necrotizing typhlitis and colitis. Clinical and pathologic findings are most frequent in swine. During periods of drought (Farleigh, 1966a), whipworms apparently increase and may be found in large numbers in the cecum and colon of sheep. Death may result under these conditions.

Beer, R.J., and Rutter, J.M.: Spirochaetal invasion of the colonic mucosa in a syndrome resembling swine dysentery following experimental *Trichuris suis* infection in weaned pigs. Res. Vet. Sci., 13:593–595, 1972.

Beer, R.J.S.: Experimental infection of man with pig whipworm. Br. Med. J., 2:44, 1971.

———: Studies on the biology of the life-cycle of *Trichuris suis* Schrank, 1788. Parasitology, 67:253–262, 1973.

Beer, R.J.S., and Lean, I.J.: Clinical trichuriasis produced experimentally in growing pigs. I. Pathology of infection. Vet. Rec., 93:189–195, 1973.

Farleigh, E.A.: Observations on the pathogenic effects of *Trichuris ovis* in sheep under drought conditions. Aust. Vet. J., 42:462–463, 1966a.

———: Whip worm (*Trichuris ovis*) of sheep. Vet. Insp. N.S.W., 30:70–71, 1966.

Hall, G.A., Rutter, J.M., and Beer, R.J.S.: A comparative study of the histopathology of the large intestine of conventionally reared, specific pathogen free and gnotobiotic pigs infected with *Trichuris suis.* J. Comp. Pathol., 86:285–292, 1976.

Onchocerciasis

A chronic infection of the skin and subcutis, with the formation of parasitic nodules, onchocerciasis is a serious disease of man in tropical regions of Africa and Central America. Involvement of the uveal tract and retina by larvae of *Onchocerca volvulus* is a prominent cause of blindness in humans. Different species affect domestic animals; for example, *Onchocerca gutturosa* is found in cattle, and *O. cervicalis* and *O. reticulata* in horses.

The adults of all species produce microfilariae, which live in the dermis and are ingested by biting insects, particularly simuliid and culicoid flies, which transport them to new hosts. For example, *Onchocerca gibsoni* is transmitted by *Culicoides pungens; O. gutturosa* by *Simulium ornatum,* and *O. cervicalis* by *Culicoides nubeculosus.*

In the horse, the adults of *O. cervicalis* are slender, filariform worms ranging from 27 to 75 mm in length, which are found in the ligamentum nuchae and occasionally in nodular cutaneous lesions. The microfilariae concentrate in the skin of the abdomen adjacent to the umbilicus, the flank, or in the eyelids and other ocular tissues. *O. cervicalis* is common in horses, and the worms have been thought to have some etiologic relationship to "poll evil," "fistulous withers," periodic ophthalmia, and remittent dermatitis; however, there is no sound evidence to attribute these maladies to onchocerciasis. *O. reticulata* inhabits the suspensory ligaments of the forelimbs of horses. The adults of *O. gutturosa* in cattle reside in connective tissue adjacent to the nuchal ligament or between the spleen and rumen, and the microfilariae concentrate in the skin around the umbilicus. Neither the adults nor the larvae elicit any significant pathologic change. *Onchocerca armillata* is particularly frequent in cattle in Ghana. The adults of this parasite form tunnels, nodules, and cysts in the aortic

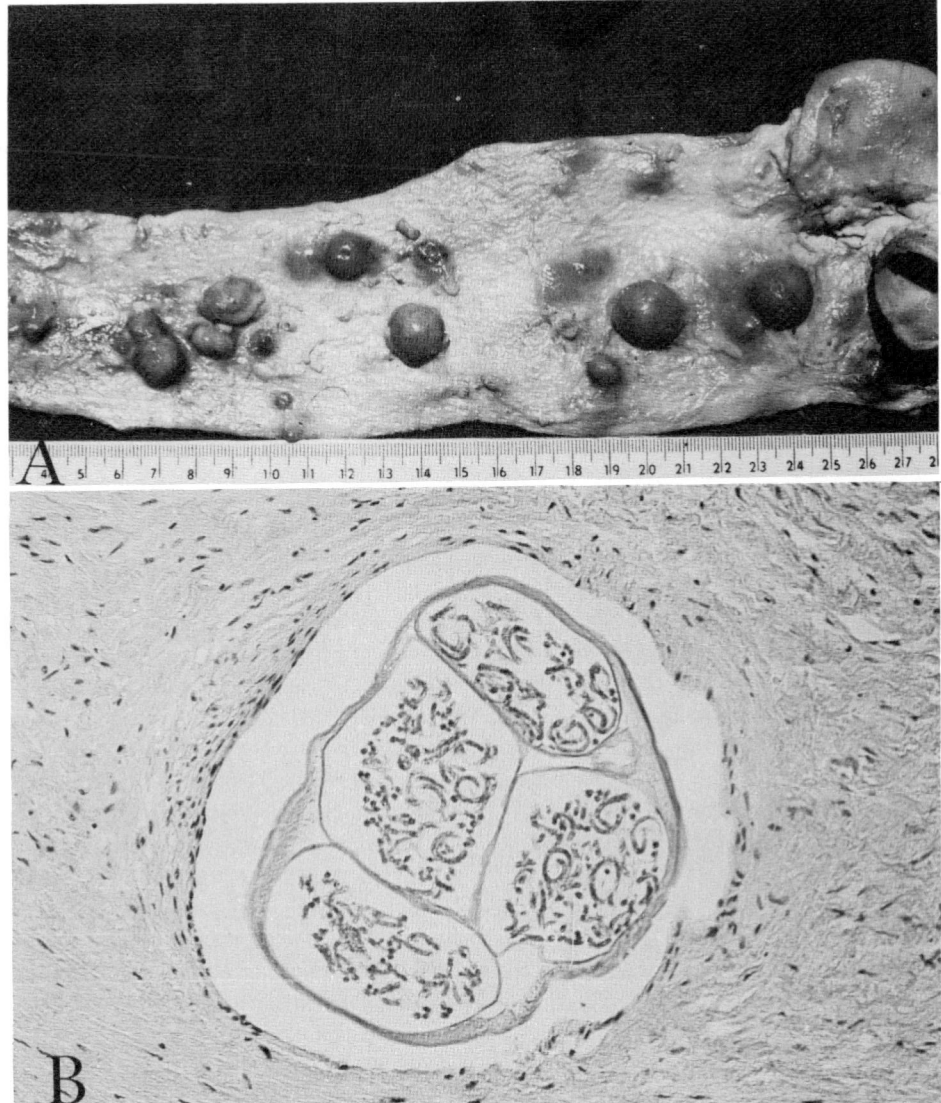

Fig. 14–23. Bovine onchocerciasis. *A*, Nodules in the adventitia of the aorta produced by *Onchocerca armillata*. *B*, Cross section of *O. armillata* in the media of the aorta. (Courtesy of Dr. A. H. Cheema and *Veterinary Pathology*.)

wall of affected cattle (Chadnik, 1958), and microfilariae concentrate in the skin.

Chadnik, K.S.: Histopathology of the aortic lesions in cattle infected with *Onchocerca armillata*. Ann. Trop. Med. Parasitol., *52*:145–148, 1958.

Dikmans, G.: Skin lesions of domestic animals in the United States due to nematode infestation. Cornell Vet., *38*:3–23, 1948.

Eichler, D.A., and Nelson, G.S.: Studies on *Onchocerca gutturosa* (Neumann, 1910) and its development in *Simulium ornatum* (Meigen, 1818). I. Observations on *O. gutturosa* in cattle in Southeast England. J. Helminthol., *45*:245–258, 1971.

ElBihari, S., and Hussein, H.S.: Location of the microfilariae of *Onchocerca armillata*. J. Parasitol., *61*:656, 1975.

Gunders, A.E., and Neumann, E.: Parasitology and diagnosis of onchocerciasis with special reference to the outer eye. Isr. J. Med. Sci., *8*:1139–1142, 1972.

Hilmy, N., Khamis, M.Y., and Selim, M.K.: The role of *Onchocerca reticulata* as the cause of fistulous withers and ulcerative wounds of the back in solipeds, and its treatment. Vet. Med. J. Giza, 14:149–164, 1967. VB 39:2979, 1969.

Ivanov, I.V.: Histological changes in the skin of cattle with onchocerciasis. Trudy vses. Inst. Gel'mint., 11:59–61, 1964. VB 36:1477, 1966.

Marolt, J., Zukovic, M., and Molan, M.: Onchocerciasis in horses. Dtsch. Tierarztl. Wochenschr., 73:130–134, 1966. VB 36:3555, 1966.

Mellor, P.S: Studies on *Onchocerca cervicalis* Railliet and Henry 1910. II. Pathology in the horse. J. Helminthol., 47:111–118, 1973.

Rabalais, F.C., Eberhard, M.L., Ashley, D.C., and Platt, T.R.: Survey for equine onchocerciasis in the midwestern United States. Am. J. Vet. Res., 35:125–126, 1974.

Rabalais, F.C., and Votava, C.L.: Cutaneous distribution of microfilariae of *Onchocerca cervicalis* in horses. Am. J. Vet. Res., 35:1369–1370, 1974.

Stannard, A.A., and Cello, R.M.: *Onchocerca cervicalis* infection in horses from the western United States. Am. J. Vet. Res., 36:1029–1031, 1975.

Elaeophoriasis (Filarial Dermatosis of Sheep)

Elaeophora schneideri, the "arterial worm," is a filarial parasite of deer and sheep, which produces "filarial dermatosis" in the skin of the latter species. The adult worms, found in the carotid, mesenteric, and iliac arteries, are slender, thread-like, and glossy white, and 6 to 12 cm in length. From 1 to 12 worms may be found in each infected sheep. Microfilariae, measuring 18 by 270 μ, are found in the dermis in specific areas of the skin. Cutaneous lesions, consisting of a circumscribed dermatitis, are found over the head, poll, and face in most cases. The skin of the abdomen and hind feet may be involved, as well as the cornea and oral and nasal mucosae. The lesion is apparently accompanied by considerable pruritus; vesicles and small pustules form in the skin; epilation and crust formation follow. There is sometimes proliferation of the horns in normally hornless rams.

Adcock and Hibler (1969) have described lesions in the blood vessels, skin, eye, and brain associated with infection of elk (*Cervus canadensis*). They found proliferation of the intima of the common carotid artery and its branches in which adult *Elaeophora schneideri* were present. Dead nematode larvae resulted in a granulomatous reaction that often occluded the artery. Thrombosis was detected in cerebral vessels particularly, where small infarcts of the brain resulted. Blindness was the result of such infarcts in the optic nerve, retina, occipital cortex, optic radiations, or lateral geniculate bodies. Similar vascular lesions were found to underlie malformed antlers, necrosis of the muzzle, nostrils, and tips of ears.

Horse flies, especially *Hybomitra laticornis*, *H. rubrilata*, and *Tabanus eurycerus*, have been shown to be vectors of *E. schneideri* (Clark and Hibler, 1973). The parasite has been reported in sheep and deer from New Mexico, Arizona, Colorado, Utah, and California, and from deer in British Columbia.

Lesions. The microscopic changes in the skin in this disease have been studied by Davis and Kemper (1951) and Jensen and Seghetti (1955). The affected epithelium is covered with a thick hyperkeratotic or parakeratotic layer variously infiltrated with cell debris and exudative fluid, and shows severe localized acanthosis with clubbing of the rete pegs. Areas of ulceration are associated with hemorrhagic and serous exudation. Superficial vesicles or bullae in the epithelium are common, and some are filled with serum or an admixture of serum, red blood cells, and eosinophils. The dermis is severely involved in an inflammatory process of granulomatous nature, centering around microfilariae in vascular channels or enclosed in the inflammatory exudate. In some foci of inflammation, histiocytes and giant cells predominate, with some lymphocytes and plasma cells in the surrounding tissue; in others, eosinophils are predominant. These changes are undoubtedly influenced by the age of the lesion, death of larvae, and sensitization of the host. The dermis is often completely involved to the level of the musculature.

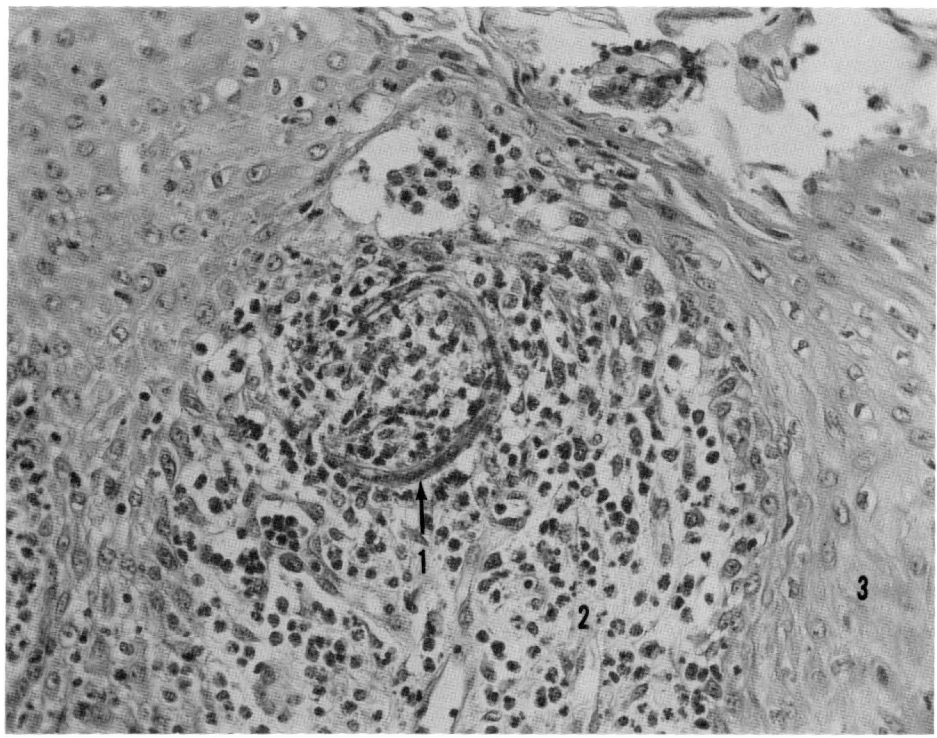

Fig. 14-24. Elaeophoriasis, skin of sheep (× 260). Larva of *Elaeophora schneideri (1)* in dermal papilla *(2)* which is congested and infiltrated with lymphocytes and eosinophils. The epidermis *(3)* is acanthotic. (Courtesy of Armed Forces Institute of Pathology.) Contributor: Bureau of Animal Industry, U.S. Department of Agriculture.

Localization of the larvae in skin and mucous membranes exposed to the external environment suggests a tropism for such localities. The adult worms may cause thrombosis of the arteries in which they are found.

Diagnosis. Diagnosis can be made by finding characteristic microfilariae in microscopic sections of affected skin or in smears of skin scrapings. The adult worms are found only at necropsy.

Adcock, J.L., and Hibler, C.P.: Vascular and neuro-ophthalmic pathology of elaeophorosis in elk. Pathol. Vet., 6:185–213, 1969.

Bindernagel, J.A.: *Elaeophora poeli* (Nematoda: Filaroidea) in African buffalo in Uganda, East Africa. J. Wldlf. Dis., 7:296–298, 1971

Clark, G.G., and Hibler, C.P.: Horse flies and *Elaeophora schneideri* in the Gila National Forest, New Mexico. J. Wldlf. Dis., 9:21–25, 1973.

Davis, C.L., and Kemper, H.E.: The histopathologic diagnosis of filarial dermatosis in sheep. J. Am. Vet. Med. Assoc., 118:103–106, 1951.

Douglas, J.R., Cordy, D.R., and Spurlock, G.M.: *Elaeophora schneideri*, Wehr and Dikmans, 1935 (Nematoda, filarioidea) in California sheep. Cornell Vet., 44:252–258, 1954.

Foreyt, W.J., and Foreyt, K.M.: *Elaeophora schneideri* in a White-Tailed deer from Texas. J. Wldlf. Dis., 15:55–56, 1979.

Hibler, C.P., Gates, G.H., and Donaldson, B.R.: Experimental infection of immature mule deer with *Elaeophora schneideri*. J. Wldlf. Dis., 10:44–46, 1974.

Hibler, C.P., Gates, G.H., White, R., and Donaldson, B.R.: Observations on horseflies infected with larvae of *Elaeophora schneideri*. J. Wldlf. Dis., 7:43–45, 1971.

Hibler, C.P., and Metzger, C.J.: Morphology of the larval stages of *Elaeophora schneideri* in the intermediate and definitive hosts with some observations on their pathogenesis in abnormal definitive hosts. J. Wldlf. Dis., 10:361–369, 1974.

Jensen, R., and Seghetti, L.: Elaeophoriasis in sheep. J. Am. Vet. Med. Assoc., 127:499–505, 1955.

Kemper, H.E.: Filarial dermatosis of sheep. North Am. Vet., *19*:36–41, 1938.

Robinson, R.M., Jones, L.P., Galvin, T.J., and Harwell, G.M.: Elaeophorosis in Sika deer in Texas. J. Wldlf. Dis., *14*:137–141, 1978.

Titche, A. R., Prestwood, A. K., and Hibler, C. P.: Experimental infection of White-Tailed deer with *Elaeophora schneideri*. J. Wldlf. Dis., *15*:273–280, 1979.

Worley, D.E.: Observations on epizootiology and distribution of *Elaeophora schneideri* in Montana ruminants. J. Wldlf. Dis., *11*:486–488, 1975.

Rhabditis Dermatitis

Pustular dermatitis resulting from the invasive effects of larvae of nematodes known as *Rhabditis strongyloides* has been described in dogs (Chitwood, 1932) and cattle (Rhode et al., 1953). The parasites are ordinarily free-living nematodes found in water and moist soil or organic matter, but under certain conditions, they penetrate the skin or invade the hair follicles to produce lesions. In one outbreak in dairy cattle, large areas of the skin of the legs and abdomen were affected by a pustular dermatitis, larvae being demonstrable in microscopic sections of hair follicles. The larvae were found in large numbers in the moist rice hulls used as bedding for these animals.

Chitwood, B.G.: The association of *Rhabditis strongyloides* with dermatitis in dogs. North Am. Vet., *13*:35–40, 1932.

Chitwood, M., and Lichtenfels, J.R.: Parasitological review. Identification of parasitic metazoa in tissue sections. Exp. Parasitol., *32*:407–519, 1972.

Georgi, J.R.: Parasitology for Veterinarians. 2nd ed. Philadelphia, W. B. Saunders, 1974.

Jibbo, J.M.C.: Bovine parasitic otitis. Bull Epizoot. Dis. Afr., *14*:59–63, 1966.

Rhode, E.A., et al.: The occurrence of *Rhabditis* in cattle. North Am. Vet., *34*:634–637, 1953.

Schlotthauer, C.F., and Zollman, P.E.: The occurrence of *Rhabditis strongyloides* in association with dermatitis in a dog. J. Am. Vet. Med. Assoc., *127*:510–511, 1955.

Stephanofilariasis

Nematode dermatitis occurring in cattle in widely scattered parts of the world is caused by several related filarial worms. *Stephanofilaria stilesi*, originally recognized by Stiles and described by Dikmans (1948),

has been reported in skin lesions of cattle in most of the western and midwestern states, as well as Louisiana. This filarid causes a circumscribed dermatitis usually located on the abdomen near the midline. *S. dedoesi* has been reported from Java, Sumatra, Celebes, and Indonesia; it produces lesions on the sides of the neck, withers, dewlap, shoulders and around the eyes. *S. assamensis*, occurring in Assam and other parts of India, causes a chronic dermatitis in Zebu cattle, known as "hump sore." In Malaya, a fourth species, *S. kaeli*, is reported to produce "filarial sores" on the lower legs of cattle. An apparently new species of *Stephanofilaria* has been identified (Kono, 1965) in the Ryukyu Islands as the cause of pruritic lesions on the muzzle of cattle. These lesions result in erosion of the epidermis over zones of infiltration of papillary and reticular layers of the dermis by lymphocytes, plasma cells, macrophages, and eosinophils in relation to adult nematodes. In the United States, Hibler (1966) has shown that the horn fly, *Haematobia irritans*, is an intermediate host for *Stephanofilaria stilesi*. Other flies may have a similar role for *Stephanofilaria* in other parts of the world.

Lesions. The adult forms of *Stephanofilaria stilesi* are found either in small cysts with epithelial linings in the base of hair follicles or in the dermis near the epidermis (Fig. 14–25). In either site, the worms are surrounded by a zone of inflammation containing eosinophils, lymphocytes, some neutrophils, and histiocytes, and often a layer of connective tissue. The microfilariae are found a short distance from the adults in spaces in the dermal papillae. The adults and microfilariae can often be seen in the same field when the low power of the microscope is used (Fig. 14–25). Hyperkeratosis and parakeratosis may be noted in the epidermis of parasitized areas, and crusts of exuded serum and detritus may collect on the surface. Death of the parasites and sensitization of the host result in a rather severe dermatitis.

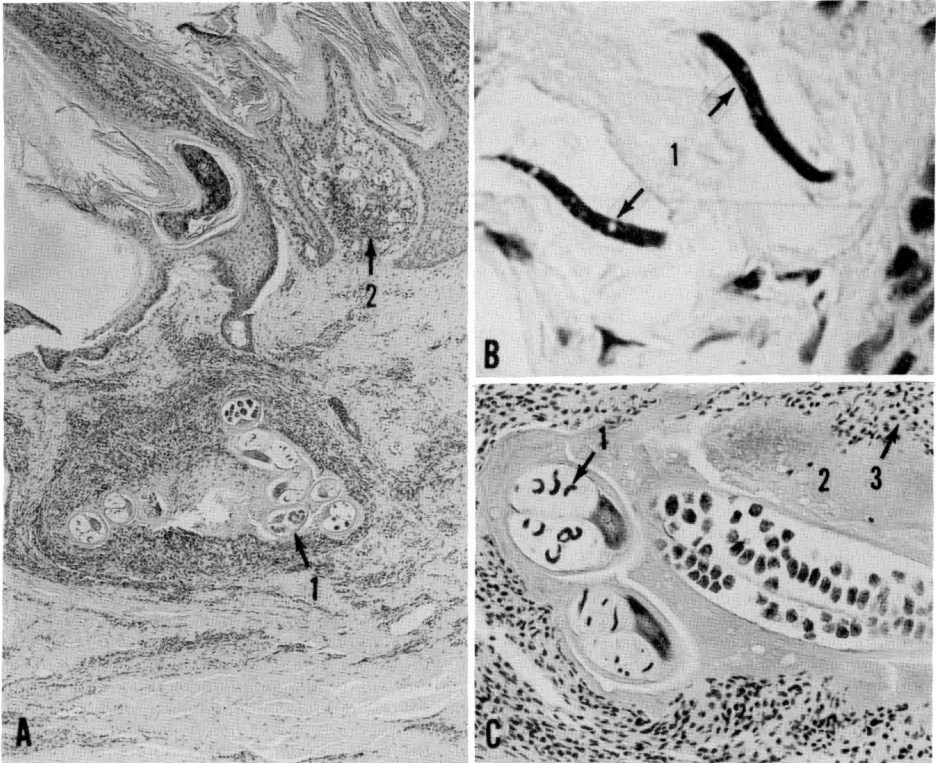

Fig. 14–25. Stephanofilariasis, bovine skin. *A*, Section of skin (× 75) containing coiled adult *Stephanofilaria stilesi (1)* deep in a hair follicle and larvae in the dermal papillae *(2)*. Note acanthosis and hyperkeratosis. *B*, Larvae *(1)* (× 900) in papilla. *C*, Adult (× 150) worm with larvae in uterus *(1)*, hyaline material *(2)* surrounding it, and zone of inflammation *(3)*. (Courtesy of Armed Forces Institute of Pathology and Dr. C. L. Davis.)

Diagnosis. The diagnosis may be established by the demonstration of adults and microfilariae in biopsy or necropsy specimens of affected skin. The parasites can also be collected by deep scrapings of skin and identified by microscopic examination.

Chitwood, M., and Lichtenfels, J.R.: Parasitological review. Identification of parasitic metazoa in tissue sections. Exp. Parasitol., *32*:407–519, 1972.

Dewan, M.L., and Rahman, M.M.: Isolation of microorganisms from stephanofilariasis (humpsore) and their roles in the initiation of the disease. Bangladesh Vet. J., *4*:25–30, 1970. VB, *42*:1972; art. #6983.

Dikmans, G.: Skin lesions of domestic animals in the United States due to nematode infestation. Cornell Vet., *38*:3–23, 1948.

Georgi, J.R.: Parasitology for Veterinarians. 2nd ed. Philadelphia, W. B. Saunders, 1974.

Hibler, C.P.: Development of *Stephanofilaria stilesi* in the horn fly. J. Parasitol., *52*:890–898, 1966.

Kono, I., and Fukuyoshi, S.: Leucoderma of the muzzle of cattle induced by a new species of *Stephanofilaria*. II. Jpn. J. Vet. Sci., *29*:301–313, 1967. VB *38*:4627, 1968.

Levine, N.D., and Morrill, C.C.: Bovine stephanofilarial dermatitis in Illinois. J. Am. Vet. Med. Assoc., *127*:528–530, 1955.

Loke, Y.W., and Ramachandran, C.P.: Histopathology of *Stephanofilaria kaeli* lesions in cattle. Med. J. Malaya, *20*:348–353, 1966. VB *37*:931, 1967.

Mia, A.S., and Haque, A.: Skin diseases in cattle. Pakist. J. Vet. Sci., *1*:76–83, 1967. VB *39*:1271, 1969.

Oduye, O.O.: Stephanofilarial dermatitis of cattle in Nigeria. J. Comp. Pathol., *81*:581–583, 1971.

Pal, A.K., and Sinha, P.K.: *Stephanofilaria assamensis* as the cause of common chronic ulcerated growth at the base of the dewclaws in cattle in West Bengal. Ind. Vet. J., *48*:190–193, 1971.

Ramachandran, C.P., Loke, Y.W., and Nagendram, C.: Studies on *Stephanofilaria kaeli* in cattle. Med. J. Malaya, *20*:344–347, 1966.

Sharma Deorani, V.P.: Studies on the pathology of *Stephanofilariasis assamensis* in cattle. Curr. Sci., 34:410–411, 1965.

Thelaziasis

"Eye worms" have been reported from the conjunctival sac, tear duct, the bulbar and tarsal conjunctiva and membrana nictitans of animals. Several species are of interest: *Thelazia californiensis* has been reported in the United States from sheep dogs, deer, and rarely, cats and man. *T. callipaeda* occurs in Asia in the membrana nictitans of the dog, less frequently in the rabbit and man. *T. gulosa* occurs in cattle (France, Sumatra, and recently in Kentucky); *T. alfortensis,* in cattle (France); *T. skrjabini,* in calves; and *T. lacrymalis,* in the horse. *T. rhodesii* has been reported from Asia, Africa, and Europe in the conjunctival sac of buffaloes, cattle, goats, and sheep.

The life cycle (Soulsby, 1968) of these spiruroid worms depends upon flies as intermediate hosts and vectors. The larvae move from the gut to develop first in the ovary of the fly, where they penetrate and develop in ovarian follicles. They spend their second and third stages in the ovary, then as third-stage, infective larvae, they migrate to the mouth parts of the fly, ready to be transferred to the conjunctivae of cattle.

The intermediate hosts are as follows: for *T. rhodesii*—*Musca larvipara, M. convexifrons;* for *T. skrjabini*—probably *M. amica;* for *T. gulosi*—*M. amica* and *M. larvipara;* for *T. lacrymalis*—probably *M. autumnalis.* The intermediate hosts and vectors for *T. californiensis, T. callipaeda,* and *T. alfortensis* are at present unknown.

Their presence in the conjunctival sac results in considerable photophobia and excessive lacrimation; if not removed, they are reported to cause blindness, presumably through production of corneal opacity. The diagnosis is made by finding and identifying the parasites in the conjunctiva.

Barker, I.K.: *Thelazia lacrymalis* from the eyes of an Ontario horse. Can. Vet. J., 11:186–189, 1970.
Fitzsimmons, W.M.: Verminous ophthalmia in a cow in Berkshire—a review of Thelazia infections as a veterinary problem. Vet. Rec., 75:1024–1027, 1963.
Lyons, E.T., and Drudge, J.H.: Two eyeworms, *Thelazia gulosa* and *Thelazia skrjabini,* in cattle in Kentucky. J. Parasitol., 61:1119–1122, 1975.
Soulsby, E.J.L.: Helminths, Arthropods and Protozoa of Domesticated Animals, (Mönnig). 6th ed. Philadelphia, Lea & Febiger, 1968, pp. 274–276.

Stephanuriasis (Kidney Worm Disease)

The swine kidney worm, *Stephanurus dentatus,* is a stout parasitic nematode, 20 to 40 mm in length, found principally in the perirenal fat and adjacent tissues. It is especially common in the southern United States. These worms form cystic cavities that communicate with the lumen of the ureter and permit the discharge of ova with the urine. The larvae hatch only in moist, shaded soil, and remain infective for some time unless exposed to direct sunlight and desiccation. The infective larvae may be ingested by the host or penetrate the mud-caked skin. The larvae lose their sheaths to reach the fourth stage in one of two sites, depending upon the route of entry. Orally ingested worms molt in the wall of the stomach, while those that penetrate the skin undergo this change in the abdominal muscles. The fourth-stage larvae soon migrate to the liver, where they remain for two or three months, their movements exciting severe tissue reaction. Eventually the larvae break out of the liver into the peritoneal cavity and wander extensively, most of them eventually reaching the perirenal fat. Here the successful adults copulate and the female lays her eggs in a cyst, which empties into the ureter. This life cycle requires about six months. Infected swine are commonly emaciated in spite of a good appetite, and ascites is frequent as a result of liver damage. Death may occur following secondary infection, extensive tissue destruction, or urinary obstruction. The condemnation of livers and carcasses of infected animals slaughtered for food makes the disease an important economic problem.

Lesions. Both the larvae and the adult forms of this nematode produce severe effects upon the host. Nodules and edema in the subcutis and transitory enlargement of superficial lymph nodes are produced by the passage of larvae, but their most serious effect is upon the liver. Not only do these worms burrow into the liver, but during their relatively long stay they move about aggressively. This restive sojourn in the liver eventually results in extensive portal fibrosis, which may spread to obliterate many liver lobules. The fibrotic change is accompanied by intense tissue eosinophilia, foci of coagulation necrosis, and infiltration by other leukocytes. The lesions are often so severe as to render the liver totally unfit for human food.

This parasite, to a greater extent than most others, wanders through the host's tissue producing widespread damage. Although the successful worms find their way to the vicinity of the ureters, many wander to other sites where they excite a local purulent tissue reaction. *S. dentatus* has been found in the kidney, lumbar muscles, myocardium, lungs, pleural cavity, spleen, and even the spinal canal. Paralysis may result from destruction of the lumbar spinal cord by the migrations of these worms.

Diagnosis. The diagnosis may be made by demonstrating the ova in the urine or by finding the worms at necropsy. Leukocytic infiltration and fibrosis in the liver are usually much more intense and extensive than the changes in this organ caused by other larvae (e.g., ascarids), a point which may be used in histologic differentiation.

Ashizawa, H., Nosaka, D., Tateyama, S., and Saito, I.: Pathological findings in stephanuriasis in pigs. I. Route of penetration of worms into the urinary passages. II. Pathological changes in the kidneys, ureters, and adjacent tissues. Bull. Fac. Agricul., Miyazaki, *19*:155–165, 167–178, 1972.

Ashizawa, H., Nosaka, D., Tateyama, S., and Murakami, T.: Pathological findings in stephanuriasis in pigs. III. Pathological changes in the liver and lungs. Bull. Fac. Agricul., Miyazaki, *19*:179–192, 1972.

Batte, E.G., Moncol, D.J., and Barber, C.W.: Prenatal infection with the swine kidney worm (*Stephanurus dentatus*) and associated lesions. J. Am. Vet. Med. Assoc., *149*:758–765, 1966.

Peneyra, R.S., and Naui, V.C.: Observations on the incidence and pathology of kidney-worm infection in swine (slaughterhouse material). Philipp. J. Vet. Med., *4*:129–140, 1967.

Gongylonemiasis

These tiny worms are of interest because of their habitat in the stratified squamous epithelium of the esophagus, the rumen, and stomach. They are often encountered in histologic sections of these organs, coiled in the epithelium (Fig. 14–26), apparently inciting little or no host reaction. *Gongylonema pulchrum* occurs in sheep, cattle, goats, pigs, buffalo, and occasionally the horse, camel, wild boar, and donkey. It has been reported in man. *G. verrucosum* inhabits the rumen of sheep, goats, cattle, deer, and zebu. It is known in the United States, India, and South Africa. *G. monnig* infects sheep and goats in South Africa. Other species infect the rat *(G. neoplasticum)* and nonhuman primates (Fig. 14–26).

Chitwood, M., and Lichtenfels, J.R.: Parasitological review. Identification of parasitic metazoa in tissue sections. Exp. Parasitol., *32*:407–519, 1972.

Georgi, J.R.: Parasitology for Veterinarians. 2nd ed. Philadelphia, W. B. Saunders, 1974.

Lichtenfels, J.R.: Morphological variation in the gullet nematode, *Gongylonema pulchrum* Molin, 1857, from eight species of definitive hosts with a consideration of gongylonema from *Macaca spp.* J. Parasitol., *57*:348–355, 1971.

Soulsby, E.J.L.: Helminths, Arthropods and Protozoa of Domesticated Animals, 6th ed. Philadelphia, Lea & Febiger, 1968.

Zinter, D.E., and Migaki, G.: *Gongylonema pulchrum* in tongues of slaughtered pigs. J. Am. Vet. Med. Assoc., *157*:301–303, 1970.

Acanthocephalan Infections

Acanthocephalan or thorny-headed worms have important pathogenic effects

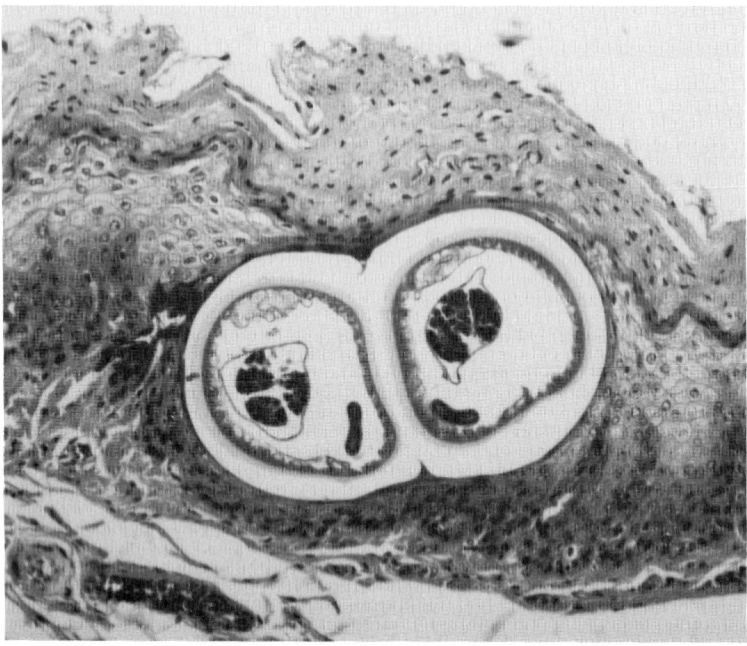

Fig. 14–26. *Gongylonema sp.* Cross sections of a parasite embedded in the epithelium of the tongue of a rhesus monkey (*Macaca mulatta*). (Courtesy New England Regional Primate Research Center, Harvard Medical School.)

upon their host because of their tendency to burrow into and attach to the intestinal wall. These worms are classified in a separate phylum **(Acanthocephala)** and have

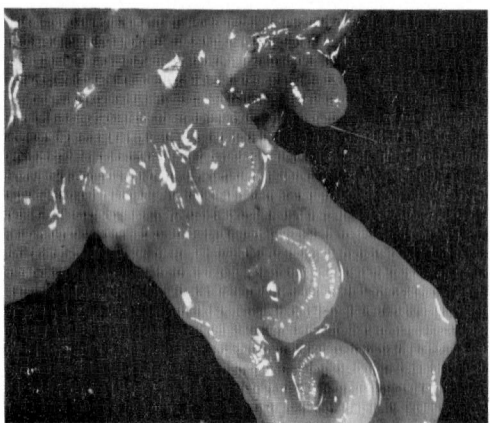

Fig. 14–27. *Prosthenorchis elegans,* marmoset (*Saguinus oedipus*). These acanthocephalids characteristically embed their thorny heads in the mucosa of the terminal ileum. (Courtesy New England Regional Primate Research Center, Harvard Medical School.)

parasitic representatives in many species of mammals, birds, and fishes. They invariably attach to the intestinal wall of the host, and in the host have somewhat flattened bodies that tend to round up after removal. The arrangement and number of "thorns" on the head parts are used to identify individual species. *Macracanthorhynchus hirudinaceus* is the thorny-headed worm that infects domestic swine and incidentally provides young veterinary students with a "jawbreaker" name which, when mastered in pronunciation and spelling, somehow makes it easier to cope with other scientific names. It utilizes various coprophagous beetles as intermediate hosts.

Prosthenorchis elegans (Figs. 14–27, 14–28) is found in the small intestine and colon of South American monkeys, such as the squirrel monkey (*Saimiri sciureus*) and marmosets (*Tamarinus, Saguinus, Cebuella*). One of its intermediate hosts is the cockroach. *Acanthocephalus jacksoni* is

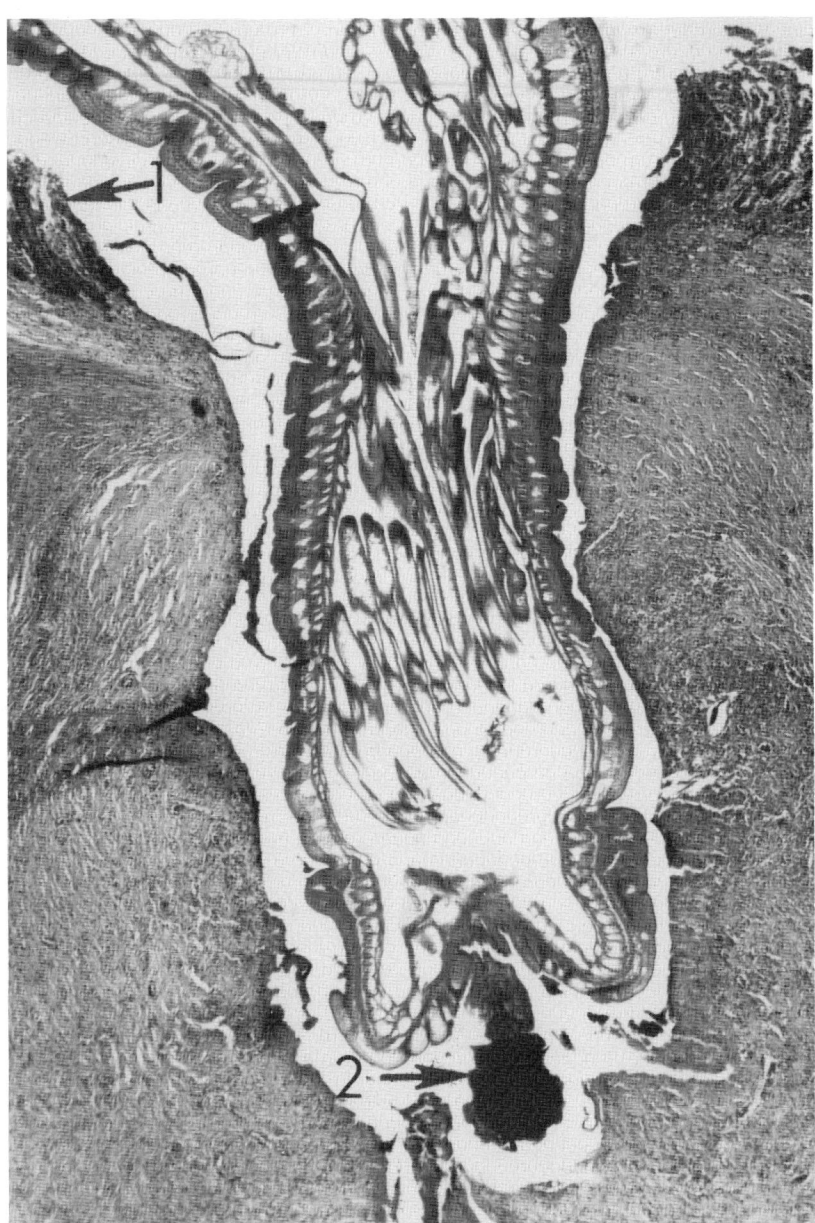

Fig. 14–28. Acanthocephalid in a marmoset *(Saguinus oedipus). Prosthenorchis elegans* which has penetrated through the mucosa of the ileum *(1)* assisted by its thorny proboscis *(2).* (Courtesy New England Regional Primate Research Center, Harvard Medical School.)

known to parasitize several species of freshwater fish in New England.

The acanthocephalids bury the thorny proboscis into the mucosa of the small intestine, resulting in a small ulcer surrounded by neutrophils and granulation tissue. Rarely, the parasites penetrate the wall, leading to peritonitis.

Arambulo, P.V., III, and Blanea, M.R.: The occurrence of *Macracanthorhynchus hirudinaceus* in swine in the Philippines with a note on its zoonotic implications. Kajian Veterinaire, Malaysia-Singapore, 4:5–8, 1972.

Bullock, W.L.: Intestinal histology of some salmonid fishes with particular reference to histopathology of acanthocephalan infections. J. Morphol., 112:23–44, 1963.

Chaicharn, A., and Bullock, W.L.: The histopathology of acanthocephalan infections in suckers with observations on the intestinal histology of two species of catostomid fishes. Acta Zool., 48:19–42, 1967.

Chitwood, M., and Lichtenfels, J.R.: Parasitological review. Identification of parasitic metazoa in tissue sections. Exp. Parasitol., 32:407–519, 1972.

Dunn, F.L.: Acanthocephalans and cestodes of South American monkeys and marmosets. J. Parasitol., 49:717–722, 1963.

Georgi, J.R.: Parasitology for Veterinarians. 2nd ed. Philadelphia, W. B. Saunders, 1974.

Moore, J.G.: Epizootic of acanthocephaliasis among primates. J. Am. Vet. Med. Assoc., 157:699–705, 1970.

Richart, R., and Benirschke, K.: Causes of death in a colony of marmoset monkeys. J. Pathol. Bact., 86:221–223, 1963.

Sloss, M.W., and Kemp, R.L.: Veterinary Clinical Parasitology. 5th ed. Ames, Iowa State Univ. Press, 1978.

Takos, M.J., and Thomas, L.J.: The pathology and pathogenesis of fetal infections due to an acanthocephalid parasite of marmoset monkeys. Am. J. Trop. Med. Hyg., 7:90–94, 1958.

Van Cleave, H.J.: Acanthocephala of North American Mammals. Illinois Biol. Monograph, 23:(1–2):1–179, 1953.

Cestodiasis (Tapeworm Disease, Taeniasis)

Cestodes, or tapeworms (phylum: Platyhelminthes, class: Cestoda), are common parasites of all vertebrate animals, including man. An exception occurs in the United States at least, where the pig seems to be singularly free of tapeworms. The adult forms in the intestinal tract of the definitive host are flat worms made up of a chain of independent, hermaphroditic segments (proglottides) fastened together, and usually attached to the intestinal mucosa by a specialized segment (scolex) at the anterior end. Each proglottid contains male and female genitalia and is complete in other respects; hence the tapeworm is in reality a colony of individuals attached to one another in a tape-like chain. As proglottides of most tapeworms mature, those at the caudal end are shed and expelled from the body with the feces, to release their innumerable ova.

All tapeworms have one or more larval stages through which they pass in various intermediate hosts, including insects and mammals; some tapeworms require more than one intermediate host. Only one tapeworm, *Hymenolepis nana*, a parasite of rodents, has a direct life cycle, the definitive host serving also for the stages of development usually completed within the intermediate host. These larval forms invade animal tissues, and by replacing vital cells can produce serious effects upon the host. Certain tapeworm larvae were recognized for a long time before their connection with the adult form was appreciated. For this reason, the larval form may have a separate, well-established name—for example, *Cysticercus cellulosae*, the bladderworm of "measly pork," is the larval form of *Taenia solium*, a tapeworm of man.

The class Cestoda is usually divided into eleven orders, nine of which include parasites of fishes, annelids, reptiles, or amphibia, and two, Pseudophyllidea and Cyclophyllidea, in which are classified all tapeworms parasitic for man and other mammals. The Pseudophyllidea are largely parasites of fish; the adult of only one species, *Diphyllobothrium latum*, is parasitic in mammals. Species of this order have a scolex which has no hooks and narrow, deep grooves, **bothria,** instead of suckers. The eggs are usually operculated, resembling those of trematodes. All of the rest of the species of

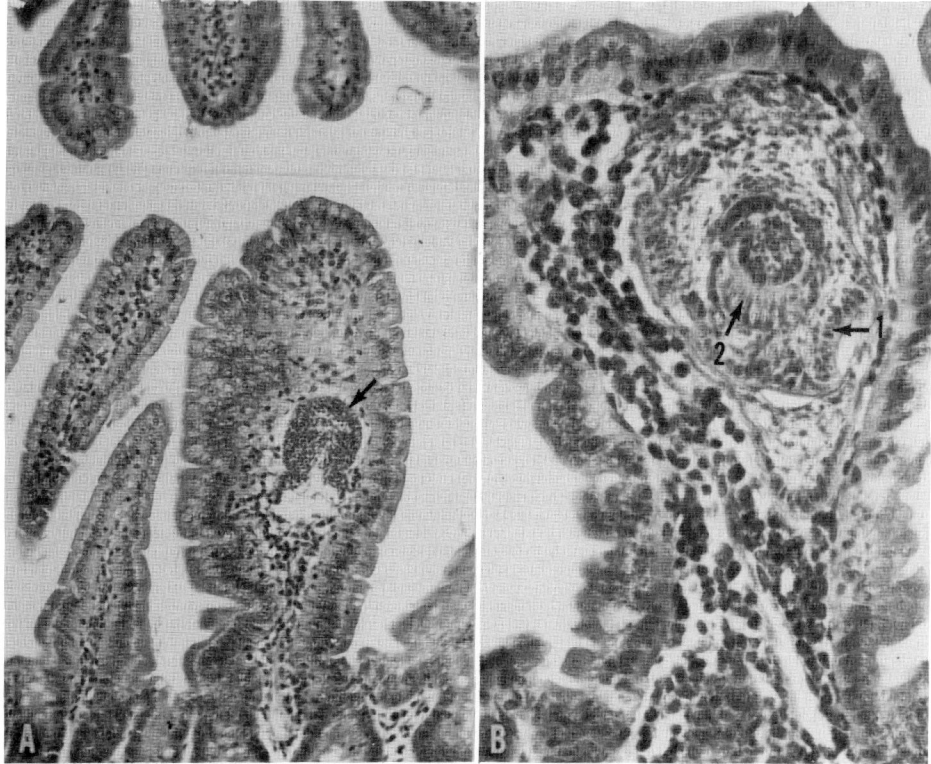

Fig. 14–29. Cestodiasis. *A*, Cysticercoid larva (arrow) of *Hymenolepis nana* (× 45) in intestinal villus of a mouse. *B*, Later stage in larval development (× 395). Note sucker *(1)* and hooklets *(2)* of the larva encysted in the lamina propria of the intestinal villus. (Courtesy of Armed Forces Institute of Pathology.) Contributor: Dr. W. S. Bailey.

tapeworms parasitic for mammals are classified in the order Cyclophyllidea.

Life Cycles. The adult tapeworms apparently produce little serious effect upon the host except in very heavy infections, in which they interfere with digestion or cause partial obstruction. The adults all reside in the intestine, with the exception of a few species, such as *Thysanosoma actinoides* and *Stilesia hepatica* (limited to Africa), which inhabit bile ducts in ruminants, and *Hymenolepis microstoma,* in bile ducts of rodents.

The parasites in their intermediate stages produce more important effects upon the host. The pathologist may encounter these intermediate stages of tapeworms in animal tissues; therefore the identifying features of the different types

are of diagnostic significance. The larvae usually develop in one of two possible ways, to become (1) solid larvae and (2) bladder larvae. In the first (solid) type, the ovoid, operculate ovum is passed out of the uterus to hatch into a ciliated motile embryo, the **coracidium,** which escapes through the operculum and becomes free-living. The coracidium is ingested by a freshwater crustacean, in whose tissues it develops into an elongated form, the **procercoid** larva. Development of this larva continues after the arthropod is swallowed by a second intermediate host (often a fish), until it becomes an elongated solid larva **(plerocercoid; sparganum)** with a head resembling that of the mature tapeworm. The broad fish tapeworm (*Diphyllobothrium latum*) provides an

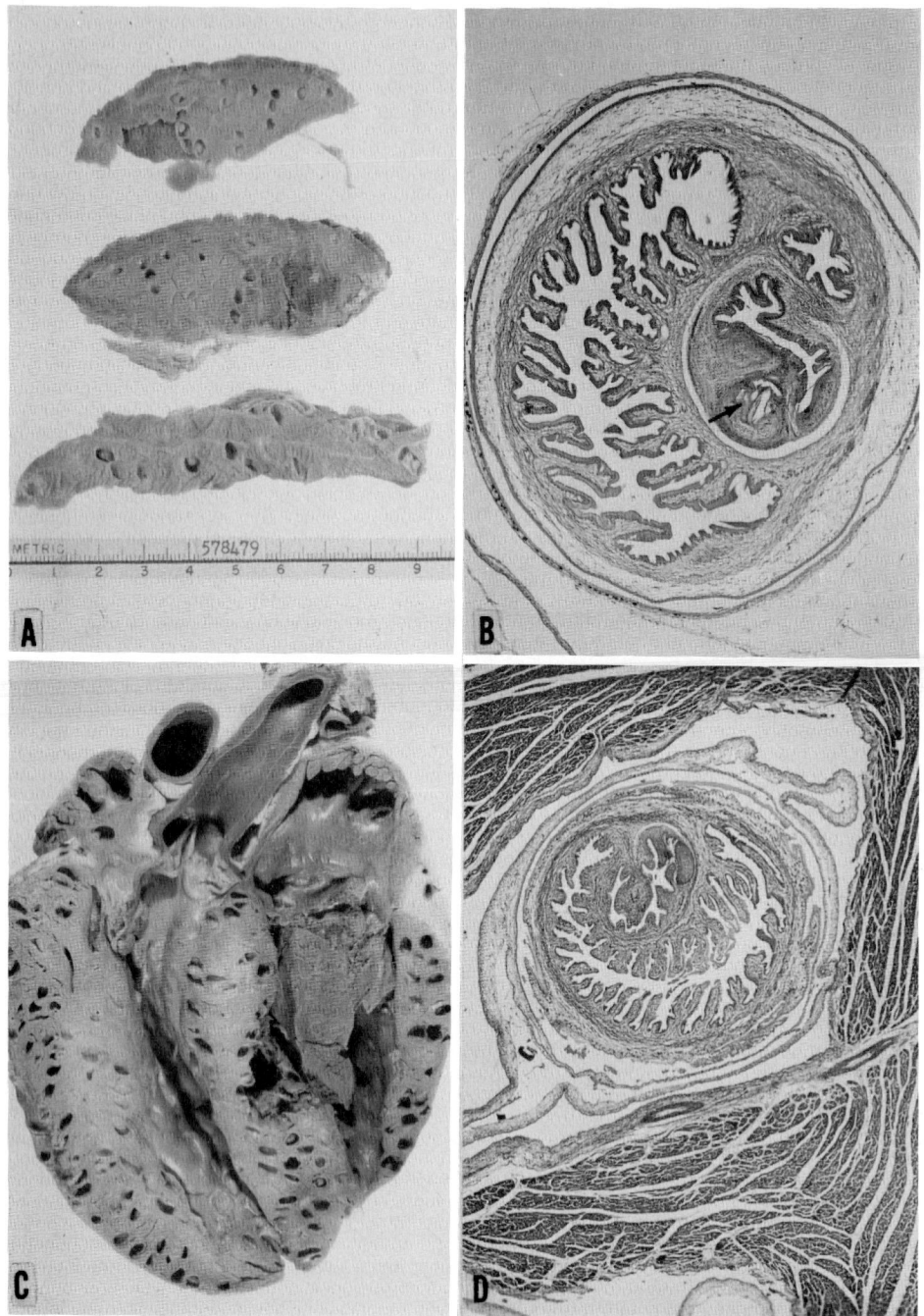

Fig. 14–30. Cestodiasis. An unusual bovine infection with the pork tapeworm *Cysticercus cellulosae* *(Taenia solium). A,* Skeletal muscles containing cysticerci. *B,* A single inverted scolex (× 38). Note hooklets (arrow) which distinguish this larva from that of the more common beef tapeworm, *Cysticercus bovis (Taenia saginata). C,* Cysticerci in the myocardium. *D,* A single cysticercus (× 21) in the heart muscle. (Courtesy of Armed Forces Institute of Pathology.) Contributor: Major C. N. Barron.

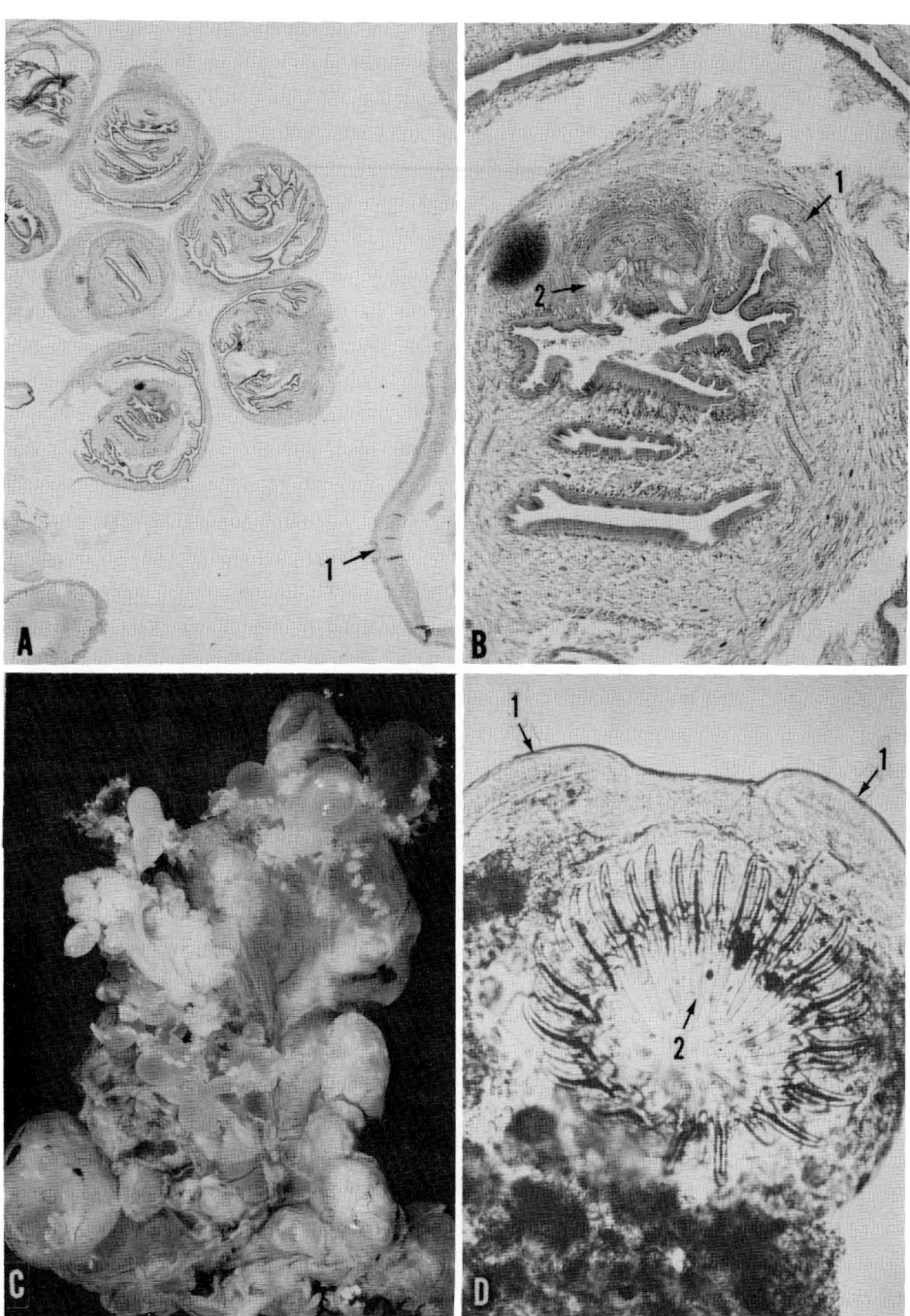

Fig. 14–31. Cestodiasis. *A,* Coenurus of *Multiceps serialis* (× 12) in muscle of a rabbit. Note several scolices and wall of cyst *(1). B,* A single inverted scolex of *M. serialis* (× 50). Note sucker *(1)* and hooklets *(2).* Contributor: Capt. Morris Schneider, V.C. *C, Multiceps serialis,* larvae from the subcutis of a monkey. Contributor: National Zoological Park. *D,* Everted scolex (× 150) of *Taenia pisiformis,* larva from the peritoneum of a deer. Note suckers *(1)* and hooklets *(2).* (Courtesy of Armed Forces Institute of Pathology.) Contributor: Capt. James R. Prine.

Table 14–7. Outline of Features of Some Important Tapeworms

Name of Tapeworm	Adult Host	Anatomic Site	Intermediate Stage	
			Type of Larva	Intermediate Hosts
Taenia saginata	Man	Heart, skeletal muscle	Cysticercus (bovis)	Cattle
T. solium	Man	Muscle, heart, viscera	Cysticercus (cellulosae)	Swine, cattle
Echinococcus granulosus	Man, dog, fox, wolf, jackal	Liver, lungs, other viscera	Echinococcus (granulosus)	Man, cattle, swine, sheep, deer, horse, moose, etc.
E. multilocularis	Man, dog, fox, wolf, jackal	Liver, lungs, other viscera	Echinococcus (multilocularis)	Man, cattle, swine, sheep, deer, horse, moose, etc.
Taenia hydatigena	Dog	Liver, mesentery, etc.	Cysticercus (tenuicollis)	Squirrels, cattle, wild ruminants, sheep, goats, swine
T. ovis	Dog, fox, wolf, coyote	Muscles	Cysticercus (ovis)	Sheep
T. pisiformis	Dog, cat, fox, wolf	Liver capsule, peritoneum	Cysticercus	Rabbit, squirrel, other small rodents
T. taeniaeformis (syn.: T. crassicollis)	Cat, dog, fox	Liver	Cysticercus (fasciolaris)	Rats, mice, rabbits

Species	Host	Location	Larval form	Intermediate host
Multiceps multiceps	Dog	Brain, spinal cord	Coenurus (cerebralis)	Sheep, goats
M. serialis	Dog, other carnivores	Subcutis	Coenurus (serialis)	Rabbit
Diphyllobothrium latum	Man, bear, dog, cat, pig, fox	Muscles	Procercoid and plerocercoid	Microcrustacea, freshwater fish
Spirometra (Diphyllobothrium) mansonoides	Dog, cat	Peritoneal cavity	Procercoid and plerocercoid (sparganum)	Snakes, man, monkeys, dog
Mesocestoides corti, M. lineatus	Dog, cat, wild carnivore, man	Peritoneal and pleural cavities, liver, lung, other organs	Tetrathridium	Mites and wild rodents, dogs, cat, other mammals, reptiles
Dipylidium caninum	Dog, cat		Cysticercoid	Dog flea, biting lice
Moniezia expansa	Sheep, goats, cattle	—	Cysticercoid	Mites: *Galumna, Scheloribates, Scutovertex minutus*
M. benedeni	Sheep, goats, cattle	—	Cysticercoid	*Scutovertex minutus*
Anoplocephala magna	Equines	—	Cysticercoid	Mites of family *Oribatidae*
A. perfoliata	Equines	—	Cysticercoid	*Oribatidae*
Paranoplocephala mammillana	Equines	—	Cysticercoid	*Oribatidae*
Thysanosoma actinioides	Sheep, cattle, goats, deer	—	Cysticercoid	*Oribatidae*

example of larval development of this type. "Spargana" is a term applied to certain plerocercoid larvae of other pseudophyllidae and the larvae of *Mesocestoides spp.*, cestodes somewhat intermediate between pseudophyllidae and cyclophyllidae. The latter larvae, however, are most commonly termed **tetrathridia**.

In development of the second type, the bladder larvae arise from eggs that are usually round or nearly square, released from the uterus by disintegration of the proglottid or by discharge through one or more uterine pores by those species which have them. These eggs are fully developed when they escape from the uterus, in that they contain a larva, the **onchosphere** or **hexacanth embryo,** surrounded by a dense membrane. In the intestine of the intermediate host, the onchosphere is released to migrate through the intestinal mucosa and enter the lymph or blood, by which it is carried to other tissues, where it becomes transformed into a bladder-shaped structure with one or more inverted scolices in an invaginated portion of the wall. If the larva has a solid caudal portion and a bladderlike proximal portion, it is called a **cysticercus**. Modifications of the cysticercus include the **strobilocercus,** with an invaginated scolex attached to a small bladder by a segmented portion; the **coenurus** or **multiceps,** with a germinal layer capable of producing multiple scolices beneath the bladder wall; and the **echinococcus** or **hydatid cyst,** with a germinal layer that produces brood capsules within which scolices develop. **Cysticercoid,** a form usually found in invertebrates, consists of a small vesicle with a tiny cavity and one scolex. The scolices in all of these larval stages possess suckers and (in armed species) hooklets identical to those of the adult stage. When ingested by the definitive host, the scolex evaginates and attaches itself to the intestinal mucosa; growth of the tapeworm then proceeds by proliferation of segments at the posterior extremity.

Some of the features of important tapeworms of domestic animals are outlined in Table 14–7.

Cysticercosis. The presence of larvae of certain tapeworms in the tissues of man or animals results in a disease known as **cysticercosis** (beef or pork "measles," bladderworm disease). The effect upon the host depends largely upon the organs involved and the degree of parasitism. In some sites, such as peritoneum and subcutis, the cysticerci are tolerated with little reaction, but those species that invade and displace tissue in critical organs (liver, heart, brain) may produce grave signs or death.

Cysticercus bovis (larva of *Taenia saginata*, beef bladderworm), which may be found in muscle, liver, heart, lungs, diaphragm, lymph nodes, and other parts of the body of cattle, is of importance because the bovine parasite is the intermediate stage of a human tapeworm. Few symptoms are produced in cattle, but in some cases of massive infection death may occur following a febrile course. The cysticerci are usually found on postmortem inspection as small cysts, up to 9 mm in diameter, in musculature or (in the heart) partly embedded and partly projecting from the surface. The cysts are white or gray, with a small yellowish spot representing the scolex, which is unarmed (without hooklets). As a rule, the principal tissue change is displacement of normal cells, with little inflammatory reaction surrounding the viable bladderworm. In long-standing cases, however, death of the parasite is followed by dense encapsulation with eventual formation of a scar. Microscopic sections through the lesion may disclose the thin bladder wall and the invaginated scolex of the cysticercus bearing hooklets. The adult *T. saginata* has four suckers, but lacks a rostellum and has no hooks.

Cysticercus cellulosae, the pork bladderworm, or worm of "pork measles," is the intermediate stage of *Taenia solium,* the adult that occurs in the small intestine of man. In some instances this bladderworm has been found in cattle, sheep, deer, and man. The cysticerci resemble *C. bovis* and are most frequent in striated muscles, particularly of the neck, cheek, shoulder, and tongue, but the heart, abdominal wall, liver, lungs, brain, and eye may be involved. This bladderworm is very like *Cysticercus bovis*, except that the scolex bears a double row of hooklets. This tapeworm is of serious import in man because of the possibility of autoinfection, with cysticerci developing in the tissues. Diagnosis in man is often possible by radiography because of the frequent calcification of mature cysts.

Cysticercus ovis, the intermediate stage of *Taenia ovis*, a tapeworm of dogs, foxes, wolves, coyotes, and other carnivores, is the cause of sheep "measles," or ovine cysticercosis. The bladderworms are found in the connective tissue of the heart, voluntary muscles, diaphragm, esophagus, and rarely, the lungs of sheep and goats. The effect of this parasite on its intermediate host is similar to that of the other cysticerci that invade the same tissues. Experimental feeding of large numbers of gravid proglottides of *Taenia ovis* has caused death in sheep. Heavy infections are also the cause of condemnation of animals slaughtered for food.

Coenurus cerebralis, the larval stage of a dog tapeworm, *Multiceps multiceps*, is the causative agent of a rather uncommon disease of the central nervous system of sheep known as "gid" or "sturdy." It may also infect other herbivorous animals and rarely carnivores, monkeys, and man. Symptoms indicating central nervous involvement depend upon localization of the bladderworms in the brain or spinal cord, and vary from incoordination to paralysis. The larvae wander through the body before localizing in nervous tissue in the form of cysts, which reach a diameter of 50 mm or more. Each cyst is filled with clear fluid and contains as many as 500 scolices, visible through the thin walls of the cyst as small white foci. The **coenurus** is a modified cysticercus with a germinal layer and the ability to produce many scolices. The disease has not been recognized in sheep in the United States for several decades. A relatively recent report described a coenurus in the brain of a cat in New York (Georgi et al., 1969).

Cysticercus tenuicollis, the intermediate stage of a tapeworm of dogs and other carnivores, *Taenia hydatigena*, is found chiefly in the liver, mesentery, and omentum of squirrels, cattle, wild ruminants, sheep, and swine. The cysticerci may be large, often attaining a diameter of 80 mm, but they contain only a single scolex armed with a double row of hooklets. The effect upon the intermediate host may not be obvious, the cysticerci merely being noted during postmortem examination. The migration of the larvae through the liver results in necrotic tracts similar to those caused by *Fasciola hepatica*.

Other cysticerci that may be encountered by the veterinary pathologist include *Cysticercus pisiformis*, which occurs on the peritoneum and liver capsule of rabbits, squirrels, and other small rodents. The adult stage of this parasite (*Taenia pisiformis*) is attained in the small intestine of the dog, cat, fox, wolf, and other carnivores. A similar parasite, *Cysticercus fasciolaris* (or *crassicollis*), is found embedded in the liver of rats, mice, and other rodents; the adult form (*Taenia taeniaeformis*) being a tapeworm of the cat, less often of the dog, fox, and other carnivores. *Cysticercus fasciolaris* is of particular interest because of the undifferentiated sarcoma that often develops in the rat liver adjacent to the parasites. A bladderworm found in the subcutis of rabbits is known as *Coenurus serialis* and is the intermediate stage of *Multiceps serialis*, a tapeworm of the dog and closely related carnivores.

Sparganosis is a term used to designate infection with the larva (**sparganum**) of certain Pseudophyllidea; the adults occur in mammals. The sparganum is an elongated, solid larva (**plerocercoid**) which may increase in number by transverse division. The first intermediate hosts are species of *Cyclopidae* and the second are frogs, snakes, and mammals. In some, the sparganum is recognized but the adult form has not been identified. *Sparganum proliferum* occurs in the muscles and connective tissues of man in Taiwan and Japan, and the adult stage is thought to be *Spirometra ranarum*, parasitic in frogs. *Spirometra mansoni*, found in dogs and cats in Asia, produces spargana which are found in the connective tissues of frogs and snakes. *Sparganum mansoni* may infect the eye of man through the practice of applying the flesh of frogs to treat eye disease, or by the consumption of infected *Cyclops sp.*, frogs, or snakes.

Spirometra mansonoides parasitizes the cat, bobcat, and dog in North America. Larvae (procercoids) infect various *Cyclops* species (*C. leukarti*, *C. bicuspidatus*, and *C. viridis*), and the second intermediate hosts are wild mice, rats, and snakes. Experimental infection of man has been demonstrated.

Spirometra erinacei has been found in the intestine of foxes and cats in Asia and Australia.

Wild pigs infected with spargana have been found in the same habitat and are believed to have acquired them from infected crustaceans or frogs. The precise association and identification of the larvae and adult forms of these parasites are not clearly established.

Tetrathridiosis is an infection with the intermediate stages of *Mesocestoides spp.* These stages resemble spargana and are often referred to as such. The adult tapeworms, which are of little consequence, parasitize dogs, cats, man, and other mammals. Although imperfectly understood, the life cycle uses two intermediate hosts: a mite, followed by dogs, cats, wild mammals, or reptiles. In the second intermediate host, tetrathridia develop in the peritoneal and pleural cavities, lung, liver, and other organs, where they may incite an intense purulent and necrotizing inflammatory response, which ultimately progresses to a granulomatous reaction. *M. corti* occurs in North and Central America, and *M. lineatus*, in Europe and Asia.

Banerjee, D., and Singh, K.S.: Studies on *Cysticercus fasciolaris*. III. Histopathology and histochemistry of rat liver in cysticerciasis. Indian J. Anim. Sci., *39*:242–249, 1969.

Becklund, W.W.: Current knowledge of the gid bladder worm, *Coenurus cerebralis* (=*Taenia multiceps*), in North American domestic sheep, *Ovis aries*. Proc. Helminthol. Soc. Wash., *37*:200–203, 1970.

Clark, J.D.: Coenurosis in a Gelada baboon (*Theropithecus gelada*). J. Am. Vet. Med. Assoc., *155*:1258–1263, 1969.

Corkum, K.C.: Sparganosis in some vertebrates of Louisiana and observations on human infection. J. Parasitol., *52*:444–448, 1966.

Dinnik, J.A., and Sachs, R.: Cysticercosis, echinococcosis and sparganosis in wild herbivores in East Africa. Vet. Med. Rev. Leverkusen, No. 2. 104–114, 1969.

Gemmell, M.A.: Hydatidosis and cysticercosis. 2. Distribution of *Cysticercus ovis* in sheep. Aust. Vet. J., *46*:22–24, 1970.

Georgi, J.R., DeLahunta, A., and Percy, D.H.: Cerebral coenurosis in a cat. Report of a case. Cornell Vet., *59*:127–134, 1969.

Greve, J.H., and Tyler, D,E.: *Cysticercus pisiformis* (Cestoda: Taenidae) in the liver of a dog. J. Parasitol., *50*:712–716, 1964.

Hernández-Jáuregui, P.A., Márquez-Monter, H., and Sastré-Ortiz, S.: Cysticercosis of the central nervous system in hogs. Am. J. Vet. Res., *34*:451–453, 1973.

Irfan, M., and Hatch, C.: The pathology of *Taenia hydatigena* infection in Irish lambs. Irish Vet. J., *23*:62–66, 1969.

Ivens, V., Conroy, J.D., and Levine, N.D.: *Taenia pisiformis* cysticerci in a dog in Illinois. Am. J. Vet. Res., *30*:2017–2020, 1969.

Kassai, T., and Mahunka, S.: Vectors of *Moniezia*. Magy. Allatorv. Lap., *19*:531–538, 1964. VB 35:4282, 1965.

Larsh, J.E., Jr., Race, G.J., and Esch, G.W.: A histopathologic study of mice infected with the larval stage of *Multiceps serialis*. J. Parasitol., *51*:45–52, 1965.

Lloyds, T.S.: Hepatitis cysticercosa causing sudden death in a pig. Vet. Rec., *76*:1080, 1964.

McIntosh, A., and Miller, D.: Bovine cysticercosis, with special reference to the early developmental stages of *Taenia saginata*. Am. J. Vet. Res., *21*:169–177, 1960.

Migaki, G., and Zinter, D.E.: Hepatic lesions caused

by *Cysticercus tenuicollis* in sheep. J. Am. Vet. Med. Assoc., *164*:618–619, 1974.

Norman, L., Sadum, E.H., and Allain, D.S.: A bentonite flocculation test for the diagnosis of hydatid disease in man and animals. Am. J. Trop. Med. Hyg., *8*:46–50, 1959.

Pawlowski, Z., and Schultz, M.G.: Taeniasis and cysticercosis *(Taenia saginata)*. Adv. Parasitol., *10*:269–343, 1972.

Rees, G.: Pathogenesis of adult cestodes. Helminth Abstr., *36*:1–23, 1967.

Schiefer, B.: Sudden death of pigs caused by *Cysticercus tenuicollis*. Tierarztl. Umsch, *21*:276–278, 281, 1966. VB 36:4819, 1966.

Schultz, M.G., Hermos, J.A., and Steele, J.H.: Epidemiology of beef tapeworm infection in the United States. Publ. Health Rep., *85*:169–176, 1970.

Silverman, P.H., and Hulland, T.J.: Histological observations on bovine cysticercosis. Res. Vet. Sci., *2*:248–252, 1961. VB 4022–61.

Tazieva, A. K.: Histological differences between cysticerci of small ruminants. Parazity sel'skokhoz zhivotnykh Kazakhstan, *3*:7–29, 1964. VB 35:975, 1965.

Thompson, J.E.: Some observations on the European broad fish tapeworm *Diphyllobothrium latum*. J. Am. Vet. Med. Assoc., *89*:77–86, 1936.

Todd, K.S., Jr., Simon, J., and DiPietro, J.A.: Pathological changes in mice infected with tetrathyridia of *Mesocestoides corti*. Lab. Anim., *12*:51–53, 1978.

Vickers, J.H., and Penner, L.R.: Cysticercosis in four rhesus brains. J. Am. Vet. Med. Assoc., *153*:868–871, 1968.

Voge, M., and Berntzen, A.K.: Asexual multiplication of larval tapeworms as the cause of fatal parasitic ascites in dogs. J. Parasitol., *49*:983–988, 1963.

Wardle, R.A., and McLeod, J.A.: The Zoology of Tapeworms. Minneapolis, University of Minnesota Press, 1952.

Echinococcosis

The intermediate stages of *Echinococcus granulosus* and *E. multilocularis*, tapeworms of dogs, cats, foxes, wolves, and other carnivores, are important because of the effects of the larvae upon their intermediate hosts, which include sheep, goats, cattle, horses, deer, moose, swine, monkeys, rodents, and man. In man, **echinococcosis** or **hydatid disease** is particularly serious because the cysts may reach any part of the body, especially the liver and lung, but also the brain, where their large size (up to 200 mm diameter) and tendency to produce endogenous daughter cysts may displace vital tissues. The cysts grow slowly, often

being encapsulated by dense fibrous tissue of the host. The larva has an outer dense laminated wall without nuclei, which encloses a germinal layer. From this layer numerous spherical brood capsules arise, which may be attached by a short stalk or may be free in the bladder. Each brood capsule contains germinal epithelium from which as many as 40 scolices arise. Each scolex is ovoid and bears a crown of 32 to 40 hooklets, 21 to 29 μ in length. In addition to producing brood capsules, the germinal epithelium of the larva may give rise to daughter cysts, which may remain free within the parent cyst or grow outside the parent cyst.

The ability to form exogenous daughter cysts is limited to *Echinococcus multilocularis (alveolaris)*, according to the work of Rausch (1954). His observations indicate that the "alveolar form" of the disease is caused by *E. multilocularis*, a distinct species with a separate but overlapping host and geographic distribution. Daughter cysts may produce additional brood capsules containing scolices. Individual scolices also may arise within the brood capsules or directly from the germinal layers of parent or daughter cysts. It is readily apparent that the potential of the intermediate stage of either *Echinococcus granulosus* or *multilocularis* for growth and reproduction is considerable. The effect upon the intermediate host therefore depends upon the organ parasitized and the size attained by the hydatid cysts. In experimentally infected mice, it has been demonstrated that male mice are more susceptible than females, and that exogenous testosterone can increase the susceptibility of female mice (Frayha et al., 1971). Greater susceptibility of males to several different forms of parasites has been noted in a number of different species of animals. In some parts of the world, hydatidosis is a major problem in public health.

Several subspecies of *E. granulosa* have been described from South Africa (Verster, 1965). The host range of these parasites has

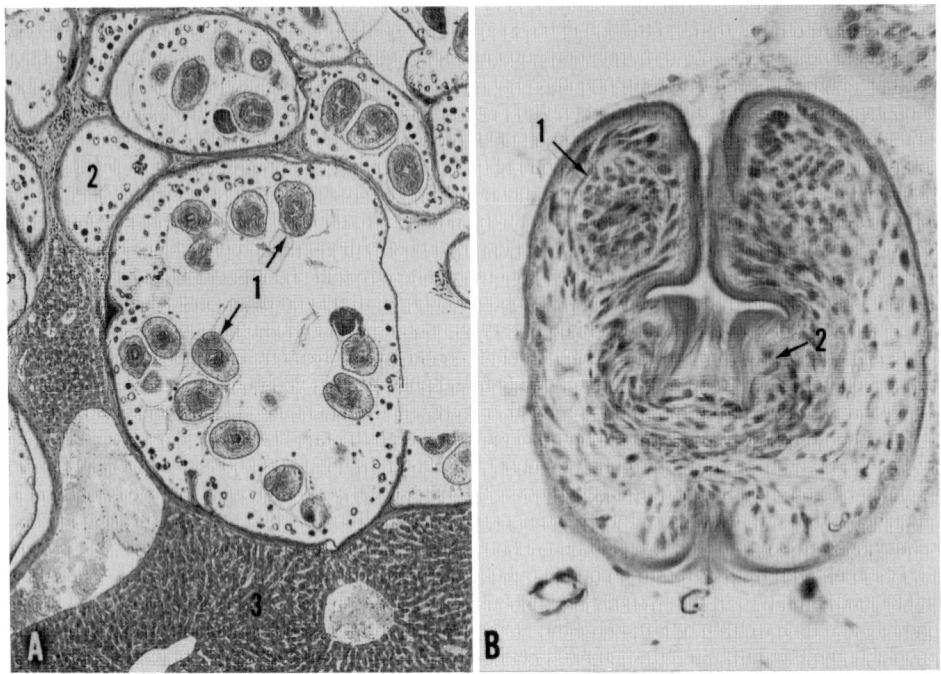

Fig. 14–32. Echinococcosis. A, *Echinococcus multilocularis* (× 50) in the liver of a vole. Note many inverted scolices *(1)*, some surrounded by a thin, brood capsule. Some daughter cysts *(2)* do not yet contain fully developed scolices. Liver parenchyma *(3)* is displaced by the cysts. B, A single scolex (× 525). Note part of inverted sucker *(1)* and hooklets *(2)*. (Courtesy of Armed Forces Institute of Pathology.) Contributor: Dr. Robert Rausch.

not been defined. They have been named as follows: *Echinococcus granulosus, E. g. africanus, E. g. felidus, E. g. lycaontis,* and *E. g. ortleppi.*

Diagnosis. The presence of the adult worm in the intestinal tract can be verified by the demonstration of segments and ova in the feces, but the intermediate stage presents more difficulties. The hydatid cysts may be identified by pathologic examination of tissue removed at exploratory laparotomy or at necropsy. Complement fixation test, delayed hypersensitivity tests, hemagglutination tests, fluorescent antibody test, and other immunologic procedures have been used with varying results (Gore et al., 1970).

Crosby, W. M., Ivey, M.H., Shaffer, W.L., and Holmes, D.D.: Echinococcus cysts in the Savannah baboon. Lab. Anim. Care, *18*:395–397, 1968.

Dent, C.H.R.: Cerebral hydatids in a cow. Aust. Vet. J., *42*:28–30, 1966.

Frayha, G.J., Lawlor, W.K., and Dajani, R.M.: *Echinococcus granulosus* in albino mice: effect of host sex and sex hormones on the growth of hydatid cysts. Exp. Parasitol., *29*:255–262, 1971.

Gore, R.W., Sadun, E.H., and Hoff, R.: *Echinococcus granulosus* and *E. multilocularis:* soluble antigen fluorescent antibody test. Exp. Parasitol., *28*:272–279, 1970.

Hatch, C.: Hydatidosis in Irish horses. Irish Vet. J., *26*:74–77, 1972.

Healy, G.R., and Hayes, N.R.: Hydatid disease in rhesus monkeys. J. Parasitol., *49*:837, 1963.

Hutchison, W.F.: Studies on *Echinococcus granulosus.* III. The rhesus monkey (*Macaca mulatta*) as a laboratory host for the larval stage. J. Parasitol., *52*:416, 1966.

Ilievski, V., and Esber, H.: Hydatid disease in a rhesus monkey. Lab. Anim. Care, *19*:199–204, 1969.

Kostyak, J., and Adam, T.: Experimental echinococcosis in pigs. Magy. Allatorv. Lap., *20*:166–169, 1965. VB *36*:1861, 1966.

Leiby, P.D.: Cestode in North Dakota: echinococcus in field mice. Science, *150*:763, 1965.

Leiby, P.D., and Kritsky, D.C.: *Echinococcus mul-*

tilocularis: a possible domestic life cycle in central North America and its public health implications. J. Parasitol., *58*:1213–1215, 1972.

Leiby, P.D., and Olsen, O.W.: The cestode *Echinococcus multilocularis* in foxes in North Dakota. Science, *145*:1066, 1964.

Matoff, K., and Yanchev, Y.: The fox as definitive host of *Echinococcus granulosus.* Acta Vet. Hung., *15*:155–160, 1965. VB *36*:640, 1966.

Myers, B.J., Kuntz, R.E., and Vice, T.E.: Hydatid disease in captive primates (*Colobus* and *Papio*). J. Parasitol., *51*(Suppl.):22, 1965.

Powers, R.D., Price, R.A., Houk, R.P., and Mattlin, R.H.: Echinococcosis in a drill baboon. J. Am. Vet. Med. Assoc., *149*:902–905, 1966.

Rausch, R.: Studies on the helminth fauna of Alaska. XX. The histogenesis of alveolar larvae of *Echinococcus* species. J. Infect. Dis., *94*:178–186, 1954.

Rausch, R., and Schiller, E.L.: Studies on the helminth fauna of Alaska. XXIV. *Echinococcus sibiricensis* N. Sp. from St. Lawrence Island. J. Parasitol., *40*:659–662, 1954.

Simitch, T.: (*Echinococcus multilocularis* and *E. granulosus:* world incidence and distribution.) Bull. Off. Int. Epizoot., *62*:1031–1061, 1964.

Smyth, J.D., and Smyth, M.M.: Some aspects of host specificity in *Echinococcus granulosus.* Helminthologia, *9*:519–529, 1968.

Verster, A.J.M.: Review of echinococcus species in South Africa. Onderstepoort. J. Vet. Res., *32*:7–118, 1965.

Ward, J.W.: Additional records of *Echinococcus granulosus* from dogs in the lower Mississippi region. J. Parasitol., *51*:552–553, 1965.

Distomiasis (Fascioliasis, Liver Fluke Disease, Liver Rot, Fascioloidiasis, Dicrocoeliasis)

The liver flukes recognized as significant pathogens in domestic animals are presently classified within the order Digenea under the class Trematoda, and are limited to two families, Fasciolidae and Dicrocoeliidae. Four species are of particular importance as the cause of distomiasis in animals: *Fasciola hepatica* (common liver fluke), *Fasciola gigantica* (large African liver fluke), *Fascioloides magna* (large liver fluke), and *Dicrocoelium dendriticum* (lancet fluke).

Fasciola hepatica in its adult form is found in the liver, bile ducts, and gallbladder of cattle and sheep, but it may also parasitize the horse (rarely), goat, dog, rabbit, guinea pig, squirrel, deer, beaver, pig, and man. The adult fluke is 20 to 30 mm long and about 13 mm wide, flattened and leaf-like, and usually reddish-brown. It is hermaphroditic and reproduces by depositing ova in the biliary passages, through which they reach the intestine and are expelled with the feces. Each ovum produces a free-living form, a miracidium, which penetrates the body of one of several varieties of snails, where encystment and asexual reproduction take place through several stages. The parasites finally emerge from the snail in motile forms known as cercariae, which usually encyst on plants or other vegetation. In this form, called **metacercariae,** the parasites are ingested by cattle or other hosts; when they reach the intestines they excyst, penetrate the wall and migrate to the liver, eventually developing to maturity in the biliary passages.

Fasciola gigantica resembles *Fasciola hepatica* but is larger, the adult measures up to 75 mm in length and is about 12 mm wide. The eggs measure 156 to 197 microns by 90 to 104 microns. These flukes are common parasites of cattle and sheep in Africa and are reported to occur in India, Taiwan, Hawaii and the Philippines. The intermediate hosts (Kendall and Parfitt, 1965) are different races of the snail *Lymnaea auricularia.* The effects of this trematode on the adult host are similar to those caused by *Fasciola hepatica.*

Clinical Manifestations. The signs of distomiasis are hardly specific, since they consist of weakness, anemia, emaciation, and at times, icterus. Diarrhea and constipation have been observed. Severe infection, particularly of sheep and young calves, may result in prostration and death. Pregnant animals may abort.

Lesions. The lesions produced by the common liver fluke are most constant and important in the liver, although occasional parasites may wander into the lungs or other tissues, where they are usually found within abscesses. Infective metacercariae of *Fasciola hepatica,* upon

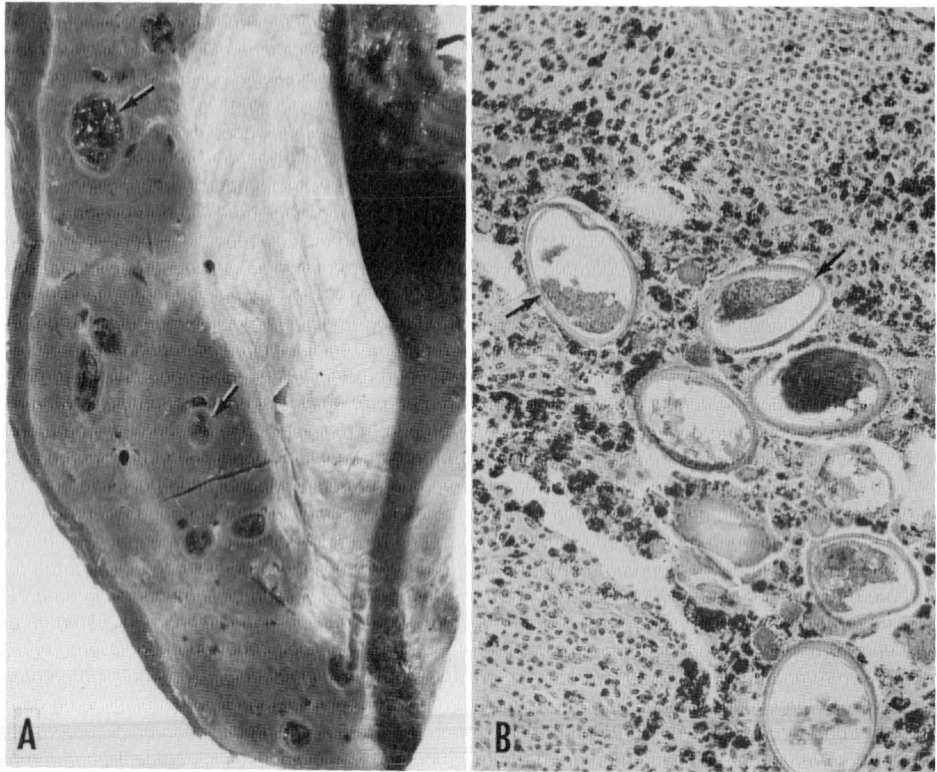

Fig. 14–33. Distomiasis. *A*, Liver of a sheep with distended, thick-walled bile ducts (arrows) containing *Dicrocoelium dendriticum.* Contributor: Dr. G. Dikmans. *B*, Ova of *Fascioloides magna* (arrows) in a bovine liver (× 150). Note black granular pigment interspersed among the ova. (Courtesy of Armed Forces Institute of Pathology.) Contributor: Dr. Henry J. Griffiths.

ingestion by a definitive host, pass through the intestinal wall into the peritoneal cavity, thence migrating into the liver parenchyma. The immature flukes spend about six weeks in the liver parenchyma, starting to reach the bile ducts during the seventh week. As the larvae migrate through the liver parenchyma, they result in damage to the liver, which depends upon the number of parasites, their survival or death at this site, and the tissue reaction of the host. After the initial penetration of the liver parenchyma by the flukes, hepatic cells are destroyed, and the larvae lie in a pool of blood, fibrin, and cellular debris. As some larvae die and the host apparently develops sensitivity to the parasite, neutrophils, eosinophils, and lymphocytes be-

come part of the infiltrate. Macrophages and epithelioid cells become increasingly numerous in older lesions, particularly around dead larvae.

If exposed to large numbers of metacercariae, either naturally or experimentally, this early migration results in extensive damage to the liver leading to an acute syndrome characterized by anemia, eosinophilia, peritonitis, and sudden death. This acute syndrome is more frequent in sheep than cattle.

Flukes that reach the bile ducts start producing eggs by the tenth week following oral infection. The presence of these parasites in the biliary passages excites considerable tissue reaction. The biliary epithelium is stimulated to papillary and glandular hyperplasia in some places and

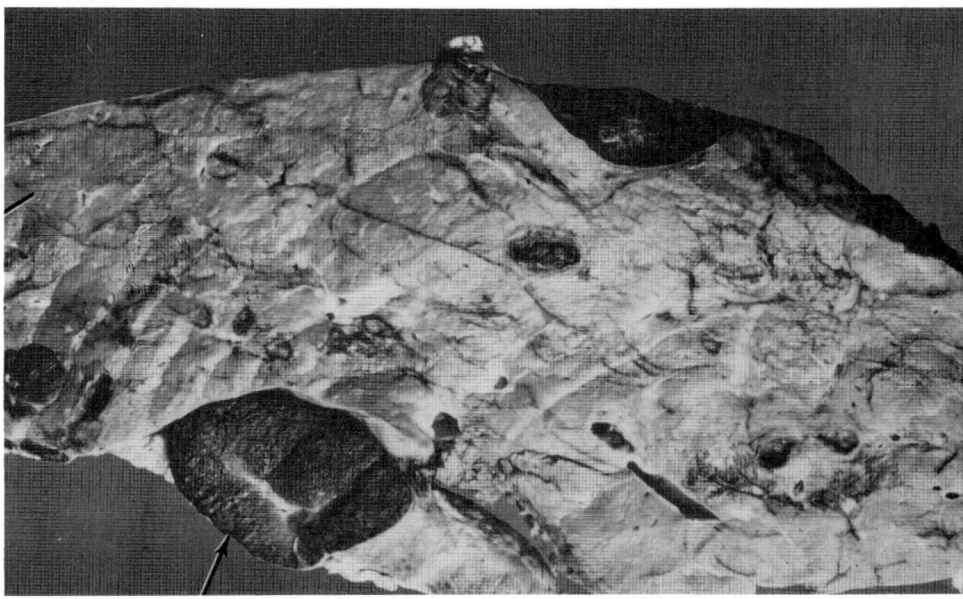

Fig. 14–34. Circumscribed zones of black pigment in the liver of a deer infected with *Fascioloides magna*, the large liver fluke. The adjacent lymph nodes contained similar pigment.

is eroded in others. Partial or complete occlusion of bile ducts is a frequent effect. Globule leukocytes resembling mast cells occur in the hyperplastic epithelium. The origin or significance of these cells is not known, but they have been recognized within mucous membranes of many species in association with various parasitisms. Hyperplasia of the mucosa of the gallbladder has been described by Cheema (1974). The walls of involved bile ducts eventually become greatly thickened from fibrous proliferation, and calcification may take place in the fibrotic areas. The scarring around bile ducts often extends deep into the hepatic lobules, producing severe fibrosis in the perilobular connective tissue. Scarring and calcification may affect large parts of the liver. In longstanding infections, fibrosis and occasional occlusion of bile ducts interferes with liver function, leading to weight loss or failure to gain normally. Elevated serum hepatic enzymes, eosinophilia, hypoproteinemia, and progressive anemia are

usual findings. The hypoproteinemia is a result of low serum albumin due to plasma leakage through bile ducts. Albumin synthesis is not impaired. The anemia is usually normocytic normochromic, but may be macrocytic hypochromic and associated with anisocytosis, poikilocytosis, polychromasia, and basophilic stippling. The pathogenesis of the anemia has been the subject of considerable debate. Interference with vitamin B_{12} and defective erythropoiesis have been suggested, but it appears that hemorrhage into the bile ducts is the principal mechanism.

Fascioloides magna, the large liver fluke, occurs in the liver of cattle, deer, sheep, moose, horse, wapiti, yak, bison and rarely swine, and has also been reported in the lungs of some of these hosts. Rabbits and guinea pigs are susceptible to experimental infection. This fluke is similar in appearance to the common liver fluke, except that it is larger, 30 by 80 mm in greatest dimension, and has more rounded ends. It is hermaphroditic and its life cycle is similar to that of *Fasciola hepatica*, snails being required as intermediate hosts. The infective forms penetrate the intestinal wall and wander around in the peritoneal cavity before invading the liver. Within the liver parenchyma, the migrations of this fluke produce severe damage in some hosts, less in others. In the "true" hosts (deer, wapiti, moose), the parasite is reasonably well tolerated. Although it soon becomes encysted, the cyst wall is thin and its lumen communicates with bile ducts. Thus, ova of the fluke escape with its excreta into the intestinal lumen of the host, a factor that favors the completion of the life cycle of the parasite.

In **Bovidae** (cattle, bison, yak), however, the flukes wander briefly through the liver parenchyma, destroying tissue and eliciting a reaction of the host which encapsulates the parasites. A cyst soon forms, but its lumen rarely communicates with the bile ducts; hence, excreta and ova accumulate around the fluke. Black granular pigment collects in the cyst and is phagocytized by the macrophages of the host. This distinctive pigment is believed to be part of the excrement of the fluke, because similar material can be found within its alimentary tract. The black, sooty pigment is often grossly visible in affected liver. The failure of the fluke to establish and maintain continuity with the bile ducts in these hosts prevents the ova from escaping. For this reason, cattle and bison are unfavorable hosts for the propagation of the parasite.

In **sheep,** the migration of this large liver fluke through the liver is almost entirely unchecked; hence, severe tissue destruction and marked clinical disease result. A severe neutrophilic tissue reaction with little attempt at encapsulation is

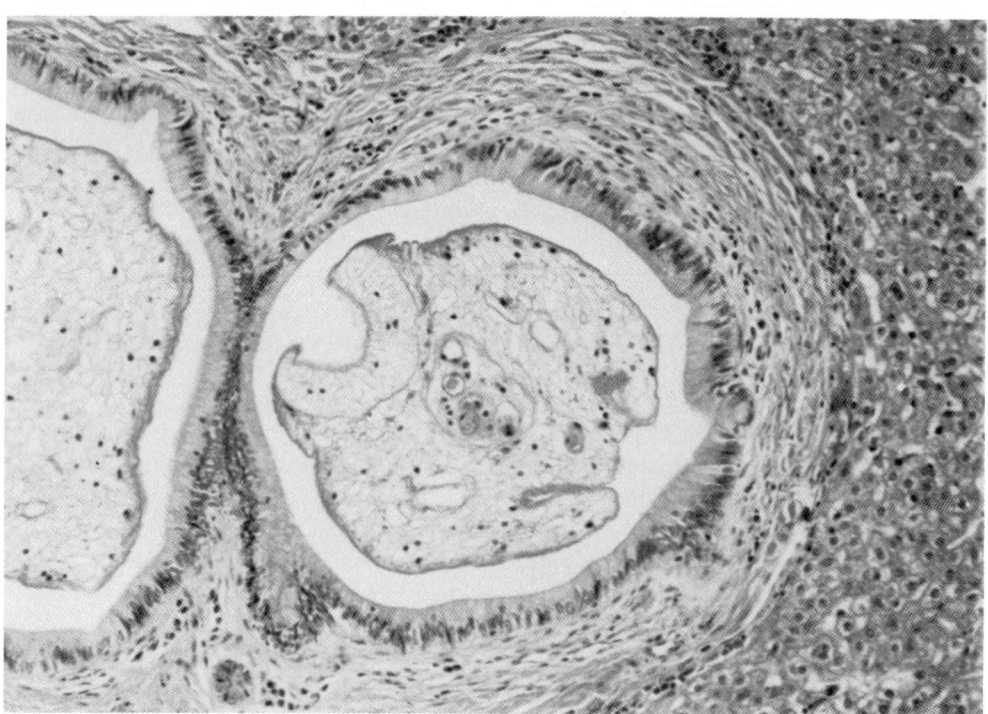

Fig. 14–35. A typical trematode *(Athesmia foxi)* within a bile duct of a *Cebus albifrons* monkey. The infestation is accompanied by slight periductal fibrosis.

the rule in the liver of infected sheep. Even a few flukes may, by their wanderings through the liver, produce severe symptoms and death in sheep. The death of this host brings to a halt the life cycle of the parasite; therefore, the sheep is not considered a true host for *Fascioloides magna*.

Dicrocoelium dendriticum, the Old World, or lancet, fluke, is capable of infecting cattle, sheep, goats, horses, camels, deer, elk, pigs, rabbits, and man. This parasite, smaller than the other flukes, is 5 to 12 mm long and about 1 mm wide. It is slender, flat, and lancet-shaped, with pointed ends.

The life cycle of the lancet fluke has been elucidated by the work of Krull and Mapes (1953), who found that this parasite requires not only a snail as intermediate host, but also an ant (*Formica fusca*) as a second intermediate host. The final hosts are infected by the ingestion of ants containing encysted metacercariae. A fascinating bit of biologic knowledge lies in the report of Anokhin (1966), who confirmed Hohorst's observation that encysted metacercariae in the brains of ants (*Formica nigricans*) cause the ants to remain on herbage after normal ants return to their nest. This presumably increases the possibility that infected ants will be ingested by a grazing cow or sheep. The adult flukes are found in the bile ducts of the definitive host. The infection is less severe than that of *Fasciola hepatica;* and being smaller, they may be found in smaller bile ducts. There is hyperplasia of bile duct epithelium, and although superficial erosions are present, plasma or blood loss is not extensive. The walls of the bile ducts become thickened, and general periportal fibrosis may be produced by the parasite. There is little tendency for destruction of liver parenchyma.

Diagnosis. Distomiasis can be recognized in the living host by the identification of characteristic ova in the feces (Fig. 14–33). At necropsy or biopsy of the liver,

the lesions in the liver are typical and the parasite can usually be found in the liver parenchyma or affected biliary system.

Anokhin, I.A.: The diurnal rhythm of ants invaded by *Dicrocoelium lanceatum* metacercariae. Dokl. Akad. Nauk. SSSR, *166*:757–759, 1966.
Ashizawa, H.: Pathological studies on fascioliasis. I. The liver of goats. II. The liver of sheep. III. The liver of cattle. IV. The liver of experimentally infected goats, rabbits and guinea pigs. Bull. Fac. Agric. Univ. Miyazaki, *9*:1–44, 143–191; *10*:1–40, 189–221, 1963/65. VB 35:3886, 1965.
———: Pathological studies on fascioliasis. V. Parasitic bronchiectasis in cattle caused by *Fasciola sp.* Bull. Fac. Agric. Univ. Miyazaki, *12*:1–57, 1966. VB 37:4779, 1967.
Bailenger, J., et al.: Hares and rabbits as reservoirs of *Fasciola hepatica* and *Dicrocoelium dendriticum*. Ann. Parasit. Hum. Comp., *40*:51–54, 1965. VB 35:4644, 1965.
Baker, D.W., and Nelson, S.K.: *Dicrocoelium dendriticum* infections in New York State cattle. Cornell Vet., *33*:250–256, 1943.
Bengtsson, E., et al.: Infestation with *Dicrocoelium dendriticum*—the small liver fluke—in animals and human individuals in Sweden. Acta Path. Microbiol. Scand., *74*:85–92, 1968.
Beresford, O.D.: A case of fascioliasis in man. Vet. Rec., *98*:15, 1976.
Cheema, A.H.: Adenomatous cholecystitis in cattle with chronic fascioliasis. Vet. Pathol., *11*:407–416, 1974.
Dawes, B., and Hughes, D.L.: Fascioliasis: the invasive stages in mammals. Adv. Parasitol., *8*:259–274, 1970.
Dow, C., Ross, J.G., and Todd, J.R.: The pathology of experimental fascioliasis in calves. J. Comp. Pathol., *77*:377–385, 1967.
———: The histopathology of *Fasciola hepatica* infections in sheep. Parasitology, *58*:129–135, 1968.
Hatch, C.: *Fasciola hepatica* infection in donkeys. Irish Vet. J., *20*:130, 1966.
Holmes, P.H., et al.: Albumin and globulin turnover in chronic ovine fascioliasis. Vet. Rec., *83*:227–228, 1968.
Hjerpe, C.A., Tennant, B.C., Crenshaw, G.L., and Baker, N.F.: Ovine fascioliasis in California. J. Am. Vet. Med. Assoc., *159*:1266–1271, 1971.
Keck, G., and Supperer, R.: Studies on the large liver fluke. I. The x-ray picture of isolated ox livers. II. The course of infection of the bovine liver. Wien. tierarztl. Mschr., *53*:29–33, 328–331, 1966. VB 36:3548, 1966.
Kendall, S.B.: Host specificity as evidenced by species of *Fasciola*. Helminthologia, *8*:223–233, 1968.
Kendall, S.B., and Parfitt, J.W.: The life-history of some vectors of *Fasciola gigantica* under laboratory conditions. Ann. Trop. Med. Parasitol., *59*:10–16, 1965.
Konrad, J.: The biochemical picture in bovine hepatic cirrhosis due to fascioliasis. Tierärztl. Umsch., *23*:369–372, 375–376, 1968. VB 39:215, 1969.

Krull, W.H., and Mapes, C.R.: Studies on the biology of *Dicrocoelium dendriticum* (Rudolphi, 1819) Looss 1899—including its relation to the intermediate host, *Cionella lubrica* (Müller). III. Observations on the slimeballs of *Dicrocoelium dendriticum*. Cornell Vet., *42*:253–276, 1952.

———: Studies on the biology of *Dicrocoelium dendriticum* (Rudolphi, 1819) Looss 1899—including its relation to the intermediate host, *Cionella lubrica* (Müller). IV. Infection experiments involving definitive hosts. Cornell Vet., *42*:277–285, 1952.

———: Studies on the biology of *Dicrocoelium dendriticum* (Rudolphi, 1819) Looss 1899—including its relation to the intermediate host *Cionella lubrica*. IX. Notes on the cyst, metacercaria, and infection in the ant, *Formica fusca*. Cornell Vet., *43*:389–410, 1953.

Migaki, G., Zinter, D.E., and Garner, F.M.: Fascioloides magna in the pig—3 cases. Am. J. Vet. Res., *32*:1417–1421, 1971.

Nansen, P.: Albumin metabolism in chronic *Fasciola hepatica* infections of cattle. Acta Vet. Scand., *12*:335–343, 1971.

Nansen, P., Andersen, S., and Hesselholt, M.: Experimental infection of the horse with *Fasciola hepatica*. Exp. Parasitol., *37*:15–19, 1975.

Nansen, P., et al.: Chronic fascioliasis in sheep. II. Metabolism of ^{131}I-labelled albumin and ^{125}I-labelled immunoglobulin-G. Nord. Vet. Med., *20*:651–656, 1968.

Pinkiewicz, E., and Madej, E.: Changes in the peripheral blood of Ca, P, K, Na, Mg and AP in the course of experimental fascioliasis in sheep. Acta Parasitol. Polon., *15*:225–229, 1967. VB *39*:217, 1969.

Poljakova-Krusteva, O., et al.: The morphogenesis of experimental fascioliasis. J. Helminthol., *42*:367–372, 1968.

Pullan, N.B., Sewell, M.M.H., and Hammond, J.A.: Studies on the pathogenicity of massive infections of *Fasciola hepatica* in lambs. Br. Vet. J., *126*:543–558, 1970.

Rahko, T.: The pathology of natural *Fasciola hepatica* infection in cattle. Pathol. Vet., *6*:244–256, 1969.

Rahko, T.: Globule leukocyte and mast cell in bile ducts of cattle naturally infected with liver flukes. Acta Vet. Scand., *11*:219–227, 1970.

Robinson, V.B., and Ehrenford, F.A.: Hepatic lesions associated with liver fluke (*Platynosomum fastosum*) infection in a cat. Am. J. Vet. Res., *23*:1300–1303, 1962.

Ross, J.G., Dow, C., and Todd, J.R.: A study of *Fasciola hepatica* infections in sheep. Vet. Rec., *80*:543–546, 1967.

———: The pathology of *Fasciola hepatica* infection in pigs. A comparison of the infection in pigs and other hosts. Br. Vet. J., *123*:317–322, 1967.

Ross, J.G.: Experimental infections of cattle with *Fasciola hepatica*: a comparison of low and high infection rates. Nature (Lond.), *208*:907, 1965.

Ross, J.G., and Dow, C.:The problem of acute fascioliasis in cattle. Vet. Rec., *78*:670, 1966.

Rossow, N., et al.: The liver in bovine fascioliasis:

biopsy and function tests. Arch. Exp. Vet. Med., *20*:307–321, 1966. VB *37*:602, 1967.

Rubaj, B., and Furmaga, S.: Pathomorphological and histochemical studies of livers of sheep experimentally infected with the liver fluke. Acta Parasitol. Polon., *16*:77–81, 1969. VB *39*:5048, 1969.

Sewell, M.M.H.: The immunology of fascioliasis. II. Qualitative studies on the precipitin reaction. Immunology, *7*:671–680, 1964.

———: The pathogenesis of fascioliasis. Vet. Rec., *78*:98–105, 1966.

———: Serum enzyme activities in acute ovine fascioliasis. Vet. Rec., *80*:577–578, 1967.

Simesen, M.G., et al.: Chronic fascioliasis in sheep. I. Clinical, clinical-pathological and histological studies. Nord. Vet. Med., *20*:638–650, 1968. VB *39*:2100, 1969.

Sinclair, K.B.: Iron metabolism in ovine fascioliasis. Br. Vet. J., *121*:451–461, 1965.

———: The pathogenicity of *Fasciola hepatica* in pregnant sheep. Br. Vet. J., *128*:249–259, 1972.

———: Studies on the anaemia of chronic ovine fascioliasis. Res. Vet. Sci., *13*:182–184, 1972.

Sofrenovic, D., et al.: Pathology, incidence and diagnosis of liver flukes in pigs. (In Serbian.) Acta Vet., Belgrade, *11*:31–40, 1961. VB 186–62.

Stemmermann, G.N.: Human infestation with *Fasciola gigantica*. Am. J. Pathol., *29*:731–753, 1953.

Swales, W.E.: The life cycle of *Fascioloides magna* (Bassi, 1875). The large liver fluke of ruminants in Canada. Can. J. Res., *12*:177–215, 1935.

———: Further studies on *Fascioloides magna* (Bassi, 1875), Ward 1917, as a parasite of ruminants. Can. J. Res., *14*:83–95, 1936.

Symons, L.E.A., and Boray, J.C.: The anaemia of acute and chronic ovine fascioliasis. Z. Tropenmed. Parasitol., *19*:451–472, 1968. VB *39*:1648, 1969.

Thorpe, E., and Ford, E.J.H.: Serum enzyme and hepatic changes in sheep infested with *Fasciola hepatica*. J. Pathol., *97*:619–629, 1969.

Tsvetaeva, N.P., and Gumen'shchikova, V.P.: Pathology and histochemistry of the liver of sheep with acute or chronic fascioliasis following single infection, superinfection and reinfection. Mater. Konf. Vses. Obshch. Gel'mint., *2*:255–259, 1965. VB *37*:2693, 1967.

Schistosomiasis

Studies of ancient Egyptian records and mummies indicate that since the pre-Christian era the people of the Middle East have been subject to a disease in which hematuria, dysentery and cirrhosis were prominent features. It was not until 1851 that Bilharz observed adult flukes in the veins of an Egyptian, and even later before he demonstrated the relation of the orga-

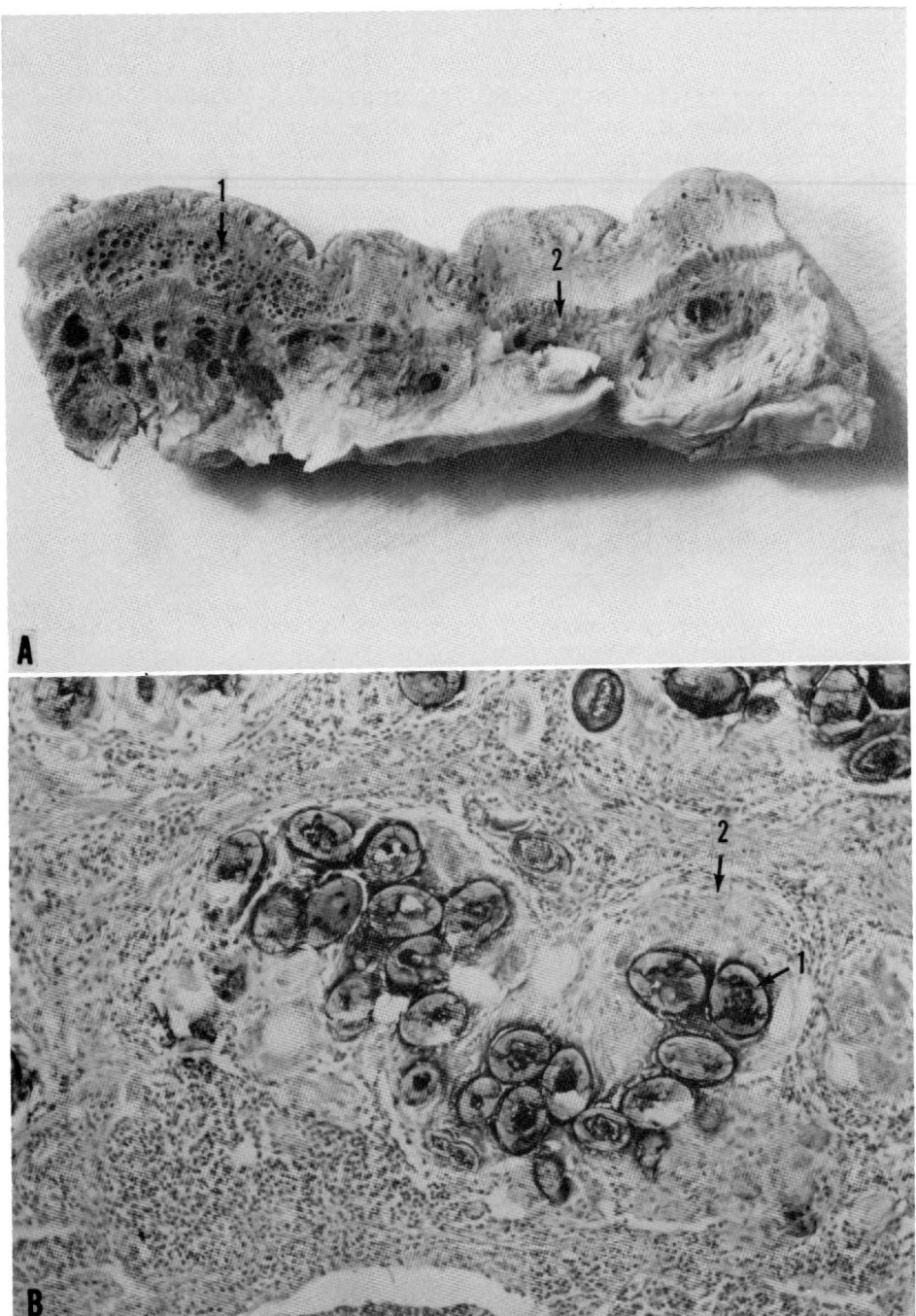

Fig. 14-36. Schistosomiasis. *A,* Small intestine of a dog, with thickened submucosa *(1)* and muscularis. The inner part of the muscularis is marked *(2). B,* Ova of *Schistosoma japonicum* in a lymph node ($\times$ 135) of a dog. The ova *(1)* are surrounded by epithelioid cells *(2)* and fibrous stroma. (Courtesy of Armed Forces Institute of Pathology.) Contributor: 36th Evacuation Hospital.

nisms to this prevalent and historic disease. Many more years elapsed before Leiper, in 1918, demonstrated experimentally that two separate parasites were responsible for the human disease, and that snails were necessary intermediate hosts for the blood flukes.

Although schistosomiasis is today an important parasitic disease in man and animals in many parts of the world, it is not prevalent in the United States, except for some infections of wild birds and mammals.

These worms are small trematodes that live in the blood vessels of their hosts; their ova, which circulate as emboli and lodge in tissue as foreign bodies, produce the principal pathologic changes in the host. The females are slender round worms, 1.4 to 2.0 cm in length; the distinctive feature of the slightly shorter male is a long gynecophoric canal, a canoe-shaped structure in which the female is held during coitus. The blood flukes are classified as Trematoda within the suborder Strigeata, with the parasites of birds and mammals grouped in the fam-

Table 14–8. Schistosomiasis

Species	Natural Definitive Hosts	Anatomic Site of Adult Fluke	Geographic Distribution
Schistosoma japonicum	Man, dog, cat, rat, cattle, sheep, water buffalo, goat, horse, swine	Mesenteric and portal veins, hemorrhoidal plexus	China, Japan, Taiwan, Celebes, Philippines
S. hematobium	Man, monkey	Pelvic veins, esp. vesical and mesenteric, vesicoprostatic, pubic, and uterine plexus	Africa, Western Asia, Southern Europe, Australia
S. mansoni	Man, monkey	Mesenteric and portal veins, hemorrhoidal plexus	Africa, South America, West Indies
S. bovis	Cattle, sheep, goat, horse, mule, antelope, baboon	Portal and mesenteric veins	Africa, Southern Asia, Sardinia
S. spindale	Cattle, sheep, goat, horse, antelope, water buffalo	Mesenteric and portal veins	India, Sumatra, Africa
S. hippopotami	Hippopotamus	Cardiovascular system generally	South Africa
S. incognitum	Dog, pig	Mesenteric and portal veins	India
S. nasalis	Cattle, goats, horses	Nasal veins	India
S. indicum	Cattle, sheep, goats, horse, camels	Mesenteric, portal, and pelvic veins	India
S. intercalatum	Man	Mesenteric and portal veins	Africa
S. mattheei	Cattle, sheep, goats, horses, and rarely man	Mesenteric and portal veins	Africa
Schistosomatium douthitti	Meadow mouse, vole, hare, muskrat	Mesenteric veins	North America
Trichobilharzia ocellata	Wild and domesticated ducks	Mesenteric veins	Europe and North America
T. stagnicolae	Canaries, other birds (?)	Mesenteric veins	North America
T. physellae	Ducks, teal	Mesenteric veins	North America
Heterobilharzia americana	Dog, raccoon, bobcat, rabbit, nutria	Mesenteric veins	North America
Orientobilharzia harinasutai	Water buffalo	Portal and mesenteric veins	Thailand

ily Schistosomatidae. Table 14–8 summarizes certain characteristics of important blood flukes of man and animals.

Life Cycle. All blood flukes have similar life cycles. The adult female, after copulation with the male within the lumen of a vein, moves against the venous blood stream into small venules, where she deposits the ova. Schistosomes that live in the mesenteric veins (*S. bovis, S. japonicum, Heterobilharzia americana,* and *S. mansoni*) deposit their ova in venules of the intestine, while those that dwell in the vesical and other pelvic veins (*S. hematobium* and occasionally *S. mansoni*) utilize venules of the urinary bladder. The ova so deposited secrete cytolytic fluid through pores of the egg shell, which, assisted by the movement of the host's tissues, permits them to rupture the capillary walls and move through the tissues toward the lumen of the intestine or the urinary bladder. The successful ova leave the body of the host with the feces (*S. japonicum, S. bovis, H. americana,* and *S. mansoni*) or the urine (*S. hematobium, S. mansoni*). Unsuccessful ova may remain in any tissue through which they are unable to pass, or they may be transported via the blood stream to other organs, where they produce lesions. Fertile ova will not hatch in the tissues of the host, but upon reaching a favorable external environment, a single, ovoid ciliated organism, a **miracidium,** quickly escapes from the ovum. The miracidium swims about in water until it finds a suitable intermediate host, a snail, whose body it penetrates by a head-on boring action with the aid of proteolytic enzymes secreted by its cephalic glands.

Each schistosome has an affinity for one or more species of snail, which it utilizes as an intermediate host. The availability of suitable gastropod hosts thus influences the geographic distribution of schistosomiasis.

Within the body of the snail, the miracidium soon becomes a thin-walled saccular sporocyst which reproduces several daughter sporocysts. Each of these secondary sporocysts releases thousands of tiny fork-tailed organisms, **cercariae,** which wander through the tissues of the snail, occasionally killing it, and finally emerge into the surrounding water. These cercariae must find a suitable definitive host in order to carry their life cycle further. Upon meeting with such a host, the cercariae penetrate the skin, usually between the hair follicles, undergo certain structural changes, become **metacercariae** and enter small peripheral veins. The metacercariae are carried by the venous circulation to the lungs, where, it is believed they either break through the lung parenchyma, migrating directly to the liver, or reach the arterial system to be carried to the liver. Within the intrahepatic portal system the flukes grow in size, then eventually migrate to the portal, mesenteric, or pelvic veins, depending upon the species, where they attain their adult form and continue the reproductive cycle.

Lesions. It is obvious from the life cycle of parasites of this group that injury to the definitive host can result from the presence of (1) adults in the veins, (2) ova in veins or tissues, (3) cercariae as they penetrate the skin, or (4) metacercariae as they migrate through the tissues.

The adult blood flukes living within the veins may produce some phlebitis, with intimal proliferation and occasionally venous thrombosis. Vascular lesions are most likely to be severe when the adult worms die or are trapped in unusual sites. The adult schistosomes also consume erythrocytes and discharge blood pigment, which is engulfed by macrophages and may be found in reticuloendothelial tissues in the liver and spleen. This pigment appears in the cytoplasm of macrophages as black granules, not unlike that seen in association with certain liver flukes.

The ova of the blood flukes are the most important factors in the production of lesions. The ova deposited in the venules reach venous capillaries, adhere to and become embedded within the endothelium, rupture the basement membrane by means of enzymes secreted through the pores of the egg shell by the miracidium within, and escape into the tissues to make their way to the lumen of the intestine or urinary bladder. This migration leads to small hemorrhagic ulcers, which in extensive infestations may lead to overt hemorrhage, anemia, and hypoproteinemia. Within the tissues, the ovum may stimulate considerable inflammatory reaction upon the part of the host. A microabscess containing neutrophils and eosinophils may surround the ovum at the outset, but if it remains long at the site, a granuloma with foreign body giant cells soon replaces the abscess. This granuloma, or "pseudotubercle," is a characteristic feature of the microscopic findings in schistosomiasis. In sections, ova can be seen within these granulomas, often engulfed by large, foreign-body giant cells. These schistosome eggs are ovoid with a thick, hyaline, unstained, or yellow wall. Sometimes a single spine may be seen protruding from this wall. The spine is located along the lateral surface in ova of *S. mansoni* and at one terminal pole in *S. hematobium, S. bovis, S. indicum, S. intercalatum, S. nasalis,* and *S. spindale;* it is lateral, small and inconspicuous on the ova of *S. japonicum*. The nature and location of the spine can be utilized in identifying the type of infection in some cases. Microscopic sections of ova may contain recognizable parts of the miracidium, but in older lesions only the egg shell may be left. It is often ruptured in such situations, and only a fragment may be present, but the tissue reaction and microscopic appearance of the egg shell are characteristic. The Ziehl-Neelsen stain is useful in differentiating some schistosome eggs. Eggs of *S. mansoni, S. nasalis,* and *S. intercalatum* are acid-fast, whereas *S. spindale, S. indicum, S. hematobium, S. mattheei, S. japonicum,* and *S. bovis* are negative.

As the disease progresses, fibrosis around the granulomas leads to further destruction of tissue and interference with function. Ova in the submucosa or lamina propria of the intestine or the submucosa of the urinary bladder may be assumed to be on their way out of the body of the host. However, many ova are not successful in continuing the life cycle because they gain access to the blood and are circulated widely throughout the body. These ova may cause endarteritis, periarteritis, or phlebitis, or become entrapped in capillaries, which they rupture to escape into the tissues and produce the typical foreign-body granulomas. These embolic ova may reach the liver, spleen, lungs, lymph nodes, skin, testes, brain, or any other organ of the body. In the liver, the cirrhosis in long-standing cases is the result of periportal fibrosis that follows formation of granulomas around embolic ova brought to this site by the portal radicles.

Cutaneous lesions develop in man and animals as a result of penetration of the skin by the cercariae of schistosomes. The intensity of the tissue reaction depends to some extent upon the sensitivity and resistance of the host to the parasite. As the cercariae reach the dermis, a leukocytic reaction of varying intensity is elicited, including neutrophils, lymphocytes, and eosinophils. This is accompanied by urticaria, itching, and formation of tiny nodules that elevate the epidermis. In sensitized animals or man, a severe tissue reaction is provoked, and death of the parasite in the dermis may set up a prolonged local tissue reaction. Cercariae have the ability to penetrate the epidermis of hosts in which complete development of the fluke does not occur, the cercariae dying in the dermis. This is the basis of **cercarial dermatitis** ("swimmer's itch," "collector's itch," "swamp itch"), a problem to individuals exposed to infested waters (e.g., agricultural workers, swimmers). Numerous schistosomes of birds and mammals have been demonstrated to cause cercarial dermatitis, but the most important appear to be *Trichobilharzia* *stagnicolae,* a blood fluke of canaries; *Trichobilharzia ocellata,* a parasite of ducks; *Trichobilharzia physellae* (wild ducks and teal), *Schistosomatium douthitti* (meadow mouse, muskrat) and *Schistosoma spindale* (cattle, sheep, goat, horse, antelope, and water buffalo).

A schistosome of some importance in parts of southern United States is *Heterobilharzia americana.* This parasite, reported for the first time by Malek et al., (1961), to be a parasite of the dog, usually has other definitive hosts: bobcat *(Lynx rufus),* rabbit *(Sylvilagus aquaticus),* raccoon *(Procyon lotor)* and the nutria *(Myocastor coypus).* The life cycle of this schistosome is essentially the same as others described previously. The free-swimming miracidium is released from an ovum to penetrate a snail *(Lymnaea cubensis* or *Pseudosuccinea columella),* in whose digestive gland it undergoes development to a mature cercaria, which in turn penetrates the skin of its mammalian host. After periods of maturation in the lung and liver, the adults move to the mesenteric veins and undergo copulation. Ova reach the intestine, liver, and other viscera, and incite the tissue reaction described previously for *S. japonicum* and *S. mansoni.* Ova appear in the feces about 68 days after cercariae penetrate the skin (the prepatent period). *Schistosomatium douthitti* is the only other schistosome that infests mammals in the United States.

In human beings, carcinoma of the urinary bladder is a not infrequent complication of vesicular schistosomiasis. The carcinomas are often squamous cell types arising in metaplastic epithelium. The exact causal relationship has not been established. Experimentally, neoplasms have developed in nonhuman primates infected with *S. hematobium* and *S. intercalatum;* however, these have been composed of transitional epithelium and not squamous. Glomerulonephritis is also frequently associated with schistosomiasis in human beings, and has been induced experimen-

tally in chimpanzees (Cavallo et al., 1974). Available evidence suggests an immune complex origin, but this has not been firmly established.

Diagnosis. The clinical diagnosis of schistosomiasis can be confirmed by demonstration of schistosome ova in the feces or by histologic examination of biopsy specimens of rectal mucosa, liver, or other affected organs. The adult parasite may be found in veins at necropsy, and the typical ova in granulomas are demonstrable by histologic examination of specimens collected at necropsy or biopsy.

Barbosa, F.S., Barbosa, I., and Malgalhães-Filho, A.: Natural infection of cattle with *Schistosoma mansoni.* Proc. 1st Int. Congr. Parasit. Roma, 2:703–710, 1964. VB 37:2698, 1967.

Bartsch, R.C., and Ward, B.C.: Visceral lesions in raccoons naturally infected with *Heterobilharzia americana.* Vet. Pathol., 13:241–249, 1976.

Brackett, S.: Pathology of schistosome dermatitis. Arch. Dermat. Syph., 42:410–418, 1940.

Cavallo, T., Galvanek, E.G., Ward, P.A., and Von Lichtenberg, F.: The nephropathy of experimental hepatosplenic schistosomiasis. Am. J. Pathol., 76:433–450, 1974.

Cheever, A.W., et al.: Animal model of human disease: carcinoma of the urinary bladder in *Schistosoma haematobium* infection. Proliferative urothelial lesions in nonhuman primates infected with *Schistosoma haematobium.* Am. J. Pathol., 84:673–676, 1976.

Cheever, A.W., Kuntz, R.E., Moore, J.A., and Huang, T.C.: Proliferative epithelial lesions of urinary bladder in cynomolgus monkeys *(Macaca fascicularis)* infected with *Schistosoma intercalatum.* Cancer Res., 36:2928–2931, 1976.

Dargie, J.D., and MacLean, J.M.: Pathophysiology of ovine schistosomiasis. III. Study of plasma protein metabolism in experimental *Schistosoma mattheei* infections. J. Comp. Pathol., 83:543–557, 1973.

Dargie, J.D., and Preston, J.M.: Patho-physiology of ovine schistosomiasis. VI. Onset and development of anaemia in sheep experimentally infected with *Schistosoma mattheei*—ferrokinetic studies. J. Comp. Pathol., 84:83–91, 1974.

Dinnik, J.A., and Dinnik, N.N.: The schistosomes of domestic ruminants in eastern Africa. Bull. Epizoot. Dis. Afr., 13:341–359, 1965. VB 36:3138, 1966.

Fenwick, A.: Baboons as reservoir hosts of *Schistosoma mansoni.* Tr. R. Soc. Trop. Med. Hyg., 63:557–567, 1969.

Hsu, H.F., Davis, J.R., and Hsu, S.Y.L.: Histopathological lesions of Rhesus monkeys and chimpanzees infected with *Schistosoma japonicum.* Z. Tropenmed. Parasitol., 20:184–205, 1969.

Hsu, S.Y.L., Hsu, H.F., Lust, G.L., and Davis, J.R.: Organized epithelioid cell granulomata elicited by schistosome eggs in experimental animals. J. Reticuloendothel. Soc., 12:418–435, 1972.

Hussein, M.F.: The pathology of experimental schistosomiasis in calves. Res. Vet. Sci., 12:246–252, 1971.

Kruatrachue, M., Bhaibulaya, M., and Harinasuta, C.: *Orientobilharzia harinasutai sp. nov.*, a mammalian blood-fluke, its morphology and lifecycle. Ann. Trop. Med. Parasitol., 59:181–188, 1965.

Kuntz, R.E., Cheever, A.W., and Myers, B.J.: Proliferative epithelial lesions of the urinary bladder of non-human primates infected with *Schistosoma haematobium.* J. Natl. Cancer Inst., 48:223–235, 1972.

MacHattie, C., and Chadwick, C.R.: *Schistosoma bovis* and *S. mattheei* in Iraq with notes on development of eggs of *S. haematobium* pattern. Tr. Roy. Soc. Trop. Med. Hyg., 26:147–156, 1932.

Malek, E.A., Ash, L.R., Lee, H.F., and Little, M.D.: *Heterobilharzia* infection in the dog and other mammals in Louisiana. J. Parasitol., 47:619–623, 1961.

Muller, R.L., and Taylor, M.G.: On the use of the Ziehl-Neelsen technique for specific identification of schistosome eggs. J. Helminthol., 46:139–142, 1972.

Olivier, L., and Weinstein, P.P.: Experimental schistosome dermatitis in rabbits. J. Parasitol., 39:280–291, 1953.

Penner, L.R.: Possibilities of systemic infection with dermatitis-producing schistosomes. Science, 93:327–328, 1941.

Perrotto, J.L., and Warren, K.S.: Inhibition of granuloma formation around *Schistosoma mansoni* eggs. IV. X-irradiation. Am. J. Pathol., 56:279–292, 1969.

Pierce, K.R.: *Heterobilharzia americana* infection in a dog. J. Am. Vet. Med. Assoc., 143:496–499, 1963.

Preston, J.M., and Dargie, J.D.: Patho-physiology of ovine schistosomiasis. V. Onset and development of anaemia in sheep experimentally infected wtih *Schistosoma mattheei*—studies with ^{51}Cr-labelled erythrocytes. J. Comp. Pathol., 84:73–81, 1974.

Price, H.F.: Life history of *Schistosomatium douthitti* (Cort). Am. J. Hyg., 13:685–727, 1931.

Saeed, A.A., Nelson, G.S., and Hussein, M.F.: Experimental infections of calves with schistosomes. Trans. R. Soc. Trop. Med. Hyg., 63:15, 1969.

Sharma, D.N., and Dwivedi, J.N.: Pulmonary schistosomiasis in sheep and goats due to *Schistosoma indicum* in India. J. Comp. Pathol., 86:449–454, 1976.

Tewari, H.C., Dutt, S.C., and Iyer, P.K.R.: Observations on the pathogenicity of experimental infection of *Schistosoma incognitum* Chandler (1926) in dogs. Indian J. Vet. Sci., 36:227–231, 1966.

Thrasher, J.P.: Canine schistosomiasis. J. Am. Vet. Med. Assoc., 144:1119–1126, 1964.

Von Lichtenberg, F., Erickson, D.G., and Sadun, E.H.: Comparative histopathology of schistosome granulomas in the hamster. Am. J. Pathol., 72:149–178, 1973.

Warren, K.S.: The pathology of schistosome infections. Helminthol. Abs., 42A:591–633, 1973.

Wu, K.: Cattle as reservoir hosts of *Schistosoma japonicum* in China. Am. J. Hyg., 27:290–297, 1938.

Paragonimiasis

Small reddish-brown, egg-shaped flukes of the genus *Paragonimus* are important parasites of man and animals. These flukes are 8 to 12 mm long, 4 to 6 mm in diameter, hermaphroditic, and have a spiny cuticle. They are currently classified in the family Troglotrematidae, which includes the intestinal fluke of salmon-poisoning *Nanophyetus (Troglotrema) salmincola* (see p. 531). Two species are of particular interest: *Paragonimus westermani*, parasitic in man, and *P. kellicotti*, whose adult host may be mink, dog, cat, pig, muskrat, or opposum.

The adult flukes, *P. kellicotti*, are found in cysts in the lung, where their presence may result in cough, blood-stained sputum (man), mild anemia, and slight fever. The hermaphroditic flukes produce ova which escape from ruptured cysts in the lung parenchyma to reach the bronchi or to enter the circulation and thereby reach the spleen, liver, brain, urinary system, intestinal wall muscles, or other tissues. In these tissue sites, the thick-walled, anisotropic, yellowish-brown ova, which measure 80 to 118 μ in length and 48 to 60 μ in width, incite the production of characteristic epithelioid granulation tissue. The resulting lesion is similar in microscopic appearance to the lesion caused by ova of liver flukes or schistosomes.

Life Cycle. The life cycle of *P. kellicotti* is rather complex. Ova that reach the bronchi are coughed up, swallowed, and reach the exterior with the feces. Under most conditions, miracidia develop slowly in these ova, hatch into water, and then burrow into the tissues of various snails.

In the United States, the fresh-water snail, *Pomatiopsis lapidaria* is most frequently the first intermediate host. Within the snail, the miracidia change into sporocysts, which each produce about 12 first generation **rediae,** which in turn produce a similar number of second generation rediae. These result in 30 to 40 fully developed cercariae about 78 days after infestation of the snail. The cercariae creep or float with the current until contact is made with the second intermediate host. On the North American continent these hosts are usually species of crayfish of the genus *Cambarus,* which live in small sluggish streams. In China, Japan, and the Philippines, freshwater crabs are the usual second intermediate hosts, but in Korea, crayfish may play this role.

The fully developed cercariae pierce the cuticle of the crayfish and make their way to the heart or pericardium, where they encyst and in six weeks or more develop into infective metacercariae. If ingested with uncooked crayfish (or crab), the young flukes bore through the wall of the duodenum of their adult host, wander about in the peritoneal sac, then penetrate the diaphragm and lung. The tissue reaction to the fluke in the lung parenchyma results in the formation of a cyst, usually lined in part by bronchial epithelium and surrounded by a granulomatous inflammatory reaction.

Ameel, D.J.: Paragonimiasis, its life history and distribution in North America and its taxonomy. Am. J. Hyg., 19:279–317, 1934.

Comfort, C.F., and Axelson, R.D.: Two reports of unusual parasites diagnosed in dogs. Can. Vet. J., 3:22–24, 1962.

Greve, J.H., et al.: Paragonimiasis in Iowa. Iowa State Univ. Vet., 26:21–28, 1963–64. (No. 1.)

Herman, L.H., and Helland, D.R.: Paragonimiasis in a cat. J. Am. Vet. Med. Assoc., 149:753–757, 1966.

LaRue, G.R., and Ameel, D.J.: The distribution of *Paragonimus.* J. Parasitol., 23:382–388, 1937.

Nielson, S.W.: Canine paragonimiasis. North Am. Vet., 36:657–662, 1955.

Rendano, V.T., Jr.: Paragonimiasis in the cat: a review of five cases. J. Small Anim. Pract., 15:637–644, 1974.

Seed, J.R., Sogandares-Bernal, F., and Mills, R.R.: Studies on American paragonimiasis. II. Serological observations of infected cats. J. Parasitol., 52:358–362, 1966.

Other Flukes

A small red fluke, *Eurytrema pancreaticum,* is found in the pancreatic duct of sheep, goats, cattle, and buffalo in Eastern Asia and Brazil. These flukes are only about 1 cm long, but when present in large numbers, they may result in fibrosis of the duct and the acinar tissue as well. Erosion of the mucosa may allow eggs to enter the tissue, where they incite granulomas. (See Figure 14–37.)

Other liver flukes include *Metarchis conjunctus* of dogs and cats in North America; *Opisthorchis caninus, O. noverca, O. felineus,* and *O. (Clonorchis) sinensis* of dogs, cats, and occasionally other species, including man, in Europe and Far East; *Pseudoamphistomum truncatum* of dogs and cats in Europe and the Far East; *Platynosomum concinnum* in cats in the Far East, Latin America, and southern United States; *Amphimerus pseudofelineus* in cats in the United States, and species of *Athesmia* in monkeys. Several species of *Paramphistoma* parasitize the forestomachs or small intestine of ruminants, which in heavy infection leads to erosion or ulceration. Species of *Alaria* are parasitic in the small intestines of dogs, foxes, wolves, and coyotes.

Allen, J.R., and Mills, J.H.L.: *Alaria arisaemoides* in Saskatchewan dogs. Can. Vet. J., 12:24–28, 1971.

Basch, P.F.: Completion of the life cycle of *Eurytrema pancreaticum* (Trematoda: Dicrocoeliidae). J. Parasitol., 51:350–355, 1965.

Cosgrove, G.E.: The trematodes of laboratory primates. Lab. Anim. Care, 16:23–39, 1966.

Faust, E.C.: Athesmia (Trematoda: Dicrocoeliidae) Odhner, 1911 liver fluke of monkeys from Colombia, South America, and other mammalian hosts. Trans. Am. Microsc. Soc., 86:113–119, 1967.

Horak, I.G.: Paramphistomiasis of domestic ruminants. Adv. Parisitol., 9:33–72, 1971.

Nosaka, D., Ashizawa, H., and Nagata, Y.: Pathological studies on *Eurytrema* infection in cattle. III. Behaviour of *Eurytrema* eggs in the wall and

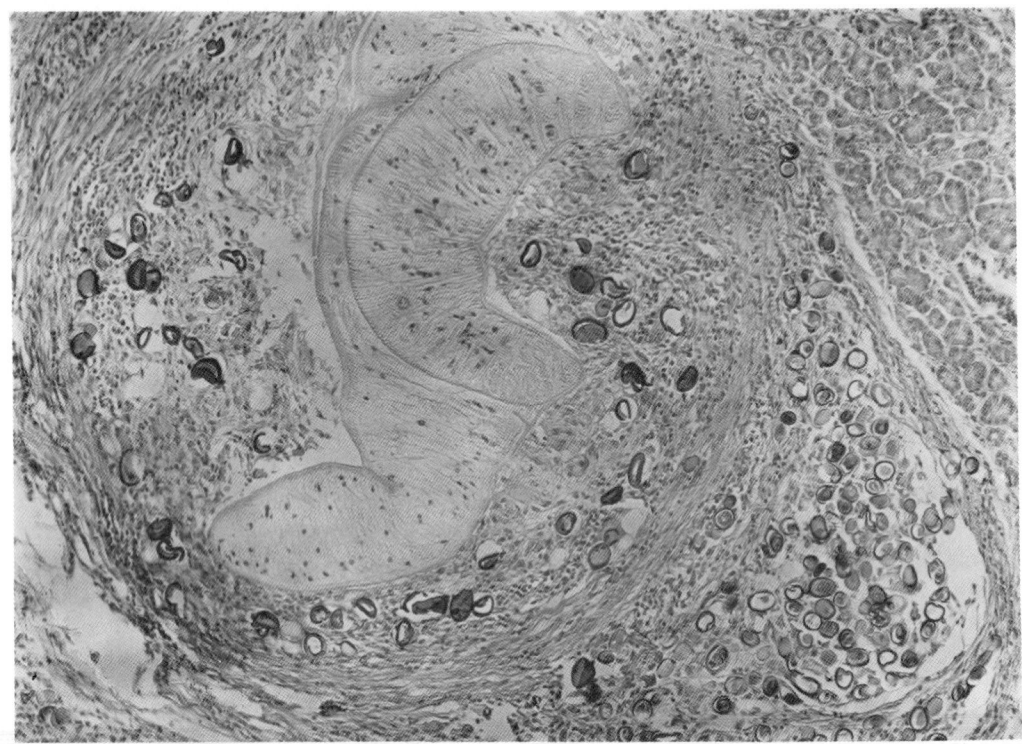

Fig. 14–37. A fluke, *Eurytrema pancreaticum*, in the pancreatic duct of a Brazilian cow. Note the large numbers of ova and the inflammation in the duct. Contributor: Dr. A. V. Machado, University of Munas Gervais.

surrounding tissue of bovine pancreatic ducts infected with *Eurytrema* species. Bull. Fac. Agric. Miyazaki Univ., *17*:104–132, 1970.

Palumbo, N.E., et al.: Cat liver fluke, *Platynosomum concinnum*, in Hawaii. Am. J. Vet. Res., *35*:1445, 1974.

Pande, B.P., and Shukla, R.P.: Experimentally induced *Opisthorchis caninus* infection in hamsters and rhesus monkey with a note on role of larval digeneans in fisheries production. Indian J. Exp. Biol., *12*:184–191, 1974.

Rothenbacher, H., and Lindquist, W.D.: Liver cirrhosis and pancreatitis in a cat infected with *Amphimerus pseudofelineus* (a fluke). J. Am. Vet. Med. Assoc., *143*:1099–1102, 1963.

Sahai, B.N., and Srivastava, H.D.: Pathology of liver and pancreas in *Opisthorchiasis noverca* in dogs and pigs. Br. Vet. J., *127*:239–243, 1971.

Singh, C.D.N., and Lakra, P.: Pathologic changes in naturally occurring *Cotylophoron cotylophorum* infection in cattle. Am. J. Vet. Res., *32*:659–663, 1971.

Strauss, J.M., and Heyneman, D.: Fatal ectopic fascioliasis in a guinea pig breeding colony from Malacca. J. Parasitol., *52*:413, 1966.

Taylor, D., and Perri, S.F.: Experimental infection of cats with the liver fluke *Platynosomum concinnum*. Am. J. Vet. Res., *38*:51–54, 1977.

Todd, K.S., Jr., Bergeland, M.E., and Hickman, G.R.: *Amphimerus pseudofelineus* infection in a cat. J. Am. Vet. Med. Assoc., *166*:458–459, 1975.

Zwicker, G.M., and Carlton, W.W.: Fluke (*Gastrodiscoides hominus*) infection in a rhesus monkey. J. Am. Vet. Med. Assoc., *161*:702–703, 1972.

PARASITIC ARTHROPODS

Veterinary entomology is generally regarded as the science that deals with all parasitic arthropods of animals, although many members of the phylum are not insects. The phylum **Arthropoda** is in general made up of organisms characterized by bilateral symmetry, metameric segmentation, the presence of jointed appendages and a hardened exoskeleton. It is divided into five classes as follows:

Crustacea: crabs, crayfish, shrimp, copepods

Onychophora: *Peripatus*

Myriapoda: centipedes and millipedes

Insecta: six-legged insects (mosquitoes, flies, etc.)

Arachnida: spiders, scorpions, ticks, and mites

The classes **Insecta and Arachnida** contain most of the parasitic species and the vectors of disease-producing viruses, protozoa, nematodes, rickettsia, and spirochetes. Each of these vectors is considered briefly in the part of this text devoted to the disease which it transmits. In the class **Insecta,** there are many orders, some of which contain species that are parasitic to animals, but those of most interest are the Diptera (flies), Hemiptera (bugs), Siphonaptera (fleas), and suborders Anoplura and Mallophaga (lice). Other orders contain species of less interest which may act as vectors of disease, but these will not be discussed here. Fleas, lice, and bugs, although vexing and sometimes injurious parasites, do not often have a serious portent from the pathologist's viewpoint; hence, will not be considered further. Flies, however, do incite specific and severe pathologic changes, thus are pathogens in their own right.

Myiasis

Myiasis results from the invasion of the living tissues of animals by the larval stage of flies of the order **Diptera.** The sites of invasion of these larvae provide a basis for their clinical classification: (1) cutaneous—the larvae live in or under the skin, e.g., ox warble; (2) intestinal—in the stomach or intestines, e.g., horse "bots"; (3) atrial—in the oral, nasal, ocular, sinusal, vaginal, and urethral cavities, e.g., *Oestrus ovis*; (4) wound invading—"screw-worm larvae"; and (5) external—bloodsucking larvae. Some fly larvae occupy more than one of these sites during the course of development in the host.

Many fly larvae are specific parasites of a certain host; others are accidental or nonspecific parasites in that they are deposited in or near diseased or wounded tissues in which they find a favorable environment.

Botflies. The genus *Gasterophilus* contains three species whose larvae are parasitic for equines in the United States. *Gasterophilus intestinalis* (syn. *G. equi*), DeGeer, 1776, the most common botfly in the United States, is a brown fly that deposits its eggs on hair of horse's fetlocks or forelegs, occasionally also in the scapular region. The female fly darts in quickly and attaches her pale yellow eggs to the hair with a tenacious material. These eggs are ready to hatch in five to ten days, but actual hatching requires licking or rubbing by the horse. This action also helps the larvae to reach the animal's mouth, where they penetrate the mucosa and wander beneath it as far as the pharynx. The developing larvae remain in the cheek or tongue for 21 to 28 days, then migrate to the stomach, and with their mouth parts attach to the mucosa in its cardiac portion. These bot larvae at this stage have a reddish color and are quite selective in their location; only rarely are they found attached to the fundic or pyloric portion of the stomach. Each larva causes a small unbilicated ulcer at its site of attachment. Large numbers of bots obviously interfere with function in the affected part of the stomach, but only occasionally do they produce general debility in the host. Surprisingly often they are tolerated without recognizable effect. The larvae remain attached to the mucosa, living on blood and tissue, for 10 to 12 months. After this period, they loosen their hold and pass out with the feces; the larvae pupate in soil for three to five weeks and then emerge as adults.

Gasterophilus hemorrhoidalis, Linne, 1761, the "nose botfly," is a small red-tailed fly that lays its eggs on hairs around

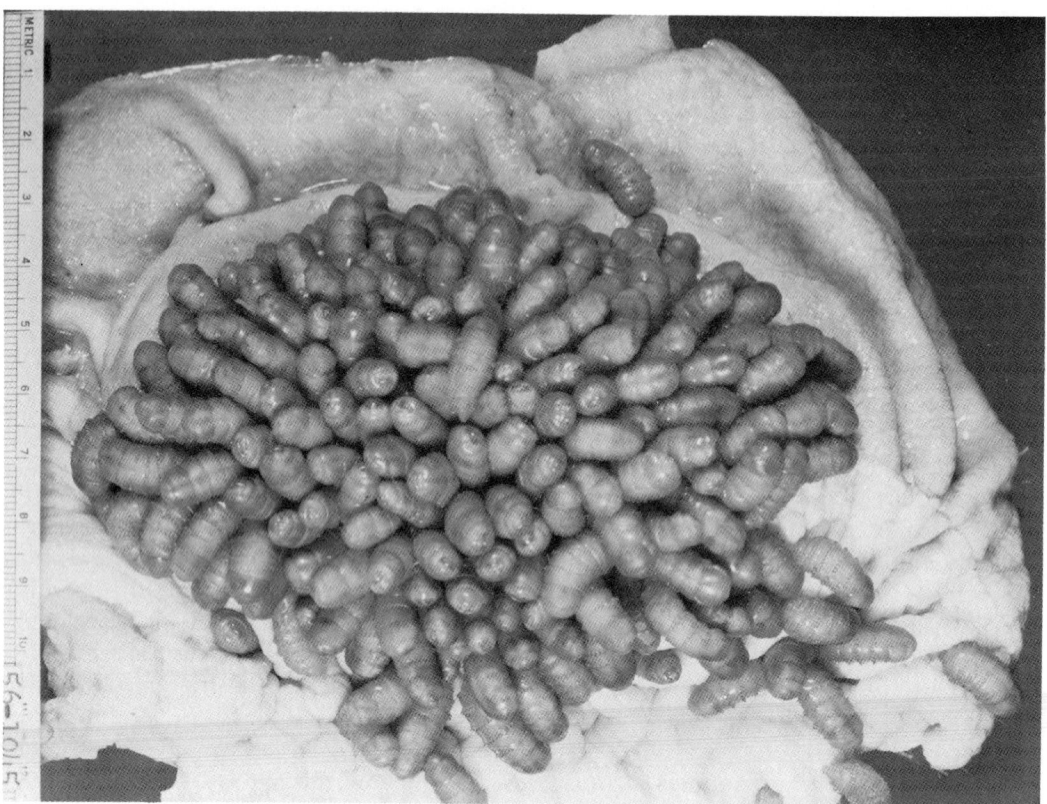

Fig. 14–38. Larvae of *Gasterophilus intestinalis*, "bots," attached to the stomach of a two-year-old gelding. (Courtesy of Dr. C. R. Cole, Ohio State University.)

the mouth, nose, and cheeks of horses. The eggs of this species are dark brown or black in color, elongated and pointed at one end with an operculum at the other. The larvae hatch from these eggs, then pierce the skin of the face and wander into the mouth. The young red-colored larvae are sometimes found in the pharynx, but eventually become attached at the cardia of the stomach. Here they have a similar effect to that of *G. intestinalis*, and remain for 10 to 12 months at this site before passing to the rectum, where they again attach for a few days before passing out with the feces. The rest of their life cycle is similar to that of *G. intestinalis*.

Gasterophilus nasalis, Clark, 1897, (Synonym: *G. veterinus*, Linne, 1761), the "chin" or "throat" fly, lays it eggs on hairs in the intermandibular region of horses.

The larvae are pale yellow and migrate to eventually become attached to the mucosa of the pylorus and duodenum. Otherwise, their life cycle and effect upon the host are similar to that of *G. intestinalis*.

Gasterophilus pecorum, Fabricus, 1794, is a botfly found in Europe, but not in the United States. The female fly deposits her eggs on the hoofs on horses and on inanimate objects such as food and other materials. The eggs are dark colored and must be rubbed or licked by the host before the larvae can emerge. The larvae penetrate the mucosa of the cheeks and soon assume a blood-red color. The third-stage larvae attach to the stomach mucosa, and before leaving the host in the spring, attach to the rectal mucosa for a few days.

Gasterophilus inermis, Braurer, 1858, is principally a botfly of Europe but has been observed in North America. The adult fly deposits her eggs on hairs around the mouth and cheeks. The larvae may penetrate the skin and leave tracks as they wander toward the mucosa. The third-stage larvae attach to the mucosa of the rectum. Otherwise the life history is similar to that of *G. intestinalis.*

Oestrus ovis, the botfly or "head grub" of sheep, deposits its larvae in the nose of sheep; the larvae migrate into the nasal cavity and nasal sinuses, where they attach and undergo further development. Growth and migration of these larvae in these sites result in serious damage to the tissue and may cause death. The successful larvae eventually drop to the ground, where they pupate and later emerge as adult flies.

Heel Flies. The genus *Hypoderma* contains two species of interest, *H. bovis* and *H. lineatum,* the hairy yellow and black

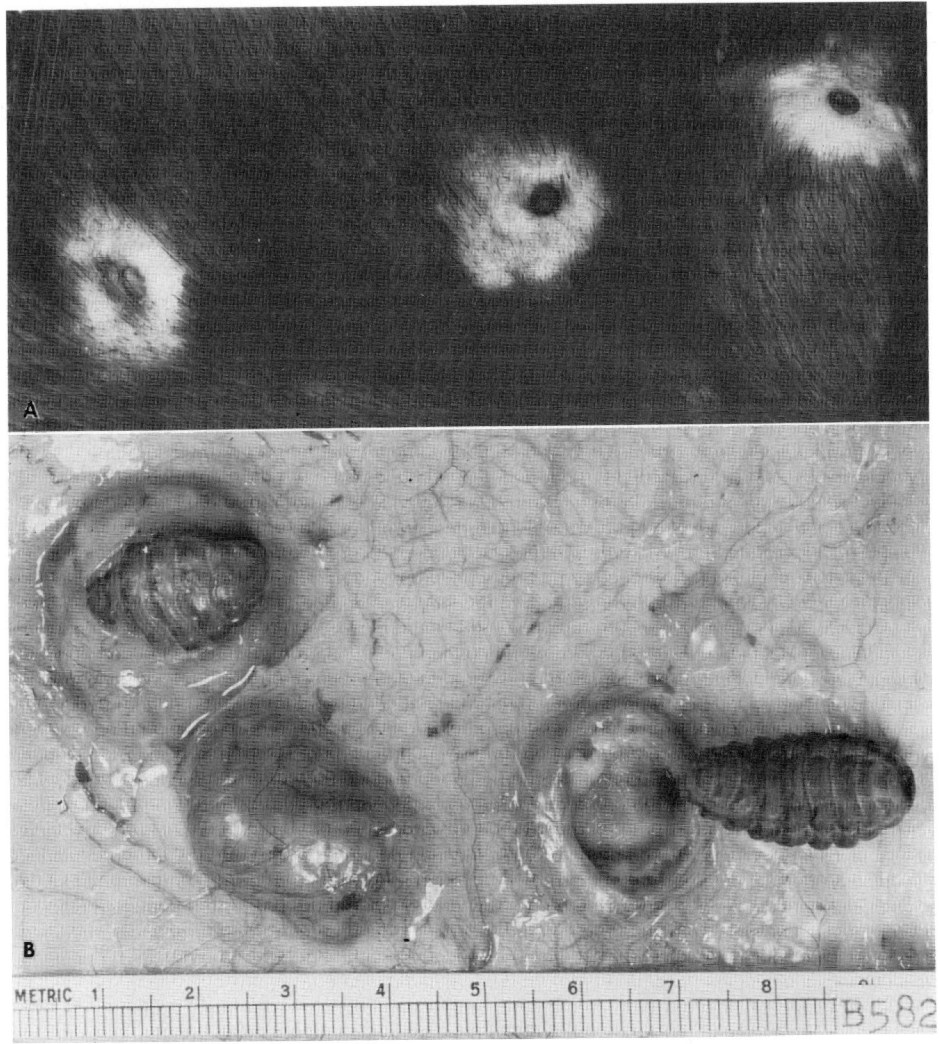

Fig. 14–39. *Hypoderma bovis,* "ox warble," in the bovine skin. *A,* Three holes viewed from the external surface of the skin. The larvae lie under these holes, which eventually enlarge to permit escape of the larvae. *B, H. bovis* larvae from the deep surface of the bovine skin. (Courtesy of Dr. C. R. Cole, Ohio State University.)

"warble" or heel flies of cattle, which occasionally attack horses and rarely, man. The female fly deposits her eggs on the hairs of the legs, flanks, or dewlap of cattle, producing much irritation and excitement in their victims while so doing. The larvae from these eggs hatch and penetrate the skin, migrate through the tissues into the thoracic and abdominal cavities, and eventually reach the subcutaneous tissues of the back. Occasionally these larvae invade the central nervous system and cause death. Surprisingly enough, the migration pathway of these larvae is usually sterile, even though there is considerable tissue destruction along the way. The larvae remain in an encapsulated nodule in the subcutis of the back during the winter months. In the spring, they gradually produce a large hole in the epidermis, through which the grub eventually emerges. Heavy infestation leaves holes in the skin that make the hide unfit for use. The larvae pupate after reaching the ground, emerging as adult flies 40 to 50 days later.

Screw-worm Fly. In some parts of the United States the "screw-worm" fly, *Callitroga (Cochliomyia) americana,* can be an important problem in animal agriculture and may also cause a serious disease in man. The pathogenic effects of this fly are produced by the larvae, which feed upon living tissues and thereby may produce serious effects upon their hapless host. In man, deleterious effects have been produced by the maggots' invasion of the nasopharynx (nasopharyngeal myiasis). In animals, the larvae attack any wounds in which they can gain entrance. In sheep and lambs, "needle" grass may produce wounds that the maggots can invade, although cuts in the skin made by shearing can also be troublesome. In cattle, the screw-worm larvae may invade the umbilicus of the newborn calf or the vagina of its mother. Dehorning and castration may also provide wounds that invite the assault of this parasite.

The adult fly has a dark greenish-blue metallic abdomen with an orange or reddish face and three stripes on the surface of the thorax. The female deposits her eggs in large numbers near wounds, and after 11 to 21 hours, the larvae emerge to feed voraciously for three to five days. A prepupal stage lasts for a few hours to 3 days, and the pupal stage about 7 days. The entire cycle from egg to adult is completed in about 11 days.

Cutaneous Myiasis. This disease may also be caused by larvae of flies of the subfamily Cuterebrinae. Two genera are of particular interest: *Dermatobia* and *Cuterebra. Dermatobia hominis* may infect man, cattle, dogs, sheep, cats, rabbits, and other animals, particularly in tropical America. The adults do not feed, surviving on food stores obtained during the larval period. The adult female, about 12 mm long, with a dark blue thorax and short broad abdomen with a brilliant blue color, glues her ova to the abdomen of a mosquito or blood-sucking fly. The larvae hatch on this transport host and penetrate the skin of a warm-blooded host, upon which the transport host feeds. The larvae of *D. hominis* develop in the subcutis, producing a painful enlargement with a pore opening to the surface. The larvae require up to ten weeks to mature to about 25 mm in length, with rows of strong spines on their surface. They escape from the skin to the ground, where they pupate to produce the mature fly.

The genus *Cuterebra* is made up of large flies with bee-like bodies, 20 mm or more in length. The adult flies oviposit near the mouths of burrows of rodents and rabbits. Larvae hatch to penetrate the skin of the host, mature in about a month, and produce large, subcutaneous lesions. The larvae pupate on the ground and also are covered with bands of characteristic spines. *Cuterebra buccata, C. americana,* and *C. lepivora* are usually parasitic in rabbits, but these and other species may also infect dogs, cats, and man. Another species, *C. emasculator,* usually parasitizes mice and chipmunks, but may involve other species. Larvae may invade the brain, scrotum, or other tissues, as well as the subcutis.

Beesley, W.N.: Recent work on the ox warble flies (*Hypoderma*). Vet. Bull., 35:1–6, 1965.

————: Further observations on the development of *Hypoderma lineatum* de Villiers and *Hypoderma bovis,* Degeer (*Diptera, Oestridae*) in the bovine host. Br. Vet. J., 122:91–98, 1966.

Cunningham, D.G., and Zanga, J.R.: Myiasis of the external auditory meatus. J. Pediatr., 84:857–858, 1974.

Davis, C.L., and Leadbetter, W.A.: Fatal brain hemorrhage in the bull caused by the cattle grub (*Hypoderma bovis*). North Am. Vet., 33:703–705, 1952.

Greve, J.H., and Cassidy, D.R.: Aberrant *Hypoderma bovis* infection in a cow. J. Am. Vet. Med. Assoc., 150:627–628, 1967.

Hatziolos, B.C.: Cuterebra larva in the brain of a cat. J. Am. Vet. Med. Assoc., 148:787–793, 1966.

————: Cuterebra larva causing paralysis in a dog. Cornell Vet., 57:129–145, 1967.

Olander, H.J.: The migration of *Hypoderma lineatum* in the brain of a horse. A case report and review. Pathol. Vet., 4:477–483, 1967.

Roberts, I.H., and Colbenson, H.P.: Larvae of *Oestrus ovis* in the ears of sheep. Am. J. Vet. Res., 24:628–630, 1963.

Simmons, S.W.: Some histopathological changes caused by *Hypoderma* larvae in the esophagus of cattle. J. Parasitol., 23:376–381, 1937.

Zumpt, F.: Myiasis in Man and Animals. London, Butterworth, 1965.

Acariasis

Within the class Arachnida, the order Acarina includes the ticks and mites, both of which are at times parasitic in their relation to animals. These and other exoparasites, such as fleas and lice, usually are not associated with serious disease except when present in large numbers. All of these parasites cause variable degrees of inflammation at the site of attachment or bite, which results from mechanical irritation, immediate hypersensitivity reactions (localized anaphylaxis or arthus-type reaction), delayed hypersensitivity reaction (contact dermatitis), or the introduction of secondary bacteria.

Ticks are particularly important as vectors of disease-producing agents, but except when present in large numbers or in particular sites, as in the ears, do not produce any immediate or serious effect upon the host. An important exception is **tick paralysis,** a dramatic paralytic disease observed in man, sheep, dogs, cats, and other species. Twenty-two species of ticks have been associated with paralysis in various parts of the world. In the United States, *Dermacentor andersoni* (wood tick) is the most important, and in Australia, *Ixodes holocyclus.* The paralysis ensues within about one week after one or more ticks are attached to the skin, and may disappear dramatically when the offending ticks are removed or slowly abate in several days. Young and small animals are more susceptible to the condition, with fewer ticks required to induce paralysis. Death occurs in animals and man when the ticks are not detected and removed in time. The paralysis is believed to result from a neuroparalytic toxin secreted by the tick, but its mode of action has not been elucidated, although it is thought to interfere with release of acetylcholine. A short-lived immunity follows exposure, and immune serum can be made from hyperimmunized animals.

The tissue-burrowing habits of mites cause them to produce more obvious lesions in animals than do ticks. Common mites that are pathogenic for animals are listed in Table 14–9. These mites may be appropriately considered in groups arranged in accord with the body system which they attack, i.e., pulmonary, cutaneous, intestinal, and urinary.

Pulmonary Acariasis. The frequent occurrence of pulmonary lesions caused by a lung mite, *Pneumonyssus simicola,* and related species, in monkeys is of some interest in connection with the experimental use of these animals. Nearly all imported rhesus monkeys are infected with lung mites, whose presence in the bronchiolar system incites rather characteristic lesions. Clinical manifestations are not usually observed. The life cycle is not understood, but the occurrence of pulmonary

Table 14–9. Acarid (Mite) Parasites of Animals

Name	Anatomic Site	Disease	Hosts
Demodex folliculorum (demodectic mange mite)	Hair follicles, sebaceous glands	Demodectic or "red" mange	Dog, cat, man, swine, sheep, cattle
Demodex phylloides	Hair follicles, sebaceous glands	Demodectic mange	Swine
Sarcoptes scabiei var. *suis, bovis,* etc. (sarcoptic mange mite)	Epidermis generally	Scabies, sarcoptic mange	Cattle, sheep, dog, cat, man, swine, horse
Notoedres sp.	Epidermis, especially of neck	Notoedric mange	Cat, others
Psoroptes communis var. *equi, ovis,* etc.	Epidermis of ears and generally	Psoroptic mange, sheep scab	Sheep, cattle, horse, rabbit
Otodectes cynotis	External ear canal	Otitis externa	Dog, cat
Chorioptes sp.	Epidermis, feet, base of tail	Chorioptic mange	Cattle, sheep, horse, goat
Myobia musculi	Epidermis	Mange	Mice
Mycoptes musculinus	Epidermis	Mange	Mice
Cytoleichus nudus (air sac mite)	Air sacs, respiratory tract	Air sac mite infection	Bird
Pneumonyssus caninum	Paranasal sinuses	Mite infection	Dog
Pneumonyssus simicola	Bronchioles, alveoli of lung	Pulmonary acariasis	*Macaca mulatta*
Rhinophaga sp.	Nasal and respiratory passages	Nasal or pulmonary acariasis	Monkeys
Dermanyssus gallinae (common red mite)	Epidermis generally	Anemia, mite dermatitis	Poultry
Cnemidocoptes mutans (scaly leg mite)	Scales of legs	Scaly leg disease	Chicken
Cnemidocoptes gallinae (feather mite)	Feather follicles	Depluming mite infestation	Chicken
Linguatula serrata (tongue "worm," pentastoma worm)	Nasal and respiratory passages	Pentastomiasis or linguatuliasis	Dog, fox, wolf, man, horse, goat, sheep
Tyroglyphus sp. (cereal mite)	Urinary and intestinal tract	"Grocer's itch"	Man, dog
Psorergates simplex	Epidermal cysts in skin	"Mouse mange"	Mice
Psorergates ovis	Same	Mange	Sheep
Cheyletiella parasitivorax	Epidermis	"Mange"	Dog, rabbit, cat
Cheyletiella yasguri	Epidermis	Mange	Dogs, man

acariasis in monkeys born in captivity (United States) suggests direct transmission.

These acarids, barely large enough to be seen with the unaided eye, are found in the bronchi and bronchioles. Apparently they move down the bronchial tree until the lumen becomes small enough to impede their progress. Their presence results in accumulation of mucus, localized bronchiolitis, peribronchiolitis and occasional bronchiectasis. The mites can often be found in a pool of mucus and cellular debris, surrounded by the thickened remnants of the bronchiolar wall, which is largely replaced by lymphoid cells. The nodule thus formed can be recognized grossly. A characteristic crystalline pig-

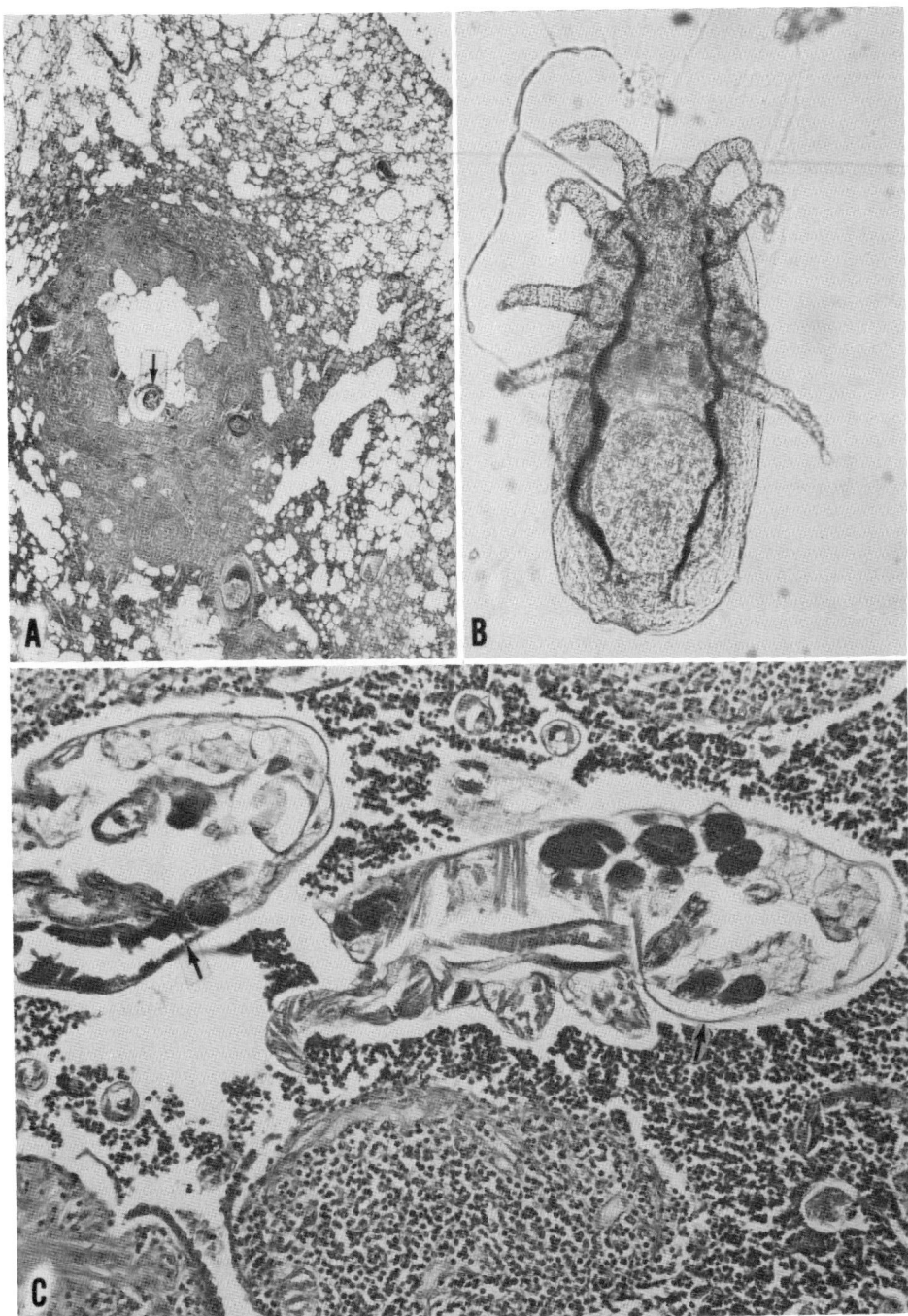

Fig. 14–40. Pulmonary acariasis. *A, Pneumonyssus simicola* (arrow) in a dilated bronchiole with thickened wall, lung of a rhesus monkey *Macaca mulatta. B,* A female, egg-bearing mite teased from a lesion. *C,* Section of two mites in a bronchiole. (Courtesy of Dr. J. R. M. Innes.)

ment that is microscopically demonstrable accumulates in affected lungs, sometimes at points rather distant from the parasite. This pigment occurs as golden brown, coarsely granular or needle-like, anisotropic crystals in lymphatic spaces, or in the form of finely granular, phagocytized or free, light-brown refractile and anisotropic crystals. The pigment is difficult to analyze, but it contains iron and lipofuscin and is probably derived from the excreta of the mites.

A related mite, *Pneumonyssus caninum,* is encountered occasionally in the paranasal sinuses and upper respiratory tract of dogs. The presence of these mites may result in purulent sinusitis, but this is rarely recognized in the living animal. Mites of another genus, *Cytoleichus,* are found in the air sacs of birds.

Pentastomiasis. Organisms related to the mites and grouped in the class Pentastomida include several genera which are parasitic in mammals. All have indirect life cycles. *Linguatula serrata (Pentastomum taenioides)* is a tongue-shaped, worm-like arthropod which inhabits the respiratory passages of the fox, dog, wolf, horse, goat, sheep, and man. The adults are slightly convex dorsally, flattened ventrally, males up to 2.0 cm and females up to 13 cm in length. The cuticle is transversely striated. Eggs expelled from the nostrils are ingested by a suitable intermediate host, most usually sheep or cattle, but swine, horses, rabbits, and other species can be infected. They hatch in the digestive tract, penetrate the intestinal wall to localize in mesenteric lymph nodes or other tissues where larvae grow to the infective stage. Dogs presumably become infected by eating tissues containing larvae.

The larvae of a related species, *Armillifer armillatus* have been reported to infect viscera of cattle, monkeys, swine, and man (du Toit and Sutherland, 1968; Challier, Gidel and Traore, 1967).

Cutaneous Acariasis (Mange, Scabies, Scab, Mite Infestation). A wide variety of

mites parasitize the skin of animals; many of them produce lesions of serious import. In general, each species of mite has its preferred host and will not flourish on any other; however, some species are harbored by one host with little harm but can cause serious lesions in another. Such a mite is *Demodex folliculorum,* a cigar-shaped mite, commonly demonstrable in normal human hair follicles, where it survives with no visible effect upon the host. Morphologically identical parasites are the cause of **demodectic** or **red mange** in dogs, a persistent and disfiguring skin disease in that species. These mites burrow into the hair follicles of the canine skin, producing intense itching accompanied by alopecia and scaling of the epidermis. The itching causes the animal to rub the affected part, accentuating the symptoms and promoting exudation of serum and scab formation on the denuded surface. The mites may burrow into sebaceous or sweat glands or to the depths of hair follicles, causing proliferation and then necrosis of the epithelium, followed by intense inflammation of the underlying dermis, which takes the form of small abscesses, granulomas with giant cells, and diffuse infiltration of lymphocytes. In some cases, the mites migrate even deeper and may reach lymph nodes. Secondary pyogenic infections can result in death. The deep folliculitis and dermatitis can be readily recognized in tissue sections and the offending parasites easily demonstrated. Deep scrapings of affected skin may also be examined microscopically for the mites.

A similar, but morphologically distinguishable mite, *Demodex phylloides,* occasionally causes lesions in the hair follicles and sebaceous glands of the skin of swine. It is common for the parasite to produce dilatation of the skin adnexa with the formation of epithelial-lined cysts filled with the mites. These lesions have somewhat the same effect as an epidermal inclusion cyst, exciting little inflammation

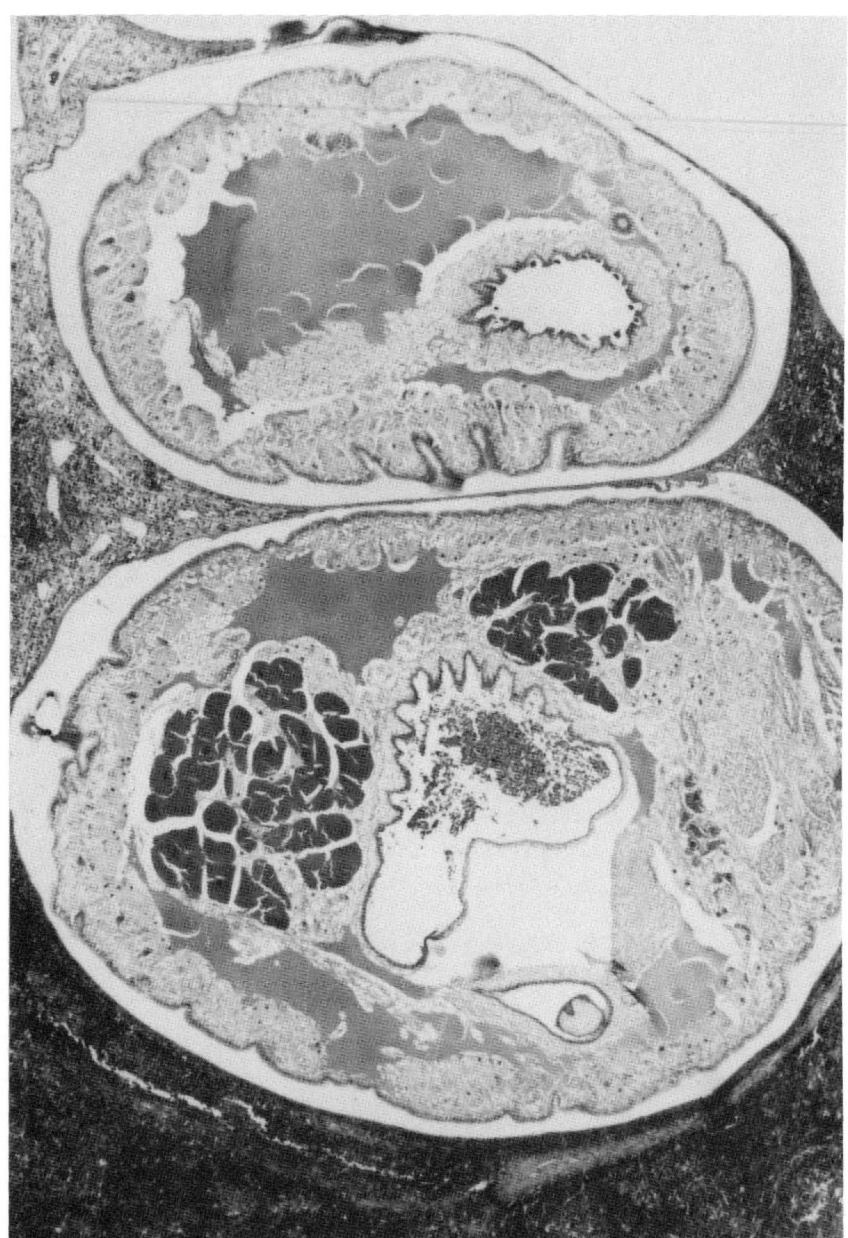

Fig. 14-41. Pentastomiasis, rhesus monkey *(Macaca mulatta)*. Pentastome nymphs *(Armillifera armillatus)* embedded in the spleen. (Courtesy of New England Regional Primate Research Center, Harvard Medical School.)

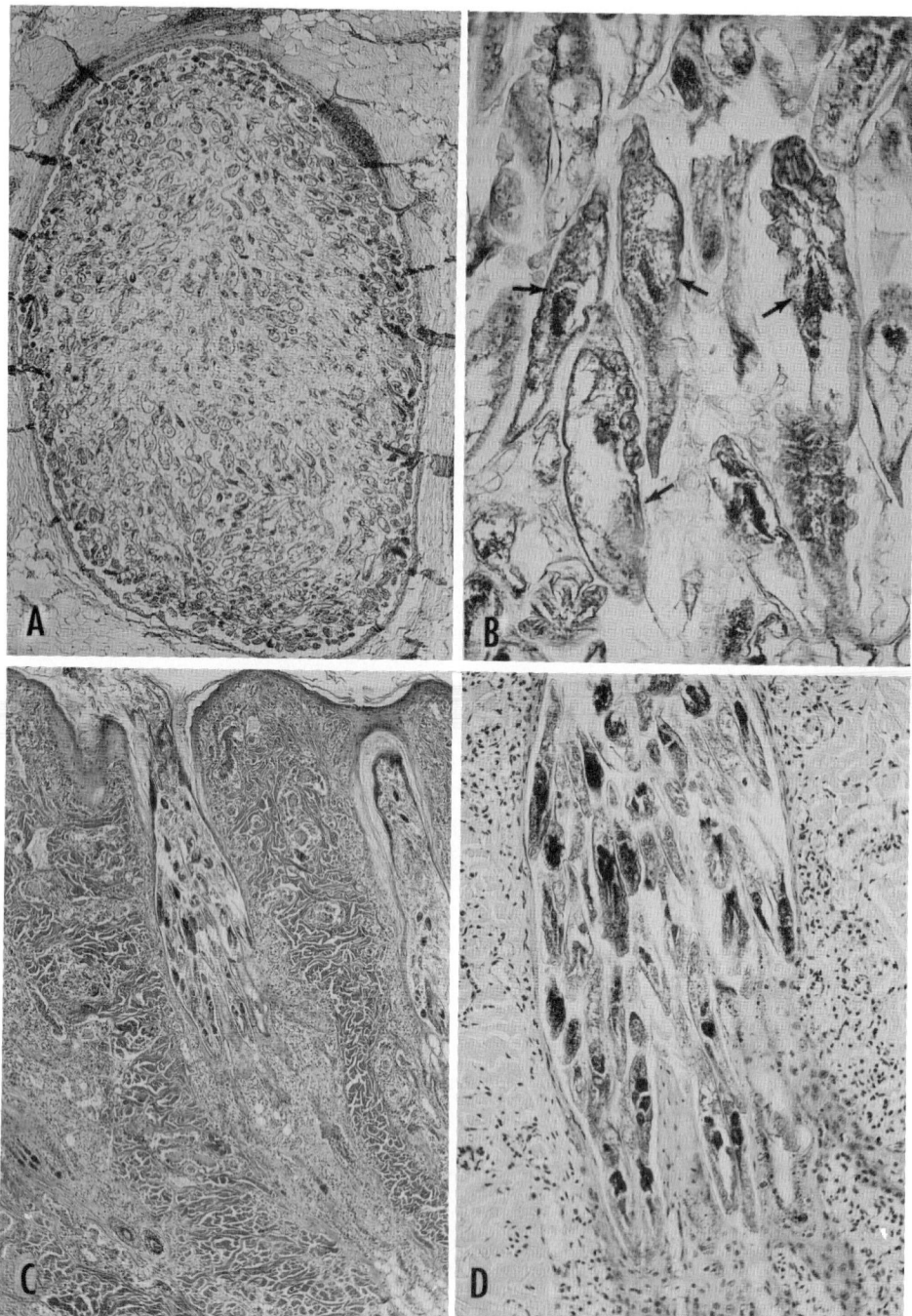

Fig. 14–42. Cutaneous acariasis. *A,* Demodectic mange in the skin of a pig (× 35). Large dilated hair follicle filled with *Demodex phylloides. B,* Higher magnification (× 210) of *A,* to show detail of sections of mites (arrows). Contributor: Dr. C. L. Davis. *C,* Demodectic mange, skin of a dog (× 35). Note the acanthosis and prominent, distended hair follicles. *D,* A single follicle (× 115) from *C,* containing many *Demodex folliculorum.* (Courtesy of Armed Forces Institute of Pathology.) Contributor: Dr. R. D. Turk.

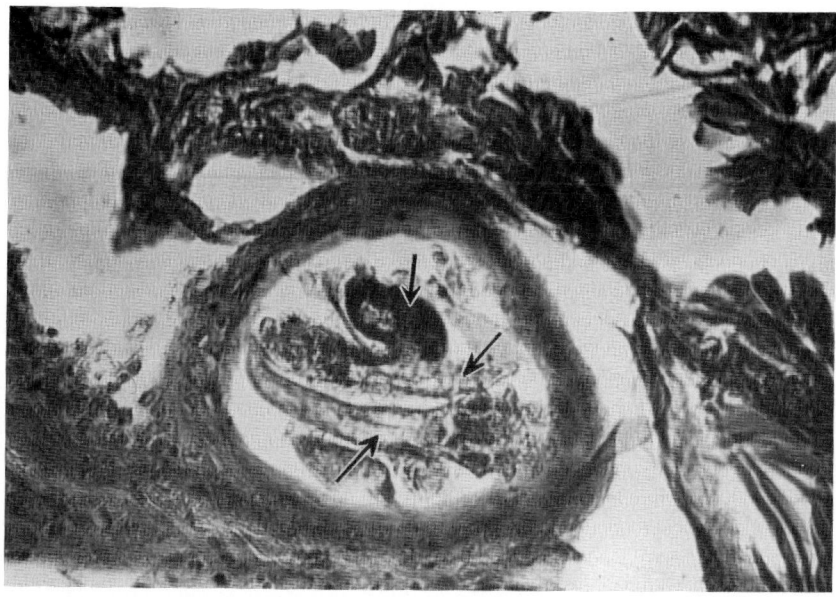

Fig. 14-43. *Demodex folliculorum*, acarid mites (arrows) in a hair follicle cut in cross section, skin of a dog. (H & E × 250.)

unless it ruptures and causes a reaction of foreign-body type. It is possible for *Demodex* mites to be present in hair follicles or sebaceous glands in the skin, particularly in man and the dog, without exciting any inflammation. Species of *Demodex* also affect laboratory rodents and nonhuman primates, usually without significant dermatitis. The factors that make these mites pathogenic are unknown.

Sarcoptic mange is caused by a specific mite, *Sarcoptes scabiei* (sarcoptic mange mite), which may attack many species, including cattle, sheep, dogs, swine, horses, and man. Morphologically indistinguishable varieties of *S. scabiei (bovis, suis*, etc.) are found in each host species, each variety of mite having its definite host preference; cross infection of heterologous species rarely occurs. The sarcoptic mange mite burrows in the deeper parts of the stratum corneum or the superficial layers of the stratum malpighii of the skin, and rarely goes deeper. Even in this superficial position, however, the mites cause severe itching, hyperkeratosis and

acanthosis, with resultant loss of hair or wool. The intense pruritus results in rubbing of the skin, which in turn causes loss of epithelium and secondary infection of the dermis. In dogs at least, the pruritus is much more intense in sarcoptic than in demodectic mange.

Species of other genera, *Notoedres, Psoroptes,* and *Chorioptes,* produce similar lesions, but with slightly different host range and anatomic site of preference. The diseases caused by these mites are known, respectively, as **notoedric, psoroptic,** or **chorioptic mange.** The offending mites can be seen in tissue sections, but it is necessary to tease them out and mount them under a cover slip in order to identify them. This can be done as readily with fixed specimens of skin as with fresh skin scrapings.

Of particular interest to laboratory investigators is the rabbit ear mite, *Psoroptes communis* var. *cuniculi,* which lives in the external auditory meatus of rabbits, where it produces severe lesions that may lead to middle or inner ear infection and death.

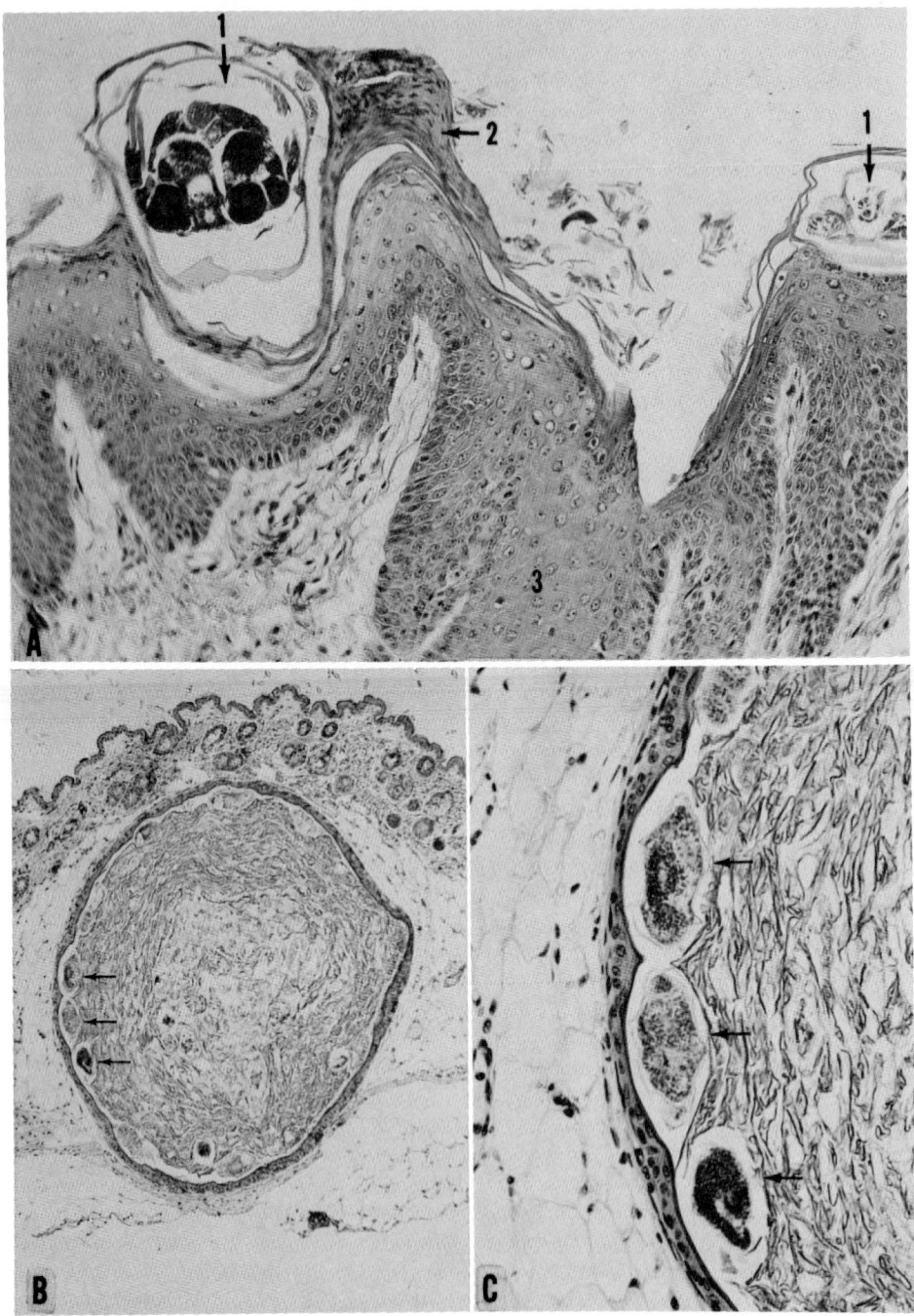

Fig. 14–44.   Cutaneous acariasis. *A,* Sarcoptic mange. The mites *(1)* are in the superficial epidermis, resulting in parakeratosis *(2)* and acanthosis *(3).* Contributor: Col. J. H. Rust, V.C. *B,* Acariasis in the skin of a mouse (× 70). The mites *(Psorergates simplex)* (arrows) cause the formation of epidermal inclusion cyst. *C,* The mites (arrows) in the cyst (× 250). (Courtesy of Armed Forces Institute of Pathology.) Contributor: Dr. Robert J. Flynn.

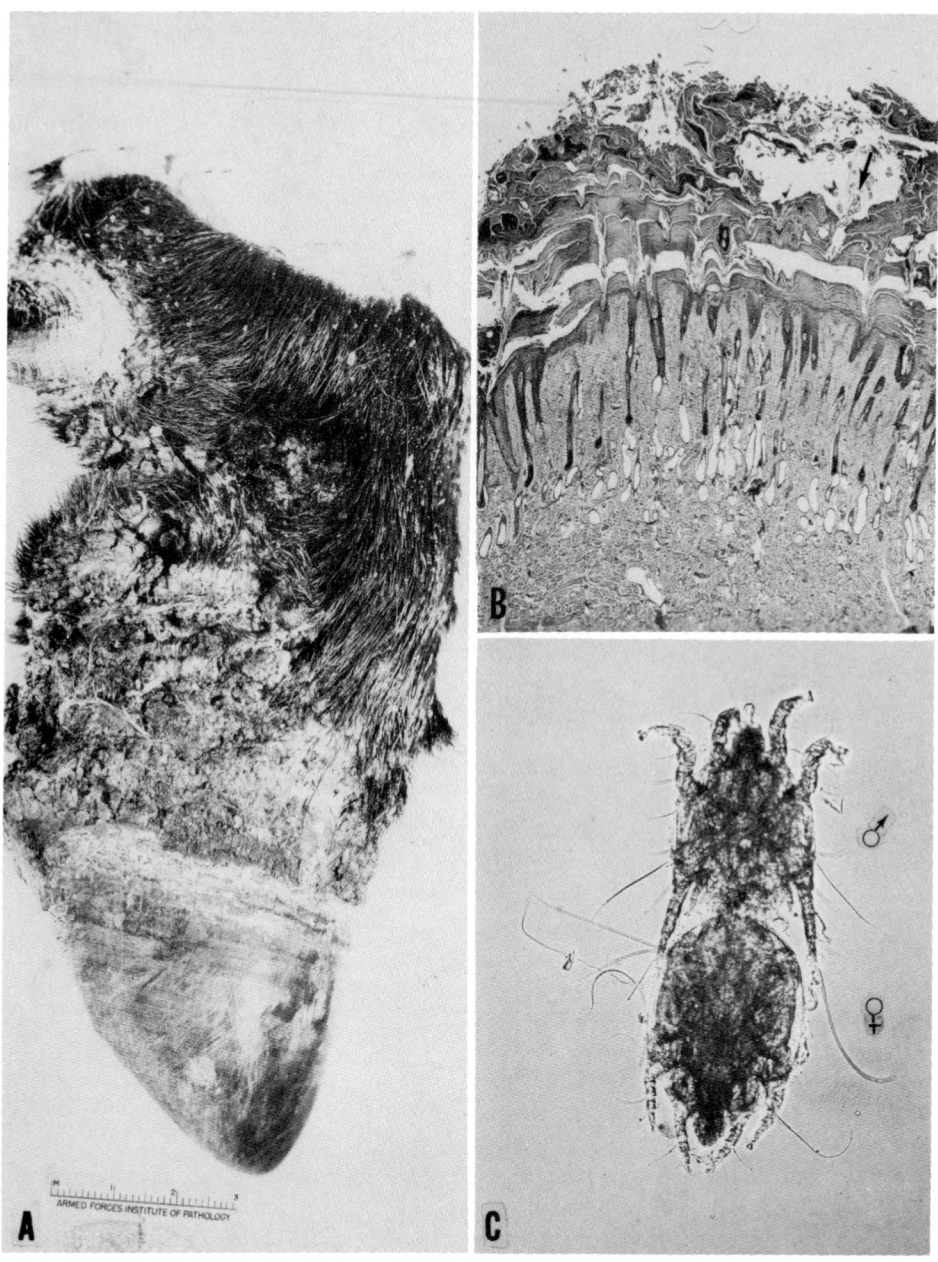

Fig. 14–45. Chorioptic mange, fetlock region of an Angus steer. *A,* Tenacious, thick scales adhering to hairs. *B,* Section (× 10) of the affected skin. Note thick exudate adhering to epidermis. Arrow points to the mites. *C,* Pair of mites in coitus, teased from the fixed specimen and cleared in phenol (× 75). (Courtesy of Armed Forces Institute of Pathology.) Contributor: Dr. E. R. Derflinger.

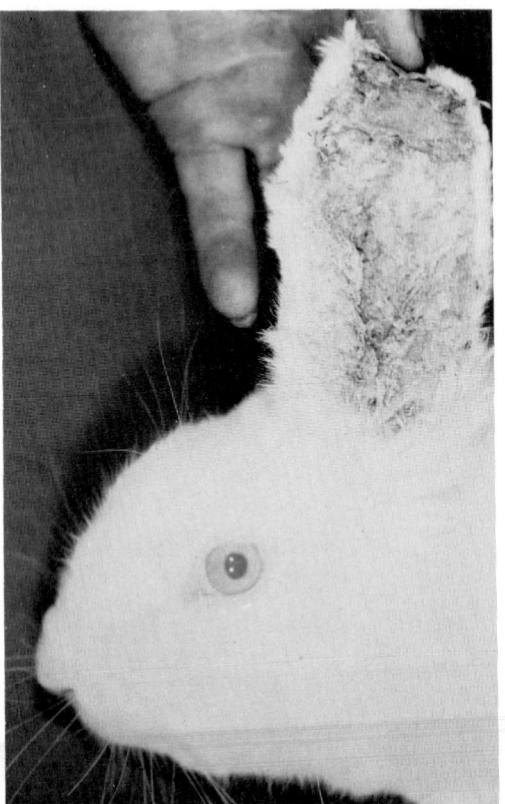

Fig. 14–46. Lesions of ear mites *(Psoroptes communis v. cunuliculi)* in the ear of a New Zealand white rabbit.

The mites tunnel into the superficial layers of the stratum malpighii, producing hyperkeratosis and exfoliation of keratin and debris which accumulates in the ear canal. The ear mite of the domestic cat, *Felis catus*, is also of interest, as it produces similar lesions. The usual parasite is *Notoedres cati*.

Intestinal and Urinary Acariasis. Certain mites live normally in cereal products and are not pathogenic but may produce dermatitis ("grocer's itch"), enteritis, or urethritis in man or animals if they gain access to these structures. Of interest are the cereal mites, *Tyroglyphus sp.*, which have been reported in feces of dogs fed infested cereal products. Few symptoms are produced and the mites do not multi-ply in the intestinal tract, but their close resemblance to mange mites may at times be confusing when they are encountered upon microscopic examination of fecal specimens.

Baker, E.W.: Ectopic ear mite infestation in the dog. J. Am. Vet. Med. Assoc., *164*:1125–1126, 1974.

Baker, E.W., et al.: A Manual of Parasitic Mites of Medical or Economic Importance. New York, National Pest Control Assn., Inc., 1956.

Baker, D.W., and Nutting, W.B.: Demodectic mange in New York State sheep. Cornell Vet., *40*:140–142, 1940.

Baker, K.P.: The histopathology and pathogenesis of demodecosis of the dog. J. Comp. Pathol., *79*:321–327, 1969.

————: Infestation of domestic animals with the mite *Cheyletiella parasitivorax*. Vet. Rec., *84*:561, 1969.

Beresford-Jones, W.P.: Occurrence of the mite *Psorergates simplex* in mice. Aust. Vet. J., *41*:289–290, 1965.

Carter, H.B.: A skin disease of sheep due to an ectoparasitic mite, *Psorergates ovis*, Womersley, 1941. Aust. Vet. J., *17*:193–201, 1941.

Challier, A., Gidel, R., and Traore, S.: Porocephalosis caused by *Armillifer (Nettorhynchus) armillatus*, Wyman 1847, in a bull and pig. Revue Elev. Med. Vet. Pays Trop., *20*:255–259, 1967.

Danilov, I.: Lethal infestation of goats with juvenile forms of *Linguatula serrata*. Vet. Sbir., *56*:24–25, 1959. VB 3513–59.

du Toit, R., and Sutherland, R.J.: *Armillifer armillatus* (Wyman) (Order: Pentastomida) from slaughter stock. J. S. Afr. Vet. Med. Assoc., *39*:77–79, 1968.

Dodd, K.: *Cheyletiella yasguri*: widespread infestation in a breeding kennel. Vet. Rec., *86*:346–347, 1970.

Doube, B.M.: Cattle and the paralysis tick *Ixodes holocyclus*. Aust. Vet. J., *51*:511–515, 1975.

Doube, B.M., and Kemp, D.H.: Paralysis of cattle by *Ixodes holocyclus* Neumann. Aust. J. Agric. Res., *26*:635–640, 1975.

Ewing, S.A., Mosier, J.E., and Foxx, T.S.: Occurrence of *Cheyletiella spp.* on dogs with skin lesions. J. Am. Vet. Med. Assoc., *151*:64–67, 1967.

Flatt, R.E., and Patton, N.M.: A mite infestation in squirrel monkeys (*Saimiri sciureus*). J. Am. Vet. Med. Assoc., *155*:1233–1235, 1969.

Flynn, R.J., and Jaroslow, B.N.: Nidification of a mite (*Psorergates simplex*, Tyrrell, 1883: Myobiidae) in the skin of mice. J. Parasitol., *42*:49–52, 1956.

Foxx, T.S., and Ewing, S.A.: Morphologic features, behavior, and life history of *Cheyletiella yasguri*. Am. J. Vet. Res., *30*:269–285, 1969.

French, F.E.: *Demodex canis* in canine tissues. Cornell Vet., *54*:271–290, 1964.

Friedman, S., and Weisbroth, S.H.: The parasitic ecology of the rodent mite *Myobia musculi*. II. Genetic factors. Lab. Anim. Sci., *25*:440–445, 1975.

Gething, M.A.: Cheyletiella infestation in small animals. Vet. Bull., 43:63–69, 1973.

Griffin, C.A., and Dean, D.J.: Demodectic mange in goats. Cornell Vet., 34:308–311, 1944.

Grono, L.R.: Studies of the ear mite, *Otodectes cynotis*. Vet. Rec., 85:6–8, 1969.

Innes, J.R.M., Colton, M.W., Yevich, P.P., and Smith, C.L.: Pulmonary acariasis as an enzootic disease caused by *Pneumonyssus simicola* in imported monkeys. Am. J. Pathol., 30:813–835, 1954.

Khalil, G.M., and Schacher, J.F.: *Linguatula serrata* in relation to halzoun and the Marrara syndrome. Am. J. Trop. Med. Hyg., 14:736–746, 1965.

Kim, C.S., and Bang, B.G.: Nasal mites parasitic in nasal and upper skull tissues in the baboon (*Papio sp.*). Science, 169:372–373, 1970.

Kirkwood, A., and Kendall, S.B.: Demodectic mange in cattle. Vet. Rec., 78:33–34, 1966.

Leerhoy, J., and Jensen, H.S.: Sarcoptic mange in a shipment of cynomolgus monkeys. Nord. Vet. Med., 19:128–130, 1967.

Lindquist, W.D., and Cash, W.C.: Sarcoptic mange in a cat. J. Am. Vet. Med. Assoc., 162:639–640, 1973.

Martin, H.M., and Deubler, M.J.: Acariasis (*Pneumonyssus sp.*) of the upper respiratory tract of the dog. Univ. of Pa. Bull., 43:21–27, 1943.

McConnell, E.E., Basson, P.A., and de Vos, V.: Laryngeal acariasis in the chacma baboon. J. Am. Vet. Med. Assoc., 161:678–682, 1972.

McKeever, P.J., and Allen, S.K.: Dermatitis associated with Cheyletiella infestation in cats. J. Am. Vet. Med. Assoc., 174:718–720, 1979.

McLennan, H., and Oikawa, I.: Changes in function of the neuromuscular junction occurring in tick paralysis. Can. J. Phys. Pharmacol., 50:53–58, 1972.

Miller, J.K., Tompkins, V.N., and Sieracki, J.C.: Pathology of Colorado tick fever in experimental animals. Arch. Pathol., 72:149–157, 1961.

Nelson, W.A., and Bainborough, A.R.: Development in sheep of resistance to the ked, *Melophagus ovinus* (L.). III. Histopathology of sheep skin as a clue to the nature of resistance. Exp. Parasitol., 13:118–127, 1963. VB 3570–63.

Nemeseri, L., and Szeky, A.: Demodecicosis in cattle. Zctz. Vet. Acad. Sci. Hung., 11:209–221, 1961. VB 493–62.

———: Demodicosis in sheep. Acta Vet. Hung., 16:53–63, 1966. VB 36:4809, 1966.

———: Demodicosis of swine. Acta Vet. Hung., 16:251–261, 1966. VB 37:1720, 1967.

Prathap, K., Lau, K.S., and Bolton, J.M.: Pentastomiasis: a common finding at autopsy among Malaysian aborigines. Am. J. Trop. Med. Hyg., 18:20–27, 1969.

Savov, N.: Death of a heifer caused by massive infestations with juvenile forms of *Linguatula serrata*. Vet. Sbir., 56:22–24, 1959. VB 3512–1959.

Schaffer, M.H., Baker, N.F., and Kennedy, P.C.: Parasitism by Cheyletiella parasitivorax. A case report of the infestation in a female dog and its litter. Cornell Vet., 48:440–447, 1958.

Schnelle, G.B., and Jones, T.C.: Occurrence of the cereal mite in war dogs. J. Am. Vet. Med. Assoc., 104:213–214, 1944.

Sharma Deorani, V.P., and Chaudhuri, R.P.: On this histopathology of the skin lesion of goats affected by sarcoptic mange. Indian J. Vet. Sci., 35:150–156, 1965.

Sheahan, B.J.: Pathology of *Sarcoptes scabiei* infection in pigs. I. Naturally occurring and experimentally induced lesion. II. Histological, histochemical and ultrastructural changes at skin test sites. J. Comp. Pathol., 85:87–95, 97–110, 1975.

Sloan, C.A.: Mortality in sheep due to *Ixodes species*. Aust. Vet. J., 44:527–528, 1968.

Smith, E.B., and Claypoole, T.F.: Canine scabies in dogs and in humans. J. Am. Med. Assoc., 199:59–64, 1967.

Whitney, R.A., and Kruckenberg, S.M.: Pentastomid infection associated with peritonitis in Mangabey monkeys. J. Am. Vet. Med. Assoc., 151:907–908, 1967.

Yasgur, I.: Parasitism of kennel puppies with the mite Cheyletiella parasitivorax. Cornell Vet., 54:406–407, 1964.

CHAPTER 15

Pathologic Effects of Ionizing Radiations

An understanding of the pathologic effects of radiation has increased in importance over the past several years, and its significance will continue to grow with the expanding development of nuclear energy. The explosion of a nuclear bomb produces huge quantities of radioactive substances which may be scattered widely by blast and wind with possible hazard to man and animals. The use of nuclear energy as a controlled source of power in reactions and atomic "piles" presents the potential hazard of accidental exposure. Hopefully, these two sources of radiation will remain controlled. Radiation, however, will continue to increase in importance in the diagnosis and treatment of disease, and in its many forms, will be a valuable tool to animal research. It is important, therefore, to study the biologic effects of radiation, from whatever source.

Radiation of the types to be considered, which exists in both electromagnetic and particulate form, gives up its energy and in general produces its effect upon cells and tissues by the process of ionization. This property, the ionization of matter, also provides the usual means for detection of radiation of this type; thus, the term **ionizing radiation** is appropriate and useful to differentiate it from radiation of other types (heat, light), which also produce

biologic effects. Ionization is the production of ions (atoms or molecules that possess an electrical charge) by a sequence of atomic events leading to displacement of electrons and transfer of energy.

Details of atomic physics lie outside the scope of this book, but some of the nomenclature must be used in studying the lesions produced by ionizing radiation. Therefore, a few terms will be discussed prior to considering the biologic effects of ionizing radiation.

TYPES OF IONIZING RADIATION

As indicated previously, ionizing radiation may be either electromagnetic or particulate.

Electromagnetic Radiation

Electromagnetic radiation includes a broad spectrum of energy waves: radio waves, infrared waves, ultraviolet waves, visible light, gamma rays, x-rays (roentgen rays), and cosmic rays. All have their specific wavelengths and frequencies and travel at the speed of light. Those with short wavelengths and high frequencies are ionizing radiations, and include gamma, x-, and cosmic rays. Ionization results from the ejection of electrons from the target molecules.

Gamma rays (γ) are electromagnetic radiations of short wavelengths emitted from the nucleus of radioisotopes. They are essentially similar to x-rays but usually of higher energy, and generally come from different sources. Gamma rays have long range and deep penetration in tissues, but low ionization per unit of matter penetrated. These rays may penetrate deep into the body and produce an effect upon the entire body (total body effect).

X-rays or **roentgen rays** are penetrating electromagnetic radiations having wavelengths less than those of visible light. Although similar to gamma rays, they usually are of much lower energy and are produced by the bombardment of a metallic target by fast-moving electrons in a high vacuum. Their biologic effects are similar to those of gamma rays.

Cosmic rays are complex radiation phenomena that originate in outer space and are largely absorbed by the earth's atmosphere. Some constituents of cosmic rays are capable of extremely deep penetration, even in dense matter such as rock.

Particulate Radiation

A variety of discrete particles, which may be released from radioisotopes or accelerated artificially, comprise particulate radiation. As particles, they all have lesser penetrability into tissues than electromagnetic radiations, but possess greater capacity for ionization.

The **alpha particle** (α) is a helium nucleus consisting of two protons and two neutrons with a double positive charge and having a definite mass. A stream of alpha particles (so-called alpha ray) has high ionizing but very low penetrating properties and a short range, since a thin sheet of paper, the keratin layer of the skin, or other material of comparable thickness will prevent its passage. It has little biologic effect except when alpha-emitting isotopes (such as radium) are deposited in tissues, where prolonged effects are produced.

The **beta particle** (β) is a charged particle (negative or positive) emitted from the nucleus of an atom; its mass and charge are equal in magnitude to those of the electron. A positive electron is called a positron (β+). Depending on its energy, a beta particle has a longer range and deeper penetration than an alpha particle, but causes only a medium degree of ionization. Radioactive isotopes that emit beta particles ("beta emitters") may produce lesions in the skin upon continued contact and may be particularly dangerous when concentrated in bone (as in radioactive isotopes deposited in bone, i.e., "bone seekers").

Neutrons (n) are elementary nuclear particles that bear no electrical charge and have a mass approximately the same as that of hydrogen atoms. Neutrons have very long range, deep penetration, and may induce radioactivity. They may be artificially accelerated in the form of a beam, which provides a useful means of tissue analysis by induction of radioactivity (neutron activation analysis).

Protons are also constituents of atomic nuclei with the same mass as a neutron but bearing a positive charge equal and opposite to that of an electron. They have high ionizing capacity and may induce radioactivity. Proton beams can also be artificially created and used to induce radioactivity for tissue analysis (proton activation analysis). Proton beams are more definable in outline than the more diffuse neutron beams.

MEASUREMENT OF RADIATION

The **roentgen** (r) is a unit of x- or gamma radiation used, as a rule, in measuring dosage. It is defined as that quantity of x- or gamma radiation which is of such magnitude that its associated corpuscular emission per 0.001293 gram of air produces in air ions carrying one electrostatic unit of electricity of either sign. The intensity of the roentgen (r) is measured in air; hence it is not an accurate indication of radioactivity absorbed by the tissues. In order to overcome this discrepancy, a unit of measurement of absorbed dosage of radiation, the **rad,** was adopted by the International Commission on Radiologic Units at the Seventh International Congress of Radiology, Copenhagen, in 1953. The rad is a measure of the energy (100 ergs per gram) imparted to matter by ionizing particles per unit mass of unit material at the place of interest. Another unit, the **Gray,** is an absorbed dose 100 times larger than one rad. In biologic systems, the matter irradiated is usually stated as a specific tissue.

The **curie** (Ci) is that quantity of radioactive material having associated with it 3.7 $\times$ 10^{10} disintegrations per second. It is therefore a measure of radioactivity and is most commonly used in biology as millicurie (mc) or microcurie (μc) units.

The **specific activity** of radioactive material is the activity of a sample per unit mass.

The **half life** of a radioactive substance is the length of time (in seconds, hours, days, or years) required for the substance to lose 50% of its radioactivity by decay. The **biologic half life** of a substance is the time required for the body to eliminate one-half of an administered dose of the substance by the usual process of elimination. The **lethal dose** (LD) of radiation is usually stated as the amount required to kill a given number of animals within a specified period of time. Thus, LD 50/30 is the dosage of radiation required to kill 50% of a group of animals in 30 days.

An **electron volt** (eV) is a unit of energy equivalent to the amount of energy gained by an electron passing through a potential difference of one volt. Large multiples of this unit are commonly used, viz., *kev* (thousand electron volts), *mev* (million electron volts), and *bev* (billion electron volts).

Linear energy transfer (LET) is a term used to express the quality of radiation. It concerns the spatial distributions of energy transfers which occur along and within the tracks of particles as they penetrate matter. These energy transfers influence the effectiveness of an irradiation in producing physical, chemical, or biological changes, and are independent of other physical factors, such as **total energy dissipated, absorbed dose, absorbed dose rate,** and **absorbed dose fractionation. Relative biological effectiveness** (RBE) is used to compare the absorbed dose of two forms of radiation to produce the same biologic effect. The precise, technical definition of these terms may be found in the report of the International Commission on Radiation Units and Measurements (1970).

RADIOISOTOPES

An isotope of an element is one of several nuclides of that element having the same number of protons in their nuclei, hence the same atomic number, but differing in the number of neutrons and consequently in mass number. Isotopes of a particular element have almost identical chemical properties, and may be stable or unstable. Unstable isotopes undergo radioactive decay, and are therefore called **radioactive isotopes** or **radioisotopes.** Only a few radioisotopes occur in nature and generally these do not constitute a large source of radioactivity. The fission reaction in the atomic bomb or the neutron bombardment of stable isotopes in a nuclear reactor can produce large quantities of artificial radioisotopes which have wide use in science, industry, and medicine. Isotopes are usually designated by their chemical symbol and mass number; thus, radium-223 (^{223}Ra), potassium-40 (^{40}K), uranium-238 (^{238}U) are naturally occurring radioisotopes; iodine-131 (^{131}I), and phosphorus-32 (^{32}P) are artificially produced radioisotopes; while potassium-39 (^{39}K), carbon-13 (^{13}C) and oxygen-16 (^{16}O) are stable isotopes. These symbols may be written with left (^{32}P) or right (P^{32}) superscripts. The convention using the left superscript for the mass number and a left subscript for the atomic number of the element may also be encountered—i.e., $^{1}_{1}$H for hydrogen and $^{2}_{1}$H for heavy hydrogen (deuterium). The student is referred to the texts listed under references for further information on this vitally important subject.

International Commission on Radiation Units and Measurements (ICRU). Linear Energy Transfer, ICRU Report No. 16, 1970. Washington, D.C.

Lapp, R.E., and Andrews, H.L.: Nuclear Radiation Physics, 2nd ed. New York, Prentice-Hall, 1954.

National Council on Radiation Protection and Measurements. Radiation Protection in Veterinary Medicine. NCRP Report No. 36, 15 August 1970, Washington, D.C.

Upton, A.C.: Radiation Injury, Chicago, Univ. Chicago Press, 1969.

EFFECTS OF RADIATION ON BIOLOGIC SYSTEMS

Direct Effects

Direct effects of radiation may be explained on the basis of the target theory; particularly in relation to viruses, genes, and chromosomes (Florey, 1970). The target is visualized as one of relatively large molecular dimensions, and the effect is attributed to a single ionization, or a small number of ionizations, anywhere within the structure. It is presumed that a chemical change is produced in a molecule when ionization occurs directly within it. A larger molecule is more likely to be hit than a smaller one, thus the dose required to change a quantity of a substance by radiation will be inversely proportional to its molecular weight. A method based upon this principle has been used to determine the molecular weight of some proteins.

Quantitation of direct effects depends upon the target size, type of radiation, and intensity of radiation dosage.

Indirect Effects

Indirect action of radiation is particularly applicable in aqueous solution and depends upon ionization, which produces free radicals, which in turn may react chemically. These free radicals (for example, hydroxyl [OH−] and perhydroxyl [HO_2] radicals) are highly reactive and may become responsible for chemical changes in other molecules in the solution. This indirect effect upon molecules would depend upon the number of free radicals released and not upon molecular size or concentration. If a single substance in solution is radiated, changes in that solute will increase linearly with the dose of radiation. If two or more substances are present in the irradiated solution, one may have a protective effect by competing for the free radicals.

Enzymes and Enzyme Systems

The inactivation of vital enzymes or enzyme systems in cells has been postulated as one of the possible means by which radiant energy could injure cells. Purified enzymes, such as ribonuclease, in the solid state may be partially inactivated by x-radiation if very large doses are used (i.e., 20×10^6 rads). This appears to be due to a direct effect of the radiation. In dilute aqueous solution, a purified enzyme is inactivated more readily, but increased concentrations appear to be protective, suggesting an indirect effect of the radiation. Many compounds, particularly those such as cysteine and glutathione which have an affinity for reaction with oxidizing radicals, exert a protective effect upon enzymes radiated in solution. Oxidative phosphorylation in biologic systems results in the generation of adenosine triphosphate (ATP) from adenosine diphosphate (ADP) or monophosphate (AMP). This generation of ATP in cells is accomplished principally in the mitochondria. Radiation of isolated mitochondria, in vitro, has little effect on their phosphorylation potential unless very high doses are used (10,000 rads). On the other hand, mitochondria from spleen or thymus of irradiated rats (700 rads), have decreased phosphorylating capacity. Isolated calf thymic nuclei, in vitro, have phosphorylating activity which can be inactivated by radiation. Phosphorylation of nuclear histone is also depressed by gamma irradiation. Synthesis of deoxyribonucleic acid (DNA) is also inhibited in plant cells following irradiation, particularly if done prior to the onset of mitosis.

Viruses

The direct effect of radiation on viruses appears to be most significant in purified, dry, or concentrated solution, or in the presence of protective substances. The mean lethal dose may be correlated with the size of some plant and phage viruses. However, with the larger vaccinia virus, the target volume appears to be smaller than the virus itself, perhaps indicating a more radiosensitive component of the virus complex.

Bacteria

The survival of bacteria has been studied following ionizing radiation in the dry state or suspended in water or nutrient media. Curves prepared of the logarithmic numbers of surviving bacteria usually indicate an exponential relationship to dose, but in some instances an increasing percentage of bacteria are killed by each increment of radiation dosage before this exponential relationship is reached. In some conditions, bacteria are protected from the lethal effects of radiant energy by freezing or by the presence of reducing agents in the solution.

Mammalian Cells

The radiosensitivity of cells, in vitro, has been demonstrated for many types of neoplastic and normal animal cells. Many neoplastic murine cells (lymphoma, Ehrlich ascites, sarcoma, mammary carcinoma, and squamous cell carcinoma) have been exposed, in vitro, to x-rays or gamma rays under varying experimental conditions. Of interest is the observation that most of these tumor cells are much more radiosensitive in the oxygenated as compared to the anoxic state. The sensitivity of these cells also varies widely in relation to the stage of mitotic cycle in which they are irradiated. All cells are most radiosensitive during mitosis, then are resistant for a period, until the start of DNA synthesis. After completion of DNA synthesis, these cells remain radioresistant until mitosis again is resumed.

Some heritable changes have been demonstrated to occur in cultures of irradiated mammalian cells (Abraham and Berry, 1970). The nucleus of most cells is clearly more sensitive to radiation than the cytoplasm. Although most cells irreparably injured by radiation are unable to reproduce subsequently, many functions of the cell are not impaired until the cell actually undergoes necrosis. A few cells, particularly oocytes and lymphocytes, are quite sensitive in interphase, undergoing necrosis shortly after receiving a small dose.

Nonlethal doses of radiant energy may produce lesions in **chromosomes** which are of particular interest. Gamma irradiation is of greatest significance in whole body irradiation, but if radioisotopes are introduced into tissues through whatever means, alpha-emitters are 15 to 20 times more damaging to chromosomes than either gamma- or beta-emitters. Modern cytogenetic techniques make it possible to examine chromosomes in metaphase and to detect anomalies in number and morphology. These effects have been observed in human patients who were irradiated for treatment of one of various disorders and in radiation workers whose circulating lymphocytes were subsequently studied by cytogenetic methods (Court-Brown et al., 1965). These abnormalities have also been seen in many animal karyotypes. Certain lesions in chromosomes are considered unstable in that they are usually lost as the cell undergoes mitosis. These include: chromatid breaks (fracture of one arm of the chromosome), acentric fragments (bits of chromosome with no centromere, resulting from fracture), dicentric chromosomes (with two centromeres, resulting from fracture and rejoining at centromere), tricentric chromosomes (three centromeres), and aneuploidy (more or less than the normal diploid number). Stable, or permanent, lesions include: reciprocal translocations (exchange transfer of parts of chromatids between two chromosomes), ring chromosomes (breaks with fusion of telomeric ends of chromosomes), and aneuploidy (trisomy especially, may also be unstable).

Lesions in chromosomes occur in increased numbers in lymphocytes of patients and experimental animals following x-ray treatment. Similar breaks occur in unirradiated subjects, but usually in less than 1% of the cells examined. Following irradiation, these may constitute as much as 37% of the cells karyotyped. These defects undoubtedly change the metabolism of the affected cells, but have not been shown to affect germ cells and thus influence the genetic makeup of offspring.

Genes

The rearrangement, loss, or addition of parts of a chromosome doubtlessly has an effect upon the metabolism and progeny of the affected cell. It is also possible for radiant energy to cause chemical alteration in the DNA of cells, resulting in **mutation**. The mutagenic effect of ionizing radiation has been clearly demonstrated in such organisms as the bread mold, *Neurospora*, and fruit fly, *Drosophila*. The evidence for such mutagenic effects in mammals, such as mice, is not as convincing. It is possible that mutagenic effects do occur in mammalian germ cells, but resulting gametes are less viable, resulting in fewer zygotes carrying the mutant gene.

Carcinogenesis

Several clear-cut examples exist to indicate that some forms of neoplasia appear with increased frequency in animals and man following exposure to ionizing radiation. (See Neoplasia.) The possible interaction of certain oncogenic viruses in some neoplasms is yet to be explained. Leukemia in Japanese people who were exposed to irradiation at Hiroshima or Nagasaki clearly became more frequent than in their unirradiated countrymen. Irradiated mice also have significant in-

creased frequency of lymphoma (so-called leukemia). The appearance of squamous cell carcinomas on the hands of radiologists and veterinarians following x-ray injury also is acceptable evidence. Clearly, ionizing radiation may be an antecedent event in certain types of malignant disease, although the precise etiologic relationship and pathogenetic mechanisms are not yet established.

Environmental Pollution

Some forms of radioactivity, particularly resulting from atomic explosions, may become concentrated by biologic processes and therefore represent a special kind of pollutant. Radioiodine is one example, the ^{131}I is concentrated in the thyroid of animals after consumption of contaminated forage. Radiostrontium is more important in this respect because it is metabolized as a chemical analogue of calcium and is concentrated by aquatic plants and animals. Here it becomes part of the food chain of animals and man and therefore a hazard. Radiostrontium (^{90}Sr) is stored in bones of animals and excreted in milk. However, specific biologic discrimination by the cow (i.e., intestinal absorption of only part of the ^{90}Sr, deposit of some of it in bone and subsequent urinary excretion with calcium) makes milk one of the safest sources of calcium in an area contaminated by radioactive fallout. In other words, foods directly contaminated would provide relatively more ^{90}Sr to be absorbed and metabolized as calcium (Comar, 1965).

Abraham, E.P., and Berry, R.J.: Some biological effects of radiant energy. Chapters 25 and 26. *In* General Pathology, 4th ed. edited by H. W. Florey, Philadelphia, W. B. Saunders Co., 1970.

Barnett, M.H.: The biological effects of ionizing radiation. Conn. Med., 43:75–80, 1979.

Bender, M.A., and Gooch, P.C.: Persistent chromosome aberrations in irradiated human subjects. Radiation Res., 16:44–53, 1962.

Bischoff, F., Ullman, H.J., and Ingraham, L.P.: The influence of irradiation of the ovaries upon estrus and neoplastic development in Marsh-Buffalo mice. Radiology, 43:55–58, 1944.

Blumenfeld, H., and Thomas, S.F.: Chronic massive pericardial effusion following roentgen therapy for carcinoma of the breast. Radiology, 43:335–340, 1945.

Brill, A.B., and Forgotson, E.H.: Radiation and congenital malformations. Am. J. Obstet. Gynecol., 90:1149–1168, 1964.

Brooks, A.L.: Chromosome damage in liver cells from low dose rate alpha, beta, and gamma irradiation: derivation of RBE. Science, 190:1090–1092, 1975.

Case, M.T., and Simon, J.: Whole-body gamma irradiation of newborn pigs: hematologic changes. Am. J. Vet. Res., 33:1217–1222, 1972.

Comar, C.L.: Radioisotopes in Biology and Agriculture. New York, McGraw-Hill, 1955.

Court-Brown, W.M., Buckton, K.E., and McLean, A.S.: Quantitative studies of chromosome aberrations in man following acute and chronic exposure to x rays and gamma rays. Lancet, 1:1239–1241, 1965.

Florey, H.W. (ed.): General Pathology. Philadelphia, W. B. Saunders, 1970.

Furth, J., and Lorenz, E.: Carcinogenesis by ionizing radiations. In Radiation Biology, edited by A. Hollaender. New York, McGraw-Hill, 1954.

Hollaender, A.: Radiation Biology. New York, McGraw-Hill, 1954.

Hugon, J., and Borgers, M.: Fine structure of the nuclei of duodenal crypt cells after x-irradiation. Am. J. Pathol., 52:701–723, 1968.

Hutchinson, F.: The molecular basis for radiation effects on cells. Cancer Res., 26:2045–2052, 1966.

Kochupillai, N., Verma, I.C., Grewal, M.S., and Ramalingaswami, V.: Down's syndrome and related abnormalities in an area of high background radiation in coastal Kerala. Nature, 262:60–61, 1976.

Loutit, J.F.: Irradiation of Mice and Men. Chicago, Univ. Chicago Press, 1962.

Luxton, R.W.: Radiation nephritis. Quart. J. Med., 22:215–242, 1953.

MacLeod, J., Hotchkiss, R.S., and Sitterson, B.W.: Recovery of male fertility after sterilization by nuclear radiation. J. A. M. A., 187:637–641, 1964.

McDonald, L.W., and Hayes, T.L.: The role of capillaries in the pathogenesis of delayed radionecrosis of brain. Am. J. Pathol., 50:745–758, 1967.

Moore, W., Jr., and Gillespie, L.J.: Persistence of chromosomal damage following in utero irradiation of the dog. Am. J. Vet. Res., 28:890–891, 1967.

Murphree, R.L., Whitaker, W.M., Wilding, J.L., and Rust, J.H.: Effects of whole body exposure to irradiation upon subsequent fertility of male rabbits. Science, 115:709–711, 1952.

Russell, W.L.: The effect of radiation dose rate and fractionation on mutation in mice. In Repair from Genetic Radiation Damage, edited by F. H. Sobels. Oxford, Pergamon Press, 1963, pp. 205–217.

Sasser, L.B., Bell, M.C., and Cross, F.H.: Hematologic response of sheep and cattle to whole-body gamma irradiation and gastrointestinal and skin beta irradiation. Am. J. Vet. Res., 34:1555–1560, 1973.

Spalding, J.F., Brooks, M.R., and Archuleta, R.F.: Genetic effects of x-irradiation of 10, 15 and 20 generations of male mice. Health Phys., 10:293–296, 1964.

Wolff, S.: Some postirradiation phenomena that affect the induction of chromosome aberrations. J. Cell Comp. Physiol., 58: (Supp. 1) 151–162, 1961.

RADIOSENSITIVITY OF TISSUES

The susceptibility of tissues to radiation varies widely even in the same species. In general, those tissues undergoing the most rapid growth are most susceptible to the injurious effects of ionizing radiation; conversely, cells that have a slower rate of reproduction are most resistant. Also, tissues with the least degree of differentiation are more sensitive than those that are highly differentiated. Thus, cells may be listed in order of their susceptibility to radiation:

Extreme Radiosensitivity

Lymphocytes
Immature hematopoietic cells
Intestinal epithelium
Germinal cells

High Radiosensitivity

Urinary bladder epithelium
Gastric epithelium
Epithelium of the skin
Epithelium of mouth, pharynx, and esophagus

Intermediate Radiosensitivity

Endothelium
Connective tissue cells
Cartilage and growing bone cells
Renal epithelium
Hepatic epithelium
Pancreatic epithelium
Thyroid epithelium
Adrenal epithelium
Pulmonary epithelium

Low Radiosensitivity

Skeletal muscle cells
Mature bone cells
Mature connective tissue
Neurons
Mature hematopoietic cells

SUSCEPTIBILITY OF DIFFERENT SPECIES

The susceptibility of various animal species to ionizing radiation differs within wide limits. In large animals, the LD 50/30 is also influenced by the source of the radiation and the dosage rate (Rust et al., 1954). The following list from Bond et al., 1965, indicates the approximate lethal dose (LD 50/30) of x- or gamma radiation given in one dose over the total body:

Species	rad
Sheep	200–300
Swine	200–300
Dog	240–320
Goat	250–300
Burro	250–300
Guinea pig	400–500
Rhesus monkey	500–600
Mouse	525–775
Rabbit	700–800
Rat	700–820

Simpler forms of life are, in general, much more resistant to the lethal effects of radiation. For example, 750,000 r are required to kill all bacteria in milk; sporulating bacteria may require as much as 500,000 r to kill all spores; tobacco mosaic virus is killed by 1,800,000 r, and although some enzyme systems show measurable effects after this large amount of radiation, many times this dose is required to destroy all enzyme systems in tissues.

Bond, V.P., Fliedner, T.M., and Archambeau, J.O.: Mammalian Radiation Lethality: A Disturbance in Cellular Kinetics. New York, Academic Press, 1965.
Gleiser, C.A.: The determination of the lethal dose 50/30 of total body x-radiation for dogs. Am. J. Vet. Res., 14:284–286, 1953.
Rust, J.H., et al.: The lethal dose of whole-body tantalum 182 gamma irradiation for the burro (Equus asinus asinus). Radiology, 60:579–582, 1953.
Rust, J.H., Trum, B.F., and Kuhn, U.S.G., III: Physiological aberrations following total body irradiation of domestic animals with large doses of gamma rays. Vet. Med., 49:318, 1954.

WHOLE BODY RADIATION

In contrast to radiation delivered to a specific part of the body (as in radium or x-ray therapy), whole body radiation is the exposure of the entire surface of the body so as to give a uniform dose of ionizing radiation to all parts of the body. This type of radiation injury may be produced experimentally by x- and gamma rays and may occur following the detonation of an atomic blast. If dosages are sufficiently high, several systems of the body will be affected, resulting in the syndrome of **radiation sickness.**

Clinical Manifestations

The clinicopathologic changes in animals exposed to whole body radiation include immediate and severe lymphopenia with a slow recovery in surviving animals. Within a few days, the polymorphonuclear cells in the circulating blood decrease. Thrombocytes in the blood are progressively reduced and return slowly to the circulation. This thrombocytopenia undoubtedly underlies the hemorrhagic phenomena that follow. Anemia slowly becomes evident, probably due to the reduction of the red cell precursors; blood clot retraction is delayed, and blood levels of alkaline phosphatase are reduced. The iodine uptake by the thyroid may be decreased, the respiratory quotient is reduced, and urea excretion is slightly increased.

The **signs** observed in animals exposed to lethal doses of ionizing radiation depend to some extent upon the dose as well as the dose rate. A few dogs which receive twice a 100% lethal dose (2 × LD 100/30) of total body radiation may die suddenly within 72 hours without manifesting significant symptoms. Diarrhea may develop in some animals, and after a time the stools may become tarry or bloody. Other animals receiving similar doses may not show symptoms for seven to nine days following radiation; then hemorrhages may be observed in visible mucosae, septicemia follows the severe agranulocytosis, and death soon supervenes. Animals exposed to a very high dosage may suddenly exhibit severe disturbances of locomotion and die within 72 hours. The symptoms that might be observed, therefore, are not specific, and easily could be mistakenly attributed to any one of several causes. **Infection and septicemia** are common following high or lethal doses of radiation and are often responsible for death. The killing of leukocyte stem cells is of primary importance in this regard, but high doses also impair chemotaxis and phagocytosis of fully differentiated neutrophils.

Gross Lesions

The most prominent gross changes in animals dying after lethal doses of whole body radiation are hemorrhages, which may occur anywhere in the body, but most frequently involve the heart, the gastrointestinal, and the genitourinary systems. In early stages, congestion of small blood vessels of heart, brain, lungs, mesentery, intestine, and subcutis may be the only findings, but later, scattered petechiae also may be found in these organs. The hemorrhages observed in severely affected animals vary from small petechiae to extensive extravasations with occasional hematomas. In goats and pigs, petechiae have been described in the renal cortices and pelves, with large blood clots in the pelves.

Hemorrhages may be seen in the musculature of the back, abdomen, legs, thorax, and diaphragm. This is particularly common in guinea pigs, rare in rats, and occasionally seen in goats and pigs. The lymph nodes and tonsils are characteristically hemorrhagic, edematous, enlarged, and dark red; on cut surfaces, hemolytic areas are interspersed with gray, moist-appearing lymphoid tissue. Hemorrhages and ulcerations are the predominant lesions in the gastrointestinal tract. The ulcers are most common in the large intestine and are superficial. Fibrinous membranes, stained with feces, may be removed from the mucosal surface with difficulty, leaving raw, eroded areas in the underlying mucosa. The bone marrow usually loses its deep red color and appears pale and often gelatinous with a yellowish tint.

Microscopic Lesions

The microscopic findings in lethal whole body radiation generally can be correlated with the gross as well as the clinical manifestations. The degree of injury to tissues depends to some extent upon dosage, but to a greater extent upon the radiosensitivity of the tissue. Lymphoid cells, being most susceptible, will manifest the most severe changes, while mature bone will be least affected.

In general, the lesions resulting from radiation at the level of the cell or the body as a whole are not unique. This is exemplified by the reference to effects of certain drugs and even viruses as radiomimetic. Following irradiation, cells may undergo degenerative changes and necrosis similar to those described in Chapter 2. Nuclear chromatin becomes clumped and the nucleus may swell or become pyknotic and fragment (karyorrhexis). The entire cell becomes swollen and vacuolated (see acute cellular swelling, p. 14), as do individual cytoplasmic organelles. These events and cell death may not occur until after mitosis or until after several divisions, indicative of chromosomal damage. The loss of cells or necrosis leads to the varying consequences of necrosis caused by other injurious agents, e.g., impairment of function, atrophy, regeneration, repair, fibrosis. Thus, a spectrum of chronic histopathologic lesions may be seen even years subsequent to the initial injury.

Changes in the reproductive capacity of a cell is another effect of radiation on cells. Although an irradiated cell may appear morphologically normal, it may lose its ability to divide, or it may replicate without cellular division, leading to the formation of multinucleated giant cells. Multinucleated giant cells, particularly in fibroblasts, are a clue to radiation damage. Other causes, such as certain viral infections, must of course be excluded.

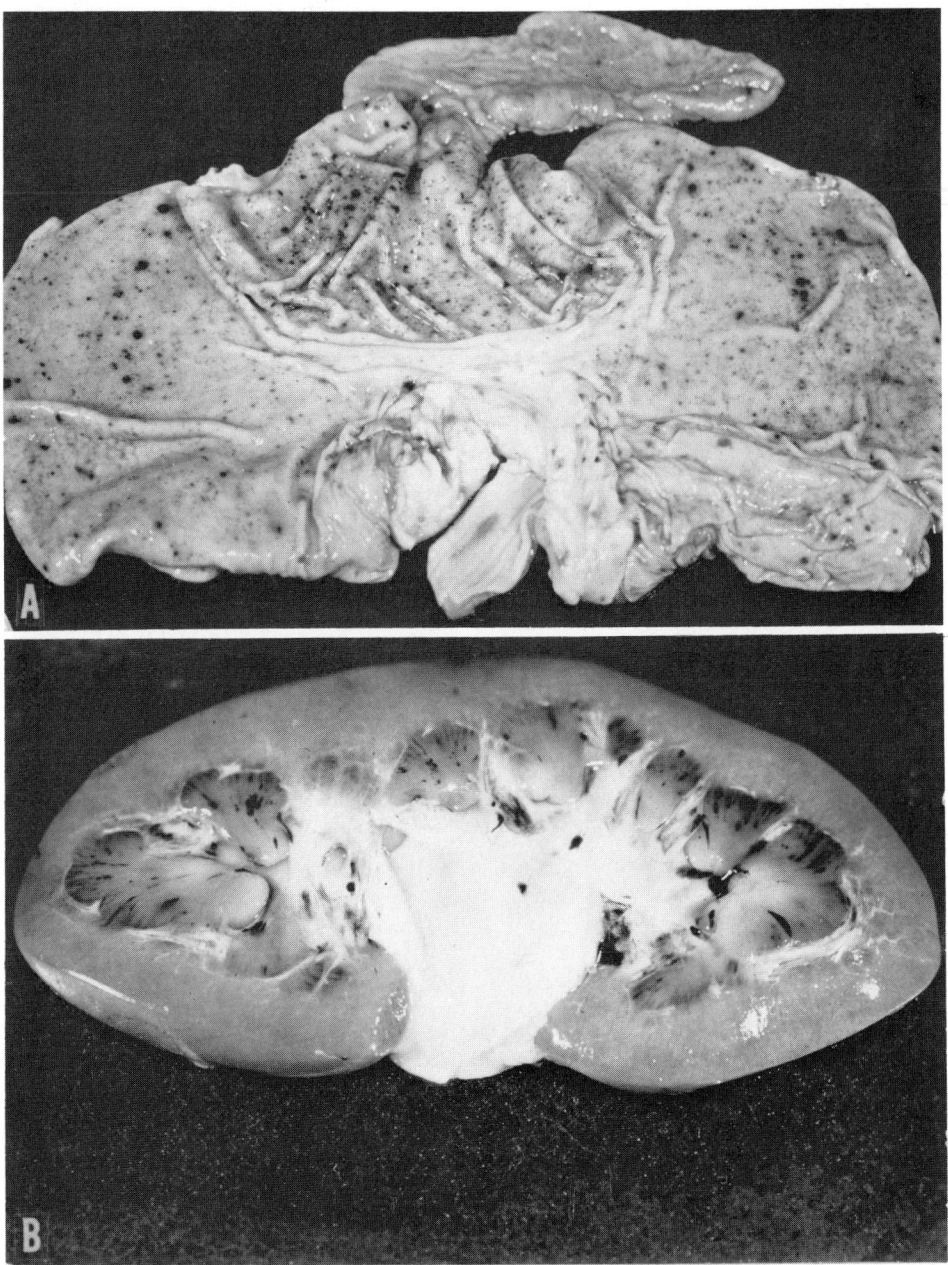

Fig. 15–1. *A,* Whole body radiation. Hemorrhages in the stomach of a pig. *B,* Whole body radiation. Hemorrhages in the renal medulla, kidney of a pig. Contributor: Medical Section, Joint Task Force No. 1, Operation Crossroads. (Courtesy of Armed Forces Institute of Pathology.)

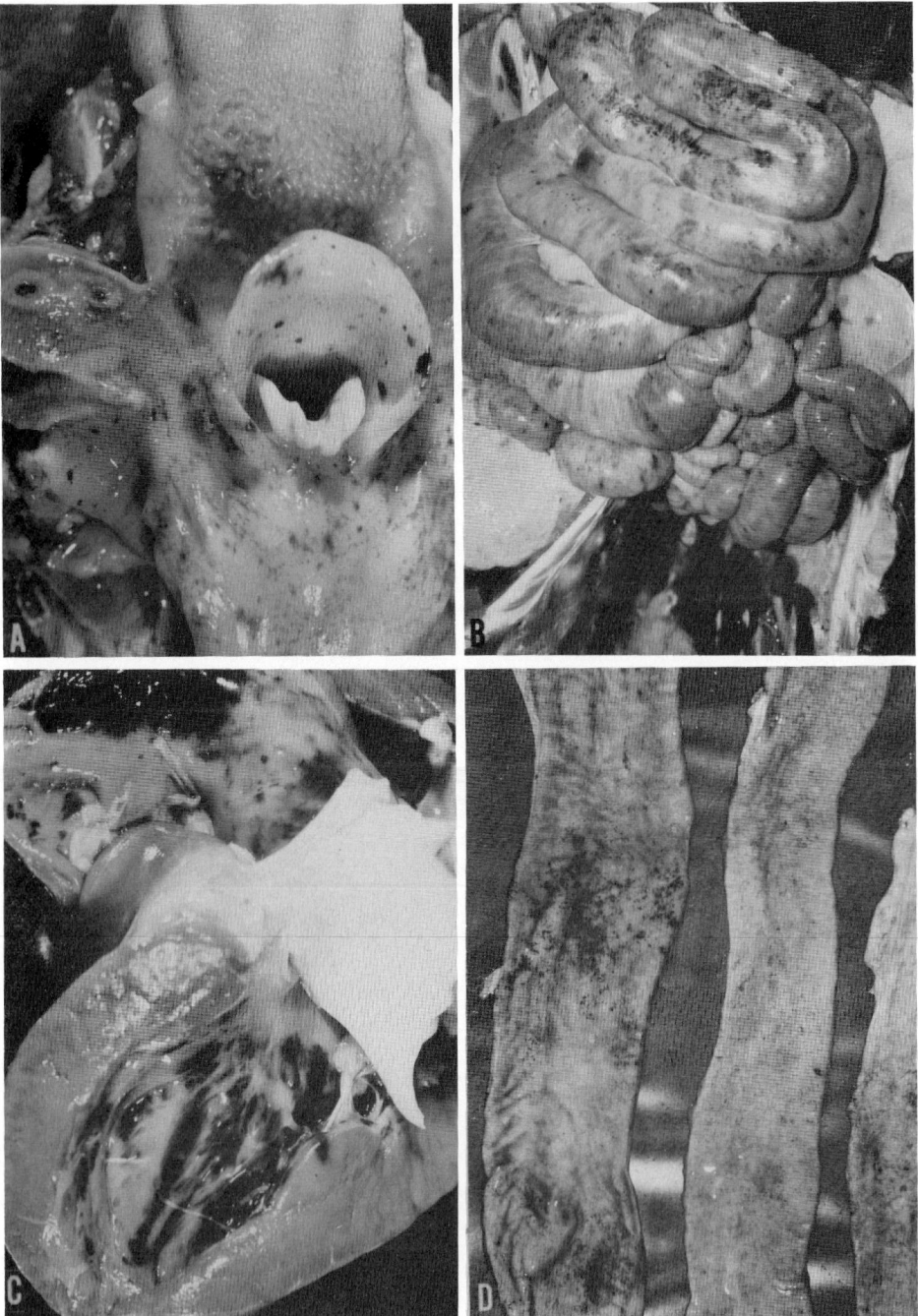

Fig. 15–2.   Whole body radiation. *A*, Hemorrhages in the mucosa of the pharynx and epiglottis of a pig. *B*, Hemorrhages in the intestinal serosa of a pig. *C*, Subendocardial hemorrhages, heart of a pig. *D*, Hemorrhages in the intestinal wall of a pig. Contributor: Medical Section, Joint Task Force No. 1, Operation Crossroads. (Courtesy of Armed Forces Institute of Pathology.)

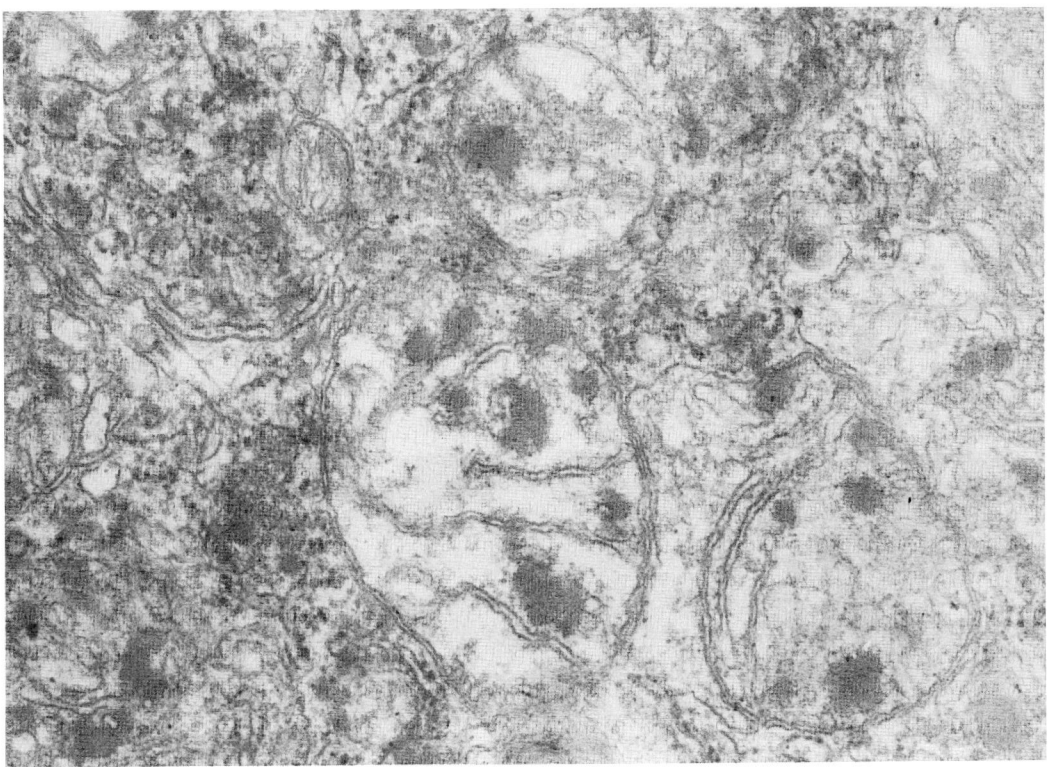

Fig. 15–3. Mitochondrial swelling and disruption of cristae in the kidney of a mouse following 2.01×10^6 rads of x-ray exposure. These changes develop within two minutes after exposure. (Courtesy of Scott W. Jordan, M.D.)

Damage to blood vessels account for some of the acute effects of irradiation and is responsible for a number of chronic sequelae. Initially there is vascular dilation leading to hyperemia, which is believed to result from release of various chemicals, as in inflammation. Subsequently, endothelial cells become swollen and vacuolated, leading to increased permeability and egress of plasma and cells. Over a period of months, the walls of arteries and arterioles become sclerotic and hyalinized, and the number of lining endothelial cells increases. Resultant reduction of blood flow leads to further functional impairment and fibrosis of affected organs.

Lymphoid Tissue. Lymphoid tissues, such as lymph nodes, spleen, thymus, and tonsils, are affected promptly, and this is reflected in the microscopic alterations.

Necrosis of lymphocytes, as evidenced by pyknosis, karyorrhexis, and karyolysis of nuclei, is the earliest and most significant finding. As a result, the germinal centers soon appear "washed out," leaving only the reticuloendothelial cells. The sinuses are dilated and filled with macrophages, some of which have engulfed erythrocytes as well as tissue debris. Recent hemorrhages may be evident, and in cases of longer duration, collections of blood pigment. Secondary changes due to abscesses, ulcers, hemorrhages, or other lesions in the organs drained by a particular lymph node may occur in animals with prolonged survival time.

Bone Marrow. Microscopically, detectable lesions occur in the bone marrow within a few hours after heavy doses of radiation. Necrosis of hematopoietic cells, particularly the most immature, occurs very early. The myelocytes appear most susceptible, the megakaryocytes and erythrocytes less so, and the reticular cells quite resistant. The sinuses become dilated with plasma or red blood cells. Within a week or two, most radiosensitive elements disappear from the bone marrow, leaving aplastic, acellular marrow that contains only fat cells, reticular cells, edema, and hemorrhage. Secondary infection may be the means by which colonies of fungi or bacteria are transplanted in the marrow, where they grow, usually without apparent inflammatory reaction to their presence. Bloom (1948) has described a change in irradiated small animals in which the bony trabeculae on the diaphyseal side of the epiphyseal cartilage disappear and are replaced by fibrillar stroma. The resulting separation of the epiphyseal cartilage from the spongy bone on the diaphyseal side has been referred to as "severance" of the epiphyseal plate.

Digestive System. Shallow ulcers with little or no underlying leukocytic infiltration are common in the oral and pharyngeal mucous membranes, especially along the margins of the tongue and adjacent to the tonsillar crypts. These shallow ulcers have a necrotic base, but only if the animal is beginning to recover from agranulocytosis do leukocytes appear. The mucous membrane of the digestive tract from the esophagus to the anus is severely affected by whole body radiation. Edema of the submucosa and subserosa is common throughout the tract, and is usually associated with necrosis of the mucosal epithelium and frequent hemorrhages in all parts of the wall. The necrosis of the epithelium rarely extends deeper than the submucosa, and perforation seldom occurs. Blood vessels of the lamina propria and submucosa adjacent to ulcers may be dilated and contain fibrin thrombi. Individual epithelial cells may be seen to have undergone several changes; namely, vacuolization of cytoplasm or nuclei, and dis-

tortion in size and shape. Hyaline changes in the submucosal stroma may occur late in association with formation of bizarre fibroblasts and fibrocytes. Strictures may result from the fibrosis, causing intestinal obstruction.

Genital System. The germinal cells of the testis and ovary are among the more radiosensitive cells of the animal body, hence are readily destroyed by radiation. In the acute stage, hemorrhage and edema may be seen, but the most specific effect is the destruction of spermatogonia as well as spermatocytes, with little effect upon spermatozoa. Whole body radiation in sufficient dosage to destroy germinal cells would be enough to kill the animal; hence, sterility would be an academic problem. If the same dosage were applied only to the gonads, the whole body effect would be nil, but sterility of temporary or permanent duration would result.

Skin. Radiation injury to the skin is frequent after radiation therapy of tumors and is one of the principal tissues affected by radioactive fallout. The lesions are discussed in detail in the next section.

Respiratory System. Respiratory epithelium is relatively resistant to radiation damage. High doses will lead to swelling and desquamation of alveolar lining cells and epithelium of the bronchial tree. Most of the acute and chronic effects result from vascular damage, resulting in pulmonary edema in the acute stage and alveolar fibrosis and consolidation as chronic manifestations. Pulmonary edema may account for the immediate cause of death following whole body irradiation. A hyaline material free in alveoli and within alveolar macrophages and proliferation of granular pneumocytes have been described in human beings and dogs.

Urinary System. Renal epithelium is intermediate in its radiosensitivity, and as with the lung, the most important change in the kidney results from chronic vascular sclerosis. The glomeruli become hyalinized; the tubules, atrophic; and the interstitium, fibrotic. In man, hypertension is associated with the chronic nephritis. The transitional epithelium of the urinary bladder is very radiosensitive, and in contrast to the kidney, the lesions are acute. The epithelial cells become necrotic and slough, leading to ulcers. Infection is a frequent complication. Fibrosis from healing may result in distortion of the bladder.

Bone and Cartilage. Mature osteocytes and chondrocytes are very radioresistant, and lesions in these tissues are of little consequence in adults. Proliferating osteoblasts and chondroblasts, however, are more radiosensitive. In growing animals, damage to these cells will result in retarded or distorted growth.

Heart. Although the myocardium has been generally considered relatively radioresistant, radiation-induced heart disease has been reported in a number of human patients following radiation therapy and has been experimentally produced in animals. It is characterized by fibrous pericarditis, interstitial fibrosis of the myocardium, and perivascular accumulations of mononuclear cells. In monkeys, the extent of the myocardial fibrosis suggests healed infarcts. All these lesions probably result from ischemia caused by vascular damage.

Other Tissues and Lesions. Chronic vascular lesions may result in impaired circulation to many tissues, with the resultant lesions of anoxia. Therefore, chronic effects may be encountered even in very radioresistant tissues such as the nervous system. During embryogenesis, when all tissues are less differentiated and rapidly dividing, irradiation may cause a variety of congenital abnormalities. Cataract formation is not infrequent following irradiation of the lens. Carcinogenesis is one of the most serious of the chronic sequelae following irradiation; a variety of different neoplasms have been associated with radiation. This is discussed in Chapter 4.

Barratt, N.P.: The effect of cobalt-60 and neutron irradiation upon the immune response of tumour bearing dogs. Dissert. Abstr. Intl., 36B:2148–2149, 1975.

Behrens, C.F.: Atomic Medicine, New York, Thomas Nelson & Sons, 1949.

Case, M.T., and Simon, J.: Whole-body gamma irradiation of newborn pigs: pathologic changes. Am. J. Vet. Res., 33:1223–1230, 1972.

Cogan, D.G., Martin, S.F., and Kimura, S.J.: Atom bomb cataracts. Science, 110:654–655, 1949.

Dagle, G. E., Filipy, R.E., Adee, R.R., and Stuart, B.O.: Pulmonary hyalinosis in dogs. Vet. Pathol., 13:138–142, 1976.

Fajardo, L.F., and Stewart, J.R.: Pathogenesis of radiation-induced myocardial fibrosis. Lab. Invest., 29:244–257, 1973.

Faulkner, C.S., II, and Connolly, K.S.: The ultrastructure of ⁶⁰Co radiation pneumonitis in rats. Lab. Invest., 28:545–553, 1973.

Geeraets, W.J.: Radiation cataract: biomicroscopic observations in rabbit, monkey, and man. Med. College Virginia Q., 8:259–263, 1972.

Gleiser, C.A.: A review of some basic concepts of the biology and pathogenesis of acute ionizing body radiation. J. Am. Vet. Med. Assoc., 124:220–224, 1954.

———: The pathology of total body radiation in dogs which died following exposure to a lethal dose. Am. J. Vet. Res., 15:329–335, 1954.

Guttman, P.H., and Kohn, H.I.: Progressive intercapillary glomerulosclerosis in the mouse, rat, and Chinese hamster, associated with aging and x-ray exposure. Am. J. Pathol., 37:293–307, 1960.

Haymaker, W., Rubinstein, L.J., and Miquel, J.: Brain tumors in irradiated monkeys. Acta Neuropathol. (Berl.), 20:267–277, 1972.

Holley, T.R., et al.: Effect of high doses of radiation on human neutrophil chemotaxis, phagocytosis and morphology. Am. J. Pathol., 75:61–72, 1974.

Jordan, S.W., Dean, P.N., and Ahlquist, J.: Early ultrastructural effects of ionizing radiation. I. Mitochondrial and nuclear changes. Lab. Invest., 27:538–549, 1972.

Kato, H.: Review of thirty years study of Hiroshima and Nagasaki atom bomb survivors. II. Biological effects. B. Genetic effects. 1. Early genetic surveys and mortality study. J. Radiat. Res. (Tokyo), 16(Suppl.):67–74, 1975.

Leibow, A.A., Warren, S., and DeCoursey, E.: Pathology of atomic bomb casualties. Am. J. Pathol., 25:853–1027, 1949.

Mayhew, C.J., et al.: Bacterial permeation of the gut wall in irradiated burros. Am. J. Vet. Res., 16:525–528, 1955.

McLean, F.C., Rust, J.H., and Budy, A.M.: Extension to man of experimental whole-body irradiation studies; some military and civil defense considerations. Mil. Surg., 112:174–182, 1953.

Mewissen, D.J., Comar, C.L., Trum, B.F., and Rust, J.H.: A formula for chronic radiation dosage versus shortening of life span: application to a large mammal. Radiat. Res., 6:450–459, 1957.

Pfleger, R.C., et al.: Biological alterations resulting from chronic lung irradiation. I. The pulmonary lipid composition, physiology and pathology after inhalation by Beagle dogs of ¹⁴⁴Ce-labeled fused clay aerosols. Radiat. Res., *63*:275–298, 1975.

Phillips, S.J., Macken, D.L., and Rugh, R.: Pathologic sequelae of acute cardiac irradiation in monkeys. Am. Heart J., *81*:528–542, 1971.

Ragan, H.A., Clarke, W.J., and Bustad, L.K.: Radiation-induced cutaneous neoplasm in a sheep. Am. J. Vet. Res., *32*:167–172, 1971.

Rust, J.H., Folmar, G.D., Jr., Lane, J.J., and Trum, B.F.: The lethal dose of total body cobalt-60 gamma radiation for the rabbit. Am. J. Roentgen., *74*:135–138, 1955.

Rust, J.H., et al.: Effect of 200 roentgens fractional whole body irradiation in the burro. Proc. Soc. Exp. Biol. Med., *85*:258–261, 1954.

———: Effects of 50 roentgens and 25 roentgens fractional daily total-body *r*-irradiation in the burro. Radiat. Res., *2*:475–482, 1955.

———: Lethal dose studies with burros and swine exposed to whole body cobalt-60 irradiation. Radiology, *62*:569–574, 1954.

Slauson, D.O., et al.: Inflammatory sequences in acute pulmonary radiation injury. Am. J. Pathol., *82*:549–572, 1976.

Snider, R.S., and Raper, J.R.: Histopathological effects of single doses of total-surface beta radiation of mice. In Effects of External Beta Radiation, edited by R. E. Zirkle. New York, McGraw-Hill, 1951, Chap. 9, pp. 152–178.

Trum, B.F., et al.: Effect of 400 fractional whole body gamma irradiation in the burro (*Equus asinus asinus*). Am. J. Physiol., *174*:57–60, 1953.

Trum, B.F., Rust, J.H., and Wilding, J.L.: Clinical observations upon the response of the burro to large doses of external whole body gamma irradiation. The Auburn Veterinarian, *8*:131–136, 1952.

Warren, S.: Effect of radiation on normal tissues. Arch. Pathol., *34*:443–450, 917–1084, (with C. E. Dunlap) 562–608 (with N. B. Friedman) 749–788, 1942.

———: The histopathology of radiation lesions. Physiol. Rev., *24*:225–238, 1944.

Wise, D., and Turbyfill, C.L.: The acute mortality response of the miniature pig to pulsed mixed gamma-neutron radiations. Radiat. Res., *41*:507–515, 1970.

RADIOACTIVE FALLOUT

The explosion of a thermonuclear weapon releases not only vast quantities of

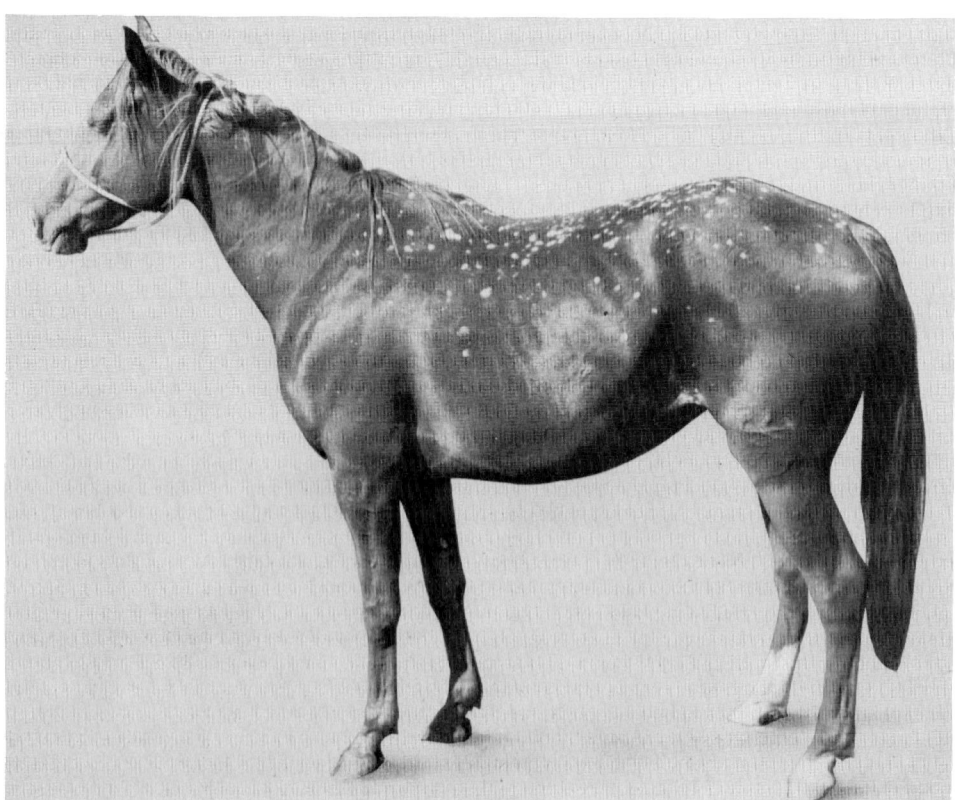

Fig. 15–4.   Effect of radioactive fallout. The lesions are discrete and located on the dorsal portions of the body of this horse. (Courtesy of Lt. Col. B. F. Trum, V.C.)

energy in the form of heat, light, and blast, but also great amounts of radioactivity. Part of this radioactivity is released instantaneously in the form of neutrons and gamma rays, which can produce radiation effects within their range. This range, or distance through which these radiations travel and thus produce biologic effects, depends upon the energy of the explosion, but is not great, even in the most powerful explosions. However, fast-moving neutrons can penetrate deeply into matter and induce radioactivity in otherwise stable substances. This **induced,** or **secondary,** radioactivity, under certain circumstances, can be an important source of ionizing radiation.

Of far greater significance in an explosive fission reaction is the release of radioactive substances in particulate form. These particles consist of radioactive fission products, matter (sea water, air, soil) in which radioactivity has been induced, and perhaps, remnants of the original fissionable material. The explosive power of the bomb may send great quantities of these radioactive materials high into the earth's atmosphere, wind currents move them as clouds over great distances, then rain or other atmospheric conditions cause the particulate matter to fall back to the earth. This **fallout** may constitute serious hazard to man, plants, and animals in areas downwind from the point of detonation. The areas of serious radioactivity would vary in size according to such factors as yield and height of burst, the nature of the surface over which the burst occurs, and the meteorologic conditions present. The radioactive material may lodge on the skin of the backs of animals which are out in the open, or may fall on pasture or animal feed,

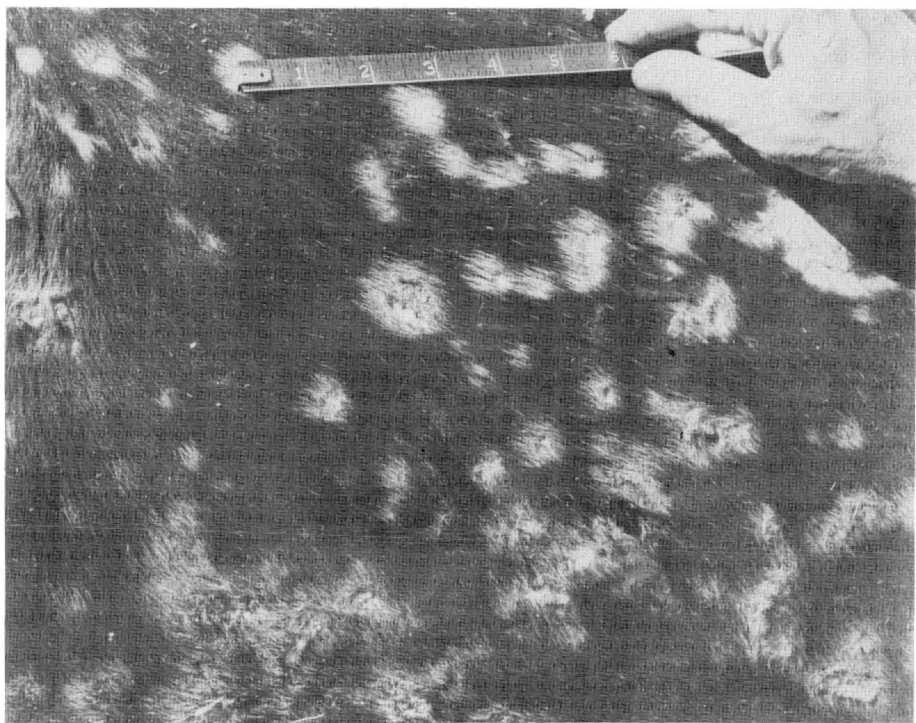

Fig. 15-5. Radioactive fallout. Lesions in the skin of the back of a horse. Depigmentation of hair in sharply circumscribed areas with alopecia and ulceration in the center of some of them. (Courtesy of Lt. Col. B. F. Trum, V.C.)

where it may be ingested and cause **internal radiation,** a condition that will be discussed later.

The fallout of radioactive materials may occur as a shower of dry flaky material or as minute invisible particles, perhaps accompanied by rain. The fact that radioactivity is associated with particles has an important influence upon skin lesions resulting from contact with this material. The chemical nature of material in radioactive fallout depends upon the composition of the bomb as well as the medium in which it was exploded (air, sea, underground). Most radioisotopes of importance in such radioactive clouds decay by emission of beta particles and gamma rays. Alpha particle emitters are a possibility, but because of their low penetrability would have little effect upon the skin.

The effect of radioisotopes on the skin depends upon (1) their energy and type of emission, (2) duration of their contact with the skin, (3) their radioactive half-life, (4) any irritating effect due to their chemical nature.

Lesions

Lesions will develop in the skin of animals exposed to radioactive fallout, provided the material is in contact with the skin for a sufficient length of time. As indicated previously, alpha particles do not penetrate the keratin layer, hence produce no effect upon the skin; gamma rays penetrate deeply but have low specific ionization in the superficial layers, therefore produce little direct effect upon the skin; beta particles, on the other hand, penetrate most layers of the skin, have high specific ionization, and produce severe effects. The skin lesions caused by beta particles have been called "beta burns," but they are not strictly burns since no heat is involved.

The sequence of changes resulting from contact with beta-emitting radioisotopes has been studied by Moritz and Henriques (1952), who placed beta-emitting plaques in contact with the skin of swine. These

workers used radioisotopes of different energies—sulfur-35 (0.17 MeV), cobalt-60 (0.31 MeV), cesium-137 (0.55 MeV), yttrium-91 (1.53 MeV), and strontium-yttrium-90 (0.61 and 2.2 MeV)—to demonstrate the relationships between the energy of the isotope and the surface, or transepidermal, dose to the resultant radiation injury. These studies provide information on the development of changes following radiation of this type; some of these changes have been observed in "field" cases of injury due to radioactive fallout. The remarks that follow are based on the reports of Moritz and Henriques.

The first observable change in swine skin following exposure to these radioactive isotopes is **erythema,** which may appear within 24 hours. If erythema persists 72 hours or more, it is indicative of injury severe enough to result in chronic radiation dermatitis. Edema of dermal papillae, if recognizable within 48 hours following irradiation, will be followed by transepidermal necrosis. Death of cells in the basal and deeper malpighian layers of the epidermis, demonstrated by increase in staining intensity of their nuclei, occurs within 24 hours following high dosage, but with lower dosage may not appear for 10 to 14 days.

Epidermal atrophy, one of the least severe changes, is recognized in microscopic sections only and is seen one to two weeks following radiation. This change is evidenced by thinning of the rete, presumably as a result of depression of cell division in the basal layer plus continued desquamation of surface layers. It persists for two to four weeks and appears to be completely reversible, since there are no residua. **Exfoliation** and crust formation follow more severe injury, begin during the second week, and may be precursors of chronic radiation dermatitis. A scaling brown crust is shed for weeks or months, apparently because of accelerated maturation of malpighian cells without loss of their nuclei, thus resulting in **parakeratosis.** Death of individual cells in the deeper parts of the epidermis may continue for many weeks after irradiation.

Epidermal necrosis and exfoliation follow higher dosages of radiation. The first indication of probable irreversible injury is swelling and vacuolation of cytoplasm of epidermal cells, which may appear ragged or coagulated into round, acidophilic hyaline masses. There is also disorganization of the basal and malpighian layers, with vesicles appearing at the dermal-epidermal interface. **Transepidermal necrosis,** with ulceration of the entire target area, follows still higher dosage, and may be complete within 48 hours. With lower dosage, several weeks may elapse before necrosis of the epidermis is complete. Radiation of lower energy (sulfur-35, 0.17 MeV) produces shallow ulcers with little damage to the dermis, while higher energy beta radiation—from strontium-yttrium-90 (0.61 and 2.2 MeV), cobalt-60 (0.31 MeV), and cesium-137 (0.55 MeV)—results in deep injury to the dermis and is followed by chronic radiation dermatitis.

Changes in the **dermis** and **subcutis** are observed only if the epidermis is damaged. The earliest lesion is hyperemia of the capillaries in the dermal papillae, followed by edema, asteroid swelling of fibrocytes, and exudation of lymphocytes and neutrophils in relation to the ulceration of epidermis. Edema, capillary ectasia, and degenerative changes in arterioles may persist after regeneration of epithelium, but the dermis in this state apparently cannot support the growth of epithelium, therefore ulceration recurs.

Epilation takes place when the dosage of higher energy beta particles is sufficient to produce recognizable injury in the epidermis; lower energy beta radiation from sulfur-35, however, does not produce epilation. When dermal papillae receive sufficient radiation to cause loss of hair, they become atrophic and contracted, particularly in length. Atrophy occurs in epithelial cells of the hair matrix, including the inner root sheath, and may or may not be associated with swelling and squamous metaplasia. Sometimes columns of cells from hair follicles may persist, but they undergo central dissolution, producing epithelial-lined cysts, which may or may not communicate with the surface. In severe injury, hair follicles are permanently destroyed.

Other **skin adnexa,** sebaceous and sweat glands, may disappear without a trace after high energy beta radiation in sufficient dosage to destroy the epidermis. These structures are not replaced. Less severely affected tubular glands may become atrophic and be surrounded by a dense hyaline membrane.

In **chronic radiation dermatitis,** characterized clinically by persistent exfoliation with crust formation of one- to three-months' duration, the microscopic findings are parakeratosis with atrophy (or less often, hyperplasia) of the epidermis associated with chronic inflammation in the dermis. In some instances, there is proliferation and downward growth of the epithelium, with pleomorphism, loss of polarity, and increased numbers of mitotic figures. This change suggests a trend toward neoplasia.

The skin of cattle studied several years after exposure to severe doses of radiation from fallout presented irregular areas of scarring, surrounded by zones of epilation and white hair. The scarred areas were partially covered by dense layers of tough horny material several centimeters in thickness. Microscopically, these scarred areas were covered by thick stratified squamous epithelium with an overlying dense layer of keratin. The rete pegs, hair follicles, sebaceous, and sweat glands were absent under the affected epithelium, but occasionally were present, although atrophic, at the edges of lesions (Fig. 15–6).

In horses exposed to radioactive fallout, focal areas of ulceration surrounded by a wide zone of white hair (Fig. 15–5) have been reported. Because radioactivity emit-

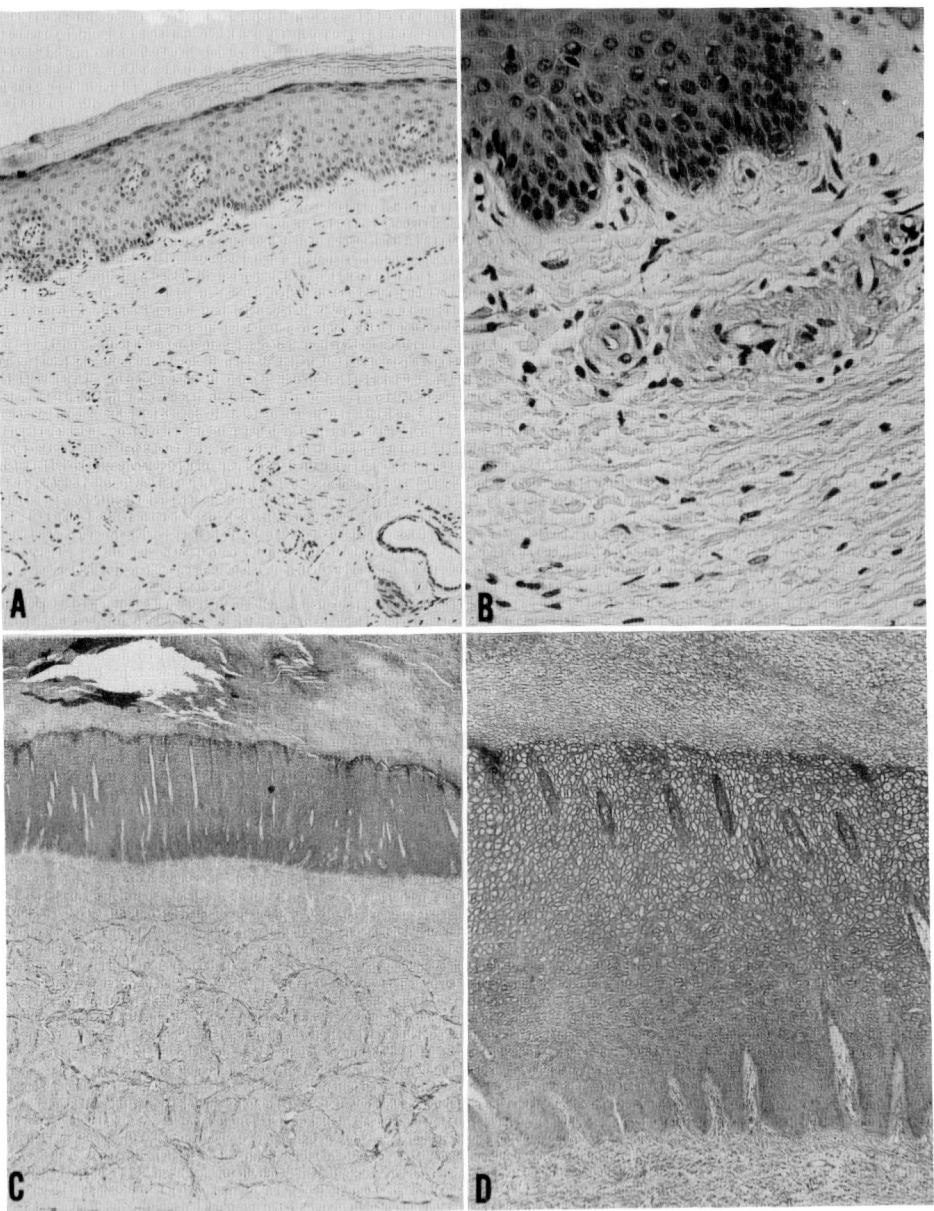

Fig. 15–6. *A,* Radioactive fallout, bovine skin (× 75). Note absence of sebaceous glands and remnant of sweat gland in dermis. *B,* Radioactive fallout, bovine skin (× 250). Thickened hyaline wall in capillary of dermis. Specimen taken several years after exposure. *C,* Radioactive fallout, bovine skin (× 11). Several years after exposure. Severe hyperkeratosis, acanthosis and loss of adnexa. *D,* Higher magnification of *C* (× 48), illustrating acanthosis and part of the layer of hyperkeratosis. (Courtesy of Armed Forces Institute of Pathology.) Contributor: Dr. Cyril Comar.

ted from particulate fallout usually arises from a point source and is given off nearly equally in all directions, the volume of skin affected will be roughly hemispherical in depth, while the surface lesion will be round.

Solar radiation results in similar but less rapidly progressive precancerous lesions in the skin (see page 132).

Archambeau, J.O., Fairchild, R.G., and Commerford, S.L.: Response of skin of swine to increasing exposures of 250 KVP x-ray. *In* Swine in Biomedical Research, edited by L. K. Bustad and R. O. McClellan. Richland, Wn, Battelle Memorial Institute, 1966, pp. 463–489.

Ballard, R.V., et al.: Iodine 129 in thyroids of grazing animals. Health Phys., 30:345–350, 1976.

Bogen, D.C., et al.: "Fallout tritium" distribution in the environment. Health Phys., 30:203–208, 1976.

Brown, D.G., Reynolds, R.A., and Johnson, D.F.: Late effects in cattle exposed to radioactive fallout. Am. J. Vet. Res., 27:1509–1514, 1966.

George, L.A., and Bustad, L.K.: Comparative effects of beta irradiation of swine, sheep and rabbit skin. *In* Swine in Biomedical Research, edited by L. K. Bustad and R. O. McClellan. Richland, Wn., Battelle Memorial Institute, 1966, pp. 491–500.

Henriques, F.W., Jr.: Effect of beta rays on the skin as a function of the energy intensity and duration of radiation. I. Physical considerations. Preparation and calibration of beta-emitting plaques. Lab. Invest., 1:153–166, 1952.

Moritz, A.R., and Henriques, F.W., Jr.: Effect of beta rays on the skin as a function of the energy, intensity and duration of radiation. II. Animal experiments. Lab. Invest., 1:167–185, 1952.

Tessmer, C.F.: Radioactive fallout effects on skin. I. Effects of radioactive fallout on skin of Almagordo cattle. Arch. Pathol., 72:175–190, 1961.

Tessmer, C.F., and Brown, D.G.: Carcinoma of skin and bovine exposed to radioactive fallout. J. Am. Med. Assoc., 179:210–214, 1962.

Tullis, J.L., and Warren, S.: Gross autopsy observation in the animals exposed at Bikini; preliminary report. J. Am. Med. Assoc., 134:1155–1158, 1947.

Tullis, J.L., Lawson, B.C., and Madden, S.C.: Pathology of swine exposed to total body gamma radiation from an atomic bomb source. Am. J. Pathol., 31:41–51, 1955.

INTERNAL RADIATION

Radioactive isotopes may gain access to the human or animal body by inhalation, ingestion, parenteral injection, or absorption through wounds in the skin. The effect produced by these isotopes depends upon many factors, the most important of which are the following: the quantity, specific ionization, and energy of radioactivity taken into the body; its deposition in critical or radiosensitive tissues; the biologic half-life of the isotope; and the size and importance to life of the organ in which the isotope is deposited. Except in the immediate region of an explosion and close-in areas of fallout, internal radiation is a much greater hazard than external radiation, since the isotope is in contact with the animal tissues for longer periods of time, and even if of low energy, may be deposited in critical tissues (bone, thyroid) in intimate enough contact to cause serious damage. Sources of radioactivity that possibly could become internal radiation hazards to animals include fallout following explosions of atomic weapons, with contamination of animal feeds, water, or pastures, and contamination of feed or water by inadequate disposal of radioactive wastes from atomic "piles," power reactors, or industrial and medical facilities in which radioisotopes are used.

Radioactive isotopes are metabolized in the body in exactly the same manner as are nonradioactive isotopes of the same element. Therefore, radioiodine (^{131}I) is rapidly concentrated in the thyroid exactly as is stable iodine (^{127}I). Radiocalcium (^{45}Ca) is deposited in bone as are its nonradioactive isotopes (^{40,42}Ca, etc.), and is eliminated not only in feces and urine but in milk. Radiosodium (^{24}Na) is distributed more widely through the tissues and is eliminated rather rapidly, hence is not as great a hazard as ^{131}I or ^{45}Ca.

Many radioisotopes are not ordinarily metabolized by the body but are deposited in tissues in much the same way as are similar chemical elements. The most important of these are the **"bone seekers,"** which include strontium-90, radium-226, uranium, radioactive rare earths, and plutonium. Bone-seeking radioisotopes are deposited in growing bone, at first most heavily concentrated in the metaphysis, particularly adjacent to the epiphyseal line, where they remain in

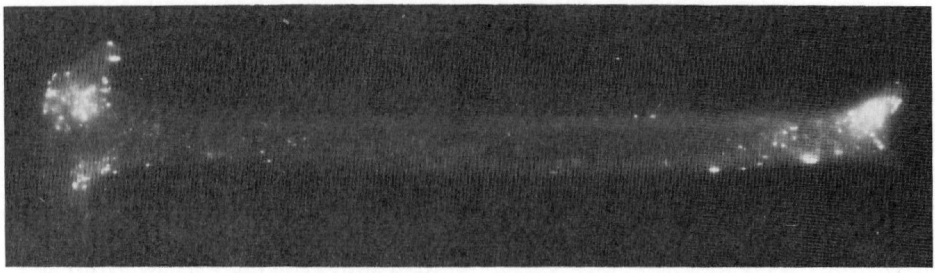

Fig. 15–7.   Positive print of an autoradiograph of the femur of a dog which had received strontium-90. (Courtesy of Dr. Arthur Lindenbaum, Argonne National Laboratory.)

greatest concentration. After a time, radioactivity can be demonstrated also in the diaphyses of the long bones by radioautographs (Fig. 15–7), prepared by placing slabs of affected bone in contact with photographic film for a period of time, then developing the film. Radioactive components darken the film, indicating their site of deposition in the tissue.

The deposition of radioactivity in the bones may destroy the hematopoietic elements, thus producing aplastic anemia, and may adversely affect the growing bone, predisposing to osteogenic sarcoma. Aside from these effects upon the individual, radioactive bones in meat-producing animals could become a food hazard to man or to other animals.

Radioiodine (^{131}I) in sufficient dosage can cause enough destruction of thyroid tissue to interfere seriously with the function of the gland. Internal radiation from these isotopes has especially deleterious effects on young animals.

Bloom, W.: Histopathology of Irradiation from External and Internal Sources. New York, McGraw-Hill Book Co., 1948.

Freire-Maia, A., et al.: Human genetic studies in areas of high natural radiation. IX. Effects on mortality, morbidity and sex ratio. Health Phys., *34*:61–65, 1978.

Graupera, B.B.: Osteoradionecrosis of the mandible. Radiol. Technol., *49*:132–142, 1977.

Krumholz, L.A., and Rust, J.H.: Osteogenic sarcoma in a muskrat from an area of high environmental radiostrontium. Arch. Pathol., *57*:270–278, 1954.

Prosser, C.L., et al.: Plutonium project; clinical sequence of physiological effects of ionizing radiation in animals. Radiology, *49*:299–312, 1947.

Sobells, F.H.: Repair from Genetic Radiation Damage, Oxford, Pergamon Press, 1963.

CHAPTER *16*

Diseases Due to Extraneous Poisons

Some poisons are produced by pathogenic microorganisms in the course of an infection and a few are generated by disorders of body metabolism, but the majority are formed outside the body, which they enter through the digestive canal, by inhalation, through the skin, or occasionally by other routes.

Poisons entering the body produce their effects in a large variety of ways. Many poisons, when in sufficient concentration, kill the tissues with which they come in contact (necrosis), or if the action is milder, injure the tissues and initiate an acute inflammatory reaction. Poisons in this category are those that have a strong chemical action on organic matter: strong acids, strong alkalies, or compounds with a highly active ion such as fluorine. If the poison has been ingested, the alimentary mucous membranes suffer the necrosis or inflammation. The most powerful ones, such as lye, destroy the lining of the mouth or esophagus as they are swallowed and then carry their effect to the stomach. Others pass through the stomach with little damage and cause superficial necrosis and inflammation in the upper or lower intestine, presumably because they remain longer in contact with the injured part. In speaking of the intestine, it may be interjected here that some poisons (such as mercury), after absorption into the blood, are

excreted into the large intestine, producing inflammation as they pass through the mucous membrane.

Poisons of a second and very important group have little or no immediate action, but after absorption from the alimentary mucosa, other mucous membrane or the skin, affect the delicate epithelial cells of such parenchymatous organs as the liver or kidneys, which they reach by way of the blood stream. This group includes most of the poisons of the first group when diluted sufficiently that they do not kill by direct local destruction. It also includes most of the plant poisons as well as bacterial toxins.

Other poisons owe their effect to interference with some vital nervous function, and often leave no visible pathologic change to betray their harmful handiwork. Strychnine is an example.

Certain poisons owe their effects to, or at least reveal their presence by, numerous petechiae or ecchymoses, the result of injury to the endothelium of capillaries. Some poisons hemolyze the circulating erythrocytes; a few destroy the hematopoietic powers of the bone marrow. Certain poisons produce their effects by blocking vital enzyme systems, usually without any identifying lesions. Many combine several of the above and other actions.

It is hoped here to summarize such in-

Table 16–1. Extraneous Poisons

Group (page)	Pathologic Feature	Poisons	
A (904)	Local injury	Venoms Phenol	Lewisite Mustard gas
B (906)	Gastroenteritis	Arsenic Salt Petroleum Sodium fluoroacetate Ground glass Dynamite Urea Nicotine Nightshades	Castor beans Locust tree Tung oil tree Flourensia cernua Oaks Oleander Milkweeds Red squill Blister beetle
C (919)	Hepatotoxicity; often nephrotoxicity	Phosphorus Phosphates Copper Tannic acid Carbon tetrachloride Tetrachloroethylene Phenothiazine Phenanthridinium Clay pigeons (Pitch) Hydrogen sulfide Gossypol Cocklebur Senecios	Crotalaria Heliotrope Tarweed Lantana Sacahuiste Drymaria Lechuguilla Phyllanthus Mushrooms Lupines Vetch Algae Hepatotoxic mycotoxins (p. 704)
D (944)	Nephrotoxicity	Turpentine Sulfonamides Oxalates Broomweed	Chloroform Chinese tallow tree Bitterweed Nephrotoxic mycotoxins (p. 704)
E (952)	Cardiac insufficiency	Selenium Death camas Aconite	Baileya Jimson weed Pimelea
F (957)	Extensive hemorrhage	Dicoumarin Bracken fern	Trichloroethylene- extracted soybean meal Aspirin (p. 1028)
G (963)	Hemolytic anemia	Molybdenum Naphthalene	Onions
H (965)	Production of methemo-globin and chocolate-colored blood	Nitrates Nitrites	Chlorates
I (968)	Production of car-boxyhemoglobin and cherry red blood	Carbon monoxide	Cyanides

Table 16–1. Extraneous Poisons (Cont'd)

Group (page)	Pathologic Feature	Poisons	
J (969)	Edema	Alpha-naphthyl thiourea (ANTU)	
K (970)	Pulmonary disease	Rape Kale	Paraquat
L (972)	Gangrene of extremities	Fescue grass	
M (972)	Lesions of bone and teeth	Fluorine	
N (978)	Hypercalcemia	*Solanum malacoxylon*	*Cestrum diurnum*
O (979)	Loss of hair or wool	Thallium	Jumbay tree
P (982)	Epithelial hyperplasia	Chlorinated dibenzodioxins Chlorinated naphthalenes	Polychlorinated biphenyls Polybrominated biphenyls
Q (988)	Nervous malfunction	Strychnine Nitrogen trichloride Loco Vetch-like Astragali Atropine Equisetum Hemlocks Lathyrus Larkspur Yellow Star Thistle Botulinus	Anguina Carbon disulfide Ortho-tricresyl phosphate Lead Mercury Chlorinated hydrocarbons Organic phosphates Cycada Arsanilic acid
R (1017)	Degeneration of cardiac and skeletal muscles	Coffee senna Coyotillo	Hairy vetch (p. 942)
S (1019)	Teratogenic or other effects on embryo or fetus	Veratrum californicum Thalidomide Pine needles	Lupin (p. 941) Selenium (p. 952) Lathyrus (p. 995)
T (1022)	Miscellaneous or unclassified	Smallhead sneezeweed Box Grasstree Stinkwood Pokeweed Yew Phalaris grass Sorghum Sesbania Djenkol bean Estrogen Nitrogen dioxide	Cobalt Hexachlorophene Chloroquine Zinc Zinc phosphide Gidyea tree Wild everlasting Chinaberry tree Aspirin Benzoic acid Cadmium Carpet weed Fish, shellfish

formation as is available concerning the tissue changes resulting from those poisons commonly involving domestic animals. Unfortunately, many of the poisons have not been adequately studied from the standpoint of their pathologic effects, diagnosis, therefore, being unnecessarily difficult.

Despite the length of this chapter, it is by no means a complete list of poisonous substances. We have purposely avoided including many poisonous plants not found in the Americas, and the scores of plants identified as toxic by isolated reports concerning one or two animals. Also, the rapid expansion of industrial chemicals precludes complete coverage of these compounds. Only those associated with natural poisonings are discussed. Finally, there is hardly any drug (both pharmaceutical and biologic) which will not, under some circumstances, produce an adverse reaction. Although some drugs are included here, we leave a more detailed treatment to pharmacology.

Having ourselves been pupils at one time (and still being students), we suspect that considerable effort may be necessary if the reader is to keep clearly in mind the characteristic symptoms and lesions that accompany each of the poisonings described in this chapter. To facilitate this somewhat painful process, we have grouped the various poisons in accordance with some outstanding lesion which, upon being encountered, might afford a clue to the diagnosis. To effect such a grouping is by no means easy, not only because the manifestations of a given poisoning vary in different individuals, but more so because many of the poisons attack the patient by several mechanisms and produce a number of lesions, no one of which is salient among the others. It thus becomes most difficult to decide to which pathologic family a particular poison belongs. Nevertheless, we hope that a grouping of this nature may facilitate fixing in mind at least one important pathologic feature of each poison, thus

providing assistance in problems of differentiation. We have an exception to this approach with respect to mycotoxins. These are discussed as a group at the conclusion of Chapter 12.

Whenever it is possible to use pathologic and clinical features to decrease the number of suspected etiologic agents, further investigation is simplified. Chemical identification of the poison or clear demonstration of its ingestion or contact should always be attempted when the situation permits. In only a few poisonings are lesions characteristic enough to permit definitive diagnosis. As with infectious diseases, it is important to demonstrate the etiologic agent in association with the lesions that it is expected to cause.

Many poisonous plants are referred to in this chapter by their common and scientific names. No further effort is made to identify the plants. This identification is admirably accomplished by John M. Kingsbury in his book, Poisonous Plants of the United States and Canada, Prentice-Hall, 1964.

Extraneous poisons will be taken up in the sequence shown in Table 16–1.

GROUP A: LOCAL INJURY

Poisons that produce local injury (necrosis and inflammation) to the tissues with which they come in contact are included in this group. Obviously, an appropriate degree of concentration is essential to produce this effect. As mentioned earlier, strong acids and alkalies fall in this group, but are not discussed here.

Venoms of Snakes and Other Creatures

Snake bites, at least those of the North American rattlesnakes, copperheads, and moccasins, promptly cause an extremely rapid though weakening heart beat, but their most spectacular effect is tremendous local swelling, which is well under way within minutes after the bite is inflicted. The swelling is the result of inflammatory edema, or more precisely, of serous inflammatory exudation. Within three or four hours the maximum is reached, and if the bite is on the nose, as it usually is in horses and may be in the case of dogs and cattle, suffocation may ensue from closing of the nostrils or glottis. If the animal survives, the swelling subsides in four to seven days, but the toxic injury is sometimes so severe that necrosis and sloughing of a large mass of tissue may supervene. Hemolysis is another effect of the venom, perhaps to the extent that hemoglobinuria and hemolytic icterus may be noticeable. There is also interference with clotting of the blood. Certain venoms are also strongly neurotoxic, leading to restlessness, irritability, and trembling followed by paralysis. Postmortem findings include the foregoing changes plus extreme passive congestion of all organs and hemorrhages in the region of the bite. Local gas gangrene or tetanus occasionally supervenes, initiated by the bacterial contamination of the serpent's mouth.

Many species of **toads** (*Bufo sp.*) throughout the world produce toxins (venoms) in their parotid glands that are responsible for poisoning animals, especially dogs and occasionally cats and human beings. Poisoning usually follows when a dog plays with the toad and absorbs the toxin through the buccal and gastric mucosa. The toxins are digitalis-like, leading to irregularities in cardiac function, which may result in death.

The **stings of bees** and various other insects are similar to snake bites in causing an extreme degree of serous exudation. This fluid in either type of poisoning exerts a valuable protective effect by diluting the poison and causing so much local pressure that circulation of the blood and the consequent dissemination of the poison are inhibited. The severity of the reaction to the stings of bees and scorpions and the bites of ants varies greatly in different individuals of any species, apparently on an allergic basis. Even horses have died from multiple bee stings, methemoglobinemia and bilirubinemia being noted.

The **black widow spider** (*Latrodectus mactans*), according to Pritchard (1940), requires careful consideration in the diagnosis of sudden canine illnesses in practically all parts of the United States and many other countries. While some dogs appear to be entirely immune (whether from a previous exposure is unknown), the bite of this black spider with the red "hour-glass" spot on its abdomen may well be fatal to a dog or, presumably, to a cat. The period of illness may terminate fatally in two hours or it may continue for two or three days with recovery or death. Early symptoms commence with pain at the site of the bite, which may be severe. Edema (serous inflammatory exudate) also develops around the bite. The whole integument becomes painful and hypersensitive to slight pressure; the abdominal wall becomes rigid through reflex contraction of the muscles. In some cases, hyperesthesia, which appears to reside in the articular surfaces, causes fleeting but pronounced pain which, in a matter of minutes, may shift from one limb to another. If the intoxication persists, a gradually increasing paralysis may appear on the second or third day, and become so extensive as to produce death, the pain, meanwhile, having subsided. Postmortem, there is little to be seen but venous congestion.

Baerg, W.J.: The black widow: its life history and the effects of the poison. Scient. Monthly, *17*:535–547, 1923.

Bedford, P.G.C.: Toad venom toxicity and its clinical occurrence in small animals in the United Kingdom. Vet. Rec., *94*:613–614, 1974.

Comstock, J.H.: The Spider Book. Ithaca, New York, Comstock Pub. Co., Inc., 1948.

Crimmins, M.L.: Facts about Texas snakes and their poisons. J. Am. Vet. Med. Assoc., *71*:704–712, 1927.

Ditmars, R.L.: Snake bites among domestic animals. J. Am. Vet. Med. Assoc., *94*:383–388, 1939.

Fitzgerald, W.E.: Snakebite in the horse. Aust. Vet. J., *51*:37–39, 1975.

McNellis, R.: Rattlesnake bite. J. Am. Vet. Med. Assoc., *114*:145–146, 1949.

Nighbert, E.M.: Effects of bites of poisonous snakes on dogs. North Am. Vet., *24*:363–364, 1943.

Palumbo, N.E., Perri, S., and Read, G.: Experimental induction and treatment of toad poisoning in the dog. J. Am. Vet. Med. Assoc., *167*:1000–1005, 1975.

Parrish, H.M., Scatterday, J.E., and Pollard, C.B.: The clinical management of snake venom poisoning in domestic animals. J. Am. Vet. Med. Assoc., *130*:548–551, 1957. (Includes pathology.)

Perry, B.D., and Bracegirdle, J.R.: Toad poisoning in small animals. Vet. Rec., *92*:589–590, 1973.

Pritchard, C.W.: Black widow spider and snake venom in small animals. J. Am. Vet. Med. Assoc., *96*:356–358, 1940.

Schöll, G.: Todlicher Kreuzotterbiss bei einem Dackel. (Necropsy findings in a Dachshund bitten by a common viper.) Die Kleintierpraxis, *13*:113–115, 1968.

Wirth, D.: Bienenstichvergiftung beim Pferd. (Bee sting poisoning in horses.) Wien. Tierärztl. Monatschr., *30*:129–134, 1943.

Phenol

Phenol, or carbolic acid, is used in medicine much less than formerly, but poisoning through accidental ingestion or by absorption through the skin is still occasionally seen. In general, symptoms are those of nervous shock and nervous depression, paralysis, and coma. The salient lesion results from the action of all but high dilutions of phenol as a potent tissue fixative. Mucous membranes (mouth, stomach) with which it comes in contact promptly become firm and white, a state of coagulative necrosis. Microscopically, the white, coagulated tissue is found to be perfectly preserved, while adjoining areas may show postmortem autolysis in keeping with the time between death and preservation of the tissue.

Lewisite

This war gas, chlorovinyldichloroarsine or a mixture of closely related compounds, is vesicant and necrotizing on the skin or other tissues with which it comes in contact. The eyes and air passages suffer severely when the gas is inhaled; the mouth and whole gastrointestinal tract, when it is ingested. There is also absorption of the material, with the result that the blood-borne poison produces the usual changes of acute toxic hepatitis and a less severe toxic nephrosis. The epithelium of the bile ducts and gallbladder may suffer necrosis as the result of elimination of some of the poison in the bile. Shock, comparable to that which results from ordinary burns, may develop after a few days, with a fatal termination.

Cameron, G.R., Carlton, H.M., and Short, R.H.D.: Pathological changes induced by lewisite and allied compounds. J. Pathol. Bact., *58*:411–422, 1946.

Mustard Gas

Animals have been poisoned by eating forage or pasturage contaminated with this deadly war gas, which chemically is B, B^1-dichloroethyl sulfide. Clinical signs described are profuse salivation, lacrimation and conjunctivitis, mucous rhinitis, refusal to eat, pain in the mouth and pharynx, nausea, and rapid pulse and respiration. Lesions are chiefly due to the local irritant and necrotizing action upon the mucous membranes of the mouth, esophagus, and stomach. These could lead to confusion with "mucosal disease" (p. 420), or in sheep, with contagious ecthyma (p. 303), or possibly with other viral infections. Hemorrhages and focal prenecrotic degeneration are reported in the myocardium. Burns, of course, can occur on the skin when the poisonous liquid or vapor comes in contact with it. Coagulative necrosis is the fundamental change, with ulceration supervening. In fatal cases, death after several days is partly attributable to secondary infection of the ulcerated surfaces.

Koschnick, H.: Gelbkreuz-(Lost-) vergiftungen bei Pferden. Z. Veterinärk., *55*:57–63, 1943.

Pullinger, B.D.: Some characters of coagulation necrosis due to mustard gas. J. Pathol. Bact., *59*:255–259, 1947.

Watson, J.F.: Mustard gas poisoning in the horse. Vet. Rec., *55*:338, 1943.

Young, L.: Effects of mustard gas on the rat. Can. J. Res., Sect. E, *25*:141–151, 1947.

GROUP B: GASTROENTERITIS

Poisons in group B have **gastroenteritis** as their prominent pathologic feature. However, lesions in other organs are present in most of these poisonings and clinical signs may be diverse.

Arsenic

Animals rather frequently acquire arsenic in poisonous quantities through the accidental ingestion of such compounds as lead arsenate and Paris green, which are kept on the farm for use as insecticidal sprays, and lead arsenite, which is used as a cutaneous parasiticide (dips) for ticks and mites. Another frequent accident consists of animals eating plants and weeds that have been sprayed with arsenicals intentionally, to kill the plants, or inadvertently, while the spray was being applied to fruit trees. Poisoning occurs readily through cutaneous absorption if animals are dipped in a solution that is too concentrated. Occasional poisoning results from excessive administration of arsenical medicaments, such as Fowler's solution or neoarsphenamine. Chronic poisoning also occurs in animals grazing on the land subject to precipitated fumes from smelters and blast furnaces using arsenic-containing ores. Arsenous acid, in the experience of one of the authors (Jones), has accidentally contaminated commercial dog food, with numerous fatalities. Arsanilic acid (an organic arsenical) is used in poultry and swine feeds as a stimulant to growth. It is also occasionally used to control dysentery in swine. These practices have added to the possibility of causing arsenic poisoning by error in compounding feed or by contamination of feeds intended for other species.

The outstanding lesion of acute arsenical poisoning is severe gastritis or gastroenteritis, often hemorrhagic. The usual signs of severe abdominal pain, vomiting (in the dog and pig), purgation, and tenesmus obviously depend upon this lesion, and the same may well be true of the acceleration of pulse and respiration and general collapse. The gastroenteritis is said to occur regardless of the route by which the poison enters the body. There is dehydration of the tissues with abundant fluid in the bowels (diluting the irritant).

In less acute poisonings, diarrhea usu-

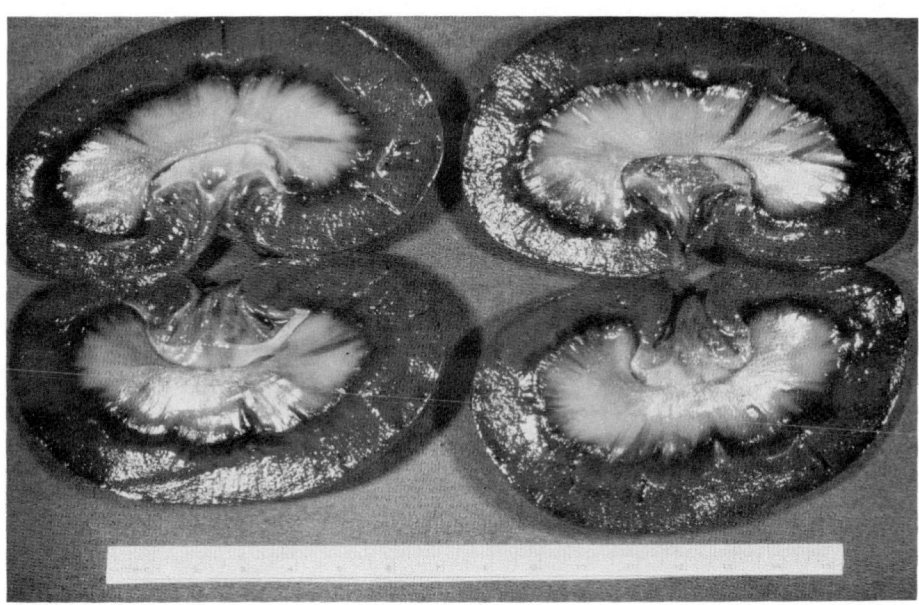

Fig. 16–1. Arsenic poisoning, kidneys of a four-year-old male foxhound. Note dark congested cortico-medullary junction and blanched medulla. (Courtesy of Angell Memorial Animal Hospital.)

ally marks the presence of a moderately severe gastroenteritis. In these cases there are stupor, incoordination, convulsions, and subnormal temperature. Such cases in cows have been mistaken for milk fever.

The chronic form is more rare now than in past years, when arsenicals were often used in treatment of several obscure diseases. The principal lesions are (1) toxic hepatitis (hydropic degeneration, fatty change, and necrosis), (2) chronic dermatitis with excessive pigmentation (in white skins) and extreme hyperkeratosis, and (3) a "neuritis" causing atrophy of the optic nerve and blindness. Peripheral motor nerves and their neurons in the cord may also be destroyed, leading to paraplegia and dysphagia. (4) In cattle, there is sometimes an unexplained periarticular fibrosis, producing stiffness and asymmetric enlargements of hocks or other joints of the limbs.

Arsenic is chemically rather indestructible, and can be detected in the liver and other tissues years after death and burial. The element is also detectable in the urine.

Arsanilic acid poisoning is characterized by neurologic signs and lesions and is discussed under Group Q.

Byron, W.R., et al.: Pathologic changes in rats and dogs from two-year feeding of sodium arsenite and sodium arsenate. Toxicol. Appl. Pharmacol., 10:132–147, 1967.

Darraspen, E., Tapernoux, A., and Vuillaume, R.: Contribution a l'étude de l'intoxication arsenicale chez le cheval. Rev. méd. vét., Lyon et Toulouse, 101:281–293, 1950. Abstr. Vet. Bull. No. 1793, 1951.

Harding, J.D.J., Lewis, G., and Done, J.T.: Experimental arsanilic acid poisoning in pigs. Vet. Rec., 83:560–564, 1968.

Maas, E.E.: Arsenic content of urine from cattle dipped in arsenical solutions. J. Am. Vet. Med. Assoc., 110:249–251, 1947.

McCulloch, E.C., and St. John, J.L.: Lead-arsenate poisoning of sheep and cattle. J. Am. Vet. Med. Assoc., 96:321–326, 1940.

Moxham, J.W., and Coup, M.R.: Arsenic poisoning of cattle and other domestic animals. NZ Vet. J., 16:161–165, 1968.

Nockolds, C.: Paris green poisoning. Am. Vet. Rev., 20:343–345, 1896.

Oliver, W.T., and Roe, C.K.: Arsanilic acid poisoning in swine. J. Am. Vet. Med. Assoc., 130:177–178, 1957.

Peoples, S.A.: Arsenic toxicity in cattle. Ann. NY Acad. Sci., 111:644–649, 1964.

Pritchett, H.D.: Acute arsenic poisoning in a dog. North Am. Vet., 22:627–628, 1941.

Smith, I.D., Perdue, H.S., and Kolar, J.A.: Tolerance of swine to varying levels of arsanilic acid in the feed. J. Anim. Sci., 21:1014, 1962.

Stumpff, C.: Arsenic poisoning in cows. Vet. Med., 39:393, 1944.

Vorhies, M.W., Sleight, S.D., and Whitehair, C.K.: Toxicity of arsanilic acid in swine as influenced by water intake. Cornell Vet., 59:3–9, 1969.

White, C.B.: Sodium arsenate (acid) poisoning in cattle. North Am. Vet., 10:38, 1929.

Salt

Swine and poultry are sometimes poisoned by sodium chloride when the very salty (60%) brines used for the preservation of meats on the farm are discarded in such a manner that animals have access to them. Other animals are occasionally poisoned by consuming too much when the usual free supply of salt, with or without other minerals, has been unavailable for some time and then is abruptly replenished. Other forms of accidental ingestion of excessive amounts have been reported.

Chickens and other farm birds are most susceptible, by far, to poisoning by sodium chloride. Swine are next most susceptible. For baby chicks, physiologic salt solution (0.9% NaCl) as the exclusive source of drinking water is regularly fatal in a few days. A concentration of 0.5% administered in the same way may also kill, but 0.25% does not (Edwards, 1918). Adult hens are able to consume appreciably more, especially if the salt is administered dry, mixed with the food. In the latter form of administration, Blaxland (1946) found that 30% in the ration was sometimes fatal, but 20% evoked no unfavorable signs. In young pigs, salt amounting to 2.5% of the ration and mixed with the feed caused severe nervous symptoms but no fatalities, unless the supply of water was restricted (Larsen et al., 1955). Cattle are sometimes poisoned, as mentioned previously, but on the other hand, they have been unharmed by the prolonged consumption of two pounds (900 g) of salt per day as long as the large consumption of water that resulted remained unrestricted. It can be said with respect to all species that it is not easy to produce poisoning so long as animals are allowed all the water they wish to drink.

The signs are those of nervous derangement and hyperirritability. Blindness, stumbling, walking backward or in circles, and convulsive seizures are most frequently mentioned. Smith (1957) in experimental cases reported deranged consciousness, blindness, epileptiform seizures beginning with twitching of the nose and progressing clonus of the neck muscles, circling or running movements, retropulsion, pleurothotonos, opisthotonos, and sialorrhea. As the effects become more severe, signs of abdominal pain become paramount. Thirst is always excessive.

Lesions following the sudden ingestion of excessive amounts of salt, especially if unlimited water has not been available, consist of severe acute inflammation of the gastric and upper intestinal linings. Sometimes crystals of undissolved salt adhere to the inflamed mucosa. In cases of continued consumption of moderately excessive amounts over a period of days, usually experimental, the principal lesion is edema of both tissues and body cavities. A microscopic lesion that appears to be pathognomonic in swine, but not necessarily in poultry, has been called eosinophilic meningoencephalitis. It is characterized by a startlingly extensive infiltration of eosinophils into the perivascular (Virchow-Robin) spaces of the brain, along with edema and sometimes encephalomalacia. Experimental work by Smith (1957) indicates that sodium becomes concentrated in the brain tissue, its high osmotic pressure then being responsible for the edema. Sodium is also a strong inhibitor of anaerobic glycolysis in the brain. Sodium and chloride of the blood are elevated.

In poultry, salt poisoning causes a form of nephritis which is thought by many to be the same as a disease known by such names as nephrosclerosis of poultry or pullet disease.

Blaxland, J.D.: Toxicity of sodium chloride for fowls. Vet. J., 102:157–173, 1946.

Bohosiewicz, M.: Experimental sodium chloride poisoning in pigs. Méd vét., Varsovie. 9:498–501, 1953. Abstr. Vet. Bull. No. 2134, 1955.

Bohosiewicz, M.: Laboratory diagnosis of poisoning by sodium chloride. Méd. Vét., Varsovie. 13:478–481, 1957. Abstr. Vet. Bull. No. 888, 1958.

Bohstedt, G., and Grummer, R.H.: Salt poisoning in pigs. J. Anim. Sci., 13:933–939. 1954.

Bryant, J.B.: An unusual case of salt poisoning. J. Am. Vet. Med. Assoc., 93:41, 1938.

Doll, E.R., Hull, F.E., and Insko, W.M., Jr.: Toxicity of sodium chloride solution for baby chicks. Vet. Med., 41:361–363, 1946.

Done, J.T., Harding, J.D.J., and Lloyd, M.K.: Meningo-encephalitis eosinophilica of swine. II. Studies of the experimental reproduction of the lesions by feeding sodium chloride and urea. Vet. Rec., 71:92–96, 1959.

Edwards, J.T.: Salt poisoning in pigs and poultry. J. Comp. Pathol. Therap., 31:40–43, 1918.

Hofferd, R.M.: Salt poisoning in hogs. J. Am. Vet. Med. Assoc., 94:55–56, 1939.

Lames, H.S.: Salt poisoning in swine (water deprivation syndrome). Vet. Med. Small Anim. Clin., 63:882–883, 1968.

Larsen, N.B., Moller, T., and Thordal-Christensen, A.A.: Meningoencephalitis eosinophilica in pigs. Nord. Vet. Med., 7:653–659, 1955.

Madejski, Z.: Some aspects of acute sodium chloride poisoning in animals. Polskie Archwm wet., 8:463–483, 1964. VB 35:2304, 1965.

Michalska, Z.: Histopathology of experimental salt poisoning in pigs (TT). Weterynaria, Wroclaw., 11:45–68, 1962.

Mocsy, J.: Sodium chloride poisoning in pigs. Magyar Allatorvosok Lapja, 4:66–67, 1949. Abstr. Nutritional Abstr. Rev., 19:494, 1949, and in Vet. Bull. No. 1047, 1950.

Rac, R., Bray, J.H., and Lynch, J.: Meningoencephalitis eosinophilica of pigs. Vet. Rec., 71:688–692, 1959.

Sautter, J.H., Sorenson, D.K., and Clark, J.J.: Symposium on salt poisoning: salt poisoning in swine. J. Am. Vet. Med. Assoc., 130:12–22, 1957.

Smith, D.L.T.: Poisoning by sodium salt. A cause of eosinophilic meningoencephalitis in swine. Am. J. Vet. Res., 18:825–850, 1957.

Szeky, A., and Szabo, I.: Diagnosis and pathogenesis of sodium chloride poisoning in pigs, and the occurrence of eosinophilic meningitis and en-

910   *DISEASES DUE TO EXTRANEOUS POISONS*

cephalitis. Acta Vet. Acad. Sci. Hung., 12:319–341, 1962.

Trainer, D.O., and Karstad, L.: Salt poisoning in Wisconsin wildlife. J. Am. Vet. Med. Assoc., 136:14–18, 1960.

Petroleum

When one observes the utter lack of gustatory discrimination shown by most bovine animals, he is not too greatly astonished to see cattle drinking crude petroleum that has escaped from an oil tank or pipeline and is standing in a pool on the ground or floating on the surface of a pond or stream. Just how toxic a given specimen of crude oil is remains subject to determination. Well-purified petroleum oil constitutes the liquid petrolatum of the Pharmacopeia and is practically inert in the digestive tract. On the other hand, the volatile fractions of petroleum are irritating and definitely poisonous. It can be said with certainty that fresh oil is consequently more toxic than that which has been out of the ground long enough for much of the volatile material to have evaporated. Parker and Williamson (1951) found one specimen of crude oil used as tractor fuel to be lethal at the rate of 1 gallon (3800 ml) for a bovine weighing 450 pounds (200 kg). While other species are not immune, their different habits usually protect them.

Signs have usually included fetid and hemorrhagic diarrhea, although constipation has been noted, probably as an initial change. Oil is usually detectable in the feces and it may be regurgitated. Bloating commonly occurs. The temperature is somewhat elevated; respiration and heart beat are accelerated. Terminally there are dilated pupils and muscular incoordination. Some animals recover in a few days.

Postmortem lesions include acute enteritis with marked enteric edema, renal hyperemia, perhaps with hemorrhages, and acute cystitis. Pulmonary congestion and edema are prominent if the oil contained much volatile material.

Kerosene is occasionally administered accidentally and more often is given by the laity for some supposed medicinal effect. Not all of the victims die, but in those that do, pneumonia is usually an outstanding lesion, presumably because of inhalation of irritant fumes. The central nervous system dysfunction, which is a well recognized sequela to kerosene poisoning in man, is believed to result from hypoxia. It is sometimes applied externally (for lice, etc.) and has caused loss of hair in the horse. In cattle, severe dermatitis and hematuria have been reported.

Bottarelli, A.: Grave forma di intossicazione da sabbie petrolifere in un allevamento suino. (Poisoning of pigs by crude oil-bearing sand from an oil well.) Atti. Soc. Ital. Sci. Vet., 5:208–212, 1951.

Foley, J.C., et al.: Kerosene poisoning in young children. Radiology, 62:817–829, 1954.

Gibson, E.A., and Linzell, J.L.: Diesel oil poisoning in cattle. Vet. Rec., 60:60–61, 1948.

McConnell, W.C.: Salt water and oil pollution and its relation to livestock losses. North Am. Vet., 26:600–601, 1945.

Parker, W.H., and Williamson, T.F.: Paraffin [crude petroleum] poisoning in cattle. Vet. Rec., 63:430–432, 1951.

Richardson, J.A., and Pratt-Thomas, H.R.: Toxic effects of varying doses of kerosene administered by different routes. Am. J. Med. Sci., 221:531–536, 1951.

Rowe, L.D., Dollahite, J.W., and Camp, B.J.: Toxicity of two crude oils and of kerosene to cattle. J. Am. Vet. Med. Assoc., 162:61–66, 1973.

Strober, M.: Toxicity for cattle of crude and heating oil. Dtsche. tierarztl. Wochenschr., 69:386–390, 1962.

Wolfsdorf, J.: Kerosene intoxication: an experimental approach to etiology of CNS manifestations in primates. J. Pediatr., 88:1037–1040, 1976.

Woldsdorf, J., and Kundig, H.: Kerosene poisoning in primates. S. Afr. Med. J., 46:619–621, 1972.

Sodium Fluoroacetate

This compound of fluorine, sometimes sold as "Formula 1080," inhibits the citric acid cycle. It is used as a poison for destroying rats. It is sometimes accidentally eaten by dogs when it is placed in meat as a bait and by cattle which may ingest contaminated forage or grain. Signs include increasing weakness and rapidity of the heart beat; the heart eventually becomes exhausted. Signs of severe abdominal pain and nausea are prominent in dogs and swine (experimentally). Nervous disturbances terminate in opisthotonos and convulsions, with death in a few or several hours after ingestion of the poison. It is said that the prognosis is hopeless once symptoms have appeared. Lesions are few, but there is ordinarily severe inflammation of the small intestine. As a result of cardiac failure and anoxia, the blood is dark and there are subepicardial and subendocardial petechiae. Studies of the nervous tissues have not been reported.

Jensen, R., Tobiska, J.W., and Ward, J.C.: Sodium fluoroacetate poisoning in sheep. Am. J. Vet. Res., 9:370–372, 1948.
Murphy, S.D.: Pesticides. *In* Toxicology: The Basic Science of Poisons, edited by J. Doull, C.D. Klaasen, and M.O. Amdur. New York, Macmillan, 1980, pp. 395–396.
Nichols, H.C., et al.: Poisoning of two dogs with 1080 rat poison (sodium fluoroacetate). J. Am. Vet. Med. Assoc., 115:355–356, 1949.
Schnautz, J.O.: Sodium fluoroacetate poisoning in cattle. J. Am. Vet. Med. Assoc., 114:435, 1949.
Schwarte, L.H.: Toxicity of sodium monofluoroacetate for swine and chickens. J. Am. Vet. Med. Assoc., 111:301–303, 1947.

Ground Glass

More or less finely shattered glass is administered from time to time to man or animals with felonious intent. In a majority of cases, no effects are noticed. In some instances, there is transient abdominal discomfort, diarrhea, and mild gastroenteritis.

Mayo, N.S.: Effect of "ground glass" on the gastrointestinal tract of dogs. J. Am. Vet. Med. Assoc., 55:202–203, 1919.
Simmons, J.S., and Von Glahn, W.C.: Effect of "ground glass" on the gastro-intestinal tract of dogs. J. Am. Med. Assoc., 71:2127, 1918.

Dynamite

Incredible as it may seem, cattle are sometimes poisoned by eating dynamite or the wrappings thereof. One suspects that the native bovine curiosity, which is sometimes manifested in most incongruous ways, has more to do with the animal's eating a substance of this kind than has the actual appetite. Nitroglycerine, of course, is available as a drug, and would have the same effect as dynamite if ingested in excessive amounts.

Signs are polyuria and polydipsia, nausea, colic, and perhaps coma. In fatal cases, death comes in 24 to 36 hours. Postmortem lesions are acute gastroenteritis, acute toxic tubular nephritis, dark or chocolate-colored blood due to the formation of methemoglobin, and often petechiae due to terminal anoxia.

Buffington, R.M.: Nitroglycerine (dynamite) poisoning in cattle. Vet. Bull., 21:197–198, 1928.
Holm, L.W., et al.: Experimental poisoning of cattle and sheep with dynamite. Cornell Vet., 42:91–96, 1952.
Kinnell, G.N.: Dynamite poisoning. Am. Vet. Rev., 17:554–556, 1894.

Urea (Ammonia)

Since the practice has developed of feeding to cattle and other ruminants artificially concocted feeds containing urea as a substitute for protein nitrogen, deaths attributed to poisoning by this substance have ceased to be rare. It appears that 2 to 3% of the total ration (dry-weight basis) can safely be urea, but that larger amounts are likely to produce poisoning. Urea is much better tolerated when mixed with plentiful amounts of other feeds than when, for any reason, it enters the digestive tract less well diluted; hence, the occurrence of poisoning is erratic. Poisoning is due to the local and generalized effects of ammonia released by hydrolysis of the urea by urease. Ammonium salts are also used in feeds, and their use in fertilizer provides another source of exposure. The effects of urea and ammonium salts are comparable.

Signs arise suddenly and may lead to death in one or two hours or less. However, illness does not necessarily develop at the first ingestion of the urea-containing feed, but apparently occurs whenever, through intestinal inactivity or other functional irregularity, a sufficient amount of ammonia is released at one time and (judging from experimental administration via the stomach tube [Dinning et al., 1948]) in the same region of the digestive canal.

Signs are attributable to the effect of ammonia on the nerve centers, and include twitching of eyelids, lips and tail, ataxia in locomotion, and convulsions. Salivation may be prominent, with frothing at the mouth. Pulse and respirations become progressively slower and death follows. The resemblance to strychnine poisoning is often marked. Blood-urea nitrogen, as well as ammonia-nitrogen in the rumen, are elevated. The pH of the blood and urine are abnormally high.

Postmortem lesions are not extensive. There is usually rather severe acute catarrhal or, at times, hemorrhagic enteritis. In the experience of some, the inflammation has been found in the stomach (abomasum); in the experience of Hilton Smith, there has always been severe inflammation in the last third of the small intestine. Mild toxic hepatitis and toxic tubular nephrosis accompany the enteric injury. In the lungs, there may be hemorrhages, either peribronchial or intra-alveolar, as well as mild acute catarrhal bronchitis. The central nervous lesions, consisting of neuronal degenerations, pial hemorrhages, and congestion, are probably attributable to the direct effects of ammonia.

Clark, R., Oyaert, W., and Quinn, J.I.: The toxicity of urea to sheep under different conditions. Onderstepoort J. Vet. Sci., 25:73–78, 1951.

Davis, G.K., and Roberts, H.F.: Urea toxicity in cattle. Bul. Fla. Agric. Expt. Sta., No. 611, pp. 16, 1959.

Dinning, J.S., et al.: Effect of orally administered urea. Am. J. Physiol., 153:41–46, 1948.

Engels, O.: Ist Handelsdünger Gift für die Tiere? Ztschr. f. Schafzucht., 31:137–138, 1942.

Fujimoto, Y., and Tajima, M.: Pathological studies on urea poisoning. Jpn. J. Vet. Sci., 15:125–134, 1953. (English summary.) Abstr. Vet. Bull., No. 1769, 1955.

Green, D.F.: Urea feeding. North Am. Vet., 36:733–736, 827–833, 1955.

Hale, W.H., and King, R.P.: Possible mechanisms of urea toxicity in ruminants. Proc. Soc. Exp. Biol. Med., 89:112–114, 1955. Abstr. Vet. Bull., No. 4104, 1955.

Koval, M.P., and Vas'ko, I.V.: (Poisoning of cows with carbamide [urea]). Veterinariya (Moscow), 41:49–50, 1964.

Osebold, J.W.: Urea poisoning in cattle. North Am. Vet., 28:89–91, 1947.

Singer, R.H., and McCarty, R.T.: Acute ammonium salt poisoning in sheep. Am. J. Vet. Res., 32:1229–1238, 1971.

————: Pathologic changes resulting from acute ammonium salt poisoning in sheep. Am. J. Vet. Res., 32:1239–1246, 1971.

Nicotine

Poisoning by nicotine occurs in animals almost exclusively from the improper use of insecticidal solutions on the skin or nicotine sulfate as an anthelmintic internally. One of the most deadly poisons known, nicotine is promptly absorbed from mucous membrane or skin and acts rapidly, producing at first nervous stimulation and then depression. If swallowed, there is local pain in the throat and stomach. Muscular tremors and weakness cause the animal to fall. Convulsions are followed in a matter of minutes by loss of voluntary movement, so that the patient lies quietly. Concurrently with vomiting and purging, the pulse and respiration become weaker and slower, with death from respiratory failure and collapse, all within two or three hours. A case of a dog being poisoned by eating cigarette stubs (equivalent of 15 to 20 cigarettes per day) is on record (Boissière, 1938). Depression and polyuria were followed by vomition and then by diarrhea lasting four days. Another reported fatality, in a three-month-old puppy, resulted from eating a pack of cigarettes (Kaplan, 1968).

As would be expected from the rapidity of the poisonous action, lesions are minimal. Acute inflammation of the stomach (abomasum) and intestines is likely to be pronounced, even when the mode of entry is by cutaneous absorption. Mesenteric vessels are severely hyperemic, the blood being bright red.

Boissière: Intoxication du chien par le tabac. Rec. méd. vét., 114:35, 1938.

Crawshaw, H.A.: Nicotine poisoning in lambs. Vet. Rec., 56:276–277, 1944.

Fincher, M.G.: Blackleaf 40 poisoning. Cornell Vet., 24:86, 1934.

Kaplan, B.: Acute nicotine poisoning in a dog. Vet. Med. Small Anim. Clin., 63:1033–1034, 1968.

Nightshades (Genus Solanum)

For the pathology of deadly nightshade, see Belladonna, page 993.

In the genus *Solanum* are included the following: the common or black nightshade (*S. nigrum*); the "bitter apple" (*S. incanum*), a plant similar in appearance to the common tomato, its close relative; the "apple of Sodom" (*S. panduraeforme*); the "Jerusalem berry" (*S. pseudocapsicum*); the white "horse nettle" (*S. eleagnifolium*); the "buffalo bur" (*S. rostratum*); and the common potato (*S. tuberosum*). All of these and various other, less toxic species contain the poisonous glycoalkaloid, solanin, either constantly or transiently, in the whole or certain parts of the plant, their poisonous actions being similar. In the case of potatoes, the growing sprouts on stored tubers are more or less poisonous, as is also the skin of a tuber that has grown partly exposed at the surface of the ground, so that its skin becomes thickened and green.

Gastrointestinal signs, salivation, stomatitis, vomiting, tympanites, and diarrhea are usually overshadowed by nervous depression, apathy, narcosis, and paralysis. A mild degree of poisoning may exhibit only an exanthematous form. Lesions in the digestive tract are acute catarrhal or hemorrhagic gastritis and enteritis, sometimes accompanied by ulcers that extend to or through the muscularis propria. There is rarely desquamation of patches of buccal mucosa. Tissue changes accounting for the nervous symptoms have not been described, and apparently histopathological studies of the brain have not been made. Since the poison usually acts within a matter of hours, such studies possibly would yield little. In the exanthematous form, which is relatively chronic and benign, the more tender areas of skin show vesicles and hyperemia. Conjunctivitis is a frequent accompaniment. The degree of toxicity of these plants varies greatly from time to time.

The possible association between potato tubers and malformation of the neural tube leading to anencephaly and spina bifida has raised considerable concern and discussion, but the association has not been proven.

Solanum malocoxylon poisoning is discussed on page 978.

Andrade, S.O.: Estudos sobre a toxicidade de *Sessea brasiliensis (Solanaceae)*. Arq. Inst. Biol. S. Paulo, 27:191–196, 1960.

Casselberry, N.H.: Nightshade poisoning of swine. Vet. Med., 34:444–445, 1939.

Eckell, O.A.: Acción Toxica del *Solanum glaucum*, Dun (Duraznillo blanco). An. Fac. Med. Vet. Univ. La Plata, 5:9–91, 1942.

Koslowski, B.: Dermatitis in unweaned pigs from feeding green potatoes to the sows. Méd. vét., Varsovie, 9:505, 1953. Abstr. Vet. Bull. No. 3290, 1954.

Sever, J.L.: Potatoes and birth defects: summary. Teratology, 8:319–320, 1973.

Simic, W.J.: Solanine poisoning in swine. Vet. Med., 38:353–354, 1943.

Steyn, D.G.: Toxicology of Plants in South Africa. Johannesburg, The Central News Agency, Ltd., 1934.

Castor Beans (Ricinus communis)

The meal remaining after the extraction of oil from castor beans contains ricin, an extremely potent poison that is water-soluble, hence not found in the castor oil. Ricin resembles bacterial exotoxins in that an animal can be hyperimmunized to it so that the serum has high antitoxic properties. As in the case of bacterial toxins, heat (about 56°C) destroys a toxic fraction (toxophore) and leaves an immunizing fraction (haptophore). Boiling the meal or the whole seeds definitely renders them nonpoisonous.

Signs appear a few hours after ingestion of small amounts of meal or the whole seeds. They consist chiefly of vomiting, violent diarrhea, signs of severe abdominal pain (grinding of teeth, humping of back), tumultuous heart action, slightly elevated temperature, and collapse. Horses show profuse sweating, and tetanic spasms have occurred. Lesions are severe acute gastritis (abomasitis in ruminants), with the reddening and edema continuing into the upper small intestine, where they are accompanied by petechiae. Free blood may be found in the bowel. Microscopically, the epithelium of the affected gastrointestinal areas is necrotic, although sometimes still present. Hepatocytes undergo hydropic degeneration, fatty change, and areas of necrosis (acute toxic hepatitis). The renal epithelium displays a less severe fatty degeneration and necrosis (acute toxic nephritis). There is a striking destruction of lymphocytes in the lymphoid organs (possibly simulating that seen in rinderpest and in irradiation). Necrosis has been demonstrated in the brain. In horses, severe edema is reported in the lungs, with a less severe degree in bronchial, mesenteric, and hepatic nodes and elsewhere. There is much fluid in the inflamed digestive tract. Treatment is symptomatic unless serum from a previously hyperimmunized animal should be available.

Clarke, E.G.C.: Poisoning by castor seed. Vet. J., *103*:273–278, 1947.
Geary, T.: Castor bean poisoning. Vet. Rec., *62*:472–473, 1950.
McCunn, J., Andrew, H., and Clough, G.W.: Castor-bean poisoning in horses. Vet. J., *101*:136–138, 1945.

Locust Tree

The seeds, leaves, bark, and roots of the black locust tree (*Robinia pseudoacacia*) have long been known to be poisonous, several different alkaloidal or glycosidal poisonous principles having been described. The clammy locust (*Robinia viscosa*) is also known to be poisonous, and presumably the same is true of other locusts. Horses and also humans have been poisoned by chewing the bark of young trees; chickens, by eating leaves and young sprouts.

Signs appear several hours after the poisonous material is ingested and include extreme muscular weakness, mental depression and maximum dilatation of the pupils. There is serious cardiac depression. The beat may be weak, but in the terminal stages it is frequently reported as being characterized by a loud thump, au-

dible for some distance. There may be signs of abdominal pain, and humans report nausea, but rarely, if ever, is there purgation. Salivation and bleeding from the mouth have been described in the horse. Many patients, man and animal, recover after a few days and gradually regain their strength.

Necropsy of those that die shows mucous inflammation of the gastrointestinal tract and occasionally more severe gastroenteritis. Gardiner (1903) found that the "stomach and intestine contained nearly all the fluids of the body." There is venous congestion, and some have described a yellowish discoloration of the mucous membranes "similar to" icterus.

Some experimental evidence indicates that the toxicity is seasonal (early and midsummer), or at least that locust trees are not constantly poisonous (Barnes, 1921).

Barnes, M.F.: Black locust poisoning of chickens. J. Am. Vet. Med. Assoc., *59*:370–372, 1921,
Gardiner, W.W.: Locust-tree bark poisoning. Am. Vet. Rev., *27*:599–600, 1903.
Pammel, L.H.: The toxicity of black locust. North Am. Vet., *8*:41–43, 1927.
Waldron, C.A.: Poisoning from locust bark. Am. Vet. Rev., *33*:456–459, 1908.

Tung Oil Tree

The tung tree (*Aleurites fordi*) is cultivated in warm countries for its oil, which is valuable in paints and varnishes. Poisoning of farm animals, including chickens, has resulted from attempts to feed the meal that remains after extraction of the oil from the tung nuts and from ingestion of foliage, not from the tree directly, but in the form of cut leaves and branches, which have considerable palatability to cattle.

Profuse watery or bloody diarrhea occurs after an interval of a few days and is the chief sign. Illness lasts from one to three weeks before terminating fatally. Lesions are severe hemorrhagic gastroenteritis, severe congestion of the splanchnic organs, and early toxic changes in the liver.

Davis, G.K., et al.: Tung meal in rations for growing chicks. Poult. Sci., *25*:74–79, 1946.

Emmel, M.W., et al.: Toxicity of foliage of *Aleurites fordi* for cattle. J. Am. Vet. Med. Assoc., 101:136–137, 1942.

Hurst, E.: The Poison Plants of New South Wales. 1942. Univ. of Sydney and N.S.W. Dept. Agric., Sydney.

Fluorensia Cernua

Known popularly as **blackbush** or **tarbush,** this plant is indigenous to the arid areas of the southwestern United States and Mexico. Poisoning occurs almost exclusively in sheep and goats, which eat the berry-like fruit, sometimes merely in the course of being driven through an infested area.

Symptoms are salivation, grinding of teeth, and signs of severe abdominal pain, such as groaning and arching of the back. Muscular twitchings are not infrequent. If the animal lives for some time, there is likely to be mucous rhinitis. Death frequently occurs in 24 to 48 hours; animals that survive five days usually recover. Lesions are severe inflammation of the abomasum and duodenum. In cases of some standing, the inflammatory infiltration of fluid and leukocytes extends into the muscularis.

Mathews, E.P.: Toxicity of the ripe fruit of blackbrush, tarbush *(Fluorensia cernua).* Exp. Sta. Bull. 644, 1944. Texas A. & M. College, College Station.

Oaks

Several hundred species of oak trees or shrubs are known, and poisoning by members of this genus (*Quercus*) has been recognized for a long time, but is not fully understood. The principal toxins of oaks are tannins (gallotannins), which are broken down into gallic acid and pyrogallol, both of which are toxic.

The usual form of oak poisoning occurs when the young leaf-buds and flowers are making their annual springtime appearance, and accordingly is often called "oak-bud poisoning." The usual outbreaks of the disease result from the ingestion of the buds and young leaves of certain small shrub-like species known as shin-oak or shinnery oak, *Quercus havardi,* indigenous to the southwestern United States, and it may well be that this species is more poisonous than others. However, typical oak-bud poisoning has occurred when budding branches of large oak trees have been made accessible to cattle or sheep in the course of lumbering operations. To what extent some or all oaks are more poisonous during the budding and early leafing stage, and to what extent the occurrence of poisoning at that time may be related to the contemporary shortage of other green feed and an appetite for the oaks, are questions that have not been answered. Oak poisoning may also result from consuming acorns in large quantity. In contrast to oak-bud poisoning, acorn poisoning occurs in the fall. Green acorns are more toxic than mature acorns.

Signs of oak-bud poisoning are chiefly alimentary and urinary in nature. While a few animals have diarrhea from the outset, the great majority have severe constipation with tenesmus. The frequent efforts at defecation produce small, hard balls of mucus-covered feces, to which blood is sometimes adherent. After several days, the constipation commonly gives way to a fetid and hemorrhagic diarrhea. A blood-stained nasal exudate is a frequent sign. Ventral edema of renal origin is also characteristic, especially in sheep. The severe injury to the kidneys, which appears always to be a part of the syndrome, is evidenced by polydipsia and polyuria, clear urine of low specific gravity being voided at frequent intervals. The illness may terminate fatally in 24 hours, after several days, or may yield to slow recovery in two or three weeks. New cases may appear for approximately a week after the herd or flock has been removed from access to the budding oaks.

The lesions are those that would be predicted from the signs. Mucous enteritis involves the last half of the digestive canal and becomes partly or eventually almost entirely hemorrhagic. The mesenteric lymph nodes are edematous. In addition to the subcutaneous edema already mentioned, there are usually hydropericardium and hydroperitoneum. The liver is congested and shows a moderate degree of acute toxic hepatitis. The gallbladder is distended with viscid, brownish bile. The kidneys are of the large, pale type, but rather uniformly sprinkled with petechiae 2 or 3 mm in diameter. The medulla is congested. The microscopic renal picture is almost pathognomonic. Numerous proximal convoluted tubules contain dense casts of albumin, their pink color being stained with brown, doubtless from bile pigment and possibly also from hemoglobin. The necrotic epithelial lining cells are usually so intimately mixed with the proteinaceous contents of the lumen that the whole forms a dense, homogeneous mass limited by the basement membrane and interstitial tissue. Adjacent to such a tubule are others that appear quite uninjured. The glomeruli show little change, and the medulla remains nearly normal in appearance except for congestion. In our experience, this type of tubular damage has not been duplicated in any other disease.

Begovic, S., et al.: Poisoning of cattle by oak leaves. Vet. Glasn., 11:673–679, 1957. (In Croat., Ger. summary.) Abstr. Vet. Bull. No. 3725, 1958.

Boughton, I.B., and Hardy, W.T.: Oak poisoning in range cattle and sheep. J. Am. Vet. Med. Assoc., 89:157–162, 1936.

Cedervall, A., Johansson, H.E., and Jönsson, L.: Acorn poisoning in cattle. Nord. Vet. Med., 25:639–644, 1973.

Kingrey, B.W., Richter, W.R., and Dingel, R.M.: Acorn poisoning in cattle. Iowa State Univ. Vet., 22(No. 1):30–31, 1959.

Marsh, C.D., Clawson, A.B., and Marsh, H.: Oak-leaf poisoning of domestic animals. U.S. Dept. Agric. Bull., 767, 1919.

Sandusky, G.E., Fosnaugh, C.J., Smith, J.B., and Mohan, R.: Oak poisoning of cattle in Ohio. J. Am. Vet. Med. Assoc., 171:627–629, 1977.

Smith, H.A.: The diagnosis of oak poisoning. Southwestern Vet., 13:343–349, 1959.

Oleander

The oleander (*Nerium oleander*), native to most of the warmer parts of the world and grown as an ornamental plant in the southern United States, has been known for its extreme toxicity since ancient times. Human beings have been fatally poisoned not only by eating a few leaves, but even when oleander twigs were used as skewers in meat (Hurst, 1942). Horses, cattle and sheep usually do not eat it; most cases of poisoning occur when cuttings from a garden are thoughtlessly thrown into a dry lot, especially where animals are accustomed to having forkfuls of hay placed before them. Although the presenting signs and lesions focus on the gastrointestinal tract, death is the result of heart failure. The toxic principles of oleander are cardiac glycosides (oleandrin, neriine), similar in action to digitalis.

The signs are abdominal pain, nausea, vomiting, diarrhea, and tenesmus, plus a digitalis-like stimulation of the heart and constriction of vessels. As a result, extremities are cold, while the general body temperature is raised. Respirations are augmented both in rate and depth. There may be bradycardia or tachycardia associated with various arrhythmias. Tremors and tetanic stiffness give way to paralysis and death, usually without convulsions. The duration of symptoms is usually less than 24 hours.

Lesions are chiefly those of severe catarrhal or hemorrhagic gastroenteritis, the irritation even beginning in the pharynx in some cases. Terminal petechial and ecchymotic hemorrhages are common on the heart, serous and mucous membranes, including the gallbladder and the meninges. Blood-stained or clear fluid is frequent in the serous cavities. In a case studied by Hilton A. Smith, there were petechiae in the renal cortex and hematuria. The case also showed early toxic hepatitis and toxic tubular nephrosis. The cortical tubules were largely in a state of coagulative necrosis and contained casts of hemoglobin-stained albumin.

Hurst, E.: The Poison Plants of New South Wales. 1942. Univ. of Sydney and N.S.W. Dept. Agric., Sydney.

Novara, V.: Avvelenamento naturale da oleandro (Nerium oleander) nei Bovini. Vet. Ital., 9:18–24, 1958. Abstr. Vet. Bull. No. 3381, 1958.

Panisset, L.: Noxiousness of rhododendron (oleander). North Am. Vet., 4:255–256, 1923.

Ratigan, W.J.: Oleander poisoning in a bear. J. Am. Vet. Med. Assoc., 60:96–98, 1921.

Schwartz, W.L., et al.: Toxicity of Nerium oleander in the monkey (Cebus apella). Vet. Pathol., 11:259–277, 1974.

Steyn, D.G.: The Toxicology of Plants in South Africa. 1934, Johannesburg, The Central News Agency, Ltd.

Szabuniewicz, M., et al.: Experimental oleander poisoning and treatment. Southwest Vet., 25:105–114, 1972.

Milkweeds

The plants known as milkweeds, at least in North America, belong to the genus *Asclepias*. The common broad-leafed milkweeds, *A. eriocarpa* and *A. latifolia* (Baxter, 1944), have caused fatalities, and *A. speciosa*, a similar species, is considered moderately poisonous. The whorled milkweed, *A. subverticillata* (syn. *A. galioides*) and *A. verticillata,* and the dwarf *A. pumila* are much more common causes of poisoning. These latter have slender leaves and an appearance quite different from that of the common broad-leafed milkweeds. *A. crispa, A. fruticosa,* and *A. physocarpa* are narrow-leafed species that have been reported as poisoning animals in South Africa (Steyn, 1934).

The effects on all species seem to be much the same. Signs are nervous and gastrointestinal. Depression and apathy, great weakness, loss of mucular control, falling, dilated pupils, and respiratory paralysis represent the former group; intestinal stasis and fermentation, foul odors from the mouth, and occasionally a terminal fetid diarrhea belong to the latter. All species of farm animals, including chickens, are susceptible. Depending on the degree of toxicity and the amount eaten, signs commence in 2 to 14 hours after ingestion of the plants and continue for 1 or 2 to several hours. Lesions are acute catarrhal gastroenteritis and congestion of the lungs. The kidneys may also show acute congestion. Terminal dilation of the ventricles of the heart is frequent.

Baxter, C.M.: Broadleaf milkweed poisoning. Cornell Vet., 34:256–259, 1944.

Campbell, H.W.: Poisoning in chickens with whorled milkweed. J. Am. Vet. Med. Assoc., 79:102–104, 1931.

Steyn, D.G.: Toxicology of Plants in South Africa. Johannesburg, The Central News Agency, Ltd., 1934.

Tunnicliff, E.A., and Cory, V.L.: Broad-leafed milkweed poisonous for sheep and goats. J. Am. Vet. Med. Assoc., 77:165–168, 1930.

Red Squill

Also known as the sea onion, *Urginea maritima*, red squill is notably emetic, as well as nauseating, for many species. The red varity is used to poison rats, which like it and do not vomit. Most other animals do not eat it, but dogs have been known to do so. Swine have eaten red squill when it was accidentally mixed with their feed. Dogs usually vomit promptly, hence are not likely to be killed by it. Cats dislike it but have been poisoned by it.

The signs are vomition in the dog, usually not in other species, depression, collapse, incoordination, twitching, and convulsions in severe cases. Death may come in two to three days. Lesions include hyperemia and inflammation of gastric and intestinal mucosae, often with terminal bronchopneumonia. In most cases, there are toxic changes in the liver and kidney, but large experimental doses killed swine before these changes had become pronounced.

Gwatkin, R., and Plummer, P.J.G.: Toxicity of red squill for swine and rats. Can. J. Comp. Med., 7:244–249, 1943.

Nagle, A.C.: Red squill poisoning in a dog. J. Am. Vet. Med. Assoc., 112:139, 1948.

Rietz, J.H., and Moore, E.N.: Red squill poisoning in swine. J. Am. Vet. Med. Assoc., 102:120–121, 1943.

Blister Beetle

Striped blister beetles of the genus *Epicauta* gain their name from the action of **cantharidin,** a substance in their hemolymph which, when applied topically, causes acantholysis leading to

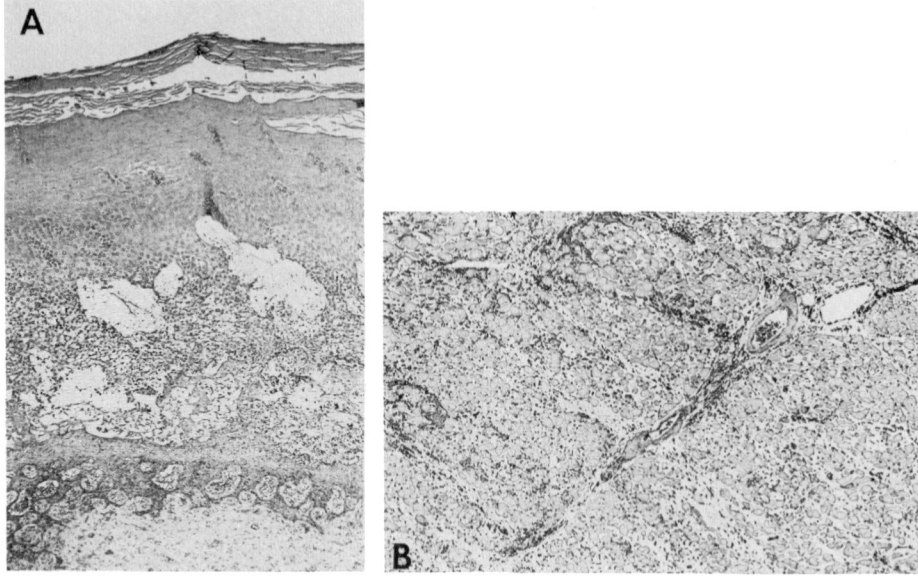

Fig. 16–2. Blister beetle poisoning in a horse. *A,* Acantholysis of the squamous gastric mucosa. *B,* Necrosis, edema and hemorrhage of the myocardium. (Courtesy of Dr. T. R. Schoeb.)

formation of intraepidermal vesicles. The beetles feed on alfalfa, and dead beetles may be incorporated into alfalfa hay which, if consumed by horses, leads to acute poisoning. Although the geographic range of the beetles is wide, reports of poisoning in horses have been limited to Tennessee, Texas, and Oklahoma. The clinical and pathologic features of natural poisoning in horses have recently been reviewed by Schoeb and Panciera (1979) who also experimentally reproduced the disease. The most consistent clinical signs include abdominal pain, fever, depression, frequent urination, and increased pulse and respiration rates. Laboratory findings indicate hemoconcentration, and there is a slight increase in blood urea nitrogen, decrease in serum calcium and hematuria. The tissue changes appear to result from local action of the toxin on the gastrointestinal tract as well as systemic effects following absorption, but the biochemical action of cantharidin is unknown.

Erosion and ulceration of the mucosa of the distal esophagus and esophageal part of the stomach are frequent, which results from separation of epithelial cells and their necrosis. There is little inflammatory reaction at these sites, but the glandular stomach, small intestine and colon are hyperemic and edematous. The contents are watery. Mild toxic tubular nephritis is evident, but rarely is there extensive necrosis. Grossly, the urinary bladder is hyperemic and contains petechiae or larger hemorrhages. Microscopically, focal necrosis of transitional epithelium, erosion, and ulceration are evident. Discrete gray-red or pale yellow patches of necrosis up to 5 cm in greatest dimension in the ventricular myocardium are visible on the epicardial, endocardial, and cut surfaces. Histologically, the muscle fibers are swollen, have increased eosinophilia, and lose their striations. The lungs are hyperemic and edematous, and there is centrilobular congestion of the liver. These lesions apparently result from myocardial failure.

None of these lesions is pathognomonic,

but this combination of findings should suggest blister beetle poisoning, and the beetles should be sought in hay.

Schoeb, T.R., and Panciera, R.J.: Blister beetle poisoning in horses. J. Am. Vet. Med. Assoc., 173:75–77, 1978.
———: Pathology of blister beetle (*Epicauta*) poisoning in horses. Vet. Pathol., 16:18–31, 1979.

GROUP C: HEPATOTOXICITY; OFTEN NEPHROTOXICITY

Poisons in Group C are primarily **hepatotoxic**, resulting in fatty change, necrosis, and acute or chronic hepatitis. Many hepatotoxins are also nephrotoxic and clinical signs may reflect damage to both organ systems. Signs of central nervous system derangement such as depression, hyperirritability, and convulsions, in the absence of morphologic changes in the brain, are frequent.

Phosphorus

Owing to changes in manufacturing methods and popular customs, the traditional poisoning by phosphorus matches has all but disappeared, and that due to the accidental ingestion of fireworks is not far behind. Animals (dogs, pigs) are poisoned most often by eating preparations intended for the consumption of rats, ants, or other pests. Phosphorus poisoning has also occurred in herbivorous animals pastured on former battlefields where certain weapons have been used.

While a peracute poisoning marked by coma, convulsions, and fatal central nervous depression has been described, the usual case is characterized by abdominal signs, which appear some hours after ingestion of the fatal potion. Nausea, vomiting, and abdominal pain then appear, and are succeeded by fever, polydipsia, and polyuria. The appearance of jaundice is followed by delirium, convulsion, and coma, the whole illness lasting usually from two to five days.

At autopsy, there may be mild inflammation of parts of the gastrointestinal tract, but the principal lesions consist of degenerative changes in the liver and kidneys. Icterus is prominent and is said to be due in many cases to obstructive swelling of the bile duct. However, the outstanding lesion is fatty change, for which phosphorus poisoning is one of the classic causes through interference with protein synthesis. In the liver, the majority of the cells are filled with fat droplets, centrilobular necrosis supervening if the patient lives for a while. Fatty change of the kidney and heart is pronounced, and smaller amounts of fat can be demonstrated in other tissues. In the kidney of a dog, at least, most of the fat appears in the epithelium of the ascending loops of Henle in the medullary rays. The distal convoluted tubules contain the second largest amount of fat; other structures of the kidney may have slight amounts. The accumulation of lipids is due to interference with lipoprotein synthesis and excretion. Hydropic degeneration is marked in the proximal convoluted tubules. The spleen is regularly small and atrophic. Hydrothorax and more or less generalized edema occur in some cases, doubtless because of gradual failure of the degenerating heart muscle. One of us has seen severe hemorrhagic enteritis, cholecystitis, and urinary cystitis in an experimental dog. Ecchymotic hemorrhages sometimes occur in the heart and elsewhere.

A chronic form of phosphorus poisoning occurs in humans, characterized by a necrotizing purulent osteomyelitis of the mandible and maxilla, with multiple draining sinuses and deformity. This usually results from inhalation of phosphorus-containing fumes in industrial plants, to which animals are unlikely to be exposed.

Phosphates

Cattle are poisoned rarely by eating commerical fertilizers, which are usually mixtures of phosphates, nitrates, potassium, and ammonium. It appears, however, that these poisonings are chiefly attributable to nitrates or potassium rather than phosphates. Ammonium nitrate is surprisingly harmless; nitrates are considered on page 965 and potassium on page 1061. Chickens and other birds have been poisoned by zinc phosphate, which is used as a treatment for seed-wheat. Characteristic features were dullness, anorexia, thirst, and terminal nervous effects, ending fatally a few hours after ingestion. A garlic-like odor of $Zn_3(PO_4)_2$ was noted in the contents of the crop. (See also organic phosphates, Group Q.)

Adutskevich, V.A., and Zaitseva, A.G.: Phosphorus poisoning in animals and birds. Veterinariya (Moscow), 8 and 9:40–43, 1944. Abstr. Vet. Bull. No. 1653, 1948.
Bubien, Z., and Miedzobrodzki, K.: Zinc phosphate poisoning in birds. Méd. Vét., Varsovie, 13:422–425, 1957. Abstr. Vet. Bull. No. 887, 1958.
Smith, H.A.: Renal lipidosis. Thesis, University of Michigan, Ann Arbor, 1949. (Three phosphorus experiments.)
Swan, J.B., and McIntosh, I.G.: Toxicity of North African phosphate and superphosphate to milking cows. Proc. NZ Soc. Anim. Prod., 12:83–88, 1952.

Copper

While ingestion or cutaneous absorption of adequate amounts of copper salts is able to produce acute gastroenteric poisoning with greenish tinged, fluid feces, the usual poisoning in domestic animals is a chronic disorder that terminates precipitously in acute symptoms when copper stored in the liver reaches a critical level. Herbivorous animals, especially sheep, become poisoned by eating herbage growing on soils too rich in copper. Included are soils naturally so afflicted and those of old orchards that have been contaminated by heavy spraying (e.g., Bordeaux mixture). Poisoning has occurred where copper sulfate has been used in wet pastures to control snails, which are one of the hosts for liver flukes. Contamination of pastures from mines and smelters has also been responsible. Most often, poisoning has resulted from the misapplication of copper medication, especially when copper sulfate is mixed with the animals' salt for anthel-

mintic purposes, or when solutions used in treating "foot-rot" are ingested. Vaginal bougies containing copper sulfate have also been incriminated. Miller and Nelson (1978) have described copper poisoning in sheep grazing on pastures fertilized with chicken litter from birds whose ration was supplemented with copper oxide and copper sulfate.

Molybdenum deficiency increases copper retention and thereby susceptibility to copper poisoning. Conversely, molybdenum exerts a protective action against excessive copper. Hepatic damage from other causes, such as by pyrrolizidine alkaloids, increases susceptibility to copper poisoning.

Signs last 24 to 48 hours and include weakness and exhaustion (trembling), arching of the back (renal pain), icterus, and hemoglobinuria. The last two are so constant and pronounced that the disease was known as **icterohemoglobinuria** before its cause was discovered. At autopsy, the icterus proves to be both toxic and hemolytic. The liver is yellow and friable grossly, with centrilobular fatty change and necrosis and a possible increase of reticuloendothelial cells (acute toxic hepatitis). Terminally there is pronounced hemolytic anemia, with counts as low as 2,000,000/cmm, and erythrocytic changes characteristic of hemolytic destruction and myeloid regeneration (Allen and Harding, 1962). The kidneys show toxic degenerative changes (acute toxic nephrosis), plus blocking of the tubules by erythrocytes and hemoglobin. Severe hemorrhagic nephritis has been described. The spleen is markedly enlarged and crowded with whole or fragmented erythrocytes. Grossly, it is often a "blackberry-jam" spleen, resembling that of anthrax. Analysis of the liver shows a high content of copper, above 500 ppm. The amount of copper in the blood is also high when symptoms appear, for example, 250 ppm.

The abnormal accumulation of copper in the tissues and blood is a point of similarity with a disease of man known as **hepatolenticular** or **hepatocerebral degeneration** or **Wilson's disease.** This disease, inherited as an autosomal recessive trait, is characterized by a defect in excretion of copper and excessive deposition of copper in the liver, basal ganglia, cerebral cortex, kidney, and cornea. Lesions and functional changes are produced in each of these organs. Hepatic cirrhosis with nodular regeneration in the liver is accompanied by icterus and decreased liver function. Neurologic abnormalities appear to result from injury to the basal ganglia and cerebrum, where cavitation, increase in size and number of astrocytes, and decrease in neurons occur. Deposits of copper-bearing pigment in the renal tubular epithelium is often accompanied by glycosuria, aminoaciduria, phosphaturia, and uricosuria. A characteristic brown or gray-green precipitation at the limbus of the cornea is considered specific, and is called the **Kayser-Fleischer ring**.

In patients with Wilson's disease, the normal hepatic copper-binding protein (copperthionein) has a much greater affinity for copper than normal. Levels of serum copper and ceruloplasmin are low, but the exact defect is not known. A disorder with some similarities to Wilson's disease occurs in a high percentage of Bedlington Terriers. Twedt et al. (1979) reported accumulations of toxic excesses of copper in the liver leading to focal hepatitis and cirrhosis in 68 of 90 Bedlington Terriers. In contrast to Wilson's disease, central nervous sytem dysfunction has not been described in these dogs.

Ultrastructural lesions that closely resemble the changes in human patients with Wilson's disease have been observed in hepatocytes of rats poisoned with copper (Barka et al., 1964). Electron-dense structures corresponding to copper-bearing lipofuscin pigment appear to be specific. Other changes were observed in mitochondria, endoplasmic reticulum, sinusoidal borders, and Golgi apparatus.

The pigment formation, changes in histochemical distribution of acid phosphatase, and mobilization of Kupffer cells are common features of Wilson's disease and experimental copper intoxication.

Lesions described as spongy transformation in myelinated tracts in the midbrain, pons, and cerebellum of sheep poisoned by long-term feeding of a diet containing 80 ppm of copper have been described by Doherty et al. (1969) and others. This is of interest in comparison with hepatolenticular degeneration of man.

Allen, M.M., and Harding, J.D.J.: Experimental copper poisoning in pigs. Vet. Rec., 74:173–179, 216, 248, 277, 304, and 306, 1962.

Barka, T., Scheuer, P.J., Schaffner, F., and Popper, H.: Structural changes of liver cells in copper intoxication. Arch. Pathol., 78:331–349, 1964.

Boughton, I.B., and Hardy, W.T.: Chronic copper poisoning in sheep. Bull. 499. Division of Vet. Science, Texas Agric. Exper. Sta., 1934.

Cunningham, I.J.: The toxicity of copper to bovines. NZ J. Sci. Tech. (Sec. A), 27:372–376, 1946.

Cunningham, I.J., Hogan, K.G., and Lawson, B.M.: The effect of sulphate and molybdenum on copper metabolism in cattle. NZ J. Agric. Res., 2:145–152, 134–144, 1959.

Doherty, P.C., Barlow, R.M., and Angus, K.W.: Spongy changes in the brains of sheep poisoned by excess dietary copper. Res. Vet. Sci., 10:303–304, 1969.

Fincham, I.H.: Copper poisoning in sheep. Vet. Rec., 57:581, 1945.

Gopinath, C., and Howell, J. McC.: Experimental chronic copper toxicity in sheep. Changes that follow the cessation of dosing at the onset of haemolysis. Res. Vet. Sci., 19:35–43, 1975.

Miller, S., and Nelson, H.A.: Copper poisoning in sheep grazing pastures fertilized with chicken litter. J. Am. Vet. Med. Assoc., 173:1587–1589, 1978.

Muth, O.H.: Chronic copper poisoning in sheep. J. Am. Vet. Med. Assoc., 120:148–149, 1952.

Pierson, R.E., and Aanes, W.A.: Treatment of chronic copper poisoning in sheep. J. Am. Vet. Med. Assoc., 133:307–311, 1958. (Includes pathology, experimental.)

St. George-Grambauer, T.D., and Rac, R.: Hepatogenous chronic copper poisoning in sheep in South Australia due to consumption of *Echium plantagineum* L. Aust. Vet. J., 38:288–293, 1962.

Sutter, M.D., et al.: Chronic copper toxicosis in sheep. Am. J. Vet. Res., 19:890–892, 1958.

Todd, J.R., and Thompson, R.H.: Studies on chronic copper poisoning. III. Effects of copper acetate injected into the blood stream of sheep. J. Comp. Pathol., 74:542–551, 1964.

————: Studies on chronic coppper poisoning. IV. Biochemistry of the toxic syndrome in the calf. Br. Vet. J., *121*:90–97, 1965.

Twedt, D.C., Sternlief, I., and Gilbertson, S.R.: Clinical, morphologic, and chemical studies on copper toxicosis of Bedlington Terriers. J. Am. Vet. Med. Assoc., *175*:269–275, 1979.

Weiss, E., Baur, P., and Plank, P.: Chronic copper poisoning in calves. Vet. Med. Nachr., 35–51, 1967. No. 1. VB *38*:301, 1968.

Wolff, S.M.: Copper deposition in the rat. Arch. Pathol., *69*:217–223, 1960.

Tannic Acid

The astringent action of tannic acid interferes so much with absorption from the digestive mucosa that poisoning by this route is quite unlikely and is even difficult to produce experimentally. The same cannot be said when the substance is introduced into the animal body parenterally. The usual form of poisoning by tannic acid appeared contemporaneously with the use of this drug in the treatment of burns, and results from applying it over too large an area, whence it is extensively absorbed. There is one outstanding lesion, namely, acute toxic hepatitis with centrilobular necrosis. Several days are usually required to produce death, during which there are symptoms of depression, inappetence, and other signs traceable to hepatic impairment. Liver function tests usually show decreased hepatic function. There are also experimental indications that tannic acid leads to "increased permeability of capillaries" and loss of fluid from the blood. This contributes to the anhydremia and shock that are often serious complications developing approximately three days after severe burns. However, this syndrome is not infrequent in burns without treatment with tannic acid; toxic hepatitis is not usual from the burn alone.

Barnes, J.M., and Rossiter, R.J.: Toxicity of tannic acid. Lancet, *245*:218–222, 1943.

Cameron, G.R., Milton, R.F., and Allen, J.W.: Toxicity of tannic acid, an experimental investigation. Lancet, *245*:179–186, 1943.

Clark, E.J., and Rossiter, R.J.: Liver function in rabbits after injection of tannic acid. Lancet, *245*:222–223, 1943.

Handler, P., and Baker, R.D.: Toxicity of orally administered tannic acid. Science, *99*:393, 1944.

Carbon Tetrachloride and Tetrachloroethylene

Human beings become poisoned by carbon tetrachloride through inhalation of its vapor, as in the clothes-cleaning industry. In animals, poisoning is not altogether infrequent as the result of the use of this substance as an anthelmintic. Such poisoning is ordinarily acute. Symptoms include loss of appetite, gastrointestinal pain, diarrhea (after a few hours), and blood-stained feces. Icterus is often but not always present. Collapse and death come in about 24 hours.

Lesions are acute catarrhal or hemorrhagic gastritis and enteritis, and acute toxic changes in the liver and kidneys. The hepatic changes are those usually found in acute toxic hepatitis, namely hydropic degeneration, fatty change, and necrosis with cellular infiltrations, if the animal lives long enough. Often there is little but necrosis at the time of death. The necrosis tends to be central, but often becomes massive, involving whole groups of lobules in their entirety. In the kidney, the changes are often less pronounced, but consist principally of fatty change and necrosis of the epithelium of the tubules. Nevertheless, in some cases, death must be attributed to renal failure. Petechiae, said to be due to thrombocytopenia, may be present in various organs and tissues. In chronic cases, which are unusual, the acute toxic hepatitis becomes chronic toxic hepatitis; in other words, cirrhosis.

The endoplasmic reticulum is the primary site of injury. Carbon tetrachloride is believed to be converted by microsomal enzymes to a highly potent product with strong peroxidant effects. Toxicity is enhanced by conditions promoting proliferation of endoplasmic reticulum and increased activity of microsomal enzymes. These include high-protein diets and such drugs as phenobarbital; thus, animals on a good plane of nutrition are more susceptible. Decreased protein synthesis by hepatocytes is one of the earliest manifestations of carbon tetrachloride poisoning, and accounts for the early and extensive fatty change by preventing lipoprotein formation. The hepatic necrosis is not related to decreased protein synthesis, but rather to peroxidation of membrane lipids. Antioxidants protect against these effects.

Tetrachloroethylene is considerably less toxic than carbon tetrachloride, hence more desirable as an anthelmintic, but the two have similar actions. Gallagher and Simmonds (1959) found a preventive effect in nicotinic acid or tryptophane. These substances are precursors of the respiratory cofactors, pyridine nucleotides.

Poisonings have been reported in several rather unique situations. One of the most interesting is the high sensitivity of male mice of certain inbred strains. A minute amount of carbon tetrachloride, released into an animal room, may cause the death of many adult male mice (Meshorer and Benhar, 1966). Male mice of the inbred strains Balb/c, A/He, C_3H, and Swiss are susceptible in that order. Inbred strains C58, DBA/2, SJL, AKR, and RF are apparently quite as resistant as all females and young. This sensitivity in mice is similar to that observed with chloroform.

Robinson and Harper (1967) exposed dogs, monkeys, rats and mice to carbon tetrachloride vapor under varying simulated altitudes, and concluded that the higher altitudes (with 100% oxygen) had an additive effect upon the toxicity of carbon tetrachloride on these species.

Chandler, A.C., and Chopra, R.N.: The toxicity of carbon tetrachloride for cats. North Am. Vet., 7:49, 1926.

Fairfax, R.E.: Carbon Tetrachloride Poisoning of Sheep. New South Wales, Yearb. Inst. Insp. Lystk, 1948, p. 73.

Gallagher, C.H., and Simmonds, R.A.: Prophylaxis of poisoning by carbon tetrachloride. Nature. Lond., *184*, Suppl. No. *18*:1707–1708, 1959.

Harper, D.T., Jr., and Robinson, F.R.: Comparative pathology of animals exposed to carbon tetrachloride in oxygen at 258mm. Hg and in ambient air. Aerospace Med., *38*:784–788, 1967.

Harris, F.H.: Acute carbon tetrachloride poisoning. U.S. Armed Forces Med. J., *3*:1023–1028, 1952.

Hase, T.: Development of portahepatic venous shunts and cirrhosis in carbon tetrachloride poisoning in rats. Am. J. Pathol., *53*:83–98, 1968.

Kondos, A.C., and McClymont, G.L.: Enchanced toxicity of carbon tetrachloride in sheep on high protein intakes. Aust. Vet. J., *41*:349–351, 1965.

Levine, S.: A case of tetrachlorethylene poisoning in an English Setter. Vet. Med., *33*:171–172, 1938.

Meshorer, A., and Benhar, E.: Accidental poisoning of inbred male mice by carbon tetrachloride. Lab. Anim. Care, *16*:198–201, 1966.

Muth, O.H.: Carbon tetrachloride poisoning of ewes on a low selenium ration. Am. J. Vet. Res., *21*:86–87, 1960.

Setchell, B.P.: Poisoning of sheep with anthelmintic doses of carbon tetrachloride. Chemical pathology. Aust. Vet. J., *38*:580–582, 1962.

Woods, W.W.: The changes in the kidneys in carbon tetrachloride poisoning, and their resemblance to the "crush syndrome." J. Pathol. Bact., *58*:767–777, 1946.

Phenothiazine

This important anthelmintic drug produces highly variable toxic effects, principally in horses. There appears to be two important factors that determine whether poisoning will result from a dose of given size. The first and most crucial is the diet and nutritional state of the patient. As is the case with many hepatotoxic drugs, a well-nourished animal on a high-protein diet with ample stores of glycogen in the liver is much less apt to suffer ill effects than an animal in the opposite condition. The second factor is the degree of refinement of the phenothiazine and the presence or absence of diphenylamine, which is a contaminant of the crude drug. Poisoned animals show more or less severe anemia, which reaches its height a few days after the drug is ingested. This is an hemolytic anemia, and it is occasionally rapid enough to cause hemoglobinuria. There are also acute toxic hepatitis and nephrosis of varying degrees of severity. The hepatic injury is of such a nature that photosensitization occasionally arises. Symptoms include depression, dullness, weakness, and coma, in addition to the derangements directly traceable to the pathologic changes. Many animals recover from the depressive symptoms after some hours, and from the anemia and hepato-renal symptoms after several days.

Phenothiazine is also a cause of primary photosensitizational dermatitis, which is described in Chapter 3.

Baird, J.D., Hutchins, D.R., and Lepherd, E.E.: Phenothiazine poisoning in a Thoroughbred horse. Aust. Vet. J., 46:496–499, 1970.

Biswal, G., and Patnaik, B.: Photosensitized keratitis in calves and kids following administration of phenothiazine. Indian Vet. J., 38:400–403, 1961.

Bolton, J.: A case of phenothiazine poisoning in young bovines. Vet. Rec., 60:479, 1948.

Britton, J.W.: Phenothiazine poisoning in pigs. Cornell Vet., 33:368–369, 1943.

Carter, C.D., et al.: Tetrachlorodibenzodioxin: an accidental poisoning episode in horse arenas. Science, 188:738–740, 1975.

Chopra, P., Roy, S., Ramalingaswami, V., and Nayak, N.C.: Mechanism of carbon tetrachloride hepatotoxicity: an in vivo study of its molecular basis in rats and monkeys. Lab. Invest., 26:716–727, 1972.

Eichelberger, L., and Roma, M.: Phenothiazine poisoning in a farm dog. Vet. Med., 42:302–303, 1947.

Hebden, S.P., and Setchell, B.P.: Phenothiazine toxicosis. Aust. Vet. J., 38:399, 1962.

Jha, G.J., and Iyer, P.K.R.: Pathology of phenothiazine intoxication in cattle—clinical pathology. Indian Vet. J., 44:457–466, 1967.

————: Pathology of phenothiazine intoxication in cattle and sheep—changes in endocrine organs. Indian J. Vet. Sci., 37:165–171, 1967.

McSherry, B.J., Roe, C.K., and Milne, F.J.: The hematology of phenothiazine poisoning in horses. Can. Vet. J., 7:3–12, 1966.

Mitrovic, M.: Due casi di avvelenamento ad esito letale in cavalli trattati con dosi terapeutiche di fecondita. Zootec. Vet., Milan, 3:157–160, 1948. (English summary.)

Reynolds, E.S., and Ree, H.J.: Liver parenchymal cell injury. VII. Membrane denaturation following carbon tetrachloride. Lab. Invest., 25:269–278, 1971.

Westermarck, H.: Toxicity of phenothiazine for horses. Suom. Eläinlääkäril., 54:43–72, 1948. (English summary.)

Woolf, F.P., and Simms, B.T.: Studies of the toxicology of phenothiazine in horses and mules. North Am. Vet., 24:595–599, 1943.

Phenanthridinium and other Trypanocidal Drugs

Certain compounds of phenanthridinium, especially 2:7-diamino-9-phenyl-10 methyl phenanthridinium bromide, commonly called dimidium bromide, and ethidium bromide, which is identical except that it has an ethyl group instead of the methyl radical, are currently used parenterally to free animals of trypanosomal infections. Quinapyramine sulfate and chloride, usually in a mixture bearing the common name of antrycide, have the same therapeutic use. Of these, dimidium bromide is toxic and poisoning may occur when the amount administered is too great or too frequently repeated. The effects of a single or repeated dose are commonly delayed for five to seven weeks, during which the animal, usually a bovine, loses weight severely. The van den Bergh reaction and other tests show impaired hepatic function. The principal lesion is an acute toxic hepatitis, beginning with hydropic or vacuolar degeneration of the hepatic cells at the periphery of the lobule. This is followed by fatty change, which spreads toward the center of the lobule. Photosensitization follows in some individuals, especially if the dose is later repeated. In the case of antrycide, toxic tubular nephritis is more severe than the hepatitis and is accompanied by anemia. Many animals recover from the toxicity of either drug.

Burdin, M.L., and Plowright, W.: Toxic effects of four trypanocidal substances for East African type of zebu cattle. Vet. Rec., 64:635–639, 1952.

Gretillat, E.H.: Observations sur les accidents toxiques survenus a la suite du traitement de la trypanosomiase bovine par le bromure de dimidium dans quelques troupeaux du Kwango. Bull. Agric. Congo belge., 44:787–812, 1953.

Plowright, W., Burdin, M.L., and Thorold, P.W.: Delayed toxicity due to dimidium bromide. J. Comp. Pathol. Ther., 62:136–140, 178–195, 1952.

"Clay-Pigeon" Poisoning—Coal-Tar Pitch

It has happened more than once that a club of trap-shooters has rented a small piece of ground for their shooting contests and then turned it back to the farmer. The "clay pigeons" that are used as targets to be shattered in the air by the marksman are constructed of an amalgam held together by a kind of pitch derived from coal tar, a heterogeneous and variable mixture in which a number of poisonous chemical compounds have been identified. The fragments remain in the soil and are tasty to pigs, which may be pastured on the contaminated ground. At least a few days are required for illness to develop, depending on the amount of the material consumed. There are usually only a few hours of nonspecific symptoms.

The principal postmortem lesion consists of severe centrilobular necrosis of the liver with blood replacing the lost cells and filling the center of the lobule. The supporting reticular tissue of the lobule appears to remain intact. Since involvement of the liver tends to be patchy, the organ is grossly spotted with reddish and yellowish areas. There may be a limited fibrinous or adhesive perihepatitis. Other lesions include a well-marked anemia, with erythrocyte counts and hemoglobin often approximating half the normal, jaundice, edema of lymph nodes, and ascites. Blood glucose is also reduced prior to death, and thymol turbidity, serum chloride, and phosphorus are increased, according to Davis and Libke (1968). White cell counts, sedimentation rate, serum protein, calcium and creatinine are not changed.

Davis, J.W., and Libke, K.G.: Hematologic studies in pigs fed clay pigeon targets. J. Am. Vet. Med. Assoc., *152*:382–384, 1968.
Graham, R., Hester, H.R., and Henderson, J.A.: Coal-tar pitch poisoning in pigs. J. Am. Vet. Med. Assoc., *96*:135–140, 1940.
Giffee, J.W.: Clay pigeon poisoning in swine. Vet. Med., *40*:97, 1945.
Rummler, H.J.: Pigsty flooring materials containing tar and bitumen. Mh. Vet. Med., *17*:482–487, 1962.

Hydrogen Sulfide

Animals have been poisoned by the inhalation of H_2S in the atmosphere of stables so constructed that the gases from manure pits could enter them. (In some cold countries, the excreta are collected and stored in underground pits, where decomposition processes reduce it to a semi-liquid mass, useful as fertilizer.) A concentration of as much as 0.03% H_2S in the air is dangerous. While harmless in medicinal amounts, the accidental feeding of a large quantity of sulfur has resulted in a similar type of poisoning, H_2S being formed as a decomposition product.

Signs, which may last for a few hours, are dyspnea, cyanosis, mucous exudate from the upper respiratory passages, depression, and apathy, or in some species, convulsions. Lesions include severe pulmonary edema, hyperemia, and catarrhal inflammation of the air passages, acute toxic hepatitis and nephrosis, and subendocardial and other hemorrhages. The tissues of the gastrointestinal tract are edematous but not congested. There is also edema of the brain. The blood is dark brown due to formation of sulfhemoglobin.

Blaser, E.: Ein Beitrag zur Kenntnis der Schwefelwasserstoffvergiftung beim Tier durch Jauchegase. Schweiz. Arch. f. Tierheilk, *88*:401–413, 433–446, 1946.
Coghlin, C.L.: Hydrogen sulphide poisoning in cattle. Can. J. Comp. Med., *8*:111–113, 1944.
Dougherty, R.W., Wong, R., and Christensen, B.E.: Studies on hydrogen-sulfide poisoning. Am. J. Vet. Res., *4*:254–256, 1943.
O'Donoghue, J.G.: Hydrogen sulphide poisoning in swine. Can. J. Comp. Med., *25*:217–219, 1961.
Skrypnik, E.I.: (Poisoning of cattle by water containing H_2S, chlorine, and chlorides.) Veterinarii, Moscow, *10*:42–44, 1945. (In Russian).

Gossypol

A byproduct of the cotton industry, cottonseed meal is a valuable protein concentrate for cattle and other farm animals. A small amount of a poisonous substance, gossypol, remains in the meal which is made from the seeds after cottonseed oil has been extracted from them. The processor endeavors to keep the gossypol at a level approximating 0.02 to 0.04%, but owing to variations in temperature with the hydraulic-press process and to undesirable solvents in other processes, this amount may be greatly exceeded.

Swine are much more susceptible to poisoning than other species, and it is usually recommended that cottonseed meal not exceed 9% of the total ration of these animals. Signs commonly develop after pigs have been fed from one to three months on rations containing excessive amounts of gossypol. They consist principally of dyspnea, panting, weakness, and anorexia, and last commonly for several, rarely for many, days before death occurs.

The lesions account readily for the signs. Most conspicuous are hydrothorax, hydropericardium, hydroperitoneum, and edema of the lungs, many or all lymph nodes, and often the subcutaneous tissues. Edema of the wall and attachments of the gallbladder is conspicuous in half the cases. Passive congestion is prominent in the lungs, liver, and kidneys. All this is readily explained as cardiac edema and congestive heart failure when the heart is examined. Dilatation of the ventricles is readily demonstrable in nearly all cases, with well-marked hypertrophy in the more prolonged ones. "White muscles," a definite paleness of various skeletal muscles, exist in two-thirds of the affected individuals. Icterus is noticeable in a minority of cases. The livers are most often redder than normally, because of the congestion, but some, containing less blood, show the paleness indicative of necrosis and other changes. In either case, the lobular architecture is more distinct even than that which is normal for the pig, so that the experienced prosector has little doubt grossly of the existence of some form of toxic hepatitis.

Microscopic changes are in accord with

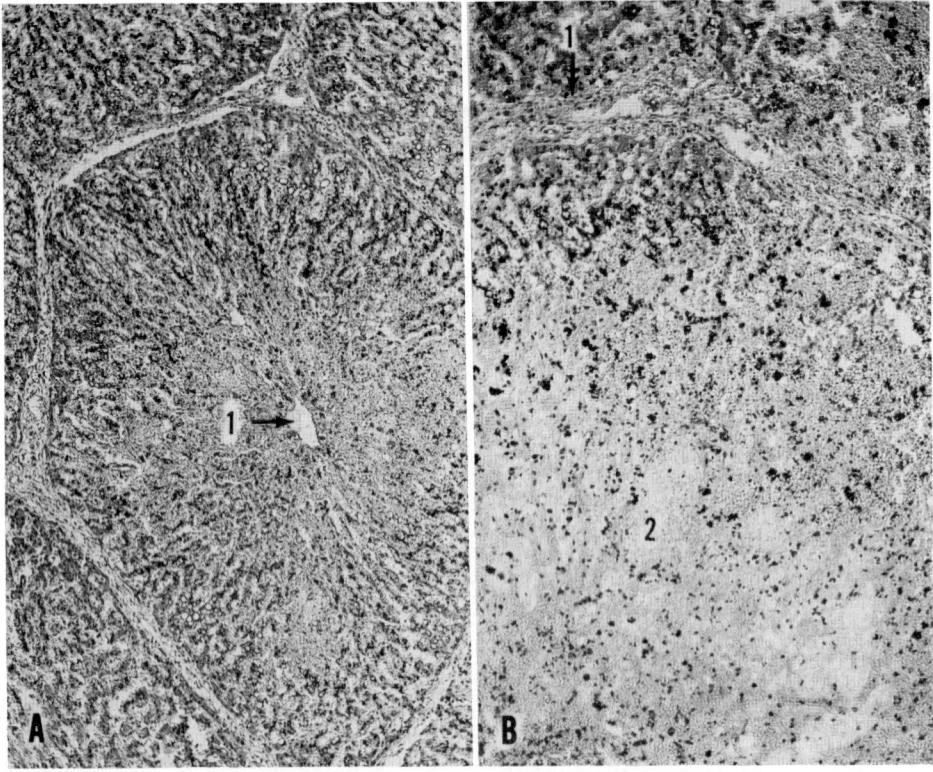

Fig. 16–3. Liver of a pig poisoned by gossypol. *A,* Necrosis of hepatic cells around central vein (*1*) (× 60). *B,* Same liver (× 100). Portal area (*1*) is relatively unaffected, but necrosis and hemorrhage are extensive in the center of the lobule (*2*).

what is seen grossly, those in the liver and heart requiring especial mention. The fundamental hepatic lesion is centrilobular necrosis. The space left by the lost parenchymal cells is filled with blood, the scanty reticulum of Kupffer cells remaining, at least for a time. In 80% of the livers, the necrosis in practically all lobules is so extensive that hepatic cells remain in only a narrow peripheral zone, perhaps only three or four cells wide, the rest of the lobule being filled with blood. This condition is obviously responsible for the red color of these livers grossly. In a minority of livers, a limited zone of cells in a state of fatty degeneration exists between the peripheral living zone and the blood-filled central area. Whether the centrilobular necrosis should be attributed to direct toxic injury by the gossypol or to anoxia resulting from cardiac insufficiency is difficult to determine. Both conditions are present, but the extent of necrosis is greater than that which usually results from cardiac disease alone. Microscopic examination of the heart reveals necrosis or degeneration of numerous myocardial fibers; some are without the normal number of nuclei; in some there are large and poorly outlined vacuoles in the cytoplasmic areas; some are greatly atrophied. Except in the hearts of pigs that die early, fibers showing compensatory hypertrophy mingle with those that have degenerated. The hypertrophy is evidenced by a limited increase in the size of the fiber, but more especially by a marked increase in both the size and the number of nuclei in the hypertrophic fiber.

Diagnosis can be made with considerable assurance on the basis of the combination of cardiac changes, the marked edema, and the hepatic changes, the clinical history being important if available. (It is usually inconclusive as to the amount of gossypol consumed.) Poisoning by coal-tar pitch occurs in swine and produces comparable hepatic changes, but there is no cardiac injury. In hepatosis diaetetica, the hepatic necrosis is not uniform.

Dinwiddie, R.R., and Short, A.K.: Cottonseed poisoning of livestock. Exp. Sta. Bull. 108, Univ. Arkansas, Fayetteville, 1911, pp. 395–410.

Hove, E.L., and Seibold, H.R.: Liver necrosis and altered fat composition in vitamin E-deficient swine. J. Nutr., 56:173–186, 1955.

Lambert, R.A., and Allison, B.R.: Types of lesion in chronic passive congestion of the liver. Bull. Johns Hopkins Hosp., 27:350–356, 1916.

Obel, A.L.: Studies on the morphology and etiology of so-called toxic liver dystrophy (hepatosis diaetetica) in swine. Acta Path. Microbiol. Scand., Suppl., 94:1–87, 1953.

Rogers, P.A.M., Henaghan, T.P., and Wheeler, B.: Gossypol poisoning in young calves. Irish Vet. J., 29:9–13, 1975.

Smith, H.A.: Pathology of gossypol poisoning. Am. J. Pathol., 33:353–365, 1957.

West, J.L.: Lesions of gossypol poisoning in the dog. J. Am. Vet. Med. Assoc., 96:74–76, 1940.

Withers, W.A., and Carruth, F.E.: Gossypol, the toxic substance in cottonseed meal. J. Agric. Res., 5:261–288, 1916.

Cocklebur

Cockleburs (*Xanthium italicum et spp.*) are most poisonous, as well as more palatable, at or shortly after the two-leaf seedling stage. Pigs are more often poisoned than other species, but cattle and sheep have also suffered. Signs appear several hours after ingestion of the plants and are those of gastrointestinal pain and irritation and of cardiac and muscular weakness. There are also opisthotonos and convulsions. The failing heart, with weak and rapid pulse, is responsible for death after an illness of a few hours.

Lesions include subepicardial and other subserous hemorrhages, and a moderate degree of gastritis and enteritis, but toxic injury to the liver, kidneys, and heart is more important. The liver shows the usual changes of acute toxic hepatitis, with fatty change predominant in some individuals, necrosis in others. The necrosis is preceded by acute cellular swelling and narrowing of the hepatic cords; it is centrilobular at first, but may extend throughout all but the most peripheral parts of the lobule. Fatty change, of patchy distribution and demonstrable only by fat stains, is present in various parts of the myocardium. In the kidney, fat is prominent in the ascending loops of Henle, and incipient necrosis of

928

the proximal convoluted tubules is usually present. The lower tubules often contain albuminous casts. Changes in the central nervous system appear not to have been investigated.

Xanthium pungens, the Noogoora bur, causes a similar form of poisoning in Australia.

Forrest, G.P.: Cocklebur poisoning. J. Am. Vet. Med. Assoc., 93:42–43, 1938.
Kenny, G.C., Everist, S.L., and Sutherland, A.K.: Noogoora bur poisoning of cattle. Queensland Agric. J., 70:172–177, 1950.
Pribicevic, S., and Sevkovic, N.: Experimental study of poisoning by *Xanthium saccharatum* in pigs. Acta Vet. Belgrade, 4:58–64, 1954. Abstract from English summary, Vet. Bull. No. 3371, 1955.

Pyrrolizidine Alkaloids

The toxicity of several unrelated plants results from their content of pyrrolizidine alkaloids, which are esters of the amino-alcohols derived from the heterocyclic pyrrolizidine nucleus. These include plants of the genera *Senecio, Crotalaria, Amsinckia, Heliotropium, Echium,* and *Trichodesma.* Although there is variance in the alkaloids between the plants and in the conditions of poisoning of man and domestic animals, the lesions produced by these alkaloids are remarkably similar. They are all hepatotoxic, causing varying degrees of hepatocellular necrosis, megalocytosis, fibrosis, and bile ductule proliferation. Many of the alkaloids also cause occlusive lesions of veins, especially in the liver, leading to a syndrome referred to as Budd-Chiari syndrome in human beings, and in the lung leading to cor pulmonale or right heart failure. Megalocytosis of renal tubular epithelium and glomerulosclerosis resulting from endothelial damage are also frequent findings. Descriptions of major pyrrolizidine alkaloid poisonings of domestic animals follow.

Adam, S.E.I.: Hepatotoxic activity of plant poisons and mycotoxins in domestic animals. Vet. Bull., 44:767–776, 1974.
Jago, M.V.: The development of the hepatic megalocytosis of chronic pyrrolizidine alkaloid poisoning. Am. J. Pathol., 56:405–421, 1969.
McLean, E.K.: The toxic actions of pyrrolizidine (*Senecio*) alkaloids. Pharmacol. Rev., 22:429–483, 1970.

Senecios

Plants of the genus *Senecio* are of almost worldwide distribution. Characteristically, they are woody herbs with terminal clusters of yellow flowers, bushy, and commonly reaching a height between 20 to 50 cm. Like most poisonous plants, they are eaten only when more palatable pasturage is not available. Certain species are popularly known in many localities as ragworts or groundsels. In Europe, South Africa, New Zealand, or the plains region of the United States and Canada, at least the following species are known to be poisonous: *S. aquaticus, burchelli, ilicifolius, integerrimus, jacobaea, longilobus, plattensis, riddellii,* and *scleratus.* Chemically, it has been shown that pyrrolizidine alkaloids, retrorsine, and seneciophylline are responsible for the toxicity.

Poisoning involves horses and cattle chiefly, sheep being much less susceptible. In earlier times what is now known to be poisoning by senecios was described as several different diseases before their true nature was recognized. Of these, the principal ones were **Molteno disease** (Chase, 1904) of cattle in Cape Colony (Africa), **Winton disease** (Gilruth, 1905) of horses and cattle in New Zealand, **Pictou disease** (Pethick, 1906) of cattle in Canada and **Van Es' walking disease** (Van Es et al., 1929) of horses in Nebraska. **Zd'ar disease** of horses in Bohemia and probably **Schweinsberger disease** in Bavaria have also been added to this list (Vanek, 1958).

Signs appear after the animal has consumed varying amounts of the plant for a number of days or as long as three weeks. A disturbance of consciousness causes the animal to walk aimlessly but stubbornly, and to press the head continually against an object with which it collides. In the later stages of the illness, which usually lasts a few days, there may be mania. The

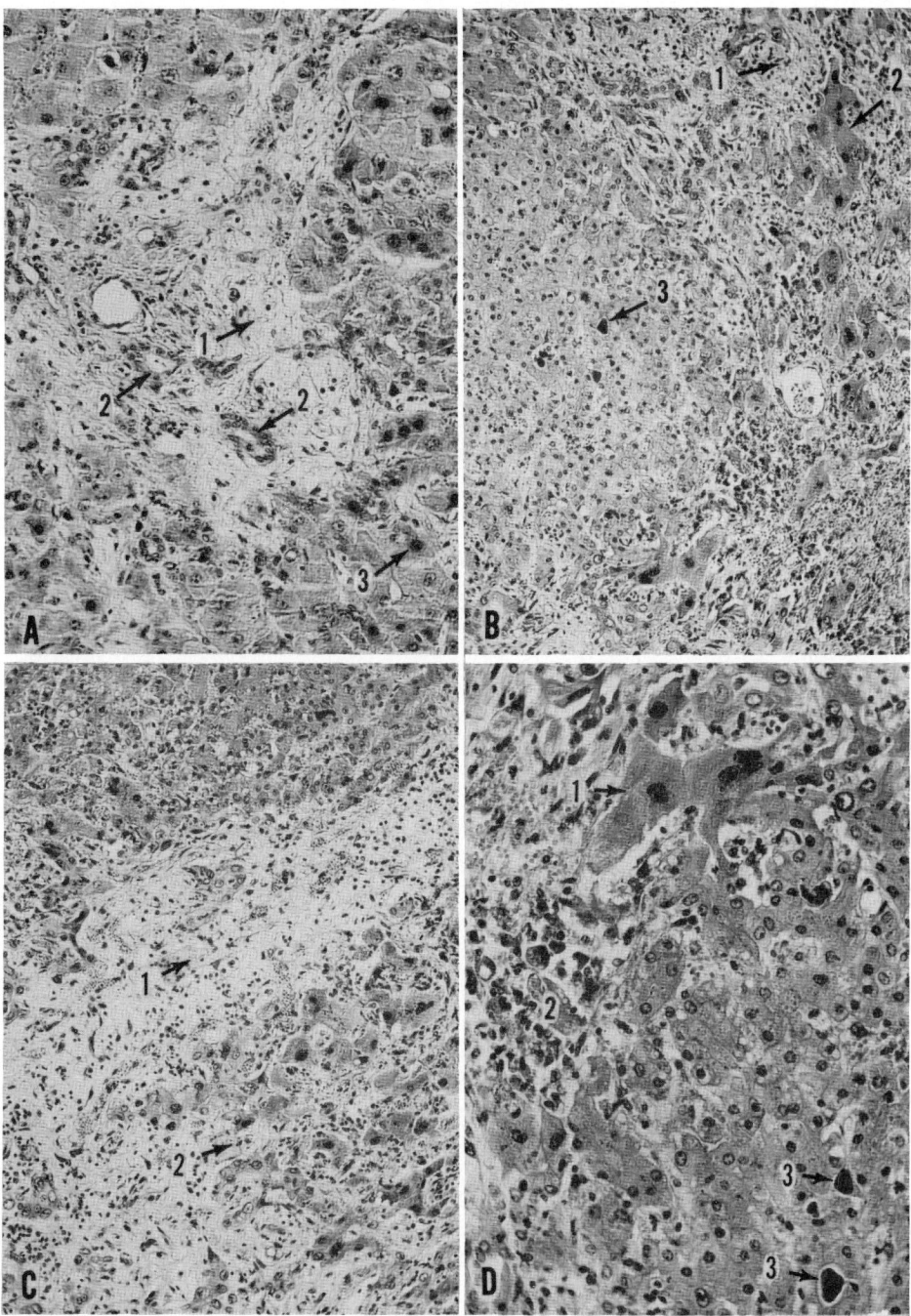

Fig. 16–4. *A,* Bovine liver (× 150) in Senecio poisoning. Periportal fibrosis (*1*), hyperplasia of bile ducts (*2*), and hyperchromatism in hepatic nuclei (*3*). (Photograph courtesy of Dr. C. L. Davis.) *B,* Equine liver in crotalaria poisoning (× 100). Periportal fibrosis (*1*), regenerating liver cells (*2*), and distended bile canaliculi (*3*). *C,* Another field, equine liver in *B* (× 100). Note portal fibrosis (*1*), which extends into the lobule (*2*). *D,* Equine liver (same as *B* and *C*) (× 210). Regenerating liver cells (*1*), leukocytes in portal region area (*2*), and distended bile canaliculi (*3*). (Courtesy of Dr. H. R. Seibold.)

semidomesticated cattle of the western ranges, especially, may become dangerously belligerent, with a behavior suggestive of rabies but without the terminal paralysis that characterizes the latter disease. In addition, there is jaundice and severe intestinal irritation, which results in frequent watery defecations with marked tenesmus and even eversion of the rectum.

Senecios can be classed among the stronger hepatotoxic poisons. Postmortem lesions are those of a chronic toxic hepatitis, with actively acute inflammation usually still in progress, and the jaundice and abdominal edema incident thereto. Hepatic changes vary from megalocytosis and necrosis of the hepatic cells to full-fledged portal cirrhosis, depending on the duration of the disease, its severity, and rapidity of its progress. The fibrous tissue tends to spread into the lobule in an irregular fashion, differing in this respect from the typical portal, or atrophic, cirrhosis. Proliferation of new bile ducts is prominent in many areas, perhaps somewhat more so than in the usual examples of portal cirrhosis. With the necrosis of the hepatic parenchymatous cells, there are frequently conspicuous attempts at regeneration. Such areas are recognized by the unusually large size of the cells and their nuclei and the relative frequency of cells with more than one nucleus. As a result of the architectural derangement, the bile canaliculi are occluded in various areas. Such areas show considerable deposits of bile pigment microscopically; grossly, there is the greenish-brown discoloration of icteric liver tissue. Since there is also considerable congestion in the less fibrotic areas, the typical liver shows a totally irregular mottling grossly, and is unduly hard in proportion to the amount of cirrhosis. The hepatic lymph nodes may be enlarged due to reticuloendothelial proliferation (Mathews, 1933). The lumens of hepatic veins, especially the central veins, become constricted as a result of reticulum and collagenous tissue proliferation,

edema, and endothelial hypertrophy. It is believed that endothelial cells become metaplastic and contribute to the reticulum and collagen fiber deposition. Passive congestion results from the cirrhosis and veno-occlusive disease.

The generalized toxic jaundice is usually of conspicuous severity and is stated by Mathews (1933) to be invariably present. The abdominal edema is widely diffused in the subserosa of the intestines and often of the stomach. The mesenteries are often markedly thickened with fluid. The gallbladder not only has a highly edematous wall, but also is distended with unused bile, sometimes to enormous proportions. The bile is stated to be of normal quality; hence, the condition is presumed to represent a combination of edema based upon intrahepatic obstruction and the usual accumulation of bile that occurs in the absence of cholecystikinetic stimuli from the intestine. There is commonly considerable edema in the mucosa and submucosa of the stomach and intestine. Since this is not proportional to the subserosal edema, and since a certain degree of catarrhal enteritis is demonstrable on the basis of hyperemia and other changes, the submucous fluid should doubtless be considered inflammatory. While the toxic action of the senecio plants mainly affects the liver, there is also a noticeable degree of toxic tubular nephrosis with megalocytosis, as seen in the liver. Petechiae and ecchymoses are rather prominent on the heart, mesentery, and omentum, and are doubtless attributable to toxic injury of capillaries.

Pulmonary lesions have been produced in experimental poisoning in rats. They are not well described in natural poisonings, but probably are a consistent finding. They are discussed in more detail under Crotalaria poisoning.

There appear to be no extensive studies of the brain that would determine whether the manic symptoms are based upon cerebral lesions or merely upon the tendency for nervous hyperirritability, which so frequently accompanies hepatic diseases. The violent behavior has been reported chiefly by Mathews and to those familiar with the untamed range cattle with which he worked; their belligerency is rather understandable merely as an expression of the bodily discomfort which they undoubtedly felt. Even these cattle, Mathews points out, commonly showed no bellicose symptoms when, during the course of experimental studies, they were fed the plants while confined in a small pen.

Hepatic tumors have been reported in experimentally poisoned rats.

Diagnosis must be based upon a combination of presence of the plant, symptoms, and lesions. There are no specific tests; neither are there many other equally hepatotoxic substances that are likely to be encountered under circumstances where senecio plants would be ingested.

Burns, J.: The heart and pulmonary arteries in rats fed on *Senecio jacobaea*. J. Pathol., 106:187–194, 1972.

Chase, W.H.: The Molteno cattle disease. Agric. J. of Cape of Good Hope, 25:675–678, 1904.

Crawford, M.: Mycotoxicosis in veterinary medicine. Vet. Bul., 32:415–420, 1962.

Dienzer, M.L., Thomson, P.A., Burgett, D.M., and Isaacson, D.L.: Pyrrolizidine alkaloids: Their occurrence in honey from tansy ragwort *(Senecio jacobaea L)*. Science, 195:497–499, 1977.

Evans, W.C.: Poisoning of farm animals by the marsh ragwort. Nature (Lond.), 164:30–31, 1949.

Gilruth, J.A.: Hepatic cirrhosis or Winton disease. Thirteenth Rept., Dept. of Agriculture, New Zealand, 1905, p. 178. (Cited by Mathews.)

Harding, J.D.J., et al.: Experimental poisoning by *Senecio jacobaea* in pigs. Pathol. Vet., 1:204–220, 1964.

Harris, P.N., and Chen, K.K.: Development of hepatic tumors in rats following ingestion of *Senecio longilobus*. Cancer Res., 30:2881–2886, 1970.

Mathews, F.P.: Poisoning of cattle by species of groundsel. Exp. Sta. Bull., 481, Texas A. & M. College, College Station, Texas, 1933.

Pethick, W.H.: Special report on Pictou cattle disease. Canadian Dept. Agriculture, No. 8, 1906. (Cited by Mathews.)

Selzer, G., and Parker, R.G.F.: Senecio poisoning exhibiting as Chiari's syndrome. Am. J. Pathol., 27:885–907, 1951.

Van der Watt, J.J., Purchase, I.F.H., and Tustin, R.C.: Chronic toxicity of retrorsine, a pyrrolizidine alkaloid, in vervet monkeys. J. Pathol., 107:279–287, 1972.

Vanek, J.: Poisoning with *Senecio erraticus* as the cause of Zd'ár disease of horses. Schweiz. Z. Allg. Pathol., 21:821–848, 1958. Abstr. Vet. Bull. No. 3724, 1959.

Van Es, L., Cantwell, L.R., Martin, H.M., and Kramer, J.: Nature and cause of the "walking disease" of northwestern Nebraska. Exp. Sta. Bull. No. 43, Univ. of Nebraska, Lincoln, 1929.

Crotalaria

The *Crotalaria* genus includes several leguminous plants which are used as soil-building cover crops or, in some cases, to provide hay or forage of rather questionable value. Some species are weeds in other parts of the world, particularly South Africa and Australia. *Crotalaria spectabilis* is probably the most poisonous species. With certain other, less toxic species, it is grown rather extensively in the southeastern United States. Human beings and all species of farm animals are susceptible, including chickens and turkeys.

In general, there are acute and chronic forms of poisoning. In the former, the period of illness is at most a few days, although the poison has usually been accumulating as the result of repeated ingestion over weeks or months. Symptoms are those of gastrointestinal disturbance accompanied by salivation, weakness, and relatively nonviolent nervous malfunction, such as staggering, incoordination, and ultimately inability to stand. Diarrhea with severe tenesmus and partial eversion of the rectum have been prominent in bovines. In the more chronic cases, the illness persists for a few weeks or several months, with anorexia, inactivity, and terminal emaciation. Horses may press against solid objects, the so-called "blind staggers." Icterus is noticeable in chronic cases, especially. Emphysema, pulmonary and later subcutaneous, is characteristic.

In North America, the outstanding postmortem lesion is hemorrhage, which appears in the form of petechiae or large ecchymoses. These hemorrhages, characterized by as yet unexplained bright red color, involve serous and mucous surfaces.

All organs are congested; many are edematous, especially the abomasum, omasum, and gallbladder. The severely congested liver in the acute case may progress to cirrhosis if the poisoning is prolonged. The lesions resemble those of *Senecio* poisoning. In the lungs, emphysema alternates with atelectasis and hemorrhages.

In South Africa, *Crotalaria dura* and *C. globifera*, both known as wild lucerne, cause chronic poisoning having many of the features just outlined, but also affect horses and sheep with repeated febrile episodes of pulmonary disease and eventually fatal termination. Early in the course of the disease, pulmonary emphysema, alveolar and interstitial, is the salient feature. Spreading from the lungs via the hilus, air appears in the mediastinal tissues and ultimately in the subcutaneous tissues of the neck. Terminally, the lungs undergo a chronic proliferative process involving all parts. The proliferated cells are largely epithelioid, probably originating from the alveolar walls. There are also gland-like proliferations of the bronchial epithelium resembling "jaagsiekte," and indeed, sometimes called by that name. Partial to complete occlusion of pulmonary capillaries and arterioles, apparently on the same basis as in veno-occlusive disease in the liver, may be seen in natural poisoning and has been reproduced in experimental animals. This leads to pulmonary hypertension and cardiac hypertrophy.

Also in South Africa, *Crotalaria burkeana*, the "rattle bush," causes bovine "stiff-sickness," in which the animal suffers at first from a generalized stiffness and then from laminitis in all four feet. The latter condition is prolonged, the hoofs become greatly elongated and horizontally wrinkled (compare with selenium poisoning, p. 952), and a layer of granulation tissue fills the space between the separated sensitive and insensitive laminae. Experimentally, the laminitis has appeared in as little as six days after feeding of the toxic plant. Its pathogenesis is probably related to an

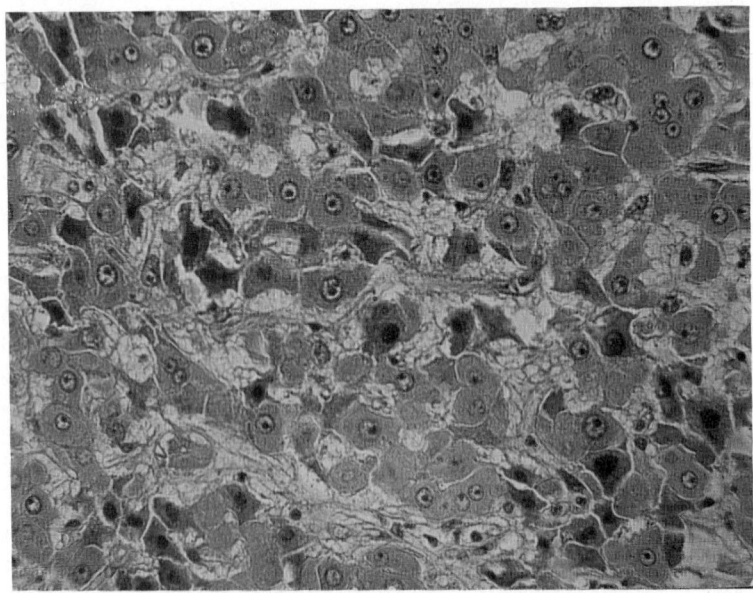

Fig. 16–5. Poisoning due to *Crotalaria spectabilis* seed. Liver of rhesus monkey (*Macaca mulatta*). Variation in cell size, staining of nuclei, and distortion of nuclei. (Courtesy of Dr. J. R. Allen and *American Journal of Veterinary Research*.)

inflammatory enteric disorder, as is believed to be true of laminitis under other circumstances.

In Northern Australia, *Crotalaria retusa* and *C. crispata* have been incriminated as the cause of "walkabout" or "Kimberly horse disease." This disease is characteristic of crotalaria poisoning, although cases due to *C. crispata* usually are more acute.

Swine poisoned by *Crotolaria spectabilis* develop typical hepatic lesions and extensive nephrosis characterized by glomerulosclerosis resulting from endothelial cell damage. Megalocytosis of tubular epithelium, as seen in many species, is also a feature.

In children, **infantile cirrhosis**, in which occlusion of intrahepatic veins is a significant feature, has been described in Jamaica, and is associated with ingestion of "bush-tea" made from *Crotalaria fulva* or other plants (Bras et al., 1957). The similarity of the lesions in fatal cases in children and in animals suggested the possibility of *Crotalaria* poisoning. Pulmonary lesions have not been reported in man. Simian primates (*Macaca mulatta*) are susceptible to acute poisoning (Allen et al., 1965), with lesions essentially similar to those observed in other species. *Crotalaria spectabilis* seeds, finely ground and added to the diet of *M. mulatta* at the level of 0.25 to 1%, result in ascites, hydrothorax, subcutaneous edema, leukopenia, decrease in serum albumin, acute toxic hepatitis, pulmonary edema, and occasional leukocytic infiltration of the adventitia of pulmonary arteries.

In guinea pigs, a naturally-occurring disease due to contamination of feed with seeds of *Crotalaria* has been recognized and reproduced experimentally (Carlton, 1967). Seeds of *Crotalaria spectabilis* added to the guinea pig diet at the level of 5% resulted in disease typical of crotalaria poisoning.

Several active toxic agents which are capable of causing the lesions ascribed to the poisoning have been identified from *Crotalaria* plants. A pyrrolizidine alkaloid, **monocrotaline,** is present in most of the species examined (*C. retusa, C. spectabilis, C. mitchelli* and *C. crispata)* (Culvenor and Smith, 1963). Two other alkaloids, **fulvine** (originally isolated from *C. fulva*) and **cris-**

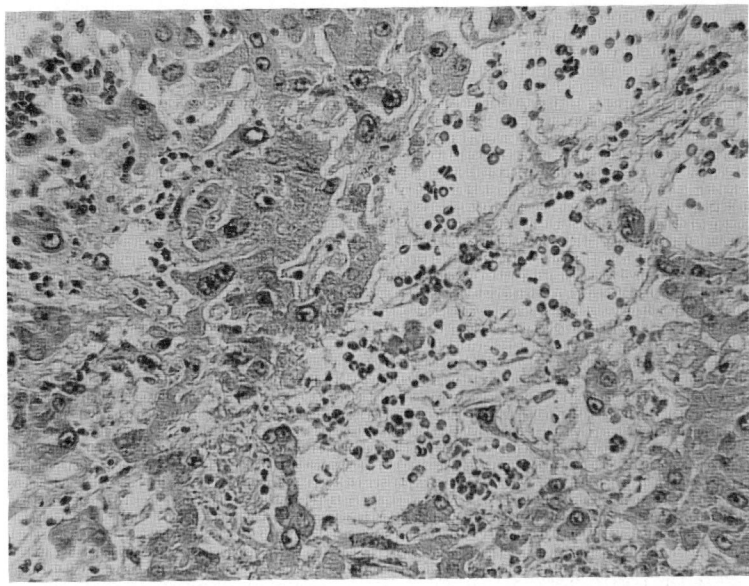

Fig. 16–6. Poisoning due to *Crotalaria spectabilis* seed. Liver of *Macaca mulatta*. Focal necrosis with loss of hepatocytes. (Courtesy of Dr. J. R. Allen and *American Journal of Veterinary Research*.)

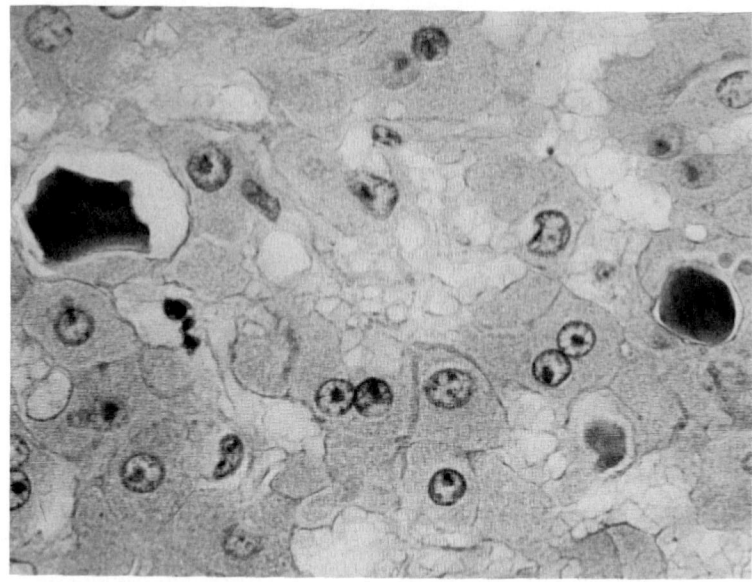

Fig. 16–7. Poisoning due to *Crotalaria spectabilis*. Liver of *Macaca mulatta*. Vacuoles in hepatocytes and bile stasis. (Courtesy of Dr. J. R. Allen and *American Journal of Veterinary Research*.)

patine *(C. crispata)*, have been isolated, identified as macrocyclic esters of retrorsine, which is also a toxic factor in plants of the genus *Senecio*.

Among the three alkaloids from *Crotalaria*, fulvine appears to be most toxic to rabbits; monocrotaline and crispatine, in order, are slightly less toxic. Each of these produces slightly different lesions when fed in pure form to rabbits (Gardiner et al., 1965). Monocrotaline poisoning in rabbits results in enlargement of most hepatic cells, with much variation in size and shape of nuclei. Abnormal mitotic figures are frequent in hepatocytes, and marginated or depleted chromatin is common. Proliferation of small cholangioles and bile ductules with portal fibrosis is also conspicuous. Frank necrosis is infrequent. The lungs are not affected.

Crispatine in rabbits produces lesions essentially similar to those caused by monocrotaline, but subcutaneous injection is often followed by tonic and clonic convulsions, lasting 15 to 20 minutes. Lesions of centrilobular fibrosis suggesting veno-occlusive disease are seen infrequently.

Fulvine administered subcutaneously to rabbits produces centrilobular necrosis and fibrosis of the liver. Hypertrophy of liver cells and proliferation of bile ducts are much less conspicuous. At the lower doses, changes in the lung with thickened fibrotic alveolar walls, proliferation and desquamation of alveolar phagocytes and fibroblasts are conspicuous features.

Widespread vascular lesions have been described in rats fed upon ground seeds of *Crotalaria spectabilis* for several months (Lalich and Merkow, 1961, Carstens and Allen, 1970). The ultrastructural features of the hyaline lesions in glomeruli and renal arteries have been reported to be the result of deposition of amorphous and fibrillar material structurally identical to basal lamina. This material obliterated lumens of glomerular capillaries and distorted endothelial and mesangial cells.

Allen, J.R., Carstens, L.A., and Knezevic, A.L.: *Crotalaria spectabilis* intoxication in rhesus monkeys. Am. J. Vet. Res., 26:753–757, 1965.
Allen, J.R., Childs, G.R., and Cravens, W.W.: *Crotalaria spectabilis* toxicity in chickens. Proc. Soc. Exp. Biol. Med., 104:434–436, 1960.

Allen, J.R., Lolich, J.J., and Schmittle, S.C.: *Crotalaria spectabilis* induced cirrhosis in turkeys. Lab. Invest., *12*:512–517, 1963.

Berry, D.M., and Bras, G.: Venous occlusion of the liver in crotalaria and senecio poisoning. North Am. Vet., *38*:323–326, 1957.

Bras, G., Berry, D.M., and György, P.: Plants as aetiological factor in veno-occlusive disease of the liver. Lancet, *1*:960–962, 1957.

Carlton, W.W.: Crotalaria intoxication in guinea pigs. J. Am. Vet. Med. Assoc., *151*:845–855, 1967.

Carstens, L.A., and Allen, J.R.: Arterial degeneration and glomerular hyalinization in the kidney of monocrotaline-intoxicated rats. Am. J. Pathol., *60*:75–91, 1970.

Chesney, C.F., and Allen, J.R.: Endocardial fibrosis associated with monocrotaline-induced pulmonary hypertension in non-human primates (*Macaca arctoides*). Am. J. Vet. Res., *34*:1577–1581, 1973.

Cox, D.H., et al.: Chemical identification of crotalaria poisoning in horses, J. Am. Vet. Med. Assoc., *133*:425–426, 1958.

Culvenor, C.C.J., and Smith, L.W.: Alkaloids of *Crotalaria crispata* F. Muell ex Benth. The structures of crispatine and fulvine. Aust. J. Chem., *16*:239–245, 1963.

Gardner, C.A.: The wedge-leaved rattlepod (*Crotalaria retusa*), a poison plant of tropical Australia. J. Dept. Agric. W. Aust., *1*:641–647, 1952.

Gardiner, M.R., Royce, R., and Bokor, A.: Studies on *Crotalaria crispata*, a newly recognized cause of Kimberly horse disease. J. Pathol. Bact., *89*:43–53, 1965.

Lalich, J.J., and Merkow, L.: Pulmonary arteritis produced in rats by feeding *Crotalaria spectabilis*. Lab. Invest., *10*:744–750, 1961.

Laws, L.: Toxicity of *Crotalaria mucronata* to sheep. Aust. Vet. J., *44*:453–455, 1968.

McGrath, J.P.M., Duncan, J.R., and Munnell, J.F.: *Crotalaria spectabilis* toxicity in swine: characterization of the renal glomerular lesion. J. Comp. Pathol., *85*:185–194, 1975.

Peckham, J.C., Sangster, L.T., and Jones, O.H., Jr.: *Crotalaria spectabilis* poisoning in swine. J. Am. Vet. Med. Assoc., *165*:633–638, 1974.

Piercy, P.L., and Rusoff, L.L.: *Crotalaria spectabilis* poisoning in Louisiana livestock. J. Am. Vet. Med. Assoc., *108*:69–73, 1946.

Sanders, D.A., Shealy, A.L., and Emmel, M.W.: Pathology of *Crotalaria spectabilis*: roth poisoning in cattle. J. Am. Vet. Med. Assoc., *89*:150–156, 1936.

Sippel, W.L.: Crotalaria poisoning in livestock and poultry. Ann. NY Acad. Sci., *111*:562–570, 1964.

Stalker, M.: Crotalism—a new disease among horses. Rept. Iowa Agric. College: Dept. Botany. 1884, pp. 114–115.

Thomas, E.F.: Toxicity of certain species of Crotalaria seed for the chicken, quail, turkey and dove. J. Am. Vet. Med. Assoc., *85*:617–622, 1934.

Heliotrope

The wild heliotrope (*Heliotropium europaeum*) is eaten by sheep and is poisonous by virtue of a slowly progressive toxic hepatitis, symptoms of illness appearing perhaps months after access to the plant has ceased. Jaundice is the salient feature. The usual fatty and other changes of acute toxic hepatitis progress to cirrhosis and a shrunken and "hob-nailed" liver. The effect of this plant is due to pyrrolizidine alkaloids (lasiocarpine, heliotrine), and is thus similar to that of the senecios and a number of other plants. It is especially important in Australia. Intestinal atrophy has been induced in sheep, rats, and mice injected with lasiocarpine or heliotrine.

Hooper, P.T.: Experimental acute gastrointestinal disease caused by the pyrrolizidine alkaloid, lasiocarpine. J. Comp. Pathol., *85*:341–349, 1975.

McKenna, C.T., and Orchard, H.E.: Heliotrope poisoning in sheep. J. Dept. Agric. S. Aust., *52*:436–437, 1949.

Tarweed

Tarweed, *Amsinckia intermedia*, is a weed that often seriously contaminates the wheat fields of the Pacific region of the United States and occasionally other areas. The rather small seeds are harvested with the crop and are separated from the wheat at the flour mill, going into the cull portion known as "screenings." The latter are commonly returned to the farm to be used as feed for animals, chiefly swine. After a few or many weeks on a diet containing considerable amounts of the seeds, icterus and other signs of toxic hepatitis appear. As evidence of alimentary irritation and disturbance, small ulcers often appear in the mouth. Mild ataxia and the central nervous disturbances characteristic of many hepatic disorders appear in the later stages. The behavior of horses is comparable to that seen in Van Es' walking disease, in other words, senecio poisoning. As in *Senecio*, the toxic principles are pyrrolizidine alkaloids. Swine often reach marketable age with no more conspicuous disturbance than general unthriftiness, and at slaughter are found to be victims of "hard-liver disease." As the reader has already surmised, the lesions are those of acute or chronic toxic hepatitis or, most often, of both together.

McCulloch, E.C.: Hepatic cirrhosis of horses, swine and cattle due to ingestion of seeds of the tarweed, *Amsinckia intermedia*. J. Am. Vet. Med. Assoc., 96:5–17, 1940.

———: Use of grain containing tarweed seed as poultry feed. J. Am. Vet. Med. Assoc., 101:481–483, 1942.

Woolsey, J.H., Jasper, D.E., Cordy, D.R., and Christensen, J.F.: Two outbreaks of hepatic cirrhosis in swine in California, with evidence incriminating tarweed. Vet. Med., 47:55–58, 1952.

Lantana

Lantana camara, a plant closely related to the common verbena of the flower-garden, and one or two other similar species have poisoned cattle in the southern United States, Australia, Mexico, and Africa. Certain other related species have little toxicity; all of them are unpalatable. The toxicity is principally manifest by hepatotoxic photosensitivity, icterus, and varying degrees of gastrointestinal irritation. The lips and muzzle are particularly affected by photosensitivity dermatitis. The mildest form of poisoning to be noticed is the "pink nose" of Australian cattle. In this condition, the hairless parts of the muzzle are merely inflamed and red. In many of the more severe cases, the visible lesions are almost exclusively those of photosensitization. The skin of the muzzle and surrounding regions becomes inflamed, thickened, and cracked, and tends to peel off, leaving severely inflamed ulcerated areas. The same condition affects the mouth, producing ulcerative stomatitis, with drooling of saliva and, of course, refusal to eat. There is mild dermatitis with itching over various other areas of the integument. Such cases recover after several weeks.

The most severe forms are acute, often being fatal after three or four days of illness. Clinically there are symptoms of gastrointestinal disturbances, with bloody feces, icterus, and marked weakness. At necropsy, the principal lesions are acute hemorrhagic gastroenteritis with blood clots and pseudomembranes in the gut. Icterus is marked. There are also subcutaneous edema and subepicardial hemorrhages. The usual changes of acute toxic hepatitis, varying from barely discernible to extensive necrosis, are seen in the liver. Photosensitization is present in those animals that live a few days. No doubt there is always some injury to hepatic cells, accounting for the photosensitization.

Seawright has studied the lesions in sheep (1964) and cattle (1972) produced by the ingestion of predetermined amounts of powdered leaves of *Lantana camara*. Icterus, photosensitization, swollen, ochre-colored livers, distended gallbladders, dry feces in the colon anterior to the ansa spiralis and excessive mucus in the remainder of the large intestine, ascites, and pulmonary edema were the principal findings at necropsy. Microscopic lesions in the liver in the less severely affected sheep were limited to vacuolization of hepatic cells in the portal region of the lobules, with proliferation of bile ductules. Hepatocytes in the center of the lobules were apparently unaffected. In severely affected sheep, necrosis involved most of the liver cells, with disorganization of lobular architecture, proliferation of bile ductules, and regeneration of liver cells. In the kidney, necrosis of proximal convoluted tubules was the essential feature, which resulted in proteinuria, bilirubinuria, and in some cases, uremia. Some necrosis of isolated cardiac muscle fibers suggested a possible direct effect of *Lantana* on the heart muscle.

Ultrastructural changes in hepatocytes from sheep poisoned with *Lantana camara* have also been described by Seawright (1965a). These changes usually start with distention of the bile canaliculi and proliferation of the villi into the canaliculi (Fig. 16–8). A space containing new microvilli forms between plasma membranes of adjacent hepatocytes at points where the

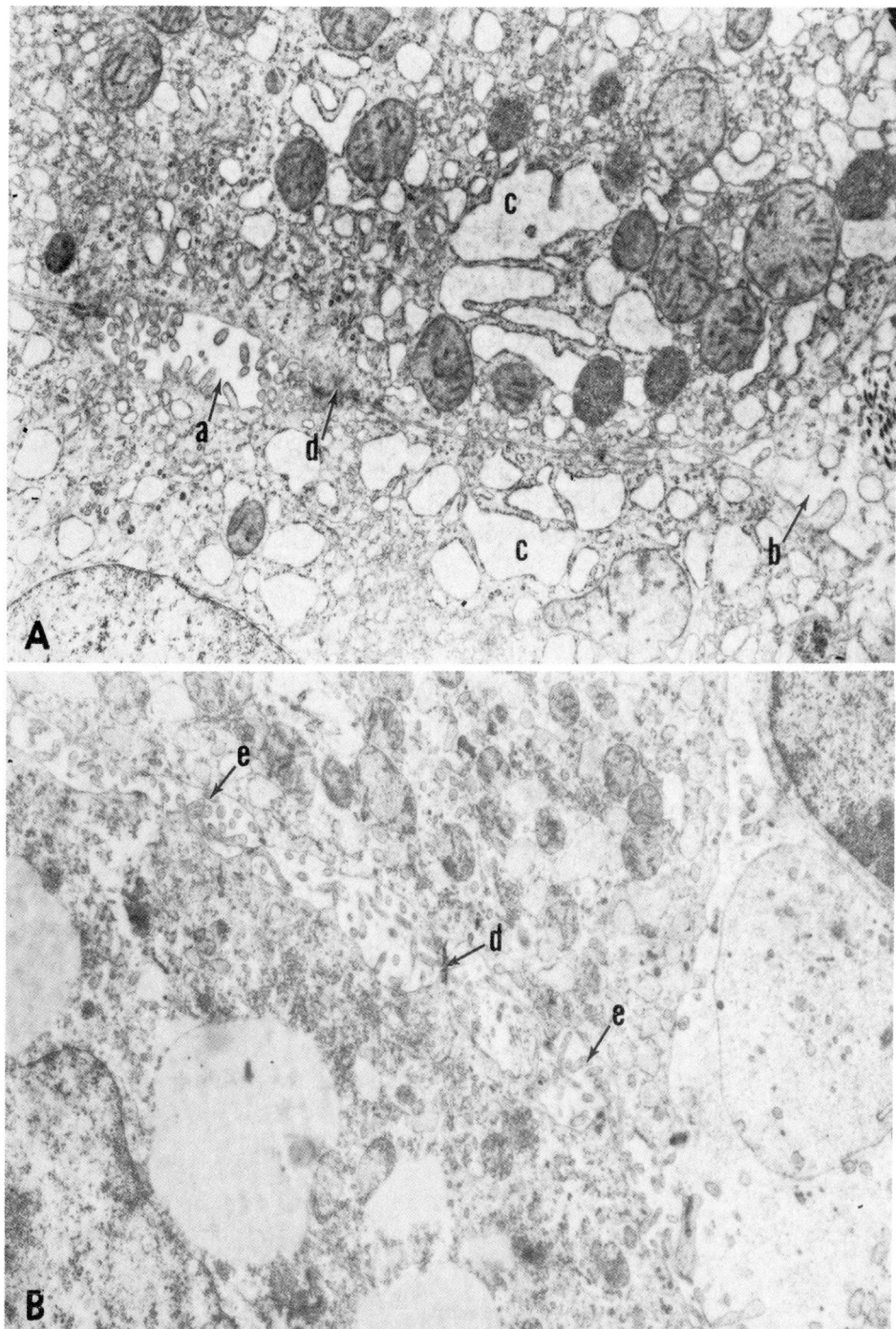

Fig. 16–8. *Lantana* poisoning, sheep. *A,* Electron micrograph of liver cells of normal, fasted sheep. Note the intercellular membrane between hepatocytes, extending from the bile canaliculus (*a*) to the space of Dissé (*b*). The endoplasmic reticulum (*c*) is distended, the terminal bar (*d*) is intact.

B, Electron micrograph of liver cells of sheep poisoned by *Lantana*. Note intercellular space (*e*) formed by microvilliform changes in the plasma membranes of contiguous hepatocytes. The terminal bar (*d*) indicates the location of the modified plasma membranes. (Courtesy of Dr. A. A. Seawright and *Pathologia Veterinaria*.)

plasma membranes are normally contiguous and parallel. Only at the terminal bars do the plasma membranes remain in contact. Characteristic blebs often form as modification of the wall of the canaliculus. These changes are believed by Seawright to be characteristics of lantana poisoning. In severely damaged hepatocytes, the endoplasmic reticulum is often fragmented and dispersed. The nuclear membrane many disintegrate or lose its definition. The mitochondria remain intact. In some severely affected cells, rounded masses formed from the plasma membranes may be seen in the newly formed intercellular spaces. Deposits of bile may surround the distended endoplasmic reticulum. Invagination of nuclear membrane containing cytoplasmic organelles was sometimes seen. Large pinocytic vesicles, deposits of bile, and distended or fragmented endoplasmic reticulum occupied the cytoplasm of severely affected hepatocytes.

In an additional publication, Seawright (1965b) has proposed that the hepatocytes at the periphery of the lobules are so damaged by lantana poisoning to permit the bile to regurgitate from the canaliculi to the sinusoids. This would account for the biliary retention and accumulation of bile in the peripheral blood without microscopic evidence of bile stasis in the hepatocytes or bile ducts.

Hurst, E.: The Poison Plants of New South Wales. 1942, Univ. of Sydney and N.S.W. Dept. of Agric., Sydney.

Sanders, D.A.: Lantana poisoning in cattle. J. Am. Vet. Med. Assoc., *109*:139–141, 1946.

Seawright, A.A.: Studies on the pathology of experimental lantana (*Lantana camara*, L.) poisoning of sheep. Pathol. Vet., *1*:504–529, 1964.

———: Electron microscopic observations of the hepatocytes of sheep in lantana poisoning. Pathol. Vet., *2*:175–196, 1965a.

———: A possible mechanism of intrahepatic obstruction in lantana poisoning. Aust. Vet. J., *41*:116–119, 1965b.

Seawright, A.A., and Allen, J.G.: Pathology of the liver and kidney in lantana poisoning in cattle. Aust. Vet. J., *48*:323–331, 1972.

Sacahuiste

Sacahuiste, sacahuista, or beargrass (*Nolina texana*) is a perennial plant that grows in the moderately arid parts of the southwestern United States, principally in central and western Texas. Because of its extremely long, blade-like leaves (60 to 160 cm long, 2 to 5 mm wide), which rise to a height of 50 to 75 cm, then bend and droop on all sides, the plant resembles a very large tuft of grass. In early spring, it sends up flowering stems, which bear panicles of fine flowers of inconspicuous grayish color. Only the flowering panicles and the buds are poisonous, according to the experimental work of Mathews (1940). Sheep and goats more frequently eat poisonous amounts than cattle.

This is one of the photosensitizing plants, and if the animal at the same time eats adequate amounts of chlorophyll-containing material and is exposed to sunlight, the usual edema and necrosis of the unpigmented skin result. These changes are most prominent in the face and ears. The ears of sheep may swell to a thickness of 2 or 3 cm, drooping because of the added weight. Dermatitis is frequently characterized by severe pruritus. Necrosis of areas of skin may or may not supervene, depending on the severity of this phase of the disease. Other outstanding signs of poisoning by sacahuiste include icterus, which appears within a day or two after the first loss of appetite, a discharge of tenacious, yellow exudate from the nostrils, and a copious conjunctival exudate, which is serous at first and later purulent. The urine is dark yellow or sometimes reddish. The latter discoloration appears to be due to hemoglobin; at least there is no hematuria. A band of purplish discoloration encircling the hoof just below the coronary band is thought by Mathews to represent an aspect of the photosensitization. Poisoned animals usually live a week or more after the appearance of symptoms, seeking water and shade meanwhile. A few recover.

The lesions are those of acute toxic hepatitis, so that grossly the liver has a greenish paleness and greasy feeling. Upon incision, greenish casts of inspissated bile can be expressed from the severed ducts. Microscopically, the hepatic changes are disorganization of the hepatic cords, fatty change, chiefly centrilobular, biliary casts containing cholesterol clefts, and a minimal amount of necrosis. The other principal changes are those of toxic tubular nephrosis, the large, pale kidney grossly, hydropic degeneration and fatty change being most prominent microscopically. As in the liver, actual necrosis is minimal. Albuminous casts are numerous and may extend into Bowman's capsules. Bile pigment tends to produce a greenish-brown discoloration macroscopically, which is carried over into the microscopic sections to temper the usual staining reactions of the cells.

In diagnosis, the absence of marked changes in the gallbladder and the frequent presence of photosensitization help to differentiate this poisoning from that caused by senecios and possibly from those due to some other plants having the same geographical habitat. It is doubtful that any of the chemical poisons produce exactly this combination of changes.

Mathews, F.P.: Poisoning in sheep and goats by sacahuiste (Nolina texana) buds and blooms. Exp. Sta. Bull. 585. Texas A. & M. College, College Station, Texas, 1940.

Drymaria Pachyphylla

This plant, found on the arid ranges of the southwestern United States, has been shown by Mathews (1933) to be highly poisonous to sheep and somewhat less so to cattle and goats. A member of the "chickenweed" group, it grows flat on the ground, reaching a width of as much as 40 cm. Its rather sparse, trailing branches bear ovate leaves about a centimeter in length, which are thick and juicy. (Pachyphylla means thick-leaved.) Its fruits and seeds are quite tiny and are borne where the short leaf-stalks come off from the branches.

Signs appear in a little less than 24 hours after ingestion of the plant (experimentally) and may be followed by death in two hours or possibly by recovery in about two days. They consist of diarrhea and evidence of mild abdominal pain. Lethargy, coma, and death tend to follow rapidly, depending on the severity of the poisoning. Pulse and respiration remain practically normal.

Lesions include hemorrhagic inflammation, at least of the ileum, and at times of higher portions of the intestine. This is accompanied by severe serous and often hemorrhagic cholecystitis, with edematous pericholecystitis and pericholangitis. Ecchymotic hemorrhages are described as numerous in the diaphragm, epicardium, and outer myocardium. The liver and spleen are congested. The liver also undergoes centrilobular necrosis, usually coagulative, with acidophilic staining of the cytoplasm. More peripherally, there is fatty change. Toxic changes in the kidneys are much more limited and without casts.

Diagnosis is not likely to be possible on the basis of lesions alone, but should become reasonably certain if the availability of the plant and the unavailability of normal and palatable forage are known to exist. The poison may be classified as enteritis-producing and hepatotoxic.

Mathews, F.P.: The toxicity of Drymaria pachyphylla for cattle, sheep and goats. J. Am. Vet. Med. Assoc., 83:255–260, 1933.

Lechuguilla

Agave lechuguilla is a plant of the arid southwestern United States, Mexico, and similar regions; it is eaten, upon necessity, by sheep and goats. In addition to the usual signs of general illness, such as weakness and emaciation, symptoms include a yellow tenacious mucous exudate from the eyes and nose, icterus, and high blood urea nitrogen or nonprotein nitrogen. The latter change can be detected by examination as early as the eighth day after ingestion of the plant begins. If the patient is exposed to bright summer sunlight, photosensitization manifests itself by edematous swelling ("bighead") of the ears and face, the overlying skin sometimes becoming necrotic. Leukocytosis is then added to the hematologic abnormalities. A short period of coma usually precedes death.

Postmortem lesions are those that would be expected from the symptoms: acute toxic hepatitis and acute toxic tubular nephrosis. Fatty change of the liver is marked and is principally responsible for its pale or yellow color grossly. Centrilobular necrosis is of moderate degree. Lymphocytic infiltrations in or around the islands of Glisson (portal spaces) are usually noticeable. There is considerable retention and inspissation of bile, which forms precipitated masses in some of the intrahepatic bile ducts. In the kidneys, dilation of the tubules is pronounced. This distention is probably due to obstruction by large albuminous casts in the case of some nephrons, but there are also evidences of hypertrophic dilation and also of regeneration of epithelium. Fatty change occurs in the ascending loops of Henle. In addition to the rather frequent, obstructing casts, a precipitate of albumin is to be seen in most of the proximal convoluted tubules. In individuals that develop photosensitization, the edema, cutaneous necrosis, and subsequent inflammatory exudation are typical.

Mathews, F.P.: Lechuguilla poisoning in sheep and goats. J. Am. Vet. Med. Assoc., 93:168–175, 1938.

Phyllanthus

A plant popularly classed as a spurge, *Phyllanthus abnormis* or *P. drumondii*, has poisoned cattle in the southern and western parts of Texas. It produces a slowly progressive intoxication, characterized by depression, inappetence, and cachexia, with diarrhea and slight icterus. Postmortem lesions show this to be another example of hepatotoxic and nephrotoxic poisoning. The usual changes of acute toxic hepatitis progress, in chronic cases, to cirrhosis. The renal damage is in the necrosis and degenerative epithelial changes characteristic of acute toxic tubular nephrosis, together with albuminous material in the tubules, which is perhaps more in the nature of proteinaceous debris from disintegrating cells than of albuminous excretion.

Mathews, F.P.: Toxicity of a spurge (*Phyllanthus abnormis*) for cattle, sheep and goats. Cornell Vet., 35:336–346, 1945.

Mushrooms

Certain species of mushrooms, especially *Amanita phalloides*, *A. pantherina*, and *A. verna* (popularly called the "destroying angel"), are well known to be poisonous, human fatalities being only too frequent. Cattle may develop a notable liking for these mushrooms when they are numerous in the pasture, as they may be in warm, humid climates, and cases of fatal poisoning have been reported.

Signs include vomiting, painful defecation, sometimes with eversion and ulceration of the rectal mucosa, muscular spasms, drowsiness and death. In man there are hallucinations. Illness begins several hours after ingestion of the mushrooms and is likely to last for several days. Principal lesions are acute catarrhal gastroenteritis throughout the tract, and hemorrhages on the heart, liver, and other organs. Gross appearances indicate a considerable degree of acute toxic hepatitis and toxic tubular nephrosis. In humans poisoned by *Amanita phalloides*, the hepatic and renal toxic changes are the principal lesions, with marked fatty change of these organs and the heart. Complete microscopic studies appear not to have been made in animals.

Burton, H.A.: Mushroom poisoning in cattle. Vet. Med., *39*:290, 1944.

Piercy, P.L., Hargis, G., and Brown, C.A.: Mushroom poisoning in cattle. J. Am. Vet. Med. Assoc., *105*:206–208, 1944.

Ridgway, R.L.: Mushroom (*Amanita pantherina*) poisoning. J. Am. Vet. Med. Assoc., *172*:681–682, 1978.

Lupines

Lupines are leguminous plants of the pea family, native to most of the temperate regions of the world. Most of the 100 or more species of the genus *Lupinus* are native to the western United States, but have also been incriminated in poisoning of livestock in Australia, South Africa, and Central and Western Europe. In Europe, the plants were for the most part introduced as a means of providing nitrogenous forage and improving poor soils. The Greeks and Romans used the seeds of certain lupines for making flour after first loosening the hulls by cooking, and then soaking out the bitter and poisonous principles in running water.

Several species have been identified with losses of livestock. In the western United States, these are: *L. sericeus, L. leucophyllus, L. argenteus, L. caudatus, L. perennis, L. pusillus, L. laxifloris,* and *L. onustus.* In South Africa, *L. angustifolius,* widely used as a cover crop and feed for sheep, has upon occasion been the cause of severe losses in sheep, cattle, and sometimes swine. In Australia, *L. digitatus* is the commonest variety, widely cultivated and naturalized after its introduction during the late nineteenth century. This blue lupine is usually involved in livestock losses from lupines in Australia.

Certain alkaloids found in lupines have been identified as the cause of illness in animals; in fact, development of new genetic strains ("sweet lupines"), which do not contain these alkaloids, has eliminated losses due to this cause. The following alkaloids have been isolated from lupine species: **lupinine, lupinidine** or **l-sparteine, d-lupanine, hydroxy-(oxy)** **lupanine,** and **spathulatine.** The toxic effects of these lupine alkaloids have been grouped under the terms **lupine poisoning, American lupinosis, alkaloidal poisoning,** or **lupine madness.** Gardiner (1967) has proposed that the term **lupine poisoning** be used for lupine alkaloid poisoning, to differentiate it from another syndrome associated with lupines but unrelated to toxic alkaloids. This latter syndrome Gardiner calls **lupinosis** or **European lupinosis,** and is due to a mycotoxin produced by the fungus *Phomopsis leptostomiformis,* which may grow on sweet and bitter lupines. This is discussed elsewhere with other mycotoxicoses.

Lupine poisoning, due to the effects of one or more of the lupine alkaloids, is manifest by severe effects on nerve centers, especially respiratory and vasomotor centers, which are first stimulated, then paralyzed. This effect results in fall of blood pressure, a slow heart rate, dilation of pupils, and death by asphyxia associated with convulsions. All mammals are susceptible, but natural poisonings have been observed in sheep, horses, cattle, goats, swine, and deer. Signs of poisoning may appear a few hours after ingesting poisonous lupines. In sheep, nervous manifestations predominate, with erratic behavior, confused running about, dyspnea, excessive frothy salivation, convulsions, stupor, or coma leading to death. The gross and microscopic lesions in this type of poisoning due to lupine alkaloids apparently are not distinctive.

A distinctive congenital syndrome, **crooked calf disease,** occurs in range cattle in certain western states and Alaska and has been shown by Shupe et al. (1967) to be caused by the teratogenic effect of lupines consumed by cows between the fortieth to seventieth days of pregnancy. The disease is seen in newborn calves from cows that have access to lupines on the range (Shupe, James, and Binns, 1967), and has been reproduced by feeding pregnant cows dried lupine plants, especially *Lupinus sericeus.*

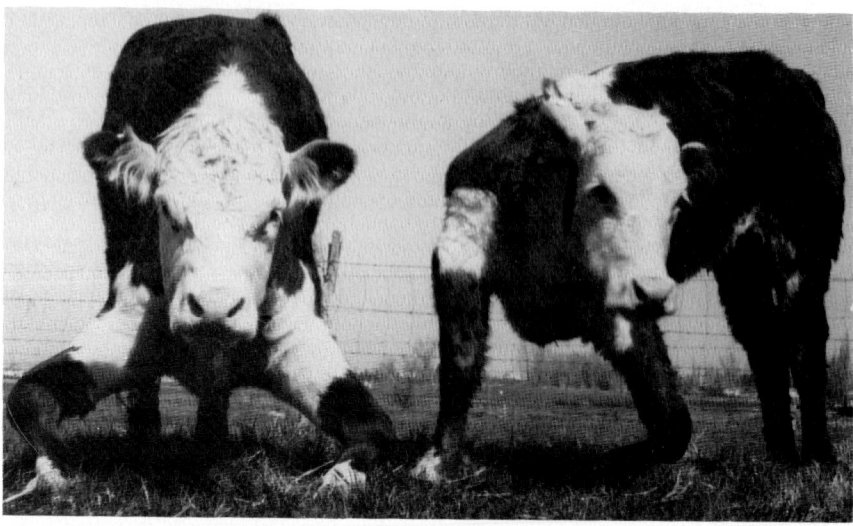

Fig. 16–9. Arthrogryposis and scoliosis of calves following lupine poisoning. (Courtesy of Dr. J. L. Shupe and *Journal of the American Veterinary Medical Association*.)

The cows exhibit lethargy, nervousness, incoordination, muscular twitching, and dry, rough hair coat as a result of feeding on lupines months before delivery of the deformed calves.

Affected calves are born with any or all of several anomalies (Fig. 16–9), including **arthrogryposis, scoliosis, torticollis,** and **cleft palate.** Most calves are viable and may survive to become adults, but some abortions are recorded among affected cattle. This disease, known by cattlemen for many years in certain regions, was originally thought to be hereditary, but the genetic evidence was not convincing and the experimental data now clearly point toward lupines as the cause. The toxic principle, at this writing, has not been identified.

Gardiner, M.R.: Lupinosis. Adv. Vet. Sci., *11*:85–138, 1967.

Gardiner, M.R., and Parr, W.H.: Pathogenesis of acute lupinosis of sheep. J. Comp. Pathol., *77*:51–62, 1967.

Shupe, J.L., James, L.F., and Binns, W.: Observations on crooked calf disease. J. Am. Vet. Med. Assoc., *151*:191–197, 1967.

Shupe, J.L., et al.: Lupine, a cause of crooked calf disease. J. Am. Vet. Med. Assoc., *151*:198–203, 1967.

Shupe, J.L., James, L.F., and Binns, W.: Cleft palate in cattle. Cleft Palate J., *1*:346–355, 1968.

Shupe, J.L., Balls, L.F., and James, L.F.: Changes in blood serum transaminase associated with lupine and larkspur poisoning in cattle. Cornell Vet., *58*:129–135, 1968.

Vetch

The vetches *(Vicia spp.)* are leguminous plants related to the lupines genetically and also in their toxicology. Several species, especially *Vicia sativa*, the "common vetch," are raised, like certain lupines, as proteinaceous forage or as nitrogen-fixing soil-builders. The seeds of this and some other species contain poisonous amounts of prussic acid, especially before maturity. However, the toxic effects of the vetches in hay or forage are in most cases of a different nature. The illness, which usually extends over several days or longer, is characterized especially by vague digestive disturbances and icterus. In more acute forms, there are muscular twitchings and definite signs of gastroenteritis. In the case of *Vicia faba*, the "broad bean" or "horse bean," hemolytic anemia and hemoglobinuria are also symptoms. Lesions are those of acute

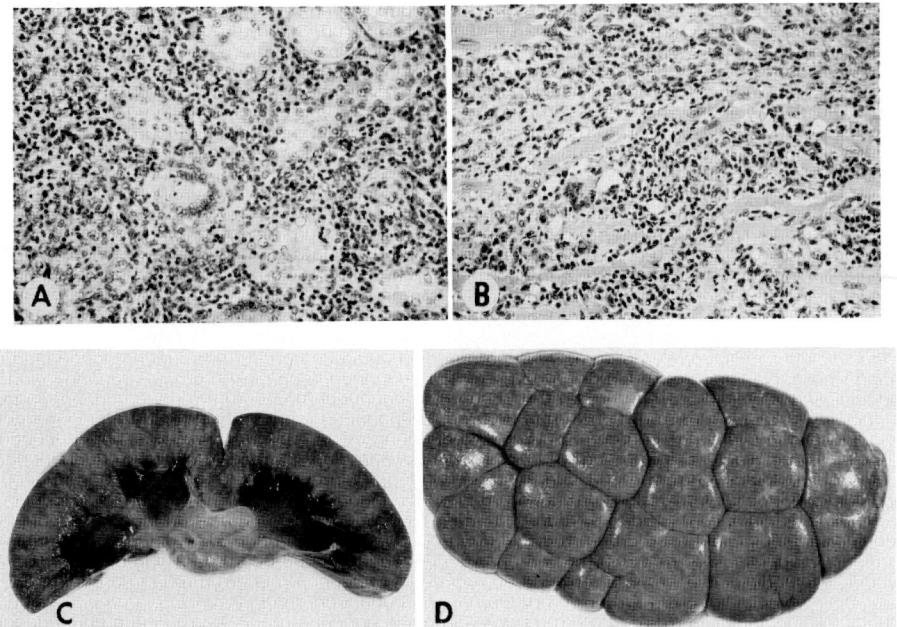

Fig. 16–10. Poisoning by hairy vetch (*Vicia villosa*) of cattle. *A*, Kidney. Distortion of tubules and leukocytic infiltration. *B*, Myocardium. Necrosis and calcification of muscle fibers, proliferation of sarcolemma, regeneration of muscle cells and leukocytic infiltration. *C*, Cross section of kidney. Grayish, infiltration of cortex. *D*, Kidney. Grayish foci disseminated through cortex. (Courtesy of Dr. Roger J. Panciera and *Journal of the American Veterinary Medical Association*.)

toxic hepatitis with or without gastroenteritis.

Panciera et al. (1966) have associated a syndrome in cattle with feeding upon pastures containing hairy vetch (*Vicia villosa*). This disease differs in several ways from that usually associated with other vetch poisoning. The disease was observed in 13 herds, in which dermatitis, conjunctivitis, and diarrhea were the principal signs of illness. Approximately 800 cattle were observed, about 7% of them were sick, and about half of these sick cattle died. The affected skin became thickened, folded, and in places, denuded of hair. The lesions occurred in pigmented as well as nonpigmented areas of the skin. A few pregnant cows aborted.

The lesions in fatal cases were distributed through the myocardium, kidney, adrenal, lymph nodes, and thyroid, and appeared grossly as focal or confluent grayish infiltrations, usually moderately firm and sharply demarcated from the adjacent tissue. Microscopically, these focal lesions were formed by necrosis of parenchyma and infiltration by macrophages, multinucleated giant cells, eosinophils, and lymphocytes. Myocardial fibers were necrotic, sometimes mineralized (Fig. 16–10), and the sarcoplasma was often absent, leaving sarcolemmal nuclei and many giant cells. Necrosis of renal tubules was also observed in this syndrome, accompanied by replication of tubular epithelial cells, intense infiltration by leukocytes, principally lymphocytes, and peculiar membranous thickening of the glomerular tufts.

A specific hemolytic anemia, **favism,** in certain human subjects depends upon a genetic factor and the ingestion of the broad bean, *Vicia faba*. The inherited defect in susceptible human patients results in a deficiency of the enzyme glucose-6-

phosphate dehydrogenase. Deficiency of this enzyme (G-6-PD) is reflected in reduced glutathione in the red blood cells. Extracts of beans of *Vicia faba* have been shown to have a destructive effect upon the erythrocytes of susceptible individuals in vitro, and it is therefore believed that the beans may act similarly on the susceptible red blood cells in vivo, resulting in hemolytic anemia.

Bowman, J.E., and Walker, D.G.: Action of *Vicia faba* on erythrocytes: possible relation to favism. Nature, *189*:555–556, 1961.
Panciera, R.J., Johnson, L., and Osburn, B.I.: A disease of cattle grazing hairy vetch pasture. J. Am. Vet. Med. Assoc., *148*:804–808, 1966.
Steyn, D.G.: Toxicology of Plants in South Africa. Johannesburg, The Central News Agency, 1934.

Algae

Certain kinds of green or blue-green algae, usually not identified as to species, some of which grow beneath rather than on the surface of waters of lakes and rivers, are at times extremely poisonous to all species of animals that drink the water. Poisoning has usually occurred when winds have blown much of this material to the shore at which cattle drink, especially during midsummer.

Death occurs suddenly within approximately an hour or two after drinking the water. Symptoms are acute prostration followed by convulsions, or else rapidly developing general paralysis. Postmortem lesions are usually stated to be absent, excepting possibly the presence of hydroperitoneum. On the other hand, subacute and chronic cases are reported in South Africa. In the former, there is acute toxic hepatitis with icterus, the liver being yellow and friable. There are bloody or yellowish fluid in the serous cavities, acute swelling of the spleen, and sometimes hemorrhagic enteritis. In a few chronic cases, the liver is described as hard, presumably cirrhotic. In cattle which have recovered, severe cutaneous lesions characteristic of photosensitization have developed. Toxicity of the water can be demonstrated in experimental animals orally or parenterally, but toxic conditions in the lakes may change quickly, with the "water-bloom" being blown elsewhere, or by other means.

Brandenburg, T.O., and Shigley, F.M.: "Water Bloom" as a cause of poisoning in livestock in North Dakota. J. Am. Vet. Med. Assoc., *110*:384–385, 1947.
Deem, A.W., and Thorp, F., Jr.: Toxic algae in Colorado. J. Am. Vet. Med. Assoc., *95*:542–544, 1939.
Fitch, C.P., Bishop, L.M., and Boyd, W.L.: "Water Bloom" as a cause of poisoning in domestic animals. Cornell Vet., *24*:30–38, 1934.
Francis, G.: Poisonous Australian lake. Nature, *18*:11–12, 1878.
Gorham, P.R.: Toxic waterblooms of blue-green algae. Can. Vet. J., *1*:235–245, 1960.

GROUP D: NEPHROTOXICITY

Poisons in Group D are primarily **nephrotoxic.** Some of these poisonings may also affect other organ systems, but in general, less so than with the hepatotoxins discussed in the previous section.

Turpentine

Turpentine is a local as well as diffusible irritant. Skin is readily blistered within one or two hours after a single topical application. Ingested without adequate dilution, turpentine causes severe gastroenteritis, in addition to stomatitis and esophagitis. When it is inhaled, the result is bronchopneumonia. A considerable amount, however, is tolerated in the digestive tract if properly diluted. Fatalities result from acute toxic tubular nephrosis, which develops within a few days. Most cases of poisoning result from attempts by stockmen to use the substance for therapeutic purposes. An unusual case of fatal nephritic poisoning came to our attention when a dog walked upon a freshly painted floor and the owner used turpentine to wash the animal's feet. Giffee (1939) reports sudden fatal poisoning when turpentine was applied to castration wounds in little pigs. Symptoms of acute peritonitis appeared within minutes and death of several came within an hour or two.

Giffee, J.W.: Turpentine poisoning in pigs. J. Am. Vet. Med. Assoc., 95:509, 1939.

Sulfonamides

The usual toxic effects of the sulfonamide drugs, as seen in domestic animals, depend upon obstruction of renal tubules by precipitated crystals of the sulfonamide in question. With the unaided eye, masses of the yellowish crystals can often be seen in the renal papillae and pelvis, or even forming pale radial lines, which mark distended medullary tubules. It is said that their amount is sometimes so great as to act as obstructive calculi in the ureter. Microscopically, the crystals in the papillae are seen to lie within the ducts of Bellini and collecting tubules, which they commonly obstruct and whose lining their sharp points mechanically irritate. Fatalities appear to be possible from these effects alone, but in some instances the obstructive changes may be accompanied by the formation of albuminous casts, suggesting a more subtle renal injury. This is accompanied by mild degenerative changes in the cells of the proximal convoluted tubules.

In human beings, the kidneys often contain foci of necrosis, in and around which the heavy accumulation of reticuloendothelial and other inflammatory cells amounts to a granulomatous reaction. This is the so-called nephrotoxic reaction; it is considered an allergic process, supposedly depending on previous sensitization. The rarity or nonexistence of this phenomenon in animals might be attributable to the infrequency with which an animal patient has more than one illness treated by sulfonamides. However, when one considers the alacrity and nonchalance with which stockmen administered sulfonamide drugs (until antibiotics replaced them) for illnesses of all sorts, such an explanation seems doubtful.

Other disorders that have resulted from the administration of sulfonamides include temporary nervous dysfunctions, such as blindness, failure of optical adaptation and accommodation, hyperesthesia, incoordination, ataxia, and convulsions. These usually follow a single excessive dose of the drug. Demyelinization of nerves has also resulted, and serious or fatal results have attended the application of sulfonamide medications where they came into contact with central or peripheral nervous tissue.

The therapeutic administration of sulfonamides occasionally leads to detectable porphyrinuria in human patients. We do not find reports of accompanying photosensitization, but the situation might well be different in case a farm animal, normally exposed to much sunlight, were to suffer the provocative hepatic damage. Experimentally, in rats, sulfonamides administered to the pregnant mother have inhibited ossification of the bones of the fetus. In young chickens, as little as 0.06% of sodium sulfaquinoxaline in the drinking water for four days has produced a hemorrhagic syndrome of serious import.

In spite of the several dangerous possibilities, however, the sulfonamides remain highly useful therapeutic agents. Crystallization in the renal tubules as the glomerular filtrate is concentrated into urine, the most likely catastrophe, is rendered improbable by promoting alkalinity in those species having an acid urine, and even more by a copious intake of water.

Benesch, R., Chance, M.R.A., and Glynn, L.E.: Inhibition of bone calcification by sulphonamides. Nature (Lond.), 155:203–204, 1945.

Davies, S.F.M.: Sulphonamide poisoning in chickens treated for coccidiosis. Papers Presented to Tenth World's Poultry Congr., Edinburgh, 1954. pp. 275–278.

Delaplane, J.P., and Milliff, J.H.: Gross and micropathology of sulfaquinoxaline poisoning in chickens. Am. J. Vet. Res., 9:92–96, 1948.

Figge, H., Carey, T.N., and Weiland, G.S.: Porphyrin-excretion by a patient treated with sulfadiazine and later with sulfanilamide. J. Lab. Clin. Med., 31:752–756, 1946.

French, A.J.: Hypersensitivity in the pathogenesis of histopathologic changes associated with sulfonamide chemotherapy. Am. J. Pathol., 22:679–701, 1946.

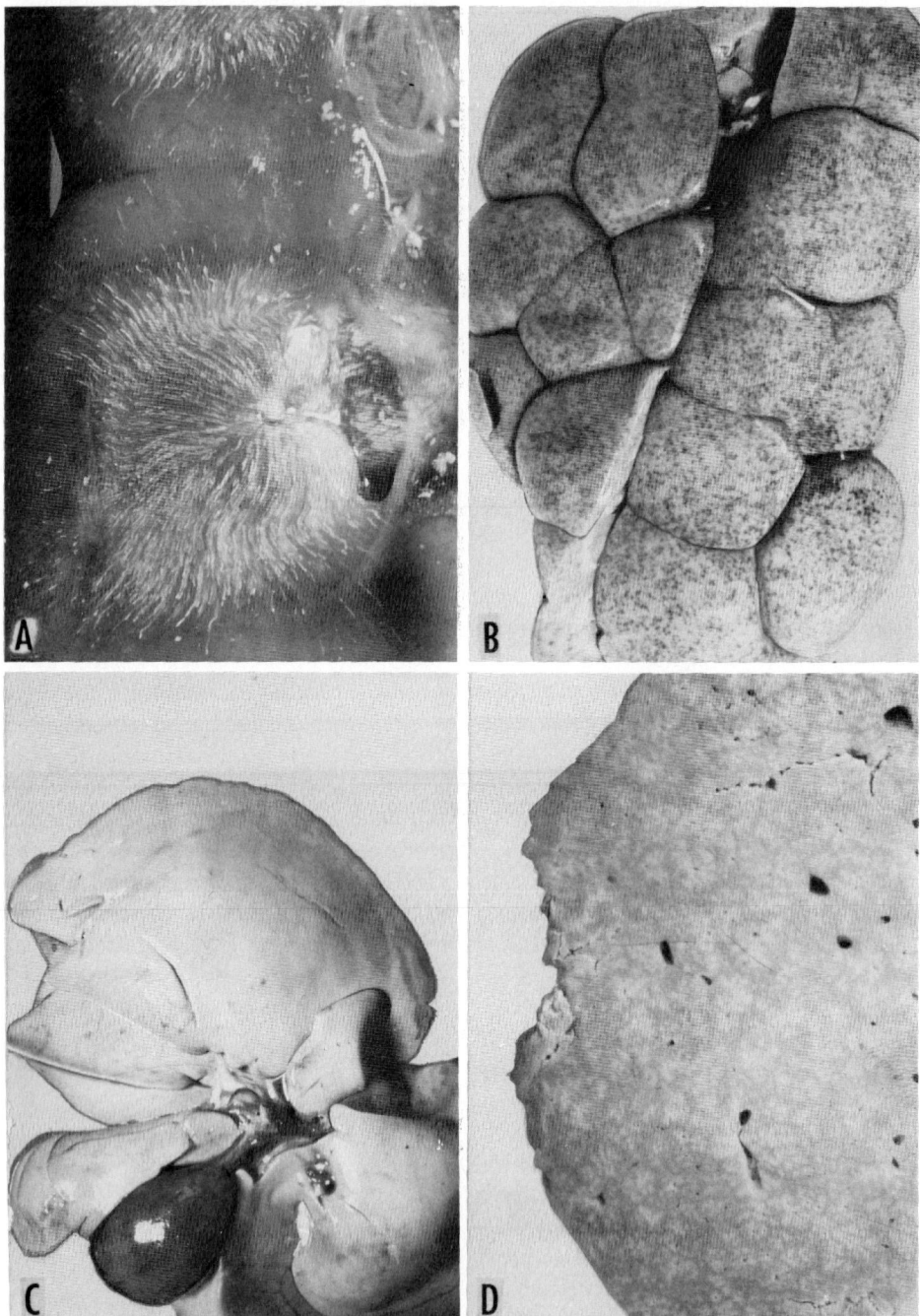

Fig. 16–11. *A*, Poisoning by sulfathiazole, kidney of a three-week-old calf. Crystals fill collecting tubules. (Case at Texas Sch. Vet. Med.) *B*, Kidney of a Brahman heifer poisoned by eating oak buds. (Case at Texas Sch. Vet. Med.) *C*, Liver of a dog which survived three days after being poisoned by phosphorus. The liver was pale yellowish in color. (Case at Iowa Sch. Vet. Med.) *D*, Liver of a horse with toxic hepatitis, probably due to crotalaria poisoning.

Jones, L.M., Smith, H.A., and Roepke, M.H.: Effects of large doses of various sulfonamides injected in dairy cattle. Am. J. Vet. Res., *10*:318–326, 1949.

Moore, R.H., McMillan, G.C., and Duff, G.L.: Pathology of sulfonamide allergy in man. Am. J. Pathol., *22*:703–735, 1946.

Oxalate-Bearing Plants and Ethylene Glycol

Oxalate poisoning may result from ingestion of (1) plants that contain toxic levels of oxalate, (2) ethylene glycol, (3) oxalate salts, or (4) plants infected with fungi that produce oxalates. Ordinary garden rhubarb (*Rheum rhaponticum*) is one of the oxalate-containing plants, but of more significance in causing losses of livestock are halogeton (*Halogeton glomeratus*) and greasewood (*Sarcobatus vermiculatus*), both of which grow in the Rocky Mountain region of the United States. In dry weather, halogeton has been known to contain oxalates, largely sodium and potassium oxalate, equivalent to 19% of anhydrous oxalic acid. Soursob (*Oxalis cernua*), indigenous to South Australia, is another plant that owes its poisonous qualities to its content of oxalates, as is also the common sorrel, *Rumex acetosa* and other members of the genus *Rumex.*

Another plant demonstrated by analysis (Marshall et al., 1967) to contain high levels of oxalate is *Amaranthus retroflexus*, pigweed, redroot, or careless weed. The leaves of this plant may contain as much as 30% of total oxalate on a dried weight basis. Oxalate poisoning from ingestion of these plants is primarily a disease of sheep. Cattle and horses are relatively resistant.

The poisonous effects of calcium oxalates are also produced in some species (man, dog, cat) by the ingestion of toxic amounts of **ethylene glycol.** This colorless, odorless, slightly viscous, dihydric alcohol has a sweetish taste and is widely used as a solvent in manufacturing (Kersting and Nielsen, 1965). Its common use as a nonvolatile antifreeze makes it available in many households, and its taste appeals to some people, cats, and dogs. Ethylene glycol is metabolized in the liver by **alcohol dehydrogenase,** which results in the formation of oxalates. This enzyme is also necessary for the degradation of ethyl alcohol. The simultaneous administration of ethyl alcohol competes for this enzyme in the liver and decreases the formation of oxalate. This fact is utilized in the treatment of ethylene glycol poisoning (Wacker et al., 1965).

The initial effect of oxalate poisoning is hypocalcemia, resulting from the formation of insoluble calcium oxalate. Serum calcium levels may drop to less than half of normal. The signs of acute poisoning are observed within two to four hours. In sheep, these include depression, anorexia, slight to moderate bloating, weakness, restlessness, frequent attempts to urinate, occasional reddish-brown urine and brownish-black feces, blood-tinged nasal exudate, and coma, followed by death. Ethylene glycol poisoning in dogs results in the rapid development of ataxia, polydipsia, depression, miosis, tachycardia, tachypnea, hyperpnea, bradycardia, and coma. Convulsions and vomiting are frequent. In most cases, death follows the administration of 6.6 ml/kg of body weight or more.

The neurologic signs are believed to be the result of hypocalcemia. Precipitation of calcium oxalate in cerebral blood vessels, however, may contribute in some manner.

Calcium oxalate is precipitated in the renal tubules during the process of elimination, and a fatal outcome may occur from renal insufficiency and uremia after the earlier symptoms have abated. Recovery, on the other hand, is possible, with blood urea levels slowly subsiding after about a month. Cystitis and urethritis may be a part of this syndrome.

Postmortem diagnosis can usually be made in these cases by the presence of numerous nearly transparent crystals in the renal tubules. Visible when the light is sharply reduced, these may be single, irregularly rhomboidal, and 30 or 40 μ long.

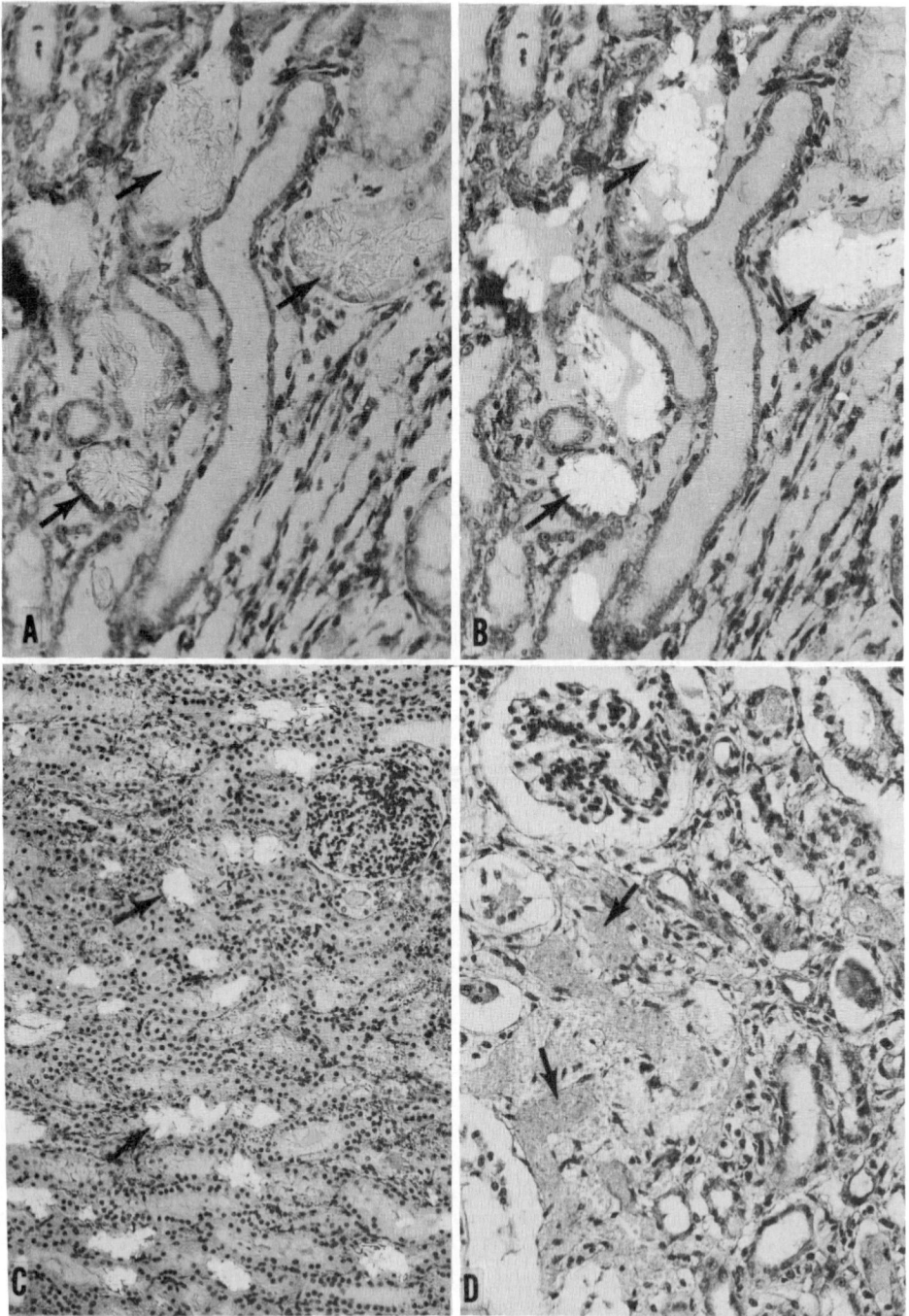

Fig. 16–12. *A,* Kidney of a kitten poisoned by ethylene glycol (antifreeze) (× 210). Note oxalate crystals (arrows) in tubules. *B,* Same section as *A,* photographed under polarized light. Note brilliance of oxalate crystals (arrows). (Courtesy of Dr. Wm. J. Hadlow.) *C,* Kidney of a sheep poisoned by eating Halogeton plants (× 125). Note oxalate crystals (arrows), photographed under polarized light. (Courtesy of Dr. Wayne C. Anderson.) *D,* Kidney of a steer poisoned by eating buds of an oak tree (× 210). Necrosis (arrows) of certain convoluted tubules.

Often, however, the crystals lie closely packed in a radial arrangement, the whole rosette-like structure more than filling the lumen of the tubule and occupying space at the expense of the epithelial cells (Fig. 16–12). The latter eventually become necrotic, although the extent of cellular damage depends upon whether death occurred early or late. There is also severe congestion of all parts of the kidney, moderate increase in cellularity of the glomeruli, and marked albuminous precipitate in the tubules. Those epithelial cells not directly affected by the crystals show little toxic injury. Oxalate nephrosis has been reported in fetal kidneys of sheep exposed to oxalic acid during pregnancy.

The widespread hemorrhages and edema found at postmortem, particularly in the rumen of sheep poisoned by halogeton, are associated with deposits of calcium oxalate in the walls of blood vessels. The presence of the oxalate at these sites appears to damage the blood vessel wall, but the interference with clotting due to hypocalcemia is probably of greater significance.

The **diagnosis** is usually established, postmortem, by the demonstration of characteristic birefringent crystals in renal tubules and cerebral blood vessels (Fig. 16–12). Nonfatal doses do not appear to produce permanent damage to renal tubules.

Studies (Roberts and Seibold, 1969) of the toxicity of ethylene glycol administered to three species of Old World monkeys (*Macaca mulatta, M. fascicularis*, and *M. radiata*) reveal lesions similar to those described in other species. The toxic dose in these species is believed to be similar to that in man, 1.6 ml/kg of body weight.

Amaranthus retroflexus is believed to be one of the causes of an entity called **perirenal edema disease** of swine. This syndrome has been observed (Buck et al., 1966) in swine given access to pastures bearing heavy growth of common piglot weeds, such as *Amaranthus retroflexus*, or the weed called lambs' quarters (*Chenopodium album*). Other weeds, such as black nightshade (*Solanum nigrum*), buffalo burr (*Solanum rostratum*), and Jimson weed (*Datura stramonium*), have also been suspected as causative.

The signs in perirenal edema syndrome are trembling, weakness, incoordination, sternal recumbency, and coma, followed by death. The characteristic postmortem lesion is the presence of a large amount of edema surrounding the kidney between the renal capsule and the perirenal peritoneum. Sometimes this edema fluid is tinged with blood, but the affected kidneys are usually pale and normal in size. Edema in the wall of the abdomen, around the rectum, and in the wall of the stomach may also be present. Clear, transparent, or straw-colored fluid may distend the peritoneal and pleural cavities. The renal capsule usually is not affected, although the edema may extend into the renal parenchyma. Microscopic evidence of toxic tubular nephrosis with interstitial edema in the renal cortex has been described. The pathogenesis of the syndrome has not been elucidated. A similar syndrome is described in cattle, also associated with *Amaranthus* poisoning (Stuart et al., 1975; Jeppesen, 1966).

The lesions are not typical of oxalate poisoning; oxalate crystals are not readily identifiable in tissue section; hence the exact pathogenetic mechanisms are not settled. The possibility that nitrate is an etiologic factor is still open, because it is known that *A. retroflexus* may contain elevated levels of nitrate. Feeding of this plant appears to have produced this syndrome in swine (Bennett, 1964).

Andrews, E.J.: Oxalate nephropathy in a horse. J. Am. Vet. Med. Assoc., 159:49–52, 1971.

Bennett, P.C.: Edema disease. *In* Diseases of Swine, edited by H. W. Dunn. Ames, Iowa State University Press, 1964.

Bennett, B., and Rosenblum, C.: Identification of calcium oxalate crystals in patients with uremia. Lab. Invest., 10:947–955, 1961.

Buck, W.B., et al.: Perirenal edema in swine: a disease caused by common weeds. J. Am. Vet. Med. Assoc., *148*:1525–1531, 1966.

Dickie, C.W., Hamann, M.H., Carroll, W.D., and Chow, F.-h: Oxalate (*Rumex venosus*) poisoning in cattle. J. Am. Vet. Med. Assoc., *173*:73–74, 1978.

Dodson, M.E.: Oxalate ingestion studies in the sheep. Aust. Vet. J., *35*:225–233, 1959.

Dunn, J.S., Haworth, A., and Jones, N.A.: Urea retention in oxalate nephritis. J. Pathol. Bact., *27*:377–400, 1924.

Hadlow, W.J.: Acute ethylene glycol poisoning in a cat. J. Am. Vet. Med. Assoc., *130*:296–297, 1957.

James, L.F.: Serum electrolyte, acid-base balance, and enzyme changes in acute *Halogeton glomeratus* poisoning in sheep. Can. J. Comp. Med., *32*:539–543, 1968.

James, L.F.: Locomotor disturbance of cattle grazing *Halogeton glomeratus*. J. Am. Vet. Med. Assoc., *156*:1310–1312, 1970.

Jeghers, H., and Murphy, R.: Practical aspects of oxalate metabolism. N. Engl. J. Med., *233*:208–215, 238–246, 1945.

Jeppeson, Q.E.: Bovine perirenal disease associated with pigweed. J. Am. Vet. Med. Assoc., *149*:22, 1966.

Jonsson, L., and Rubarth, S.: Ethylene glycol poisoning in dogs and cats. Nord. Vet. Med., *19*:265–276, 1967.

Kersting, E.J., and Nielsen, S.W.: Ethylene glycol poisoning in small animals. J. Am. Vet. Med. Assoc., *146*:113–118, 1965.

———: Experimental ethylene glycol poisoning in the dog. Am. J. Vet. Res., *27*:574–582, 1966.

Littledike, E.T., James, L., and Cook, H.: Oxalate (*Halogeton*) poisoning of sheep: certain physiopathologic changes. Am. J. Vet. Res., *37*:661–666, 1976.

Marshall, V.L., Buck, W.B., and Bell, G.L.: Pigweed (*Amaranthus retroflexus*); an oxalate-containing plant. Am. J. Vet. Res., *28*:888–889, 1967.

Maymone, B., et al.: Oxalic acid metabolism in ruminants on prolonged diet of *Oxalis cernua* Thunb. 8th Int. Congr. Anim. Prod. Hamburg., *2*:54–55, 1961.

Nunamaker, D.M., Medway, W., and Berg, P.: Treatment of ethylene glycol poisoning in the dog. J. Am. Vet. Med. Assoc., *159*:310–314, 1971.

Roberts, J.A., and Seibold, H.R.: Ethylene glycol toxicity in the monkey. Toxicol. Appl. Pharmacol., *15*:624–631, 1969.

Schiefer, B., Hewitt, M.P., and Milligan, J.D.: Fetal renal oxalosis due to feeding oxalic acid to pregnant ewes. Zentralbl. Veterinärmed., *23A*:226–233, 1976.

Shupe, J.L., and James, L.F.: Additional physiopathologic changes in *Halogeton glomeratus* (oxalate) poisoning in sheep. Cornell Vet., *59*:41–55, 1969.

Smith, W.S.: Soursob poisoning in sheep. J. Dept. Agric. S. Aust., *54*:377–378, 1951.

Stuart, B.P., Nicholson, S.S., and Smith, J.B.: Perirenal edema and toxic nephrosis in cattle, associated with ingestion of pigweed. J. Am. Vet. Med. Assoc., *167*:949–950, 1975.

Wacker, W.E.C., et al.: Treatment of ethylene glycol poisoning with ethyl alcohol. JAMA, *194*:1231–1233, 1965.

Watts, P.S.: Effects of oxalic ingestion by sheep. I. Small doses to chaff-fed sheep. II. Large doses to sheep on different diets. J. Agric. Sci., *52*:244–255, 1959.

Wilson, B.J., and Wilson, C.H.: Oxalate formation in mouldy feedstuffs as a possible factor in livestock toxic disease. Am. J. Vet. Res., *22*:961–969, 1961.

Broomweed

The broomweeds (*Xanthocephalum*, or *Gutierrezia spp*.) are plants that grow on the arid ranges of the western United States, are eaten by cattle and sheep under stress of necessity, and are commonly, but judging by experimental results, not always poisonous. It is probable that the different degrees of toxicity may be related to variations in growing conditions, although they do not appear to depend upon the stage of maturity of the plant. The plant is a somewhat herbaceous perennial which makes a very bushy growth to a height of about 1 foot (30 cm). It has fine foliage, covered with a sticky exudate, and large numbers of tiny yellow flowers.

Signs appear after an animal has been eating appreciable amounts of the plant for at least a few days, and begin with anorexia, listlessness, arched back, and drooping head. There is a noticeable degree of icterus. Appropriate tests reveal uremia, and in severe acute cases, there is also hematuria. Abortion often occurs in pregnant sheep or cattle.

The lesions can be summarized as those of acute toxic tubular nephrosis and a rather unsual form of toxic hepatitis. The proximal and distal convoluted tubules and the ascending loops of Henle suffer from hydropic degeneration and disintegration of the cytoplasm of their epithelial cells, with ultimate necrosis if the animal lives long enough. In the more acute cases, there are hemorrhages into the Bowman's capsules and the tubules, as well as into the intertubular tissue, while in animals with a more prolonged course (one to two weeks), there is a considerable degree of lymphocytic infiltration. The hepatic changes consist of hydropic degeneration and necrosis, diffusely distributed without regard to any particular zone in the lobule. While there are many diseases characterized by toxic nephrosis and hepatitis, it would seem that the hemorrhages into the nephron and the hydropic degeneration of the liver cells would serve to distinguish broomweed poisoning from many of the other nephrotoxic and hepatotoxic poisonings.

The toxic principle in broomweed appears to be saponin, which produces the clinical signs, including abortion, when administered orally to pregnant rabbits, cows, and goats (Dollahite et al., 1962). This saponin isolated from broomweed has no estrogenic properties, but stimulates contractions of isolated uterine muscle (Shaver et al., 1964) under laboratory conditions.

Dollahite, J.W., and Anthony, W.V.: Poisoning of cattle with *Gutierrezia microcephala*, a perennial broomweed. J. Am. Vet. Med. Assoc., *130*:525–530, 1957.
Dollahite, J.W., Shaver, T., and Camp, B.J.: Injected saponins as abortifacients. Am. J. Vet. Res., *23*:1261–1263, 1962.
Mathews, F.P.: Toxicity of broomweed (*Gutierrezia microcephala*) for sheep, cattle and goats. J. Am. Vet. Med. Assoc., *88*:55–61, 1936.
Shaver, T.N., Camp, B.J., and Dollahite, J.W.: The chemistry of a toxic constituent of *Xanthocephalum* species. Ann. NY Acad. Sci., *111*:737–743, 1964.

Chloroform

Chloroform toxicity serves to emphasize specific sexual dimorphisms and genetically determined sensitivity in certain inbred strains of laboratory mice. Experience has taught laboratory workers to avoid opening a bottle of chloroform in a room in which inbred mice are kept. Even a slight exposure to chloroform vapor will cause the death of male mice. The following inbred strains are particularly susceptible: CBA-p, DBA, C_3H, A, and HR. Immature males, adult females and castrated males are relatively insusceptible. Cas-

trated males become sensitive after administration of testosterone.

Inhalation of chloroform vapor by these susceptible mice results in necrosis of liver cells, glomeruli and proximal convoluted tubules. Animals that survive sublethal doses may later be demonstrated to have many calcified deposits in glomeruli and tubules in the renal cortex (Dunn, 1965).

Bennet, R.A., and Whigham, A.: Chloroform sensitivity of mice. Nature (Lond.), *204*:1328, 1964.
Christensen, L.R., et al.: Accidental chloroform poisoning of Balb/cAnNIcr mice. Z. Versuchstierkd., *2*:135–140, 1963.
Deringer, M.K., Dunn, T.B., and Heston, W.E.: Results of exposure of strain C_3H mice to chloroform. Proc. Soc. Exp. Biol. Med., *83*:474–479, 1953.
Dunn, T.B.: Spontaneous lesions of mice. *In* The Pathology of Laboratory Animals, edited by W. E. Ribelin, and J. R. McCoy. Springfield, Charles C Thomas, 1965, pp. 303–329.
Eschenbrenner, A.B., and Miller, E.: Induction of hepatomas in mice by repeated oral administration of chloroform, with observations on sex differences. J. Nat. Cancer Inst., *5*:251–255, 1945.
———: Sex difference in kidney morphology and chloroform necrosis. Science, *102*:302–303, 1945.
Hewitt, H.B.: Renal necrosis in mice after accidental exposure to chloroform. Br. J. Exp. Pathol., *37*:32–39, 1956.
Jacobsen, L., Andersen, E., and Thorborg, J.V.: Accidental chloroform nephrosis in mice. Acta Path. Microbiol. Scand., *61*:503–513, 1964.
Shubik, P., and Ritchie, A.C.: Sensitivity of male dba mice to the toxicity of chloroform as a laboratory hazard. Science, *117*:285, 1953.

Chinese Tallow Tree

The Chinese tallow tree (*Sapium sebiferum, Croton sebiferum,* or *Stillingia sebifera*), originally imported from China, is grown in the United States as an ornamental plant. It is quite abundant along the Atlantic coast from South Carolina to Florida and along the Gulf Coast west to Texas and Oklahoma, and it is suspected to cause poisoning in cattle. Leaves and fruit from these trees have been shown experimentally to be toxic to cattle, but less so for sheep and goats (Russell et al., 1969). Administration of material from this tree to cattle was followed by severe diarrhea, weakness, and dehydration within 12 hours. Usual hematologic values (packed cell volume, hemoglobin) were not affected, nor were total serum protein or serum glutamic oxaloacetic transaminase changed. Blood urea nitrogen and serum creatine phosphokinase levels were elevated in some animals.

Gross lesions were found in the intestines, which were thickened and irregularly hyperemic. The kidneys were slightly swollen, and one liver had a yellow oily appearance. The principal lesion appeared to be toxic tubular nephrosis.

The Chinese tallow tree does appear to have a potential for poisoning cattle, although differing conditions of growth may affect its toxic properties.

Russell, L.H., Schwartz, W.L., and Dollahite, J.W.: Toxicity of Chinese tallow tree (*Sapium sebiferum*) for ruminants. Am. J. Vet. Res., *30*:1233–1238, 1969.

Bitterweed

Hymenoxys odorata, known as bitterweed or rubberweed, is a weed native to southwestern United States which has caused considerable losses among sheep. *H. richardsonii* (Colorado rubberweed or Pingue) is also poisonous. The manifestations of bitterweed poisoning have recently been studied by Witzel et al. (1977), who dosed sheep with 1 g of dried *H. odorata* per kilogram body weight per day. Signs, which developed within four to five days, included anorexia, depression, mucoid nasal discharge, and weakness. Most animals died within two weeks.

The principal gross lesions were gaseous and liquid distention of the gastrointestinal tract, edema and congestion of the gastrointestinal tract, ascites, hydropericardium, and hemorrhage in the mucosa of the gallbladder. Microscopically, there was necrosis of the superficial third of the ruminal papillae. Others have reported erosions of the rumen, reticulum, and abomasum. Toxic hepatitis and hepatocellular necrosis were seen in the liver. The authors considered the renal lesions distinctive; these included epithelial degeneration of the proximal and distal convoluted tubules, dilation of tubules, intense congestion, especially through the medullary rays and inner medulla, and proteinaceous casts. The toxic principle has been isolated by Ivie et al. (1975), who termed it hymenovin, a sesquiterpene lactone (see also sneezeweed, page 1022).

Ivie, G.W., et al.: Hymenovin. Major toxic constituent of western bitterweed (*Hymenoxys odorata* DC). J. Agric. Food Chem., *23*:841–845, 1975.
Rowe, L.D., Dollahite, J.W., Kim, H.L., and Camp, B.J.: *Hymenoxys odorata* (bitterweed) poisoning in sheep. Southwestern Vet., *26*:287–293, 1973.
Witzel, D.A., Jones, L.P., and Ivie, G.W.: Pathology of subacute bitterweed (*Hymenoxys odorata*) poisoning in sheep. Vet. Pathol., *14*:73–78, 1977.
Witzel, D.A., Rowe, L.D., and Clark, D.E.: Physiopathologic studies on acute *Hymenoxys odorata* (bitterweed) poisoning in sheep. Am. J. Vet. Res., *35*:931–934, 1974.

GROUP E: CARDIAC INSUFFICIENCY

Poisons of Group E have **cardiac insufficiency** as their prominent clinical sign. The pathogenesis may be direct injury to the myocardium with conspicuous lesions, but more usually it is alkaloids that interfere with cardiac action without causing morphologically demonstrable myocardial lesions (see also Group Q).

Selenium

The rare element selenium exists in appreciable concentrations in the soil of certain areas in the arid western part of North America and in similar situations in other parts of the world. All plants able to grow in such soils tend to incorporate the element in their tissues. This amounts to 20 or 30 ppm in the case of most of the common cereal and forage plants, but certain uncultivated plants which thrive in selenium areas commonly harbor as much as 5000 to 15,000 ppm. In the latter group are species of the genus *Astragalus,* including the common loco weed and milk vetch (*A. bisulcatus*), as well as the woody aster (*Aster parryi*) and saltbush (*Atriplex nuttallii*). (This is not to imply that loco poisoning is due to selenium.) Appreciable amounts of selenium in plants can be detected by a sulfurous odor when the plants are crushed in the hand.

Acute selenium poisoning occurs in herbivorous animals as the result of eating one or several meals of some of the strongly seleniferous weeds, such as those mentioned. Another source of acute poisoning is the administration of overdoses of selenium in the therapeutic or preventative treatment of animals suspected of being deficient in selenium. As little as 10 mg of sodium selenite given orally to young lambs has resulted in fatalities (Morrow, 1968). Differences in susceptibility between species may be considerable, and many other factors, such as nature of the diet, chemical form of the selenium, and rate of administration, have been shown to modify the toxic effects (Muth and Binns, 1964). This form of poisoning is largely an acute congestive and enteric disease, with gastrointestinal symptoms and collapse from respiratory and myocardial failure in a few hours or a day or two. Postmortem lesions include hemorrhagic enteritis and proctitis, passive congestion of the lungs and abdominal viscera, early toxic changes in the liver and kidneys (acute toxic hepatitis and toxic tubular nephrosis), and terminal anoxic hemorrhages in the epicardium and elsewhere. Mucosae of both the bladder and gallbladder, as well as that of the folds of the omasum, are commonly inflamed, probably because the poisonous substance is eliminated through them.

Chronic selenium poisoning has been described under two rather distinct syndromes, "blind staggers" and "alkali disease."

A rather violent termination of slow, cumulative poisoning is picturesquely, though inaccurately, designated by the name, **blind staggers.** This is a reversion to the layman's terminology of a century ago, when mad staggers meant violently painful spasmodic colic, blind staggers, any of the toxic or infectious nervous disturbances

characterized by a desire to press forward, and staggers in general suggested the antics of a horse in severe abdominal pain. This form of selenium poisoning, however, has been seen most commonly in cattle. Somewhat as in Van Es' "walking disease" of horses, which is simply toxic hepatitis caused by senecio poisoning, the animal is impelled to seek relief from constant abdominal discomfort by continuous walking; as the condition worsens, there is actual nervous impairment of vision as well as of other functions, and the animal tries to walk through obstacles that he would normally avoid. He frequently stands pressing his forehead against some solid object, possibly gaining some relief thereby. Great weakness and paralysis supervene, being most severe in the forelimbs, and dyspnea, cyanosis, and death follow as the result of respiratory failure.

The form of chronic selenium poisoning known as **alkali disease** was once attributed to excessive ingestion of soil alkali (e.g., sodium carbonate, sulfate), which is commonly plentiful in the same arid areas where selenium is concentrated. It is now known to result from consumption of mildly seleniferous plants over a period of weeks or months. It is characterized by falling hair, especially of the mane and tail **(bob-tail disease)**, and a related malnutrition of the hoofs. The latter develop deep encircling grooves parallel to the coronary band that are more pronounced than those of laminitis. In the more severe cases, the groove may become a painful crack that causes partial separation of the hoof. Occasionally, one or more hoofs become detached from the sensitive laminae and slough. More often, the distorted hoof remains attached and, with the amount of wear reduced by painful locomotion, the toe grows to an inordinate length, which deforms it with an anterior concavity. This applies to the hooves of either cattle or horses. Eroded joints also make walking difficult, and the animal may die from inability to get food and water. Erosions of the articular surfaces of the long bones, especially of the distal end of the tibia and the proximal end of the metatarsus, are common.

The lesions are basically similar in the two clinical syndromes of chronic selenium poisoning. Myocardial insufficiency accounts for chronic passive congestion of the lungs and splanchnic viscera, and is itself based upon focal necroses in the heart muscle and a reaction that has been described as serofibrinous and spreading into the muscle from the endocardium. Lymphocytic infiltrations accompany these changes in advanced cases. Edema of the pericardial, thoracic, and peritoneal cavities, and of the lungs, brain, and lymph nodes, is doubtless traceable to a cardiac origin as well.

Petechiae and ecchymoses on the external and internal cardiac surfaces and in various other organs are apparently attributable to a direct toxic origin, as are the comparatively mild toxic changes in the liver and kidneys. In the liver, these are described as hydropic degeneration, fatty change and necrosis with eventual fibrous scarring. In sheep, the hepatic damage may attain the status of acute yellow atrophy; in the slowly developing alkali disease of cattle, some livers become truly cirrhotic. In the kidney, there is swelling of the renal epithelium, and hyaline changes and hyaline casts appear in the convoluted tubules.

Widespread hyaline degeneration and fibrinoid necrosis of arterioles, which were believed to be the basis for the edema, hemorrhages, and visceral degenerative changes, have been described in experimental selenium poisoning in swine (Herigstad et al., 1973). In affected swine, there were also edema and necrosis of the cerebral and cerebellar cortices and gray matter of the spinal cord.

The gastrointestinal mucosa suffers from rather mild inflammatory changes in the omasum and upper intestine, which be-

come less conspicuous in proportion to the duration of the illness. Apparently due to a depressant action on smooth muscle, there is nearly always impaction of a dilated rumen and even of the omasum. Hemorrhage and necrosis of the pancreas has been reported in swine. The accumulation of hemosiderin in the spleen in the most chronic (alkali disease) cases probably rests entirely upon the chronic passive congestion, although the possiblity of a hemolytic action seems not to have been fully investigated. Hemolytic anemia has been induced in rats fed sodium selenite (Halverson et al., 1970).

The fetus shares in the deposition of selenium and malformations are common (another example of nongenetic developmental anomalies). Eggs from selenium-fed hens show a constant and severe impairment of hatchability directly proportional to the amount of selenium ingested. Those chicks which do hatch have little vitality.

Gardiner, M.R.: Chronic selenium toxicity studies in sheep. Aust. Vet. J., 42:442–448, 1966.
Glenn, M.W., Jensen, R., and Griner, L.A.: Sodium selenate toxicosis: the effects of extended oral administration of sodium selenate on mortality, clinical signs, fertility and early embryonic development in sheep. Am. J. Vet. Res., 25:1479–1485, 1964.
———: Sodium selenate toxicosis: pathology and pathogenesis of sodium selenate toxicosis in sheep. Am. J. Vet. Res., 25:1486–1494, 1964.
Glenn, M.W., Martin, J.L., and Cummins, L.M.: Sodium selenate toxicosis: the distribution of selenium within the body after prolonged feeding of toxic quantities of sodium selenate to sheep. Am. J. Vet. Res., 25:1495–1499, 1964.
Halverson, A.W., Tsay, D.-t., Triebwasser, K.C., and Whitehead, E.I.: Development of hemolytic anemia in rats fed selenite. Toxicol. Appl. Pharmacol., 17:151–159, 1970.
Herigstad, R.R., Whitehair, C.K., and Olson, O.E.: Inorganic and organic selenium toxicosis in young swine: comparison of pathologic changes with those in swine with vitamin E-selenium deficiency. Am. J. Vet. Res., 34:1227–1238, 1973.
Jacobsson, S.O., and Oksanen, H.E.: The placental transmission of selenium in sheep. Acta Vet. Scand., 7:66–76, 1966.
Morrow, D.A.: Acute selenite toxicosis in lambs. J. Am. Vet. Med. Assoc., 152:1625–1629, 1968.
Muth, O.H., and Binns, W.: Selenium toxicity in

domestic animals. Ann. NY Acad. Sci., *111*:583–590, 1964.

Neethling, L.P., Brown, J.M.M., and de Wet, P.J.: The toxicology and metabolic fate of selenium in sheep. J. S. Afr. Vet. Med. Assoc., *39*:25–33, 1968.

Rosenfeld, I., and Beath, O.A.: Selenium: Geobotany, Biochemistry, Toxicity and Nutrition. New York, Academic Press, 1964.

Death Camas

Zygadenus gramineus, Z. nuttallii, and other closely related species are known by the name of death camas or by the descriptive synonym of wild onion. These are among the most poisonous plants, toxic to all species but eaten most often by sheep. The signs usually do not appear for several hours after the plant is eaten. They consist of nausea and salivation, failing heart and respiration, and great weakness and nervous depression. Terminal coma may be of several hours' duration. Postmortem lesions are usually limited to the congestions of anoxic heart failure and to early changes of acute toxic hepatitis and tubular nephrosis, demonstrable microscopically.

Marsh, C.D., Clawson, A.B., and Marsh, H.: Zygadenus, or death camas. U. S. Dept. Agric. Bull. 125, 1915.

Morris, M.D.: Nuttall death camas poisoning in horses. Vet. Med., *39*:462, 1944.

Nieman, K.W.: Death camas poisoning in fowls. J. Am. Vet. Med. Assoc., *73*:627–631, 1928.

Aconite

Aconitum columbianum, a flowering and ornamental plant known either as monkshood or aconite, is similar to, and often confused with, larkspur. Animals are occasionally poisoned by it, either on the ranges or through contact with garden plants. Therapeutically, the drug is used to slow the heart. In poisonous doses, it not only slows but weakens the cardiac action. The signs are those of restlessness and anxiety, nausea, salivation, abdominal pain, increasing weakness and prostration, a weakening and terminally rapid heart rate, and final asphyxia. Of special diagnostic significance are continual swallowing movements, due to a peculiar irritation of the throat, and a pronounced risus sardonicus, the lips being maximally retracted and displaying the foam-covered teeth as the horse or other animal lies helpless on the ground. Cats and rabbits jump vertically into the air, topple over backwards and go into convulsions. Death is seldom delayed more than an hour or two, so that few lesions can be expected beyond the hemorrhages and congestions incident to asphyxia.

Baileya Multiradiata

This is a plant of the arid Southwest, from Texas to California, which sheep eat reluctantly with poisonous results. Its many slender stalks reach a height of 50 to 60 cm, bear elongated, tongue-shaped leaves on their lower parts, and terminate each in a single yellow flower-head at the top.

Signs include the usual arched back, loss of weight, and disinclination to move. Excessive salivation appears early. If the animal is forced to exercise, cardiac embarrassment, which is the fundamental disturbance, is revealed by a rapid, pounding heart action audible at a distance of several feet.

The lesions are those of congestive heart failure, including venous congestion of the liver, spleen, kidneys, and other abdominal viscera. Zenker's necrosis and preliminary degenerative changes proceed in the myocardium, commonly involving muscle cells individually here and there. Pursuant to the congestive and anoxemic state, the parenchymatous cells of the liver and renal cortical tubules undergo hydropic degeneration and fatty change. If the illness continues for several days, acute dilatation of the damaged ventricles develops. On the other hand, if the cardiac failure brings a more sudden anoxic death, widespread hemorrhages over the epicardium, diaphragm, and other areas result, as is usual in terminal anoxia.

A considerable proportion of animals slowly recover after several days, during which all food is refused.

Mathews, F.P.: Toxicity of *Baileya multiradiata* for sheep and goats. J. Am. Vet. Med. Assoc., *83*:673–679, 1933.

Jimson Weed, Thornapple

Datura stramonium and a few other closely related species, known as Jimson weed, thornapple, mad apple, stinkweed, stinkwort, Jamestown lily, and some others, are of worldwide distribution. While ordinarily unpalatable, the ingested plant has considerable toxicity, which is due to the powerful alkaloids, atropine and hyoscyamine. The domesticated herbivora, birds, and humans are sometimes poisoned.

Signs are chiefly nervous, with excitement which may deepen into insane delirium somewhat suggestive of rabies, and which is usually followed by incoordination, coma, and death. Dilated pupils are of considerable diagnostic significance. Inhibition of salivary and related secretions leads to extreme thirst with consequent polyuria. The heart beat, no longer restrained by the paralyzed vagus, becomes rapid and weak, and death is from anoxia. The signs appear within minutes or after only a few hours. Recovery, if it occurs, requires several days. Lesions include marked congestion and edema of the lungs, hydrothorax, congestion of the meninges, and dilation of the ventricles. Hemorrhages characteristic of asphyxia occur, as well as petechiae in the brain, stomach, and upper intestine. Recognizable fragments of the large leaves or of the "thornapples" may be found in the stomach or forestomachs.

Jimson weed has been associated with congenital arthrogryposis in swine, but the causal relationship has not been firmly established.

Behrens, H., and Horn, M.: Tolerance of pigs to *Datura stramonium* seeds (TT). Prakt Tierarzt., No. 2:43–44, 1962.

King, E.D., Jr.: Jimson weed poisoning. J. Am. Vet. Med. Assoc., *64*:98–99, 1923.

Leipold, H.W., Oehme, F.W., and Cook, J.E.: Congenital arthrogryposis associated with ingestion of jimsonweed by pregnant sows. J. Am. Vet. Med. Assoc., *162*:1059–1060, 1973.

Pimelea

An obscure disease of cattle in Australia termed **St. George disease** has been recognized for several decades, but the cause of the syndrome has remained in doubt. Recent outbreaks of the disease have been associated with the presence of *Pimelea simplex* (desert rue flower), a small perennial herb native to Queensland. Feeding trials with the plant have reproduced most of the clinical and pathologic features of field cases of St. George disease. Although principally a disease of cattle, losses of horses have also been attributed to *Pimelea*, and experimentally the plant has been demonstrated to be toxic to horses.

Clinically, there is diarrhea (which may be tinged with blood), weakness, anemia, and signs of circulatory failure. There is a jugular pulse and pronounced subcutaneous edema, especially in the submaxillary and pharyngeal regions extending to the brisket, ventral abdomen, and to a lesser degree, the limbs. Pathologically, the most striking finding is extensive edema and congestion of all organs and tissues, but especially the subcutis and gastrointestinal tract. There is hydrothorax. Histologically, villous atrophy and small ulcers and hemorrhages may be present in the intestine, but the changes are minimal when compared to the extent of the diarrhea. The heart is dilated without hypertrophy and small foci of myocardial necrosis are present. The liver is enlarged and dark purple. Hepatic sinusoids are dilated and hepatocytes are atrophic. The anemia, which is a consistent finding, may be characterized by hemoglobin levels as low as 5.5 g/100 ml. The pathogenesis is obscure: the bone marrow is neither suppressed nor hyperplastic, and hemorrhage rarely extensive. It is postulated that it is primarily the result of hemodilution.

Roberts et al. (1975) have isolated a toxin called **simplexin** which is capable of causing cardiac insufficiency. The mechanism of action in experimental poisoning and the pathogenesis of the natural disease, however, remain obscure.

Hill, M.W.M.: Toxicity of *Pimelea decora* in horses. Aust. Vet. J., *46*:287–289, 1970.

Kelly, W.R.: The pathology and haematological changes in experimental *Pimelea spp.* poisoning in cattle ("St. George disease"). Aust. Vet. J., *51*:233–243, 1975.

Kelly, W.R.: [59]Fe utilisation and excretion in anaemia of cattle caused by *Pimelea trichostachya* intoxication. Aust. Vet. J., *51*:504–510, 1975.

McClure, T.J., and Farrow, B.R.H.: Chronic poisoning of cattle by desert rice flower (*Pimelea simplex*) and its resemblance to St. George disease as seen in north-western New South Wales. Aust. Vet. J., *47*:100–102, 1971.

Roberts, H.B., and Healy, P.J.: *Pimelea simplex* and St. George disease of cattle. Aust. Vet. J., *47*:123–124, 1971.

Roberts, H.B., et al.: The isolation and structure of the toxin of *Pimelea simplex* responsible for St. George disease of cattle. Aust. Vet. J., *51*:325–326, 1975.

Rogers, R.J., and Roberts, K.H.: *Pimelea altior* poisoning of cattle. Aust. Vet. J., *52*:193–194, 1976.

GROUP F: EXTENSIVE HEMORRHAGE

Dicoumarin

Sweet clover hay (not pasturage) contains a substance called coumarin, which not infrequently undergoes change into a related compound, known as dicoumarin or dicumarol. This substance is such a potent anticoagulant for the blood that it has been adopted as a drug for use when reduced coagulability of the blood is desired, and has been utilized as a rat poison in the commercial product called warfarin. The anticoagulant action, although not completely understood, results primarily from depressing the synthesis of prothrombin and factors VII, IX, and X, all of which require vitamin K for their formation. Vitamin K inhibits the anticoagulant effect, but apparently is not a complete antidote for the poisoning (Collentine and Quick, 1951). The interference with the synthesis of clotting factors results from the accumulation of a natural metabolite inhibitory to vitamin K (a naphthoquinone

[Vitamin K]-2, 3-epoxide). Normally, this epoxide is reduced to vitamin K, but in the presence of warfarin, the reductase is inhibited. Apparently capillary permeability is also affected by warfarin independently from its anticoagulant activity. Loss of endothelial ground substances and organelles and degeneration of smooth muscle and elastic fibers have been described (Kahn et al., 1971). Horses are not affected by this hay. Rabbits are very susceptible and may be used to test the safety of a given supply of hay, since they die from hemorrhages in a much shorter time than cattle (6 to 12 days). Warfarin is poisonous to dogs and doubtless to all species.

Historically, the development of dicoumarin as an important anticoagulant drug started with the studies of Schofield (1924) on a new disease of cattle. Schofield described this disease as manifest by large hemorrhages that occurred in animals recently fed on hay made from sweet clover. He aptly named the disease **sweet clover poisoning** and correctly ascribed the signs and lesions to the anticoagulant effect of something in the sweet clover. Roderick (1929, 1931) demonstrated that this substance was water-soluble and easily extracted from sweet clover hay. Campbell and Link (1941) eventually isolated, crystallized, and identified the active ingredient as dicoumarin.

Signs arise after cattle have consumed the poisonous hay for about a month, and consist of uncontrollable hemorrhage from accidental or operative wounds and slow internal hemorrhages as the result of bruises and minor injuries. Postmortem lesions take the form of "hematomas" in the subcutis, between the muscles, or beneath the capsules of organs. Ecchymoses occur in many places, commonly beneath the endocardium. The liver lobule is likely to contain petechiae and may show fatty change or hydropic degeneration. Necrosis and hyaline-droplet degeneration involve the renal tubules; scattered small foci of necrosis may be found in the heart.

Newborn calves may be affected, be-

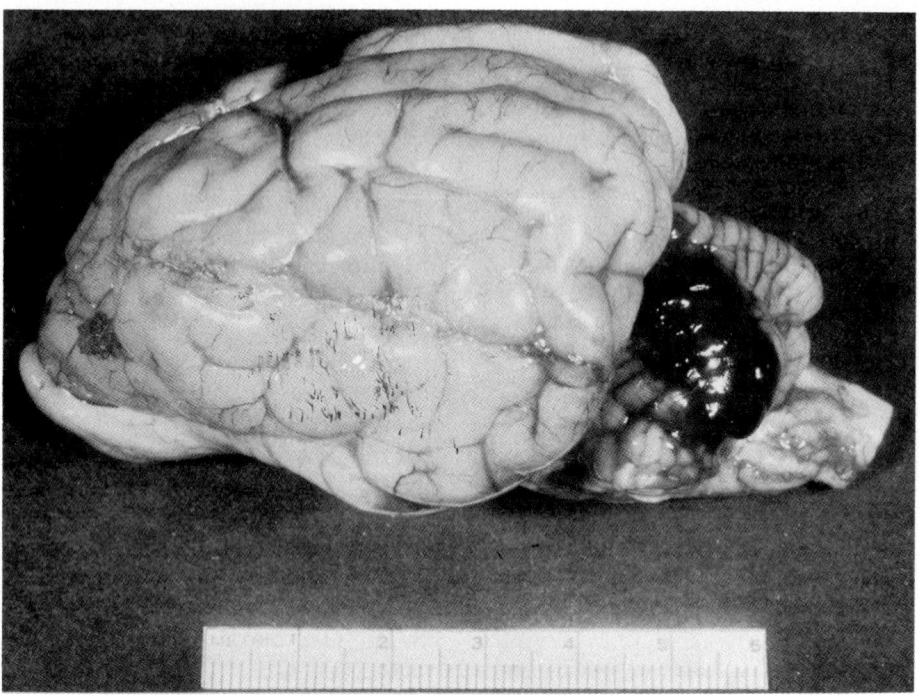

Fig. 16–13. Hemorrhage in the leptomeninges due to warfarin (dicoumarin) poisoning in a 15-year-old male mongrel collie. (Courtesy of Angell Memorial Animal Hospital.)

cause dicoumarin crosses the placenta, even though their dams do not manifest clinical signs at the time of parturition. This apparently results from a transient hypoprothrombinemia in calves, which is intensified by the transplacental passage of dicoumarin. Cows that produce such calves may be shown to be feeding on sweet clover hay, and the clotting time of their blood is prolonged.

Broman, U.: The postmortem findings in dicoumarol poisoning in dogs and cats. Nord. Vet. Med., 13:604–611, 1961.

Campbell, H.A., et al.: Studies on the hemorrhagic sweet clover disease. I. The preparation of hemorrhagic concentrates. J. Biol. Chem., 136:47–55, 1940.

Campbell, H.A., and Link, K.P.: Studies on the hemorrhagic sweet clover disease. IV. The isolation and crystallization of the hemorrhagic agent. J. Biol. Chem., 138:21–33, 1941.

Campbell, H.A., et al.: Studies on the hemorrhagic sweet clover disease. II. The bioassay of hemorrhagic concentrates by following the prothrom-

bin level in the plasma of rabbit blood. J. Biol. Chem., 138:1–20, 1941.

Clark, W.T., and Halliwell, R.E.W.: The treatment with vitamin K preparations of warfarin poisoning in dogs. Vet. Rec., 75:1210–1213, 1963.

Collentine, G.E., and Quick, A.J.: The interrelationship of vitamin K and dicoumarin. Am. J. Med. Sci., 222:7–12, 1951.

Forbes, C.D., et al.: Experimental warfarin poisoning in the dog. Platelet function, coagulation and fibrinolysis. J. Comp. Pathol., 83:173–180, 1973.

Fraser, C.M., and Nelson, J.: Sweet clover poisoning in newborn calves. J. Am. Vet. Med. Assoc., 135:283–286, 1959.

Kahn, R.A., Johnson, S.A., and DeGraff, A.F.: Effects of sodium warfarin on capillary ultrastructure. Am. J. Pathol., 65:149–156, 1971.

Prier, R.F., and Derse, P.H.: Evaluation of the hazard of secondary poisoning by warfarin-poisoned rodents. J. Am. Vet. Med. Assoc., 140:351–354, 1962.

Roderick, L.M.: The pathology of sweet clover disease in cattle. J. Am. Vet. Med. Assoc., 74:314–324, 1929.

———: A problem in the coagulation of the blood. "Sweet clover disease in cattle." Am. J. Physiol., 96:413, 1931.

Stahmann, M.A., Huebner, C.F., and Link, K.P.: Studies on the sweet clover disease. V. Identification and synthesis of the hemorrhagic agent. J. Biol. Chem., 138:513–527, 1941.

Schofield, F.W.: Damaged sweet clover: the cause of a new disease in cattle simulating hemorrhagic septicemia and blackleg. J. Am. Vet. Med. Assoc., 64:553–575, 1924.

Wignell, W.N.: Dicoumarol poisoning of cattle and sheep in South Australia. Aust. Vet. J., 37:456–459, 1961.

Zimmermann, A., and Matschiner, J.T.: Biochemical basis of hereditary resistance to warfarin in the rat. Biochem. Pharmacol., 23:1033–1040, 1974.

Bracken Fern

This common fern, *Pteris aquilina (Adlerfarn,* German), grows in most humid parts of the world. Poisoning of cattle has been reported form the eastern and far northwestern United States, Central Europe, Great Britain, Central and South America, the Middle East, Southern India, Java, and the Philippines. Illness appears after the plant has been consumed in quantity for several months. The manifestations of bracken fern poisoning in monogastric animals and ruminants differ.

In cattle and sheep, bracken fern causes severe hypoplasia or aplasia of the hematopoietic tissue, to which most signs and lesions can be ascribed. The illness may start suddenly with high fever, hemorrhages from any and often several body openings, delayed clotting time, thrombocytopenia, neutropenia, anemia, and death in one to three days. Diarrhea or upper respiratory inflammation may be noted. The hemorrhage results from the thrombocytopenia as well as increased levels of anticoagulant substances in the blood. Secondary infection follows the neutropenia, resulting in the high fever. Under experimental conditions, as long as 15 months may be required before signs of toxicity ensue. The acute, and usually terminal, episode may occur weeks after removal from access to the plant. The active principle responsible for the depression of bone marrow has not been identified.

Experimental evidence (Rosenberger, 1960) supports the idea that **bovine enzootic hematuria** is a part of the syndrome resulting from poisoning by bracken fern. Although the active principle is not yet clearly established, prolonged feeding of bracken fern to cattle is followed by lesions in the bladder and the generalized hemorrhagic syndrome.

Autopsy lesions include widespread petechiae and ecchymoses, especially on the heart and other serous surfaces, on mucous membranes, and in muscles and the subcutaneous tissues. Abomasal ecchymoses in cattle may lead to ulceration. The large bowel often contains clotted blood. Necrotic areas in the liver have been described by some. Thrombocytopenia is marked and is the cause of the hemorrhages. Neutropenia and terminal anemia accompany the thrombocytopenia and are due to destruction of the early myeloid cells. Megakaryocytes disappear.

The lesions in the urinary system most often involve the bladder, but may also occur in the ureters or renal pelvis, and appear to represent a chronic but violently hyperplastic and hemorrhagic inflammation that leads to frank neoplasia. The transitional epithelium undergoes localized proliferation with metaplasia to mucinous columnar or stratified squamous types or a mixture of the two (Fig. 16–14). In many cases, the hyperplastic epithelium acquires neoplastic properties, developing into a squamous cell or adenocarcinoma, which is locally invasive and may metastasize to the regional lymph nodes and lungs. The capillaries of the inflammatory lesion also participate in the hyperplasia, sometimes to the extent of forming hemangiomas in the stroma or projecting from the mucosal surface. These hemangiomas may be the source of much of the hemorrhage into the urine, and are capable of developing malignant qualities.

The carcinogenic properties of bracken fern have been demonstrated experimentally in cattle as well as laboratory animals, in which a variety of neoplasms have resulted, including intestinal adenocarcinomas in rats and quail, malignant lym-

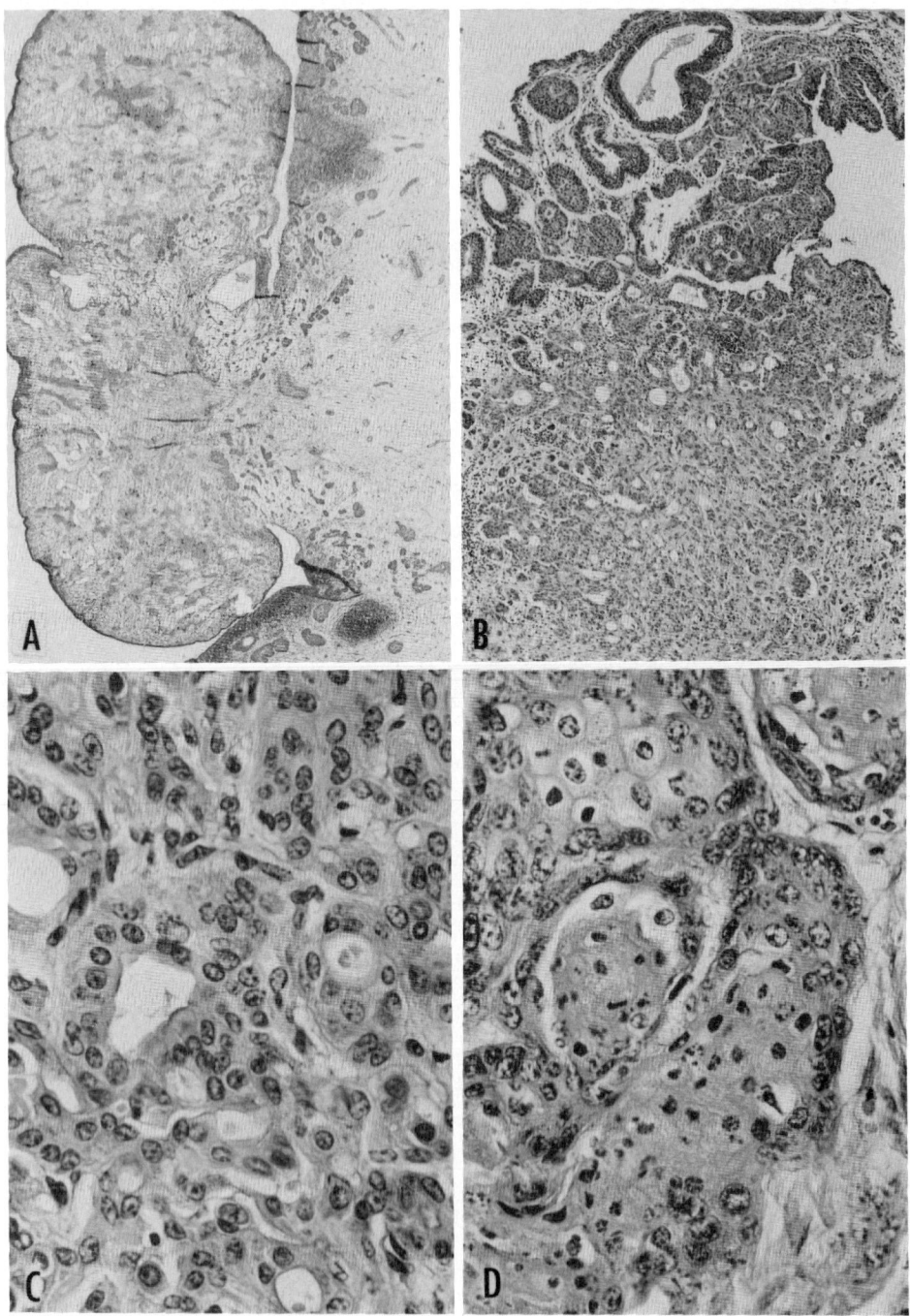

Fig. 16–14. Bovine enzootic hematuria. *A,* Papillomatous hemangioma in the urinary bladder (× 24). *B,* Neoplastic transformation in the urinary bladder (× 50) with transitional cell carcinoma and adenocarcinoma in juxtaposition. *C,* Adenocarcinoma (× 350), higher magnification of *B. D,* Squamous cell carcinoma (× 350) in bovine urinary bladder. (*A, C* and *D* courtesy of Armed Forces Institute of Pathology.) Contributor: Dr. Sati Baran.

phoma and pulmonary adenomas in mice, and bladder tumors in guinea pigs.

In Great Britain, bracken fern has been associated with a form of **retinal atrophy** in sheep known as **bright blindness.** The condition, which has been experimentally reproduced, develops in the absence of the changes just described. It is characterized by loss of rods and cones and reduction in the width of the outer nuclear layer. The lesions are most extensive in the tapetal region, and when advanced, the layer of rods and cones and outer nuclear layer are completely destroyed. The factor responsible has not been identified.

In differential diagnosis, it is to be noted that in sweet clover poisoning the hemorrhages are very large, with hematomas often forming in the tissues, and there is no fever. Blood transfusions are promptly curative in sweet clover poisoning. In crotalaria poisoning, the hemorrhages may show no differential features, but the liver usually shows considerable fibrosis, the gallbladder is distended, and there is often edema of the abomasal and duodenal tissues. In poisoning by trichloroethylene-extracted soybean meal, hemorrhages and anemia are the principal lesions, and differentiation may depend on the history. Anaplasmosis has to be considered, but can usually be distinguished by the large spleen and by finding the causative organism in the erythrocytes. Leptospirosis causes fever and hemorrhages, but the latter are much less extensive. Icterus should be present with both these infections. Demonstration of a high serologic titer or of the leptospirae in the kidney or liver by silver techniques is decisive. In none of the above conditions, except at one stage of leptospirosis, is there neutropenia comparable to that of bracken poisoning.

In horses and in experimental rats, the usual bracken poisoning is cured by administration of thiamine (Cordy, 1952), but this is not so in cattle. Thiaminase appears to be one of the active toxic principles. Presumably cattle synthesize

adequate thiamine and other B-vitamins, and the toxicity of the bracken fern is based upon other actions. In horses, therefore, bracken poisoning is similar to poisoning by equisetum and the lesions are those of thiamine deficiency. Affected horses become incoordinated and ataxic, develop tremors, may fall, and ultimately are recumbent. Although there is thrombocytopenia and depression of other hematopoietic elements, the neuropathologic sequelae overshadow these lesions. Presumably the hematopoietic changes are based upon the same toxic principles as in cattle, but their relationship to thiamine deficiency is not resolved. In swine, focal myocardial necrosis, comparable to that caused by thiamine deficiency in this and other species, has been described in experimentally poisoned animals.

Barnett, K.C., and Watson, W.A.: Bright blindness in sheep. A primary retinopathy due to feeding bracken (Pteris aquilina). Res. Vet. Sci., 11:289–290, 1970.

Beran, G.W.: Bovine cystic hematuria in the Philippines: a report on an enzootic area. J. Am. Vet. Med. Assoc., 149:1686–1690, 1966.

Bryan, G.T., Brown, R.R., and Price, J.M.: Studies on the etiology of bovine bladder cancer. Ann. NY Acad. Sci., 108:924–937, 1963.

Caine, R., Albert, D.M., Lahav, M., and Bullock, J.: Oxalate retinopathy: an experimental model of a flecked retina. Invest. Ophthalmol., 14:359–363, 1975.

Cordy, D.R.: The pathology of experimental bracken poisoning in rats. Cornell Vet., 42:108–117, 1952.

Döbereiner, J., et al.: Metabolites in urine of cattle with experimental bladder lesions and fed bracken fern. Pesquisa agropec. bras., 1:189–199, 1966. VB 38:1133, 1968.

Dzuvic, A.: Bovine chronic haematuria: histopathology of the bladder in spontaneous and experimental cases. Dtsch. Tierarztl. Wschr., 76:260–263, 1969. VB 39:4763, 1969.

Evans, I.A., and Mason, J.: Carcinogenic activity of bracken. Nature, 208:913–914, 1965.

Evans, I.A., et al.: Studies on bracken poisoning in cattle. Part V. Br. Vet. J., 114:253–267, 1958.

Evans, W.C., Widdop, B., and Harding, J.D.J.: Experimental poisoning by bracken rhizomes in pigs. Vet. Rec., 90:471–475, 1972.

Georgiev, R., and Antonov, S.: Aetiology of chronic bovine haematuria. II. The presence of carcinogenic metabolites in the urine of a healthy cow fed on hay from a haematuria region. Vet.

Med. Nauki, Sofia, 1:29–32, 1964. VB 35:293, 1965.

Georgiev, R., et al.: Aetiology of bovine chronic hematuria. I. Its cancerous nature. Vet. Med. Nauki, Sofia, 1:21–35, 1964. VB 35:292, 1965.

Gorisek, J., and Marzan, B.: Changes in blood picture and blood coagulation in calves with bracken poisoning. Wien. Tierarztl. Mschr., 52:530–538, 1965. VB 36:744, 1966.

Hagan, W.A.: Bracken poisoning of cattle. Cornell Vet., 15:326–332, 1925.

Hirono, I., et al.: Comparative study of carcinogenic activity in each part of bracken. J. Natl. Cancer Inst., 50:1367–1371, 1973.

Nandi, S.N.: Histopathology of enzootic bovine haematuria in the Darjeeling district of India. Br. Vet. J., 125:587–590, 1969.

Pamukcu, A.M., Ertürk, E., Price, J.M., and Bryan, G.T.: Lymphatic leukemia and pulmonary tumors in female Swiss mice fed bracken fern (Pteris aquilina). Cancer Res., 32:1442–1445, 1972.

Pamukcu, A.M., Olson, C., and Goksoy, S.K.: Influence of a papilloma vaccine on chronic bovine enzootic haematuria. Cancer Res., 27:2197–2200, 1967.

Pamukcu, A.M., Price, J.M., and Bryan, G.T.: Assay of fractions of bracken fern (Pteris aquilina) for carcinogenic activity. Cancer Res., 30:902–905, 1970.

———: Naturally occurring and bracken fern-induced bovine urinary bladder tumors. Clinical and morphological characteristics. Vet. Pathol., 13:110–122, 1976.

Parker, W.H., and McCrea, C.T.: Bracken (Pteris aquilina) poisoning of sheep in the North York moors. Vet. Rec., 77:861–866, 1965.

Parodi, A.: Lesions in idiopathic haematuria of cattle. Revue Path. Comp., 66:589–591, 1966. VB 37:4867, 1967.

Rosenberger, G.: Uber die Ursache der Haematuria Vesicalis Bovis. Proc. 17th World Vet. Congr. Hanover, 2:1167–1170, 1963.

———: Prolonged feeding of bracken (Pteris aquilina), as cause of bovine chronic haematuria. Wien. Tierarztl. Mschr., 52:415–421, 1965. VB 36:743, 1966.

Rosenberger, G., and Heeschen, W.: Adlerfarn (Pteris aquilina)—die Ursache des sog. Stallrotes der Rinder (Haematuria vesicalis bovis chronica.) Dtsch. Tierarztl. Wschr., 67:201–208, 1960.

Sippel, W.L.: Bracken fern poisoning. J. Am. Vet. Med. Assoc., 121:9–13, 1952.

Stamatovic, S., Bratanovic, U., and Sofrenovic, D.: The clinical picture of haematuria in cattle, experimentally produced by feeding of bracken (Pteris aquilina). Wien Tierarztl. Mschr., 52:589–596, 1965. VB 36:321, 1966.

Watson, W.A., Barnett, K.C., and Terlecki, S.: Progressive retinal degeneration (bright blindness) in sheep: a review. Vet. Rec., 91:665–670, 1972.

Watson, W.A., et al.: Experimentally produced progressive retinal degeneration (bright blindness) in sheep. Br. Vet. J., 128:457–469, 1972.

Yamane, O., et al.: Studies on hemorrhagic diathesis of experimental bovine bracken poisoning. I. Detection of circulating anticoagulants. II. Heparin-like substance level in blood. Jpn. J. Vet. Sci., 37:335–347, 1975.

Trichloroethylene-Extracted Soybean Meal

Soybean meal derived from soybeans, the oil of which was extracted by trichloroethylene, has been known to produce poisoning of livestock, chiefly ruminants and horses (Stockman, 1916). Owing to the infrequent use of that method of extraction losses attracted little attention until the period of increased production following World War II. The disease probably can now be relegated to the past. Soybean meal prepared by this process ceased to be used in 1952, following demonstration of the causative role of trichloroethylene. Apparently trichloroethylene reacts with soybean protein to produce a toxic ingredient. Trichloroethylene itself is also toxic, but causes a different syndrome. Names applied earlier to this syndrome before its true nature was known are Stockman disease, Duren disease, and Brabant disease.

The signs and lesions result from suppression (aplasia) of all elements of the bone marrow, and thus mimic bracken fern poisoning of ruminants.

Depending upon the amount fed and the toxicity of the particular sample of meal, symptoms appear after from 1 to 9 months of feeding and usually last for from 5 to 10 days (rarely 20 days), before they are terminated by death. New cases continue to arise for some time after the offending meal has been removed from the diet. In the usual acute cases, the first positive signs of the disease are (1) a serous nasal exudate, later becoming viscous and hemorrhagic, (2) sudden high fever, possibly due to secondary infection, (3) petechiae on the visible mucous membranes, and (4) slight or copious hemorrhages from any of the body openings, including the anus. Signs of abdominal pain are prominent in a few. Subcutaneous or deeper hematomas are not infrequent, sometimes causing lameness. Depression and emaciation are terminal. A minority of affected bovines experience a more chronic form, with weakness, ataxia, anemic paleness of mucous membranes, jaundice, and irregularity of the bowels, but with few hemorrhages.

Blood studies reveal the fundamental myeloaplastic nature of the disease. Thrombocytopenia with platelet counts dropping from the normal 250,000 to 20,000 is the cause of the widespread hemorrhages, the clotting times showing only inconstant variations. Extreme neutropenia, with lymphocytes constituting almost the whole of the white cells, is shortly followed by severe normochromic and normocytic anemia, the erythrocyte counts descending to 3,000,000 and the hemoglobin to 5 or 6 g/100 ml. The postmortem lesions consist of spectacular hemorrhages, which are likely to be found in almost any location or tissue in the animal's body. In the stomach and intestines, the hemorrhagic areas are often hemorrhagic ulcers (bacterial invasion); liver, kidneys, and brain do not escape. Microscopically, the arterioles are frequently necrotic and ruptured. This explains how the hemorrhages start; the lack of platelets explains why they are not limited to small sizes. There is also extensive necrosis in the liver, centrilobular or massive. Fibrous proliferation constitutes a healing reaction around many of the ruptured vessels. The bone marrow is highly aplastic, with few normal erythroblasts and fewer granulocytes.

Trichloroethylene is still used as an industrial solvent, degreasing agent, and anesthetic. Poisoning in man (and presumably animals) may result from inhalation or ingestion, and is characterized by neurologic signs (confusion, incoordination, dizziness, headache, convulsions, coma), nausea, vomiting, and occasionally death from respiratory failure or cardiac arrhythmias. Impure trichloroethylene may decompose to chlorine, hydrochloric acid, phosgene, and other compounds that are highly irritant to the skin and respiratory passages.

Eveleth, D.F., and Holm, G.C.: Feed toxicity similar to that caused by trichloroethylene-extracted soybean oil meal. J. Am. Vet. Med. Assoc., 122:377–378, 1953.

Huff, J.E.: New evidence on the old problems of trichloroethylene. Industr. Med. Surg., 40:25–33, 1971.

Kleinfeld, M., and Tabershaw, I.R.: Trichloroethylene toxicity (in man); five fatal cases. Arch. Ind. Hyg., 10:134–141, 1954.

Menzani, C.: La malattia di Düren o malattia dei Brabante. (Intossicazione da trichloroetilene). Atti soc. ital. sci. vet., 3:493–499, 1949.

Pritchard, W.R., Rehfeld, C.E., and Sautter, J.H.: Aplastic anemia of cattle associated with trichloroethylene-extracted soybean oil meal. J. Am. Vet. Med. Assoc., 121:1–8, 1952.

Sautter, J.H., Rehfeld, C.E., and Pritchard, W.R.: Necropsy findings: aplastic anemia of cattle associated with ingestion of trichyloroethylene-extracted soybean meal. J. Am. Vet. Med. Assoc., 121:73–79, 1952.

Stockman, S.: Poisoning in cattle on meal from soybean after extraction of the oil. J. Comp. Pathol. Ther., 29:95–107, 1916.

Twiehaus, M.J., and Leasure, E.E.: A hemorrhagic factor in soybean pellets extracted with trichloroethylene. Vet. Med., 46:428–431, 1951.

GROUP G: ANEMIA

Clearly, most poisonings characterized by hemorrhage, discussed in the preceding group, are also characterized by anemia.

Molybdenum

In Florida, in California, and in other areas of the western United States and in England, certain muck or shale soils ("teart" soils in England) contain enough molybdenum that green pasture plants, but not cured hay, contain toxic amounts of the element. Ruminants are almost exclusively affected, principally cattle.

Signs include unthriftiness or emaciation, a faded and rough hair coat, apathy, anemia, foul and gaseous diarrhea, sterility, and evidence of painful locomotion. Lesions are hypochromic, microcytic anemia and emaciation. Enlargement of the epiphyses of the long bones and of the costochondral articulations, comparable to those of ordinary rickets, may occur in the young; in older animals, there is rarefaction of bone with a susceptibility to fractures. Aspermatogenesis, likely to be permanent, occurs in bulls; in cows, there is reversible cessation of ovarian function. Among the progeny of affected animals, there is an unusually high percentage of developmental anomalies.

Chemically, molybdenum appears to facilitate the excretion of phosphorus, which may be the mechanism of the disorders of bone, although the levels of blood phosphorus and calcium are usually normal. Molybdenum poisoning usually occurs in animals whose intake of copper is low, and for reasons unknown, increasing the copper in the diet (copper sulfate, 1 or 2 g daily) prevents the deleterious effects of a surprising amount of molybdenum. Copper deficiency has also been noticed to have a more pronounced effect in the presence of molybdenum in the bovine diet. We may ask whether the anemia given as a characteristic of molybdenum poisoning is not due to lack of utilizable copper.

Britton, J.W., and Goss, H.: Chronic molybdenum poisoning in cattle. J. Am. Vet. Med. Assoc., *108*:176–178, 1947.
Cook, G.A., et al.: Interrelationship of molybdenum and certain factors to the development of the molybdenum toxicity syndrome. J. Anim. Sci., 25:96–101, 1966.
Gardner, A.W., and Hall-Patch, P.K.: An outbreak of industrial molybdenosis. Vet. Rec., *74*:113–116, 1962.
Muir, W.R.: The teart pastures of Somerset. Vet. J., *97*:387–400, 1941.

Naphthalene

Poisoning by naphthalene (naphthol, not naphtha) has occurred in humans from the accidental ingestion of moth-balls, and in dogs experimentally (Zuelzer and Apt, 1949). While symptoms include anorexia and nausea, the principal effect is the destruction within a few days of a majority of the erythrocytes with hemoglobinuria and hemolytic jaundice. The liver and kidneys develop toxic degenerative changes. The contrast with the pathologic effects of the *chlorinated* naphthalenes is interesting.

Abelson, S.M., and Henderson, A.T.: Moth ball poisoning. U.S. Armed Forces Med. J., 2:491–493, 1951.
Zuelzer, W.W., and Apt, L.: Acute hemolytic anemia due to naphthalene poisoning. J. Am. Med. Assoc., *141*:185–190, 1949.

Onions

In onion-growing districts, it is not unusual for cattle and sheep to be given cull or unsalable onions *(Allium cepa)* as a major part of their diet. Even when somewhat decomposed, onions appear to be palatable and commonly harmless. Nevertheless, poisoning, often fatal, does occur unexpectedly in these animals and in horses, and in dogs experimentally. Wild onions *(A. canadense, A. validum)* are also toxic and occasionally poison horses, cattle, and sheep grazing on pastures containing these plants. The toxic principle (hemolysin) of onions is n-propyl disulfide, which alters glucose-6-phosphatase, resulting in denaturation and precipitation of hemoglobin.

Both symptoms and lesions can be summarized as hemolytic anemia, hemolytic icterus, and hemoglobinuria. The signs may arise within a few days of the onion diet; the anemia, as estimated by hemoglobin determinations, may be extreme, but clinical recovery occurs in a few days if the animal, not yet moribund, is given a change in diet. The breath, urine, and tissues have a strong odor of onions, making diagnosis easy. Wild onions, of which there are several species, have the same propensities, but animals are not likely to get sufficient quantities to do more than flavor the milk, in the case of dairy cows. Experimental feeding of one species of wild onion *(Allium validum)* to pregnant ewes resulted in loss of appetite and weight, plus depression of erythropoietic tissues, but had no effect on fetal development (James and Binns, 1966).

Goldsmith, W.W.: Onion poisoning in cattle. J. Comp. Pathol. Therap., 22:151, 1909.
James, L.F., and Binns, W.: Effect of feeding wild

onions (*Allium validum*) to bred ewes. J. Am. Vet. Med. Assoc., 149:512–514, 1966.

Kirk, J.H., and Bulgin, M.S.: Effects of feeding cull domestic onions (*Allium cepa*) to sheep. Am. J. Vet. Res., 30:397–399, 1979.

Koger, L.M.: Onion poisoning in cattle. J. Am. Vet. Med. Assoc., 129:75, 1956.

Pierce, K.R., Joyce, J.R., England, R.B., and Jones, L.P.: Acute hemolytic anemia caused by wild onion poisoning in horses. J. Am. Vet. Med. Assoc., 160:323–327, 1972.

Sebrell, W.H.: Anemia of dogs produced by feeding onions. Pub. Health Rep., 45:1175–1191, 1930.

Thorp, F., Jr., and Harshfield, G.S.: Onion poisoning in horses. J. Am. Vet. Med. Assoc., 94:52–53, 1939.

Van Kampen, K.R., James, L.F., and Johnson, A.E.: Hemolytic anemia in sheep fed wild onion (*Allium validum*). J. Am. Vet. Med. Assoc., 156:328–332, 1970.

GROUP H: METHEMOGLOBIN

Poisons in Group H are characterized by production of **methemoglobin** with chocolate-colored blood and the associated inability of hemoglobin to function as a carrier of oxygen.

Nitrates and Nitrites

Human beings, as well as animals, have been poisoned by drinking or ingesting with the food, water containing nitrates in solution. Such water always comes from shallow, surface wells (or possibly from ponds or pools). Waters causing poisoning usually have contained between 1000 and 3000 ppm of nitrate; however, since the presence of nitrates indicates organic pollution, water containing any amount of nitrate is undesirable even if within the limits of chemical safety. Another possible source of poisoning is the swallowing of lubricating oil to which nitrites have been added by the manufacturer. This has happened in a human being. The release of nitric oxide and nitrogen dioxide from automobile exhausts and other combustion sources provides another means of exposure. Herbivorous animals will also lick or eat commercial fertilizers left in their way and are poisoned by the nitrates contained therein. Sheep are especially prone to eat such salty-tasting compounds, even when

adequately supplied with sodium chloride. "Salting the range" was the spreading of salt-petre (potassium nitrate) in places where sheep would eat it, a practice which our pioneer cattlemen are said to have used in an effort to drive sheep-raisers and their flocks from an area of free range in the public domain of the then unsettled western United States.

But the usual source of nitrate and nitrite poisoning in veterinary practice is in plants, growing or cured, which have derived a large amount of nitrate, chiefly KNO_3, from a soil excessively rich in that substance. Among the plants that have been found at one time or another to contain poisonous amounts of nitrates are oats, either green, as hay, straw or stubble, barley, wheat, millets, flax, cornstalks (maize), sorghums, sugar-beet leaves, and a number of weeds, including pigweed (*Amaranthus retroflexus*) and variegated (or "bull") thistle (*Silybum marianum*). Some species of *Astragalus* that synthesize aliphatic nitro compounds may also cause nitrite poisoning. *Astragalus* species are also the cause of locoweed poisoning and selenium poisoning. The application of weed killers such as "2, 4-D," 2, 4-dichlorophenoxyacetic acid, sometimes causes a marked increase in the nitrate content of some plants, such as sugar beets, the harvested leaves of which are a standard feed for ruminants. The sorghums, of course, are noted for the development of hydrocyanic acid, but occasionally appear to have been poisonous through an excessive content of nitrate. To what extent the rather frequent **"corn-stalk poisoning"** has been poisoning by nitrates is a difficult question, but evidence indicates that some of the outbreaks may be explainable on this basis.

Nitrates are irritants to the kidneys and urinary tract; potassium nitrate was at one time used as a diuretic. Poisoning by ingestion of excessive amounts of this chemical results in severe hemolytic anemia despite active hematopoiesis, as well as toxic injury to the renal parenchyma (Whitehead, 1953). There is localized gastroenteritis, and probably because of sensations originating in the gastrointestinal disorder, dogs show mental disturbances and depression. Decomposition of the nitrate into the nitrite is insignificant, and consequently methemoglobinemia is minimal or absent.

Quite the opposite is true of the nitrates contained in the tissues of plants. In the presence of moisture and possibly with the aid of bacteria, the phytogenous nitrates are rather easily reduced to nitrites (and eventually to ammonia). This occurs either in the stomach, and especially the rumen, or externally, as in stacks of hay that have become wet from rain or snow. In the experiments of Riggs (1945), the process (in oat hay) reaches a maximum in 20 hours after the application of moisture. Poisoning from excessive nitrates in the various plants, hay, and straw, then, is poisoning by nitrites, the principal effect of which is the formation of methemoglobin, sometimes from more than half of the total hemoglobin. The process involves transformation of the Fe atom from the ferrous to the ferric state, and hemoglobin so deranged has no oxygen-carrying capacity. Nitrites also markedly dilate the arterioles, thereby lowering blood pressure and accelerating the pulse.

The lethality of ingested nitrates is influenced by the manner and rate of administration. The LD_{50} for nitrate fed to cattle with forage is about 45 g/100 pounds of body weight. About a third of this amount would produce lethality when administered in a drench (Crawford et al., 1966).

Signs of nitrite poisoning that have attracted most attention include cyanosis, dyspnea, extremely rapid pulse (150/minute), great weakness and recumbency, diarrhea, and the voiding of colorless urine every few minutes. Some mention terminal convulsions, but coma seems to be more usual.

The outstanding lesion is the dark, brownish color of the blood, the effect of methemoglobin. It is commonly described as chocolate-colored, but this must not be taken too literally. Clotting remains approximately normal. The mucous membranes are cyanotic, except those of the stomach and intestines, which show more or less hyperemia and inflammation. There may be a few petechiae, as in most anoxemias. Blood-stained pericardial fluid is a frequent finding. The discoloration of the blood should be diagnostic, but tests for methemoglobin can be performed, remembering that small amounts are demonstrable in healthy cattle (Householder, et al., 1966).

Andersen, H.K.: Methaemoglobinaemia in pigs due to drinking nitrite-containing water that condensed in ventilating shafts in piggeries (TT). Nord. Vet. Med., 14:16–28, 1962.

Asbury, A.C., and Rhode, E.A.: Nitrite intoxication in cattle: the effects of lethal doses of nitrite on blood pressure. Am. J. Vet. Res., 25:1010–1013, 1964.

Bodansky, O.: Methemoglobinemia and methemoglobin-producing compounds. Pharmacol. Rev., 3:144–196, 1951.

Campbell, J.B., Davis, A.N., and Myhr, P.J.: Methemoglobinenia of livestock caused by high nitrate contents of well water. Can. J. Comp. Med., 18:93–101, 1954.

Campbell, D.J., and Wetherell, G.D.: Parasitic bronchitis in adult cattle. J. Am. Vet. Med. Assoc., 131:273–275, 1957.

Crawford, R.F., Kennedy, W.K., and Davison, K.L.: Factors influencing the toxicity of forages that contain nitrite when fed to cattle. Cornell Vet., 56:3–17, 1966.

Diven, R.H., Reed, R.E., and Pistor, W.J.: The physiology of nitrite poisoning in sheep. Ann. NY Acad. Sci., 111:638–643, 1964.

Diven, R.H., et al.: The determination of serum or plasma nitrate and nitrite. Am. J. Vet. Res., 23:497–499, 1962.

Dobai, A.A.: Investigations and observations on pigs concerning methemoglobinemia. Proc. XVIth Int. Vet. Congr. Madrid, 2:251–252, 1959.

Householder, G.T., Dollahite, J.W., and Hulse, R.: Diphenylamine for the diagnosis of nitrate intoxication. J. Am. Vet. Med. Assoc., 148:662–665, 1966.

Jainudeen, M.R., Hansel, W., and Davison, K.L.: Nitrate toxicity in dairy heifers. 3. Endocrine responses to nitrate ingestion during pregnancy. J. Dairy Sci., 48:217–221, 1965.

Jensen, C.W., and Anderson, H.D.: Rate of formation

and disappearance of methemoglobin following oral administration or injection of sodium nitrite. Proc. S. Dakota Acad. Sci., 21:37–40, 1941.

Kendrick, J.W., Tucker, J., and Peoples, S.A.: Nitrate poisoning in cattle due to ingestion of variegated thistle, Silybum marianum. J. Am. Vet. Med. Assoc., 126:53–56, 1955.

Lewis, D.: The reduction of nitrate in the rumen of the sheep. Biochem. J., 48:175–180, 1951.

Li Chuan Wang, Garcia-Rivera, J., and Burris, R.H.: Metabolism of nitrate by cattle. Biochem. J., 81:237–242, 1961.

Michel, J.F., and Shand, A.: A study of the epidemiology and clinical manifestations of parasitic bronchitis in adult cattle. Vet. Rec., 67:249, 1955.

Riggs, C.W.: Nitrite poisoning from ingestion of plants high in nitrate. Am. J. Vet. Res., 6:194–197, 1945.

Rubin, R., and Lucker, J.T.: The course and pathogenicity of initial infections with Dictyocaulus viviparus, the lungworm of cattle. Am. J. Vet. Res., 17:217–226, 1956.

Schneider, N.R., and Yeary, R.A.: Nitrite and nitrate pharmacokinetics in the dog, sheep, and pony. Am. J. Vet. Res., 36:941–947, 1975.

Seerley, R.W., et al.: Effect of nitrate or nitrite administered continuously in drinking water for swine and sheep. J. Anim. Sci., 24:1014–1019, 1965.

Sinclair, B.K., and Jones, D.I.H.: Nitrate toxicity in sheep. J. Sci. Fd. Agric., 15:717–721, 1964.

Stahler, L.M., and Whitehead, E.I.: Effect of 2, 4-D on potassium nitrate levels in leaves of sugar beets. Science, 112:749–751, 1950.

Taylor, E.R.: Parasitic bronchitis in cattle. Vet. Rec., 63:859–873, 1951.

Whitehead, J.E.: Potassium nitrate poisoning in a dog. J. Am. Vet. Med. Assoc., 123:232–233, 1953.

Williams, M.C., James, L.G., and Bond, B.O.: Emory milkvetch (Astragalus emoryanus var emoryanus) poisoning in chicks, sheep, and cattle. Am. J. Vet. Res., 40:403–406, 1979.

Winter, A.J., and Hokanson, J.F.: Effects of long-term feeding of nitrate, nitrite, or hydroxylamine on pregnant dairy heifers. Am. J. Vet. Res., 25:353–361, 1964.

Chlorates

Sodium chlorate, a strong oxidizing agent, is used to kill noxious weeds, being sprayed on the foliage and on the ground in a concentration amounting to 4 pounds/sq. rod (72 g/M^2). Trials indicate that animals are not poisoned by eating any ordinary amount of sprayed foliage, especially if a few days have elapsed since the spraying, nor from the soil, but poisoning has occurred when animals accidentally gained access to supplies of the chemical, which is palatable because of its salty taste. The minimum lethal dose for sheep and probably for other farm mammals approximates 2 or 3 g/kg of body weight, death coming in 6 to 48 hours.

Signs are somnolence and dyspnea, the temperature being normal. If small, sublethal amounts are ingested over a period of time, icterus and a dark or brownish discoloration of the conjunctivae can be expected. Postmortem lesions are those of methemoglobinemia, ably described for sheep and cattle by McCulloch and Murer, 1939. The musculature is dark or almost black, cut surfaces becoming somewhat lighter on exposure to air. The blood is very dark or blackish but clots readily. The liver is almost black; the lungs have the color of normal liver. The heart is flabby and dark. The spleen is dark but not enlarged. The abomasum contains ulcerated areas that are very black; all other parts of the alimentary tract were without lesions in the experience of these writers. In addition to these changes, hemolytic anemia has been described in dogs. Concentrations of the chemical in ingesta or blood are too slight to respond to the ordinary chemical tests.

Fitch, C.P., Boyd, W.L., and Hewitt, E.A.: Toxicity of sodium chlorate (NaClO$_3$) for cattle. Cornell Vet., 19:373–375, 1929.

Heywood, R., Sortwell, R.J., Kelley, P.J., and Street, A.E.: Toxicity of sodium chlorate to the dog. Vet. Rec., 90:416–418, 1972.

Holzer, F.J., and Stöhr, R.: Eine Massenvergiftung von Schafen durch das Unkrautvertilgungsmittel Natriumchlorat. Schweiz. Arch. Tierheilkd., 92:339–354, 1950.

Joubert, L., Magat, A., and Oudar, J.: Intoxication pseudo-charbonneuse par ingestion de cheddite (chlorate de soude et trinitrotoluène) chez le Mouton. Bul. Soc. Sci. Vet. Lyon, 63:327–332, 1961.

McCulloch, E.C., and Murer, H.K.: Sodium chlorate poisoning. J. Am. Vet. Med. Assoc., 95:675–682, 1939.

Moore, G.R.: Sodium chlorate poisoning in cattle. J. Am. Vet. Med. Assoc., 99:50–52, 1941.

Seddon, H.R., and McGrath, T.T.: Toxicity of sodium chlorate. Agric. Gaz. New S. Wales, 41:765–766, 1930.

Sheahan, B.J., Pugh, D.M., and Winstanley, E.W.: Experimental sodium chlorate poisoning in dogs. Res. Vet. Sci., 12:387–389, 1971.

Skjerven, O.: Sodium chlorate poisoning in cattle. Norsk. Vet. tidsskr., *56*:274–276, 1944.

GROUP I: CARBOXYHEMOGLOBIN

These poisons are characterized by production of **carboxyhemoglobin** and inability of hemoglobin to transfer oxygen.

Carbon Monoxide

An important form of poisoning in humans, carbon monoxide poisoning, in veterinary practice, is ordinarily limited to pet animals which may chance to be confined in houses or basements where defective heating equipment may permit accidental accumulation of the gas.

Signs include incoordination and ataxia, vomiting, involuntary urination and defecation, and unconsciousness. In humans, the fatal drowsiness often overcomes the victim so stealthily that he is unaware of the danger from which he could at first easily remove himself. The one salient and usually diagnostic lesion is the bright cherry-red color of the blood and tissues. This color is due to the formation of carboxyhemoglobin. The CO radical replaces the O of hemoglobin, which has greater affinity for CO. Inability of the blood to transport oxygen leads to fatal asphyxia. If death occurs quickly, few or no lesions of significance are encountered aside from petechiae on serosal surfaces and white matter of the cerebral hemispheres. In patients surviving several days, there is bilateral necrosis of cerebral white matter, basal ganglia, and cortical gray matter (laminar necrosis), which may be visible grossly. In human beings, focal subendocardial myocardial necrosis has also been described. The leuko- and polioencephalopathy are believed to result primarily from hypoxia, but acidosis may also play a role in their pathogenesis. The lesions are not pathognomonic and may be encountered in other conditions characterized by hypoxia. Diagnosis should be based upon analysis for carboxyhemoglobin.

Barondes, R. de R.: Carbon monoxide poisoning in a dog. Vet. Med., *34*:105, 1939.

Eckardt, R.E., et al.: The biologic effect from long term exposure of primates to carbon monoxide. Arch. Environ. Health, *25*:381–387, 1972.

Finck, P.A.: Exposure to carbon monoxide: review of the literature and 567 autopsies. Milit. Med., *131*:1513–1539, 1966.

Ginsberg, M.D., and Myers, R.E.: Experimental carbon monoxide encephalopathy in the primate. I. Physiologic and metabolic aspects. Arch. Neurol., *30*:202–208, 1974.

Ginsberg, M.D., Myers, R.E., and McDonagh, B.F.: Experimental carbon monoxide encephalopathy in the primate. II. Clinical aspects, neuropathology, and physiologic correlation. Arch Neurol., *30*:209–216, 1974.

Poppenhouse, G.C.: Carbon monoxide poisoning in a dog. Vet. Med., *34*:324–325, 1939.

Sterling, J.R.: Acute carbon monoxide poisoning in a dog. Vet. Med., *33*:66–68. 1938.

Cyanides

While accidents with chemical preparations of cyanides are possible, the usual cause of cyanide poisoning in animals is ingestion of cyanogenic plants, such as sorghums of all kinds, Sudan, Johnson, arrow, and velvet grasses, African or giant star grass *(Cynodon plectostachyum)*, a plant of Australia and certain southern parts of Africa, flax, suckleya *(Suckleya suckleyana)*, reed sweetgrass *(Poa aquatica)*, hydrangea, wild or domesticated members of the cherry family (including cherry pits eaten by chickens), and a number of others.

Death may be instantaneous, but usually effects last for some minutes or an hour. The animal falls, with convulsions, frothing at the mouth, unconsciousness, and infrequent gasping respirations. Pupils are dilated and involuntary defecation and micturition occur. Respiration ceases while the heart still beats. Acute cases are without lesions in the organs, but a bright red, arterial color of the venous blood is a diagnostic change. It is seen best by putting a small amount of blood over a dark background; the bright red persists for several hours despite drying. The proverbial odor of almonds or cherry pits is seldom detectable. There is seldom any erosion or inflammation of the alimentary mucosa. In animals surviving longer or repeatedly exposed to cyanide, focal necrosis of gray and white matter in the brain may be seen. The lesions are similar to those of carbon monoxide poisoning and are believed to result from hypoxia.

The poison acts by preventing the intracellular oxidative process, although the blood does not lack for oxygen. This action is the reason for the bright red blood, which is prevented from losing its oxygen to the tissues.

Ruminants may convert cyanide to the less toxic thiocyanate, which is goitrogenic.

Hadley, F.B.: Sudan grass poisoning problem. Can. J. Comp. Med., 2(6):169–170, 1938.

Haymaker, W., Ginzler, A.M., and Ferguson, R.L.: Residual neuropathological effects of cyanide poisoning. (A study of the central nervous system of 23 dogs exposed to cyanide compounds.) Milit. Surg., 3:231–246, 1952.

Henrici, M.: Occurrence of HCN in the grasses of Bechuanaland. 11th and 12th Rept., Director Vet. Ed. and Research, U. of So. Africa, 1926, pp. 495–498.

Levine, S., and Geib, L.W.: Leukoencephalopathy in a cat due to accidental cyanide poisoning. Pathol. Vet., 3:190–195, 1966.

Maitai, C.K., Gondwe, A.T.D., and Kamau, J.A.: Toxicity of Kiliambiti plant (Adenia volkensii): identification and estimation of toxic principle. Am. J. Vet. Res., 35:829–830, 1974.

Manges, J.D.: Cyanide poisoning. Vet. Med., 30:347–349, 1935.

Mathews, F.P.: Johnson grass (Sorghum halepense) poisoning. J. Am. Vet. Med. Assoc., 81:663–666, 1932.

Peters, A.T., Slade, H.B., and Avery, S.: Poisoning of cattle by common sorghum and Kafir corn (Sorghum vulgare). Expt. Sta. Bull. 77, Univ. Nebr., Lincoln. 1903.

Reber, K.: Hydrocyanic acid content of flaxseed. (Abstr. from Schweiz. Apoth. Ztg., 76:229, 1938.) J. Am. Pharm. Assoc., 5:82–83, 1939.

Rose, C.L., et al.: Cobalt salts in acute cyanide poisoning. Proc. Soc. Exp. Biol. Med., 120:780–783, 1965.

Schubel, E.C.W.: Poisoning by hydrocyanic acid. J. Am. Vet. Med. Assoc., 95:371–373, 1939.

Sharman, J.R.: Cyanide poisoning of cattle grazing "reed sweet-grass." N.Z. Vet. J., 15:7–8, 1967.

Shaw, C-M., Papayannopoulou, T., and Stamatoyannopoulos, G.: Neuropathology of cyanate toxicity in rhesus monkeys. Preliminary report. Pharmacol., 12:166–176, 1974.

Timson, S.D.: Prussic acid content of the giant star grasses (Cynodon plectostachyum) and of Kavirondo sorghum. Rhod. Agric. J., 40:371–373, 1943.

GROUP J: EDEMA

Poisons in Group J cause marked and conspicuous edema.

Alpha-Naphthyl Thiourea (ANTU)

This compound is popular for killing rats; it is usually mixed with meat or grain for that purpose. It was originally heralded as not dangerous to dogs because it was thought they would rid themselves of the substance by vomiting. Experience has proved otherwise, in spite of the fact that vomition does occur. Symptoms include cardiac and respiratory embarrassment, with imperceptible but rapid pulse and rapid, shallow respiration. Vomitus is frothy and may become bloody. Diarrhea is severe, becoming bloody. Weak and comatose, the dog commonly lies in the sternal recumbent position, fluid from the lungs often running out from his mouth. The temperature becomes markedly subnormal before death. As a rule, all this transpires and death occurs in one to four hours after the ANTU is eaten.

Postmortem lesions of poisoning by alpha-naphthyl thiourea are practically diagnostic. Hydrothorax is present in nearly all cases. If the thorax is opened carefully and without contaminating hemorrhage from the vessels, it is found to be full to overflowing with clear watery fluid. Extremely severe edema of the lungs occurs almost without exception, fluid often running out the trachea, if the thoracic organs are raised posteriorly. The lungs also show severe congestion, with diapedesis of erythrocytes into numerous alveoli. In the stomach, the fundic mucosa is severely inflamed and reddened in more than half the cases, moderately so in most of the remainder. Microscopically, the stomach shows considerable mucous exudate, as well as hyperemia. The surface epithelium is intact, but the chief cells are inconspicuous in appearance and numbers as compared to the parietal cells. This catarrhal inflammation continues into the small intestine and subsides gradually in the large bowel. Considerable amounts of bile are found in the upper intestine, although the gallbladder is not completely emptied. The kidneys are severely congested, often deep red. In the cortex and some of the medullary rays, fatty change of the epithelial cells is demonstrable. In the liver, the light color of vacuolization and central necrosis alternates in spots with the red of acute congestion. Fatty change, however, is absent. The spleen is small and empty of blood.

Poisoning by alpha-naphthyl thiourea has also occurred in horses through the accidental ingestion of poison bait.

Anderson, W.A., and Richter, C.P.: Toxicity of alpha naphthyl thiourea for chickens and pigs. Vet. Med., *41*:302–303, 1946.
Frick, E.J., and Fortenberry, J.D.: Equine ANTU poisoning. Vet. Med., *43*:107–108, 1948.
Jones, L.M., Smith, D.A., and Smith, H.A.: Alpha-naphthyl (ANTU) thiourea poisoning in dogs. Am. J. Vet. Res., *10*:160–167, 1949.
Hesse, F.E., and Loosli, C.G.: The lining of the alveoli in mice, rats, dogs, and frogs following acute pulmonary edema produced by ANTU poisoning. Anat. Rec., *105*:299–324, 1949.
Latta, H.: Pulmonary edema and pleural effusion produced by acute alpha-naphthyl thiourea poisoning in rats and dogs. Bull. Johns Hopkins Hosp., *80*:181–197, 1947.
Lopes, A.C.: Pathology and histology of experimental poisoning of dogs with ANTU, alpha-naphthyl thiourea. Pesquisa agropec. bras., *2*:287–291, 1967. VB *39*:334, 1969.

GROUP K: PULMONARY DYSFUNCTION

Pulmonary dysfunction is the principal feature of rape, kale, and paraquat poisoning, the only three included in this group.

Rape, Kale and other Plants of Genus Brassica

The disease recognized as rape poisoning commonly makes its appearance in a herd seven to ten days after the cattle or sheep have been placed in a pasture of this kind. Luxuriant growth, wet weather, and possibly, frosting, appear to increase the danger. In Schofield's experience, it is more likely to occur on certain farms than on others (1948).

Signs include (1) more or less digestive disturbance, usually absence of peristalsis and constipation, occasionally the reverse with fetid diarrhea; (2) respiratory difficulties including dyspnea with open mouth and a thumping sound at each respiration; (3) gradually increasing anemia, usually with hemoglobinuria and mild icterus. Whether the icterus is hemolytic or toxic has not been made clear. The anemia has been described as hyperchromic and macrocytic (Rosenberger, 1943). Weakness, ataxia, and nervous abnormalities, as well as blindness, are also described. If the cow is recently postparturient, the condition has been found to be indistinguishable from the poorly understood disorder called puerperal hemoglobinuria.

Of the lesions, a severe and destructive pulmonary emphysema, accompanied by congestion and edema and involving all parts of both lungs, is the most spectacular in the experience of Schofield and other Canadian investigators. Microscopically, rupture of the pulmonary alveoli is uniformly widespread, and both the emphysema and edema also involve the interlobular septa. Emphysema of the mediastinal and even subcutaneous tissues also develops in some cases when the pulmonary emphysema has existed for a few days. There may be hemorrhages in the trachea and bronchi; it is not clear whether bronchiectasis is also present. There is moderate acute toxic hepatitis, shown chiefly by centrilobular necrosis. The gallbladder regularly shows the distention with viscid bile which is characteristic of alimentary inactivity.

The pathogenetic mechanisms have been the subject of considerable speculation and study. Some suspect that the condition has an allergic basis. Schofield has found in a number of instances a heavy invasion of the contents of the alimentary canal by *Clostridium perfringens*, with evidence of toxin similar to that of the enterotoxemia that develops under other circumstances and is associated with other species of clostridia. The concept of a specific poisonous substance is supported, not only by the variety of lesions produced, but to some extent, by the fact that rape seed has been found poisonous to fowls. Wild cabbage *(Brassica oleracea)* has been reported as poisoning cattle when in the seed stage only (Angelo, 1951). Rape-seed cake has a locally irritant action with the production of vesicles. (See also the pulmonary emphysema-adenomatosis syndrome.)

Experimentally feeding kale to cattle, sheep, and goats has regularly induced anemia.

Angelo, M.: [Anaemia and Hemoglobinuria in Dairy Cattle Caused by Wild Cabbage *(Brassica oleracea)* Gone to Seed.] Zooprofilassi. 6:361–363, 1951.

Clegg, F.G., and Evans, R.K.: Haemoglobinemia of cattle associated with the feeding of Brassica species. Vet. Rec., 74:1169–1176, 1962.

Cote, F.T.: Rape poisoning in cattle. Can. J. Comp. Med., 8:38–41, 1944.

Crawshaw, H.A.: Rape blindness. Vet. Rec., 65:254, 1953; and Dalton, P.J.: *Ibid.* p. 298.

Evans, E.T.R.: Kale and rape poisoning in cattle. Vet. Rec., 63:348–349, 1951.

Grant, C.A., et al.: Kale anaemia in ruminants. I. Survey of the literature and experimental induction of kale anaemia in lactating cows. Acta Vet. Scand., 9:126–140, 1968.

Grant, C.A., et al.: Kale anaemia in ruminants. II. Observations on kale fed sheep. Acta Vet. Scand., 9:141–150, 1968.

Greenhalgh, J.F.D., Sharman, G.A.M., and Aitken, J.N.: Kale anaemia. I. The toxicity to various species of animal of three types of kale. Res. Vet. Sci., 10:64–72, 1969.

Greenhalgh, J.F.D., Sharman, G.A.M., and Aitken, J.N.: Kale anaemia. II. Further factors concerned in the occurrence of the disease under experimental conditions. Res. Vet. Sci., 11:232–238, 1970.

Patrizi, F., and Moriconi, M: Deaths of cattle from rape seed cake poisoning. Atti Soc. Ital. Sci. Vet., 5:225–227, 1951.

Penny, R.H.C., David, J.S.E., and Wright, A.I.: Observations on the blood picture of cattle, sheep, and rabbits fed on kale. Vet. Rec., 76:1053–1059, 1964.

Rosenberger, C.: Kohlanämie des Rindes. Dtsch. Tierärztl. Wochenschr., 51:63–67, 1943.

Schofield, F.W.: Acute pulmonary emphysema of cattle. J. Am. Vet. Med. Assoc., 112:254–259, 1948.

Stamp, J.T., and Stewart, J.: Haemolytic anemia with jaundice in sheep. J. Comp. Pathol. Ther., 63:48–52, 1953.

Tucker, E.M.: The onset of anaemia and the production of haemoglobin C in sheep fed on kale. Br. Vet. J., 125:472–479, 1969.

Paraquat

Paraquat (1,1-dimethyl-4, 4-dipyridylium dichloride) is a broad-spectrum herbicide responsible for poisonings in man and domestic animals. The lung is the principal site of injury. Following a single large dose, regardless of route, pulmonary edema and hemorrhage develop within hours and may lead to death. In animals that recover from a single exposure or experience repeated smaller exposures, paraquat induces fatal progressive interstitial inflammation and fibrosis of the lung. Based on experimental poisoning in rats, type I alveolar epithelial cells are target cells in acute and chronic poisoning. Type II cells are less affected, and proliferate to replace defects left by necrosis of type I cells. Endothelial cell damage contributes to the acute edema and hemorrhage. The mechanism leading to progressive fibrosis is not understood. Alveoli contain numerous macrophages, of which many contain hemosiderin.

The clinical signs focus on pulmonary distress, but signs resulting from local contact toxicity to the oral cavity and gastrointestinal tract may be the first to be encountered. Oral and gastrointestinal tract ulcers may be present following acute toxicity. Signs related to renal and hepatic failure have been reported, and focal hepatic and renal necrosis have been described in some but not all experimental studies. Rabbits are relatively resistant to the pulmonary effects of paraquat.

Butler, C., II: Pulmonary interstitial fibrosis from paraquat in the hamster. Arch. Pathol., 99:503–507, 1975.

Johnson, R.P., and Huxtable, C.R.: Paraquat poisoning in a dog and cat. Vet. Rec., 98:189–191, 1976.

Murray, R.E., and Gibson, J.E.: A comparative study of paraquat intoxication in rats, guinea pigs and monkeys. Exp. Mol. Pathol., 17:317–325, 1972.

Restuccia, A., Foglini, A., and Nannini, D. de A.: Paraquat toxicity for rabbits. Vet. Italiana, 25:555–561, 1974.

Rogers, P.A.M., Spillane, T.A., Fenlon, M., and Henaghan, T.: Suspected paraquat poisoning in pigs and dogs. Vet. Rec., 93:44–45, 1973.

GROUP L: GANGRENE

Group L contains only fescue poisoning, which is characterized by **gangrene**. Poisoning by ergot, a mycotoxin, is very similar, and limited evidence suggests fescue poisoning may also be mycotoxic.

Fescue Grass

In Australia and in the United States, there has been reported poisoning of cattle characterized by gangrene of the extremities entirely comparable to the usual case of ergotism. Commencing within two weeks after the animals start eating this grass, there are lameness, local heat, swelling, and severe pain involving a digit and extending upward to a line of demarcation in the phalanges or at or above the fetlock joint. The dried and shriveled extremity may then separate at this line.

The causative grass is a kind known as fescue grass, usually tall fescue, *Festuca arundinacea*, but a shorter, improved variety was incriminated in one instance. The toxic principle has not been identified, but apparently it is a vasoconstrictive substance that becomes concentrated in the grass as it dries. The possibility that these effects are caused by a mycotoxin produced by an associated microorganism has not been eliminated. Cows appear to be most susceptible when they graze on dry fescue meadows and receive no supplemental feed or protection from the cold weather.

The signs and lesions are similar and must be differentiated from those of ergotism, selenium poisoning, or cold injury. Arterioles at the coronary band have been reported to have thickened walls and constricted lumens in experimental fescue poisoning (Williams et al., 1975).

Cunningham, I.J.: A note on the cause of tall fescue lameness in cattle. Aust. Vet. J., 25:27–28, 1949.
Farnell, D.R., et al.: Field studies on etiology and control of fescue toxicosis. J. Environ. Qual., 4:120–122, 1975.
Goodman, A.A.: Fescue foot in cattle in Colorado. J. Am. Vet. Med. Assoc., 121:289–290, 1952.
Jacobson, D.R., and Miller, W.M.: Fescue toxicity. J. Anim. Sci., 20:960–961, 1961.
Pulsford, M.F.: A note on lameness in cattle grazing on tall meadow fescue (Festuca arundinacea) in South Australia. Aust. Vet. J., 26:87–88, 1950.
Stearns, T.J.: Fescue foot or ergot-like disease in cattle in Kentucky. J. Am. Vet. Med. Assoc., 122:388–389, 1953.
Williams, G.F.: Epidemiology of fescue toxicity. J. Dairy Sci., 48:1135, 1965.
Williams, M., et al.: Induction of fescue foot syndrome in cattle by fractionated extracts of toxic fescue hay. Am. J. Vet. Res., 36:1353–1357, 1975.

GROUP M: BONES AND TEETH

Fluorine is the single poison included in Group M and is characterized by lesions in **bones and teeth**.

Fluorine

Fluorosis may occur in chronic or acute forms.

Chronic Fluorine Poisoning. Chronic fluorosis occurs in animals receiving more than a minute amount of fluorine in the diet over a long period of time. The minimum amount of fluorine in the form of soluble fluorides required to produce evidence of injury in cattle and other farm animals lies between 1 and 2 mg/kg of body weight per day, or between 12 and 27 ppm of the diet. As a partially soluble contaminant of rock phosphate, a somewhat larger amount may possibly be harmless. In human beings, the amount tolerated without lesions (in the teeth) is said to be much less. Chronic poisoning of this nature occurs in animals eating pasturage or forage contaminated by air-borne residues from aluminum manufacturers, phosphate refineries, and similar industrial installations, or drinking well-water containing soluble fluorides to the extent of 10 ppm or more. In Iceland, fluorosis has been noted to follow volcanic eruptions. Following the Hekla eruption of May 5, 1970, volcanic ash was demonstrated to have up to 2000 ppm fluoride, and grass up to 4300 ppm fluoride. The concentration rapidly dropped, but remained at toxic levels for several weeks. When, as is commonly the case, both water and forage contain considerable amounts of fluorine, the safe level for the water alone is less than the figure given.

Clinical Manifestations. The clinical signs of chronic fluorine poisoning in catttle according to Shupe et al. (1964) include (1) mottling and abrasion of teeth, (2) intermittent lameness, (3) periosteal hyperostosis, demonstrable radiographically, and (4) demonstration of more than 6 ppm of fluorine in the urine. In fluorosis, as much as 30 ppm of fluorine may be present in the

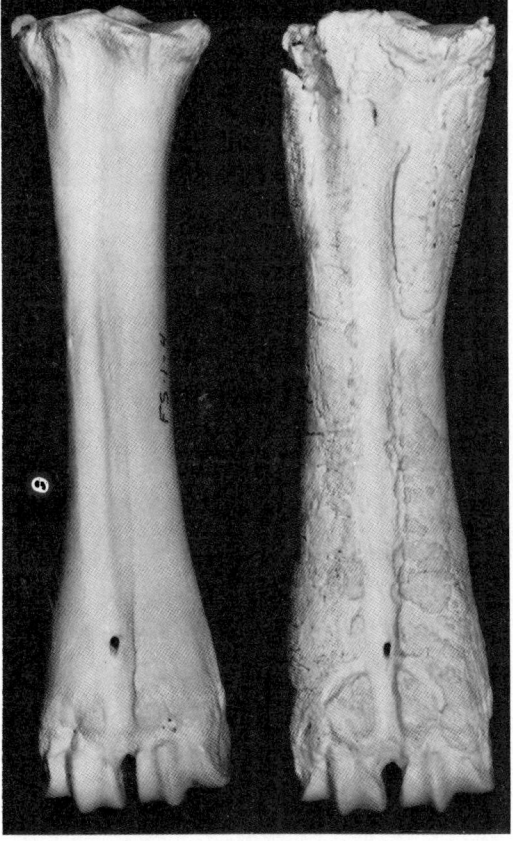

Fig. 16–15. Chronic bovine fluorosis Left: normal metatarsal bone of a dairy cow after ingesting 12 ppm fluorine in the diet for about seven years. Right: Hyperostosis and roughened periosteum of metatarsal bone of a dairy cow after consuming 93 ppm fluorine for approximately seven years. (Courtesy of Dr. J. L. Shupe and *American Journal of Veterinary Research*.)

urine, depending upon the age of the animal, specific gravity of the urine and length of time the animal has ingested fluorine.

Lesions. The pathognomonic lesions of chronic fluorine poisoning involve the teeth, the bones, and possibly the kidneys. The principal changes in the teeth are (1) "chalky" areas, (2) "mottling," (3) excessive attrition, and (4) hypoplastic pitting of the enamel. The chalky areas have received this description because the enamel has lost its shiny, translucent appearance and has assumed the dull, white opacity characteristic of chalk. Slight degrees of this condition are best detected by placing a light behind the tooth. The mottling consists of spots of yellow, brown, or greenish black. The pigmentation is in the enamel and cannot be removed from it, but may tend to be accentuated at the site of hypoplastic defects.

The excessive attrition results from an abnormal softness of the enamel and perhaps also of the dentine. Affected teeth are short because of rapid wear, which may reduce them to the level of the gums in the worst cases. The pitting consists of punctate or linear depressions on the side of the tooth due to deficient deposition of enamel at those places. The distribution of the hypoplastic "pits" may follow a horizontal pattern, considered to represent a chronologic period in the development of the tooth. Note that these dental lesions develop only if the fluorosis is present and active when the tooth is being formed. Once the tooth is fully formed, it is not affected by fluorosis. For this reason, the deciduous teeth do not develop lesions, and the permanent teeth which are formed earliest in life show the least damage. The more lateral incisors, as well as the later arriving molars and premolars, having been subjected to the fluorine over a longer period in most naturally occurring cases, are more worn and discolored than the older teeth, a situation quite contrary to the wear pattern of normal teeth.

The bony changes are most pronounced

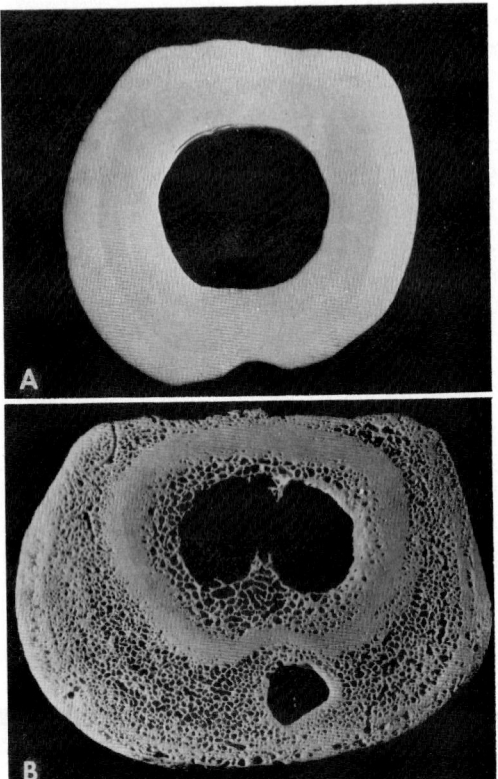

Fig. 16–16. Chronic bovine fluorosis, ground cross sections of metatarsus. *A*, Osteosclerosis, in a cow which received slightly elevated levels of fluorine for several years. *B*, Osteoporosis, with periosteal hyperostosis and endosteal resorption, in a cow which received high levels of fluorine in its diet for several years. (Courtesy of Dr. J. L. Shupe and *Annals of New York Academy of Sciences.)*

but that sodium fluoride causes the opposite condition of osteoporosis. Another view (Shupe et al., 1964) is that osteosclerosis occurs in animals receiving low doses of fluorine over a long time. Osteoporosis, with endosteal resorption and periosteal hyperostosis, on the other hand, is believed to result in animals receiving high doses of fluorine over a similarly prolonged period. The periosteal proliferation may result in microscopically demonstrable subperiosteal thickening and often, in the more severely affected individuals, is accompanied by the formation of sessile exostoses, seldom more than .5 cm in height. These may or may not be detectable clinically but, in company with the general periosteal disturbance, result in stiffness and lameness. Chemically the bones of appreciably poisoned animals contain fluorine to the extent of 4000 to 15,000 ppm (1.5%). The concentration has been developed slowly over a period of years and could conceivably represent absorption of fluorine from environmental sources no longer present; the same, of course, is true of the dental changes.

In the kidneys of experimental rats, degenerations and disintegration of the tubular epithelium, slight glomerular changes, thickened arterioles and terminal fibrosis are described. The fibrotic areas are radially arranged and are devoid of alkaline phosphatase. Polydipsia, polyuria, and poorly concentrated urine are concomitant signs.

The general health of the animal is not necessarily affected when mild dental changes are the only sign of fluorosis, but in more severe cases, there are lameness, anorexia, loss of weight, decreased production of milk, general unthriftiness, and perhaps intermittent diarrhea. Fluorine passes through the placenta and may accumulate in the bones of the fetus, but no significant direct effect upon fertility has been demonstrated.

The exact mechanisms involved in chronic fluorosis are unknown. One

in the metacarpals, metatarsals, and mandible, although all bones, like the teeth, store considerable amounts of fluoride and suffer from it. The bones become thicker and heavier than normal, the marrow cavity often being diminished in size, and the periosteal layer, in severe cases, is thickened. Microscopically, the bony trabeculae are thickened at the expense of the intertrabecular marrow spaces. The trabeculae have a dense appearance, with sharp, heavy outlines. However, it has been claimed that osteopetrotic changes, such as these, are due to calcium fluoride,

hypothesis is that fluoride ions replace hydroxyl radicals in the apatite crystal and that this in some way results in abnormal osteoid. This in turn is thought to be responsible for the poor bony matrix, which is defective and irregularly mineralized. It is evident that osteoblastic activity is abnormal, as judged by the defective new bone and dentine.

Chronic fluorosis in the guinea pig has been identified by Hard and Atkinson (1967) as the underlying factor in a syndrome referred to in Australia as "slob-

bers." This descriptive name comes from the characteristic excessive salivation that results from abnormal teeth. The teeth grow irregularly, become elongated or wear excessively, and the enamel is eroded and often encrusted with tartar. The irregularly shaped teeth are thought to interfere with swallowing, resulting in drooling of saliva. Affected animals eventually die unless the diet is corrected. At necropsy, lesions in the teeth are most significant. Elevated levels of fluorine in bones of naturally and experimentally affected animals

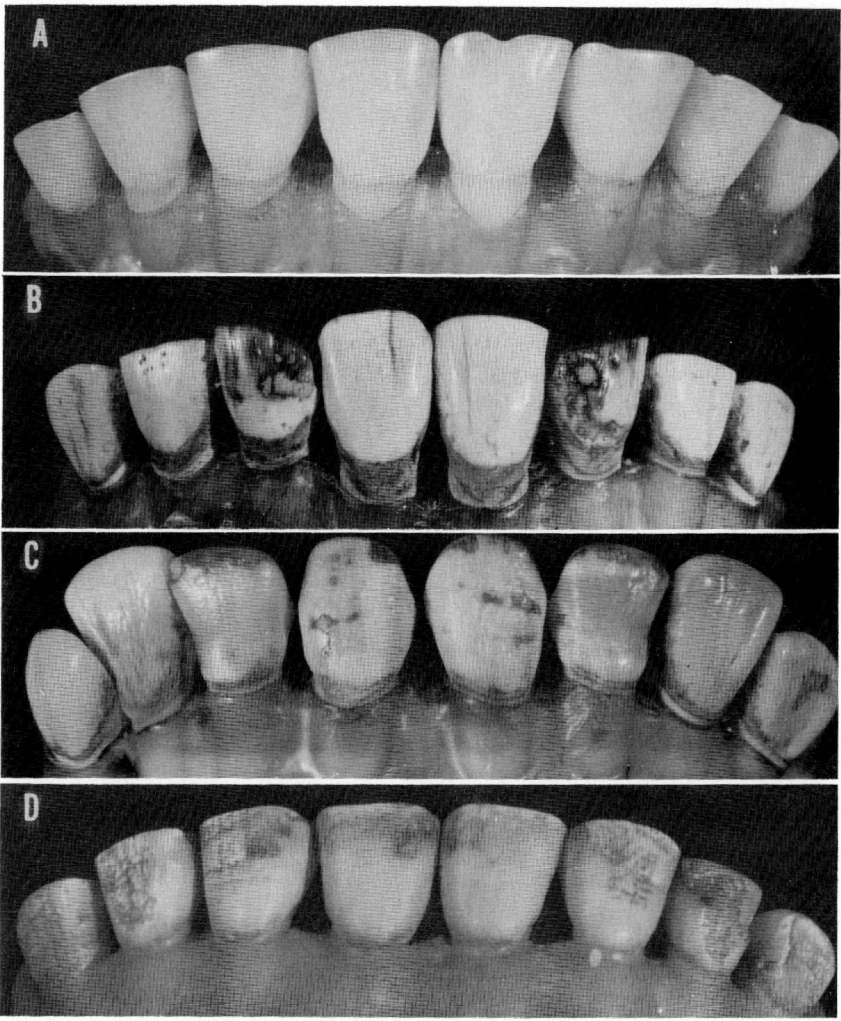

Fig. 16-17. Teeth in chronic bovine fluorosis. A, Normal incisors. B–D, Varying degrees of mottling of enamel of incisor teeth. (Courtesy of Dr. J. L. Shupe.)

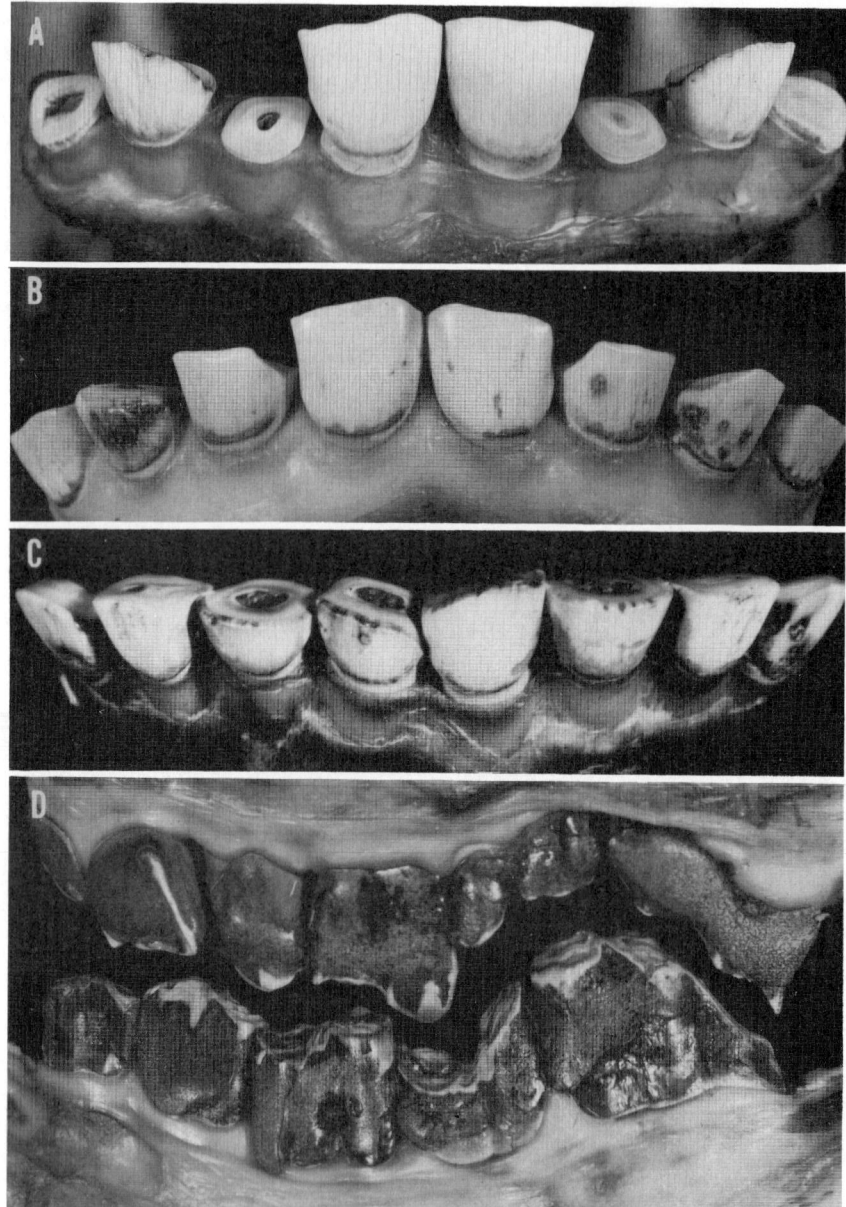

Fig. 16–18. Teeth in chronic bovine fluorosis. *A,* Irregular wear of incisors. *B,* Irregular mottling of incisors. *C,* Excessive wear of incisors. *D,* Irregular wear and stained enamel of molar teeth. (Courtesy of Dr. J. L. Shupe.)

corroborate the diagnosis. Levels of up to 6700 ppm in naturally affected guinea pigs and over 5700 ppm in experimentally poisoned animals have been recorded, in contrast to levels of not over 160 ppm of fluorine in normal animals.

One source of fluorine in guinea pig feed appears to have been rock phosphate of high content used as a component of pelleted feed.

Acute Fluorine Poisoning. This results from accidents or the improper use of sodium fluoride, which is employed as a vermifuge in swine and externally for lice in poultry. It also occurs in dogs that eat dead rats poisoned by the rodenticide, **sodium monofluoroacetate** ("compound 1080"), or when a domestic animal eats the bait itself. Lasting a few hours or a day or two, the symptoms are extreme abdominal pain, convulsions, and frenzy alternating with weakness and lethargy. Diarrhea develops shortly. Collapse is followed by death from respiratory and myocardial arrest. The postmortem lesions are those of acute gastroenteritis.

The anesthetic agent methoxyflurane is recognized as nephrotoxic in man and experimental animals. Prolonged exposure may lead to severe mitochondrial swelling and necrosis of proximal convoluted tubules mediated through inorganic fluoride released by metabolism of the anesthetic. Halothane, which is also a fluorinated anesthetic agent, is also recognized as nephrotoxic, but to a much lesser degree. In man, repeated exposure to halothane may, in a small number of subjects, result in acute hepatic necrosis. This is believed to result from an "allergic" basis and is not related to fluoride poisoning (Carney and Van Dkye, 1972). Fluorinated hydrocarbons used in aerosol propellants (Freons) have generally been considered to be inert. Recently, cardiac irregularities which may lead to death have been associated with these agents. The mechanism of action is not known (Harris, 1973).

Atkinson, F.F., and Hard, G.C.: Chronic fluorosis in the guinea-pig. Nature (Lond.), *211*:429–430, 1966.

Bond, A.M., and Murray, M.M.: Kidney functions and structure in chronic fluorosis. Br. J. Exp. Pathol., *33*:168–176, 1952.

Carney, F.M.T., and Van Dyke, R.A.: Halothane hepatitis: a critical review. Anesth. Analg. (Cleve.), *51*:135–160, 1972.

Faccini, J.M., and Care, A.D.: Effect of sodium fluoride on the ultrastructure of the parathyroid glands of the sheep. Nature (Lond.), *207*:1399–1401, 1965.

Garlick, N.L.: Dental fluorosis. Am. J. Vet. Res., *16*:38–44, 1955.

Georgsson, G., and Pétursson, G.: Fluorosis of sheep caused by Hekla eruption in 1970. Fluoride, *5*:58–66, 1972.

Hard, G.C., and Atkinson, F.F.: "Slobbers" in laboratory guinea pigs as a form of chronic fluorosis. J. Pathol. Bact., *94*:95–102, 1967.

———: The aetiology of "slobbers" (chronic fluorosis) in the guinea pig. J. Pathol. Bact., *94*:103–112, 1967.

Harris, W.S.: Toxic effects of aerosol propellants on the heart. Arch. Intern. Med., *131*:162–166, 1973.

Hoogstratten, B., et al.: Effect of fluorides on hematopoietic system, liver and thyroid gland in cattle. J. Am. Med. Assoc., *192*:26–32, 1965.

Jensen, R., Tobiska, J.W., and Ward, J.C.: Sodium fluoroacetate poisoning in a sheep. Am. J. Vet. Res., *9*:370–372, 1948.

Kosek, J.C., Mazze, R.I., and Cousins, M.J.: The morphology and pathogenesis of nephrotoxicity following methoxyflurane (penthrane) anesthesia: an experimental model in rats. Lab. Invest., *27*:575–580, 1972.

Narozny, J.: Dental fluorosis in cattle. Vet. Med Praha., *7*:421–424, 1965. VB *36*:273, 1966.

Neeley, K.L., and Harbaugh, F.G.: Effects of fluoride ingestion on a herd of dairy cattle in the Lubbock, Texas, area. J. Am. Vet. Med. Assoc., *124*:344–350, 1954.

Newell, G.W., and Schmidt, H.J.: The effects of feeding fluorine, as sodium fluoride, to dairy cattle. Am. J. Vet. Res., *19*:363–376, 1958.

Nichols, H.C., Thomas, E.F., Brawner, W.R., and Lewis, R.Y.: Poisoning of two dogs with 1080 rat poison (sodium fluoroacetate). J. Am. Vet. Med. Assoc., *115*:355–356, 1949.

Rand, W.E., and Schmidt, H.J.: The effect upon cattle of Arizona waters of high fluoride content. Am. J. Vet. Res., *13*:50–61, 1952.

Reinhard, H.: Die Fluorschaden im unteren Fricktal. Schweiz. Arch. Tierheilk., *101*:1–14, 1959.

Schmidt, H.J., and Rand, W.E.: A critical study of the literature on fluoride toxicology with respect to cattle damage. Am. J. Vet. Res., *13*:38–49, 1952.

Schmidt, H.J., Newell, G.W., and Rand, W.E.: The controlled feeding of fluorine, as sodium fluoride, to dairy cattle. Am. J. Vet. Res., *15*:232–239, 1954.

Shupe, J.L., et al.: Relative effects of feeding hay atmospherically contaminated by fluoride residue, normal hay plus calcium fluoride, and normal hay plus sodium fluoride to dairy heifers. Am. J. Vet. Res., *23*:777–787, 1962.

———: The effect of fluorine on dairy cattle. V. Fluorine in the urine as an estimator of fluorine intake. Am. J. Vet. Res., *24*:300–306, 1963.

———: The effect of fluorine on dairy cattle. II. Clinical and pathologic effects. Am. J. Vet. Res., *24*:964–979, 1963.

Shupe, J.L., Miner, M.L., and Greenwood, D.A.: Clinical and pathological aspects of fluorine toxicosis in cattle. Ann. NY Acad. Sci., *111*:618–637, 1964.

Shupe, J.L., and Olson, A.E.: Clinical aspects of fluorosis in horses. J. Am. Vet. Med. Assoc., *158*:167–174, 1971.

Suttie, J.W.: Vertebral biopsies in the diagnosis of bovine fluoride toxicosis. Am. J. Vet. Res., 28:709–712, 1967.

Weatherell, J.A., and Weidmann, S.M.: The skeletal changes of chronic experimental fluorosis. J. Pathol. Bact., 78:233–241, 243–255, 1959.

Zipkin, I., Eanes, E.D., and Shupe, J.L.: Effect of prolonged exposure to fluoride on the ash, fluoride, citrate, and crystallinity of bovine bone. Am. J. Vet. Res., 25:1595–1597, 1964.

GROUP N: HYPERCALCEMIA

Group N contains two poisonous plants that induce **hypercalcemia,** mimicking hypervitaminosis D.

Solanum Malacoxylon

A severe generalized calcifying arteriosclerotic disease of cattle and sheep has been recognized from certain tropical areas, particularly Jamaica, British West Indies, Argentina, and Hawaii. Its colloquial names in these places are, respectively, "Manchester wasting disease," "enteque seco," and "Naalehu disease." This latter term comes from the name of the district in Hawaii meaning "covered with gray ashes" (Lynd et al., 1965). Only recently has each of these diseases been considered to represent the same syndrome and to be caused by the consumption of leaves and stems of the plant *Solanum malacoxylon* (syn: *S. glaucum* Dun.). The plant contains a molecule similar or identical to 1,25-dihydroxy vitamin D_3 combined with one or more carbohydrate moieties. The glycoside is believed to be cleaved in vivo to release the active form of vitamin D_3 (Peterlik et al., 1976). Thus, the toxicity of *S. malacoxylon* is analogous to vitamin D toxicity. The disease occurs naturally in cattle and sheep, but experimentally other domestic animals and laboratory animals are susceptible. Calves are less susceptible than adult cows.

The disease is manifest by progressive emaciation, stiffness of joints, and weakness. The clinicopathologic findings are those of vitamin D toxicity. Serum calcium is greatly elevated and serum phosphorus moderately increased. There is extensive calcification of the media and intima of the aorta and all major and minor blood vessels, as well as calcification of the kidney, heart, lung, and other tissues. Bones may be thickened due to hyperostosis. A dark basophilic band separates new bone growth from pre-existing bone. Its composition is not known, but presumably it is a mucopolysaccharide.

Poisoning by other species of *Solanum* is discussed on page 913.

Bingley, J.B., Ruksan, B.E., and Carrillo, B.J.: Serum calcium fractions in sheep treated with *Solanum malacoxylon.* Res. Vet. Sci., 21:121–122, 1976.

Cabrejas, M., Ladizesky, M., and Mautalen, C.A.: Calcium kinetics in the *Solanum malacoxylon*-treated rat. J. Nutr., 105:1562–1566, 1975.

Camberos, H.R., Davis, G.K., Djafar, J.I., and Simpson, C.F.: Soft tissue calcification in guinea pigs fed the poisonous plant *Solanum malacoxylon.* Am. J. Vet. Res., 31:685–696, 1970.

Carrillo, B.J.: The pathology of *Enteque seco* and experimental *Solanum malacoxylon* toxicity. Dis. Abstr. Intern., 32B:4955–4956, 1972.

Döbereiner, J., Done, S.H., and Beltran, L.E.: Experimental *Solanum malacoxylon* poisoning in calves. Br. Vet. J., 131:175–185, 1975.

Done, S.H., Tokarnia, C.H., Dämmrich, K., and Döbereiner, J.: *Solanum malacoxylon* poisoning in pigs. Res. Vet. Sci., 20:217–219, 1976.

Lynd, F.T., et al.: Bovine arteriosclerosis in Hawaii. Am. J. Vet. Res., 26:1344–1349, 1965.

Peterlik, M., et al.: Further evidence for the 1,25-dihydroxyvitamin D-like activity of *Solanum malacoxylon.* Biochem. Biophys. Res. Comm., 70:797–804, 1976.

Cestrum Diurnum

This plant, also known as day-blooming jessamine, wild jasmine, day cestrum or Chinese inkberry, is a member of the nightshade family *(Solonaceae),* but in contrast to most toxic plants in this group, *Cestrum diurnum* owes its toxicity to its content of 1,25-dihydroxyvitamin D_3-glycoside. Its effect, therefore, resembles *Solanum malacoxylon* poisoning. The plant, introduced from the West Indies, is grown as an ornamental in warmer parts of the United States, including Florida, Texas, and California, as well as in India and Hawaii. It is especially abundant in southern Florida, where Krook et al. (1975) have recently described poisoning in horses and cattle.

The disease was first recognized in 1970 in horses, in which most examples of poisoning have been observed. Affected horses lose weight over a period of months, become stiff and reluctant to move, and develop a short, choppy gait. Flexor tendons and the suspensory ligament are sensitive to palpation. The animals become progessively debilitated and are ultimately destroyed. Serum calcium is elevated (11.4 to 16.7 mg/100 ml), but serum phosphorus is normal. Pathologic soft tissue calcification resulting from hypervitaminosis D is widespread in arteries, tendons, and ligaments. Calcification of the kidneys and lungs was not a feature of the disease. Generalized osteopetrosis (hyperostosis) was described by Krook et al. (1975) as resulting from retarded osteocytic osteolysis.

Hughes, M.R., et al.: Presence of 1,25-dihydroxy-vitamin D_3-glycoside in the calcinogenic plant, *Cestrum diurnum*. Nature, 268:347–349, 1977.

Kasali, O.B., Krook, L., Pond, W.G., and Wasserman, R.H.: *Cestrum diurnum* intoxication in normal and hyperparathyroid pigs. Cornell Vet., 67:190–221, 1977.

Krook, L., et al.: *Cestrum diurnum* poisoning in Florida cattle. Cornell Vet., 65:557–575, 1975.

———: Hypercalcemia and calcinosis in Florida horses: implication of the shrub, *Cestrum diurnum*, as the causative agent. Cornell Vet., 65:26–56, 1975.

Wasserman, R.H., Corradino, R.A., and Krook, L.: *Cestrum diurnum*: a domestic plant with 1,25-dihydroxycholecalciferol-like activity. Biochem. Biophys. Res. Comm., 62:85–91, 1975.

GROUP O: LOSS OF HAIR OR WOOL

Thallium

A heavy metal with toxic effects and atomic weight similar to lead and mercury, thallium may be involved in poisonings of man and animals. The thallous form, particularly thallous sulfate, is most active pharmacologically and is odorless, colorless, and tasteless; each of these characteristics favors its use as a pesticide. Although banned by federal law from sale to the general public for household use, acci-

dental poisonings of children, dogs, and cats still occur. Cattle and sheep have also been reported to have eaten poisoned bait. Poisonings from industrial wastes and use of thallium as a depilatory seem to be decreasing.

The clinical signs reflect involvement of several body systems and depend to some extent on the amount of thallium ingested. According to Zook and Gilmore (1967), dogs exhibit these signs in order of frequency: vomiting, cutaneous alterations, depression, anorexia, nervous signs, diarrhea, respiratory distress, conjunctivitis, dehydration, and esophageal paralysis. The cutaneous lesions first appear as localized areas of erythema from the third to seventh day after poisoning. Serum oozes from these lesions, and in a few days they become covered with thick crusty material. Hair may be plucked easily in early stages, later it may fall readily from large areas of skin. Necrosis and sloughing of skin may eventually occur.

Clinical laboratory findings in dogs, in order of frequency, include: lymphopenia, neutrophilia, eosinopenia, left shift of neutrophils, hemoconcentration, and circulating immature red blood cells. Blood urea nitrogen often is elevated. Serum glutamic pyruvic transaminase may be elevated, and serum glutamic oxaloacetic transaminase is usually elevated. Proteinuria and bilirubinuria may be present. Elevated specific gravity is characteristic of the urine, presumably due to dehydration. Glycosuria may be evident, and granular casts, erythrocytes, leukocytes, and epithelial cells are usually excessive in the urine sediment.

The microscopic lesions of thallotoxicosis are found in most systems of the body. The changes in the skin are striking and characteristic (Fig. 16–19A), consisting of severe acanthosis and parakeratosis involving epidermis and hair follicles, occasional intraepithelial abscesses, and congestion of epidermal capillaries. Necrosis of isolated renal convoluted tubules is also

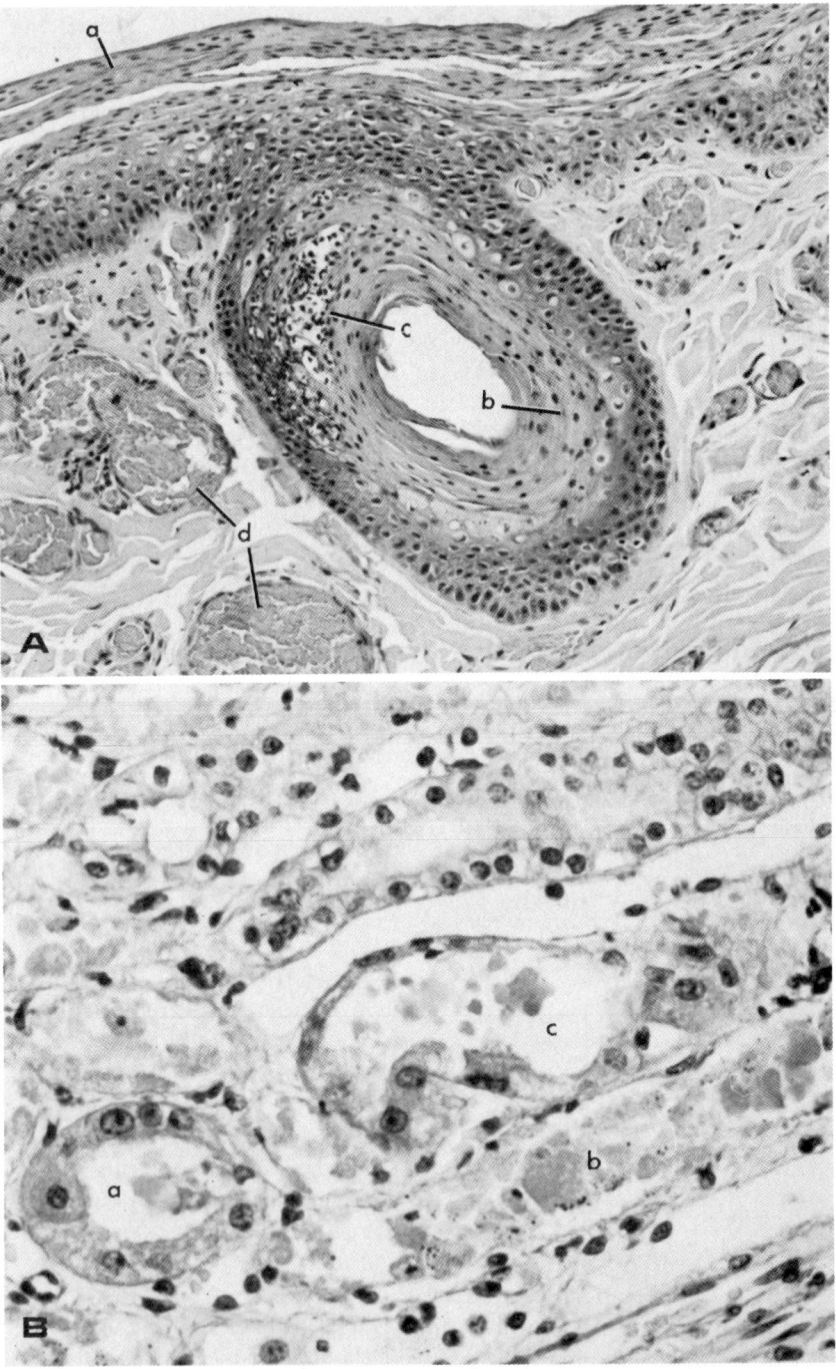

Fig. 16-19. Thallium poisoning. *A,* Thallium poisoning in a one-year-old male Scottish terrier. Note: *(a)* parakeratosis and acanthosis in the epidermis and the hair follicle *(b)*; intraepithelial abscess *(c),* and congestion of capillaries *(d). B,* Kidney of a two-year-old castrated male collie which died of thallium poisoning. Note: *(a)* renal tubule with slightly affected cells (cytoplasm swollen, cells partially individualized); tubule with completely necrotic epithelium *(b),* and part of tubule with some necrotic cells *(c).* (Courtesy of Angell Memorial Animal Hospital.)

typical (Fig. 16–19B), with proteinaceous material in some Bowman's spaces. In later stages, some leukocytic infiltration may occur, completing the picture of toxic tubular nephrosis. Edema of the lungs is usual, and purulent bronchopneumonia may be found in about a third of the cases. Disseminated focal necroses of skeletal and cardiac muscle fibers are constant, with the expected leukocytic infiltration at the sites of necrosis. Spleens and lymph nodes are often edematous and enlarged with hyperplasia of reticuloendothelial elements. Some myelinated nerves may have some degenerated axons with enlarged, empty myelin sheaths. Aspermatogenesis with formation of multinucleated masses of spermatids is evident in the testes. Ulceration of the esophagus, with focal necrosis in nearby muscle fibers, is a constant finding. Hepatic lesions are usually limited to early toxic hepatitis, with necrosis and distention of sinusoids near central veins. In the brain, lesions may be found in animals in which neurologic involvement is indicated by the clinical signs. These consist of disseminated early necrotic lesions (with chromatolysis and neuronophagia), and edema throughout the cerebellum and cerebrum.

The gross lesions, as may be judged from the clinical signs and microscopic findings, consist of patchy or diffuse areas of cutaneous erythema, alopecia, or dermatitis, cardiac hypertrophy, subendocardial hemorrhages, severe congestion of the kidneys, edema and consolidations of the lungs, edema and enlargement of lymph nodes, enlargement of the spleen, and dilation, erosion, or ulceration of the esophagus.

The pathologic diagnosis is established by the microscopic lesions, particularly those in the skin, and by the chemical demonstration of thallium in urine or tissues.

Egyed, M.: Distribution of thallium in the body fluids and organs of experimentally poisoned sheep. Refuah Vet., 25:81–82, 108–110, 1968. VB 39:824, 1969.
Gabriel, K.L., and Dubin, S.: A method for the detection of thallium in canine urine. J. Am. Vet. Med. Assoc., 143:722–724, 1963.
Newsom, I.E., Loftus, J.B., and Ward, J.C.: The toxicity of thallium sulphate for sheep. J. Am. Vet. Med. Assoc., 76:826–832, 1930.
Pile, C.H.: Thallium poisoning in domestic felines. Aust. Vet. J., 32:18–20, 1956.
Schulte, F.: Thalliumvergiftung beim Hund. Dtsch. Tierarztl. Wochenschr., 57:92–93, 1950.
Schwartzman, R.M., and Kirschbaum, J.O.: The cutaneous histopathology of thallium poisoning. J. Invest. Dermatol., 39:169–173, 1962.
Skelley, J.F., and Gabriel, K.L.: Thallium intoxication in the dog. Ann. NY Acad. Sci., 111:612–617, 1964.
Vacirca, G., and Agosti, M.: (Thallium poisoning in dogs). Veterinaria, Milano, 16:171–196, 1967. VB 37:4897, 1967.
Vismara, E.: Reperti dell'avvelenamento spontaneo da tallio nel cane. Atti. Soc. Ital. Sci. Vet., 15:523–530, 1961.
Wenger, P., and Rusconi, I.: A new specific reaction for the identification of thallium. Helv. Chim. Acta., 26:2263–2264, 1943.
Willson, J.E.: Thallotoxicosis (thallium poisoning). J. Am. Vet. Med. Assoc., 139:1116–1119, 1961.
Zook, B.C., and Gilmore, C.E.: Thallium poisoning in dogs. J. Am. Vet. Med. Assoc., 151:206–217, 1967.
Zook, B.C., Holzworth, J., and Thornton, G.W.: Thallium poisoning in cats. J. Am. Vet. Med. Assoc., 153:285–299, 1968.

Jumbay Tree (Leucaena glauca)

A chronic poisoning of horses in the Bahamian Islands has been reported by Mullenax. It is due to the consumption for several weeks of the leaves and twigs of a small leguminous tree, *Leucaena glauca*, commonly known as the jumbay. *Leucaena glauca* is known as "ipil-ipil" in the Philippines, as "lamtoro" in Indonesia, "cow bush" in Australia. In Hawaii, where it is cultivated extensively, it is called "kao haole," or "ekoa" or "white popinac." It is able to grow in the worst kinds of soil and with little water, has good value as forage, may contain up to 30% protein (dry weight) and twice as much carotene as alfalfa. Toxicity is due to an unbound amino acid called mimosine (the plant belongs to the family Mimosaceae). Horses and pigs are most frequently affected; ruminants are less susceptible than monogastric animals. The most striking symptom is partial to complete loss of the long hair of the mane, tail, and forelock; if the case is severe, a patchy loss above and below the knees and hocks and in the flanks and neck occurs. Experimental feeding of high levels has produced severe stomatitis, hemorrhagic enteritis, proctitis, edema of the hind legs and genitals, and chronic laminitis with rings in the hoof. Recovery occurs after feeding is discontinued and possibly some tolerance develops.

The feeding of *Leucaena* to swine reportedly causes fetal death and resorption, and polypodia of the forelimbs.

Mullenax, C.H.: A dietary cause of hair loss in Bahamian livestock. J. Am. Vet. Med. Assoc., *131*:302, 1957.
————: Observations on *Leucaena glauca*. Aust. Vet. J., *39*:88–91, 1963.
Wayman, O., Iwanaga, I.I., and Hugh, W.I.: Fetal resorption in swine caused by *Leucaena leucocephala* (Lam.) de Wit. in the diet. J. Anim. Sci., *30*:583–588, 1970.

GROUP P: EPITHELIAL HYPERPLASIA

Group P contains several chlorinated compounds which have **epithelial hyperplasia** as their most prominent pathologic feature.

Chlorinated Dibenzodioxins (TCDD, Dioxin, Toxic Fat)

Several chlorinated dibenzodioxins are known to be toxic, with 2, 3, 7, 8-tetrachlorodioxin (TCDD), commonly referred to as dioxin, being one of the most toxic compounds known. Dioxins originate from various chlorophenol compounds, especially if treated with alkali, and may therefore contaminate products containing or derived from chlorophenols. Chlorophenols are widely used as antiseptics, disinfectants, fungicides, herbicides, hide preservatives, and wood preservatives. Dioxin has also been found as a contaminant of polychlorinated biphenyls.

Poisoning by dioxin in human beings and a variety of animals has been well documented and may account for many mysterious illnesses. Dioxin may also be the active principle in chlorinated naphthalene poisoning, discussed following this section.

The first identification of dioxin as an important toxin took place in 1962, when it was shown to be the responsible cause of a mysterious disease of chickens first recognized in 1957. The disease in poultry was first named "edema disease," "water belly," and "ascitic disease" by poultrymen and veterinarians, indicating the common postmortem findings. Following the recognition of a toxic factor in the unsaponifiable fraction of certain fats, it was labeled **toxic fat poisoning.** After five years of research, dioxin or TCDD was shown to be the cause. The source was shown to be fleshing grease from hides that had been treated with commerical pentachlorophenol. Millions of broilers died in the 1957 "outbreak." A subsequent outbreak occurred in 1969, which was traced to contaminated vegetable oil by-product fatty acids used in the feed. The vegetable oil refinery also formulated antimicrobial products that contained chlorophenols.

Subsequent to recognition of "edema disease" in poultry, poisoning by dioxin has been confirmed in other animal species and human beings exposed to chemicals containing dioxin as a contaminant. Industrial accidents have occurred in Ludwigshafen, West Germany, the Netherlands, Derbyshire, England, and Seveso, Italy, and exposure of workers at a chemical plant in the United States have all been associated with human illness. The use of waste oil to control dust in riding arenas has also resulted in human and animal poisoning by dioxin. Currently, there is considerable attention focused on the use of the herbicide, 2-4,5 trichlorophenoxyacetic acid (2-4,5-T or agent orange), which was widely sprayed in Vietnam as well as in other countries, such as Colombia, and which contains dioxin as a contaminant.

Chloracne, a persistent and disfiguring form of acne, is the principal outward sign of toxicity in human beings, and comparable lesions of the skin occur in animals experimentally or naturally exposed. These lesions closely resemble those described in greater detail in the following sections on chlorinated naphthalene and PCB poisonings.

Lesions of the skin, however, are by no means the only effect of dioxin toxicity. Other lesions include necrosis of the liver, edema, thrombocytopenia and prothrombin deficiency leading to bleeding, conjunctivitis, abortion, congenital malformations, chromosomal aberrations, and carcinoma of the liver. The mortality rate may be low or high, but death occurs remarkably late after exposure, ranging from one month to one year.

The mechanism of toxicity of dioxin is not known, but it is speculated to be related to the fact that it is a potent inducer of aryl hydrocarbon hydroxysynthetase.

Allen, J.R.: The role of "toxic fat" in the production of hydropericardium and ascites in chickens. Am. J. Vet. Res., 25:1210–1219, 1964.

Allen, J.R., and Carstens, L.A.: Electron microscopic alterations in the liver of chickens fed toxic fat. Lab. Invest., 15:970–979, 1966.

————: Light and electron microscopic observations in *Macaca mulatta* monkeys fed toxic fat. Am. J. Vet. Res., 28:1513–1526, 1967.

Anonymous: Seveso. Lancet, 2:297, 1976.

Carter, C.D., et al.: Tetrachlorodibenzodioxin: an accidental poisoning episode in horse arenas. Science, 188:738–740, 1975.

Firestone, D.: Etiology of chick edema disease. Environmental Health Perspectives. Issue #5:59–66, 1973.

Gupta, B.N., Vos, J.G., Moore, J.A., Zinkl, J.G., and Bullock, B.C.: Pathologic Effects of 2,3,7,8-Tetrachlorodibenzo-p-dioxin in Laboratory Animals. Environ. Health Perspect., No. 5:125–140, 1973.

Holden, C.: Agent orange furor continues to build. Science, 205:770–772, 1979.

Kearney, P.C., Woolson, E.A., Isensee, A.R., and Helling, C.S.: Tetrachlorodibenzodioxin in the environment: sources, fate, and decontamination. Environ. Health Perspect., No. 5:273–277, 1973.

Laporte, J.R.: Effects of dioxin exposure. Lancet, 1:1049–1050, 1977.

Poland, A., and Glover, E.: Studies of the mechanism of toxicity of the chlorinated dibenzo-p-dioxins. Environ. Health Perspect., No. 5:245–251, 1973.

Robbins, A.: Dioxin studies. Science, 205:1332, 1979.

Schmittle, S.C., Edwards, H.M., and Morris, D.: A disorder of chickens probably due to a toxic feed—preliminary report. J. Am. Med. Assoc., 132:216–219, 1958.

Chlorinated Naphthalenes

A disease entity, known as hyperkeratosis previous to the discovery of its etiology, has been traced to the presence of highly chlorinated naphthalenes (five or more Cl ions, probably), which gain access to the animal metabolism either through ingestion or cutaneous absorption. While the disease was first described in connection with a wood preservative used on stables in which cattle were kept, a more common source of the naphthalene compounds has been lubricating oils. Such compounds have been found to improve the lubricating properties of the oil, but minute amounts from the bearings of machines used in the process have contaminated commercially produced feeds, especially those made into pellets. Animals have also absorbed the poison through contact with farm machinery so lubricated. Cattle are ordinarily involved, although sheep have been poisoned experimentally.

Signs include lacrimation, which may develop within a week after the first contact with the poison, often salivation, afebrile depression, anorexia, emaciation, terminal diarrhea, and death after several weeks.

Lesions can be summarized as an overgrowth of epithelium. This includes an increase of the cornified layer (hyperkeratosis) on those surfaces where the epithelium is already stratified squamous, and squamous metaplasia in many places where it is normally of the columnar type. This results in marked thickening of the skin, especially over the neck and withers, with coarse, deep wrinkling, scaliness, and loss of hair. Microscopically, there is some degree of acanthosis with deepening of the rete pegs, but most of the increased thickness is in the cornified layer. The keratohyaline of this layer extends deep into the hair follicles, compressing the surrounding zone of cellular epithelium. The corium commonly shows a noticeable infiltration with lymphocytes.

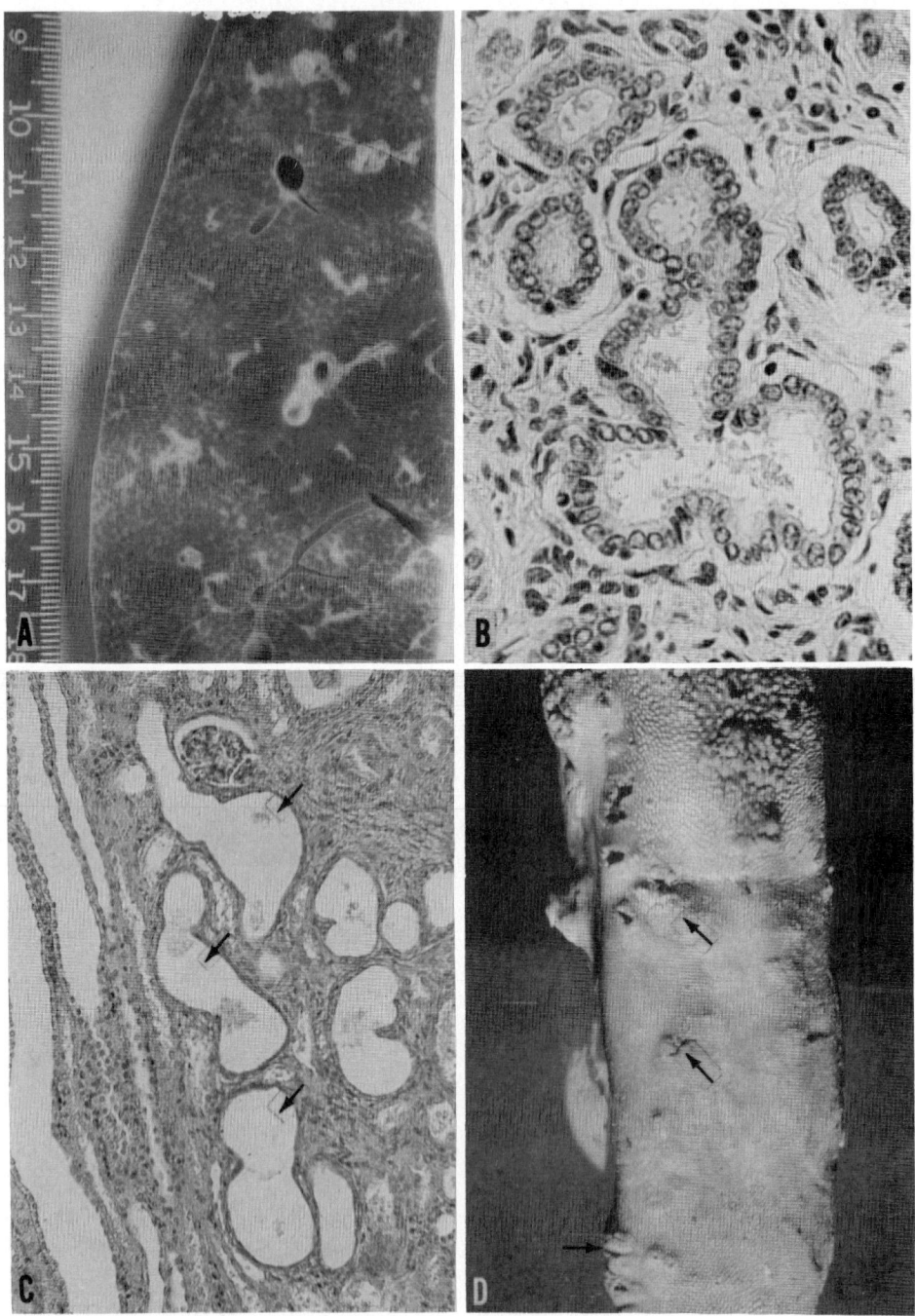

Fig. 16–20. Poisoning caused by chlorinated naphthalene (bovine hyperkeratosis). *A*, Bovine liver with prominent biliary system. *B*, Hyperplasia of bile ducts (× 485) in portal region. Contributor: Dr. J. F. Ryff. *C*, Hyperplasia and dilatation of renal tubules (arrows) in a bovine kidney (× 100). (Courtesy of Armed Forces Institute of Pathology.) Contributors: Drs. Kenneth McEntee and Peter Olafson. *D*, Tongue of an affected cow. Note elevated lesions in epithelium (arrows). (Case at Iowa Sch. Vet. Med.)

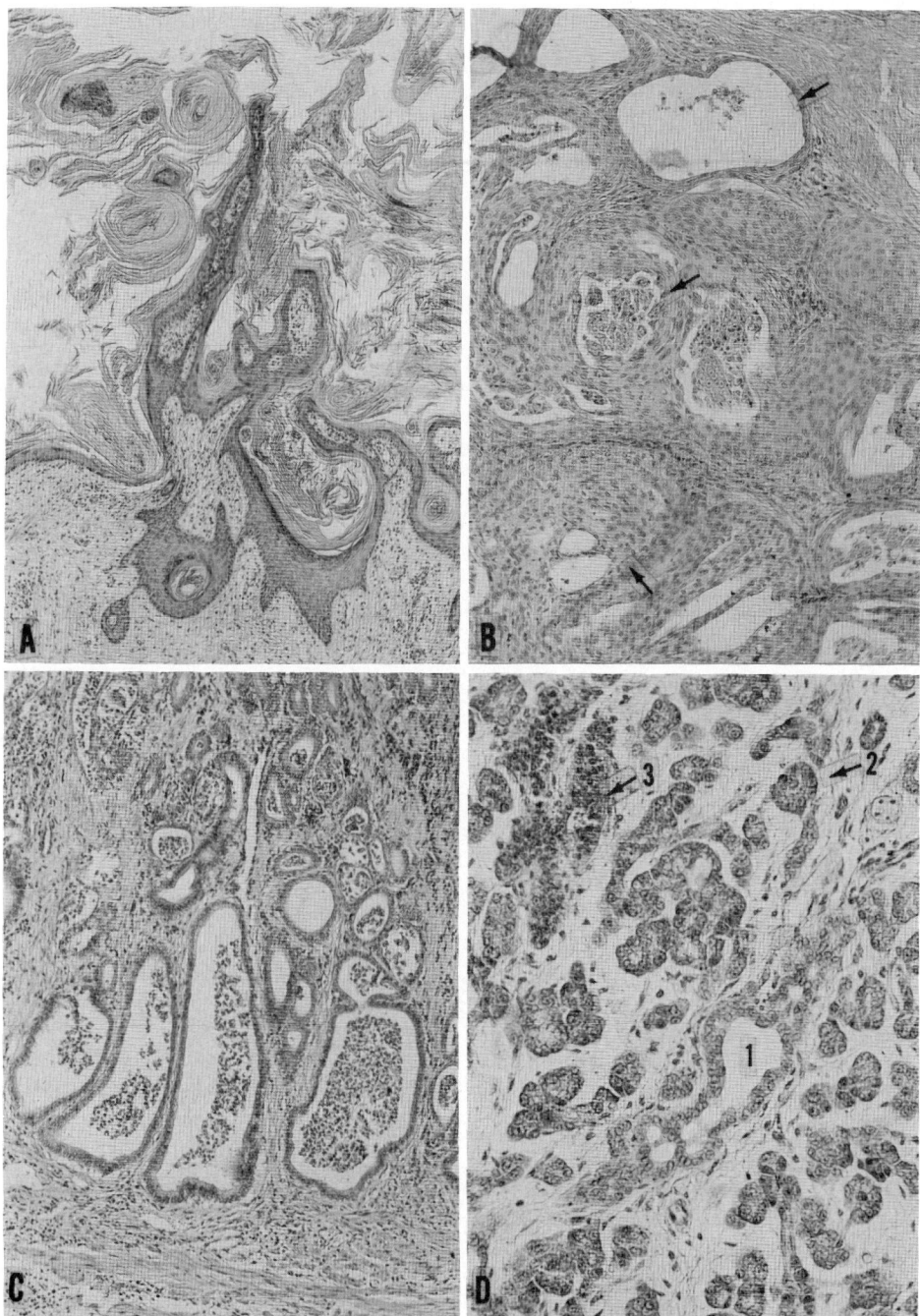

Fig. 16–21. Poisoning from chlorinated naphthalene (bovine hyperkeratosis). *A,* Severe hyperkeratosis in bovine skin (× 56). Contributor: Dr. J. F. Ryff. *B,* Squamous metaplasia of tubular epithelium (arrows) of epididymis (× 100). Contributors: Drs. Kenneth McEntee and Peter Olafson. *C,* Hyperplasia and cystic dilatation of epithelium in crypts of small intestine (× 70). Contributor: Dr. J. F. Ryff. *D,* Hyperplasia of ductal epithelium, bovine pancreas (× 195). Duct (*1*), stroma (*2*) and island of Langerhans (*3*). This is more severe than usual. (Courtesy of Armed Forces Institute of Pathology.) Contributor: Dr. J. F. Ryff.

On the mucosa of the mouth and lips and especially on the tongue, there are likely to be raised "plaques" of thickened, hyperkeratotic epithelium. These average a centimeter or more in diameter. Judging from early experimental cases, they apparently are preceded by shallow ulcers. Similar but smaller nodular proliferations are likely to be found in the esophagus. The same tendency toward nodular increase of epithelium extends through the digestive tract, where thickened spots or areas occasionally develop through hyperplasia of the columnar epithelium, forming cysts filled with mucus and cell debris. This general tendency is more likely to be seen in the gallbladder and in the extrahepatic and intrahepatic bile ducts. The latter often develop thickenings characterized by irregular epithelial-lined cysts, which vary from microscopic size up to a diameter of a centimeter. Within the liver, such ducts are encircled by increased fibrous tissue. In a few instances, the changes approach those of biliary cirrhosis. The ducts of the salivary glands and pancreas sometimes show metaplastic changes similar to those in the bile ducts.

In the kidneys, the same tendency toward epithelial hyperplasia reveals itself in enlargement and dilatation of tubules, chiefly the collecting tubules of the medullary rays. The epithelium of these tubules is not compressed but hyperplastic, even to the extent that small papillary projections extend into the lumen. A certain amount of fibrosis accompanies these tubular changes if they are marked.

Squamous metaplasia and cornification are likely to be found in the tubular and glandular organs of the male genitalia, especially in the seminal vesicles.

In sheep, similar squamous metaplasia has been found in the endometrial lining and glands. The epithelium of the cervix may be hyperplastic in both cattle and sheep.

It is not to be expected that all of the above lesions will be found in the same animal. Usually any of them, if unequivocally developed, are sufficient for a diagnosis.

A milder degree of epithelial hyperplasia and hyperkeratosis is characteristic of avitaminosis-A. Investigations have shown that in poisoning by chlorinated naphthalenes the amount of vitamin A in the blood declines sharply within five days after the first ingestion of the poison. It falls as low as 25 μg/100 ml, but does not reach zero as it almost does in experimental deprivation of the vitamin. This antivitamin-A effect persists for at least a month after ingestion of the poison has ceased. Feeding five times the normal requirement of vitamin A (5 × 5000 IU vitamin A per 100 pounds of body weight per day) maintains a satisfactory amount of the vitamin in both blood and liver against a limited amount of the toxic feed, but this effect is transient and it does not appear that larger amounts of the vitamin are able to keep pace with increases of the poison. If administration of the vitamin is continued adequately beyond the period of ingestion of the poison, some animals recover and some do not. The question of just how the chlorinated naphthalene neutralizes the effect of vitamin A has baffled investigators. There is evidence that it interferes with conversion of carotene to vitamin A, doubtless through impairment of the liver, but this is by no means the only toxic action, nor is it possible to duplicate the lesions by deprivation of the vitamin, no matter how complete. The similarity of the lesions to dioxin poisoning raises the possibility that chlorinated naphthalenes are contaminated with dioxins.

Since the epithelial hyperplasia of this disease sometimes reaches such proportions to suggest neoplasia, the question arises as to whether chlorinated naphthalenes could possibly have carcinogenic actions. The answer, to date, is entirely in the negative, and is supported by extensive experimentation. To the question whether any other substances can have the same effects as chlorinated naphthalenes, the answer is possibly less certain, but apparently also negative.

Hansel, W., McEntee, K., and Olafson, P.: The effects of two causative agents of experimental hyperkeratosis on vitamin-A metabolism. Cornell Vet., 41:367–376, 1951.

Hoekstra, W.G., Hall, R.E., and Phillips, P.H.: Relationship of vitamin-A to the development of hyperkeratosis (X disease) in calves. Am. J. Vet. Res., 15:41–46, 1954.

Knocke, K.W.: Hyperakeratose in einem Rinderbestand 13 Jahre nach Anwendung eines Holzschutmittels. Dtsche. Tierärztl., 68:701–703, 1961.

Olafson, P.: Hyperkeratosis (X disease) of cattle. Cornell Vet., 37:279–291, 1947.

Pallaske, G.: Zur pathologischen Anatomie der Chlornaphthalinvergiftung der Rinder. Monatsheft. Veterinärmed., 11:677–678, 1956.

Schmidt, H., and Franklin, T.E.: Hyperkeratosis investigations in Texas, 1946–56. Bul. MP-316, Texas Agric. Exp. Sta., 1958.

Sikes, D., and Bridges, M.E.: Experimental production of hyperkeratosis ("X disease") of cattle with a chlorinated naphthalene. Science, 116:506–507, 1952.

Teuscher, R.: Ein seltener klinischer Fall von zweimaliger Vergiftung eines Rinderbestandes durch chloriente naphthaline. Monatsheft. Veterinärmed., 11:675–677, 1956.

Wagener, K.: Hyperkeratosis of cattle in Germany. J. Am. Vet. Med. Assoc., 119:133–137, 1951.

Polychlorinated Biphenyls (PCB) and Polybrominated Biphenyls (PBB)

Polychlorinated biphenyls (PCB), polychlorinated triphenyls (PTB), and polybrominated biphenyls (PBB) are relatively chemically inert compounds that resist high temperatures and are used in the manufacture of plastics, lubricants, wood coatings, and other products in which heat resistance is desired. The toxicity of PCB was first recognized in human beings in Japan, where contaminated cooking oil caused an acneiform dermatitis termed "Yusko." Isolated reports of poisoning in animals have appeared in the past decade, and probably many poisonings have gone unrecognized. The most recent experience occurred in Michigan in 1973, in which a PBB fire retardant ("Firemaster") was inadvertently used in the preparation of cattle feeds. Nearly 30,000 cattle and thousands of other farm animals were destroyed or quarantined, causing estimated losses of between $75 and $100 million.

The most consistent outward signs include swelling of the eyelids, which be-

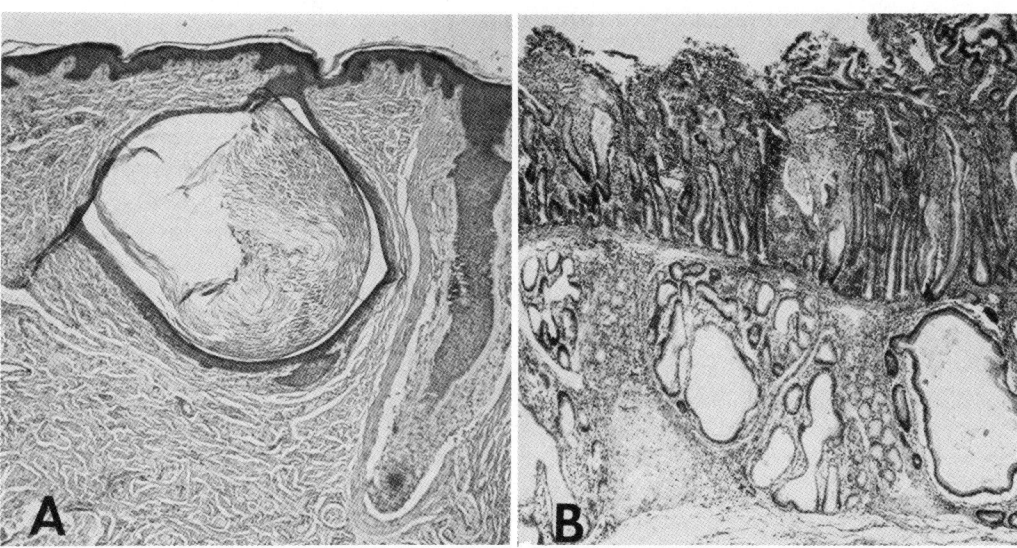

Fig. 16–22. Polychlorinated biphenyl intoxication. *A*, Keratin-filled cyst in skin. *B*, Adenomatous hyperplasia of gastric mucosa. (Courtesy of Dr. J. R. Allen.)

come encrusted with exudate, loss of hair, particularly about the face and neck, but also on the back and thorax, and thickened and wrinkled skin. In cattle, there may be abnormal growth of the hoofs, causing them to grow long and curl upward and inward. Weight loss, subcutaneous edema, diarrhea, shrinking of the udder, drop in milk production, embryonic resorption, and prolonged gestation are other reported signs.

Pathologically, the predominant finding is epithelial hypertrophy, hyperplasia, and metaplasia, especially of the skin and gastrointestinal tract. The epidermis is thickened and hyperkeratotic. Hair follicles become distorted into large, keratin-filled cysts. Squamous metaplasia of sebaceous glands and Meibomian glands leads to their enlargement, ultimately to large keratin-filled cysts. The gastric mucosa undergoes hyperplasia and mucous metaplasia. Large cysts develop in the mucosa, and the epithelium invades extensively through the muscularis mucosa into the submucosa. Hyperplasia of the mucosa of the gallbladder and bile ductule proliferation and fibrosis may or may not be prominent. Focal hepatic necrosis and renal tubular necrosis are often present, especially in the more acute stages. Hepatocellular hypertrophy may lead to gross enlargement of the liver.

The mechanism by which PCB and PBB bring about these changes is unclear at present. As with chlorinated naphthalenes, reduction in vitamin A levels has been noted, but it is doubtful that the lesions are solely related to this effect. Dioxin is a contaminant of PCB and may in part explain its toxicity.

Allen, J.R., Abrahamson, L.J., and Norback, D.H.: Biological effects of polychlorinated biphenyls and triphenyls on subhuman primates. Environ. Res., 6:344–354, 1973.

Allen, J.R., and Carstens, L.A.: Long-term effects on monkeys of limited exposure to the polychlorinated biphenyls. Am. J. Pathol., 74:24a–25a, 1974.

Bruckner, J.V., Khanna, K.L., and Cornish, H.H.: Biological responses of the rat to polychlorinated biphenyls. Toxicol. Appl. Pharmacol., 24:434–448, 1973.

Carter, L.J.: Michigan's PBB incident: chemical mix-up leads to disaster. Science, 192:240–243, 1976.

Cecil, H.C., Harris, S.J., Bitman, J., and Fries, G.F.: Polychlorinated biphenyl-induced decrease in liver vitamin A in Japanese quail and rats. Bull. Environ. Contam. Toxicol., 9:179–185, 1973.

Dunckel, A.E.: An updating on the polybrominated biphenyl disaster in Michigan. J. Am. Vet. Med. Assoc., 167:838–841, 1975.

Jackson, T.F., and Halbert, F.L.: A toxic syndrome associated with the feeding of polybrominated biphenyl-contaminated protein concentrate to dairy cattle. J. Am. Vet. Med. Assoc., 165:437–439, 1974.

Koller, L.D., and Zinkl, J.G.: Pathology of polychlorinated biphenyls in rabbits. Am. J. Pathol., 70:363–378, 1973.

McNulty, W.P., and Griffin, D.A.: Possible polychlorinated biphenyl poisoning in rhesus monkeys (Macaca mulatta). J. Med. Primatol., 5:237–246, 1976.

Moorhead, P.D., Willett, L.B., Brumm, C.J., and Mercer, H.D.: Pathology of experimentally induced polybrominated biphenyl toxicosis in pregnant heifers. J. Am. Vet. Med. Assoc., 170:307–313, 1977.

Peakall, D.B.: PCB's and their environmental effects. Crit. Rev. Environ. Control, 5:469–508, 1975.

Platonow, N.S., and Karstad, L.H.: Dietary effects of polychlorinated biphenyls on mink. Can. J. Comp. Med., 37:391–400, 1973.

Sleight, S.D., and Sanger, V.L.: Pathologic features of polybrominated biphenyl toxicosis in the rat and guinea pig. J. Am. Vet. Med. Assoc., 169:1231–1235, 1976.

GROUP Q: NERVOUS MALFUNCTION

These poisons cause **nervous malfunction** with or without demonstrable lesions in the tissues. Note that many poisons in other groups, for example hepatotoxins, may also be characterized by nervous malfunction.

Strychnine

The intermittent tonic spasms, initiated by noises or other external stimuli, provide a well-known symptomatology that is practically diagnostic. Strychnine binds to synaptic membranes and antagonizes the hyperpolarizing action of glycine (a major inhibitory neurotransmitter), resulting in hyperirritability and lack of normal inhibitory restraint in the spinal part of the reflex arc. There are no postmortem lesions, except possibly petechiae resulting from the anoxia incident to arrest of respiration during the spasms. The very absence of lesions often has diagnostic significance when associated with typical symptoms. The drug can be identified by chemical procedures or by microscopic identification of typical crystals, but both methods are complicated. An infusion of suspected ingesta or urine can be inoculated either into the dorsal lymph space or the peritoneum of frogs or into the peritoneum of mice, with the result that the test animals show the characteristic tonic spasms when irritated by touch. This should occur within 20 minutes. The test is regarded as highly sensitive; the urine of any dog fatally poisoned is stated to contain sufficient strychnine at death for a positive test. In addition to malicious poisoning, accidents in the use of strychnine-containing rodent and grasshopper poisons afford instances of poisoning.

Cox, D.H.: Isolation and identification of strychnine and other alkaloids in veterinary toxicology. Am. J. Vet. Res., 18:929–931, 1957.

McConnell, E.E., van Rensburg, I.B.J., and Minne, J.A.: A rapid test for the diagnosis of strychnine poisoning. J. S. Afr. Vet. Med. Assoc., 42:81–84, 1971.

Thienpont, D., and Vandervelden, M.: Dichapetalum michelsonii Hauman, Nouvelle Plante Toxique pour le Betail du Ruanda-Burundi. Rev. Elev., 14:209–211, 1961.

Young, A.B., and Snyder, S.H.: Strychnine binding associated with glycine receptors of the central nervous system. Proc. Natl. Acad. Sci. USA, 70:2832–2836, 1973.

Nitrogen Trichloride

Under the trade name of **Agene,** nitrogen trichloride, NCl_3, has been used extensively as a bleaching agent in the production of white flour from wheat. At least as early as the 1920s, dogs have been afflicted with a nervous disorder called **fright disease, hysteria,** or **running fits.** Some dogs become sullen, but a larger number have spells when they suddenly appear frightened. With a wild and unnatural expression, the dog may run off for a considerable distance, returning after 5 to 30 minutes in an exhausted and depressed condition. This may be repeated on subsequent occasions, and before many days, incoordination and ataxia become prominent. Such a "running fit" may begin and quickly terminate in convulsions of one or two minutes' duration. Ultimately death may ensue.

The observation made in Europe that this syndrome appeared to be restricted to dogs fed biscuits made from certain flours imported from the United States during the years immediately following World War II led to the discovery that the cause was the toxic effect of this bleaching agent in the flour. Nitrogen trichloride has been found toxic to dogs, ferrets and rabbits but not to guinea pigs, cats, monkeys and humans. Several nontoxic bleaching agents, particularly chlorine dioxide, ClO_2, have now largely replaced the earlier product.

The lesions have been studied by Lewey (1950) and found to consist chiefly of patchy necrosis in the deeper parts of the cerebral cortex, with beginning liquefaction and rather similar changes in the hippocampus. The nerve cells show the usual changes of necrosis, shrinking, distortion, loss of structure and eventual disappearance. These changes are not obvious grossly.

Impey, S.G., Moore, T., and Sharman, I.M.: Effect of flour treatment on the suitability of bread as food for dogs. J. Sci. Food Ag., 12:729–732, 1961.

Lewey, F.H.: Neuropathological changes in nitrogen trichloride intoxication of dogs. J. Neuropathol. Exp. Neurol., 9:396–405, 1950.

Loco

A nervous disorder (loco, Spanish for madness) related to consumption of certain plants (loco weeds) was first recognized in the horses of De Soto and other Spanish conquistadores during their explorations of the New World. The offending plants grow particularly in the western United

States and are classified in the genus *Astragalus,* such as *A. earlei, A. mollissimus* (purple woolly loco), *A. pubentissimus,* and *A. lentiginosus,* or in the genus *Oxytropis,* such as *O. sericea* and *O. lambertii.* In Australia, plants such as *Swainsona luteola, S. greyana,* and *S. galegifolia* are known as the cause of a similar disease ("pea struck") in sheep (Kater, 1965), which has been reproduced experimentally in guinea pigs (Huxtable, 1969). The active principle in all loco weeds appears to be **locoine.** *Astragalus* species are also poisonous through two other mechanisms, discussed previously. Some concentrate selenium and cause selenium poisoning, and others synthesize aliphatic nitro compounds which results in nitrite poisoning.

The disease develops slowly in cattle; consumption over a period of 60 days of an amount equal to 90% of the body weight is necessary to produce symptoms; 98 days and 3.2 times the animal's weight are the minimum likely to cause death. In the horse, however, consumption equivalent to only 30% of the animal's weight during a period of 49 days has been fatal experimentally. As a cumulative poison, signs may not develop until after ingestion of the plants has ceased. In the horse, hyperexcitability, fright, and violent reactions to slight stimuli are the early signs of loco poisoning. Much of this may be due, however, to inability to see clearly. The same impaired vision and disordered judgment cause a cow to perform all the movements of drinking while her mouth is 6 inches above the water. The sensory and motor derangements increase until the animal is unable to get food for itself. A slowly increasing ataxia of the limbs has by this time become an ascending paralysis, so that

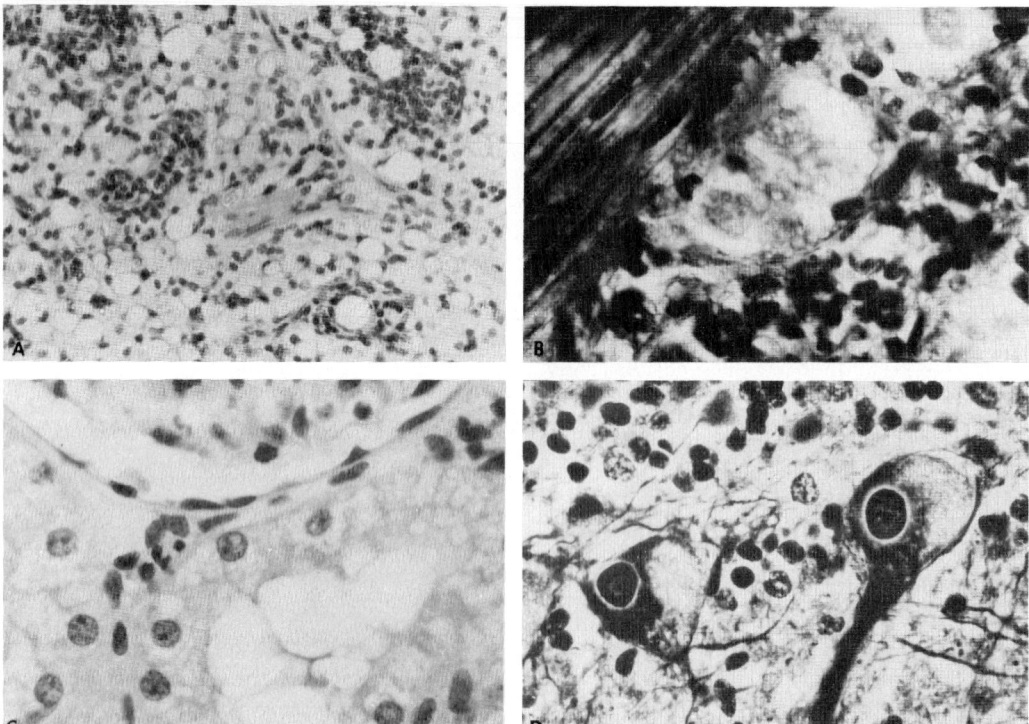

Fig. 16–23. Locoweed poisoning in sheep. *A,* Vacuolated cells in lymph node. *B,* Vacuolated neurons in Auerbach's plexus, *C,* Vacuoles in cells of convoluted tubule, kidney. *D,* Cytoplasmic vacuolation in Purkinje cells. (Courtesy of Dr. Kent R. Van Kampen and *Pathologia Veterinaria.*)

death results from a combination of nervous failure and starvation. Sheep are depressed from the start; goats suffer from posterior paresis and ascending paralysis beginning in the initial stages, with opisthotonos at the last. In all species, the terminal aspects are similar.

Lesions. The microscopic lesions, described in detail by Van Kampen and James (1969) in sheep experimentally poisoned with *Oxytropis sericea, Astragalus pubentissimus* or *A. lentiginosus,* tend to explain the clinical signs. The principal lesion is the result of accumulation of vacuoles in the cytoplasm of cells of various tissue. The nature of this cytoplasmic lesion has not been determined, but the accumulated material, which imparts the vacuolated appearance in sections seen by light microscopy, is not lipid or glycoprotein as indicated by negative reactions to oil-red-O and PAS stains. The material does accumulate in the cytoplasm, displacing the nucleus to one side and eventually, at least in neurons, leads to necrosis. Ultrastructurally, the vacuoles are bound by a single membrane, but bear no relationship with normal organelles. They may represent lysosomes storing an unidentified substance.

Damage to neurons is most significant and may be found in any part of the central and peripheral nervous systems, including those in Meissner's and Auerbach's plexuses in the gastrointestinal tract. In late stages, karyolysis, karyorrhexis, or cytolysis leads to loss of neurons or mineralization of the necrotic remnants. Axonal degeneration may be found, but myelin is not significantly altered. Gliosis and neuronophagic nodules are not conspicuous. Perivascular edema is usually evident throughout the central nervous system. Spheroids (swollen axons) develop following neuronal necrosis.

Accumulations of material similar to that noted in neurons have been described in many other organs, including the follicular epithelium of the thyroid, chief cells of parathyroid, adrenal cortical cells, serous cells of salivary glands, hepatocytes, reticuloendothelial cells of lymph nodes and spleen, epithelial cells of renal convoluted tubules, transitional epithelium of the urinary tract, spermatogonia, and chorionic epithelium. Widespread cytoplasmic vacuolation is also seen in fetuses of ewes which have consumed locoweed. In ewes experimentally fed *A. lentiginosus,* vacuoles appeared within four days in renal tubular epithelium and by eight days in neurons, and neuronolysis was evident by the sixteenth day (Van Kampen and James, 1972). The vacuolated, sometimes foamy appearance of affected cells has been compared to some lipid storage diseases of man, but of course, the cytoplasmic material is not the same. Perhaps further studies with electron microscopy or histochemistry will reveal the precise nature of this lesion and give a clue to the exact effect of the toxin on cells.

Nearly identical vacuolar lesions in neurons and renal epithelium were encountered by Laws and Anson (1968) in sheep poisoned naturally and experimentally by eating *Swainsona luteola* and *S. galegifolia.* James, Van Kampen, and Hartley (1970) compared the toxic effects on pregnant ewes of *Swainsona galegifolia, Astragalus pubentissimus,* and *A. lentiginosus,* and concluded that the active poisonous principle in each of these plants may be the same.

The gross lesions are not diagnostic, but the enlargement of thyroids, emaciation, golden color of liver and renal cortex, generalized edema, and focal erosions in the mucosa of the abomasum near the pylorus have been described. In pregnant cows, the severe edema may resemble **hydrops amnii.** Similarities in clinical signs and chemical interrelationships have suggested that some of the toxins in locoweeds are related to those of lathyrus.

Teratogenic effects have been observed in nature and reproduced experimentally in sheep (James et al., 1969). Feeding of

Astragalus pubentissimus to pregnant sheep results in frequent occurrence of congenital anomalies in the offspring. The type of anomaly appears to depend upon the stage of pregnancy during which the locoweed is eaten. If this locoweed is consumed by the ewes during the twenty-fifth to the forty-ninth days of pregnancy, aplasia of the lower jaw is the dominant congenital anomaly in the lambs. Ingestion of *A. pubentissimus* between the fortieth to sixtieth days of pregnancy often results in hypermobility of the hock and stifle joints in affected lambs. Feeding the plant between the sixtieth and ninetieth days of gestation results in offspring with flexures of carpal joints. Lambs born of ewes which ingested loco between the one-hundredth and one-hundred-twentieth days of pregnancy are apt to have relaxed pastern joints. Abortions are common and some ewes die from this plant poisoning. *Oxytropis sericea* has also been fed to ewes between the eighty-second and one-hundred-second days of gestation, leading to contracted flexor tendons (or muscles) in the offspring. A few cases of arthrogryposis (see lupines) have been associated with locoweed poisoning.

Fraps, G.S., and Carlyle, E.C.: Locoine, the poisonous principle of loco weed. Exp. Sta. Bull. 537, 1936, Texas A. & M. College, College Station.

Hartley, W.J., and James, L.F.: Microscopic lesions in fetuses of ewes ingesting locoweed (*Astragalus lentiginosus*). Am. J. Vet. Res., 34:209–212, 1973.

Huxtable, C.R.: Experimental reproduction and histo-pathology of *Swainsona galegifolia* poisoning in the guinea-pig. Aust. J. Exp. Biol. Med. Sci., 47:339–347, 1969.

Huxtable, C.R.: Ultrastructural changes caused by *Swainsona galegifolia* poisoning in the guinea pig. Aust. J. Exp. Biol. Med. Sci., 48:71–80, 1970.

James, L.F., Keeler, R.F., and Binns, W.: Sequence in the abortive and teratogenic effects of locoweed fed to sheep. Am. J. Vet. Res., 30:377–380, 1969.

James, L.F., and Van Kampen, K.R.: Effects of locoweed intoxication on the genital tract of the ram. Am. J. Vet. Res., 32:1253–1256, 1971.

James, L.F., Van Kampen, K.R., and Hartley, W.J.: Comparative pathology of *Astragalus* (locoweed) and *Swainsona* poisoning in sheep. Pathol. Vet., 7:116–125, 1970.

Laws, L., and Anson, R.B.: Neuronopathy in sheep fed *Swainsona luteola* and *S. galegifolia*. Aust. Vet. J., 44:447–452, 1968.

Nockolds, C.: Poisoning by loco weed. Am. Vet. Rev., 20:569–571, 1896.

Schwartzkopf, D.: Effects of "loco weed." Am. Vet. Rev., 12:160–163, 1888.

Shupe, J.L., et al.: The effect of loco plant on libido and fertility in rams. Cornell Vet.,58:59–66,1968.

Van Kampen, K.R., and James, L.F.: Pathology of locoweed poisoning in sheep. Pathol. Vet., 6:413–423, 1969.

———: Ophthalmic lesions in locoweed poisoning of cattle, sheep, and horses. Am. J. Vet. Res., 32:1293–1295, 1971.

———: Ovarian and placental lesions in sheep from ingesting locoweed (*Astragalus lentiginosus*). Vet. Pathol., 8:193–199, 1971.

———: Pathology of locoweed (*Astragalus lentiginosus*) poisoning in sheep. Sequential development of cytoplasmic vacuolation in tissues. Pathol. Vet., 7:503–508, 1970.

Vetch-Like Astragali

A number of small leguminous plants that resemble the true vetches and sometimes receive that designation produce poisoning on the ranges of the Rocky Mountain region of the United States. They are classified, however, in the genus *Astragalus*, which is notable because of locoweeds, which are also included in it. The form of poisoning produced, like loco, involves the nervous system principally, and does not resemble the hepatotoxic effects of the true vetches.

Under the name of timber milkvetch, we may include *Astragalus decumbens*, *A. convallarius*, *A. hylophilus*, and *A. campestris*, which are similar or identical species. The *red-stemmed peavine*, *A. emoryanus*, is a similar plant; it grows in the more southern regions, whereas the timber milkvetch reaches north into Canada.

Another classification of these plants (Williams et al., 1969) places several varieties in a single genus, *Astragalus miser*. These are: *A. miser var oblongifolius, serotinus, hylophilus, miser, tenuifolius, praeteritus, decumbens,* and *crispatus*. The first three have been incriminated in poisoning of livestock. Cattle appear to be most susceptible, sheep much less so; rabbits and chickens may be poisoned experimentally. The basic sign is nervous weakness and incoordination involving the hindlimbs. When mild, this may be shown only by a momentary sinking of the hindquarters at the start of a forward movement. Later, there is distinct incoordination, such as crossing of the legs and weakness, shown by "knuckling over" of the fetlock joints. Ultimately, the animal falls frequently and rises with difficulty. In the cattle poisoned by milkvetch, the metatarsal and phalangeal joints are abnormally relaxed and poorly controlled, so that in walking the dewclaws (first metatarsal rudiments) strike the hoofs with a flapping sound. This has resulted in the nickname of "cracker-heel" for the disease. In sheep, another prominent, and at times primary, symptom is dyspnea accompanied by a loud rasping noise at inspiration and a cough frequently at expiration. The morphologic basis for this seems not to have been determined. It may be presumed the complete microscopic studies of the nervous system would reveal degenerative changes that would account for the posterior weakness. On the other hand, the fact that a considerable number of victims die suddenly from acute dilatation of the heart, while the usual difficulties are yet at an early stage, raises the suspicion of interference with the metabolic processes of muscle. It should be noted that, while the posterior weakness and paraplegia are much like the corresponding effects of the closely related locoweeds *(Astragalus mollissimus et spp.)*, there are no disturbances of sensation or of the sensorium in the presently considered poisonings.

One toxic agent has been identified as **miserotoxin,** the β glucoside of 3-nitro-1-propanol. This toxin is catabolized in vivo to two toxic fractions, inorganic nitrite and a 3-carbon nitro side chain (Williams et al., 1969). Nitrite (NO_2) produces methemoglobinemia, particularly in rabbits.

Mathews, F.P.: Toxicity of red-stemmed peavine for cattle, sheep, and goats. J. Am. Vet. Med. Assoc., 97:125–134, 1940.
Newsom, I.E., et al.: Timber milk vetch as a poison-ous plant. Exper. Sta. Bull. 425, 1936. Colorado State College, Fort Collins.
Williams, M.C., Van Kampen, K.R., and Norris, F.A.: Timber milkvetch poisoning in chickens, rabbits, and cattle. Am. J. Vet. Res., 30:2185–2190, 1969.

Atropine (Deadly Nightshade, Belladonna)

The foliage and unripe berries of the belladonna plant *(Atropa belladonna)* poison swine and rarely other animals by virtue of the atropine (and other alkaloids) which they contain. Symptoms are largely those of loss of nervous control with incoordination, shortly followed by convulsions and death, usually within 12 hours after the plant is eaten. There are typically mydriasis, falling temperature, and a failing heart. Postmortem lesions are not diagnostic, but may include subserous serofibrinous exudations, perhaps tinged with blood, especially around the kidneys and gallbladder. Of prime importance in diagnosis is the mydriatic action of belladonna. Not only are the patient's pupils dilated, but instillation of a small amount of the patient's urine into the conjunctival sac of a small experimental animal, particularly a cat, dog, or rabbit, should dilate the pupil within a few minutes.

Smith, H.C., Taussig, R.A., and Peterson, P.C.: Deadly nightshade poisoning in swine. J. Am. Vet. Med. Assoc., 129:116–117, 1956.

Equisetum

Known by such names as **horsetail,** mare's tail and jointed rush, several species of equisetum, of which E. *arvense* is the most common, are poisonous, chiefly to horses. Signs are those of nervous disorder and muscular weakness, the latter probably related to faulty innervation. Incoordination gradually increases until there are staggering, reeling, and ultimately inability to stand. Progressive muscular rigidity reaches the point where the animal can only lie on its side with the four limbs stiffly outstretched. Constipation and tenesmus are marked. Large amounts of watery urine are voided. The pupils are dilated; the animal's expression and actions reveal a state of apprehension, which deepens into fright as the result of noises or other stimuli. In a recumbent state, the horse continues to live for several days, maintaining a good appetite until too weak to eat.

Lesions found postmortem include a pale and flabby state of the skeletal musculature, frequently hydroperitoneum, and congestion and inflammatory edema (serous exudate) of the cerebellar and spinal meninges. Microscopic studies are needed, especially of the nervous tissues and the kidneys, which from the polyuria appear to be damaged.

Poisoning by equisetum is prevented and usually cured by the administration of large amounts of thiamine (vitamin-B_1), but not by other components of the B-complex. From this it is inferred that equisetum owes its toxicity to a powerful opponent of thiamine; indeed, an extract of the plant has been shown to neutralize thiamine in vitro. Biochemical studies by Forenbacher have shown that carbohydrate metabolism was impaired in equisetum poisoning in the same way that it is in thiamine deficiency. Glycolysis by the blood in vitro was diminished. Glucose tolerance in the living animal was depressed, as were the amounts of glycogen in liver and muscle. The pyruvic acid in the blood rose to 1.52 mg/100 ml, with oxalic acid behaving similarly; phosphates reached levels of 13 mg, and potassium, 50 mg. The levels of alkaline phosphatase and cholesterinase also rose. (See thiaminase, p 1036, and polioencephalomalacia, Chap. 27.)

Lesions in the central nervous system should be comparable to those of thiamine deficiency or bracken fern poisoning.

Forenbacher, S.: Equisetum poisoning of horses and the vitamin B Complex. Vet. Archiv., 20:405–471, 1950, and 21:497–547, 1951. (English summary.) Abstr. Vet. Bull. No. 2671, 1953; also in Schweiz. Arch. Tierheilkd., 94:153–171, 1952.
Henderson, J.A., et al.: The antithiamine action of equisetum. J. Am. Vet. Med. Assoc., 120:375–378, 1952.
Lott, D.G.: The use of thiamin in mare's tail poisoning of horses. Can. J. Comp. Med., 15:274–276, 1951.
Rich, F.A.: Equisetum poisoning. Am. Vet. Rev., 26:944–954, 1903.

Hemlocks

Poisoning by deadly hemlock, *Conium maculatum*, has been recognized since the dawn of history. Ancient Greeks compelled condemned prisoners (Socrates the most famous) to drink an infusion of this plant, causing a relatively painless death. Herbivorous animals, including swine, occasionally eat the plant in spite of unpalatability and an offensive odor which it releases when bruised. After a mild and transient stimulation, the plant acts as a nerve depressant, and it is upon this nervous depression that the signs are based. While varying somewhat in different species, they involve loss of muscular strength and gradual loss of the power of locomotion, the hindlimbs, as is usual in nervous and paralytic disorders, being the most severely affected. In some cases, there are tremors and rarely generalized trembling, but more often the animal's activities quietly subside into a sort of coma, in which consciousness appears to be greatly depressed but not disordered. Death may come in an hour or thereabouts, but many animals remain comatose for one or several hours and then quietly recover. In cattle, lacrimation, salivation, dyspnea, and fetid or bloody diarrhea have been described. Signs usually commence within an hour or two after the plants are eaten and last for several hours or a day or two.

The postmortem lesions are based upon the cardiac depressant action of the poison, which is an alkaloid called coniine. As a consequence of the slow cardiac failure there is widespread passive congestion, most noticeable in the lungs and liver and the vessels that nourish the heart muscle. It would appear from descriptions of "watery blood" that there is probably hemolysis or decreased clotting power, or both, but opportunities for systematic studies have seldom arisen. Severe localized catarrhal or hemorrhagic enteritis have been described in cattle. Recognizable fragments of leaves or stems may be found in the forestomachs of ruminants and true stomachs of other species, constituting a valuable aid in diagnosis. Congenital malformation of the hindlimbs characterized by lateral deviation and marked rotation has been associated with hemlock poisoning in swine. Whether the *Conium* alkaloids induced these abnormalities is not known (Edmonds et al., 1972).

There is also a similar plant, *Cicuta douglasii et spp.*, which grows in wet places in the Rocky Mountain region of the United States, and which is known as hemlock, **water hemlock,** or poison hemlock. Its large, chambered primary stem and the adjoining roots are especially poisonous. It differs from *Conium maculatum* in causing convulsions of the greatest violence, which are almost always fatal.

Also of interest are the poisonous quails of North America, which in both biblical and modern times have poisoned people who ate their flesh. Evidence indicates that the meat of the quails contained the poisonous principle of hemlock plants which the birds had eaten. The much greater resistance of birds to many poisons than that possessed by mammals is a well-known phenomenon.

Aggio, C.: Two interesting outbreaks of vegetable poisoning. Am. Vet. Rev., 32:368–369, 1907.
Buckingham, J.L.: Poisoning in a pig by hemlock (*Conium maculatum*). Vet. J., 92:301–302, 1936.
Durrel, L.W., et al.: Poisonous and injurious plants in Colorado. Exper. Sta. Bull. 412-A, Colorado A. & M. College, Fort Collins, 1950.
Edmonds, L.D., Selby, L.A., and Case, A.A.: Poisoning and congenital malformations associated with consumption of poison hemlock by sows. J. Am. Vet. Med. Assoc., 160:1319–1324, 1972.
Gunn, A.: Cattle poisoned by hemlock. Vet. J. and Ann. Comp. Pathol., 13:233–235, 1881.
MacDonald, H.: Hemlock poisoning in horses. Vet. Rec., 49:1211–1212, 1937.
Sergent, E.: Les cailles empoisonneuses dans la Bible, et an Algérie de nos jours. Aperçu historique et recherches expérimentales. Arch. Inst. Pasteur D'Algérie, 19:161–192, 1941.
———: Les cailles empoisonneuses en france. (Toxicity of flesh after ingestion of seeds of *Conium maculatum* or *Oenanthe crocata*.) Arch Inst. Pasteur D'Algérie, 26:249–252, 1948.

Lathyrus

Although there are several other closely related toxic species, the principal one is *Lathyrus sativus*. Several common names are in use, including Indian pea, dogtooth pea, flat pea and Singletary pea. *Lathyrus odoratus* is the common sweet pea grown in flower gardens for its fragrance. *L. sativus* is also known in some English-speaking countries as "chickling vetch," but it is not to be confused with the usual vetches, which belong to a different genus, although they are indeed, leguminous plants of generally similar appearance. *Lathyrus sativus*, frequently in mixture with the closely related *L. cicera* and *L. clymenum*, are grown as forage plants especially in Mediterranean countries and India, and the seeds are a frequent article of human food. Under the name of "lathyrism," poisoning from excessive consumption of the seeds is well known in humans and domestic animals, especially horses. Since, in limited amounts, it is a nutritious legume rich in protein, and because of its hardiness, it has been introduced into the agricultural regions of Africa, Canada, and the mountainous ranges of the United States.

Poisoning only occurs when large amounts of seeds are eaten over a period of at least a few weeks, more often months. In man and animals, the one outstanding effect is gradually increasing paralysis of the posterior (inferior) limbs. This is said to depend upon degeneration and disappearance of neurons in the spinal cord accompanied by gliosis and ultimate atrophy of the cord. Since many well-established cases recover, human and animal, it is difficult to believe that irreversible changes occur until the late stages of illness. Some refer to the changes in the cord as inflammatory rather then degenerative. Paralysis of the recurrent laryngeal nerve with the production of "roaring" has been noted several times in horses. In cattle, blindness, torticollis, and anesthesia of the skin are additional symptoms that have been recorded. In any species, the pulse becomes rapid and weak because of incipient vagal paralysis. Constipation and mild digestive disturbances occur occasionally. Death is from respiratory paralysis.

In addition to the lesions of the spinal cord, there are mild chronic enteritis, perhaps with cecal or other impactions, terminal subepicardial hemorrhages (asphyxiative), and pulmonary congestion. A neurotoxin, β-N-oxalyl-L-α, β-diaminopropionic acid (ODAP), has been isolated from seeds of *L. sativus*. The mode of action is suggested to be due to interference with ammonia metabolism in the brain, leading to chronic ammonia toxicity.

Ground sweet pea seeds (*Lathyrus odoratus*) fed to growing rats result in striking skeletal deformities and changes in other mesodermal tissues. Periosteal new bone formation, kyphoscoliosis, and dissecting aneurysms of the aorta occurred, presumably as a result of severe disturbance of the growth of cartilage, bone, or elastic tissues. Paralysis in these rats appeared to result either from pressure upon segments of the spinal cord, as a consequence of the severe scoliosis, or from specific destruction of neurons in the cord. The effect upon bone, cartilage and tendons is considered by Levene (1962) to be the result of impairment of cross-linkage of collagen molecules. The active principles are often referred to as osteolathyrogens or neurolathyrogens, depending upon their effects. Some evidence has accrued (Mennin and Thomas, 1970) that some of these compounds may affect both bone and nervous tissue. The principal lathyrogenic compounds now known are: aminoacetonitrile, a,r-diaminobutyric acid, β-aminopropionitrile, β-cyanoalanine, β-N-oxalyl-L-2,3 diaminopropionic acid, r-glutamyl-β-cyanoalanine, and r-glutamyl-β-aminopropionitrile.

Poisoning of pregnant animals, particularly sheep, has been shown by Keeler et al. (1967) to result in abortions, intrauterine death, contracted tendons, and aplasia of the lower jaw in the offspring. Thus this group of plant toxins has a teratogenic potential.

In turkeys, lathyrism is associated with dissecting aneurysms of the aorta.

Bachauber, T.E., and Lalick, J.J.: The effect of sweet pea meal on the rat aorta. Arch Pathol., 59:247–253, 1955.

Bachauber, T.E., et al.: Lathyrus-factor activity of beta-aminopropionitrile and related compounds. Proc. Soc. Exp. Biol. Med., 89:294–297, 1955.

Cameron, J.M.: Lathyrism-like changes in chicks. J. Pathol. Bact., 82:519–521, 1961.

Cheema, P.S., Padmanaban, G., and Sarma, P.S.: Mechanism of action of β-N-oxalyl-L-α, β-diaminopropionic acid, the *Lathyrus sativus* neurotoxin. J. Neurochem., 18:2137–2144, 1971.

Cleary, E.G.: Lathyrism in swine. Aust. J. Exp. Biol. Med. Sci., 46:8–9, 1968.

Huang, T.C., Cunha, T.J., and Ham, W.E.: Deleterious effects of flat pea seeds for rats. Am. J. Vet. Res., 11:217–220, 1950.

Keeler, R.F., et al.: An apparent relationship between locoism and lathyrism. Can. J. Comp. Med., 31:334–341, 1967.

Lee, J.G.: Experimental lathyrism produced by feeding singletary pea (*Lathyrus pusillus*) seed. J. Nutr., 40:587–594, 1950.

Levene, C.I.: Studies on the mode of action of lathyrogenic compounds. J. Exp. Med., 116:119–133, 1962.

Levene, C.I., and Gross, J.: Alterations in state of molecular aggregation of collagen induced in chick embryos by β-aminopropionitrile (lathyrus factor). J. Exp. Med., 110:771–789, 1959.

McKay, G.F., and Lalich, J.J.: A crystalline "lathyrus factor" from *Lathyrus odoratus*. Arch. Biochem., 52:313–322, 1954.

Mennin, S., and Thomas, D.W.: Comparative effects of an osteolathyrogen and a neurolathyrogen on brain and connective tissues. Proc. Soc. Exp. Biol. Med., 134:489–491, 1970.

Petri, E.: Pathologische Anatomie und Histologie der Vergiftungen. *In* Handbuch der speziellen pathologischen Anatomie und Histologie, Vol. 10. edited by O. Lubarsch and F. Henke. Berlin, J. Springer, 1930.

Ponseti, I.V., and Shepard, R.S.: Lesions of the skeleton and other mesodermal tissue in rats fed sweet-pea seeds. J. Bone Joint Surg., 36-A:1031–1058, 1954.

Selye, H.: Lathyrism. Rev. Can. Biol., 16:1–82, 1957.

Steffek, A.J., and Hendrickx, A.G.: Lathyrogen-induced malformations in baboons: a preliminary report. Teratol., 5:171–180, 1972.

Yeager, V.L., and Taylor, J.J.: Lathyrism and aging. Proc. Soc. Exp. Biol. Med., 129:44–46, 1968.

Zahor, Z., and Machova, M.: Dissecting aneurisms of the large arteries of chick embryos due to (sweet pea) lathyrism. Nature, Lond., 192:532–533, 1961.

Larkspur (Delphinium sp.)

Larkspurs of several different species cause considerable poisoning of cattle and horses on the ranges of the western United States. Symptoms appear in a short time after the plant is eaten and terminate favorably or unfavorably usually within 24 hours. While there are salivation, repeated swallowing and signs of nausea, the most prominent symptoms are related to extreme neuromuscular weakness with sprawling gait, staggering, and finally falling and inability to rise. Muscular quivering is followed toward the end by convulsions and death. The postmortem lesions are acute catarrhal gastroenteritis (hyperemia chiefly) and the widespread venous congestion typical of gradual cardiac failure. Congestion is especially prominent in the kidneys, as well as in the vena cava and large veins.

Marsh, C.D., Clawson, A.B., and Marsh, H.: Larkspur poisoning of livestock. Bull. 365. U.S. Dept. Agr., 1916.
Olsen, J.D.: Tall larkspur poisoning in cattle and sheep. J. Am. Vet. Med. Assoc., 173:762–765, 1978.

Yellow Star Thistle

A plant that grows abundantly in dry, weedy pastures in the northern valleys of the state of California, *Centaurea solsitialis*, popularly known as the yellow star thistle, is credited, on the basis of clinical and experimental studies, with causing an equine central nervous disorder called **"chewing disease"** by stockmen and **nigropallidal encephalomalacia** by pathologists.

Signs appear suddenly after the animal has been eating the plant for one to three months and has consumed several hundred pounds of it. They consist essentially of hypertonicity of the muscles of the face, lips, and tongue due to hyperirritability of the nervous mechanism controlling them, the whole being dependent upon loss of central control from the higher centers. Local reflexes and sensation remain intact. The horse performs involuntary chewing movements, but is unable effectively to obtain food or swallow it. The lips are rigid and the skin is puckered, although the angles of the mouth are not necessarily retracted as in the risus sardonicus of some other nervous disorders. The mouth may be held half open with the tongue protruding, although the animal is able to withdraw the latter and there is no (flaccid) paralysis. A mild degree of somnolence usually prevails, and some disturbance of gait, but death eventually results from starvation or thirst in horses so severely affected that they are unable to drink.

Postmortem, the dorsum of the tongue is regularly coated with the dried salivary and other material that accumulates with cessation of swallowing, and there is often a tendency to local edema and buccal ulceration, perhaps from injury in efforts to eat. Some cases develop enterocolitis, which may or may not be due directly to the poison. The fundamental lesion was found by Cordy (1954) to consist in localized encephalomalacia (necrosis) involving the anterior portions of the globus pallidus and substantia nigra. The necrotic areas were sharply demarcated, roundly elongated, and as much as 10 to 15 mm in greatest dimension. Slightly yellowish or buff in color, the areas were gelatinous and bulging in the early stages, distinctly soft at one or two weeks of age, and cavities filled with semifluid debris at three weeks. The lesions were usually bilaterally symmetrical; when they were unilateral, the peripheral disturbances were contralateral. Microscopically, the early lesions (two to five days) showed pyknosis and karyolysis of neuroglial nuclei and gradual disappearance of neurons, with a limited glial proliferation and slight accumulation of scavenger cells (gitterzellen). With time, the proliferated neuroglia increased (gliosis), as well as the number of scavenger cells, until at three to six weeks, a definite glial capsule had formed and some of the scavenger cells had developed into bizarre forms and giant cells. While there were minute hemorrhages in the dead areas, hyperemia was not a feature. Cordy summarized the changes under the name of nigropallidal encephalomalacia.

A similar disease with essentially the same lesions has been seen in Colorado, and has been produced in horses by feeding dried Russian knapweed (*Centaurea repens*) (Young et al., 1970). They also described necrosis in the nucleus of the inferior colliculus, the mesencephalic nucleus of the trigeminal nerve, and the dentate nucleus.

Cordy, D.R.: Nigropallidal encephalomalacia in horses, associated with ingestion of yellow star thistle. J. Neuropathol. Exp. Neurol., *13*:330–342, 1954.

Fowler, M.E.: Nigropallidal encephalomalacia in the horse. J. Am. Vet. Med. Assoc., *147*:607–616, 1965.

Gard, G.P., Sarem, W.G., and De Ahrens, P.J.: Nigropallidal encephalomalacia in horses in New South Wales. Aust. Vet. J., *49*:107–108, 1973.

Mettler, F.A., and Stern, G.M.: Observations on the toxic effects of yellow star thistle. J. Neuropathol., *22*:164–169, 1963.

Young, S., Brown, W.W., and Klinger, B.: Nigropallidal encephalomalacia in horses fed Russian knapweed *Centaurea repens*, L. Am. J. Vet. Res., *31*:1393–1404, 1970.

———: Nigropallidal encephalomalacia in horses caused by ingestion of weeds of the genus *Centaurea*. J. Am. Vet. Med. Assoc., *157*:1602–1605, 1970.

Botulism

Botulism, or poisoning by the toxin of *Clostridium botulinum*, figures prominently in veterinary diagnoses; especially those made in the earlier decades of this century. The existence of the condition in chickens is well established, the complete flaccid paralysis being graphically described by the popular name of "limberneck." Wild ducks die of a similar condition caused by toxins developed in vegetation decaying in the anaerobic conditions of stagnant pools. The condition was formerly known as **alkali disease** (Quortrup, 1941). Cattle die from a paralytic toxemia known as **loin disease,** which Schmidt has shown to result indirectly from phosphorus deficiency. The cattle, lacking adequate dietary phosphorus, chew the bones of their deceased herd-mates. Bits of decomposed flesh still adhering to the bones frequently harbor soil-borne *Clostridia* and their toxins. **Lamsiekte** in South Africa is a similar disorder.

Symptoms of botulism in horses, as in other species, are those of a gradually increasing paralysis, the functions of swallowing and vision being among the first to suffer. Paralytic prostration follows and ends after a total course of 24 hours, more or less, in death from failure of the respiratory muscles. However, most cases of equine "botulism," as of "forage poisoning," have been reclassified as equine encephalomyelitis with advancing knowledge, so that serious doubts may be entertained about any appreciable frequency of botulinus poisoning occurring in horses. In dogs and cats, as well as sheep and swine, the disease probably does not occur, although a certain experimental susceptibility can be demonstrated. Gastroenteritis has been given as a prominent postmortem lesion, but commonly the true diagnosis has been open to question in the cases showing this lesion. It is doubtful that there are any gross lesions of botulism beyond the petechiae and congestion characteristic of terminal anoxia. Except in typical cases of "limberneck," it is unsafe to render a diagnosis of botulism unless symptoms are produced by oral administration of the suspected material to a guinea pig, while a control previously immunized by antitoxin remains healthy. (See page 584.)

Allen, T.: Botulism in cattle. J. Am. Vet. Med. Assoc., *106*:163–164, 1945.

Quortrup, E.R., and Holt, A.L.: Botulism type C in minks. J. Am. Vet. Med. Assoc., *97*:167–168, 1940.

———: Botulinus-toxin producing areas in western duck marshes. J. Bact., 41:363–372, 1941.

Anguina (Rye Grass Poisoning; Rye Grass Staggers)

Anguina agrostis is one of the many species of minute nematodes that infest plants. In the case of this species, microscopic larvae invade the seeds of certain grasses, causing the seed to become an enlarged reactive mass known as a gall. The multitudinous larvae remain dormant in the gall until it is softened by moisture, when they escape and reproduce. Among the species of grass liable to be infested by this parasite are Chewings fescue, creeping red fescue, various kinds of bent grass, orchard grass, buffalo grass, red top, creeping timothy, sweet vernal grass, velvet grass, annual blue grass, and Kentucky blue grass. *Anguina lolii* has been identified as a parasite on Wimmera rye grass (*Lolium rigidum*) in Australia. This parasite acts as a vector for a *Corynebacterium sp.*, which grows as a yellow slime on the plants and in the galls. It is thought that the source of the toxicity is from the *Corynebacterium sp.*

As has been shown by Galloway, working on the irrigated grass fields of arid central Oregon (USA), horses and cattle, as well as experimental rats and chickens, are poisoned when they consume sufficient amounts of infested grass seeds, either mixed with the hay or in "screenings," the discarded imperfect seeds separated from harvested grass seed. The grass in which this occurred in Galloway's experience was Chewings fescue grass (*Festuca rubra v. commutata*).

Formerly viewed as manifestations of forage poisoning, the signs indicate that the toxic substance, which can be extracted with boiling alcohol, is a nerve poison. Prominent among these symptoms are staggering, knuckling of the feet, tucking the head between the forelegs, falling, and clonic spasms. The illness may arise when the toxic material has been consumed for two weeks, more or less. Death may follow in a matter of hours or the nervous symptoms may continue for a week or more. Gross lesions are not discernible; microscopic changes apparently have not been studied. Diagnosis is made by soaking the suspected seeds and galls and demonstrating the microscopic larvae, which are numerous.

Berry, P.H., and Wise, J.L.: Wimmera rye grass toxicity in western Australia. Aust. Vet. J., 51:525–530, 1975.

Galloway, J.H.: Grass seed nematode poisoning in livestock. J. Am. Vet. Med. Assoc., 139:1212–1214, 1961.

Haag, J.R.: Toxicity of nematode infested Chewings fescue seed. Science, 102:406–407, 1945.

Lanigan, G.W., Payne, A.L., and Frahn, J.L.: Origin of toxicity in parasitized annual ryegrass (*Lolium rigidum*). Aust. Vet. J., 52:244–246, 1976.

Latch, G.C.M., Falloon, R.E., and Christensen, M.J.: Fungi and ryegrass staggers. NZ J. Agric. Res., 19:233–242, 1976.

Shaw, J.N., and Muth, O.H.: Some types of forage poisoning in Oregon cattle and sheep. J. Am. Vet. Med. Assoc., 114:315–317, 1949.

Carbon Disulfide

This highly volatile liquid has a number of industrial and laboratory uses, but domestic animals come in contact with it when it is administered as a treatment against gastric or intestinal parasites, chiefly in horses and swine. Serious excesses in dosage have been rare, but a more frequent accident has been the breaking of a capsule in the patient's pharynx. Violent spasm of the regional musculature is the result, and fatal arrest of respiration is a possibility. Signs of poisoning include transient local pain and inflammation, but are largely related to its nerve-depressant action, dullness and lethargy being followed by lower neuron paralysis and coma. Lesions, other than localized gastritis and enteritis in areas of contact, are neurologic. Nerve cells are destroyed here and there in the brain and cord, and fiber tracts and peripheral nerves suffer demyelinization.

Ortho-Tricresyl Phosphate

This substance, contained in a type of synthetic rubber used for shoe soles, scraps of which were eaten by chickens, was shown clinically and experimentally to be highly fatal. Signs in chickens were inappetence, fetid diarrhea, and progressive paralysis of the legs. Sensation, at least of pain, was not lost. The poisoning was invariably fatal in three or four weeks. Lesions consisted principally of enteritis with atrophy of the unused gastrointestinal tract and a full gallbladder. There was wallerian degeneration of the myelin sheaths of peripheral nerves, principally the sciatic and lumbosacrals, which resembled histologically the lesion of thiamine deficiency.

Hartwigk, H.: Lähmungen bei Hühnern durch Weichigelit. Monatsh. Veternirm., 5:53–55, 1950.

Lead

Animals are sometimes poisoned by lead salts through licking painted surfaces, which is a habit of calves especially, or through the ingestion of paint or putty left in cans or otherwise discarded. Puppies are most often poisoned by chewing or eating objects painted with lead-base paints, old paint chipped from surfaces to be repainted, linoleum containing lead, and less frequently, broken wet cell batteries, plumber's lead compounds, or lead-containing roofing material (Zook et al., 1969). Children may be poisoned from these same sources or possibly from lead-glazed cooking ware. Waterfowl have been poisoned by metallic lead shot ingested from the sludge of lake-bottoms, in which the discharges from the guns of many hunters had accumulated (Trainer and Hunt, 1965). Fumes from burning storage batteries, cutaneous absorption from gasoline containing tetra-ethyl lead, and other mechanisms have been rarely incriminated. Habitual exposure to fumes from lead smelters has poisoned horses working in or near them. The lead in wind-borne contamination of pastures in

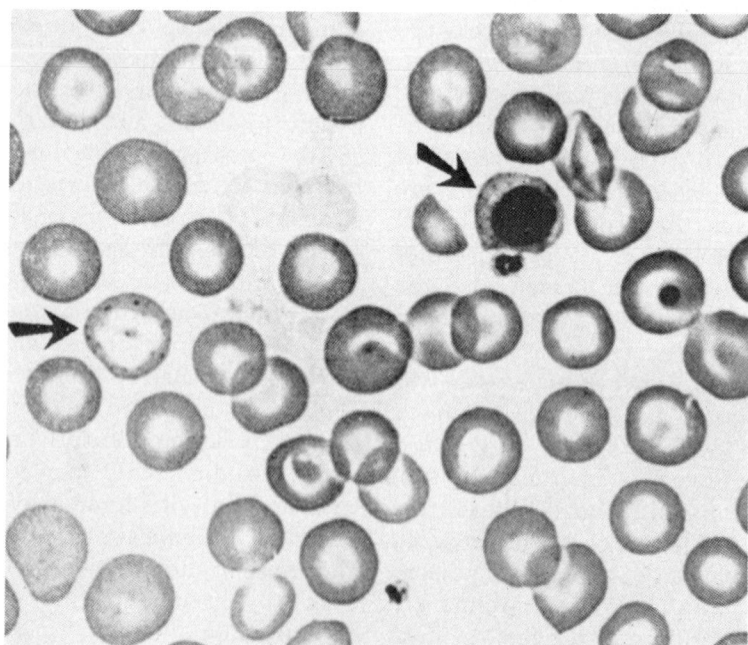

Fig. 16–24. Lead poisoning of a dog. Punctate basophilic stippling in nucleated and non-nucleated erythrocytes (arrows) in a smear of peripheral blood stained with Wright-Giemsa's stain. Note anisocytosis, poikilocytosis, hypochromia, "target" cells, and polychromatophilia involving red blood cells. (Courtesy of Dr. B. C. Zook and *Journal of the American Veterinary Medical Assocation*.)

the vicinity of such smelters may reach 130 mg/kg of dry forage, and accumulations of lead in the soil to levels reaching 1000 ppm have been associated with poisoning of cattle and horses. Orchard sprays frequently contain lead arsenate, but the arsenical ion is the one of principal importance. In calves and sheep, a single dose of 200 to 400 mg/kg of body weight is regularly fatal, but a daily intake of about 6 mg/kg of

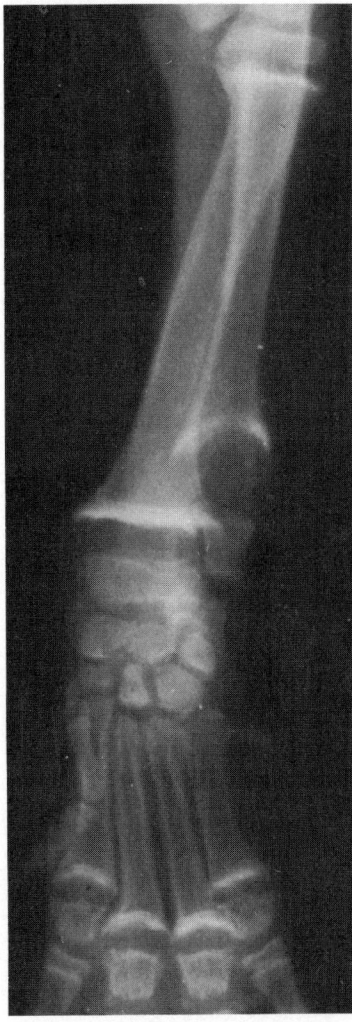

Fig. 16–25. Lead poisoning of a young dog. Radiograph of a foreleg. Radiographically dense bands in the distal metaphysis of radius, ulna and metacarpal bones and proximal metaphysis of the radius. (Courtesy of Dr. B. C. Zook and *Journal of the American Veterinary Medical Association.*)

body weight is necessary to produce cumulative poisoning in an adult cow. Horses appear to be somewhat more susceptible (Hammond and Aronson, 1964). The minimum lethal dose of lead in waterfowl has been found to approximate 8 mg/kg of body weight (Coburn et al., 1951). Lead poisoning is rarely seen in swine, which seem to be more tolerant than other domestic species (Lassen and Buck, 1979).

Signs and Lesions. The signs and lesions of lead poisoning in general focus on its effects on red blood cells, the nervous system, kidney, and bone. There is, however, great variation in the extent of the lesions in these tissues from one example of lead poisoning to another and between species. The explanation for these variations is not clear, but in part, is related to the duration of exposure. Young animals and children appear to be more susceptible. High environmental temperature and vitamin D accentuate the poisoning. Undoubtedly, there are many more factors that influence the toxicity and development of lesions.

Red Blood Cells. Anemia develops in almost all species. In dogs, the anemia is usually slight, but there are regularly large numbers of nucleated red blood cells in peripheral circulation, often up to 100 or more per 100 white blood cells. Basophilic stippling occurs in almost all examples. The appearance of immature red blood cells with little anemia is a strong indication of lead poisoning in the dog. Lead inhibits two enzymes involved in hemoglobin synthesis: d-aminolevulinic acid dehydratase and ferrochelatase. Inability to synthesize hemoglobin is in part the basis of anemia. This also leads to increased urinary excretion of porphyrins and d-aminolevulinic acid, two measurements which can be useful as diagnostic aids. Erythrocytes accumulate protoporphyrin IX, which causes them to fluoresce red when exposed to 320 to 400 nm ultraviolet light. Inhibition of nucleotidase is believed to result in the basophilic stippling as well as the increased fragility of red cells. The resultant shortened erythrocyte lifespan also contributes to anemia. Bone marrow, as to be expected, is hyperplastic.

Nervous System. The neuropathologic effects of lead poisoning are of the greatest concern and have received the greatest attention, but are still not clearly understood. Signs in most species include restlessness, head pressing, hyperesthesia, colic, tremors, ataxia, convulsions, and blindness. Horses most often exhibit gradual paralysis. Laryngeal paralysis is quite characteristic, resulting in noisy respiration (roaring).

Lesions may be minimal or absent even in the presence of neurologic signs. Microscopically the most consistent findings are cerebral edema and marked distention of many arterioles, venules, and capillaries. Endothelial cells are swollen and hyperplastic and occasionally pyknotic. In dogs, arteriolar walls may be hyalinized or contain hyalin thrombi. Laminar necrosis in the deeper cortical gray matter is often a feature that is believed to develop independently of vascular lesions. It is accompanied by astrocytosis. Astrocytosis may also be evident diffusely throughout both gray and white matter. Focal necrosis of basal nuclei and brain stem nuclei may also be encountered. A demyelinating encephalopathy has been associated with lead poisoning in nonhuman primates, but this is not consistent with the findings in other species, in which necrosis is principally confined to gray matter, nor has the lesion been seen in experimentally poisoned monkeys (Sauer et al., 1970; Hopkins and Dayan, 1974; Clasen et al., 1974).

Peripheral neuropathy leading to motor weakness is one of the common manifestations of lead poisoning in human beings,

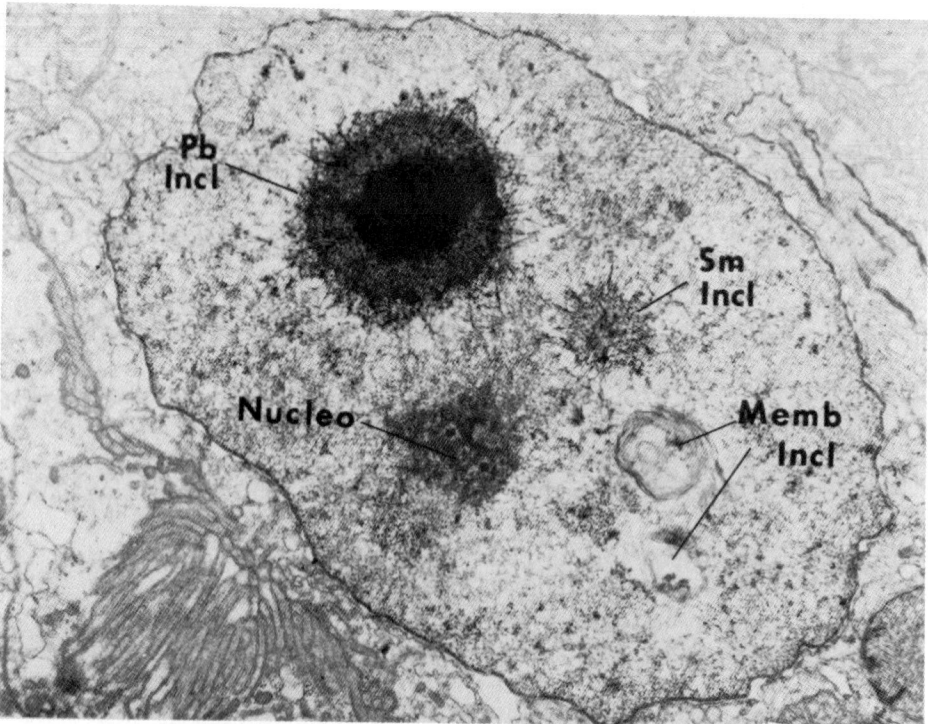

Fig. 16–26.   Lead poisoning of a rat. Electron micrograph of nucleus of a proximal renal tubular epithelial cell. Inclusion body (*Pb incl*); nucleolus (*nucleo*); small, possibly incipient inclusion body (*sm incl*), and nonspecific invaginations of cytoplasmic fragments (*memb incl*). (Courtesy of Dr. Robert A. Goyer and *Laboratory Investigation*.)

and may account for the paralysis seen in horses. The peripheral nerves have not been studied extensively in animals, but the lesion in man is wallerian degeneration of nerve roots. Segmental degeneration of axons and myelin have been reproduced in laboratory rats and guinea pigs.

Kidney. One of the most well known lesions of lead poisoning is the occurrence of intranuclear inclusion bodies in tubular epithelial cells of the kidney. Similar inclusion bodies develop in hepatocytes and osteoclasts. These inclusions are recognized by light microscopy by their acid-fast character when stained with carbol-fuchsin, and their failure to stain for DNA by the Feulgen reaction. In electron micrographs (Goyer et al., 1970), the inclusion is a distinctive discrete body with a dense central core surrounded by a zone of fibrillar structures (Fig. 16–26). Inclusions isolated from cells after digestion with trypsin are seen as a dense homogeneous core surrounded by a membrane (Fig. 16–28). Chemical analysis of isolated inclusions reveals them to contain lead and protein in relatively constant ratios. Although the presence of these inclusion bodies is considered pathognomonic for exposure to lead, caution should be used in assessing their usefulness to diagnose lead poisoning. They develop within hours of exposure and may be present in the absence of any clinical signs or other lesions of lead poisoning. Moreover, they are not invariably present in lead poisoning. Cytoplasmic inclusion bodies may also be present.

Renal tubular dysfunction, as indicated

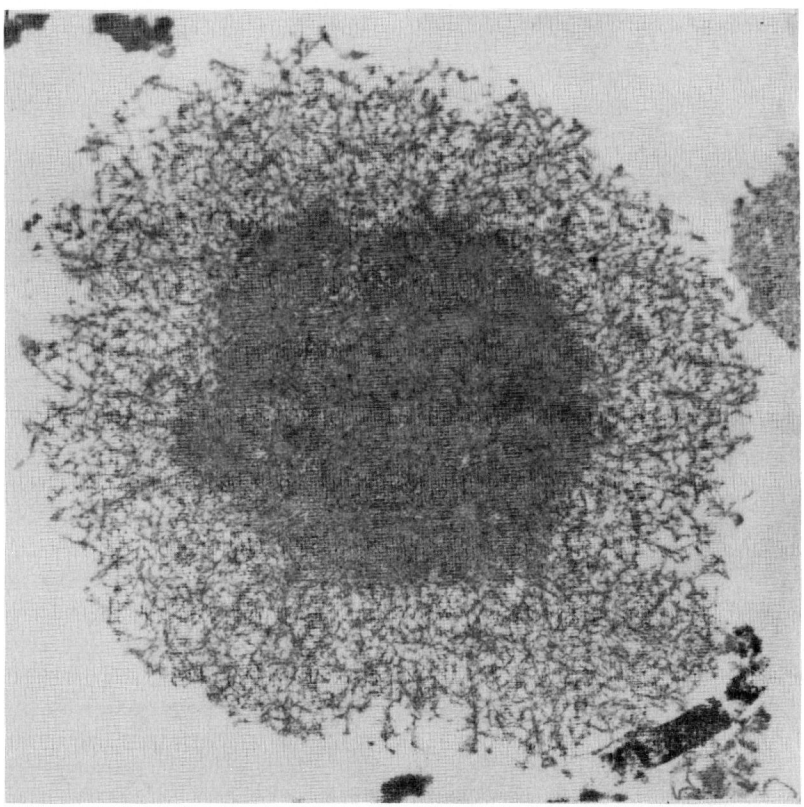

Fig. 16–27. Lead poisoning. Electron micrograph (× 30,000) of an isolated inclusion body from renal tubular epithelium of a rat. Note fibrillar outer zone with attached granules. (Courtesy of Dr. Robert A. Goyer and *Laboratory Investigation*.)

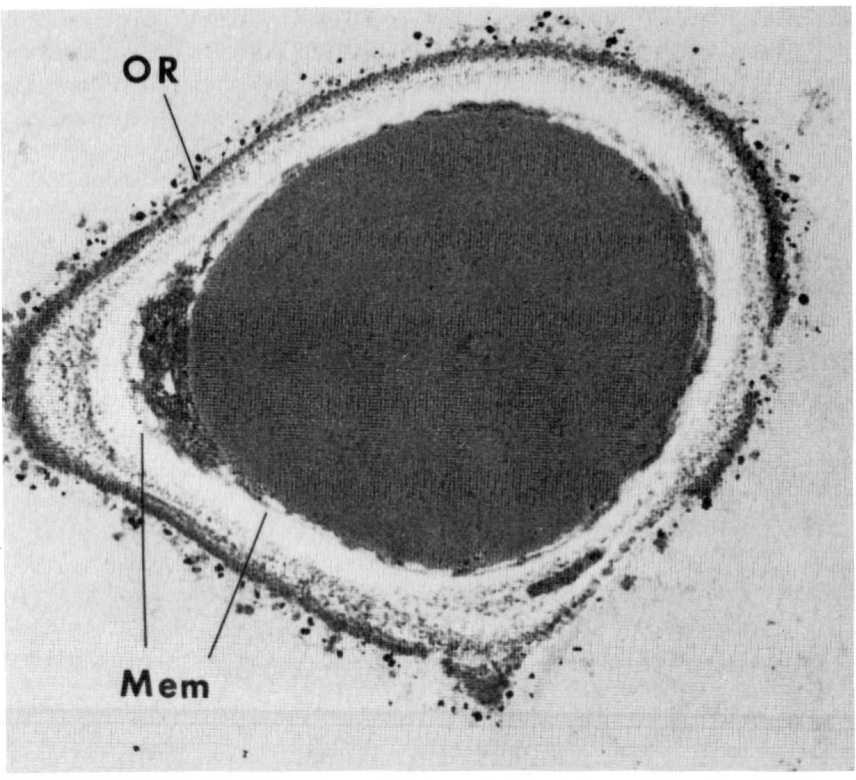

Fig. 16–28. Lead poisoning. Isolated inclusion body after digestion with trypsin. Electron micrograph (× 35,200). Note central core bounded by a membrane (Mem), probably consisting of hydrated phospholipids. A clear zone separates this membrane from a granular outer rim (OR). (Courtesy of Dr. Robert A. Goyer and *Laboratory Investigation.*)

by proteinuria or aminoaciduria, has been noted in human beings, dogs, and experimentally poisoned rats; however, tubular lesions have been described in almost all species. The acute lesions are principally restricted to the proximal convoluted tubule, whose epithelial cells have enlarged nuclei, become swollen, and may undergo necrosis and slough. Chronic nephropathy is described as an outcome of lead poisoning in man and has been reproduced in rats and rabbits. It is characterized by tubular dilatation and fibrosis. The exact causal relationship to lead poisoning, however, deserves further study.

Bone. The lead line, a linear metaphyseal density seen on radiographs, is another well-recognized lesion of lead poisoning in growing animals. Microscopically, this band is composed of trabeculae of calcified cartilage covered by a thin layer of bone. The bars of mineralized cartilage, which results from impaired resorption by osteoclasts, are wider than normal and project further into the metaphyseal marrow cavity than normal. Although numerous multinucleated giant cells surround these spicules, they are apparently incapable of digesting the mineralized matrix. Many such cells bear acid-fast intranuclear inclusion bodies. Bone formation appears to be depressed, which is consistent with reports of osteoporosis resulting from lead poisoning. Lameness is a not infrequent clinical sign, and may result from the metaphyseal lesion.

Other Tissues. A variety of changes have been reported in other tissues, but the lesions are less consistent and their relationship to lead poisoning not clear. These include pancreatic fibrosis, interstitial pneumonia, retarded embryonic development, oligospermia, focal myocardial necrosis, hepatic fatty change, and toxic hepatitis. Night blindness has been reported in experimentally poisoned monkeys, and a degenerative retinopathy, in rabbits (Bushnell et al., 1977; Hughes and Coogan, 1974).

Diagnosis. It is frequently difficult to diagnose lead poisoning with certainty. The demonstration of lead in fluids and tissues is of value, but extreme variations are encountered. Zook et al. (1972) consider the following levels of significance: blood lead 35 μg or more/100 ml; urine lead, 75 μg or more/L; urine lead 24 hours after starting chelation therapy, 821 μg or more/L; hair lead, 88 μg or more/g; liver lead (wet weight), 3.6 μg or more/g. Reference has already been made to the usefulness of urinary excretion of porphyrins, d-aminolevulinic acid, and erythrocyte fluorescence. The occurrence of nucleated and other immature red blood cells in peripheral circulation, out of proportion to anemia, is one of the best diagnostic clues, especially in the presence of neurologic signs.

Pathologically, the lesions in the central nervous system, kidney, and bone are of greatest consistency. Lead-containing foreign bodies (e.g., paint, linoleum) may sometimes be demonstrated radiographically in the gastrointestinal tract. The classic "lead line," a dark bluish discoloration of the gingival mucosa adjacent to the teeth, is less useful and frequent in animals than, reportedly, it is in man. This lead line is the result of precipitation of lead sulfide following interaction with blood-borne lead and hydrogen sulfide arising from decaying particles of food. In young dogs, increased radiographic density may be demonstrated at the epiphysis of long bones (Fig. 16–25).

Allcroft, R.: Lead poisoning in cattle and sheep. Vet. Rec., *63*:583–590, 1951.

Anderson, C., and Danylchuk, K.D.: The effect of chronic low level lead intoxication on the haversian remodeling system in dogs. Lab. Invest., *37*:466–469, 1977.

Bushnell, P.J., Bowman, R.E., Allen, J.R., and Marlar, R.J.: Scotopic vision deficits in young monkeys exposed to lead. Science, *196*:333–335, 1977.

Choie, D.D., and Richter, G.W.: Lead poisoning: rapid formation of intranuclear inclusions. Science, *177*:1194–1195, 1972.

Christian, R.G., and Tryphonas, L.: Lead poisoning in cattle: brain lesions and hematologic changes. Am. J. Vet. Res., *32*:203–216, 1971.

Clasen, R.A., et al.: Experimental acute lead encephalopathy in the juvenile rhesus monkey. Environ. Health Perspect., *7*:175–185, 1974.

Cordy, D.R.: Osteodystrophia fibrosa accompanied by visceral accumulations of lead. Cornell Vet., *47*:480–490, 1957.

de Bruin, A.: Certain biological effects of lead upon the animal organism. Arch. Environ. Health, *23*:249–264, 1971.

Donawick, W.J.: Chronic lead poisoning in a cow. J. Am. Vet. Med. Assoc., *148*:655–661, 1966.

Eisenstein, R., and Kawanoue, S.: The lead line in bone: a lesion apparently due to chondroclastic indigestion. Am. J. Pathol., *80*:309–316, 1975.

Fenstermacher, R., Pomeroy, B.S., Roepke, M.H., and Boyd, W.L.: Lead poisoning in cattle. J. Am. Vet. Med. Assoc., *108*:1–4, 1946.

Fullerton, P.M.: Chronic peripheral neuropathy produced by lead poisoning in guinea-pigs. J. Neuropathol. Exp. Neurol., *25*:214–236, 1966.

Goyer, R.A.: The renal tubule in lead poisoning. I. Mitochondrial swelling and aminoaciduria. Lab. Invest., *19*:71–77, 1968.

Goyer, R.A., and Krall, R.: Ultrastructural transformation in mitochondria isolated from kidneys of normal and lead-intoxicated rats. J. Cell. Biol., *41*:393–400, 1969.

Goyer, R.A., and Rhyne, B.C.: Pathological effects of lead. Int. Rev. Exp. Pathol., *12*:1–77, 1973.

Goyer, R.A., et al.: Lead and protein content of isolated intranuclear inclusion bodies from kidneys of lead-poisoned rats. Lab. Invest., *22*:245–251, 1970.

Hammond, P.B., and Aronson, A.L.: Lead poisoning in cattle and horses in the vicinity of a smelter. Ann. NY Acad. Sci., *111*:595–611, 1964.

Harbourne, J.F., McCrea, C.T., and Watkinson, J.: An unusual outbreak of lead poisoning in calves. Vet. Rec., *83*:515–517, 1968.

Hopkins, A.P., and Dayan, A.D.: Pathology of experimental lead encephalopathy in baboon (*Papio anubis*). Br. J. Ind. Med., 31:128–133, 1974.

Hsu, F.S., et al.: Lead inclusion bodies in osteoclasts. Science, 181:447–448, 1973.

Hughes, W.F., and Coogan, P.S.: Pathology of the pigment epithelium and retina in rabbits poisoned with lead. Am. J. Pathol., 77:237–254, 1974.

Knight, H.D., and Burau, R.G.: Chronic lead poisoning in horses. J. Am. Vet. Med. Assoc., 162:781–786, 1973.

Kowalczyk, D.F.: Lead poisoning in dogs at the University of Pennsylvania Veterinary Hospital. J. Am. Vet. Med. Assoc., 168:428–432, 1976.

Lassen, E.D., and Buck, W.B.: Experimental lead toxicosis in swine. Am. J. Vet. Res., 40:1359–1364, 1979.

Link, R.P., and Pensinger, R.R.: Lead toxicosis in swine. Am. J. Vet. Res., 27:759–763, 1966.

MacKintosh, P.G.: Clinical manifestations and surgical treatment of lead poisoning in the horse. J. Am. Vet. Med. Assoc., 14:193–195, 1929.

McIntosh, I.G.: Lead poisoning in animals. Vet. Rev. Annotations, 2:57–60, 1956. (A review.)

Muro, L.A., and Goyer, R.A.: Chromosome damage in experimental lead poisoning. Arch. Pathol., 87:660–663, 1969.

Park, E.A., Jackson, D., Goodwin, T.C., and Kadji, L.: X-ray shadows in growing bones produced by lead: their characteristics, cause, anatomical counterpart in the bone and differentiation. J. Pediatr., 3:265–298, 1933.

Richter, G.W.: Evolution of cytoplasmic fibrillar bodies induced by lead in rat and mouse kidneys. Relation to clusters of ferritin. Am. J. Pathol., 83:135–148, 1976.

Richter, G.W., Kress, Y., and Cornwall, C.C.: Another look at lead inclusion bodies. Am. J. Pathol., 53:189–217, 1969.

Roscoe, D.E., Nielsen, S.W., Eaton, H.D., and Rousseau, J.E.,Jr.: Chronic plumbism in rabbits: a comparison of three diagnostic tests. Am. J. Vet. Res., 36:1225–1229, 1975.

Sauer, R.M., Zook, B.C., and Garner, F.M.: Demyelinating encephalomyelopathy associated with lead poisoning in nonhuman primates. Science, 169:1091–1093, 1970.

Stowe, H.D., Goyer, R.A., Krigman, M.M., Wilson, M., and Cates, M.: Experimental oral lead toxicity in young dogs. Arch. Pathol., 95:106–116, 1973.

Thomson, R.G.: Reliability of acid-fast inclusions in the kidneys of cattle as an indication of lead poisoning. Can. Vet. J., 13:88–89, 1972.

Trainer, D.O., and Hunt, R.A.: Lead poisoning of whistling swans in Wisconsin. Avian Dis., 9:252–264, 1965.

Wells, G.A.H., Howell, J.McC., and Gopinath, C.: Experimental lead encephalopathy of calves. Histological observations on the nature and distribution of the lesions. Neuropathol. Appl. Neurobiol., 2:175–190, 1976.

White, E.G., and Cotchin, E.: Natural and experimental cases of poisoning of calves by flaking lead paint. Vet. J., 104:75–91, 1948.

Zook, B.C.: The pathologic anatomy of lead poisoning in dogs. Vet. Pathol., 9:310–327, 1972.

Zook, B.C.: Lead intoxication in urban dogs. Clin. Toxicol., 6:377–388, 1973.

Zook, B.C., Carpenter, J.L., and Leeds, E.B.: Lead poisoning in dogs. J. Am. Vet. Med. Assoc., 155:1329–1342, 1969.

Zook, B.C., et al.: Lead poisoning in dogs: analysis of blood, urine, hair, and liver for lead. Am. J. Vet. Res., 33:903–909, 1972.

Zook, B.C., and Sauer, R.M.: Leucoencephalomyelosis in nonhuman primates associated with lead poisoning. J. Wildl. Dis., 9:61–63, 1973.

Mercury

Acute mercurial poisoning may result from the accidental ingestion of mercury compounds, chiefly the extremely poisonous mercuric chloride (bichloride of mercury) or the organic mercurial fungicides. It may also occur as the result of excessive absorption from bichloride antiseptic solution, or possibly from mercuric iodide (red biniodide of mercury) used as a counterirritant or due to inhalation of mercury vapor from metallic mercury. In such cases, symptoms, arising within a period of some hours, include severe colicky pains, vomiting, and diarrhea. The chief lesion is severe and perhaps hemorrhagic gastroenteritis. The gastric mucosa undergoes coagulative necrosis, a change comparable to what happens to tissues subjected to mercurial fixatives in the pathology laboratory.

If the patient lives a few days, a severe and stubborn ulcerative colitis develops, for absorbed mercury is extensively eliminated through the colonic mucous membrane. About this time, too, anuria and uremia develop because of destruction of the renal tubules. The proximal convoluted tubules and, to a lesser degree, the other tubules undergo hydropic degeneration and necrosis of their epithelium, the necrotic cytoplasm being desquamated and sometimes congealed to form albuminous casts in the lumen. If the patient manages to survive, a new epithelial lining, at first very low and flat, is regenerated after about ten days.

The employment of mercurial drugs by

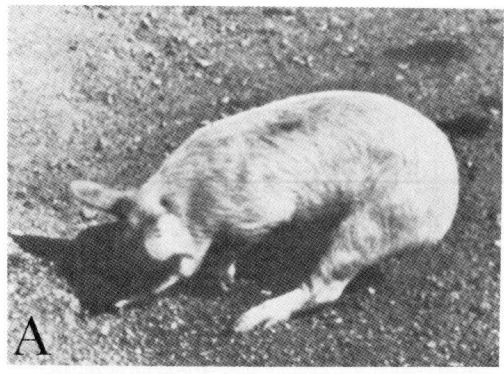

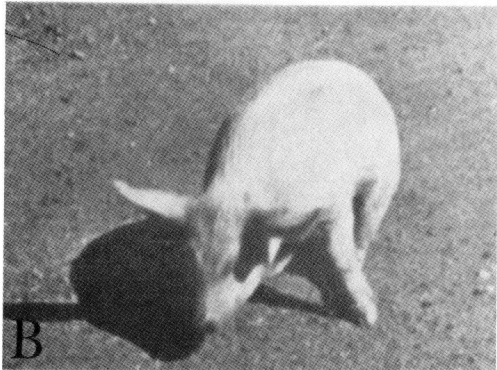

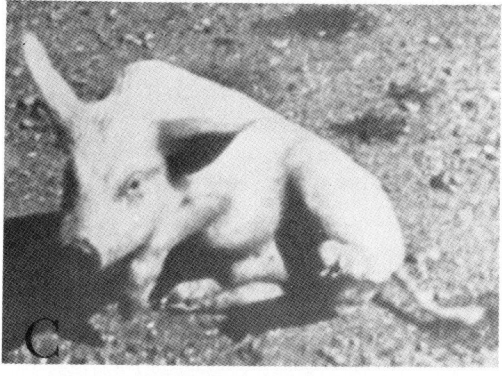

Fig. 16–29. Organo-mercurial poisoning. This affected pig demonstrates paresis, manifest by *A*, knuckling of fetlocks, and *B*, and *C*, falling backwards. (Courtesy of Dr. L. Tryphonas.)

ingestion or in ointment, douches or other preparations, or exposure to metallic mercury, if continued for a time, produces a slower type of poisoning, with soreness, swelling, bleeding, and ultimately, ulceration of the gums, tongue, and buccal mu-

cosa generally. Necrosis may extend to the jaw bones; anemia, edema (doubtless of renal origin), cachexia, and terminal infections lead to death. Nervous disorders based upon injury essentially similar to the nervous changes, presently to be described, accompany this form of poisoning, the whole syndrome sometimes being known as **mercurialism.** Local poisoning, characterized by paralysis of the hand and forearm involved, is reported in a man who rubbed an ointment containing mercuric iodide into the skin of cattle.

The usual mercurial poisoning encountered in domestic animals at the present time results from using as feed for animals, chiefly swine, grains (e.g., wheat, oats, barley, rice) that had been set aside for seed and treated with an organic mercurial, such as methylmercury, arylmercury, ethylmercury phosphate, and mercury p-toluene sulfonanilide, as a means of controlling fungous diseases in the germinating plants. The use of such seed grains for feed is not always accidental, the temptation to avoid waste being great. Industrial plants that discharge mercurial waste products into streams or rivers present a potent hazard to man and animals.

At least one report has been made concerning mercury poisoning in a family that involved an eight-year-old girl, her thirteen-year-old brother, and their twenty-year-old sister (Storrs, 1970; Curley et al., 1971). All were ill with similar signs of decreased vision, ataxia, and depression leading to coma. Toxic amounts of mercury were demonstrated in the urine of each patient. Each of these children, and four other members of the family, had eaten pork from swine slaughtered on their farm. Fourteen of seventeen swine on the farm had been ill with blindness and disturbance of gait. Twelve of the fourteen swine died. The swine had been fed seed grain treated with mercury dicyandiamide; mercury was demonstrated chemically in the pork and in the seed grain. This report appears to establish mercury poisoning of

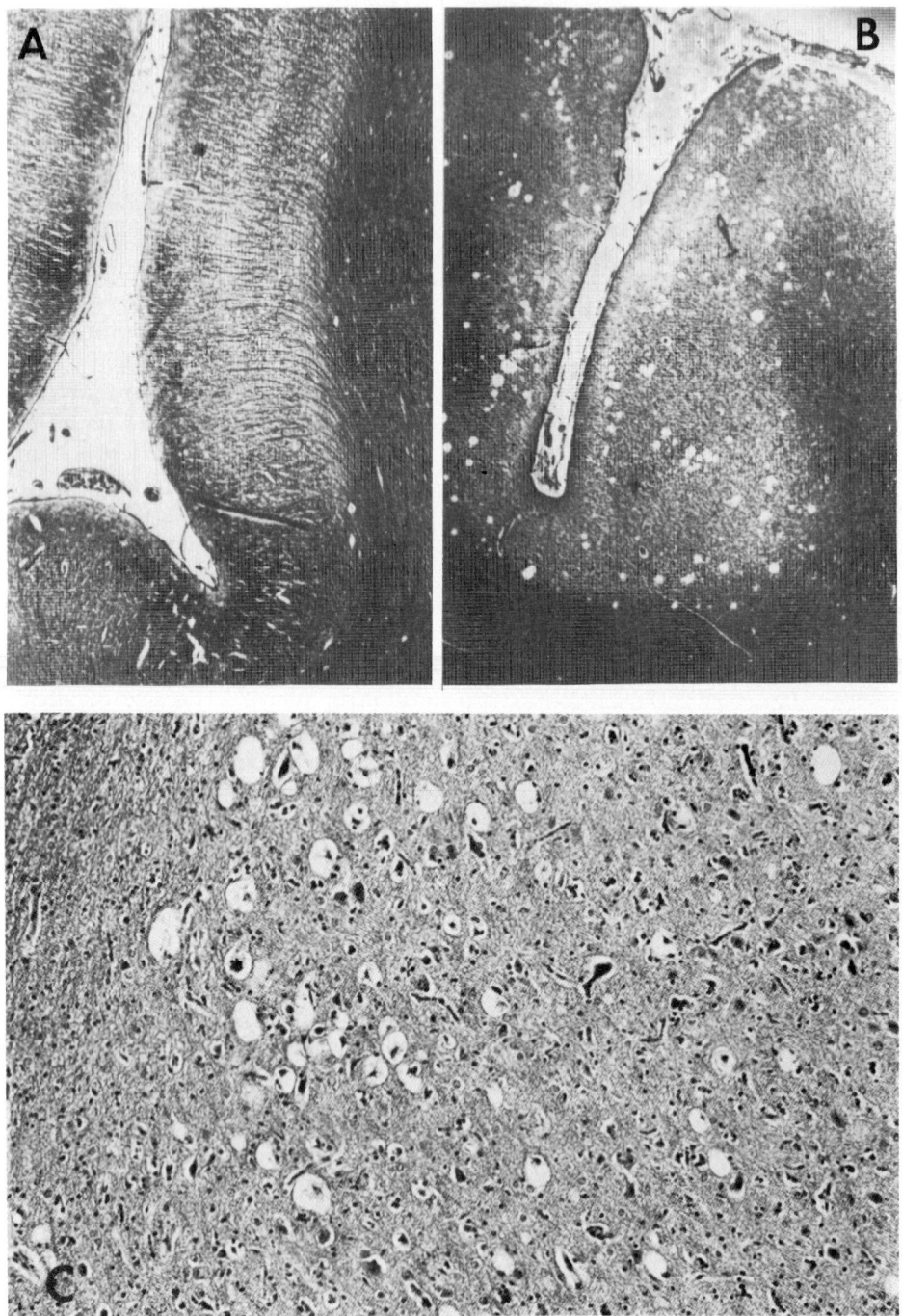

Fig. 16–30. Organomercurial poisoning, swine. *A* and *B*, Necrosis of the occipital cerebral cortex. Bielchowsky stain. (Courtesy of Dr. L. Tryphonas.) *C,* Cerebrocortical neuronal necrosis in experimental swine methylmercury poisoning. (Courtesy of Dr. T. S. Davies and Dr. S. W. Nielsen.)

swine as a potential hazard to public health.

The signs and lesions of this form of mercurial poisoning are related almost entirely to the nervous system. After 15 to 50 days on a diet of the treated grain, pigs become blind without ocular lesions, lose their appetites, become weak and incoordinated, and shortly can no longer stand. The usual experience with experimental pigs receiving minimal toxic amounts of treated seed has been that the animals then sink into a coma of increasing depth. They often live several days, lying on the side, with the head drawn backward but with the back arched and with the forelegs drawn rigidly backward against the sternum. They perform convulsive running movements periodically or when irritated, but ultimately lie still with slower and slower respirations and little evidence of life. In clinical cases, death usually comes after an illness considerably shorter than the period of a week or more which was characteristic of the experimental poisonings.

There are scarcely any gross lesions. Microscopically, the glandular organs (e.g., salivary glands, pancreas) show more conspicuous hydropic degeneration than does the liver. The renal tubules show hydropic degeneration or early necrosis. The lumens of the proximal convoluted tubules are commonly obliterated by the swelling. Albuminous precipitate is seen in some of the tubules still patent. There is commonly a well-marked increase of reticuloendothelial tissue in the spleen and lymph nodes.

The nervous system is most severely affected. Throughout the brain, many nerve-cell bodies show the usual changes of degeneration and necrosis, and there is a diffuse increase of microglia, including rod-shaped nuclei. Demyelinization of nerve tracts extends into the cord, and occasionally encephalomalacia and myelomalacia are seen. Neuronal necrosis is usually most extensive in the cerebral cortex, but may also develop in the cerebellar cortex or any other gray matter. Dorsal root ganglia are also affected, and wallerian degeneration of peripheral sensory nerves is a frequent finding. Often many peripheral nerve fibers are reduced to hollow cylinders containing only irregular globules of red-staining (hematoxylin-eosin) necrotic material. Perivascular cuffing with lymphocytes may be extensive in the brain. In some species (notably cattle, swine, and rats), varying degrees of fibrinoid necrosis of the media of leptomeningeal arteries is a nearly consistent finding, and has been suggested to contribute to the cortical necrosis through ischemia. This vascular lesion, however, does not accompany the neuropathologic sequelae of experimental organomercurial poisoning in most species.

Hyaline degeneration of Purkinje fibers and cardiac muscle fibers occurs in cattle. Zenker's necrosis of skeletal muscle has been described in experimentally poisoned animals, but this may not be a primary lesion. In chronic organomercurial poisoning, hair concentrates the greatest amount of mercury, followed by the liver, gallbladder and kidney. Other tissues, including the brain, contain considerably less. Clearly, tissue sensitivity to the toxic effects of mercury is more important than concentration of the metal in some tissues.

Mercury remains in tissues for a considerable period of time. Following a single oral dose of methylmercury, about 35% (23% excluding hair) remains after 156 days (Hollins et al., 1975). The concentration of methylmercury in the brain resulting in neurologic signs is about 10 ppm.

Tryphonas and Nielsen (1970) have pointed out that certain organomercurials, such as arylmercury, are metabolized more rapidly than others, and that poisoning by such compounds more closely resembles mercuric chloride poisoning, with colitis and renal tubular necrosis as the principal lesions without injury to the central nervous system.

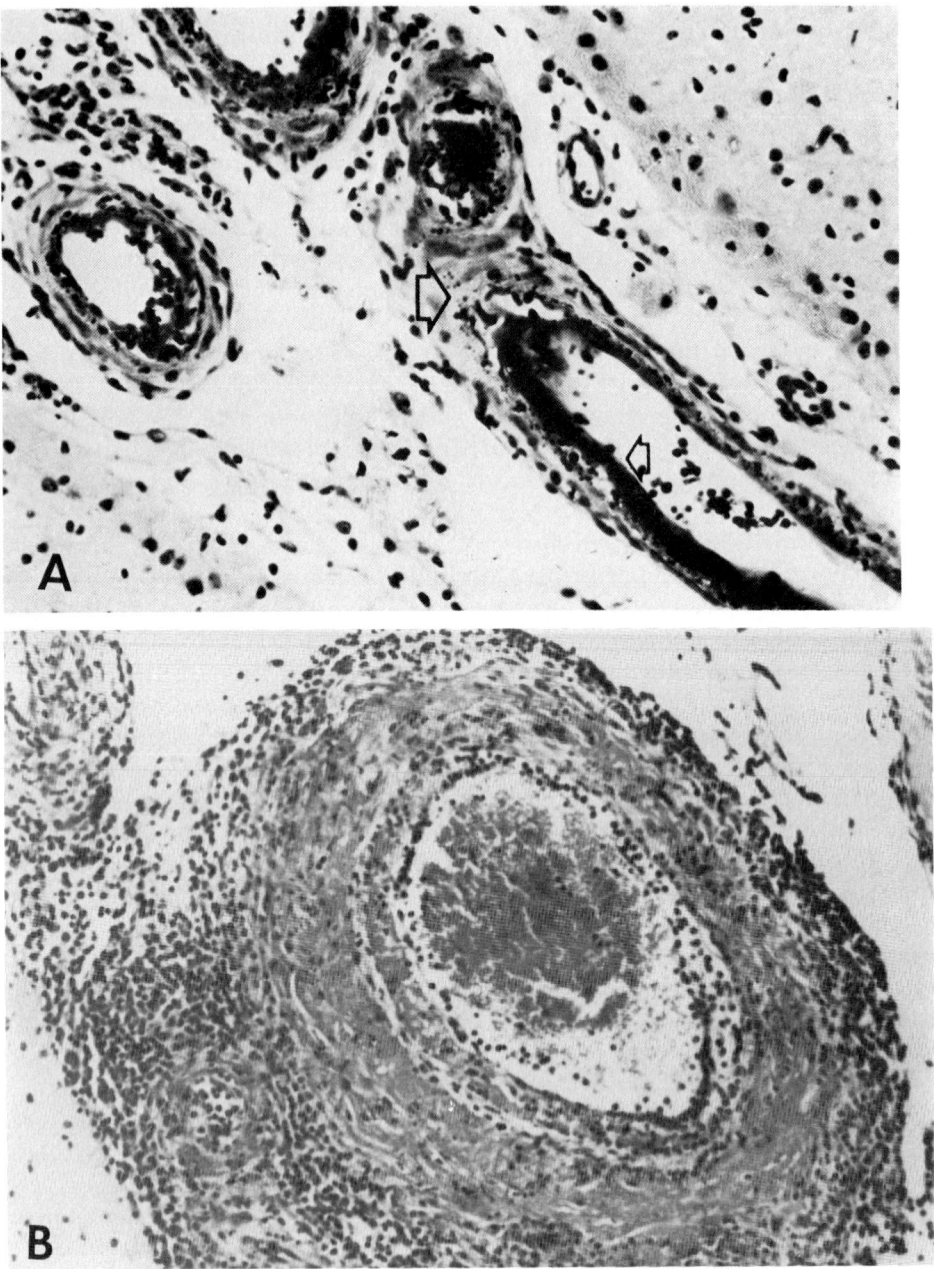

Fig. 16–31. Organomercurial poisoning, swine. *A*, Arterial fibrinoid necrosis in experimental swine methylmercury poisoning. Note fibrinoid deposits (small arrow) and medial necrosis (large arrow). (Courtesy of Dr. T. S. Davies and Dr. S. W. Nielsen.) *B*, Necrosis and vasculitis of a small cerebral artery. (Courtesy of Dr. L. Tryphonas.)

Berlin, M., et al.: Neurotoxicity of methylmercury in squirrel monkeys. Arch. Environ. Health, 30:340–348, 1975.

Chang, L.W., Yamaguchi, S., and Dudley, A.W., Jr.: Neurological changes in cats following long-term diet of mercury contaminated tuna. Acta Neuropathol., 27:171–176, 1974.

Charlton, K.M.: Experimental alkylmercurial poisoning in swine. Lesions in the peripheral and central nervous systems. Can. J. Comp. Med., 38:75–81, 1974.

Curley, A., et al.: Organic mercury identified as the cause of poisoning in human and hogs. Science, 172:65–67, 1971.

Davies, T.S., and Nielsen, S.W.: Pathology of subacute methylmercurialism in cats. Am. J. Vet. Res., 38:59–67, 1977.

Davies, T.S., Nielsen, S.W., and Kircher, C.H.: The pathology of subacute methylmercurialism in swine. Cornell Vet., 66:32–55, 1976.

Diamond, S.S., and Sleight, S.D.: Acute and subchronic methylmercury toxicosis in the rat. Toxicol. Appl. Pharmacol., 23:197–207, 1972.

Garman, R.H., Weiss, B., and Evans, H.L.: Alkylmercurial encephalopathy in monkey (*Saimiri sciureus* and *Macaca arctoides*): histopathologic and autoradiographic study. Acta Neuropathol., 32:61–74, 1975.

Herigstad, R.R., et al.: Chronic methylmercury toxicosis in calves. J. Am. Vet. Med. Assoc., 160:173–182, 1972.

Hollins, J.G., et al.: The whole body retention and tissue distribution of (^{203}Hg) methylmercury in adult cats. Toxic. Appl. Pharmacol., 33:438–449, 1975.

Irving, F., and Butler, D.G.: Ammoniated mercury toxicity in cattle. Can. Vet. J., 16:260–264, 1975.

Kahrs, R.F.: Chronic mercurial poisoning in swine. A case report of an outbreak with some epidemiological characteristics of hog cholera. Cornell Vet., 58:67–75, 1968.

Loosmore, R.M., Harding, J.D.J., and Lewis, G.: Mercury poisoning in pigs. Vet. Rec., 81:268–269, 1967.

Miyakawa, T., et al.: Experimental organic mercury poisoning. I. Regeneration of peripheral nerves. II. Pathological changes in muscles. Acta Neuropathol., 17:6–13, 80–83, 1971.

McEntee, K.: Mercurial poisoning in swine. Cornell Vet., 40:143–147, 1950.

Oliver, W.T., and Platonow, N.: Studies on the pharmacology of N-(ethylmercury) p-toluenesulfonanilide. (Ceresan M.) Am. J. Vet. Res., 21:906–916, 1960.

Palmer, J.S.: Tolerance of sheep to the organic-zinc fungicide, Zineb. J. Am. Vet. Med. Assoc., 143:994–995, 1963.

———: Mercurial fungicidal seed protectant toxic for sheep and chickens. J. Am. Vet. Med. Assoc., 142:1385–1387, 1963.

Storrs, B.: Epidemiologic notes and reports; organic mercury poisoning. Morbidity and Mortality Weekly Report, U.S. Dept. Health, Education & Welfare, 19:25–26, 1970.

Taylor, E.L.: Mercury poisoning in swine. J. Am. Vet. Med. Assoc., 111:46–47, 1947.

Tryphonas, L., and Nielsen, N.O.: The pathology of arylmercurial poisoning in swine. Can. J. Comp. Med., 34:181–190, 1970.

———: Pathology of chronic alkylmercurial poisoning in swine. Am. J. Vet. Res., 34:379–392, 1973.

Turner, J.P.: Mercurial poisoning of cattle. Am. Vet. Rev., 28:669–671, 1904.

Insecticides of the Chlorinated Hydrocarbon Group

The original and still important member of this group is DDT, dichloro, diphenyl trichloroethane. The discovery of this substance and its insecticidal powers marked the advent of a series of insecticidal substances which is still growing, and whose total value to the human race is beyond our power to estimate. Other prominent members of the group are chlordane, lindane (which is the gamma isomer of benzene hexachloride), toxaphene, strobane, endrin, heptachlor (epoxide), methoxychlor, TDE, aldrin, and dieldrin. All these are rather closely related hydrocarbons to which several chlorine atoms have been joined. Only the first four of the 11 compounds listed are commonly used on the skin of animals; all may be used against plant pests that prey upon farm crops and pastures. The limits of safety in the employment of these insecticides have been well established by extensive research, and as long as they are used as intended, either upon parasitized animals, feed crops, or buildings, poisoning is unlikely. However, errors in mixing or application and downright accidents are all too numerous. By the latter term, which is perhaps too mild, we mean such incidents as one in which a farmer mixed his DDT spray in the bucket used for calf feed, forgot the fact, mixed calf feed with what remained of the spraying solution and fed it to the calves with fatal results (Radeleff, 1948). In another "accident," a stockman dipped a large herd of cattle in the proper dilution of a hydrocarbon insectide, as he thought, to free them of ticks. All died within a few hours. He complained to the manufacturer, but when it was demonstrated that his dipping fluid contained arsenic, he discovered that he had filled the vat with an arsenical intended for the cotton field. Baffling diagnostic problems are obviously presented in such cases, and unfortunately, they cannot be solved entirely by the observable aspects of the animals' illnesses.

A serious objection to the use of these insecticides is that they are not degraded by natural biologic processes, and therefore become a permanent part of the environment. They make their way into the water supply, are taken up by aquatic animals, and become part of the food chain because they are accumulated and concentrated, usually in fat, by many such animals. Deleterious effects on wildlife, especially birds, are reported. These effects include soft eggshells and loss of hatchability, which probably result from the known estrogenic actions of DDT. Decreased reproductive performance has also been noted in mammals, apparently on the same basis.

The signs of these poisonings are more informative from the diagnostic standpoint than the lesions. The earlier signs, which may appear within minutes and almost always within a few hours, are those of nervous hyperirritability and stimulation. Spasmodic twitching and quivering of various groups of muscles, including those of the eyelids, increase in extent and frequency until almost the whole body is trembling. Apprehensiveness or occasionally belligerency deepens into frenzy; incoordination and various abnormal stances are replaced by convulsions. The animal may press its head against solid objects (blind staggers), may plunge headlong into an obstacle of any sort, or without warning, jump as if stung by the sudden lash of a whip and then fall in a convulsion. As in tetanus or strychnine poisoning, these symptoms are initiated or augmented by slight external stimuli, such as a sharp

noise. A minority of animals become depressed, drowsy, and eventually comatose. Occasionally an animal licks continually at a certain spot of the body surface, simulating Aujeszky's disease. Many of these patients die, others recover suddenly and completely after nervous seizures lasting a few minutes or a few hours. Simultaneously with the appearance of convulsions, the body temperature soars to unbelievable heights, perhaps 115° F. This rise is more than can be attributed to muscular activity and must depend on derangement of the heat-regulating center. Dyspnea and cyanosis accompany the convulsive seizures. There may be groaning, grunting, and grinding of teeth; some have interpreted these as signs of severe pain, but to others they have appeared to stem from the nervous derangement.

Lesions at necropsy include petechiae and ecchymoses on and in the heart and in many other places. These occur especially in association with convulsions and are explainable on the basis of dyspneic anoxia. Pulmonary congestion and edema, diffuse or localized, are the rule. The heart usually stops in systole. In spite of the startling symptoms of central nervous disorder, there are few changes in the central nervous cells and tissues. This, of course, is in conformity with the rapid and complete recovery that may follow some of the most violent symptoms. Some have reported Nissl's degeneration and necrosis of neurons, especially in the ganglia of the medulla, cerebellum, and brain stem; others have found no central nervous lesions beyond congestion and increased cerebrospinal fluid. In the few cases in which symptoms have been prolonged for a day or two, the usual changes of acute toxic hepatitis and acute toxic tubular nephrosis have been noted, centrilobular necrosis being especially prominent. Focal necroses have been noticed in the skeletal muscles. Enteritis is noticeable only if the poison has been eaten. Dehydration and rapid depletion of depot fat are usual in these cases. The biochemist can demonstrate accumulation of chlorinated compounds in the body tissues, chiefly the stored fat.

The pharmacologic actions of chlorinated hydrocarbons has been the subject of an extensive review by Hrdina, Singhal, and Ling (1975).

Anonymous: Pesticide, chemicals, established tolerance levels in meat, and acceptability for use in slaughter animals and on agricultural premises. J. Am. Vet. Med. Assoc., 147:616, 1965.

Baxter, J.T.: Some observations on the histopathology of aldrin poisoning in lambs. J. Comp. Pathol., 69:185–191, 1959.

Ely, R.E., et al.: Lindane poisoning in dairy animals. J. Am. Vet. Med. Assoc., 123:448–449, 1953.

Haber, W.G., and Link, R.P.: Toxic effects of hexachloronaphthalene on swine. Toxicol. Appl. Pharmacol., 4:257–262, 1962.

Harrison, D.L., et al.: Dieldrin poisoning of dogs. II. Experimental studies. N.Z. Vet. J., 11:23–31, 1963.

Hayes, W.J., Jr.: Review of the metabolism of chlorinated hydrocarbon insecticides especially in mammals. Annu. Rev. Pharmacol., 5:27–52, 1965.

Haymaker, W., Ginzler, A.M., and Ferguson, R.L.: The toxic effects of prolonged ingestion of DDT on dogs with special reference to lesions in the brain. Am. J. Med. Sci., 212:423–431, 1946.

Hrdina, P.D., Singhal, R.L., and Ling, G.M.: DDT and related chlorinated hydrocarbon insecticides: pharmacological basis of their toxicity in mammals. Adv. Pharmacol. Chemother., 12:31–88, 1975.

Judah, J.D.: Metabolism and mode of action of DDT. Br. J. Pharmacol., 4:120–131, 1949.

Kitselman, C.H.: Long-term studies on dogs fed aldrin and dieldrin in sublethal dosages, with reference to the histopathological findings and reproduction. J. Am. Vet. Med. Assoc., 123:28–30, 1953.

Lillie, R.D., and Smith, M.I.: Pathology of experimental poisoning in cats, rabbits and rats with 2,2 bis-parachlorphenyl-1,1,1 trichloroethane. Pub. Health Rep., 59:979–984, 1944.

Link, R.P., Bruce, W.N., and Decker, G.C.: The effects of chlorinated hydrocarbon insecticides on dairy cattle. Ann. NY Acad. Sci., 111:788–792, 1964.

McEnerney, P.J.: Accidental poisoning of dairy calves by benzene hexachloride. Cornell Vet., 41:292–295, 1951.

Nelson, A.A., et al.: Histopathological changes following administration of DDT to several species of animals. Pub. Health Rep., 59:1009–1020, 1944.

Pearson, J.K.L., et al.: An outbreak of aldrin poisoning in suckling lambs. Vet. Rec., 70:783–785, 1958.

Radeleff, R.D., et al.: The acute toxicity of chlorinated hydrocarbon and organic phosphorus insecticides to livestock. U.S. Dept. Agr. Tech. Bull. No. 1122, 1955.

Radeleff, R.D.: Chlordane poisoning: symptomatology and pathology. Vet. Med., 43:343–347, 1948.

———: Toxaphene poisoning, symptomatology and pathology. Vet. Med., 44:436–442, 1949.

Ressang, A.A., et al.: Aldrin, dieldrin and endrin intoxication in cats. Commun. Vet., Bogor., 2:71–88, 1959. (In Engl.) Abstr. Vet. Bull. No. 3266, 1959.

St. Omer, V.V.: Chronic and acute toxicity of the chlorinated hydrocarbon insecticides in mammals and birds. Can. Vet. J., 11:215–226, 1970.

Organic Phosphates

Under the group name of **organic phosphates** are included certain "nerve gases" devised for use in warfare and a number of valuable insecticides, anthelmintics, and defoliants. Tetra-ethyl pyrophosphate (TEPP) is one belonging to both categories. The insecticides and antihelmintics are usually best known by specific trade names, the more important of which are currently parathion, o,o-diethyl p-nitrophenyl thiophosphate, and malathion, o,o-diethyl dithiophosphate. Others in this group are: carbaryl (Sevin), carbophenothion (Trithion), ciodrin, coumaphos (Co-rad), demetron, diazinon, dichlorvos (DDVP), trichlorfon, phosalone, dioxathion, disyston, endosulfan, ENP, ethion, guthion, methyl parathion, mevinphos (Phosdrin, naled (Dibrom), phorate (Thiomet), ronnel, and trichlorophon (Dipterex). Others, such as triaryl phosphate, have industrial use in lubricants.

Known as anticholinesterases, these organic phosphates have essentially similar effects, which depend upon an ability to prevent or inhibit the action of cholinesterase. This leaves the acetylcholine of the sympathetic and parasympathetic nerve endings free to act continuously and without release of the effectors at the end of each stimulus. The oral lethal dose of parathion for dogs is estimated by Tsaggare (1967) as 25 to 35 mg/kg body weight; for cats, 15 mg/kg; for rabbits, 40 mg/kg body weight. Signs include excessive salivation, the

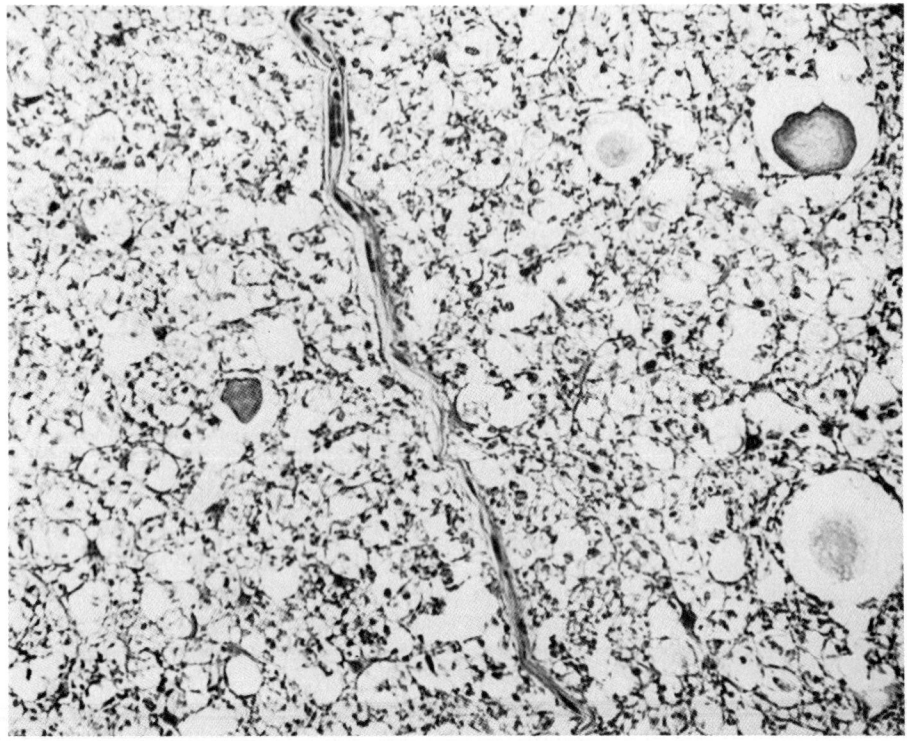

Fig. 16–32.   Triaryl phosphate poisoning. Axonal degeneration in the spinal cord of a poisoned cow. Note swollen axons or spheroids. (Courtesy of Dr. B. E. Beck and *Veterinary Pathology*.)

saliva being copious but watery. There is respiratory difficulty, with labored and exaggerated respiratory movements, the mouth often being held partially open. Before death, there are loud pulmonary rales and soft grunts. Twitching and fasciculation of muscles and ataxia occur, but only exceptionally, convulsions. Asphyxia is the main cause of death. Signs commonly arise within an hour or two after a single contact with the poison, which may occur by inhalation or cutaneous absorption more often than by ingestion. Somewhat exceptionally, death has come within five minutes after tetra-ethyl pyrophosphate was sprayed on the skin of cattle (Radeleff, 1954). Nonfatal cases recover within 48 hours, as a rule. Susceptibility varies greatly among individuals of any species, and can be increased by frequently repeated mild exposure. The greater susceptibility appears to be due to exhaustion of the body's store of cholinesterase.

Postmortem lesions are decidedly minor. Hemorrhages appear in various locations, especially the heart, lungs, and gastrointestinal tube. Pulmonary congestion with edema is a prominent, but not necessarily constant, lesion. The most specific lesion is axonal degeneration, characterized by marked swelling up to 20 times normal (Beck et al., 1977; Cavanaugh and Patangia, 1965). Beck and colleagues ascribed the pathogenesis of the lesion to inhibition of esterases necessary to transport nutrients from the nerve cell body to more distal portions of the axon. The longest axons are affected first. Ultrastructurally, there is mitochondrial swelling, vacuolation of axoplasm, and separation of myelin lamellae.

Parenchymatous degeneration of the

liver and kidneys has been reported but is probably exceptional.

Berger and Bayliss (1952) described a histochemical method for the detection of cholinesterase at motor end plates in teased preparations of skeletal muscles, which should be useful to detect fatal accumulations of anticholinesterase.

Decrease in the level of cholinesterase in circulating red blood cells is considered to be good evidence of toxicity by organic phosphates (Anderson et al., 1969).

Flea collars impregnated with the organic phosphate, dichlorvos, are also associated with allergic dermatitis.

Ahmed, M.M.: The ultrastructure of tricresylphosphate poisoning in primates. I. Studies on axonal alterations in the spinal cord. Arch. Histol. Jpn., 35:283–288, 1973.

Anderson, P.H., Machin, A.F., and Hebert, C.N.: Blood cholinesterase activity as in index of acute toxicity of organophosphorus pesticides in sheep and cattle. Res. Vet. Sci., 10:29–33, 1969.

Beck, B.E., Wood, C.D., and Whenham, G.R.: Triaryl phosphate poisoning in cattle. Vet. Pathol., 14:128–137, 1977.

Bell, R.R., Price, M.A., and Turk, R.D.: Toxicity of malathion and chlorthion to dogs and cats. J. Am. Vet. Med. Assoc., 126:302–303, 1955.

Bell, T.G., Farrell, R.K., Padgett, G.A., and Leendertsen, L.W.: Ataxia, depression, and dermatitis associated with the use of dichlorvos-impregnated collars in the laboratory cat. J. Am. Vet. Med. Assoc., 167:579–586, 1975.

Bello, T.R., Amborski, G.F., and Torbert, B.J.: Effects of organic phosphorus anthelmintics on blood cholinesterase values in horses and ponies. Am. J. Vet. Res., 35:73–78, 1974.

Berger, A.D., and Bayliss, M.W.: Histochemical detection of fatal anticholinesterase poisoning. U.S. Armed Forces Med. J., 3:1637–1644, 1952.

Cavanagh, J.B., and Patangia, G.N.: Changes in the central nervous system in the cat as the result of tri-o-cresyl phosphate poisoning. Brain, 88:165–180, 1965.

Cox, D.H., and Baker, B.R.: A diagnostic test for organic phosphate insecticide poisoning in cattle. J. Am. Vet. Med. Assoc., 132:485–487, 1958. (Also swine, Ibid. 133:329–330, 1958.)

Denz, F.A.: Poisoning by P-nitrophenyl diethyl thiophosphate (E605): a study of anticholinesterase compounds. J. Pathol. Bact., 63:81–91, 1951.

Dzhurov, A.: Pathology of acute parathion poisoning in cattle. Nauchni. Trud. Vissh. Vet. Med. Inst., 16:59–66, 1966. VB, 37:1398, 1967.

Gallo, M.A.: Chronic toxicologic investigations of phosalone in the dog and rat. Toxicol. Appl. Pharmacol., 36:561–568, 1976.

Holmstedt, B., Krook, L., and Rooney, J.R.: The pathology of experimental cholinesterase-inhibitor poisoning. Acta Pharmacol. Toxicol., 13:337–344, 1957.

McCoy, J.W.: A case of parathion poisoning. Southwest. Vet., 16:196, 1963.

Mukula, A.L.: Detection of parathion poisoning. In Engl. Acta Pharm. Tox. Kbh., 17:304–314, 1960.

Palmer, J.S., and Schlinke, J.C.: Oral toxicity of tributyl phosphorotrithioite, a cotton defoliant, to cattle and sheep. J. Am. Vet. Med. Assoc., 163:1172–1174, 1973.

Petty, C.S.: Histochemical proof of organic phosphate poisoning. Arch. Pathol., 66:458–463, 1958.

Radeleff, R.D.: TEPP (tetra-ethyl pyrophosphate) poisoning of cattle. Vet. Med., 49:15–16, 1954.

Smalley, H.E.: Diagnosis and treatment of carbaryl poisoning in swine. J. Am. Vet. Med. Assoc., 156:339–344, 1970.

Snow, D.H.: The acute toxicity of dichlorvos in the dog. 2. Pathology. Aust. Vet. J., 49:120–125, 1973.

Snow, D.H., and Watson, A.D.J.: The acute toxicity of dichlorvos in the dog. 1. Clinical observations and clinical pathology. Aust. Vet. J., 49:113–119, 1973.

Tsaggare, Th.A.: (Pathological changes in animals poisoned with parathion.) Epistem. epet. kteniatrik. Skhol. (Ann. Rep. Vet. Fac. Thessaloniki), 6:245–315, 1967. VB 37:5311, 1967.

Yasnova, G.P., Abbasov, T.G., and Tsaregorodtseva, G.N.: Pathological and histochemical changes in organs and tissues of calves given certain organophosphorous insecticides over a long period. Probl. Veterinaroi Sanitarii, 29:228–233, 1971.

Younger, R.L.: Toxicity studies of certain organic phosphorus compounds in horses. Am. J. Vet. Res., 26:776–779, 1965.

Cycada

Plants of the order Cycadales, particularly *Zamia integrifolia*, *Z. portoricoensis*, *Z. latafoleatus*, *Cycas circinalis*, *C. media*, *Bowenia serrulata*, *Macrozamia lucida*, and *M. reidlei*, are coarse, woody, fern-like, and grow in Australia, New Guinea, Puerto Rico, Dominican Republic, and Florida. The fruit and nuts have been used as a source of feed for man and animals and the leaves are consumed by grazing stock. Both contain two toxins: a neurotoxin, which is resistant to drying, and hepatotoxin, which is readily destroyed by drying. Cattle and sheep are susceptible. In cattle, neurologic sequelae are the usual outcome, whereas in sheep, acute or chronic liver disease is more frequent. Although the plants grow in Florida, no poisonings of this type have been reported in the United States.

Poisoning of cattle, associated with these plants, results in nervous signs which have prompted such colloquial names as: "wobbles," "rickets," "zamia paralysis," cycad ataxia, derriengue (Dominican Republic) and ranilla (Puerto Rico). The clinical signs are chiefly neurologic, with ataxia involving the hindquarters initially. A peculiar involvement of the hind legs results in swaying, flexion of the hock and fetlock joints, wobbling, and malpositioning of the legs. The lesions are concentrated in the spinal cord. Degeneration of myelin is evident in nerve fibers of all funiculi of the cord throughout its length. The Marchi and Guillery silver-staining methods are particularly useful in demonstrating these lesions (Hall and McGavin, 1968). Swollen axons, appearing as large, eosinophilic spheroids 10 to 50 μ in diameter, are present within the spinal tracts and medulla oblongata.

Hepatic necrosis in sheep has most often followed consumption of *Macrozamia reidlei*. Acute poisoning is characterized by jaundice, ascites, hydrothorax, serosal hemorrhages, and extensive centrilobular hemorrhagic necrosis of the liver. Hepatic fibrosis is the predominant finding in chronic poisoning in sheep. The hepatotoxin is methylazoxymethanol, a compound similar in structure to dimethylnitrosamine, which inhibits hepatic protein synthesis.

Gabbedy, B.J., Meyer, E.P., and Dickson, J.: Zamia palm *(Macrozamia reidlei)* poisoning of sheep. Aust. Vet. J., 51:303–305, 1975.

Gardiner, M.R.: Chronic ovine hepatosis following feeding of *Macrozamia reidlei* nuts. Aust. J. Agric. Res., 21:519–526, 1970.

Hall, W.T.K., and McGavin, M.D.: Clinical and neuropathological changes in cattle eating the leaves of *Macrozamia lucida* or *Bowenia serrulata* (family Zamiaceae). Pathol. Vet., 5:26–34, 1968.

Hooper, P.T., Best, S.M., and Campbell, A.: Azonal dystrophy in the spinal cords of cattle consuming the cycad palm, *Cycas media*. Aust. Vet. J., 50:146–149, 1974.

Mason, M.M., and Whiting, M.G.: Caudal motor weakness and ataxia in cattle in the Caribbean area following ingestion of cycads. Cornell Vet., 58:541–554, 1968.

Arsanilic Acid

Arsanilic acid poisoning in swine is not characterized by gastroenteritis as is arsenic (Group B), but rather almost entirely by neurologic signs and lesions. Harding et al. (1968) have experimentally induced poisoning in pigs by adding arsanilic acid to the feed at the rate of 611, 1000, or 2000 g to each (English) ton of feed. (The usual recommended dose as a growth stimulant is 100 g/ton, or for treatment of dysentery, 250 g/ton.) At all dose levels, signs of intoxication were produced. Clinical signs appeared earlier in pigs receiving the higher dosages. Tremors, incoordination, progressively developing blindness, and eventual inability to stand were the principal signs. Poisoned animals remained alert with good appetites in spite of these severe signs. The principal lesions were microscopic and consisted of wallerian degeneration of optic nerves, optic tracts, and peripheral nerves. Ledet et al. (1973) described similar signs and lesions in pigs fed 1000 ppm arsanilic acid in their ration. The neuropathologic changes were limited

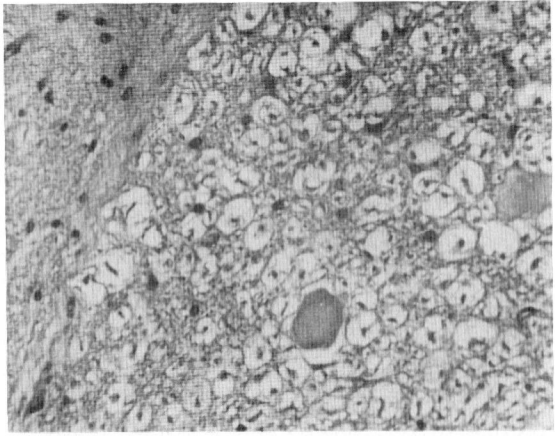

Fig. 16–33. Cycad palm poisoning. Spheroids and demyelination in the dorsolateral white matter of the cervical spinal cord in a steer poisoned by *Cycas armstrongii* (*C. media*). (Courtesy of Dr. P. T. Hooper and *Australian Veterinary Journal.*)

to the same three sites and were characterized by necrosis of myelin-supporting cells and degeneration of myelin sheaths and axons. Cutaneous hyperemia and hyperesthesia were described as the earliest signs, appearing within five days. More severe neurologic signs appeared in almost two weeks.

Harding, J.D.J., Lewis, G., and Done, J.T.: Experimental arsanilic acid poisoning in pigs. Vet. Rec., 83:560–564, 1968.

Ledet, A.E., Duncan, J.R., Buck, W.B., and Ramsey, F.K.: Clinical, toxicological, and pathological aspects of arsanilic acid poisoning in swine. Clin. Toxicol., 6:439–457, 1973.

Oliver, W.T., and Roe, C.K.: Arsanilic acid poisoning in swine. J. Am. Vet. Med. Assoc., 130:177–178, 1957.

Smith, I.D., Perdue, H.S., and Kolar, J.A.: Tolerance of swine to varying levels of arsanilic acid in the feed. J. Anim. Sci., 21:1014, 1962.

Vorhies, M.W., Sleight, S.D., and Whitehair, C.K.: Toxicity of arsanilic acid in swine as influenced by water intake. Cornell Vet., 59:3–9, 1969.

GROUP R: DEGENERATION OF CARDIAC AND SKELETAL MUSCLE

Poisons in Group R produce necrosis of **cardiac and skeletal muscles** as their principal lesions. Similar lesions may also be found in some other poisonings such as selenium (Group E) and gossypol (Group C).

Coffee Senna

Coffee senna (*Cassia occidentalis*, L.) received its common name because of the use of the bean as a substitute for coffee. The plant is an annual shrub that grows natively in the southeastern United States as well as in many other parts of the world. The plant has drab green leaves and bright golden yellow flowers. The seed pods are green with brown transverse bars when immature, and become brown when mature. Other sennas are known to have cathartic properties and some may be toxic to animals (Kingsbury, 1964). Among these plants are: *Cassia fistula* (senna of commerce), *C. lindheimeriana*, *C. fasciculata* (partridge pea) and *C. tora* (sicklepod). Reported as poisonous to livestock first in 1911 (O'Hara et al., 1969), episodes of toxicity in horses, cattle, and sheep have been recorded over the years. Experimental poisoning has also been recorded in cattle, rabbits, sheep, and goats.

Calves given daily oral doses of ground beans of *Cassia occidentalis* at the dose rate of 0.5% or more of their body weight survive at a rate inversely proportional to the dosage (O'Hara et al., 1969). Signs of poisoning are anorexia and diarrhea, followed by hyperpnea, tachycardia, and progressive muscular incapacitation, with stumbling and ataxic gait. Elevated levels of serum glutamic oxaloacetic transaminase and phosphocreatine kinase are constant, and hemoglobin appears in the urine of about half of these cases. Death follows prostration and recumbency by a few hours due to heart failure.

The gross lesions consist of focal or diffuse pallor of skeletal muscles, generally distinguishable from the chalky whiteness and granular consistency observed in white-muscle disease. Stippling of pale muscles may be seen in calves. The myocardium is usually mottled or streaked with pale or yellow zones. These areas may be diffusely distributed or concentrated adjacent to the endocardium. Subepicardial hemorrhages may be seen, particularly along the course of the coronary arteries. Effusion into the pericardial sac sometimes occurs. The lungs are usually diffusely dark red, partially airless and heavy. The interlobular septa are thickened by edema. Trachea and bronchi are filled with serous fluid, which is white and frothy in part. Blood flows freely from the cut surface of the lung.

The earliest lesions seen with the light microscope in cardiac muscle (Read et al., 1968) consist of numerous small indistinct vacuoles among the myofibrils, in some cases giving them a distinctly fenestrated appearance. These vacuoles are demonstrated with electron microscopy to be due to swelling of the mitochondria, with loss of their matrix and fragmentation and dis-

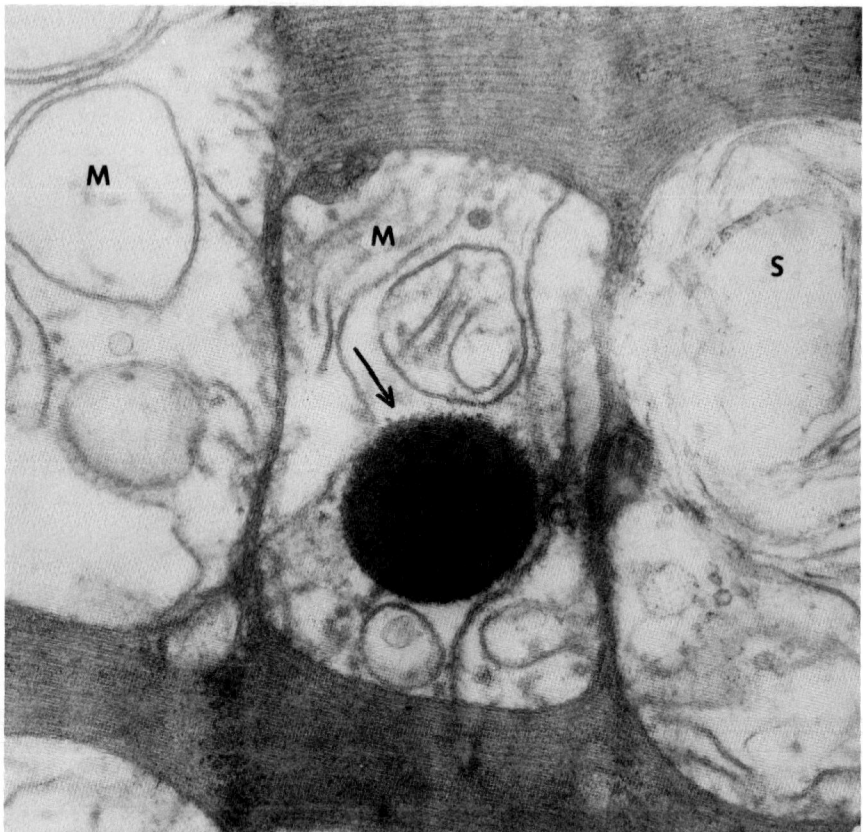

Fig. 16–34. Poisoning due to coffee senna. Electron micrograph of myocardium of a calf poisoned with *Cassia occidentalis* (× 43,200). Note electron dense spherule (arrow) in swollen mitochrondrion of myocardial muscle cell. Note disorganized cristae and spheromembranous structure(s) in mitochondrion. (Courtesy of Dr. W. Kay Read and *Laboratory Investigation*.)

organization of cristae. Electron-dense spherical inclusions sometimes appear in these dilated mitochondria (Fig. 16–34). With loss of mitochondrial energy production, cellular swelling ensues, with loss of glycogen and degeneration of the sarcotubular system.

The lesions of skeletal muscles seen by light microscopy (Henson et al., 1965) are compatible with classic Zenker's necrosis of muscle. The affected muscle fibers are swollen, eosinophilic (amorphous), and sometimes fragmented. Occasional nuclei are necrotic and some proliferation of sarcolemmal nuclei is evident. Calcification is not reported.

Brocq-Rousseau, and Bruere, P.: Accidents Mortels sur des cheveaux due a la graine de *Cassia occidentalis*, L. Compt. Rend. Soc. Biol., 92:555–557, 1925.

Dollahite, J.W., and Henson, J.B.: Toxic plants as the etiologic agent of myopathies in animals. Am. J. Vet. Res., 26:749–752, 1965.

Henson, J.B., et al.: Myodegeneration in cattle grazing *Cassia* species. J. Am. Vet. Med. Assoc., 147:142–145, 1965.

Kingsbury, J.M.: Poisonous Plants of the United States and Canada. Englewood Cliffs, New Jersey, Prentice-Hall, 1964.

Mercer, H.D., et al.: *Cassia occidentalis* toxicosis in cattle. J. Am. Vet. Med. Assoc., 151:735–741, 1967.

Moussu, R.: L'Intoxication par les graines de *Cassia occidentalis* L., est due à une Toxalbumine. Compt. Rend. Soc. Biol., 92:862–863, 1925.

O'Hara, P.J., and Pierce, K.R.: A toxic cardiomyopathy caused by *Cassia occidentalis*. I.

Morphologic studies in poisoned rabbits. II. Biochemical studies in poisoned rabbits. Vet. Pathol., *11*:97–109, 110–124, 1974.

O'Hara, P.J., Pierce, K.R., and Read, W.K.: Degenerative myopathy associated with ingestion of *Cassia occidentalis* L.: clinical and pathologic features of the experimentally induced disease. Am. J. Vet. Res., *30*:2173–2180, 1969.

Read, W.K., Pierce, K.R., and O'Hara, P.J.: Ultrastructural lesions of an acute toxic cardiomyopathy of cattle. Lab. Invest., *18*:227–231, 1968.

Coyotillo

The coyotillo plant (*Karwinskia humboldtiana*) is a spineless shrub with pinnately veined leaves, small greenish flowers, and ovoid, brown-black fruit (Dewan et al., 1965). The fruit has been shown to cause, in sheep and goats, a toxicosis called **limberleg**, which is manifest by progressive weakness of legs, muscular incoordination, recumbency, and death (Marsh et al., 1928). In 1789, Indian children reportedly lost the use of their limbs, and some died after eating the fruit of the coyotillo (Clavergo, cited by Marsh et al., 1928).

This shrub is native to southwest Texas and Mexico, and in some regions it grows profusely (Sperry et al., 1955).

The lesions in this toxicosis are found in cardiac and skeletal muscle, peripheral nerves and liver. In the myocardium, disseminated focal lesions of coagulation necrosis involve a few muscle fibers in each location. A few fibers lose their sarcoplasma. In skeletal muscle, any or all muscles may be involved, and the microscopic lesions are typical of Zenker's necrosis. The isolated muscle fibers are swollen, eosinophilic, often fragmented, and occasionally associated with infiltration of lymphocytes and macrophages and proliferation of sarcolemmal cells (Dewan et al., 1965). Toxic hepatitis is also a feature, with focal necroses of small numbers of hepatic cells, usually at the center of the lobules, plus some mild fatty change. Peripheral neuropathy with swollen Schwann cells, segmental demyelination, and wallerian degeneration has been found in goats (Charlton and Pierce, 1969, 1970).

Associated with these lesions are severe increases in the serum concentration of glutamic oxaloacetic transaminase and moderate increases in glutamic pyruvic transaminase. The serum alkaline phosphatase may be slightly decreased.

Charlton, K.M., and Pierce, K.R.: Peripheral neuropathy in experimental coyotillo poisoning in goats. Texas Rpts. Biol. Med., *27*:389–399, 1969.

———: A neuropathy in goats caused by experimental coyotillo (*Karwinskia humboldtiana*) poisoning. II. Lesions in the peripheral nervous system—teased fiber and acid phosphatase studies. Pathol. Vet., *7*:385–407, 1970.

———: A neuropathy in goats caused by experimental coyotillo (*Karwinskia humboldtiana*) poisoning. III. Distribution of lesions in peripheral nerves. Pathol. Vet., *7*:408–419, 1970.

———: A neuropathy in goats caused by experimental coyotillo (*Karwinskia humboltiana*) poisoning. IV. Light and electron microscopic lesion in peripheral nerves. Pathol. Vet., *7*:420–434, 1970.

Charlton, K.M., et al.: A neuropathy in goats caused by experimental coyotillo (*Karwinskia humboldtiana*) poisoning. V. Lesions in the central nervous system. Pathol. Vet., *7*:435–447, 1970.

Dewan, M.L., et al.: Toxic myodegeneration in goats produced by feeding mature fruits from coyotillo plant (*Karwinskia humboldtiana*). Am. J. Pathol., *46*:215–226, 1965.

Dollahite, J.W., and Henson, J.B.: Toxic plants as the etiologic agent of myopathies in animals. Am. J. Vet. Res., *26*:749–752, 1965.

Marsh, C.D., Clawson, A.B., and Roe, G.C.: Coyotillo (*Karwinskia humboldtiana*) as a poisonous plant. U.S. Dept. Agr. Tech. Bull., *29*, 1928.

Sperry, O.E., et al.: Texas range plants poisonous to animals. Texas Agric. Exp. Sta. Bull., *796*:23–24, 1955.

GROUP S: TERATOGENS

These poisons cause teratogenic or other effects on the embryo or fetus. Other poisons are also teratogenic but are classified elsewhere as this effect is not the most outstanding finding.

Veratrum Californicum

This impressive perennial plant grows profusely in eleven western states, reaching 3 to 8 feet in height. Its common names include: skunk cabbage, western helibore, false helibore, and wild corn. It is included in the lily family (Lileacea), in which seven other species in this genus are classified and are indigenous to North America. *Veratrum veride,* which grows in the eastern United States, and *V. album,* a European species, are the source of several alkaloids, some of which are used medicinally. Among these specific alkaloids are: veratridine, protoveratrine, veratrine, cevadine, and jirvine.

A striking and grotesque congenital malformation of lambs was first described by Binns et al. (1969) as occurring in sheep pastured on mountain ranges in southern Idaho, located at altitudes up to 10,000 feet (Fig. 16–35). The deformed lambs were

usually born alive singly or with a living or dead twin which may or may not have been affected. The malformations are limited to the head and represent several defects, the commonest being partial or complete cyclopia. A single eye or two fused eyes usually occupy a single orbit. The two fused eyes give the startling appearance that caused the sheepmen to call them "monkey-faced lambs." The upper jaw may be slightly distorted with a cleft palate or almost totally absent. The nose is distorted in varying degrees, and the lower jaw usually protrudes drastically. A large

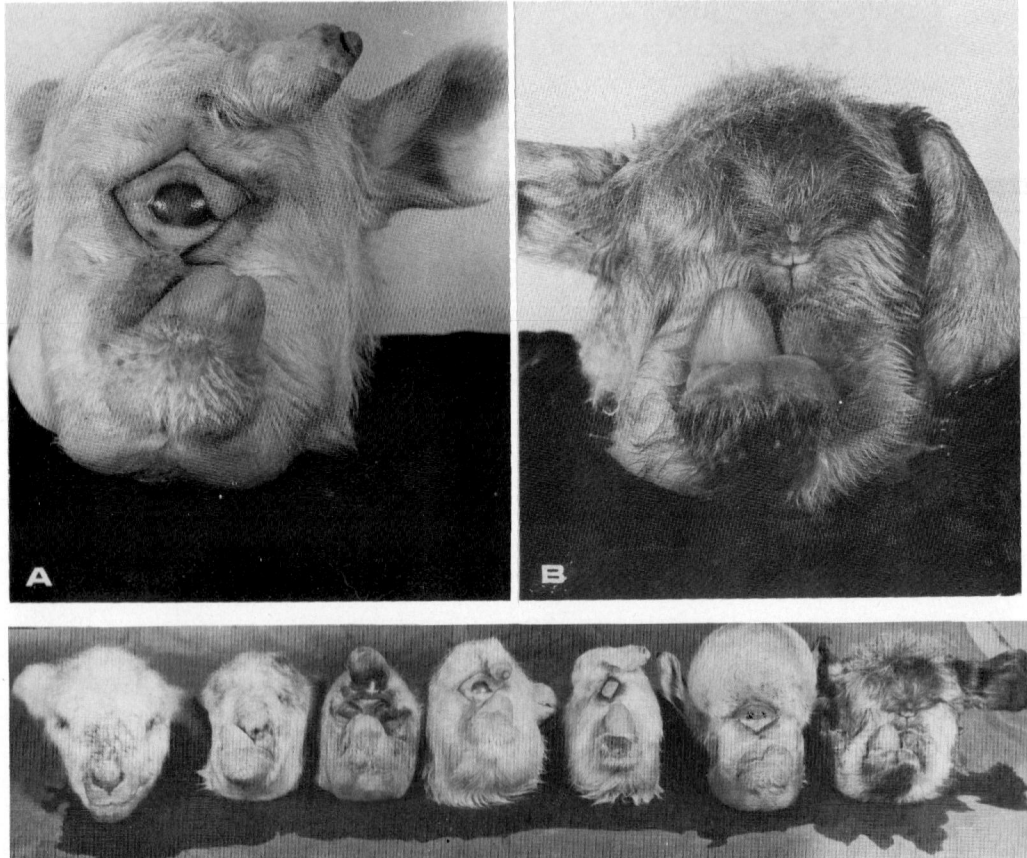

Fig. 16–35. Congenital malformations in newborn lambs resulting from feeding their mothers a plant, *Veratrum californicum* (false helibore) on the fourteenth day of gestation. *A,* A lamb's head with cyclopia and other anomalies. *B,* A lamb with anophthalmia and other defects. *C,* Several lambs' heads with varying congenital deformities. Normal lamb at left. (Courtesy of Dr. Wayne Binns, United Stated Department of Agriculture.)

median cutaneous protuberance often occurs over the single eye. The cerebral hemispheres are frequently fused, and hydrocephalus involves the lateral ventricles. The optic nerves may be fused.

In many cases the pituitary of the fetus is absent, and this is associated with **prolonged gestation** and a large fetus, which is not delivered except by hysterotomy.

In a series of carefully conducted experiments, Binns and co-workers have clearly established that this congenital malformation results from the consumption of the fresh or dried plant *Veratrum californicum*, or extracts thereof, by the ewe during her thirteenth to fifteenth days of pregnancy. Several steroidal alkaloids (cyclopamine, veratramine, veratrosine, muldamine) have been isolated from *V. californicum* and have been demonstrated to cause the teratogenic effects just described, as well as other malformations (Binns et al., 1972). When the plant or certain of the alkaloids are fed to sheep on the thirteenth and fourteenth days of pregnancy, the cyclopian deformity results. Exposure on days 17 and 18 results in motor nerve paralysis, whereas a multiplicity of abnormalities followed exposure from days 12 through 30, including cleft palate, hare-lip, brachygnathia, syndactylism, decrease in length and diameter of all bones, or shortening only of metacarpals and metatarsals and a decrease in number of coccygeal vertebrae. Exposure after day 30 only resulted in hypoplasia of the metacarpal and metatarsal growth plates. Some of the malformations have also been experimentally produced in cattle, goats, rabbits, and chickens.

Binns, W., Keeler, R.F., and Balls, L.D.: Congenital deformities in lambs, calves, and goats resulting from maternal ingestion of *Veratrum californicum*: hare-lip, cleft palate, ataxia, and hypoplasia of metacarpal and metatarsal bones. Clin. Toxicol., 5:245–261, 1972.

Binns, W., et al.: A congenital cyclopian-type malformation in lambs. J. Am. Vet. Med. Assoc., 134:180–183, 1969.

Binns, W., et al.: Cyclopian-type malformation in lambs. Arch. Environ. Health, 5:106–108, 1962.

Binns, W., et al.: A congenital cyclopian-type malformation in lambs induced by maternal ingestion of a range plant, *Veratrum californicum*. Am. J. Vet. Res., 24:1164–1175, 1963.

Binns, W., et al.: Toxicosis of *Veratrum californicum* in ewes and its relationship to congenital deformity in lambs. Ann. NY Acad. Sci., 111:571–576, 1964.

Bryden, M.M., Perry, C., and Keeler, R.F.: Effects of alkaloids of *Veratrum californicum* on chick embryos. Teratology, 8:19–28, 1973.

Keeler, R.F.: Teratogenic compounds in *Veratrum californicum* (Durand). IX. Structure-activity relation. X. Cyclopia in rabbits produced by cyclopamine. Teratology, 3:169–174, 175–180, 1970.

Keeler, R.F., and Binns, W.: Chemical compounds of *Veratrum californicum* related to congenital ovine cyclopian malformations: extraction of active material. Proc. Soc. Exp. Biol. Med., 116:123–127, 1964.

————: Possible teratogenic effects of veratramine. Proc. Soc. Exp. Biol. Med., 123:921–923, 1966.

Van Kampen, K.R., and Ellis, L.C.: Prolonged gestation in ewes ingesting *Veratrum californicum*: morphological changes and steroid biosynthesis in the endocrine organs of cyclopic lambs. J. Endocrinol., 52:549–560, 1972.

Thalidomide

This tranquilizing drug, introduced in Germany in the late 1950s, was eventually associated with a large number of congenitally malformed babies whose mothers had taken the drug during early pregnancy (days 21 to 36 postconception). The most striking malformations in these infants were absence of limbs (amelia) or shortening of the arms or legs to the point at which they resembled a seal's flippers (phocomelia, phoke = seal, melos = extremity). Other anomalies have also been described in these children (Toms, 1962).

Although not a naturally-occurring teratogen for animals, thalidomide has been shown to produce congenital anomalies comparable to those seen in children in several species. Nonhuman primates develop the same anomalies as described in human beings. The susceptible period is also comparable to man, ranging from 22 through 30 days of gestation at dose levels of 5 to 50 mg/kg/day. Administration of 50 to 200 mg thalidomide daily to female rhesus monkeys (*Macaca mulatta*) started after mating appeared to kill the embryo or prevent implantation, since no young were born. Administration of the drug to rabbits (150 mg/kg body weight daily) from day 8 to day 16 of pregnancy resulted in stillborn and deformed offspring. Rats apparently reabsorbed fetuses in utero, but produced no deformed offspring when placed on a similar regimen. Congenital abnormalites in tail vertebrae, sternebrae and extremities also occur in puppies whose mothers are given thalidomide during pregnancy.

Thalidomide also may produce phocomelia in the armadillo (*Dasypus novemcinctus mexicanus*), and a choriocarcinoma of the uterus with metastases has been associated with its administration (Marin-Padilla and Benirschke, 1963). Injury to the myocardium of armadillo embryos has also been demonstrated (Marin-Padilla and Benirschke, 1965).

Hendrickx, A.G., Axelrod, L.R., and Clayborn, L.D.: "Thalidomide" syndrome in baboons. Nature (Lond.), *210*:958–959, 1966.
Lucey, J.F., and Behrman, R.E.: Thalidomide: effect on pregnancy in the rhesus monkey. Science, *139*:1295–1296, 1963.
Marin-Padilla, M., and Benirschke, K.: Thalidomide-induced alterations in the blastocyst and placenta of the armadillo, *Dasypus novemcinctus mexicanus*, including a choriocarcinoma. Am. J. Pathol., *43*:999–1016, 1963.
———: Thalidomide injury to the myocardium of armadillo embryos. J. Embryol. Exp. Morphol., *13*:235–241, 1965.
Somers, G.F.: Thalidomide and congenital malformations. Lancet, *1*:912–913, 1962.
Toms, D.A.: Thalidomide and congenital malformations. Lancet, *2*:400, 1962.
Vickers, T.H.: The thalidomide embryopathy in hybrid rabbits. Br. J. Exp. Pathol., *48*:107–117, 1967.
Weidman, W.H., Young, H.H., and Zollman, P.E.: The effect of thalidomide on the unborn puppy. Staff Meeting Mayo Clinic, *38*:518–522, 1963.
Wilson, J.G.: An animal model of human disease: thalidomide embryopathy in primates. Comp. Pathol. Bull., *5*:3–4, 1973.

Pine Needles

The consumption of the needles of yellow ponderosa pine (*Pinus ponderosa*) may lead to birth of weak calves or abortion in cattle. It is principally a problem of range cattle in western United States and Canada, the habitat of the ponderosa pine.

Sheep appear to be resistant. In cattle, pine needle abortion most often occurs in late fall, winter, or early spring during the last trimester of pregnancy. Prior to abortion, cattle become depressed, and there is a rapid edema of the vulva and udder. Retention of the placenta is common following abortion. Histopathologic studies are limited, but necrosis of proximal convoluted tubules of the kidney of the aborted fetuses has been reported. The toxic principle in pine needles has not been specifically identified, but a heat-labile water-soluble toxin and a heat-stable water-insoluble toxin are recognized. The former has been suggested to be a mycotoxin, but is not considered the toxin of importance. An antiestrogenic factor in pine needles has been suggested to be the cause, but the pathogenesis of abortion is not clearly established.

Anderson, C.K., and Lozano, E.A.: Pine needle toxicity in pregnant mice. Cornell Vet., *67*:227–235, 1977.
Call, J.W., and James, L.F.: Pine needle abortion in cattle. *In* Effects of Poisonous Plants on Livestock, edited by R. F. Keeler, K. R. Van Kampen, and L. F. James. New York, Academic Press, 1978, pp. 587–590.
James, L.F., Call, J.W., and Stevenson, A.H.: Experimentally induced pine needle abortion in range cattle. Cornell Vet., *67*:294–299, 1977.

GROUP T: MISCELLANEOUS POISONS

Within the group of **miscellaneous poisons** are included a variety of poisonous plants and inorganic and organic chemicals which, for the most part, are not encountered with any frequency. Although for some a single most conspicuous lesion or clinical sign could be selected, we have chosen not to do so, in order to keep the number of poisons in each group to a minimum as a modest attempt to aid the student's memory.

Smallhead Sneezeweed (Helenium microcephalum). This plant, with such intriguing and descriptive common and scientific names, grows in Texas and Mexico. Many losses of cattle, sheep, and goats have been attributed to eating this plant.

Dollahite et al. (1964) have demonstrated this toxicity by feeding studies with calves, goats, rabbits, and sheep. The flowering plants were more toxic than those in earlier stages of growth. Experimentally poisoned animals exhibited signs of excess salivation, nasal discharge, bloating, and severe abdominal pain within an hour, and died within 24 hours after eating these plants. Accelerated pulse and respiratory rates, vomiting, and diarrhea were often exhibited. The gross lesions consisted of pulmonary edema, hydrothorax, ascites, hyperemia, and edema in the submucosa of the rumen and reticulum. Microscopically, edema of nervous tissue, lung, submucosa of rumen and reticulum was conspicuous. Mild toxic tubular nephritis was seen occasionally, plus some fatty change in cardiac muscle. The toxic principle has been identified as helenatin, a sesquiterpene lactone (Witzel et al., 1976).

Box (Buxus sempervirens). The common box, boxwood, or boxtree is native to Europe and Asia and is widely grown in the warmer climates of the United States as an ornamental or hedge. Losses of sheep, horses, pigs, cattle, and camels have been reported as a result of eating the leaves and stems of this plant. Severe gastroenteritis, sometimes with bloody diarrhea, are reported, with death in a short time. Several alkaloids have been extracted from the plant, including boxine—a severe emetic or purgative (Couch, 1937; Kingsbury, 1964; van Soest et al., 1965; Reynard and Norton, 1942).

Grasstree (Xanthorrhoea resinosa, X. hastile). This plant has been reported to cause poisoning of cattle only in Australia. The animals apparently eat this plant only when other feed is not available. The principal signs are "lurching to one side" and dribbling urine. In some animals, signs appear or are exacerbated two to three weeks after they have stopped eating the plant (Hall, 1965).

Stinkwood (Zieria arborescens). This is another Australian poisonous shrub that may cause death of cattle. The principal signs and lesions are related to massive pulmonary edema (Munday, 1968). The disease has been experimentally reproduced in rabbits (Munday et al., 1974).

Pokeweed (Phytolacca americana). Although boiled young shoots of this plant have been recommended for human consumption, poisoning has resulted in swine from eating the roots and in cattle from eating the tops of the plant or its fruit (**pokeberries**) (Kingsbury and Hillman, 1965). Signs of poisoning have appeared overnight after feeding green plants cut with corn silage. The signs were severe diarrhea and purgation, subnormal temperature, severe drop in milk flow, and convulsions and paralysis, which may lead to deaths from respiratory failure.

Yew (Taxus cuspidata, T. baccata, T. canadensis). These ornamental shrubs are rarely eaten by animals, but severe toxicity has been ascribed to them. The European variety, *T. baccata,* is a more frequently reported cause of poisoning on that continent, principally affecting cattle. The Japanese yew, *T. cuspidata,* a popular ornamental shrub in the United States, has been incriminated in deaths of horses, deer, reindeer, and burros. Cattle have been reported to die after eating *T. canadensis,* but the toxicity of *T. brevifolia* has been imputed but not confirmed.

Signs of poisoning may be missed; the animals may simply be found with the offending plant in mouth and stomach. Nervous manifestations, such as trembling, dyspnea, and collapse, may be evident during a short course. Lesions have not been recognized (Lowe, 1970; Kingsbury, 1964; Alden et al., 1977).

Phalaris grass (Phalaris tuberosa). This pasture plant, introduced into Australia from South Africa, has been occasionally incriminated as the cause of an acute death or chronic "phalaris staggers" in sheep. Sheep may die suddenly a few hours after grazing on a pasture of phalaris, with no signs or lesions evident. Others may exhibit convulsive movements, staggering, hyperexcitability, tremors, or convulsions before death. The toxic principles are believed to be tryptamine alkaloids. Green pigment, chemically related to tryptamine, is deposited in the kidneys and in neurons (Gallagher et al., 1966). The pigment is believed to accumulate within and ultimately to destroy mitochondria.

Sorghum (Sorghum sudanese, Sudan Grass). Horses grazing in pastures rich in sudan grass have been observed to develop chronic cystitis and occasionally ataxia. The urinary bladder in prolonged cases becomes thick-walled due to fibrosis; the epithelium is ulcerated, and abscesses may occur in the wall. The vagina may also be ulcerated and presumably infected, and abortion may occur. The urine may contain deposits of calcium carbonate (a common finding in equine urine), and in one case, *Streptococcus zooepidemicus* was recovered. The basis for the ataxia described in some cases has not been explained (Knight, 1968; Romane, 1966).

Sesbania (Sesbania punicea, Purple Sesbane, Purple Rattlebox). This South African shrub or small tree has been reported to be toxic to most domestic animals and poultry. The whole plant is poisonous; the seeds, flowers, and leaves each contain the toxic element. The poisoning is manifest by irritation of the gastrointestinal tract and cardiac failure. Terminal renal failure has been noted in some cases (Terblanche et al., 1966). Several North American species are also known to be poisonous (Kingsbury, 1964). These are known under various scientific and common names. *Sesbania vesicaria*, bagpod, bladderpod, or coffeebean, is a vigorous annual that grows especially in damp soils in the coastal plain from North Carolina and Florida to Texas.

Sesbania drummondii, coffeebean, rattlebush or rattlebox, is a perennial shrub or small tree with a distribution similar to *S. vesicaria*. Sheep and goats have been poisoned under natural conditions; cattle, experimentally. *S. punicea* has been de-

scribed as growing in Florida to Louisiana after its introduction as an ornamental from Mexico. The toxic principle in these plants is suspected to be saponin, but has not been clearly identified.

Djenkol bean (Pithecellobium jiringa, P. lobatum). Beans of the djenkol tree are used as food in the Far East. Cooking apparently renders them safe, but poisoning is occasionally encountered in human beings. The toxic principle is djenkolic acid, which crystallizes in the kidney, leading to tubular necrosis. Signs include dysuria, anuria, hematuria, and spasmodic pain in the loin.

Estrogens. These hormones have been known to cause poisoning under two generally different conditions. Synthetic estrogen, diethylstilbestrol, is used in feed for cattle to stimulate economical growth and usually causes no overt ill effects in these animals. On occasion, however, the "premix" containing the synthetic estrogen has been erroneously mixed with feed under preparation for laboratory mice (Hadlow, 1955, 1957). Certain inbred strains of mice are very sensitive to estrogens, and the effect upon a breeding colony is dramatic. In one incident in such a breeding colony of white mice, the number of pregnancies declined rapidly from 1000 a week to 20 per week. Litter size was reduced and many young were stillborn. About 90% of the adult males suddenly exhibited scrotal hernias, and sections of testes revealed complete azoospermia. After removal of the offending adulterated feed, reproduction gradually resumed in the mouse colony (Fig. 16–36).

A second source of estrogens is in natural plants, such as subterranean clover (*Trifolium subterraneum*). This clover poisoning is a major problem to sheep in certain parts of Australia. Different strains of clover vary in estrogen content and toxicity. The effects include stillbirths, neonatal deaths, dystocia, prolapse of uterus, and infertility in ewes. Virgin ewes may undergo precocious mammary development and lactation. Castrated males (wethers) may also

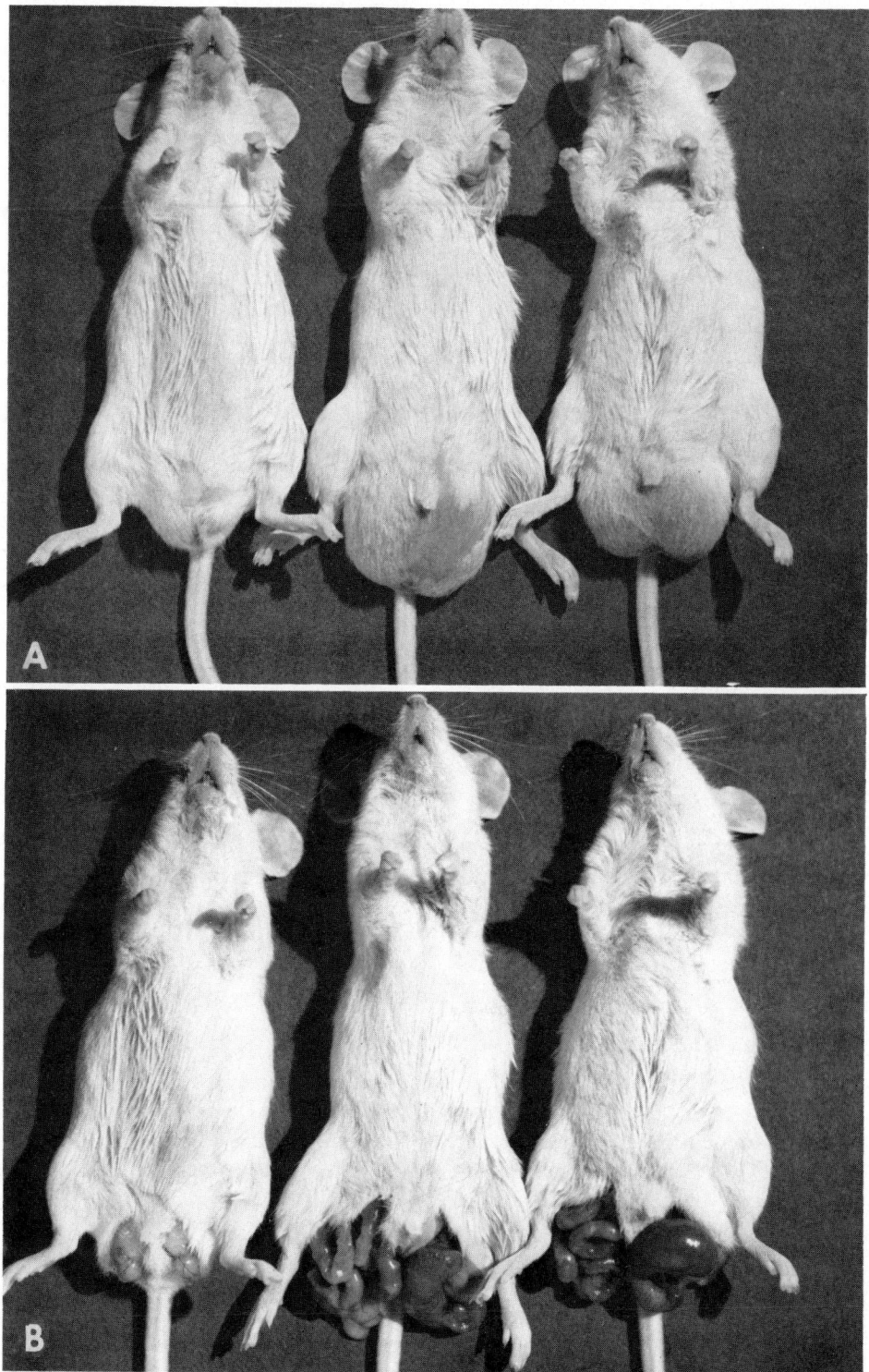

Fig. 16–36. Poisoning by diethylstilbestrol. Scrotal hernias in adult male mice. Normal mouse on the left. *A*, Intact mice. *B*, Scrotum incised to reveal intestinal content in two affected mice. (Courtesy of Dr. W. J. Hadlow and Proceedings of *The Animal Care Panel.*)

lactate. White clover (*T. repens*) has also been shown to have estrogenic effects. Estrogenic mycotoxins are another source of exogenous estrogenic compounds; these are discussed elsewhere.

Nitrogen Dioxide. This gas has been incriminated as a cause of "silo-fillers disease" in man (Lowry and Schuman, 1956) and pulmonary adenomatosis in cattle (Seaton, 1958; Cutlip, 1966). Intratracheal instillation of nitrogen dioxide gas in controlled doses into cattle results in severe respiratory distress, methemoglobinemia, and death. Animals that survive for 11 to 14 days following this exposure exhibit severe pulmonary consolidation and emphysema of the lungs. The respiratory epithelium undergoes squamous metaplasia in the trachea and proliferation in the rest of the bronchial tree. The alveolar epithelium proliferates and fills alveoli in some lobules; in others, fibrin precipitates in alveoli to form a hyaline membrane. The bronchiolar epithelium becomes redundant, and subepithelial fibrosis is conspicuous. Invasion by leukocytes into affected lungs may be extensive.

Cobalt. Cobalt is necessary for bacterial synthesis of vitamin B_{12} in the rumen, and some soils are deficient in this element. This has led to application of cobalt sulfate to the soil, and sometimes to injudicious dosing of ruminants with this salt (MacLaren, et al., 1964). Overdoses have led to death of cattle within a few hours. The principal findings at necropsy indicate severe congestion of the abomasal mucosa and microscopic evidence of toxic nephrosis. Cobalt may be demonstrated by spectrographic analysis to be present in liver and kidney.

In human beings, an endemic cardiomyopathy in heavy beer drinkers has been ascribed to cobalt (a beer additive). Necrotizing cardiomyopathy has been reproduced in rats given cobalt sulfate. Protein deficiency augmented the lesion. Many rats also developed vegetative endocarditis (Rona, 1971).

Hexachlorophene (2,2 methylene bis [3,5,6-trichorophenol]). This bactericidal chlorinated biphenol is widely used in surgical and germicidal soaps, ordinarily without any side effects. However, frequent exposure, especially in infants, may lead to demyelination of the white matter in the cerebral hemispheres and the medulla, which has led to fatal respiratory distress. The neurotoxicity has been experimentally reproduced in laboratory animals, in which peripheral nerve demyelination has also been noted. Optic nerve lesions and secondary retinopathy have also been described in rats. Hexachlorophene has caused periportal fatty change in the liver of sheep following oral dosing. Hexachlorobenzene, a fungicide, causes porphyria in human beings and is hepatotoxic in rats (Mollenhauer et al., 1975; Cam and Nigogosyan, 1963). Hexachlorophene is also used to treat sheep infected with *Fasciola hepatica*. Thorpe (1969) has demonstrated that single doses of hexachlorophene (25 or 50 mg/kg body weight) administered to sheep cause a significant effect upon spermatogenesis. Similar effects have been found in male rats (Thorpe, 1967). Following a single oral dose, spermatozoa and spermatids disappear from the testis, leaving only spermatogonia and spermatocytes. This effect may be transitory, but could cause a significant decrease in conceptions if it occurred during the breeding season. Hexachlorophene has also been shown to inhibit activity of certain enzymes in the liver, namely adenosine triphosphatase, succinic dehydrogenase, and glutamic dehydrogenase. Fatty change may also occur in the liver.

Chloroquine. Chloroquine has been used for the suppression or treatment of malaria in man as well as for treatment of systemic or discoid lupus erythematosus and rheumatoid arthritis. Tests of this drug in swine have revealed some interesting toxicologic effects (Gleiser et al., 1968). Daily oral doses of 25 mg/kg body weight were not lethal, but pigs were killed by doses of 50 to 100 mg/kg per day. The significant pathologic lesions included a diffuse myopathy of skeletal muscles, degenerative changes in neurons of the central nervous system and retina, necrosis of lymphocytes, and edema of the retina. The changes in skeletal muscles resemble Zenker's necrosis. By light microscopy, the changes in neurons appeared as swollen, foamy cytoplasm with displacement of nuclei. Electron micrographs disclosed this foamy cytoplasm to contain numerous lamellated, membranous bodies.

Zinc. Deficiency of this element associated with parakeratosis of swine and its necessity in metabolism are discussed elsewhere (p. 1070). It seems inevitable that poisoning with zinc will occur as a result of overzealous administration of zinc compounds. Experimentally, toxicity has been demonstrated in sheep and cattle (Ott et al., 1966). Depressed or depraved appetites result in cattle that have been fed zinc oxide in the diet at the rate of 0.9 g or more per kilogram of feed. Zinc accumulates in the blood, liver, pancreas, kidney, and bone, and in lesser amounts in hair, spleen, lung, and heart. After prolonged periods, hemoglobin and packed cell volumes in the blood are decreased.

Zinc Phosphide. A gray-black powder, used as a rodenticide, which releases phosphine (PH_3) when mixed with water has caused poisoning in a variety of animal species in Europe, but only recently has poisoning been described in the United States (Stowe et al., 1978). The histopathological changes have not been well described, but clinically poisoning is characterized by vomiting, abdominal pain, lethargy, and convulsions.

Gidyea Tree. The leaves and pods of this tree (*Acacia georginae*) contain a poisonous principle which may be lethal to sheep and cattle (Whittem and Murray, 1963). This poisoning is reported from the Georgina River basin in eastern Northern Territory and western Queensland of Australia,

where it is known as **Georgina River poisoning.** Of particular interest is the finding that the active poison is the fluoroacetate ion. It is possible that this tree may concentrate fluoroacetate in its leaves and pods, under specific conditions, from soils rich in fluorine. Monofluoroacetic acid in significant quantities has been isolated from the "gifblaar" plant (*Dichapetalum cymosum*) in South Africa where severe losses of livestock have been associated with eating this plant. See also sodium monofluoroacetate poisoning, page 910.

The most significant lesion is reported (Whittem and Murray, 1963) to occur in the myocardium. Focal necroses of myocardial fibers, usually followed by leukocytic infiltration and in some cases fibrosis, are seen microscopically. These are associated with gross petechiae and ecchymoses under the endocardium and epicardium, and occasional focal scars in the myocardium.

Helichrysum argyrosphaerum (Wild Everlasting, "Proprosie," "Sewejarrtjie"). This plant, native to Africa, long suspected as toxic, has recently been shown to cause a disease characterized by blindness and paralysis in sheep and cattle. Most field cases occur in sheep. The lesions, which have been reproduced experimentally (Basson et al., 1975), are characterized by marked demyelination and necrosis of white matter in the brain, optic nerves and chiasm, spinal cord, and peripheral nerves. There is also degeneration of the retina, commencing in the layer of rods and cones and extending to the inner nuclear layer. Cataracts characterized by necrosis of lens epithelium and lens cortex have been associated with natural outbreaks, but have not been reproduced.

Melia azedarch (Chinaberry Tree, White Cedar). Poisoning of livestock, principally sheep and swine, have been reported in Africa, Australia, and India from consumption of the fruits of this tree. Although the tree is naturalized in southern United States, examples of poisoning are rare. The signs of poisoning are those of gastroenteritis (principally diarrhea) and nervous dysfunction (trembling, depression, paralysis). The lesions have not been described in detail. Kwatra et al. (1974) reported hemorrhagic gastroenteritis, focal necrosis of the liver, kidney, myocardium, lymph nodes, and spleen, meningeal congestion, cerebral hemorrhage, and perivascular cuffing.

Aspirin. Aspirin (acetylsalicylic acid) is one of the most widely used drugs in human medicine, as an analgesic, antiphlogistic, and anticoagulant. In most species there is an extremely wide margin of safety, but intolerance reflected as hypersensitivity reactions (atopy, anaphylaxis) are reported, and its anticoagulant properties may lead to hemorrhage if used in high doses for prolonged periods. Cats are extremely intolerant of aspirin. Toxicity leads to hemorrhagic and ulcerative gastritis and toxic hepatitis with centrilobular necrosis. The principal effect of aspirin lies with its interference with the modulating role of prostaglandins on platelet aggregation and release of their contents. Aspirin, which inhibits cyclooxygenase, an enzyme necessary for prostaglandin production, leads to defective platelet aggregation and release. Other nonsteroid anti-inflammatory drugs have similar actions. Acetaminophen (metabolic product of phenacetin), another analgesic, is also toxic to cats and reported to induce hemolytic anemia and methemglobinemia.

Benzoic Acid. Benzoic acid is commonly used as a preservative in some dog and cat foods. Poisoning has been suspected in cats, which appear to be more sensitive to its effects than dogs. Bedford and Clarke (1972) reported an experimental poisoning of cats with meat containing 0.5 to 1.0% benzoic acid. The syndrome was characterized by aggression, hyperesthesia, convulsions, and death. The pathogenesis of these signs is unknown.

Cadmium. Cadmium is not a documented health hazard to animals. Environmental contamination with cadmium is increasing and its potential hazard is real. Shellfish and plants may concentrate cadmium. Experimental poisoning results in damage to endothelial cells at restricted sites, leading to hemorrhagic testicular necrosis, necrotizing enteritis, and intestinal atrophy. In Japan, cadmium poisoning in women was characterized by a malabsorption syndrome.

Kallstroemia. Poisoning by carpet weed or hairy caltrop (*K. hirsutissima*) has been documented in cattle and sheep respectively (Mathews, 1944; Dollahite, 1975). The plants are native to western United States. Poisoning is characterized by a peculiar knuckling over of the hind legs at the fetlock joints, which progresses to posterior paralysis and death. The forelimbs are unaffected. The basis for these unusual signs or death is not known. Severe gastroenteritis is reported in sheep.

Fish and Shellfish Poisoning. Poisoning from consumption of certain fishes and shellfish under appropriate conditions is well recognized in human beings. Although most mammals are believed to be susceptible, few examples exist. Most probably similar poisonings in animals go unrecognized. There are many different types of fish poisoning in man. **Ciguatera and scombroid poisoning** are the most common (Hughes and Merson, 1976.)

Ciguatera (from Spanish—poisonous snail) is most often associated with barracuda, red snapper, amberjack, and grouper. The heat-stable toxin is referred to as ciguatoxin, which is believed to enter fish through the food chain. It is a cholinesterase inhibitor, but its action is believed to be more complex. Signs of poisoning, which develop within a few minutes to 30 hours after ingestion, include abdominal cramps, nausea, vomiting, diarrhea, and paresthesia, particularly of the lips, tongue, and throat.

Scombroid fish poisoning is associated with tuna, mackerel, bonito, and shipjack, and the nonscombroid fish, mahi-mahi. The toxin, formed by bacteria on fish flesh, is called **scombrotoxin,** and is believed to consist of histamine and other heat-stable substances. Symptoms begin within a few minutes to a few hours after ingestion, and include flushing, headache, dizziness, burning of the mouth and throat, abdominal cramps, nausea, vomiting, diarrhea, urticaria, and pruritus.

Shellfish poisoning results from ingestion of bivalve mollusks contaminated with neurotoxins of the dinoflagellates *Gonyaulax catenalla* or *Go. tamarensis,* which results in a paralytic disease commencing within 30 minutes, or *Gymnodinium breve,* which is associated with neurologic signs such as ataxia but not with paralysis. In both forms there is also nausea, vomiting, and diarrhea. The toxins are heat-stable. Mussels, clams, oysters, and scallops are the main vehicles. When in abundance, these and other toxic dinoflagellates as well as nontoxic dinoflagellates impart a reddish brown color to the water, usually called a **red tide**.

Alden, C.L., Fosnaugh, C.J., Smith, J.B., and Mohan, R.: Japanese yew poisoning of large domestic animals in the midwest. J. Am. Vet. Med. Assoc., *170*:314–316, 1977.

Areekul, S., Kirdudom, P., and Chaovanapricha, K.: Studies on djenkol bean poisoning (djenkolism) in experimental animals. Southeast Asian J. Trop. Med. Public Health., *7*:551–558, 1976.

Basson, P.A., et al.: Blindness and encephalopathy caused by *Helichrysum argyrosphaerum* DC (Compositae) in sheep and cattle. Onderstepoort J. Vet. Res., *42*:135–148, 1975.

Beck, A.B., and Gardiner, M.R.: Clover disease of sheep in western Australia. J. Dept. Agric. West. Aust., *6*:390–392 and 395–400, 1965. VB *36*:3330, 1966.

Bedford, P.G.C., and Clarke, E.G.C.: Suspected benzoic acid poisoning in the cat. Vet. Rec., *88*:599–601, 1971.

————: Experimental benzoic acid poisoning in the cat. Vet. Rec., *90*:53–58, 1972.

Call, J.W., and James, L.F.: Effect of feeding pine needles on ovine reproduction. J. Am. Vet. Med. Assoc., *169*:1301–1302, 1976.

Cam, C., and Nigogosyan, G.: Acquired toxic porphyria cutanea tarda due to hexachlorobenzene. J. Am. Vet. Med. Assoc., *143*:88–91, 1963.

Cook, H., and Kitts, W.D.: Anti-oestrogenic activity in yellow pine needles (*Pinus ponderosa*). Acta Endocrinol., *45*:33, 1964.

Couch, J.F.: The chemistry of stock-poisoning plants. J. Chem. Educ., *14*:16–24, 1937.

Cutlip, R.C.: Experimental nitrogen dioxide poisoning in cattle. Pathol. Vet., *3*:474–485, 1966.

Davis, L.E., and Donnelly, E.J.: Analgesic drugs in the cat. J. Am. Vet. Med. Assoc., *153*:1161–1167, 1968.

Dollahite, J.W.: Toxicity of *Kallstroemia parviflora* (warty caltrop) to sheep, goats, and rabbits. Southwestern Vet., *28*:135–139, 1975.

Dollahite, J.W., Hardy, W.T., and Henson, J.B.: Toxicity of *Helenium microcephalum* (smallhead sneezeweed). J. Am. Vet. Med. Assoc., *145*:694–696, 1964.

Finco, D.R., Duncan, J.R., Schall, W.D., and Prasse, K.W.: Acetaminophen toxicosis in the cat. J. Am. Vet. Med. Assoc., *166*:469–472, 1975.

Gabbiani, G., Badonnel, M.-C., Mathewson, S.M., and Ryan, G.B.: Acute cadmiun intoxication: early selective lesions of endothelial clefts. Lab. Invest., *30*:686–695, 1974.

Gaines, T.B., Kimbrough, R.D., and Linder, R.E.: The oral and dermal toxicity of hexachlorophene in rats. Toxicol. Appl. Pharmacol., *25*:332–343, 1973.

Gallagher, C.H., Koch, J.H., and Hoffman, H.: Disease of sheep due to ingestion of *Phalaris tuberosa.* Aust. Vet. J., *42*:279–284, 1966.

————: Poisoning by grass. New Scientist, 25 Aug. 1966:412–414, 1966.

Gleiser, C.A., et al.: Study of chloroquine toxicity and a drug-induced cerbrospinal lipodystrophy in swine. Am. J. Pathol., *53*:27–45, 1968.

Hadlow, W.J., Grimes, E.F., and Jay, G.E., Jr.: Stilbestrol contaminated feed and reproductive disturbances in mice. Science, *122*:643–644, 1955.

Hadlow, W.J., and Grimes, E.F.: Influence of stilbestrol-contaminated feed on reproduction in a colony of mice. Proc. Anim. Care Panel, *6*:19–25, 1955.

Hadlow, W.J.: Stilbestrol poisoning in mice. J. Am. Vet. Med. Assoc., *130*:300–303, 1957.

Hall, W.T.K.: Grasstree poisoning of cattle. Qd. Agric. J., *91*:504–506, 1965.

Herrgesell, J.D.: Aspirin poisoning in the cat. J. Am. Vet. Med. Assoc., *151*:452–455, 1967.

Hughes, J.M., and Merson, M.H.: Current concepts: fish and shellfish poisoning. N. Engl. J. Med., *295*:1117–1120, 1976.

Kingsbury, J.M.: Poisonous Plants of the United States and Canada. Englewood Cliffs, N.J., Prentice-Hall, 1964.

Kingsbury, J.M., and Hillman, R.B.: Pokeweed (*Phytolacca*) poisoning in a dairy herd. Cornell Vet., *55*:534–538, 1965.

Knight, P.R.: Equine cystitis and ataxia associated with grazing of pastures dominated by sorghum species. Aust. Vet. J., *44*:257, 1968.

Koppang, N.: Dimethylnitrosamine—formation in fish meal and toxic effects in pigs. Am. J. Pathol., *74*:95–108, 1974.

Kwatra, M.S., Singh, B., Hothi, D.S., and Dhingra, P.N.: Poisoning by *Melia azedarach* in pigs. Vet. Rec., *95*:421, 1974.

Larson, E.J.: Toxicity of low doses of aspirin in the cat. J. Am. Vet. Med. Assoc., *143*:837–840, 1963.

Lowe, J.E., et al.: *Taxus cuspidata* (Japanese yew) poisoning in horses. Cornell Vet., *60*:36–39, 1970.

Lowry, T., and Schuman, L.M.: Silo-filler's disease—a syndrome caused by nitrogen dioxide. JAMA, *162*:153–160, 1956.

MacLaren, A.P.C., Johnston, W.G., and Voss, R.C.: Cobalt poisoning in cattle. Vet. Rec., *76*:1148–1149, 1964.

Mathews, F.P.: The toxicity of *Kallstroemia hirsutissima* (carpetweed) for cattle, sheep and goats. J. Am. Vet. Med. Assoc., *95*:152–155, 1944.

Mollenhauer, H.H., Johnson, J.H., Younger, R.L., and Clark, D.E.: Ultrastructural changes in liver of the rat fed hexachlorobenzene. Am. J. Vet. Res., *36*:1777–1781, 1975.

Munday, B.L.: *Zieria arborescens* (stinkwood) intoxication in cattle. Aust. Vet. J., *44*:501–502, 1968.

Munday, B.L., Cummings, R., and Wilson, B.J.: Experimental *Zieria arborescens* (stinkwood) poisoning in rabbits. Res. Vet. Sci., *17*:270–272, 1974.

Ott, E.A., et al.: Zinc toxicity in ruminants. IV. Physiological changes in tissues of beef cattle. J. Anim. Sci., *25*:432–438, 1966.

———: Zinc toxicity in ruminants. III. Physiological changes in tissues and alterations in rumen metabolism in lambs. J. Anim. Sci., *25*:424–431, 1966.

———: Zinc toxicity in ruminants. II. Effect of high levels of dietary zinc on grains, feed consumption and field efficiency of beef cattle. J. Anim. Sci., *25*:419–423, 1966.

———: Zinc toxicity in ruminants. I. Effect of high levels of dietary zinc on grains, feed consumption, and feed efficiency of lambs. J. Anim. Sci., *25*:414–418, 1966.

Pate, F.M., Johnson, A.D., and Miller, W.J.: Testicular changes in calves following injection with cadmium chloride. J. Anim. Sci., *31*:559–564, 1970.

Reid, I.M., and Hall, G.A.: An ultrastructural and biochemical study of hexachlorophane-induced fatty liver in sheep. J. Pathol., *115*:33–43, 1975.

Reynard, G.B., and Norton, J.B.S.: Poisonous plants of Maryland in relation to livestock. Univ. of Maryland, Agric. Exper. Station. Tech. Bull. A10, 1942.

Richardson, M.E., and Fox, M.R.S.: Dietary cadmium and enteropathy in the Japanese quail: histochemical and ultrastructural studies. Lab. Invest., *31*:722–731, 1974.

Robinson, G.R., Wagstaff, D.J., Colaianne, J.J., and

Ulsamer, A.G.: Experimental hexachlorophene intoxication in young swine. Am. J. Vet. Res., *36*:1615–1618, 1975.

Romane, W.M., et al.: Equine cystitis associated with grazing of sudan grass. J. Am. Vet. Med. Assoc., *149*:1171, 1966.

Rona, G.: Experimental aspects of cobalt cardiomyopathy. Br. Heart J., *33*(Suppl):171–174, 1971.

Schlaepfer, W.W.: Sequential study of endothelial changes in acute cadmium intoxication. Lab. Invest., *25*:556–564, 1971.

Scott, D.W., Bolton, G.R., and Lorenz, M.D.: Hexachlorophene toxicosis in dogs. J. Am. Vet. Med. Assoc., *162*:947–949, 1973.

Seaton, V.A.: Pulmonary adenomatosis in Iowa cattle. Am. J. Vet. Res., *19*:600–609, 1958.

Stevenson, A.H., James, L.F., and Call, J.W.: Pine-needle (*Pinus ponderosa*)-induced abortion in range cattle. Cornell Vet., *62*:519–524, 1972.

Stowe, C.M., et al.: Zinc phosphide poisoning in dogs. J. Am. Vet. Med. Assoc., *173*:270, 1978.

Terblanche, M., et al.: A toxicological study of the plant *Sesbania punicea*, Benth. J. S. Afr. Vet. Med. Assoc., *37*:191–197, 1966. VB 37:1817, 1967.

Thorpe, E.: Some pathological effects of hexachlorophene in the rat. J. Comp. Pathol., *77*:137–142, 1967.

———: Some toxic effects of hexachlorophene in sheep. J. Comp. Pathol., *79*:167–171, 1969.

Towfighi, J., Gonatas, N.K., and McCree, L.: Hexachlorophene neuropathy in rats. Lab. Invest., *29*:428–436, 1973.

———: Hexchlorophene retinopathy in rats. Lab. Invest., *32*:330–338, 1975.

Van Soest, H., Gotink, W.M., and v.d. Vooren, L.J.: Poisoning in pigs and cows by boxtree leaves (*Buxus sempervirens*). Tijdschr. Diergeneesk., *90*:387–389, 1965. VB 35:2732, 1965.

Ward, B.C., Jones, B.D., and Rubin, G.J.: Hexachlorophene toxicity in dogs. J. Am. Anim. Hosp. Assoc., *9*:167–169, 1973.

Whittem, J.H., and Murray, L.R.: The chemistry and pathology of Georgina River poisoning. Aust. Vet. J., *39*:168–173, 1963.

Witzel, D.A., Ivie, G.W. and Dollahite, J.W.: Mammalian toxicity of helenalin, the toxic principle of *Helenium microcephalum* DC (smallhead sneezeweed). Am. J. Vet. Res., *37*:859–861, 1976.

Wong, E., Flux, D.S., and Latch, G.C.M.: The oestrogenic activity of white clover (*Trifolium repens* L). NZ J. Agric. Res., *14*:639–645, 1971.

CHAPTER *17*

Nutritional Deficiencies

It is possible to demonstrate the indispensability of a large number of dietary substances by depriving experimental animals of them. While the usefulness of fundamental research is not questioned, a casual perusal of the long list of abnormalities, which can be shown experimentally to follow withholding of various vitamins, minerals, or amino acids, tends to confuse more than to enlighten and accords to deficiencies a prominence they do not possess in actual diagnosis and therapy. Therefore, those deficiencies that are known to occur under conditions of veterinary medical practice will be emphasized. Most of these deficiencies arise as the result of the restricted diets often imposed upon domestic animals by their caretakers through either ignorance or greed. The current tendency to feed livestock various artificially manufactured products and by-products, as well as certain unnatural substances (hormones, antibiotics, synthetics) designed to cause abnormal gains in weight or excessive production of milk or eggs, serves to introduce a continuous succession of new diseases, the diagnosis of which is often far from simple.

Deficiency of a single nutrient is rare as a natural disease, although some examples can be cited: iodine deficiency leading to goiter; iron deficiency leading to anemia; ingestion of thiaminase leading to thiamine deficiency; molybdenum toxicosis leading to copper deficiency. But in general, nutritional diseases in both man and lower animals are multiple deficiencies. This creates a more complex disease state which is often difficult to analyze, and also makes it difficult to make comparisons with the single nutrient deficiencies produced in the laboratory. The bulk of nutritional research has concerned single nutrient deficiency.

Obviously, lack of a specific nutrient(s) in the diet is the simplest and most easily understood cause of nutritional disease. But other and more usual causes include: (1) The diet may be of generally poor quality (e.g., predominantly roughage) or volume may be inadequate (simple starvation). (2) **Interference with intake** arising from anorexia, mechanical obstruction, dental disease, and so forth have the same net effect as inadequate supply. (3) Other conditions can lead to deficiency states by **interfering with absorption of nutrients.** Lack of digestive secretions from hepatic or pancreatic disease, hypermotility of the intestinal tract, and formation of insoluble complexes such as between calcium and phytate are examples. (4) **Interference with storage or utilization** of a nutrient may have the same effect as a simple dietary deficiency. As example, in thyroiditis, insufficient normal tissue may be available for the proper utilization of iodine. (5) **Increased excretion** represents another mechanism leading to deficiency disease. Loss of potassium associated with diarrhea or calcium loss in hyperparathyroidism are examples. (6) **Increased requirements** associated with pregnancy, lactation, or hyperthyroidism can lead to deficiency states if the diet is not adjusted. (7) **Inhibition of nutrients** by specific inhibitors or analogs also results in deficiency. Analogs are known for several of the B vitamins.

Dobbing, J.: Under-nutrition and the developing brain: the use of animal models to elucidate the human problem. Psychiatr. Neurol. Neurochir., 74:433–442, 1971.

Follis, R.H.: Deficiency Disease. Springfield, Charles C Thomas, 1958.

Gortner, R.A., Jr.: Some recent advances in human nutrition research. Fed. Proc., 33:2263–2269, 1974.

Kerr, G.R., Allen, J.R., and Scheffler, G.: Malnutrition studies in the rhesus monkey. I. Effect on physical growth. Am. J. Clin. Nutr., 23:739–748, 1970.

Newberne, P.M., and Wilson, R.B.: Prenatal malnutrition and postnatal responses to infection. Nutr. Rep. Interntl., 5:151–158, 1972.

Newberne, P.M.: The influence of nutrition response to infectious disease. Adv. Vet. Sci. Comp. Med., 17:265–289, 1973.

HYPOVITAMINOSIS A

Herbivorous animals obtain their vitamin A (retinol) in the form of carotene, a yellow pigment (or group of pigments) that occurs with chlorophyll in all green plants. By a slight chemical change, one molecule of carotene is converted into two molecules of vitamin A, the change taking place in the intestinal mucosa. Vitamin A is then

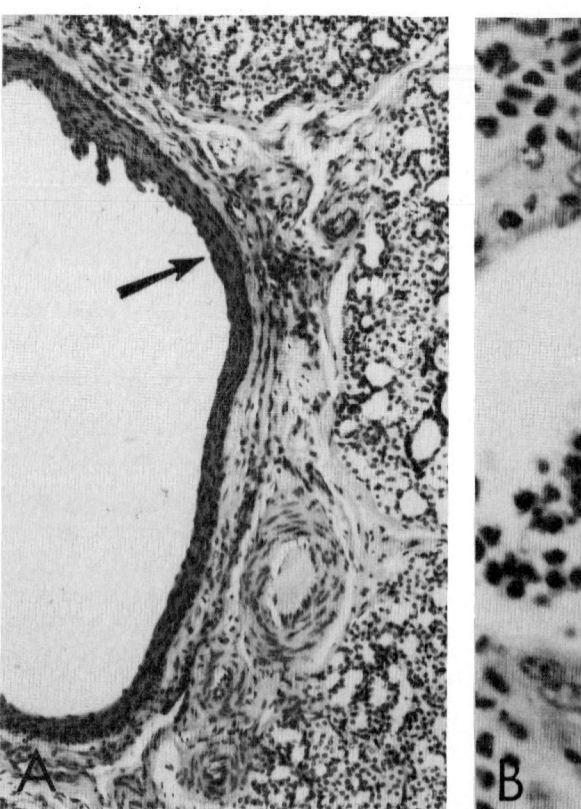
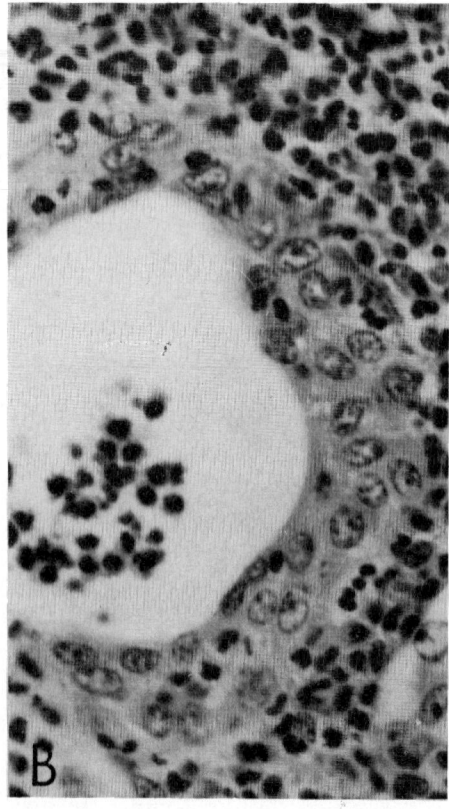

Fig. 17–1. Vitamin A deficiency. *A*, Squamous metaplasia of a major duct in the salivary gland of a calf. *B*, Squamous metaplasia of a collecting tubule in the kidney of a mink. Also note purulent exudate in the lumen of the tubule and interstitium.

transported via the lymph to the general circulation and ultimately to the liver, where it is stored. Carnivorous animals usually depend upon animal tissues for their food, the liver obviously being especially desirable in this respect. The vitamin is fat-soluble and, since certain fishes store large amounts of it, cod-liver oil and shark-liver oil constitute concentrated sources of this vitamin. Certain species such as man and bovines can also absorb carotenoids directly and subsequently convert them to vitamin A in the liver. In all species, bile salts and pancreatic juice are necessary for the absorption of vitamin A and carotenoids.

The biochemical events of absorption, transport and storage of vitamin A and its precursors have recently been reviewed by Olson (1969) and Goodman (1980).

The earliest sign of deficiency of vitamin A is **night blindness** (nyctalopia). The animal is unable to see as well as it should in partial darkness, as can be determined by placing obstructions in front of it under nocturnal conditions. Changes in cellular morphology consist of retinal degenerations not easily detected, but it has been determined that night vision depends upon a continuous chemical interchange involving the light-induced bleaching of a pigment in the rods of the retina, known as rhodopsin or visual purple, and its restoration. Rhodopsin is composed of vitamin A aldehyde (retinene) and the protein opsin. Descriptions of morphologic alterations in the retina have varied from the absence of lesions to accumulation of eosinophilic debris and macrophages between the rods and pigmented epithelium with thinning of the outer nuclear layer in rabbits, to degeneration of rods and the outer nuclear, outer molecular and inner nuclear layers in rats.

While nyctalopia is not likely to be noticed unless sought, the classic early sign is xerophthalmia, which means dryness of the eye. The deficiency of lacrimal secretion responsible for this dryness is due to interference with the glands and partial obstruction of their ducts by squamous metaplasia and thickened linings. Apparently because of the lack of the protective tears, animals, especially horses and cattle, when suffering from this deficiency, are subject to recurrent episodes of conjunctivitis and keratitis. The latter are doubtless precipitated by dust, foreign particles, and infection. The keratitis may or may not be of such severity as to lead to ulceration and opacity, but healing is the rule, subsequent attacks being not improbable.

The epithelial changes in the lacrimal glands are an index to the fundamental disorder of vitamin A deficiency, which is squamous metaplasia and pronounced cornification of many columnar and cuboidal epithelial surfaces. A demonstrable quantitative atrophy or even necrosis often precedes the metaplasia. These changes involve the digestive tract and especially the glands that open into it, the respiratory mucous membranes, where the protective cilia are lost, and practically all genitourinary surfaces and glands. Partially or wholly as the result of impairment of epithelial protection, respiratory infections are unusually frequent. Mastitis of unusual frequency and severity has been observed in deficient dairy herds.

Ultrastructural studies reveal that the metaplasia of columnar epithelial cells to stratified squamous type results from changes in the differentiation of cells growing from the basal layer, followed by loss of preexisting cells. This change in the growth pattern of the columnar cells starts from single cells in the basal layer and eventually spreads to all cells in the epithelium involved. This metaplasia may also be produced in tissue culture systems of bronchial epithelium, for example, and the squamous metaplasia may be prevented or reversed by adding vitamin A to the culture medium.

In birds, the mucous glands that open into the esophagus and pharynx become distended with inspissated secretion because their ducts are occluded by the increased thickness of their epithelial linings, which have undergone squamous metaplasia and hyperkeratosis. The spherical nodules, 1 to 2 mm in diameter, spaced at rather wide but regular intervals over the mucosa, are pathognomonic of hypovitaminosis A. Accompanied by coryza and other upper respiratory inflammations, doubtless infectious, and by general malaise and inanition, this condition goes by the name of **nutritional roup.**

Probably the most important effect of this epithelial dysplasia is to be found in the urinary tract. Practically all male cattle, sheep, and goats subjected to prolonged severe deficiency of vitamin A die of urinary obstruction caused by urinary calculi lodged at the sigmoid flexure. Desquamated clumps of epithelial cells from the renal pelves or other urinary surfaces are considered to form nuclear granules upon which mineral salts precipitate. Females escape the effects of this **urolithiasis** because of the less constricted urethra.

Also of importance is interference with maternal reproduction. Excessive cornification is at least sufficient to upset the cycle of epithelial changes as shown by the vaginal smear, cornified epithelium being constantly present. It is known that in experimentally deficient rats, the embryo undergoes implantation but is resorbed a short time later. While difficult to prove, strong clinical evidence supports the view that the same happens in other species, including cattle, and that this defect, based upon imperfect endometrial function, is an important cause of infertility in the bovine. Atrophy of seminiferous epithelium is demonstrable in deficient rats, but it is doubtful that testicular function deteriorates in domestic animals; however, more thorough studies are needed on this point.

Severe deficiency of this vitamin also alters normal bone growth and remodeling, especially of cranial bones, resulting in a disparity between growth of the nervous system and its bony enclosure. This apparently results from a replacement of subperiosteal resorption by osteoblastic activity. Probably the only noticeable effects of this, as far as domestic animals are concerned, are to be seen in occasional fetal malformations and, as found in certain experimental work, in a failure of the optic foramina to grow to sufficient diameter. This is believed by some to be the cause, through constriction of the optic nerve, of the frequent blindness in newborn calves from experimentally deficient mothers. One hypothesis concerning the defect in growth of bone in calves is that deficiency of vitamin A leads to slower rates of osteolytic and osteoclastic resorption of bone, while synthesis of bone proceeds at a normal rate (Davis et al., 1970).

Increased cerebrospinal fluid pressure regularly follows vitamin A deficiency. In part, reduction in size of the cranial vault may explain the increased pressure; however, in that pressure returns to normal levels when adequate dietary vitamin A is provided, other mechanisms undoubtedly participate. Present evidence suggests that absorption of cerebrospinal fluid via arachnoid villi is impeded. In experimentally deficient calves, the dura mater is thickened over the anterior cerebellum and tentorium cerebelli, where arachnoid villi are abundant.

Comparable to differentiation of periosteal cells, odontogenic epithelium also fails to differentiate in experimentally deficient animals, resulting in a reduction in the deposition of enamel. Although similar lesions may occur spontaneously, the role of vitamin A deficiency and dental disease has not been assessed in domestic animals.

Lastly, fetal malformations must be mentioned. In addition to blindness at birth, the exact pathogenesis of which is often obscure, calves have been born with an island of hairy skin in the middle of the cornea (dermoid), with jaws that did not fit each other, and with other deformities. Litters of pigs have been born without eyes. These and similar developmental anomalies have occurred among animals experimentally deprived of vitamin A with a frequency altogether too great to be explained by the laws of chance. Surprisingly, developmental anomalies have also been reported to result from great excesses of the vitamin. Prolonged gestation has also been reported in hypovitaminosis A in cattle. This may be related to fetal anomalies.

Except through the secondary development of some fatal disorder such as urinary obstruction, deficiency of vitamin A does not cause death. Deficient animals fatten as well as any and have been maintained in a condition of marketable obesity for indefinite periods. The tissue changes are reversible, and complete return to normal can be expected if the deficiency is corrected. In any species, the liver stores an amount ample for a considerable period, during which total dietary deprivation produces no effect. This period is usually five or six months in cattle and probably horses, two or three months in sheep and goats. Dogs and cats are susceptible to this deficiency, but suffer from it only when kept under very unusual conditions. In cats, squamous metaplasia of the respiratory tract, conjunctiva, salivary glands, and endometrium have been reported. These animals appear to be unable to convert carotene to vitamin A.

Davis, T.E., Krook, L., and Warner, R.G.: Bone resorption in hypovitaminosis A. Cornell Vet., 60:90–119, 1970.

Dreizen, S., Levy, B.M., and Bernick, S.: Studies on biology of periodontium of marmosets. II. Histopathologic manifestations of spontaneous and induced vitamin-A deficiency in oral structures of adult marmosets. J. Dent. Res., 52:803–809, 1973.

Dutt, B.: Effect of vitamin A deficiency on the testes of rams. Br. Vet. J., 115:236–238, 1959.

Dutt, B., and Vasudevan, B.: Clinical syndromes and histopathological changes in vitamin "A" deficiency in cow calves. Indian Vet. J., 39:584–587, 1962.

Eaton, H.D.: Chronic bovine hypo- and hypervitaminosis A and cerebrospinal fluid pressure. Am. J. Clin. Nutr., 22:1070–1080, 1969.

Eaton, H.D., Lucas, J.J., Nielsen, S.W., and Helmboldt, C.F.: Association of plasma or liver vitamin A concentrations with the occurrence of parotid duct metaplasia or of ocular papilledema in Holstein male calves. J. Dairy Sci., 53:1775–1779, 1970.

Felix, E.L., Loyd, B., and Cohen, M.H.: Inhibition of the growth and development of a transplantable murine melanoma by vitamin A. Science, 189:886–888, 1975.

Frier, H.I., et al.: Formation and absorption of cerebrospinal fluid in adult goats with hypo- and hypervitaminosis A. Am. J. Vet. Res., 35:45–55, 1974.

Gallina, A.M., et al.: Bone growth in the hypovitaminotic A calf. J. Nutr., 100:129–142, 1970.

Goodman, D.S.: Vitamin A metabolism. Fed. Proc., 39:2716–2722, 1980.

Hayes, K.C., McCombs, H.L., and Faherty, T.P.: The fine structure of vitamin A deficiency. I. Parotid duct metaplasia. Lab. Invest., 22:81–89, 1970.

Hayes, K.C., Nielsen, S.W., and Eaton, H.D.: Pathogenesis of the optic nerve lesion in vitamin A-deficient calves. Arch. Ophthal., 80:777–787, 1968.

Marchok, A.C., Cone, M.V., and Nettesheim, P.: Induction of squamous metaplasia (vitamin A deficiency) and hypersecretory activity in tracheal organ cultures. Lab. Invest., 33:451–460, 1975.

Marsh, H., and Swingle, K.F.: The calcium, phosphorus, magnesium, carotene and vitamin A content of the blood of range cattle in eastern Montana. Am. J. Vet. Res., 21:212–221, 1960.

Mills, J.H.L., et al.: Experimental pathology of dairy calves ingesting one-third the daily requirement of carotene. Acta Vet. Scand., 8:324–346, 1967.

Muto, Y., Smith, F.R., and Goodman, D.S.: Comparative studies of retinol transport in plasma. J. Lipid Res., 14:525–532, 1973.

Newberne, P.M.: Vitamin A deficiency hydrocephaly in the rabbit. Comp. Pathol. Bull., 5:3–4, 1973.

Nielsen, S.W., et al.: Parotid duct metaplasia in marginal bovine vitamin A deficiency. Am. J. Vet. Res., 27:223–233, 1966.

Noell, W.K., and Albrecht, R.: Irreversible effects of visible light on the retina: role of vitamin A. Science, 172:76–80, 1971.

Noell, W.K., Delmelle, M.C., and Albrecht, R.: Vitamin A deficiency effect on retina: dependence on light. Science, 172:72–75, 1971.

Olson, J.A.: Metabolism and function of vitamin A. Fed. Proc., 28:1670–1677, 1969.

O'Toole, B.A., Fradkin, R., Wilson, J.G., and Warkany, J.: Vitamin A deficiency and reproduction in rhesus monkeys. Teratology, 7:A24–A25, 1973.

O'Toole, B.A., et al.: Vitamin A deficiency and reproduction in rhesus monkeys. J. Nutr., 104:1513–1524, 1974.

Palludan, B.: The teratogenic effect of vitamin A deficiency in pigs. Acta Vet. Scand., 2:32–59, 1961.

Schmidt, H.: Vitamin A deficiencies in ruminants. Am. J. Vet. Res., 2:373–389, 1941.

Smith, J.C., McDaniel, E.G., Fan, F.F., and Halsted, J.A.: Zinc: a trace element essential in vitamin A metabolism. Science, 181:954–955, 1973.

Sorsby, A., Reading, H.W., and Bunyan, J.: Effect of vitamin A deficiency on the retina of the experimental rabbit. Nature (Lond.), *210*:1011–1015, 1966.

Spratling, F.R., et al.: Experimental hypovitaminosis-A in calves. Clinical and gross post-mortem findings. Vet. Rec., *77*:1532–1542, 1965.

Wong, Yong-Chuan, and Buck, R.C.: An electron microscopic study of metaplasia of the rat tracheal epithelium in vitamin A deficiency. Lab. Invest., *24*:55–66, 1971.

HYPOVITAMINOSIS B

The original vitamin B is now known to include a number of specific chemical compounds, thiamine (vitamin B_1), riboflavin (B_2), nicotinic acid ("niacin"), pantothenic acid, pyridoxine (B_6), and cyanocobalamin (B_{12}). A number of other factors, such as folic acid, biotin, and para-aminobenzoic acid are also usually included in the vitamin B group. Since these substances have largely the same source (yeast, grains, and seeds) and since the lesions resulting from their deficiency tend to overlap, all can be considered together, the term B-complex being in common use for the group. The long used descriptive name of "the antineuritic vitamin" gives an insight into many aspects of the B-group.

Thiamine (Vitamin B_1) Deficiency

Thiamine is essential to health in most animals and man. Deficiency may result in any of several situations: (1) The diet may lack sufficient thiamine. (2) The vitamin may be destroyed by thiamine analogues, such as amprolium. (3) Destruction may result from the action of thiaminases in the diet, such as found in bracken fern (*Pteridium aquilinum*), horse tail (*Equisetum aroena*), and the flesh of certain fishes, or by thiaminase produced by certain organisms growing in the gastrointestinal tract (*Bacillus thiaminolyticus*, *B. aneurinolyticus*, *Clostridium thiaminolyticum*, or *Cl. sporogenes*). The precipitating situation varies in different species. In cats, dogs, mink, and foxes, deficiency usually results from lack of thiamine in the diet or from feeding certain thiaminase-containing fish. This fish diet is also responsible for thiamine deficiency in captive pinnipeds (sea lions, harp seals, harbor seals). Birds are also susceptible to a deficient diet.

Adult ruminants, such as cattle and sheep, do not require thiamine in the diet because the vitamin is produced by bacteria in the forestomachs. Calves and lambs, however, have no such activity in the forestomachs early in life, and are therefore susceptible to dietary deficiency at this time. Adult cattle and sheep may become deficient by consuming plants containing thiaminase (such as bracken fern) or by the activity of thiaminase-producing bacteria. Horses on rare occasions may also exhibit the deficiency after eating plants bearing thiaminase. In foxes, the disease was originally designated **Chastek paralysis; Wernicke encephalopathy** is applied to the human disease.

Signs. The signs of thiamine deficiency are essentially mediated by the nervous system. Opisthotonos, ascending paralysis, torticollis, and mydriasis are the principal features.

Lesions. The lesions in monogastric animals are usually limited to bilaterally symmetric zones of malacia involving various nuclei in the brain. Ruminants, on the other hand, usually manifest diffuse lesions in the cerebral cortex (polioencephalomalacia or cerebrocortical necrosis). The lesions are described more fully in Chap. 27.

Baggs, R.B., deLahunta, A., and Averill, D.R.: Thiamine deficiency encephalopathy in a specific-pathogen-free cat colony. Lab. Anim. Sci., *28*:323–326, 1978.

Draper, H.H., and Johnson, B.C.: Thiamine deficiency in the lamb and calf. J. Nutr., *43*:413–422, 1951.

Evans, W.C., et al.: Induction of thiamine deficiency in sheep, with lesions similar to those of cerebrocortical necrosis. J. Comp. Pathol., *85*:253–268, 1975.

Geraci, J.R.: Thiamine deficiency in seals and recommendations for its prevention. J. Am. Vet. Med. Assoc., *165*:801–803, 1974.

Jubb, K.U., Saunders, L.Z., and Coates, H.V.:

Thiamine deficiency encephalopathy in cats. J. Comp. Pathol., *66*:217–227, 1956.

Loew, F.M., et al.: Naturally-occurring and experimental thiamin deficiency in cats receiving commercial cat food. Can. Vet. J., *11*:109–113, 1970.

Loew, F.M., and Dunlop, R.H.: Induction of thiamine inadequacy and polioencephalomalacia in adult sheep with amprolium. Am. J. Vet. Res., *33*:2195–2205, 1972.

Markson, L.M., and Terlecki, S.: The aetiology of cerebrocortical necrosis. Br. Vet. J., *124*:309–315, 1968.

Markson, L.M., Edwin, E.E., Lewis, G., and Richardson, C.: The production of cerebrocortical necrosis in ruminant calves by the intraruminal administration of amprolium. Br. Vet. J., *130*: 9–16, 1974.

Pill, A.H.: Evidence of thiamine deficiency in calves affected with cerebrocortical necrosis. Vet. Rec., *81*:178–181, 1967.

Read, D.H., Jolly, R.D., and Alley, M.R.: Polioencephalomalacia of dogs with thiamine deficiency. Vet. Pathol., *14*:103–112, 1977.

Robertson, D.M., Wasan, S.M., and Skinner, D.B.: Ultrastructural feature of early brain stem lesions of thiamine-deficient rats. Am. J. Pathol., *52*:1081–1097, 1968.

Robertson, D.M., Manz, H.J., Haas, R.A., and Meyers, N.: Glucose uptake in the brainstem of thiamine-deficient rats. Am. J. Pathol., *79*:107–118, 1975.

Saunders, L.Z.: Thiamine deficiency encephalopathy in cats. *In* Comparative Neuropathology, edited by J. R. M. Innes and L. Z. Saunders. New York, Academic Press, 1962.

Shreeve, J.E., and Edwin, E.E.: Thiaminase-producing strains of *Clostridium sporogenes* associated with outbreaks of cerebrocortical necrosis. Vet. Rec., *94*:330, 1974.

Tellez, I., and Terry, R.D.: Fine structures of the early changes in the vestibular nuclei of the thiamine-deficient rat. Am. J. Pathol., *52*:777–794, 1968.

Blacktongue

Blacktongue, or canine pellagra, is a supposed entity characterized by severe cyanosis of the distal portion of the tongue which, in severe cases, makes it practically black. In milder forms, which include those usually produced experimentally, the tongue shows only superficial ulceration along its borders. Regularly, there are petechial or ecchymotic hemorrhages throughout the digestive canal, with patches of hemorrhagic enteritis or gastritis. The symptomatologic entity resulting includes precipitous anorexia, salivation, foul-smelling ulceration of the buccal mucosa, vomiting, and bloody diarrhea with resultant dehydration and emaciation. Death is usually stated to be preceded by fever, presumably from terminal bacterial infection.

Rather extensive experimental studies have seemed to show that this syndrome, like human pellagra, results from a diet consisting largely of Indian corn (maize) and foods made from it. Experimentally, the same syndrome has been produced by various diets lacking nicotinic acid and the amino acid, tryptophan, both of which are almost nonexistent in corn. The experimental disorder is considered to have been prevented by feeding yeast or meat, but in one experiment, cod-liver oil had to be given in addition. The interpretation is current that both canine and human pellagra result from a deficiency of nicotinic acid of the B complex coupled with a low level of tryptophan, but the possibility of an "antivitamin" or direct toxic action from corn has not been excluded.

The experimental disease is rarely observed under "field" conditions and it is likely that many early cases were actually due to leptospirosis. Canine pellagra should be kept in mind, however, as a disease that might appear spontaneously due to errors in preparing diets.

Chittenden, R.H., and Underhill, F.P.: The production in dogs of a pathological condition which closely resembles human pellagra. Am. J. Physiol., *44*:13–17, 1917.

Denton, J.: A study of the tissue changes in experimental blacktongue of dogs compared with similar changes in pellagra. Am. J. Pathol., *4*:341–347, 1928.

Dreizen, S., Levy, B.M., and Bernick, S.: Studies on the biology of the periodontium of marmosets. XIII. Histopathology of niacin deficiency stomatitis in the marmoset. J. Periodontol., *48*:452–455, 1977.

Goldberger, J., and Wheeler, G.A.: Experimental blacktongue of dogs and its relation to pellagra. Publ. Health Rep., *43*:172–177, 1928.

Gopalan, C., and Narasinga Rao, B.S.: Experimental niacin deficiency. Methods Achiev. Exp. Pathol., *6*:49–80, 1972.

Smith, D.T., Pearsons, E.L., and Harvey, H.L.: On the identity of the Goldberger and Underhill types of canine blacktongue. Secondary spirochaetal infection in each. J. Nutr., *14*:373–377, 1937.

Riboflavin (Vitamin B₂) Deficiency

Deficiency of this vitamin has been well-studied experimentally. Spontaneous deficiency under natural conditions is rarely reported in animals. The characteristic lesion is vascularization of the cornea (Fig. 28–2). This lesion may be encountered in animals maintained on experimental diets. Large doses of riboflavin have been shown to prevent initial attacks of equine periodic ophthalmia.

Heywood, R., and Partington, H.: Ocular lesions induced by vitamin B₂ deficiency. Vet. Rec., 88:251–252, 1971.

Jones, T.C., Roby, T.O., and Maurer, F.D.: The relation of riboflavin to equine periodic ophthalmia. Am. J. Vet. Res., 7:403–416, 1946.

Jones, T.C.: Riboflavin and the control of equine periodic ophthalmia. J. Am. Vet. Med. Assoc., 64:326–329, 1949.

Tandler, B., Erlandson, R.A., and Wynder, E.L.: Riboflavin and mouse hepatic cell structure and function. I. Ultrastructural alterations in simple deficiency. Am. J. Pathol., 52:69–95, 1968.

Pantothenic Acid Deficiency

This essential nutrient has been recognized as deficient in the diet of growing swine under field conditions. The deficiency usually appears when corn (maize) is a significant part of the diet. The clinical signs are gradual loss of flesh and dirty, scaly skin, fluid feces, followed by stiffness in the rear legs and apparent weakness in the loin muscles. The muscular weakness progresses and eventually the animals rest their weight on their hocks. Later the pigs assume a sitting position, with the hindlegs extended forward and to the side. The pigs eventually drag themselves about with their forelegs. Supplementation with pantothenic acid in the diet stops the appearance of new cases.

Experimental deficiency of pantothenic acid in swine results in mucous, hemorrhagic, and necrotizing colitis with consequent diarrhea. Necrosis of neurons in the dorsal spinal ganglia plus degeneration of myelin and axons in brachial and sciatic nerves result in an ataxic gait and terminal recumbency. Experimental deficiency can also be produced in dogs, monkeys, rats, chicks, and other animals. Naturally occurring deficiencies are rare because of the many sources of this vitamin.

Oakley, G.A.: Pantothenic acid deficiency in a commercial herd of pigs. Vet. Rec., 86:252–253, 1970.

Cobalamin (Vitamin B₁₂) Deficiency

This vitamin is deficient in man and monkeys under certain conditions in nature. The disease has been called "cage paralysis" in rhesus monkeys who manifest blindness and posterior paralysis under conditions of long-time cage confinement. Depressed levels of vitamin B_{12} in serum were first noted in affected monkeys by Krohn, Oxnard, and Chalmers (1963). The lesions in cage paralysis were first described by Rothman in 1906, and later compared to the human lesions of subacute combined degeneration by Scherer (1940). Agamanolis and associates (1976) have described the lesions in rhesus monkeys after maintenance on a diet deficient in vitamin B_{12} for as long as four years.

Lesions. The lesions may be described briefly as consisting of sharply delimited demyelinizing lesions in white matter in the optic nerve, optic tracts, spinal cord, and some other myelinated tracts. "Biochemical megaloblastosis" has been described, but anemia was not a feature in deficient rhesus monkeys.

Ruminant animals do not usually require a dietary source of vitamin B_{12} because it is synthesized by certain bacteria growing in the rumen. These bacteria require minute amounts of cobalt to thrive and produce vitamin B_{12}. Lack of cobalt in the diet leads to vitamin B_{12} deficiency. This is discussed further under cobalt.

Agamanolis, D.P., et al.: Neuropathology of experimental vitamin B₁₂ deficiency in monkeys. Neurology, 26:905–914, 1976.

Goodman, A., Harris, J.W., and Hines, J.D.: Biochemical megaloblastosis in B-12 deficient monkeys. Clin. Res., 26:347A, 1978.

Hogan, K.G., Lorentz, P.P., and Gibb, F.M.: The diagnosis and treatment of vitamin B_{12} deficiency in young lambs. NZ Vet. J., *21*:234–237, 1973.

Kark, J.A., et al.: Nutritional vitamin B_{12} deficiency in rhesus monkeys. Am. J. Clin. Nutr., *27*:470–478, 1974.

Krohn, P.L., Oxnard, C.E., and Chalmers, J.N.M.: Vitamin B_{12} in the serum of the rhesus monkey. Nature, *197*:186, 1963.

Marston, H.R.: The requirements of sheep for cobalt or for vitamin B_{12}. Br. J. Nutr., *24*:615–633, 1970.

Oxnard, C.E.: Some variations in the amount of vitamin B_{12} in the serum of the rhesus monkey. Nature (Lond.), *201*:1188–1191, 1964.

Oxnard, C.E., and Smith, W.T.: Neurological degeneration and reduced serum vitamin B_{12} levels in captive monkeys. Nature, *210*:507–509, 1966.

Rothman, M.: Über eine tabes-artige Erkrankung beim Affen. Monatschr Psychiat. Neurol., *20*:204–221, 1906.

Scherer, H.J.: Degeneration of the papillomacular bundles in apes and its significance in human neuropathology. J. Neurol. Neurosurg. Psychiatry, *3*:37–48, 1940.

Van Bogaert, L.V., and Innes, J.R.M.: Neurologic diseases of apes and monkeys. *In* Comparative Neuropathology, edited by J. R. M. Innes and L. Z. Saunders. New York, Academic Press, 1962, pp. 55–139.

Willigan, D.A., Cronkite, E.P., Meyer, L.M., and Noto, S.L.: Biliary excretion of Co^{60} labeled vitamin B_{12} in dogs. Soc. Exp. Biol. Med., *99*:81–84, 1958.

Folic Acid Deficiency

Several metabolic processes utilize folic acid as a coenzyme. The purine and pyrimidine bases required for DNA and RNA synthesis are included in these metabolic pathways. Thus, this vitamin is necessary for all cell proliferation; and the hematopoietic system is particularly sensitive. Signs of folic acid deficiency in man and other animals therefore include leukopenia, macrocytic anemia, and megaloblastic cytologic changes in the bone marrow. The cat and cebus monkey are susceptible to experimental deprivation. Anemia due to folic acid deficiency is confirmed by adding folic acid to the diet, resulting in correction of the anemia.

Rasmussen, K.M., Hayes, K.C., and Thenen, S.W.: Folic acid deficiency in cebus monkey. Fed. Proc., *36*:1121, 1977.

Thenen, S.W., and Rasmussen, K.M.: Megaloblastic erythropoiesis and tissue depletion of folic acid in the cat. Am. J. Vet. Res., *39*:1205–1207, 1978.

Pyridoxine (Vitamin B_6) Deficiency

This deficiency has been produced experimentally in dogs, pigs, monkeys, and rodents. It is manifest by cutaneous hyperkeratosis and acanthosis, anemia, and signs of nervous disturbances. To quote our late colleague, Dr. Hilton A. Smith: "Since its production involves removal of the natural ingredients of foods by alcoholic extraction, the advent of this deficiency among clinical diseases does not appear imminent!"

HYPOVITAMINOSIS C

Scurvy or **scorbutus** in man was known in the eighteenth century to be prevented by eating fresh fruit or green vegetables. Lime juice was required in the daily ration of sailors on British ships-of-war, hence their nickname of "Limeys." It is now known that most animals synthesize adequate amounts of vitamin C (ascorbic acid). A few species, including man, other primates, and flying mammals (bats), lack an enzyme, L-gulonolactone oxidase, and depend upon a dietary source of this essential vitamin. Also, insects, invertebrates, and fish generally do not synthesize vitamin C.

Ascorbic acid is synthesized in the liver of most mammals and in the kidney of reptiles and the amphibians. Most birds produce the vitamin in the liver, but in a few the kidney serves this function.

Vitamin C is found in all tissues of the mammalian body and is involved in many metabolic processes. Some of the important functions involve the production of collagen, wound healing, integrity of endothelial cells, and detoxification of histamine.

Signs. The signs of scurvy include gingivitis and bleeding gums, failure of wounds to heal, inappetence, dermatitis, loss of weight, and sudden death. Guinea

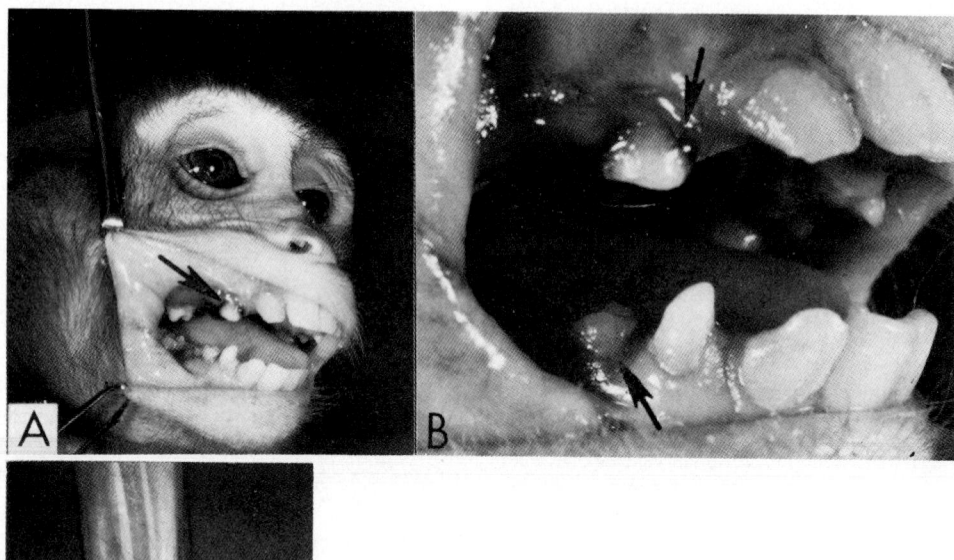

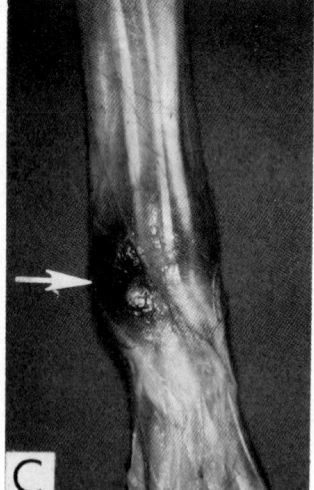

Fig. 17–2. Scurvy, rhesus monkey *(Macaca mulatta)*. *A* and *B*, Loosening of teeth and gingival hemorrhage (arrows). *C*, Subperiosteal hemorrhage at distal tibia (arrow). (Courtesy of New England Regional Primate Research Center, Harvard Medical School.)

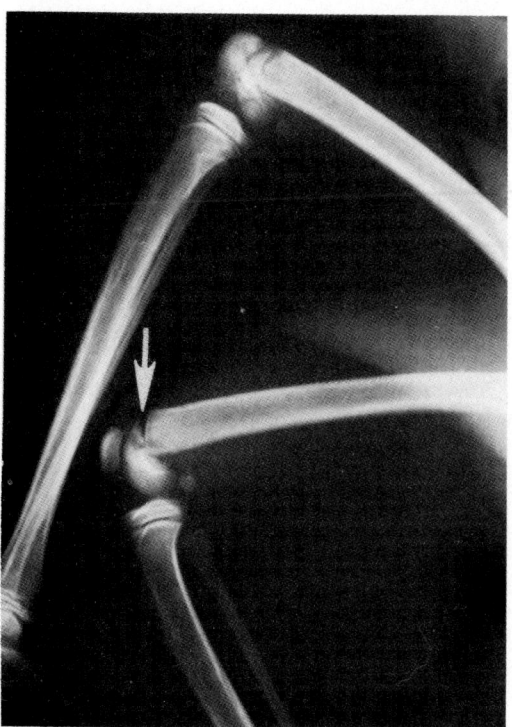

Fig. 17–3. Scurvy, rhesus monkey (*Macaca mulatta*). Epiphyseal fracture (arrow) of the distal femur. (Courtesy of New England Regional Primate Research Center, Harvard Medical School.)

pigs succumb within three to four weeks after ascorbic acid is withdrawn from their diet; longer intervals usually are required in Old and New World monkeys and man.

Lesions. The lesions consist chiefly of subperiosteal hemorrhages, abnormal ossification of long bones, and gingivitis. The fundamental disturbance is the inability of fibroblasts to form collagen or osteoid. This accounts for the failure of wounds to heal and for the pathologic changes in bones. The epiphysis is usually widened, due to a zone of calcified but unossified cartilage at the site of endochondral bone formation. The cartilaginous side of the epiphyseal junction is convex and bulges into the disordered osseous side (Fig. 17–4B). Focal necroses in the myocardium sometimes occur, accounting for sudden death.

Diagnosis. The diagnosis is arrived at from the clinical signs and lesions, and may be confirmed in living animals by the prompt response to the addition of ascorbic acid to the diet.

Baker, E.M., et al.: Metabolism of ascorbic acid and ascorbic-2-sulfate in man and subhuman primate. Ann. NY Acad. Sci., *258*:72–80, 1975.

Chatterjee, I.B., Majumder, A.K., Nandi, B.K., and Subramanian, N.: Synthesis and some major functions of vitamin C in animals. Ann. NY Acad. Sci., *258*:24–47, 1975.

deKlerk, W.A., et al.: Vitamin C requirements of the vervet monkey (*Cercopithecus aethiops*) under experimental conditions. S. Afr. Med. J., *47*: 705–708, 1973.

Demaray, S.Y., Altman, N.H., and Ferrell, T.L.: Suspected ascorbic acid deficiency in a colony of squirrel monkeys (*Saimiri sciureus*). Lab Anim. Sci., *28*:457–460, 1978.

DiFilippo, N.M., and Blumenthal, H.J.: Cholelithiasis in the scorbutic guinea pig. J. Am. Osteopath. Assoc., *72*:284–287, 1972.

Hsu, C.-K.: Vitamin C and immune response in rhesus monkeys. Fed. Proc., *36*:1177, 1977.

Jukes, T.H.: Further comments on the ascorbic acid requirement. Proc. Natl. Acad. Sci. USA, *72*:4151–4152, 1975.

Kotze, J.P.: The effects of vitamin C on lipid metabolism. S. Afr. Med. J., *49*:1651–1654, 1975.

Lehner, N.D.M., Bullock, B.C., and Clarkson, T.B.: Ascorbic acid deficiency in the squirrel monkey. Proc. Soc. Exp. Biol. Med., *128*:512–514, 1968.

MacKenzie, I.C., Kolar, G., Kashani, H., and Dahlberg, S.: Periodontal changes in ascorbic acid deficient rhesus monkeys. J. Dent. Res., *56*:B111, 1977.

Sulkin, N.M., and Sulkin, D.F.: Tissue changes induced by marginal vitamin C deficiency. Ann. NY Acad. Sci., *258*:317–328, 1975.

HYPOVITAMINOSIS D

Vitamin D is formed from steroid precursors or provitamins, of which two have been found in nature; ergosterol (provitamin D_2) is found in plants, and 7-dehydrocholesterol (provitamin D_3) is found in animal tissues. To be effective, these steroids, either in the skin of the animal or its food, must be exposed to the radiant action of violet and ultraviolet light, ordinarily of sunlight, which converts ergosterol to vitamin D_2 (ergocalciferol), and 7-dehydrocholesterol, to vitamin D_3 (cholecalciferol). In case the vitamin is not available in the food, a comparatively short exposure

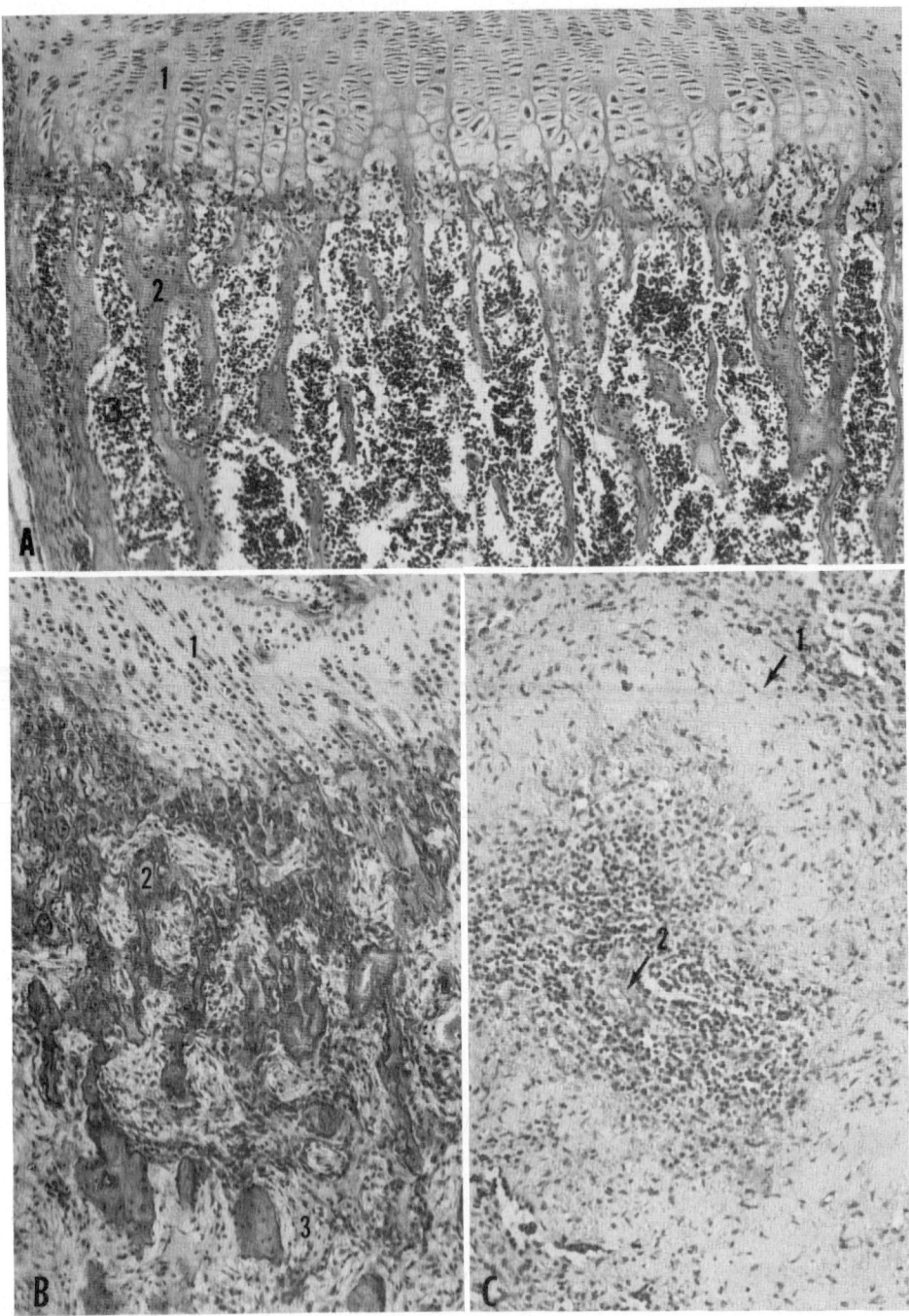

Fig. 17–4. Scurvy in the guinea pig. *A*, Femur of normal guinea pig (× 90). Epiphyseal cartilage *(1)*, new-formed bone *(2)*, and hematopoietic marrow *(3)*. *B*, Femur of scorbutic guinea pig (× 100). Distorted epiphyseal cartilage *(1)*, disrupted spicules of new bone *(2)*, and fibrous marrow *(3)*. *C*, Amyloidosis of spleen of scorbutic guinea pig (× 150). Amyloid *(1)* surrounds and displaces lymphocytes of the splenic corpuscle. Central artery *(2)*. (Courtesy of Armed Forces Institute of Pathology.) Contributor: Army Medical Nutrition Laboratory.

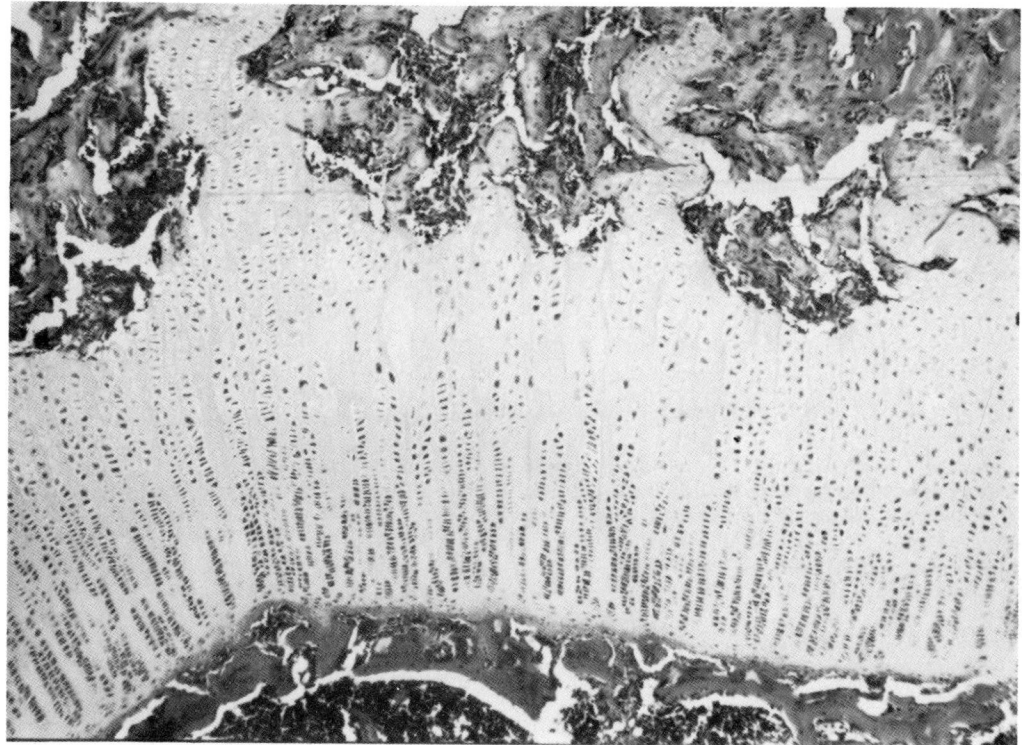

Fig. 17–5. Rickets. The cartilaginous growth plate is disorganized and extends irregularly into the metaphysis. The cartilage does not mineralize or die. There is no defect in osteoid formation.

to direct sunlight (two minutes per day for chickens in midsummer) is adequate for normal health.

The principal role of vitamin D is to maintain serum calcium at optimal levels for its numerous physiologic functions. Two vitamin-D-dependent processes serve to elevate serum calcium: (1) calcium transport across the intestine, and (2) mobilization of calcium from bone. The latter function depends upon parathyroid hormone. Great progress has recently been made which explains in part how vitamin D mediates these functions. It is now known that following ingestion or formation in the skin, vitamin D is transported to the liver by means of an α_2-globulin, where it is converted to 25-hydroxycholecalciferol (25-HCC). The 25-HCC is then carried by an $\alpha_2$globulin to the kidney where it is oxygenated. The resultant product, 1,25-

dihydroxycholecalciferol, is believed to be the principal calcium-mobilizing hormone. This hormone circulates, and at the level of bone and intestine, acts on DNA to make messenger RNA, which is coded for the production of specific proteins or enzymes responsible for calcium transport. The hormone (1,25 dihydroxycholecalciferol) has now been synthesized in an active form (Holick et al., 1975). The recent demonstration of the role played by the kidney in producing the active vitamin D metabolite may explain, in part, certain metabolic bone diseases associated with chronic renal failure.

Young chickens provide a means for precise studies of this deficiency; they are hatched with enough vitamin for the first two weeks of life; if more is not received from the food, chicks kept in darkness die between the eighteenth and twenty-first days of life (so-called leg-weakness). Although other metabolic disorders may also cause it, the disease resulting from deficiency of vitamin D is **rickets,** which will be described with the other diseases of bone. There is also retarded and abnormal dentition.

Briggs, M.H., and Briggs, M.: Vitamin D hormones: Part I. Med. J. Aust., 1:838–843, 1974.

DeLuca, H.F.: The kidney as an endocrine organ for the production of 1,25-dihydroxyvitamin D_3, a calcium-mobilizing hormone. N. Engl. J. Med., 289:359–365, 1973.

————: The kidney as an endocrine organ involved in the function of vitamin D. Am. J. Med., 58:39–47, 1975.

Fraser, D.R., and Kodicek, E.: Unique biosynthesis by kidney of a biologically active vitamin D metabolite. Nature, 228:764–766, 1970.

Holick, M.F., et al.: Synthesis of (6-^{3}H)-1 α-hydroxyvitamin D_3 and its metabolism in vivo to (^{3}H)-1α,25-dihydroxyvitamin D_3. Science, 190:576–578, 1975.

Lam, H.-Y.P., Schnoes, H.K., and DeLuca, H.F.: 1α-Hydroxyvitamin D_2: A potent synthetic analog of vitamin D_2. Science, 186:1038–1040, 1974.

Lee, S.W., Russell, J., and Avioli, L.V.: 25-Hydroxy-cholecalciferol to 1,25-dihydroxycholecalciferol: conversion impaired by systemic metabolic acidosis. Science, 195:994–996, 1977.

Norman, A.W.: Evidence for a new kidney-produced hormone, 1,25-dihydroxycholecalciferol, the proposed biologically active form of vitamin D. Am. J. Clin. Nutr., 24:1346–1351, 1971.

Norman, A.W., Mitra, M.N., Okamura, W.H., and Wing, R.M.: Vitamin D: 3-deoxy-1α-hydroxyvitamin D_3, biologically active analog of 1α, 25-dihydroxyvitamin D_3. Science, 188:1013–1015, 1975.

Wong, G.L., Luben, R.A., and Cohn, D.V.: 1,25-Dihydroxycholecalciferol and parathormone: effects on isolated osteoclast-like and osteoblast-like cells. Science, 197:663–665, 1977.

HYPOVITAMINOSIS E

Vitamin E consists chemically of an alcohol, or a group of closely related alcohols, named tocopherols (Gr. *tokus* = childbirth; *phero* = to carry). Four naturally occurring tocopherols have been discovered, alpha-, beta-, delta-, and eta-tocopherol. Alpha-tocopherol is the most active biologically. Alpha-tocopherol occurs especially in the germs of seeds and extracts thereof (wheat-germ oil).

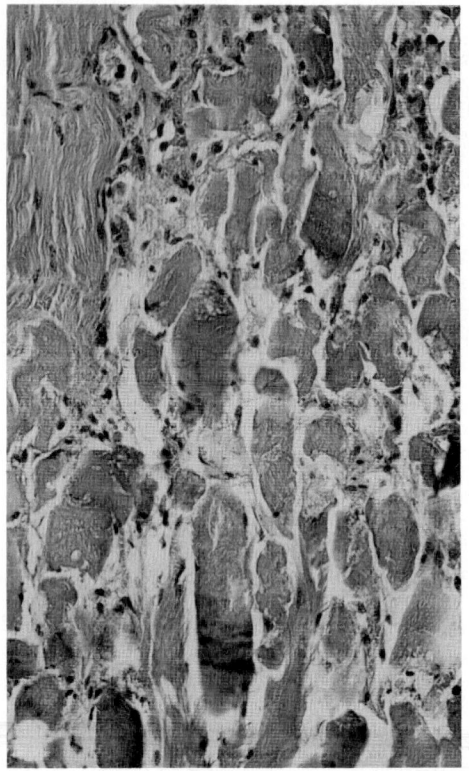

Fig. 17–6. Nutritional myopathy, white-muscle disease, skeletal muscle of a cow ($\times$ 195). Fragmentation of muscle fibers with swelling and early calcification. (Courtesy of Armed Forces Institute of Pathology.) Contributor: Dr. J. F. Ryff.

Vitamin E deficiency has been held responsible for a variety of pathologic processes in domestic animals. Based on experimentally induced deficiency and clinical observations, the following conditions are believed to result:

Rats: Necrosis of the germinal cells of the seminiferous tubules and aspermatogenesis; necrosis of skeletal and cardiac muscle; retarded development, death, and resorption of embryos; axonal degeneration in the central nervous system; hepatic necrosis; deposition of ceroid in adipose tissue.

Mice: Necrosis of skeletal and cardiac muscle; hepatic necrosis; renal necrosis.

Rabbits: Necrosis of skeletal muscle; steatitis (yellow fat disease).

Calves and Lambs: Necrosis of skeletal and cardiac muscle (white muscle disease).

Pigs: Necrosis of skeletal and cardiac muscle (**Herztod**); hepatic necrosis (**hepatosis dietetica**);

steatitis (yellow fat disease); exudative diathesis; anemia.

Cats: Steatitis (yellow fat disease).

Dogs: Ceroid deposition in smooth muscle; necrosis of skeletal muscle; testicular degeneration; axonal degeneration in the central nervous system.

Monkeys: Necrosis of skeletal muscle; anemia.

Chicks: Exudative diathesis; necrosis of skeletal, cardiac, and gizzard muscle; encephalomalacia; decreased egg production, fertility and hatchability.

Mink: Necrosis of skeletal muscle; steatitis (yellow fat disease).

Guinea pig: Necrosis of skeletal muscle.

The exact function of vitamin E at the molecular level is not understood, a fact which makes it exceedingly difficult to explain the diverse group of lesions attributed to its deficiency. A complex physiologic link between selenium, sulfur-containing amino acids, and vitamin E has been demonstrated. It appears that certain of the lesions listed above are the result of vitamin E deficiency, others from selenium deficiency, and a third group due to a combined deficiency. Selenium has reportedly been used successfully to treat muscular dystrophy of sheep, calves, and chicks, hepatosis dietetica in pigs and exudative diathesis of poultry.

Vitamin E is an integral part of cell membrane structure and is a lipid-soluble antioxidant. It protects the erythrocyte plasma membrane from peroxidative action, which leads to hemolysis. Selenium is an essential component of the enzyme glutathione peroxidase, which is important in destroying hydrogen peroxide and organic hydroperoxides. This enzyme, therefore, protects against damage to membranes and other cell structures by oxidants. This prevention of oxidant damage forms the basis for a theory to account for the interaction between vitamin E, selenium, unsaturated lipids, sulfur-containing amino acids, and toxicants such as silver and tri-o-cresyl phosphate (Hoekstra, 1975).

Deficiencies of vitamin E and selenium have been associated with **nutritional myopathy** or **white muscle disease** in several species. This condition has also been referred to as muscular dystrophy, an inappropriate term because it is a degenerative process, not a disturbance of growth. In suckling lambs, this entity has been referred to as **stiff-lamb disease**, a term indicating one of the conspicuous signs. The signs are similar to those seen in polyarthritis resulting from low grade pyosepticemia neonatorium. The affected muscles of horses that succumb to azoturia and those of swine poisoned by gossypol have similar gross and microscopic appearances. It is clear that all cases of "white muscle disease" are not due to the same cause.

Acute myodegeneration in swine, which has been called **Herztod,** has also been attributed to vitamin E deficiency. In this condition there is acute necrosis of skeletal and cardiac muscle, which results in sudden death. Acute hepatic necrosis or **hepatosis dietetica** (dietary hepatic necrosis) of swine has been more clearly related to vitamin E deficiency, although selenium and sulfur-containing amino acids afford protection. The lesions of the liver are characterized by massive necrosis of entire lobules. Dietary hepatic necrosis is frequently associated with myodegeneration, generalized edema (exudative diathesis), and yellow pigmentation of fat.

The yellow pigment occurs in what is known as **yellow fat disease or steatitis.** The disorder has been encountered in mink and swine that were fed considerable amounts of fish meal, fish offal, or other products of like origin. After a month, more or less, on such a diet, the animals come to have a body fat that is strangely yellowish or brownish in color, although but little changed in other respects. Microscopic examination of such fat, subcutaneous or visceral, reveals droplets or amorphous bodies of a brown or yellow substance at the interstices of the adipose cells. The substance appears to be oily or waxy in nature and, for this reason, has received the name of **ceroid.** It is insoluble

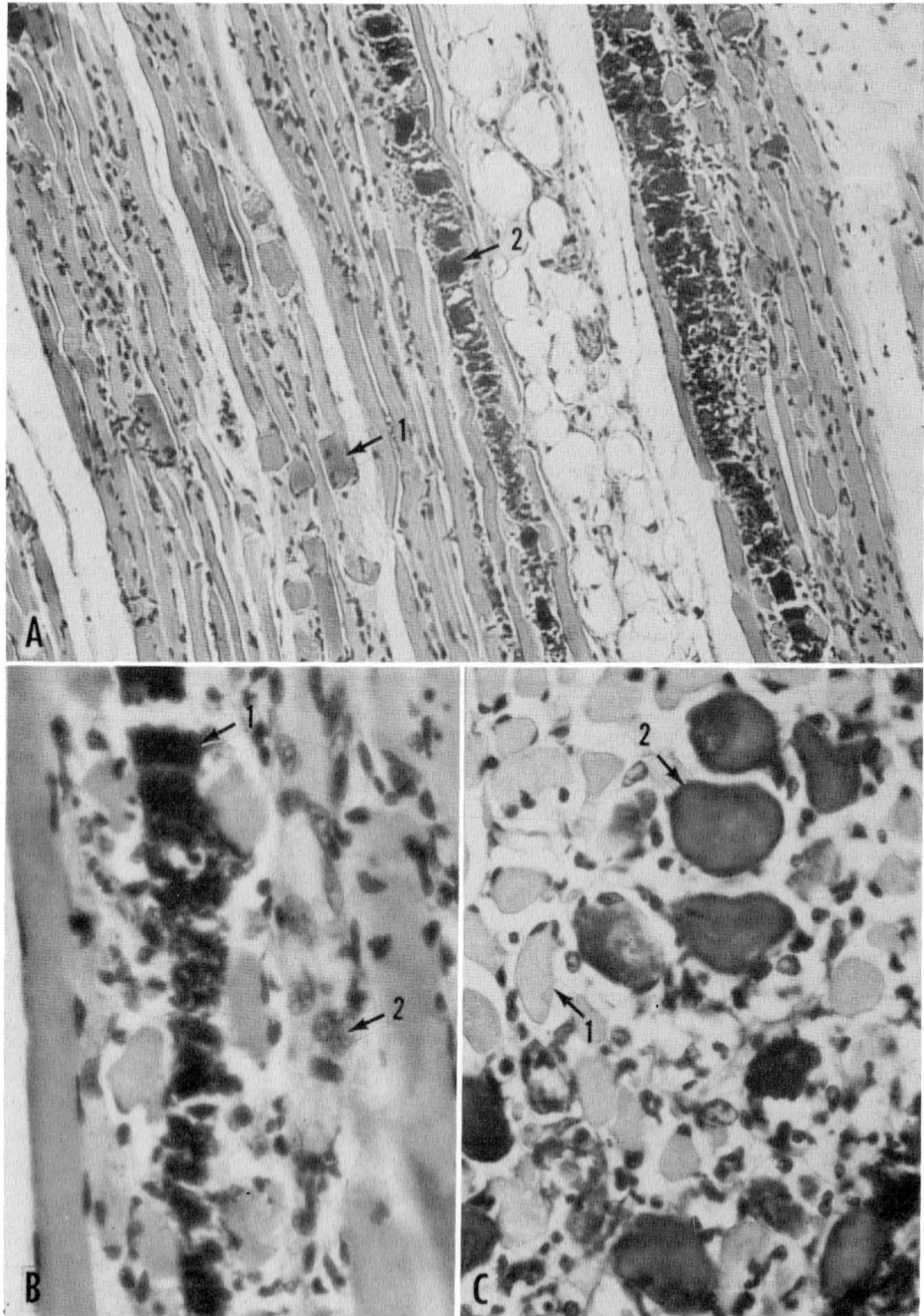

Fig. 17–7. Nutritional myopathy, white-muscle disease, in the tongue of a newborn foal. *A,* Low power (× 150) to show fragmentation of muscle bundles *(1)* and calcification *(2)*. *B,* Longitudinal section (× 500) of muscle bundles. Calcification within muscle bundles *(1)*, proliferation of sarcolemmal nuclei *(2)*. *C,* Cross section of mucle fibers (× 500). Note normal *(1)* and calcified *(2)* muscle bundles. (Courtesy of Armed Forces Institute of Pathology.) Contributor: Dr. W. O. Reed.

in fat solvents, does not respond to stains for iron, but does take and retain the red fuchsin when the usual stain for acid-fast bacteria is applied. With hematoxylin and eosin or similar tissue stains, the substance is relatively basophilic. The amount at any one interstice may be so large as to approach the volume of an adipose cell, but this material is outside those cells. Ceroid may, however, be within phagocytic cells, and these macrophages occasionally develop to form foreign body giant cells. The ceroid is also found in the Kupffer cells of the liver, and sometimes small particles of it can be stained in the cytoplasm of the hepatic epithelial cells themselves. Phagocytes containing it occasionally migrate to the regional lymph nodes and even to the spleen. In the areas of adipose tissue it excites a slight infiltration of inflammatory leukocytes.

While the fishy odor that sometimes causes condemnation of meat from swine fed on fish meal may not be ameliorated, the formation of ceroid and the yellow discoloration are inhibited and usually prevented by increased amounts of alpha-tocopherol in the diet. Since unsaturated fatty acids have notable oxidizing properties through their attraction for H-ions, and since alpha-tocopherol appears to owe its effect chiefly to its antioxidant powers, it is believed that the ceroid is a byproduct of oxidative processes that are inhibited by a larger supply of the vitamin. Conversely, it may conceivably be formed as a degradation product in the interaction of the tocopherol and the oxidant fatty acids.

A similar or identical pigment has occurred in experimental animals fed large amounts of cod-liver oil for its content of vitamin D. Apparently the oily vehicle of vitamin D exerted a similar antagonistic effect on the limited amount of vitamin E available, although signs of deficiency did not extend beyond the formation of ceroid pigment.

Steatitis in cats occurs after some weeks on certain fish diets, arising suddenly with fever and general malaise. There is severe pain when the cutaneous region is disturbed either by manipulation or by the patient's own movements, and palpation reveals an abnormal denseness and lumpiness of the subcutaneous fat. These effects, together with a pronounced neutrophilia, a marked "shift to the left," and often moderate eosinophilia, tend to persist for many days and may terminate fatally unless relieved by suitable treatment. By biopsy or necropsy it is seen that the fat, in addition to being markedly discolored by the yellow or brown pigment, is heavily infiltrated with neutrophils accompanied by a few leukocytes of other kinds and perhaps by Langhans giant cells. Typical deposits of acid-fast ceroid are plentiful, and it has been suggested that, as irritant foreign bodies, they are the direct cause of the inflammatory reaction (Fig. 17–8).

An apparently comparable steatitis, cause unknown, has been reported in the muscles of foals in New Zealand. Rarely similar fatty deposits have been found to be fluorescent, and accompanied by photosensitizational dermatitis.

Although yellow fat disease has not been reported in dogs, a histologically and histochemically identical pigment has been described in smooth muscle cells, particularly of the small intestine and spleen, often imparting a grossly visible brown color to the small intestine. The condition has been called "brown dog gut" and the pigment, "leiomyometoplasts." However, experimental evidence indicates that the pigment is a lipofuscin similar, if not identical to, ceroid, and can be induced by vitamin E deficiency.

Axonal degeneration, principally in the brain stem, which follows vitamin E deficiency in rats and dogs, is not infrequently encountered in clinically normal dogs, suggesting that vitamin E deficiency may be more frequent in this species than usually suspected. The degenerating axons form eosinophilic spherical bodies up to 150 μ in diameter.

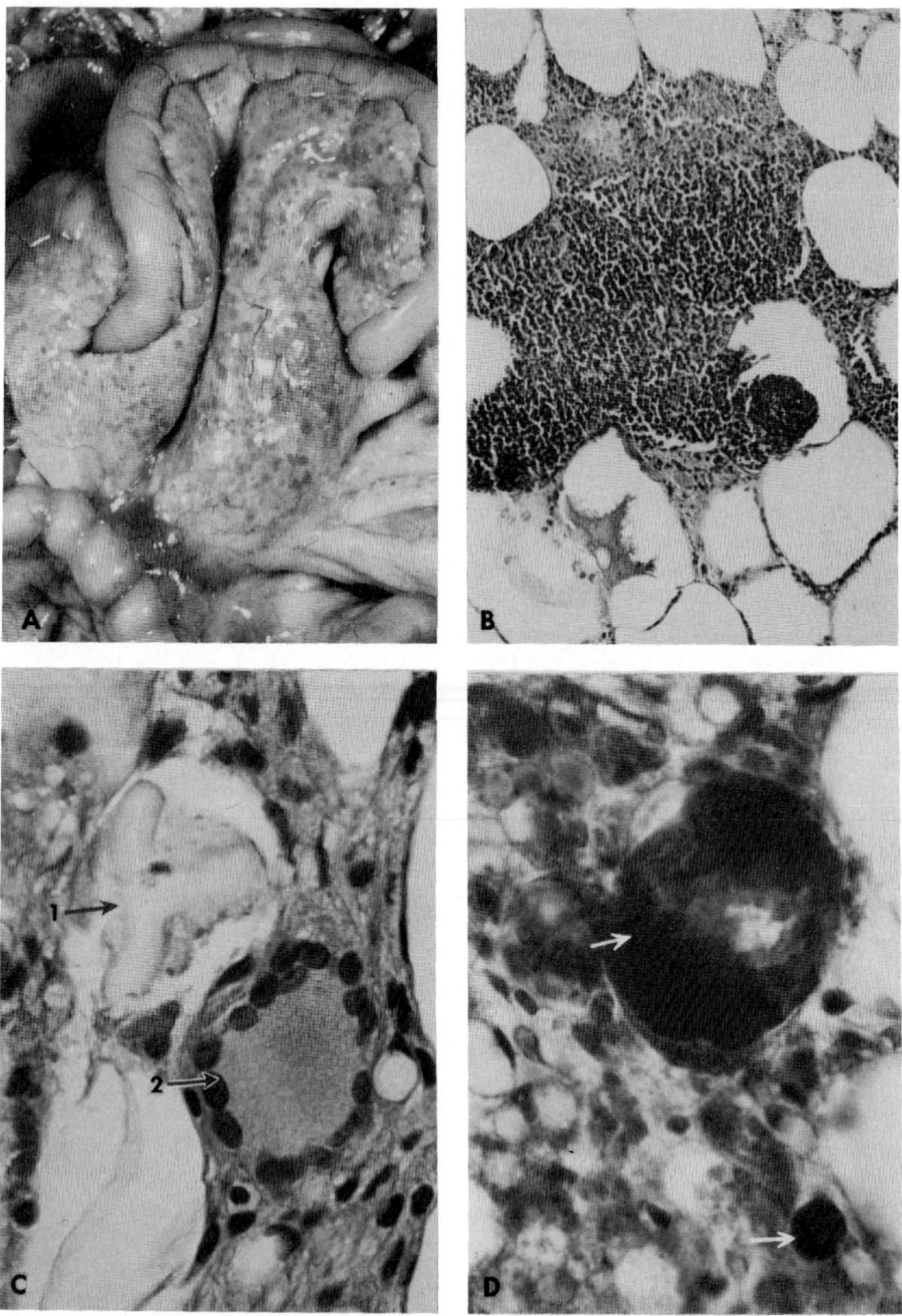

Fig. 17–8. Steatitis in the cat. *A,* Mesenteric fat of a 1½-year-old castrated male cat. The dark spots were bright yellow color, the rest of the abundant mesenteric fat was yellowish tan. *B,* Neutrophils in adipose tissue of a young obese cat which exhibited fever and severe neutrophilic leukocytosis. (H & E, × 110.) *C,* Adipose tissue of a cat in a late stage of the disease with altered fat *(1)* and Langhans' type giant cell *(2).* (H & E, × 540.) *D,* A section of adipose tissue from the same cat as C, with globules of acid-fast ceroid pigment (arrows). (Ziehl-Neelsen's Acid Fast Stain, × 540.) (Courtesy of Angell Memorial Hospital and *Journal of the American Veterinary Medical Association.*)

Ausman, L.M., and Hayes, K.C.: Vitamin E deficiency anemia in Old and New World monkeys. J. Clin. Nutr., 27:1141–1151, 1974.

Baustad, B., and Nafstad, I.: Haematological response to vitamin E in piglets. Br. J. Nutr., 28:183–190, 1972.

Bieri, J.G., and Poukka Evarts, R.H.: Vitamin E nutrition in the rhesus monkey. Proc. Soc. Exp. Biol. Med., 140:1162–1165, 1972.

Cheville, N.F.: The pathology of vitamin E deficiency in the chick. Pathol. Vet., 3:208–225, 1966.

Danse, L.H.J.C., and Steenbergen-Botterweg, W.A.: Enzyme histochemical studies of adipose tissue in porcine yellow fat disease. Vet. Pathol., 11:465–476, 1974.

Danse, L.H.J.C., and Verschuren, P.M.: Fish oil-induced yellow fat disease in rats. I. Histological changes. Vet. Pathol., 15:114–124, 1978.

Danse, L.H.J.C., and Steenbergen-Botterweg, W.A.: Fish-oil-induced yellow fat disease in rats. II. Enzyme histochemistry of adipose tissue. Vet. Pathol., 15:125–132, 1978.

Danse, L.H.J.C., and Verschuren, P.M.: Fish oil-induced yellow fat disease in rats. III. Lipolysis in affected adipose tissue. Vet. Pathol., 15:544–548, 1978.

Davis, C.L., and Gorham, J.R.: The pathology of experimental and natural cases of "yellow fat" disease in swine. Am. J. Vet. Res., 15:55–59, 1954.

Dodd, D.C., et al.: Muscle degeneration and yellow-fat disease in foals. NZ Vet. J., 8:45–50, 1960.

Droneman, J., and Wensvoort, P.: Muscular dystrophy and yellow fat disease in Shetland pony foals. Neth. J. Vet. Sci., 1:42–48, 1968.

Endicott, K.M.: Similarity of the acid-fast pigment ceroid and oxidized unsaturated fat. Arch. Pathol., 37:49–53, 1944.

Ewan, R.C., Wastell, M.E., Bicknell, E.J., and Speer, V.C.: Performance and deficiency symptoms of young pigs fed diets low in vitamin E and selenium. J. Anim. Sci., 29:912–915, 1969.

Ewan, R.C., and Wastell, M.E.: Effect of vitamin E and selenium on blood composition of the young pig. J. Anim. Sci., 31:343–350, 1970.

Fitch, C.D.: The hematopoietic system in vitamin E-deficient animals. Ann. NY Acad. Sci., 203:172–176, 1972.

Gershoff, S.N., and Norkin, S.A.: Vitamin E deficiency in cats. J. Nutr., 77:303–308, 1962.

Gorham, J.R., Boe, N., and Baker, G.A.: Experimental "yellow-fat" disease in pigs. Cornell Vet., 41:332–338, 1951.

Hayes, K.C., Nielsen, S.W., and Rousseau, J.E., Jr.: Vitamin E deficiency and fat stress in the dog. J. Nutr., 99:196–209, 1969.

Hayes, K.C., Rousseau, J.E., Jr., and Hegsted, D.M.: Plasma tocopherol concentrations and vitamin E deficiency in dogs. J. Am. Vet. Med. Assoc., 157:64–71, 1970.

Hayes, K.C.: Animal model of human disease: hemolytic anemia of premature infants associated with vitamin E deficiency. Am. J. Pathol., 77:123–126, 1974.

———: Pathophysiology of vitamin E deficiency in monkeys. Am. J. Clin. Nutr., 27:1130–1140, 1974.

———: Retinal degeneration in monkeys induced by deficiencies of vitamin E or A. Invest. Ophthalmol., 13:499–510, 1974.

Hidiroglou, M., Jenkins, K.J., Lessard, J.R., and Carson, R.B.: Metabolism of vitamin E in sheep. Br. J. Nutr., 24:917–928, 1970.

Hoekstra, W.G.: Biochemical function of selenium and its relation to vitamin E. Fed. Proc., 34:2083–2089, 1975.

Jones, D., Howard, A.N., and Gresham, G.A.: Aetiology of "yellow fat" disease (pansteatitis) in the wild rabbit. J. Comp. Pathol., 79:329–334, 1969.

Leach, R.M., Jr.: Biochemical function of selenium and its inter-relationships with other trace elements and vitamin E. Fed. Proc., 34:2082, 1975.

Lohr, J.E., and Mclaren, R.D.: Yellow fat disease (pansteatitis) in wild hares in New Zealand. NZ Vet. J., 19:266–269, 1971.

Lynch, R.E., Hammar, S.P., Lee, G.R., and Cartwright, G.E.: The anemia of vitamin E deficiency in swine: an experimental model of the human congenital dyserythropoietic anemias. Am. J. Hematol., 2:145–158, 1977.

Machlin, L.J., Meisky, K.A., and Gordon, R.S.: Production of encephalomalacia in chickens fed aerated heated fats. Fed. Proc., 18:535, 1959.

Michel, R.L., Whitehair, C.K., and Keahey, K.K.: Dietary hepatic necrosis associated with selenium-vitamin E deficiency in swine. J. Am. Vet. Med. Assoc., 155:50–59, 1969.

Moustgaard, J., and Hyldgaard-Jensen, J. (eds.): Cellular membranes in vitamin E-deficiency: an ultrastructural and biochemical study of isolated outer and inner mitochondrial membranes. Acta Agriculturae Scand. (Suppl.), 19:192–203, 1973.

Munson, T.O., et al.: Steatitis ("yellow fat") in cats fed canned red tuna. J. Am. Vet. Med. Assoc., 133:563–568, 1958.

Nafstad, I., and Nafstad, H.J.: An electron microscopic study of blood and bone marrow in vitamin E-deficient pigs. Pathol. Vet., 5:520–537, 1968.

Nafstad, I.: Studies of hematology and bone marrow morphology in vitamin E-deficient pigs. Pathol. Vet., 2:277–287, 1965.

Nafstad, I., and Tollersrud, S.: The vitamin E-deficiency syndrome in pigs. I. Pathological changes. Acta Vet. Scand., 11:452–480, 1970.

Nafstad, I.: The vitamin E-deficiency syndrome in pigs. III. Light and electron microscopic studies on myocardial vascular injury. Vet. Pathol., 8:239–255, 1971.

Nair, P.P., and Kayden, H.J. (eds.): Vitamin E and its role in cellular metabolism. Ann. NY Acad. Sci., 203:1–247, 1972.

Newberne, P.M., and Hare, W.V.: Axon dystrophy in clinically normal dogs. Am. J. Vet. Res., 23:403–411, 1962.

Platt, H., and Whitwell, K.E.: Clinical and pathological observations on generalized steatitis in foals. J. Comp. Pathol., 81:499–506, 1971.

Raychaudhuri, C., and Desai, I.D.: Ceroid pigment formation and irreversible sterility in vitamin E deficiency. Science, 173:1028–1029, 1971.

Ringler, D.H., and Abrams, G.D.: Nutritional muscular dystrophy and neonatal mortality in a rabbit breeding colony. J. Am. Vet. Med. Assoc., 157:1928–1934, 1970.

Ringler, D.H., and Abrams, G.D.: Laboratory diagnosis of vitamin E deficiency in rabbits fed a faulty commercial ration. Lab. Anim. Sci., 21:383–388, 1971.

Ruth, G.R., and Van Vleet, J.R.: Experimentally induced selenium-vitamin E deficiency in growing swine: selective destruction of type I skeletal muscle fibers. Am. J. Vet. Res., 35:237–244, 1974.

Sharp, B.A., Young, L.G., and van Dreumel, A.A.: Dietary induction of mulberry heart disease and hepatosis dietetical in pigs. 1. Nutritional aspects. Can. J. Comp. Med., 36:371–376, 1972.

Stowe, H.D., and Whitehair, C.K.: Gross and microscopic pathology of tocopherol-deficient mink. J. Nutr., 81:287–300, 1963.

Sweeny, P.R., and Brown, R.G.: Ultrastructural changes in muscular dystrophy. I. Cardiac tissue of piglets deprived of vitamin E and selenium. Am. J. Pathol., 68:479–492, 1972.

Sweeny, P.R., et al.: Ultrastructure of muscular dystrophy. II. A comparative study in lambs and chickens. Am. J. Pathol., 68:493–510, 1972.

Trapp, A.L., Keahey, K.K., Whitenack, D.L., and Whitehair, C.K.: Vitamin E-selenium deficiency in swine: differential diagnosis and nature of field problem. J. Am. Vet. Med. Assoc., 157:289–300, 1970.

Van Vleet, J.F., Hall, B.V., and Simon, J.: Vitamin E deficiency: a sequential study by means of light and electron microscopy of the alterations occurring in regeneration of skeletal muscle of affected weanling rabbits. Am. J. Pathol., 51:815–830, 1967.

Van Vleet, J.F., Meyer, K.B., and Olander, H.J.: Control of selenium-vitamin E deficiency in growing swine by parenteral administration of selenium-vitamin E preparations to baby pigs or to pregnant sows and their baby pigs. J. Am. Vet. Med. Assoc., 163:452–456, 1973.

Van Vleet, J.F.: Experimentally induced vitamin E-selenium deficiency in the growing dog. J. Am. Vet. Med. Assoc., 166:769–774, 1975.

Van Vleet, J.F., Ruth, G., and Ferrans, V.J.: Ultrastructural alterations in skeletal muscle of pigs with selenium-vitamin E deficiency. Am. J. Vet. Res., 37:911–922, 1976.

Van Vleet, J.F., Ferrans, V.J., and Ruth, G.R.: Ultrastructural alterations in nutritional cardiomyopathy of selenium-vitamin E deficient swine. I. Fiber lesions. Lab. Invest., 37:188–200, 1977.

Van Vleet, J.F., Ferrans, V.J., and Ruth, G.R.: Ultrastructural alterations in nutritional cardiomyopathy of selenium-vitamin E deficient swine. II. Vascular lesions. Lab. Invest., 37:201–211, 1977.

Van Vleet, J.F., and Ferrans, V.J.: Ultrastructural alterations in skeletal muscle of ducklings fed selenium-vitamin E-deficient diet. Am. J. Vet. Res., 38:1399–1405, 1977.

Wensvoort, P.: (I) Morphogenesis of the altered adipose tissue in generalized steatitis in equidae. (II) Age-linked features of generalized steatitis in equidae. Tijdschr. Diergeneeskd., 99:1060–1066, 1067–1069, 1974.

Wilson, T.M., et al.: Myodegeneration and suspected selenium-vitamin E deficiency in horses. J. Am. Vet. Med. Assoc., 169:213–216, 1976.

HYPOVITAMINOSIS K

Vitamin K, a fat-soluble vitamin synthesized as 2-methyl-1, 4-naphthaquinone and closely related compounds, is necessary for the proper formation of prothrombin and clotting factors VII, IX, and X and other proteins. However, since it is prevalent in nature and is freely synthesized by intestinal bacteria, no clinical deficiency occurs in healthy animals. An exception to this statement may possibly arise as the result of prolonged dosing with salicylates or certain bacteriostatic drugs. In obstructive jaundice and possibly in severe and long-continued diarrhea, there may not be enough bile in the digestive canal for successful absorption of the vitamin, and under such circumstances it needs to be administered to prevent hypoprothrombinemia. (See hemorrhage, p. 157.) It is at least a partial antidote for coumarin, the active substance in poisoning by sweet clover, and by "warfarin." A hemorrhagic disease in swine has been reported to be associated with some defect in the feed. Substances interfering with vitamin K are suspected (Osweiler, 1970).

Caldwell, P.T., Ren, P., and Bell, R.G.: Warfarin and metabolism of vitamin K. Biochem. Pharmacol., 23:3353–3362, 1974.

Osweiler, G.D.: Investigation of feed related porcine hemorrhagic disease. Proc. 74th Ann. Meeting US Anim. Health Asssoc., 1970, pp. 522–526.

Suttie, J.W.: Vitamin K—introduction to symposium. Fed. Proc., 37:2598, 1978.

———: Control of clotting factor biosynthesis by vitamin K. Fed. Proc., 28:1696–1701, 1969.

———: The metabolic role of vitamin K. Fed. Proc., 39:2730–2735, 1980.

HYPERVITAMINOSIS

Large doses of most vitamins may be given to animals without any deleterious

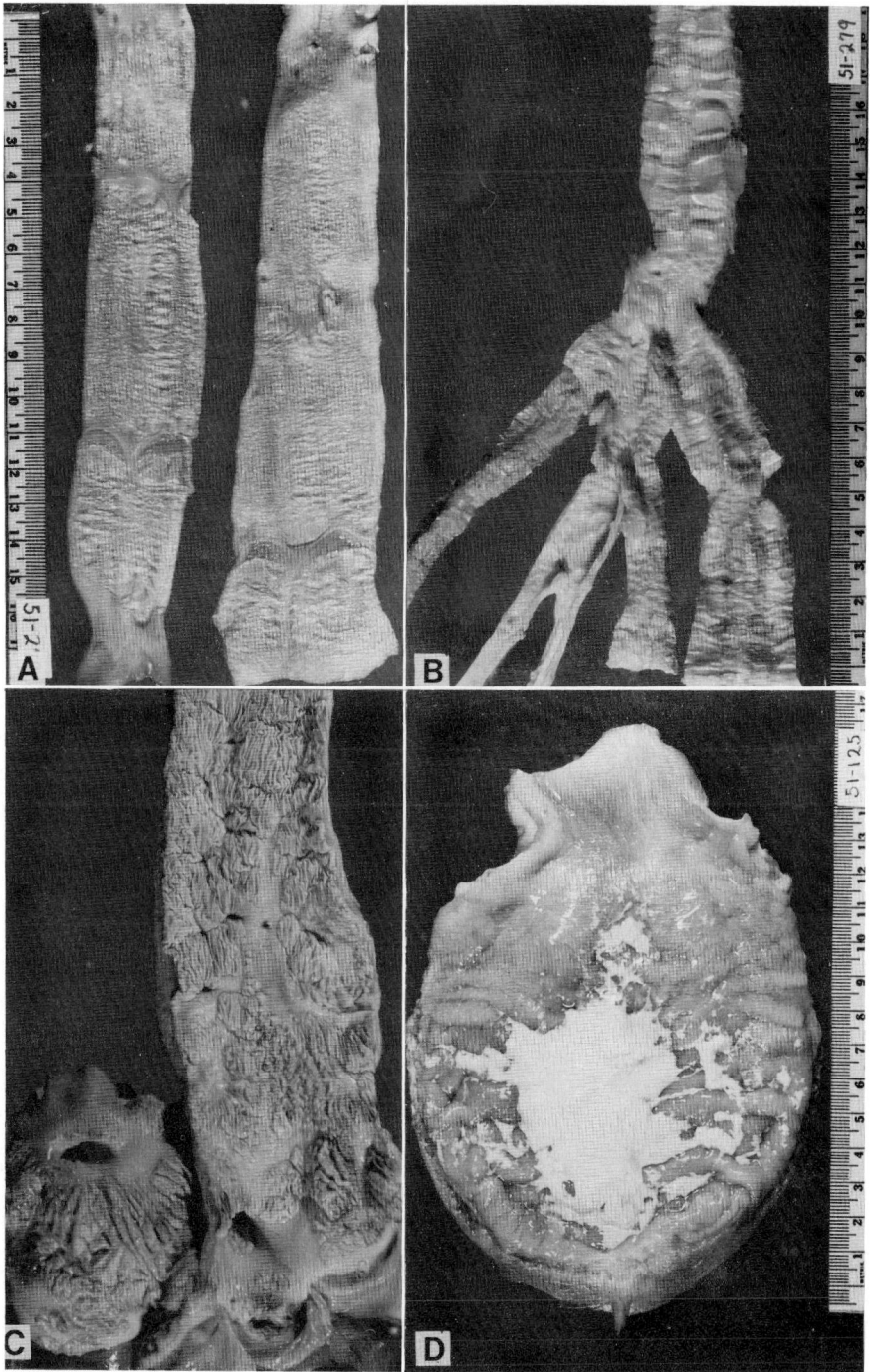

Fig. 17–9. Hypervitaminosis D. Lesions in a pregnant Jersey cow, six years, which had been given 30 million IU of vitamin D (viosterol) for 20 days preceding parturition, and killed one day later. *A,* Jugular vein with transverse corrugations in roughened intima. *B,* Terminal aorta and its branches with mineralization of media, resulting in loss of contractility and elasticity and irregular plaques visible from the intimal surface. *C,* Aortic valves and aortic arch. Raised, rugose plaques of calcareous material are conspicuous from the intimal surface. *D,* Urinary bladder, containing white granular material. (Courtesy of Dr. C. R. Cole, Ohio State University.)

effect. The exceptions are vitamins D and A. Both of these vitamins produce significant toxic effects when consumed or administered in large doses.

Hypervitaminosis D

Although several times the normal requirement is necessary to produce toxicity, hypervitaminosis D is occasionally encountered in man and animals. The deleterious effects are due to hypercalcemia resulting from increased intestinal absorption of calcium, and increased mobilization of calcium from the skeleton. The predominant tissue change is metastatic calcification as phosphate salts, comparable to hydroxyapatite crystals of normal bone. The mineral deposits often contain histochemically demonstrable iron and are usually PAS-positive. Tissues most frequently affected are the intima and media of large arteries (where the lesions resemble Mönckeberg's arteriosclerosis), myocardium, gastric mucosa, lung, and kidney. There is bone resorption with fibrous replacement and excessive deposition of osteoid, which has been termed "hypervitaminosis D rickets." Although once considered a paradox, bone resorption is a direct effect of vitamin D in maintaining serum calcium.

Poisoning by vitamin D in children usually results from overzealous (and ignorant) medication of the child by one or both parents. A specific situation in cattle causes severe hypervitaminosis D. This

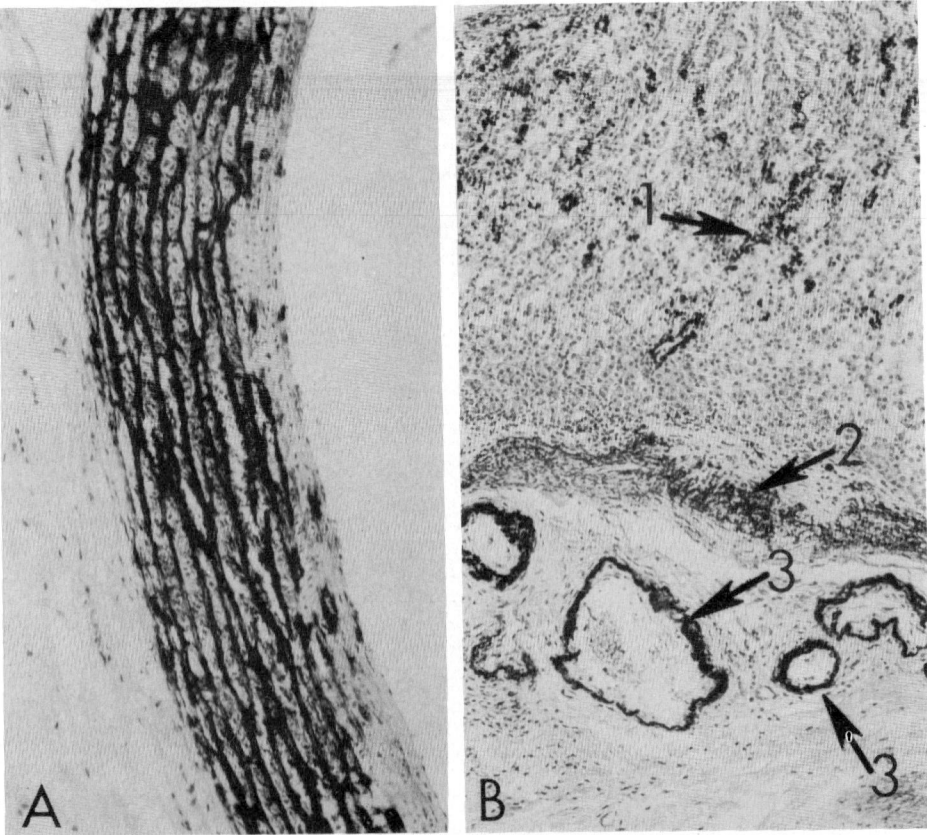

Fig. 17-10. Hypervitaminosis D, cebus monkey. *A*, Metastatic calcification of the aorta. *B*, Metastatic calcification of the gastric mucosa*(1)*, muscularis mucosa*(2)*, and arteries*(3)* in the muscularis. (Courtesy of New England Regional Primate Research Center, Harvard Medical School.)

poisoning has resulted from the administration of large doses (as much as 30 million IU per day) of vitamin D_3 for a prolonged time to prevent parturient hypocalcemia (milk fever).

A disease of cattle manifest by widespread calcification of soft tissues, especially the cardiovascular system, is known in several parts of the world. It is called "enteque seco" in South America, "Manchester wasting disease" in Jamaica, and "Naalehu disease" in Hawaii. The South American disease (enteque seco) is associated with ingestion of a plant, *Solanum malacoxylon*. This plant contains an active principle that causes increased absorption of calcium and phosphorus. It acts as a biologically active substance that mimics the action of 1,25-dihydroxycholecalciferol, the active hormonal form of vitamin D_3.

A similar disease of sheep, described in India as "enzootic calcinosis," is evidenced by metastatic calcification, but the etiology is presently unknown (Gill et al., 1976). Calcinosis in young piglets, possibly associated with overdoses of vitamin D, has been described in Switzerland and Great Britain (Häni and Rossi, 1975; Penn, 1970). Cervical scoliosis and metastatic calcification have been associated with overdoses of vitamin D given to young sheep (Clegg and Hollands, 1976).

Arnold, R.M.: The interaction of calcium, magnesium, phosphorus, other minerals and vitamin D in the aetiology of Manchester wasting disease. Trop. Anim. Health Prod., 1:75–84, 1969.

Burgisser, H., Jacquier, C., and Leuenberber, M.: Hypervitaminosis D in pigs. Schweiz. Arch. Tierheilk., 106:714–718, 1964.

Capen, C.C., Cole, C.R., and Hibbs, J.W.: The pathology of hypervitaminosis D in cattle. Pathol. Vet., 3:350–378, 1966.

Capen, C.C., and Young, D.M.: Fine structural alterations in thyroid parafollicular cells of cows in response to experimental hypercalcemia induced by vitamin D. Am. J. Pathol., 57:365–382, 1969.

Clegg, F.G., and Hollands, J.G.: Cervical scoliosis and kidney lesions in sheep following dosage with vitamin D. Vet. Rec., 98:144–146, 1976.

Gill, B.S., Singh, M., and Chopra, A.K.: Enzootic calcinosis in sheep: clinical signs and pathology. Am. J. Vet. Res., 37:545–552, 1976.

Häni, H., and Rossi, G.L.: Zur Calcinose des Jungferkels. Schweiz. Arch. Tierheilkd., 117:19–30, 1975.

Hunt, R.D., Garcia, F.G., and Hegsted, D.M.: Hypervitaminosis D in New World monkeys. Am. J. Clin. Nutr., 22:358–366, 1969.

Penn, G.B.: Calciphylactic syndrome in pigs. Vet. Rec., 86:718–721, 1970.

Wasserman, R.H.: Calcium absorption and calcium-binding protein synthesis: *Solanum malacoxylon* reverses strontium inhibition. Science, 183:1092–1094, 1974.

Hypervitaminosis A

In man, acute vitamin A intoxication has been described following ingestion of a single massive dose and following consumption of large quantities of polar bear liver. Chronic hypervitaminosis A has occurred in food faddists and individuals using large daily doses of vitamin A for dermatologic conditions. In animals there are several reports of experimentally induced hypervitaminosis A, but few examples of natural poisoning. Skeletal lesions have received the greatest attention, but descriptions of the changes have been conflicting. It appears that, in part, species variation is responsible for the conflicting reports. Osteoporosis and retarded bone growth due to decreased osteoblastic activity and destruction of the cartilaginous growth plate are described as the predominant changes in pigs, rats, and cattle. The striking abnormality in man and cats is the development of multiple exostoses of the skeleton. Seawright and co-workers (1964, 1965, 1967) have presented evidence to indicate that hypervitaminosis A is the cause of a naturally occurring skeletal disease of cats termed **deforming cervical spondylosis.** The exostoses in this condition, which principally develop on the cervical and thoracic vertebrae, forelimbs and ribs, are histologically irregular masses of cartilage and new subperiosteal bone. In the experimentally induced disease, collections of large foamy macrophages occur in the liver, lungs, spleen, and lymph nodes, and lipoid material is present in renal tubular epithelium. These changes are believed

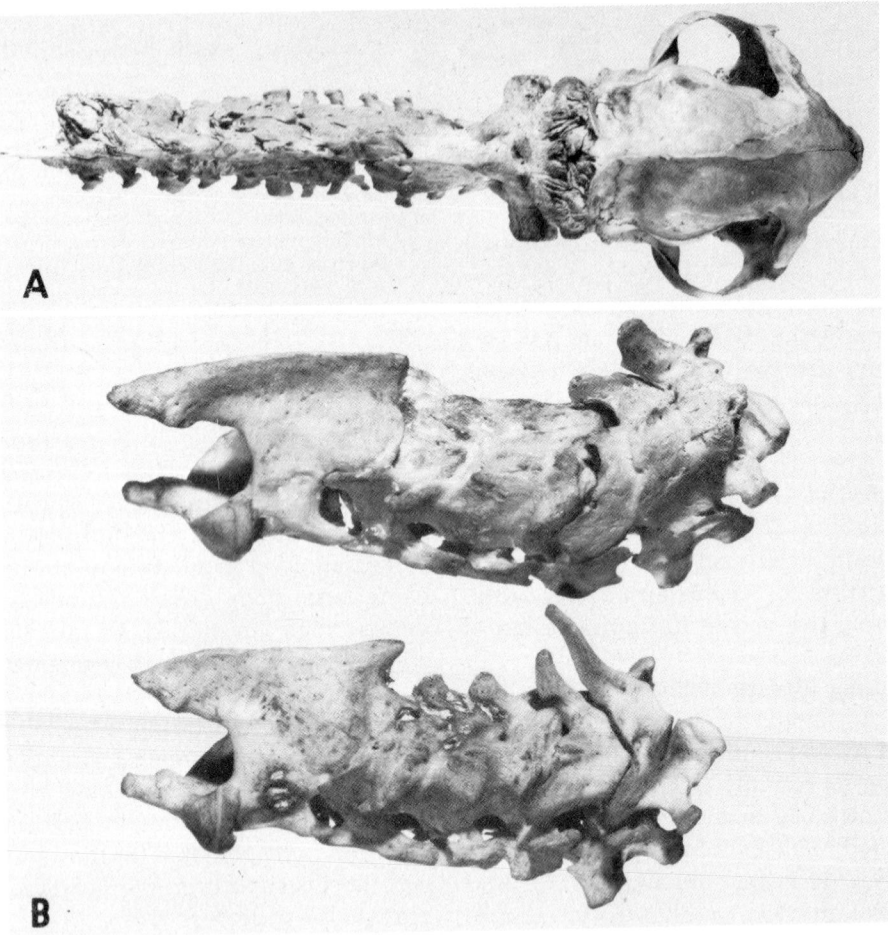

Fig. 17–11. Hypervitaminosis A, feline. *A,* Dorsal aspect of vertebral column and cranium in a natural case of the disease. Exostoses have resulted in fusion of vertebrae and fusion of the atlas to the occipital bone. *B,* Fusion of vertebrae in an experimentally induced case. (Courtesy of Dr. A. A. Seawright.)

to represent storage sites of excess vitamin A. In experimentally treated kittens, severe reduction in length of long bones of the hind legs also resulted from overdoses of vitamin A. The phalanges were also disparate in length. This failure to grow in length appears to be due to arrest of growth of the epiphyseal cartilages. Some epiphyseal plates actually disappear completely (Clark and Seawright, 1968). Retarded growth and retention of incisors were also noted in kittens fed on a diet of sheep liver with a high vitamin A content (Seawright and Hrdlicka, 1974).

In contrast to hypovitaminosis A, excess vitamin A results in a drop in cerebrospinal fluid pressure, believed to result from a decreased formation of cerebrospinal fluid. Toxic levels of vitamin A administered by parenteral routes induce calcification of arteries, heart, and kidney comparable to the changes seen in hypervitamosis D. It is of interest that the toxicity and lesions of hypervitaminosis D can be ameliorated in part by the administration of relatively large amounts of vitamin A.

Calhoun, M.C., Rousseau, J.E., Jr., and Hall, J.J.: Cisternal cerebrospinal fluid pressure during development of chronic bovine hypervitaminosis. Am. J. Dairy Sci., 48:729–732, 1965.

Cho, D.Y., Frey, R.A., Guffy, M.M., and Leipold, H.W.: Hypervitaminosis A in the dog. Am. J. Vet. Res., 36:1597–1603, 1975.

Clark, L., and Seawright, A.A.: Skeletal abnormalities in the hindlimbs of young cats as a result of hypervitaminosis A. Nature (Lond.), 217:1174–1176, 1968.

Clark, L., Seawright, A.A., and Hrdlicka, J.: Exostoses in hypervitaminotic A cats with optimal calcium-phosphorus intakes. J. Small Anim. Pract., 11:553–561, 1970.

Clark, I., and Smith, M.R.: Effects of hypervitaminosis A and D on skeletal metabolism. J. Biol. Chem., 239:1266–1271, 1964.

Eaton, H.D.: Chronic bovine hypo- and hypervitaminosis A and cerebrospinal fluid pressure. Am. J. Clin. Nutr., 22:1070–1080, 1969.

Frier, H.I., et al.: Rates of formation and absorption of cerebrospinal fluid in mild chronic bovine hypervitaminosis. J. Dairy Sci., 53:1051–1057, 1970.

Gallina, A.M., et al.: Bone lesions in mild chronic bovine hypervitaminosis A. Arch. Exp. Veterinaermed., 24:1091–1100, 1970.

Gorgacz, E.J., et al.: Morphologic alterations associated with decreased cerebrospinal fluid pressure in chronic bovine hypervitaminosis A. Am. J. Vet. Res., 36:171–180, 1975.

Grey, R.M., et al.: Pathology of skull, radius and rib in hypervitaminosis A in young calves. Pathol. Vet., 2:446–467, 1965.

Irwin, C., and Bassett, A.L.: The amelioration of hypervitaminosis D in rats with vitamin A. J. Exp. Med., 115:147–156, 1962.

Lucke, V.M., et al.: Deforming cervical spondylosis in the cat associated with hypervitaminosis A. Vet. Rec., 82:141–142, 1968.

Meyer, V., and Prutkin, L.: An ultrastructural study of the effect of hypervitaminosis A acid on the cartilage of the rabbit's ear. J. Comp. Pathol., 82:237–240, 1972.

Seawright, A.A., and English, P.B.: Cervical spondylosis—cats. J. Pathol. Bact., 88:503–509, 1964.

Seawright, A.A., English, P.B., and Gartner, R.J.W.: Hypervitaminosis A and hyperostosis of the cat. Nature, Lond., 206:1171–1172, 1965.

————: Hypervitaminosis A and deforming cervical spondylosis of the cat. J. Comp. Pathol., 77:29–39, 1967.

Seawright, A.A., and Hrdlicka, J.: Pathogenetic factors in tooth loss in young cats on a high daily oral intake of vitamin A. Aust. Vet. J., 50:133–141, 1974.

————: Severe retardation of growth with retention and displacement of incisors in young cats fed a diet of raw sheep liver high in vitamin A. Aust. Vet. J., 50:306–315, 1974.

Strebel, R.F., Girerd, R.J., and Wagner, B.M.: Cardiovascular calcification in rats with hypervitaminosis A. Arch. Pathol., 87:290–297, 1969.

Wolke, R.E., Nielsen, S.W., and Rousseau, J.E., Jr.: Bone lesions of hypervitaminosis A in the pig. Am. J. Vet. Res., 29:1009–1024, 1968.

Wolke, R.E., et al.: Qualitative and quantitative osteoblastic activity in chronic porcine hypervitaminosis. Am. J. Pathol., 97:677–686, 1969.

CALCIUM

In considering the disorders of calcium metabolism, two separate aspects are presented—the mobilized calcium in the blood and the organized calcium in the bones. Disorders involving the bones include rickets, osteomalacia, and osteitis fibrosa cystica, which are discussed in the section on bones and in connection with parathyroid disorders. In general, in case the assimilation of calcium from the food is deficient for any reason, the concentration of the element in the circulating blood is maintained at or near the normal level by its withdrawal from the bones, a process which is under the control of parathyroid hormone, vitamin D, and calcitonin (thyrocalcitonin). Hence, when signs of hypocalcemia (deficiency in the blood) arise, we do not ordinarily expect to find the cause in a shortage of the element in the diet.

The classic signs and symptoms of **hypocalcemia** are displayed when all the parathyroids are removed experimentally and are known as **parathyroid tetany**. Arising about two days after the removal are intermittent tonic spasms with tremors, paresthesias, and muscular pain, the whole syndrome being referable to hyperirritability of the peripheral nervous system. However, tetany can also occur in connection with various other disorders, apparently unrelated, such as gastrointestinal disturbances, pregnancy, and thyroidectomy. (In the last instance it seems possible that the parathyroids may have been unintentionally extirpated along with the thyroid lobes.) Tetany may develop whenever the amount of calcium in the blood falls below a certain critical level, which, for most species, is about 7 mg/100 ml, or when the calcium present is not adequately ionized. Theoretically, such tetany can result from excessive phosphorus in the blood, alkalosis, or failure of a sufficient supply of calcium in the diet. Actually, however, the normally functioning parathyroid supplies deficits of this kind from the bones.

Interference with the normal flow of bile, coupled with a diet rich in fats, may produce steatorrhea and the formation of calcium soaps in the intestine to the point that hypocalcemia results and leads to **celiac rickets**. Likewise, there are kidney disorders (nephrosis, nephritis) sufficiently severe that, due to inability to excrete phosphates in the urine, hyperphosphatemia develops, which causes hypocalcemia. Cases are known in the human where tetany has resulted from severe loss of calcium (below 7 mg/100 ml) in connection with these disorders. Persistence of such renal drain upon the calcium reserves leads to **renal rickets** and also to a certain degree of compensatory hyperplasia of the parathyroids. The so called "rubber jaw" of dogs is one way in which this disturbance is manifested. Nephrosis may also lead to hypocalcemia by causing marked loss of protein, which leads to a lowering of total serum protein and the protein-bound or nondiffusible fraction of serum calcium. Recent findings may indicate that renal lesions could interfere with the production of the calcium-mobilizing hormone of vitamin D (1,25-dihydroxycholecalciferol), and this could lead to withdrawal of calcium and phosphate from the bones.

Hypocalcemia often occurs in acute pancreatitis. Presumably calcium is rapidly depleted in extracellular fluids by its fixation as insoluble calcium soaps, with fatty acids released during fat necrosis accompanying acute pancreatitis.

Hypocalcemic tetany may also accompany alkalosis, which causes a reduction in serum ionized calcium.

Contrary to what occurs in parathyroid tetany, there are instances where hypocalcemia appears to depress nervous and general body activity. This is regularly seen in milk fever.

Hypocalcemia is a principal or subordinate factor in milk fever of cows, probably in the so-called eclampsia of lactating bitches, and with hypomagnesemia in grass tetany.

Hypercalcemia

Hypercalcemia occurs in severe hypervitaminosis D, as mentioned in the preceding section. It also occurs in hyperparathyroidism from parathyroid tumors or in hyperparathyroidism compensatory to nephritis, and even to rickets and similar disorders when the cause is not an actual deficiency of elemental calcium. Hypercalcemia tends to cause metastatic calcification and urolithiasis as the excess of calcium is eliminated in the urine.

Barlet, J.P.: Role of the thyroid gland in magnesium-induced hypocalcemia in the bovine. Horm. Metab. Res. (Stuttgart), 3:63–64, 1971.

——: Calcium homeostasis in the normal and thyroidectomized bovine. Horm. Metab. Res. (Stuttgart), 4:300–303, 1972.

Barrett, C.P., Donati, E.J., Volz, J.E., and Smith, E.: Variations in serum calcium between strains of inbred mice. Lab. Anim. Sci., 25:638–640, 1975.

Chisari, F.V., Hochstein, H.D., Kirschstein, R.L., and Seligmann, E.B.: Parathyroid necrosis and hypocalcemic tetany induced in rabbits by L-asparaginase. Am. J. Pathol., 68:461–468, 1972.

Hellman, B., Sehlin, J., and Taljedal, I.B.: Calcium and secretion: distinction between two pools of glucose-sensitive calcium in pancreatic islets. Science, 194:1421–1423, 1976.

Kirk, G.R., Breazile, J.E., and Kenny, A.D.: Pathogenesis of hypocalcemia tetany in the thyroparathyroidectomized dog. Am. J. Vet. Res., 35:407–408, 1974.

Krook, L., Lutwak, L., and McEntee, K.: Dietary calcium ultimobranchial tumors and osteopetrosis in the bull. Syndrome of calcitonin excess? Am. J. Clin. Nutr., 22:115–118, 1969.

Oberc, M.A., and Engel, W.K.: Ultrastructural localization of calcium in normal and abnormal skeletal muscle. Lab. Invest., 36:566–577, 1977.

Posner, A.S.: Problems in calcium metabolism. Bone mineral on the molecular level. Fed. Proc., 32:1933–1937, 1973.

Rahaman, H., Srihari, K., and Krishnamoorthy, R.V.: Changes in calcium and phosphate levels in bones of baby and adult loris, Loris tardi-gradus. Curr. Sci., 44:52–53, 1975.

Reddy, B.S.: Calcium and magnesium absorption: role of intestinal microflora. Fed. Proc., 30:1815–1821, 1971.

Resnick, S.: Hypocalcemia and tetany in the dog. Vet. Med. Small Anim. Clin., 67:637–641, 1972.

Schryver, H.F., Hintz, H.F., and Craig, P.H.: Calcium metabolism in ponies fed a high phosphorus diet. J. Nutr., *101*:259–264, 1971.

Schryver, H.F., Hintz, H.F., and Lowe, J.E.: Calcium metabolism, body composition and sweat losses of exercised horses. Am. J. Vet. Res., *39*:245–248, 1978.

Swartzman, J.A., Hintz, H.F., and Schryver, H.F.: Inhibition of calcium absorption in ponies fed diets containing oxalic acid. Am. J. Vet. Res., *39*:1621–1623, 1978.

Wysocki, A.A., and Klett, R.H.: Hair as an indicator of the calcium and phosphorus status of ponies. J. Anim. Sci., *32*:74–78, 1971.

Parturient Hypocalcemia (Milk Fever, Parturient Paresis, Parturient Apoplexy, Eclampsia, Paresis Puerperalis, Hypocalcemia Puerperalis)

Dairy cows and sometimes sheep and other species, at or shortly after parturition, may suddenly become recumbent, somnolent and often comatose. The animal lies on its sternum with the head characteristically turned toward the flank. The cow is unable to get to her feet and may die in a day or so if not treated. The signs are consistently accompanied by severe hypocalcemia (as low as 3.0 mg Ca^{++} per 100 ml blood; normal levels are 9 to 11 mg/100 ml blood) and hyperglycemia. In some cases, significant hypophosphatemia and hypokalemia may be detected.

Prior to the advent of modern treatments, most cases were fatal after a number of hours, but in 1897 Schmidt began achieving a high percentage of cures by the intramammary injection of a solution of potassium iodide, theorizing that some toxin was elaborated in the udder. Later this was changed to the injection of oxygen into each teat orifice until the udder was rather tensely inflated, and then it was found that inflation with air would suffice just as well. Recovery in a few hours was the rule.

Little and Wright, in 1925, and Dryerre and Greig, in 1928, as well as many others showed that milk fever is characterized by a level of blood calcium equal to about half the normal (mean 5.13, minimum 3.00 mg/100 ml), and that the severity of the symptoms was proportional to the degree of hypocalcemia. In most cases there is also hypophosphatemia and slight hypermagnesemia. The present-day treatment consists of the intravenous injection of perhaps 50 g of calcium borogluconate (other salts of calcium have been used) in appropriate solution, and disappearance of the signs is sometimes only a matter of minutes. Treatment with high levels of vitamin D$_3$ has also been used satisfactorily in some cases.

The involvement of calcium and relation to secretion of colostrum seems apparent from the blood analyses, the spectacular success of treatment, and also from the historical fact that the disease first began to be recognized contemporaneously with the development of the heavily producing dairy breeds, the earliest references to it, according to Hutyra et al. (1938), being those of Eberhardt in 1793, Price in 1806, Jorg in 1808, and Fabe in 1837. However, the reason for the disturbed calcium homeostasis has not been answered satisfactorily. Comparative studies between cows with parturient paresis and healthy postpartum cows have not elucidated the basic disturbance. Calcium loss in milk or urine is not greater in cows with paresis. Disturbed endocrine function has been a tempting conclusion, but to date investigations have not revealed a clearly defined abnormality in parathormone, thyroxin, estrogen, or adrenal cortical steroid metabolism.

Most emphasis has been directed to parathormone. It has been hypothesized that the basic defect lies in the parathyroid gland, which fails to cause mobilization of sufficient calcium to meet demands of lactation. This hypothesis has not been proved. Studies by Capen and Young (1967) offer a different approach, which includes the hypothesis that the basic defect in milk fever is a sudden release of thyrocalcitonin at parturition. Although the stimulus for the apparent release is unknown, their data demonstrated degranulation of parafollicular cells (origin of thyrocalcitonin) and reduced thyrocalcitonin activity in the thyroid glands of cows with parturient paresis. Their data and that of Sherwood and co-workers (1966) suggest hyperactivity of parathormone synthesis rather than hypoactivity.

Experimental induction of parturient hypocalcemia in pregnant dairy cows was accomplished for the first time (Yarrington et al., 1976). This was done by giving three pregnant cows disodium ethane-1-hydroxy-1, 1-diphosphonate, which selectively inhibits the resorption of bone. Serum total calcium decreased to below 6.0 mg/100 ml, and ionized calcium, to less than 1.0 mg/100 ml in treated cows that simultaneously manifest clinical signs of the natural disease. These studies suggest a new approach to investigation of this disease by blocking the reabsorption of calcium from the bones. The exact mechanisms involved in parturient hypocalcemia are not yet fully understood.

Two other disease conditions of cattle may be confused with parturient hypocalcemia: acetonemia and grass tetany. The essential findings in acetonemia are ketosis and hypoglycemia; in grass tetany, hypomagnesemia and hypocalcemia.

Although the majority of cows with milk fever respond rapidly to therapy, some individuals do not get to their feet after calcium treatment. These cases may represent a complication of milk fever or other poorly understood maladies associated with parturition and grouped under the term "downer cow syndrome."

Gross lesions, in those which die, are practically nil, and the same is presumably true microscopically, as well, but extensive microscopic studies have not been reported.

Black, H.E., Capen, C.C., Yarrington, J.T., and Rowland, G.N.: Effect of a high calcium prepartal diet on calcium homeostatic mechanisms in thyroid glands, bone and intestine of cows. Lab. Invest., 29:437–448, 1973.

Blum, J.W., Ramberg, C.F., Jr., Johnson, K.G., and Kronfeld, D.S.: Calcium (ionized and total), magnesium, phosphorus, and glucose in plasma from parturient cows. Am. J. Vet. Res., 33:51–56, 1972.

Blum, J.W., Mayer, G.P., and Potts, J.T., Jr.: Parathyorid hormone responses during spontaneous hypocalcemia and induced hypercalcemia in cows. Endocrinology, 95:84–92, 1974.

Bowen, J.M., Blackmon, D.M., and Heavner, J.E.: Neuromuscular transmission and hypocalcemic paresis in the cow. Am. J. Vet. Res., 31:831–839, 1970.

Capen, C.C., and Young, D.M.: The ultrastructure of the parathyroid glands and thyroid parafollicular cells of cows with parturient paresis and hypocalcemia. Lab. Invest., 17:717–737, 1967.

————: Thyrocalcitonin: evidence for release in a spontaneous hypocalcemic disorder. Science, 157:205–206, 1967.

Carlstom, G.: Studies on parturient paresis in dairy cows. V. On the composition and calcium binding capacity of two bovine serum protein fractions, with special regard to parturient paresis. Acta Vet. Scand., 11:89–102, 1970.

Dryerre, H., and Greig, R.: Further studies on etiology of milk fever. Vet. Rec., 8:721–728, 1928.

Fish, P.A.: Physiology of milk fever; blood phosphates and calcium. Cornell Vet., 19:147–160, 1929.

Greig, J.R.: Calcium gluconate as a specific in milk fever. Vet. Rec., 10:115–120, and 301–305, 1930.

Hutyra, F., Marek, J., and Manninger, R.: Special Pathology and Therapeutics of the Diseases of Domestic Animals. Vol. III, Engl. translation. Chicago, Alex Eger, 1938, p. 454.

Kronfeld, D.S.: Parturient hypocalcemia in dairy cows. Adv. Vet. Sci. Comp. Med., 15:133–135, 1971.

Little, W.L., and Wright, N.C.: The aetiology of milk fever in cattle. Br. J. Exp. Pathol., 6:129–134, 1925–26. Vet. Rec., 5:631–633, 1925.

Littledike, E.T., Whipp, S.C., and Schroeder, L.: Studies on parturient paresis. J. Am. Vet. Med. Assoc., 155:1955–1962, 1969.

Littledike, E.T.: Parturient hypocalcemia, hypomagnesemia, mastitis-metritis-agalactia complex of swine. In Lactation, A Comprehensive Treatise, Vol. II, edited by B. L. Larson and V. R. Smith. New York, Academic Press, 1974.

Mullen, P.A.: Clinical and biochemical responses to the treatment of milk fever. Vet. Rec., 97:87–92, 1975.

Olsen, W.G., Jorgensen, N.A., Schultz, L.H., and Deluca, H.F.: 25 hydroxycholecalciferol (25-OHD$_3$) II. Efficacy of parenteral administration in prevention of parturient paresis. J. Dairy Sci., 56:889–895, 1973.

Reitz, R.E., Mayer, G.P., Deftos, L.J., and Potts, J.T., Jr.: Endogenous parathyroid hormone response to thyrocalcitonin-induced hypocalcemia in the cow. Endocrinology, 89:932–935, 1971.

Sherwood, L.M., et al.: Intravenous infusions of calcium and ethylenediamine tetraacetic acid in the cow and goat. Nature (Lond.), 209:52–55, 1966.

Yarrington, J.T., et al.: Experimental parturient hypocalcemia in cows following prepartal chemical inhibition of bone resorption. Am. J. Pathol., 83:569–588, 1976.

MAGNESIUM

Magnesium in animal systems is the most abundant intracellular bivalent cation. It is known to be the activator of many enzyme systems, including alkaline phosphatase and most enzymes that utilize adenosine triphosphatase (ATP) or catalyze transfer of phosphate. Since ATP is involved in most biologic systems that require energy, magnesium is likely involved in many biologic activities, including membrane transport, the activation of amino acid, acetate, or succinate, the synthesis of protein, nucleic acid, fat, or coenzymes, the generation and transmission of nerve impulses, the contraction of muscle and oxidative phosphorylation. It is also involved in systems that use thiamine pyrophosphate as a coenzyme. Thus, magnesium is known to be involved in many individual, isolated systems, but a great deal still is to be learned about its role in physiologic activities in the animal body.

Magnesium ions are present in the blood at the approximate level of 2.0 mg/100 ml. Dietary deficiency is believed to be the principal cause of lowered levels in the blood. Levels below 0.7 mg/100 ml cause nervous hyperirritability. Excessively high levels cause depression, coma, and death. This effect is readily demonstrated when euthanasia is accomplished by intravenous injection of a solution of magnesium sulfate.

Two clinical syndromes are associated with hypomagnesemia: grass tetany of adult cattle and hypomagnesemia of calves. Clinically, the two syndromes are similar, however, their pathogenesis differs.

Hypomagnesemia in Calves

Hypomagnesemia in calves occurs in animals raised on a low magnesium diet, usually milk, the disease representing a nutritional deficiency. Serum magnesium falls from 2.0 mg to 0.7 mg/100 ml and bone ash magnesium is reduced to about one-third of normal. Serum calcium and phosphorus remain within normal limits. Clinical signs focus on hyperirritability and tetany. Early signs include opisthotonus, frequent movement or fixed depression of the ears, greatly exaggerated scratching, kicking at the belly or twitching of the skin in response to slight stimuli, spastic extreme flexion of the carpus in walking, salivation, exophthalmos, and apprehensiveness. These signs are intermittent and initiated by excitement or exercise. After days or weeks, terminal tonic-clonic convulsions, lasting one or two hours, are fatal at the first or second attack.

Postmortem lesions in the experimental cases of Blaxter and co-workers (1954) were largely limited to agonal hemorrhages (heart, intestinal and mesenteric serosae) and congestion of viscera. Contraction of segments of stomach (abomasum) and intestines persisted after death. Microscopically, thrombosis of venules of the heart, surrounded by necrosis and inflammatory reaction, was seen. Beyond this and the hemorrhages and congestion, there were no microscopic lesions of note. Neither the central nervous tissue nor muscles contained lesions of significance.

On the other hand, Moore and co-workers (1938) performed autopsies on 38 calves that had died from experimentally produced hypomagnesemia and found rather extensive lesions, the most prominent of which was calcification of the intimal layer of the heart and large blood vessels. This calcification was apparently an example of metastatic calcification rather than that due to previous necrosis. The lesions took the form of slightly raised, light-colored plaques, a few millimeters in diameter, on the intimal surfaces, in which there was an increase of fibrous and elastic elements. These animals also showed toxic degeneration of the renal tubules and early cirrhotic tendencies. The amount of calcium in the diet of these calves was reported as low or normal, but it would appear that the conditions of metastatic calcification were somehow met. Similar calcification of the endocardium and blood vessels, as well as of muscle and kidney, has since been reproduced by other investigators in calves, rats, and dogs. However, evidence from experimental studies indicates that necrosis of myofibers precedes calcification. Natural incidents have also been reported in which calves fed on a low magnesium diet succumbed with lesions of metastatic calcification (Haggard et al., 1978).

Grass Tetany

Although also characterized by low serum magnesium, hypomagnesemia in adult cattle is not analogous to the deficiency disease described previously in calves. When cattle, sheep, and rarely, horses have been pastured for some time exclusively on lush and succulent grasses of various kinds, they are likely to undergo sudden tetanic convulsive seizures. Premonitory hyperirritability, apprehensiveness, or incoordination are often overlooked. Such an attack is commonly fatal, perhaps after a period of terminal recumbency in a state of partial coma or paresis. **Grass staggers** is a colloquial synonym based on the incoordination of the limbs. If the grass in question happens to be young and vigorously growing wheat which is being used for pasturage, a common practice in wheat-growing areas, the condition is often called **wheat poisoning**. The terminal convulsive attack may be initiated by excitement and exercise. If these are incident to the animal's being transported by rail or truck, the terms "railroad sickness" or "lorry disease" may be heard (lorry, motor truck).

The signs are obviously similar to those of experimental hypomagnesemia. Postmortem lesions may be nonexistent or there may be, as in experimental hypomagnesemia, agonal hemorrhages associated with a convulsive death (really an asphyxiative death due to immobilization of the respiratory muscles; see hemorrhage). A similarity to milk fever is also obvious in the more comatose cases. Hypocalcemia and much more severe hypomagnesemia may also be detected. Bone ash magnesium is not reduced. Increase of the potassium level may also be noted. Grass tetany is usually considered to be due primarily to the low magnesium, with hypocalcemia playing a prominent secondary part. Calcium gluconate given intravenously often cures the acute attack.

High dietary intake of potassium by ruminants leads to reduced effective absorption of magnesium. The use of fertilizers containing much potassium increases the potassium content of the forage. Consumption of this forage with its increased level of potassium inhibits the absorption of magnesium and can lead to hypomagnesemia and tetany. Increased levels of nitrogen given to plants also appear to have the effect of reducing absorption of magnesium. This appears to be the result of changes in the forage plant because feeding nitrogen directly does not lower the blood level of magnesium (Fontenot et al., 1973).

Another tetanic condition is the **winter tetany** occurring in cows. As has been stated, many cows in apparently normal health have only half the normal blood magnesium when wintered on fresh bluegrass. Some of these do sicken with typical tetanic signs, which are fatal in many instances. Pronounced hypocalcemia accompanies the hypomagnesemia, and calcium gluconate is more often curative than are magnesium compounds. Coupled with the fact that a majority of the cows are recently postparturient, these features suggest a confusing similarity to milk fever. Indeed it may be questioned whether there is any fundamental difference. Both the abrupt onset of lactation and disorders of dietary metabolism seem capable of causing serious depletion of the blood's supply of calcium or magnesium or of both. However, in contrast to grass tetany, the hypomagnesemia of winter tetany appears to be the result of prolonged nutritional deficiency.

Hypomagnesemia also occurs in sheep. Both the winter tetany type due to magnesium-deficient diets, the acute grass tetany type, and "transport tetany" have been described. Experimental metastatic calcification has also been produced in foals with a ration deficient in magnesium.

Alcock, N.W., and Shils, M.E.: Comparison of magnesium deficiency in the rat and mouse. Proc. Soc. Exp. Biol. Med., 146:137–141, 1974.

Ashton, D.G., Jones, D.M., and Gilmour, J.S.: Grain-sickness in two non-domestic equines. Vet. Rec., 100:406–407, 1977.

Blaxter, K.L., and Rook, J.A.F.: The magenisum requirements of calves. J. Comp. Pathol. Ther., 64:176–186, 1954.

Christian, K.R., and Williams, V.J.: Attempts to produce hypomagnesaemia in dry non-pregnant sheep. NZ J. Agric. Res., 3:389–398, 1960.

Dick, H.J., and Prior, J.T.: Experimental acute metastatic calcification in the kidney of rats. Am. J. Clin. Pathol., 21:409–422, 1951.

Flink, E.B., and Jones, J.E. (eds).: The pathogenesis and clinical significance of magnesium deficiency. Ann. NY Acad. Sci., 162:705–984, 1969.

Fontenot, J.P., Wise, M.B., and Webb, K.E., Jr.: Interrelationships of potassium, nitrogen and magnesium in ruminants. Fed. Proc., 32:1925–1928, 1973.

Haggard, D.L., Whitehair, C.K., and Langham, R.F.: Tetany associated with magnesium deficiency in suckling beef calves. J. Am. Vet. Med. Assoc., 172:495–497, 1978.

Hall, R.F., and Reynolds, R.A.: Concentrations of magnesium and calcium in plasma of Hereford cows during and after hypomagnesemic tetany. Am. J. Vet. Res., 33:1711–1714, 1972.

Harrington, D.D.: Pathologic features of magnesium deficiency in young horses fed purified rations. Am. J. Vet. Res., 35:503–513, 1974.

Heggtveit, H.A., Herman, L., and Mishra, R.K.: Cardiac necrosis and calcification in experimental magnesium deficiency. A light and electron microscopic study. Am. J. Pathol., 45:757–782, 1964.

Herd, R.P.: Grass tetany in sheep. Aust. Vet. J., 42:160–164, 1966.

Herd, R.P., and Peebles, R.M.: Hypomagnesaemia and grass tetany in sheep. Austr. Vet. J., 38:455–456, 1962.

Hughes, J.P., and Cornelius, C.E.: An outbreak of grass tetany in lactating beef cattle. Cornell Vet., 50:26–33, 1960.

Kemp, A.: (Agricultural aspects of hypomagnesemic tetany.) Tijdshr. Diergeneesk., 84:469–484, 1959. Abstr. Vet. Bull., No. 2899, 1959.

Kemp, A., et al.: Hypomagnesemia in milking cows: intake and utilization of magnesium from herbage by lactating cows. Neth. J. Agric. Sci., 9:134–149, 1961.

Marsh, H., and Swingle, K.F.: The calcium, phosphorus, magnesium, carotene and vitamin A content of the blood of range cattle in eastern Montana. Am. J. Vet. Res., 21:212–221, 1960.

Marshak, R.R.: Some metabolic derangements associated with magnesium metabolism in cattle. J. Am. Vet. Med. Assoc., 133:539–542, 1958.

Mayo, R.H., Plumlee, M.P., and Beeson, W.M.: Magnesium requirement of the pig. J. Anim. Sci., 18:264–274, 1959.

Mershon, M.M.: Tetany in cattle on winter rations. II. Stresses and mineral metabolism. J. Am. Vet. Med. Assoc., 135:435–439, 1959.

Moore, L.A., Hallman, E.T., and Sholl, L.B.: Cardiovascular and other lesions in calves fed diets low in magnesium. Arch. Pathol., 26:820–838, 1938.

Owen, J.B., and Sinclair, K.B.: The development of hypomagnesaemia in lactating ewes. Vet. Rec., 73:1423–1424, 1961.

Patterson, R., and Crichton, C.: Grass staggers in large scale dairying on grass. J. Br. Grass Soc., 15:100–105, 1960.

Rook, J.A.F.: Spontaneous and induced magnesium deficiency in ruminants. Ann. NY Acad. Sci., 162:727–731, 1969.

———: Rapid development of hypomagnesaemia in lactating cows when given artificial rations low in magnesium. Nature (Lond.), 191:1019, 1961.

Todd, J.R., and Horvath, D.J.: Magnesium and neuromuscular irritability in calves, with particular reference to hypomagnesaemic tetany. Br. Vet. J., 126:333–346, 1970.

Udall, R.H.: Low blood magnesium and associated tetany occurring in cattle in the winter. Cornell Vet., 37:314–324, 1947.

Unglaub, I., Sylim-Rapoport, I., and Strassburger, I.: Pathologisch-anatomische Befunde bei experimentellem Magnesium-Mangel des Hundes. Virchow's Arch., 32:122–131, 1959.

Wacker, W.E.C.: The biochemistry of magnesium. Ann. NY Acad. Sci., 162(2):717–726, 1969.

Wilcox, G.B., and Hoff, J.E.: Grass tetany: an hypothesis concerning its relationship with ammonium nutrition of spring grasses. J. Dairy Sci., 57:1085–1089, 1974.

POTASSIUM

Experimental deficiency of potassium has been shown in rats to cause necrotic foci in the heart with infiltration of reticuloendothelial cells and subsequent scarring. It also causes fatty change and necrosis of the epithelium of the renal tubules. The cardiac changes are similar to those produced by deficiency of thiamine and not altogether different from those that result from deficiency of vitamin E or experimental magnesium deficiency in rats. Paralyses of skeletal muscles have been reported in the dog in experimentally produced potassium deficiency. Physiologic actions of potassium are known to be related to relaxation of cardiac muscle and to certain metabolic aspects of skeletal muscle and of nerve. Recorded examples of potassium deficiency are few; however, it may be encountered in patients with chronic diarrhea and hyperadrenalism or as a result of medication with deoxycorticosterone, which enhances the excretion of potassium with corresponding retention of sodium, and which has resulted in cardiac and renal lesions like those just described. In view of the frequent occurrence of chronic diarrhea in animal diseases, greater attention should be given to the effects of potassium deficiency.

Belman, A.S., and Schwartz, W.B.: The nephropathy of potassium depletion. N. Engl. J. Med., *255*:195, 1956.

SODIUM AND CHLORINE

Both ions are indispensable, but neither is the basis of a separate clinical deficiency. Practically speaking, the metabolism of these two elements is the metabolism of sodium chloride. Carnivorous animals obtain sufficient sodium chloride from the animal tissues that they eat, but the need for salt on the part of humans and domestic and wild herbivora is such that access to the substance has been the basis of taxation, has occasioned wars, and has governed the strategy of generals and of hunters.

Nevertheless, experiments depriving animals of salt over considerable periods of time have shown that such deprivation leads to poor growth, rough coat, and general unthriftiness, as well as to poor reproduction, but indicate that it would be quite difficult to kill an animal by withholding salt. To a limited degree, other basic and acidic ions can substitute for the sodium and chloride respectively in maintaining the proper status of the body fluids. Considerable amounts of all such ions are, of course, acquired in any food.

In a few instances, deficiency of sodium chloride in the diet of dairy cows has resulted in salt hunger, pica, weight loss, decreased milk production, polydipsia, and polyuria. These signs disappeared promptly after addition of salt to the ration (Whitlock et al., 1975).

Transient depletion of sodium chloride or of the chloride ion, the result of loss through excessive sweating, is thought to be important in heat prostration of men and horses, but it must not be assumed that an increased intake of salt is complete protection against excessive heat.

Sudden heavy excesses of salt cause salt poisoning in swine and chickens. A cow, on the other hand, can consume as much as 2 pounds of sodium chloride daily over an indefinite period. Large amounts of water are consumed, but no ill effects are detected either clinically or postmortem.

McDougall, J.G., Coghlan, J.P., Scoggins, B.A., and Wright, R.D.: Effect of sodium depletion on bone sodium and total exchangeable sodium in sheep. Am. J. Vet. Res., *35*:923–930, 1974.

Sato, K., Dobson, R.L., and Mali, J.W.H.: Enzymatic basis for the active transport of sodium in the eccrine sweat gland. J. Invest. Dermatol., *57*:10–16, 1971.

Schrier, R.W., and de Wardener, H.E.: Tubular reabsorption of sodium ion: Influence of factors other than aldosterone and glomerular filtration rate (first of two parts). N. Engl. J. Med., *285*:1231–1243, 1971.

———: Tubular reabsorption of sodium ion: Influence of factors other than aldosterone and glomerular filtration rate (second of two parts). N. Engl. J. Med., *285*:1292–1303, 1971.

Turpeinen, O.: The effects of deprivation of sodium on young puppies. Am. J. Hyg., *18*:104–109, 1938.

Whitlock, R.H., Kessler, M.J., and Tasker, J.B.: Salt (sodium) deficiency in dairy cattle: polyuria and polydipsia as prominent clinical features. Cornell Vet., *65*:512–526, 1975.

FLUORINE

There is no evidence to indicate that fluorine deficiency is an important problem in domestic animals, although it is generally accepted that fluorine is an essential nutrient. Female mice fed a diet low in fluoride over two generations are reported to have reduced fertility, which is restored by the addition of fluoride to the diet.

We are more concerned with excessive intakes of fluorine. These are treated under the heading of Fluorine Poisoning.

In recent years, there is great interest in the possibility that rather minute amounts of fluorine may render the teeth of humans more resistant to caries. Fluorine is being added to many public water supplies for this purpose. This practice is vehemently protested by some citizens. An excess of fluorine, such as 50 or 100 ppm in the total diet, produces noticeable changes in the teeth, consisting of brownish discoloration, chalkiness, and hypoplastic pitting of the enamel.

Messer, H.H., Armstrong, W.D., and Singer, L.: Fertility impairment in mice on a low fluoride intake. Science, *177*:893–894, 1972.

PHOSPHORUS

The inorganic phosphorus of the blood plasma of the domestic herbivora varies normally between 4 and 8 mg/100 ml, approaching the higher limit in the young and declining in the aged. In the dog, considerably lower figures are said to be normal. Three-fourths of the amount present in the body is in the bones as calcium phosphate. Deficiency of phosphorus is much more likely to be encountered in herbivora, being due to an abnormally low amount in the plants consumed. Plants lack phosphorus when grown on the deficient soils of certain well-recognized localities, especially under conditions of drought.

The most characteristic sign of aphosphorosis (deficiency) is a tendency to chew or lick bones or to eat dirt, all being manifestations of a depraved and abnormal appetite known as **pica**. However, it must be borne in mind that animals eat dirt when suffering from other deficiencies or from anemia, such as that caused by trichostrongyle worms.

A deficiency of phosphorus in the diet is one of the causes of rickets (and osteomalacia), but since phosphorus, like calcium, can be replenished in the blood by reducing the amount in the bones, there is only a limited degree of **hypophosphatemia**. The symptoms and lesions are entirely comparable to those of rickets or osteomalacia from other causes, but in some cases they were originally recognized as separate diseases, their true pathogenesis not being understood. Pain in walking was responsible for the colloquial designation of "creeps," which is prevalent in some localities. In the "loin disease" of the coastal plain along the Gulf of Mexico and in **lamsiekte** in South Africa, the phosphorus-deficient cattle often chew the bones of animals dead on the range, to which there still cling shreds of decaying musculature. In these cases, the symptoms of aphosphorosis are complicated by paraplegia and other paralytic signs due to toxins of *Clostridium botulinum* or closely related soil-borne anaerobes which have contaminated the putrid flesh. In sheep, aphosphorosis is considered the most common cause of rickets; in other species, that disease is more frequently due to other disorders.

Hyperphosphatemia can arise in two different ways. In "bran disease" of horses, the animals receive an excess of phosphorus because of unduly large amounts of wheat bran (the outer hull-like layers of the wheat kernel, rejected in the milling of white flour). This useful feed contains a high percentage of phosphorus and little calcium. The symptoms and lesions are those of adult rickets or osteomalacia, the jaw bones as well as those of the limbs being weakened and painful, with loosening and soreness of the teeth. Similarly, meat diets in cats and dogs may result in hyperphosphatemia due to their high phosphorus, low calcium content.

Hyperphosphatemia also occurs as the secondary effect of some forms of severe nephritis. The kidney is unable to excrete phosphates. These accumulate in the blood, reaching a level two to four times the normal, amounting to a form of acidosis. The rise in serum inorganic phosphate, whether of dietary or renal origin, causes hypocalcemia, which in turn results in secondary parathyroid hyperplasia. To maintain serum calcium, parathyroid hormone extracts calcium from the skeleton, thus the bones suffer the changes of fibrous osteodystrophy when the blood phosphorus is excessively high or when it is excessively low. The hypocalcemia arising in this way, even to the point of tetany, has been mentioned in connection with the metabolism of calcium.

Hypophosphatemia occurs in postparturient hemoglobinuria of cattle; however, the relationship of the low serum phosphorus to the occurrence of hemolytic anemia has not been established.

Eicher, E.M., Southard, J.L., Scriver, C.R., and Glorieux, F.H.: Hypophosphatemia: mouse model for human familial hypophosphatemic (vitamin D-resistant) rickets. Proc. Natl. Acad. Sci. USA, 73:4667–4671, 1976.
Morrow, D.A.: Phosphorus deficiency and infertility in dairy heifers. J. Am. Vet. Med. Assoc., 154:761–768, 1969.
Symonds, H.W.: The effect of thyroidectomy and thyroparathyroidectomy upon phosphorus homeostasis in the goat: a hypothesis for the cause of hypophosphataemia. Res. Vet. Sci., 11:260–269, 1970.

SULFUR

Deficiency of sulfur, as such, does not occur, nor is the animal mechanism able to use inorganic sulfur to synthesize or replace the sulfur-containing amino acids, methionine or cystine, deficiency of which is sometimes experienced. **Sulfur rickets** is known, sulfur being able to replace phosphorus in the mineral of bones. This has happened when animals have been fed large amounts of sulfur, as for instance when sulfur is used as an anticoccidial drug in chickens.

SELENIUM

For many years, the toxic role of selenium in animals has been emphasized (see Chapter 17). It is now clear that selenium is an essential nutrient to animals, birds, and probably man. An important recent discovery was that selenium is an essential component of the enzyme glutathione peroxidase (glutathione: H_2O_2, oxidoreductase). Deficiency of selenium in the rat, chick, and sheep causes a severe decrease in glutathione peroxidase in the tissues. This enzyme acts to prevent peroxidative damage to erythrocytic plasma cell membranes. Dietary selenium therefore protects against hemolysis of red blood cells and oxidation of hemoglobin. By destroying hydrogen peroxide and organic hydroperoxides in the tissues, glutathione peroxidase prevents damage to the cell membrane and other membrane-bound structures (mitochondria, lysosomes, microsomes). The relation of selenium to vitamin E is discussed further on page 1045.

The dietary requirement of selenium for most species is 0.1 to 0.3 ppm of diet (mg/kg). Toxic levels range from 2 to 10 ppm and greater amounts are rapidly lethal. Toxic levels may be exceeded in some situations by parenteral use of commercial selenium-vitamin E preparations (Van Vleet, Meyer and Olander, 1974).

Ammerman, C.B., and Miller, S.M.: Selenium in ruminant nutrition; a review. J. Dairy Sci., 58:1561–1577, 1975.
Herigstad, R.R., Whitehair, C.K., and Olson, O.E.: Inorganic and organic selenium toxicosis in young swine: comparison of pathologic changes with those in swine with vitamin E-selenium deficiency. Am. J. Vet. Res., 34:1227–1238, 1973.
Hidiroglou, M., Jenkins, K.J., Wauthy, J.M., and Proulx, J.G.: A note on the prevention of nutritional muscular dystrophy by winter silage feeding of the cow or selenium implantation of the calf. Anim. Prod., 14:115–118, 1972.
Jenkins, K.J., Hidiroglou, M., Mackey, R.R., and Proulx, J.G.: Influence of selenium and linoleic acid on the development of nutritional muscular dystrophy in beef calves, lambs, and rabbits. Can. J. Anim. Sci., 50:137–146, 1970.
National Academy of Sciences: Selenium in Nutrition. Washington, D.C., 1971.
Noguchi, T., Langevin, M.L., Combs, G.F., Jr., and Scott, M.L.: Biochemical and histochemical studies of the selenium deficient pancreas in chicks. J. Nutr., 103:444–453, 1973.
Rotruck, J.T., et al.: Selenium: biochemical role as a component of glutathione peroxidase. Science, 179:588–590, 1973.

Scott, M.L.: The selenium dilemma. J. Nutr., *103*:803–810, 1973.

Van Vleet, J.F., Carlton, W., and Olander, H.J.: Hepatosis dietetica and mulberry heart disease associated with selenium deficiency in Indiana swine. J. Am. Vet. Med. Assoc., *157*:1208–1219, 1970.

Van Vleet, J.F., Meyer, K.B., and Olander, H.J.: Acute selenium toxicosis induced in baby pigs by parenteral administration of selenium-vitamin E preparations. J. Am. Vet. Med. Assoc., *165*:543–547, 1974.

Van Vleet, J.F., Ruth, G., and Ferrans, V.J.: Ultrastructural alterations in skeletal muscle of pigs with selenium-vitamin E deficiency. Am. J. Vet. Res., *37*:911–922, 1976.

Van Vleet, J.F., and Ruth, G.R.: Efficacy of supplements in prevention of selenium-vitamin E deficiency in swine. Am. J. Vet. Res., *38*:1299–1305, 1977.

IRON

Absorption and excretion of iron are accomplished through the mucosal cells of the small intestine. The iron status of the body, depending upon the erythropoietic needs of the host and other factors, is regulated by homeostatic mechanisms, which may act by regulating the production of specific iron receptors in the mucosal cell. Ionic iron in the intestinal lumen is absorbed to these specific receptors in the brush border of mucosal epithelial cells of the small intestine. The iron is transferred to the cytoplasm of the mucosal cell by an active energy-dependent process. This absorbed iron appears to be in small molecular weight form—possibly chelated to amino acids, and in equilibrium with iron-poor ferritin. Transfer to the plasma involves attachment to transferrin and utilizes receptors, but may be independent of cell energy.

If not transferred to plasma, iron remains in the mucosal cell, later to be returned to the intestinal lumen when the mucosal cell is shed from the tip of the villus. This process is one of the means of maintaining the homeostatic level of iron in the body. A second process involves the return of iron from the plasma to the mucosal cell, to be shed into the intestinal lumen. A third process involves the migration and exocytosis of iron-laden macrophages into the intestinal lumen. This alternative appears to operate in pathologic conditions involving iron overload or hemosiderosis (Linder and Munro, 1977).

Dietary deficiency of iron has long been known as a potent cause of anemia. This anemia is hypochromic and microcytic in type. Deficiency usually means that the amount available in the diet is inadequate, or absorption may be seriously impaired by long-standing diarrhea or by achlorhydria (lack of hydrochloric acid in the gastric juice). Achlorhydria interferes because an acid medium is essential to copious absorption of iron. In veterinary practice, however, anemia due to insufficient iron is seldom seen except in little pigs raised without access to the soil. It should be noted, nevertheless, that when there is unusually rapid production of erythrocytes in compensation for hemorrhagic or hemolytic anemia from some other cause, such as ancylostomiasis, the amount of iron required for rapid regeneration of blood cells is correspondingly increased, so that without a fully adequate supply iron-deficiency anemia may develop. The postmortem lesions of anemia have been given.

The ultrastructural and enzymatic changes in the spleen, resulting from dietary iron-deficiency anemia induced experimentally in rabbits, have been described (Rodvien et al., 1974). Fragmentation and phagocytosis of erythrocytes and platelets is a conspicuous feature. The macrophages undergo changes in their endoplasmic reticulum, membranes, and mitochondria. The membranes are segmentally dilated, with accumulation of floccular material in perinuclear spaces. The outer segment of the nuclear membrane is studded with ribosomes. The nuclear membrane buds off to form vesicles or sacs of rough endoplasmic reticulum. The mitochondria undergo focal dilation of cristae and loss of integrity of internal structure. Profiles of rough endoplasmic reticulum form around the mitochondria.

Glutathione peroxidase is deficient in the affected red blood cells. The changes in membranes suggest the effect of lipid peroxidation. It has been proposed that the effect of the iron deficiency may result in deficiency of enzymes responsible for protection against peroxidation injury. A similar role has been suggested for selenium.

A hereditary, sex-linked gene in mice (gene symbol **sla**) results in a hypochromic anemia resembling anemia due to dietary deficiency of iron. The gene-controlled defect leads to failure of transfer of iron in the intestinal mucosal cell to the plasma. Ferritin therefore accumulates in the absorptive cell, in vacuoles, and free in the cytoplasm. Accumulation of this ferritin is associated with a decrease in the rough endoplasmic reticulum and an increase in the smooth endoplasmic reticulum (Bedard et al., 1971).

Tremendously excessive amounts of iron are stored in various tissues in hemochromatosis, a disease in which control and limitation of absorption appear to have been lost. Whether it be the excessive storage that accompanies hemochromatosis or the limited and transient splenic storage that occurs in hemolytic anemia or other blood destruction, stored iron appears in the form of hemosiderin.

Like sulfur, iron is able to enter the calcium phosphate compound of the bone and cause rickets (osteomalacia). The compound thus formed is $Fe_3(PO_4)_2$. The disorder has occurred in poultry. A similar displacement is also theoretically possible when aluminum, magnesium, or beryllium are in excess.

As will be seen, minute amounts of copper and cobalt are necessary for the successful utilization of iron in hematopoiesis.

Amine, E.K., and Hegsted, D.M.: Iron deficiency lipemia in the rat and chick. J. Nutr., 101:1575–1582, 1971.
Bedard, Y.C., Pinkerton, P.H., and Simon, G.T.: Ul-

trastructure of the duodenal mucosa of mice with a hereditary defect in iron absorption. J. Pathol., 104:45–51, 1971.
Bedard, Y.C., Clarke, S., Pinkerton, P.H., and Simon, G.T.: Effect of cycloheximide on iron absorption. Lab. Invest., 30:155–160, 1974.
Burger, P.C., and Klintworth, G.K.: Experimental retinal degeneration in the rabbit produced by intraocular iron. Lab. Invest., 30:9, 1974.
Cook, J.D.: Absorption of food iron. Fed. Proc., 36:2028–2032, 1977.
Cusak, R.P.,and Brown, W.D.: Achromotricia in iron-deficient rats. Nature, 204:582–583, 1964.
d'Arcy, P.F., and Howard, E.M.: The acute toxicity of ferrous salts administered to dogs by mouth. J. Pathol. Bact., 83:65–72, 1962.
Ender, F., Dishington, I.W., Madsen, R., and Helgebostad, A.: Iron-deficiency anemia in mink fed raw marine fish. A five year study. In Advances in Animal Physiology and Animal Nutrition, No. 2. Oslo (Vet. College), 1972.
Jacobs, A.: Serum ferritin and iron stores. Fed. Proc., 36:2024–2027, 1977.
Linder, M.C., and Munro, H.N.: The mechanism of iron absorption and its regulation. Fed. Proc., 36:2017–2023, 1977.
Lindvall, S., Moberg, G., and Nordblom, B.: Studies on sudden fatalities among piglets following parenteral iron therapy. Acta Vet. Scand., 13:206–217, 1972.
Moore, R.W., Redmond, H.E., and Livingston, C.W., Jr.: Iron deficiency anemia as a cause of stillbirths in swine. J. Am. Vet. Med. Assoc., 147:746–748, 1965.
Munro, H.N.: Iron absorption and nutrition. Fed. Proc., 36:2015–2016, 1977.
Nath, I., Sood, S.K., and Nayak, N.C.: Experimental siderosis and liver injury in the rhesus monkey. J. Pathol., 106:103–112, 1970.
Osbaldiston, G.W., and Griffith, P.R.: Serum iron levels in normal and anemic horses. Can. Vet. J., 13:105–108, 1972.
Rodvien, R., Tavassoli, M., and Crosby, W.H.: The structure of spleen in experimentally induced iron deficiency anemia. Am. J. Pathol., 75:243–254, 1974.
Vandijk, J.P.: Iron metabolism and placental transfer of iron in term rhesus monkey (Macaca mulatta): compartmental analysis. Europ. J. Obstet. Gynecol., 7:127–139, 1977.
Wong, C.T., and Morgan, E.H.: Source of foetal iron in the cat. Aust. J. Exp. Biol. Med. Sci., 52:413–416, 1974.

COPPER

Copper occurs in most tissues of the animal body, including the central nervous system, which contains some 20 to 30 mg/kg of dry matter. Minute amounts are essential to the utilization of iron in hematopoiesis. Thus, in copper deficiency, anemia is a usual development. In most species, this occurs as a microcytic hypochromic anemia.

Herbivorous animals raised in a few localities where the soil is almost devoid of this element have been found to suffer from disorders of the blood-forming tissue, of the hair or of the central nervous system. The anemia that occurs is often of subclinical degree. In Florida, a disease characterized by anemia and unthriftiness and colloquially called "salt sick" is cured by giving copper plus iron.

Copper is also an essential component of the enzyme tyrosinase, which is required for the normal production of melanin. Therefore achromotrichia represents another feature of deficiency. The condition is not related to the graying of human hair. A disorder expressively described as **steely wool** is considered to be due to copper deficiency. Changes in the physical nature of hair and wool also develop. Wool loses its crimp and becomes more hair-like.

As indicated, disorders of the central nervous system also follow copper deficiency. In England and Australia, sheep and sometimes goats have a disease called **enzootic ataxia** or "swayback," which occurs on copper-deficient soils and is considered to be due to a shortage of that element in the animal's metabolism. As the names imply, the signs are chiefly incoordination and weakness of the posterior limbs. Spastic paralysis and sometimes blindness occur. The lesions are most pronounced in newborn lambs and consist of demyelinization, and even extensive softening, necrosis, and disappearance of much of the white matter in the central portions of the cerebral hemispheres and spinal cord. In the severest cases, there is little left of the hemispheres but the cortical shell of gray matter. Such a lesion is distinguished from internal hydrocephalus by the irregular and obviously necrotic lining of the cavity and the absence of histologic structures there. Milder forms involve only areas of demyelinization, symmetrically located, with "gitter" cells and necrotic

nerve cells. There is no inflammatory reaction. Innes and Shearer (1940) suspected a relationship between this condition and Schilder's disease of humans. The condition is further discussed in Chapter 27.

A disease considered to be due also to deficiency of copper occurs in adult cattle in Australia and the United States, known as **falling disease** because the cows commonly fall and die very suddenly. Anemia and loss of weight occur, but there are usually no definite premonitory symptoms. Lesions include marked hemosiderosis of the spleen, liver, and kidneys, presumably as the result of the anemia, and diffuse fibrous scarring of the heart muscle. The latter, no doubt, accounts for the sudden death. The details of the pathogenesis of this condition have not been fully elucidated, but copper has been shown to be essential for the maintenance of the structural elements of the myocardium and arteries. In swine, rabbits, and chicks fed low copper diets, there is defective elastogenesis resulting in fragmentation, disruption, and elimination of elastic fibers in the cardiovascular system. The disorder has been shown to result from a decrease in intramolecular crosslinkage of elastin.

Copper deficiency also results in extensive skeletal changes. Although reference is made to "rickets," fractures, and impaired gaits, the nature of the lesions has not been studied under conditions of natural deficiency. In experimental animals, a form of osteoporosis develops that is remarkably similar to the osseous lesions of scurvy. The epiphyseal cartilage is normal or thicker than normal, and it calcifies normally but it does not degenerate. There is cessation of, or reduced, osteoblastic activity with reduced formation of osteoid. Bone resorption is apparently not impaired. These features are in direct opposition to the changes of rickets.

An excessive amount of molybdenum in the pasturage or forage necessitates much larger amounts of copper in the diet. This situation arises on some soils.

An excess of copper is treated under the heading of Copper Poisoning.

Wilson's disease (hepatolenticular degeneration) in man is caused by deranged copper metabolism, presumably a defect in ceruloplasmin (an α-globulin transport system) synthesis. It is characterized by low ceruloplasmin levels, high nonbound plasma copper, increased tissue copper concentration, hepatic necrosis and cirrhosis, and progressive cerebral damage, particularly of the basal ganglia. Lesions in the central nervous system have been described in copper poisoning in sheep. Copper poisoning is discussed in Chapter 16.

Barlow, R.M., Field, A.C., and Ganson, N.C.: Measurement of nerve cell damage in the spinal cord of lambs affected with swayback. J. Comp. Pathol., 74:530–541, 1964.

Bull, L.B., et al.: Ataxia in young lambs. Bull. Council Sci. Indust. Res., Australia, 113:72, 1938.

Cancilla, P.A., and Barlow, R.M.: Structural changes of the central nervous system in swayback (enzootic ataxia) of lambs. II. Electron microscopy of the lower motor neuron. Acta Neuropathol., 6:251–259, 1966.

———: Structural changes of the central nervous sytem in swayback (enzootic ataxia) of lambs. III. Electron microscopy of the cerebral lesions. Acta Neuropathol., 6:260–265, 1966.

———: Experimental copper deficiency in miniature swine. Biochemistry, histochemistry and pathology of the central nervous system. J. Comp. Pathol., 80:315–319, 1970.

Chalmers, G.A.: Swayback (enzootic ataxia) in Alberta lambs. Can. J. Comp. Med., 38:111–117, 1974.

Cordy, D.R., and Knight, H.D.: California goats with a disease resembling enzootic ataxia or swayback. Vet. Pathol., 15:179–185, 1978.

Coulson, W.F., et al.: Cardiovascular system in naturally occurring copper deficiency and swayback in sheep. Am. J. Vet. Res., 27:815–818, 1967.

Doherty, P.C., Barlow, R.M., and Angus, K.W.: Spongy changes in the brain of sheep poisoned by excess dietary copper. Res. Vet. Sci., 10:303–304, 1969.

Everson, G.J., Hyan-Chang Chow Tsai, and Tong-In Wang: Copper deficiency in the guinea pig. J. Nutr., 93:533–540, 1967.

Fisher, G.L.: Effects of disease on serum copper and zinc values in the beagle. Am. J. Vet. Res., 38:935–940, 1977.

Goodrich, R.D., and Tilman, A.D.: Copper, sulfate and molybdenum interrelationships in sheep. J. Nutr., 90:76–80, 1966.

Gumbrell, R.C.: Suspected copper deficiency in a group of full sib Samoyed dogs. NZ Vet. J., 20:238–240, 1972.

Howell, J.McC., et al.: Chronic copper poisoning and changes in the central nervous system of sheep. Acta Neuropathol. (Berl.), 29:9–24, 1974.

Howell, J., Davison, A.N., and Oxberry, J.: Observations on the lesions in the white matter of the spinal cord of swayback sheep. Acta Neuropathol., 12:33–41, 1969.

Huisingh, J., Gomez, G.G., and Matrone, G.: Interactions of copper, molybdenum, and sulfate in ruminant nutrition. Fed. Proc., 32:1921–1924, 1973.

Innes, J.R.M., and Shearer, G.D.: "Swayback" a demyelinating disease of lambs with affinities to Schilder's encephalitis in man. J. Comp. Pathol. Ther., 53:1–41, 1940.

Irwin, M.R., Poulos, P.W., Jr., Smith, B.P., and Fisher, G.L.: Radiology and histopathology of lameness in young cattle with secondary copper deficiency. J. Comp. Pathol., 84:611–621, 1974.

Keen, C.L., and Hurley, L.S.: Copper supplementation in quaking mice: reduced tremors and increased brain copper. Science, 193:244–245, 1976.

Leigh, L.C.: Changes in the ultrastructure of cardiac muscle in steers deprived of copper. Res. Vet. Sci., 18:282–287, 1975.

Lewis, G., Terlecki, S., and Parker, B.N.J.: Observations on the pathogenesis of delayed swayback. Vet. Rec., 95:313–316, 1974.

Lewis, G., Terlecki, S., and Allcroft, R.: The occurrence of swayback in the lambs of ewes fed a semi-purified diet of low copper content. Vet. Rec., 81:415–416, 1967.

McGavin, M.D., Ranby, P.D., and Tammemagi, L.: Demyelination associated with low liver copper levels in pigs. Aust. Vet. J., 38:8–14, 1962.

Owen, E.C., et al.: Pathological and biochemical studies of an outbreak of swayback in goats. J. Comp. Pathol., 75:241–251, 1965.

Pryer, W.J.: The liver copper levels of foetal and maternal pigs. Aust. J. Sci., 25:498, 1963.

Rucker, R.B., Parker, H.E., and Rogler, J.C.: Effect of copper deficiency on chick bone collagen and selected bone enzymes. J. Nutr., 98:57–63, 1969.

Savage, J.E., et al.: Comparison of copper deficiency and lathyrism in turkey poults. J. Nutr., 88:15–25, 1966.

Schwarz, F.J., and Kirchgessner, M.: Untersuchungen zum Ort der intestinalen Cu-Absorption. Zentralbl. Veterinaermed., 20A:734–741, 1973.

Shields, G.S., et al.: Studies on copper metabolism. XXXII. Cardiovascular lesions in copper-deficient swine. Am. J. Pathol., 41:603–621, 1962.

Simpson, C.F., and Harms, R.H.: Pathology of the aorta of chicks fed a copper-deficient diet. Exp. Molec. Pathol., 3:390–400, 1964.

Suttle, N.F., Field, A.C., and Barlow, R.M.: Experimental copper deficiency in sheep. J. Comp. Pathol., 80:151–162, 1970.

Waisman, J., Carnes, W.H., and Weissman, N.: Some properties of the microfibrils of vascular elastic membranes in normal and copper-deficient swine. Am. J. Pathol., 54:107–119, 1969.

Waisman, J., and Carnes, W.H.: Cardiovascular

studies on copper-deficient swine. X. The fine structure of the defective elastic membranes. Am. J. Pathol., 51:117–135, 1967.

Wiener, G.: Genetic and other factors in the occurrence of swayback in sheep. J. Comp. Pathol., 76:435–447, 1966.

COBALT

Small amounts of cobalt, usually provided by the soil and the herbage that grows upon it, are necessary in ruminants only. Without sufficient cobalt, the numbers of bacteria in the rumen decline and the prevailing species change unfavorably. Since vitamin B_{12} is synthesized by ruminal bacteria and since cobalt is an essential constituent (4%) of that substance, it appears that the lack of adequate cobalt is deleterious to the bacteria, preventing their growth, and to the host animal through absence of vitamin B_{12}. The latter is essential in erythropoiesis, in growth, and probably in other ways. Attempts to produce cobalt deficiency disease in experimental animals have failed, although the element does stimulate erythropoiesis, even to the extent of producing polycythemia.

"Grand Traverse disease" of the American Great Lakes region, "pine" in England (so-called because animals pine away and die), "hill sickness" in New Zealand, and "coast disease," "wasting disease," and **enzootic marasmus** in Australia are examples of a cachectic syndrome in which cattle or sheep, after grazing on a certain pasturage for several months, lose their appetites, waste away, and die while still in the midst of ample amounts of the same food plants. Since affected animals were anemic, attempts were naturally made to cure them by giving iron. It was found that certain impure iron salts would effect a cure, but that the curative properties of such salts ("limonite" in Australia) were not proportional to their iron content. Further study showed that cobalt, existing as an impurity, was the effective ingredient. Iron, indeed, is stored in excess in the tissues of the sick animals. In the "coast disease" of Australian sheep, both cobalt

and copper have been found to be lacking, the symptoms and lesions combining those characteristic of enzootic marasmus with demyelinization and destruction of certain tracts in the spinal cord.

The lesions of enzootic marasmus are anemia and marked hemosiderosis of the liver, spleen, kidneys, and other organs. The hemosiderin, or material indistinguishable from it, probably represents a storage of iron which should be, but cannot be, utilized. Fatty change of the liver is also prominent.

Cobalt has been described in one report as effective in prevention of cerebrocortical necrosis in sheep. This effect is presumed to work through stimulation of rumenal bacteria, which produce thiamine or inhibit production of thiaminase.

Andres, E.D., Hart, L.I., and Stephenson, B.J.: Vitamin B_{12} and cobalt concentrations in livers from healthy and cobalt-deficient lambs. Nature (Lond.), 182:869–870, 1958.

Decker, D.E., and Smith, L.E.: The metabolism of cobalt in lambs. J. Nutr., 43:87–100, 1951.

Filmer, J.F.: Enzootic marasmus of cattle and sheep. Aust. Vet. J., 9:163–179, 1933.

Filmer, J.F., and Underwood, E.J.: Enzootic marasmus; treatment with limonite fractions. Aust. Vet. J., 10:83–87, 1934.

Gardiner, M.R., and Nicol, H.: Cobalt-selenium interactions in the nutrition of the rat. Aust. J. Exp. Biol. Med. Sci., 49:291–296, 1971.

Ibbotson, R.N., Allen, S.H., and Gurney, C.W.: An abnormality of the bone-marrow of sheep fed cobalt-deficient hay chaff. Aust. J. Exp. Biol. Med. Sci., 48:161–169, 1970.

Keener, H.A., Percival, G.P., and Morrow, K.S.: Cobalt deficiency in New Hampshire with sheep. J. Anim. Sci., 7:16–25, 1948.

MacPherson, A., Moon, F.E., and Voss, R.C.: Biochemical aspects of cobalt deficiency in sheep with special reference to vitamin status and a possible involvement in the aetiology of cerebrocortical necrosis. Br. Vet. J., 132:294–308, 1976.

O'Moore, L.B., and Smyth, P.J.: The control of cobalt deficiency in sheep by means of a heavy pellet (containing cobaltic oxide). Vet. Rec., 70:773–774, 1958.

Tokarnia, C.H., et al.: Cobalt deficiency in cattle in the state of Ceara, Brazil (TT). Arq. Inst. Biol. Anim. Rio de J., 4:195–202, 1963.

Underwood, E.J., and Filmer, J.F.: The determination of the biologically potent element cobalt in limonite. Aust. Vet. J., 11:84–92, 1935.

Underwood, E.J.: Cobalt. Nutr. Rev., 33:65–69, 1975.

Wessels, C.C.: Cobalt in relation to ruminant nutrition in South Africa. J. S. Afr. Vet. Med. Assoc., 32:289–312, 1961.

Rojas, M.A., Dyer, I.A., and Cassatt, W.A.: Manganese deficiency in the bovine. J. Anim. Sci., 24:664–667, 1965.

MANGANESE

Small amounts of manganese are essential for several mechanisms of the body. Experimental deficiency in rats on artificially concocted diets results in aspermatogenesis, weak and defective offspring, and retarded growth. In rats, rabbits, swine, cattle, and avians, there is suppression of epiphyseal cartilage cell proliferation and reduced osteoblastic activity resulting in decreased growth, rarefaction of bone, bowing and fractures, joint deformities, and tendon slippage. However, deficiency of this element does not occur clinically except in birds, although it has been suggested as a cause of spontaneous lameness and joint deformity in swine. In chickens and turkeys, a deformity of the hock joint known as **perosis** or "slipped tendon" is frequent at an age of several weeks. In this condition, the epiphyseal cartilage fails to ossify, as it normally should at 12 weeks in chickens; the epiphysis loosens and the tendon of the gastrocnemius slips medially. Deficiency of choline has also been blamed for this disorder. Many deformed chicks, having short, thick legs and wings and globular heads, are hatched from eggs of manganese-deficient hens, an interesting example of a developmental defect due to malnutrition.

Amdur, M.O., Norris, L.C., and Heuser, G.F.: The need for manganese in bone development by the rat. Proc. Soc. Exp. Biol. Med., 59:254–255, 1945.

Barnes, L.L., Sperling, G., and Maynard, L.A.: Bone development in the albino rat on a low manganese diet. Proc. Soc. Exp. Biol. Med., 46:562–565, 1941.

Miller, R.C., et al.: Manganese as a possible factor influencing the occurrence of lameness in pigs. Proc. Soc. Exp. Biol. Med., 45:50–51, 1940.

Neher, G.M., et al.: Radiographic and histopathological findings in the bones of swine deficient in manganese. Am. J. Vet. Res., 17:121–128, 1956.

Oliver, J.W.: Interrelationships between athyreotic and manganese-deficient states in rats. Am. J. Vet. Res., 37:597–600, 1976.

ZINC

Zinc was recognized as a dietary essential to the animal economy in very small amounts over three decades ago, but clinical deficiency has only recently been described. **Parakeratosis** of swine, first described by Kernkamp and Ferrin (1953), is now accepted as the result of zinc deficiency. Although the exact circumstances that bring about zinc deficiency in swine are not entirely understood, it has been established that excess dietary calcium interferes with zinc absorption. Addition of zinc to the ration and adjusting calcium intake dramatically cures or prevents parakeratosis. Available evidence suggests that calcium in conjunction with either phytate or phosphate forms a complex with zinc, making it unavailable for absorption.

Parakeratosis usually appears in young swine 10 to 20 weeks of age and is manifested by circumscribed erythematous areas, 3 to 5 cm in diameter, particularly in the skin of the abdomen and medial surfaces of the thighs. An elevated, scaly character is soon assumed by these affected areas, and the lesions become widespread with a symmetric distribution. The surface layer of keratin becomes increasingly thick, rough, horny, and fissured. The hairs are not lost, but are often entangled and matted in the superficial horny material. The appetite may be impaired and the rate of gain somewhat reduced, but often signs are inconstant and probably not specific.

The microscopic appearance of the affected skin is dominated by parakeratosis and acanthosis, with elongation and congestion of dermal papillae and disappearance of the stratum granulosum. In the thick, horny parakeratotic layer, retained nuclei are usually seen in undulating, irregular rows and sometimes are mixed with cellular debris. In some areas, the stratum germinativum is thinner than normal, but acanthosis appears to be the rule.

Experimental zinc deficiency was first induced in rats and mice, but has also been described in lambs, calves, dogs, and monkeys. In each of these species, the ensuing disease is dominated by loss of hair or wool and acanthosis and parakeratosis of the skin, esophagus, and oral mucosa. Lesions have also been reported in the testicle and bone, but it has not clearly been shown whether they result from zinc deficiency or inanition.

Facial eczema, a disease of cattle described in New Zealand, is manifest by eczema on the face and other parts of the body, weight loss, and occasionally death. This condition responds quite favorably, at least in one report, to dietary supplementation with zinc sulfate in the drinking water (Rickard, 1975). **Infectious pododermatitis**, involving dermatitis in the cleft between the digits in cattle, is also reported to respond favorably to feeding of zinc (Demertzis and Mills, 1973).

Hereditary thymic hypoplasia (adema disease) as seen in newborn calves, which have cutaneous exanthema and gastroenteric lesions as well as immunodeficiency, also responds well to zinc therapy. A similar disease in human infants, **acrodermatitis enteropathica,** is also inherited as an autosomal recessive lethal disease, but responds dramatically following oral feeding of zinc. In both of these conditions there is a genetic inability to absorb zinc through the gastrointestinal tract. The mechanism leading to thymic hypoplasia is not entirely clear but thought to relate to the role of zinc in various metalloenzymes necessary for DNA synthesis. Another different heritable anomaly in adult human beings is inherited as a dominant trait and is manifest by high levels of zinc in the blood (Smith et al., 1976).

Brummerstedt, E., Flagstad, T., Basse, A., and Andresen, E.: The effect of zinc on calves with heredi-

tary thymus hypoplasia. Acta Pathol. Microbiol. Scand., 79A:686–687, 1971.

Dahmer, E.J., Coleman, B.W., Grummer, R.H., and Hoekstra, W.G.: Alleviation of parakeratosis in zinc deficient swine by high levels of dietary histidine. J. Anim. Sci., 35:1181–1189, 1972.

Demertzis, P.N., and Mills, C.F.: Oral zinc therapy in the control of infectious pododermatitis in young bulls. Vet. Rec., 93:219–222, 1973.

Gainer, J.H.: Effects of heavy metals and of deficiency of zinc on mortality rates in mice infected with encephalomyocarditis virus. Am. J. Vet. Res., 38:869–872, 1977.

Hanson, L.J., Sorensen, D.K., and Kernkamp, H.C.H.: Essential fatty acid deficiency—its role in parakeratosis. Am. J. Vet. Res., 19:921–930, 1958.

Kernkamp, H.C.H., and Ferrin, E.F.: Parakeratosis in swine. J. Am. Vet. Med. Assoc., 123:217–220, 1953.

Kienholz, E.W., et al.: Effects of zinc deficiency in the diets of hens. J. Nutr., 75:211–221, 1961.

Kroneman, J., van der Mey, G.J.M., and Helder, A.: Hereditary zinc deficiency in Dutch Friesian cattle. Zentralbl. Veterinaermed., 22A:201–208, 1975.

Macapinlaf, M.P., et al.: Production of zinc deficiency in the squirrel monkey (Saimiri sciureus). J. Nutr., 93:499–510, 1967.

McKenzie, J.M., Fosmire, G.J., and Sandstead, H.H.: Zinc deficiency during the latter third of pregnancy: effects on fetal rat brain, liver and placenta. J. Nutr., 105:1466–1475, 1975.

Miller, W.J., Blackman, D.M., Gentry, R.P., and Pate, F.M.: Zinc distribution in various tissues of zinc-deficient and normal bull calves with time after single intravenous or oral dosing. J. Anim. Sci., 31:149–156, 1970.

Miller, W.J.: Dynamics of absorption rates, endogenous excretion, tissue turnover, and homeostatic control mechanisms of zinc, cadmium, manganese, and nickel in ruminants. Fed. Proc., 32:1915–1920, 1973.

Mills, C.F., et al.: The production and signs of zinc deficiency in the sheep. Proc. Nutr. Soc., 24:21–22, 1965.

Norrdin, R.W., Krook, L., Pond, W.G., and Walker, E.F.: Experimental zinc deficiency in weanling pigs on high and low calcium diets. Cornell Vet., 63:264–290, 1973.

Oberleas, D., Muhrer, M.E., and O'Dell, B.L.: Effects of phytic acid on zinc availability and parakeratosis in swine. J. Anim. Sci., 21:57–61, 1962.

Pierson, R.E.: Zinc deficiency in young lambs. J. Am. Vet. Med. Assoc., 149:1279–1282, 1966.

Prasad, A.S. (ed.): Zinc Metabolism. Springfield, Charles C Thomas, 1966.

Rickard, B.F.: Facial eczema: zinc responsiveness in dairy cattle. NZ Vet. J., 23:41–42, 1975.

Robertson, B.T., and Burns, M.J.: Zinc metabolism and the zinc-deficiency syndrome in the dog. Am. J. Vet. Res., 24:997–1002, 1963.

Sandstead, H.H., et al.: Zinc deficiency in pregnant

rhesus monkeys: effects on behavior of infants. Am. J. Clin. Nutr., 31:844–849, 1978.

Shaw, N.A., et al.: Zinc deficiency in female rabbits. Lab. Anim., 8:1–7, 1974.

Shrader, R.E., and Hurley, L.S.: Enzyme histochemistry of peripheral blood and bone marrow in zinc-deficient rats. Lab. Invest., 26:566–571, 1972.

Smith, J.C., Jr., Zeller, J.A., Brown, E.D., and Ong, S.C.: Elevated plasma zinc: a heritable anomaly. Science, 193:496–498, 1976.

Stevens, M.D., MacKenzie, W.F., and Anand, V.D.: Influence of cage material on amount of zinc in blood of the rhesus monkey (Macaca mulatta). Vet. Pathol., 14:508–509, 1977.

Tucker, H.F., and Salmon, W.D.: Parakeratosis or zinc deficiency disease in the pig. Proc. Soc. Exp. Biol. Med., 88:613–616, 1955.

Vallee, B.L.: Biochemistry, physiology and pathology of zinc. Physiol. Rev., 39:443–490, 1959. (359 references.)

Van Preenen, H.J., and Patel, A.: Tissue zinc and calcium in chronic disease. Arch. Pathol., 77:53–56, 1964.

Weisman, K., and Flagstad, T.: Hereditary zinc deficiency (adema disease) in cattle, an animal parallel to acrodermatitis enteropathica. Acta Derm. Venereol. (Stockh.) 56:151–154, 1976.

IODINE

Iodine received into the circulation is, even within minutes, stored in the thyroid gland, where it is gradually converted into the active principle of the thyroid hormone, thyroxin.

Deficiency of iodine causes **goiter**. The usual type of goiter seen in animals makes its appearance with birth and is the hyperplastic type characteristic of cretinism in the human. As has been seen in the case of a number of other elements, the amount of iodine available to the animal depends on the amount in the soil. Certain areas (e.g., the Great Lakes region and the Pacific Northwest in the United States, the Swiss Alps) are known as endemic, goiter-producing regions because of their iodine-deficient soils and water.

The goiters in newborn colts, calves, lambs, and pigs are often of conspicuous size. In swine, there is a strong tendency for the pigs to be born with little or no hair—**hairless pigs**. Untreated, such animals either develop poorly or die. The condition is easily avoided by administration of minute amounts of iodine to the pregnant mother. After birth, the same treatment applied to the offspring is only moderately successful.

A great excess of absorbed iodine produces the condition known as **iodism**. This occurs when iodine or its compounds are administered internally or externally in maximal dosages over a period of time. It is characterized by lacrimation and exfoliation of dandruff-like epidermal scales and possibly cutaneous eruptions and pharyngitis.

Andrews, F.N., et al.: Iodine deficiency in new-born sheep and swine. J. Anim. Sci., 7:298–310, 1948.

Evvard, J.M.: Iodine deficiency symptoms and their significance in animal nutrition and pathology. Endocrinology, 12:539–590, 1928.

PROTEINS AND AMINO ACIDS

The usual difficulty here is simply a lack of total protein, which results in slow growth and poor reproductive and other functions. About ten of the amino acids are known to be indispensable, and a variety of symptoms and lesions have been produced by experimental exclusion of various ones. However, such deprivations do not occur except experimentally.

Several common farm feeds are moderately deficient in certain essential amino acids and may cause difficulty if fed alone. Indian corn (maize) is especially deficient in lysine and tryptophan; other grains, linseed meal, and cotton-seed meal are less so in descending order. Peanuts are deficient in methionine and soybeans are less so. The principal signs of deficiency of amino acids in general are hypoproteinemia, anemia, poor growth, and delayed healing of wounds. Any of these disorders have other more frequent causes.

Even in experimentally induced protein deficiency the lesions are not specific. The major pathologic changes include cessation of cell proliferation of epiphyseal cartilages, reduced osteoblastic activity, failure of collagen formation, atrophy of endocrine glands including testicle and ovary, atrophy of thymus and lymphoid tissues, anemia, hypoproteinemia, and edema. These lesions develop in animals following protracted periods of inanition, which accompany many diseases including nutritional deficiencies. The pathologist must exert extreme caution in assigning these changes to a specific nutrient deficiency or other cause.

Interest in protein nutrition has intensified because of the increased frequency of a protein-caloric deficiency, which results in diseases of children called **kwashiorkor** or **marasmus.** Many questions about the human diseases have led to experimental studies on animals, especially nonhuman primates, in an effort to determine the short- and long-term effects of this deprivation. The details of the numerous findings attributed to dietary deficiency of protein and calories are outside the scope of this book, and in many instances require confirmation. The appended references will start one on the search of the literature on this subject.

Specific effects have been attributed to certain amino acid deficiencies. Experimental deficiency of tryptophan, a precursor of niacin, results in alopecia, cataracts, corneal vascularization, necrosis of skeletal muscle, and fatty change in the liver. Methionine deficiency also results in fatty change of the liver, presumably owing to its role in choline synthesis. Lysine deficiency in rats causes achromotrichia.

Ausman, L.M., et al.: Acute erythroid hypoplasia in malnourished infant squirrel monkeys fed isolated soy protein. Am. J. Clin. Nutr., 30:1713–1720, 1977.

Bhuyan, U.N., and Ramalingaswami, V.: Lymphopoiesis in protein deficiency. Stathmokinetic and tritiated thymidine uptake studies of the mesenteric lymph node of the guinea pig. Am. J. Pathol., 75:315–328, 1974.

Deo, M.G., and Mathur, M.: Immune and nonimmune defense mechanisms in protein deficiency. Indian J. Pathol. Bacteriol., 17:79–90, 1974.

Enwonwu, C.O., Worthington, B.S., and Jacobson, K.L.: Protein energy malnutrition in infant nonhuman primates *(Macaca nemestrina)*: I. Correlation of biochemical changes with fine structural alterations in liver. Br. J. Exp. Pathol., 58:78–94, 1977.

Felsenfeld, O., Gyr, K., and Wolf, R.H.: Malnutrition and susceptibility to infection with *Vibrio cholerae* in vervet monkeys *(Cercopithecus aethiops)*. 1. Induction of protein, B-vitamin complex and calorie malnutrition. J. Med. Primatol., 5:186–194, 1976.

——: Malnutrition and susceptibility to infection with *Vibrio cholerae* in vervet monkeys *(Cercopithecus aethiops)*: 2. Response of vervet monkeys on protein, B-vitamin complex and calorie-deficient diets to infection. J. Med. Primatol., 5:305–311, 1976.

Fleagle, J.G., Samonds, K.W., and Hegsted, D.M.: Physical growth of cebus monkeys, *Cebus albifrons* during protein or calorie deficiency. Am. J. Clin. Nutr., 28:246–253, 1975.

Gallina, D.L., and Ausman, L.M.: Diabetic-like syndrome associated with protein malnutrition in squirrel monkeys. Fed. Proc., 34:921, 1975.

Geist, C.R., Zimmermann, R.R., Smith, O.W., and Geist, E.M.: Emergence of a kwashiorkor-like syndrome associated with protein-calorie malnutrition in the developing rhesus monkey *(Macaca mulatta)*. Psychol. Rep., 40:1330–1344, 1977.

Hillman, N.M., and Riopelle, A.J.: Protein deprivation in primates: VII. Food preferences of juvenile rhesus monkeys. Percept. Mot. Skills, 45:3–10, 1977.

Isoun, T.T.: The influence of infectious diarrhoea on plasma phenylalanine and tyrosine values in experimental protein-calorie malnutrition in pigs. West Afr. J. Biol. Appl. Chem., 16:23–28, 1973.

Jacobson, H.N.: Protein deficiency in primates. Am. J. Clin. Nutr., 28:801–802, 1975.

LaMotte, G.B.: Total serum protein, serum protein fractions and serum immunoglobulins in colostrum-fed and colostrum-deprived calves. Am. J. Vet. Res., 38:263–268, 1977.

Lombardi, B., and Oler, A.: Choline deficiency fatty liver. Protein synthesis and release. Lab. Invest., 17:308–321, 1967.

Manocha, S.L.: Experimental protein malnutrition in primates: histochemical studies on dorsal root ganglion cells of healthy and malnourished squirrel monkeys, *Saimiri sciureus*. Acta Histochem. (Jena), 47:220–232, 1973.

Manocha, S.L., and Olkowski, Z.L.: Experimental protein malnutrition in primates—cytochemistry of the nervous system. Am. J. Phys. Anthropol., 38:439–445, 1973.

——: Experimental protein malnutrition in primates: cytochemical studies on cerebellum of the squirrel monkey, *Saimiri sciureus*. Histochem. J., 5:105–118, 1973.

Olkowski, Z., and Manocha, S.L.: Experimental protein malnutrition in squirrel monkeys: reaction of the Nissl substance in the motor neurons of the spinal cord. Histochemie, 30:281–288, 1972.

Platt, B.S., and Stewart, R.J.C.: Experimental protein-calorie deficiency: histopathological changes in the endocrine glands of pigs. J. Endocrinol., 38:121–143, 1967.

Portman, O.W., et al.: Effects of perinatal malnutrition on lipid composition of neural tissues from rhesus monkeys. J. Nutr., *107*:2228–2235, 1977.

Riopelle, A.J., et al.: Protein deficiency in primates. IV. Pregnant rhesus monkey. Am. J. Clin. Nutr., *28*:20–28, 1975.

Roberts, E.D., Gallo, J.T., and Maner, J.H.: Protein deficiency in swine and use of opaque-2 corn to prevent changes in bone: Light, fluorescence, and electron microscopy study. Am. J. Vet. Res., *33*:1985–1994, 1972.

Schalm, O.W.: Hypoproteinemia in the dog. Calif. Vet., *28*:6–14, 1974.

Slocum, S.V., and Strobel, D.: Rehabilitation of protein deficient rhesus macaques. Am. J. Phys. Anthropol., *47*:161, 1977.

Vijai, K.K., and Manocha, S.L.: Maternal protein malnutrition of squirrel monkeys during pregnancy and biochemical alteration of nucleic acids and proteins in cerebellar cortex of neonates. Anat. Rec., *181*:500, 1975.

LIPID

Fat is an important dietary component because it supplies essential fatty acids, serves as a carrier for fat-soluble vitamins, has high caloric value, and adds palatability to food. Deficiency of fat per se probably does not exist in domestic animals. Deficiency of essential fatty acids (linolenic, arachidonic, and linoleic) has been produced and studied in experimental animals and is often suggested as a cause of ill-defined dermatoses in animals. Dietary supplementation with fats occasionally results in improvement of certain skin disorders, but virtually no sound study has demonstrated fatty acids to be specific for the "cure." For changes to take place in the skin of dogs, experimental fatty acid deficiency requires months to years. The earliest change is dryness, followed by alopecia and scaling. Microscopically, the epidermis is thickened due to an increase in cells and hyperkeratosis. Hair follicles become hypercellular and plugged with keratin, and sebaceous glands increase in size. The dermis becomes edematous and infiltrated with mononuclear cells.

Armstrong, M.J., Nicolosi, R.J., and Hayes, K.C.: Substrate availability for LCAT in cebus monkeys fed saturated fat. Clin. Res., *25*:A534, 1977.

Brady, R.O.: The abnormal biochemistry of inherited disorders of lipid metabolism. Fed. Proc., *6*:1660–1667, 1973.

Crawford, M.A., Rivers, J.P.W., and Hassam, A.G.: Comparative studies on the metabolic equivalence of linoleic and arachidonic acids. Nutr. Metab., *21*:189–190, 1977.

Dietschy, J.M., and Wilson, J.D.: Regulation of cholesterol metabolism. N. Engl. J. Med., *282*:1128–1138, 1970.

———: Regulation of cholesterol metabolism (second part of three). N. Engl. J. Med., *282*:1179–1184, 1970.

———: Regulation of cholesterol metabolism (third of three parts). N. Engl. J. Med., *282*:1241–1250, 1970.

Hansen, A.E., and Wiese, H.F.: Fat in the diet in relation to nutrition of the dog. I. Characteristic appearance and gross changes of animals fed diets with and without fats. Texas Rep. Biol. Med., *9*:491–515, 1951.

Hansen, A.E., Holmes, S.G., and Wiese, H.F.: Fat in the diet in relation to nutrition of the dog. IV. Histologic features of skin from animals fed diets with or without fat. Texas Rep. Biol. Med., *9*:555–570, 1951.

Hansen, A.E., Sinclair, J.G., and Wiese, H.F.: Sequence of histologic changes in skin of dogs in relation to dietary fat. J. Nutr., *52*:541–554, 1954.

Hoilund, L.J., et al.: Essential fatty acid deficiency in the rat. I. Clinical syndrome, histopathology, and hematopathology. Lab. Invest., *23*:58–70, 1970.

Jones, D.C., Lofland, H.B., Clarkson, T.B., and St. Clair. R.W.: Plasma cholesterol concentrations in squirrel monkeys as influenced by diet and phenotype. J. Food Sci., *40*:2–7, 1975.

McCullagh, K.G.: Are African elephants deficient in essential fatty acids? Nature, *242*:267–268, 1973.

Percy, D.H., and Jortner, B.S.: Feline lipidosis. Arch. Pathol., *92*:136–144, 1971.

Rivers, J.P.W., Sinclair, A.J., and Crawford, M.A.: Inability of the cat to desaturate essential fatty acids. Nature, *258*:171–173, 1975.

Rivers, J.P.W., Hassam, A.G., and Crawford, M.A.: The comparative nutrition of essential fatty acid metabolism. Nutr. Metab., *20*:193, 1976.

Seiler, M.W., et al.: Hyperlipemia in the gerbil: effect of diet on serum lipids and hepatic glucokinase. Am. J. Physiol., *221*:548–553, 1971.

Sinclair, A.J., et al.: Linolenic acid deprivation in capuchin monkeys. Proc. Nutr. Soc., *33*:A49–A50, 1974.

Turton, J.A., et al.: Composition of the milk of the common marmoset (*Callithrix jacchus*) and milk substitutes used in hand-rearing programmes, with special reference to fatty acids. Folia Primatol., *29*:64–79, 1978.

Wensing, T., van Gent, C.M., Schotman, A.J.H., and Kroneman, J.: Hyperlipoproteinaemia in ponies: mechanisms and response to therapy. Clin. Chim. Acta, *58*:1–15, 1975.

WATER

Unfortunately, many veterinary patients, ill with various diseases, actually die because of excessive loss and inadequate replacement of water. Clinicians learn to detect this situation (dehydration) partly by a slight wrinkling of the skin, which seems just a bit too big for the body it covers, and of course, by a gauntness of the flanks and abdomen. Frequently, the patient is too weak or apathetic to get water in the usual way and injections of water or physiologic saline solution are necessitated. A blood-cell count made on such a patient gives an abnormally high count of both white and red cells—relative polycythemia. Conditions tending to cause dehydration are (1) fever, (2) diseases accompanied by vomiting or diarrhea, (3) severe hemorrhage, (4) polyuria, as in diabetes. Dehydration resulting from renal disease, protracted diarrhea or vomiting, and metabolic disturbances such as diabetes mellitus are obviously complicated by other deficiencies, such as sodium loss and potassium loss, and by altered acid-base balance. Pathologic findings in dehydration are minimal. Little or no fluid will be evident in the pericardial, pleural, and thoracic cavities, and the serosal membranes are dry and appear to have lost their usual glistening character.

Deprivation of water is more common in animals than the published literature indicates. Animals may be herded into a lot without water and overlooked for days (Lindley, 1977). The attendant may fail to give water to animals kept in enclosed quarters. The automatic drinking device or water bottle may become occluded for some reason and deprive laboratory animals of water. "Everyone" knows that all animals require water from some source, but it is an alert husbandman who never fails to provide this essential.

Deprivation of water, by freezing for example, is always a hazard to livestock. Affected swine respond to lack of water in much the same way as to salt poisoning.

Lindley, W.H.: Water deprivation in cattle. J. Am. Vet. Med. Assoc., *171*:439–440, 1977.
Shimamura, T., and Trojanowski, S.: Effects of repeated deprivation of drinking water on the structure of renal medulla of rats. Am. J. Pathol., *84*:87–92, 1976.
Sinha, R.P., and Ganapathy, M.S.: Studies on experimental dehydration in canines with particular reference to clinical picture, haemoglobin concentration, hematocrit, specific gravity of the plasma and plasma sodium concentration. Indian Vet. J., *44*:127–136, 1967.

KETOSIS

Ketosis, also known as **acetonemia**, is a condition in which "ketone bodies," or "acetone bodies," appear in the blood and thence in the urine. The ketone substances are the three chemical compounds, beta-hydroxybutyric acid, acetoacetic acid, and acetone. Numerous theories have been advanced to explain the biochemical events leading to ketosis, but the pathogenesis of ketosis, especially the "specific disease" termed bovine ketosis, remains in a state of confusion. No attempt will be made here to discuss the various hypotheses and experimental data available, our intention being to concentrate on the salient features of the disease; however, certain biochemical events deserve brief comment. In all species, ketosis develops in response to a decrease in the availability of blood glucose, whether from hypoglycemia or inability to utilize glucose as in diabetes mellitus. To compensate for the "lack" of glucose, oxidation of fatty acids provides an alternate source of energy. This is accompanied by production of ketone bodies, which serve as a source of cellular energy. If the serum levels of ketone bodies do not reach a "pathologic" level, the process is considered a normal physiologic process of supplying tissues with a readily utilizable fuel when glucose is not available. However, in the face of a high rate of gluconeogenesis which accompanies clinical ketosis, oxaloacetate becomes unavailable to allow the incorporation of fatty acids into the tricarboxylic acid cycle, which results in continual production of ketone bodies, which eventually reach harmful levels.

The symptoms of ketosis include anorexia, depression, and terminal coma.

The animal often has a sickly sweet smell derived from ketone bodies.

Lesions. Lesions are primarily chemical. The **ketone substances** are detected in the blood serum by appropriate tests, but the usual diagnostic procedure is a test for acetone in the urine. If this is strongly positive, it can be assumed that the acetoacetic and beta-hydroxybutyric acids are also present. In cows, it may be more convenient to test the milk for acetone than the urine. The concentration of acetone in the milk is comparable to that in the blood; in the urine, it is several times greater. A noticeable degree of **hyperlipemia** accompanies the mobilization of stored body fat. The increased presentation of free fatty acids to the liver leads to accumulation of neutral fat in the hepatocytes, i.e., fatty change. **Acidosis,** a depletion of the body's reserve of alkaline ions, chiefly those in $NaHCO_3$, results from the neutralization of the two ketone acids. This loss of alkali is thought to be mainly responsible for the symptoms manifested. **Hypoglycemia** and a reduction in hepatic glycogen are also consistent findings in bovine ketosis.

Causes. The usual cause of ketosis in animals is **starvation**. The animal then derives its necessary energy by oxidation of its stored fats, later of proteins of the muscles. The usual clinical case of ketosis in bovines results from loss of appetite and failure to eat. It thus depends upon the presence of some other disorder, most often rumenal indigestion or atony. Some of the coarser roughages, such as straw, contain little digestible carbohydrate, so that the development of ketosis becomes easy. Coarse dry roughages contain carbohydrate mostly in the form of cellulose. This is to some extent digestible with the aid of the lytic activities of bacteria normally growing in the rumen. Rather minor functional disturbances of the rumen often cause an environment unfavorable for bacterial growth with an abrupt shortage of carbohydrate and development of ketosis. Digestive disorders that prevent assimila-

tion cause it in any species. These forms of ketosis, whether in the bovine or monogastric animals, have been termed **primary nutritional ketosis** (simple starvation) and **secondary ketosis** (starvation on account of some other disease).

Primary spontaneous ketosis is a phrase applied to bovine ketosis which develops in cattle under a good plane of nutrition and in the absence of another recognizable disorder that interferes with appetite or nutrient utilization. A hereditary predisposition has been presumed, but adequate proof is lacking. This form of bovine ketosis is most frequent in cows during the first few weeks after parturition.

Ketosis is also caused by diabetes mellitus and by severe toxic damage to the liver, as from phosphorus or carbon tetrachloride, which prevents the metabolism and storage of glycogen. It is possible to produce ketosis in carnivora and omnivora by a **ketogenic diet**, that is one containing much fat and little carbohydrate. This is sometimes done with a view to producing acidosis and a more acid urine, which is unfavorable to the formation of certain kinds of urinary calculi or the growth of certain pathogenic bacteria. Temporary deficiency of adrenal glucocorticoids has also been advocated as a cause.

Pregnancy Disease of Ewes

Known also as "pregnant-ewe paralysis" and toxemia of pregnancy, this disease is at once an outstanding example of ketosis and of a toxemia of pregnancy. The symptoms are depression, somnolence, and coma, but not true paralysis. These are characteristic of ketosis and hypoglycemia, and verification is furnished by chemical examination of the blood. However, the disease, which is frequently seen and usually fatal in a few days, occurs only in the last weeks of pregnancy, and usually in ewes carrying twins or triplets. Birth or abortion is likely to be curative if not postponed too long. The lesions are severe fatty change of the liver, kidneys and heart (ketosis) with terminal subepicardial petechiae and ecchymoses (toxemia).

Causes. The causes are a combination of the toxic waste products of mother and fetuses, plus dietary difficulties of the kind that cause ketosis. Sometimes these are plain starvation, but more often there is semistarvation on a non-nutritious ration such as corn stalks or wheat straw. If the ewe was previously well supplied with stored fat, ketosis is even more likely to arise. An abrupt diminution in the accustomed amount of exercise is also contributory. Some believe this is because ketone substances are consumed in the muscles, a physiologic concept that is not altogether proved. Since the disease rarely occurs in nonpregnant sheep, it is evident that either set of causes without the other can usually be endured.

Pregnancy toxemia is also known in guinea pigs and nonhuman primates. In guinea pigs, the disease usually appears in the later stages of pregnancy and is usually relieved by parturition. The clinical signs are rapid onset of acidosis, proteinuria, hyperexcitability (followed by coma), severe hyperlipidemia, ketosis, and death within five days. Parturition often interrupts the course of the disease. The disease may be induced in obese guinea pigs, whether pregnant or not, by a period of starvation.

Ketosis has also been described in South American monkeys *(Callicebus moloch)* and chimpanzees *(Pan troglodytes)*. In these nonhuman primates, depression and terminal coma were observed. Ketone bodies were found in the urine. Pathologic lesions included fatty change in the liver, kidneys, and myocardium (Seibold, 1969).

Ambo, K., et al.: Studies on ketosis in ruminants. II. Principal site of ketone body formation (TT). Jpn. J. Vet. Sci., 23:265–273, 1961.

Ganaway, J.R., and Allen, A.M.: Obesity predisposes to pregnancy toxemia (ketosis) of guinea pigs. Lab. Anim. Sci., 21:40–44, 1971.

Jasper, D.E.: Acute and prolonged insulin hypoglycemia in cows. Am. J. Vet. Res., 14:184–191, 1953.

——: Prolonged insulin hypoglycemia in sheep. Am. J. Vet. Res., 14:209–213, 1953.

Krebs, H.A.: Bovine ketosis. Vet. Rec., 78:187–192, 1966.

Kronfeld, D.S.: The hypoglycemia of bovine ketosis: its metabolic origin and clinical effects. Proc. 17th World Vet. Congr., Hanover, 2:1315–1317, 1963.

Pehrson, B.: Studies on ketosis in dairy cows. Acta Vet. Scand. Suppl., 15:1–59, 1966.

Procos, J.: Ovine ketosis. I. The normal ketone body values. Onder. J. Vet. Res., 28:557–567, 1961.

Reid, I.M.: An ultrastructural and morphometric study of the liver of the lactating cow in starvation ketosis. Exp. Mol. Pathol., 18:316–330, 1973.

Reid, R.L.: The physiopathology of undernourishment in pregnant sheep, with particular reference to pregnancy toxemia. Adv. Vet. Sci., 12:163–238, 1968.

Roderick, L.M., Harshfield, G.S., and Hawn, M.C.: The pathogenesis of ketosis: pregnancy disease of sheep. J. Am. Vet. Med. Assoc., 90:41–50, 1937.

Saba, N., et al.: Some biochemical and hormonal aspects of experimental ovine pregnancy toxaemia. J. Agric. Sci. Camb., 67:129–138, 1966.

Sampson, J.: The significance of hypoglycemia. J. Am. Vet. Med. Assoc., 112:350–352, 1948.

Seibold, H.E.: Ketosis in subhuman primates. Lab. Anim. Care., 19:826–830, 1969.

Van Den Hende, C., Oyaert, W., and Bouckaert, J.H.: I. Fermentation of glutamic acid by rumen bacteria. II. Metabolism of glycine, valine, leucine, and isoleucine by rumen bacteria. Res. Vet. Sci., 4:367–381 and 382–389, 1963.

CHAPTER 18

The Skin and Its Appendages

Consideration is given in this chapter to those diseases of the skin and adnexa which are of unknown or uncertain etiology; diseases of known causation are described elsewhere in this book. Especial attention is invited to Chapter 4 (neoplasms), Chapter 8 (inherited diseases), Chapter 9 (pox, vesicular exanthema, aphthous fever, vesicular stomatitis, contagious ecthyma, papillomatosis), Chapter 11 (staphylococcal infections), Chapter 12 (dermatomycoses, epizootic lymphangitis, blastomycosis, maduramycosis), Chapter 13 (dourine), Chapter 14 (helminth and arthropod parasites), Chapter 15 (ionizing radiation) and Chapter 16 (photosensitization, hyperkeratosis), and Chapter 17 (parakeratosis or zinc deficiency). The mammary glands are anatomically part of the integument but are considered with the reproductive system of which they are a functional part.

ANATOMY AND HISTOLOGY

The skin of animals presents particular problems to the pathologist, not only because of the complexity of its components in various parts of the body, but also because of the many differences between species. Knowledge of normal histology is therefore particularly important to the interpretation of lesions of the skin.

The skin has three principal layers: the epidermis, dermis (or derma), and sub-cutis (or hypodermis), each of which has definite structure and function and is subject to specific pathologic changes. The **epidermis**, the most superficial layer, is made up of stratified squamous epithelium in which the following layers can be distinguished in those parts of the body in which the skin is thickest:

Stratum corneum, or horny layer, is the most superficial and consists of flattened cells that have lost their nuclei and consist principally of keratin.

Stratum lucidum, or clear layer, lies just under the stratum corneum, is present only in some regions of the skin, and consists of a layer two or three cells thick which appears as a clear wavy stripe in histologic sections. It contains eleidin, which comes from the dissolution of keratohyaline granules found in the deeper adjoining layer. The cells have lost their nuclei.

Stratum granulosum, or granular layer, is made up of rows two to five epithelial cells in depth in which the cells are rhomboid-shaped and whose cytoplasm is filled with dark-staining basophilic keratohyalin granules. The origin of these granules is unknown. The nuclei are pale or shrunken.

Stratum germinativum, malpighian layer, or stratum spinosum is made up of polyhedral cells, which are cylindrical in the deeper portions and flattened toward the surface. The deepest row of cells in this stratum, the **basal layer**, consists of distinctive cuboidal cells with hyperchromatic nuclei in which mitotic figures are frequent. The bulk of this malpighian layer contains nucleated cells which are joined by spines, which suggested the name spiny, spinose, or prickle-cell layer. These spines (formerly called "intercellular bridges") consist of fine cytoplasmic filaments (tonofibrils), which end at desmosomes attaching adjacent cell surfaces, giving the false impression of continuity between cells. In some parts of the skin, the stratum germinativum is widened at regularly spaced intervals, forming the **rete ridges** which extend into the dermis. Melanin pigment can be present in the basal layer and cells superficial to it. The melanin is formed by melanoblasts located beneath the basal layer and is transferred to the epidermal cells by long cellular processes. Within the epidermis, there are peculiar dendritic or stellate-shaped cells called Langerhan's cells. The cells, which are of unknown significance, stain black with gold chloride and are not seen in usual preparations.

The **dermis**, which is separated from the epidermis by a thin basement membrane, is made up of connective tissue rich in collagen and elastic fibers. It provides strength and elasticity to the skin and brings nutrients to the epidermis through its vasculature. It may be divided into two indistinctly separable papillary and reticular layers. The **papillary layer** is most clearly distinguishable in the dermal papillae, which lie between the rete pegs. The most superficial part of the dermis is made up of the fine meshwork of connective tissue fibrils, among which are found elastic fibrils, capillaries, and lymphatics. The deeper **reticular layer** of the dermis makes up its bulk and consists principally of dense collagenous connective tissue in which are distributed elastic fibers, blood and lymphatic vessels, and the adnexa of the epidermis. Large individual cells (melanophores) laden with granules of melanin

pigment may be found in any part of the dermis, particularly in dark-skinned animals. Other individual cells may also be normally present, such as mast cells, histiocytes, plasma cells, and occasionally eosinophils.

The **adnexa** include the specialized structures that arise from the epidermis. They are for the most part contained in the dermis, but may extend into the subcutis in some situations. The adnexa include:

1. Sudoriferous or sweat glands ("merocrine" glands)
2. Apocrine glands
3. Specialized tubular glands, such as lacrimal and mammary glands
4. Sebaceous glands and modified sebaceous glands, e.g., perianal glands
5. Hair follicles of two types, those of common or "guard" hairs and tactile hairs.

Tactile follicles are distinguished in tissue sections by the large surrounding vascular spaces and the sensory nerve, which can usually be seen.

The **subcutis** or hypodermis is not always sharply demarcated from the dermis, but is usually distinguished by its loose areolar connective tissue, large nerves and blood vessels, adipose tissue (panniculus adiposus), and muscular layer (panniculus muscularis). It contains some elastic fibers, but is generally poor in collagen.

The nails, claws, hoofs, and horns develop from the epidermis in particular, although the dermis may contribute supporting elements for some of the larger structures (horns, hoofs).

The pathologist must be fully aware of normal variations in the components of the skin in different body regions in order to interpret accurately any deviations from the normal. The skin is generally thinnest in the axillae and over the abdomen, and thickest over the back and loins. The dermis contributes most to the difference in thickness, whether it involves different anatomic sites or different species. The elephant's skin, for example, has a heavy dermal layer; the epidermis is not much thicker than that of other species. Most animals are fully covered with hair, but hairless areas do occur, particularly inside the flanks and on the abdomen. The long tactile hairs, which are found around the lips and nostrils of many animals, are distinguished by a specialized hair follicle, which has large blood sinuses in its wall and especially prominent nerve fibers. The guard or common hairs always emerge from the skin at an angle, and in carnivores several hair shafts emerge through the mouth of one follicle, although each has its separate root. The fine wool hairs of sheep emerge vertically from the skin, and the follicles are richly supplied with plump sebaceous glands.

Apocrine glands, which are found only in certain regions of the human skin, are the predominant tubular gland in many animals and may be found in any skin region. The ducts of these apocrine glands empty into the hair follicles in contrast to the sudoriferous glands, whose ducts emerge through the epidermis between hair follicles. The deep secretory portion of the apocrine glands of the dog, cow, and goat have a serpentine arrangement, whereas in the horse, sheep, pig, and cat, this portion is wound up into a ball (glomiform). In the dog, sac-like diverticula may normally occur.

These differences, here briefly outlined, emphasize the particular importance of the normal anatomy in the exact skin region that is being studied. It is highly advisable to have "control" sections available for comparison whenever possible.

Archambeau, J.O.: Histologic parameters and elemental composition of skin of swine. J. Invest. Dermatol., 52:399, 1969.

Bloom, W., and Fawcett, D.W.: A Textbook of Histology, 9th ed. Philadelphia, W. B. Saunders Co., 1968.

Creed, R.F.S.: Histology of mammalian skin, with special reference to the dog and cat. Vet. Rec., 70:1–7, 1958.

Goldsberry, S., and Calhoun, M.L.: The comparative histology of the skin of Hereford and Aberdeen-Angus Cattle. Am. J. Vet. Res., 20:61–68, 1959.

Kozlowski, G.P., and Calhoun, M.L.: Microscopic anatomy of the integument of sheep. Am. J. Vet. Res., 30:1267–1279, 1969.

Lovell, J.E., and Getty, R.: The hair follicles, epidermis, dermis and skin glands of the dog. Am. J. Vet. Res., 18:873–885, 1957.

Lyne, A.G., and Hollis, D.E.: The skin of the sheep: a comparison of body regions. Aust. J. Biol. Sci., 21:499–527, 1968.

Montagna, W.: Cutaneous comparative biology. Arch Dermatol., 104:577–591, 1971.

Montagna, W., and Yun, J.S.: The skin of the domestic pig. J. Invest. Dermatol., 43:11–21, 1964.

Nielsen, S.W.: Glands of the canine skin. Am. J. Vet. Res., 14:448–454, 1953.

Searle, A.G.: Comparative Genetics of Coat Colour in Mammals. London, Logos Press, 1968.

Speed, J.G.: Sweat glands of the dog. Vet. J., 97:252–256, 1941.

Strickland, J.H., and Calhoun, M.L.: The integumentary system of the cat. Am. J. Vet. Res., 24:1018–1029, 1963.

Talukdar, A.H., Calhoun, M.L., and Stinson, A.W.: Sweat glands of the horse: a histologic study. Am. J. Vet. Res., 31:2179–2190, 1970.

Trautman, A., and Fiebiger, J.: Fundamentals of the Histology of Domestic Animals. Translated and Revised by Habel, R.E., and Biberstein, E.L., Ithaca, N.Y., Comstock Publishing Co., 1952.

Webb, A.J., and Calhoun, M.L.: The microscopic anatomy of the skin of mongrel dogs. Am. J. Vet. Res., 15:274–280, 1954.

DEFINITIONS

Certain terms are used by the pathologist in consideration of lesions of the skin that are not necessarily applicable to the rest of the human or animal body. Definitions of some commonly used terms in gross or histologic description follow:

Acanthosis—thickening of the epidermis as a result of hyperplasia of the malpighian layer, especially the prickle cell layer. This may occur with or without hyperkeratosis.

Ballooning degeneration—isolation of the cells of the epidermis from one another, particularly in the deeper layers, following intracytoplasmic edema and vacuolization; leading to vesiculation. Often seen in viral diseases.

Bulla (bleb)—cavitation in the epidermis, similar to but generally larger than a vesicle.

Dyskeratosis—an abnormality of development with distinctive alterations in epidermal cells. Two types are distinguished: **benign**—disorganization of epidermal cells, especially in the granular layer, with swollen, eosinophilic cytoplasm, sometimes containing elementary viral particles (pox, contagious ecthyema); **malignant**—anaplastic changes in the epidermis manifest by hyperchromatism, changes in polarity, increase in mitotic activity, and enlargement of nuclei. This is generally considered a step toward carcinoma.

Erosion (excoriation)—superficial loss of epithelium, usually produced mechanically.

Fissure—a linear defect in the epidermis, which may be crusted and tender. Most often occurs at points of cutaneous mobility and at mucocutaneous junctions.

Hyperkeratosis—thickening of the keratin layer (stratum corneum), usually but not invariably associated with thickening of the granular layer (stratum granulosum).

Liquefactive degeneration—obliteration of the dermal-epidermal junction by edema and leukocytic infiltration in the basal layer of epidermis and the adjacent dermis.

Parakeratosis—the retention of nuclei in the keratin layer (stratum corneum), usually with diminution or absence of the granular layer (stratum granulosum). This change is more frequent on moist surfaces and is characterized grossly by scaling of flaky, loosely adherent material (dandruff).

Pseudoepitheliomatous hyperplasia—severe acanthosis with downward growth of the epidermis. This occurs at the margins of indolent ulcers and burns, and might be mistaken for carcinoma.

Pustule—a vesicle filled with pus.

Reticular colliquation—a change in the epidermis in which nuclei become pyknotic or karyorrhectic and the cytoplasm of several cells becomes granular, coalescent, partially disintegrated, and edematous, with the remaining cytoplasm forming reticulated septa separating lobules of fluid. This lesion occurs in viral diseases in which vesicles are a feature.

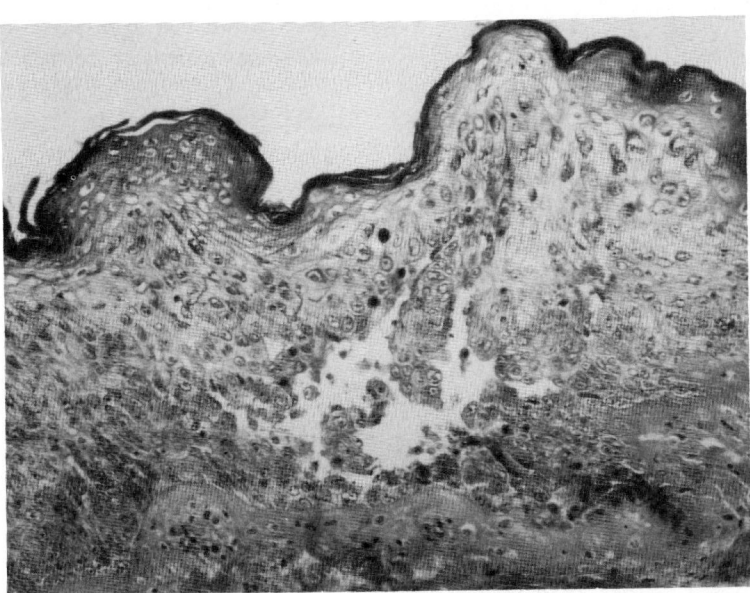

Fig. 18-1. Epithelial viral vesicle in the skin of a patas monkey (*Erythrocebus patas*) affected with herpesvirus. (Courtesy of Dr. H. R. Seibold.)

Spongiosis—intercellular edema of the epidermis. Severe spongiosis leads to vesiculation, as in eczema.

Ulcer—a break in the continuity of the epidermis, with exposure of the underlying dermis.

Urticaria—a circumscribed area of edema and swelling involving principally the papillary layer of the dermis. In urticaria pigmentosa, a rare disease of man, aggregation of mast cells gives the lesions some resemblance to mast cell tumors of dogs.

Vesicle—a circumscribed cavity in the epidermis filled with serum, plasma, or blood, and covered by a thin layer of epidermis, which is greatly elevated above the surface. Vesicles may be single or multiple and may coalesce to form larger bullae.

Allen, A.C.: The Skin, a Clinicopathologic Treatise. St. Louis, C. V. Mosby Co., 1954.

Anderson, W.D.: Pathology, 5th ed. St. Louis, C. V. Mosby Co., 1966.

Muller, G.H., and Kirk, R.W.: Small Animal Dermatology. Philadephia, W. B. Saunders, 1976.

CONGENITAL AND HEREDITARY DISEASES OF SKIN

The conditions included in this section do not have any particular pathologic relationship to one another, other than that they are congenital or hereditary diseases.

Vegetative Dermatosis (Dermatosis Vegetans) in Swine. Hjärre (1953) has described in young swine in Sweden a syndrome involving vegetating dermatosis of unknown etiology associated with a specific type of pneumonia. The cutaneous lesions usually appeared in newborn animals, which occasionally survived for as long as a year but usually were dead by the seventh week. Usually only one pig in a litter was involved, and no abnormalities were evident in the parents or siblings of the same litter, but subsequent litters frequently contained an affected piglet.

The lesions usually appeared first on the distal parts of the extremities, but frequently spread to the rest of the body, particularly the inner surfaces of the legs and the abdomen. The lesions appeared as elevated, roughened, hairless plaques, which sometimes assumed a papillomatous character. Involvement of the growing hoof often resulted in some deformity.

Microscopically, the cutaneous lesions in the early stages consisted principally of acanthosis and hyperkeratosis in the epidermis with elongation of the rete pegs. Microabscesses occurred in the elongated dermal papillae and in the epidermis. Older lesions consisted of severe acanthosis involving broad areas of the epidermis, often with moderate to severe hyperkeratosis. In some instances, the dermis was thrown up into papillary folds. In some, the sweat glands were cystic, presumably as a result of occlusion of their ducts by the acanthotic epidermis.

The lungs were often consolidated by the presence of many mononuclear cells and multinucleated giant cells in the alveoli. Fetalization of the alveolar lining was also recognized.

The inheritance as an autosomal recessive of the underlying factors in this disease was originally reported by Larsson (1953) in Sweden and confirmed by Percy and Hulland (1967) in Canada. The gene appears to be carried only by swine of the Landrace breed, and common ancestors in Sweden appear to be responsible for the gene demonstrated in swine in Norway, England, and Canada.

Hjärre, A.: Vegetierende Dermatosen mit Riesenzellem-pneumonien bei Schwein. Dtsch. Tierarztl. Wochenschr., 60:105–110, 1953.

Larsson, E.L.: Klumpfotgrisar. Svenska Svinavelsför Tidskr., 1:1–15, 1953.

Percy, D.H., and Hulland, T.J.: Dermatosis vegetans (vegetative dermatosis) in Canadian swine. Can. Vet. J., 8:3–9, 1967.

———: Evolution of multinucleate giant cells in dermatosis vegetans in swine. Pathol. Vet., 5:419–428, 1968.

———: The histopathological changes in the skin of pigs with dermatosis vegetans. Can. J. Comp. Med., 33:48–54, 1969.

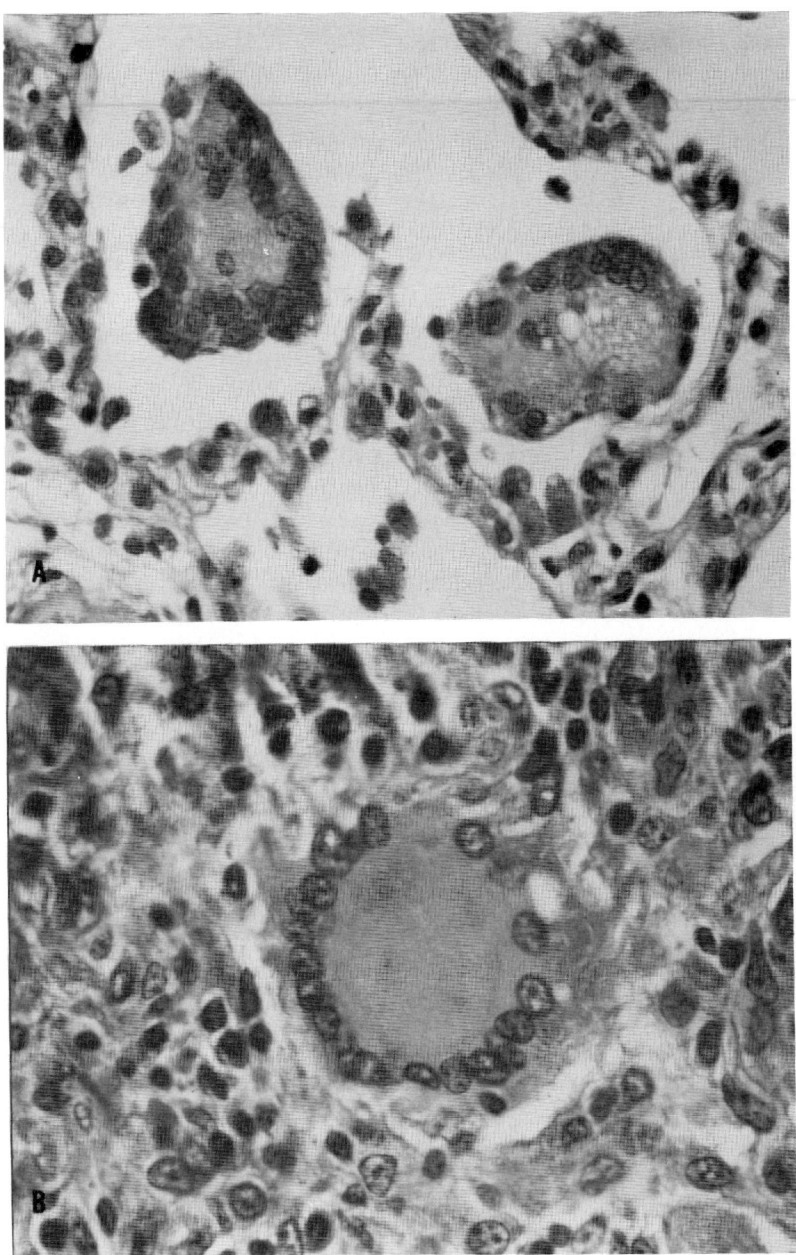

Fig. 18–2. Vegetative dermatosis of swine. *A,* Multinucleated giant cells with vacuolated cytoplasm in alveoli of lung. *B,* Langhan's type of multinucleated giant cell in bronchial lymph node. (Courtesy of Drs. Dean H. Percy, Thomas J. Hulland, and *Pathologia Veterinaria.*)

Congenital Ichthyosis. A rare congenital disease of newborn infants, ichthyosis is sometimes encountered in calves and has been recently recognized in dogs. The name ichthyosis was suggested by the scaly epidermis, which resembles the skin of fish. The severe form, ichthyosis congenita fetalis (Harlequin fetus, from the grotesque garb of Harlequin clown), astounding in appearance, was first described more than one and one-half centuries ago, and still is incompletely explained. The animal counterpart is infrequently recorded in the literature, although accounts are found in the old literature, and most veterinary museums in Europe have at least one skin from an affected calf. Jones has studied pathologic material from calves in a herd in which several cases reportedly occurred. Hutt (1934) considers this condition in cattle to be due to a simple autosomal recessive gene, homozygous in the affected calf, and

Muller (1976) has suggested a similar mode of inheritance in dogs. A recessive mutant mouse (ic/ic) provides a laboratory tool to study the syndrome.

Ichthyosis is recognized at birth, and in severely affected infants and calves survival is rarely more than a few hours or days. The condition as described in dogs is not associated with early death, but the disease is chronic and at present incurable.

The entire skin is hairless or nearly so and is covered with thick, scaly, horny epidermis, which is divided into plates by deep fissures. These fissures are often wide, with a red, raw-appearing base, and follow a pattern that corresponds to the cleavage planes of the skin. The skin is everted around the lips, eyes, and other body orifices, giving the impression of being too small for the body which it encases. One explanation offered for the appearance of the skin is that a defect in keratinization inhibits the proper expan-

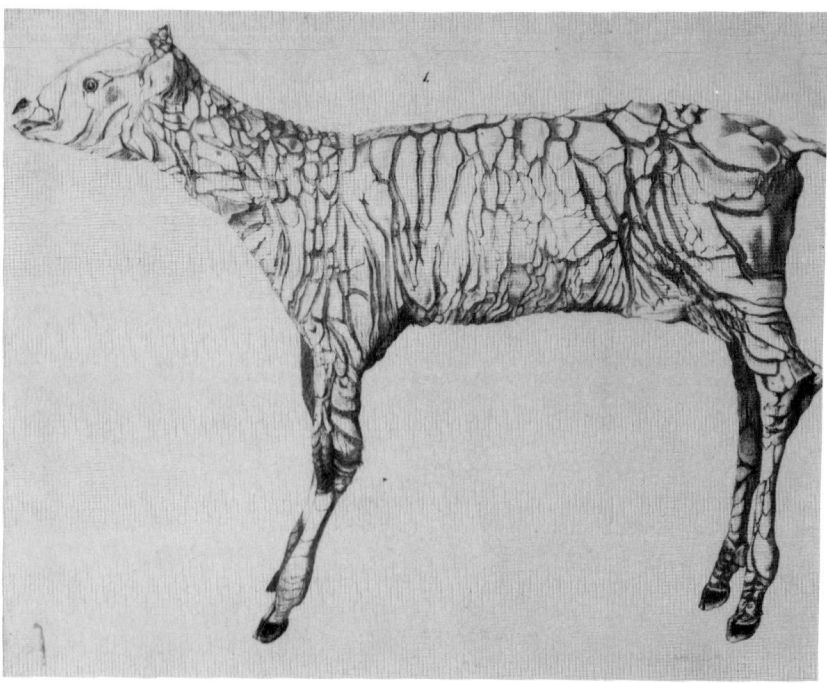

Fig. 18–3. Congenital ichthyosis, skin of a newborn calf. (Courtesy of Armed Forces Institute of Pathology.)

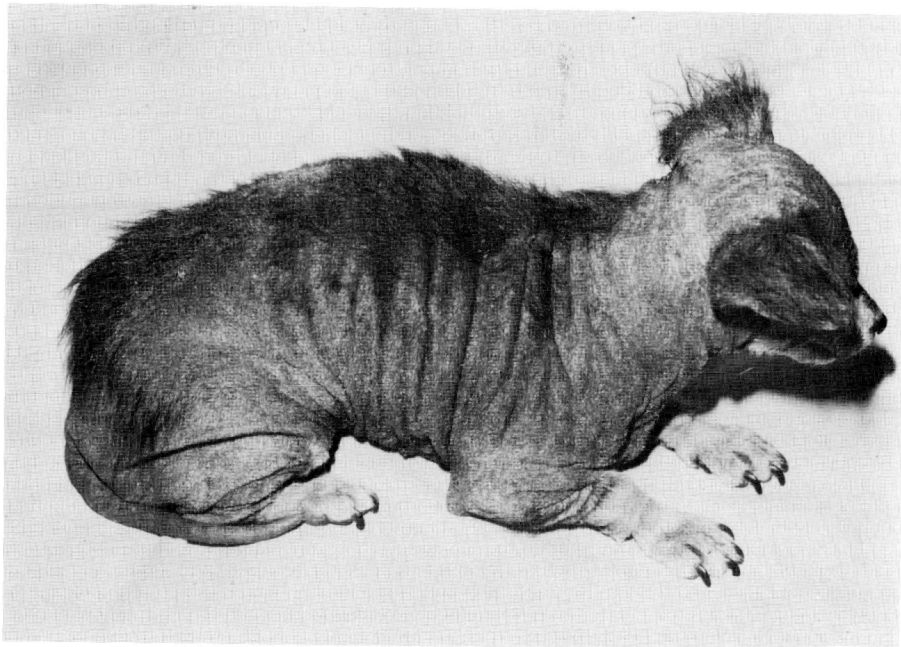

Fig. 18–4. Canine ichthyosis. There is little body hair, the skin is thickened and covered with keratin scales. (Courtesy of Dr. G. H. Muller and *Journal of the American Veterinary Medical Association*.)

sive growth of the epidermis, preventing it from keeping pace with growth of the rest of the body.

Microscopic sections reveal the epidermis to be covered by an extremely thick, dense, and tightly adherent layer of keratin. The rete pegs are elongated; the dermis is moderately thickened and contains congested capillaries, particularly in areas underlying the fissures. The fissures extend through the hyperkeratotic stratum corneum and separate the upper layers of the stratum germinativum, but the basal layer is usually intact.

Other types of congenital and adult ichthyosis are known in man, but apparently have not been recognized in animals.

Edmonds, H.W., and Dolan, W.D.: Ichthyosis congenita fetalis, severe type (harlequin fetus). Bull. Internat. Assoc. Med. Mus., 32:1–21, 1951.
Hutt, F.B.: Inherited lethal characters in domestic animals. Cornell Vet., 24:1–25, 1934.
Jensen, J.E., and Esterly, N.B.: The ichthyosis mouse: histologic, histochemical, ultrastructural and au-
toradiographic studies of interfollicular epidermis. J. Invest. Dermatol., 68:23–31, 1977.
Julian, R.J.: Ichthyosis congenita in cattle. Vet. Med., 55:35–41, 1960.
Muller, G.H.: Ichthyosis in two dogs. J. Am. Vet. Med. Assoc., 169:1313–1317, 1976.
Tuff, P., and Gledish, L.A.: Ichthyosis congenita hos Kalveren arvelig letal defekt. Nord. Vet. Med., 1:619–627, 1949.

Congenital Dermal Asthenia. Collagenous tissue dysplasias that result in cutaneous asthenia, hyperelasticity, and fragility of the skin and hypermobility of joints have been reported in man, dogs, cats, mink, cattle, and sheep. The condition is called **Ehlers-Danlos syndrome** in man, **cutaneous asthenia** in the dog, cat, and mink, and **dermatosparaxis** in cattle and sheep. Dogs, cats, and mink have a dominant pattern of inheritance, whereas in cattle and sheep, it is a recessive trait. In man there are seven forms of the syndrome. It is not certain at this writing whether these are identical pathologic processes in each species, as the biochemical

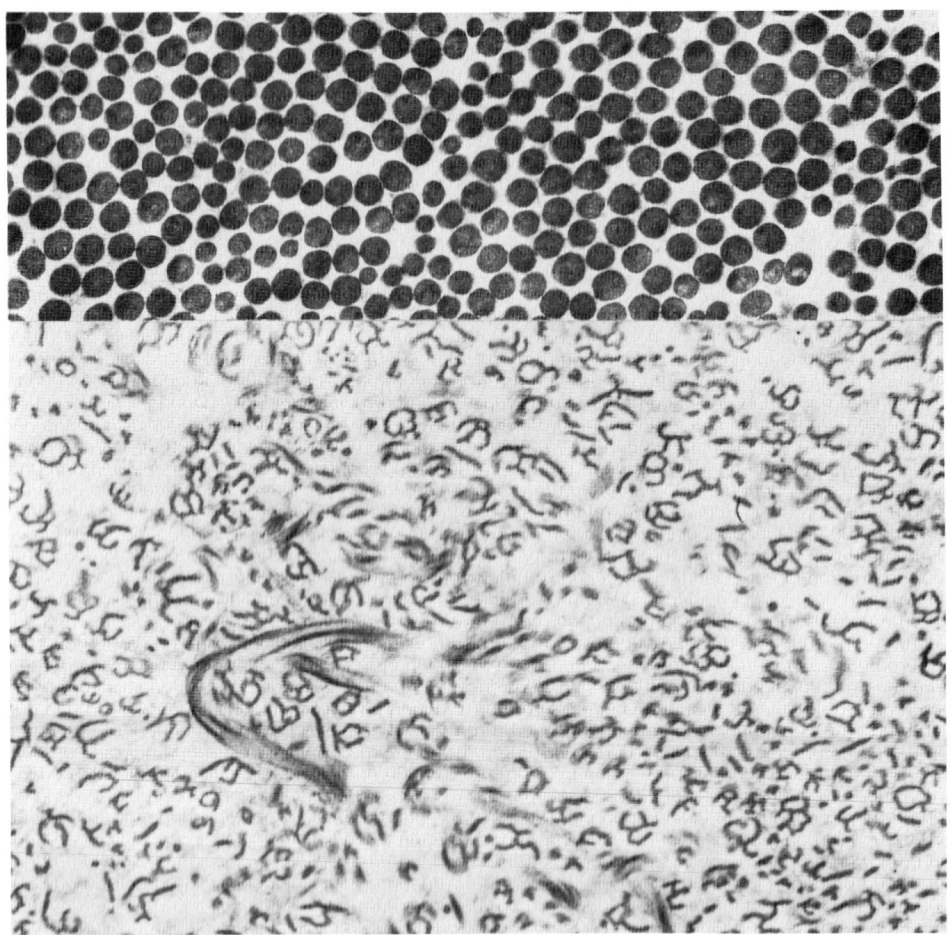

Fig. 18–5.   Bovine dermal collagen (× 49,400.) *Top*, Normal collagen fibers in cross section. *Bottom*, Collagen of calf affected with dermatosparaxis. (Courtesy of Dr. W. Kay Read and *Laboratory Investigation*.)

basis for the defect is not established in each. Current evidence, however, points toward several differing defects in collagen metabolism, each of which results in fragility and hyperextensibility of the skin. In cattle and sheep, light microscopy indicates deficiency in the amount of collagen in the dermis and its fine fibrillar and disorganized nature. Ultrastructural studies (Fig. 18–5) indicate that the collagen fibrils are inadequately packed and fail to form the orderly, uniform, cylindrical fibers characteristic of normal collagen, but rather exist as flattened, twisted ribbons. The basis is believed to be a deficiency in

the activity of procollagen peptidase, which precludes the formation of mature collagen.

In dogs, mink, and cats, the collagen fibers are irregular in size, lack orientation, and are fragmented. Collagen fibrils are disorganized within the fibers.

Ansay, M., Gillet, A., and Hanset, R.: (Hereditary dermatosparaxia [fragility of the skin] in cattle. I. Biochemical constitution of the skin. II. Additional observations on collagen and acid mucopolysaccharides.) Ann. Med. Vet., *112*:449–464 and 465–478, 1968. V.B. *39*:2636, 1969.

Butler, W.F.: Fragility of the skin in a cat. Res. Vet. Sci., *19*:213–216, 1975.

Fjølstad, M., and Helle, O.: A hereditary dysplasia of collagen tissues in sheep. J. Pathol., *112*:183–188, 1974.

Hanset, R., and Ansay, M.: (Dermatosparaxia [fragility of the skin]–a new hereditary defect of connective tissue in cattle.) Ann. Med. Vet., *111*:451–470, 1967. V.B. *38*:2079, 1968.

Hanset, R., and Lapiere, C.M.: Inheritance of dermatosparaxis in the calf. A genetic defect of connective tissues. J. Heredity, *65*:356–358, 1974.

Hegreberg, G.A., and Padgett, G.A.: Ehlers-Danlos syndrome in animals. Bull Pathol., *8*:247, 1967.

Hegreberg, G.A., et al.: A connective tissue disease of dogs and mink resembling the Ehlers-Danlos-syndrome of man. J. Hered., *60*:249–254, 1969.

Hegreberg, G.A., Padgett, G.A., and Henson, J.B.: Connective tissue disease of dogs and mink resembling Ehlers-Danlos syndrome of man. III. Histopathologic changes of the skin. Arch. Pathol., *90*:159–166, 1970.

Helle, O., and Nes, N.N.: A hereditary skin defect in sheep. Acta Vet. Scand., *13*:443–445, 1972.

O'Hara, P.J., Read, W.K., Romane, W.M., and Bridges, C.H.: A collagenous tissue dysplasia of calves. Lab. Invest., *23*:307–314, 1970.

Patterson, D.F., and Minor, R.R.: Hereditary fragility and hyperextensibility of the skin of cats: a defect in collagen fibrillogenesis. Lab. Invest., *37*:170–179, 1977.

Epitheliogenesis Imperfecta.

A congenital defect characterized by discontinuity of squamous epithelium is recognized in man and many species of animals, including several breeds of cattle, swine, horses, dogs, and cats. It is most common in cattle, where it is inherited as an autosomal recessive trait. Affected calves may be aborted or they succumb to infection shortly after birth. The epithelial defects most often affect the feet and claws, but may exist anywhere, including the oral mucosa. Microscopically, the normal epithelium terminates abruptly at the affected site.

Crowell, W.A., Stephenson, C., and Gosser, H.S.: *Epitheliogenesis imperfecta* in a foal. J. Am. Vet. Med. Assoc., *168*:56–58, 1976.

Gupta, B.N.: *Epitheliogenesis imperfecta* in a dog. Am. J. Vet. Res., *34*:443–444, 1973.

Leipold, H.W., Mills, J.H.L., and Huston, K.: *Epitheliogenesis imperfecta* in Holstein-Friesian calves. Can. Vet. J., *14*:114–118, 1973.

Munday, B.L.: *Epitheliogenesis imperfecta* in lambs and kittens. Br. Vet. J., *126*:47, 1970.

Congenital Hypotrichia and Atrichia.

Hairlessness (alopecia) of part or all of the body may be encountered in most species of animals. In some animals, these hereditary defects under some circumstances are recognized as breeds (Chinese Crested dog, Mexican Hairless, Chihuahua) or strains (nude mouse). When incomplete, the hairless sites follow regular patterns, or may be restricted to certain colored areas in multicolored animals. Hair follicles may be completely lacking in some forms, or present but not functional in others.

Becker, R.B., Simpson, C.F., and Wilcox, C.J.: Hairless Guernsey cattle: hypotrichosis—a non-lethal character. J. Hered., *54*:3–7, 1963.

Conroy, J.D., Rasmusen, B.A., and Small, E.: Hypotrichosis in Miniature Poodle siblings. J. Am. Vet. Med. Assoc., *166*:697–699, 1975.

Eldridge, F.E., and Atkesan, F.W.: Streaked hairlessness in Holstein-Friesian cattle. J. Hered., *44*:265–271, 1953.

Hutt, F.B., and Saunders, L.Z.: Viable genetic hypotrichosis in Guernsey cattle. J. Hered., *44*:97–103, 1953.

Letard, E.: Hairless Siamese cats. J. Hered., *29*:173–175, 1931.

Roberts, E., and Carroll, E.: The inheritance of hairlessness in swine. J. Hered., *22*:125–132, 1931.

Schleger, A.V., Thompson, B.J., and Hewetson, R.W.: Histopathology of hypotrichosis in calves. Aust. J. Biol. Sci., *20*:661–668, 1967.

Selmanowitz, V.J., Markofsky, J., and Orentreich, N.: Black-hair follicular dysplasia in dogs. J. Am. Vet. Med. Assoc., *171*:1079–1081, 1977.

Thomsett, L.F.: Congenital hypotrichia in the dog. Vet. Rec., *73*:915–917, 1961.

Pigmentary Abnormalities.

Albinism is a complete lack of pigmentation resulting from a deficiency of tyrosinase, which is necessary for melanin synthesis. Melanocytes are, however, present. The condition is encountered sporadically and is believed to be a recessive trait in most species. Focal or localized absence or loss of pigmentation is seen in scars and for poorly understood reasons on the nose, lips, and other sites of certain breeds of dogs. Loss of melanin in previously pigmented skin in man and dogs is known as **vitiligo**. Although the pathogenesis is unknown, an autoimmune disease has been suggested, with humoral antibodies directed against melanocytes. Vitiligo occurs in association with melanomas in human beings and swine, and in horses there is an association

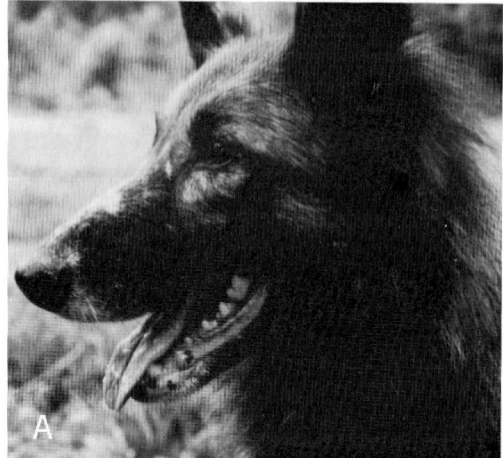

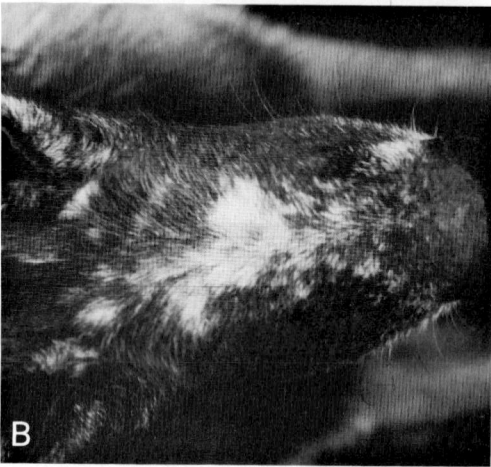

Fig. 18–6. Hypopigmentation of the face and mouth of the Belgian Tervuren dog. The condition, which usually becomes manifest during young adulthood, is believed to be hereditary and resembles vitiligo in man. (Courtesy of Dr. M. B. Mahaffey.)

between melanomas and graying. The only microscopic finding in any form of hypopigmentation is the lack of pigment. Secondary solar dermatitis is discussed elsewhere (p. 1092). Copper deficiency and hypopigmentation are discussed on page 1067. Hyperpigmentation is not frequent, but may be encountered in hormonal disturbances, acanthosis nigricans, or as focal, raised macules (freckles) of no appreciable significance aside from their differentiation from melanomas.

Hertz, K.C., Gazze, L.A., Kirkpatrick, C.H., and Katz, S.I.: Autoimmune vitiligo. Detection of antibodies to melanin-producing cells. N. Engl. J. Med., *297*:634–637, 1977.

Mahaffey, M.B., Yarbrough, M., and Munnell, J.F.: Focal loss of pigment in the Belgian Tervuren dog. J. Am. Vet. Med. Assoc., *173*:390–396, 1978.

ALLERGIC DERMATITIS

Many antigens (allergens) can be responsible for initiating immunologically mediated inflammatory reactions in the skin. The terms allergy (allergic) or hypersensitivity encompass all of the various forms of this type of dermatitis. The mechanisms and kinds of hypersensitivities are discussed in Chapter 7, and will only briefly be reviewed here. Both immediate and delayed hypersensitivity reactions may lead to dermatitis; however, both mechanisms may be operant simultaneously.

Immediate reactions are most often those of localized anaphylaxis, but cytotoxic reactions and Arthus type reactions may also cause dermatitis. Immediate reactions are referred to as **atopy** or **atopic dermatitis**, and delayed reactions, as **contact dermatitis**.

Offending antigens potentially responsible for atopic dermatitis include pollens and other plant products, feathers, dust, wool, and foods. The most common route of entry is by inhalation, although ingestion and direct contact may also lead to atopic dermatitis. Contact dermatitis is associated with soaps, detergents, and organic chemicals, including dichlorvos (flea collar dermatitis). Ectoparasites, particularly fleas, are responsible for allergic dermatitis in which both immediate and delayed reactions occur.

The lesions of atopic and contact dermatitis are similar, and the two are not readily distinguishable. The principal differentiating feature is the distribution of lesions, which tend to be localized in contact dermatitis, and usually are generalized or involve multiple sites in atopic dermatitis. In both, there is an erythematous

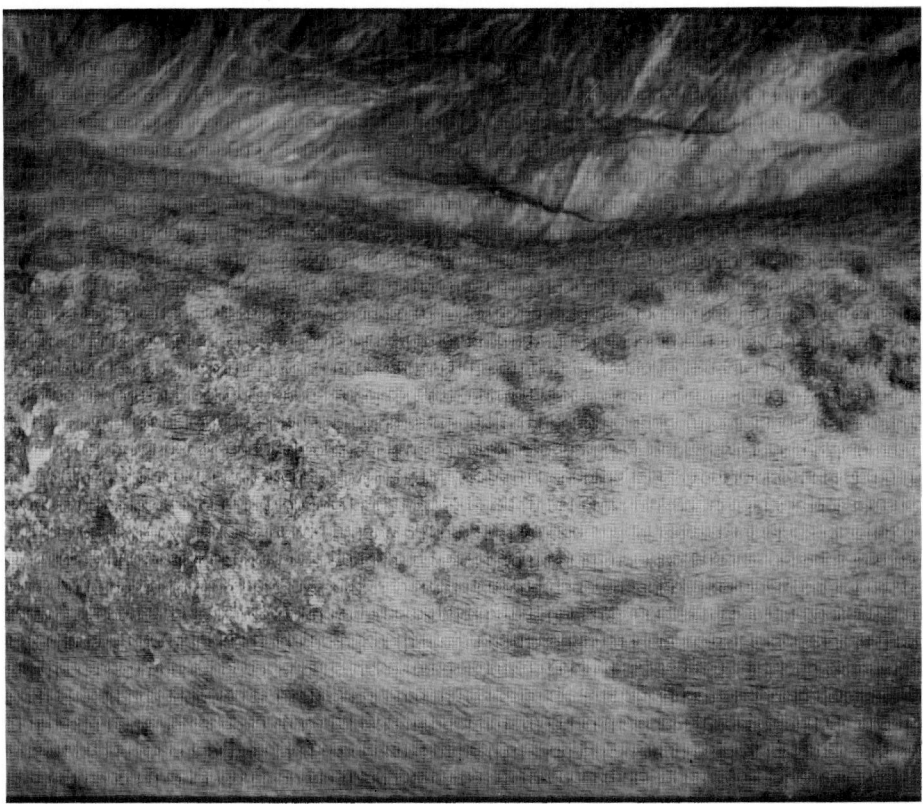

Fig. 18–7. Eczematous dermatitis, skin of the abdomen of a female collie, age five years. (Courtesy of Angell Memorial Animal Hospital.)

papular and/or vesicular rash, which may weep a serous exudate. Pruritus leads to self-inflicted trauma, which considerably exaggerates the severity of the lesions. With repeated or chronic exposure, the skin becomes thickened and hairless. Microscopically, the lesions reflect the clinical findings, with hyperemia, edema, and vesiculation in the early stages, and acanthosis and parakeratosis in examples of long standing. Cellular infiltrations, principally lymphocytic, accompany the vascular changes. Mast cells and eosinophils are frequently present.

Eczema is a term commonly applied in a broad and somewhat loose sense to cutaneous lesions of obscure etiology. Eczema is generally thought to represent one or another form of allergic dermatitis. Unfortunately, offending antigens are often not identified, nor the lesions submitted for microscopic study, which makes it difficult to establish an allergic basis in most examples.

Booth, B.H., Patterson, R., and Talbot, C.H.: Immediate-type hypersensitivity in dogs: cutaneous, anaphylactic, and respiratory responses to *Ascaris*. J. Lab. Clin. Med., 76:181–189, 1970.
Halliwell, R.E.W., and Schwartzman, R.M.: Atopic disease in the dog. Vet. Rec., 89:209–214, 1971.
Nesbitt, G.H.: Canine allergic dermatitis: a review of 230 cases. J. Am. Vet. Med. Assoc., 172:55–60, 1978.

Other Potentially Immunity-Mediated Vesicular Diseases

Pemphigus Vulgaris. Pemphigus vulgaris is one of several diseases of man characterized by extensive blistering. Dogs are subject to a similar syndrome, which was

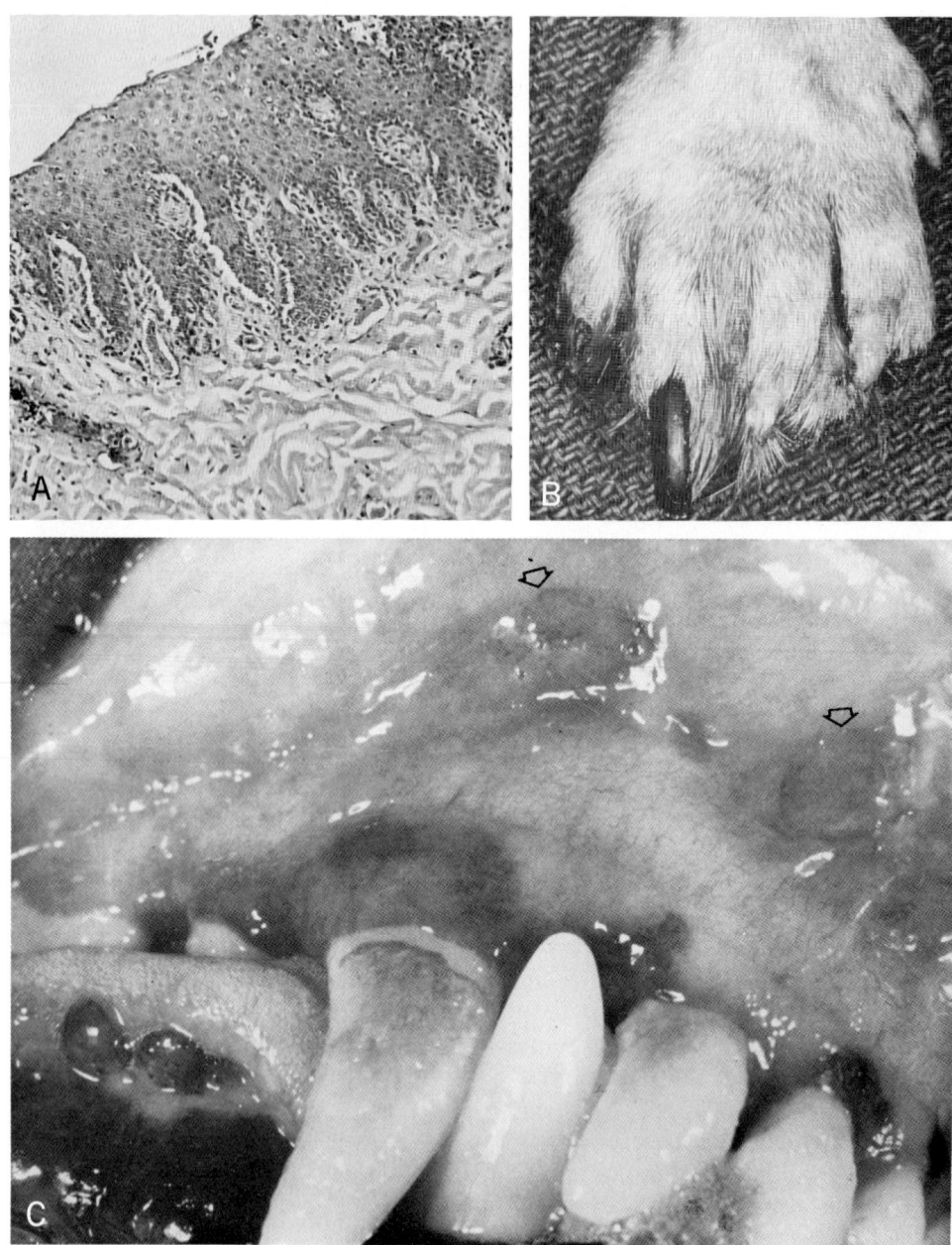

Fig. 18–8.   Canine pemphigus vulgaris. *A*, Sub-basal acantholysis. *B*, Loss of claws and exposure of ungual processes. *C*, Erosions of oral mucous membrane (arrows). (Courtesy of Dr. A. I. Hurwitz and *Journal of the American Veterinary Medical Association*.)

described by Hurvitz and Feldman (1975), Stannard et al. (1975), and Austin and Maibach (1976). The disease is characterized by bullae that rapidly progress to ulcers in the oral cavity, mucocutaneous junctions, and skin. The essential lesion is acantholysis, the separation of epidermal cells from one another due to degeneration of the intercellular space substance, and loss of intercellular bridges. This leads to clefts and ultimately bullae. The condition is believed to result from autoantibodies directed against intercellular space substance. These antibodies can be demonstrated by immunofluorescent staining. Without therapy, pemphigus is progressive and fatal.

Variant forms of pemphigus with similar immunopathologic findings have been described in dogs. These include *pemphigus vegetans*, which is accompanied by papillomatous proliferations of the epidermis; *pemphigus foliaceus*, in which the oral cavity is usually spared and which regularly involves hair follicles; and *pemphigus erythematosus*, which resembles the former but is confined to the head and neck. A condition of unknown cause, termed *bullous pemphigus*, characterized by subepidermal vesicles, has also been seen in dogs.

Similar vesicular diseases have been described in Angus calves as familial acantholysis (Jolly et al., 1973), and sheep and dogs as epidermolysis bullosa (Alley et al.,

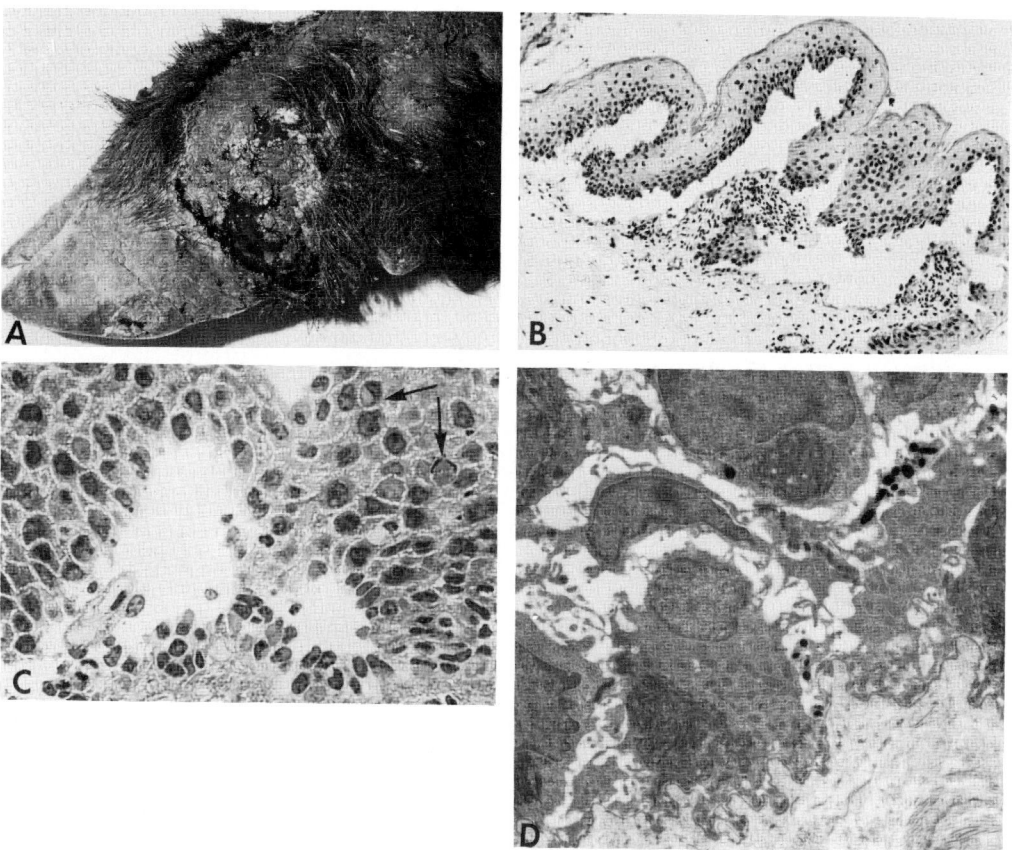

Fig. 18–9. Familial acantholysis of Angus calves. *A,* Ulceration of skin of hind foot. *B,* Acantholysis and vesiculation of mucosa of hard palate. *C,* Separation of prickle cells of the nasolabium. *D,* Separation of basal cells and prickle cells. Tonofilaments are aggregated in the cytoplasm, and desmosome-tonofilament complexes are deficient. (Courtesy of Dr. R. D. Jolly and *Veterinary Pathology.*)

1974; Scott et al., 1980). In these disorders, vesicle formation is predominantly confined to the basal epidermis with separation of the epidermis from the dermis. As of this writing, their pathogenesis has not been determined. *Dermatitis herpetiformis*, which is recognized in human beings and dogs, is also characterized by subepidermal vesicles, but in addition there are microabscesses and collections of eosinophils. In man, IgA and complement have been demonstrated at the dermoepidermal junction, but such has not been demonstrated in dogs.

Alley, M.R., O'Hara, P.J., and Middleberg, A.: An epidermolysis bullosa of sheep. NZ Vet. J., 22:55–59, 1974.

Austin, V.H., and Maibach, H.I.: Immunofluorescence testing in a bullous skin disease of a dog. J. Am. Vet. Med. Assoc., 168:322–324, 1976.

Hurvitz, A.I., and Feldman, E.: A disease in dogs resembling human pemphigus vulgaris: case reports. J. Am. Vet. Med. Assoc., 166:585–590, 1975.

Jolly, R.D., Alley, M.R., and O'Hara, P.J.: Familial acantholysis of Angus calves. Vet. Pathol., 10:473–483, 1973.

Lund, J.E., and Park, J.F.: Focal mastocytosis in lymph nodes from a Beagle dog. Vet. Pathol., 15:64–67, 1978.

Scott, D.W., and Schultz, R.D.: Epidermolysis bullosa simplex in the Collie dog. J. Am. Vet. Med. Assoc., 171:721–727, 1977.

Scott, D.W., Wolfe, M.J., Smith, C.A., and Lewis, R.M.: The comparative pathology of non-viral bullous skin diseases in domestic animals. Vet. Pathol., 17:257–281, 1980.

Stannard, A.A., Gribble, D.H., and Baker, B.B.: A mucocutaneous disease in the dog, resembling pemphigus vulgaris in man. J. Am. Vet. Med. Assoc., 166:575–582, 1975.

SOLAR DERMATITIS (ACTINIC DERMATOSIS)

Prolonged exposure to sunlight and its ultraviolet radiation results in chronic premalignant lesions in unprotected skin. The association of sunlight, chronic dermatitis, and neoplasia is well recognized in human beings, where it is most frequent in middle-aged individuals with fair complexions. The incidence is highest in the southwestern United States and other sunny geographic locations in the world. The lesions resemble those induced in the skin by other forms of irradiation. Grossly, these are rough, slightly raised papules or plaques, which microscopically consist of hyperkeratosis, parakeratosis, acanthosis, epithelial atypism or dysplasia, and pseudoepitheliomatous hyperplasia. The dermis may also be thickened and contain scattered foci of chronic inflammation. In human beings, solar dermatitis is associated with squamous cell carcinoma, basal cell carcinoma, and malignant melanoma. The mechanism is presumably through damage to DNA. The same mechanism is believed to be the primary cause of squamous cell carcinoma of the eye of white faced Hereford cattle, and of the ear in white cats. Solar dermatitis associated with squamous cell carcinoma has also been described in dogs (Hargis, et al., 1977).

Hargis, A.M., Thomassen, R.W., and Phemister, R.D.: Chronic dermatosis and cutaneous squamous cell carcinoma in the Beagle dog. Vet. Pathol., 14:218–228, 1977.

DERMATOSES OF UNKNOWN ETIOLOGY

Any disease of the skin may be considered a dermatosis, but those to be discussed in this section include only those of unknown or uncertain etiology, or which are not discussed elsewhere in this book.

Acanthosis Nigricans. A dermatosis of obscure etiology, acanthosis nigricans is recognized in man and in the dog. It is most frequent in dachshunds. The principal clinical features in the dog are the presence of symmetric patches of heavily pigmented, rough, thick skin, particularly in the flanks, axillae, inguinal, circumanal, and abdominal regions. These changes are persistent, gradually spread to other parts of the body, and may produce a disagreeable odor. The lesions are usually poorly circumscribed, vary in diameter from 1 to 8 cm, but surprisingly result in little epilation in most cases, although in some instances this becomes a prominent feature. The cutaneous lesions are in some in-

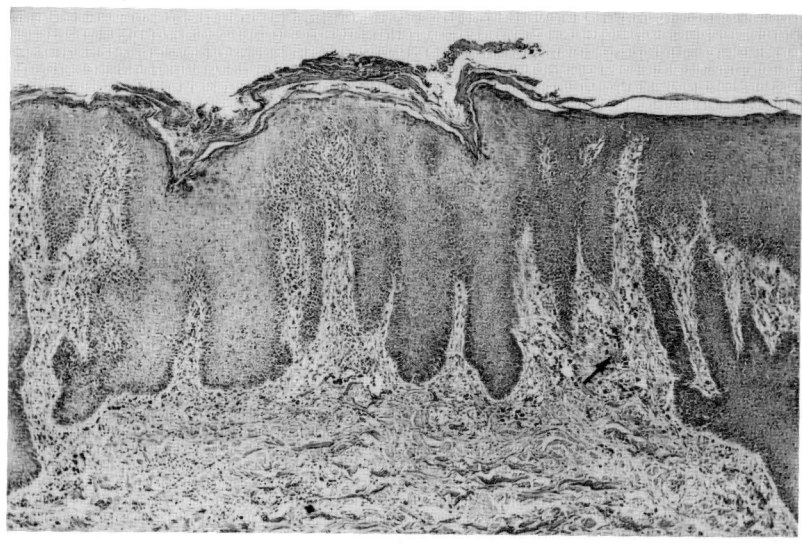

Fig. 18–10. Ancanthosis nigricans, skin of a dog. Thick epidermis (× 50) with elongated rete pegs. Melanin is increased in the epidermis and dermis (arrows). (Courtesy of Armed Forces Institute of Pathology.) Contributor: Dr. M. A. Troy.

stances associated in man and in animals with adenocarcinomas, particularly involving the liver, but any causal relationship to such neoplasia is not established. A causal relation to deficiency of pituitary thyroid stimulating hormone is indicated by the work of Bornfors (1959).

The microscopic appearance of the involved skin is dominated by acanthosis and hyperkeratosis of the epidermis. The dermal papillae are elongated in relation to the overlying acanthotic epidermis and may be congested, but the dermis is otherwise not affected. Hair follicles and adnexa may be slightly decreased in number or unchanged. Cystic dilatation of apocrine or sweat glands may occur. Increased amount of melanin, suspected from the gross appearance, is not always easily measured in histologic sections. This is especially difficult to assess in animals, which normally have a deeply pigmented skin. However, careful comparison with adjoining unaffected skin will usually disclose excessive amounts of melanin in the epidermis and dermis of the involved areas.

Bornfors, S.: Acanthosis nigricans in dogs. Acta Endocr. Copenhagen, Suppl No. 37, 63, 1959.

Curth, H.O., and Slanetz, C.A.: Acanthosis nigricans and cancer of the liver in a dog. Am. J. Cancer, 37:216–223, 1939.

Montgomery, H.: Dermatopathology. New York, Harper & Row, 1967.

Nesbitt, G.H.: Canine allergic dermatitis: a review of 230 cases. J. Am. Vet. Med. Assoc., 172:55–60, 1978.

Subcorneal Pustular Dermatosis. This disease, recognized in man and dogs (in particular, Miniature Schnauzers), is characterized by the appearance of pustules immediately beneath the stratum corneum. The pustules, which are sterile, often rupture resulting in annular or gyrate lesions with irregular borders. The cause is unknown.

McKeever, P.J., and Dahl, M.V.: A disease in dogs resembling human subcorneal pustular dermatosis. J. Am. Vet. Med. Assoc., 170:704–708, 1977.

Scott, D.W., Wolfe, M.J., Smith, C.A., and Lewis, R.M.: The comparative pathology of non-viral bullous skin diseases in domestic animals. Vet. Pathol., 17:257–281, 1980.

Parakeratosis of Swine. This is an afebrile dermatosis of young swine and has been named parakeratosis from one out-

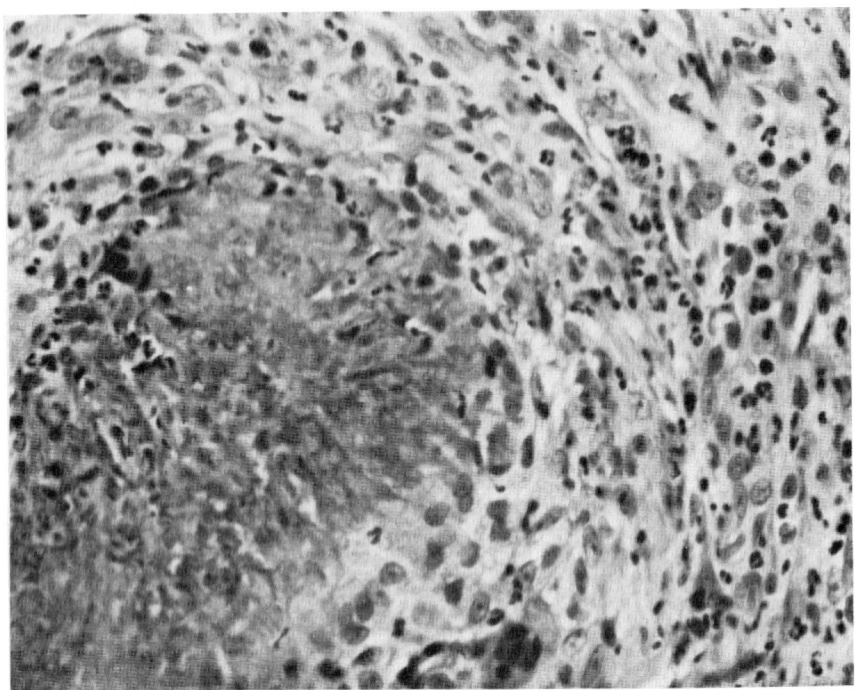

Fig. 18–11. Eosinophilic granuloma, tongue of a cat. A central core of brightly eosinophilic degraded collagen is surrounded by macrophages, epithelioid cells, and eosinophils. (Courtesy of Dr. N. W. King, Jr.)

standing feature. This is described as a deficiency of zinc (see Chapter 17).

Keloid. A keloid is a hypertrophic scar of the dermis that results from certain types of injury, particularly burns. It occurs more frequently in certain people, such as the Japanese and blacks, and sometimes is seen in animals. The hypertrophic scar tissue elevates the epidermis, which frequently becomes ulcerated. Histologically, the keloid is made up of heavy bands of eosinophilic collagen in which thinner collagen fibers and fibroblasts are rather haphazardly mixed. The skin adnexa are usually absent and the epidermis may be atrophied or excoriated. Elastic fibers are usually sparse.

Eosinophilic Granuloma (Feline Intradermal Granuloma, Feline Linear Granuloma). A peculiar granulomatous inflammation associated with necrosis and degeneration of collagen and infiltration of eosinophils is a relatively common lesion in cats. These lesions appear on the skin of any site, elevating it with nodular or linear configurations. Ulceration may occur and some lesions appear to be self-limiting. Ulcerative lesions in the lips and oral and pharyngeal mucosae are often associated with cutaneous lesions, particularly on the feet or legs. The lesions on the lips are often referred to as "rodent ulcer." The term "linear granuloma" is used to describe the elongated lesions in the dermis, which are often bilaterally symmetrical, involving lateral or medial surfaces of both legs or both axillae. More than one disease entity may be involved, but the histologic features in biopsy specimens are similar, justifying consideration of this to be one entity until more can be learned. The cause is at present undetermined, although allergy is suspected to be a component. Microorganisms have not been demonstrated.

The lesions are limited for the most part to the dermis. In early lesions, foci of necrosis of collagen may be found, and the inflammatory reaction is evidently the result of this necrosis. Epithelioid cells, giant cells, and leukocytes (eosinophils often in great numbers) make up this cellular reaction. The necrotic collagen often forms discrete masses surrounded by epithelioid and foreign-body giant cells.

We have seen an identical lesion in Siberian Huskies.

Bucci, T.J.: Intradermal granuloma associated with collagen degeneration in three cats. J. Am. Vet. Med. Assoc., 148:794–800, 1966.
Conroy, J.D.: Diseases of the skin. In Feline Medicine and Surgery, edited by E. J. Catcott. Wheaton, Ill., Amer. Vet. Public, 1964, pp. 346–347.
Scott, D.W.: Observations on the eosinophilic granuloma complex in cats. J. Am. Anim. Hosp. Assoc., 11:261–270, 1975.

Equine Cutaneous Granulomas. The horse especially is prone to develop chronic, ulcerated, and bloody granulomas, chiefly on the limbs. Commonly, they are known to have originated as wire-cuts or similar cutaneous injuries. The granulation tissue in many instances grows unceasingly and results in large, raw masses that are cured only by radical surgery, if at all. Clinically, they have to be differentiated from equine sarcoids and other tumors.

It has long been accepted that the reasons for such intractable wound-healing are an unusual susceptibility of the equine species, coupled with the continued irritation of uncontrolled movement and unavoidable contamination of the raw surfaces with bacteria and dirt. For some of these cases, this concept is still retained, but in the warmer parts of the world, where these granulomas are often known as **summer sores, bursatti**, or colloquially as "leeches," other causes have been discovered.

In the latter group of cases, complete gross examination of the granulation tissue should reveal here and there a limited number of yellowish-white specks, mostly visible to the naked eye, which consist of a denser and more-or-less separable material. The presence of these bodies appears to be diagnostic.

Microscopically, the granulomas of this group are composed of rather loosely arranged, newly formed fibrous tissue, with large numbers of hyperemic capillaries and an active inflammatory process in which eosinophils tend to be predominant among the other leukocytes. The characteristic bodies prove to be sharply bound, necrotic masses, which with hematoxylin and eosin take a startlingly conspicuous deep red color, although interspersed with necrotic nuclei. Cellular remnants suggest that many may have been eosinophils; peripherally the other cells, fibroblastic in nature, with much red cytoplasm, are often radially oriented, forming a minutely spinous fringe.

In some patients, distorted sections of helminths are readily seen within some of these necrotic masses, and the lesion is accepted as cutaneous habronemiasis. In other individuals, no evidence of helminths is discoverable, but careful observation reveals coarse, septate hyphae of a fungus. Pale and practically unstained by hematoxylin-eosin, they are faintly visible in the red-staining mass of necrotic cells. Stains such as the Gridley fungus stain show that the mycelial fragments are numerous, especially around the periphery of the necrotic bodies. Bridges et al. (1961, 1962) have identified two organisms from such lesions: *Hyphomyces destruens* and *Entomorphthora coronata*, the former from the leg and the latter from the skin of the nostril.

It would appear, then, that these troublesome lesions of the horse may signify any one of three entities: a nonspecific granulation tissue, cutaneous habronemiasis, or a "phycomycosis." To date, the two etiologic agents have never been found in the same individual. Differentiation should be readily possible by histopathologic methods. Similar lesions with similar fungal pathogenesis occur occasionally in other species, but habronemiasis is limited to the horse.

Bridges, C.H., and Emmons, C.W.: A phycomycosis of horses caused by *Hyphomyces destruens*. J. Am. Vet. Med. Assoc., *138*:579–589, 1961.

Bridges, C.H., Romane, W.M., and Emmons, C.W.: Phycomycosis of horses caused by *Entomophthora coronata*. J. Am. Vet. Med. Assoc., *140*:673–677, 1962.

Exudative Epidermitis of Swine. A specific pustular dermatitis was described and reproduced experimentally by Hjärre (1948), who named it **contagious pyoderma** or **impetigo contagiosa suis**. The currently favored name in the United States, **exudative epidermitis**, was first used by Jones (1956). Other names are apparently synonyms: "seborrhea oleosa" (Kernkamp, (1948), "greasy pig disease," and "acute or chronic generalized dermatitis" (Mebus et al., 1968).

Staphylococcus hyos, described by Underdahl et al. (1965), has been isolated repeatedly from natural cases and has been used to reproduce the disease experimentally. It is possible that natural outbreaks are made more severe by the presence of other organisms, particularly viruses. An antecedent viral infection has been postulated, but no evidence produced for it.

The disease usually affects only young swine during their first month of life. It has been reported from most places where swine are raised on a large scale, including Germany, Holland, Ireland, Norway, Sweden, United States, Canada, and Australia (Obel, 1968). The cutaneous manifestations usually appear suddenly around the eyes and ears, and soon spread to the trunk and other parts of the body. The lesions appear first as sharply delineated patches, red- or yellow-tinged, which soon become covered by a greasy exudate that may be removed easily, revealing hyperemic skin underneath. In chronic cases, the exudate eventually sloughs, leaving congested, healing skin underneath.

Microscopically, in the early lesion, the epidermis becomes acanthotic, with severe spongiosus in the upper layers of the stratum spinosum. A superficial parakeratotic layer is soon formed and covers a vesicle. Granules are lost in the stratum granulosum, the cells become swollen and vacuolated, and desmosomes and tonofibrils are reduced in number. The papillary layer of the dermis is hyperemic. Acanthosis and intercellular edema tend to persist in the epidermis, and vesicles become pustules. Coccoid organisms are usually demonstrable in these pustules. Periodic acid Schiff (PAS)-positive material appears in epithelial cells and intercellular spaces. Some microabscesses may extend into hair follicles. The dermis in late stages becomes intensely infiltrated by leukocytes as the overlying epidermis contains abscesses or becomes excoriated.

One reported complication in spontaneous and experimentally induced cases is a severe ureteritis, with edema of the ureter sufficient to produce occlusion. Hydronephrosis is reported to follow, and pyelonephritis might be an expected result.

Hjärre, A.: Kontagious pyodermi hos svin (Impetigo contagiosa). Skand. Vet. Tidskr. *38*:662–682, 1948.

Jones, L.D.: Exudative epidermitis of pigs. Am. J. Vet. Res., *17*:178–193, 1956.

Kernkamp, H.C.H.: Seborrhea oleosa in pigs. North Am. Vet., *29*:438–441, 1948.

L'Ecuyer, C.: Exudative epidermitis in pigs. Clinical studies and preliminary transmission trials. Can. J. Comp. Med., *30*:9–16, 1966.

Mebus, C.A., Underdahl, N.R., and Twiehaus, M.J.: Exudative epidermitis. Pathogenesis and pathology. Pathol. Vet., *5*:146–163, 1968.

Obel, A.L.: Epithelial changes in porcine exudative epidermitis. The light-microscopical picture. Pathol. Vet., *5*:253–269, 1968.

Obel, A.L., and Nicander, L.: Epithelial changes in porcine exudative epidermitis. An ultrastructural study. Pathol. Vet., *7*:329–345, 1970.

Schmidt, U., Bollwahn, W., and Amtsberg, G.: Exudative epidermitis of pigs: pathology. Berl.

Muench. Tieraerztl. Wochensch., 85:181–184, 1972.
Underdahl, N.R., Grace, O.D., and Twiehaus, M.J.: Porcine exudative epidermitis: characterization of bacterial agent. Am. J. Vet. Res., 26:617–624, 1965.

Folliculitis (Pyoderma). Inflammation of the hair follicles (folliculitis) is common, especially in the dog. Aside from the parasitic and mycotic infections described in Chapters 14 and 12, respectively, folliculitis of unknown etiology is encountered with moderate frequency by the veterinary pathologist. The lesions are usually localized in irregular areas and the skin appears grossly thickened, indurated, and hairless. Ulceration of the overlying epidermis is frequent, usually as a result of prolonged gnawing or scratching of the part by the animal. Surgical specimens are usually submitted because of a suspected neoplasm.

Histologically, the lesions are related to inflammatory and necrotizing changes in the deep parts of the hair follicles. Necrosis of the epithelium results in the isolation of bits of hairs or contents of sebaceous glands; either of these evokes an intense local foreign body reaction. The dermis adjacent to these items of debris may contain microabscesses, or more frequently, aggregates of epithelioid cells and foreign-body type giant cells. The surrounding dermis becomes quite thick as the result of proliferation of collagenous connective tissue. The overlying epidermis may be unchanged, acanthotic, or ulcerated.

In **acne**, a type of folliculitis, the sealed-off hair follicles or sebaceous glands become enlarged, filled with pus, and surrounded by intense inflammation. In **furunculosis,** abscesses in the dermis, hair follicles, or sebaceous glands may reach rather large size, then rupture through the epidermis. This leaves a rounded hole in the epidermis and a pit or canal leading down into the dermis. *Staphylococcus aureus* is the most frequently recovered organism in folliculitis, acne, and furunculosis.

Pustules may, of course, also form in the dermis or epidermis unrelated to adnexa.

McKeever, P.J., and Dahl, M.V.: A disease of dogs resembling human subcorneal pustular dermatosis. J. Am. Vet. Med. Assoc., 170:704–708, 1977.
Quadros, E.: Furunculosis in dogs. Aetiology, pathogenesis and treatment. A clinical study. Acta Vet. Scand., Suppl., 52:114, 1974.

Seborrhea. A chronic dermatosis characterized by oily or greasy skin with patchy alopecia and a rancid odor is seen in dogs and occasionally cats. The pathogenesis is not understood. Microscopically, it is not distinctive, although the number or size of sebaceous glands is increased. There are acanthosis and hyperkeratosis, but little or no inflammation.

Rojko, J.L., Hoover, E.A., and Martin, S.L.: Histologic interpretation of cutaneous biopsies from dogs with dermatologic disorders. Vet. Pathol., 15:579–589, 1978.

"Brand Papillomas." Exuberant growth of epidermis with a thick overlying layer of keratin is sometimes observed in the skin of cattle adjacent to the site of a brand. Squamous cell carcinomas rarely arise at these injured sites. These lesions (Fig. 18–12) have some resemblance to those seen in the bovine skin several years after injury by beta radiation following radioactive fallout (Fig. 15–6).

Cutaneous Amyloidosis. Amyloid has been described by Hjärre and Nordlund (1942) in the skin of the horse. It appears as multiple, hard, elevated spherical nodules 5 to 25 mm in diameter, located particularly in the skin of the head, neck, and pectoral regions. The amyloid is seen microscopically in masses in the dermal papillae and in collars surrounding the sweat and sebaceous glands, as well as around blood vessels. This type of amyloidosis is not associated with deposition of amyloid in the visceral organs. Its cause is unknown.

Hjärre, A., and Nordlund, I.: Om atypisk amyloidos hos djuren. Skand. Vet. Tidskr., 32:385–441, 1942.

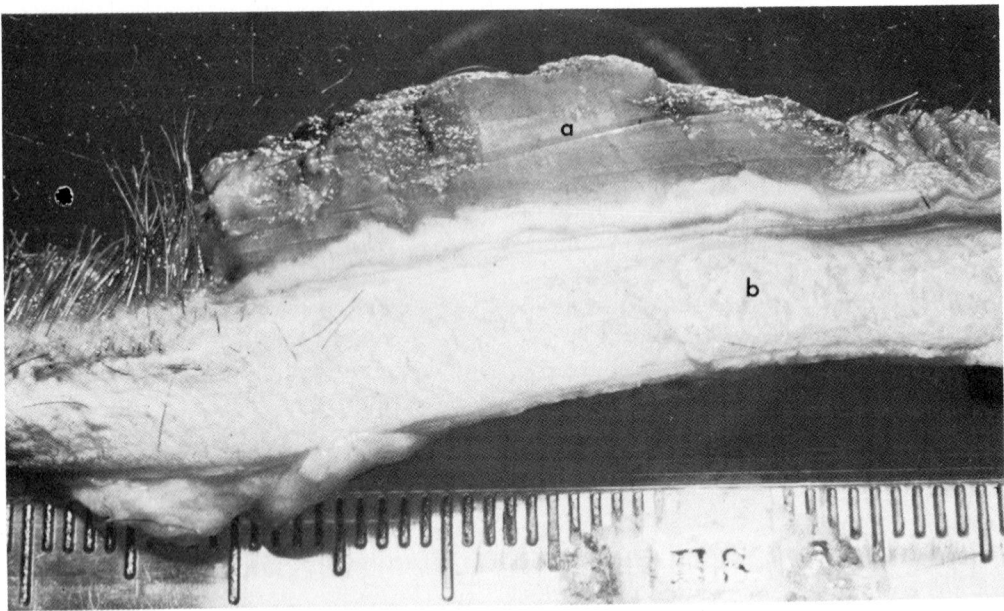

Fig. 18–12. "Brand papilloma" in the skin of a six-year-old male Hereford. Note the thick keratin layer (a) at the site of the scar caused by a hot-iron brand; dermis (b).

Lipogranulomatous Inflammation. A chronic inflammatory reaction within subcutaneous adipose tissue is occasionally encountered which is apparently unrelated to steatitis (yellow fat disease) due to vitamin E deficiency or traumatic necrosis of fat. The lesion is characterized by granulation tissue and mononuclear inflammatory cells surrounding and separating islands of adipose tissue. Macrophages contain neutral fat, and there are usually foci of typical fat necrosis. The lesions are usually multiple and unexplained. Identical lesions are sometimes seen in abdominal or mediastinal adipose tissue, especially in the bovine, where the term "lipomatosis" has been applied.

Xanthomatosis. Collections of histiocytic cells laden with lipid substances are occasionally encountered in the dermis and subcutis of animals. It is presumed that this finding is associated with some defect in lipid metabolism, but studies have been so limited that its significance is not understood. The lesions are recognized in microscopic sections only. Diffuse or nodular accumulations of large cells with abundant "foamy"-appearing cytoplasm are most frequent. In some cases, the presence of cholesterol is indicated by characteristic clefts in the tissue. Multinucleated giant cells are occasionally seen. Special stains of frozen sections reveal the lipid content of the cells.

The occurrence of familial diseases characterized by defects in lipid metabolism, as are known in man, has not yet been reported in animals. However, a disease of chickens has been described in which cutaneous xanthomatosis was a prominent feature.

Peckham, M.C.: Xanthomatosis in chickens. Am. J. Vet. Res., 16:580–583, 1955.
Sanger, V.L., and Lagace, A.: Avian xanthomatosis. Etiology and pathogenesis. Avian Dis., 10:103–111, 1966.
Thoonen, J., Hoorens, J., and Van Mierhaeghe, E.: Xanthomatosis beim Huhn. Arch. Gelflügelk., 23:314–318, 1959.

Laminitis. This inflammatory disease of the foot of solipeds usually has an acute onset following some event such as parturition or digestive upset. The affected horse has a fever and may be slightly lame in mild cases or may refuse to walk if severely affected.

The pathogenesis is poorly understood, but there is general agreement that the basis is cellular damage to the corium of the sensitive laminae (the laminated structure of the epithelium and its underlying dermis, which gives rise to and supports the hoof) resulting from altered circulation. There are, however, conflicting views regarding the nature of the initial vascular events. Early reports held that an increased blood flow due to vascular shock preceded cellular damage and inflammation. Currently the evidence indicates that the initial event is arteriolar constriction as a component of hypertension. Horses, lame from acute and chronic laminitis, have been demonstrated to be hypertensive. The resulting hypoxia then leads to tissue damage and inflammation, and possibly to a reduced availability of methionine, a necessary metabolite for synthesis of keratin. The cause of the hypertension, however, remains unknown.

Laminitis is known to occur in association with (1) sudden acute indigestion resulting from overeating of a concentrated grain ration. Diarrhea and presumably a severe acute enteritis are present in these cases. (2) It occurs following the use of irritant purgatives, especially aloes. It also occurs (3) following a sudden drink of cold water, or even exposure to a sudden cold rain, when the horse is hot from strenuous exercise in hot weather. Particularly when related to these gastrointestinal disturbances, the disease is often called **founder**. (4) It occurs in connection with septicemic infections, such as postparturient metritis (parturient laminitis), infected castration wounds, and possibly valvular endocarditis. (5) Laminitis develops from local causes, including the effects of an unusually hard drive on paved roads, or standing still too long while being transported on board ship. Standing with the pressure continually placed on one foot because of lameness in the other causes a unilateral laminitis in the foot subjected to this continuous pressure. Cattle also occasionally have laminitis from these local stresses.

The highly specialized epidermal and dermal structures of the hoof form layers of epithelium, corium, and keratin, which have orderly and intimate relationships to one another. Primary layers of epithelium are arranged in elongated, parallel fronds separated by thin bands of vascular stroma. The keratinized layer is specialized in that it forms primary and secondary onychogenic fibrils, which are bound together to form the horny part of the hoof. According to Obel (1948), the primary lesion in laminitis involves the epithelium, particularly the keratogenic zones. The keratohyalin granules disappear, and the onychogenic fibers are disorganized and lost. Eventually necrosis occurs in the epithelium, and this is presumed to lead to the severe hyperemia and occasionally to eventual separation of the hoof from the laminae.

If the congestion and inflammation subside within three or four days, laminitis may leave no permanent injury. If the condition persists longer, permanent deformity is likely to be the result, evidenced by the separated and downward pointing os pedis and the convex "dropped sole." Also, the normally straight anterior contour of the hoof becomes concave from the coronet to the toe, which is unduly prolonged, and the unevenly growing hoof forms a series of bulging rings parallel to its coronary origin, each representing a different phase of growth.

Ackerman, N., Garner, H.E., Coffman, J.R., and Clement, J.W.: Angiographic appearance of the normal equine foot and alterations in chronic laminitis. J. Am. Vet. Med. Assoc., 166:58–62, 1975.

Coffman, J.R., Johnson, J.H., Guffy, M.M., and Finocchio, E.J.: Hoof circulation in equine laminitis. J. Am. Vet. Med. Assoc., 156:76–83, 1970.

Garner, H.E., et al.: Equine laminitis and associated hypertension: a review. J. Am. Vet. Med. Assoc., 166:56–57, 1975.

Maclean, C.W.: The histopathology of laminitis in dairy cows. J. Comp. Pathol., *81*:563–570, 1971.
Obel, N.: Studies on the Histopathology of Acute Laminitis. Uppsala, Sweden, Almqvist and Wiksells, 1948.

Foreign Bodies in Skin. Foreign bodies usually reach the skin through some type of wound and may consist of any material or substance. Tissue reactions vary, depending on the anatomic site and the nature of the foreign body. Keratin and hair in the dermis or subcutis may stimulate intense inflammation. This is often observed when an inclusion cyst, hair matrix tumor, or keratoacanthoma ruptures, exposing its keratinaceous contents directly to the dermis or subcutis. This is the usual reason for sudden increase in size, ulceration, and inflammation associated with these lesions.

Other foreign bodies are found in the skin of animals upon occasion. Nettles and thorns of plants are among these. Schumacher and Majno (1967) reported thorns, believed to be from the palm (*Bactris minor*), in the skin and joints of a New World monkey, *Cebus albifrons*. These thorns, recognized in microscopic sections, produced little inflammation in the dermis, but provoked an intense granulomatous response in the synovial membrane of these animals. These have been compared to blackthorn (*Prunus spinus*) described in human skin and joints by Kelly (1966).

Kelly, J.J.: Blackthorn inflammation. J. Bone Joint Surg., *48*:474–477, 1966.
Schumacher, R.H., and Majno, G.: Thorns in the skin and joints of the monkey. Arch. Pathol., *84*:536–538, 1967.

Endocrine Alopecia. Certain changes in the skin characterized by bilateral symmetry, loss of hair, and atrophy of epidermis have for many years been ascribed to "endocrine dysbalance" or "deficiency," with scant knowledge of the causative factors involved. This view, while not wholly incorrect, is not accurate nor specific enough to permit understanding of the etiologic or therapeutic aspects of the disease. Much still needs to be learned, but at least three specific endocrine disturbances are now known to cause "endocrine alopecia."

The first of these is hyperestrogenism, resulting from the prolonged administration of estrogens, such as diethylstilbestrol, or from the presence of an estrogen-secreting **Sertoli cell tumor** of the testicle. The estrogen elaborated by this tumor not only produces changes in the skin, but causes redistribution of body fat, gynecomastia, squamous metaplasia of the prostate, and other evidence of feminization. This tumor is most common in cryptorchid testes of dogs. The skin in this condition loses its hair over broad, bilaterally symmetric areas of the legs, neck, buttocks, flanks, and occasionally the entire body. The hairs become brittle and are easily pulled or rubbed out and are not replaced. Depletion of hair follicles and sebaceous glands are evident in microscopic sections, as is moderate atrophy of the epidermis.

The second condition in which endocrine alopecia is a prominent feature is **hypothyroidism**. In this disease, hair loss is gradual but has the usual bilateral symmetry. The skin in involved areas is thin, smooth, and sometimes irregularly pigmented. Hair that remains over the rest of the body is usually fine and sparse. Administration of thyroxin results in improvement in vigor and return of the normal hair coat. The microscopic changes in the skin are essentially similar to those seen in hyperestrogenism.

A third syndrome in which endocrine alopecia occurs has been descibed by Coffin and Munson (1953), and named by them a **pituitary-adrenal state** or **canine Cushing's syndrome**. This disease is recognized in dogs, particularly Boston Terriers, and is manifest by gradual onset of abdominal enlargement, roughness of the hair coat, and symmetric alopecia. The legs develop bare areas that extend to involve the flanks, buttocks, and thighs. The hair

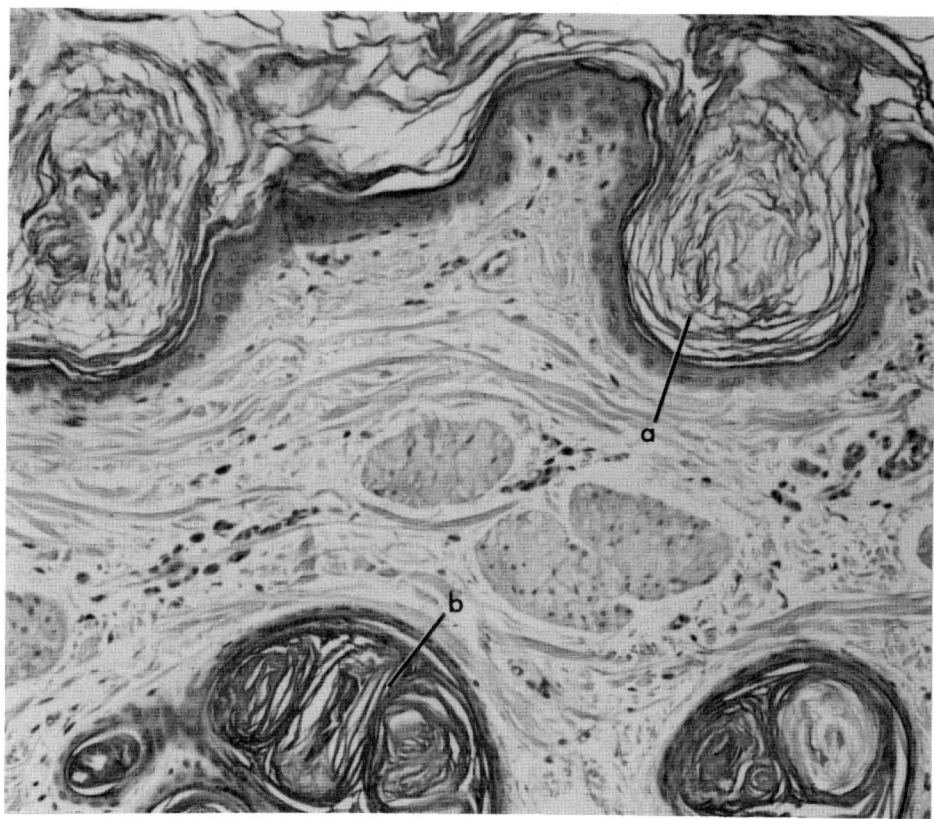

Fig. 18–13. The skin in canine hypothyroidism. A seven-year-old female Chihuahua with characteristic clinical signs. Note hyperkeratosis involving epidermis (*a*) and the hair follicles (*b*). (Courtesy of Angell Memorial Animal Hospital.)

becomes rough, dry, and is easily broken or pulled out. The skin may be rough and scaly and bear small pustules, which appear sporadically. These pustules rupture, leaving a scaly margin and a dark pigmented center. The skin is often cool to the touch. Muscular relaxation and weakness may appear, resulting in trembling and assumption of straight-legged posture. Diabetes insipidus occurs in some cases, evidenced by polydipsia, polyuria, and low specific gravity of the urine. Lymphopenia and eosinopenia are also characteristic features.

The lesions in the skin are described as atrophy of the hair follicles, sebaceous glands, and epidermis, with loss of dermal fat, condensation of collagen and elastic fibers, and hyperkeratosis. In some severely affected animals, the dermis becomes calcified, replaced by new bone over rather large areas of the body. The pathologic findings in the rest of the body consist of enlargement of the pituitary with hyperplasia of basophil cells and formation of multiple cysts, and symmetric hyperplasia of the adrenal cortices, which causes enlargement of the adrenals to four to eight times their normal size.

Amoroso, E.C., and Ebling, F.J.: Allergic and endocrine dermatoses in the dog and cat—II. Hormones and skin. J. Small Anim. Pract., 7:755–775, 1966.

Coffin, D.L., and Munson, T.O.: Endocrine diseases of the dog associated with hair loss. J. Am. Vet. Med. Assoc., 123:402–408, 1953.

Gardner, W.U., and DeVita, J.: Inhibition of hair

growth in dogs receiving estrogen. Yale J. Biol. Med., *13*:312–315, 1940.

Montgomery, H.: Dermatopathology, Vol. 1 and 2. New York, Harper & Row, 1967.

Thomsett, L.R.: Allergic and endocrine dermatoses in the dog and cat. III. Endocrine disorders and hair loss in the dog. J. Small Anim. Pract., *7*:777–780, 1966.

Walton, G.W.: Symposium on allergic and endocrine dermatoses in the dog and cat. I. Allergic dermatoses of the dog and cat. J. Small Anim. Pract., *7*:749–754, 1966.

HELMINTH AND ARTHROPOD DISEASES OF SKIN

Helminths and arthropods frequently parasitize the integument of animals, producing a variety of pathologic manifestations. These parasites and the diseases they cause are described in Chapter 14, but because of their importance, Table 18–1 was prepared to permit the student to visualize the variety of such parasites that affect domestic animals, and to provide a convenient reference.

NON-NEOPLASTIC CYSTS

Epidermal Inclusion Cyst. Epidermal inclusion cysts are most frequently encountered in the dog. They usually are firmly attached within the dermis and appear as small nodules, which slowly increase in size. The overlying skin usually remains covered with hair until the nodule attains a large size. Incision of the nodules reveals one or more spherical cysts with a thin wall and a gray, grumous, somewhat desiccated content. These cysts usually are cured by surgical excision; occasionally they may become ulcerated and infected. (See Fig. 18–14.)

Microscopic examination discloses the cyst wall to be made up of flattened squamous epithelium surrounded by a dense collagenous capsule. Skin adnexa are not present in association with the cyst wall. The cyst contains concentrically and irregularly laminated masses of keratin, occasionally mixed with amorphous tissue debris. Sometimes the epithelial wall of the cyst ruptures, stimulating an intense foreign body reaction around the extruded cyst contents.

The origin of these epidermal inclusion cysts is not entirely explained, but in the dog at least they appear to result from the occlusion of the mouth of hair follicles and subsequent isolation of the involved epithelium. The continuous desquamation of keratin by the stratified squamous epithelium which makes up the cyst wall soon fills the internal space and forces the cyst to expand.

Epidermoid or Dermoid Cyst. The epidermoid cyst is grossly similar to the epidermal inclusion cyst but is differentiated by the character of the cyst wall, which is made up of epidermis supplied with skin adnexa. Sebaceous glands, hair follicles, and sweat glands may be present singly or in combination. In some instances, in addition to the keratinaceous and oily debris found in the cyst, fragments of hairs may be present. Epidermoid and epidermal inclusion cysts have essentially the same biologic significance. The epidermoid cyst has no connection with the teratomatous "dermoid" of the ovary (Chapter 25) nor with congenital "dermoid" of the eye (Chapter 28).

Complex epidermoid cysts occur quite often in the midline of the back of one breed of dog—the Rhodesian Ridgeback. These are elongated sacs lined by stratified squamous epithelium with adnexa (hair, sebaceous, and apocrine glands) and extend deep into the tissues, often reaching to the bodies of the vertebrae (Fig. 18–17). These have been compared to **trichostasis spinulosa** (Hare, 1932, Stratton, 1964) and may have some relationship to spina bifida.

Epidermoid cysts must be distinguished from the **hair matrix tumor** (benign calcifying epithelioma, epithelioma of Malherbe), which is somewhat similar in appearance but has a different significance. This lesion can be distinguished microscopically by its content, which has a

Table 18–1. Parasitic Diseases of the Skin

Hosts	Parasite	Location of Lesion
Cattle, sheep, dog, man, swine, horse	*Sarcoptes scabiei,* var. *bovis, ovis, canis, suis,* etc.	Epidermis generally (scabies or sarcoptic mange)
Dog, cat, man, swine, sheep, cattle	*Demodex folliculorum*	Hair follicles, sebaceous glands, dermis, lymph nodes (demodectic mange)
Sheep, cattle, horses, rabbits	*Psoroptes communis,* var. *ovis, bovis, equi,* and *cuniculi*	Epidermis of ears and elsewhere
Cattle, sheep, horses, goats	*Chorioptes bovis*	Epidermis of feet and base of tail
Swine	*Demodex phylloides*	Hair follicles and sebaceous glands
Dogs, cats, sheep, deer, rarely man	*Thelazia californiensis*	Conjunctiva, membrana nictitans
Dogs, cattle	larvae of *Rhabditis strongyloides*	Dermis and hair follicles
Cat	*Notoedres cati*	Epidermis, esp. of neck (notoedric mange)
Cattle	larvae of *Hypoderma bovis* and *lineatum* (ox warble)	Subcutis and dermis of back
Cattle	*Thelazia rhodesi*	Conjunctiva, membrana nictitans
Cattle	*Onchocerca gutturosa*	Dermis and subcutis
Cattle	*Onchocerca gibsoni*	Subcutis
Cattle (U.S.)	*Stephanofilaria stilesi*	Hair follicles and dermis, usually of abdomen
Cattle (Indonesia)	*Stephanofilaria dedoesi*	Hair follicles and dermis of shoulders, eyelids, neck, withers, dewlap
Cattle (India)	*Stephanofilaria assamensis*	Dermis of shoulders and elsewhere
Cattle (Malaya)	*Stephanofilaria kaeli*	Dermis and epidermis of lower parts of legs
Cattle	*Parafilaria bovicola*	Subcutis
Sheep, deer	microfilaria of *Elaeophora schneideri*	Dermis of head, face, poll
Sheep	*Psorergates ovis*	Epidermis generally
Horses	microfilaria of *Onchocerca cervicalis*	Dermis of abdomen and pectoral region
Horses	larvae of *Habronema majus*	Dermis, pectoral region
Horses	larvae of *Draschia megastoma*	Dermis, pectoral region
Horses	larvae of *Habronema muscae*	Dermis, pectoral region
Horses, asses, mules	*Parafilaria multipapillosa*	Nodules, subcutis
Horses, asses, mules	*Onchocerca reticulata*	Subcutis, dermis
Man	larvae of *Schistosomes* of birds and mammals	Dermis ("swimmer's itch")
Man	larvae of *Ancylostoma*	Dermis ("creeping eruption")
Mice	*Psorergates simplex*	Epidermis generally
Poultry	*Dermanyssus gallinae*	Epidermis generally
Chicken	*Cnemidocoptes mutans*	Scales of legs
Chicken	*Cnemidocoptes gallinae*	Feather follicles
Dog, rabbit, cat	*Cheyletiella parasitivorax*	Epidermis generally
Dog, mink, otter, raccoon	*Dracunculus insignis*	Subcutis of limbs

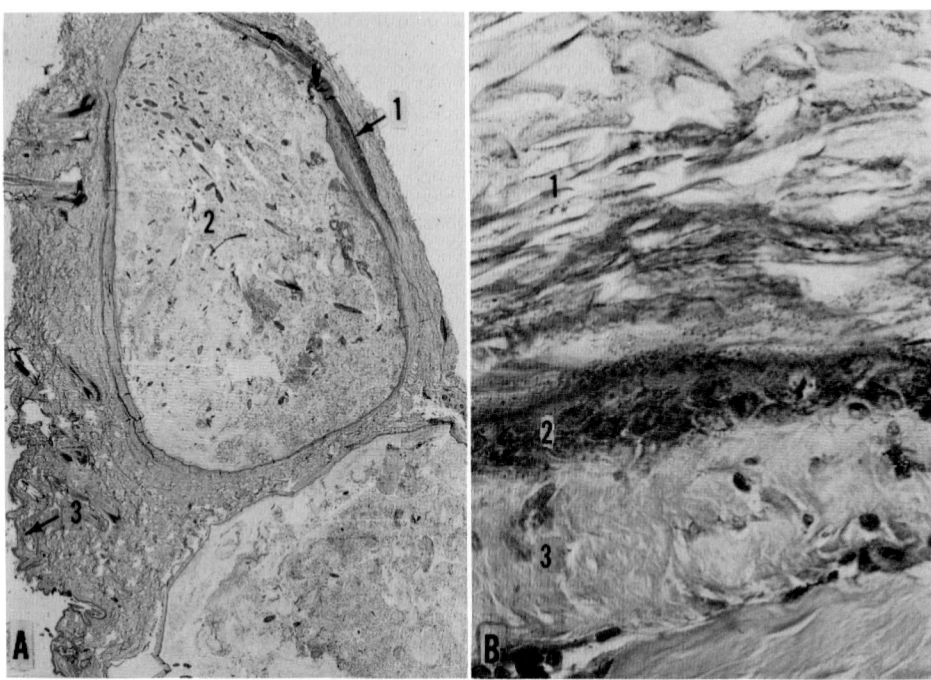

Fig. 18–14.   Epidermal inclusion cysts in the skin of a dog. *A,* Cyst (× 9) in dermis, with squamous wall (*1*), keratinous contents (*2*). Epidermis (*3*). *B,* Same lesion as *A* (× 490). Flakes of keratin (*1*) in the center of the cyst, stratified squamous epithelium (*2*), and dense collagen (*3*) in the cyst wall. (Courtesy of Armed Forces Institute of Pathology.) Contributor: Dr. Edward Baker.

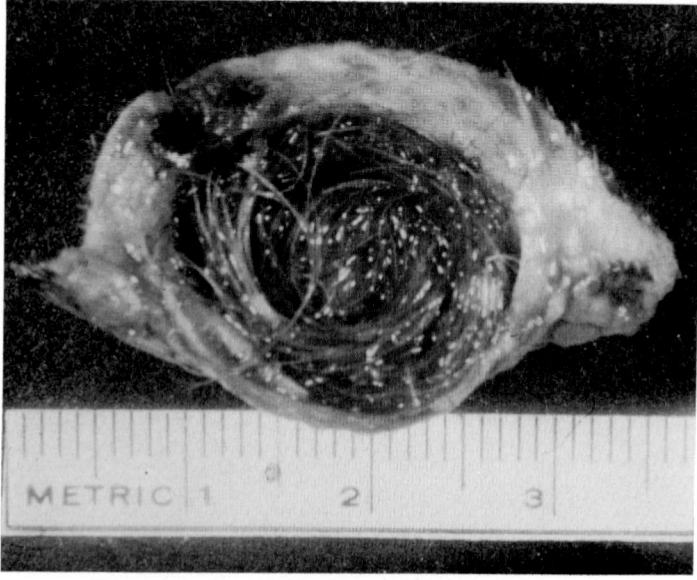

Fig. 18–15.   Epidermoid cyst in the skin of the tail of a seven-year-old castrated male bloodhound. Note hair in cyst. (Courtesy of Angell Memorial Animal Hospital.)

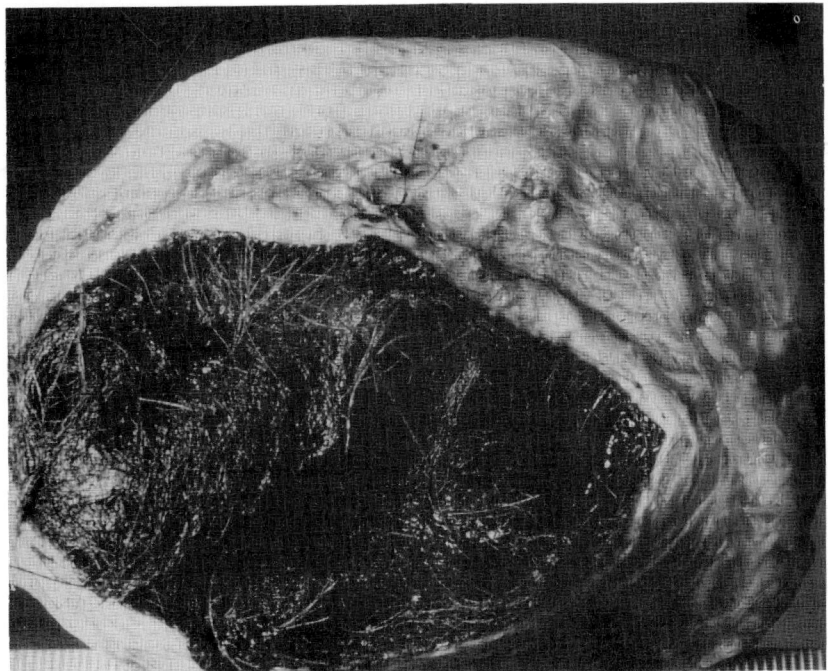

Fig. 18–16. Dermoid cyst, skin of cervical region, bovine.

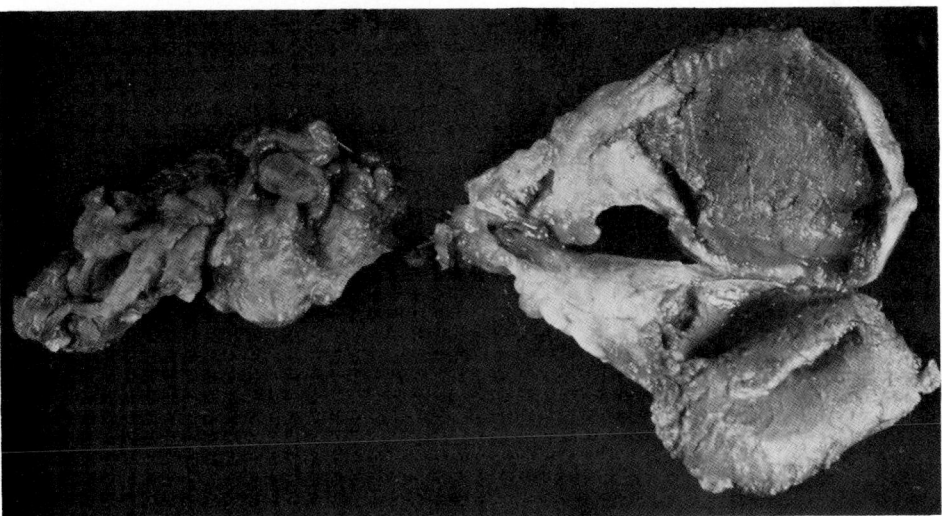

Fig. 18–17. Epidermoid cyst removed surgically from the midline of the back of a male Rhodesian Ridgeback dog, age one year. The opened sac at the right was near the skin, the tissue at the left extended down to the vertebra. (Courtesy of Angell Memorial Animal Hospital.)

definite pattern of multiple whorls, suggesting hair follicles, even though nuclei and all details are lost. It is apparent that the contents develop from the outer rim of viable cells by loss of nuclei and differential staining, but have a much more definite structure than the concentrically laminated pattern in the epidermal inclusion or cyst, which results from extrusion of keratin from its wall. The wall of the hair matrix tumor is also more complex, consisting mostly of basal cells, which often form abortive hair follicles. Calcification is apt to occur in the contents of the hair matrix tumor.

Sebaceous Cyst. A sebaceous cyst arises from dilatation of a sebaceous gland or its duct and is essentially similar to an epidermal cyst, except that the contents are even more rich in sebaceous material and may contain cholesterol clefts.

Sudoriferous Cyst. Cysts of sweat glands arise on the basis of occlusion of their ducts, usually as the result of changes in the epidermis. They may be single or multiple, are filled with watery fluid, and lined by a single layer of simple columnar or cuboidal epithelium. They usually do not become large.

Calcinosis Circumscripta. Circumscribed masses of calcium salts are sometimes recognized in the dermis of the dog, most often in the larger breeds, and occasionally in horses. Similar deposits that occur in human skin have been designated as "calcinosis circumscripta," a term which is descriptive of the animal lesion to which the name may be applied, at least until more is known about its cause and significance. The lesion appears as a mass 1 to 10 cm in diameter, containing a cluster of chalky-white granular foci separated by thin strands of connective tissue. The entire nodule thickens the dermis and ele-

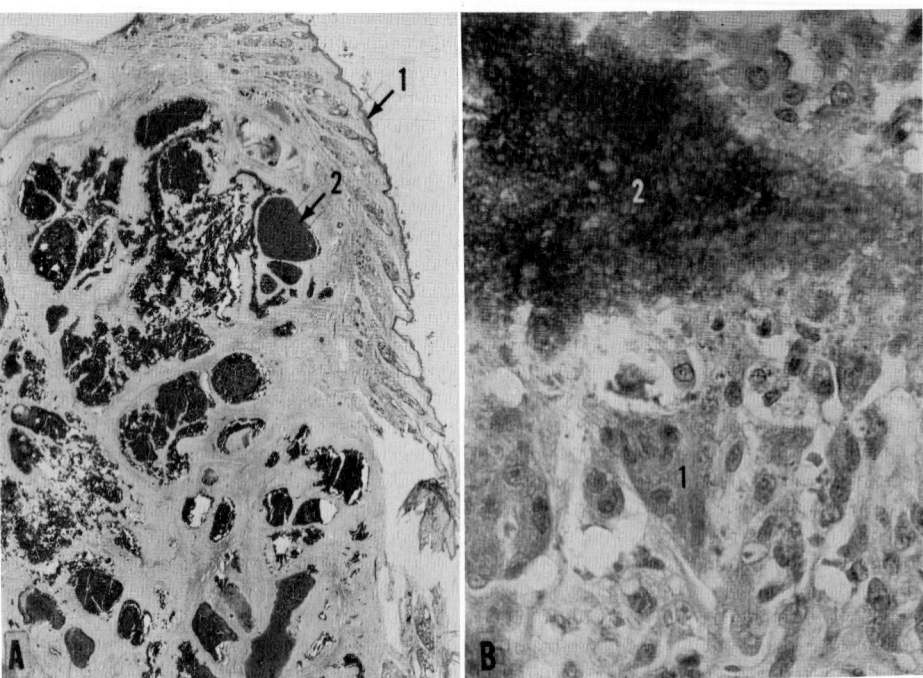

Fig. 18–18. Calcinosis circumscripta, skin of a dog. *A,* Low magnification (× 7). Epidermis (*1*), circumscribed deposits (*2*) of calcium salts in the dermis. *B,* Same specimen as *A* (× 440). Epithelioid cells (*1*) surrounding calcium salts (*2*). (Courtesy of Armed Forces Institute of Pathology.) Contributor: Dr. S. W. Stiles.

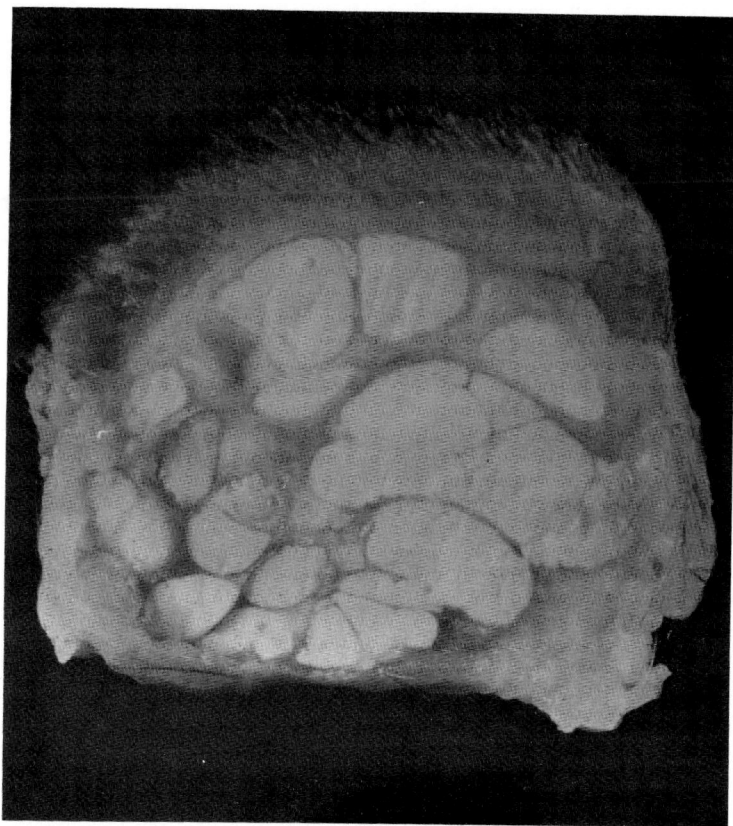

Fig. 18–19. Calcinosis circumscripta, skin of a male, three-year-old dachshund. Freshly cut specimen. (Courtesy of Angell Memorial Animal Hospital.)

vates the epidermis. The cut surface reveals its chalky appearance and gritty consistency. (See Figs. 18–18 and 18–19.)

Microscopically, the lesion is composed of multiple spherical loculi sharply demarcated from the adjacent stroma and from one another. In early stages these loculi contain amorphous material which is basophilic in hematoxylin and eosin stained sections, PAS-positive, stains deeply with alcian blue, and is occasionally metachromatic. Calcification in the form of fine granules extends inward from the outer borders of these loculi. The border first consists of stroma, but eventually is made up of epithelioid and multinucleated giant cells.

Christie and Jabara (1964) propose that the lesion of calcinosis circumscripta arises

from cystic apocrine sweat glands and therefore should be called "cystic apocrine calcinosis." This appears plausible and may eventually prove to be correct, but does not explain the identical lesions that we have observed in the tongue. Further, in early lesions studied by Jones, it was not possible to demonstrate a morphologic relation to apocrine glands. We consider that the question of the pathogenesis of this lesion is not yet settled.

Antin, I.P.: Dermoid sinus in a Rhodesian Ridgeback dog. J. Am. Vet. Med. Assoc., 157:961–962, 1970.

Christie, G.S., and Jabara, A.G.: Apocrine cystic calcinosis: the sweat gland origin of calcinosis circumscripta in the dog. Res. Vet. Sci., 5:317–322, 1964.

Cordy, D.R.: Apocrine cystic calcinosis in dogs and its relationship to chronic renal disease. Cornell Vet., 57:107–118, 1967.

Dodd, D.C., and Raker, C.W.: Tumoral calcinosis (calcinosis circumscripta) in the horse. J. Am. Vet. Med. Assoc., 157:968–972, 1970.

Hare, T.: A congenital abnormality of hair follicles in dogs resembling trichostasis spinulosa. J. Pathol. Bact., 35:569–572, 1932.

Howell, J. McC. and Ishmael, J.: Calcinosis circumstripta in the dog with particular reference to lingual lesions. Pathol. Vet., 5:75–80, 1968.

Kunge, A.: Über multiple Kalkeinlagerung in der Unterhaut der Extremitäten des Hundes. Arch wiss. prakt. Thierheilk., 54:462–478, 1926.

Stratton, J.: Dermoid sinus in the Rhodesian Ridgeback. Vet. Rec., 76:846–848, 1964.

Thompson, S.W., II., Sullivan, D.J., and Pedersen, R.A.: Calcinosis circumscripta. A histochemical study of the lesions in man, dogs and monkey. Cornell Vet., 49:265–285, 1959.

NEOPLASMS

Neoplasms of the skin are of particular interest in veterinary medicine for they are not only common, but usually accessible for surgical excision or other means of treatment. The general and identifying features of neoplasms are discussed in Chapter 4. Included here are primary neoplasms of the epidermis and the adnexae, and the neoplasms of the dermis that are most frequent in the skin or restricted to this location. Neoplasms that arise in specialized epidermal structures (e.g., mammary gland, ceruminous gland) are discussed elsewhere, as are neoplasms of supporting structures covered in other systems (e.g., hemangioma, neurofibroma). Table 18–2 lists cutaneous neoplasms by site of origin and indicates which are discussed in other sections of this book. The relative frequency of neoplasms of the skin in dogs and cats is listed in Table 18–3. The skin is the most common site for neoplasia in dogs, and second only to malignant lymphomas in cats.

Neoplasms of Epidermis

Papilloma. The term "papilla" denotes a small projection; a papilloma is a tumor consisting of papillary projections, usually a large number of them. It is a benign epithelial neoplasm, but since epithelium always rests upon a connective tissue base, which provides the blood vessels supply-

Table 18–2. Neoplasms of the Skin

Neoplasm	Chap.
Epidermis	
Papilloma	
Squamous cell carcinoma	
Keratoacanthoma	
Basal cell carcinoma	
Malignant melanoma	
Adnexa	
Adenoma and adenocarcinoma of sweat and apocrine glands	
Adenoma and adenocarcinoma of sebaceous glands	
Adenoma and adenocarcinoma of perianal gland	
Hair matrix tumor (benign calcifying epithelioma)	
Trichoepithelioma	
Adenoma and adenocarcinoma of ceruminous glands	28
Mammary gland neoplasms	25
Dermis and Subcutis	
Fibroma and fibrosarcoma	
Equine sarcoid	
Mast cell tumor	
Canine cutaneous histiocytoma	
Venereal tumor	25
Hemangioma, hemangiosarcoma	21
Lymphangioma, lymphangiosarcoma	21
Hemangiopericytoma	
Neurofibroma, neurofibrosarcoma	27
Lipoma, liposarcoma	
Tumor of brown fat (hibernoma)	
Xanthoma	
Myxoma, myxosarcoma	

ing necessary nutrients, the epithelial tumor always has a core of fibrous connective tissue. As the epithelial cells grow and multiply, their excess population finds room by bulging and folding outward from the surface. As these bulges grow into more and more complicated papillary projections, the underlying connective tissue grows with them. It is believed that the true neoplastic process resides in the epithelium, however. Papillomas of known viral etiology and the bovine fibropapilloma are discussed in Chapter 9.

Papillomas of the skin are covered with stratified squamous epithelium, cornified but usually unpigmented, and always

Table 18–3.   Relative Frequency (%) of Neoplasms of Skin, Subcutis, and Adnexa in Dogs and Cats*

	Dog	Cat
1. Mast cell tumor	18.2	15.6
2. Hemangiopericytoma	9.1	0
3. Lipoma	8.3	3.9
4. Adenoma, perianal gland	8.3	0
5. Canine cutaneous histiocytoma	8.2	0
6. Adenoma of sebaceous gland	6.8	2.6
7. Hair matrix tumor	6.5	1.3
8. Malignant melanoma	5.3	3.9
9. Keratoacanthoma	3.8	1.3
10. Hemangioma	3.4	0
11. Papillomatosis	3.4	0
12. Basal cell tumor	2.9	23.4
13. Adenocarcinoma of sebaceous gland	2.3	2.6
14. Adenocarcinoma of perianal gland	2.0	0
15. Fibrosarcoma	2.0	5.2
16. Adenoma of sweat gland	1.7	3.9
17. Adenocarcinoma of sweat gland	1.5	5.2
18. Hemangioendothelioma	1.5	7.8
19. Melanoma, benign	1.2	0
20. Tumor, unclassified	1.1	6.5
21. Squamous cell carcinoma	1.0	6.5
22. Ganglioneuroma	0.6	3.9
23. Fibroma	0.5	3.9
24. Neurofibroma	0.3	2.6
25. Liposarcoma	0.1	0
26. Tumor of brown fat	0.1	0
27. Mixed tumor of sweat gland	0.1	0
Total %	100	100
Total (No.)	(1370)	(77)

* Modified from Jones, 1971.

without accessory skin structures and rete pegs. The epithelium is clearly demarcated from the underlying dermis. They may be small rounded elevations, but more usually they are papillary, with a characteristic cauliflower-like appearance. The surface may be smooth but generally is rough and horny. The head and neck are the most common sites, but they may arise anywhere, particularly in cattle. Papillomas are illustrated in Chapter 9.

Smaller but similarly formed papillomas near the corneoscleral junction constitute an early stage of squamous-cell carcinoma of the bovine eye. Whether the malignant change is to be attributed to the original or to some further carcinogenic stimulus is not known.

Squamous papillomas may also occur in the oral cavity, esophagus, and rumen (Chapter 23); transitional cell papillomas, in the urinary bladder (Chapter 24); and papillary growths (called polyps), covered with cuboidal or columnar epithelium, in the intestine and ducts of glands (Chapter 23).

Squamous Cell Carcinoma. This, the commonest form of carcinoma, is characterized by and derived from stratified squamous epithelium. Its epithelium cornifies or not, in accordance with the epithelium from which it was derived.

Pigmentation and papillation (formation of rete pegs), however, are not carried over into the neoplasm. In a reasonably well-differentiated tumor of this type, the usual succession of layers is preserved from the underlying connective-tissue stroma, the dark, basal stratum germinativum, the larger and paler cells of the stratum spinosum or prickle-cell layer, gradually flattening out to join the stratum corneum or cornified (keratinized) layer. However, this epithelium is by no means restricted to the outer surface of the neoplasm, as would be the case in a papilloma. On the contrary, epithelial masses and columns extend promiscuously into and through the neoplastic mass. Cross sections of these masses present themselves as islands of epithelium surrounded by stroma. The basal layer of epithelial cells thus comes to lie at the periphery of such an island, with

what would normally be the most superficial epithelium occupying the center of the mass. In the case of a cornifying tumor, the red-staining keratin of the stratum corneum comes to lie at the center of the epithelial mass, becomes quite dense from the pressure of growing cells, and forms a rounded, laminated structure known as an **epithelial pearl**. The presence of intercellular bridges between adjacent cells (prickle cells) provide an easy means of identifying the origin of the tumor. Epithelial pearls and intercellular bridges, however, may be lacking in poorly differentiated squamous cell carcinomas.

The term **epidermoid carcinoma** is sometimes used to designate these tumors, inasmuch as they are derived from the epidermis. The tongue, esophagus, rumen, ocular surfaces, and vagina also bear cornifying squamous-cell carcinomas.

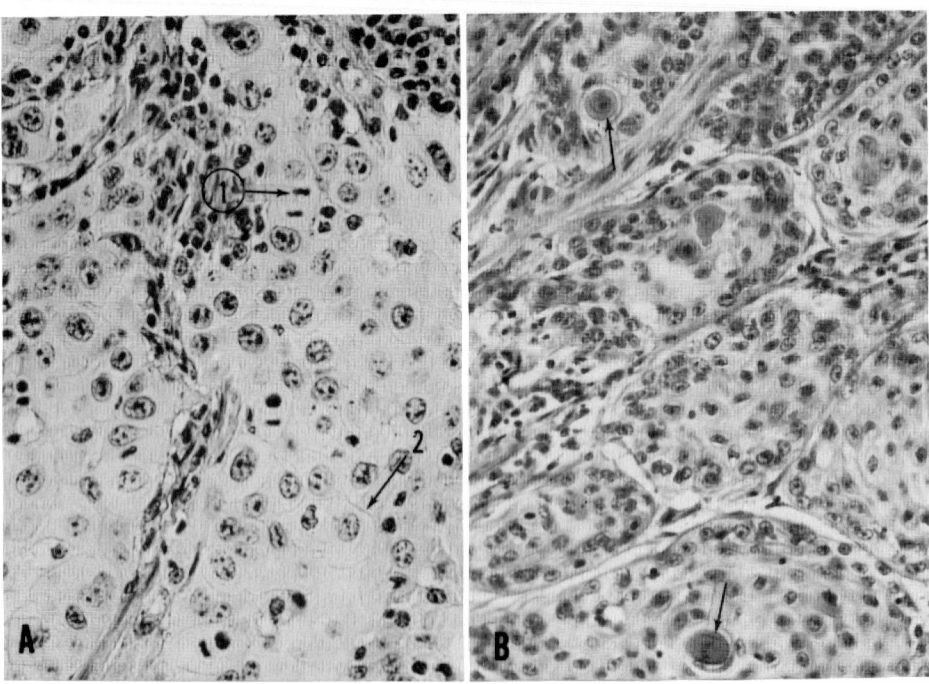

Fig. 18–20. Squamous cell carcinoma. *A,* From the corneal epithelium of a four-year-old Hereford cow. Mitotic figures (*1*) are frequent and cell borders (*2*) are prominent (× 335). Contributor: Drs. C. N. Barron and G. T. Easley. *B,* Primary tumor in the vulva of a six-year-old Hereford cow. (× 224). Keratinized centers of epithelial "pearls" are indicated by arrows. Contributor: Dr. C. L. Davis. (Courtesy of Armed Forces Institute of Pathology.)

The more anaplastic squamous-cell carcinomas lack differentiation into layers,
and the epithelial masses consist of cells
that are all more nearly uniform, with dark,
hyperplastic nuclei, sometimes in the
process of mitosis. Occasionally, the
epithelial cells of a highly anaplastic carcinoma (squamous-cell or adenocarcinoma) may assume a fusiform or spindle
shape, so that it becomes difficult even to
make the primary determination whether
the tumor is a carcinoma or sarcoma. Of
some assistance is the fact that the cells of a
sarcoma, being relatives of endothelium,
can and usually do form the walls of the
blood vessels in the tumor. Epithelial cells
cannot do this, but must be provided with
at least enough interstitial tissues to form
an endothelium for the blood vessels.
These endothelial cells almost always have
a different appearance from the neoplastic
cells. Also, among the cells of an anaplastic
sarcoma, there almost always run minute
fibrils of stroma; carcinoma cells are merely
in juxtaposition. Of course, carcinoma cells
must always rest upon a fibrous stroma
somewhere, and in all but the most anaplastic the difference between the tumor
cells and their stroma is readily perceived.

Squamous-cell carcinomas arise from the
skin and the stratified squamous epithelium of all body openings, and are rather
frequent in all domestic species. These,
like other carcinomas, are especially liable
to metastasize to the regional lymph nodes,
thence to visceral organs. As with most
neoplasms, the cause is not known, but
there is a relationship to solar irradiation
with the occurrence of squamous cell carcinoma of the eyelid (and corneoscleral
junction) in cattle, the ear of white cats, and
nose and skin in lightly pigmented dogs.
An unusual form of squamous cell carcinoma called **carcinoma of the horn** or
horn cancer arises at the junction of the
skin and the horn. It is seen in Zebu cattle
in India and Sumatra, where it is most
common in castrated bulls, rare in cows,
and nonexistent in intact bulls, except for

one report in a cryptorchid bull (Naik et al.,
1970).

Pseudoepitheliomatous hyperplasia, as
the name implies, must be differentiated
from squamous cell carcinoma. The former
is noninvasive, but the architectural relationships may be obscured by inflammation. The morphology of squamous cell
carcinomas is also frequently complicated
by secondary inflammatory reactions arising from ulcerated surfaces, or by an intense lymphocytic infiltration, presumably
a T-cell response.

Keratoacanthoma. In recent years an increasingly frequent lesion in the human
skin has been recognized under various
names, including "nonmetastasizing
squamous-cell carcinoma" and "keratoacanthoma," the latter being most favored.
A corresponding entity occurs in the dog
and rarely in other animals. The lesion is
not a true neoplasm, but rather a keratinaceous cyst surrounded by hyperplastic epithelium which may mimic squamous cell
carcinoma. The appearance suggests an
origin from hair follicles or adnexa, but
from study of early lesions the process starts
as a downgrowth of epidermis between
hair follicles. The thickened, downward-
growing epidermis forms a crypt, which
eventually becomes a multiloculated cyst
crowded with persistent keratin. Continued
folding of this epithelium produces few or
many concentrically laminated masses of
keratin surrounded by a uniform layer of
squamous epithelium, whose cells maintain
their usual polarity and orderly arrangement. As the epithelial mass continues to
expand, the central collections of keratin
may become conspicuous. In most, but not
all cases, columns of cuboidal cells grow
out from the basal surface of the epithelium
into the dermal stroma and in some instances join one another to form interlacing
cords or columns (Fig. 18–22). This feature
sometimes suggests an abortive attempt to
form sweat glands, but such an interpretation is by no means established. Inflammation may become a prominent feature in

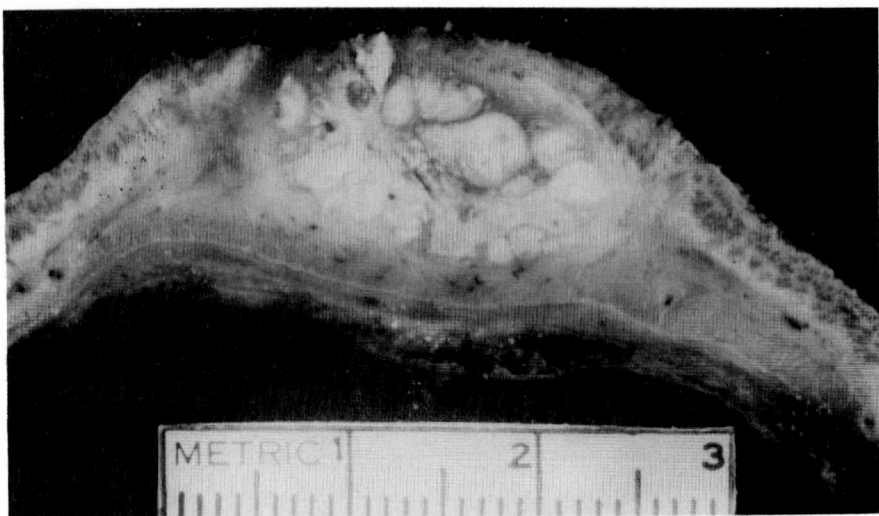

Fig. 18–21. Keratoacanthoma, skin of a four-year-old German Shepherd. Note ulceration of the epidermis and the multilobulated masses in the dermis and subcutis. (Courtesy of Angell Memorial Animal Hospital.)

the surrounding dermis, especially if any keratin or other detritus escapes through a rupture in the epidermis.

All available evidence indicates that the keratoacanthoma in the dog, as in man, is a self-limiting disease, although multiple tumors and recurrent lesions are common. Stannard and Pulley (1975) observed up to 40 growths on one dog, and suggested that Norwegian Elkhounds were more prone to this generalized form of the disease. Keratoacanthomas appear to be more frequent in males and occur in a younger population than most other cutaneous tumors.

Basal-cell Tumor. The adjective, "basal-cell," is applied to this clinically homogeneous group of epithelial neoplasms in the belief that they arise from the basal, or germinal layer (stratum germinativum), of the epidermis. The classic name for these tumors is "basal cell carcinoma," but their proclivity to remain localized seems to make it inconsistent to call them carcinomas. Other terms used to indicate the character of this tumor include **basal cell epithelioma** and **basiloma**. While some pathologists make certain distinctions and

subdivisions, it may be said in general that basal cell tumors arise from the basal layer of the epidermis proper or basal cells of hair follicles, sebaceous glands, or sweat glands (which have only one epithelial layer).

Clinically, basal-cell tumors in man are locally and persistently invasive, but rarely metastasize. They are also highly sensitive to roentgen rays. Sufficient numbers have scarcely received careful study to justifiy conclusions on all phases of their clinical behavior in animals, but indications are that this is about the same in animals as in man. In the dog, as in man, the head, neck, and shoulder are favorite sites of localization. Grossly, the tumors are likely to remain small, but with the exception of the trichoepithelioma, tend to ulcerate early. They frequently recur after surgical removal, but metastasis is exceptionally rare.

The arrangement of the tumor cells varies in different cases, but the cells themselves are rather constantly of small or medium size, ovoid, and closely packed. The nuclei are small, ovoid, or round and darkly stained, like those of the normal stratum germinativum. The cytoplasm is

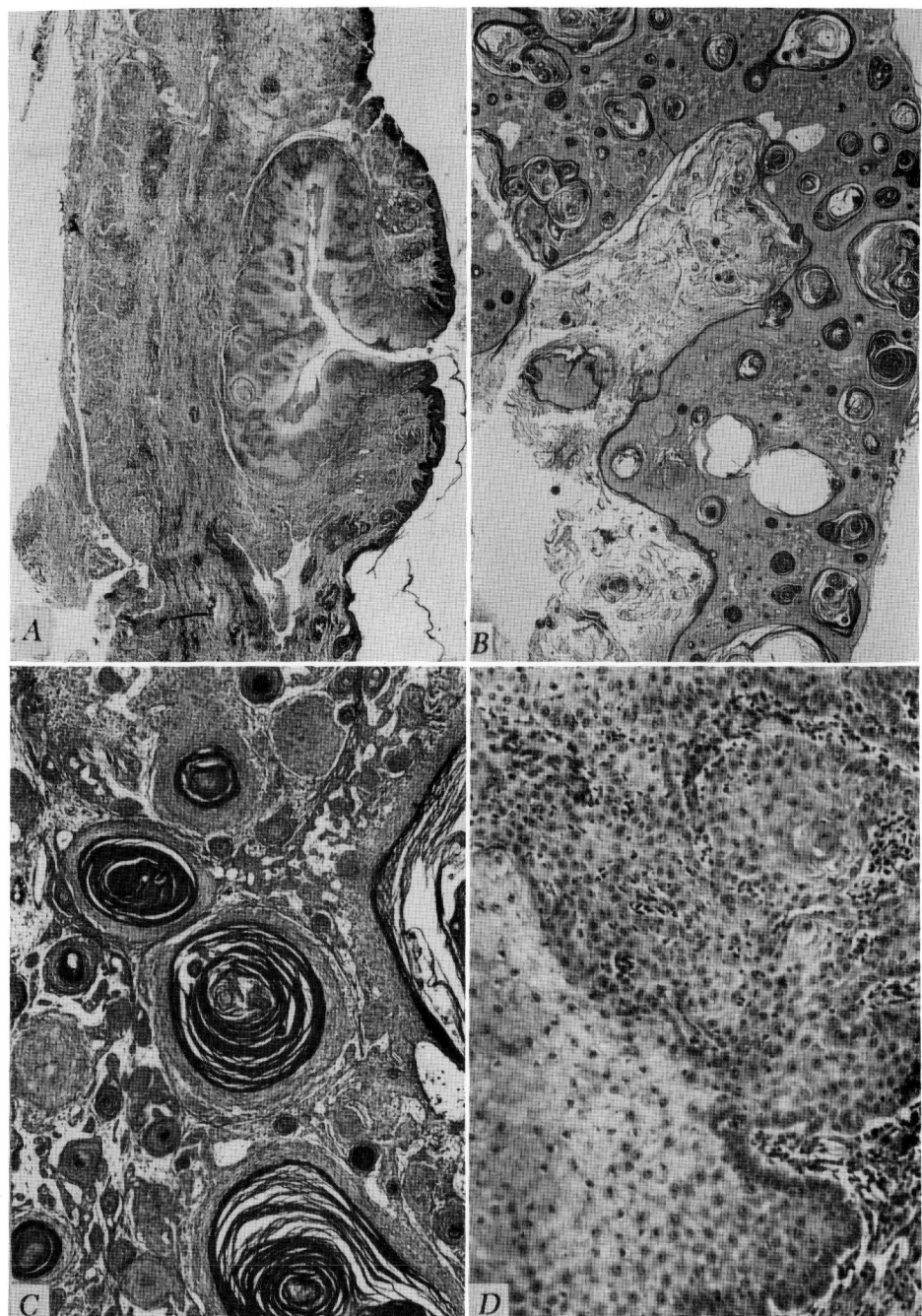

Fig. 18–22. Keratoacanthoma (canine). *A,* Early lesion (× 9) arising from epidermis which is thickened and forced downward into the dermis. *B,* A more fully developed lesion (× 9) with multiple keratin nests and a cystic center. *C,* Another lesion, with many epithelial nests filled with keratin and cords of cells between them (× 50). *D,* Solid zones of epithelium in the early development of the lesion. (H & E, × 150.) (Courtesy of Angell Memorial Animal Hospital.)

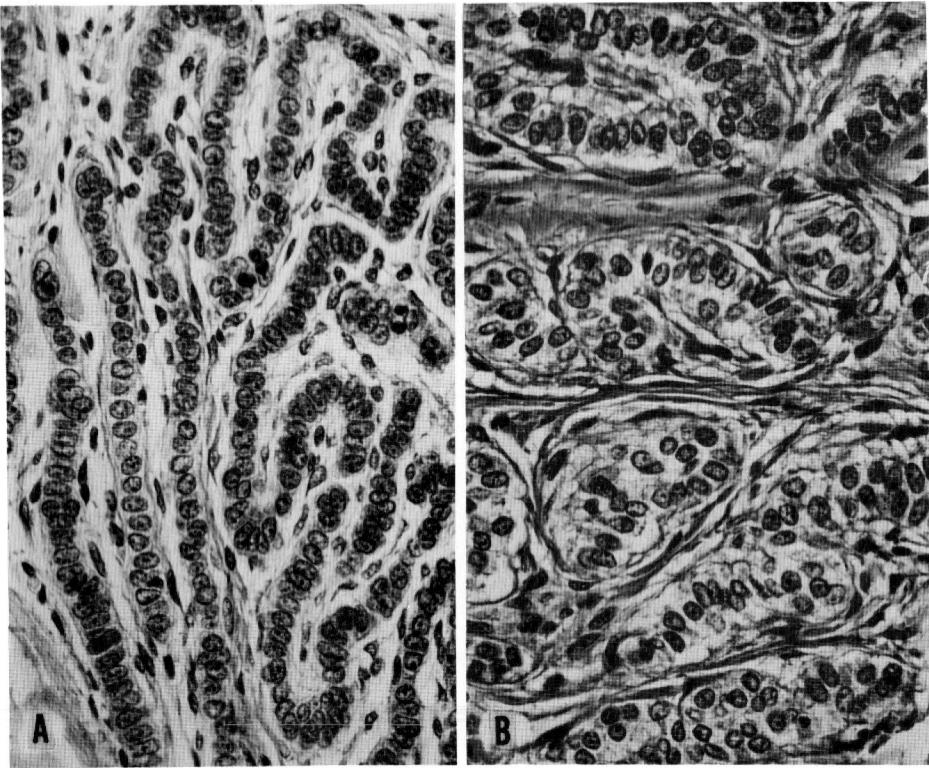

Fig. 18–23. Basal-cell tumor, skin of nose of a four-year-old male, mongrel dog. *A*, Characteristic long, tortuous cord of cells with elongated nuclei perpendicular to length of cord. (× 400). *B*, Another area in same tumor (× 400), with tumor cells forming nests. (Courtesy of Armed Forces Institute of Pathology.) Contributor: Dr. W. H. Cowan.

scanty and pale and may contain melanin. Projecting spines, prickles, or intercellular bridges, as they are variously designated, are absent, which again relates the neoplasm to the germinal rather than the more superficial layers of epidermis. Mitoses are usually scarce.

In most basal-cell tumors, the cells form **solid masses**, rounded and sharply contoured, which lie just beneath the epidermis but are separated from it by a zone of dermal connective tissue. Occasionally, a place may be found where the two epithelia join; such a spot is considered one of the points of origin of the neoplastic process. Like the basal layer in normal skin, the outermost layer of cells of the mass is often unusually dark (hyperchromatic), with its individual cells elongated in a direction perpendicular to the base line. These tumors are differentiated from squamous-cell carcinomas by the lack of any gradation or transition from basal cells to larger and paler prickle cells, and by the absence of any semblance of the cornification that characterizes cutaneous and some other squamous-cell carcinomas. (Rarely, intermediate types are reported that have limited formation of cornified foci and a clinical behavior that is also intermediate between that of the basal-cell and the more malignant squamous-cell carcinomas.) These tumors may, on occasion, contain melanin.

Some basal-cell tumors form small or large **cystic spaces**. These often resemble glands and possibly should be so considered, although the cells lining the

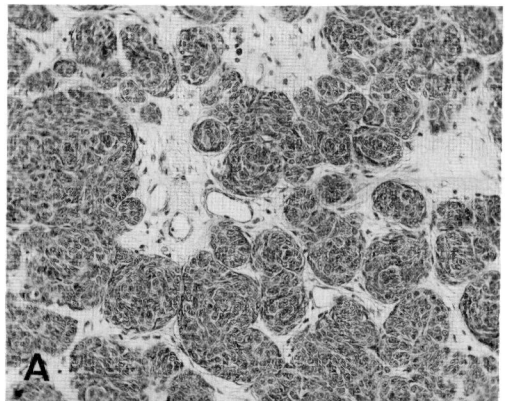

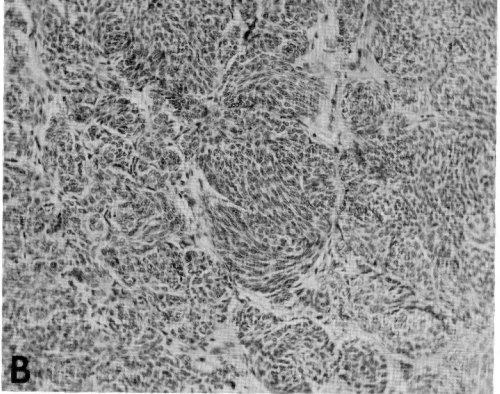

Fig. 18–24. Basal-cell tumor, skin of a cat. *A*, Discrete interconnecting islands of oval cells in a connective tissue stroma. *B*, From another area of the same neoplasm, the cells are more fusiform in shape. (Courtesy of Armed Forces Institute of Pathology.)

glands usually are not different in appearance from their neighbors at some distance from the gland-like space. This situation has led to the belief that such tumors arise in sweat glands, justifying a separate classification of sweat-gland carcinoma or adenoma, or such special terms as syringocarcinoma, syringadenoma, and others. Some authorities also ascribe a sweat-gland origin to a type in which the basal cells insinuate themselves into the stroma in **long, twisting lines** composed of just one or two rows of transversely elongated cells, thus resembling the single layer of cells that lines a normal sudoriferous gland. However, this type and the solid type first described both occur in the same tumor.

The confusion that exists in the classification and nomenclature of the basal-cell group is illustrated by the fact that for one form that constitutes a rather definite entity in human medicine the following synonyms exist: turban tumor, cylindroma, multiple sarcoma, nevoepithelioma adenoides, sweat-gland carcinoma, epithelioma adenoides cysticum, syringoma, syringocystadenoma, plexiform sarcoma, angiosarcoma, endothelioma capitis, and tomato tumors (Cooper, 1946). Various authors attribute the origin of this tumor to sweat glands, sebaceous glands, and basal cells. It is probable that all are correct, depending on the variety encountered in the individual case.

Hair matrix tumor and trichoepithelioma are often considered variants of basal cell tumors. These are discussed under neoplasms of adnexa.

Melanomas. Melanomas arise from melanin-forming cells. They are malignant or, at least only temporarily, benign. Cells that have the ability to produce melanin (melanoblasts) arise embryologically in the neural crest, which originates from the neuroectoderm. Early in embryonic life, these cells migrate to other positions in the body, particularly the skin, where they eventually produce melanin. This pigment enters into other tissue cells (e.g., dermis, epidermis, choroid, retina, ciliary processes, meninges) adjacent to the melanoblast. It is not surprising, therefore, that tumors of melanin-producing cells are most common in the skin but may originate elsewhere. Their nature and chemistry have been discussed in connection with melanin. Since some melanomas consist of cells formed and arranged like epithelium and others equally resemble undifferentiated fibrous or supporting tissue, they have been called melanocarcinomas and melanosarcomas respectively. Present usage employs neither of those terms.

Melanomas of the skin are common tumors in most species, even in fishes. Their mode of origin has been the subject of much speculation and study. In human beings, many cutaneous melanomas arise in the small raised, brown spots present in almost everyone's skin known as **pigmented moles** or **nevi** (singular—nevus). Fortunately, most nevi do not undergo malignant transformation. Lesions morphologically somewhat similar to human nevi occur in dogs (and probably other species), but there have been few studies to determine whether their clinical behavior is the same as that in man. If in fact nevi do occur in animals, they are usually diagnosed as benign or malignant melanomas. The types of nevi seen in human beings have been classified into three principal morphologic types (for which there is further subdivision). These are **junctional nevus, intradermal nevus** and **compound nevus**.

A junctional nevus is composed of roughly spherical clusters of large round cells in the basal and prickle cell layer of the epidermis. The cells are separated from one another due to acantholysis, and the cytoplasm may or may not be pigmented. If the cells are anaplastic, the lesion is believed to be malignant. A histologically similar finding is seen in the epidermis overlying melanomas in man as well as animals. This is referred to as a **junctional change** and essentially is diagnostic of malignant melanomas in dogs. An intradermal nevus is composed of nests of cells sometimes forming cords within the upper dermis. The mass is not clearly demarcated from the dermis and the cells may or may not be pigmented. In a compound nevus, there are both features of junctional nevus and intradermal nevus. The majority of pigmented spots in dogs are foci of *circumscribed epidermal hyperpigmentation* (Kraft and Frese, 1976), and not analogous to nevi.

The histologic appearance of melanomas varies considerably. The cells may be so filled with the brown pigment that little else can be seen, or at the other extreme, there may be no melanin at all, an amelanotic melanoma. The shape of the cells varies in different tumors, or sometimes within the same tumor, from round or polyhedral forms resembling epithelium to elongated, fusiform cells which one would take for fibroblasts. Typically the latter type predominates, and the spindle-shaped cells fit together somewhat like the segments of an orange, to fill compartments clearly or vaguely marked off by thin fibrous trabeculae. The cytoplasm tends to be basophilic, and typically, when stained with the milder hematoxylin preparations (Mayer's hemalum), the nuclei have a distinctive violet hue which is not seen in other than melanoma cells. The nucleoli are large and prominent. In most cases the large amounts of melanin in the cytoplasm of the tumor cells, as well as that phagocytized by melanophores in the vicinity, leave no doubt regarding the diagnosis, but some melanomas are so amelanotic that the diagnosis must be made on the morphologic features of the cells. A particularly useful if not pathognomonic feature is the occurrence of a junctional change in the epidermis overlying a dermal melanoma. This change is similar in appearance to a junctional nevus as described previously, but the islands of separated epidermal cells are more anaplastic and usually contain melanin. The basement membrane is lost and the altered epithelium blends with the dermal neoplasm and extends upward into the epidermis. Some rete ridges may be entirely replaced by junctional change. In human beings, this altered epithelium is believed to be the origin of malignant melanoma. The change is not seen in melanoma metastatic to the skin.

Although we incline to the view that all melanomas are potentially malignant, many follow a course that can be considered benign for months or even years, the patient perhaps dying of some other cause. Attempts to separate the malignant

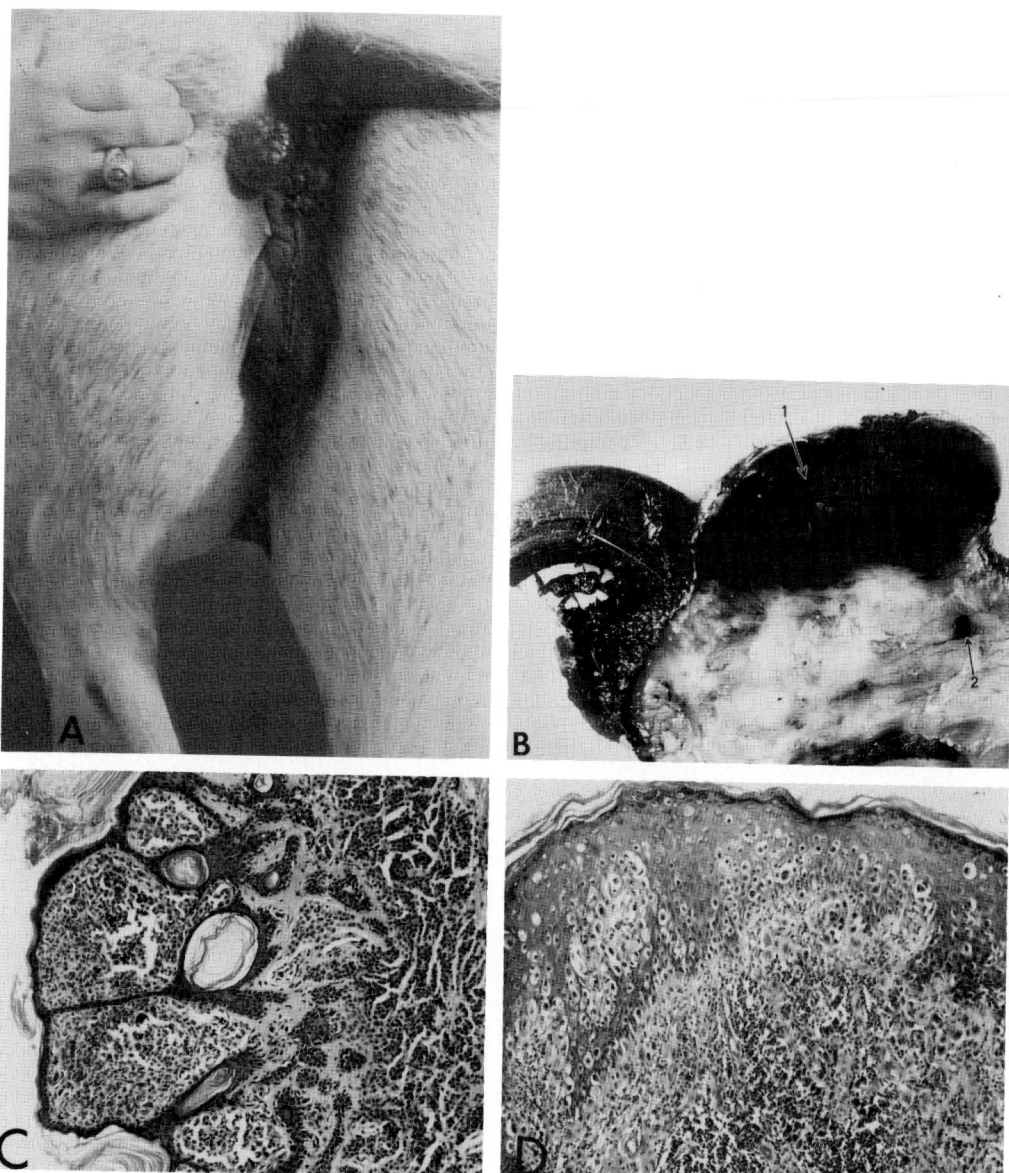

Fig. 18–25. *A,* Melanoma in the perineum of an aged mule. (Courtesy of Dr. Thomas Hardy.) *B,* Malignant melanoma arising at base of toe nail of a 16-year-old male dachshund-collie crossbred dog. The tumor mass (*1*) is not encapsulated and a small mass is separated from it (*2*). (Courtesy of Angell Memorial Animal Hospital.) *C,* Compound nevus in the skin of a human being. Although not infrequent in man, such lesions are rare to nonexistent in animals. *D,* Junctional change of the epidermis overlying a malignant melanoma. Epithelial cells of the basal and prickle cell layer are separated from one another, swollen, and disorganized.

from the benign by histologic examination depend on the general criteria of malignancy already given. These include large, hyperchromatic nuclei, bizarre forms, and mitotic figures. An underlying lymphocytic infiltration is considered a sign of malignancy, as is also invasion of lymphatics. However, highly differentiated melanomas (heavily pigmented, noninvasive, low mitotic index) may behave as malignant neoplasms. These cannot be readily differentiated from those melanomas that follow a benign course.

Grossly, the melanoma is ordinarily recognized by its deep black color and by the inky pigment that diffuses from it into any watery medium with which the cut surface may come in contact. The true nature of an amelanotic melanoma may be discoverable only by microscopic examination.

Melanomas occur in so many forms and locations that generalization is difficult. Quiescent or actively malignant melanomas are especially frequent in old gray horses, although they are by no means nonexistent in horses of other colors. Their location is especially likely to be in the perianal and perineal regions (Fig. 18–25), from where they spread to perirectal and other pelvic lymph nodes. In one case, the first symptom in a brown mare was complete inability to use one hind leg. Investigation showed that an intrapelvic melanoma had spread along the femoral canal and had enveloped the sciatic nerve. In some equine cases, death results from metastases to the spleen, lungs, or other internal organs without the primary lesion having been found. One case is recalled in which half a mare's mammary gland was replaced by melanoma, probably by direct extension from a tumor of the overlying skin.

The association of graying or loss of pigmentation (known as vitiligo) with melanoma is also recognized in human being and in Sinclair swine (Millikan et al., 1974). In man, vitiligo occurs in patients with melanoma 10 to 20 times more frequently than in the general population. This is thought to result from destruction of normal melanocytes through an immune mechanism stimulated by a melanoma. In Sinclair swine, which reportedly have an incidence of multiple melanomas over 20%, there is depigmentation of normal skin as well as of the tumors, most of which ultimately regress. In horses, graying appears to precede development of melanoma, but this deserves more careful attention.

In cattle, melanomas arise in the skin at various locations. In swine, cutaneous melanomas varying in diameter from a few millimeters to several centimeters and usually somewhat elevated are common. The smaller ones usually remain until the pig is slaughtered; larger ones are often removed surgically, a perfect cure usually resulting. They are most frequent on the posterior half of the body. In the meat-producing animals, there is little opportunity to observe the ultimate outcome of these tumors. In the dog, cutaneous melanomas arise in various parts of the body and are one of the commonest neoplasms of the lip and oral cavity in breeds having pigmented oral mucosa. In dogs, melanomas in the latter location have a more rapidly malignant course than those arising in the skin.

As indicated, most melanomas arise in the skin; those arising in the meninges and eyes are discussed in Chapters 27 and 28 respectively.

Neoplasms of Adnexa

Adenomas and Adenocarcinomas of Sweat and Apocrine Glands. Most neoplasms of sweat and apocrine glands are probably diagnosed as basal cell tumors (excluding certain specialized neoplasms, e.g., those of mammary gland); however, in the dog, neoplasms are encountered that are clearly glandular in structure or whose cells have the morphologic characteristics of apocrine glands. Most such tumors, as would be expected, are of apocrine gland

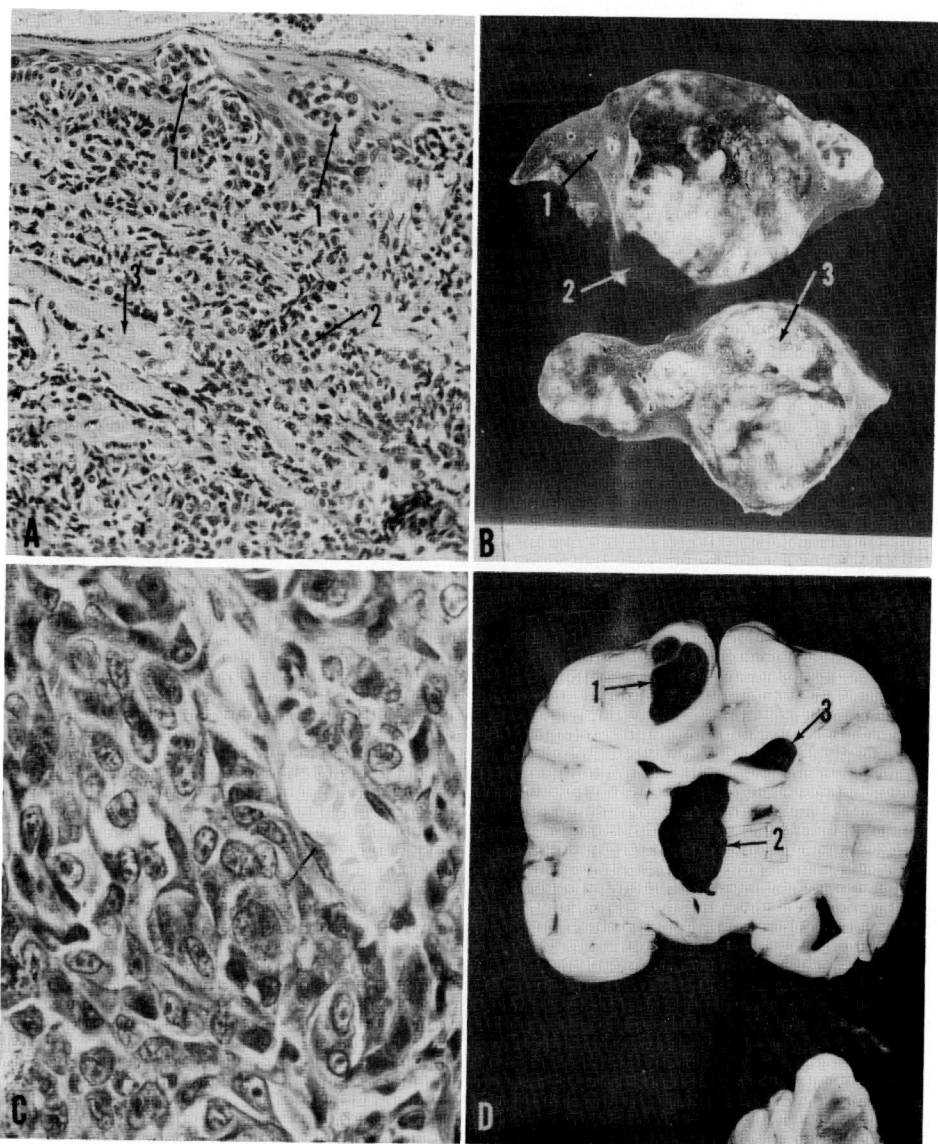

Fig. 18–26. Malignant melanoma. *A,* Primary lesion in tongue of a dog (× 160). Note neoplastic cells in epidermis (*1*) and dermis (*2*), displacing collagen fibers (*3*). *B,* Metastatic malignant melanoma in lung (*1*) of a dog. Note melanotic (*2*) and amelanotic (*3*) areas. Contributor: Dr. M. L. Povar. *C,* High magnification (× 574) of tumor in *A*. Large cells laden with melanin (arrow). Contributor: Dr. Leo L. Lieberman. *D,* Metastatic malignant melanoma (*1*) and (*2*) in brain of a dog. Note slight internal hydrocephalus (*3*). (Courtesy of Armed Forces Institute of Pathology.) Contributor: Dr. C. L. Davis.

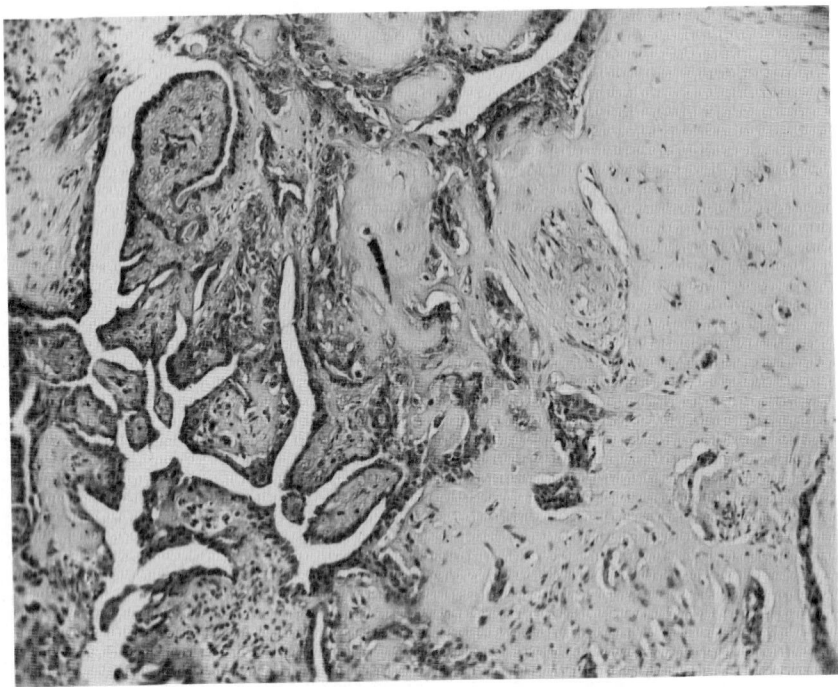

Fig. 18–27. Mixed tumor of sweat gland. The neoplasm contains cartilage and glandular epithelium. (Courtesy of Armed Forces Institute of Pathology.)

origin. The benign neoplasms resemble normal apocrine glands, but have more variation in size or papillary projections into the lumens. They are usually surrounded by abundant dense collagenous connective tissue. Adenocarcinomas have the usual features of malignancy, and the cells may form solid masses with little or no attempt to form glands, in which case their histologic origin is difficult to ascertain. Rarely, the tumors may contain cartilage and resemble mixed tumors of the canine mammary gland (**"mixed tumor" of sweat glands**).

Adenomas and Adenocarcinomas of Sebaceous Glands. A rather common benign tumor closely simulating the normal sebaceous gland histologically is readily recognized in dogs. Often there is little but size to distinguish it from the normal glands, and the question of mere hyperplasia arises. The adenomas tend to be sharply localized in the dermis but are not encapsulated. Hyperplasia is more apt to be a diffuse process, with many enlarged, hypercellular sebaceous glands spread over a larger part of the dermis.

Adenocarcinomas, which occur in the dog, are much more anaplastic than adenomas, with many undifferentiated cells and few cells with vacuolated cytoplasm resembling sebaceous cells. They often extend haphazardly into the dermis, are not sharply circumscribed or encapsulated, and may metastasize. In dogs, tumors of sebaceous glands are most frequent in the skin of the hindquarters, abdomen, and thorax.

Adenomas and Adenocarcinomas of Perianal Glands. The perianal or circumanal glands in the dog are paired, modified sebaceous glands located in the subcutis on each side of the anus. Their excretion is discharged into two epithelial-lined sacs, lateral to the anus, which communicate with the anus through a small opening near the mucocutaneous junction. The glands are composed of irregular columns of large, closely packed polyhedral cells with eosinophilic cytoplasm rich in finely particulate lipid. The cells extrude their holocrine secretion through ducts lined by modified perianal gland cells, emptying into perianal sacs.

Benign tumors (adenomas) are common, particularly in male dogs, and are usually sharply circumscribed, thinly encapsulated, spherical masses of varying size. Their cut surface is usually orange-tinted and greasy in texture, sometimes altered by dark hemorrhage or ulceration of the overlying skin. Histologically, the adenoma closely resembles the normal gland, except that the glands are usually larger and more closely packed; the epithelial cells, hyperplastic and hypertrophic; and ducts, irregular in numbers and location. Ulceration and hemorrhages due to external trauma are frequent. The modified sebaceous cells cling together and usually have an orderly relationship to their scant stroma (Fig. 18–28).

Adenocarcinomas are much less frequent, but surprisingly, are apt to arise in aged spayed females, in which the benign form is rare. This malignant form may metastasize to the iliac lymph nodes (Fig. 18–29) and thence to sublumbar and other intraabdominal lymph nodes, and eventually reach the general circulation. The identifying feature of this malignant variety is the isolation of individual tumor cells and small irregular groups of these cells in the stroma, which is apparently invaded. This is the only reliable histologic criterion for malignancy in this tumor. To the uninitiated who has not studied and followed the biologic behavior of the neoplasm, many adenomas may appear to be malignant from their histologic appearance.

Hair Matrix Tumor (Benign Calcifying Epithelioma). One type of benign epidermal growth thought to arise from the hair follicle is recognized under the name "hair

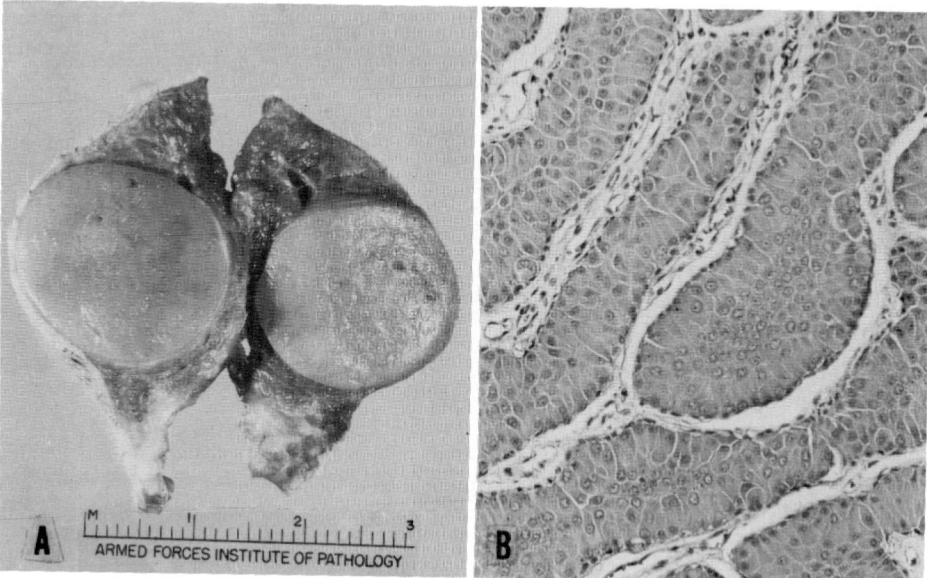

Fig. 18–28. Adenoma of perianal gland of a six-year-old male beagle. *A,* Gross specimen with its spherical outline and orange-tinted, greasy cut surface. *B,* Photomicrograph (× 150) of the new growth. Irregular columns of large polyhedral cells supported by delicate stroma. (Courtesy of Armed Forces Institute of Pathology.) Contributor: Major C. N. Barron.

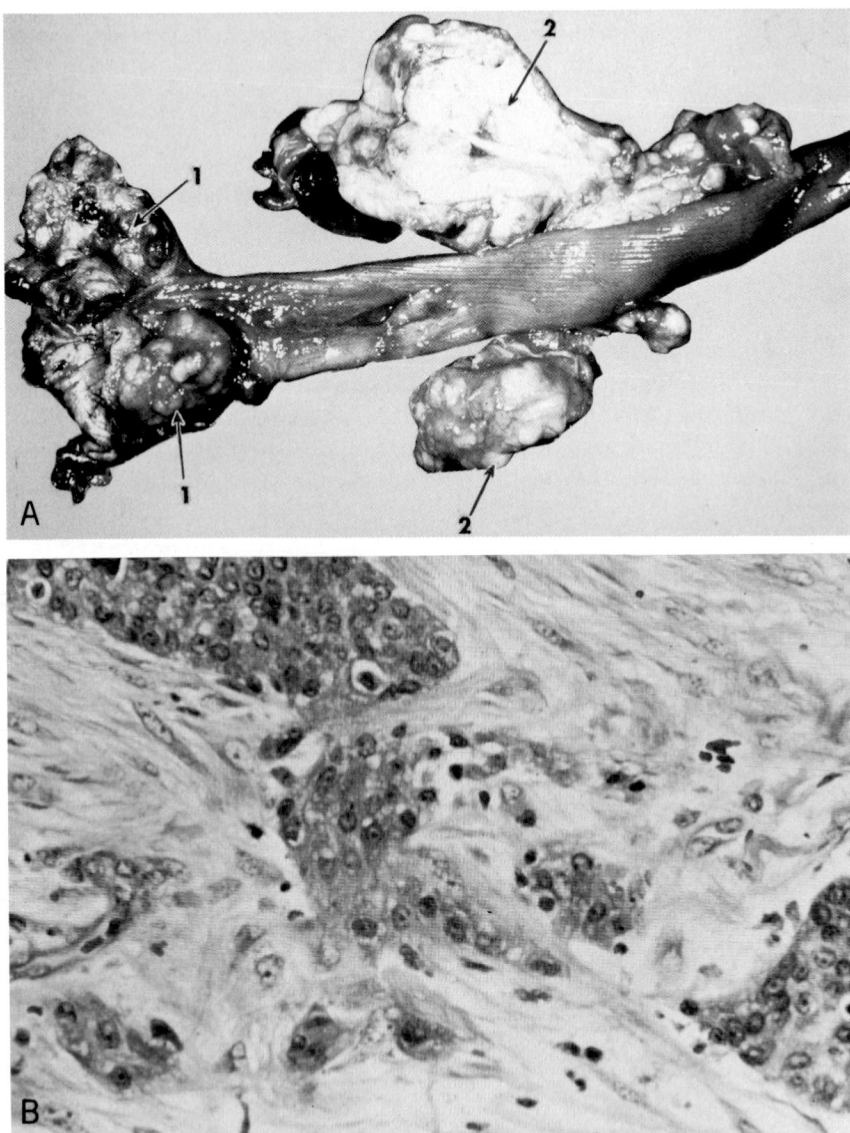

Fig. 18–29.   Adenocarcinoma of perianal gland of a ten-year-old spayed female Cocker Spaniel. *A,* Two tumor masses *(1)* near anus, and metastatic tumors in iliac lymph nodes *(2)* adherent to the rectum. (Courtesy of Angell Memorial Animal Hospital.) *B,* Microscopic appearance of malignant cells of adenocarcinoma of perianal gland. Note irregular bizarre shape of the cells and their isolation into small groups in the cellular stroma.

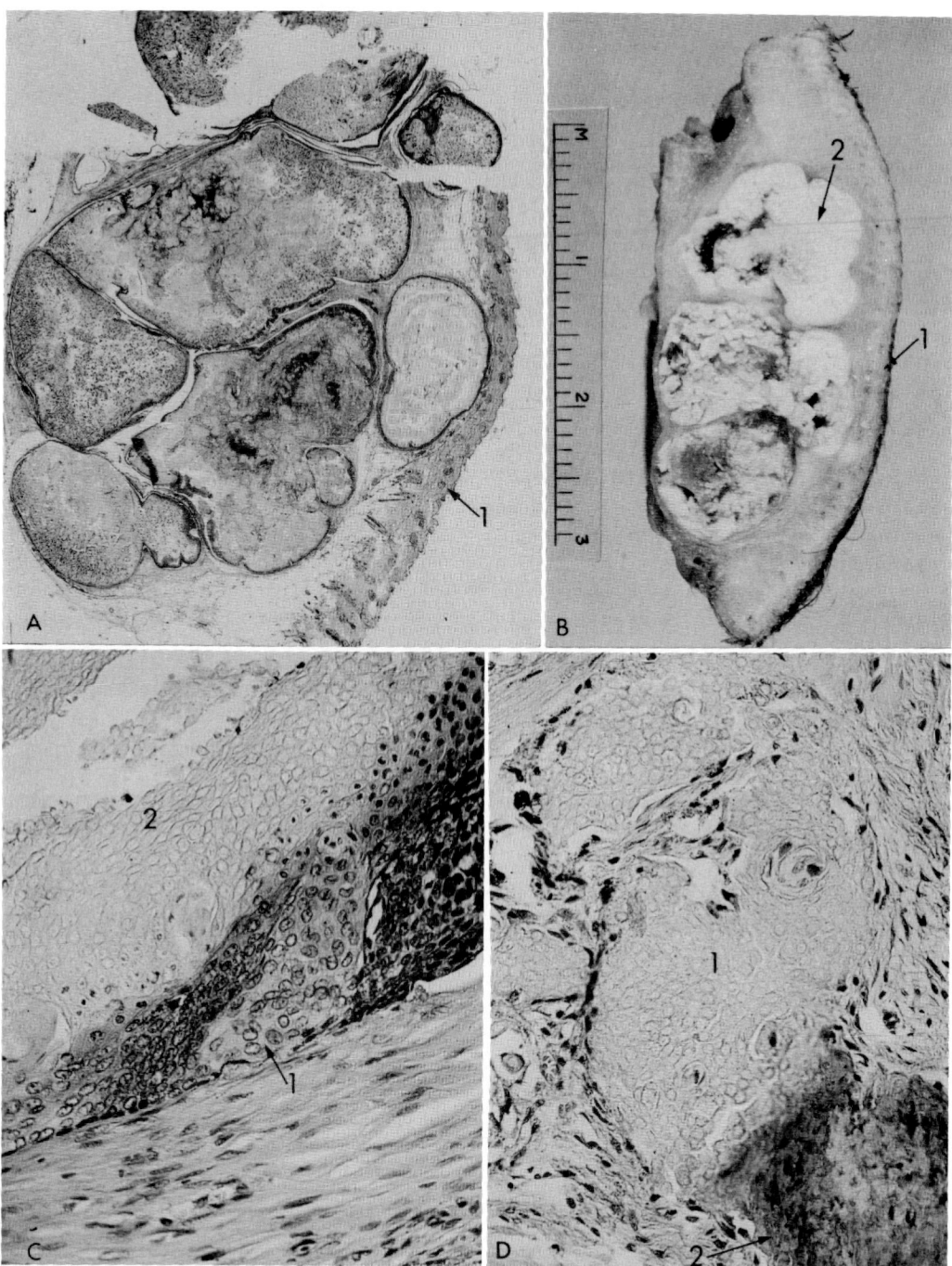

Fig. 18–30. Hair matrix tumor (benign calcifying epithelioma). *A*, Tumor (× 4) in dermis and subcutis of right prescapular region of a three-year-old female French Poodle. Note the lobulated nature of the new growth. Epidermis *(1)*. *B*, Gross appearance of the same tumor. Epidermis *(1)* chalky, granular, and lobulated tumor *(2)*. Contributor: Dr. M. G. Rhoades. *C*, A similar tumor from the dermis of a two-year-old Kerry Blue Terrier (× 250). Epithelial cells *(1)* simulating hair matrix, and cells *(2)* in center of lesion, which stain poorly but maintain their outline ("shadow" or "ghost" cells). *D*, Another area of same tumor as C (× 200). Outlines of cells *(1)* in center of lesion; calcification is present *(2)*. (Courtesy of Armed Forces Institute of Pathology.) Contributor: Dr. G. A. Goode.

matrix tumors." This neoplasm is made up of lobules of epithelial tissue (Fig. 18–30), the outer rim of which contains groups of cells that resemble the hair matrix. The interior of these lobules is usually made up of masses of cells resembling those at the periphery, but which are necrotic, as evidenced by their failure to take the usual hematoxylin stain. The outlines of the cells may be seen, however, causing some to call them "ghost cells"—an apt description. These tumors thus resemble cysts. In contrast to epidermal inclusion cysts, the walls are entirely composed of undifferentiated basal cells with an abrupt junction with the ghost cells. Calcification often starts in the center of the tumor lobules and may involve much of the necrotic tumor. These tumors are benign, but they may be multiple and may ulcerate the overlying skin, and if their necrotic contents escape into the dermis, it incites much inflammatory reaction. Only rarely are malignant hair matrix tumors encountered.

Trichoepithelioma. This tumor, also thought to arise from hair follicles, consists of multiple, varying sized cysts lined with stratified squamous epithelium and filled with keratin, but without hairs. Basal cells proliferate and mature from the outer rims of the cysts. The lesion is rare and benign.

Neoplasms of the Dermis and Subcutis

Fibroma; Fibrosarcoma. In the skin, fibromas and fibrosarcomas are the most frequent mesenchymal tumors in all species, except the dog, in which the mast-cell tumor is the most frequent of all cutaneous neoplasms. In general, fibrosarcomas occur with about the same or slightly higher frequency as fibromas. The tumors arise from fibrous connective tissue in its ubiquitous locations and resemble it in appearance. The cells with their collagenous fibrils run aimlessly in a variety of directions. Fasciculi of cells lying in the same plane are often seen (Fig. 18–32B), and are of value in distinguishing the fibrosarcoma from the hemangiopericytoma,

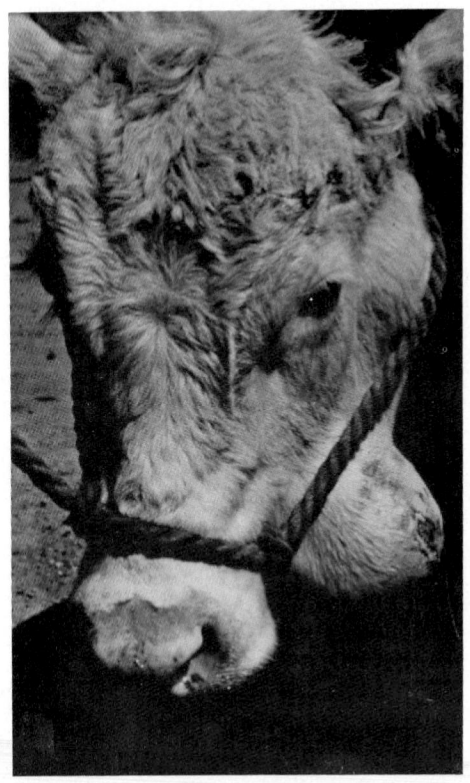

Fig. 18–31. Fibrosarcoma involving mandible of a Hereford steer. This neoplasm could easily be confused clinically with actinomycosis.

in which this is not a feature. If the fibrous material predominates at the expense of the nuclei and plump cell bodies, the tumor is hard and is called a **fibroma durum**. If cell bodies and nuclei predominate, with fewer fibrils, the tumor is softer and is called a **fibroma molle**. All degrees of malignancy exist. Among the criteria of malignancy in general, a high degree of cellularity, hyperchromatic staining of the nuclei, and a tendency for the nuclei to be plump, rounded, or even stellate are especially significant in the fibrosarcoma. Highly undifferentiated carcinomas may be mistaken for fibrosarcomas. Virus-caused fibropapillomas are discussed in Chapter 9.

Equine Sarcoid. A cutaneous growth peculiar to equines was first recognized

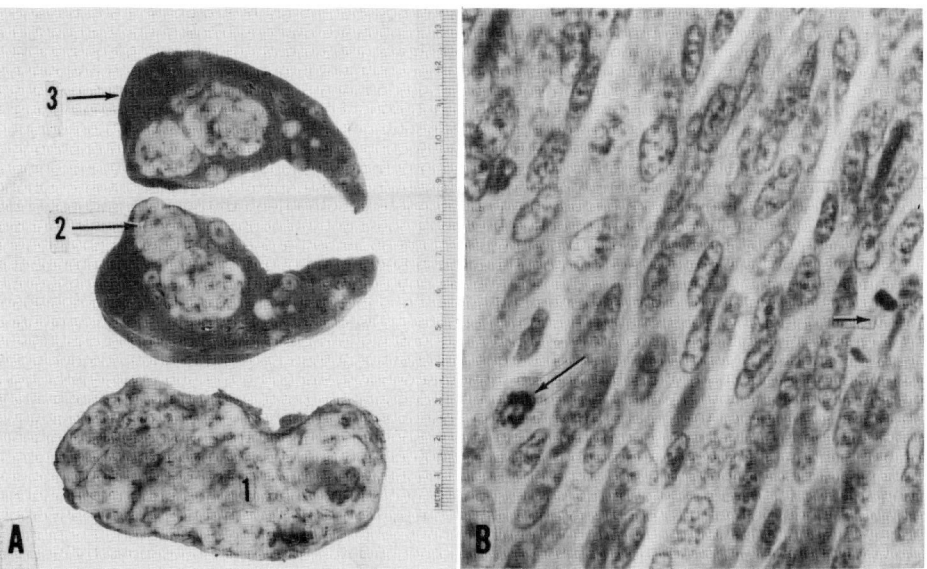

Fig. 18–32. *A*, Fibrosarcoma, primary (*1*), in cheek of a 12-year-old male Scottish terrier, with metastases (*2*) to lung (*3*). *B*, Photomicrograph of same tumor (× 700). Note spindle-shaped cells with ovoid nuclei and mitotic figures (arrows). (Courtesy of Armed Forces Institute of Pathology.) Contributor: Dr. John E. Craige.

by Jackson (1936), who named it equine sarcoid because, despite contrary clinical behavior, its histologic appearance is certainly that of a sarcoma of moderate malignancy. The lesion, often multiple, is most frequently found on the lower legs, head, and prepuce. It occurs perhaps even more frequently in mules and donkeys than in the horse. The growths may reach the size of a man's fist, variable in shape and in extent of the base, and bulging under the skin, which is thickened and roughened (acanthotic), and which sooner or later becomes ulcerated and infected. The growing mass may extend into the dermis, especially when it recurs after incomplete removal, but the underlying muscle is not invaded.

Microscopically, the new growth is made up principally of interlacing bundles of spindle-shaped cells which may form whorls and bundles suggestive of a neurofibroma. It is not surprising that most pathologists, confronted with the lesion for the first time, consider it a neurofibroma, neurofibrosarcoma, fi-broma or fibrosarcoma. The proportion of collagen fibrils to nuclei varies, but it is not so high that the sarcoid is likely to be mistaken for a keloid. Inflammatory infiltration is, of course, present near an ulcerated surface; a few lymphocytes and eosinophils may appear anywhere among the fibroblastic cells, but these are so few that there is no likelihood of mistaking the lesion for inflammatory granulation tissue. Neither is the number of capillaries great enough to favor such an error. The real difficulty is in distinguishing the sarcoid from a sarcoma. Usually there is less anaplasia of nuclei and fewer mitoses than in a sarcoma, but in borderline cases differentiation may not be possible on histologic grounds alone. Indeed, when the day comes that everything is known about neoplasia, it may be found that there is no real distinction. The overlying epidermis often sends long fronds deep into the mass, a feature which Jackson thought more or less confirmed his opinion that the epithelium participated in the neoplastic process. However, this bizarre epithelial

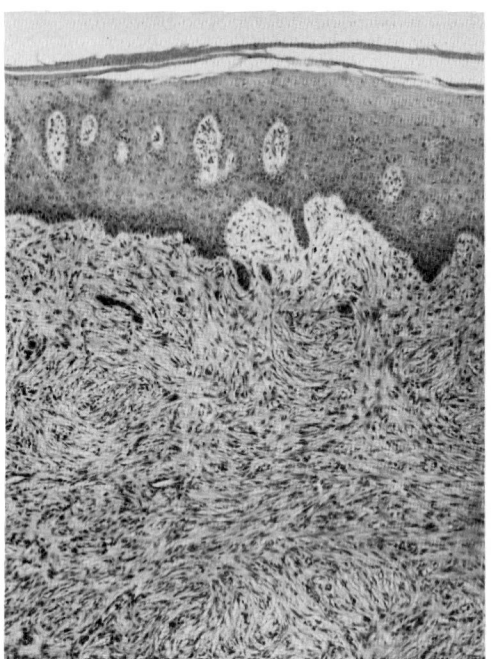

Fig. 18–33. Equine sarcoid, skin of a horse. Hyperplastic epithelium covers the mass within the dermis. The neoplasm resembles a neurofibrosarcoma.

proliferation is not unusual in any epidermis which is struggling under difficulties to cover a stubborn subcutaneous enlargement of any sort.

Anything less than complete removal is followed invariably by a recurrent growth that tends to be more richly cellular, the spindle-shaped cells being increased in size, with large, hyperchromatic nuclei and more frequent mitotic figures. Metastasis, however, does not occur, the situation being reminiscent of the diagnosis of "sarcoma of local malignancy only." The apparently viral etiology of this growth is discussed with the tumor-forming viruses (Chapter 9).

Lipoma; Liposarcoma. Lipomas, often multiple, occur in a great variety of locations as masses of adipose tissue of various sizes and shapes. They are most frequently encountered in the subcutis. The fat may be yellowish. These benign tumors are distinguished grossly from the excessive fat of obesity, which they frequently accompany, by the fact that they form discrete lumps or masses in contrast to the diffuse distribution of ordinary adipose tissue. Microscopically, close comparison shows a greater variation in the size and shape of the fat cells than occurs in normal adipose tissue. The liposarcoma, which is rare, is characterized by areas of anaplastic fibrous tissue in company with adipose tissue and an intermediate tissue in which only rudimentary fat cells with small vacuoles exist.

A particular type of fatty tumor occurs in the subcutis in the midline of the back over the thorax or in the axilla. This is called a **"tumor of brown fat"** or **"hibernoma."** It forms solid masses of cells which resemble those of the "brown fat" or "hibernating gland" of many animals. This fat is brownish grossly and the lipid in the cytoplasm is in the form of tiny droplets uniformly distributed throughout the rather dark brownish cytoplasm. These fat cells contain much more potential energy than do ordinary fat cells. The tumors may reach large sizes but are usually benign. Dogs, rats, and wild animals have been found with these tumors.

Myxoma; Myxosarcoma. These tumors are composed of connective tissue that forms mucin; in other words, connective tissue of embryonal type. The nuclei tend to be round or stellate; the intercellular fibrils are bluish (hematoxylin and eosin) and show little parallelism. These tumors are always more or less malignant, but the term myxoma is generally used in spite of that fact. They are encountered with some frequency in veterinary medicine. Some effort must be made to distinguish this neoplasm from a fibrosarcoma with myxomatous degeneration.

The Mast-Cell Tumor. The mast cell has been considered synonymous with the basophilic granulocyte of the blood. However, the mast cells seen in canine pathology, with their rounded, primitive-appearing nuclei, have little save the basophilic granules in the cytoplasm to tie them to the basophils of the blood, which are never numerous in the dog. Similar cells occur here and there among the varied mesodermal types found in the cutaneous tissues, omentum, and mesentery.

The term "mastocytoma" often appears in the literature in reference to tumors composed largely of tissue mast cells. The prefix "mast" in this context comes from the German, meaning fattened or stuffed, and "cyte" comes from the Greek, *kytos*, meaning a hollow cell. The combining form "mast" from the Greek *mastos* (breast) has quite a different meaning. In deference to the sensitivities of our classical scholarly colleagues, we chose not to use this incorrect combination of two languages.

Mast-cell tumors are one of the most frequent neoplasms of the skin of the dog, where they arise in the dermis. Mast-cell tumors are not uncommon in the skin of the cat and are rare lesions in swine and cattle. They are seen occasionally in laboratory animals, including monkeys. The tumor cells are of the large round type, rather loosely put together, forming shapeless masses beneath the bulging epidermis. They infiltrate among the coarse collagen fibers of the region, the fibers often persisting for some time, so that a marginal area of the tumor might be mistaken for an inflammatory infiltration.

From the standpoint of diagnosis, the cells of the mast-cell tumor differ from those of a malignant lymphoma in that the nuclei of the former are more dense and dark-staining, with less tendency to show individual chromatin granules. The mast cells have more cytoplasm than is the case with the lymphocytic type of malignant lymphoma. The mast-cell tumor nearly always contains mature eosinophils, often in considerable abundance, and on occasion there may be irregular eosinophilic foci of collagen necrosis (see also eosinophilic granuloma). Its individually discrete cells are less uniform in size and shape, while the nuclei are more deeply staining than

those of the transmissible venereal tumor, with which it may be confused. It also lacks the rather frequent mitotic figures (nuclei in various stages of mitosis) which are seen in the transmissible tumor. The proof of the diagnosis of mast-cell tumor lies in the demonstration of the dark cytoplasmic granules. In some specimens of the tumor, these are so numerous that the nucleus is obscured in a black smudge around it. More frequently, the granules are hard to find. They are much more evident by the Giemsa or a similar metachromatic stain than when hematoxylin and eosin are used, and it is commonly necessary to resort to such a procedure for diagnosis.

The mast-cell tumor is most likely to be located on the posterior part of the animal's body. It produces a bulging cutaneous tumor commonly reaching a diameter of 2 to 5 cm and a height of 1 to 3 cm. Ulceration is common.

Metastases are rare but the tumor has definite local malignancy, so that wide excision is imperative. This neoplasm has only a rare counterpart in the human species, although urticaria pigmentosa presents similar aggregations of mast cells.

In the cat, a **generalized mast-cell tumor** is encountered with equal or greater frequency than those localized to the skin. Most often the neoplasms affect the spleen and may also involve lymph nodes, the liver, bone marrow, lungs, kidneys, and skin. The spleen is usually much enlarged, with a characteristic deep mahogany color and fleshy consistency. Mast cells are usually found in small numbers in the peripheral circulation in such cases, and the term *mast cell leukemia* has been used by some authors. These circulating cells are morphologically identical to tissue mast cells rather than basophils. An interesting concomitant feature is the presence of small, sharply demarcated ulcers in the mucosa of the pylorus or duodenum. These ulcers are probably the result of excess histamine (or possibly serotonin) produced by the mast cells.

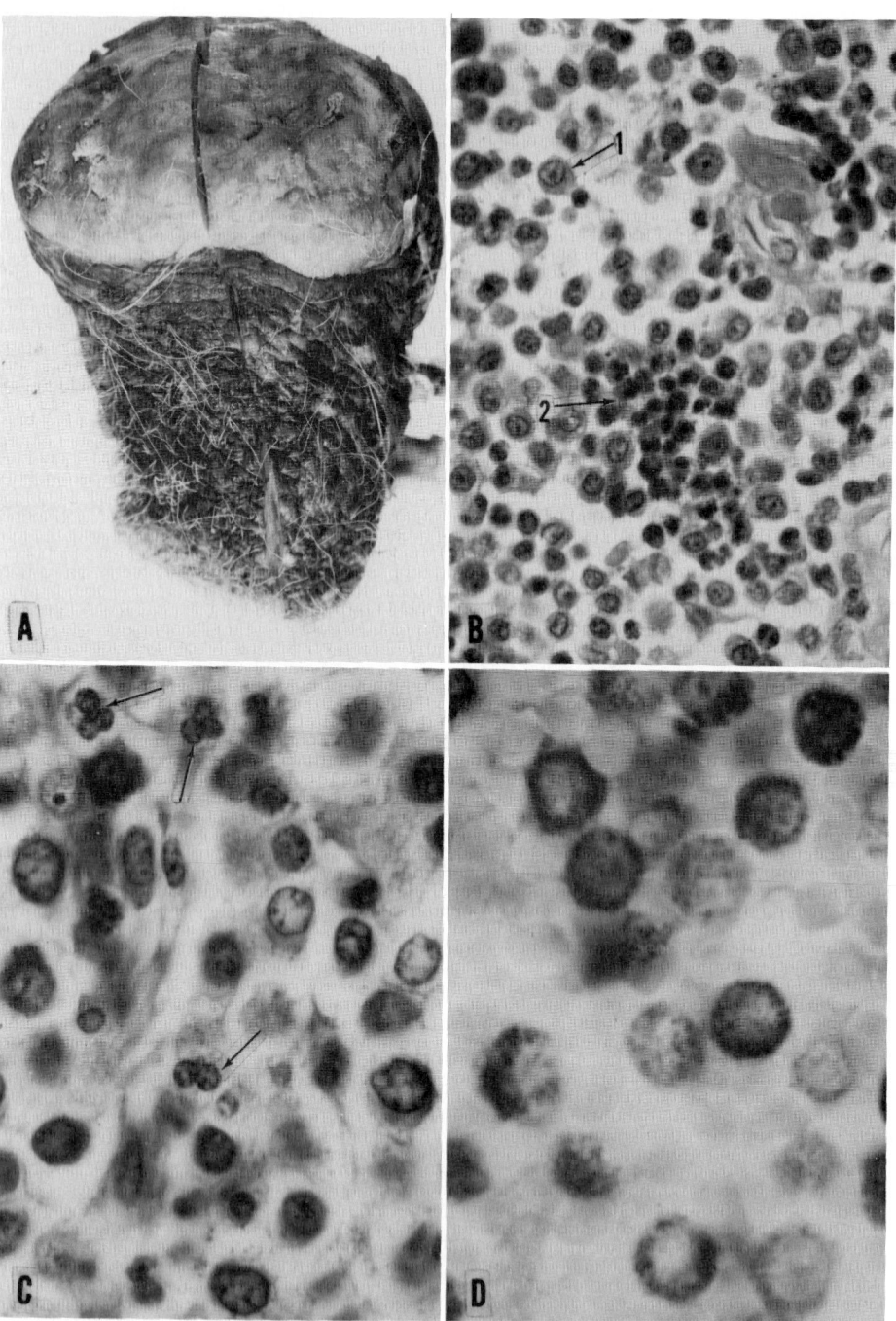

Fig. 18–34. Mast-cell tumor. *A*, Ulcerated tumor involving the skin of the scrotum of a thirteen-year-old male Spitz dog. Contributor: Dr. S. W. Stiles. *B*, Photomicrograph (× 545) of a mast-cell tumor from the cheek of a ten-year-old male Cocker Spaniel. Mast cells (*1*) and nests of eosinophils (*2*) are present. (H & E.) Contributor: Dr. W. H. Riser. *C*, Higher magnification of a mast-cell tumor from the skin of the leg of a 12-year-old male Boston terrier. (H & E, × 650.) A few mast cells contain cytoplasmic granules. Eosinophils (arrows) are common. Contributor: Army Veterinary School. *D*, Section with Giemsa stain (× 1200) to demonstrate metachromatic granules in the cytoplasm of the neoplastic mast cells. (Courtesy of Armed Forces Institute of Pathology.) Contributor: Dr. C. L. Davis.

An apparently third form of mast-cell tumor occurs in the intestine of cats. Intestinal mast-cell tumors arise in the small intestine, less often in the colon, resulting in a segmental thickening of the wall not sharply demarcated from adjacent tissue. The bulk of the mass is confined to the muscularis, although it may extend into the mucosa. Metastasis is frequent. The cells have finely granular or vacuolated cytoplasm, but usually are more clear than other forms of mast cell tumors. These neoplasms were once thought to arise from enterochromaffin cells and likened to carcinoid tumors of man. The studies of Alroy et al. (1975), however, have demonstrated that they are in fact mast-cell tumors. Interestingly, intestinal ulcers do not occur in association with these tumors.

In horses, Altera and Clark (1970) described a rare condition termed **equine cutaneous mastocytosis**, which closely resembles mast-cell tumors of dogs. Diffuse or sharply defined collections of mast cells associated with mature eosinophils and collagen necrosis with calcification were described in the skin from varied sites. It has been suggested (Cheville et al., 1972) that the cells are basophils and not mast cells and that the condition resembles urticaria pigmentosa of human beings. It does not appear to be a true neoplasm.

Canine Cutaneous Histiocytoma. This lesion of the dermis of the dog has been known for many years as one of the commonest "tumors" of the skin of that species. It has borne a number of names over the years, each indicating a lack of knowledge about the exact nature of the lesion. Such names as "round cell tumor," benign lymphoma, "extragenital venereal tumor" and "histiocytoma" have been applied, the last by Mulligan, who believed it was identical to the venereal tumor described elsewhere. This lesion bears no resemblance to the human lesion, which is usually called histiocytoma, and some evidence indicates it may not be a neoplasm at all. Nevertheless, for want of a better label, we shall use this appellation, "canine cutaneous histiocytoma" to label a specific entity. Ultrastructural studies also support the view that the cell type is a histiocyte, although clearly separable from macrophages and monocytes. The histiocytoma is not the same as the canine venereal tumor, although at one time they were considered variants of the same neoplasm.

This lesion occurs for the most part in young dogs. It appears within a week or two as an elevated mass, movable in the dermis, 1 to 3 cm in diameter. It apparently irritates the canine patient, who licks and rubs it until it may become ulcerated. Simple excision usually results in complete cure, although no interference at all also usually is followed by disappearance of the lesion. Apparently, no recurrence or further lesions appear once the initial lesion is healed. Transmission attempts have uniformly failed. This cutaneous lesion apparently still occurs in regions in the United States where the canine venereal tumor has not been encountered for many years.

The canine cutaneous histiocytoma is seen with the light microscope to be composed of rather large, individually discrete cells closely packed in the dermis, separating fibers of dermal collagen and elevating the epidermis. These cells may extend into the subcutis, infiltrating fat and connective tissue (Fig. 18–35). The typical cells have round or ovoid, finely stippled to vesicular nuclei, and distinct, nongranular cytoplasm. They are not phagocytic. Mitoses may be found and the cells appear to be actively invasive. The benign course of the lesion is in contrast to its "malignant" histologic appearance.

Subtle differences in cell morphology and the normal karyotype of these cells differentiate the lesion from the venereal tumor. Epizootiologic data and failure of transmission are also different. It is quite possible that this lesion is not a "neoplasm" at all, but more data are required to settle this point. It is a common lesion

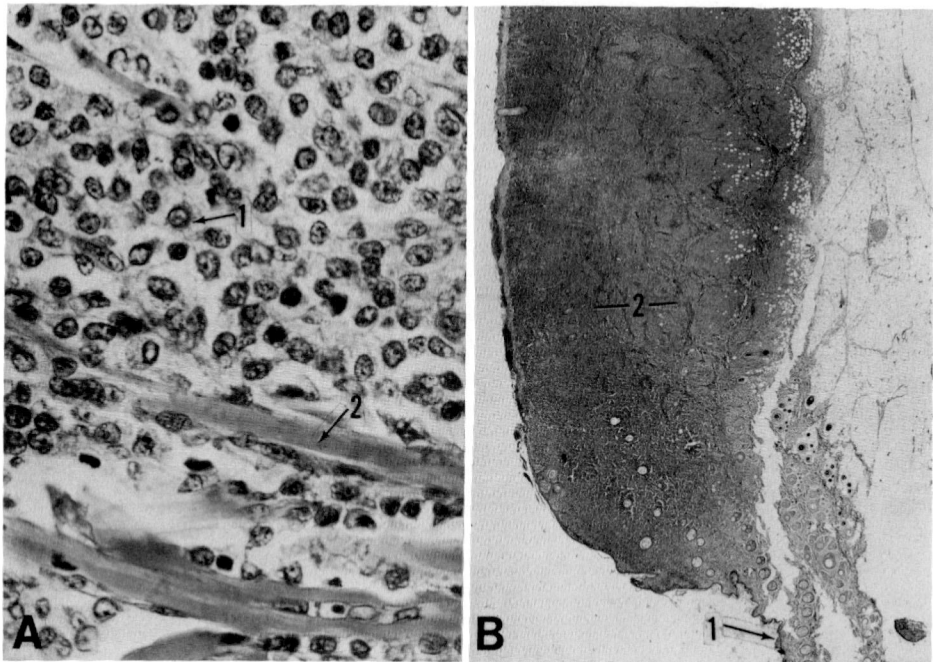

Fig. 18–35. Canine cutaneous histiocytoma. *A,* Cells of the new growth (*1*) infiltrating collagen bundles (2) of the dermis (× 440). *B,* Low power view of the cutaneous nodule (× 8). The epidermis (*1*) is elevated by the mass (2), which also infiltrates the subcutis. (Courtesy of Armed Forces Institute of Pathology.) Contributor: Dr. Elihu Bond.

which the veterinary pathologist or clinician must be able to recognize.

Hemangiopericytoma. The hemangiopericytoma (Mulligan, 1955; Stout and Murray, 1942; Yost and Jones, 1958) originates from blood vessels but is included here because it is essentially restricted to the skin. It is a common tumor of dogs, but rare in other species. It consists, in general, of spindle-shaped cells with ovoid or elongated nuclei and considerable cytoplasm, which frequently becomes fibrillar. The tumor thus bears a superficial resemblance to "spindle-celled sarcoma," neurofibroma, and hemangioendothelioma, with which many specimens of this type have doubtless been classed in the past. The distinguishing characteristic, however, is the presence of numerous small capillaries, open or collapsed, which are lined by endothelium but closely encircled by the more or less anaplastic and pleomorphic "spindle" cells, which are considered to be pericytes. In some specimens, encircling cells are flattened and extended in a circumferential direction; in others, their relationship to the vessel wall is less obvious, but the cells tend to form whorls or clusters around a capillary space. By suitable reticulum stains, large and numerous reticular fibers can be demonstrated in concentric layers around the vessels. The tumor is always subcutaneous. It recurs after many months, and in the course of several years, metastasizes. In our experience, this is one of the most common neoplasms encountered in surgically removed specimens from dogs.

The term **perithelioma** has been applied to this tumor, or one similar to it, by European writers. Histologists are poorly agreed on just what constitutes a pericyte. Just how widely the concept of this neoplastic type will be accepted, only time will

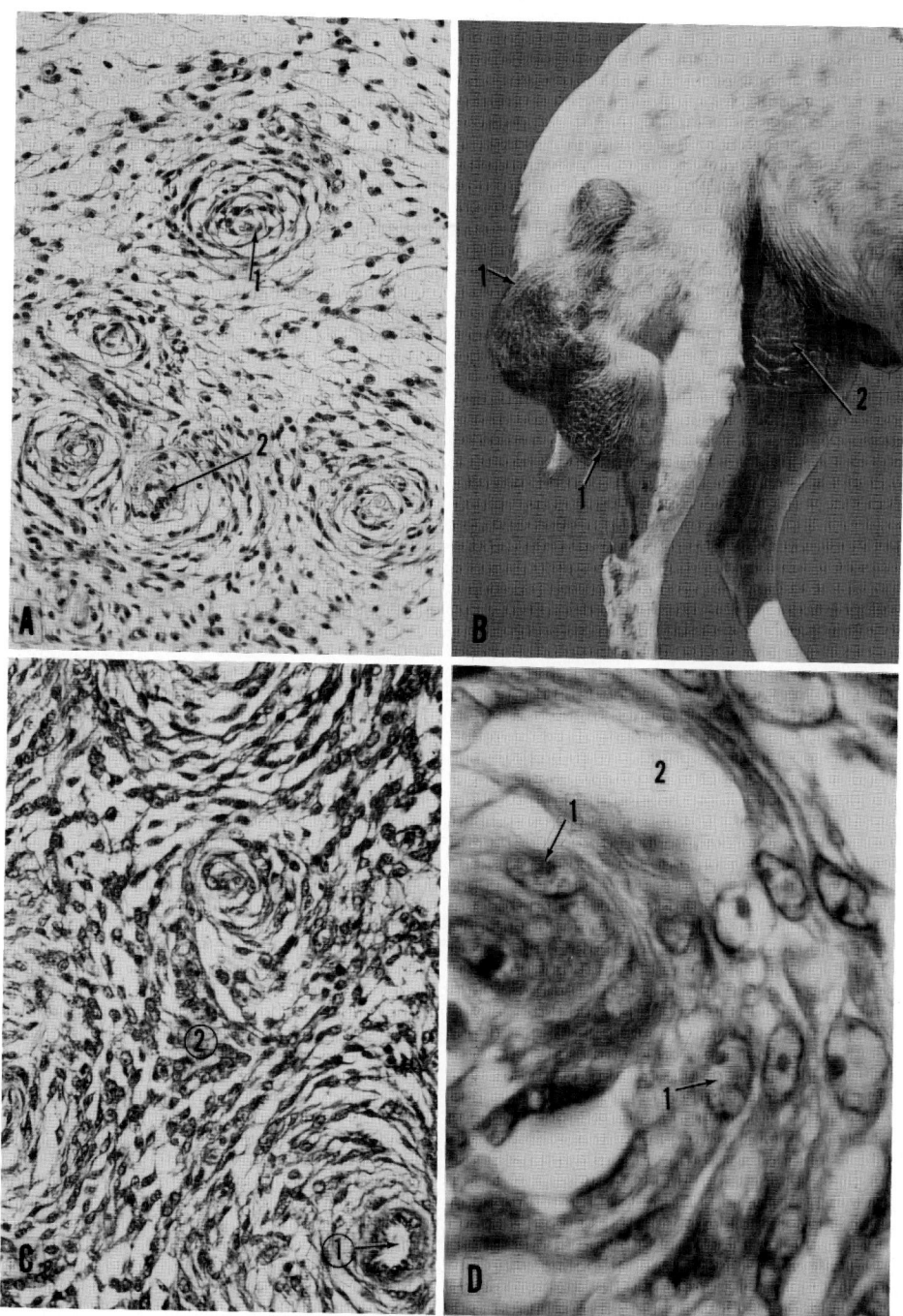

Fig. 18–36. Hemangiopericytoma of the subcutis of the dog. *A*, Photomicrograph (× 160) with whorl arrangement of tumor cells around occult*(1)* and overt capillaries*(2)*. Contributor: Dr. S. W. Stiles. *B*, Large subcutaneous hemangiopericytoma (*1*) in a 15-year-old terrier dog. Note metastasis to inguinal region (*2*). Contributor: Dr. W. J. Zontine. *C*, Section (× 210) in a densely cellular area with capillaries (*1*) and spindle-shaped cells (*2*) concentrically arranged around them. Contributor: Dr. W. H. Riser. *D*, High magnification (× 1080) of another tumor. Note ovoid nuclei (*1*), which are often vesicular and contain a single nucleolus. Clear, empty spaces (*2*) are common. (Courtesy of Armed Forces Institute of Pathology.) Contributor: Phillips Veterinary Hospital.

tell. It must be admitted that the designation of whorl-forming tumors as being of perineural origin (neurofibromas) has often been grounded more on habit than on proof.

Xanthoma. This term refers to tiny yellowish nodules that form on the skin of the eyelids and on tendons and tendon sheaths in man. They consist of collections of large, pale "foam cells," doubtless of reticuloendothelial origin, whose extensive cytoplasm is made granular by many minute droplets of cholesterol and other lipids. With them are fibroblasts and other phagocytes. This is not truly a neoplasm, but a reactive lesion. It possibly bears some significant relation to cholesterol metabolism.

Rather wide-based, sessile proliferations called xanthomas have been encountered subcutaneously in chickens. They consist mostly of connective tissue and "foamy," cholesterol-containing phagocytes similar to those in human xanthomas. The proliferations are quite irregular in contour but do not grow to extensive heights. They are not true neoplasms. A typical xanthoma also occurs with some frequency in subcutis of the shell parakeet (budgerigar) (Petrak and Gilmore, 1969).

Alroy, J., Leav, I., DeLellis, R.A., and Weinstein, R.S.: Distinctive intestinal mast cell neoplasms of domestic cats. Lab. Invest., 33:159–167, 1975.

Altera, K., and Clark, L.: Equine cutaneous mastocytosis. Pathol. Vet., 7:43–55, 1970.

Anderson, L.J., and Sandison, A.T.: Tumours of connective tissues in cattle, sheep, and pigs. J. Pathol., 98:253–263, 1969.

Baker, J.R., and Leyland, A.: Histological survey of tumours of the horse, with particular reference to those of the skin. Vet. Rec., 96:419–422, 1975.

Bloom, F.: Spontaneous solitary and multiple mast-cell tumors in dogs. Arch. Pathol., 33:661–676, 1942.

Borland, R., and Webber, A.J.: An electron microscope study of squamous cell carcinoma in Merino sheep associated with keratin-filled cysts of the skin. Cancer Res., 26:172–182, 1966.

Bostock, D.E.: The prognosis following surgical removal of mastocytomas in dogs. J. Small Anim. Pract., 14:27–40, 1973.

———: Prognosis after surgical excision of canine melanomas. Vet. Pathol., 16:32–40, 1979.

Brown, N.O., et al.: Soft tissue sarcomas in the cat. J. Am. Vet. Med. Assoc., 173:744–749, 1978.

Burdin, M.L.: Squamous-cell carcinoma of the vulva of cattle in Kenya. Res. Vet. Sci., 5:497–505, 1964.

Cheville, N.F., Prasse, K., van der Maaten, M., and Boothe, A.D.: Generalized equine cutaneous mastocytosis. Vet. Pathol., 9:394–407, 1972.

Christie, G.S., and Jabara, A.G.: Canine sweat gland tumors. Res. Vet. Sci., 5:237–244, 1964.

Cooper, D.L.: Cylindroma; report of an unusually extensive case. J. A. M. A., 132:575–577, 1946.

Cotchin, E.: Further observations on neoplasms in dogs, with particular reference to site of origin and malignancy. I. Cutaneous, female genital and alimentary systems. Br. Vet. J., 110:218–232, 1954.

———: Melanotic tumours of dogs. J. Comp. Pathol., 65:115–129, 1955.

Crowell, W.A., Chandler, F.W., Jr., and Williams, D.J.: Melanoma in cattle: fine structure and a report of two cases. Am. J. Vet. Res., 34:1591–1593, 1973.

Dodd, D.C.: Mastocytoma of the tongue of a calf. Pathol. Vet., 1:69–72, 1964.

Drommer, W.: Submikroskopische untersuchungen am Basaliom des Hundes. Pathol. Vet., 5:174–185, 1968.

Drommer, W., and Schultz, L.-Cl.: Vergleichende licht- und electromen-mikroskopische Untersuchungen am übertragbaren venerischen Sarkom und Histiozytom des Hundes. Pathol. Vet., 6:273–286, 1969.

Fezer, G.: Histologische Klassifizierung der Hautdrüsentumoren bei Hund und Katze. Inaug. Diss. Tierarztl. Fak., Munchen, 1968. V.B. 39:262, 1969.

Flatt, R.E., et al.: Pathogenesis of benign cutaneous melanomas in miniature swine. J. Am. Vet. Med. Assoc., 153:936–941, 1968.

Fowler, E.H., Kasza, L., and Koestner, A.: Enzyme histochemical comparison of the canine mastocytoma cell in vivo and in vitro. Am. J. Vet. Res., 29:853–862, 1968.

Fox, J.G., Snyder, S.B., and Campbell, L.H.: Connective tissue nevus in a dog. Vet. Pathol., 10:65–68, 1973.

Frese, K.: Statistical studies on skin tumours in domestic animals. Zentrabl. Veterinaermed., 15A:448–459, 1968. V.B. 39:745, 1969.

Fujimoto, Y., and Olson, C.: The fine structure of the bovine wart. Pathol. Vet., 3:659–684, 1966.

Garner, F.M., and Lingeman, C.H.: Mast-cell neoplasms of the domestic cat. Pathol. Vet., 7:517–530, 1970.

Goto, N., et al.: Pathological observations of feline mast cell tumor. Jpn. J. Vet. Sci., 36:483–494, 1974.

Greve, J.H., and Moses, H.E.: Histopathologic changes in xanthomatosis in chickens. J. Am. Vet. Med. Assoc., 139:1106–1110, 1961.

Hamilton, D.P., and Byerly, C.S.: Congenital malignant melanoma in a foal. J. Am. Vet. Med. Assoc., 164:1040–1041, 1974.

Hargis, A.M., Thomassen, R.W., and Phemister, R.D.: Chronic dermatosis and cutaneous squamous cell carcinoma in the Beagle dog. Vet. Pathol., 14:218–228, 1977.

Head, K.W.: Skin diseases. Neoplastic diseases. Vet. Rec., 65:926–929, 1953.

Holzinger, E.A.: Feline cutaneous mastocytomas. Cornell, Vet., 63:87–93, 1973.

Hottendorf, G.H., and Nielsen, S.W.: Collagen necrosis in canine mastocytomas. Am. J. Pathol., 49:501–513, 1966.

———: Pathologic report of 29 necropsies on dogs with mastocytoma. Pathol. Vet.,5:102–121,1968.

Hottendorf, G.H., Nielsen, S.W., and Kenyon, A.J.: Canine mastocytoma. I. Blood coagulation time in dogs with mastocytoma. Pathol. Vet., 2:129–141, 1965.

———: Ribonucleic acid in canine mast cell granules and the possible interrelationships of mast cells and plasma cells. Pathol. Vet., 3:178–189, 1966.

Howard, E.B., et al.: Mastocytoma and gastroduodenal ulceration. Gastric and duodenal ulcers in dogs with mastocytoma. Pathol. Vet., 6:146–158, 1969.

Ivascu, I., Simu, G., Muresan, E., and Papay, Z.: Clinical and pathological observations on five cases of equine sarcoidosis identified in Romania. Zentralbl. Veterinaermed. (A), 21:815–823, 1974.

Jabara, A.: Two cases of mammary neoplasms arising in male dogs. Aust. Vet. J., 45:476–480, 1969.

Johnson, R.M., and Sanger, V.L.: Lipids in avian xanthomatous lesions. Am. J. Vet. Res., 24:1280–1282, 1963.

Jones, S.R., MacKenzie, W.F., and Robinson, F.R.: Comparative aspects of mastocytosis in man and animals with report of a case in a baboon. Lab. Anim. Sci., 24:558–562, 1974.

Jones, T.C.: Tumors of specialized sebaceous glands of dogs. Bull. Internat. Assoc. Med. Museums (now Lab. Invest.), 28:66–72, 1948.

Jones, T.C.: Comparative pathology of skin. Int. Acad. Pathol. Monogr., 10:597–605, 1971.

Kelly, D.F.: Canine cutaneous histiocytoma. A light and electron microscopic study. Pathol. Vet., 7:12–27, 1970.

Kraft, I., and Frese, K.: Histological studies on canine pigmented moles. The comparative pathology of the naevus problem. J. Comp. Pathol., 86:143–155, 1976.

Lerner, A.B., and Cage, G.W.: Melanomas in horses. Yale J. Biol. Med., 46:646–649, 1973.

Lindley, W.H.: Malignant verrucae of bulls. Vet. Med. Small Anim. Clin., 69:1547–1550, 1974.

Liu, S.K., and Hohn, R.B.: Squamous cell carcinoma of the digit of the dog. J. Am. Vet. Med. Assoc., 153:411–424, 1968.

Lombard, L.S., and Moloney, J.B.: Experimental transmission of mast cell sarcoma in dogs. Fed. Proc., 18:490, 1959.

Masson, P.: Les naevi pigmentaires, tumeurs nerveuses. Ann. d. Anat. Pathol., 3:417–453, and 656–696, 1926.

Mawdesley-Thomas, L.E. and Bucke, D.: Squamous cell carcinoma in a gudgeon (*Gobio golio,* L). Pathol. Vet., 4:484–489, 1967.

McClelland, R.B.: Benign neoplasms of the skin glands of dogs. Cornell Vet., 30:67–72, 1940.

Migaki, G., and Langheinrich, K.A.: Mastocytoma in a pig. Pathol. Vet., 7:353–355, 1970.

Millikan, L.E., Boylon, J.L., Hook, R.R., and Manning, P.J.: Melanoma in Sinclair swine: a new animal model. J. Invest. Dermatol., 62:20–30, 1974.

Millikan, L.E., Hook, R.R., and Manning, P.J.: Immunobiology of melanoma. Gross and ultrastructural studies in a new melanoma model: the Sinclair swine. Yale J. Biol. Med., 46:631–645, 1973.

Mills, J.H.L., and Nielsen, S.W.: Canine haemangiopericytomas—a survey of 200 tumours. J. Small Anim. Pract., 8:599–604, 1967.

Mulligan, R.M.: Neoplastic diseases of dogs: mast cell sarcoma, lymphosarcoma, histiocytoma. Arch. Pathol., 46:477–492, 1948.

———: Hemangiopericytoma in the dog. Am. J. Pathol., 31:773–789, 1955.

Mustafa, I.E., Cerna, J., and Cerny, L.: Melanoma in goats. Sudan Med. J., 4:113–118, 1966. V.B. 37:2244, 1967.

Naik, S.N., Randelia, H.P., and Dabholkar, R.D.: Carcinoma of the horn in a cryptorchid bull. Pathol. Vet., 7:265–269, 1970.

Nielsen, S.W., and Aftosmis, J.: Canine perianal gland tumors. J. Am. Vet. Med. Assoc., 144:127–135, 1964.

Nielsen, S.W., and Cole, C.R.: Canine mastocytoma—a report of one hundred cases. Am. J. Vet. Res., 19:417–432, 1958.

———: Cutaneous epithelial neoplasms of the dog. A report of 153 cases. Am. J. Vet. Res., 21:931–948, 1960.

Nomura, Y., et al.: Porcine melanomas of skin in a serial occurrence. I. Eighteen pig cases with melanotic tumor discovered in the early stage of survey. Bull. Azabu Vet. Col., 28:55–62, 1974.

Olson, C., Jr.: Equine sarcoid, a cutaneous neoplasm. Am. J. Vet. Res., 9:333–341, 1948.

Olson, C., Jr. and Cook, R.H.: Cutaneous sarcoma-like lesions of the horse caused by the agent of bovine papilloma. Proc. Soc. Exp. Biol. Med., 77:281–284, 1951.

Orkin, M., and Schwartzman, R.M.: A comparative study of canine and human dermatology. II. Cutaneous tumors, the mast cell and canine mastocytoma. J. Invest. Dermatol., 32:451–466, 1959.

Patnaik, A.K., Liu, S.-K., Hurvitz, A.I., and McClelland, A.J.: Nonhematopoietic neoplasms in cats. J. Natl. Cancer Inst., 54:855–860, 1975.

Peckham, M.C.: Xanthomatosis in chickens. Am. J. Vet. Res., 16:580–583, 1955.

Peters, J.A.: Canine mastocytoma: excess risk as related to ancestry. J. Nat. Cancer Inst., 42:435–443, 1969.

Petrak, M.L., and Gilmore, C.E.: *In* Diseases of Cage and Aviary Birds, edited by M. L. Petrak. Philadelphia, Lea & Febiger, 1969, pp. 459–489.

Ragan, H.A., Clarke, W.J., and Bustad, L.K.: Radiation-induced cutaneous neoplasms in a sheep. Am. J. Vet. Res., 32:167–172, 1971.

Ragland, W.L., Keown, G.H., and Gorham, J.R.: An epizootic of equine sarcoid. Nature (Lond.), 210:1399, 1966.

Rosenberg, J.C., et al.: The malignant melanoma of hamsters. I. Pathologic characteristics of a transplanted melanotic and amelanotic tumor. Cancer Res., *21*:627–631, and 632–635, 1961.

Sakurai, Y.: Adenoid cystic epithelioma ("Brooke's tumor") in a dog. J. Jpn. Vet. Med. Assoc., *13*:206–208, 1960.

Schäffer, E.: Histologische Klassifizierung epithelialer Hauttumoren bei Hund und Katze. Inaug. Diss. tierarztl Fak. Munchen, pp. 139, 1967. V.B. *38*:242, 1968.

Schulz, K.C.A., and Schutte, J.A.: Multiple acanthoma in the skin of swine. J. S. Afr. Vet. Med. Assoc., *31*:437–442, 1960.

Sells, D.M., and Conroy, J.D.: Malignant epithelial neoplasia with hair follicle differentiation in dogs. J. Comp. Pathol., *86*:121–129, 1976.

Shope, R.E., et al.: An infectious cutaneous fibroma of the Virginia White-Tailed deer *(Odocoileus virginianus)*. J. Exp. Med., *108*:797–802, 1958.

Smit, J.D.: Skin lesions in South African domestic animals with special reference to the incidence and prognosis of various skin tumors. J. S. Afr. Vet. Med. Assoc., *33*:363–376, 1962.

Stannard, A.A., and Pulley, L.T.: Intracutaneous cornifying epithelioma (keratoacanthoma) in the dog: a retrospective study of 25 cases. J. Am. Vet. Med. Assoc., *167*:385–388, 1975.

Stout, A.P., and Murray, M.R.: Hemangiopericytoma: a vascular tumor featuring Zimmermann's pericytes. Ann. Surg., *116*:26–33, 1942.

Strafuss, A.C.: Squamous cell carcinoma in horses. J. Am. Vet. Med. Assoc., *168*:61–62, 1976.

————: Basal cell tumors in dogs. J. Am. Vet. Med. Assoc., *169*:322–324, 1976.

————: Sebaceous gland carcinoma in dogs. J. Am. Vet. Med. Assoc., *169*:325–326, 1976.

————: Sebaceous gland adenomas in dogs. J. Am. Vet. Med. Assoc., *169*:640–642, 1976.

Strafuss, A.C., Cook, J.E., and Smith, J.E.: Squamous cell carcinoma in dogs. J. Am. Vet. Med. Assoc., *168*:425–427, 1976.

Strafuss, A.C., et al.: Cutaneous melanoma in miniature swine. Lab. Anim. Care, *18*:165–169, 1968.

Testi, F.: Epithelial tumours of the skin in domestic animals. Acta Med. Vet. Napoli., *9*:479–517, 1963.

Trautwein, G., and Stober, M.: (Leucaemic mast cell reticulosis in a cow: a contribution to non-lymphatic leucosis in cattle). Zentbl. Vet. Med., *12A*:211–231, 1965. V.B. *35*:3088, 1965.

Ward, J.M., and Hurvitz, A.I.: Ultrastructure of normal and neoplastic mast cells of the cat. Vet. Pathol., *9*:202–211, 1972.

Weiss, E.: Intranukleäre und intrazytoplasmatische Glycogenablagerungen in Mastzellentumoren des Hundes. Pathol. Vet., *2*:514–519, 1965.

Weiss, E., and Fezer, G.: Histologische Klassifizierung der Schweissdrusentumoren von Hund und Katze. Berl. Münch. Tierarztl. Wochenschr., *81*:249–254, 1968.

Weiss, E., Rudolph, R., and Deutschlander, N.: Untersuchungen zur Ultrastruktur und Ätiologie der mastzellentumoren des Hundes. Pathol. Vet., *5*:199–211, 1968.

West, G.B.: Pharmacology of the tissue mast cell. Br. J. Dermatol., *70*:409–417, 1958.

Yost, D.H., and Jones, T.C.: Hemangiopericytoma in the dog. Am. J. Vet. Res., *19*:159–163, 1958.

CHAPTER *19*

The Musculoskeletal System

Most of the skeletal muscles function by providing movement to parts of the skeleton, but also depend on the nervous system for the stimuli that cause the muscles to contract. We have arbitrarily chosen to consider the muscular system in connection with the skeletal system. The cardiac muscles (except in conditions involving both skeletal and cardiac muscles) will be discussed with the cardiovascular system. Diseases of smooth (nonstriated) muscle will be taken up in connection with the systems in which these muscles function: digestive, urinary, genital.

THE SKELETAL MUSCLES

The methods that the pathologist most often uses to study diseases of skeletal muscle encompass the gross, microscopic, and ultrastructural morphology as well as histochemical features. Careful dissection of the muscles and detailed inspection of their surfaces, attachments, and cut sections are necessary to adequately distinguish gross features. Careful fixation and inclusion of both cross and longitudinal sections are vital to avoid distracting artifacts in histologic sections. Precise technics are particularly necessary for the correct interpretation of lesions in muscle (Dubowitz and Brooke, 1973).

Structure

A brief review of the structure of skeletal muscle follows. The reader is encouraged to study other references, particularly Dubowitz and Brooke (1973) and Pearson and Mostofi (1973).

The contractile function of muscle is provided by interaction of the structural proteins actin and myosin, under the influence of several regulatory proteins. Actin and myosin may be seen under the electron microscope as parallel interdigitating thick (myosin) and thin (actin) filaments. Several hundred of these filaments make up the myofibril, which along its length may be seen to have alternating transverse bands and lines. The darker A band contains thick myosin filaments surrounded in a hexagonal array by thin actin filaments. The less dense I band contains actin filaments only, which are attached in the dense, transversely oriented Z line (*Zwischenscheibe*). The actin filaments extend from this Z line in the I band into part of the A band.

The center of the A band, slightly less dense than the rest of the A band, is called the H (Hensen's) zone, and contains only myosin filaments. In the middle of the H zone is an additional transverse line, the M (*Mittelscheibe*) line, where the myosin filaments are slightly thickened. That part of the filamentous myosin and actin array extending between one Z line and the next is called a **sarcomere.**

The **myofibril** is formed by the repetitive sequence of many sarcomeres. Each myofibril is separated from the adjacent one by the **intermyofibrillar** space, which contains aqueous sarcoplasm and organelles such as mitochondria and glycogen granules. These mitochondria are seen in longitudinal sections to occupy the I band and extend to the margin of the A band. Glycogen granules, electron dense bodies 150 to 300 Å in diameter, may be seen in any part of the muscle fiber but are concentrated in the I band.

The **transverse tubular system** is interwoven across the muscle to contact many myofibrils. This tubular structure has an outer limiting membrane which is continuous with the external sarcolemma. The **sarcoplasmic reticulum** forms a fenestrated sheath around each myofibril, and small sacs are found where it comes into contact with a transverse tubule.

The **muscle fiber** consists of thousands of myofibrils, each surrounded by interfibrillar material which, using the light microscope, may be demonstrated as a network in cross sections of muscle. Each muscle fiber is surrounded by a plasma membrane, the sarcolemma, and within it, elliptical nuclei with their long axis parallel to the length of the fiber. The muscle cell is thus an elongated, multinucleated unit. Each muscle fiber is surrounded by an endomysial connective tissue which contains capillaries and terminal ramifications of the nerve fibers. Groups of muscle fibers form fasciculi, which are surrounded by perimysial connective tissue. These fasciculi, grouped together, make up the individual muscles.

The **muscle spindles** may occasionally be seen in sections of muscle. These consist of specialized muscle fibers within a connective tissue sheath in the perimysial stroma. Blood vessels are readily recognized, and nerves may be demonstrated in the perimysium with Verhoeff–van Gieson's stain. Their terminal ramifications enter the endomysium at the neuromuscular junctions.

Cross striations, demonstrable with the light microscope, are the cumulative effect of the A and I bands, with their included zones and lines, seen with the electron microscope.

Types of Muscle

The earliest observations on different types of muscle are credited by Ciaccio (1898) to Stephano Lorenzini, who in 1698 noted differences in animal muscles and suggested, on the basis of their color, they be called red or white. This is still part of the foundation for the **anatomic classification** of muscle. This system takes into consideration such features as (1) red versus white muscle or fibers, (2) dark versus light, (3) high or low granularity under the light microscope, (4) fibers rich or poor in protoplasm, and (5) ultrastructural differences such as size, number of mitochondria and cristae, width of Z bands, content of H band region.

Physiologic behavior also provides a basis for classifying muscle, based on two features: (1) slow versus fast response to stimulation and (2) high or low resistance to fatigue. **Biochemical properties,** based upon differential centrifugation of muscle cell components followed by chemical analyses, have also indicated differences in muscle. High or low respiratory activity, for example, is clearly based upon the mitochondrial content. White muscle generally has lower content of mitochondria and low respiratory activity; red muscle is high in mitochondria and thus has higher respiratory activity. High or low enzyme activity could also be ascribed to different muscles by these methods.

Histochemistry

All skeletal muscle fibers are not the same, and enzyme histochemistry makes it possible to tell the difference. More than 70 enzymes have been identified in muscle, but fortunately, only a few need to be utilized to gain useful information about diseased muscle. Identification is complicated, however, because the histochemical types of muscle fibers are subject to several methods of classification. Also, the terminology is confused by use of terms based upon anatomic, biochemical, or physiologic characteristics described previously.

Histochemical features of muscle are utilized to identify individual muscle fibers and have recently been recognized as useful in the study of muscle and muscle disease. With histochemical methods, the individual muscle fibers may be identified and classified on the basis of high or low content of specific enzymes. The quantity and presence or absence of specific enzymes in individual fibers is also of interest in understanding the function of individual fibers. Terminology and classification schemes of muscle fiber types are still evolving. We choose to use the system proposed by Dubowitz and Brooke (1973) for human muscle as most appropriate to the study of diseased muscle and most useful for comparative purposes.

Dubowitz and Brooke have devised a two-fiber system, distinguishing the fibers by either the enzyme activity of an oxidative enzyme such as succinic dehydrogenase or reduced nicotinamide adenine dinucleotide–tetrazolium reductase (NADH–TR), or by the standard adenosine triphosphatase (ATPase) reaction (pH 9.4). These reactions distinguish fiber types 1 and 2 without ambiguity, fiber type 1 giving a strong reaction with NADH–TR and a weak reaction with ATPase (pH 9.4). Fiber types 2, A and B, give an intermediate to weak reaction with NADH–TR and a strong reaction with ATPase. Other enzyme reactions which are useful in classifying and studying diseased muscle fibers include modified ATPase (pH 4.6 and 4.3), alpha glycerophosphate–dihydrogenase (menadione-linked), periodic acid Schiff (PAS) and phosphorylase. (See Table 19–1.)

Neuromuscular Interrelations

Skeletal muscles are innervated by nerve fibers originating in the neurons of the ventral horn of the spinal cord. Each

Table 19–1.   Histochemical Classification of Muscle Fibers—Human and Canine

| Histochemical Reaction | Intensity of Reaction in Muscle Fibers | | | | | | | |
| | Type 1 | | Type 2A | | Type 2B | | Type 2C | |
	Human	Canine	Human	Canine	Human	Canine	Human	Canine
Routine ATPase (pH 9.4)*	+	+	+++	+++	+++	—	+++	+++
Modified ATPase (pH 4.5 or 4.6)	+++	+++	0	0	+++	—	+++	++
Modified ATPase (pH 4.3)	+++	+++	0	0	0	—	++	++
NADH–TR	+++	+++	++	++	+	—	++	++

— = no fibers found
 0 = no reaction
 + = low reaction
++ = intermediate reaction
+++ = high reaction

* Indicates preincubation pH

Adapted from Dubowitz and Brooke (1973) and Braund, Hoff and Richardson (1978)

neuron in this ventral gray matter has a single axon which eventually branches into nerve fibers supplying many muscle fibers. This functional-anatomic relationship between neuron, axon, and muscle fibers is known as the **motor unit.** This relationship is the key to understanding both physiologic and pathologic processes. Necrosis of the motor neuron results in neurogenic atrophy of the muscle fibers supplied by that neuron.

Evidence also indicates that the peripheral nerve influences or determines the type of muscle fiber that it innervates. Experimental crossing of the nerves of a cat from one muscle, for example, a slow muscle such as the soleus, to a fast muscle such as the flexor hallucis longus—changes the contractile properties of these muscles. The slow muscle becomes fast, the fast becomes slow. Also, histochemical fiber types may be changed by reinnervation. Types 1, 2A, and 2B appear to be separately innervated. Type 2C fibers do not have this characteristic and appear to be primitive fibers, capable of differentiatng into types 2A or 2B.

Pathologic Changes In Muscle

Dubowitz and Brooke (1973) have recognized a large number of changes in biopsy specimens of human muscle studied by histologic and histochemical methods. Some of these changes have been identified in animal muscle, and others may be found by further study. A brief review of the definitions and descriptions of these changes seems indicated. The interpretation of these changes is considered in other sections in connection with specific diseases. The original reference should be consulted for more detail. It appears likely that the ability to recognize all such details would be useful in the study of experimental and natural diseases in animals.

Changes in Fiber Size. Muscle fibers change their cross-sectional diameter under several conditions. Exercise results in increased size (**work hypertrophy**); inactivity leads to decreased size (**disuse at-**rophy). If the change in fiber size is uniform, it may be difficult to recognize, but if some fibers are clearly smaller than others, the change is readily apparent. It is useful to measure the smallest cross-sectional diameter of a number of muscle fibers with an ocular micrometer, followed by the preparation of a histogram. Both type 1 or type 2 fibers may be atrophied or hypertrophied. Increased variability in fiber size may also be determined by this approach. Adult men normally have greater mean fiber diameters than women.

Abnormalities of Distribution of Fibers. Pathologic changes may not be uniformly distributed throughout a muscle. In **small group atrophy,** a small collection of atrophied fibers is observed among normal sized fibers. This is characteristic of denervation. Atrophy of a large number of fibers, **large group atrophy,** involves large units of muscle (fasciculi), adjacent to relatively normal fasciculi. This involves denervation of affected fasciculi. **Perifascicular atrophy** is used to describe decrease in fiber size at the periphery of the muscle fasciculus. **Type grouping** involves the occurrence of large clusters of fibers of one type as distinguished from the usual mosaic distribution. This change is seen in reinnervated muscle. **Fiber type predominance** is used to describe what may be an extreme form of type grouping. Fibers of one or another type may become more numerous than expected. Careful comparison with control sections of the same muscle from the same species, age, and sex is necessary. Less than 10% of the fibers may be of one type, a condition called **fiber type deficiency.**

Changes in Sarcolemmal Nuclei. Individual nuclei may migrate in large or small numbers from their usual sarcolemmal position at the periphery of the fiber. These internal nuclei may form long chains clearly evident in longitudinal sections. Individual nuclei may also become vesicular. The nucleus becomes swollen and rounded, with the nucleoplasm transparent and the nucleolus conspicuous. The chromatin material, usually finely dispersed, may become granular or clumped—the so-called **tigroid nucleus.** **Pyknotic nuclei** may be recognized by their dark stain and shrunken appearance. They also tend to occur in clumps.

Degeneration and Regeneration. The muscle fiber may become pale-staining ("liquified") or uniformly eosinophilic (hyaline), indicating necrosis of the fiber. Other necrotic fibers may be filled with coarse, granular, bluish staining (with hematoxylin and eosin) material. With Gomori's trichrome stain, these fibers are red, and hence have been called "ragged-red fibers." Basophilic fibers, bluish when stained with hematoxylin and eosin, are thought to represent regenerative attempts. Fiber splitting is the partial division of a fiber into one or more smaller fibers. This may be evident in transverse or longitudinal sections. This is apparently a normal phenomenon at myotendinous junctions.

Cellular Reactions. Infiltration of leukocytes into the muscle usually is evident between the muscle fibers. Macrophages were mentioned previously in connection with phagocytosis of muscle cells. Polymorphonuclear leukocytes, lymphocytes, and plasma cells may also appear in muscle tissue. Fibrosis may be seen as connective tissue proliferation involving the endomysium between muscle fibers or the perimysium surrounding muscle fasciculi. It is usually considered secondary to necrotizing or inflammatory processes.

Changes in Architecture of Individual Fibers. The **target fiber** is best seen in sections following the oxidative enzyme reactions. The affected fiber has a periphery which is essentially normal, but the center contains an unstained zone surrounded by a densely stained intermediate zone. This gives the fiber the appearance of a three-zone target. Target fibers are most often type 1. **Central cores** are demonstrated with oxidative enzymes but are also seen in sections stained with a trichrome stain. Central cores have been described as consisting of two types: structured and unstructured. With ATPase, the **structured core** is strongly reactive, and the group of myofibrils in the center of the fiber is densely colored. Most are type 1 fibers, although type 2 (usually 2C) fibers may be affected. The **unstructured core** differs from the structured in the distortion of the architecture and loss of cross striations within the core. It does not react with most histochemical techniques and appears as a pale, usually central, area of the fiber. **Moth-eaten fibers** are the result of whorling of the intermyofibrillar network, associated with areas that do not react with the oxidative enzymes. **Tubular aggregates** (microsomal aggregates) are limited to type 2B fibers. With the exception of succinic dehydrogenase and menadione-linked α-glycerophosphate dehydrogenase (which do not react), oxidative enzyme reactions cause tubular aggregates to appear as dense masses replacing part of the fiber. With Gomori's trichrome stain they are red, and with hematoxylin and eosin, bluish. With the ATPase reaction they appear unstained. These structures occur under many circumstances and their specificity is as yet undetermined.

In the **ring fiber,** the orientation of the myofibrils is distorted by a bundle of myofibrils with its axis at right angle to the main body of the fiber. This gives the appearance of a ring or annulus around or running through the fiber. Ring fibers are demonstrated readily by the periodic acid Schiff reaction, and their specific significance is not yet established. **Cytoplasmic bodies** may assume different shapes but usually consist of an eosinophilic center (with trichrome) surrounded by a halo. When numerous, they have been associated with collagen vascular disease, but their significance is not clearly established. **Rod bodies** or **nemaline bodies** have been associated with myopathy variously called "rod," "nemaline," or "myogranular" myopathy. The bodies are most readily demonstrated with Gomori's trichrome stain, which colors them red or purple. They are not demonstrated with hematoxylin and eosin or routine histochemical stains. Ultrastructurally, they appear to be continuous with the Z lines and have a crystalline structure. They occur in familial cases of nonprogressive myopathy and in other situations, including experimental tenotomy in cats. Mitochondrial abnormalities may give isolated muscle fibers a granular appearance when mitochondria are abnormal in size, number, or distribution. Electron microscopy is needed to demonstrate the precise status of mitochondria.

Aberle, E.D., et al.: Fiber types and size in equine skeletal muscle. Am. J. Vet. Res., 37:145–148, 1976.

Ariano, M.A., Armstrong, R.B., and Edgerton, V.R.: Hindlimb muscle fiber populations of five mammals. J. Histochem. Cytochem., 21:51–55, 1973.

Ashmore, C.R., and Doerr, L.: Comparative aspects of muscle fiber types in different species. Exp. Neurol., 31:408–418, 1971.

Barnard, R.J., Edgerton, V.R., Furukawa, T., and Peter, J.B.: Histochemical, biochemical, and contractile properties of red, white and intermediate fibers. Am. J. Physiol., 220:410–414, 1971.

Braund, K.G., Hoff, E.J., and Richardson, K.E.Y.: Histochemical identification of fiber types in canine skeletal muscle. Am. J. Vet. Res., 39:561–565, 1978.

Brooke, M.H., and Kaiser, K.K.: Use and abuse of muscle histochemistry. Ann. NY Acad. Sci., 228:121–144, 1974.

Burke, R.E., et al.: Mammalian motor units: Physiological-histochemical correlation in three types in cat gastrocnemius. Science, 174:709–712, 1971.

Burke, R.E., et al.: Physiological types and histochemical profiles in motor units of the cat gastrocnemius. J. Physiol., 234:723–748, 1973.

Cardinet, G.H., III: Skeletal muscle. In Clinical Biochemistry of Domestic Animals, Vol II. 2nd Ed., edited by J.J. Kaneko and C.E. Cornelius. New York, Academic Press, 1971. pp. 155–177.

Cardinet, G.H., Fedde, M.R., and Tunell, G.L.: Correlates of histochemical and physiological properties of normal and hypotrophic pectineus muscles of the dog. Lab. Invest., 27:32–38, 1972.

Ciaccio, G.V.: La découverte des muscles blancs et des muscles rouges, chez la lapin, revendiquée en faveur de S. Lorenzini. Archiv. Ital. de Biol., 30:287, 1898.

Davies, A.S., and Gunn, H.M.: Histochemical fiber types in the mammalian diaphragm. J. Anat., 112:41–60, 1972.

Dubowitz, V., and Brooke, M.H.: Muscle Biopsy: A Modern Approach. Phila., W.B. Saunders Co., 1973. pp. 5–33, 89.

Guth, L., Samaha, F.J., and Albers, R.W.: The neural regulation of some phenotypic differences between the fiber types of mammalian skeletal muscle. Exp. Neurol., 26:126–135, 1970.

Guth, L.: Fact and artifact in the histochemical procedure for myofibrillar ATPase. Exp. Neurol., 41:440–450, 1973.

Montgomery, C.A.: Muscle diseases. In Pathology of Laboratory Animals, edited by K. Benirschke, F.N. Garner, and T.C. Jones. New York, Springer Verlag, 1978. pp. 821–887.

Padykula, H.A., and Herman, E.: The specificity of the histochemical method for adenosine triphosphatase. J. Histochem. Cytochem., 3:170–176, 1955.

Pearson, C.M., and Mostofi, F.K. (editors): The Striated Muscle. Baltimore, Williams and Wilkins, 1973.

Trevino, G.S., Demaree, R.S., Jr., Sanders, B.V., and O'Donnell, T.A.: Needle biopsy of skeletal muscle in dogs: light and electron microscopy of resting muscle. Am. J. Vet. Res., 34:507–514, 1973.

Inherited Diseases of Muscle

A growing number of inherited diseases of muscle are becoming known in man and animals. We have chosen to present a summary of current knowledge by means of tabulation (Table 19–2). Several congenital disease entities, for which the evidence of inheritability is not convincing, will be discussed separately. The inherited diseases in different species often have similar lesions and clinical manifestations. At this writing, the mechanisms that underlie the abnormal manifestations are for the most part unknown. It seems likely that once the deficient enzyme systems are identified, a better understanding of the relationships of these muscular diseases will be at hand. It is now possible to distinguish each entity among most of these diseases listed in Table 19–2 by their clinical or pathologic features, but at present the significance of their relationships is unknown.

It is generally believed that these inherited diseases are primary, that they result from abnormalities in the muscle itself, not as a secondary effect of some disorder of the nervous system. It is well to keep an open mind on this point. At least one study

Table 19–2. Inherited Diseases of Muscles

Species	Name of Disease	Mode of Inheritance	Features of Disease	References
Mouse	Muscular dystrophy	dy/dy A,R LG IV	Weakness and atrophy of muscles begin to show at about 3 weeks of age; most die before 10th week. Histology: decrease in size of muscle fibers; increase in connective tissue and fat; some coagulation necrosis of muscle fibers; nuclei fall into closely-packed chains. Ultrastructure: loss of myofibrils, mitochondria often enlarged; endoplasmic reticulum swollen and lost.	Banker, 1969 Hadlow, 1962 Forbes and Sperelakis, 1972 Meier et al., 1965 Davidowitz et al., 1976 Pachter et al., 1976 Jones, 1978
Mouse	Muscular dysgenesis	mdg/mdg A,R	Homozygote born dead; lesions limited to skeletal muscle; myoblasts differentiate into myotubules and cross striations appear, then development ceases; necrosis of muscle cells eventually with pyknotic and karyorrhectic nuclei and dissolution of cytoplasm; macrophages engulf degenerated cell detritus.	Gluecksohn-Waelsch, 1963 Pai, 1965a,b Platzer and Gluecksohn-Waelsch, 1972
Mouse	Muscular dystonia	dt/dt LG XIII Chr 1 A,R	Atrophy of muscles secondary to degeneration of peripheral nerves, dorsal root ganglia, and gray matter of spinal cord.	Duchen et al., 1963 Duchen and Strich, 1964 Duchen et al., 1966
Chicken	Muscular dystrophy	A,R	Mild progressive disease; first sign is failure of fowl to right itself when placed on its back. Lesions: variation in muscle size; vacuolation of fibers; loss of fibers and replacement by adipose tissue.	Asmundson and Julian, 1956 Ashmore, 1968 Julian, 1973 Sweeny et al., 1972 Cardinet et al., 1972
Mink	Muscular dystrophy	A,R	Manifest as early as 2 months of age by locomotor dysfunction; dysphasia and atrophy especially of muscles of head, pectoral, and pelvic girdles. Histology: striking variation in size of muscle fibers; hyaline degenerative changes; nuclei centralized; often regenerating multinucleated nuclei; increase of connective tissue. Serum enzymes elevated include: creatine phosphokinase, aldolase, glutamic-oxalacetic transaminase.	Hegreberg, et al., 1974, 1975, 1976

Table 19–2. Inherited Diseases of Muscles (Cont'd)

Species	Name of Disease	Mode of Inheritance	Features of Disease	References
Hamster	Cardiomyopathy; muscular dystrophy; myopathy	A,R	Disease appears at about 30 days of age in skeletal and cardiac muscle. Histology: progressive necrosis and some repair of muscle cells; nuclei become centrally placed in fibers and fall into long chains; coagulation necrosis of muscle fibers; focal fibrosis in myocardium.	Nixon et al., 1962 Homburger et al., 1963, 1966 Gertz, 1973
Swine	Hereditary metabolic myopathy; malignant hyperthermia	A,D (?) polygenic (?)	Inherited susceptibility to halothane, etc., which triggers severe muscular rigidity, very high temperature, elevated electrolytes and muscle enzymes in serum.	See Chapter 6
Sheep	Progressive ovine muscular dystrophy	A,R	In Merino sheep in Australia, recognized as early as 1 month of age by reduced flexion of femorotibial and tibial-tarsal joints and stiff gait. Bilaterally symmetrical lesions occur, particularly in vastus intermedius muscles. Progressive loss of muscle fibers with irregular size, central rows of nuclei, replacement over years by adipose cells.	McGavin and Baynes, 1969 McGavin, 1974
Dog	Progressive muscular dystrophy; myopathy with myotonia	S,R	Recognized in Irish Terriers by stiff gait and difficulty in swallowing; high muscle tone; decreased stamina. Progresses with gross atrophy of muscles and myotonia. Histology: normal and abnormal fibers are mixed; Zenker's degeneration often; phagocytosis of some fibers; nuclei often fall into rows.	Whitney, 1958 Wentink et al., 1972 Wentink et al., 1974 Duncan and Griffiths, 1975
Cattle	Congenital hyperplasia ("double muscles"); hereditary muscular hypertrophy	A,D (?)	Calves are born with muscles in the shoulder and rump much larger than normal; may cause dystocia; fat deposits are reduced by about 60% from normal. Microscopic features: Hyperplasia of muscle fibers; increased proportion of white muscle fibers, decrease in red type; virtual absence of fat between fiber bundles.	Ashmore and Robinson, 1969 Holmes and Robinson, 1970 Holmes et al., 1972

Species	Disease	Inheritance	Description	References
Calves	Hereditary myopathy associated with hydrocephalus	A,R	Newborn Hereford calves are alive but unable to stand; limbs mobile and joints normal; hydrocephalus accompanied also by microphthalmia and cerebellar hypoplasia; muscles are atrophied, pale, soft, sometimes spongy. Histology: thin muscles with few myofibers scattered in connective tissue; some hyalinization and necrosis of myofibrils, little regeneration and few fat cells.	Baker et al., 1961; Hadlow, 1962; Rhodes et al., 1962; Urman and Grace, 1964; Greene et al., 1974
Turkey	Muscular dystrophy	A,R	Seen in broad-breasted Bronze breed; atrophy of pectoral and wing muscles is evident first at 8 to 16 weeks of age; other muscles not affected. As in chickens, first sign is inability of fowl to right itself when placed on back. Lesions: variations in size of myofibrils, necrosis of individual fibers, mild deposition of fat cells.	Harper and Parker, 1964, 1967
Dogs	"Muscle disorder"	A,R	Seen in Labrador Retrievers. Onset at less than 6 months of age. Features include abnormal head and neck posture; stiff, hopping gait; loss of muscle mass; myotonia indicated by electromyotonic studies. Some relief with diazepam. Lesions: progressive loss of myofibrils, especially red type; usual destruction and partial repair similar to other muscle dystrophies.	Kramer et al., 1976
Mouse	Hereditary motor end-plate disease (MED); myopathy; hereditary myopathy	A,R	Considered a new form of hereditary myopathy; appears 11–14 days after birth, increased muscle weakness especially in hind legs, to almost complete loss of movement; no atrophic or dystrophic changes in motor end-plates. In muscle: focal myofibrillar disorganization, enlarged mitochondria, autophagic vacuoles, engulfing sarcoplasm; increased acid phosphatase in membranes; possible diminished protein synthesis.	Duchen and Searle, 1967; Duchen, 1970; Sheff and Zacks, 1977; Zacks et al., 1969
Dog	"Scottie cramp," muscular hypertonicity	A,R	Scottish Terrier breed affected. Episodes of muscular hypertonicity result in arching of back, then forelimbs and neck, causing head to lower; sometimes somersaults. No functional defect in peripheral axon myoneural junction, myomembrane, or contractile proteins. No morphologic lesion in muscle, nervous tissue, or parenchyma. Believed to originate in central nervous system.	Klarenbeek et al., 1942; Meyers et al., 1969, 1971; Meyers, Padgett and Dickinson, 1970

(Peterson, 1974) points to the possibility of an abnormality as yet unidentified in the central nervous sytem of dystrophic (*dy 2J*) mice.

Ashmore, C.R., Doerr, L., and Somes, R.G.: Microcirculation: loss of an enzyme activity in chickens with hereditary muscular dystrophy. Science, 160:319–320, 1968.

Ashmore, C.R., and Robinson, D.W.: Hereditary muscular hypertrophy in the bovine. I. Histological and biochemical characterization. Proc. Soc. Exp. Biol. Med., 132:548–554, 1969.

Asmundson, V.S., and Julian, L.M.: Inherited muscle abnormality in the domestic fowl. J. Hered., 47:248–250, 1956.

Baker, M.L., Payne, L.C., and Baker, G.N.: The inheritance of hydrocephalus in cattle. J. Hered., 52:135–137, 1961.

Banker, B.Q.: A pathological study of muscular dystrophy in the Bar Harbor 129 house mouse with particular reference to the ultrastructural features. In Modern Neurology, edited by S. Locke. Boston, Little, Brown and Co., 1969. pp. 241–259.

Cardinet, G.H., III, Freedland, R.A., Tyler, W.S., and Julian, L.M.: Morphologic, histochemical and quantitative enzyme study of hereditary avian muscular dystrophy. Am. J. Vet. Res., 33:1671–1684, 1972.

Davidowitz, J., Pachter, B.R., Phillips, G., and Breinin, G.M.: Structural alterations of the junctional region in extraocular muscles of dystrophic mice. I. Modifications of sole-plate nuclei. Am. J. Pathol., 82:101–110, 1976.

Duchen, L.W.: Hereditary motor end-plate disease in the mouse: light and electron microscopic studies. J. Neurol. Neurosurg. Psychiatry, 33:238–244, 1970.

Duchen, L.W., Falconer, D.S., and Strich, S.J.: Dystonia muscularum. A hereditary neuropathy of mice affecting mainly sensory pathways. J. Physiol., 165:7–9, 1963.

Duchen, L.W., Falconer, D.S., and Strich, S.J.: Hereditary progressive neurogenic muscular atrophy in the mouse. J. Physiol., 183:53p–55p, 1966.

Duchen, L.W., Searle, A.G., and Strich, S.J.: An hereditary motor end-plate disease in the mouse. J. Physiol. (Lond.), 189:4p–6p, 1967.

Duchen, L.W., and Strich, S.J.: Clinical and pathological studies of an hereditary neuropathy in mice. (*dystonia muscularum*). Brain, 87:367–378, 1964.

Duncan, I.D., and Griffiths, I.R.: A myopathy associated with myotonia in the dog. Acta Neuropath., 31:297–303, 1975.

Forbes, M., and Sperelakis, N.: Ultrastructure of cardiac muscle from dystrophic mice. Am. J. Anat., 134:271–289, 1972.

Gertz, E.W.: Cardiomyopathy in Syrian hamster. Am. J. Pathol., 70:151–154, 1973.

Gluecksohn-Waelsch, S.: Structural genes and analysis of differentiation. Science, 142:1269–1279, 1963.

Green, H.J., Leipold, H.W., and Hibbs, C.M.: Bovine congenital defects. Variations of internal hydrocephalus. Cornell Vet., 64:596–600, 1974.

Hadlow, W.J.: Diseases of skeletal muscle. In Comparative Neuropathology by J.R.M. Innes and L.Z. Saunders. New York, Academic Press, 1962. pp. 147–243.

Hamilton, M.J., Hegreberg, G.A., and Gorham, J.R.: Histochemical muscle fiber typing in inherited muscular dystrophy of mink. Am. J. Vet. Res., 35:1321–1324, 1974.

Harper, J.A., and Parker, J.E.: Hereditary muscular dystrophy in the domestic turkey (*Meleagris gallopavo*). Poultry Sci., 43:1326–1328, 1964.

Harper, J.A., and Parker, J.E.: Hereditary muscular dystrophy in the domestic turkey. J. Hered., 58:189–190, 1967.

Hegreberg, G.A., Camacho, Z., and Gorham, J.R.: Histopathologic description of muscular dystrophy of mink. Arch. Pathol., 97:225–229, 1974.

Hegreberg, G.A., Padgett, G.A., Prieur, D.J., and Johnson, M.I.: Genetic studies of a muscular dystrophy of mink. J. Hered., 66:63–66, 1975.

Hegreberg, G.A., Norton, S.L., and Gorham, J.R.: Muscular dystrophy of mink. Am. J. Pathol., 85:233–236, 1976.

Holmes, J.H.G., and Robinson, D.W.: Hereditary muscular hypertrophy in the bovine: metabolic response to nutritional stress. J. Anim. Sci., 31:776–780, 1970.

Holmes, J.H.G., et al.: A condition resembling "azoturia" in a "double muscled" heifer. Vet. Rec., 90:625–630, 1972.

Homberger, F., et al.: Further morphologic and genetic studies on dystrophy-like primary myopathy of Syrian hamsters. Fed. Proc., 22:195–197, 1963.

Homberger, F., et al.: Hereditary dystrophy-like myopathy. The histopathology of hereditary dystrophy-like myopathy in Syrian hamsters. Arch. Pathol., 81:302–307, 1966.

Jones, T.C.: Hereditary Disease. In Pathology of Laboratory Animals, edited by K. Benirschke, F.N. Garner, and T.C. Jones. New York and Berlin, Springer-Verlag, 1978 (2 vol). pp. 1981–2064.

Julian, L.M.: Herditary muscular dystrophy of chickens. Am. J. Pathol., 70:273–276, 1973.

Klarenbeek, A., Koopmans, S., and Winser, J.: Eeen Aavalsgewijs Optrendende Stoornes in de Regulatie van de Spiertonus: Waagenomen bij Schotsche Terriers. T. Diergeneesh, 69:14–21, 1942.

Kramer, J.W., Hegreberg, G.A., Bryan, G.M., Meyers, K., and Ott, R.L.: A muscle disorder of Labrador Retrievers characterized by deficiency of Type II muscle fibers. J. Am. Vet. Med. Assoc., 169:817–820, 1976.

McGavin, M.D., and Baynes, I.D.: A congenital progressive ovine muscular dystrophy. Pathol. Vet., 6:513–524, 1969.

McGavin, M.D.: Progressive ovine muscular dystrophy. In Handbook, Animal Models of Human Disease, Model no. 51, 1974, edited by T.C. Jones, D.B. Hackel, and G. Migaki. Reg. Comp. Pathol., AFIP, Wash., D.C.

Meier, H., West, W.T., and Hoag, W.G.: Preclinical histopathology of mouse dystrophy. Arch. Pathol., *80*:165–170, 1965.

Meyers, K.M., Lund, J.E., Padgett, G.A., and Dickson, W.M.: Hyperkinetic episodes in Scottish Terrier dogs. J. Am. Vet. Med. Assoc., *155*:129–133, 1969.

Meyers, K.M., Padgett, G.A., and Dickson, W.M.: The genetic basis of a kinetic disorder of Scottish Terrier dogs. J. Hered., *61*:189–192, 1970.

Meyers, K.M., Dickson, W.M., Lund, J.E., and Padgett, G.A.: Muscular hypertonicity. Episodes in Scottish Terrier dogs. Arch. Neurol.,*25*:61–68, 1971.

Nixon, C.W., Whitney, R., Baker, J.R., and Homburger, F.: Primary myopathy in an inbred line of Syrian golden hamsters. Fed. Proc.,*21*:313, 1962.

Pachter, B.R., Davidowitz, J., and Breinin, G.M.: Structural alterations of the junctional region in extraocular muscle of dystrophic mice. II. Hypertrophy of the neuromuscular junctional apparatus. Am. J. Pathol., *82*:111–118, 1976.

Pai, A.C.: Developmental genetics of a lethal mutation, muscular dysgenesis (*mdg*) in the mouse. I. Genetic analysis and gross morphology. Develop. Biol., *11*:82–92, 1965a.

Pai, A.C.: Developmental genetics of a lethal mutation, muscular dysgenesis (*mdg*) in the mouse. II. Developmental analysis. Develop. Biol., *11*:93–109, 1965b.

Peterson, A.C.: Chimaera mouse study shows absence of disease in genetically dystrophic muscle. Nature, *248*:561–564, 1974.

Platzer, A.C., and Gluecksohn-Waelsch, S.: Fine structure of mutant (muscular dysgenesis) embryonic mouse muscle. Develop. Biol., *28*:242–252, 1972.

Rhodes, M.B., Urman, H.K., Marsh, C.L., and Grace, O.D.: Serum enzyme studies of a hydrocephalic syndrome of newborn calves. Proc. Soc. Exp. Biol. Med., *111*:735–737, 1962.

Sheff, M.F., and Zacks, S.I.: Muscle protein synthesis in MED myopathy. Lab. Invest., *37*:216–222, 1977.

Sweeny, P.R., Buchanan-Smith, J.G., Petit, J.R., and Moran, E.T.: Ultrastructure of muscular dystrophy. II. A comparative study in lambs and chickens. Am. J. Pathol., *68*:493–510, 1972.

Urman, H.K. and Grace, O.D.: Hereditary encephalomyopathy. A hydrocephalus syndrome in newborn calves. Cornell Vet., *54*:229–232, 1964.

Wentink, G.H., et al.: Myopathy with a possible recessive X-linked inheritance in a litter of Irish Terriers. Vet. Pathol., *9*:328–349, 1972.

Wentink, G.H., Meijer, A.E.F.H., van der Linde–Sipman, J.S., and Hendriks, H.J.: Myopathy in an Irish Terrier with a metabolic defect of the isolated mitochondria. Zbl. Vet. Med. A., *21*:62–74, 1974.

Whitney, J.C.: Progressive muscular dystrophy in the dog. Vet. Rec., *70*:611–613, 1958.

Zacks, S.I., Sheff, M.F., Rhoades, M.A., and Saito, A.: MED myopathy: A new hereditary myopathy. Lab. Invest., *21*:143–153, 1969.

Equine Rhabdomyolysis (Azoturia, Monday Morning Disease, Paralytic Myoglobinuria, Tying-up)

In a typical case of azoturia, the horse begins his morning's work in fine spirits following a holiday period of one or several days on a full diet and no exericse. (Hence the name, Monday-morning disease.) It may well be a colder morning than usual, and the patient is likely to be an animal hardened and conditioned by previous hard work. Suddenly, in the course of a few steps the horse becomes practically unable to move and stands transfixed, trembling and sweating in extreme pain. Examination shows certain muscles or groups of muscles, usually but not necessarily one of the large muscles of the femoral or gluteal groups, to be slightly swollen and as hard as wood. These muscles are in a state of extreme cramp or tonic spasm. Anyone who has experienced transient cramping of the muscles of the calf of the leg (systremma) has no difficulty in understanding the animal's inability to move. Azoturia may result also from abnormal and strained positions of muscles while the horse is restrained in a casting harness: a normally ambulatory animal is thrown to the ground; a seriously crippled one arises or perhaps does not rise.

The preceding paragraph, written by Hilton A. Smith in a earlier edition of *Veterinary Pathology*, describes the characteristic clinical features of this age-old but poorly understood equine disease. We have accepted Lindholm's (1974) suggestion that the disease be called equine rhabdomyolysis instead of azoturia to more accurately reflect its known features. The problem is quite prevalent among Standardbred and Thoroughbred horses in training. Acute episodes appear in these animals after a few days of rest (often over the weekend) on full feed, followed by resumption of exercise.

In addition to the clinical signs described, levels of serum glutamic oxaloacetic transaminase and creatine phosphokinase are increased, roughly in proportion to the severity of the disease.

Lesions. The lesions in the muscle consist of necrosis of large or small groups of fibers. Such areas, seen one to several days after the onset, are white, usually with some increase of tissue fluid. With the light microscope, the change may at first qualify as what many call hyaline degeneration, but shortly all the changes of Zenker's necrosis are present, and eventually the complete picture of necrosis is attained with absence of all but the sarcolemma and stromal elements. Thus, if the animal survives, severe disease results in atrophy of the affected muscles, which is slowly resolved with regeneration of the sarcoplasm. Except that they are larger, the degenerated and necrotic areas are not particularly different from those seen in the so-called white-muscle disease of nutritional origin. Affected muscle fibers have been shown to be type 1 (fast twitch) fibers as identified by negative staining for myofibrillar adenosine triphosphatase.

The **ultrastructural lesions,** according to Lindholm, et al. (1974), start with "myofibrillar waving" followed by alterations in mitochondria (enlargement, dilated matrix of low electron density, indistinct cristae, focal electron-dense deposits) and sarcotubules (dilated sarcoplasmic reticulum, dissolution of myofibrils, complete loss of myofibrils due to condensation), leading to degeneration of myofibrils and necrosis. This latter event is followed by invasion of the sarcolemma by monocytes and macrophages.

The urine is usually darkened to a shade of brown with excreted myoglobin. This myoglobinuria must be distinguished

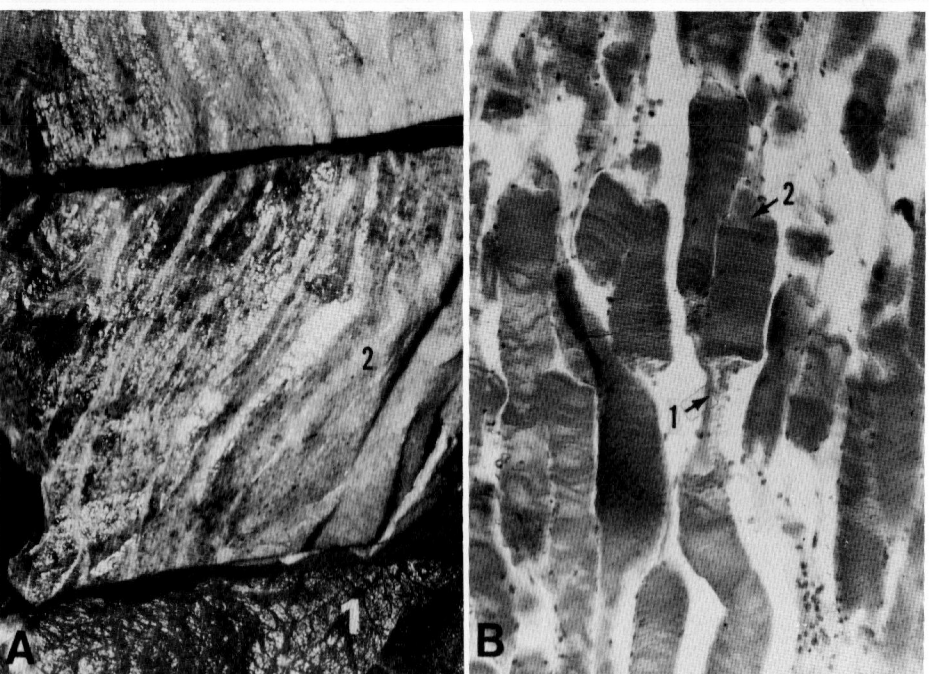

Fig. 19–1. Equine rhabdomyolysis. *A,* Muscle of a year-old colt tangled in halter rope (lived three days). Normal dark red muscle (*1*) can be compared with white and degenerating muscle (*2*). (Courtesy College of Vet. Med. Iowa State University.) *B,* Microscopically (× 180), note atrophy (*1*) and distention (*2*) of muscle fibers. The latter appeared dark red and shiny in the section stained with hematoxylin and eosin. (Courtesy College of Vet. Med. Iowa State University.)

from hemoglobinuria. The kidneys suffer considerable injury which becomes increasingly apparent as the patient survives a few or several days. The epithelium of the proximal convoluted tubules passes through a stage of degeneration and becomes necrotic. That of the distal convoluted tubules is more prone to desquamate, and the same is true of the straight tubules. Some tubules fill with a brownish pigmented material that resembles hemoglobin but is actually the closely related myoglobin. This does not appear to form the solidified casts that are characteristic of the hemoglobin of the human "crush syndrome."

Biochemical changes in affected muscle include low concentrations of glycogen, adenosine triphosphatase, and creatine phosphatase, plus elevated concentrations of lactate and glucose. Serum creatine phosphokinase and glutamic oxaloacetic transaminase are both elevated during the disease due to release of enzymes by necrotic muscle.

Cause. The cause of equine rhabdomyolysis is in doubt. The acute renal tubular necrosis apparently is the result of hypotensive shock and renal arteriolar constriction leading to renal ischemia and not directly related to the myoglobinuria. The lesions and their pathogenesis are comparable to what occurs when muscles are extensively injured, as is seen in the well-known "crush syndrome," and other conditions leading to hypotensive shock in human beings.

But the original injury to the muscle is not easily explained. Ordinary muscular cramps, such as occur in man, are commonly attributed to an insufficient blood supply to the muscle, but the basic chemical difficulty is not greatly clarified by this information. From the clinical circumstances that usually precede an attack of azoturia, it is easy to believe that something accumulates in the muscles during the antecedent period of abnormal inactivity. This something can scarcely be anything but glycogen, which all muscles normally store. As a muscle performs work, lactic acid ($CH_3CHOHCOOH$) is known to accumulate in it. The accepted concept is that the stored glycogen is changed by a series of intermediate steps into pyruvic acid ($CH_3COCOOH$), approximately one-fifth of which is oxidized to $CO_2 + H_2O$ with the production of energy. When the amount of oxygen immediately available is limited, the remaining four-fifths is converted to lactic acid, which may be oxidized later. Pursuant to the above conception it may well be that the amount of lactic acid formed is especially large when the supply of stored glycogen is large, not being directly proportional to the amount of work done.

Confirmation of this view is found in the work of Paris (1958), who showed more than 1% of lactic acid in the urine of horses after a strenuous race. Lactic acid artificially injected into the tissues in sufficient concentration is both painful and irritant in other ways. The amount of lactic acid accumulating in the muscles of a fresh, vigorously exercising horse must be considerable. This is in accord with data and beliefs concerning azoturia that have been prevalent for a long time. Likewise, if the blood supply to a muscle is inadequate, as in cramps, there must be a deficiency of oxygen and an accumulation of lactic acid. So, shall we conclude that accumulating lactic acid irritates or stimulates the muscle to extreme contraction in equine azoturia and perhaps in human systremma and other forms of cramps? The severe contraction of the cramped muscle (hard and board-like, as already stated) certainly does not favor the free flow of blood through it, which is essential for increasing the oxygen supply and oxidation of the lactic acid. If this theory be correct, a "vicious cycle" is obviously instituted: less oxygen causes more accumulation of lactic acid, which causes more severe spasmodic contraction of the muscle, which excludes the blood even more and causes a still greater shortage of oxygen. And, let us remember, the cramped, or spasmodically contracted muscle is continuing to do work, which still further augments the shortage of oxygen and the accumulation of lactic acid. The lack of blood supply and lack of oxygen are, as we well know, among the most prominent causes of necrosis, which is the end result. As a further explanation of the severe pain, we should recall that insufficient blood supply and insufficient oxygenation were seen to be the cause of an extremely painful condition in another equine disease, thrombosis of the iliac arteries.

The evidence for increased glycogen storage in the early stages of the disease and for accumulation of lactate caused Lindholm, et al. (1974) to suggest that increased anaerobic energy demands may be present due to decreased oxygen pressure in the mitochondria. Hypoxia is suggested as an antecedent event. Further studies are needed on the mechanisms involved and may lead to better understanding of this disease.

A disease in man, called exertional rhabdomyolysis, or "march myoglobinuria," has many features similar to the equine condition. The signs appear after strenuous exercise; skeletal muscles are severely affected and myoglobinuria is frequent. Myopathy associated with severe exercise and myoglobinuria has also been reported in cattle and one nonhuman primate.

Barton, C.R.Q., and Allen, W.M.: Possible paralytic myoglobinuria of unknown aetiology in young cattle. Vet. Rec., 92:288–290, 1973.

Bywaters, E.G.L., and Dible, J.H.: Acute paralytic myohaemoglobinuria in man. J. Pathol. Bact., 55:7–15, 1943.

Cardinet, G.H., Litterell, J.F., and Friedland, R.A.: Comparative investigations of serum creatine phosphokinase and glutamic oxaloacetic transaminase activities in equine paralytic myoglobinuria. Res. Vet. Sci., 8:219–226, 1967.

Geller, S.A.: Extreme exertion rhabdomyolysis. A histopathological study of 31 cases. Hum. Pathol., 4:241–250, 1974.

Greenberg, J., and Arneson, L.: Exertional rhab-

domyolysis with myoglobinuria in a large group of military trainees. Neurology, 17:216–222, 1967.

Holmes, J.H.G., et al.: A condition resembling "azoturia" in a "double muscled" heifer. Vet. Rec., 90:625–630, 1972.

Johnston, W.S., and Murray, I.S.: Myopathy in young cattle associated with possible myoglobinuria. Vet. Rec., 97:176–177, 1975.

Lindholm, A., Johansson, H.-E., and Kjaersgaard, P.: Acute rhabdomyolysis ("tying up") in Standardbred horses: a morphological and biochemical study. Acta Vet. Scand., 15:325–339, 1974.

McLean, J.G.: Equine paralytic myoglobinuria ("azoturia"): A review. Aust. Vet. J., 49:41–43, 1973.

Paris, R.: Lactic acid in the urine of Thoroughbred racehorses after exercise. Austr. Vet. J., 34:111–115, 1958.

Ribelin, W.E.: Azoturia and the crush syndrome. J. Am. Vet. Med. Assoc., 119:284–288, 1951.

Scarpelli, D.G., Greider, M.H., and Frajola, W.J.: Idiopathic recurrent rhabdomyolysis. A clinical, chemical and morphologic study. Am. J. Med., 34:426–433, 1963.

Seibold, H.R., Roberts, J.A., and Wolf, R.H.: Idiopathic muscle necrosis with apparent myoglobinuria in Macaca arctoides. Lab. Anim. Sci., 21:242–246, 1971.

Sova, Z., and Jicha, J.: "Determination of serum glutamic oxalacetic acid and serum glutamic pyruvic acid transaminase in horses with myoglobinaemia (TT)." Berl. Münch. Tieraerztl. Wochenschr., 76:385–387, 1963.

Steyn, D.G.: Paralytic myoglobinuria (Kimberley horse disease, "Bewerasiesiekte") in horses and mules under field conditions. J. So. Afr. Vet. Med. Assoc., 19:200–220, 1948.

Exertional Rhabdomyolysis in Wild Animals (Muscular Dystrophy, Capture Myopathy, Overstraining Disease, White Muscle Disease, Muscle Necrosis, Idiopathic Muscle Necrosis)

Conservation efforts involving capture and transport of large wild mammals has led to the recognition of an apparently new disease. The condition becomes evident following the severe physical exertion associated with capture, and obviously involves the musculature and is often accompanied by myoglobinuria. The signs vary: some animals undergo severe depression, others fever and muscular fibrillation; the animal may be reluctant to move or continually shifts its weight from one leg to another. Convulsions, torticollis, or opisthotonos may be followed by paralysis and death in two to four days. Less severely affected animals may survive for two weeks to a month and then succumb. In some species (zebras), severe acidosis has been recognized immediately following capture. This has led to the recommendation of antiacidotic therapy (intravenous bicarbonate) in this species.

Lesions. The lesions observed grossly in the muscles consist of sharply demarcated zones of hemorrhage and pale muscle which may be soft and gelatinous. The lesions are usually bilateral but rarely symmetric. The kidneys are swollen, and dark brown, and myoglobin may be demonstrated in the urinary bladder. Hemorrhages are evident in all layers of the adrenal cortex. Levels of creatine phosphokinase, glutamic oxaloacetic transaminase, and lactic dehydrogenase in the serum are all elevated. Blood pH in zebras may be decreased (pH 6.5 to 6.45).

The microscopic lesions in the skeletal muscles are characteristic of Zenker's necrosis, with calcification. The renal lesions consist of tubular necrosis and acute glomerular degeneration and necrosis.

Cause. The features of this syndrome in wild animals clearly resemble those of exertional rhabdomyolysis of equines and man. Whether the precise causal mechanisms are the same can only be answered by further research.

Bartsch, R.C., McConnell, E.E., Imes, G.D., and Schmidt, J.M.: A review of exertional rhabdomyolysis in wild and domestic animals and man. Vet. Pathol., 14:314–324, 1977.

Harthoorn, A.M., van der Walt, K., and Young, E.: Possible therapy for capture myopathy in captured wild animals. Nature, 247:577, 1974.

Roach, R.W., and Windsor, R.S.: Degenerative polymyopathies in East African domestic and wild animals. Vet. Rec., 81:445, 1967.

Wilson, T.M.: Diffuse muscular degeneration in captive harbor seals. J. Am. Vet. Med. Assoc., 161:608–610, 1972.

Wobester, G., et al.: Myopathy and myoglobinuria in a white-tailed deer. J. Am. Vet. Med. Assoc., 169:971–974, 1976.

Young, E.: Muscle necrosis in captive red hartebeeste (*Alcelaphus buselaphus*). J. S. Afr. Vet. Med. Assoc., 37:101–103, 1966.

Nutritional Muscular Degeneration (Nutritional Muscular Dystrophy; White Muscle Disease of Sheep, Cattle, Swine; Dietetic Microangiopathy [Swine]; Mulberry Heart Disease; Hepatosis Dietetica; Toxic Liver Dystrophy of Swine; Dietary Hepatic Necrosis; Nutritional Anemia)

After years of confusion and controversy over the origin of the problem, which led to the proliferation of descriptive names, evidence from the laboratory and the field indicates that specific lesions result from the dual dietary deficiency of selenium and vitamin E. Nutritional muscular degeneration has been observed for many years in its natural occurrence and has been reproduced experimentally. The disease is most conspicuous in lambs, calves, piglets, and ducklings, but may occur in nature or be reproduced experimentally in many species.

The dual role of selenium and vitamin E has been demonstrated repeatedly and is now explained on the following basis. Selenium is a natural element in most soils, but may be deficient in many parts of the United States. It is taken up by a large number of plants (sometimes in toxic amounts—see Chapter 16) and thereby reaches the diet of man and animals. Selenium in the animal body becomes an essential part of a selenoenzyme, glutathione peroxidase, which in tissues reduces lipid peroxides to hydroxy acids, eliminating their toxic potential to cellular membranes.

Vitamin E (alpha-tocopherol) functions as an antioxidant to protect cellular membranes, especially those rich in fatty acids, from exposure to high concentrations of lipoperoxides. It has been clearly demonstrated that affected muscles contain decreased levels of vitamin E, selenium, and

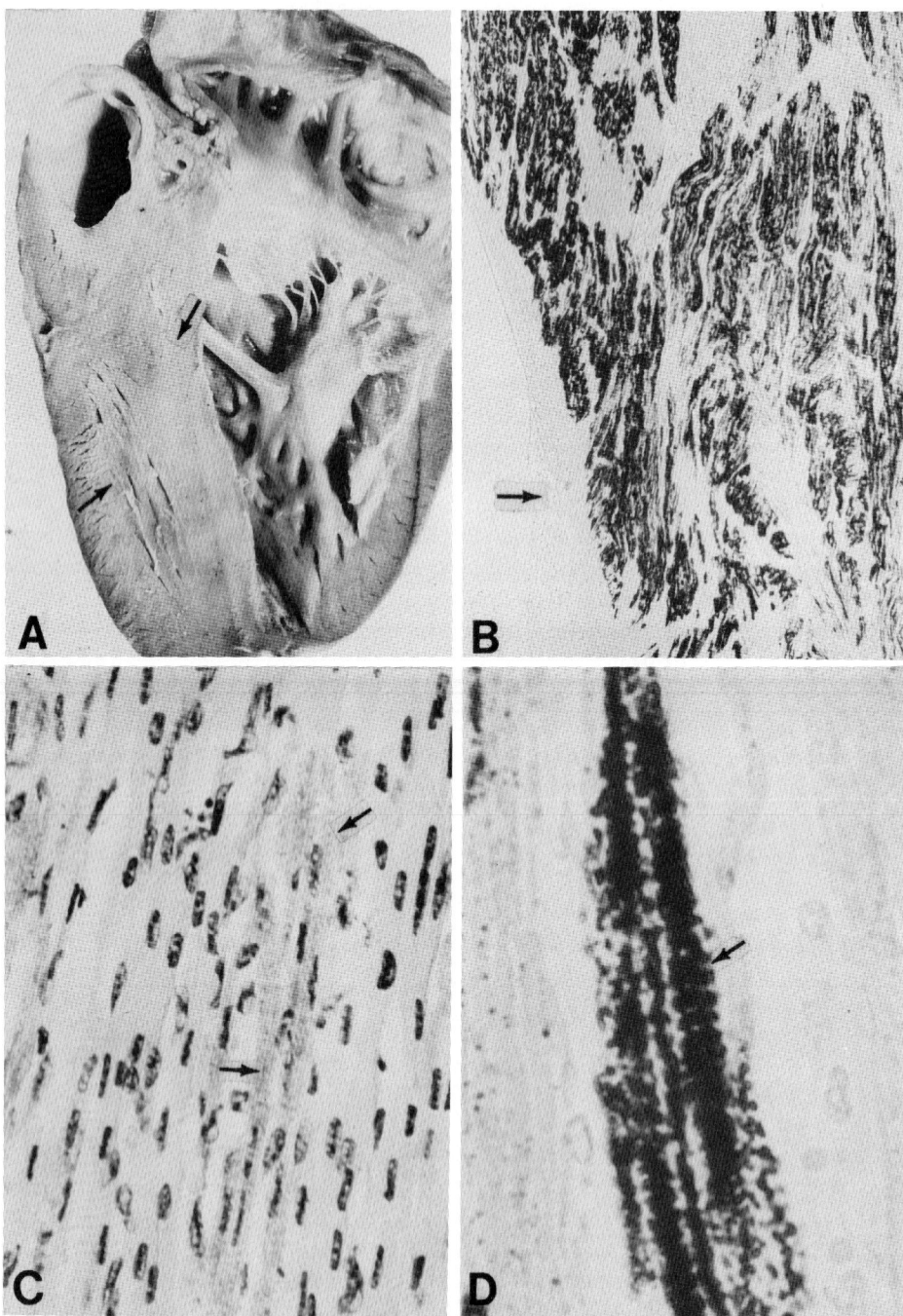

Fig. 19–2. Nutritional muscular degeneration in the heart of a newborn lamb. *A,* Gray areas in the myocardium (arrows). *B,* Section of myocardium (× 45) stained with von Kossa's method to demonstrate salts of calcium (black). Arrow indicates the endocardium. *C,* Another section (× 515) stained with hematoxylin and eosin. Note dark granules (arrows) in fibers of cardiac muscle. *D,* Another section (× 600) stained with von Kossa's method. Note calcium salts (arrow), which outline the cross striations. (Courtesy of Armed Forces Institute of Pathology.) Contributor: Dr. O.H. Muth.

glutathione peroxidase and increased concentration of lipoperoxides.

Some evidence indicates that dietary sulfur-containing amino acids may act as a source of glutathione, which has a sparing effect upon vitamin E/selenium deficiency. In the natural disease, some selenium antagonists, such as silver, cadmium, copper, or zinc, in the diet may have an accentuating effect upon selenium/vitamin E deficiency.

Lesions. Lesions have been described in cardiac and skeletal muscles, in the liver (*hepatosis dietetica*), the brain (avian encephalomalacia), and the bone marrow (anemia) as a result of this dietary deficiency of selenium/vitamin E. We shall consider the changes seen in cardiac and skeletal muscle, leaving the others to the appropriate chapters.

Gross Appearance. The **gross lesions** in the heart consist of edema in the pericardial sac and scattered pale or white streaks in the myocardium. Hemorrhage in the experimental disease is not conspicuous, contrasting with the natural disease in swine ("mulberry heart disease"). In skeletal muscle, pale or white streaks seldom involve a whole muscle, but rather segments of it, and run parallel to the direction of the muscle fibers.

Microscopic Appearance. The microscopic lesions in cardiac muscle consist of hyaline degeneration in various stages, culminating in necrosis of individual muscle fibers. Groups of fibers may be affected, especially in the atrial myocardium. Calcification is a conspicuous feature in early stages (Fig. 19–2). Necrosis of the fibers is manifest by hyaline change in myofibers, pyknosis of nuclei, and invasion of the sarcolemma by macrophages. Lysis of myofibrils follows. These lesions are found throughout the heart, but tend to be concentrated in the atria.

In skeletal muscles, the microscopic lesions are similar in appearance and follow a course resembling that of cardiac muscle. Both necrosis and repair and regeneration may be observed in the same section, involving different myofibers. Regeneration involves proliferation of myoblasts with nuclear fusion, production of myofibrils, and eventual replacement of the sarcolemma.

The ultrastructural lesions in the myocardium are described as involving myofibrillar degeneration with occasional condensation into hypercontraction bands, myofibrillar lysis, swelling of mitochondria, disruption, and mineralization. The myofibrils become more dense, and the condensed fibrils then are lysed and disrupted. The Z bands are smeared or dispersed, leaving dense, tangled masses of filamentous debris. The fibrils, although condensed and homogeneous, maintain a persistent fibrillar pattern. The mitochondria become scattered among the damaged myofibrils and develop swollen, disrupted outer and cristae membranes. Occasionally, matrically dense bodies accumulate. The injured muscle fibers have disrupted plasma membranes, but the external laminae or basement membranes usually persist. The skeletal muscles undergo similar ultrastructural changes, such as myofibrillar lysis and disruption, disorganization of mitochondria, sarcoplasmic reticulum, and plasma membranes in muscle fibers with these myofibrillar alterations. Macrophages are active in phagocytosis of the debris. The basal lamina of the sarcolemma remains after destruction of the enclosed sarcolemma. This serves as a scaffold for later regeneration. The stages of regeneration include: myoblastic proliferation, fusion into cords and myotubules, followed by fibrillogenesis to restore contractile material.

Arterioles in the myocardium are involved during late stages of the process and are not believed to cause the degeneration by producing ischemia. The entire arteriolar wall in certain segments is replaced by fibrinoid degeneration and is later invaded by fibroblastic cells and surrounded by macrophages.

Bird, J.W.C., and Szabo, N.A.B.: Lipid peroxidation in nutritional muscular dystrophy. Proc. Soc. Exp. Biol. Med., 117:345–347, 1964.

Burton, V., et al.: Nutritional muscular dystrophy in lambs—selenium analysis of maternal, fetal and juvenile tissues. Am. J. Vet. Res., 23:962–965, 1962.

Cheville, N.F.: The pathology of vitamin E deficiency in the chick. Pathol. Vet., 3:208–225, 1966.

Combs, G.F., Jr., Naguchi, T., and Scott, M.L.: Mechanisms of action of selenium and vitamin E in protection of biological membranes. Fed. Proc., 34:2090–2092, 1975.

Cotchin, E.: Muscular dystrophy in lambs ("stiff-lamb disease") in a flock in Berkshire. Vet. J., 104:102–108, 1948.

Dam, H., Prange, I., and Søndergaard, E.: Muscular degeneration (white striation of muscles) in chicks reared on vitamin-E deficient, low-fat diets. Acta Pathol. Microbiol. Scand., 31:172–184, 1953.

Dodd, D.C., et al.: Muscle degeneration and yellow fat disease in foals. N.Z. Vet. J., 8:45–50, 1960.

Ekman, L., Orstadius, K., and Aberg, B.: Distribution of Se[75]-tagged sodium selenite in pigs with nutritional muscular dystrophy. Acta Vet. Scand., 4:92–96, 1963.

Gardiner, M.R.: White muscle disease (nutritional muscular dystrophy) of sheep in Western Australia. Aust. Vet. J., 38:387–391, 1962.

Hartley, W.J.: White muscle disease and muscular dystrophy. Aust. Vet. J., 39:338–339, 1963.

Hogue, D.E.: Selenium and muscular dystrophy. J. Am. Vet. Med. Assoc., 133:568, 1958.

Kaspar, L.V., and Lombard, L.S.: Nutritional myodegeneration in a litter of Beagles. J. Am. Vet. Med. Assoc., 143:284–288, 1963.

Keeler, R.F., and Young, S.: Electrophoretic and histological evidence for muscle regeneration in ovine muscular dystrophy. Nature, 193:338–340, 1962.

Muth, O.H.: White muscle disease (myopathy) in lambs and calves. I. Occurrence and nature of the disease under Oregon conditions. J. Am. Vet. Med. Assoc., 126:355–361, 1955.

Muth, O.H., et al.: White muscle disease (myopathy) in lambs and calves. VI. Effects of selenium and vitamin E on lambs. Am. J. Vet. Res., 20:231–234, 1959.

Muth, O.H., and Allaway, W.H.: The relationship of white muscle disease to the distribution of naturally occurring selenium. J. Am. Vet. Med. Assoc., 142:1379–1384, 1963.

Muth, O.H., Whanger, P.D., Weswig, P.H., and Oldfield, J.E.: Occurrence of myopathy in lambs of ewes fed added arsenic in a selenium-deficient ration. Am. J. Vet. Res., 32:1621–1624, 1971.

Oksanen, A., and Poukka, R.: An electron microscopical study of nutritional muscular degeneration (NMD) of myocardium and skeletal muscle in calves. Acta Pathol. Microbiol. Scand. (A), 80:440–448, 1972.

Proctor, J.F., et al.: Relation of selenium, vitamin E and other factors to muscular dystrophy in the rabbit. Proc. Soc. Exp. Biol. Med., 108:77–79, 1961.

Ruth, G.R., and Van Vleet, J.F.: Experimentally induced selenium-vitamin E deficiency in growing swine: selective destruction of Type I skeletal muscle fibers. Am. J. Vet. Res., 35:237–244, 1974.

Van Vleet, J.F., Hall, B.V., and Simon, J.: Vitamin E deficiency. A sequential light and electron microscopic study of skeletal muscle degeneration in weanling rabbits. Am. J. Pathol., 52:1067–1079, 1968.

Van Vleet, J.F., Ruth, G., and Ferrans, V.J.: Ultrastructural alterations in skeletal muscles of pigs with selenium-vitamin E deficiency. Am. J. Vet. Res., 37:911–922, 1976.

Van Vleet, J.F., Ferrans, V.J., and Ruth, G.R.: Ultrastructural alterations in nutritional cardiomyopathy of selenium-vitamin E deficient swine. I. Fiber lesions. Lab. Invest., 37:188–200, 1977a.

Van Vleet, J.F., Ferrans, V.J., and Ruth, G.R.: Ultrastructural alterations in nutritional cardiomyopathy of selenium-vitamin E deficient swine. II. Vascular lesions. Lab. Invest., 37:201–211, 1977b.

Vawter, L.R., and Records, E.: Muscular dystrophy (White muscle disease) in young calves. J. Am. Vet. Med. Assoc., 110:152–157, 1947.

Vracko, R.: Basal lamina scaffold—anatomy and significance for maintenance of orderly tissue structure. Am. J. Pathol., 77:314–346, 1974.

West, W.T., and Mason, K.E.: Histopathology of muscular dystrophy in the vitamin E deficient hamster. Am. J. Anat., 102:323–349, 1958.

Young, S., et al.: Nutritional muscular dystrophy in lambs—morphologic and electrophoretic studies on preparations of fetal and juvenile muscle; selenium analysis of maternal, fetal and juvenile tissue; the effect of muscular activity on the symmetrical distribution of lesions. Am. J. Vet. Res., 23:955–971, 1962.

Myodegeneration due to Other Causes

Nutritional muscular degeneration due to dietary deficiency of selenium and vitamin E is undoubtedly the most frequent disorder of this type affecting skeletal and cardiac muscles of animals. It should not be assumed that it is the only cause of myodegeneration.

At least two plant poisonings produce grossly visible white color to muscle fibers, which are seen microscopically as hyalinization and necrosis of muscle fibers. These poisonous plants, coyotillo (*Karwinskia humboldtiana*) and coffee senna (*Cassia occidentalis*) and their effects, are discussed more fully in Chapter 16. Both plants are native in the southwestern United States.

Dollahite, J.W., and Henson, J.B.: Toxic plants as the etiologic agents of myopathies in animals. Am. J. Vet. Res., 26:749–752, 1965.

Canine Eosinophilic Myositis

Under the name of eosinophilic myositis, a rare disease involving the masseter, temporalis, and pterygoid muscles of the dog has been recognized since about 1940. A number of cases have been reported in Northern Europe and a few in the Northern United States, usually but not invariably in the German Shepherd breed. The muscles named show prominent acute swelling, which is painful and prevents mastication. In most cases, tonsillitis and inflammation and erosion of the mucosa of the tonsillar region are present. The mandibular lymph nodes are secondarily inflamed, swollen, and hard. Considerable exophthalmos results from retrobulbar pressure. The blood shows a moderate increase of white cells, but the most significant change is an eosinophil count of 15 to 20 per cent. In one case, the eosinophils amounted to 63 per cent. Irfan (1971) has indicated circulating eosinophilia in only 15% of 20 affected dogs and points out the importance of the total eosinophil count. It may be that increased numbers of eosinophils in the circulation are related to the acute stage of the muscular lesion. Further studies are needed on this point. Some individuals have a slight fever and there is regularly depression and loss of weight, largely, perhaps, because eating is difficult. The above is the picture of an acute attack, which subsides gradually in two or three weeks, to be followed by a similar one after a few months or weeks. While the dog may show no ill effects between the earlier exacerbations, the eosinophil count remains at its high level and ultimately residual atrophy of the muscles becomes so pronounced that eat-

ing is impossible and the dog dies of general inanition.

Gross and Microscopic Examination. Gross and microscopic examination of the muscles shows the swelling to be due to a very extensive infiltration with eosinophils and "mononuclear" cells, which insinuate themselves between the muscle fibers. The latter show few or no degenerative changes. The gross appearance of the swollen muscles is described as a streaking of gray and red with a yellowish mottling superimposed, all of which is of course attributable to the infiltrated cellular exudate. The changes in the lymph nodes are similar in nature. After several attacks, the muscles show considerable chronic inflammatory fibrosis.

The cause of the disease is unknown. Searches for parasites have always been fruitless. Current theories relate the condition to some localized allergic state, although the failure of antihistaminic drugs to influence the condition has caused some to question this.

Atrophic myositis of the masticatory muscles has been described in dogs as a distinct entity, however, the lesions are nearly identical to the chronic phase of eosinophilic myositis. The disorder is rapidly progressive and lacks eosinophilia.

Berg, O.A., Erichsen, S., and Gjestvang, P.: Myositis eosophilica et atrophicans canis. Nordiske Vet., 7:347–348, 1954.
Clare, M.: Three year history of a case of eosinophilic myositis. Vet. Rec., 68:202–203, 1956.
Harding, H.P., and Owen, L.N.: Eosinophilic myositis in the dog. J. Comp. Pathol., 66:109–122, 1956.
Irfan, M.: The peripheral blood picture in myositis and atrophy of head muscles in dogs. Irish Vet. J., 25:189–193, 1971.
Kuscher, A.: Eosinophile muskelentzündurg beim Hund. Wien Tierärzl Monatschr, 27:177–186, 1940.
Moon, C., and Wood, A.C.: Eosinophilic myositis in a dog. J. Am. Vet. Med. Assoc., 125:312–313, 1954.
Whitney, J.C.: Atrophic myositis in a dog: the differentiation of this disease from eosinophilic myositis. Vet. Rec., 69:130–131, 1957.
Wintor, H., and Stephenson, H.C.: Eosinophilic myositis in a dog. Cornell Vet., 42:531–537, 1952.

Bovine Eosinophilic Myositis

Eosinophilic myositis has been reported in cattle and sheep and appears likely to be caused by *Sarcosporidia* under certain circumstances. The disorder is most frequently encountered by meat inspectors in cuts of beef from animals that appeared normal clinically. Gross changes consist of grayish, sometimes green-tinged areas in otherwise red muscle. The affected areas are usually well circumscribed although irregular in shape, several centimeters in diameter, and tend to follow the course of muscle fibers.

Microscopic examination reveals the change in color to be due to extensive infiltration of eosinophils between remaining muscle fibers (Fig. 19–3). Monocytes and macrophages may occur in some places,

and frank granulomas may be present in others. In some cases degenerating sarcosporidial cysts in muscle may form the nidus for the granulomas.

Experimental infection of calves with many sporocysts derived from feces of dogs fed sarcocystic-infected meat, resulted in severe myositis 26 to 33 days after infection. Schizonts of sarcocystis were numerous throughout the lesions (Johnson, et al., 1975).

Under most conditions, sarcosporidial cysts are found in muscle fibers surrounded by a dense capsule with no inflammatory cells in the adjacent muscle. Under conditions yet to be identified, severe inflammatory reaction results from the presence of *Sarcosporidia*.

Chronic eosinophilic myositis has been described in a Rhesus monkey (*Macaca*

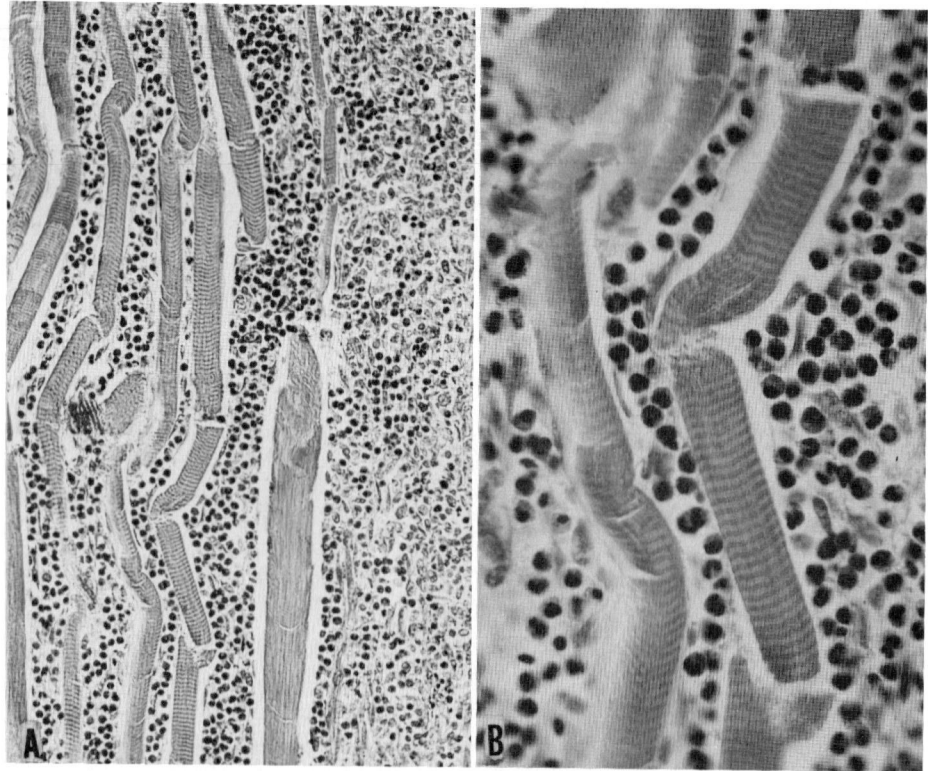

Fig. 19–3. Eosinophilic myositis, psoas muscles of a cow. *A,* Eosinophilic leukocytes isolating and replacing muscle bundles (× 195). *B,* Detail of *A* (× 460). Distention and rupture of muscle bundles and replacement by eosinophils. (Courtesy of Armed Forces Institute of Pathology.) Contributor: Dr. C.L. Davis.

mulatta) in association with sarcosporidial infection. The causal relation of the parasites is not as well established in this case, although degenerating cysts were found in some of the granulomas.

Fayer, R., and Johnson, A.J.: *Sarcocystis fusiformis:* Development of cysts in calves infected with sporocysts from dogs. Proc. Helminthol. Soc. Wash., *41*:105–108, 1974.

Hamilton, W.J., and McCance, C. McB.: Eosinophilic myositis in cattle. Vet. Rec., *83*:471–472, 1968.

Harcourt, R.A., and Bradley, R.: Eosinophilic myositis in sheep. Vet. Rec., *92*:233–234, 1973.

Johnson, A.J., Hildebrandt, P.K., and Fayer, R.: Experimentally induced sarcocystis infection in calves: Pathology. Am. J. Vet. Res., *36*:995–999, 1975.

Munday, B.L., and Rickard, M.D.: Is *Sarcocystic tenella* two species? Aust. Vet. J., *50*:558–559, 1974.

Rommel, M., and Heydorn, A.O.: Beiträge zum Lebenzyklus der Sarcosporidien. III. *Isospora hominus* (Railliet and Luceet, 1891). Wenyon, 1923, eine Dauerform der Sarkosporidian des Rindes und der Schweins. Berlin und München Tierärztl Wochenschr, *85*:143, 145, 1972.

Terrell, T.G., and Stookey, J.L.: Chronic eosinophilic myositis in a rhesus monkey infected with sarcosporidiosis. Vet. Pathol., *9*:266–271, 1972.

Steatosis

The term steatosis has been used to designate a variant condition in the musculature of beef cattle. It is usually recognized at slaughter as an extensive increase in intramuscular fat, particularly in the muscles of the loin and back. This gross change is the result of replacement of many muscle fibers by adipose tissue cells (Fig. 19–4). In this respect it resembles the type of muscular dystrophy ("pseudohypertrophic") in which the end stage is replacement of muscle fibers by fat cells, resulting in grossly apparent enlargement of the muscle. The cause is unknown. It may be under genetic control but insufficient data are available at this writing to establish this point.

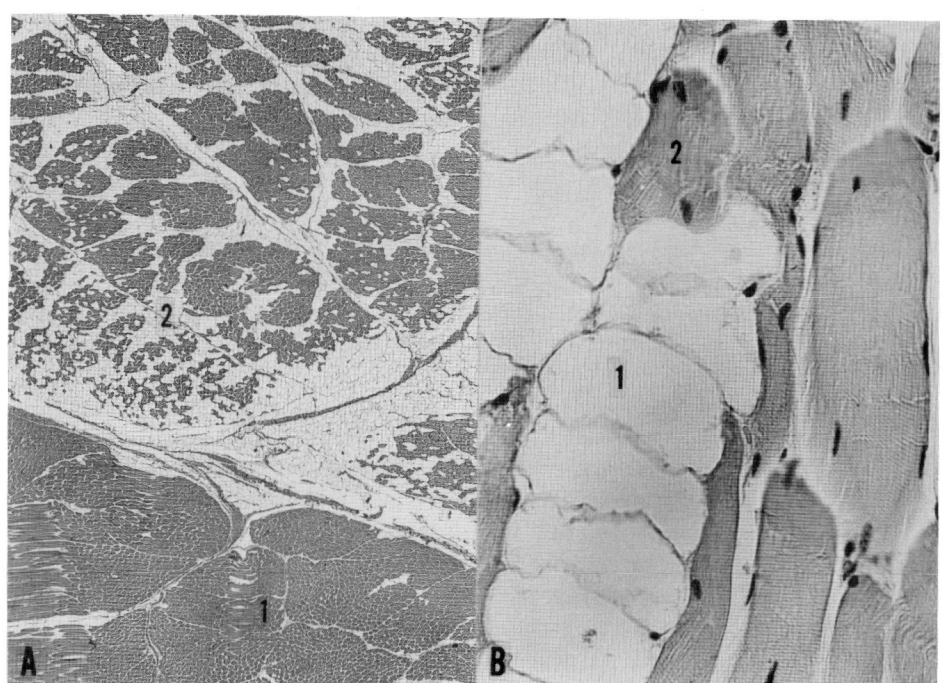

Fig. 19–4. *A*, Steatosis, psoas muscle (× 10) of a steer. Normal muscle (*1*) is infiltrated and replaced by fat (*2*). *B*, The same muscle as *A* (× 330). Note fat cells (*1*) replacing muscle bundles (*2*). (Courtesy of Armed Forces Institute of Pathology.) Contributor: Colonel Russell McNellis, V.C.

Myasthenia

An uncommon disease, manifested by muscular weakness, increased fatigue and response to anticholinesterase drugs, has in recent years been recognized in dogs and a cat. This disease has similarities to human **myasthenia gravis,** which is evident by the following clinical signs: excessive muscular fatigue and reduced tolerance to exercise, alleviated by rest or administration of anticholinesterase drugs (such as prostigmin). The defect involves a functional disturbance at neuromuscular junctions and is confirmed by administration of the anticholinesterase drug mentioned above plus demonstration of characteristic electromyographic response.

Characteristic features of myasthenia gravis have been induced in mice by the prolonged administration of serum immunoglobins (IgG) from patients with myasthenia gravis. The experimental mice become weak, manifest reduced amplitude of miniature end-plate potentials, have a reduced number of receptor sites, and typical electromyographic response. It appears that myasthenia results from a neuromuscular blockade on the postsynaptic side and involves antibody in some way.

Lesions. The lesions have not been reported extensively, but the presence of a flaccid, dilated esophagus has been confirmed at postmortem examination. The presence of a thymoma in the anterior mediastinum was noted in some cases. Aspiration pneumonia was a feature in some animals. Microscopic studies of skeletal muscle with routine technics have revealed no abnormalities such as myositis, hemorrhages, lymphocytic infiltration, muscle necrosis, or neurogenic muscle atrophy. In one case, however (Darke, et al., 1975) degenerative changes in muscle fibers were found. These were associated with lymphocytic infiltration and some fibrosis. In this case, a thymoma was present in the anterior mediastinum.

Darke, P.G.G., McCullagh, K.G., and Geldart, P.H.: Myasthenia gravis, thymoma and myositis in a dog. Vet. Rec., 97:392–394, 1975.

Dawson, D.M.: Human disease transferred to mice: Myasthenia gravis. N. Engl. J. Med., 296:168–169, 1977.

Fraser, D.C., Palmer, A.C., Senior, J.E.B., Parkes, J.D., and Yealland, M.F.T.: Myasthenia gravis in the dog. J. Neurol. Neurosurg. Psychiatr., 33:431–437, 1970.

Hall, G.A., Howell, J. McC., and Lewis, D.G.: Thymoma with myasthenia gravis in a dog. J. Pathol., 108:177–180, 1972.

Jenkins, W.L., van Dyk, E., and McDonald, C.B.: Myasthenia gravis in a Fox Terrier litter. J. S. Afr. Vet. Assoc., 47:59–62, 1976.

Johnson, R.P., Watson, A.D., Smith, J., and Cooper, B.J.: Myasthenia in Springer Spaniel littermates. J. Small Anim. Pract., 16:641–647, 1975.

Palmer, A.C., and Barker, J.: Myasthenia in the dog. Vet. Rec., 95:452–454, 1974.

Toyka, K.V., Drachman, D.B., Pestronk, A., and Kao, I.: Myasthenia gravis: passive transfer from man to mouse. Science, 190:397–399, 1975.

Myofibrillar Hypoplasia

Congenital myofibrillar hypoplasia or splayleg has been studied best in piglets, but a similar condition is seen in other species, particularly in puppies. The newborn animal is unable to stand on its feet due to weakness of the adductor muscles. The hind legs are most frequently affected; both of them extend (splay) outward or forward, and the weight rests on the pubis. The forelimbs may be similarly affected. The newborn piglet thus affected is at a serious disadvantage and may succumb to trauma or starvation. If the legs can be held together and the animal nursed carefully, recovery may occur.

The basic defect appears to be immaturity of particular skeletal muscles. The muscle fibers have not reached an adequate stage of development at the time of birth. The disease is often reported to be hereditary, but the evidence for its inheritance is not entirely convincing.

Lesions. The microscopic lesions in affected muscle fibers consist of reduced numbers of myofibrils, particularly in the muscles of the trunk and limbs. Not only are the myofibrils few in number, but they are small in diameter and tend to be concentrated in one part of the fiber within the endomysium.

Ultrastructural lesions are described as having: (1) reduced number of myofibrils occupying only a part of the fiber; (2) myofibrils generally smaller than in normal fibers, with some longitudinal splitting and imperfect alignment of transverse bands and (3) granular material occupying the remaining space within affected fibers (Deutsch and Done, 1971).

Splayleg is also applied to a condition with similar signs in rabbits. This is considered to be due to defects in the coxofemoral joints. The muscles, however, may not have been studied adequately.

Deutsch, K., and Done, J.T.: Congenital myofibrillar hypoplasia of piglets. Ultrastructure of affected fibres. Res. Vet. Sci., 12:176–177, 1971.

Dobson, K.J.: Failure of choline and methionine to prevent splayleg in piglets. Aust. Vet. J., 47:587–590, 1971.

Lax, T.: Herditary splayleg in pigs. J. Hered., 62:250–252, 1971.

Thurley, D.C., Gilbert, F.R., and Done, J.T.: Congenital splayleg of piglets: myofibrillar hypoplasia. Vet. Rec., 80:302–304, 1967.

Myotonia

Myotonia is used to describe the manifestations which occur when a muscle continues to contract actively after the stimulus (voluntary effort or electrical-stimulation) has ceased. It may be recognized by the signs or by use of the electromyograph. A repetitive high frequency discharge which tends to increase and then decrease in amplitude and frequency is demonstrated by this instrument. The loudspeaker emits a sound that waxes and wanes, resembling the sound of a dive-bomber.

Myotonia is not due to any primary neural dysfunction, but is a result of a hyperexcitable muscle cell membrane. The persistent discharge continues after neuromuscular block with depolarizing and non-depolarizing muscle relaxants. Local procaine injection may stop the discharge, but anticholinesterases have no effect.

This condition has been reported in man, goats, dogs, mice, a horse, and a calf. The lesions described have varied to some extent from severe Zenker's degeneration to little or no reaction. It appears that several lesions in muscle may result in myotonia or that several forms occur. It is of interest that in two hereditary muscular dystrophies in dogs (Kramer, et al., 1976; Wentink, et al., 1974), the affected animals exhibit myotonia.

Brown, G.L., and Harvey, A.M.: Congenital myotonia in the goat. Brain, 62:341–363, 1939.

Duncan, I.D., Griffiths, I.R., and McQueen, A.: A myopathy associated with myotonia in the dog. Acta Neuropathol., 31:297–303, 1975.

Griffiths, I.R., and Duncan, I.D.: Myotonia in the dog: a report of four cases. Vet. Rec., 93:184–188, 1973.

Kramer, J.W., Hegreberg, G.A., Bryan, G.M., Meyers, K., and Ott, R.L.: A muscle disorder of Labrador Retrievers characterized by deficiency of type II muscle fibers. J. Am. Vet. Med. Assoc., 169:817–820, 1976.

McComas, A.J., and Mossawy, S.J.: Research in Muscular Dystrophy. Proceedings III Symposium of the Muscular Dystrophy Group, London, Pitman Med. Publ., 1965.

Steinberg, S., and Botelho, S.: Myotonia in a horse. Science, 137:979–980, 1962.

van Neikerk, I.J.M., and Jaros, G.G.: Myotonia in the calf; a case report. S. Afr. Med. J., 44:898–899, 1970.

Wentink, G.N., Meijer, A.E.F.H., van der Linde–Sipman, J.S., and Hendriks, H.J.: Myopathy in an Irish Terrier with a metabolic defect of the isolated mitochondria. Zbl. Vet. Med. Assoc., 21:62–74, 1974.

Calcification and Ossification of Muscle

Dystrophic calcification may accompany degenerative lesions of muscle, as noted under white-muscle disease. Calcification of unknown cause may be seen in animals with Cushing's disease. Ossification of muscle or myositis ossificans, which is heterotopic bone formation in muscle and not ossification of muscle fibers, may follow trauma. A generalized form of myositis ossificans of unknown cause has been described by Seibold and Davis (1967) in pigs. Myositis ossificans, confined to single muscles or muscle groups, has been reported in dogs and a cat. The lesions must be differentiated from osteosarcoma, which may not always be a simple matter; but of great importance if the fate of a life or limb depends on interpretation of a biopsy. Myositis ossificans is not neoplastic.

Adams, O.R.: Fibrotic myopathy and ossifying myopathy in the hindlegs of horses. J. Am. Vet. Med. Assoc., *139*:1089–1092, 1961.

Barrett, R.B.: Radiography in trauma of the musculocutaneous soft tissue of dogs and cats. J. Am. Vet. Rad. Soc., *12*:5, 1971.

Liu, S.K., Dorfman, H.D., and Patnaik, A.K.: Primary and secondary bone tumors in the cat. J. Small Anim. Pract., *15*:141–156, 1974.

Liu, S.K., and Dorfman, H.D.: A condition resembling human localized myositis ossificans in two dogs. J. Small Anim. Pract., *17*:371–377, 1976.

Seibold, H.R., and Davis, C.R.: Generalized myositis ossificans (familial) in pigs. Pathol. Vet., *4*:79–88, 1967.

Infectious Myositis

Many infectious diseases are characterized by myositis, but only a few represent primary forms of myositis. Clostridial myositis is a classic example of primary myositis. The several species of the genus *Clostridium* which induce myositis in animals are discussed in Chapter 11. Myositis is a usual finding in penetrating wounds, where a variety of bacterial organisms may be implanted in muscle or extend from the skin. *Staphylococcus spp., Streptococcus spp.,* and *Corynebacterium spp.* are of particular importance in wound infections of domestic animals. Actinobacillosis is a cause of primary myositis of the tongue. Other infectious processes may extend from contiguous tissues to produce myositis as in actinomycosis of the mandible.

Myositis is a component of many systemic infectious diseases of domestic animals including foot and mouth disease, blue tongue, *Hemophilus agni* infection in sheep, Chagas' disease, and toxoplasmosis.

Parasitic infestations which predominantly involve muscle include sarcosporidiosis, trichinosis, and cysticercosis.

Bohan, A., and Peter, J.B.: Polymyositis and dermatomyositis. N. Engl. J. Med., *292*:344–347; 403–407, 1975.

Currie, S.: Experimental myositis: the in-vivo and in-vitro activity of lymph-node cells. J. Pathol., *105*:169–185, 1971.

Despommier, D.: Adaptive changes in muscle fibers infected with *Trichinella spiralis*. Am. J. Pathol., *78*:477–496, 1975.

Laguens, R.P., et al.: Immunopathologic and morphologic studies of skeletal muscle in Chagas disease. Am. J. Pathol., *80*:153–162, 1975.

Sato, T., Walker, D.L., and Peters, H.A.: Chronic polymyositis and myxovirus-like inclusions. Electron microscopic and viral studies. Arch. Neurol., *24*:409–418, 1971.

Neoplasms

Rhabdomyoma or **rhabdomyosarcoma** are names given respectively to benign or malignant neoplasms arising from striated muscle, skeletal or cardiac. Although known in many animal species, they are quite infrequent. The benign variety is essentially unknown in animals. Rhabdomyosarcoma has been reported to arise from skeletal muscle, the tongue, pharynx, panniculis muscle, myocardium, and urinary bladder. They have been reported most often in the dog and are locally invasive but slow to metastasize.

Microscopic Features. The microscopic features of rhabdomyosarcoma present great variety and are often difficult to identify with certainty. (See Fig. 19–5.) More differentiated tumors may have histologic features that clearly resemble those of immature striated muscle, with incompletely or completely developed muscle fibers with identifiable myofibrils and cross striations. These are more easily identified. Others may be highly undifferentiated, containing pleomorphic cells, often with bizarre, giant, and multiple nuclei. The cytoplasm may be abundant but somewhat amorphous. Sometimes small amounts of eosinophilic cytoplasm may be seen in cylindrical form. Special stains, such as phosphotungstic acid hematoxylin, may be required to demonstrate the cross striations which provide definitive identification.

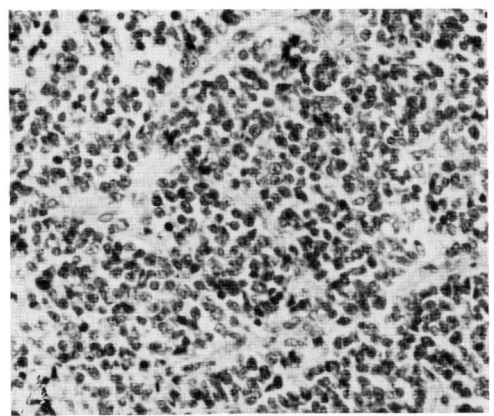

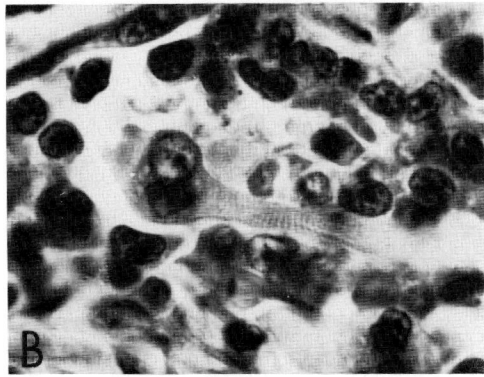

Fig. 19-5. Juvenile rhabdomyosarcoma in a dog. *A*, Undifferentiated region of tumor. *B*, Multinucleated "racquet" cell with cross striations. (Courtesy of Dr. H.R. Seibold and *Veterinary Pathology*.)

Fibrosarcomas that invade and displace striated muscle sometimes present a problem in differential diagnosis. The disturbed or displaced muscle cells may undergo regenerative changes which simulate neoplastic growth. In general, the neoplastic cells in this case are clearly fibroblastic, and the bizarre cells which are sometimes identifiable as poorly-formed muscle cells are not present.

Granular Cell Myoblastoma. This is a microscopically startling growth consisting principally of large, or even huge, polyhedral and spherical cells of epithelioid appearance which have a comparatively small central nucleus and an extensive, pale, granular cytoplasm. There is more or less collagen-bearing stroma. In the human tongue, especially, these cells appear related to, and derived from striated muscle, and this conception is responsible for the name applied to the tumor. However, these growths have also been described in structures, such as the human mammary gland and hypophysis, where there is no striated muscle. One school of thought places the origin of the peculiar cells in nervous tissue; another considers them as altered fibroblasts. Whatever their nature, the tumor constitutes a readily recognizable entity, and its metastasis is known to be highly unlikely. Hyperplastic changes (acanthosis) of the overlying epidermis are likely to accompany it. There are those who believe the large cells to be degenerative or possibly regenerative and not truly neoplastic. Such a tumor has been recorded in the subcutaneous tissue of a dog. Some foreign material of plant origin was found embedded in the overlying dermis, which may or may not be significant. The tumor was excised with an apparent cure. Additional cases have been reported in the horse, mouse, and tongue of a dog.

Secondary neoplasms involve striated muscle by direct extension or expansion of tumors of adjacent or component tissues (fibrosarcoma, neurofibrosarcoma, hemangioendothelioma). Malignant neoplasms of the skin very often involve the panniculus carnosus and may extend to other muscles. Malignant lymphoma often invades skeletal muscle by metastasis or direct extension. Neoplasms of bone (osteosarcoma, chondrosarcoma) and mammary gland (adenocarcinoma, medullary carcinoma, undifferentiated carcinoma) also may involve the muscles by metastasis or direct extension.

Ladds, P.W., and Webster, D.R.: Pharyngeal rhabdomyosarcoma in a dog. Vet. Pathol., 8:256–259, 1971.

Misdorp, W., and Nauta-van Gelder, H.L.: "Granular cell myoblastoma" in the horse: a report of 4 cases. Pathol. Vet., 5:385–394, 1968.

Osborne, C.A., Low, D.G., Perman, V., and Barnes, D.M.: Neoplasms of the canine and feline urinary bladder: Incidence, etiologic factors, occurrence and pathologic features. Am. J. Vet. Res., 29:2041–2055, 1968.

Peter, C.P., and Kluge, J.P.: An ultrastructural study of a canine rhabdomyosarcoma. Cancer, 26:1280–1288, 1970.

Seibold, H.R.: Juvenile alveolar rhabdomyosarcoma in a dog. Vet. Pathol., 11:558–560, 1974.

Troy, M.A.: Granular cell myoblastoma in a dog. J. Am. Vet. Med. Assoc., 126:397, 1955.

Wyand, D.S., and Wolke, R.E.: Granular cell myoblastoma of the canine tongue: Case reports. Am. J. Vet. Res., 29:1309–1313, 1968.

ARTHROGRYPOSIS (NEUROMYODYSPLASIA CONGENITA)

Arthrogryposis is a term used to designate a congenital situation in which one or more joints are fixed in distorted position and cannot be moved in any way. Surviving animals have grossly distorted legs throughout their lives. The fixation of the joints and the grotesque distortion of the limbs is the result of severe atrophy of large groups of muscles. In many cases, concomitant necrosis or loss of neurons in the ventral gray matter are a significant part of the lesions. The manifestations vary considerably in severity and extent of involvement of limbs. Arthrogryposis is also often associated with other congenital anomalies such as hydranencephaly, cleft palate, hydrocephalus, scoliosis, kyphosis, torticollis, ocular defects, and imperforate anus. It has been described in children, calves, piglets, lambs, kids, and kittens (Fig. 16–9).

The etiology appears to be varied. Large-scale losses of newborn or aborted calves in Japan have been demonstrated to be associated with infection by the Akabane virus, an arbovirus isolated originally from mosquitoes in Japan by Oya, et al. (1961). The virus was demonstrated serologically to be associated with arthrogryposis in New South Wales by Hartley et al. (1975), and the virus was recovered from affected calves in Japan by Kurogi, et al., 1976. More than 30,000 abortions are reported due to this infection in one prefecture of Japan in the course of one breeding season.

The disease has been reported in cattle in several parts of the United States, where it has been associated with poisoning due to *Lupinus sericeus,* to heredity factors or infection by bluetongue and bovine viral diarrhea viruses. The clinical features have been reproduced in guinea pig fetuses in association with hyperthermia (Edwards, 1971). The disease in swine has been putatively ascribed to feeding of tobacco plants (*Nicotiana tabacum*). Outbreaks involving calves, lambs, and kids have been reported in Israel. It is likely that it will eventually be recognized worldwide.

Crowe, M.W., and Pike, H.T.: Congenital arthrogryposis associated with ingestion of tobacco stalks by pregnant sows. J. Am. Vet. Med. Assoc., 162:453–455, 1973.

Crowe, M.W., and Swerczek, T.W.: Congenital arthrogryposis in offspring of sows fed tobacco (*Nicotiana tabacum*). Am. J. Vet. Res., 35:1071–1074, 1974.

Edwards, M.J.: The experimental production of arthrogryposis multiplex congenita in guinea-pigs by maternal hyperthermia during gestation. J. Pathol., 104:221–229, 1971.

Greene, H.J., Leipold, H.W., Huston, K., and Guffy, M.M.: Bovine congenital defects: Arthrogryposis and associated defects in calves. Am. J. Vet. Res., 34:887–892, 1973.

Hamana, K., et al.: Outbreaks of the abortion-arthrogryposis-hydranencephaly syndrome in cattle in Japan, 1972–1973. II. Clinical findings in affected calves. Bulletin of the Faculty of Agriculture, Miyazaki Univ., 20:292–310, 1973.

Hartley, W.J., and Wanner, R.A.: Bovine congenital arthrogryposis in New South Wales. Aust. Vet. J., 50:185–188, 1974.

Hartley, W.J., Wanner, R.A., Della-Porta, A.J., and Snowden, W.A.: Serological evidence for the association of Akabane virus with epizootic bovine congenital arthrogryposis and hydranencephaly syndromes in New South Wales. Aust. Vet. J., 51:103–104, 1975.

Herzog, A., and Adam, R.: Der Neuromyodysplasia congenita (Kongenitallie Arthrogrypose) der Hintergliedmassen beim Kalb. Dtsch. Tierärztl. Wschr., 75:237–243, 1968.

Kurogi, H., et al.: Epizootic congenital arthrogryposis-hydranencephaly syndrome in cattle: isolation of Akabane virus from affected fetuses. Arch. Virol., 51:67–74, 1976.

Leipold, H.W., Green, H.J., and Huston, K.: Arthrogryposis and Palatoschisis in neonatal Charolais calves. Vet. Med. Small Anim. Clin., October, 1140–1146, 1973.

Markusfeld, O., and Mayer, E.: An arthrogryposis and hydranencephaly syndrome in calves in Israel, 1969/70. Epidemiological and clinical aspects. Refuah Vet., 28:51–61, 1971.

Nobel, T.A., Klopfer, U., and Neumann, F.: Pathology of an arthrogryposis-hydranencephaly syndrome in domestic ruminants in Israel, 1969/70. Refuah Vet., 28:144–151, 1971.

Nosaka, D., et al.: Outbreaks of the abortion-arthrogryposis-hydranencephaly syndrome in cattle, in Japan, 1972/1973. III. Pathological findings in affected calves. Bulletin of the Faculty of Agriculture, Miyazaki University, 20:311–344, 1973.

Oya, A., et al.: Akabane, a new arbor virus isolated in Japan. Jpn. J. Med. Sci. Biol., 14:101–108, 1961.

Shupe, J.L., et al.: Probable hereditary skeletal deformity in Hereford cattle. J. Hered., 58:311–313, 1967.

THE SKELETAL SYSTEM

The Normal Development of Bone

As is explained in textbooks of histology, bone is formed in two different situations by somewhat differing processes. The flat bones develop by the process known as **intramembranous bone formation,** in which the fibroblastic-appearing cells of the inner or "cambium" layer of the periosteum gradually differentiate into osteoblasts, or bone-forming cells, and osteocytes, which are completely differentiated bone cells, each locked in its particular lacuna. The transition is gradual so that it is impossible to say exactly where the fibrous tissue of the periosteum ends and the bone begins. This type of bone formation is not only responsible for the formation of the flat bones of the head and pelvis, but also occurs along the periosteal surfaces of the shafts (diaphyses) of the long bones as these latter grow in width.

Increase in length of the long bones, however, is achieved by **endochondral bone formation** which goes on at the epiphyseal cartilage, which joins the epiphysis to its respective end of the diaphysis. This endochondral bone formation occurs only on one side of the epiphyseal cartilage, the side toward the diaphysis. On the other, or articular side, the epiphyseal cartilage abruptly joins the cancellous bone of which the epiphysis consists. As for the epiphysis, its growth is by means of a rather inconspicuous transition from cartilage to bone along the base of the articular cartilage on the diaphyseal side.

Returning to the principal growth process, the endochondral bone development on the diaphyseal side of the epiphyseal cartilage, we find a series of consecutive changes represented by successive zones in this region, the so-called metaphysis. Proceeding from the normal, inactive cartilage of the epiphysis, we encounter a zone of (1) proliferating cartilage, where the cells in their lacunae are close together and darkly stained, (2) columnar cartilage, the cells being arranged in distinct longitudinal columns, (3) swollen cartilage cells with extensive but nearly colorless cytoplasm, a degenerative stage, no doubt, and (4) calcified cartilage where the intercellular matrix takes a deep blue or purple stain because of calcium salts deposited in it. Invaded by capillaries reaching from the adjacent marrow spaces and apparently carrying lytic substances, the cartilage is reduced in the next zone (5) to minute longitudinal trabeculae. A bit farther on (6) osteoblasts appear along the edges of these cartilaginous trabeculae, surrounding them and replacing them by pink-staining osteoid which is subsequently calcified (blue-staining). As more material is brought in via the capillaries, more osteoid is deposited, burying the osteoblasts and their lacunae in primary trabeculae of bone. These primary trabeculae of bone or circumferential lamellae of the cortex are ultimately replaced by more mature bone. Resorption by osteoclasts (see below) cuts through primary bone, forming tunnels or "cutting cones," which are then filled in centripetally by osteoblasts forming successive layers of bone which constitute the Haversian system or osteones. This form of remodeling continues throughout life, producing successive generations of osteones. Preexisting lamellar bone or preexisting osteones lie between adjacent osteones forming what is termed interstitial lamellae.

It is to be noted that in this metaphyseal region of a long bone the bony cortex or outer wall of compact bone is missing, even the marrow spaces being in direct connection with the fibrous periosteum. This permits continual rebuilding and remodeling of the bone here, a process necessitated as continued growth pushes what was the metaphysis into a diaphyseal position. The marrow in this region of active growth is at first fibrous but soon develops the usual myeloid and fatty pattern. Since the deposition of the bone-forming ingredients depends upon their being brought in by the blood, newly formed bone tends to lie in encircling layers a short distance from the capillary which nourishes it. This is, indeed, the reason for the architectural arrangement into Haversian systems. The continual remodeling, thus, is dependent upon the rearrangement of capillaries.

Mineralization of osteoid to bone does not occur immediately following its deposition; there is a lag of five to ten days before calcium salts are deposited. Apparently osteoid must "mature" in some manner in order to calcify. Although details of the process of maturation and subsequent calcification are unknown, it is under control of osteoblasts, and not directly related to serum levels·of calcium. Failure of osteoblasts to cause maturation of osteoid is a basic defect in osteomalacias (see below). Remodeling obviously proceeds at a more rapid pace in growing animals, because with growth, bones increase in size, but retain a rather constant shape. For this reason, if bone formation is upset from any cause the pathological effects are more severe or proceed more rapidly in the young animal.

Remodeling obviously implies bone resorption, a process also of significant importance to the pathogenesis of many of the diseases to be discussed shortly. Classi-cally the osteoclast, a large multinucleated cell, is the physiological antagonist of the osteoblast. By mechanisms poorly understood, osteoclasts cause resorption of bone. They do not engulf bone as a foreign body giant cell ingests particulate matter but rather initiate enzymatic reactions which result in the breakdown of bone. It should be noted that unmineralized bone (osteoid) is not resorbed by osteoclasts. Osteoclasts are restricted to the surface of bone spicules and, therefore, osteoclasia is a surface phenomenon. The mature osteocyte is also responsible for bone resorption. The process, termed osteolysis or onchosis, is a major factor in many resorptive bone diseases and in contrast to osteoclasia, is operative within spicules of bone where the osteocytes are entrapped. Osteoclasia and osteolysis are stimulated by parathyroid hormone and vitamin D and inhibited by thyrocalcitonin.

In bone diseases characterized by malacia or increased resorption of bone there is often an associated increased osteoblastic activity with osteoid formation. The stimulus to the osteoblast under these circumstances is poorly understood. Parathyroid hormone, which stimulates bone resorption, is believed to inhibit bone formation, but this is either counteracted by mechanical stress or it may be that prolonged parathormone action actually stimulates bone formation.

From this discussion it should be obvious that a diversity of endogenous and exogenous factors is necessary to maintain bone formation, growth, and remodeling in homeostatic balance. These include *nutrients* such as calcium, phosphorus, magnesium, copper, vitamins D, A, and C (see Chapter 17); *hormones* such as parathyroid hormone, thyrocalcitonin, thyroxin, growth hormone, adrenal cortical steroids, estrogens, and androgens (see Chapter 27); *mechanical forces;* and a diversity of other influencing factors such as acid-base balance, citrate, numerous enzymes, and so forth.

Before we consider specific disorders of bone, a few introductory comments on **metabolic bone diseases** may help the student's understanding of a group of diseases which are often baffling. To be certain, these disorders are complicated, but the frequent and continued unnecessary misuse of such terms as rickets, osteomalacia, and osteoporosis has led to as much confusion as has the complexity of the diseases. Metabolic bone diseases can be conveniently divided into three general types: (1) those principally characterized by porosis, (2) those principally characterized by malacia, and (3) those principally characterized by petrosis. **Osteoporosis** is simply a generalized atrophy of bone, i.e., there is too little bone present, but what bone remains is properly calcified. Although osteoporosis is the most important metabolic bone disease in man, it is not frequent in domestic animals. The cause is usually not known, but may follow defects in bone formation or excessive resorption.

Osteomalacia (softening of bones) is characterized by failure to mineralize (calcify) osteoid into true bone. In most disorders resulting in osteomalacia there is a disturbance in calcium and phosphorus balance. The mechanism of calcification of osteoid still remains to be elucidated but the process is under control of osteoblasts which for reasons poorly understood are defective when serum calcium and/or phosphorus levels are lowered. Osteomalacia is the predominant feature of rickets and osteomalacia. In both of these conditions there is no defect in forming osteoid, in fact excess osteoid formation is the rule. Fibrous osteodystrophy represents a third disorder characterized by osteomalacia, but this condition differs from rickets or osteomalacia in that a marked increase of bone resorption is a constant feature. Fibrous osteodystrophy results from a prolonged and excessive stimulation of bone by parathyroid hormone. This may result from primary hyperpara-

thyroidism which is rare in animals, or secondary hyperparathyroidism in response to hypocalcemia. Secondary hyperparathyroidism is not infrequent in animals with chronic renal disease or chronic nutritional imbalance, such as vitamin D deficiency, calcium deficiency or excess dietary phosphorus. Thus, fibrous osteodystrophy obviously begins as a simple osteomalacia which is subsequently altered due to increased bone resorption stimulated by parathyroid hormone. It should be clear that both rickets and osteomalacia may progress to fibrous osteodystrophy.

Osteopetrosis is characterized by an excess of calcified bone (not to be confused with an excess of osteoid). Although it occurs in animals, it is infrequent.

The following classification should aid the student's understanding:

1. Too little bone, *e.g.* osteoporosis.
2. Defective calcification of matrix, *e.g.* rickets, osteomalacia.
3. Increased resorption of bone (usually associated with defective mineralization), *e.g.* fibrous osteodystrophy.
4. Too much calcified bone, *e.g.* osteopetrosis.

Although the classification is helpful, the student will be quick to realize that in most metabolic disorders of bone he may find features of more than one process within a particular case. For example, with increased resorption of bone the first feature will be too little bone, *i.e.* osteoporosis; but as osteoblasts respond and produce new osteoid which fails to mineralize the disease becomes osteomalacia.

Anderson, C., and Danylchuk, K.D.: Bone-remodeling rates of the Beagle: a comparison between different sites on the same rib. Am. J. Vet. Res., 39:1763–1765, 1978.
Boyde, A., Howell, P.G., and Jones, S.J.: Measurement of lacunar volume in bone using a stereological grid counting method evolved for the scanning electron microscope. J. Microsc., 101:261–266, 1974.
Brown, M.P., and MacCallum, F.J.: A system of grading ossification in limbs of foals to assist in radiologic interpretation. Am. J. Vet. Res., 36:655–661, 1975.

Carter, E.R., and Hayes, W.C.: Bone compressive strength: the influence of density and strain rate. Science, 194:1174–1175, 1976.

Gomes, B.C., Hausmann, E., Weinfeld, N., and de Luca, C.: Prostaglandins: bone resorption stimulating factors released from monkey gingiva. Calcif. Tiss. Res., 19:285–293, 1976.

Kelley, S.T., Bucci, T.J., and Silverman, S.: Skeletal maturation in owl monkeys (Aotus sp). Fed. Proc., 37:356, 1978.

McCarthy, T.C., Wells, M.K., and Gorman, H.A.: Bone-methyl methacrylate interfacial shear strength: an experimental study in dogs. Am. J. Vet. Res., 38:75–80, 1977.

Miller, S.S., Wolf, A.M., and Arnaud, C.D.: Bone cells in culture: morphologic transformation by hormones. Science, 192:1340–1342, 1976.

Momeni, M.H., and Pool, R.R.: Bone and bone marrow spaces in dosimetry of Beagle skeletons. Health Physics, 29:877–881, 1975.

Mundy, G.R., et al.: Direct resorption of bone by human monocytes. Science, 196:1109–1111, 1977.

Sage, M., et al.: Bone metabolism in thyroidectomized young pigs. Cornell Vet., 60:547–559, 1969.

Schryver, H.F.: Bending properties of cortical bone of the horse. Am. J. Vet. Res., 39:25–28, 1978.

Storey, E.: Tissue response to the movement of bones. Am. J. Orthodont., 64:229–247, 1973.

Weisbrode, S.E., Capen, C.C., and Nagode, L.A.: Ultrastructural evaluation of the effects of Vitamin D and uremia on bone in the rat. Am. J. Pathol., 76:359–376, 1974.

Wilsman, N.J., and Van Sickle, D.C.: Histochemical evidence of a functional heterogeneity in neonatal canine epiphyseal chondrocytes. Histochem. J., 3:311–318, 1971.

Young, D.R., Howard, W.H., and Cann, C.: Noninvasive measures of bone bending rigidity in the monkey. Fed. Proc., 37:216, 1978.

Zimmerman, R.E., Griffiths, H.J., and D'Orsi, C.: Bone mineral measurement by means of photon absorption. Radiol., 106:561–564, 1973.

Rickets

Rickets, sometimes called **rachitis,** is a disease characterized by failure of adequate deposition of calcium (chiefly calcium phosphate) in the bones of growing animals and children. As **adult rickets** the term is often used to include the essentially similar osteomalacia in older animals.

Gross Appearance. Outstanding are enlargement of the ends of the long bones and of the costochondral articulations. The former are observable during life, and in severe cases the bones of the limbs become permanently bent under the weight of the animal's body, producing "bow legs" and other skeletal deformities. Due to weakening of the muscles and tendons the abdomen is pendulous, "pot-bellied." At autopsy the same changes are seen; the enlarged costochondral articulations, viewed collectively from the inner side, have been likened to a string of beads, the "rachitic rosary." This condition persists even after healing, the enlarged articulations becoming permanently calcified without regressing. Even the intestine may appear relaxed and dilated. When a long bone is sawed longitudinally the epiphyseal cartilage is seen to be abnormally wide, the result of unimpaired proliferation of the cartilage. The bones are abnormally soft and can often be cut with a knife. Routine necropsy procedure should include determination of this point by an attempt to slice a rib with a knife. In birds a crooked sternum with deviation to one side or the other is of frequent occurrence and exhibits a mild degree of rickets in early life.

Microscopic Appearance. The principal microscopic changes are (1) an increase in the depth of the zone of proliferating cartilage adjacent to the area of ossification (zone of the metaphysis); and (2) disorderly arrangement of this cartilage, as well as a crookedness and irregularity of this zone or line as it stretches from one side of the bone to the other. Normally the cartilage cells form regular rows running lengthwise of the bone; in rickets no such rows exist. Since the whole bone is widened at this point, the cartilage is correspondingly increased in the transverse direction also. (3) Disorderly penetration of the cartilage by blood vessels. (4) Defective calcification and failure of normal degeneration of the cartilage. (5) A great excess of uncalcified osteoid in the metaphysis. (6) The marrow areas tend to be fibrosed with a corresponding reduction of myeloid cells. Evidence of increased resorption is usually not a feature of rickets, in fact osteoclasts are fewer in number than one might expect. If, however, secondary hyperparathyroidism in response to hypocalcemia is of sufficient degree, bone resorption and fibrous replacement become features of rickets, and the microscopic appearance, especially in the diaphysis, resembles fibrous osteodystrophy. Since vitamin D is necessary for this action of parathyroid hormone, an absolute deficiency of vitamin D would preclude the development of these changes. The absence of active resorption in the usual case of rickets might well be explained by the dependency of parathyroid hormone on vitamin D. As indicated earlier, osteoid itself is resistant to the action of osteoclasts, therefore, active osteoclastic resorption, if present in rickets, is limited to mineralized bone.

Causes of Rickets and Osteomalacia. (1) Vitamin D deficiency is the classic cause of rickets in children or young animals. In fact, many pathologists restrict the use of the term rickets to vitamin D deficiency. However, the microscopic lesions described above, which develop as a result of an inadequate availability of calcium, are duplicated by any disorder favoring hypocalcemia. Thus, other causes of rickets include the following. (2) Dietary lack of calcium is a fundamental cause but in actual practice this seldom occurs, the daily requirement of new calcium being very small. (3) Since calcium is less soluble in an alkaline solution than at an acid pH, a continued excessive alkalinity of the intestinal contents is a cause, but is seldom of more than theoretical importance. The same may be said of (4) continued escape of calcium in combination with fatty acids from unassimilated fat (celiac rickets), and (5) formation of other insoluble complexes between calcium and oxalate or phytate which prevents calcium absorption. (6) Deficiency of phosphorus obviously is able to cause rickets, since this element is essential in forming calcium phosphate. Phosphorus deficiency occurs in herbivorous animals in certain parts of the world (Gulf Coast of the United States and in South Africa) where the soil, and consequently the plants, are deficient in this element. As a rule, however, other signs, such as chewing bones or clostridial intoxication therefrom, usually direct attention to the deficiency before the impaired condition of the bones becomes apparent. In addition to simple dietary lack, phosphorus deficiency can arise from steatorrhea, formation of insoluble complexes, and changes in the pH of intestinal contents. (7) A severely unbalanced calcium-phosphorus ratio in the diet is entirely capable of causing rickets, and such cases are encountered especially where inexperienced persons supply mineral mixtures to livestock. If the diet contains an excessive amount of phosphorus, as when animals are fed wheat bran as a large part of their ration, or too much bone meal, such an imbalance develops for the reason that either the Ca ion or PO_4 ion tends to be excreted with the feces in combination with its counterpart, as $Ca_3(PO_4)_2$. (8) **Strontium rickets** is a special, usually experimentally induced, type of rickets. Strontium interferes with the conversion, by the kidneys, of 25-hydroxycholecalciferol to the most active form of vitamin D, 1,25-dihydroxycholecalciferol. The metabolism of vitamin D is discussed further in Chapter 17.

Significance and Effect. Supporting weight on the poorly calcified bones is painful, and results in lameness or disinclination to move. Pathological fractures, even of the vertebral column, are not infrequent. Normal chicks, experimentally raised without sunlight or vitamin D, regularly develop rickets, called leg weakness by poultrymen, on the eighteenth or nineteenth day after hatching and shortly die.

When the cause is corrected, normal ossification promptly begins. The strength and hardness of the bone become normal, although the deformities tend to persist for life. The roentgenologist readily detects the lack of calcification in the diseased bone, as well as the restoration which occurs during healing.

While there may be a slight (10%) lowering of the serum calcium level of the blood in rickets, symptomatically and functionally speaking, the action of the parathyroids maintains the blood calcium at the proper level, even at the expense of the bones. Only rarely is there severe hypocalcemia in rickets. In these cases tetany may occur. Serum alkaline phosphatase levels are elevated. As indicated earlier, in longstanding rickets, the parathyroids undergo hypertrophy, perhaps to twice or thrice their normal size. This may be looked upon as a compensatory hypertrophy. In cases of hyperparathyroidism, as from a parathyroid tumor, the bones lose calcium but the picture is somewhat different from that of rickets, the condition being known as fibrous osteodystrophy.

The changes in bone which are characteristic of avitaminosis C need to be distinguished in some species from those of rickets. They are mentioned in the section dealing with that vitamin.

Bennett, D.: Nutrition and bone disease in the dog and cat. Vet. Rec., *98*:313–321, 1976.

Brion, A.J., and Fontaine, M.: A hemorrhagic and rachitic-like syndrome in chickens due to nitrofural-medicated feed. Poultry Sci., *37*:1071–1074, 1958.

Charan, K., Iyer, P.K.R., and Dutt, B.: Pathological studies on osteorenal syndrome in goats. Indian Vet. J., *49*:743–750, 1972.

Duckworth, J., et al.: Dental mal-occlusion and rickets in sheep. Res. Vet. Sci., *2*:375–380, 1961.

Groth, A.H., Jr.: The comparative histopathology of rickets and an osteodystrophy in immature Iowa swine. Am. J. Vet. Res., *19*:409–416, 1958.

Hidiroglou, M., Dukes, T.W., Ho, S.K., and Heaney, D.P.: Bent-limb syndrome in lambs raised in total confinement. J. Am. Vet. Med. Assoc., *173*:1571–1574, 1978.

Malherbe, W.D.: Some observations on rickets and allied bone diseases in South African domestic animals. Ann. N.Y. Acad. Sci., *64*:128–146, 1956.

McRoberts, M.R.: A dental malocclusion associated with rickets in growing lambs. Proc. Nutr. Soc., *20*:37–38, 1961.

Osteomalacia

Osteomalacia occurs in the bones of adults through the same mechanisms as rickets in the young and is often called **adult rickets.** Since normal bone is continually being made over through the for-

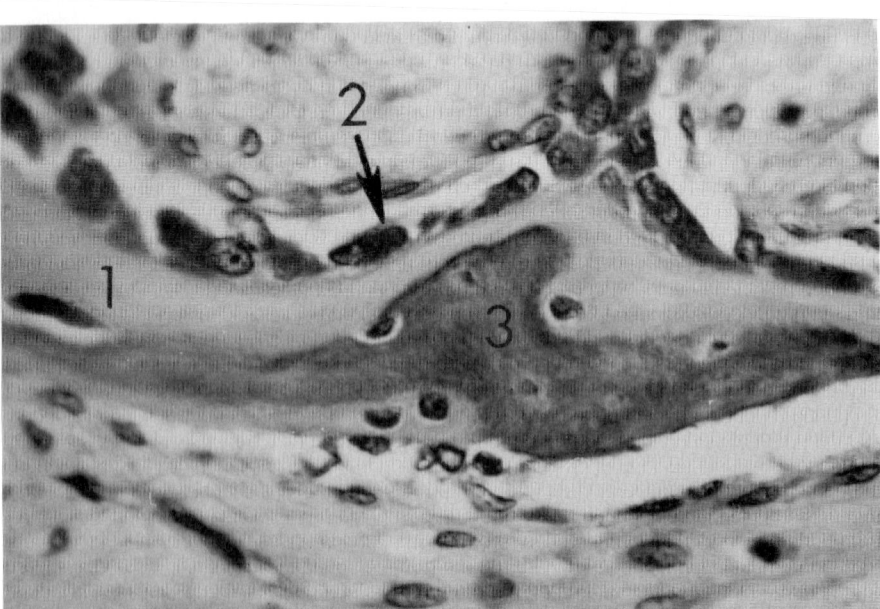

Fig. 19–6. Osteoid seam in osteodystrophia fibrosa in a monkey. The light staining osteoid (*1*) immediately beneath a layer of osteoblasts (*2*) overlays a mature spicule of bone (*3*). Osteoid seams are the hallmark of osteomalacia.

mative action of the osteoblasts, and at the same time is being destroyed by the osteoclasts, the failure of calcification and accumulation of osteoid is chiefly just beneath the periosteum and, to a lesser degree, the endosteum. As in rickets of the young, there is too much pink-staining osteoid, usually in the form of wide borders around a blue-staining calcified central portion in each bony trabecula. These osteoid borders which are lined by prominent osteoblasts are the so-called "osteoid seams" upon which the histopathological diagnosis of osteomalacia is based. As in rickets, osteoid is resistant to osteoclastic resorption which allows its continual buildup. Osteoclasia of calcified bone may be apparent but it is seldom a striking finding unless secondary hyperparathyroidism ensues. In the latter event, resorption and fibrous replacement of bone become paramount, and the pathological picture progresses to that of fibrous osteodystrophy.

Irregular diffuse thickening of the bones occurs all along the diaphysis but the bone is soft, easily cut or sawed, and may become permanently deformed. As growth is no longer in progress the epiphyseal changes are absent or minimal. Enlargement at the carpal and tarsal regions occurs, nevertheless, at least in the horse. The flat bones of the head and pelvis share prominently in the thickening and distortion. Due to the stresses of weight-bearing, marked deformity of the pelvis often develops.

Causes have been given under Rickets. Significance and effect are also much the same.

Nisbet, D.I., Butler, E.J., Robertson, J.M., and Bannatyne, C.C.: Osteodystrophic diseases of sheep. IV. Osteomalacia and osteoporosis in lactating ewes on West Scotland hill farms. J. Comp. Pathol., *80*:535–542, 1970.

Fibrous Osteodystrophy

Also known by the Latin names **osteitis fibrosa cystica** and **osteodystrophia fibrosa,** fibrous osteodystrophy is characterized by marked bone resorption, fibrous replacement, accelerated osteoid formation which does not become mineralized (osteomalacia), and the formation of cysts. It is the direct result of the continuous and excessive action of parathyroid hormone on bone. In man, the disease has also been called **von Recklinghausen's disease.** The bones in general, and especially the larger ones, gradually soften and become flexible and deformed. At the same time they are easily fractured and are painful when bearing weight. Roentgenological examination shows widespread areas of rarefaction, sometimes with cystic spaces in them.

Gross and Microscopic Examination. Gross and microscopic examination of affected bones shows a marked disappearance of bone tissue, which begins at the greatly enlarged Haversian canals and spreads outward from each one. The space formerly occupied by calcified bone is filled by fibrous connective tissue, with osteoclasts and osteoclastic giant cells lining receding bone in some places, and the smaller osteoblasts attempting to replace the lost bone in others. The fibrous tissue may undergo cystic degeneration in places, probably because of insufficent blood supply. The bones, in addition to being deformed, may be so soft that they can be cut with a knife.

As indicated, the **cause** of this startling disorder is hyperparathyroidism. The marked osteoclastic and osteolytic resorption of bone is a direct effect of parathyroid hormone. The stimulus for increased osteoblastic activity and fibrosis is less well understood though it would appear that it is a compensatory mechanism. Mechanical stress is believed to be of primary importance in initiating these attempts at healing. Parathyroid hormone itself may play a role in this stimulus but this hormone is also known to depress osteoblastic activity. Parathyroid hormone also inhibits the mineralization of osteoid even in the presence of hypercalcemia, which is the usual

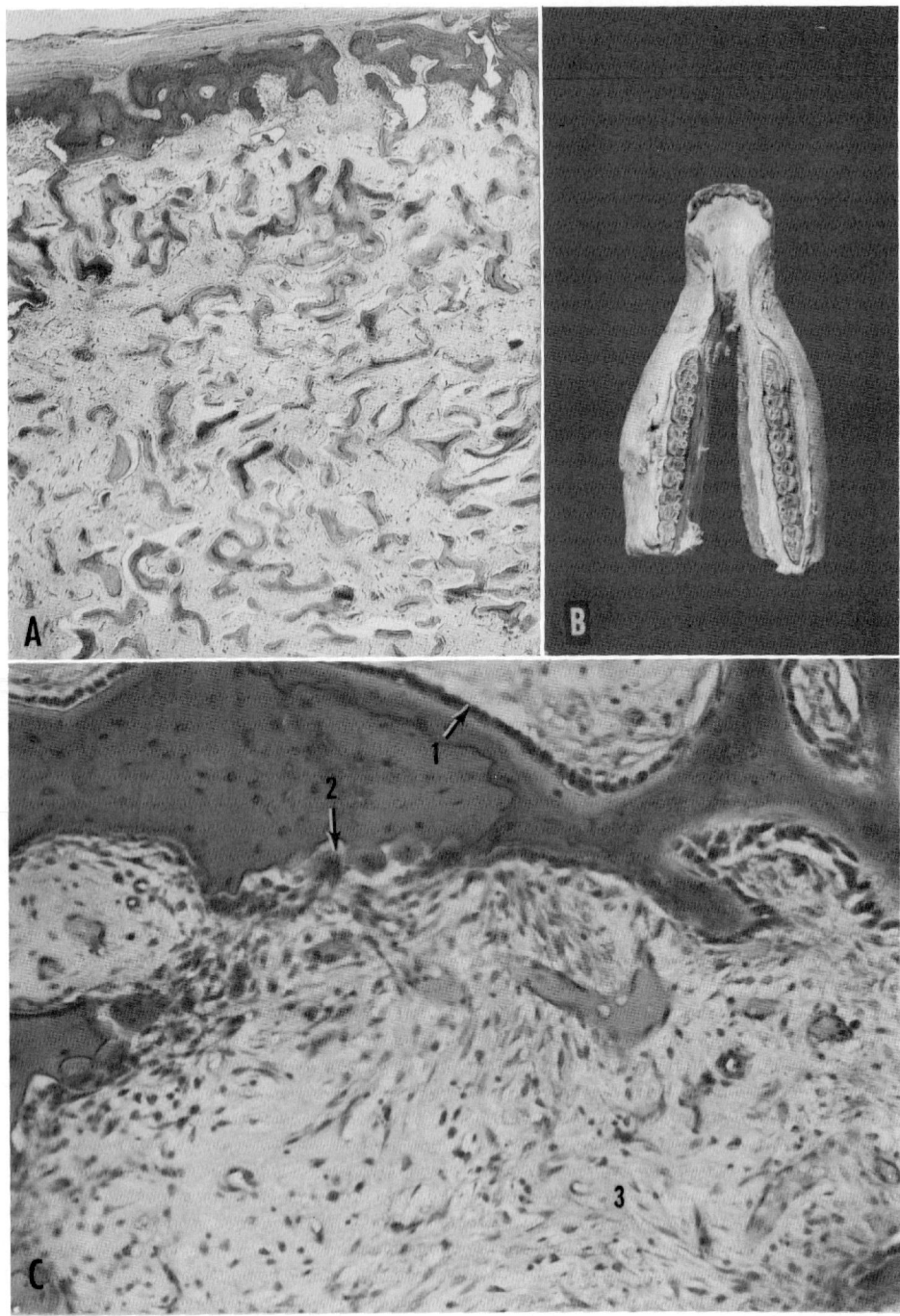

Fig. 19–7. Equine fibrous osteodystrophy. *A,* Section of mandible (× 50) showing replacement of marrow and cortex with irregular spicules of poorly calcified bone supported by a fibrous stroma. *B,* Mandible of an affected horse. Note great thickness of mandible, which was soft and easily cut with a knife. *C,* Higher magnification of *A* (× 200). Note active osteoblasts (*1*), osteoclasts (*2*), and fibrous replacement of the marrow (*3*). (Courtesy of Armed Forces Institute of Pathology.) Contributors: Colonels John J. Kintner and Rufus L. Holt.

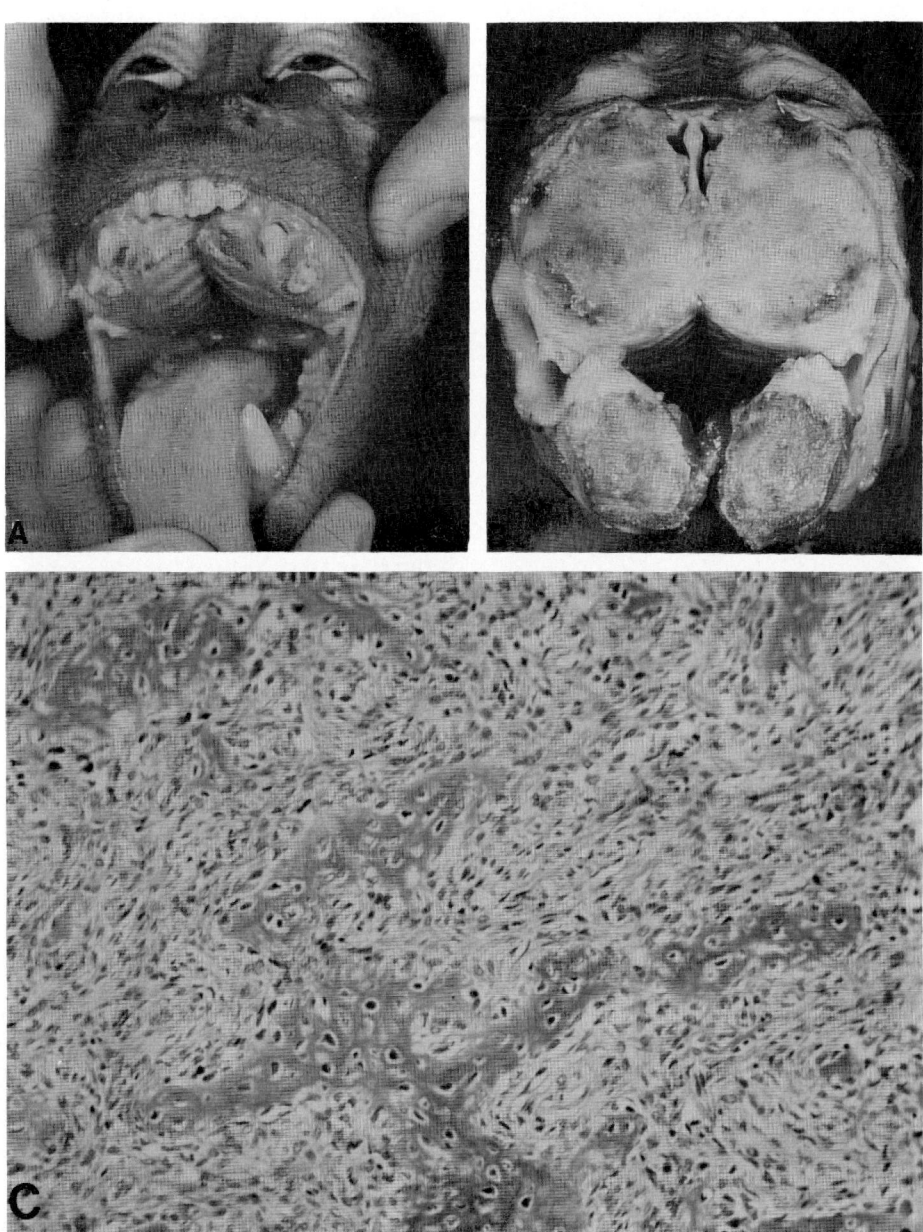

Fig. 19–8. Fibrous osteodystrophy in a male spider monkey, 1½ years old. *A,* Thickened maxilla and deeply-embedded teeth in the living animal. *B,* Mandibles and maxillae, softened and thickened and encroaching on the nasal cavity. *C,* Section of the maxilla with zones of osteoid interspersed in fibrous marrow. (H & E, × 150.) (Courtesy of Angell Memorial Animal Hospital.)

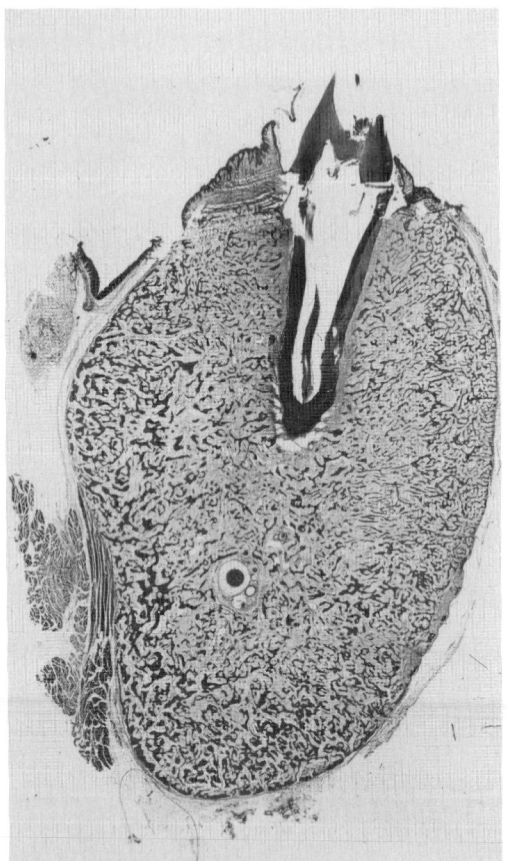

Fig. 19-9. Fibrous osteodystrophy, wooly monkey. The cortex, lamina dura and medullary cavity of the mandible have been entirely replaced with trabecular bone in a loose fibrous stroma. (Courtesy of New England Regional Primate Research Center, Harvard Medical School.)

phatase. Metastatic calcification of soft tissues is a consistent finding.

Secondary hyperparathyroidism is without question the most common cause of fibrous osteodystrophy in animals. Hypocalcemia regardless of cause is the stimulus for the increased activity of the parathyroid glands. In animals secondary hyperparathyroidism occurs in nutritional deficiencies (nutritional secondary hyperparathyroidism) and in chronic renal disease.

Renal secondary hyperparathyroidism is most common in the dog in which the disorder has been termed **renal rickets** or **rubber-jaw.** Inability to excrete phosphates causes these ions to accumulate in the blood, which causes a lowering of the serum calcium concentration. The inability of the damaged kidney to produce the active metabolite of vitamin D is of equal or greater importance to the development of hypocalcemia. Hyperparathyroidism in

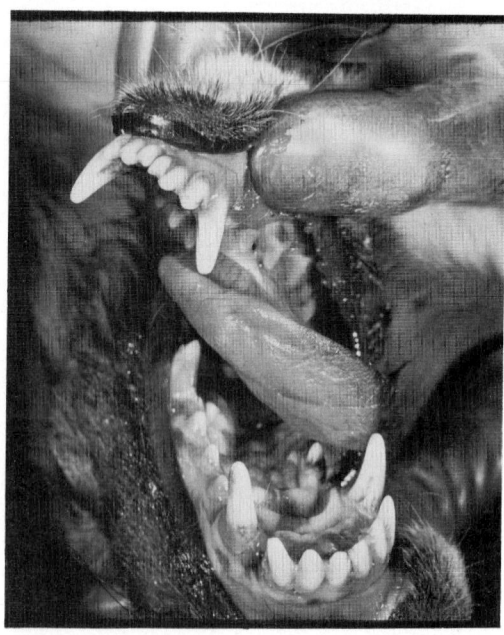

Fig. 19-10. The flexible "rubber jaws" of a 5½-year-old male terrier with chronic interstitial nephritis. Normal jaws cannot be distorted in this manner. (Courtesy of Angell Memorial Animal Hospital.)

finding in primary hyperparathyroidism. A separate function of parathyroid hormone is to increase renal loss of phosphate.

Hyperparathyroidism may be primary or secondary, but in either event the pathologic picture in bone is identical.

Primary hyperparathyroidism is usually the result of a functioning parathyroid adenoma which is rare in animals. Parathyroid adenomas have been reported in horses, cattle, and dogs. In primary hyperparathyroidism there is hypercalcemia, hypophosphatemia (renal loss), and marked elevation of serum alkaline phos-

response to hypocalcemia induces resorption of bone, but owing to primary renal disease the hormone does not increase urinary loss of phosphate, which continues to rise in the serum. Hyperphosphatemia is present throughout the course of the disease; serum alkaline phosphatase is also elevated. Serum calcium is usually low, but is partially compensated for by the continued release of calcium from bone. In the dog the bones of the head show pronounced softening, enlargement, and roentgenologically detectable rarefaction, the jaws becoming "rubbery." Microscopically the lesions are those of fibrous osteodystrophy with osteoclastic and osteolytic resorption, fibrous replacement, and active osteoblasts producing osteoid which fails to mineralize. All bones are affected to varying degrees, but the lesions are most striking in the facial bones and the mandible. Metastatic calcification of soft tissues is a regular feature. The parathyroids are grossly enlarged. Tests for renal function are indicative of severe renal insufficiency.

Nutritional secondary hyperparathyroidism has been described in most domestic animals as well as many exotic species. The usual nutritional imbalances associated with the development of fibrous osteodystrophy are dietary deficiency of calcium and/or dietary excess of phosphorus, and vitamin D deficiency. As indicated under rickets and osteomalacia, secondary parathyroid hyperplasia may develop, causing these diseases to progress to fibrous osteodystrophy.

Fibrous osteodystrophy, described under the name **Bran disease,** has occurred when horses, owned by flour-millers, to whom bran was a cheap by-product, were fed almost exclusively on that substance. Changes in the head and facial outlines are commonly the first signs of the disease; it has therefore been described under the expressive designation of **big head.** The sharp features of the head, especially in the region of the zygomatic arch and upper and lower jaws, become rounded and indefinite, giving the appearance of more swelling than really exists. Dissection shows a rather uniform thickening and rounding due to diffuse proliferation of imperfect bone in the subperiosteal region. The teeth may loosen and fall out. There is also lameness and a general tenderness of the joints. Microscopically, classic lesions of fibrous osteodystrophy are most obvious in facial bones and the mandible but the lesions are generalized throughout the skeleton. The disorder is the result of feeding diets low in calcium and high in phosphorus. Clinicopathologic findings may reveal hyperphosphatemia and hypocalcemia, but compensation may occur through the action of parathyroid hormone on bone and the kidneys. Serum alkaline phosphatase is elevated.

In young cats a diet consisting almost exclusively of beef hearts (low in calcium, high in phosphorus) has been found to cause fibrous osteodystrophy. The lesions in cats are often distinct from those seen in other species especially with respect to the amount of new bone (osteoid) formation by osteoblasts and fibrous replacement which has accounted for the disorder to be termed **osteogenesis imperfecta** and **juvenile osteoporosis.** To be certain there is often less bone, but the disorder in no way resembles osteogenesis imperfecta as seen in man, which is an hereditary disease (it was once thought to be hereditary in cats). The disease is caused by a nutritional imbalance of calcium and phosphorus, which results in hypocalcemia and secondary hyperparathyroidism. Unless compensated there is hypocalcemia, hyperphosphatemia, and elevated serum alkaline phosphatase. The signs of the disease are nervousness and hyperirritability (hypocalcemia?), reluctance to move, abnormal stance and gait, and spontaneous fractures. Microscopically in the usual case the lesions are characteristic of fibrous osteodystrophy, but rarely is there a significant production of new osteoid. Osteoblasts are present, however, and they do form osteoid but there is not the marked osteoid production leading to an increase in the overall dimensions of the bones except in rare examples. Krook (1963) refers to this expression of the disease as hypostotic type fibrous osteodystrophy in contrast to the hyperostotic type seen in horses (big head). Jowsey and co-workers (1964, 1968) have fed adult cats beef heart for 13 months and described the resultant bone disease as osteoporosis without any evidence of fibrous osteodystrophy. They clearly showed that parathyroid activity was necessary for the development of the skeletal abnormality but suggested that the absence of fibrous osteodystrophy indicated that severe hyperparathyroidism had not developed. These findings and similar results in mice (Ulmansky, 1965) suggest that the level of hyperparathyroidism and the age of the animal may influence the pattern of the disease, which emphasizes caution in interpreting pathogenesis of bone disease based on morphological features alone. Osteoporosis presumably of similar pathogenesis has also been described as a spontaneous disease in young cats and dogs on meat diets.

Fibrous osteodystrophy is a frequent disorder of the pet and laboratory monkey. The disease is almost exclusively encountered in New-World monkeys (*i.e.* those from Central and South America) and has been the recipient of numerous inappropriate and misleading terms such as goundou, Paget's disease, simian bone disease and cage paralysis. In monkeys the disease is characterized by facial deformity, reluctance to move, bending of long bones, and multiple fractures leading to distortion of the limbs. Microscopically the lesions are classical of fibrous osteodystrophy, with marked production of new bone causing gross enlargement of the skeleton, especially of the skull bones. The cause is not clear in each example, but in most cases it is the result of vitamin D deficiency. Hunt, et al. (1967, 1969) have clearly demonstrated

that in New-World monkeys vitamin D_2 is relatively ineffective in promoting intestinal absorption of calcium and that these species require vitamin D_3 in their diet or access to ultraviolet radiation or sunshine. The substitution of vitamin D_3 for vitamin D_2 in commercial primate diets has greatly reduced the incidence of fibrous osteodystrophy in laboratory monkeys, but it still remains a frequent disorder of the pet monkey. No doubt lack of vitamin D is important to the development of the disease in the pet monkey, but the condition is also aggravated by unusual dietary programs which often contain foods high in phosphorus and low in calcium such as cereal grains (baby foods) and bananas.

Brown, et al. (1966) have proposed that atrophic rhinitis of swine is an expression of generalized fibrous osteodystrophy.

In addition to the specific examples cited, fibrous osteodystrophy of nutritional origin has been described in cattle, goats, dogs, and birds. Both renal and nutritional osteodystrophy are not uncommon in rats and hamsters.

As a rule, in all species with nutritional or renal fibrous osteodystrophy, the parathyroid glands are grossly enlarged. Microscopically the enlargement is the result of an increase in size and number of light chief cells. Many chief cells become vacuolated and the number of water clear cells increases.

We have stated several times in this chapter that rickets and osteomalacia may progress to fibrous osteodystrophy if severe hyperparathyroidism develops in the course of the disease. There is little difficulty in understanding this progression, but what often appears as a dilemma is the presence of fibrous osteodystrophy in a young animal in the absence of rickets which in some species is a frequent finding. Apparently rickets only develops if the ion product of calcium and phosphorus is low, and in many cases of fibrous osteodystrophy the ion product is maintained at a normal level due to the action of parathyroid hormone or is actually elevated due to hyperphosphatemia. Calcification of cartilage (which fails in rickets) is directly dependent on calcium availability; rachitic cartilage will calcify *in vitro*. Calcification of osteoid, however, requires maturation under control of osteoblasts and is not directly related to calcium availability; osteoid from animals with osteomalacia or fibrous osteodystrophy does not calcify *in vitro*. However, it seems likely that other physiological factors and possibly other dietary deficiencies or excesses which may be present in certain diets (such as a 100% beef heart diet) influence the course of both rickets and fibrous osteodystrophy in young animals.

Bienfet, V., et al.: A primary parathyroid disorder. Osteofibrosis caused by parathyroid adenoma in a shetland pony. Recovery after surgical removal. Ann. Med. Vet., *108*:252–265, 1964.

Brody, R.S.: Renal osteitis fibrosa cystica in a wire-haired Fox Terrier. J. Am. Vet. Med. Assoc., *124*:275–278, 1954.

Brown, W.R., Krook, L., and Pond, W.G.: Atrophic rhinitis in swine. Etiology, pathogenesis and prophylaxis. Cornell Vet., *56*:Suppl. No. 1, 1–108, 1966.

Carda-Aparici, P., Gallego-Garcia, E., and Rodriguez, S.E.: Osteodystrophia fibrosa in the goat. Zootechnia, *21*:425–426, 1972.

Chakrabarti, A., Basak, D.K., Shom, R.N., and Banerjee, A.K.: Studies on osteodystrophia fibrosa in Black Bengal goats. Indian J. Anim. Health, *14*:95–97, 1975.

duBoulay, G.H., and Crawford, M.A.: Nutritional bone disease in captive primates. Symp. Zool. Soc. Lond., *21*:223–236, 1968.

duBoulay, G.H., Hime, J.M., and Verity, P.M.: Spondylosis in captive wild animals. A possible relationship with nutritional osteodystrophy. Br. J. Radiol., *45*:841–847, 1972.

Flom, J.O., Brown, R.J., and Jones, R.E.: Fibrous osteodystrophy in a wild dolphin. J. Am. Vet. Med. Assoc., *173*:1124–1126, 1978.

Freedman, M.T., Bush, M., Novak, G.R., et al.: Nutritional and metabolic bone disease in a zoological population: a review of radiologic findings. Skeletal Radiol., *1*:87–96, 1976.

Fujimoto, Y., et al.: Electron microscopic observations of the equine parathyroid glands with particular reference to those of equine osteodystrophia fibrosa. Jpn. J. Vet. Res., *15*:37–51, 1967.

Griffiths, H.J., Zimmerman, R.E., Bailey, G., and Snider, R.: The use of photon absorptiometry in the diagnosis of renal osteodystrophy. Radiology, *109*:277–281, 1973.

Griffiths, H.J., Hunt, R., Grindle, T., Anderson, M., and Sandor, T.: The use of a primary magnification technic in metabolic bone disease. J. Am. Vet. Radiol. Soc., *28*:12–18, 1977.

Groenendyk, S., and Seawright, A.A.: Osteodystrophia fibrosa in horses grazing *Setaria sphacelata*. Aust. Vet. J., *50*:131–132, 1974.

Groenewald, J.W.: Osteofibrosis in equines. Onderstepoort, J. Vet. Sci. Anim. Indust., *9*:601–621, 1937.

Hintz, H.F., and Schryver, H.F.: Nutrition and bone development in horses. J. Am. Vet. Med. Assoc., *168*:39–44, 1976.

Hogg, A.H.: Osteodystrophic disease in the dog, with special reference to rubber jaw (renal osteodystrophy) and its comparison with renal rickets in the human. Vet. Rec., *60*:117–122, 1948.

Hunt, R.D., Garcia, F.G., and Hegsted, D.M.: A comparison of Vitamin D_2 and D_3 in New World primates. I. Production and regression of osteodystrophia fibrosa. Lab. Anim. Care, *17*:222–234, 1967.

———: Hypervitaminosis D in New World monkeys. Am. J. Clin. Nutr., *22*:358–366, 1969.

Jaffe, H.L., and Bodansky, A.: Experimental fibrous osteodystrophia in hyperparathyroid dogs. J. Exp. Med., *52*:669–694, 1932.

Jowsey, J., and Gershon-Cohen, J.: Effect of dietary calcium levels on production and reversal of experimental osteoporosis in cats. Proc. Soc. Exp. Biol. Med., *116*:437–441, 1964.

Jowsey, J., and Raisz, L.G.: Experimental osteoporosis and parathyroid activity. Endocrinology, *82*:384–396, 1968.

Kinter, J.H., and Holt, R.L.: Equine osteomalacia. Philippine J. Sci., *49*:1–89, 1932.

Krook, L., Barrett, R.B., Usui, K., and Wolke, R.E.: Nutritional secondary hyperparathyroidism in the cat. Cornell Vet., *53*:224–240, 1963.

Krook, L., and Lowe, J.E.: Nutritional secondary hyperparathyroidism in the horse, with a description of the normal equine parathyroid gland. Pathol. Vet., *1*:Suppl. 1–98, 1964.

Krook, L., and Barrett, R.B.: Simian bone disease—a secondary hyperparathyroidism. Cornell Vet., *52*:459–492, 1962.

Krook, L.: Dietary calcium-phosphorus and lameness in the horse. Cornell Vet., *58*:Suppl. 59–73, 1968.

Nielsen, S.W., and McSherry, B.J.: Renal hyperparathyroidism (rubber-jaw syndrome) in a dog. J. Am. Vet. Med. Assoc., *124*:270–274, 1954.

Nisbet, D.I., et al.: Osteodystrophic diseases of sheep. I. An osteodystrophic condition of hoggs known as double scalp or cappi. J. Comp. Pathol., *72*:270–280, 1962.

Nisbet, D.I., Butler, E.J., and Smith, B.S.: Osteodystrophic diseases of sheep. J. Comp. Pathol., *76*:159–169, 1966.

Omar, A.R.: Osteogenesis imperfecta in cats. J. Pathol. Bact., *82*:303–314, 1961.

Platt, H.: Canine chronic nephritis. III. The skeletal system in rubber jaw. J. Comp. Pathol., *61*:197–204, 1951.

Riser, W.H.: Juvenile osteoporosis (osteogenesis imperfecta)—a calcium deficiency. J. Am. Vet. Med. Assoc., *139*:117–119, 1961.

Rowland, G.N., Capen, C.C., and Nagode, L.A.: Experimental hyperparathyroidism in young cats. Pathol. Vet., *5*:504–519, 1968.

Scott, P.P., McKusick, V.A., and McKusick, A.B.: The nature of osteogenesis imperfecta in cats. Evidence that the disorder is primarily nutritional, not genetic, and therefore not analogous to the disease in man. J. Bone Joint Surg. (Amer.), *45-A*:125–134, 1963.

Scott, P.P.: Osteodystrophies. Vet. Rec., *84*:333–335, 1969.

Storts, R.W., and Koestner, A.: Skeletal lesions associated with a dietary calcium and phosphorus imbalance in the pig. Am. J. Vet. Res., *26*:280–294, 1965.

Theiler, Sir Arnold: Osteodystrophic diseases of animals. Vet. J., *90*:183–206, 1934.

Trevino, G.S.: Renal osteitis fibrosa cystica in a Cocker Spaniel, the "rubber-jaw" syndrome. Southwestern Vet., *8*:338–340, 1955.

Ulmansky, M.: The effect of "meat diet" on long bones of mice. Am. J. Pathol., *47*:435–445, 1965.

Wallach, J.D., and Flieg, G.M.: Nutritional secondary hyperparathyroidism in captive psittacine birds. J. Am. Vet. Med. Assoc., *151*:880–883, 1967.

Williamson, W.M., Lombard, L.S., and Firfer, H.S.: Fibrous dysplasia in a monkey and a kudu. J. Am. Vet. Med. Assoc., *147*:1049–1052, 1965.

Osteoporosis

Osteoporosis, properly speaking, is an atrophic disorder in which the bones are less resistant to cutting and sawing, but at the same time brittle and porous. The porosity is due to widening of the Haversian canals, possibly in connection with an increased blood supply, and fragility is augmented by a diminution in the thickness of the bony trabeculae and the whole zona compacta. There is no failure of, or deficiency in, calcification in what remains of the trabeculae and no increase of osteoid, as there is in osteomalacia. Normally throughout life there is continual rearrangement of the trabeculae, osteoblasts forming new bone, osteoclasts dissolving it (apparently through the action of an enzyme, acid phosphatase). In osteoporosis, the destructive phase of this process exceeds production. The levels of serum calcium and serum phosphorus are usually normal.

Causes are not fully understood. The disorder occurs in senility, disuse atrophy, as when surgical fixation of a limb is necessitated in the treatment of some injury of bone or joint, in a variety of obscure hormonal imbalances involving the adrenals, thyroid or pituitary, and in some other conditions. Causative mechanisms are thought to include absence of the stimulation coming from the stresses and strains of movement, malnutrition, especially with respect to proteins, and possibly deficiency of estrogen (human post-menopausal), excessive adrenal cortical hormone, hyperpituitarism, and hyperthyroidism. Vitamin C deficiency, and copper deficiency also result in osteoporosis. Considerable attention is presently being directed toward calcium deficiency as a cause of osteoporosis. We have already indicated the role of calcium deficiency in rickets, osteomalacia, and fibrous osteodystrophy. The role of calcium deficiency in osteoporosis is yet to be defined, but osteoporosis has been produced experimentally in cats (Jowsey, 1964) and mice (Ulmansky, 1965) by feeding meat diets which are low in calcium. Also, osteoporosis is seen spontaneously in cats subsisting on such a diet, however, as previously indicated, in many cats rather than leading to osteoporosis, meat diets lead to fibrous osteodystrophy.

Osteoporosis, as here defined, is rare but not unknown in animals. The cases that have been designated by that name have usually proved to depend on inadequate calcium deposition and, hence, come under the heading of osteomalacia. In contrast to diseases characterized by malacia (*i.e.*, rickets, osteomalacia, and fibrous osteodystrophy) in most examples of osteoporosis there is no obvious increase in resorption, no increase in osteoblastic activity, no fibrous replacement, and no excess of osteoid. To the contrary, the bone appears quiescent.

Jowsey, J., and Gershon-Cohen, J.: Effect of dietary calcium levels on production and reversal of experimental osteoporosis in cats. Proc. Soc. Exp. Biol. Med., *116*:437–441, 1964.

Manzke, E., et al.: Relationship between local and

total bone mass in osteoporosis. Metabolism, 24:605–615, 1975.

El-Najjar, M.Y., and Robertson, A.L.: Spongy bones in prehistoric America. Science, 193:141–143, 1976.

Nordin, B.E.C.: The pathogenesis of osteoporosis. Lancet, May 13, 1961, pp. 1011–1015.

Platt, B.S., and Steward, R.C.J.: Transverse trabeculae and osteoporosis in bones in experimental protein-calorie deficiency. Br. J. Nutr., 16:483–495, 1962.

Ulmansky, M.: The effect of "meat diet" on long bones of mice. Am. J. Pathol., 47:435–445, 1965.

Wu, K., and Frost, H.M.: Bone formation in osteoporosis. Arch. Pathol., 88:508–510, 1969.

Inherited Diseases of the Skeletal System

A large number of genes have been identified in the laboratory mouse which affect the development of the skeleton. Many of these effects are minor and are useful as markers for linked genes, while others produce serious lethal or sublethal effects. These have been recently summarized (Woodard, 1978; Jones, 1978) and will not be repeated here. An increasing number of skeletal defects in domesticated animals, many known for years, are being identified as under genetic control. A partial listing of these are found in Chapter 8. Descriptions of some of the more prevalent hereditary diseases of the skeleton follow.

Achondroplasia. An autosomal recessive factor in cattle has been known for many years. The Dexter breed of cattle is generally heterozygous for this gene, although it does occur in other breeds. The homozygous affected fetus is usually aborted during the fourth to sixth month of pregnancy. The prognathia, domed skull, and shortened legs are responsible for the name, "Bull-dog calf," often given to the affected fetus. Other features include anasarca, phocomelus, protruding tongue, and generalized abnormal growth of epiphyseal cartilage.

An achondroplasia also occurs in the rabbit, controlled by an autosomal recessive gene (symbol, *ac*). Also called chondrodysplasia, affected animals die shortly after birth and are recognized by their short limbs and domed, prominent skull.

The growth plate of cartilage contains irregularly arranged cells and loss of cells in the capsule of the cartilage.

A nonlethal type of achondroplasia is also well known as a breed characteristic of Basset Hounds and Dachshunds, but may appear in other breeds. The joints have the usual enlargement, long bones are severely shortened, and a quantitative decrease in endochondral growth is apparent. Central ossification in long bones is also retarded, although periosteal and membranous formation of bone is normal. This type of bone growth is also called hypochondroplastic dwarfism, chondrodystrophia fetalis, endochondral chondrodystrophy, and hypochondroplasia. The unsatisfactory and incomplete understanding of the mechanisms underlying this defect is underscored by the plethora of descriptive names.

Cartilaginous Exostoses. Multiple protuberances of bone and cartilage, predominately arising from bones, at or near epiphyseal cartilage, have been described in man, horse, dog and cat. Many names have been ascribed to this lesion: hereditary multiple exostoses, chondrodysplasia, diaphyseal aclasis, osteogenic disease, and hereditary deforming chrondrodysplasia. Multiple masses of varying size occur in attachment to the bone. Cartilaginous growth seems to be the initial factor, followed by ossification. The cartilage usually persists around the periphery of the masses, and the center becomes ossified. Inheritance in man and horse is clearly due to a single dominant gene. In the dog and cat, the genetic basis is not clearly established.

Chondrodysplasia. The Alaskan Malamute dog carries a recessive gene (symbol: *dan*) which is expressed in the homozygous state by developmental defects in bone growth and anemia. Stunted growth becomes evident at about three months of age. All bones which undergo endochondral ossification are affected, thus the long bones are shortened. The epiphyseal plates and ends of long bones are thickened. The cartilage in the growth plate is not adequately ossified. The macrocytic hemolytic anemia appears to be a pleiotrophic effect of the gene.

Dysplasia of Acetabulum (Hip Dysplasia). Under the name of "hip dysplasia" a disorder has been described in growing dogs, most notably German Shepherds, which usually first manifests itself as an unexplained luxation of the coxofemoral articulation. At autopsy it is found that the acetabular cavity is extremely and abnormally shallow, its lips being flattened and atrophic. It has been logically assumed that the luxation resulted because of the shallowness of the cavity so that the head of the femur was inadequately supported. There is evidence that this dysplasia (the shallowness) is inherited. On the other hand, most of the necropsies have been performed after the dislocation has been in existence for some weeks, and it has been shown experimentally that dislocation, uncorrected for as little as four weeks, can, in growing pups, produce dysplasia even to the extent that the acetabular cavity is almost obliterated (disuse atrophy). It has been noted that in the dogs subject to the dysplasia, the several muscles concerned with pressing the head of the femur into the cavity and holding it there are much smaller, lighter in weight, and therefore weaker than in normal dogs. This again leads to a concept of disuse atrophy as far as the bony tissues are concerned. The degree of development of these muscles may be the inherited characteristic. The best evidence currently indicates that polygenic factors are involved in the inheritance of hip dysplasia.

Elbow Dysplasia. This disease, involving the elbow joint and occurring most frequently in German Shepherds, may or may not be associated with hip dysplasia. The disease is reported in many large breeds of

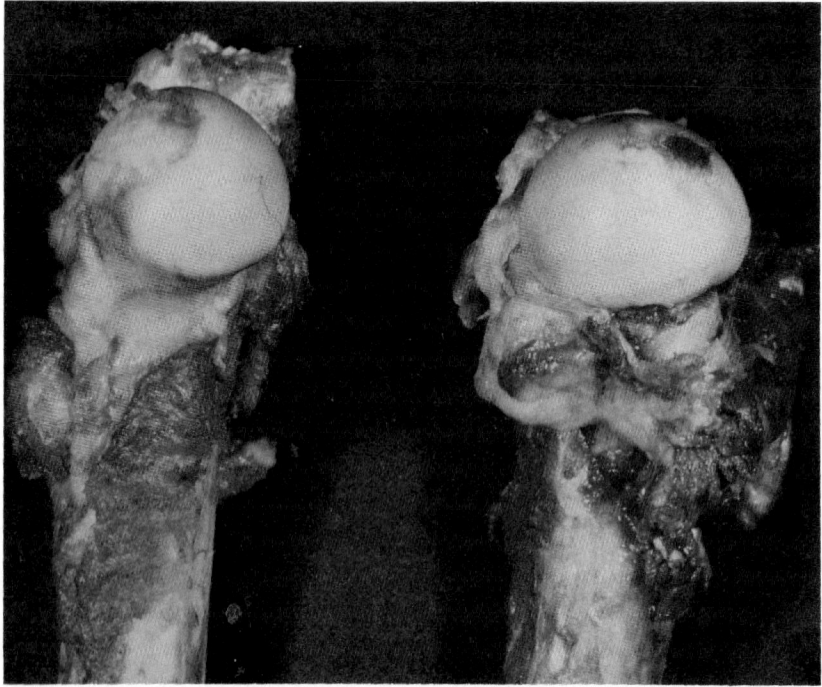

Fig. 19–11. Osteoarthritis of the femoral heads subsequent to hip dysplasia in a ten-year-old male German Shepherd. The femoral heads are flattened and the articular surfaces eroded. (Courtesy of Angell Memorial Animal Hospital.)

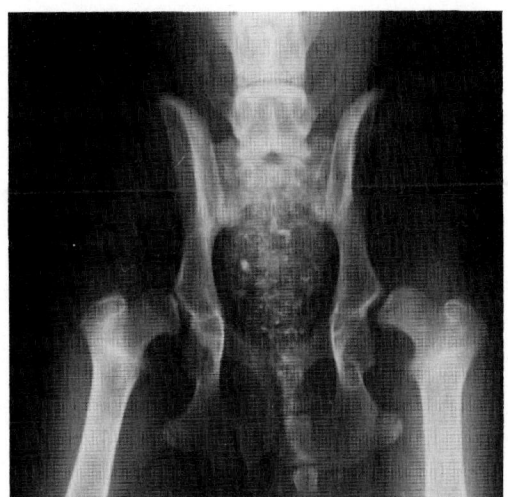

Fig. 19–12. Hip dysplasia. Radiograph of severe dysplasia (grade IV) in a six-month-old male German Shepherd. Note that the acetabula are shallow, the femoral heads are not within the acetabulum on either side. The articular surface of the femoral head on the right is flattened. (Courtesy of Dr. G.B. Schnelle, Angell Memorial Animal Hospital.)

dogs (as is hip dysplasia). The lesions involve failure of the anconeal process to be united and osteoarthritis of the elbow joint. Polygenic factors appear to be involved.

Epiphyseal Dysplasia. A congenital lesion detected radiographically in young children and puppies may be inherited, and is variously called "multiple epiphyseal dysplasia," "stippled epiphyses," or *chondrodystrophia calcificans congenita*. The lesions are seen radiographically as punctal densities in the epiphyses or as a pronounced mottled appearance. Histologic sections contain either acellular masses of tissue containing calcium, or abnormal punctate calcifications of epiphyseal cartilage. The lesions are usually multiple, involving the epiphyses of femur and humerus most consistently, but affecting many other bones as well.

Osteopetrosis

A frequently used synonym for osteopetrosis in human patients is marble-bone disease. In this rare disease, those bones which are of endochondral origin are enlarged to the point of deformity, heavy and dense with calcium but surprisingly brittle. Not only are their outside dimensions increased, but the marrow cavity is reduced or all but obliterated. Microscopically, it is seen that the cartilage does not disappear, as it must do in normal bone development, but persists, is calcified, and is surrounded by osteoid which becomes heavily calcified. Owing to the virtual absence of marrow space, there is severe myelophthisic anemia with extramedullary hematopoiesis.

In addition to its rare occurrence in humans, in whom it is inherited as an autosomal recessive trait, it has been reported in cattle, dogs, rabbits, mice, and rats in which it is also described as due to hereditary factors. On the basis of transmission experiments, as well as the concomitant presence of typical lesions in the soft tissues, it is considered to be one form of avian leukosis. Another form of osteopetrosis is a feature of fluorosis.

Polyostotic Fibrous Dysplasia. Under this name, a familial disease in Doberman Pinscher dogs has been described. The inherited nature of the disease has not been established. The lesions may be evidenced radiographically by enlargements and cysts in distal metaphyses of radius or ulna. The histologic appearance suggests fibrous osteodystrophy with osteoid and fibrous marrow. Cysts may also be seen.

Short Spine. Chondrodystrophy of vertebrae is of interest because it was known in ancient times in dogs of Japan and Europe, although it is apparently rare today. A single autosomal gene, with recessive expressivity, determines the disease. The thoracic and lumbar vertebral columns are shortened and crooked, giving high shoulders with a sharp decline to the tail. The tail is screw-shaped or kinked.

Spina Bifida. This congenital anomaly is known to occur in man and many other species. The defect (rachischisis) consists of various degrees of failure of closure of the dorsal part of the spinal column, and may extend from the sacral region to the occipital bone or may just involve a few segments of the sacral bones. The open spinal canal usually is covered by skin, but may be completely open. Nonhereditary intrauterine factors can be responsible for the anomaly, but genetically-determined cases are clearly known in rabbits and cats.

In the domestic rabbit, spina bifida is manifest as described above, detected at birth, and often associated with harelip, cleft palate, kyphosis and deviations of the tail. Autosomal recessive inheritance (gene symbol: *sb*) has been identified in this species.

In the domestic cat (*Felis catus*) spina bifida is one of the expressions of the dominant Manx gene (gene symbol: *M*) which is characteristic of the tailless breed, known as Manx. Genetically tailless cats are heterozygous for the Manx gene (*M/m*). Variations of expression of the homozygous state (*M/M*) occur, but homozygosity is generally lethal. In addition to spina bifida and absence of coccygeal vertebrae, anomalous defects of the sacrum and spinal cord may also occur.

Subluxation of Carpus. This anomaly has been described in dogs and has been shown to be due to a recessive sex-linked gene. It appeared in the course of studies on the inheritance of the genes for hemophilia A and B. The condition is manifest by dislocations, bilaterally, of the carporadial joints in the forelegs, which gradually appear at about three weeks of age. The flexor tendons fail to bear weight, allowing the weight to fall upon the posterior surface of the carpus. Trauma on the joint may lead to fractures of the distal aspect of the radius.

Banks, W.C., and Bridges, C.H.: Multiple cartilaginous exostoses in a dog. J. Am. Vet. Med. Assoc., 129:131–135, 1956.
Beachley, M.C., and Graham, F.H. Jr.: Hypochondroplastic dwarfism (enchondral chondrodys-

trophy) in a dog. J. Am. Vet. Med. Assoc., 163:283–284, 1973.
Bowen, J.M., et al.: Progression of hip dysplasia in German Shepherd dogs after unilateral pectineal myotomy. J. Am. Vet. Med. Assoc.,161:899–904, 1972.
Brown, R.J., Trevethan, W.P., and Henry, V.L.: Multiple osteochondroma in a Siamese cat. J. Am. Vet. Med. Assoc., 160:433–435, 1972.
Cardinet, G.H., Guffy, M.M., and Wallace, L.J.: Canine hip dysplasia: effects of pectineal tenotomy on the coxofemoral joints of German Shepherd dogs. J. Am. Vet. Med. Assoc., 164:591–598, 1974.
Carrig, C.B., and Seawright, A.A.: A familial canine polyostotic fibrous dysplasia with subperiosteal cortical defects. J. Small Anim. Pract., 10:397–405, 1969.
Chester, D.K.: Multiple cartilaginous exostoses in two generations of dogs. J. Am. Vet. Med. Assoc., 159:895–897, 1971.
Corley, E.A., Sutherland, T.M., and Carlson, W.D.: Genetic aspects of elbow dysplasia. J. Am. Vet. Med. Assoc., 153:543–547, 1968.
Cotton, W.R., and Gaines, J.F.: Osteopetrosis with associated unerupted dentition in the albino rat. J. Dent. Res., 53:935, 1974.
Crary, D.D., Fox, R.R., and Sawin, P.B.: Spina bifida in the rabbit. J. Hered., 57:236–243, 1966.
Dingwall, J.S., Pass, D.A., Pennock, P.W., and Cawley, A.J.: Case report. Multiple cartilaginous exostoses in a dog. Can. Vet. J.,11:114–119,1970.
Fletch, S.M., and Pinkerton, P.H.: An inherited anaemia associated with hereditary chondrodysplasia in the Alaskan Malamute. Can. Vet. J., 13:270–271, 1972.
Fletch, S.M., Smart, M.E., Pennock, P.W., and Subden, R.E.: Clinical and pathologic features of chondrodysplasia (dwarfism) in the Alaskan Malamute. J. Am. Vet. Med. Assoc.,162:357–361, 1973.
Fox, R.R., and Crary, D.D.: A new recessive chondrodystrophy in the rabbit. Teratology, 4:245–246, 1971.
Fox, R.R., and Crary, D.D.: Hereditary chondrodystrophy in the rabbit: genetics and pathology of a new mutant, a model for metatropic dwarfism. J. Hered., 66:271–276, 1975.
Gambardella, P.C., Osborne, C.A., and Stevens, J.B.: Multiple cartilaginous exostoses in the dog. J. Am. Vet. Med. Assoc., 166:761–768, 1975.
Gardner, D.L.: Familial canine chondrodystrophia foetalis (achondroplasia). J. Pathol. Bact., 77:243–247, 1959.
Gardner, E.J., Shupe, L.L., Leone, N.C., and Olson, A.E.: Hereditary multiple exostosis. A comparative genetic evaluation in man and horses. J. Hered., 66:318–322, 1975.
Gee, B.R., and Doige, C.E.: Multiple cartilaginous exostoses in a litter of dogs. J. Am. Vet. Med. Assoc., 156:53–59, 1970.
Greene, H.J., Leipold, H.W., Hibbs, C.M., and Kirkbride, C.A.: Congenital osteopetrosis in angus calves. J. Am. Vet. Med. Assoc., 164:389–395, 1974.

Hanselka, D.V., Roberts, R.E., and Thompson, R.B.: Equine multiple cartilaginous exostoses. Vet. Med. Small Anim. Clin., 60:979–983, 1974.

Hansen, H.J.: Historical evidence on a rare malformation in the dog ("short-spine dog"). Nord. Vet. Med., 17:44–49, 1965.

Henricson, B., and Olsson, S.E.: Hereditary acetabular dysplasia in the German Shepherd dog. J. Am. Vet. Med. Assoc., 135:207–210, 1959.

Hoag, G.N., Brown, R.G., Smart, M.E., and Subden, R.E.: Alaskan Malamute chondrodysplasia. I. Bone composition studies. Growth, 40:3–11, 1976.

Hoag, G.N., Brown, R.G., Smart, M.E., and Subden, R.E.: Alsakan Malamute chondrodysplasia. II. Urinary excretion of hydroxyproline, uronic acid, and acid mucopolysaccharides. Growth, 40:13–18, 1976.

Hoorens, J., and De Sloovere, J.: Osteogenesis imperfecta bij de Hond. Diergeneeskundig Tijedschrift, 41:515–521, 1972.

Howell, J.M., and Siegel, P.B.: Phenotype variability of taillessness in Manx cats. J. Hered., 54:167–169, 1963.

Howell, J.M., and Siegel, P.B.: Morphological effects of the Manx factor in cats. J. Hered., 57:100–104, 1966.

Hurst, R.E., Cezayirli, R.C., and Lorincz, A.E.: Nature of the glycosaminoglycanuria (mucopolysaccahariduria) in brachycephalic "snorter" dwarf cattle. J. Comp. Pathol., 85:481–486, 1975.

Huston, K., and Leipold, H.W.: Hereditary osteopetrosis in Aberdeen Angus calves. II. Genetical aspects. Ann. Génét. Sél. Anim., 3:419–423, 1971.

Hutt, F.B.: Inherited lethal characters in domestic animals. Cornell Vet., 24:1–25, 1934.

Hutt, F.B.: Genetic selection to reduce the incidence of hip dysplasia in dogs. J. Am. Vet. Med. Assoc., 151:1041–1048, 1967.

Hutt, F.B.: Developments in veterinary science. Advances in canine genetics, with special reference to hip dysplasia. Can. Vet. J., 10:307–311, 1969.

Innes, J.R.M.: "Inherited dysplasia" of the hip joint in dogs and rabbits. Lab. Invest., 8:1170–1177, 1959.

Innes, J.R.M., and Saunders, L.Z.: Comparative Neuropathology. New York, Academic Press, 1962.

James, C.C.M., Lassman, L.P., and Tomlinson, B.E.: Congenital anomalies of the lower spine and spinal cord in Manx cats. J. Pathol., 97:269–276, 1969.

Jones, T.C.: Hereditary Disease. In Pathology of Laboratory Animals (2 vol.), edited by K. Bernirschke, F.N. Garner, and T.C. Jones. New York, Springer Verlag, 1978, Chapter 22.

Julian, L.M., Tyler, W.S., and Gregory, P.W.: The current status of bovine dwarfism. J. Am. Vet. Med. Assoc., 135:104–109, 1959.

Larsen, J.S.: Report on canine hip dysplasia. J. Am. Vet. Med. Assoc., 162:662–668, 1973.

Leighton, E.A., Linn, J.M., Williams, R.L., and Castleberry, M.W.: A genetic study of canine hip dysplasia. Am. J. Vet. Res., 38:241–244, 1977.

Leipold, H.W., Doige, C.E., Kaye, M.M., and Cribb, P.H.: Congenital osteopetrosis in Aberdeen Angus calves. Can. Vet. J., 11:181–185, 1970.

Leipold, H.W., Huston, K., Dennis, S.M., and Guffy, M.M.: Hereditary osteopetrosis in Aberdeen-Angus calves: I. Pathological changes. Ann. Génét. Sél. Anim., 3:245–253, 1971.

Leipold, H.W., Huston, K., Blauch, B., and Guffy, M.M.: Congenital defects of the caudal vertebral column and spinal cord in Manx cats. J. Am. Vet. Med. Assoc., 164:520–523, 1974.

Leipold, H.W., and Cook, J.E.: Animal model of human disease: osteopetrosis, Albers-Schönberg disease, marble bone disease. Am. J. Pathol., 86:745–748, 1977.

Ljunggren, G., Cawley, A.J., and Archibald, J.: The elbow dysplasias in the dog. J. Am. Vet. Med. Assoc., 148:887–891, 1966.

Lust, G., Craig, P.H., Geary, J.C., and Ross, G.E., Jr.: Changes in pelvic muscle tissues associated with hip dysplasia in dogs. Am. J. Vet. Res., 33:1097–1108, 1972.

Lust, G., Craig, P.H., Ross, G.E., Jr. and Geary, J.C.: Studies on pectineus muscles in canine hip dysplasia. Cornell Vet., 62:628–645, 1972.

Lust, G., Pronsky, W., and Sherman, D.M.: Biochemical studies on developing canine hip joints. J. Bone Joint Surg., 54A:986–992, 1972.

Lust, G., Geary, J.C., and Sheffy, B.E.: Development of hip dysplasia in dogs. Am. J. Vet. Res., 34:87–92, 1973.

Mansson, J., and Norberg, I.: Dysplasia of the hip in dogs. Hormonally induced flaccidity of the ligaments followed by dysplasia of the acetabulum in puppies. Medlemsbl. Sverig. Vet. Forb., 13:330–332, 335–339, 1961.

Marks, S.C., Jr., and Lane, P.W.: Osteopetrosis, a new recessive skeletal mutation on chromosome 12 of the mouse. J. Hered., 67:11–18, 1976.

Marks, S.C., Jr., and Walker, D.G.: The role of the parafollicular cell of the thyroid gland in the pathogenesis of congenital osteopetrosis in mice. Am. J. Anat., 126:299–314, 1969.

Marks, S.C., Jr.: Pathogenesis of osteopetrosis in the ia rat: Reduced bone resorption due to reduced osteoclast function. Am. J. Anat., 138:165–190, 1975.

Martin, A.H.: A congenital defect in the spinal cord of the Manx cat. Vet. Pathol., 8:232–238, 1971.

Morgan, J.P., Carlson, W.D., and Adams, O.R.: Hereditary multiple exostosis in the horse. J. Am. Vet. Med. Assoc., 140:1320–1322, 1962.

Morgan, J.P.: Hip dysplasia in the Beagle: A radiographic study. J. Am. Vet. Med. Assoc., 164:496–498, 1974.

Murphy, H.M.: A review of inherited osteopetrosis in the mouse: man and other mammals also considered. Clin. Orthop., July-Aug:97–109, 1969.

Ojo, S.A., Leipold, H.W., Cho, D.Y., and Guffy, M.M.: Osteopetrosis in two Hereford calves. J. Am. Vet. Med. Assoc., 166:781–783, 1975.

Owen, L.N., and Nielsen, S.W.: Multiple cartilaginous exostoses (diaphyseal aclasis) in a Yorkshire Terrier. J. Small Anim. Pract., 9:519–521, 1968.

Parker, A.J., Park, R.D., Byerly, C.S., and Stowater,

J.L.: Spina bifida with protrusion of spinal cord tissue in a dog. J. Am. Vet. Med. Assoc., 163:158–160, 1973.

Pearce, L.: Hereditary osteopetrosis of the rabbit. J. Exp. Med. 92:601–624, 1950.

Pool, R.R., and Carrig, C.B.: Multiple cartilaginous exostoses in a cat. Vet. Pathol., 9:350–359, 1972.

Pool, R.R., and Harris, J.M.: Feline osteochondromatosis. Feline Pract., 5:24–30, 1975.

Priester, W.A., and Mulvihill, J.J.: Canine hip dysplasia. Relative risk by sex, size, and breed, and comparative aspects. J. Am. Vet. Med. Assoc., 160:735–739, 1973.

Rasmussen, P.G.: Multiple epiphyseal dysplasia in a litter of Beagle puppies. J. Small. Anim. Pract., 12:91–97, 1971.

Rasmussen, P.G., and Reimann, I.: Multiple epiphyseal dysplasia with special reference to histologic findings. Acta. Pathol. Microbiol. Scand. (A), 81:381–389, 1973.

Riser, W.H.: The dog as a model for the study of hip dysplasia. Growth, form, and development of the normal and dysplastic hip joint. Vet. Pathol., 12:235–238, 1975.

Schnelle, G.B.: Congenital dysplasia of the hip (canine) and sequelae. Proc. Am. Vet. Med. Assoc., pp. 253–258, 1954.

Schnelle, G.B.: Canine hip dysplasia. Lab. Invest., 8:1178–1189, 1959.

Seer, G., and Hurov, L.: Elbow dysplasia in dogs with hip dysplasia. J. Am. Vet. Med. Assoc., 154:631–637, 1969.

Smart, M.E., and Fletch, S.: A hereditary skeletal growth defect in purebred Alaskan Malamutes. Can. Vet. J., 12:31–32, 1971.

Snavely, J.G.: The genetic aspects of hip dysplasia in dogs. J. Am. Vet. Med. Assoc., 135:201–207, 1959.

Sprinkle, T.A., and Krook, L.: Hip dysplasia, elbow dysplasia, "eosinophilic" panosteitis. Three clinical manifestations of hyperestrinism in the dog. Cornell Vet., 50:476–490, 1970.

Stevens, D.R., and Sande, R.D.: An elbow dysplasia syndrome in the dog. J. Am. Vet. Med. Assoc., 165:1065–1069, 1974.

Subden, R.E., Fletch, S.M., Smart, M.A., and Brown, R.G.: Genetics of the Alaskan Malamute chondrodysplasia syndrome. J. Hered., 63:149–152, 1972.

Todd, N.B.: The inheritance of taillessness in Manx cats. J. Hered., 52:228–232, 1961.

Todd, N.B.: The Manx factor in domestic cats. J. Hered., 55:225–230, 1964.

Tomlinson, B.E.: Abnormalities of the lower spine and spinal cord in Manx cats. J. Clin. Pathol., 24:480, 1971.

Ueshima, T.: A pathological study on deformation of the vertebral column in "short-spine dog." Jpn. J. Vet. Res., 9:155–178, 1961.

Wiesner, E.: Die Erbschöden der landwertschaftlichen Nutztiere. Jena, Gustaf Fischer, 1960.

Woodard, J.C.: Bones. In Pathology of Laboratory Animals (2 vol.), edited by K. Benirschke, F.N. Garner, and T.C. Jones. New York, Springer Verlag, 1978.

Pulmonary Osteoarthropathy

Also known as Marie's disease for its discoverer (in man, 1890), this rather rare disease occurs in the dog and in man, and has been reported in sheep, deer, cat, gibbon, horse, and lion. Often preceded a few months earlier by a cough, dyspnea, or other pulmonary disturbances, the characteristic lesions are chronic proliferation of new bone producing marked thickening and deformity of the limbs. The new bone is formed just beneath the periosteum, which is pushed outward, but the osteophytic growths are irregular, so that the bone is made extremely rough. The bones usually affected are those of all four limbs from the femorotibial and shoulder joints to the phalanges. The joint surfaces are not involved, although there is much periarticular proliferation and enlargement. Occasionally, a bone may attain twice its normal diameter. There is considerable pain on movement and ultimately on palpation. Terminal effects of the osseous and pulmonary lesions together are fatal.

There are ordinarily important and extensive lesions in the lungs, most often either a bronchogenic carcinoma or other primary neoplasm. In some countries, advanced pulmonary tuberculosis is frequently present; chronic bronchiectatic, purulent processes are occasionally found. Hilton A. Smith had seen one case occasioned (presumably) by a large esophageal sarcoma which compressed and incapacitated a considerable portion of one lung. In humans, chronic heart diseases and insufficiencies have been concomitant with osteoarthropathy. In one canine case, there were several heartworms (*Dirofilaria immitis*) impeding the circulation. In a few human cases, there have been lesions outside the thorax which apparently obstructed circulation to the limbs.

In view of the above circumstance, the **cause** has been postulated as a longstanding anoxia, although some have suspected the presence of an obscure toxemia. Ac-

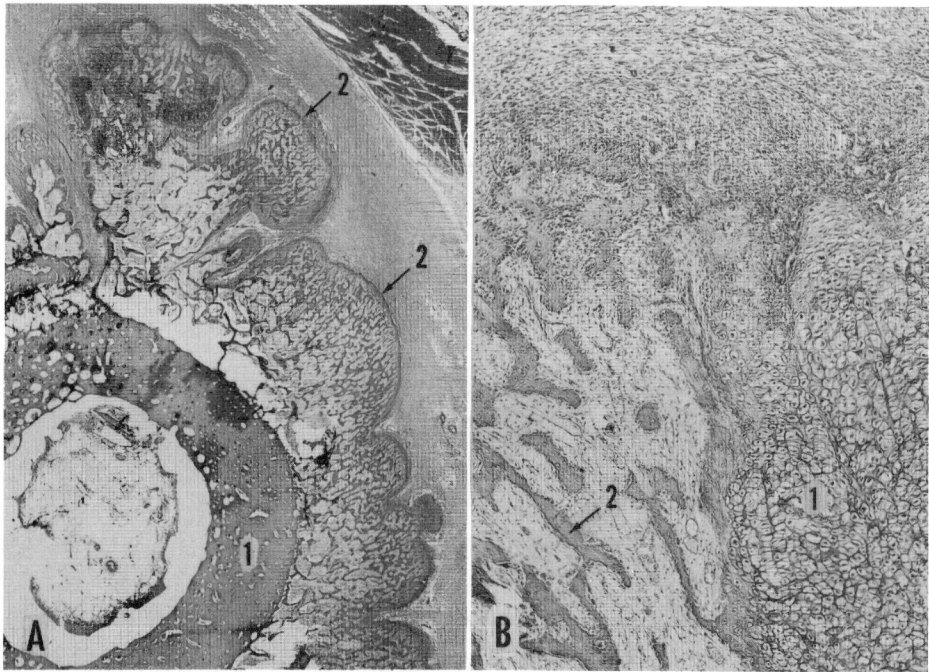

Fig. 19–13. Hypertrophic pulmonary osteoarthropathy. *A,* Cross section of tibia of a dog (× 3¾). Note cortex of bone (*1*) and bulbous new bone (*2*) on its exterior surface. *B,* Higher magnification (× 40). Note cartilaginous (1) and osseous (2) components. (Courtesy of Armed Forces Institute of Pathology.) Contributor: Dr. H.R. Seibold.

cordingly, an experimental anastomosis shunting a part of the blood past the lungs is stated to have produced the osteoarthropathy. It has also been theorized that increased pulmonary circulation without a corresponding demand for blood in the systemic circulation has resulted in excessive flow of blood in the extremities and consequent proliferation. It has been demonstrated that severing the vagus nerve has quickly cured the disorder; the fundamental mechanism is still under study. Vagotomy results in a prompt fall in blood flow to the limbs, which supports the hypothesis that increased peripheral blood flow is responsible for the bony growths. Presumably, the intrathoracic lesions induce a neural reflex involving the vagus and resulting in abnormal peripheral blood flow. There is agreement that the bony growth is in no way neoplastic, neither do metastatic neoplasms in the lungs appear to be associated invariably with pulmonary osteoarthropathy.

Ball, V.H.: L'ostéo-arthropathie hypertrophiante pneumonique chez les fauves en captivité. Rev. gén. de méd vét., *35*:417–432, 1926.

Brodey, R.S.: Hypertrophic osteoarthropathy in the dog: A clinicopathologic survey of 60 cases. J. Am. Vet. Med. Assoc., *159*:1242–1256, 1971.

Brodey, R.S., Riser, W.H., and Allen, H.: Hypertrophic pulmonary osteoarthropathy in a dog with carcinoma of the urinary bladder. J. Am. Vet. Med. Assoc., *162*:474–478, 1973.

Carroll, K.B., and Doyle, L.: A common factor in hypertrophic osteoarthropathy. Thorax, *29*:262–264, 1974.

Cotchin, E.: Marie's disease associated with tuberculosis in a horse. Brit. Vet. J., *100*:261–267, 1944.

Flavell, G.: Reversal of pulmonary hypertrophic osteoarthropathy by vagotomy. Lancet, *1*:260–262, 1956.

Gerbode, F., Birnstingl, M., and Braimbridge, M.: Experimental hypertrophic osteoarthropathy. Surgery, *60*:103–105, 1966.

Goodbary, R.F., and Hage, T.J.: Hypertrophic pulmonary osteoarthropathy in a horse. J. Am. Vet. Med. Assoc., *137*:602–605, 1970.

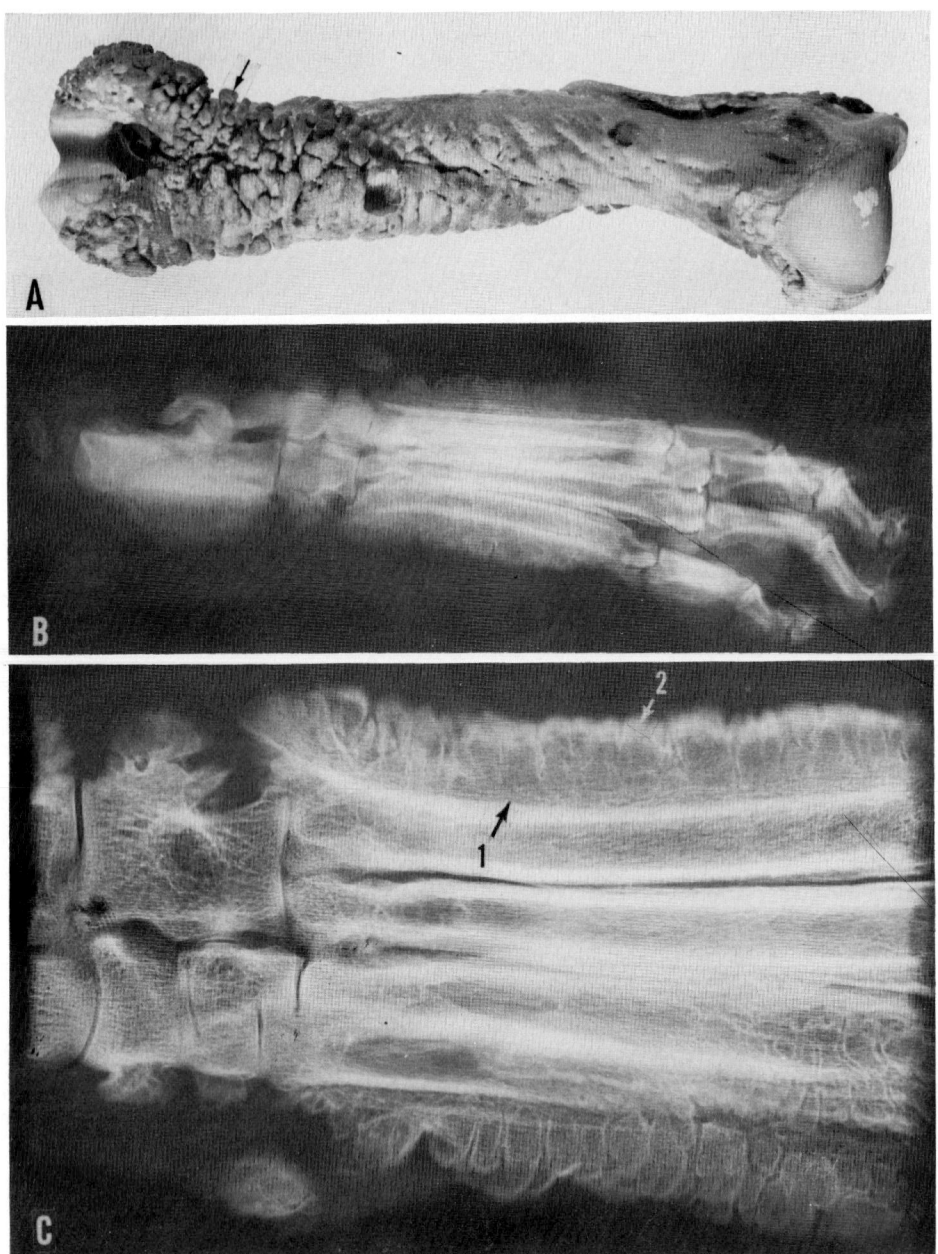

Fig. 19–14. Hypertrophic pulmonary osteoarthropathy. *A,* Humerus of a dog with severe exostosis. Note knob-like projections of bone from the cortex. Contributor: Dr. H.R. Seibold. *B,* Roentgenograph of the forelimb of a dog. Note severe exostosis on external surfaces of metacarpal bones, phalanges and carpus. *C,* Roentgenograph of the specimen collected at necropsy from *B.* The cortex of the bone is sharply demarcated at (*1*) and the new bone growth (*2*) is all external to the cortex. (*A* and *C,* Courtesy of Armed Forces Institute of Pathology.) Contributor: Dr. H.R. Seibold.

Holling, H.E., Brodey, R.S., and Boland, H.C.: Pulmonary hypertrophic osteoarthropathy. Lancet, 2:1269–1276, 1961.

Jones, T.C., and Schnelle, G.B.: Pulmonary hypertrophic osteoarthropathy in dogs. Lab. Invest., 8:1287–1303, 1959.

Kersjes, A.W., van de Watering, C.C., and Kalsbeek, H.C.: Hypertrophic pulmonary osteoarthropathy (Marie-Bamberger Disease). Neth. J. Vet. Sci., 1:55–68, 1968.

Lord, G.H.: Hypertrophic osteoarthropathy in a dog. A clinicopathological report. J. Am. Vet. Med. Assoc., 134:13–17, 1959.

Mather, G., and Low, D.: Chronic pulmonary osteoarthropathy in the dog. J. Am. Vet. Med. Assoc., 122:167–171, 1953.

Mendlowitz, M., and Leslie, A.: The experimental simulation in the dog of the cyanosis and hypertrophic osteoarthropathy which are associated with congenital heart disease. Am. Heart J., 24:141–152, 1942.

Poley, P.P., and Taylor, J.S.: Hypertrophic pulmonary osteoarthropathy associated with bronchogenic giant-cell tumor on the left lung of a dog. J. Am. Vet. Med. Assoc., 100:346–352, 1942.

Ryder-Davies, P., and Hine, J.M.: Hypertrophic osteoarthropathy in a gibbon (*Hylobates lar*). J. Small Anim. Pract., 13:655–658, 1972.

Smythe, A.R.: Some clinical aspects of tuberculosis in the dog (osteoarthropathy). Vet. Rec., 9:421–433, 1929.

Trum, B.F.: Pathogenesis of osteoarthritis in the horse (particularly as related to nutritional aspects). Lab. Invest., 8:1197–1208, 1959.

Verge, J.: Les ostéopathies hypertrophiantes: étude de deux cas chez le lion. Rev. gen. de méd. Vét., 43:1–22, 1934.

Exostoses

Whenever injured, bone, like other connective tissues, may react with a chronic proliferative inflammation. This results in a bony growth, in reality a granulation tissue composed of bone instead of the usual fibrous tissue which is seen in other locations. Such proliferations are usually rather strictly localized and are called exostoses, or osteophytes. The horse is especially subject to exostoses on the limbs, just as he is to excessive fibrous granulation tissue arising in the soft tissues. An exostosis or group of exostoses arising on the second or, less commonly, on the first phalanx is a ringbone. It causes serious and painful periarthritis. Small exostoses at the ends of the second and fourth metacarpal (rarely metatarsal) bones are called splints. Because of their less sensitive surroundings, they usually do not cause lameness. Exostoses frequently form on the medial portions of the distal bones of the tarsus. Such a lesion is called a (bone) spavin. Though small, it is a serious and stubborn cause of lameness.

Microscopically, an exostosis is seen to consist of compact bone of the usual appearance except it is not arranged into Haversian systems. The outer limit of original normal bone is usually visible as a slender line; the new bone appears as an added layer. In some cases, the extreme tip of an exostosis is formed of hyaline cartilage. Adjacent soft tissue may show inflammatory changes. The mature and orderly microscopic structure of an exostosis serves to distinguish it from a bony neoplasm.

The cause of an isolated exotosis is usually a single local trauma. The exostoses on the horse's legs are causally related to the continued strains and stresses of the horse's physical exertions. Some equine families are considered to be more susceptible to these disorders than others, but to a considerable extent, at least, this situation is based upon mechanically disadvantageous conformation of the bones, joints and tendons. The possibility that increased susceptibility to the formation of exostoses is related to suboptimal nutrition has been advocated but never proved.

Canine Cortical Hyperostosis. A disease described in a young dog (Baker and Lewis, 1975) resembles human infantile cortical hyperostosis or Caffey's disease. The single reported canine case involved an 18-month-old West Highland White Terrier which exhibited pain on movement and when joints were manipulated and a fever of 104.8°F. Slight evidence of periosteal changes, seen initially, progressed to extensive new bone formation on periosteal surfaces of all long bones, pelvis and scapulae. The lesions at necropsy, involving most of the bones, consisted of subperiosteal growth of new bone

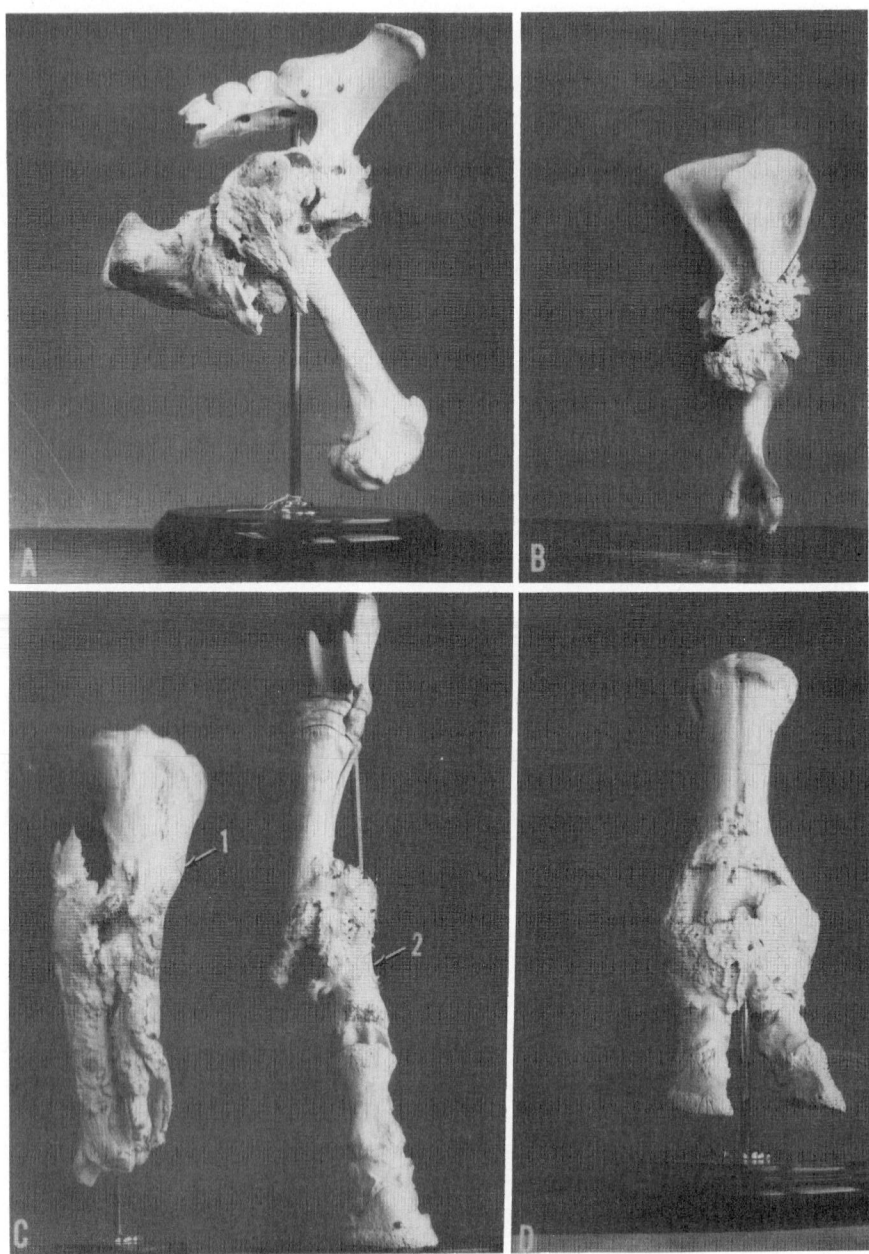

Fig. 19–15. *A*, Periarthritis and long-standing luxation of the coxofemoral joint of a cow. *B*, Exostosis following arthritis of the scapulohumeral joint in a pig. *C*, Attempted healing of two unreduced fractures in the tibia (*1*) and metatarsus (*2*) of two different horses. *D*, Exostosis involving the metacarpophalangeal joint in a cow. (Mark Francis Collection, Texas School Veterinary Medicine.)

which gave the surface of the bones a roughened appearance. The new growth of bone resembled that seen in pulmonary hypertrophic osteodystrophy, except for its distribution. The etiology of this rare disease is presently unknown.

Schlumberger (1959) has found exostoses developing at various sites in 21 female parakeets, but in no males. Similar changes have been seen in pigeons, probably in some other birds (not chickens), and possibly in women. Excess of estrogens has been thought to be the cause, perhaps due to faulty inactivation of estrogens by the liver, a belief partially supported by experimental evidence. Possibly a residuum of estrogen develops following active egg-laying.

Seawright and co-workers (1964, 1967) have demonstrated that a disorder of cats called deforming cervical spondylosis and characterized by multiple exostoses is the result of hypervitaminosis A.

Baker, J.R., and Lewis, D.G.: Bone disease in a dog similar to infantile cortical hyperostosis (Caffey's disease). Vet. Rec., *97*:74–75, 1975.

Bane, A., and Hansen, H.J.: Spinal changes in the bull and their significance in serving inability. Cornell Vet., *52*:362–384, 1962.

Kaye, M.M.: Hyperostosis in new born pigs. Can. J. Comp. Med., *26*:218–221, 1962.

Roberts, E.D., et al.: Pathologic changes of porcine suppurative arthritis produced by *Streptococcus equisimilis*. Am. J. Vet. Res., *29*:253–262, 1968.

Schlumberger, H.G.: Polyostotic hyperkeratosis in the female parakeet. Am. J. Pathol., *35*:1–24, 1959.

Schryver, H.F.: Symposium on equine bone and joint diseases. Cornell Vet., *58*:Suppl., 1968.

Seawright, A.A., and English, P.B.: Cervical spondylosis—cat. J. Pathol. Bact., *88*:503–509, 1964.

———: Hypervitaminosis A and deforming cervical spondylosis of the cat. J. Comp. Pathol., *77*:29–39, 1967.

Craniomandibular Osteopathy

Craniomandibular osteopathy ("lion jaw") is a disease of dogs of unknown cause characterized by multiple bilateral exostoses of the mandible and tympanic bullae of the temporal bone. Less regularly, exostoses occur on the occipital, frontal, lacrimal, and maxillary bones and in some instances involve bones of the limbs. The disease is most frequent in Scottish and West Highland White Terriers, but has also been seen in the Boston Terrier, Cairn Terrier, Labrador Retriever and other breeds. Exostoses of the mandibular processes and tympanic bullae mechanically obstruct the motion of the jaw, causing difficulty in eating, which is usually the first sign of the disease. Distortion of the mandible is rarely the first recorded observation owing to the long shaggy hair around the head of the breeds usually affected. As the lesions advance, it may not be possible to open the mouth more than 1 or 2 cm., and the mandible may approach twice its normal thickness. The exostoses are tender to the touch, and there is often intermittent fever up to 104°F, but aside from pain and inability to eat, the condition does not cause other systemic signs. The disease is usually first seen in dogs four to seven months of age and runs a course of intermittent progression and regression of the exostosis until 11 to 13 months of age when the disease ceases to progress and may recede completely.

Lesions. The gross lesions involve the maxilla, tympanic bullae, occasionally parietal and frontal bones, and single long bones. The long bones usually have exostoses extending outward from the preexisting cortex. The mandible is thickened through its width and longitude, usually from the middle mental foramen caudally. The greatest change appears in the region of the angular process. The lesions are, in general, bilaterally symmetrical. The tympanic bullae are enlarged 3 to 4 times normal diameter and are filled with new bone. Each bulla is usually fused with the adjacent angular process of the mandible. This fusion obviously interferes with the movement of the mandible.

The microscopic lesions (Riser, et al., 1967) in the mandible consist of: osteoclastic resorption of existing lamellar bone; replacement of lamellar bone by a primitive

coarse-type bone which extends beyond the normal periosteal boundaries; loss of marrow spaces between the coarse trabecular bone and replacement by highly vascular fibrous stroma; invasion of the periphery of new bone by inflammatory cells (lymphocytes, plasma cells, neutrophils) and formation of coarse new trabecular bone with a mosaic pattern of irregular cement lines.

These lesions and the clinical features of this canine disease have some similarities to cortical hyperostosis of infants (Caffey-Silverman Syndrome).

Adequate genetic evidence on the canine disease has not at this time been reported.

Burk, R.L., and Broadhurst, J.J.: Craniomandibular osteopathy in a Great Dane. J. Am. Vet. Med. Assoc., 169:635–636, 1976.

Caffey, J.: Infantile cortical hyperostosis: a review of the clinical and radiographic features. Proc. R. Soc. Med., 50:347–354, 1957.

Holman, G.H.: Infantile cortical hyperostosis: a review. Q. Rev. Pediatr., 17:24–31, 1962.

Littewort, M.C.G.: Tumor-like exostoses on the bones of the head in puppies. Vet. Rec., 70:977–978, 1958.

Pool, R.R., and Leighton, R.L.: Craniomandibular osteopathy in a dog. J. Am. Vet. Med. Assoc., 154:657–660, 1969.

Riser, W.H., Parkes, L.J., and Shirer, J.F.: Canine craniomandibular osteopathy. J. Am. Vet. Rad. Soc., 8:23–31, 1967.

Riser, W.H.: Hypertrophic osteopathy of the mandibles and cranium in West Highland Terriers. J. Am. Vet. Med. Assoc., 148:1543–1547, 1966.

Strasser, H., and Brunk, R.: Gehäuftes Auftreten einer nekrotisierenden Panostitis der Kieferknochen bei Beagle-Hunden. Dtsch. Tierarztl. Wochen., 78:304–307, 1971.

de Vries, H.W., and van de Watering, C.C.: Prednisone in the treatment of canine craniomandibular osteopathy. Neth. J. Vet. Sci., 5:123–131, 1973.

Watkins, J.D., and Bradley, R.: Craniomandibular osteopathy in a Labrador puppy. Vet. Rec., 79:262–264, 1966.

Watson, A.D.J., Huxtable, C.R.R., and Farrow, B.R.H.: Craniomandibular osteopathy in Doberman Pinschers. J. Small Anim. Pract., 16:11–19, 1975.

Enostosis

Enostosis, like an exostosis, is a bony proliferation, but rather than projecting from the surface outward an enostosis projects into the medullary cavity. It may originate from either trabecular bone or the cortex. Obviously such proliferations will not interfere with tendons, joints or other adjacent tissues. Few examples are recorded; enostosis is either uncommon or rarely produces clinical signs. An exception lies in a disease of dogs characterized by multiple enostoses of the long bones of the limbs, particularly the radius and ulna. The disease as described by Cotter and associates (1968) appears to be analogous to eosinophilic panostitis described by Zeskov (1961). In both reports, the disease was almost exclusively limited to the German Shepherd breed, although it was also recorded in other large breeds. Affected dogs first present lameness of the affected limb or limbs at six to 12 months of age. Usually only one limb is involved. No sign of systemic illness is apparent nor is there swelling or heat at the site of the enostosis, although a pain reaction can be elicited by deep palpation. Lameness may subside and reappear in the same or another limb and spontaneous recovery invariably follows a course of two to nine months. Radiographs are required to depict the lesions which appear as irregular, circumscribed areas of increased density of the endosteum in the diaphyses. In an occasional case periosteal proliferation (exostoses) is also present. Microscopically, the density is composed of trabecular bone surrounded by osteoclasts embedded in a fibrous stroma. Zeskov (1961) observed eosinophils within the lesion and a circulating eosinophilia, however, these changes are not observed in Cotter's (1968) series. The cause of the disease is unknown, but Zeskov claims artificial transmission by intramedullary injection of filtered bone marrow into young German Shepherd dogs.

Bohning, R.H., Jr., Suter, P.F., Hohn, R.B., and Marshall, J.: Clinical and radiologic survey of canine panosteitis. J. Am. Vet. Med. Assoc., 156:870–883, 1970.

Bruyere, P.: Clinical and radiographic features of eosinophilic panosteitis in the dog. Ann. Med. Vet., 118:9–20, 1974.

Cotter, S.M., Griffiths, R.C., and Leav, I.: Enostosis of young dogs. J. Am. Vet. Med. Assoc., *153*:401–410, 1968.

Herron, M.R.: Eosinophilic panosteitis diagnosis and therapy. S. West. Vet., 23:103–105, 1970.

Scott, D.W., and DeLahunta, A.: Eosinophilic polymyositis in a dog. Cornell Vet., *64*:47–56, 1974.

Zeskov, B.: A contribution to "eosinophilic panostitis" in dogs. Zentralbl. Veterinaermed., 7:671–680, 1960. VB, 31:#222, 1961.

Fractures of Bones

A clean break, separating a bone into two parts, is called a simple fracture. If there are many parts, it is a comminuted fracture. When, as rarely happens, one piece of bone is forcibly driven into another, the lesion is an impacted fracture. If in addition to the break in the bone, there is an opening in the overlying skin, the lesion is a compound fracture. The latter is much more dangerous because infection is able to enter. A fracture in which the periosteum remains intact and holds the ends of bone in place is a greenstick fracture. The term, pathological fracture, is used to designate one which occurs, not as the result of any unusual trauma, but because the bone was previously weakened by some other disease (such as fibrous osteodystrophy.)

Healing of a Fracture. When a bone is broken, its blood vessels and usually those nearby suffer the same fate, so that hemorrhage occurs into the area. The escaped blood forms a clot, which fares the same here as elsewhere: Its fibrin affords an attractive field for the proliferation of fibroblasts, mostly from the periosteum, which convert the clot into fibrous connective tissue. The fibrous mass receives blood via capillaries which build into it from the adjoining tissue. Some of the fibroblasts differentiate into an imperfect kind of cartilage cells. This happens especially if there is interference with healing by movement. This structure holds the ends of the bone with reasonable firmness and is called the provisional callus (*callus*, a hard structure.) The periosteal fibroblasts begin to show their true nature after about two weeks by developing osteoblastic characteristics, and the callus is gradually changed into osteoid. Calcium phosphate and carbonate are deposited in the osteoid and it becomes bone, the true callus. This bony callus not only replaces the broken structure, but fills

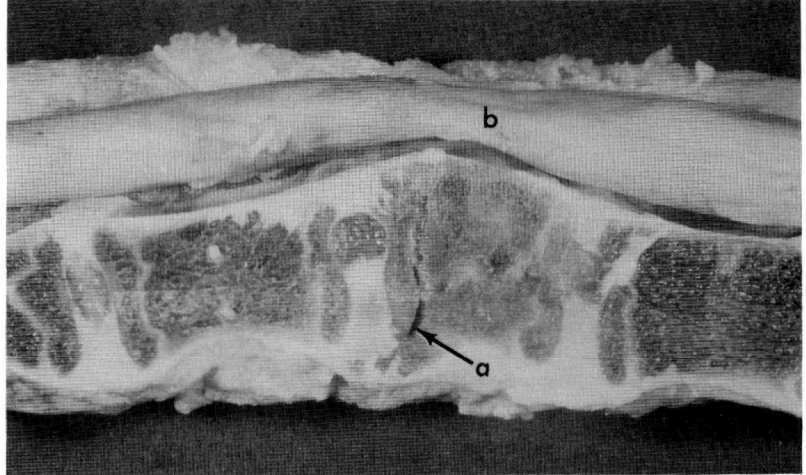

Fig. 19–16. Fracture of a vertebra through the epiphysis (*a*), resulting in compression of the spinal cord (*b*). A nine-month-old female German Shepherd which had been hit by a car. (Photograph courtesy of Angell Memorial Animal Hospital.)

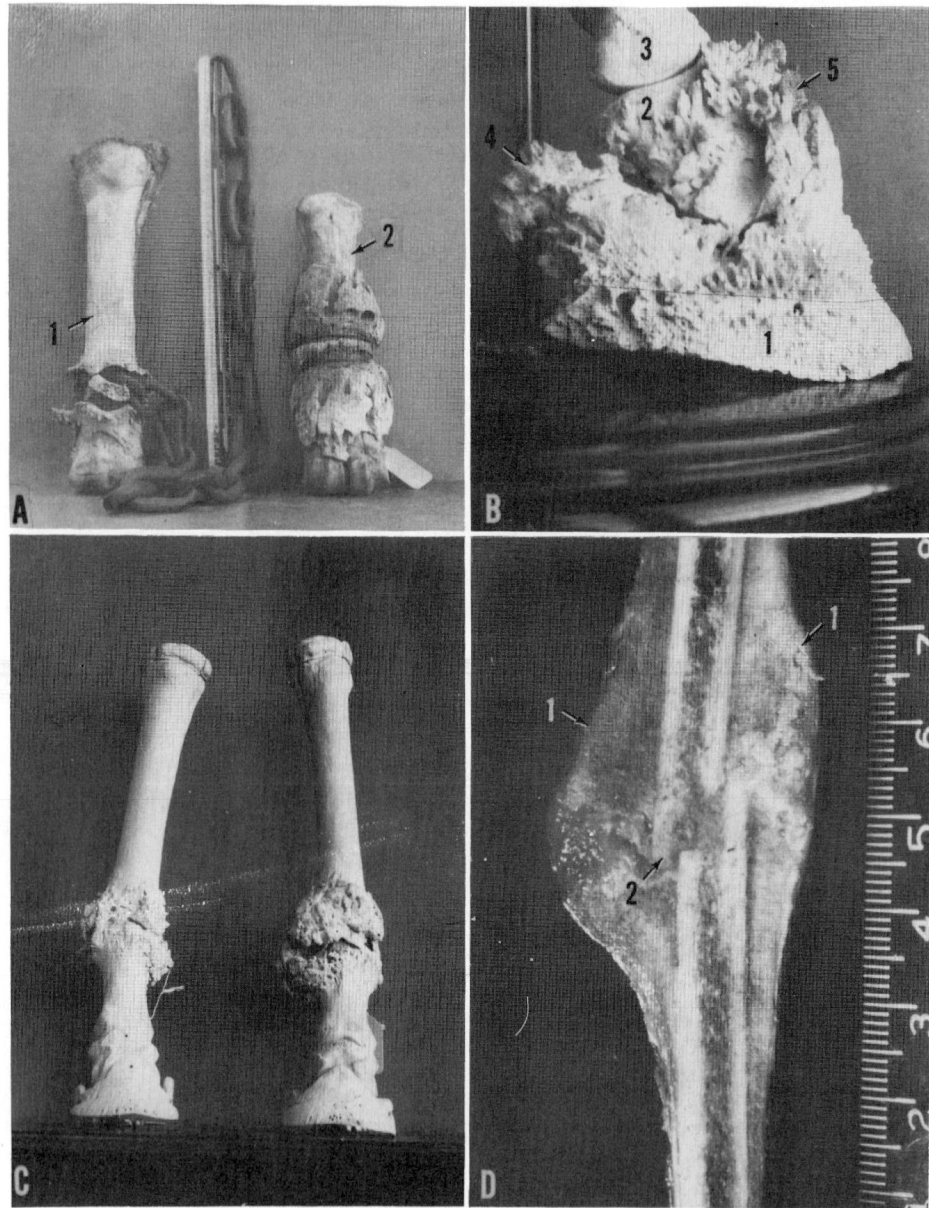

Fig. 19–17. *A*, Chronic proliferative osteitis resulting from forgotten hobbles used in pioneer days. A chain around an equine (*1*) and two wires around a bovine metatarsus (*2*). *B*, Ossification of lateral cartilage (sidebone) and low ringbone in a horse. Third phalanx (*1*), second phalanx (*2*), first phalanx (*3*), ossified lateral cartilage (*4*), and exostosis of second phalanx (*5*). *C*, Exostosis around fetlock joint (high ringbone) in both legs of a saddle horse. (*A*, *B* and *C* from: Mark Francis Collection, Texas School Veterinary Medicine.) *D*, Fracture of rib of a year-old Guernsey calf. Note bony callus (*1*) surrounding the fracture (*2*). (Courtesy of College of Veterinary Medicine, Iowa State University.)

the marrow cavity, and also protrudes outwardly, forming a considerably larger mass than the original bone. For some months or even years afterward, this bone is repeatedly digested by osteoclasts and replaced by more perfect bone with normal Haversian systems, more nearly duplicating the original in structure, dimensions, and restoration of the marrow cavity. Until the latter is accomplished, the bone formed in this or other healing processes, which are essentially reactions to injury and, therefore, akin to proliferative inflammation, has the structure of cancellous (spongy) bone, the bony trabeculae being numerous but very irregular, the marrow initially fibrous. In the external layers of the bony callus this cancellous bone is seen attached to the outside of the layer of compact bone which formed the original shaft. In those rather frequent cases where the healing segments are not fixed in absolute rigidity during the healing process, a cartilaginous union often precedes the formation of bone. The more lateral ends of the line of union, where a tilting movement would be most pronounced, may thus show areas of hyaline cartilage, in contrast to the proliferating bone which constitutes normal healing.

Alcantara, P.J., and Stead, A.C.: Fractures of the distal femur in the dog and cat. J. Small Anim. Pract., 16:649–659, 1975.
Gleeson, L.N., and Larkin, H.A.: Fracture of the occipital bone with cerebellar compression in a dog. J. Am. Vet. Med. Assoc., 161:1113–1116, 1972.
Thrall, D.E., Lebel, J.L., and O'Brien, T.R.: A five-year survey of the incidence and location of equine carpal chip fractures. J. Am. Vet. Med. Assoc., 158:1366–1368, 1971.

Epiphyseal Necrosis

Epiphyseal necrosis, most often of the head of the femur or humerus, is occasionally encountered in domestic animals and laboratory rats and mice. It regularly follows fracture of the femoral neck which interferes with the vascular supply to the epiphysis, but it is also encountered without a clearly defined pathogenesis; although vascular interference is most likely the underlying cause in all examples.

Aseptic necrosis of the femoral head of the latter type is most frequent in dogs where, like its human counterpart, it has often gone by the eponym *Legg-Perthes* disease and *Calvé-Perthes* disease. Osteochondritis of the hip, juvenile osteochondrosis of the hip, and coxa plana have also been applied to this condition, which as indicated is not associated with fractures or obvious interference with the vascular supply to the femoral head. The disease is restricted to miniature breeds such as the miniature Pinscher, Lakeland Terrier, toy and miniature Poodle, Fox Terrier, Pug and Griffin. The disease has been reviewed in detail by Ljunggren (1967), who examined 238 spontaneous cases. Her observations revealed that the disease develops in adolescent dogs with initial symptoms of lameness appearing between 4 and 11 months of age. The affected leg is painful, especially upon abduction, and there may be crepitation of the hip joint, shortening of the affected leg, and muscle atrophy. In radiographs, the earliest changes are a widening of the joint space and the presence of single or multiple foci of decreased density of the femoral head which, as the disease progresses, become more numerous and larger, giving a "moth-eaten" appearance to the head of the femur. The head of the femur eventually develops an irregular contour and fragments. Gross lesions, which are best observed after midsagittal sectioning, vary from subtle changes in shape of the femoral head to fragmentation; the articular cartilage is often brownish and roughened. Ljunggren (1967) described the microscopic changes as commencing with excessive production of endosteal bone followed by osteonecrosis and necrosis of marrow. Subsequent to necrosis, there is obviously fibroplasia, osteoclasis, and additional new bone formation. Ljunggren theorized that the development of *Legg-Perthes* disease was related to premature closure of cartilaginous growth plates and that miniature breeds were predisposed to the disease due to earlier sexual maturity.

Osteochondritis Dissecans (Idiopathic Avascular Necrosis, Osteochondrosis Dissecans). This condition was first described in man by Sir James Paget in 1870 and named by König in 1888. The disease conditions described in animals meet many of the diagnostic criteria for the human disease. The name has been used widely to indicate specific disease conditions in dogs and horses. Canine osteochondritis dissecans is differentiated from aseptic necrosis of the head of the femur (*Legg-Perthes disease*) by the fact that it occurs in larger breeds of young dogs and affects particularly the shoulder joint (scapulohumeral) and sometimes the stifle or other joints. Young dogs 4 to 12 months are affected with a painful process. The head of the humerus is particularly involved, but other bones may be as well.

Radiographs reveal free bodies in the joint cavity amid indications that they arose from the articular cartilage. Microscopically, early cleavage lines may be detected in the growing articular cartilage which eventually separates the cartilage, plus some bone, from the underlying epiphyseal bone. The free body in the joint cavity can cause damage to the articular surface. The bone and cartilage at the point of detachment can be remodeled by the growth of granulation tissue, bone, and cartilage. Surgical intervention by removing the free bodies or partially detached cartilage may prove therapeutically effective.

The cause is unknown. The known controlling influences of certain hormones (thyroxin, somatostatin, estrogens, and testosterone) on the epiphyseal growth of bone and cartilage, suggests that these endocrine factors should be investigated.

Leg Weakness, Osteochondrosis, Arthrosis. These names have been used to indicate a problem encountered in young, fast-growing, well-fed swine. Locomotor defects are seen in as many as 30% of certain breeds of swine as the growing pigs reach about 50 to 65 kg body weight. The affected pigs are otherwise healthy and the condition is not associated with any systemic or infectious disease. Awkward gait and inability to bear weight on front or hind legs are the principal signs.

Several lesions have been described in the epiphyseal growth plates. Separation of the cartilage of the plate between the proliferative and calcified zones is one such lesion. A second is a fracture through the zone of provisional calcification with hemorrhage into the cartilaginous lattice, with accumulation of fibrin, fibrosis, and a tendency of the cartilage to separate from the epiphysis. Repair of the horizontal defect in the cartilage is attempted. Normal fibrosis, cartilage growth, and ossification can occur, reducing the lesion to a fibrous band or nodule among the bony trabeculae. Complete resorption can occur. In some cases, separation of the caput of the femur is also described, not unlike the effect of so-called aseptic necrosis. Here again, necrosis occurs through the growth plates and adjacent bone, splitting through and detaching it through the middle of the epiphyseal plate.

The cause of this condition is also unknown. The comments made earlier on the possible significance of endocrine factors to osteochondritis dissecans seem to apply to "leg weakness" as well.

Birkeland, R.: Osteochondritis dissecans in the humeral head of the dog. Nord. Vet. Med., *19*:294–305, 1967.

Birkeland, R., and Haakenstad, L.H.: Intracapsular fragments of the distal tibia of the horse. J. Am. Vet. Med. Assoc., *152*:1526–1529, 1968.

Bouchaert, A., and Mattheeuws, D.: Avascular necrosis of the head of the femur in dogs: Radiographic aspects of 50 cases. Vlaams Diergeneeskd Tijdschr., *43*:125–133, 1973.

Cordy, D.R., and Wind, A.P.: Transverse fracture of the proximal humeral articular cartilage in dogs (so-called osteochondritis dissecans). Pathol. Vet., *6*:424–427, 1969.

Griffiths, R.C.: Osteochondritis of the canine shoulder. J. Am. Vet. Med. Assoc., *153*:1733–1735, 1968.

Grondalen, T.: Osteochondrosis, arthrosis, and leg weakness in pigs. Nord. Vet. Med., 26:534–537, 1974.

Grondalen, T.: Leg weakness in pigs. I. Incidence and relationship to skeletal lesions, feed level, protein and mineral supply, exercise, and exterior conformation. II. Litter differences in leg weakness, skeletal lesions, joint shape, and exterior conformation. Acta Vet. Scand., 15:555–573, 574–586, 1974.

Grondalen, T.: Osteochondrosis and arthrosis in pigs. I. Incidence in animals up to 120 kg live weight. II. Incidence in breeding animals. III. A comparison of the incidence in young animals of the Norwegian Landrace and Yorkshire breeds. Acta Vet. Scand., 15:1–25, 26–42, 43–52, 1974.

Grondalen, T., and Grondalen, J.: Osteochondrosis and arthrosis in pigs. IV. Effect of overloading on the distal epiphyseal plate of the ulna. Acta Vet. Scand., 15:53–60, 1974.

Grondalen, T., and Vangen, O.: Osteochondrosis and arthrosis in pigs. V. A comparison of the incidence in three different lines of the Norwegian Landrace breed. Acta Vet. Scand., 15:61–79, 1974.

Grondalen, T.: Osteochondrosis and arthrosis in pigs. VI. Relationship to feed level and calcium, phosphorus, and protein levels in the ration. Acta Vet. Scand., 15:147–169, 1974.

Grondalen, T.: Osteochondrosis and arthrosis in pigs. VII. Relationship to joint shape and exterior conformation. Acta Vet. Scand. (Suppl.), 46:1–32, 1974.

Hogg, A., Ross, R.F., and Cox, D.F.: Joint changes in lameness of confined swine. Am. J. Vet. Res., 36:965–970, 1975.

Johansson, H.E., and Rejno, S.: Light and electron microscopic investigation of equine synovial membrane. A comparison between healthy joints and joints with intraarticular fractures and osteochondrosis dissecans. Acta Vet. Scand., 17:153–168, 1976.

Knecht, C.D., et al.: Osteochondrosis of the shoulder and stifle in 3 of 5 Border Collie littermates. J. Am. Vet. Med. Assoc., 170:58–60, 1977.

König, F.: Ueler freie Körper in den Gelenken. Dtsch. Z. Chirirgie., 27:90–100, 1888.

Ljunggren, G.: Legg-Perthes disease in the dog. Acta Orthoped. Scand. Suppl., 95:1–79, 1967.

Moor, A. de, et al.: Osteochondritis dissecans of the tibio-tarsal joint in the horse. Equine Vet. J., 4:139–143, 1972.

Oliver, J.W., and Neher, G.M.: Experimentally induced athyreosis in swine: clinical signs, radiographic changes and necropsy observations. Am. J. Vet. Res., 32:905–911, 1971.

Oliver, J.W., and Neher, G.M.: Athyreotic arthropathy in swine. Am. J. Vet. Res., 34:1539–1547, 1973.

Paatsama, S., Rokkanen, P., Jussila, J., and Sittnikow, K.: A study of osteochondritis dissecans of the canine humeral head using histological, OTC bone labelling, microradiographic, and microangiographic methods. J. Small Anim. Pract., 12:603–611, 1971.

Paget, J.: On the production of some of the loose bodies in joints. Saint Bartholomew's Hospital Reports, 6:1–12, 1870.

Palmer, C.S.: Osteochondritis dissecans in Great Danes. Vet. Med. Small Anim. Clin., 65:994–1000 & 1002, 1970.

Punzet, G., Walde, I., and Arbesser, E.: Zur osteochondrosis dissecans genu des hundes. Kleinter-Praxis, 20:88–98, 1975.

Reiland, S.: Osteochondrosis in the pig. A morphologic and experimental investigation with special reference to the leg weakness syndrome. Akademisk Avhandling, Veter. Stockholm, 118 pp, 1975.

Van Pelt, R.W., Riley, W.F., and Tillotson, P.J.: Stifle disease (gonitis) in horses: clinicopathologic findings and intra-articular therapy. J. Am. Vet. Med. Assoc., 157:1173–1186, 1970.

Vaughan, L.C.: Leg weakness in pigs. Vet. Rec., 89:81–85, 1971.

Walker, T., et al.: Observations on "leg weakness" in pigs. Vet. Rec., 79:472–479, 1966.

Infections of Bone

The infections which occasionally localize in bone include brucellosis, tuberculosis, actinomycosis, and coccidioidomycosis. Brucellosis ordinarily forms an intra-osseous abscess, or sometimes a focus of caseation necrosis encapsulated by fibrous tissue with a mixture of leukocytes including many eosinophils. In swine and calves, a fairly frequent location is within one or two adjoining vertebrae, the condition being called **spondylitis.** Each of the other three diseases produces its typical granulomatous lesion, which is able to grow and proliferate by destroying the bony tissue around it. The bone tissue reacts with a reparative proliferation at the same time that adjoining areas are being dissolved. The result is a pronounced local enlargement which proves to be very much honey-combed when the soft tissues are removed by maceration. This type of lesion is especially conspicuous in actinomycosis as it involves the jaw bones of cattle. In the case of tuberculosis, the bone lesion is usually part of a generalized process; in the few reported cases of coccidioidomycosis, the same may be true; in actinomycosis and brucellosis, the bone lesion is usually the only manifestation. The marrow may or may not be invaded in any of these conditions.

Metastatic abscesses occasionally occur in the vertebrae of animals and may produce paraplegia due to pressure on or infection of the spinal cord. In a study of such abscesses in cattle, sheep, and swine, Finley (1975) reported *Corynebacterium pyogenes* to be most frequently isolated from all three species. *Spheropherous necrophorus* was isolated next in frequency from bovines. In swine, streptococci were recovered second in frequency. Other organisms isolated from isolated cases included *Staphylococcus sp., Pseudomonas sp., Pasteurella haemolytica,* and *Escherichia coli.*

Osteomyelitis, infection of the bone marrow, is now less frequent due to the application of antibiotic therapy, but still occurs and may result in prolonged infection and severe changes in the bone. The infection usually reaches the bone by the hematogenous route but can arrive at the site through direct injury, compound fracture, or penetrating wounds. Persistent pyogenic infection results in destruction, replacement, and excessive growth of new bone adjacent to the infected part.

Caywood, D.D., Wallace, L.J., and Braden, T.D.: Osteomyelitis in the dog: a review of 67 cases. J. Am. Vet. Med. Assoc., *172*:943–946, 1978.

Finley, G.G.: A survey of vertebral abscesses in domestic animals in Ontario. Can. Vet. J., *16*:114–117, 1975.

Nall, J.D., and Bartels, J.E.: Spondylitis in Diana guenon monkey. J. Zoo. Anim. Med., *4*:22–23, 1973.

Norden, C.W.: Experimental osteomyelitis. I. A description of a model. J. Infect. Dis., *122*:410–418, 1970.

Pichard, R.: Chronic traumatic osteitis of the diaphysis of the humerus in the dog. Recueil de Medecine Veterinaire, *147*:1362–1387, 1971.

Waldvogel, F.A., Medoff, G., and Swartz, M.: Osteomyelitis: a review of clinical features, therapeutic considerations, and unusual aspects. N. Engl. J. Med., *282*:198–206, 1970.

Protrusion of Intervertebral Discs

The intervertebral discs consist of a central semi-solid mucoid connective tissue, the nucleus pulposus, enclosed in a thick fibrous zone, the annulus fibrosus. In old age, the disc becomes fibrocartilaginous. In response to sudden strains and, it is thought, following a certain degree of degeneration which is possibly of hereditary origin, the annulus fibrosus may be partially ruptured so that a bulging mass protrudes into the spinal canal (Fig. 19–18). The lumbar or last thoracic discs are most likely to suffer this accident, although the cervical discs are not immune. In many instances, no symptoms are produced, but in other cases severe and rather sudden pain and reflex immobility result from pressure upon nervous elements. In humans, there is ordinarily impingement upon one of the spinal nerves as it passes through the intervertebral foramen, and the symptoms are severe pain referred to the area of distribution of the nerve involved. Since this is usually one of those making up the sciatic nerve, the condition is often called sciatica. In the dog, the spinal cord extends caudally past the sacrum, and the protruding mass usually presses directly upon the spinal cord. Symptoms then are those of partial or complete paralysis of the innervated regions, often the whole of the hind quarters. In severe cases, there may be local hemorrhage and necrosis of the area under pressure, with eventual wallerian degeneration of fibers coming from the destroyed nerve cells. Fortunately, many cases, even of complete posterior paralysis, are not quite so severe and, with adequate nursing, slowly recover as the protruding nucleus pulposus is resorbed. Although the protrusions usually occur dorsally, ventral protrusion of degenerated discs is also encountered, but obviously protrusion in this direction is of less importance. With healing, the ventral protrusion causes the development of osteophytes which may progress to ankylosing spondylitis (spondylosis deformans).

The pathologist needs to realize that a very careful examination of the floor of the spinal canal is necessary to establish with certainty the presence or absence of this lesion. It is claimed that some ruptures merely cause bulging of the dorsal longitudinal ligament, which overlies them, and this subsides during the manipula-

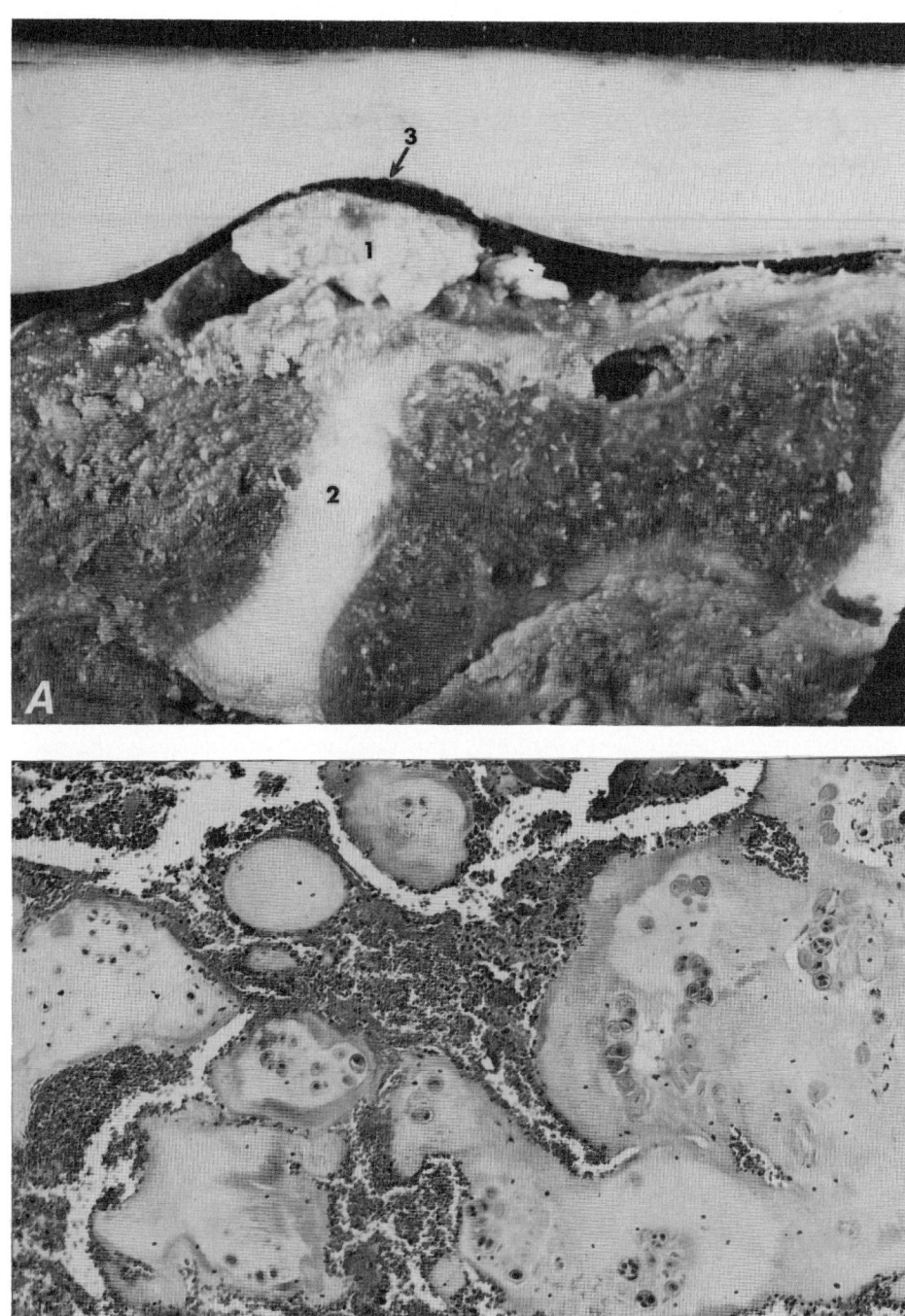

Fig. 19–18. *A,* Protrusion of intervertebral disc in a five-year-old male Dachshund. The protruded material *(1)* from cervical disc 5–6 *(2)* has compressed the spinal cord at *(3).* The vertebral column and spinal cord were fixed in formalin, then cut sagittally. *B,* Chondroid material, hemorrhage, and debris from the nucleus pulposus, which has undergone "chondroid" degeneration and has been expelled into the vertebral canal through a diseased annulus fibrosus. (H & E, × 150.) (Courtesy of Angell Memorial Animal Hospital.)

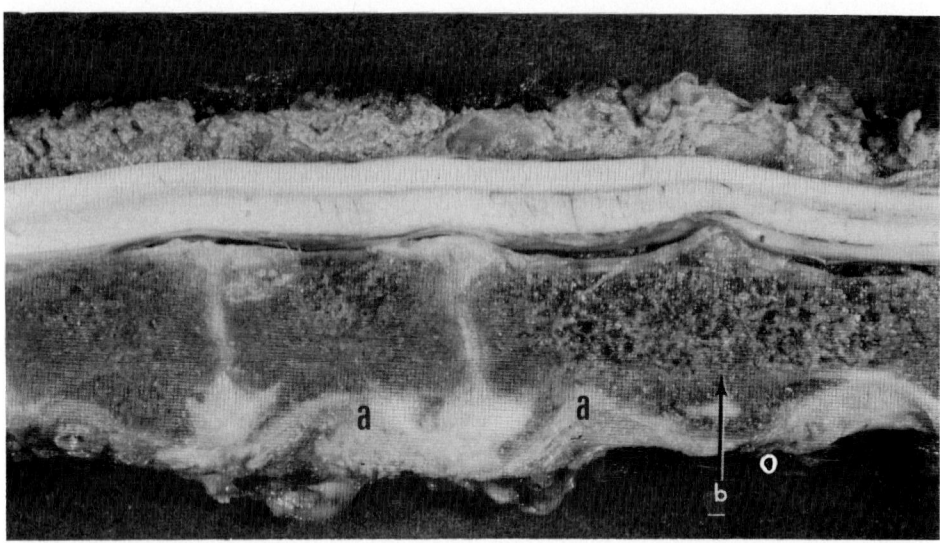

Fig. 19–19. Ankylosing spondylitis (a) fusing lumbar vertebrae of a 15-year-old cross breed terrier. Note loss of intervertebral disc (b). (Courtesy of Angell Memorial Animal Hospital.)

tions of the autopsy. On the other hand, roentgenologists frequently demonstrate a mild calcification of a degenerated disc even when no protrusion or any acute symptoms are attributable to it.

As far as known this condition is rare in domestic animals other than the dog and is less frequent in the cat. As indicated in the dog, protrusion of intervertebral discs is preceded by degenerative changes in the annulus fibrosus and nucleus pulposus. Two morphologically distinct degenerative processes are apparent in dogs. One in dogs of chondrodystrophoid breeds (Dachshunds, Pekinese, French Bulldogs) develops at an early age, and the other occurs in aged dogs of all breeds. In the former type, the changes are characterized by chondroid metaplasia of the nucleus pulposus followed by calcification. Granular amorphous material accumulates between the fibers of the annulus fibrosus, which leads to disruptions of its normal lamellated structure. The lamellae themselves undergo hyaline degeneration and fragmentation. In nonchondrodystrophoid breeds the changes in the annulus fibrosus are similar to those seen in chondrodystrophoid breeds, however, in the nucleus pulposus the degenerative change is characterized by a collagenization, described as fibroid degeneration, rather than chondroid metaplasia and calcification is rare.

In some cases the injury to the spinal cord is not limited to one or two segments near the point of disc protrusion, but involves a large segment or most of the cord. The affected cord undergoes severe necrosis, which is very likely due to ischemia. The mechanism which results in this ischemia has not yet been clearly demonstrated, hence is a matter of speculation. Embolism of material from the degenerated disc is one of the possibilities. This lesion has been called "the ascending syndrome," hemorrhagic myelomalacia, or ascending cord necrosis.

In cats the condition is analogous to that seen in nonchondrodystrophoid dogs.

Bojrab, M.J.: Disc disease. Vet. Rec., *89*:37–41, 1971.

Butler, W.F., and Smith, R.N.: Age changes in the annulus fibrosus of the non-ruptured intervertebral disc of the cat. Res. Vet. Sci., *6*:280–289, 1965.

Ghosh, P., Taylor, T.K.F., Braund, K.G., and Larsen, L.H.: A comparative chemical and histochemical study of the chondrodystrophoid and nonchondrodystrophoid canine intervertebral disc. Vet. Pathol., 13:414–427, 1976.

Goggin, J.E., and Franti, C.E.: Canine intervertebral disc disease: characterization of age, sex, breed, and anatomic site of involvement. Am. J. Vet. Res., 31:1687–1692, 1970.

Griffiths, I.R.: The extensive myelopathy of intervertebral disc protrusions in dogs (the ascending syndrome). J. Small Anim. Pract., 13:425–438, 1972.

Griffiths, I.R.: Some aspects of the pathogenesis and diagnosis of lumbar disc protrusion in the dog. J. Small Anim. Pract., 13:439–447, 1972.

Hansen, H.J.: Comparative views on the pathology of disc degeneration in animals. Lab. Invest., 8:1242–1265, 1959.

Hayes, M.A., Creighton, S.R., Boysen, B.G., and Holfeld, N.: Acute necrotizing myelopathy from nucleus pulposus embolism in dogs with intervertebral disc degeneration. J. Am. Vet. Med. Assoc., 173:289–295, 1978.

Hoerlein, B.F.: Intervertebral-disc protrusions in the dog. Am. J. Vet. Res., 14:260–283, 1953.

Hoerlein, B.F.: Canine Neurology. Philadelphia, W.B. Saunders, 1971.

Hurov, L., Troy, G., and Turnwald, G.: Diskospondylitis in the dog: 27 cases. J. Am. Vet. Med. Assoc., 173:275–281, 1978.

Lahunta, A.De, and Alexander, J.W.: Ischemic myelopathy secondary to presumed fibrocartilaginous embolism in nine dogs. J. Am. Anim. Hosp. Assoc., 12:37–48, 1976.

Palmer, A.C.: Clinical and pathological aspects of cervical disc protrusion and primary tumours of the cervical spinal cord in the dog. J. Small Anim. Pract., 11:63–67, 1970.

Parker, A., Park, R.D., and Henry, J.D., Jr.: Cervical vertebral instability associated with cervical disk disease in two dogs. J. Am. Vet. Med. Assoc., 163:1369–1371, 1973.

Pettit, G.D. (ed.): Intervertebral Disc Protrusion in the Dog. New York, Appleton-Century-Crofts, 1966.

Swaim, S.F., and Vandevelde, M.: Clinical and histologic evaluation of bilateral hemilaminectomy and deep dorsal laminectomy for extensive spinal cord decompression in the dog. J. Am. Vet. Med. Assoc., 170:407–413, 1977.

Vaughan, L.C.: Studies on intervertebral disc protrusion in the dog. III. Pathological features. Brit. Vet. J., 114:350–355, 1958.

Arthritis and Periarthritis

Acute inflammation of a joint is commonly serous, fibrinous, or purulent. The serous form is equivalent to an excessive formation of synovia, which distends the joint capsule and forms a "puffy" swelling. The articular and synovial surfaces show nothing more than a slight hyperemic redness. This type of arthritis is usually due to mild, and often, to repeated trauma; when infection is present the intracapsular exudate is fibrinous or, in the presence of pyogenic organisms, purulent. In such cases, the articular surfaces are likely to be eroded and there is extreme pain. The surrounding tissues are edematous.

In chronic arthritis, which is also known as osteoarthritis and degenerative joint disease, there tends to be proliferation of the mesothelium and soft tissues lining the non-articular surfaces of the joint capsule. The proliferated tissue takes very irregular forms, often projecting into the joint cavity as bizarre but smooth, mesothelial-covered "synovial fringes." Such a projecting "tag" may be caught between the articulating surfaces and produce sudden severe pain, which slowly subsides after the projecting tissue escapes from the compression. Not too infrequently, some of the more pedunculated projections may be broken off, or may become detached because of atrophy of the narrow neck. These bits of tissue remain alive by absorption of nutrients from the joint fluid and are slowly kneaded into rounded or elliptical bodies of tissue, to which are given such names as **corpora libra,** free bodies, melon-seed bodies, or joint-mice. Being subject to impingement between the articulating surfaces, they also may at any moment be responsible for sharp pain by placing undue pressure upon an area of joint surface. Rarely, such free bodies may be formed of compressed, unorganized fibrin or of fragments of cartilage.

If the inflammatory process has destroyed much of the smooth articular surface of a joint (eburnation), fibrous and osseous adhesions between the apposed surfaces tend to form, and marginal osteophytes (exostoses) develop. After some time, for instance several months, the two bones will be completely joined together by a union of solid bone. This process of bony fusion is called **ankylosis** and the obliterated joint is said to be ankylosed. It is interesting to note that after a few years (in the human) two ankylosed bones are

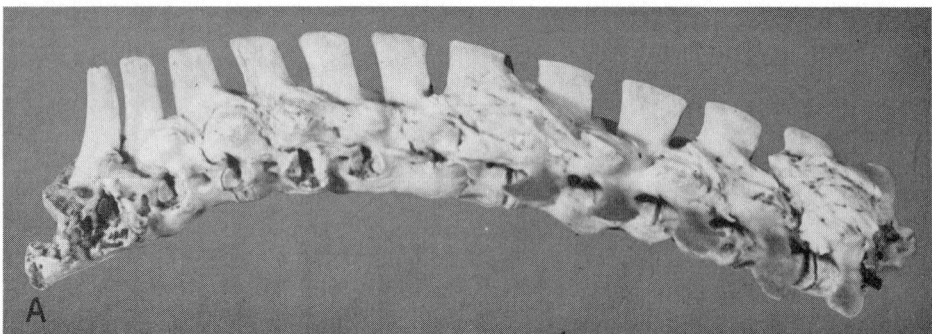

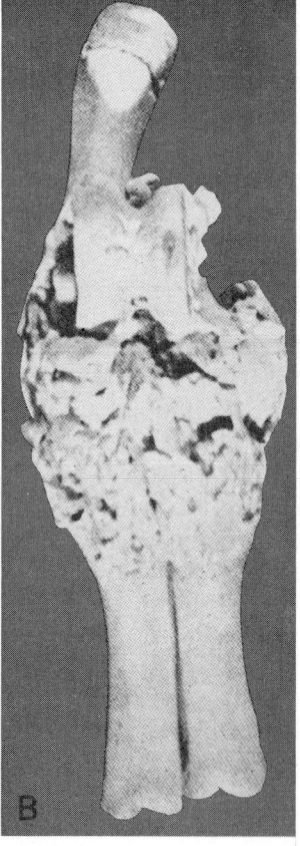

Fig. 19–20. *A*, Thoracic and lumbar spondylitis in a swine which, at the age of three months, was inoculated with a pure culture of *Erysipelothrix rhusiopathiae*. Most of the joints developed a proliferative and ankylosing inflammation which was continuously progressive until euthanasia at three years of age. (Courtesy of Dr. Dennis Sikes, Georgia Sch. Vet. Med.) *B*, Tarsometatarsal arthritis in same animal as *A*. (Courtesy of Dr. Dennis Sikes.)

united as a single bone, the marrow cavity passing completely through what was formerly the epiphyses and the joint cavity.

Chronic proliferative or ankylosing arthritis, like the mild serous type, may be due to trauma, such as repeated strains, and the concussion of severe work on hard surfaces in the case of horses. Chronic arthritis may also follow infectious processes such as swine erysipelas and may develop from an acute arthritis. However, chronic arthritis is more frequently seen without an association with trauma or infection, in which case it has been termed primary chronic arthritis or primary osteoarthritis. The cause is not usually known, but structural defects, congenital or acquired, predispose to osteoarthritis. For example, osteoarthritis is a feature of hip dysplasia in dogs, "wobbles" in horses, necrosis of the femoral head in dogs, and canine elbow dysplasia. The latter disorder, which is believed to be of hereditary origin, is most frequent in German Shepherd dogs and is associated with an ununited anconeal process.

Acute suppurative or acute fibrinous arthritides (which may progress to chronic arthritis) may be due to wounds which open the joint cavity to infective microorganisms, but they are more frequent as articular localizations of generalized septicemic or pyemic infections. The most common of these is the pyosepticemia of the newborn (pyosepticemia neonatorum, "joint-ill") resulting from infection of the umbilicus at birth. A variety of microorganisms may be associated with infectious arthritis in both newborn and adult animals. In foals, *Shigella equirulus* is the most common organism recovered, but other organisms such as *Streptococcus spp.*, *Salmonella spp.*, and *Escherichia coli* are also recovered with frequency. *Erysipelas rhusiopathiae* is notable for causing a chronic low grade arthritis and periarthritis in swine, lambs, and turkeys. *Corynebacterium ovis*, *Escherichia coli*, and *Streptococcus spp.* are also frequent causes of arthritis in sheep. *Mycoplasma spp.* are important causes of arthritis in swine, sheep, goats, and cattle. A member of the psittacosis-lymphogranuloma group of agents is a cause of arthritis in sheep. *Hemophilus suis* produces polyserositis with arthritis in swine. *Brucella spp.* and *Streptococcus spp.* also not infrequently cause a suppurative arthritis in swine. Tuberculous arthritis which may develop in any species and which often localizes in the vertebral column is characterized by the usual granulomatous reaction, which in a joint is of very limited extent. In rats, mycoplasma, *Streptobacillus moniliformis*, *Diplococcus pneumoniae*, and *Corynebacterium kutscheri* are frequent causes of arthritis. It should be clear from this list that arthritis is an important manifestation of many infectious diseases, but noticeably absent are generalized infections of dogs and cats. Aside from occasional joint involvement in infections such as cryptococcosis, there is little information about infectious joint disease in these species. Most examples of infectious arthritis in dogs and cats are the result of penetrating wounds in which case the ordinary pyogenic bacteria are responsible.

Canine Rheumatoid Arthritis. Rheumatoid arthritis is an important debilitating disease of undetermined etiology involving human patients. A canine disease with many critical similarities to the human disease is now known. The canine disease is manifest by severe polyarthritis with swollen, painful joints, fever and neutrophilia (in initial stages), radiographic and pathologic evidence of arthritis, and a positive test for rheumatoid factor. In some cases, evidence for presence of systemic lupus erythematosus may also be present. The lesions in the joints include pitting and erosion of the articular cartilages, fibrinous exudate in synovial fluid, and thickening of the synovial membrane and its underlying stroma with aggregations of plasma cells within the synovium. Villous tags, coated with fibrin, project into the joint space. Adjacent arterioles are surrounded by neutrophils, and nearby collagen bundles are often necrotic. Radiographically, a jagged "saw-tooth" image is seen at the joint surface due to erosions of the apposing articular surfaces. Some joints involved become fixed in position (*ankylosis*).

Progressive Feline Polyarthritis. This disease entity, described by Pederson, et al. (1975) appears to be a specific entity in cats. The etiology is at present unknown. The clinical signs include swollen painful joints, particularly the carpal and tarsal joints, fever, lymphadenopathy, neutrophilia, and sometimes lymphocytosis. Tests for lupus erythematosus (LE) factor and rheumatoid (R) factor are negative.

The joint fluid, removed by aspiration, is

turbid, yellowish, and contains greatly increased numbers of neutrophils and lymphocytes. Cultures so far have not yielded mycoplasma or bacteria. No organisms have yet been demonstrated with the electron microscope. Feline syncytial-forming virus has been isolated, but appears to be non-pathogenic.

Radiographic findings include a radiolucent zone around the affected articulation, presence of periarticular new bone, and periarticular osteophytes.

The gross lesions are often found with symmetrical distribution in paired joints and are sometimes accompanied by tenosynovitis. In early stages, the lesions in the joints involve the synovial membrane which is thickened and often covered with fibrinous exudate infiltrated by numerous neutrophils. In older lesions, the joint capsule is infiltrated by lymphocytes, plasma cells, and neutrophils, and is both hyperemic and hyperplastic. Granulation tissue becomes evident, particularly at the margin of the joint. This inflammatory exudate may bridge the articular surfaces and lead to early ankylosis. Ossification completes the bony ankylosis.

Glomerulonephritis is also described in affected cats. Its significance is as yet unknown, but believed related to the immunologic processes involved in the polyarthritis.

Polyarthritis in Greyhounds. This appears to be an enzootic disease of unknown etiology in young Greyhounds in Australia (Huxtable and Davis, 1976). The significant gross lesions described so far are limited to the affected joints and their draining lymph nodes. In the joints, an excessive amount of turbid, cloudy to opaque yellowish-brown fluid is present, containing shreds or clots of fibrin. The synovial membrane is thickened, yellowish-brown, and may have fibrin adhering to its surface. Hemorrhages may be evident in the membrane. The articular cartilage is involved by several or many deep erosions, sometimes coalescent into large areas of erosion.

The microscopic lesions include mild to severe involvement of the synovial membrane, with fibrovascular villi, infiltration by neutrophils, plasma cells, and lymphocytes. In some cases, fibrinous exudate attached to the villi may contain hemorrhages.

Enzootic Polyarthritis of Goats. This problem has been reported from Switzerland and Japan. The disease, more prevalent in summer months, affects young animals initially and may persist throughout the life of the animal. Swollen, painful joints with lameness are usually the first signs seen. The carpal joints are most frequently affected and both joints are similarly involved. The etiology has not been established.

In the early stages, the synovial fluid is excessive and may be clear, turbid, or blood-tinged. The synovial membranes are edematous, thickened, and hyperemic. The regional lymph nodes are swollen and may occasionally contain multiple abscesses. Microscopically, exudation of lymphocytes, histiocytes, and plasma cells into the hyperemic and edematous villous synovia, is usually seen. Lymphoid nodules are often formed in the underlying stroma. The villi are elongated, infiltrated by cellular exudate, and often covered by fibrinous exudate. In some cases, diffuse necrosis of the synovial membrane may be found. The enlarged joints may eventually be ankylosed by exostoses.

Ankylosing Spondylitis. Also known as spondylosis deformans, this disease is most frequent in dogs, cats, cattle, and swine and relatively rare in other domestic animals. It results from the formation and ultimate fusion of osteophytes (exostoses) on the ventral aspect of adjacent vertebral bodies. In dogs and possibly other species, ventral prolapse of intervertebral discs is believed to be the cause. Infectious spondylitis can also lead to ankylosis of vertebrae. It has been described as an occupational hazard of stud bulls, but the cause has not been established. The disease in cats is usually due to hypervitaminosis A.

Hemophilia. Hemophilic arthropathy is not common owing to the fact that many animals with hemophilia die at an early age. However, hemophilic joint disease has been reported in dogs, and the lesions include hemarthrosis and hemosiderosis, fibrosis, and proliferation of synovial tissues. In advanced cases, degeneration of articular cartilage and osteoarthritis are present.

Navicular Disease. This is a bursitis and terminal arthritis involving the equine distal sesamoid, or navicular bone, usually in a foreleg. The earlier changes are hyperemia and inflammation of the lining surfaces of the bursa podotrochlearis; these are soon followed by erosion and ulceration of the cartilage which serves as a bearing surface for the deep flexor tendon; the latter becomes frayed and will eventually rupture. The bone itself becomes rarefied and inflamed and has been known to disintegrate.

Ackerman, N., Johnson, J.H., and Dorn, C.R.: Navicular disease in the horse: risk factors, radiographic changes, and response to therapy. J. Am. Vet. Med. Assoc., *170*:183–187, 1977.

Cross, G.M., Penny, R.H.C., and Claxton, P.D.: The abattoir incidence of polyarthritis in pigs in Australia. Aust. Vet. J., *47*:126, 1971.

Cutlip, R.C., and Cheville, N.F.: Structure of synovial membrane of sheep. Am. J. Vet. Res., *34*:45–50, 1973.

Halliwell, R.E.W., Lavelle, R.B., and Butt, K.M.: Canine rheumatoid arthritis—a review and a case report. J. Small Anim. Pract., *13*:239–248, 1972.

Hoopes, P.J., et al.: Suppurative arthritis in an infant orangutan. J. Am. Vet. Med. Assoc., *173*:1145–1147, 1978.

Hough, A.J., Banfield, W.G., Mottram, F.C., and Sokoloff, L.: The osteochondral junction of mammalian joints: an ultrastructural and microanalytic study. Lab. Invest., *31*:685–695, 1974.

Huxtable, C.R., and Davis, P.E.: The pathology of polyarthritis in young Greyhounds. J. Comp. Pathol., *86*:11–21, 1976.

Imrie, R.C.: Animal models of arthritis. Lab. Anim. Sci., *26*:345–351, 1976.

Lewis, R.M., and Hathaway, J.E.: Canine systemic lupus erythematosus presenting as a symmetrical polyarthritis. J. Small Anim. Pract., *8*:273–284, 1967.

Lust, G., Pronsky, W., and Sherman, D.M.: Biochemical and ultrastructural observations in normal and degenerative canine articular cartilage. Am. J. Vet. Res., *33*:2429–2440, 1972.

Nakagawa, M., Motoi, Y., Iizuka, M., and Azuma, R.: Histopathology of enzootic chronic polyarthritis of goats in Japan. Natl. Inst. Anim. Health Q., *11*:191–200, 1971.

Nemeth, F., Morgan, J.P., and Badoux, D.M.: Equine sesamoiditis. Tijdschr. Diergeneeskd, *98*:988–994, 1973.

Newton, C.D., et al.: Rheumatoid arthritis in dogs. J. Am. Vet. Med. Assoc., *168*:113–120, 1976.

Nickels, F.A., Grant, B.K., and Lincoln, S.D.: Villonodular synovitis of the equine metacarpophalangeal joint. J. Am. Vet. Med. Assoc., *168*:1043–1046, 1976.

Pedersen, N.C., et al.: Chronic progressive polyarthritis of the cat. Feline Pract., *5*:42–51, 1975.

Pedersen, N.C., Pool, R.C., Castles, J.J., and Weisner, K.: Noninfectious canine arthritis: rheumatoid arthritis. J. Am. Vet. Med. Assoc., *169*:295–303, 1976.

Pedersen, N.C., et al.: Noninfectious canine arthritis: the inflammatory nonerosive arthritides. J. Am. Vet. Med. Assoc., *169*:304–310, 1976.

Persson, L.: On the synovia in horses. A clinical and experimental study. Acta. Vet. Scand. (Suppl.), *35*:1–77, 1971.

Sikes, D., Hayes, F.A., Prestwood, A.K., and Smith, J.F.: Ankylosing spondylitis and polyarthritis of the dog: Physiopathologic changes of tissues. Am. J. Vet. Res., *31*:703–712, 1970.

Sikes, D., Fletcher, O.J., Jr., and Jones, T.J.: Agglutinating factor eluted from the erythrocytes of swine with rheumatoid arthritis. Am. J. Vet. Res., *31*:2191–2196, 1970.

Sokoloff, L., Snell, K.C., and Stewart, H.L.: Spinal ankylosis in old rhesus monkeys. Clin. Orthop., *61*:285–293, 1968.

Stünzi, H., Büchi, H.F., Le Roy, H.L., and Leemann, W.: Endemische arthritis chronica bei Ziegen. Schweiz. Arch. Tierheilkd., *106*:778–788, 1964.

Thomson, R.G.: Vertebral body osteophytes in bulls. Suppl. Pathol. Vet., *6*:1–65, 1969.

Van Pelt, R.W., and Langham, R.F.: Synovial fluid changes produced by infectious arthritis in cattle. Am. J. Vet. Res., *29*:507–516, 1968.

Van Pelt, R.W., and Langham, R.F.: Degenerative joint disease of the carpus and fetlock in cattle. J. Am. Vet. Med. Assoc., *157*:953–961, 1970.

Van Pelt, R.W., Riley, W.F., Jr., and Tillotson, P.J.: Stifle disease (gonitis) in horses: clinicopathologic findings and intra-articular therapy. J. Am. Vet. Med. Assoc., *157*:1173–1186, 1970.

Van Pelt, R.W.: Monarticular idiopathic septic arthritis in horses. J. Am. Vet. Med. Assoc., *158*:1658–1673, 1971.

Van Pelt, R.W.: Idiopathic septic arthritis in dairy

cattle. J. Am. Vet. Med. Assoc., *161*:278–284, 1972.

Van Pelt, R.W.: Idiopathoic tarsitis in postparturient dairy cows: clinicopathologic findings and treatment. J. Am. Vet. Med. Assoc., *162*:284–290, 1973.

Van Pelt, R.W.: Interpretation of synovial fluid findings in the horse. J. Am. Vet. Med. Assoc., *165*:91–95, 1974.

Van Pelt, R.W.: Tarsal degenerative joint disease in cattle; blood and synovial fluid changes. Am. J. Vet. Res., *36*:1009–1014, 1975.

Watt, D.A., Bamford, V., and Nairn, M.E.: *Actinobacillus seminis* as a cause of polyarthritis and posthitis in sheep. Aust. Vet. J., *46*:515, 1970.

Wiltberger, H., and Lust, G.: Ultrastructure of canine articular cartilage: comparison of normal and de- generative (osteoarthritic) hip joints. Am. J. Vet. Res., *36*:727–740, 1975.

Neoplasms of Bone and Cartilage

Osteosarcoma (Osteogenic Sarcoma, Periosteal Sarcoma). Malignant neoplasms, identified as osteosarcomas, are known in most species, but are more frequent in the dog, especially in the giant breeds. These tumors usually originate near the epiphysis of long bones, but may arise from periosteum at any site (Fig. 19–21.) Two extra-osseous sites of origin are

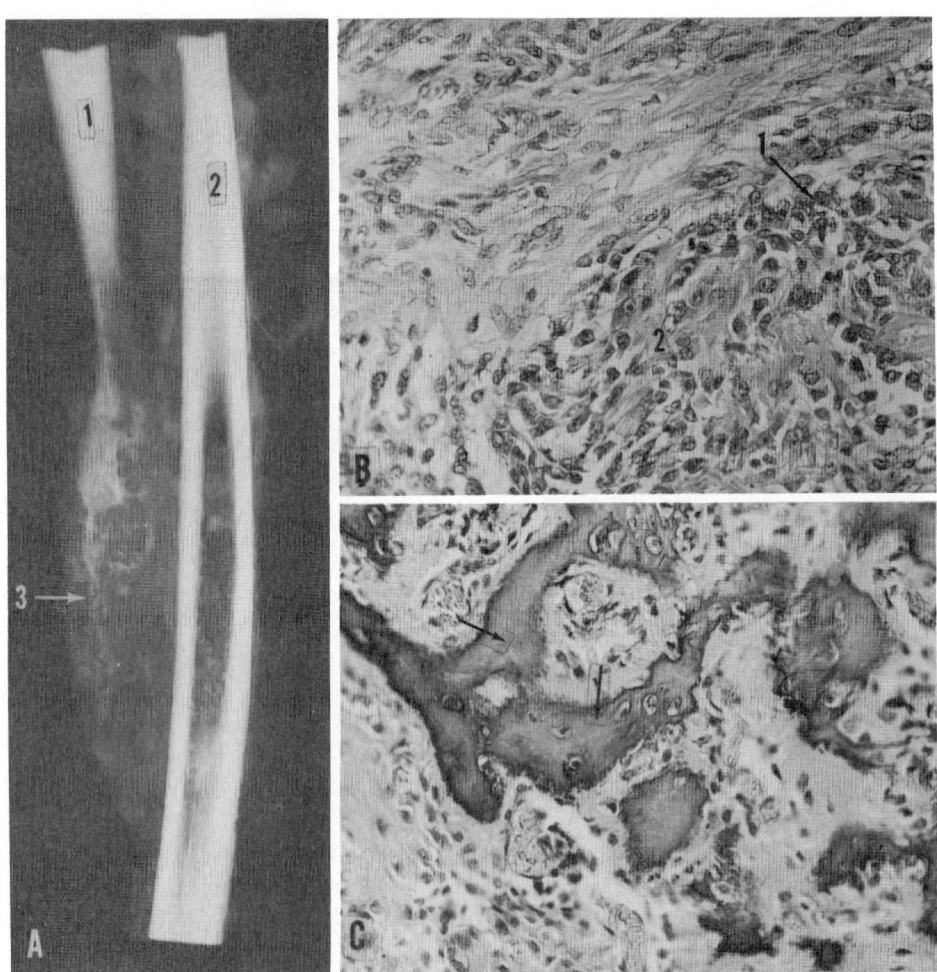

Fig. 19–21. Osteosarcoma of the ulna of a ten-year-old female Golden Retriever. *A,* Radiograph of the neoplasm (*3*) in the distal third of the ulna (*1*). The radius (*2*) is not directly involved. *B,* Photomicrograph (× 250) in an area of the neoplasm made up of densely packed cells (*1*) which form osteoid (*2*). *C,* Photomicrograph (× 250) of the same tumor from an area with irregular spicules of new bone (arrows). (Courtesy of Armed Forces Institute of Pathology.) Contributor: Fourth Medical Field Laboratory, U.S. Army.

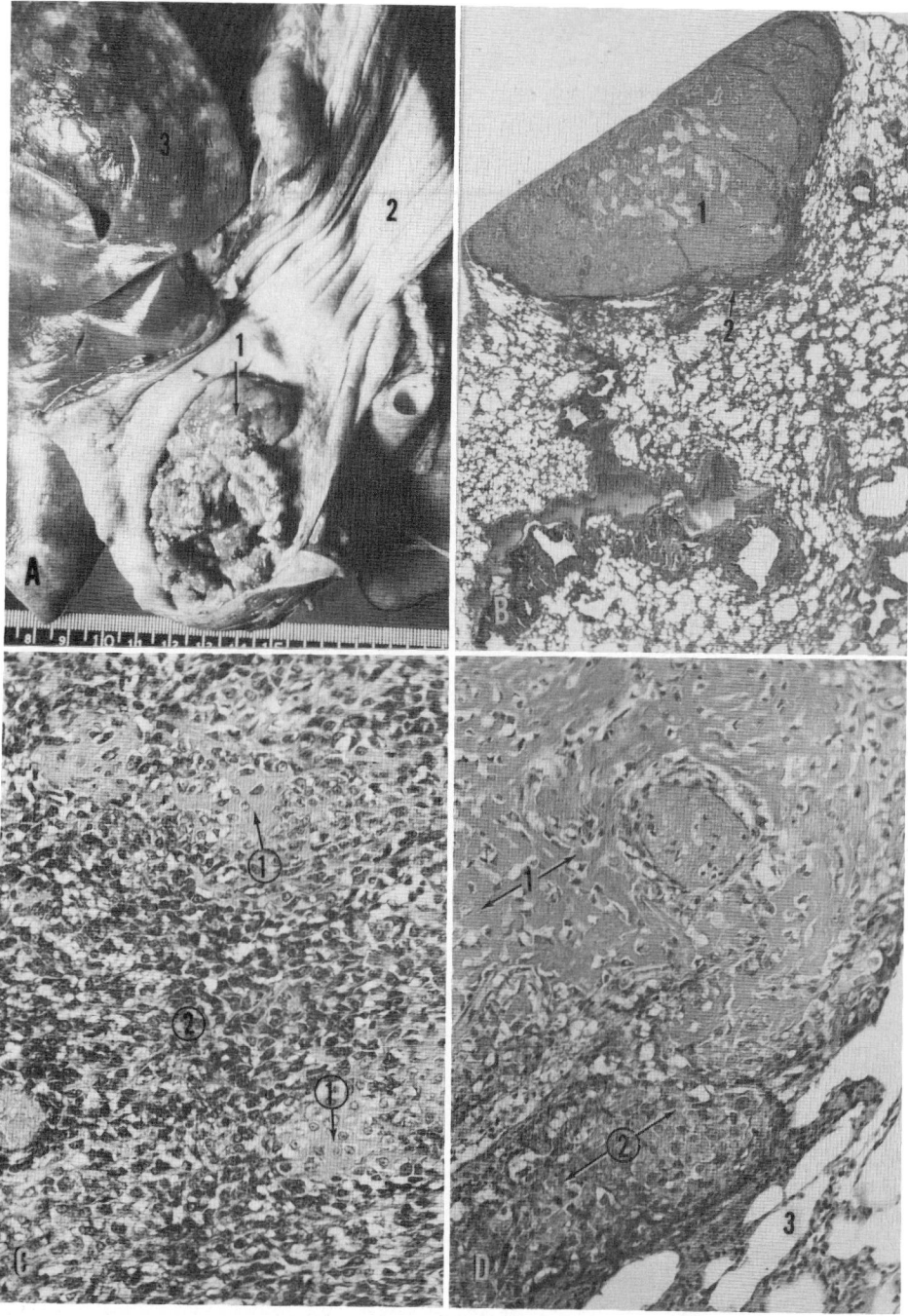

Fig. 19–22. Osteosarcoma, primary, in the esophagus of a seven- year-old male hound. The neoplasm was associated with long-standing infection of the esophagus by *Spirocerca lupi. A,* The tumor *(1)* involves the terminal esophagus *(2).* The lung is identified at *(3). B,* Metastasis *(1)* of osteosarcoma to lung (× 12). *C,* An area of the tumor (× 150) in which osteoid *(1)* is formed by the densely packed hyperchromatic cells *(2). D,* Higher magnification (× 150) of *B,* showing osteoid *(1),* spindle-shaped cells *(2),* and alveolus *(3).* Bone was formed in other parts of this tumor. (Courtesy of Armed Forces Institute of Pathology.) Contributor: Dr. H.R. Seibold.

known in dogs. One such site is in the esophagus (Fig. 19–22), as a part of the lesion produced by the spirurid worm, *Spirocerca lupi*. The second extra-osseous site is the canine mammary gland as one component of a mixed tumor. The radiographic appearance of osteosarcoma in bone usually features a radio-translucent mass originating near the epiphysis of a long bone, invading nearby bone and contiguous tissues. Metastasis occurs readily, particularly to the lungs.

Osteosarcoma is the most frequent primary neoplasm of bone in the dog. In one study (Ling, et al., 1974), among 133 primary tumors of bone was the following distribution: Osteosarcomas 64.6%; chondrosarcomas 11.3%; fibrosarcomas 9.0%; hemangiosarcomas 6.0%; osteomas 6.0% and chondromas 3.0%. The other malignant tumors of bone (chondrosarcoma, fibrosarcoma, and hemangiosarcoma) have a similar tendency to metastasize, especially to lung, as does the osteosarcoma.

The characteristic feature of the osteosarcoma is the presence of neoplastic osteoblasts which are seen histologically as short, spindle- or triangular-shaped cells with plump ovoid nuclei, usually closely packed together. They are oriented to point in various directions, and do not lie parallel to one another in bundles. The critical identifying characteristic of these cells is their ability to produce **osteoid**, the ground substance or matrix of bone, which may or may not become calcified to form bone. Newly formed osteoid is extracellular, dense, darkly eosinophilic staining material which may be somewhat fibrillar. Osteocytes may be trapped within it (Fig. 19–21)—a feature also of normal bone. Multinucleated cells may also be present. Poorly formed, unorganized cartilage may also be formed in some osteosarcomas.

Osteoma. From its name, osteoma is identified as a benign tumor of bone. Rarely occurring in animals, it may be confused with inflammatory or hereditary exostoses. This tumor is most often iden-

tified arising in the skull, and is made up of irregular spicules of bone, usually forming a spherical mass. It grows slowly by expansion and does not contain undifferentiated osteoblasts.

Chondrosarcoma. This tumor is made up of irregular, disorderly masses of immature cartilage which invade tissue and metastasize through the lymphatic and blood circulation. The cartilage cells in lacunae of cartilaginous matrix vary in size and do not maintain any orderly polarity. Malignancy is evident by its invasiveness and tendency to metastasize to the lungs and elsewhere. Bone is not formed. This neoplasm tends to arise from anatomic sites where normal cartilage exists, such as near rib cartilage, scapular cartilage, pelvis, and the nasal turbinates or septum (Fig. 19–23).

In the dog, most often affected with bone tumors, chondrosarcomas are second in frequency to osteosarcomas. They are also quite malignant and tend to recur when excised. Slightly more success following surgical removal is experienced, however, with chondrosarcoma when compared to osteosarcoma.

Chondroma. Benign forms of cartilaginous tumor are not frequent, but are reported and are distinguished from chondrosarcoma by their lack of local invasiveness, more orderly arrangement of the cartilage cells, and closer resemblance to normal mature cartilage. Cartilage growth in inherited chondromatosis and multiple exostosis may be distinguished by their multiple sites of growth, inherited features, and biologic behavior.

Cartilage Analogue of Fibromatosis (Juvenile Aponeurotic Fibroma). A disease entity which has some features of chondrosarcoma has been described in dogs under the above names. Radiographic study reveals rather diffuse nodular or stippled densities in soft tissues around the skull. These are accompanied by rarefaction of the underlying cranial bones. Microscopic examination reveals islands of chondroid tissue surrounded by spindle-

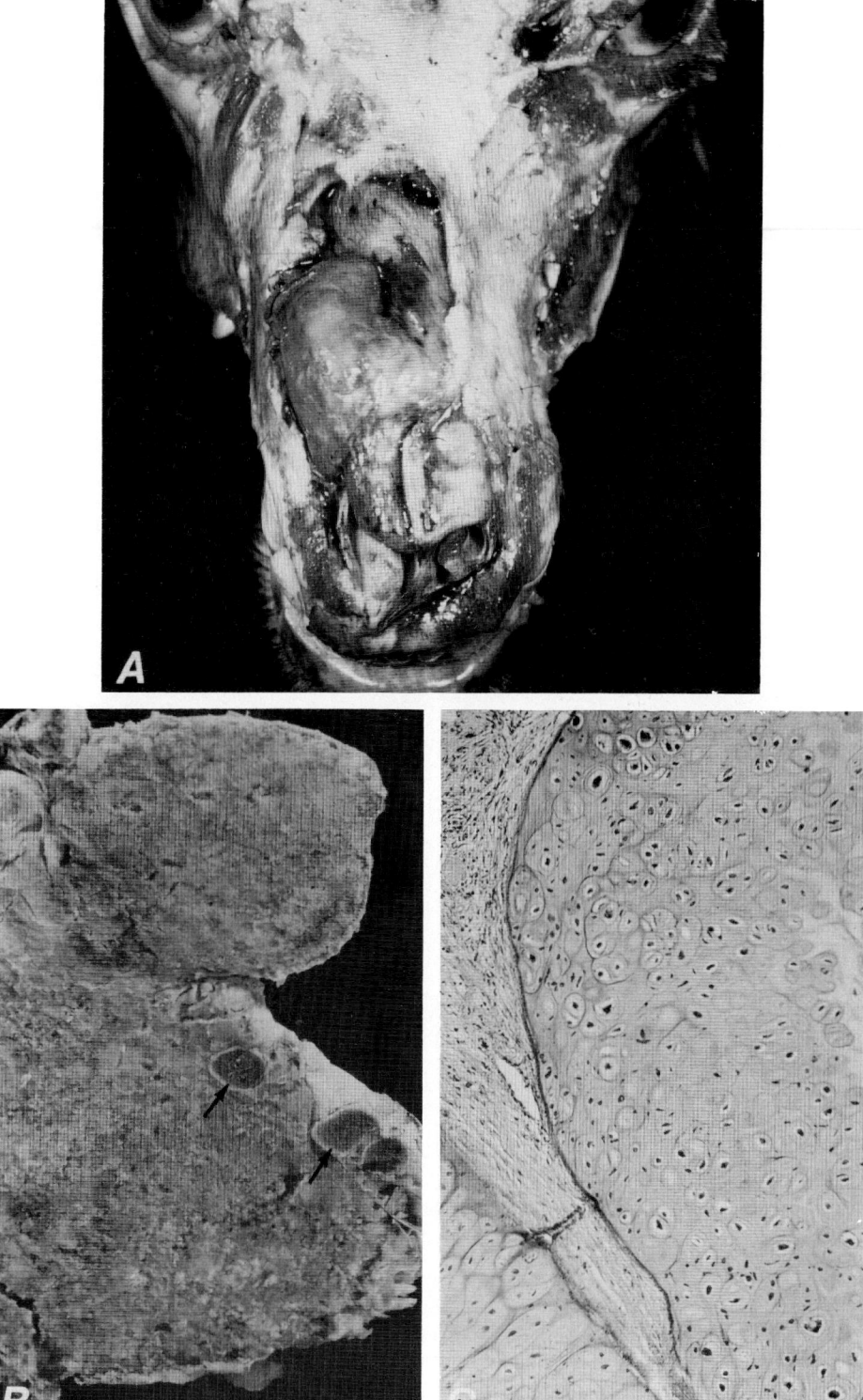

Fig. 19–23. *A*, Chondrosarcoma of nasal septum of a seven-year-old male pointer. (Courtesy of Angell Memorial Animal Hospital.) *B*, Chondrosarcoma of the ribs of a five-year-old ewe. The tumor metastasized to the lung. Contributor: Dr. C.L. Davis. *C*, Chondrosarcoma (× 120) of the ribs of an aged ewe. Note cells with irregular polarity and variable size in cartilaginous matrix. Metastasis to lungs also occurred in this case. (Courtesy of Armed Forces Institute of Pathology.) Contributor: Dr. C.L. Davis.

shaped cells in connective tissue. Foci of calcification may be seen in the fibroblastic cells. This lesion is differentiated from chondrosarcoma by the absence of nuclear atypia of the cartilage cells and by the presence of a conspicuous fibrous element (Liu and Dorfman, 1974). This disease does not result in metastasis, but the skull and brain may be invaded in some cases. The etiology of this lesion is unknown.

Fibrosarcoma. This tumor may arise from connective tissue anywhere in the body and occasionally is primary in bone. The cells are pleomorphic and vary from high undifferentiated, roughly spindle-shaped cells with round to ovoid nuclei, often in mitosis, to elongated cells in interlacing bundles resembling immature connective tissue. This tendency for groups of cells to be parallel to one another is a feature of value in identifying the fibrosarcoma.

Fibromas. These tumors are extremely infrequent as primary tumors of bone, but have been reported. They are circumscribed, usually encapsulated, and made up of more mature collagenous connective tissue. Their course is benign, although they may be locally disfiguring.

Hemangiosarcoma (Malignant Hemangio-endothelioma). A tumor arising from endothelium, the hemangiosarcoma may be primary in almost any tissue, but in most species it more frequently originates in spleen, liver, heart muscle (atrium), and bone. The histologic features include neo-

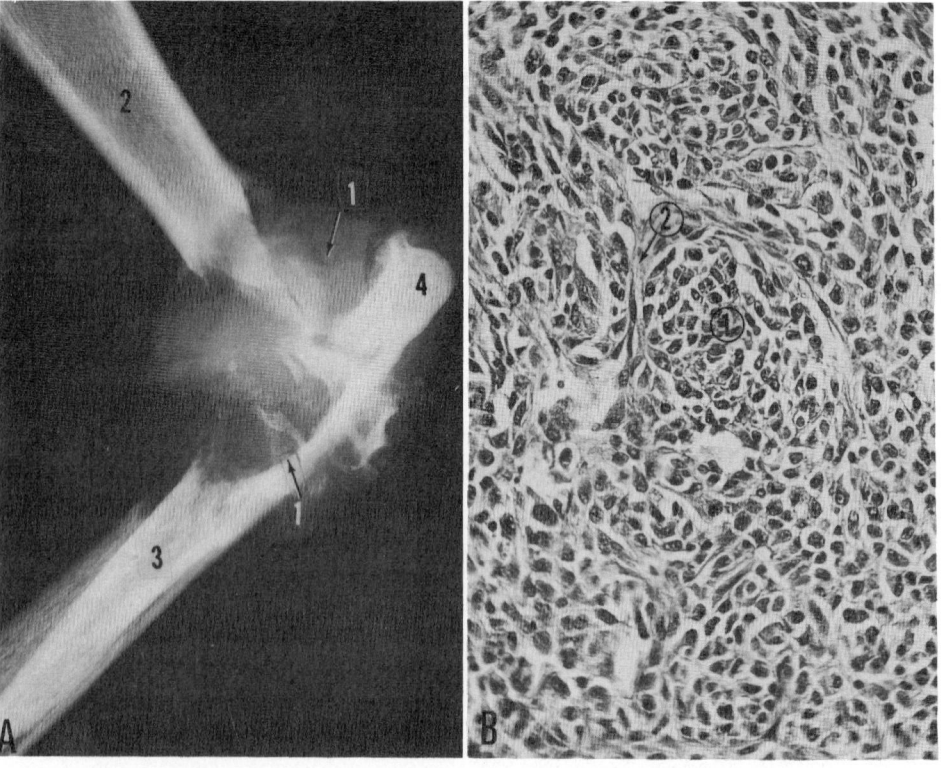

Fig. 19–24. Malignant synovioma involving elbow joint, humerus, radius and ulna of an 11-year-old female Spitz dog. *A,* Radiograph of the tumor (*1*), which replaces the joint and destroys the distal part of the humerus (*2*), proximal part of the radius (*3*) and ulna (not shown). The olecranon (*4*) is partially invaded. *B,* Photomicrograph (× 330) of the highly cellular neoplasm (*1*) with indistinct stroma (*2*). (Courtesy of Armed Forces Institute of Pathology.) Contributor: Dr. Leo L. Lieberman.

plastic cells with large hyperchromatic nuclei and scant cytoplasm. The cells tend to form vascular spaces, often quite large, which may be distended with blood. The blood vessels are clearly formed by tumor cells and are not part of the supporting stroma. Mitoses are common, multiple sites may occur, and metastases can be expected. These tumors destroy bone locally as do osteosarcomas and chondrosarcomas and metastasize just as readily.

Hemangiomas. These tumors are more frequent in the subcutis and dermis of most species, but are rarely seen in bone. Vascular spaces, growth by expansion, and few if any solid nests of neoplastic epithelial cells are histologic features of these tumors.

Synovioma. Locally destructive and metastasizing tumors infrequently arise from the synovial membrane of a joint (Fig. 19–24). The tumor is made up of solid masses of cells with round to ovoid nuclei and irregularly stellate cytoplasm. A radiolucent mass usually invades and replaces bone on both sides of an articulation. In this respect, synovioma differs from osteosarcoma and chondrosarcoma.

Giant Cell Tumor of Bone, Osteoclastoma. Not too infrequently there occurs on the end of one of the long bones of the human limbs a tumor of very bizarre microscopic structure consisting chiefly of large, dark-staining, fusiform nuclei in a moderately fibrous stroma. With these are large multi-nucleated giant cells in great numbers. The histologic picture is highly bizarre and suggestive of malignancy, but clinical experience shows the tumor to be practically always benign. A growth of similar histological structure occurs on the gums and is called an epulis. Epulides have been reported occasionally in the dog.

In general, this tumor is rarely encountered in animals, although multinucleated osteoclasts in an osteosarcoma may cause

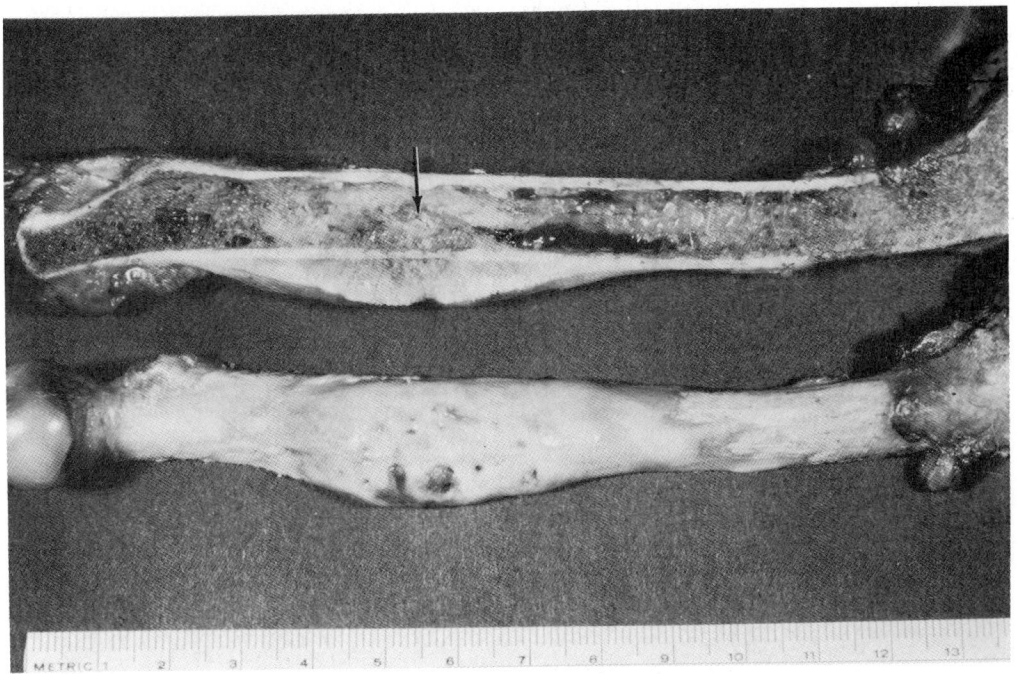

Fig. 19–25. Secondary, metastatic tumor in femur of a 12-year-old spayed female Kerry Blue Terrier. The primary was a bronchiolar-alveolar cell carcinoma of the lung. (Courtesy of Angell Memorial Animal Hospital.)

this diagnosis to be considered. The epulis in the gums of the dog must be differentiated from the much more common non-neoplastic lesion called "fibrous hyperplasia of the gum," "fibrous epulis" or "gingival hypertrophy."

Secondary Tumors of Bone. Malignant neoplasms of man and animals may metastasize to bone from such primary sites as mammary gland, lung, oral mucosa, skin and subcutis, and thyroid, among others. Surprisingly, reports of secondary bone tumors in the literature include only man, dog, cat, and one lion, leading to the likely conclusion that most secondary neoplasms in bone of animals have not been recognized or reported.

The clinical manifestations of secondary tumors in bone include: lameness, pain, swelling, and less frequently, paraplegia. The radiographic appearance is often indistinguishable from a primary tumor. For example, secondary (metastatic) tumors may localize near the epiphysis, expand extensively, and be radiolucent. Sometimes they may contain spicules of bone. Definitive diagnosis is based upon identification of the tissue in histologic sections.

Some neoplasms, arising adjacent to bone, may either invade the bone or alter it by compression. Squamous cell carcinomas arising in the oral or pharyngeal mucosa may invade the mandible or maxilla, although their usual route is to the lymph nodes and then to lungs. Epidermal inclusion cysts and epidermoid cysts may be found deep in bone as in the case of the Rhodesian Ridgeback. In this instance, squamous epithelium extends deep into the vertebrae at the midline, sometimes forming cysts at this site. Neoplasms of hemopoietic cells may originate in and displace the bone marrow.

Benjamin, S.A., et al.: Occurrence of hemangiosarcomas in Beagles with internally deposited radionuclides. Cancer Res., *35*:1745–1755, 1975.

Brodey, R.S., Reid, C.F., and Sauer, R.M.: Metastatic bone neoplasms in the dog. J. Am. Vet. Med. Assoc., *148*:29–43, 1966.

Brodey, R.S., Misdorp, W., Riser, W.H., and van der Heul, R.O.: Canine skeletal chondrosarcoma: a clinicopathologic study of 35 cases. J. Am. Vet. Med. Assoc., *165*:68–78, 1974.

Cello, R.M., and Olander, H.: Cord compression and paraplegia in a dog secondary to pancreatic carcinoma. J. Am. Vet. Med. Assoc., *142*:1407–1409, 1963.

Charles, R.T., and Turusov, V.S.: Bone tumours in CF-1 mice. Lab. Anim., *8*:137–144, 1974.

Chesney, S.C., and Allen, J.R.: Spontaneous osteogenic sarcoma in a stumptail (*Macaca arctoides*) monkey. J. Natl. Cancer Inst., *49*:139–146, 1972.

Diaz, E.E., Bianchi, C.F., and Maulion, A.F.: Tarsal synovioma in a dog. Gac. Vet., *36*:526–528, 1974.

Ford, G.H., Empson, R.N., Plopper, C.G., and Brown, P.H.: Giant-cell tumor of soft parts: A report of an equine and a feline case. Vet. Pathol., *12*:428–433, 1975.

Goedegebuure, S.A.: Secondary bone tumors in the dog. Vet. Pathol., *16*:520–529, 1979.

Kas, N.P., van der Heul, R.O., and Misdorp, W.: Metastatic bone neoplasms in dogs, cats, and a lion (with some comparative remarks on the situation in man). Zentralbl. Vet. Med., *17A*:909–919, 1971.

Knecht, C.D., and Greene, J.A.: Osteoma of the zygomatic arch in a cat. J. Am. Vet. Med. Assoc., *171*:1077–1078, 1977.

Ling, G.V., Morgan, J.P., and Pool, R.R.: Primary bone tumors in the dog: a combined clinical radiographic, and histologic approach to early diagnosis. J. Am. Vet. Med. Assoc., *165*:55–67, 1974.

Linnabary, R.D., Holscher, M.A., Page, D.L., and Fitzpatrick, D.: Primitive multipotential primary sarcoma of bone in a cat. Vet. Pathol., *15*:432–434, 1978.

Liu, S.K., and Dorfman, H.D.: The cartilage analogue of fibromatosis (juvenile aponeurotic fibroma) in dogs. Vet. Pathol., *11*:60–67, 1974.

Liu, S.K., and Dorfman, H.D.: Intra-osseous epidermoid cysts in two dogs. Vet. Pathol., *11*:230–234, 1974.

Liu, S.K., Dorfman, H.D., and Patnaik, A.K.: Primary and secondary bone tumors in the cat. J. Small Anim. Pract., *15*:141–156, 1974.

Misdorp, W., and Den Herder, E.A.: Bone metastasis in mammary cancer. A report of 10 cases in the female dog and some comparison with human cases. Br. J. Cancer, *20*:496–501, 1966.

Owen, L.N.: Bone Tumours in Man and Animals. London, Butterworth, 1969.

Pool, R.R., and Wolf, H.G.: An unusual case of canine osteosarcoma. Cancer, *34*:771–779, 1974.

Quigley, P.J., et al.: Two cases of hemangiosarcomas of the radius in the dog. Vet. Rec., *77*:1207–1209, 1965.

Quigley, P.J., Leedale, A., and Dawson, I.M.P.: Carcinoma of mandible of cat and dog simulating osteosarcoma. J. Comp. Pathol., *82*:15–18, 1972.

Riser, W.H., Brodey, R.S., and Biery, D.N.: Bone infarctions associated with malignant bone tumors in dogs. J. Am. Vet. Med. Assoc., *160*:411–421, 1972.

Salm, R., and Field, J.: Osteosarcoma in a rabbit. J. Pathol. Bact., *89*:400–402, 1965.

Sullivan, D.J.: Cartilaginous tumors (chondroma and chondrosarcoma) in animals. Am. J. Vet. Res., *21*:531–535, 1960.

Thurman, G.B., et al.: Growth dynamics of Beagle osteosarcomas. Growth, *35*:119–125, 1971.

Tjalma, R.A.: Canine bone sarcoma: estimation of relative risk as a function of body size. J. Natl. Cancer Inst., *36*:1137–1150, 1966.

Wolke, R.E., and Nielsen, S.W.: Site incidence of canine osteosarcoma. J. Small Anim. Pract., *7*:489–492, 1966.

CHAPTER 20

The Respiratory System

Our approach to the respiratory system in this chapter will be to consider disease processes of undetermined etiology and others not described elsewhere in this book. In general, pathologic entities due to specific causes are considered in earlier chapters. Several conditions that have profound effects on the respiratory system include: disturbances of circulation (Chap. 5), viral infections (Chap. 9), bacterial and fungal infections (Chaps. 11 and 12), infections due to mycoplasma, rickettsia, and spirochaetes (Chap. 10), protozoal diseases (Chap. 13), parasitic helminths and arthropods (Chap. 14), and extraneous poisons (Chap. 16).

The pathogenetic mechanisms will be discussed in those cases in which they are reasonably well established; lesions and diagnostic criteria will be described in as succinct a manner as possible. Anatomic and species differences will be referred to in those conditions in which they are significant factors.

UPPER AIR PASSAGES

The mucous membrane of the nares, paranasal sinuses, pharynx, larynx, trachea, and bronchi is subject to injury by chemical and infectious agents brought to it in the inspired air. Chemical injury is infrequent, being due to accidental inhalation of such gases as ammonia and chlorine, as well as war gases; injury by

infectious microorganisms, including viruses, is frequent and often severe. As might be expected, the more external of the respiratory passages are more accessible to such injurious agents; the deeper structures, such as the bronchi, are less often attacked, but the effects of infections here are most severe and more ominous than in the upper part of the respiratory tract. It is entirely possible, however, for these mucous membranes to be attacked via the hematogenous route by infections which have an affinity for them. For instance, when material containing the virus of bovine malignant catarrhal fever is injected subcutaneously, the respiratory mucous membranes become the principal seat of disease just as if the infection had gained primary access to them.

Inflammations

Rhinitis (inflammation of the nasal mucosa), **sinusitis, pharyngitis, laryngitis, tracheitis,** and **bronchitis** usually commence as acute mucous (catarrhal) inflammations of the respective mucous membranes. They tend somewhat later to become purulent or fibrinous, depending on the nature of the infectious agent, and fulfill the descriptions already given in the general study of inflammation. In most cases the infectious process, like the human "cold," starts as a rhinitis, and the extent to which it spreads into the lower air passages depends upon its virulence and the susceptibility of the patient. Some of them reach the lung parenchyma itself, causing pneumonia. Among the acute infections localizing in the upper air passages are strangles (*Streptococcus equi*), equine rhinopneumonitis, and influenza in the horse; pasteurellosis, malignant catarrhal fever, infectious bovine rhinotracheitis, and calf diphtheria in cattle; pasteurellosis, influenza, and inclusion body rhinitis in swine; the distemper virus and probably the bronchisepticus organism (*Bordetella, Alcaligenes,* or *Brucella bronchiseptica*) in the dog; feline viral rhinotracheitis and probably other viruses in cats; and the various coryza-producing viruses and bacteria in poultry. Several of the chronic granulomatous infections may be localized in these structures, particularly glanders, bovine nasal granuloma, rhinosporidiosis, and tuberculosis. The lesions are those characteristic of each specific disease. *Cryptococcus neoformans* is occasionally encountered as a cause of rhinitis in animals, especially cats.

Frontal sinusitis occurs in cattle from infection of the wound produced by dehorning. Extension of infection to the cranial cavity is similarly possible. Maxillary sinusitis, especially in the horse, results from disease of the molar teeth and the walls of the dental alveoli, which are surprisingly thin.

Infectious inflammations of the nasopharynx occasionally spread up the mucosa of one or both eustachian tubes in man, more or less completely closing the lumen by the swelling produced, and in some cases spreading into the middle ear to produce **otitis media.** Called eustachitis, the condition may occur in domestic animals but, since the symptoms are chiefly subjective (interference with hearing, etc.), it is seldom diagnosed in veterinary practice.

In the horse, **catarrh of the guttural pouches** occurs as a continuation of a similar eustachitis. The pouches are filled and often distended with exudate, which is most often mucopurulent and tenacious. Since swelling of the tube, as well as its position, interferes with drainage, the catarrh is likely to become chronic, and the desiccated exudate may develop into caseous or even more solid concrements. **Tympanites of the guttural pouches** occurs as a bulging pneumatic swelling, usually bilateral, apparently related to the head being held downward, as in grazing. The more or less swollen tube appears to have a valve-like action permitting air to be pumped in but not expelled as the animal chews. This is comparable to the development of subcutaneous emphysema from a wound in the axillary region. A similar meteorism of the guttural pouches is said to exist as the result of their distension by gases derived from putrefaction of the exudate in chronic catarrh, mentioned previously.

Arthropod and Helminthic Parasites

In sheep, the larvae of the **bot-fly,** *Oestrus ovis,* some 2 cm long when fully grown, migrate up the nares, usually into the frontal sinus, sometimes into the recesses of the turbinate bones. They cause the formation of a tenacious mucopurulent exudate, in which they are more or less buried. Naturally such a sinusitis is the cause of much suffering and interference with the general health. It is occasionally fatal by extension to the cranial cavity via the ethmoid. *Linguatula serrata* is a parasite which infects the nasal passages of dogs and, rarely, other species. Also in dogs, the paranasal sinuses and nasal passages may be infested with the mite *Pneumonyssus caninum.*

The nasal passages of Old-World nonhuman primates as well as man are occasionally infested with the nematodes *Anatrichosoma cutaneum* and *A. cynomolgi.* Two new species of *Anatrichosoma, A. rhina* and *A. nacepobi,* have been described from the nasal mucosa of Rhesus monkeys (*Macaca mulatta*) (Conrad and Wong, 1973). The anatrichosomes are somewhat rare and incompletely understood trichuroid worms, which are found in nasal passages of many Asian and African monkeys. The adult, egg-laying females inhabit the upper nasal passages and burrow into the squamous epithelium, which becomes hyperplastic. Their eggs reach the surface of the epithelium through tunnels and can be demonstrated by swab collection and microscopic examination. Mites identified as *Rhinophagus papionis* have been identified in the nasal fossae of the baboon (*Papio spp.*).

Leeches are distributed worldwide and may become parasitic on man, domestic animals, or nonhuman primates that come in contact with them in their water habitat. They are most common in Sri Lanka, Thailand, Taiwan, India, Burma, and China. *Dinobdella ferox* is reported from nasal cavities of domestic cattle, buffalo, yak, deer, dogs, and monkeys (*Macaca mulatta* and *M. cyclopis*). This leech has a dorsoventrally flattened body, blackish-brown in color, and varies in length from 35 to 60 mm. An anterior sucker is somewhat smaller than the posterior sucker. Their life cycle is direct, but apparently they do not reproduce during their sojourn in the nasal cavity. They can induce inflammation and impede breathing, as well as suck blood from their hosts.

Amyloidosis

Nodular amyloidosis of the nasal mucosa is occasionally seen in horses, albeit rarely. The amyloid is deposited surrounding blood vessels and glands and within the connective tissue. The cause is not known, but it is not associated with generalized amyloidosis.

Air Sacs

Air sacs are mucosa-lined diverticula from the larynx or trachea occurring in several species of nonhuman primates including orangutan (*Pongo pygmaeus*), howler monkey (*Alouatta*), baboon (*Papio*), macaques (*Macaca*), and gibbons (*Hylobates*), as well as others. These air sacs may become infected, usually with several species of bacteria and lead to septicemia or aspiration pneumonia.

Nasal Polyps

Nasal polyps (polypi) are inflammatory new growths which resemble true neoplasms. They are often pedunculated or elongated so that a single polypus fills most of the nasal lumen in which it lies. They are smoothly covered with mucous membrane. The inner tissue is fibrous and myxomatous with a generous infiltration of leukocytes, chiefly neutrophilic granulocytes and lymphocytes, the presence of which does not depend on any ulceration of the surface. These, together with numerous capillaries, suffice to indicate an inflammatory pathogenesis which puts polypi in the same category as the granulation tissue of wound healing, although the exact etiology is often not discernible. They have to be differentiated from nasal granuloma of bovines, rhinosporidiosis, granulomatous growths caused by the blood fluke, *Schistosoma nasalis* (at least in India), and by the larvae of the equine stomach worm, *Habronema sp.*, and probably by other occasional parasites, as well as true neoplasms, which are encountered rarely. In horses, nasal inflammatory polyps may be a source of hemorrhage (Platt, 1975). Feline nasal polyps are occasionally attached to similar inflammatory polyps which extend into the external auditory meatus (Fig. 20–1).

Epistaxis

Expistaxis, or **nosebleed,** occurs infrequently in domestic animals. If not caused by some trauma such as a heavy blow or the passing of a stomach tube, it is likely to be an indication of an ulcerative infection or neoplasm, a hemangioma (rare), or possibly a fractured bone which has lacerated a blood vessel in the region.

A study of epistaxis in horses (Cook, 1974) indicates that the site of the hemorrhage depends to some extent upon the

Laryngeal Hemiplegia

Normally at each inspiration the arytenoid cartilages of the larynx are drawn outward by their muscles, as two double doors might be swung open, to admit air. In this disease of the horse there is a paralysis, usually partial, of one of the arytenoid cartilages which leaves it vapid in the rushing air currents. Commonly the muscles have enough strength to hold it open during ordinary breathing but not during the more violent respiration which goes with vigorous exercise, when the air current draws the flap of tissue into midstream. The result is that at each inspiration this fluttering obstruction not only limits the amount of air which can reach the lungs, but also sets up a considerable sound, which is responsible for the disease being called **roaring.**

The affected crico-arytenoideus muscle shows atrophy of many of its fibers, which progresses until they disappear completely, with replacement by fibrous tissue. This latter often shows considerable mucoid degeneration, so that grossly the degenerated muscle is said to look like fish flesh. The recurrent laryngeal nerve supplying the muscle shows the successive stages of demyelinization and wallerian degeneration.

It is almost always the left arytenoid cartilage, crico-arytenoideus muscle, and recurrent laryngeal nerve which are involved in this disorder. This is believed to be because of the unique course of the left nerve around the arch of the aorta and along the deep face of that vessel. Causes of certain infrequent cases which may be on either side include pressure by enlarged granulomatous lymph nodes, tumors, abscesses, aneurysms, and esophageal swelling. Congenital defects have been suspected. Many cases follow pneumonia.

Pharyngeal Diverticulitis

In the pig, the diverticulum pharyngeum lies just dorsal to the origin of the

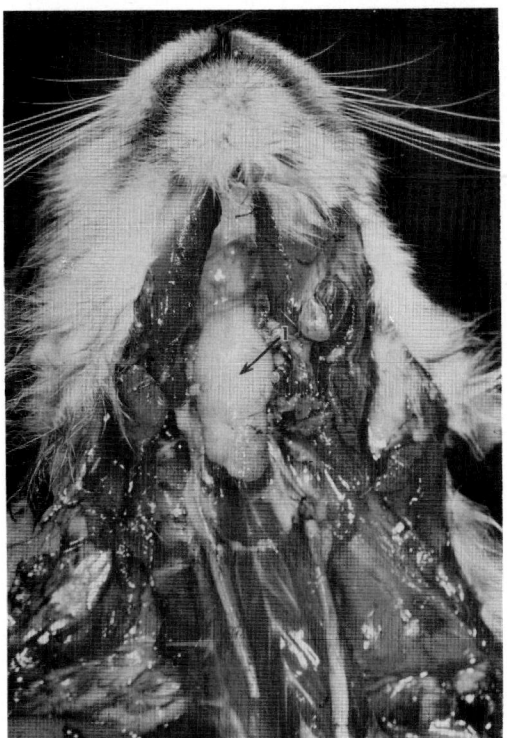

Fig. 20–1. A nasal polyp (*1*) extending from the nasopharynx of a nine-year-old female cat. A similar fibrinous, inflammatory mass extended through the eustachian tube and connected with another in the external auditory canal. (Courtesy of Angell Memorial Animal Hospital.)

occupation of the horse. About 28% of 174 cases were bilateral and occurred in racehorses following competitive exercise, and the source was considered to be the lungs. Spontaneous hemorrhage appearing while the horse was at rest was usually unilateral and originated in the nasal cavity (10%) following viral infection or in the paranasal sinuses and labyrinth of the ethmoid (27%) due to hematoma (which may be bilateral) in the ethmoid region. Auditory tube diverticulum was the site of 34% of the hemorrhages, which were usually unilateral and due to erosion of blood vessels. Hemorrhage from nasopharynx, larynx, and trachea were not encountered in this series.

esophagus. It is rather frequently the site of lodgement of capsules incorrectly administered for the treatment of intestinal helminthiasis or other diseases. Depending on the nature of the contained medicaments, severe inflammation or fatal gangrene may result from release of the drug in the diverticulum. Prosectors must not overlook a lesion of this kind.

Allen, A.M.: Occurrence of the nematode *Anatrichosoma cutaneum* in the nasal mucosa of *Macaca mulatta* monkeys. Am. J. Vet. Res., 21:389–392, 1960.

Binn, L.N., et al.: Viral antibody patterns in laboratory dogs with respiratory disease. Am. J. Vet. Res., 31:697–702, 1970.

Binn, L.N., et al.: Upper respiratory disease in military dogs: bacterial, mycoplasma and viral studies. Am. J. Vet. Res., 29:1809–1815, 1968.

Campbell, R.S.F., et al.: Respiratory adenovirus infection in the dog. Vet. Rec., 83:202–203, 1968.

Conrad, H.D., and Wong, M.M.: Studies of *Anatrichosoma* (Nematoda-Trichinellida) with descriptions of *Anatrichosoma rhina* sp. n. and *Anatrichosoma nacepobi* sp. n. from nasal mucosa of *Macaca mulatta*. J. Helminth., 47:289–302, 1973.

Cook, W.R.: Epistaxis in the racehorse. Equine Vet. J., 6:45–48, 1974.

Crandell, R.A., Cheatham, W.J., and Maurer, F.D.: Infectious bovine rhinotracheitis—the occurrence of intranuclear inclusion bodies in experimentally infected animals. Am. J. Vet. Res., 20:505–509, 1959.

Ditchfield, J., MacPherson, L.W., and Zbitnew, A.: Association of a canine adenovirus (Toronto A21–61) with an outbreak of laryngotracheitis (kennel cough). Can. Vet. J., 3:238–247, 1962.

Doyle, L.P., Donham, C.R., and Hutchings, L.M.: Report on a type of rhinitis in swine. J. Am. Vet. Med. Assoc., 105:132–133, 1944.

Fairchild, G.A., Medway, W., and Cohen, D.: A study of the pathogenicity of a canine adenovirus (Toronto A26/61) for dogs. Am. J. Vet. Res., 30:1187–1193, 1969.

Fox, J.G., and Ediger, R.D.: Nasal leech infestation in the Rhesus monkey. Lab. Anim. Care, 20:1137–1138, 1970.

Guilloud, N.B., and McClure, H.M.: Air sac infection in the Orangutan *(Pongo pygmaeus)*. Recent Adv. Primatol., 3:143–147, 1969.

Harding, J.D.J.: Inclusion body rhinitis of swine in Maryland. Am. J. Vet. Res., 19:907–912, 1958.

Hilloowala, R.A.: Laryngeal air sacs and air spaces in certain primates. Anat. Rec., 169:340, 1971.

Kim, C.S., and Bang, G.F.: Nasal mites parasitic in nasal and upper skull tissues in the baboon (*Papio* sp.). Science, 169:372–373, 1970.

Knezevich, A.L., and McNulty, W.P., Jr.: Pulmonary acariasis (*Pneumonyssus simicola*) in colony-bred *Macaca mulatta*. Lab. Anim. Care, 20:693–696, 1970.

Lewis, J.C., Montgomery, C.A., Jr., and Hildebrandt, P.K.: Air-sacculitis in the baboon. J. Am. Vet. Med. Assoc., 167:662–663, 1975.

Leyland, A., and Baker, J.R.: Lesions of the nasal and paranasal sinuses of the horse causing dyspnoea. Br. Vet. J., 131:339–346, 1975.

Loliger, H.C., Alberti, V., and Matthes, S.: Pathological anatomy and histology of contagious coryza of rabbits. Dtsch. Tieraerztl. Wochenschr., 79:126–131, 1972.

Mason, B.J.E.: Laryngeal hemiplegia: a further look at Haslam's anomaly of the left recurrent nerve. Equine Vet. J., 5:150–155, 1973.

Neumann-Kleinpaul, K., and Tabbert, B.: Zur aetiologie und pathologie der recurrenslahmung des pferdes. Arch. Tierheilk., 70:413–416, 1936.

Orihel, T.C.: Anatrichosomiasis in African monkeys. J. Parasitol., 56:982–985, 1970.

Platt, H.: Haemorrhagic nasal polyps of the horse. J. Pathol., 115:51–55, 1975.

Rooney, J.R., and Delaney, F.M.: An hypothesis on the causation of laryngeal hemiplegia in horses. Equine Vet. J., 2:35–39, 1970.

Smith, J.E.: The aerobic bacteria of the nose and tonsils of healthy dogs. J. Comp. Path., 71:428–433, 1961.

Wheat, J.D.: Tympanites of the guttural pouch of the horse. J. Am. Vet. Med. Assn., 140:453–454, 1962.

Porcine Atrophic Rhinitis

This insidious disease of swine was first recognized in North America about 1940 (Doyle et al., 1944), although what was probably the same disease attracted attention in Northern Europe early in the nineteenth century. Commencing in young pigs with slight catarrh, nasal irritation, and sneezing, the disease progresses slowly over many months, with increasing dyspnea and anorexia and eventual death from inanition.

The earliest lesions usually described are small, depressed, and congested foci on the mucosa of the turbinate bones. Erosion and disappearance of the mucous membrane follow and are accompanied by a heavy infiltration of inflammatory cells, chiefly lymphocytes and monocytes. Areas of the turbinate bones begin to soften, grossly. Microscopically, this appears first as a rarefaction and fading of the bony tissue. As destruction of the bone continues, large numbers of fibroblastic cells proliferate in the periosteal region. These are interpreted as osteoblasts, but no

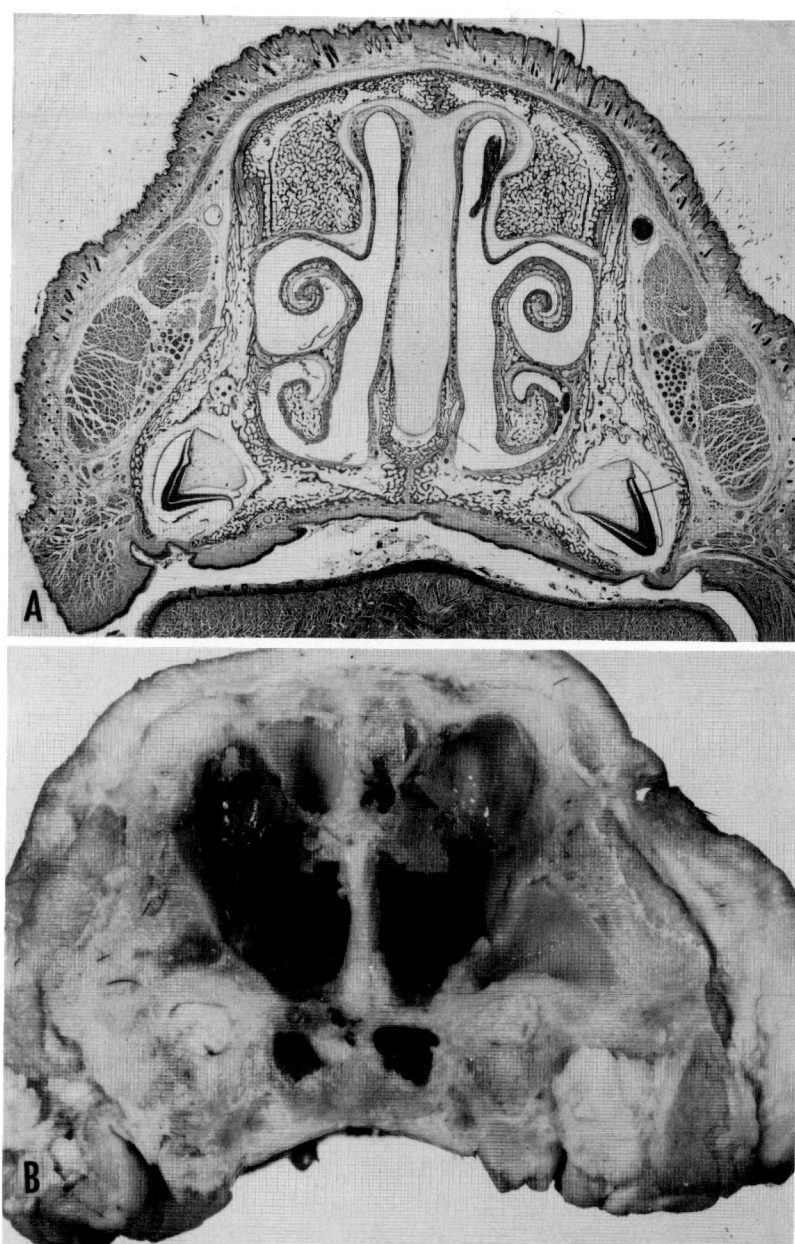

Fig. 20–2. Porcine atrophic rhinitis. *A,* Stained section through nose of a normal pig (× 4). (Courtesy of Armed Forces Institute of Pathology.) Contributor: Lt. Col. T.C. Jones. *B,* Transverse section (gross specimen) through the nose of a pig with atrophic rhinitis. Except for part of the ethmoids, all the turbinates have been destroyed. (Courtesy of Armed Forces Institute of Pathology.) Contributor: Dr. C.L. Davis.

new bone is formed. Osteoclasts are never numerous. Bone resorption is believed to result from osteolysis. Schofield and Jones (1950) found that the turbinate bones disappear in 2 to 4 weeks following apparent experimental inoculation, leaving only a dense, fibrous band to mark their place of attachment. A tenacious mucopurulent exudate clings in the recesses of the turbinates as long as they remain, and in the cells of the ethmoid. Late in the course of the disease, the nasal septum likewise disappears, a process requiring some months. Growth of the snout is retarded so that its dorsal aspect becomes short and concave. Often the interference with growth is greater on one side than on the other, so that the snout curves slightly toward the most severely affected side. In the nasal passages of some advanced cases, little remains but the inflamed walls of the passages, bearing perhaps a coating of dried and clotted blood. In other cases, the nares are more or less plugged by solidified and inspissated exudate and dead tissue. In spite of the slow progress and rather low virulence of the disease, it does not appear that recovery ever occurs.

Etiology. The best evidence now indicates that the principal cause of atrophic rhinitis is infection due to *Bordetella bronchiseptica.* The evidence may be summarized as follows: (1) Infection of the nasal cavity of experimental pigs with *Bordetella bronchiseptica* results in typical lesions of atrophic rhinitis. (2) Naturally occurring lesions of atrophic rhinitis are usually accompanied by infection by *B. bronchiseptica.* (3) Diets low in calcium and high in phosphorus do not lead to typical lesions nor do high levels of calcium protect swine from the effects of *B. bronchiseptica.* (4) Ultrastructural study of thyroid parafollicular cells of pigs with naturally occurring atrophic rhinitis reveals no difference from controls. (5) Progressive degenerative changes in osteoblasts and osteoclasts are seen in turbinates of infected pigs (swollen mitochondria, distention of

cysternae of endoplasmic reticulum), and bacteria (probably *B. bronchiseptica*) are observed in the cytoplasm of osteoblasts and close to the bone surface (Fetter, Switzer, and Capen, 1975).

Not all factors are clearly defined, nor has the possibility of inherited susceptibility or nutritional deficiency been completely eliminated, although the weight of the evidence appears against nutritional factors. Selection of infected adult swine by cultural methods and eliminating them from the herd appears to be one way of reducing the frequency of atrophic rhinitis (Farrington and Switzer, 1977).

Harris, Switzer, and Harris (1971) have developed a theoretic mechanism for the pathogenesis of atrophic rhinitis. Their studies indicate that extracts of *B. bronchiseptica* inhibited or uncoupled the energized processes of mitochondria from bovine or pig hearts. Energy-dependent accumulation of calcium phosphate by these mitochondria was inhibited by the extracts. The idea was broached that the extracts of *B. boviseptica* contain the membrane-damaging component responsible for atrophic rhinitis. The active component has not yet been isolated.

Baustad, B., Teige, J., Jr., and Tollersrud, S.: The effect of various levels of calcium, phosphorus and vitamin D in the feed for growing pigs with special reference to atrophic rhinitis. Acta Vet. Scand. 8:369–389, 1967.

Brion, A.J., and Fontaine, M.P.: Étude sur la rhinite atrophique du porc. Les lésions nerveuses. Essai d'interprétation étiologique et pathogénique. Can. J. Comp. Med., 22:88–95, 1958.

Brown, W.R., Krook, L., and Pond, W.G.: Atrophic rhinitis in swine, etiology, pathogenesis, prophylaxis. Cornell Vet., 56:Suppl. 1,1–108, 1966.

Doyle, L.P., Donham, C.R., and Hutchings, L.M.: Report on a type of rhinitis in swine. J. Am. Vet. Med. Assoc., 105:132–133, 1944.

Duncan, J.R., Ramsey, F.K., and Switzer, W.P.: Pathology of experimental *Bordetella bronchiseptica* infection in swine: Pneumonia. Am. J. Vet. Res., 27:467–472, 1966.

Duncan, J.R., et al.: Pathology of experimental *Bordetella bronchiseptica* infection in swine: atrophic rhinitis. Am. J. Vet. Res., 27:457–466, 1966.

Edington, N., Smith, I.M., Plowright, W., and Watt,

R.G.: Relationship of porcine cytomegalovirus and *Bordetella bronchiseptica* to atrophic rhinitis in gnotobiotic piglets. Vet. Rec., *98*:42–45, 1976.

Farrington, D.O., and Switzer, W.P.: Evaluation of nasal culturing procedures for the control of atrophic rhinitis caused by *Bordetella bronchiseptica* in swine. J. Am. Vet. Med. Assoc., *170*:34–38, 1977.

Fetter, A.W., and Capen, C.C.: Ultrastructural evaluation of thyroid parafollicular cells of pigs with naturally occurring atrophic rhinitis. Pathol. Vet., *7*:171–185, 1970.

Fetter, A.W., and Capen, C.C.: Ultrastructural evaluation of bone cells in pigs with experimental turbinate osteoporosis (atrophic rhinitis). Lab. Invest., *24*:392–403, 1971.

Fetter, A.W., and Capen, C.C.: Fine structure of bone cells in the nasal turbinates of pigs with naturally occurring atrophic rhinitis. Am. J. Pathol., *62*:265–282, 1971.

Fetter, A.W., Switzer, W.P., and Capen, C.C.: Electron microscopic evaluation of bone cells in pigs with experimentally induced *Bordetella* rhinitis (turbinate osteoporosis). Am. J. Vet. Res., *36*:15–22, 1975.

Harris, D.L., Switzer, W.P., and Harris, R.A.: A suggested mechanism for the pathogenesis of infectious atrophic rhinitis. Can. J. Comp. Med., *35*:318–323, 1971.

Kang, B.K., Koshimizu, K., and Ogata, M.: Studies on the etiology of infectious atrophic rhinitis of swine. II. Agglutination test on *Bordetella bronchiseptica* infection. Jpn. J. Vet. Sci., *32*:295–305, 1970.

Kemeny, L.J., Littledike, E.T., and Cheville, N.F.: Experimental transmission of atrophic rhinitis in pigs. Effect of diet. Cornell Vet., *60*:502–517, 1970.

Kemeny, L.J.: Experimental atrophic rhinitis produced by *Bordetella bronchiseptica* culture in young pigs. Cornell Vet., *62*:477–485, 1972.

Koshimizu, K., Kodama, Y., and Ogata, M.: Studies on the etiology of infectious atrophic rhinitis of swine. V. *Bordetella bronchiseptica* infection in conventional piglets. Jpn. J. Vet. Sci., *35*:223–229, 1973.

Koshimizu, K., et al.: Studies on the etiology of infectious atrophic rhinitis of swine. VI. Effect of vaccination against nasal establishment of *Bordetella bronchiseptica*. Jpn. J. Vet. Sci., *35*:411–418, 1973.

Logomarsino, J.V., Pond, W.G., Sheffy, B.E., and Krook, L.: Turbinate morphology in pigs inoculated with *Bordetella bronchiseptica* and fed high or low calcium diets. Cornell Vet., *64*:573–583, 1974.

Maeda, M., Inui, S., and Konno, S.: Lesions of nasal turbinates in swine atrophic rhinitis. Nat. Inst. Anim. Health Quart. (Tokyo), *9*:193–202, 1969.

Maeda, M.: Nasal turbinate atrophy in newborn rabbit infected with *Alcaligenes bronchisepticus* of pig origin. Natl. Inst. Anim. Health Q. (Tokyo), *13*:229–230, 1973.

Maeda, M., and Shimizu, T.: Lesions of experimental swine atrophic rhinitis and *Alcaligenes bronchisepticus* antigen detected by fluorescent antibody technique. Natl. Inst. Anim. Health Q. (Tokyo), *14*:188–198, 1974.

Nakagawa, M., Shimizu, T., and Motoi, Y.: Pathology of experimental atrophic rhinitis in swine infected with *Alcaligenes bronchisepticus* or *Pasteurella multocida*. Natl. Inst. Anim. Health Q. (Tokyo), *14*:61–71, 1974.

Ogata, M., et al.: Studies on the aetiology of porcine atrophic rhinitis. II. Relationship between the disease and bacterial flora of the nasal cavity of pigs. Jpn. J. Vet. Sci., *32*:185–199, 1970.

Schofield, F.W., and Jones, T.L.: The pathology and bacteriology of infectious atrophic rhinitis in swine. J. Am. Vet. Med. Assoc., *116*:120–123, 1950.

Shimizu, T., Nakagawa, M., Shibata, S., and Suzuki, K.: Atrophic rhinitis produced by intranasal inoculation of *Bordetella bronchiseptica* in hysterectomy-produced colostrum-deprived pigs. Cornell Vet., *61*:696–705, 1971.

Switzer, W.P.: Studies on infectious atrophic rhinitis of swine. J. Am. Vet. Med. Assn., *123*:45–47, 1953; Vet. Med., *46*:478–481, 1951; *48*:392–394, 1953; Am. J. Vet. Res., *16*:540–544, 1955; *17*:478–484, 1956.

Bovine Nasal Granuloma

Granulomatous inflammation in the mucosa of the bovine nasal cavity is not infrequent and appears to be due to several causes. In the United States, a form due to mycotic infection has been described. In India, a type of granulomatous reaction in the nasal mucosa has been ascribed to a blood fluke, *Schistosoma nasalis*. Actinobacillosis may also occur in the bovine nasal cavity, tiny abscesses in the nasal mucosa simulating some of the clinical features and gross lesions. A fourth type of nasal granuloma has been described from Australia and New Zealand. The published reports on this disease merit summarizing.

The Australasian form of nasal granuloma (called chronic granular rhinitis in New Zealand) appears to be more frequent in the Jersey breed of cattle. The usual course starts with gradual onset over a period of weeks with a nasal discharge, at first mucous, then mucopurulent. Nasal pruritus is evident from the earliest stages. Exacerbation of the signs is observed in the summer months, remission in the winter. The anterior third of the nasal mucosa becomes elevated by tiny nodules which give it a roughened "cobblestone" appearance.

The histologic features of the involved nasal mucosa are characteristic. The mucosa is altered by many closely-packed tiny polyps covered by acanthotic squamous epithelium projecting into the lumen. The underlying lamina propria is edematous, filled with capillaries, fibroblasts, eosinophils, mast cells, and plasma cells. The necks of the ducts of mucous glands are also made up of metaplastic pseudostratified columnar epithelium, but deeper structures are not affected. Epithelioid macrophages of typical granulomas are not a feature of this lesion.

An acute lesion is also recognized by infiltration of the lamina propria by eosinophils, "globule" leukocytes, edema, and increased numbers of mast cells.

The nature of the lesion plus other evidence, points toward the idea that this disease is caused by episodic type I hypersensitivity reaction to unidentified antigens. The granulation tissue is identifiable with type III hypersensitivity. Specific allergens responsible for this disease have not, at this time, been identified but affected cows are definitely hypersensitive to many disease antigens. These include a large number of plant pollens, tree pollens, fungi, and miscellaneous items such as mites (Pemberton and White, 1976). In one experiment, nasal lesions have been associated with induced hypersensitivity to hen egg albumen (Pemberton, et al., 1974).

Carbonell, P.L.: Bovine nasal granuloma: a review. Aust. Vet. J., *52*:158–165, 1976.

Carbonell, P.L.: Bovine nasal granuloma. Gross and microscopic lesions. Vet. Pathol., *16*:60–73, 1979.

Hore, D.E., et al.: Nasal granuloma in dairy cattle: distribution in Victoria. Aust. Vet. J., *49*:330–334, 1973.

James, M.P., Lake, D.E., and Sinclair, C.G.: Bovine nasal granuloma. N.Z. Vet. J., *23*:63–64, 1975.

Pemberton, D.H., White, W.E., and Hore, D.E.: The experimental reproduction of nasal granuloma by repeated acute episodes of immediate hypersensitivity. Aust. Vet. J., *50*:233–234, 1974.

Pemberton, D.H., and White, W.E.: Bovine nasal granuloma in Victoria. 1. Histological comparison of the nasal mucosa of clinically normal Jersey and Hereford cattle. Aust. Vet. J., *50*:85–88, 1974.

Pemberton, D.H., and White, W.E.: Bovine nasal granuloma in Victoria. 2. Histopathology of

nasal, ocular, and oral lesions. Aust. Vet. J., *50*:89–97, 1974.

Pemberton, D.H., and White, W.E.: Bovine nasal granuloma in Victoria—a search for the causative allergens. Aust. Vet. J., *52*:155–157, 1976.

Pemberton, D.H., White, W.E., and Hore, D.E.: Bovine nasal granuloma (atrophic rhinitis) in Victoria. Experimental reproduction by the production of immediate type hypersensitivity in the nasal mucosa. Aust. Vet. J., *53*:201–207, 1977.

Congenital Anomalies

Congenital malformations that involve the respiratory system are usually secondary. For example, malformations of the head and face (cyclopia, anencephalia, campylognathia, cebocephalus, among others) result in anomalies of the upper respiratory tract. Lesions in the thorax such as diaphragmatic hernia, occurring during gestation, lead to hypoplasia or atelectasis of the lung. Intrauterine poisoning of lambs due to *Veratrum californicum* is one of the serious causes of congenital malformations of the respiratory tract. In most instances, however, the cause is unknown, although hereditary factors have been identified in some types of malformations.

Dennis, S.M.: Congenital respiratory tract defects in lambs. Aust. Vet. J., *51*:347–350, 1975.

Heider, L., et al.: Nasolacrimal duct anomaly in calves. J. Am. Vet. Med. Assoc., *167*:145–147, 1975.

Huston, R., Saperstein, G., Schoneweis, D., and Leipold, H.W.: Congenital defects in pigs. Vet. Bull., *48*:645–675, 1978.

Thomson, F.G.: Congenital bronchial hypoplasia of calves. Pathol. Vet., *3*:89–109, 1966.

THE TRACHEA AND BRONCHI

Lining Cells of Trachea, Bronchi and Bronchioles

The nasal epithelium nearest the nares is lined by stratified squamous epithelium, which toward the pharynx becomes typical pseudostratified respiratory epithelium. This type of epithelium extends to the origin of the bronchiole, where it becomes simple columnar. Nine types of epithelial cells have been identified in the tracheobronchial epithelium, these are: ciliated, goblet, epithelial serous, brush, basal, intermediate, Kultschitzky-like (K type), special type, and Clara cells. One important function of the tracheobronchial epithelium is the production of mucus. This is accomplished by the epithelial serous cells, goblet cells, and mucous glands in the lamina propria, which are lined by serous and mucous cells and communicate with the lumen.

The ultrastructural features of the cells lining the upper airways has been reviewed by Breeze, et al. (1976).

The **tracheal rings** occasionally suffer permanent deformity, usually by upward compression. This condition is often asymptomatic and discovered only at autopsy. **Ossification** of the laryngeal and tracheal cartilages has been mentioned.

Bronchiectasis

This is a dilation of one or more bronchi. During violent or forced respiration, the bronchi and bronchioles dilate to full capacity and become round in cross section, but at other times all but the largest bronchi are contracted by their encircling musculature so that the mucosa is thrown into folds. In cross sections, these folds give the smaller and medium bronchi a star-like appearance. In bronchiectasis, they are dilated and the folds stretched out to a full circle, a position which persists after death. This inelasticity and failure to return to the normal contracted state are due to small amounts of fibrous tissue in and around the bronchial wall, which has proliferated as the result of chronic inflammation. Commonly a number of leukocytes and reticulo-endothelial cells are still visible in the peribronchial zone. The scar tissue also acts to keep the lumen distended by fixing the wall to surrounding structures. Bronchiectasis is thus an indication of a present or previous inflammation. The peribronchial tissue commonly shares in the inelasticity, so that the ability of the lung to collapse is impaired, and its functional efficiency diminished. Continued irritation results from these structural derangements, as is generally evidenced by catarrhal exudation and cough. This exudative state may be enhanced by continuing or recurrent infections of low virulence. Owing to chronic irritation, squamous metaplasia of the bronchial epithelium is a frequent finding. A striking example of bronchiectasis is a consistent feature of chronic murine pneumonia. A specific type of bronchiectasis has been described (Jensen, et al., 1976) in yearling feedlot cattle. This lesion is limited to single lobules, but involves all of the bronchial branches in the lobule. This lesion was encountered in 32 (1.6%) of 1988 necropsies of yearling cattle. Many bacterial organisms (*Pasteurella haemolytica, P. multocida, Corynebacterium pyogenes, Escherichia coli, Salmonella anatum, Staphylococcus spp.*) and one mycoplasma (*Mycoplasma arginini*) were isolated from these bronchi. The pathogenetic mechanisms remain obscure.

Bronchitis

Bronchitis has been mentioned in common with the upper respiratory diseases. It is most often an extension of one of these infections, but may rarely represent an extension of a pneumonic process which originated in the pulmonary parenchyma. The mild or early forms are characterized by catarrhal inflammation; later the exudate usually becomes fibrinous or purulent. The virulence and the importance of an upper respiratory infection can usually be gauged by how far it extends from the nares toward the lungs, bronchitis being the most formidable of the subpneumonic infections.

Canine tracheobronchitis or "kennel cough" is a clinical designation for a disease characterized by intermittent coughing. Although clinically the disease may appear as a single entity, there is little reason to consider it a specific disease with a single cause, anymore so than the human cold. Various viruses, including adenoviruses, influenza viruses, and herpes viruses have been reported to induce tracheobronchitis in dogs, but their respective roles in the natural disease are not established. There are few reports describing the gross or histopathologic features as the disease is not fatal. Inclusion bodies in tracheal and bronchial epithelium, similar to those produced by adenoviruses and herpes viruses, are occasionally encountered in dogs with a history of coughing.

Chronic bronchitis has been described in dogs, particularly from Great Britain (Wheeldon et al., 1974), manifest particularly by a cough which persists for months to years. The findings at postmortem examination consist of mucous plugs in the tracheobronchial tree, thickened and hyperemic bronchial mucosae, occasional polypoid lesions in mucosa, and often moderately extensive subpleural emphysema. Microscopically, mucous exudate may be seen in the lumen of bronchioles, goblet cells are increased in number, and the lamina propria is infiltrated with inflammatory cells (lymphocytes and plasma cells). At severely affected sites, epithelial cells may lose cilia, undergo excessive proliferation or may be sloughed, leaving an ulcerated zone. Some degree of pneumonia may be associated with the bronchitis. The principal bacterial inhabitant appears to be *Bordetella bronchiseptica*.

A similar chronic bronchitis has been reproduced in Beagles by prolonged exposure to sulfur dioxide gas in closed chambers (Chakrin and Saunders, 1974).

Adams, L.E., et al.: An epizootic of respiratory tract disease in Sprague-Dawley rats. J. Am. Vet. Med. Assoc., 161:656–660, 1972.
Amis, T.C.: Tracheal collapse in the dog. Aust. Vet. J., 50:285–289, 1974.
Bienenstock, J., Johnston, N., and Perey, D.Y.E.: Bronchial lymphoid tissue. I. Morphologic characteristics. Lab. Invest., 28:686–692, 1973.
Bienenstock, J., Johnston, N., and Perey, D.Y.E.: Bronchial lymphoid tissue. II. Functional characteristics. Lab. Invest., 28:693–698, 1973.
Booth, B.H., Talbot, C.H., and Patterson, R.: Bronchial secretions in dogs with IgE mediated respiratory responses. Arch. Allergy Appl. Immunol., 40:639–642, 1971.

Breeze, R.G., Wheeldon, E.B., and Pirie, H.M.: Cell structure and function in the mammalian lung: the trachea, bronchi, and bronchioles. Vet. Bull., 46:319–337, 1976.
Chakrin, L.W., and Saunders, L.Z.: Experimental chronic bronchitis: pathology in the dog. Lab. Invest., 30:145–154, 1974.
Dill, G.S., Jr., Stookey, J.L., and Whitney, G.D.: Nodular amyloidosis in the trachea of a dog. Vet. Pathol., 9:238–242, 1972.
Jensen, R., et al.: Bronchiectasis in yearling feedlot cattle. J. Am. Vet. Med. Assoc., 169:511–514, 1976.
Splitter, G.A., Butcher, W.I., and Stevens, M.D.: Tracheal basement membrane thickening in Rhesus monkeys. Vet. Pathol., 11:278–288, 1974.
Wheeldon, E.B., Pirie, H.M., Fisher, E.W., and Lee, R.: Chronic bronchitis in the dog. Vet. Rec., 94:466–471, 1974.

THE LUNG

The lung in all mammals has similar functions, but some differences in anatomy among various species affect the nature of pathologic lesions. The respiratory function, involving exchange of gases, particularly oxygen and carbon dioxide, between the bloodstream and the ambient air, is preeminent, but the lung has other, nonrespiratory functions. These functions include self-cleansing mechanisms that deal with inadvertent intake of contaminated air; a water-drainage system that prevents flooding of the gas-exchanging surfaces; elaboration of essential biological products, such as surfactant, and other metabolic activities that keep the lungs continuously viable. The functions are influenced by autacoids (prostaglandins), catecholamines, and steroids.

The distribution and nature of pathologic lesions in the lung are influenced to some extent by anatomic features. A brief outline of some of these differences between species is given in Table 20–1.

The Alveolus

The terminal air saccule of the lung is shaped by a skeleton of connective tissue which contains a network of capillaries and is lined by an uninterrupted layer of cells, in turn covered by a film (surfactant) which

Table 20–1. Comparative Pulmonary Anatomy*

Species	Pleura	Lobules	Distal Airways
Man, horse	Thick	Extensive interlobular stroma; lobules incompletely separated	Terminal bronchiole; respiratory bronchioles poorly developed
Rhesus monkey (Macaca mulatta), dog, cat	Thin	Poorly defined; little interlobular stroma	Respiratory bronchiole; terminal bronchioles short or absent; muscle conspicuous in dog
Cattle, sheep, swine	Thick	Completely separated by extensive interlobular stroma	Terminal bronchiole; respiratory bronchioles are rare
Rat, mouse, rabbits	Thin	Poorly defined; little interlobular connective tissue	Terminal bronchiole; respiratory bronchioles are poorly developed; cardiac muscle in rats and mice follows pulmonary vein into lung

* In part after McLaughlin, Tyler, Canada, 1961

separates them from the air. Three kinds of epithelial lining cells have been described.

The **type I pneumonocyte** covers most of the alveolar surface. Its shape resembles that of a fried egg: the yolk corresponds to the nucleus and the peripheral egg white to the cytoplasm of the cell which extends around the alveolus into contact with other lining cells. Ribosomes are concentrated around the nucleus, but few organized structures occupy the thin part of the cell. The cell has sparse endoplasmic reticulum and a Golgi complex. Many vesicles occupy this type I cell, some contained entirely within the cell, others appearing to open to the surface. These vesicles serve to carry macromolecules across the epithelium between alveolar and interstitial spaces.

The **type II cell (granular pneumonocyte or giant alveolar cell)** is interspersed among the type I cells and is apt to be located near the points where adjacent alveoli intersect. This cell is roughly cuboidal, is known to undergo rapid proliferation under some conditions, and is thought to be the progenitor of the type I cell. The cytoplasm contains numerous organelles, including cytosomes, mitochondria, and peroxisomes. The cytosomes are the most distinctive organelles, consisting of osmiophilic lamellae arranged in layers or whorls 0.2 to 1.0 μ in diameter. These lamellar bodies are the sites of storage and elaboration of surfactant.

Secretory activity is indicated by the presence of numerous mitochondria, a well-developed Golgi apparatus, and many multivesicular bodies. Histochemistry and cytochemistry studies have demonstrated the presence of many different enzymes, including hydrolases, esterases, catalase, and phosphatases. This is the cell that proliferates to give the alveolar lining its cuboidal appearance under many circumstances, a feature called by many names: "fetalization," "epithelialization," "adenomatosis," etc.

A **type III pneumonocyte,** the "alveolar brush cell," has been described in rat lung but at this writing its functions have not been uncovered.

Alveolar Macrophages. These cells, important to the defense functions of the lung, are derived from monocytes from the bone marrow that migrate through the alveolar wall to reach the lumen of the alveolus. They are active phagocytes and contain hydrolases, such as lysozyme, acid phosphatase, and cathepsin, which enable them to digest bacteria and neutralize other material. Lymphocytes and plasma cells are also present in small numbers in the alveolar wall and can increase greatly in numbers when the circumstances warrant.

Mast Cells. The distribution of these important cells varies between species. Their functional components are contained in large metachromatic granules which contain heparin, lipids (slow-reacting substances of anaphylaxis), prostaglandins, amines (histamine and, in rat and mouse, serotonin), polypeptides (bradykinin and eosinophil leukocyte chemotactic factor of anaphylaxis), proteins (kallikrein), and other substances.

Surfactant. The surface of the alveoli of the lungs becomes covered in postnatal life by surface-active material generally referred to as surfactant. This material forms an insoluble film at the air-liquid interface of the alveolus, modifies surface tension depending upon the alveolar surface area, and prevents atelectasis. The source of this material is the type II pneumonocyte. The cytoplasm of these cells contain membrane-bound inclusions which are ultrastructurally visible as laminated osmiophilic bodies. In fortuitous sections, these bodies may be seen open to the exterior and contributing their contents to the overlying surfactant layer.

The chemical content of surfactant at the time this is written is believed to consist of several fractions. The first consists of 50% saturated dipalmitoyl phosphatidylcholine, which contributes the unusual surface properties that lower the surface tension to less than 10 dynes/cm. A second component, made up of monoenoic phosphatidylcholines in combination with a small amount of cholesterol, is believed to give surfactant increased molecular mobility and increase its rate of adsorption to the alveolar interface. Other components, whose functions are as yet unknown, include phosphatidylethanolamines, acidic phosphatides, and one or more proteins.

Type II pneumonocytes become able to produce and extrude surfactant at a critical time in late prenatal life. In the rabbit this time occurs within a 24-hour period at about the 29th day of pregnancy. The respiratory distress experienced by premature infants is believed to be for the most part due to the absence or incompetence of surfactant. Its role in other pulmonary diseases is yet to be elucidated.

Adamson, I.Y.R., and Bowden, D.H.: Derivation of Type 1 epithelium from Type 2 cells in the developing rat lung. Lab. Invest., *32*:736–745, 1975.

Bradley, P.A., Bourne, F.J., and Brown, P.J.: The respiratory tract immune system in the pig. I. Distribution of immunoglobulin-containing cells in the respiratory tract mucosa. Vet. Pathol., *13*:81–89, 1976.

Breeze, R.G., Wheeldon, E.B., and Pirie, H.M.: Cell structure and function in the mammalian lung: the trachea, bronchi and bronchioles. Vet. Bull., *46*:319–337, 1976.

Brunner, P., and Petsch, M.: Superficial structure of the bronchus mucosa. Comparative morphological studies. Lung, *154*:103–119, 1977.

Clements, J.A.: Symposia: Biochemical aspects of pulmonary function: Introductory remarks. Fed. Proc., *33*:2231, 1974.

Creasey, J.M., Pattle, R.E., and Schock, C.: Ultrastructure of inclusion bodies in type II cells of lung, human and sub-simian. J. Physiol. (Lond.), *237*:35P–37P, 1974.

Diglio, C.A., and Kikkawa, Y.: The type II epithelial cells of the lung. IV. Adaptation and behavior of isolated type II cells in culture. Lab. Invest., *37*:622–631, 1977.

Evans, M.J., Cabral-Anderson, L.J., and Freeman, G.: Role of the Clara Cell in renewal of the bronchiolar epithelium. Lab. Invest., *38*:648–655, 1978.

Fishman, A.P., and Pietra, G.G.: Handling of bioactive materials by the lung. N. Engl. J. Med., *291*:884–890; 953–959, 1974.

Kikkawa, Y., et al.: The type II epithelial cells of the lung. II. Chemical composition and phospholipid synthesis. Lab. Invest., *32*:295–302, 1975.

King, R.J.: The surfactant system of the lung. Fed. Proc., *33*:2238–2247, 1974.

Lauweryns, J.M., Cokelaere, M., and Theunynck, P.: Neuroepithelial bodies in the respiratory mucosa of various mammals. A light optical, histochemical and ultrastructural investigation. Z. Zellforsch, *135*:569–592, 1972.

Mathe, A.A., Hedqvist, P., Strandberg, K., and Leslie, C.A.: Aspects of prostaglandin function in the lung (first and second of two parts). N. Engl. J. Med., *296*:850–855; 910–914, 1977.

McLaughlin, R.F., Tyler, W.S., and Canada, R.O.: A study of the subgross pulmonary anatomy in various mammals. Am. J. Anat., *108*:149–160, 1961.

Meyrick, B., and Reid, L.: The alveolar brush cell in rat lung—a third pneumonocyte. J. Ultrastruct. Res., *23*:71–80, 1968.

Parra, S.C., Gaddy, L.R., and Takaro, T.: Ultrastructural studies of canine interalveolar pores (of Kohn). Lab. Invest., *38*:8–13, 1978.

Robertson, B., and Enhorning, G.: The alveolar lining

of the premature newborn rabbit after pharyngeal deposition of surfactant. Lab. Invest., 31:54–59, 1974.

Smith, F.B., and Kikkawa, Y.: The type II epithelial cells of the lung. III. Lecithin synthesis: A comparison with pulmonary macrophages. Lab. Invest., 38:45–51, 1978.

Stuart, B.O.: Selection of animal models for evaluation of inhalation hazards in man. Proc. 20th Ann. OhOLO Biol. Confer. Air Pollution and the Lung. New York, Wiley and Ames, 1975, pp. 268–292.

Stupfel, M.: Choix des modeles animaux pour l'etude des nuisances respiratoires. Sci. Tech. Anim. Lab., 1:45–51, 1976.

Sueishi, K., Tanaka, K., and Oda, T.: Immuno-ultrastructural study of surfactant system: distribution of specific protein of surface active material in rabbit lung. Lab. Invest., 37:136–142, 1977.

Pneumonia, Pneumonitis

Pneumonitis can properly refer to any inflammatory disease of the lungs, but its use usually is restricted to new infectious diseases of the lung, such as immunologically mediated pneumonitis and a more or less chronic reaction in which a prominent part is taken by fibroblasts of the interstitial tissue and the lining cells of the alveoli (reticuloendothelial cells, epithelioid cells, septal cells). The term pneumonia is usually reserved to apply to one of the acute infectious inflammations with copious exudate filling the alveoli.

Pneumonia

Acute inflammation of the lung, which is pneumonia, occurs in all species, but from a variety of causes. In many instances the gross and microscopic lesions are (to the diagnostician) disconcertingly similar regardless of what particular bacterium or virus is the cause.

It is traditional and somewhat advan-

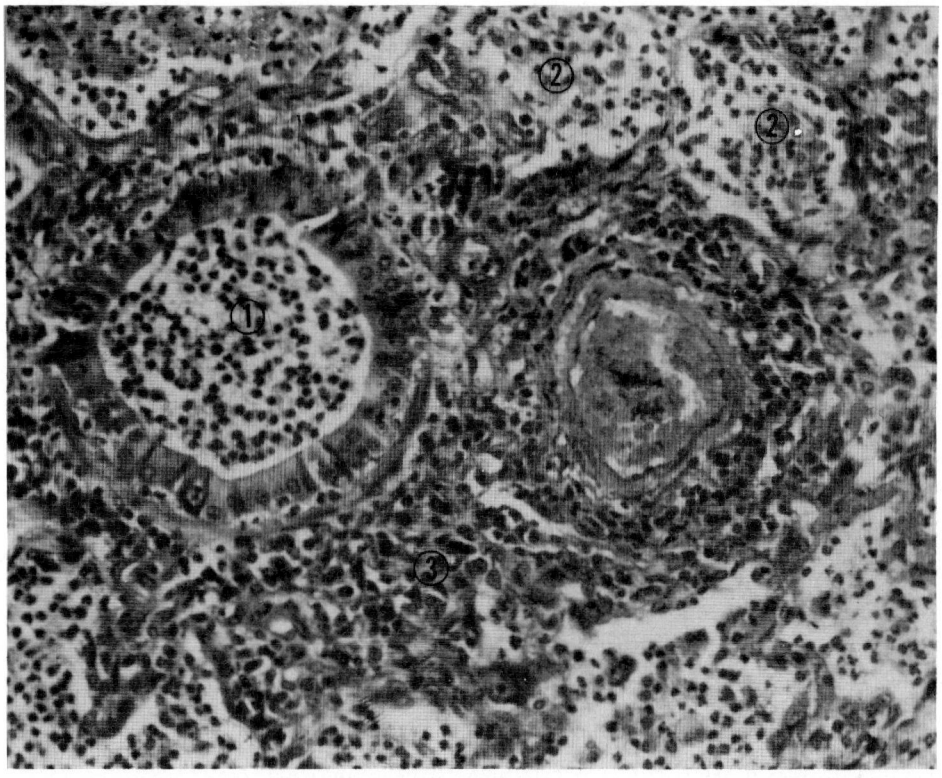

Fig. 20–3. Pneumonia associated with equine rhinopneumonitis. Lung of a young horse (× 280). Mononuclear and polymorphonuclear cells fill the bronchioles (1), alveoli (2), and interstitial stroma (3). (Courtesy of Armed Forces Institute of Pathology.) Contributor: Army Veterinary Research Laboratory.

tageous to consider the disease in four successive stages, congestion, red hepatization, gray hepatization, and resolution, although there certainly are no clear demarcations between any of these stages. The classsical **stage of congestion** involves what we have defined as active hyperemia plus inflammatory edema. The capillaries are distended with blood, and the alveoli are filled with serous fluid (recognized microscopically by a pink-staining, homogeneous precipitate). The fluid is really a serous inflammatory exudate as has been previously stated, but custom decrees the term edema. When the cause is a chemical irritant, this stage is attained in less than 2 minutes after its application. When the cause is an infectious agent, its development requires a very few hours.

In the **stage of red hepatization,** the affected area of lung is consolidated or hepatized so that it has about the same degree of firmness as liver tissue (*hepar,* liver). Completely hepatized lung tissue sinks in water. It is still red because of a certain amount of hyperemia and hemorrhage into the alveoli. While a considerable quantity of serous fluid may still remain in the alveoli, the hepatization results from the filling of the alveoli with a cellular exudate. mixed, in some cases, with fibrin. With the erythrocytes there are neutrophils, lymphocytes, and large mononuclear cells, the proportions depending upon the type and virulence of the causative agent. This stage of pneumonia is reached in about 2 days. (See Fig. 20–8A.)

The **stage of gray hepatization** follows. The lung tissue is still hepatized, and, perhaps, its color, rather than gray, is better described as merely less red than it was earlier. Microscopically, the hyperemia is somewhat less in evidence, and the erythrocytes have disappeared from the alveolar contents, giving way to white cells and fibrin. The proportions of the different components of the exudate vary, chiefly with the causative organisms. If pyogenic bacteria are prominent invaders, the exudate

consists largely of polymorphonuclear neutrophils, and we speak of a purulent pneumonia. In human lobar pneumonia, the causative organism is *Diplococcus pneumoniae,* and the exudate is almost exclusively fibrinous. A predominantly fibrinous pneumonia is seen, particularly in cattle, but we are not prepared to generalize as to the causative infection. In a considerable proportion of animal pneumonias, the predominant reactive cell is a large cell with a rounded central nucleus and a rather extensive cytoplasm. Some of these must be monocytes from the blood, others doubtless come from the reticulo-endothelial system, and there is considerable evidence that many are descendants of proliferating cells of the lining of the alveolus. Partly because of this presumed origin, and partly because they often bear a startling resemblance to individualized epithelial cells, they often go by the name of **epithelioid cells**. Regardless of their origin, these cells serve as macrophages and probably have other functions characteristic of reticulo-endothelial cells. A number of lymphocytes are usually mixed with the other cell types.

In favorable cases, the **stage of resolution** supervenes in about a week after the onset of pneumonia. The invading pathogens having been overcome and destroyed, and, the hyperemia having subsided, the cells and fibrin which filled the alveoli are gradually but rather rapidly liquefied, it is believed, by lytic substances produced by neutrophils. In a matter of a very few days, the material which filled the alveoli is coughed up as a semi-solid material or drained away by the veins and lymphatics in a completely liquefied state. The lining cells of the alveoli, most of which perished during the inflammatory period, are regenerated within a few days, and the lung returns to morphological, and soon thereafter, functional normality.

As a general concept, it is well to think of any pneumonia, or any given pneumonic area of lung, as passing through these successive stages. It must be recognized, however, that some pneumonias, especially those caused by viruses, show little tendency toward suppuration and tend to terminate, either by recovery or by death, from toxicity without advancing beyond a stage of sero-fibrinous exudate ("edema") accompanied by a limited number of septal or epithelioid cells.

Along with these fundamental exudative changes several other features require attention. While pneumonia itself is a reaction taking place in the alveoli and their walls, the interlobular septa and other connective tissue structures are also distended with exudate, especially with the serous fluid. There is usually, but not always, a discernible bronchitis in the pneumonic area. This is recognized by desquamation and disappearance of the epithelial lining cells, by an infiltration of lymphocytes and other leukocytes in the wall of the bronchus or bronchiole, and an accumulation of exudate, usually polymorphonuclear, in the lumen. However, if a bronchial lumen contains pus or other exudate while the epithelium and wall still appear normal, it may be concluded that the exudate came from some other area, the bronchus merely serving as a drainage way.

The pleura over the pneumonic area may or may not share in the inflammatory process. If pleuritis (see below) is present, the exudate is usually fibrinous or fibrinopurulent on its surface and the causative organism or secondary invaders can be isolated there.

In some pneumonias, it is only in the immediate vicinity of the bronchi and bronchioles that the inflammatory changes and consolidation are in evidence, the infection having entered by the bronchial route. Such a form is known as **peribronchial** pneumonia, or even as **peribronchitis** and peribronchiolitis.

In the vicinity of the pneumonic changes, there are almost sure to be areas of atelectasis and areas of emphysema. The former are due to plugging of the bronchioles which served them by masses of exudate. The emphysema involves alveoli which expand unduly because of decreased space occupied by neighboring alveoli which are either atelectatic or consolidated.

Unfortunately, the prompt and complete resolution described above does not always occur and complications develop. One of these is the spreading of the pneumonic process to new areas of lung tissue. These must then proceed through the same series of stages, recovery of the patient being delayed by the time required for these stages. This is characteristic of lobular pneumonia (see below) in debilitated individuals. Of considerable import also is the fact that areas of lung adjoining the pneumonic parts usually suffer from marked inflammatory edema, which may represent spread of the pneumonia but which, at any rate, interferes seriously with pulmonary function.

With delayed resolution in a given area, certain **chronic changes** may develop. The type II alveolar lining cells may undergo hyperplasia and resemble cuboidal epithelium. Their nuclei are very dark and the cells are conspicuous, sometimes being known as **cells of Tripier.** The condition has also been called **pulmonary adenomatosis** or **fetalization** of the lining cells, since they resemble those of the fetal lung. In Marsh's ovine chronic progressive pneumonia, this change becomes extreme, so that the area of lung may strikingly resemble an adenoma.

If a fibrinous or partially fibrinous exudate remains long (2 to 3 weeks) in the alveoli, the same thing happens that occurs when fibrin persists in a thrombus or in a fibrinous exudate elsewhere: the fibrin is organized by fibroblasts which build into it from surrounding tissues. Such an area is then converted permanently into fibrous tissue, a process known as **carnification** (*caro, carn,* flesh). Similarly, if the offending organism destroys pulmonary parenchyma (necrosis), healing is by scarring.

Lesions. The distribution and extent of lesions deserve attention. From statements in the preceding description, it will be inferred that the areas of pneumonic consolidation do not necessarily involve a major portion of the pulmonary tissue, and this is true. It is unusual for more than a third of the total of the two lungs to be hepatized, and frequently the process is much more limited. In the great majority of pneumonias, which are bronchogenous in origin, the anterior and ventral portions of the lungs are first and most extensively affected. These are the apical and cardiac lobes in those species whose lungs are divided into lobes. Evidence indicates that this is because infective particles, when inhaled, fall most readily into the bronchial system of these lobes. The pneumonic process commonly progresses centrally in these lobes and may eventually involve the anterior part of the diaphragmatic lobes, not to mention the intermediate lobe in species which have it. The disease may be localized in one lung but more frequently it attacks both.

There are two routes by which pathogenic organisms may enter the lungs, via the bronchi, the **bronchogenous** route, and via the blood stream, the **hematogenous** route. The former is the more frequent. Coming down the arborization of the bronchial system, it is obvious that infected particles may drop into certain bronchioles and not into others. Around each infected bronchiole, a pneumonic area forms and extends to the limits of the histologic lobule supplied by the bronchiole in question. Other lobules become infected in the same way, with the result that the affected portion of the lung is spotted with hepatized and relatively normal lobules in an irregular pattern. This form constitutes **lobular pneumonia.** Since its origin is by way of the bronchial passages, it is also known as **bronchial pneumonia** or bronchopneumonia. While in some instances, infected particles fall or are sucked through a normal bronchial passageway, in other cases,

the infection and the inflammation spread along the lining of the bronchus, infecting it bit by bit. In this case, the bronchopneumonia is accompanied by bronchitis and bronchiolitis.

Hematogenous pneumonia arises when the blood carries pathogenic organisms to produce, at least temporarily, a condition of septicemia. This happens in the case of certain viral infections, like psittacosis. It also occurs with bacterial septicemias. Pasteurellosis, while often bronchogenous, may reach the lungs in this way as is proven by the fact that the causative organisms often invade the pericardial space, which can be reached in no other way than by the blood. Pneumonia of hematogenous origin may be lobular or it may be **lobar,** meaning that it involves not a lobule here and lobule there, but that it affects all lobules in a considerable area, even a whole lobe. The term **fibrinous pneumonia** is often used synonymously with lobar pneumonia, but fibrinous describes the character of the exudate rather than the anatomical distribution, and should not be considered as a substitute for the term lobar. The virulence of the invading pathogen is of greater importance than the route by which the pathogen reaches the lung in determining if the resultant pneumonia is lobular or lobar. Many pneumonias arising by the bronchogenous route are lobar in distribution, if the offending organism is highly virulent or the host lacks resistance; in fact many examples of lobar pneumonia in animals are aerogenous in origin.

The distinction between lobar and lobular pneumonia is less important in veterinary than in human medicine, where lobar pneumonia is a specific disease with a specific cause, the *Diplococcus pneumoniae,* a fibrinous reaction, and a specific course and treatment. Most pneumonias in animals are lobular.

Causes. The causes of pneumonia are infections; bacterial, viral, and exceptionally, fungal. Chemical irritants, such as gases like chlorine, sulfur dioxide, mustard gas,

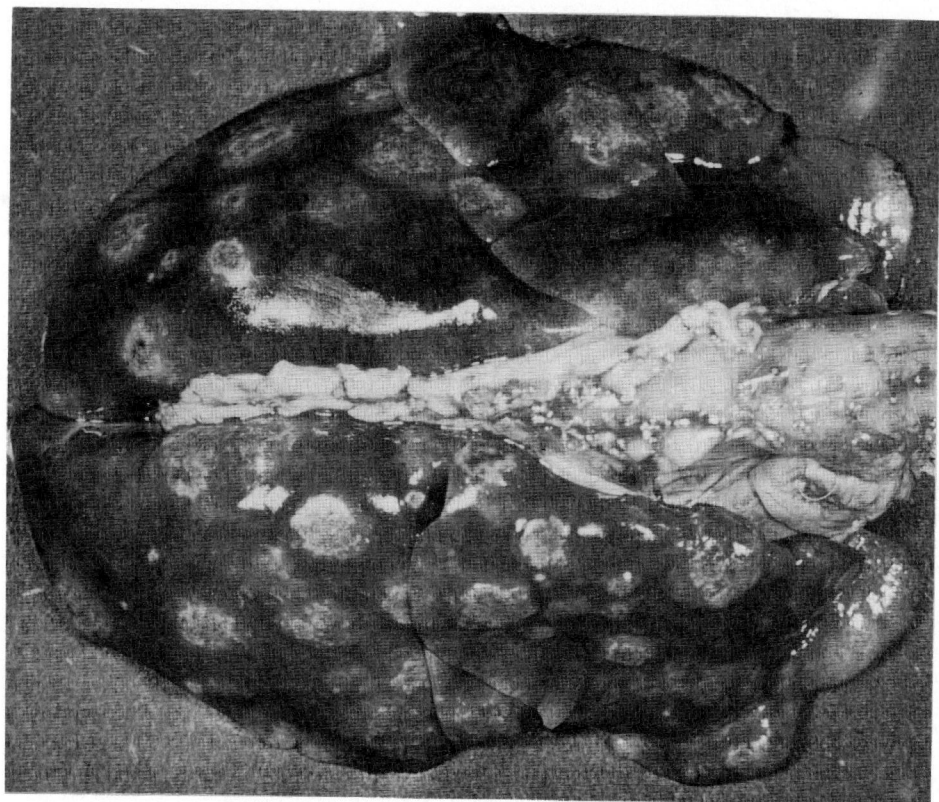

Fig. 20–4. Purulent pneumonia in the lungs of a one-year-old female tortoiseshell cat. (Courtesy of Angell Memorial Animal Hospital.)

and ether vapor used as an anesthetic, and various irritating medicinal substances accidentally introduced via the trachea when intended for the esophagus, should be added to the list of causes conditionally. They are frequent inciting causes, but usually they merely produce an area of injury or necrosis with a distinctly limited inflammatory reaction. Inhaled bacteria, finding a fertile field of growth in the injured and debilitated area, then continue the irritation and are responsible for most of the pneumonic process. Chemicals do not reproduce themselves; bacteria multiply indefinitely. Likewise, metazoan parasites produce an initial injury, the injured area then becoming infected with inhaled bacteria which would not be able to colonize the healthy tissue.

An outline of the types of infectious agents that have been identified in pneumonic lungs is included in Table 20–2. This table undoubtedly does not include all such agents but may give a perspective to the complex susceptibility of the lung to infection.

It would be a matter of great diagnostic convenience if a characteristic type of pneumonic reaction could be attributed to each individual causative agent but only a few generalities are possible. In foals, a distinctly suppurative exudate with neutrophil polymorphs filling the alveoli is likely to be due to *Corynebacterium equi.* In other hosts a strongly suppurative reaction may be seen at times but can hardly be used to identify the offending pathogen. A reaction that is strongly fibrinous is sug-

Table 20-2. Putative Infectious Causes of Pneumonia (Organisms Identified in Pneumonic Lungs)

Bacteria: (see Chapter 10)	Principal Hosts:
Pasteurella multocida	many species
Pasteurella hemolytica	ruminants
Streptococcus spp.	several species
Corynebacterium pyogenes	ruminants, several species
Corynebacterium equi	horses
Bordetella bronchiseptica	dogs, swine, nonhuman primates
Hemophilus suis	swine
Hemophilus influenzae	nonhuman primates
Klebsiella pneumoniae	nonhuman primates, dogs
Staphylococcus spp.	dogs
Pseudomonas aeruginosa	cats, rabbits, several others
Diplococcus pneumoniae	nonhuman primates, rats
Corynebacterium pseudotuberculosis	sheep, rabbits
Mycobacterium tuberculosis	primates, all other species
Actinobacillus lignieresi	cattle

Viruses: (see Chapter 9)	Principal Hosts:
Equine Influenza A	horses, mules, donkeys
Equine herpesvirus, 1–4	horses, mules, donkeys
Equine rhinovirus	horses, mules, donkeys
Equine parainfluenza-3	horses, mules, donkeys
Equine adenovirus	horses
Equine viral arteritis	horses
Equine horse-sickness	horses
Canine distemper	dogs, mink, ferrets
Canine herpesvirus	dogs
Canine adenovirus 1,2	dogs, foxes
Parainfluenza, SV5	dogs
Canine reovirus-1	dogs
Infectious bovine rhinotracheitis	cattle
Bovine parainfluenza–3	cattle
Bovine respiratory syncytial	cattle
Bovine mucosal disease	cattle, sheep
Bovine reovirus	cattle
Feline herpesvirus	cats

Mycoplasma: (Chapter 10)	Principal Hosts:
Mycoplasma dispar	ruminants
Ureaplasma	ruminants
Mycoplasma bovirhinis	ruminants
Mycoplasma mycoides	ruminants
Mycoplasma spp.	ruminants, swine
Mycoplasma pulmonis	rats

Chlamydia: (Chapter 10)	Principal Hosts:
Chlamydia spp.	cattle
Chlamydia spp.	cats
Chlamydia psittaci	parrots and other birds, man

Higher bacteria and fungi: (Chapter 12)	Principal Hosts:
Aspergillus fumigatus, flavus, niger, nidulans	birds, mammals
Coccidioides immitis	many mammals
Blastomyces dermatidis	dogs, man
Histoplasma capsulatum	man, dogs
Cryptococcus neoformans	cats, man
Haplosporangium parvum	rodents, armadillo
Actinomyces bovis	cattle, swine
Nocardia spp.	several species
Sphaeropherus necrophorus	swine, cattle
Geotrichum candidum	dog

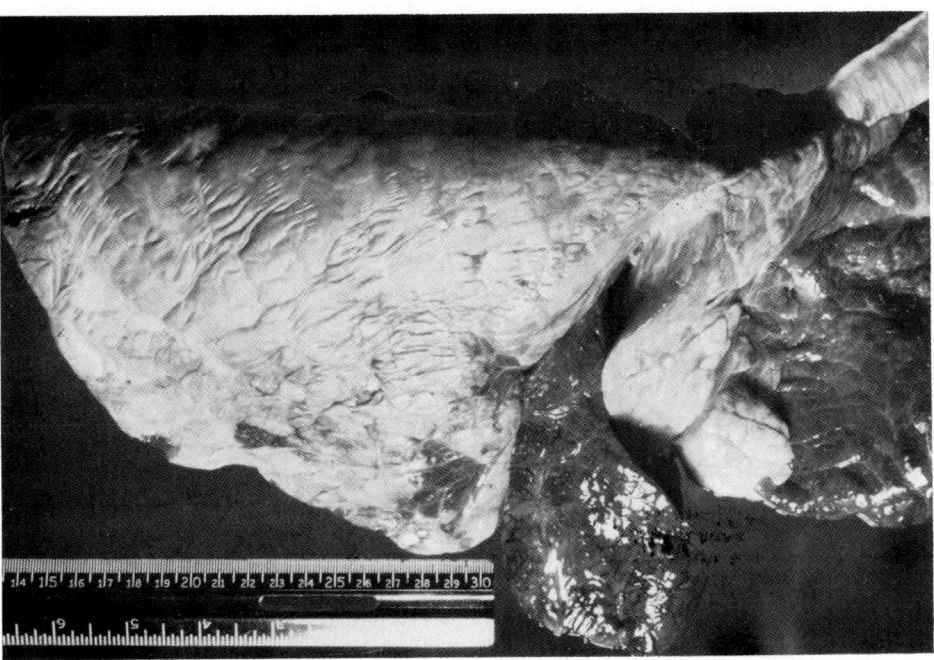

Fig. 20–5. Pneumonia involving apical and cardial lobes of the right lung of a male calf, four months of age. *Pasteurella spp.* was isolated from the affected lobes.

gestive of *Pasteurella sp.*, although not all *Pasteurella* pneumonias are fibrinous by any means. Streptococcal pneumonias are likely to be fibrinous.

It is possible to make the general statement that pneumonia having a virus as its cause is usually characterized by a serous and mononuclear reaction, whereas most pneumonias of bacterial causation produce an exudate in which both the granulocytes and fibrin predominate. A number of viruses, mycoplasma, and members of the psittacosis-lymphogranuloma group of agents, either cause pneumonia independently or predispose to one or more of the bacterial invaders so that pneumonia becomes a feature of the typical syndrome produced by them. These include the agents of equine rhinopneumonitis, bovine contagious pleuropneumonia, canine distemper, feline pneumonitis, a contagious mycoplasma pleuropneumonia of pigs, and contagious pleuropneumonia of goats. For the most part, pneumonias

produced by these agents, in the absence of secondary bacterial invaders (and excluding bovine and caprine pleuro-pneumonia), are not comparable to the exudative lobular and lobar pneumonias described above. Instead the inflammatory reaction is predominantly interstitial, and appropriately the lesion is termed **interstitial pneumonia,** which is characterized by exudation within the interalveolar septa. The septa become greatly thickened by infiltrating lymphocytes, macrophages, and plasma cells, the accumulation of serum or fibrin, and by an increase in connective tissue fibers. Hyperplasia of alveolar lining cells is a frequent finding. Exudation of neutrophils into the alveoli is not a usual feature, however, free-lining cells and macrophages may occupy the alveoli. These features are also characteristic of **hypersensitivity pneumonitis.** In some infections, such as canine distemper, measles, and parainfluenza-3 in calves, multinucleated giant cells are a component

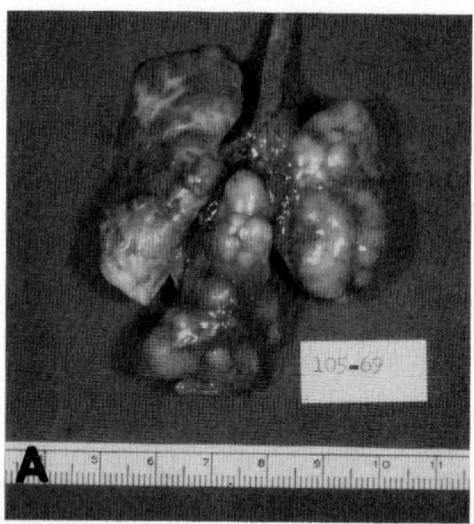

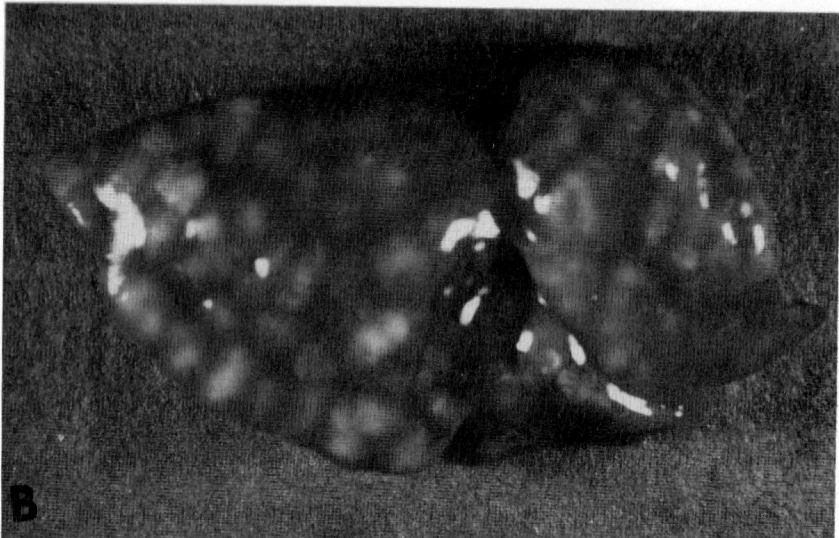

Fig. 20–6.   Chronic murine pneumonia, rat. *A,* Bronchiectatic nodules. *B,* Focal consolidation. (Courtesy of Animal Research Center, Harvard Medical School.)

of the exudate in the septa and the alveolar lumens. Focal accumulation of lymphocytes often producing distinct nodules with germinal centers is a feature of many interstitial pneumonias, such as those in swine, calves, sheep, and rats caused by mycoplasmas and chlamydiae.

Chilling of the body or a part of it lowers resistance and predisposes to pneumonia as it does to other respiratory infections. Extreme fatigue and severe hunger lower resistance to most infections, respiratory as well as others. How chilling and fatigue lower resistance is somewhat of a mystery; but how often have most of us associated our own "colds" (or other afflictions) with wet feet, a chill, or being tired?

Effects. Many cases of pneumonia are fatal. The pneumonia may be accompanied by morbid changes in other organs, as, for instance, in pasteurellosis. When the pulmonary disease alone is responsible for death, it may occur because too many of the alveoli are filled and unable to do their part in aerating the blood. This happens especially if non-hepatized areas are in a state of congestion and edema, conditions which also prevent the erythrocytes from getting and purveying oxygen. However, pneumonia is often fatal with very considerable portions of the lung tissue still functional. In such cases, death is attributed to toxic effects from the microorganisms and their products.

Bronchiectasis and carnification have been mentioned as unfavorable sequelae. In a few cases in which the invading organisms belong to the pyogenic group and are of high virulence, **abscesses** may form in the hepatized tissue. More frequently, however, pulmonary abscesses are of embolic origin in an otherwise healthy lung. In a few other pneumonias from non-pyogenic pathogens of high virulence, areas of tissue are killed by the toxins produced and gangrene results, but pulmonary gangrene usually has other causes.

Bitsch, V., Friis, N.F., and Krogh, H.V.: A microbiological study of pneumonic calf lungs. Acta Vet. Scand., 17:32–42, 1976.

Chattopadhyay, S.K., et al.: Studies on the incidence and pathology of suppurative pneumonia in sheep. Indian J. Anim. Sci., 41:692–697, 1971.

Coggins, L.: Viral respiratory infections of horses: host resistance and immunity. J. Am. Vet. Med. Assoc., 166:78–80, 1975.

Coggins, L., and Kemen, M.J.: Viral respiratory infections of horses: some specific viruses affecting the horse. J. Am. Vet. Med. Assoc., 166:80–83, 1975.

Done, S.H.: Some aspects of pathology of the lower respiratory tract of the dog: review. J. Small Anim. Pract., 11:655–668, 1970.

Fulton, R.W., Ott, R.L., Duenwald, J.C., and Gorham, J.R.: Serum antibodies against canine respiratory viruses: prevalence among dogs of eastern Washington. Am. J. Vet. Res., 35:853–856, 1974.

Good, R.C., and May, B.D.: Respiratory pathogens in monkeys. Infect. Immunol., 3:87–93, 1971.

Jang, S.S., Demartini, J.C., Henrickson, R.V., and Enright, F.M.: Focal necrotizing pneumonia in cats associated with a gram-negative eugonic fermenting bacterium. Cornell Vet., 63:446–454, 1973.

Jensen, R., et al.: Shipping fever pneumonia in yearling feedlot cattle. J. Am. Vet. Med. Assoc., 169:500–506, 1976.

Martin, G.V., and Heath, R.B.: Further studies on induced respiratory viral infection of vervet monkeys (Cercopithecus aethiops). Lab. Anim., 6:181–187, 1972.

McChesney, A.E.: Viral respiratory infections of horses: structure and function of lungs in relation to viral infection. J. Am. Vet. Med. Assoc., 166:76–77, 1975.

McChesney, A.E.: Viral respiratory infections of horses: pathogenesis. J. Am. Vet. Med. Assoc., 166:77–78, 1975.

Nielsen, S.W.: Comparative pathology of pulmonary diseases. In The Lung, Int. Acad. Pathol. Monograph No. 8. Baltimore, Williams and Wilkins, 1967, Chapter 15, pp. 226–244.

Platt, H.: The role of respiratory viruses in equine disease. Vet. Rec., 91:33–36, 1972.

Powell, D.G.: Equine infectious respiratory disease. Vet. Rec., 96:30–34, 1975.

Ramachandran, K.M., and Sivadas, C.G.: Pathology of pneumonia in pigs. 1. Studies on natural cases and a report on the incidence of enzootic pneumonia of pigs in India. Kerala J. Vet. Sci., 2:29–37, 1971.

Rathore, B.S., and Singh, N.P.: Pneumonia in buffaloes—a pathological study. Indian J. Anim. Sci., 40:499–507, 1970.

Rathore, B.S., Singh, N.P., and Singh, V.B.: Lymphoid pneumonia in buffaloes. Indian J. Anim. Sci., 41:667–671, 1971.

Rybicka, K., Daly, B.D.T., Migliore, J.J., and Norman, J.C.: Intravascular macrophages in normal calf lung. An electron microscope study. Am. J. Anat., 139:353–367, 1974.

Singh, S.P., and Singh, N.P.: Studies on mortality in bovine calves due to pneumoenteritis. Indian J. Anim. Sci., 42:798–802, 1972.

Thomas, L.H., and Swann, R.G.: Influence of colostrum on the incidence of calf pneumonia. Vet. Rec., 92:454–455, 1973.

Thomas, L.H.: Observations on the role of viruses in pneumonia of calves. Vet. Rec., 93:384–388, 1973.

Thompson, H., Wright, N.G., and Cornwell, H.J.C.: Contagious respiratory disease in dogs. Vet. Bull., 45:479–488, 1975.

Velo, G.P., and Spector, W.G.: The origin and turnover of alveolar macrophages in experimental pneumonia. J. Pathol., 109:7–19, 1973.

Special Types of Pneumonia

A number of types of pneumonia commonly receive special recognition because of peculiar characteristics.

Embolic Pneumonia

This is characterized by numerous pneumonic foci which are rather evenly scattered through all lobes of both lungs, the greatest number of foci being near the pleural surface until they become confluent and their site of origin becomes obscured. The sub-pleural location is attributable to the fact that this area contains the largest proportion of small arteries and arterioles in which an embolus may be lodged. In contrast, the hematogenous pneumonia which accompanies septicemic diseases is diffuse. However, it is more frequent that lodged emboli produce individualized abscesses (rarely other types of reaction, such as specific granulomas) rather than areas of hepatization. Microscopically, embolic pneumonia can be seen in its earlier stages to differ from bronchopneumonia in that the foci spread out from blood vessels and not from bronchi.

Verminous Pneumonia

Verminous pneumonia is another form in which there is departure from the usual anteroventral distribution of lesions. In verminous pneumonia, the diaphragmatic lobes have their full share of pneumonic areas because these depend upon the localization of the worms. The larvae of ascarid worms pass through the lungs, especially in swine, but may leave only negligible lesions. The inflamed areas in verminous pneumonia are usually small, scattered, and in different chronological stages, a fact of diagnostic value. The adult nematodes are usually found in the bronchi and bronchioles, where they incite a mucopurulent bronchitis. However, the exact site of localization of the adult nematodes varies among lungworms. Their embryonated ova or larvae are conspicuous in the bronchial exudate, by which they leave the lungs for the extraneous part of their existence. True pneumonic lesions develop when the tissue which the worms have injured is attacked by inspired pathogens from the throat region. Each individual inflammatory focus, small, large, or perhaps confluent, thus has the usual characteristics of bronchopneumonia, some of the usual organisms being demonstrable. However, there is considerable tendency to chronicity, not only through the consecutive development of different foci, but also within the individual lesions. These heal with difficulty or not at all until the worm lives its life span and disappears (several weeks), and there is often considerable reaction of the foreign-body type and fibrous encapsulation. In the meantime, an extensive and fatal bacterial pneumonia may or may not develop. The immunologic aspects of repeated infections by lungworms are referred to in Chapter 7.

Gangrenous Pneumonia

Gangrenous pneumonia is in veterinary medicine almost synonymous with what is variously called **aspiration pneumonia, foreign-body pneumonia, medication pneumonia, lipid pneumonia** and others of similar import. As previously stated it is possible for some pneumonia-producing pathogens of high virulence to kill tissue outright, which then becomes subject to invasion by putrefactive saprophytes, thus fulfilling the specifications of gangrene, but such cases are rare. Pulmonary embolism and infarction with saprophytic invasion of the dead infarct are also possible but rare.

The usual cause of gangrenous pneumonia is the introduction into the lungs of medicines intended for the esophagus. Henceforth, what happens is largely dependent on the nature and quantity of the material introduced. Many drugs are highly irritant and entirely capable of producing necrosis of the pulmonary tissue, which is much less resistant than the mucus-protected lining of the stomach. Oily drugs are especially harmful, not because of their immediately irritating properties, but because the oil, especially mineral oil, is not capable of being absorbed and cannot be eliminated. In any case, these medicines are not sterile, nor is the pharyngeal mucosa over which they pass. We thus have an irritant chemical substance and a rather massive concentration of various kinds of bacteria in the same place. The result is very often, but not invariably, necrosis of the area followed by gangrene. In animals whose cough reflexes are impaired by anesthesia, paralysis, or coma, there is always the possibility of aspiration of drops of exudate, particles of food or vomitus. Indeed whole grains, heads of wheat, or parts of ears of corn are occasionally found in the lungs of the herbivorous animals (see Fig. 20–7). These usually carry high concentrations of bacteria of many kinds. Gangrene of the area involved is a common result, preceded by a very intense inflammation.

The definitive lesion of gangrenous pneumonia is death of tissue. It is accompanied by intense hyperemia and exudative and even hemorrhagic inflammation in the surrounding living tissue. The dead tissue soon liquefies (liquefaction necrosis) so that it can almost be said that the characteristic lesion is cavitation. Like other necrotic tissue, the remaining dead tissue may be white or black depending on the amount of blood in it. As putrefying bacteria multiply, foul odors appear. The liquefied material may be of pasty consistency at one stage, but ultimately becomes entirely fluid. These changes are commonly well established in a course of 2 or 3 days, although death may come earlier. Numerous foreign bodies have been reported to cause focal or diffuse pneumonic lesions. These include foreign feed or plant material inhaled by swine; hair fragment emboli reaching the lungs of rats via the vasculature from the skin—introduced by a needle through the skin into a vein; and inhaled vegetable products that often reach the lung of brachiocephalic dogs.

Hyaline-membrane Disease

This designation has been applied to a fatal respiratory distress syndrome of premature infants in which one of the features is the presence, at postmortem, of hyaline membranes within alveoli. These membranes are probably the result of fibrinous and other debris in alveoli. This syndrome is associated with surfactant deficiency due to prematurity, disturbance of the fibrinolytic system, atelectasis, and pulmonary hypoperfusion, possibly induced by perinatal asphyxia. The exact cause is unknown.

Homologues of the human disease have been produced experimentally in premature lambs and nonhuman primates. A few natural cases have been reported in animals. These may or may not involve the same mechanisms seen in the human disease.

Pneumonia of "Shipping Fever"

This respiratory disease syndrome in young cattle is usually associated in time by transport from one place to another—often from the farm to a feedlot. The signs may be overlooked, but usually involve upper respiratory disease, which ends in recovery or fatal pneumonia. In a study of 1988 necropsies of cattle in feedlots, Jensen, et al. (1976), found that 64% had lesions of the respiratory tract. "Shipping fever pneumonia" was identified in 75% of the necropsies involving respiratory disease. The lesions tended to be localized in the lower parts of the cardiac and intermediate lobes. The pneumonic areas were associated with bronchitis, accumulation of fibrinous exudate, lymphatic clots, intravascular clots, thrombosis, and focal necrosis. *Pasteurella spp.*, *Mycoplasma*, and infectious bovine rhinotracheitis virus were isolated most frequently.

Hypothetical pathogenic processes, proposed by Jensen, et al. (1976), are initiated by viral, *Pasteurella,* or other microbial growth in the upper respiratory system, which has a deleterious effect on the ciliated cells and mucous coating of the trachea, bronchi, and bronchioles. Pathogenic *Pasteurella* and other microorganisms from the nasopharynx reach the ventral bronchi and alveoli by gravitational drainage along the tracheal floor. *Pasteurella* endotoxin, produced by growth of the organisms in infected lobules, causes thrombosis of veins, capillaries, and lymphatics. This causes ischemic necrosis. Fibrinous exudate predominates in the alveoli but leukocytes and bacteria are also present. It is useful to have a hypothesis concerning pathogenetic mechanisms; such a theory often forms the basis for future study.

Hypostatic Pneumonia

Hypostatic congestion has been described. The porous nature of pulmonary tissue is especially conducive to hypostatic congestion, as a result of which edema of the area is likely to develop. Tissue devitalized by these two circulatory disorders may well fall prey to inhaled upper respiratory pathogens which would be promptly destroyed in a healthy lung. Pneumonia thus develops, in recumbent patients, in the lower parts of the lower lung as a feature, all too frequently terminal, of many diseases.

Granulomatous Pneumonia

A group of infectious organisms often localize in the lung and do not induce pneumonia comparable to the acute exudative pneumonias or interstitial pneumonitis already described. These include many of the higher bacteria and fungi. Although tuberculous pneumonia occurs rarely as an acute febrile pulmonary inflammation which is clinically and pathologically much like the pneumonia already described, the usual tuberculous involvement of the lung is a very different matter, having a much slower course and being characterized by granulomatous rather than exudative lesions. This latter is well termed tuberculous pneumonia.

In the same group are other granulomatous infections that involve the lungs: actinomycosis, actinobacillosis, coccidioidomycosis, histoplasmosis, glanders, chronic aspergillosis, the usual chronic form of blastomycosis, and rarely mucormycosis and others. *Blastomyces dermatitidis* occasionally causes diffuse pneumonia in the dog, although granulomatous lesions are more usual.

Pneumoconiosis

Chronic inflammatory reaction to several inhaled mineral contaminants results in forms of granulomatous pneumonia. Such substances include various dusts from mines, quarries, grinding, sand-blasting, and other industries, the most formidable being silica (SiO_2), beryllium, and asbestos. Bauxite (impure Al_2O_3), graphite, and carbon are less important. Large quantities inhaled over a period of time are usually necessary to cause important disease, but eventual fatalities are not uncommon. The reaction to silicon dioxide is typically in the form of dense fibrous nodules, the condition being known as **silicosis. Asbestosis** is characterized by a more cellular and a more diffuse reaction and by "asbestos bodies" which can be found microscopically in the lesions. These are brownish, club-shaped filaments bearing some resemblance in size and shape to the broken mycelial filaments seen in mucormycosis. The "beryllium granuloma" resembles a non-caseating tubercle, even including Langhans' giant cells. Asteroid inclusion bodies of unique appearance are occasionally seen in the giant cells. The pneumoconioses are largely limited to humans and experimental animals for the reason that domestic animals are seldom exposed to the dusts which cause them. Horses and mules used in quarries and mines are subject to the same atmospheric contamination as the men and develop the same lesions, but such use of draft animals is largely past. The dust pneumonia of pigs belongs with the acute pneumonias. Anthracosis is frequent in dogs required to sleep in coal bins. Pneumonia due to *Pneumocystis carinii* has been described in Chapter 13. Chronic murine pneumonia is considered as a mycoplasmosis in Chapter 10, as is enzootic pneumonia of swine, sheep and calves.

Alley, M.R., and Manktelow, B.W.: Alveolar epithelialization in ovine pneumonia. J. Pathol., 103:219–224, 1971.

Billups, L.H., Lui, S.K., Kelly, D.F., and Garner, F.M.: Pulmonary granulomas associated with PAS-positive bodies in brachycephalic dogs. Vet. Pathol., 9:294–300, 1972.

Bils, R.F.: Effects of nitrogen dioxide and ozone on monkey lung ultrastructure. Pneumonologie, 150:99–111, 1974.

Castleman, W.L., Dungworth, D.L., and Tyler, W.S.: Hyperplastic and inflammatory lesions in pulmonary airways of primates following subacute exposure to low levels of ozone (0.2 PPM). Bull. Int. Union Tuberc., 51:561–563, 1976.

Conway, D.A.: Canine lung changes associated with air pollution. Irish Vet. J., 25:143–147, 1971.

Corner, A.H., and Jericho, K.W.F.: Pneumonia associated with inhaled plant material in swine. Vet. Pathol., 9:384–391, 1972.

Dayan, A.D., Morgan, R.J.I., Trefty, B.T., and Paddock, T.B.B.: Naturally occurring *Diatomaceous pneumoconiosis* in subhuman primates. J. Comp. Pathol., 88:321–325, 1978.

Dodd, D.C., Marshall, B.E., Soma, L.R., and Leatherman, J.: Experimental acid-aspiration pneumonia in the rabbit. Vet. Pathol., 13:436–448, 1976.

Egberts, J.: Spontaneous hyaline membrane disease in mature newborn lambs. Tijdschr. Diergeneeskd., 95:401–406, 1970.

Egberts, J., and Rethmeier, H.B.: Hyaline membrane disease in lambs: a changing morphology. Pathol. Eur., 8:299–306, 1973.

Giddens, W.E., Jr., Whitehair, D.K., and Sleight, S.D.: Nitrogen dioxide (silo gas) poisoning in pigs. Am. J. Vet. Res., 31:1779–1786, 1970.

Gois, M., Sisak, F., Kuksa, F., and Sovadina, M.: Incidence and evaluation of the microbial flora in the lungs of pigs with enzootic pneumonia. Zentralbl. Veterinarmed., 22B:205–219, 1975.

Goldstein, B., Webster, I., and Vanas, A.: Use of nonhuman primates in pneumoconiosis and other industrial disease research. Environ. Res., 7:320–329, 1974.

Gooding, C.A., Gregory, G.A., Taber, P., and Wright, R.R.: An experimental model for the study of meconium aspiration of the newborn. Radiology, 100:137–140, 1971.

Jensen, R., et al.: Atypical interstitial pneumonia in yearling feedlot cattle. J. Am. Vet. Med. Assoc., 169:507–510, 1976.

Jericho, K.W.F.: Inhaled feed particles in experimental pigs with and without vitamin A deficiency. Vet. Pathol., 12:415–427, 1975.

Jones, R., Bakerville, A., and Reid, L.: Histochemical identification of glycoproteins in pig bronchial epithelium: (a) normal and (b) hypertrophied from enzootic pneumonia. J. Pathol., 116:1–11, 1975.

Liu, C.I., Chang, C.F., and Cheng, C.M.: A study on the porcine pneumonias in the slaughter houses. Taiwan J. Vet. Med. Anim. Husb., No. 20, 18–36, 1972.

Long, G.G., White, J.D., and Stookey, J.L.: *Pneumocystis carinii* infection in splenectomized owl monkeys. J. Am. Vet. Med. Assoc., 167:651–654, 1975.

Ludwin, S.K., Northway, W.H., and Bensch, K.G.: Oxygen toxicity in the newborn: necrotizing bronchiolitis in mice exposed to 100% oxygen. Lab. Invest., 31:425–435, 1974.

Mieog, W.H.W., and Egberts, J.: Spontaneous hyaline membrane disease in a kitten. Vet. Rec., 88:264, 1971.

Murphy, J., et al.: Hyaline membrane disease in the premature monkey. Am. Rev. Resp. Dis., 113:44, 1976.

Pattison, I.H.: A histological study of a transmissible pneumonia of pigs characterized by extensive lymphoid hyperplasia. Vet. Rec., 68:490–494, 1956.

Resnick, J.S., Brown, D.M., and Vernier, R.L.: Oxygen toxicity in fetal organ culture. II. The developing lung. Lab. Invest., 31:665–677, 1974.

Richter, C.B., Humason, G.L., and Godbold, J.H.: Endemic *Pneumocystis carinii* in a marmoset colony. J. Comp. Pathol., 88:171–180, 1978.

Robinson, F.R.: Toxicity of beryllium and other elements in missile propellants. Clin. Toxicol., 6:497–502, 1973.

Takeli, S.: Occurrence of hair-fragment emboli in the pulmonary vascular system of rats. Vet. Pathol., 11:482–485, 1974.

Pneumonitis

There is considerable diversity in the use of this term, which literally means an inflammation of the lungs. In general, it has been used for inflammatory conditions of the lung to which one hesitates to apply the term pneumonia. The latter we have already described in the classic way as an acute exudative filling of the lung alveoli, with a rather typical febrile clinical course. Many consider the term pneumonitis synonymous with interstitial pneumonia. Several special types of pneumonitis are now recognized in animals and it appears most useful to consider them in connection with their etiology.

Hypersensitivity Pneumonitis (allergic alveolitis)

Exposure to specific antigens, particularly products of mold growth, results in a hypersensitive immune state which is precipitated by reexposure into a severe tissue reaction. If the lung is the target organ, the tissue reactions and clinical signs are grouped under this term, hypersensitivity pneumonitis. This phenomenon has been demonstrated repeatedly in animals under experimental conditions and is also recognized in man and animals as a disease phenomenon in nature.

A large number of antigens have been found to produce hypersensitivity upon inhalation by man or animals. These antigens have been identified particularly in vegetable, animal, insect, bacterial, or viral products, particularly if contaminated by molds. The disease conditions have been long identified with the affected worker's occupation: "farmer's lung," "mushroom-worker's disease," "malt-worker's lung," "paprika-slicer's lung," "thatched-roof disease," "pigeon-breeder's disease," "miller's lung," etc. Some of the specific antigens have been identified. "Farmer's lung" was initially associated (Campbell, 1932) with farmers who had been working with moldy hay. The antigens are now associated with certain thermophilic actinomycetes, particularly *Micropolyspora faeni* and *Thermoactinomyces vulgaris*. Many other sensitizing organisms have been tentatively identified (Wessels et al., 1973; Salvaggio, 1976; Olenchock, 1977).

Equine Pulmonary Emphysema (chronic diffuse alveolar emphysema, heaves, broken wind)

An equine disease long associated with moldy, dusty hay, and compared with chronic allergic bronchitis—asthma in man—as early as 1887 (Stömmer), its cause is not completely known. Sensitization to products of some common contaminants of a horse's environment has been demonstrated (Eyre, 1972). *Aspergillus spp., Alternaria spp.,* and *Hormodendrum spp.* have been used as antigens to demonstrate sensitivity in affected horses by direct skin tests and passive cutaneous anaphylactic skin tests (Prausnitz-Küstner). Affected horses have also been shown to be sensitized to chickens (Mansmann, et al., 1975).

Horses with pulmonary emphysema have a characteristic sign which consists of two successive expiratory movements, with the second forcibly expelling the last portion of tidal air. The lesions include diffuse and rather evenly distributed alveolar emphysema, which is identified by gross inspection of the lung. The emphysema appears to be secondary to chronic bronchiolitis, which may be associated with bronchiospasms that occlude the alveolar ducts. Hyperplasia of the bronchiolar musculature and peribronchiolar leukocytic infiltration has been noted in association with mucous and purulent exudate in bronchiolar lumens.

Bovine Allergic Alveolitis (bovine-farmer's lung, bovine hypersensitivity pneumonitis)

If a farmer, while feeding moldy hay to his cows, becomes hypersensitive to the molds, it should be no surprise that the cows also become sensitized to the same molds, which is exactly what does happen. Typically, the bovine disease occurs during the winter months when the adult cows are housed indoors and fed last year's crop of hay. Affected cows cough frequently, have an increased rate of respiration, and a decrease in milk yield, weight, and appetite. The number of affected animals increases and severity of signs intensifies as the winter progresses. After some months, chronically affected animals may die.

Using double-diffusion tests, precipitating antibodies may be detected in antigen prepared from cultures of *Micropolyspora faeni*. Skin tests are also of value in detecting the antigen of *M. faeni* in affected cows. Induration of the skin at the site of antigenic inoculation may be present 2 to 4 hours after injection. Exposure of sensitized animals to aerosol suspensions of mold by way of the respiratory tract, will accentuate the clinical signs.

Lesions. The gross lesions in chronic cases are concentrated in the lungs. Lobules in all lobes may contain small gray foci, and peripheral alveoli are grossly distended. Excessive yellow mucus may be found in some bronchi. Microscopically, the bronchioles are particularly affected. Some are obliterated by protrusion of inflammatory exudate into the lumen, carrying the epithelium with it. The interstitial exudate contains macrophages, monocytes, lymphocytes, plasma cells, and occasional fibroblasts; a few multinucleated giant cells may be present. The affected bronchioles are surrounded by lymphocytes, plasma cells, globule cells, and occasionally eosinophils. These cells are numerous in the alveolar septa and may form small, discrete granulomas. In many areas, this interstitial exudate is accompanied by hyperplasia of cuboidal, sometimes ciliated cells, lining the alveoli.

Equine Allergic Pneumonitis

A syndrome with many similarities to bovine and human "farmer's lung" has been described in horses by Pauli, Gerber, and Schatzmann (1972). This disease is manifest by attacks of dyspnea and coughing associated with eosinophilia of peripheral blood and nasal secretions. Intracutaneous response was demonstrated to allergenic mixtures of dust from food and bedding. Precipitins develop for *Micropolyspora faeni* and *Aspergillus fumigatus.*

The lesions began as acute interstitial pneumonitis with interalveolar edema, intravascular fibrin masses, fibrillar hyaline membranes in alveoli, and extensive infiltration of interstitium and alveoli with monocytes and macrophages. Hyperplasia of the alveolar epithelium and fibrosis of interstitial tissues were seen in late stages.

Bronchial Asthma

This disease is characterized by attacks lasting from one to many hours of very difficult, wheezing respiration, especially expiration, due to spasmodic contraction of the encircling musculature of the bronchioles and smaller bronchi, as well as to the production of large amounts of viscid mucous exudate which is strongly inclined to adhere to the bronchial walls. While some cases are secondary to a bronchial infection, the majority are allergic reactions to a great variety of inhaled organic substances to which the individual has become hypersensitive. That contraction of smooth muscle is an outstanding manifestation of the anaphylactic state has been demonstrated many times by suitable laboratory experiments.

Lesions. The principal lesions in fatal cases include extensive infiltration of the bronchial and bronchiolar walls with lymphocytes, monocytes and usually large numbers of eosinophils, accumulation of dense mucous exudate in the lumens, as well as in the epithelial cells which produce it, and frequently an astonishing hyaline thickening of the bronchial basement membranes. The mucus sometimes condenses in peculiar spiral strings called Curschmann's spirals. There is marked secondary emphysema.

Causes. Asthma is chiefly a human disease, but it has possibly occurred in cattle and certainly, though rarely, in cats and dogs. In the latter, it has been produced artificially in experimental work. The similarities in etiology and lesions causes us to consider asthma in relation to hypersensitivity pneumonitis. The antigens which affect animals have not yet been adequately studied. Hypersensitivity to pollens in the dog results from exposure through the respiratory tract, but the effects are manifest principally in the skin (atopy, atopic skin disease). Susceptibility appears to be inherited.

Hypersensitivity in Lungworm Infection

Reinfection of previously infected cattle with the lungworm, *Dictyocaulus viviparous,* has been considered to produce acute respiratory distress. This situation can be differentiated from acute interstitial emphysema or "fog fever" on the basis of the clinical and pathologic features. It is known that initial infections with lung-worms produce almost no tissue reaction in the lung until immune reactions have had sufficient time to appear. Animals (cattle or sheep especially) which were infected with lungworms one season and then reinfected at the beginning of the second season may exhibit signs of severe respiratory distress, and death may occur. Severe tissue reaction to the parasites is a constant feature of the pulmonary lesions. It appears that immunologic factors are important in this disease and require further study.

Brentjens, J.R., et al.: Experimental immune complex disease of the lung. The pathogenesis of a laboratory model resembling certain human interstitial lung diseases. J. Exp. Med., 140:105–125, 1974.

Campbell, J.M.: Acute symptoms following work with hay. Brit. Med. J., 2:1143, 1932.

Eyre, P.: Equine pulmonary emphysema: a bronchopulmonary mould allergy. Vet. Rec., 91:134–140, 1972.

Gillespie, J.R., and Tyler, W.S.: Chronic obstructive lung disease in horses. In Research Animals in Medicine, edited by L.T. Harmison. Washington, D.C., U.S. Government Printing Office, 1973. pp. 223–227.

Halliwell, R.E.W., and Schwartzman, R.M.: Atopic disease in the dog. Vet. Rec., 89:209–214, 1971.

Harbourne, J.F., Luery, K.W., Wallace, J.C., and Threlkeld, J.M.: Farmer's lung hay antibodies in cattle. Vet. Rec., 87:559–560, 1970.

Jensen, R., et al.: Atypical interstitial pneumonia in yearling feedlot cattle. J. Am. Vet. Med. Assoc., 169:507–510, 1976.

Major, P.C., Lapp, N.L., and Burrell, R.: Immunopathology and pathophysiology in experimental hypersensitivity pneumonitis. Fed. Proc., 31:664, 1972.

Mansmann, R.A., Osburn, B.I., Wheat, J.D., and Frick, O.: Chicken hypersensitivity pneumonitis in horses. J. Am. Vet. Med. Assoc., 166:673–677, 1975.

Moore, V.L., Hensley, G.T., and Fink, J.N.: An animal model of hypersensitivity pneumonitis in the rabbit. J. Clin. Invest., 56:937–944, 1975.

Olenchock, S.A.: Animal models of hypersensitivity pneumonitis: a review. Ann. Allergy, 38:119–126, 1977.

Patterson, R., Pruzomsky, J.J., and Chang, W.W.Y.: Hypersensitivity to ragweed. Characterization of the serum factor. Transferring skin, bronchial, and anaphylactic sensitivity. J. Immunol., 90:35–42, 1963.

Pauli, B., Gerber, H., and Schatzmann, U.: "Farmer's Lung" beim Pferd. Pathol. Microbiol., 38:200–214, 1972.

Peckham, J.C., Mitchell, F.E., Jones, O.H., Jr., and

Doupnik, B., Jr.: Atypical interstitial pneumonia in cattle fed moldy sweet potatoes. J. Am. Vet. Med. Assoc., 160:169–172, 1972.

Pirie, H.M., et al.: A bovine disease similar to farmer's lung: extrinsic allergic alveolitis. Vet. Rec., 88:346–350, 1971.

Richerson, H.B., Cheng, F., and Bauserman, S.C.: Acute experimental hypersensitivity pneumonitis in rabbits. Am. Rev. Respir. Dis., 104:568–575, 1971.

Richerson, H.B.: Acute experimental hypersensitivity pneumonitis in the guinea pig. J. Lab. Clin. Med., 79:745–757, 1972.

Salvaggio, J.: Animal models in the pathogenesis of immunologically mediated pulmonary disease. Bull. Int. Union Tuberc., 51:443–449, 1976.

Stömmer, O.: Über das chronische vesikuläre Emphysem namentlich der Pferdelunge. Deutsche Z. Thiermed. (Lpz), 13:93–118, 1887.

Wessels, F., Salvaggio, J., and Lopez, M.: Animal models of hypersensitivity pneumonitis. J. Am. Anim. Hosp. Assoc., 9:588–597, 1973.

Wilkie, B.N., Gygax, M., and Pauli, B.: Immunofluorescent studies of bovine hypersensitivity pneumonitis. Can. J. Comp. Med., 38:475–479, 1974.

Wiseman, A., Selman, I.E., Dawson, C.O., Breeze, R.G., and Pirie, H.M.: Bovine farmers' lung: a clinical syndrome in a herd of cattle. Vet. Rec., 93:410–417, 1973.

Zaidi, S.H., and Chandra, S.V.: Experimental farmer's lung in guinea pigs. J. Pathol., 105:41–48, 1971.

Pleuritis

Inflammation of the pleura is known as pleuritis or by the older name of pleurisy. The ordinary forms of pleuritis belong to the acute exudative inflammations, usually being either serous, fibrinous, or purulent. If the pleuritis accompanies pneumonia, the pleuritic area overlies the hepatized portions of lung parenchyma, the condition being called **pleuropneumonia.** But there are many cases of pneumonia without pleuritis, and it is entirely possible for pleuritis to exist without pneumonia. The pulmonary pleura is first involved, as a rule, but the infection and the inflammatory reaction promptly spread to the contiguous areas of parietal pleura.

The usual attack of pleurisy begins with acute hyperemia and swelling of the thin covering membrane. During this stage, the friction of the visceral and parietal surfaces at each respiratory movement is very painful, causing a typical kind of breathing. After about 2 days a serous exudate appears, which lubricates and separates the two surfaces, and the pain is assuaged. The exudate may remain serous, filling the pleural cavity and compressing the lungs, or it may become fibrinous or purulent. Often all forms coexist, resulting in a sero-fibrino-purulent pleuritis. Microscopically, the pleural layer is infiltrated with lymphocytes and other inflammatory cells. Its thickness is increased several fold by edema fluid which fills the intercellular spaces and distends the numerous but previously unseen lymph vessels. Capillaries are numerous and greatly dilated. The surface layer of mesothelial cells is largely destroyed, and the surface is covered with a thin or thick layer of fibrin or with adherent dead neutrophils and other elements characteristic of a purulent exudate.

With the lapse of a few days the amount of seropurulent exudate collecting in the pleural cavity may become so great as to interfere seriously with expansion of the lungs, requiring drainage by thoracocentesis. In such cases, the exudate is very likely to become fibrinous, depending largely on the kind of organism that is causing it. The layers of fibrin on each of the two apposing surfaces tend to become organized by immigrating fibroblasts, and the two surfaces often become tied together by strands of fibrous connective tissue. These are known as **adhesions;** the inflammatory process is then called **adhesive pleuritis.** It is not unusual to find large areas of lung surface inseparably joined to the chest wall. Most animals so affected die while the process is still active. Some survive the causative infection with adhesions of limited extent. These adhesions cause pain with respiratory movement, but this diminishes as the anatomical structures adjust themselves. There is no permanent disability in most cases.

Causes. The causes of pleuritis are usually infectious, and, in general, they are the same kinds of organisms which cause pneumonia. Infection of the pleura may result by direct extension from the lung, but many cases of pleuritis arise by the hematogenous route without involvement of the lungs, especially in septicemic diseases of young animals. An important variant is seen in those bovines in which a swallowed metallic foreign body penetrates from the reticulum into the pleural cavity, carrying infection with it. A majority of these, however, penetrate the pericardium and produce "traumatic pericarditis" rather than pleuritis. **Tuberculous pleuritis** is a fairly common accompaniment of tuberculosis of other parts. It manifests itself as "pearly disease," in which pleural surfaces, especially those of the thoracic wall, become studded with protruding, irregularly spherical tubercles, dense, white and shiny and thus reminiscent of pearls. They commonly approximate a diameter of 3 to 10 mm. Tuberculous infection may be hematogenous or it may be a direct extension from a tuberculous lung or possibly from a thoracic lymph node. In swine, pleuritis is part of a generalized serositis in two infections, Glasser's disease, caused by *Hemophilus suis,* and a serositis, caused by mycoplasma.

A considerable accumulation of purulent exudate (pus) in the pleural cavity is known as **empyema. Hydrothorax** denotes accumulation of (non-inflammatory) edema fluid in the pleural cavity. The watery fluid has the low specific gravity (1.017 or less) and the low protein content (4% or less) characteristic of a transudate. Hydrothorax is one of the manifestations of generalized edema, usually cardiac or renal. **Chylothorax** denotes the presence of chyle in the pleural cavity. This rare condition results from rupture or erosion of the thoracic duct. The chyle has a milky appearance. However, it is possible for edema fluid or serous exudate to appear milky from a high content of emulsified fat or albumin. Exudates may also accompany intrathoracic neoplasms. **Pneumothorax** is a rare condition in which air gains access to

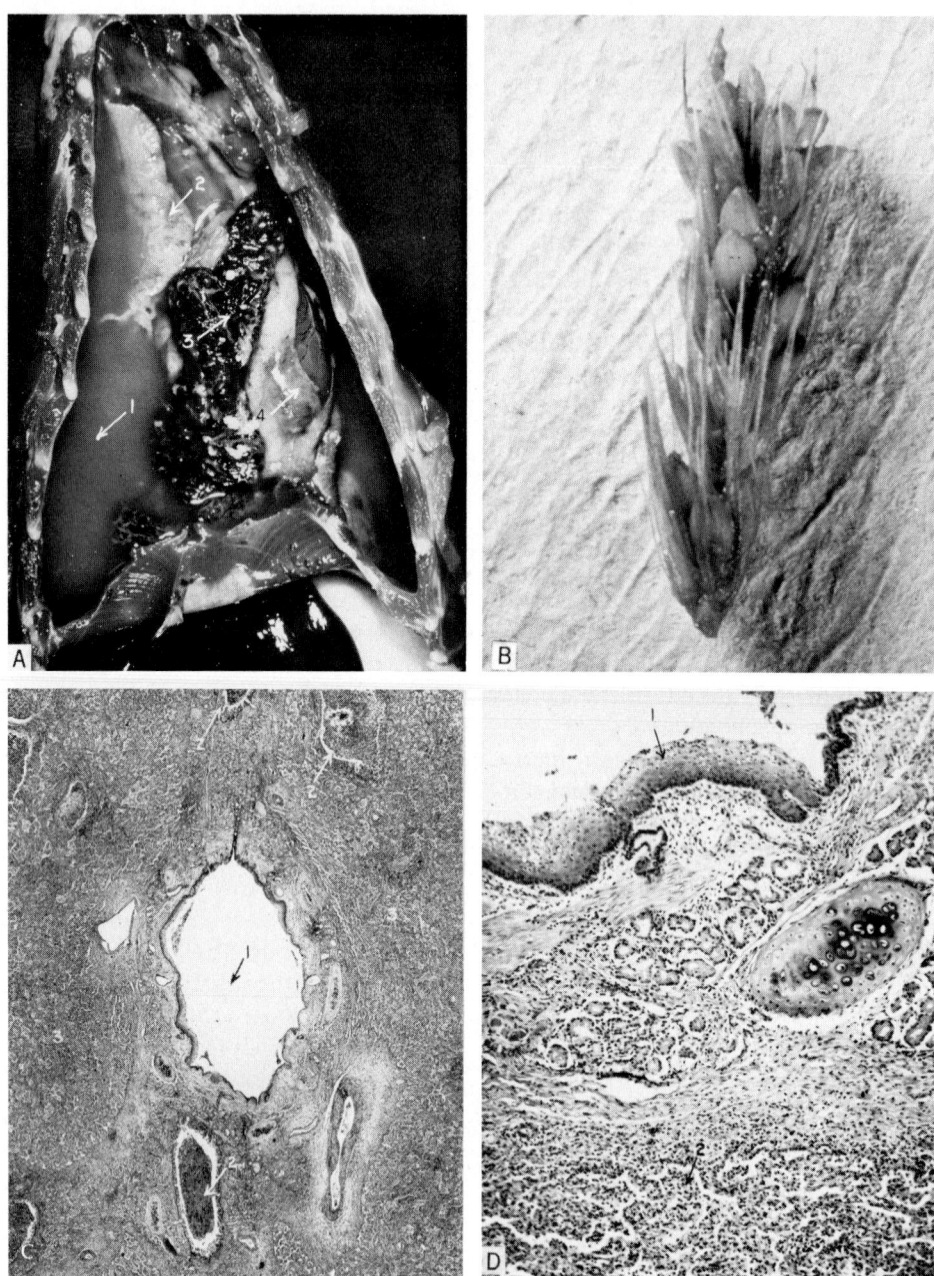

Fig. 20–7. Pyothorax and pneumonia secondary to aspiration of a grass awn by a male cat, age 1½ years. *A,* The thorax at necropsy, containing purulent fluid (*1*), cardiac lobe of lung (*2*), fibrinous exudate in mediastinum (*3*), and fibrinous exudate on pericardium (*4*). *B,* Grass awn found in major bronchus at necropsy. *C,* Bronchus (*1*) in which the grass awn was found, secondary bronchi (*2*) and alveoli (*3*) are filled with purulent exudate. *D,* Higher magnification of *C*. Squamous metaplasia of bronchial epithelium (*1*) and consolidation (*2*) of alveoli. (H & E, × 125.) (Courtesy of Angell Memorial Animal Hospital.)

the pleural cavity. This may occur through a rupture of the chest wall, or through rupture of an emphysematous "bulla" or of some other air-containing lesion of the lung. If large amounts of air enter the pleural sac, the lung on the affected side collapses; pain and dyspnea result. In the horse, such an accident is likely to be fatal, for the right and left pleural cavities usually communicate, and the pneumothorax becomes bilateral. Cases are on record, nevertheless, of recovery from penetrating thoracic wounds.

Among the non-inflammatory disorders which may involve the lung, congestion, edema, infarction, thrombosis, and embolism have been treated at the appropriate places in the section on General Pathology.

Hemorrhages, usually recent, but sometimes old, with clotted fibrin occur in the lungs not only from septicemias and the other causes listed in the discussion of hemorrhage, but also as a result of uremia, presumably because of toxic injury to capillary walls. This may be an important explanation of the hemorrhages of leptospirosis.

While the lungs share in any generalized **passive congestion,** usually acute and terminal, due to a failing heart muscle, it will be remembered that the usual chronic passive congestion is a result of interference with the prompt passage of blood through the left side of the heart. The resulting brown induration with its "heart-failure cells" due to phagocytized hemosiderin has been described. The possibility of hypostatic pneumonia supervening was mentioned under that heading.

In those cases in which recent and relatively acute pulmonary congestion and edema are prominent at autopsy, there is always the question whether one is dealing with active hyperemia and inflammatory edema which would have developed into full-fledged pneumonia if the patient had lived a few hours longer. The relative scarcity of pathogenic organisms when such lungs are submitted to bacterial culture suggests that most of these cases are the result of a failing heart rather than pneumonia. The tendency for the accumulation of fluid to be greatest in the more dependent portions of the lungs and the presence of congested vessels elsewhere in the body tend to confirm this interpretation. Acute hypersensitivity reactions may account for pulmonary edema, but in these examples there is diffuse involvement in all lobes. Anaphylaxis is a classic example, but hypersensitivity also plays a role in hypersensitivity pneumonitis of cattle.

The gross differentiation of the lung that is congested and edematous from one that is pneumonic may confuse the inexperienced. The former is voluminous with little or no tendency to collapse, well rounded and grayish pink, especially in the dorsal parts of the diaphragmatic lobes. It is doughy and "pits on pressure," but it does yield to pressure of the finger, while the hepatized lung is incompressible save for a slight "give" which lets the finger descend just a bit before it comes to an abrupt standstill. From the cut surface, a watery fluid, clear or blood stained, runs out either freely or upon the application of pressure, depending on the degree of severity. The microscopic differentiation is obvious from the nature of the processes involved.

Fibrin **emboli** lodge in the lungs if they are released into the circulation elsewhere but, on the whole, this is not frequent in animals. Fatty emboli are even more rarely recognized. Thrombi form in the vessels of the lungs during the course of severe pneumonias.

As has already been explained, infarction of the lung is unlikely to occur when the pulmonary and bronchial circulations are of normal force. Large infarcted areas tend to become gangrenous upon the advent of saprophytic bacteria, which are sure to be inhaled from time to time.

Atelectasis

This term means failure of the alveoli to open or to remain open; in other words, the empty alveoli are collapsed and do not contain air. The usual atelectasis involves one or more relatively small areas of lung. Such an area is slightly depressed and shrunken as compared to the surrounding tissue, and is sharply demarcated from it. The atelectatic area is dull red in color and has the feeling and consistency which one would expect, for instance, in liver. However, the hepatized tissue of pneumonia is swollen and not shrunken. Atelectatic, as well as hepatized, tissue sinks in water, or almost sinks if it still contains a bit of air. No fluid can be squeezed from its cut surface. Microscopically, the alveoli are compressed into scarcely recognizable slits, all lying parallel in a direction determined by adjacent pressures. Careful inspection will reveal that the cells are those which normally compose lung tissue. While well-filled capillaries may be seen, the total content of blood is less than the same tissue would have contained normally. The bronchioles are collapsed as far as their structure permits.

Cause. The cause of the usual atelectatic area is occlusion of the bronchus or bronchiole which supplies it. This results most often from a plug of mucous or purulent exudate. The air contained at the time the bronchus is closed is absorbed in a short time as is regularly the case with entrapped gases. The airless alveoli then collapse under surrounding pressures.

A lung collapsed because of pneumothorax is also obviously atelectatic, but the usual reference is merely to a portion of lung so affected. The collapse of the alveoli is scarcely so complete when it is the result of pneumothorax since the external pressure does not exceed that within the still patent bronchi. The same is true of areas of atelectasis resulting when pleural fluid occupies some of the space belonging to the lungs. Atelectasis also accompanies space-occupying lesions in the thoracic cavity and the accumulation of transudates and exudates when their volume is great.

Atelectasis neonatorum describes the non-aerated condition of the lungs of a newly born animal which has never breathed. The appearances are not remarkably different from those of atelectasis under other circumstances. The whole lung sinks in water. Determination of this condition may have legal import in settling controversies over breeding fees which are contingent upon the birth of living young. However, caution must be exercised in relying solely on whether the lung sinks in water, for such is occasionally the case in animals born alive, but dying in the perinatal period.

Emphysema

With a literal meaning of inflation, emphysema designates a condition in which there is air in the tissues. This may be, for instance, subcutaneous as the result of a cutaneous wound in such a location that movements exert a sucking or pumping action. It should not be confused with postmortem gas formation, which sometimes causes much gas to accumulate in the tissues as the result of bacterial action. Many times more frequent is pulmonary emphysema. Pulmonary emphysema is of two kinds, alveolar and interstitial.

Alveolar Pulmonary Emphysema

Without qualifying adjectives, it is alveolar pulmonary emphysema that is meant when reference is made to emphysema. In this ordinary emphysema, certain areas of lungs are unduly distended with air. They are thereby distorted so that they project somewhat beyond the surrounding tissue, pale or almost white in color, dry, easily compressed by the finger, but not very resilient. This is because the compressing finger forces air out of the area through narrow openings and devious passageways; its movement can sometimes be recognized by the sensation in the finger. Then, upon removal of the finger the air returns slowly by the same route.

Microscopically, many alveoli are too large and many have wide openings into each other or into a common space due to

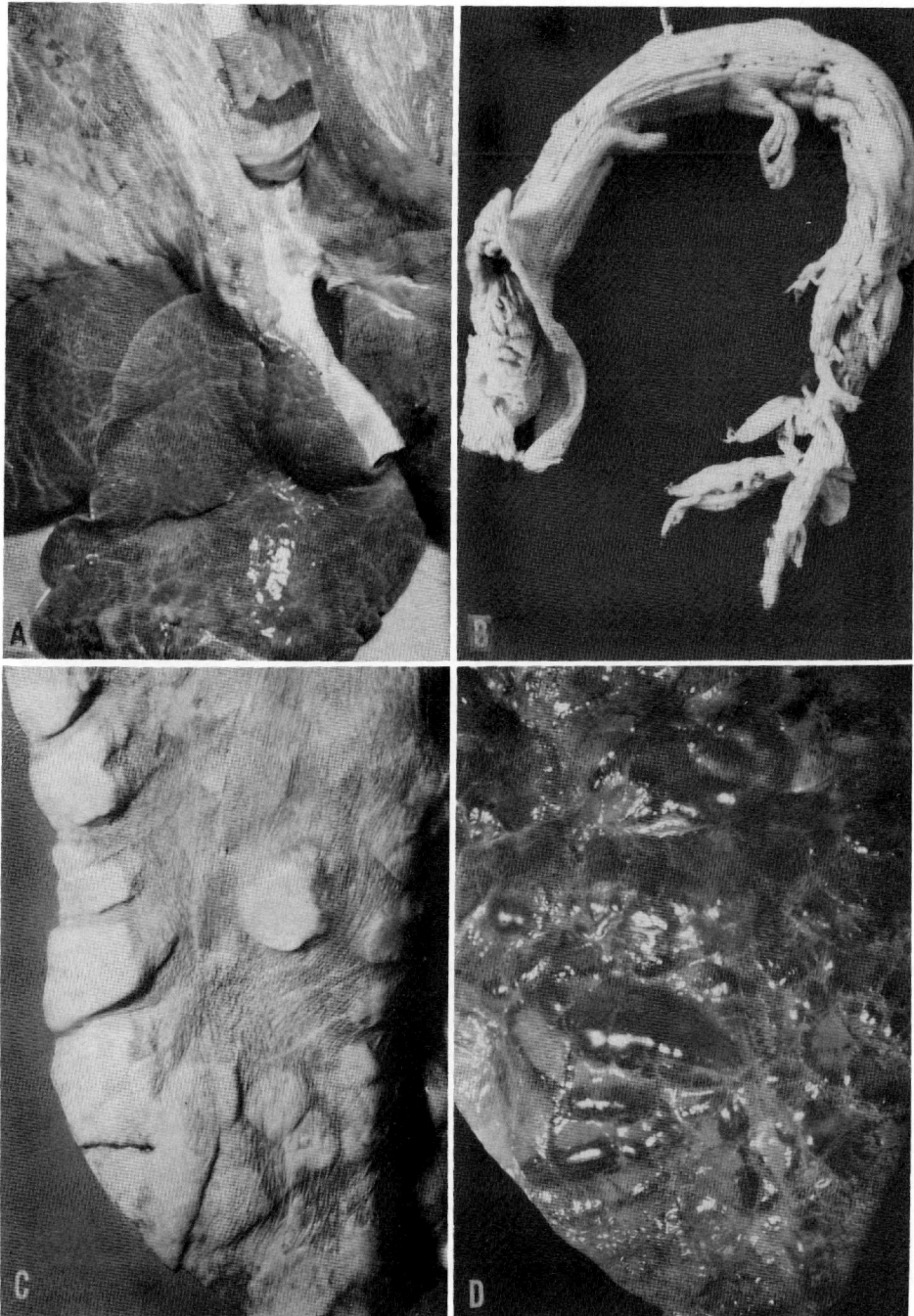

Fig. 20–8. *A*, Early red hepatization in the lung of a calf. *B*, A fibrinous cast from a bronchus and its branches. This was coughed up by a calf whose owner had noticed no sign of illness. *C*, Alveolar emphysema (raised pale areas) in the lung of a swine which died of swine erysipelas. *D*, Interstitial emphysema in the lung of a cow. Death was the result of pyelonephritis.

rupture of alveolar walls. This situation is thus the exact opposite of atelectasis. The blunt ends of alveolar walls which have been broken often persist and become thickened and hyperplastic rounded knobs. Some of the walls are slightly thickened—hence, inelastic—but others are stretched and very thin. Blood-filled capillaries are scarce. The smooth muscle of the alveolar ducts is often hyperplastic.

Cause. Frequently emphysematous areas of lung are seen near, or alternating with, areas of atelectasis. Such examples of emphysema represent areas of lung which have expanded unduly, under the pressure of inhaled air, to occupy the space left vacant by the collapsed, atelectatic portions. In doing this, some alveoli have been stretched beyond their capacity and have burst.

In other cases where there is difficult and forced respiration, a plug of mucus may have seriously but not completely impeded the passage of air in a given bronchus. At inspiration, the area connected with this bronchus slowly fills with air; then, by the forcible expiration which accompanies some acute respiratory diseases, the area in question is put under considerable pressure. The air cannot pass out through the bronchus as fast as this is accomplished in certain neighboring areas; the general pressure tends to force the full alveoli into space being vacated by neighboring emptying alveoli, and the full one is ruptured. The healing of ruptured alveoli involves enough light fibrosis to interfere with their elasticity, although it usually fails to restore the continuity of their walls.

Interstitial Pulmonary Emphysema

This is a condition in which air collects in the interlobular septa, beneath the pleura and wherever there is interstitial tissue in the lungs. Probably because of anatomical peculiarities, the condition is most often seen in necropsies on cattle. In these animals, various interlobular septa as much as 0.5 cm in thickness are seen in criss-crossing straight lines, usually at wider intervals than would be the case if every lobular wall were so thickened. The septum is shiny, well outlined, usually filled with large and small bubbles, and obviously distended with air. Microscopically, the increased width of the septum is seen to be due to separation and distention of the fibers without any increase of tissue elements. It is reported that air from these emphysematous tissues sometimes finds its way into the mediastinal structures and even into the dorsal part of the neck.

Cause. The air gains access to the interstitial tissues from alveoli which have ruptured during violent respiratory efforts. For this reason, this type of emphysema is most often seen as a terminal phenomenon when death from some other cause has been accompanied by violent efforts to compensate for growing anoxia. One of the most familiar situations of this sort is death from loss of blood. This type of emphysema is clearly associated with severe respiratory efforts which appear to be caused by some impediment to the exchange of gases in the alveoli.

Goldring, I.P., et al.: Histopathology and mechanical properties of the lung in experimental emphysema. Pathol. Microbiol., 35:176–180, 1970.

Kuhn, C., III, and Tavassoli, F.: The scanning electron microscopy of elastase-induced emphysema: a comparison with emphysema in man. Lab. Invest., 34:2–9, 1976.

Kuhn, C., et al.: The induction of emphysema with elastase. II. Changes in connective tissue. Lab. Invest., 34:372–380, 1976.

McLauthlin, R.R., Jr., and Edwards, D.W.: Naturally occurring emphysema, the fine, gross and histopathologic counterpart of human emphysema. Am. Rev. Resp. Dis., 93:22–29, 1966.

Port, C.D., Ketels, K.V., Coffin, D.L., and Kane, P.: A comparative study of experimental and spontaneous emphysema. J. Toxicol. Environ. Health, 2:589–604, 1977.

Pushpakom, R., et al.: Experimental papain-induced emphysema in dogs. Am. Rev. Respir. Dis., 102:778, 1970.

Strawbridge, H.T.G.: Chronic pulmonary emphysema. Historical review. Am. J. Pathol., 37:161–174, 1960.

———: Chronic pulmonary emphysema—an experimental study. Am. J. Pathol., 37:391–412, 1960.

Bovine Acute Pulmonary Emphysema (acute pulmonary edema and emphysema, "fog fever," "atypical interstitial pneumonia")

This syndrome, described from many parts of the world, has often been confused with acute respiratory distress due to other diseases. Although diverse causes have been demonstrated, it appears that this syndrome has some fundamental features which merit considering it one disease, at least for the present. This disease appears abruptly, usually in adult cattle 2 to 10 days after they have been moved from dry, sparse grazing to lush, nutritious pasture. In Great Britain, beef-type adult cattle are usually affected during the fall months (August–November), after they have been moved to pasturage consisting of new growth which followed a recent cutting of hay. According to Breeze, et al. (1976), this grass that has regrown from an earlier cut for hay, is known by the ancient words "aftermath" or "foggage." Thus the name "fog fever" comes from "foggage" and has nothing to do with the event of nature that activates foghorns and sometimes closes airports.

The clinical onset is typically sudden in its severest form, with severe dyspnea, frothing at the mouth, mouth breathing, tachypnea and a loud expiratory grunt. Auscultation usually reveals inspiratory and expiratory sounds, occasionally with rales, and sometimes with the crackling sounds of emphysema. Death occurs within 2 days in about one-third of the severely affected animals. The herd usually includes less severely affected animals that survive.

Gross Lesions. The gross lesions are essentially limited to the lungs, although severe congestion and hemorrhages are usually seen in tracheal and bronchial mucosa. The lumens of trachea and bronchi are filled with white frothy edema fluid. This fluid in terminal bronchi may be tinged with blood. Edema and emphysema are the most conspicuous lesions in the lungs. In severe cases, gas bubbles are seen in interlobular fascia in most lobes (most severe in diaphragmatic) of the lungs and form subpleural bullae up to 15 cm in diameter. The air also may extend into the mediastinum, mediastinal lymph nodes, and subcutis of the shoulders and back. Edema fluid often accompanies the gas bubbles. The lung is uniformly dark, congested and edematous, but not collapsed. The cut surface is smooth, homogeneous and exudes much edematous fluid.

Microscopic. The microscopic features of the lesions include edema and hyaline membranes in most alveoli and alveolar ducts. The alveolar septae are edematous and congested. Alveolar epithelial cells are often conspicuous and type II pneumocytes are increased in number, usually lying in short rows. In non-fatal cases, sacrificed several days after onset, proliferation of alveolar lining cells (type II pneumocytes) and accumulation of large monocytes in the alveoli are conspicuous features. This gives the lung an "edematous" or "fetalized" appearance. Monocytes and macrophages are numerous in the thickened, edematous septae, and some may be seen in alveoli. Emphysematous bullae may be seen under the pleura. The mediastinal lymph nodes are characteristically enlarged, congested, edematous, and filled with gas bullae.

Etiology. At present writing, the etiology appears to consist of many factors, all perhaps acting through a common mechanism. The disease has been associated with lush pastures and specific types of plants including rape, turnips, *Brassica*, spoiled sweet potatoes, and other plants such as *Perilla frutescens*. Of particular interest is the experimental production of the signs and lesions of this syndrome with several substances.

The amino acid, DL tryptophan has been shown to produce this disease following oral administration. One ruminal fermentation product of tryptophan, 3-methylindole (skatole), has been shown to be even more active following intravenous or oral administration to cattle. Sheep and goats have also been reported to be susceptible to this experimental disease. A natural disease of sheep with many similarities to the bovine disease has been described. Demonstration of increased levels of tryptophan or 3-methylindole in the forage of naturally affected cattle has not been accomplished at this writing.

Spoiled sweet potatoes, infected with a mold *Fusarum solani,* have been demonstrated to produce fatal pulmonary edema and emphysema in cattle. Two toxic compounds have been isolated from these spoiled sweet potatoes: a furanoterpenoid, ipomeanarone, is a hepatoxin in mice; the second compound, 4-ipomeanol, a "lung edema factor" in mice, produces typical signs and lesions of acute pulmonary edema and emphysema when administered per os to cattle. The synthetic compound is also similarly toxic.

It seems likely that other toxic compounds may be demonstrated in connection with this bovine syndrome characterized by acute pulmonary edema and atelectasis.

Blake, J.T., and Thomas, D.W.: Acute bovine pulmonary emphysema in Utah. J. Am. Vet. Med. Assoc., *158*:2047–2052, 1971.

Bradley, B.J., Carlson, J.R., and Dickinson, E.O.: 3-Methylindole-induced pulmonary edema and emphysema in sheep. Am. J. Vet. Res., *39*:1355–1358, 1978.

Breeze, R.G., Pirie, H.M., Selman, I.E., and Wiseman, A.: Fog fever: provocation tests with *Dictyocaulus viviparus.* J. Comp. Pathol., *84*:577–588, 1974.

Breeze, R.G., Pirie, H.M., Selman, I.E., and Wiseman, A.: Acute respiratory distress in cattle. Vet. Rec., *97*:226–229, 1975.

Breeze, R.G., Pirie, H.M., Selman, I.E., and Wiseman, A.: Fog fever in cattle: cytology of the hyperplastic alveolar epithelium. J. Comp. Pathol., *85*:147–156, 1975.

Breeze, R.G., Pirie, H.M., Selman, I.E., and Wiseman, A.: Fog fever (acute pulmonary emphysema) in cattle in Britain. Vet. Bull., *46*:243–251, 1976.

Caldwell, E.J., Powell, R.D., Jr., and Mullooly, J.P.: Interstitial emphysema: a study of physiologic factors involved in experimental induction of the lesion. Am. Rev. Respir. Dis., *102*:516–525, 1970.

Carlson, J.R., Yokoyama, M.T., and Dickinson, E.O.: Tryptophan-induced interstitial pulmonary emphysema in cattle. II. 3-methylindole as a cause of pulmonary edema and emphysema in cattle and goats. Fed. Proc., *31*:681, 1972.

Carlson, J.R., Dickinson, E.O., Yokoyama, M.T., and Bradley, B.: Pulmonary edema and emphysema in cattle after intraruminal and intravenous administration of 3-methylindole. Am. J. Vet. Res., *36*:1341–1348, 1975.

Dickinson, E.O., Spencer, G.R., and Gorham, J.R.: Experimental induction of an acute respiratory syndrome in cattle resembling bovine pulmonary emphysema. Vet. Rec., *80*:487–489, 1967.

Doster, A.R., Mitchell, F.E., Farrell, R.L., and Wilson, B.J.: Effects of 4-Ipomeanol, a product from mold-damaged sweet potatoes, on the bovine lung. Vet. Pathol., *15*:367–375, 1978.

Eyre, P.: Acute bovine pulmonary emphysema. Vet. Rec., *91*:38–40, 1972.

Gronstol, H., and Ulvund, M.J.: A "fog-fever"-like disease in sheep. Vet. Rec., *96*:383, 1975.

MacKenzie, A., Ford, J.E., and Scott, K.J.: Pasture levels of tryptophan in relation to outbreaks of fog fever. Res. Vet. Sci., *19*:227–228, 1975.

Moulton, J.B., Harrold, J.B., and Horning, M.A.: Pulmonary emphysema in cattle. J. Am. Vet. Med. Assoc., *139*:669–677, 1961.

Pasco, R.R., and McGavin, M.D.: Atypical interstitial pneumonia. Vet. Rec., *85*:376–377, 1969.

Peterson, D.R.: Bovine pulmonary emphysema caused by the plant *Perilla frutescens.* Symposium on acute bovine pulmonary emphysema. Univ. of Wyoming, Laramie, 1965.

Pirie, H.M., Breeze, R.G., Selman, I.E., and Wiseman, A.: Fog fever in cattle: pathology. Vet. Rec., *95*:479–483, 1974.

Roberts, H.E., Benson, J.A., and Jones, D.G.H.: Fog fever (acute bovine pulmonary emphysema) in mid-Wales, 1971: features of occurrence. Vet. Rec., *92*:558–561, 1973.

Schiefer, B., Jayasekara, M.U., and Mills, J.H.L.: Comparison of naturally occurring and tryptophan-induced bovine atypical interstitial pneumonia. Vet. Pathol., *11*:327–339, 1974.

Schofield, F.W.: Acute pulmonary emphysema of cattle. J. Am. Vet. Med. Assoc., *112*:254–259, 1948.

Selman, I.E., Wiseman, A., Pirie, H.M., and Breeze, R.G.: Fog fever in cattle: clinical and epidemiological features. Vet. Rec., *95*:139–146, 1974.

Tucker, J.O., and Maki, L.R.: Acute pulmonary emphysema of cattle. Experimental production, etiology. Am. J. Vet. Res., *23*:821–826, 1962.

Ossification in the Lungs

In cows and in old dogs, cases occur from time to time in which considerable areas of lung are found with spicules or tiny plates of bone extensively distributed in the alveolar walls. These may reach a length of a millimeter or more. They lie entirely within the alveolar septum, which is thickened to accommodate them. Blood vessels are not involved. The bony formations never appear in the pleura nor in the peribronchial areas.

Severe ossification may occur in the lungs of cattle suffering from Manchester wasting disease (p. 978).

Pires (1942) found the spicules of bone to be closely related to the alveolar epithelium and pointed out that, if we adopt the view that this lining "epithelium" is of mesenchymal origin, the ossification can be explained as metaplasia of the lining cells. There appear to be no objective data on accompanying disorders or circumstances which would cast light on the underlying cause, but this may well be chronic irritation of some sort or a metabolic deficiency. The condition, of course, is not to be confused with simple calcification of tissue. This shows no bone cells and no lacunae.

Equine habronemiasis sometimes results in small, hard, yellowish-gray nodules with a caseous or calcified center. These hard centers are only lightly joined to the surrounding thin layer granulation tissue and are easily separated from it. Eosinophils are usually numerous in the granulation tissue. A microscopic larva is sometimes demonstrable in them, identified as belonging to one of the *Habronema* stomach worms.

Creech, G.T.: Arteriosclerosis in cattle associated with pulmonary ossification. Am. J. Vet. Res., 2:400–406, 1941.

Pires, R.E.: Ossificação em pulmao de bovino. Rev. Fac. méd. vét., Univ. São Paulo, 2:(Fasc. 2):77–84, 1942.

NEOPLASMS

Nasal Passages and Paranasal Sinuses

Neoplasms may arise from structures in the wall of the upper respiratory tract. In one study (Madewell, et al., 1976), 300 nasal tumors were identified among 12,300 microscopically confirmed neoplasms in dogs, cats, and horses. The estimated rate of occurrence (number per 100,000 patient years) of neoplasms arising from nasal or sinus walls were as follows:

Species	Origin of tumors	
	Nasal	Sinus
Canine	65	16
Feline	38	1
Equine	15	11

In this study, the histologic diagnosis of the canine tumors were in this order: (1) adenocarcinoma, (2) carcinoma (not otherwise specified), (3) chondrosarcoma, (4) squamous cell carcinoma, (5) fibrosarcoma, (6) adenoma, (7) mast cell tumor, (8) fibropapilloma, (9) osteosarcoma, (10) others. Among the feline tumors, squamous cell carcinomas were most frequent, adenocarcinoma second, and fibrosarcoma third. In this group, equine tumors were most often squamous cell carcinomas, second were adenocarcinomas.

Adenocarcinoma of nasal or sinus epithelium is recognized by the columnar or cuboidal cells which make up the tumor mass. These cells are often pseudostratified, suggesting the nasal epithelium from which they arose. Rosettes, acini, and papillary growths of the tumor cells may be seen in these tumors. Tumor cells which arise in the ethmoid region often resemble those of the olfactory epithelium and have a tendency to grow through the cribriform part of the ethmoid bone into the olfactory lobe of the brain. Adenocarcinomas arising from the nasal or sinus epithelium tend to invade and displace the nasal turbinates and maxilla. Metastases to pharyngeal and anterior cervical lymph nodes may also occur.

A special type of adenomatous tumor has been described from the nasal passages of sheep and cattle. These have been designated as adenopapillomas or ethmoid carcinomas and appear to be less invasive than the adenocarcinomas found in dogs. The ovine disease appears to be transmissible, but the etiologic agent has not been identified at the time this is written.

Squamous cell carcinomas arising from upper respiratory epithelium are made up of undifferentiated squamous epithelial cells. Invasion and replacement of contiguous bone and other structures is a consistent feature of this neoplasm. Metastases to regional lymph nodes are to be expected.

Chondrosarcomas appear to arise from the nasal septum and are made up of solid masses of undifferentiated cartilage cells which produce immature cartilage.

Mucoepidermoid carcinomas, consisting of squamous cell elements and glandular cells with mucous secretion, are occasionally encountered. Other tumors (fibrosarcoma, adenoma, mast cell tumor, fibropapilloma, malignant lymphoma, hemangioma, sarcoma, and osteosarcoma) are much less frequent and are described in the chapter concerned with the system from which they most often arise.

Neoplasms of the larynx and trachea are rarely reported in animals. Two cases of osteochondroma arising from the mid-thoracic trachea of dogs have been described. Osteosarcomas which develop in association with lesions produced by *Spirocerca lupi* may also involve the trachea.

Brown, R.J., et al.: Nasal adenocarcinoma in a Taiwan macaque. Vet. Pathol., *14*:294–296, 1977.

Brownstein, D.G., Montali, R.J., Bush, M., and James, A.E.: Nasal carcinoma in a captive Eld's deer. J. Am. Vet. Med. Assoc., *167*:569–571, 1975.

Cho, D.Y., Bahr, R.J., and Leipold, H.W.: Adenocarcinoma in the nasal cavity and brain of a dog. J. Am. Vet. Med. Assoc., *165*:350–351, 1974.

Confer, A.W., and DePaoli, A.: Primary neoplasms of the nasal cavity, paranasal sinuses, and nasopharynx in the dog. A report of 16 cases from the files of the AFIP. Vet. Pathol., *15*:18–30, 1978.

Correa, P., Dalgard, D.W., and Adamson, R.H.: Olfactory neuroepithelioma in a cynomolgus monkey (*Macaca fascicularis*). J. Med. Primatol., *4*:51–61, 1975.

Duncan, I.R., Tyler, D.E., Van der Maaten, M.I., and Anderson, I.R.: Enzootic nasal adenocarcinoma in sheep. J. Am. Vet. Med. Assoc., *151*:732–734, 1967.

Gourley, L.M.G., Morgan, J.P., and Gould, D.H.: Tracheal osteochondroma in a dog. A case report. J. Small Anim. Pract., *11*:327–335, 1970.

Gussmann, H.J.: Endemic infectious adenopapillomatosis of the nasal mucosa in sheep. Mh. Vet. Med., *17*:529–532, 1962.

Hänichen, T., and Schiefer, B.: Zur Morphologie und Häufigheit primärer Geschwulste der Nasenhöhlen und Nasennebenhöhlen bei Hund und Katze. Z. Krebsforsch., *71*:255–266, 1968.

Hough, J.D., et al.: Tracheal osteochondroma in a dog. J. Am. Vet. Med. Assoc., *170*:1416–1418, 1977.

Legendre, A.M., Carrig, C.B., Howard, D.R., and Dade, A.W.: Nasal tumor in a cat. J. Am. Vet. Med. Assoc., *167*:481–484, 1975.

Madewell, B.R., Priester, W.A., Gillette, E.L., and Snyder, S.P.: Neoplasms of the nasal passages and paranasal sinuses in domesticated animals as reported by 13 veterinary colleges. Am. J. Vet. Res., *37*:851–856, 1976.

Njoku, C.O., Shannon, D., Chineme, C.N., and Bida, S.A.: Ovine nasal adenopapilloma: Incidence and clinico-pathologic studies. Am. J. Vet. Res., *39*:1850–1852, 1978.

Pospischil, A., Haenichen, T., and Schaeffler, H.: Histological and electron microscopic studies of endemic ethmoidal carcinomas in cattle. Vet. Pathol., *16*:180–190, 1979.

Rajan, A., Sivadas, C.G., Nair, M.K., and Maryamma, K.I.: Incidence and pathology of tumors of the paranasal sinuses in domestic animals. Kerala J. Vet. Sci., *3*:89–101, 1973.

Rubaj, B., and Woloszyn, S.: Enzootic adenopapilloma of the nasal cavity in sheep. Medycyna Wet., *23*:226–229, 1967.

Sande, R.D., and Alexander, J.E.: Turbinate bone neoplasms in dogs. Mod. Vet. Pract., *51*:23–29, 1970.

Vohradsky, F.: Adenocarcinoma of the olfactory mucosa of sheep and pigs in Ghana. Acta. Vet. Brno., *43*:243–249, 1974.

Yonemichi, H., et al.: Intranasal tumor of the ethmoid olfactory mucosa in sheep. Am. J. Vet. Res., *39*:1599–1606, 1978.

Zaki, F.A., and Liu, S.K.: Adenocarcinoma of the olfactory gland in the dog. Vet. Pathol., *11*:138–143, 1974.

Neoplasms of the Lung

Secondary (metastatic) neoplasms in the lung are more frequent than primary neoplasms of the lung, but fortunately not many histologic types occur in animals, and they can be distinguished by careful microscopic study. Note that primary tumors are designated as being "of" the lung, secondary tumors are "in" the lung—a tiny detail that's significant to note. Secondary tumors in the lung may include almost any malignant neoplasm of any part of the body. If malignant cells be-

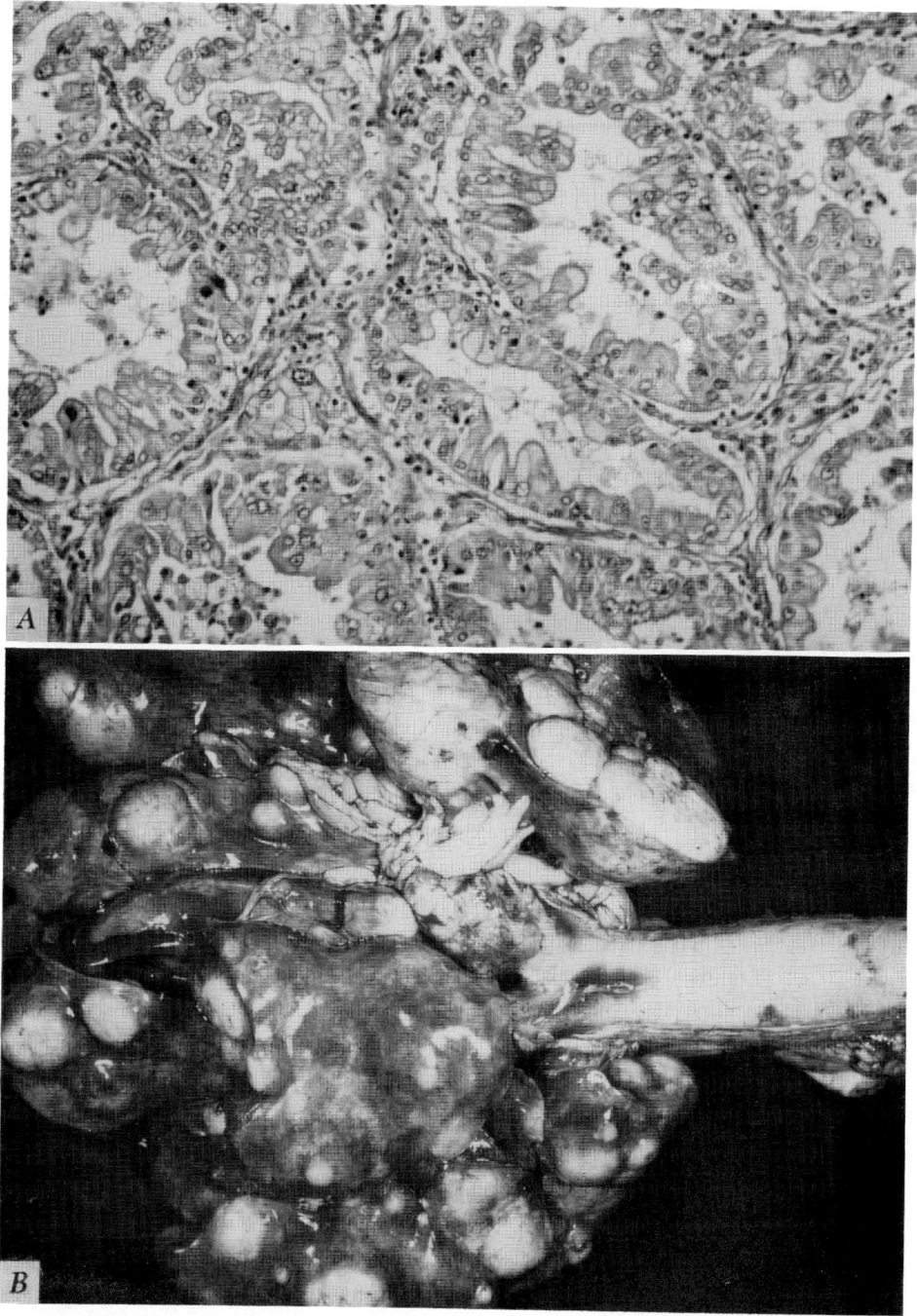

Fig. 20–9. Primary adenocarcinoma or bronchiolar-alveolar carcinoma of the lung of a Cocker-Dachshund, male, nine years old. *A,* Section of one of the tumor nodules. (H & E, × 200.) *B,* The gross lung. (Courtesy of Angell Memorial Animal Hospital.)

come detached from the primary growth and are swept into lymphatics or veins, they soon reach the pulmonary circulation. The capillaries of the lungs form a fine screen through which all of the blood circulates. Tumor cells are readily entrapped and often find the lung a suitable place in which to grow.

Primary tumors of the lungs of animals described in the literature, include the following:

Neoplasm:	Species affected:
Adenocarcinoma (bronchiolar- alveolar cell carcinoma)	Dogs, cats, horses, cattle, sheep, mice, rats, wild animals
Squamous cell carcinoma (bronchogenic carcinoma)	Dogs, cats, horses, cattle, sheep, wild animals
Chondromas and chondrosarcomas	Dogs, horses, cattle
Lipomas, fibrosarcomas, teratomas, hemangiosarcomas	Dogs, horses, cattle, cats

Adenocarcinoma of the lung apparently arises from the epithelial cells of the alveoli, although some contend that their origin is bronchiolar epithelium. It is clear that these neoplastic cells grow into alveoli and tend to maintain the structural outline of the alveoli. The cells are usually columnar or cuboidal, but may be tall columnar with cilia and protruding cytoplasm (Fig. 20–9). Acini are formed frequently and cells may become detached, but usually remain in contact with adjacent epithelial tumor cells.

Pulmonary adenomatosis of sheep (jaagsiekte) is a viral-induced lesion that resembles adenocarcinoma of the lung and may be difficult to distinguish in some circumstances.

Metastasis of adenocarcinoma to bronchial lymph nodes does occur. If the malignant cells get into the efferent lymphatics, they are carried to the thoracic duct, the right atrium, right ventricle, and thence back to the lungs. Thus metastasis of pulmonary tumors to other parts of the lung is readily accomplished.

Squamous cell carcinoma is much less

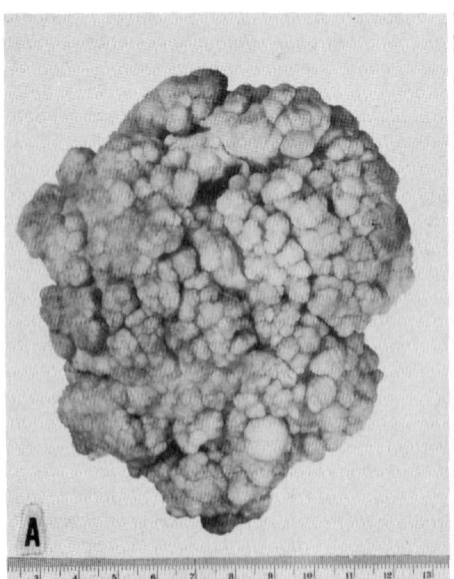
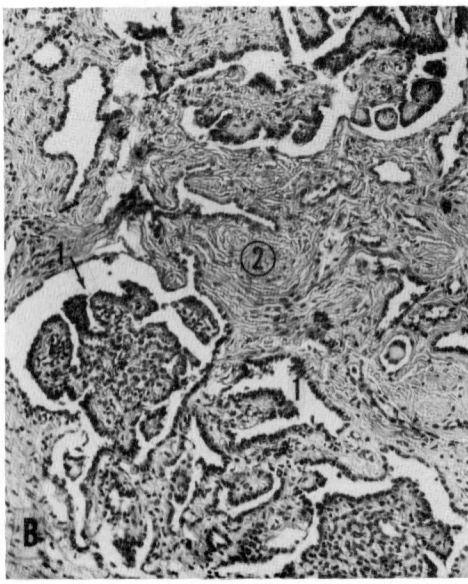

Fig. 20–10. Mesothelioma of the pleura of a six-year-old cow. *A*, Gross appearance of the nodular pleura. *B*, Photomicrograph (× 105) showing papillary growth of mesothelium (*1*) and supporting stroma (*2*). (Courtesy of Armed Forces Institute of Pathology.) Contributor: Dr. C.L. Davis.

frequent than adenocarcinoma in most animal species. This tumor resembles the bronchiogenic carcinoma (squamous cell carcinoma), which has increased in the human population in recent decades. The tumor appears to arise from the epithelium of the terminal bronchi, which undergoes squamous metaplasia and neoplasia. It extends from its central position peripherally, eventually to involve much of the affected lobule, then the lobe of the lung.

Chondromas and chondrosarcomas appear to arise from cartilage in the terminal bronchi, but are much less frequent than epithelial tumors.

Other tumors may arise primarily from tissues within the lung. They are infrequent but include lipoma, fibrosarcoma, teratoma, and hemangioma. These are described elsewhere in connection with the tissues from which they more frequently originate.

Mesothelioma of the Pleura. The pleura may be host to metastatic tumors that reach the lung or arise in the mediastinum (lymphoma), but the only primary tumor is the mesothelioma. This tumor arises from the mesothelial lining of the pleural sac and resembles its parent cells (Fig. 20–10). They are usually benign, but may interfere with respiration by their location and by the accompanying hydrothorax.

Altman, N.H., et al.: Primary pulmonary mucoepidermoid tumours in the goat. Cancer, 26:726–732, 1970.

Amaral-Mendes, J.J.: Histopathology of primary lung tumours in the mouse. J. Pathol., 97:415–427, 1968.

Brandly, P.J., and Migaki, G.: Types of tumors found by federal meat inspectors in an eight-year survey. Ann. N.Y. Acad. Sci., 108:872–879, 1963.

Brody, R.S., and Craig, P.H.: Primary pulmonary neoplasms in the dog: a review of 29 cases. J. Am. Vet. Med. Assoc., 147:1628–1643, 1965.

Davis, C.L.: Primary carcinoma of the lung of a sheep. J. Am. Vet. Med. Assoc., 94:237–240, 1939.

Deerberg, F., Pittermann, W., and Rapp, K.: Der Lungentumor der Maus: ein progressiver tumor. Vet. Pathol., 11:430–441, 1974.

Kauffman, S.: Kinetics of alveolar epithelial hyperplasia in lungs of mice exposed to urethane. Lab. Invest., 30:170–175, 1974.

Kharole, M.U., Gill, B.S., Gupta, P.P., and Singh, B.: Bronchogenic carcinoma in Indian water buffaloes (Bubalus bubalis). Vet. Pathol., 12:462–463, 1975.

Koller, L.D., and Olson, C.: Pulmonary fibroblastomas in a deer with cutaneous fibromatosis. Cancer Res., 31:1373–1375, 1971.

Leipold, H.W., Noordsy, J.L., and Cook, J.E.: Bronchogenic carcinoma in a cow. J. Am. Vet. Med. Assoc., 165:628–632, 1974.

Migaki, G., Helmboldt, C.F., and Robinson, F.R.: Primary pulmonary tumors of epithelial origin in cattle. Am. J. Vet. Res., 35:1397–1400, 1974.

Monlux, W.S.: Primary pulmonary neoplasms in domestic animals. Southwestern Vet. (College Station, Texas), 6:131–133, 1952.

Nielsen, S.W., and Horava, A.: Primary pulmonary tumors of the dog. A report of sixteen cases. Am. J. Vet. Res., 21:813–830, 1960.

Schepers, G.W.H.: Lung tumors of primates and rodents. Parts I, II, and III. Industr. Med., 40:8–26; 23–31; 48–53, 1971.

Sevei, I.: Lung Tumors in Animals. Perigia, Div. of Cancer Res., 1966.

Stewart, H.L.: Pulmonary cancer and adenomatosis in captive wild mammals and birds from the Philadelphia Zoo. J. Natl. Cancer Inst., 36:117–138, 1966.

Stünzi, H.: The histopathology of feline lung cancer. In Lung Tumors in Animals, edited by I. Sevei. Perigia, Div. of Cancer Res., 1966.

Stünzi, H.: Sinn and Unsinn der Krebsstatistik beim Hund. Schweiz. Arch. Tierheilkd., 112:420–427, 1970.

Stünzi, H.: Das epidermoide Lungenkarzinom des Hundes als Vergleichsobjekt für das Raucherkarzinom des Menschen. Schweiz. Arch. Tierheilkd., 113:311–319, 1971.

Stünzi, H.: Das anaplastische Lungenkarzinom des Hundes. Vet. Pathol., 10:102–113, 1973.

Stünzi, H.: Das epidermoide Karzinom der Bronchialdrüsen bei Hund und Katze. Vet. Pathol., 13:277–285, 1976.

Swoboda, R.: Über das Lungenkarzinom bei Tieren mit besonderer Berücksichtigung des Rindes. Pathol. Vet., 1:409–422, 1964.

Tomlinson, M.J., et al.: Adenocarcinoma of the lung with secondary pericardial effusion and leukemoid response in a dog. J. Am. Vet. Med. Assoc., 163:257–258, 1973.

CHAPTER 21

The Cardiovascular System

CONGENITAL CARDIOVASCULAR ANOMALIES

Anomalies which occur during the embryologic development of the heart, blood, and lymphatic vessels are well known in human infants and in every other species that has been adequately studied. Present methods of diagnosis utilizing cardiac catheterization and contrast radiography, particularly cineradiography, have made it possible to recognize many anomalies during life. In some cases, corrective surgical procedures have been very successful. Most anomalies of the heart are recognized grossly by their anatomic features, which serve as a convenient method of classification. Careful, systematic gross examination of the heart at necropsy is necessary to recognize these lesions.

Patent Ductus Arteriosus

In the fetus, blood is diverted from the lung by means of the ductus arteriosus, a short blood vessel which leads from the pulmonary artery to the aorta. Following birth, the flow of blood to the lungs through the pulmonary artery is suddenly magnified, and the diversion through the ductus is no longer required. Within a few days after birth, the lumen of the ductus is closed and eventually permanently sealed, the remnant remaining as the ligamentum arteriosum. In this common congenital cardiac defect of man and animals, the lumen remains open, and blood continues to be shunted between the pulmonary artery and aorta (Fig. 21–1). This anomaly often occurs in association with other defects which will be described later. In severe cases, the defect leads to congestive heart failure, pulmonary hypertension, and mixture of venous and arterial blood resulting in cyanosis. A review of 532 examples of patent ductus arteriosus in dogs identified the anomaly most frequently in miniature and toy Poodles (Ackerman, et al., 1978).

Pulmonary Stenosis

The lumen of the pulmonary artery is narrowed near its origin from the right ventricle by fibrous connective tissue. The weir or "jet" effect on the blood forced through this narrow orifice results in somewhat bullous distortions of the pulmonary artery (Fig. 21–1). The increased resistance also results in hypertrophy of the right ventricle.

Subaortic Stenosis

This not infrequent congenital cardiac defect in animals results from the formation of a constricting band of dense fibrous connective tissue at a point in the left ventricle just below the aortic semilunar valves

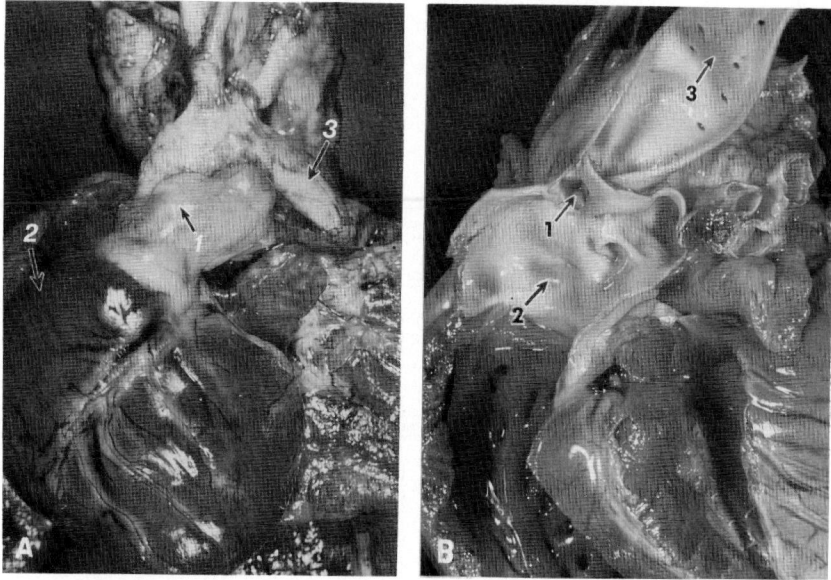

Fig. 21–1.   Congenital cardiac anomalies. *A*, Pulmonary stenosis in a seven-month-old German Shepherd. The pulmonary artery (*1*) is dilated due to the "jet effect" of the blood flow through the stenotic aperture at the level of the pulmonary valves. The right atrium (*2*) is hypertrophied. Aorta (*3*). *B*, Aortic-pulmonary communication through a patent ductus arteriosus (*1*) between the pulmonary artery (*2*) and aorta (*3*). A male Cocker Spaniel, 6½ months old. (Courtesy of Angell Memorial Animal Hospital.)

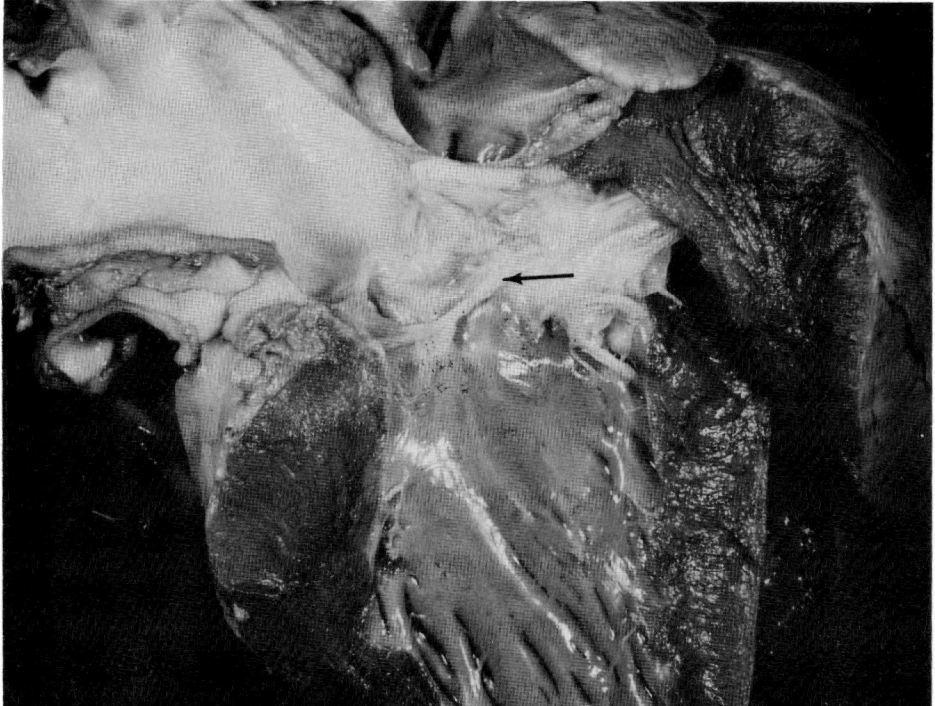

Fig. 21–2.   Congenital subaortic stenosis in a six-month-old male German Shepherd. Note subaortic constricting band (arrow). (Courtesy of Angell Memorial Animal Hospital.)

(Fig. 21–2). The valves may be essentially normal or slightly distorted by the fibrous band which restricts the outflow of blood into the aorta. The left ventricle usually undergoes hypertrophy. In dogs, dilation of the aorta above the valves has been described (Flickinger and Patterson, 1967). Intramural arteries in the adjacent myocardium have been described by Flickinger and Patterson as having thickened intima with increased numbers of elastic fibers and in some cases fibrosis. The human and canine anomalies appear to be quite similar. In neither is the pathogenesis clearly understood.

Defects in aortic semilunar valves, arising congenitally, may also produce aortic stenosis. These are rare in man and not yet recognized in animals.

Coarctation of Aorta

This is a narrowing of the aorta, which is usually localized to a short segment near or immediately before the attachment of the ductus arteriosus, although occasionally longer sections may be affected. It is usually associated with other cardiac anomalies which result in insufficient blood passing through the left ventricle and hence the aorta, leading to hypoplasia. This form is referred to as **infantile coarctation**. A second form called **adult-type coarctation** is believed to result from extension of the normal obliterative process of the ductus arteriosus into the adjacent aorta.

Interventricular Septal Defects

Early in embryonic life, the ventricles consist of a single chamber which is eventually divided into the left and right ventricles by the growth of the interventricular septum. The muscular wall grows upward from the apex of the heart toward the atrioventricular partition. Fusion with the membranous portion of the septum growing downward from the bulbus arteriosus (which eventually divides the aorta and pulmonary artery) results in closure of the communication between the ventricles. Failure of this fusion results in a ventricular septal defect which may be occult (probe patent) or quite large (Fig. 21–3A). Because of the origin of the membranous part of the interventricular septum, defects in it are often associated with anomalies in the aorta and pulmonary artery.

Thickening and roughening of the endocardium may occur due to turbulence around the orifice between the ventricles, and the endocardium of the right ventricle opposite the opening may also be thickened as a result of the jet stream of blood from the orifice. In some cases, continued overload of the right heart and pulmonary hypertension may lead to reversed flow of blood from the right into the left ventricle, resulting in cyanosis.

Persistent Right Aortic Arch

This is in the strict sense an anomaly of the aorta rather than of the heart, but for convenience shall be described at this point. The aortic arches are formed early in embryonic life as paired structures, some of which atrophy, others which develop to become part of the cardiovascular system of the fetus and adult. The aorta normally develops from one of the left aortic arches. This places the aorta and the ductus arteriosus on the same (left) side of the trachea and esophagus. If the aorta develops by persistence of a right arch, the aorta will be on the right side of the trachea and esophagus. The ductus arteriosus, by connecting to the aorta and pulmonary artery, forms a vascular ring around the trachea and esophagus. As the young animal develops, the esophagus, and, later, trachea will be partially occluded by the vascular ring (Fig. 21–3B). Other anomalies of the aortic arch system may also result in such vascular rings, but this one has been more frequently observed in animals.

Interatrial Septal Defects

In embryonic life, the common atrial chamber is divided by the growth of a

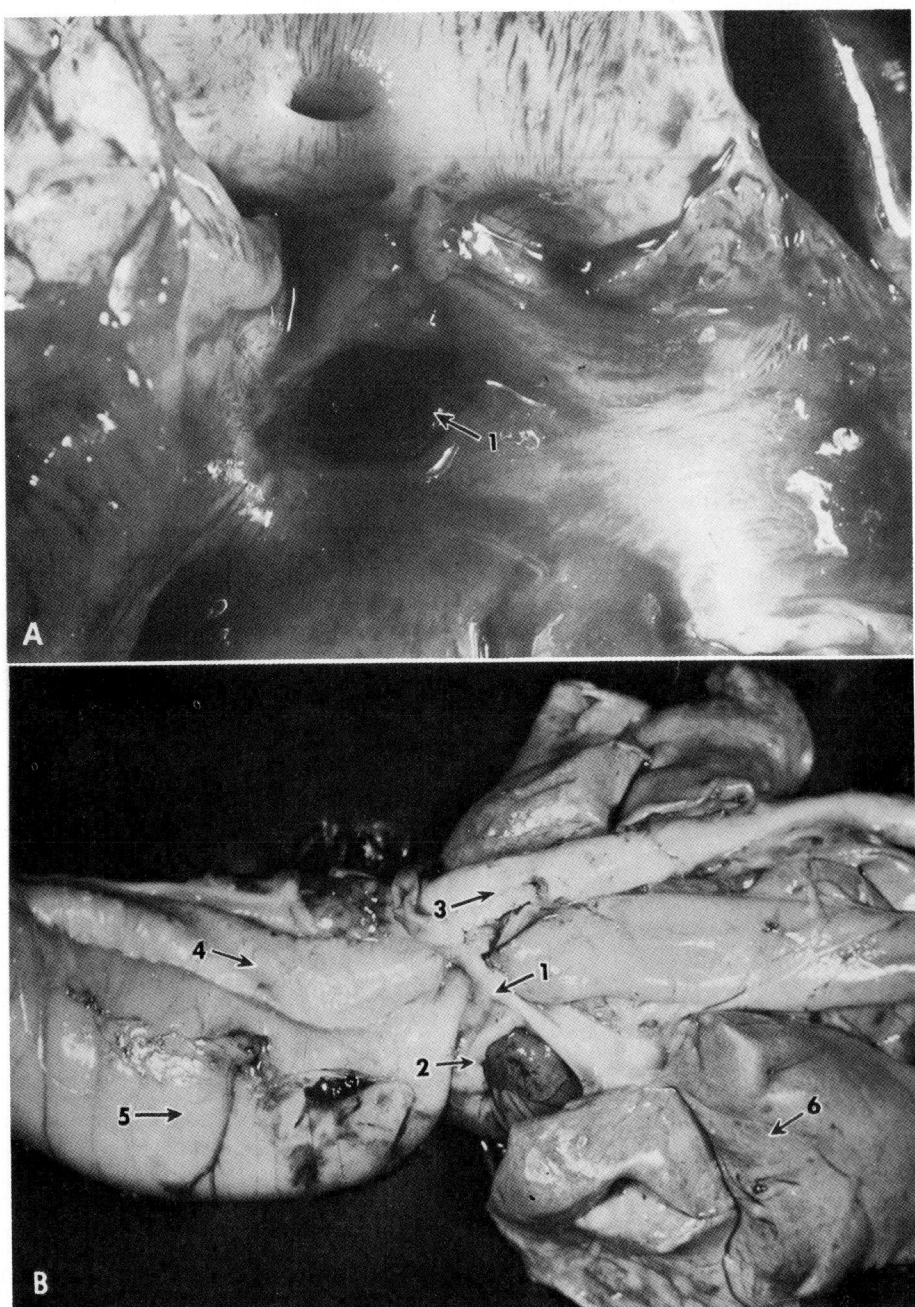

Fig. 21–3.   Congenital cardiac anomalies. *A,* Interventricular septal defect (*1*) in a seven-month-old male German Shepherd puppy (same animal with pulmonary stenosis, Fig. 21–1, *A*). *B,* Persistent right aortic arch. The ductus arteriosus (*1*) completes a vascular ring with the pulmonary artery (*2*) and aorta (*3*). This ring encircles and compresses the trachea (*4*) and esophagus (*5*), which is dilated. The lung is also labeled (*6*). This lesion was found a a ten-week-old male German Shepherd. (Courtesy of Angell Memorial Animal Hospital.)

membranous structure from its wall. This membrane attaches to the atrioventricular partition incompletely, leaving an opening, the **ostium primum.** A second defect later appears in the dorsal portion of this membrane, known as the **ostium secundum.** Later in fetal life, a second membrane grows upward on the right side of the first membrane, usually closing the ostium primum and partially closing the ostium secundum. The orifice formed by these two membranes and ostia is called the **foramen ovale.** It is usually functionally closed in the young animals by the differential in pressure between the right and left atria, but may remain as a potential orifice which can be detected with a probe at necropsy. The patent foramen ovale may result from incomplete formation of the membrane which normally closes it. Other defects in the membrane may result in septal defects involving the ostium primum.

The effect of an interatrial septal defect is usually to produce continued overload of the right side of the heart by blood flowing through the defect into the right atrium. Hypertrophy of the right heart and pulmonary hypertension may result. Should pressure in the right side of the heart exceed that of the left, mixture of venous blood into the aorta may lead to recognizable cyanosis. On the other hand, small defects in the septum may persist into adult life without significant effect on the health of the animal.

Transposition of the Great Vessels

It is possible for the aorta and pulmonary artery to be transposed, the aorta arising from the right ventricle and the pulmonary artery from the left. This may be simply a shift in position, with the arterial side of the heart on the right and the venous side on the left. This has no significant clinical effect. On the other hand, should the aorta originate from the venous ventricle, and the pulmonary artery from the arterial side, only a large shunting defect such as an interventricular septal defect, patent foramen

ovale, or persistent ductus arteriosus will permit enough communication of blood for survival. Sometimes the aorta and pulmonary artery fail to divide, persisting as a large single blood vessel: the **persistent truncus arteriosus.** Less frequently, the aorta and pulmonary artery may both arise from the right ventricle (**double outlet right ventricle**). A large ventricular septal defect makes the anomaly compatible with life. Transpositions of the aorta and pulmonary arteries are among the more frequent cardiac anomalies in cattle.

Tetralogy of Fallot

The grammatically correct name for this complex is **tetrad of Fallot.** It consists of the following individual anomalies occurring together: (1) interventricular septal defect; (2) transposition of the aorta; (3) pulmonic or subpulmonic stenosis; and (4) hypertrophy of the right ventricle. The ductus arteriosus is also persistent in those animals which survive birth; in fact it is essential for survival. It is believed that this tetrad of anomalies results initially from embryologic failure to form the interventricular septum. Malpositioning of the septum is thought to affect the development of the aorta and pulmonary artery as well as the septum. This complex results in severe clinical cyanosis. Patterson, et al. (1974) reported an unusually high frequency of an anomaly resembling tetralogy of Fallot in Keeshonds.

A related combination of cardiac defects, the **Eisenmenger complex,** has been reported in man and animals. This complex differs from the tetrad of Fallot in that pulmonic stenosis is not present. Thus, it consists of: (1) interventricular septal defect; (2) transposition of the aorta; and (3) hypertrophy of the right ventricle. Some cyanosis usually results from this set of anomalies.

Ectopia Cordis

In this rare condition, the entire heart lies outside the thorax under the subcutis.

In human infants, the dislocation is caudad and related to defects in the sternum and soft tissues of the thorax. In cattle, the dislocation is cranial; the heart lies in the subcutis of the lower cervical region (Fig. 4–4). In the bovine, the anomaly is not always fatal; we have seen young adult animals with this condition among the living bovine patients at several veterinary schools.

Endocardial Fibroelastosis

This appears as a rare congenital malformation in man and animals (dog, cat, cattle). The name describes the lesion well: the endocardium is thickened many times by layers of fibrous and elastic tissue, giving the endocardial surface a white to silvery glistening appearance. It usually involves the left atrium and left ventricle to the level of the aortic valves. There is left and right ventricular hypertrophy and dilation. The condition leads to signs and lesions of heart failure. Paasch and Zook (1980) have described degeneration of Purkinje fibers, which was suggested to be of importance to heart failure. In cats it is most common in Siamese and Burmese. Endocardial fibroelastosis often accompanies **round heart disease** of turkeys, a cardiomyopathy of unknown etiology accompanied by left ventricular hypertrophy and dilatation leading to a rounded shape. A form of endocardial fibroelastosis may also occur in poisoning by pyrrolizidine alkaloids.

Other Cardiac Anomalies

Among those reported in animals are such things as mitral insufficiency, tricuspid insufficiency, double outlet from right ventricle and **Ebstein's anomaly** of the tricuspid valve. The anomaly is manifest by the congenital downward displacement of the tricuspid valve into the right ventricle. A cardiomyopathy inherited by an autosomal recessive gene is recognized in Syrian hamsters (Gertz, 1973). It is charac-terized by focal myocardial degeneration leading to congestive heart failure.

Anomalies of Pericardium

The pericardium may be totally or partially absent in rare cases. The most striking anomaly is the presence of an orifice in pericardium extending through the diaphragm into the peritoneal sac. Herniation of liver and intestines through such an orifice may lead to dramatic clinical consequences. We have seen this in the dog and cat.

Arterial and Venous Anomalies

The persistent right aortic arch with formation of a vascular ring has been referred to. Other anomalies of the vasculature include: persistent left cranial vena cava, anomalous pulmonary veins, retroesophageal right subclavian artery, arteriovenous fistulae, anomalous origin of various branches of the ascending and descending aorta, and postcaval shunts.

Congenital Hereditary Lymphedema

This is a rare disorder resulting from abnormal morphogenesis of the peripheral lymphatic system, resulting in failure to establish connections with the more central lymphatic system. It is recognized in man (Milroy's disease), dogs, Ayrshire cattle, and swine. In man and dogs, the inheritance is an autosomal dominant trait with variable expression, whereas in cattle and swine, it is an autosomal recessive trait. Edema may be generalized, in which case neonatal death is the usual outcome, but more usually, edema is restricted to the hind limbs. Other parts, for example the ears, may also be affected. In mildly affected pups, the edema gradually disappears by about the age of 3 months. Microscopically, lymphatics in the dermis and subcutis are markedly dilated. In dogs, regional lymph nodes, most often the popliteal and/or axillary, are absent.

Frequency and Etiology of Cardiovascular Anomalies

Although cardiovascular anomalies have been recognized in almost all species of animals, based on reports they are most frequent in dogs, cats, and cattle. The studies of Detweiler, et al. (1960) and Patterson (1968) contribute to the understanding of these anomalies in dogs. According to these authors, the prevalence rate of cardiovascular malformations among dogs studied in a large university veterinary clinic was 6.8 per 1000 admissions. Purebred dogs have higher, breed-specific prevalence rates than mongrels, and patent ductus arteriosus in the dog (as in man) is more prevalent in females than males.

These workers present evidence that genetic factors have a bearing on the occurrence of several such cardiovascular anomalies. The frequency of many can be increased by selective matings in certain families of dogs.

Patterson (1968) has reported cardiovascular anomalies in 290 dogs studied over a 13-year period. His data are summarized in Table 21–1.

Ackerman, N., Burk, R., Hahn, A.W., and Hayes, H.M., Jr.: Patent ductus in the dog: a retrospective study of radiographic, epidemiologic, and clinical findings. Am. J. Vet. Res., *39*:1805–1810, 1978.

Barrett, R.E., et al.: Four cases of congenital portacaval shunt in the dog. J. Small Anim. Pract., *17*:71–85, 1976.

Table 21–1. Cardiovascular Malformations in 290 Dogs (Patterson, 1968)

Malformation	Number	Percentage of Total
Patent ductus arteriosus	82	25.3
Pulmonic stenosis	57	17.5
Subaortic stenosis	40	12.3
Persistent right aortic arch	23	7.1
Ventricular septal defect	20	6.2
Tetralogy of Fallot	11	3.4
Atrial septal defect (ostium secundum inc. patent foramen ovale)	12	3.7
Persistent left cranial vena cava	13	4.0
Mitral insufficiency	9	2.8
Pericardial anomalies:		
Pericardiodiaphragmatic hernia	3	.9
Absent pericardium	1	.3
Incomplete pericardium	1	.3
Arterial anomalies:		
Retro-esophageal right subclavian artery	1	.3
Separate origin of right subclavian artery from ascending aorta	2	.6
Ebstein's anomaly of tricuspid valve	1	.3
Tricuspid insufficiency	1	.3
Double outlet, right ventricle	1	.3
Anomalous pulmonary venous drainage	1	.3
Conduction disturbance—without gross malformations:		
Right bundle branch block	2	.6
Wolff-Parkinson-White syndrome	1	.3
Arteriovenous fistula	1	.3
Incompletely diagnosed	42	12.9
Total	325	100

Note: In 32 dogs, more than one malformation was found.

Belling, T.H., Jr.: Ventricular septal defect in the bovine heart—report of three cases. J. Am. Vet. Med. Assn., 138:595–598, 1961.

Bolton, G.R., Ettinger, S.J., and Liu, S.-K.: Tetralogy of Fallot in three cats. J. Am. Vet. Med. Assoc., 160:1622–1631, 1972.

Breznock, E.M.: Spontaneous closure of ventricular septal defects in the dog. J. Am. Vet. Med. Assoc., 162:399–403, 1973.

Burt, J.H.: Anomalous posterior vena cava of a dog. J. Am. Vet. Med. Assn., 108:152, 1946.

Bush, M., et al.: Tetralogy of Fallot in a cat. J. Am. Vet. Med. Assoc., 161:1679–1686, 1972.

Cordy, D.R., and Ribelin, W.E.: Six congenital cardiac anomalies in animals. Cornell Vet., 40:249–256, 1950.

Dawes, G.S., et al.: Patent ductus arteriosus in newborn lambs. J. Physiol., 128:344–361, and 361–383, 1955.

Dear, M.G., and Price, E.K.: Complex congenital anomaly of a bovine heart. Vet. Rec., 36:219–222, 1970.

Dennis, S.M., and Leipold, H.W.: Congenital cardiac defect in lambs. Am. J. Vet. Res., 29:2337–2340, 1968.

Detweiler, D.K.: Genetic aspects of cardiovascular diseases in animals. Circulation, 30:114–127, 1964.

Detweiler, D.K., Hubben, K., and Patterson, D.F.: Survey of cardiovascular disease in dogs. Am. J. Vet. Res., 21:329–359, 1960.

Donald, H.P., Deas, D.W., and Wilson, A.L.: Genetic analysis of the incidence of dropsical calves in herds of Ayrshire cattle. Br. Vet. J., 108:227, 1952.

Easley, J.C., and Carpenter, J.L.: Hepatic arteriovenous fistula in two Saint Bernard pups. J. Am. Vet. Med. Assoc., 166:167–171, 1975.

Eliot, T.S., et al.: First report of the occurrence of neonatal endocardial fibroelastosis in cats and dogs. J. Am. Vet. Med. Assn., 133:271–274, 1958.

Eyster, G.E., et al.: Ebstein's anomaly: A report of three cases in the dog. J. Am. Vet. Med. Assoc., 170:709–713, 1977.

Eyster, G.E., et al.: Coarctation of the aorta in a dog. J. Am. Vet. Med. Assoc., 169:426–428, 1976.

Flickinger, G.L., and Patterson, D.F.: Coronary lesions associated with congenital subaortic stenosis in the dog. J. Path. Bact., 93:133–140, 1967.

Freigang, B., and Knobil, E.: Patent ductus arteriosus with pulmonary hypertension and arteritis in a Rhesus monkey. Yale J. Biol. Med., 40:239–242, 1967.

Gaag, I., Van Der, and Luer, R.J.T., Van Der: Eight cases of pericardial defects in the dog. Vet. Pathol., 14:14–18, 1977.

Gertz, E.W.: Cardiomyopathy in Syrian hamsters. Am. J. Pathol., 70:151–154, 1973,

Greene, H.J., Wray, D.D., and Greenway, J.A.: Two equine congenital cardiac anomalies. Irish Vet. J., 29:115–117, 1975.

Hackel, D.B., et al.: Interatrial septal defect in a chimpanzee. Lab. Invest., 2:154–163, 1952.

Hamlin, R.L., Smetzer, D.L., and Smith, R.C.: Inter-ventricular septal defect (Roger's disease) in the dog. J. Am. Vet. Med. Assn., 145:331–340, 1964.

Hare, T.: Patent interventricular septum of a dog's heart. Vet. Rec., 55:103–107, 1943.

Hueper, W.C.: Aortic abnormalities in dogs used for experimental purposes. Arch. Path., 39:375–380, 1945.

Jeraj, K., et al.: Double outlet right ventricle in a cat. J. Am. Vet. Med. Assoc., 173:1356–1360, 1978.

Kast, A.: Angeborene transpositionen von aorta und A. pulmonalis beim rind. (Congenital transposition of the aorta and pulmonary artery in cattle.) Zentbl. Vet. Med., 17A:780–795, 1970.

Kemler, A.G., and Martin, J.E.: Incidence of congenital cardiac defects in bovine fetuses. Am. J. Vet. Res., 33:249–251, 1972.

Kitchell, R.L., Stevens, C.E., and Turbes, C.C.: Cardiac and aortic arch anomalies, hydrocephalus and other abnormalities in newborn pigs. J. Am. Vet. Med. Assn., 130:453–457, 1957.

Legendre, A.M., Krahwinkel, D.J., Carrig, C.B., and Michel, R.L.: Ascites associated with intrahepatic arteriovenous fistula in a cat. J. Am. Vet. Med. Assoc., 168:589–591, 1976.

Lev, M., Neuwelt, F., and Necheles, H.: Congenital defect of the interventricular septum, aortic regurgitation and probable heart block in a dog. Am. J. Vet. Res., 2:91–94, 1941.

Linde-Sipman, J.S., van der: Hypoplasia of the left ventricle in four ruminants. Vet. Pathol., 15:474–480, 1978.

Linde-Sipman, J.S., van der, Ingh, T.S.G.A.M., van den, and Koeman, J.P.: Congenital heart abnormalities in the cat. A description of sixteen cases. Zentralbl. Veterinaermed., 20A:419–425, 1973.

Linton, G.A.: Anomalies of the aortic arches causing strangulation of the esophagus and trachea. J. Am. Vet. Med. Assn., 129:1–5, 1956.

Liu, S.-K., and Tilley, L.P.: Dysplasia of the tricuspid valve in the dog and cat. J. Am. Vet. Med. Assoc., 169:623–630, 1976.

Ljunggren, G., et al.: Four cases of congenital malformation of the heart in a litter of eleven dogs. J. Small Anim. Pract., 7:611–623, 1966.

Luer, R.J.T., van der, and Linde-Sipman, J.S., van der: A rare congenital cardiac anomaly in a foal. Vet. Pathol., 15:776–778, 1978.

Luginbuhl, H., Chacko, S.K., Patterson, D.F., and Medway, W.: Congenital hereditary lymphoedema in the dog. II. Pathological studies. J. Med. Genet., 4:153–165, 1967.

McLeod, W.M.: Unusual bovine left coronary artery. J. Am. Vet. Med. Assn., 128:39, 1956.

Meyerowitz, B.: Defectus interventricularis septi in heart of pig. Am. J. Vet. Res., 3:368–372, 1942.

Monti, F.: Le cardiopatie congenite in pathologia comparata. Nuova Vet., 27:33–43, 65–79, 107–111, and 146–150, 1951.

Morris, B., et al.: Congenital lymphatic oedema in Ayrshire calves. Aust. J. Exp. Biol. Med. Sci., 32:265, 1954.

Naylor, J.R.: Regurgitation in pups. I. Persistent aortic arches. J. Am. Vet. Med. Assn., 130:283–284, 1957.

Olafson, P.: Congenital cardiac anomalies in animals. J. Tech. Meth. & Bull. Inter. Assn. Med. Mus., 19:129–134, 1939.

Paasch, L.H., and Zook, B.C.: The pathogenesis of endocardial fibroelastosis in Burmese cats. Lab. Invest., 42:197–204, 1980.

Parker, G.W., Jackson, W.F., and Patterson, D.F.: Coarctation of the aorta in a canine. J. Am. Anim. Hosp. Assoc., 7:353–355, 1971.

Patterson, D.F.: Epidemiologic and genetic studies of congenital heart disease in the dog. Circulation Res., 23:171–202, 1968.

Patterson, D.F.: Canine congenital heart disease: epidemiology and etiological hypotheses. J. Small Anim. Pract., 12:263–287, 1971.

Patterson, D.F., Medway, W., Luginbuhl, H., and Chacko, S.: Congenital hereditary lymphoedema in the dog. I. Clinical and genetic studies. J. Med. Genet., 4:145, 1967.

Patterson, D.F., et al.: Hereditary patent ductus arteriosus and its sequelae in the dog. Circ. Res., 29:1–13, 1971.

Patterson, D.F., et al.: Hereditary defects of the conotruncal septum in Keeshond dogs. Am. J. Cardiol., 34:187–205, 1974.

Perkins, R.L.: Multiple congenital cardiovascular anomalies in a kitten. J. Am. Vet. Med. Assoc., 160:1430–1431, 1972.

Prickett, M.E., Reeves, J.T., and Zent, W.W.: Tetralogy of Fallot in a Thoroughbred foal. J. Am. Vet. Med. Assoc., 162:552–555, 1973.

Prior, J.T., and Wyatt, T.C.: Endocardial fibroelastosis. Amer. J. Path., 26:969–987, 1950.

Pyle, R.L., and Patterson, D.F.: Multiple cardiovascular malformation in a family of boxer dogs. J. Am. Vet. Med. Assoc., 160:965–976, 1972.

Roberts, S.J., et al.: Persistent right aortic arch in a Guernsey bull. Cornell Vet., 43:537–543, 1953.

Rooney, J.R., and Franks, W.C.: Congenital cardiac anomalies in horses. Path. Vet., 1:454–464, 1964.

Rooney, J.R., II, and Watson, D.F.: Persistent right aortic arch in a calf. J. Am. Vet. Med. Assn., 129:5–7, 1956.

Sandusky, G.E., and Smith, C.W.: Anomalous left coronary artery in a calf. J. Am. Vet. Med. Assoc., 173:475–477, 1978.

Sass, B., and Albert, T.F.: A case of Eisenmenger's complex in a calf. Cornell Vet., 60:61–65, 1970.

Seibold, H.R., and Evans, L.E.: A complex cardiac anomaly in a calf. J. Am. Vet. Med. Assn., 130:99–101, 1957.

Stowens, D.: Pediatric Pathology, 2nd ed. Baltimore, The Williams & Wilkins Co., 1966.

Van Nie, C.J.: Congenital malformations of the heart in cattle and swine. A survey of a collection. Acta Morph. Neerl. Scand., 6:387–393, 1966.

———: Anomalous origin of the coronary arteries in animals. Path. Vet., 5:313–326, 1968.

Vitums, A.: Origin of the aorta and pulmonary trunk from the right ventricle in a horse. Pathol. Vet., 7:482–491, 1970.

Wegelius, O., and von Essen, R.: Endocardial fibroelastosis in dogs. Acta Path. Microbiol. Scand., 77:66–72, 1969.

THE HEART

Cardiac Failure

Cardiac failure is the inability of the heart to maintain adequate circulation. It is a leading cause of death in adult human beings, owing to the high incidence of coronary vascular disease, particularly atherosclerosis and resultant myocardial infarction. Although domestic animals may develop coronary vascular disease, the frequency and severity do not approach the proportions seen in man. Other mechanisms may lead to heart failure in man and domestic animals, however, and heart failure is the usual immediate cause of death in many acute infectious diseases, as well as in many poisonings.

Acute Cardiac Failure

Acute cardiac failure is the result of a sudden cessation of effective cardiac contraction leading to "brain death" within minutes. It may result from anoxia, the action of certain drugs or poisons, myocardial necrosis (especially of the conducting system), shock, cardiac tamponade, or sudden occlusion of the pulmonary artery or aorta. It may also follow repeated chronic injury to the myocardium which the heart had, until the final insult, compensated for; or compensated injury which becomes uncompensated due to increased demands from exercise. In the absence of a primary lesion such as cardiac tamponade or an occlusive thrombus, the lesions of acute cardiac failure are minimal. Pulmonary and/or systemic congestion may be prominent. Edema is not a feature because of the acute failure of circulation.

The right and/or left ventricles may be acutely dilated (acute dilatation of the heart). As the name implies, this is a pathologic enlargement of one or more of the cardiac chambers, most frequently of the right ventricle. The left ventricle, because of its thicker wall, offers more resistance to the dilatative force; the atria expand less noticeably and less extensively, because the absence of an "intake" valve prevents the development of any great internal pressure. Cardiac dilatation is recognized by a rounded bulging of one or both ventricles; the line from the atrioventricular level to the apex, which normally is almost straight, assumes an outward curvature that is often noticeable. Palpation reveals the muscular wall to be yielding and flexible, a condition to which the adjective flabby is conventionally applied. Rarely a weakened, sac-like aneurysm develops.

The primary cause may not be discernible even in the case of myocardial necrosis, as insufficient time elapses for autolytic processes to proceed, allowing the cells to be recognized morphologically as necrotic. Should acute cardiac failure not result in immediate death, but rather extend for one to several days, the congestion will be more pronounced and will be accompanied by edema. Degenerative changes may develop in the passively congested organs, particularly the liver, where centrilobular necrosis ("nutmeg" liver) may be striking. Damaged myocardium will also now have had time to become evident grossly and microscopically.

Chronic Cardiac Failure

Chronic cardiac failure, often referred to as **congestive heart failure,** is the result of the inability of cardiac output to keep pace with venous return. It is usual to divide chronic heart failure into **left-sided heart failure** and **right-sided heart failure,** which may exist independently of one another; but in time, failure of one side leads to increased strain on the other, resulting in total heart failure.

Left-Sided Heart Failure. Left-sided heart failure may follow damage to the myocardium, aortic and mitral valve disease, various congenital defects, or hypertension. The latter is particularly common in man, but appears to be much less frequent in

animals. Aside from the primary heart disease, the most striking pathologic lesions are in the lungs. Increased pressure in the pulmonary veins and, ultimately, alveolar capillaries results in congestion and alveolar edema. Alveolar lining cells become hypertrophied, and fibrosis develops in alveolar walls. Alveolar hemorrhage leads to the presence of hemosiderin-laden alveolar macrophages, the so-called "heart failure cells." Clinically, there is dyspnea and shortness of breath. Decreased renal circulation results in reduced glomerular filtration rate, increased tubular resorption of sodium, and, therefore, increased blood volume compounding the load on the myocardium. In man and presumably in animals, plasma renin and angiotensin are elevated.

There is **chronic dilatation** of the heart which is readily distinguished from the acute disorder by the myocardial hypertrophy that accompanies it.

Right-Sided Heart Failure. Right-sided heart failure follows impedance of pulmonary circulation and therefore obviously follows left-sided failure. Primary disease of the lung or pulmonary vasculature may lead to primary right-sided failure which is sometimes called **cor pulmonale.** In this "pure" form, the secondary lesions focus on the visceral and portal circulation rather than the lung, which does not become congested or develop the lesions described in left-sided failure. The liver develops the characteristic "nutmeg" appearance due to centrilobular congestion, atrophy, necrosis, and fibrosis. Other abdominal organs are also congested. The increased venous pressure leads to edema, especially of the subcutis, and ascites, and if severe, a venous pulse, which is best recognized in the jugular veins (jugular pulse). Although increased hydrostatic pressure contributes to edema, retention of water and sodium are also of importance due to reduced glomerular filtration and increased tubular reabsorption of sodium. In human beings with congestive heart failure, there is also increased secretion of aldosterone, but the responsible mechanism is not understood.

High-Altitude Disease

Since it is essentially a condition of slow cardiac failure, we may consider a disease which arises in cattle and less frequently in sheep and horses, which are pastured on mountainous ranges at an elevation above 2500 meters (7600 feet). A corresponding condition known as "miners' disease" occurs in men laboring in the high Andes. Dyspnea and weakness occur, as in any cardiac insufficiency, but frequently the first sign of illness noticed by the stockman is subcutaneous and more deeply placed edema of the ventral body wall. This is usually most prominent in the sternal region, or brisket; hence, the disease is often called **"brisket disease."** Animals may be gradually acclimatized to the low oxygen-content of the rarefied atmosphere at these altitudes, their erythrocyte count reaching a level well above the usual normal, and the oxygen-carrying capacity increasing so that normal health is maintained. With careful nursing and removal to a lower altitude, recovery may ensue in those which do become ill but, under common husbandry conditions, the disease is usually eventually fatal.

Lesions in fatal cases include dilatation and hypertrophy, generally of both ventricles, and chronic passive congestion. The latter is notable in the large veins, the spleen, and especially in the liver, where the typical "nutmeg liver" usually develops. Cardiac edema develops, as mentioned. Polycythemia is often found. Blood pressure in the pulmonary artery and its branches is increased (pulmonary arterial hypertension) with a corresponding enlargement of the heart. Replacing the inhaled air with oxygen causes the hypertension to subside. Will, et al. (1975) have suggested that susceptibility of cattle to high-altitude disease is genetically transmitted. Cattle native to high altitudes suffer a 0.5 to 2% incidence of the disease, whereas 10 to 40% of cattle native to low altitudes will develop the disease when taken to high altitudes.

Polycythemia, pulmonary hypertension, and cardiac hypertrophy can be induced in most animal species by exposure to high altitude. In dogs, polycythemia and pulmonary hypertension develop, but interestingly, cardiac hypertrophy does not follow (Vogel, et al., 1971).

Myocardium

Atrophy of the Myocardium

Atrophy of the myocardium is recognized grossly by a heart that is smaller than normal and microscopically by a decrease in size of muscle fibers. The latter may be best recognized by an apparent increase in number of nuclei in proportion to fibers. Lipofuscin may be abundant within the myofibers near the poles of nuclei, giving use to the term brown atrophy of the heart. Myocardial atrophy is seen in chronic wasting diseases and malnutrition.

Hypertrophy of the Myocardium

Hypertrophy develops in either ventricle when conditions arise requiring the accomplishment of more work in the form of a greater output of blood per unit of time or the development of a greater pressure in order to force the blood along its normal channels. The hypertrophic cardiac wall is thicker, often much thicker, than normal; if there has been dilatation of the ventricle, it is also larger both in external and internal dimensions. The weight of such a heart is abnormally great. However, in veterinary practice, where animals of different breeds and species vary tremendously with respect to what is normal, the increased thickness and a rubbery firmness are the best gross indices of cardiac hypertrophy. Microscopically, the individual myocardial fibers are increased in thickness; their nuclei are numerous, enlarged and tend to be especially plump and square-ended.

Causes. The cause of cardiac hypertrophy may lie within the heart itself in the form of stenosis or insufficiency (leaking) of the valve through which the ejected blood must pass, or it may be found in leakage of the valve through which the blood enters. In the valvular insufficiencies, when functionally compensated, there is also dilatation of the ventricle in question. In this way, it may hold a volume large enough to permit a certain portion to leak backward and still to propel the normal amount forward. Such a cardiac disorder is said to be "fully compensated." Extra-cardiac causes of ventricular hypertrophy are those disorders which oblige the ventricle to pump against abnormally high resistance. The right ventricle, there-fore, undergoes hypertrophy when there are obstructive processes in the lungs, such as the diffuse increase of fibrous tissue that thickens the alveolar walls in some chronic inflammatory processes (including "heaves"), in chronic passive congestion (brown induration), pneumoconiosis, or pulmonary stenosis. Hypertrophy of the left ventricle results from aortic stenosis, arterial hypertension in general, and especially from nephrosclerotic changes of whatever nature. An adherent pericardium tends to cause hypertrophy of the part involved as an aid in overcoming the immobilizing effect of the adhesions.

Cardiac hypertrophy may occur in the absence of any obvious cause (idiopathic). Several forms of idiopathic cardiac hypertrophy (**hypertrophic cardiomyopathy; cardiomegaly**) are recognized in man and occasionally encountered in dogs and cats. Liu and associates (1979) reported on several examples in which there was particularly striking hypertrophy of the ventricular septa.

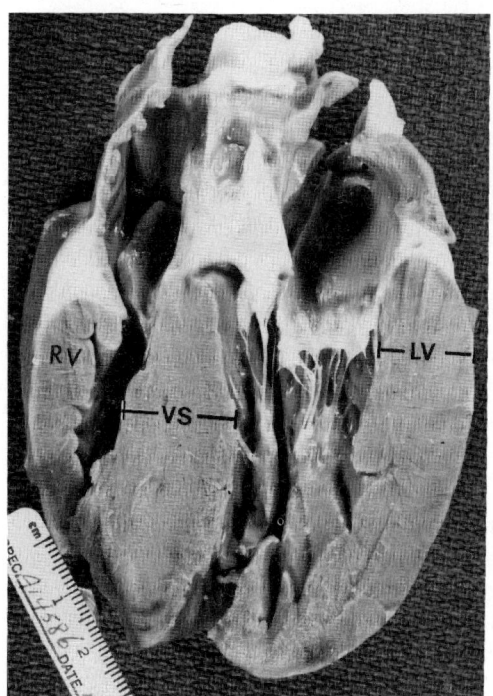

Fig. 21-4. Canine hypertrophic cardiomyopathy. The ventricular septum (VS) is greatly thickened. *LV*, left ventricular wall; *RV*, right ventricular wall. (Courtesy of Dr. S. Liu and *Journal of the American Veterinary Medical Association.*)

Degenerative Changes

Several of the degenerations described in Chapter 2 occur in the heart, but the details given there need not be repeated. Albuminous degeneration is described by some, but is not easily recognized either grossly or microscopically. Mucoid degeneration is not rare in the subepicardial fat of the coronary border, resulting from cachexia and malnutrition. Hyaline degeneration of muscle fibers occurs as a prenecrotic change and a part of the picture of the "toxic myocarditis" of myocardial exhaustion, and in company with the lesions of the deficiencies mentioned in that section. Fatty infiltration, it will be recalled, is excessive extension of the coronary adipose tissue among the cardiac muscle fibers. Fatty change leads to the appearance of minute droplets of lipid within the muscle fibers. It is detected with certainty only by fat stains. The pigment of brown atrophy

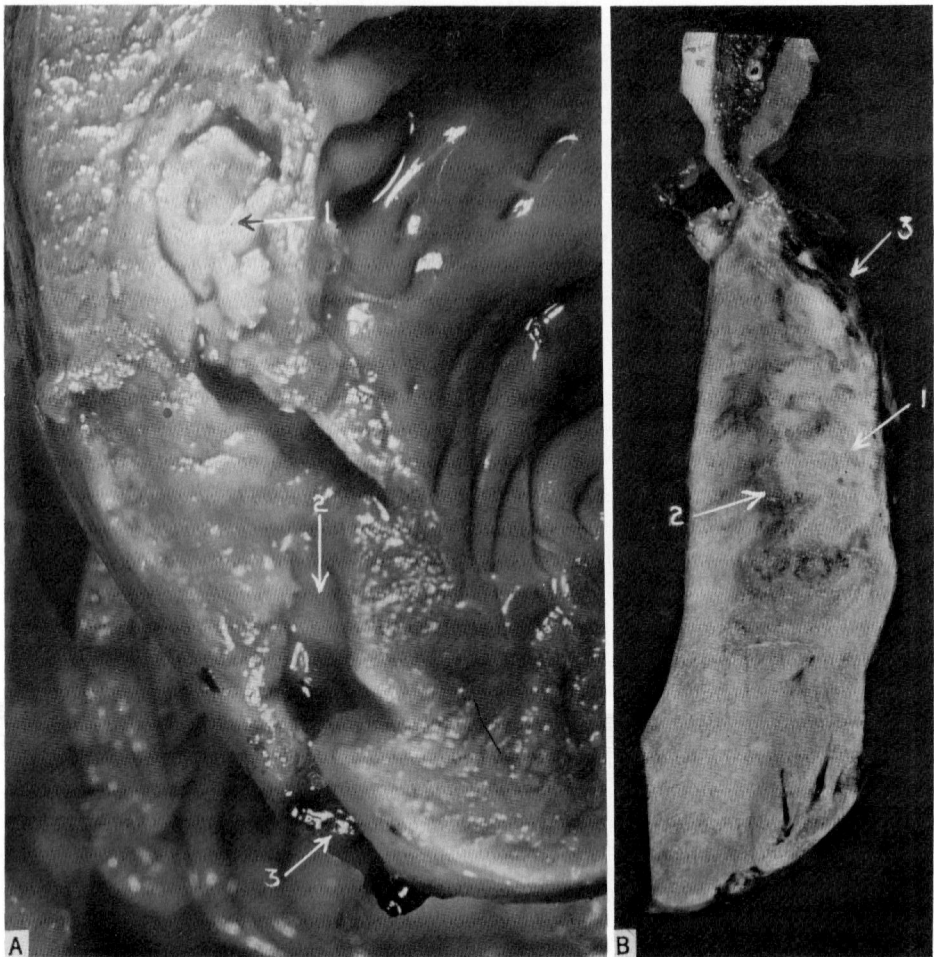

Fig. 21–5. Infarction of the heart. *A*, Infarction of left ventricle of a 12-year-old male mongrel terrier. Necrosis of myocardium (*1*) has led to formation of a channel (*2*) in the left ventricle and rupture (*3*). Death followed this cardiac tamponade and hemopericardium. *B*, Infarction of the intraventricular septum of a four-year-old spayed female Poodle. The gray-colored necrotic myocardium (*1*) is separated from the normal myocardium by a zone of hemorrhage (*2*). Subendocardial hemorrhage is seen at (*3*). (Courtesy of Angell Memorial Animal Hospital.)

has the myocardial fibers as a favorite site of localization. Melanosis rarely involves epicardial or endocardial surfaces, especially those on or near the heart valves.

Infarcts of the myocardium are all too common in humans, sudden infarction constituting the usual "heart attack." The cause ordinarily is arteriosclerotic or atherosclerotic obstruction of a coronary artery, or thrombosis of one of those vessels. The extent of the infarct depends on the location of the obstruction; many of them slowly heal with replacement of the necrotic area of muscle by a fibrous scar. Lesions of this kind are quite uncommon in veterinary patients, although it is possible to produce them experimentally.

Congestion and hyperemia follow the usual laws. Edema fluid tends to drain into the pericardial cavity, so that edema of the heart muscle itself is rare. Both the external and internal surfaces of the heart are common sites for the hemorrhages of anoxia, toxemias, and septicemias. The subepicardial hemorrhages tend to be petechial; the subendocardial are usually ecchymoses. They conform to the general statements already made on the subject of hemorrhages.

Necrosis of the myocardium unrelated to vascular disease is the more usual finding in domestic animals. Microscopically, it is characteristically hyaline necrosis (hyaline degeneration). Focal myocardial necrosis is seen in deficiency of potassium, thiamine and tocopherol, and several poisonings such as gossypol, coffee senna, coyotillo, and vetch.

Myocarditis

Myocarditis, as a diffuse exudative inflammation of the heart muscle, is an uncommon disease in animals. Infections, which are the usual inciters of such inflammations, usually localize in the outer or inner coverings of the myocardium, rather than in the muscle itself, or take the form of abscesses or similarly circumscribed foci. This may well be attributable to the dense and solid character of the myocardium, which renders it less favorable for the growth and spread of microorganisms than the adjacent surfaces and spaces.

Occasionally, a heart is seen in which there is an appreciable degree of proliferation of the interstitial reticulum in the form of cells of reticulo-endothelial type, with large, pale vesicular nuclei. A few lymphocytes are also present in most cases. The cause of this mild subacute inflammation is seldom readily identifiable but is probably toxic, coupled perhaps with a mild allergic state. Foci of such cells sometimes bear a superficial resemblance to the Aschoff nodule of human rheumatic fever, but no clearly comparable rheumatic heart disease exists in animals.

A special type of reactive cell peculiar to the heart is known as the **Anitschkow cell** (sometimes called the myocardial reticulocyte or the Aschoff cell, but never to be confused with the Aschoff body). With inconspicuous cytoplasm, this cell is characterized by an elongated, ellipsoidal nucleus, along the center of which lies a longitudinally placed rod of deeply staining chromatin. The diameter of this rod is very close to one-third of that of the whole nucleus; on each side of it is another third which remains clear and unstained. The periphery of the rod bears minute projections from some of which fine lines of chromatin, barely visible, extend across the clear zone to tie the rod to the nuclear membrane, which, though thin, is also distinctly stained.

Unless seen in longitudinal section, the Anitschkow cell may be confused with other kinds of cells, but the true Anitschkow cell is held to be of histiocytic (reticulocytic) origin and is restricted to the heart. In spite of the fact that it may be seen in the cellular aggregate known as the Aschoff body of (human) rheumatic heart disease, it occurs in many forms of injury to the myocardium and many (presumably all) mammalian species. It is occasionally seen congregated into syncytial giant cells and can be shown to have phagocytic properties.

Along with the cells characteristic of inflammation in general, the earlier stages of inflammatory reactions in cardiac and striated muscle also include the presence of "myogenic" or "sarcolemma cells" whose nuclei have a prominent central nucelolus with a resultant similarity to the appearance of the Anitschkow cell in cross section. These often form syncytial giant cells, but the nuclear characteristics serve to differentiate such giant cells from the foreign-body giant cells that may be present, but which have dense, homogeneous nuclei.

Certain of the infectious granulomatous diseases, especially tuberculosis and caseous lymphadenitis, rarely localize in the heart and initiate their characteristic lesions, which may be single or multiple, the intervening areas being free of abnormalities. Such lesions are the result of hematogenous spread of the infection in question from a focus somewhere else. Similar hematogenous spread occurs in the case of infections by the pyogenic cocci, although invasion of the heart is exceptional. The lesions resulting are **abscesses;** they may be large or small, many or few, thickly or thinly encapsulated. The site of origin may be in any infected region of the body, the uterus, a joint or an infected umbilicus in the newborn being especially likely locations. Similar metastasis of the necrophorus organism leads to a circumscribed area of coagulative necrosis, more or less completely encapsulated as in the case of abscesses and granulomas. This also is rare in the heart. Myocarditis (and necrosis) is a relatively consistent finding in several other infectious diseases such as listeriosis, clostridial infections, toxoplasmosis, Chagas' disease, and encephalomyocarditis. It may also be a prominent finding in other infectious diseases, such as foot-and-mouth disease, bluetongue, canine parvovirus, and coxsackie virus infection. Eosinophilic myocarditis of cattle is discussed under eosinophilic myositis.

Scars of white fibrous tissue are occasionally seen in the myocardium. While such a scar might well represent a healed myocardial infarct in the human, in animals, a healed abscess or parasitic lesion is a more likely explanation. The size, shape and location should afford a clue to previous events.

Parasites

Heartworms (*Dirofilaria immitis*) occupy the right ventricle and pulmonary artery, sometimes filling the available space with astonishing completeness. It is remarkable how long life may continue despite the obvious interference with function. *Cysticercus cellulosae*, the intermediate stage of the pork tapeworm of man, forms cystic cavities about 3 or 4 by 10 mm, elongated in the direction of the muscular fibers. The cysts may be few or so numerous as to riddle the myocardium. *Cysticercus bovis* is much less prone to involve the heart, but

may do so. Sarcosporidial cysts are common in the heart muscle of ruminants.

Neoplasms

Primary neoplasms of the myocardium are rare. **Rhabdomyoma** and **rhabdomyosarcoma** are neoplasms of myofibers that are not common in any species. They are usually grayish nodules within the atrial or ventricular myocardium, and often project into the lumen. Microscopically, the neoplastic fibers may resemble normal myocardium, but generally the cells are disorganized and anaplastic with large nuclei and thin cytoplasmic extensions, or so-called strap cells. Multiple cytoplasmic processes may emanate from a single enlarged hyperchromatic nucleus. Multinucleated tumor cells are frequent. A benign lesion called the **congenital rhabdomyoma** has been described in several species, but is most frequent in swine and guinea pigs. It is believed to result from focal arrest of maturation of cardiac muscle and not represent a true neoplasm. These are usually multiple, discrete, nonencapsulated masses of swollen myofibers filled with glycogen.

Aortic Body Tumor-Carotid Body Tumor. Tumors of the aortic body or carotid body are not neoplasms of the heart, but are discussed here because those of the aortic body, the more frequent of the two, occur at the base of the heart. They are sometimes called **heart-base tumors.** These bodies are chemoreceptors, sensitive to blood pH, oxygen, and carbon dioxide, and they help in the regulation of respiration and circulation. Based on this function, neoplasms of the aortic body and carotid body are also known as **chemodectomas.** There is dispute as to whether aortic and carotid body tumors belong to the chromaffinoma or paraganglioma group. The term **paraganglioma** is applied to chromaffin tumors outside the adrenal glands. Some refer to this group of tumors as **nonchromaffin paragangliomas.** Rarely, similar tumors may develop at other sites.

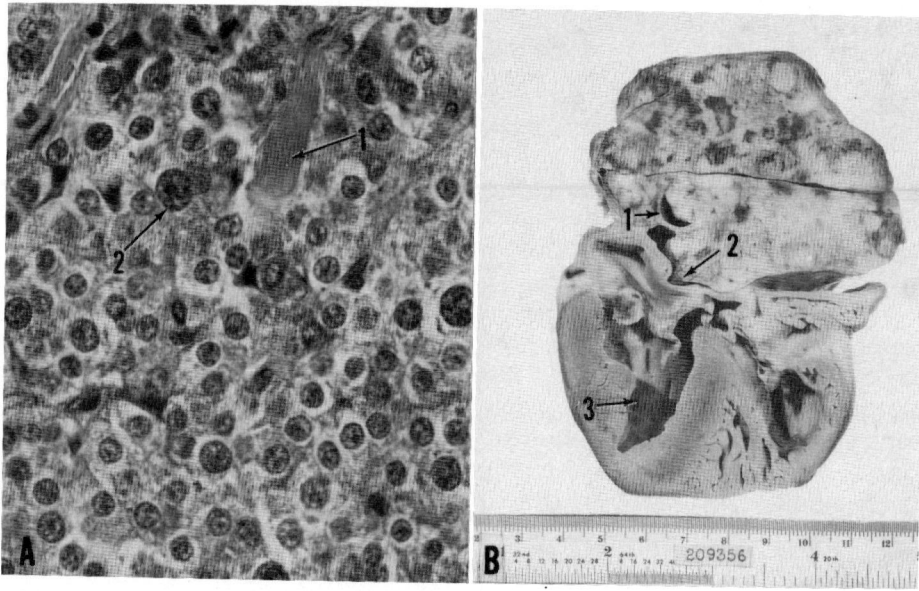

Fig. 21–6. Aortic body tumor. *A*, Photomicrograph (× 500). Collagen-rich supporting stroma (*1*) and polyhedral cells with spherical nuclei, some large and hyperchromatic (*2*). *B*, The gross tumor at the base of the heart of a ten-year-old English bulldog. Tumor invades the aorta (*1*), compresses the atrium (*2*). Left ventricle (*3*). (Courtesy of Armed Forces Institute of Pathology.) Contributor: Dr. W.H. Riser.

The aortic body tumor is located at the base of the heart, usually intimately related to both the aorta and pulmonary artery. This anatomic relationship corresponds to that described by Bloom (1943) for the normal aortic body of the dog. The media of both the pulmonary artery and aorta is often infiltrated by tumor cells, occasionally with encroachment upon the lumen. The anatomic site is of importance because the morphology of the tumors cells could be confused with that seen in a number of other tumors. The tumor cells are usually polyhedral in shape, with vacuolated or granular cytoplasm and spherical, finely stippled nuclei. Very large hyperchromatic nuclei are often scattered through the neoplasm. It is divided into lobules of irregular size by fine strands of connective tissue; blood vessels are in close proximity to the tumor cells. The tumors rarely metastasize, but are usually locally invasive.

Apparently without any endocrine function, aortic body tumors have ordinarily been found only in the dog, most frequently in brachiocephalic breeds (Bulldog, Boston Terrier, Boxer). However, there are isolated reports in many other species, including birds.

A few carotid body tumors of dogs have been seen in the experience of the authors and have also been reported by others (Scotti, 1958; Cheville, 1972). Dean and Strafuss (1975) indicated in their review that 9 of 22 dogs with carotid body tumors simultaneously had aortic body tumors. Others have been reported in a cow (Nordstoga, 1966) and in a cat (Buergelt and Das, 1968).

Other Neoplasms. Neoplasms at the base of the heart may arise from other tissues as demonstrated by von Bomhard, et al. (1974). They studied 69 "heart base tumors" in dogs and found that 45 arose from aberrant thyroid tissue, 20 were true aortic body tumors, and 4 could not be classified. Aberrant parathyroid tumors may also occur at the base of the heart.

Cheville (1972) has described the ultra-structure of these various heart base tumors.

Hemangioendothelioma is occasionally found in the right atrium of the canine heart either as a primary tumor or as a metastasis from the spleen or other site. Hemangioendothelioma is discussed in another section of this chapter.

The most frequently encountered neo-plasm in the heart is the **malignant lymphoma.** A considerable proportion of these neoplasms involve the heart in cattle. Some result in the formation of one or more discrete masses, but many infiltrate among the muscle bundles. An area of rather faint white streaks parallel to the course of the muscle fibers should be considered malignant lymphoma until shown to be otherwise. (See Chapter 22.)

Pericardium

Pericarditis

Pericarditis includes inflammation of both the parietal and visceral surfaces of the pericardial cavity, in other words, the inner surface of the sac and the outer surface of the heart, the epicardium. The exu-date formed naturally accumulates in the lumen of the pericardial sac. Although, for reasons not clearly understood, moderate amounts of serum and fibrin sometimes accumulate in the sac as a result of **uremia,** true pericarditis is always infectious and nearly always exudative. The source of infection may be regarded as always hematogenous except when it enters by direct extension, the latter form constituting the common "traumatic pericarditis" of bovines. It is doubtful that extension from an infected pleural cavity or surface ever occurs, for the membrane of the pericardial sac, covered with pleural mesothelium on the outside and pericardial on the inside, the whole scarcely thicker than a sheet of paper, forms an effective barrier between the two cavities. Similarly, infection involving the epicardial surface seldom shows any appreciable spread into the underlying myocardium.

Hematogenous Pericarditis

The pericardial surfaces are commonly involved, with the pleura and lungs, in pasteurellosis (including fowl cholera) and less commonly, in certain viral diseases, among which are hog cholera, equine viral

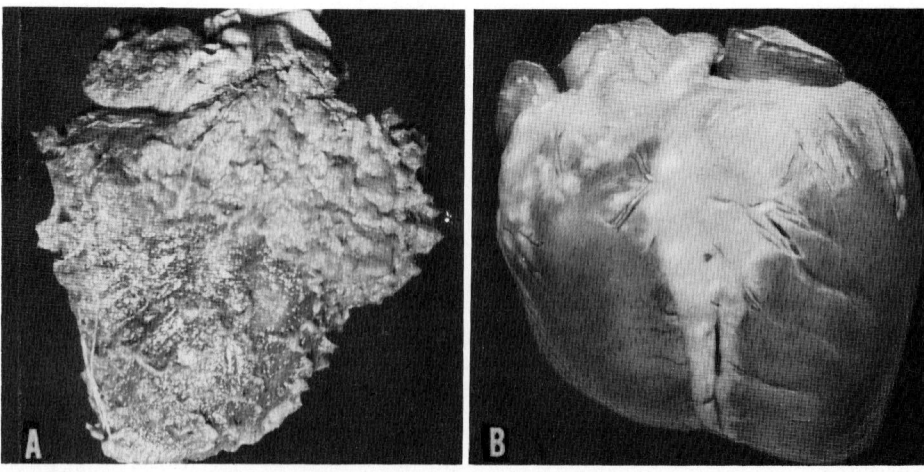

Fig. 21–7. *A,* Chronic organizing fibrinous pericarditis in a sow. *B,* Acute dilatation of the right heart of a young Guernsey cow which died with circulatory collapse following cesarean operation. Note rounded outline of the heart, viewed from its anterior aspect. (Courtesy of College of Veterinary Medicine, Iowa State University.)

pneumonitis, and psittacosis. Just how often the pericarditis itself is due to a virus and how often to a secondary bacterial invader has not been adequately investigated. As is usual on serous membranes, the inflammation tends to be of the fibrinous or sero-fibrinous type unless caused by pyogenic organisms such as staphylococci or streptococci, in which case it is purulent. The amount of exudate accumulating in the pericardial cavity may be considerable, but it can usually be distinguished from hydropericardium both grossly and microscopically by the presence of fibrin, leukocytes, or even erythrocytes. In other instances, the exudate is chiefly fibrinous, appearing at the very first as a cloudiness of the epicardial surface and shortly as a thin mesh-work of fine fibrin. This conforms to the usual course of fibrinous inflammations, but in these cardiac diseases it is more common for either death or recovery to supervene before the exudate advances to organization or adhesions.

Traumatic Pericarditis

This form is ordinarily a disease of bovine animals, and in cows kept in frequent and close proximity to stables and the usual activities of the farmstead, it is all too frequent. In such places, there are almost sure to be old nails, bits of wire, and similar hardware which cattle swallow as a result of their not-too-discriminatory feeding habits. Many of these sharp metallic objects penetrate the wall of the reticulum and slowly move, encompassed in reactive granulation tissue, through the diaphragm and into the pericardial sac (a distance of only a few centimeters). Carrying cocci or other common bacteria with them, they initiate acute infectious pericarditis. The exudate is most often fibrinous or fibrinopurulent in nature and copious in amount. Cattle usually live for a number of days or weeks after the start of the process, so that the exudate has time to become extensive, organized in its deeper zones and adherent to the formative surface.

A common picture at time of death is the **cor rugosum,** or "shaggy heart." Such a heart is covered with a layer of white or blood-stained fibrin several millimeters thick, of which the deeper part is being organized into vascular fibrous tissue. The more superficial unorganized portion is of indefinite depth with irregular shreds and strings of fibrin hanging from it. More or less seropurulent fluid may distend the pericardial space, or the cavity may be empty and collapsed. In the latter case, the organizing fibrin reaches from the epicardial to the outer pericardial surface, joining the two inseparably over a large part of their area—adhesive pericarditis. Obviously such an exudate exerts pressure, and if adhesive, it tends to immobilize the heart muscle more or less rigidly. In spite of attempts at compensatory hypertrophy, the mechanical interferences, coupled with the toxic effect of the pathogenic organisms and their products, eventually bring the master pump to a standstill, and death ensues.

Lesions. Accompanying lesions are those of chronic venous congestion or of toxemia, depending upon the rapidity or slowness of the developing process. The granulation tissue with its fistulous tract reaching from the diaphragm and reticulum may be extensive or slender. The wire or similar object is commonly still present, reaching into or through the wall of the sac and not infrequently penetrating into the myocardium itself at time of death. On the other hand, iron rusts and dissolves rather quickly in the body fluids and may have completely disintegrated before death occurs, only the narrow sinus tract, its lining blackened by iron sulfide, remaining as evidence of the fatal accident.

Hydropericardium

Hydropericardium is the accumulation of fluid (lymph) in the pericardial sac. It can be distinguished from inflammatory edema, which is a serous exudate, by the absence of other aspects of an inflamma-

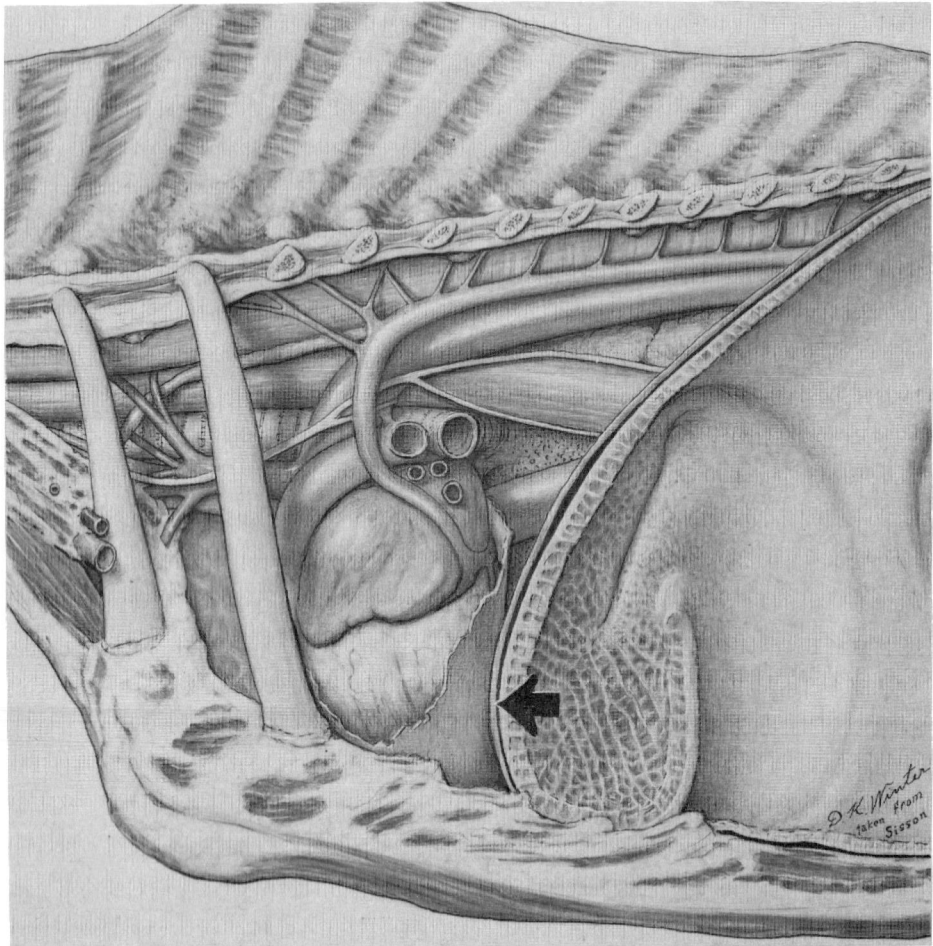

Fig. 21-8. The anatomic relationships in traumatic pericarditis. Foreign bodies penetrate the wall of the reticulum, diaphragm, and pericardium in the direction indicated by the arrow. (Modified after Sisson.)

tory process, for hydropericardium is true noninflammatory edema of the pericardium and heart. The amount of fluid encountered naturally varies greatly; in a general way, it might be stated that a quantity equal to about one-half the capacity of a ventricle of the same heart would represent a pronounced case of hydropericardium. The causes are any of the usual causes of edema, cardiac and nutritional edema probably being somewhat more important in this respect than renal edema. The effect is to interfere with the flow of venous blood returning to the heart, but this is commonly overshadowed by other effects of the basic disease.

Hemopericardium

In hemopericardium, hemorrhage fills the sac with blood. The sudden escape of blood into the pericardial sac, perhaps through rupture of an atrial or myocardial wall, is sometimes referred to as **cardiac tamponade.** Its effect is similar to, although more dramatic than, hydropericardium, because it also interferes with venous return to the heart.

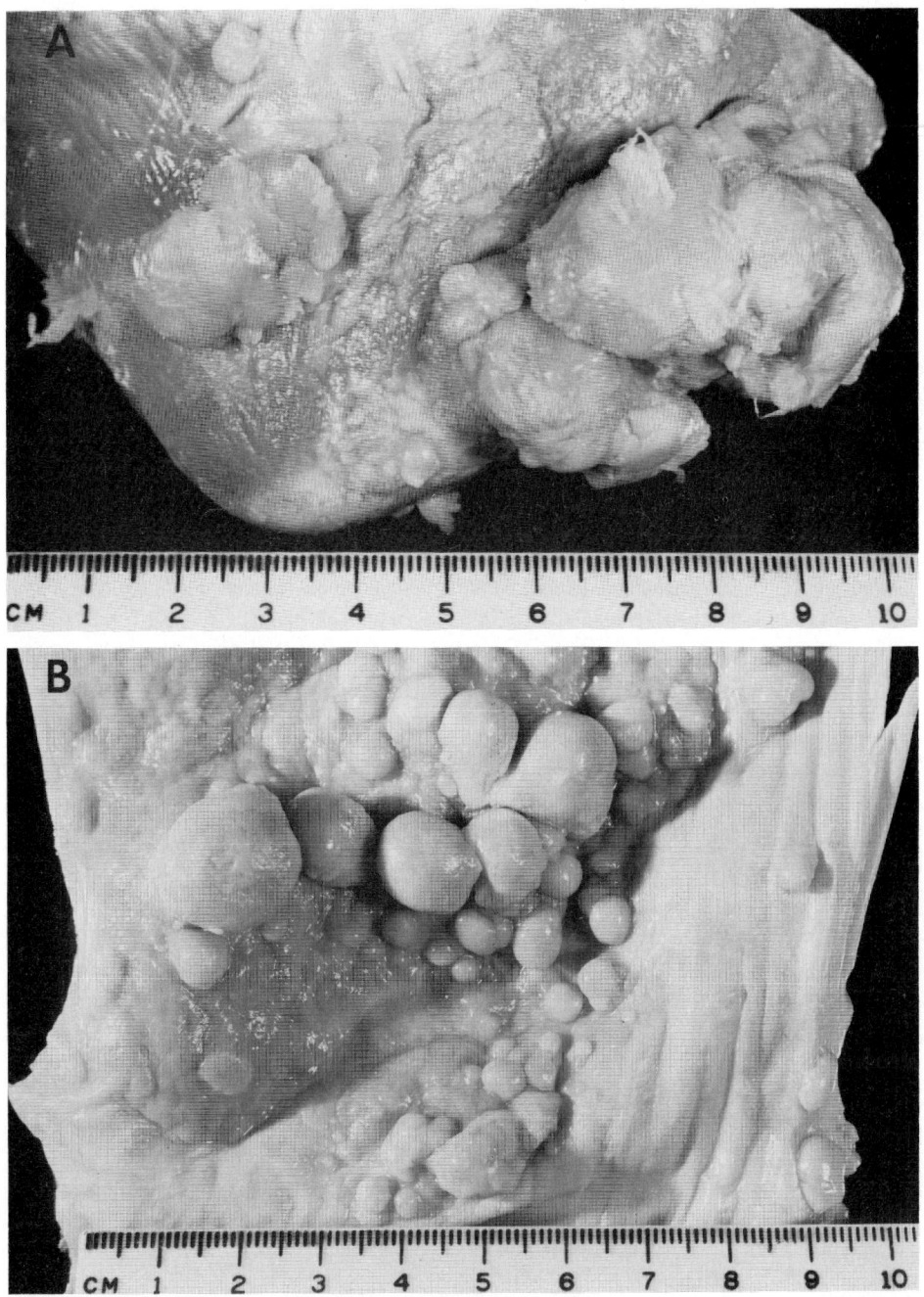

Fig. 21-9. Multiple mesothelioma of pericardium of a 27-year-old quarter horse mare. *A,* Nodular growth on the epicardium of the apex of the heart. *B,* Multiple mesotheliomas on the pericardial sac of the same horse. (Courtesy of Dr. H.W. Leipold and *Veterinary Pathology.*)

Neoplasms

Neoplasms of the pericardium are infrequent. Fibromas, leiomyomas, and hemangioendotheliomas may arise in the pericardium, but the most frequent primary neoplasms are the **mesotheliomas** (Fig. 21–9). They resemble mesotheliomas arising in the pleura and peritoneum.

Endocardium

Endocarditis

Another usually infectious disease of the heart is endocarditis, inflammation of the endocardial lining. Endocarditis may be **mural** (*murus,* wall), when the lesions are located on the lining of an atrium or ventricle, but it is much more frequently **valvular,** the lesions being located on the valves. Doubtless because of the greater pressure and mechanical strains to which the structures are subjected, valvular endocarditis is much more frequent on the left side of

the heart than on the right, and also more frequent and more extensive on the atrioventricular than on the semilunar valves. Bovines are an exception to this statement, according to the statistics of Winqvist (1945) and of Evans (1957), the reasons being obscure. Species and age affect the incidence only in accordance with the various susceptibilities to the several infections of which endocarditis is a manifestation.

Lesions. The lesion of endocarditis involves death and disappearance of the endothelium, although this may be preceded by hyperemia and infiltration of inflammatory cells and fluid in the affected area. Upon the raw surface left by the destroyed endothelium, a thrombus forms. Like other thrombi, it is initiated by the lodgment of platelets and the deposition of fibrin. As the days pass, the thrombus grows continually in size and, like other thrombi, its deeper parts are organized by

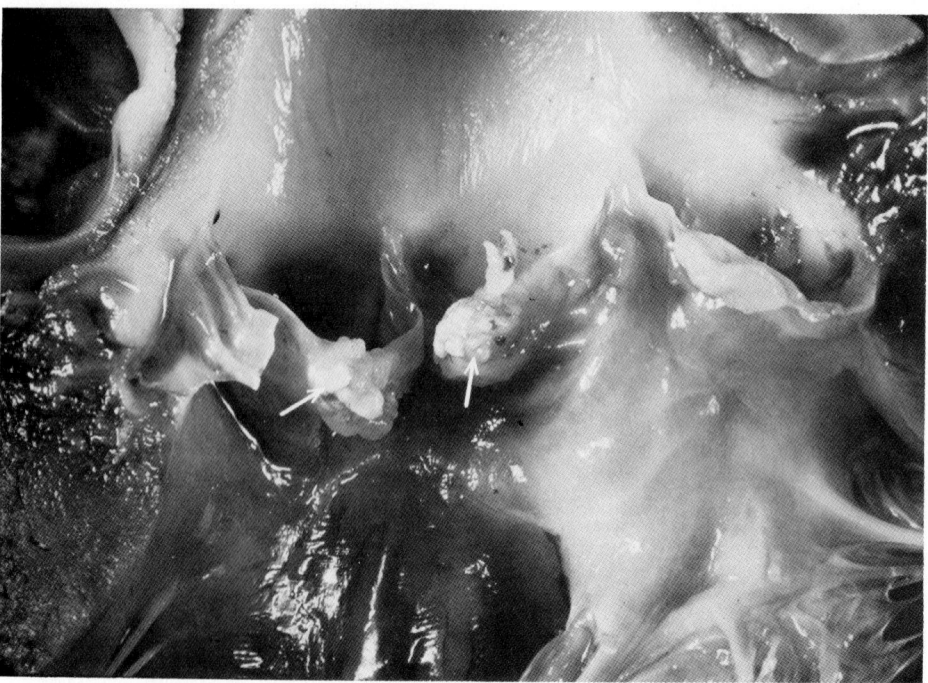

Fig. 21–10. Endocarditis of aortic semilunar valves of an eight-year-old spayed female Dachshund. Nodular lesions (arrows) on margin and surface of valves. (Courtesy of Angell Memorial Animal Hospital.)

fibrous tissue. Thus the mass becomes essentially inflammatory granulation tissue, which, under a covering zone of still unorganized exudate, may attain considerable size (one to several centimeters) and a totally irregular and bizarre shape (Fig. 21–11). Such growths are often called "vegetations," presumably because of their similarity in shape to the head of a cauliflower, or, if small and wart-like, they are called verrucae, the corresponding **"vegetative endocarditis"** and **"verrucous endocarditis"** being in use. In the case of some species and infections, healing is possible, the uneven surface being covered by regenerated endothelium. Thereupon the vascular, fibrous structure, like other granulation tissue, slowly matures into a denser, non-vascular, scar-like mass. In mural locations, lesions which are not too protuberant may subside into a flat, shiny white scar of fibrous tissue.

As can be readily imagined, the effect of one or more nodules of new tissue, when located on the wall of a ventricle or an atrium, might not be too serious, but when on a valve, as they almost always are, there is important and often disastrous interference with function. The "vegetations" or verrucae tend to form at points of contact of the valve cusps with each other, hence there is every probability that their location will be such as, not only to obstruct the lumen, but also to prevent perfect closure of the valve. They may also induce contraction of the cusp or occasionally tie it down to the heart wall or to the chordae tendineae. Mere inflammatory thickening of the cusps lessens their flexibility and ability to close properly. Valvular stenoses or insufficiencies are the result to be expected from any of these changes.

Causes. As to the causes of endocarditis in animals, generally, it may be said that the disease is a feature of certain specific infections, mostly septicemias. In horses, streptococci, chiefly *Strep. equi*, the cause of strangles, *Shigella equirulis (Bacterium viscosum equi, B. nephritidis equi)*, and possibly other organisms found in umbilical infections (pyosepticemia neonatorum) of foals, have been held responsible for endocarditis. The meningococcus (*Neisseria meningitidis*) has had this effect in horses used for the production of antiserum for meningitis. In cattle, streptococci of undetermined species, *Staphylococcus aureus, Corynebacterium pyogenes,* and paracoliform organisms causing diarrhea ("white scours") of calves have been incriminated. Endocarditis is rare in sheep, but *Streptococcus faecalis* has been found in the blood and hearts of affected lambs. A rather frequent disease in swine, endocarditis is due to the organism of swine erysipelas or to streptococci with about equal frequency. *Corynebacterium pyogenes* is a much less important cause in swine.

Hypercoagulability of the blood may lead to valvular thrombosis in the absence of infection. These thrombi, however, provide excellent sites for bacteria introduced through wounds or by surgical procedures

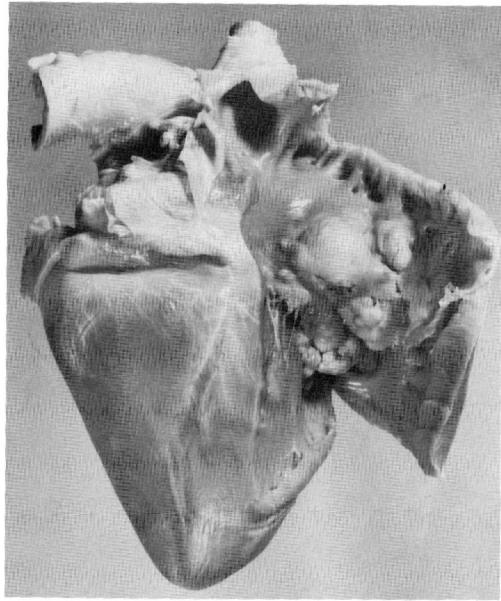

Fig. 21–11. Bacterial endocarditis affecting the tricuspid valve and mural endocardium in a five-year-old white-tailed deer. (Courtesy of Dr. W.J. Hadlow.)

to lodge and proliferate, leading to endocarditis secondary to thrombosis.

Uremia is probably the most common cause of endocarditis (and vasculitis) in the dog. The lesion is usually confined to the left atrium but may also extend into the left ventricle from uremic aortitis. The endocardium becomes edematous, which is followed by endocardial necrosis and thrombosis. Necrosis of the underlying myocardium and mineralization frequently accompany the lesion.

The most common endocardial lesion in dogs is fibrous thickening of the atrioventricular valves. Both valves may be affected, but the mitral is usually more extensively involved. The lesion has been variably referred to as chronic valvular endocarditis, chronic valvular disease, and **valvular endocardiosis** (Fig. 21–12). The cause is unknown. The valvular cusps are rather evenly reduced in height, white, and glistening, with their outer margins smoothly but markedly thickened. Microscopically, the thickening is observed to be the result of proliferation of collagenous and elastic connective tissue smooth muscle cells and the accumulation of mucinous ground substance. There is no cellular or vascular inflammatory reaction. Valvular amyloidosis is occasionally seen in dogs.

An important form of endocarditis in humans is that which accompanies rheumatic fever and rheumatic heart disease. The valvular lesions typically consist of small verrucae and are accompanied by a myocarditis characterized by focal reticuloendothelial proliferations, just visible to the naked eye, which are known as Aschoff bodies. This disease appears to have no natural counterpart in animals, although similar lesions have resulted in

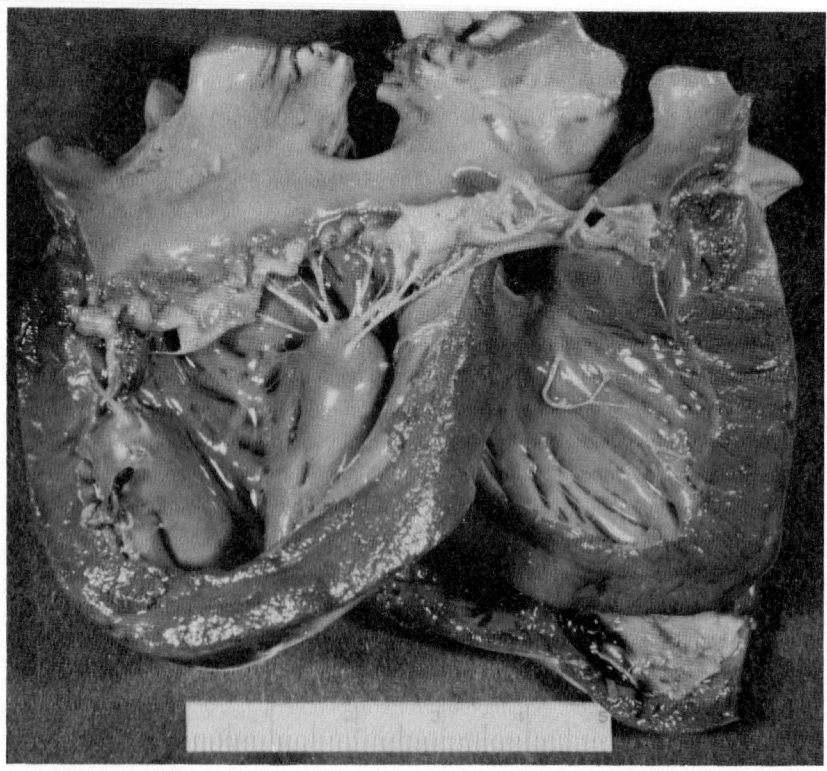

Fig. 21–12. Thickened, nodular left atrioventricular valve. The valve and the left ventricle were also dilated. From a ten-year-old female, crossbreed "Spitz" dog. (Courtesy of Angell Memorial Animal Hospital.)

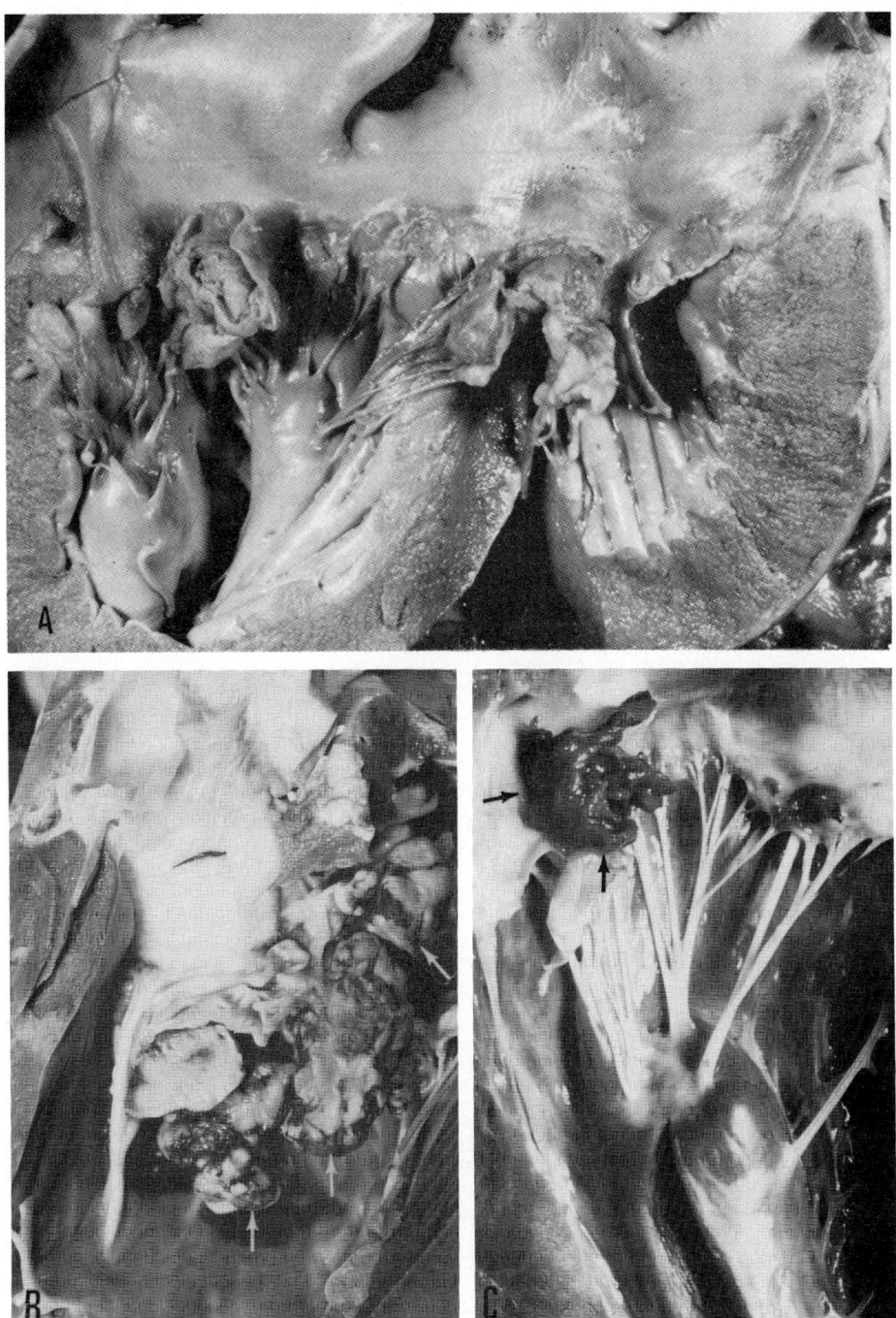

Fig. 21-13. *A*, Acute bacterial endocarditis involving the left atrioventricular valves of a 15-year-old male crossbreed terrier. (Courtesy of Angell Memorial Animal Hospital.) *B*, Valvular endocarditis in a cow. Note thick, irregular masses firmly attached to the bicuspid valve (arrows). (*B*, Courtesy of Armed Forces Institute of Pathology.) Contributor: Dr. C.L. Davis. *C*, Smaller lesions (arrows) in the bicuspid valve of a cow; *Corynebacterium pyogenes* was isolated from the lesions.

dogs experimentally infected under suitable conditions with the streptococcus derived from the human disease. Naturally occurring endocarditides in animals show no evidence of an allergic origin, nor are they accompanied ordinarily by arthritis, both of which are features of the human disease. (The swine erysipelas organism is capable of causing both endocarditis and nonexudative periarthritic proliferations, but these are very seldom found together.) The proliferative (vegetative) valvular lesions of some size usually seen in animals have much more in common with human "subacute bacterial endocarditis" than with rheumatic heart disease.

Mulberry Heart Disease. Mulberry heart disease designates a poorly understood syndrome which brings death to young pigs in a matter of hours. The whole heart at death is in a state of firm contraction and spotted with hemorrhages, thus suggesting the appearance of a mulberry. Edema is the most impressive lesion, however, with hydropericardium, limited hydroperitoneum, and pronounced pulmonary edema. The edema fluid may clot owing to its high protein content. The gastrointestinal tract is inactive, its contents dry, although there may be marked hyperemia of the fundic portion of the stomach. If death is delayed for perhaps a day, softening of the white matter in the cerebral gyri may be detected. The cause is not known but may well be an unknown toxic substance in the food, although a limited amount of experimental work has failed to reveal it. A relationship to *Escherichia coli* enterotoxemia, with or without hypersensitivity, has been suggested but not proven. This disease has also been called "dietetic microangiopathy" (Mouwen, 1965).

Alexander, A.F., et al.: Pulmonary hypertension and right ventricular hypertrophy in cattle at high altitude. Am. J. Vet. Res., 21:199–204, 1960.

Alexander, A.F., and Jensen, R.: Gross cardiac changes in cattle with high mountain (brisket) disease and in experimental cattle maintained at high altitudes. Am. J. Vet. Res., 20:680–689, 1959.

————: I. Pulmonary arteriographic studies of bovine high mountain disease. II. Pulmonary vascular pathology of high altitude-induced pulmonary hypertension in cattle. Am. J. Vet. Res., 24:1094–1097, 1112–1122, 1963.

Arango, J.E.: Alrededor de la llamada enfermedad de las alturas. Rev. Fac. méd. vet. Bogota, 18:141–144, 1949.

Benbrook, E.A.: Serofibrinous pericarditis in a dog. (Symposium, Am. Col. Vet. Path.) J. Am. Vet. Med. Assn., 127:521–522, 1955.

Bishop, S.P., and Cole, C.R.: Ultrastructural changes in the canine myocardium with right ventricular hypertrophy and congestive heart failure. Lab. Invest., 20:219–229, 1969.

Blake, J.T.: I. Certain hematopathologic conditions associated with brisket disease. II. Cardiac structural changes in cattle with brisket disease. Am. J. Vet. Res., 26:68–75 and 76–82, 1965.

————: Etiology of brisket disease. Cornell Vet., 58:305–314, 1968.

Bloom, F.: Structure and histogenesis of tumors of the aortic bodies in dogs. Arch. Pathol., 36:1–12, 1943.

Bobb, J.R.R., et al.: Experimental endocarditis and other changes in dogs with arteriovenous fistulas and bacteremia. Am. J. Path., 28:523–524, 1952.

Bomhard, D.V., Luderer, M., Hanichen, T., and Sandersleben, J.V.: Zur histogenese der herzbasistumoren beim hund. Eine histologische, histochemische, und elektronenmikroskopische studie. (Histogenesis of heart base tumors in the dog. A histological, histochemical and electron microscope study.) Zentralbl. Veterinaermed., 21A:208–224, 1974.

Bragdon, J.H., and Levine, H.D.: Myocarditis in vitamin E deficient rabbits. Am. J. Path., 25:265–272, 1949.

Buergelt, C.D., and Das, K.M.: Aortic body tumor in a cat. A case report. Pathol. Vet., 5:84–90, 1968.

Byrne, M.J.: Coronary thrombosis leading to auricular fibrillation in a Thoroughbred gelding. Irish Vet. J., 4:90–92, 1950.

Carnine, B.L., Schneider, G., Cook, J.E., and Leipold, H.W.: Pericardial mesothelioma in a horse. Vet. Pathol., 14:513–515, 1977.

Cheville, N.F.: Ultrastructure of canine carotid body and aortic body tumors. Comparison with tissues of thyroid and parathyroid origin. Vet. Pathol., 9:166–189, 1972.

Clarkson, T.B.: Animal models for atherosclerosis. A review. North Carolina Med. J., 32:88–96, 1971.

Cotchin, E., and Hayward, A.: Streptococcal endocarditis in a pig following intravenous infection of an organism from a natural case. J. Comp. Path. and Therap., 63:68–73, 1953.

Coulson, W.F., and Carnes, W.H.: Cardiovascular studies on copper-deficient swine. V. The histogenesis of the coronary artery lesions. Amer. J. Path., 43:945–954, 1963.

Crawshaw, G.R., et al.: Mitral incompetence in the dog. S. African J. Med. Sci., 18:79–83, 1953.

Dean, M.J., and Strafuss, A.C.: Carotid body tumors in the dog: A review and report of four cases. J. Am. Vet. Med. Assoc., 166:1003–1006, 1975.

Dick, G.F., and Swartz, W.B.: Experimental endocarditis of dogs. Arch. Path., 42:159–162, 1946.

Donald, D.E., and Elliott, F.J.: Auricular fibrillation in horses. Vet. Rec., 60:473–477, 1948.

Dow, C., Lawson, G.H.K., McFerran, J.B., and Todd, J.R.: Mulberry heart disease. Vet. Rec., 75:76, 1963.

Epling, G.P.: Electron microscopy of bovine cardiac muscle: the transverse sarcotubular system. Am. J. Vet. Res., 26:224–238, 1965.

———: Electron microscopy of the bovine heart in congestive failure of high mountain disease. Am. J. Vet. Res., 29:97–109, 1968.

Ernst, E., Schneider, P., and Trautwein, G.: Aetiology and pathogenesis of endocardiosis and endocarditis of the dog. II. Pathological findings. Deutsche Tierarztliche Wochenschrift, 80:315–332, 1973.

Evans, E.T.R.: Bacterial endocarditis of cattle. Vet. Rec., 69(Pt. 2):1190–1202, 1957.

Faccincani, F., and Carati, M.: Gli ematonoduli delle valvole cardiache. Riv. med. vet., Parma, 6:407–408, 1954.

Finestone, A.J., and Geschickter, C.F.: Bone formation in the heart. Am. J. Clin. Path., 19:974–980, 1949.

Follis, R.H., Jr., et al.: Myocardial necrosis in thiamine deficiency in pigs. Am. J. Path., 19:341–357, 1943.

French, A.J., and Weller, C.V.: Interstitial myocarditis following the clinical and experimental use of sulfonamide drugs. Am. J. Path., 18:109–122, 1942.

Gerriets, E.: Zur aetiologie des enzootischen herztodes der hühner. Monatschr. Vet. Med., 10:416–418, 1955.

Geurden, L.M.G., and Thoonen, J.: Onderzoekingen over round heart disease. Vlaam. diergeneesk. Tijdschr., 19:29–39, 1950.

Glasser, K.: Die seuchenartige (enzootische) herzmuskelentartung des Schweines. Tierarztl. Umsch., 4:151–154, 1949.

Glover, G.H., and Newsom, I.E.: Brisket disease. Exper. Sta. Bull. 229, Colorado State Univ., 1933.

Gullickson, T.W., and Calverley, C.E.: Cardiac failure in cattle; relation to vitamin E. Science, 104:312–313, 1946.

Harding, J.D.J.: Some observations on the histopathology of mulberry heart disease in pigs. Res. Vet. Sci., 1:129–132, 1960.

Hartroft, W.S., and Hartroft, P.M.: New approaches in the study of cardiovascular disease—aldosterone, renin hypertension and juxtaglomerular cells. Fed. Proc., 20:845–854, 1961.

Hayashi, Y., Hussa, J.F., and Lalich, J.J.: Cor pulmonale in rats. Lab. Invest., 16:875–881, 1967.

Hont, S., and Banks, A.W.: Streptococcal endocarditis in young pigs. Australian Vet. J., 20:206–210, 1944.

Innes, J.R.M., et al.: Subacute bacterial endocarditis with pulmonary embolism in a horse associated with Shigella equirulis. Brit. Vet. J., 106:245–250, 1950.

Jamieson, S., and Stuart, J.: Streptococcal endocarditis in lambs. J. Path. and Bact., 62:235–239, 1950.

Jensen, R.: Right heart failure. Calif. Vet., 5:18–19, 1952.

Jensen, R., et al.: Brisket disease in yearling feedlot cattle. J. Am. Vet. Med. Assoc., 169:515–517, 1976.

Jorgensen, L., et al.: Adenosine diphosphate-induced platelet aggregation and myocardial infarction in swine. Lab. Invest., 17:616–644, 1967.

Kahler, J., and Aicher, J.: Der galtstreptokokkus als erreger einer ulzero-polypösen endokarditis beim menschen. Zentralbl. f. allg. Path. Anat., 88:312–317, 1952.

Karpas, A.: (Histopathological examination of a spontaneous case of a left bundle branch block in the heart of a young dog.) Zentralbl. Veterinaermed., 12A:197–210, 1965. V.B. 35:2719, 1965.

Kent, S.P., and Diseker, M.: Early myocardial ischemia; histochemical changes in dogs. J. Lab. Invest., 4:398–405, 1955.

Kersten, U., and Brass, W.: Aetiology and pathogenesis of endocardiosis and endocarditis in dogs. I. Introduction and clinical findings. Deutsche Tierarztliche Wochenschrift, 80:315–332, 1973.

Kleine, L.J., Zook, B.C., and Munson, T.O.: Primary cardiac hemangiosarcomas in dogs. J. Am. Vet. Med. Assoc., 157:326–337, 1970.

Ladds, P.W., and Daniels, P.W.: Aortic body tumour in an ox. Aust. Vet. J., 51:43, 1975.

Lentz, R.W.: Der plötzliche herztod der schweine. Dtsch. Tierärztl. Wochenschr. u. Tierärztl. Rdsch., 52:345–349, 1944.

Lentz, W.J.: Canine heart diseases. Vet. Ext. Quart., Univ. Pa., 48:7–17, 1948.

Liu, S.-K.: Acquired cardiac lesions leading to congestive heart failure in the cat. Am. J. Vet. Res., 31:2071–2088, 1970.

Liu, S.-K., Maron, B.J., and Tilley, L.P.: Canine cardiac cardiomyopathy. J. Am. Vet. Med. Assoc., 174:703–713, 1979.

Luke, D.: "Round heart disease" in poultry. Vet. J., 103:17–20, 1947.

Lumb, G., Shacklett, R.S., and Dowkins, W.A.: The cardiac conduction tissue and its blood supply in the dog. Amer. J. Path., 35:467–487, 1959.

Lumb, G., and Singletary, H.P.: Blood supply to the atrioventricular node and bundle of His: A comparative study in pig, dog and man. Amer. J. Path., 41:65–76, 1962.

Meyling, H.A., and Ter Borg, H.: The conducting system of the heart in hoofed animals. Cornell Vet., 47:419–455, 1957.

Mouwen, M.V.M.: (Mulberry heart disease [dietetic microangiopathy].) Tijdschr. Diergeneeskd., 90:77–93, 1965. V.B. 35:2285, 1965.

Murray, J.D., and Strafuss, A.C.: Carotid body tumors in the dog: a review and report of four cases. J. Am. Vet. Med. Assoc., 166:1003–1006, 1975.

Niederehe, H.: Parasiten als ursache von allergischen herzveränderungen bei schafen. Berl. Muench. Tieraerztl. Wochenschr., 7:77–79, 1948.

Nordstoga, K.: Carotid body tumor in a cow. Pathol. Vet., 3:412–420, 1966.

Omar, A.: Congenital cardiac rhabdomyoma in a pig. Pathol. Vet., 6:469–474, 1969.

Osebold, J.W., and Cordy, D.R.: Valvular endocarditis associated with listeria monocytogenes infections in sheep. J. Am. Vet. Med. Assn., 143:990–993, 1963.

Patnaik, A.K., Lord, P.F., and Liu, S.-K.: Chemodectoma of the urinary bladder in a dog. J. Am. Vet. Med. Assoc., 164:797–800, 1974.

Peery, T.M., and Belter, L.F.: Brucellosis and heart disease. II. Fatal brucellosis: a review of the literature and report of new cases. Am. J. Path., 36:673–679, 1960.

Povar, M.L., and Brownstein, B.: Valvular endocarditis in the fowl. Cornell Vet., 37:49–54, 1947.

Puntriano, G.O.: Physiological basis of "brisket disease" in cattle. J. Am. Vet. Med. Assn., 125:327–329, 1954.

Quiring, D.P., and Baker, R.J.: The equine heart. Am. J. Vet. Research, 14:62–67, 1953.

Raggi, L.: Histopathology of the heart, brain, liver and kidneys in a case of endocarditis caused by Bact. coli in a pig. Zooprofillassi., 3:1–9, 1948.

Ratcliffe, H.L.: Environmental factors and coronary disease. Circulation, 27:481–483, 1963.

Read, W.K., Pierce, K.R., and O'Hara, P.J.: Ultrastructural lesions of an acute toxic cardiomyopathy of cattle. Lab. Invest., 18:227–231, 1968.

Roemmele, O.: Rotlauf-endokarditis bei schlachtrindern. Lebensmitteltierarzt., 3:43–45, 1952. Abstr. Vet. Bull. No. 821, 1953.

Romagnoli, A.: Metodi diretti ed indiretti di misurazione della pressione arteriosa nel cane. Ann. Fac. med. vet., Pisa, 5:158–182, 1952.

———: Comparative study of blood pressure measurements in dogs. Cornell Vet., 43:161–174, 1953.

———: Sull'impiego dell'eletromanometro e dell'elettropletismografo in medicina veterinaria. Atti Soc. Ital. Sci. Vet., Sanremo, 6:334–338, 1953.

Ryff, J.F.: Brisket disease syndrome. J. Am. Vet. Med. Assn., 131:425–429, 1957.

Saphir, O., and Lowenthal, M.: Changes in the endocardium of pigs simulating the rheumatic stigmata of man. Am. J. Path., 27:211–229, 1951.

Schneider, P., Ernst, E., and Trautwein, G.: Amyloidose der Herzklappen beim hund. (Amyloidosis of the heart valves of the dog.) Vet. Pathol., 8:130–145, 1971.

———: Enzymhistochemie der atrioventrikularklappen bei endokardiose des hundes. Vet. Pathol., 10:281–294, 1973.

Schofield, F.W.: Sudden death in calves associated with myocardial degeneration. Canad. J. Comp. Med., 11:324–329, 1947.

Scotti, T.M.: The carotid body tumors in dogs. J. Am. Vet. Med. Assoc., 132:413–419, 1958.

Sheridan, J.P.: The canine heart. Results of 100 random autopsies. J. Small Anim. Pract., 8:373–381, 1967.

Shouse, C.L., and Meier, H.: Acute vegetative endocarditis in the dog and cat. J. Am. Vet. Med. Assn., 129:278–289, 1956.

Spörri, H., and Scheitlin, M.: Klinisch-physiologische und pathologisch-anatomische Untersuchungen an zwei Fällen von persistierendem Ductus arteriosus (Botalli). Schweiz. Arch. f. Tierheilk, 94:387–402, 1952.

Svenkerud, R.R., and Iversen, L.: Shigella equirulis (S. viscosum equi) som arsak til klappeendocarditis hos hest. (S. equirulis isolated from a horse with vegetative endocarditis.) Nord. Vet. Med., 1:227–232, 1949.

Syvurud, R.: Rhabdomyoma in the cat. Western Vet. (Washington State University, Pullman, Wash.), 6:49–50, 1959.

Szcsech, G.M., Blevins, W.E., Carlton, W.W., and Cutlan, G.R.: Chemodectoma with metastasis to bone in a dog. J. Am. Vet. Med. Assoc., 162:376–378, 1973.

Tilley, L.P., et al.: Primary myocardial disease in the cat. A model for human cardiomyopathy. Am. J. Pathol., 86:493–522, 1977.

Trevino, G.S., and Nessmith, W.B.: Aortic body tumor in a white rat. Vet. Pathol., 9:243–248, 1973.

Velasquez, Q.J.: Enfermedad de las alturas. Rev. med. vet., Bogotá, 16:53–70, 1947.

Vogel, J.A., et al.: Cardiac size and pulmonary hypertension in dogs exposed to high altitude. Am. J. Vet. Res., 32:2059–2066, 1971.

Wallace, C.R., and Hamilton, W.F.: Study of spontaneous congestive heart failure in the dog. Circulation Res., 11:301–314, 1962.

Will, D.H., Hicks, J.L., Card, C.S., and Alexander, A.F.: Inherited susceptibility of cattle to high altitude pulmonary hypertension. J. Appl. Physiol., 38:491–494, 1975.

Willigan, D.A., and Beamer, P.D.: Isolation of a transmissible agent from pericarditis of swine. J. Am. Vet. Med. Assn., 126:118–122, 1955.

Winqvist, G.: Topografisk och etiologisk sammanställning av de fibrinösa och ulcerösa endokarditerna hos en del av vara husdjur. (Fibrinous and ulcerative endocarditis in domestic animals.) Skandinav. Vet. Tidskr., 45:575–585, 1945. (Engl. summary.)

Zook, B.C.: Some spontaneous cardiovascular lesions in dogs and cats. Adv. Cardiol., 13:148–168, 1974.

BLOOD VESSELS AND LYMPHATIC VESSELS

Arteries

Arteriosclerosis

In considering disease of the arteries, the disorder or group of disorders recognized as arteriosclerosis confronts us with universal preeminence. This disease is of infinitely more importance in man than it is in animals and has been studied principally in relation to the human species. Let us summarize, then, as briefly as possible, what is known or believed about arteriosclerosis in man before proceeding to consider its various aspects in animals.

Under the general term arteriosclerosis, which literally means hardening of the arteries, are included three different lesions, which probably are distinct etiologic entities.

The first is **atherosclerosis,** the first half of the word being derived from a Greek word *athere,* which means a mushy substance. Earlier writings called the lesions **atheromas.** Atherosclerosis is the most frequent and most important vascular disease of human beings. It chiefly affects large elastic and muscular arteries, such as the aorta and coronary and cerebral arteries, entirely sparing the smaller branches and arterioles.

Lesions. The earliest lesions are fatty streaks running parallel to the direction of the artery. These yellowish lines are composed of collections of mononuclear cells whose cytoplasm is filled with lipid droplets. The cells which lie beneath the endothelium in the intima resemble macrophages, but are in fact altered smooth muscle cells. The proliferation of altered smooth muscle cells is believed by many to precede lipid deposition. The accumulated lipids include cholesterol, fatty acids, triglycerides, and phospholipids.

As the lesion progresses, fibrous connec-

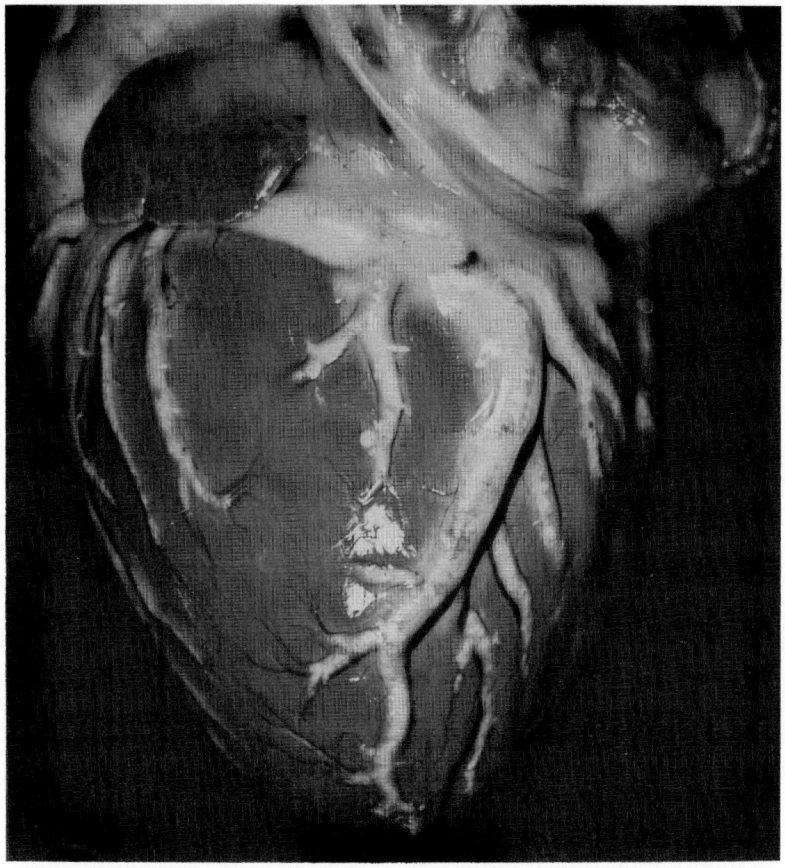

Fig. 21–14. Atherosclerosis of coronary arteries of a nine-year-old German Shepherd. The major branches of these arteries are yellowish and thickened due to lipid in the media. See Figure 21–15 for microscopic appearance. (Courtesy of Angell Memorial Animal Hospital.)

tive tissue surrounds the lipid-laden cells, giving rise to the designation **fibrous plaque.** This would appear to be an attempt at healing, although unsuccessful. With further lipid deposition and fibrosis the plaques become confluent and may involve the entire arterial wall. Lipid also accumulates outside cells, especially near the centers of plaques. Presumably lipid-filled cells rupture, but direct extracellular deposition is not ruled out. This is seen as a clear, hazy area, often with the cholesterol taking on crystalline form as shown by cholesterol clefts. A number of other features may accompany the advanced lesions including hyalinization of fibrous connective tissue, necrosis of small to large areas of the plaques, calcification, and osseous metaplasia. The endothelium may be destroyed (ulcerated), exposing the plaque to the lumen leading to atheromatous emboli and local thrombosis. The lesion is restricted to the intima, but secondary thinning of the media and fragmentation of the elastica are associated with advanced lesions. The reduced strength of the wall may result in an aneurysm. Although the lumen may be narrowed, the most serious consequence of atherosclerosis in man is thrombosis which often results in myocardial or cerebral ischemia and infarction.

Causes. Extensive studies have given rise to several theories on the causation of atherosclerosis, but no single causative factor has been identified. It appears that the formation of atheromatous plaques is affirmatively related to a high level of cholesterol and of total lipids in the blood and also to a high ratio of cholesterol to phospholipids. The formation of such plaques is also favored by hypertension (high blood pressure). On the basis of these facts and considerable experimentation in rabbits, monkeys, dogs, pigeons, and other species, not to mention pertinent clinical evidence, the theory that diets too high in saturated fats and cholesterol are causative has many adherents, although some incongruities have yet to be explained. Cer-

tain other theories deserve attention in a complete presentation of the matter but will be omitted here.

The second of the arteriosclerotic entities is known as the **medial sclerosis** of Mönckeberg, also as **medial calcification.** Instead of affecting the large, elastic arteries of the body, it involves the medium-sized, muscular arteries. There are hyaline and fatty degenerative changes in the muscular tissue of the media, leading to necrosis. The process is gradual and, as a typical sequence to necrosis, calcification regularly supervenes. Rarely, ossification occurs in the vessel wall. This form of arteriosclerosis goes with advancing age but not necessarily with hypertension. It is thought to be related causally to prolonged or habitual over-stimulation of the medial musculature by the vasomotor (sympathetic) nerves. Experimentally, a similar calcification has been produced in dogs and rabbits by excessive administration of epinephrine (adrenalin). Nicotine is said to have a similar effect. Hyperparathyroidism and vitamin D toxicity are other well known causes of medial calcification of arteries. Poisoning by *Solanum malacoxylon* and *Cestrum diurnum* also lead to arterial calcification. Deposition of calcium and iron salts in the walls of cerebral arterioles (cerebrovascular siderosis) is occasionally encountered in many species, but is of unknown significance (Fig. 21–16). Extensive calcification of the aorta and large thoracic arteries (media only) has been seen in young cattle, otherwise normal, when slaughtered for beef (Gailiunas, 1958).

The third entity of arteriosclerotic disease is **diffuse arteriolar sclerosis,** or **arteriolosclerosis.** The term hyperplastic sclerosis has been used and is suggestive of some of the changes that occur in the small peripheral arteries called arterioles, located especially in the kidney, spleen, and pancreas. The hyperplasia consists of proliferation of the cells of the intima, producing concentric lamellations which nearly or

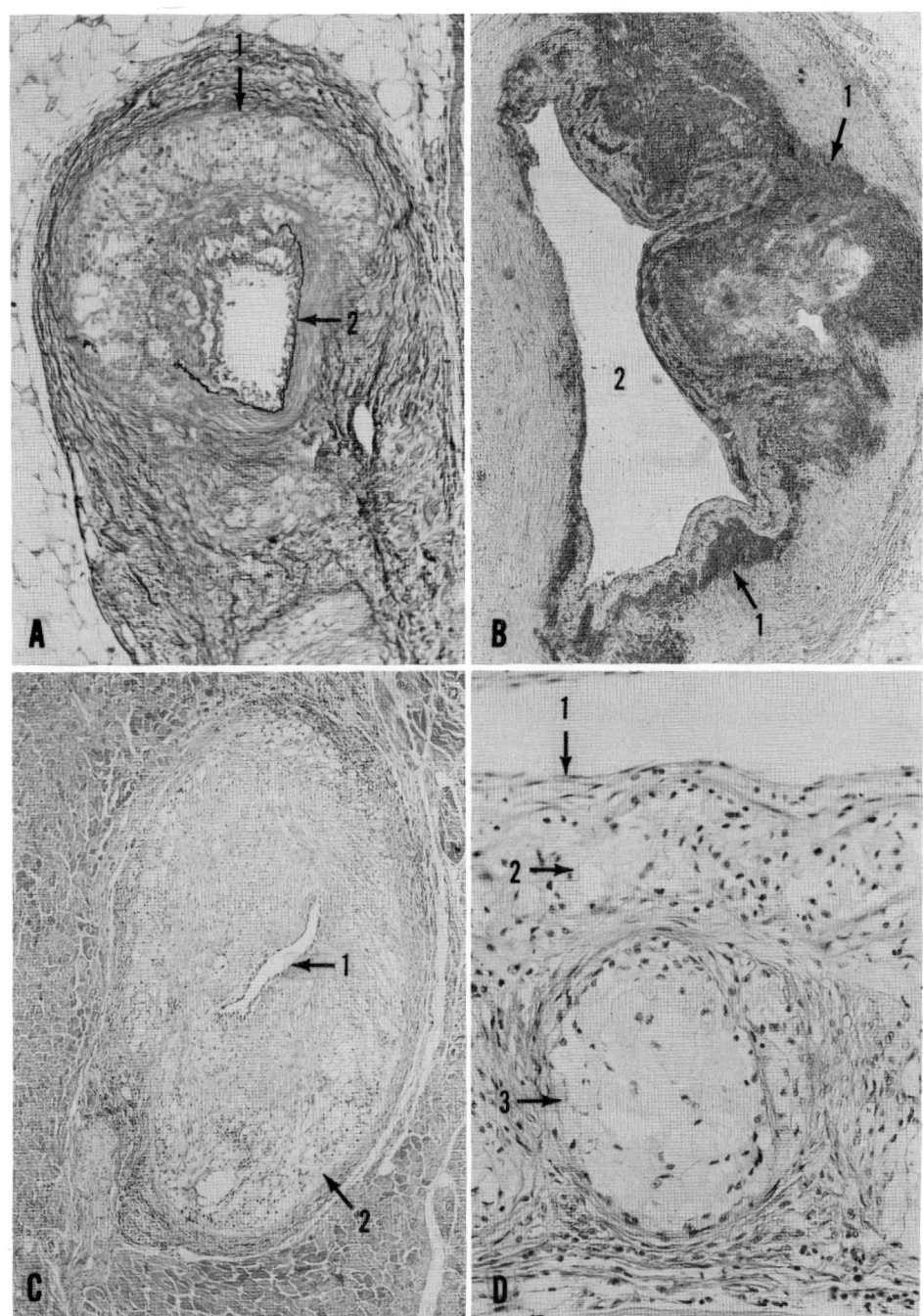

Fig. 21–15.   Xanthomatosis or atherosclerosis in the coronary arteries of a dog. *A,* Cross section of a coronary artery (× 80). Elastica stain. Lipid-laden cells in media (*1*) and intima. Note rupture of internal elastic membrane (*2*). *B,* A section (× 35) of another segment of the same coronary artery, stained for lipid by Sudan III. Note sudanophilic material (*1*) particularly in the media. The lumen is indicated by (*2*). *C,* A branch of the coronary artery. Endothelium at (*1*), lipid-laden foam cells in media (*2*). (H & E, ×55.) *D,* Higher magnification (× 175) of a wall of a coronary artery. Endothelium (*1*), lipid-laden macrophages in subintima (*2*), and in media (*3*). (Courtesy of Armed Forces Institute of Pathology.) Contributor: Dr. Wayne H. Riser.

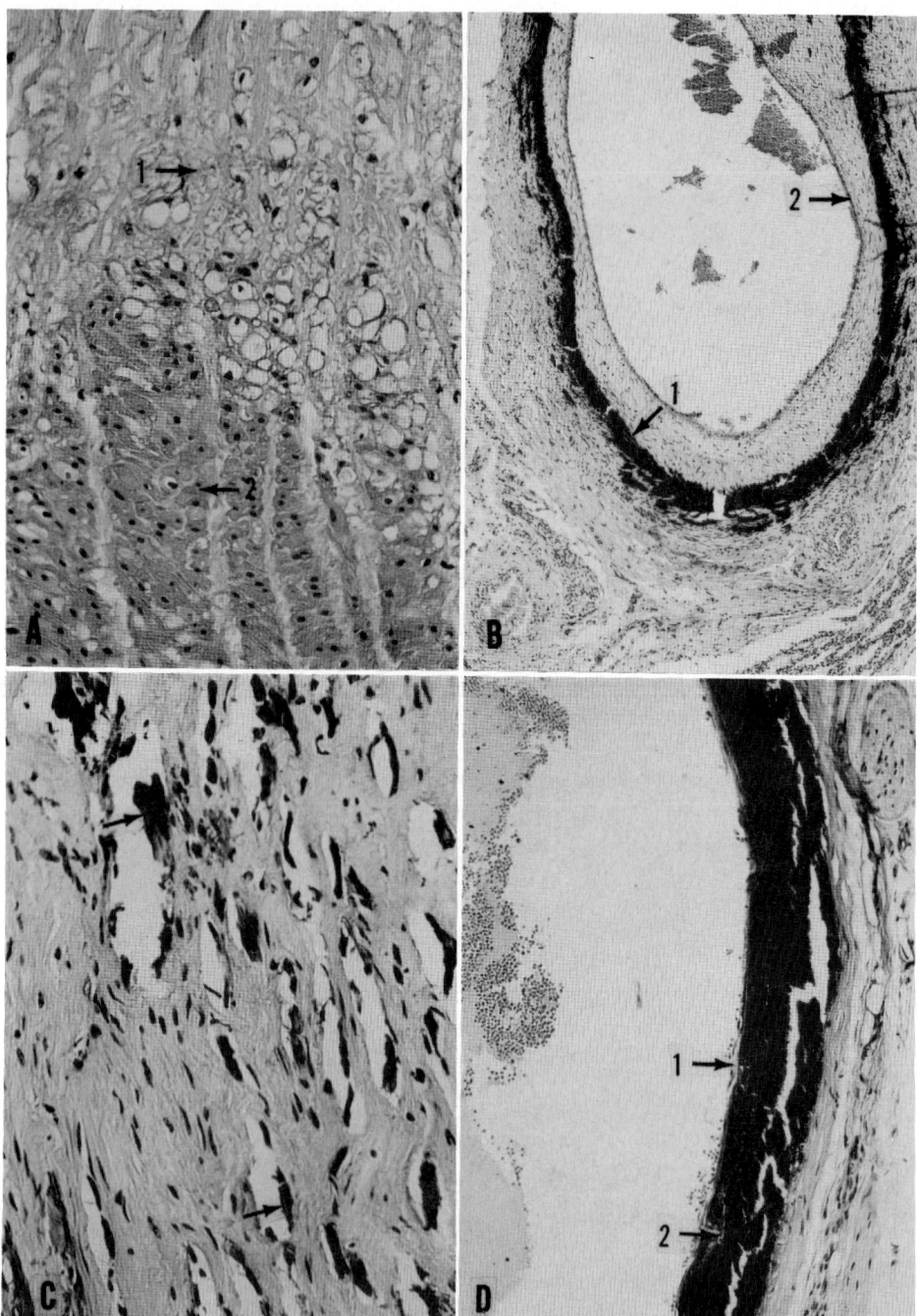

Fig. 21–16. *A*, Medial sclerosis of aorta (× 300) of a cow. Scarred but not yet calcified area (*1*) is distinguishable from the normal media (*2*). Contributor: Dr. E.L. Stubbs. *B*, Medial calcification (*1*) in a bovine pulmonary artery (× 45). Intima (*2*). Contributor: Dr. J.F. Ryff. *C*, Calcification (arrows) of the media of a bovine aorta (× 300). Contributor: Dr. E.L. Stubbs. *D*, Calcification (*2*) in an artery (× 130) of a cat which died of uremia. Intima (*1*). (Courtesy of Armed Forces Institute of Pathology.) Contributor: Dr. Edward Baker.

completely fill the lumen. The intima may be replaced with connective-tissue hyalin or there may be swelling and necrosis of the medial layers with marked compression of the lumen. The latter change occurs when the disease is of rapid development and may be considered related to "malignant hypertension," a rapidly developing increase of blood pressure. Hyperplastic reduplication of the lamina elastica interna is also a frequent finding.

All of the above changes are counted, not only as lesions of arteriosclerosis, but of hypertension, which is one of the commoner disorders with which the human race contends. The two conditions are not always coexistent but are inextricably interrelated: primary hypertension will lead to arteriolar sclerosis, and arteriolar sclerosis, when affecting the kidney, leads to hypertension. Neither can we claim, in spite of wide acceptance, that agreement is entirely universal on the classification of the lesions as we have described them or on the propriety of considering them all as manifestations of a single disease.

Arteriosclerosis in Animals

None of the three forms of arteriosclerosis are common in animals, but examples of each are seen sporadically in most domestic and captive wild animals.

In attempting to evaluate the features and even the existence of arteriosclerotic disease in the domestic animals, it is necessary to remember that the thickening of arterial walls, especially through proliferation of the intimal tissue (endarteritis), occurs frequently in the vicinity of many chronic inflammatory processes, whatever their cause. Such localized arterial lesions should not be interpreted as signs of arteriosclerosis without confirmation in other areas. Similarly, calcification of the walls of arteries may well have local or metabolic causes not concerned with true arteriosclerotic disease. It is not safe to speculate, in the absence of much precise data on blood pressures in our animal pa-

tients, that hypertension is not a feature of either of these conditions.

Irregular thickenings of the intima of the aorta, coronary, and other large arteries are seen in cattle, dogs, swine, and other species, and these have been compared with human arteriosclerotic changes. The incidence of arteriosclerosis is relatively high in most species, but unlike atherosclerosis in man, it is essentially unimportant to health. The interest focuses primarily on a search for animal models for the disease in man. In dogs, arteriosclerotic plaques are common in the aorta, coronary, and other arteries. They consist of intimal thickenings composed mainly of smooth muscle cells and a fibrillar matrix. Medial thickening due to hyperplasia, fibrosis, hyaline change, or amyloid deposition may also be present. Unlike atherosclerosis in man, intracellular or extracellular lipid is only rarely seen. It may, however, be induced by modifications in diet and other experimental manipulations. An exception is seen in hypothyroidism in dogs, which may be accompanied by extensive atherosclerosis. In domestic animals, the vascular lesions of swine most clearly resemble atherosclerosis of man. The intimal lesions are composed of aggregations of smooth muscle cells, which undergo transformation to lipid-laden foam cells with ultimate extracellular lipid deposition characteristic of atherosclerosis in man. Nonhuman primates of various species also develop atherosclerosis comparable in structure to the human disease. Again it is not important to their health but has provided a good experimental model. Descriptions of the spontaneous and experimentally induced disease in monkeys can be found in several reviews (Strong, 1976; Clarkson, et al., 1976).

The importance of considering animals of all ages, particularly those toward the end of the life span, is emphasized by the finding of advanced lesions in aged animals (Fankhauser, Luginbuhl, and McGrath, 1965; Jones and Zook, 1965; Mar-

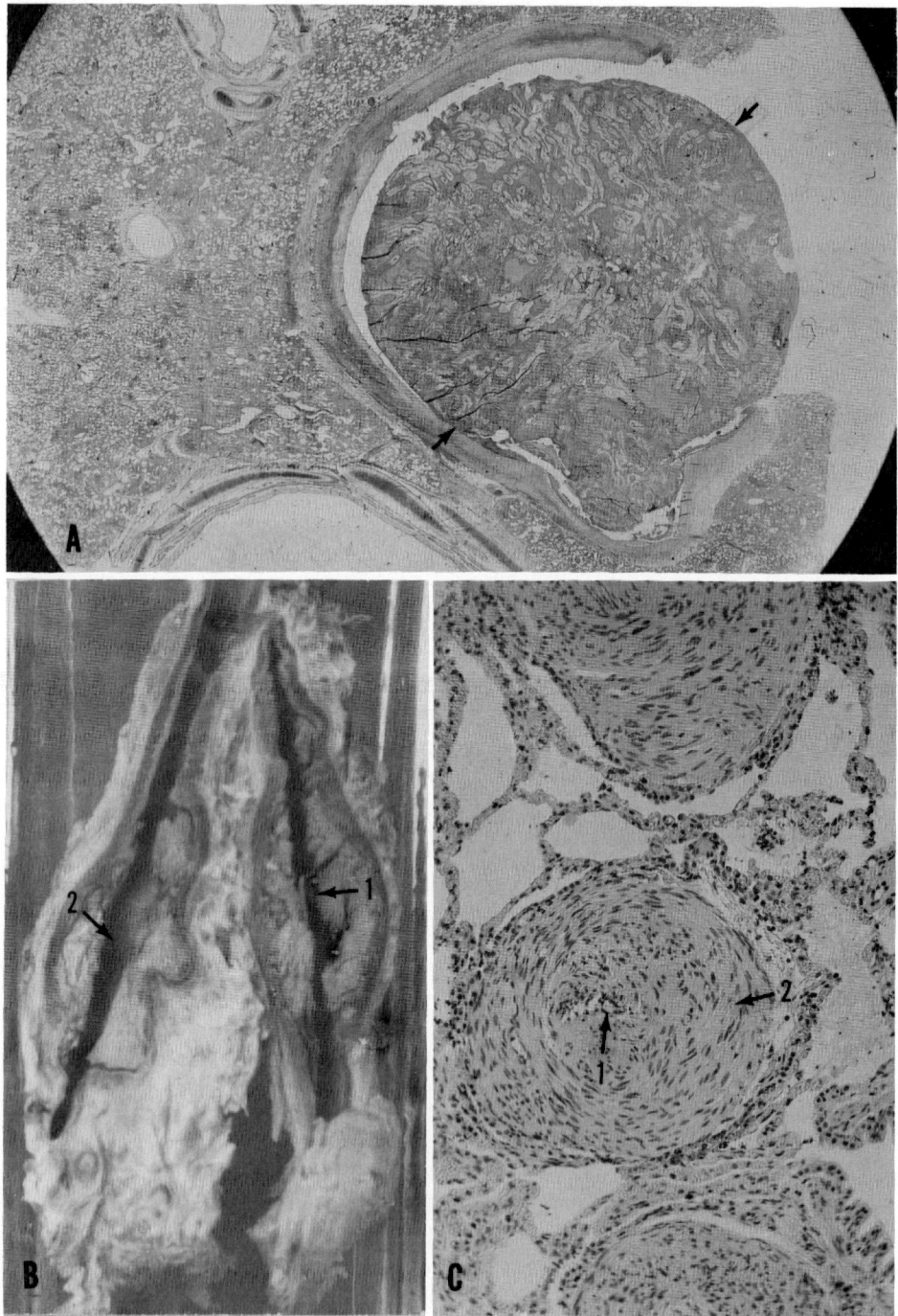

Fig. 21–17. *A,* Thrombosis of the pulmonary artery (× 5) of a horse. Contributor: Dr. J.R.M. Innes. *B,* Verminous arteritis, anterior mesenteric artery of a horse. A single larva of *Strongylus vulgaris* is seen at (*1*) and, although the wall is necrotic and thickened by inflammation, the lumen (*2*) appears reasonably patent. (Specimen in Mark Francis Collection, Texas Sch. Vet. Med.) *C,* Medial hypertrophy, branches of the pulmonary artery (× 130) of a cat. Intima (*1*) is surrounded by some sclerosis, but the greatest increase in diameter is due to the thickened media (*2*). (*A* and *C,* Courtesy of Armed Forces Institute of Pathology.) Contributor: Dr. Leo L. Lieberman.

cus and Ross, 1967; Luginbuhl, et al., 1977). Too often, experimental samples do not include the appropriate older age groups.

Arteritis

Arteritis is characterized by the presence of inflammatory exudate, usually neutrophilic or other leukocytes, within the layers of the vessel wall. Chronic fibrosis is also to be include provided it is within the wall and not merely perivascular. This inflammatory state may arise in an artery which passes through inflamed and infected surroundings or which contains an infected thrombus or embolus, but it is remarkable how well the vessel walls usually resist infection under such circumstances.

Causes. The causes of arteritis are multiple. Deposition of immune complexes may lead to localized or generalized vasculitis. Several metazoan parasites inhabit or pass part of their life cycle in arteries and elicit varying degrees of inflammation and necrosis. These include *Strongylus vulgaris* in horses, *Dirofilaria immitis* in dogs, *Schistosoma* sp. in many species, *Elaeophora schneideri* in sheep, and *Onchocerca armillata* in cattle.

A specific arteritis of medium-sized muscular arteries is known in the horse infected with the agent of equine viral arteritis. Border disease of sheep may be associated with arteritis, particularly in the central nervous system. Another inflammatory disease of arteries occurs in rats of some strains. The mesenteric artery and its branches are particularly involved. This is often referred to as **polyarteritis nodosa** (Young, 1965; Cutts, 1966). A similar lesion has been described in mice (Conklin, et al., 1967; Wigley, et al., 1970).

Lesions similar to those described in man as **periarteritis nodosa** have been de-

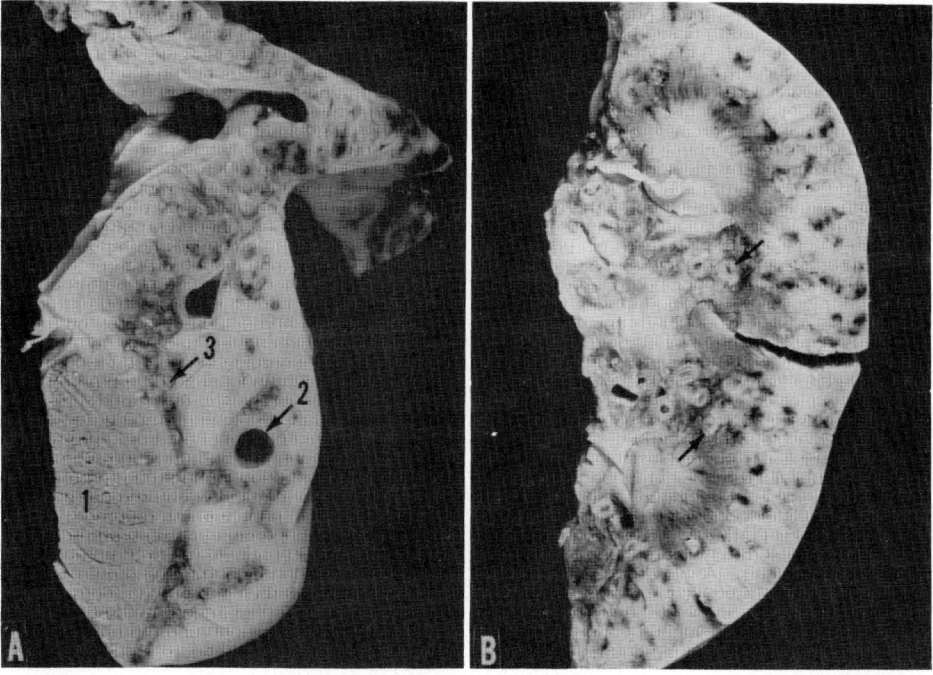

Fig. 21–18. Periarteritis nodosa or generalized arteritis in a bovine. *A,* Myocardium (*1*), large unaffected coronary artery (*2*), and many thick-walled arteries (*3*) in epicardium. *B,* The kidney, with many redundant, thick-walled arteries (arrows). (Courtesy of Armed Forces Institute of Pathology.) Contributor: Dr. C.L. Davis.

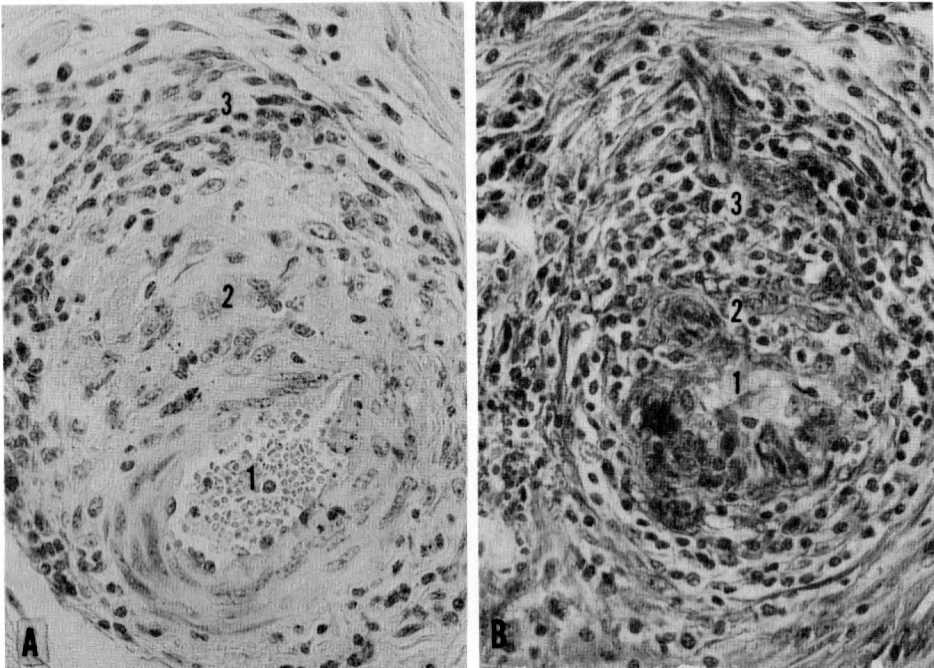

Fig. 21–19.   Periarteritis nodosa in bovine arteries. *A,* A mildly affected artery (× 330). The arterial lumen (*1*), media (*2*), and adventitia (*3*). *B,* A severely affected artery. Lumen (*1*), media (*2*), and adventitia (*3*). (Courtesy of Armed Forces Institute of Pathology.) Contributor: Dr. C.L. Davis.

scribed in several species (Figs. 21–17 to 21–19), although their etiology is not known nor is any relationship to the human disease established.

Aneurysm

An aneurysm is a pathologic dilatation of an artery (or a cardiac chamber), usually, but not invariably, saccular in shape and definitely circumscribed. A true aneurysm results from weakening of the vessel wall, which is stretched beyond its capacity to resist, and certain layers, ordinarily the intima and media, will be found to have been wholly or partly ruptured. If the development has been gradual, replacement of the damaged tissues by an excess of fibrous tissue is the rule.

A second form is the **dissecting aneurysm** or **false aneurysm.** This is due to fracture or necrosis in the medial layer of the aorta or some other large artery.

Through an interruption of the inner coat or sometimes apparently through the vasa vasorum, the blood current gains access to the medial defect. Under the considerable arterial pressure, the blood then splits the inner cylindrical layer from the outer, much as the intact cylinder of bark can sometimes be separated from the inner wood of a twig. The blood thus flows in two tubes, one inside the other. Once started, this arrangement may extend for a considerable distance or even for the length of the aorta, the blood returning to its normal channel when one of the main arterial branches is encountered.

The causes of aneurysms are damage done by inflammatory or arteriosclerotic and degenerative disease. Syphilitic aortitis is a classical, but by no means the unique, cause in humans. However, there are evidences of nutritional causes for dissecting aneurysm in rats, where it accompanies poisoning by the sweet pea (*Lathyrus odoratus*) (Bachhuber and Lalich, 1954), and in turkeys, where a diet containing aflatoxin has appeared to have a causative relationship (Carnaghan, 1955; McSherry, et al., 1954; Pritchard, Henderson and Beall, 1958). Aneurysms of the pulmonary artery in cattle may result from infectious emboli lodging at this site and weakening the wall. The emboli originate from thrombi in the vena cava secondary to hepatic abscesses. The injurious effects of aneurysms lie chiefly in the danger of rupture of the vessel or in the formation of a thrombus on the damaged and roughened intimal wall.

Mucoid Medial Degeneration

Also known as **Erdheim's disease** or **idiopathic cystic medionecrosis,** mucoid medial degeneration is a disease of the aorta of unknown cause. It is associated with a genetic defect in Marfan's syndrome in human beings, but is also seen independently of this disorder. A similar degeneration is occasionally encountered in domestic animals, especially dogs and cattle, and has been described in poultry. The lesion resembles, in many respects, that seen in the aorta in lathyrism. Histopathologically, there is diffuse or patchy fragmentation and loss of muscle and elastic fibers and a marked increase in mucopolysaccharide ground substance. The resultant weakening of the wall may lead to aneurysms.

Atrophy of Arteries

Atrophy of arteries and arterioles occurs in ergotism and the similar poisoning by fescue grass. Continuously contracted, the bloodless arteries grow smaller and accompany the surrounding tissues to their gangrenous destruction.

The natural atrophy that occurs in those vessels which normally change into ligaments with the advent of postnatal life is a more gradual process than might be expected. For instance, the closing of the umbilical arteries begins when they are severed at birth, but may require as much as 2 months for completion (in the calf). The lumen is contracted, but remains filled with hemolyzed and eventually with clotted blood; its slow recession can be followed inch by inch from the umbilicus to the bladder, as a central core of fibrous tissue progresses upward. This may be viewed as disuse atrophy, similar to the change that occurs when a vessel is ligated.

Hypertrophy

Medial hypertrophy of branches of the pulmonary artery is frequently recognized in the domestic cat. The affected arteries have thick, hyperplastic muscular walls and often intimal fibrosis, which effectively narrows the lumen (Fig. 21–17C). The cause and pathogenesis have been subject to considerable debate, but to date not elucidated. Evidence indicates that this lesion is related to prior infection with *Aleurostrongylus abstrusus* or *Toxocara cati* (Stunzi, et al., 1966; Hamilton, 1966); however, others have observed the condition in specific-pathogen-free cats in which there was no evidence of *A. abstrusus* infection (Rogers, et al., 1971).

Thrombosis

Two of the more frequently encountered examples are thrombosis of the anterior mesenteric artery in horses, associated with *Strongylus vulgaris* migration, and aortic saddle thrombosis at the iliac bifurcation in cats. Saddle thrombi result in paraplegia, loss of femoral pulse, cold rear extremities, pain, and ultimately, muscle atrophy. These signs have been presumed to result from ischemia from inadequate collateral circulation. Ischemia is undoubtedly the cause of the signs, but the pathogenesis of the ischemia is not simply the result of occlusion of the aorta.

Butler (1971) and others have shown that neither single nor double aortic ligation in cats results in paralysis despite loss of femoral pulse. Butler was able to induce

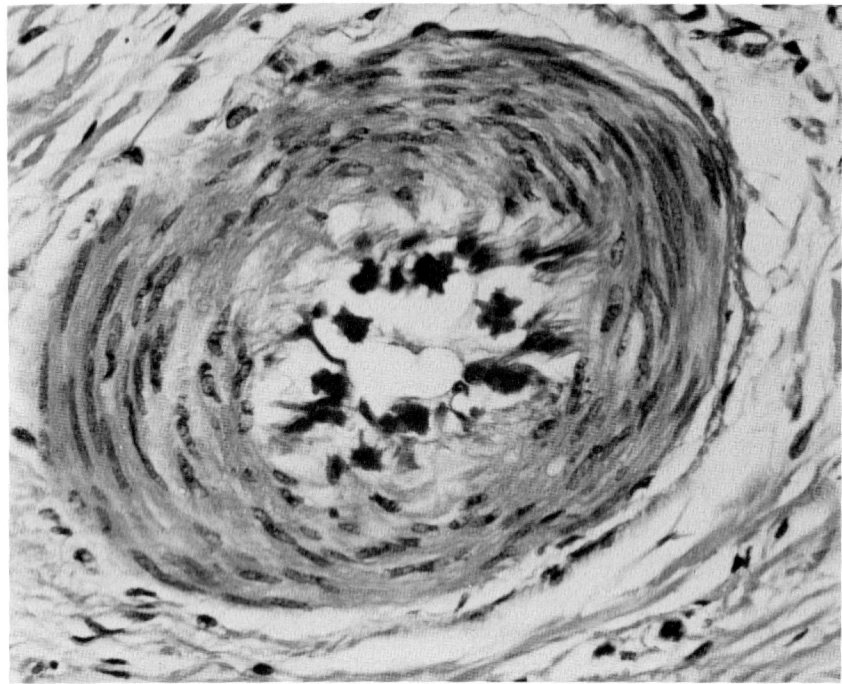

Fig. 21–20. Equine intimal bodies. Irregularly shaped dense bodies in intima of an arteriole. (Courtesy of Dr. Richard J. Montali and *Laboratory Investigation*.)

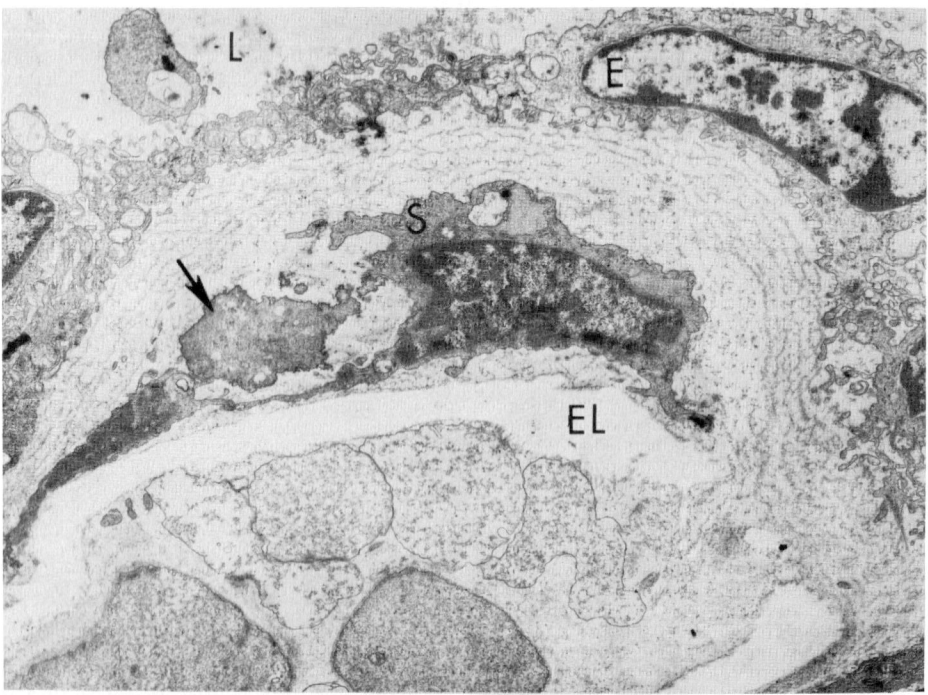

Fig. 21–21. Equine intimal body. Electron micrograph (× 8,200). L, lumen of arteriole; E, nucleus of endothelial cell; EL, internal elastic lamina; S, subendothelial cell; arrow, irregular dense mass associated with cytoplasm of subendothelial cell. (Courtesy of Dr. Richard J. Montali and *Laboratory Investigation*.)

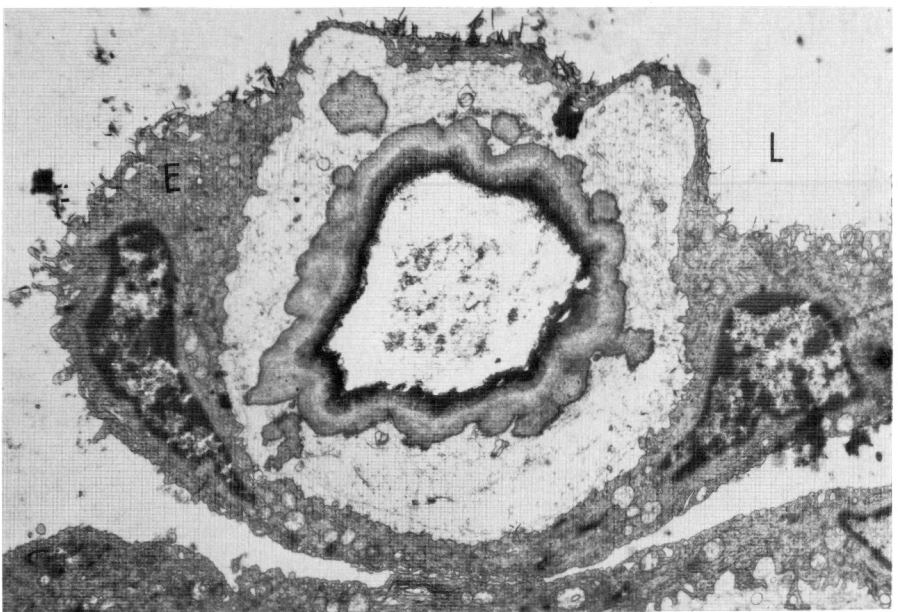

Fig. 21–22. Equine intimal body with a hollow core (× 8,000). E, endothelial cell, surrounding central mass; L, lumen of arteriole. (Courtesy of Dr. Richard J. Montali and *Laboratory Investigation.*)

paralysis, however, if 5-hydroxytryptamine was injected into the aorta between the double ligatures. He suggested that the release of 5-hydroxytryptamine by platelets in the thrombus interfered with collateral circulation by causing contraction of vascular smooth muscle.

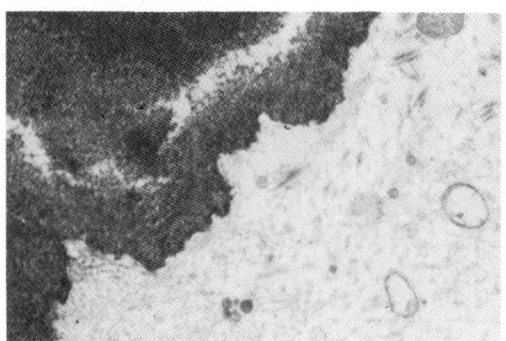

Fig. 21–23. Equine intimal body. Membranous debris, collagen fragments, bits of altered elastica, and basement membrane in light area on right; electron dense central mass on left. (Courtesy of Dr. Richard J. Montali and *Laboratory Investigation.*)

Amyloidosis

Amyloid is often deposited in vessels. Amyloidosis of coronary arteries is not infrequent in aged dogs. Intramural arteries and arterioles are affected, often with obstruction of the lumens and resultant myocardial necrosis and fibrosis.

Equine Intimal Bodies

Mineralized hyaline bodies have been noted from time to time in the intima of arterioles of horses (Marcus and Ross, 1967). In ordinary paraffin-embedded sections these bodies appear as pleomorphic, densely stained bodies in the vascular endothelium. The exact pathologic significance of these structures is unknown, but they have been characterized morphologically at light and electron microscopic levels by Montali, Strandberg, and Squire (1970). This work indicates that these bodies are "mineralized, degenerate cellular and intercellular elements that arise from subendothelial cells and intercellular material of the vascular wall" (Figs. 21–20 to 21–23).

Veins

Phlebitis

Phlebitis is inflammation of a vein and is characterized by the presence of any of the usual inflammatory exudates. Most frequently neutrophilic leukocytes predominate; in chronic forms, inflammatory fibrous tissue surrounds the vein. These can hardly be expected to be confined within the thin wall of a vein, but phlebitis occurs usually within a more extensive inflamed and infected area through which the vein passes. Or, it may represent spread of the inflammatory process to the wall when an infected embolus lodges in the lumen or a thrombus forms there. Commonly the term phlebitis is employed, with its emphasis on the venous lesion, when there is especial concern for the spread of the infectious inflammation along the venous passageway, or perhaps when the process starts by virtue of injury incurred by the vein itself, as in the case of repeated, unsterile and unskillfully made therapeutic venipunctures. Phlebitis involving the smaller veins is a regular feature of extensively infected wounds, of septic metritis, or of similar processes. The principal dangers from such inflamed (and usually infected) veins are two: necrosis resulting in local hemorrhage, and formation of thrombi, parts of which may become detached as emboli.

Varicose Veins

Varicose veins are those that are markedly dilated and, at the same time, elongated so that, in order to find a place for the excess length, they follow an irregular, tortuous course. They thus hold an abnormal amount of blood, which tends to become static. Local anoxia and malnutrition result, together with a certain amount of pain. The condition also favors thrombosis within the vein, although this is not a frequent complication unless there is operative or other intervention. In animals, they occur chiefly in the hind legs, the saphenous and other superficial veins being involved. The usual cause is trauma or traumatic hindrance of return flow at some point in advance of the varicose area.

Telangiectasis

Telangiectasis is a marked dilatation of each of an abnormal cluster of blood vessels. The structure of their walls usually characterizes them as capillaries, although occasionally the more complicated structure of veins may be present. A type occurring beneath the skin or mucous membrane and elsewhere in humans is considered to be hereditary. The usual telangiectasis in veterinary parlance is a similar dilatation of a group of sinusoidal capillaries in one or more lobules of the bovine liver. The gross appearance is that of a small (one to several millimeters), irregular spot which is slightly depressed and so dark with venous blood as to be almost black. The lesions are often numerous in livers of animals slaughtered for food and cause condemnation of the affected parts. They are thought to be causally related to infection of the liver with the necrophorus organism. Extreme examples of telangiectasis may simulate hemangioma.

Lymphatic Vessels

Lymphangitis

Lymphangitis is diagnosed under much the same circumstances as phlebitis, that is, when we are concerned with an infectious inflammatory process which may spread by way of lymphatic vessels. The extremely thin vascular wall is, in itself, scarcely capable of harboring any significant inflammatory exudate; the disease process belongs originally to the surrounding tissues. The specific lymphangitides, such as equine epizootic lymphangitis, cause the subcutaneous and other lymphatic vessels to be visibly distended and

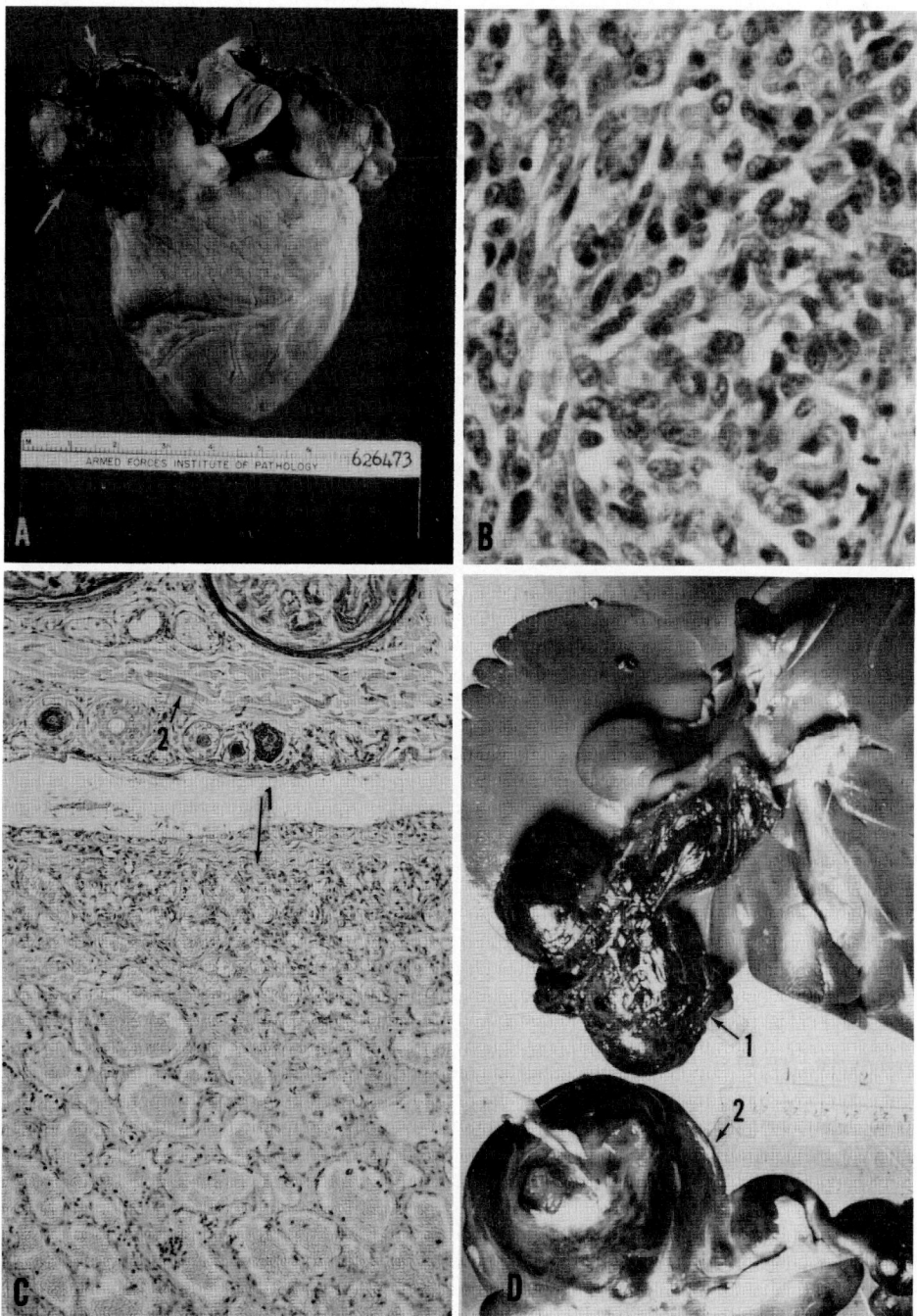

Fig. 21–24. *A*, Hemangioendothelioma (arrows), primary in the myocardium of the right atrium of a seven-year-old female Beagle dog. Contributor: Dr. Leo L. Lieberman. *B*, Hemangioendothelioma (× 300), primary in spleen of a dog. The tumor cells have elongated nuclei and frequently form vascular channels. *C*, Hemangioma (× 75) in the subcutis of tarsal region of a 2½-year-old wire-haired Fox Terrier. The new growth is encapsulated (*1*) and separated from the dermis (*2*). (Courtesy of Armed Forces Institute of Pathology.) Contributor: Dr. Leo L. Lieberman. *D*, Hemangioendothelioma involving liver (*1*) and spleen (*2*) of a dog.

somewhat thickened, but the lesions are principally in the contiguous tissues, including the normally microscopic lymphoid aggregates which are interspersed along the vessels. *Corynebacterium ovis*, the cause of caseous lymphadenitis, also causes lymphangitis in horses as does *Sporotrichum schenkii*. Failure of drainage of lymphatics, of course, leads to edema of the part in question.

Lymphatic vessels are regenerated or reinforced by the formation of collateral vessels within a few (4 to 10) days following operative or traumatic destruction, their function of drainage being only very transiently interrupted.

Neoplasms of Blood and Lymphatic Vessels

Nomenclature of neoplasms of blood and lymphatic vessels is somewhat confusing owing to the recognition of vascular growths in man once considered tumors as not being true neoplasms. This has resulted in using the term capillary hemangioma and cavernous hemangioma in the human literature for benign congenital abnormalities most common in the skin (red birthmarks). Similar clinical and pathologic correlations have not yet been made for animals, but it is wise to bear in mind that some apparent neoplasms of blood vessels may represent anomalous growths.

Hemangioma; Hemangioendothelioma

These tumors arise from the endothelial cells that line blood vessels. The tumor consists of a mixture of cellular areas, the endothelial cells resembling short, plump fibroblasts, and of endothelium-lined blood spaces filled with normal, circulating blood. The hemangioma having small to medium-sized blood spaces and no great amount of cellular tissue is designated **capillary hemangioma;** the one with large blood spaces, **hemangioma cavernosum;** and the opposite type, with a large amount of cellular tissue and minimal blood spaces, **hemangioma hypertrophicum.** The great majority are benign. In fact an area of tumor sufficiently anaplastic to be malignant would be unlikely to have any features distinguishing it from other sarcomas, although other areas of the same tumor may be sufficiently well differentiated to betray its origin. Logically or not, those forms considered malignant are usually called **hemangioendotheliomas, malignant hemangiomas,** or **hemangiosarcomas.**

In the dog, hemangioendotheliomas with malignant potentialities are encountered arising from the spleen, right atrium, and occasionally from the subcutis. These neoplasms consist of ovoid cells with hyperchromatic nuclei and scanty cytoplasm. The cells form or tend to form many small capillaries, the distinguishing feature of the growth. Cutaneous hemangiomas have been produced in ducks by the application of methylcholanthrene (Rigdon, 1952), and an association between hemangioendothelioma of the liver and vinyl chloride has been made in human beings.

Lymphangioma; Lymphangioendothelioma

These tumors are entirely comparable to the hemangiomas, except that the vascular spaces are connected to the lymphatic system and contain lymph instead of blood. They are much less frequent than their blood-containing counterparts.

Altera, K.P., and Bonasch, H.: Periarteritis nodosa in a cat. J. Am. Vet. Med. Assn., *149*:1307–1311, 1966.

Andrews, E.J., and Kelly, D.F.: Naturally occurring aortic medial necrosis in a dog. Am. J. Vet. Res., *31*:791–795, 1970.

Bachhuber, T.E., and Lalich, J.J.: Production of dissecting aneurysms in rats fed *Lathyrus odoratus*. Science, *120*:712–713, 1954.

Bishop, S.P., Cole, C.R., and Smetzer, D.L.: Functional and morphologic pathology of equine aortic insufficiency. Path. Vet., *3*:137–158, 1966.

Bloom, F.: Xanthomatosis of the arterial media in a dog. Amer. J. Path., *22*:519–537, 1946.

Bostroem, B., and Schoedel, W.: Uber die durchblutung der arteriovenosen anastomosen in der hinteren extremität des hundes. Arch. f. d. ges Physiol., *256*:371–380, 1953.

Breeze, R.G., Pirie, H.M., Selman, I.E., and Wiseman, A.: Thrombosis of the posterior vena cava in cattle. Vet. Ann., 16:52–59, 1976.

Butler, H.C.: An investigation into the relationship of an aortic embolus to posterior paralysis in the cat. J. Small Anim. Pract., 12:141–158, 1971.

Carlström, D., et al.: Chemical composition of normal and abnormal blood vessel walls. Chemical nature of vascular calcified deposits. Lab. Invest., 2:325–335, 1953.

Carnaghan, R.B.A.: Atheroma of the aorta associated with dissecting aneurysms in turkeys. Vet. Rec., 67:568–569, 1955.

Clarkson, T.B., Hamm, T.E., Bullock, B.C., and Lehner, N.D.M.: Atherosclerosis in Old World monkeys. Primates Med., 9:66–89, 1976.

Clarkson, T.B., et al.: Atherosclerosis in New World monkeys. Primates Med., 9:90–144, 1976.

Clarkson, T.B., et al.: Pathogenesis of atherosclerosis: some advances from using animal models. Exp. Molec. Pathol., 24:264–286, 1976.

Columbo, S., and Cerioli, A.: Endocardial thickening in cattle. Atti Soc. Ital. Sci. Vet., 19:388–392, 1966. V.B. 37:343, 1967.

Conklin, J.W., et al.: Necrotizing polyarteritis in aging RF mice. Lab. Invest., 16:483–487, 1967.

Cutts, J.H.: Vascular lesions resembling polyarteritis nodosa in rats undergoing prolonged stimulation with oestrogen. Brit. J. Exp. Path., 47:401–404, 1966.

Dahme, E.G.: Atherosclerosis and arteriosclerosis in domestic animals. Ann. New York Acad. Sci., 127:657–670, 1965.

Das, K.M., and Tashjian, R.J.: Chronic mitral valve disease in the dog. (A preliminary report of 550 consecutive necropsies.) Vet. Med. Small Anim. Clin., 60:1209–1216, 1965.

Davies, A.P., et al.: Primary lymphedema in three dogs. J. Am. Vet. Med. Assoc., 174:1316–1320, 1979.

Engelke, J.: Endemisches vorkommen der periarteritis nodosa beim schwein. Inaug. Diss. Hanover. Path. Inst. der Tierarztl. Hochschule., pp. 16, 1949.

Fankhauser, R., Luginbuhl, H., and McGrath, J.T.: Cerebrovascular disease in various animal species. Ann. New York Acad. Sci., 127:817–859, 1965.

Farrelly, B.T.: Pathogenesis and significance of parasitic endarteritis and thrombosis in the ascending aorta of the horse. Vet. Rec., 66:53–61, 1954.

Finlayson, R., Symons, C., and Fiennes, R.N.T.W.: Atherosclerosis: a comparative study. Brit. Med. J., Feb. 24, 1962, pp. 501–507.

French, J.E., Jennings, M.A., and Florey, H.W.: Morphological studies on atherosclerosis in swine. Ann. New York Acad. Sci., 127:780–799, 1965.

French, J.E., et al.: Intimal changes in the arteries of aging swine. Proc. Roy. Soc. Ser. B., 158:24–42, 1963.

Fry, R.J.M., Hamilton, K.H., and Lisco, H.: Thrombi in the left atrium of the heart in mice. Arch. Path., 80:308–313, 1965.

Gailiunas, P.: Calcification of arteries in young cattle. Case Report. J. Am. Vet. Med. Assn., 132:533, 1958.

Geer, J.C., et al.: Fine structure of the baboon aortic fatty streak. Amer. J. Path., 52:265–286, 1968.

Goman, E.M., Feigenbaum, A.S., and Schenk, E.A.: Spontaneous aortic lesions in rabbits. Part 3. Incidence in genetic factors. J. Atheroscler. Res., 7:131–141, 1967.

Gottlieb, H., and Lalich, J.J.: Occurrence of arteriosclerosis in the aorta of swine. Amer. J. Path., 30:851–855, 1954.

Gresham, G.A., et al.: Atherosclerosis in primates. Brit. J. Exp. Pathol., 46:94–103, 1965.

Gupta, P.P., Tandon, H.D., and Ramalingaswami, V.: Spontaneous vascular lesions in Indian pigs. J. Path., 99:19–28, 1969.

Gyorkey, F., and Reiser, R.: Experimental dietary arteriosclerosis in young swine: a histopathological, histochemical and biochemical study. Acta Morph. Hung., 12:415–427, 1964. V.B. 35:1017, 1965.

Hamilton, J.M.: Pulmonary arterial disease of the cat. J. Comp. Path., 76:133–145, 1966.

———: Experimental lung-worm disease of the cat. Association of the condition with lesions of the pulmonary arteries. J. Comp. Path., 76:147–157, 1966.

Harding, J.D.J.: A cerebrospinal angiopathy in pigs. Path. Vet., 3:83–88, 1966.

Helmboldt, C.F., Jungherr, E.L., and Hwang, J.: Polyarteritis in sheep. J. Am. Vet. Med. Assn., 134:556–561, 1959.

Hofmann, W.: Medionecrosis aortae idiopathica microcystica als ursache spontaner aortenrupturen beim hund. (Idiopathic microcystic medionecrosis of the aorta as a cause of spontaneous aortic ruptures in dogs.) Tierarztliche Umschau, 26:308–312, 1971.

Holzworth, J., et al.: Aortic thrombosis with posterior paralysis in the cat. Cornell Vet., 45:468–487, 1955.

Humphreys, E.M.: Atherosclerosis in the coronary arteries of rats. J. Atheroscler. Res., 4:416–434, 1964.

Jensen, R., et al.: Embolic pulmonary aneurysms in yearling feedlot cattle. J. Am. Vet. Med. Assoc., 169:518–520, 1976.

Jones, T.C., and Zook, B.C.: Aging changes in the vascular system of animals. Ann. New York Acad. Sci., 127:671–684, 1965.

Jonsson, L.: Senile cardiac amyloidosis in the dog. Acta Vet. Scand., 15:206–218, 1974.

Jordan, G.L., DeBakey, M.E., and Halpert, B.: Coronary atheromatous change induced by chronic hypercholesterolemia in dogs. Amer. J. Path., 35:867–875, 1959.

Kammermann, K.L., Luginbuhl, H., and Ratcliffe, H.L.: Intramural coronary arteriosclerosis of normal and dwarfed swine. Vet. Pathol., 13:104–109, 1976.

Kelley, F.B., Jr., Taylor, C.B., and Hass, G.M.: Experimental atheroarteriosclerosis. Arch. Path., 53:419–436, 1952.

Knieriem, H.J.: Electron-microscopic study of bovine arteriosclerotic lesions. Amer. J. Path., 50:1035–1065, 1967.

Kohler, H.: Endarteritis obliterans der zehenarterien beim pferde. Frankf. Ztschr. f. Path., 62:326–344, 1951.

Krause, C.: Zur frage der arteriosklerose bei Rind, pfered und hund. Beitr. Z. Path. Anat. u.z. allg. Path., 70:121–178, 1922.

Landi, A.: Su di un particolare caso di calcificazione nell aorta di un cane. Atti Soc. Ital. Sci. Vet., Sanremo, 6:202–205, 1952.

Likar, I.N., and Robinson, R.W.: Bovine arterial disease. I. Localization of lipids in the abdominal aorta in relation to bovine atherosclerosis. Arch. Path., 82:555–560, 1966.

——: Lipid distribution and pattern in abdominal aorta with and without naturally occurring lesions. Arch. Path., 82:561–565, 1966.

Lindsay, S., and Chaikoff, I.L.: Coronary arteriosclerosis of birds; comparison of spontaneous and experimental lesions. Arch. Path., 49:434–446, 1950.

Lindsay, S., Chaikoff, I.L., and Gilmore, J.W.: Arteriosclerosis in the dog, spontaneous lesions in the aorta and coronary arteries. Arch. Path., 53:281–300, 1952. In the cat; Arch. Path., 60:29–38, 1955.

Lindsay, S., et al.: "Arteriosclerosis in the dog." II. Aortic, cardiac, and other vascular lesions in thyroidectomized-hypophysectomized dogs. Arch. Path., 54:573–591, 1952.

Lindsay, S., Chaikoff, I.L.: Naturally occurring arteriosclerosis in nonhuman primates. J. Atheroscler. Res., 6:36–61, 1966.

Lloyd, H.E.D.: Arteriosclerosis in certain wild animals dying in captivity. J. Comp. Path. & Therap., 69:98–104, 1959.

Lucké, V.M.: Renal polyarteritis nodosa in the cat. Vet. Rec., 82:622–624, 1968.

Luginbuhl, H.: Angiopathien im zentralnervensystem bei tieren. Schweiz. Arch. Tierheilkd., 104:694–700, 1962.

Luginbuhl, H.: Spontaneous atherosclerosis in swine. In Swine in Biomedical Research, edited by L.K. Bustad and R. McClellan. Richland, Washington, Battelle Memorial Institute, 1966, pp. 347–363.

Luginbuhl, H., Pauli, B., and Ratcliffe, H.L.: Atherosclerosis in swine and swine as a model of the study of atherosclerosis. Adv. Cardiol., 13:119–126, 1974.

Luginbuhl, H., Rossi, G.L., Ratcliffe, H.L., and Muller, P.: Comparative atherosclerosis. Adv. Vet. Sci. Comp. Med., 21:421–448, 1977.

Lynd, F.T., et al.: Bovine arteriosclerosis in Hawaii. Am. J. Vet. Res., 26:1344–1349, 1965.

McAllister, W.B., Jr., and Waters, L.L.: Vascular lesions in the dog following thyroidectomy and viosterol feeding. Yale J. Biol. & Med., 22:651–700, 1950.

Marcus, L.C., and Ross, J.N.: Microscopic lesions in the hearts of aged horses. Path. Vet., 4:162–185, 1967.

McCombs, H.L., Zook, B.C., and McGandy, R.B.:

Fine structure of spontaneous atherosclerosis of the aorta in the squirrel monkey. Amer. J. Path., 55:235–252, 1969.

McCully, K.S.: Vascular pathology of homocysteinemia: implications for the pathogenesis of arteriosclerosis. Amer. J. Path., 56:111–128, 1969.

McGrath, J.M., and Stewart, G.J.: The effects of endotoxin on vascular endothelium. J. Exp. Med., 129:833–848, 1969.

McSherry, B.J., et al.: Dissecting aneurysm in internal hemorrhage in turkeys. J. Am. Vet. Med. Assn., 124:279–283, 1954.

Montali, E.J., Strandberg, J.D., and Squire, R.A.: A histochemical and ultrastructural study of intimal bodies in horse arterioles. Lab. Invest., 23:302–306, 1970.

Moore, L.A., Hallman, E.T., and Sholl, L.B.: Cardiovascular and other lesions in calves fed diets low in magnesium. Arch. Path., 26:820–838, 1938.

Moorehead, R.P., and Little, J.M.: Changes in the blood vessels of apparently healthy mongrel dogs. Amer. J. Path., 21:339–353, 1945.

Neumann, F., and Ungar, H.: Cystic medial degeneration of the aorta in poultry. J. Comp. Pathol., 82:147–150, 1972.

Oka, M., Brodie, S.S., and Angrist, A.A.: Sex-dependent vascular changes in young, adult, aged and hypertensive rats. Amer. J. Path., 53:127–147, 1968.

Prasad, M.D., Rajya, B.S., and Mohanty, G.C.: Caprine arterial diseases. I. Spontaneous aortic lesions. Exp. Mol. Pathol., 17:14–28, 1972.

Prior, J.T., and Hutter, R.V.P.: Intimal repair of the aorta of the rabbit following experimental trauma. Amer. J. Path., 31:107–123, 1955.

Pritchard, W.R., Henderson, W., and Beall, C.W.: Experimental production of dissecting aneurysm in turkeys. Am. J. Vet. Res., 19:696–705, 1958.

Ratcliffe, H.L., and Luginbuhl, H.: The domestic pig: a model for experimental atherosclerosis. Atherosclerosis, 13:133–136, 1971.

Ratcliffe, H.L., Luginbuhl, H., and Pivnik, L.: Coronary, aortic and cerebral atherosclerosis in swine of 3 age-groups: implications. Bull. WHO, 42:225–234, 1970.

Ratcliffe, H.L., Luginbuhl, H., Schnarr, W.R., and Chacko, K.: Coronary arteriosclerosis in swine: evidence of a relation to behavior. J. Comp. Physiol. Psychol., 68:385–392, 1969.

Ratcliffe, H.L., and Snyder, R.L.: Coronary arterial lesions in chickens: origin and rates of development in relation to sex and social factors. Circ. Res., 17:403–413, 1965.

Rigdon, R.H.: Tumors produced by methylcholanthrene in the duck. Arch. Pathol., 54:368–377, 1952.

Rinehart, J.F., and Greenberg, L.D.: Arteriosclerotic lesions in pyridoxine-deficient monkeys. Amer. J. Path., 25:481–491, 1949.

Roberts, J.C., and Straus, R. (ed.): Comparative Atherosclerosis. New York, Harper & Row, 1965.

Rogers, W.A., Bishop, S.P., and Rohovsky, M.W.: Pulmonary artery medial hypertrophy and hyperplasia in conventional and specific-pathogen-free cats. Am. J. Vet. Res., *32*:767–774, 1971.

Rooney, J.R., Prickett, M.E., and Crowe, M.W.: Aortic ring rupture in stallions. Path. Vet., *4*:268–274, 1967.

Rubin, L.F., and Patterson, D.F.: Arteriovenous fistula of the orbit in a dog. Cornell Vet., *55*:471–481, 1965.

Schenk, E.A., Gaman, E., and Feigenbaum, A.S.: Spontaneous aortic lesions in rabbits. I. Morphologic characteristics. II. Relationship to experimental atherosclerosis. Circulation Res., *19*:80–95, 1966.

Simpson, C.F., and Harms, R.H.: Pathology of aortic atherosclerosis and dissecting aneurysms of turkeys induced by diethylstilbestrol. Exp. & Molec. Path., *5*:183–184, 1966.

Skold, B.H., Getty, R., and Ramsey, F.K.: Spontaneous atherosclerosis in the arterial system of aging swine. Am. J. Vet. Res., *27*:257–273, 1966.

Slavin, R.E., and Gonzalez-Vitale, J.C.: Segmental mediolytic arteritis: a clinical pathologic study. Lab. Invest., *35*:23–29, 1976.

Stambaugh, J.E., Harvey, C.E., and Goldschmidt, M.H.: Lymphangioma in four dogs. J. Am. Vet. Med. Assoc., *173*:759–761, 1978.

Steiner, A., and Kendall, F.E.: Atherosclerosis and arteriosclerosis in dogs following ingestion of cholesterol and thiouracil. Arch. Path., *42*:433–434, 1946.

Stout, C.: Atherosclerosis in exotic carnivora and pinnipedia. Amer. J. Path., *57*:673–687, 1969.

Strauch, C.: Zur kenntnis der spontanen arterienveranderungen beim hunde mit besonderer berucksichtigung der arteriosklerose. Beitr. Pathol. Anat. allg. Pathol., *61*:532–549, 1916.

Strong, J.P.: Atherosclerosis in primates. Introduction and overview. Primates Med., *9*:1–15, 1976.

Stunzi, H., Teuscher, E., and Pericin-Rauhur, D.: Die hyperplasia der arteria pulmonalis bei feliden. Path. Vet., *3*:461–473, 1966.

Suzuki, M., et al.: "Experimental atherosclerosis in the dog: a morphologic study." Exp. Molec. Path., *3*:455–467, 1964.

Wigley, R.D., Couchman, K.G., and Maule, R.: Polyarteritis nodosa: the natural history of a spontaneously occurring model in outbred mice. Aust. Ann. Med., *19*:319–327, 1970.

Wilens, S.L., and Plair, C.M.: The relationship between cortical hyperplasia of the adrenals and arteriosclerosis. Amer. J. Path., *41*:224–232, 1962.

Willers, E.H., et al.: Experimental studies of bovine arteriosclerosis in Hawaii. Am. J. Vet. Res., *26*:1350–1355, 1965.

Wissler, R.W.: Recent progress in studies of experimental primate atherosclerosis. Prog. Biochem. Pharm., *4*:378–392, 1968.

Young, Y.H.: Polyarteritis nodosa in lab rats. Lab. Invest., *14*:81–88, 1965.

Zeek, P.M.: Periarteritis nodosa and other forms of necrotizing angitis. N.E. J. Med., *248*:764–772, 1953.

Zinserling, W.D.: Uber bindegewebige intimaverdickungen und spontane lipoidose der aorta und anderer organe bei hunden. Beitr. Pathol. Anat. allg. Pathol., *88*:241–314, 1932.

CHAPTER 22

The Hemic and Lymphatic Systems

BONE MARROW

When one hears the term bone marrow, it is the red marrow to which reference is made. The fatty marrow is inert with respect to hematopoiesis and merely fills space left by the functional red marrow. In early life all marrow is red; by the time of maturity, this has normally been replaced by fatty marrow in the long bones, beginning at the distal ends of the limbs and leaving, perhaps, a bit of red marrow at the proximal epiphyses of the humerus and femur. Even the red marrow commonly contains some adipose cells, the functional myeloid and related cells being scattered among them, all held together by a reticulum of connective tissue, with numerous blood vessels.

The cells of the bone marrow form a series of graduations from the large, round myeloblast with its central spherical nucleus and very limited basophilic cytoplasm to the polymorphonuclear leukocytes, neutrophilic, eosinophilic, or basophilic, or to the nucleated erythroblast with its acidophilic cytoplasm and its successor, the non-nucleated erythrocyte. Many intermediate types are recognized by hematologists, but they can seldom be identified in sections. Megakaryocytes, also called bone-marrow giant cells, are huge, irregularly nucleated cells scattered among the others. Mononuclear reticulo-endothelial cells form a part of the supporting framework. While the great majority of the cells are engaged in the formation of more blood cells, a process called hematopoiesis, the reticulo-endothelials have, among others, the function of converting into bilirubin the hemoglobin from red blood cells which have completed their life span and disintegrated. In birds and lower forms, the erythrocytes retain their nucleus, as the student is aware. In these creatures, birds, reptiles, and amphibians, the erythrocytes are formed within vascular sinuses and the granulocytes develop outside such spaces. In mammals, granulopoiesis also takes place outside the blood stream, but the location of erythropoiesis has not been positively determined, although it is apparently extravascular.

Bone-marrow cells deteriorate rapidly after death. They are usually studied from biopsies obtained during life. A segment of the sternum is usually punctured by means of a fine cannula, but in horses and cattle, puncture of a rib has been found more feasible. The iliac crest has also been used with success in most animals as well as in man. Smears obtained from biopsies are essential to cellular identification and determination of myeloid:erythroid ratios. Tissue sections prepared from autopsy material are necessary to evaluate aplasia, hypoplasia, or hypertrophy and to identify focal lesions such as granulomas or metastatic neoplasms.

Erythropoiesis

The production of erythrocytes (red blood cells) in the bone marrow is regulated in order to maintain the level of circulating erythrocytes or hemoglobin at optimum for the transport of oxygen. Red blood cell production and maturation in the bone marrow depends upon (1) **erythropoietin,** which stimulates growth and differentiation of erythrocytes; (2) an adequate supply of iron, and (3) normal erythroid generating cells in the marrow. Erythropoietin, the marrow-stimulating hormone, is produced in the kidney, which thus serves, in part at least, as the regulating center. The production of erythropoietin varies with the oxygen content of the arterial blood and the oxygen-affinity of its hemoglobin. This second factor may be altered in certain hemoglobinopathies.

The level of hemoglobin and number of red blood cells in an individual are maintained within a narrow range, although the variation between individuals is much greater. Testosterone also has an effect upon the number of erythrocytes, males having a greater number than females. The life span of the erythrocyte is about 120 days in man and most mammals, and its generation time in the marrow is about 1 week. This gives the mass of red blood cells considerable stability; changes in the red cell count occur slowly under most circumstances. For example, after ascent to 15,000 feet altitude, 2 to 3 months are required before the hematocrit changes from 45 to 62%.

The effects of erythropoietin in regulating erythropoiesis may be summarized as follows: (1) precursor cells of the bone marrow divide more rapidly, nucleated red blood cells increase in number, and young cells enter the circulation; (2) production of hemoglobin in red blood cells is augmented, cell volume increases, and the hemoglobin content of erythrocytes increases; (3) marrow reticulocytes are released in greater numbers into the circulation, as evidenced by the greater proportion of reticulocytes in the blood smear (reticulocyte count).

Erythrocyte production and maturation in the bone marrow occurs in an extravascular syncytium of cells, which can increase production of erythrocytes four to five times under erythropoietin stimulation. Further increase in production requires extension of the hematopoietic marrow into unused (fatty) portions of the marrow, a process which requires some time. This capacity to expand may be impaired by (1) disease or replacement (by tumor) of the stroma; (2) inadequate nutritional supply, or (3) abnormalities in the erythroid cells themselves.

The availability of iron, which is incorporated into the hemoglobin molecule, sets the upper production limit of erythrocytes. Other limiting nutritional factors may be the presence of vitamins B_{12} and E, folic acid, and selenium. These substances may affect the viability of the red cells, but are not incorporated into the hemoglobin. Human beings are vulnerable to overload of iron because of their limited capacity to excrete it. In this species, most body iron is confined to the erythron by maintenance of a low plasma level and by transferrin saturation. These low stores of iron place a low ceiling on the rate of erythropoiesis because marrow production of erythrocytes is limited to the iron available. Iron-deficient erythropoiesis is clinically indicated by: (1) decrease in sideroblasts within the bone marrow; (2) increase in red-cell protoporphyrin; (3) with time, changes in red blood cell size and hemoglobin content.

Granulopoiesis

The study of the regulation of the production and maturation of granulocytes (neutrophils, eosinophils, basophils), monocytes and thrombocytes (platelets) by hematopoietic bone marrow has not progressed as far as studies on regulation of erythropoiesis by erythropoietin. However, at this point, it appears that factors similar to erythropoietin are involved in this regulation. Cultures of bone marrow cells (usually from mice) have been shown to produce colonies (clones) of granulocytic cells or macrophages when exposed to certain factors, called "culture-stimulating factors." These have been demonstrated in serum, urine, some tissues (of man and animals), and culture medium in which certain cells have grown. These factors vary in physical characteristics and effects, depending on their source and the species of the target cells. However, partially purified preparations have in them sialic acid-containing glycoproteins with molecular weight of 45,000 to 60,000 daltons, which migrate electrophoretically between alpha-1 globulin and albumin.

Colony-stimulating factors have been shown to increase in the serum of animals and man following infection and antigen administration. Also, administration of partially-purified colony-stimulating factors to mice causes increased maturation of granulocytic and monocytic precursor cells, leading to elevated numbers of granulocytes and monocytes in the peripheral blood. It thus appears likely that colony-stimulating factors may serve to regulate granulopoiesis in a similar manner to the regulation of erythropoiesis by erythropoietin.

Cerami, A.: Blood cell differentiation. Humoral factors of blood cell differentiation. Fed. Proc., 34:2271, 1975.

Golde, D.W., and Martin, J.C.: Regulation of granulopoiesis. N. Engl. J. Med., 291:1388–1396, 1974.

Goldwasser, E.: Erythropoietin and the differentiation of red blood cells. Fed. Proc., 34:2285–2292, 1975.

Hillman, R.S., and Finch, C.A.: Erythropoiesis. N. Engl. J. Med., 285:99–102, 1971.

Lewis, J.P., et al.: Response in mice to erythropoiesis regulatory factors. Am. J. Vet. Res., 34:1367–1368, 1973.

Louwagie, A.C.: Haemopoietic stem cells. II. Properties, regulation, and identity. Acta Clin. Belg., 31:136–143, 1976.

Prasse, K.W., Kaeberle, M.L., and Ramsey, F.K.: Blood neutrophilic granulocyte kinetics in cats. Am. J. Vet. Res., 34:1021–1026, 1973.

Prasse, K.W., Seagrave, R.C., Kaeberle, M.L., and Ramsey, F.K.: A model of granulopoiesis in cats. Lab. Invest., 28:292–299, 1973.

Shahidi, N.T.: Androgens and erythropoiesis. N. Engl. J. Med., 289:72–80, 1973.

Stanley, E.R., Hansen, G., Woodcock, J., and Metcalf, D.: Colony stimulating factor and the regulation of granulopoiesis and macrophage production. Fed. Proc., 34:2272–2278, 1975.

Till, J.E., Price, G.B., Mak, T.W., and McCullough, E.A.: Regulation of blood cell differentiation. Fed. Proc., 34:2279–2284, 1975.

Tsuchiya, J., and Maekawa, T.: Cytokinetic studies on hematopoietic cells of the bone marrow. Acta Haemat. Jpn., 36:641–660, 1973.

Zanjani, E.D., Gordon, A.S., Wong, K.K., McLaurin, W.D.: The renal erythropoietic factor (REF). X. The question of species and class specificity. Proc. Soc. Exp. Biol. and Med., 131:1095–1098, 1969.

Hyperplasia

Hyperplasia of bone marrow is recognized grossly in the form of an increase in the amount of red marrow and a decrease of the fatty marrow, as compared with the normal for a given age. In pronounced hyperplasias which have existed for a considerable time, the red marrow greatly replaces adult fatty marrow of long bones, beginning at the proximal ends of the femur and humerus and extending distally through the extremities. The finer bony trabeculae which reach from the endosteal zone into the marrow cavity tend to disappear before the advancing hyperplastic marrow tissue. In judging the degree of hyperplasia of bone marrows an accurate knowledge of the normal is necessary. In general, at the time a normal animal is half grown there is practically no red marrow in the marrow cavity of the radius, tibia, and bones distal to them. Toward the proximal end of the humerus and femur, a minimal amount of marrow can be expected at this age. As the animal approaches maturity even this disappears. Red marrow, of course, fills the marrow spaces of the spongy, or cancellous, bone of the epiphysis proper at all ages, as well as that of the flat bones, namely the ribs, sternum, and bones of the skull and pelvis. In case a biopsy of bone marrow is to be made, the sternum or iliac crest are the customary sites, although many find the tuber coxae more readily feasible in large animals. There are two principal varieties of **myeloid hyperplasia,** as the condition is synonymously designated.

Erythroblastic hyperplasia is characterized by red marrow which microscopically is found to consist principally of the precursors of erythrocytes, namely erythroblasts and normoblasts. This occurs in and is a reaction to most of the anemias except toxic aplastic anemia, which owes its existence to inability of the marrow to function. In human pernicious anemia, with its deficient erythrocyte-maturing factor, and in the similar anemia due to the fish tapeworm, *Diphyllobothrium latum,* megaloblasts become numerous, and the terms megaloblastic anemia and megaloblastic hyperplasia are applicable.

Leukoblastic hyperplasia, on the other hand, is characterized by a predominance of the precursors of leukocytes, usually mature and immature neutrophilic granulocytes and their predecessors, the myelocytes and myeloblasts. This variety of hyperplasia occurs in consequence of those infections which are accompanied by leukocytosis and a vigorous pyogenic reaction. If, however, the pyogenic disease is prolonged for several weeks, the myeloid cells and their progeny become exhausted, leaving little but erythroblastic cells and some lymphoid cells. The leukocytosis is naturally replaced by a leukopenia.

A leukoblastic reaction with large numbers of eosinophilic granulocytes and their predecessors is found in many human cases of ancylostomiasis and trichinosis, and the same may be presumed to be true in animals. In lymphoid leukemia (malignant lymphoma), areas of marrow may be largely replaced by lymphoid cells. In myeloid leukemia, the neoplastic cells take possession of many areas of the marrow. In these cases, as well as in leukoblastic hyperplasia, the marrow grossly tends toward a grayish color without the yellowish tinge of fat.

Hypoplasia

Hypoplasia of the bone marrow occurs in connection with toxic aplastic anemia, being, indeed, the cause of it. The proportion of fatty marrow is greater than normal, and frequently such hematopoietic tissue as remains is scattered in little islands through the fatty marrow. Microscopically, it may be principally the erythropoietic forms of developing cells that are missing or the deficiency may involve all cell types. In **leukopenia,** which results from the marrow-depressant action of certain infections, the more mature forms of the leukoblastic series of cells, especially the neutrophilic granulocytes and their predecessors, are largely or entirely absent.

Agranulocytosis

Agranulocytosis must be mentioned here. The term refers to a more or less complete absence of granulocytes from the circulating blood. This, in turn, is due to a complete aplasia of the leukoblastic cells of the bone marrow. It is thus related to aplastic anemia and is probably attributable to similar toxic causes. A number of commonly used medicines are known to have a depressant action on the bone marrow and are cited under the latter type of anemia. Since the tissues are deprived of the protection of leukocytes, the condition is usually fatal in a few weeks at most as the result of some infection which would be trivial in a normal individual. Agranulocytosis is diagnosed with a fair degree of frequency in human medicine. In animals, it doubtless occurs when the same causes are operating but this is apparently rather seldom.

Osteomyelitis

Osteomyelitis is an inflammatory process in the bone marrow due to infection, which gains access to the marrow through a local wound (fracture, etc.) or by hem-

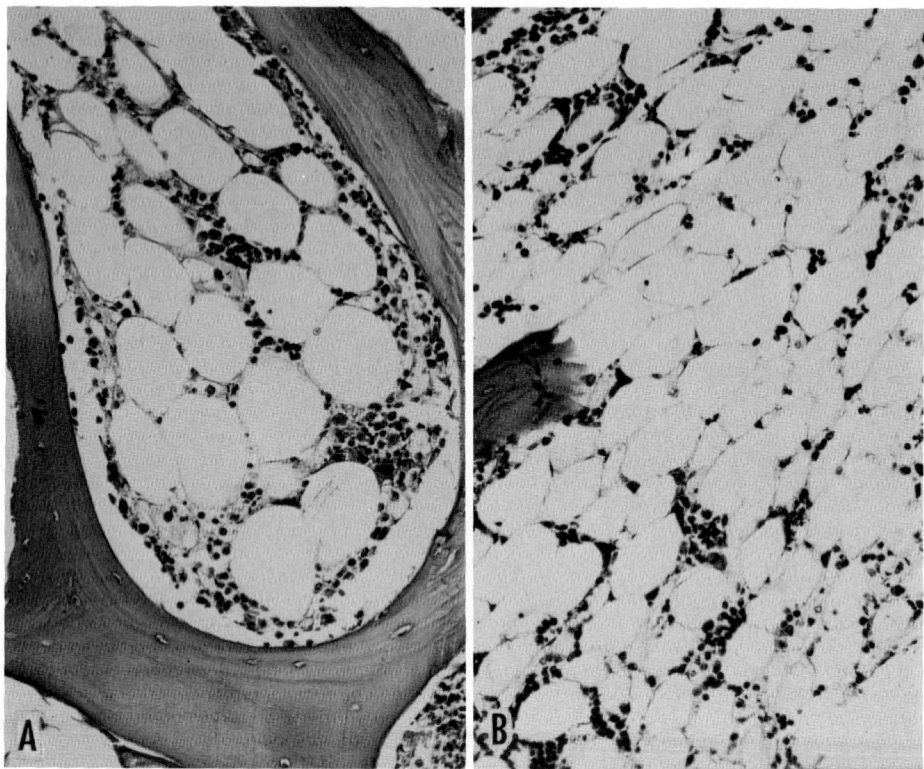

Fig. 22–1.   Hypoplasia of the bone marrow in a dog with hypochromic microcytic anemia. *A*, A rib (× 195). *B*, Sternum (× 195). Note paucity of hematopoietic cells as in rib. (*B*, Courtesy of Armed Forces Institute of Pathology.) Contributor: Dr. E.E. Ruebush.

atogenous metastasis. It is thus a localized process, involving usually a single bone, in contrast to the widespread character of hyperplasia, hypoplasia, and aplasia. The infection is usually pyogenic and the reaction purulent, although specific infections such as tuberculosis and coccidioidomycosis also produce their typical lesions in the bone marrow. Owing to the difficulty of drainage and other anatomic considerations, osteomyelitis was feared prior to the advent of modern antibiotics and is still difficult to treat. The condition is recognized grossly by a painful accumulation of pus, which eventually causes softening and necrosis of the overlying bony wall and makes its way to the body surface. Microscopically, accumulation of neutrophilic polymorphonuclear leukocytes, and perhaps fibrin and other

inflammatory elements at times almost to the exclusion of the myeloid cells, reveals the nature of the condition.

Fibrosis

Fibrosis of the bone marrow, with or without **myxomatous degeneration**, occurs as a rare accompaniment of or sequel to hypoplasia or aplasia. The cause is obscure: possibly some forms represent exhaustion of a previously active marrow. Myxomatous degeneration is prominent in starvation.

NEOPLASMS OF HEMOPOIETIC AND LYMPHOPOIETIC TISSUES

Neoplasms of these tissues are recognized by their resemblance to normal cells, or their precursors, produced by cells of the bone marrow or lymphocytic tissues.

Many confusing names have been introduced in the past to indicate some postulated function or history of origin of the tumors cells. Some primitive precursor or stem cells are not readily identified, causing further confusion and difficulties in recognition of the tumors they produce.

The point of encounter in the life history of a neoplastic disease in this system must also be kept in mind. Some neoplasms develop simultaneously in several organs, others start in a single organ, for example, the thymus, then eventually spread to other organs and the blood. Changes in the morphologic features of the cells may also occur, particularly in cells from the bone marrow. Certain viruses, such as the feline leukemia virus, produce a panoply of effects upon cells in bone marrow and lymph nodes. Consideration of the entire disease complex, in so far as possible, throughout its course is vital to the understanding of hemopoietic neoplasms.

The World Health Organization has engaged specialists over the world to develop standard classification schemes and nomenclature that could be used worldwide as a basis for comparison, epizootic studies, communication, and further research. The histologic classification scheme for tumors of this organ system developed by WHO consultants is outlined in Table 22–1 (Jarrett and Mackey, 1974). The information in this table has been taken from the cited publication, translated into American English for the purposes of this text. We shall adhere to the system proposed by the WHO consultants not because it meets all of our prejudices and favorite names concerning these neoplasms or that we agree with all the concepts proposed, but because we think it provides a sound basis for communication and future research. Other systems, for example, functional (B cell, T cell) or etiologic, are also of value. We shall endeavor to keep the numbers of synonyms to a minimum, although some will be use-

Table 22–1.   Neoplastic Diseases of Hemopoietic and Lymphopoietic Tissues*

LYMPHOID NEOPLASMS:	MYELOID NEOPLASMS:

A. *Lymphosarcoma* (multicentric, alimentary, thymic, and other anatomic forms)
  1. Poorly differentiated
  2. Lymphoblastic
  3. Lymphocytic and prolymphocytic
  4. Histiocytic, histioblastic, and histiolymphocytic
B. *Lymphoid leukemia*
  1. Poorly differentiated
  2. Lymphoblastic
  3. Lymphocytic and prolymphocytic
C. *Nodular lymphoid hyperplasia of the canine spleen*
D. *Tumors of immunoglobulin-forming cells*
  1. Solitary plasmacytoma
  2. Myeloma
  3. Primary macroglobinemia (Waldenström)
E. *Thymoma*
  1. Predominantly epithelial
  2. Predominantly lymphocytic
	A. *Myeloid leukemia*
	  1. Poorly differentiated
	  2. Well differentiated
	    (a) neutrophilic
	    (b) eosinophilic
	B. *Erythroleukemia*
	C. *Acute erythremia* (di Guglielmo)
	D. *Polycythemia vera*
	E. *Megakaryocytoid leukemia*
	F. *Panmyelosis*
	G. *Myelosclerosis*
	H. *Myeloproliferative disease*
	I. *Monocytic (monocytoid) leukemia*
	
	MAST CELL TUMORS (considered elsewhere)

*After Jarrett and Mackey, 1974

ful to the student because not everyone in the profession will accept this international classification and nomenclature.

The etiologies of neoplasms are discussed in Chapter 4. It should be kept in mind that some neoplasms of blood cells are known to be caused by viruses. For example, the feline leukemia virus is clearly associated with lymphosarcoma; mouse lymphomas are caused by an RNA virus; experimental lymphoproliferative disease in marmosets, owl monkeys, and rabbits is produced by *Herpesvirus saimiri* and *Herpesvirus ateles.* In man and most other species, a specific viral or other causative agent has not been identified.

Lymphoid Neoplasms

Lymphosarcoma (Malignant Lymphoma)

Lymphocytic cells and their precursors form the most frequent neoplasms in most animal species. Lymphosarcomas form solid masses of white, uniformly textured tumors in lymph nodes, spleen, thymus, and other lymphocytic organs especially, but may occur in any organ system. The tendency for tumor masses to be distributed in various anatomic sites is one characteristic used to classify them. When initially recognized, lymphosarcomas may be **multicentric,** involving most of the lymph nodes as well as other organs (this applies to about 65% of canine cases). In the **thymic** form (seen in about 20% of feline cases and often involved in the bovine, canine, porcine, and ovine species), the thymus is replaced and greatly enlarged by lymphosarcoma. The **alimentary** form is seen especially in the cat, dog, and horse. The tumors appear to arise in Peyer's patches but invade submucosa and muscularis. A **leukemic** form occurs upon occasion, the lymphocytic tumor cells replacing the bone marrow and other visceral organs.

Four cytologic types are recognized in animal species, especially domesticated species; these are: (1) poorly differentiated; (2) lymphoblastic; (3) lymphocytic and pro-lymphocytic; and (4) histiocytic, histioblastic, and histiolymphocytic. (See Table 22–1.)

Poorly Differentiated Type. The poorly differentiated type of lymphosarcoma is made up of individually discrete cells, with irregularly outlined, somewhat eosinophilic cytoplasm. The nuclei are large, round or oval with a centrally placed nucleolus surrounded by an essentially clear halo.

Lymphoblastic Type. The lymphoblastic histologic type is made up of a rather uniform population of cells with scant somewhat basophilic cytoplasm and large, round to ovoid nuclei. The nuclear chromatin tends to be clumped, and a single nucleolus is usually conspicuous.

Lymphocytic and Prolymphocytic Type. In the lymphocytic and prolymphocytic type, the cells resemble differentiated lymphocytes closely. The cytoplasm is closely confined to the nuclear margin and is often not distinguishable in histologic sections. The nuclei contain coarsely clumped chromatin, may be irregular in outline and occasionally contain recognizable nucleoli.

Histiocytic, Histioblastic, or Histiolymphocytic Type. These types of lymphosarcoma are made up of cells closely resembling the normal cells which line the cortical sinuses of lymph nodes. The cells of the histiocytic type vary in size and often have a large amount of eosinophilic cytoplasm. Phagocytic activity may be in evidence. Their nuclei are large, round to ovoid, and contain one or more conspicuous nucleoli. In the histioblastic type, the cells tend to be binucleate and the nuclei tend to have sharp outlines and a large nucleolus. The cytoplasm is less abundant than in the histiocytic type. A mixture of histiocytic and lymphocytic types is called histiolymphocytic and is encountered most frequently in the viral-induced disease in young cats.

These histologic types may not always be clearly separable; in some cases two types may occur together and in some instances

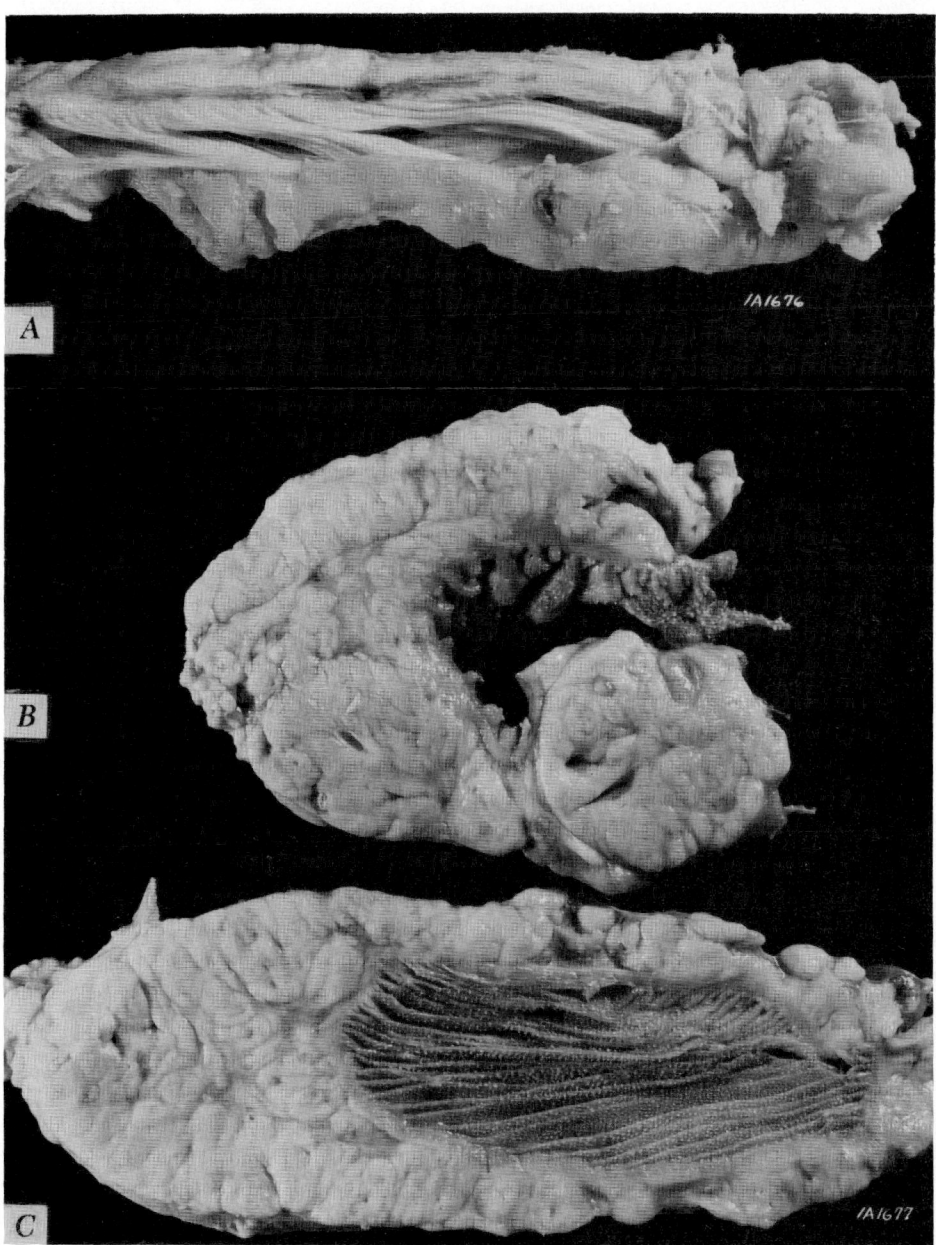

Fig. 22–2. Bovine lymphosarcoma (malignant lymphoma) illustrating neoplastic invasion of cauda equina (A), reticulum (B), and omasum (C). (Courtesy of Dr. M.J. Twiehaus.)

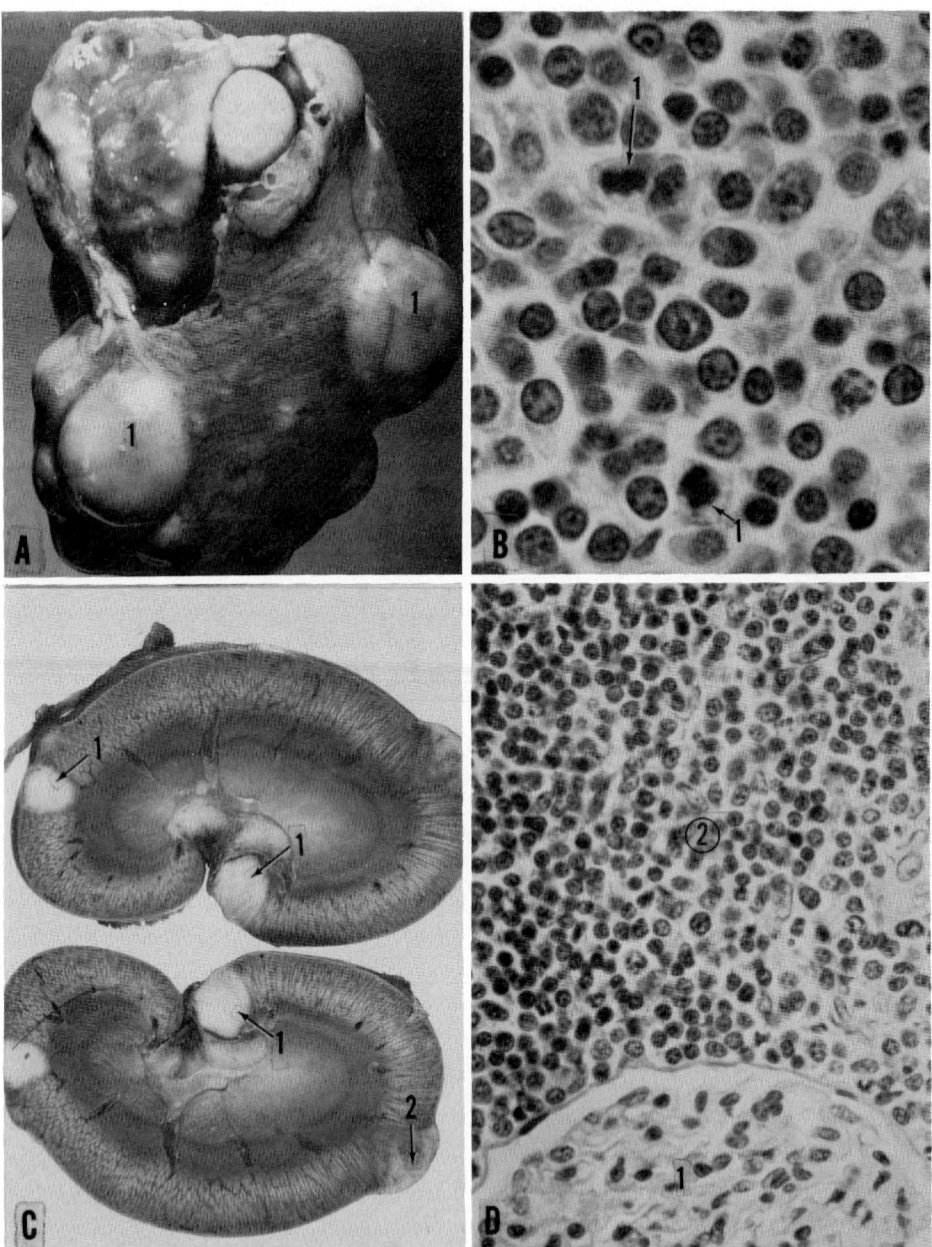

Fig. 22–3. Lymphosarcoma (malignant lymphoma). *A*, Lesions (*1*) in the kidney of a dog. *B*, Photomicrograph (× 1190) of lesion in *C*. Note individually discrete tumor cells and mitotic figures (*1*). *C*, Kidney of a five-year-old male German Shepherd. Lymphosarcoma tumor masses (*1*) and (*2*) in renal cortex. *D*, Neoplastic cells (× 500); same case as *C*. Note infiltration of renal cortex by tumor cells (*2*). The glomerulus (*1*) is not yet invaded by tumor. (Courtesy of Armed Forces Institute of Pathology.) Contributor: Dr. Leo L. Lieberman.

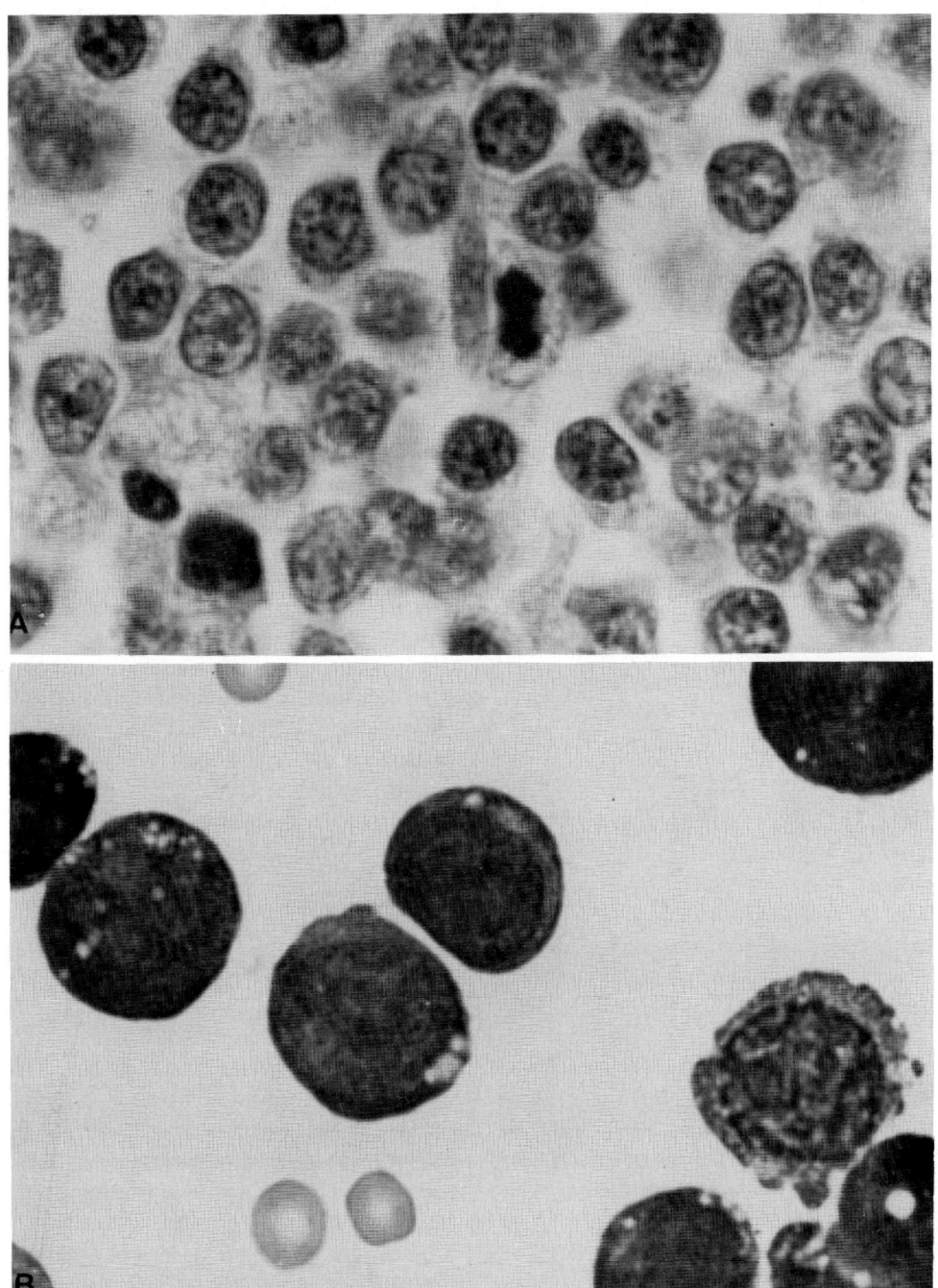

Fig. 22–4. Lymphosarcoma (malignant lymphoma) involving thymus and pleura of a cat. *A*, Section of pleura. (H & E, × 1600.) *B*, Smear of fluid aspirated from pleural cavity. (Wright-Giemsa's stain, × 1600,) Note the apparent difference in size of the tumor cells prepared by sectioning and smear techniques.

the prevailing type of cell may change during the course of the disease.

Lymphoid Leukemia

The disease called lymphoid leukemia is manifest by replacement of bone marrow and invasion of the blood by malignant lymphoid cells conforming to three of the histologic types described under lymphosarcoma (poorly differentiated, lymphoblastic, or lymphocytic and prolymphocytic). Although the anatomic distribution of the lesions is different, one might question whether this is not simply one form of lymphosarcoma. In cases of solid lymphocytic tumors, conforming to the description of lymphosarcoma, the blood picture may be leukopenic or anemic in the early stages but eventually, malignant cells appear in the circulation, often in very large numbers.

Nodular lymphoid hyperplasia of the canine spleen will be described in this chapter in the section on the spleen.

Tumors of Immunoglobulin-Forming Cells

These are made up of neoplastic plasma cells which are differentiated to the extent that they maintain their function of producing immunoglobulins.

Solitary Plasmacytoma. The solitary plasmacytoma is made up of plasma cells which are usually well-differentiated with eccentric nuclei and eosinophilic, amphophilic, or weakly basophilic cytoplasm. Some less well differentiated tumors may be encountered with pleomorphic cells, occasional multinucleated cells mixed with some plasma cells or plasmablasts.

Myeloma. Myeloma is occasionally encountered in animals. The malignant cells resemble plasma cells and are found in large numbers in bone marrow and often in spleen, lymph nodes, and viscera. These cells may form discrete masses or may diffusely replace preexisting structures. These cells usually produce monoclonal gamma globulins which are demonstrable in the blood as Bence Jones protein (light chain complexes).

Primary Macroglobulinemia (Waldenström). A lymphoproliferative disorder is responsible for the production of 19S immunoglobulin, which is identified as primary macroglobulinemia (Waldenström). A mixture of plasma cells and lymphocytes are usually seen in lymph nodes and spleen. The immunoglobulins usually have high viscosity which may produce a characteristic syndrome.

Thymoma

This is described as a localized benign tumor which is made up primarily of epithelial or lymphocytic cells. These proliferated cells simulate the appearance of normal thymic lymphocytes and epithelium, including Hassall's corpuscles. Thymomas are infrequent and are considered benign. Lymphosarcoma of the thymus is much more frequent and may be distinguished by the florid replacement of the thymus by malignant cells conforming to any of the histologic types described under lymphosarcoma.

Myeloid Neoplasms

Myeloid Leukemia

Neoplasms involving cells that are precursors of leukocytes of the granulocytic series (neutrophils, eosinophils and possibly basophils) are referred to as myeloid leukemia (myelogenous leukemia, myelocytoma, myeloblastoma, myelosarcoma) in the undifferentiated form. When differentiated, immature leukocytes can be recognized, and the designation neutrophilic or eosinophilic leukemia is used. Basophilic leukemia has been reported rarely in animals, but is difficult to distinguish from generalized mast cell tumors.

Myeloid leukemias arise in the bone marrow, which is generally replaced by the neoplastic cells. Some of these tumors have a grossly visible greenish hue. These were called **chloromas** in older literature.

Leukemic cells usually abound in the circulating blood and may invade liver, spleen, lymph nodes, and other organs as well. In these tissue sites it may be difficult to distinguish the lesion from extramedullary hemopoiesis, but the presence of erythroblastic cells, normoblasts, and megakaryocytes is helpful in distinguishing extramedullary hemopoiesis.

Myeloid cells are recognizable as resembling the myelogenous cells of the bone marrow with all their variations in size and tinctorial features. They are individually discrete, rounded cells with abundant cytoplasm and a centrally-placed, round and vesicular nucleus. Cytoplasmic granules in tissue sections can usually only be recognized in eosinophils and basophils. Neutrophilic granules are distinguishable usually in impression smears stained with Giemsa's or Wright-Giemsa's stains. The polymorphonuclear feature of these cells is usually indicated by early lobation of the nuclei. Only in completely mature cells are the nuclei divided into several lobes.

Erythroleukemia

This term has been applied to neoplasms of the bone marrow in which cells of the erythrocytic and granulocytic series both participate. Neoplastic cells replace the bone marrow and invade the blood and other organs as well, particularly liver, lymph nodes, and spleen. Differentiation from extramedullary hemopoiesis (myeloid metaplasia) is sometimes difficult. Abnormal red cell precursors, often with many megaloblastic cells, are a striking feature of this tumor.

Acute Erythremia (di Guglielmo)

Proliferation of erythrocytic cells and their precursors is characteristic of this neoplasm. Blast cells, erythroblasts, and normoblasts can be recognized. The bone marrow and circulating blood are the prin-

cipal sites of the malignant cells, but they may be seen in the vascular system of organs such as liver and spleen. Abnormal red cell precursors are commonly seen. In order to distinguish this neoplastic condition from severe deficiency anemia, it is necessary to demonstrate negative response to dietary supplementation with folic acid, vitamin B_{12}, and other vitamins (Chapter 17).

Polycythemia Vera

This type of polycythemia is not related to anoxia or to reduced plasma volume, but to an absolute increase in the erythrocyte mass. Leukocytosis, thrombocytosis, and hypervolemia usually accompany this disease, which may terminate in erythroid-leukemia or myeloid leukemia. Familial polycythemia is described in children.

Tennant, et al. (1967) described a disease in Jersey cattle which appears to be an inherited polycythemia, controlled by a single autosomal recessive gene. In these cattle, polycythemia developed during the second month of life, persisted throughout the first year and disappeared at maturity. This may not be related to the disease considered to be neoplastic.

McGrath (1974) has summarized the findings in reported cases of polycythemia vera in dogs. Presenting signs usually include: polydipsia, polyuria, nocturia, pica, posterior weakness, ataxia, vaginal discharge, enlarged mammary glands, intolerance to heat, and seizures. The consistent hematologic findings include elevated packed cell volume (65 to 82); increased hemoglobin concentration (21.6 to 28.3 g/100 ml); elevated red blood cell counts, red blood cell mass, and total blood volume. Aortic thrombosis is often encountered.

Polycythemia related to anoxia or reduced plasma volume is discussed on page 1320.

One case of polycythemia vera has been reported in the cat (Reed, et al., 1970).

Megakaryocytoid Leukemia

This rare tumor of megakaryocyte precursors, mainly megaloblasts and promegakaryocytes, starts in the bone marrow and may spread to other organs. Neoplastic megakaryocytes are not usually recognized in the blood. Promegakaryocytes are very large cells with partially lobulated nuclei containing nucleoli. Aberrant mitoses may be seen in these cells. Megakaryoblasts are indistinguishable morphologically from other hemocytoblasts.

Panmyelosis

This term denotes a neoplasm of the bone marrow cells including cells of the erythrocytic, granulocytic, and megakaryocytic series. Tumor cells replace the marrow, appear in the blood, and proliferate in hemopoietic sites such as liver, spleen, and lymph nodes. Panmyelosis is difficult to distinguish from combined myeloid leukemia with extramedullary hemopoiesis, except that it occurs where extramedullary hemopoiesis ordinarily does not and consists predominately of erythrocytic and megakaryocytic cells.

Myelofibrosis (Intramedullary Fibrosis)

Some forms of myeloid leukemia may be accompanied or followed by fibrosis of the bone marrow. Myeloid metaplasia or osteosclerosis may be associated with myeloid leukemia or possibly be a primary disease of marrow. This latter point is not established.

Myeloproliferative Disease

This general term is used to designate those situations in which neoplasms of bone marrow do not appear to fit any of the terms described previously. Some cases may have certain features of myelosclerosis, myeloid metaplasia, and granulocytic leukemia.

Monocytic (Monocytoid) Leukemia

Monocytes and precursors of monocytes may undergo neoplastic change. The precursor cells and malignant monocytes are difficult to identify precisely, and, therefore, some neoplasms of this type may go unrecognized. Monocytes are now established as the cells which become macrophages, and some malignant monocytes exhibit the faculty of phagocytosis—a point which may be helpful in their identification.

Monocytes are quite large (15 to 18 μ) and have abundant finely granular or translucent cytoplasm, which may at times contain fine azurophilic granules. The nucleus is oval, sometimes indented, contains one or more nucleoli and is located in the center of the cell.

The term "myelomonocytic leukemia" is used occasionally to describe neoplasms which cannot be distinguished as principally consisting of myeloid or monocytic cells.

Bone marrow and lymph nodes are infiltrated by these tumor cells, which may also infiltrate lung, liver, spleen, gall bladder, kidney, and brain. White blood cell counts may exceed 200,000 per mm³ due to malignant monocytes in the circulation. The clinical disease may be expressed also by anemia, thrombocytopenia, enlarged lymph nodes, splenomegaly, and pulmonary thromboses containing tumor cells.

Hodgkin's Disease (Malignant Lymphoma, Hodgkin's Type)

The true nature of this obscure human disease has not been entirely settled. It has been linked with infectious granulomas, but prevailing opinions place it with the lymphomas. Cases in animals are reported from time to time with the proposed diagnosis of Hodgkin's disease. Most of these are not accepted as analogous to the human disease by the most critical specialists. The veterinary pathologist needs to be aware of the criteria which would justify this diagnosis in animals.

Characterized by slowly enlarging lymph nodes, especially in the thoracic and cervical regions, Hodgkin's disease involves continuous proliferation of four kinds of cells in varying proportions: lymphoid cells, histiocytes, fibroblasts, and eosinophils. If the embryologic precursors of these cells are traced back far enough they all have the same parent cell, hence it may be that Hodgkin's disease should be viewed as a disorder arising in prelymphoid and premyeloid stem cells.

The histologic picture may be difficult to distinguish from that of a lymphoma (histiocytic type, especially) or from that of inflammatory granuloma, depending on the predominant cell types. In this dilemma, consideration is given to the giant cell known as the Sternberg-Reed cell, which can be found after some searching in all cases. This giant cell, which is fundamentally a syncytium of at least two, and usually more, incompletely divided histiocytes, has a multilobar or at least bilobate nucleus or a piled-up, overlapping group of single vesicular nuclei. Each nucleus or nuclear lobe has a single prominent acidophilic (reddish) nucleolus near its center. At least one or two of these nucleoli must be visible in the plane of the microscopic section under study. Less than these specifications does not permit interpretation of a giant cell as a Sternberg-Reed cell, and without Sternberg-Reed cells, Hodgkin's disease cannot be diagnosed with certainty.

Adamson, R.H., et al.: Nonhuman primate models for lymphoma, leukemia, and other neoplasms. Bibl. Haematol., 40:723–730, 1973.

Alroy, J.: Basophilic leukemia in a dog. Vet. Pathol., 9:90–95, 1972.

Barthel, C.H.: Acute myelomonocytic leukemia in a dog. Vet. Pathol., 11:79–86, 1974.

Bostock, D.E., and Owen, L.N.: Porcine and ovine lymphosarcoma: a review. J. Natl. Cancer Inst., 50:933–939, 1973.

Brown, R.J., Kupper, J.L., Trevethan, V.P., and Britz, W.E.: Malignant lymphoma in a Rhesus monkey. Vet. Pathol., 8:289–291, 1971.

Cohen, H., et al.: Pathogenesis of a transplanted canine lymphocytic leukemia. Cancer, 33:1313–1324, 1974.

Cole, N.: Polycythemia in a dog. No. Am. Vet., 35:601, 1954.

Cotter, S.M., and Essex, M.: Animal model of human disease: acute lymphoblastic leukemia, aplastic anemia. Am. J. Pathol., 87:265–268, 1977.

Crighton, G.W.: Clinical aspects of lymphosarcoma in the cat. Vet. Rec., 81:122–125, 1968.

Crowley, L.V.: A diffuse plasma-cell disease in a golden hamster (Cricitus auratus). Pathol. Vet., 7:135–138, 1970.

De Paoli, A., Johnsen, D.O., and Noll, W.W.: Granulocytic leukemia in whitehanded gibbons. J. Am. Vet. Med. Assoc., 163:624–628, 1973.

Donovan, E.F., and Loeb, W.F.: Polycythemia rubra vera in the dog. J. Am. Vet. Med. Assoc., 134:36–37, 1959.

Dunkel, V.C., and Myers, S.L.: Continuous lymphoblastoid cell line from a Rhesus monkey with myelogenous leukemia. J. Natl. Cancer Inst., 48:777–782, 1972.

Fowler, M.E., Cornelius, C.E., and Baker, N.F.: Clinical and erythrokinetic studies on a case of bovine polycythemia vera. Cornell Vet., 54:153–159, 1964.

Fox, R.R., et al.: Lymphosarcoma in the rabbit: genetics and pathology. J. Natl. Cancer Inst., 45:719–729, 1970.

Fraser, C.J., Joiner, G.N., Hardine, J.H., and Gleiser, C.A.: Acute granulocytic leukemia in cats. J. Am. Vet. Med. Assoc., 165:355–359, 1974.

Frye, F.L., and Carney, J.D.: Acute lymphatic leukemia in a boa constrictor. J. Am. Vet. Med. Assoc., 163:653–656, 1973.

Garman, R.H., et al.: Lymphoma associated with an epizootic of lymphocytic choriomeningitis in Syrian hamsters (Mesocricetus auratus). Am. J. Vet. Res., 38:497–502, 1977.

Griner, L.A.: Malignant leukemic lymphoma in two harbor seals (Phoca vitulina geronimensis). Am. J. Vet. Res., 32:827–830, 1971.

Gupta, B.N.: Lymphosarcoma in a rabbit. Am. J. Vet. Res., 37:841–843, 1976.

Head, K.W., et al.: Hereditary lymphosarcoma in a herd of pigs. Vet. Rec., 95:523–527, 1974.

Henness, A.M., Crow, S.E., and Anderson, B.C.: Monocytic leukemia in three cats. J. Am. Vet. Med. Assoc., 170:1325–1328, 1977.

Holmberg, C.A., Manning, J.S., and Osburn, B.I.: Feline malignant lymphomas: comparison of morphologic and immunologic characteristics. Am. J. Vet. Res., 37:1455–1460, 1976.

Holmberg, C.A., Manning, J.S., and Osburn, B.I.: Canine malignant lymphomas: comparison of morphologic and immunologic parameters. J. Natl. Cancer Inst., 56:125–135, 1976.

Holmberg, C.A., Manning, J.S., and Osburn, B.I.: Malignant lymphoma with B-lymphocyte characteristics in dogs. Am. J. Vet. Res., 38:1877–1879, 1977.

Holscher, M.A., Collins, R.D., Glick, A.D., and Griffith, A.D.: Megakaryocytic leukemia in a dog. Vet. Pathol., 15:562–565, 1978.

Hurvitz, A.I., MacEwen, E.G., Middaugh, C.R., and Litman, G.W.: Monoclonal cryoglobulinemia with macroglobulinemia in a dog. J. Am. Vet. Med. Assoc., 170:511–515, 1977.

Jarrett, W.F.H., and Mackey, L.J.: International histological classification of tumors of domestic animals. II. Neoplastic diseases of the hematopoietic and lymphoid tissues. Bull. WHO, 50:21–34, 1974.

Johnsen, D.O., Wooding, W.L., Tanticharoenyos, P., and Bourgeois, C.H., Jr.: Malignant lymphoma in the gibbon. J. Am. Vet. Med. Assoc., 159:563–566, 1971.

Johnstone, A.C., and Manktelow, B.W.: The pathology of spontaneously occurring malignant lymphoma in sheep. Vet. Pathol., 15:301–312, 1978.

Loeb, W.F., Rininger, B., Montgomery, C.A., and Jenkins, S.: Myelomonocytic leukemia in a cat. Vet. Pathol., 12:464–467, 1975.

Lukes, R.J., and Tindle, B.H.: Immunoblastic lymphadenopathy: a hyperimmune entity resembling Hodgkin's disease. N. Engl. J. Med., 292:1–8, 1975.

Mackey, L.J., Jarrett, W.F.H., and Wiseman, A.: Monocytic leukaemia in a cow. Res. Vet. Sci., 13:287–289, 1972.

Mackey, L.J., Jarrett, W.F.H., and Lauder, I.M.: Monocytic leukaemia in the dog. Vet. Rec., 96:27–30, 1975.

Martinsson, K., Jonsson, L., and Johansson, H.E.: Multiple myeloma of IgA type in a dog. Zentralbl. Veterinaermed., 20A:826–835, 1973.

McGrath, C.J.: Polycythemia vera in dogs. J. Am. Vet. Med. Assoc., 164:1117–1122, 1974.

Meier, H., Fox, R.R., and Crary, D.D.: Myeloid leukemia in the rabbit (Oryctolagus cuniculus). Cancer Res., 32:1785–1787, 1972.

Meincke, J.E., Hobbie, W.V., Jr., and Hardy, W.D., Jr.: Lymphoreticular malignancies in the cat: clinical findings. J. Am. Vet. Med. Assoc., 160:1093–1100, 1972.

Michel, R.L., O'Handley, P., and Dade, A.W.: Megakaryocytic myelosis in a cat. J. Am. Vet. Med. Assoc., 168:1021–1025, 1976.

Miller, J.M.: Animal model of human disease: malignant lymphoma. Animal model: lymphosarcoma in cattle, sheep, horses, and pigs (malignant lymphoma, leukosis, leukemia). Am. J. Pathol., 75:417–420, 1974.

Miller, L.D., and Olson, C.: Regression of bovine lymphosarcoma. J. Am. Vet. Med. Assoc., 158:1536–1541, 1971.

Morita, M.: An autopsy case of malignant lymphogranulomatosis (so-called Hodgkin's disease) in Cercopithecus aethiops. Primates, 15:47–53, 1974.

Neufeld, J.L.: Lymphosarcoma in a mare and review of cases at the Ontario Veterinary College. Can. Vet. J., 14:149–153, 1973.

Nielsen, S.W.: Spontaneous hematopoietic neoplasms of the domestic cat. Natl. Cancer Inst., Monograph No. 32, Hematopoietic Neoplasms. Presented at Symp. on Comp. Morph. of Hemat. Neoplasms, AFIP, Wash., D.C., March 11 & 12, 1968.

O'Gara, R.W., Adamson, R.H., Kelly, M.G., and Dalgard, D.W.: Neoplasms of the hematopoietic system in nonhuman primates: report of one spontaneous tumor and two leukemias induced by procarbazine. J. Natl. Cancer Inst., 46:1121–1130, 1971.

O'Gara, R.W., and Adamson, R.H.: Spontaneous and induced neoplasms in nonhuman primates. In Pathology of Simian Primates, edited by R.N. T-W. Fiennes. New York, S. Karger, 1972, pp. 191–238.

Onions, D.E.: B and T cells in canine lymphosarcoma. Vet. Rec., 97:108, 1975.

Page, R.C., Schectman, L., Ammons, W.F., and Dillingham, L.: Spontaneous malignant lymphoma in a New World primate. Vet. Pathol., 11:52–59, 1974.

Port, C.D., and Richter, W.R.: Eosinophilic leukemia in a Syrian hamster. Vet. Pathol., 14:283–286, 1977.

Rabin, H., et al.: Rhesus monkey lymphosarcoma. Study of one case. In Medical Primatology, Part III, edited by E.I. Goldsmith, and J. Moor-Jankowski. Basel, Karger, 1972, pp. 169–175.

Rabin, H., et al.: Studies on spontaneous lymphosarcomas of rhesus monkeys. In Vitro, 7:257–258, 1972.

Ragan, H.A., Hackett, P.L., and Dagle, G.E.: Acute myelomonocytic leukemia manifested as myelophthisic anemia in a dog. J. Am. Vet. Med. Assoc., 169:421–425, 1976.

Rangan, S.R.S., Calvert, R.C., and Vitols, K.: Fibrillar bundles in canine lymphosarcomas: an ultrastructural study. J. Ultrastruct. Res., 36:425–436, 1971.

Reed, C., et al.: Polycythemia vera in a cat. J. Am. Vet. Med. Assoc., 157:85–91, 1970.

Rhim, J.S., and Green, I.: Guinea pig L₂C leukemia: immunological, virological, and clinical aspects. Fed. Proc., 36:2247–2332, 1977.

Richter, C.B., Estes, P.C., and Tennant, R.F.W.: Spontaneous stem cell leukemia in young Sprague-Dawley rats. Lab. Invest., 26:419–428, 1972.

Ripps, C.R., and Hurvitz, A.I.: Myeloproliferative disorder in two cats: cytogenetic studies. Am. J. Vet. Res., 32:93–98, 1971.

Schneider, P., and Bilerach, F.R.G.: Malignant lymphoma in a Rhesus monkey: light and electron microscopic investigations. Vet. Pathol., 11:449, 1974.

Schultz, D.R., and Yunis, A.A.: Immunoblastic lymphadenopathy with mixed cryoglobinemia. N. Engl. J. Med., 292:8–12, 1975.

Shepard, V.J., Dodds-Laffin, W.J., and Laffin, R.J.: Gamma A myeloma in a dog with defective hemostasis. J. Am. Vet. Med. Assoc., 160:1121–1127, 1972.

Sheriff, D., and Newlands, R.W.: A case of foetal leukaemia in a calf. Vet. Rec., 98:174, 1976.

Shifrine, M., Chrisp, C.E., Wilson, F.D., and Heffernon, U.: Lysozyme (Muramidase) activity in canine myelogenous leukemia. Am. J. Vet. Res., 34:695–696, 1973.

Sonoda, M., and Marshak, R.R.: Electron microscopic observations on the mononuclear cells in the peripheral blood of the clinically normal and lymphosarcoma cows. Jpn. J. Vet. Res., *18*:9–20, 1970.

Squire, R.A., et al.: Clinical and pathologic study of canine lymphoma: clinical staging, cell classification, and therapy. J. Natl. Cancer Inst., *51*:565–574, 1973.

Stowell, R.E., Smith, E.K., Espana, C., and Nelson, V.G.: Outbreak of malignant lymphoma in Rhesus monkeys. Lab. Invest., *25*:476–479, 1971.

Tennant, B., et al.: Familial polycythemia in cattle. J. Am. Vet. Med. Assoc., *150*:1493–1509, 1967.

Ubertini, T.R.: Etiological study of a lymphosarcoma in a domestic rabbit. J. Natl. Cancer Inst., *48*:1507–1509, 1972.

Weiden, P.L., Storb, R., and Tsoi, M.S.: Marrow origin of canine alveolar macrophages. J. Reticuloendothel. Soc., *17*:342–345, 1975.

Wells, G.A.H.: Hodgkin's disease-like lesions in the dog. J. Pathol., *112*:5–10, 1974.

THE CIRCULATING BLOOD

Anemia

Anemia is defined as a reduction below normal of the number of erythrocytes and/or hemoglobin concentration per unit volume of blood. With rare exception, anemia is not a primary disease, but rather develops secondary to another disorder. For example, anemia following the rupture of an aortic aneurysm is secondary to the primary disease of the aorta; and anemia following lead poisoning is secondary to the toxic effects of lead and only represents one facet of the primary disease. Anemia, therefore, is usually a sign of another disorder and as such, the term does not represent a specific diagnosis. Anemia does, however, lead to the development of clinical signs which are secondary to the anemia. In chronic anemia, these include pallor of the mucous membranes, cardiac hypertrophy, and dyspnea. Edema may occur secondary to loss of plasma proteins in blood loss anemia. In anemia resulting from acute massive hemorrhage, the clinical signs are referable to those of hemorrhagic shock.

Anemias can be classified as to their cause and on the basis of morphologic characteristics of the erythrocytes. Obviously an etiologic classification is more meaningful and useful in that anemia is a secondary lesion, but morphologic characteristics are often extremely helpful in ascertaining the primary disorder.

Morphologic Classification

Two features of the red blood cell are used to classify an anemia on a morphologic basis—their size and their hemoglobin content. The size is expressed as **mean corpuscular volume (MCV),** which is determined by dividing the packed cell volume (PCV) in per cent by the erythrocyte count in millions per cu mm and multiplying by 10. The answer is expressed in cubic microns. For example for a PCV of 42% and an erythrocyte count of 6,000,000/mm^3, the MCV is 70 cu μ

$$\left(\frac{42}{6} \times 10 = 70\right).$$

The hemoglobin content is expressed as the **mean corpuscular hemoglobin concentration (MCHC),** which is determined by dividing the hemoglobin in grams per 100 ml of blood by the PCV in per cent and multiplying by 100. The answer is expressed as per cent hemoglobin per cell. For example, for a hemoglobin of 14 gm% and a PCV of 42, the MCHC is 33.3%

$$\left(\frac{14}{42} \times 100 = 33.3\right).$$

Based on MCV and MCHC, anemias can be classified as macrocytic, normocytic, or microcytic and either normochromic or hypochromic. Hyperchromic anemias do not exist in that there is a limit to the percentage of hemoglobin that can exist in an erythrocyte. This is generally accepted as 33.3% (normochromic). However, an abnormally large erythrocyte in a macrocytic anemia may contain more hemoglobin by weight than a cell of normal size, even though both are normochromic. The amount of hemoglobin in micromicrograms per erythrocyte is termed **mean corpuscular hemoglobin (MCH)** and is calculated by dividing hemoglobin in grams per 100 ml of blood by erythrocytes in millions per cu mm and multiplying by 10. As example, for a 14 gm% hemoglobin and an erythrocyte count of 6,000,000/mm³, the MCH is 23.3 micro-micrograms $\left(\frac{14}{6} \times 10 = 23.3\right)$. However, in the classification of anemias MCH is not used to determine hypochromasia or normochromasia.

Macrocytic anemias are most frequent following acute blood loss or acute hemolysis. The outpouring of less mature erythrocytes (reticulocytes) in response to the anemia accounts for the increase in MCV. These cells are usually hypochromic. Macrocytic normochromic anemias result from deficiency of vitamin B_{12}, folic acid, and niacin.

Normocytic normochromic anemias are the most frequently encountered anemias in animals. They result from depression of erythrogenesis and are, therefore, often referred to as aplastic anemia. Neoplastic diseases, irradiation, and certain toxicities may produce this form of anemia.

Microcytic hypochromic anemia is the classical iron deficiency anemia or "tired blood" to the modern generation. It may follow dietary deficiency of iron or chronic blood loss. Nutritional deficiencies of copper and pyridoxine also produce microcytic hypochromic anemias. Copper is necessary for the utilization of iron in the production of hemoglobin.

Other Features of Anemia

While the enumeration of erythrocytes, the determination of hemoglobin, and the calculation of MCV and MCHC are the correct and certain way to establish the presence or absence of anemia, certain other signs afford strong presumptive evidence of the disorder. In the blood film, or smear, stained as for making the white-cell differential count, anemic blood is likely to show one or several of the following changes: In **anisocytosis,** the erythrocytes are not of

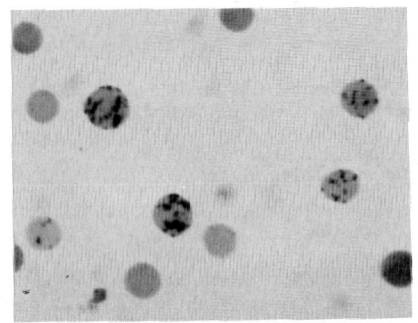

Fig. 22–5. Reticulocytosis following acute blood loss in a rhesus monkey (*Macaca mulatta*). (Courtesy of New England Regional Primate Research Center, Harvard Medical School.)

sufficiently uniform size, some are markedly larger than others. One should observe by practice how much variation occurs in normal blood, which is not very much. In **poikilocytosis,** some of the erythrocytes have bizarre and abnormal shapes, being elongated, angular, ovoid or irregularly distorted. The blood film may show occasional **nucleated erythrocytes.** These cells, because of the abnormal demand for replenishment of losses in the circulating blood, were hurried out of the bone marrow before they were completely mature. By a somewhat similar mechanism, **rubriblasts** occasionally are found in the blood smear, although normally they never leave the bone marrow. In **basophilic stippling,** minute dark specks appear in the erythrocyte, usually several or many in one cell. This feature is especially common following acute blood loss in cattle and sheep. In **polychromatophilia,** the erythrocytes do not stain uniformly, either as one is compared to another or within the boundaries of the same cell. One should be cautious, however, in attaching significance to paleness in cells which take a weak, but uniform stain. Polychromatophilic erythrocytes are generally reticulocytes which have entered the peripheral blood in response to blood loss and are evidence of active erythrogenesis.

Other evidences of anemia to be found in the tissues include hyperplasia of the bone marrow, a proliferation of red marrow in places where fatty marrow is normal for a given age. Sections of spleen or liver may rarely show erythropoietic centers in severe and prolonged anemia, these organs regaining some of the hematopoietic functions which they had during embryonic life. Such hematopoietic centers consist of a variety of hyperchromatic cells which are essentially myeloblasts, but which may be confused with foci of inflammatory leukocytes. The finding of nucleated erythrocytes in these collections of dark cells is the needed assurance as to their true nature. Megakaryocytes may also be present in these foci. Extramedullary hematopoiesis is not always indicative of a response to anemia. In most species, it is normal for varying periods of time in the liver and spleen and in certain animals such as rodents, hematopoiesis occurs in the spleen throughout life.

In certain hemolytic anemias denaturation and precipitation of hemoglobin results in the occurrence of supravitally stainable, refractile, purplish granules near the erythrocyte membrane known as **Heinz bodies.**

Gross Appearance. The mucous membranes are unusually pale during life. After death, the same is seen to be true of these membranes and the tissues generally. At autopsy, the blood may be noticeably pale and watery, but one must not let his enthusiasm run away with his judgment in this observation. Distinct gray dots in the liver may possibly be hematopoietic centers, although they are much more likely to be minute foci of necrosis. The hyperplastic bone marrow is, of course, a gross, as well as a microscopic, observation. With the exception of the last, all these gross indications of anemia are equivocal and have led many observers into error.

Causes. Like our bank accounts, the body's store of erythrocytes can be depleted either because of too heavy withdrawals or through failure of replenishment. Anemia can result from loss or destruction of excessive numbers of circulating erythrocytes or from functional failure of the hematopoietic tissue of the bone marrow. On the basis of the causative mechanism, anemias can be classified under five types.

Hemorrhagic Anemia

Hemorrhagic anemia results from severe hemorrhages. Acute hemorrhagic anemia is that which follows single or multiple severe hemorrhages. The color and cell-volume indices are normal. As stated under the subject of hemorrhage, regeneration is complete in a month or 6 weeks. In addition to traumatic causes, acute bleeding may accompany idiopathic thrombocytopenic purpura, sweet clover and warfarin poisoning, bracken fern poisoning, and poisoning from trichlorethylene-extracted soybean oil meal.

Chronic hemorrhagic anemia results from continued loss of blood in a series of small hemorrhages. The hemorrhages may be due to unhealed ulcers, such as the human peptic ulcer, but in animals they are much more frequently due to heavy infestations with blood-sucking parasites of which hookworms, the stomach worm of ruminants, *Hemonchus contortus,* and the intestinal strongyles of the horse are outstanding. This type of anemia tends to be hypochromic and slightly macrocytic or normocytic. Poikilocytosis is prominent, as is hyperplasis of the bone marrow. After some time, iron stores of the body approach exhaustion, and this type of anemia becomes the microcytic anemia of iron deficiency. Hemophilia and vitamin C deficiency also result in chronic hemorrhagic anemia.

Hemolytic Anemia

Hemolytic anemia results from excessive destruction of the circulating erythrocytes, occurring within the blood stream. Accompanying disturbances which assist in identifying this type of anemia are hemolytic icterus, which may be detected by a high bilirubin level in the blood as well as by the physical signs, hemoglobinuria in the acute forms, and, in more chronic forms, stimulation of the bone marrow, shown in the blood picture by nucleated red cells and reticulocytes.

The causes are infectious, toxic, and immunologic. They include several infections of the erythrocytes themselves such as (1) piroplasmosis, (2) anaplasmosis, (3) eperythrozoonosis of swine and cattle, (4) hemobartonellosis of dogs and cats, (5) malaria of humans, monkeys, and birds. Among the piroplasmoses are not only the North American tick fever caused by *Babesia (Piroplasma) bigemina,* now extinct in the United States, but also similar tick-borne infections caused by other species of *Babesia,* and also piroplasmoses in other species of hosts, particularly the dog. (6) Certain viral diseases, such as equine infectious anemia, also destroy erythrocytes. (7) The trypanosomiases destroy large numbers of erythrocytes, presumably by the action of toxins; in dourine the red-cell count is said to reach a figure as low as one-tenth of the normal. Several acute bacterial infections, including those due to (8) *Streptococcus "hemolyticus,"* (9) *Clostridium hemolyticum bovis,* (10) *Clostridium welchii,* and (11) *Leptospirae* cause rapid destruction of erythrocytes and severe anemia, although this aspect of the disease is likely to be overshadowed by more startling symptoms and lesions. The same may be said about most (12) snake venoms. Certain chemical poisons have a similar effect, including (13) potassium and sodium chlorate (used to sterilize the soil of weeds and sometimes eaten by cattle), (14) lead, usually as a chronic poisoning, and (15) chronic copper poisoning, formerly known as ictero-hemoglobinuria of sheep. (16) Ricin, the toxic principle of castor beans, (17) phenylhydrazine, and, to a lesser extent, (18) saponin are other strongly hemolytic poisons. (19) The anemia which often accompanies poisoning by kale and rape is believed to be of hemolytic origin.

To this list of causes of hemolytic anemia should be added what is best called **hemolytic disease of the newborn,** also known as **erythroblastosis fetalis,** and **neonatal isoerythrolysis.** This type of hemolytic anemia is discussed further elsewhere in this chapter.

Autoimmune hemolytic anemia represents another immunologic hemolytic anemia. Well known for years in man, and more recently in dogs, this disease results from the failure of an individual to recognize "self" with the formation of antibodies against autogenous tissues. Autoimmune diseases are treated in greater detail elsewhere.

Deficiency Anemias

These can be caused by deficiencies of several compounds or vitamins.

(1) Deficiency of Iron: Anemia caused by a deficiency of iron compounds in the diet, or rarely perhaps by defective assimilation of that element, is rather common in the human family and is a form easily understood, since hemoglobin cannot be made unless the elementary ingredients are available. It may be for this reason that many of us, when we think of how a case of anemia might be caused, think first of iron.

The disorder is rather frequent in nursing pigs born in the winter in cold climates, for under those circumstances the sow and her litter often spend the first several weeks in a hog house with a concrete or other type of floor. If pigs can have access to the soil their rooting will, in almost any locality, provide the minute amount of iron which is necessary. Swine management systems, designed to prevent infection by helminths and microorganisms, do not allow access to soil and therefore require that some source of iron be provided. Without this or some artificial source of the element, deficiency anemia is likely to develop, for mother's milk, the much heralded "perfect food," does not contain adequate amounts of iron.

This is the traditional example of hypochromic, microcytic anemia. Poikilocytosis is also prominent.

Anemia reported to result from the (experimental) feeding of certain kinds of raw fish (coal-fish, *Gadus virens,* and raw whiting, *G. merlangus,* and not other kinds) to mink was prevented by cooking the fish and cured by feeding 16 mg of organic iron per week.

(2) Deficiency of Copper: Minute traces of copper are also essential to avoid deficiency anemia. Natural deficiency is not common in that most soils contain an adequate amount of this element. However, usual amounts of copper become insufficient in the presence of excessive molybdenum. Copper is necessary for hematopoiesis by virtue of the fact that it is required for the proper utilization of iron in the production of hemoglobin. As in iron deficiency, the anemia is microcytic hypochromic.

(3) Deficiency of Cobalt: This deficiency is only of concern in ruminant species. Ruminants enjoy the unique position of not requiring a dietary source of B vitamins including vitamin B_{12}. Instead, they depend upon the rumen flora which synthesize these essential metabolites. Synthesis obviously cannot proceed without certain basic raw ingredients. Cobalt being an integral component of vitamin B_{12} (cobalamin) is therefore a dietary requirement for the ruminant and deficiency of this mineral is in essence a vitamin B_{12} deficiency.

(4) Vitamin B_{12} Deficiency: This results in a macrocytic normochromic anemia. Deficiency of this vitamin is the basic defect of cobalt deficiency of ruminants. It is required in erythropoiesis for normal development and maturation of erythrocytes, although its exact mechanism of action is not understood. Deficiency is not a commonly encountered clinical problem.

(5) Folic acid deficiency also results in a macrocytic anemia. Although it is essential for maturation of erythrocytes, an understanding of its exact biochemical function is still incomplete. The actions of vitamin B_{12} and folic acid in erythropoiesis are closely related.

(6) Pyridoxine Deficiency: Experimentally induced in dogs, cats, and swine, this deficiency results in a microcytic hypochromic anemia. This is the prototype of **sideroblastic anemia,** described in animals and men. Siderotic cells are erythroid cells which contain granules of Prussian-blue reactive material recognizable under the light microscope. These granules may be identified in bone marrow in normoblasts (sideroblasts), reticulocytes (reticulatedsiderocytes), and in erythrocytes (siderocytes). Ultrastructurally, these granules may be seen to consist of two types. The first consists of cytoplasmic aggregates of ferritin, usually without a limiting membrane. These are normal structures which occur in metabolic processes involving ferritin. Almost none of these cells reach the circulation except in situations involving rapid blood production.

The second type of siderotic cells, distinguished by electron microscopy, contain granules of iron, not in the form of ferritin, localized within mitochondria. These cells are part of a defective heme synthesis found in sideroblastic anemias of man and animals. In addition to pyridoxine-deficiency, a natural hereditary anemia of mice is known among the sideroblastic anemias. This disease of mice (Grüneberg, 1941) was the first in which the siderocyte was recognized.

(7) Deficiencies of riboflavin, ascorbic acid, vitamin E (alpha-tocopherol), and selenium may also result in anemia in susceptible species: In the case of ascorbic acid (vitamin C) human and nonhuman primates and guinea pigs are susceptible to scurvy and the associated anemia. Human infants and certain nonhuman primates (*Macaca fascicularis* and *Aotus trivirgatus*) develop anemia due to insufficient selenium and alpha-tocopherol. Both of

these substances contribute to the stability of plasma membranes, and their absence is believed to result in disintegration of the membranes of red blood cells.

(8) Pernicious Anemia: While this type of anemia may be chiefly of academic importance in veterinary medicine, the monumental achievements of Whipple (1935), Peabody (1927), and Minot and Murphy (1926), in solving the riddle of human pernicious anemia is worth the attention of anyone in the medical sciences. When Hilton A. Smith was in college, a needy student could replenish his finances by selling a pint of his blood to be used as a transfusion to keep alive some unfortunate person afflicted with pernicious anemia. Then came the discovery that the liver (of man or beast) contained a substance, the "erythrocyte-maturing factor," which, if continuously provided, would relieve the patient of all his symptoms. The demand for beef livers became such that liver changed from what was almost a waste-product to one of the more highly priced cuts of meat.

Eating 2 pounds of raw liver a day had its disadvantages but, fortunately, scientists soon learned how to make concentrated extracts, which could be injected at intervals. It was also learned that the mysterious "erythrocyte-maturing factor" in the liver is a storage product made by the action of an unidentified fraction of the gastric juice upon protein (of animal origin) in the food. Vitamin B_{12} is now known to be the essential constituent of the protein, and to become the erythrocyte-maturing factor upon absorption. Pernicious anemia, macrocytic and normochromic, results when this chain is broken. Usually the fault is failure of the stomach to provide its contribution, the "intrinsic factor," in the gastric juice. Many such stomachs have very atrophic glands and secrete almost no gastric juice (achylia gastrica); in others, only the hydrochloric acid is demonstrably absent (achlorhydria). The intrinsic factor is a glycoprotein secreted by parietal cells, which binds to vitamin B_{12}, creating a stable complex that is absorbed in the ileum. Occasionally, the chain is broken through shortage of the "extrinsic factor," apparently through failure of assimilation in certain chronic diarrheic diseases such as sprue or an actual dietary lack of animal protein, as in pellagra. Rarely the liver is so badly damaged, usually cirrhotic, that it fails in its part of the process, which is to serve as a storage reservoir for the finished erythrocyte-maturing substance.

Humans have an anemia of the same macrocytic type when parasitized by the tapeworm *Diphyllobothrium latum*, apparently because of impaired assimilation of the extrinsic factor. Perhaps the anemia which dogs show when harboring this worm represents a parallel condition, although the presence of a hemolytic toxin has been reported. Beyond this, human pernicious anemia appears to have no counterpart in animals.

Toxic Aplastic Anemias

In aplastic anemia (meaning no growth), the hematopoietic tissues of the bone marrow are injured in such a way that their ability to produce erythrocytes is impaired or destroyed. There is nothing remarkable about the size, shape, or color of the cells which remain in the circulating blood during their life span. There is an absence of normoblasts, megaloblasts, reticulated erythrocytes, and polychromasia (basophilic staining of the cytoplasm approaching that of early myeloid cells), all of which are signs of active erythropoiesis in the marrow. The formation of the granulocytic leukocytes is also depressed, leading to more or less severe **agranulocytosis.** The bone marrow in aplastic anemia is predominantly fatty, with scattered islands of hematopoietic cells, or sometimes it is sclerotic. Myelopoiesis is utterly destroyed in severe cases of feline panleukopenia.

Causes. To the extent that they are known, the causes are either toxic radiations or toxic substances brought to the marrow cells in the circulating blood. These latter include benzol poisoning, which is the classical example, trinitrotoluene and, in the case of hypersensitized humans at least, the sulfonamides. A number of proprietary medicines highly advertised for human self-medication are reported to be almost equally toxic. The Bracken fern owes some of its poisonous effects to production of toxic aplastic anemia, as does poisoning by trichlorethylene-extracted soybean meal. Irradiation, whether by x-rays, radium, or the more recently developed radioactive isotopes, is highly destructive of the hematopoietic tissues and this action is the chief reason that significant dosages are lethal. Anemia from an imperfectly understood disorder of hematopoiesis occurs in association with nephritis and uremia, apparently through direct toxic action of the retained waste products. Interference with the production in the kidney of erythropoietin has been reported as the explanation. Anemia develops in various chronic infections apparently because of the effects of toxins upon the mechanism of formation of hemoglobin. Neoplastic diseases may also result in a selective depression of erythrogenesis.

Myelophthisic Anemia (myelo, the marrow; phthisis, a wasting disease)

This type of anemia results from physical destruction of the erythropoietic tissue, usually from its replacement by metastatic tumor tissues. Various carcinomas are prone to fill the marrow cavities with neoplastic tissue in their advanced stages, leaving no room for the normal tissue, which undergoes pressure atrophy and pressure necrosis. This also applies to the anemia which usually accompanies leukemia and malignant lymphoma. Os-

teopetrosis is similarly destructive to the marrow space.

Significance and Effect of Anemia

Anoxia of the tissues is the most important product of anemia. This leads to fatty change of the myocardium, liver, and other susceptible organs and even necrosis. It explains the principal symptoms of rapid and perhaps irregular pulse, shortness of breath, and muscular weakness. In hemolytic anemia, the spleen contains much phagocytized hemosiderin. A tendency toward hemorrhage, which is characteristic of anemia, can presumably be explained on the basis of anoxic damage to capillary endothelium. When edema accompanies anemia, it is conceivably related to increased permeability, but in hemorrhagic anemias, protein loss is also contributory and, in those cases which go with helminthiasis the continued drain of erythrocytes offers some explanation. Removal of the cause cures anemia except in the case of the toxic aplastic anemias, where the changes soon become irreversible.

In perusing the causes of hemolytic anemia, it is noted that they largely duplicate the list given for hemolytic icterus. It is obvious that if erythrocytes are hemolyzed excessively, there tends to be both a shortage of erythrocytes and an accumulation of the products of their destruction. If the rate surpasses the rate at which the liver can eliminate bilirubin, jaundice will result. If the rate of erythrocytic destruction exceeds the capacity of the reticulo-endothelium to convert hemoglobin to bilirubin, hemoglobinemia results, and then hemoglobinuria, as the excess is excreted in the urine.

One characteristic lesion of anoxia in the liver is paracentral necrosis.

Ausman, L.M., and Hayes, K.C.: Vitamin E deficiency anemia in Old and New World monkeys. Am. J. Clin. Nutr., 27:1141–1151, 1974.
Ausman, L., Gallina, D., and Camitta, B.: Hypoplas-

tic anemia in infant squirrel monkeys fed low soy diets. Fed. Proc., 35:502, 1976.

Cartwright, G.E., and Deiss, A.: Sideroblasts, siderocytes, and sideroblastic anemia. N. Engl. J. Med., 292:185–193, 1975.

Cramer, D.V., and Lewis, R.M.: Reticulocyte response in the cat. J. Am. Vet. Med. Assoc., 160:61–67, 1972.

Fox, A.E., and Plescia, O.J.: Viral etiology of autoimmune hemolytic anemia. Fed. Proc., 31:765, 1972.

Giles, R.C., Berman, A., Hildebrandt, P.K., and McCaffrey, R.P.: Use of Fe for sheep erythrocyte kinetic studies. Am. J. Vet. Res., 38:535–538, 1977.

Grünberg, H.: The anemia of the flex-tailed mice (Mus musculus L.). II. Siderocytes. J. Genet., 44:246–271, 1942.

Harvey, J.W., and Kornick, H.P.: Phenazopyridine toxicosis in the cat. J. Am. Vet. Med. Assoc., 169:327–331, 1976.

Helgebostad, A., and Martinsons, E.: Nutritional anemia in mink. Nature, 181:1660–1661, 1958.

Jain, N.C., and Keeton, K.S.: Scanning electron microscopy of Heinz bodies in feline erythrocytes. Am. J. Vet. Res., 36:1691–1696, 1975.

Lokhorst, H.M., and Breukink, H.J.: Auto-immune hemolytic anemia in two horses. Tijdschr. Diergeneeskd., 100:752–757, 1975.

Lombardi, M.H.: Plasma iron-59 clearance and plasma iron turnover rate in dogs. Am. J. Vet. Res., 34:1437–1440, 1973.

Mackenzie, C.P.: Idiopathic (acquired) haemolytic anaemia in the dog. Vet. Rec., 85:356–361, 1969.

Maede, Y., and Nigi, H.: A case of megaloblastic anemia in the gibbon (Hylobates hoolock). Jpn. J. Vet. Res., 19:81–84, 1971.

Martinovich, D., and Woodhouse, D.A.: Postparturient haemoglobinuria in cattle: A Heinz body haemolytic anaemia. NZ Vet. J., 19:259–263, 1971.

Mauk, A.G., Whelan, H.T., Putz, G.R., and Taketa, F.: Anemia in domestic cats: effect on hemoglobin components and whole blood oxygenation. Science, 185:447–449, 1974.

Minot, G.R., and Murphy, W.P.: Treatment of pernicious anemia by a special diet. J. Am. Med. Assoc., 87:470–476, 1926.

Mizuno, N.S., et al.: The life span of thrombocytes and erythrocytes in normal and thrombocytopenic calves. Blood, 14:708–719, 1959.

Osbaldiston, G.W., Coffman, J.R., and Kruckenbuer, S.M.: Biochemical differentiation of equine anemias. J. Am. Vet. Med. Assoc., 157:322–325, 1970.

Peabody, F.W.: Pathology of the bone marrow in pernicious anemia. Am. J. Pathol., 3:179–202, 1927.

Penny, R.H.C., Carlisle, C.H., Prescott, C.W., and Davidson, H.A.: Further observations on the effect of chloramphenicol on the haemopoietic system of the cat. Br. Vet. J., 126:453–458, 1970.

Pond, W.G., Walker, E.F., Jr., and Kirtland, D.: Cadmium-induced anemia in growing pigs: protective effect of oral or parenteral iron. J. Anim. Sci., 36:1122–1124, 1973.

Schalm, O.W., and Ling, G.V.: Hematologic characteristics of autoimmune hemolytic anemia in the dog. Calif. Vet., 23:19–24, 1969.

Schechter, R.D., Schalm, O.W., and Kaneko, J.J.: Heinz body hemolytic anemia associated with the use of urinary antiseptics containing methylene blue in the cat. J. Am. Vet. Med. Assoc., 162:37–44, 1973.

Shull, R.M., Bunch, S.E., Maribei, J., and Spaulding, G.L.: Spur cell anemia in a dog. J. Am. Vet. Med. Assoc., 173:978–982, 1978.

Siddons, R.C.: The experimental production of vitamin B_{12} deficiency in the baboon (Papio cynocephalus). Br. J. Nutr., 32:219–228, 1974.

Simpson, C.F.: The ultrastructure of Heinz bodies in horse, dog, and turkey erythrocytes. Cornell Vet., 61:228–238, 1971.

Venn, J.A.J., and Davies, E.T.: Piglet anaemia. Vet. Rec., 77:1004–1005, 1965.

Watson, A.D.J., Duff, B.C., and Allan, G.S.: Erythrocyte aplasia in a dog. Aust. Vet. J.,51:94–96,1975.

Weide, K.D., and Twiehaus, M.J.: Hematological studies of normal, ascarid-infected, and hog cholera-vaccinated swine. Am. J. Vet. Res., 20:562–567, 1959.

Weiden, P.L., and Baese, R.M.: Hemolytic anemia in agammaglobulinemic chickens: a model of autoimmune disease in immune deficiency. J. Immunol., 107:1004–1013, 1971.

Whipple, G.H.: Hemoglobin regeneration as influenced by diet and other factors. Nobel Prize Lecture. J. Am. Med. Assoc., 104:791–793, 1935.

Wolcott, G.J., Valentine, J.A., and Cebul, R.D.: Induction of anaemia in monkeys. Lab. Anim., 7:297–303, 1973.

Hereditary Anemia

Genetically determined defects in erythropoiesis or in viability of red blood cells result in anemias that may be considered as distinct entities. The effects of the anemia are not significantly different from those resulting from anemia due to other causes. A brief description of these anemias will follow, using the gene-designation to identify them.

Hertwig's anemia of the mouse (an, autosomal recessive, chromosome 4, linkage group VIII) is a macrocytic anemia of varying severity, depending upon the genetic background. It results from defective hemopoiesis and is manifest by the twelfth day of gestation. It is accompanied by leukopenia.

Tail short anemia of the mouse (Ts, autosomal dominant, unknown linkage group) is associated with short, kinked tails, and other skeletal anomalies. Deficient hemopoiesis is demonstrable in the yolk sac at 8 days of gestation. The prenatal anemia is thought to result in other abnormalities.

Steel, Steel-Dickie, Grizzle-belly, and **Sooty** are names used to identify four allelic genes in the mouse (Sl, Sl^d, Sl^{ab}, Sl^{so}, autosomal recessive, linkage group IV), each causing similar defects. Homozygotes are white, infertile, black-eyed, and anemic. The hemopoietic cells appear to be normal because they reproduce and differentiate normally when transferred into mice with Dominant, Spotting (W^b). On the other hand neither normal or W cells will cure the anemia of steel mice. The defect appears not to be in the stem cells but in their environment.

Dominant Spotting in the mouse (W, W^v, W^b, W^j, and W^a, chromosome 5, linkage group XVII) is made up of five autosomal recessive alleles at the W locus; any two alleles result in severe macrocytic, hypoplastic anemia. Hemopoiesis is deficient in the liver, and the severity of the anemia depends upon the genetic background and genotype. The mutant mice are sterile and have black eyes and white hair. The names and symbols of these five alleles are: Dominant Spotting (W); Viable Dominant spotting (W^v); Ballantyne's spotting (W^b); Jay's dominant spotting (W^j), and Ames dominant spotting (W^a). Increasing degrees of anemia may be demonstrated in these genotypes: $W/+$, $W^j/+$, W^v/W^v, W/W^v, W/W, W/W^j, and W^j/W^j. Transfusion of normal or *steel* mouse bone marrow cells into mice affected with Dominant Spotting, cures their anemia, indicating that the stem cells are likely to be defective. Erythropoietic cells are not able to respond to erythropoietin stimulation.

Diminutive in the mouse (dm, chromosome 2, linkage group V, autosomal recessive) is a microcytic anemia which occurs in mice with small body size, short kinked tails, accessory ribs, and presacral vertebrae, malformed vertebrae, and fused ribs.

Microcytic in the mouse (mk, autosomal recessive) results in a microcytic, hypochromic anemia and is associated with anomalies of the skin.

Flex-tailed in the mouse (f, autosomal recessive, chromosome 13, linkage group XIV) is associated with siderocytic anemia. This disease led to the identification of siderocytes for the first time (Grüneberg, 1942). The anemia is transient and is associated with axial skeletal deformity and white spotting on the belly. The anemia is most severe on the fifteenth day of gestation, still severe at birth, but absent by 2 weeks of age. The percentage of siderocytes among the red blood cells may reach 80%, significantly higher than in normal mice, which have about 5% siderocytes. The defect is one of fetal hepatic hemopoiesis; the capacity of fetal (f/f) erythroblasts to incorporate iron into hemoglobin is delayed but eventually becomes normal. The capacity of fetal but not adult reticulocytes is impaired. The defect appears to be identified with erythropoietic progenitors, but it is not clear whether the defect in heme synthesis is primary or secondary to abnormal erythroid differentiation.

Sex-linked anemia in the mouse (sla, sex-linked recessive, chromosome X, linkage group XX) is hypochromic anemia with reticulocytosis and apparent deficient marrow. It is manifest in hemizygous males or homozygous females. Growth is retarded in both sexes but they usually survive. This anemia results from a deficiency of iron due to faulty absorption from the intestine. Parenteral administration of iron cures the anemia which tends to disappear as the animals become older.

Studies on iron transport in everted intestinal loops indicate that intestinal epithelial cells take up iron but fail to pass it on. The excess iron is held in the epithelial cells in association with rough endoplasmic reticulum and with lysosomes, some of it in the form of ferritin. Other studies indicate a possible transfer defect in the placenta—less iron reaches the fetus in the *sla* mice than in normal controls.

Belgrade in the rat (*b*, autosomal recessive, linkage group unknown) is a severe, often lethal anemia of the rat. The red cells are quite hypochromic, containing only 5 μg of hemoglobin compared to 15 μg which is normal for rats and mice. Plasma iron values are usually high, plasma iron clearance is slower than normal, and the electrophoretic pattern of the hemoglobin is normal. Intestinal iron absorption appears to be impaired and red-cell–free erythrocyte protoporphyrin is elevated. Intracellular iron deficiency or a block in hemoglobin synthesis is suspected.

Hemoglobin deficit in the mouse (*hbd*, autosomal recessive, linkage unknown) identifies a hypochromic macrocytic anemia.

Jaundiced in the mouse (*ja*, autosomal recessive, linkage group unknown) involves intense hemolysis and is usually lethal. An intrinsic red cell defect is suspected. Anemia is detectable at 14 days gestation; jaundice appears a few hours after birth. Death occurs in the neonatal period with kernicterus, bilirubin toxicity, or anoxia. Microcytic reticulocytes and nucleated erythrocytes appear in the circulation.

Normoblastic in the mouse (*nb*, autosomal recessive, linkage group unknown) is another hemolytic anemia with an intrinsic red cell defect. Hemoglobinuria may occur.

Basenji in the dog (no gene symbol, linkage unknown, autosomal recessive) denotes an anemia limited to the Basenji breed and due to an intrinsic red cell defect (pyruvate kinase deficiency). Known also as congenital hemolytic anemia and familial anemia of Basenjis, this disease is usually recognized during the first year of life, and most dogs succumb before 3 years of age unless treated by repeated blood transfusions. The anemia is hemolytic; the erythrocytes have osmotic fragility and a diminished life span; severe reticulocytosis is conspicuous as is splenomegaly. Defective erythrocyte pyruvate kinase may be differentiated by any of several chemical methods (Standerfer, et al., 1975). Several affinities to the human disease have been described.

Spherocytosis of the mouse (*sph*, linkage group unknown, autosomal recessive) is manifest as hemolytic anemia, spherocytosis, hyperbilirubinemia, and death shortly after birth. This mutant's effects are suspected to be due to an intrinsic red cell defect.

Spherocytosis of the deer mouse (*sp*, autosomal recessive, linkage group unknown) is characterized by spherocytosis of the erythrocytes, but the effect on the host appears not to be severe or, at least, is compensated by some mechanism.

Alaska Malamute, a mutant in this breed of dogs (*dan*, autosomal recessive, linkage group unknown), identifies an anemia associated with dwarfism. The dwarfism and anemia are believed to be pleiotrophic effects of one gene. This anemia is characterized by macrocytosis, decreased MCHC, increased osmotic fragility, diminished red cell survival time, reticulocytosis, erythroid hyperplasia, and increased iron turnover. Stomatocytosis is recognized in some red cells by a linear unstained area across their center. This suggested a mouth-like orifice to those who first recognized this feature in human red blood cells. Stomatocytosis has been observed in human erythrocytes in both acquired and inherited anemias. Red blood cell concentration of sodium and water are increased in anemic dogs. Glutathione deficiency is also present. The canine anemia resembles several human hemolytic anemias with similar characteristics.

Hemolytic in the mouse (*ha*, autosomal recessive, linkage group unknown) identifies a hemolytic anemia which is present on the 14th day of gestation and at birth. Anemic newborn mice have severe neonatal jaundice and hemoglobinuria and usually die within a week. An intrinsic red cell defect is suspected.

Luxoid in the mouse (*lst,* autosomal recessive, linkage group unknown) is associated with luxation of limbs, polydactyly, and anemia. The anemia is normocytic and hemorrhagic.

Lethal Anemia in the rat (*an,* autosomal recessive, linkage unknown) identifies a microcytic and spherocytic anemia.

Fetal erythroblastic anemia in the mouse (no gene symbol, linkage group unknown) is lethal in utero and accompanied by hydrops.

Cribriform in the mouse (*cri,* autosomal recessive, chromosome 4, linkage group VIII) is a gene associated with demyelination and electrolyte disturbance, as well as macrocytic anemia.

Bannerman, R.M., Edwards, J.A., and Pinkerton, P.H.: Hereditary disorders of the red cell in animals. Prog. Hematol., 8:131–179, 1974.

Bannerman, R.M., and Edwards, J.A.: Hereditary anaemias in laboratory animals. Br. J. Haematol., 32:299–307, 1976.

Chandler, F.W., Jr., Prasse, K.W., and Callaway, C.S.: Surface ultrastructure of pyruvate kinase-deficient erythrocytes in the Basenji dog. Am. J. Vet. Res., 36:1477–1480, 1975.

Edwards, J.A., and Bannerman, R.M.: Hereditary defect of iron transport in mice with sex-linked anemia. J. Clin. Invest., 49:1869–1872, 1970.

Edwards, J.A., and Bannerman, R.M.: Animal models of human disease. Inherited hypochromic anemias of rodents. Comp. Pathol. Bull., 4:3–4, 1972.

Ewing, G.O.: Familial nonspherocytic hemolytic anemia of Basenji dogs. J. Am. Vet. Med. Assoc., 154:503–507, 1969.

Fletch, S.M., Brueckner, P.J., and Pinkerton, P.H.: Hereditary hemolytic anemia and chondrodysplasia in the dog. Fed. Proc., 32:821, 1973.

Grüneberg, H.: The anemia of flex-tailed mice (*Mus musculus*). II. Siderocytes. J. Genet., 44:246–254, 1942.

Jones, T.C.: Hereditary Disease. *In* Pathology of Laboratory Animals, edited by K. Bernischke, R.N. Garner, and T.C. Jones. New York, Springer Verlag, 1978 (2 vol).

Loeb, W.F., Bannerman, R.M., Reninger, B.F., and Johnson, A.J.: Hematologic Disorders. *In* Pathology of Laboratory Animals, edited by K. Bernischke, R.N. Garner, and T.C. Jones. New York, Springer Verlag, 1978, (2 vol).

Pinkerton, P.H., Fletch, S.M., Brueckner, P.J., and Miller, D.R.: Hereditary stomatocytosis with hemolytic anemia in the dog. Blood, 44:557–567, 1974.

Prasse, K.W., et al.: Pyruvate kinase deficiency anemia with terminal myelofibrosis and osteosclerosis in a Beagle. J. Am. Vet. Med. Assoc., 166:1170–1175, 1975.

Searcy, G.P., Miller, D.R., and Tasker, J.B.: Congenital hemolytic anemia in the Basenji dog due to erythrocyte pyruvate kinase deficiency. Can. J. Comp. Med., 35:67–70, 1971.

Standerfer, R.J., Templeton, J.W., and Black, J.A.: Anomalous pyruvate kinase deficiency in the Basenji dog. Am. J. Vet. Res., 35:1541–1544, 1974.

Standerfer, R.J., et al.: Canine erythrocyte pyruvate kinase. II. Properties of the abnormal enzyme associated with hemolytic anemia in the Basenji dog. Biochem. Genet., 13:341–351, 1975.

Tasker, J.B., Severin, G.A., Young, S., and Gillette, E.L.: Familial anemia in the Basenji dog. J. Am. Vet. Med. Assoc., 154:158–165, 1969.

Immunohemolytic Anemias

Isoimmune hemolytic anemia (erythroblastosis fetalis) has been considered. What remains to be discussed here is autoimmune hemolytic anemia. A general discussion of autoimmunity will be found in Chapter 7. Autoimmune hemolytic anemia, which has been documented in dogs (Lewis, et al., 1963, 1965) and apparently in horses (Farrelly, et al., 1966), results from an immune response directed against the animals' own erythrocytes (and other tissues). Erythrocytes coated with the autoantibody directed against them, become spherical in shape (spherocytes; spherocytosis), become more fragile, may agglutinate, and are actively destroyed by the spleen, leading to anemia. The coated erythrocytes are detected by the direct Coomb's test, which is necessary to establish the diagnosis. The Coomb's test employs a specific anti-canine-globulin (or anti-horse, anti-human, etc.), usually prepared in rabbits, which when mixed with washed erythrocytes coated with autoantibody (globulin) causes agglutination.

In the series of dogs with autoimmune hemolytic anemia reported by Lewis, the disorder had features remarkably similar to systemic lupus erythematosus in man, and the "LE cell test" (lupus induction test) also proved of diagnostic value (Lewis, 1965).

In addition to anemia and spherocytosis, peripheral blood changes consistent with active erythropoiesis are evident as well as thrombocytopenia. Other clinical and pathological features may include splenomegaly, lymphadenopathy, purpura, and glomerulonephritis. Lameness is seen in some affected dogs which may be the result of a "rheumatoid arthritis" (Lewis and Hathaway, 1967). A disease resembling lupus erythematosus also occurs in NZB/BL mice. The disease in mice and man has been suggested to be a viral infection. Ultrastructural studies of affected mice and men have revealed viral particles in tissue, but their etiological importance has not been established.

Farrelly, B.T., Collins, J.D., and Collins, S.M.: Autoimmune haemolytic anemia (AHA) in the horse. Irish Vet. J., 20:42–45, 1966.

Lewis, R.M.: Clinical evaluation of the lupus erythematosus cell phenomenon in dogs. J. Am. Vet. Med. Assoc., 147:939–943, 1965.

Lewis, R.M., et al.: A syndrome of autoimmune hemolytic anemia and thrombocytopenia in dogs. Sci. Proc. AVMA, pp 140–163, 1963.

Lewis, R.M., and Hathaway, J.E.: Canine systemic lupus erythematosus presenting with symmetrical polyarthritis. Br. J. Small Anim. Pract., 8:273–284, 1967.

Lewis, R.M., Swartz, R., and Henry, W.B.: Canine systemic lupus erythematosus. Blood, 25:143–160, 1965.

Polycythemia

Polycythemia is an excess of circulating erythrocytes. In the great majority of cases, an excessive number of erythrocytes noted in the blood-cell count is purely relative; the total number of cells is not increased, but the total volume of plasma is decreased. This is the result, ordinarily, of dehydration, the bane of the clinician, the importance and frequency of which are not always realized. Dehydration may result from severe vomiting, diarrhea, or hemorrhage, but usually it is due to the fact that the animal patient is too weak to get to its source of water. It is in such cases purely a nursing problem, but one of prime importance to the welfare and comfort of the patient. Death from disease may not be always preventable, but death from thirst should be avoided.

An absolute, rather than relative, polycythemia, also known as erythrocytosis, results from prolonged but mild anoxemia. This occurs as a feature of life in high altitudes and compensates for the fact that a "lung-full" of air at a high altitude is considerably less (by weight) than it is at sea level. A sufficient degree of anoxia to cause erythrocytosis also sometimes occurs in such diseases of the heart as patent foramen ovale and patent ductus arteriosus, as well as in severe pulmonary emphysema, fibrosis, or other disorders interfering with oxygenation of the blood.

Polycythemia vera is discussed on page 1305.

Reticulo-endotheliosis

Reticulo-endotheliosis as described by Gilmore, Gilmore, and Jones (1964) is a myeloproliferative disease of cats characterized by proliferation of undifferentiated (reticulum) cells in bone marrow, spleen, liver, and lymph nodes and their entrance into peripheral blood. The principal clinical signs are anorexia, listlessness, loss of weight, fever, splenomegaly, hepatomegaly, and enlargement of lymph nodes. Hematologic findings include anemia and usally leukocytosis. Total leukocyte counts as reported in Gilmore's series of 10 cats ranged from 6,100 to 53,000/mm^3 of blood. In each example reticulum cells accounted for up to 55% of the circulating leukocytes and up to 76.8% of cells in the bone marrow. The cells have large round red-purple eccentric nuclei with a fine chromatin pattern, a single pale-blue nucleolus and abundant dull-blue cytoplasm with azurophilic granules. There is no evidence of maturation to another cell type. The disease is rapidly progressive, leading to death in 2 to 4 weeks after clinical signs are first noted. Gross findings are dominated by marked splenomegaly and enlargement of the liver and lymph nodes. Microscopically, undifferentiated myeloid cells fill the vascular and lymphatic spaces in these organs, remaining individually discrete without forming solid sheets or invading connective tissues. Extramedullary hematopoiesis was found by Gilmore and associates in the liver, spleen, and lymph nodes.

The cause of reticulo-endotheliosis is not known. It is distinguishable from malignant lymphoma with leukemia, but no doubt the two have often been confused. Whether the disease is malignant is not clearly established. The disorder is mimicked to some extent by vitamin B_{12} and folic acid deficiency. The relation, if any, to feline leukemia viral infection has not been established. The interpretation of many reticuloproliferative diseases of man and animals vacillates between neoplastic and proliferative inflammation depending on who is doing the interpretation and the prevailing fashion. No doubt, in reticuloproliferative disorders, a broad gray zone exists between simple proliferation and malignancy.

Crow, S.E., Madewell, B.R., and Henness, A.M.: Feline reticuloendotheliosis: a report of four cases. J. Am. Vet. Med. Assoc., 170:1329–1332, 1977.

Gilmore, C.E., Gilmore, V.H., and Jones, T.C.: Reticulo-endotheliosis, a myeloproliferative disorder of cats: a comparison with lymphocytic leukemia. Pathol. Vet., 1:161–183, 1964.

Harvey, J.W., Shields, R.P., and Gaskin, J.M.: Feline myeloproliferative disease. Changing manifestations in the peripheral blood. Vet. Pathol., 15:437–448, 1978.

Purpura Hemorrhagica

Purpura hemorrhagica denotes a syndrome characterized by many hemorrhages, petechial or ecchymotic in size, in the skin and external and internal mucous membranes. In the horse, there is usually much subcutaneous edema, perhaps localized about the head or commonly in the form of numerous subcutaneous swellings several centimeters in diameter suggestive of urticaria. The cutaneous hemorrhages frequently bleed into these plaque-like collections of edema fluid. The disease is afebrile throughout most of its stormy course, of variable severity, but frequently fatal. Practically all reported cases have supervened when the patient appeared to be recovering from some infectious or necrotizing disease, such as equine strangles or other respiratory infection, often with streptococcal organisms as the cause.

The Latin word, purpura, refers merely to the purple color of the hemorrhagic spot (in a white skin). Hence, in some quarters there has been a confusing tendency to designate as "purpura" any disease characterized by multiple hemorrhages into the tissues. Such confusion can at least be avoided in veterinary medicine with its frequently encountered and usually well-defined acute hemorrhagic diseases. Classically, purpura hemorrhagica is the result of a severe deficiency of platelets in the circulating blood (thrombocytopenia). This form of purpura is appropriately termed thrombocytopenic purpura and is discussed below, but limited studies on horses with purpura hemorrhagica have usually shown no thrombocytopenia, nor defects in coagulation. Marked neutrophilia and mild icterus have been reported and in one study (King, 1949) hemorrhagic focal necroses were found in the voluntary muscles. Possibly from the resultant release of myoglobin, there were also renal lesions comparable to those seen in the "crush syndrome" of humans and experimental animals and in azoturia. The most striking feature of purpura in horses is edema of subcutaneous tissues.

That edema and hemorrhage by diapedesis, such as occurs in this disease, could result from injury to the capillaries seems self-evident. While the degree of permeability or impermeability of capillary walls has defied accurate elucidation, the concept of increased permeability in inflammation is well founded, if not understood. There is no reason to discredit the possibility of a similar state of increased permeability in equine purpura hemorrhagica, and in many examples of this disorder, such an injurious change in capillary walls must be thought to exist, for as indicated above the thrombocytopenia proves to be minor or absent.

How, then, do the non-thrombocytopenic examples of purpura hemorrhagica differ from the numerous hemorrhagic disorders attributed to infections, toxic substances, or anoxia? The identifying characteristic of purpura hemorrhagica is that it appears in company with, but late in the course of, an infection such as those mentioned, developing when convalescence had seemed to be well established. Etiologically speaking, this fact seems to tie it to a hypersensitization or anaphylaxis developing as a reaction to, but not a primary feature of, the original infection. That the manner of pathogenesis involves injury to capillary walls seems probable but is not proven. The other feature distinguishing purpura hemorrhagica from one of the primary hemorrhagic diseases is the fact that one of the latter with hemorrhagic lesions as extensive as those typically seen in purpura hemorrhagica would prove promptly fatal, probably within hours. The course of purpura hemorrhagica, even in fatal cases, is seldom less than several days.

In domestic species other than the equine, this disease is certainly rare. There are reports of purpuric lesions in swine and one of the production of such lesions in dogs by the administration of sesame oil as a vehicle for estradiol benzoate (Cruz, et al., 1945). The equine species has long shown a strong propensity for developing antibodies; just possibly the preponderance of purpura hemorrhagica in this species is a further indication for an immunologic origin for the disease.

Thrombocytopenic Purpura

A reduction in number of circulating platelets results in purpura hemorrhagica owing to a prolongation of bleeding time. Edema and hemorrhage of subcutaneous tissues, mucous membranes, and internal organs similar to equine purpura hemor-

rhagica described above characterize the clinical and pathologic findings. In animals, thrombocytopenia is most often associated with disorders which cause extensive destruction of bone marrow, such as may result from lymphomatous or other neoplastic invasion, ionizing radiations, or the various inciters of aplastic anemia (bracken fern poisoning, trichlorethylene-extracted soybean meal poisoning). Not to be overlooked as a cause of thrombocytopenia is the simple hypothesis of exhaustion of supply in the course of repeated attempts to seal leaking capillaries. Thrombocytopenia may also develop in the course of bacterial and viral infections. For example, thrombocytopenia is a regular finding in equine infectious anemia, and transient thrombocytopenia has been reported (Foster and Cameron, 1968) in sheep with experimental tick-borne fever. Tick-borne fever is usually a mild transient infection of sheep and cattle in Great Britain caused by *Rickettsia phagocytophilia*. Thrombocytopenia of unknown cause (idiopathic thrombocytopenia) is encountered on occasion in animals, but reports are few. Very possibly, certain examples of idiopathic thrombocytopenia are immunologic in origin.

Immunologic thrombocytopenia has been recognized in baby pigs, caused by maternal isoimmunization and in a horse and dogs as an autoimmune disease. The disorder in pigs which has been described in Norway, Sweden, Finland, England, and Canada is analogous to isoimmune hemolytic anemias (erythroblastosis fetalis, hemolytic disease of newborn). Following numerous pregnancies, antibodies against platelets of the offspring are developed in the sow during gestation, resulting from mating with a boar possessing platelet antigens different from those of the sow. Purpura which may lead to death develops in the pig 8 to 72 hours after birth, apparently receiving the antithrombocyte antibodies in the colostrum. In addition to the usual lesions of purpura, megakaryocytes may be absent from the bone marrow. Autoimmune hemolytic anemia with thrombocytopenia has been reported in dogs (Lewis, et al., 1963, 1965) and limited evidence suggests its occurrence in horses (Farrelly, et al., 1966).

Anderson, S., and Nielsen, R.: Pathology of isoimmune purpura thrombocytopenia in piglets. Nord. Vet. Med., 25:211–219, 1973.

Biggers, J.D., Ingram, P.L., and Murray, C.B.: Studies on equine purpura hemorrhagica. Brit. Vet. J., 105:191–200, 1949.

Brodey, R.S., and Schalm, O.W.: Hemobartonellosis and thrombocytopenic purpura in a dog. J. Am. Vet. Med. Assoc., 143:1231–1236, 1963.

Cottereau, P.: Le flux de sang du Charolais ou purpura hemorrhagique. Encycl. Vet. Period., 22:33–42, 1965.

Cruz, W.O., Da Silva, E.M., and De Mello, R.P.: Manifestaçoes purpuricas na pele em caes anemiados com benzoato de estradiol. Rev. Brazil. Biol., 5:367–376, 1945.

Farrelly, B.T., Collins, J.D., and Collins, S.M.: Autoimmune haemolytic anemia (AHA) in the horse. Irish Vet. J., 20:42–45, 1966.

Foster, W.N.M., and Cameron, A.E.: Thrombocytopenia in sheep associated with experimental tick-borne fever infection. J. Comp. Pathol., 78:251–254, 1968.

Jennings, A.R., and Highet, D.R.: Some cases of purpura haemorrhagica in the horse. Vet. J., 103:369–376, 1947.

Joshi, B.C.: An investigation of immunologic thrombocytopenia in dogs. Diss. Abs. Int., 36B:4934–4935, 1976.

King, A.S.: Studies on equine purpura haemorrhagica: morbid anatomy and histology. Br. Vet. J., 105:35–54, 1949.

Lewis, R.M., et al.: A syndrome of autoimmune hemolytic anemia and thrombocytopenia in dogs. Sci. Proc. AVMA, pp. 140–163, 1963.

Lewis, R.M., Swartz, R., and Henry, W.B.: Canine systemic lupus erythematosus. Blood, 25:143–160, 1965.

Lie, H.: Thrombocytopenic purpura in baby pigs. Clinical studies. Acta Vet. Scand., 9:285–301, 1968.

Medway, W., and Rapp, J.P.: A case of granulocytic leukemia with thrombocytopenic purpura in a dog. Cornell Vet., 52:247–260, 1962.

Saunders, C.N., and Kinch, D.A.: Thrombocytopenic purpura of pigs. J. Comp. Pathol., 78:513–523, 1968.

Saunders, C.N., Kinch, D.A., and Imlah, P.: Thrombocytopenic purpura in young pigs. Vet. Rec., 79:549–550, 1966.

Stormorken, H.R., et al.: Thrombocytopenic bleedings in young piglets due to maternal isoimmunization. Nature, 198:1116–1117, 1963.

Weiss, H.J.: Platelet physiology and abnormalities of platelet function (first of two parts). N. Engl. J. Med., 293:531–541, 1975.

Weiss, H.J.: Platelet physiology and abnormalities of platelet function (second of two parts). N. Engl. J. Med., 293:580–588, 1975.

Wilkins, R.J., Hurvitz, A.I., and Dodds-Laffin, W.J.: Immunologically mediated thrombocytopenia in the dog. J. Am. Vet. Med. Assoc., 163:277–282, 1973.

Diseases of Leukocytes

Other abnormalities of the circulating blood include excesses of leukocytes, which are **leukocytosis** if inflammatory and **leukemia** if neoplastic. An abnormally low number of leukocytes constitutes **leukopenia.** In tissues, leukocytes of one type or another participate in most inflammatory reactions and are victims of certain specific infections and poisons. Aside from these "general" degenerative inflammatory and neoplastic reactions of leukocytes, few specific diseases focus on the leukocyte.

Genetic factors have been demonstrated to control at least three diseases of animals involving the leukocytes. These are: Chediak-Higashi syndrome, cyclic neutropenia, and Pelger-Huët anomaly.

Chediak-Higashi Syndrome

Although this disorder involves many tissues and cell types, most attention has focused on abnormal granules in peripheral leukocytes, and accordingly we will briefly consider this rare syndrome under circulating blood. Described in man, cattle, mink, mice, cats, and a killer whale, the Chediak-Higashi syndrome is characterized by the presence of giant granules or cytoplasmic inclusions in neutrophils, eosinophils, basophils, monocytes, and lymphocytes, as well as in many other cell types, such as hepatocytes, renal tubular epithelium, neurons, endothelial cells, and melanocytes. Ultrastructural studies indicate that the granules are abnormal lysosomes, but their exact significance is unknown. In man, cattle, and mink the disease is inherited by an autosomal recessive gene. All affected individuals are partial albinos; in mink, the coat color of this partial albinism is known as Aleutian or "blue" and all Aleutian mink have the Chediak-Higashi syndrome. Other characteristics of the disease include photophobia (albinism), hemorrhagic tendencies, and a marked susceptibility to infections, which usually accounts for the cause of death. In mink, there is increased susceptibility to the virus of Aleutian disease, which may, of course, affect mink of any coat color.

The basis for the partial albinism seems to be the redistribution of melanin granules by the fusion of granules with lysosomes. The melanin deposits are thus in larger granules and farther apart.

The hemorrhagic tendency in mice and cattle has been related to the reduced uptake and storage of serotonin and adenosine nucleotide by the platelets of affected animals. The serotonin content of affected platelets is about 10% of normal and is associated with reduced numbers of osmiophilic bodies in the platelets. Adenosine nucleotide is reduced to about 18% of normal in platelets. The increased susceptibility to infection appears to be related to decreased chemotaxis of the leukocytes and to their diminished bactericidal capacity. Microphagocytosis appears to be normal.

The significance of the enlarged lysosomes in the distal segment of the proximal convoluted tubules has not yet been established.

Bedoya, V., Grimley, P.M., and Duque, O.: Chediak-Higashi Syndrome. Arch. Pathol., 88:340–349, 1969.

Bell, T.G., Camacho, Z., Meyers, K., and Padgett, G.: Platelet storage disease in Chediak-Higashi syndrome animals. Fed. Proc., 34:861, 1975.

Blume, R.S., Padgett, G.A., Wolff, S.M., and Bennett, J.M.: Giant neutrophil granules in the Chediak-Higashi Syndrome of man, mink, cattle, and mice. Can. J. Comp. Med., 33:271–274, 1969.

Brandt, E.J., and Swank, R.T.: The Chediak-Higashi (Beige) mutation in two mouse strains. Am. J. Pathol., 82:573–588, 1976.

Davis, W.C., Spicer, S.S., Greene, W.B., and Padgett, G.A.: Ultrastructure of bone marrow granulocytes in normal mink and mink with the homolog of the Chediak-Higashi trait of humans. I. Origin of the abnormal granules present in the neutrophils of mink with the C-HS trait. Lab. Invest., 24:303–318, 1971.

Essner, E., and Oliver, C.: A hereditary alteration in kidneys of mice with Chediak-Higashi syndrome. Am. J. Pathol., 73:217–228, 1973.

Essner, E., and Oliver, C.: Lysosome formation in hepatocytes of mice with Chediak-Higashi syndrome. Lab. Invest., 30:596–607, 1974.

Essner, E., Oliver, C., and Haimes, H.: Fate of exogenous peroxidase in renal lysosomes of mice with Chediak-Higashi syndrome. Am. J. Pathol., 77:407–422, 1974.

Gallin, J.I., Klimerman, J.A., Padgett, G.A., and Wolff, S.M.: Defective mononuclear leukocyte chemotaxis in the Chediak-Higashi syndrome of humans, mink, and cattle. Blood, 45:863–870, 1975.

Hirano, A., Zimmerman, H.M., Levine, S., and Padgett, G.A.: Cytoplasmic inclusions in Chediak-Higashi and wobbler mink. An electron microscopic study of the nervous system. J. Neuropathol. Exp. Neurol., 30:470–487, 1971.

Holland, J.M.: Serotonin deficiency and prolonged bleeding in beige mice. Proc. Soc. Exp. Biol. Med., 151:32–39, 1976.

Kramer, J.W., Davis, W.C., and Prieur, D.J.: The Chediak-Higashi syndrome of cats. Lab. Invest., 36:554–562, 1977.

Levine, S., Padgett, G.A., and Leader, R.W.: Allergic encephalomyelitis in Chediak-Higashi mink. Arch. Pathol., 82:234–241, 1966.

Lutzner, M.A., Lowrie, C.T., and Jordan, H.W.: Giant granules in leukocytes of the beige mouse. J. Hered., 58:299–300, 1967.

McGarry, M.P., Brandt, E.J., and Swank, R.T.: Eosinophil and neutrophil granulocyte exudation in the Chediak-Higashi (beige) mouse. Am. J. Pathol., 85:685–692, 1976.

Oliver, C., and Essner, E.: Formation of anomalous lysosomes in monocytes, neutrophils, and eosinophils from bone marrow of mice with Chediak-Higashi syndrome. Lab. Invest., 32:17–27, 1975.

Padgett, G.A.: Neutrophilic function in animals with the Chediak-Higashi syndrome. Blood, 29:906–915, 1967.

Padgett, G.A.: Comparative studies of the Chediak-Higashi syndrome. Am. J. Pathol., 51:553–571, 1967.

Padgett, G.A.: The Chediak-Higashi syndrome. Adv. Vet. Sci., 12:239–284, 1968.

Padgett, G.A., et al.: Comparative studies of susceptibility to infection in the Chediak-Higashi syndrome. J. Pathol. Bact., 95:509–522, 1968.

Padgett, G.A., Holland, J.M., Davis, W.C., and Henson, J.B.: The Chediak-Higashi syndrome: a comparative review. Cur. Top. Pathol., 51:175–194, 1970.

Phillips, L.L., et al.: Comparative studies on the Chediak-Higashi syndrome. Coagulation and fibrinolytic mechanisms of mink and cattle. Am. J. Vet. Clin. Pathol., 1:1–6, 1967.

Prieur, D.J., Holland, J.M., Bell, T.G., and Young, D.M.: Ultrastructural and morphometric studies of platelets from cattle with the Chediak-Higashi syndrome. Lab. Invest., 35:197–204, 1976.

Renshaw, H.W., Davis, W.C., Fundenberg, H.H., and Padgett, G.A.: Leukocyte dysfunction in the bovine homologue of the Chediak-Higashi syndrome of humans. Infect. Immun., 10:928–937, 1974.

Robison, W.G., Jr., Kuwabara, T., and Cogan, D.G.: Lysosomes and melanin granules of the retinal pigment epithelium in a mouse model of the Chediak-Higashi syndrome. Invest. Ophthalmol., 14:312–317, 1975.

Sung, J.H., and Okada, K.: Neuropathological changes in mink with Chediak-Higashi disease. J. Neuropathol. Exp. Neurol., 30:33–62, 1971.

Windhorst, D.B., and Padgett, G.A.: The Chediak-Higashi syndrome and the homologous trait in animals. J. Invest. Dermatol., 60:529–537, 1973.

Cyclic Neutropenia

Also known as "gray Collie syndrome," cyclic neutropenia is confined to the collie breed and only occurs in dogs with a gray (dark pewter gray to silver) coat color. A similar cyclic neutropenia is known in man. Not all gray collies suffer from cyclic neutropenia, a fact clearly illustrated by the studies of Ford (1969), who demonstrated that at least three types of gray or silver collies exist which are controlled by separate genes. Dominant gray or slate gray is inherited as a dominant gene and only appears if observable in one parent. Dominant gray collies are normal. Maltese gray collie pups appear in litters of nongray parents. The controlling gene is recessive, and the dogs are normal. Lethal gray which is light silvery gray (almost white) is also inherited as a recessive gene which is apparently not an allele to maltese gray. Lethal gray collies suffer from cyclic neutropenia and generally die before maturity.

As its name suggests, the outstanding characteristic of this disease is a periodic neutropenia occurring at regular intervals of 8 to 12 days. Neutrophils may completely disappear from the peripheral blood at 10.5 to 11.5 day intervals, only to reappear with a "rebound" neutrophilia. The cause of the neutropenia is apparently a failure of maturation of stem cells. The controlling mechanism is not known, nor do we have an explanation for the periodic-

ity of this failure. The dogs are extremely susceptible to infections, which if not controlled lead to their death. Whether other primary abnormalities are associated with the disease and contribute to death has not been determined. Cheville (1968) described fundic ectasia with incomplete pigmentation of the retina, maladsorption, diarrhea, and failure of maturation of the gonads as part of the picture. As a result of study of 8 gray Collies and 5 controls, he further reported (1970) clinical signs in addition to the cyclic neutropenia and gray hair color; these included diarrhea, lameness, and chronic ulceration of oral and genital mucosae.

Microscopic Lesions. Microscopic lesions included lymphoid atrophy, amyloidosis, enteritis, aseptic bone necrosis, and acute and chronic purulent inflammation in several organs. Serum albumin and gamma and alpha-2 globulins were elevated. Ultrastructural study of spleen revealed amyloid fibers deposited chiefly at the periphery of the splenic follicle and within the central artery.

The mechanism controlling this phenomenon is not clearly understood. A defect in stem cells is suspected because transplantation of affected bone marrow to a normal recipient will result in cyclic neutropenia in the recipient. Conversely, transplantation of normal marrow into a radiated affected dog results in alleviation of all the clinical signs, including the cyclic neutropenia. These studies suggest that such transplants of normal marrow to affected human patients might be effective.

Cheville, N.F.: The gray collie syndrome. J. Am. Vet. Med. Assoc., 152:620–630, 1968.

Cheville, N.F.: Amyloidosis associated with cyclic neutropenia in the dog. Blood, 31:111–114, 1968.

Cheville, N.F., Cutlip, R.C., and Moon, H.W.: Microscopic pathology of the gray collie syndrome. Cyclic neutropenia, amyloidosis, enteritis, and bone necrosis. Pathol. Vet., 7:225–245, 1970.

Dale, D.C., Brown, C.H., Carbone, P., and Wolff, S.: Cyclic urinary leukopoietic activity in gray collie dogs. Science, 173:152–153, 1971.

Dale, D.C., and Graw, R.G., Jr.: Transplantation of allogeneic bone marrow in canine cyclic neutropenia. Science, 183:83–84, 1974.

Ford, L.: Hereditary aspects of human and canine cyclic neutropenia. J. Hered., *60*:293–299, 1969.

Jones, J.B., Jones, E.S., and Lange, R.D.: Early life hematologic values of dogs affected with cyclic neutropenia. Am. J. Vet. Res., *35*:849–852, 1974.

Jones, J.B., Lange, R.D., and Jones, E.S.: Cyclic hematopoiesis in a colony of dogs. J. Am. Vet. Med. Assoc., *166*:365–367, 1975.

Jones, J.B., et al.: Canine cyclic neutropenia: erythropoietin and platelet cycles after bone marrow transplantation. Blood, *45*:213–219, 1975.

Joyce, R.A., Boggs, D.R., and Chervenick, P.A.: Neutrophil kinetics in hereditary and congenital neutropenias. N. Engl. J. Med., *295*:1385–1390, 1976.

Lange, R.D., et al.: Erythropoiesis and erythrocytic survival in dogs with cyclic hematopoiesis. Am. J. Vet. Res., *37*:331–334, 1976.

Lund, J.E., Padgett, G.A., and Ott, R.L.: Cyclic neutropenia in gray collie dogs. Blood, *29*:452–461, 1967.

Lund, J.E., Padgett, G.A., and Gorham, J.R.: Additional evidence on the inheritance of cyclic neutropenia in the dog. J. Hered., *61*:47–49, 1970.

Page, A.R., and Good, R.A.: Studies on cyclic neutropenia. Am. J. Dis. Child., *94*:623–661, 1957.

Patt, H.M., Lund, J.E., and Maloney, M.A.: Cyclic hematopoiesis in gray collie dogs: a stem-cell problem. Blood, *42*:873–884, 1973.

Renshaw, H.W., et al.: Canine granulocytopathy syndrome: neutrophil dysfunction in a dog with recurrent infections. J. Am. Vet. Med. Assoc., *166*:443–448, 1975.

Renshaw, H.W., and Davis, W.C.: Canine granulocytopathy syndrome. An inherited disorder of leukocyte function. Am. J. Pathol., *95*:731–744, 1979.

Reynolds, H.Y., Dale, D.C., Wolff, S.M., and Johnson, J.S.: Serum immunoglobulin levels in gray collies. Proc. Soc. Exp. Biol. Med., *136*:574–577, 1971.

Scott, R.E., Dale, D.C., Rosenthal, A.S., and Wolff, S.M.: Cyclic neutropenia in gray collie dogs: ultrastructural evidence for abnormal neutrophil granulopoiesis. Lab. Invest., *28*:514–526, 1973.

Weiden, P.L., et al.: Canine cyclic neutropenia: a stem cell defect. J. Clin. Invest., *53*:950–953, 1974.

Windhorst, D.B., et al.: Intestinal malabsorption in the gray collie syndrome. Fed. Proc., *26*:260, 1967.

Yang, T.J., Jones, J.B., Jones, E.S., and Lange, R.D.: Serum colony-stimulating activity of dogs with cyclic neutropenia. Blood, *44*:41–48, 1974.

Pelger-Huët Anomaly

This inherited anomaly in the development of granulocytic nuclei has been described in man, rabbit, and dog. In each species, the gene acts as an autosomal dominant, although the effects on the phenotype are varied. The anomaly is recognized in the circulating neutrophilic and eosinophilic granulocytes, which have single, indented, or bilobular nuclei rather than their normal segmented polymorphic nuclei. In man, the nuclei in the homozygous affected state are predominantly oval, spherical, and indented. In the heterozygote, bilobular nuclei are frequent. These often have the shape of pince-nez glasses. In the human patient, the anomaly has little clinical effect, but is of importance to differentiate affected cells from nonsegmented neutrophils.

Pelger-Huët Anomaly has been recognized particularly in Foxhounds. Approximately 50 to 67% of the neutrophils and eosinophils of heterozygotes have nonsegmented nuclei, and migration of these leukocytes appears to be obstructed. A slight reduction in number of pups weaned (63 vs 81%) in an outbred colony carrying the gene has been recorded. The trait is inherited as a single autosomal dominant gene in dogs, and homozygotes are reported to die at birth. It has been postulated that an abnormal substance in the serum affects lymphocytic blastogenesis. After transfusion to a normal dog, affected neutrophil leukocytes disappear from the circulation in about 5 hours. Eosinophils with the anomaly disappear from the circulation within about 30 minutes.

Bowles, C.A., Alsaker, R.D., and Wolfle, T.L.: Studies of the Pelger-Huët anomaly in Foxhounds. Am. J. Pathol., *96*:237–248, 1979.

Carper, H.A., and Hoffman, P.L.: The intravascular survival of transfused canine Pelger-Huët neutrophils and eosinophils. Blood, *27*:739–743, 1966.

Huët, G.J.: Familial anomaly of leukocytes. Nederl. T. Geneesk., *75*:5956–5959, 1931.

Klein, A., Hussar, A.E., and Bornstein, S.: Pelger-Huët anomaly of the leukocytes. N. Engl. J. Med., *253*:1057–1063, 1955.

Loeb, W.F., Bannerman, R.M., Rininger, B.F., and Johnson, A.J.: Hematologic Disorders. *In* Pathology of Laboratory Animals, edited by K. Benirschke, F.N. Garner, and T.C. Jones. New York, Springer-Verlag, 1978 (2 vol.).

Nachtsheim, H.: The Pelger anomaly in man and rabbits. J. Hered., *41*:131–137, 1950.

Pelger, K.: Demonstratie van een paar zeldzam vorkomende typen van bloedlichampjes en bespreking der patienten. Nederl. T. Geneesk., *72*:1178, 1928.

Blood Groups

Blood groups are identified by the occurrence on red blood cells of specific antigens (agglutinogens or hemolysinogens), which interact with the corresponding antibody (hemagglutinin or hemolysin) to produce agglutination of the red cells and/or hemolysis. These interactions may occur in vivo and produce disease, or in vitro and be used to detect blood groups.

Antibodies (agglutinins) against specific red-cell antigens may occur spontaneously in the serum of an animal or man without prior immunization. In this instance, the agglutinins are present in the serum of an individual in the absence of the specific antigen (agglutinogen) in the red blood cells. For example, in the A,B,O system in man—when a (antigen) is present in the serum of an individual, anti-a agglutinin is absent.

A blood group system in a single species is made up of red cell antigenic factors which are controlled by genes inherited at the same or closely-linked genetic loci and are inherited independently of other systems. The specific gene (which may be dominant, codominant, or recessive) determines the nature of the agglutinogen on the red-cell membrane.

Each agglutinogen has one or more serologic specificity, called a blood factor. Agglutination of red blood cells may be demonstrated in the test tube by adding specific antiserum to a suspension of washed erythrocytes in physiologic saline. Hemolysis occurs only in the presence of complement and is the preferred indicator in some systems (all bovine, some swine, porcine, and canine systems). Both hemagglutination and hemolysis may occur in living animals and result in significant disease (hemolytic disease of newborn, transfusion reactions and chemically-induced sensitization of red blood cells).

Isoantibodies are those found naturally or which can be induced by introduction of specific red-cell antigens (isoantigens) from other individuals of the same species. ABO blood factors occur naturally. The Rh (Rhesus) system and many other systems are activated by immunization: for example, by blood transfusions or experimental immunization with erythrocytes; in pregnancy, by antigens of fetal red blood cells crossing the placenta and stimulating the mother to produce antibodies; and through certain drugs which increase sensitivity to agglutination or lysis of red blood cells.

Hetero-agglutinins are produced in one species by the injection of red-cell antigens of another species. The first description of such antigenic determinants was written by Ehrlich and Morganroth (1899). These authors injected individual goats with pooled blood of other goats and demonstrated the appearance of isolysins in the serum of the injected goats. Four antiserums so developed, named A, B, C and D, were shown to each have a different lytic specificity against goat and sheep cells.

Blood Group Systems in Various Species

Human

The ABO blood group system was the first to be demonstrated in the human species (Landsteiner, 1900) and has widespread clinical applications. The agglutinogens A and B were demonstrated on the red blood cells of persons who did not have the corresponding anti-A or anti-B agglutinin in their sera. Thus the antigen was present in the absence of antibody and reciprocally, absent when the antibody was present. Persons who carried neither A or B antigens are designated O; persons who have both A and B antigens are designated AB. The two antigenic factors, A and B, were found to be determined by two allelic genes which are inherited as codominants (both are expressed when present). The gene for O appears not to be expressed. The phenotypes in this blood group system are A, B, AB, and O. The genotypes (symbolized in italics) are: *OO*,

AA, AO, BB, BO and *AB*. It is now known that the ABO locus occupies human chromosome number 9 (McKusick and Ruddle, 1977).

The second human blood group system to be discovered (Landsteiner and Wiener, 1940) is of particular interest because it was identified in human red blood cells by their agglutination when exposed to serum of a rabbit which had been immunized by red blood cells of a Rhesus monkey (*Macaca mulatta*). This system is now designated as the Rh-Hr (Rh from Rhesus) blood group system (Landsteiner and Wiener, 1940) or the CDE blood group system (Race and Sanger, 1975). Both of these terminologies are in use at the present time. Twelve blood factors are currently known to make up this system, which, of course, is of importance to the causation of erythroblastosis fetalis in human infants. The genetic locus for this human blood group system is on chromosome 1.

A large number of additional blood group systems have been established in man and others have been tentatively identified. These include systems named Duffy, Kell, Kidd, P, MNSs, I-i, Lutheran, Xg, Diego, Cartwright, Auberger, and Dombrock. Further details outside the scope of this text may be found in Huestis, Bove, and Busch, 1976, and in Race and Sanger, 1975.

Nonhuman Primates

Blood groups of nonhuman primates (apes, monkeys, and prosimians) are of particular interest because many of the blood factors are identical to those found in human blood group systems. The same reagents used to identify human hemagglutinogens may therefore be used to identify antigens in lower primates, and the blood group systems are similar in many species.

For example, chimpanzees (*Pan paniscus* and *P. troglodytes*) have homologues of factors O and A, A_1 and A_2 of the ABO system. Orangutans (*Pongo pygmaeus*) have factors

A, A_1, B, and AB, as do gibbons (*Hylobates lar, H. agilis, H. moloch, H. hoolock, H. concolor, H. klossii*). B-type factors have been demonstrated in gorillas (*Gorilla gorilla gorilla*). Baboons (*Papio papio, P. anubis, P. cynocephalus, P. ursinus, P. hamadryas*) and crab-eating macaques (*Macaca fascicularis*) have been shown to have factors A, B, AB, and rarely, O. Several other species have similar homologous human blood factors of the ABO system, evidence of the evolutionary relationships of these species. Apes and monkeys have also been shown to have some of the blood factors of the human MN and Rh-Hr systems (Moor-Jankowski, 1973).

Many simian-type blood factors have been identified in gibbons, baboons, geladas, rhesus and crab-eating macaques, and Celebese black apes, using isoimmune and heteroimmune reagents. These may be analogous to human factors but are not homologous since they differ in antigenic specificity. None of these has been studied sufficiently at this writing to place it in a blood group system.

It is surprising to learn that homologies exist in blood groups of several disparate species (Stormont, 1973). For example, anti-J antibodies of cattle cross react and identify A of man, the J or J-Oc system of cattle, the R-O groups of sheep, the AO groups of pigs, and Tr factor of dogs. Thus it is evident that the antigens of each of these systems are homologous. Similar homologies exist respectively between the B and C systems of sheep and cattle, the S system of cattle, and the M system of sheep.

Mice

Blood group factors have been demonstrated in many species of laboratory animals. It appears that isoagglutinogens occur in all vertebrates (Cohen, 1962). Of particular interest are the histocompatibility antigens which are found not only in red blood cells but in many other body cells. Those which occur at the histocompatibility locus two (H2) in the mouse are of special significance. A large number of specific isoantigens have been demonstrated to be determined by genes at the H2 locus in mice. The gene products are found on macrophages, epithelial and reticuloendothelial tissues, as well as in skin, mammary glands, lungs, and red blood cells. These isoantigens are demonstrated by various technics including agglutination, hemolysis, complement-fixation, and lysis of tumor cells (which bear the antigens of their cells of origin).

Canines

Only nine blood factors (A, A_1, B, C, D, E, F, G, and Tr) have been identified in dogs, and these have not been organized into blood group systems. Most have low reactivity and repeated immunization is necessary to produce potent antisera. The exception appears to be factor A_1, which also produces hemolysis. The blood type becomes of importance when repeated transfusions are necessary.

Cattle

Bovine species have been found so far to have 80 blood factors in 12 blood grouping systems. Many of these systems contain multiple allelic phenotypes—the B system more than 500 (Stormont, 1973). These are only detected by demonstrating hemolysis in the testing system: agglutination of red cells is not a reliable indicator. Complement is of course necessary in the hemolytic reaction. These blood groups are useful in determining parentage and in exploring the taxonomic relationships among species of Bovidae and other families (Stormont, 1973).

Sheep

Seven blood group systems and 50 factors have been identified in sheep. Except for blood group system D, in which agglutination occurs, each factor is recognized by the presence of hemolysins.

Numerous blood-group homologies exist between cattle and sheep.

Swine

Fifteen phenotype blood group systems and 60 blood factors have been identified in pigs. Some systems have so-called incomplete agglutinins, which require the presence of antiglobulins to produce hemagglutination; others are based on hemolysins, which always require complement. Some systems are effective only in dextran solution. Hemolytic disease of newborn piglets is described and has an interesting feature: not all piglets in one litter are affected with the disease due to segregation of blood group phenotypes in the individuals in the litter. Only those offspring with red-cell antigens against which the mother produces antibodies would be affected by hemolysis.

Equines

Twenty blood group factors have been identified so far among eight systems in equine species. Hemolysis and agglutination are utilized as reactions to detect specific factors. These systems may be used to decide parentage and are of importance in hemolytic disease of the foal. Blood typing is of value also in situations requiring multiple blood transfusions.

Agergaard, N., and Larsen, B.: Bovine plasma alkaline phosphatase activity in relation to age, J substance and betalactoglobulin phenotypes. Anim. Blood Groups Biochem. Genet., 5:11–19, 1974.

Bouw, J., and Oosterlee, C.C.: Blood groups in animals. The research in genetically determined characters in animal cells and fluids. Neth. J. Vet. Sci., 2:91–116, 1969.

Bowdler, A.J., Bull, R.W., Slating, R., and Swisher, S.N.: Tr: a canine red cell antigen related to the A antigen of human red cells. Vox Sang., 20:542–544, 1971.

Cohen, C. (ed.): Blood Groups in Infrahuman Species. Ann. N.Y. Acad. Sci., 97:1–328, 1962.

Duggleby, C.R., and Stone, W.H.: Immunogenetic studies of rhesus monkeys. I. The G blood group system. Vox Sang., 20:109–123, 1971.

Duggleby, C.R., Blystad, C., and Stone, W.H.: Immunogenetic studies of rhesus monkeys. II. The H, I, J, K, and L blood group systems. Vox Sang., 20:124–136, 1971.

Edwards, R.H.: The G and H Rhesus monkey blood group systems. J. Heredity, 62:79–86, 1971.

Ehrlich, P., and Morganroth, J., 1899. Contributions to the theory of lysin action. In Studies in Immunity, 2nd ed., edited by C. Ehrlich: translated by C. Bolduan. New York, John Wiley and Sons, 1910, Chapter 1.

Froehlich, J.W., et al.: Blood groups of the mantled howler monkey. J. Med. Primatol., 6:219–231, 1977.

Gengozian, N., and Patton, M.L.: Identification of three blood factors in the marmoset, Saguinus fuscicollis, ssp. In Medical Primatology, 1972, Part I, edited by E.I. Goldsmith, J. Moor-Jankowski. Basel, S. Karger, 1972, pp. 349–360.

Hall, D.E.: A naturally occurring red cell antigen-antibody system in Beagle dogs. J. Small Anim. Pract., 11:543–551, 1970.

Healy, P.J.: Serum alkaline phosphatase activity in sheep. Aust. J. Exp. Biol. Med. Sci., 52:375–385, 1974.

Hirose, Y., and Balner, H.: Red cell isoantigens of Rhesus monkeys. Blood, 34:661–681, 1969.

Huestis, D.W., Bove, J.R., and Busch, S.: Practical Blood Transfusion, 2nd Ed. Boston, Little, Brown, 1976.

Ikemoto, S., Sakurai, Y., Watanabe, Y., and Ejima, H.: Comparsion of blood groups between primates Pan troglodytes and Macaca fascicularis by use of human blood grouping antisera. Jpn. J. Vet. Sci., 40:349–351, 1978.

Landsteiner, K., and Wiener, A.S.: An agglutinable factor in human blood recognized by immune sera for rhesus blood. Proc. Soc. Exp. Biol. Med., 43:223, 1940.

La Salle, M., and de Lannoy, C.W., Jr.: Immunologic responses to blood transfusions in subhuman primates. Am. J. Vet. Res., 30:429–434, 1969.

McDermid, E.M., Vos, G.H., and Downing, H.J.: Blood groups, red cell enzymes and serum proteins of baboons and vervets. Folia Primatol., 19:312–326, 1973.

McKusick, V.A., and Ruddle, F.H.: The status of the gene map of the human chromosomes. Science, 196:390–405, 1977.

Moor-Jankowski, J., and Wiener, A.S.: Blood groups of nonhuman primates: summary of the currently available information. Primates in Med., 1:49–67, 1968.

Moor-Jankowski, J.: Blood groups of apes and monkeys: human and simian types. In Research Animals in Medicine, edited by L.T. Harmison. Washington, D.C., U.S. Dept. HEW Publication No. (NIH) 72-333, 1973.

Moor-Jankowski, J., Wiener, A.S., Socha, W.W., and Valerio, D.A.: Blood groups of crab-eating macaques (Macaca fascicularis) demonstrated by isoimmune Rhesus monkey sera. J. Med. Primatol., 6:76–86, 1977.

Race, R.R., and Sanger, R.: Blood Groups in Man, 6th Ed. Oxford, Blackwell, 1975.

Rasmusen, B.A., and Christian, L.L.: H blood types in pigs as predictors of stress susceptibility. Science, 191:947–948, 1976.

Rosenfield, R.E., Allen, F.H., Jr., and Rubinstein, P.: Genetic model for the Rh blood-group systems. Proc. Natl. Acad. Sci. USA, 70:1303–1307, 1973.

Socha, W.W., Wiener, A.S., Moor-Jankowski, J., and Valerio, D.: The first isoimmune blood group system of Rhesus monkeys (Macaca mulatta): the graded D^{rh} system. Int. Arch. Allergy Appl. Immunol., 52:355–363, 1976.

Sandberg, K.: The D blood group system of the horse. Anim. Blood Groups Biochem. Genet., 4:193–205, 1973.

Stormont, C., and Suzuki, Y.: Genetic systems of blood groups in horses. Genetics, 50:915–929, 1964.

Stormont, C., Suzuki, Y., and Rhode, E.A.: Serology of horse blood groups. Cornell Vet., 54:439–452, 1964.

Stormont, C.: The language of phenogroups. Haematologia, 6:73–79, 1972.

Stormont, C.J.: A survey of blood groups in several species of large animals used in medical research. In Research Animals in Medicine, edited by L.T. Harmison. Washington, D.C., U.S. Dept. HEW Publication No. (NIH) 72-333, 1973.

Sullivan, P.T., Duggleby, C.R., Blystad, C., and Stone, W.H.: Immunogenetic studies of Rhesus monkeys. V. Transplacental immunization. Immunogenetics, 3:473–479, 1976.

Sullivan, P.T., Blystad, C., and Stone, W.H.: Immunogenetic studies of Rhesus monkeys. VII. A simple hemagglutination technique for blood typing. J. Immunol. Methods, 14:31–36, 1976.

Sullivan, P.T., Blystad, C., and Stone, W.H.: Immunogenetic studies of Rhesus monkeys. IX. The M and N blood group systems. Immunogenetics, 5:415–421, 1977.

Sullivan, P.T., Blystad, C., and Stone, W.H.: Immunogenetic studies on the Rhesus monkey (Macaca mulatta): XI. Use of blood groups in problems of parentage. Lab. Anim. Sci., 27:348–351, 1977.

Swisher, S.N., Young, L.E.,and Trabold, N.: In vitro and in vivo studies of the behavior of canine erythrocyte-isoantibody systems. Ann. N.Y. Acad. Sci., 97:15–25, 1962.

Wiener, A.S., Moor-Jankowski, J., Balner, H., and Gordon, E.B.: Blood groupings in monkeys demonstrated with antisera produced by combined skin transplantation and isoimmunization with red cells. Int. Arch. Allergy Appl. Immunol., 34:386–391, 1968.

Wiener, A.S., et al.: The AP-BP blood groups of baboons. Am. J. Phys. Anthropol., 33:433–438, 1970.

Hemolytic Disease of Newborn (Erythroblastosis Fetalis, Neonatal Isoerythrolysis, Icterus Neonatorum, Neonatal Jaundice)

This disease is fundamentally the result of incompatible blood group antigens in male and female parents, causing the destruction of erythrocytes in their offspring. In the usual case, the female does not have the antigen, but her fetus inherits it from its male parent. In some cases, the mother may be immunized by an incompatible blood transfusion. The red-cell antigen, through placental exchange, immunizes the mother. The antibodies resulting in the maternal circulation cause hemolysis of the fetal erythrocytes, *in utero,* in species with a placenta permeable to the antibodies (human, nonhuman primates, and rabbits). In some species (horse, swine, dog), the antibodies do not pass through the placenta, and hemolysis occurs only after the newborn suckles and receives antibody in the colostrum.

In human beings, incompatibility in the Rh system is the most frequent cause of hemolytic disease of the newborn. The father is Rh-positive, the mother Rh-negative. The Rh-positive cells of the fetus immunize the mother, who develops antibodies which cause hemolysis of red cells of her fetus. Usually the first pregnancy results in immunization of the mother with little or no effect on the fetus, but in subsequent pregnancies, the fetus is severely affected before birth. Intrauterine effects on the fetus are dependent upon the titer of antibody in the mother. In severe cases, hemolytic anemia and kernicterus result in death *in utero* or if the fetus survives, in severe mental retardation. Incompatibility in other blood group systems (ABO, etc.) may also result in this disease in human beings, although much less frequently.

The blood group systems involved in hemolytic disease of the newborn have not been identified in all species in which the disease has been reported. Some work on the identity of antigens has been reported, however, and research seems to be continuing. Anti-Ba and anti-Ea antibodies have been demonstrated in swine to cause changes in fetal osmotic fragility and hemolysis in erythrocytes if the maternal titer is high enough.

Natural cases of the disease have been observed in marmosets (*Tamarinus nigricollis*) and baboons (*Papio spp.*), but macaques (*Macaca mulatta* and *M. fascicularis*) seem to be protected against this disease, although blood-group incompatibility does occur.

In cattle, isoimmunization does not appear to occur between fetus and mother, but immunized females have resulted from receiving incompatible blood in certain vaccines (for babesiasis and anaplasmosis). Hemolytic disease has resulted after suckling, in the newborn of such animals. Artificial immunization and production of the disease has been demonstrated in dogs.

Abe, T., et al.: A subclinical case of hemolytic disease of newborn pigs caused by anti Ea. Jpn. J. Vet. Sci., *32*:139–145, 1970.

Dimmock, C.K., and Bell, K.: Haemolytic disease of the newborn in calves. Aust. Vet. J., *46*:44–47, 1970.

Gengozian, N., Lushbaugh, C.G., Humason, G.L., and Kniseley, R.M.: Erythroblastosis fetalis in the primate, *Tamarinus nigricollis.* Nature, *209*:731–732, 1966.

Hall, S.A., Rest, J.R., Linklater, K.A., and McTaggart, H.S.: Concurrent haemolytic disease of the newborn and thrombocytopenic purpura in piglets without artificial immunization of the dam. Vet. Rec., *91*:677–678, 1972.

Langford, G., Knott, S.G., Dimmock, C.K., and Derrington, P.: Haemolytic disease of newborn calves in a dairy herd in Queensland. Aust. Vet. J., *47*:1–4, 1971.

Linklater, K.A., and Imlah, P.: Haemolytic disease of the newborn, thrombocytopenic purpura and neutropenia occurring concurrently in a litter of piglets. Br. Vet. J., *129*:36–46, 1973.

Meyer, R.C., Rasmusen, B.A., and Simon, J.: A hemolytic neonatal disease in swine associated with blood group incompatibility. J. Am. Vet. Med. Assoc., *154*:531–537, 1969.

Noda, H., and Watanabe, Y.: Relationships between blood groups and hemolytic disease of newborn foal. Jpn. J. Zootec. Sci., *46*:180–184, 1975.

Sonoda, M., Noda, H., Kobayashi, K., and Maede, Y.: Clinical and hematological studies on hemolytic icterus of foals. Exp. Rep. Equine Health Lab., *9*:103–111, 1972.

Stormont, C.J.: Hemolytic diseases of newborn calves. Fed. Proc., *31*:761, 1972.

Wiener, A.S., Socha, W., Niemann, W., and Moor-Jankowski, J.: Erythroblastosis models: a review and new experimental data in monkeys. J. Med. Primatol., *4*:179–187, 1975.

Wiener, A.S., Socha, W.W., and Moor-Jankowski, J.: Erythroblastosis models. 11. Materno-fetal incompatibility in chimpanzee. Folia Primatol., 27:68–74, 1977.

Wilson, J.S., and Trace, J.C.: Neonatal isoerythrolysis of the bovine. Proc. 74th Ann. Meet. U.S. Anim. Health Assoc., 1970, 115–119, 1971.

Inherited Disorders of Coagulation

Several inherited diseases involve the clotting mechanisms described in Chapter 5. The list has grown over the past few years, and it seems likely that more such disorders will be recognized in the future. In each case, the defect in coagulation described in animals has a counterpart in human patients.

Fibrinogen Deficiency (Hypofibrinogenemia, Afibrinogenemia, Factor I Deficiency)

Deficiency of factor I, fibrinogen, has been reported in dogs and goats. The defect is manifest by severe bleeding episodes and low fibrinogen levels in the plasma. One canine family with this defect has been documented (Kammerman, et al., 1971), but it has been observed on at least two other occasions (Dodds, 1974).

Hereditary afibrinogenemia has been studied in a family of Saanen goats (Breukink, et al., 1972). This is a severe hemorrhagic disorder in newborn and young goats with bleeding from the mucous membranes and umbilicus and into joints and subcutaneous tissues. The inheritance pattern is compatible with a single autosomal incompletely dominant gene. Fibrinogen levels in heterozygotes, as measured by bioassay or by immunologic methods, were recorded as a trace or completely absent. Prolonged bleeding time and decreased platelet retention in glass filters were also observed.

Hypoproconvertinemia (Factor VII Deficiency)

Deficiency of coagulation factor VII has been observed in dogs by several authors since the original description by Mustard, et al. (1962). The effects of this deficiency are mild; hemorrhages following surgery and bruises from trauma are the essential manifestations. Most reported cases have been in laboratory Beagles, probably because of effective monitoring of these animals, and the widespread use of Beagles in experimental work. Other breeds are susceptible. Heterozygous dogs may be distinguished from homozygous dogs deficient in factor VII by prothrombin time determinations. The most clearly defined differences are detected by using human brain thromboplastin as a reagent.

Factor VII deficient canine plasma has proved to be a useful reagent in diagnostic tests for hemorrhagic disorders in man and animals. It is also used in testing the quality of tissue thromboplastins which are needed for monitoring anticoagulant therapy. In this assay system, the prothrombin clotting time in heterozygous dogs with hereditary factor VII deficiency was 17.9 ($\pm$1.8) seconds; homozygotes were 60.9 ($\pm$14.7) seconds, and normal dogs 11.7 ($\pm$1.8) seconds (Dodds, 1974).

Classic Hemophilia (Hemophilia A, Factor VIII Deficiency)

In humans, this disease is of historical fame as the tragic affliction of many male members of European and Russian royal families. The same basic disorder was first identified in dogs (Taskin, 1935) and is now known to affect horses (Archer, 1961) and cats (Cotter, et al., 1978). Research on the canine disease was greatly intensified by Brinkhous, et al. (1950), who followed up the report of natural cases in Setters (Field, et al., 1946) by establishing breeding colonies and research programs using this animal model.

Canine hemophilia A continues to be the most commonly reported hemorrhagic disorder in dogs. Inherited as a sex-linked recessive gene, the usual event is for carrier (heterozygous) females to pass the gene to half of their male and female offspring. The females inheriting the gene become carriers, and the hemizygous males are affected with hemophilia. Homozygous affected females have been produced by selective mating of hemophiliac males to heterozygous females (Brinkhous and Graham, 1950).

The hemorrhages in the canine disease may vary in severity depending upon the level of factor VIII which may be measured by a specific assay. Hemophilic dogs have very low or undetectable levels of anti-hemophilia factor (factor VIII, AHF). On the other hand, the level of factor VIII-related antigen is normal or elevated. This antigen is measured by a precipitin assay using specific heterologous antibodies. Primary bleeding time may be normal; secondary bleeding time is prolonged. Mild, moderate, or severe bleeding diathesis may be present. Moderate to severe hemarthrosis is observed, particularly in larger breeds. Heterozygous females have reduced (about 50%) levels of factor VIII, but normal levels of factor VIII antigen (Dodds, 1974).

A severe form of hemophilia A has been described in Thoroughbred and Standard-bred horses in England, Australia, and the United States. Inheritance is through a sex-linked gene. The disease appears to closely resemble the human and canine diseases (Archer, 1961; Archer, et al., 1959; Hutchins, et al., 1967; Sanger, et al., 1964).

Hemophilia A has also been confirmed in several unrelated cats (Cotter, et al., 1978). These cats were detected initially by their severe protracted bleeding after minor surgery. This hemorrhage was controlled by transfusion of fresh whole blood. Laboratory studies revealed prolonged whole blood clotting time and prothrombin consumption time plus deficiency of factor VIII coagulant activity. Other analyses, including fibrinogen, Russell's viper time, activated partial thromboplastin time, and levels of factors VII, IX, X, and XI were in normal range.

Hemophilia B (Christmas Disease, Factor IX Deficiency)

A canine disease, analogous in many respects to the human disease, was originally described in Cairn Terriers (Rowsell, et al., 1960; Mustard, et al., 1960). The disease was subsequently described in two other breeds of dogs: Black and Tan Coonhounds and Saint Bernards (Dodds, 1969; Dodds and Kaneko, 1971; Rowsell, 1969). This disease is quite similar to hemophilia A in its inheritance, laboratory data (except that Factor IX is deficient), and clinical bleeding episodes. In general, the bleeding is more uniformly severe than in hemophilia A. Homozygous females can be produced by mating hemophilic males to carrier females, and their hemophilia is essentially like the hemizygous affected male.

The plasma from factor IX-deficient dogs has proved useful as a reagent in the quantitative bioassay of factor IX in man and other species (Aronson, et al., 1972). This plasma has also proved useful in developing a new two-stage assay system for factor IX (Dodds, 1974).

Stuart-Prower Factor Deficiency (Factor X Deficiency)

This coagulation factor was reported to be deficient in Cocker Spaniel dogs by Dodds (1973). At this time, it has not been reported in other breeds or species. The disease is manifest in newborn or young adult dogs by severe bleeding and in adult animals by a mild bleeding disorder, usually prolonged estrual bleeding or bleeding intensified by surgery. Rectal bleeding and hemoptysis may be exhibited.

Laboratory data reveal severely to mildly reduced levels of factor X activity and some prolongation of thromboplastin and Stypven times (Dodds, 1974). Inheritance is autosomal and probably dominant with lethality in the homozygous state.

Plasma Thromboplastin Antecedent (PTA) Deficiency (Factor XI Deficiency)

Two reports of this deficiency indicate that it occurs in cattle (Kociba et al., 1969) and Springer Spaniel dogs (Dodds, 1971). Two bovine animals that were half siblings were found to be severely deficient in PTA. One of these was also afflicted with lymphoblastic leukemia. The bovine affected plasma has been found to be suitable as a substrate for PTA assay in man or other species. The canine PTA deficiency was encountered in a single female during a routine ovariohysterectomy. Heterozygotes were detected in three offspring of this female (two females and one male) as indicated by PTA levels between 23 and 40% of normal. The inheritance is not established, but appears to be autosomal.

Von Willebrand's Disease

This bleeding disorder in man is manifest by low factor VIII levels, prolonged bleeding times, reduced platelet retention in glass-bead filters, a paradoxical increase in circulating factor VIII after transfusion with plasma from normal or hemophilia-A patients, and autosomal inheritance. Canine and porcine disorders have been described which have these same characteristics (Chan, et al., 1968; Dodds, 1970; Cornell and Muhrer, 1964; Cornell, et al., 1969; Kahn, et al., 1970).

According to Jaffe (1977), factor VIII is a glycoprotein which is present in normal human plasma in trace amounts, 5–10 micrograms per milliliter of plasma. Its functions include the initiation of coagulation and platelet functions. Factor VIII is believed to have three functional components: (1) an antigen which may be demonstrated by precipitin assay using specific heterologous antibodies (this component is normal in hemophiliacs); (2) a clot-promoting or anti-hemophilia factor which corrects the coagulation defects in plasma of hemophilia and von Willebrand's disease; (3) a von Willebrand factor which is deficient in von Willebrand's disease but normal in hemophilia A. This factor is detected by an abnormal bleeding time or by *in vitro* analysis of platelet function.

In vivo analyses with a monospecific rabbit antihuman factor VIII antibody demonstrate that factor VIII antigen is found only in endothelial cells, platelets, and megakaryocytes. These and other studies suggest that endothelial cells may be a site of synthesis of factor VIII antigen but not antihemophilic factor or von Willebrand factor.

The inheritance of von Willebrand's disease in man and dog appears to be via an autosomal dominant gene. The porcine disease has been reported to be an autosomal recessive. Both heterozygous and homozygous states appear to be expressed in man, swine, and dogs, based upon differing degrees of clinical severity, factor VIII activity, and platelet adhesiveness. The term codominant might be used in this case to express the situation in which heterozygous and homozygous states may be detected.

Thrombopathia (Thrombasthenia or Glanzmann's Disease)

A canine disorder of platelet function was described by Dodds (1967) in a family of Otterhounds. The disease was termed thrombasthenic thrombopathia because of manifest characteristics of both disorders. The canine disease has a hereditary functional platelet disorder which is similar, except for platelet morphology, to Glanzmann's thrombasthenia. Platelet function tests indicate poor clot retraction; long bleeding time; low platelet retention (in glass-bead filters); defective platelet aggregation with adenosine phosphate, thrombin, or collagen; reduced platelet fibrinogen; and failure of intact platelets to support normal thromboplastin generation. Other laboratory data, including the abnormal platelet factor III release and giant bizarre platelets, suggest that the defect is also thrombopathic. In severely affected dogs, more than 80% of the platelets are giant forms. It was suggested (Dodds, 1974) that the platelets may consist of two populations: one (20% of the platelets) being thrombasthenic; the other (consisting of 80% giant platelets) being thrombopathic.

Canine thrombasthenic thrombopathia is inherited as an autosomal dominant;

both heterozygotes and homozygous affected animals can be detected by laboratory tests.

A hereditary platelet function defect has been described in a group of fawn-hooded rats (Tschopp and Zucker, 1972). The affected rats have long bleeding times (greater than 15 minutes), reduced platelet retention, defective platelet aggregation, and reduced serotonin release with connective tissue. Aggregation with ADP is normal, washed platelets aggregated with thrombin fail to release adenosine triphosphate (ATP) or adenosine phosphate (ADP). The platelets contain only one-third as much serotonin as those from normal rats.

Hageman Factor Deficiency (Factor XII Deficiency)

Deficiencies of factor XII have been observed in animals, but none were associated with a bleeding disorder. Further evidence that Hageman factor is not essential for normal hemostasis is its complete absence in marine mammals (dolphins, killer whales, and porpoises); in fowl (ducks, geese, chickens, turkeys, and pigeons); and in most reptiles (lizards, turtles, and tiger snakes) (Ratnoff, 1966).

Factor XII deficiency and defective plasma thromboplastin formation have been described in horses, none of them with any bleeding tendency (Ollendorff, 1960).

Archer, R.K., and Bowden, R.S.T.: A case of true hemophilia in a Labrador dog. Vet. Rec., 71:560–561, 1959.

Archer, R.K.: True haemophilia (haemophilia A) in a Thoroughbred foal. Vet. Rec., 73:383–386, 1961.

Archer, R.K., and Allen, B.V.: True haemophilia in horses. Vet. Rec., 91:655–656, 1972.

Aronson, D.L., Dodds, W.J., and Mustafa, A.J.: A quantitative two-stage assay for factor IX (Christmas factor) using plasma from dogs with Christmas Disease. Thromb. Diath. Haemorrh., 27:529–533, 1972.

Benson, R.E., and Dodds, W.J.: Autosomal factor VIII deficiency in rabbits: size variations of rabbit factor VIII. Thromb. Haemost., 38:380–383, 1977.

Bogart, R., and Muhrer, M.E.: The inheritance of a hemophilia-like condition in swine. J. Hered., 33:59–64, 1942.

Bowie, E.J.W., et al.: Tests of hemostasis in swine: normal values and values in pigs affected with von Willebrand's Disease. Am. J. Vet. Res., 34:1405–1407, 1973.

Breukink, H.J., et al.: Congenital afibrinogenemia in goats. Zentralbl. Veterinaermed., 19A:661–676, 1972.

Brinkhous, K.M., Morrison, F.C., Jr., and Muhrer, M.E.: Comparative study of clotting defects in human, canine, and porcine hemophilia. Fed. Proc., 11:409–411, 1952.

Brinkhous, K.M., and Graham, J.B.: Hemophilia in the female dog. Science, 111:723–724, 1950.

Brinkhous, K.M., Davis, P.D., Graham, J.B., and Dodds, W.J.: Expression and linkage of genes for X-linked hemophilias A and B in the dog. Blood, 41:577–585, 1973.

Brock, W.E., et al.: Canine hemophilia. Arch. Pathol., 76:464–469, 1963.

Capel-Edwards, K., and Hall, D.E.: Factor VII deficiency in the Beagle dog. Lab. Anim., 2:105–112, 1968.

Chan, J.Y.S., et al.: Von Willebrand disease "stimulating factor" in porcine plasma. Am. J. Physiol., 214:1219–1224, 1968.

Cornell, C.N., and Muhrer, M.E.: Coagulation factors in normal and hemophiliac-type swine. Am. J. Physiol., 206:926–931, 1964.

Cornell, C.N., Cooper, R.G., Kahn, R.A., and Garb, S.: Platelet adhesiveness in normal and bleeder swine as measured in a Celite system. Am. J. Physiol., 216:1170–1175, 1969.

Cotter, S.M., Brenner, R.M., and Dodds, W.J.: Hemophilia A in three unrelated cats. J. Am. Vet. Med. Assoc., 172:166–168, 1978.

Dodds, W.J., Packham, M.A., Rowsell, H.C., and Mustard, J.F.: Factor VII survival and turnover in dogs. Am. J. Physiol., 213:36–42, 1967.

Dodds, W.J.: Familial canine thrombocytopathy. Thromb. Diath. Haemorrh., 26:241–248 (Suppl.), 1967.

Dodds, W.J.: Current concepts of hereditary coagulation disorders in dogs. Experimentation Animale, 1:243–252, 1969.

Dodds, W.J.: Canine von Willebrand's Disease. J. Lab. Clin. Med., 76:713–721, 1970.

Dodds, W.J., and Kull, J.E.: Canine factor XI (plasma thromboplastin antecedent) deficiency. J. Lab. Clin. Med., 78:746–752, 1971.

Dodds, W.J., and Kaneko, J.J.: Hemostasis and blood coagulation. In Clinical Biochemistry of Domestic Animals, Vol. 2, 2nd Ed. Edited by J.J. Kaneko, C.E. Cornelius. New York, Academic Press, 1971, pp. 179–206.

Dodds, W.J.: Hemorrhagic disorders. In Current Veterinary Therapy IV, edited by R.W. Kirk. Philadelphia, W.B. Saunders Co., 1971, pp. 247–254.

Dodds, W.J.: Canine factor X (Stuart-Prower factor) deficiency. J. Lab. Clin. Med., 82:560–566, 1973.

Dodds, W.J.: Blood coagulation: hemostasis and thrombosis. In Handbook of Laboratory Animal Science, Vol. II, edited by E.C. Melby, Jr. and N.H. Altman. Cleveland, CRC Press, 1974, pp. 87–116.

Dodds, W.J.: Hereditary and acquired hemorrhagic disorders in animals. *In* Progress in Hemostasis and Thrombosis, Vol. II, edited by T.H. Spaet. New York, Grune and Stratton, 1974, pp. 215–247.

Dodds, W.J.: Further studies of canine von Willebrand's disease. Blood, *45*:221–230, 1975.

Dodds, W.J.: The diagnosis, management, and treatment of bleeding disorders, parts 1 and 2. Mod. Vet. Pract., *58*:680–684, 756–762, 1977.

Dodds, W.J.: First international registry of animal models of thrombosis and hemorrhagic diseases. ILAR News, *21*:A1–A23, 1977.

Fass, D.N., et al.: Factor VIII (Willebrand) antigen and ristocetin-Willebrand factor in pigs with von Willebrand's disease. Thromb. Res., *8*:319–327, 1976.

Field, R.A., Rickard, C.G., and Hutt, F.B.: Hemophilia in a family of dogs. Cornell Vet., *36*:283–300, 1946.

Forbes, R.D.C., Guttmann, R.D., and Bazin, H.: Hyperacute rejection of cardiac allografts in a rat strain with a hereditary platelet function defect. Lab. Invest., *37*:158–161, 1977.

Gentry, P.A., Crane, S., and Lotz, F.: Factor XI (plasma thromboplastin antecedent) deficiency in cattle. Can. Vet. J., *16*:118–120, 1975.

Graham, J.B., Buckwalter, J.A., Hartley, L.J., and Brinkhous, K.M.: Canine hemophilia. Observations on the course, the clotting anomaly, and the effect of blood transfusions. J. Exp. Med., *90*:97–111, 1949.

Gralnick, H.R., Sultan, Y., and Coller, B.S.: Von Willebrand's disease: Combined quantitative abnormalities. N. Engl. J. Med., *296*:1024–1030, 1977.

Green, R.A., and White, F.: Feline factor XII (Hageman) deficiency. Am. J. Vet. Res., *38*:893–896, 1977.

Hawkey, C.M.: Relationship between blood coagulation and thrombosis and atherosclerosis in man, monkeys, and carnivores. Thromb. Diath. Haemorrh., *31*:103–118, 1974.

Hogan, A.G., Muhrer, M.E., and Bogart, R.: A hemophilia-like disease in swine. Proc. Soc. Exp. Biol. Med., *48*:217–219, 1941.

Hovig, T., et al.: Experimental hemostasis in normal dogs and dogs with congenital disorders of blood coagulation. Blood, *30*:636–668, 1967.

Howell, J., and Lambert, P.S.: A case of hemophilia A in the dog. Vet. Rec., *76*:1103–1105, 1964.

Hutchins, D.R., Lepherd, E.E., and Crook, I.G.: A case of equine haemophilia. Aust. Vet. J., *43*:83–87, 1967.

Hutt, F.B., Rickard, C.G., and Field, R.A.: Sex-linked hemophilia in dogs. J. Hered., *39*:2–9, 1948.

Jaffe, E.A.: Endothelial cells and the biology of factor VIII. N. Engl. J. Med., *296*:377–383, 1977.

Kahn, R.A., Cooper, R.G., Cornell, C.N., and Muhrer, M.E.: Electron microscopy of bleeder swine platelets. Am. J. Vet. Res., *31*:679–684, 1970.

Kammerman, B., Gmür, J., and Stunzi, H.: Afib-rogenämie beim hund. Zentralbl. Veterinaermed., *18*:192–194, 1971.

Kaneko, J.J., Cordy, D.R., and Carlson, G.: Canine hemophilia resembling classic hemophilia A. J. Am. Vet. Med. Assoc., *150*:15–21, 1967.

Kociba, G.J., et al.: Bovine plasma thromboplastin antecedent (factor XI) deficiency. J. Lab. Clin. Med., *74*:37–39, 1969.

Lewis E.F., and Holman, H.H.: Haemophilia in a Saint Bernard dog. Vet. Rec., *63*:666–667, 1951.

Mustard, J.F., et al.: Canine hemophilia B (Christmas Disease). Br. J. Haematol., *6*:259–264, 1960.

Mustard, J.F., et al.: Canine factor VII deficiency. Br. J. Haematol., *8*:43–47, 1962.

Norman, J.C.: Splenic homotransplantation for hemophilia. N. Engl. J. Med., *283*:435, 1970.

Norman, J.C., Covelli, V.H., and Sise, H.S.: Experimental transplantation of the spleen for classical hemophilia A: rationales and long-term results. Bibl. Haemat., *34*:187–199, 1970.

Ollendorff, P.: Defects in and variability of the thromboplastic system in horse plasma. Thromb. Diath. Haemorrh., *4*:45–49, 1960.

Osbaldiston, G.W., Stowe, E.C., and Griffith, P.R.: Blood coagulation: comparative studies in dogs, cats, horses, and cattle. Br. Vet. J., *126*:512–521, 1970.

Ratnoff, O.D.: The biology and pathology of the initial stages of blood coagulation. *In* Progress in Hematology, Vol. 5, edited by E.B. Brown, and C.J. Moore. New York, Grune and Stratton, 1966, p. 204.

Rowsell, H.C., et al.: A disorder resembling hemophilia B (Christmas Disease) in dogs. J. Am. Vet. Med. Assoc., *137*:247–250, 1960.

Rowsell, H.C., and Mustard, J.F.: Blood coagulation disorders in some common laboratory animals. Lab. Anim. Care, *13*:752–762, 1963.

Rowsell, H.C.: The hemostatic mechanisms of mammals and birds in health and disease. Adv. Vet. Sci., *12*:337–410, 1968.

Rowsell, H.C.: Blood coagulation and hemorrhagic disorders. *In* Textbook of Veterinary Clinical Pathology, edited by W. Medway, J.E. Prier, and J.S. Wilkinson. Baltimore, Williams and Wilkins, 1969, pp. 247–281.

Sanger, V.L., Mairs, R.E., and Trapp, A.L.: Hemophilia in a foal. J. Am. Vet. Med. Assoc., *144*:259–264, 1964.

Spurling, N.W., Peacock, R., and Pilling, T.: The clinical aspects of canine factor VII deficiency including some case histories. J. Small Anim. Pract., *15*:229–239, 1974.

Stevens, R.W.C., and Crane, S.: Canine haemophilia: blood clotting time of X⁸X⁹ bitches. Genetics, *60*:229–233, 1968.

Taskin, J.: Un cas grave d'hemophilia chez une chienne. Bull. Acad. Vet. Fr., *8*:595, 1935.

Tschopp, T.B., and Zucker, M.B.: Hereditary defect in platelet function in rats. Blood, *40*:217–226, 1972.

Weiss, H.L. (ed.): Platelets and their role in hemostasis. Ann. N.Y. Acad. Sci., *201*:3–450, 1972.

White, J.G., and Gerrard, J.M.: Ultrastructural features of abnormal blood platelets. A review. Am. J. Pathol., *83*:590–632, 1976.

Wurzel, H.A., and Lawrence, W.C.: Canine hemophilia. Thromb. Diath. Haemorrh., *6*:98–103, 1961.

Hemoglobinemia and Hemoglobinuria

The presence of free hemoglobin in the blood or in the urine is a sign, but is sometimes carelessly considered as if it were a disease in itself. For instance, there was an inclination formerly to use hemoglobinuria as a longer (and more sophisticated?) name for the disease of muscles known as azoturia. Even if the pigment in the urine were hemoglobin, instead of myoglobin, the colored urine is only one sign of the disease, as it is of various others.

Hemoglobin occurs normally in the erythrocytes, and only there. From the principles set forth in connection with anemia, we learn its history in case it is released from disintegrating erythrocytes, and that when the amount of hemoglobin in the blood plasma passes a certain level (the renal threshold), it is excreted in the urine, giving to the latter a reddish or brownish color. It follows that whenever there is hemoglobinemia of any considerable degree there is also hemolytic anemia, not to mention hemolytic icterus, which develops if the rapid destruction of erythrocytes continues.

Hemoglobinuria is diagnosed tentatively, but with considerable reliability by the brownish color of the urine. A microscopic examination of the urinary sediment, separated preferably by centrifugation, otherwise by settling in a tall vessel, is necessary to eliminate hematuria, which is the presence of whole blood and blood cells in the urine. This latter is essentially hemorrhage into the urinary passages anywhere from the glomerulus to the external meatus. Its causes and significance are obviously quite unrelated to the presence in the urine of hemoglobin without blood cells. Simple chemical tests serve to eliminate other possible sources of brownish discolorization, as well as to detect minute amounts of hemoglobin which escape visual observation.

Hemoglobinemia of a degree insufficient to produce hemoglobinuria, of course, may exist and can be detected only by an appropriate test upon the blood serum.

Causes. The causes of hemoglobinemia and hemoglobinuria are to be sought first among the causes already given for hemolytic anemia. Prominent among the infections are bovine bacillary hemoglobinuria (which should rarely be diagnosed without bacteriological confirmation), severe forms of leptospirosis in the bovine, and piroplasmoses. Anaplasmosis, on the other hand, is said never to reach a sufficiently violent state to cause hemoglobinuria.

Hemoglobinuria is probably more often a symptom of toxic diseases than it is of infections. Some hemoglobinuria toxins probably remain unknown, but we do recognize in this category poisoning by copper, chlorates, the pasture plant, rape, and, in some cases, by ricin (castor beans). Poisonous mushrooms, eaten by humans, produce marked hemoglobinuria. In humans, severe hemolysis with icterus and hemoglobinuria results from eating a bean, *Vicia flava.* Venoms of most snakes and some of the more poisonous scorpions and spiders belong in the same class. The toxemic state which results from the decomposition of large amounts of dead tissue following extensive burns or freezing causes notable hemoglobinuria as does also severe crushing trauma (the "crush syndrome") (myoglobin?). The hemolysis which follows transfusions of incompatible blood, of course, results in hemoglobinuria.

Postparturient Hemoglobinuria

The term **postparturient hemoglobinuria** has been applied to an obscure toxic disorder which is often fatal in cattle in the western United States, Australia, and other localities. It appears usually but not invariably in cows that have given birth to calves a few weeks previously. The hemoglobin in blood and urine results from severe hemolysis of circulating erythrocytes, the red-cell count often being less than 2,000,000 in spite of active hematopoiesis (nucleated red cells, etc.). Hemolytic jaundice develops except in peracute cases. Marked hypophosphatemia is an accompaniment. Acute toxic hepatitis is suggested by centrilobular necrosis and midzonal fatty change, although these changes are attributed by some merely to anoxia resulting from the severe anemia. The lesions of hemoglobinuric nephropathy may be mild to severe. Suspected causes range from a deficiency of phosphorus in the diet and in the soil to accumulation of toxic products which the parturient uterus failed to discharge. Some cases possibly have been confused with plant poisonings, including a diet excessive in the leaves of the sugar beet, which is a plentiful farm crop in some of the affected regions.

Myoglobinuria

Although completely unrelated to disorders of the hemic and lymphatic systems, hemoglobinuria must be differentiated from myoglobinuria. The causes of myoglobinuria are discussed in Chapter 19. The molecular weight of myoglobin is approximately one-fourth the weight of hemoglobin, which accounts for a much lower renal clearance. Myoglobin appears in the urine when plasma levels reach approximately 20 mg/100 ml, whereas hemoglobin does not appear in the urine until plasma levels approach 100 mg/100 ml. As a result of this difference, plasma is generally not colored by myoglobin, whereas in those diseases causing hemoglobinuria the plasma is red. Obviously caution must be used to prevent mechanical hemolysis in obtaining blood specimens. Both myoglobin and hemoglobin react to the usual tests for occult blood. The two pigments can be distinguished by spectroscopic techniques.

Farquharson, J., and Smith, K.W.: Post-parturient hemoglobinuria of cattle. J. Am. Vet. Med. Assoc., 93:37–39, 1938.
Madsen, D.E., and Nielsen, H.M.: Parturient hemoglobinuria of dairy cows. J. Am. Vet. Med. Assoc., 94:577–586, 1939.
Madsen, D.E., and Nielsen, H.M.: The production of hemoglobinemia by low phosphorus intake. J. Am. Vet. Med. Assoc., 105:22–25, 1944.
Mullins, J.C., and Ramsay, W.R.: Hemoglobinuria and anaemia associated with aphosphorosis. Aust. Vet. J., 35:140–147, 1959.
Parkinson, B., and Sutherland, A.K.: Post-parturient haemoglobinuria in dairy cows. Aust. Vet. J., 30:232–236, 1954.
Penny, R.H.C.: Post-parturient haemoglobinuria (haemoglobinaemia) in cattle. Vet. Rec., 68:238–241, 1956.

THE SPLEEN

By far the most common problem which confronts pathologists as they examine the spleen has to do with its size, for, as with soldiers' uniforms, there appear to be two sizes: too large and too small. While we shall presently mention some pathological enlargements, the great majority of spleens encountered at autopsy are essentially normal. It is well to remember that the spleen is a "great reticulo-endothelial sponge" (Boyd) which holds a large but varying amount of blood. From the arterioles, the blood slowly percolates through the multitudinous, ill-defined spaces of the splenic pulp, and is collected into the venous sinuses. This is by no means accidental, but serves to expose the blood to the action of the reticulo-endothelial and lymphoid cells, which are the principal components of the splenic parenchyma, and which perform such functions as destruction of decadent erythrocytes, conversion of hemoglobin, elaboration of antibodies, and many others. There is evidence, indeed, that the flow of blood through the maze of poorly recognizable compartments among the cells of the splenic pulp is controlled by little vascular sphincters which open and close at the proper time.

Obviously the spongy organ can hold a considerable amount of blood, varying with the state of the sphincters, if they exist, and, at any rate, with the degree of contraction or relaxation of the muscular trabeculae and capsule (muscular in animals). Furthermore, the concentration of blood cells varies, doubtless according to changing needs of the body, and the stored blood is often highly cellular.

It is entirely understandable, then, that when an animal dies of hemorrhage, the spleen is small, "dry," and "atrophic," in other words simply empty, for no living thing perishes without exhausting every resource that might counteract the attack which threatens it. The same is generally true when death comes from one of the many diseases which destroy blood cells (hemolytic anemias), although the picture in such cases is influenced by accumulation of various white cells if the cause is an infection, by the presence of hematopoietic cells in some anemias, by an increase in phagocytic reticulo-endothelial cells needed to dispose of fragmented erythrocytes or other waste particles, by the augmentation of reticulo-endothelium for the production of antibodies, by enlargement of the splenic (Malpighian) corpuscles in lymphoid hyperplasia, by fibrosis, congestion, and other changes.

Evaluation of the net results thus becomes more than a little complicated, and this situation is enhanced by the difficulty of recognizing each cell type and the total impossibility of ascertaining the functions and purposes of the cells by means of microscopic sections. While the term **splenitis** is in use by some to refer to some of the cellular accumulations to which allusion has just been made, we prefer to limit the concept of splenic inflammation to those infrequent cases where the spleen itself is the object of attack and to view its various reactions to generalized disease as functional changes designed or fitted, as

they certainly are, to counteract certain disorders of the body as a whole through the medium of its circulating blood.

Splenic Enlargements, Splenomegaly

In a broad sense, the latter term can be used to indicate any abnormal increase in size of the spleen, the following different kinds existing.

Acute Congestion of the Spleen

The acutely congested spleen is enlarged, but not excessively so, and somewhat soft. Its cut surface is dark and bulges moderately, with blood oozing from it. Microscopically, there may be little change beyond a large number of erythrocytes in the pulp and sinuses, or the lesion may be combined with others, such as a decrease or increase of splenic cells.

The most frequent example of acute splenic congestion encountered in veterinary pathology is that which results from the use of Nembutal or similar barbiturates for procuring a humane death, the usual procedure when pet animals have to be given euthanasia. One of the actions of the drug is to relax smooth muscle, including that of the spleen, with the result that the organ fills with dark, venous blood at the moment of death.

Acute congestion is also common as a part of the picture of generalized venous congestion which accompanies a failing heart. The immediate cause of death in a great variety of diseases is this congestive heart failure.

Chronic Passive Congestion

The spleen is moderately enlarged and filled with blood, but is firm or a little tough because of the increase of fibrous tissue.

Microscopic Lesions. The microscopic lesions, which result from long continued venous pressure, are (1) distention of the sinusoids and pulp-spaces with blood, (2) often an appreciable hyperplasia of the endothelium of the sinusoids so that the lining cells resemble cuboidal epithelium, (3) marked diffuse fibrosis throughout the pulp, the fibrous tissue being an attempt to strengthen the walls of the sinusoidal spaces, (4) even a thickening of the trabeculae with additional fibrous strands, and (5) accumulation of phagocytized hemosiderin from erythrocytes which have been entrapped in the nearly static blood and hemolyzed in excessive numbers.

Causes. Chronic passive congestion of the spleen is comparatively infrequent in animals owing to the infrequency of the causative disorders. The latter include anything which will produce increased pressure, or back pressure, in the splenic vein, such as thrombotic obstructions in, or pressure of tumors or abscesses upon, the vascular drainage system anywhere from the spleen to the heart. Cirrhosis constricts the venules through which the splenic blood must traverse the liver and causes congestion of the spleen as well as the other structures drained by the portal vein. Even right-sided valvular lesions of the heart and fibrosis of the lungs leave their marks upon the spleen in the form of venous back-pressure.

In humans, a poorly understood condition known as **Banti's disease** simulates chronic passive congestion with respect to its diffuse fibrosis. Banti's disease, however, produces a more startling picture with marked enlargement of the total size of the organ, peculiar "siderotic nodules" thought to result from old hemorrhages and the ultimate accompaniment of cirrhosis and gastric hemorrhages. In the opinion of many, Banti's disease is related to chronic passive congestion also in being a result of increased venous pressure in the spleen. The condition is not known in animals.

Acute Splenic Swelling

This form of splenic enlargement is associated with infectious inflammations and by some is called acute splenitis, although the primary inflammation is not in the spleen. The increase in size is moderate. The organ is mushy in consistency, and the purplish pulp bulges from the cut surface, from which the protruding surplus is easily removed by scraping. The enlargement is found microscopically to be due to an augmentation of the pulp, in which there are increased numbers of lymphocytes, reticulo-endothelial cells, neutrophilic granulocytes, and erythrocytes in varying proportions. The accumulation of blood cells, which is less than that seen in severe congestion, has been explained on the basis of obstructive pressure on the venules and sinuses by proliferated reticulo-endothelial tissue, a postulate which is perhaps only occasionally applicable. However implemented, it is theorized that thus delaying the blood in its passage through the spleen serves a useful purpose by exposing it longer to the actions of the several kinds of leukocytes and to humoral antibodies produced there.

In a majority of cases, the most numerous of the reactive cells are lymphocytes. In a few instances, there is a proliferation of masses of reticulo-endothelial cells which develop almost an epithelioid appearance. Some cases of brucellosis furnish an example of this, although such a change is usually more prominent in the lymph nodes. In cases of septicemia from pyogenic bacteria, areas of heavy neutrophilic infiltration occur; such a spleen is often called a **septic spleen.** In anthrax, the swelling is greater than in most other inflammatory diseases, and the considerable amount of blood in the organ makes it unusually soft, the **"blackberry-jam spleen."** However, the spleen is softened rapidly as a result of postmortem autolysis, and some humiliating diagnostic errors have been made through overlooking this fact.

Fat-storage Diseases

In the human spleen, great enlargement occurs in a group of rare diseases known variously as lipid-storage disease, reticulo-endothelial granulomas, and by other names. Gaucher's disease is the best known member of the group. All are characterized by proliferation of reticuloendothelial cells which phagocytize lipoid substances and swell to huge dimensions thereby.

Splenomegaly in Anemia

The spleen is usually enlarged and filled with blood in cases of hemolytic anemia. This appears to be a feature of the mechanism for the final disposal of the injured or disintegrating erythrocytes. It is possible that the hypothetical sphincters play a part in holding the blood in the spleen longer than the usual time. There is a varying degree of hyperplasia of the reticuloendothelial tissue, whose cells perform the function of final hemolysis, and this hyperplasia contributes also to the enlargement of the organ. What causes a certain erythrocyte to be phagocytized and destroyed while its fellows escape is an intriguing question. Presumably some cellular injury, visible as in piroplasmosis, or invisible as in some other disease, renders the erythrocyte both vulnerable and attractive to the phagocytes. In one form of hemolytic anemia (autoimmune), the cells swell and become relatively spherical (spherocytes) before they are phagocytized, a change presumably indicative of injury to them. It has also been suspected that in hemolytic anemias, the phagocytic reticulo-endothelial cells become more voracious through some change in their chemical constituents. In such spleens, there is also a marked accumulation of hemoglobinogenous pigment in the form of phagocytized hemosiderin. When the amount of hemosiderin is great, giant cells of the foreign-body type may also be numerous in the splenic pulp. These have to be distinguished from megakaryocytes, which appear in extramedullary hematopoiesis. The latter have very irregularly multilobed nuclei; the foreign-body giant cells tend to have multiple nuclei clustered together in the central portion of the cell

and not infrequently piled one upon another.

Reticulo-endothelial hyperplasia leading to splenic enlargement may also accompany diseases which are not characterized by anemia. Such is the case in histoplasmosis, leishmaniasis, and East Coast fever.

Splenic Hematopoiesis. An entirely different basis for splenic enlargement is splenic hematopoiesis. The total increase in size is only moderate. Microscopically, there are clumps and areas of cells recognizable as members of the myeloid and hematopoietic groups, myelocytes, hemocytoblasts, nucleated and mature erythrocytes, and megakaryocytes. Myelocytes are also scattered through the pulp in some cases but are recognized with difficulty.

These hematopoietic changes occur in connection with myelophthisic anemias, the bone marrow being unable to function because it is wholly or partially nonexistent. Splenic hematopoiesis also occurs in other chronic forms of anemia, especially in the young, when, without any deficiency of the essential raw materials, the normal marrow is unable to meet the demands for new cells. In other forms of anemia, the size of the spleen is not directly affected. At times caution must be exercised in judging the significance of extramedullary hematopoiesis, as it is to be expected in most perinatal animals and persists throughout life in species such as rats and mice.

Abscesses, large or small, numerous or few, form in the spleen as the result of blood-borne pyogenic infections. Abscesses or encapsulated areas of necrosis or liquefaction occasionally result from infection brought in on penetrating foreign bodies which chance to wander into the spleen from the reticulum instead of pursuing their usual course toward the heart. In such cases, there usually are extensive fibrous adhesions along the path taken by the nail, wire, or other body. Especially in

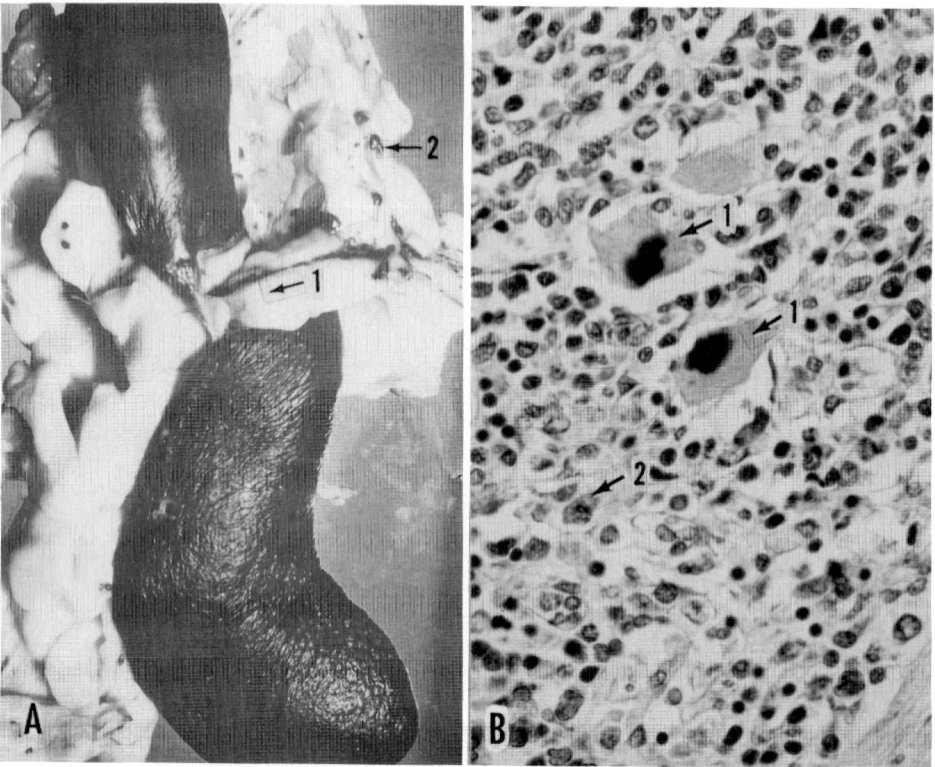

Fig. 22–6. *A*, Rupture of the spleen (*1*) of a seven-year-old Scottish Terrier, with implants of spleen (*2*) in the mesentery. The dog was hit by a car one year prior to necropsy. *B*, Extramedullary hematopoiesis, spleen of a dog. Megakaryocytes (*1*) and myeloid cells (*2*) are evident. (*B*, Courtesy of Armed Forces Institute of Pathology.) Contributor: Dr. John Mills.

the experimental animals and birds, some infections of septicemic distribution produce myriads of minute gray spots in or on the spleen. Sometimes these prove to be minute abscesses or lymphocytic foci; more often they are foci of necrosis.

Tuberculosis and other **granulomas** produce their typical lesions in the spleen when the specific organisms happen to be carried there from other regions. While tuberculosis of the bovine spleen is rare it will be noted that metastasis to the spleen is always via the systemic circulation, a consideration which is often of importance in tracing the origin of infectious or neoplastic lesions in the spleen, as in meat inspection.

Lymphoid Hyperplasia

The general aspects of the increase of lymphoid tissues of the body which accompanies many infectious processes of some duration have been described. In the spleen, this frequently encountered reaction takes the form of enlargement of the individual splenic corpuscles (Malpighian bodies). The increase is principally in the zone of densely packed lymphocytes but occasionally in young animals large, pale germinal centers develop within the splenic corpuscle. Grossly, the corpuscles appear as bulging, fuzzy, whitish nodules from 1 to 3 mm in diameter scattered through the splenic pulp. The latter is usually increased in amount and dark red or purple in color (acute splenic swelling) in these same spleens, and from the same cause, which is still acutely active.

Upon complete recovery from the causative infection, the enlarged corpuscles gradually return to normal size. Just how great a part increased lymphoid tissue has in overcoming the infection is, of course, not susceptible to precise measurement, but to the diagnostic pathologist, the lymphoid reaction is a valuable clue to the existence of a sometimes poorly evidenced infection such as canine distemper or its sequelae. Lymphoid hyperplasia need not involve all Malpighian corpuscles.

Other Disorders of the Spleen

Infarctions occur occasionally in the spleen, usually being hemorrhagic but not invariably so. They tend to be conical with the base at the capsule, as explained in the general discussion of infarcts, but may be so large as to occupy a whole end or a considerable segment of the spleen (Fig. 22–7). Infarcted areas in the dog spleen may become quite large, and consist of a mixture of elements, such as necrosis, repeated hemorrhages, blood pigments, and or-

ganization by fibrous connective tissue. Some of the hemorrhages may rupture the splenic capsule and cause death by exsanguination into the peritoneal sac.

A lesion consisting of a raised, subcapsular area, almost black in color and usually multiple, occurs in 50% of cases of hog cholera (swine fever). These have been classed as hemorrhagic infarcts, although some have been confused with mere hemorrhages. The obstruction of blood essential to infarction is considered to be due to thickening of capillary walls and minute thrombi in them.

Amyloidosis involves the splenic corpuscles, as previously explained. It is rare except in animals which have been used for the production of hyperimmune serums.

In old dogs, **siderotic plaques** or **Gandy-Gamna nodules** are frequently found on the splenic capsule. They appear as yellow, dry encrustations. Microscopically yellow-brown, iron positive pigment in trabeculae and capsule is mixed with deep blue (with hematoxylin) fibers which react to the usual stains for calcium salts. Although usually considered a senile change, the significance is not known; it may be that they are sites of previous hemorrhages.

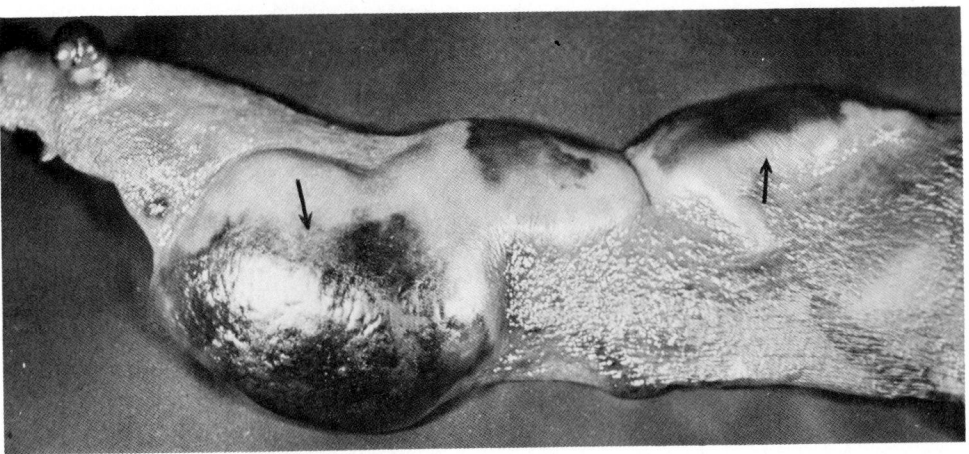

Fig. 22–7.   Infarction of the spleen of a ten-year-old female Springer Spaniel. The infarcts (arrows) near the apex are elevated and partially hemorrhagic. (Courtesy of Angell Memorial Animal Hospital.)

Cysts in the spleen may prove to contain the scolices of *Echinococcus granulosus* in the herbivorous and omnivorous species. However, this parasite is practically nonexistent in the United States.

Rupture of the spleen is a not infrequent accident in the dog for reasons which must be evident in a world of automotive transportation. A considerable number of dogs so injured survive, and the two or more healed fragments of the spleen are found at autopsy years later. There are even cases in which several small fragments of spleen are spattered over the adjoining areas and become implanted in the mesentery to live and carry on such functions as do not require anatomically normal vascular connections. Infarction of the spleen and malignant tumors (hemangioendothelioma) may also lead to rupture of the capsule and exsanguination. Accessory spleens of varying sizes originate also as congenital malformations but these are rare.

Neoplasms of the Spleen

Lymphosarcoma, Malignant Lymphoma

Solitary lesions of lymphosarcoma may occasionally be found in the spleen of many species, but usually such tumors are present as a part of the generalized neoplastic disease. Sharply demarcated lesions may be seen, made up of lymphocytic cells. In some cases, more diffuse invasion and replacement of the spleen may be evident.

Canine Nodular Hyperplasia, "Splenoma"

Not infrequently in old dogs this lesion may be encountered as an incidental finding at necropsy. The lesion consists of one or more sharply demarcated nodules which elevate the splenic capsule (Fig. 22–8). Microscopically, the lesion is made up of most of the elements of the spleen, except that the lymphocytic cells are quite hyperplastic. Some structures of hyperplastic cells are spherical and resemble splenic corpus-

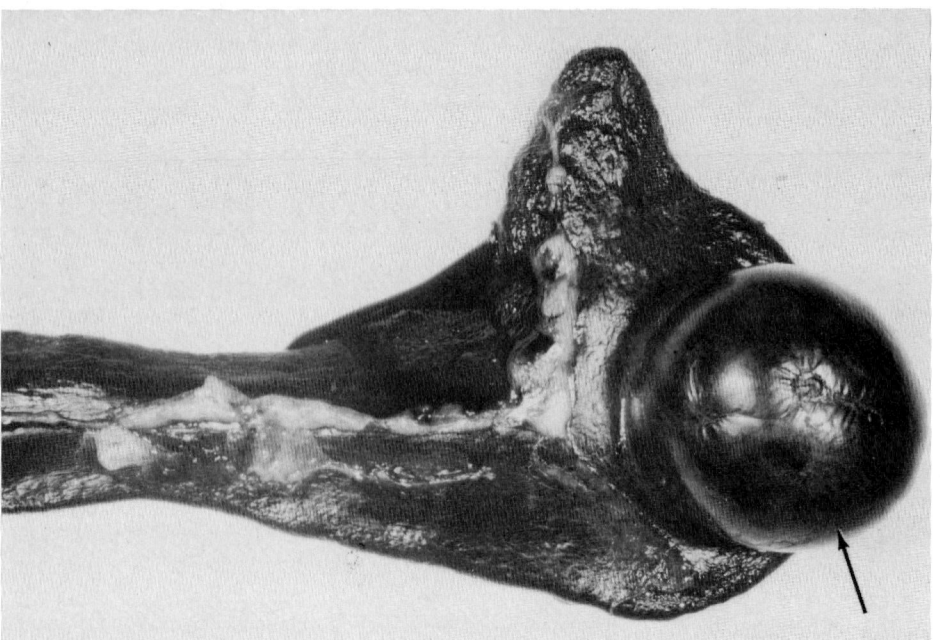

Fig. 22–8. Nodular hyperplasia ("splenoma") of the spleen of a 14-year-old male Collie. (Courtesy of Angell Memorial Animal Hospital.)

cles except that the central artery is absent. The significance of this lesion is unknown. It may or may not be neoplastic but its course is assumed to be benign. Grossly, this lesion may be distinguished by its uniform smooth surface and globoid shape from long standing infarcts of the spleen. Microscopically, the lymphoid nature of the mass is clearly different than the necrosis, hemorrhage, and fibrous organization found in old infarcts.

Hemangioendothelioma, Hemangiosarcoma

This is among the most frequently encountered primary tumors of the spleen, especially in the dog. The essential feature is the presence of pleomorphic masses of tumor cells resembling endothelial cells. These cells have large, ovoid hyperchromic nuclei and cytoplasm which may be fused with contiguous cells. Mitoses are frequent. The tumor cells may be seen to form blood-filled vascular spaces, a distinguishing characteristic. Sometimes the tumor cells form sheets which suggest the littoral cells and their sinusoids.

Repeated hemorrhages, necrosis, and organization may make this tumor difficult to distinguish from long-standing infarction of the spleen. The critical item in the diagnosis of hemangioendothelioma is the presence of typical vascular-forming malignant endothelial cells. These are usually found at the periphery of the lesion and sometimes are dwarfed by large amounts of hemorrhage, necrosis, and organization.

These tumors sometimes rupture the splenic capsule and lead to fatal bleeding into the peritoneal sac. If this hemorrhage is not fatal, tumor cells may be seeded and grow on peritoneal surfaces. They may also be associated with multicentric or metastatic hemangioendotheliomas in the liver and atrium of the heart.

Leiomyosarcoma

These tumors presumably arise from the smooth muscle cells of the splenic trabeculae. Light-colored, irregular, single or multiple masses are present in the spleen, often accompanied by hemorrhage. The tumor cells are immature smooth muscle cells with elongated cytoplasm arranged in interwoven sheets and masses with some cells in parallel arrays. The nuclei are ovoid, their long axis parallel to the length of the cells, and mitoses are frequent.

These tumors are considered malignant and may metastasize via the blood stream or become seeded in the peritoneal cavity.

Metastatic Neoplasms

Although not a frequent event, any malignant neoplasm whose cells reach the bloodstream could metastasize to the spleen. It appears that the lung filters out most such circulating malignant cells, but a few are deposited and grow in the spleen. Myeloid leukemia may involve the spleen, presenting a problem in distinguishing it from extramedullary hemopoiesis. A myelolipoma, with myeloid and lipomatous elements, has been described in a cat.

Dennis, S.M.: Congenital splenic defects in newborn lambs. Cornell Vet., *62*:473–476, 1972.

Ishmael, J., and Howell, J. McC.: Neoplasia of the spleen of the dog with a note on nodular hyperplasia. J. Comp. Path., *78*:59–67, 1968.

Jacobsen, G.: Morphological-histochemical comparison of dog and cat splenic ellipsoid sheaths. Anat. Rec., *169*:105–113, 1971.

Jolly, R.D.: Nodular hyperplasia of the ovine spleen. N.Z. Vet. J., *15*:91–94, 1967.

Lau, D.T.L.: Ectopic splenic nodules in the pancreas of a Capuchin monkey (*Cebus albifrons*). J. Med. Primatol., *2*:67–70, 1973.

Sander, C.H., and Langham, R.F.: Myelolipoma of the spleen in a cat. J. Am. Vet. Med. Assoc., *160*:1101–1103, 1972.

THE LYMPH NODES

Reactive Hyperplasia

The alert student will recognize the error in the designation *adenitis* for inflammatory lesions involving lymph nodes which are not glands. However, the use of the term "lymphadenitis" is so well entrenched in the literature and vocabulary of veterinarians as well as physicians that it has become the accepted (although erroneous) way to communicate inflammatory lesions of lymph nodes. The term reactive hyperplasia is in many instances more suitable and correct for describing the changes lymph nodes undergo in inflammation. More specific designations are also recommended, such as "abscess in the lymph node," "edematous lymph node," "granulomatous reaction in the lymph node." We are not able to bury the old misnomer, "lymphadenitis" because of its widespread usage, but we can and shall continue to push it toward a well-deserved grave.

By far the most frequent disorder of lymph nodes to concern the veterinary pathologist is the acute swelling which is characteristic of most of the acute septicemic diseases. Prominent among these are anthrax, pasteurellosis, hog cholera, swine erysipelas, and others. In septicemias such as these, the infection is rather generally spread throughout the body and, accordingly, the reaction usually involves many, or perhaps nearly all of the nodes with little regard for anatomic location.

A comparable process is seen when a particular organ or region of the body is involved in an acute infectious inflammation, for the lymph nodes which drain the affected part undergo a similar acute inflammatory swelling. For instance, the bronchial lymph nodes are enlarged in the presence of pneumonia, the mandibular and pharyngeal nodes swell in the case of rhinitis or an infected tooth, and the supramammary nodes respond similarly to mastitis. The reason for this is obviously that the infectious irritant is drained into the regional lymph nodes. It produces approximately the same effects in the node as it did in its original location, including pain as well as the other aspects of inflammation. The total results are frequently beneficial by virtue of the filtering capacity of the node to prevent further progress of the pathogenic organisms. If this fails, the filtering attempt is repeated at the next group of lymph nodes along the lymph-vascular route.

Lesions. The lesion which accounts for the swelling is a combination of exudation with proliferation of the lymphoid and reticular (reticulo-endothelial) tissues of the node. The exudate most frequently is chiefly serous, and the lymph nodes are described grossly as edematous (inflammatory edema). They are swollen and somewhat soft, and the cut surface bulges slightly. There is always hyperemia, and in some of the septicemias the nodes are "hemorrhagic." This means that considerable amounts of blood accompany the incoming lymph so that the node is red grossly, and microscopically contains large numbers of erythrocytes in the lymph sinuses. In a minority of cases when the infecting organism is in the pyogenic group, the exudate in the regional lymph nodes is clearly purulent, the sinuses containing large numbers of neutrophilic granulocytes. Abscesses develop rarely and will be mentioned later.

The proliferative part of the reaction is always considerable, the lymph sinuses being narrowed or filled with lymphocytes among which are mixed a certain number of reticulo-endothelial mononuclears, a few plasma cells, and a scattering of blood-borne leukocytes.

In many acute generalized infections, especially those caused by viruses, necrosis of lymphocytes is a major feature of acute lymphadenitis. This in part may be due to the depressant effect of adrenal corticosteroids on lymphocytes, but many viruses specifically destroy lymphocytes, for example, rinderpest virus and most herpesviruses.

If the outcome of the infectious process is favorable, the nodes return to normal with recovery from the primary disease process.

Abscesses develop in acutely inflamed lymph nodes less frequently than would be expected, even though the reaction be of

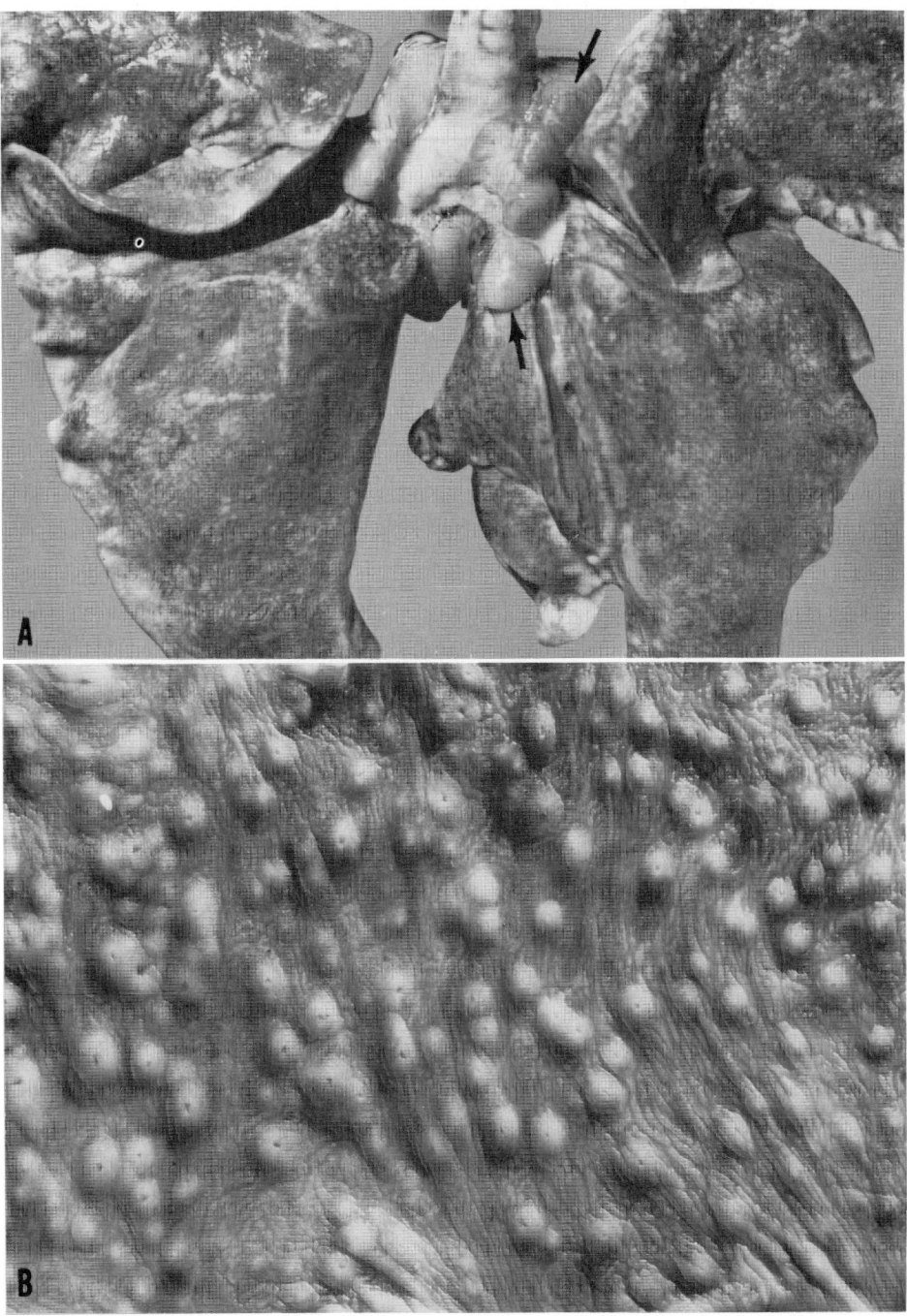

Fig. 22–9. *A*, Hyperplasia of bronchial lymph nodes (arrows) in a dog with "salmon disease." *B*, Hyperplasia of the lymph nodules in colon of a dog with "salmon disease." (Courtesy of Dr. Wm. J. Hadlow.)

the purulent type. When this change does occur, the whole node is usually transformed into a single abscess, the capsule of the node becoming the capsule of the abscess. These abscesses usually rupture to the exterior, sometimes into a body cavity. This process is the rule in equine strangles, the submaxillary (mandibular) nodes regularly forming a single large abscess.

Lymphoid Hyperplasia

Lymphoid hyperplasia, general or regional, is the usual reaction to a number of less virulent and less rapidly progressive infections, like canine distemper, chronic pneumonitis and chronic enteritides. The affected nodes are moderately enlarged, firm and dry, but neither fibrous nor calcified. Microscopic examination shows the increase in size to be due to lymphocytes almost exclusively. Germinal centers are numerous and surrounded by a wide zone of closely packed and darkly staining lymphocytes. In cases of generalized lymphoid hyperplasia, the lymphocyte count of the blood shows some increase from the previous level for the individual animal, but does not necessarily exceed the normal maximum. A frequent picture when death comes from one of the diseases in this group is a node containing many germinal centers which are very large, but with only a narrow and inconspicuous zone of mature lymphocytes around them. The germinal centers proper are large and pale because of the very active proliferation of the pale maternal lymphoblasts, even though the accumulation of mature lymphocytes is slight. This condition has the very suitable name of lymphoid hyperplasia with lymphoid exhaustion. The lymph nodes return to the normal state if the cause of the disease is overcome.

Granulomatous Reactions

Granulomatous reactions usually represent one of the specific infectious granulomatous infections. The lesion in the lymph node is that which is typical for the disease in question regardless of location. Among the more prominent granulomatous infections of lymph nodes are tuberculosis, Johne's disease, glanders, "caseous lymphadenitis," and actinobacillosis.

A diffuse and extensive proliferation of solid masses of reticulo-endothelial cells is occasionally seen. The large pale cells with their expansive cytoplasm fill the lymphoid sinuses, especially in the medulla of the node. This reaction is typical of, but not limited to, **brucellosis** in swine. Rarely, the reticulo-endothelial cells assume bizarre forms and develop into giant cells with multilobar central nuclei. If they are accompanied by some fibrosis and a variable number of eosinophilic granulocytes, the proliferated tissue comes to resemble the tissue of **Hodgkin's disease** as seen in human patients. The latter is usually thought to be a variant of lymphoblastic neoplasia (malignant lymphoma), although the theory that it is inflammatory has also had numerous supporters.

Other Disorders of the Lymph Nodes

Other disorders found to affect lymph nodes include amyloidosis and certain pigmentations. Anthracosis of the nodes occurs when carbon pigment is carried to them from the lungs. Hemosiderosis, hemochromatosis, and melanosis occur rarely. A brownish discoloration of the medullary portion, especially, seen frequently in bovine lymph nodes does not indicate ill health. It may be related to porphyrinemia.

Aberrant parasites, including the mange mite, *Demodex folliculorum*, are seldom found in lymph nodes.

Neoplasms of the Lymph Nodes

Primary Neoplasms

Primary neoplasms of lymph nodes include lymphosarcoma (malignant lymphoma), hemangioendothelioma, and lymphangiosarcoma. The latter tumor is rare and may arise at other sites, but is usually seen in lymph nodes. The tumor arises from cells of the lymphatic vessels and therefore tends to form cystic spaces lined with endothelium, but not containing blood. Most individual tumors are benign.

The problem of malignant lymphogranulomatosis (Hodgkin's Disease) in animals is referred to earlier in this chapter.

Metastatic Neoplasms

Metastatic neoplasms in lymph nodes are a frequent occurrence and present challenges as well as opportunities to the pathologist. All malignant neoplasms have the potential of metastasis to lymph nodes. Those neoplasms most often seen as metastases to lymph nodes of animals include: adenocarcinomas (mammary especially), squamous cell carcinomas, mast cell tumors, hemangiopericytoma, and hemangioendotheliomas. One important point for the histopathologist to remember is that the afferent lymphatics lead to the lymph node's cortex and empty into the cortical sinuses. Malignant cells will initially be seen, therefore, in the cortical sinuses. As the tumor cells proliferate, they involve the cortex of the lymph node. When tumor growth reaches the hilus of the lymph node, malignant cells have the opportunity to metastasize further via the efferent lymphatics. This is true in all domestic animals except the pig in which the cortical and medullary tissues of lymph nodes are reversed. In swine, the afferent lymphatics penetrate deep into the nodes where the lymphatic nodules are located, and the lymph filters to the peripheral sinuses and exits via efferent lymphatics.

If an epithelial neoplasm, such as adenocarcinoma or squamous cell carcinoma, is found in viable state in a lymph node, it is clearly malignant, no matter how differentiated the tumor cells may appear.

Thymus

The role of the thymus in determining the immunologic functioning of lymphocytes is described in Chapters 6 and 7. The occurrence of lymphosarcoma and benign epithelial and lymphocytic thymomas in the thymus is recorded previously in this chapter. A thymoma consisting of epithelial cells with clear, vacuolated cytoplasm has been reported (Mackey, 1975). It appears that thymomas occur with more frequency in cattle and dairy goats than in other species, although reported in many species, including dog, cat, and mastomys (Praomys (Mastomys) natalensis). The association of thymoma and myasthenia gravis in man and animals has been referred to in Chapter 19.

Thymic hyperplasia, or failure of involution, is occasionally recorded in animals, although its significance is not at this time understood.

Hadlow, W.J.: High prevalence of thymoma in the dairy goat. Report of seventeen cases. Vet. Pathol., 15:153–169, 1978.

Loveday, R.K.: Thymoma in a Siamese cat. J. So. Afr. Vet. Med. Assoc., 30:33–34, 1959.

Mackey, L.: Clear-cut thymoma and thymic hyperplasia in a cat. J. Comp. Pathol., 85:367–371, 1975.

Robinson, M.: Malignant thymoma with metastases in a dog. Vet. Pathol., 11:172–180, 1974.

Sandison, A.T., and Anderson, L.J.: Tumors of the thymus in cattle, sheep, and pigs. Cancer Res., 29:1146–1150, 1969.

Stewart, H.L., and Snell, K.C.: Thymomas and thymic hyperplasia in Praomys (Mastomys) natalensis. Concomitant myositis, myocarditis, and sialodacryoadenitis. J. Natl. Cancer Inst., 40:1135–1159, 1968.

CHAPTER 23

The Digestive System

MOUTH AND ADNEXA

The mucous surface of the buccal cavity, the gums, tongue, and pharynx are subject to acute exudative inflammations of the usual kinds. Caustic medicines are occasionally administered and cause severe inflammation or necrosis in the mouth or pharynx. Physical trauma from sharp awns of plants may act as an inciting cause in the mouths of herbivora; sharp bones may play a similar role in dogs and cats. However, all extensive or prolonged forms of **stomatitis,** as inflammation of the buccal mucosa is called, owe their existence to the activity of pathogenic microorganisms or viruses. The buccal lesions of aphthous fever, vesicular stomatitis, vesicular exanthema, rinderpest, and malignant catarrhal fever are discussed in the descriptions of those diseases. Nonspecific infections may be caused by the various pyogenic bacteria or the necrophorus organism, with inflammatory lesions characteristic of those pathogens, but only in the event that the involved area has previously suffered traumatic or chemical injury or has been otherwise devitalized. An example of severe stomatitis is seen in experimental or natural niacin deficiency.

Ulcers

Ulcers of variable latitude but of minimal depth are encountered with some frequency in the mouth of the dog, many of them on the less heavily epithelialized parts of the tongue. The majority of these are manifestations of uremia, constituting one aspect of the injury done to the whole alimentary mucosa in the course of the partial elimination of toxic urinary wastes through the mucous membrane. Buccal ulcers are a part of the syndrome of canine leptospirosis, but the pathogenetic mechanism is still that of uremia. Ulcers on the tongue and necrosis of the tip have also been considered characteristic of canine pellagra, or blacktongue.

Many infectious diseases result in ulceration of the oral mucosa. These include those listed above under stomatitis as well as most herpesvirus infections, bluetongue, papular stomatitis of cattle, and the virus diarrhea : mucosal disease complex. Actinobacillosis in bovines frequently involves the tongue.

The epithelial hyperplasia and hyperkeratosis of poisoning by chlorinated naphthalenes in bovines are commonly evident on the mucosa of the tongue, lips, and other buccal surfaces.

Feline Eosinophilic Granuloma

A specific ulcerative lesion is not infrequent in the oral mucosa of domesticated cats. The lesions may appear in cats of any age upon the lips at the mucocutaneous junction, buccal or pharyngeal mucosa, or in mucosa at the base of the tongue. The ulcers are irregular in shape, sharply demarcated, and not very deep. They heal with cortisone administration, but the cause is unknown. A familial disease is also known in Siberian Husky dogs.

The microscopic lesion is distinctive. The underlying collagen fibers are frequently necrotic and associated with a dense leukocytic reaction. Eosinophilic leukocytes predominate in the exudate and may be seen in the stroma around the ulcerated zone.

Developmental Anomalies

Two developmental anomalies of the tongue merit mention here. The first is *epitheliogenesis imperfecta lingua bovis* (smooth tongue). In this defect, the small filiform papillae on the surface of the tongue are reduced in size, leaving the surface abnormally smooth. The defect is believed to be inherited as an autosomal recessive factor. It affects bovine animals of the Friesian breed.

The second anomaly is called "lethal glossopharyngeal defect" in the dog. This is manifest by a malformed small pointed tongue in newborn puppies. They cannot suckle and die soon after birth.

Periodontium

The periodontium consists, as its name implies, of those structures of the mandible and maxilla which surround and give support to the teeth. Specifically, the alveolar bone, periodontal ligament, and gingiva are components of the periodontium. The periodontal ligament is made up of collagenous connective tissue which binds the alveolar bone to the cementum of the tooth. The periodontium of many species has been studied in detail by investigators interested in human dentistry, and the literature on the subject continues to grow.

Periodontal Disease

Periodontal disease or periodontitis is applied to the rather specific inflammatory processes in the periodontium which eventually lead to loss of teeth. This disease is considered to be the most common cause of loss of teeth in people in the United States. Comparable changes have been described in several nonhuman primates (chimpanzee, baboon, marmosets, galago, squirrel monkey, and Rhesus monkey). The process in chimpanzees most closely mimics the human disease. Periodontitis has also been described in dogs, cats, ferrets, hamsters, guinea pigs, least shrew, and rat. It mainly affects people in the 30- to 50-year-old group and is also more common in older animals.

The pathogenic process is believed to start in the gingiva with localized gingivitis at the junction of tooth and gum where dental plaques have formed. The capillaries in the subepithelial stroma of the gingiva become dilated and congested, and often are filled with neutrophils. Leukocytes (lymphocytes, monocytes, and macrophages) and fibroblasts become numerous in the stroma, which eventually becomes edematous and contains proliferating endothelial cells of capillaries, fibroblasts, and fragmented collagen.

The crevicular epithelium migrates deeper along the cementum of the tooth. The sulcus between tooth and gingiva is expanded and filled with bacterial plaque and calculus along with leukocytes and tissue debris. This inflammation and increased vascular flow is accompanied by destruction of alveolar bone with osteolytic packets in the bone. The continued destruction of bone and periodontal ligament leads to increased mobility, tilting, and drifting of the teeth. Eventually, the periodontal inflammation leads to loss of the teeth. This somewhat simplified, as well as abbreviated, description of the visualized pathologic processes may be enhanced by the student from the references which follow.

A troublesome problem in sheep which results in loss of incisor teeth has been described in New Zealand under the term

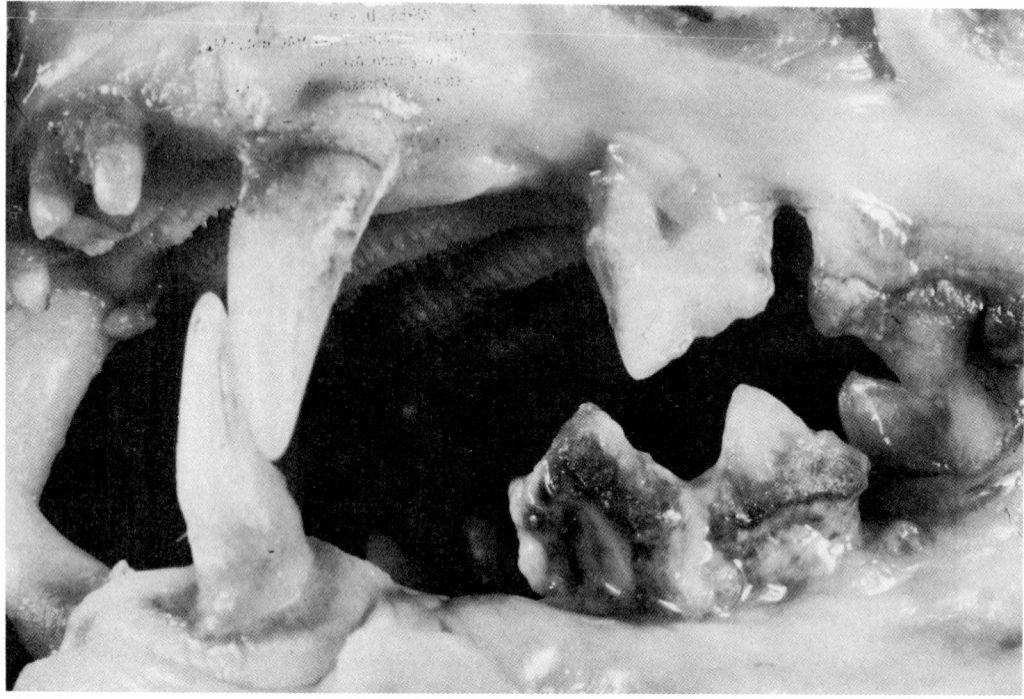

Fig. 23–1. Periodontal disease resulting in receding gums and exposure of roots of teeth of a three-year-old female tortoiseshell and white cat. (Courtesy of Angell Memorial Animal Hospital.)

periodontosis (Cutress, et al., 1972). This disease appeared to differ in pathogenetic mechanism from periodontitis and was associated with deficiency of serum calcium, albumin, alkaline phosphatase, and citrate. The calcium:phosphorous ratio was generally lower in affected animals than in normal controls on a nearby farm. This disease was concluded to have, in all probability, a nutritional basis.

Another serious antecedent to loss of teeth is fibrous osteodystrophy (Figure 19–8). Infections such as actinomycosis and actinobacillosis may also displace teeth. Neoplasms in the mandible or maxilla may also have this effect.

Ammons, W.F., Schectman, L.R., and Page, R.C.: Host tissue response in chronic periodontal disease. I. The normal periodontium and manifestations of dental and periodontal disease in the marmoset. J. Periodont. Res., 7:131–143, 1972.

Arnold, L., and Baram, P.: Periodontal disease in chimpanzees. J. Periodont., 44:437–442, 1973.

Cutress, T.W., et al.: Periodontal disease in sheep. II. The composition of sera from sheep with periodontosis. J. Periodontol., 43:668–676, 1972.

Dreizen, S., Levy, B.M., and Bernick, S.: Studies on biology of periodontium of marmosets. X. Cortisone induced periodontal and skeletal changes in adult cotton top marmosets. J. Periodont. Res., 42:217–224, 1971.

Dreizen, S., Levy, B.M., and Bernick, S.: Studies on the biology of the periodontium of marmosets. XII. Effect of an experimentally produced malabsorption syndrome on marmoset periodontium. J. Periodont. Res., 7:251–254, 1972.

Dreizen, S., Levy, B.M., and Bernick, S.: Studies on the biology of the periodontium of marmosets. XIII. Histopathology of niacin deficiency stomatitis in the marmoset. J. Periodont., 48:452–455, 1977.

Dreizen, S., and Levy, B.M.: Monkey models in dental research. J. Med. Primatol., 6:133–144, 1977.

Grant, D., and Bernick, S.: Formation of the periodontal ligament. J. Periodontol., 43:17–25, 1972.

Grant, D.A., Chase, J., and Bernick, S.: Biology of the periodontium in primates of the Galago species. J. Periodontol., 44:540–550, 1973.

Hershkovitz, P.: Dental and periodontal diseases and abnormalities in wild-caught marmosets (primates-Callithricidae). Am. J. Phys. Anthropol., 32:377–394, 1970.

Hodosh, M., Povar, M., and Shklar, G.: Periodontitis in baboon (*Papio anubis*). J. Peridont., 42:594–596, 1971.

Hull, P.S., Soames, J.V., and Davies, R.M.: Periodontal disease in a Beagle dog colony. J. Comp. Pathol., 84:143–150, 1974.

Kennedy, J.E., and Polson, A.M.: Experimental marginal periodontitis in squirrel monkeys. J. Periodont., 44:140–144, 1973.

Levy, B.M.: Nonhuman primate as an analog for study of periodontal disease. J. Dent. Res., 50:246–253, 1971.

Levy, B.M., Dreizen, S., and Bernick, S.: Effect of aging on the marmoset periodontium. J. Oral Pathol., 1:61–65, 1972.

Levy, B.M.: Prevention of periodontal disease—a pathologist's view. Int. Dent. J., 23:476–480, 1973.

Levy, B.M.: Animal model of human disease. Chronic destructive periodontitis in marmosets. Am. J. Pathol., 83:637–640, 1976.

Schectman, L.R., Ammons, W.F., Simpson, D.M., and Page, R.C.: Host tissue response in chronic periodontal disease. II. Histologic features of the normal periodontium, and histopathologic and ultrastructural manifestations of disease in the marmoset. J. Periodont. Res., 7:195–212, 1972.

Teeth and Palate

The teeth of animals are much less subject to caries (dental decay) than are those of humans. The comparative absence of readily fermentable carbohydrates in the diets of animals may well be credited for this fortunate difference, in the light of current doctrines on this important human disorder. Supernumerary teeth, usually rudimentary in size and development, are not rare in the horse ("wolf teeth") and occur occasionally in other species. Developmental anomalies in the form of teeth misplaced in the middle of the hard palate have been seen in the horse especially. In rickets, the development and emergence of the teeth may be greatly delayed. Rather specific changes are present in the teeth in fluoride poisoning. Infectious diseases, such as canine distemper and rat virus, in the neonate may result in severe alterations in the growth of permanent or deciduous teeth. These teeth are often small, distorted, and discolored.

One of the most frequent congenital anomalies is the **cleft palate.** This results from the failure of the primitive oral-nasal cavity to be divided, leaving a cleft of varying length in the approximate center of the hard palate (Figure 4–5). The defect may extend cranially to involve the lip, leaving a cleft which produces the so called "hare lip" anomaly. Failure of teeth to develop is a rare anomaly, known in sheep and rats as hereditary defects.

Another developmental anomaly involving the teeth is "enamel pearls." These are displaced excrescences of enamel which are infrequently found on human teeth at the bifurcation of the roots of the permanent molar teeth. One case in a dog has been reported (Schneck, 1973) that involved both lower first molars. The layers of enamel lying partially over the dentine resulted in collection of food particles and purulent gingivitis.

Dennis, S.M., and Leipold, H.W.: Agnathia in sheep: external observations. Am. J. Vet. Res., 33:339–348, 1972.

Friedman, L.A., Levy, B.M., and Ennever, J.: Epidemiology of gingivitis and calculus in a marmoset colony. J. Dent. Res., 51:803–806, 1972.

Gardner, A.F., Darke, B.H., and Keary, G.T.: Dental caries in domesticated dogs. J. Am. Vet. Med. Assoc., 140:433–436, 1962.

Hock, J., and Nuki, K.: A vital microscopy study of the morphology of normal and inflamed gingiva. J. Periodont. Res., 6:81–88, 1971.

Horowitz, S.L., and Chase, H.B.: A microform of cleft palate in dogs. J. Dent. Res., 49:892, 1970.

Hutt, F.B., and de Lahunta, A.: A lethal glossopharyngeal defect in the dog. J. Hered., 62:291–293, 1971.

Kenney, E.B.: A histopathologic study of incisal dysfunction and gingival inflammation in Rhesus monkey. J. Periodont., 42:3–7, 1971.

Lawson, D.D., et al.: Dental anatomy and histology of the dog. Res. Vet. Sci., 1:204–210, 1960.

Noble, H.W.: Comparative aspects of amelogenesis imperfecta. Proc. R. Soc. Med., 62:1295–1297, 1969.

Schneck, G.W.: A case of enamel pearls in a dog. Vet. Rec., 92:115–117, 1973.

Swindler, D.R., and Merrill, O.M.: Spontaneous cleft lip and palate in a living nonhuman primate. *Macaca mulatta*. Am. J. Phys. Anthropol., 34:435–440, 1970.

Weinreb, M.M., and Sharav, Y.: Tooth development in sheep. Am. J. Vet. Res., 25:891–908, 1964.

Weisman-Hammerman, Z.M.: Some aspects of the hereditary defect epitheliogenesis imperfecta linguae bovis (smooth-tongue): studies on differentiation and keratinization in tongue epithelium. Praefschrift Vet. Fak., Utrecht, Rijksuniv., p. 135, 1970.

Tumors in the Oral Cavity

Primary tumors in the oral cavity and pharynx may originate from one of three tissue sources: the oral mucosa, the periodontium, or odontogenic tissues. The neoplasms which are reported to occur in animals from these tissues are listed in Table 23–1. It may be questioned whether the epulides from the periodontium or some odontogenic new growths are actually neoplasms, but until the matter is settled we shall consider all new growths together.

The periodontium, from which certain new growths arise, has been described. The embryonic development of the tooth needs to be understood in order to grasp the probable nature and origin of odontogenic tumors. In the mammalian embryo, the tooth starts as a focal proliferation of the entoderm along a part of the foregut which will eventually become oral mucosa adjacent to the mandible or maxilla. The growth of the entoderm (odontogenic epithelium) is met by specific proliferation of the mesoderm; together these tissues soon resemble the eventual shape of the tooth. The two tissues, epithelium and mesenchyme, appear to interact with one another to cause specific differentiation or specialization by both. This interaction is referred to as "reciprocal induction" in tooth formation. It is used as a basis for the classification scheme of odontogenic tumors proposed by the World Health Organization's "International Histological Classification of Tumors."

Thus, the development of the normal tooth is believed to depend upon inductive influences exerted by one tissue upon another. The main inductive effect appears to be exerted by the odontogenic epithelium on the adjacent mesenchymal tissues (mesoderm). This interaction results in formation of the dental papilla from which are formed odontoblasts which produce dentin. The dentin appears to instigate the formation of ameloblasts from the odontogenic epithelium, which eventually differentiate to the extent that they produce the enamel organ, and eventually the enamel of the crown of the tooth.

Dentin normally has a structure of parallel tubules, which makes it easy to identify in histologic sections. If this tubular arrangement is absent, as may occur in tumors, the dentin may be difficult to distinguish from bone or osteoid. The cementum is also produced by the mesodermal tissues of the dental papilla, and it is deposited on that part of the tooth to become the root. In abnormal conditions, cementum may also be difficult to distinguish histologically from dentin or osteoid. Abnormal growth of this already complex odontogenic apparatus may add even more complexity. Tumors of this origin are rare in man and even more rarely reported in animals. Future progress in the understanding of the neoplasms or other lesions in the odontogenic apparatus may be stimulated by an orderly, international classification scheme for these lesions. For this reason we have chosen to follow, insofar as possible, the World Health Organization proposal.

Odontogenic Tumors

Ameloblastoma. The most frequently reported of this rare group of tumors in animals is the ameloblastoma (adamantinoma). See Fig. 23–2. This is a benign lesion which usually arises deep in the mandible or maxilla. It is usually radiolucent, sometimes multiloculated, and an embedded tooth may be included in the lesion. It is made up of proliferated odontogenic epithelium in a fibrous stroma and may have many variant histologic features. The **follicular variant** contains many irregular nests of epithelial cells, which in the basal layer are made up of tall columnar cells with elongated, closely packed nuclei arranged perpendicular to the basement membrane. These resemble the internal dental epithelium or preameloblasts. The central mass of epithelial cells is usually

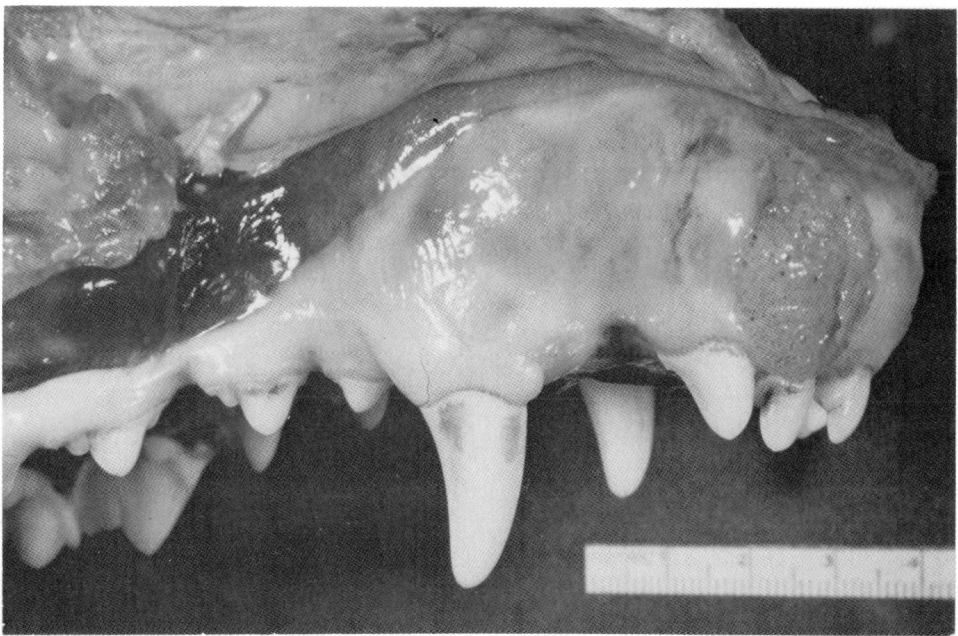

Fig. 23–2. Ameloblastoma of maxilla of a 14-month-old standard poodle. (Courtesy of Angell Memorial Animal Hospital.)

stellate or polyhedral and often vesiculated. The **acanthomatous form** resembles the follicular except that squamous cells are conspicuous in the center of many of the epithelial masses. In the **plexiform variant,** the supporting stroma is scant, and the epithelium is bounded by the usual columnar cells with characteristic basal arrangement, but the enclosed epithelial cells are irregular, often stellate, and sometimes absent. Cysts in the stroma may be seen. The **basal cell type,** although arising deep in the jaw, resembles basal cell tumor of the skin. The **granular cell type** may have some epithelial cells suggesting ameloblasts, but many epithelial cells are enlarged and polyhedral, and their cytoplasm is filled with coarse acidophilic granules. The resemblance of this tumor to the "granular-cell myoblastoma," which arises at the base of the tongue, may be striking.

Other variations which may be seen in histologic sections of ameloblastomas may include sharply demarcated hyalinized stroma, large blood-filled spaces in the stroma, and, rarely, association with a neuroma.

The ameloblastoma, often reported as an adamantinoma, has been recorded in dogs; cattle; horses; cats; a Rhesus, cebus, and a spider monkey; and a Bengal tiger.

Ameloblastic Fibroma. The ameloblastic fibroma has been described in a few animals (cattle, cats). It is seen histologically as containing large areas of cellular stroma, some part of which may be hyalinized, with an array of odontogenic epithelium scattered through it. In some cases, the epithelium consists of spherical masses with columnar cells radiating around the periphery, in other cases, the epithelium may appear as multiple branching strands of double rows of epithelium.

These tumors grow by expansion and may reach relatively large size. Metastasis has not been reported.

Ameloblastic Odontoma. Ameloblastic odontoma has been recorded on rare occasions in the equine and bovine species. This tumor is made up of mesodermal tissue which resembles that of the dermal papilla and odontogenic epithelium which has undergone proliferation. Odontoblasts are not formed.

Complex Odontoma. Complex odontoma is reported rarely in animals (dogs, sheep, cattle, rats). It is histologically, by the presence of all of the dental tissues, essentially well formed, but with a disorderly arrangement. Complete teeth are not formed. The lesion is considered a malformation.

Compound Odontoma. Compound odontoma is distinguished from the complex odontomas by the presence of teeth with enamel, dentin, cementum, and pulp. The tooth-like structures vary in size and arrangement and may replace normal teeth. These are also rare, but have been reported in horses, cattle, dogs, and rats.

Odontogenic Myxoma. Odontogenic myxoma is a rare lesion in animals (dogs).

This lesion is described as being locally invasive and consists of angular and rounded cells in an abundant stroma rich in mucoid material. A few strands of odontogenic epithelium may be scattered through the mass.

Cementoma. Cementoma is a term used for confluent masses of cementum, usually found around the base of a tooth. Part of the cementum may be mineralized, other parts not. The variant called "cementifying fibroma" has a dense fibrous stroma with many islands of irregular cementum scattered through it. These lesions have been reported in the horse and dog.

Periodontal Tumors

These lesions are most frequently seen growing as single or multiple masses from the gingiva of dogs. Boxers and Boston Terriers are more frequently involved, according to some studies. Dubielzig, et al., (1979) have suggested that these lesions be

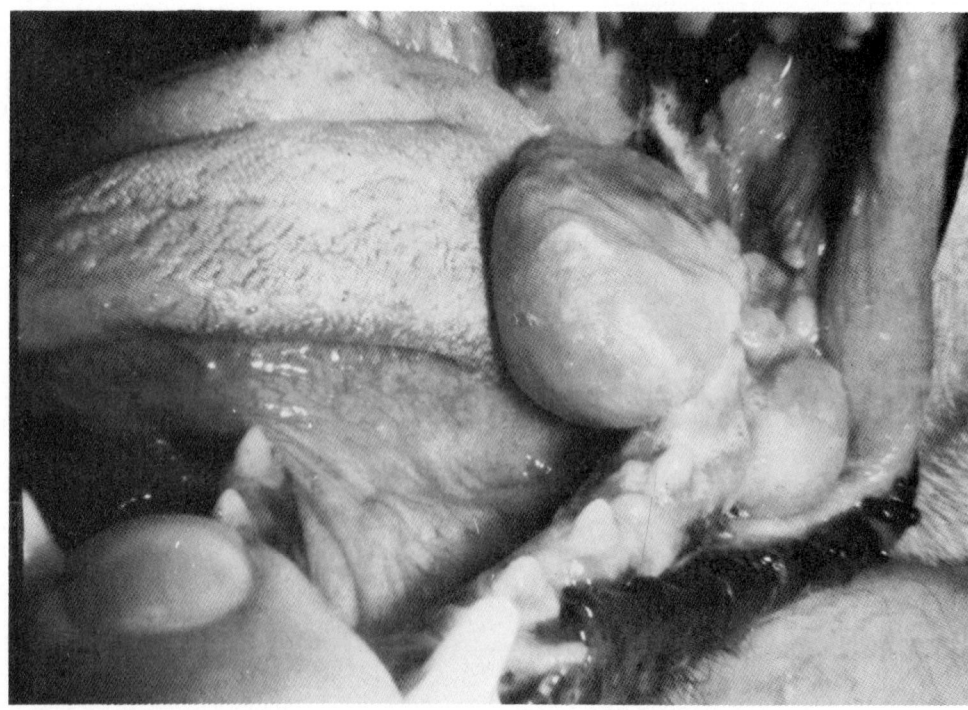

Fig. 23–3. Fibromatous epulis of periodontal origin on mandible. (Courtesy of Dr. R. R. Dubielzig and *Veterinary Pathology*.)

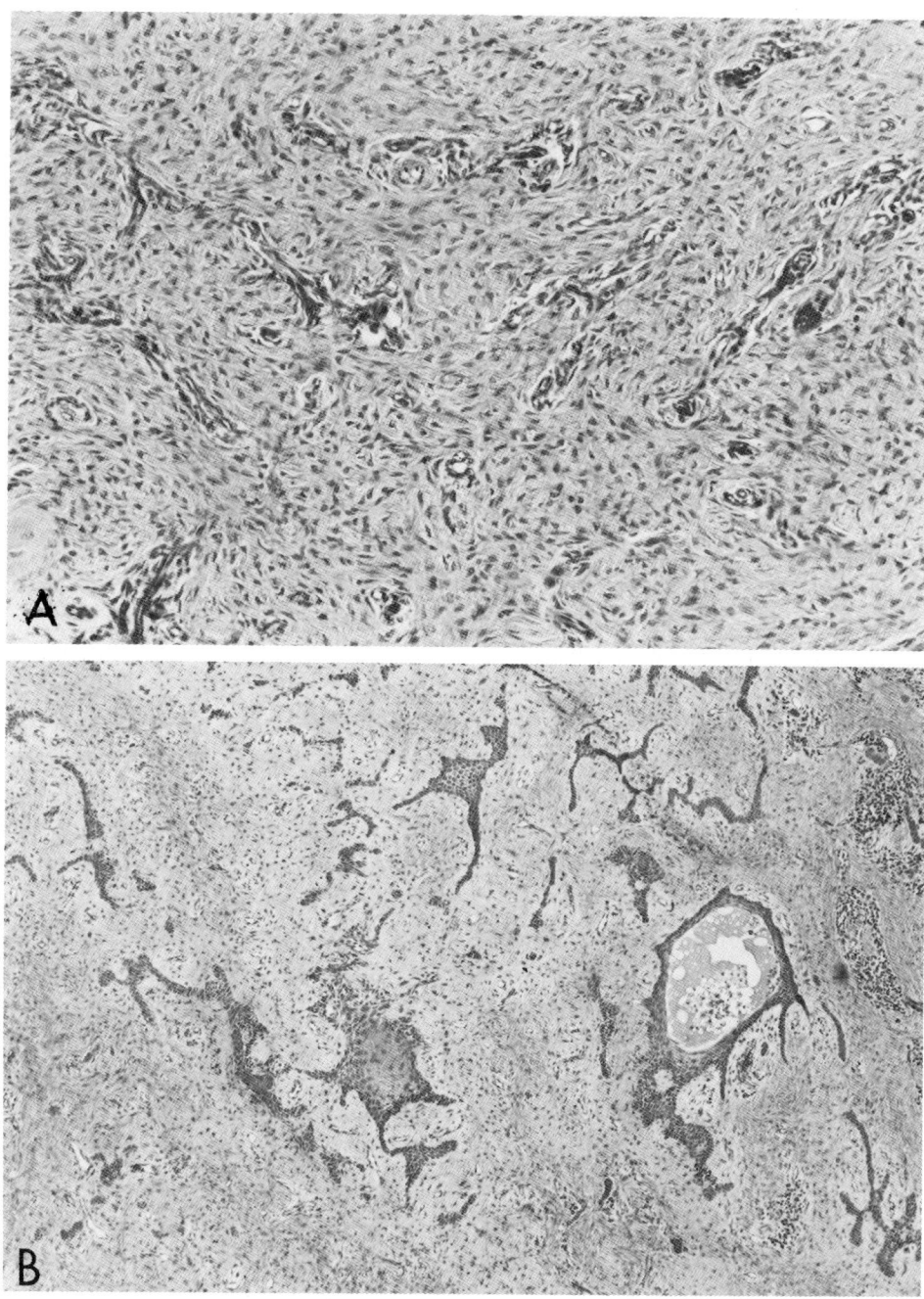

Fig. 23–4. Fibromatous epulis, dog. *A,* Dense fibrillar stroma containing tightly packed stellate cells and blood vessels. *B,* Branching cords of epithelial tissue resembling odontogenic epithelium. (Courtesy of Dr. R.R. Dubielzig and *Veterinary Pathology*.)

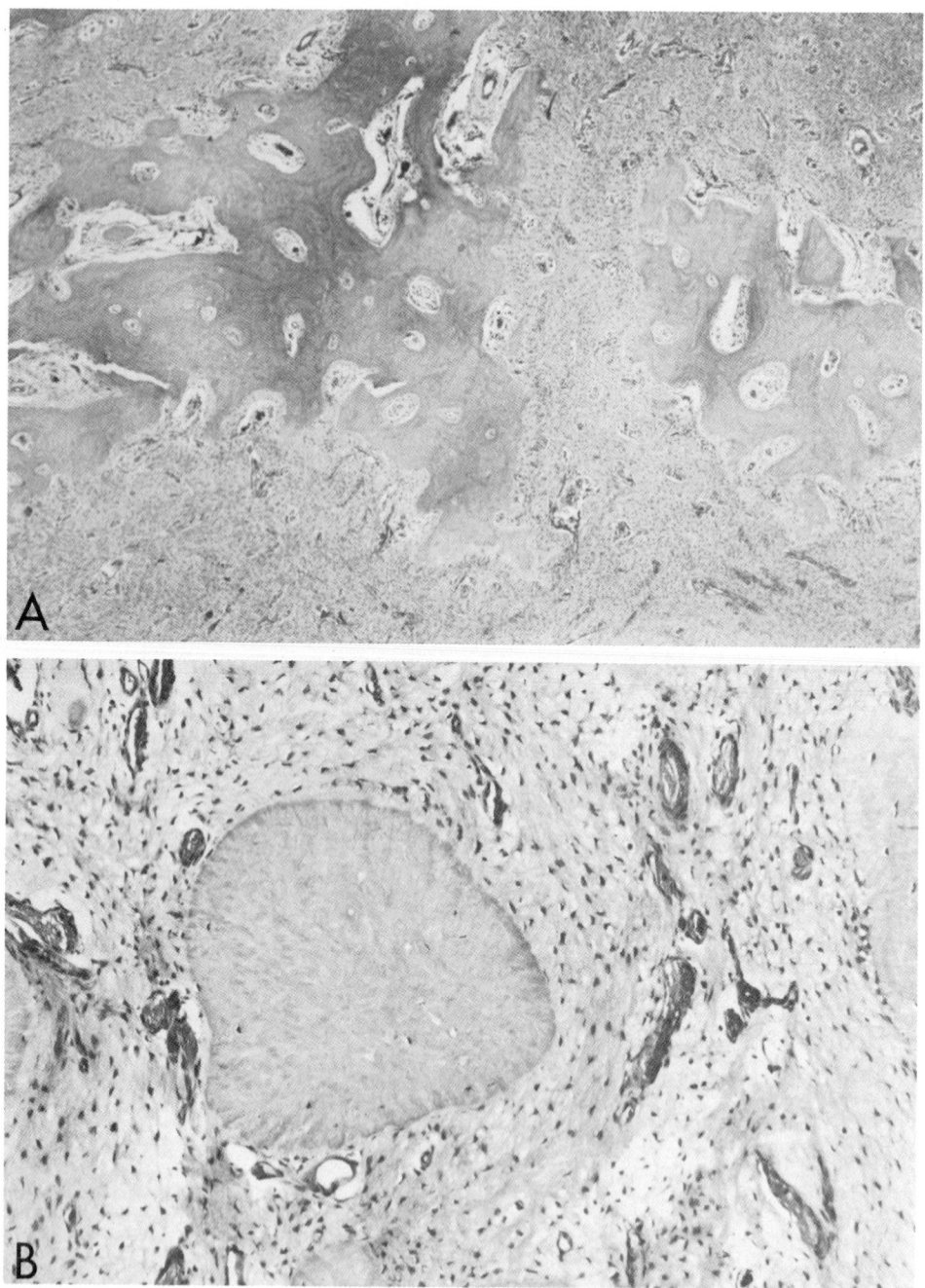

Fig. 23–5. *A,* Ossifying epulis, dog. Bone within a stroma resembling fibromatous epulis. *B,* Cementum or dentin-like material in a fibromatous epulis. (Courtesy of Dr. R.R. Dubielzig and *Veterinary Pathology*.)

designated by three names, which we shall follow.

Fibromatous Epulis. Fibromatous epulis (fibromatosis gingivae, gingival hypertrophy, fibrogingivae hyperplasia) is seen as single or multiple solid lesions protruding from the gums. These may become large enough to interfere with mastication, are not invasive, but may recur following surgical excision. The lesions are solid, firm, and white on cut section. Microscopically, they consist largely of a dense fibrillar stroma, rich in collagen and blood vessels and covered with noncornified, stratified squamous epithelium. The overlying epithelium may send branching fronds of epithelium into the mass in a manner resembling pseudoepitheliomatous hyperplasia. This epithelium often has a stellate structure, suggestive of odontogenic epithelium, and may occasionally form cysts. The stroma closely resembles that of the gingiva and is continuous with the periodontal ligament.

Diphenylhydantoin sodium is a drug used as an anticonvulsant in man and animals. One of its side effects is the production of gingival hyperplasia in several species, including experimental administration to *Macaca arctoides* (stump-tailed macaque). This hyperplasia involves the epithelium more than does the fibromatous epulis, and the lesions regress when administration of the drug is discontinued.

Ossifying Epulis. Ossifying epulis is a term applied to gingival lesions in the dog, in all respects identical to the fibromatous epulis except that the stroma also contains considerable osteoid, cementum, or dentin. In the past, we have considered this as one variable feature in the fibromatous epulis, but it may be useful to so distinguish this histologic feature. It may have some as yet unknown significance in the biology of the lesion.

Acanthomatous Epulis. This is a diagnostic term used to distinguish those canine gingival lesions, similar to fibro-

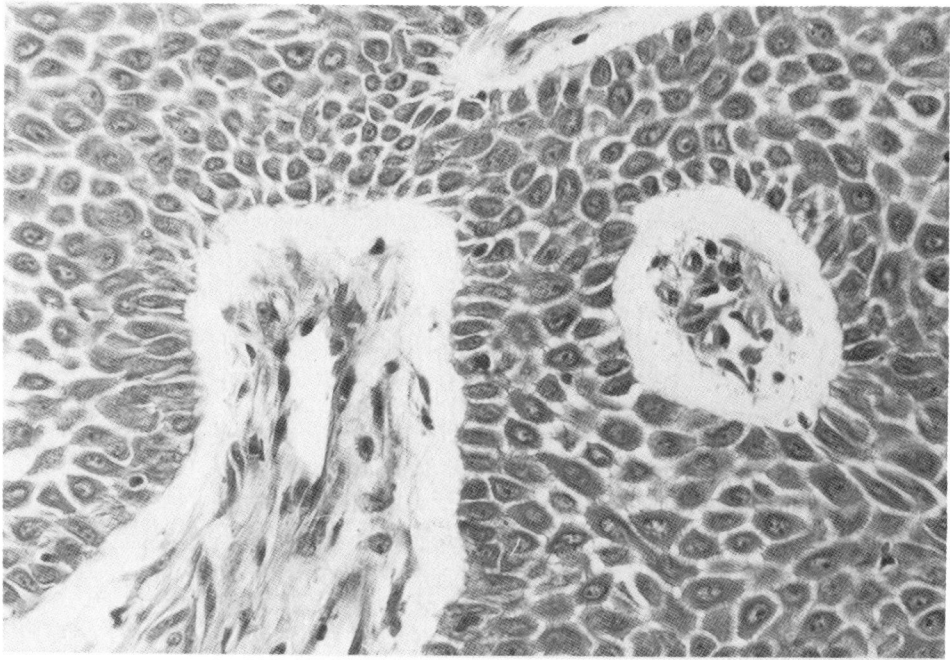

Fig. 23–6. Acanthomatous epulis, dog. The epithelial cells resemble basal or prickle cells with prominent intracellular bridges. (Courtesy of Dr. R.R. Dubielzig and *Veterinary Pathology*.)

matous epulis with its abundant stroma, vessels, and some pseudoepitheliomatous hyperplasia, from those lesions which in addition have an abundant and characteristic epithelial component. This epithelium occurs in bands and solid sheets of squamous epithelial cells, with conspicuous intercellular bridges in the center and tall columnar cells along the periphery, perpendicular to the basement membrane and nearest the stromal vessels. This lesion differs in behavior from the two other epulides: the tumor often invades the bone locally. The mandible is usually involved, but the maxilla also may be the site of origin (Fig. 23–6).

Neoplasms of the Oral Mucosa

In addition to those new growths that may arise in odontogenic or periodontal tissues, other neoplasms may also originate in the oral mucosa. These are listed in Table 23–1 and will be described briefly.

Squamous Cell Carcinoma. The squamous cell carcinoma may be primary in the oral epithelium at any site, but is more frequent in the tonsillar crypt in the dog. It tends to produce an ulcerous lesion, depressed in the center, with firm new growth around the periphery (Fig. 23–7). Metastasis usually occurs to the retropharyngeal and anterior cervical lymph nodes. The histologic appearance differs little from the squamous cell carcinoma of other sites except that it tends not to be cornified.

Malignant Melanoma. This is the most frequent tumor in the oral mucosa of the dog, occurring more often in partially pigmented mucous membranes. The ventral and lateral surfaces of the tongue as well as the mucosa of cheek and pharynx may be the site of origin of this malignant neoplasm. The tumor cells have characteristic appearance, are typically in clusters and may be present in epithelium and adjacent stroma (junctional change). Usually the cells contain cytoplasmic melanin, but in some instances large parts of a tumor may be amelanotic. Usually, with some diligent searching, one may find melanin-containing cells in some part of the otherwise amelanotic malignant melanoma. Metastasis usually is by way of veins, with most secondary tumors in the lung.

Fibrosarcoma. Fibrosarcoma may occur as a primary neoplasm in the mouth. The buccal mucous membrane appears to be the preferred site of origin. This malignant tumor may metastasize widely, usually following the blood vascular route. The tumor is identified by the elongated cells with spindle shaped nuclei, which occur in fasciculi of cells, lying in many directions, sometimes in interlacing bundles. Mitoses are frequent; necrosis and hemorrhage are common.

Adenocarcinoma of Oral Salivary Glands. This tumor is an infrequent lesion in the oral cavity that tends to form ducts or acini resembling those of the salivary glands in the oral mucosa. They are malignant and invade locally as well as metastasize to the lungs.

Granular Cell Myoblastoma. The granular cell myoblastoma has been described

---

Table 23–1. Tumors of Mouth and Pharynx by Tissue of Origin

Oral Mucosa	Periodontium	Odontogenic Tissues
Squamous cell carcinoma	Fibromatous epulis	Ameloblastoma
Malignant melanoma	Ossifying epulis	Ameloblastic fibroma
Fibrosarcoma	Acanthomatous epulis	Ameloblastic odontoma
Adenocarcinoma of oral salivary glands		Complex odontoma
Granular cell myoblastoma (tongue)		Compound odontoma
Lymphosarcoma (tonsil)		Odontogenic myxoma
Craniopharyngioma		

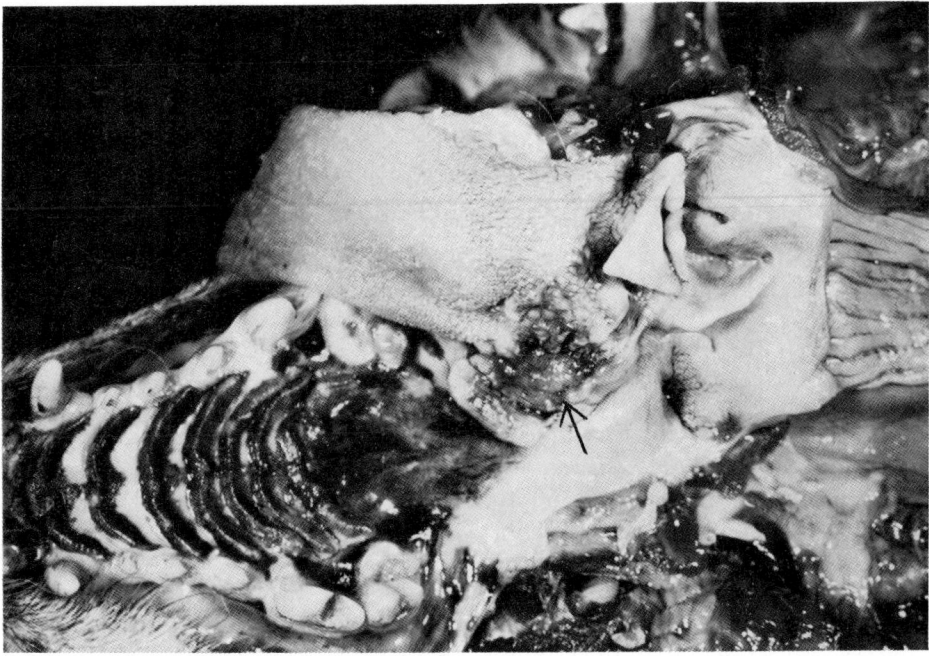

Fig. 23-7. Squamous-cell carcinoma in tonsillar crypt (arrow) of a Spaniel-type dog, aged eight years, spayed female. Note that lesion is eroded and depressed. The left retropharyngeal lymph node was infiltrated by the tumor. (Courtesy of Angell Memorial Animal Hospital.)

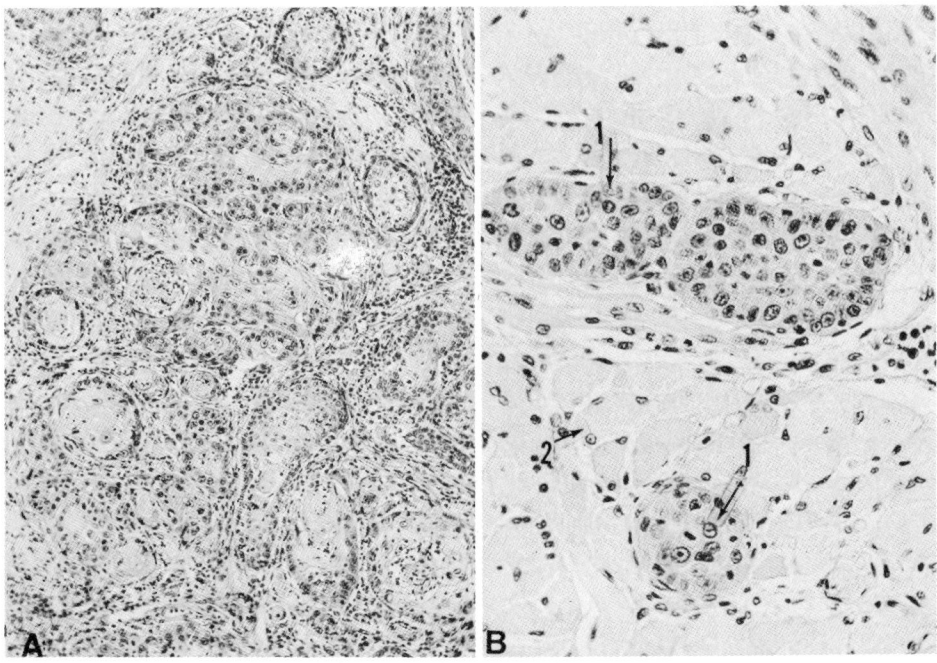

Fig. 23-8. Squamous-cell carcinoma. *A*, Primary tumor (× 90) from epithelium of tongue of a 13-year-old male cat. Note inflammation surrounding irregular nests of tumor cells. *B*, Extension of tumor (*1*) deep into the musculature (*2*) of the tongue. These are probably tumor emboli in lymphatics (× 235). (Courtesy of Armed Forces Institute of Pathology.) Contributor: Dr. Edward Baker.

and is known to be rare, but may arise from the base of the tongue. Its giant-sized cells packed with coarse eosinophilic granules are distinctive. Their resemblance to the cells of the granular cell ameloblastoma has been noted.

Lymphosarcoma (Malignant Lymphoma). This tumor may originate in the tonsil or may be secondary in the oral mucosa. Usually, lesions of this type in the mouth are associated with lesions elsewhere.

Craniopharyngioma. Craniopharyngioma is a rare but specific lesion, arising in remnants of Rathke's pouch. This is an embryonic structure which extends as a stalk of epithelium from the primitive pharynx in the midline to the pituitary, supplying the progenitor cells of the anterior and intermediate lobes of the pituitary. Rathke's pouch usually disappears completely as the animal develops, but in a few instances, remnants left behind give rise to a neoplasm. The histologic features may be of squamous-cell or basal-cell type. Degenerative cysts often occur. The tumor may cause pituitary deficit by pressure upon the gland or the hypothalamus. Craniopharyngioma has been reported in the dog.

An epidemiologic study of malignant neoplasms of oral and pharyngeal origin in dogs, cats, horses, and cattle is of interest (Dorn and Priester, 1976). Malignant tumors of the mouth and pharynx, collected by several veterinary schools in the United States, were most frequent in dogs. The estimated rate per 100,000 patient years of all such malignancies was for dogs, 129.77; cats, 45.43; horses, 27.98; and cattle, 2.53. This study included 550 tumors, of which dogs accounted for 469, cats 50, horses 29, and cattle 2. It must be remembered that this study is based upon those cases examined in veterinary college hospitals and does not reflect the frequency of these tumors in the general animal population. The relative frequency of different histologic types of malignant neoplasms in the dog is of interest. The order of frequency was: (1) malignant melanoma, (2)

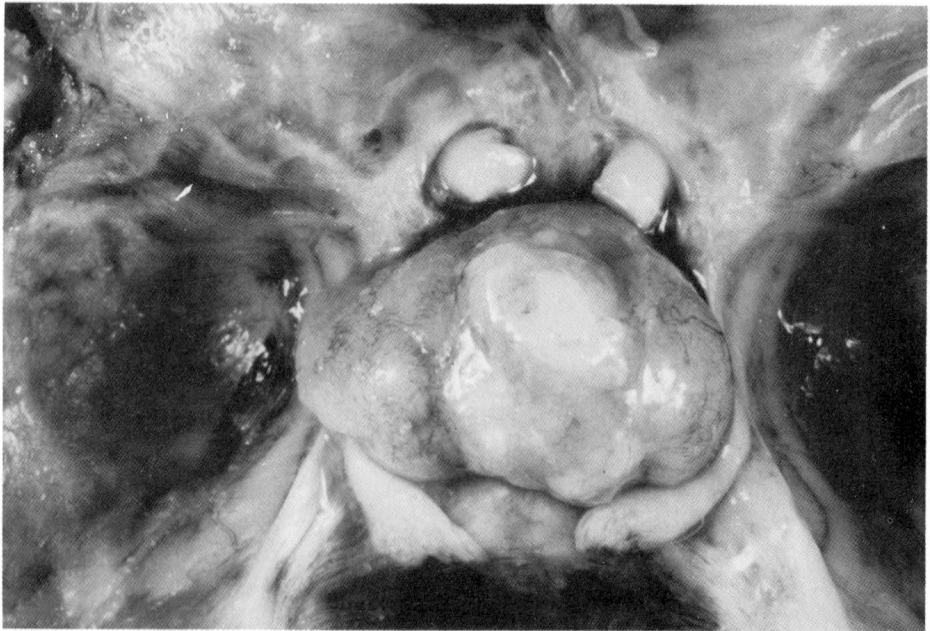

Fig. 23–9.   Craniopharyngioma involving the pituitary of a ten-year-old female boxer. (Courtesy of Angell Memorial Animal Hospital.)

squamous cell carcinoma, (3) fibrosarcoma, (4) adamantinocarcinoma, (5) sarcoma not otherwise specified, (6) carcinoma, not otherwise specified, (7) ameloblastoma, malignant, (8) adenocarcinoma, (9) hemangiosarcoma, and (10) other.

Benjamin, S.A., and Lang, C.M.: An ameloblastic odontoma in a cebus monkey (Cebus albifrons). J. Am. Vet. Med. Assoc., 155:1236–1240, 1969.

Cheema, A.H., and Shanin, H.: Congenital ameloblastoma in a calf. Vet. Pathol., 11:235–239, 1974.

Dorn, C.R., and Priester, W.A.: Epidemiologic analysis of oral and pharyngeal cancer in dogs, cats, horses, and cattle. J. Am. Vet. Med. Assoc., 169:1202–1206, 1976.

Dubielzig, R.R., Goldschmidt, M.H., and Brodey, R.S.: The nomenclature of periodontal epulides in dogs. Vet. Pathol., 16:209–214, 1979.

Gaag, I. van der, and Gruys, E.: Adamantinoma in a cat and a cow and odontomas in two cows. Tijdschr. Diegeneeskd., 97:22–37, 1972.

Giles, R.C., Jr., Montgomery, C.A., Jr., and Izen, L.: Canine lingual granular cell myoblastoma: a case report. Am. J. Vet. Res., 35:1357–1359, 1974.

Gorlin, R.J., Barron, C.N., Chaudhry, A.P., and Clark, J.J.: The oral and pharyngeal pathology of domestic animals. A study of 487 cases. Am. J. Vet. Res., 20:1032–1061, 1959.

Gorlin, R.J., Meskin, L.H., and Brodey, R.: Odontogenic tumors in man and animals: pathologic classification and clinical behavior: a review. Ann. N. Y. Acad. Sci., 108:722–771, 1963.

Head, K.W.: Tumors of the upper alimentary tract: international histologic classification of tumors of domestic animals, part 2, WHO, 1976, page 152.

Jasper, D.E., and Kanegis, L.A.: Adamantinoma in the bovine. Cornell Vet., 36:262–267, 1946.

Langham, R.F., Keahey, K.K., Mostosky, U.V., and Shirmer, R.G.: Oral adamantinoma in the dog. J. Am. Vet. Med. Assoc., 146:474–480, 1965.

Rao, A.T., Nayak, B.C., and Chaudhury, C.H.: A case of adamantinoma in a newly born cross-bred male calf. Indian J. Anim. Sci., 42:353–354, 1972.

Saunders, L.Z., and Rickard, C.G.: Craniopharyngioma in a dog with apparent adiposogenital syndrome and diabetes insipidus. Cornell Vet., 42:490–494, 1952.

Sheldon, W.G.: Fibrous gingival hyperplasia of a mustached guenon monkey (Cercopithecus cephus). Lab. Anim. Care, 17:140–143, 1967.

Shmidl, J.A., and Holmes, D.D.: Undifferentiated salivary gland carcinoma in a baboon. J. Am. Vet. Med. Assoc., 163:617–618, 1973.

Splitter, G.A., Pryor, W.H., Jr., and Casey, H.W.: Ameloblastic odontoma in a Rhesus monkey. J. Am. Vet. Med. Assoc., 161:710–713, 1972.

Staple, P.H., Reed, M.J., and Mashimo, P.A.: Diphenylhydantoin gingival hyperplasia in Macaca arctoides: a new human model. J. Periodont., 48:325–336, 1977.

Tate, C.L., Conti, P.A., and Nero, E.P.: Focal epithelial hyperplasia in the oral mucosa of a chimpanzee. J. Am. Vet. Med. Assoc., 163:619–621, 1973.

Tontis, A., and Luginbühl, H.: Plattenepithelkarzinom am zahnfleisch eines rindes. Schweiz. Arch. Tierheilkd., 118:535–537, 1976.

Ulland, B.M., Siblinovic, S., and Innes, J.R.M.: Gingival hyperplasia in a Macaca mulatta. Lab. Anim. Care, 20:756–758, 1970.

White, E.G.: A suprasellar tumour in a dog. J. Pathol. Bacteriol., 47:323–326, 1938.

Williams, C.S.F., Murray, R.E., McGovney, R.M., and Cockrell, B.Y.: Adamantinoma in a spider monkey (Ateles fusciceps). Lab. Anim. Sci., 23:273–275, 1973.

Pharyngitis (p. 1208) occurs in connection with infection of the air passages, as does tonsillitis. Foreign bodies in the supra-esophageal diverticulum of swine have been mentioned (p. 1211). Actinobacillosis occasionally involves the parapharyngeal lymph nodes, causing swelling which interferes with deglutition and respiration.

SALIVARY GLANDS

The salivary glands may participate in infectious inflammatory processes arising in their vicinity, usually from trauma. In domestic animals, there is no specific infection, comparable to mumps, which has a predilection for salivary tissue. It should be recalled, however, that the cytomegaloviruses have a predilection for the salivary gland, however, they rarely induce sialadenitis. In rats, there are specific forms of transmissible sialadenitis and sialodacryoadenitis caused by a virus. It is possible, but quite unusual, for infection to ascend the duct of a parotid or other salivary gland. Foreign bodies, such as kernels of grain or awns of plants, rarely find their way up a parotid or submaxillary duct, causing inflammation and possibly obstruction or dilatation of the duct.

Sialoliths, or salivary calculi, form in a duct or in the gland itself as a result of chronic inflammation which provides desquamated cells or consolidated exudate as a minute nidus upon which calcium salts precipitate. Foreign bodies may also serve to start the precipitation of salts. Since the salivary secretion contains but little dissolved mineral, the process of formation of salivary calculi is possibly more akin to calcification of tissue than it is to the formation of urinary or biliary stones. At any rate sialoliths may reach astonishing dimensions, parotid calculi several centimeters in diameter and length occurring in the horse.

When its duct is occluded, a salivary gland undergoes atrophy, but before this process is complete, a **cyst** may form in the obstructed duct due to the dilating effect of the imprisoned secretion. Such a cyst in the sublingual duct, located in the frenum linguae, has the special name of **ranula.** A salivary fistula occasionally forms when an injury has made an opening from the duct to the outside of the body, proper healing being prevented by the flow of saliva through the opening.

Neoplasms of Salivary Glands

Primary neoplasms of the major (parotid, mandibular, sublingual) and minor (palate, tongue, lip, gingiva) salivary glands are infrequent in animals. However, Koestner and Buerger (1965) have assembled and tabulated 43 cases from the literature, 1875 through 1959, and described an additional 30 cases from their own collection. The histologic diagnoses used by these authors will be listed and described briefly.

Three **mucoepidermoid tumors** were described (one mucoepidermoid cystodermoma in the parotid of a Hamadryas baboon, and two mucoepidermoid carcinomas— one parotid, one palatal— in dogs). This new growth consists of squamous epithelial elements plus adenomatous cells which secrete mucus. One case involved a **squamous cell carcinoma** arising in the sublingual gland of a cat. The possibility of its origin being the oral mucosa could not be excluded. Six tumors were classified as **mixed tumors** made up of cells with morphologic features of epithelial and mesenchymal cells. Myoepithelial cells were recognized in these tumors, as well as carti-

lage, bone, squamous, and glandular epithelium. Two equine cases involved the parotid salivary glands. Of three canine cases, two arose in the mandibular, and one in the parotid salivary glands. One mixed tumor originated in the sublingual salivary gland of a guinea pig.

Adenoid-cystic carcinoma (cylindroma) is a variety characterized by small dark-staining cells arranged in an adenoid and cystic as well as solid pattern. This tumor occurs in human salivary glands but is not represented among the animal tumors. **Acinic cell tumor (acinic cell carcinoma)** is described as consisting of acinar structures made up of small, rather uniform carcinomatous cells arranged in solid complexes as well as in adenoid and adenoid-cystic patterns. Twelve animal tumors were classified in this category, 11 in dogs and 1 in the parotid of a horse. All were locally invasive. The 11 canine tumors were distributed in the major salivary glands (parotid, 5 cases; mandibular, 2 cases) and in the minor salivary glands (4 cases).

Adenocarcinomas were classified as ductular (papillary) or trabecular. In the first (ductular) category, two tumors were encountered in dogs; one arose from the parotid, the other from a minor salivary gland of the tongue. Three trabecular adenocarcinomas were identified in a cat, a dog, and a horse. All arose in the parotid, were malignant, and metastasized to lymph nodes and lung. **Anaplastic (undifferentiated carcinomas)** were found in two dogs, one in the mandibular and the other in the sublingual salivary gland. Both metastasized to lymph nodes and elsewhere. The **papillary cystadenoma lymphomatosum** (Warthin tumor), which is a benign lesion developing in people, is described as consisting of an epithelial and a lymphoid component. No example has yet been found in animals.

In addition to the series described above from the work of Koestner and Buerger, a single case of a mixed tumor in a cat has been thoroughly described by Wells and

Robinson (1975). This malignant mixed tumor in a 12-year-old neutered female cat arose from the parotid salivary gland and metastasized to the submandibular lymph nodes and skeletal muscle. The tumor contained epithelial elements, sarcomatous cells (some producing osteoid), bone, and cartilage.

Glen, J.B.: Canine salivary mucocoeles. Results of sialographic examination and surgical treatment of fifty cases. J. Small Anim. Pract., 3:515–526, 1972.

Harrison, J.D., and Garrett, J.R.: An ultrastructural and histochemical study of a naturally occurring salivary mucocele in a cat. J. Comp. Pathol., 85:411–416, 1975.

Harrison, J.D., and Garrett, J.R.: Histological effects of ductal ligation of salivary glands of the cat. J. Pathol., 118:245–254, 1976.

Knecht, C.D., and Phares, J.: Characterization of dogs with salivary cyst. J. Am. Vet. Med. Assoc., 158:612–613, 1971.

Koestner, A., and Buerger, L.: Primary neoplasms of the salivary glands in animals compared to similar tumors in man. Pathol. Vet., 2:201–226, 1965.

Wells, G.A.H., and Robinson, M.: Mixed tumour of salivary gland showing histological evidence of malignancy in a cat. J. Comp. Pathol., 85:77–85, 1975.

ESOPHAGUS

Inflammation of the esophagus is infrequent but, like that of the mouth, results from trauma produced by foreign objects, from caustic chemicals or from infection. Because of the heavy and impervious epithelial lining, injury from elimination of toxic substances through the esophageal mucous membrane probably never occurs.

Reddened streaks of catarrhal inflammation may extend up and down the tops of the longitudinal ridges which form in the relaxed esophagus. In cattle, these suggest the presence of "mucosal disease."

Any considerable injury, chemical or traumatic, to the esophageal lining is much to be feared because of its tendency to produce **stenosis** of the esophageal lumen. The mechanism depends upon the production of scar tissue, which is very likely to form as such an injury heals. The scar tissue, contracting as it ages, draws the lumen into a **stricture,** or inordinate narrowing of the lumen. Injury from the swallowing of highly irritant or caustic chemicals including lye is the common cause. In one memorable case, a German Shepherd dog stole a hot hamburger from the family outdoor grill and gulped it down. The hamburger lodged at the midpoint of the esophagus long enough to produce a severe burn, which in a few weeks resulted in complete stenosis of the esophagus. Surgical operations on the esophagus are formidable because of the same effect of contracting cicatricial tissue.

Choke, a complete or partial obstruction of the esophagus by foreign material, is all too common in cattle as the result of trying to swallow such things as beets, turnips, apples, or small ears of corn without reducing them to small pieces. The horse practically never makes such a mistake as this, but does become choked by the gradual accumulation of ground or whole grain or tough grasses that fail to continue their passage through the whole length of the esophagus. Dogs and cats become choked by sharp pieces of bone which lodge usually in the thoracic esophagus. Contrary to popular belief, choking, as long as it is in the esophagus and not the pharynx or larynx, does not interfere seriously with respiration, although in the cow it prevents regurgitation of gas formed in the rumen with tympanites of that organ, which may well be fatal in some hours. Without this complication, if choke cannot be relieved, death is likely in about 3 days because of local gangrene (from pressure and from compressed blood vessels) and resultant sapremia·and toxemia.

Sometimes choking on a single foreign body results in only partial obstruction of the esophageal passageway. A common result then, especially in the dog, is that food is eaten, but after some minutes is returned by vomition, only small amounts or none at all reaching the stomach. In a few weeks, the repeated stretching of the wall just above the obstruction produces a sac-like dilatation, usually asymmetric and unilateral, known as an **esophageal diverticulum.** Perforation is another possible outcome in the case of sharp bones or similar objects.

In dogs and doubtless in related wild species, the spirurid worm *Spirocerca lupi* penetrates the mucosa and submucosa of the lower esophagus and causes a reaction in the form of subepithelial fibrous nodules as it develops there. The smoothly covered and perhaps coalescent nodules bulge into the lumen as much as 0.5 cm. Interference with esophageal function appears to be minimal (unless a sarcoma is formed, see below) and the lesions are usually found incidentally postmortem. Other parasites of the esophagus include *Gongylonema spp.* in ruminants and nonhuman primates, and sarcosporidia in ruminants and, rarely, other species.

Amand, W.B., O'Brien, J.A., and Tucker, J.A.: Dysphagia in a wooly monkey (*Lagothrix lagotricha*) following a caustic esophageal burn. J. Am. Vet. Med. Assoc., *157*:706–711, 1970.

Clifford, D.H., Soifer, F.K., and Freeman, R.G.: Stricture and dilatation of the esophagus in the cat. J. Am. Vet. Med. Assoc., *156*:1007–1014, 1970.
Rogers, W.A., and Donovan, E.F.: Peptic esophagitis in a dog. J. Am. Vet. Med. Assoc., *163*:462–464, 1973.

Mega-esophagus

Extensive, nonlocalized dilatation of the esophagus with food has been described in dogs, cats, and man. The condition is suspected in cases involving postprandial vomition and is confirmed by radiographic study. More than one cause has been demonstrated. **Persistent right aortic arch** is one cause of mega-esophagus. In this congenital anomaly, the right aortic arch (which usually disappears in embryonic life) persists into postnatal life, causing the trachea and esophagus to be surrounded by a vascular ring made up of aorta, pulmonary artery and ductus arteriosus. When the newborn begins to eat, this vascular ring prevents expansion of the

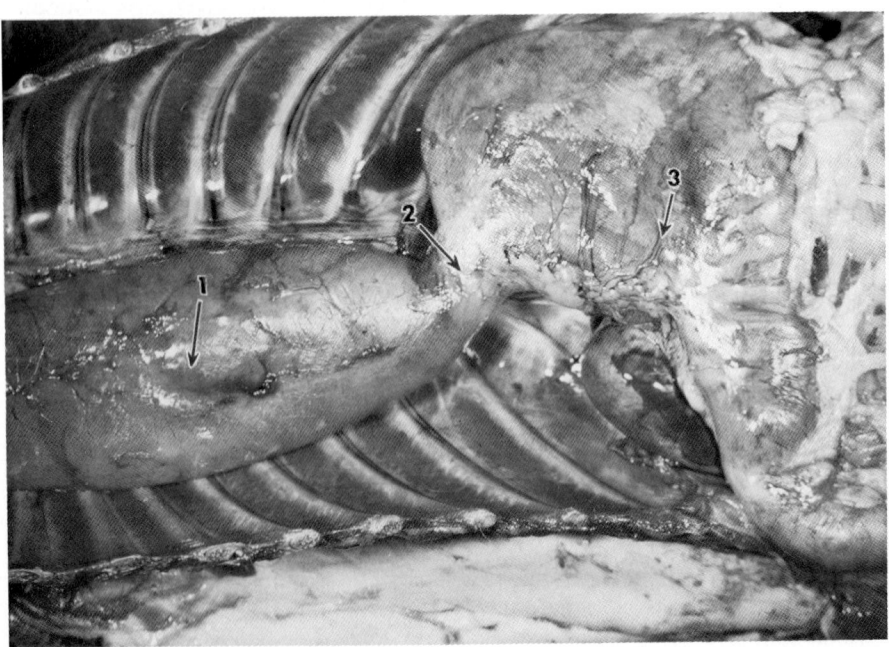

Fig. 23–10. Megaesophagus, nine-month-old female collie, due to unknown cause. The thoracic viscera and diaphragm have been removed, leaving the esophagus and stomach *in situ*. The esophagus (*1*) was not obstructed at the cardia (*2*) of the stomach (*3*). (Courtesy of Angell Memorial Animal Hospital.)

esophagus and causes food to be obstructed at a point above the base of the heart.

Achalasia of the esophagus is usually used to describe a second form of mega-esophagus. Other terms used to denote this condition include: cardiospasm, simple ectasia, idiopathic dilatation, phenospasm, and dystonia of esophagus. In this condition, the point of occlusion of the esophagus appears to be in the esophagus just outside the stomach, within the thorax. In affected animals, puppies or kittens usually, the esophagus becomes dilated and filled with food proximal to the cardia of the stomach. No anatomic defect at this point is apparent, and evidence generally points toward a failure of reflex dilatation of the esophageal sphincter during deglutition. Aside from the distension, no gross or microscopic lesion has been demonstrated in the esophageal musculature, mucosa, or myenteric plexuses. The absence of such lesions led to physiologic studies, which revealed that the reflex could be restored by stimulation of the vagus. The site of the lesion in the central nervous system appears to be confirmed by experimental production of lesions in the medulla oblongata (nucleus of tractus solitarius), which result in mega-esophagus. The specific nucleus in the medulla appears also to be involved in tracheal reflex as well as in the swallowing reflex; both defects are demonstrable in animals with achalasia.

Young animals are most frequently affected, and in one study, females more often than males. German Shepherds and Great Danes appear to be most prone of any breed. The disease has a familial pattern, both in dogs and cats, but the genetic evidence does not yet meet critical standards.

Cricopharyngeal achalasia has been described in the dog. In this instance, food is retained in the pharynx due to inadequate relaxation of the cricopharyngeal sphincter. According to one report, the signs were relieved by cricopharyngeal myotomy.

Clifford, D.H., and Gyorkey, F.: Myenteric ganglial cells in dogs with and without achalasia of the esophagus. J. Am. Vet. Med. Assoc., *150*:205–211, 1967.

Clifford, D.H., Ross, J.N., Jr., Waddell, E.D., and Wilson, C.F.: Effect of persistent aortic arch on the ganglial cells of the canine esophagus. J. Am. Vet. Med. Assoc., *158*:1401–1410, 1971.

Clifford, D.H., et al.: Congenital achalasia of the esophagus in four cats of common ancestry. J. Am. Vet. Med. Assoc., *158*:1554–1560, 1971.

Clifford, D.H., and Pirsch, J.G.: Myenteric ganglial cells in dogs with and without hereditary achalasia of the esophagus. Am. J. Vet. Res., *32*:615–619, 1971.

Clifford, D.H., et al.: Management of esophageal achalasia in miniature Schnauzers. J. Am. Vet. Med. Assoc., *161*:1012–1021, 1972.

Clifford, D.H.: Myenteric ganglial cells of the esophagus in cats with achalasia of the esophagus. Am J. Vet. Res., *34*:1333–1336, 1973.

Gray, G.W.: Acute experiments on neuroeffector function in canine esophageal achalasia. Am. J. Vet. Res., *35*:1075–1082, 1974.

Harvey, C.E., et al.: Megaesophagus in the dog: a clinical survey of 79 cases. J. Am. Vet. Med. Assoc., *165*:443–446, 1974.

Higgs, B., Kerr, F.W.L., and Ellis, F.H.: The experimental production of esophageal achalasia by electrolytic lesions in the medulla. J. Thorac. Cardiovasc. Surg., *50*:613–625, 1965.

Morgan, J.P., and Lumb, W.V.: Achalasia of the esophagus in the dog. J. Am. Vet. Med. Assoc., *144*:722–726, 1964.

Nakayama, S., Neya, T., Watanabe, K., and Tsuchiya, K.: Effects of electrical stimulation and local destruction of the medulla oblongata on swallowing movements in dogs. Rendic. Gastroenter., *6*:6–11, 1974.

Osborne, C.A., Clifford, D.H., and Jessen, C.: Hereditary esophageal achalasia in dogs. J. Am. Vet. Med. Assoc., *151*:572–581, 1967.

Rosin, E., and Hanlon, G.F.: Canine cricopharyngeal achalasia. J. Am. Vet. Med. Assoc., *160*:1496–1499, 1972.

Sokolovsky, V.: Achalasia and paralysis of the canine esophagus. J. Am. Vet. Med. Assoc., *160*:943–955, 1972.

Strombeck, D.R., and Troya, L.: Evaluation of lower motor neuron function in two dogs with megaesophagus. J. Am. Vet. Med. Assoc., *169*:411–414, 1976.

Neoplasms of the Esophagus

Papillomas of the skin, caused by *Papillomavirus* in cattle are occasionally accompanied by papillomas in the mouth, pharynx, esophagus, and rumen. These papillomas in the digestive system are presumably caused by the same virus. Reports from Kenya and Scotland indicate rather frequent association of **squamous cell carcinomas** with the papillomas of the digestive system. Two causative factors are suspected: first, the bovine *Papillomavirus*; second, chronic poisoning due to ingestion of bracken fern (*Pteridium aquilinum*). The synergistic effect of these two factors is strongly suggested, but has not been established experimentally. Transitional cell carcinoma of the urinary bladder has also been associated with chronic bracken fern poisoning of cattle.

Osteosarcoma of the esophagus of dogs has clearly been associated with long standing lesions of *Spirocerca lupi*.

Secondary (metastatic) tumors of the esophagus are rare. Tumors of adjacent structures (lymph nodes or thyroid) usually do not spread to the esophagus. A rather large epidermal inclusion cyst has been reported as removed surgically from the mucosa of the esophagus of a horse.

Jarrett, W.F.: Oesophageal and stomach cancer in cattle: a candidate viral and carcinogen model system and its possible relevance to man. Br. J. Cancer, *28*:93, 1973.

Pirie, H.M.: Unusual occurrence of squamous carcinoma of the upper alimentary tract in cattle in Britain. Res. Vet. Sci., *15*:135–138, 1973.

Plowright, W.: Malignant neoplasia of the esophagus and rumen of cattle in Kenya. J. Comp. Pathol. Therap., *65*:108–114, 1955.

Ribelin, W.E., and Bailey, W.S.: Esophageal sarcoma associated with *Spirocerca lupi* infection in the dog. Cancer, *2*:1242–1246, 1958.

Schutte, K.H.: Esophageal tumors in sheep: some ecological observations. J. Natl. Cancer Inst., *41*:821–824, 1968.

Scott, E.A., et al.: Intramural esophageal cyst in a horse. J. Am. Vet. Med. Assoc., *171*:652–654, 1977.

Seibold, H.R., et al.: Observations on the possible relation of malignant esophageal tumors and *Spirocerca lupi* lesions in the dog. Am. J. Vet. Res., *16*:5–14, 1955.

Thorsen, J., Cooper, J.E., and Warwick, G.P.: Oesophageal papillomata in cattle in Kenya. Trop. Anim. Health Prod., *6*:95–98, 1974.

Yoshida, S.: Contribution to the study on *Gnathostoma spinigerum*, Owen, 1836: Cause of esophageal tumor in the Japanese mink, with special reference to its life history. Trans. 9th Congress, Far East Assoc. Trop. Med., Nanking, China, *1*:625–630, 1934.

FORESTOMACHS OF RUMINANTS

The rumen, reticulum, and omasum are called stomachs only because of their general shape and size. They store food in a manner similar to that of the crop (ingluvies) of a chicken; bacterial decomposition proceeds in them, but there is no secretory function such as characterizes a true stomach. References to the stomach, in this work, apply only to the true, secretory stomach.

Tympanites or Bloat

Tympanites of the rumen, or bloat, consists in the accumulation of excessive quantities of gas in the organ, distending it to a dangerous degree. The gas, which can often be ignited with a match, consists largely of methane, carbon dioxide, carbon monoxide, and small amounts of various others including the poisonous hydrogen disulfide (H_2S). These gases are the usual products of bacterial decomposition of carbohydrates and proteins and result from the action of many kinds of saprophytic bacteria upon ingested plant tissues. These fermentational processes are normal and go on continuously, but normally the gas is discharged in the form of frequent belchings or eructations through the esophagus and mouth.

Pathologic bloating can obviously arise as the result of any interference with the normal eructations or from the production of gas at a rate beyond the capacity of esophageal eructations to discharge it. We do not know what mechanisms, if any, limit the amount of gas that can pass up the esophagus in a given period of time, but the escape, rather than being a passive process, requires active reverse peristaltic waves on the part of the esophagus and hence is under control of the (autonomic) nervous system. The amount of gas produced, of course, depends upon the rapidity of bacterial fermentational processes, and these are greatly favored when the food ingested is fresh, succulent, green legumes such as clovers and alfalfa.

We can suspect, but cannot say with certainty, that the habitual capacity for repeated eructation may be exceeded at such times. There are various other theories on this point, however. One is that this green succulent material is very soft and that the initiation of expulsive ruminal contractions requires the mechanical irritation of rough stems and stalks upon the lining of the rumen. This explanation seems only slightly attractive when we consider that when the animal is on a diet of coarse, dry, and largely indigestible straw, the rumen is well filled yet develops but little gas, with few eructations.

Another theory is that the gases developed from the fresh green legumes include sufficient amounts of hydrogen disulfide to exert a toxic depressant action upon the local nervous structures. This is as yet unproved, either that important amounts of that gas are absorbed or that the H_2S would have that effect if the absorption did, indeed, occur. It is doubtful that the phenomenon of imprisoned gas in the bovine rumen is much different from that in the equine stomach or cecum (see below), where spasmodic contractions of adjacent segments of the alimentary canal are known to exert a sphincter-like action. It is common human experience that excessive fermentation in the intestine induces a certain degree of spasmodic action of the bowel. It seems not improbable that similar reflex spasms of the esophageal tube or orifice are responsible for the impounding of ruminal gases, and that the increased pressure is sufficiently irritant to stimulate further spasm, a vicious circle being created. Certain it is that upon the passing of a stomach tube the excess of gas promptly escapes.

"Frothy bloat" constitutes an exception to the last statement and is a form of tympanites complicated by other factors than the mere excessive production of gas and its inability to escape through the tightly contracted esophagus. In this disorder, the gas is finely mixed with the fluid in the rumen in the form of very small bubbles, like the foam that one gets when shaking an emulsion with air. The inability of the gas to escape from the foamy mixture is dependent on the surface tension of the liquid and doubtless of the colloidal state of dissolved solids. Liquids added to the mixture which reduce its surface tension tend to release the bubbles, but the chemical changes responsible for the original rise have not been satisfactorily ascertained. Possibly there is release from the ingested plant material of too much saponin, a soap-like emulsifying agent, but clinically, the rapid ingestion of a large amount of succulent plants, usually leguminous, is the inciting cause.

Bloating of the preceding types is acute, arising suddenly and often causing death within an hour or two. The second form of tympanites is that which results from some physical obstruction of the esophageal or pharyngeal passageways. Choke has been mentioned earlier in this chapter as a cause of such obstruction. Strictures may have the same effect but are rare. Other causes include pressure upon the esophagus by tumors, abscesses, swollen lymph nodes, and similar enlargements. Except in the case of a completely obstructing choke, these forms of bloating arise more gradually and often they are chronic or intermittent depending upon the cause.

One of the effects of severe bloating is to push the diaphragm forward, seriously limiting the respiratory capacity. The increase of pressure within the rumen causes it to expand and thereby compress the abdominal viscera and occlude the caudal vena cava. This shunts the blood from caudal to cephalic parts of the body. These mechanisms result in anoxia, which is the immediate cause of death in those cases which are fatal. If the excessive pressure is relieved by surgical or other form of intervention the above effects promptly subside.

Sheep, as well as cattle, are susceptible to bloating, but, because of their more conservative eating habits, are less commonly involved. Specific types of forage may be incriminated. For example, in Australia, the wild gooseberry plant (*Nicandra physaloides*) has been demonstrated to cause fatal bloat in sheep under specific conditions.

Clarke, R.T.J., and Reid, C.S.W.: Foamy bloat of cattle. A review. J. Dairy Sci., 57:753–785, 1974.
Cohen, R.D.H.: Bloat in sheep grazing wild gooseberry, *Nicandra physaloides*. Aust. Vet. J., 46:559, 1970.
Dougherty, R.W.: Pathophysiology of the ruminant digestive tract. *In* Dukes' Physiology of Domestic Animals, 8th ed., edited by M.J. Swenson. Ithaca, Comstock Publishing Associates, a division of Cornell University Press, 1970, pp. 516–525.
Dougherty, R.W.K., Hill, K.J., Cook, H.M., and Riley, J.L.: Electromyographic and pressure studies of the esophagus of the sheep. Am. J. Vet. Res., 32:1247–1251, 1971.
Head, M.J.: Bloat in cattle. Nature, 183:757, 1959.
Howarth, R.E.: A review of bloat in cattle. Can. Vet. J., 16:281–294, 1975.
Leng, R.A., and McWilliam, J.R. (ed.): Bloat. Proceedings of a symposium held at the University of New England, Armidale, NSW, Australia, August 1973, 103 pp.
Mills, J.H.L., and Christian, R.G.: Lesions of bovine ruminal tympany. J. Am. Vet. Med. Assoc., 157:947–952, 1970.
Wright, D.E., and Curtis, M.W.: Bloat in cattle. XLII. The action of surface-active chemicals on ciliated protozoa. N. Z. J. Agri. Res., 19:19–23, 1976.

Ruminal Atony and Intoxication

In most cases, weak and atonic musculature is seen in a rumen which is tightly impacted with undigested roughage, although there are a few cases in which the rumen is nearly empty, except, perhaps, for an accumulation of sand or similar foreign substance. The essential feature is that the rumen stops working; there are no more contractions of sufficient force to move the contents forward along the normal digestive course nor to regurgitate them for "chewing the cud." There is little or no gas in the rumen, and this fact affords a clue to what is at least an important aspect of the pathogenesis of this disorder, namely, a failure of bacterial growth. Present knowledge of just what bacterial species are involved and the pertinent aspects of their physiologic processes (production of gas, acid, etc.) is not complete, nor can we always point to the exact reason why desirable species stop growing and disappear, but the absence of fermentational processes is evident in the condition of the ruminal contents. They are dull in color, soggy, and solid in consistency, like unleavened bread dough. Unleavened it is, indeed, for the fermentation has stopped. Putrefactive bacteria begin, at least, to produce their characteristic odors. The wall, at autopsy, is thin and "lifeless," easily folded in any direction. Microscopically, it is difficult to describe specifically any change in the tissues other than a certain degree of quantitative atrophy.

The disease is gradual and insidious in its onset, and for a day or two after symptoms become manifest, the changes are reversible; later, it is unlikely that any known treatment will be availing. There is clinical evidence that potent toxins are absorbed from the decomposing mass, and at death toxic changes are discernible in the liver. However, both the clinical and pathologic pictures are likely to be complicated, at the end, by ketosis due to lack of assimilation of food.

Nichols, R.E., and Penn, K.E.: Simple methods for the detection of unfavorable changes in ruminal ingesta. J. Am. Vet. Med. Assoc., 133:275–279, 1958.
Vestweber, J.G.E., and Leipold, H.W.: Experimentally induced ovine ruminal acidosis: Pathologic changes. Am. J. Vet. Res., 35:1537–1540, 1974.
Wienand, F.: Beobactungen zur parakeratosé der pansenschliemhaut von schlachtkälbern. Giessener Beitr. Erbpath. Zuchthyg., 6:45–52, 1974.
Zumpt, I.: Impaction of the rumen in cattle due to the ingestion of the cocoons of the Molopo caterpillar, *Gonometa postica* (Walker). J. S. Afr. Vet. Med. Assoc., 42:315–318, 1971.

Rumenitis and Ulcers of the Rumen

The mucosa of the rumen is subject to the formation of frequent and extensive ulcers, but they are seldom seen by other than meat inspectors for the reason that they occur ordinarily in young cattle fattened for market and in excellent health as far as can be determined by clinical standards. It is not unusual for a majority of a pen of animals fattened for "prime, heavy beef" on a concentrated ration such as corn and alfalfa hay to show one or more ruminal ulcers each, when slaughtered. Limited to the papillated areas, the ulcers are of entirely irregular shape but may be as large as a person's outspread hand. They are often multiple, but always superficial, usually reaching no deeper than the mucosa, and have no true similarity to the human peptic ulcer. They have been found to originate in an area where the villi are somewhat swollen and loosely glued together with a slightly sticky substance.

Microscopically, this substance proves to be an inflammatory exudate of seropurulent nature and quite limited in amount. The affected villi die, become detached and disappear, leaving a smooth, raw surface. A mild leukocytic infiltration, which is composed chiefly of lymphocytes and neutrophilic granulocytes, is found in the underlying submucosa. The ulcer, now completely formed, begins to heal by proliferation of new epithelium at the outer edges. The proliferating epithelium, in a period which may be estimated as several weeks, eventually covers the largest ulcer, which meantime has shrunk greatly. At first the new epithelium is white, contrasting with the normal ruminal lining, which is black in a majority of cattle. As time goes on, nothing remains but a narrow, angular or stellate scar. This becomes a mere line and eventually disappears completely, the process probably requiring several months or a year. Bacteriologic examination of the ulcer usually reveals the necrophorus organism as the principal if not the only invader.

What we believe to be a variant of the ulcerative process is the formation of a clump of little spherical white nodules attached to the mucosal surface. Diameters of 1 to 2 cm are common. Frequently they occur on the pillars, as well as in the papillated areas. The epithelium is nonpigmented, comparatively thin, and always smooth, like that of the healing scars. It is underlaid by fibrous tissue which constitutes the inner bulk of the nodule. We look upon the nodules as representing an inflammatory hyperplasia rather than neoplasms, which they have been called. One reason for this view is that after examining large numbers we have seen none which reached large size; their potentialities of growth appear to be definitely limited. We have seen the nodules forming in connection with and as parts of the more usual flat scars.

The cause and pathogenesis of ulcers in the rumen are only partly clear, but they have been shown to have an important relation to a sudden shift from a diet of range grasses to the too luxurious ration of the feedlot. Their possible connection with abscesses in the liver is discussed in the study of that organ.

Exceptionally, localized areas of acute rumenitis and possibly ulceration have been encountered in the vicinity of slowly dissolving capsules or boluses of such mildly stomachic drugs as tartar emetic (potassium-antimony tartrate). A more or less essential provocative factor appears to be cessation of ruminal motility so that the chemical is left concentrated in one spot.

A disorder descibed as **parakeratosis of the rumen** has been encountered in sheep whose diet consisted largely of "pelleted" feeds, the ground material being formed into small cylinders by a feed mill. The cornified (keratinized) layer and the underlying Malpighian layer of the epithelium are each far thicker than normal, and the keratinized cells retain vestiges of their nuclei rather than losing their cellular identity in the pink-staining homogeneity which is normally expected. Whether this is wholly a retardation of a normal maturation, a failure of the aging cells to wear off and disappear, or whether there is also involved a reactive hyperplasia with more rapid production of new epithelium may well be inquired. The latter is known to occur as the result of some irritant substances in feeds (chlorinated naphthalenes), and the existence of other irritants, presently unknown, may well be suspected.

Jensen, R., Connell, W.E., and Deem, A.W.: Rumenitis and its relation to rate of change of ration and the proportion of concentrate in the ration of cattle. Am. J. Vet. Res., 15:425–428, 1954.

Jensen, R., et al.: Rumenitis-liver abscess complex in beef cattle. Am. J. Vet. Res., 15:202–216, 1954.

Jensen, R., et al.: Parakeratosis of the rumens of lambs fattened on pelleted feed. Am. J. Vet. Res., 19:277–282, 1958.

Smith, H.A.: Ulcerative lesions of the bovine rumen and their possible relation to hepatic abscesses. Am. J. Vet. Res., 5:234–243, 1944.

Foreign Bodies in the Reticulum

The bovine species is not equipped with highly sensitive prehensile organs nor a delicate sense of taste. As a consequence, cattle that are kept in farmyards, stables, or in other proximity to the various mechanized activities of humans are prone to swallow metallic objects like nails, screws, and bits of wire that have been carelessly allowed to get into their mangers or feed boxes. Probably some of these objects are even licked up from the surface of the ground as the cow wraps her tongue around a choice tuft of grass.

These objects almost invariably remain in the reticulum, retarded, no doubt, by the baffle-like action of the criss-crossing folds of its lining. No especial harm results from the presence of smooth foreign bodies, but the sharp ones either become entrapped in perforations they have made in one or more of the lining folds or penetrate the wall of the organ. The perforation of a fold is a relatively harmless accident as shown by the fact that many healthy cattle are slaughtered and found to have nails or wires embedded horizontally in the reticulated mucous folds with small white, scarred areas around them. Those which penetrate the wall proper are gradually pushed through it by the recurrent peristaltic movements of the organ.

While migration in any direction is possible, the great majority of the objects move anteriorly. They pass through the diaphragm and into the pericardium and heart muscle, carrying infectious organisms with them, and producing the condition known as traumatic pericarditis. Movement is usually slow, so that a dense fibrous wall encircles the path of the wire or similar object. It is not unusual for the ordinary iron wire to become completely rusted out by the time pericardial infection reaches its usually fatal culmination. In such a case, the diagnosis can still be made by finding the dense fibrous encapsulating mass of highly variable size and shape, but with a slender, blackened tract usually demonstrable along the path taken by the penetrating body. The anterior surface of the reticulum is usually adherent to the diaphragm and examination for adhesions in this region should constitute a part of every bovine necropsy. Not infrequently, there are also heavily encapsulated abscesses in the vicinity. If the foreign body has chanced to take a different direction, there is localized (rarely generalized) peritonitis with abscesses anywhere among the abdominal viscera or there may be penetration of the liver or spleen. If the infection transported happens to be other than pyogenic, the lesion shows changes characteristic of the organism involved, usually caseous or liquefactive necrosis.

Omasum

The omasum and the esophageal groove are seldom the seat of important pathologic processes. Actinobacillosis rarely localizes in the region, producing the characteristic granulomatous reaction. Malignant lymphomas may develop neoplastic masses in any of the local tissues, but are more likely to infiltrate the wall of the rumen or abomasum. A rare but curious disorder is

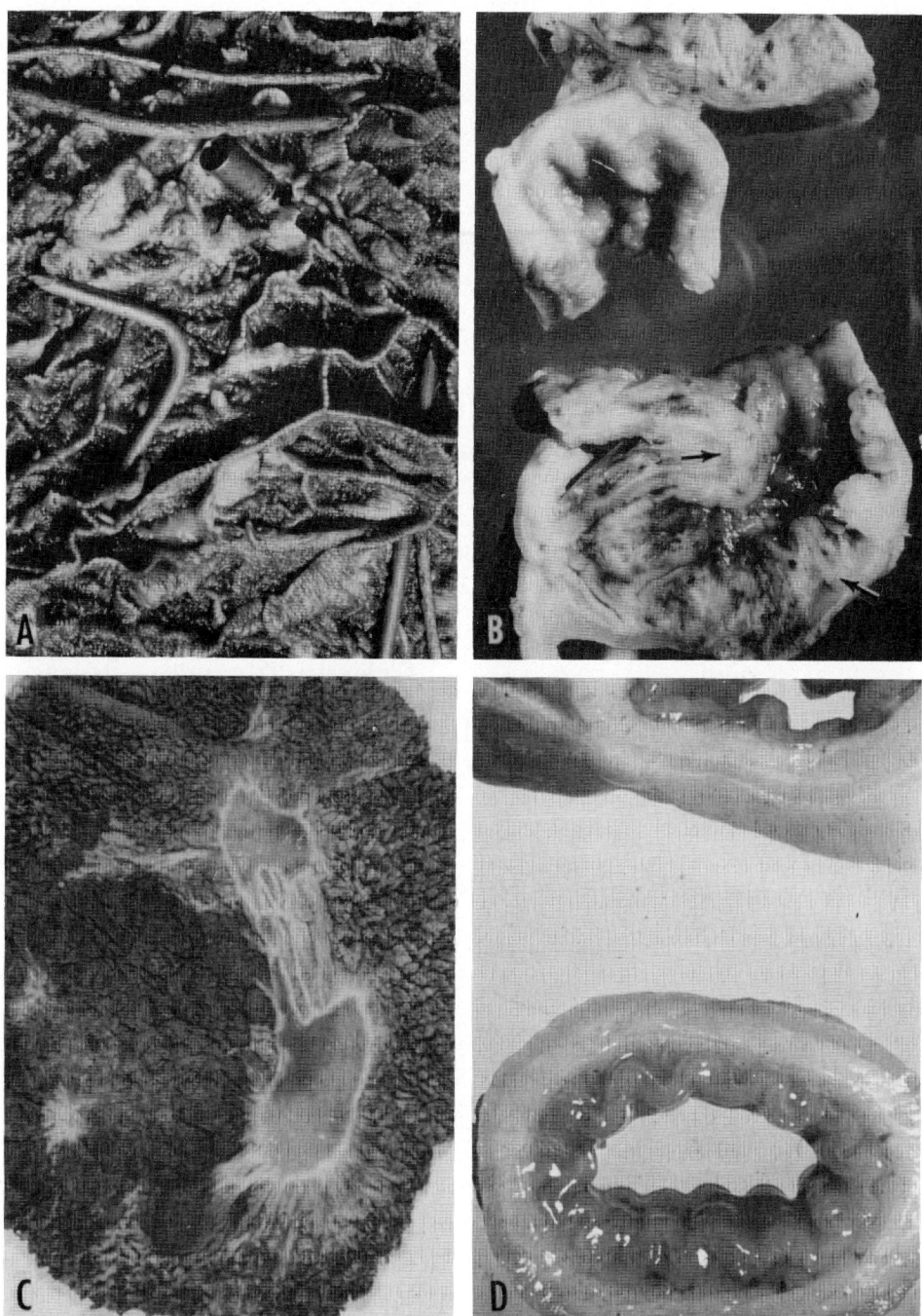

Fig. 23–11. *A,* Foreign bodies in the reticulum of a cow. Note that one nail (lower right) has penetrated the wall. Objects such as these may lead to traumatic gastritis. (Courtesy College of Veterinary Medicine, Iowa State University.) *B,* Regional cicatrizing enterocolitis in a two-year-old dog given euthanasia because of severe diarrhea for six months. (Courtesy Texas School of Veterinary Medicine.) *C,* Ulcers in the rumen of a fattened steer which was slaughtered in apparently normal health. The large dark area at left is undergoing necrosis and would have sloughed. (Courtesy of Colorado School of Veterinary Medicine.) *D,* Edema of the mucosa and submucosa of the ileum incarcerated in an umbilical hernia in a four-year-old mule. Death followed laparotomy and attempted relief. (Courtesy College of Veterinary Medicine, Iowa State University.)

1373

the formation of horn-like protruding growths several millimeters in diameter and some 2 to 4 cm in height, arising on the edges of the esophageal groove, on nearby portions of the pillars of the rumen or at the opening of the omasum. They are essentially papillomas but of no clinical importance.

Awadhiya, R.P., Kolte, G.N., and Vegad, J.L.: Cardiac tamponade—fatal complication of traumatic reticulitis—cattle. Vet. Rec., 95:260–262, 1974.

Frandson, R.D., and Davis, R.W.: Partial strangulation of bovine abomasum. J. Am. Vet. Med. Assoc., 124:267, 1954.

Said, A.H.: Rumenotomy and experimental traumatic reticulitis in the camel. Vet. Rec., 75:966–969, 1963.

Neoplasms of the Forestomachs

The association of bovine fibropapillomatosis (papillomavirus) and chronic bracken fern poisoning with papillomas and squamous cell carcinomas in the upper digestive tract (esophagus, rumen, reticulum, and omasum) has been discussed. An unusual occurrence in a guanaco, born and raised in a zoo, was the occurrence of a squamous cell carcinoma in the rumen and amyloidosis in the thymus. Lymphosarcoma may occasionally involve the wall of the forestomachs, particularly the omasum and reticulum (see Figure 22–2).

Altman, N.H., Small, J.D., and Squire, R.A.: Squamous cell carcinoma of the rumen and thymic amyloidosis in a guanaco. J. Am. Vet. Med. Assoc., 165:820–823, 1974.

STOMACH

The abomasum of ruminants is essentially similar in anatomic and physiologic features to the glandular stomach of most other mammals. Some animals, such as the rat and horse, have a part of the stomach lined with stratified squamous epithelium. This is continuous with the esophageal epithelium and forms the cardia of the stomach. The fundus is lined by thick secretory epithelium which contains both parietal and chief cells. The pyloric epithelium is continuous with that of the duodenum and is lined by serous and mucous secreting cells. In each species, the relative size of these distinct anatomic and specialized parts of the stomach is somewhat different and may affect the kind and frequency of lesions in the stomach. In general, however, the stomachs of most nonruminants may be considered as having similar functions and lesions.

Gastritis

Inflammation of the stomach is essentially an affection of its mucous lining. The symptoms, in general, are pain, anorexia, and vomiting. The latter sign is invariably present in gastritis, but may also be induced by reverse peristalsis initiated lower in the gastrointestinal tract, as well as by central nervous disturbances. Gastritis is usually catarrhal or hemorrhagic in type.

Acute catarrhal gastritis is recognized by an increased reddening and thickening of the entire surface or parts of it, the fundic area usually being most severely involved. There is an increase of the mucous secretion, which may or may not be sufficient to be recognizable grossly. Under the microscope, one sees that the redness is due to a combination of hyperemia and desquamation of the epithelium. It is often difficult to decide whether some of the desquamation is attributable to postmortem autolysis. In company with these changes, there is a limited amount of lymphocytic or, less commonly, neutrophilic infiltration of the mucosa and submucosa. Lymphoid hyperplasia of the normally minute lymphocytic foci in the gastric mucous membrane may result in microscopically large or even grossly recognizable nodules in the case of inflammatory processes of some days' duration.

Acute hemorrhagic gastritis is also common and is to be distinguished grossly by deeper reddening and by the presence of free blood on the surface or in the gastric contents. It should be noted that blood which has remained for any considerable time exposed to the gastric juice turns brown; commonly it is mixed with mucus as a slimy and viscid brownish substance, clinging more or less to the gastric surface. In the exact microscopic distinction as to whether an inflammation is hemorrhagic or merely catarrhal, it must be recognized that the extravascular blood may be within the tissues as well as on the surface. Since these two types of gastritis differ mainly in degree, the distinction is usually academic. Of course, the presence of extravasated blood without other signs of inflammation is to be interpreted as hemorrhage.

Catarrhal or hemorrhagic gastritis is a typical effect of various locally destructive poisons, but is also a characteristic lesion of certain infectious diseases, including swine erysipelas. The bites or points of attachment of several kinds of parasitic helminths, especially the trichostrongyles of ruminants, leave tiny hemorrhages or inflamed spots. With large numbers of parasites, the tiny spots become more or less confluent.

Serous fluid (serous exudate), usually termed **inflammatory edema,** may be a prominent part of the picture of gastritis, causing marked thickening of the mucosa and submucosa. The other varieties of acute inflammation are unusual in the stomach, although a fibrinous exudate may be formed in response to certain infections of a mucosa previously devitalized. Certain poisons exert specific effects upon the gastric lining when ingested in concentrated form. Mercuric chloride produces coagulative necrosis and at the same time acts as a fixative, preserving the tissue from postmortem changes. Carbolic acid has a similar effect and turns the surface white or gray.

Chronic hypertrophic gastritis ("giant rugal gastritis," "gastritis hypertrophia gigantica") has been described in dogs affected with a condition resembling Menet-rier's disease in man. So far, the disease has been described in Boxer and Basenji dogs. The etiology is unknown. It is manifest by lethargy, emaciation, vomiting, prolonged anorexia, and anemia. Protein is lost, resulting in hypoalbuminemia in late stages of the disease. The lesions consist of elevation and folding of the mucosa due to severe local epithelial hyperplasia, particularly in the fundus around the greater curvature. Inflammatory cells are present in the superficial parts of the lamina propria. Cystic glands are seen at the base of the crypts.

Gastritis glandularis and **gastritis cystica profunda** are terms used to designate a gastropathy observed in nonhuman primates (*Macaca mulatta*) (Scotti, 1973). The gross lesions were diffuse, involving much of the gastric mucosa, but varying in individual cases. The mucosa folds were large in some cases, small and inconspicuous in others. Hyperemia and petechiae were common in the mucosa, and ulcers were occasionally noted. The microscopic lesions included hyperplasia of the mucosa with many mucus-filled cysts in both mucosa and submucosa. The causes of this lesion are unknown but it seems likely that ingestion of some chemical irritants, such as polychlorinated biphenyls, should be suspected.

Eosinophilic gastritis is used to name severe inflammatory lesions of the stomach, in which eosinophil leukocytes are a conspicuous component. This chronic gastritis may result in fibrosis of the stomach wall, with fibrinoid necrosis of the wall of muscular arteries. Eosinophilia is usually manifest. Polyarteritis may be observed in omentum and reticulo-endothelial hyperplasia may be severe in the spleen. Lymph nodes and liver may be involved, with similar exudates. These lesions resemble those described in visceral larva migrans in dogs, except that the helminth larvae are not usually seen. It seems not unlikely, but is not established, that this lesion may result from repeated infection of a dog with helminth larvae (possibly *Toxocara canis*), after the animal has already been immunized by prior infection.

Barron, C.N., and Saunders, L.Z.: Visceral larva migrans in a dog. Pathol. Vet., 3:315–330, 1966.

Hayden, D.W., and Van Kruiningen, H.J.: Eosinophilic gastroenteritis in German Shepherd dogs and its relationship to visceral larva migrans. J. Am. Vet. Med. Assoc., 162:379–384, 1973.

Hayden, D.W., and Fleischman, R.W.: Scirrhous eosinophilic gastritis in dogs with gastric arteritis. Vet. Pathol., 14:441–448, 1977.

Kipnis, R.M.: Focal cystic hypertrophic gastropathy in a dog. J. Am. Vet. Med. Assoc., 173:182–194, 1978.

Scotti, T.M.: Simian gastropathy with submucosal glands and cysts. Gastritis glandularis or cystica profunda. Arch. Pathol., 96:403–408, 1973.

Van Der Gaag, I., Happé, R.P., and Wolvekamp, W.T.C.: A Boxer dog with chronic hypertrophic gastritis resembling Menetrier's disease in man. Vet. Pathol., 13:172–185, 1976.

Van Kruiningen, H.J.: Giant hypertrophic gastritis of Basenji dogs. Vet. Pathol., 14:15–18, 1977.

Hemorrhages

Large and small hemorrhages may occur in the gastric mucosa under any of the circumstances listed as causative in the general discussion of hemorrhage, but localized and generalized toxic conditions occupy a prominent place among them. Uremia is among the latter, as well as canine "blacktongue." Outstanding among the hemorrhage-producing infections likely to involve the gastric mucosa are hog cholera (swine fever), anthrax, and leptospirosis. Numerous small or punctate hemorrhages, some being old and faded, should lead to a search for helminth parasites, especially for the trichostrongyles of cattle and sheep. On the peritoneal surface, hemorrhages signify either hemorrhagic poisons or infections.

Chronic passive congestion, with or without (noninflammatory) edema, represents the effect upon the stomach of the circulatory impairment which results from cirrhosis or cardiac insufficiency.

Dilatation and Torsion

Acute distension of the stomach with gas occurs in several species including man, dog, horse, swine, rabbit, cat, and Rhesus monkey (*Macaca mulatta*). This life-threatening condition appears to have been studied most in the dog, hence the following remarks will apply especially to the canine disease: the canine disorder is manifest by obvious discomfort, abdominal pain, distension of the abdomen, and reluctance to move about. Larger breeds of dogs are more apt to be affected, including German Shepherds, Great Danes, Irish Setters, Weimaraners, Doberman Pinschers, Saint Bernards, and Boxers. Toy and standard-sized breeds are rarely affected.

The cause is generally unknown, although many events have been associated with dilatation, including parturition, overeating, pica, abdominal surgery, and trauma. Most observers are convinced that acute gastric dilatation precedes torsion of the stomach, which is a common sequel. The stomach becomes turned 190 or 300° around its long axis, resulting in twisting of the gastrosplenic omentum.

The effects of the gastric dilatation have been confirmed by experimental inflation of the stomach with a balloon. This results in mechanical obstruction of the caudal vena cava and portal vein, resulting in shunting of blood into the intervertebral and azygos veins. The common iliac, deep circumflex iliac, and renal veins also are distended by this obstruction. Cardiac output is decreased, arterial hypotension results; cellular catabolism is increased, and renal function is decreased.

Impaired renal function is indicated by rapid elevation of serum urea nitrogen, phosphorus, and creatinine. Serum glucose is elevated, as is serum glutamic oxaloacetic transaminase activity. Metabolic acidosis is evident from decrease in arterial HCO_3 values.

The lesions found following sudden death, or death during the night, are principally the greatly enlarged stomach, distended with gas and some ingesta. Torsion may result in twisting of the gastrosplenic omentum. Veins in the caudal aspect of the body are usually intensely engorged and the associated tissues congested. The stomach may have ruptured, spilling its contents into the peritoneal cavity. The cranial aspect of the body is usually ischemic, pale. The liver may be pale and friable; the spleen engorged with blood. Petechiae and ecchymoses may be seen in peritoneum and elsewhere. Sometimes subcutaneous edema is evident.

Acute dilatation in the horse usually leads to rupture of the stomach. The condition in the macaque closely resembles the canine disease. Rabbits may also be afflicted by similar events. The disorder also has been reported in swine, usually in breeding-age sows.

Betts, C.W., Wingfield, W.E., and Greene, R.W.: A retrospective study of gastric dilation-torsion in the dog. J. Small Anim. Pract., 15:727–734, 1974.

Blackburn, P.W., McCrea, C.T., and Randall, C.J.: Torsion of the stomach in sows. Vet. Rec., 94:578, 1974.

Cedervall, A.: Gastric torsion in swine. Acta Vet. Scand., 12:142–144, 1971.

Chapman, W.L., Jr.: Acute gastric dilation in *Macaca mulatta* and *Macaca speciosa* monkeys. Lab. Anim. Care, 17:130–136, 1967.

Newton, W.M., Beamer, P.D., and Rhoades, H.E.: Acute bloat syndrome in stumptailed macaques (*Macaca arctoides*): a report of four cases. Lab. Anim. Sci., 21:193–196, 1971.

Soave, O.A.: Observations on acute gastric dilatation in nonhuman primates. Lab. Anim. Sci., 28:331–334, 1978.

Turner, A.E., and Cowey, A.: Bloat syndrome in captive Rhesus monkeys: report on twelve cases. J. Inst. Anim. Tech., 22:181–186, 1971.

Wingfield, W.E., Cornelius, L.M., and DeYoung, D.W.: Pathophysiology of the gastric dilation-torsion complex in the dog. J. Small Anim. Pract., 15:735–739, 1974.

Wingfield, W.E., Cornelius, L.M., and DeYoung, D.W.: Experimental acute gastric dilation and torsion in the dog. 1. Changes in biochemical and acid-base parameters. J. Small Anim. Pract., 16:41–53, 1975.

Wingfield, W.E., Cornelius, L.M., Ackerman, N., and DeYoung, D.W.: Experimental acute gastric dilation and torsion in the dog. 2. Venous angiographic alterations seen in gastric dilation. J. Small Anim. Pract., 16:55–60, 1975.

Impaction of the stomach in the horse as the result of rapid ingestion of an excessive amount of ground feed or heavy grains (wheat, Indian corn) is especially dangerous. Even without gaseous fermentation, which is usual, absorption of toxic products of partial digestion, circulatory derangement and shock may be fatal in a number of hours or may cause laminitis.

Parasites

A variety of parasites may infest the stomach. In horses *Gastrophilus spp.* larvae are common. The roundworm, *Hyostrongylus rubidus,* invades the mucosa in swine. In ruminants, stomach worms are a major problem. The more common nematodes are *Hemonchus spp., Ostertagia spp.,* and *Trichostrongylus axei.*

Ulcers

Some of the infectious or toxic inflammations are ulcerative, especially in the later stages, and some of the hemorrhages owe their origin to erosions or ulcerations, but all these ulcers are acute and superficial. Ulceration of the gastric mucosa is now recognized in most domesticated species. Some differences between species are apparent, and the etiology may not be the same in each species.

In cattle, ulcers in the abomasum are apparently observed more frequently in recent years. Necropsies of 1988 yearling cattle in feedlots (Jensen, et al., 1976) disclosed 31 (1.6%) cattle with fatal outcome due to perforation or hemorrhage of ulcers. About an equal number of cattle were found to have ulcers which had not perforated. These discrete ulcers were found largely in the pylorus of the abomasum. A study of adult cattle (Aukema and Breukink, 1974) revealed most ulcers to be in the ventral part of the fundus with few in the pylorus. Among 1370 presumed normal cattle, 1% were found at slaughter to have ulcers; in 1200 cows brought in for "emergency slaughter" (due to some illness), 9.1% were found to have abomasal ulcers. In this same study, 141 cows were identified with fatal hemorrhages from abomasal ulcers.

The cause or causes of abomasal ulcers are not known. Several environmental conditions have been associated with the

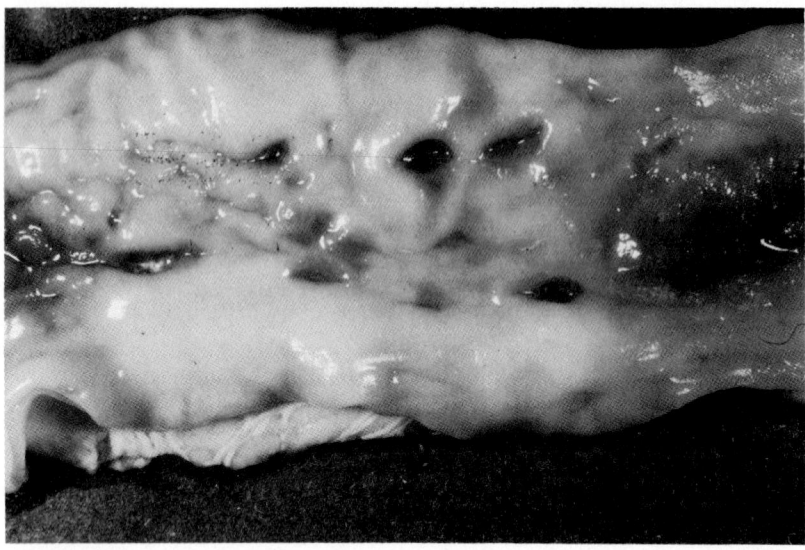

Fig. 23–12. Ulcers in duodenum of a five-year-old spayed female cat. Neoplastic mast cells invaded the spleen. (Courtesy of Angell Memorial Animal Hospital.)

disease but the evidence is not convincing that they are significant etiologic factors.

Ulceration of the nonglandular (stratified squamous epithelium) stomach in swine is a frequent and often serious disease. The ulcers are irregular in shape and may be single or multiple, varying in size from a few millimeters to several centimeters in diameter. Histologically, the ulcers extend into the submucosa, but rarely beyond and are associated with edema, arteritis, infiltration of neutrophils and eosinophils, and hyperplasia of submucosal lymphoid follicles. Adjacent epithelium is acanthotic and parakeratotic: changes which are believed to develop prior to erosion and ulceration. Blood in varying quantities may be admixed with the stomach contents. Healed ulcers leave contracted scars. Depending on the degree of ulceration, clinical signs may be inapparent as death may result from acute gastric hemorrhage without premonitory signs. More often the affected animals are weak, pale (anemia), and dyspneic. Vomiting may occur, and the feces may be tarry. The cause of gastric ulceration in swine is

not known. The most promising hypothesis suggests vitamin E deficiency, but the pathogenesis is not clear. Diets deficient in vitamin E and high in unsaturated fatty acids have been shown experimentally to be ulcerogenic. Ulcers have been seen in association with hepatosis dietetica. Deficiencies of vitamins A and D, zinc, and copper have also been suggested, as has hyperacidity, but all are unproved. Gelatinized corn and finely ground grain rations have been associated with ulceration.

Stress of confinement and transportation may also play a role in the development of ulcers. No doubt ulcers may be incited by more than a single factor, but the syndrome in swine suggests that most gastric ulcers are part of a single disease process. Ulceration of the glandular stomach of swine is much less frequent and not associated with ulceration of the nonglandular stomach.

The role of inheritance was examined in an interesting study by Grondalen and Vangen (1974). Three lines of swine were established by selection of breeding stock on the basis of backfat thickness (measured with ultrasound) and under standard conditions a mean daily rate of gain. The "low backfat line" was selected for low backfat and high rate of gain; the "high backfat line" was selected for high backfat and low rate of gain. A control line was maintained without apparent selection. After four or five generations, stomachs were examined for ulcers in the pars esophagea of these swine, and the following results obtained:

Line	Number of Stomachs Examined	Stomachs with Ulcers	
		Numbers	Per cent
Low backfat	96	16	16.7
High backfat	38	4	10.5
Control	73	4	5.5

From these results, it was concluded that genetic factors are significant in gastric ulcers of swine.

Ulceration of the nonglandular portion of the stomach is occasionally encountered in foals. Rooney (1964) believes they are related to mechanical trauma by *Gastrophilus intestinalis* larvae, stones, etc. Ulceration of the glandular mucosa also occurs in horses and is common in calves. Trauma and stress are believed to be causative factors, but vitamin E deficiency has also been suggested. In calves, mucormycosis commonly develops in gastric ulcers as well as in ulcers of the colon.

Ulcers of the pylorus and proximal duodenum are often associated with generalized mast cell tumors ("mast cell leukemia") in cats.

Chronic gastric ulcers have been associated with ingestion of aspirin by people and by experimental administration of aspirin (acetylsalicylic acid) to rats. These animals develop ulcers in the esophageal (squamous) part of the stomach when given 250 to 500 mg aspirin per day; with slightly smaller doses, multiple erosions appear in the mucosa of the fundus.

Angus, K.W., and Bannatyne, C.C.: Abomasal ulceration in adult sheep: a report of two contrasting cases. Vet. Rec., 86:531–533, 1970.

Aukema, J.J., and Breukink, H.J.: Abomasal ulcer in adult cattle with fatal haemorrhage. Cornell Vet., 64:303–317, 1974.

Baustad, B., and Nafstad, I.: Gastric ulcers in swine. 4. Effects of dietary particle size and crude fiber contents on ulceration. Pathol. Vet., 6:546–556, 1969.

Berruecos, J.M., Robison, O.W.: Inheritance of gastric ulcers in swine. J. Anim. Sci., 35:20–24, 1972.

Bivin, W.S., De Barros, C.L., De Barros, S.S., and Dos Santos, M.N.: Gastric ulcers in Brazilian swine. J. Am. Vet. Med. Assoc., 164:405–407, 1974.

Grondalen, T., and Vangen, O.: Gastric ulcers in pigs selected for leanness or fatness. Nord. Vet. Med., 26:50–53, 1974.

Ito, T., Miura, S., and Tanimura, I.: Pathological studies on proventricular ulcer in swine. Jpn. J. Vet. Sci., 36:263–272, 1974.

Jensen, R., et al.: Fatal abomasal ulcers in yearling feedlot cattle. J. Am. Vet. Med. Assoc., 169:524–526, 1976.

Nair, M.K.: The incidence and pathology of peptic ulcer in domestic animals. Kerala J. Vet. Sci., 4:120–123, 1973.

Norton, L.P., Nolan, J.E., Sales, L., and Eiseman, B.: A swine stress ulcer model. Ann. Surg., 176:133–138, 1972.

O'Brien, J.J.: Gastric ulceration (of the pars oesophagea) in the pig—a review. Vet. Bull., 39:75–82, 1969.

Penny, R.H.C., Edwards, M.J., and Mulley, R.: Gastric ulcer in the pig: a new South Wales abattoir survey of the incidence of lesions of the pars oesophagea. Br. Vet. J., 128:43–49, 1972.

Rooney, J.R.: Gastric ulceration in foals. Pathol. Vet., 1:497–503, 1964.

St. John, D.J., Yeomans, N.D., and DeBoer, W.G.: Chronic gastric ulcer induced by aspirin: an experimental model. Gastroenterology, 65:634–641, 1973.

Tasker, J.B., Roberts, S.J., Fox, F.H., and Hall, C.E.: Abomasal ulcers in cattle—recovery of one cow after surgery. J. Am. Vet. Med. Assoc., 133:365–368, 1958.

Displacement of Abomasum

Under certain conditions, as yet poorly defined, the abomasum may be displaced from its ventral and right-sided position in the anterior abdomen to the left side of the abdomen, displacing the rumen to the right. The abomasum moves along the abdominal floor to the left then between the left abdominal wall and the rumen. The cause is unknown although the condition is believed to be preceded by atony and gaseous distention of the abomasum. It is more apt to occur in older dairy cows and is associated with feeding of rations containing high proportions of concentrates rather than roughage. It often follows recent parturition and metritis. Less frequently, the displaced abomasum is found in the right flank rather than the left. More frequent occurrence in certain families has been cited as evidence of genetic factors.

The signs are anorexia, depression, and dehydration, distended abdomen, particularly protrusion in the left paralumbar fossa. The history often includes recent parturition. Auscultation and percussion are used to detect the abnormal position of the abomasum. If the displacement is not corrected immediately, death will occur.

Baker, J.S.: Displacement of the abomasum in dairy cows. Pract. Vet., Spring–Summer, 1973.

Coppock, C.E.: Displaced abomasum in dairy cattle: etiological factors. J. Dairy Sci., 57:926–933, 1974.

Jones, B.E.V., and Poulsen, J.S.D.: Abomasal emptying rate in goats and cows measured by external counting of radioactive sodium chromate injected directly into the abomasum. Nord. Vet. Med., 26:13–21, 1974.

Martin, W.: Left abomasal displacement: an epidemiological study. Can. Vet. J., 13:61–68, 1972.

Poulsen, J.S.D.: Clinical chemical examination of a case of left-side abomasal displacement, changing to a right-sided displacement. Nord. Vet. Med., 26:91–96, 1974.

Poulsen, J.S.D.: Variations in the metabolic acid-base balance and some other clinical chemical parameters in dairy herds during the year. Nord. Vet. Med., 26:1–12, 1974.

Poulsen, J.S.D.: Right-sided abomasal displacement in dairy cows: Pre- and postoperative clinical chemical findings. Nord. Vet. Med., 26:65–90, 1974.

Robertson, J. McD.: Left displacement of the bovine abomasum: epizootiologic factors. Am. J. Vet. Res., 29:421–434, 1968.

Smith, D.F.: Right-side torsion of the abomasum in dairy cows: Classification of severity and evaluation of outcome. J. Am. Vet. Med. Assoc., 173:108–111, 1978.

Stöber, M., Wegner, W., and Lünebrink, J.: Untersuchungen über familiäre disposition zur linksseitigen labmagenverlagung beim Rind. Dtsch. Tieraerztl. Wochenschr., 81:430–433, 1974.

Stöber, M., and Saratsis, Ph.: Vergleichende massung am rumpf von schwarzbunten küchen mit und ohne linksseitiger labmagenverlagung. Dtsch. Tieraerztl. Wochenschr., 81:564–565, 1974.

Stöber, M., Wegner, W., and Lünebrink, J.: Research on the familial occurrence of left-side displacement of the abomasum in cattle. Bovine Pract., 10:59–61, 1975.

Foreign Bodies

Foreign bodies are occasionally encountered, for instance, a rubber ball in the stomach of a dog. Piliconcretions may be in the stomach but are more likely to be found in the intestine.

Neoplasms of the Stomach

The statement is often recorded that tumors of the stomach of animals are rare. Certainly not many cases have been reported, but it appears likely that many cases are not recognized or not reported. We will of necessity confine our remarks to information in the literature or from our own experience.

Adenocarcinoma of the stomach has been reported in several species (bony fish, tortoise, birds, rats, hamsters, rabbit, cats, dogs, bovines, rhinoceros, macropus, and monkeys) but is most frequently recorded in the dog (Lingeman, et al., 1971). (Fig. 23–13.) Most canine gastric adenocarcinomas arise in the pyloric antral segment along the lesser curvature. The tumors tend to invade the wall of the stomach and often produce large ulcers in the center of a crater, with raised edges. Metastases occur to lymph nodes, liver, and lung.

The most frequent type in the dog is described as diffuse with epithelial cells diffusely infiltrating the stomach wall. The tumor cells obviously arise from columnar epithelium of the gastric mucosa, but may, in some species, be papillary, tubular, mucinous, or signet ring cell types (Head, 1976). In the papillary type, the epithelium forms frond-like layers of cells, similar to those seen in papillary adenomas. Tubular

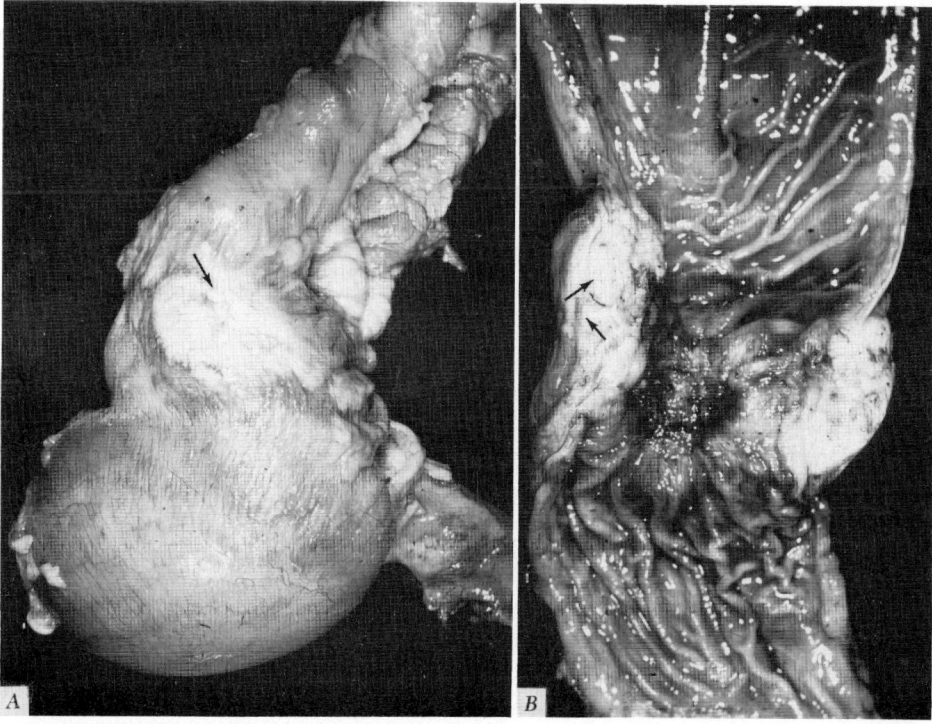

Fig. 23–13. *A*, Adenocarcinoma of stomach of an Irish setter, female, age 12 years. Note white scar (arrow) on serosal surface. A large ulcer was found on the opposing mucosal surface. *B*, Adenocarcinoma (arrow) of the rectum of an eight-year-old male Springer Spaniel. The tumor encircled the rectal wall, causing partial obstruction. (Courtesy of Angell Memorial Animal Hospital.)

structures may predominate in some tumors in other species. Mucinous secreting tumor cells may be a feature in some cases. Signet ring cells get their characteristic shape by the accumulation of mucus in the cytoplasm, which pushes the nucleus to one side of the cell. All of these cells characteristically invade the gastric submucosa and muscularis and eventually metastasize by way of the lymphatics.

Adenomas characteristically project from the mucosa into the lumen. They consist of hyperplastic epithelial cells which form elongated villi (papillary or villous form) or irregular tubules (adenomatous polyp). Some tumors may have both features (papillotubular). Some papillomas have been described in the stomach of monkeys (*Macaca fascicularis* and *M. arctoides*) in association with helminths

(*Nochtia nochti*). The parasites may be seen in microscopic sections, hence should be easily associated with this type of polyp.

Undifferentiated carcinomas (carcinoma simplex, medullary carcinoma, solid carcinoma) are occasionally seen and may be identified by their component of large epithelial cells with many mitoses, in solid nests or masses of cells. Tubules and squamous cells are not present.

Squamous cell carcinomas arise from the squamous epithelium of the stomach in the cardia. In those species which have a large cardiac component to the stomach (horse, pig, rat), squamous cell carcinoma is more frequent than adenocarcinoma. The tumor is made up of squamous epithelial cells which have in many places lost their normal polarity in relation to each other and the basement membrane. Mitoses are frequent and may be seen at sites outside the basal cell layer. Invasion of stroma is characteristic, and occasionally clumps of cells may be seen in lymphatics. Metastasis occurs by way of the lymphatics.

Leiomyoma and **leiomyosarcoma** may occasionally originate from the muscularis of the stomach, although more frequently appear in the small or large intestine. The tumor cells resemble those of the muscularis except for irregular arrangement, mitoses, and occasionally very immature cells. The malignant form (leiomyosarcoma) may be distinguished by its more undifferentiated cells, mitotic figures, and tendency to invade adjacent tissues. In both varieties, the tumor cells are apt to be arranged in interlacing bundles of parallel cells. Extension to adjacent tissues or organs and metastasis can be expected of the leiomyosarcoma.

Carcinoid tumors have been reported in the stomach of mastomys (*Mastomys natalensis*) and rarely in the dog, but are more apt to be found in the small intestine in the cat or bovine. These tumors are made up of epithelial cells in small nests or pockets; the cells have a centrally placed vesicular nucleus and finely granular cytoplasm. They are believed to arise from enterochromaffin cells which contain acidophilic cytoplasmic granules. In one type, the argentaffin tumor, the cells have the ability to reduce ammoniacal silver to metallic silver. In nonargentaffin tumors, the cells do not give the argentaffin reaction, but are argyrophilic. Granules may be demonstrated in these cells by using silver impregnation methods with reducers.

These tumors are primary in the mucosa, but spread to the submucosa. In the mastomys, these tumors have been shown to produce histamine but not serotonin.

Secondary tumors of the stomach may include lymphosarcoma, mast cell tumors, and metastatic tumors from liver or pancreas. Mesotheliomas of the peritoneum may occasionally involve the stomach wall.

Brody, R.S.: Alimentary tract neoplasms in the cat. A clinicopathologic survey of 46 cases. Am. J. Vet. Res., 27:74–80, 1966.

Conroy, J.D.: Multiple gastric adenomatous polyps in a dog. J. Comp. Pathol., 79:465, 1969.

Damodaran, S., and Ramachandran, P.V.: Gastric carcinoma in equines. Indian Vet. J., 47:118–120, 1970.

Davis, C.L., and Naylor, J.R.: Carcinoma in the stomach of a dog. J. Am. Vet. Med. Assoc., 102:286–288, 1943.

Fukushima, Y., Kawachi, T., Makanishi, M.: Histamine formation in spontaneous gastric carcinoids of *Praomys (mastomys) natalensis*. Gann, 65:279–280, 1974.

Hayden, D.W., and Nielsen, S.W.: Canine alimentary neoplasia. Zentralbl. Veterinaermed., 20A:1–22, 1973.

Head, K.W.: International histological classification of tumors of domestic animals. XII. Tumors of the lower alimentary tract. Bull. WHO, 53:167–186, 1976.

Krahnert, R.: Zum magenkrebs des pferdes. Monatsh. Vet. Med., 7:399–404, 1952.

Krook, L.: On gastrointestinal carcinoma in the dog. Acta Pathol. Microbiol. Scand., 38:43–57, 1956.

Lapin, B.A., and Krylova, R.I.: Gastric polyps in monkeys of Sukhumi Colony. Z. Versuchstierkd., 16:286–292, 1974.

Lingeman, C.H., Garner, F.M., and Taylor, D.O.N.: Spontaneous gastric adenocarcinomas of dogs. A review. J. Natl. Cancer Inst., 47:137–153, 1971.

Meagher, D.M., Wheat, J.D., Tennant, B., and Osburn, B.I.: Squamous cell carcinoma of the equine stomach. J. Am. Vet. Med. Assoc., 164:81–84, 1974.

Murray, M., et al.: Primary gastric neoplasia in dogs: a clinicopathological study. Vet. Rec., 91:474–489, 1972.

Patnaik, A.K., Hurvitz, A.I., and Johnson, G.F.: Canine gastrointestinal neoplasms. Vet. Pathol., 14:547–555, 1977.

Patnaik, A.K., Hurvitz, A.I., and Johnson, G.F.: Canine gastric adenocarcinoma. Vet. Pathol., 15:600–607, 1978.

Sautter, J.H., and Hanlon, G.F.: Gastric neoplasms in the dog: a report of 20 cases. J. Am. Vet. Med. Assoc., 168:691–696, 1975.

Stewart, H.L.: Experimentally induced gastric adenocarcinomas. Lab. Invest., 25:672–674, 1971.

Szepsenwol, J.: Tumors of the glandular stomach in mice of the BALB/c strain fed raw egg yolk or hard-boiled egg white. Fed. Proc., 31:926, 1972.

Titis, R.S., Leipold, H.W., and Anderson, N.V.: Gastric carcinoma in a mare. J. Am. Vet. Med. Assoc., 161:270–274, 1972.

SMALL INTESTINE

Enteritis

The term enteritis commonly refers to inflammation of any or all parts of the intestinal tract, but often it is used to refer only to the small intestine. Other terms may be used when inflammation involves more than one part of the gastrointestinal tract, such as: gastroenteritis (the entire tract), typhlitis or cecitis (involving cecum), duodenitis, jejunitis, ileitis, colitis, and proctitis. We shall consider specific diseases of each part of the tract separately, but it is well to remember that several parts of the digestive system may be affected simultaneously.

Acute enteritis may conform to any one of the five types of acute exudative inflammation, and subacute lymphocytic and chronic proliferative forms are by no means lacking. The whole small intestine may be rather uniformly inflamed, or even the small and large intestines together, but it is more usual that the inflammation be more pronounced toward one end or the other of the small intestine or perhaps relatively localized. The location of the reaction, of course, coincides with the site of greatest concentration of the irritant, be it chemical or infectious. Toxic substances which are ingested may be held for some time in the stomach so that their principal effect is a gastritis. Other toxic substances are of such a nature that the stomach rather quickly advances them to the intestine, where most of their effect is felt. Most enterotoxins (products of bacteria) are destroyed by gastric juice. There is also the factor of solubility; those which dissolve slowly may progress to the intestine before becoming extensively dissolved. The rather high acidity in the stomach and the relative alkalinity in the intestine are also important influences on solubility and absorption. If the irritant is of infectious nature, the time required for adequate multiplication of the organisms may be instrumental in determining where their harm is greatest. A rather common situation is for the upper small intestine to be severely inflamed, with the ileum remaining relatively normal. This is ordinarily

attributable to the injurious substance having been dissipated or at least diluted before it reached the lower portions of the bowel. The length of time during which the ingesta remain in a given place is also important and may be responsible for a cecitis or colitis with little or no damage in the more rapidly emptying small intestine.

When inflammation is principally in the colon, the possibility of its being caused by a toxic substance in process of elimination there should be entertained. Numerous toxic substances of endogenous or exogenous origin are eliminated from the blood into the bowel, some of them principally in the large bowel (mercury, uremic products), causing injury and an inflammatory reaction in the mucous membrane through which they pass. Lastly, the peculiar affinities of a particular infecting organism have to be considered: the coccidia of most mammals confine themselves almost entirely to the last part of the large bowel although certain species localize in the small intestine; the various avian coccidia have different sites of predilection, the cecum or the upper small intestine, depending on the species of coccidium. Some microorganisms depend upon metazoan parasites to provide a mode of entry, and hence localize in the area favored by the metazoan species.

Specific viruses have a predilection for precise cells in the intestinal epithelium. For example, the coronavirus of transmissible gastroenteritis of swine grows in and destroys most of the epithelium of the villus; sparing the cells in the crypts; rotaviruses of calf diarrhea and enzootic diarrhea in mice attack the most mature epithelium near the apex of the villus; the parvovirus of feline panleukopenia thrives in the dividing cells in the crypt of the intestinal mucosa, causing total collapse of the mucosa and impaired regeneration.

In **catarrhal enteritis,** acute or chronic, the changes simulate those of catarrhal gastritis: death of epithelium and perhaps the underlying stroma in the more exposed structures, moderate hyperemia and moderate lymphocytic infiltration in the deeper parts of the mucosa. Enteritis of this kind is a common accompaniment of many infectious diseases as well as the result of toxic substances. The multitudinous bites occurring in an extensive infestation of hookworms cause confluent hemorrhages and catarrhal or hemorrhagic enteritis in the small intestine of the dog. Somewhat less conspicuous injury is done to the cecum and large colon of the horse in the case of severe strongylosis. In canine autopsies, a mild degree of catarrhal duodenitis and jejunitis is found with such frequency as to be almost routine.

Occasionally, a truly mucous exudate is encountered, of such intensity that the microscopic section reveals streams of blue-staining epithelial mucin stretching out from the intestinal glands (crypts). Clinically, this type of reaction, occurring in the large bowel, is revealed by sheets or strings of white, inspissated mucus on the formed feces. The soft fecal discharges of the bovine are an obvious exception, but in the constipation, which often accompanies benign and transitory enteric disturbances, formed feces flecked with visible aggregations of solidified mucus sometimes appear even in cattle.

Like its gastric counterpart, **hemorrhagic enteritis** is chiefly a violent form of the acute catarrhal. Its distribution is practically always patchy for the simple reason that an animal could scarcely remain alive until a hemorrhagic enteritis had become widespread. This form is usually the enteric manifestation of a locally destructive poison in concentrated form or of one of the highly virulent infections, such as anthrax. Salmonella species, commonly S. enteritidis or S. typhimurium, have been reported as causing acute catarrhal, and often hemorrhagic enteritis in cattle, horses and monkeys. In swine, Salmonella cholerae suis is the common cause of acute enteritis, but there are numerous reports of a spirochete (Treponema hyodysenteriae) causing severe and fatal enteritis in young pigs. Shigellosis is an important cause of hemorrhagic enteritis in most species of nonhuman primates. Viruses have also been incriminated.

Purulent enteritis is infrequent, but occasionally occurs where mechanical injuries from helminth parasites (e.g., hookworms, nodular worms) have opened the tissues to invasion by pyogenic bacteria. Chronic mucopurulent enteritis in the dog, apparently of nonspecific origin, is characterized by dense, slightly tenacious, semi-solid, whitish exudate lying to a depth of 2 or 3 mm over the duodenal and jejunal surfaces.

Acute **fibrinous enteritis** is probably more frequent in the large intestine of cattle. The fibrinous exudate is often of the pseudomembranous type, and as the inflammation subsides, the pseudomembrane may be loosened to pass out with the feces in the form of a long, hollow cast bearing an uncanny resemblance to the lining of a stretch of intestine.

A more diphtheritic form of acute fibrinous inflammation sometimes involves either the small or large intestine of the pig. Limited data indicate that it is due to the activities of the organism, Salmonella cholerae suis (suipestifer).

The much more usual fibrinous enteritis in the pig is chronic, the well-known **necrophorus enteritis,** or "necro." The term "necrotic enteritis" has also been used, but the careful pathologist will naturally suspect that it is the tissue rather than the enteritis which undergoes necrosis! The lesions occur in the large intestine and, to some extent, in the last portion of the ileum. They consist of patches, large or small, of thick, rough, brownish or grayish diphtheritic exudate which is tightly adherent to the dead and living tissue beneath. As is usual with diphtheritic exudates, the underlying cells undergo coagulative necrosis, and the fibrils of the exudate extend into and among them, tying the whole into a crust-like layer. Fecal material becomes mixed with the superficial portions of the exudate. The exudative areas may line a considerable portion of the bowel, or they may be limited to raised patches here and there. Not infrequently they form rather perfect circular structures known as "button ulcers." Since necrophorus enteritis frequently accompanies severe outbreaks of hog cholera, the button ulcers were at one time considered diagnostic of that viral disease.

As the name implies, the necrophorus organism (presently *Spherophorus necrophorus*) plays an important part in producing the lesions of this disease, but it is generally believed to be a secondary invader, supervening upon primary injury caused by some other infection, possibly the *Salmonella* just mentioned. Whatever its precise bacteriological status may be, necrophorus enteritis is a disease which belongs to filthy or long-used and contaminated pig pens; adequate sanitation and husbandry eliminate it. Deficiency of nicotinic acid in the diet may have predisposing importance but cannot be accepted as fundamental.

Chronic proliferative enteritis is seen in those granulomatous infections which involve the intestine, notably Johne's disease, tuberculosis, colibacillosis (Hjärre's disease) of fowls, histoplasmosis, and others. The proliferative enteric reaction is that characteristic of each disease. Partial obstructions or other mechanical factors are occasionally responsible for localized chronic inflammations of the same general variety.

Many of the specific infections which produce enteritis, gastroenteritis, or enterocolitis have been considered elsewhere in this text and will not be considered at length in this chapter. Viral enteritides such as caused by *Rotavirus, Coronavirus,* and *Parvovirus* are discussed in Chapter 9. Bacterial diseases, including colibacillosis, shigellosis, salmonellosis, versiniosis, pasteurellosis, and infections due to *Clos-*tridium perfringens, Bacillus piliformis* (Tyzzer's Disease), and *Campylobacter sputorum* are taken up in Chapter 11. Other specific enteric infections, such as paratuberculosis, avian tuberculosis, mucormycosis, and swine dysentery are described in Chapter 12. Protozoal enteric pathogens (coccidiosis, amebiasis, giardiasis) and the diseases they produce are considered in Chapter 13.

Anon: Colloquium on selected diarrheal diseases of the young. J. Am. Vet. Med. Assoc.,*173*:511–676, 1978.
Bywater, R.J.: Pathophysiological aspects of unidirectional water and sodium transport in calf intestine. Ann. Rech. Vet., *4*:125–133, 1973.
Ferney, J.: Disease of the digestive system of monkeys. Zool. Gart. Leipzig, *37*:197–223, 1969.
Grady, G.F., and Keusch, G.T.: Pathogenesis of bacterial diarrheas (2 parts). N. Engl. J. Med., *285*:831–841; 891–900, 1971.
Kent, T.H., and Moon, H.W.: The comparative pathogenesis of some enteric diseases, based on cases presented at the 22nd annual seminar of the Am. College of Vet. Pathol. Vet. Pathol., *10*:414–469, 1973.
Mebus, C.A., Newman, L.E., and Stair, E.L.: Scanning electron, light, and transmission electron microscopy of intestine of gnotobiotic calf. Am. J. Vet. Res., *36*:985–994, 1975.
Moon, H.W.: Vacuolated villous epithelium of the small intestine of young pigs. Vet. Pathol., *9*:3–21, 1972.
Moon, H.W., Kohler, E.M., and Whipp, S.C.: Vacuolation: a function of cell age in porcine ileal absorptive cells. Lab. Invest., *28*:23–28, 1973.
Moon, H.W.: Mechanisms in the pathogenesis of diarrhea: A review. J. Am. Vet. Med. Assoc., *172*:443–448, 1978.
Mottet, N.K.: On animal models for inflammatory bowel disease. Gastroenterol., *62*:1269–1271, 1972.
Mukherjee, T.M., and Williams, A.W.: A comparative study of the ultrastructure of microvilli in the epithelium of small and large intestine of mice. J. Cell Biol., *34*:447–461, 1967.
Orlic, D., and Lev, R.: An electron microscopic study of intraepithelial lymphocytes in human fetal small intestine. Lab. Invest., *37*:554–561, 1977.
Takeuchi, A.: Penetration of the intestinal epithelium by various microorganisms. Curr. Top. Pathol., *54*:1–27, 1971.

Regional Cicatrizing Enterocolitis

Regional cicatrizing enterocolitis, regional ileitis, or Crohn's disease, was established as an entity in humans in 1932.

An entirely comparable disease was recognized in the dog by Strande et al. (1954). In the general vicinity of the ileo-cecal orifice and sometimes both above and below it, the mucosa and submucosa are rather irregularly involved in asymmetrical thickening which reaches as much as 6 cm, and is strongly suggestive of mucosal neoplasia. Microscopically, the suspected neoplasm proves to consist of fibrous and reticulo-endothelial granulation tissue with many bizarre epithelioid and even multinucleated giant cells. In places, the mucous surface is ulcerated, with an acute purulent reaction. Fistulas may reach the serosal side of the bowel. Dense fibrous scarring marks attempted healing. The regional mesenteric lymph nodes may undergo a similar granulomatous enlargement. The ultimate result is partial or complete obstruction of the intestinal lumen. The cause appears to be a chronic infection, but rather extensive search has failed to identify one in either man or animal. A chronic granulomatous enteritis has been described in horses and compared to Crohn's disease. The lesions are somewhat alike in man, dog, and horse, but until the etiology is clearly understood, the identity of these lesions remains clouded.

Cave, D.R., Mitchell, D.N., Kane, S.P., and Brooks, B.N.: Further animal evidence of a transmissible agent in Crohn's disease. Lancet, 2:1120–1122, 1973.

Cave, D.R., Mitchell, D.N., and Brooks, B.N.: Experimental animal studies of the etiology and pathogenesis of Crohn's disease. Gastroenterol., 69:618–624, 1975.

Cimprich, R.E.: Equine granulomatous enteritis. Vet. Pathol., 11:535–547, 1974.

Menard, D.B., et al.: Granulomatous myositis and myopathy associated with Crohn's colitis. New Engl. J. Med., 295:818–819, 1976.

Merritt, A.M., Cimprich, R.E., and Beech, J.: Granulomatous enteritis in nine horses. J. Am. Vet. Med. Assoc., 169:603–609, 1976.

Sachar, D.B., Taub, R.N., and Janowitz, H.D.: A transmissible agent in Crohn's disease? New pursuit of an old concept. N. Engl. J. Med., 293:354–355, 1975.

Strande, A., Sommers, S.C., and Petrak, M.: Regional enterocolitis in Cocker Spaniel dogs. Arch. Pathol., 57:357–362, 1954.

Muscular Hypertrophy of the Ileum in Swine

An apparently unrelated condition of swine, characterized by marked hypertrophic thickening of the muscularis propria in the last portion of the ileum, has been confused with the above granulomatous disease under the name of **terminal ileitis.** The great thickening of the intestinal wall and stenosis of the lumen are similar although usually less abrupt. Microscopically, the thickening is not granulomatous and does not involve the mucosa and submucosa but is, rather, an extensive but orderly increase in both layers of the muscularis. This is probably to be explained, as pointed out by Nielsen (1955), on a functional basis, an adaptive hypertrophy gradually developing as the result of impaction or spasmodic contraction lower in the tract. With increasing stenosis, ingesta actually become lodged at the site of narrowing. Local pressure brings venous obstruction and edema, with bacterial and gangrenous invasion of the devitalized mucosa. Nielsen suggested the name "muscular hypertrophy of the ileum" in place of terminal ileitis.

There is a single report of segmental hypertrophy of a 5½ cm length of the transverse colon of a Rhesus monkey (*Macaca mulatta*) (Casey, et al., 1969). In this animal the hypertrophy was principally of the muscularis.

Casey, H.W., et al.: Segmental hypertrophy of colon in a Rhesus monkey. J. Am. Vet. Med. Assoc., 155:1245–1248, 1969.

Nielsen, S.W.: Muscular hypertrophy of the ileum in relation to "terminal ileitis" in pigs. J. Am. Vet. Med. Assoc., 127:437–441, 1955.

Regional Ileitis of Swine

A varied pattern of clinical signs and pathologic lesions, interpreted by many authors scattered throughout the world, has resulted in many names for this syndrome. It may be that the confusion may now be lessened based upon the demonstration of an organism, *Campylobacter sputorum* ss *mucosalis* in the cytoplasm of ileal mucosal epithelial cells of affected pigs.

A brief review of the historical development of the literature may be helpful in understanding what seem to be divergent views. Biester and Schwarte (1931) described proliferation of undifferentiated epithelium in the terminal ileum of young swine and called the disease "intestinal adenoma." Crohn et al. (1932) published a report on "regional ileitis" of man which established this disease as a clinical and pathologic entity ("Crohn's disease"). Subsequent writers have often compared ileitis in swine, horses, and other species with Crohn's disease. Emsbo (1951) described a "terminal or regional ileitis" in swine in which he recognized hyperplasia of the ileal muscularis ("stiff as a garden hose") associated with hyperplasia of Peyer's patches, severe inflammation and thickening of the mucosa, and downgrowth of undifferentiated epithelium. This adenomatous hyperplasia may be seen in Emsbo's photomicrographs, but he gave this aspect of the lesions scant credence. Dodd (1968) apparently redescribed the lesions originally recognized by Biester and Schwarte and introduced the terms "adenomatous intestinal hyperplasia" or "proliferative ileitis" of swine.

In 1967, Jones described from South Wales an "intestinal haemorrhage syndrome" in pigs. This disease sporadically affected young pigs, but did occasionally involve adults. The principal lesions were the presence of large amounts of fresh blood in the small intestine, extending from a point 50 to 60 cm from the pylorus to the cecum. Aside from severe vascular congestion in the wall of the affected small intestine, no significant microscopic lesions were described. This syndrome or something akin to it was subsequently called "haemorrhagic bowel syndrome" by other writers (O'Neill, 1970; Rowland and Rowntree, 1972; Chu and Hong, 1973).

Rowland and Rowntree (1972), Rowland,

et al. (1973), and later Rowland and Lawson (1973) described the possible relationship of "porcine intestinal adenomatous" to "necrotic enteritis," "regional ileitis," and "proliferative haemorrhagic enteropathy." Rowland and Lawson (1974) reported the demonstration of unidentified bacteria by electron microscopy and immunologic methods in affected epithelial cells of the ileum. In a subsequent paper, Lawson and Rowland (1974) identified the intracellular organisms as *Campylobacter sputorum* ss *mucosalis*. The relationship of this organism to natural cases of this many-faceted disease or diseases was confirmed by Gunnarsson, et al. (1976) in Sweden, but experimental reproduction of the disease had not been reported at the time this text was written. The lesions of "proliferative haemorrhagic enteropathy" in pigs have been more recently described by Love and Love (1979).

Additional features of infection with *Campylobacter* spp. are described in Chapter 11.

Biester, H.E., and Schwarte, L.H.: Intestinal adenoma in swine. Am. J. Pathol., 7:175–185, 1931.

Chu, R.M.R., and Hong, C.B.: Haemorrhagic bowel syndrome in pigs in Taiwan. Vet. Rec., 93:562–563, 1973.

Crohn, B.B., Ginsburg, L., and Oppenheimer, G.D.: Regional ileitis, a pathologic and clinical entity. J. Am. Med. Assoc., 99:1323–1329, 1932.

Dodd, D.C.: Adenomatous intestinal hyperplasia (proliferative ileitis) of swine. Pathol. Vet., 5:333–341, 1968.

Emsbo, P.: Terminal or regional ileitis in swine. Nord. Vet. Med., 3:1–28, 1951.

Gunnarsson, A., et al.: Regional ileitis in pigs. Isolation of *Campylobacter* from affected ileal mucosa. Acta Vet. Scand., 17:267–269, 1976.

Jones, J.E.T.: An intestinal haemorrhage syndrome in pigs. Br. Vet. J., 123:286–294, 1967.

Lawson, G.H.K., and Rowland, A.C.: Intestinal adenomatosis in the pig: a bacteriological study. Res. Vet. Sci., 17:331–336, 1974.

Love, D.N., and Love, R.J.: Pathology of proliferative haemorrhagic enteropathy in pigs. Vet. Pathol., 16:41–48, 1979.

O'Hara, P.J.: Intestinal haemorrhage syndrome in the pig. Vet. Rec., 91:517–518, 1972.

O'Neill, P.A.: Observations on a haemorrhagic bowel syndrome involving pigs on three associated premises. Vet. Rec., 87:742–747, 1970.

Rahko, T., and Saloniemi, H.: Regional ileitis in pigs

in Finland. 1. Pathological changes. Suomen. Lehti, *78*:318–327, 1972.

Rahko, T., and Saloniemi, H.: On the pathology of regional ileitis in the pig. Nord. Vet. Med., *24*:132–138, 1972.

Rowland, A.C., and Lawson, G.H.K.: Intestinal hemorrhage syndrome in the pig. Vet. Rec., *93*:402–404, 1973.

Rowland, A.C., and Lawson, G.H.K.: Intestinal adenomatosis in the pig: immunofluorescent and electron microscopic studies. Res. Vet. Sci., *17*:323–330, 1974.

Rowland, A.C., and Lawson, G.H.K.: Porcine intestinal adenomatosis: a possible relationship with necrotic enteritis, regional ileitis and proliferative haemorrhagic enteropathy. Vet. Rec., *97*:178–181, 1975.

Rowland, A.C., and Lawson, G.H.K.: Intestinal adenomatosis in the pig: a possible relationship with a haemorrhagic enteropathy. Res. Vet. Sci., *18*:263–268, 1975.

Rowland, A.C., Lawson, G.H.K., and Maxwell, A.: Intestinal adenomatosis in the pig: occurrence of a bacterium in affected cells. Nature, *243*:417, 1973.

Rowland, A.C., and Rowntree, P.G.M.: A haemorrhagic bowel syndrome associated with intestinal adenomatosis in the pig. Vet. Rec., *91*:235–241, 1972.

Smith, W.J., and Shanks, P.L.: Intestinal haemorrhage syndrome. Vet. Rec., *89*:55–56, 1971.

Proliferative Ileitis in Hamsters

This disease has been given several names, based on interpretations as to its probable cause. It was first called "enzootic intestinal adenocarcinoma" (Jonas, et al., 1965), later "proliferative ileitis" (Boothe and Cheville, 1967), and also has been called "regional enteritis," "atypical ileal hyperplasia," and "hamster enteritis." The diarrhea which occurs in this disease, probably not specific, is sometimes referred to as "wet tail." Most evidence indicates this is probably an infectious disease.

In the report of Boothe and Cheville, the disease spread slowly, had a morbidity rate of 25 to 60% and a mortality rate of 90%. The lesions develop in the ileum, less often in the jejunum, and rarely in the colon. Grossly, the ileum is dilated, thickened, studded with small white subserosal foci and often adhered to other viscera. Microscopically, there is hyperplasia of the intestinal epithelium, accompanied by purulent inflammation and coagulation necrosis extending into the submucosa. The hyperplastic epithelium extends into the submucosa, muscularis, and often to the serosa, forming small glands or cysts which remain after healing. Diffuse and focal collections of large histiocytes occur on the lamina propria, submucosa, muscularis and serosa as well as in mesenteric lymph nodes.

Tomita and Jonas (1968) have isolated two viruses (which may be herpesviruses) from affected hamsters, but their relationship in this disease is not established at present. Lussier and Pavilanis (1969) described eosinophilic intranuclear inclusion bodies in the ileal epithelium, which may add support to the hypothesis of a viral etiology.

A bacterial organism identified as *Shigella boydii* has been demonstrated ultrastructurally in hyperplastic intestinal epithelial cells of the hamster, but no other evidence indicates it to be an etiologic agent (Wagner, et al., 1973). Additional electron microscopic studies (Frisk and Wagner, 1977) identified *Escherichia coli* in early lesions and *Campylobacter* species in later lesions in the natural disease. Although the disease may be transmitted with suspensions of tissue from affected ileum, reproduction of the disease with pure cultures of any organism appears not to have been accomplished.

Amend, N.K., Loeffler, D.G., Ward, B.C., and Van Hoosier, G.L., Jr.: Transmission of enteritis in the Syrian hamster. Lab. Anim. Sci., *26*:566–572, 1976.

Boothe, A.D., and Cheville, N.F.: The pathology of proliferative ileitis of the Golden Syrian Hamster. Pathol. Vet., *4*:31–44, 1967.

Frisk, C.S., and Wagner, J.E.: Experimental hamster enteritis: an electron microscopic study. Am. J. Vet. Res., *38*:1861–1869, 1977.

Jacoby, R.O., Osbaldiston, G.W., and Jonas, A.M.: Experimental transmission of atypical ileal hyperplasia of hamsters. Lab. Anim. Sci., *25*:465–473, 1975.

Jonas, A.M., Tomita, Y., and Wyand, D.S.: Enzootic intestinal adenocarcinoma in hamsters. J. Am. Vet. Med. Assoc., *147*:1102–1108, 1965.

Lussier, G., and Pavilanis, V.: Presence of intranuclear inclusion bodies in proliferative ileitis of the hamster (*Mesocricetus auratus*). A preliminary report. Lab. Anim. Care, *19*:387–390, 1969.

Tomita, Y., and Jonas, A.M.: Two viral agents isolated from hamsters with a form of regional enteritis. A preliminary report. Am. J. Vet. Res., 29:445–453, 1968.

Wagner, J.E., Owens, D.R., and Troutt, H.F.: Proliferative ileitis of hamsters: electron microscopy of bacteria in cells. Am. J. Vet. Res., 34:249–252, 1973.

Spontaneous Ileitis in Rats

Also described as "megaloileitis," this disease of unknown cause occurs in young rats less than 2 months of age. Clinically, there is marked distention of the abdomen, rough hair coat, and occasionally diarrhea. Approximately 50% of affected rats die, the others recovering over a period of about a week. At necropsy, the most striking lesion is a severe dilatation of the ileum with 7 to 10 cm segments distended up to 1.5 cm. The distention generally terminates at or near the ileocecal junction. The contents of the ileum vary from a frothy semi-fluid to a

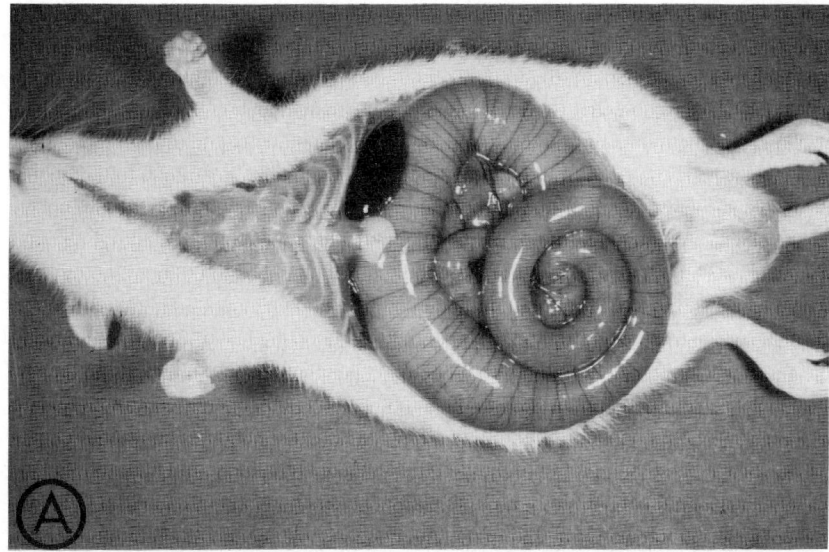

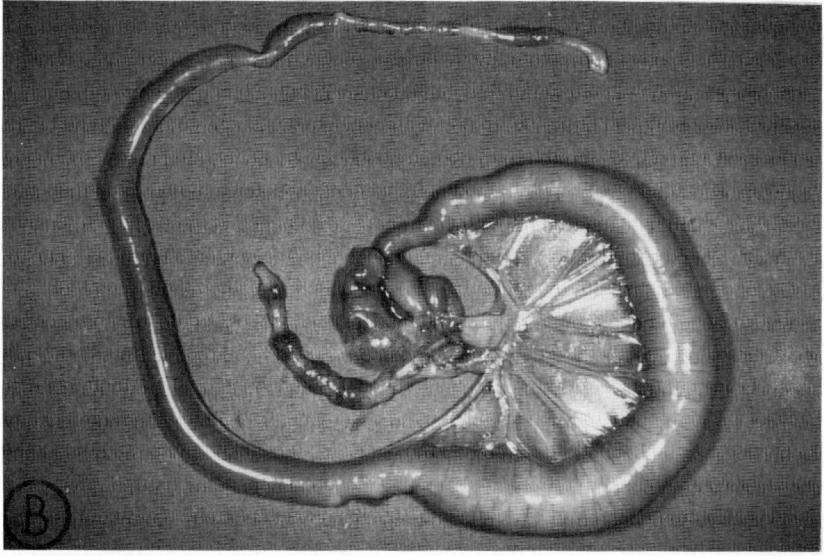

Fig. 23–14. Regional ileitis, rat. There is marked dilation of the ileum. (Courtesy Animal Research Center, Harvard Medical School.)

pasty consistency. Microscopically, the lesions are not striking. There is hydropic degeneration and coagulation necrosis of both layers of the muscularis associated with an inflammatory cell infiltration composed of lymphocytes, macrophages, and a lesser number of neutrophils. In the mucosa, a lymphocytic infiltration occurs in the lamina propria, and many of the crypts of Lieberkühn are occluded with amorphous eosinophilic material. In the healing stages of the condition, fibrovascular proliferation repairs the lesions in the muscularis. Occasionally, the distended ileum becomes adhered to the abdominal wall or other viscera. In some rats with this disease there is also a necrotizing and lymphocytic myocarditis and hepatitis.

Geil, R.G., Davis, C.L., and Thompson, S.W.: Spontaneous ileitis in rats. Am. J. Vet. Res., 22:932–936, 1961.
Hottendorf, G.H., Hirth, R.S., and Peer, R.L.: Megaloileitis in rats. J. Am. Vet. Med. Assoc., 155:1131–1135, 1969.

Terminal Ileitis in Lambs

Terminal ileitis in lambs has been described in one report. The disease involved lambs 4 to 6 months of age which had shown a poor rate of growth. The terminal 50 to 75 mm of the ileum was involved with thickened rugae resulting from hyperplasia of the mucosa. In one lamb, submaxillary edema was also seen. Some of the affected lambs had bleeding ulcers in the ileum. Aerobic and anaerobic cultures failed to disclose any bacterial organisms. The lesions were not believed to resemble paratuberculosis (Johne's disease).

Cross, R.F., Smith, C.K., and Parker, C.F.: Terminal ileitis in lambs. J. Am. Vet. Med. Assoc., 162:564–566, 1973.

Diverticulosis in the Small Intestine

Diverticulosis in the small intestine has been recorded in horses, pigs, and sheep. This lesion is seen as small, epithelial-lined cavities projecting into the muscularis and often reaching the serosa. The serosal surface is elevated by spherical balloonings, which on occasion rupture into the peritoneal cavity. This usually results in death from peritonitis. In the horse, the duodenum is most apt to be involved. Hypertrophy of the muscularis often accompanies this diverticulosis, although both may occur independently. Adult horses are usually affected. In pigs, the site of diverticulosis is the terminal ileum in young pigs. Rupture with peritonitis has been recorded. The suggestion has been made that its frequency in certain familial groups points toward hereditary origin in this species, however, no relevant data are available on this point.

In sheep, adults appear to be most frequently affected, although reports are sparse. The duodenum and terminal ileum are involved.

Cordes, D.O., and Dewes, H.F.: Diverticulosis and muscular hypertrophy of the small intestine of horses, pigs, and sheep. N. Z. Vet. J., 19:108–111, 1971.
Gill, D.A.: Multiple diverticula of the duodenum in sheep. Vet. Rec., 9:638, 1929.
Hancock, J.L.: Muscular hypertrophy of the ileum in the horse. Vet. Rec., 83:304, 1968.
Hodgson, J.: Animal models in the study of diverticular disease. Clin. Gastroenterol., 4:201–219, 1975.
Rooney, J.R., and Jeffcott, L.B.: Muscular hypertrophy of the ileum in a horse. Vet. Rec., 83:217–219, 1968.

Winter Dysentery of Cattle

Winter dysentery of cattle is a comparatively mild and transient enteritis, which has at times been considered to be caused by *Vibrio jejuni*. Although a virus was suspected, this has not been confirmed. Known viruses of cattle, infectious bovine rhinotracheitis, bovine viral diarrhea, parvoviruses, and enteroviruses do not appear to be involved. It is highly contagious in stabled herds in northern lands. The outstanding lesion is an acute mucous ileitis and jejunitis, which in exceptionally severe cases becomes hemorrhagic.

Kahrs, R.F., Scott, F.W., and Hillman, R.B.: Epidemiologic observations on bovine winter dysentery. Bovine Pract., 8:36–39, 1973.

MacPherson, L.W.: Bovine virus enteritis (winter dysentery). Can. J. Comp. Pathol., 21:184–192, 1957.

Scott, F.W., Kahrs, R.F., Campbell, S.G., and Hillman, R.B.: Etiologic studies of bovine winter dysentery. Bovine Pract., 8:40–43, 1973.

Staphylococcal Enteritis in Chinchillas

A severe enteritis in these animals has followed long-term feeding of a mixture containing antibiotics. The normal gram-negative bacterial flora of the intestine were found to have disappeared and to have been replaced by hemolytic *Staphylococcus aureus* in huge numbers. The animals returned to normal when the feeding was changed to more ordinary ingredients. This experience is comparable to staphylococcal infections elsewhere accompanying the indiscriminate use of antibiotics.

Wood, J.S., Bennett, I.L., and Yardley, J.H.: Staphylococcal enterocolitis in chinchillas. Bull. Johns Hopkins Hosp., 98:454–463, 1956.

Eosinophilic Enteritis of Dogs

A chronic enteritis or gastroenteritis is recognized in dogs by the occurrence of repeated episodes of diarrhea associated with eosinophilia. The lesions in the intestine consist of chronic inflammatory reaction in which eosinophil leukocytes are conspicuous. The cause is unknown, but it is suspected, as in similar gastric lesions, that the inflammatory response is mediated by immunologic factors, which result from repeated infection by helminth larvae in a hypersensitive individual.

Easley, J.R.: Gastroenteritis and associated eosinophilia in a dog. J. Am. Vet. Med. Assoc., 161:1030–1032, 1972.

Legendre, A.M., and Krehbiel, J.D.: Eosinophilic enteritis in a Chesapeake Bay retriever. J. Am. Vet. Med. Assoc., 163:258, 1973.

Edema Disease of Swine

First reported by Shanks in Ireland in 1938, this disease has been encountered with some frequency in most of the swine-producing countries of the world. It attacks previously thrifty animals without warning, produces incoordination and paralyses of the limbs, pain and coma and is commonly, but not invariably, fatal within a number of hours or a day or two. It is not highly contagious, but herd morbidity may approach 35%. Mortality may reach 100%.

The edema is typically but not invariably found in the wall of the stomach, where it may involve the cardiac region or the greater curvature, or the whole organ. The thickness of the gastric wall may be increased just perceptibly or it may reach 3 cm. The coiled portion of the colon, with its mesentery, is another common location of the edema, but these regions are by no means the only sites which may be involved. The body cavities usually contain small or large amounts of fluid; other parts of the intestinal tract sometimes are involved. The face and eyelids are edematous in a high proportion of cases, as can be observed during life. Less frequently, the tarsal and carpal regions and the ventral belly wall contain an excess of fluid. The parenchymatous organs of the abdomen usually appear normal, as do the brain and, usually, the lungs. Subepicardial hemorrhages sometimes occur, but inflammatory changes are typically absent from all organs. Although not noted by other investigations, Kurtz and associates (1969) have described lesions in the brain and arterioles which help to explain the clinical and pathologic features of edema disease. They noted a necrotizing arteritis in most all organs and tissues of the body. They also described focal symmetrical encephalomalacia, presumably secondary to arteritis, involving the thalamus, basal ganglia, and nuclei of the brain stem. These findings are the first pathologic observations which correlate with the clinical signs of the disease.

Luke and Gordon (1950) found evidence of hypoproteinemia in cases studied by them, but, in general, metabolic and physiologic studies have not been made. A number of transmission experiments indicate that the intravenous injection of supernatant fluids or bacteria-free filtrates from the edematous gastrointestinal structures or their contents will reproduce the disease. This fact, plus the erratic and unpredictable occurrence of individual cases, has led to the prevalent belief that the disease is an endogenous toxemia similar to the "enterotoxemia" of sheep, possibly with hypersensitivity to the toxic substance. The findings of several investigators that beta hemolytic strains of *Escherichia coli* can be regularly isolated from pigs with edema disease, and more recently, the reproduction of the disease by oral administration of these strains of *E. coli* (Smith and Halls, 1968), provides very strong evidence incriminating *E. coli* as the cause.

Gastrointestinal edema in other species has occasionally been seen. Severe edema of the ileum has been encountered in the horse, without adequate explanation. Priouzeau (1954) has reported a chronic edematous gastritis affecting cattle which was recurrent and eventually continuous, with death from diarrhea and cachexia.

The action of some unrecognized locally destructive poison probably cannot be entirely excluded in such cases.

Dorn, K., et al.: Studies on pigs. V. Chemical studies on pigs with edema disease. Arch. Exp. Vet. Med., 16:1187–1203, 1962.
Gitter, M., and Lloyd, M.K.: Haemolytic *Bact. coli* in the bowel edema syndrome. II. Transmission and protection experiments. Brit. Vet. J., 113:212–218, 1957.
Jones, J.E.T., and Smith, H.W.: Histological studies on weaned pigs suffering diarrhea and oedema disease produced by oral inoculation of *Escherichia coli*. J. Pathol., 97:168–172, 1969.
Kernkamp, H.C.H., et al.: Epizootiology of edema disease in swine. J. Am. Vet. Med. Assoc., 146:353–357, 1965.
Kurtz, H.J., et al.: Pathologic changes in edema disease of swine. Am. J. Vet. Res., 30:791–806, 1969.
Luke, D., and Gordon, W.A.M.: Oedema of the bowel in pigs. Nature, (Lond.), 165:286, 1950.
Mushin, R., and Basset, C.R.: Haemolytic *Escherichia coli* and other bacteria in oedema disease of swine. Aust. Vet. J., 40:315–320, 1964.
Nielsen, N.O., Moon, H.W., and Roe, W.E.: Enteric colibacillosis in swine. J. Am. Vet. Med. Assoc., 153:1590–1606, 1968.

Philip, J.R., and Shone, D.K.: Some observations on oedema disease and a possibly related condition in pigs in Southern Rhodesia. J. S. Afr. Vet. Med. Assoc., 31:427–434, 1960.
Priouzeau, M.: Gastrite oedémateuse des bovidés. Res. Med. Vet., 130:377–380, 1954.
Smith, H.W., and Halls, S.: The production of oedema disease and diarrhea in weaned pigs by the oral administration of *E. coli*. Factors that influence the course of the experimental disease. J. Med. Microbiol., 1:45–59, 1968.
Thomlinson, J.R., and Buxton, A.: Anaphylaxis in pigs and its relationship to the pathogenesis of oedema disease and gastroenteritis associated with *Escherichia coli*. Immunology, 6:126–139, 1963.
Underdahl, N.R., Stair, E.L., and Young, G.A.: Transmission and characterization of edema disease of swine. J. Am. Vet. Med. Assoc., 142:27–30, 1963.

Malabsorption Syndrome

Failure of absorption of nutrients from the intestinal tract results in clinical manifestations, collectively called malabsorption syndrome. The clinical signs most evident in man and animals are: persistent gastrointestinal upset (vomiting, diarrhea), change in eating habits, loss of weight, and steatorrhea (in some cases). Diagnostic laboratory procedures are outlined in Table 23–2. The causal types of malabsorption currently recognized in animals and man include the following.

1. **Pancreatic insufficiency,** due to chronic pancreatitis or malignant neoplasia, results in a lack of pancreatic enzymes in the small intestine. Since these (trypsin, especially) are involved in the emulsification of fats, the appearance of undigested fats in the feces (steatorrhea) is a conspicuous clinical sign. In dogs, chronic pancreatic disease is often accompanied by destruction of pancreatic islets, resulting in an associated diabetes mellitus.

2. Disease involving the **mucosal epithelium** of the small intestine may result in defects in transport of glucose, amino acids, or lipids across the epithelial cells. Among the identified entities of this nature is *nontropical sprue* of adult human patients who are sensitized to gluten. The lesions in the small intestine are flattened

Table 23–2. Laboratory Screening Tests in Canine Malabsorption Syndrome*

Types of Lesions	Fat Assimilation	Fecal Trypsin	Xylose Absorption Test	Glucose Tolerance Test	Starch Tolerance Test	Lactose Tolerance Test
Pancreatic insufficiency	Severely reduced	Very low	Normal	Abnormal	Abnormal	
Mucosal defect, small intestine	Reduced	Very low or high activity	Reduced	Abnormal	Abnormal	
Lactose or milk intolerance	Normal	Normal	Normal	Normal	Normal	Abnormal
Pancreatic insufficiency and mucosal disease, small intestine	Severely reduced	Very low	Reduced	Abnormal	Abnormal	
Liver disease	Reduced	Normal				

* Adapted after Hill (1972)

villi (villous atrophy), elongated crypts, and increased cell turnover (mitoses are increased). These lesions are accompanied by increased lability of lysosomal membranes and loss of acid hydrolases. The disease in infants is called "coeliac sprue." Removal of gluten from the diet is curative.

Tropical sprue is caused by folic acid deficiency, which leads to macrocytic anemia as well. Dietary supplementation with folic acid is usually curative.

Transmissible gastroenteritis of swine is caused by a virus that attacks mucosal epithelial cells below the apex of the villi and results in villous atrophy and malabsorption. Other viral, bacterial, or toxic enteritides not clearly identified may have a similar effect on intestinal absorption.

Protein-losing enteropathy of unknown cause, associated with dilatation of lymphatics in villi (lymphangiectasia), has also been associated with intestinal malabsorption.

3. **A combination of pancreatic insufficiency and mucosal malabsorption** may be encountered in animals, especially dogs.

4. **Intolerance to lactose** contained in milk may appear in man or animals due to genetic or acquired deficiency of the enzyme lactase. Removal of lactose from the diet usually relieves the signs of this type of malabsorption.

5. **Gastric malfunction,** due to neoplasia or chronic gastritis, may also lead to intestinal malabsorption.

6. **Liver malfunction,** particularly bile stasis, has also been associated with intestinal malabsorption. Icterus and other evidence of liver dysfunction are present in these cases.

Lesions. Lesions associated with malabsorption syndrome include chronic pancreatitis, and biliary stasis. Lesions found in the small intestine include villous atrophy; the villi are shortened due to loss of epithelium and broadened due to infiltration of leukocytes into the lamina propria. Accelerated proliferation of the epithelial cells in the crypts results in hyperplasia of the epithelium nearest the muscularis mucosa. Increased rate of cell turnover is evidenced by the increased numbers of mitoses in the crypt epithelium.

An essential structure involved in the absorption of materials from the intestinal lumen is the brush-border of the mucosal cells of the small intestinal epithelium. This is recognized at the ultrastructural level as made up of myriad microvilli on the lumenal surface. The microvilli project into the lumen about 2 μ in parallel arrays and are covered by a membrane. The interior of each microvillus contains fine parallel contractile fibrils, probably actin, which extend down into the cell to intertwine and form the terminal web. Contraction of these filaments serves to shorten the microvilli. At the apex of the microvilli on the surface of the brush-border membrane is a structure called the glycocalyx. This is probably a product of the epithelial cells and is rich in neutral and amino sugars. The brush-border contains many hydrolytic enzymes (disaccharidases, peptidases, and phosphatases) as well as nonenzymatic proteins such as the intrinsic-factor-vitamin B_{12} complex and the soluble calcium-binding protein that is dependent upon vitamin D.

Study of ultrastructural aspects of the brush-border of mucosal cells of animals with malabsorption syndrome appears, at this writing, yet to be done.

Other intestinal lesions which have been associated with malabsorption syndrome in the dog include purulent, eosinophilic, and histiocytic enteritis; lymphosarcoma involving the intestine; and intestinal lymphangiectasia. Lesions in the liver have been described as including fatty change, cirrhosis, proliferation of bile ducts, and intrahepatic cholestasis.

An intriguing malabsorptive effect has been demonstrated in marmosets (*Saguinus oedipus oedipus*) fed a diet high in cholesterol and coconut oil but otherwise adequate. The result was a jejunal lipodystrophy (accumulation of fat particles in epithelial cells) steatorrhea, and osteomalacia (Dreizen, et al., 1971).

Alpers, D.H., and Seetharam, B.: Pathophysiology of diseases involving intestinal brush-border proteins. N. Engl. J. Med., 296:1047–1050, 1977.

Campbell, R.S.F., Brobst, D., and Bisgard, G.: Intestinal lymphangiectasia in a dog. J. Am. Vet. Med. Assoc., 153:1050–1054, 1968.

Dreizen, S., Levy, B.M., and Bernick, S.: Diet-induced jejunal lipodystrophy in the cotton-top marmoset (*Saguinus oedipus*). Proc. Soc. Exp. Biol. Med., 138:7–11, 1971.

Finco, D.R., et al.: Chronic enteric disease and hypoproteinemia in 9 dogs. J. Am. Vet. Med. Assoc., 163:262–271, 1973.

Haeltermann, E.O.: On the pathogenesis of transmissible gastroenteritis of swine. J. Am. Vet. Med. Assoc., 160:534–540, 1972.

Hill, F.W.G., Osborne, A.D., and Kidder, D.E.: Pancreatic degenerative atrophy in dogs. J. Comp. Pathol., 81:321–330, 1971.

Hill, F.W.G., Malabsorption syndrome in the dog: a study of 38 cases. J. Small Anim. Prac., 13:575–594, 1972.

Kaneko, J.J., Moulton, J.E., Brodey, R., and Perryman, V.D.: Malabsorption syndrome resembling nontropical sprue in dogs. J. Am. Vet. Med. Assoc., 146:463–473, 1965.

Maronpot, R.R., and Whitehair, C.K.: Experimental sprue-like intestinal lesions in pigs. Can. J. Comp. Med., 31:309–316, 1967.

Mouwen, J.M.V.M., and Schotman, A.J.H.: Steatorrhoea in piglets. Vet. Rec., 87:172–173, 1970.

Olson, N.C., and Zimmer, J.F.: Protein-losing enteropathy secondary to intestinal lymphangiectasia in a dog. J. Am. Vet. Med. Assoc., 173:271–274, 1978.

Robinson, J.W.L.: Intestinal malabsorption in the experimental animal. Gut, 13:938–945, 1972.

Seibold, H.R., Clewe, T.H., and Wolf, R.H.: Enteropathy resembling sprue in nonhuman primates. Lab. Anim. Sci., 33:353–362, 1972.

Strober, W., Wochner, R.D., Carbone, P.P., and Waldmann, T.A.: Intestinal lymphangiectasia: a protein-losing enteropathy with hypogammaglobulinemia, lymphocytopenia, and impaired homograft rejection. J. Clin. Invest., 46:1643–1656, 1967.

Vernon, D.G.: Idiopathic sprue in a dog. J. Am. Vet. Med. Assoc., 140:1062–1067, 1962.

Windhorst, D.B., Lund, J.E., Decker, J., and Swatez, I.: Intestinal malabsorption in the Gray Collie syndrome. Fed. Proc., 26:260, 1967.

Intestinal Obstruction

The small intestine not infrequently suffers complete obstruction by foreign bodies, such as rubber balls, rubber nipples, nuts, or peach stones in the dog, or piliconcretions (hairballs) in calves. **Strangulated hernias** (umbilical or scrotal, usually) cause complete obstruction in any species, being most frequent in horses and pigs. The long and tenuous intestine of the horse is subject to obstruction because of accidents resultant from its tortuosity and the length of the mesentery which suspends it. These are **torsion,** or twisting upon itself, or **volvulus,** in which a loop of

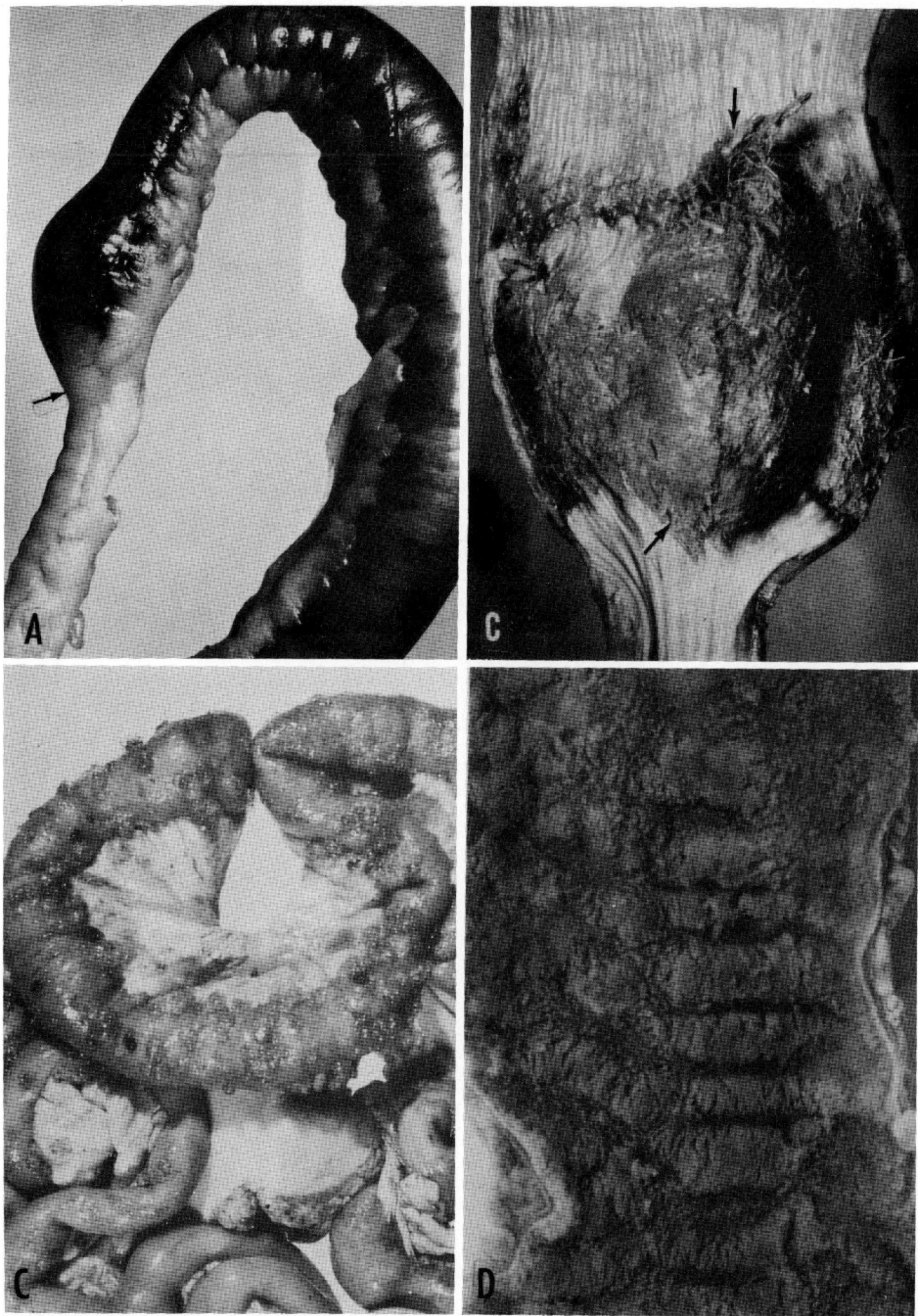

Fig. 23–15. *A,* Obstruction of the small intestine of a dog. A large peach stone was lodged just above the arrow. *B,* Obstruction of the esophagus (choke) in a horse which died on the third day from severe toxic hepatitis and toxic tubular nephritis. The site of the large obstructing mass of ingesta is indicated by arrows. *C,* Intestinal emphysema, small intestine of swine. Note bubbles of air under serosa. *D,* Necrotizing enteritis of swine. Dark, thick, tenacious exudate consisting largely of fibrin and necrotic cells on intestinal mucosa. (Courtesy of College of Veterinary Medicine, Iowa State University.)

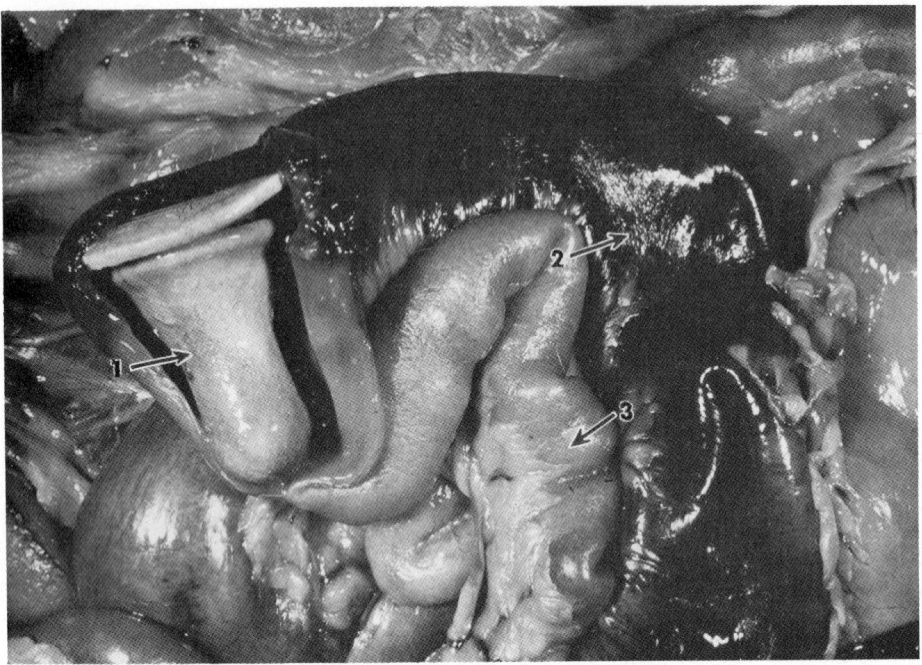

Fig. 23–16. Obstruction of the duodenum of an eight-month-old male Doberman Pinscher puppy. The foreign body was a rubber nipple (*1*) from a nursing bottle. Note hemorrhagic wall of duodenum (*2*) proximal to the obstruction, and normal-appearing intestine distal to it (*3*). (Courtesy of Angell Memorial Animal Hospital.)

intestine passes through a tear in the mesentery or similar abnormality.

Intussusceptions occur in any species. In this accident, excessive peristaltic movement forces a segment of the bowel inside the segment just below it, as the smaller tube of a telescope slides into the slightly larger tube just ahead of it. In the intestine, there is actually no difference in the diameters of the outer and inner tubes. As a consequence of this fact, and of the attached mesentery, the outermost of the three layers which make up the intussusception is greatly stretched, the innermost greatly compressed. Interference with the flow of blood being greater in the thin-walled veins than it is in the less compressible arteries, venous stasis and edema promptly develop and lead, in a matter of hours, to adhesive inflammation, which binds the layers together, or to necrosis and gangrene. The absence of these several features serves to differentiate from true pathological intussusceptions, brought about by excessive peristalsis in diarrheic and similar conditions, others which occur rather frequently near the moment of death, even in slaughtered animals. Because of the pressure, an intussusception is usually completely obstructive to passage of the intestinal contents. **Neoplasms,** chiefly carcinomas, in the intestinal wall tend to assume an annular (ring-shaped) form and more slowly, but scarcely less surely, stop the movement of the ingesta.

While the effects of a gradually developing obstruction may be mitigated by hypertrophy of the local muscularis (see terminal ileitis, above), complete blocking of the intestinal canal has definite and constant results. The lumen of the bowel for a considerable distance above the obstruction becomes greatly distended with fluid which is chiefly that of inflammatory

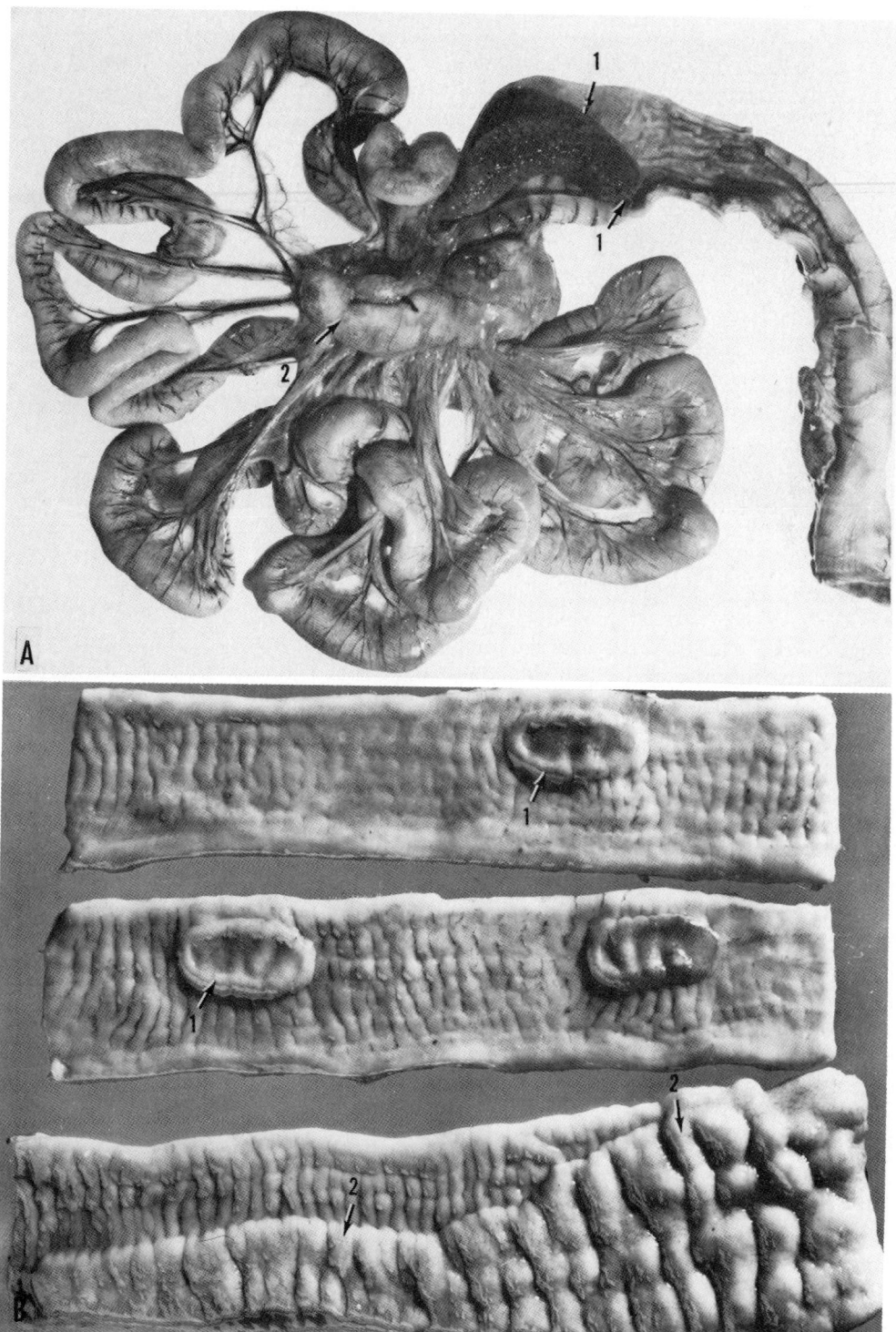

Fig. 23–17. *A*, Intussusception of the ileum (*1*) into the colon of a dog with "salmon disease." Note also hyperplastic lymph node (*2*). *B*, Hyperplasia of Peyer's patches (*1*) and lymphoid tissue in terminal ileum (*2*) in a dog with rickettsiosis of "salmon disease." (Courtesy of Dr. Wm. J. Hadlow.)

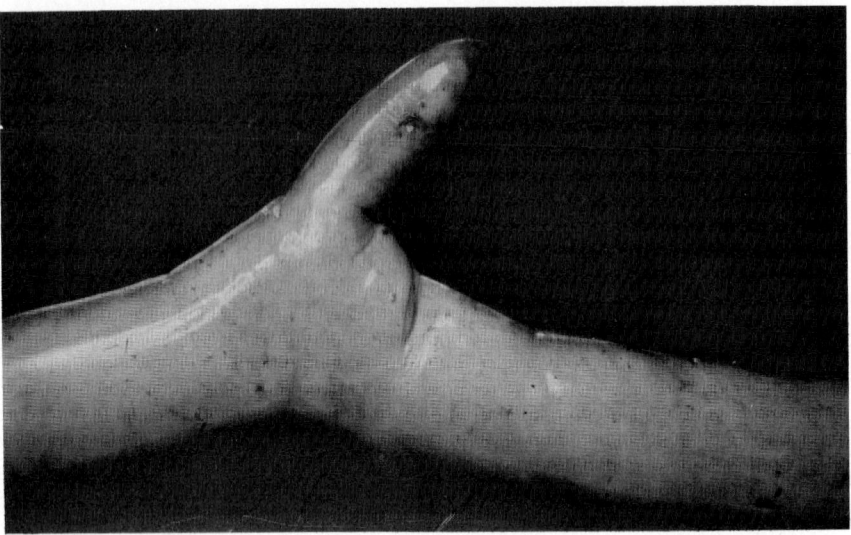

Fig. 23–18.   Meckel's diverticulum in the ileum of a pony.

edema (serous exudate), the accumulated ingesta constituting a minor portion. The wall is not only edematous but red with hyperemia and infiltrated with leukocytes. These changes are most marked just above (anterior to) the obstruction and gradually fade out with increasing distance from it. Below the obstruction, the bowel is empty and normal. While pathogenic and saprophytic bacteria would bring havoc to the involved section of the bowel and eventually spread to the peritoneum, usually with gangrene (and this sometimes occurs), the regular outcome of complete obstruction of the bowel is death after some hours or, in some species, a day or two unless it is surgically relieved. This is earlier than such changes would ordinarily be fatal and, on the basis of the course and symptoms, death is attributed to endotoxic shock. If the obstruction involves the upper small intestine, vomiting is the principal sign, and loss of electrolytes constitutes the greatest danger.

Meckel's diverticulum is rarely encountered as a small tube branching from the ileum and terminating after several centimeters (in the horse) in a rounded closed end. It is a congenital anomaly representing persistence of the omphalo-enteric duct of the embryo and has, in a rudimentary way, the histologic structure of the intestine. Stasis of ingesta occurs in it only exceptionally. This anomaly sometimes forms a nidus for intussusception, and tumors may also originate there.

Grant, B.D., and Tennant, B.: Volvulus associated with Meckel's diverticulum in the horse. J. Am. Vet. Med. Assoc., 162:550–551, 1973.

Moon, V., and Morgan, D.R.: Shock: the mechanism of death following intestinal obstruction. Arch. Surg., 32:776–788, 1936.

Pearson, H.: Intussusception in cattle. Vet. Rec., 89:426–437, 1971.

Pollock, W.B., and Hagan, T.R.: Two cases of torsion of the cecum and ileum in rats. Lab. Anim. Sci., 22:549–551, 1972.

Rooney, J.R.: Volvulus, strangulation, and intussusception in the horse. Cornell Vet., 55:644–653, 1965.

Schoenbaum, M., Klopfer, U., and Egyed, M.N.: Spontaneous intussusception of the small intestine in guinea pigs. Lab. Anim., 6:327–330, 1972.

Wilson, G.P., and Burt, J.K.: Intussusception in the dog and cat: a review of 45 cases. J. Am. Vet. Med. Assoc., 164:515–519, 1974.

Wolfe, D.A.: Recurrent intestinal intussusception in the dog. J. Am. Vet. Med. Assoc., 171:553–556, 1977.

Intestinal Emphysema

Intestinal emphysema is occasionally seen in healthy swine at slaughter. Numerous small air-filled vesicles from 1 mm to 2 cm in diameter are found in the serosa, submucosa, and mucosa of the small intestine and in the mesentery and mesenteric lymph nodes. Microscopically, the gas bubbles occupy lymphatics. The cause is not known. Occasionally, intestinal emphysema is seen in sheep with enterotoxemia.

Biester, H.E., Evaleth, D.F., and Yamashiro, Y.: Intestinal emphysema in swine. J. Am. Vet. Med. Assoc., 88:714–731, 1936.

Sofrenovic, D., Matic, G., and Zigic, B.: Intestinal emphysema of pigs, in the past and at present. Veterinarski Glasnik, 29:119–124, 1975.

Neoplasms of the Small Intestine

The World Health Organization's International Histologic Classification of Tumors of Domestic Animals (Head, 1976) provides a framework for classifying neoplasms of the small intestine on a worldwide basis. For the most part, neoplasms of nonhuman primates, man, and laboratory animals may also be accommodated by this classification. A brief description of these histologic types follows.

Adenoma, a benign tumor of epithelial cells, is made up of cells that closely resemble those of normal intestinal mucosa, but is more cellular, has generally hyperchromic nuclei, and is demarcated from the adjacent normal mucosa. Adenomas usually project toward the lumen and may be polypoid. They are not readily distinguished from inflammatory polyps, but the increased amount of inflammatory tissue or the presence of foreign bodies or nematodes may be helpful. The "adenomatosis" of the ileum of swine with regional ileitis may be distinguished by its diffuse distribution. In all cases, this tumor does not invade the submucosa, muscularis mucosa, muscularis, or lymphatics.

Descriptive terms may be used to indicate predominant patterns of growth, such as: papillary (villous), tubular (adenomatous) and papillotubular (tubulovillous)— a combination of the first two.

Adenocarcinoma is a malignant tumor arising from the epithelial cells of the intestinal mucosa. Although some part of the tumor may project into the lumen, its predominant feature is its growth from the mucosa through the muscularis mucosa into the submucosa and muscularis to the serosa. Invasion of lymphatics is common, and metastases to regional (mesenteric) lymph nodes and to distant organs (lung, liver, etc.) are to be expected. Adenocarcinomas have a tendency to grow in an annular form around the wall of the intestine. This trait as well as the fibrous component of the tumor usually result in obstruction of the intestinal lumen.

Several morphologic types may be distinguished, sometimes more than one in a single neoplasm, and may be useful in characterizing a specific tumor. **Papillary adenocarcinoma** has finger-shaped fronds of epithelial-covered stroma resembling villi, but more elongated, undifferentiated, and cellular. **Tubular adenocarcinoma** is descriptive of a tumor consisting of branching tubules lined by flattened, cuboidal, or columnar epithelial cells and supported by a fibrous stroma. **Mucinous adenocarcinoma** distinguishes one in which large amounts of mucin are produced by the tumor cells, causing the formation of grossly visible cysts filled with mucin. **Signet ring** cell carcinoma is made up largely of individualized tumor cells with a globule of mucin in their cytoplasm, with the acentrically placed nucleus giving the cell its characteristic appearance of a signet ring.

Adenocarcinoma of the small intestine is an infrequent tumor in most animal species, but nevertheless has been reported as a spontaneous occurrence in many species. A singular exception appears to be its more frequent occurrence in aged sheep in New Zealand, first reported by Dodd (1960) and subsequently documented further by Simpson (1972), Simpson and Jolly (1974), and Webster (1966). This increased frequency in sheep appears to be associated with forage which may be carcinogenic, but experimental reproduction of the disease has not yet been reported. After sheep, the frequency of reported cases appears to follow in turn: cats, cattle, mice, dogs, hamsters, rats, and other species.

Undifferentiated carcinoma (carcinoma simplex, medullary carcinoma, or solid carcinoma) is made up of epithelial cells which do not form any glandular or papillary structure. This is an even more uncommon type of carcinoma, but may be encountered in domestic, laboratory, or wild animals.

Carcinoid tumors of argentaffin or nonargentaffin types as described in the stomach have been reported in the small intestine of the dog, cat, ox, and elephant. Solid nests of epithelial cells with finely stippled cytoplasm present a characteristic histologic appearance.

Leiomyoma and **leiomyosarcoma,** the benign and malignant varieties respectively of tumors of smooth muscle, may originate from the muscularis or (rarely) the muscularis mucosa of the small intestine. The tumor cells resemble smooth muscle cells which are elongated, usually in parallel or interlacing bundles. Their nuclei are elongated with blunt, rounded ends. The malignant variety is distinguished by its lack of cell differentiation, less circumscribed and more irregular borders, more aggressive invasion of neighboring structures, and metastasis. Either tumor may cause intestinal obstruction or serve as the nidus for intussusception.

Cavernous hemangioma, a benign lesion made up of blood vascular spaces, has been recorded in the small intestine of most domestic species. The malignant variety, hemangioendothelioma does not appear to have been reported as primary from the small intestine of domesticated or other species.

Lipomas are benign, circumscribed masses made up of mature adipose tissue. They may occur in the wall of the intestinal tract or in the mesentery. In some species, especially the horse, these tumors are pedunculated and may rarely become twisted around the intestine to produce obstruction. Twisting of the pedicle more often leads to necrosis of the adipose tissue. The lipoma should be distinguished from lipomatosis or fibrolipomatosis, which is the deposition of normal fat in thick layers in the mesentery, omentum, and retroperitoneum. This may result in as much as 10 cm of fat in the wall of the ileum and colon, between the muscularis and serosa. Fat necrosis and fibrosis may occur, but the effect on the animals appears minimal. Jersey and Guernsey breeds of cattle seem to be most prone to this condition.

Liposarcoma is the malignant tumor made up of undifferentiated fat cells. It has been reported on rare occasions in the wall of the small intestine of dogs.

Lymphosarcomas are not infrequent in the wall of the small intestine and presumably arise from lymphoid structures (Peyer's patches), but eventually involve the entire wall. The cat is especially prone to this tumor, which may be the presenting lesion in about 20% of feline lymphosarcomas. Single tumors may cause intestinal obstruction or intussusception.

Mast cell tumors may be primary in the small intestine of dog or cat, presumably arising from the mast cells found normally in the subserosa and submucosa of the intestine.

Secondary tumors may involve the small intestine by direct extension from adjacent organs (pancreas), by implantation on the serosa as a consequence of seeding of the peritoneal cavity (for example, hemangioendothelioma from a ruptured splenic neoplasm), or by metastasis via the general circulation (usually in disseminated carcinomatosis or lymphosarcoma). Mesotheliomas of the peritoneum may also extend, rarely, into the wall of the small intestine.

An **osteosarcoma** has been reported (Eckerlin, et al., 1976) in the jejunum of a dog. This tumor, believed to be primary in the jejunum, occurred in a 10-year-old castrated male mongrel.

A single case, designated as a **neoplasm of globule leukocytes,** has been reported in a 12-year-old, castrated, short-haired male cat (Finn and Schwartz, 1972). This tumor was presumed to arise from "globule leukocytes," cells with large non-metachromatic globulin-containing cytoplasmic granules of unknown origin and function, found normally in the wall of the intestine of several species (Takeuchi, et al., 1969).

Coop, K.L., Sharp, J.G., Osborne, J.W., and Zimmerman, G.R.: An animal model for the study of small bowel tumors. Cancer Res., 34:1487–1494, 1974.

Dodd, D.C.: Adenocarcinoma of the small intestine of sheep. N. Z. Vet. J., 8:109–112, 1960.

Eckerlin, R.H., Garman, R.H., and Fowler, E.H.: Chondroblastic osteosarcoma in the jejunum of a dog. J. Am. Vet. Med. Assoc., 168:691–693, 1976.

Finn, J.P., and Schwartz, L.W.: A neoplasm of globule leukocytes in the intestine of a cat. J. Comp. Pathol., 82:323–328, 1972.

Giles, R.C., Jr., Hildebrandt, P.K., and Montgomery, C.A., Jr.: Carcinoid tumor in the small intestine of a dog. Vet. Pathol., 11:340–349, 1974.

Lingeman, C.H., and Garner, F.M.: Comparative study of intestinal adenocarcinomas of animals and man. J. Natl. Cancer Inst., 48:325–346, 1972.

Howard, D.R., Schirmer, R.G., Mostosky, U.V., and Michel, R.L.: Adenocarcinoma in the ileum of a young dog. J. Am. Vet. Med. Assoc., 162:956–958, 1973.

Head, K.W.: International histological classification of tumours of domestic animals. XII. Tumours of the lower alimentary tract. Bull. WHO, 53:137–304, 1976.

Kolaja, G.J., and Fairchild, D.G.: Leiomyosarcoma of the duodenum in a dog. J. Am. Vet. Med. Assoc., 163:275–276, 1973.

McDonald, J.W., and Leaver, D.O.: Adenocarcinoma of the small intestine of Merino sheep. Aust. Vet. J., 41:269–271, 1965.

Palumbo, N.E., and Perri, S.F.: Adenocarcinoma of the ileum in a cat. J. Am. Vet. Med. Assoc., 164:607–608, 1974.

Patnaik, A.K., Liu, S.K., and Johnson, G.F.: Feline intestinal adenocarcinoma. A clinicopathologic study of 22 cases. Vet. Pathol., 13:1–10, 1976.

Patnaik, A.K., Hurvitz, A.I., and Johnson, G.F.: Canine gastrointestinal neoplasms. Vet. Pathol., 14:547–555, 1977.

Simpson, B.H.: The geographic distribution of carcinomas of the small intestine in New Zealand sheep. N. Z. Vet. J., 20:24–28, 1972.

Simpson, B.H.: An epidemiological study of carcinoma of the small intestine in New Zealand sheep. N. Z. Vet. J., 20:91–97, 1972.

Simpson, B.H., and Jolly, R.D.: Carcinoma of the small intestine in sheep. J. Pathol., 112:83–92, 1974.

Takeuchi, A., Jervis, H.R., and Sprinz, H.: The globule leukocyte in the intestinal mucosa of the cat: A histochemical and electron microscopic study. Anat. Rec., 164:79–99, 1969.

Tontis, A., and Luginbühl, H.: Jejunumkarzinom bei zwei kühen. Schweiz. Arch. Tierheilkd., 118:543–545, 1976.

Tontis, A., and Luginbühl, H.: Gallertkarzinom im jejunum bei einer kuh: Operation, patholizische befunde und verlauf. Schweiz. Arch. Tierheilkd., 118:539–541, 1976.

Webster, W.M.: Neoplasia in food animals with special reference to the high incidence in sheep. N.Z. Vet. J., 14;203–214, 1966.

Werle, E., Haendle, H., and Schmal, A.: Ein fall von carcinoid bei einem elefonten. Pathol. Vet., 5:81–83, 1968.

THE CECUM

Impaction of Cecum

Impactions cause fatal obstruction in the horse. Cecal impaction is the most frequent and results when older animals are forced to subsist on coarse, dry roughage such as wheat straw. The cecum becomes progressively more atonic as it is filled with increasing amounts of undigested stalks and stems, until it is distended to unbelievable dimensions with little chance of recovery. Impaction of segments of the small colon results from one or more unusually large boluses of undigested roughage, frequently coarse alfalfa hay. The irritated intestine contracts spasmodically around the lodged bolus, tightening the obstruction.

Tympanites of the cecum is the usual form of alimentary bloating in the horse and is scarcely less formidable than its counterpart in the bovine rumen. Spasmodic or other disorders interfering with peristaltic movement through the colon and rectum appear to be causative without much relation to the kind of feed.

Dilatation of Cecum

Dilatation of cecum is a relatively uncommon abdominal disease in cattle believed to follow atony of the cecum, usually as a consequence of a change to a more concentrated diet. One study (Svendsen and Kristensen, 1970) indicates that change from a ration of hay to one containing ½ kg hay and 7½ kg rolled barley resulted in an increase in concentration of volatile fatty acids and decrease in pH in the cecum. These events led to an increase in the concentration of undissociated ions and a concomitant decrease in frequency of cecal contractions. This study may present a partial explanation of the cecal atony which is believed to precede cecal dilatation.

In germfree rats, the cecum becomes dilated to about five times the cecal volume of rats with conventional bacterial flora. The dry weight of the cecal contents is increased more than twice. The epithelial cells of the cecum of the germfree rat are taller and have larger nuclei and microvilli than similar cells in conventional rats. The crypts of Lieberkühn are more varied in shape than in conventional rats, the lamina propria is almost devoid of plasma cells, but rich in mast cells. The tunica muscularis externa is hypertrophied. The crypts of Lieberkühn contain what appear to be pure cultures of elongated bacilli in large numbers. The cecal lumen, on the other hand, contains large numbers of varied organisms. This finding led to the postulate that the cecum is important in symbiotic relationships, and the crypts of Lieberkühn are the sites of this interaction.

Intussusception of the Cecum

Rarely in the dog and cat, the cecum becomes inverted into the colon, projecting into the latter for a considerable distance and acting as a partial obstruction. Naturally a variable degree of edema, inflammation, and perhaps chronic fibrosis results locally, but the disorder is not necessarily fatal.

Neoplasms of the Cecum

Neoplasms of the cecum are not often reported, but lymphosarcoma is known to occur, and adenocarcinomas have been recorded in the cecum of the rat, mouse, dog, cat (Fig. 23–19), horse, and genet. Leiomyosarcomas have been reported in the cecum of dogs. These tumors correspond in most respects to those arising in the small intestine.

Gustafsson, B.E., and Maunsbach, A.B.: Ultrastructure of the enlarged cecum in germfree rats. Z. Zellforsch. Mikro. Anat., *120*:555–578, 1971.
Kolata, R.J., and Wright, J.H.: Inflammation and inversion of the cecum in a cat. J. Am. Vet. Med. Assoc., *162*:958, 1973.
Lingeman, C.H., and Garner, F.N.: Comparative study of intestinal adenocarcinomas of animals and man. J. Natl. Cancer Inst., *48*:325–346, 1972.
Patnaik, A.K., Liu, S.K., and Johnson, G.F.: Feline intestinal adenocarcinomas. A clinicopathologic study of 22 cases. Vet. Pathol., *13*:1–10, 1976.
Patnaik, A.K., Hurvitz, A.I., and Johnson, G.F.: Canine gastrointestinal neoplasms. Vet. Pathol., *14*:547–555, 1977.
Svendsen, P., and Kristensen, B.: Cecal dilatation in cattle. An experimental study of the etiology. Nord. Vet. Med., *22*:578–583, 1970.

THE COLON

Congenital and Hereditary Anomalies

Congenital and hereditary anomalies are not numerous in the recorded literature. A few should be mentioned. **Megacolon** has been studied in the dog and mice. The lesion is recognized by severe distension of the colon with fecal content, terminating abruptly at the rectum. This lesion appears to be a failure to dilate, the result of absence of myenteric ganglia in the terminal part of the colon distal to the dilated portion. The disease is considered to be inherited in both puppies and young mice. The defect is linked with mutant genes piebald-lethal (Sl) and lethal spotting (ls) in mice.

Situs inversus viscerum, recognized in rats and man as a rare inherited defect, probably polygenic, results in transposition of all abdominal viscera from right to left. No functional defect has been iden-

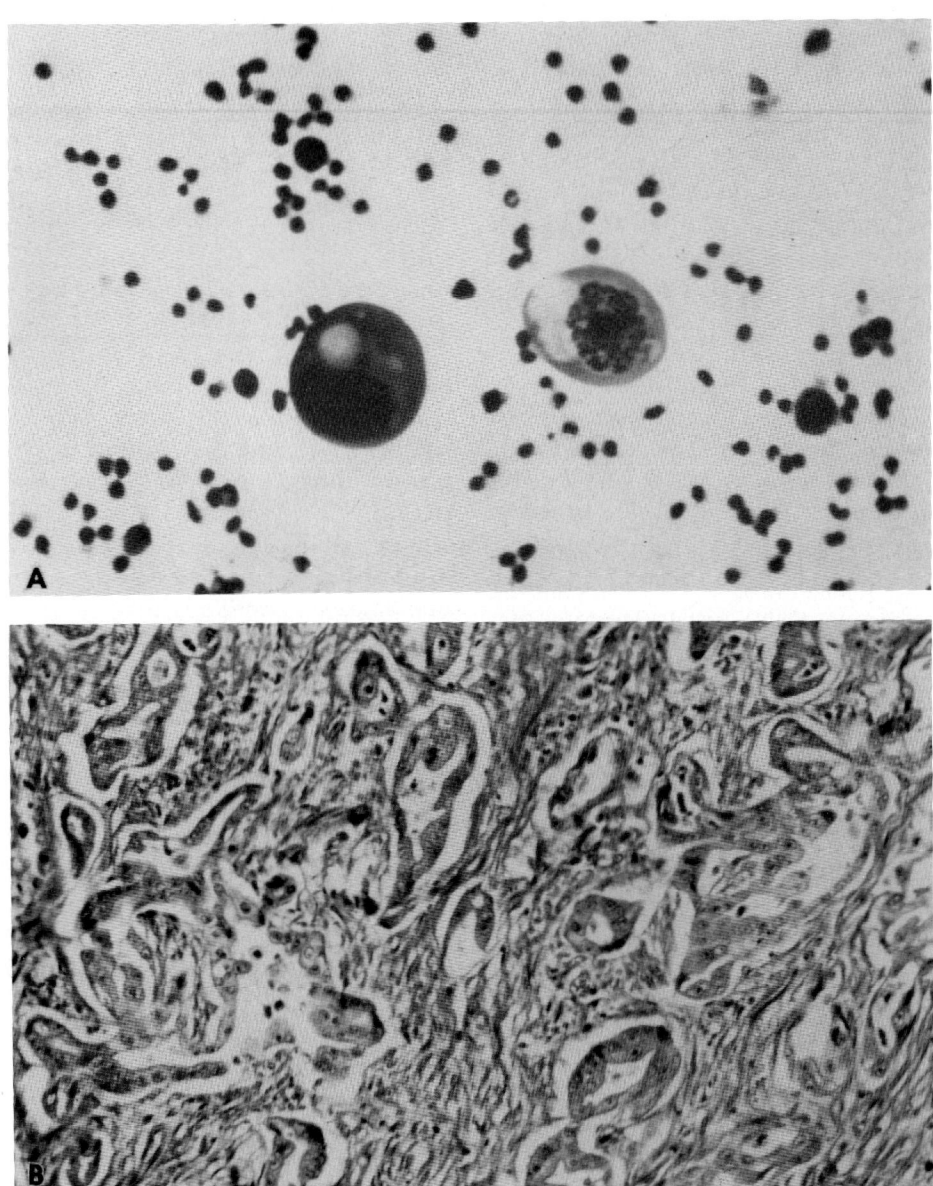

Fig. 23–19. Adenocarcinoma of the cecum of a 14-year-old castrated male cat, with metastases to diaphragm, abdominal wall, liver and spleen. *A,* Smear of ascitic fluid containing large malignant cells, Giemsa's stain (× 400). *B,* Section of metastatic tumor in diaphragm. (H & E, × 250.) (Courtesy of Angell Memorial Animal Hospital.)

tified in association with this transposition.

Duplication of the colon has been described in a dog in association with malformations of the bodies of vertebrae T4 and T5. In this case in a 9-week-old Labrador Retriever, the colon was equally duplicated from the cecum to the rectum, with which the two colons connected. **Atresia coli** is another rarely recorded anomaly. In one reported case in an identical twin Simmental calf, the colon was absent, the intestine terminating in a blind cecum. The other identical twin was normal. The monozygosity of these calves was established by identifying identical blood types, electrophoretic patterns, transferrin, and amylase. From this, it was concluded that the atresia coli was not inherited, since each twin should have the same genome.

Bolande, R.P., and Towler, W.F.: Ultrastructural and histochemical studies of murine megacolon. Am. J. Pathol., 69:139–162, 1972.

Hoffsis, G.F., and Bruner, R.R., Jr.: Atresia coli in a twin calf. J. Am. Vet. Med. Assoc., 171:433–434, 1977.

Jakowski, R.M.: Duplication of colon in a Labrador Retriever with abnormal spinal column. Vet. Pathol., 14:256–260, 1977.

Webster, W.: Aganglionic megacolon in piebald-lethal mice. Arch. Pathol., 97:111–117, 1974.

Histiocytic Ulcerative Colitis of Boxer Dogs

Confined to dogs of the Boxer breed, this disorder, also termed granulomatous colitis, is similar in many respects to Whipple's disease of man. Affected dogs, which are usually less than 2 years of age, pass soft tan feces often mixed with blood, with great frequency (up to 15 times a day). Profuse diarrhea does not occur, and throughout the course the disease is afebrile, and weight is usually maintained. Significant gross lesions are confined to the colon, cecum, and mesenteric lymph nodes. The wall of the colon and cecum is thickened and the mucosa is ulcerated often to the extent that little intact mucosa remains. Microscopically, the surface of the ulcers is composed of fibrin and neutrophils, but the striking feature throughout the colonic mucosa as well as the submucosa is a marked infiltration by large macrophages, which may be accompanied by lymphocytes, plasma cells, and collagen. The macrophages have pink foamy cytoplasm which is PAS positive and stains lightly with fat stains. Ultrastructural studies by Van Kruiningen (1967) have demonstrated the cells to be filled with packets of phagocytized material composed of membranes often arranged in whorls. In one dog, he saw structures suggesting a psittacoid agent. Enlargement of mesenteric lymph nodes results from lymphocytic hyperplasia and aggregates of macrophages similar to those in the colon and cecum. In advanced cases peripheral lymph nodes may also be enlarged and contain similar macrophages. The cause of this disease is not known.

Cockrell, B.Y., and Krehbiel, J.D.: Ultrastructural changes in histiocytic ulcerative colitis in a Boxer. Am. J. Vet. Res., 33:453–459, 1972.

Russell, S.W., Gomez, J.A., and Trowbridge, J.O.: Canine histiocytic ulcerative colitis. The early lesion and its progression to ulceration. Lab. Invest., 25:509–515, 1971.

Van Kruiningen, H.J., et al.: A granulomatous colitis of dogs with histologic resemblance to Whipple's disease. Pathol. Vet., 2:521–544, 1965.

Van Kruiningen, H.J.: Granulomatous colitis of Boxer dogs. Comparative aspects. Gastroenterol., 53:114–122, 1967.

Van Kruiningen, H.J.: Canine colitis comparable to regional enteritis and mucosal colitis of man. Gastroenterol., 62:1128–1142, 1972.

Van Kruiningen, H.J.: The ultrastructure of macrophages in granulomatous colitis of Boxer dogs. Vet. Pathol., 12:446–459, 1975.

Infections

Infections of the colon which have been identified with a causal organism are described in other chapters: for example, balantidiasis and amebiasis in Chapter 13; protothecosis and histoplasmosis in Chapter 12; and yersiniosis and salmonellosis in Chapter 11. Swine dysentery, an acute infection of young pigs, also called hemorrhagic enteritis and vibrionic dysentery, is characterized by bloody diarrhea and failure to grow. *Vibrio coli* was for many years alleged to be the cause, but the presence of *Vibrio coli* in many normal pigs and failure to produce the disease consistently cast doubt on this organism as the etiologic agent. More recent evidence points toward an anaerobic spirochete, *Treponema hyodysenteriae* in concert with one or two anaerobic gram-negative bacteria as being causative. This is discussed further in Chapter 12.

Ulcerative Colitis

Ulcerative colitis of unknown etiology has been described in many species. Although the inflammatory and ulcerative features are common, the lack of common etiology makes it difficult to make rational comparisons. Ulcerative disease has been produced in laboratory animals (guinea pigs and rabbits) by addition of pepsin inhibitors (sodium lignosulfonate or sulfated amylopectin) in drinking water. Carrageenan will also produce ulcerative lesions in the colon of guinea pigs and has been associated with squamous metaplasia of the rectal mucosa of the rat. Ulcerative disease also occurs naturally in apes (gibbons) and has been associated with "emotional stress" and shigellosis. Colitis in the mouse and hamster is not uncommon as a natural disease and may result in rectal prolapse.

Anver, M.R., and Cohen, B.J.: Animal model of human disease: ulcerative colitis induced in guinea pigs with degraded carrageenan. Am. J. Pathol., *84*:431–434, 1976.

Ediger, R.D., Kovatch, R.M., and Rabstein, M.M.: Colitis in mice with a high incidence of rectal prolapse. Lab. Anim. Sci., *24*:488–494, 1974.

Fabian, R.J., Abraham, R., Coulston, F., and Golberg, L.: Carrageenan-induced squamous metaplasia of the rectal mucosa in the rat. Gastroenterol., *65*:265–276, 1973.

Marcus, R., and Watt, J.: Ulcerative disease of the colon in laboratory animals induced by pepsin inhibitors. Gastroenterol., *67*:473–483, 1974.

Mullink, J.W.M.A.: Colitis in the mouse. Z. Versuchstierkd., *15*:217–228, 1973.

Pollock, W.B.: Prolapse of invaginated colon through the anus in Golden hamsters (*Mesocricetus auratus*). Lab. Anim. Sci., *25*:334–336, 1975.

Scott, G.B.D., and Keymer, I.F.: Ulcerative colitis in apes: a comparison with the human disease. J. Pathol., *115*:241–244, 1975.

Scotti, T.: Colitis cystica profunda in Rhesus monkeys. Lab. Anim. Sci., *25*:55–61, 1975.

Stout, L.C.: Ulcerative colitis-like lesions in siamang gibbons. Digest. Dis., *16*:371–372, 1971.

Watt, J., and Marcus, R.: Experimental ulcerative disease of the colon in animals. Gut, *14*:506–510, 1973.

Murine Colonic Hyperplasia

Murine colonic hyperplasia is a naturally occurring, transmissible disease of laboratory mice, caused by *Citrobacter freundii*. The signs most often seen in young mice include ruffled fur, retarded growth, soft feces, occasional rectal prolapse, and death of some affected animals. The lesions consist of striking hyperplasia of distal colonic epithelium 2 to 3 weeks after inoculation with cultures of *C. freundii*. The colonic mucosa becomes several times thickened, with great increase in epithelial cells and mitoses, but decrease in number of goblet cells. In young animals, inflammatory and necrotizing changes in the mucosa appear to contribute to higher mortality. In animals destined to recover, the hyperplasia of mucosal epithelium gradually subsides and goblet cells return dramatically, contributing to the formation of mucus-filled cysts deep in the mucosa.

Barthold, S.W., et al.: Transmissible murine colonic hyperplasia. Vet. Pathol., *15*:223–236, 1978.

Barthold, S.W., et al.: The etiology of transmissible murine colonic hyperplasia. Lab. Anim. Sci., *26*:889–894, 1978.

Brennan, P.C., et al.: *Citrobacter freundii* associated with diarrhea in laboratory mice. Lab. Anim. Care, *15*:266–275, 1965.

Silverman, J., Chovannes, J.M., Rigotty, J., and Ornaf, M.: A natural outbreak of transmissible murine colonic hyperplasia in A/J mice. Lab. Anim. Sci., *29*:209–218, 1979.

Neoplasms of the Colon

Benign and malignant neoplasms may be classified according to the WHO histologic criteria described for the small intestine. Some rather striking differences in frequency of colonic tumors have been described in different species. Adenocar-

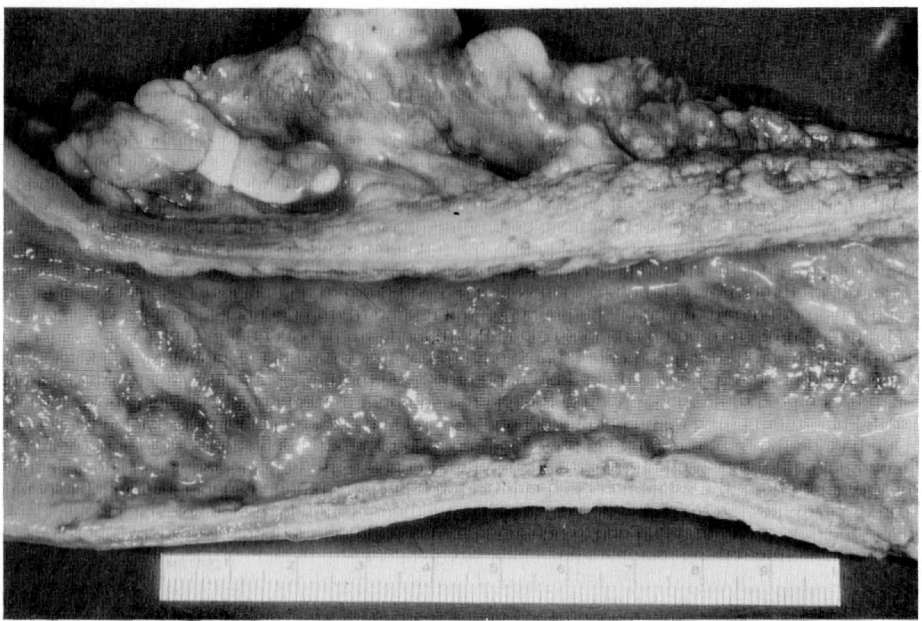

Fig. 23–20. Adenocarcinoma of the colon of a seven-year-old male German Shepherd. Note that the mucosa is eroded and the lumen is partially stenotic due to the invasion of the wall by the tumor. (Courtesy of Angell Memorial Animal Hospital.)

cinomas of the colon are one of the important neoplastic diseases of man. All animals have a lower frequency of adenocarcinoma of the colon than man, although several studies have demonstrated that chemical carcinogens (azoxymethane, 1,2-dimethylhydrazine) will induce adenocarcinomas of the colon in a high proportion of animals exposed. Naturally occurring tumors of the colon are generally less frequent than those of the small intestine.

Adenocarcinoma of the colon is recognized in the dog more often than in any other species (Fig. 23–20). Colonic tumors are more common than gastric, but are less frequent than adenocarcinomas of the rectum in this species. Adenocarcinoma in the "W" strain of rats reportedly was seen in 28 out of 3000 necropsies (Miwa et al., 1976). This tumor appears to be much less frequent in cats, hamsters, and mice. In sheep and oxen, the lesions usually involve the spiral colon rather than the rectum and are less frequent than in the dog.

Adenocarcinoma of the colon is quite unusual in most nonhuman primates, but the laboratory-maintained cotton-top marmoset (*Saguinus oedipus oedipus*) has been found (Lushbaugh, et al., 1978) to be quite susceptible to naturally occurring adenocarcinoma of the colon. In a colony of about 500 marmosets, 13 cases were discovered in *Saguinus oedipus oedipus*, and one case in a Goeldi's marmoset (*Callimico goeldi*). The frequency of this lesion obviously is increasing as animals become older. These adenocarcinomas arise in the mucosa, invade the submucosa, muscularis, and lymphatics; metastasis to the colonic lymph nodes is frequent. The lungs occasionally bear metastatic tumors.

Evans, J.T., Lutman, G., and Mittleman, A.: The induction of multiple large bowel neoplasms in mice. J. Med., 3:212–215, 1972.

Head, K.W.: International histological classification

of tumours of domestic animals. XII. Tumours of the lower alimentary tract. Bull. WHO, *53*:137–304, 1976.

Lushbaugh, C.C., et al.: Spontaneous colonic adenocarcinoma in marmosets. Primates Med., *10*:119–134, 1978.

Martin, M.S., et al.: An experimental model for cancer of the colon and rectum. Intestinal carcinoma induced in the rat by 1,2-dimethylhydrazine. Digestion, *8*:22–34, 1973.

Miwa, M., et al.: Spontaneous colon tumor in rats. J. Natl. Cancer Inst., *56*:615–617, 1976.

Newberne, P.M., and Rogers, A.E.: Adenocarcinoma of the colon. Animal model. DMH-induced adenocarcinoma of the colon in the rat. Am. J. Pathol., *72*:541–544, 1973.

Swartzendruber, D.C., et al.: Ultrastructural abnormalities of marmoset colon cancer cells. Fed. Proc., *34*:825, 1975.

Ward, J.M., et al.: Experimentally induced cancer of the colon in rats and mice. J. Am. Vet. Med. Assoc., *164*:729–732, 1974.

THE RECTUM AND ANUS

Atresia ani is a failure of development of the anal opening. Often there is little more than the skin and subcutis remaining imperforate, and it may be possible to establish surgically a satisfactory opening, the muscular sphincter and the rectum being adequately developed.

Prolapse of the rectum occurs probably in any species, but especially in cattle and swine. The exposed portion of the bowel becomes traumatized and inflamed, as well as filled with venous blood confined there by pressure of the rectal sphincter. Here, as elsewhere, venous flow is often stopped by a degree of pressure which permits the arterial circulation to continue. Hemorrhoids, which consist, when severe, of slightly, prolapsed hemorrhoidal veins and mucosa, do not occur in domestic animals.

Stricture of the rectum is a frequent problem in young swine. According to the work of Wilcock and Olander (1977 a,b), the natural disease is clearly associated with salmonellosis and can be reproduced experimentally with pure cultures of *Salmonella typhimurium*. This organism produces an ulcerative fibronecrotic colitis and proctitis in susceptible pigs. The rectum is believed to be particularly vulnerable to deep ischemic injury due to the precarious blood supply of the rectum. The cranial hemorrhoidal artery of the pig provides almost the total blood supply to the rectum. Fibrinous thrombi in the submucosal arteries in the rectum are associated with necrosis in mucosa and submucosa. At the site 2 to 5 cm cranial to the anorectal junction, the deep ulceration is eventually healed by scar formation which contracts and severely constricts the lumen of the rectum. The accumulation of feces in the colon causes severe dilatation of the colon and compression atrophy of abdominal and thoracic viscera. The affected pig fails to grow and develops a distended abdomen.

Rectal and vaginal constriction in certain herds of Jersey cattle have been described as occurring together, presumably the result of inherited factors (Leipold and Saperstein, 1975).

Anal sac disease occurs in dogs frequently. The anal sacs are paired blind pouches, lined with stratified squamous epithelium, which lie on either side of the anus in the subcutis. The anal sacs communicate with the anus through small orifices at the anocutaneous junction. Occlusion of these orifices results in distension of the sac with exudate and occasionally in purulent debris. This causes a great deal of discomfort to the dog until the pressure is relieved.

Squamous metaplasia of the rectal mucosa has been recorded in the rat in association with the feeding of degraded carrageenan. The carrageenans are a group of sulfated polysaccharides extracted from seaweeds (*Rhodophyceae*). Native carrageenan is extracted from the seaweed *Chondrus crispus* and used to suspend particles in chocolate milk, milk puddings, and infant formulas. The degraded carrageenan is extracted from *Eucheuma spirosum* and has been used in the treatment of ulcers. This latter type has been implicated in the causation of ulcers in the cecum and colon of guinea pigs, rats, and rabbits. The squamous metaplasia, produced in rats (Fabian, et al., 1973), is accompanied by severe chronic inflammation in the mucosa and submucosa; occasionally, adenomatous polyps may also appear.

Neoplasms of the Rectum and Anus

Adenocarcinomas of the rectal mucosa are the most frequent gastrointestinal neoplasm in the dog and in fact appear more frequently in this species than any other. The canine rectum is affected with this neoplasm about three times as frequently as any other part of the gastrointestinal tract. Some of these malignant adenocarcinomas appear to develop from benign adenomas in the dog rectum.

Squamous cell carcinomas occasionally originate at the mucocutaneous junction of the anus. These are more frequently reported in dogs but may appear in any species.

Adenomas and, less frequently, **adenocarcinomas** of the **perianal glands** are the most frequent neoplasms of this perianal region. These are described more fully in Chapter 18 in connection with tumors of the skin. **Adenocarcinomas of apocrine glands** may also occur in this region and are also considered in Chapter 18.

Dennis, S.M., and Leipold, H.W.: Atresia ani in sheep. Vet. Rec., *91*:219–222, 1972.

Fabian, R.J., Abraham, R., Coulston, F., and Golberg, L.: Carrageenan-induced squamous metaplasia of the rectal mucosa in the rat. Gastroenterol., *65*:265–276, 1973.

Harvey, C.E.: Incidence and distribution of anal sac disease in the dog. J. Am. Anim. Hosp. Assoc., *10*:573–577, 1974.

Head, K.W.: International histological classification of tumours of domestic animals. XII. Tumours of the lower alimentary tract. Bull. WHO, *53*:167–186, 1976.

Leipold, H.W., and Saperstein, G.: Rectal and vaginal constriction in Jersey cattle. J. Am. Vet. Med. Assoc., *166*:231–232, 1975.

Lingeman, C.H., and Garner, F.M.: Comparative study of intestinal adenocarcinomas of animals and man. J. Natl. Cancer Inst., *48*:325–346, 1972.

Saunders, C.N.: Rectal stricture syndrome in pigs: a case history. Vet. Rec., *94*:61, 1974.

Schäffer, E., and Schiefer, B.: Incidence and type of canine rectal carcinoma. J. Small Anim. Pract., *9*:491–496, 1968.

Wilcock, B.P., and Olander, H.J.: The pathogenesis of porcine rectal stricture. I. The naturally occurring disease and its association with salmonellosis Vet. Pathol., *14*:36–42, 1977.

Wilcock, B.P., and Olander, H.J.: The pathogenesis of porcine rectal stricture. II. Experimental salmonellosis and ischemic proctitis. Vet. Pathol., *14*:43–55, 1977.

PERITONEUM

Peritonitis

Peritonitis is nearly always infectious. Acute inflammation of the peritoneum may be localized to a given area or may be generalized over the whole peritoneal surface. This depends upon the mode of entrance of the infection and the relative resistance of the patient. The latter is largely a matter of species; dogs seldom have serious peritonitis; in horses, the introduction of any appreciable amount of infectious material into the peritoneal cavity is practically a death sentence, although antibiotics

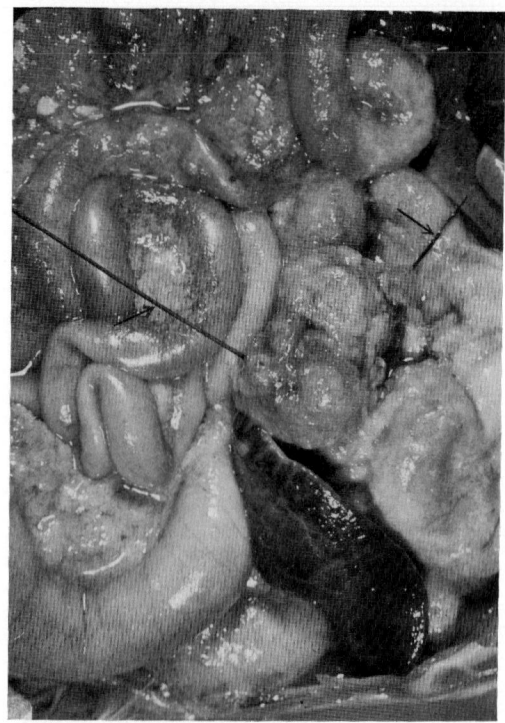

Fig. 23–21. Chronic peritonitis in a cat following ingestion of broom straws (arrows) which penetrated the stomach.

have mitigated the danger somewhat. Cattle not infrequently die of generalized peritonitis but, on the other hand, have sufficient resistance to maintain localization of many infections.

The infecting organisms are various, and many cases represent invasion by more than one pathogen. Prominent among the possible causative species are the colon bacillus and its relatives and streptococci of different types and species. Corynebacteria and staphylococci may be the offenders, and occasionally the clostridium of malignant edema and other anaerobes are responsible.

The inflammatory exudate is most often serofibrinous or fibrinous, although suppurative peritonitis results when the invaders are exclusively pyogenic species. Certain of the granuloma-producing organisms also thrive on the peritoneal surfaces, as will be explained shortly.

The principal routes by which infections enter are (1) operative incisions through the abdominal wall, (2) rupture or perforation of the stomach, intestines, or uterus, (3) direct extension through the more or less necrotic wall of one of these organs during the course of a severe infectious inflammation of its lining, and (4) by the bloodstream in the case of certain specific infections, such as bovine viral encephalitis and feline infectious peritonitis. Other routes are possible, such as via the ostium abdominale of the Fallopian tube, from an infected umbilicus in the newborn, or by direct extension from an infected kidney.

The peritoneum constitutes one of the large absorptive surfaces of the body, even when compared with the gastrointestinal mucous membrane or the total of the pulmonary alveolar or renal tubular surfaces. If its thin mesothelial lining becomes coated with toxin-producing microorganisms, the consequences are sure to be of a most serious nature. The victim's best chance of survival depends upon keeping the infection localized near its portal of entry, to which end several mechanisms are

well adapted. Fibrin tends to seal off infected areas and cover the invading pathogens. In those species which have a well-developed and flexible omentum, that membrane moves through some unknown attraction to cover an infected or injured area almost within minutes, becoming glued to the diseased surface. Through reflexes partly the result of pain, movements are kept to a minimum; peristalsis ceases; the abdominal wall becomes rigid; the breathing is limited to thoracic movements.

These mechanisms are not without their disadvantages. Paralytic ileus may develop in the motionless and nondigesting intestine. In this condition, the bowel becomes distended with gas and the shock-like accompaniments of intestinal obstruction (see above) are likely to develop. If the patient survives, the fibrin, like fibrin elsewhere, tends to become organized by fibroblasts and to tie the various abdominal organs to each other and to the diaphragm and abdominal wall. This process begins if the inflammation is not resolved in 6 to 10 days. The adhesions commonly interfere considerably with peristalsis and the digestive process and may bring it almost to a standstill.

Tuberculous peritonitis is common enough that, in cattle, it has received the popular name of "pearly disease" from the large numbers of shiny gray spheres constituting individual tubercles on the diaphragmatic or other peritoneal surfaces. In countries in which bovine or human tuberculosis is prevalent, young dogs may contract a severe tuberculous peritonitis. **Actinobacillosis** occasionally involves the peritoneal surfaces of cattle with a multitude of tiny nodular excrescences of granulation tissue, the mode of entry of the infection being obscure. Diagnosis of this condition hinges upon microscopic features.

Actinobacillosis, as well as tuberculosis, has to be differentiated from **neoplastic transplantations.** Occasionally a malignant neoplasm, usually a carcinoma arising in the digestive mucosa, a malignant hemangioendothelioma from a ruptured spleen, or (in human patients) an adenocarcinoma from the ovary, gains access to the peritoneal cavity, and its cells are transplanted through movement of the surfaces and fluids to form myriads of tiny nodular growths over many peritoneal areas, both parietal and visceral.

Feline infectious peritonitis, a viral disease, is described in Chapter 9.

Necrosis of abdominal fat regularly accompanies necrotizing pancreatitis, and is occasionally encountered in most animal species as small plaques or nodules in the abdominal cavity. The cause of the latter is not known. A peculiar form of abdominal fat necrosis of unknown cause occurs in cattle, characterized by extremely large masses of necrotic fat in the omentum, mesentery, and retroperitoneal tissues. Casts of necrotic fat may encircle the intestine leading to obstruction.

Hydroperitoneum, Ascites

Accumulation of watery fluid in the peritoneal cavity, in the broadest sense, is called hydroperitoneum. If, as is often the case, the fluid represents a true (noninflammatory) edema, the term ascites is applicable. Fluid in the peritoneal cavity may, however, represent an inflammatory edema (serous peritonitis) or it may be the result, especially in male cattle and sheep, of severe acute urinary obstruction with, or even without, rupture of the bladder. With the possible exception of the inflammatory form, the amount of fluid which accumulates may be tremendous, causing great distension of the abdomen and all the symptoms that go with great abdominal pressure.

Ascites, or true edema of the peritoneal cavity, may form a part of the syndrome of generalized edema and be referable to any of the causes of that condition. Such cases betray themselves by the presence of edema in other places, which need not be listed here. But ascites more typically results from chronic passive congestion of the portal venous system. The special causes of that congestion are conditions which obstruct (incompletely) the flow of the portal vein, most commonly cirrhosis. Other causes of obstruction include pressure of neoplasms, abscesses, granulomas, and enlarged lymph nodes upon the vein, as well as thrombosis within it.

Like any edema fluid, this is a true transudate, with a specific gravity less than 1.017 and with a protein content usually below 3%.

Inflammatory accumulation of fluid is distinguished by the presence of other signs of inflammation and by other elements of inflammatory exudation, chiefly leukocytes and fibrin. The specific gravity and level of protein are correspondingly higher.

Urinary fluid, whether it came directly from a ruptured bladder or as a transudate concomitant with the gradual uriniferous infiltration of the tissues of the periurethral region, has the odor and other characteristics of urine. Evidence of urinary obstruction is present in the form of calculi, cystitis, hydronephrosis, or related lesions.

The effects of hydroperitoneum are those of pressure, interfering with the abdominal organs and also, through pressure upon the diaphragm, with respiration. If the fluid is surgically withdrawn, more soon accumulates. The causal disorders, of course, produce other characteristic effects, such as uremia in the case of urinary obstruction.

Neoplasms of the Peritoneum

Neoplasms of the peritoneum are rare events, and only a few primary tumors are known in animals: the mesothelioma, fibrosarcoma, lipoma, and liposarcoma. The mesothelioma arises from the mesothelial cells lining the peritoneum and is made up of these flattened to cuboidal cells supported by a fibrous stroma. In some cases, the cells form tubules or solid masses of epithelial cells, in others, the fibrous cells predominate, suggesting fibroma or fibrosarcoma. The tumors may become implanted at various sites in the peritoneum and are usually associated with ascites. Cases have been reported in man, cattle, buffalo, horses, rats, mice, dogs, fowl, sheep, hamsters, and cats.

Lipomas and liposarcomas have been described in connection with tumors of the small intestine.

Raflo, C.P., and Nernberger, S.P.: Abdominal mesothelioma in a cat. Vet. Pathol., 15:781–783, 1978.
Ricketts, S.W., and Peace, C.K.: A case of peritoneal mesothelioma in a Thoroughbred mare. Equine Vet. J., 8:78–80, 1976.

LIVER

Structure

The liver is surrounded by a thick connective tissue membrane, Glisson's capsule. This capsule extends to and surrounds the portal vein, hepatic artery, and common bile duct at the porta hepatis and forms a sheath around these structures extending throughout the liver. These together form the portal triad, a characteristic feature seen with the light microscope. The portal vein is larger than the hepatic artery, which in appropriate preparations may be seen to entwine the portal vein throughout its length.

The liver may be seen with the light microscope or even naked eye to be divided into many lobules, about 2.0 mm in diameter, with the shape of an irregular pyramidal hexahedron. The center of each such classic lobule is formed by the central efferent or intralobular vein. Four or five portal triads are arranged around the periphery of the hepatic lobule at regular intervals. The functional lobule as defined by Rappaport (1973) is described as the **liver acinus**, having at its center a portal triad, surrounded by the margins of several classic lobules. It is advantageous to understand this functional concept, which has a bearing on the

nature of lesions in some instances, but the classic lobule is more readily identified and is used in most descriptions of pathologic lesions of the liver.

Liver cells (hepatocytes) are radially arranged around the central veins between sinusoids, which empty into the central vein. These hepatocytes are so placed that at least two cells at their poles opposite the sinusoids are joined to form a bile canaliculus. Each liver cell is also in contact with a hepatic sinusoid. This provides a sinusoidal system, which carries blood from the portal blood vessels to the central vein and a bile canalicular system. These canaliculi form an interlacing network that is in contact with at least one side of every hepatic cell and leads into larger channels, which join bile ductules at the margin of the lobule.

The sinusoids are arranged in a radial network that allows every hepatic cell to be in contact with blood as it flows toward the central vein. Kupffer's cells line the sinusoids but do not completely cover them, making it possible for plasma, but not blood cells, to circulate freely between the sinusoidal wall and a space formed by the plasma membrane of the liver cells. This is called the space of Disse. The Kupffer's cells are active phagocytes and contain abundant rough endoplasmic reticulum, mitochondria, lysosomes, and vacuoles.

Liver cells are large, polyhedral, with abundant cytoplasm, and each has one round nucleus containing a fairly prominent nucleolus. Each cell is in contact with its neighbor at the bile canaliculus and is separated from the sinusoid by the space of Disse. Adjacent liver cells are also separated by a narrow space, but desmosomes are present along these lateral borders. Near the canaliculus, tight junctions are formed by the fusion of external leaflets of adjacent plasma membranes. These plasma membranes also form short microvilli that project into the lumen of the bile canaliculus. Along the side of the hepatocyte near the bile canaliculus, histochemical and electron microscopic methods have demonstrated strong activity of nucleoside triphosphatase. The plasma membrane along the sinusoidal surface of the liver cell has strong activities of alkaline phosphatase and nucleoside monophosphatase.

The cytoplasm of each liver cell contains many mitochrondria, with proportionally more in cells in the periphery of the lobule in comparison to those in centrilobular zones. Endoplasmic cisternae form a system which is believed to distribute nutrients to all parts of the cell. Golgi's apparatus, consisting of membranes arranged with a concave and convex surface, is located between the nucleus and bile canaliculus. It is considered to be the apparatus which places a membrane around ("packages") material to be excreted from the cell. Glycogen is present in small electron-dense granules throughout the cytoplasm. Lysosomes are numerous in the functioning liver cell; vesicles and vacuoles of varying sizes are seen near Disse's space. Vesicular invaginations of the plasma membrane occur between the bases of villi that project into the space of Disse.

The blood supply of the liver comes from the hepatic artery and portal vein, the former supplying about 40 to 50% of the oxygen and less than half of the circulating blood to the liver. Some small amount of the blood from the hepatic artery flows directly, at arterial pressure, into the peripheral sinusoids. Most arteriolar branches of the hepatic artery enter a perpendicular plexus which lowers the blood pressure before it enters the peripheral sinusoids. An intermittent flow is apparently regulated by the tonus of the hepatic arteriolar system and by precapillary sphincters. The portal vein supplies little more than half the blood supply, containing 50 to 60% of the oxygen. This blood is at low pressure (8–10 mm Hg in man) and is 80% saturated with oxygen.

The intralobular vein, which courses through the center of the lobule, empties into a sublobular vein. These sublobular veins have a special connective tissue wall and are not accompanied by an artery or bile duct. These sublobular veins unite to form the hepatic veins which empty into the caudal (inferior) vena cava.

Function

The liver has several functions, which may be measured to determine the functional state of the organ. These include:

1. secretion of bile and other substances
2. intermediate metabolism of proteins, lipids, and carbohydrates
3. storage of certain minerals and foodstuffs
4. detoxification of various compounds
5. metabolism of hormones and drugs
6. production of certain proteins

The rough endoplasmic reticulum of the liver cells produces several important proteins with specific functions. These include: albumin; prothrombin (factor II); labile factor (VII); fibrinogen (factor I); plasma thromboplastin component (PTC, factor IX); plasma thromboplastin antecedent (PTA, factor XI); and Stuart factor (X).

Quantitative coagulation tests to determine prothrombin time are commonly used to assess the presence of liver disease. The synthesis of prothrombin factors V and VII is dependent upon the availability of vitamin K, which is normally stored in the liver. Available vitamin K may be reduced by several factors: malabsorption syndromes, pancreatic insufficiency, impaired bile flow, and chronic use of mineral oil will interfere with its absorption from the intestine; sterilization of intestinal contents by prolonged use of antibiotics will reduce production of vitamin K by intestinal bacteria; and coumarin will block the utilization of this vitamin.

Normal flow of bile promotes emulsification of lipids in the intestine, which is necessary for esterification and absorption of lipids, including vitamin K. Therefore chronic biliary obstruction of liver cell disease results in low prothrombin levels. Parenteral administration of vitamin K will result in prompt increase in prothrombin levels if the decrease is due to biliary obstruction, but not if it is due to liver cell disease.

The origin of alkaline phosphatase is not entirely from the liver, but its determination is of value as a liver-function test because it is elevated in (1) liver disease (especially biliary obstruction), (2) bone abnormalities, (3) bone growth, and (4) late pregnancy (Edmondson and Peters, 1977).

Transaminases, particularly glutamic pyruvic transaminase (GPT), are present in large quantities in liver cells (man, primates, dogs, cats, rats) and are released into the serum when hepatocytes are destroyed. Measurement of serum levels of GPT provides a useful clinical test of liver cell disease in species with high normal levels in the liver. In species with low normal levels (pigs, sheep, cattle, and horses) of hepatic glutamic pyruvic transaminase, its determination in serum is of no value in detecting liver disease. Other enzymes, such as glutamic oxaloacetic transaminase (GOT), occur in liver cells, but also in other tissues and therefore their quantitation does not provide as specific a test.

The determination of conjugated and unconjugated bilirubin is of value in detecting hyperbilirubinemia of various causes. The clearance of sulfobromophthalein is also of value in detection of uptake and excretion of various substances (e.g., bilibrubin, sulfobromophthalein, phylloerythrin, etc.) by the liver.

Necrosis of liver cells may at times have unique characteristics and may be described with distinctive names. *Lytic* necrosis is the result of lysis and disappearance of individual or groups of liver cells, leaving a space until regeneration can replace the missing cells. *Acidophilic* necrosis is used to describe the unicellular death of hepatocytes which become globular and small in size and lose their pyknotic nucleus by extrusion. These cells are also called "Councilman bodies" or "shrinkage necrosis." They are seen in human viral hepatitis, yellow fever, and ischemic necrosis. This "Councilman body" may be extruded into the sinusoid and engulfed by Kupffer cells. *Caseous* or *liquefactive* necrosis may be seen in the liver in granulomatous infections. *Hyaline* necrosis is believed to often follow hyaline degeneration of liver cells. The affected individual cells become deeply eosinophilic, relatively insoluble, and are most frequently seen in human alcoholic liver disease. They are also referred to as "alcoholic hyaline bodies" or "Mallory's bodies."

Disassociation of liver cells is one characteristic feature of certain diseases, particularly canine leptospirosis, which precedes other evidence of widespread necrosis of liver cells. The liver cells, although still in place, become detached from one another, individualized, and somewhat rounded. Their cytoplasm may become more acidophilic. This striking picture is believed to depict one of the early manifestations of death of liver cells.

Cornelius, C.E., Arias, I.M., and Osburn, B.L.: Hepatic pigmentation with photosensitivity: a syndrome in Corriedale sheep resembling Dubin-Johnson syndrome in man. J. Am. Vet. Med. Assoc., 146:709–713, 1965.

Cornelius, C.E.,and Gronwall, R.R.: Congenital photosensitivity and hyperbilirubinemia in Southdown sheep in the United States. Am. J. Vet. Res., 29:291–295, 1968.

Cornelius, C.E.: Animal model for human disease. Gilbert's syndrome. Comp. Pathol. Bull., 11:2–4, 1970.

Cornelius, C.E.: Congenital hyperbilirubinemia, Gilbert's syndrome. In Handbook: Animal Models of Human Disease. Washington, D.C., Armed Forces Institute of Pathology, 1972 a, model no. 8.

Cornelius, C.E.: Congenital hyperbilirubinemia, Dubin-Johnson syndrome. In Handbook: Animal Models of Human Disease. Washington, D.C., Armed Forces Institute of Pathology, 1972 b, model no. 2.

Cornelius, C.E., and Arias, I.M.: Congenital hyperbilirubinemia, Crigler-Najjar syndrome. In Handbook: Animal Models of Human Disease. Washington, D.C., Armed Forces Institute of Pathology, 1973, model no. 26.

Cornelius, C.E.: Rates of choleresis in various species. Am. J. Dig. Dis., 21:426–428, 1976.

Edmondson, H.A., and Peters, R.L.: Liver. In Pathology, edited by W.A.D. Anderson, and J.M. Kissane. St. Louis, Mosby, 1977 (7th Edition), pp. 1321–1438.

Engelking, L.R., Gronwall, R., and Anwer, M.S.: Effect of bile acid on hepatic excretion and storage of bilirubin in ponies. Am. J. Vet. Res., 37:47–50, 1976.

Forssmann, W.G., and Ito, S.: Hepatocyte innervation in primates. J. Cell Biol., 74:299–313, 1977.

Hammond, K.D., Balinsky, D., Bersohn, I., and Jersky, J.: Kinetic studies on alkaline phosphatase from liver of baboon, Papio ursinus. Int. J. Biochem., 4:511–520, 1973.

Javitt, N.B.: Hepatic bile formation (two parts). N. Engl. J. Med., 295:1464–1469, 1511–1516, 1976.

Jones, T.C.: Pathology of the liver of rats and mice. In Pathology of Laboratory Rats and Mice, edited by E. Cotchin, and F.J.C. Roe. Oxford and Edinburgh, Blackwell Science Public., 1967, pp. 1–23.

Matas, A.J., et al.: Hepatocellular transplantation for metabolic deficiencies: decrease of plasma bilirubin in Gunn rats. Science, 192:892–894, 1976.

Misra, M.K., et al.: Acute hepatic coma: a canine model. Surgery, 72:634–642, 1972.

Naughton, B.A., et al.: Hepatic regeneration and erythropoietin production in the rat. Science, 196:301–302, 1977.

Rappaport, A.M.: Microcirculatory hepatic units. Microvasc. Res., 6:212–228, 1973.

Strombeck, D.R., and Qualls, C.: Hepatic sulfobromophthalein uptake and storage defect in a dog. J. Am. Vet. Med. Assoc., 172:1423–1426, 1978.

Wiggers, K.D., French, S.W., French, B.A., and Carr, B.N.: The ultrastructure of Mallory body filaments. Lab. Invest., 29:652–658, 1973.

Infectious Hepatitis

For this term to apply, the infective organisms must invade the liver and be rather diffusely distributed in it. Infections of other organs, for instance of the uterus, often cause a toxic hepatitis because of toxic substances absorbed and carried by the blood, without the metastasis of pathogens into the liver, which is essential if the hepatitis is to be classed as infectious.

The infections that may attack the liver include a few which are peculiar to the liver and several which localize elsewhere with equal or greater facility. In the former group are Rubarth's canine viral hepatitis (hepatitis contagiosa canis) or canine adenovirus infection, leptospirosis, equine rhinopneumonitis (equine herpesvirus), murine hepatitis (mice), viral hepatitis of ducks, yellow fever (monkeys), herpesvirus T and simplex in marmosets, and infectious hepatitis or acute liver atrophy of horses.

In man, acute **viral hepatitis A** (infectious hepatitis, catarrhal jaundice, epidemic hepatitis) is a relatively mild infection transmitted by fecal-oral means and usually ending in recovery. The marmoset is susceptible to experimental infection with this virus. Fulminant **viral hepatitis B** (acute red atrophy, acute yellow atrophy, subacute yellow atrophy) on the other hand, is more severe, often prolonged, and fatal in as many as 73% of the cases. Some patients have a prolonged course and die as the result of cirrhosis. This infection is often associated with contaminated syringes or serum products. Chimpanzees may be infected in nature and are experimentally susceptible until immunized by prior infection. Another viral disease of man, **hepatitis, non-A, non-B,** is less common and poorly understood but is differentiated from hepatitis A and B. Animals have not been infected.

Other human diseases involving infectious hepatitis include: yellow fever, leptospirosis (Weil's disease), typhoid fever, and infectious mononucleosis (Epstein-Barr virus).

In laboratory animals experimentally inoculated, a number of other infections such as brucellosis and tularemia localize in the liver as minute foci widely disseminated. The more prominent members of the latter group are tuberculosis, syphilis (humans), coccidioidomycosis, histoplasmosis, toxoplasmosis (rarely other granulomas), necrobacillosis, and the pyogenic infections. The features of a given case of hepatitis due to such an infection are those characteristic of the disease itself. In fact, while it is not erroneous to speak of tuberculous hepatitis, for instance, tuberculosis of the liver is more usual and possibly more meaningful. One also considers to what extent these infections are diffuse or localized in the liver. Often the granulomatous lesions are decidedly restricted and the pyogenic infections much more commonly form localized and encapsulated abscesses than diffuse infectious processes. All of the above infections are treated individually elsewhere and their characteristics need not be repeated here.

Of more importance in appreciating the general aspects of infectious hepatitis is a consideration of the routes by which infections of any sort gain access to the liver. These are, more or less in order of frequency, (1) the portal vein, (2) the hepatic artery, (3) the umbilical vein in the newborn, (4) the bile-duct system, (5) the hepatic vein, and (6) direct extension. The importance of the portal blood as a carrier of infectious material is obvious in view of its large volume and the fact that it drains the extensively exposed intestinal area. Entrance of infective material via the hepatic artery occurs when the microorganisms, as emboli or otherwise, are in the general systemic circulation. In farm animals, infection of the umbilical structures by contact soon after birth is by no means unusual. The umbilical vein, filled with partially clotted blood, affords an excellent route of access to the liver. Coming from contaminated soil, the infections entering in this way are usually the necrophorus bacillus or the pyogenic organisms, and necrotic areas or abscesses are the usual results. Infections may ascend the biliary passages either through static secretion consequent upon obstruction or by continuous spread of the infectious inflammatory process from the duodenum and up the ductal tissues. Usually the two processes are combined. Spread of infection to the liver via the hepatic vein would appear impossible, but it occurs very rarely due to momentary reversal of the current in right-sided valvular disease, the primary source of infection usually being the diseased valve itself. A retrograde thrombus may form, reaching backward into the hepatic vein and its tributaries, the distance involved being really very short. Direct extension of infec-

tion from adjoining tissues and organs is, of course, possible. It usually depends upon a traumatic origin, such as that due to foreign bodies in the bovine reticulum.

Serum Hepatitis of Horses

Known by such names as **serum hepatitis, equine viral hepatitis, Theiler's disease,** and possibly confused with Kimberly horse disease (*Crotalaria retusa*), or merely acute yellow atrophy, a suddenly occurring and usually fatal disease of horses has been recognized since as early as 1919 (Theiler). Symptoms of acute indigestion, including those of "blind staggers," develop in the course of a few hours, accompanied by marked icterus. Death in a day or two reveals a swollen, typical "nutmeg liver," all parts being uniformly involved. Microscopic examination shows that the "nutmeg" appearance is due to centrilobular necrosis with replacement by blood, often to the extent that only a narrow rim of hepatic cells survives around the periphery of the blood-filled lobule. The picture differs from that of the usual acute toxic hepatitis in that in the portal areas (islands of Glisson) and throughout whatever hepatic parenchyma remains there is a liberal infiltration of inflammatory cells, chiefly lymphocytes and neutrophils.

The etiology is unknown, and it may well be that a number of intoxications have been confused to form what has been considered a single syndrome but it is of interest that many of the afflicted horses have a history of having received a few months previously a therapeutic agent consisting of horse serum. Among such agents are immunizing sera directed against several equine infections such as African horse-sickness in South Africa and equine encephalomyelitis in North America, as well as tetanus antitoxin. Also occupying a prominent place in the list is the serum of pregnant mares, which has been injected in liberal amounts in the hope of assisting placentation in brood mares. This situation has led to a widespread suspicion that the equine species may be plagued with a virus hidden in the serum of apparently normal horses, transferable in therapeutic sera, comparable to the "serum hepatitis" of man. On the other hand, it must be noted (1) that in many instances the administration of the supposedly causative therapeutic agent occurred several months previous to the sudden development of this disease, (2) that of thousands of horses receiving therapeutic sera only a minute proportion have ever shown this disease, (3) that numerous experimental attempts to produce a hepatitis in horses by the administration of horse serum have given uniformly negative results.

The symptomatology of nervous disorder ("staggers") when the hepatitis followed the use of an anti-encephalomyelitis serum has led to a theory that the supposed virus also attacked the brain. However, convincing lesions have been uniformly lacking.

Lorenz, D., et al.: Hepatitis in the marmoset, *Saguinus mystax*. Proc. Soc. Exp. Biol. Med., *135*:348, 1970.

Gerin, J.L., Ford, E.C., and Purcell, R.H.: Biochemical characterization of Australia antigen. Evidence for defective particles of hepatitis B virus. Am. J. Pathol., *81*:651–668, 1975.

Hinthorn, D.R., et al.: Outbreak of chimpanzee associated hepatitis. J. Occup. Med., *16*:388–391, 1974.

Maynard, J.E.: Hepatitis A. Perspectives and recent advances. Am. J. Pathol., *81*:683–694, 1975.

Popper, H.: Clinical pathologic correlation in viral hepatitis. Effect of the virus on the liver. Am. J. Pathol., *81*:609–628, 1975.

Purcell, R.H., Alter, H.J., and Dirstag, J.L.: Non-A, Non-B Hepatitis. Yale J. Biol. Med., *49*:243–250, 1976.

Robinson, M., Gopinath, C., Hughes, D.L.: Histopathology of acute hepatitis in the horse. J. Comp. Pathol., *85*:111–118, 1975.

Strombeck, D.R., Krum, S., and Rogers, Q.: Coagulopathy and encephalopathy in a dog with acute hepatic necrosis. J. Am. Vet. Med. Assoc., *169*:813–816, 1976.

Szmuness, W.: Recent advances in the study of the epidemiology of hepatitis B. Am. J. Pathol., *81*:629–650, 1975.

Theiler, A.: Acute liver atrophy and parenchymatous hepatitis in horses. Rep. Dir. Vet. Res., U. So. Afr., *5*:6–7, 1919.

Thomsett, L.R.: Acute hepatic failure in the horse. Equine Vet. J., *3*:15–19, 1971.

Acute Toxic Hepatitis

Acute toxic hepatitis is characterized by death of hepatic cells and the changes which precede and follow cell death, in other words, by hydropic degeneration, fatty change, and necrosis.

Microscopic Appearance. Microscopically, the necrosis is most often coagulative in type, recognized by pyknosis and acidophilic cytoplasm. Disintegration and disappearance of the cells follow.

From the standpoint of location, necrosis in the liver may take any one of five forms: (1) **Diffuse necrosis,** in which the change spreads over considerable areas without regard to lobular boundaries. This is simply a very severe manifestation of the lobular forms listed below. (2) **Focal necrosis,** in which minute necrotic areas, or foci, of sublobular size, appear here and there, occupying any part of any lobule. These are characteristic of disseminated infections, often in laboratory animals. Included here are livers of equine fetuses aborted because of rhinopneumonitis (equine herpesvirus). (3) **Peripheral necrosis,** in which the peripheral zones of the lobules are regularly necrotic. This form is not common, but results when strong toxic substances are brought to the lobule by the bloodstream without any impairment in circulation of the blood and oxygenation of the cells. The peripheral cells receive the toxic blood first and suffer most from its effects. (4) **Midzonal necrosis,** in which the most pronounced necrotic changes involve the cells halfway between the periphery and the center of the lobule. This form is unusual but is characteristic of human eclampsia and a few other diseases. (5) **Centrilobular necrosis,** in which the cells nearest the central vein suffer both from bloodborne toxins and from a stagnation of the circulation with consequent anoxia. This is the usual form of necrosis as seen in acute toxic hepatitis, the primary disorder being responsible for both production of toxic substances and impairment of circulation. (6) **Paracentral necrosis** is an unusual form in which the necrotic area adjoins the central vein on one side but does not surround it. Attributed to local circulatory disorder, it is a characteristic of Rift Valley fever and is also seen in some anemic diseases. The affected necrotic zone may be demonstrated to involve the cells whose blood supply comes from the blood vessels (hepatic artery and portal vein) of one hepatic acinus. Thus, the affected cells may be part of one physiologic acinus and also within several contiguous classic lobules.

The typical (but not invariable) microscopic picture of acute toxic hepatitis may then be described as centrilobular necrosis with disappearance of a considerable number of the most centrally located cells, blood taking their place. More peripherally in the lobule, there are most typically hepatic cells in a state of fatty change and, peripheral to these and commonly comprising the remainder of the lobule, hydropic degeneration. When the condition is several days old, a moderate infiltration of lymphocytes into the periportal connective tissue (islands of Glisson) usually begins. The typical picture, however, is often incomplete, with the fat, or the necrosis or other elements missing.

Gross Appearance. The gross appearance of a liver affected by acute toxic hepatitis involves the changes already described for hydropic degeneration, fatty change, and necrosis. Such a liver is usually lighter in color, even to the tan of severe fatty degeneration. It is also likely to be redder because of an increased content of blood. The majority probably are best described as showing **accentuation of the lobular markings.** In the normal liver (except that of the pig), lobules are not readily discernible with the naked eye. In the livers under consideration, the lobules can usually be seen because of a difference in color between the centers and the peripheries of the lobules. If the central part of the lobule is seriously congested, it will have the redder color of blood. The more peripheral part then is relatively more yellow and often decidedly pale, because of cellular swelling, fat, or necrosis in this zone. At another stage, however, the coagulated necrotic cells of the center may be the palest part of the lobule, the more nearly normal cells of the peripheral zone retaining their natural deep brown.

It is seldom possible to decide the exact status grossly, but there should be little difficulty in detecting that some of these changes are present. The size of the liver tends to be decreased as some of its parenchymal cells undergo necrosis and disappear, but the influx of blood and the accumulation of fat tend to augment its volume. Thus, no positive statement can be made as to size, although severely affected livers are usually smaller than they were during health.

Acute yellow atrophy was formerly listed as a disease entity, usually of unknown cause. During an acute illness, the liver became yellow because of fatty change and necrosis and became smaller because of disappearance of many of its cells. We now know these cases to represent acute toxic hepatitis, a fact which affords at least some clue to their causes. **Acute red atrophy** was an essentially similar condition, the red of severe congestion overwhelming the yellow of the damaged cells.

Causes. The causes of acute toxic hepatitis are toxic substances of great variety, many of them not clearly identified. They may be divided into three groups:

(1) Chemical poisons. Included are copper, arsenic, and the arsenical drugs, phosphorus (if the patient survives 3 days or more), mercury (unless chronic), chloroform (delayed poisoning developing 2 or 3 days after anesthesia), tannic acid (used in treatment of burns), cincophen (a proprietary drug), tetrachloroethane (industrial), trinitrotoluene (industrial), tet-

rachloroethylene, and carbon tetrachloride. The last two are of especial interest in veterinary medicine because they are commonly used as anthelmintic drugs. Their toxicity to the patient is due to their destructive action on the liver. Coal-tar pitch and gossypol cause a severe destructive type of toxic hepatitis.

(2) Plant poisons. Among those recognized at present are species of the genera *Senecio* (Nebraska, Texas, Nova Scotia, South Africa), *Amsinckia* (tar weed of Pacific Northwest), *Phyllanthus* (Texas); and, under certain circumstances of growth and preservation, the wild and cultivated lupines, vetches, velvet beans (*Macuna utilus*), and other legumes. Other forage crops are said to have similar effects when they have undergone certain types of spoilage or fermentation. Certain of the latter toxicities are not based on poisons in the plant itself, but rather toxins produced by various fungi. A notable example is the hepatic injury in aflatoxin poisoning.

(3) Metabolic poisons. Certain types of gastroenteritis are believed to generate toxic substances of this nature. Mild degrees of toxic injury accompany many of the acute infectious diseases. Toxemias of pregnancy are important in humans. The outstanding example in veterinary medicine is the so-called "pregnancy disease" of ewes, which depends upon the combined effects of pregnancy and ketosis.

It has been found that hepatic necrosis and icterus can be produced in experimental animals by administration of extremely high doses of follicular hormones. Also vitamin E and selenium deficiencies may result in acute hepatic necrosis. Alcohol poisoning, a frequent cause of acute and chronic hepatitis in man, is not encountered in animals, except in the experimentally induced disease.

Significance and Effect. The severe acute cases are fatal within a few days, with most of the hepatic parenchymal cells necrotic and disappearing. It is such cases that constitute the classical "acute yellow atrophy."

In less severe cases, the patient recovers completely, the hepatic epithelium being regenerated with considerable facility after removal of the toxic substances. All too frequently in animals the unsuspected toxic component of the feed or pasturage is continuously or repeatedly ingested in moderate amount, and the acute condition just described is superseded or accompanied by cirrhosis, the chronic form of toxic hepatitis.

Allen, J.R., and Carstens, L.A.: Monocrotaline induced Budd-Chiari syndrome in monkeys. Am. J. Dig. Dis., 16:111–113, 1971.
Bull, L.B.: Liver disease of livestock from intake of hepatotoxic substances. Aust. Vet. J.,37:126–130, 1961.
Gocke, D.J., Morris, T.Q., and Bradley, S.E.: Chronic hepatitis in the dog: the role of immune factors. J. Am. Vet. Med. Assoc., 156:1700–1705, 1970.
Gyorgy, P., et al.: Prevention of experimental dietary hepatic injury by extracts of some tropical plants. Proc. Soc. Exp. Biol. Med., 113:203–206, 1963.
Heimberg, M., et al.: The action of carbon tetrachloride on the transport and metabolism of triglycerides and fatty acids by the isolated perfused rat liver and its relationship to the etiology of fatty liver. J. Biol. Chem., 237:3623–3627, 1962.
Lieber, C.S., and DeCarli, L.M.: An experimental model of alcohol feeding and liver injury in the baboon. J. Med. Primatol., 3:153–163, 1974.
Lieber, C.S.: Liver disease and alcohol: fatty liver, alcoholic hepatitis, cirrhosis, and their interrelationships. Ann. N. Y. Acad. Sci., 252:63–84, 1975.
McCulloch, E.C.: Hepatic cirrhosis of horses, swine, and cattle due to seeds of the tarweed, *Amsinckia intermedia*. J. Am. Vet. Med. Assoc., 96:5–18, 1940.
Michel, R.L., Whitehair, C.K., and Kealey, K.K.: Dietary hepatic necrosis associated with selenium-vitamin E deficiency in swine. J. Am. Vet. Med. Assoc., 155:50–59, 1969.
Nath, I., Sood, S.K., and Nayak, N.C.: Experimental siderosis and liver injury in the Rhesus monkey. J. Pathol., 106:103–111, 1972.
Rogers, A.E., and Newberne, P.M.: Animal model: fatty liver and cirrhosis in lipotrope-deficient male rats. Am. J. Pathol., 73:817–820, 1973.
Rogers, W.A., and Ruebner, B.H.: A retrospective study of probable glucocorticoid-induced hepatopathy in dogs. J. Am. Vet. Med. Assoc., 170:603–606, 1977.
Ruebner, B.H., et al.: Nutritional cirrhosis in Rhesus monkeys: electron microscopy and histochemistry. Exp. Mol. Pathol., 11:53–70, 1969.
Schaffner, F.: Drug metabolism and adverse hepatic drug reactions. Vet. Pathol., 12:145–156, 1975.
Setchell, B.P., and Littlejohn, I.R.: Poisoning of sheep with anthelmintic doses of carbon tetrachloride.

PLATE II

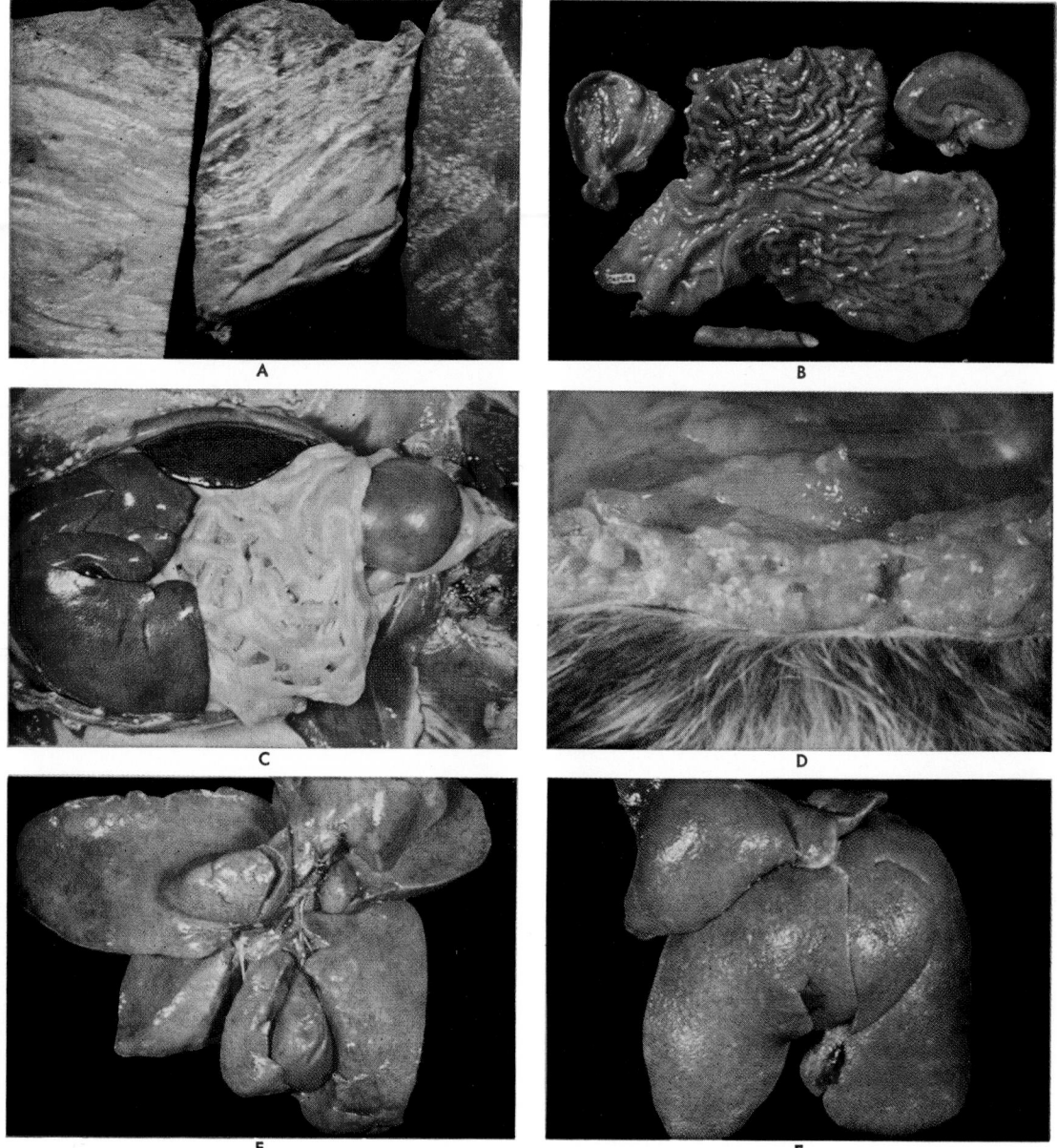

A, Azoturia in a yearling Palomino colt which became entangled in a halter rope and was unable to rise from a recumbent position. The colt was sacrificed after three days. Specimens of biceps femoris and latissimus dorsi muscles are illustrated, with normal muscle for comparison. (Case from Iowa School Vet. Med.)

B, Icterus due to acute leptospirosis in a male Springer Spaniel, nine months old. The yellow color is pronounced in tissues that are naturally pale (aorta, gastric and bladder mucosa) and is discernible in darker tissues (kidney, prostate)

C, Acute hemolytic icterus and hemolytic anemia due to *Hemobartonella felis*, affecting a two-year-old male cat. Note the yellow-colored omentum contrasting with the white intestines, the pale and swollen liver, and the enlarged, congested spleen. Most of this splenic enlargement is due to extramedullary hematopoiesis. The bluish object is the urinary bladder filled with hemoglobin-stained urine. (Courtesy of Angell Memorial Animal Hospital)

D, Steatitis involving the subcutaneous fat of a one-year-old spayed female cat. This cat's diet consisted almost exclusively of canned red tuna. (Courtesy of Angell Memorial Animal Hospital)

E, Severe fatty infiltration of the liver, secondary to diabetes mellitus in a spayed female terrier, age 12 years. (Courtesy of Angell Memorial Animal Hospital)

F, Toxic hepatitis, following exposure to benzene, in a 12-year-old castrated male cat. Microscopic sections revealed severe focal necrosis, fatty degeneration and bile retention. The greenish color in the gross specimen results from oxidation of bilirubin to biliverdin. (Courtesy of Angell Memorial Animal Hospital)

III. Liver histopathology, Aust. Vet. J., *39*:49–50, 1963.

Strombeck, D.R., Rogers, W., and Gribble, D.: Chronic active hepatic disease in a dog. J. Am. Vet. Med. Assoc., *169*:802–804, 1976.

Cirrhosis

The word "cirrhosis" originally came from the Greek, *kirrhos,* which meant tawny or orange-colored. This relation to the color of the affected liver has over the years lost its meaning. Systems of classification and nomenclature of the disease in man and animals, based upon incomplete or incorrect knowledge, have risen and disappeared over the years. The present prevailing view is that cirrhosis is the result of a series of pathologic events leading to increase in dense fibrous connective tissue in the liver. This fibrous tissue growth may extend from the portal connective tissue, from that around the venous outflow tract, or both. The definition (Report of Board for Classification and Nomenclature of Cirrhosis of Liver, 1956) most commonly used includes the concept of nodular regeneration as a part of cirrhosis. A pro-

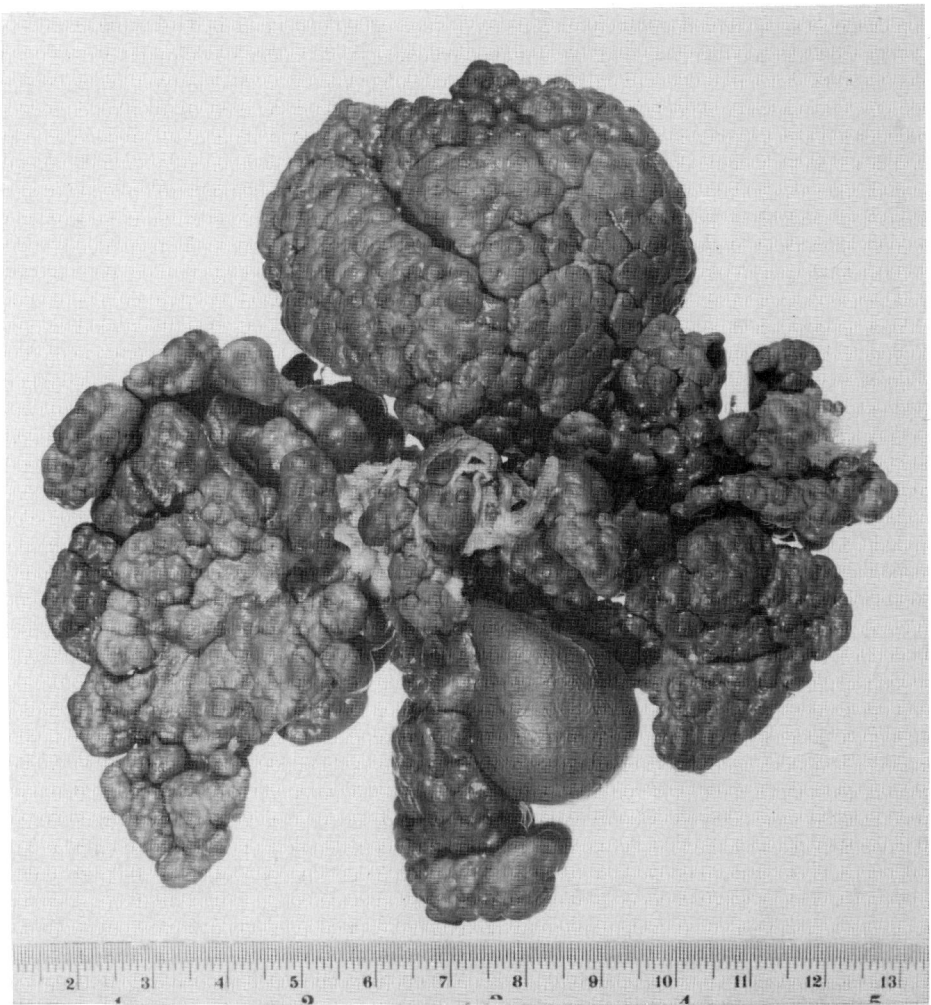

Fig. 23–22. Cirrhosis of liver of a dog. Note extensive nodularity and atrophy. (Courtesy of Armed Forces Institute of Pathology.) Contributor: Dr. Robert Ferber.

posed classification and nomenclature system for human cirrhosis (Edmondson and Peters, 1977) suggests a classification based upon etiology, morphology, and the functional state of the liver. This appears to be most useful in relation to clinical problems and their management.

Alcoholic cirrhosis, the most common type of the disease in humans, is used to designate lesions associated with alcoholism. Older terms such as "gin drinker's liver," "Laennec's cirrhosis," "nodular" and "atrophic cirrhosis," "hobnail liver," and "postnecrotic cirrhosis" are no longer recommended (Edmondson and Peters, 1977). Hepatitis B virus is known to be one cause of cirrhosis in human patients.

The classification system advocated for cirrhosis in animals by Hilton A. Smith in earlier editions of *Veterinary Pathology* included the view that cirrhosis was synonymous with chronic toxic hepatitis; it had the advantage of simplicity and made use of most knowledge available. It is still apparent that most cases of cirrhosis in animals result from the effects of ingestion of toxic substances, but infectious agents may also be causative in animals as in man. It is often not possible to determine the antecedent lesions in livers in advanced stages of cirrhosis nor to pinpoint the etiology. The duration of the disease also makes a difference in the nature of the lesions seen at necropsy.

Microscopic Appearance. The outstanding microscopic feature of cirrhosis is proliferation of fibrous connective tissue, which begins at the islands of Glisson (portal areas) and increases to surround the lobules, which are irregularly reduced in size. The change may vary from a slight increase of the normally fibrous portal areas to a condition where the interstitial connective tissue exceeds the parenchymatous tissue of the lobules. The connective tissue may be young and cellular, but is more often of the mature, fibrous variety. There is usually more or less infil-

tration with lymphocytes and mononuclear leukocytes, chiefly in the islands of Glisson. These indicate that the inflammatory process is still active. Newly formed (nonfunctioning) bile ducts are often seen in the connective tissue. They are recognized as tiny circles (or in longitudinal section as double lines) of small epithelial cells with darkly staining nuclei. Necrosis and the other changes described under acute toxic hepatitis may still be active within the lobules. There is often considerable regeneration of new hepatic epithelium. This usually results in marked distortion of lobular architecture. In addition, regenerative hyperplasia of individual hepatic cells may result in bizarre forms with tremendously large and hyperchromatic nuclei.

Causes. Frequently the cause in an individual case of cirrhosis cannot be ascertained, but in general the causes of portal cirrhosis are the same as those of acute toxic hepatitis. They act more slowly, doubtless because the amount of toxic substance ingested in a given period is less. Some, perhaps many cases, represent the end result of an attack of acute toxic hepatitis. In the farm animals, chronic poisoning by plants, known and unknown, should be suspected as the most likely cause. Thus, the "walking disease" of horses described by Van Es (1929) in Nebraska proved to be cirrhosis caused by a plant of the *Senecio* genus, while walking disease of the horses in the Pacific Northwest is a cirrhosis produced by seeds of the plant *Amsinckia intermedia* (tarweed). "Hard-liver disease" of swine and cattle in that region is due to the same plant. Hard-liver disease of sheep in many parts of the world (Texas, South Africa), Pictou disease of cattle in Canada, and Winton's disease of horses and cattle in New Zealand have been traced to other poisonous senecios, the essential lesion being cirrhosis. It is probable that other plants, presently unrecognized, have similar toxic properties. However, cirrhosis is occasionally seen in dogs, showing that some cases in animals must be attributed to other causes than plant toxins.

Biliary cirrhosis is distinguishable from portal cirrhosis only with difficulty; this form of cirrhosis has an entirely unrelated cause, namely, chronic inflammation of the intrahepatic bile ducts. With the cholangitis there is usually an obstruction somewhere in the extrahepatic ductal system (pressure of tumors, etc.), but the inflammatory process may have an infectious basis. While parasites (flukes, ascarids) are named as causes of biliary cirrhosis in humans, it is noteworthy that in animals liver flukes practically never cause more than an encircling fibrosis in the immediate vicinity of the invaded ducts, which are the relatively larger ones.

Microscopically, well-advanced biliary cirrhosis presents a perilobular fibrosis similar to that of atrophic cirrhosis, but careful observation reveals that the process is marked especially by fibrous tissue which encircles the various bile ducts. Its spread through the portal areas and around the lobules is incidental to the anatomical position of the structures. Newly formed (nonfunctional) bile ducts are especially numerous in this form of cirrhosis, and the infiltration of inflammatory cells (lymphocytes and monocytes usually) is especially prominent, also. Since there is almost always some obstruction of the ductal system, from local swelling if nothing else, bile pigment collects in the liver and jaundice is almost always present.

Grossly, the liver in this form of cirrhosis is completely or nearly smooth. It is enlarged and is of a greenish hue because of the retained bile.

Glissonian cirrhosis presents a picture in the microscopic section quite similar to that of portal cirrhosis, but grossly, the fibrous change is found to be confined to areas extending only a short distance beneath the capsule. It represents the spread of a chronic fibrosing inflammation of Glisson's capsule (the covering of the liver), hence of a regional peritonitis. It is not a true cirrhosis since the latter term applies to a condition involving the liver as a whole.

Central, or **cardiac, cirrhosis** refers to an increase of fibrous tissue around the central veins incident to chronic passive congestion. This proliferative phenomenon is characteristic of long-standing congestion in any vessel. The fibrous tissue is rarely extensive.

Pigment cirrhosis refers to the form which occurs in connection with hemochromatosis.

Parasitic cirrhosis is occasionally seen in domestic animals, but not with the frequency that hepatic parasitism is encountered. Of greatest significance is the migration of the larvae of the swine kidney worm (*Stephanurus dentatus*) and *Ascaris lumbricoides* which if their number are great, may result in hepatic necrosis leading to cirrhosis. Infestation with liver flukes rarely leads to cirrhosis. Schistosomiasis in man may result in parasitic cirrhosis and can be anticipated to lead to cirrhosis in affected nonhuman primates, but this has not been reported.

Effects of Cirrhosis. Owing to the large reserve capacity of the liver, impaired hepatic function is not a common accompaniment of cirrhosis. In humans, the liver may fail in its function of inactivating estrogens with resultant atrophy of the testes and feminization. Presumably, the same could occur in intact male animals. Rarely, there is inadequate formation of prothrombin and other clotting factors and interference with clotting. Porphyrinemia and photosensitization may also result. Decreased levels of blood protein and of vitamin A have been reported.

The principal effect of cirrhosis (ordinary portal but not biliary) is interference with the flow of the portal blood through the many hepatic ramifications on its way to the heart. The result is chronic passive congestion of the spleen and of the digestive organs. Mild digestive disturbances and discomfort follow, but the chief effect

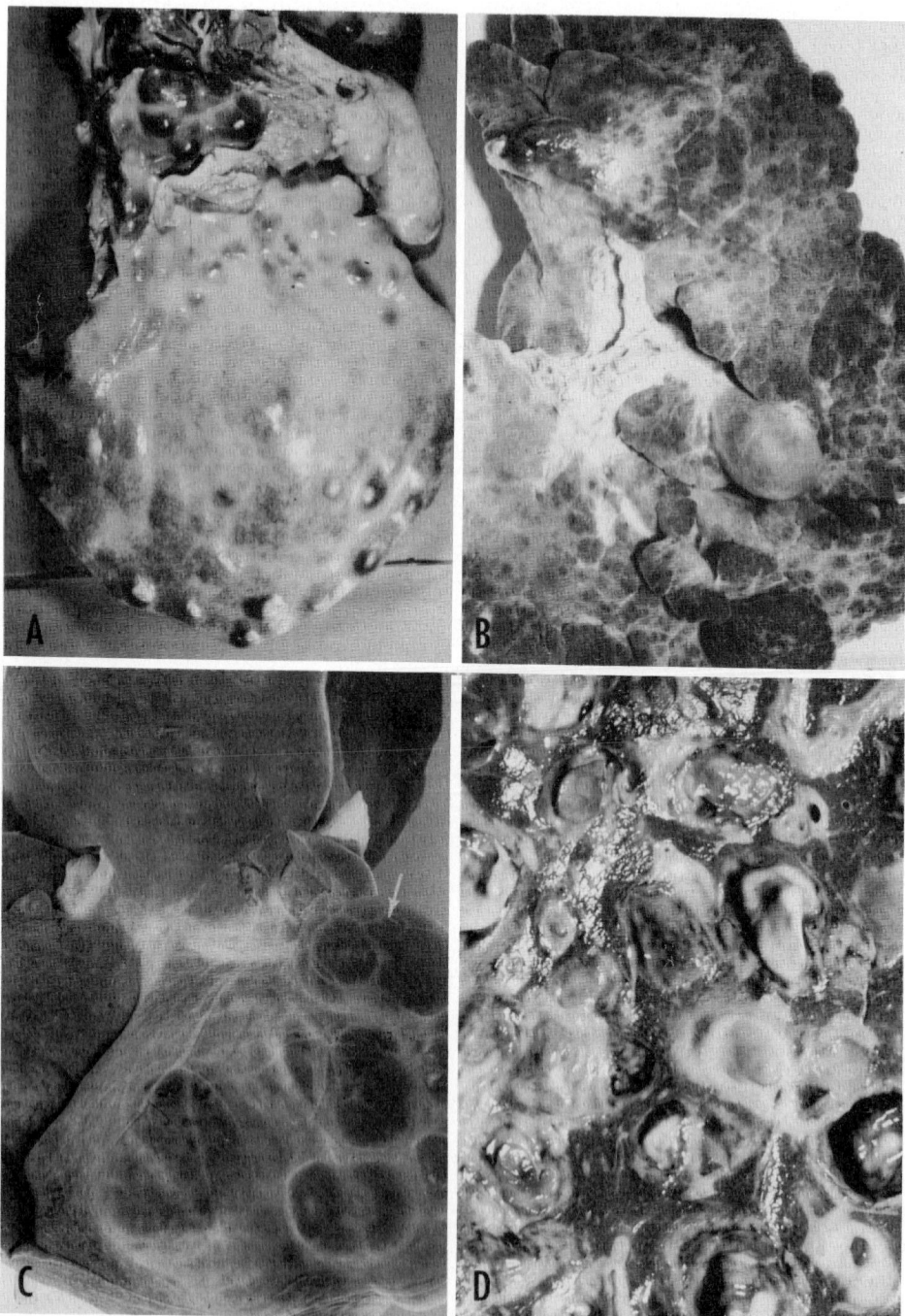

Fig. 23–23.   *A,* Cirrhosis of liver of a two-year-old steer. *B,* Cirrhosis, liver of a four-month-old pig. *C,* Large cysts in the liver of a ten-year-old female Spaniel dog. *D,* Abscesses in a bovine liver. Ordinarily they are much less numerous. (Courtesy of College of Veterinary Medicine, Iowa State University.)

of the retarded venous flow is ascites, the collection of edema fluid in the peritoneal cavity. Jaundice is the rule in biliary cirrhosis, but occurs only terminally in portal cirrhosis. On the other hand, interference with the portal circulation goes with portal but not biliary cirrhosis.

An unfortunate feature of cirrhosis is the fact that the presence of the proliferated fibrous tissue itself appears to have an irritant effect, stimulating the production of more fibrosis. Thus, the condition tends to continue to an eventually fatal termination even if the original cause is removed.

Anonymous: Report of board for classification and nomenclature of cirrhosis of the liver. Fifth Pan-American Congress of gastroenterology, La Habana, Cuba, Jan. 1956. Gastroenterol., 31:213–216, 1956.

Edmondson, H.A., and Peters, R.L.: Liver. In Pathology, 7th ed., edited by W.A.D. Anderson, and J.M. Kissane. St. Louis, Mosby Co., 1977, pp. 1321–1438.

Gaisford, W.D., and Zuidema, G.D.: Nutritional Laennec's cirrhosis in the Macaca mulatta monkey. J. Surg. Res., 5:200–206, 1965.

Giovonelli, N.E.: Estudio de una enfermedad in equinos con lesion de cirrhosis hepatica. Rev. Med. Vet. B. Aires, 42:173–185, 1961.

Smetana, H.F., and Greer, W.E.: Experimental study of the histiogenesis of nutritional cirrhosis in primates. Recent Adv. Gastroenterol., 3:25–29, 1967.

Van Es, L., Cantwell, L.R., Martin, H.M., and Kramer, J.: Nature and cause of the "walking disease" of northwestern Nebraska. Exp. Sta. Bull. No. 43, University of Nebraska, Lincoln, 1929.

Hepatic Abscesses and Related Conditions

Abscesses occasionally form in the liver of all species as the result of the entrance of microorganisms by any of the routes mentioned under Infectious Hepatitis. Important among these in newly born or young animals is the umbilical vein, which affords a route of metastasis or direct extension from the umbilicus. As the metastatic lesions develop in the liver, the primary site of infection at the umbilicus may even heal, without affecting the hepatic disease. Abscesses also occur in the livers of old dairy cows and others living under barn-yard conditions, these being the result of extension from the wounds of penetrating foreign bodies in the reticulum. Abscesses under any of the above circumstances are regularly due to the entrance of pyogenic cocci or other well-recognized pus-producing species. They practically always play a central role in the generalized and fatal disease. But the much more frequent and important cause of hepatic abscesses in veterinary medicine is a disease of fattening cattle and is of a much more subtle nature. Before discussing this, it is desirable to present briefly two disorders of the bovine liver which are often concurrent and probably predisposing to the former condition.

"Sawdust Livers." This descriptive bit of professional slang refers to bovine livers seen frequently (and condemned) by meat inspectors. They come most often from well-fattened young cattle which appear clinically to be in perfect health. The livers contain several or many minute yellowish foci of necrosis, as if the same number of granules of sawdust had been scattered over them. The necrotic foci, 1 or 2 mm in diameter, are scattered without grossly apparent relation to the lobular architecture. They consist of collections of hepatic epithelial cells in a state of coagulative necrosis or in the process of disappearing, mingled with or surrounded by a thin sprinkling of neutrophils and lymphocytes. They are often concomitant with telangiectasis and hepatic abscesses, and there is at least statistical evidence to link them etiologically with those conditions. It is suspected that "sawdust" foci may be the forerunners of telangiectatic spots and possibly of abscesses. It may be said with confidence, however, on purely numerical grounds that there are tremendous numbers of "sawdust" foci which never become abscesses. Vitamin E deficiency (which has been blamed for innumerable idiopathic lesions in most organs and tissues) has been suggested as the cause of "sawdust." Todd and Krook (1966) ex-

perimentally induced lesions similar to spontaneous "sawdust" using a diet high in polyunsaturated fatty acids and poor in protein, vitamin E and selenium.

Telangiectasis. This term denotes a dilatation of functioning blood vessels anywhere. In the liver, the lesion consists of a small group of sinusoidal capillaries within any part of a lobule which are greatly widened. The cells of the hepatic cords between the dilated sinusoids have partially or completely disappeared. Jarrett (1956) believes that the early lesion of telangiectasis consists of an accumulation of glycogen between the hepatic cell and the sinusoidal epithelium. When the glycogen penetrates the sinusoid its place is taken by blood, which erodes the column of hepatic cells. He feels there is evidence that absorption of hydrogen sulfide from the bowel may be responsible for the lesion. Grossly, the result is a dark red spot, irregular in shape, from one to several millimeters in diameter. Seen from the surface of the organ these spots tend to be slightly depressed. Appearances indicate that a telangiectatic spot may well represent a stage superseding the necrotic "sawdust" granule and, as stated above, the two often occur together in the same liver. However, telangiectasis is of some frequency not only in heavily fattened beef cattle, but also in old and debilitated cattle, some of which come to the autopsy room rather than the abattoir. While there is no detectable effect on the general health of the animal, telangiectatic livers are not passed for human food.

A similar lesion in the liver described under the term **peliosis hepatis** (*pelios* from Greek, meaning blue-black) has been described in cattle in Australia with "St. George disease" (Seawright and Francis, 1971). This disease is manifest by subcutaneous edema, particularly in the neck and brisket region. The lesions in the liver closely resemble telangiectasis described above. However, the two diseases may not be related, in spite of the similarity of the lesions. Peliosis hepatis has also been seen in a cat (Torry and Walton, 1975) due to unknown cause, and in rats infected with a specific (9H) virus (Bergs and Scotti, 1967). This lesion has also been associated in people with pulmonary tuberculosis, chronic wasting disease due to carcinomatosis, and in patients receiving therapeutic doses of androgens. Peliotic lesions have also been observed in mice after transplantation of ovarian or testicular tumors. In this species the lesions may be associated with hypervolemia.

Abscesses. Occasionally, an animal of the bovine or other species dies of abscesses of the liver, after a few days of acute but vague digestive symptoms. The liver of such an animal usually contains a dozen abscesses at least, often several times this number. Their cause is often, but not necessarily, apparent from other lesions revealed by the necropsy. But, as previously stated, the usual hepatic abscesses occur in heavily fattened cattle which are slaughtered in apparently perfect health. The incidence of these abscesses approximates 5% of the cattle slaughtered throughout the United States, reaches 10% in the Rocky Mountain area, and approaches 100% in some shipments from certain feedlots. Postmortem examination reveals no other abnormalities beyond, perhaps, the "sawdust" and telangiectasis just noted, possibly localized diaphragmatic adhesions over certain abscesses and, quite frequently, the ulcerative lesions of the rumen already described as bearing a noteworthy relation to these abscesses. Bacteriological studies have incriminated the necrophorus organism (which has received with the changing times the successive appellations of *Bacillus necrophorus, Actinomyces necrophorus,* and *Spherophorus necrophorus,* and which in Europe is very logically known as *Fusiformis necrophorus*). In nearly all cases in the United States, it is found in pure culture.

The number of abscesses in the liver of one of these animals may vary from one to many but a number between 3 and 8 is typical. In size, the abscesses range typically from 2 to 5 cm in diameter. We must hasten to explain that many, probably a majority, of these "liver abscesses" are not true abscesses but circumscribed areas of coagulative necrosis.

Observation has long suggested that the early lesion is one of coagulative necrosis (the usual result of infection with the necrophorus organism), and that the true abscesses consisting of encapsulated pus represent older processes. This is confirmed by the work of Jensen et al. (1954), who produced typical lesions by the experimental introduction of necrophorus organisms into the portal blood. They found the lesion to be entirely coagulative for the first 6 to 8 days, with a gradual change to pus commencing beneath the fibrous capsule, the development of which began at about the same time. The central mass of coagulated necrotic tissue continued to enlarge until the thirtieth day, but by the one hundredth day it had been completely replaced by pus. By this time, the capsule had grown to considerable thickness, consisting of mature fibrous tissue on the outside and immature fibrous tissue shading into reticulo-endothelial and individual mononuclear macrophages centrally. Polymorphonuclear neutrophils were fairly numerous surrounding the central necrotic area. It is thus seen that the "abscesses" are at first necrotic areas (nodular necroses of Hutyra and Marek, 1926), and later, chronic abscesses with the granulomatous reticulo-endothelioid type of reaction playing an important part. The fact that the abscesses eventually heal was also confirmed by Jensen's work, in which fibrous scars had replaced the abscesses at stages varying from 45 to 180 days after the inoculation. The scars themselves ultimately disappear.

As we have stressed, clinical disease is rarely associated with hepatic abscesses in cattle. Occasionally, however, depressed, emaciated cattle slaughtered for salvage are found to have hepatic abscesses, and there is little reason not to suspect that these abscesses lead to the chronic wasting condition. Erosion and perforation of the wall of the posterior vena cava with entrance of the bacteria-rich abscess contents into the circulation is a sporadic complication, which leads to sudden and unexpected death in an apparently healthy animal. Rubarth (1960), in a report of 56 cases with rupture into the posterior vena cava, described the abscesses as invariably present on the dorsal portion of the liver immediately ventral to the vena cava. Necropsy findings in such cases include emphysema, edema, and hemorrhages in the lungs, subendocardial and subepicardial petechiae, congestion of the spleen, and edema, hyperemia, and hemorrhage of lymph nodes. Bacterial emboli occlude capillaries in the lung, liver, kidney, and myocardium. *Corynebacterium pyogenes animalis* was the most frequent bacterial isolate in Rubarth's series of Swedish cattle.

Causes. It would be difficult indeed to explain these abscesses except as the result of hematogenous metastasis. Jensen has demonstrated that this metastasis is via the portal vein. While occasionally abscesses of the liver have been observed subsequent to a necrophorus infection such as foot-rot, these coincidences seem to have been accidental. An infection picked up by the peripheral venous circulation should reach the lungs and then be disseminated to all susceptible organs and tissues. While conceivably the lungs might not provide the ánaerobic environment needed by this organism, certainly other organs than the liver should receive their share of abscesses. Thus the absence of involvement elsewhere than in the liver is in conformity with Jensen's experimental findings. Smith (1944), at the suggestion of Gooch, was the first to call attention to ulcers of the rumen as a probable source of infection for the portal blood, and this theme has been further developed by Jensen and his colleagues (1954). The latter investigators have presented evidence strongly supporting the prevalent clinical impression that the ruminal disturbances accompany the highly concentrated grain diets of the fattening pen, and have also shown a relation to the suddenness of the change from pasturage or roughage to the ration high in concentrates. The exact mechanism by which the dietary indiscretions produce their pathological effects has not been elucidated, but the chain of causative events seems clear. In one report, a controlled study involved replacement of the roughage component of the diet with oak sawdust and resulted in disappearance of liver abscesses (Rothenbacher, et al., 1972).

Andersen, A.C.: The pathogenesis of telangiectasis in the bovine liver. Am. J. Vet. Res., 16:27–34, 1955.

Bergs, V.V., and Scotti, T.M.: Virus-induced peliosis hepatis in rats. Science, 158:377–378, 1967.

Getty, R.: The histopathology of a focal hepatitis and of its termination ("sawdust" and "telang") in cattle. Am. J. Vet. Res., 7:437–449, 1946.

Huytra, F., and Marek, J.: Special Pathology and Therapeutics of the Diseases of Domestic Animals. 3rd Am. edition. Translated by J.R. Mohler and A. Eichhorn. Chicago, Alexander Eger, 1926. Vol. II. pp. 428, 430, 438, 448.

Jarrett, W.F.H.: Bovine hepatic disease. Vet. Rec., 68:825, 1956.

Jensen, R., Frey, P.R., Cross, F., and Connell, W.E.: Telangiectasis, "sawdust," and abscesses in the liver of beef cattle. J. Am. Vet. Med. Assoc., 110:256–261, 1947.

Jensen, R., Flint, J.C., and Griner, L.A.: Experimental hepatic necrobacillosis in beef cattle. Am. J. Vet. Res., 15:5–14, 1954.

Rothenbacher, H., El-Sabban, F.F., Long, T.A., and Baumgardt, B.R.: Prevention of stomach and liver pathology in feeder steers by sawdust roughage replacer. Vet. Med. Small Anim. Clin., 67:1127–1131, 1972.

Rubarth, S.: Hepatic and subphrenic abscesses in cattle with rupture into vena cava caudalis. Acta Vet. Scand., 1:363–382, 1960.

Seawright, A.A., and Francis, J.: Peliosis hepatis—a specific liver lesion in St. George disease of cattle. Aust. Vet. J., 47:91–99, 1971.

Smith, H.A.: Ulcerative lesions of the bovine rumen and their possible relation to hepatic abscesses. Am. J. Vet. Res., 5:234–243, 1944.

Todd, G.C., and Krook, L.: Nutritional hepatic necrosis in beef cattle. "Sawdust liver." Pathol. Vet., 3:379–400, 1966.

Torry, J.M., and Walton, R.M.: Peliosis hepatis in a cat. Br. Vet. J., 131:716–719, 1975.

Hepatosis Dietetica

Hepatosis dietetica is a disorder of swine characterized by massive liver necrosis. All evidence indicates it is caused by vitamin E: selenium deficiency, and is often associated with other lesions of this deficiency complex to include: yellow fat disease, necrosis of skeletal muscle and myocardium, and ulceration of the nonglandular stomach.

Parasitic Diseases of the Liver

Echinococcus or Hydatid Cysts

Echinococcus or hydatid cysts occur in the livers of the farm animals (and man) in those countries where the corresponding adult tapeworm, Echinococcus granulosus (Taenia echinococcus), is prevalent in dogs. Unilocular cysts commonly reach a diameter of 4 or 5 cm, developing over a period of months or years. During the first several months, while the cystic embryo is only a few millimeters in diameter, the surrounding tissue presents a considerable reaction, with reticulo-endothelial, fibroblastic, and foreign-body giant cells, and a marked infiltration of eosinophils. The more mature cyst is tightly surrounded by a dense fibrous capsule, but with little evidence of a more vigorous reaction. The cyst itself has an outer zone of hyaline, non-nucleated material approaching 1 mm in thickness, beneath which is an inner layer of embryonal-appearing cells. From the latter, unless the cyst is sterile, which is not unusual, several minute papillary structures project into the clear fluid of the lumen. These are in the process of development into brood capsules with very thin-walled vesicles whose inner lining produces embryonal scolices some 100 microns in diameter. Typical hooklets can (with patience and good fortune) be demonstrated in the scolex, but the echinococcus cyst can be differentiated from other cysts by its general structure.

If the host lives several years, the cyst dies and degenerates into a pulpy mass, of which the capsule, at least, becomes calcified. Occasionally in cattle (and man), the young cyst, for reasons which are in doubt (possibly the parasite is of a different species), pursues an abnormal form of growth, failing to attain a diameter of more than, perhaps, a centimeter, but producing a spreading mass of new subsidiary cysts. Known as an **alveolar cyst**, this formation grows indefinitely in spite of a surrounding granulomatous and fibrous reaction, and parts of it may even be carried by hematogenous metastasis to establish a new growth in some other organ. A moderate eosinophilia (6%) usually exists during the active phases of hydatidosis. Humoral antibodies of diagnostic value are also produced.

Liver Flukes

These parasites of sheep, cattle, and, rarely, horses and other species include the common *Fasciola hepatica (Distomum hepaticum)* and some other species of flatworms *(Trematoda)*. The adult flukes live in the lumens of the intrahepatic bile ducts and reach considerable size, for example, 2 by 1 by 0.2 cm in the case of *F. hepatica*. Before attaining their permanent domicile, the flukes, as larvae of gradually increasing size, migrate through the hepatic tissue, in many cases having penetrated the perihepatic capsule from the peritoneal cavity. In severe infestations, the local damage from the migrating larvae results in necrosis and considerable escape of blood, and abscesses or other secondary infections are possible.

However, in the average case, it is not until the flukes approach their mature size in the bile ducts that clinical signs appear. These include cachexia, weakness, constipation, jaundice, anemia, and edema ("bottle-jaw," ascites). The usual lesions in the liver are those which result from the mechanical and toxic irritation of these large parasites. The lumen of the duct is necessarily dilated as the fluke grows, the wall is greatly thickened by proliferation of

encircling fibrous tissue, and there is a limited infiltration of lymphocytes and eosinophils. The fibrosis extends for a short distance among the liver lobules, but does not constitute a true cirrhosis. Extensive calcification of the injured walls is common. The lumen of the duct becomes more or less completely closed by the body of the fluke and an accumulation of amorphous, blood-stained exudate and debris. The jaundice which develops in severe infestations is thus explainable on an obstructive basis but may be in part hemolytic, since hemolytic toxins are produced. If the patient survives, the flukes die, and pass out with the bile after about 9 months. Severe infestations are fatal but, in spite of the dark picture here portrayed and various other possible complications that might be mentioned, the usual outcome is that the animal fattens sufficiently well to go to slaughter, where its liver is condemned because of a number of flukes. In many parts of the country, as many as 25% of sheep's livers are condemned for this reason; in cattle, the liver condemnations vie in number with those made for abscesses.

Fascioloides magna, a rather rare fluke of large size found in the livers of ruminants in northern North America and northern Europe, causes the deposition of large amounts of a deep black pigment in the liver and hepatic lymph node. The nature of the pigment appears not to have been determined.

Dicrocoelium dendriticum in cattle produces changes similar to those induced by *Fasciola magna,* but less severe. Many other flukes infest animals but they are usually of little clinical or pathological significance.

Other Parasites

In addition to the adults of *Capillaria hepatica* in monkeys, dogs, and rats, a number of parasites wander through the liver during their larval migrations, including the kidney worm of swine *(Stephanurus dentatus),* which leaves slight scars on the visceral surface, but the only one requiring much further attention is the ascarid of swine. It is known that these larvae pass through the liver, as well as through the lungs. It is common to see livers of pigs from 3 to 10 months of age in which the diaphragmatic and other surfaces bear poorly outlined, diffuse white spots from 1 to 3 cm in diameter. These spots have no definite limits nor typical shapes, appearing possibly as if they had been applied with a paint brush. Microscopic sections show that the white spots consist of a thin layer of excess fibrous tissue underlying the capsule and extending along the interlobular septa for a depth equal to the width of two or three lobules. These scars are commonly attributed to damage done by larval ascarids. If anyone has proved or disproved this belief, we have overlooked the fact. Tentatively, we accept this explanation of this frequent lesion.

Other hepatic parasites include *Eimeria stiedae, Hepatocystis kochi*, and schistosomes.

Harcourt, R., and Costema, P.: Hepatic ascariasis in lambs. Vet. Rec., 92:482–483, 1973.

Miscellaneous Hepatic Disorders

Cysts

Cysts, other than hydatid cysts, are assumed to represent a congenital malformation in which one or more primitive bile ducts lack an outlet or connection with the main biliary system. They are lined with cuboidal epithelium, but contain a clear fluid having little resemblance to bile. Solitary or multiple, they are of varying sizes, even in the same liver, diameters of 2 to 5 cm being common. They appear to be less rare in dogs, cats, and swine than in other domestic species. While considered to be congenital, they are not necessarily encountered in the young. Most often they are found incidentally upon death from some other cause. The hepatic parenchyma suffers heavily from pressure atrophy and

pressure necrosis when the cysts are numerous and large.

In poisoning by chlorinated naphthalenes, the hyperplastic epithelium of the intrahepatic bile ducts occasionally becomes so irregular as to form a series of cystic spaces as much as 5 or 6 mm in diameter along the wall of the duct.

Congestion

Congestion of the liver is frequent. If acute, it is usually the consequence of terminal myocardial failure, which occurs in many diseases. Chronic hepatic congestion is also traceable with rare exceptions to cardiac disease, either myocardial or valvular (right-sided insufficiency or stenosis). A striking example of chronic hepatic congestion due to myocardial weakness is the so-called "brisket-disease" which cattle have at high altitudes. Another important example exists in gossypol poisoning in swine. Chronic pericarditis as seen in the "traumatic" pericarditis from a penetrating foreign body in bovines leads to similar congestion in the liver. Rarely, pulmonary emphysema and fibrosis cause similar impairment of the venous circulation.

Grossly, the congested liver is dark red, somewhat swollen with rounded edges, and considerable blood escapes from the severed vessels when it is incised. Microscopically, the dilated sinusoids indicate congestion whether or not they are filled with erythrocytes when examined. Chronic passive congestion leads to the fibrous proliferation around the central veins which has been called central cirrhosis. It also leads to anoxic centrilobular necrosis, the spaces left by the destroyed cells being filled by blood. As a result, the centers of the lobules are very dark. Frequently, the less severely anoxic cells in the peripheral parts of the lobule suffer from fatty degeneration, hence are lighter in color. There is thus produced a fine sprinkling of dark brown and gray reminiscent of the outside of a nutmeg. Such a liver is called, by professional tradition, a **"nut-meg liver."**

Infarction

The rarity of infarcts in the liver has already been pointed out and attributed to the double blood supply of that organ.

Pigmentation

Under this heading, the accumulation of dissolved (bilirubin) or precipitated (bile pigment) biliary coloring matter first comes to mind. Carotenosis must be differentiated from this discoloration as seen grossly. The liver is the most common site of the pigment of brown atrophy. It harbors large amounts of iron-containing pigment in hemachromatosis. Melanosis is occasionally seen in the liver. The blood-containing spots in telangiectasis are almost as black, when seen grossly, as if they contained melanin, but are depressed and shrunken. Infestations with *Fascioloides magna* and schistosomes are associated with a peculiar black pigmentation. Arias, et al. (1964) have described a disorder in sheep similar to the Dubin-Johnson syndrome of man which is associated with a peculiar melanin-like pigment in hepatocytes. A similar disorder has been described in howler monkeys (Maruffo, et al., 1966). All these conditions are discussed under "Pigments" in Chapter 3. In cadavers which have undergone considerable postmortem autolysis, that part of the liver which has lain in contact with the gallbladder is often stained a deep green or yellow, especially in the dog.

Hyperbilirubinemia from inherited or acquired causes has been described elsewhere.

Hepatic Disease and Encephalopathy

The association of hepatic disorders and nervous signs or symptoms has been recorded in medical and nonmedical literature for many years. The offending material was often considered to be retained bile (cholemia), an idea which has not been supported by evidence. Bile seems only to be harmful to the nervous system in neonatal infants and animals (see kernicterus). Clearly, however, hepatic insufficiency is associated with nervous signs, varying from hepatic coma to malaise, disorientation, and uncontrolled nervous stimulation.

Elevated levels of ammonia (NH_3) in the blood and of glutamine in the cerebrospinal fluid have been associated with nervous signs and spongy degeneration of the brain (status spongiosus). Experimental poisoning of sheep with the pyrrolizidine alkaloid lasiocarpine results in severe necrosis of hepatic cells. This hepatic failure leads to accumulation of ammonia in the blood and is believed to be the principal cause of encephalopathy (Hooper, 1972; Hooper, et al., 1974). Similar signs and lesions (spongy degeneration) may be produced in the brain of sheep by intravenous infusion of ammonia. It must be kept in mind that spongy degeneration is difficult to distinguish from histologic artefact, especially in brains of young animals. Ammonia is likely to be at least one of the causative factors in encephalopathy due to hepatic failure. This appears to be the case in man and many other species. Several other toxic substances found in plants, such as *Senecio quadridentata* (pyrrolizidine), *Senecio jacobaea*, *Crotalaria retusa*, and *Echium lycopsis*, have been shown to produce hepatic failure and encephalopathy (Hooper, 1972).

The mechanism involved in this increase in ammonia in the blood is believed to be a failure of liver cells to metabolize ammonia, received by way of the portal vein, into urea. It is believed that glutamine may be a byproduct of ammonia metabolism in the brain; alpha-ketoglutarate, an intermediate metabolite of the citric acid cycle, combines with ammonia to form glutamic acid or glutamate. Elevated glutamate, on this basis, appears in increased amounts in the cerebrospinal fluid of animals poisoned with ammonia.

Situations other than those involving destruction or malfunction of liver cells have been shown to have the effect of increasing ammonia in the peripheral blood. These include congenital anomalies of the portal vein such as (1) persistent patency of the fetal ductus venosus, (2) atresia of the portal vein with portosystemic shunts, (3) anomalous course of portal to azygos vein, and (5) drainage of portal vein and caudal vena cava into the ayzgos vein. These anomalies have been demonstrated in dogs by angioradiographic studies and are shown to result in ascites and signs of disturbances of the central nervous system (Ewing, et al., 1974; Cornelius, et al., 1975). An inherited deficiency of arginosuccinate synthetase, a urea cycle enzyme, also has been shown in two dogs to result in hyperammonemia in the absence of portal venous shunts bypassing the liver (Strombeck, et al., 1975).

Nuclear Inclusions

Nuclear inclusions of a crystalline nature called *acidophilic crystalline intranuclear (ACN) inclusions* are frequently encoun-

tered in hepatocytes and renal tubular epithelium of dogs. They are usually rectangular, up to 15 μ long, and distort the nuclear membrane. Although their significance is not known, they are believed to be crystallized protein and are not related to viral infections. Invagination of cytoplasm into the nucleus produces peculiar membrane-bound intranuclear inclusions. They are encountered most frequently in the hepatocytes of aged rodents but may also be found in dogs and monkeys. In addition to the liver, cytoplasmic invaginations are occasionally seen in other tissues, such as corpus luteum, interstitial cell tumors of the testes, and adenocarcinoma of the lung. Normal cytoplasmic organelles can be demonstrated within the inclusion with electron microscopy.

Torsion

Torsion of lobes of the liver occurs occasionally, especially in rats, mice, and rabbits. The lesion is usually encountered at necropsy and is recognized by the ischemic necrosis of an entire lobe of the liver. The nature of the lesion is usually evident from

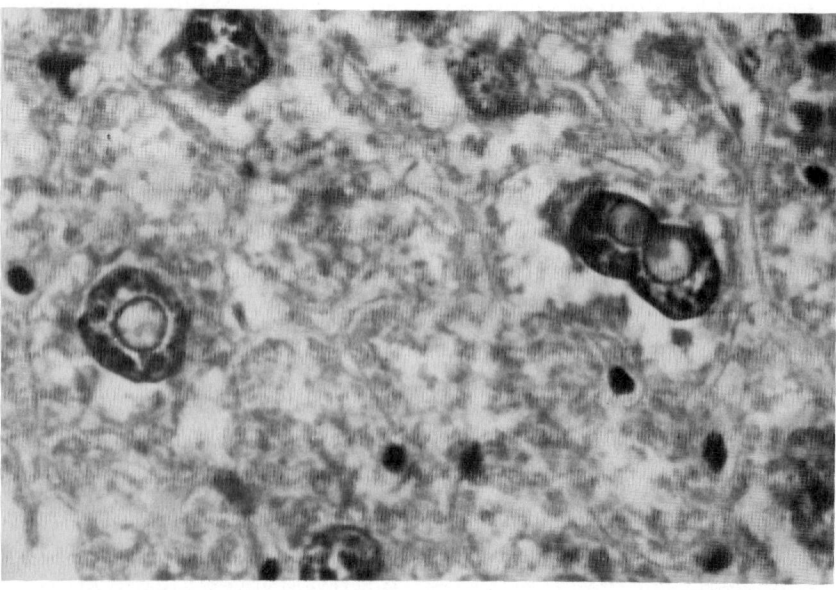

Fig. 23–24. Cytoplasmic invaginations into hepatocyte nuclei in a mouse. (Courtesy of Animal Research Center, Harvard Medical School.)

the pregnant uterus, mesentery, or omentum twisted around the lobe at the base of the ischemic portion. It is not usually a lethal lesion.

Arias, I., et al.: Black liver disease in Corriedale sheep: a new mutation affecting hepatic excretory function. J. Clin. Invest., 43:1249–1250, 1964.

Brobst, D.F., and Schall, W.D.: Needle biopsy of the canine liver and correlation of laboratory data with histopathologic observations. J. Am. Vet. Med. Assoc., 161:382–388, 1972.

Cornelius, L.M., et al.: Anomalous portosystemic anastomoses associated with chronic hepatic insufficiency in six young dogs. J. Am. Vet. Med. Assoc., 167:220–228, 1975.

Doige, C.E., and Furneaux, R.W.: Liver disease and intrahepatic portal hypertension in the dog. Can. Vet. J., 16:209–214, 1975.

Ewing, G.O., Suter, P.F., and Bailey, C.S.: Hepatic insufficiency associated with congenital anomalies of the portal vein in dogs. J. Am. Anim. Hosp. Assoc., 10:463–476, 1974.

Fischer, J.E.: Hepatic coma in cirrhosis, portal hypertension, and following portacaval shunt: its etiologies and the current status of its treatment. Arch. Surg., 108:325–336, 1974.

Hooper, P.T.: Spongy degeneration in the brain in relation to hepatic disease and ammonia toxicity in domestic animals. Vet. Rec., 90:37–38, 1972.

Hooper, P.T., Best, S.M., and Murray, D.R.: Hyperammonaemia and spongy degeneration of the brain in sheep affected with hepatic necrosis. Res. Vet. Sci., 16:216–222, 1974.

Maruffo, C.A., et al.: Pigmentary liver disease in Howler monkeys. Am. J. Pathol., 49:445–456, 1966.

Schleger, A.V.: Histopathology of melanotic sheep liver. 1. Histology and nonenzymic histochemistry. 2. Enzymic histochemistry. Aust. Vet. J., 46:48–54 and 55–61, 1970.

Strombeck, D.R., Weiser, M.G., and Kaneko, J.J.: Hyperammonemia and hepatic encephalopathy in the dog. J. Am. Vet. Med. Assoc., 166:1105–1108, 1975.

Strombeck, D.R., Meyer, D.J., and Freedland, R.A.: Hyperammonemia due to a urea cycle enzyme deficiency in two dogs. J. Am. Vet. Med. Assoc., 166:1109–1111, 1975.

Weisbroth, S.H.: Torsion of the caudate lobe of the liver in the domestic rabbit (Oryctolagus). Vet. Pathol., 12:13–15, 1975.

Neoplasms of the Liver

Liver cell adenoma (hepatocellular adenoma) has been described in domestic animals and some laboratory and exotic species. These tumors are sharply circumscribed, usually single and tan-colored, and compress, but do not invade, adjacent liver tissue. They may reach a large size but do not metastasize. Most have a trabecular or acinar pattern made up of cells resembling normal hepatocytes, but often contain glycogen and fat droplets. Well differentiated adenomas may be difficult to distinguish from normal liver except that they have no portal triads. In young animals, tumors have been seen in which extramedullary hematopoiesis was a conspicuous feature.

Intrahepatic bile duct adenoma (or cystadenoma) is a circumscribed tumor made up of irregular-sized tubules lined with cuboidal epithelium resembling epithelium of intrahepatic bile ducts. The stroma may be conspicuous. The cystic variety is somewhat more frequent. Cysts containing clear fluid may vary in size and the lining cells may be flattened. Mitoses are rarely seen.

Cholangiocarcinoma or intrahepatic bile duct carcinoma, is a malignant tumor made up of epithelial cells resembling those of the intrahepatic bile ducts. These tumors may occur in any part of the liver and commonly spread along the biliary tract, sometimes into the liver capsule. Metastasis may occur by spread to the liver serosa and via the lymphatics to the lungs. The tumor cells are cuboidal or columnar and have clear or granular cytoplasm. They usually form small acini, but when less differentiated may appear in solid cords with rare formation of lumina. Papillary arrangement of tumor cells may be seen, and mucous secretion in some cases may lead to accumulation of collections of mucin. Bile may occasionally be seen in tumor acini but is not recognizable in cells.

In some cases, accompanying proliferation of connective tissue (desmoplasia) gives the tumors a grossly apparent, dense white fibrous consistency. A few cases containing squamous as well as adenosarcomatous elements are reported, presumably due to metaplasia of adenomatous to squamous epithelial tumor cells.

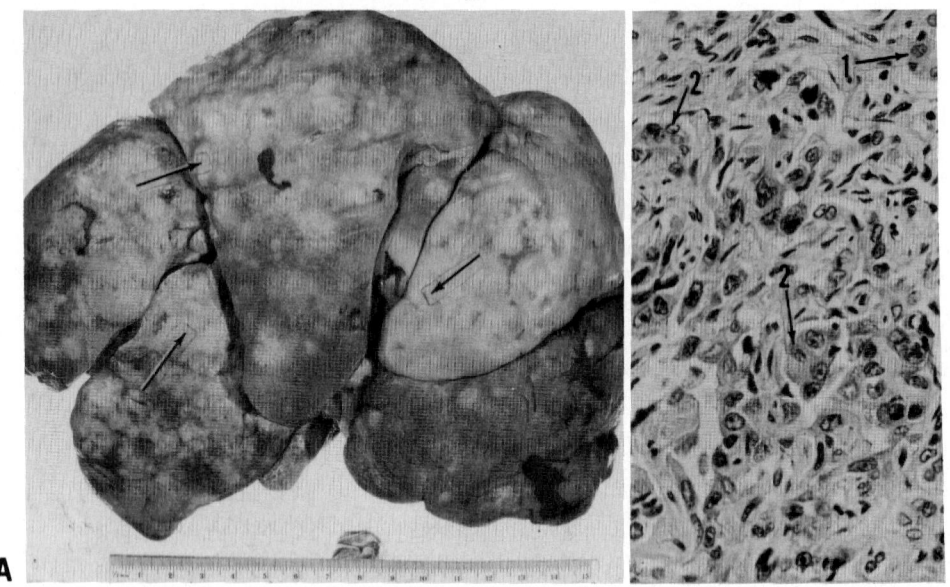

Fig. 23–25. *A,* Adenocarcinoma of intrahepatic bile ducts, liver of a fifteen-year-old male Beagle. Masses of tumor (arrows) enlarge the liver and elevate the capsule. *B,* Photomicrograph of the neoplasm in *A* (× 300). The neoplastic cells form structures resembling bile ducts (*1*) in some places, but in others they are undifferentiated (*2*). (Courtesy of Armed Forces Institute of Pathology.) Contributor: Dr. D.N. Bader.

Hepatocellular carcinoma (liver cell carcinoma) is made up of cells that resemble liver cells, but vary considerably in degree of differentiation. The cells may be arranged in trabecular or acinar patterns or mixtures of both. In some cases plates of cells may be a few cells thick and separated by sinusoids. In differentiated parts, the tumor cells are polyhedral and clearly resemble hepatocytes, but no hepatic triads are present. The tumor compresses and may invade adjacent liver. Many cells are undifferentiated in some tumors, with variation in size, tinctoral features, and cytoplasmic content such as fat and glycogen. Mitoses and enlarged nuclei may be frequent. Some are so undifferentiated that the tumor cells are difficult to identify as coming from liver cells. Occasionally, acini and cysts are formed. These tumors may reach rather large size before spreading by metastasis to hepatic lymph nodes and lung. An association between hepatocellular carcinoma and biliary cirrhosis due to

fascioliasis has been made by Vitovec (1974).

Hepatoblastoma is an unusual type, made up of granular cells which resemble the smaller hepatocytes of the fetus. Nests of hematopoietic cells always accompany this tumor and are essential to the diagnosis.

Hemangiomas may also be primary in the liver, occurring as benign, circumscribed, solitary or multiple nodules of vascular architecture with a fine supporting stroma between endothelial-lined vascular channels. These tumors may compress adjacent liver cells, but do not invade or metastasize.

Hemangiosarcoma (hemangioendothelioma, angiosarcoma) is a malignant vascular tumor with many immature, pleomorphic, endothelial cells which form blood-filled vascular spaces or solid masses of cells. The nuclei are hyperchromatic, often in mitosis, and closely packed. Hemorrhage frequently occurs within these tumors and ischemic necrosis is apt to occur. Hemangiosarcomas are clearly invasive and tend to metastasize to the lung. Rupture into the peritoneal sac may result in implantations of tumor on the peritoneal surface.

Carcinoid tumor of the liver may also occur as a rare primary neoplasm. This tumor is identified by the argentaffin granules in the cells, similar to these tumors found in the gastrointestinal tract.

Secondary neoplasms of the liver of animals are in general more frequent than primary. Lymphosarcoma and mast cell tumors may be either primary or metastatic in the liver. The portal vein provides the means for malignant tumors of the intestine and pancreas to metastasize to the liver. A pancreatic adenocarcinoma, metastatic in the liver, may present some difficulties in distinguishing it from a primary adenocarcinoma of intrahepatic bile ducts. The presence of the tumor in the pancreas is helpful, and one can clearly distinguish an adenocarcinoma of acinar pancreas by identifying zymogen granules in the cytoplasm of tumor cells. Tumors, which implant and grow in the peritoneal sac after escaping from spleen (hemangiosarcoma), intestine (adenocarcinoma), or ovary (adenocarcinoma), may randomly grow on the liver capsule and possibly invade the liver parenchyma.

Ashley, L.M.: Animal model: liver cell carcinoma in rainbow trout. Am. J. Pathol., 72:345–348, 1973.

Blumberg, B.S., et al.: The relation of infection with hepatitis B agent to primary hepatic carcinoma. Am. J. Pathol., 81:669–682, 1975.

Clark, J.D., and Olsen, R.E.: Hepatoma in a Mangabey (Cercocebus atys). Vet. Pathol., 10:89–93, 1973.

Dunning, W.F., and Curtis, M.R.: Malignancy induced by Cysticercus fasciolaris: its dependence on age of the host when infested. Am. J. Cancer, 37:312–328, 1939.

Dunning, W.F., and Curtis, M.R.: Multiple peritoneal sarcoma in rats from intraperitoneal injection of washed, ground Taenia larvae. Cancer Res., 6:668–670, 1946.

Feldman, B.F., Strafuss, A.C., and Gabbert, N.: Bile duct carcinoma in the cat: three case reports. Feline Pract., 6:33–39, 1976.

Gyorkey, F., et al.: Experimental carcinoma of liver in macaque monkeys exposed to diethylnit-

rosamine and hepatitis B virus. J. Natl. Cancer Inst., 59:1451–1467, 1977.

Hueper, W.C., and Payne, W.W.: Observations on the occurrence of hepatomas in rainbow trout. J. Natl. Cancer Inst., 27:1123–1142, 1961.

Jeffcott, L.B.: Primary liver-cell carcinoma in a young Thoroughbred horse. J. Pathol., 97:394–397, 1969.

Johnstone, A.C.: Two cases of hepatic mastocytoma in sheep. Vet. Pathol., 9:159–163, 1972.

Kanahara, H., Soga, J., and Tazawa, K.: Hepatic tumors of the mastomys. Spontaneous and experimental production: a preliminary report. Acta Med. Biol., 20:91–96, 1972.

Krishna, L., Chattopadhyay, S.K., Iyer, P.K.R., and Sharma, R.M.: A pathological study of hepatocellular carcinoma in sheep. Indian J. Anim. Sci., 43:34–37, 1973.

Manktelow, B.W.: Hepatoblastomas in sheep. J. Pathol. Bact., 89:711–714, 1965.

Marier, R.J., Cook, J.E., Samuelson, M.L., and Kennedy, G.A.: Intrahepatic bile duct carcinoma with metastasis to bone in a dog. Vet. Pathol., 14:516–518, 1977.

McClure, H.M., Chang, J., and Golarz, M.N.: Cholangiocarcinoma in a Margay (Felis wiedii). Vet. Pathol., 14:510–512, 1977.

Ponomarkov, V., and Mackey, L.J.: International histological classification of tumours of domestic animals. XIII. Tumours of the liver and biliary system. Bull. WHO, 53:187–194, 1976.

Salmon, W.D., and Newberne, P.M.: Occurrence of hepatomas in rats fed diets containing peanut meal as a major source of protein. Cancer Res., 23:571–575, 1963.

Squire, R.A., and Levitt, M.H.: Report of a workshop on classification of specific hepatocellular lesions in rats. Cancer Res., 35:3214–3223, 1975.

Strafuss, A.C., Vestwever, J.G.E., Njoku, C.O., and Ivoghli, B.: Bile duct carcinoma in cattle: three case reports. Am. J. Vet. Res., 34:1203–1206, 1973.

Strafuss, A.C.: Bile duct carcinoma in dogs. J. Am. Vet. Med. Assoc., 169:429, 1976.

Strombeck, D.R.: Clinicopathologic features of primary and metastatic neoplastic disease of the liver in dogs. J. Am. Vet. Med. Assoc., 173:267–269, 1978.

Vitovec, J.: "Hepatozelluläre karzinome beim rind und ihre beziehung zur biliären zirrhose fasciolären ursprungs." Vet. Pathol., 11:548–557, 1974.

Wettimuny, S.G. de S.: Primary liver tumors of cattle in Ceylon. J. Comp. Pathol., 79:355–362, 1969.

Williams, A.O.: Ultrastructure of liver cell carcinoma in Macaca mulatta monkey. Exp. Mol. Pathol., 13:359–361, 1970.

Woodruff, J.M., and Johnson, D.K.: Hepatic hemangioendothelioma in a Rhesus monkey. Pathol. Vet., 5:327–332, 1968.

GALLBLADDER

Cholecystitis and Cholangitis

Inflammation of the gallbladder (cholecystitis) or common bile duct (cholangitis) may result from blood-borne metastasis of infectious organisms or by their ascent from the duodenum. Such infections are rarely recognized in animals. Cholecystitis may also result from the action of retained and concentrated bile or from the presence of choleliths. Experimentally, cholecystitis is claimed to have been produced in poultry and dogs by diets high in fat and low in protein, but this has no known clinical significance. Any of the ordinary types of exudative inflammation are possible, but the usual kinds are mucous (catarrhal), characterized by excessive secretion of the mucous glands, or serous, characterized by inflammatory edema. Leukocytic infiltration is seldom extensive.

More puzzling to the student may be the proper interpretation of the degree of fullness of the organ and the character of its contents. Bile is secreted continually and stored in the gallbladder (except in the horse, rat, and other species that have no gallbladder), to be discharged when a full meal begins to reach the intestine (action of cholecystokinin). Throughout the period of storage, water is resorbed from the bile by the mucosa, and concurrently the mucous glands scattered through the mucous membrane add a small amount of mucus, so that the organ tends slowly to become distended. At the same time, fluid continues to be resorbed, leaving the solids. These, together with the slow accumulation of mucus, make the bile more and more viscous. A catarrhal cholecystitis sometimes coexists, resulting in a markedly increased flow of mucus. With rare exceptions, such as obstruction of the common duct, these mechanisms and failure of the sick animal to eat explain the enlarged gallbladders and viscous, "inspissated bile" so often given prominence in descriptions of disease.

If the ingress of bile to the gallbladder is prevented by swelling of the cystic duct or

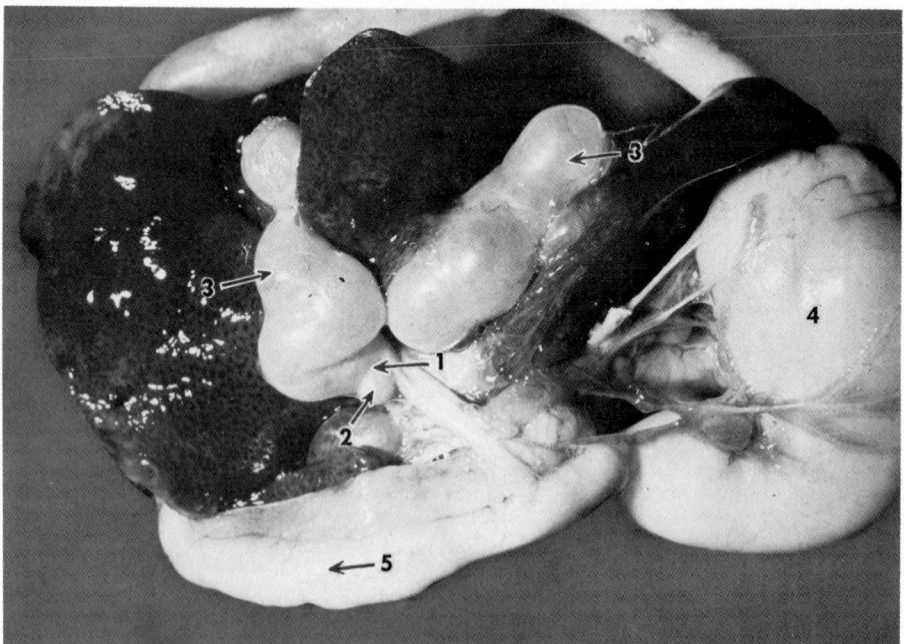

Fig. 23–26. Obstruction of the gallbladder, presumably congenital, in a ten-week-old female Siamese kitten. The obstruction (1) was related to a small adenoma (2). The distended gallbladder was double (3) in this animal, an occasional occurrence in this species. The stomach (4) and duodenum (5) were not affected. (Courtesy of Angell Memorial Animal Hospital.)

other obstruction, the epithelium of the gallbladder secretes a clear watery fluid, filling the cavity with what has been called "white bile."

Cystic Hyperplasia

Also known as cystic mucinous hypertrophy, papillary adenomatous hypertrophy, and other descriptive phrases, this lesion is frequently encountered in dogs. The mucosa of the gallbladder is thickened by numerous fronds and cysts lined by squamous to columnar epithelium. The epithelial cells and the cysts contain mucin which stains blue in hematoxylin- and eosin-stained tissue sections. Grossly, the wall of the gallbladder is thickened and numerous multilocular, gelatinous, translucent cysts of varying size are evident. The cause and significance of the lesion are not known. Hyperplastic cholecystitis has been observed in the gallbladder of cattle in connection with liver fluke (*Fasciola gigantica* and *F. hepatica*) infection.

Diverticulosis, probably not related to hyperplasia, has been observed in the Rhesus monkey.

Cheema, A.H.: Adenomatous cholecystitis in cattle with chronic fascioliasis. Vet. Pathol., *11*:407–416, 1974.

Kovatch, R.M., Hildebrandt, P.K., and Marcus, L.C.: Cystic mucinous hypertrophy of the mucosa of the gallbladder in the dog. Pathol. Vet., *2*:574–584, 1965.

Rosenquist, C.J., and Silverman, S.: Diverticulosis of gallbladder in a Rhesus monkey. J. Am. Vet. Radiol. Soc., *19*:38–40, 1978.

Yoshida, T., et al.: Plasma alkaline phosphatase and experimental cholestasis of squirrel monkeys (*Saimiri sciureus*). Acta Hepat. Jpn., *18*:913–918, 1977.

Witzleben, C.L., Buck, B.E., Schnaufer, L., and Brzosco, W.J.: Studies on the pathogenesis of biliary atresia. Lab. Invest., *38*:525–532, 1978.

Cholelithiasis

Biliary calculi, gallstones, or choleliths, as they may be called, occur with rarity in all of the usual domestic species, having been reported even in the chicken. They appear to be less rare in bovines than in the other farm or pet animals. They may be of minute size, like grains of sand, several hundred having been found in the bile ducts of a horse, or they may be few or single, a length of 11.5 cm having been reported. Depending upon their composition, three types of stones are known, one being the cholesterol stone which is large, white, light in weight and contains glistening crystals of cholesterol radially arranged. This cholesterol stone has been seen frequently in squirrel monkeys and baboons maintained on diets containing elevated levels of cholesterol.

The second type, called the "pigment stone," consists of dried and precipitated bilirubin as its principal ingredient. These stones are almost black in color, friable and usually small but multiple in a given patient. Hilton Smith has observed gallstones of this type up to 2 cm in diameter in cattle and swine. The third type is a heavy, pale stone consisting largely of calcium phosphate and carbonate. These are less common, but such a stone 2.5 cm in diameter has been seen from a bovine animal.

The usual gallstones, however, are composites of these several ingredients, commonly being yellow to dark brown in color, light in weight, somewhat fragile, sometimes concentrically laminated, and often faceted, that is, flattened on each of several sides where the stones lay side by side in the gallbladder. Commonly all the stones are of nearly identical size, presumably because they are of the same age.

Cause. The cause of gallstones of this, the ordinary type, is almost without question cholecystitis of infectious origin. Such infectious processes are by no means frequent in animals and have been studied only occasionally, but the pyocyaneus organism (*Pseudomonas aeruginosa*) has been isolated from cases of cholelithiasis in sheep. The mechanism of formation is doubtless similar to that responsible for urinary calculi, solid particles of dead cells or inspissated material serving as the starting point for a process of crystallization. In the case of gallstones, however, changes in the water content and colloidal state are certainly of considerable importance. It is probable that some constituents of bile are reabsorbed in the event of biliary stasis more easily than others, leaving highly desiccated residues.

Many gallstones are "silent," that is, produce no signs. Others, in man, cause episodes of severe pain, dyspepsia and nausea, and other gastric symptoms based upon the closely related innervation of both gallbladder and stomach. The accompanying cholecystitis is doubtless more responsible for the symptoms than are the stones themselves. Presumably similar effects occur at times in animal patients, but they have seldom been recognized clinically. Cholelithiasis has more frequently been discovered at autopsy incidental to icterus and hepatic disease of a more general nature. Obstruction of the biliary flow as the result of choleliths is possible but not usual.

Decker, R.A., and Krohn, A.F.: Cholelithiasis in an Indian elephant. J. Am. Vet. Med. Assoc., 163:546–547, 1973.

France, V.M., and Wood, J.R.: Gallstones in foetal sheep. J. Physiol., 233:13–14, 1973.

Geistfeld, B.L., Bond, M.G., and St. Clair, R.W.: Cholelithiasis in a male Rhesus monkey (Macaca mulatta) fed a cholesterol-containing diet. J. Med. Primatol., 6:237–244, 1977.

Ghanadian, R., et al.: Cholelithiasis in a male Rhesus monkey. Urol. Res., 5:169–173, 1977.

Gurll, N., and DenBesteu, L.: Animal models of human cholesterol gallstone disease: a review. Lab. Anim. Sci., 28:428–432, 1978.

Lofland, H.B., Bullock, B.C., and Clarkson, T.B.: Cholelithiasis in African green monkeys (Cercopithecus aethiops). Fed. Proc., 34:862, 1975.

O'Brien, T.R., and Mitchum, D.G.: Cholelithiasis in a cat. J. Am. Vet. Med. Assoc., 156:1015–1017, 1970.

Osuga, T., Portman, O.W., Mitamura, K., and Alexander, M.: A morphologic study of gallstone development in the squirrel monkey. Lab. Invest., 30:486–493, 1974.

Osuga, T., et al.: A scanning electron microscopic study of gallstone development in man. Lab. Invest., 31:696–704, 1974.

Portman, O.W., Osuga, T., and Tanaka, N.: Biliary lipids and cholesterol gallstone formulation. Adv. Lipid Res., 13:135–194, 1975.

Redinger, R.N., and Grace, D.M.: Cholesterol gallstones and biliary lipid metabolism in the primate. Gastroenterol., 74:201–204, 1978.

Schall, W.D., et al.: Cholelithiasis in dogs. J. Am. Vet. Med. Assoc., 163:469–472, 1973.

Scott, D.W., Hoffer, R.E., Amand, W.B., and Roenigk, W.J.: Cholelithiasis in a dog. J. Am. Vet. Med. Assoc., 163:254–259, 1973.

Wood, J.R., France, V.M., and Sutor, D.J.: Occurrence of gallstones in foetal sheep. Lab. Anim., 8:155–159, 1974.

Neoplasms of the Gallbladder

Primary neoplasms of the gallbladder and common bile duct are uncommon in most animal species. Adenomas and adenocarcinomas appear to be the only such tumors reported in domestic species. Secondary tumors in the liver may occasionally involve the gallbladder by extension.

Adenomas of the gallbladder are benign, localized tumors that occur in most species and originate from the epithelium. The tumor cells form acinar or papillary patterns of tall columnar cells, the tumor mass projects into the lumen and does not infiltrate the deeper parts of the wall. Adenomas or adenomatous polyps (Fig. 23–27) reported in the gallbladder of cattle are distinctive due to the presence of parietal and chief cells similar to those of the gastric mucosa. Mucin-secreting cells are also present.

Adenocarcinoma of the gallbladder is distinguished from its benign counterpart, the adenoma, by its tendency to invade the gallbladder wall, to form incomplete tubules and undifferentiated cells, and to undergo necrosis. Some of these tumors may contain a papillary arrangement in parts of the tumor. Mucin-secreting cells are usually present. Extension to liver and adjacent peritoneum may occur, and metastasis to the lungs and elsewhere can happen in advanced cases. Early evidence of malignancy may be recognized by the invasion of perineural lymphatics.

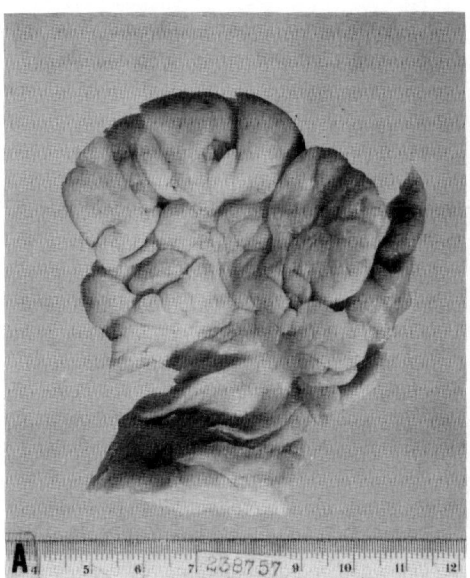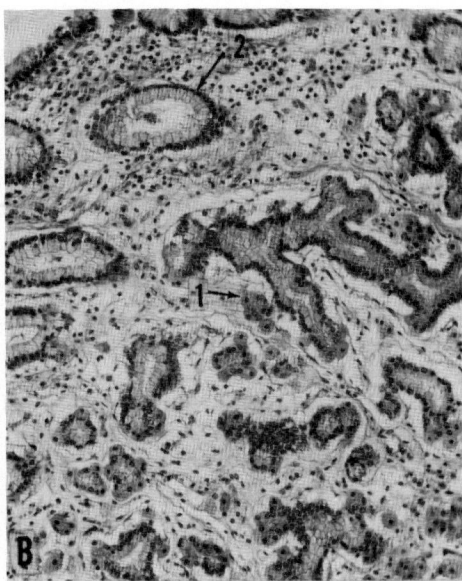

Fig. 23–27. Adenomatous polyp or adenoma in the gallbladder of a seven-year-old cow. *A,* The gross specimen, attached by its sessile stalk (bottom of photograph) in the neck of a gallbladder. *B,* Photomicrograph (× 160) of a tumor. Note "parietal" (*1*) and "chief" (*2*) cells resembling those of the gastric mucosa. These cells are normally present in the neck of the bovine gallbladder. (Courtesy of Armed Forces Institute of Pathology.) Contributor: Dr. C.L. Davis.

Anderson, W.A., Monlux, A.W., and Davis, C.L.: Epithelial tumors of the bovine gallbladder. A report of eighteen cases. Am. J. Vet. Res., *19*:58–65, 1958.

Ivoghli, B., and Cheema, A.H.: Bile duct carcinoma in a goat. Vet. Pathol., *14*:538, 1977.

O'Gara, R.W., Kelley, M.G., and Kerber, W.T.: A spontaneous metastasizing carcinoma of the gallbladder in a Rhesus monkey. Folia Primatol., *6*:284–291, 1967.

Ponomarkov, V., and Mackey, L.J.: XIII. Tumours of the liver and biliary system. International Histological Classification of Tumours of Domestic Animals. Bull. WHO, *53*:187–194, 1976.

Stalker, L.K., and Schlotthauer, C.F.: Papillary adenoma of the gallbladder in two dogs: intrahepatic gallbladder in one. J. Am. Vet. Med. Assoc., *89*:207–212, 1936.

PANCREAS

Structure

The pancreas in all mammalian species is located in the anterior or upper abdomen. It is covered in part by the mesentery and omentum, but in some species part of the gland is retroperitoneal. The principal excretory duct in some species (man, dog) joins the common bile duct near the wall of the duodenum, forming a combined duct which pierces the duodenal wall at an angle and empties into the lumen through the ampulla of Vater. A secondary duct from the pancreas enters the duodenum through a smaller ampulla a few centimeters caudal to the ampulla of Vater. In some cases this secondary duct is absent, in others, the principal duct is absent.

The pancreatic lobules are rhomboidal, formed by many acini and a single ductule. The blood vessels, nerves, lymphatics, and interlobular ducts are seen in a delicate connective tissue stroma which surrounds the lobules. The acini are made up of pyramidal-shaped cells which, in their apical portion, contain characteristic large, eosinophilic spherical granules, the zymogen granules. These are produced by the ergastoplasm of the pancreatic cells, mature (surrounded by membrane) in the

Golgi region, and eventually fuse with the plasma membrane and rupture to discharge their contents into the lumen of the acinus.

Important structures in the pancreas are the islands (islets) of Langerhans or pancreatic islets, which are specialized epithelial nodules derived from, but not communicating with, the ductal epithelium. These are the endocrine components of the pancreas and will be considered further in Chapter 26.

Function

The exocrine function of the pancreas is to accomplish certain digestive functions in the intestinal tract. This is carried out by digestive enzymes produced in the pancreatic cell, packaged in zymogen granules, and delivered to the duodenum with the pancreatic juice. A brief summary of the nature and functions of these enzymes follows.

Pancreatic amylase is a complex of enzymes which hydrolyze polysaccharides to simple carbohydrates: dextrins, maltose, and glucose. This enzyme, in contrast to all other pancreatic enzymes, exists in the pancreas in an active state. **Chymotrypsinogen,** activated by trypsin to **chymotrypsin,** is a proteolytic endopeptidase which acts on peptide bonds to produce polypeptides. **Carboxypeptidase** (activated from procarboxypeptidase by trypsin) is an exopeptidase which acts on peptide bonds to produce polypeptides and amino acids. **Elastase** is an enzyme which acts to hydrolyze elastic tissue. **Lipase** is a lipolytic enzyme which hydrolyzes fat to glycerol and fatty acids, and which also forms di- and triglycerides. Lipase is activated by bile salts, and the emulsifying activity of bile acts to potentiate digestive activity of this enzyme. **Trypsinogen** is activated initially to trypsin by enterokinase; this trypsin so activated can itself activate trypsinogen. Trypsin is an endopeptidase,

acting on interior peptide bonds of proteins, resulting in polypeptides.

Acute Necrotizing Pancreatitis (Acute Pancreatic Necrosis)

This is a clinical and pathologic entity which has been observed in dogs, cats, horses, mice, pigs, nonhuman primates, and man. As far as we can ascertain, the disease has not been reported in ruminants. The dog is the most commonly affected animal and may be used as a prototype of the animal disease. The clinical signs in the dog are initiated suddenly with decreased appetite, dullness, vomiting, diarrhea, thirst, weak pulse, and severe abdominal pain. The affected dog often has a history of being a scavenger and may have recently eaten a meal rich in fats. Amylase content of the serum is greatly increased in the early stages of this disease. In some instances, the blood levels of sugar and nonprotein nitrogen may be elevated.

Many dogs succumb to this acute disease, others may survive and have repeated acute episodes, finally resulting in chronic fibrosing pancreatitis.

Causes. The cause in an individual case may be difficult to identify, although it appears likely that the lesions result from release or activation of pancreatic enzymes within the pancreas. Experimental disease has been produced in the dog following many procedures, including ligation of the pancreatic duct and injection of trypsin into it; injection of a mixture of trypsin, bile, or bile salts into the pancreatic duct and injection of chloroform into the pancreas. The disease has been observed in mice with DL ethionine and choline dietary deficiency and in mice experimentally infected with encephalomyocarditis virus, reovirus, Coxsackievirus B1, and foot-and-mouth-disease viruses. Acute pancreatitis has also been studied in a Rhesus monkey naturally infected with simian adenovirus 31. Swine are also susceptible to experimental induction of the disease by

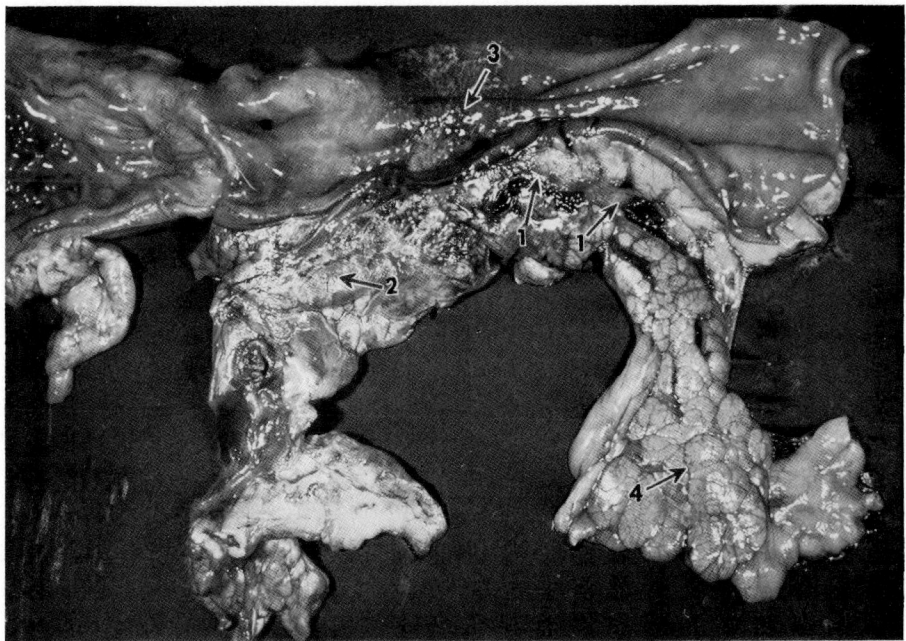

Fig. 23–28. Necrotizing and hemorrhagic pancreatitis in a male Beagle dog, age seven years. Interstitial hemorrhage (*1*), gray necrotic areas (*2*), and congestion in duodenal mucosa (*3*). The head of the pancreas (*4*) is not affected. (Courtesy of Angell Memorial Animal Hospital.)

infusion of a mixture of bile salts and trypsin into the pancreatic duct.

Lesions. The lesions center around focal necrosis, involving large or small areas and usually starting near the main pancreatic duct and its orifice into the duodenum. The necrosis is accompanied by hemorrhages, thrombosis, and local edema, followed by limited infiltration of leukocytes. Pancreatic necrosis of fat is almost always present and may extend for some distance into the mesenteric or omental fat. Small lesions may result in local fibrosis and prompt recovery. Larger lesions or repeated episodes may lead to extensive fibrosis and destruction of both exocrine and endocrine tissues of the pancreas. These changes lead to pancreatic insufficiency and diabetes mellitus.

Chronic Fibrosing Pancreatitis

Severe acute pancreatic necrosis is believed in some cases to be a prelude to chronic fibrosing pancreatitis. The latter is manifest in the dog by loss of body weight; increased volume of foul-smelling, fat-laden feces; intermittent diarrhea; and frequently, diabetes mellitus, indicated by polydipsia, polyuria, hyperglycemia, and glucosuria.

Lesions. The lesions are recognized in the pancreas by its fibrous, nodular, and atrophied appearance grossly and by the fibrous replacement of most exocrine and endocrine cells. Some zones of active necrosis may be identified and are usually accompanied by leukocytic response. Other lesions of diabetes mellitus and malabsorption syndrome may be found. Extreme fatty infiltration of the liver is one of the outstanding findings in such cases.

Angiolelli, R.F., and Rio, G.J.: Infectious pancreatic necrosis virus-induced pancreatic lesion in Swiss albino mice: electron microscopy. Am. J. Vet. Res., 33:1513–1520, 1972.

Bass, V.D., Hoffman, W.E., and Dorner, J.L.: Normal canine lipid profiles and effects of experimentally induced pancreatitis and hepatic necrosis on lipids. Am. J. Vet. Res., 37:1355–1357, 1976.

Bhattacharyya, H.M., Das, S.K., Dhar, M.M., and Roy, A.K.: Acute necrotic pancreatitis in pigs. Indian Vet. J., 50:850–852, 1973.

Bockman, D.E., et al.: Fine structure of early experimental acute pancreatitis in dogs. Lab. Invest., 28:584–592, 1973.

Craighead, J.E.: Pathogenicity of the M and E variants of the encephalomyocarditis (EMC) virus: II. Lesions of the pancreas, parotid, and lacrimal glands. Am. J. Pathol., 48:375–386, 1966.

Creutzfeldt, W., and Schmidt, H.: Aetiology and pathogenesis of pancreatitis (current concepts). Scand. J. Gastroent., 5:47–62, 1970.

Greve, T., Dayton, A.D., and Anderson, N.V.: Acute pancreatitis with coexistent diabetes mellitus: an experimental study in the dog. Am. J. Vet. Res., 34:939–946, 1973.

Hartman, H.A., Robison, R.L., and Visscher, G.E.: Naturally occurring intracytoplasmic inclusions in the canine exocrine pancreas. Vet. Pathol., 12:210–219, 1975.

Holroyd, J.B.: Canine exocrine pancreatic disease. J. Small Anim. Pract., 9:269–281, 1968.

Janigan, D.T., Nevalainen, T.J., MacAulay, M.A., and Vethamany, V.G.: Foreign serum-induced pancreatitis in mice. I. A new model of acute pancreatitis. Lab. Invest., 33:591–607, 1975.

Lombardi, B., Estes, L.W., and Longnecker, D.S.: Acute hemorrhagic pancreatitis (massive necrosis) with fat necrosis induced in mice by DL4 ethionine fed with a choline-deficient diet. Am. J. Pathol., 79:465–480, 1975.

Lombardi, B., and Rao, N.K.: Acute hemorrhagic pancreatic necrosis in mice. Influence of the age and sex of the animals and of dietary ethionine, choline, methionine, and adenine sulfate. Am. J. Pathol., 81:87–100, 1975.

McClure, H.M., Chandler, F.W., and Hierholzer, J.C.: Necrotizing pancreatitis due to simian adenovirus type 31 in a Rhesus monkey. Arch. Pathol. Lab. Med., 102:150–153, 1978.

Mia, A.S., Koger, H.D., and Tierney, M.M.: Serum values of amylase and pancreatic lipase in healthy mature dogs and dogs with experimental pancreatitis. Am. J. Vet. Res., 39:965–969, 1978.

Musa, B.E., et al.: A model to study acute pancreatitis in the dog. J. Surg. Res., 21:51–56, 1976.

Papadimitriou, J.M., and Walters, M.N.I.: Studies on the exocrine pancreas: II. Ultrastructural investigation of reovirus pancreatitis. Am. J. Pathol., 51:387–403, 1967.

Platt, H.: The occurrence of pancreatic lesions in adult mice infected with the virus of foot-and-mouth disease. Virology, 9:484–486, 1959.

Thorpe, C.D., and Frey, C.F.: Experimental pancreatitis in pigs. Arch. Surg., 103:720–723, 1971.

Tsui, C.Y., Burch, G.E., and Harb, J.M.: Pancreatitis in mice infected with Coxsackievirus B1. Arch. Pathol., 93:379–389, 1972.

Wanke, M.: Experimental acute pancreatitis. Curr. Top. Pathol., 52:64–142, 1970.

Juvenile Pancreatic Atrophy (or Hypoplasia)

This entity is recognized in young dogs (usually less than 13 months old), particularly German Shepherds, by signs of chronic exocrine pancreatic insufficiency. The signs include some loss of weight in spite of a voracious appetite; increased volume of gray, foul-smelling feces (steatorrhea); and laboratory evidence of decreased pancreatic enzymes (trypsin and chymotrypsin, especially) in the feces. Signs of diabetes mellitus are not a feature of this disease. The disease may be inherited, but definitive evidence is yet to be developed on this point.

Lesions. The lesions are characteristic. The glandular pancreas is essentially absent; only remnants of the pancreatic ducts may be seen in the mesentery at the usual site of the pancreas. Microscopic examination reveals a few poorly formed groups of pancreatic acini along the course of the pancreatic duct. Islets of Langerhans appear to be unaffected by this massive loss or failure of development of the exocrine pancreas. Inflammation is minimal. It is not clearly evident whether the exocrine pancreas fails to develop (hypoplasia) or has developed then disappeared for some reason (atrophy). The evidence available for either mechanism is not convincing at the time this was written.

Freudiger, U., and Berger, G.: Über die bestimmung der trypsin und chymotrypsin—activität im kot von hunden und ihre bedeutung für die diagnose der chromischen exokrinin pankreasinsuffizienz. Schweiz. Arch. Tierheilkd., 113:169–183, 1971.

Freudiger, U.: Die erkrankungen des exokrinin pankreas des hundes. Kleintierpraxis, 16:201–211; 229–234, 1971.

Freudiger, U.: Die diagnose der chromischen exokrinen pankreasinsuffizienz. Schweiz. Arch. Tierheilkd., 114:476–487, 1972.

Freudiger, U., and Bigler, B.: Die diagnose der chromischen exokrinen pankreasinsuffizienz mit dem PABA test. Kleintier Praxis, 22:73–79, 1977.

Gyr, K., Wolf, R.H., and Felsenfeld, O.: Exocrine pancreatic function tests in Patas monkeys (*Erythrocebus patas*). Am. J. Vet. Res., 35:1361–1364, 1974.

Hashimoto, A., Kita, I., Okada, K., and Fujimoto, J.:

Juvenile acinar atrophy of the pancreas of a dog. Vet. Pathol., 16:74–80, 1979.

Hill, R.W.G., Osborne, A.D., and Kidder, D.E.: Pancreatic degenerative atrophy in dogs. J. Comp. Pathol., 81:321–330, 1971.

Strombeck, D.K.: New method for evaluation of chymotrypsin deficiency in dogs. J. Am. Vet. Med. Assoc., 173:1319–1323, 1978.

Weber, W., and Freudiger, U.: Erbanalytische untersuchungen die chromische exocrine pankreasinsuffizienz beim Deutschen Schäferhund. Schweiz. Arch. Tierheilkd., 119:257–263, 1977.

Parasites

Small red flukes, *Eurytrema pancreaticum*, usually less than 1 cm in length, may be numerous in the pancreatic ductal system of cattle, buffalo, sheep, and goats, causing chronic fibrosing pancreatitis of mild or minimal nature. They occur commonly in Brazil and Asia. Rarely *Ascaris lumbricoides* may invade the pancreatic ducts, as well as the bile duct. A minute spirurid nematode, *Trichospirura leptostoma*, has been found in nearly 30% of necropsied marmosets (*Saguinus spp*). These parasites were associated with inflammation of the pancreatic duct in one marmoset and chronic fibrosing pancreatitis in three others (Cosgrove, et al., 1970).

Pancreatic Calculi

Pancreatic calculi are found rarely in the pancreatic ducts of cattle. They are usually hard, white, and numerous, but small. They are reported to consist of carbonates and phosphates of calcium and magnesium, in company with organic substances. In one study in Denmark (Velling, 1975), pancreoliths were found in 279 cattle (0.43%) out of 65,471 examined post mortem at slaughter. No clinical signs or other pathologic changes were found except for some inflammation in the wall of ducts containing calculi. Older cattle were more often affected and the Red Danish breed was more often affected than the Holstein-Friesian or Jersey breeds, based on relation to total populations. The first report of bovine pancreolithiasis is believed to have been made by Furstenberg (1846).

Ectopic Pancreatic Tissue

Ectopic pancreatic tissue is rarely observed in dogs in the submucosa or muscularis of the gastrointestinal tract and gallbladder or in the mesentery. Ectopic pancreatic tissue has also been reported in the liver and the duodenal submucosa of two rats, from the principal hepatic canal in a monkey embryo, and from the spleen of a cat.

Barron, C.N.: Ectopic pancreas in the rat. Report of a case. Pathol. Vet., 7:81–83, 1970.

Briziarelli, G., and Tornaben, J.A.: Ectopic pancreas in the liver of a rat. Vet. Pathol., 9:263–265, 1972.

Cosgrove, G.E., Humason, G., and Lushbaugh, C.C.: *Trichospirura leptostoma*, a nematode of the pancreatic ducts of marmosets (*Saguinus spp.*). J. Am. Vet. Med. Assoc., 157:696–698, 1970.

Furstenberg, K.: Von den steinen und concrementen in körper der haussäugetiere. Magazin ges Tierheilkd., 12:113–124, 1846.

Gianelli, F.: Contributo all conoscenza della calcolosi pancreatiche dei bovini. Atti Soc. Ital. Sci.,Vet., 5:218–224, 1951.

Smith, W.N., and Chitwood, M.B.: *Trichospirura leptostoma*, gen, et sp. m (Nematoda: Thelazioidea) from the pancreatic ducts of the white-eared marmoset, *Callithrix jacchus*. J. Parasitol., 53:1270–1272, 1967.

Velling, K.: Bovine pancreolithiasis in Denmark. Acta Vet. Scand., 16:327–340, 1975.

Verine, H.J.: An animal model of human disease: bovine pancreatolithiasis. Comp. Pathol. Bull., 5:3–4, 1973.

Neoplasms of the Exocrine Pancreas

Consideration will be given here to neoplasms primary in the exocrine part of the pancreas. Tumors arising from the pancreatic islets (islands of Langerhans) are discussed in Chapter 26. Neoplasms of the supporting tissues such as hemangiosarcomas, fibrosarcomas, and liposarcomas are quite rare in the pancreas and are described elsewhere. The two neoplasms of the exocrine (zymogen) cells of the pancreas are classified as adenoma and adenocarcinoma of the pancreas.

Adenocarcinoma of the pancreatic acinar cells is the most frequent neoplasm of the pancreas in all species. Reported cases are more numerous from dogs, but this tumor is also recognized in cats, cattle, sheep, swine, snakes, rats, mice, and other laboratory and zoo animals. Pancreatic adenocarcinomas have also been induced with carcinogens in mice, rats, and hamsters.

This tumor is made up of epithelial cells, which usually form small or large tubules or acini or are undifferentiated and hence rarely form tubules. The key feature in identification of adenocarcinoma of acinar origin is the presence, in at least a few cells, of zymogen granules characteristic of normal pancreatic exocrine cells. These granules are spherical, eosinophilic in hematoxylin and eosin stain, and acidophilic with Masson's trichrome stain. These tumors may have a dense fibrous stroma in some cases, but usually have a rather delicate connective tissue framework. Invasion of stroma and adjacent normal pancreas is usually extensive, and in advanced cases the pancreas may be essentially destroyed, leading to clinical expression of pancreatic insufficiency. Metastasis to adjacent duodenum, liver, spleen, lymph nodes, mesenteric fat, and lung may be expected rather early in the life of the tumor.

Adenoma of exocrine pancreas is known in several species and is recognized by its ductal or acinar pattern of cells, with an expanding growth pattern and rather complete encapsulation. Cystic spaces may be created by the tumor cells, which may also project in a papillary pattern into the lumen of the cysts. The cytoplasm of the cells near the lumen of tubules may contain zymogen granules which may be less intensely stained than in normal acini. Hyperplastic nodules may be seen in the pancreas of many older animals. They are usually less well encapsulated than are adenomas, but may be difficult to distinguish with certainty.

Anderson, N.V., and Johnson, K.H.: Pancreatic carcinoma in the dog. J. Am. Vet. Med. Assoc., 150:286–295, 1967.

Banner, B.F., Alroy, J., and Kipnis, R.M.: Acinar cell carcinoma of the pancreas in a cat. Vet. Pathol., 16:543–547, 1979.

Dissin, J., et al.: Experimental induction of pancreatic adenocarcinoma in rats. J. Natl. Cancer Inst., 55:857–864, 1975.

Gans, J.H.: Carcinoma of the pancreas in the dog. Cornell Vet., 48:372–377, 1958.

Kircher, C.H., and Nielsen, S.W.: International histological classification of tumours of domestic animals. XIV. Tumours of the pancreas. Bull. WHO, 53:195–202, 1976.

Pour, P., et al.: Cancer of the pancreas induced in the Syrian golden hamster. Am. J. Pathol., 76:349–358, 1974.

Priester, W.A.: Data from eleven United States and Canadian colleges of veterinary medicine on pancreatic carcinoma in domestic animals. Cancer Res., 34:1372–1375, 1974.

Ratcliffe, H.L.: Carcinoma of the pancreas in Say's pine snake, *Pituophus sayi*. Am. J. Cancer, 24:78–79, 1935.

Ratcliffe, H.L.: Neoplastic disease of the pancreas of snakes (*Serpentes*). Am. J. Pathol., 19:359–369, 1943.

Rowlatt, U.: Pancreatic neoplasms of rats and mice. In Pathology of Laboratory Rats and Mice, edited by E. Cotchin, and F.J.C. Roe. Oxford, Blackwell Scientific Publications, 1967, pp. 85–103.

Rowlatt, U.: Spontaneous epithelial neoplasms of the pancreas of mammals. Brit. J. Cancer, 21:82–107, 1967.

Slye, M., Holmes, H.F., and Wells, H.G.: The comparative pathology of carcinoma of the pancreas with report of two cases in mice. Am. J. Cancer, 23:81–86, 1935.

CHAPTER 24

The Urinary System

KIDNEYS

Anatomy and Physiology

Nephron

The essential anatomic and functional unit of the kidney is the nephron. Each kidney contains many nephrons, depending upon the species (the human kidneys are estimated to contain between one and two million). Each nephron is made up of the **glomerulus,** a spherical body which is formed by invagination of branching segments of an afferent arteriole into a terminal bud of a **renal tubule.** The renal tubule has distinct segments known as (1) the proximal convoluted tubule, (2) the loop of Henle, with descending and ascending limbs, and (3) the distal convoluted tubule, which connects with a collecting duct, which in turn empties into a duct of Bellini and then to the renal pelvis and ureter.

In the glomerulus, the afferent artery branches and re-anastomoses to form a capillary tuft which is intimately associated with the epithelial cells of the tubule and the visceral layer of Bowman's capsule. The glomerular space surrounds the capillary tuft, communicates with the proximal convoluted tubule, and is surrounded by an epithelial layer and a thin fibrous capsule—the parietal layer of Bowman's capsule.

At light microscopic magnification, the capillary endothelium may be seen to be closely applied to the tubular epithelium, separated only by a basement membrane, which can be best demonstrated with the periodic acid-Schiff reaction or silver-staining methods. Ultrastructurally, the basement membrane is composed of three layers—an electron-dense layer (lamina densa) separating two less compact layers (lamina rara externa, lamina rara interna). The endothelial cell which lines the capillary lumen is stretched out with only a thin layer of cytoplasm over most of the surface of the basement membrane. The endothelial lining is not continuous, but contains multiple fenestrae approximately 1000 Å in diameter where the basement membrane is bare. The cells of the visceral layer of Bowman's capsule are in contact with the basement membrane by means of long extensions of the cytoplasm known as foot processes, giving a name to these cells: **podocytes**. The space between the foot processes is bridged by a thin line called the slit membrane, or diaphragm.

In addition to the endothelial and epithelial cells, a third cell, the **mesangial** or **intercapillary** cell, is found in the glomerulus. This cell is located centrally within the capillary loops, one side of the capillary always facing the mesangial cell. The cytoplasm of the mesangial cell is similar to that of the epithelial cell, but adjacent extracellular spaces contain fine reticular filaments and material similar to basement membrane (**mesangial matrix**). The function of mesangial cells has received considerable attention, and evidence indicates that they are (1) phagocytic and may clear debris from the mesangium, (2) contractile by virtue of cytoplasmic myofibrillar bundles and may influence glomerular blood flow, and (3) contribute to the formation of glomerular basement membrane.

The **proximal convoluted tubule** leaves the glomerulus as a short segment called the neck piece. The tortuous tubule is lined by a single layer of cuboidal cells which have a brush border on their luminal surface. Under the electron microscope, this brush border is seen to consist of microvilli that increase the absorptive surface of the cells. Infoldings of the cell membrane also extend deep into the cell from the base of the microvilli. Similar membranes extend into these cells from their basal surface. Mitochondria are often found between these membranes. The tubule then assumes a straight course descending toward the medulla where it becomes the **thin descending limb** of the **loop of Henle,** continuing the renal tubule into the renal medulla. The epithelial cells lining this segment are flattened and contain few mitochondria. The loop is completed, usually in the peripheral medulla, and the lining cells of this ascending limb are cuboidal and contain numerous mitochondria. Their cytoplasm is for this reason usually darker when viewed by light microscopy. At the point where the ascending limb returns to the cortex, the tubule becomes the **distal convoluted tubule.** The epithelial cells lining this segment are columnar, but have clear cytoplasm and no brush border. A few microvilli may be demonstrated with the electron microscope in these cells. Their basal surface bears deeply infolded cell membranes, which are closely aligned with many mitochondria.

At the point where the ascending limb joins the distal convoluted tubule, the tubule lies in contact with its own afferent arteriole, near the hilus of the glomerulus. The epithelial cells at this point, called the **macula densa,** are uniformly cuboidal and arranged in an easily recognized palisade adjacent to the afferent arteriole. Cells in the media of the arteriole in this zone are enlarged and resemble cells of the aortic or carotid body. These are believed to be modified smooth muscle cells. Together with the **macula densa,** these cells of the arteriole form the **juxtaglomerular apparatus,** which is considered the source of **renin.**

Glomeruli, once destroyed, do not regenerate, although those that remain may undergo some compensatory hypertrophy. Fortunately, the total number of nephrons is considerably in excess of requirements, so that many of them, or even a whole kidney, may be lost without fatal effects providing the remaining renal tissue is uninjured.

Destroyed tubular epithelium regenerates readily. The new cells have hyperchromatic nuclei but may be less columnar than their predecessors. It is not unusual to encounter tubules whose epithelium is flattened and whose lumens are large. These are variously interpreted as dilated because of obstruction, regenerated or hypertrophic with increased functional requirements compensatory to destruction of other tubules, or merely hyperplastic. Although tubular epithelium can undergo hypertrophy and hyperplasia, new nephrons cannot be formed. Thus, hyperplasia of tubular epithelium may repair or enlarge a nephron, but cannot increase the number of nephrons.

In certain species, particularly the dog, rat, and cat, the orifice in Bowman's capsule through which the neck piece of the proximal convoluted tubule passes may be widened under certain circumstances. This permits part of the tubule to protrude into Bowman's space and presents a puzzling feature in histologic sections. This phenomenon has been variously named "protrusions of tubular epithelium" or "infraglomerular epithelial reflux." Mullink and Feron (1967) present evidence that this histologically recognized feature is the result of postmortem change.

Anatomic differences between species are of some consequence in interpreting lesions in the kidneys. A few might be mentioned: Bovine animals have lobulated kidneys, similar to fetal lobulation in other species. Each lobule has multiple calices, a separate ureter, and its blood is supplied through a single artery entering at the hilus. The kidney of the dog has a single renal ridge which extends the length of the kidney to form what amounts to a single papilla. The capsule is apt to be adherent, and fat is normally present in tubular epithelium. The cat also frequently has fat in renal tubular epithelium and the kidneys are more moveable in the abdomen. The horse has many compound mucous glands in the renal pelvis.

The kidney of newborn and young animals may be recognized histologically by glomeruli which are small with hyperchromic epithelial and endothelial nuclei. The tubules are less well developed than in the adult, and fewer nephrons have tubules which dip into the medulla. The young animal therefore has much less capacity to concentrate urine than does the adult.

Blood Supply

The renal vasculature is complex, with two capillary networks, one in the glomeruli and the other surrounding the tubules. As a result of the dual nature of the vasculature, lesions affecting one site ultimately affect the other. After entering the hilus, the renal arteries branch into large segmental arteries, which at the corticomedullary junction give rise to the arcuate arteries. From these, interlobular arteries originate and run parallel to collecting tubules. These tend to lie in groups so that when congested, each group is represented by a red streak, radial in direction, which is readily visible to the naked eye. The interlobular arteries are end arteries with no anastomoses with each other. For this reason, infarction of the renal cortex readily occurs. The infarcted areas take the form of pyramids with their bases at the capsule.

The afferent arteriole originates from the interlobular artery, each one supplying a single glomerulus, where it forms a tuft of capillaries, which in turn join to form the efferent arteriole leaving the glomerulus. The wall of the afferent arteriole is considerably thicker than the efferent arteriole. Small arteries may directly connect afferent and efferent arterioles, bypassing the glomerulus, but they are few in number and apparently insufficiently developed to provide protective anastomoses.

The efferent arteriole then subdivides into a capillary network that surrounds the tubules. The tubular capillary plexus forms venules, which ultimately form intertubular veins, arcuate veins, and ultimately the renal vein. Thus, the delicate epithelial cells of the tubules are dependent for their blood supply upon the free movement of blood through the tortuous passageways of the glomerulus. As will be explained, the glomerulus is, unfortunately, vulnerable to a number of lesions that interfere with this free flow of blood, and death and destruction of tubules as the result of such lesions are of frequent occurrence. The glomeruli are almost equally dependent on proper conditions in the tubular regions, and there are situations, such as swelling of the epithelium of the tubules or other lesions, which will lead to stasis of blood flow with loss of glomerular function.

Physiology

It is computed that about one-third of the cardiac output of blood goes to the kidney at each circuit, and that nearly 10% of blood, equivalent to 16% of the plasma, which passes through the glomerulus, filters freely into Bowman's capsule as the "glomerular filtrate." Only about 1% of this is believed to be excreted as urine, the remaining 99% being reabsorbed through the epithelium of the tubules. Substances with a molecular weight above about 70,000 do not pass into the glomerular filtrate, thus most proteins and, of course, cells are retained in the blood stream.

Electrolytes such as chlorides, carbonates and bicarbonates, phosphates, silicates (herbivorous animals), and sulfates of ammonium, sodium, potassium, and calcium, as well as various organic substances including glucose and urea, pass freely into the glomerular filtrate, either to be excreted in the urine or to be reabsorbed more or less selectively by the epithelial cells. At the same time that many are reabsorbed, some substances are excreted by the epithelium of the tubules. These include creatinine in man, but not apparently in the dog.

As indicated, compounds with large molecules, especially the proteins, do not pass through the healthy glomerular filter, which is comparable to a dialyzing membrane, and do not appear in the normal urine. The presence of protein in the urine is a readily determined clinical sign of injury to the glomeruli and a serious renal malfunction.

Glucose is absent from normal urine, because it is completely reabsorbed in the tubules unless its concentration in the blood is above a certain critical level, called the renal threshold. The latter situation arises in diabetes mellitus, in which the glucose of the blood cannot be utilized, and at times, immediately following an excessively large meal of carbohydrates.

Formation of urine can be prevented completely (anuria) or partially (oliguria) by various lesions in the glomeruli, by renal ischemia, or by the excessive swelling of the tubular epithelium previously mentioned. When this occurs, profound changes appear constituting the condition of uremia.

Anonymous: (Symposium) Kinins, renal function and blood pressure regulation. Fed. Proc., 35:172–206, 1976.

Bharadwaj, M.B., and Calhoun, M.L.: Histology of the urethral epithelium of domestic animals. Am. J. Vet. Res., 20:841–851, 1959.

Brenner, B.M., and Humes, H.: Mechanics of glomerular ultrafiltration. N. Engl. J. Med., 297:148–154, 1977.

Camazine, S.M., Ryan, G.B., Unanue, E.R., and Karnovsky, M.J.: Isolation of phagocytic cells from the rat renal glomerulus. Lab. Invest., 35:315, 326, 1976.

Christensen, G.C.: Circulation of blood through the canine kidney. Am. J. Vet. Res., 13:236–245, 1952.

Crowell, W.A., Duncan, J.R., and Finco, D.R.: Canine glomeruli: light and electron microscopic change in biopsy, perfused, and in situ autolyzed kidney from normal dogs. Am. J. Vet. Res., 35:889–896, 1974.

Fisher, E.R., Copeland, C., and Fisher, B.: Correlation of ultrastructure and function following hypothermic preservation of canine kidneys. Lab. Invest., 17:99–120, 1967.

Friedman, M., and Byers, S.O.: Causes of the excess excretion of uric acid in the Dalmatian dog. J. Biol. Chem., 175:727–735, 1948.

Griffith, L.D., Bulger, R.E., and Trump, B.F.: The ultrastructure of the functioning kidney. Lab. Invest., 16:220–246, 1967.

Hays, R.M.: Antidiuretic hormone. N. Engl. J. Med., 295:659–665, 1976.

Huber, G.C.: The arteriolae rectae of the mammalian kidney. Amer. J. Anat., 6:391–406, 1906–1907.

Jamison, R.L., and Maffly, R.H.: The urinary concentrating mechanism. N. Engl. J. Med., 295:1059–1067, 1976.

Jorgensen, F.: Electron microscopic studies of normal glomerular basement membrane. Lab. Invest., 17:416–424, 1967.

Latimer, H.B.: The growth of the kidneys and the bladder in the fetal dog. Anat. Rec., 109:1–12, 1951.

Marshall, M.E., and Deutsch, H.F.: Clearances of some proteins by the dog kidney. Amer. J. Physiol., 163:461–467, 1950.

Mayer, E., and Ottolenghi, L.A.: Protrusion of tubular epithelium into the space of Bowman's capsule in kidneys of dogs and cats. Anat. Rec., 99:477–510, 1947.

Mottram, V.H.: Fat infiltration of the cat's kidney. J. Biol. Chem., 24:11–12, 1916.

Moustgaard, J.: Variation of the renal function in normal and unilaterally nephrectomized dogs. Am. J. Vet. Res., 8:301–306, 1947.

Mullink, J.W.M.A., and Feron, V.J.: Infraglomerular epithelial reflux as a postmortem phenomenon in the kidneys of dog and rat. Path. Vet., *4*:366–377, 1967.

Oparil, S., and Haber, E.: The renin-angiotensin system. N. Engl. J. Med., *291*:446–457, 1974.

Rhodin, J.A.G.: An Atlas of Ultrastructure. Philadelphia, W.B. Saunders Co., 1963.

Wolfson, W.Q., Cohn, C., and Shore, C.: The renal mechanism for urate excretion in the Dalmatian Coach-hound. J. Exper. Med., *92*:121–128, 1950.

Yadava, R.P., and Calhoun, M.L.: Comparative histology of the kidney of domestic animals. Am. J. Vet. Res., *19*:958–968, 1958.

Congenital and Hereditary Anomalies

Anomalies of the kidney have been reported in man and many other species. Some are known to be caused by inherited factors, others are of unknown etiology.

Aplasia or Agenesis. The most frequently reported anomaly involves aplasia or agenesis of one or both kidneys. Absence of both kidneys of course is incompatible with life and would be encountered only in the fetus, newborn, or stillborn animal. On the other hand, aplasia of one kidney results in compensatory hypertrophy of the remaining kidney, and the individual may cope with life quite well. Agenesis of one or both kidneys has been reported in most species of domestic animals. Unilateral agenesis is most common in swine, dogs, and cattle and is less frequent in cats, horses, sheep, and other animals.

Renal Hypoplasia. Renal hypoplasia describes kidneys in newborn or young animals, which are markedly smaller than normal with little or no function. Cordes and Dodd (1965) described bilateral renal hypoplasia in 19 swine, 12 of which were born dead or died within 2 days of birth. Varying degrees of hypoplasia were found, from tiny almost unrecognizable kidneys to bilobate kidneys or kidneys with distinct fetal lobulation. All affected piglets were sired by the same boar, and the evidence indicated probable control of the defect by a single recessive autosomal gene. This condition has also been recognized in the dog (Fig. 4–1) and cat.

Horseshoe Kidney. This descriptive name is applied to the appearance of kidneys which are fused at one pole to produce a horseshoe-shaped structure centered roughly in the midline of the abdomen. The ureters are usually intact, and the kidneys function adequately in most instances. This condition has been reported in man and cat.

Vascular Anomalies. Congenital variations in origin and course of renal arteries and veins are sometimes observed, usually at time of necropsy. These have no deleterious effects, except in those instances in which their position partially occludes the ureter. In this instance, hydronephrosis might result.

Displacement. The anatomic position of the kidneys is retroperitoneal in all species, but the exact position varies between species and to some extent between individuals. In the cat, for example, the kidneys during life may be quite moveable if the blood vessels are longer than usual. This so-called "floating kidney" appears to have little pathologic significance.

Cysts in the Kidney. Simple cysts, presumably acquired, are not infrequently seen in the kidneys of various species, but are considerably more common in swine and dogs than in the other domestic animals. They may be solitary or very numerous, varying in size from those just visible to the eye up to a diameter of about a centimeter in the case of multiple cysts of the pig and dog, or of several centimeters in the case of a single cyst. Their walls are usually thin and transparent, their contents clear and watery, perhaps tinged with yellow. They may bulge from the surface or lie buried in the depths of the parenchyma. Cysts may arise from gradual distention of a nephron whose outlet has been closed, usually by the pressure of exudates or fibrous tissue. But if the kidney contains a considerable number of cysts, the disorder is usually that designated as the **congenital polycystic kidney.** In man, Osathanondh and Potter (1964) have described three types of polycystic renal disease, each arising from abnormal fetal development, as follows. Type I, or infantile polycystic kidney, is due to dilatation and hyperplasia of collecting tubules, with saccular or cylindrical dilatations developing in all collecting tubules. This results in a bilaterally symmetrical, sponge-like appearance of the kidneys. The dilated channels lie at right angles to the surface of the cortex, completely replacing the medulla and cortex. The cysts are lined with uniform cuboidal epithelium. This type is found only in infants because it is not compatible with prolonged survival. Cystic bile ducts are also often present. The condition is believed to be inherited as an autosomal recessive trait.

Type II congenital polycystic renal disease is considered to be due to inhibition of ureteral ampullary activity. It is believed that failure of the ureteral ampullary regions to branch results in the absence of collecting tubules and consequent failure of nephrons to develop. The cysts tend to be asymmetrical, but may involve one or both kidneys. The cysts are usually large and thick-walled and separated by dense connective tissue in which few nephrons and irregular blood vessels may be embedded. This type is compatible with life unless large parts of both kidneys are involved.

Type III, or adult polycystic kidneys, according to Osathanondh and Potter (1964) are due to multiple abnormalities of development. Normal and cystic nephrons are admixed in involved kidneys, and survival is possible to adulthood, depending on the number of functional nephrons. This type is always bilateral and results in masses of cysts greatly enlarging the kidneys. The cysts contain clear or sometimes bloody fluid (Fig. 24–1). The cysts are thought to arise from tubules or parts of nephrons. When Bowman's capsules are involved, remnants of glomeruli may be found in some cysts. This human type has been seen in cats.

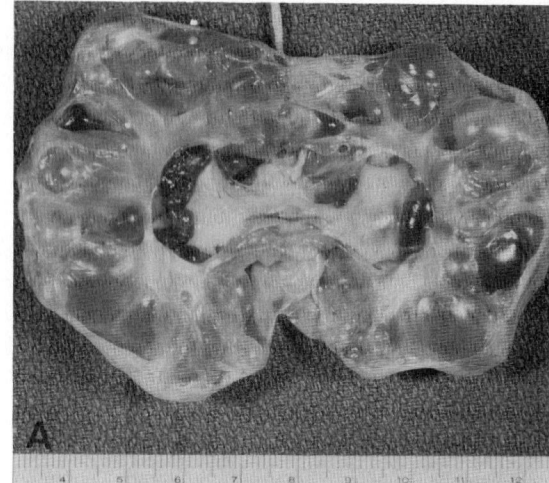

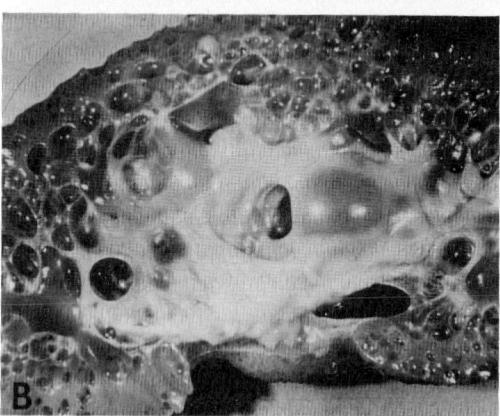

Fig. 24–1. A, Polycystic kidney from an eight-year-old spayed female cat. (Courtesy of Angell Memorial Animal Hospital.) B, Polycystic kidney in a hog. (Courtesy of Dr. C. L. Davis.)

Medullary cystic disease represents yet another form of cystic kidney described in man. Two types with differing clinical sequelae are recognized: medullary sponge kidney, in which renal function is usually normal, and uremic medullary cystic disease, in which renal failure develops in adolescents or young adults. The pathogenesis is unknown. The cysts result from dilatation of collecting ducts in the renal medulla. In the uremic form, there is glomerular sclerosis, interstitial fibrosis, and tubular atrophy causing the kidney to be contracted and granular.

Cysts, whether of the congenital type or not, tend to enlarge slowly and, by pressure atrophy, to cause progressive loss of functioning renal parenchyma, so that in early or middle life, renal insufficiency develops with lethal results. This is true in dogs and cats as well as in human beings; in swine, the cystic kidney is usually revealed at slaughter. Cysts are also known in the peripelvic tissues arising from nephrogenic vestiges or obstruction of the lymphatic vessels there; these are very rare.

Polycystic disease can be induced in rabbits and rats by the injection of steroids.

Cordes, D.O., and Dodd, D.C.: Bilateral renal hypoplasia of the pig. Path. Vet., 2:37–48, 1965.

Crocker, J.F.S., Stewart, A.G., Sparling, J.M., and Bruneau, R.T.: Steroid-induced polycystic kidneys in the newborn rat. The electrolyte and chemical requirements. Am. J. Pathol., 82:373–380, 1976.

Evan, A.P., and Gardner, K.D., Jr.: Comparison of human polycystic and medullary cystic kidney disease with diphenylamine-induced cystic disease. Lab. Invest., 35:93–101, 1976.

Hofliger, H.: Zur kenntnis der knogenitalen unilateralen nierenagenesie bei haustieren. II. Beitrag: ihr vorkommen bei den einzelnen tierarten. (Congenital Unilateral Renal Agenesis in Domestic Animals. II. Occurrence in the Various Animal Species.) Schweiz. Arch. Tierheilkd., 113:330–337, 1971.

Hunt, H.R.: Absence of one kidney in the domestic cat. Anat. Rec., 15:221–223, 1918.

Johnson, C.E.: Pelvic and horseshoe kidneys in the domestic cat. Anat. Anz., 46:69–78, 1914.

Kardevan, A.: Cystic kidneys in cattle, originating from Bowman's capsule. Magy. Allatorv. Lap., 19:444–446, 1964. V.B. 35:3967, 1965.

Klopfer, U., Neumann, F., and Trainin, R.: Renal cortical hypoplasia in a Keeshond litter. Vet. Med. Sm. Anim. Clin., 70:1081–1083, 1975.

Leighton, C.: Canine nephrosis associated with absence of the other kidney. J. Comp. Path. and Therap., 16:171–173, 1903.

Lyon, M.F., and Hulse, E.V.: An inherited kidney disease of mice resembling human nephronophthisis. J. Med. Genet., 8:41–48, 1970.

Mack, C.O., and McGlothlin, J.H.: Renal agenesis in the female cat. Anat. Rec., 105:445–450, 1949.

Maruffo, C.A., and Cramer, D.L.: Congenital renal malformations in monkeys. Folia Primat., 5:305–311, 1967.

McClure, C.F.W.: Abnormalities in connection with the post-caval vein and its tributaries in the domestic cat. Am. Naturalist, 34:185–198, 1900.

McCraw, A.P., Rotheram, K., Sim, A.K., and Warwick, M.H.: Unilateral renal aplasia in the baboon. J. Med. Primatol., 2:249–251, 1973.

McFarland, L.Z., and Deniz, E.: Unilateral renal agenesis with ipsilateral cryptorchidism and perineal hypospadias in a dog. J. Am. Vet. Med. Assoc., 139:1099–1100, 1961.

Osathanondh, V., and Potter, E.: Pathogenesis of polycystic kidneys. Arch. Pathol., 77:466–509, 1964.

Robbins, G.R.: Unilateral renal agenesis in the Beagle. Vet. Rec., 77:1345–1347, 1965.

Safouh, M., Crocker, J.F.S., and Vernier, R.L.: Experimental cystic disease of the kidney. Sequential, functional, and morphologic studies. Lab. Invest., 23:392–400, 1970.

Solomon, S.: Inherited renal cysts in rats. Science, 181:451–452, 1973.

Story, H.E.: A case of horseshoe kidney and associated vascular anomalies in the domestic cat. Anat. Rec., 86:307–319, 1943.

Tannreuther, G.W.: Abnormal urogenital system in the domestic cat. Anat. Rec., 25:59–62, 1923.

Vlachos, J.D.: A new experimental model of polycystic kidneys. Similarity to a human variety. Am. J. Dis. Child., 123:118–120, 1972.

Vymetal, F.: Renal aplasia in Beagles. Vet. Rec., 77:1344–1345, 1965.

DISEASES OF GLOMERULI

Glomerulonephritis

The term glomerulonephritis is usually restricted to primary inflammation of the glomeruli. Glomeruli may also suffer damage secondarily to tubular disease or pyelonephritis, but these forms of glomerular disease are not included as primary glomerulonephritis. As indicated earlier, glomerular disease may lead to changes in renal tubules. Several differing systems of classification of glomerulonephritis have appeared over the years and further changes can be anticipated as the causative factors and pathogenesis become better known. We will consider glomerulonephritis under the following headings: acute proliferative glomerulonephritis; membranous glomerulonephritis; membranoproliferative glomerulonephritis; chronic (sclerosing) glomerulonephritis; focal embolic glomerulonephritis. The pathologic features of these forms of glomerulonephritis will be described first,

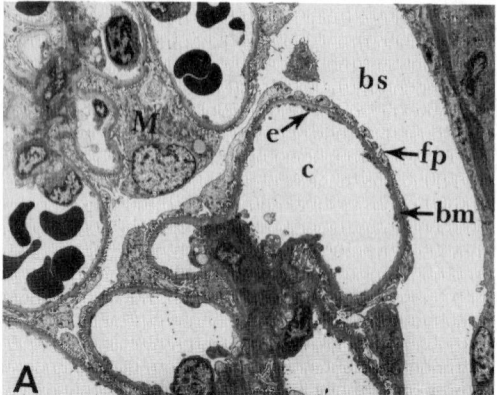

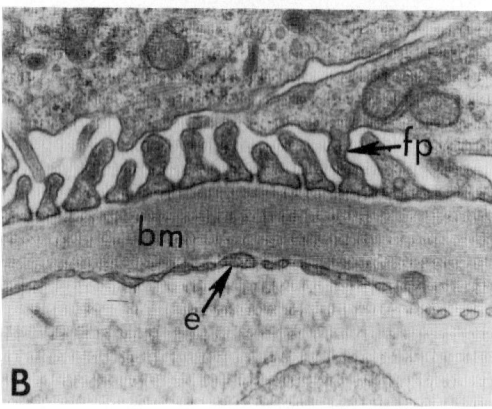

Fig. 24-2. Normal renal glomerulus. A, The lumens of glomerular capillaries (c) separated from Bowman's space (bs) by fenestrated endothelium (e), basement membrane (bm), and foot processes of epithelial cells (fp). M, mesangial cell. B, Higher magnification illustrating fenestrated endothelium (e), the three component laminae of the basement membrane (bm), and epithelial foot processes (fp). (Courtesy of Dr. N. W. King, Jr.)

and then we will discuss the immunologic mechanisms of injury.

Acute Proliferative Glomerulonephritis. This form of glomerulonephritis is the classic poststreptococcal glomerulonephritis known in children for many years and recently identified as a spontaneous and experimentally induced disease entity in animals.

The human disease, which characteristically affects young children, but may appear in adults, typically follows by 2 weeks or more an acute upper respiratory

infection by streptococci. The onset of the renal disease is sudden, with fever, nausea, weakness, subcutaneous edema, and excretion of brown or bloody urine in scant amounts. The fever may abate in about a week, but abnormalities in the urine may persist, and some cases may continue as a chronic disease. The lesions may heal or progress to chronic glomerulonephritis.

Lesions. The lesion in glomeruli is characteristic under the light microscope. Although not recognizable definitively in the gross specimen, the kidney may be en-

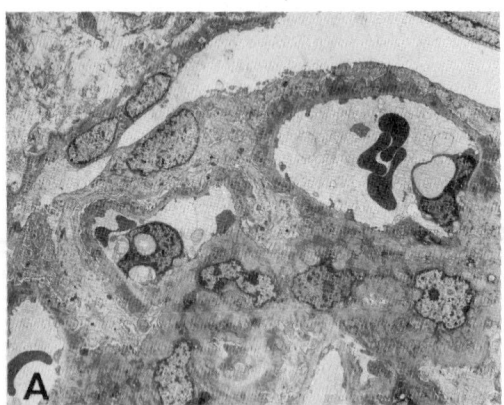

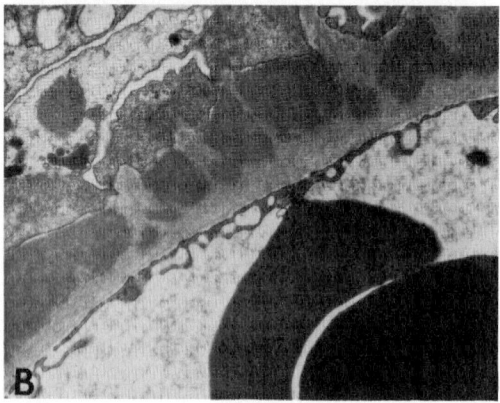

Fig. 24-3. Immune complex glomerulonephritis. A, Dense deposits are present in the basement membrane and in an exuberant mesangial matrix. B, Higher magnification of a glomerular tuft containing discrete dense deposits in the basement membrane. These correspond to the spikes seen in silver and immunofluorescent preparations. (Courtesy of Dr. N. W. King, Jr.)

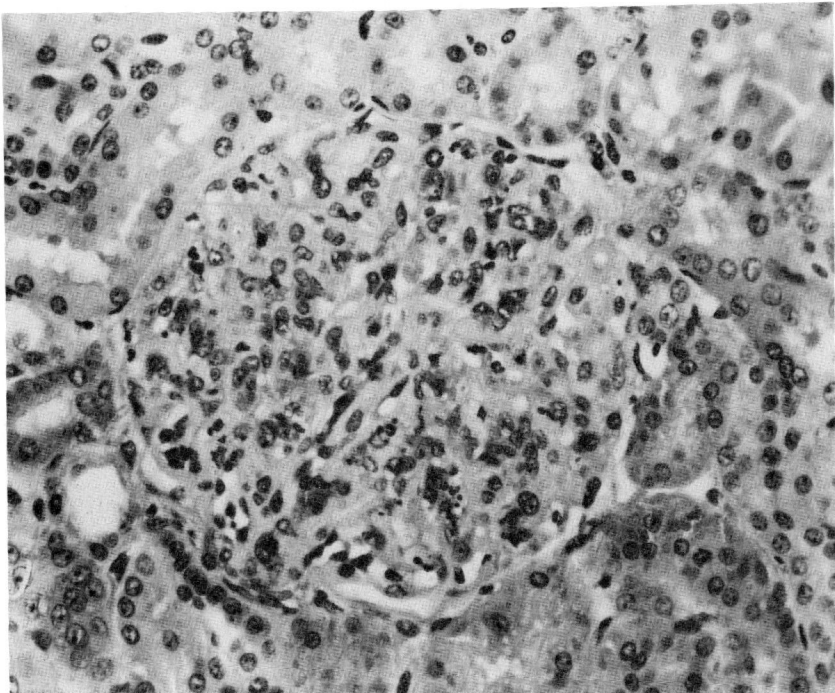

Fig. 24–4. Proliferative glomerulonephritis. Nine-year-old male dog. Glomerulus fills Bowman's space and contains numerous nuclei, including leukocytes. The basement membrane may also be thickened. (Courtesy of Armed Forces Institute of Pathology.)

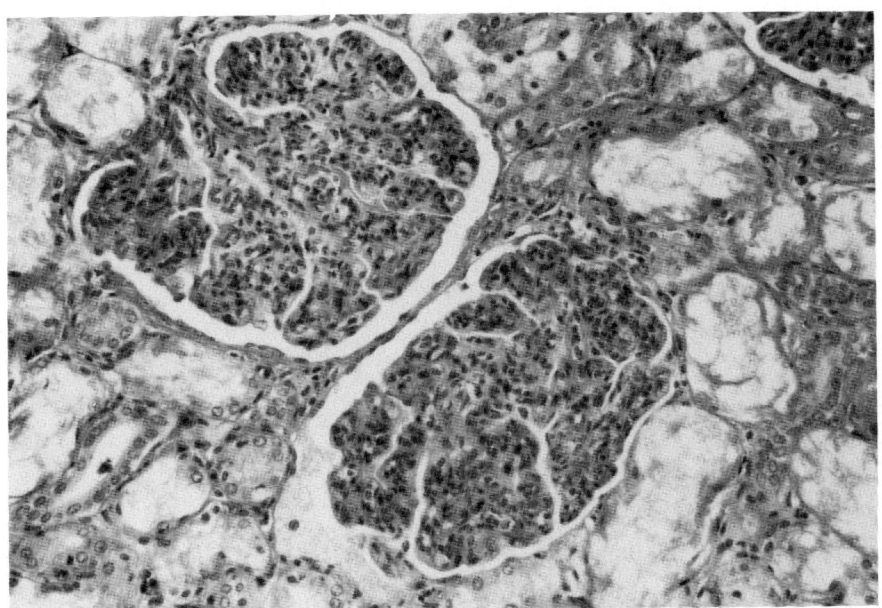

Fig. 24–5. Proliferative glomerulonephritis. Two-year-old Holstein cow. Increased cellularity obscures individual capillary loops. (Courtesy of Drs. R. M. Lewis and D. O. Slauson and *Veterinary Pathology*.)

larged and pale, with petechiae outlining the glomeruli. The glomeruli are initially congested or edematous and conspicuous at low magnification. The glomerular tufts are increased in size, with increased numbers of endothelial and mesangial cells. In this early stage, leukocytes, particularly neutrophils and monocytes, appear in the glomerulus. This influx and proliferation of cells result in compression of the capillaries and the absence of red blood cells. As the disease progresses, epithelial cells also proliferate, and some may adhere to the parietal layer of Bowman's capsule. These eventually form the epithelial "crescents" seen in subacute or chronic forms. Thrombosis and necrosis of glomerular capillaries may occur, with subsequent hemorrhage into the glomerulus. No obvious thickening of the basement membrane or alteration in the foot processes of epithelial cells is found by examination with the electron microscope.

The most characteristic ultrastructural finding is the presence of deposits or "humps" of immune complex on the epithelial side of the basement membrane. These deposits are usually less than a micron in diameter, but may be large and project between podocytes. Occasionally, the deposits may be present within the lamina densa and in the subendothelial portion of the basement membrane. When stained with silver techniques or the periodic acid-Schiff reaction, the basement membrane is disrupted by these deposits, giving it the characteristic "lumpy-bumpy" appearance.

Leukocytic infiltration may occur adjacent to glomeruli or in nearby interstitial tissues. Tubular changes are not pronounced in acute stages of disease aside from proteinaceous casts and red cells in tubular lumens and hyalin droplets in proximal convoluted tubular epithelium.

Membranous Glomerulonephritis. Rather clearly distinguishable from proliferative glomerulonephritis in man, membranous glomerulonephritis also occurs naturally as a distinct entity in other animals. In individual cases, however, differentiation is not always simple, and it is possible for

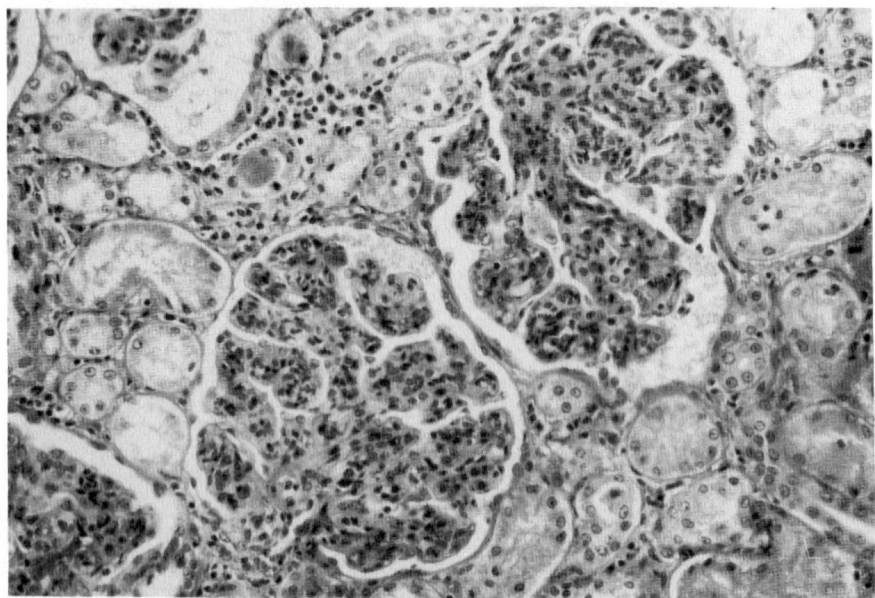

Fig. 24–6. Proliferative glomerulonephritis with a lobular pattern in a horse. There is an increase in overall glomerular cellularity. (Courtesy of Drs. R. M. Lewis and D. O. Slauson and *Veterinary Pathology*.)

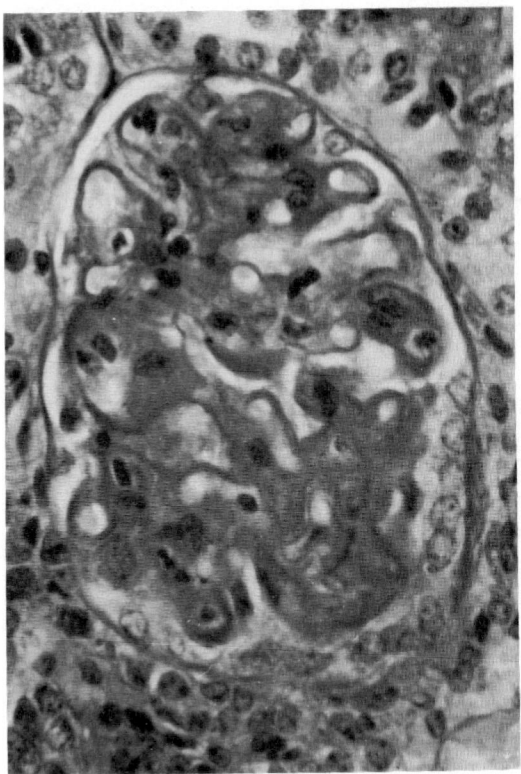

Fig. 24–7. Diffuse membranous glomerulone-phritis in mouse with chronic allogeneic disease. Note thickened basement membranes and mesangium. (Courtesy of Dr. Robert M. Lewis and *The Journal of Experimental Medicine*.)

both forms to occur simultaneously. Membranous glomerulonephritis is distinguished in the final analysis by certain features detected by study of sections with light and electron microscopy, and also by some distinguishing clinical characteristics. It is believed to be the most frequent cause of the nephrotic syndrome in man and usually has an insidious onset and prolonged course in man or animals. Early studies in children associated the clinical disease with deposits of lipid in epithelial cells of proximal convoluted tubules, but changes in glomeruli were overlooked, resulting in the application of the now obsolete name "lipoid nephrosis."

Lesions. The morphologic changes that identify membranous glomerulonephritis

are (1) thickening, splitting, and reduplication of the glomerular basement membrane, and (2) loss of the foot processes of the podocytes (epithelial cells) of the glomerulus. With the electron microscope, the earliest detectable lesions appear to be the loss of the foot processes and spaces between glomerular basement membrane and epithelial cells by the application of broad segments of the epithelium to the external surface of the basement membrane. Later in the course of the disease, the glomerular basement membrane becomes irregularly thickened with scalloped portions along its external (epithelial) border. This thickening of the basement membrane becomes severe enough to be recognized by light microscopy and is particularly evident in sections stained by periodic acid-Schiff (PAS) and silver impregnation methods. The basement membrane may develop the "lumpy-bumpy" appearance described in the preceding section, and ultrastructurally, dense deposits of immune complex are encountered in the epithelial side of the basement membrane. These deposits are not dissimilar from those described for proliferative glomerulonephritis. The thickened basement membrane is sometimes described as resembling a "wire loop" in microscopic section. The epithelial cells in the glomerulus may become swollen and laden with fat, giving the glomerulus a hypercellular appearance. Similar lipid vacuoles in the cells of the proximal convoluted tubules may be expected.

After a prolonged course, the glomerulus may become enlarged and hypercellular and distend Bowman's capsule. The glomerular space is rarely obliterated, however, and epithelial crescents and adhesions are not usual. The glomerulus is not only dense and cellular, but is essentially bloodless at this stage.

Grossly, the kidney affected with membranous glomerulonephritis is usually enlarged and pallid ("large pale kidney"), presumably due to the fatty changes and

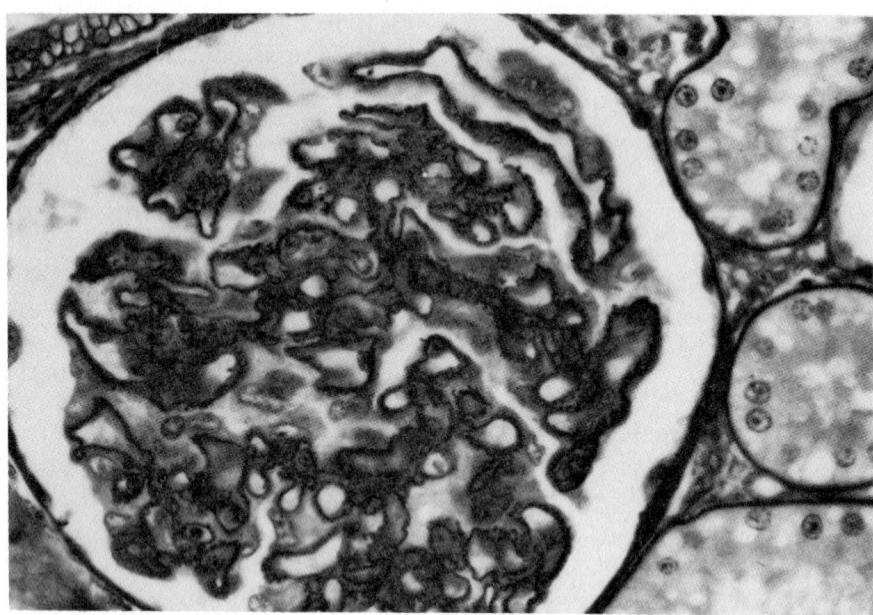

Fig. 24–8.   Diffuse membranous glomerulonephritis in a cat. Brushlike "spikes" on outside of basement membranes imply immune complex disease. (PAS-methenamine silver stain.) (Courtesy of Drs. R. M. Lewis and D. O. Slauson and *Veterinary Pathology*.)

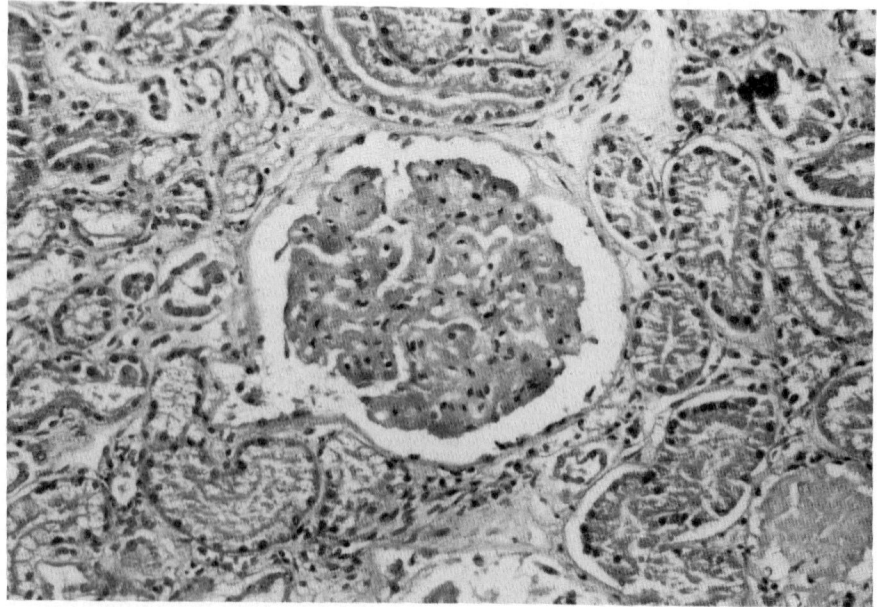

Fig. 24–9.   Chronic membranous glomerulonephritis in a dog. The capillary walls are greatly thickened. Note absence of cellular proliferation. (H&E stain.) (Courtesy of Drs. R. M. Lewis and D. O. Slauson and *Veterinary Pathology*.)

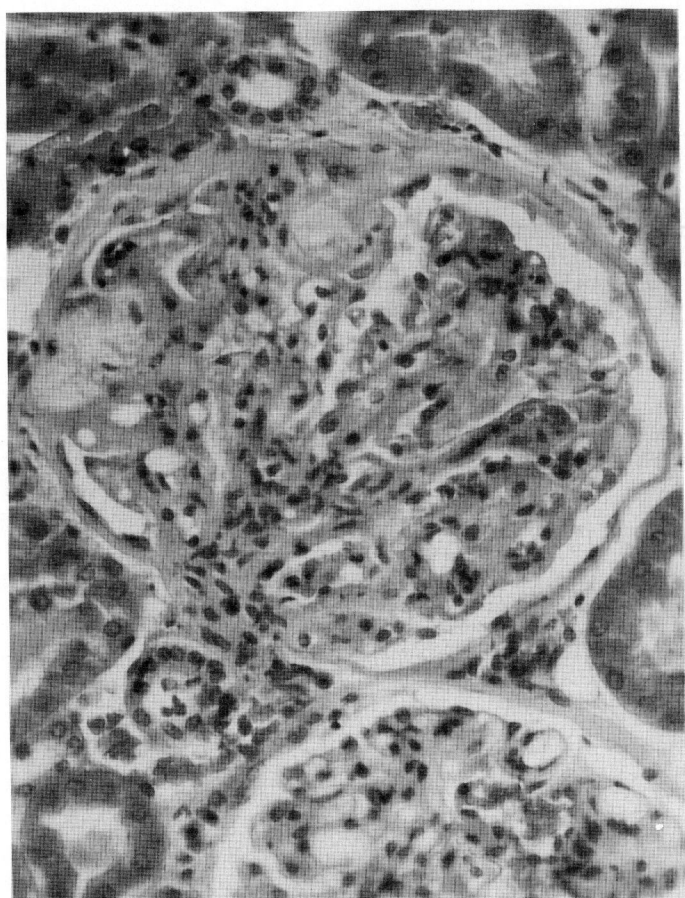

Fig. 24–10.   Membranous glomerulonephritis in an aged dog. Basement membranes thickened and adhesions to Bowman's capsule. (Courtesy of Armed Forces Institute of Pathology.)

increase in interstitial fluid caused by generalized edema. In some stages, the kidney may become contracted and fibrous as an end stage. The possibility of chronic glomerulonephritis resulting from this entity must also be considered.

Membranoproliferative Glomerulonephritis (Mesangiocapillary Glomerulonephritis, Mesangioproliferative Glomerulonephritis). Often glomerular disease in man and animals is characterized by both proliferative and membranous changes. The pathologic features represent a combination of the lesions already described including a marked increase in mesangial cells and mesangial basement membrane

substance, thickened basement membranes, and often splitting of basement membranes. It appears to be a distinct entity and not a combination of the other two forms.

The condition has been subgrouped into two types based on two patterns of immunoglobulin deposition. In one, granular deposits of immune globulin are present on the subendothelial side of the basement membrane and in the mesangium, and in the other, a more linear, dense deposit containing little immunoglobulin but significant amounts of complement (see alternate pathway glomerulonephritis) within the basement membrane. A membranoprolif-

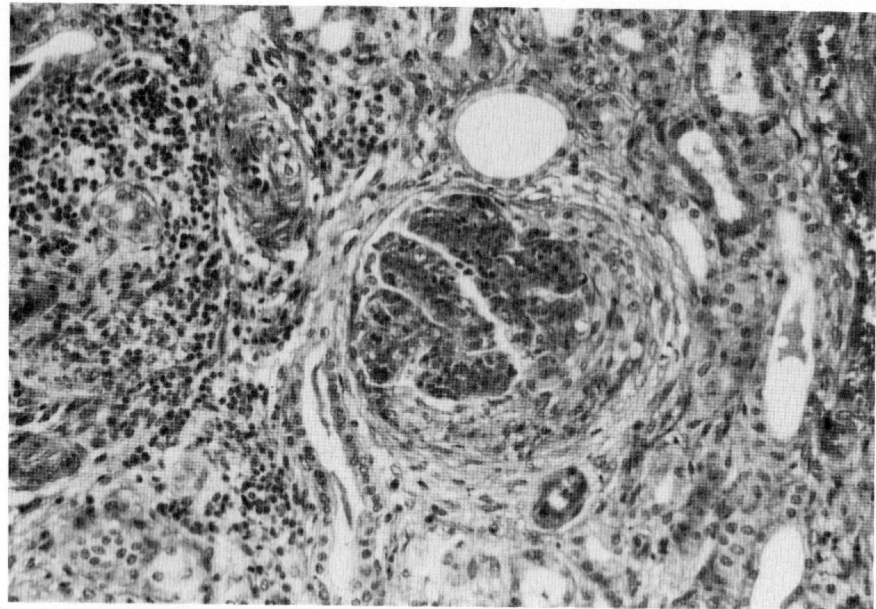

Fig. 24–11. Mesangioproliferative glomerulonephritis in a Finnish Landrace lamb. There are proliferative changes in tufts and marked epithelial crescent formation. (Courtesy of Drs. R. M. Lewis and D. O. Slauson and *Veterinary Pathology*.)

erative (mesangiocapillary) glomerulonephritis has been recognized in Finnish Landrace sheep and is believed to resemble the disease as seen in man (Angus, et al., 1973, 1974; Gardiner, 1976). Affected sheep are deficient in the third component of complement from birth, as are human patients. Glycoprotein deposits, presumably immunoglobulin, are also present in the choroid plexus, associated with focal malacia and edema of the brain.

If the proliferative component is principally mesangial, the term mesangioproliferative glomerulonephritis is applied. This also appears to be a distinct entity and has been associated with mesangial IgM deposition in man.

Chronic Glomerulonephritis. This lesion currently appears to be the late stage of one or more of the various forms of glomerulonephritis. At this writing it is not known which forms of glomerular disease are most often responsible for this lesion. This end stage of glomerular disease may be encountered at necropsy and is

often the lesion which results in terminal uremia. The clinical manifestations are variable and depend upon the number of glomeruli affected as well as the degree of malfunction in involved glomeruli.

Lesions. Microscopically, the lesions in glomeruli include increased numbers of cells (endothelial, mesangial, and epithelial) in the glomerulus with disorganization and occlusion of the lumens of glomerular capillaries. The proliferating epithelial cells may accumulate along the parietal layer of Bowman's capsule to form the so-called epithelial crescents. Adhesions of the glomerulus to Bowman's capsule may occur, and Bowman's space is often obliterated. Electron micrographs confirm the proliferation of epithelial and endothelial cells and disclose reduplication, thickening, and disorganization of the glomerular basement membrane. The lumen of capillaries is usually occluded. In advanced stages, the entire glomerulus is replaced by hyaline connective tissue.

Interference with the circulation through

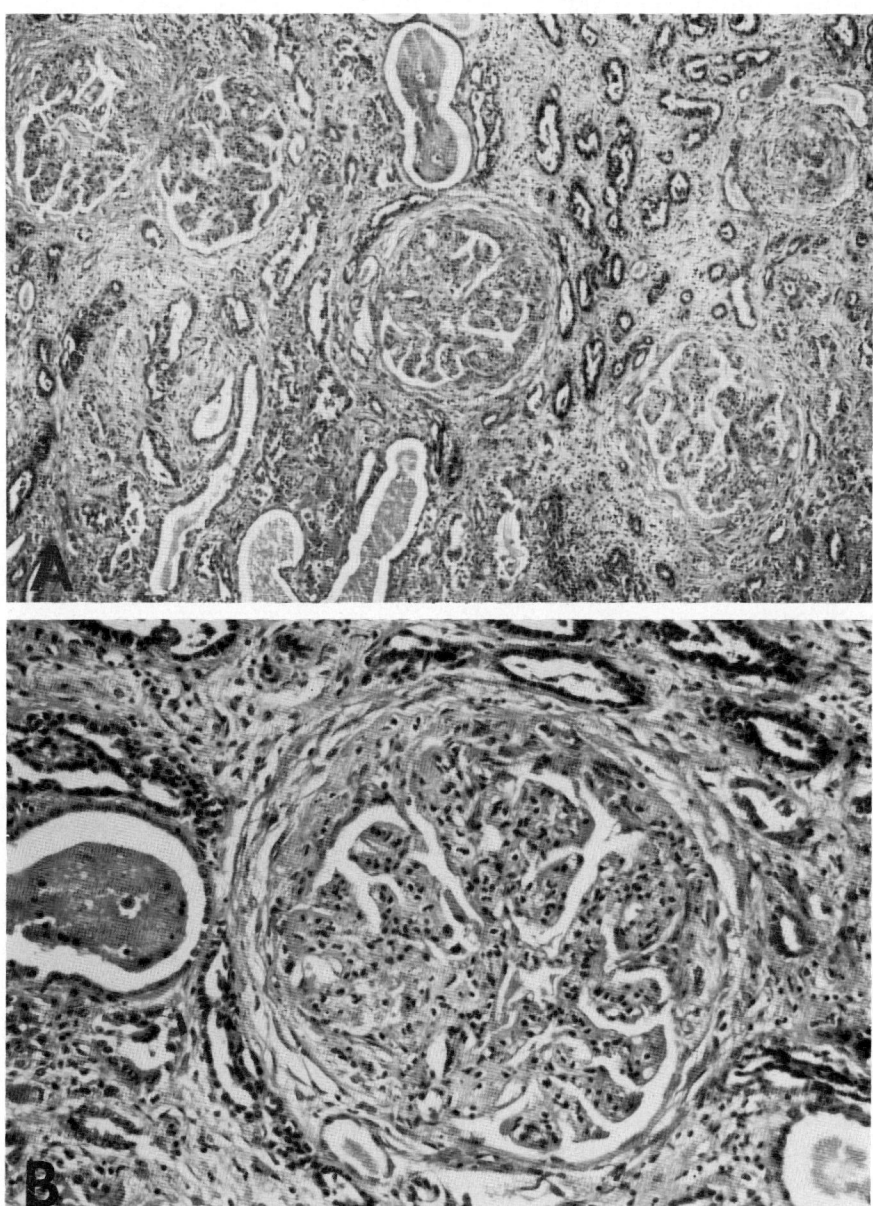

Fig. 24–12. Chronic glomerulonephritis in a dog. *A,* There are proliferative and sclerotic changes within the glomeruli, and concentric periglomerular fibrosis. Tubules are atrophied and replaced by interstitial fibrosis. *B,* Higher magnification of a single glomerulus. (Courtesy of Drs. R. M. Lewis and D. O. Slauson and *Veterinary Pathology*.)

the glomerulus obviously decreases the blood supply to the tubular parts of the nephron and leads to their degeneration. Severe fibrosis of the interstitium results from this ischemia, and many tubules atrophy.

As the fibrous connective tissue contracts, the kidney tends to decrease in size and increase in density. At this end stage it is difficult to reconstruct the events in glomeruli, tubules, or interstitium that may have led to this combination of lesions. Such kidneys are usually smaller than normal, rough or pitted on the surface, and tough to cut, often with a coarse, granular, or cystic cut surface.

It is evident that chronic glomerulonephritis, from the pathologist's viewpoint, represents a definite combination of lesions which obviously seriously interfered with renal function during life, but whose etiology and pathogenesis cannot be discerned in each individual case. This lesion has been reported in many mammalian and reptilian species (Zwart, 1964). Presumably, it would be found in all mammals by adequate study of these species.

Etiology and Pathogenesis. With the exception of embolic glomerulonephritis, the cause and mechanisms involved in glomerulonephritis are generally unknown. Most evidence, however, suggests that proliferative, membranous, and membranoproliferative glomerulonephritis result from immunologically mediated injury. Slauson and Lewis (1979) have recently reviewed these mechanisms in glomerulonephritis in animals. Two principal types of immunologic injury are recognized: immune complex glomerulonephritis and antiglomerular basement membrane antibody disease.

Immune complex glomerulonephritis results from the deposition in glomeruli of antigen-antibody complexes. The complexes most often become entrapped within the glomerular basement membrane on the epithelial side, but may also occur in the lamina densa, on the endothe-

lial side, or in the mesangium. The deposits are characteristically focal, giving rise to a "lumpy-bumpy" appearance of the glomerular basement membrane when stained with silver or periodic acid-Schiff techniques. The complexes contain IgG (and sometimes other immunoglobulins), complement, and antigen. Complement activation is the principal mechanism for initiating the damaging inflammatory sequelae. The offending antigen is most often not identified, but may be foreign or autologous.

Many different foreign antigens, most often infectious agents, have been identified. These include: streptococcal antigens in poststreptococcal glomerulonephritis in human beings; lactic dehydrogenase virus; lymphocytic choriomeningitis virus; equine infectious anemia virus; Aleutian mink disease virus; murine leukemia and sarcoma viruses; hog cholera virus; African swine fever virus; canine adenovirus; *Dirofilaria immitis;* and *Plasmodium* sp. Many more agents are suspected of leading to similar immune complexes. Immune complexes of noninfectious origin that lead to glomerulonephritis are encountered in acute and chronic serum sickness; recently, tumor antigen-antibody complexes have been identified in glomerular disease. Pyometra in dogs is associated with a high incidence of glomerulonephritis, but the offending antigen has not been identified.

Autologous immune complex glomerulonephritis is similar to that resulting from viral or other foreign antigen, but in this case, the immune complexes are a combination of antibody with autologous antigens. The disease was first experimentally induced in rats by Heyman, et al. (1959) by the injection of homologous renal tissue and Freund's adjuvant. In this model, the glomerular lesions result from deposition of circulating immune complexes composed of auto-antibody and an autologous antigen which is normally present in proximal convoluted tubular cells. The disease has also been induced in rabbits with

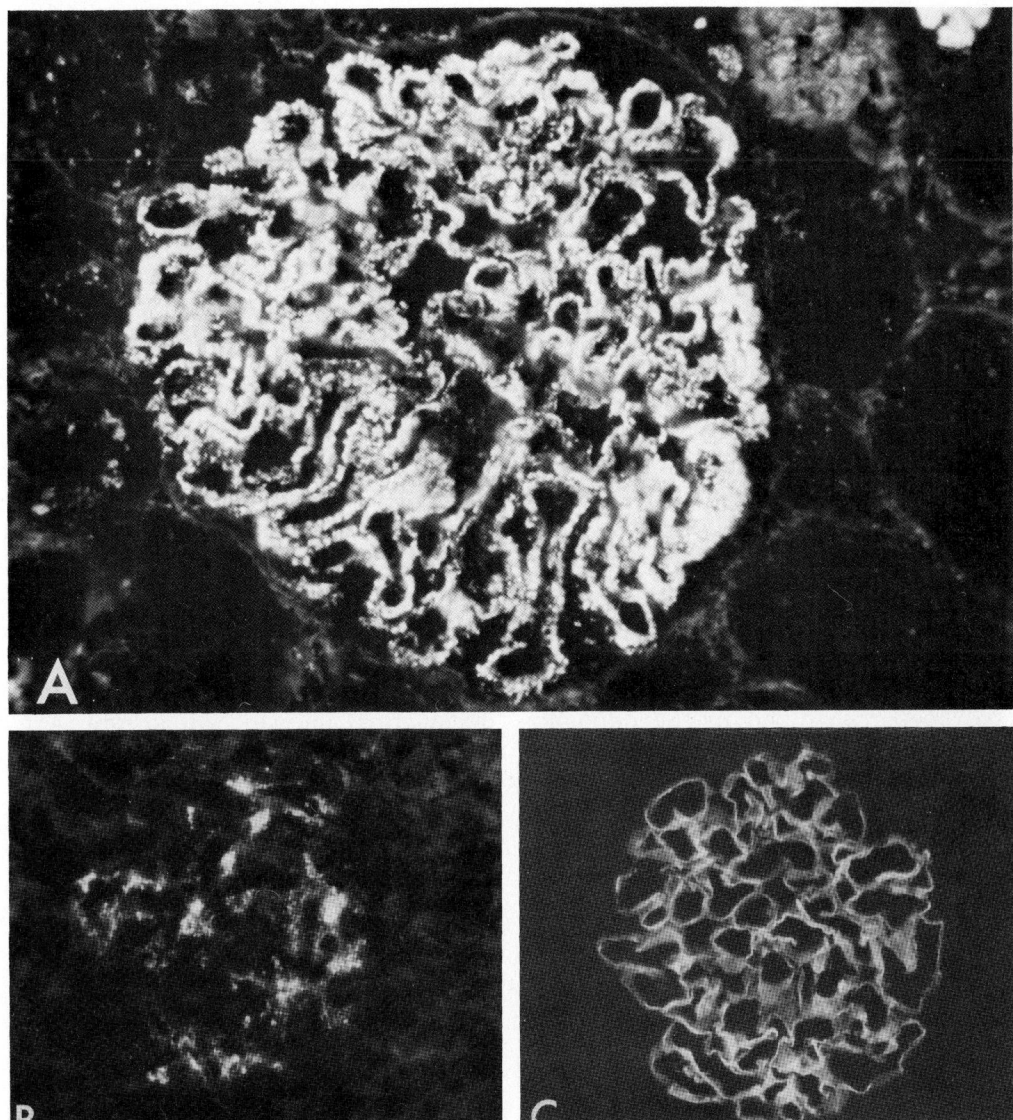

Fig. 24-13. Immunofluorescent patterns in glomerulonephritis. *A*, Chronic membranoproliferative glomerulonephritis in a three-year-old female miniature Schnauzer. Focal discrete deposits of canine immunoglobulins and complement along glomerular capillary basement membranes. This is the classic lumpy-bumpy deposition characteristic of immune complex glomerulonephritis. (Courtesy of Dr. R. M. Lewis.) *B*, Granular deposits of immune complexes confined almost exclusively to the mesangial regions. This is from a rat injected four hours earlier with soluble immune complexes. *C*, Anti-GBM disease in a rat following injection of rabbit anti-rat GBM serum. There is a completely continuous smooth (linear) staining for IgG along the glomerular basement membrane. (*B* and *C* courtesy of Dr. A. Bernard Collins, Department of Pathology, Massachusetts General Hospital.)

thyroglobulin (Weigle and Nakamura, 1969).

Autologous immune complex glomerulonephritis is a much less common cause of immune complex disease, but does represent the major mechanism in two animal diseases: New Zealand Black (NZB) mice disease and canine lupus erythematosus. Bielchowsky et al. (1966) first described an autoimmune hemolytic anemia in NZB mice in 1959. Hybrids with a "normal" strain (NZW) were found to have a spontaneous disease in which weight loss, progressive anemia, hepatosplenomegaly, alopecia, positive lupus erythematosus (LE) preparations, and circulating autoantibody—free and on red blood cells— were conspicuous features. Death occurred from renal failure at 8 to 10 months of age. The glomerular disease is both membranous and proliferative and characterized ultrastructurally by nodular deposits of immune complex within and on either side of the basement membrane. Three antibodies have been recognized in the deposits: antinuclear antibody, antibody to Gross leukemia virus, and antibody directed against erythrocyte antigens. The disease resembles systemic lupus erythematosus of man but differs in some minute details.

Canine lupus erythematosus, described by Lewis, et al. (1963, 1965), is another animal disease complex which closely simulates the human syndrome. The canine disease is manifest by recurring episodes of hemolytic anemia and thrombocytopenia, positive Coombs test and LE (lupus erythematosus) preparations; it has an autoimmune basis, the antigen being nuclear deoxyribonucleic acid (DNA). The antinuclear antibody immune complex leads to membranous or membranoproliferative glomerulonephritis. Some canine patients are affected with a type of arthritis typical of the rheumatoid type, and most eventually die from membranous glomerulonephritis. The renal lesions are typical of those described previously in this chapter.

Antiglomerular basement membrane antibody disease results from antibodies directed against glomerular basement membrane. Masugi (1934) first produced an experimental model of this type of glomerulonephritis by injecting rats with an antiserum prepared by immunizing rabbits with preparations of rat kidney. This antibody localized in the glomerular basement membranes and resulted in a glomerulonephritis sometimes referred to as "nephrotoxic nephritis." It has been found subsequently that the antigen in this system is glomerular basement membrane, and that its antigenicity is not species specific. In the natural disease it is possible that some autoimmune mechanism may make the animal's basement membrane antigenic to its own immune mechanisms, or that bacteria or viruses may contain common antigens which are selectively deposited with antibody on basement membranes. Antiglomerular basement membrane (anti-GBM) disease has been documented in man, but is rare. Aside from rare reports in horses (Banks and Henson, 1972) and dogs (Wright, et al., 1976), the disease has not been described as a natural disease of animals.

The pattern of antibody deposits in anti-GBM disease differs from that seen in immune complex disease. Fluorescent microscopy reveals a linear deposition rather than granular, and ultrastructurally, there is a thin linear layer of fluffy material between the capillary endothelium and basement membrane.

In man and to a lesser extent in animals, a third immunologic mechanism has been described called **alternate pathway disease.** In this membranoproliferative glomerulonephritis, immunofluorescence demonstrates deposits of complement and properdin with little immunoglobulin. This mechanism is particularly important in membranoproliferative glomerulonephritis.

In human patients a glomerulonephritis is recognized in which large amounts of

IgA (with lesser amounts of IgG) are deposited in the mesangium and capillary loops. This **immunoglobulin A glomerulonephritis** is usually focal and nonprogressive.

Anderson, L.J., and Jarrett, W.F.H.: Membranous glomerulonephritis associated with leukaemia in cats. Res. Vet. Sci., 12:179–180, 1971.

Angus, K.W., Gardiner, A.C., Sykes, A.R., and Davison, A.M.: A rapidly progressing mesangiocapillary glomerulonephritis in Finnish Landrace lambs. Vet. Rec., 92:337–338, 1973.

Angus, K.W., et al.: Mesangiocapillary glomerulonephritis in lambs. II. Pathological findings and electron microscopy of the renal lesions. J. Comp. Pathol., 84:319–330, 1974.

Banks, K.L., Henson, J.B., and McGuire, T.C.: Immunologically mediated glomerulitis of horses. I. Pathogenesis in persistent infection by equine infectious anemia virus. Lab. Invest., 26:701–707, 1972.

Banks, K.L., and Henson, J.B.: Immunologically mediated glomerulitis of horses. II. Antiglomerular basement membrane antibody and other mechanisms in spontaneous disease. Lab. Invest., 26:708–715, 1972.

Ben-Ishay, Z., et al.: Fine structure alterations in the canine kidney during hemorrhagic hypotension. Effects of osmotic diuresis. Lab. Invest., 17:190–210, 1967.

Bhasin, H.K., Abuelo, J.G., Nayak, R., and Esparza, A.R.: Mesangial proliferative glomerulonephritis. Lab. Invest., 39:21–29, 1978.

Bielchowsky, M., Helyer, B.J., and Howie, J.B.: Spontaneous haemolytic anaemia of mice of the NZB/Bl strain. Blood, 27:435, 1966.

Bradfield, J.W.B., and Cattell, V.: The mesangial cell in glomerulonephritis. I. Mechanisms of hypercellularity in experimental immune complex glomerulonephritis. Lab. Invest., 36:481–486, 1977.

Burkholder, P.M.: Ultrastructural demonstration of injury and perforation of glomerular capillary basement membrane in acute proliferative glomerulonephritis. Am. J. Pathol., 56:251–266, 1969.

Burkholder, P.M., Marchand, A., and Krueger, R.P.: Mixed membranous and proliferative glomerulonephritis. Lab. Invest., 23:459–479, 1970.

Casey, H.W., and Splitter, G.A.: Membranous glomerulonephritis in dogs infected with *Dirofilaria immitis*. Vet. Pathol., 12:111–117, 1975.

Comerford, F.R., Cohen, A.S., and Desai, R.G.: The evolution of the glomerular lesion in NZB mice. A light- and electron-microscopic study. Lab. Invest., 19:643–651, 1968.

Davis, B.K., and Cavallo, T.: Membranoproliferative glomerulonephritis. Am. J. Pathol., 84:283–298, 1976.

Finlayson, G., et al.: Immunoglobulin A glomerulonephritis: a clinicopathologic study. Lab. Invest., 32:140–148, 1975.

Fisher, E.R., and Fisher, B.: Glomerular lipoidosis in the dog. Am. J. Vet. Res., 15:285–286, 1954.

Foley, W.A., et al.: A renal lesion associated with diuresis in the aging Sprague-Dawley rat. Lab. Invest., 13:439–450, 1964.

French, J.: Glomerulonephrosis. A morphologic manifestation of renal cortical ischemia in toxic oliguria and lower nephron nephrosis. Arch. Pathol., 49:43–54, 1950.

Gardiner, A.C.: Mesangiocapillary glomerulonephritis in lambs. III. Quantitative and qualitative aspects of immunopathology. J. Pathol., 119:11–19, 1976.

Grishman, E., et al.: Lupus nephritis with organized deposits in the kidneys. Lab. Invest., 16:717–725, 1967.

Gude, W.D., and Upton, A.C.: A histologic study of spontaneous glomerular lesions in aging RF mice. Am. J. Pathol., 40:699–709, 1962.

Guttman, P.H., and Kohn, H.I.: Progressive intercapillary glomerulosclerosis in the mouse, rat, and Chinese hamster, associated with aging and x-ray exposure. Am. J. Pathol., 37:293–307, 1960.

Helyer, B.J., and Howie, J.B.: Renal disease associated with positive lupus erythematosus tests in a cross-bred strain of mice. Nature, 197:197, 1963.

Henson, J.B., Gorham, J.R., and Tanaka, Y.: Renal glomerular ultrastructure in mink affected by Aleutian disease. Lab. Invest., 17:123–139, 1967.

Heyman, W., et al.: Production of nephrotic syndrome in rats by Freund's adjuvant and rat kidney suspension. Proc. Soc. Exp. Biol. Med., 100:660, 1959.

Kajima, M., and Pollard, M.: Ultrastructural pathology of glomerular lesions in gnotobiotic mice with congenital lymphocytic choriomeningitis (LCM) virus infection. Am. J. Pathol., 61:117–140, 1970.

Kindig, D., Spargo, G., and Kirsten, W.H.: Glomerular response in Aleutian disease of mink. Lab. Invest., 16:436–443, 1967.

Krohn, K., Jokelainen, P.T., and Sandholm, M.: Light and electron microscopic observations on glomerular changes in canine interstitial nephritis. Acta Pathol. Microbiol. Scand., 81A:461–473, 1973.

Kurtz, J.M., et al.: Naturally occurring canine glomerulonephritis. Am. J. Pathol., 67:471–482, 1972.

Lambert, P.H., and Dixon, F.J.: Pathogenesis of the glomerulonephritis of the NZB/W mice. J. Exp. Med., 127:507–521, 1968.

Lerner, R.A., and Dixon, F.J.: Induced and spontaneous glomerulonephritis in sheep. Fed. Proc., 25:660, 1966.

Lerner, R.A., and Dixon, F.J.: Spontaneous glomerulonephritis in sheep. Lab. Invest., 15:1279–1289, 1966.

Lerner, R.A., Dixon, F.J., and Lee, S.: Spontaneous glomerulonephritis in sheep. II. Studies on natural history, occurrence in other species, and pathogenesis. Am. J. Pathol., 53:501–512, 1968.

Lewis, R.M., et al.: A syndrome of autoimmune hemolytic anemia and thrombocytopenia in dogs. Sci. Proc. AVMA, 140–163, 1963.

Lewis, R.M.: Clinical evaluation of the lupus erythematosus cell phenomenon in dogs. J. Am. Vet. Med. Assoc., *147*:939–943, 1965.

Lewis, R.M., et al.: Chronic allogeneic disease. I. Development of glomerulonephritis. J. Exp. Med., *128*:653–679, 1968.

Lewis, R.M., Schwartz, R.S., and Gilmore, C.E.: Autoimmune diseases in domestic animals. Ann. N.Y. Acad. Sci., *124*:178–200, 1965.

Lewis, R.M., Schwartz, R.S., and Henry, W.B.: Canine systemic lupus erythematosus. Blood, *25*:143–160, 1965.

Margolis, G., et al.: Glomerulonephritis occurring in experimental brucellosis in dogs. Am. J. Pathol., *23*:983–993, 1947.

Masugi, M.: Uber die experimentelle glomerulonephritis durch das specifische antinierenserum. Beitr. Path. Anat., *92*:429–440, 1934.

McCoy, R.C., Abramowsky, C.R., and Tischer, C.C.: IgA Nephropathy. Am. J. Pathol., *76*:123–144, 1974.

McFadyean, J.: Nephritis in animals. J. Comp. Pathol. Therap., *42*:58–71, 141–162, 231–241, 1929.

Merrill, J.P.: Glomerulonephritis (1, 2, and 3 of 3 parts). N. Engl. J. Med., *290*:257–266, 313–319, 374–380, 1974.

Morrison, W.I., Nash, A.S., and Wright, N.G.: Glomerular deposition of immune complexes in dogs following natural infection with canine adenovirus. Vet. Rec., *96*:522–524, 1975.

Muller-Peddinghaus, R., and Trautwein, G.: Spontaneous glomerulonephritis in dogs. I. Classification and immunopathology. Vet. Pathol., *14*:1–13, 1977.

Murray, M., and Wright, N.G.: A morphologic study of canine glomerulonephritis. Lab. Invest., *30*:213–221, 1974.

Osborne, C.A., and Vernier, R.L.: Glomerulonephritis in the dog and cat: a comparative review. J. Am. Anim. Hosp. Assoc., *9*:101–127, 1973.

Pascal, R.R., Koss, M.N., and Dassel, R.L.: Glomerulonephritis associated with immune complex deposits and viral particles in spontaneous murine leukemia: an electron microscopic study with immunofluorescence. Lab. Invest., *29*:159–165, 1973.

Porter, D.D., Dixon, F.J., and Larsen, A.E.: Metabolism and function of gamma globulin in Aleutian disease of mink. J. Exp. Med., *121*:889–900, 1965.

Recher, L., et al.: Further studies on the biological relationship of murine leukemia viruses and on kidney lesions of mice. With leukemia induced by these viruses. Natl. Cancer Inst. Monogr., *22*:459–479, 1966.

Saegusa, S., Shimizu, F., Hasegawa, A., and Usui, K.:Some clinical and immunological aspects on contracted kidney in cats. Jpn. J. Exp. Med., *45*:403–413, 1975.

Slauson, D.O., and Lewis, R.M.: Comparative pathology of glomerulonephritis in animals. Vet. Pathol., *16*:135–164, 1979.

Sun, S.-C., et al.: Coxsackie B₄ viral nephritis in mice and its autoimmunelike phenomena. Proc. Soc. Exp. Biol. Med., *126*:882–885, 1967.

Weigle, W.O., and Nakamura, R.M.: Perpetuation of autoimmune thyroiditis and production of secondary renal lesions following periodic injections of aqueous preparations of altered thyroglobulin. Clin. Exp. Immunol., *4*:645–647, 1969.

Weksler, M.E., et al.: Nephrotic syndrome in malignant melanoma: demonstration of melanoma antigen-antibody complexes in kidney. Kidney Int., *6*:112A, 1974.

Wright, N.G., et al.: Chronic renal failure in dogs: a comparative clinical and morphological study of chronic glomerulonephritis and chronic interstitial nephritis. Vet. Rec., *98*:288–293, 1976.

Wright, N.G., Morrison, W.I., Thompson, H., and Cornwell, H.J.C.: Mesangial localization of immune complexes in experimental canine adenovirus glomerulonephritis. Br. J. Exp. Pathol., *55*:458–465, 1974.

Zwart, P.: Studies on renal pathology in reptiles. Path. Vet., *1*:542–556, 1964.

Focal Embolic Glomerulonephritis. This lesion is most often a sequel to a localized bacterial infection elsewhere in the body. In man, acute bacterial endocarditis is the most common antecedent—a situation which also occurs in other species, particularly in cattle, swine and dogs. Other sources of infection may also be possible, such as bacterial pneumonia, reticulitis, and other localized infections. Emboli of infected necrotic tissue are presumed to reach the glomeruli to initiate the lesion, although the presence of organisms is not always demonstrable.

In some instances, however, colonies of bacteria may be demonstrable in glomeruli (Fig. 24–14) and some of these may lead to frank abscesses (Fig. 24–16C).

The lesion is recognized by light microscopy as a focal zone of necrosis, usually involving part of the glomerulus, with neutrophil infiltration and occasionally hemorrhage. Affected glomeruli are patchily scattered throughout the kidneys. In some, proliferation of epithelial cells and formation of "crescents" may occur, making the lesion difficult to distinguish from proliferative glomerulonephritis. In this latter situation, necrosis is not as conspicuous and larger numbers of glomeruli are involved nearly simultaneously.

Affected kidneys may bear scattered petechiae and occasionally multiple tiny

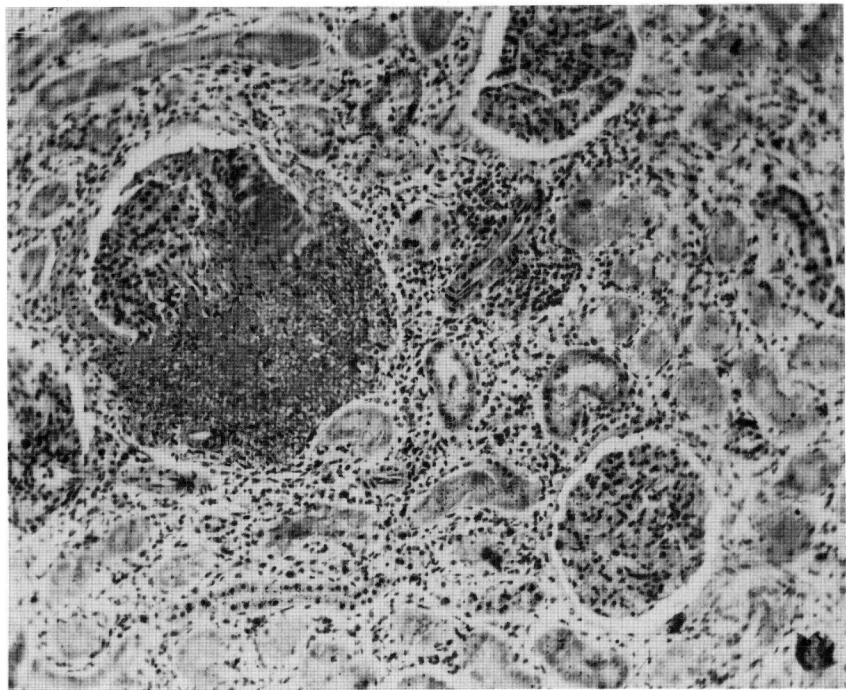

Fig. 24–14. Focal embolic glomerulonephritis in a dog. (Courtesy of Armed Forces Institute of Pathology.)

abscesses. In the bovine, one or more renal lobules may be affected with most of the kidney free of gross involvement. Although frank embolism is not demonstrable in each case, it seems expedient to consider this lesion in animals to be most often the result of bacterial embolism.

Other Glomerular Lesions

Amyloid in the Kidney. The kidney is one of the most frequently affected organs in both primary and secondary amyloidosis. The glomeruli are the usual and most important site of deposition in most species, but there is, in addition, usually some deposition in arterial walls and surrounding tubules as well. For reasons unknown, in cats with renal amyloidosis, the glomeruli are usually less affected than are the tubules, especially those in the medulla. The medulla is also frequently affected in bovine renal amyloidosis. Medullary deposits in cats have been associated with papillary necrosis, presumably by interfering with circulation.

Microscopically, the amount of amyloid is seen to be small in the early stages, but eventually many renal corpuscles are almost completely replaced by amyloid. The amyloid usually remains more or less lobulated, however, which facilitates distinguishing amyloidosis from hyaline scarring of glomeruli. Grossly, the change is not easily detected, but the application of an iodine solution such as Lugol's to a slice of fresh kidney which has previously been exposed to a weak acid brings out affected glomeruli as conspicuous brown spots visible to the naked eye.

Extensive glomerular amyloidosis leads to glomerular inefficiency, proteinuria, and renal failure. A high incidence of thrombosis, particularly of pulmonary arteries, has been reported in dogs with renal amyloidosis by Slauson and Gribble (1971).

Nephrotic Syndrome. This is a clinical syndrome, best known in human patients, but also occurring in animals. It should not be confused with **nephrosis,** a term used to refer to specific pathologic entities. The nephrotic syndrome is manifest by (1) proteinuria, principally albuminuria, (2) hypoproteinemia, (3) generalized edema (anasarca), (4) hyperlipemia (especially hypercholesterolemia), and (5) lipiduria. The syndrome may result from any of the disseminated diseases of glomeruli (membranous glomerulonephritis, proliferative glomerulonephritis, amyloidosis, nodular glomerulosclerosis), thrombosis of renal veins, or rarely toxic tubular nephritis.

The syndrome is believed to result from increased permeability of the glomeruli to protein, permitting it to be lost with the urine. The exact mechanism is unknown but present theories include the concepts that (1) the glomerular basement membrane is chiefly responsible for the filtration or (2) the podocytes are responsible for this function. Lesions in one or the other of these structures could account for increased permeability, resulting in the loss of protein.

Arakawa, M.: A scanning electron microscopy of the glomerulus of normal and nephrotic rats. Lab. Invest., 23:489–496, 1970.

Gruys, E.: Bovine renal amyloidosis. I. Incidence, macroscopical and microscopical features. Tijdschr. Diergeneeskd., 99:715–728, 1974.

Osborne, C.A., et al.: Clinicopathologic progression of renal amyloidosis in a dog. J. Am. Vet. Med. Assoc., 157:203–219, 1970.

Platt, H.: A case of generalized amyloidosis in the dog. J. Comp. Path. and Therap., 59:91–96, 1949.

Slauson, D.O., and Gribble, D.H.: Thrombosis complicating renal amyloidosis in dogs. Vet. Pathol., 8:352–363, 1971.

Diseases of Renal Tubules and the Interstitium

In this section we shall consider primary degeneration and inflammatory diseases of the renal tubules and interstitium in the absence of glomerular disease. We have already stressed that tubular and interstitial disease may be secondary to glomerular damage. Primary tubulointerstitial disease, or interstitial nephritis, is characterized by degeneration and necrosis of tubular epithelium, edema, cellular infiltration, and other components of the inflammatory reaction in the interstitium. Depending on the severity of the insult and its duration, the lesion may progress to chronic interstitial nephritis characterized by marked interstitial fibrosis, absence of tubules and dilated tubules. The end stage may be a fibrotic kidney containing relatively normal glomeruli. Several systems of classification have evolved for primary tubulointerstitial disease, none of which is completely satisfactory. In part, this results from the diversity of causes. We shall consider this group as follows.

1. Acute Interstitial Nephritis
   a. Toxic Tubular Nephritis
   b. Hypoxic (lower nephron) Nephrosis
   c. Immunologic Tubulointerstitial Nephritis
   d. Infectious Interstitial Nephritis
2. Chronic Interstitial Nephritis
3. Pyelonephritis
4. Miscellaneous Tubular Disorders

Acute Interstitial Nephritis

Toxic Tubular Nephritis. In this condition, various irritant toxic substances act directly and without any previous hypersensitization to produce fatty change and necrosis of the delicate epithelial cells lining the tubules, a sequence of degenerative changes which have already been seen to result from the actions of similar toxins on the epithelium of the liver. There are also hyperemia and, somewhat later, limited infiltrations of lymphocytes and neutrophils and proliferation of fibrous tissue. The inflammatory reaction may be minimal, especially if the insult leads to early death. For this reason, the term **nephrosis** (acute toxic tubular nephrosis) is often used to describe the lesion. Toxic tubular nephritis and toxic tubular nephrosis should be considered synonymous.

The proximal convoluted tubules, with their large and highly specialized epithelial cells, suffer most, especially with respect to necrosis, which may, in some toxemias (as poisoning from the budding leaves of certain oaks), leave these tubules as solid, dense-appearing masses of coagulated protoplasm. The lipidosis may be most extensive in these tubules or it may appear chiefly or exclusively in the epithelium of the ascending loops of Henle, especially in the medullary rays. This difference may well have diagnostic significance, but the exact distinctions have not been elucidated. Calcification, usually in the form of granules no larger than one or two cells, is not unusual in tubules which persist after a limited amount of necrosis. The gross appearance of toxic tubular nephrosis is that of the large, pale kidney.

If degeneration and necrosis have not become too extensive, regeneration of the epithelial lining cells is possible upon removal of the cause. Hence, a most important aspect of treatment in the case of acute nephrotoxic poisonings is the adoption of measures (the "artificial kidney") designed to avoid a fatal uremia before regeneration and restoration of tubular function can occur, a period of 10 days or more. In fatal cases, the proximal tubules, at least, suffer complete destruction; the other parts of the nephron follow the same course less rapidly. In the surviving patient, the fibrous tissue of chronic inflammation partially takes the place of lost tubules, producing the "small, white, granular, contracted kidney." The glomeruli may survive, and, with the loss of most of the intervening tubular structures, they come to lie very close together, giving the erroneous impression that their number has been increased. All of the above changes may advance rapidly in one segment of the kidney, but leave an adjacent part untouched. This is probably because of a physiologic tendency of one group of nephrons to function while another rests, the nonfunctioning group often escaping a transient severe concentration of the blood-borne poison. It is this mechanism which sometimes permits survival of the patient, although with permanent loss of segments of his renal parenchyma. In such a case, the remaining tubules tend to undergo a compensatory hypertrophy characterized by increase in size, with or without increase in height of their epithelial linings. Such patients secrete large volumes of poorly concentrated urine of low specific gravity.

Causes. The causes of toxic tubular nephritis are toxic irritant substances brought to the kidney by the circulating blood, the previously stated facts being borne in mind by the reader that the tubules commonly suffer a limited amount of toxic injury from locally elaborated toxins in the vicinity of lesions of infectious nephritis, and, also, that ischemia from occlusion of the glomerular capillaries can cause the same types of degenerative tubular injury. The blood-borne toxic substances can conveniently be divided into classes as follows:

1. "Chemical" poisons. In general, the same poisons that cause toxic effects on the liver produce toxic nephritis to some degree. More or less in order of declining importance are the soluble salts of mercury (mercuric chloride, excessive doses of calomel, mercurial fungicides used to disinfect seed, such as Ceresan), of chromium (potassium bichromate), uranium (uranium nitrate), copper (copper sulfate used as a parasiticide, fungicide, molluscicide), bismuth (excessive "BIPP," bismuth-iodoform-petrolatum paste used in the treatment of wounds), cadmium, arsenic, and phosphorus. Organic nephrotoxic chemicals, also somewhat in order of declining importance to the renal lesions include carbon tetrachloride (solvent, anthelmintic), tetrachloroethylene (anthelmintic), various chlorinated-hydrocarbon insecticides such as "Toxaphene," sulfonamide allergy, oxalic acid and oxalates, usually of plant origin, turpentine, cantharides,

iodoform, phenol, pyrogallic acid, alpha-naphthyl thiourea (ANTU rat-poison), and others. Sodium monofluoroacetate (the rodenticide "1080") and other fluorine compounds probably belong in this group. In the case of many of these substances, the direct toxic effect is reinforced by the anoxia of renal congestion and failing circulation.

A startling picture of **hydropic degeneration** of practically 100% of the epithelial cells of the kidney is produced in poisoning by dioxane, by ethylene glycol (used as "antifreeze" in automobiles), and by diethylene glycol (formerly used as a vehicle for sulfonamide drugs). The cytoplasm is distended with fluid so that in ordinary microscopic sections the enlarged and crowded cells are strikingly clear and empty. The change is sometimes called **vacuolar degeneration.** It leads to necrosis, and the patient is likely to die, but the change is promptly reversible if the cause is removed. A similar picture can result from the experimental injection intravenously of concentrated solutions of sucrose, although this is transitory. A vacuolar change in the epithelium of the proximal tubules is stated to be characteristic of potassium deficiency.

2. Plant poisons, many of which undoubtedly have not been identified in accurate relation to renal pathology. Included are poisoning by the young buds of certain species of oaks, young plants of cockleburs, which are eaten by pigs, sacahuiste, broomweed of the Southwestern United States, called snakeweed in the Great Plains (*Gutierrezia microcephala*), *Baileya multiradiata, Drymaria pachyphylla*, lupines, aspidium (male fern), used as a teniacide, senecios, mushrooms, and moldy feeds. Oxalate-containing plants injure the kidney by deposition of crystals in the tubules.

3. Mycotoxins are also recognized as causing toxic nephrosis. Of particular interest are ochratoxins and atrinin as causes of mould nephrosis of swine.

4. Endogenous toxemias are usually produced in the course of other diseases. Here belongs the necrosis characteristic of most of the acute infections. In the ketosis of "pregnant-ewe toxemia," severe lipidosis of the renal tubules, as well as of the liver, is a prominent lesion.

The term **hepatorenal syndrome** has been applied to the simultaneous occurrence of hepatic and renal dysfunction in the human or animal patient. The assumption that the lesions in the kidney were caused by those in the liver has not been supported by satisfactory evidence. For this reason the term has little meaning in the field of pathology.

Hypoxic (Hemoglobinuric, Shock, Lower Nephron) Nephrosis. A syndrome differing both in tissue changes and in etiology from the ordinary toxic disorders just described exists in the form of the rather poorly understood condition which Lucké (1946) has called "lower nephron nephrosis." While this condition has some aspects in common with the toxic tubular nephrosis just discussed, particularly the ultimate necrosis of tubular epithelium, there are two essential characteristics which mark "lower nephron nephrosis" as a different entity. These are (1) the fact that the epithelial damage is primarily in the "lower nephron," that is, the last part of Henle's loop and the distal convoluted tubule, rather than in the usually vulnerable proximal tubule, and (2) the presence of dense and conspicuous casts in many of these lower nephrons. The casts stain a dirty, almost brownish red when submitted to hematoxylin and eosin, a shade quite different from the bright pink of the ordinary hyalin casts of albuminuria. While the exact chemical changes have not been elucidated, the different appearance is due to derivatives of hemoglobin (or myoglobin) and the casts are called **hemoglobin casts.** Lesions which accompany these two pathognomonic changes, at least in the late stages, include cytoplasmic disintegration and necrosis of epithelium in other than the lower parts of the nephron, and localized infiltrations of lymphocytes and other inflammatory cells in the interstitial tissue. The proximal tubules are often markedly dilated, as if from obstruction lower down in the nephron.

Symptomatically, the syndrome presents itself with oliguria, anuria, and uremia. Shock or a shock-like condition is a preceding or accompanying derangement contributing to the seriousness of the situation. Obstruction of the lower parts of the nephron by the hemoglobin casts is one postulated cause of the cessation of urinary secretion, but the number of casts is scarcely sufficient to account entirely, or even principally, for the loss of function. The accompanying hypotension and inadequate glomerular hydrostatic pressure are believed to be the principal basis of renal shutdown and ischemic injury to renal tubules. Increased renin excretion further restricts blood supply, augmenting tubular damage.

The extra-renal disorders leading to "lower nephron nephrosis" are numerous and diverse, although the inexact boundaries assigned to this syndrome cause some variations in the list of acceptable causes. The large crushing and bruising injuries, azoturia, and the extensive hemolysis which follows a transfusion with incompatible blood are the most important causes in animals. They all result directly in the accumulation of free hemoglobin or myoglobin in the blood and therefore in the kidneys. Similar renal changes are said to occur in certain rare myoglobinurias resembling azoturia, but affecting other species than the equine. A practically identical syndrome, either histopathologically or clinically, also follows extensive burns and perhaps some other forms of tissue destruction.

The urine in humans suffering this affliction is highly acid, and the suggestion has been made that this acidity is important in precipitating the hemoglobin. Whether the same acidity is present in similar cases in the herbivorous animals, whose urine is normally alkaline, we are not able to say. Lower nephron nephrosis has followed experimental transfusions in dogs, but only when the urine was made highly acid and the blood was hemolyzed in considerable amounts previous to introduction into the animal's circulation. The disorder was, however, more easily produced in dogs whose renal circulation was already impaired by preexisting chronic nephritis or by the low hydrostatic pressure incident to a state of shock. It may well be that in most naturally occurring cases in man or animal, both hemoglobinemia and renal ischemia operate synergistically to produce the renal damage and insufficiency (De Gowin, et al., 1938; Yuile, et al., 1949).

Immunologic Tubulointerstitial Nephritis. Immunologically mediated tubular disease can be induced in experimental animals and is recognized as a rare mechanism in renal disease of human beings. Immune complex disease (foreign and autologous) and antitubular basement membrane disease similar to their glomerular counterparts, as well as injury mediated by cytotoxic antibodies and cell-mediated mechanisms, have been identified. **Immune complex tubular disease** is comparable to immune complex glomerulonephritis, the antigen-antibody complexes being deposited in a granular fashion. Granular immune complex may also be present in the glomeruli. By light microscopy, the lesion is characterized by mononuclear interstitial nephritis and degeneration of tubular epithelial cells.

Antitubular basement membrane nephritis is analogous to antiglomerular basement membrane disease glomerulonephritis, but results from antibodies directed against tubular basement membrane. The disease has been experimentally induced in several laboratory animals, and a similar form of disease has been recognized in man. The immunofluorescent findings are characterized by linear accumulation of IgG and, sometimes, C3 along the tubular basement membrane. Histologically, degenerative changes in the tubular epithelium include vacuolation, swelling, increased cytoplasmic acidophilia, and nuclear pyknosis. The cellular infiltrate early in the course of the disease is predominately composed of lymphocytes, macrophages, and multinucleated giant cells with peripheral nuclei. As the disease progresses, tubular necrosis and cellular infiltration become more extensive and accompanied by fibrosis, eventually destroying the overall renal architecture. The relative importance of this autoimmune tubular disease in spontaneous renal disease of animals is not at present known.

In human beings, certain drug-associated tubular damage is recognized as being mediated through immune mechanisms and is not the result of direct toxic action. The toxicity of several antibiotics is believed to result from an immune response to tubular basement membrane (TBM). It is believed that the drugs act like haptens, combining with TBM protein and eliciting the production of anti-TBM antibodies.

Infectious Interstitial Nephritis. Many organisms, but most notably the Leptospira, cause extensive interstitial nephritis. These organisms are found in renal tubular epithelium, but the inflammatory reaction to their presence is confined to the interstitium. Red blood cells, plasma, and neutrophils make up the exudate in early stages but are gradually replaced by plasma cells, lymphocytes, and epithelioid cells as the disease progresses. Interstitial fibrosis and thickening of Bowman's capsule (periglomerular fibrosis) are also believed to be long-term effects (Fig. 24–16A).

Other organisms may also localize in the kidney, resulting in tubular damage and interstitial nephritis. If the organisms are pyogenic, the resulting lesion is acute purulent interstitial nephritis. Certain viruses, such as canine herpesvirus, may also cause tubular damage and interstitial nephritis.

Chronic Interstitial Nephritis

Characterized by marked fibrosis, chronic interstitial nephritis marks the end result of acute interstitial nephritis. Most of the causes of acute interstitial nephritis lead to chronic fibrosing lesions, including chronic bacterial infection, poisons, and immunologic injury. Other mechanisms include ischemia, obstructions, and radiation. The lesion is characterized by marked fibrosis, loss of tubules, and foci of mononuclear infiltration. The glomeruli are relatively unaffected.

Chronic interstitial nephritis was once the most common designation for sclerosing nephritis in dogs; however, most evidence indicates this disorder represents the results of chronic glomerulonephritis.

Pyelonephritis

Pyelonephritis represents one of the more frequent and important forms of interstitial and tubular disease. The word signifies inflammation of the renal pelvis and parenchyma of the kidney. Infection is believed to reach the kidney by ascending through the urinary tract or by dissemination through the vasculature. The latter is the so-called descending route of infection, and although feasible, it is not considered the usual mechanism. In human beings as well as animals, most evidence indicates that the ascending route following cystitis is the more usual. This does not imply a progressive inflammatory reaction of the ureters, which indeed is not a regular finding, but rather a *vesicoureteral reflux* which carries organisms from the bladder to the renal pelvis and even into the renal tubules (*intrarenal reflux*). Pyogenic organisms account for most examples of pyelonephritis. *Escherichia coli* and *Staphylococcus aureus* have been incriminated experimentally in dogs, and *Corynebacterium renale* and *C. pyogenes* are well known pathogens in bovine animals, and *C. suis* in swine.

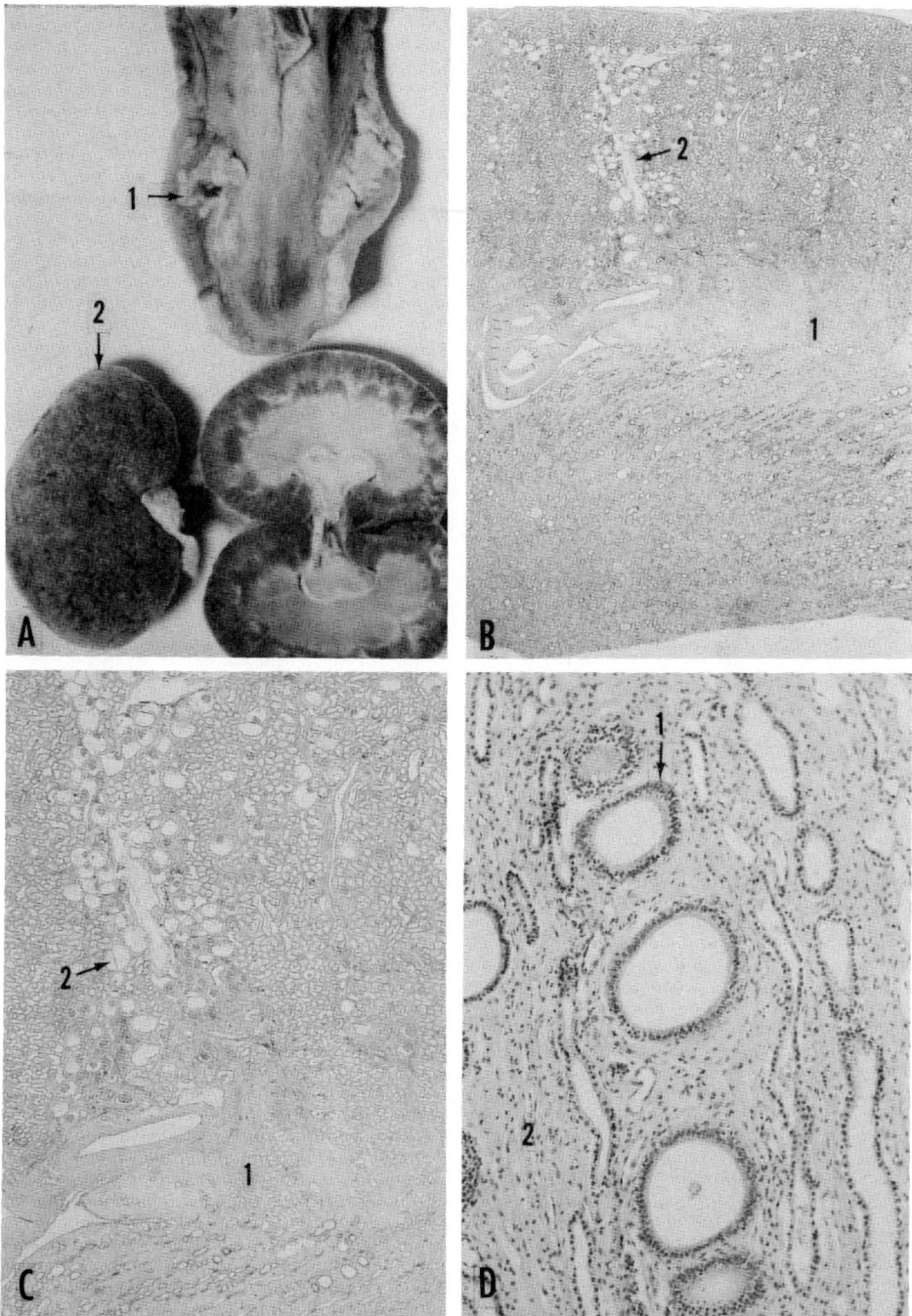

Fig. 24–15. *A,* Nephrosclerosis, granular contracted kidney of chronic nephritis in a nine-year-old dog. Uremic ulcers of the tongue (*1*) and the pitted, contracted kidney (*2*). *B,* Nephrosclerosis, concentrated at the cortico-medullary junction (*1*), kidney of a dog (× 5). Note dilated tubules (*2*) in one nephron. *C,* The renal cortex of *B* (× 10). Scarring at corticomedullary junction (*1*) and dilatation of Bowman's space (*2*). *D,* The renal medulla in *B* and *C* (× 100). Collecting tubules are lined with multiple rows of cells (*1*) and are spherical in outline. Note connective tissue (*2*). (*B, C* and *D* courtesy of Armed Forces Institute of Pathology.) Contributor: Base Veterinarian, Barksdale AFB.

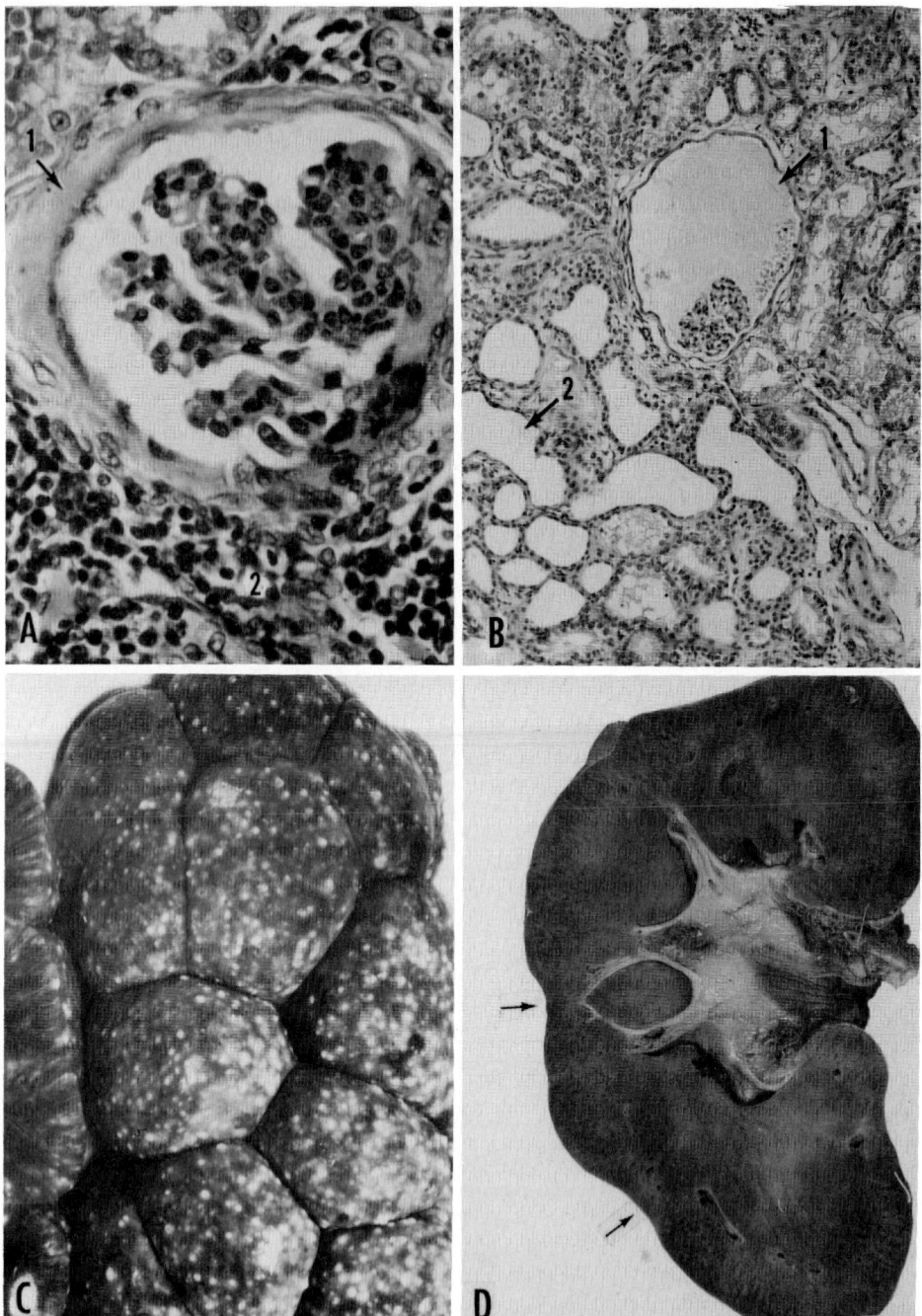

Fig. 24–16. *A*, Thickened Bowman's capsule (*1*) and lymphoid cells in interstitial stroma (*2*) in kidney (×
450) of a dog with chronic leptospirosis. Contributor: Army Veterinary Research Laboratory. *B*, Dilated
Bowman's space (*1*) and renal tubule (*2*) in the kidney (× 100) of a dog with scarring at the cortico-medullary
junction. (See Fig. 24–15, *B, C, D.*) *C*, Metastatic abscesses in the kidney of a Jersey cow. The primary lesion
was a foreign body reticulitis. *Corynebacterium pyogenes* was isolated from lesions of valvular endocarditis.
D, Depressions of the capsular surface due to old healed infarcts (arrows) in the kidney of a dog. (*A* and *D*,
courtesy of Armed Forces Institute of Pathology.) Contributor: Dr. Elihu Bond.

Shigella equerulis infection of foals is almost always associated with localization in the kidney (hematogenous route). Embolic spread from bacterial endocarditis is another source of infection, but this usually begins as a glomerulitis. In man, *E. coli* is the commonest pathogen; others include: *Enterobacter (Aerobacter) aerogenes, Proteus vulgaris,* alpha hemolytic streptococci, hemolytic staphylococci, *Pseudomonas aeruginosa* and *Klebsiella pneumoniae.*

Lesions. The lesions in the acute form of pyelonephritis consist of purulent inflammation and necrosis, which involve renal parenchyma and extend into collecting ducts, calyces, and renal pelvis. Classically, glomeruli and nephrons are spared, but they may become entrapped in the widespread inflammation. The lesions may be focal or diffuse, involving one or both kidneys or a single lobule (in bovines). Some lesions may be sharply circumscribed and consist essentially of abscesses. Sometimes the lesions are distributed around a single calyx, suggesting ascending infection from the renal pelvis. Extension of infection into nephrons usually results in neutrophils and granular or leukocytic casts in nephrons or collecting ducts. Purulent exudate may be found in the pelvis or just outside the pseudostratified epithelium which lines the pelvis.

Grossly, acute pyelonephritis is recognized by congestion, hemorrhages, and sometimes abscesses in the renal cortex, with severe congestion and pus in the pelvis—usually involving the ureters and possibly urethral and bladder mucosae.

Pyelonephritis may be accompanied by fever and malaise and often is preceded by localized or generalized infections (prostatitis, pneumonia). **Pyuria** (pus in the urine) and **bacteriuria** are constant findings, and **dysuria** with frequent urination may occur. Microscopic examination of urine reveals neutrophils, granular and leukocytic casts, red blood cells, and bacteria in large numbers. The acute signs may

abate shortly, but persistence of pus and bacteria in the urine indicates active infection which may result in active lesions characteristic of chronic pyelonephritis.

In the chronic form of pyelonephritis, usually but not always preceded by acute pyelonephritis, the kidneys become grossly scarred and contracted. These scarred areas may be single, with a depressed base located adjacent to the capsule, or may be multiple, giving the kidneys a coarsely nodular appearance. In extreme cases, the kidney may be small, fibrous, and contracted. Microscopically, at this stage, the interstitium contains lymphocytes, plasma cells, and neutrophils; tubules may be atrophic and contain casts and pus (sometimes bacteria); glomerular capsules are thickened by fibrosis (periglomerular fibrosis), and blood vessels may have thickened walls with fibrinous material in the media. In the most advanced stages, fibrous connective tissue replaces the exudate in the interstitium and contraction eventually results. The tubules may be dilated and contain proteinaceous casts. Some lymphocytes and plasma cells usually persist in the interstitium. This stage usually results in death due to uremia.

Miscellaneous Tubular Disorders

Tubular Transport Diseases. Excess amounts of inorganic and organic compounds not normally present in appreciable quantity may make their appearance in urine through one of several mechanisms. If there are unusually high levels in the blood, the substance may exceed its normal renal threshold and appear in the urine. Glycosuria of diabetes mellitus is an example. If the integrity of the glomerular filtration mechanism is impaired, larger molecules will enter the filtrate and exceed the ability of the tubules to reabsorb them. Proteinuria of glomerulonephritis is an example of this mechanism. Tubular damage through poisons, such as mercury or other mechanisms, will result in tubular dysfunction and the appearance of many abnormal urinary constituents. What remain are specific metabolic defects in tubular function which interfere with tubular transport or metabolism of specific compounds.

In humans, a number of specific tubular transport diseases, most of them concerning one or more amino acids or glucose, collectively known as aminoaciduria or glycosuria, have been identified. For some, analogous entities have been recognized in dogs. The best known is uric acid secretion by dogs of the Dalmatian breed. In contrast to other breeds, there is a defect in tubular reabsorption of uric acid, however, the Dalmatian does possess the enzyme uricase. The defect predisposes to uric acid calculi. Cystinuria has been described in several species of male dogs as a sex-linked hereditary disease in which there is a high incidence of cystine uroliths. In addition to decreased tubular reabsorption of cystine, the amino acids lysine, arginine and ornithine are also affected. Aside from calculi, no other renal lesion or other abnormality has been associated with the disease. Glycosuria has been reported in Basenji dogs. A syndrome resembling the Faconi syndrome in human beings has been described in dogs, particularly Basenji's by Bovee, et al. (1979). In the latter condition, there was aminoaciduria, glycosuria, polydipsia, and polyuria. In their report, some affected dogs died of renal failure. There was no characteristic lesion.

Vacuolar (Osmotic) Nephrosis. This term has been applied to a lesion in tubular epithelium in which large vacuoles displace much of the cytoplasm. The vacuoles contain fluid but not fat, glycogen, mucus, or other foreign substances. The presence of this fluid is believed related to disturbances in the osmotic relationships within these cells. It is associated with disturbances in fluid balance, such as gastrointestinal and other disorders which result in severe vomiting or diarrhea. Most characteristically, this lesion is associated with

severe hypokalemia (hypokalemic nephropathy). Potassium deficiency is believed to be a most significant cause, but the exact mechanism involved is not clear. The lesion does not appear to have a prolonged effect upon renal function, provided that the potassium stores are restored promptly.

Glycogen Nephrosis. Glycogen may accumulate in the epithelium of proximal convoluted tubules and the loops of Henle in diabetes mellitus and glycogen-storage disease such as von Gierke's disease in human patients. The former disease, of course, is not infrequent in animals. The presence of glycogen in the renal tubular epithelium gives the cytoplasm a uniformly vacuolated appearance. These changes are reversible and apparently do not cause significant functional impairment of the kidneys.

Cholemic Nephrosis. Bile pigments may be found in the epithelium of proximal convoluted tubules or loop of Henle in animals with obstructive icterus or severe liver disease. The bile is seen in these tubular cells as yellow granules of irregular size. Formalin-fixed gross specimens of kidney are green in color due to the change of bilirubin to biliverdin (Plate II). The fresh specimen may be yellow (icteric). Moderate degeneration of tubular epithelium may occur, but severe interference with renal function is not usual. The pathogenesis of this lesion is not clearly understood, although it appears that toxic products released by the liver or not detoxified by the liver may be the cause. Unconjugated bile at elevated levels may be toxic, but bilirubin glucuronide (conjugated bilirubin) does not appear to be injurious to renal cells. Hepatic injury may result in excretion of large amounts of amino acids, such as cystine, arginine, histidine, and tryptophan, which experimentally have been shown to damage renal tubular epithelium.

Uric Acid Precipitates. Extensive deposits of urate crystals may sometimes impart a yellowish color to the renal pyramids. The presence of these crystals in collecting tubules may give a radial pattern to the yellowish streaks. Microscopically, the collecting tubules are seen to be filled with yellow crystals. Urates may also be found (especially in birds) in the interstitial stroma where the crystals have a radial pattern. The urates in tubules presumably result from destruction of cells, particularly erythroblasts in newborn animals, and are most likely to be seen in pigs. This change also may occur in gout. (See Fig. 3–5.)

Cloisonné Kidney. An interesting pigmented thickening of tubular basement membranes has been described in goats (Zahawi, 1957; Light, 1960). The pattern of these thickened basement membranes around renal tubules under low magnification suggests the inlay of metal wire in porcelain using the cloisonné technique (cloisonné, Fr. *cloison* = partitioned; Latin, *claudere* = shut, close). The thickened basement membrane surrounds only the proximal convoluted tubules and has dark brown or grayish-brown color even in unstained sections. The chemical nature of the material in these basement membranes has not been established, although it does not appear to be either hemosiderin or melanin. Iron-positive material has been demonstrated in some places, but for the most part the involved basement membranes do not contain iron. Antecedent hemosiderosis has been postulated as a possible means of staining these basement membranes. The lesion appears to be limited to goats and does not interfere with renal function.

The gross appearance of this change is striking. The renal cortex in both kidneys, in severe cases, is dark brown, almost black. This color extends through the entire

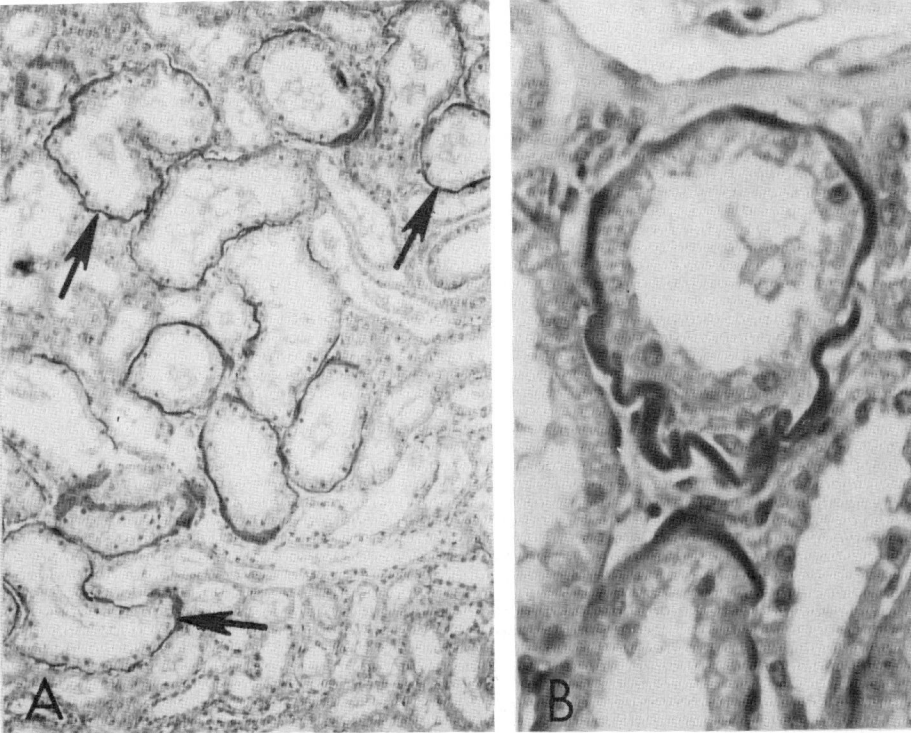

Fig. 24–17. Cloisonné kidney, Angora goat. *A,* Deeply pigmented basement membranes (arrows) encompass renal tubules. *B,* Higher magnification of a single tubule.

cortex, but is abruptly interrupted at the corticomedullary junction.

The lesion has been identified in living goats by histologic examination of specimens of kidney obtained by percutaneous biopsy (Altman, et al., 1970). These authors confirmed the absence of significant change in renal function and speculated that low levels of erythrocytic glucose-6-phosphate dehydrogenase and glutathione in normal and affected goats, plus elevated serum-iron-binding saturation, predispose to fragility of erythrocytes. The presence of ferritin deposits in affected basement membranes and hemosiderin in tubular epithelial cells in electron micrographs (Altman, et al., 1968) is also presented as evidence for intravascular hemolysis as the antecedent lesion. Further studies are needed to firmly establish the pathogenesis of this lesion.

Sulfonamides in the Kidney. Sulfonamide medication, especially if accompanied by a limited intake of water and an acid condition of the urine, may damage the kidney in various ways, often with lethal results. The lesions include toxic tubular degeneration and necrosis, commonly with marked inflammatory infiltrations around the tubules that are involved. As previously stated, the degeneration of tubular epithelium may be of the hydropic type; the changes may also resemble those described for "lower nephron nephrosis." Other changes apparently based on hypersensitivity may occur, such as glomerulonephritis, periarteritis nodosa, and necrosis of areas of peripelvic tissue. Some of these changes have been produced experimentally in dogs. The more usual lesion, however, has been, in dogs and cattle, a plugging of the lower collecting tubules with masses of fine crystals (Fig. 16–11A), a fatal anuria resulting. The crystals of most of the sulfonamides now in use are elongated, acicular, anisotropic, and yellowish in color. Since they are soluble in water, many or perhaps all of them may be dissolved out in the routine preparation of microscopic sections.

Fat in the Kidney. Lipids or lipoids stainable by ordinary techniques can be demonstrated in the epithelium of the several parts of the tubules, the glomerular tufts, the walls of Bowman's capsules, the interstitial tissue, the walls of blood vessels, the epithelium of the pelvic lining, and the tubular lumens of the kidneys of the various species of domestic animals and man (Smith, 1949). In normal cats, the epithelium of the proximal convoluted tubules contains an abundant amount of neutral lipid (triglycerides), which increases with age. The significance of this species variation is not known.

In all other species, any appreciable amount of lipid in the renal tubular epithelium represents a toxic or anoxic change comparable to that in the liver. As in the liver, lipid is deposited in epithelial cells in diabetes mellitus and ketosis, which characterize ovine toxemia of pregnancy and similar conditions.

The gross appearance of renal lipidosis is pathognomonic only in canine cases of severe fatty change of the ascending arms of Henle's loops. In these instances, the medullary rays stand out as prominent white streaks, radially directed, evenly spaced and reaching from the corticomedullary junction nearly, but not quite, to the capsule. In other species and in other localizations of the fat, little more can be detected grossly than a certain degree of paleness of the cortex and a hazy distinction between the alternating cortical labyrinths and medullary rays, as one views a cut surface traversing the cortex. In many kidneys with the latter appearance, the paler band represents not the medullary ray but the labyrinth, in which the proximal tubules especially have undergone swelling with or without fatty degeneration and necrosis, the picture of toxic tubular nephrosis in general. Microscopically, the fat is in the form of clear cytoplasmic droplets as explained under the general heading of Fatty Change.

Rarely in the dog, a portion of the glomerular area has been taken over by large reticuloendothelial cells filled with fat. Other parts of the glomerulus appear normal. The condition has been called glomerular xanthomatosis in some quarters (Fisher and Fisher, 1954). In some examples of pyelonephritis, large lipid filled cells may form small nodules, leading to the term xanthogranulomatous pyelonephritis.

Dilated Renal Tubules. The interpretation of this common abnormality deserves a moment of consideration. First of all, the investigator must make sure that the tubules are really dilated. It is possible to mistake enlargement of the tubular lumens resulting from atrophy or flattening of the epithelial lining cells for true enlargement of the whole tubule. Dilatation usually involves a group of tubules, or in some cases, the same nephron is seen several times in cross section, in the same area. They may be either convoluted tubules, the loops of Henle, or collecting tubules, or a combination of these. The degree of dilatation may be slight or the tubule may be enlarged to two or three times its normal diameter. An epithelial-lined space, seen in a single cross section, may give rise to the question whether it is a greatly dilated tubule or a cyst. The lining cells are most frequently, but not always, flattened; this depends on the cause of the dilatation. In many instances, the condition is due to back pressure caused by closure, from external pressure or otherwise, of the nephron at some lower point in its course. The increased internal pressure naturally tends to compress and flatten the epithelial lining. Such internal pressure must be mild, slowly developed, and long continued, for sudden and marked increase of intratubular pressure merely stops the filtration process by counterbalancing the "hydrostatic" pressure of the blood within the glomerular

capillaries. It appears from careful study, however, that not infrequently, nephrons become dilated through a process of hypertrophy. In such a case, the lining cells may be stretched and flattened or they may be of normal height. If they have recently proliferated or regenerated, the cells tend to be hyperchromatic, like other young cells, even though they have not yet developed to normal height. Such hypertrophy appears to be common in certain nephrons that survive when their neighbors have been destroyed through some pathologic process. It is compensatory hypertrophy, the nephron adding to its own some of the load formerly carried by its departed brethren. Obviously, hypertrophic nephrons of this kind are likely to be located in or near areas of fibrosis.

Peripelvic Necrosis

Known as **papillitis necroticans,** a necrotizing and at the same time inflammatory change affecting one or, more often, several of the renal papillae occurs in the human kidney. The distal half or two-thirds of the renal papilla is a yellowish gray and is sharply demarcated from the normal adjacent tissue by a narrow inflammatory zone and, except for its position, resembles an anemic infarct. Microscopically, the tissue is in a state of coagulative necrosis. Some of these lesions occur in connection with pyelonephritis (and concurrent diabetes in the human); others result from urinary obstruction. In the former case, the pressure of intrarenal exudates is thought to compress and close the blood vessels supplying this rather distant and isolated part of the kidney; in the case of urinary obstruction, the back pressure of the urine, acting from several directions on the protruding papilla, is supposed to produce a similar ischemia. The disorder tends to cause anuria and is likely to be fatal. A corresponding change has been seen at least in the dog, in which it involves the renal crest rather than a papilla because of anatomic differences. In one such case, amyloidosis in the basal region of the pyramids appeared to be responsible for compression of the blood vessels.

Papillary necrosis can be produced experimentally in rats by a single intravenous injection of bromoethylamine hydrobromide (Murray, et al., 1972).

Bilateral Renal Cortical Necrosis

Complete or almost complete necrosis of the renal cortices is a rare finding in human beings, which is also rarely seen in dogs, cattle, swine, horses, and cats. In man, the condition is most frequently associated with complications of pregnancy, but is also associated with various infections and traumatic events. In animals, no clearly established associated illness has been recognized. Microscopically, there is necrosis of all cortical structure with sparing of the medulla. The pathogenesis is not well understood, but believed to result from either vascular spasm or widespread fibrin and platelet thrombi in renal arterioles. It has been induced with injections of bacterial endotoxin, leading to arteriolar thrombi as a component of the generalized Shwartzman reaction. Natural exposure to bacterial toxins is a likely cause, but other conditions which lead to disseminated intravascular coagulation must also be considered. Nordstoga and Fjolstad (1967) produced bilateral renal cortical necrosis in swine with killed *Hemophilus influenza* organisms and suggested the pathogenesis was due to a generalized Shwartzman reaction.

Nephrosclerosis

Whether secondary or primary, the condition of chronic fibrosis of the kidney is often called nephrosclerosis. As discussed earlier, it may result from glomerulonephritis or any of the causes of interstitial nephritis. An important cause in man, occasionally encountered in animals, is arteriolarsclerosis. Constriction of arteries and arterioles leads to ischemia, tubular atrophy, necrosis and, ultimately, fibrosis.

Having developed without a preceding nephritis, this form of nephrosclerosis is known as the **primary contracted kidney.** The distribution of the fibrous tissue often tends to be in the shape of numerous small, healed infarcts—narrow wedges with their base at the capsule. The presence of thick-walled, sclerotic arteries and arterioles is also important in differentiation from the postnephritic secondary contracted kidney. Hindrance of the circulation of blood through the kidneys results in an increase in blood pressure through the release of renin from the juxtaglomerular apparatus. The hypertension accentuates the vascular disease and renal ischemia creating a vicious cycle, known as **malignant hypertension** (*malignant nephrosclerosis*).

Two sclerosing renal diseases of uncertain classification have been recognized in dogs. Finco and associates (1970, 1976) have described in Norwegian Elkhound dogs a familial renal disease of uncertain cause and pathogenesis. The pups are born normal, but subsequently develop progressive renal disease characterized by loss of glomeruli and tubules and extensive fibrosis in the cortex and medulla. The kidneys ultimately become small, white, and very firm. Gribble (personal communication) has recognized a renal disease in Lhasa apso, Pekingese, and similar breeds, characterized by focal to diffuse fibrosis. In contrast to the condition in Norwegian Elkhound dogs, there are many small, unperfused glomeruli in the cortex and hyalinized afferent arterioles.

Diseases of the Renal Vasculature

Infarcts. Infarcts happen with some frequency in the kidney from the same causes as infarctions elsewhere. Most often, but not invariably, they are of the anemic type and present the picture of one or more sharply outlined wedge-shaped pale—or red, as the case may be—areas with the apex near the zone of the arcuate arteries and the base at the capsule. Given time,

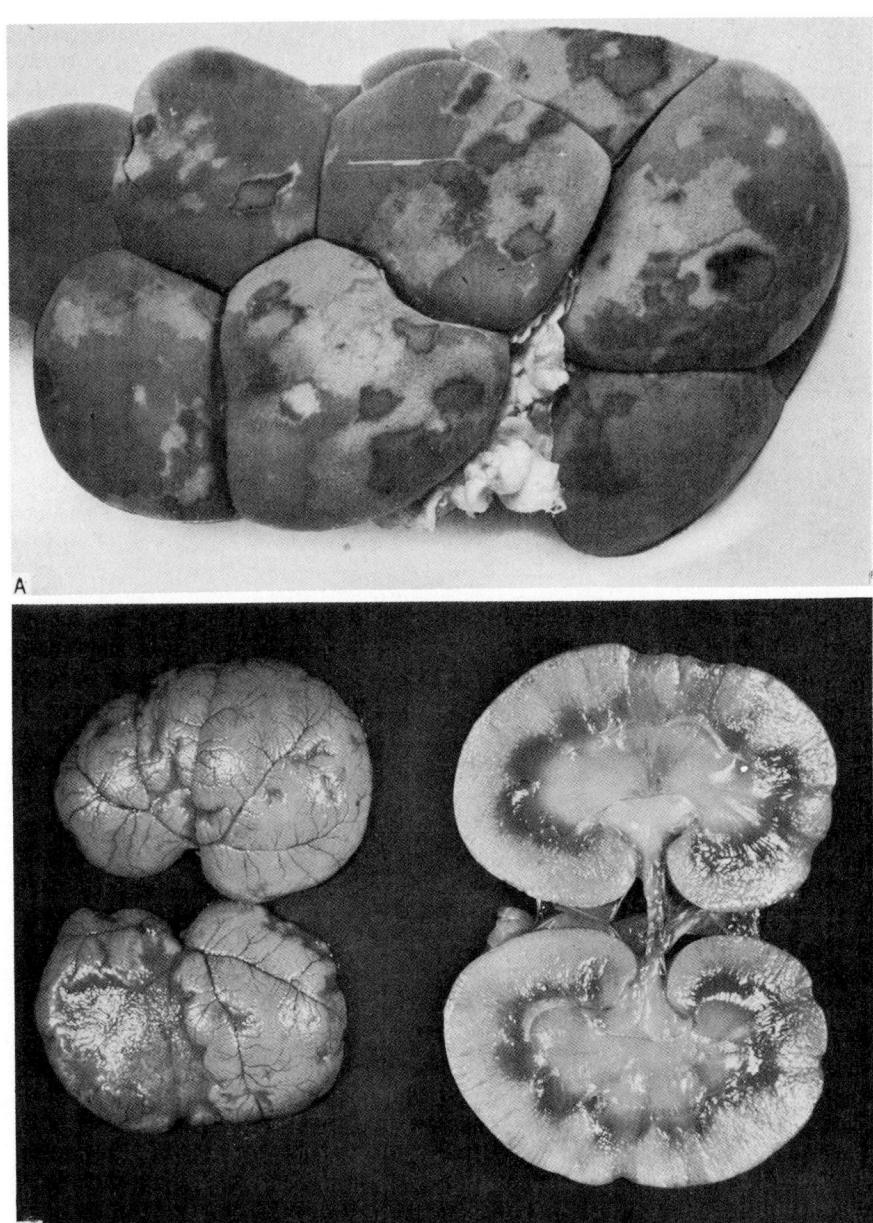

Fig. 24–18. Infarction of the kidney. *A*, Kidney of an 11-year-old cow with septic infarcts secondary to suppurative mastitis and pneumonia. Sharply demarcated anemic gray and hemorrhagic red infarcts are present in this lobulated kidney. *B*, Old infarcts in the kidneys of a seven-year-old castrated male cat. Note depressed zones in cortex in kidney on the left and the wedge-shaped contracted zones which extend from the capsule toward the pelvis of the kidney on the right. (Courtesy of Angell Memorial Animal Hospital.)

they heal with disappearance of the parenchymatous tissue, excepting possibly a few atrophic glomeruli, and with partial replacement by a narrow scar of white fibrous tissue. Due to shrinking of the scar, the capsule comes to be indented at this point. Multiple scarred infarcts of this kind may be indicative of a slowly developing nephrosclerosis but this is very exceptional in animals (Figs. 24–16D, 24–18B). Bilateral renal cortical necrosis is discussed earlier.

Hemorrhages. Hemorrhages, usually **petechial** in size, located just beneath the capsule and visible through it, or in the intertubular connective tissues, are frequent in septicemic diseases, especially hog cholera, and in many types of poisoning, including those from crotalarias and "oak-buds." Commonly, death occurs within a number of hours after their formation so that microscopic examination shows the erythrocytes to be well pre-served, but if a few days intervene, the petechiae darken and become indistinct.

Hemorrhages may also open into the glomerular capsules, the tubules, or the renal pelves, producing varying, but usually minor, degrees of hematuria. Extensive hemorrhage into the pelves, or peripherally with separation and distention of the capsule, has occurred, as in poisoning by sweet-clover (coumarin) and lye (NaOH), but ordinarily the hemorrhages are significant as aids in diagnosis rather than for their effect on the patient. Extensive hemorrhage, usually the result of trauma, may occur under the renal capsule. Such hemorrhage may result in ischemia and severe impairment of renal function.

Hyperemia. Active hyperemia and passive congestion occur, the former as a feature of acute inflammation, the latter as a part of generalized passive congestion, but neither reaches spectacular proportions in

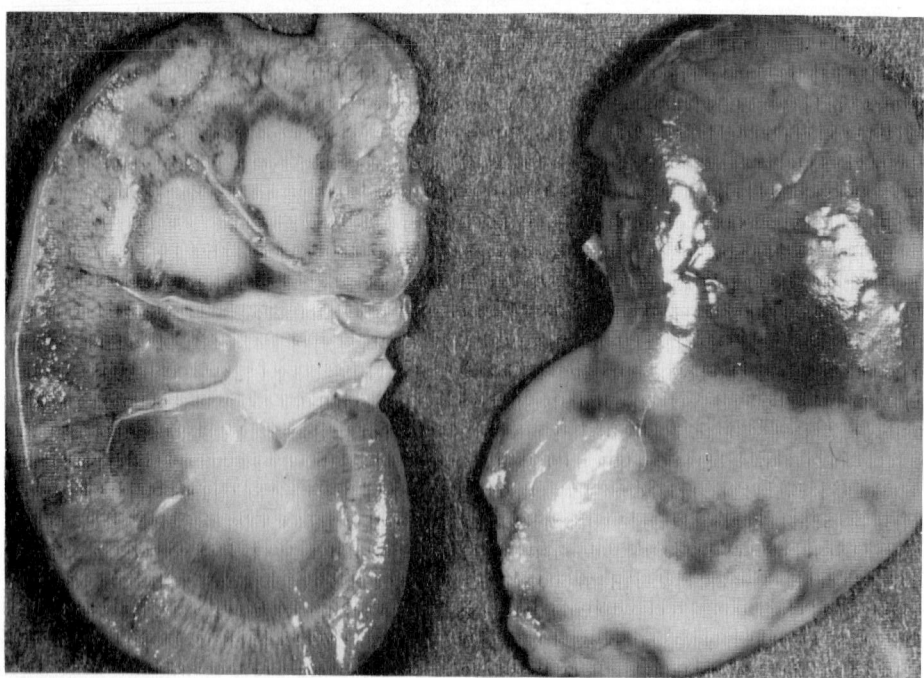

Fig. 24–19. Infarcts of the kidney of a spayed-female crossbreed dog, age five years. The light, blanched areas were found to be ischemic and generally necrotic upon microscopic examination. (Courtesy of Angell Memorial Animal Hospital.)

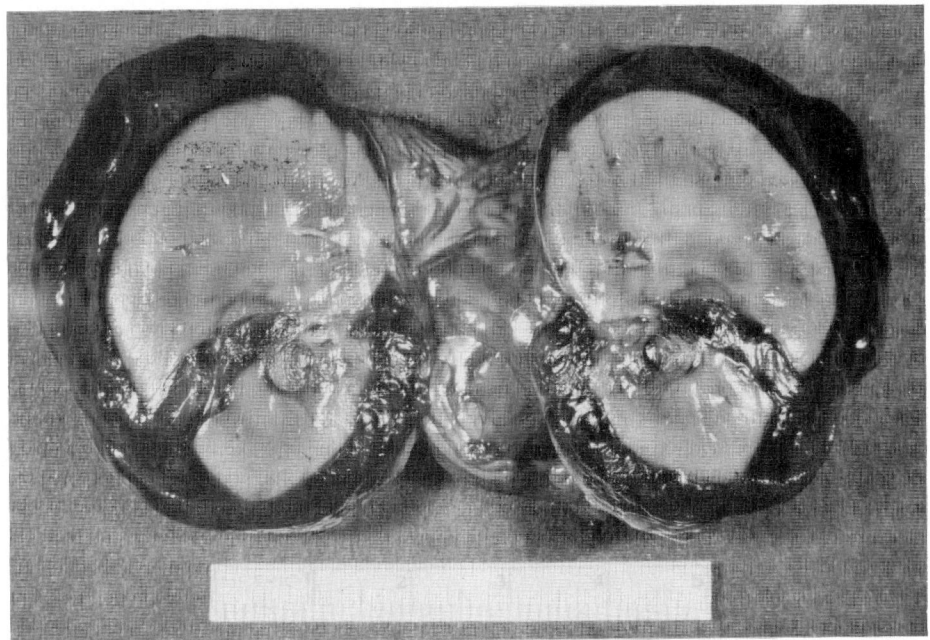

Fig. 24–20. Subcapsular hemorrhage, kidney of a four-year-old female black cat. Kidney has been incised in the horizontal plane. (Courtesy of Angell Memorial Animal Hospital.)

the kidney because of the dense and unyielding character of the organ. Congestion is most evident in the medulla, where the capillaries (venulae rectae) running in groups produce radial red lines, which are often strikingly conspicuous at autopsy.

Anemia. Anemia, general or local, tends to produce a kidney of paler color than normal. This sometimes results in the renal pyramids being practically white. Information is needed on the exact pathogenesis of this latter condition and the reasons for it. Attention may be called here to the fact that without a sufficient blood pressure in the glomeruli, secretion of urine is impossible, a situation which arises in shock and similar conditions, and which must be considered in therapy.

Edema. Edema of the kidney is described, but the kidney takes little part in generalized edema because of the inelastic character of its capsule and firmness of its parenchyma. Since drainage from the kidney is in the form of urine, local edema is represented by hydronephrosis.

Altman, N.H., Grossman, I.W., and Jernigan, N.B.: Electron microscopy of caprine cloisonné renal proximal tubular basement membranes. Proc. 26th Ann. Mtg. Electron Micro. Soc. Amer., Claitors, Baton Rouge, La. 192–193, 1968.

———: Caprine cloisonné renal lesions. Clinicopathological observations. Cornell Vet., *60*:83–90, 1970.

Anderson, L.J.: Experimental reproduction of canine interstitial nephritis. J. Comp. Path., *77*:413–418, 1967.

Battifora, H.A., and Markowitz, A.S.: Nephrotoxic nephritis in monkeys. Amer. J. Path., *55*:267–281, 1969.

Bloom, F.: A clinical and pathological study of nephritis in dogs. J. Am. Vet. Med. Assn., *91*:679–699, 1937.

Bloom, F.: The histopathology of canine leptospirosis. Cornell Vet., *31*:266–288, 1941.

Boyd, W.L.: Pyelonephritis in cattle. Cornell Vet., *8*:120–121, 1918.

———: Pyelonephritis in cattle. Cornell Vet., *17*:45–56, 1927.

Boyd, W.L., and Bishop, L.M.: Pyelonephritis of cattle and horses. J. Am. Vet. Med. Assn., *90*:154–162, 1937.

Border, W.A., et al.: Antitubular basement-membrane antibodies in methicillin-associated interstitial nephritis. N. Engl. J. Med., 291:381–384, 1974.

Bovee, K.C., et al.: Characterization of renal defects in dogs with a syndrome similar to the Fanconi syndrome in man. J. Am. Vet. Med. Assoc., 174:1094–1099, 1979.

DeGowin, E.L., Warner, E.D., and Randall, W.L.: Renal insufficiency from blood transfusion; anatomic changes in man compared with those in dogs with experimental hemoglobinuria. Arch. Int. Med., 61:609–630, 1938.

Easley, J.R., and Breitschwerdt, E.B.: Glucosuria associated with renal tubular dysfunction in three Basenji dogs. J. Am. Vet. Med. Assoc., 168:938–943, 1976.

Ericsson, J.L.E., Mostofi, F.K., and Lundgren, G.: Experimental hemoglobinuric nephropathy. I. Comparative light microscopic, histochemical and pathophysiologic studies. Virchows Arch. Abt. B. Zellpath., 3:181–200, 1969.

Feenstra, E.S., Thorp, F., and Clark, C.F.: Artificially induced case of pyelonephritis in a bovine. Mich. State Coll. Vet., 5:147–150, 1945.

Feenstra, E.S., and Thorp, F.: Bacteriopathology of infectious bovine pyelonephritis. Am. J. Vet. Res., 7:432–436, 1946.

Finco, D.R.: Familial renal disease in Norwegian Elkhound dogs: physiologic and biochemical examinations. Am. J. Vet. Res., 37:87–91, 1976.

Finco, D.R., Duncan, J.R., Crowell, W.A., and Hulsey, M.L.: Familial renal disease in Norwegian Elkhound dogs: morphologic examinations. Am. J. Vet. Res., 38:941–947, 1977.

Finco, D.R., Kurtz, H.J., Low, D.G., and Perman, V.: Familial renal disease in Norwegian Elkhound dogs. J. Am. Vet. Med. Assoc., 156:747–760, 1970.

Fisher, E.R., and Fisher, B.: Glomerular lipoidosis in the dog. Am. J. Vet. Res., 15:285–286, 1954.

Foote, J.J., and Grafflin, A.L.: Quantitative measurements of the fat-laden and fat-free segments of the proximal tubule in the nephron of the cat and dog. Anat. Rec., 72:169–179, 1938.

Foss, J.A.: Identification of *Corynebacterium renalis* from the kidney and bladder of a horse. J. Am. Vet. Med. Assn., 104:27, 1944.

Fuller, R.H.: Lipoids in the kidney. Arch. Path., 32:556–568, 1941.

Gold, A.C., Jeffs, R.D., and Wilson, R.B.: Experimental pyelonephritis in dogs. Canad. J. Comp. Med., 32:450–453, 1968.

Goldblatt, H., Lynch, J., Hanzal, R.F., and Summerville, W.W.: Studies on experimental hypertension: production of persistent elevation of systolic blood pressure by means of renal ischemia. J. Exper. Med., 59:347–379, 1934.

Goldman, M.L., Schroeder, H.A., and Dammin, G.J.: Morphologic alterations in the kidney during prolonged experimental renal and neurogenic hypertension in the dog. Abstr. Amer. J. Path., 28:528–529, 1952.

Hall, G.A.: Renal cortical necrosis in a cat. Vet. Pathol., 9:122–130, 1972.

Heptinstall, R.H.: Interstitial nephritis. A brief review. Am. J. Pathol., 83:214–236, 1976.

Heptinstall, R.H., and Hill, G.S.: Experimental pyelonephritis and hypertension. A study on the immunity of pyelonephritic glomeruli from hypertensive change. Lab. Invest., 16:96–111, 1967.

Jaenike, J.R.: The renal lesion associated with hemoglobinemia. J. Exper. Med., 123:523–535, 1966.

Jones, F.S., and Little, R.B.: Specific infectious cystitis and pyelonephritis of cows. J. Exper. Med., 42:593–607, 1925.

————: The organism associated with specific infectious cystitis and pyelonephritis of cows. J. Exper. Med., 44:11–20, 1926.

Jones, T.C., et al.: Control of leptospirosis in war dogs. Am. J. Vet. Res., 6:120–128, 1945.

Kaler, L.W., and Haensly, W.E.: Kidney in the aging cat: neutral lipid and adenyl cyclase histochemistry. Am. J. Vet. Res., 38:897–902, 1977.

Klassen, J., Sugisaki, T., Milgrom, F., and McCluskey, R.T.: Studies on multiple renal lesions in Heymann nephritis. Lab. Invest., 25:577–585, 1971.

Krohn, K., Mero, M., Oksanen, A., and Sandholm, M.: Immunologic observations in canine interstitial nephritis. Am. J. Pathol., 65:157–172, 1971.

Lauerman, L.H., Jr., and Berman, D.T.: Urinary tract infection in mink. II. Diethylstilbestrol as a predisposing factor. Amer. J. Vet. Res., 23:1097–1103, 1962.

Lawrence, J.A.: Intracapsular renal hygroma in the pig. Vet. Rec., 77:1171–1172, 1965.

Lee, J.C., et al.: Early morphologic changes in serum-induced renal papillary necrosis. Light and electron microscopic studies. Lab. Invest., 17:458–464, 1967.

Light, F.W., Jr.: Pigmented thickening of the basement membranes of the renal tubules of the goat ("cloisonné kidney"). Lab. Invest., 9:228–238, 1960.

Ljungqvist, A., Osvaldo-Decima, L., and Richardson, J.: Studies on the pathogenesis of serum-induced renal papillary necrosis in the rat. III. The early morphologic changes studied by light and electron microscopy. Lab. Invest., 17:447–457, 1967.

Lucke, B.C.: Lower nephron nephrosis. Milit. Surg., 99:371–396, 1946.

Lucke, V.M., and Hunt, A.C.: Interstitial nephropathy and papillary necrosis in the domestic cat. J. Path. Bact., 89:723–728, 1965.

Machado, A.V., Rangel, N.M., and Giovine, N.: Persistent urachus associated with pyelonephritis. Cornell Vet., 33:372–376, 1943.

Mahaffey, L.W.: Diffuse suppurative pyelonephritis in a sheep. Aust. Vet. J., 17:109–110, 1941.

Maisel, B., McSwain, B., and Glenn, F.: Effects of administration of sodium sulfadiazine to dogs. Arch. Surg., 46:326–335, 1943.

McIntyre, W.I.M., and Montgomery, G.L.: Renal lesions in *Leptospira canicola* infection in dogs. J. Path. & Bact., 64:145–160, 1952.

Modell, W.: Observations on the lipoids in the renal tubule of the cat. Anat. Rec., 57:13–28, 1933.

Modell, W., and Travell, J.: The role of the lipoid in the renal tubule of the cat in uranium nephritis. Anat. Rec., 59:253–263, 1934.

Monlux, A.W.: The histopathology of nephritis of the dog. Am. J. Vet. Res., 14:425–439, 1953.

Morse, E.V., and Roberts, S.J.: Bovine pyelonephritis: a concurrent infection with *Corynebacterium renale* and *Escherichia coli*. Cornell Vet., 38:429–435, 1948.

Muirhead, E.E., Vanatta, J., and Grollman, A.: Papillary necrosis of the kidney, clinical and experimental correlation. J. Am. Med. Assn., 142:627–631, 1950.

Murray, G., et al.: Experimental papillary necrosis of the kidney. I. Morphologic and functional data. Am. J. Pathol., 7:235–302, 1972.

Nagle, R.B., Johnson, M.E., and Jervis, H.R.: Proliferation of renal interstitial cells following injury induced by ureteral obstruction. Lab. Invest., 35:18–22, 1976.

Nielsen, S.W., and McSherry, B.J.: Renal hyperparathyroidism (rubber jaw syndrome) in a dog. J. Am. Vet. Med. Assn., 124:270–274, 1954.

Nordstoga, K.: Spontaneous bilateral renal cortical necrosis in animals. Path. Vet., 4:233–244, 1967.

Nordstoga, K., and Fjolstad, M.: The generalized Shwartzman reactions and haemophilus infections in pigs. Pathol. Vet., 4:245–253, 1967.

Olafson, P.: Pyelonephritis in a dog due to *Corynebacterium renalis*. Cornell Vet., 20:69–73, 1930.

————: Chronic canine nephritis. The skeletal system in "rubber jaw." J. Comp. Path. & Therap., 61:140–149, and 197–214, 1951.

Ottosen, H.E.: A case of renal sulfathiazole concretion and nephrosis in a calf. Nord. Vet. Med., 1:410–415, 1949.

Palmer, C.C.: Cystitis and pyelonephritis in cattle. Vet. Med., 26:168–177, 1931.

Rehg, J.E., Montali, R.J., and Szymkowiak, M.E.: Morphological and histochemical observations on renal microbodies in cats. Vet. Pathol., 12:186–195, 1975.

Ribelin, W.E.: Azoturia and the crush syndrome. J. Am. Vet. Med. Assn., 119:284–288, 1951.

Segal, S.: Disorders of renal amino acid transport. N. Engl. J. Med., 294:1044–1051, 1976.

Smith, H.A.: Renal lipidosis. Thesis. Univ. Mich., Ann Arbor, 1949.

Sporri, H., and Leemann, W.: Das verhalten des blutdruckes bei hunden mit chronisch-interstitieller nephritis. Abl. Vet. Med., 8:523–532, 1961.

Sugisaki, T., et al.: Immunopathologic study of an autoimmune tubular and interstitial renal disease in brown Norway rats. Lab. Invest., 28:658–671, 1973.

Szeky, A., and Miklovich, N.: Histopathological changes in the rat kidney following administration of sulphamethylthiazole. Acta Sci. Hung., 12:351–371, 1962.

Yuile, C.L., et al.: Hemolytic reactions produced in dogs by transfusion of incompatible dog blood and plasma. II. Renal aspects following whole blood transfusions. Blood, 4:1232–1239, 1949.

Zahawi, S. Al: Symmetrical cortical siderosis of the kidneys in goats. Am. J. Vet. Res., 18:861–867, 1957.

Zwieten, M.J., van, Bhan, A.K., McCluskey, R.T., and Collins, A.B.: Studies on the pathogenesis of experimental anti-tubular basement membrane nephritis in the guinea pig. Am. J. Pathol., 83:531–546, 1976.

Urinary Obstruction and Hydronephrosis

When there is severe or complete obstruction of the outflow of urine at some point below the convergence of the two ureteral streams, as for instance from calculi in the slender penile urethra (common in cattle, sheep, and goats), the result is first a severe and maximal distension of the bladder, which may or may not rupture. There follows in the course of 3 or 4 days a great distension of the abdominal cavity with fluid ("water belly," among stockmen) which has some of the characteristics of dilute urine, but which ultimately contains fibrinogen so that fibrinous deposits develop on the serous surfaces, possibly in some way akin to the fibrin-containing fluid in the pericardial sac in uremia. In some of these cases, the bladder has ruptured, releasing its contents into the peritoneal cavity, but in others no rupture or evidence of previous rupture can be found. Eventually, uriniferous fluid also seeps into the periurethral tissues and urinary region generally, above the point of obstruction. The blood urea nitrogen rises from the normal between 15 and 30 to as high as 400 mg/100 ml of blood, and the animal dies of uremia without there having been time for extensive gross changes in the kidneys.

Sudden, complete obstruction on one side may cause rapid atrophy of the corresponding kidney, reducing it almost to the vanishing point without hydronephrosis or other clinical disturbance. Such a change must be distinguished from hypoplasia. On the other hand, when there is partial obstruction, unilateral or bilateral, the patient is usually able to live, and in the course of a few months there develops in

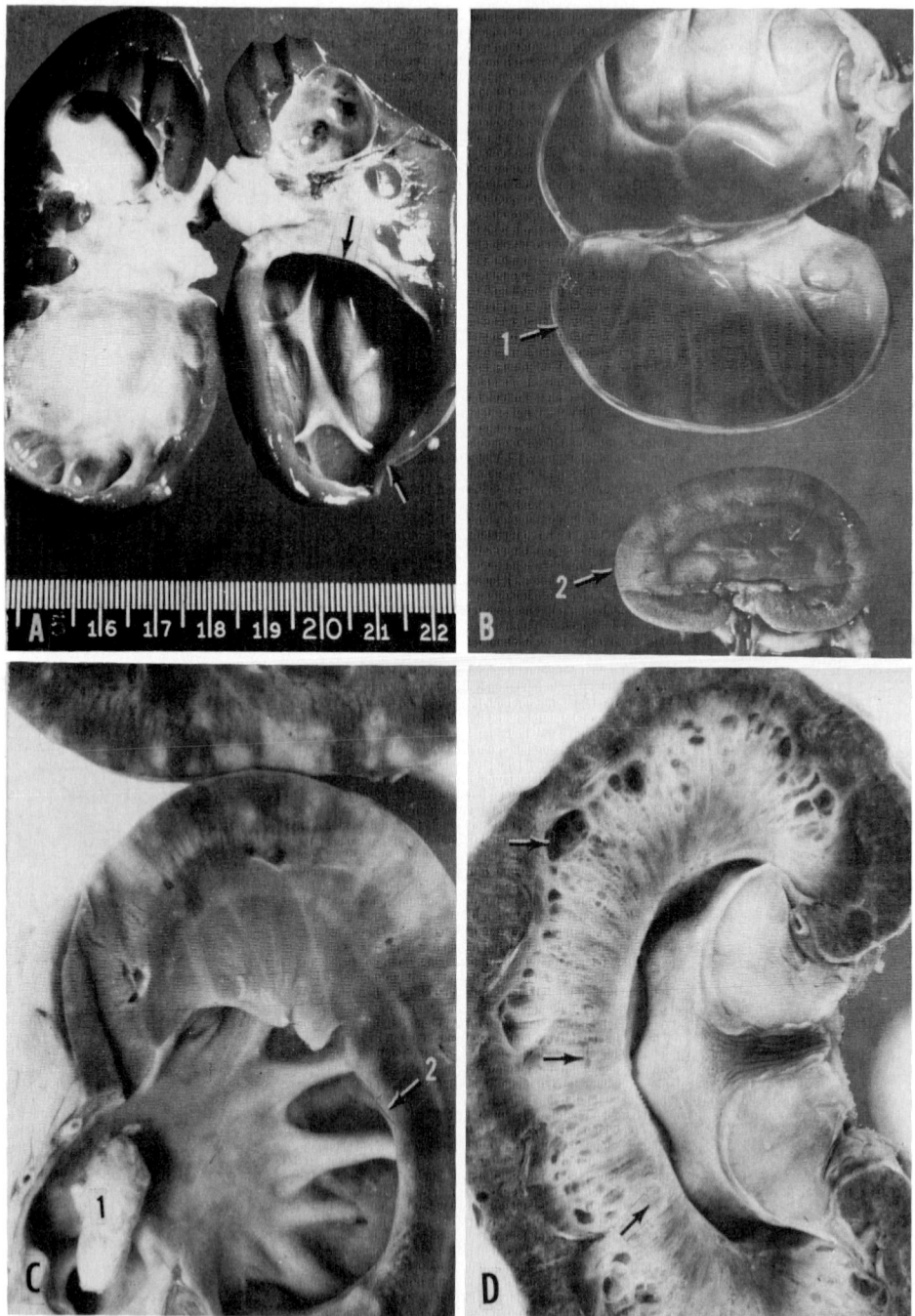

Fig. 24–21. *A,* Hydronephrosis, kidney of a pig. *B,* Severe hydronephrotic atrophy (*1*), kidney reduced to an empty capsule. Compensatory hypertrophy of the opposite kidney (*2*). One-year-old dog. *C,* Early hydronephrosis, kidney of a ten-year-old female Dachshund. Note calculus (*1*) which fitted into the urethral antrum as a stopper fits a bottle. The renal pelvis is dilated (*2*). *D,* Cysts (arrows) in the kidney of a ten-year-old male Chesapeake dog with contracted kidney.

the kidney or kidneys subjected to back-pressure the condition known as **hydronephrosis.** In hydronephrosis, the renal pelvis is gradually enlarged at the expense of the parenchyma. A considerable enlargement of the cavity of the renal pelvis can occur without much distortion of the renal parenchyma, but in time (6 months, Banks, 1952), the obstructed kidney becomes a mere hollow sac, although distended to larger outside dimensions than formerly. Ridges remain to mark the boundaries of the fetal lobules.

Microscopically, some scattered atrophic glomeruli usually remain in the thin and fibrous mass as the only vestige of kidney structure. Since the glomeruli have first access to the declining blood supply, and since their cells are somewhat less vulnerable than those of the tubules, it is only natural that glomeruli persist in the fibrous remains long after the tubules have disappeared. The fluid in the pelvic space changes from urine to a very watery liquid as the power of selective resorption declines in the dying tubules. Since an obstructed kidney is prone to become infected (see pyelonephritis), the fluid is not

infrequently pus at the time of postmortem examination; the condition is then known as **pyonephrosis.** The forms and places of obstruction to the urinary flow are numerous and varied. Calculi are the most frequent, lodging anywhere from the pelvis to the external meatus. A calculus has been observed that fitted the uretero-pelvic orifice as accurately as a stopper fits a bottle, but many start down the ureter of the urethra and lodge in the narrow passage. Strictures of either of these tubes are much rarer in animals than in humans, but have been seen. Pressure from the outside of the ureter or urethra can result from a number of things, but neoplasms are the most frequent, particularly growths of malignant lymphoma arising in the lymph nodes of the region. Carcinoma of the bladder and of the canine prostate are also noteworthy in this respect.

In uncomplicated hydronephrosis of one kidney, the other undergoes marked compensatory hypertrophy, and adequate function is usually maintained. **Hypertrophy in the kidney** involves an increase in diameter and length of the tubules, but no new nephrons are formed.

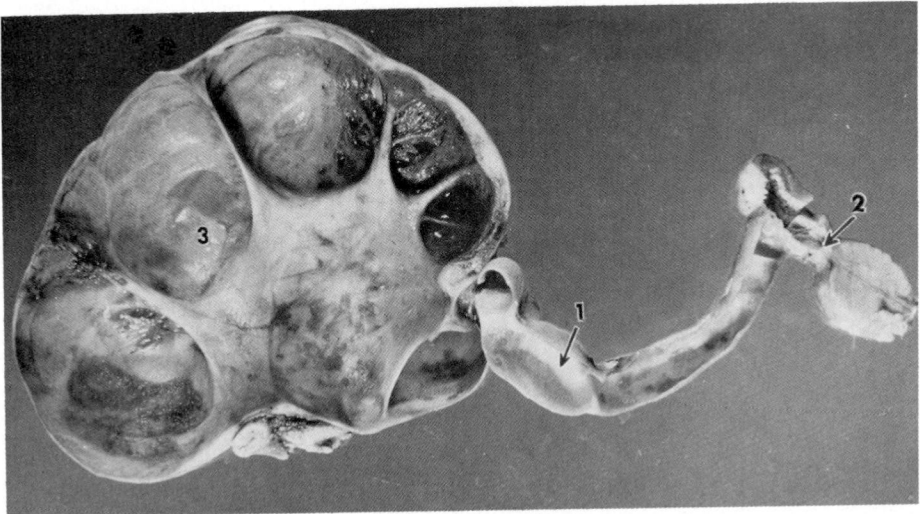

Fig. 24–22. Hydronephrosis of the kidney of a dog. The ureter (*1*) is dilated and tortuous above the obstruction (*2*) and the kidney has become a loculated sac (*3*). (Courtesy of Dr. Wayne H. Riser, Washington, D.C.)

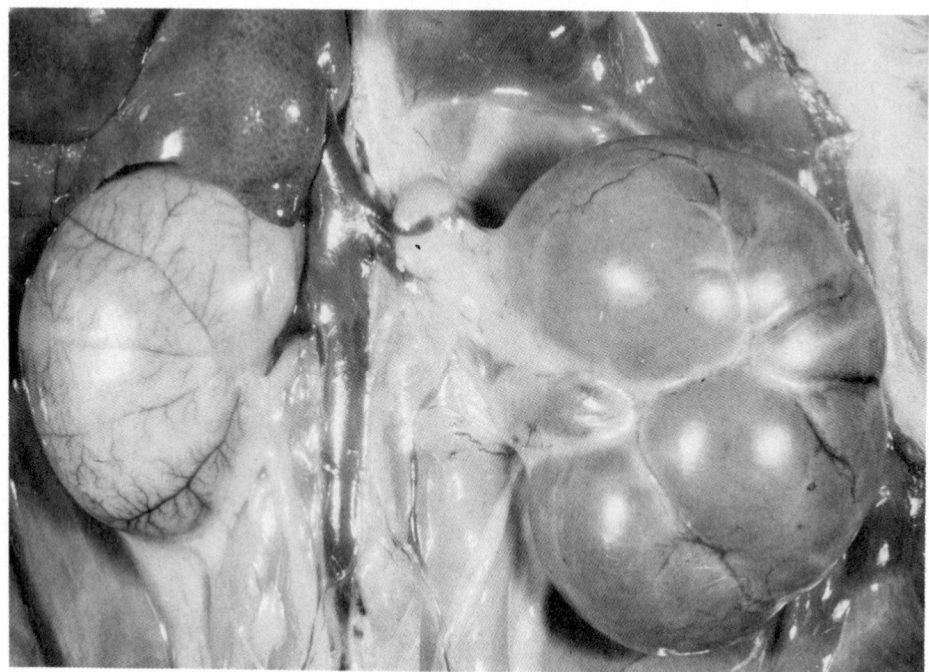

Fig. 24–23. Hydronephrosis of the left kidney of an eight-month-old male cat. (Courtesy of Angell Memorial Animal Hospital.)

One of the causes of hydronephrosis is the giant kidney worm, *Dioctophyma renale*. Hydronephrosis, possibly inherited, has been described in rats (Cohen, et al., 1970; Lozzio, et al., 1967) and inbred mice (Collins, et al., 1972; Warner, 1971).

In women and nonhuman primates, the ureter and the renal pelvis undergo a physiologic dilatation referred to as *hydronephrosis of pregnancy*. It results at least in part from endocrine effects, but it is not associated with impaired renal function and disappears after parturition. In women it predisposes to pyelonephritis.

Banks, W.C.: Intravenous urography in the dog and the pathogenesis of hydronephrosis. Thesis. A & M College of Texas, College Station, Texas, 1952.

Cohen, B.J., De Bruin, R.W., and Kort, W.J.: Heritable hydronephrosis in a mutant strain of brown Norway rats. Lab. Anim. Care, 20:489–493, 1970.

Collins, G.R., Goodheart, C.R., and Henson, D.: Spontaneous heritable hydronephrosis in inbred mice. 1. Description, incidence and distribution of lesions. Lab. Anim. Sci., 22:333–338, 1972.

Lozzio, B.B., Chernoff, A.I., Machado, E.R., and Lozzio, C.B.: Hereditary renal disease in a mutant strain of rats. Science, 156:1742–1744, 1967.

Roberts, J.A., and Wolf, R.H.: Hydronephrosis of pregnancy: a naturally occurring disorder in non-human primates closely resembling that in man. Folia Primatol., 15:143–147, 1971.

Taylor, D.M., and Fraser, H.: Hydronephrosis in inbred strains of mice with particular reference to the BRVR strain. Lab. Anim., 7:229–236, 1973.

Underwood, P.C.: Hydronephrosis in a dog. J. Am. Vet. Med. Assn., 82:256–258, 1933.

Warner, N.L.: Spontaneous hydronephrosis in the inbred mouse strain NZC. Aust. J. Exp. Biol. Med. Sci., 49:477–486, 1971.

Urolithiasis

The formation of stony precipitates anywhere in the urinary passages is called urolithiasis; the stone is called a urolith or urinary calculus. The calculi are most often found in the bladder, where the name of "cystic calculi" may be applied to them, but in other cases they are in the renal pelvis, or even in distended terminal tubules (the ducts of Bellini). One or more

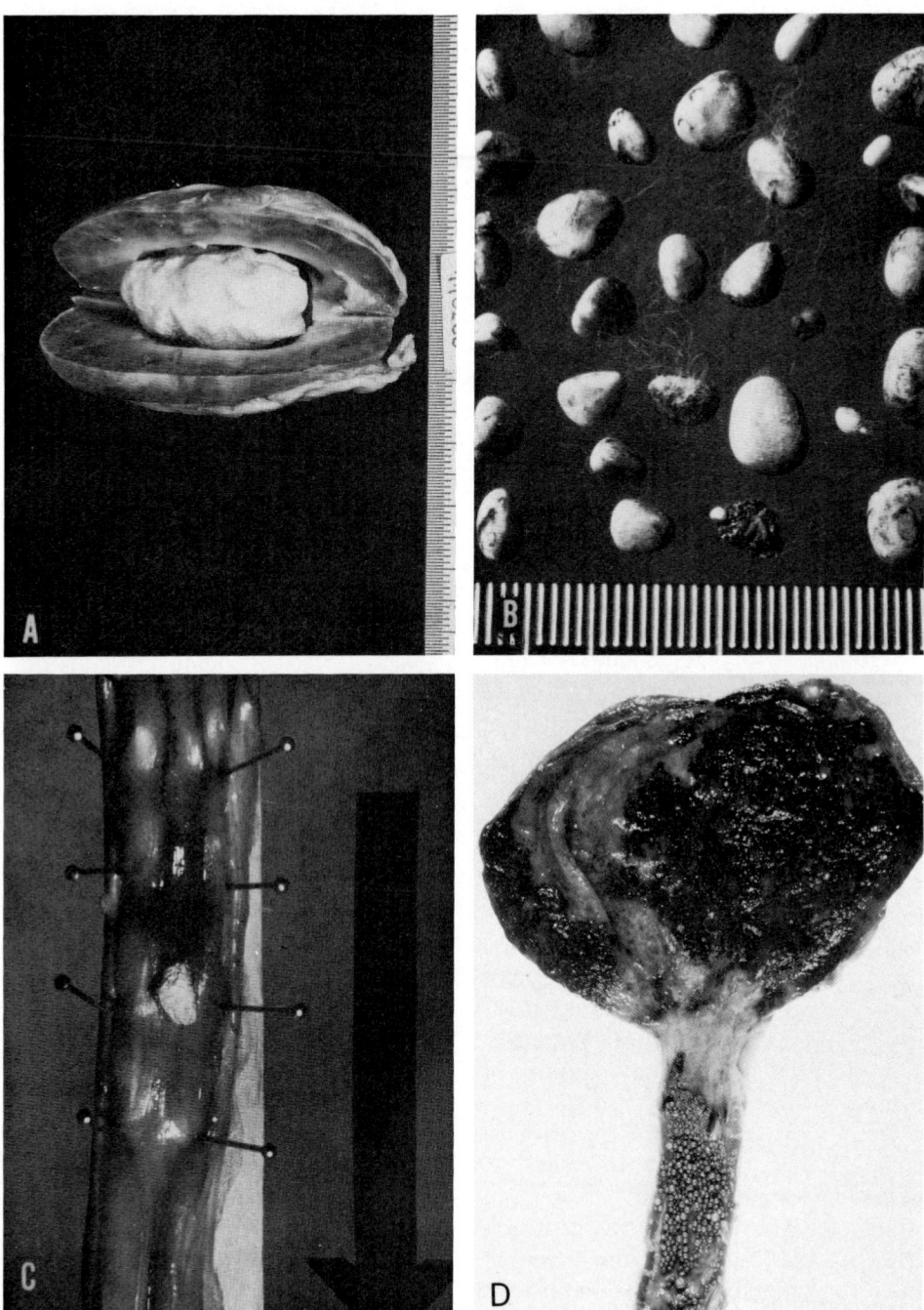

Fig. 24–24. Urolithiasis. *A,* A single large calculus filling the renal pelvis of a dog. (Courtesy of Armed Forces Institute of Pathology.) Contributor: Dr. S. Stern. *B,* Calculi removed from the prostate of a six-year-old Cocker Spaniel dog. *C,* Calculus in the urethra of a steer. *D,* Cystitis and multiple urethral calculi in a four-year-old wether. (*D,* Courtesy of Dr. W. J. Hadlow.)

uroliths may lodge in the ureter, producing excruciating pain known as ureteral colic. However, if the calculus is small enough to enter the ureter, it usually is ultimately forced into the bladder, whereupon the colic is relieved. Otherwise, the kidney involved is reduced to negligible size by pressure and disuse atrophy, or it more slowly undergoes hydronephrosis.

Calculi in the bladder are often carried out with the urine and may lodge in the narrow male urethra, usually at the sigmoid flexure in ruminants, the result being fatal obstruction unless relief is obtained. The female usually escapes this trouble because of the larger and shorter urethra.

Uroliths may be of any size from a mere collection of sand-like particles to a single stone practically filling the bladder or renal pelvis. They may be hard or relatively soft, white or yellowish, smooth or rough, rounded, or faceted (that is, with flattened sides). Siliceous stones especially are often fragile or merely collections of sandy material. However, a stone only a few millimeters in diameter is sufficient to obstruct the sigmoid urethra of a steer and must not be overlooked at autopsy.

The composition of calculi varies greatly. Chemically, the usual urinary stone of herbivorous animals contains a predominance of silicates, conjoined in a minority of cases with phosphates, carbonates, or oxalates of calcium, ammonium, and magnesium (Mathams and Sutherland, 1951; Schmidt, 1941; Swingle, 1953). Important amounts of protein are always found with these minerals, a fact which is probably of primary importance, according to the work of Swingle (1953), who analyzed calculi from 63 range steers affected with occluding urolithiasis. He found that the urine of bovine animals kept under the conditions of the western ranges of the United States (where the incidence of urolithiasis is high because of vitamin A deficiency) contains from 50 to 150 ppm of dissolved silica. He concluded that, in all probability, silica is precipitated as an insoluble complex in combination with mucoproteins in the urine. He believed that the aggregation of the dispersed insoluble material into concretions depended upon the presence of particulate nuclei (cellular fragments, organic precipitates) and upon "alterations in the quality and quantity of protective colloids in the urine." The amount of silica in the urine depends upon that in the animal's feed, some plants grown in arid areas being heavily laden with this element. In other situations, particularly in feedlots, calcium phosphate, calcium carbonate, and triple phosphate calculi occupy a more prominent position in the calculi of herbivora. The usual alkaline pH of the urine of herbivora favors the precipitation of these constituents. Occasionally calculi in herbivora may contain mixtures of both silicates and calcium salts (weddelite). Silicate and phosphate calculi are off-white in color and may be hard or crumbly. In some parts of the world (New Zealand) the nuclein derivative, xanthine (not the xanthin of plants), has been reported as a principal constituent of urinary calculi, especially in sheep. These are brownish and crumbly.

In carnivorous and omnivorous animals, the chemical constituents of uroliths are quite different. The calculi of these animals are much like those of the human, possibly because of the characteristically acid urine which is in contrast to the alkaline urine of herbivora. The **oxalate stone** is a spectacular type, very hard and heavy, white or light yellow, and typically covered with sharp, hard spines. It is usually found as a single stone in the bladder and may reach a diameter of several centimeters. It consists chiefly of calcium oxalate and has sharp edges which may damage the urinary epithelium and cause hemorrhage.

Uric acid calculi consist largely of ammonium (from decomposition of urea) and sodium urates and uric acid. They are of small or medium size, firm or moderately hard, yellow to brown in color, and either spherical or irregular in shape. They are not radiopaque. Like the oxalate calculi, they form in acid urine. They are especially common in Dalmatian dogs, which excrete large amounts of uric acid due to a defect in tubular reabsorption and subsequent oxidation of uric acid (Weiner and Fanelli, 1975) to allantoin, as is done by most mammals except primates.

Phosphate calculi are more like the calculi of herbivora, being white or gray, of chalky consistency, but often soft and friable enough that they can be crushed with little trouble. They are often multiple and may exist merely as sand-like granules. They are the most frequent form of urolithiasis in dogs despite the usual acidity of the urine. Bacterial infection with breakdown of urea to ammonia resulting in elevation of urine pH favors precipitation of phosphates. Magnesium ammonium phosphate is the commonest form of phosphate calculi in dogs.

Xanthine stones are brownish red, often concentrically laminated, fragile, and of irregular shape. They are rare.

Cystine stones are small, soft and of variable shape, and have a shiny, greasy appearance. They are yellow and become darker on exposure to air. Cystine, an amino acid, is relatively insoluble and may precipitate in the bladder of animals that excrete an increased amount through the kidneys, which results from failure of tubular reabsorption of cystine as well as other amino acids. Cystine stones in the dog have a tendency to occlude the urethra at the point where it enters the os penis. Cystine calculi have been reported in men, women, and male dogs. Cystinuria has been recognized in many different breeds of dogs in which the condition is believed to be inherited either as a sex-linked recessive trait or autosomal trait with sex-modified expression.

Siliceous calculi are rare in carnivora, but may develop if the diet contains a large amount of silicic acid.

Incidence. Urinary calculi are common in all species of animals. They are least frequently seen in swine and most often encountered in cattle, dogs, and cats. In dogs, the incidence has been reported to range from 0.6% (Krabbe, 1949) to 2.8% (Brown, et al., 1977) of all canine illnesses, with phosphate calculi accounting for 40 to 85% of all stones; cystine, 7 to 22%; urate, 2 to 8%; and oxalate, 3 to 30% (Finco, et al., 1970; Clark, 1974; Brown, et al., 1977).

Causes. While many factors have already been alluded to in the pathogenesis of urinary calculi, many examples go unexplained, as does the underlying mechanism of calculus formation. It is generally believed that an organic matrix, nucleus, or nidus is a necessary requirement for deposition of inorganic crystals and resultant stone formation. This nucleus is usually a mucopolysaccharide or mucoprotein. The nucleus could consist of dead leukocytes, fibrin, cellular debris, or agglutinated bacteria. Crystallization upon or within the nucleus does not necessarily always follow, but results when there is disruption of the colloidal system that supports the supersaturated solution of crystalloids of urine. This may result from an excess of crystalloids overwhelming the protective colloids or the presence of hydrophilic colloids. Some specific conditions associated with urinary calculi include:

1. Bacterial infection of the urinary tract, which allows for nidus formation and alteration of urinary pH. This is the principal cause of phosphate calculi in dogs.

2. Aminoaciduria leading to cystine calculi in male dogs.

3. Metabolic defect in uric acid metabolism in Dalmatian dogs, leading to urate calculi.

4. Vitamin A deficiency apparently through squamous metaplasia of urinary epithelium and increased nidus formations. Experimentally, urolithiasis has been produced repeatedly in herbivorous animals by the mere expedient of depriving them of adequate amounts of vitamin A (Higgins, 1951; Schmidt, 1941). Such experiments have explained the frequent occurrence of urinary calculi in steers,

wethers, and male goats fed upon diets of dried sorghums, cottonseed products, bleached hays, straw, corn slaths, and dried pasture grasses, none of which contain any substantial amount of vitamin A.

5. Implantation with diethylstilbestrol or grazing on estrogenic plants may lead to urinary calculi in sheep. The effect of these hormones in causing squamous metaplasia of the genitourinary epithelium is well known, as is their tendency to limit the growth in size of the genitourinary organs.

6. Hyperparathyroidism causes increased excretion of calcium, urolithiasis, and nephrocalcinosis.

7. A picornavirus has been shown to experimentally produce urolithiasis in male cats (Fabricant, et al., 1969; Rich, et al., 1971).

8. Dietary mineral imbalance and diets high in ash are attractive theories as causes of urolithiasis, but are rarely implicated. Diets with imbalances of calcium, phosphate, and magnesium may lead to either urolithiasis or nephrocalcinosis.

9. Inadequate water intake by itself is not a cause of urolithiasis; however, if the diet is high in silicates or other minerals or if other predisposing factors exist, dehydration favors calculus formation. High sodium chloride intake, provided ample water is available, will reduce the incidence of urolithiasis in cattle.

Effects. Calculi are mechanically irritating wherever they may be but only moderately so, as a rule. In the renal pelvis, the stone frequently is molded to fit the calyx or part of a calyx in which it was formed. The principal harm done by uroliths is that of obstruction when they lodge at the uretero-pelvic orifice, in the ureter or in the urethra. This has been discussed in an earlier paragraph.

Bailey, C.B.: Formation of siliceous urinary calculi in calves given supplements containing large amounts of sodium chloride. Can. J. Anim. Sci., 53:55–60, 1973.

Barker, J., and Povey, R.C.: The feline urolithiasis syndrome: a review and an inquiry into the alleged role of dry cat foods in its aetiology. J. Small Anim. Pract., 14:445–457, 1973.

Beeson, W.M., Pence, J.W., and Holm, G.C.: Urinary calculi in sheep. Am. J. Vet. Research, 4:120–126, 1943.

Blount, W.P.: Urinary calculi. Vet. J., 87:561–576, 1931.

Brown, N.O., Parks, J.L., and Greene, R.W.: Canine urolithiasis: retrospective analysis of 438 cases. J. Am. Vet. Med. Assoc., 170:414–418, 1977.

———: Recurrence of canine urolithiasis. J. Am. Vet. Med. Assoc., 170:419–422, 1977.

Bushman, D.H., Emerick, R.J., and Embry, L.B.: Incidence of urinary calculi in sheep as affected by various dietary phosphates. J. Anim. Sci., 24:671–675, 1965.

———: Experimentally induced ovine phosphatic urolithiasis: relationships involving dietary calcium, phosphorus and magnesium. J. Nutr., 87:499–504, 1965.

Butt, A.J., and Hauser, E.A.: The importance of protective urinary colloids in the prevention and treatment of kidney stones. Science, 115:308–310, 1952.

Clark, W.T.: Staphylococcal infection of the urinary tract and its relation to urolithiasis in dogs. Vet. Rec., 95:204–206, 1974.

———: Distribution of canine urinary calculi and their recurrence following treatment. J. Small Anim. Pract., 15:437–444, 1974.

Cornelius, C.E., Bishop, J.A., and Schaffer, M.H.: A quantitative study of aminoaciduria in Dachshunds with a history of cystine urolithiasis. Cornell Vet., 57:117–183, 1967.

Cornelius, C.E., Moulton, J.E., and McGowan, B.: Ruminant urolithiasis. I. Preliminary observations in experimental ovine calculosis. Am. J. Vet. Res., 20:863–871, 1959.

Djurickovic, S.M., Gankhi, D., Brown, K., and Yoon, S.: Urolithiasis in baby pigs. Vet. Med. Small Anim. Clin., 68:1151–1153, 1973.

Easterfield, T.H., Rigg, T., Askew, T.O., and Bruce, J.A.: Widespread occurrence of xanthin calculi in sheep. Vet. J., 86:251–265, 1930.

Fabricant, C.G., Gillespie, J.H., and Krook, L.: Intracellular and extracellular mineral crystal formation induced by viral infection of cell cultures. Infect. Immun., 3:416–419, 1971.

Fabricant, C.G., Krook, L., and Gillespie, J.H.: Virus-induced cholesterol crystals. Science, 181:566–567, 1973.

Fabricant, C.G., Rich, L.J., and Gillespie, J.H.: Feline viruses. XI. Isolation of a virus similar to a myxovirus from cats in which urolithiasis was experimentally induced. Cornell Vet., 59:667–672, 1969.

Finco, D.R.: Current status of canine urolithiasis. J. Am. Vet. Med. Assoc., 158:327–335, 1971.

Finco, D.R., Rosin, E., and Johnson, K.H.: Canine urolithiasis: a review of 133 clinical and 23 necropsy cases. J. Am. Vet. Med. Assoc., 157:1225–1228, 1970.

Goulden, B.E.: Clinical observations on the role of urinary infection in the aetiology of canine urolithiasis. Vet. Rec., 83:509–514, 1968.

Grünberg, W.: Vergleichende untersuchungen zur biokristallographie tierischer harnsteine. Path. Vet., *1*:258–268, 1964.

Gulati, R.L., et al.: Urolithiasis in ruminants: brief review and a preliminary survey, report I. J. Res. Ludhiana, *3*:456–462, 1966. V.B. 37:4352, 1967.

Higgins, C.C.: Experimental production of urinary calculi. J. Am. Vet. Med. Assn., *118*:81–85, 1951.

Jackson, O.F.: Oxalate calculi and oxaluria in the cat. Vet. Rec., *83*:417–419, 1968.

Jain, S.K., and Pandit, C.N.: Studies on the pathology of ovine and caprine kidneys Part III: Urolithiasis. JNKVV Res. J., *4*:37–39, 1970.

Keeler, R.F.: The internal structure and composition of siliceous calculi of bovine origin. Am. J. Vet. Res., *21*:428–436, 1960.

Kendrick, J.W.: Cystic calculi in a horse. Cornell Vet., *40*:187–188, 1950.

Krabbe, A.: Urolithiasis in dogs and cats. Vet. Rec., *61*:751–755, 1949.

Legendre, A.M.: Silica urolithiasis in a dog. J. Am. Vet. Med. Assoc., *168*:418–419, 1976.

Lewis, L.D., Chow, F.H.C., Taton, G.F., and Hamar, D.W.: Effect of various dietary mineral concentrations on the occurrence of feline urolithiasis. J. Am. Vet. Med. Assoc., *172*:559–563, 1978.

Lumb, W.W.: Prostatic calculi in a dog. J. Am. Vet. Med. Assn., *121*:14–16, 1952.

Mathams, R.H., and Sutherland, A.K.: Siliceous renal calculi in cattle. Aust. Vet. J., *27*:68–69, 1951.

McCullagh, K.G., and Ehrhart, L.A.: Silica urolithiasis in laboratory dogs fed semisynthetic diets. J. Am. Vet. Med. Assoc., *164*:712–714, 1974.

Morris, M.L., Green, D.F., Dinkel, J.H., and Brand, E.: Canine cystinuria. An unusual case of urinary calculi in the dog. North Am. Vet., *10*:16–20, 1935.

Munakata, K., Suda, H., and Ikeda, K.: Induction of the urolithiasis syndrome in cattle. Natl. Inst. Anim. Health Q. (Tokyo), *14*:31–32, 1974.

Newsom, I.E.: Urinary calculi with special reference to cattle and sheep. J. Am. Vet. Med. Assn., *92*:495–502, 1938.

Packett, L.V., and Hauschild, J.P.: Phosphorus, calcium and magnesium relationship in ovine urolithiasis. J. Nutr., *84*:185–190, 1964.

Packett, L.V., and Coburn, S.P.: Urine proteins in nutritionally induced ovine urolithiasis. Amer. J. Vet. Res., *26*:112–119, 1965.

Packett, L.V., Lineberger, R.O., and Jackson, H.D.: Mineral studies in ovine phosphatic urolithiasis. J. Anim. Sci., *27*:1716–1721, 1968.

Pearson, P.T., Jensen, E.C., and Richter, W.R.: Urinary calculi in a 2-month-old pup. J. Am. Vet. Med. Assn., *135*:329–331, 1959.

Pryor, W.H., Jr., Chang, C.-P., and Raulston, G.L.: Urolithiasis in a Taiwan monkey (*Macaca cyclopis*). A literature review and case report. Lab. Anim. Care, *19*:862–865, 1969.

Randall, A.: The initiating lesions of renal calculus. Surg. Gynec. and Obst., *64*:201–208, 1937.

Rich, L.J., and Kirk, R.W.: Feline urethral obstruction: mineral aspects. Am. J. Vet. Res., *29*:2149–2156, 1968.

Rich, L.J., and Fabricant, C.G.: Urethral obstruction in male cats: transmission studies. Canad. J. Comp. Med., *33*:164–165, 1969.

Rich, L.J., Fabricant, C.G., and Gillespie, J.H.: Virus-induced urolithiasis in male cats. Cornell Vet., *61*:542–553, 1971.

Rich, L.J., and Norcross, N.L.: Feline urethral obstruction: immunologic identification of a unique urinary protein. Amer. J. Vet. Res., *30*:1001–1005, 1969.

Robbins, J.D., Kunkel, H.O., and Crookshank, H.R.: Relationship of dietary mineral excretion and the incidence of urinary calculi in lambs. J. Anim. Sci., *24*:76–82, 1965.

Schmidt, H.: Vitamin-A deficiencies in ruminants. Am. J. Vet. Res., *2*:373–389, 1941.

Sompolinsky, D.: Urolithiasis in mink. Cornell Vet., *40*:367–377, 1950.

Stansbury, R.L., and Truesdail, R.W.: Occurrence of vesical calculi in cats receiving different diets. North Am. Vet., *36*:841–853, 1955.

Swingle, K.F.: The chemical composition of urinary calculi from range steers. Am. J. Vet. Res., *14*:493–498, 1953.

Swingle, K.F., and Marsh, H.: The relation of limited water consumption to the development of urinary calculi in steers. Am. J. Vet. Res., *14*:16–18, 1953.

Thomas, R.M., and Prier, J.E.: An experimental case of urinary calculus in a Holstein-Friesian steer. J. Am. Vet. Med. Assn., *120*:85–86, 1952.

Treacher, R.J.: Urolithiasis in the dog. II. Biochemical aspects. J. Small Anim. Pract., *7*:537–547, 1966.

Trueman, N.A., and Stacy, D.B.: Ovine urolithiasis: some mineralogic and physiologic observations. Invest. Urol., *7*:185–191, 1969.

Udall, R.H., and Chow, F.H.C.: Studies on urolithiasis. VII. The effects of sodium, potassium or chloride ions in the control of urinary calculi. Cornell Vet., *55*:538–544, 1965.

Udall, R.H., Seger, C.L., and Chow, F.H.C.: Studies on urolithiasis. VI. The mechanism of action of sodium chloride in the control of urinary calculi. Cornell Vet., *55*:198–203, 1965.

Udall, R.H., and Jensen, R.: Studies on urolithiasis. II. The occurrence in feedlot lambs following implantations of diethylstilbestrol. J. Am. Vet. Med. Assn., *133*:514–516, 1958.

Weaver, A.D.: Obstructive urolithiasis in sheep. Vet. Rec., *84*:320–324, 1969.

Weaver, A.D., and Pillinger, R.: Relationship of bacterial infection in urine and calculi to canine urolithiasis. Vet. Rec., *97*:48–50, 1975.

Weiner, I.M., and Fanelli, G.M., Jr.: Renal urate excretion in animal models. Nephron, *14*:33–47, 1975.

White, E.G.: Urinary calculi in the dog, with especial reference to cystine stone. J. Comp. Pathol. and Therap., *54*:16–25, 1944.

White, E.G.: Symposium on urolithiasis in the dog. I. Introduction and incidence. J. Small Anim. Pract., *7*:529–535, 1966.

Whiting, F., Connell, R., and Forman, S.A.: Silica urolithiasis in beef cattle. Canad. J. Comp. Med., *22*:332–337, 1958.

Neoplasms

Embryonal Nephroma, Nephroblastoma, Wilms' Tumor

This tumor arises in the kidney or occasionally outside but near it. It is the most common neoplasm in swine and occurs rarely in other species. It arises from the renal blastema, from which kidney is formed, but which in early embryonic stages is not greatly differentiated from the primitive mesenchyme. The latter is pluripotent in its capacity for differentiation into several types of mature tissue, which explains why this embryonal tumor contains more than one kind of tissue. Its structure varies, but typically involves a mixture of a certain number of gland-like acini or tubules, with large masses of cells indistinguishable from those of rather anaplastic fibrosarcoma. This led to the earlier name of **adenosarcoma,** which was in use prior to Feldman's (1932) elucidation of the embryologic origin of the neoplasm.

While the term adenosarcoma is paradoxic, it may be useful in helping the beginning student to fix the microscopic picture of the tumor in mind. It consists typically of what appears to be highly cellular fibroblastic tissue with, here and there, an inexplicable, epithelial-lined glandular acinus resembling a tubule or primitive glomerulus in its midst. In some examples, the glands are scarce and hard to find; at the other extreme are occasional tumors in which many areas consist chiefly of gland-like epithelial structures suggestive of an adenocarcinoma. The tumor is comparable to Wilms' tumor of man, which typically also contains smooth muscle, but this is

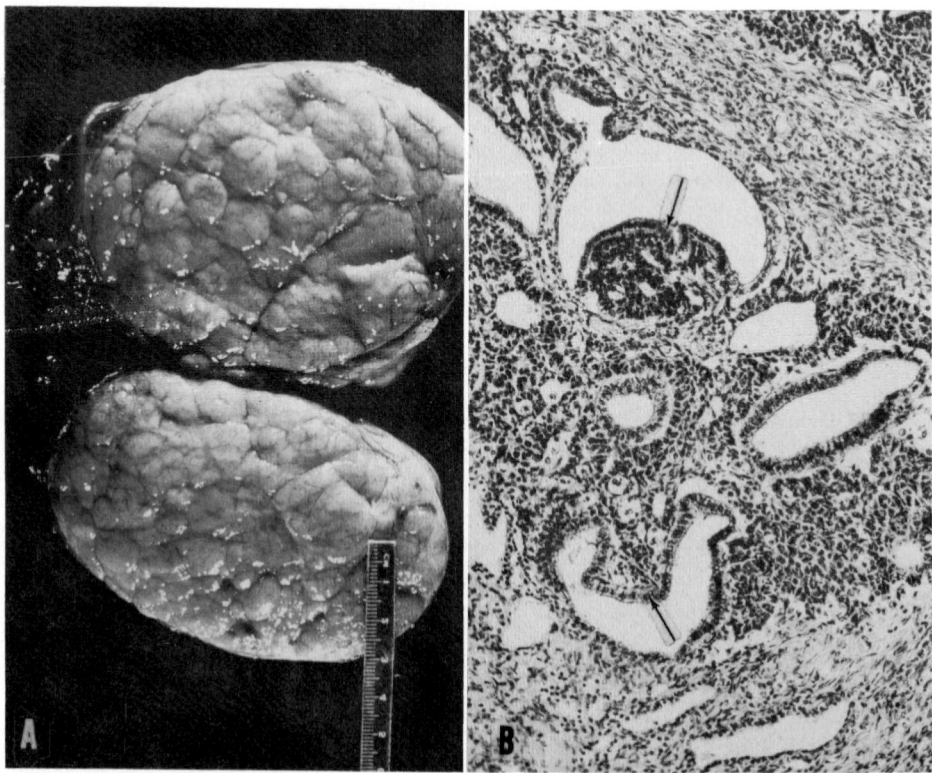

Fig. 24–25. Embryonal nephroma, kidney of a six-month-old male Fox Terrier. A, The gross specimen. B, Photomicrograph (× 100). Note structures simulating renal corpuscles. (Courtesy of Armed Forces Institute of Pathology.) Contributor: Dr. H. R. Seibold.

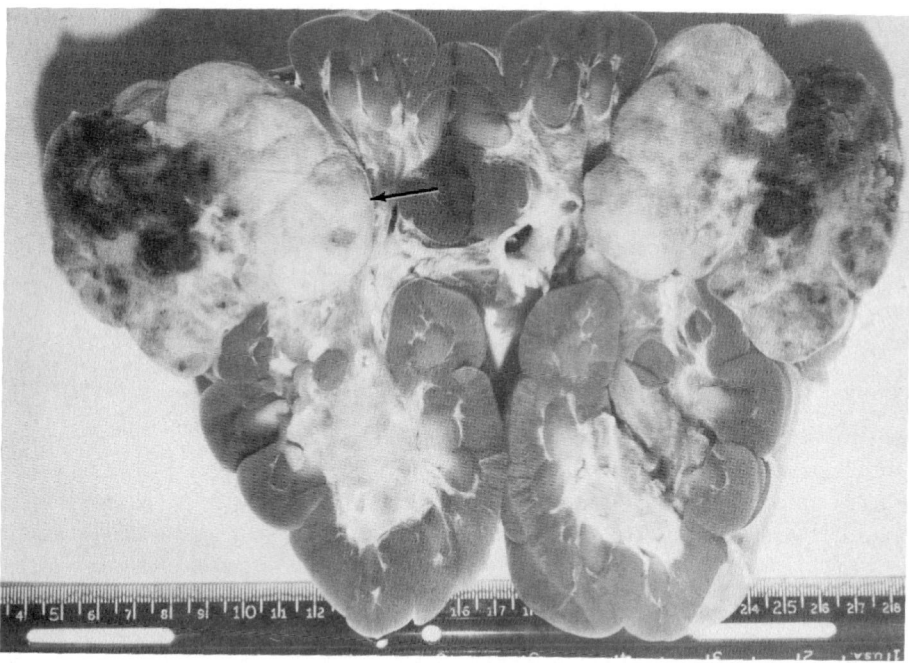

Fig. 24–26. Embryonal nephroma (arrow), kidney of an adult cow.

seldom seen in the nephroblastomas of animals. Since it has its origin in an anomaly of fetal development, it is essentially a tumor of the young. In man and animals the tumors are fatal at an early age, but pigs commonly thrive long enough to go to market in the usual way, the tumor being discovered at postmortem inspection. While still rarely seen in most species, this is one of the relatively frequent tumors of swine; it has been reported in cattle and sheep, as well as in chickens, rabbits, and other small mammalian species, becoming evident usually at an early age.

Sullivan and Anderson (1959) studied embryonal nephromas collected from meat-inspection sources, all but two being in swine. Seventy-seven percent of these occurred in pigs less than 1 year of age, but since the great majority of pigs encountered in meat inspection are of this age, it may be more significant that one occurred in a sow 6 years old. There were twice as many in females as in males, a finding which has not been explained. The tumors

were multiple in 30%, usually bilateral. Most often, but by no means invariably, arising at one pole of the kidney, they ranged from very small up to a diameter of 80 cm and a weight of 27 kg. These authors described the typical tumor as a "firm, lobulated, light-colored growth" having a "distinct capsule and numerous trabeculae of dense, mature connective tissue." While growth was described as rapid, metastases were exceptional, being chiefly to the lungs or liver. Partially calcified bone was demonstrated in one of the tumors and striated (not smooth, as in human patients) muscle was definitely recognized in five.

Other abattoir surveys (Migaki et al., 1971) have revealed incidence rates from 20/100,000 to 79/100,000 as compared to the occurrence of malignant lymphoma of about 2/100,000. In their report of 161 examples, 93% were in swine under 1 year of age, and of 147 cases, 75 were in barrows, 59 in gilts, 9 in sows, and 2 in stags. This is in contrast to the sex distribution reported by Sullivan and Anderson.

In dogs, embryonal nephroma is not common. Most examples are seen in dogs under 1 year of age, although they have been reported in dogs up to 9 years of age (Sagartz, et al., 1972).

Adenoma, Adenocarcinoma

These neoplasms arising from renal tubular epithelium usually clearly resemble their tissue of origin in microscopic sections. The tumors are most often encountered in the dog, in which they are usually malignant. An undifferentiated form of this tumor, with large, lipid-laden cells that rarely form tubules, has been called **hypernephroma,** based on an erroneous belief that its origin is in the adrenal cortex. **Undifferentiated renal carcinoma** is a preferable term. The neoplasms blend by imperceptible gradations with "clear-celled adenocarcinomas" and more ordinary adenocarcinomas and adenomas which are known to originate from the renal tubules. Benign or malignant tumors

of this general class have been found in the dog, horse, monkey, and laboratory rodent. Although carcinomas of the kidney usually metastasize by way of blood vessels, metastasis may be found in regional lymph nodes in some examples. Occasionally, squamous cell carcinoma may arise from the renal pelvis. **Transitional cell carcinoma** may originate in the renal pelvis and morphologically is similar to those which develop from the transitional epithelium of the ureter, urethra, or bladder.

Metastatic Neoplasms

The kidneys are subject to metastatic invasion by malignant neoplasms of all kinds. However, in proportion to the amount of blood which flows through them, metastases are certainly much less frequent than in the liver and lungs. The most frequent metastatic tumor, by far, is the malignant lymphoma (lymphoblastoma). It may take the form of discrete tumors of large or small size or it may in-

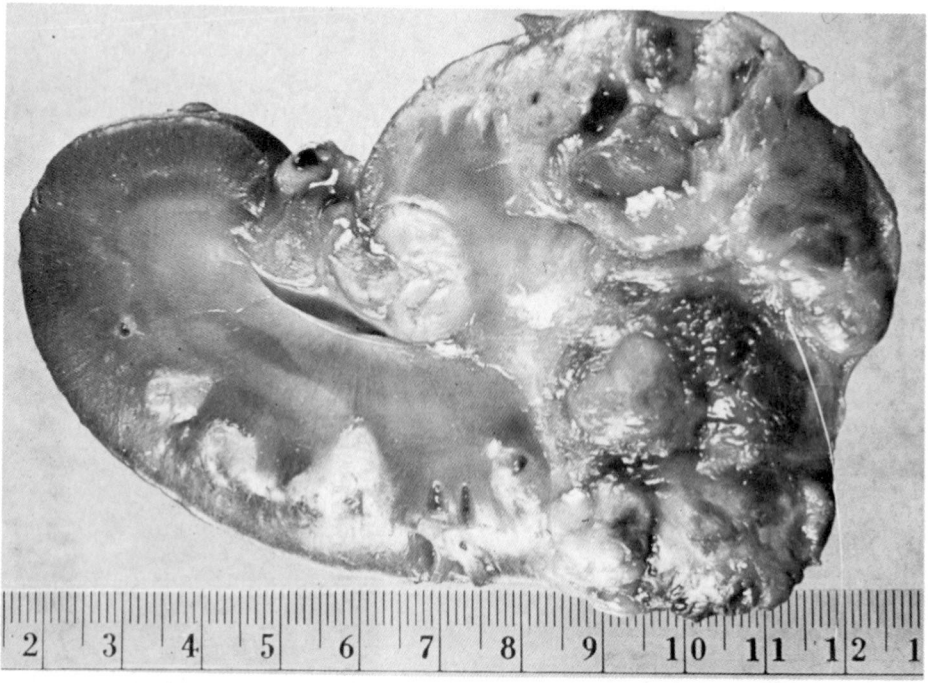

Fig. 24–27. Papillary adenocarcinoma of the kidney of an eight-year-old male Springer Spaniel.

filtrate insidiously into the intertubular interstitial tissue, with the result that irregular islets of lymphoid cells are seen microscopically here and there. The pathologist must be on guard lest these be mistaken for inflammatory infiltration; if the cells are lymphoid in character, usually somewhat larger than normal lymphocytes, and if leukocytes of other inflammatory types are not recognized, the diagnosis should be malignant lymphoma. If examination of lymph nodes and other structures is possible, the diagnosis can be confirmed. Metastatic tumors reported to occur in the kidney of animals include malignant melanoma, squamous cell carcinoma, hemangioendothelioma, and transitional cell carcinoma (from pelvis, ureter, urethra, or bladder).

Baskin, G.B., and De Paoli, A.: Primary renal neoplasms of the dog. Vet. Pathol., 14:591–605, 1977.

Burger, G.T., Moe, J.B., White, J.D., and Whitney, G.D.: Renal carcinoma in a dog. J. Am. Vet. Med. Assoc., 171:282–283, 1977.

Feldman, W.H.: Neoplasms of Domesticated Animals. Philadelphia, W.B. Saunders Co., 1932.

Kaufmann, A.F., and Quist, K.D.: Spontaneous renal carcinoma in a New Zealand white rabbit. Lab. Anim. Care, 20:530–532, 1970.

Lucke, V.W., and Kelly, D.F.: Renal carcinoma in the dog. Vet. Pathol., 13:264–276, 1976.

Migaki, G., Nelson, L.W., and Todd, G.C.: Prevalence of embryonal nephroma in slaughtered swine. J. Am. Vet. Med. Assoc., 159:441–442, 1971.

Sagartz, J.W., Ayers, K.M., Cashell, I.G., and Robinson, F.R.: Malignant embryonal nephroma in an aged dog. J. Am. Vet. Med. Assoc., 161:1658–1660, 1972.

Sullivan, D.J., and Anderson, W.A.: Embryonal nephroma in swine. Am. J. Vet. Res., 20:324–332, 1959.

Clinical Effects of Lesions in the Urinary System

Albuminuria

Albuminuria—or proteinuria because not all of the protein is albumin—is commonly revealed in the lumens of the tubules as a smoothly homogeneous, pink-staining precipitate which, at times, becomes so condensed as to form a **cast** holding the size and shape of the space in which it was molded even when voided in the urine. Epithelial cells of the proximal convoluted tubule will contain hyalin droplets which represent reabsorption of the protein by these cells. The presence of albumin (protein) in the urine is an indication of glomerular damage and ordinarily of nephritis, although moderate amounts may pass through the glomerular filter when the injury is mild and transient. Small amounts pass into the urine with the exudates of acute infectious nephritis, as previously stated.

When large amounts of blood protein continually escape into the urine, edema results because of the deficiency of protein molecules and resulting reduction of the blood's osmotic tension. Hence, in cases of generalized edema, the condition of the kidneys should always be investigated.

Hematuria is recognized and differentiated from hemoglobinuria by the microscopic demonstration of erythrocytes in a centrifuged sample of urine. If the amount of blood is large, the color of the urine becomes reddish brown. It is the result of hemorrhage anywhere from glomerulus to urethra, including hemorrhagic exudates from the kidney or bladder. Indeed, in most cases of acute exudative nephritis, small numbers of erythrocytes are demonstrable in the urine.

Hemoglobinuria is the condition in which hemoglobin, without blood cells, appears in the urine. The same brownish color as in hematuria is imparted to the urine when the condition is severe. Hemoglobinuria results from hemoglobinemia, the condition in which free hemoglobin is in solution in the blood plasma, which in turn is the result of extensive hemolysis of circulating erythrocytes by certain toxins or pathogenic microorganisms. Hemoglobin is normally eliminated through its partial decomposition by the reticuloendothelial system and excretion of the blood pigment as bilirubin. When serum levels exceed approximately 100 mg/100 ml, hemoglobin will appear in the urine; at these levels the plasma will also be red.

Hemoglobinuria must be differentiated from **myoglobinuria.** Myoglobinuria, which develops from myoglobinemia (see Azoturia, White Muscle Diseases), and hemoglobinuria are disorders identical in their superficial manifestations in the blood, but, whereas hemoglobin comes from perishing erythrocytes, myoglobin comes from damaged or destroyed muscle. Unfortunately, there is no simple chemical means of differentiating these two similar substances, only spectrographic analysis being incontrovertible. However, these two causes of brownish pigmentation of the urine can usually be distinguished on a practical basis by examination of the blood plasma. After a sample of blood has been treated with an anticoagulant and the cells allowed to settle out (accidental hemolysis being avoided) the plasma is found to be practically unstained in the case of myoglobinemia, while in hemoglobinemia the plasma shares the discoloration of the urine. The reason is that the smaller molecules of myoglobin are easily and promptly excreted from the blood into the urine, whereas in the case of hemoglobin with its large molecules, a rather high threshold must be exceeded before the pigment is released from the plasma into the urine, a considerable amount of color being constantly retained in the plasma. Myoglobin will enter the urine at levels of about 20 mg/100 ml serum. The presence of hemolytic anemia and also of hemolytic icterus affords indirect evidence of release of hemoglobin. Most cases of "red-water," as the stockman may call it, are hemoglobinuria or myoglobinuria; hematuria is much less frequently sufficient to cause marked discoloration of the urine.

Anuria

This condition of complete urinary failure and the milder oliguria, in which renal excretion is pathologically reduced but not extinguished, can arise by several different mechanisms, of which the following are of principal importance. (1) The changes described for glomerulonephritis prevent blood from flowing through the glomeruli, without which there can be no urinary secretion. (2) Since the renal capsule is quite inelastic, no great amount of intrarenal pressure is necessary to close the blood vessels which distribute blood within the kidney, thus again preventing glomerular filtration. Such pressure may result from tubular nephrosis. (3) Back pressure of urine already secreted but not discharged for any reason (hydronephrosis) prevents further secretion when the back pressure equals or closely approaches the effective filtration pressure ("hydrostatic" pressure with some modifications) of the blood within the glomeruli. (4) Similarly, when the general blood pressure in the arterial system falls below a certain level necessary to maintain filtration through the glomeruli, the formation of urine ceases. This is the mechanism responsible for the **extra-renal anuria** of shock and similar conditions. (5) Extreme dehydration prevents filtration until the volume of blood is sufficiently restored. (6) Destruction of the lining epithelium of the tubules in a later stage of tubular nephrosis than that mentioned in the second item of this series leaves the tubules with no control over resorption of the glomerular filtrate. The filtrate tends to diffuse back into the lymphatic and venous drainage as fast as it is formed. (7) Casts in general and especially the hemoglobin casts of "lower nephron nephrosis" stop the production of urine to the extent that the nephrons are occluded. Anuria is an important feature of this disease; however, the low arterial pressure of shock (item 4, above) is probably a more important causative factor than the plugging of a certain number of nephrons.

Polyuria

Physiologically, the amount of urine produced and its degree of concentration depend upon the amount of water ingested (as such or in the food) and not eliminated by such mechanisms as sweating, lactation, and respiration. The sensation of thirst ordinarily depends upon the water balance of the body and is, therefore, secondary to the extent to which water is eliminated. Hormones (pituitary, antidiuretic) also exert their influence upon the amount of urine excreted and are the decisive factor in the disease known as diabetes insipidus. As far as the kidney is concerned, polyuria is an indication of moderately injured tubules. Polyuria is often marked during the regenerative stage of tubular nephrosis, when the epithelial lining has developed to a place where it prevents the indiscriminate return of urinary fluid into the lymphatic and venous drainage, but has not yet attained its normal state of selective permeability. Similarly when numbers of tubules have disappeared, for instance through the tubular ischemia of glomerular nephritis, those remaining commonly undergo an imperfect hypertrophy which leaves their selective permeability impaired or perhaps allows the urine to pass too rapidly through a dilated and shortened nephron without adequate concentration. Waste products are, however, successfully eliminated and there is no uremia in these cases. A metabolic defect, known as **nephrogenic diabetes insipidus,** in which the tubular epithelium is unresponsive to antidiuretic hormone leading to polyuria has been recognized in dogs (Lage, 1973). There are no conspicuous light microscopic lesions, but ultrastructural studies on one dog demonstrated cytoplasmic vacuoles containing myelin in the cells of the loop of Henle (Joles and Gruys, 1979).

Uremia

Literally a condition of urine in the blood, uremia may be defined as a disorder in which a variety of harmful waste products normally eliminated in the urine remain in the circulating blood because of complete or partial failure of urinary excretion. The principal substances abnormally retained are urea, uric acid, creatinine, and ammonia, all of which are included in the nonprotein nitrogen in the ordinary laboratory examination of the blood. Also included in the list of retained substances are potassium, sulfates, chlorides, and especially phosphates. The calcium content is diminished concomitantly with the rise of phosphates. As a glance at the list of retained ions would suggest, there is a strong tendency toward acidosis. The signs cannot be attributed to any one of these hemic abnormalities. As stated by Merrill and Hampers (1970), "Efforts to discover a toxin responsible for the signs and symptoms of uremia have much in com-

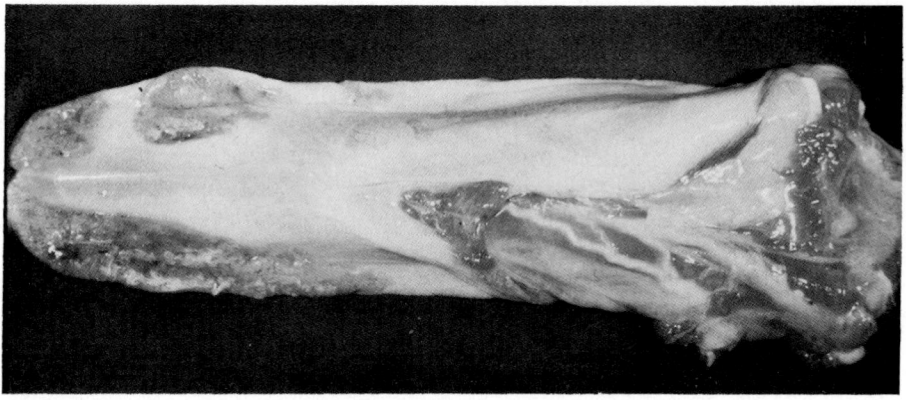

Fig. 24–28. Uremic ulcers on the tongue of a 15-year-old terrier.

mon with the attempts to identify the Yeti, or Abominable Snowman." Guanidines, which may form from a blocked urea cycle, have been shown to reproduce many of the lesions of uremia.

Symptoms such as headache are not easily evaluated in animals; vomiting can be explained on the basis of irritative lesions in the gastrointestinal tract; nervous hyperirritability, including convulsions in dogs, is usually ascribed to the lowering of calcium, although the status of the magnesium level would bear investigation in this regard. In farm animals, uremia is usually due to obstructive urolithiasis; the disease develops in the course of a very few days and, because of this and the characteristics of the species, symptoms directly attributable to the changed composition of the blood are not usually observed. In patients of any species, a urine-like odor of the breath is often present and is diagnostic. In testing for "blood urea nitrogen," it must be kept in mind that the substance is likely to be destroyed by 4 or 5 hours of postmortem autolysis.

The causes of uremia are either urinary obstruction, as noted above, or failure of renal function due to some one of the anuric diseases of the kidneys already described. Outstanding among these are the small, granular contracted kidney, whatever its cause, the tubular obstructive diseases, including obstruction by sulfonamide crystals, and extensive amyloidosis.

At the necropsy, certain extrarenal lesions may be found which are more or less characteristic of uremic death, and which, if present, have great practical significance. In the dog and also in the cat, hemorrhagic erosions or superficial ulcers are common in the buccal or pharyngeal mucosa, as is hemorrhagic gastritis, often covering a large portion of the fundic mucosa. Less frequently, the intestine may be similarly involved. In cattle, the preceding lesions seldom occur, but severe catarrhal or hemorrhagic inflammation may involve the terminal part of the large intestine. The pathogenesis of the lesions of the digestive tract is uncertain. It has been presumed to be due to elimination of some toxic substances through the affected mucous membrane. Vascular degeneration, discussed elsewhere, is particularly evident at these sites and is probably the primary basis for the degenerative and inflammatory lesions at these and other sites.

In the case of toxic tubular nephrosis or of leptospirosis (canine), it is difficult to say how much of the injury to the digestive mucosa is attributable directly to uremic products and how much to the original injurious agent. A uremic lesion which is common in man and occasional in dogs and cattle is an increase of pericardial fluid, often with a small amount of fibrin. The explanation is not apparent, but the condition has not been shown to be a true inflammation (reaction to an irritant). The so-called uremic aortitis, rather frequently seen in dogs, consists of a proliferative roughening of the intima, usually near the heart, and sometimes extending into it (the left ventricle). Microscopic areas of calcification are frequent in the intima of this and other blood vessels and beneath the endocardium. Calcification is also common in the gastric mucosa and pleura of uremic dogs. Calcification is probably preceded by necrosis at all of these sites and not directly the result of high serum inorganic phosphorous levels depressing serum calcium. If prolonged, hypocalcemia leads to secondary hyperplasia of the parathyroid glands and osteodystrophia fibrosa. Uremia is often accompanied by a noticeable degree of normochromic, normocytic anemia. The pathogenesis of anemia is not clear. There is decreased erythropoietin secretion, but the pathogenesis is probably multifactorial. Erythrocyte life span is shortened, and there is depression of production of erythrocytes by the bone marrow, although the marrow is not hypocellular and may in fact be hypercellular. Hemolysis may occur in uremia and be accompanied by hemosiderosis. Hemorrhage may also contribute to anemia, through damaged mucous membranes, and through platelet dysfunction and thrombocytopenia. Toxic injury to the bone marrow (toxic aplastic anemia) has been postulated as a cause, but the frequency of hemosiderosis in the spleen and elsewhere is suggestive of a hemolytic action. The cerebral edema which is common in humans seldom accompanies uremia in domestic animals.

URETERS, URACHUS, BLADDER, AND URETHRA

The Ureter

Anomalies of the ureter are rare. These anomalies range from aplasia to complete duplication.

Inflammation of the ureteral mucosa occurs as a part of inflammation of the whole urinary tract. Because of the dense nature of the wall of this small tubular organ, the exudative or proliferative changes are less extensive and attract less attention in the ureter than in the bladder or renal pelvis. The dilatation of the ureteral lumen and the thickening of the wall which occur in ascending pyelonephritis or pyonephrosis have been mentioned. If there is partial obstruction lower in the urinary tract, the gradual dilation of the lumen of one or both ureters (depending on location of the obstruction) can be quite remarkable. Tuberculosis and possibly certain other granulomatous infections occasionally invade the wall of the ureter, producing characteristic lesions.

Strictures in the form of an irregular fold or a gradual narrowing can occur either congenitally or as the result of previous inflammation. Such damage is most likely to be due to the temporary lodgment of

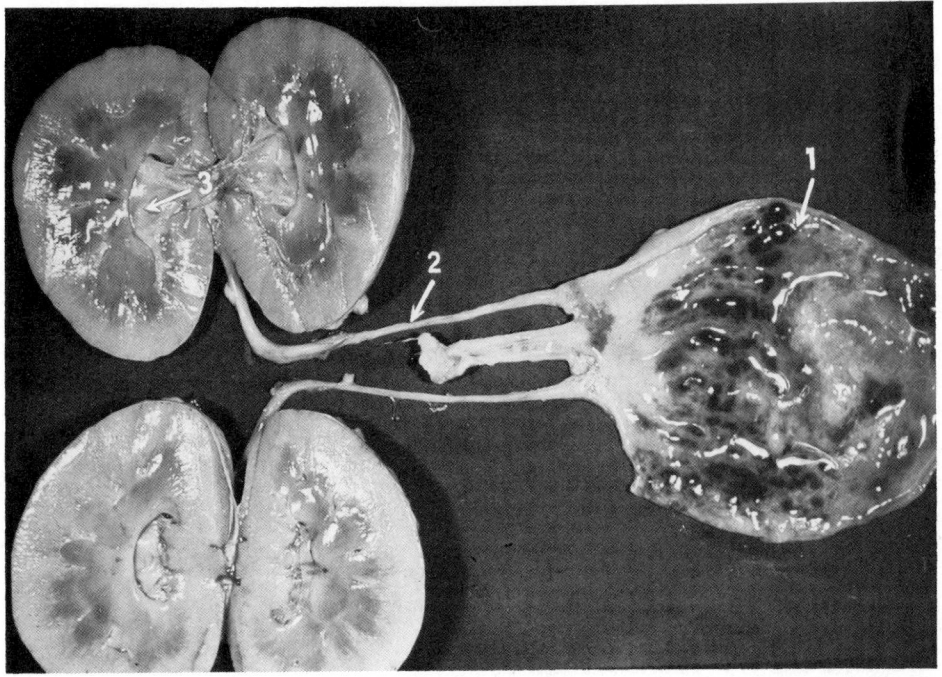

Fig. 24-29. Cystitis, ureteritis and pyelonephritis in a five-year-old male cat. The mucosa of the bladder (1) was replaced by hemorrhagic, purulent and necrotic exudates. The ureters (2) and renal pelvis (3) were found to be similarly involved when examined microscopically. (Courtesy of Angell Memorial Animal Hospital.)

calculi somewhere along the tube, although a considerable proportion of strictures are located just at the ureteral inlet.

Neoplasms, usually papillomas or carcinomas, arise from the ureteral mucosa rarely. Metastatic tumors may infiltrate the wall. Hilton A. Smith reported seeing the thickness of the wall of a bovine ureter increased to twenty times the normal by an infiltrating malignant lymphoma.

Bladder

Anomalies

"**Pervious urachus**" is a congenital failure of the fetal urachus to close, and requires surgical intervention. The occasional ascent of infection from a diseased umbilicus to the kidney has been mentioned. Cysts rarely form in the course of a urachus which closes in some parts and not in others, leaving isolated stretches of patent lumen, or they may form in the midline of the bladder. Other congenital anomalies of the urinary bladder such as aplasia, diverticula, and fistula are rare.

Cystitis

Especially when there is interference with the normal drainage of urine, the mucosa and deeper layers of the bladder are subject to infectious inflammations of the acute fibrinous, purulent, catarrhal and hemorrhagic types. The purulent form occasionally reaches phlegmonous proportions. Infection with gas-producing bacteria may lead to gas-filled vesicles in the wall of the bladder, a condition known as *emphysematous cystitis.* The latter is most frequent in the presence of glucosuria. Chronicity leads to irregular thickening of the subepithelial connective tissue and mild corrugation of the mucous side as seen grossly. A form of cystitis occurs rarely in the dog in which numerous epithelial-lined diverticula of uncertain origin become closed at their orifices and form minute cystic spaces in the inflamed and thickened wall.

Involvement by tuberculosis and possibly other infectious granulomas occurs rarely. Tubercles may be small and confined to the submucosa or may form large bulges into the lumen, with or without ulceration. Urolithiasis tends to result from long-continued cystitis of exudative type. Mucinous, adenomatous, and squamous metaplasia of the transitional epithelium is a frequent finding in chronic cystitis. This is especially evident in bovine enzootic hematuria. It is apparently related to chronic inflammation. In swine, mucinous metaplasia of the superficial transitional epithelium, especially of the renal pelvis and ureters, is seen in association with a variety of conditions, particularly exudative epidermitis. It has been called "mucinous degeneration" (Brobst et al., 1971).

Other Disorders of the Bladder

Hemorrhages, usually petechial, without inflammation are indicative of acute toxemias or septicemias. Petechiae in the mucosa are considered of diagnostic significance in hog cholera.

Hypertrophy of the muscular layer is recognized by raised parallel longitudinal ridges about 2 or 3 mm in width and height (dog) visible on the serous side. It is a compensatory (or adaptive) hypertrophy designed to provide sufficient force to expel the urine against some partial obstruction, most frequently the periurethral pressure of an enlarged canine prostate.

Two helminth parasites may inhabit the urinary bladder, *Capillaria plica* in cats and *Trichosomoides crassicaudata* in rats. These produce little or no pathologic effect. Certain schistosomes parasitize the vesicular veins, and their eggs may lead to granulomatous lesions in the wall of the urinary bladder.

Neoplasms

Papillomas of transitional epithelium are occasionally encountered neoplasms in any species. They are characterized by numerous and long, stringy papillations which resemble the flower of a dahlia. They are most frequent in cattle as part of the disorder known as bovine enzootic hematuria.

Carcinomas of the urinary bladder may be transitional cell carcinomas, squamous cell carcinomas, or adenocarcinomas. Transitional cell tumors are more frequent, and histologically, may be solid or papillary. They may be sufficiently well differentiated to resemble transitional epithelium, or they may be highly anaplastic with little resemblance to the cells from which they arose. Squamous cell carcinomas and adenocarcinomas, which may secrete mucin, arise in metaplastic epithelium. The cause of the metaplasia is often unknown, but usually ascribed to chronic cystitis or toxicity, such as in bovine enzootic hematuria.

Mesenchymal neoplasms are not common although leiomyomas, leiomyosarcomas, and rhabdomyosarcomas are seen occasionally in dogs.

Metastatic neoplasms, especially malignant lymphomas, may infiltrate the wall of the bladder, usually the submucosa or subserosa. The result is a series of diffuse or nodular thickenings consisting of smoothly homogeneous, white tissue.

Experimentally, papillomas and papillary carcinomas have been produced in the dog's bladder by prolonged administration (over several years) of such compounds as beta-naphthylamine. This was done primarily in connection with the study of certain "aniline tumors" which have de-

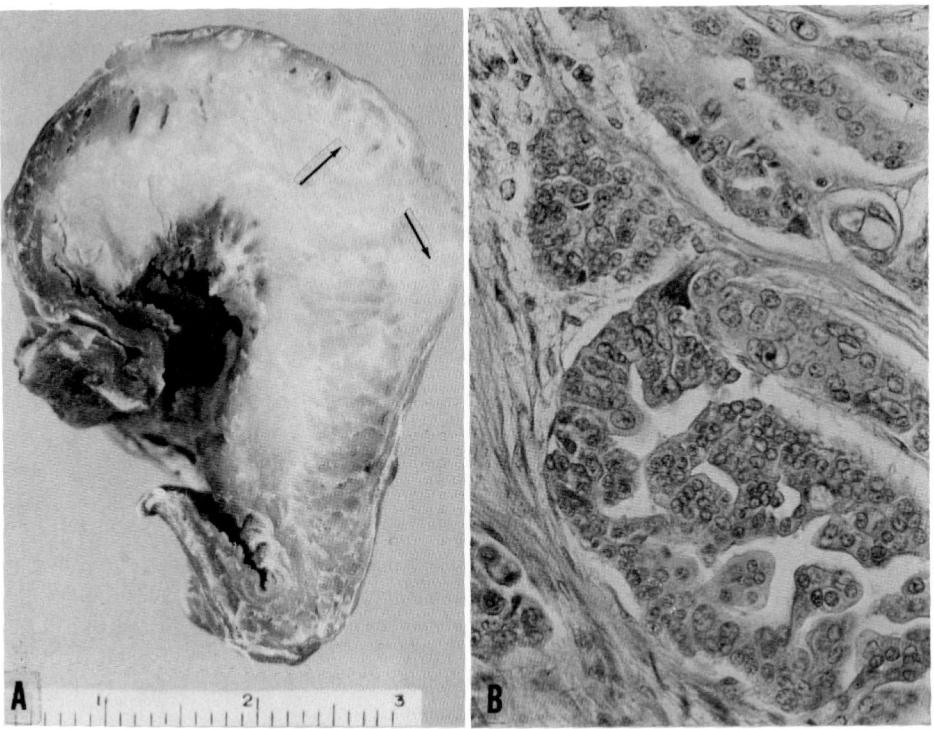

Fig. 24–30. Transitional and squamous-cell carcinoma of the epithelium of the urinary bladder of an 11-year-old male Collie-Shepherd dog. *A*, The tumor invades and replaces the mucosa as well as the muscular coat and elevates the serosa (arrows). *B*, Photomicrograph (× 305) of a part of the neoplasm in which transitional epithelium is simulated. In other areas squamous cells predominate. (Courtesy of Armed Forces Institute of Pathology.) Contributor: Dr. Leo L. Lieberman.

veloped in people working in aniline industries. There appears, however, to be nothing in the dog's bladder comparable to the human neoplasms which develop in connection with schistosomiasis. The precancerous squamous metaplasia called leukoplakia in the human patient has not been reported in animals, possibly because the prolonged episodes of chronic cystitis which appear to precede the disorder seldom occur in animals.

Urethra

The urethra almost never suffers from more than very transient inflammation as long as there is no interference with the drainage of urine. The passing of a catheter usually causes mild injury and inflammation which remains painful for a few days, especially in males. The principal lesion encountered in this organ is the lodgment of calculi. This is especially likely to occur at the sigmoid flexure in male ruminants. There is always a variable degree of hyperemia and inflammation at and above the site of lodgment, none below it. There are in animals no specific infections with a predilection for the urethra, such as gonorrheal infection in the human. The mucosa and probably its tributary glands appear to harbor such organisms as *Trichomonas fetus* in the bull, but the condition represents more a symbiosis than a pathogenesis as far as the urethra itself and its glands are concerned. A bull so infected may, however, be a source of contagion to the female, in which the infection is a cause of sterility.

Diverticula (in the female especially) and strictures (in the male chiefly) occur rarely in the urethra, being either congenital or the result of injury by stones, catheters, or compressing injuries from the outside. As in other tubular organs, a dilatation may form above a stricture as the result of pressure of accumulated fluid. The effect of obstruction in the urethra (as elsewhere) in causing hydronephrosis has been discussed.

Obstruction of the urethra of the male cat is a common clinical problem, especially in castrated males. Although uroliths are sometimes demonstrated, in many cases inflammation of the urethra appears to be the underlying factor in the obstruction. Some evidence indicates that a picornavirus may be involved (Fabricant et al., 1969).

Fistulas

Fistulous tracts can be established between adjacent pelvic organs as a result of necrotizing processes, especially if these are preceded by adhesions between the two surfaces concerned. While all such openings are rare in the domestic animals, it is possible for the rectum to become inflamed and adherent where it passes the bladder and for continuing destruction to lead to perforation into the bladder. Possible causes are trauma from foreign objects, usually surgical, caustic medicaments locally applied, cystic calculi, invasive neoplasms and some others, conceivably including lesions produced by nodular worms (*Oesophagostomum sp.*).

Rectovaginal fistulas are more frequent than the rectovesical just described. They arise from similar causes and also are at times congenital. The vesicovaginal fistula, rather common in humans, does not occur in the domestic animals to any appreciable extent, since the walls of the two organs are not contiguous as in the human female.

Bovine Enzoötic Hematuria

Reported only from certain sharply limited regions of the world, especially the northwestern United States, western Canada, Japan, New Zealand, and the Black Sea region of Turkey, Bulgaria, and Yugoslavia, this is a disease of adult cattle and also water buffalo characterized by persistent hematuria leading to (chronc hemorrhagic) anemia and death. The lesions, which arise most frequently in the bladder, but also occasionally in the ureters

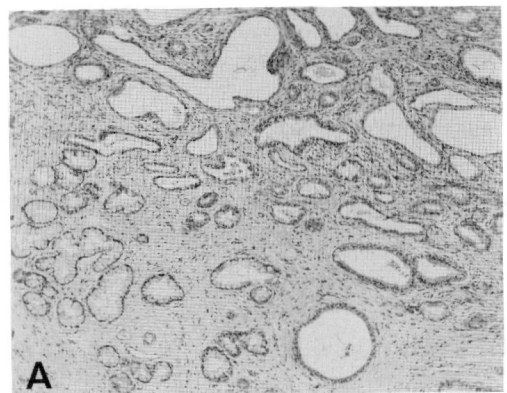

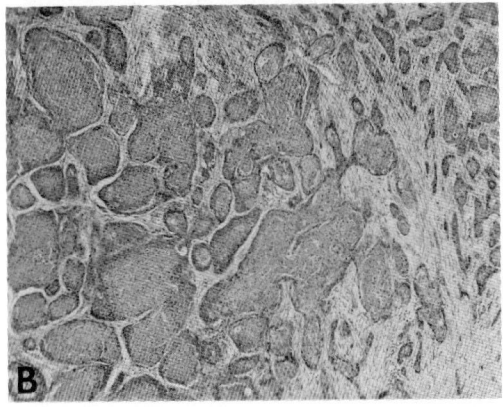

Fig. 24–31. Bovine enzootic hematuria. Mucinous adenocarcinoma, A, and squamous cell carcinoma, B, of urinary bladder. (Courtesy of Armed Forces Institute of Pathology.)

or renal pelvis, appear to represent a chronic but violently hyperplastic inflammation with severe hyperemia and recurrent hemorrhage. There is localized proliferation of epithelium with metaplasia either to mucin-forming columnar or to stratified squamous types or a mixture of the two. In certain cases, the hyperplastic epithelium acquires neoplastic properties, developing into a carcinoma (either squamous-cell or adenocarcinoma) which is locally invasive and may metastasize to the regional lymph nodes and the lungs. The capillaries of the inflammatory lesion also participate in the hyperplastic proliferation, sometimes to the extent of forming hemangiomas either in the stroma or pro-

jecting from the mucosal surface, and are capable, in themselves, of developing malignant qualities. Two or more different types of neoplasms may be encountered in a given animal. The etiology appears to be well established as one long term effect of poisoning due to bracken fern.

An **epizootic cystitis** in horses has been described in the southwestern United States and Australia. It has been associated with grazing on Sudan or hybrid Sudan grass (Romane, et al., 1966, Hooper, 1968).

Barrett, R.E., and Nobel, T.A.: Transitional cell carcinoma of the urethra in a cat. Cornell Vet., 66:14–26, 1976.

Bebko, R.L., Prier, J.E., and Biery, D.N.: Ectopic ureters in a male cat. J. Am. Vet. Med. Assoc., 171:738–740, 1977.

Brobst, D.F., Cottrell, R., and Delez, A.: Mucinous degeneration of the epithelium of the urinary tract of swine. Vet. Pathol., 8:485–489, 1971.

Burk, R.L., Meierhenry, E.F., and Schaubhut, C.W., Jr.: Leiomyosarcoma of the urinary bladder in a cat. J. Am. Vet. Med. Assoc., 167:749–751, 1975.

Chesney, C.F., and Allen, J.R.: Urinary bladder carcinoma in a Rhesus monkey (Macaca mulatta): a literature review and case report. Lab. Anim. Sci., 23:716–719, 1973.

Cheville, N.F.: Uremic gastropathy in the dog. Vet. Pathol., 16:292–309, 1979.

Dennis, S.M.: Patent urachus in a neonatal lamb. Cornell Vet., 59:581–584, 1969.

Fabricant, C.G., Rich, L.J., and Gillespie, J.H.: Feline viruses. XI. Isolation of a virus similar to a myxovirus from cats in which urolithiasis was experimentally induced. Cornell Vet., 59:667–672, 1969.

Fulton, J.D., and Armstrong, J.A.: Obstruction of the urogenital tract in some rodents. J. Reprod. Fertil., 4:309–312, 1962.

Halliwell, W.H., and Ackerman, N.: Botryoid rhabdomyosarcoma of the urinary bladder and hypertrophic osteoarthropathy in a young dog. J. Am. Vet. Med. Assoc., 165:911–913, 1974.

Hooper, P.T.: Epizootic cystitis in horses. Aust. Vet. J., 44:11–14, 1968.

Ito, T., Miura, S., Ohshima, K.-I., and Numakunai, S.: Ultrastructural studies of bovine urinary bladders with special reference to enzootic bovine hematuria. Jpn. J. Vet. Sci., 33:127–135, 1971.

Johnston, S.D., Osborne, C.A., and Stevens, J.B.: Canine polypoid cystitis. J. Am. Vet. Med. Assoc., 166:1155–1160, 1975.

Joles, J.A., and Gruys, E.: Nephrogenic diabetes insipidus in a dog with renal medullary lesions. J. Am. Vet. Med. Assoc., 174:830–834, 1979.

Kelly, D.F.: Rhabdomyosarcoma of the urinary bladder in dogs. Vet. Pathol., 10:375–384, 1973.

Lage, A.L.: Nephrogenic diabetes insipidus in a dog. J. Am. Vet. Med. Assoc., *163*:251–253, 1973.

Machado, A.V., Rangel, N.M., and Giovine, N.: Persistent urachus associated with pyelonephritis. Cornell Vet., *33*:372–376, 1943.

Marsh, H.: Urethral occlusion in lambs on feed containing stilbestrol. J. Am. Vet. Med. Assn., *139*:1019–1023, 1961.

McCully, R.M., and Lieberman, L.L.: Histopathology of a case of feline urolithiasis. Canad. Vet. J., *2*:52–61, 1961.

Merrill, J.P., and Hampers, C.L.: Uremia (1 and 2 of 2 parts). N. Engl. J. Med., *282*:953–962, 1014–1022, 1970.

Osborne, C.A., et al.: Congenital urethrorectal fistula in two dogs. J. Am. Vet. Med. Assoc., *166*:999–1002, 1975.

Romane, W.M., et al.: Cystitis syndrome of the equine. S.W. Vet., *19*:95–99, 1966.

Seely, J.C., Cosenza, S.F., and Montgomery, C.A.: Leiomyosarcoma of the canine urinary bladder, with metastases. J. Am. Vet. Med. Assoc., *172*:1427–1429, 1978.

Sherding, R.G., and Chew, D.J.: Nondiabetic emphysematous cystitis in two dogs. J. Am. Vet. Med. Assoc., *174*:1105–1109, 1979.

Skye, D.V.: Hydronephrosis secondary to focal papillary hyperplasia of the urinary bladder of cattle. J. Am. Vet. Med. Assoc., *166*:595–598, 1975.

Smith, B.L., and Beatson, N.S.: Bovine enzootic haematuria in New Zealand, N. Z. Vet. J., *18*:115–120, 1970.

Smith, B.L., and Wouden, M., van der: Bovine enzootic haematuria lesions in cattle passing through a Nelson meatworks. N.Z. Vet. J., *20*:56, 1972.

Strafuss, A.C., and Dean, M.J.: Neoplasms of the canine urinary bladder. J. Am. Vet. Med. Assoc., *166*:1161–1163, 1975.

Yoshikawa, T., and Oyamada, T.: Histopathology of papillary tumors in the bovine urinary bladder. Jpn. J. Vet. Sci., *37*:277–287, 1975.

CHAPTER 25

The Genital System

FEMALE REPRODUCTIVE ORGANS

The reader is, of course, familiar with the anatomy, histology, and physiology of the organs under consideration, but it may be advantageous to review as briefly as possible certain features that have a special bearing on their pathology.

The Estrual Cycle

Of unique importance in interpreting many failures of the reproductive process and lesions of the reproductive organs is a familiarity with the morphological changes which accompany the estrual cycle in normal, parous females of each species. Although most species of concern possess the same pituitary and ovarian hormones, their interaction and the length of the estrus cycle vary considerably. What follows is a generalization applicable to most species. If we consider a given cycle as starting just after an ovulation, which is convenient in those species which do not menstruate, we encounter a series of changes that are incited through the action of several hormones released into the blood. The pituitary secretes three reproductive hormones, the follicle-stimulating hormone, commonly abbreviated FSH, the luteinizing hormone, LH, and prolactin. The ovarian (graafian) follicle, in proportion to its size and development, liberates the hormone (or hormones), estrogen (estradiol, folliculin, theelin, etc.), which, among other actions, is believed to inhibit the production of FSH. Ovulation depends upon a massive discharge of LH, which is stimulated by high levels of estrogen. The corpus luteum owes its existence to LH. As the corpus luteum grows, it elaborates more and more of the hormone progesterone, which prevents any surge of LH and in some unknown manner prevents the developing graafian follicle from secreting estrogen.

Starting at the point in the cycle where a mature follicle has just ruptured, in other words, at ovulation, we find the production of estrogen is minimal. Peak estrogen secretion precedes ovulation by an interval of two or more days depending upon the species, and is responsible for the behavioral signs of estrus. The high level of estrogen is believed to inhibit FSH secretion and, in the absence of progesterone, causes a release of high levels of LH from the pituitary, which results in ovulation. LH also prepares the granulosa cells for their future development into a corpus luteum. With the fall in estrogen a new follicle (or follicles) begins to develop, but maturation and estrogen secretion do not commence until dissolution of the corpus luteum. Progesterone in some manner inhibits maturation of the follicle. Coinciding with ovulation, blood vessels break though the basement membrane of the follicle, and granulosa cells begin to luteinize. The cells increase in number and size, and develop a vacuolated cytoplasm containing lipid, cholesterol, and carotenoid pigments, producing a grossly visible yellow color. This is the corpus luteum, which commences to secrete progesterone.

The transition and continued secretion of progesterone depends upon LH and the pituitary hormone prolactin. Progesterone as indicated holds the developing follicle in check and also prevents any surge of LH from the pituitary. Continuation of the cycle, therefore, depends upon regression of the corpus luteum. The hormonal mechanism for this dissolution is not understood. In sheep, it depends upon an intact uterus, which under the influence of progesterone secretes a substance which in turn destroys the corpus luteum. This substance is believed to be prostaglandin F_2. Presumably pregnancy precludes this relationship and allows the persistence of the corpus luteum of pregnancy. In other species, the factors resulting in the demise of the corpus luteum are less clear. In man, the presence of the uterus is not necessary. In dogs, the corpus luteum persists for nearly the duration of a normal pregnancy whether or not the bitch conceives. This prolonged luteal phase in dogs is referred to as pseudopregnancy. In any event, the dissolution of the corpus luteum results in falling progesterone levels and subsequent maturation and estrogen secretion by the follicle, bringing the animal into estrus and ultimately causing release of LH, ovulation, and birth of another corpus luteum. Regression of the corpus luteum is characterized by loss of vascularization, gradual fatty change, atrophy, and slow necrosis of the lutein cells. By the time of the next ovulation (about 21 days in most farm animals, 28 days in human beings), the corpus luteum has receded to less than half its maximum size, and in a few more weeks there remains only a scar of hyaline connec-

tive tissue, which is called the corpus albicans.

Barring the occurrence of pregnancy, this cyclic development of follicles and corpora lutea goes on at regular intervals indefinitely in most species, including dairy cows and swine. The length of the cycle varies markedly from 4 days in rats to the long interval of 6 months in dogs. In some domestic animals and many wild animals, there is a seasonal influence, in which the length of the day is believed to be the principal environmental influence. Ewes in the Northern Hemisphere begin regular 16-day estrus cycles in the fall that cease in the spring. In some species, such as the cat, rabbit, ferret, and mink, ovulation occurs and the cycle is initiated only with the stimulation of coitus. The estrus cycle continues throughout life in animals, with the exception of some nonhuman primates, whereas in human beings the regular cycles terminate in middle or late age at the menopause.

While the ovarian cycle goes on as outlined, the other reproductive organs display cyclic changes, largely as a result of the alternating rise and fall of estrogen and progesterone, and these are of even greater significance in practical diagnostic pathology than those seen in the ovary (Fig. 25–1).

Endometrium

The variable picture encountered in the endometrium is largely cyclic and needs to be understood before endometrial disorders can be properly evaluated. Unfortunately, our knowledge of the cyclic changes in animals is far from complete in various details and is based largely on what occurs in the human species. In the cow, the only domestic animal to which much study has been given, the endometrium seems to follow much the same cycle as in the human except that the variations are less pronounced, and, of course, there is no menstruation. Cyclic changes may be observed in the lining epithelium, the glands, the

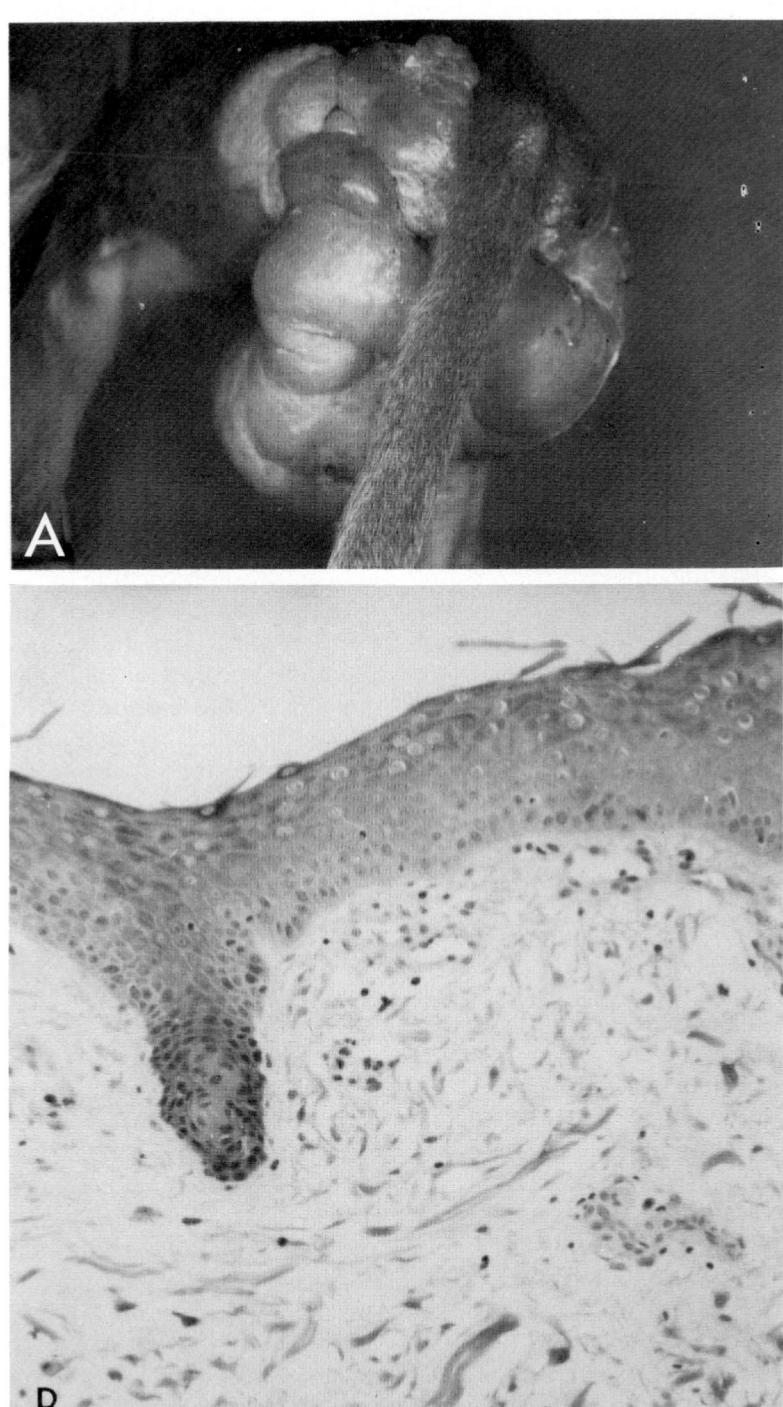

Fig. 25–1. Sex skin in a baboon. *A*, Marked swelling of the perineum recurs with each estrus cycle. *B*, Microscopically, the collagen fibers of the dermis are separated by mucopolysaccharides. (Courtesy of New England Regional Primate Research Center, Harvard Medical School.)

glandular epithelium, the stroma, and, to some extent, in the blood vessels.

A number of days previous to ovulation, in other words, at the beginning of the stage termed proestrum by physiologists, hormonal stimulation of the genital tissues may be considered at its lowest ebb. At this time, the lining epithelium of the uterus is low cuboidal and that of the glands is not much more impressive. The glands themselves are comparatively simple, straight tubular glands. The stroma consists of very closely placed, short, fibroblastic nuclei with no individual cytoplasm, but lying in a rather scanty fibrillar meshwork. The blood supply is minimal. This is not unlike the postmenstrual endometrium in the human. From here onward the tendency is toward proliferation. Indeed, the ensuing stage has been given the name of the **proliferative phase.** Since the proliferation is due to the influence of the follicular hormone, estrogen, from the growing follicle, the term "follicular phase" is used synonymously. The lining and glandular epithelial cells become taller, and mitotic figures are numerous, causing the glands to become larger and appear more numerous. Early in the proliferative phase, the glands are straight and tubular, but as they continue to grow, they become convoluted. To a slight extent, similar changes can be detected in the mucosa of the oviduct: epithelial hyperplasia with increase in the number of cilia.

As ovulation occurs (end of estrus), the endometrium falls under the predominant influence of progesterone from the corpus luteum, and enters the **secretory phase** or progesterone phase. Clear vacuoles destined for glandular secretion appear underneath the nuclei of the glandular epithelium, and push the latter toward the superficial end of the cell. These vacuoles are sharply defined and contain glycogen. Their number steadily increases until actual secretions commence, at which point supranuclear vacuoles appear as subnuclear vacuolation is lost and the nuclei sub-

side to their usual level in the cells. Colloidal secretion is evident in the glandular lumens, which over a period of several days (for most species) becomes stringy in appearance.

Under the influence of progesterone, the endometrial proliferation continues. The epithelial cells increase in number and size, causing the glands to become more tortuous with tiny folds of redundant lining. It cannot be said, however, that they reach the "saw-tooth" form which is seen in human beings at this stage. Up until the midprogestational stage, the stroma has remained relatively unchanged; however, from this point on, stromal changes predominate. The cells of the stroma tend to become more rounded and less fibrous in appearance, approaching but not attaining the predecidual type of endometrium as it exists in man. The nuclei become larger, plumper, and less deeply chromatic, and develop a little individualized cytoplasm in some cases. This alteration is particularly evident around arterioles, which are now greatly increased in number, although arteriolar proliferation commenced under stimulation by estrogen. The arterioles grow in a spiral or corkscrew pattern such that each is cut several times in any plane of section. The cells of the stroma become more separated from one another due to interstitial edema.

Each of these endometrial proliferative changes throughout all phases of the cycle occur in most animals, but their extent varies considerably between species. They are most prominent in human beings, relatively extensive in dogs, cats, and rabbits, and much less conspicuous in sheep, cattle, guinea pigs, and rodents.

At this point the uterus is prepared for implantation and pregnancy. If pregnancy occurs, this endometrial hypertrophy (and now marked myometrial enlargement) as well as growth of the corpus luteum, continues. But if there is no conception, the hypertrophic endometrium subsides in company with the regressing corpus luteum. In the human, this would be menstruation; in the domestic animals, there is no such precipitous destruction, no sloughing, no hemorrhage. Neutrophils and other leukocytes invade the endometrium in appreciable numbers to dispose of the remains of the cells that perish in the retrogressive process.

To a certain degree, the other parts of the genital tract participate in this cyclic rise and fall, this proliferation and regression, but a practical use of this fact has been limited largely to the case of the vaginal epithelium. This proliferates during the endometrial proliferative phase (proestrum) to form a thicker layer, which tends to become cornified as the more superficial cells find themselves farther from their nutrient supply. Then regression sets in, earlier than in the endometrium (early diestrum), numerous leukocytes infiltrating the stroma and epithelium. There is vaginal bleeding in the dog. Smears made from the vaginal surface reveal cells corresponding in type to those underlying it. It has been found possible to estimate the phase

of the cycle by study of such smears, at least in the canine species. In the herbivora, the period of ovulation is characterized by a copious secretion of mucus (mucus of estrum) from the glands of the cervix.

The mammary gland also undergoes cyclic changes with each estrus cycle. Prior to the onset of reproductive cycles, the gland is rudimentary; however, with the onset of regular cycles, there is proliferation of ducts, ductules, and, in some species, alveoli coincident with the proliferative and secretory phases of the endometrium. In general, the longer the cycle the greater is the degree of proliferation. In species with extremely short cycles such as the mouse, ductules are formed but not alveoli. In species with approximate monthly cycles, fine ductules and some alveoli form, and in the dog, with its long luteal phase, extensive alveolar formation occurs comparable to that seen in late pregnancy in other species.

Endometriosis. The transplantation of a bit of endometrium by embryonic or surgical displacement, to an abnormal site,

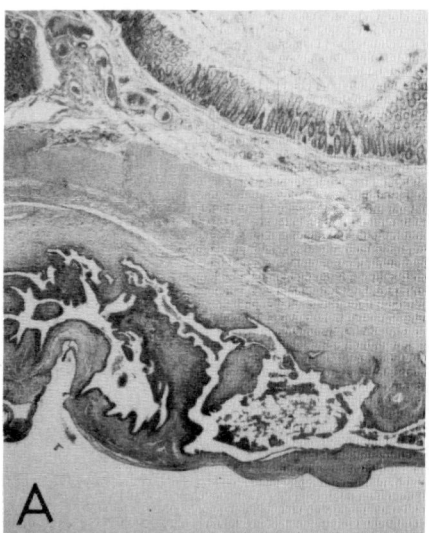 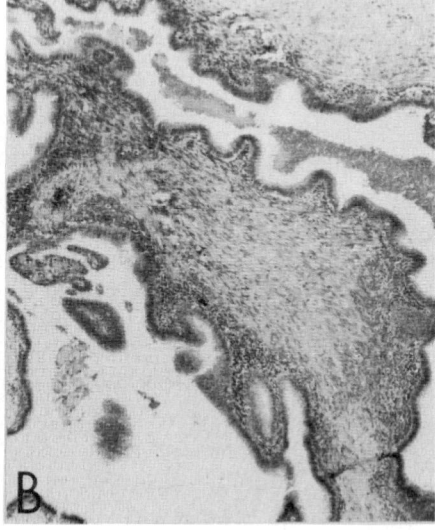

Fig. 25–2. Endometriosis, rhesus monkey *(Macaca mulatta).* A, Endometrium implanted in the wall of the colon. B, Uterine columnar epithelium accompanied by endometrial stroma differentiates endometriosis from malignancy. Note detritus which represents evidence of menstruation. Inability of menstrual fluids to escape the body results in toxemia. (Courtesy of New England Regional Primate Research Center, Harvard Medical School.)

leaves viable tissue which is subject to the effects of various hormones and has no outlet for its secretions. This may result in accumulation of secretions, possibly toxemia. It is best known in women and nonhuman primates (Fig. 25–2).

Atretic Follicles

Another normal phenomenon with which the pathologist needs to be familiar is the atresia (closing up) of follicles. Even before puberty, many primordial follicles undergo growth and maturation to vesicular follicles. This begins shortly after birth in most species and even before birth in primates. All of these prepubertal vesicular follicles undergo degeneration. With the onset of reproductive cycles, a number of follicles progress to a stage approaching complete maturity, but only one in uniparous species is able, through some unique preference which we do not understand, to attain complete maturation and send its ovum along the course designed to lead to a new life. In the case of multiple births, there is, of course, one ovum for each individual born, except identical twins. In species which are seasonably estrus, follicular development occurs during the period of long anestrus, but the follicles do not reach maturity, but rather become atretic.

After each ovulation, the remaining nearly mature follicles degenerate and disappear, no doubt because they are deprived of the follicle-stimulating hormone. This process of atresia begins with simple necrosis of the granulosa cells. Later the follicular lining is reduced to a single layer of cells of epithelial appearance or perhaps there may be no epithelial lining at all. The necrotic granulosa cells can often be seen floating uselessly in the liquor folliculi. Normally this fluid is soon resorbed, and in the bovine, the follicle is replaced temporarily by a small, circumscribed spot of fibrous tissue, the corpus fibrosum. It is denser than the surrounding stroma, but not hyaline like the corpus albicans. In some species, rounded, lipoid-containing "theca-lutein cells" precede the fibrous stage. Pathologically, resorption sometimes fails, fluid increases and the atretic follicle becomes a cystic follicle, or follicular cyst.

Placenta

While we shall refer the reader to other sources for most of our histologic details, an accurate knowledge of the placental tissues in the several species is of such importance in the practice of pathology that it is desirable to describe them briefly here. By the placenta, we mean those tissues that are concerned in the exchange of nutrients and other substances between the blood of the mother and that of the fetus. That portion which is a part of the mother's endometrium is the maternal placenta; the part which belongs to the fetal membranes is the fetal placenta. In a general way, the fetal placenta consists of minute projections from the allantochorion, called chorionic villi, which penetrate with more or less intimacy into the maternal endometrium, but there are many differences among the various species. As a matter of convenience and because of their villous appearance in the single plane of a microscopic section, the narrow strips or ridges of endometrium that fill the spaces between the chorionic villi are often called maternal villi, and this somewhat erroneous term will be indulged in here. They are also called "maternal septa" of the endometrium or "endometrial septa."

Anatomically this allantochorion, the outermost envelope of the developing embryo, early comes to fill the uterine cavity, being pressed tightly against the endometrial lining by the fetus and fluids within. Just how much of the allantochorion has placental connection with the maternal tissues depends upon the species. That part of the allantochorion which forms villi and a placental connection is called the placental area, or the chorion frondosum (fernlike); the part which merely is held in ap-position to the uterine lining is called the nonplacental area, or the chorion laeve.

In the mare and sow, the whole endometrial lining and the whole allantochorion are placental areas. This type is known as the **diffuse placenta.** In the bitch, the placental area is in the shape of a wide band which encircles the elongated elliptic fetal sac at its middle. This is the **zonary placenta.** In the human, we have a **discoid placenta,** in which only a disc-shaped area on one side of the sac is placental.

In the human and similar species, the chorion frondosum, which is the fetal component of this discoid placenta, is divided into 15 to 20 small sections, each derived from one primary villus, which are called cotyledons. In the bovine and ovine species, there is a fundamental similarity, but each cotyledon is separated from its neighbor by a wide nonplacental area, and the total number, perhaps 100 in the bovine, are scattered over the whole of the allantochorion. This is the familiar **cotyledonary placenta.**

Regardless of the anatomic distribution of the placental and nonplacental areas, placentas are classified histologically on the basis of the degree of closeness with which the fetal blood approaches that of the mother. One would expect to find interposed between the two the following six layers: fetal vascular endothelium, fetal connective tissue (mesenchymal), fetal chorionic epithelium, maternal endometrial epithelium, maternal connective tissue, and maternal vascular endothelium. This arrangement is known as an **epitheliochorial placenta.** The fetal and maternal villi dovetail with each other or, more precisely, the fetal villi are interspersed between maternal endometrial septa in simple or complex fashion.

The epitheliochorial type is found in the equine, bovine, ovine, caprine, and porcine, as well as in related species. Chorionic villi lined with one layer of epithelial cells, the trophoblast, dip into maternal crypts with one also covered by a single layer of low epithelial cells, a continuation of the normal simple columnar epithelium of the nonplacental endometrium. In the mare and sow, the trophoblast is columnar, and each cell contains a single nucleus, whereas in the cow and ewe, these cells are usually binucleate and less often syncytial (comparable to the syncytial giant cells of the human placenta), but smaller and less complicated. When chorionic epithelial cells are individual they are called **cytotrophoblasts,** whereas when they form a syncytium, characteristic of other species, the tissue is referred to as a **syncytiotrophoblast.** As indicated, the maternal epithelium is a low, simple epithelium except in sheep, in which it is a syncytium. As gestation advances, maternal and fetal capillaries come to run exceedingly close to the epithelium and even insinuate themselves between epithelial cells. This is especially conspicuous in the porcine placenta. Especially during midgestation, there are numerous tiny areas (several per square centimeter) called areolae, where the fetal and maternal surfaces are separated, the space being filled by secretion of endometrial glands which converge to open at these points. This secretion is the so-called uterine milk; fetal cells in the vicinity can be observed assimilating its solid particles.

In ruminants and especially in the bovine, the chorionic villi are large, approaching 2 cm in total length, and subdivide and branch repeatedly. Conforming to this complicated arborization, the maternal tissue forms deep crypts and saccules, correspondingly subdivided, into which the fetal villi fit. Not infrequently, the microscopic section is cut in such a direction that the maternal tissue forms hollow circles each enclosing a cross section of a chorionic villus, usually with a shrinkage space between them. The chorionic epithelium begins as a single layer of columnar cells, but as pregnancy advances, these tend to join together, forming syncytial giant cells which lie scattered at irregular intervals along the surfaces of the chorionic villi. They are comparable to the syncytial giant cells of the human placenta, but are smaller and less complicated. A majority have only two nuclei (diplokaryocytes), but cells with larger numbers are by no means nonexistent.

The three layers mentioned for the fetal side are regularly present in all species, but, owing to an invasive power possessed by the chorionic epithelium (the trophoblast or trophoderm according to the embryologists), certain maternal layers are destroyed in some species.

In the **endotheliochorial placenta,** the chorionic villi come into direct contact with the endothelium of the endometrial capillaries. This type of placenta occurs in the canine and feline species.

The chorionic villi penetrate the endometrium and destroy it to a considerable depth (down to the glandular "spongiosa"), leaving in the vicinity only the endometrial capillaries and a few stromal fibroblasts, which become large and rounded (like large mononuclears) and correspond to the specialized decidual cells of the human placenta. The chorionic villi, with their epithelium intact, thus lie in close contact with the maternal capillaries. The trophoblast is separated from the maternal endothelium by a membrane enclosing each capillary. This membrane, which may be discontinuous, is of uncertain origin; it may be basement membrane of maternal endothelium or a product of the trophoblast. The trophoblast consists of both discrete cells (cytotrophoblast) and syncytiotrophoblast. Near the edges of the zonary placenta of these species, there is considerable accumulation of maternal blood in sinus-like spaces. This, becoming stagnant, develops grossly the greenish black color of partly hemolyzed blood in the canine.

The ultimate in chorionic invasion of the maternal tissues is found in the **hemochorial** placenta of humans, monkeys, mice, rats, guinea pigs, and rabbits. In this type, the maternal tissues are destroyed to the extent that the blood escapes from ruptured endometrial capillaries, flows into sinus-like spaces surrounding chorionic villi, where the exchange of nutrients occurs with great ease, and then returns to the venous circulation of the mother. The trophoblast lining the chorionic villi is principally a syncytium.

In earlier histologic classifications of placental structure, two other types were included. The bovine, ovine, and caprine placenta were previously considered the syndesmochorial type (syndesmo refers to connective tissue), in which the trophoblast was believed to have been separated from maternal endothelium by maternal connective tissue. The placenta of rodents was thought to be hemoendothelial, with the maternal blood in direct contact with fetal capillaries. Subsequent to ultrastructural studies, both of these types have been abandoned.

Placentas are also classified as deciduate and nondeciduate. In the **deciduate placenta,** which happens to be also hemochorial or endotheliochorial, the penetrating chorionic villi produce practically a fusion of fetal and maternal structures, so that when the fetal membranes are expelled after parturition, an outer layer of the endometrium comes loose (as a deciduous tree sheds its leaves) and is expelled with them. The deciduate placenta occurs in humans and monkeys and, to a less marked degree, in the dog and cat families. In some rather primitive wild species, the placenta is not shed or expelled, but instead is slowly absorbed by the endometrium and leukocytes in it (contradeciduate placenta). This is said to be true in part in the case of the sheep. In the **nondeciduate placenta** of the mare, sow, goat, cow, and ewe (in spite of the statement in the preceding sentence), the fetal placenta is much less firmly adherent to the maternal, and there is no shedding of maternal tissue.

Anderson, J.W.: Ultrastructure of the placenta and fetal membranes of the dog. Anat. Rec., 165:15–36, 1969.

Asdell, S.A., Alba, J. De, and Roberts, S.J.: Studies on

the estrous cycle of dairy cattle; cycle length, size of corpus luteum, and endometrial changes. Cornell Vet., 39:389–402, 1949.

Assheton, Richard, VI: The morphology of the ungulate placenta, particularly the development of the organ in sheep, and some notes on the placenta of the elephant and hyrax. Phil. Tr. Roy. Soc., 198:143–220, 1906.

Barrau, M.D., Abel, J.H., Berhage, H.G., and Tietz, W.J., Jr.: Development of the endometrium during the estrous cycle in the bitch. Am. J. Anat., 142:47–65, 1975.

Bjorkman, N.: Ultrastructural features of placenta in ungulates. Fifth Inter. Congr. Anim. Reprod. Trento, 5:259–263, 1964.

————: Fine structure of the ovine placentome. J. Anat. (Lond.), 99:283–297, 1965.

————: On the fine structure of the porcine placental barrier. Acta Anat., 62:334–342, 1965.

Bjorkman, N.: An Atlas of Placental Fine Structure. Baltimore, Williams and Wilkins, 1970.

Concannon, P.W., Hansel, W., and Visek, W.J.: The ovarian cycle of the bitch: plasma estrogen, LH and progesterone. Biol. Reprod., 13:112–121, 1975.

Crotto, N.R.: Modificaciones citológicas de los epitelios vaginales en la vaca. Rev. Méd. Vet., Buenos Aires, 34:91–98, 1952.

Davies, J., and Wimsatt, W.A.: Observation on the fine structure of the sheep placenta. Acta Anat., 65:182–223, 1966.

Dawson, A.B., and Kosters, B.A.: Preimplantation changes in the uterine mucosa of the cat. Am. J. Anat., 75:1–37, 1944.

Drieux, H., and Thiéry, G.: Placentation chez les mammifères domestiques. Rec. méd. vét. Placenta des equidés., 125:197–214, 1949; des suidés, 125:437–455, 1949; des bovidés, 127:5–25, 1951; des ovidés, 128:5–18, 1952.

Fedrigo, G.: Aspetti della mucosa delle salpingi di pecora, bovina, Cavalla e cagna in periodo di gravidanza. Nuova vet., 28:95–102, 1952.

Gunther, E.: Zur Vascularisation der uterus-karunkel des schafes. Zentralbl. Veterinaermed., 5:171–196, 1958.

Hadek, R.: Morphological and histochemical study on the ovary of the sheep. Am. J. Vet. Res., 19:873–881, 1958.

————: Histochemical studies on the uterus of the sheep. Am. J. Vet. Res., 19:882–886, 1958.

Hadek, R., and Getty, R.: The changing morphology of the uterus of the growing pig. Am. J. Vet. Res., 20:573–577, 1959.

Hamilton, W.J., and Harrison,.R.J.; Cyclical changes in the uterine mucosa and vagina of the goat. J. Anat., 85:316–324, 1951.

Hansel, W., Asdell, S.A., and Roberts, S.J.: The vaginal smear of the cow and causes of its variation. Am. J. Vet. Res., 10:221–228, 1949.

Hatch, R.D.: Anatomic changes in the bovine uterus during pregnancy. Am. J. Vet. Res., 2:411–416, 1941.

Hawk, H.W., Turner, G.D., and Sykes, J.F.: Variation in the inflammatory response and bactericidal activity of the sheep uterus during the estrous cycle. Am. J. Vet. Res., 22:689–692, 1961.

Herrick, J.B.: The cytological changes in the cervical mucosa of the cow (Bos taurus) throughout the estrous cycle. Am. J. Vet. Res., 12:276–281, 1951.

Hilty, H.: Untersuchungen über die evolution und involution der uterusmucosa vom rind. Schweiz. Arch. Tierheilkd., 50:268–323, 1908.

Hodgen, G.D., Goodman, A.L., O'Connor, A., and Johnson, D.K.: Menopause in Rhesus monkeys: model for study of disorders in the human climacteric. Am. J. Obstet. Gynecol., 127:581–584, 1977.

Johnson, K.J.R.: Cyclic histological changes occurring in the endometrium of the bovine. Res. Bull. Idaho Agric. Exp. Sta., No. 63, p. 20, 1965.

Kingman, H.E.: The uterine wall of the cow. Am. J. Vet. Res., 5:223–227, 1944.

————: The placentome of the cow. Am. J. Vet. Res., 9:125–130, 1948.

McCracken, J.A.: Plasma progesterone concentration after removal of the corpus luteum in the cow. Nature, Lond., 198:507–508, 1963.

Mulligan, R.M.: Histological studies on the canine female genital tract. J. Morph., 71:431–448, 1942.

Pomeroy, R.W.: Ovulation and the passage of the ova through the fallopian tubes in the pig. J. Agric. Sci., 45:327–330, 1955.

Restall, B.J.: Histological observations on the reproductive tract of the ewe. Aust. J. Biol. Sci., 19:673–686, 1966.

Rueber, H.W., and Emmerson, M.A.: Arteriography of the internal genitalia of the cow. J. Am. Vet. Med. Assn., 134:101–109, 1959.

Sanger, V.L., Engle, P.H., and Bell, D.S.: The vaginal cytology of the ewe during the estrous cycle. Am. J. Vet. Res., 19:283–287, 1958.

Schofield, B.M.: Hormonal control of pregnancy by the ovary and placenta in the rabbit. J. Physiol., 151:578–590, 1960.

Sokolowski, J.H., Stover, D.G., and Ravenswaay, F., Van: Seasonal incidence of estrus and interestrous interval for bitches of seven breeds. J. Am. Vet. Med. Assoc., 171:271–273, 1977.

Sokolowski, J.H., Zimbelman, R.G., and Goyings, L.S.: Canine reproduction: reproductive organs and related structures of the nonparous, parous, and postpartum bitch. Am. J. Vet. Res., 34:1001–1013, 1973.

Torpin, R.: Placentation in Rhesus monkey (Macaca mulatta). Obstet. & Gynec., 34:410–413, 1969.

Van Niekerk, C.H., and Gerneke, W.H.: Persistence and parthenogenetic cleavage of tubal ova in the mare. Onderstepoort J. Vet. Res., 33:195–232, 1966.

Vollmerhaus, B.: Untersuchungen uber die normalen zychlischen veranderungen der uterusschleimhaut des rindes. Zentralbl. Veterinaermed., 4:18–50, 1957. Abstr. Vet. Bull., No. 2242, 1957.

Wagner, W.C., and Hansel, W.: Reproductive physiology of the post partum cow. I. Clinical and histological findings. J. Reprod. Fert., 18:493–500, 1969.

Wagner, W.C., Sastman, R., and Hansel, W.: Reproductive physiology of the post partum cow. II. Pituitary, adrenal, and thyroid function. J. Reprod. Fert., 18:501–508, 1969.

Weber, A.F., and Morgan, B.B.: Cyclic histological changes occurring in the endometrium of the virgin heifer. J. Animal Sci., 8:646, 1949.

Wimsatt, W.A.: New histological observations on the

placenta of the sheep. Amer. J. Anat., *87*:391–457, 1950.

Wynn, R.M., and Corbett, J.R.: Ultrastructure of the canine placenta and amnion. Am. J. Obstet. Gynecol., *103*:878–887, 1969.

Diseases of the Ovary

Anomalies

Agenesis of one or both ovaries is seen occasionally, but is rare, as are other anomalies of the ovaries. If bilateral, the oviducts and uterus are rudimentary. **Hypoplasia** of the ovaries with complete or partial lack of germ cells is also uncommon. In the Swedish Highland breed of cattle, ovarian and testicular hypoplasia occur as a hereditary disease controlled by an autosomal recessive gene with incomplete penetrance (Lagerlof and Settergren, 1953). If bilateral, there is secondary hypoplasia of the tubular genitalia. A similar genital hypoplasia has been described in pigs (Laing, 1970) and the ACEP strain of rabbits, in which an autosomal recessive gene causes hypogonadism in both sexes. In man, deletion of the second sex chromosome resulting in an XO genotype and Turner's syndrome is associated with ovarian hypoplasia. A similar anomaly has been reported in Rhesus monkeys. Interestingly, mice with an XO genotype do not have anomalous development of the ovaries. The ovary of the freemartin is hypoplastic and may contain abortive testicular elements. True hermaphrodites have either ovotestis (a gonad containing both ovarian and testicular tissue) or both ovaries and testes.

Hermaphroditism. Since the genital tracts of both sexes develop primarily from the same embryonic primordium, it is perhaps not surprising that occasionally structures characteristic of both sexes are found in the same individual. In a true hermaphrodite, which has been described in most domestic and laboratory animals, both ovarian and testicular tissue occur either in united or separate structures. When combined, the testicular tissue is lo-

cated in the medulla and usually lacks active spermatogenesis. The ovarian tissue contains oocytes and often, developing follicles. The tubular genitalia may be rudimentary or well formed, with various combinations of uterus and vas deferens. The mechanism leading to true hermaphroditism is poorly understood. Many have been demonstrated to be chimerics with both XX and XY genotypes.

In contrast to true hermaphrodites, a pseudohermaphrodite has gonadal tissue of only one sex, but some degree of genital development of the opposite sex. A male pseudohermaphrodite is a genetic male with more or less normal testes, but the accessory reproductive organs resemble those of the female. This disorder is known in most species of animals. In dogs, Miniature Schnauzers appear to be prone to male pseudohermaphroditism (Brown, et al., 1976). The female pseudohermaphrodite, which is much less common, is a genetic female with ovaries, but the tubular reproductive tract is rudimentary, and the external genitalia bear an anatomic resemblance to those of the male. A hereditary form of hermaphroditism occurs in female goats, which are homozygous for an autosomal dominant gene for polledness. These goats are called male pseudohermaphrodites in that they have testes although they are genetically female. Rarely affected goats have both ovaries and testes (true hermaphroditism). An important cause of male pseudohermaphroditism in XY individuals results from somatic tissue insensitivity to androgens due to lack of cellular androgen receptors. This condition, known as testicular feminization, is a recognized inherited defect in man, mice, and rats (and possibly in horses and swine), in which it is an X-linked recessive trait. Unexplained examples in other species, especially swine, may well be examples of testicular feminization. Failure of androgen secretion may also lead to male pseudohermaphroditism. This may result from a congenital deficiency of testicular enzymes essential for testosterone synthesis. An example of Leydig-cell agenesis has recently been described in a human male pseudohermaphrodite. Female pseudohermaphroditism can be induced by experimentally exposing the developing, genetically female, fetus to testosterone. Under natural conditions, this may occur with a fetal adrenal dysfunction, or rarely, secondary to a virilizing maternal neoplasm.

Infections

Tuberculosis and other granulomatous infections occasionally involve the ovary by virtue of hematogenous metastasis from lesions elsewhere. The ovary is much more resistant than most organs to the common pyogenic infections, neither does it often show lesions in the acute septicemias or toxemias. The ascent of infection via the oviduct is thought to be possible, but it is rare. Certain systemic viral infections may produce lesions in the ovary (e.g., herpesviruses), but none are restricted to the ovary.

Endocrine Disorders

Cystic ovaries is the common clinical term used to designate the rather frequent condition in which the ovary contains one or more clear cysts ranging in diameter from one to several centimeters.

Follicular Cysts. The ordinary type of ovarian cyst is the follicular cyst, or cystic follicle. They are most frequent in cattle, swine, and dogs. Usually acquired, they are occasionally present at birth. Such cysts arise, for reasons poorly understood, from follicles that fail to ovulate or undergo atresia. While ordinarily larger than the ripening normal follicle, they are not necessarily distinguishable on the basis of size alone. Follicular cysts may also be difficult to distinguish histologically from normally developing graafian follicles or follicles in the early stages of atresia. They usually do not contain an ovum and may be lined by several layers of normal or degenerating granulosa or by a single layer of epithelium.

The exact basis for the formation of follicular cysts is not understood but believed to result from excessive and continued secretion of FSH by the pituitary and a lack of the LH surge necessary for ovulation and luteinization. Whether the basis for abnormal hormonal balance lies in the pituitary or elsewhere is speculative. Follicular cysts have been induced in swine with ACTH.

The effect of one or more follicular cysts may be negligible; however, they may secrete estrogens in normal or excessive amounts over prolonged periods of time, leading to clinical and pathologic estrinization. Many "follicular cysts" also contain luteinized tissue and also secrete progesterone (see lutein cysts). Generally the hormonal effects are ascribed to estrogen, but may in fact result from elaboration of both hormones. Estrinization is characterized by infertility, continuous estrus, nymphomania (especially in cows), cystic endometrial hyperplasia (except in swine), and possibly an increased incidence of mammary tumors in dogs. The pathogenesis of cystic endometrial hyperplasia is discussed in greater detail elsewhere.

Like other cysts, when large, they may cause pain through pressure. Occasionally, hemorrhages occur into these cysts, and an organized clot may be the end result in accordance with the same principles that govern clotting elsewhere.

Lutein Cysts. Lutein cysts (luteal cysts) or **cystic corpora lutea** can be distinguished from follicular cysts as their wall is partially or completely luteinized. Usually, the wall contains large fat filled granulosa-luteal cells and smaller theca-luteal cells. They may be difficult to differentiate from a newly formed corpus luteum during the stage when it still possesses an antrum. They are most frequent in cows and older, multiparous bitches. Their pathogenesis is not understood, but presumably they follow abnormal pituitary function. When

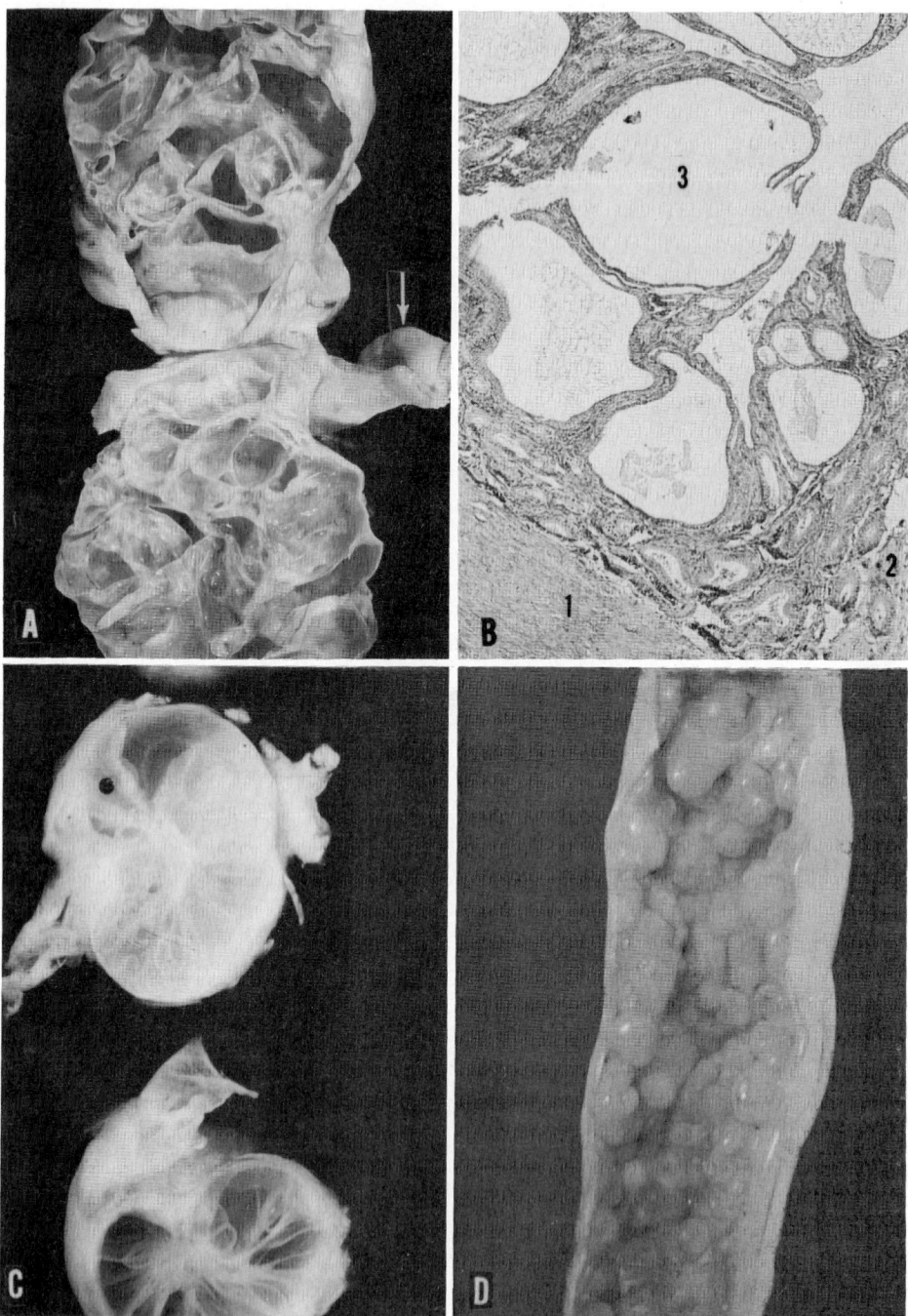

Fig. 25-3. *A,* Multiple cysts in a canine ovary. The uterine horn is indicated by the arrow. Contributor: Dr. Wayne H. Riser. *B,* Cystic glandular hyperplasia of the canine uterus (× 70), myometrium (*1*), endometrium (*2*), cyst of endometrium (*3*). (*B,* Courtesy of Armed Forces Institute of Pathology.) Contributor: Dr. C.P. Zepp, Jr. *C,* Cystic oviduct in a cow. *D,* Cystic glandular hyperplasia in the canine uterus.

functional, these cysts serve as a source of prolonged progesterone secretion, which lowers the resistance of the uterus to infection, often leading to pyometra. In dogs, cystic endometrial hyperplasia often with pyometra is frequently associated with lutein cysts.

Endometrial Cysts. Endometrial cysts, which in the human develop from ectopic endometrial tissue, have not been noted in animals. Endometriosis of man and nonhuman primates often involves the ovary.

Inclusion Cysts. Cysts occasionally develop from small isolated segments of the ovarian surface epithelium which become buried in the stroma following ovulation. These cysts are usually small, lined by a single flattened layer of epithelium, and of little consequence. They must be differentiated from follicular cysts, which may be difficult. They are most common in older animals.

Dermoid Cysts. These are discussed in connection with teratomas, and occur in the ovary. They are usually readily recognizable by the hair that they almost always contain.

Parovarian Cysts. One or several of these are frequent, especially in the bovine. They are found attached to the mesovarian or mesosalpinx, or between their two peritoneal coverings as clear spherical cysts from one to several centimeters in diameter. They are lined with simple columnar, cuboidal, or flattened epithelium. Etiologically, they arise as dilated vestigial segments of the embryonic wolffian body. The latter consists of a main duct, known as Gartner's duct, with a number of rudimentary branches. In accordance with their embryological origins, the cysts are sometimes referred to as cystic **hydatids of Morgagni.** In the herbivorous animals, it is possible for the cysts of *Taenia hydatigena* to be so located as to cause confusion in diagnosis, but the scolex of the tapeworm is, of course, absent from the parovarian cyst.

Retained Corpus Luteum

Especially in the bovine, it occasionally happens that a corpus luteum spurium fails to undergo normal involution with the advance of the cycle into its dioestrual phase. Instead it continues to enlarge, reaching the proportions (2 to 4 cm) which the corpus luteum verum normally attains in pregnancy. Apparently the normal hormonal influences necessary for involution of the corpus luteum are disturbed. As these are not understood in most species it is difficult to speculate on the pathogenesis of this lesion. The corpus luteum in dogs normally exists for about 60 days whether or not conception occurs. The effect of a retained corpus luteum is comparable to a cystic corpus luteum. The clinician, by digital expulsion of this corpus luteum per rectum, sets the normal cycle again in motion and the cow's breeding function is restored.

Tumors of the Ovary

Primary tumors of the ovary may arise from the surface epithelium, sex cord stroma (granulosa and theca-cell elements of the follicle), primordial germ cells, and supporting stroma.

Surface Epithelium. These tumors include adenomas, adenocarcinomas, cystadenomas, and cystadenocarcinomas. The latter two are the most frequent of this group and are the most common ovarian tumors of dogs. They have also been reported in cats, monkeys, and laboratory rodents. The cystadenomas and cystadenocarcinomas consist of large or small cavities lined with a single layer of epithelial cells. In one variety, the cells are cuboidal or low columnar, and the cystic fluid is serous or albuminous. In another variety, the lining cells are tall and clear, resembling goblet cells, and the fluid in the cavities is mucinous. In many cases, complicated and reduplicated papillary projections from the lining more or less fill the cystic lumens, whereupon the neoplasm is called

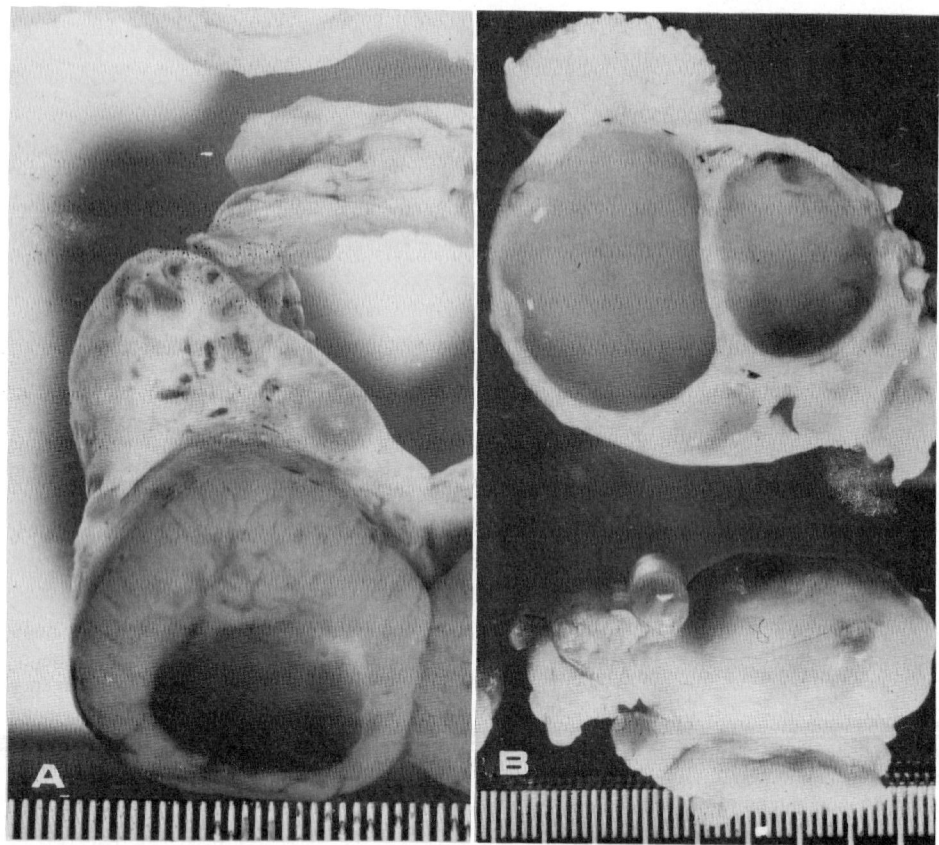

Fig. 25–4. *A,* Cystic, "retained" corpus luteum from a sterile heifer. *B,* Follicular and parovarian cysts in a bovine ovary.

a **papillary or papilliferous cystadenoma** or **cystadenocarcinoma.** This type tends toward malignancy, often with peritoneal implantation.

Solid adenomas and adenocarcinomas (medullary adenocarcinomas) are not unusual in laboratory rodents, but are rare in domestic animals. Microscopically, these neoplasms are composed of low cuboidal epithelial cells arranged in cords, tortuous tubules, small clusters, acinar structures, or diffuse sheets.

Sex Cord Stroma. The **granulosa-cell tumor** arises from the granulosa and theca-cell elements of the ovarian follicle. They occur in most all species and are the most common ovarian tumor in cattle and horses. The usual granulosa-cell tumor

consists of masses of cells of epithelial appearance with round, central nuclei and considerable cytoplasm. In some, there are fluid-filled, rounded open spaces here and there which bear a suggestive resemblance to graafian follicles. In others, there are places where a dozen or fewer cells cluster radially around a tiny open space, producing a formation called a rosette. (Rosettes are also found in ependymomas, medulloblastomas, retinoblastomas, and neuroblastomas.) Occasionally, a small spherical eosinophilic mass, the so called Call-Exner body, lies in the center of the rosette. In still others, the cells are diffusely distributed in no particular pattern except that they are held in elongated or cylindrical lobules by thin fibrous trabeculae. Grossly, the gran-

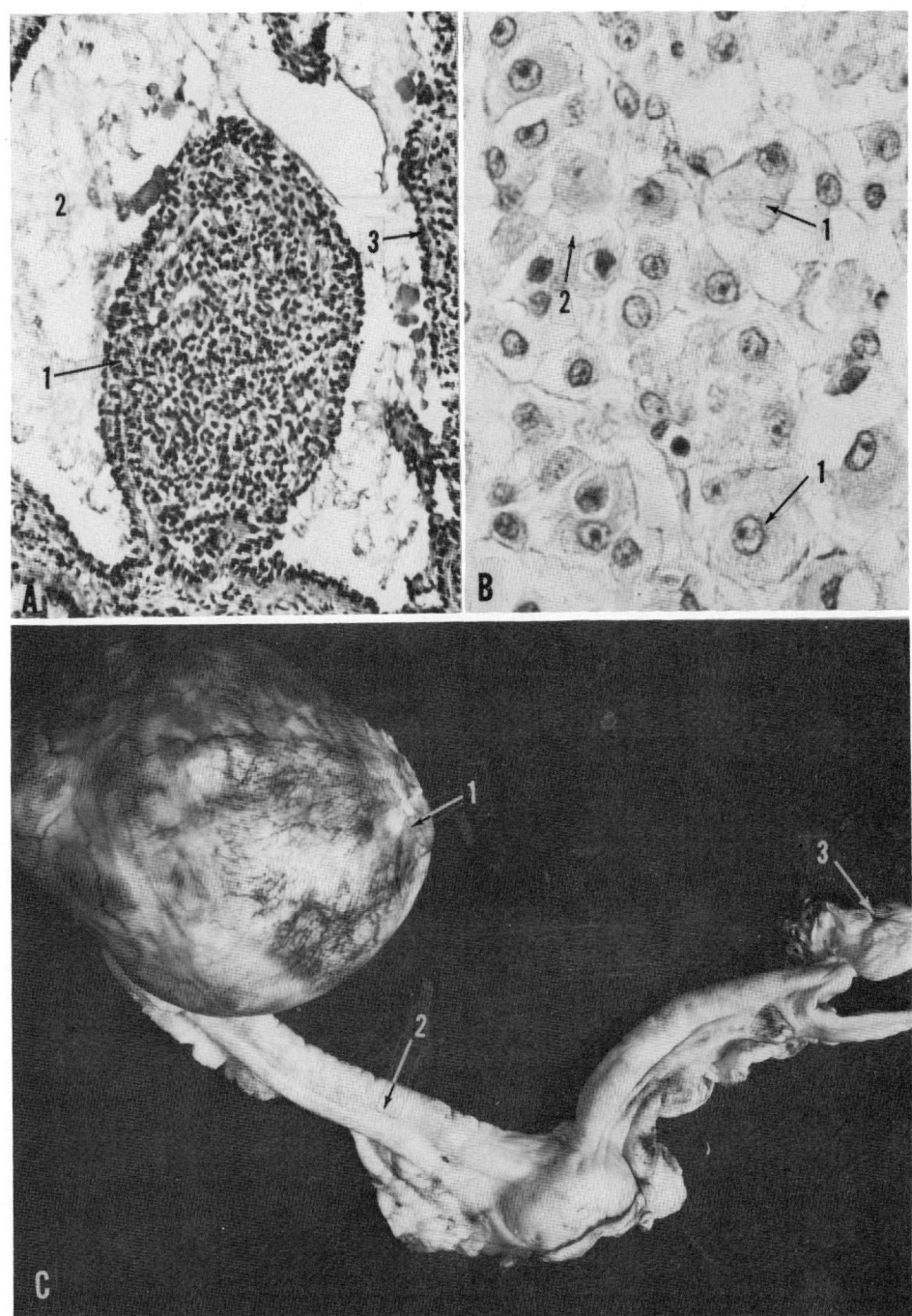

Fig. 25–5. Granulosa cell tumor. *A*, Photomicrograph (× 136) of a tumor of a mare's ovary showing cells in a nodule (*1*) with a cystic space (*2*), suggesting graafian follicle lined by granulosa cells (*3*). Contributor: Dr. F. A. Howard. *B*, Large polyhedral cells (*1*) and lipid (*2*) in a granulosa cell tumor (× 540) in ovary of a 12-year-old Wire-Haired Terrier. *C*, Gross tumor in left ovary (*1*), left cornu of uterus (*2*) and right ovary (*3*). This animal exhibited estrus for six months until the tumor was removed. (Courtesy of Armed Forces Institute of Pathology.) Contributor: Major Howard Kester.

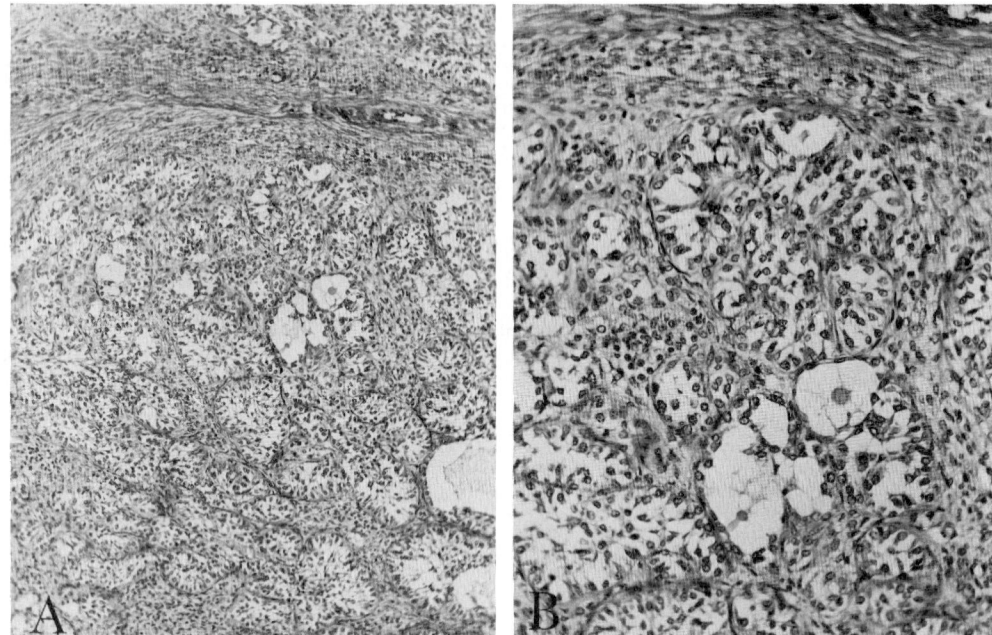

Fig. 25–6. Granulosa cell tumor, horse. *A*, The cells are slightly elongated and form small nests or radiate around tiny open spaces (rosettes). *B*, Higher magnification of same neoplasm. (Courtesy of Armed Forces Institute of Pathology.)

ulosa-cell tumor is usually rounded and smoothly encapsulated and may reach a weight of several pounds, being attached to the ovary rather than included in it. The cut surface is usually yellowish.

The **theca-cell tumor** differentiates to form spindle-shaped cells, thus resembling the theca externa of the follicle.

The **luteal-cell tumor** is similar to the usual type of granulosa-cell tumor but is even more yellow grossly, the cells containing numerous lipoidal droplets, microscopically suggestive of a corpus luteum.

The tumors of this group secrete estrogens. In the cow, this has brought relaxation of the sacrosciatic ligaments, suggestive of late pregnancy, and, more spectacularly, nymphomania. In dogs, it tends to cause cystic glandular hyperplasia of the endometrium, as in women.

The **arrhenoblastoma** is a rare masculinizing tumor arising in connection with the rete ovarii, which is considered to be the female counterpart of the testis. Its cells may be highly anaplastic, but when well differentiated, they form structures closely resembling the seminiferous tubules or the Sertoli-cell tumors of the testis. Dacorso (1947) has described an anaplastic arrhenoblastoma from a bovine ovary in which the cells varied from polyhedral to fusiform types.

Germ Cells. The **dysgerminoma** arises from undifferentiated primitive germ cells of the ovary. Its histologic picture resembles that of the seminoma, being composed of sheets of large polyhedral cells. It has no hormonal effect. The dysgerminoma has been found in cows, cats, and dogs. In the dog, they comprise about 10% of ovarian tumors.

Still more rare are the Brenner tumor and the Berger tumor, the latter arising from ovarian cells considered to be counterparts of the interstitial (Leydig) cells of the testis. Neither of these appears to have been recognized in animals.

Teratomas, including dermoid cysts, are

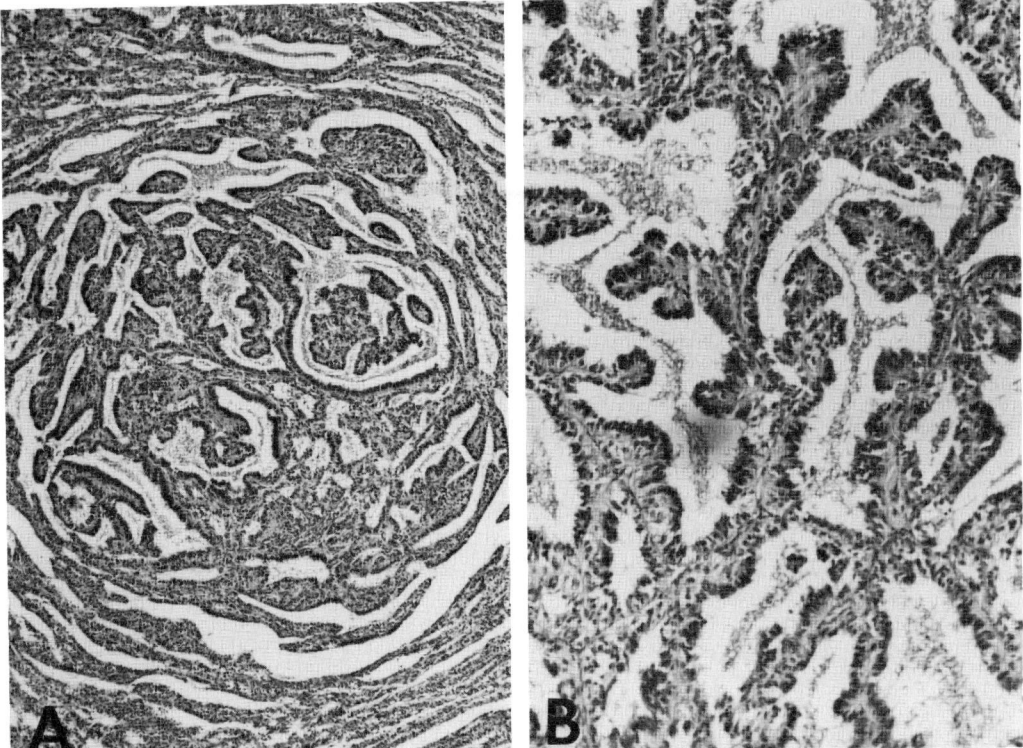

Fig. 25–7.   Papillary cystadenocarcinoma of the ovary in a 15-year-old dog. *A*, Irregular cavities containing papillary projections lined by cuboidal cells. *B*, Higher magnification of papillary projections. (Courtesy of Dr. N. W. King, Jr. and Angell Memorial Animal Hospital.)

neoplasms arising from totipotent primordial germ cells and are characterized by tissues of at least two and often all three embryonic germ layers (ectoderm, mesoderm, and endoderm). The great majority occur in either the ovary or testicle, but a few are found in the retroperitoneal region, anterior mediastinum, and other places close to the midline of the body. They are rare tumors, but have been observed in most animal species, most frequently in the dog and horse. In horses, undescended testicles are prone to develop teratomas.

In teratomas, the various tissues are in a jumbled mass and are of various kinds. Most frequently encountered are connective tissue, cartilage and bone, epithelial structures of ectodermal or entodermal type, skin, hair, and neuroglia. In one relatively common form, a cystic cavity is lined with skin and filled with an increasing amount of hair which grows from the skin. This is commonly called a dermoid cyst. Some of the cysts have one or more teeth protruding into them and are called dentigerous cysts. To qualify as true teratomas, there must be active growth. In many instances, teratomas continue slow and benign growth over a long period, the various histologic components apparently changing but little in their relative proportions. In other cases, one component or another assumes malignant qualities with rapid growth, infiltration, and metastasis, thus constituting in effect a carcinoma or a sarcoma, as the case may be.

A number of theories have been advanced on the pathogenesis of teratomas, but most have remained hypothetic with the exception that they represent par-

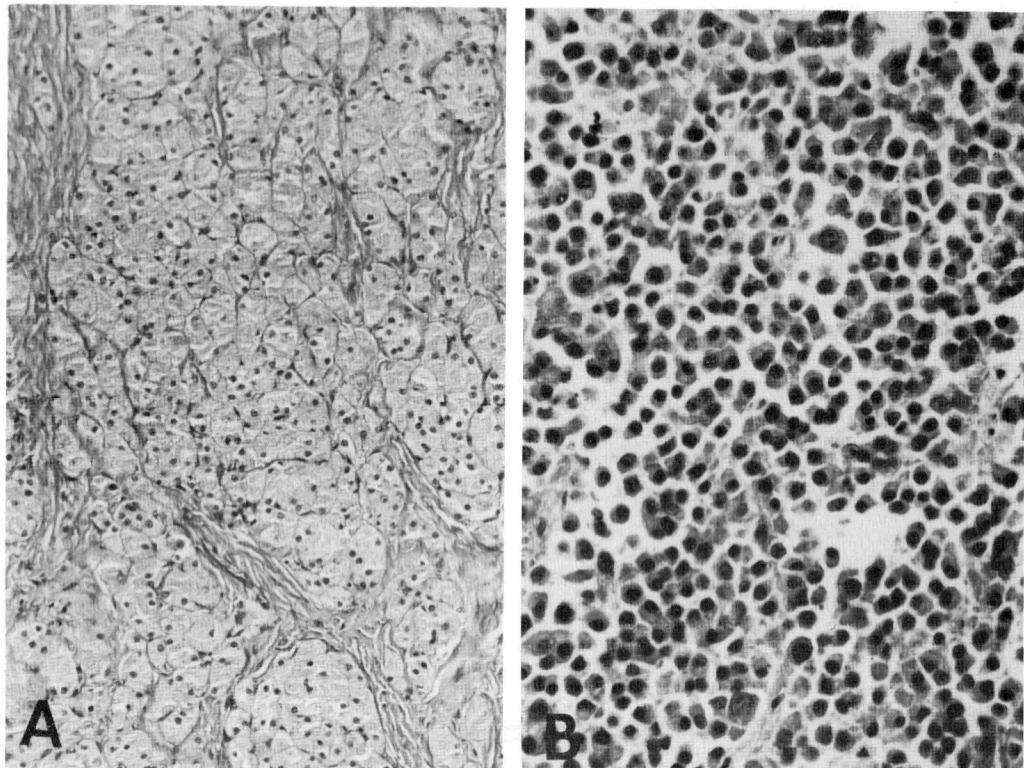

Fig. 25–8. *A,* Luteoma, ovary, dog. The cells resemble normal luteal cells. *B,* Dysgerminoma, ovary, dog. This neoplasm resembles the seminoma (Fig. 25–31). (Courtesy of Dr. N. W. King, Jr. and Angell Memorial Animal Hospital.)

thenogenetic development of germ cells. Chromosomal banding studies by Linder, et al. (1975) have demonstrated that ovarian teratomas in human beings are uniformly homozygous, indicating that they arise from a single germ cell after the first meiotic division. Testicular teratomas and teratomas at other locations have not been examined with this technique.

In view of the fact that many teratomas are discovered when the patient is a child, or even at birth, many believe that teratomas are initiated early in fetal or, more likely, embryonic life. Also, since so many histologic types of tissue make up a teratoma, tissues derived from each of the three primary layers usually being present, it must be concluded that the parent cell or cells are set apart at an extremely early stage

of embryonal development. The fact that teratomas are practically restricted in location to tissues which, in the embryo, lie close to the medial axis is construed to mean that their origin is related to abnormal development in the primitive streak.

One theory is that the teratoma develops from one ancestral cell which is the product of an abnormal mitosis at this very early stage. Such a parent cell would have the ability, as it subsequently underwent repeated subdivision, of producing practically any kind of tissue that the ovum could produce. The product of its growth would constitute essentially a twin, included within the body of the more normal descendant of the ovum itself. It would differ from ordinary identical twins, only in that the twin included within the body of the other was prevented from attaining any degree of normal development, presumably because of the limitations of its environment.

The second theory is that certain cells in the region of the primitive streak escape, by some developmental accident, from the control of certain chemical "organizers," substances which many embryologists believe exist in the normal embryo and regulate the relative development of its component structures in such a way as to develop a normal body.

In any case, it appears that if all the tissues of the teratoma are well differentiated into their respective histologic types, the teratoma remains a slowly enlarging benign mass. If the tissues, however, retain embryonal characteristics, morphologic and otherwise, they can be expected, sooner or later, to show rapid and malignant growth, stimulated by some unknown factor, possibly no different from one of the carcinogenic stimuli which incite neoplasia in other tissues.

Supporting Stroma. Primary supporting-tissue tumors are rare in the ovary. Potential neoplasms include fibromas, neurofibromas, myomas, hemangiomas, lymphangiomas, hemangiopericytomas, and their malignant counterparts.

Metastatic Tumors. Metastatic neoplasms in the ovary do not appear to be as frequent in animals as in human beings. The most frequently encountered metastatic neoplasm in animals is malignant lymphoma.

Adsell, S.A.: The genetic sex of intersexual goats and a probable linkage with the gene for hornlessness. Science, 99:124, 1944.

Amin, H.K., Ferenczy, A., and Richart, R.M.: Ovarian serous neoplasms in the rhesus monkey. Electron microscopical observations. J. Comp. Pathol., 84:161–167, 1974.

Beck, C.C., and Ellis, D.J.: Hormonal treatment of bovine cystic ovaries. Vet. Med., 55:79–81, 1960.

Berthezene, F., et al.: Leydig-cell agenesis: a cause of male pseudohermaphroditism. N. Engl. J. Med., 295:969–972, 1976.

Blackwell, W.J., Dockerty, M.B., Masson, J.C., and Mussey, R.D.: Dermoid cysts of the ovary: their

clinical and pathologic significance. Am. J. Obstet. Gynecol., 51:151–172, 1946.

Breeuwsma, A.J.: Studies on intersexuality in pigs. Proefschrift Fac. Diergeneeskunde, Rijksuniv Utrecht, 127 pp., 1970.

Brown, T.T., Burek, J.D., and McEntee, K.: Male pseudohermaphroditism, cryptorchidism, and Sertoli cell neoplasia in three Miniature Schnauzers. J. Am. Vet. Med. Assoc., 169:821–825, 1976.

Cotchin, E.: Canine ovarian neoplasms. Res. Vet. Sci., 2:133–142, 1961.

Dacorso, P.: Ovarian tumors of bovine origin. Bull. Intern. Assoc. Med. Museums (now Lab. Invest.), 27:77–83, 1947.

Dawson, F.L.M.: Bovine cystic ovarian disease: an analysis of 48 cases. Brit. Vet. J., 114:96–105, 123–142, 1958.

Dehner, L.P., Norris, H.J., Garner, F.M., and Taylor, H.B.: Comparative pathology of ovarian neoplasms. III. Germ cell tumors of canine, bovine, feline, rodent, and human species. J. Comp. Pathol., 80:299–306, 1970.

Donaldson, L.E., and Hanse, W.: Cystic corpora lutea and normal and cystic graafian follicles in the cow. Aust. Vet. J., 44:304–308, 1968.

Dow, C.: Ovarian abnormalities in the bitch. J. Comp. Path., 70:59–69, 1960.

Fox, R.R., and Crary, D.D.: Hypogonadia in the rabbit. Genetic studies and morphology. J. Hered., 62:163–169, 1971.

Garm, O.: Investigations on cystic ovarian degeneration in the cow, with special regard to etiology and pathogenesis. Cornell Vet., 39:39–52, 1949.

Goy, R.W.: Hormonally induced pseudohermaphroditism and behaviour. In International Congress Series 310, Proc. 4th Int. Conf. Vienna, Austria, edited by A. G. Motulsky, and W. Lentz. Amsterdam, Excerpta Med., 1974, pp. 155–164.

Goy, R.W.: Development of play and mounting behavior in female Rhesus virilized prenatally with esters of testosterone or dihydrotestosterone. In Recent Advances in Primatology, edited by D. J. Chivers, and J. Herbert. London, Academic Press, 1978, pp. 449–462.

Gruys, E., Dijk, J.E., van, Elsinghorst, Th. A.M., and Gaag, I., van der: Four canine ovarian teratomas and nonovarian feline teratoma. Vet. Pathol., 13:455–459, 1976.

Guarda, F.: Contributo allo studio dei tumori ovarici. L'arrhenoblastoma nella varieta di adenoma tubulare nel suino. Ann. Fac. Med. Vet. (Torino), 8:9–21, 1958.

Hamerton, J.L., et al.: Genetic intersexuality in goats. J. Reprod. Fert., Suppl, 7:25–51, 1969.

Kieffer, N.M., Burns, S.J., and Judge, N.G.: Male pseudohermaphroditism of the testicular feminizing type in a horse. Equine Vet. J., 8:38–41, 1976.

Laing, J.A.: Fertility and Infertility in the Domestic Animals. Baltimore, Williams and Wilkins, 1970.

Lagerlof, N., and Settergren, I.: Results of 17 years' control of hereditary ovarian hypoplasia in cattle of the Swedish Highland breed. Cornell Vet., 43:52–64, 1953.

Linder, D., McCaw, B.K., and Hecht, F.: Parthenogenic origin of benign ovarian teratomas. N. Engl. J. Med., 292:63–66, 1975.

Liptrap, R.M.: Oestrogen excretion by sows with induced cystic ovarian follicles. Res. Vet. Sci., 15:215–219, 1973.

Lojda, L.: The cytogenetic pattern in pigs with hereditary intersexuality similar to the syndrome of testicular feminization in man. Doc. Vet., 8:71–82, 1975.

Lyngset, O. Studies on reproduction in the goat. IV. The functional activity of the uterine horns of the goat. V. Pathological conditions and malformations of the genital organs of the goat. Acta Vet. Scand., 9:308–315, 364–375, 1968. V.B. 39:2739, 1969.

Magnusson, G.: Hermaphroditism in a rat. Pathol. Vet., 7:474–480, 1970.

Malven, P.V., et al.: Estrogenic activity in bovine luteal cyst fluid. J. Dairy Sci., 46:995–996, 1963.

McEntee, K.: Cystic corpora lutea in cattle. Int. J. Fertil., 3:120–128, 1958.

McEntee, K., and Zepp, C.P., Jr.: Canine and bovine ovarian tumors. Proc. First World Congress on Fertil. & Sterility, N.Y., 1953.

Moberg, R.: The blood picture in connection with persistency of follicles in cattle. Nord. Vet. Med., 17:232–236, 1965.

Nelson, L.W., Todd, G.C., and Migaki, G.: Ovarian neoplasms in swine. J. Am. Vet. Med. Assn., 151:1331–1333, 1967.

Norris, H.J., Garner, F.M., and Taylor, H.B.: Comparative pathology of ovarian neoplasms. IV. Gonadal stromal tumours of canine species. J. Comp. Pathol., 80:399–405, 1970.

Norris, H.J., Taylor, H.B., and Garner, F.M.: Equine ovarian granulosa tumours. Vet. Rec., 82:419–420, 1968.

Norris, H.J., Taylor, H.B., and Garner, F.M.: Comparative pathology of ovarian neoplasms. II. Gonadal stromal tumors of bovine species. Pathol. Vet., 6:45–58, 1969.

Novazzi, G.: Cystic ovaries following estrogen therapy in sows. Clin. Vet. (Milano), 86:1–8, 1963.

Patnaik, A.K., Schaer, M., Parks, J., and Liu, S.-K.: Metastasizing ovarian teratocarcinoma in dogs. A report of two cases and review of literature. J. Small Anim. Pract., 17:235–246, 1976.

Prentice, D.E., Cherry, C.P., and Wadsworth, P.F.: Ovarian teratoma in the Rhesus monkey. Toxicol. Letters, 1:187–190, 1978.

Ramamohana Rao, A., Narasimha Rao, P., and Rao, A.S.P.: Some observations on genital abnormalities of cattle. Indian Vet. J., 42:751–754, 1965.

Rohovsky, M.W., Fox, J.G., and Chalifoux, L.V.: Benign ovarian teratomas in two Rhesus monkeys (Macaca mulatta). Lab. Anim. Sci., 27:280–281, 1977.

Scott, W.J., Fradkin, R., and Wilson, J.G.: Ovarian teratoma in a Rhesus monkey. J. Med. Primatol., 4:204–206, 1975.

Soller, M., Padeh, B., Wysaki, M., and Ayalon, N.: Cytogenetics of Saanen goats showing abnormal development of the reproductive tract associated with the dominant gene for polledness. Cytogenetics, 8:51–67, 1969.

Spriggs, D.N.: Cystic ovarian disease in dairy cattle. With special reference to its treatment using a combination of chorionic gonadotrophin and progesterone. Vet. Rec., 83:231–238, 1968.

Summers, P.M.: An abattoir study of the genital pathology of cows in northern Australia. Aust. Vet. J., 50:403–406, 1974.

Thain, R.I.: Cystic ovaries and cystic endometrium in swine. Aust. Vet. J., 41:188–189, 1965.

Vyttenbroeck, F.: A study of the animal ovary (some comparisons with the human ovary). Acta Zool. Pathol. (Antwerp), 42:3–273, 1967.

Diseases of the Oviducts

Anomalies. Developmental abnormalities of the oviducts are usually associated with anomalous development of the ovaries or uterus. Agenesis is usually associated with agenesis or segmental aplasia of the uterus, and hypoplasia is associated with ovarian aplasia or atrophy. Aplasia and hypoplasia are of course seen in hermaphrodites and in the bovine freemartin. Parovarian cysts or hydatids of Morgagni are occasionally seen as pedunculated, clear cysts attached to the fimbria, the tube, or the mesosalpinx. As explained in connection with the ovary, they are vestiges of the wolffian body. Atrophy of the oviducts will follow ovarian dysfunction or ovariectomy.

Salpingitis. The fallopian tube, or oviduct, is not readily vulnerable to many of the disorders that involve the parenchymatous organs, nor is it usually accessible to the various agents that injure the exterior of the animal body. Salpingitis, or inflammation of the oviduct, is the lesion of principal importance because relatively slight inflammatory changes are incompatible with successful performance of the primary function of conveying the ovum to the uterus. Conception can be rendered impossible (1) by occlusion of the tiny lumen through acute or proliferative swelling, (2) by the lethal effect of toxic inflammatory exudates upon spermatozoa, or (3) by destruction of stretches of ciliated epithelium or contractile muscle that propel the ovum to the uterus.

The signs of inflammation are the same in the oviduct as elsewhere, but the pathologist must guard against underestimating the significance of desquamated epithelium (not postmortem), dead cells and debris in the lumen, lymphocytic infiltrations, even though scanty, and proliferation of stromal elements. This is well illustrated in Gilman's (1921) series of bovine cases in which longstanding clinical sterility could not be explained until autopsy, when the oviducts, although normal grossly, showed microscopic inflammatory changes. His diagnoses of infectious salpingitis were strikingly confirmed by the presence of virulent organisms, usually *Streptococcus viridans* or *Staphylococcus aureus*. Hirth et al. (1966) produced salpingo-oophoritis in cows by injecting semen mixed with a *Mycoplasma*.

There are occasional cases of infectious inflammations of the fallopian tubes characterized by extensive gross lesions. These include the pyogenic infections, with abscesses and **pyosalpinx,** a condition in which the tube is distended with pus entrapped within its lumen. Included also are tuberculosis and probably other chronic infections. The gonorrheal pyosalpinx of humans does not exist in animals. A pathologically mild seropurulent endosalpingitis may form a part of the syndrome of bovine trichomoniasis.

The cause of salpingitis is always an infection, with the more or less hypothetic exception of irritant medicines being introduced by uterine insufflation or by surgery. The principal causative microorganisms are mentioned above. They may gain entrance (1) by way of the bloodstream as part of a generalized infectious process, such as tuberculosis, (2) by spread of a peritonitis through the ostium abdominale, or (3) through the ostium uterinum from a progressing endometritis. Most cases of pyogenic infection represent spread from the uterus.

Sterility has been mentioned as the chief general effect or result of salpingitis. Anatomically, there may be adhesions of the fimbria of the tube to the ovary, tubo-ovarian cysts or abscesses, or local or even generalized peritonitis. Infection and inflammation of the tubal mucosa are seldom uniform throughout the length of the tube, and occlusions tend to be formed randomly rather than continuously. As a result, cysts, as well as abscesses, of microscopic or larger size, often form in the intervals of patency between occluded segments. The term **hydrosalpinx** is often used in referring to oviducts distended with secretion.

Obstruction of the lumen or stagnation of the blood vessels of the oviduct may result from mechanical displacement by local tumors, abscesses or similar enlargements.

Tubal pregnancy occurs in the human oviduct when a partial obstruction from any cause permits entry of the ascending sperm but denies egress to the much larger ovum. Development of the fertilized ovum then continues in this narrow lumen until the distended tube bursts, often with fatal hemorrhage. Tubal pregnancy seems not to have been reported in animals, perhaps because of the less invasive character of their chorionic tissues.

Tumors of the oviduct are practically nonexistent although lymphoid infiltration as a localization of generalized malignant lymphoma occurs rarely.

Diseases of the Uterus and Cervix

While in a quiescent, nongravid and nonparturient state, the uterus is usually free from disease, most of its disorders being connected in one way or another with the reproductive process. Of those illnesses to which the organ is subject, inflammatory diseases require primary attention.

Congenital Anomalies

Anomalous development of the uterus and cervix are most commonly seen in cattle and swine, though isolated reports can be found concerning most species. Complete **agenesis** is rare. When encountered, the fallopian tubes and rostral end of the vagina are also absent. **Hypoplasia** of the tubular genital tract accompanies gonadal agenesis and various intersexes. **Uterus unicornis** (or hemiuterus) is a more common anomaly. In this condition, one uterine horn is absent, being represented by a fibrous band in the broad ligament. The ovary and fallopian tube of the affected side may or may not be absent, and in many examples there is also ipsilateral renal agenesis. Uterus unicornis is often a feature of white heifer disease in Shorthorn and occasionally other breeds of cattle, as are various forms of segmental aplasia of the uterus. In segmental aplasia, only portions of one or both uterine horns are absent.

White heifer disease of cattle is characterized by partial genital aplasia. The term has been used since 1900; the disease was thought to be inherited as a single sex-linked recessive gene linked to the gene determining white coat color; thus it occurs most often, but not exclusively, in white animals. The breeding studies of Bennett et al. (1973), however, indicated that the gene for white heifer disease is not sex-linked, but rather autosomal recessive with, in all likelihood, separate genes for right and left horn abnormalities. The anatomic features of this entity usually include normal ovaries and oviducts and incompletely developed uterine horns, which may distend with fluid due to lack of communication with the cervix. The cervix is hypoplastic, as is the vagina. Failure of canalization of the distal end of the müllerian duct may occur independently of other changes, resulting in a segmental atresia of the vagina or a transverse septum across the vagina, which in turn results in the uterus filling with secretion.

Uterus didelphys is a rare anomaly resulting from failure of the müllerian ducts to fuse at their distal end, resulting in two uterine bodies, two cervices, and either a single or double vagina. Failure of fusion may affect only the cervix, leading to **cervix bifida.**

Hypertrophy and Hyperplasia

Excessive or prolonged ovarian hormonal stimulation leads to hypertrophy of the myometrium and hyperplasia of the

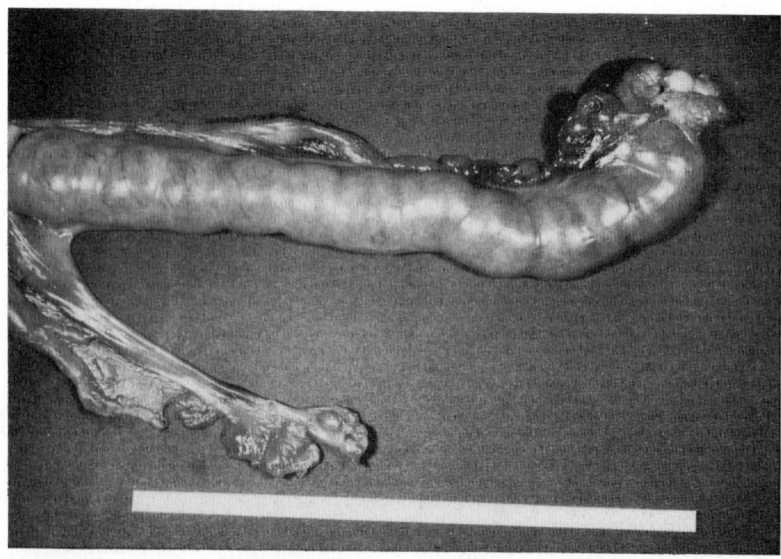

Fig. 25–9. Uterus unicornis in a five-year-old dog. Both ovaries are present. The remaining uterine horn was affected by cystic endometrial hyperplasia. (Courtesy of Drs. C. E. Gilmore and N. W. King, Jr.)

endometrium. The endometrial glands become tortuous, dilated, and usually cystic, and therefore endometrial hyperplasia is usually called **cystic glandular hyperplasia** or **cystic endometrial hyperplasia.** The mucosal surface of both horns eventually becomes filled with congeries of bulging cysts ranging up to 4 or 5 mm in diameter, most of them being much smaller and even microscopic in size. The cysts more or less fill the endometrial layer. They are lined with a single layer of epithelium which, when not too flattened by pressure from the fluid within them, resembles the cells that line the normal endometrial glands. Glands may proliferate into the myometrium, a condition called **adenomyosis.**

Cystic endometrial hyperplasia is seen in all species, but most frequently in the bitch, where it is caused by prolonged stimulation by progesterone, most usually from retained corpora lutea, luteal cysts, and rarely luteomas, and is often associated with pseudopregnancy. In contrast to cattle and laboratory rodents, hyperestrinism in dogs does not lead to endometrial hyperplasia, but low levels of estrogen may be necessary for the hyperplastic effect of progesterone. Ovarian cysts or granulosa cell tumors are encountered in some examples of the disease in dogs, but their causal relationship is uncertain. Attempts to induce cystic endometrial hyperplasia in dogs with exogenous estrogen or stilbestrol have not been successful (Teunisson, 1952; Dow, 1959), but long-term exposure to exogenous progesterone will result in the condition, indicating the importance of progesterone in its pathogenesis. The lowered resistance of the progestational endometrium to infection often leads to

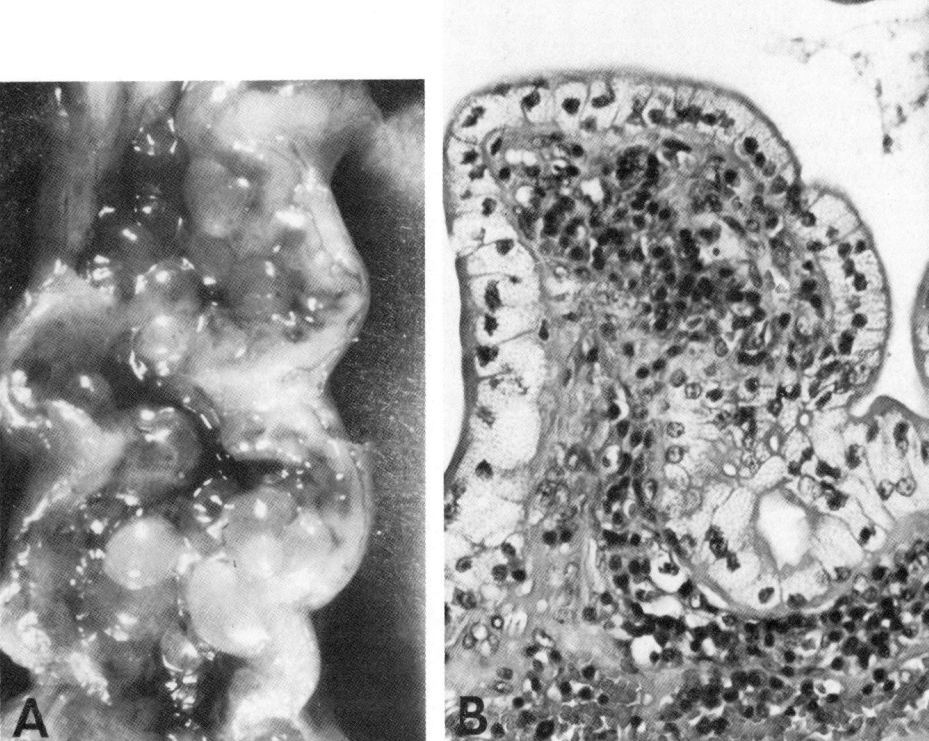

Fig. 25–10. Cystic endometrial hyperplasia in a 12-year-old bitch. *A,* Gross surface of endometrium. *B,* Vacuolated endometrial epithelium typical of progestational endometrium. (Courtesy of Drs. N. W. King, Jr. and C. E. Gilmore.)

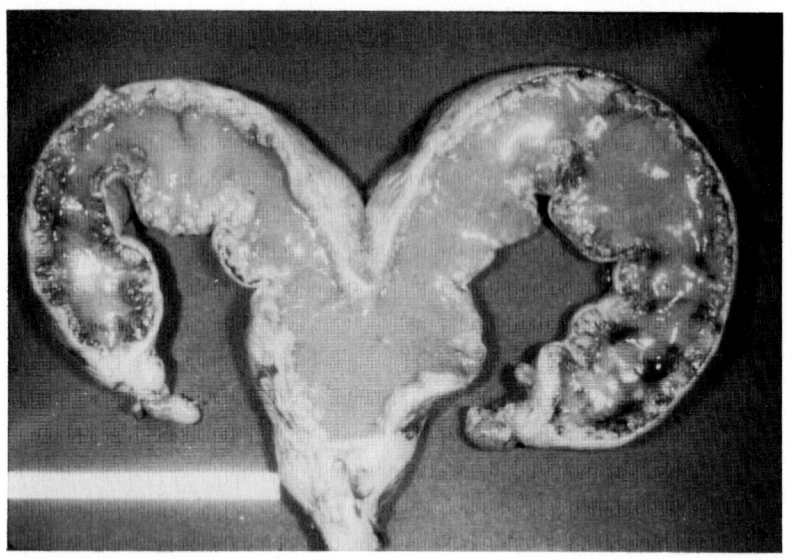

Fig. 25–11. Cystic endometrial hyperplasia and mucometria in a two-year-old bitch. (Courtesy of Drs. C. E. Gilmore and N. W. King, Jr.)

pyometra as a complication of cystic endometrial hyperplasia in dogs.

In cattle, cystic endometrial hyperplasia is most often associated with follicular cysts or granulosa cell tumors, and affected cows may show signs of continued estrus and nymphomania. The condition is therefore attributed to hyperestrinism, although the role of progesterone, if any, is uncertain. Follicular cysts in cattle may contain luteal tissue, and many follicular cysts in fact are luteal cysts. In support of estrogens as the cause in cattle is the occurrence of cystic endometrial hyperplasia in sheep grazing on certain legumes with estrogenic activity (see subterranean clover poisoning). In horses and cats, cystic endometrial hyperplasia is occasionally encountered, but the hormonal imbalance responsible for its development has not been determined. Cystic endometrial hyperplasia is uncommon in swine despite a relatively high incidence of follicular cysts. Hyperplasia of the uterus is encountered in swine exposed to certain estrogenic mycotoxins. In rabbits, cystic endometrial hyperplasia has been seen in association with pseudopregnancy due to retained corpora lutea.

Inflammation

Metritis. Inflammation of the uterus as a whole is termed metritis, while the milder and much more frequent inflammation which involves only the mucosa is endometritis. Tuberculosis and other chronic granulomatous infections may invade the uterus, the former with some frequency. In **tuberculosis** of the uterus, or tuberculous metritis, the tubercles tend to be numerous and small, being scattered through the connective tissue of the endometrium and of the intermuscular septa. They are practically always hematogenous metastases from primary infection elsewhere.

Septic metritis is a severe and often fatal inflammation of the whole uterus due ordinarily to infection introduced at or shortly after parturition. As a rule, it is the hands and instruments of an operator assisting at a difficult parturition that carry the infectious organisms into the uterine cavity. The parturient uterus is an especially susceptible field for the propagation of microorganisms during this, the puerperal (*puer*—a child), period, because of decomposing (autolyzing) bits of fetal membranes and proteinaceous fluid that remain in it, a perfect anaerobic culture medium maintained at body temperature. It also constitutes a culture flask of huge size, particularly if involution is delayed by injury of the tissues and exhaustion of the musculature suffered in the struggle of parturition.

The pathogenic organisms most likely to gain entrance and thrive in the lumen and tissues are streptococci, which are often of high virulence, staphylococci, and other pus-formers. The inflammation in such a case is suppurative in type. Less often, the organisms of tetanus, malignant edema, or blackleg are carried in, each producing its characteristic local and general disease. It happens that each of these latter infections produces a minimum of exudate, but their toxins are no less deadly, and the latter two are also necrotizing. Many streptococci also produce necrotizing (lytic) toxins, so that at the time of death the uterine wall, swollen and bloody, may scarcely have the strength to hold itself together. Other gross features include edematous and hyperemic swelling and the presence of more or less seropurulent exudate which, in acute cases, is likely to be stained with blood. If parturition was a recent event, shreds of fetal membranes may remain adherent to the swollen placentomes.

Microscopic Appearance. Microscopically, the uterine wall has the usual constituents of acute serous and purulent exudates throughout its several layers, the serous constituent (edema) being especially prominent in acute cases. In metritis of longer standing, lymphocytes are numerous. The lining epithelium is commonly missing, and the glands may contain mucus. It is interesting to note that this inflammation seldom, if ever, becomes fibrinous. The peritoneal surface of the uterus, like other peritoneal surfaces, is prone to develop a fibrinous inflammation, but this is almost always due to infection originating on the peritoneal side. The terminal period of a fatal metritis is much more likely to be accompanied by a septicemic dispersion of the infection over the body than by a direct extension through the serosa to involve the peritoneal surface. Providing there has been no mechanical perforation as the result of accident or surgery, this latter seldom occurs.

Thrombus formation in necrotic veins is a complication that should cause the veterinary pathologist to search for occluding emboli in other parts of the body when death lacks other adequate explanation.

It should not be inferred, however, that septic metritis is invariably fatal. Today's therapeutic agents present considerable hope of avoiding this outcome. In case of recovery, subsidence is gradual, and a chronic purulent endometritis commonly persists for some time.

Pyometra. Pyometra is an acute or chronic purulent infection of the uterus in which pus accumulates in the uterine cavity. Usually the cervix is closed precluding drainage of exudate, but due to the effect of gravity, exudates are also not easily expelled from the uterine lumen in the quadrupeds. The constant weight and pressure of accumulating exudate sometimes produce a gradual distention of the lumen, or impede normal involution in the event that the patient has recently given birth. The result after some days or weeks is pyometra, a condition in which the uterus is greatly distended and filled with pus. The pus usually has the color and consistency of thin cream. The uterine wall may exhibit only mild inflammatory changes. It is most common in dogs and cattle.

Pyometra almost always occurs while the uterus is under the influence of progesterone. In dogs, it is almost invariably superimposed on cystic endometrial hyperplasia resulting from persistent corpora lutea. In cattle, it most usually follows fetal death and retention. *Escherichia coli* is the most frequently isolated infectious agent in canine pyometra.

Pseudopregnancy. Also known as **pseudocyesis,** this uterine disturbance predominantly of canines represents a pathologically accentuated preparation of the endometrium for the implantation of an embryo, which, in nature's unguided processes, would normally follow estrum and ovulation. The endometrial epithelium and its stroma proliferate as illustrated in Figure 25–12, long villous extensions proceeding from what were glands, the epithelium of the more superficial villi becoming swollen with huge amounts of clear cytoplasm. Sometimes forming histologic structures suggestive of true cystic glandular hyperplasia, this is the same change that is normal in preparation for the development of the complex placental attachments in these species. The difference is that there are no fetal membranes. That these changes are indeed a manifestation of the hormonally stimulated processes of pregnancy, even though it is a false and mistaken one (*pseudo—*

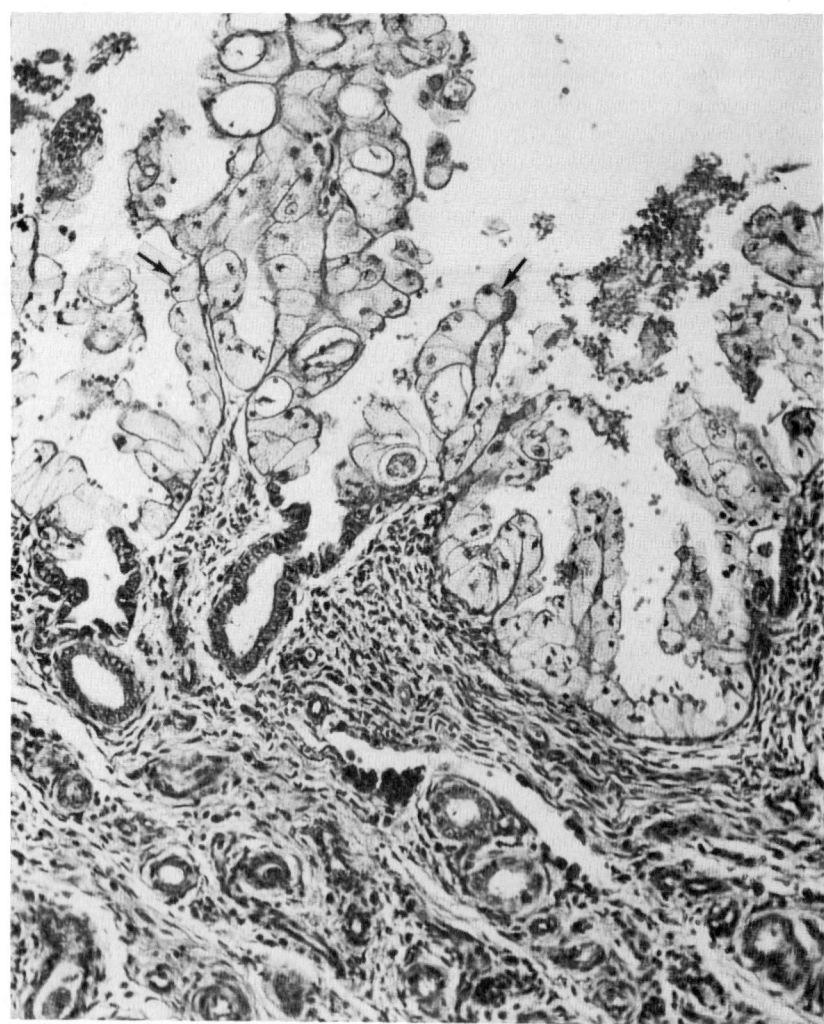

Fig. 25–12. Hypertrophy of the canine endometrium in pseudopregnancy (pseudocyesis). Note large endometrial cells with clear cytoplasm (arrow).

false), can, in the case of many bitches, be intriguingly demonstrated if one waits until the sixtieth or sixty-third day after estrus (the normal gestation period), when the expectant canine mother may be seen industriously arranging her nest for the instinctively anticipated accouchement which will not occur and the babies that will not be born.

These morphologic and physiologic characteristics of pseudocyesis would not be unhygienic or detrimental were it not for the tendency of infectious inflammatory processes to accompany them, in other

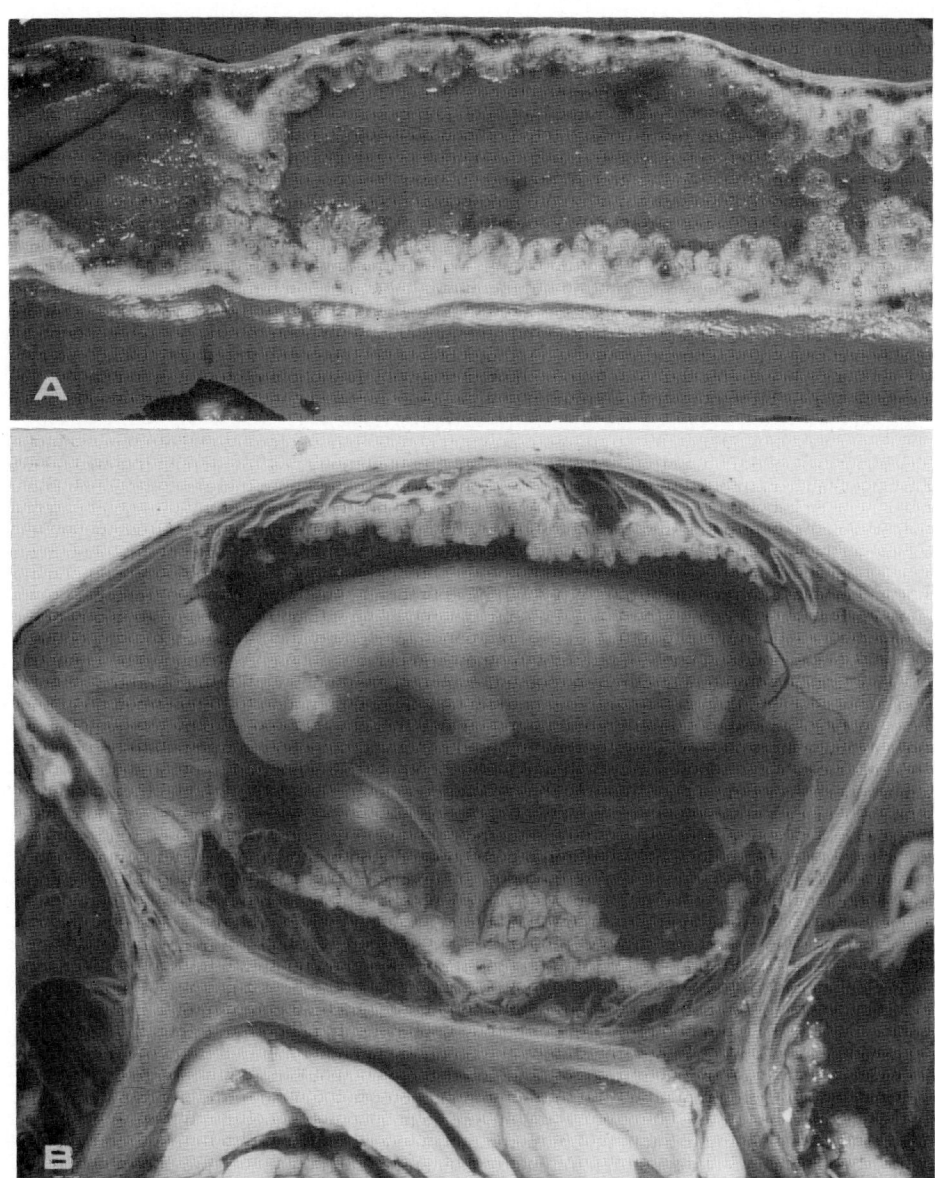

Fig. 25–13. *A,* Pseudocyesis in a canine uterus (female Cocker Spaniel, age 12 years). Compare the compartmentation and thickened endometrium with the normal pregnant uterus. *B,* Normal canine fetus *in utero* four weeks.

words, for pyometra to supervene. There is abundant evidence to show, unfortunately, that the progesterone-influenced endometrium, whether post-parturient or pseudopregnant, affords an all too favorable field for the multiplication of pyogenic and other bacteria which may chance to arrive by hematogenous or other routes.

The tendency of the (progesterone-producing) corpora lutea to persist after each ovulation, much as if pregnancy were present, is characteristic of the canine species, and this is doubtless the fundamental cause of pseudopregnancy. Normally in the dog, the corpora lutea persist for about two months after ovulation, at which time they regress; however, on occasion, especially in older, multiparous bitches, they persist longer.

In other species, pseudopregnancy is less common but does occur. Often it results from early fetal death and mummification with persistence of the corpus luteum of pregnancy. The animal then appears to remain pregnant beyond the usual time of parturition. That the changes of pseudopregnancy are the result of excessive progesteronic stimulation has been shown by experimental administration of that hormone, as well as by clinical benefits derived from expressing the corpus luteum or administration of the opposing hormone, stilbestrol.

Endometritis. As stated previously, endometritis is an inflammation of the mucous lining of the uterus, the endometrium. It may occur as a "hang-over" from a more severe, usually postparturient, metritis, in which case it is purulent in type, at least at first. A catarrhal endometritis occurs frequently in cows, without direct connection with any previous pregnancy, and even in heifers which have never been pregnant. The causative organisms appear to be some of the weaker strains of the pyogenic cocci, *Trichomonas fetus* and *Vibrio fetus.* The presence of the microorganisms may be difficult to understand, but is usually traceable to previous coitus or parturition or to ill-advised therapeutic maneuvers or artificial insemination. Not a few cases have as their cause chemical irritants in the form of applied antiseptics introduced for therapeutic purposes, but in a concentration too strong for the delicate mucous membrane of the uterus or cervix.

Visible changes in the endometrium are not impressive either grossly or microscopically. They include an excessive amount of mucous secretion in the lumen, with or without detectable hyperemia, and microscopically, a moderate or slight infiltration by lymphocytes, plasma cells, and other leukocytes; there is little more to be seen.

The principal effect of catarrhal endometritis is to prevent conception. The spermatozoa ordinarily cannot survive the toxic substances in the exudate, and the ovum, even if fertilized, would perish. There is no significant detriment to the general health as long as the endometritis is no more severe than the catarrhal type. These remarks apply to all species, but catarrhal endometritis is of principal importance as a chronic disease of cows.

Cervicitis and Endocervicitis. The dense fibrous body of the cervix is resistant to inflammatory processes as well as to their causative agents, but the cervical mucosa with its extensive development of mucous glands is peculiarly prone to develop catarrhal (mucous) inflammation. In fact many of the milder cases of catarrhal endometritis should be considered chiefly catarrhal endocervicitis, for the catarrhal mucus flows in both posterior and anterior directions. Microscopically, the condition is recognized by the hyperplastic cervical glands with tall, pale, mucin-containing epithelium and precipitated mucin in their lumens. The causes and the significance are essentially the same as for catarrhal endometritis.

Perimetritis. Inflammation of the uterine serosa and subserosa as well as of the retroperitoneal fibrosa, can exist without spreading into the muscularis or mucosa. It is usually a part of a generalized peritonitis but may result from penetrating wounds in the area, including perforations of the uterus which sometimes occur in the course of relief of dystocias. The cause is always infectious, except that large numbers of invasive parasites, such as *Dioctophyma renale* in the dog, may institute a foreign-body reaction without the presence of bacteria.

Contagious Equine Metritis. This disease emerged in the United States in 1978, although it was recognized earlier in Great Britain, Ireland, and France. It is caused by a gram-negative microaerophilic coccobacillus tentatively classified as *Haemophilus equigenitalis.* The organism is carried or transported by stallions, which indeed was the means of introducing the infection into this country. Mares may remain infected for long periods after the acute signs have abated. The acute infection in mares is characterized by a copious mucopurulent uterine discharge. Pathologic descriptions have not been reported in detail, but the primary lesion is a necrotizing and purulent endometritis, cervicitis, and vaginitis. The uterus may be distended with mucopurulent exudate (pyometra). The chronic sequelae with respect to sterility and abortion are still under investigation.

Disorders of the Gravid Uterus

Torsion of the gravid uterus is a common cause of dystocia in cattle. It is less frequent in other species. Uterine rupture is a frequent complication.

Placentitis. Infections of the placental tissues are likely to lead to early abortions, but in some types, a more or less extensive inflammatory lesion may develop previous to, or without, expulsion of the fetus. In the human, syphilis leaves its characteristic mark on the chorionic villi, and tuberculosis occasionally localizes here to produce its usual granulomatous reaction. One would not be surprised to find a tuberculous cow or other female similarly af-fected, although the more rapid course of this disease in the domestic species and their lower resistance to it would favor death of the fetus before tubercles had time to develop.

Abortion, Premature Births and Stillbirths. Abortion is usually defined as the expulsion of a dead embryo or fetus previous to the end of the full term of normal gestation. In reference to humans, abortion is considered to be the expulsion of an embryo or fetus prior to the stage of development that would enable it to survive extrauterine life. Stillbirth is defined as the expulsion of a dead fetus that has reached the stage of development that would ordinarily enable it to survive outside of the uterus. It is not always possible to distinguish these two in animals, and the legal impetus to do so is lacking. The survival of premature infants also depends upon the quality of postnatal care available. It is thought that there are numerous pregnancies in the bovine that are terminated previous to full implantation (50 to 60 days), when the expelled embryo is so small that it is usually not observed. At the other extreme, some abortions occur at any stage of pregnancy up to full term. Abortion in Bang's disease occurs typically at approximately the seventh month of gestation.

Many infectious diseases affect the uterus, placenta, or fetus leading to abortion. Those in which abortion is one of the primary manifestations are summarized here. Each is discussed more fully in other chapters.

In the active case of **brucellosis** (Bang's disease), there occurs a placentitis which is characteristic, although not entirely pathognomonic. In the usual acute form, extensive seropurulent exudate develops between the chorion and the endometrium in the interplacental areas (chorion laeve), tending to separate these two surfaces. The exudative reaction results in an (inflammatory) edema of the chorion with considerable infiltration of reticuloendothelial cells,

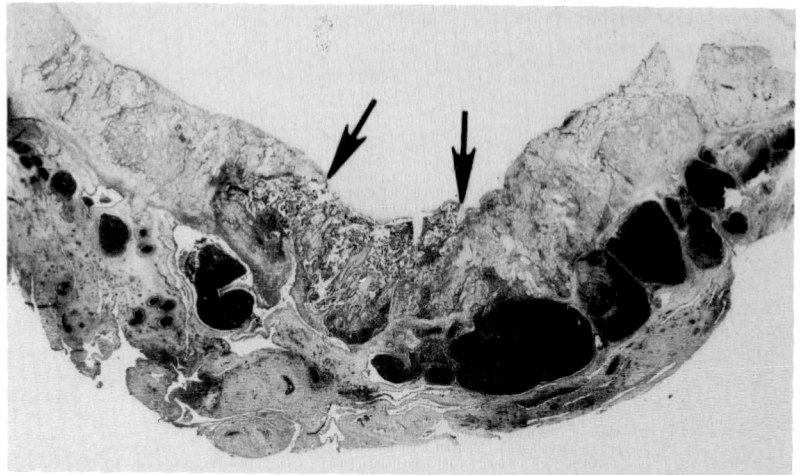

Fig. 25–14. Infarction of the placenta in a rhesus monkey *(Macaca mulatta)*. A small portion of viable tissue is evident between the arrows, the remainder is necrotic. Large thrombi fill placental vessels. (Courtesy of Drs. A. T. Hertig and N. W. King, Jr., New England Regional Primate Research Center, Harvard Medical School.)

lymphocytes, and plasma cells and, in some cases, neutrophils. Suitable stains show the chorionic epithelium to be loaded with the causative bacteria. Upon this exudative inflammation, necrosis supervenes to a variable depth in the allantochorion, producing a hyaline picture microscopically, and grossly, a brownish color and leathery consistency.

The effect of these changes is to sever, or at least impair, the placental connection between mother and fetus, with abortion as the result. Nevertheless, some cases are milder so that the calf survives to be born alive.

A chronic proliferative form of placentitis is also described in Bang's disease in which a diffuse and sparsely arranged fibrosis, aided by thickening of the tips of the chorionic villi, ties the chorion to the endometrium. This appears to be responsible for the frequent retention of the placental membranes in those cows in which the infection is not sufficiently severe to cause abortion. It is to be borne in mind that resistance to the Brucella infection gradually develops. Many cows abort only

once; a few may have three consecutive abortions.

Brucella abortus is not an important infection in sheep. In swine, infection with *B. suis* characteristically incites a more chronic granulomatous inflammatory response.

In **vibriosis** [*Vibrio (Campylobacter) fetus*], an abortifacient infection of sheep and cattle, a somewhat similar type of placentitis is encountered. The infection and its products kill the fetus, with abortion following about 2 days later, in cows between the fifth and seventh month of pregnancy, in ewes during the fifth. No permanent maternal injury results. The principal lesions include necrosis of the chorionic epithelium, serofibrinous or serous exudate (inflammatory edema) throughout the placental tissues, and infiltration of neutrophilic and other leukocytes, especially into the chorionic villi. The fetal liver contains discolored foci of necrosis a few millimeters in diameter, accompanied by perivascular neutrophilic and eosinophilic infiltration. The diagnosis can often be suspected from a notice-

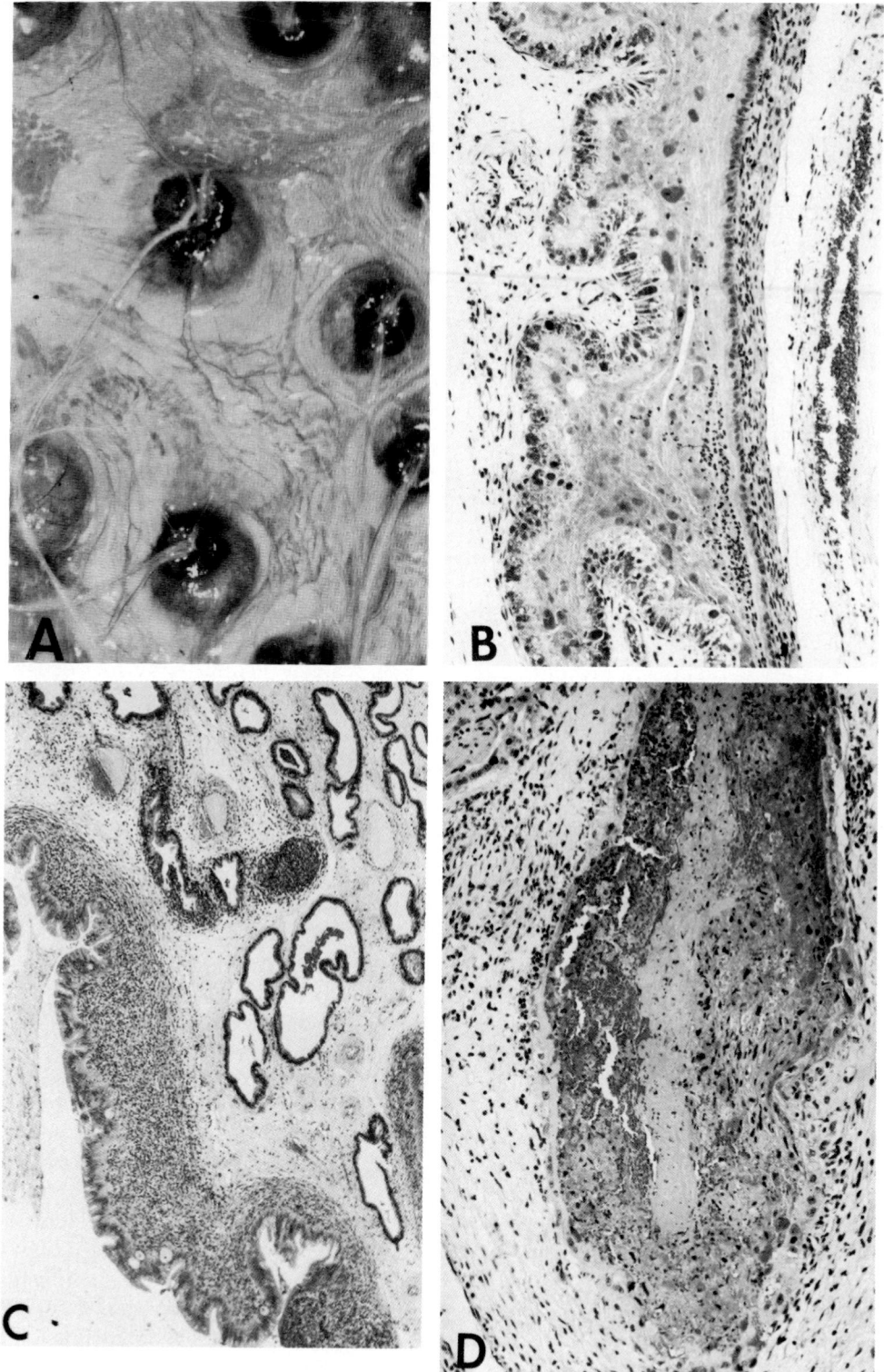

Fig. 25–15. Brucellosis. *A*, Experimental *Brucella ovis* infection in a ewe. Fetal aspect of placenta containing exudate in the periplacentomes and interplacentomes. *B*, Photomicrograph of *A*. There are exudate and bacterial colonies in the periplacentome. *C*, Experimental *Brucella melitensis* infection in a ewe. There is marked purulent endometritis. *D*, Necrosis of chorionic epithelium in a ewe experimentally infected with *B. melitensis*. (Courtesy of Dr. J. A. Molello.)

able paleness and softness of the fluid-containing cotyledons. It is confirmed by demonstration of the usually numerous curved or even comma-shaped organisms, sometimes in spiral chains. These can be shown readily in smears or sections of the placental cotyledons, preferably stained by Giemsa's or Wright's method.

In bovine **trichomoniasis** (*Trichomonas fetus*), the infection proceeds from the vagina to the uterus, where it initiates endometritis and placentitis, which range from a mild purulent reaction to a copious pyometra. The infection tends to become chronic, with retention of the fetal membranes, usually following abortion during the first half of gestation. The retention of fetal membranes is presumably due to the same mechanism of fibrosis as is the case in brucellosis. Organisms are present in the fetal membranes and fluids, but due to the difficulty of rendering trichomonads visible in tissue, they usually have to be demonstrated by methods appropriate to wet preparations.

In **paratyphoid abortion of mares** caused by *Salmonella abortus-equi*, a purulent hemorrhagic placentitis with necrosis of the chorionic villi produces abortion between the fourth and eighth months of pregnancy. *S. abortus-ovis* infection in sheep causes a diffuse endometritis and placentitis, which may result in abortion, most usually during the last 6 weeks of gestation.

In **equine virus abortion,** which is an infection of the fetus with the virus of equine rhinopneumonitis (*Herpesvirus equi*-1), the fetal membranes are said to show only edema and perhaps icterus, although a greater variety of changes are to be found in the body of the fetus. The herpesvirus of **infectious bovine rhinotracheitis** (IBR) and **Aujeszky's disease** of swine (*Herpesvirus suis*) are also causes of abortion. IBR has become one of the principal causes of abortion in cattle. Although necrosis and inflammatory changes may be

seen in the placenta, specific viral lesions are predominantly to be found in the fetus. All herpesviruses should be viewed as potential causes of abortion. Other viral infections have also been incriminated as causes of abortion, including virus diarrhea-mucosal disease, equine arteritis, Rift Valley fever, hog cholera, and swine influenza. Enteroviruses and a parvovirus have been demonstrated to cause natural and experimentally induced abortion and infertility in swine.

Epizootic bovine abortion, caused by a *Chlamydia*, has been recognized in restricted geographic localities (California, parts of Europe). Abortions usually occur during the seventh to the ninth month of gestation. Among the rather inconspicuous lesions reported in the fetus are minute, scarcely visible, gray foci of leukocytes in most of the parenchymatous organs.

Enzootic abortion of ewes, also caused by a *Chlamydia,* is associated with late abortion, with lesions similar to those of epizootic bovine abortion. Chlamydial abortion is also reported in swine (Shcherban, et al., 1972).

Listeriosis (*L. monocytogenes*) has been known to produce abortion in late pregnancy in cattle, sheep, and goats. When this involvement is present, the usual encephalitis of listeriosis is minor or absent.

Leptospirosis is another bacterial cause of abortion in several species. **Mycobacteria** (tuberculosis) may also localize in the genital tract, causing a granulomatous endometritis which may result in abortion.

Many other bacteria are isolated with frequency, although rarely proved to be the cause of abortion. *Corynebacterium pyogenes* in cattle, however, is an exception.

Toxoplasmosis may localize in the placenta and fetus, producing characteristic focal necrotizing lesions. Abortion or congenital infection follows.

Mycoplasma have been associated with metritis and vaginitis in several species and are suspected as causes of abortion in cattle, horses, cats, and humans.

Mycotic abortion is caused by several fungi, most commonly by fungi of the genera *Mucor* and *Aspergillus;* but a number of others have been isolated or identified including *Coccidioides immitis, Mortierella wolfii, Allescheria boydii,* and *Torulopsis glabrata.* Abortion usually occurs during the last half of gestation, and lesions are often striking, such as large plaques of thickened epidermis, swollen and necrotic placentomes, and a thick leathery chorion-allantois.

Abortion may, of course, be an incidental feature of many acute illnesses not fundamentally localized in the genital tract, including noninfectious disease such as poisoning. These are exemplified by ergot poisoning or consumption of pine needles by cattle (but not by sheep). Many different species of bacteria including coliform, streptococci, staphylococci, and corynebacteria are often isolated from abortuses, but their precise role is usually uncertain.

Fundamentally, the cause of most abortions is death of the fetus. The normal reaction of the uterus to a dead fetus is to expel it as a foreign body. The tissues of the placental union often are patently injured, with inflammation, necrosis, hyalinization, or other degenerative changes. Inability of the injured placenta to transmit the supply of oxygen and nutrients is the usual reason for the death of the fetus, although in some cases, such as certain blood-borne poisonings, it may well be that the fetal body itself is fatally injured by poison that has passed through the placental barrier. The same is true in some of the infections, including equine viral abortion.

An exception to the foregoing is to be found in the case of ergot, which causes expulsion of the fetus (sometimes) through the violent and abnormal contractions which it induces in the uterine smooth muscle. Abortions can also be produced, at least early in gestation, by anything that eliminates or neutralizes the progestational effect of the hormone of the corpus luteum verum. This includes manual removal of the corpus luteum from its seat and the administration of large amounts of the antagonistic hormone, estrogen.

Practically speaking, then, the primary causes of abortion are as follows:

(1) Infections that injure placental tissues and destroy their function or, in early stages, prevent the original implantation.

(2) Severe deficiencies that deprive the fetus, as well as the mother, of some substance essential to life. Deprivation of oxygen is included here, although we are more accustomed to think of deficient minerals and vitamins. If the latter deficiencies exist in the beginning, the effect will be prevention of conception rather than abortion of an embryo or fetus already conceived.

(3) Severe acute and often septicemic infections of the mother. In many cases, probably a majority, this type of abortion can be attributed to the anoxia just mentioned, which supervenes because of the generalized venous congestion characteristic of these diseases.

(4) The effect of ergot and similar abortifacient substances. Abortions have been attributed to excessive nitrates in weeds growing in fertilized lowland pastures.

(5) Hormonal disturbances resulting from artificial interference.

(6) Traumatic injury to the placental attachment, which is rare.

Mummified Fetus. As has been stated, a fetus which has died is ordinarily expelled, constituting an abortion. The reason for this is that the dead fetus acts as an irritant foreign body. This is particularly true if the fetus is invaded by pathogenic or putrefactive organisms; its continued presence then would lead to maternal infection or sapremia. But when the cervix remains closed, the uterine contents are frequently sterile; in such a case, the fetus undergoes postmortem autolysis but not putrefaction, and may not be expelled. The animal may then appear to remain pregnant (pseudo-pregnancy). The soft tissues of the fetus are gradually liquefied, and the liquid is concurrently resorbed by the maternal blood and lymph. Months later the fetus is discovered, sometimes by accident, as a mass of bones, sometimes without but usually with a covering of shrunken and wrinkled skin, a dried and shrivelled mummy.

Retained Fetal Membranes. This is a frequent postpartum result of placentitis. Either acute swelling or chronic inflammatory fibrosis appears able to prevent the timely separation of the chorionic from the maternal structures. Recent experimental evidence points to a lack of progesterone as a potent cause of the disorder, also. The visible lesions necessary for retention are often slight. Retained more than several hours the membranes undergo both postmortem autolysis and putrefaction, for they are now without a blood supply, lifeless, and exposed via the open cervix to exterior contamination. This disintegration ultimately loosens their attachment to the endometrium and, as fragments, they are expelled in the course of several days.

The mother, meanwhile, suffers more or less severely from various toxic products generated by putrefactive and pathogenic bacteria that have gained access by way of the vaginal canal. Under these circumstances, the normal involution of the uterus to its pregravid condition, which should be well advanced in a few hours, is delayed indefinitely. Such a uterus is a fertile field for the growth of bacteria, including anaerobes such as the organism of tetanus and those listed in connection with septic metritis.

Postpartum Hemorrhage. Postpartum hemorrhage is not encountered in species having the epitheliochorial placenta.

Placenta Praevia. Placenta praevia, which is the formation of the placenta in such a location that it covers the internal cervical opening, and which may, in itself, lead to severe hemorrhage in the human, is limited to species that have a discoid placenta.

Ectopic Pregnancy. The development of an embryo elsewhere than in the uterine cavity is called ectopic pregnancy. The most frequent form of this rare accidental phenomenon is tubal pregnancy, in which the embryo, fertilized in the fallopian tube and prevented by obstruction from reaching the uterus, continues its natural development in the tube. This applies to the human oviduct, where the chorionic villi make their way into the wall forming a hemochorial placenta. Unless relieved by operation, the eventual result is rupture and disastrous hemorrhage when the fetus reaches a certain size. In species having the less invasive epitheliochorial placenta, tubal pregnancy probably does not occur. There are, however, a number of reports of abdominal pregnancy in animals. In most of the reported cases, some of which have terminated in artificial delivery of living offspring, investigation has disclosed a recent rupture of the uterine musculature that allowed the fetus to slip into the peritoneal cavity. This, of course, is not true ectopic pregnancy, but fully verified abdominal pregnancy has been reported in certain domestic species. The peritoneal surfaces are obviously not a favorable site for placentation, but the development of a full-term fetus there, later becoming mummified, has been recorded in the dog.

Hydrops Amnii. This Latin term meaning edema of the amnion refers to a great excess of fluid in the amniotic cavity, a disorder that occurs occasionally. Frequently, the allantoic cavity shares in the excessive accumulation of fluid. The normal amniotic fluid in the mare and cow varies from 3 to 6 L; the allantoic, from 6 to 15 L.

The causes are not always evident but include rotation of the uterus and twisting of the umbilical cord. The mechanisms here are similar to those that cause local edema elsewhere: interference with the venous drainage by compression of veins, but not of the more resistant arteries. Hydrops amnii has been known to occur a second time in the same cow. The condition persists until parturition and may cause death of the fetus and abortion.

Neoplasms of the Uterus and Cervix

Endometriosis is not a true neoplasm and is discussed earlier in the chapter.

Polyps of the endometrium occur as sessile-based, roughly spherical masses. They are composed of endometrial glands lined with columnar epithelium within a fibrous connective tissue stroma. They are rare tumors, but are recognized in cats, rodents, and man.

Adenocarcinoma of the uterus is most common in cattle and rabbits. There are reports in most species, but it is a rare neoplasm. In cattle, the neoplasm is relatively frequent in older individuals, occurring as a firm mass within and occasionally constricting one of the uterine horns. Microscopically, they are scirrhous carcinomas with dense collagenous connective tissue often exceeding the malignant epithelial tissue. The epithelial cells occur in islands in small solid nests or in an abortive glandular pattern. Metastasis to lymph nodes and the lung is usual. Endometrial carcinoma is the most common neoplasm in rabbits. These tumors are usually multiple and readily metastasize (Ingalls, et al., 1964). Meissner, et al. (1957) have experimentally induced endometrial adenocarcinoma in rabbits by estrogen administration.

Carcinoma of the cervix is a rare tumor in animals. It is much more frequent in humans, where it typically arises in areas of squamous metaplasia.

Leiomyoma and **leiomyosarcoma** of the uterus are also more frequent in humans than animals, although they have been described in dogs, cattle, sheep, cats, rodents, and nonhuman primates. They resemble similar tumors at other sites.

Chorionepithelioma, also known as **choriocarcinoma** and **syncytioma** is a neoplasm that occurs uncommonly in man and rarely in animals; only two clearly identifiable cases have been reported, one in an armadillo (Marin-Padilla and Benirschke, 1963) and one in a Rhesus monkey (*Macaca*

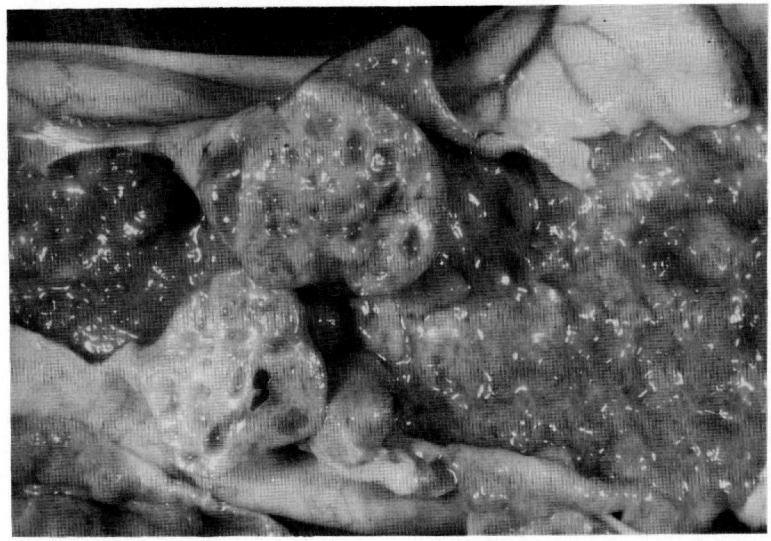

Fig. 25–16. Endometrial polyp arising in hyperplastic endometrium of a 15-year-old cat. (Courtesy of Dr. C. E. Gilmore.)

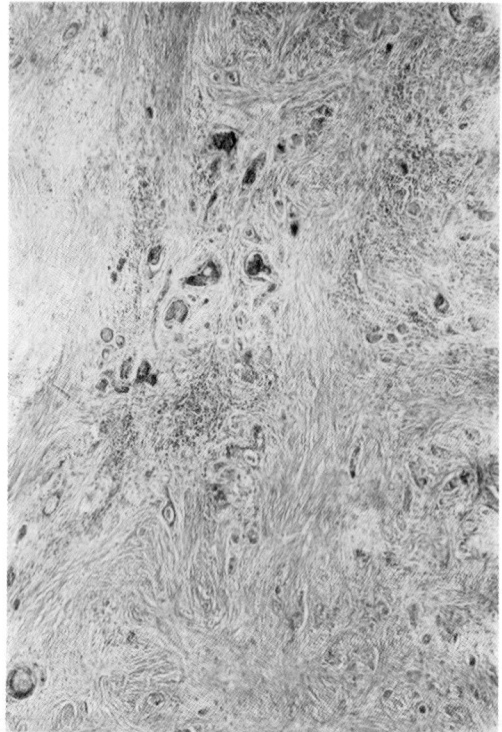

Fig. 25–17. Scirrhous adenocarcinoma of the endometrium of an eight-year-old cow.

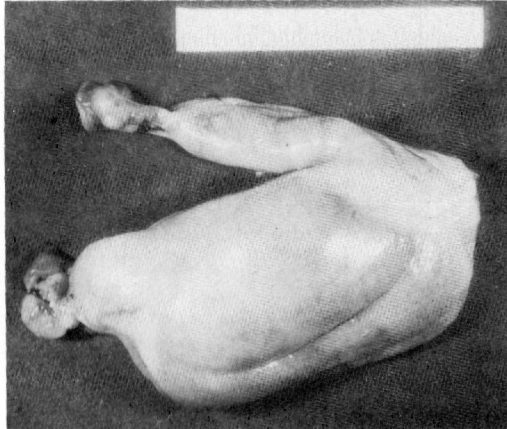

Fig. 25–18. Malignant lymphoma in the uterus of a six-year-old cat. (Courtesy of Dr. C. E. Gilmore.)

mulatta) (Lindsey, et al., 1969). In the human female, it arises in the endometrium from chorionic villi that have remained attached to the maternal tissue following parturition (or abortion) and expulsion of the bulk of the fetal membranes. The bits of chorionic tissue remain alive through absorption of nutrient materials from surrounding fluids and frequently proliferate slowly to form a botryoid, cystic structure known as a **hydatidiform mole.** Chorionic epithelial cells so retained, with or without the formation of a distinct "mole," occasionally acquire neoplastic properties from unknown causes and grow to form a highly malignant neoplasm. This tumor is characterized histologically by masses or strands of epithelial cells with lightly staining cytoplasm characteristic of the Langhans' layer of the chorionic villi. (This is less well differentiated in the domestic animals.) Mingled indiscriminately with these Langhans cells are syncytial masses of large, darkly staining epithelium corresponding to the outer, syncytial layer of chorionic epithelium. Having the same invasive power as the normal hemochorial placenta, the tumor elements tend to penetrate blood vessels and to lie in the areas of hemorrhage so produced. Like the normal chorionic tissue, these tumors secrete gonadotropic hormones, causing a positive Aschheim-Zondek test as in pregnancy. Cystic corpora lutea also results. Chorionepithelioma is occasionally found in the testis as part of a teratoma. Whatever the origin, early blood-borne pulmonary metastases are much to be feared. Comparable proliferations of retained chorionic tissue have been reported in the dog, but they have not been duplicates of the human hydatidiform mole, nor have they fulfilled the criteria of malignancy characteristic of the true chorionepithelioma. In species having the epitheliochorial placenta, such proliferations probably never occur.

Metastatic neoplasms are uncommon in the uterus or cervix except for malignant lymphoma in cattle. The invading lymphocytic neoplasm may be diffuse or nodular.

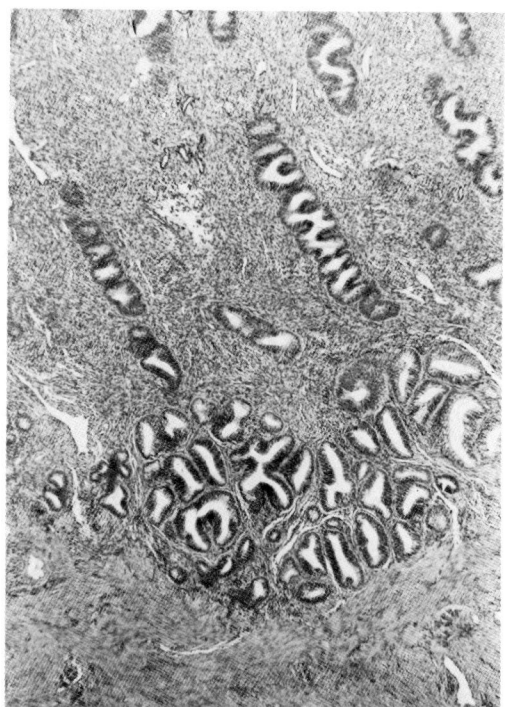

Fig. 25–19. Carcinoma *in situ*, in the uterus of a chimpanzee. A small cluster of endometrial glands at the base of the endometrium are disorganized, have hyperchromatic nuclei, and are invading adjacent tissue. Courtesy of Dr. A. T. Hertig, New England Regional Primate Research Center, Harvard Medical School.

Canine Venereal Tumor (Transmissible Lymphosarcoma, Venereal Granuloma, Infectious Sarcoma, Venereal Lymphosarcoma, Histiocytoma, Canine Condyloma). The canine venereal tumor is of great historical interest as the first neoplasm to be successfully transplanted from one host to another. A Russian veterinarian, M.A. Novinsky, was the first to demonstrate that this tumor could be transplanted to other dogs, a feat which earned him the title "Forefather of Experimental Oncology" in Russian literature. This neoplasm is readily reproduced by the experimental transfer of viable cells from one dog to another, and in nature is spread by coitus or other contact. In spite of this evidence of its infectious nature, no microbial agent has been demonstrated, nor has the tumor been transmitted by cell-free filtrate.

Diseases of the Vagina and Vulva

Anomalies of the vagina are uncommon, except for the hypoplasia seen in the bovine freemartin and various forms of hermaphroditism. Longitudinal and transverse septae may occur as developmental anomalies, as discussed under "The Uterus."

Cysts of Gartner's ducts (remnants of the wolffian ducts) and **Bartholin's glands** are occasionally encountered in cattle on the floor of the vagina. They are usually associated with cystic ovaries.

Granular venereal disease or **bovine granular vulvovaginitis** is a condition seen in cattle characterized by granular elevations of the vulvar mucosa in cows and of the penis and prepuce of bulls. Its cause is unknown, although some evidence incriminates *Mycoplasma bovigenitalium*. Microscopically, there is focal subepithelial lymphocytic accumulation. Other agents, including a picornavirus, have been associated with vaginitis in cattle.

Herpesvirus infections often localize in the mucosa of the vagina, vulva, penis, and prepuce. The best known in domestic animals is infectious pustular vulvovaginitis in cattle, caused by the bovine infectious rhinotracheitis virus. Similar infections may be seen in horses, dogs, swine, and human beings. Trichomoniasis in cattle may cause vaginitis, but is more important as a cause of endometritis. Other infections are less specific forms of vulvovaginitis caused by various bacteria including staphylococci, streptococci, and coliforms.

Neoplasms of the vagina and vulva are rare, with the exception of bovine fibropapillomas and the transmissible venereal tumor of dogs. Squamous cell carcinoma of the vulva is rare in the United States and Europe, but is reportedly not infrequent in countries near the equator such as India, Brazil, Kenya, and Sri Lanka (Wettimuny, et al., 1974). A high frequency of squamous cell carcinoma of the vulva of sheep has been reported in Australia by Vandergraff (1976) who suggested a causal relationship of short docking and exposure to sunlight.

Abou-Gabal, M., Hogle, R.M., and West, J.K.: Pyometra in a mare caused by *Candida rugosa*. J. Am. Vet. Med. Assoc., *170*:177–178, 1977.

Abusineina, M.E.: Anomalies of the cervix uteri of cattle. Br. Vet. J., *126*:347–356, 1970.

Afshar, A.: Virus disease associated with bovine abortion and infertility. Vet. Bull., *35*:735–752, 1965.

Anderson, L.J., and Sandison, A.T.: Tumours of the female genitalia in cattle, sheep, and pigs found in a British abattoir survey. J. Comp. Pathol., *79*:53–63, 1969.

Austwick, P.K.C.: Environmental aspects of *Mortierella wolfii* infection in cattle. N. Z. J. Agric. Res., *19*:25–33, 1976.

Beck, A.M., and McEntee, K.: Subinvolution of placental sites in a postpartum bitch. A case report. Cornell Vet., *56*:269–277, 1966.

Belter, L.F., Crawford, E.M., and Bates, H.R.: Endometrial adenocarcinoma in a cat. Pathol. Vet., *5*:429–431, 1968.

Bennett, R.C., Olds, D., Deaton, O.W., and Thrift, F.A.: Nature of white heifer disease (partial genital aplasia) and its mode of inheritance. Am. J. Vet. Res., *34*:13–19, 1973.

Black, W.G., et al.: Inflammatory response of the bovine endometrium. Am. J. Vet. Res., *14*:179–183, 1953.

Boyd, H.: Embryonic death in cattle, sheep, and pigs. Vet. Bull., *35*:251–266, 1965.

Boyd, W.L.: Some physiologic and pathologic aspects of sterility in cattle. Cornell Vet., *24*:138–145, 1934.

Brodey, R.S., and Fidler, I.J.: Clinical and pathologic findings in bitches treated with progestational compounds. J. Am. Vet. Med. Assn., *149*:1406–1415, 1966.

Brodey, R.S., and Roszel, J.F.: Neoplasms of the canine uterus, vagina, and vulva: a clinico-pathologic survey of 90 cases. J. Am. Vet. Med. Assn., *151*:1294–1307, 1967.

Cordes, D.O., Dodd, D.C., and O'Hara, P.J.: I. Bovine mycotic abortion. II. Acute mycotic pneumonia of cattle. N. Z. Vet. J., *12*:95–100 and 101–104, 1964.

Cotchin, E.: Spontaneous uterine cancer in animals. Br. J. Cancer, *18*:209–227, 1964.

Dawson, F.L.M.: Bovine endometritis: a review of literature to 1947, with special reference to the catarrhal type of the disease. Brit. Vet. J., *106*:104–116, 1950.

Dawson, P.J., Brooks, R.E., and Fieldsteel, A.H.: Unusual occurrence of endometrial sarcomas in hybrid mice. J. Natl. Cancer Inst., *52*:207–214, 1974.

Dennis, S.M., and Armstrong, J.M.: Ovine abortion due to *Salmonella typhimurium* in Western Australia. Aust. Vet. J., *41*:178–181, 1965.

Dennis, S.M.: The effect of bacterial endotoxin in pregnancy. Vet. Bull., *36*:123–128, 1966.

———: Comparative aspects of infectious abortion diseases common to animals and man. Int. J. Fert., *13*:191–197, 1969.

Diaz, R., Jones, L.M., and Wilson, J.B.: Antigenic relationship of the gram-negative organism causing canine abortion to smooth and rough brucellae. J. Bact., *95*:618–624, 1968.

Dow, C.: The cystic hyperplasia-pyometra complex in the bitch. J. Comp. Pathol., *69*:237–250, 1959.

Dow, C.: Experimental reproduction of the cystic hyperplasia-pyometra complex in the bitch. J. Path. Bact., *78*:267–278, 1959.

Dozsa, L.: Ein seltener fall von primärer bauch-hohlengravidität bei der katze. Schweiz. Arch. f. Tierheilk., *92*:106–110, 1950.

Dozsa, L., Olson, N.O., and Campbell, A.: The uterine biopsy technique for following the histologic changes caused by *Vibrio fetus* in the uterine mucosa. Amer. J. Vet. Res., *21*:878–883, 1960.

Ellis, W.A., Bryson, D.G., and McFerran, J.B.: Abortion associated with mixed leptospira/equid herpesvirus 1 infection. Vet. Rec., *98*:218–219, 1976.

Ellsworth, S.R., Kirkbride, C.A., Johnson, D.D., and Vorhies, M.W.: *Mycobacterium avium* abortion in a sow. Vet. Pathol., *16*:310–317, 1979.

Gardner, D.E.: Abortion associated with mycotic infection in sheep. N. Z. Vet. J., *15*:85–86, 1967.

Gibbons, W.J., et al.: The bacteriology of the cervical mucus of cattle. Cornell Vet., *49*:255–265, 1959.

Gilman, H.L.: The Diseases of the Oviduct of the Cow and Their Relation to Sterility. Ann. Rept. N.Y. State Vet. Col. (at Cornell) for 1919–20 (Legislative Document No. 8, 1921). Albany, J.B. Lyon Co., pp. 128–154.

Ginther, O.J.: Segmental aplasia of the mullerian ducts (white heifer disease) in a white shorthorn heifer. J. Am. Vet. Med. Assn., *146*:133–137, 1965.

Goudswaard, J., and van Kol, N.: *Corynebacterium uteri* (*nov. spec.*) as the probable cause of abortion in a sow. Neth. J. Vet. Sci., *2*:14–18, 1969. V.B. *39*:3678, 1969.

Griel, L.C., Jr., Kradel, D.C., and Wickersham, E.W.: Abortion in cattle associated with the feeding of poultry litter. Cornell Vet., *59*:226–235, 1969.

Hallman, E.T., Sholl, L.B., and Delez, A.L.: Pathology of *Bacterium abortus* infections. Mich. State Coll., Agric. Exp. Sta., Tech. Bull., 93, 1928.

Hardenbrook, H.: The diagnosis and treatment of nonspecific infections of the bovine uterus and cervix. J. Amer. Vet. Med. Assn., *132*:459–464, 1958.

Hellmann, E., and Raethel, S.: *Trichosporon capitatum* as cause of abortion in a cow. Berl. Munch. Tierarztl. Wschr., *77*:380–381, 1964. V.B. *35*:541, 1965.

Hillman, R.B.: Bovine mycotic placentitis in New York State. Cornell Vet., *59*:269–288, 1969.

Hillman, R.B., and McEntee, K.: Experimental studies on bovine mycotic placentitis. Cornell Vet., *59*:289–302, 1969.

Hirth, R.S., Nielsen, S.W., and Plastridge, W.N.:

Bovine salpingo-oophoritis produced with semen containing a *Mycoplasma.* Path. Vet., 3:616–632, 1966.

Hisaw, F.L., and Hisaw, F.L., Jr.: Spontaneous carcinoma of the cervix uteri in a monkey (*Macaca mulatta*). Cancer, 11:810–816, 1958.

Holland, L.A., and Knox, J.H.: Vaginal prolapse in Hereford cows. J. Anim. Sci., 26:885, 1967.

Ingalls, T.H., Adams, W.M., Lurie, M.B., and Ipsen, J.: Natural history of adenocarcinoma of the uterus in the Phipps rabbit colony. J. Natl. Cancer Inst., 33:799–806, 1964.

Jacobs, B.B., and Hureby, R.A.: Neoplasms occurring in aged Fischer rats, with special reference to testicular, uterine, and thyroid tumors. J. Natl. Cancer Inst., 39:303–309, 1967.

Jensen, R., Miller, V.A., and Molello, J.A.: Placental pathology of sheep with vibriosis. Am. J. Vet. Res., 22:169–185, 1961.

Jones, L.M., et al.: Taxonomic position in the genus *Brucella* of the causative agent of canine abortion. J. Bact., 95:625–630, 1968.

Karlson, A.G., and Mann, F.C.: The transmissible venereal tumor of dogs: observations on forty generations of experimental transfers. Ann. New York Acad. Sc., 54:1197–1213, 1952.

Kaufmann, A.F., Quist, K.D., and Broderson, J.R.: Pseudopregnancy in the New Zealand white rabbit: necropsy findings. Lab. Anim. Sci., 21:865–869, 1972.

Kendrick, J.W., Gillespie, J.H., and McEntee, K.: Infectious pustular vulvovaginitis of cattle. Cornell Vet., 48:458–495, 1958.

Kennedy, P.C., Olander, H.J., and Howarth, J.A.: Pathology of epizootic bovine abortion. Cornell Vet., 50:417–429, 1960.

Kennedy, P.C., and Richards, W.P.C.: The pathology of abortion caused by the virus of infectious bovine rhinotracheitis. Path. Vet., 1:7–17, 1964.

King, S.J., Munday, B.L., and Hartley, W.J.: Bovine mycotic abortion and pneumonia. N. Z. Vet. J., 13:76, 1965.

Kirkbride, C.A., et al.: A diagnostic survey of bovine abortion and stillbirth in the Northern Plains states. J. Am. Vet. Med. Assoc., 162:556–560, 1973.

Knudsen, O.: Partial dilatation of the uterus as a cause of sterility in the mare. Cornell Vet., 54:423–438, 1964.

Knudtson, W.U., Ruth, G.R., Kirkbride, C.A., and Tinant, M.: Pneumonia associated with *Torulopsis glabrata* in an aborted bovine fetus. Sabouraudia, 14:43–45, 1976.

Knudtson, W.U., et al.: Mycologic, serologic, and histologic findings in bovine abortion associated with *Allescheria boydii.* Sabouraudia, 12:81–86, 1974.

Langham, R.F., Beneke, E.S., and Whitenack, D.L.: Abortion in a mare due to coccidioidomycosis. J. Am. Vet. Med. Assoc., 170:178–180, 1977.

Leman, A.D., Cropper, M., and Rodeffer, H.E.: Infectious swine reproductive diseases. Theriogenol., 2:149–160, 1974.

Lindsey, J.R., et al.: Intrauterine choriocarcinoma in a Rhesus monkey. Path. Vet., 6:378–384, 1969.

Liu, K.M., et al.: Abortion associated with generalized *Corynebacterium pseudotuberculosis* infection in a mare. J. Am. Vet. Med. Assoc., 170:1086–1087, 1977.

Lombard, L., Morgan, B.B., and McNutt, S.H.: Some pathologic alterations of the oviduct. Am. J. Vet. Res., 12:69–74, 1951.

Mahaffey, L.W., and Adam, N.M.: Abortions associated with mycotic lesions of the placenta in mares. J. Am. Vet. Med. Assn., 144:24–32, 1964.

Marin-Padilla, M., and Benirschke, K.: Thalidomide-induced alterations in the blastocyst and placenta of the armadillo, *Dasypus novemcinctus Mexicanus,* including a choriocarcinoma. Am. J. Pathol., 43:999–1016, 1963.

McCann, T.O., and Myers, R.E.: Endometriosis in Rhesus monkeys. Amer. J. Obstet. Gyn., 106:516–523, 1970.

McDonald, L.E., McNutt, S.H., and Nichols, R.E.: Retained placenta—experimental production and prevention. Am. J. Vet. Res., 15:22–24, 1954.

McKercher, D.G.: Relationship of viruses to reproductive problems. J. Am. Vet. Med. Assn., 154:1184–1191, 1969.

Meissner, W.A., Sommers, S.C., and Sherman, G.S.: Endometrial hyperplasia, endometrial carcinoma, and endometriosis produced experimentally by estrogen. Cancer, 10:500–509, 1957.

Merrill, J.A.: Spontaneous endometriosis in the Kenya baboon (*Papio doguera*). Amer. J. Obstet. Gyn., 101:569–570, 1968.

Miller, F.W., and Graves, R.R.: Breeding history and gross changes found on autopsy in the genital organs of dairy cattle. J. Am. Vet. Med. Assn., 81:408–410, 1932.

Miyagi, M.: Changes in arteria uterina media of cows caused by pregnancy. Jpn. J. Vet. Res., 13:137–138, 1966.

Molello, J.A., et al.: Placental pathology. I. Placental lesions of sheep experimentally infected with *Brucella ovis.* II. With *Brucella melitensis.* III. With *Brucella abortus.* Am. J. Vet. Res., 24:897–922, 1963.

Molello, J.A., and Jensen, R.: Placental pathology. IV. Placental lesions of sheep experimentally infected with *Listeria monocytogenes.* Am. J. Vet. Res., 25:441–449, 1964.

Monlux, A.W., et al.: Adenocarcinoma of the uterus of the cow—differentiation of its pulmonary metastases from primary lung tumors. Am. J. Vet. Res., 17:45–73, 1956.

Moore, J.A., and Bennett, M.: A previously undescribed organism associated with canine abortion. Vet. Rec., 80:604–605, 1967.

Moorthy, A.R.S., Spradbrow, P.B., and McEvoy, T.: Isolation of mycoplasmas from an aborted equine foetus. Aust. Vet. J., 52:385, 1976.

Morse, E.V., et al.: Canine abortion apparently due to *Brucella abortus.* J. Am. Vet. Med. Assn., 122:18–20, 1953.

Nelson, L.W., and Kelly, W.A.: Progestogen-related gross and microscopic changes in female Beagles. Vet. Pathol., 13:143–156, 1976.

Nicholson, J.W.G., and Cunningham, H.M.: Retained placenta, abortions, and abnormal calves from beef cows fed all barley rations. Canad. Vet. J., 6:275–281, 1965.

Overgoor, G.H.A., and van Haaften, J.A.: Bovine abortion caused by *Nocardia asteroides*. Tijdschr. Diergeneesk., 90:150–154, 1965.

Palmer, W.M.: Macroscopic and microscopic changes in the reproductive tract of the lactating sow. Diss. Abstr., 26:1262–1263, 1965.

Pascoe, R.R., Spradbrow, P.B., and Bagust, T.J.: Equine coital exanthema. Aust. Vet. J., 44:485–490, 1968. V.B. 39:2010, 1969.

Pearson, H.: Uterine torsion in cattle: a review of 168 cases. Vet. Rec., 89:597–603, 1971.

Pearson, H., and Denny, H.R.: Spontaneous uterine rupture in cattle: a review of 26 cases. Vet. Rec., 97:240–244, 1975.

Platt, H., et al.: Genital infection in mares. Vet. Rec., 101:20, 1977.

Preiser, H.: Endometrial adenocarcinoma in a cat. Pathol. Vet., 1:485–490, 1964.

Ranby, P.D., and Ramsay, W.R.: A clinical note on the occurrence of oestrogen toxicity in pigs. Aust. Vet. J., 35:90–92, 1959.

Rao, P.R., et al.: Granular vulvovaginitis (GVV) in cattle—immunofluorescent studies. Vet. Rec., 96:361, 1975.

Rasbech, N.O.: A review of the causes of reproductive failure in swine. Brit. Vet. J., 125:599–616, 1969.

Ricketts, S.W., et al.: Genital infection in mares. Vet. Res., 101:65, 1977.

Rodeffer, H.E., et al.: Reproductive failure in swine associated with maternal seroconversion for porcine parvovirus. J. Am. Vet. Med. Assoc., 166:991–992, 1975.

Rowson, L.E.A., Lamming, G.E., and Fry, R.M.: The relationship between ovarian hormones and uterine infection. Vet. Rec., 65:335–340, 1953.

Sahu, S.P., Dardiri, A.H., Rommel, F.A., and Pierson, R.E.: Survival of contagious equine metritis bacteria in transport media. Am. J. Vet. Res., 40:1040–1042, 1979.

Sandholm, M., Vasenius, H., and Kivisto, A.-K.: Pathogenesis in canine pyometra. J. Am. Vet. Med. Assoc., 167:1006–1010, 1975.

Sattar, S.A., Bohl, E.H., and Senturk, M.: Viral causes of bovine abortion in Ohio. J. Am. Vet. Med. Assn., 147:1207–1210, 1965.

Schlotthauer, C.F., and Wakim, K.G.: Ectopic pregnancy in a dog. J. Am. Vet. Med. Assn., 127:213, 1955.

Schmidt, H.: Trichomoniasis or trichomonad abortion in cattle. J. Am. Vet. Med. Assn., 90:608–617, 1937.

Schutte, A.P.: Canine vaginal cytology. I. Technique and cytological morphology. II. Cyclic changes. III. Compilation and evaluation of cellular indices. J. Small Anim. Pract., 8:301–306, 307–311, 313–317, 1967.

Shcherban, G.P., et al.: Virusnyi abort svinei. ('Viral' abortion in sows.) Veterinariya, Moscow, 11:40–42, 1972.

Simon, J., et al.: Prevention of noninfectious abortion in cattle by weed control and fertilization practices on lowland pastures. J. Am. Vet. Med. Assn., 135:315–317, 1959.

Skydsgaard, J.M.: The pathogenesis of hydrallantois bovis. I. The concentration of sodium, potassium, chloride and creatinine in the foetal fluids in cases of hydrallantois and during normal pregnancy. Acta Vet. Scand., 6:193–207, 1965.

———: II. Electrical potential and chemical gradients between the allantoic fluid and the maternal blood in hydrallantois and normal pregnancy. Acta Vet. Scand., 6:193–207, 1965.

Southcott, W.H., and Moule, G.R.: Vulvitis in Merino ewes. Austr. Vet. J., 37:291–296, 1961.

Stewart, H., Snell, K., Dunham, L.J., and Schlyen, S.: Transplantable and Transmissible Tumors of Animals, Section 12, Fascicle 40, Atlas of Tumor Pathology, Washington, D.C., AFIP, 1957.

Sugimura, T., Tanaka, Y., Kita, E., and Nakahara, T.: Isolation of bacteria and viruses from aborted bovine fetuses. Natl. Inst. Anim. Health Q. (Tokyo), 14:42–47, 1974.

Swaney, L.M., and Breese, S.S., Jr.: Ultrastructure of *Haemophilus equigenitalis*, causative agent of contagious equine metritis. Am. J. Vet. Res., 41:127–132, 1980.

Talanti, S.: Observations on pyometra in dogs with reference to the hypothalamic hypophysial neurosecretory system. Am. J. Vet. Res., 20:41–43, 1959.

Tan, R.J.S., and Miles, J.A.R.: Possible role of feline T-strain mycoplasmas in cat abortion. Aust. Vet. J., 50:142–145, 1974.

Taul, L.K., Powell, H.S., and Baker, O.E.: Canine abortion due to an unclassified gram-negative bacterium. Vet. Med. Small Anim. Clin., 62:543–544, 1967.

Tennant, B., Kendrick, J.W., and Peddicord, R.G.: Uterine involution and ovarian function in the postpartum cow. A retrospective analysis of 2,338 genital organ examinations. Cornell Vet., 57:543–557, 1967.

Terlecki, S., and Watson, W.A.: Adenocarcinoma of the uterus of a ewe. Vet. Rec., 80:516–518, 1967.

Teunisson, G.H.B.: The development of endometritis in the dog and the effect of oestradiol and progesterone on the uterus. Acta Endocrinol., 9:407–420, 1952.

Ticer, J.W.: Canine infertility associated with *Pseudomonas aeruginosa* infection. J. Am. Vet. Med. Assn., 146:720–722, 1965.

Timoney, P.J., Ward, J., and Kelly, P.: A contagious genital infection of mares. Vet. Rec., 101:103, 1977.

Turner, P.D.: *Syncephalastrum* associated with bovine mycotic abortion. Nature (Lond.), 204:399, 1964.

Turner, P.D.: Simultaneous infection of a bovine foetus by two fungi. Nature (Lond.), 205:300–301, 1965.

Vandegraaff, R.: Squamous-cell carcinoma of the vulva in Merino sheep. Aust. Vet. J., 52:21–23, 1976.

Weber, A.E., Morgan, B.B., and McNutt, S.H.: A histological study of metrorrhagia in the virgin heifer. Amer. J. Anat., 83:309–327, 1948.

Westerfield, C., and Dimock, W.W.: The pathology of equine virus abortion. J. Am. Vet. Med. Assn., 109:101–111, 1946.

Wetherill, C.D.: Retained placenta in the bovine. A brief review. Canad. Vet. J., 6:290–294, 1965.

Wettimuny, S.G. de S., Wanduragala, H.H.M.L., and Pannanglia, V.S.: Neoplastic and proliferative lesions of the vulva of Ayrshire cattle in Sri Lanka. Ceylon Vet. J., 22:17–20, 1974. Vet. Bull., 45:4547, 1975.

Whitney, J.C.: The pathology of the canine genital tract in false pregnancy. J. Small Anim. Pract., 8:247–263, 1967.

———: The pathology of unilateral pyometra in the bitch. J. Small Anim. Pract., 10:223–230, 1969.

Wimsatt, W.A.: New histological observations on the placenta of the sheep. Amer. J. Anat., 87:401–459, 1950.

Winter, A.J., et al.: Variations in uterine response to experimental infection due to hormonal state of the ovaries. I. The role of cervical drainage, leukocyte numbers, and noncellular factors in uterine bactericidal activity. II. The mobilization of leukocytes and their importance in uterine bactericidal activity. Am. J. Vet. Res., 21:668–682, 1960.

Wohlgemuth, K., and Knudtson, W.U.: Abortion associated with *Mortierella wolfii* in cattle. J. Am. Vet. Med. Assoc., 171:437–438, 1977.

Young, S., Parker, H., and Firehammer, B.D.: Abortion in sheep due to virus of the psittacosis-lymphogranuloma group. J. Am. Vet. Med. Assn., 133:374–379, 1958.

MAMMARY GLAND

Bovine Mastitis

Inflammation of the udder is more commonly known by the above title, derived from the Greek word *mastos,* meaning mammary gland, than it is by the corresponding Latin term, mammitis, which is derived from *mamma,* the Latin name for the same gland. The disease may occur in any mammalian species, but is of the greatest frequency and importance, by far, in the dairy cow.

While localized and usually transitory inflammation can result here, as elsewhere, from trauma of various kinds, practically speaking, mastitis is always of infectious origin. Several different bacterial species cause the disease, and in general, it is scarcely possible to determine the causative organism by the type of reaction. The inflammation may partake of any of the acute exudative types except the catarrhal, there being no mucus-producing epithelium in the udder. Hemorrhagic in-

flammation also is exceptional. Usually acute mastitis represents a combination of the other exudative forms, serous, fibrinous, and purulent. Chronic mastitis implies the additional feature of fibrous proliferation, which is common to chronic inflammations anywhere. Since the various reactions almost always overlap in a highly variable manner, there is little to be gained by attempting to classify the multitudinous cases but, in the bovine, it may be helpful to speak of different forms on a basis related as nearly as possible to their etiologies.

In studying the lesions of mastitis, it should be remembered that this is a disease of the lactating rather than of the inactive gland, and histologic features must be appraised accordingly. The exudates, fluid and cellular, naturally follow the paths of least resistance, so that most of their component material finds its way into the alveolar lumens, but the intercellular spaces are also filled with leukocytes and fluids. It is thus not unusual to see an alveolus packed with dead or dying leukocytes (pus), but others may be distended chiefly with fluid, which is recognized in the microscopic section by a scanty albuminous precipitate. The epithelial lining of such alveoli is compressed, vacuolated, or absent. The adjoining interalveolar stroma may or may not be infiltrated and distended with leukocytes, neutrophils, monocytes, or lymphocytes, principally the latter. The capillaries are distended in the early acute forms but, in general, mastitis is more impressive for its exudation than for hyperemia. Clots of fibrin and leukocytes are not uncommonly seen in the smaller ducts. These are thought frequently to occlude the drainage of exudate and vitiated milk, thereby favoring the spread of the infective organisms with which they are heavily populated. The importance of drainage as a protective mechanism is well illustrated by the much greater prevalence of inflammatory change in the more dependent portions of the udder and its relative infrequency in the dorsal parts.

Judging from the distribution of visible organisms, most, if not all, forms of mastitis appear to be infections fundamentally of the epithelial linings rather than of the interalveolar tissues. Pattison (1952) found the early effects of *Streptococcus agalactiae* to be hyperplastic thickening and cornification of the epithelial lining of the lactiferous duct and sinus with an infiltration of reactive cells immediately beneath. As the condition improved, the extra layers of epithelial cells were shed, and the lining returned to normal. From the diseased lactiferous sinus, infection spreads up the branching ductal system to involve the alveolar epithelium and, to some extent, its supporting stroma. The rapidity and ubiquity of this spreading, which of course depends upon the relative virulence of the pathogen and the resistance of the host, are responsible for the principal distinctions between what may be called acute diffuse and chronic focal mastitis.

If the activity of the inflammatory process subsides, as it usually does either in a few days or when the lactational period has come to a normal or a premature termination, residual damage of various degrees is discernible. If the injury has been mild and of only a few days' duration, the mammary alveoli, like those of the lung in pneumonia, may return completely to normal. In the more severe forms and more virulent infections, unfortunately, the alveolar epithelium is often so thoroughly destroyed that regeneration is impossible. The alveolar walls then collapse against each other and fuse to form a firm mass of connective tissue, with or without a number of remaining lymphocytes. Despite a certain amount of fibrous proliferation which may have accompanied the process in chronic cases, the total volume of this nonalveolar residuum is considerably less than the space formerly occupied. This constitutes the terminal atrophy which is described in medical writings, the "shrunken quarter"

of the dairyman. It is difficult to predict clinically whether any regeneration will occur at the next lactation but if the alveolar destruction has been as great as that just described, regeneration is not possible.

Gross Characteristics. During life, acute inflammation of one or more of the mammary glands in any species can be recognized by the usual cardinal signs of acute inflammation. Not the least obvious of these is impaired function, for secretion of milk ceases or diminishes in proportion to the severity of the case. It may be replaced by exudative fluid of abnormal appearance as described below. If the case is of longer duration or is purely inactive and residual, the shrinking and the meaty firmness upon palpation are the decisive features. The shrinking, or atrophy, is especially evident when only one or two of the bovine quarters are so affected, the others remaining of normal size. The firmness is the result of a rather diffuse fibrous proliferation which accompanies the chronic, atrophying process and augments the preexisting fibrous tissue of the alveolar walls and interlobular septa. Occasionally, the firm tissue has a lumpy arrangement, which betrays a markedly focal form of mastitis or, possibly, old, inspissated abscesses.

Post mortem, most of the same signs are still in evidence, although heat and pain obviously no longer exist. The cut surface of normal mammary tissue in a state of active lactation is a pale pink in color. Its sharply angled and more or less rectilinear lobules are moderately conspicuous, have a diameter of several millimeters, and fit together like irregularly formed bricks in a wall. A few drops of milk commonly exude and stand upon the cut surface, but there is very little blood. By contrast, the cut surface of acutely inflamed mammary tissue is a darker pink or light red in color; its lobules are somewhat larger in average size (inflammatory swelling), but less distinct, and the cut surface is diffusely moist. Usually a few drops of blood ooze from the larger of the severed vessels; if there is any "milk," it is yellowish and resembles pus. The degree of reddening may vary from place to place. If there is chronic fibrosis, the irregularly distributed white fibrous tissue can be seen, often rather easily. Old abscesses and similar lesions of course are obvious.

Diagnosis. The diagnosis of mastitis may be accomplished in the living animal either by clinical signs discernible by careful examination of the udder, by demonstration of the causative organism or by examination of the milk. In severely acute cases, the secretion is plainly abnormal, being a yellowish, watery fluid which is little more than blood serum, a serous inflammatory exudate. In cases which are more chronic but still severe, the milk may be "stringy," "ropy," or "curdy." The ropy or stringy characteristic is due to the presence of long strands of coagulated fibrin, a fibrinous inflammatory exudate, in which numerous cells are usually entangled. The "curds" are small masses of coagulated casein, more or less pure, which results, in some cases at least, from the local production of acid, certain of the pathogenic organisms (streptococci) being strong acid-producers. This change, then, is chemically analogous to what happens in the souring and curdling of milk after it has been withdrawn and stored for human use. The milk may also contain macroscopically appreciable amounts of blood. These abnormal substances are best detected by directing the milk stream into a "strip cup," a black cloth serving to strain out and make visible such solidified substances.

A number of laboratory procedures can be applied to the milk for the more precise detection of mastitis. Foremost among these are the leukocyte count and the direct bacterial count. In these techniques, a measured amount of milk is spread on a slide and stained. The number and kinds of body and bacterial cells are readily ascertained. A total of 100 leukocytes per ml is not considered abnormal, since some leukocytes of the various kinds enter the mammary tissue physiologically. The tests by bromthymol blue and similar indicators show an increased alkalinity. In spite of the production of acid from lactose by the streptococcal, staphylococcal, and other causative organisms, if the inflammation is actively exudative, the alkalinity of the inflammatory exudate shifts the reaction in the alkaline direction. The tests for chlorides and some other substances are also tests for the presence of inflammatory exudate as an invisible contaminant of the milk. On the other hand, there are a few examples of mastitis in which little exudate is formed, and the milk shows a higher acidity, detectable by measurement of the pH or by the easier coagulation of the milk upon heating, or the addition of alcohol. The increased protein of an inflammatory exudate also favors coagulation by alcohol (or heating). However, the alcohol test is of minor importance in the diagnosis of mastitis.

The question naturally arises as to which of the several diagnostic methods are most accurate. Physical examination of the udder depends for its accuracy upon the skill of the examiner, but obviously has its limitations in the rather numerous latent and subclinical cases. The special tests upon the milk are usually considered suitable for use in conjunction with other methods of diagnosis. Culturing alone has been said to miss a very considerable proportion of cases which were detectable by leukocyte counts upon the milk and a somewhat higher proportion of those which were diagnosed post mortem by histopathological examination. However, in making the histopathological examination, it must be remembered that the presence of considerable numbers of lymphocytes is characteristic of the process of postlactational involution and not necessarily pathological.

Causes and Routes of Entry. It has already been stated that the cause of mastitis is infection by pathogenic microorganisms. While there are two routes by which pathogenic organisms theoretically may gain access to the mammary tissue, all evidence indicates that hematogenous infection almost never occurs, and that entrance through the lactiferous duct acccounts for practically all cases of mastitis. Much of this evidence is clinical and bacteriologic and will not be recounted here, but the great preponderance of cases in which one-quarter of the cow's udder becomes infected independently of the others argues for accidental contamination through the orifice of the teat. There are indications that bovine udders have been infected from the mouths of calves suckling them, at least in the case of disease caused by pasteurellae or corynebacteria. The more usual source of infection is contamination of the milker's hands, the "cups" of the milking machine, or other utensils which come in contact with the teat.

While several different pathogens are capable of causing bovine mastitis, the great majority of cases are due to *Streptococcus agalactiae (Strep. mastitidis),* a highly contagious obligate parasite of the bovine mammary gland. This organism is the cause of the usual insidiously arising, chronic form of mastitis. *Streptococcus dysgalactiae* causes an acutely arising form, sometimes apparently originating from a traumatic injury. While the infection is eventually self-limiting, its termination may apparently depend upon the exhaustion and destruction of the susceptible acinar epithelium; in other words, the affected quarter is permanently functionless. *Streptococcus uberis* also causes an acute mastitis, but the disease is typically much less severe, with early complete recovery.

Next in importance to the streptococci are staphylococci. *Staphylococcus pyogenes* causes a severe acute or fulminating infection of the gland commonly accompanied by fever and general bodily malaise. These cases are often fatal in a few days. Some go on to gangrene of the udder.

Corynebacterium pyogenes, another one of the pyogenic groups of organisms, occasionally causes mastitis. The disease is usually distinctly suppurative in type with formation of large amounts of pus, often abscesses, and sometimes extensive necrosis and sloughing of masses of tissue. There has sometimes been sloughing of whole quarters, followed ultimately by healing. Presumably, the latter phenomenon is the result of thrombosis and infarction, although there appear to be no investigations which would eliminate direct toxic action of the bacteria. Some udders rupture, others form fistulous tracts to discharge the pus. A minority of affected cows show fever and general reaction in the early stages, with signs of pain in the joints. Occasionally, the attack is fatal, but the usual result is slow recovery with functional loss of the involved quarter or quarters. This form of mastitis attacks nonlactating or even immature glands as well as those in lactation. In Europe, it has been called summer mastitis since the nonlactating cows are often affected while in summer pasture.

Pseudomonas aeruginosa (pyocyanea) is a rare cause of acutely developing mastitis. Tucker (1950) reported cases which resulted from the introduction of contaminated medicaments into the teats by a dairyman. The inflammation terminated in destruction of the affected quarters.

The Pasteurella organism (*P. multocida, P. septica*) is occasionally the cause of mastitis. It is chronic and suppurative in type.

The organism of Bang's disease, *Brucella abortus,* is thought to remain in the udder during the quiescent inter-gestational period without producing lesions. While this is doubtless true as regards clinical mastitis, Runnells and Huddleson (1925) found well-marked inflammatory changes in the form of lymphocytic infiltrations, a purulent intra-alveolar exudate, and other changes, with terminal destruction of alveoli (atrophy) in affected areas. High cell counts and other confirmatory data come from other sources. Experimental introduction of *Brucella suis* into the udders of cows produced very severe acute mastitis.

Coliform mastitis, while rare, is a rather distinct type. Acute inflammation characterized by heat, pain, and soft, edematous swelling, together with discolored, fibrinous clots in the milk, arises suddenly either without previous evidence of abnormality or as an acute exacerbation of a latent infection (determined by systematic culturing at regular intervals). The causative organisms are *Escherichia coli, Aerobacter aerogenes,* or their close relatives. Terminal effects are usually mild but vary; there is often return to normal in a few days; in other cases, persistent mastitis leads to involution of the quarter with restoration of normal function at the next lactation. A chronic form characterized by successive acute exacerbations may develop. There is also an acute form accompanied by fever, dehydration, severe toxic symptoms, and usually death (prevented by streptomycin). Histopathologic examinations of the affected glands appear not to have been made.

Aphthous fever (aftosa, foot-and-mouth disease) is accompanied by mastitis in a considerable proportion of cases. Development of this complication appears to depend upon introduction of virus into the lactiferous orifice from vesicles on nearby skin. The reaction is acute serous in type and adds considerably to the severity of the generalized disease. Infectious bovine rhinotracheitis virus may also cause mastitis. Herpes mammillitis of the teats is discussed in Chapter 9.

Although not common, *Mycoplasma* including the organism of pleuropneumonia can cause mastitis in cows, sheep, and goats.

The presence of species of *Candida* and *Trichosporon* has been reported in conjunction with mastitis in cattle, as has *Nocardia asteroides.*

Tuberculosis of the udder is among the lesions in about 20% of cows having the disease in a generalized form, the milk being correspondingly dangerous. However, tubercle bacilli have been shown to occur in milk also from external (fecal) contamination without the presence of mammary lesions. The tuberculous lesions form firm nodules, which may or may not be palpable. The histopathologic features here are the same as characterize tuberculosis elsewhere. The udder may, of course, be involved in cases of generalized tuberculosis in other species.

Gangrenous Mastitis. It is not rare for a cow to develop suddenly an acute and severe inflammation, often of all four quarters of the udder, which, in the course of a day or two progresses to gangrene. Starting in the distal portions and rising closer and closer to the attachment of the udder, the parts become cold and insensible; white skins show a bluish tinge. Commonly death supervenes about the third or fourth day. A similar disease occurs in sheep and is not necessarily precluded in other species. The tissue changes are those characteristic of any moist gangrene, often with considerable amounts of fluid, a serous inflammatory exudate, or inflammatory edema. It is noteworthy that while one group of lobules is completely necrotic and gangrenous, an adjoining area may be living and only moderately altered, with just an inflammatory line of demarcation between the two.

Many of these cases appear to be infections with highly virulent staphylococci, although Mura (1950) believed the combined action of a streptococcus and *Clostridium welchii (Cl. perfringens)* to be essential in causation. It is commonly accepted that the gangrene supervenes upon infarction resulting from thrombosis of vessels. While this is entirely plausible on the basis of pathologic principles, it is difficult to reconcile with the fact that in many cases all four quarters are synchronously affected. The possibility of a direct necrotizing action of the causative pathogen should be investigated. Numerous investigators have attributed just such an action to staphylococci.

Cryptococcal Mastitis. Rarely, the bovine udder is affected with cryptococcosis or torulosis (*Torula histolytica, Cryptococcus neoformans*), which leads to disastrous destruction of the mammary tissue. The mode of entry of the infection is accepted as being via the orifice of the teat, as in other kinds of mastitis. The number of quarters involved is variable.

The affected tissue, which is often the whole quarter, is firmer than normal and grayish or almost white in color, except for occasional small hemorrhagic areas. From the cut surface exude copious amounts of a slippery, viscid fluid which resembles mucus excepting that it is less translucent. (It contains no epithelial or connective tissue mucin.) The microscopic changes correspond to those of cryptococcosis in any location. Briefly, in the most acutely affected areas, there is replacement of the

acinar and ductal epithelium by the liquefied material just described. The yeast cells are plainly seen, but little else is visible within the relatively unchanged fibrous walls of the alveoli and ducts. In areas (or individual patients) where the infection was held to less rapid destruction, there is a limited degree of reticuloendothelial and even fibrous reaction, with large numbers of fat-filled phagocytes or small granulomatous nodules. Diagnosis is made by demonstration of the typical yeast cells, which are described elsewhere.

Mastitis in Sheep

Ewes suffer from a severe acute form of mastitis, which is often unilateral, and frequently displays considerable contagiousness. Stockmen refer to the condition as "blue bag" because of the severe venous congestion which imparts a dark bluish tinge to the exterior of the udder. Doubtless abetted by the venous stasis, the inflammatory process often is superseded by

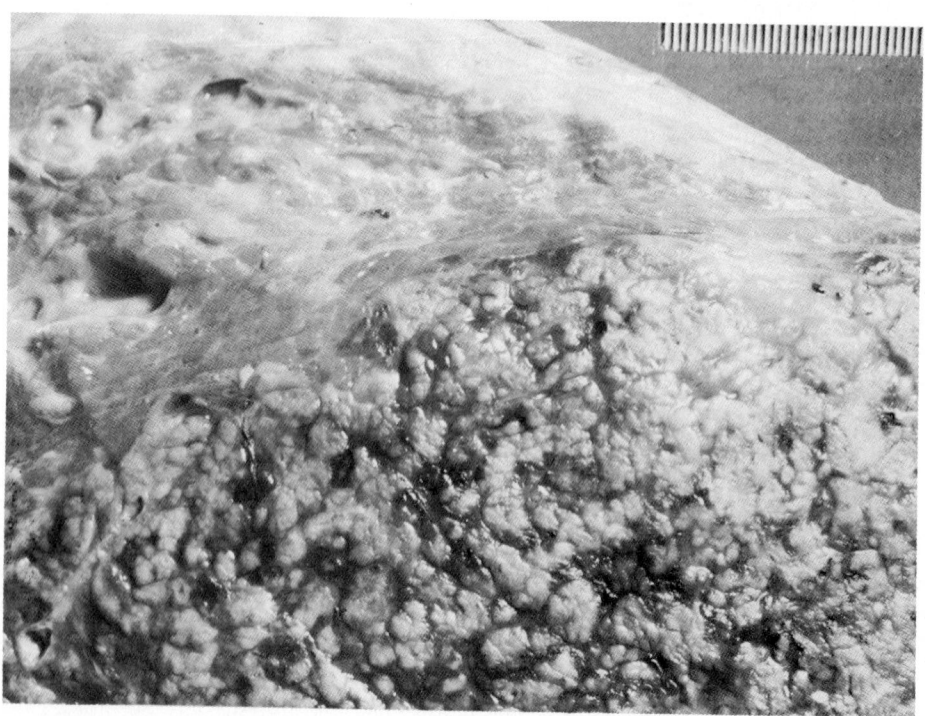

Fig. 25–20.   Gangrenous mastitis in a cow.

gangrene. In ewes, the gangrene is more prone than it is in bovines to limit its ravages to parts of a gland rather than the whole.

The microscopic picture, except in a few mild and almost subclinical cases, is that of a severe acute serofibrinopurulent inflammation. Exudate not only fills the acini but distends the interacinar walls and the interlobular septa, which are made conspicuous thereby. Many desquamated epithelial cells often mingle with the leukocytes and fluid in the alveoli. Large islands of inflamed tissue may undergo necrosis. Abscesses often form; the larger ones rupture into the lactiferous sinus or through the skin; the smaller ones become heavily encapsulated, inspissated, and fibrotic. The ultimate fate of the whole gland is usually, but not invariably, complete fibrosis and permanent loss of function.

Causes. Staphylococci, *aureus* and *albus*, have been found to cause a majority of cases. As in the cow, staphylococcal mastitis is peracute and severe. There is fever during the first few days, with a serious systemic disturbance that may prove fatal. It is this form which is most commonly terminated by gangrene. The pasteurella is probably the next most common causative organism, producing a somewhat less violent reaction. Streptococci, corynebacteria, and coliform bacteria have caused the disease in some instances. A foul odor in the affected tissue is usually attributable to the latter organism. Injuries produced by the suckling lamb are thought frequently to provide the portal of entry for organisms causing ovine mastitis.

Mastitis in Sows

While true **actinomycosis** has not been observed in the bovine udder, its occurrence in the mammary gland of the sow is not altogether rare. Commonly several, but not all, glands are involved. They are markedly enlarged, as a rule, and hard, but not hot or painful. Any secretion produced has more the qualities of pus than of milk.

The affected mammary tissue is replaced by typical actinomycotic granulation tissue: confluent areas which consist of a fibrous capsule peripherally, well-vascularized reticuloendothelial granulation tissue within this, and pus with "rosettes" centrally. The Gram stain shows that these rosettes contain pleomorphic gram-positive filaments, about 1 μ in diameter and varying in length from 1 (coccoid forms) to 20 μ, with a greater length occasionally. As in other forms of actinomycosis, the foregoing microscopic findings are diagnostic. Of equal value are Gram-stained smears of the pus showing typical gram-positive filamentous forms of the dimensions stated, provided that the presence of rosettes has been demonstrated. The latter is usually accomplished by means of a wet, unstained microscopic preparation of the pus under reduced light and low magnification (100 to 400 diameters). Rosettes are not seen in smears because smearing destroys them.

The gross appearance of the fibrous capsules and capsular trabeculae is dense and white. The reticuloendothelial tissue is yellowish and much softer. From the latter, drops or larger amounts of pus exude. The appearance often suggests a coarse and irregular honeycomb. As in actinomycosis elsewhere, large abscesses are not typical.

Melanosis occasionally produces conspicuous black discoloration of the mammary tissues of sows. It is usually unnoticed until the animal is slaughtered for food. The condition is known in packing-house circles as "seedy belly," since the black color is often localized in areas suggestive of round, black seeds. It would be interesting to know whether the condition is related to any particular breed, strain, or color of hair.

Equine Mastitis

Blastomycosis has been seen in the equine udder, but probably as a direct extension from a cutaneous infection.

Proliferative and Neoplastic Diseases of the Mammary Gland

In the dog, tumors of the mammary gland are second in frequency only to tumors of the skin. As tumors of the skin arise from extremely heterogenous cell types, tumors of mammary glands are the most common single group of tumors in the canine. Of considerable interest in the general study of neoplasia is the fact that in the bovine, where anatomic development and functional activity of the mammary gland are greater by far than in any other species, mammary neoplasms are practically unknown. The few examples have been reviewed by Povey and Osborne (1969). They occur in cats, but much less frequently than in dogs. They are rare in other domestic species.

Several systems of classification of neoplasms of the canine mammary gland have been proposed, some relatively simple with few categories, and others in our opinion overly complicated. The problem with classification in part stems from the great histologic variability encountered not only between tumors, but also within individual tumors. Within a single tissue section of a given tumor, there may be areas of papillary, tubular, and medullary adenocarcinoma; squamous cell carcinoma; myoepithelial proliferation; and cartilage. Further complicating classification is the fact that relatively benign appearing tumors may ultimately prove to be malignant. Our approach is based on the dominant histologic characteristic and presented in Table 25–1. Although there have been several recent studies to correlate biologic behavior with histologic appearance (which is after all the main purpose for classification), further studies are needed to determine the usefulness of the varied approaches to classify these neoplasms.

In dogs, neoplasms of the mammary gland are most frequent in older female dogs, and rarely are seen in males. The inguinal glands are most often affected, and multiple tumors are common. Hormones play some role in their pathogenesis as the incidence is considerably lower in bitches spayed at an early age. No positive correlation has been made with number of pregnancies or occurrence of pseudopregnancy.

In cats, mammary tumors are also most frequent in older individuals. In contrast to dogs, the anterior and posterior glands are involved with about equal frequency or with slight predilection for the anterior glands. No hormonal influence has been identified in cats.

Tumors of the mammary gland are frequent but less varied in laboratory rodents. A specific virus is the cause of adenocarcinoma of the mammary gland in mice. No infectious agent has been incriminated in domestic animals.

Hyperplasia. In older dogs, two forms of mammary gland hyperplasia are seen. **Cys-**

Table 25–1. Hyperplastic and Neoplastic Diseases of the Mammary Gland

Hyperplasia of mammary gland
  Cystic glandular hyperplasia, Fig. 25–21
  Lobular hyperplasia, Fig. 25–22A
  Feline mammary hypertrophy, Fig. 25–22B
Adenoma
  Intraductal adenoma (intraductal papilloma)
  Acinar adenoma
  Fibroadenoma (adenofibroma), Fig. 25–23A
Adenocarcinoma: simple, complex
  Papillary (ductal), Fig. 25–23B
  Tubular (ductal), Fig. 25–23C
  Lobular (acinar), Fig. 25–23D
  Scirrhous, Fig. 25–24A, B
  Adenoacanthoma, Fig. 25–24C, D
Medullary (solid) carcinoma: simple, complex, Fig. 25–25A
Undifferentiated (anaplastic) carcinoma
Mixed tumor of mammary gland, Fig. 25–26, Fig. 25–27
Sarcoma
  Osteosarcoma
  Chondrosarcoma
  Fibrosarcoma
  Combined
Myoepithelial tumor (spindle cell carcinoma), Fig. 25–25B

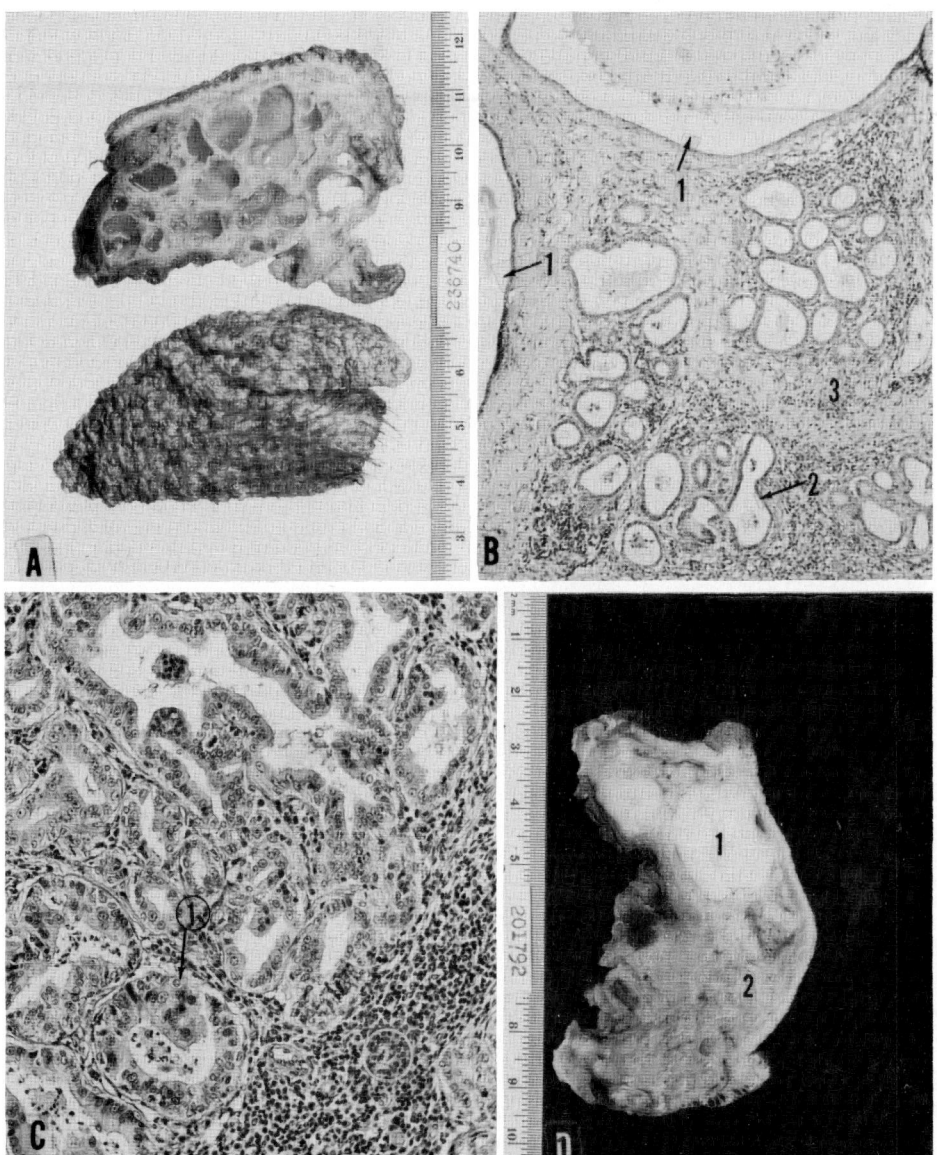

Fig. 25–21. *A*, Cystic hyperplasia of the mammary gland of a seven-year-old Coonhound. *B*, Higher magnification (× 80) of the same lesion. Cystic (*1*) and hyperplastic acini (*2*) and dense stroma (*3*) containing leukocytes. Contributor: Dr. R. F. Vigue. *C*, Adenocarcinoma (× 150) of the mammary gland of a nine-year-old female Cocker Spaniel. *D*, The gross specimen with solid areas of tumor (*1*) and diffuse neoplastic infiltration (*2*). (Courtesy of Armed Forces Institute of Pathology.) Contributor: Angell Memorial Animal Hospital.

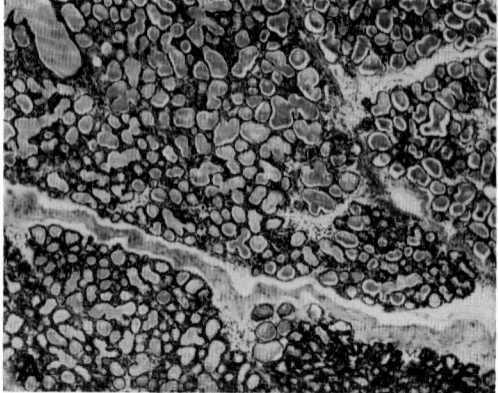
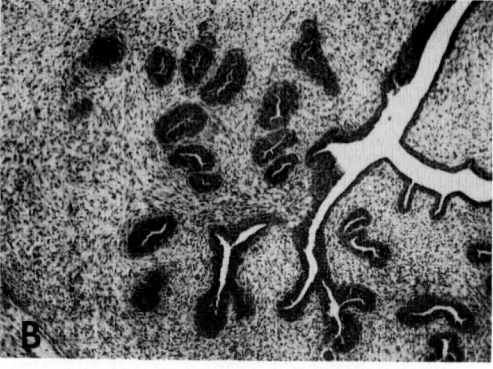

Fig. 25–22. *A,* Lobular hyperplasia, canine mammary gland. Glandular proliferation resembles normal mammary tissue. *B,* Feline mammary hypertrophy (juvenile fibroadenoma). Branching ducts and ductules within proliferating fibroblastic connective tissue.

tic **glandular hyperplasia,** sometimes called fibrocystic disease, is characterized by dilated cysts and acini embedded in a dense fibrous connective tissue containing mononuclear leukocytes. Papillary projections of epithelium may extend into the cystic lumens. The cause is unknown. **Lobular hyperplasia** is characterized by nodules (lobules) of acinar and ductular tissues, with or without any increase in connective tissue or myoepithelial proliferation. The glandular tissue may or may not be actively secreting. It is believed to result from an irregular response of individual lobules of the mammary gland during estrus.

An occasional lesion seen in young cats, termed **feline mammary hypertrophy,** is characterized by enlargement of one or several glands. Most often, multiple glands or all glands are affected. Microscopically, the enlargements are composed of branching ducts and ductules in a lobular arrangement within an abundance of proliferating fibroblastic connective tissue. The lesion has also been termed **juvenile fibroadenoma.** It is thought to result from prolonged stimulation by progesterone from retained corpora lutea. It usually regresses following ovariectomy.

Adenoma. **Intraductal adenomas (intraductal papilloma)** are composed of a well-differentiated papillary growth within a dilated or cystic interlobular duct. They are usually solitary, roughly spherical lesions projecting into a duct and well demarcated from a fibrous stroma at their base. The neoplastic cells are low cuboidal and form a single row of cells on a core of connective tissue. If the cells pile up or solid masses of cells appear within the growth, the neoplasm should be considered potentially malignant or a papillary adenocarcinoma.

Acinar adenomas arise from acinar epithelium or small intralobular ducts. They are well circumscribed nodules whose cells form well-differentiated acini or small tubules, which may be dilated or form cysts. The cells closely resemble normal acinar epithelium, and usually there is only a sparse amount of connective tissue present. Some examples in dogs are accompanied by proliferation of myoepithelial (or stromal) cells. These cells resemble plump fibroblasts with slightly vacuolated cytoplasm. When this feature is present, the lesion is termed a complex adenoma (as opposed to simple adenoma). The presence of myoepithelia is of little significance in an adenoma, but in adenocarcinomas, those accompanied by myoepithelial proliferation (complex adenocarcinomas) are of apparently lower malignancy.

In laboratory rats, the most common neoplasm of the mammary gland is the fi-

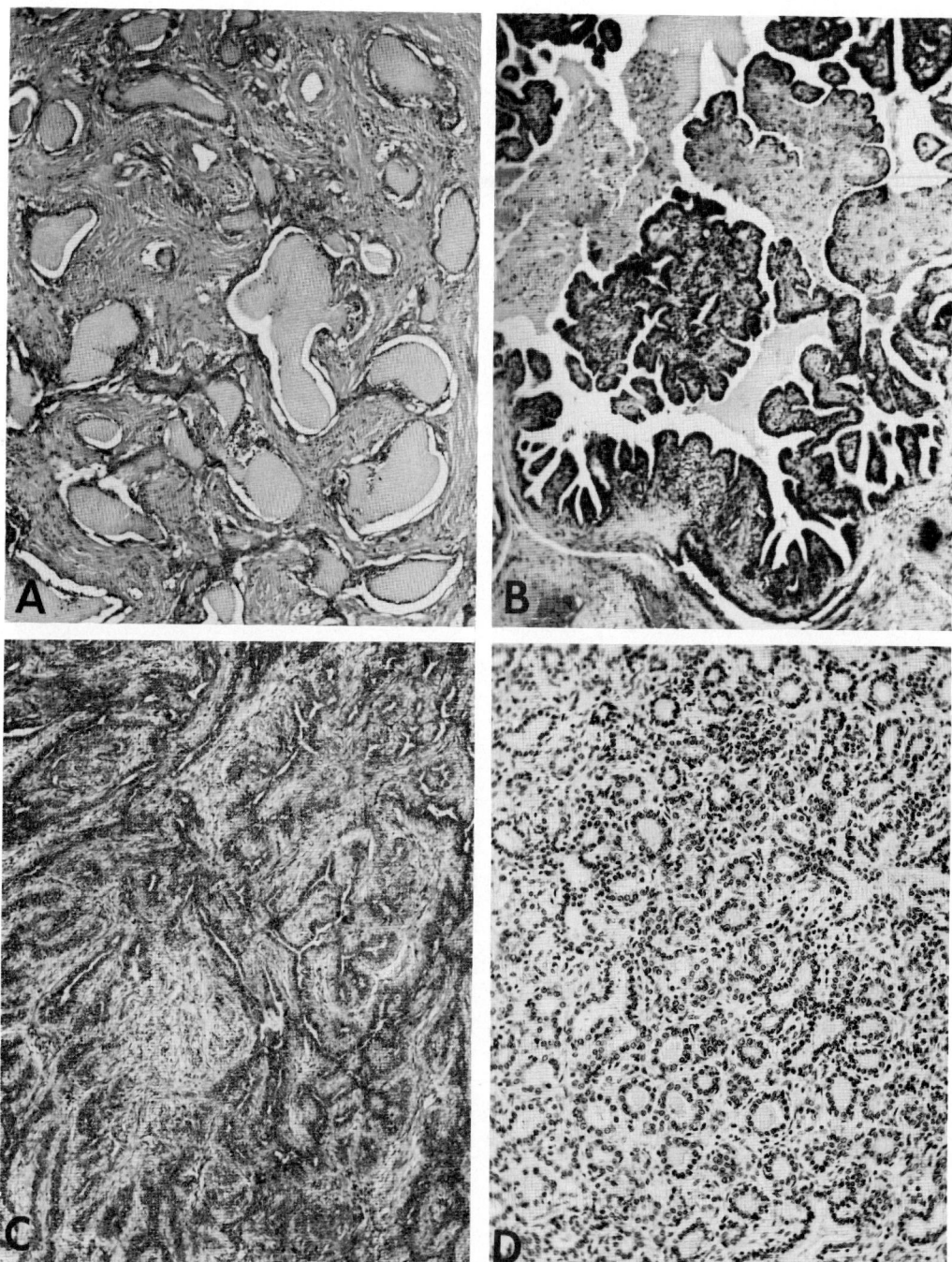

Fig. 25–23. Variations in neoplasms of the mammary gland. *A,* Fibroadenoma, cat. *B,* Papillary (ductal) adenocarcinoma, dog. *C,* Tubular (ductal) adenocarcinoma, dog. *D,* Lobular (acinar) adenocarcinoma, horse. (D, Courtesy of Armed Forces Institute of Pathology.) See text for descriptions.

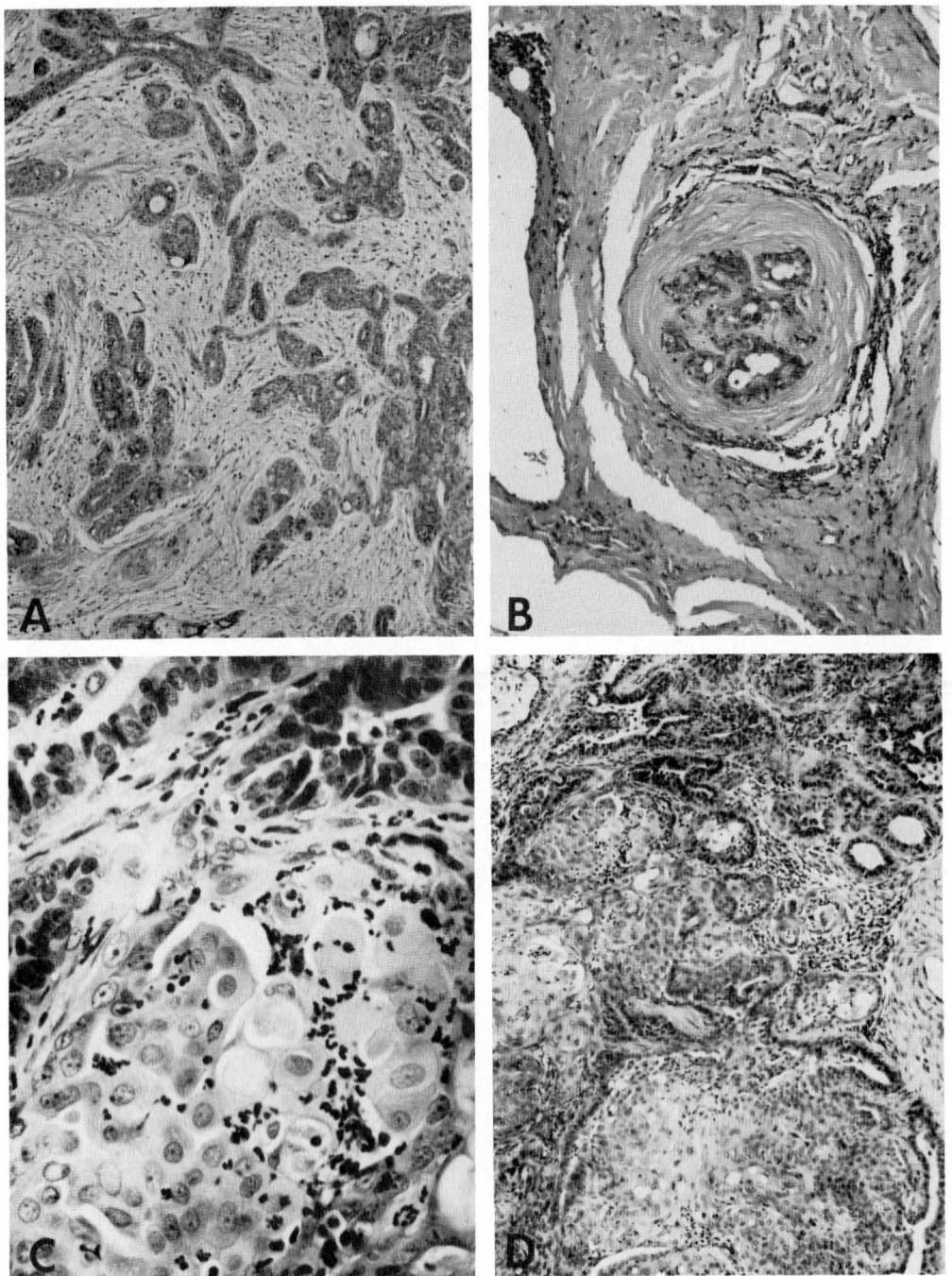

Fig. 25–24. Variations in neoplasms of the mammary gland. *A,* Scirrhous adenocarcinoma, dog. *B,* Scirrhous adenocarcinoma in a lymphatic, dog. *C, D,* Adenoacanthoma, cat. See text for descriptions.

broadenoma. This lesion is composed of well-differentiated acini, ducts, and epithelial-lined cysts embedded in a well-differentiated, relatively acellular collagenous connective tissue. The connective tissue component usually exceeds the epithelial proliferation. However, if the reverse is true, some refer to the tumors as **adenofibromas.** Similar growths are infrequently seen in dogs and other species.

Adenocarcinoma, Carcinoma. Adenocarcinomas and carcinomas may arise from the epithelium lining interlobular ducts or acinar and intralobular ductal epithelial cells. These two histogenic types may be clearly distinguishable, but in many examples, the cell of origin cannot readily be determined, and in others, examples of more than one histologic pattern or all histologic patterns may be represented. Each type may or may not be accompanied by proliferation of myoepithelial cells. If this feature is absent, the neoplasms are termed **simple adenocarcinoma (carcinoma)** and if present, **complex adenocarcinoma (carcinoma).** The complex tumors are generally considered less malignant than the simple histologic type. Invasion of stroma and lymphatics is frequent in all adenocarcinomas and carcinomas. The lymphatics are often occluded with proliferating neoplastic cells and are surrounded by dense collagenous connective tissue. At first sight, they may not resemble lymphatics.

Papillary adenocarcinomas arise from the epithelium lining interlobular or major ducts and grow for a time within their lumens. When clearly present within a duct, they are called **intraductal papillary adenocarcinomas.** In this location, they grow as papillary projections, often of complicated patterns. They differ from papillomas in that the cells are more pleomorphic and anaplastic, and are several cell layers deep over the papillary projections. Variably sized solid masses of cells are also present. The most distinguishing feature, however, is invasion. Individual cells and variably sized groups of cells can be seen extending into their own or the adjacent stroma and frequently into lymphatics. Often there are innumerable circular masses of neoplastic cells evi-

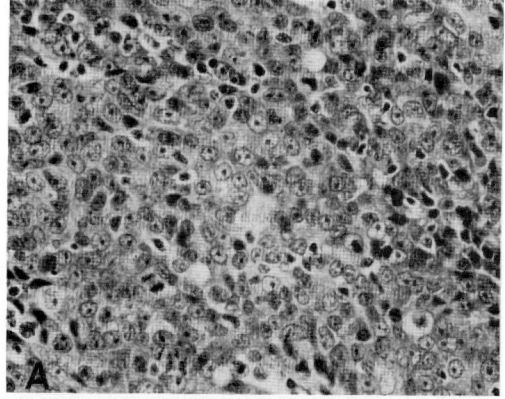
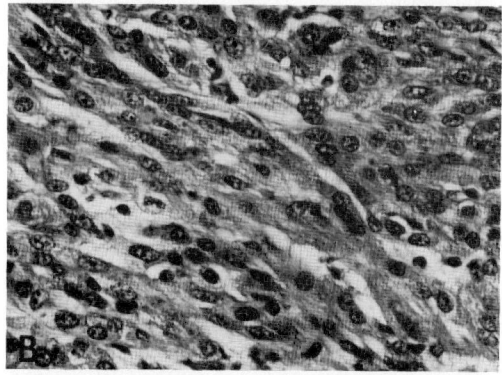
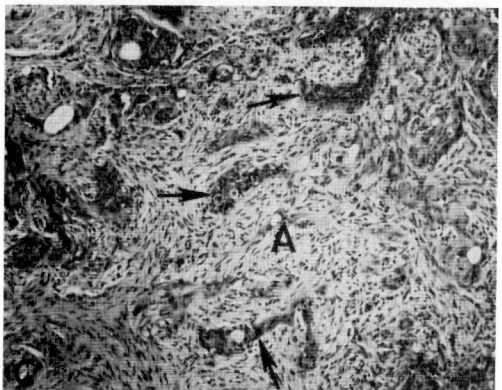

Fig. 25–25. Variations in neoplasms of the mammary gland. *A,* Medullary (solid) carcinoma, dog. *B,* Myoepithelial tumor (spindle cell carcinoma), dog. *C,* Complex tubular adenocarcinoma, dog. Neoplasms containing myoepithelial components (A) in addition to epithelial proliferation (arrows) are termed complex. See text for descriptions.

dent within lymphatics which may be difficult to distinguish from tubules. As they invade the surrounding parenchyma or metastasize to other organs, they continue the same architectural pattern by producing abortive ducts which are more or less filled with papillary projections covered by columnar or cuboidal epithelium. If myoepithelial proliferation accompanies the neoplasm, it is termed **complex,** and if absent, **simple.** Often the neoplastic tubules are cystic and this tumor is termed a **papillary cystadenocarcinoma.**

Tubular adenocarcinomas also arise from interlobular or major ducts, but their mode of growth is not papillary. They are the most frequent form of carcinoma of the mammary gland in dogs. Histologically, they are characterized by relatively uniformly sized tubules lined by single or multilayered cuboidal or columnar epithelial cells and areas of solid masses of cells. The cells may form tortuous intertwining tubules. In some, there are cystic tubules (tubular cystadenocarcinoma). The tumors may be **complex** (with myoepithelial proliferation) or **simple** (without myoepithelial proliferation). There is invasion of stroma comparable to that seen in papillary adenocarcinomas.

Lobular (acinar) adenocarcinomas resemble tubular adenocarcinomas, but the glands more closely resemble acini rather than tubules, and the neoplastic cells are smaller. Differentiation from tubular adenocarcinomas, however, may be difficult. The cells are often separated into varying sized lobules by interlacing strands of connective tissue and are therefore called **lobular adenocarcinomas.** The cells also tend to grow predominantly in sheets rather than forming glands. If this is the predominant pattern, the neoplasm should be termed medullary adenocarcinoma. They usually lack myoepithelial proliferation.

Scirrhous adenocarcinomas may be of tubular or papillary type, but are accompanied by a marked fibroblastic proliferation which differentiates to mature collagenous connective tissue. This reaction is termed a desmoplastic response and is seen in other adenocarcinomas, such as those of the gastrointestinal tract. Neoplastic cells are usually embedded within and invading the dense connective tissue.

Adenoacanthomas are adenocarcinomas admixed with squamous cell carcinoma. They are not frequent. Rarely, pure squamous cell carcinomas arise in the mammary gland. The tumors are invasive and resemble squamous cell carcinomas at other sites.

Medullary (Solid) Carcinoma. This tumor is composed of solid masses of epithelial cells without a significant ductal or acinar pattern of growth. The cells are relatively uniform in size and shape but lack any specific orientation to one another. They could be of tubular or acinar origin, but this is rarely discernible. The tumors are usually invasive into stroma and lymphatics.

Undifferentiated (Anaplastic) Carcinomas. These tumors resemble medullary carcinomas in that there is little differentiation into glandular structures, but the cell type is pleomorphic. The cells vary greatly in size, nuclei are of varying shapes and often hyperchromatic, and multinucleated tumor giant cells are frequent. The tumors invade adjacent stroma and lymphatics.

Mixed Tumors. These tumors contain neoplastic proliferation of both epithelial and mesenchymal tissue. They are the most common mammary tumor in the dog, and rare, but not nonexistent, in the cat. The neoplasms consist of varying admixtures of glandular tissue, myoepithelium, myxomatous connective tissue, cartilage, and bone. Any one of these tissues may constitute the major part of the primary tumor or of its metastases. Thus, tumors consisting principally of cartilage or bone are not rare as the culmination of this metaplastic and neoplastic process, a situation all but limited to the canine mammary gland. Although all elements may appear noninvasive and benign, all mixed tumors should be considered potentially malignant. Malignancy may, however, be clearly evident as the epithelial or mesenchymal elements may be invasive and resemble "typical" adenocarcinoma, osteosarcoma, chrondrosarcoma, etc. Some call these neoplasms **carcinosarcomas.** While ordinarily restricted to females, this tumor has been seen rarely in males. Pulley (1973) has presented evidence that the mesenchymal elements arise from myoepithelial cells,

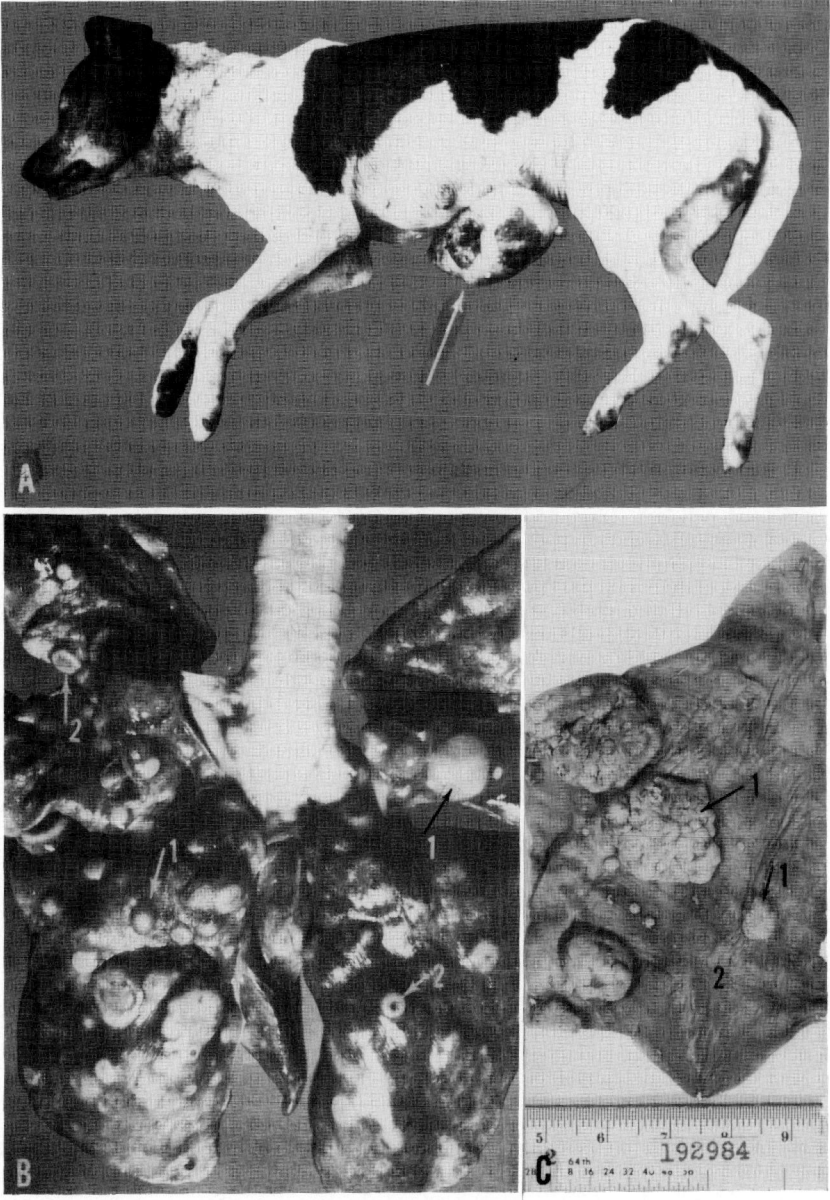

Fig. 25–26. Mixed tumor of the canine mammary gland. *A,* A single tumor of bony hardness in a five-year-old Fox Terrier. *B,* Metastatic nodules of a malignant mixed tumor from the mammary gland of a 13-year-old female Chow. *C,* Metastatic mixed tumor (*1*) on the diaphragm of a 13-year-old female Dachshund. (Courtesy of Armed Forces Institute of Pathology.) Contributor: Dr. A. M. Berkelhammer.

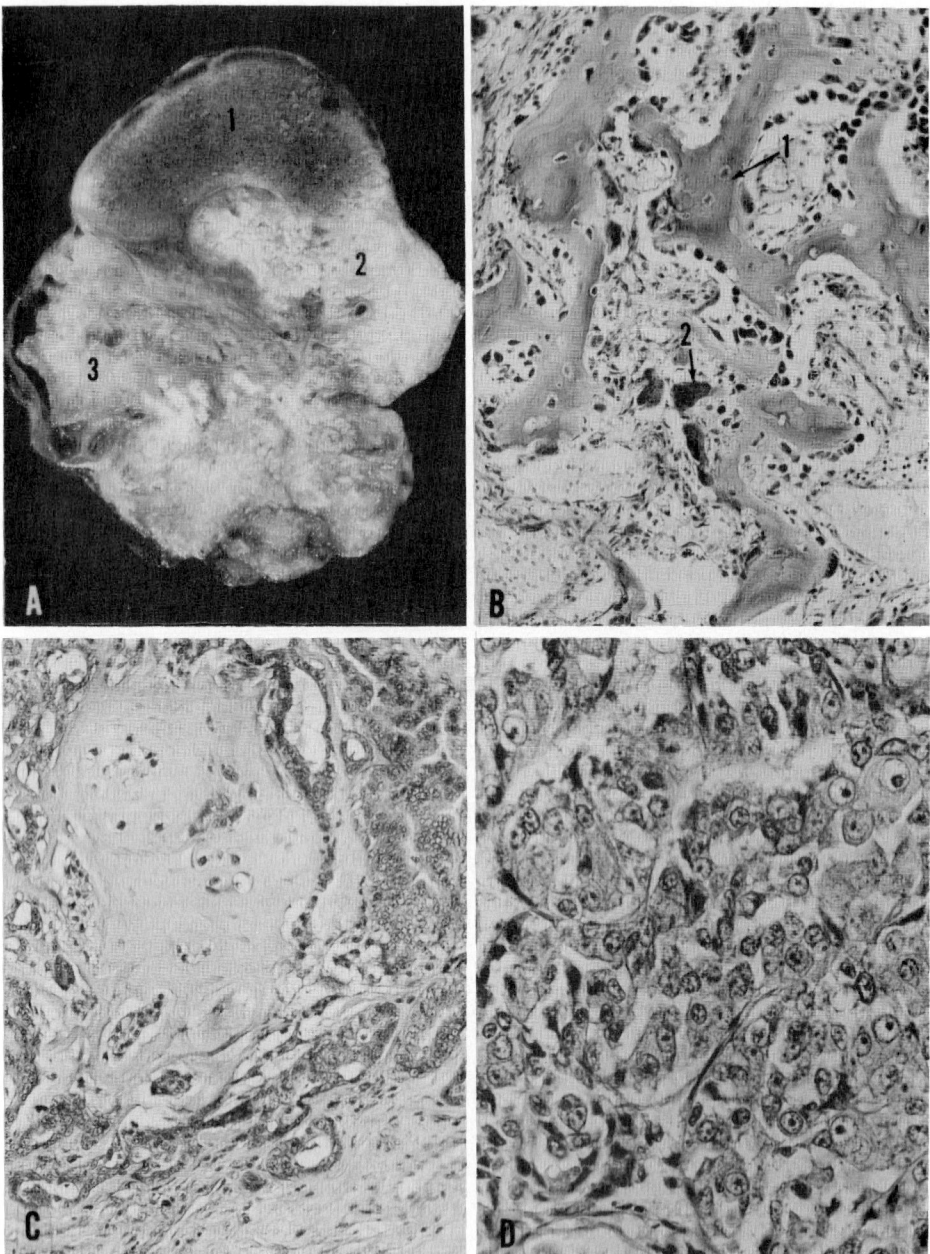

Fig. 25–27.   Mixed tumor of the canine mammary gland. *A,* A circumscribed tumor with bone (*1*), glandular tissue (*2*) and fibrous areas (*3*) recognizable grossly. *B,* Section of the osseous part in *A* (× 130). Spicules of bone (*1*) surrounded by osteoblasts and some osteoclasts (*2*). Contributor: Major Randall J. J. Foley. *C,* Cartilage (× 145) surrounded by epithelial cells in a malignant mixed tumor (see Fig. 25–26C). *D,* Undifferentiated epithelial cells (× 350) in the same tumor as *C*. (Courtesy of Armed Forces Institute of Pathology.) Contributor: Dr. A. M. Berkelhammer.

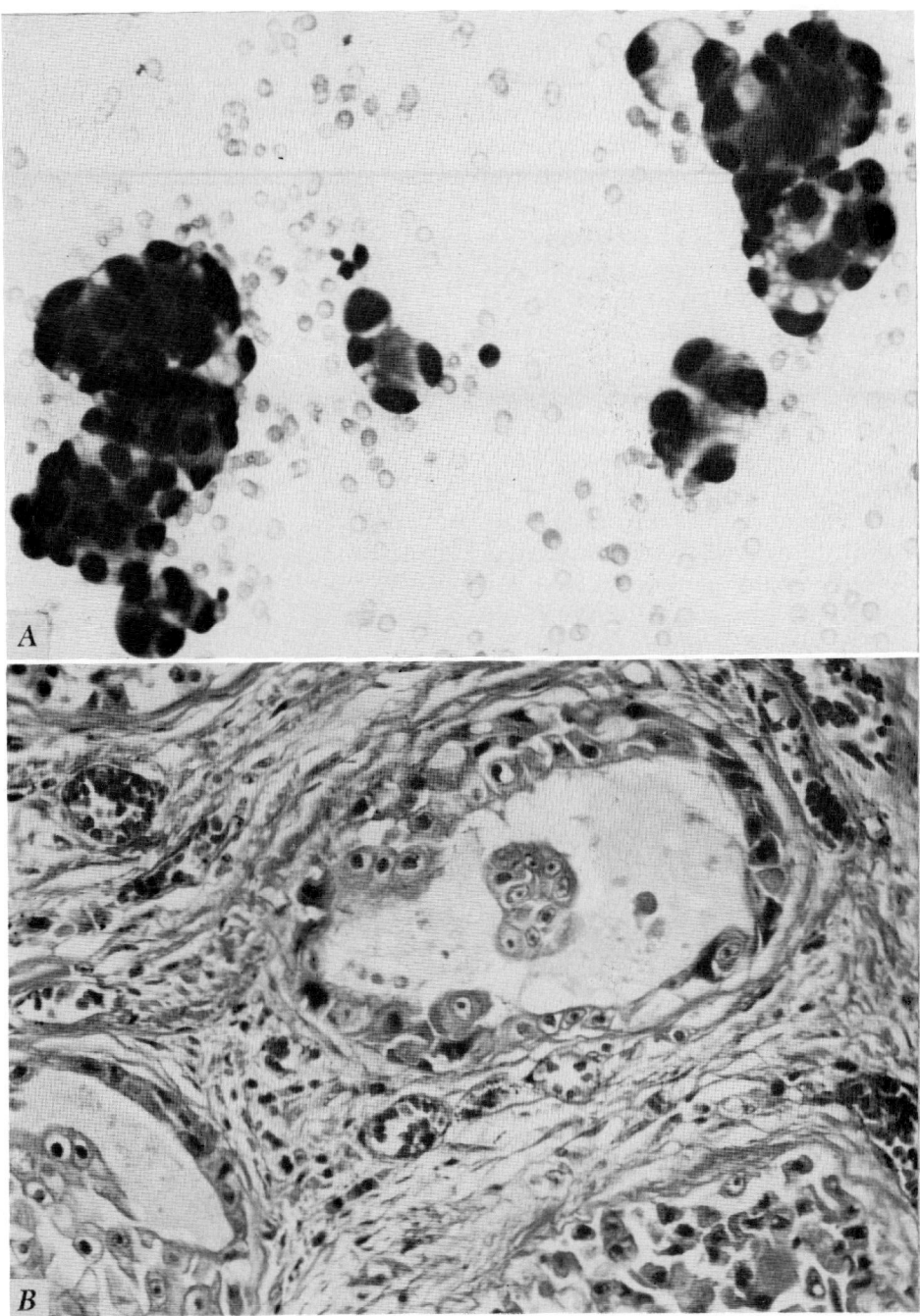

Fig. 25–28. Adenocarcinoma of the mammary gland of a 13-year-old Spitz. Metastases had occurred to the lungs, pleura, and liver. *A,* Smear of fluid aspirated from the pleural cavity. (Wright-Giemsa's stain, × 400.) *B,* Section of the primary tumor in the mammary gland. (H & E, × 400.) (Courtesy of Angell Memorial Animal Hospital.)

but metaplasia of supporting stroma remains plausible.

Sarcomas. Osteosarcomas, chondrosarcomas, fibrosarcomas, and liposarcomas are not uncommon in the mammary gland of the dog, but rare in all other species. Usually the neoplasms contain more than one type of neoplastic mesenchymal cell and are termed **combined sarcomas.** The pathogenesis of these neoplasms is probably related to mixed tumors, but for some unknown reason lack epithelial components.

Myoepithelial Tumor (Spindle Cell Carcinoma). Neoplasms of myoepithelial cells without simultaneous neoplastic transformation of mammary epithelium are occasionally encountered in the dog, but are not common. The tumors are composed of whorls and bundles of cells without any lobular pattern and completely lack any acinar or tubular structures. The cells resemble plump fibroblasts with round or elongated vesicular nuclei and slightly vacuolated cytoplasm. The stroma may have a mucinous appearance. These neoplasms may be malignant, duplicating the architecture in the metastatic neoplasm.

Adinarayanan, N., and Singh, S.B.: Caprine mastitis due to *Klebsiella pneumoniae.* Indian Vet. J., 45:373–377, 1968.

Albiston, H.E.: Actinomycosis of the mammary gland of cows in Victoria. Aust. Vet. J., 6:2–22, 1930.

Allen, A.C.: So-called mixed tumors of the mammary gland of dog and man. Arch. Pathol., 29:589–624, 1940.

Allen, H.L.: Feline mammary hypertrophy. Vet. Pathol., 10:501–508, 1973.

Appleby, E.C., Keymer, I.F., and Hime, J.M.: Three cases of suspected mammary neoplasia in nonhuman primates. J. Comp. Pathol., 84.351–364, 1974.

Bean, C.W., Miller, W.T., and Heishman, J.O.: *Corynebacterium pyogenes* as the cause of bovine mastitis. J. Am. Vet. Med. Assoc., 103:200–202, 1943.

Biggs, R.: Comparison of mixed tumors of human breast and mammary gland of the bitch. J. Pathol. Bacteriol., 59:437–444, 1947.

Bittner, J.J.: Possible relationship of the estrogenic hormones, genetic susceptibility and milk influence in the production of mammary cancer in mice. Cancer Res., 2:710–721, 1942.

Bostock, D.E.: The prognosis following the surgical excision of canine mammary neoplasms. Eur. J. Cancer, 11:389–396, 1975.

Bratlie, O.: Kolimastitis. Norsk vettidsskr., 60:241–252, 1948. Abstr. Vet. Bull. No. 2988, 1950.

Bridré, J., and Donatien, A.: Le microbe de l'agalaxie contagieuse et sa culture *in vitro.* Compt. Rend. Acad. Sci., 177:841–843, 1923.

Cherrington, V.A., and Gildow, E.M.: Bovine mastitis caused by *Pseudomonas aeruginosa.* J. Am. Vet. Med. Assn., 79:803–808, 1931.

Dahme, E., and Weiss, E.: Zur systematik der mammatumoren des hundes. Dtsch. Tieraerztl. Wochenschr., 65:458–461, 1958.

Derbyshire, J.B.: The pathology of experimental staphylococcal mastitis in the goat. J. Comp. Path. & Therap., 68:449–454, 1958.

Eales, J.D., et al.: Bovine mastitis caused by *Nocardia.* Aust. Vet. J., 40:321–324, 1964.

Easterday, B.C., Hanson, R.P., and Simon, J.: Experimental viral bovine mastitis. Am. J. Vet. Res., 20:819–824, 1959.

Eberhart, R.J.: Coliform mastitis. J. Am. Vet. Med. Assoc., 170:1160–1163, 1977.

El Etreby, M.F., and Abdel-Hamid, Y.M.: Experimental ovine mastitis. A pathologic study. Pathol. Vet., 7:246–264, 1970.

Farnsworth, R.J.: Significance of fungal mastitis. J. Am. Vet. Med. Assoc., 170:1173–1174, 1977.

Fidler, I.J., and Brodey, R.S.: A necropsy study of canine malignant mammary neoplasms. J. Am. Vet. Med. Assoc., 151:710–715, 1967.

———: The biological behavior of canine mammary neoplasms. J. Am. Vet. Med. Assoc., 151:1311–1318, 1967.

Fincher, M.G.: Mycoplasma mastitis. Rep. III. Int. Meet. Dis. Cattle, Copenhagen, 100–108, 1964.

Forbes, D.: The pathogenesis of bovine mastitis. Vet. Bull., 39:529–541, 1939.

Fowler, E.H., Wilson, G.P., and Koestner, A.: Biologic behavior of canine mammary neoplasms based on a histogenetic classification. Vet. Pathol., 11:212–229, 1974.

Gibbons, W.J.: Histopathology of mastitis. Cornell Vet., 28:240–249, 1938.

Greene, H.G.N.: Familial mammary tumors in the rabbit. J. Exp. Med., 70:147–184, 1939.

Hayden, D.W., and Nielsen, S.W.: Feline mammary tumours. J. Small Anim. Pract., 12:687–697, 1971.

Heidrich, H.J., and Renk, W.: Diseases of the Mammary Gland of Domestic Animals. Philadelphia, W.B. Saunders Co., 1967.

Innes, J.R.M., Seibold, H.R., and Arentzen, W.P.: Pathology of bovine mastitis caused by *Cryptococcus neoformans.* Am. J. Vet. Res., 13:469–475, 1952.

Jain, N.C., Jasper, D.E., and Dellinger, J.D.: Experimental bovine mastitis due to mycoplasma. Cornell Vet., 59:10–28, 1969.

Jabara, A.G.: Canine mixed tumors (mammary). Aust. Vet. J., 36:212–221, 1960.

Jasper, D.E.: Mycoplasma and mycoplasma mastitis. J. Am. Vet. Med. Assoc., 170:1167–1172, 1977.

Jasper, D.E., Jain, N.C., and Brazil, L.H.: Clinical and laboratory observations on bovine mastitis due to

Mycoplasma. J. Am. Vet. Med. Assn., 148:1017–1029, 1966.

Johnston, L.A.Y., and Connole, M.D.: A case of bovine nocardial mastitis. Austr. Vet. J., 38:462–467, 1962.

Jørgensen, K.L., and Michelsen, E.: Mund og klovesyge-mastitis. (Mastitis in cows infected with F. and M. disease.) Maanedsskr. Dyrlaeg., 58:217–233, 1946. Abstr. Vet. Bull. No. 3193, 1950.

Julian, L.M.: Multiple cisternal polyps of the bovine mammary gland. J. Am. Vet. Med. Assn., 112:238–240, 1948.

Kalra, D.S., Sharma, R.M., and Dhanda, M.R.: Mastitis in goats. Indian J. Vet. Sci., 32:181–189, 1962.

Kirschstein, R.L., Rabson, A.S., and Rusten, G.W.: Infiltrating duct carcinoma of the mammary gland of a Rhesus monkey after administration of an oral contraceptive: a preliminary report. J. Natl. Cancer Inst., 48:551–556, 1972.

Kowalski, J.J.: Microbial agents and bovine mastitis. J. Am. Vet. Med. Assoc., 170:1175–1177, 1977.

Lascelles, A.K.: The function of the mammary lymphatics in staphylococcal and streptococcal mastitis in the sheep. Brit. J. Exp. Path., 43:627–638, 1962.

Loken, K.I., et al.: Infection of the bovine udder with *Candida tropicalis.* J. Am. Vet. Med. Assn., 134:401–403, 1959.

Marsh H.: Mastitis in ewes caused by a pasteurella. J. Am. Vet. Med. Assn., 81:376–382, 1932.

McEwen, A.D., and Cooper, M.B.: Bovine mastitis. Vet. Rec., 59:655–664, 1947.

Misdorp, W., et al.: Canine malignant mammary tumours. I. Sarcomas. Vet. Pathol., 8:99–117, 1971.

————: Canine malignant mammary tumours. II. Adenocarcinomas, solid carcinomas, and spindle cell carcinomas. Vet. Pathol., 9:447–470, 1972.

————: Canine malignant mammary tumors. III. Special types of carcinomas, malignant mixed tumors. Vet. Pathol., 10:241–256, 1973.

Mitchell, L., et al.: Mammary tumors in dogs: survey of clinical and pathological characteristics. Can. Vet. J., 15:131–138, 1974.

Monlux, A.W., Roszel, J.F., MacVean, D.W., and Palmer, T.W.: Classification of epithelial canine mammary tumors in a defined population. Vet. Pathol., 14:194–217, 1977.

Morrill, C.C.: A histopathological study of the bovine udder. Cornell Vet., 28:196–210, 1938.

Moulton, J.E.: Histological classification of canine mammary tumors. Cornell Vet., 44:168–180, 1954.

Moulton, J.E., Taylor, D.O.N., Dorn, C.R., and Andersen, A.C.: Canine mammary tumors. Pathol. Vet., 7:289–320, 1970.

Mulligan, R.M.: Mammary cancer in the dog: a study of 120 cases. Am. J. Vet. Res., 36:1391–1396, 1975.

Mura, D., and Altieri, M.: Sull'etiologia, la patogenesi e la profillassi della mastite gangrenosa delle pecore e delle capre. Zooprofilassi, 5:449–465, 1950.

Mura, D.: Su di una nuova forma di mastite infettiva e contagiosa delle pecore causato dallo *Streptococcus agalactiae.* Vet. Ital., 8:417–430, 1957.

Murphy, J.M., and Stuart, O.M.: Effect of introducing small numbers of *Streptococcus agalactiae* directly into the bovine udder. Cornell Vet., 43:290–310, 1953.

Nelson, L.W., and Shott, L.D.: Mammary nodular hyperplasia in intact Rhesus monkeys. Vet. Pathol., 10:130–134, 1973.

Packer, R.A.: Bovine mastitis produced by *Corynebacteria.* J. Am. Vet. Med. Assoc., 170:1164–1165, 1977.

————: Bovine mastitis caused by *Pseudomonas aeruginosa.* J. Am. Vet. Med. Assoc., 170:1166, 1977.

Packer, R.A., and Merchant, I.A.: Bovine mastitis caused by pasteurellae. North Am. Vet., 27:496–498, 1946.

Parshall, C.J.: Natural and experimental gangrenous mastitis in cows. Cornell Vet., 24:146–155, 1934.

Pattison, I.H.: Histological examination of the teats of goats affected with streptococcal mastitis. J. Comp. Path. and Therap., 62:1–5, 1952.

Pepper, T.A., et al.: *Pasteurella septica (multocida)* mastitis in a dairy herd. Vet. Rec., 83:211–215, 1968.

Posposil, Z., and Salajka, E.: Pathogenesis of coliform mastitis in cattle. II. A comparison of morphological findings in coliform mastitis in cattle and in the experimentally induced Arthus phenomenon in the mammary gland of rabbits. Zentbl. Vet. Med., 15B:607–613, 1968. V.B. 39:461, 1969.

Povey, R.C., and Osborne, A.D.: Mammary gland neoplasia in the cow. A review of the literature and report of a fibrosarcoma. Pathol. Vet., 6:502–512, 1969.

Pulley, L.T.: Ultrastructural and histochemical demonstration of myoepithelium in mixed tumors of the canine mammary gland. Am. J. Vet. Res., 34:1513–1522, 1973.

Renk, W.:Etiology, pathogenesis and morphology of bovine mastitis. Vet. Med. Rev. Leverkusen, 3–31, 1967. V.B. 38:47, 1968.

Runnells, R.A., and Huddleson, I.F.: The nature of *Bacterium abortus* infection in the udder of the bovine. Cornell Vet., 15:376–390, 1925.

Saes, J.M.F.: (*Pasteurella multocida* mastitis in a cow.) Tijdschr. Diergeneesk., 90:37–38, 1965. V.B. 35:2059, 1965.

Salajka, E.: Pathogenesis of coliform mastitis in cattle. I. Classification of the etiologic agent (*Aerobacter aerogenes*) and "natural" immune response to its antigens in cattle. Zentbl. Vet. Med., 15B:607–613, 1968. V.B. 39:461, 1969.

Schalm, O.W.: Gangrenous mastitis in dairy cows. Vet. Med., 39:279–284, 1944.

Schalm, O.W., and Woods, G.M.: Characteristics of coliform mastitis and treatment with dihydro-streptomycin. J. Am. Vet. Med. Assn., 120:385–388, 1952.

Sharma, S.P., and Iyer, P.K.R.: Pathology of chronic lesions in mammary glands of goats (*Capra hircus*): nocardiosis and botryomycosis. Indian J. Anim. Sci., 44:41–45, 1974.

Shone, D.K., Philip, J.R., and Christie, G.J.: Agalactia of sows caused by feeding the ergot of the bulrush millet, *Pennisetum typhoides.* Vet. Rec., 71:129–132, 1959.

Singh, B., and Iyer, P.K.R.: Mammary intraductal carcinoma in goats (*Capra hircus*). Vet. Pathol., 9:441–446, 1972.

Smith, H.: Two cases of actinomycotic mastitis. J. Am. Vet. Med. Assn., 84:635–644, 1934.

Spencer, G.R., and McNutt, S.H.: Pathogenesis of bovine mastitis. Am. J. Vet. Res., 11:188–198, 1950.

Stabenfeldt, G.H., and Spencer, G.R.: The lesions in bovine udders shedding hemolytic coagulase-positive staphylococci. Path. Vet., 2:585–600, 1965.

Straub, O.C., and Kielwein, G.: (Bovine entero-viruses as agents of mastitis). Berl. Munch. Tier-arztl. Wochenschr., 78:386–389, 1965. V.B. 36:1398, 1966.

Stuart, P.: Bovine mastitis caused by *Mycoplasma*. Vet. Rec., 75:59–64, 1963.

Suveges, T.: Pasteurella as the cause of ovine mastitis. (Trans. tile.) Mag. állator. Lapia., 15:214–216, 1960.

Taylor, G.N., et al.: Mammary neoplasia in a closed Beagle colony. Cancer Res., 36:2740–2743, 1976.

Testi, F.: Eosinophilic mastitis in two cows. Nuova Vet., 38:316–324, 1962.

Testi, F., and Biavati, S.T.: (Histology and his-tochemistry of the superficial inguinal lymph nodes in bovine actinogranulomatous mastitis.) Acta Med. Vet. Napoli, 11:307–327, 1965. V.B. 36:4230, 1966.

Tucker, E.W.: Pseudomonas infection of the bovine udder apparently contracted from contaminated treatment equipment and materials. Cornell Vet., 40:95–96, 1950.

————: A case of natural *Pasteurella multocida* mas-titis. Cornell Vet., 43:378–380, 1953.

Turnbull, P.: Acute interstitial mastitis due to strains of *Staphylococcus aureus*. Vet. Rec., 62:255–256, 1950.

Uberreiter, O.: (Mammary tumours in dogs and cats.) Wien. Tierarztl. Mschr., 55:415–442, and 481–503, 1968.

Washko, F.V., and Hutchings, L.M.: Pathogenesis of *Brucella suis* for cattle. Am. J. Vet. Res., 12:165–174, 1951.

Weber, A.F.: The bovine mammary gland: structure and function. J. Am. Vet. Med. Assoc., 170:1133–1136, 1977.

Weijer, K., et al.: Feline malignant mammary tumors. II. Immunologic and electron microscopic inves-tigations into a possible viral etiology. J. Natl. Cancer Inst., 52:673–679, 1974.

Weijer, K., Hampe, J.F., and Misdorp, W.: Mammary carcinoma in cats: a model in comparative cancer research? Arch. Chir. Neer., 25:413–425, 1973.

Weijer, K., Head, K.W., Misdorp, W., and Hampe, J.F.: Feline malignant mammary tumors. I. Mor-phology and biology: some comparisons with human and canine mammary carcinomas. J. Natl. Cancer Inst., 49:1697–1704, 1972.

West, R.L.: Clinical classification of mastitis. J. Am. Vet. Med. Assn., 124:123–124, 1954.

Winslow, D.J.: Botryomycosis. Am. J. Path., 35:153–167, 1959.

Yamagiwa, S., et al.: Histopathological studies on bovine mammary gland. Jpn. J. Vet. Res., 6:51–61, 1958. (In Engl.) 11:12–25, 67–86, 1963.

MALE GENITAL ORGANS

Having a less burdensome role in the reproductive process than their female counterparts, the male genital organs are less subject to disease. This same statement can be made even of neoplastic disease. How interesting it would be to know whether the reason for this less-pro-nounced susceptibility to neoplasia is in-deed related to less complicated or less pro-longed functional processes in the male or possibly to differences in the histologic, physiologic, or genetic structure of the var-ious organs of the two sexes. Or is it that the female organs run a continuous gauntlet of exposure to physical or chemi-cal injury during the ever-changing repro-ductive cycle? Leaving those questions to be answered by the investigators and phi-losophers of the future, we do find a number of masculine diseases demanding our attention.

Testicular Tissue

Anomalies and Functional Disorders

Developmental abnormalities of the tes-tis and epididymis are rare with the exception of cryptorchidism (see below). **Hypoplasia** is seen in cryptorchidism and hermaphroditism, and in chromosomal abnormalities such as the XXY or Kline-felter's syndrome, which has been de-scribed in cats, cattle, swine, and sheep. Hereditary forms of testicular and ovarian hypoplasia have been documented in rab-bits and guinea pigs, and similar examples (often unilateral) have been reported in Swedish Highland cattle, Merino, and Romney rams. Failure of one or more of the rete mesonephric tubules to connect with the mesonephric duct (future vas deferens) may lead to blind tubules which fill with spermatozoa and are known as **spermatoceles.** Similar dilations can also be acquired and if ruptured will lead to spermatic granulomas. Rarely, the vas deferens may fail to develop in its entirety or part.

Heterotopic displacement of testicular tissue has been reported in swine (Todd, et al., 1968). The testicular tissue was found embedded in or attached to the liver, spleen, mesentery, pancreas, stomach, omentum, colon, cecum, and diaphragm. Grossly, these usually resembled neoplasms, but histologically were seen to consist of atrophic testicular tissue resembling cryptorchid testes. The origin of these testicular implants is not known. It is postulated that they may arise from displaced germ cells or possibly from surgical procedures such as castration.

Cryptorchidism. With a literal meaning of "hidden testicle," this relatively mild developmental disorder results from failure of one or both testes to descend, with their tunics, from their fetal position in the sublumbar region, through the inguinal canal, and into the scrotal sac. While normally an event of fetal life, it is not unusual for the complete descent into the scrotum to be delayed until several months after birth. Permanent retention is most important and most frequent in horses, swine, and dogs. In cattle and sheep, cryptorchidism is quite uncommon.

The cryptorchid testis fails to completely develop because of the disadvantages of its position, with its size remaining small and its consistency soft. The seminiferous tubules, if formed, are rudimentary, lacking most of the layers of reproductive cells. Only quite exceptionally is there any spermatogenesis. The interstitial cells are likely to be few and buried in much fibrous tissue, but there are cases in which these cells are unduly numerous. There have been instances where the cryptorchid testis proved to be no more than a modified vas deferens, with many tributary tubules. The reason for this hypoplasia of the cryptorchid testis appears to be less a matter of the unnatural pressures upon it than it is the higher temperature of the abdominal cavity. Experimental work indicates that the cooler environment of the scrotal sac is necessary for proper development and spermatogenesis.

The anatomic cause of cryptorchidism is often discovered in the form of a misplaced gubernaculum or shortened spermatic vessels, cremaster muscle or vas deferens, but the fundamental cause is commonly suspected to be hereditary. There is statistical support for this theory. On the other hand, Manning (1950) induced cryptorchidism in rats previously normal by a diet of egg whites (deficient in biotin). Of interest is that the testes of the elephant normally remain in the abdomen.

Testicular neoplasms arise with greater frequency in cryptorchid testes than in descended ones.

Hermaphroditism. Since the genital tracts of both sexes develop primarily from the same embryonic primordium, it is perhaps not surprising that occasionally structures characteristic of both sexes are found in the same individual. In a true hermaphrodite, both ovarian and testicular tissue occur either in united or separate structures. A male pseudohermaphrodite has more or less normal testes, but the accessory reproductive organs resemble those of the female. In the female pseudohermaphrodite, ovaries are present, but the tubular reproductive tract is rudimentary, and the external genitalia bear an anatomic resemblance to those of the male. The uterus masculinus constitutes a normal persistence in the male of parts of the female genital tract. It is usually of appreciable size in the stallion, and in some species, for instance, the guinea pig, it is a well-developed anatomic structure. Hermaphroditism represents a form of congenital malformation.

Various forms of intersexuality are discussed further in connection with chromosomal anomalies and under the "Ovary."

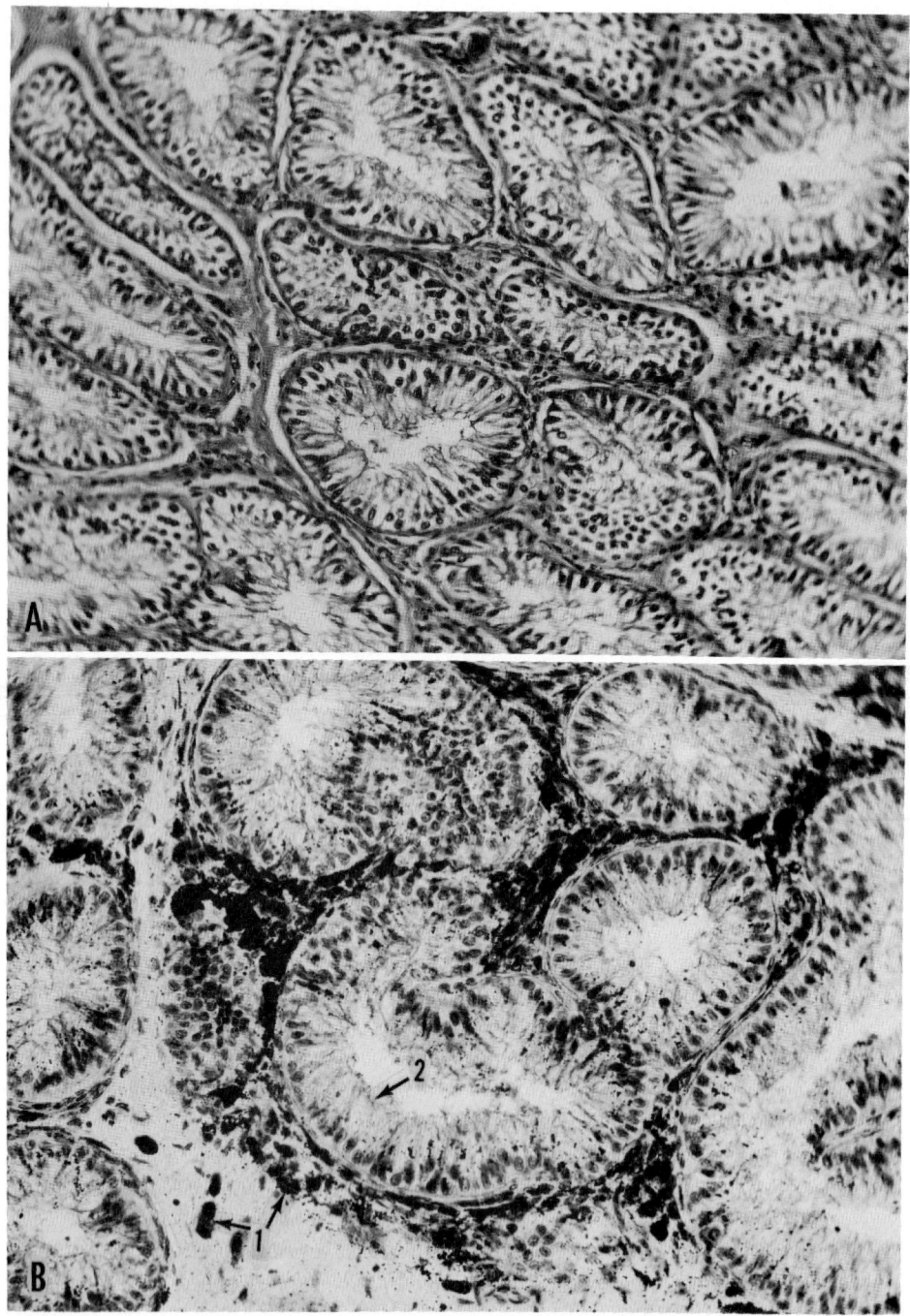

Fig. 25–29. Cryptorchid testis in a dog. *A*, Note tubules are lined completely with tall columnar Sertoli cells. (H & E stain, × 160.) *B*, Section stained with Sudan III to demonstrate lipid in interstitial cells (*1*) and Sertoli cells (*2*). (*B*, Courtesy of Armed Forces Institute of Pathology.) Contributor: Dr. Leo L. Lieberman.

Orchitis. Inflammation of the testicular tissue may occur in any species, but is probably more frequent in sheep, cattle, and swine. It is possible that many cases begin as an **epididymitis,** an infectious cause spreading up the tubular passages into the testicle proper.

Acute epididymitis, when mild in degree, may conceivably be mucous in nature, within the tubular linings. Such a change, with the exudation of considerable mucus, may possibly account for changes in viscosity of the seminal fluid, although a mucous exudate is much more likely to come from the epithelial-lined structures lower down in the genital chain. It is possible and not illogical to regard the necrotic and other degenerative changes which result from infectious and toxic agents as part of an alterative inflammatory process, as in the case of the liver. But ordinarily, acute orchitis and epididymitis are purulent or suppurative, either diffuse or localized, often with abscesses. There is usually also much acute inflammatory edema (serous exudate) of the surrounding tissues, although swelling of the testicle proper is sharply limited by its inelastic tunic.

Chronic inflammation is characterized by fibrous or reticuloendothelial proliferation here, as elsewhere, with or without the accompaniment of active exudation. The specific granulomas may involve the testes; tuberculous orchitis is not especially rare in animals already having primary lesions elsewhere. Actinomycosis of the bovine testicle has been described (Bieberdorf, 1953), although diagnosis appears to have been made on bacteriological evidence alone without identification of the lesion.

Causes. The causes of ordinary acute orchitis may be traumatic or infectious. The former are especially frequent in the ram because of the pendulous position of the testicles and their liability to injury. In such cases, the tissues of the scrotum share perhaps more violently in the acute inflammatory hyperemia, edema, and infiltration than do those of the testis proper.

Infectious orchitis may result from hematogenous metastasis or from extension of infection up the genital tract and through the epididymis, as previously mentioned. **Brucellosis** (Bang's disease) in the bull and in the boar commonly manifests itself as a severe orchitis, which may be both necrotizing and suppurative. In view of the well-known predilection which this infection has for reproductive tissue, it would be dangerous to offer an opinion as to whether entrance of the organism is hematogenous or by extension. Infections of other parts of the genital tube can often be demonstrated, but the vas deferens itself is seldom injured. In some cases, brucellosis of the testicle, most often unilateral, becomes chronic with much fibrous enlargement of the testicle, the functional tissue of which has been extensively or completely destroyed. The peritesticular and scrotal tissues usually share in the inflammatory proliferation, perhaps with pus between the layers of the tunica vaginalis.

Brucella ovis causes a specific disease known as **ram epididymitis.** It is not associated with orchitis.

An acute suppurative orchitis with or without abscesses has been described in the horse as the result of infection with the abortion-producing *Salmonella abortus-equi* (Jansen, 1946; Helmy, et al., 1966). The orchitis was accompanied by fever and general bodily reaction during its acute stage.

The other abortifacient microorganisms (*Vibrio, Trichomonas*) appear not to invade the male genital system beyond its external parts. Nonspecific hematogenous orchitis occurs occasionally in the course of various infections which assume a generalized form, such as equine strangles. An organism causing a severe purulent orchitis in rams was identified as *Pasteurella pseudotuberculosis (Corynebacterium pseudotuber-*

culosis rodentium), which is ordinarily a pathogen of guinea pigs (Jamieson and Soltys, 1947). The organism of blue-green pus (*Pseudomonas aeruginosa, Bacillus pyocyaneus*) has been identified in diseased male genital tracts, apparently without being responsible for marked lesions (Rempt and Zwanenburg, 1948). In a diagnostic test known as the **Strauss reaction,** male guinea pigs often develop periorchitis and a necrotizing and destructive suppurative orchitis a few days subsequent to intraperitoneal inoculation of small doses of the glanders bacillus as well as of the organisms which cause melioidosis, epizootic lymphangitis, ulcerative lymphangitis, and ovine caseous lymphadenitis. In humans, mumps is a disease which often includes orchitis in its manifestations when it attacks adult males.

Effects. The effects of the more severe forms of orchitis are obvious: destruction of the testis, marked pain, and in some cases a generalized febrile disease with fatal septicemia. The mildest forms result in at least temporary **aspermatogenesis.** This depends upon necrosis and destruction of the germinal cells lining the seminiferous tubules. The more superficial cells perish first; often the process continues until none but the sustentacular (Sertoli) cells remain to line the tubules. A high percentage of deformed and imperfect spermatozoa supervenes upon such injury to the germinal epithelium (Andreevskii, 1948), provided, of course, the disorder is slight so that some spermatogenesis still continues. Regeneration does not occur once the germinal tissue has been completely destroyed. In evaluating these milder lesions, it should be remembered that certain areas of aspermatogenesis may be encountered in the normal testis, as if they were in a resting or dormant state.

Torsion

Especially when the spermatic cord is unusually long or relaxed, the testicle may be rotated on its axis by trauma, exercise, or straining. In dogs, torsion of the testis occurs most often in cryptorchid testis, especially those with neoplasms. The twisting of the blood vessels produces venous and often arterial obstruction, leading to congestion and edema in mild cases. With more complete obstruction, these changes are accompanied by necrosis, at least of the delicate cells lining the seminiferous tubules. The condition is essentially that of an infarction involving the whole organ. **Infarction** of the testis or a segment of it can also occur as the result of thrombosis or embolism in the spermatic vessels, although the condition is not common.

Granuloma

Spermatic granuloma is a name given to small masses of granulation tissue, usually with a foreign-body reaction, which form around foci of escaped spermatozoa in the testis or epididymis. They are not rare (Fig. 25–30). Spermatozoa contain sequestered antigens and elicit humoral and delayed immune reactions. Their escape or release into tissues is important to the pathogenesis of orchitis and epididymitis, analogous to the release of thyroglobulin in thyroiditis.

Neoplasms

Primary tumors of the testes are seen most frequently in the dog, but in part this

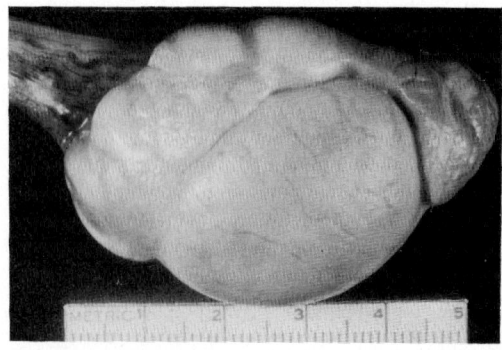

Fig. 25–30. Spermatic granulomas in epididymis of a seven-year-old male Beagle. (Courtesy of Angell Memorial Animal Hospital.)

is probably because intact males are available for observation in far larger numbers in this than in other domestic species. The Boxer breed has a higher incidence, as is the case with many other neoplasms. The types peculiar to the testicle are the seminoma, the sustentacular-cell or Sertoli-cell tumor, the interstitial-cell or Leydig-cell tumor, and the teratoma.

Seminoma. One of the three neoplasms peculiar to the testicle, the seminoma arises from the germinal epithelium of the seminiferous tubules. Seminomas occur most frequently in older dogs, although their rarity in other domestic species may well be due merely to early castration of most other species. They are often multicentric in origin, may arise in scrotal and cryptorchid testicles, and may be bilateral. They are not associated with hormonal effects. Grossly, seminomas on cut surface are soft, white to pale gray, and bulge above adjacent tissue. Microscopically, the seminoma is composed of large polyhedral cells with prominent round nuclei, cen-

trally located, not unlike spermatogonia and spermatocytes. Their nuclei contain conspicuous chromatin bodies, a feature that aids in distinguishing this tumor from some of the larger-celled malignant lymphomas and from the transmissible venereal tumors in cases in which a diagnosis is to be made without knowledge of the source of the tissue. Mitotic figures are likely to be frequent in all these tumors. Fine trabeculae divide the masses of cells into compartments. While this tumor is often deadly in men, in the dog it is much less to be feared. It tends to spread slowly along the spermatic cord (where the surgeon should seek it), but reasonably early removal is usually curative. Metastasis is rare.

A unique feature of some value in distinguishing the seminoma from other tumors encountered in the canine testicle is the rather frequent occurrence of small collections of cells, which are apparently lymphocytes, in the midst of the neoplastic cells.

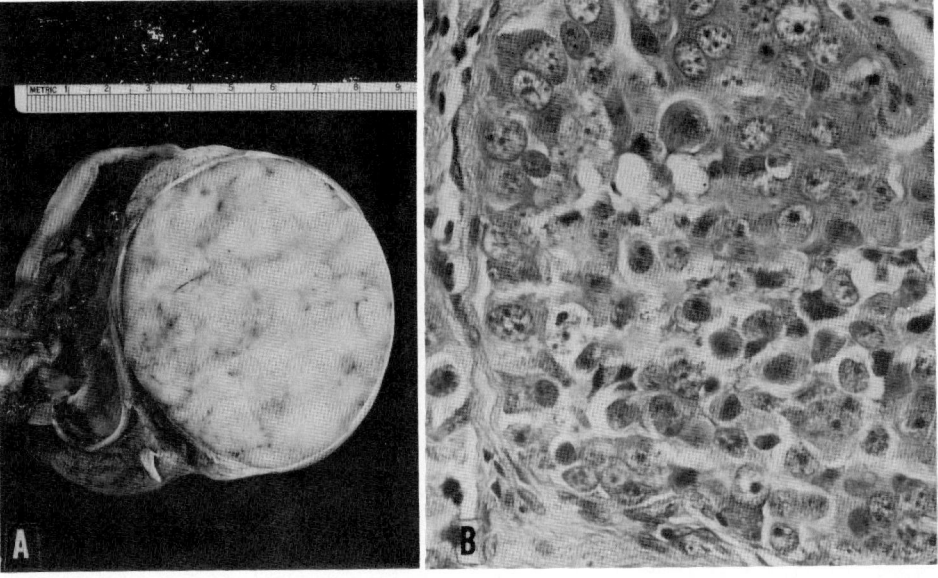

Fig. 25–31. Seminoma. *A,* Spherical mass in the testicle of a 17-year-old Chow dog. Contributor: Dr. Edward Records. *B,* Seminoma (× 355) testicle of an eight-year-old Pomeranian. Large spherical cells with hyperchromatic nuclei. (Courtesy of Armed Forces Institute of Pathology.) Contributor: Angell Memorial Animal Hospital.

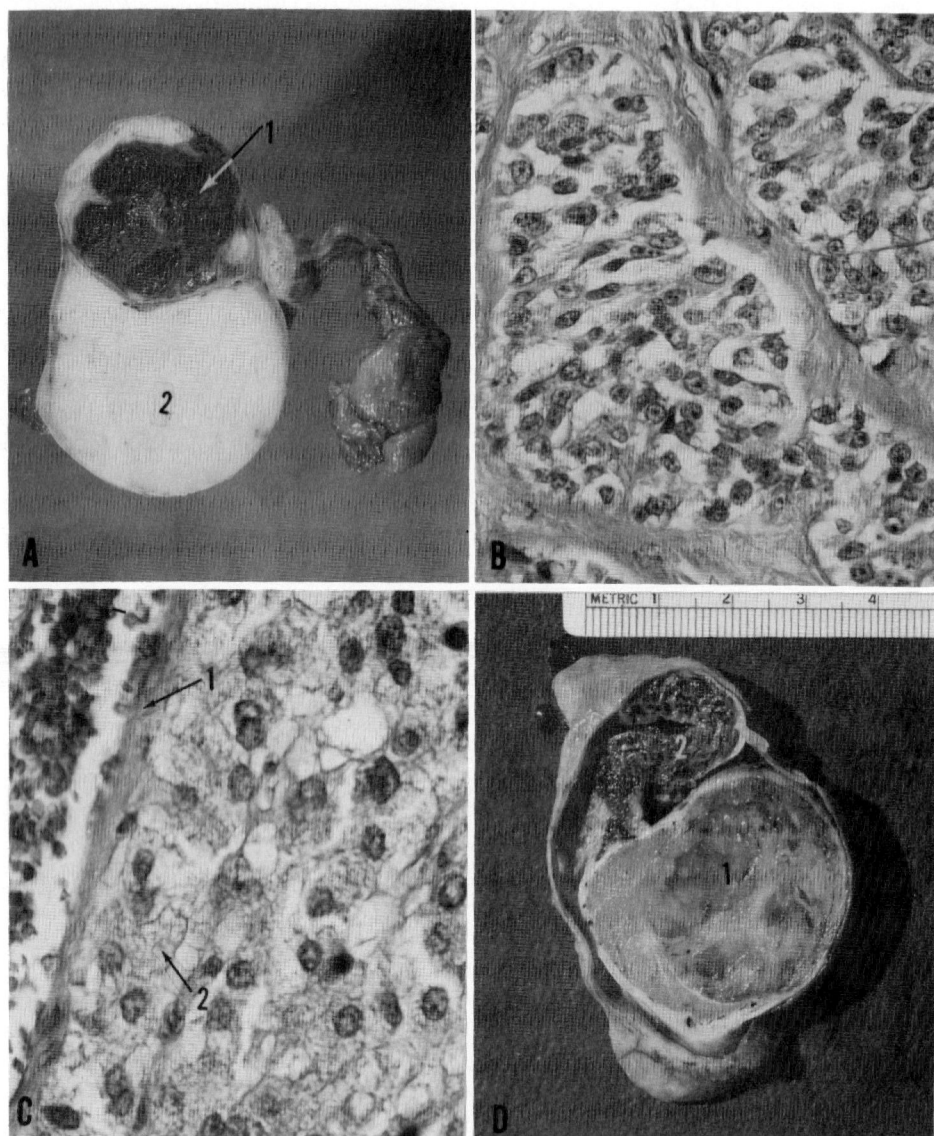

Fig. 25–32. *A,* Interstitial cell tumor (*1*) and Sertoli cell tumor (*2*), testis of a 12-year-old Dachshund. Contributor: Dr. Robert Ferber. *B,* Sertoli cell tumor (× 355), testicle of a nine-year-old Boston Terrier. Elongated, lipid-containing Sertoli cells in irregular nests. Contributor: Angell Memorial Animal Hospital. *C,* Interstitial cell tumor (× 435), testis of an eight-year-old Beagle. Blood vessels (*1*) intimately related to lipid-bearing interstitial cells (*2*). *D,* Interstitial cell tumor (*1*) displacing testicular parenchyma. Epididymis (*2*). Same case as *C.* (Courtesy of Armed Forces Institute of Pathology.) Contributor: Angell Memorial Animal Hospital.

Sertoli-cell, or Sustentacular-cell Tumor. As its name implies, this tumor arises from the sustentacular, or Sertoli cells of the seminiferous tubules. While a few may develop areas so anaplastic as to consist of solid masses of round or polyhedral cells with central nuclei, the majority of these tumors contain some areas in which continuity can be traced to seminiferous tubules of normal size and shape, but with their lining devoid of germinal cells, one or two irregular layers of tall Sertoli cells remaining. An intermediate type of structure consists of solidly filled tubules, the cells being radially elongated, angular, and with a cytoplasm that is more or less clear because of high lipid content. The common synonym of **tubular adenoma** aptly describes this, the usual appearance of the Sertoli-cell tumor.

Grossly, the Sertoli-cell tumor is likely to consist of one or more nodules which may greatly distend the tunica albuginea,

reaching several times the size of the normal testis. The cut surface bulges and is gray or light yellow. The rare anaplastic forms of this tumor spread into the surrounding structures and up the spermatic cord, and may metastasize to the sublumbar lymph nodes.

The Sertoli-cell tumor occurs almost exclusively in the dog, the human counterpart being rare. It is the most frequent tumor in the cryptorchid testicle. It commonly produces a feminizing hormone with the result that the mammae enlarge, the hair of the belly is thinned, and the dog becomes sexually attractive to other males. Squamous metaplasia of the prostate and urinary epithelium also result. This is comparable to the metaplasia noted following the feeding of stilbestrol to fattening sheep. The metaplasia has also been produced experimentally in dogs (Fig. 25–33).

Interstitial, or Leydig-cell Tumor. This

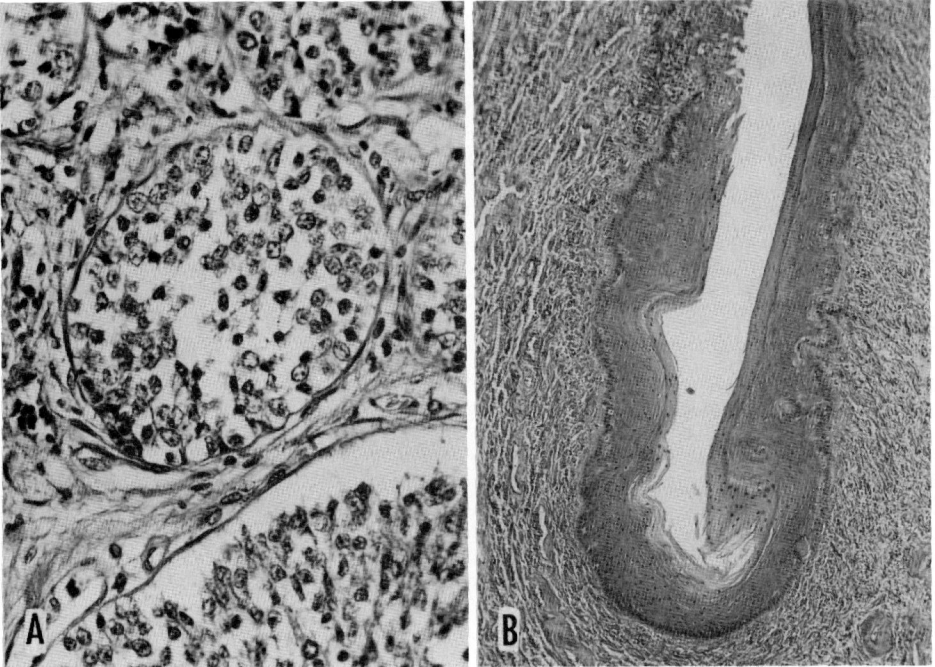

Fig. 25–33. Feminizing effect of Sertoli-cell tumor. *A,* Sertoli-cell tumor (× 350) of the testis of a dog. *B,* Squamous metaplasia of the urethra (× 70) of the same dog, one of the effects of hyperestrogenism. (Courtesy of Armed Forces Institute of Pathology.) Contributor: Rowley Memorial Animal Hospital.

neoplasm arises from the interstitial, androgen-secreting cells of the testis. Its cells are larger and have more eosinophilic cytoplasm than the two previous testicular tumors. The cytoplasm contains large amounts of lipids, which accounts for its foamy character and for a distinctly yellow color grossly. Much of the fat is anisotropic under the polarizing microscope. The cells form masses divided into compartments by fibrous trabeculae. Mitotic figures are seldom found. This tumor is the most frequent of the testicular tumors in the dog and, like the other testicular tumors, would probably be seen more frequently in other species, if the males were not castrated at an early age. It has been reported in a cryptorchid equine testicle (Smith, 1954) and in a 6-year-old bovine which had been castrated by inversion of both testes within the scrotum and torsion of their spermatic cords. McEntee (1958) reported a particularly high incidence in a strain of Guernseys. Secretion of excess androgen by the tumor can sometimes be demonstrated in early life, but at a later period, the opposite hormonal effect may be demonstrable. Usually in the dog no hormonal effects are observed clinically.

An interesting compilation from the Angell Memorial Animal Hospital shows that, of 520 canine testicular tumors, 38% were interstitial-cell tumors, 32% seminomas, and 30% Sertoli-cell tumors. In a surprisingly high number of cases, the same patient had two different testicular tumors, and in four patients, all three types were present. Among 42 cryptorchid testicles, 12 were tumorous.

Teratoma. The testicle and ovary are the most usual locations for teratomas. They are discussed under neoplasms of the ovary.

Hydrocele

Whereas hydrothorax, for example, is an accumulation of watery fluid in the thoracic cavity, hydrocele is an accumulation of watery fluid in the cavity of the scrotum. Usually the fluid lies between all adjacent layers of the tunica vaginalis and occupies all spaces between the testicle proper and the skin.

While hydrocele occurs occasionally as an accompaniment of generalized edema involving the whole ventral belly wall, it is ordinarily the result of intrascrotal disorders. These include interference with the return flow in the spermatic veins. In the majority of cases, however, hydrocele is an inflammatory edema, as shown not only by the causative circumstances, but also by the higher specific gravity and protein content of the fluid, which are such as to place it in the category of an exudate and not of a transudate. The condition is thus a histologically mild inflammatory disease of the scrotal tissues (with or without the testis proper) and is caused most often by trauma, sometimes by local infections.

Scirrhous Cord

While elephantiasis of the scrotum comparable to that seen in humans as an effect of *Filaria (Wuchereria) bancrofti* does not occur in the domestic animals, a superficially similar gross enlargement of the scrotum and its contents occurs in scirrhous cord. The disorder is merely excessive granulation tissue forming on the stump of the severed spermatic cord following castration, the cause being a chronic hyperplastic proliferative inflammation resulting from untoward operative injury and infection. It is common in pigs because of their proximity to the soil, their commonly unsanitary surroundings, and the crude sort of surgery which is sometimes performed by stockmen. The species next most frequently involved is the equine because of the horse's notoriously poor resistance to many of the ordinary infections, chiefly pyogenic.

The mass of abnormal tissue may attain startling proportions in a few weeks. It consists usually of dense fibrous tissue alternating irregularly with areas of more youthful and more active fibroblastic growth. Some areas contain much leukocytic infiltration. There are often thick-walled, chronic abscesses. Under the name of botryomycosis, a form has been described in equines in which the granulation tissue assumes a reticuloendothelial form suggestive of actinomycosis, with the formation of rosettes. This condition is in fact attributable to a staphylococcus, but it is not meant to imply that the usual case of scirrhous cord is anything more than the ordinary type of pyogenic granulation tissue. Scirrhous cords are usually terminated by operative removal.

Accessory Structures

Aplasia or lack of the epididymis is an anomaly occasionally seen in bulls but rare in other species. It represents segmental aplasia of the wolffian duct. In the Simmental breed, it has been reported to be inherited as a recessive trait (Konig, et al., 1972). Congenital cysts of the epididymis are common in rams. They may be filled with watery fluid or sperm (spermatocele), which if ruptured will lead to spermatic granuloma.

Epididymitis accompanies or may precede orchitis, in connection with which it has been mentioned.

In sheep, *Brucella ovis* causes a disease known as **ram epididymitis**, which is the most important abnormality of the male sex organs in this species. The organism invades the epididymis leading to edema, lymphocytic infiltration, epithelial hyperplasia, and fibrosis. Escape of sperm results in spermatic granuloma. Obstruction of the epididymis may follow, causing sterility if bilateral. The disease is transmitted by sexual contact between rams and recently serviced ewes, and via urine.

Epididymitis in sheep has also been ascribed to infection by *Actinobacillus seminis* by several authors (Livingston and Hardy, 1964; Simmons, et al., 1966).

Inflammation of the **vas deferens** is rare because of its simple and impervious structure and excellent drainage.

The seminal vesicles and bulbo-urethral glands (in those species which have them) tend to harbor infections because of their complicated structure and poor drainage. They are thus of some importance as sites of localization of brucellosis, vibriosis, and trichomoniasis, as well as for the locally less destructive *Pseudomonas aeruginosa (pyocyaneus)*. In the bovine seminal vesicle, pronounced metaplasia of the columnar epithelial lining to a heavily cornified stratified squamous type has been noted, apparently due to avitaminosis A. Well-marked melanosis has been seen in the bulbo-urethral (Cowper's) gland of the ram.

A syndrome involving the seminal vesicles of male bovine animals has been described and given the name **seminal vesiculitis**. An organism of the psittacosis group (*Chlamydia*) has been isolated from the semen and epididymis of affected bulls (Storz, et al., 1968; Ball, et al., 1968). *Mycoplasma bovigenitalium* as well as many bacteria such as *Corynebacterium pyogenes, C. renale, Brucella abortus*, coliform, *Pseudomonas aeruginosa*, and mycobacteria have also been associated with seminal vesiculitis.

Neoplasms of the accessory structures are rare.

Prostate

In cattle, sheep, and swine, the prostate is little more than rudimentary in size, much of its glandular tissue being disseminated in the wall of the upper urethra. The equine prostate is also relatively small; its function, limited; its diseases, rare. The dog's prostate, however, is well developed, as if to compensate for the absence of seminal vesicles and bulbo-urethral glands in this species. The diseases of the canine prostate are of importance and appear to be entirely comparable to those seen in the human being.

Acute prostatitis occurs infrequently except in the dog. It is ordinarily suppurative, often with formation of abscesses.

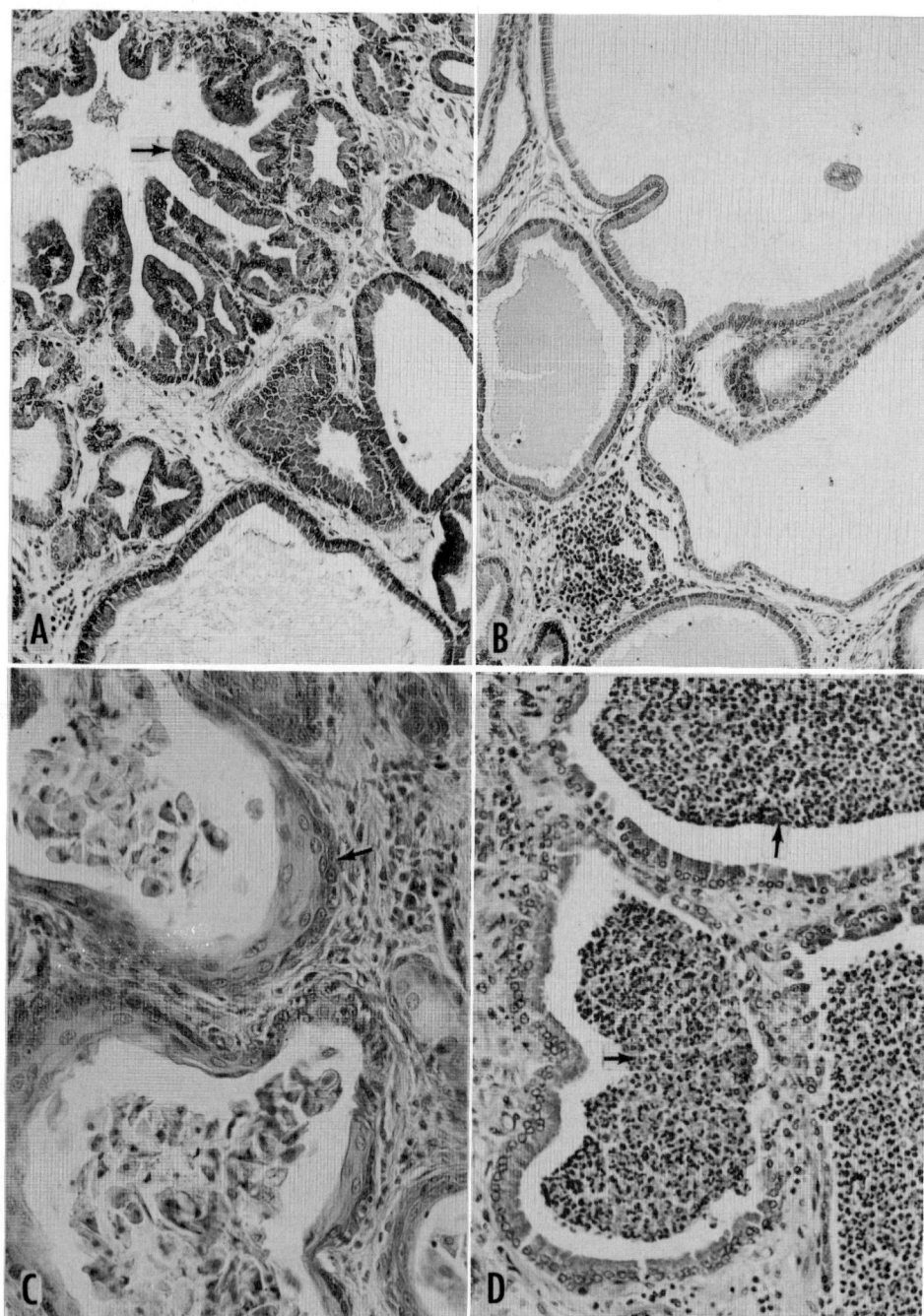

Fig. 25–34. *A,* Hyperplasia of the canine prostate. Note tall columnar cells (arrows) in long fronds extending into the lumen of prostatic acinus. Contributor: Dr. S. Pollock. *B,* Cystic glandular hyperplasia of the canine prostate. Cysts are formed in parts of the gland. Contributor: Dr. Norman G. Simels. *C,* Squamous metaplasia (arrow) of the prostate of a dog with a Sertoli cell tumor of the testis. Contributor: Dr. Wayne H. Riser. *D,* Acute purulent prostatitis in a dog. Note acini filled with neutrophils and cellular debris. (*A–D,* Courtesy of Armed Forces Institute of Pathology.) Contributor: Dr. Albert M. Berkelhammer.

There may be a number of abscesses, small or microscopic in size or there may be one or two of large size, a maximum diameter of 11 cm having been reported (Schlotthauer, 1937). With high resistance on the part of the patient, the abscess or abscesses may become heavily encapsulated; otherwise septicemia and a fatal outcome are entirely possible. One or another of the pyogenic cocci can usually be incriminated as the cause. Clinically, the acutely inflamed prostate is extremely painful when subjected to pressure, in contrast to the ordinary enlarged prostate, which is comparatively insensitive.

Hyperplasia of the Prostate

Hyperplasia of the prostate, often in association with chronic inflammation, is a common disorder in older dogs and humans. It is rare in other domestic animals. In fact, the prostate often atrophies with age in other species. In dogs, the disease is termed **benign prostatic hyperplasia.**

In prostatic hyperplasia, the organ is enlarged, often immensely, because of an increase in both the size and number of glandular acini. Accompanying this glandular proliferation there is an augmentation of the fibrous tissue and smooth muscle of the septa and supporting structures. Occasionally, this increase of the supporting tissues is the predominant change, but in

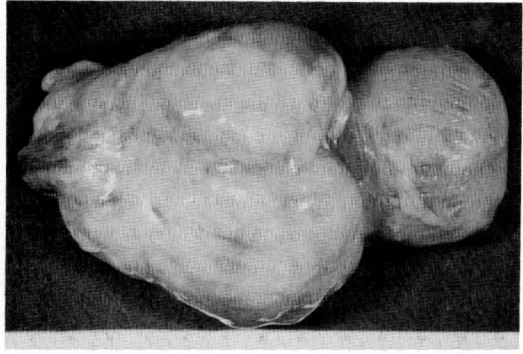

Fig. 25–35. Benign hyperplasia of the prostate of an eight-year-old male German Short-Haired Pointer dog. (Courtesy of Angell Memorial Animal Hospital.)

the great majority of cases, it merely keeps pace with the epithelial hyperplasia. The epithelial cells lining the acini increase in height, but they increase much more in numbers. As is the case with hyperplasia of the thyroid and other glands, the augmented cellular population is accommodated by the formation of tortuous folds in the acinar lining. These folds and ramifications may become very numerous and complicated so that the lumen of the acinus is filled with a complex maze of epithelial surfaces, each with its supporting fibrous stroma. It is only by carefully following the winding row of surface cells that the true arrangement is perceived, and it is only by the absence of anaplastic epithelium and its failure to penetrate through the basement membrane into the connective tissue stroma that the suspicion of neoplasia is eliminated. On the other hand, some acini dilate and fill with secreted fluid, thus forming cysts of microscopic or macroscopic size. The epithelial lining of these cysts is usually stretched and flattened. In some hyperplastic prostates the cystic changes are more or less predominant, and the condition is known as **cystic glandular hyperplasia.** Frequently, however, the cystic changes, regarded by some as degenerative in nature, and the strictly hyperplastic increase of epithelium just described occur in the same prostate. Accompanying these hyperplastic changes, there is practically always some evidence of chronic inflammation, chiefly in the form of lymphocytic infiltrations into the interstitial tissue.

Grossly, the change is a rather uniform increase in the outside dimensions of the organ without noticeable distortion in its shape. When the urethra is opened, however, it is not unusual to see a number of smooth but roundly pointed nodules projecting into its lumen. These are commonly from 1 to 4 mm in diameter and height and represent nodules of bulging prostatic tissue beneath the urethral mucosa. It is difficult to state what the dimensions of a normal prostate should be in a species whose individual members vary through the tremendously wide range of stature that is seen in dogs. Schlotthauer (1937, 1942) found that the weight of the normal canine prostate varies from 0.01 to 0.07% of the total body weight in the case of dogs less than 5 years of age. Perhaps another way of expressing the same thing would be to say that the prostate of the normal young dog extends but little beyond the width of the adjoining urethra; the diameter of the former being scarcely more than one and one-half times that of the latter. The hyperplastic prostate may easily be of a width or diameter three times the normal and, when first seen at autopsy, it not infrequently approaches or surpasses the undistended bladder in size. With the exception of a slight median furrow along the dorsal aspect, the canine prostate is not divided into lobes. Neither is there any lobe or part which tends to project into the region of the sphincter of the bladder, such as develops in the human.

Effect. As the reader probably is aware, the expected clinical effect of prostatic hyperplasia is interference with the flow of urine through the urethra. In the human male, this not infrequently becomes serious through gradual compression or invasion of the urethral lumen. The enlargement is often pronounced just at the neck and orifice of the bladder, with the formation of a "middle lobe" which actually projects into the cavity of the bladder and carries the urethral entrance with it. The "middle lobe" is said to arise as the result of hyperplasia of glandular tissue in the wall of the urethra, which must be quite comparable to the "disseminated" portions of the prostatic tissue which are normal in the several species of farm animals. There is also interference with proper closing of the sphincter, and urine may escape contrary to the patient's volition.

It is now recognized that too much has been taken for granted in applying these facts of human pathology to the dog and that enlarged prostates do not cause uri-

nary obstruction in the dog. Following the usual postmortem routine of removing the pelvic organs as an ensemble, it is commonly possible to lift the bladder by its vertex, or anterior end, and find that, by force of gravity, the urine flows unimpeded though the urethra, whatever may be the size of the prostate or however small the unfilled urethral lumen may have appeared. Whatever obstructive effect an enlarged prostate has upon the urinary flow must be due, at least in many cases, to filling and overcrowding of the nondistensible pelvic girdle. This lack of space should be more obstructive to the passage of the rectal contents than to the flow of urine and, indeed, constipation is the most frequent clinical sign of prostatic enlargement. This may be followed by perineal hernia when efforts at defecation are sufficiently forcible. Although dogs may strain on urination, incontinence is more usual. Hematuria may also be seen.

Cause. The cause of hyperplasia of the prostate is not known, either in man or dog, although a number of theoretic explanations have been proposed. In both the human and canine it is a disorder of advancing years, 50 or beyond in man, when androgen secretion is supposed to be declining. But canine prostatic enlargement was found by Schlotthauer to be commencing as early as 6 years, and there is no reason to believe that androgen secretion declines at anywhere near this age. It is known that in man or animals, castration prevents prostatic development in the young and causes pronounced atrophy of the organ when performed after puberty. Experimental injection of estrogenic substances into castrated rats produces hyperplasia of the prostate, but the addition of a suitable amount of testosterone prevents this. On the other hand, there are experiments indicating that an excess of the male hormone can cause prostatic enlargement. Part of the confusion as to the role of androgens and estrogens stems from the form in which hormones have been experimentally administered. Walsh and Wilson (1976) have produced prostatic hyperplasia in castrated male dogs with chronic administration of androstanediol in combination with estradiol. Androstanediol alone produced hyperplasia, but less consistently. The administration of dihydrotestosterone or testosterone, however, failed to lead to hyperplasia.

It has also been believed that the hyperplasia was a sequel to, and result of, chronic prostatitis. The prevalent opinion is that the lymphocytic infiltrations, fibrosis, or other evidences of chronic inflammation are the result, rather than the cause of the disturbance. On the basis of rather inconclusive statistical observations, it has been suspected that the unnatural postponement of urination required of male house-dogs was a causative factor, but our conceptions of anatomy and physiology offer little to support such a view. It seems proper to attribute hyperplasia of the prostate to imbalances in the sexual hormones, but an understanding of their precise nature awaits further elucidation. It is known that an excess of feminizing hormone will produce **squamous metaplasia** of prostatic epithelium, as in the presence of a Sertoli-cell tumor (Fig. 25–34C), or with experimental administration of estrogens.

Calculi

Stones occur in the prostate of the dog, but only with rarity. The stones are usually small (1 to 5 mm), hard, white, and spherical. They consist chiefly of phosphates and carbonates of calcium. Usually a number of them fill a cystic cavity, of which there may be one or several. The central nucleus is practically always organic material, indicating an origin in desquamated or other dead cells. They doubtless arise in connection with chronic prostatitis and hyperplasia. Since corpora amylacea are extremely rare in the prostates of domestic animals, it seems doubtful that these starch-like bodies are essential predeces-

sors of calculi. Small collections of stones are asymptomatic, others are irritant and obstructive, requiring operative removal. They can be demonstrated roentgenologically.

Neoplasms

Prostatic neoplasms are uncommon in most domestic species except older dogs, in which **adenocarcinomas of the prostate** occur with a low frequency. The neoplasms are similar in histologic appearance and clinical behavior to those which occur in man. The affected gland is enlarged and of distorted shape with firm, yellow-tan nodular tumors. Microscopically, the tumors are usually recognizable as adenocarcinomas with acinar formation within a proliferating connective tissue stroma. Papillary projections of epithelial cells and cystic glands are commonly seen. Less often, the neoplasms are undifferentiated with little or no tendency to form acini. In some, the epithelial cells are fusiform in shape with little resemblance to epithelium. Prostatic carcinomas are locally invasive and metastasize by way of lymphatics.

Fibromas and leiomyomas also originate in the prostate but are rare.

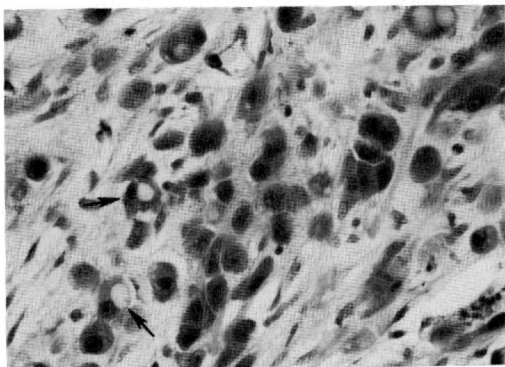

Fig. 25–36. Undifferentiated carcinoma of the canine prostate. There is no attempt to form glands. Some of the cells containing secretion assume the so-called signet ring shape (arrows). (Courtesy of Dr. N. W. King, Jr.)

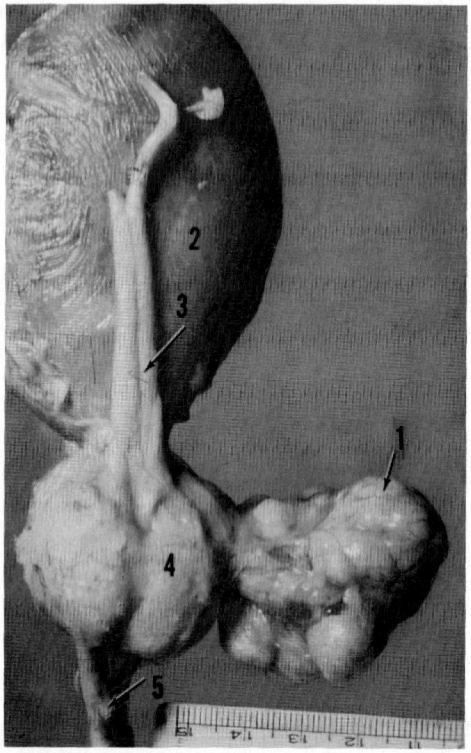

Fig. 25–37. Leiomyoma of the prostate of a dog. Tumor (*1*), urinary bladder (*2*), ductus deferens (*3*), prostate (*4*), and urethra (*5*).

Penis, Prepuce and Urethra

Anomalies of the penis and prepuce are rare, although **agenesis** and **hypoplasia** are seen in the various intersexes. **Phimosis** and **paraphimosis** may be congenital, but are more often acquired. **Hypospadias** (urethral opening on the ventral side of penis) and **epispadias** (urethral opening on dorsal side of penis) are rare in animals. In bulls, deviation of the penis (phallo-campsis) is a not too infrequent anomaly, which of course can also be an acquired disease. Depending on the form of deviation these are described as "corkscrew penis" (spiral deviation) or "rainbow penis" (ventral deviation).

The external parts of these organs are subject to trauma, leading to hematocysts, thrombosis, or the usual fibrinopurulent

reactions such as are seen in wounds generally.

Balanitis (inflammation of the glans penis or clitoris) and **posthitis** (inflammation of the prepuce) are known in most species and are considered to be caused by various pathogenic organisms. Many of the agents that cause abortion and vaginitis also cause balanoposthitis, but certain of these organisms are carried by male animals asymptomatically. *Trichomonas foetus* causes a mild balanoposthitis, but the infection soon becomes inapparent. **Infectious pustular vulvovaginitis** caused by the herpesvirus of infectious bovine rhinotracheitis has similar manifestations in bulls. It has been reported to also cause balanitis and vaginitis in swine (Onstad and Saxegaard, 1967). In horses, a herpesvirus causes **coital vesicular exanthema** which is characterized by vulvitis and vaginitis. **Dourine** is another infection of the external genitalia in equines. Experimentally, *Herpesvirus canis* has been shown to cause vaginitis and balanoposthitis, and it is likely that it does so under natural circumstances. Mycoplasmas have been recovered from vaginitis and balanoposthitis, but their causal role is uncertain. The pox virus of contagious pustular dermatitis of sheep may affect the genitalia, although it usually is confined to the lips and mouth. A troublesome infection in sheep, **ovine posthitis,** is reported by Southcott (1965) to be due to a gram-positive, diphtheroid bacterium which is carried by nondiseased animals, but under certain conditions will cause inflammation. This organism has the ability to hydrolyze urea to produce ammonia (NH_3), and its pathogenic multiplication appears related to urine stasis. The infection may be transmitted by contact or coitus. Cultural studies of the genital mucous membranes of bulls indicate that *Pseudomonas aeruginosa (pyocyaneus)* (Rempt and Zwanenburg, 1948), *Corynebacterium pyogenes,* and *C. renale* (Morgan, et al., 1946) are rather frequently present. The first of these has rarely been incriminated in abortions.

Inflammatory **phimosis** is a condition in which inflammatory swelling prevents extension of the penis from the sheath; **paraphimosis** is a similar situation, the penis being already protruded and impossible to withdraw. True congenital phimosis probably does not occur in the domestic animals because of differences in local anatomy.

The **penile urethra** is subject to lodgment of uroliths, which occur with frequency in cattle, dogs, cats, and sheep. The stone practically always lodges at the sigmoid flexure, where the lumen is narrowest. In the dog, uroliths, especially of cystine, are apt to lodge at or near the point where the penile urethra is contained by the os penis. Inflammation and limited distention occur above the stone; none below it. Strictures in the form of an irregular fold of mucous membrane have been noted at least in the bovine urethra, the cause not having been demonstrated.

Neoplasms

Neoplasms of the penis, usually on the glans, are of some frequency in horses, cattle, and dogs. Whether the males are intact or castrated appears to make no difference. In the bovine, fibropapillomas and, less frequently, fibrosarcomas predominate (see fibropapillomatosis). In the horse, most tumors of the penis arise from squamous epithelium. Although some are squamous cell carcinomas of low-grade malignancy, in our experience most resemble condyloma acuminatum of human beings. These are complex fungating papillomas characterized by upward growth and lack of invasion.

Canine Transmissible Venereal Tumor. Known by a variety of names, such as Sticker tumor, venereal granuloma, transmissible sarcoma, and transmissible lymphosarcoma, this tumor occupies a unique place among neoplastic conditions in that it is rather readily transmitted through

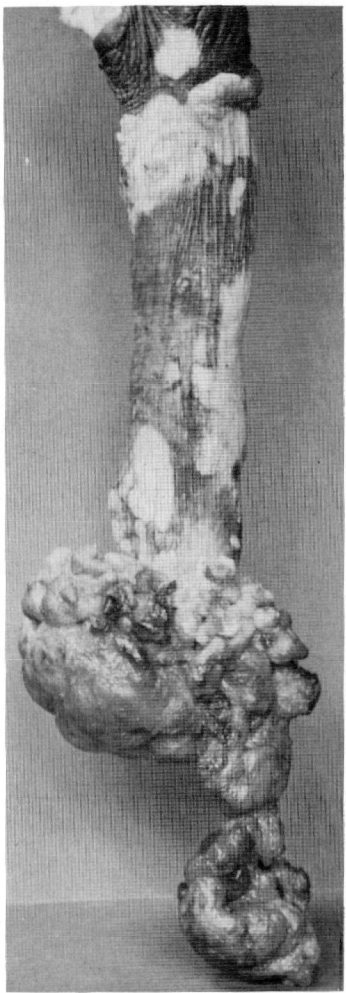

Fig. 25–38. Squamous cell carcinoma of the penis of a 25-year-old horse. The lower mass was a transplant of the tumor to the prepuce.

transplantation of cells by contact, is likely eventually to disappear spontaneously, and, having disappeared following either natural or experimental occurrence, leaves the patient in a state of appreciable immunity. Nevertheless, it appears to fulfill the criteria of malignancy in its histologic appearance and in the fact that metastases are not rare.

Historically, this neoplasm is of interest as the first frank neoplasm to be transmitted experimentally from one animal to

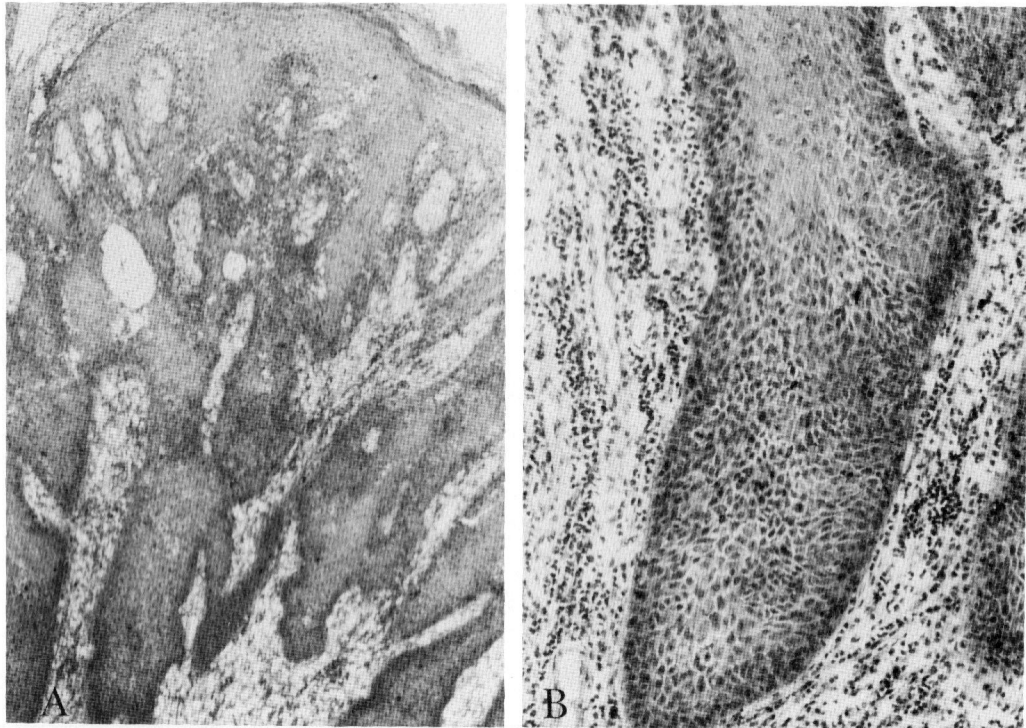

Fig. 25–39. Condyloma acuminatum, penis of a horse. *A*, The lesion is characterized by outward and downward growth of penile epithelium. The lesion is benign, although often confused with squamous cell carcinoma. *B*, Higher magnification of epithelium. Note that it does not invade the stroma. (Courtesy of Dr. N. W. King, Jr.)

another. A Russian veterinarian, M.A. Novinsky, is credited with accomplishing this feat (Stewart, et al., 1957).

Like the mast-cell tumor, the transmissible tumor consists of large round cells (polyhedral when subjected to pressure) which bear some resemblance to lymphoid cells. Both in total volume and in size of nucleus, these cells are larger than lymphocytes, being more comparable to the maternal lymphoblasts of lymph nodes. However, their nuclei, rounded or slightly indented, stain more strongly than those of lymphoblasts, both in their chromatin granules and in their nuclear membranes. In spite of these general statements, a characteristic of some value in diagnosis is a rather pronounced variation in size of individual cells and nuclei. Mitotic figures are numerous, quite out of proportion to

what one would expect from the comparatively low infiltrative and metastatic powers of the tumor.

Diagnosis is made by these characteristics after eliminating the mast-cell tumor, and by location of the (primary) tumor in close relation to the genital mucous membranes. Without a knowledge of the location, the transmissible tumor could be confused with a number of others, including the aortic-body tumor and the seminoma.

Clinically, the majority of these tumors are found on or in close proximity to the external genitalia, being transmitted by coition. They also occur, however, on the face, shoulders, and in other locations. The same dog may have a growth in two widely separated parts of the body. Commonly sessile, ulcerated, and a few centimeters in

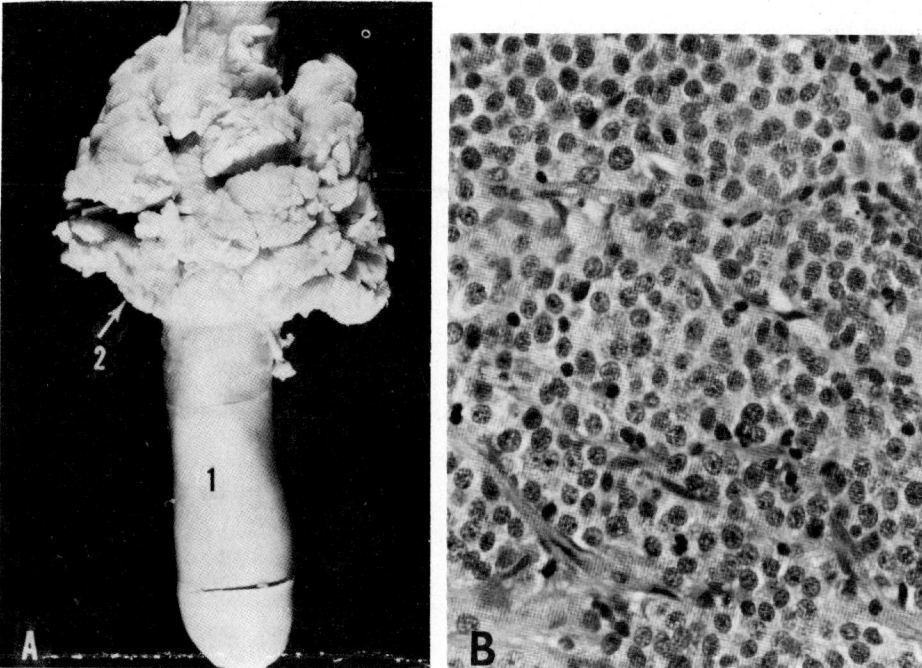

Fig. 25–40. *A,* Canine venereal tumor. Lesion (2) in the penis (1) of a dog. (Courtesy of Armed Forces Institute of Pathology.) *B,* Microscopic appearance of a venereal tumor metastatic to an inguinal lymph node.

diameter, they may attain formidable size, for instance distending and protruding from the vagina. While metastasis has been frequent enough to convince numerous experimenters of the neoplastic malignancy of this type of growth, that is not the usual clinical experience. Unmolested, it attains its considerable size in the course of several months, then remains stationary or ultimately shrinks and disappears. Probably because of its behavior as a transmissible disease, this tumor is much more common in some parts of the country than in others, and in some places where formerly frequent, it is now seldom seen. On the whole, it is the paradox among neoplasms.

It has been shown that the cells of the transmissible venereal tumor have chromosome configurations quite different from that of normal canine cells. (See Chapter 8.) Normal cells of the dog at metaphase contain 76 autosomal chromo-

somes, all of them acrocentric. The sex pair are metacentric; the X is the largest of the complement and the Y near the smallest in size. The cells of the venereal tumor, on the other hand, contain only 59 chromosomes, 17 of them metacentric and 42 acrocentric. M. Reiter, in our laboratory (T.C.J.), has demonstrated that cells of the "canine cutaneous histiocytoma" contain morphologically normal canine chromosomes in normal numbers.

Abdel-Raouf, M.: The postnatal development of the reproductive organs in bulls with special reference to puberty. (Including growth of the hypophysis and the adrenals). Acta Endocrinol., Copenhagen., Suppl. No. 49, pp. 109, 1960.

Adams, E.W., Carter, L.P., and Sapp, W.J.: Growth and maintenance of the canine venereal tumor in continuous culture. Cancer Res., 28:753–757, 1968.

Adams, E.W., and Chineme, C.M.: Canine venereal tumor. Serum protein electrophoresis, transaminase, and lactic dehydrogenase activity. Cornell Vet., 57:572–579, 1967.

Adams, E.W., Moore, E.G., and Carter, L.P.: Canine venereal tumor: biologically active deoxyribonucleic acid from canine venereal tumor. Am. J. Vet. Res., 29:1241–1244, 1968.

Adams, E.W., and Slaughter, L.J.: A canine venereal tumor with metastasis to the brain. Path. Vet., 7:498–502, 1970.

Andreevskii, V.Y.: Prichiny porochnosti spermy u baranov. (Reasons for sperm defects of rams.) Iskusst. Osemen. sel'khoz. Zhivotn., 1:36–45, 1940. Abstr. Vet. Bull., No. 997, 1948.

Ashdown, R.R.: Persistence of the penile frenulum in young bulls. Vet. Rec., 74:1464–1468, 1962.

Ashdown, R.R., and Ford, C.M.: Bilateral epididymal spermiostasis in a ram. Vet. Rec., 80:492–494, 1967.

Ashdown, R.R., and Pearson, H.: Studies on "corkscrew penis" in the bull. Vet. Rec., 93:30–35, 1973.

Bagshaw, P.A., and Ladds, P.W.: Pathology of the accessory sex glands of the bull. Vet. Bull., 44:343–348, 1974.

Ball, L., Young, S., and Carroll, E.J.: Seminal vesiculitis syndrome: lesions in genital organs of young bulls. Am. J. Vet. Res., 29:1173–1184, 1968.

Bane, A., and Nicander, L.: Electron and light microscopical studies on spermateliosis in a boar with acrosome abnormalities. J. Reprod. Fertil., 11:133–138, 1966.

Bartlett, D.E., Hasson, E.V., and Teeter, K.G.: Occurrence of Trichomonas fetus in preputial samples from infected bulls. J. Am. Vet. Med. Assn., 110:114–120, 1947.

Basset, C.R.: Ulcerative posthitis in bulls. Vict. Vet. Proc., 22:38–39, 1963/64.

Bennetts, H.W.: Metaplasia in the sex organs of castrated male sheep maintained on early subterranean clover pastures. Austr. Vet. J., 22:70–78, 1946.

Bergin, W.C., Gier, H.T., Marion, G.B., and Coffman, J.R.: A developmental concept of equine cryptorchism. Biol. Reprod., 3:82–92, 1970.

Biberstein, E.L., et al.: Epididymitis in rams. Studies on pathogenesis. Cornell Vet., 54:27–40, 1964.

Bieberdorf, F.W.: Actinomycosis of a bovine testis. J. Am. Vet. Med. Assn., 122:49–50, 1953.

Blom, E.: En hurtig-farvningsmetode til adskillelse af levende og døde spermier ved hjaelp af eosin-nigrosin. (Rapid eosin-nigrosin staining technique for differentiating living from dead spermatozoa.) Nord. Vet. Med., 2:58–61, 1950. Abstr. Vet. Bull. No. 2938, 1950.

Blom, E., and Hermansen, E.: Segmental aplasia of the wolffian duct (lack of epididymis), a sterilizing and hereditary defect in the mink. Nord. Vet. Med., 21:188–192, 1969. V.B. 39:4822, 1969.

Borthwick, R., and Mackenzie, C.P.: The signs and results of treatment of prostatic disease in dogs. Vet. Rec., 89:374–384, 1971.

Bouters, R., et al.: [Ulcerative balanoposthitis in bulls.] Vlaams Diergeneeskd. Tijdschr., 29:171–186, 1960. (In Flemish.) Abstr. Vet. Bull., No. 4086, 1960.

Brook, A.H., Southcott, W.H., and Stacy, B.D.: Etiology of ovine posthitis: relationship between urine and a causal organism. Aust. Vet. J., 42:9–12, 1966.

Bruere, A.N.: Some clinical aspects of hypo-orchidism (small testes) in the ram. N. Z. Vet. J., 18:189–198, 1970.

Chenoweth, P.J., Pascoe, R.R.R., McDougall, H.L., and McCosker, P.J.: An abnormality of the spermatozoa of a stallion (Equus caballus). Br. Vet. J., 126:476–481, 1970.

Claxton, J.H., and Yeates, N.T.M.: The inheritance of cryptorchism in a small crossbred flock of sheep. J. Hered., 63:141–144, 1972.

Fawcett, D.W.: A comparative view of sperm ultra-structure. Biol. Reprod., 2:90–127, 1970.

Flatt, R.E., and Weisbroth, S.H.: Interstitial cell tumor of the testicle in rabbits: a report of two cases. Lab. Anim. Sci., 24:682–685, 1974.

Foster, A.E.C.: Polyorchidism. Vet. Rec., 64:158, 1952.

Fraser, A.F., and Wilson, J.C.: Testicular calcinosis in domestic ruminants. Nature (Lond.), 210:547, 1966.

Garlick, N.L.: An unusual case of monorchidism in a stallion. J. Am. Vet. Med. Assn., 121:101–103, 1952.

Gerber, H.: Anatomie der prostata des hundes unter beruchsichtigung verscheidener altersstufen. Schweiz. Arch. Tierheilkd., 103, 537–567, 1961.

Girard, A., Greig, A.S., and Mitchell, D.: A virus associated with vulvitis and balanitis in the horse. . . a preliminary report. Canad. J. Comp. Med., 32:603–604, 1968.

Glover, T.D.: The semen of the pig. Vet. Rec., 67:36–40, 1955.

Greulich, W.W., and Burford, T.H.: Testicular tumors associated with mammary, prostatic and other changes in cryptorchid dogs. Am. J. Cancer, 28:496–511, 1936.

Hafez, E.S.E., and Jainudeen, M.R.: Intersexuality in farm mammals. Anim. Breed, Abst., 34:1–15, 1966.

Hanselka, D.V.: Bovine penile deviations—a review. Southwestern Vet., 26:265–271, 1973.

Hayes, H.M., Jr., and Pendergrass, T.W.: Canine testicular tumors: epidemiologic features of 410 dogs. Int. J. Cancer, 18:482–487, 1976.

Helmy, N., et al.: Orchitis and epididymo-orchitis in domesticated animals. Vet. Med. J. Giza, 11:179–209, 1966. V.B. 37:4023, 1967.

Hudson, R.C.: Thrombosis of the corpus cavernosum penis in a bull. J. Am. Vet. Med. Assoc., 159:754–756, 1971.

Innes, J.R.M.: Neoplastic diseases of the testis in animals. J. Pathol. Bact., 54:485–498, 1942.

Jabara, A.G.: Some tissue changes in the dog following stilbestrol administration. Austr. J. Exp. Biol. Med. Sci., 40:293–307, 1963.

Jamieson, S., and Soltys, M.A.: Infectious epididymo-orchitis of rams associated with Pasteurella pseudotuberculosis. Vet. Rec., 59:351–353, 1947.

Jansen, J.: Orchitis bij hengsten, abortus bij merrier (klinischbacteriologische les over Salmonella abortus-equi-infecties). (Orchitis in stallions and abortion in mares due to S. abortus-equi infection.) Tijdschr. Diergeneeskd., 71:160–167, 1946. Abstr. Vet. Bull., No. 2217, 1947.

Jensen, R., et al.: Arteriosclerosis and phlebosclerosis in testes of sheep. Am. J. Vet. Res., 23:480–488, 1962.

Julian, L.M.: The pathology of the prostate gland of man and the dog. Cornell Vet., 37:241–253, 1947.

Karlson, A.G., and Mann, F.C.: The transmissible venereal tumor of dogs; observations of forty generations of experimental transfers. Ann. N.Y. Acad. Sci., 54:1197–1213, 1952.

Kernkamp, H.C.H., Roepke, M.H., and Jasper, D.E.: Orchitis in swine due to *Brucella suis*. J. Am. Vet. Med. Assn., 108:215–221, 1946.

King, N.W., and Garvin, C.H.: Bilateral hermaphroditism in a dog. J. Am. Vet. Med. Assn., 145:997–1001, 1964.

Kodagali, S.B., and Kerur, V.K.: Gonadal hypoplasia in Gir cattle. Indian Vet. J., 45:114–118, 1968.

———: Seminal characters in testes hypoplasia. Indian J. Anim. Hlth., 7:209–212, 1968.

Konig, H.: Genital pathology of bulls. Arch. Exp. Veterinaermed., 16:501–584, 1962.

———: (An unusual form of orchitis in bulls.) Schweiz. Arch. Tierheilkd., 106:529–534, 1964. V.B. 35:423, 1965.

Konig, H., Weber, W., and Kupferschmied, H.: Zur nebenhodenaplasie beim stier und eber. (a) Darstellung von 18 fallen mit rezessivem erbgang beim simmentaler fleckvieh. (b) auftreten der anomalie bei einem eber und drei sohnen. Schweiz. Arch. Tierheilkd., 114:73–78, 1972.

Kravis, E.M., and Lorber, J.H.: Feminization syndrome associated with epididymitis in a dog. J. Am. Vet. Med. Assn., 140:803–806, 1962.

Kudo, T., Koike, T., Otomo, K., and Sakai, T.: Transplantation of canine transmissible venereal sarcoma: autoradiographic study with ³H-Thymidine. Jpn. J. Vet. Res., 22:105–110, 1974.

Lambert, G., Manthei, C.A., and Deyoe, B.L.: Studies on *Brucella abortus* infection in bull. Am. J. Vet. Res., 24:1152–1157, 1963.

Leav, I., and Ling, G.V.: Adenocarcinoma of the canine prostate. Cancer, 22:1329–1345, 1968.

Lipowitz, A.J., Schwartz, A., Wilson, G.P., and Ebert, J.W.: Testicular neoplasms and concomitant clinical changes in the dog. J. Am. Vet. Med. Assoc., 163:1364–1368, 1973.

Livingston, C.W., and Hardy, W.T.: Isolation of *Actinobacillus seminis* from ovine epididymitis. Amer. J. Vet. Res., 25:660–663, 1964.

Makino, S.: Some epidemiological aspects of venereal tumors of dogs as revealed by chromosome and DNA studies. Ann. N. Y. Acad. Sci., 108:1106–1122, 1963.

Manning, P.J., and Martin, P.D.: Metastasis of canine transmissible venereal tumor to the adenohypophysis. Path. Vet., 7:148–152, 1970.

Manning, W.K.: Biotin deficiency as the causative agent of induced cryptorchidism in albino rats. Science, 112:89, 1950.

McEntee, K.: Pathological conditions in old bulls with impaired fertility. J. Am. Vet. Med. Assn., 132:328–331, 1958.

Morgan, B.B., Johansson, K.R., and Emerson, E.Z.: Some Corynebacteria isolated from the genital tract of bulls. Mich. State College Vet., 6:68–69 and 72–74, 1946.

McMillan, K.R., and Southcott, W.H.: Aetiological factors in ovine posthitis. Aust. Vet. J., 49:405–408, 1973.

Mulligan, R.M.: Feminization in male dogs, a syndrome associated with carcinoma of the testis and mimicked by the administration of estrogens. Am. J. Pathol., 20:865–873, 1944.

Murray, M., James, Z.H., and Martin, W.B.: A study of the cytology and karyotype of the canine transmissible venereal tumour. Res. Vet. Sci., 10:565–568, 1969.

Oduye, O.O., Ikede, B.O., Esuruoso, G.O., and Akpokodje, J.U.: Metastatic transmissible venereal tumour in dogs. J. Small Anim. Pract., 14:625–637, 1973.

Oettlé, A.G., and Harrison, R.G.: The histological changes produced in the rat testis by temporary and permanent occlusion of the testicular artery. J. Pathol. Bacteriol., 64:273–297, 1952.

Onstad, O., and Saxegaard, F.: Outbreaks of vaginitis and balanitis in swine. Clinical and pathological findings. Nord. Vet. Med., 19:49–53, 1967.

Oriel, J.D., and Hayward, A.H.S.: Sexually-transmitted diseases in animals. Br. J. Vener. Dis., 50:412–420, 1974.

Palludan, B.: Vitamin A deficiency and its effect on the sexual organs of the boar. Acta Vet. Scand., 4:136–155, 1963.

———: Direct effect of vitamin A on boar testis. Nature (Lond.), 211:639–640, 1966.

Pamukcu, A.M.: Seminoma of the testicles in an Ankara goat. Vet. Facültesi dergisi, 1:42–43, 1954 (In Engl.)

Parsonson, I.M., Winter, A.J., and McEntee, K.: Allergic epididymo-orchitis in guinea pigs and bulls. Vet. Pathol., 8:333–351, 1971.

Pearson, H., and Kelly, D.F.: Testicular torsion in the dog: a review of 13 cases. Vet. Rec., 97:200–204, 1975.

Pezzoli, G.: La torsione del testiculo. Clin. Vet., Milano., 80:353–364, 1957.

Powers, R.D.: Immunologic properties of canine transmissible venereal sarcoma. Am. J. Vet. Res., 29:1637–1645, 1968.

Prier, J.E.: Chromosome pattern of canine transmissible sarcoma cells in culture. Nature, 212:724–726, 1966.

Prier, J.E., and Johnson, J.E.: Malignancy in a canine transmissible venereal tumour. J. Am. Vet. Med. Assoc., 145:1092–1094, 1964.

Rempt, D., and Zwanenburg, T.S.: *Pseudomonas aeruginosa (Ps. pyocyanea, Bac. pyocyaneus)* in het sperma van drie dekstieren. (Pseudomonas in semen of bulls.) Tijdschr. Diergeneeskd., 73:224–230, 1948. V.B. 19:356, 1949.

Rollinson, D.H.L.: Studies on the abnormal spermatozoa of bull semen. Brit. Vet. J., 107:203–214, 258–273 and 451–468, 1951.

Saxegaard, F., and Onstad, O.: Isolation and identification of IBR-IPV virus from cases of vaginitis and balanitis in swine and from healthy swine. Nord. Vet. Med., *19*:54–57, 1967. V.B. *37*:3197, 1967.

Schenker, J.: Zur functionellen anatomie der prostata des rindes. Acta Anat., *9*:89–102, 1950. V.B. *21*:3362, 1951.

Schlotthauer, C.F.: Diseases of the prostate gland in the dog. J. Am. Vet. Med. Assn., *90*:176–187, 1937.

Schlotthauer, C.F., and Bollman, J.L.: The effect of artificial cryptorchidism on the prostate gland of dogs. Am. J. Vet. Res., *3*:202–206, 1942.

Schlotthauer, C.F., McDonald, J.R., and Bollman, J.L.: Testicular tumors in dogs. J. Urol., *40*:539–550, 1938.

Simmons, G.C., and Hall, W.T.K.: Epididymitis of rams. Australian Vet J., *29*:33–40, 1953.

Simmons, G.C., Baynes, I.D., and Ludford, C.G.: Epidemiology of *Actinobacillus seminis* in a flock of Border Leicester sheep. Aust. Vet. J., *42*:183–187, 1966.

Smith, G.B., and Washbourn, J.W.: Infective venereal tumours in dogs. J. Pathol. Bact., *5*:99–110, 1898.

Smith, H.A.: Interstitial cell tumor of the equine testis. J. Am. Vet. Med. Assoc., *124*:356–359, 1954.

Smith, L.W.: Senile changes of the testis and prostate in dogs. J. Med. Res., *40*:31–51, 1919.

Southcott, W.H.: Etiology of ovine posthitis: description of a causal organism. Aust. Vet. J., *41*:193–200, 1965. V.B. *36*:45, 1966.

———: Epidemiology and control of ovine posthitis and vulvitis. Aust. Vet. J., *41*:224–234, 1965. V.B. *36*:1286, 1966.

Stewart, S.E., et al.: The induction of neoplasms with a substance released from mouse tumours by tissue culture. Virology, *3*:380–400, 1957.

Storz, J., et al.: Isolation of a psittacosis agent (*Chlamydia*) from semen and epididymis of bulls with seminal vesiculitis syndrome. Amer. J. Vet. Res., *29*:549–555, 1968.

Streett, C.S.: Sertoli cell carcinoma and multiple metastasis in a dog. Cornell Vet., *57*:597–619, 1967.

Stubbs, E.L., and Furth, J.: Experimental studies on venereal sarcoma of the dog. Am. J. Pathol., *10*:275–286, 1934.

Sullivan, D.J., and Drobeck, H.P.: True hermaphrodism in a Rhesus monkey. Folia Primat., *4*:309–317, 1966.

Swift, B.L., and Weyerts, P.R.: Ram epididymitis. A study on infertility. Cornell Vet., *60*:204–214, 1970.

Takayama, S., et al.: Cytological studies of tumors. XXV. A study of chromosomes in venereal tumors of the dog. A. Krebsforsch. Bd., *64*:253–261, 1961.

Thomas, U.P., and Raja, C.K.S.V.: Spermatic granuloma in boar. Kerala J. Vet. Sci., *5*:113–120, 1974.

Thornburn, M.J., et al.: Pathological and cytogenetic observations on the naturally occurring canine venereal tumour in Jamaica (Sticker's tumour). Br. J. Cancer, *22*:720–727, 1968.

Todd, G.C., Nelson, L.W., and Migaki, G.: Multiple heterotopic testicular tissue in the pig. A report of seven cases. Cornell Vet., *58*:614–619, 1968.

vanTonder, E.M., and Bolton, T.F.W.: Epididymitis in rams caused by *Actinobacillus seminis*. J. S. Afr. Med. Assoc., *39*:87–90, 1968.

Walsh, P.C., and Wilson, J.D.: The induction of prostatic hypertrophy in the dog with androstanediol. J. Clin. Invest., *57*:1093–1097, 1976.

Watt, D.A.: Congenital retention cysts of the epididymis in rams. Aust. Vet. J., *47*:287–288, 1971.

———: Testicular abnormalities and spermatogenesis of the ovine and other species. Vet. Bull., *42*:181–191, 1972.

Wensing, C.J.G.: Abnormalities of testicular descent. Proc. Koninklijke Nederlandse Akad Wetenschappen. Series C. Biol. Med. Sci., *76*:373–381, 1973.

White, P.T., and Johnson, P., Jr.: Strangulated hernia of a cryptorchid dog. J. Am. Vet. Med. Assn., *126*:312, 1955.

Yang, T.J., and Jones, J.B.: Canine transmissible venereal sarcoma: transplantation in neonatal and adult dogs. J. Natl. Canc. Inst., *51*:1915–1918, 1973.

Young, S.L., Hudson, R.S., and Walker, D.F.: Impotence in bulls due to vascular shunts from the corpus cavernosum penis. J. Am. Vet. Med. Assoc., *171*:643–648, 1977.

Zemjanis, R., et al.: Testicular degeneration in *Macaca nemestrina* induced by immobilization. Fertil. & Steril., *21*:335–340, 1970.

Zuckerman, S., and Groome, J.R.: Aetiology of benign enlargement of the prostate in the dog. J. Path. and Bact., *44*:113–124, 1937.

Zuckerman, S., and McKeown, T.: The canine prostate in relation to normal and abnormal testicular changes. J. Path. and Bact., *46*:7–19, 1938.

CHAPTER 26

The Endocrine System

HYPOTHALAMUS

In earlier and perhaps simpler times, the pituitary was described functionally as the "Conductor of the Endocrine Symphony." The hypothalamus might similarly be thought of as the "Board of Trustees of the Endocrine Symphony," because the pituitary receives much of its direction from the "endocrine" portion of the hypothalamus. It is now clear that the hypothalamus serves as a higher center for the regulation of functions of the pituitary. This control is facilitated by direct anatomic connections between hypothalamus and hypophysis. The neurohypophysis is connected to the hypothalamus by the hypothalamohypophyseal neural tract. This tract originates in neurons in the supraoptic and paraventricular nuclei, traverses the pituitary stalk, and terminates in the pars nervosa. Two peptide hormones, vasopressin and oxytocin, with antidiuretic and oxytocic effects respectively, are secreted in the supraoptic and paraventricular nuclei and are transported by attachment to carrier substances, neurophysins, through the axons of the hypothalamohypophyseal tract to the pars nervosa. Here they are stored until released into capillaries of the neural lobe.

The adenohypophysis is in communication with the hypothalamus through two components. The tuberohypophyseal neural tract originates from neurons in the tuberal and other nuclei in the hypothalamus and terminates in the infundibulum. Here, these axons are in contact with the primary capillary beds of the hypophyseal portal system which extend through portal veins to the sinusoids of the adenohypophysis. Releasing and inhibiting factors from the cells of the tuberal nuclei pass down the axons of the tuberohypophyseal tract, are deposited in the portal veins, and reach the sinusoids of the adenohypophysis. Here these factors control the release of hormones in the pars distalis.

The releasing and inhibiting factors produced by the hypothalamus that have been found thus far are peptides. Some of those included on a growing list of pituitary controlling factors are corticotropin-releasing factor (CRF), thyrotropin-releasing hormone (TRH), and luteotropin-releasing hormone (LRH). The inhibiting substances known at present include somatostatin or somatotropin-release-inhibiting factor (SRIF) and prolactin-inhibiting factor (PIF). The rapidly unfolding new knowledge in the field of hypothalamic and pituitary physiology is beyond the scope of this text, and much that is now written will soon be out of date. The student is therefore encouraged to read selectively in the

1583

current literature of this exciting field. This new knowledge will undoubtedly lead to a deeper understanding of disease processes affecting the endocrine system.

Hypothalamic Diabetes Insipidus

The clinical manifestations of diabetes insipidus are polydipsia, polyuria, and low specific gravity of the urine (usually less than 1.010). The disease may be *primary* as a result of excessive intake of water, *nephrogenic* as a result of chronic renal disease, or *hypothalamic* due to deficient secretion of the antidiuretic hormone, vasopressin. Diabetes insipidus has been described in many species (mice, rabbits, woolly monkey), but the hypothalamic form has been identified so far only in the dog and rat.

In the dog, diabetes insipidus is usually, but not always, manifest as a result of gross lesions that impinge upon the pituitary or hypothalamus (such as pituitary adenoma and adenocarcinoma, craniopharyngioma, ependymoma, cysts). Necrosis of neurons in hypothalamic nuclei and lesions due to nematode larval migration have also been associated with this syndrome. In many cases, the lesions in the hypothalamus have not been adequately studied. The clinical signs of diabetes insipidus are usually abated following the administration of therapeutic doses of vasopressin. Other effects of a pituitary tumor, of course, are not changed by supplying this hormone. In Jones's experience, more than half of all cases of this disease were seen in Boxer dogs.

Hypothalamic diabetes insipidus has been studied in the Brattleboro strain of rats, in which the disease is inherited as an autosomal recessive genetic factor. The affected strain of rats was developed by selective mating of rats of the hooded Long-Evans strain. Homozygous affected rats produce almost no vasopressin, and oxytocin levels are also reduced severely. Neurophysin I is also reduced in the posterior pituitary of homozygous affected rats.

Administration of vasopressin reduces the fluid turnover and restores the oxytocin levels, but has little effect on vasopressor activity or level of neurophysin I (carrier of vasopressin) in the posterior pituitary.

The fluid turnover in affected rats is astounding. Daily urine excretion is equal to about 70% of the body weight and the consumption of water is equally high. Urine osmolality is reduced and the homozygous rats are slightly smaller in body size, possibly as a result of deficiency of growth hormone. The supraoptic nuclei and the entire hypothalamoneurohypophyseal system are hypertrophied in affected rats.

Boorman, G. A., and Bree, M. M.: Diabetes insipidus syndrome in a rabbit. J. Am. Vet. Med. Assoc., *155*:1218–1220, 1969.

Brown, G. M., Schalch, D. S., and Reichlin, S.: Hypothalamic mediation of growth hormone and adrenal stress response in the squirrel monkey. Endocrinology, *89*:694–703, 1971.

Forrest, J. N., Jr., et al.: On the mechanism of lithium-induced diabetes insipidus in man and the rat. J. Clin. Invest., *53*:1115–1123, 1974.

Green, R. A., and Farrow, C. S.: Diabetes insipidus in a cat. J. Am. Vet. Med. Assoc., *164*:524–526, 1974.

Koestner, A., and Capen, C. C.: Ultrastructural evaluation of the canine hypothalamic-neurohypophyseal system in diabetes insipidus associated with pituitary neoplasms. Pathol. Vet., *4*:513–516, 1967.

Lage, A. L.: Nephrogenic diabetes insipidus in a dog. J. Am. Vet. Med. Assoc., *163*:251–253, 1973.

Moses, A. M., and Miller, M.: Accumulation and release of pituitary vasopressin in rats heterozygous for hypothalamic diabetes insipidus. Endocrinology, *86*:34–41, 1970.

Richards, M. A., and Sloper, J. C.: Hypothalamic involvement by "visceral" larva migrans in a dog suffering from diabetes insipidus. Vet. Rec., *76*:449–451, 1964.

Rogers, W. A., Valdez, H., Anderson, B. C., and Comella, C.: Partial deficiency of antidiuretic hormone in a cat. J. Am. Vet. Med. Assoc., *170*:545–547, 1977.

Saul, G. B., II., Garrity, E. G., Benirschke, K., and Valtin, H.: Inherited hypothalamic diabetes insipidus in the Brattleboro strain of rats. J. Hered., *57*:113–117, 1969.

Sawyer, W. H., Valtin, H., and Sokol, H. W.: Neurohypophyseal principles in rats with familial hypothalamic diabetes insipidus (Brattleboro strain). Endocrinology, *74*:153–155, 1964.

Sokol, H. W., and Valtin, H.: Morphology of the neurosecretory system in rats homozygous and heterozygous for hypothalamic diabetes insipidus (Brattleboro strain). Endocrinology, *77*:692–700, 1965.

Valtin, H., Schroeder, H. A., Benirschke, K., and Sokol, H. W.: Familial hypothalamic diabetes insipidus in rats. Nature, *196*:1109–1110, 1962.

Valtin, H., Sawyer, W. H., and Sokol, H. W.: Neurohypophyseal principles in rats homozygous and heterozygous for hypothalamic diabetes insipidus (Brattleboro strain). Endocrinology, *77*:701–706, 1965.

Valtin, H.: Animal model of human disease: Hereditary hypothalamic diabetes insipidus. Model 107. *In* Handbook: Animal Models of Human Disease, edited by T. C. Jones, D. B. Hackel, and G. Migaki. Washington, D. C., Registry of Comparative Pathology, AFIP, 1977.

HYPOPHYSIS OR PITUITARY GLAND

The pituitary is morphologically divisible into two distinct components, the anterior pituitary or adenohypophysis (pars distalis) and the posterior pituitary or neurohypophysis. The adenohypophysis is embryologically derived from Rathke's pouch which grows from the primitive foregut in the embryo. The neurohypophysis arises from the diencephalon. In most species, Rathke's pouch remains as a narrow cleft within the adenohypophysis, a cleft which separates the bulk of the adenohypophysis from that portion in immediate contact with the neurohypophysis, known as the pars intermedia of the adenohypophysis.

The adenohypophysis, despite its small size, secretes a minimum of seven hormones; these are follicle-stimulating hormone (FSH), luteinizing hormone (LH), thyroid-stimulating hormone (TSH), adrenocorticotropic hormone (ACTH), growth hormone (somatotropic hormone; STH), luteotropic hormone (prolactin; LTH) and melanocyte-stimulating hormone (MSH). The neurohypophysis releases two hormones, antidiuretic hormone (ADH or vasopressin) and oxytocin. Within the adenohypophysis a specific cell is responsible for the production of each hormone. With special staining techniques at least six distinct cell types can be demonstrated, but with hematoxylin and eosin only three cellular populations are evident. These are the basophils, which produce FSH, TSH, LH and MSH; acidophils, which produce STH and LTH; and chromophobes, which lack stainable granules. Chromophobes are thought to represent resting cells or basophils and acidophils that have released their granules. However, newer evidence suggests that at least in some species chromophobes produce ACTH. Identification in the cell of origin of each hormone produced by the adenohypophysis has been accomplished by means of specific immunofluorescence. The secreting cells have been further characterized by identification of the granules of secretion in the cells by electron microscopy. The evidence is more extensive in relation to the human pituitary and is gradually accumulating for other species. In the dog, corticotrophs (ACTH-producing cells) have been identified by electron microscopy as having granules of varying size and electron density, usually 170 mμ or less in diameter. These cells had well-developed rough endoplasmic reticulum (RER) and Golgi apparatus. They were identified by histologic stains and light microscopy as without granules, therefore chromophobes (Capen and Koestner, 1967). The cells and the hormones they produce are outlined further in Table 26–1.

Production and release of anterior pituitary hormones are under control of the hypothalamus which, in response to the negative feedback mechanisms, produces releasing and inhibitory factors, which pass down nerve fibers to the stalk of the pituitary, enter capillaries, and are carried to the anterior pituitary by way of the portal blood vessels. The posterior pituitary hormones are produced in the hypothalamus (principally in the supraoptic and paraventricular nuclei) and pass down nerve fibers in the hypothalamohypophyseal tract as "neurosecretory material" to the neurohypophysis, where they are released.

The endocrine role of the hypothalamus is discussed in further detail on page 1583.

Table 26–1.   Endocrine Cells and Hormones of Anterior Pituitary (Adenohypophysis)

Cells	Identified By	Hormone Produced	Effect On
Somatotrophs Acidophils Alpha cells STH cells	*H&E:* Acidophilic granules *PAS-OrG:* Orange G positive *EM:* Abundant granules, 350 nm; well-developed RER	Somatotropic or growth hormone, STH (simple protein)	Growth
Lactotrophs LTH cells	*H&E:* Acidophilic granules *PAS-OrG:* Positive *HERL-TETRA:* Erythosin positive *EM:* Sparse granules up to 750 nm; distinctive RER	Lactogenic or mammotropic hormone, prolactin, LTH (simple protein)	Lactation
Gonadotrophs FSH cells ICSH or LH cells β cells	*H&E:* Basophilic; β cells *PAS-OrG:* PAS positive *PM-AT-PAS-OR:* PAS positive; cells round *EM:* Granules with variable density, 200 to 250 nm	(1) Follicle-stimulating-hormone, FSH (mucoprotein) (2) Interstitial-cell-stimulating hormone, ICSH, or luteinizing hormone, LH (mucoprotein)	(1) Ovarian follicles (2) Interstitial cells of testis
Thyrotrophs TSH cells β_2 cells	*H&E:* Basophilic; β_2 cells *PAS-OrG:* PAS positive *PM-AT-PAS-OR:* Thionin positive; cell contour angular *EM:* Granules 150–200 nm; may be peripheral	Thyroid stimulating hormone, TSH (mucoprotein)	Thyroid
Corticomelanotrophs ACTH cells MSH cells β_1 cell	*H&E:* Basophilic; β cells *PAS-OrG:* PAS positive *PM-AT-PAS-OR:* PAS positive; cells oval *EM:* Variably dense granules, 300 to 400 nm; cytoplasmic filaments	(1) Adrenocorticotropic hormone, ACTH (polypeptide) (2) Melanocyte-stimulating hormone, MSH (polypeptide)	(1) Adrenal cortex (2) Melanocytes
Chromophobes "Resting cells"	*H&E:* Chromophobic *PAS-OrG:* no granules *PM-AT-PAS-OR:* no granules *EM:* Sparse fine granules, 150 nm or less	Note: In dog and possibly rat, some of these cells are believed to be *corticotrophs* (ACTH-secreting cells)	Possible precursors for all other cells in adenohypophysis

Abbreviations: *H&E* = Hematoxylin and eosin
PAS-OrG = periodic acid Schiff-Orange G
PM-AT-PAS-OR = Permanganate-aldehyde-thionin-periodic acid Schiff-orange G
HERL-TETRA = Herlant's tetrachrome
RER = Rough endoplasmic reticulum

Capen, C. C., and Koestner, A.: Functional chromophobe adenomas of the canine hypophysis. An ultrastructural evaluation of a neoplasm of pituitary corticotrophs. Pathol. Vet., 4:326–347, 1967.

Cutz, E., Chan, W., Wong, V. and Conen, P. E.: Endocrine cells in rat fetal lungs: Ultrastructural and histochemical study. Lab. Invest., 30:458–464, 1974.

Halmi, N. S.: Current status of human pituitary cytophysiology. NZ Med. J., 80:551–556, 1974.

Ham, A. W.: Histology, 7th ed. Philadelphia, J. B. Lippincott Co., 1974.

Herlant, M., and Pasteels, J. L.: Histophysiology of human anterior pituitary. Methods Achiev. Exp. Pathol., 3:250–305, 1967.

Hodges, J. K., and Hearn, J. P.: Positive feedback effect of estradiol on LH-release in male marmoset monkey, *Callithrix jacchus.* J. Reprod. Fertil., *52*:83–86, 1978.

Howe, A.: The mammalian pars intermedia: A review of its structure and function. J. Endocrinol., *59*:385–409, 1973.

Jubb, K. V., and McEntee, K.: The bovine pituitary gland: I. Adenohypophyseal functional cytology; II. Architecture and cytology with special reference to basophil function. Cornell Vet., *45*:576–641, 1955.

Lacy, P. E.: Endocrine secretory mechanisms. A review. Am. J. Pathol., *79*:170–188, 1975.

McGrath, P.: The pharyngeal hypophysis in some laboratory animals. J. Anat., *117*:95–115, 1974.

Paget, G. E., and Eccleston, E.: Simultaneous specific demonstration of thyrotroph, gonadotroph and acidophil cells in anterior hypophysis. Stain Technol., *35*:119–122, 1960.

Pais, C., and Hennigar, G. R.: Electron microscopy and histochemical correlation of human anterior pituitary cells. Am. J. Pathol., *59*:43–73, 1970.

Pearse, A. G. E.: Cytochemistry and cytology of the normal anterior hypophysis investigated by the trichrome-periodic acid Schiff method. J. Pathol. Bacteriol., *64*:811–826, 1952.

Pearse, A. G. E., and van Noorden, S.: The functional cytology of human adenohypophysis. Can. Med. Assoc. J., *88*:462–471, 1963.

Phifer, R. F., Midgley, A. R., and Spicer, S. S.: Immunohistologic evidence that follicle-stimulating hormone and luteinizing hormone are present in the same cell type in the human pars distalis. J. Clin. Endocrinol., *36*:125–141, 1973.

Purves, H. D., and Griesbach, W. E.: A study on the cytology of the adenohypophysis of the dog. J. Endocrinol., *14*:361–370, 1957.

von Lawzewitsch, I., Dickmann, G. H., Amezua, L., and Pardal, C.: Cytological and ultrastructural characterization of the human pituitary. Acta Anat., *81*:286–316, 1972.

von Oordt, P. G. W. J.: Nomenclature of the hormone-producing cells in the adenohypophysis. A report of the International Committee for Nomenclature of the Adenohypophysis. Gen. Comp. Endocrinol., *5*:131–134, 1965.

Warner, N. E.: Pituitary gland. *In* Pathology, 7th ed, edited by W.A.D. Anderson and J. M. Kissane. C. V. Mosby Co., St. Louis, 1977, pp. 1601–1628.

LESIONS OF THE PITUITARY

Lesions of the pituitary are of principal importance owing to their effect upon the rate of secretion of one or all of the pituitary hormones. Techniques are now available that make it possible to measure pituitary hormones in minute quantities and to identify them in cells of origin. New analytic systems for the pituitary secreting, stimulating, and inhibiting substances produced by the hypothalamus are also changing concepts of the functional interrelationships of hypothalamus and hypophysis. Excessive pituitary hormone usually results from a secreting tumor of pituitary cells or as an effect of hypothalamic neurosecretory stimulation or release of inhibitory control over the pituitary. The nature of the peripheral effects in many cases depends upon the age of the animal.

Hyperpituitarism

This term is used to describe the effect of excessive secretion of one or more pituitary hormones. One of the oldest known examples results from excessive production of growth hormone (somatotropic hormone, STH), usually due to the presence in the pituitary of an acidophilic cell adenoma. In the young person, the result is *gigantism*, with extremely lengthened long bones. In an adult whose epiphyses are closed, the bones grow heavier and thicker, producing large hands, feet, and skull bones. This is called *acromegaly*. Although acidophilic pituitary adenomas have been reported in animals, gigantism and acromegaly have not been recognized.

In another form of hyperpituitarism associated with an adenoma of corticotrophs or corticomelanotrophs, secretion of excessive amounts of adrenal cortical stimulating hormone (ACTH) leads to hyperplasia and hyperfunction of the adrenal cortex. This secondary response causes hyperadrenocorticism and excessive production of adrenal cortical hormones. These conditions will be discussed further in consideration of the adrenal gland.

Hypopituitarism

This condition may result from any lesion in the pituitary that reduces its production of hormones. One of the frequent causes of pituitary atrophy is the replacement of the gland by tumor of any type arising in the pituitary: remnants of Rathke's cleft, craniopharyngeal duct, or pharyngeal hypophysis. If the space-occupying lesion replaces the pituitary

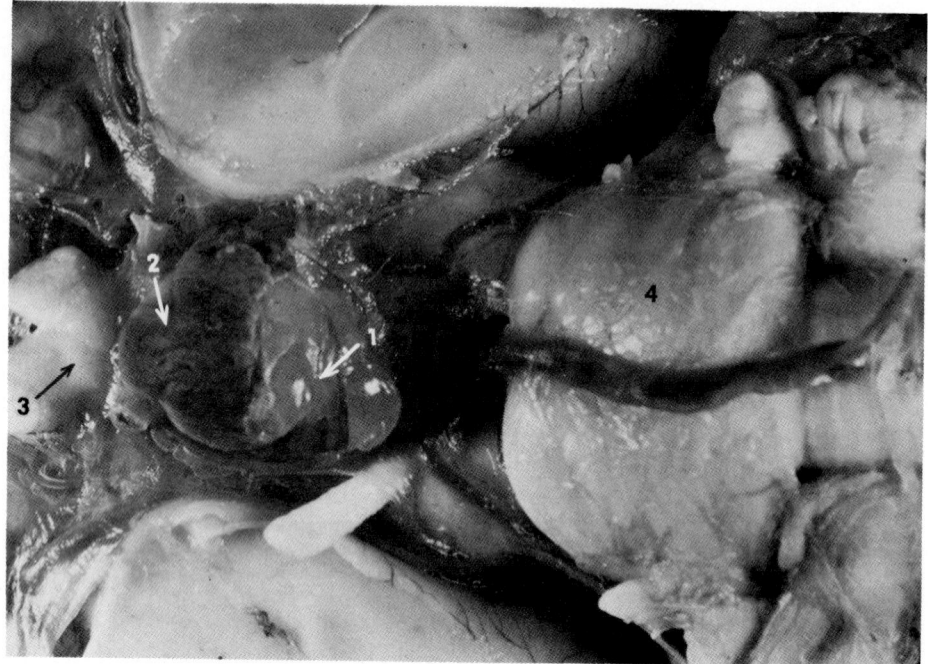

Fig. 26–1. Cyst of the intermediate lobe of the pituitary of a mongrel terrier, spayed female aged 12 years. An incidental finding. The cyst *(1)*, anterior lobe of pituitary *(2)*, optic chiasma *(3)*, pons *(4)*. (Courtesy of Angell Memorial Animal Hospital.)

only, the signs are usually limited to those resulting from pituitary deficiency. If the neoplastic mass replaces the supraoptic nuclei in the thalamus, diabetes insipidus results. Should the optic nerve, optic chiasma, or optic tract be compressed, deficiencies in vision result. Replacement of thalamic nuclei causes signs of behavioral alterations. Secondary tumors in the pituitary have similar effects.

In addition to tumors, cysts or other anomalies may result in loss of pituitary function. Cysts developing from Rathke's cleft are found in cases of pituitary dwarfism in German Shepherd dogs, for example. Other cysts, lined by ciliated columnar epithelium, may also originate in the pharyngeal hypophysis or in the craniopharyngeal duct and become large enough to cause hypopituitarism.

Aplasia or hypoplasia of the pituitary may also occur in association with gross malformations of the head, such as cyclopia and anencephaly (congenital, due to poisoning by vitamin A or *Veratrum californicum,* for example). Functional hypoplasia occurs in some gene-controlled situations, such as aplasia underlying one type of prolonged gestation in Jersey and Guernsey cattle and ateliotic dwarfism in mice.

Inflammation and infectious diseases may result in pituitary malfunction although the inflammation is usually part of a systemic disease, not limited to the hypophysis. Suppurative and lymphocytic meningitis may, on rare occasion, involve the pituitary. This may be due to any one of several viral, bacterial, helminthic, or mycotic organisms. Hemorrhage and necrosis of the pituitary have been seen in dogs with infectious canine hepatitis (adenovirus) and in swine with hog cholera. *Herpesvirus tamarinus* has produced destructive lesions in the pituitary of marmosets *(Saguinus oedipus).* Septic emboli occasionally lodge in the pituitary (especially in ruminants) and may lead to infarction and necrosis. Urate tophi may be seen in the pituitary of birds and snakes on rare occasions as a part of visceral and articular gout.

Pituitary Dwarfism. Pituitary dwarfism in dogs has been described in German Shepherds and Carelian Bear dogs, presumably the result of the same recessive autosomal gene. The lesions in the pituitary have been described only in two cases (a cyst of Rathke's cleft was found, plus a hypoplastic adenohypophysis; death at 12 weeks of age in one case was due to a patent ductus arteriosus). The evidence for its mode of inheritance is good. Of especial interest is the level of serum somatomedin, which was low in homozygous dwarf dogs, intermediate in heterozygotes, and highest in normal unrelated dogs. Somatomedins are growth-promoting proteins and their production is stimulated by growth hormone (somatotropic hormone, STH). A deficiency of somatomedin is considered a reflection of a low level of somatotropic hormone (Willeberg et al., 1975).

Affected puppies (gene symbol *d/d*) are normal at birth but grow at a rate much lower than that of their normal litter mates. By six months of age, normal dogs weigh six or more times as much as their affected littermates. The homozygous *d/d* puppy keeps its puppy hair coat for months and fails to develop sexually. It seems likely that the panhypopituitarism in dwarf German Shepherds described by Alexander (1962) is the same condition reported by Willeberg et al. (1975) and Jensen (1959), although direct comparisons apparently have not been made.

Pituitary dwarfism has been observed in three mutant strains of laboratory mice. The characteristics of the affected mice appear to be similar but were described at different times and were studied with differing techniques. The Snell dwarf, first described in 1929, is the result of a single recessive gene *(dw)* in the homozygous

state. Deficiency of anterior pituitary hormones results in a mouse about one fourth the size of normal littermates. Both males and females are sterile. Secondary myxedema due to thyroid deficiency has also been recognized. Growth at an approximately normal rate may be restored by repeated administration of a fraction of anterior pituitary.

A second pituitary dwarf mutant mouse was originally described by Schaible and Gowen (1961) and named the *Ames dwarf.* The mutant gene *(df)* is located in linkage group VII. The phenotypic characteristics are similar to Snell's dwarf. Retardation of growth is recognizable one week after birth and affected mice are greatly reduced in size at adulthood. Early treatment with bovine growth hormone results in approximately normal growth and at least the males become fertile. The anterior hypophysis (Bartke, 1964) in *df/df* mice lack acidophils and few thyrotrophs are evident.

A third mutation in mice has been described and named *little (lit)* by Eicher and Beamer (1976). This mutant recessive gene is located on chromosome 6 (linkage group XI). The homozygous mouse *(lit/lit)* is recognized by its decreased size at about 15 days of age, and is similar to the Ames *(df/df)* and Snell dwarfs *(dw/dw)* in that the size is reduced without evidence of gross malformation of bones or other structures. The size is simply reduced (ateliotic) with body proportions smaller in all systems. The females are fertile and the males sire one or two litters but rarely a third. The anterior pituitary is reduced in size in both sexes, and analyses with acrylamide gels reveal significant reduction in growth hormone (STH) and prolactin (LTH). This pituitary dwarfism of mice is believed to be similar to human isolated growth hormone deficiency, type I.

Genital Hypoplasia. Associated with a form of hypopituitarism, genital hypoplasia has been described in one of the several mutations that occur at the pink-eyed locus in mice (Johnson and Hunt, 1975). These mice, named "sterile pink-eyed mice," are homozygous for the p^{25H} gene (p^{25H}/p^{25H}). The males are sterile, small, irritable, and produce abnormal sperm. The females have low fertility; their ovaries are small with few corpora lutea; abnormal follicles contain degenerated ova. The uterus is severely hypoplastic and does not respond to estradiol. Surprisingly, no changes have been detected in the anterior pituitary, but degenerated axons have been reported in the posterior pituitary. The hypothalamus has reduced binding capacity for estradiol-17β and iodine binding in the thyroid is also decreased.

Prolonged Gestation. Prolonged gestation is now recognized as a dysfunction of the fetal pituitary. Abnormally long pregnancies were first recorded in cattle over 75 years ago, but only recently have syndromes in cattle and sheep been characterized and linked to abnormalities of the fetal pituitary. In cattle two distinct forms of prolonged gestation occur. Both are controlled by a single autosomal recessive gene. In Holstein-Friesian and Ayrshire cattle, the disease is characterized by a gestation period of up to 380 days and a calf that is abnormally large but lacks obvious deformities. The pituitary is present but there is marked degranulation of the acidophils. Adrenal cortices are hypoplastic, but other endocrine glands are normal. The calf dies in utero and is born dead (if physically possible), or if delivered by cesarean section, it may be viable but is weak, unable to nurse, and dies in 6 to 12 hours. Death is associated with severe hypoglycemia, but based on the frequent presence of meconium staining of the skin, other factors associated with intrauterine distress probably contribute.

A second type of prolonged gestation occurs in Jersey and Guernsey breeds in which the gestation periods may exceed 475 days. Normal parturition does not occur, though a dead fetus may be expelled.

Even if delivered by cesarean section, viable calves only survive a few minutes. The calf is small, has hypotrichosis and facial abnormalities such as hydrocephalus, anencephalus, and cyclopia. There is aplasia of the anterior pituitary and often hypoplasia of the neurohypophysis. The adrenal glands and thyroid gland are also hypoplastic.

Types of prolonged gestations have been observed in cattle that do not clearly fit into the two syndromes described; however, the fetuses have not been studied with the detail necessary to reach any conclusion regarding pathogenesis.

In sheep, prolonged pregnancy has been described in Karakul ewes in Southwest Africa. Gestation exceeds 200 days, the lambs are abnormally large, and if delivered survive only a few hours. The abnormally large lambs resulted in the name Grootlamsiekte (big lamb disease). The anterior pituitary is present, but acidophils are degranulated. The adrenal cortices and thymus are hypoplastic. This form of prolonged gestation is caused by consumption of the plant *Salsola tuberculata* (Joubert et al., 1972). Although the condition most frequently occurs in the Karakul breed, because they are raised where the plant is common, other breeds are susceptible.

Prolonged gestation has also been described in sheep following ingestion of *Veratrum californicum*. Ingestion of this plant in early pregnancy results in severe cranial malformations which include aplasia of the pituitary.

Alexander, J. E.: Anomaly of craniopharyngeal duct and hypophysis. Can. Vet. J., 3:83–86, 1962.

Andresen, E., Willeberg, P., and Rasmussen, P. G.: Pituitary dwarfism in German Shepherd dogs: Genetic investigations. Nord. Vet. Med., 26:692–701, 1974.

Andresen, E., and Willeberg, P.: Pituitary dwarfism in Carelian Bear dogs: Evidence of simple, autosomal recessive inheritance. Hereditas, 84:232–234, 1976.

Baker, E.: Congenital hypoplasia of the pituitary and pancreas in the dog. J. Am. Vet. Med. Assoc., 126:468, 1955.

Bartke, A.: Histology of the anterior hypophysis, thyroid and gonads of two types of dwarf mice. Anat. Rec., 149:225–235, 1964.

Carsner, R. L., and Rennels, E. G.: Primary site of gene action in anterior pituitary dwarf mice. Science, 131:829, 1960.

Eicher, E. M., and Beamer, W. G.: Inherited ateliotic dwarfism in mice. Characteristics of the mutation, *little*, on Chromosome 6. J. Hered., 67:87–91, 1976.

Green, R. A., and Farrow, C. S.: Diabetes insipidus in a cat. J. Am. Vet. Med. Assoc., 164:524–526, 1974.

Huston, K., and Gier, H. T.: An anatomical description of a hydrocephalic calf from prolonged gestation and the possible relationships of these conditions. Cornell Vet., 48:45–53, 1958.

Holm, L. W.: Prolonged pregnancy. Adv. Vet. Sci., 11:159–205, 1967.

Jensen, E. C.: Hypopituitarism associated with cystic Rathke's cleft in a dog. J. Am. Vet. Med. Assoc., 135:572-575, 1959.

Johnson, D. R., and Hunt, D. M.: Endocrinological findings in sterile pink-eyed mice. J. Reprod. Fertil., 42:51–58, 1975.

Joubert, J. P. J., Basson, P. A., Lucks, H. J., and Burger, J. H. S.: "Grootlamsiekte," a specific syndrome of prolonged gestation in sheep: further investigations. Onderstepoort J. Vet. Res., 39:59–70, 1972.

Kennedy, P. C.: Interactions of fetal disease and the onset of labor in cattle and sheep. Fed. Proc., 30:110–113, 1971.

Kennedy, P. C., Liggins, G. C., and Holm, L. W.: Prolonged gestation. In Comparative Aspects of Reproductive Failure, edited by K. Benirschke. New York, Springer-Verlag, 1967.

Kennedy, P. C., Kendrick, J. W., and Stormont, C.: Adenohypophyseal aplasia, an inherited defect associated with abnormal gestation in Guernsey cattle. Cornell Vet., 47:161–178, 1957.

Lewis, U. J.: Growth hormone of normal and dwarf mice. Mem. Soc. Endocr., 15:179–191, 1967.

Loeb, W. F., Capen, C. C., and Johnson, L. E.: Adenomas of the pars intermedia associated with hyperglycemia and glycosuria in two horses. Cornell Vet., 56:623–629, 1966.

Rogers, W. A., Valdez, H., Anderson, B. C., and Comella, C.: Partial deficiency of antidiuretic hormone in a cat. J. Am. Vet. Med. Assoc., 170:545–547, 1977.

Sawyer, W. H., Valtin, H., and Sokol, H. W.: Neurohypophyseal principles in rats with familial hypothalamic diabetes insipidus (Brattleboro strain). Endocrinology, 74:153–155, 1964.

Schaible, R. H., and Gowen, J. W.: A new dwarf mouse. Genetics, 46:896, 1961.

Shire, J. G. M., and Hambly, E. A.: The adrenal glands of mice with hereditary pituitary dwarfism. Acta Pathol. Microbiol. Scand., 81:226–228, 1973.

Snell, G. D.: Dwarf, a new Mendelian recessive character of the house mouse. Proc. Natl. Acad. Sci. USA, 15:733–734, 1929.

Sokol, H. W., and Valtin, H.: Morphology of the neurosecretory system in rats homozygous and heterozygous for hypothalamic diabetes in-

sipidus (Brattleboro strain). Endocrinology, 77:692–700, 1965.

Valtin, H.: Animal model of human disease. Hereditary hypothalamic diabetes insipidus. Am. J. Pathol., 83:633–636, 1976.

Valtin, H.: Animal model of human disease: Hereditary hypothalamic diabetes insipidus. Model 107, In Handbook: Animal Models of Human Disease, edited by T. C. Jones, D. B. Hackel, and G. Migaki. Washington, D.C., Registry of Comparative Pathology, AFIP, 1977.

Valtin, H., Schroeder, H. A., Bernirschke, K., and Sokol, H. W.: Familial hypothalamic diabetes insipidus in rats. Nature, 196:1109–1110, 1962.

Valtin, H., Sawyer, W. H., and Sokol, H. W.: Neurohypophyseal principles in rats homozygous and heterozygous for hypothalamic diabetes insipidus (Brattleboro strain). Endocrinology, 77:701–706, 1965.

Viola-Magni, M.: Cell number deficiencies in the nervous system of dwarf mice. Anat. Rec., 153:325–333, 1965.

Wegelius, O.: The dwarf mouse: An animal with secondary myxedema. Proc. Soc. Exp. Biol. Med., 101:225–227, 1959.

Willeberg, P., Kastrup, K. W., and Andresen, E.: Pituitary dwarfism in German Shepherd dogs: Studies on somatomedin activity. Nord. Vet. Med., 27:448–454, 1975.

Neoplasms of the Pituitary

Primary tumors of the pituitary have been found in all species of man and animals that have been adequately studied. Neoplasms have been most frequently reported in the pituitary of the dog, but rats are also often affected. Natural cases are rare in mice, although these animals are susceptible to experimentally induced pituitary tumors. Individual case reports may be found in the literature concerning neoplasms of the pituitary of cats, horses, nonhuman primates, sheep, and cattle. Parakeets appear to be frequently affected by thyrotropic pituitary tumors (Schlumberger, 1954).

Conventional methods of classification of pituitary tumors involve naming them in accordance with the presence of granules detectable by histologic techniques as acidophilic, basophilic, or chromophobic adenomas or adenocarcinomas. Normal and neoplastic acidophils (Tables 26–1, 26–3) are believed to be associated with the secretion of growth hor-

Table 26–2. Outline of Some Hypothalamic/Hypophyseal Lesions

Lesion(s)	Species Affected	Local Effects	Distal Effects	References
Cyst of craniopharyngeal duct	Dog, *Macaca sinica*, *Gorilla gorilla*	Compression atrophy of adenohypophysis, neurohypophysis, hypothalamus, optic chiasma, optic tracts, median eminence	Hypopituitarism: obesity, genital atrophy, hypothyroidism, hypoadrenalism; hypothalamic diabetes insipidus; visual defects; neurologic behavioral changes	Fox, 1923 Koch, 1937 Saunders and Rickard, 1952 Saunders et al., 1951
Craniopharyngioma	Dog, cat			
Chromophobe adenoma	Dog, cat, rat			Zaki and Liu, 1973 Zaki et al., 1975 Green and Farrow, 1974 Rogers et al., 1977 Boorman and Hollander, 1973
Acidophilic adenoma	Dog		No gigantism or acromegaly detected; adenomas of pancreatic islets	Capen et al., 1967b Hottendorf et al., 1966
Inherited hypothalamic defect	Rat	Decreased levels of vasopressin and oxytocin	Hypothalamic diabetes insipidus	Valtin et al., 1962, 1965 Sokol and Valtin, 1965 Sawyer et al., 1964 Valtin, 1977
Anencephaly; cyclopia (*Veratrum californicum* poisoning); hydrocephalus (viral, congenital)	Sheep, cattle	Absence or aplasia of pituitary	Prolonged gestation; hypoplasia of fetal adrenal cortex	Kennedy et al., 1967 Kennedy, 1971 Huston and Gier, 1958 Holm, 1967
Cyst of Rathke's cleft (congenital)	Dog	Pressure atrophy of pituitary; decreased production of somatotropic hormone and prolactin	Pituitary dwarfism; diabetes insipidus; hypothyroidism	Jensen, 1959

Disorder	Species	Pathophysiology	Clinical signs	Reference
Inherited disorder: degenerative lesions in pars nervosa and hypothalamus; Inherited disorder: pituitary/hypothalamic lesions unknown	Mouse (lit/lit), Mouse (dw/dw), Mouse (df/df)	Decreased production of somatotropin (STH), and prolactin (LTH)	Isolated growth deficiency (ateliotic dwarfism); pituitary dwarfism: hypothyroidism, obesity, genital aplasia, insensitivity to insulin	Eicher and Beamer, 1976; Lewis, 1967; Shire and Hambly, 1973; Chester-Jones, 1949
Basophil or chromophobe adenoma (adenoma of corticomelanotrophs, ACTH/MLM cells)	Dog, cat, horse	Excess production of ACTH/MSH by tumor; atrophy of pituitary and hypothalamus by tumor replacement	Cushing's disease, hyperadrenocorticism; serum corticosteroids increased 3.5 ×; urinary excretion of 17-hydroxycorticosteroids increased 5 ×; diabetes insipidus; hypothyroidism	Capen, et al., 1967a; Capen and Koestner, 1967; Pauli et al., 1974
Inherited deficiency of somatotrophic cells (congenital)	Dog (German Shepherd, Carelian Bear dogs)	Decreased production of somatotropin (STH, growth hormone)	Pituitary dwarfism, decreased serum levels of somatomedin	Andresen et al., 1974; Willeberg et al., 1975; Andresen and Willeberg, 1976
Chromophobe adenocarcinoma cells (not completely identified)	Bovine	Tumor spread from pituitary fossa to foramen magnum, metastasized to submaxillary lymph nodes	Atrophy of masseter muscles (cranial nerves compressed); paralysis of tongue and pharynx, difficult breathing (hypoglossal nerve compressed)	Powers and Winkler, 1977
Inherited disorder on "pink-eyed" locus; degenerated axons in pars nervosa	Mice (p^{25H}/p^{25H})	reduced binding capacity for estradiol-17β in hypothalamus	Males: sterile; small body size; abnormal sperm Females: low fecundity; ovaries atrophic; abnormal follicles, low ovulation; uterus severely hypoplastic, no response to estradiol	Johnson and Hunt, 1975

mone (somatotropin, STH), and prolactin (lactotropic hormone, LTH).

Basophils of various kind produce follicle-stimulating hormone (FSH), interstitial cell hormone (luteinizing hormone, LH, or ICSH), thyroid-stimulating hormone (TSH), adrenocorticotropic hormone (ACTH), and melanocyte-stimulating hormone (MSH). Chromophobic cells (those without demonstrable granules visible by the light microscope) have been presumed to be undifferentiated or resting cells, not secreting any hormone. However, in the dog and rat, chromophobe cells in tumors have been shown to secrete hormones and to contain secretory granules too small to be seen with the light microscope (approximately 150 nm in diameter). More precise methods of identifying these neoplastic cells and the tumors they comprise would be preferable. Such techniques are now available with the electron microscope, immunohistochemical methods, and radioimmunoassay. Nomenclature and classification of pituitary tumors in the future should take cognizance of the functional aspects of the neoplastic cells.

The effects of pituitary tumors may be exerted upon their host (1) by replacement of functional hypophyseal, hypothalamic, or thalamic tissue, or (2) by excessive secretion of specific hormones (Table 26–1). Pituitary somatotrophs produce somatotropic or growth hormone (STH, GH), which stimulates growth and also is antagonistic to the peripheral effects of insulin and, in excess, may cause diabetes mellitus. The lactotrophs stimulate mammary secretion through the action of prolactin or lactogenic hormone (LTH). The gonads are stimulated by the products of pituitary gonadotrophs, namely follicle-stimulating hormone (FSH) and interstitial-cell-stimulating (ICSH) or luteinizing hormone (LH). The pituitary thyrotrophs, through the activity of their thyroid-stimulating hormone (TSH), have a profound effect on the follicular cells of the thyroid. Corticomelanotrophs appear

to secrete two hormones: (1) adrenocorticotrophic hormone (ACTH) with its essential stimulating effect upon the adrenal cortex, and (2) melanocyte-stimulating hormone (MSH), which causes multiplication and melanin production by melanocytes.

Clearly, neoplasms of pituitary cells that secrete excessive hormone may have important effects upon other endocrine or somatic systems. These effects will be considered further as diseases of other parts of the endocrine system are taken up.

Adenomas. Adenomas of the pituitary are distinguished from their malignant counterparts (adenocarcinomas) by their circumscribed nature, growth by expansion and lack of tendency to invade adjacent tissue. The cells may have the tinctorial features of acidophils, basophils, or chromophobes, and as indicated heretofore, each of these three types may secrete hormones. Special techniques are necessary to demonstrate the hormone produced and therefore the identity of the tumor cells. A summary of the endocrine-secreting adenomas of the pituitary identified so far in humans and animals is in Table 26–3.

The differentiation of adenomas from adenocarcinomas of the pituitary has often been a matter of controversy. In our view, those neoplasms whose cells invade and destroy adjacent tissues, outgrow their blood supply and undergo necrosis, or metastasize by way of blood or lymphatics to lymph nodes or other organs should be considered malignant and, therefore, adenocarcinomas.

Chromophobe adenomas which may or may not secrete a pituitary hormone have characteristic histologic features and are the most frequent pituitary neoplasm in the dog. The tumor cell may be large or small. The large type is most frequent and is a polyhedral cell with a large vesicular nucleus containing one or two conspicuous nucleoli. The cytoplasm is distinctly outlined, abundant and eosinophilic. Cytoplasmic granules are not seen with ordi-

Functional Cell	Host Species	Hormone Produced	Origin of Tumors	Effect Upon Host	References
Somatotroph (acidophil or chromophobe)	Human	Somatotropin (STH)	Spontaneous	Gigantism; acromegaly	Warner, 1977
Somatotroph	Rat	Somatotropin (STH) and prolactin (LTH)	Induced by x ray or estrogen; transplantable	Acromegaly; galactorrhea	Ito, 1978; Furth et al., 1956, 1978
Lactotroph (acidophil or chromophobe)	Human	Lactogenic, mammotropic, or prolactin (LTH)	Spontaneous	Amenorrhea; galactorrhea	Warner, 1977
Thyrotroph (basophil or chromophobe)	Human	Thyroid-stimulating hormone (TSH)	Spontaneous	Hyperthyroidism; thyroid adenomas	Warner, 1977
Thyrotroph	Rat	Thyroid-stimulating hormone (TSH)	Experimental antithyroid diet or low iodine diet	Hyperthyroidism; thyroid adenomas	Ito, 1978; Axelrod and Lablond, 1955
Thyrotroph	Mouse	Thyroid-stimulating hormone (TSH)	Experimental antithyroid or low iodine diet	Hyperthyroidism	Dingemans, 1973
Gonadotroph	Not yet decided	Follicle-stimulating hormone (FSH) interstitial cell-stimulating hormone (ICSH), or luteinizing hormone (LH)	Not yet described	Not yet described	Ito, 1978
Corticomelanotroph (basophils or chromophobes)	Human	Adrenocorticotropic hormone (ACTH)	Spontaneous	Hyperadrenocorticism, Cushing's syndrome	Warner, 1977
Corticomelanotroph (chromophobe)	Dog	Adrenocorticotrophic hormone (ACTH)	Spontaneous	Hyperadrenocorticism	Capen and Koestner, 1967
Corticomelanotroph (chromophobe)	Rat	Adrenocorticotropic hormone (ACTH); also prolactin (LTH) and somatotropin (STH)	Experimental, induced by x-radiation; transplantable	Hyperadrenocorticism	Ito, 1978; Furth et al., 1956
Corticomelanotroph (chromophobe)	Dog	Adrenocorticotropic hormone (ACTH)	Spontaneous	Hyperadrenocorticism	Furth et al., 1953; Ito, 1978

nary histologic techniques, although secreting granules can be identified by electron microscopy. The small type of cell is about half the size of the large type and has a dark nucleus with indistinct nucleoli and scant, indistinctly demarcated cytoplasm. These cells may form two histologic patterns. In one, solid sheets of closely packed cells are formed, with few capillaries and little evident stroma; this is called the diffuse type. In the second (sinusoidal) type, the tumor contains many endothelial-lined sinusoids around which the tumor cells are closely arranged in a palisading pattern. Fine trabeculae and capillaries or small venules separate this tumor into irregularly shaped lobules. Occasionally small acini are formed by tumor cells and the lumen contains colloid material.

Adenomas of the pars intermedia are less frequent than chromophobe adenomas but may in some cases produce hormone. These tumors may be differentiated from adenomas of the pars distalis by the presence of many colloid-filled acini lined by tall columnar tumor cells. Solid arrays of cells resembling chromophobes also occur in this tumor.

Secondary Neoplasms in the Pituitary. Although infrequently encountered, metastatic neoplasms reported in the pituitary include lymphosarcoma (dogs, cattle, birds), malignant melanoma (dogs, cats, horses), adenocarcinoma of the mammary gland (dogs), osteosarcoma and ependymoma (dogs). These metastatic neoplasms may have the same destructive effects on the pituitary, hypothalamus and thalamus as primary tumors, and therefore produce similar clinical signs.

Craniopharyngioma. Craniopharyngioma is a neoplasm arising from remnants of the craniopharyngeal duct or pharyngeal pituitary and may impinge upon the pituitary or replace it. See Chapter 23 and Figure 23–9.

Anderson, M. P., and Capen, C. C.: The endocrine system. Chapter 6. *In* Pathology of Laboratory Animals, edited by K. Benirschke, F. M. Garner, and T. C. Jones. New York, Springer-Verlag, 1978.

Axelrod, A. A., and Leblond, C. P.: Induction of thyroid tumors in rats by a low iodine diet. Cancer, 8:339–367, 1955.

Berson, S. A., and Yalow, R. S.: Radioimmunoassay: General. *In* Peptide Hormones, Vol. 2A, Part 1. Methods in Investigative and Diagnostic Endocrinology, edited by S. A. Berson and R. S. Yalow. New York, Elsevier, 1973. pp. 84–120.

Boorman, G. A., and Hollander, C. F.: Spontaneous lesions in the female WAG/Rij (Wistar) rat. J. Gerontol., 28:152–159, 1973.

Capen, C. C., Martin, S. L., and Koestner, A.: Neoplasms in the adenohypophysis of the dog. A clinical and pathologic study. Pathol. Vet., 4:301–325, 1967a.

————: The ultrastructure and histopathology of an acidophil adenoma of the canine adenohypophysis. Pathol. Vet., 4:348–365, 1967b.

Capen, C. C., and Koestner, A.: Functional chromophobe adenomas of the canine adenohypophysis. An ultrastructural evaluation of a neoplasm of pituitary corticotrophs. Pathol. Vet., 4:326–347, 1967.

Clifton, K. H.: Problems in experimental tumorigenesis of the pituitary gland, gonads, adrenal cortices and mammary glands. A review. Cancer Res., 19:2–22, 1959.

Dingemans, K. P.: Development of TSH-producing pituitary tumours in mouse. Virchows Arch. (Cell Pathol.), 12:338–359, 1973.

Fitzgerald, J. E., Schardein, J. L., and Kaump, D. H.: Several uncommon pituitary tumors in the rat. Lab. Anim. Sci., 21:581–584, 1971.

Fox, H.: Diseases of Captive Wild Mammals and Birds. Incidence, Description, Comparison. Philadelphia, J. B. Lippincott, 1923.

Furth, J., Gadsden, E. L., and Upton, A. C.: ACTH secreting transplantable pituitary tumors. Proc. Soc. Exp. Biol. Med., 84:253–255, 1953.

Furth, J., Clifton, K. H., Gadsden, E. L., and Buffett, R. F.: Dependent and autonomous mammotrophic pituitary tumors in rats; their somatotrophic features. Cancer Res., 16:608–616, 1956.

Furth, J., Nakane, P. K., and Pasteels, J. L.: Pathology and pathogenesis of spontaneous and experimental pituitary tumors. *In* Pathology of Tumors in Laboratory Animals, Vol 1, Part 2. Edited by V. Turusow. Lyon, France, Internat. Agency for Research on Cancer, 1978.

Horn, H. A., and Stewart, H. L.: A review of some spontaneous tumors of noninbred mice. J. Natl. Cancer Inst., 13:591–603, 1952–1953.

Hottendorf, G. H., Nielsen, S. W., and Lieberman, L. I.: Acidophil adenoma of the pituitary gland and other neoplasms in a Boxer. J. Am. Vet. Med. Assoc., 148:1046–1050, 1966.

Ito, A., et al.: Incidence and character of the spontaneous pituitary tumors in strain CR and W/Fu male rats. J. Natl. Cancer Inst., 49:701–711, 1972.

Ito, A.: Animal model of human disease: Pituitary tumors. Model No. 121. *In* Handbook: Animal Models of Human Disease. Edited by T. C.

Jones, D. B. Hackel, and G. Migaki. Washington, D.C., Registry of Comparative Pathology, AFIP, 1978.

Chester-Jones, I.: The relationship of the mouse adrenal cortex to the pituitary. Endocrinology, 45:514–536, 1949.

Kleinberg, D. L., Noel, G. L., and Frantz, A. G.: Galactorrhea: A study of 235 cases, including 48 with pituitary tumors. N. Engl. J. Med., 296:589–600, 1977.

Koch, W.: Bericht über das Ergebnis der Obduktion das Gorilla Bobby des Zoologischen Gartens zu Berlin. Ein Beitrag zur vergleichender Konstitutions pathologie. Veroeff. Konst. Wehr. Pathol., 9:1–36, 1937.

Loeb, W. F., Capen, C. C., and Johnson, L. E.: Adenomas of the pars intermedia associated with hyperglycemia and glycosuria in two horses. Cornell Vet., 56:623–639, 1966.

Luksch, F.: Über Hypophysentumoren beim Hunde. Tierarztl. Arch., 3:1–16, 1923.

MacKenzie, W. F., and Garner, F. N.: Comparison of neoplasms in six sources of rats. J. Natl. Cancer Inst., 50:1243–1257, 1973.

Murphy, E. D.: Characteristic tumors. In The Biology of the Laboratory Mouse, edited by E. L. Green. New York, McGraw Hill, 1966.

Olivier, L., et al.: Ultrastructure of pituitary tumor cells: A critical study. In The Anterior Pituitary, edited by A. Tixier-Vidal and M. G. Farquhar. New York, Academic Press, 1975. pp. 231–276.

Pauli, B. U., Rossi, G. L., and Straub, R.: Adenoma of the pars intermedia of the hypophysis in a horse with "Cushing's disease" symptoms. Vet. Pathol., 11:417–429, 1974.

Powers, R. D., and Winkler, J. K.: Pituitary carcinoma with extracranial metastasis in a cow. Vet. Pathol., 14:524–526, 1977.

Saunders, L. Z., Stephenson, H. C., and McEntee, K.: Diabetes insipidus and adiposogenital syndrome in a dog due to an infundibuloma. Cornell Vet., 41:445–458, 1951.

Saunders, L. Z., and Rickard, C. G.: Craniopharyngioma in a dog with apparent adiposogenital syndrome and diabetes insipidus. Cornell Vet., 42:490–494, 1952.

Schlumberger, H. G.: Neoplasia in the parakeet. I. Spontaneous chromophobe pituitary tumors. Cancer Res., 14:237–245, 1954.

Sher, S. P.: Tumors of control mice. Literature tabulation. Toxicol. Appl. Pharmacol., 30:337–359, 1974.

Snell, K. C.: Spontaneous lesions of the rat. In The Pathology of Laboratory Animals, edited by W. E. Ribelin and J. R. McCoy. Springfield, Ill., Charles C Thomas, 1965. pp. 241–302.

Thompson, S. W., and Hunt, R. D.: Spontaneous tumors in the Sprague-Dawley rat: Incidence rates of some types of neoplasms as determined by serial section versus single section technic. Ann. NY Acad. Sci., 108:832–845, 1963.

Warner, N. E.: Pituitary gland. In Pathology, 7th ed., edited by W. A. D. Andersen, and F. M. Kissane. St. Louis, C. V. Mosby, 1977. pp. 1601–1628.

White, E. G.: A suprasellar tumor in a dog. J. Pathol. Bact., 47:323–326, 1938.

Zaki, F. A., and Liu, S. K.: Pituitary chromophobe adenoma in a cat. Vet. Pathol., 10:232–237, 1973.

Zaki, F., Harris, J., and Budzilovich, G.: Cystic pituicytoma of the neurohypophysis in a Siamese cat. J. Comp. Pathol., 85:467–471, 1975.

THYROID

The thyroid is an endocrine organ found in all vertebrates; in mammals it is usually a bilobed gland located just caudal to the larynx, in close proximity to the trachea. In some mammals the two lobes are connected by an isthmus which lies across the ventral (anterior) aspect of the trachea. The embryonic development of the thyroid starts from the caudal aspect of the pharynx as an outward growth of epithelium which eventually forms the thyroglossal duct. This duct usually disappears before birth but may persist into adulthood. In addition to vascular, nervous, and connective tissues, the thyroid has two types of endocrine cells. The preponderant epithelial cells are arranged into acini or follicles, which consist of cells arranged circumferentially around a central mass of colloid material. The epithelial cells may be tall columnar, cuboidal, or flattened, depending upon their secretory activity. These **follicular cells** concentrate iodide from the circulating blood and, in the course of several enzymatic reactions, form thyroglobulin, which is stored as colloid and then subsequently secreted as thyroxine (T_4) and triiodothyronine (T_3). The function of thyroxine and triiodothyronine is to stimulate the metabolism of all body cells.

The second type of endocrine cell is the "parafollicular," "light" or "C" cell, which was identified in the dog in 1932 by Nonidez, but only recently was its function discovered. These cells are found, usually few in number, along the base or between the follicular cells, within or outside the basement membrane (depending on the species). These cells have a distinct pale cytoplasm in preparations stained with periodic acid Schiff reagent (PAS) and also a similar, lightly stained cytoplasm with hematoxylin and eosin (H&E) stain. In the dog they are readily recognized in H&E preparations and may be increased in number in animals kept on a diet high in calcium. These parafollicular cells are responsible for the secretion of thyrocalcitonin, a hormone that has the effect of reducing calcium levels in the blood, and thus, in effect, is antagonistic to the action of parathyroid hormone.

The parathyroid glands in most mammals are separate endocrine glands embedded in the thyroid but functioning entirely independently. These important glands are considered separately from the thyroid.

Aberrant (ectopic) thyroid tissue is relatively frequent in most animal species. Most aberrant thyroids result from the failure of all or part of the thyroid anlage to descend from the floor of the pharynx to its normal cervical position, or from its descending beyond its normal adult position. In the first case, aberrant thyroid tissue may occur at any median point from the tongue to its normal position; in the second case it occurs caudal to the normal position, including within the thoracic cavity. Another form of aberrant thyroid results from anomalous development of fetal tissue in general. Aberrant thyroid responds to the same physiologic stimuli as the cervical gland.

A **thyroglossal cyst** is a developmental anomaly arising in the thyroglossal duct. This duct, in early embryonic life, reaches out from the lower pharyngeal mucosa to form the primitive thyroid, normally disappearing before birth. When it persists, a sinus tract or a cyst commonly develops. The cyst is always in the midline and is lined either by stratified squamous or simple columnar epithelium or by a mixture of the two. This is not a frequent anomaly in animals, but developmental anomalies are not reported with a regularity that permits statistical conclusions.

Anderson, M. P., and Capen, C. C.: The endocrine system. *In* Pathology of Laboratory Animals, edited by K. Benirschke, F. M. Garner, and T. C. Jones. New York, Springer-Verlag, 1978. pp. 423–508.

Belshaw, B. E., and Becker, D. V.: Necrosis of follicular cells and discharge of thyroidal iodine induced by administering iodine to iodine-deficient dogs. J. Clin. Endocrinol. Metab., 36:466–474, 1973.

Belshaw, B. E., Cooper, T. B., and Becker, D. V.: The iodine requirement and influence of iodine intake on iodine metabolism and thyroid function in the adult Beagle. Endocrinology, 96:1280–1291, 1975.

Blessing, M. H., and Zaborsky, F.: Über der Nachweis von intrathorakalem Schildrüsengewebe des Hundes mit I¹³¹. Frankfurter Z. Pathol., 75:14–24, 1966.

Cohrs, P.: Beitrag zur Kenntnis der intraperikardialen akzessorrischen Schildrüsen und Epithelkörperchen beim Hund *(Canis familiaris)*. Berl. Tierärztl. Wochenschr., 46:683–688, 1930.

Dämmrich, K.: Die Beeinflussung des Skeletts durch die Schilddrüse bei Tieren. Berl. Münch. Tierarztl. Wochenschr., 76:31–34, 53–56, 1963.

Eickhoff, W.: Zur Histologie und Pathologie der Wildschilddrüse. Arch. Exp. Vet. Med., 16:211–228, 1963.

Gilmore, J. W., Venzke, W. G., and Foust, H. L.: Growth changes in body organs. Part II. Growth changes in the thyroid of the normal dog. Am. J. Vet. Res., 1:66–72, 1940.

Goldwin, M. C.: The early development of the thyroid gland in the dog with especial reference to the origin and position of accessory thyroid tissue within the thoracic cavity. Anat. Rec., 66:233–251, 1936.

Hare, T.: Three cases of heterotopic deposits of thyroid tissue in the dog. Proc. Roy. Soc. Med., 25:1496–1499, 1932.

Hare, T.: Fusion of the thyroid glands in a dog. Proc. Roy. Soc. Med., 25:1500, 1932.

Hunt, R. D.: Aberrant thyroid tissue in the mouse. Science, 141:1054–1055, 1963.

Kameda, Y.: The accessory thyroid glands of the dog around the intrapericardial aorta. Arch. Histol. Jpn., 34:375–391, 1972.

Lucke, V. M.: An histological study of thyroid abnormalities in the domestic cat. J. Small Anim. Pract., 5:351–358, 1964.

Nonidez, J. F.: The origin of the parafollicular cell, a second epithelial component of the thyroid gland of the dog. Am. J. Anat., 49:479–505, 1932.

Oppenheimer, J. H.: Initiation of thyroid-hormone action. N. Engl. J. Med., 292:1063–1068, 1975.

Sansom, B. F.: Accessory thyroid tissue in the goat. Br. Vet. J., 123:162–169, 1967.

Schmidt, R. E.: Ectopic thyroid in a rhesus monkey *(Macaca mulatta)*. Lab Primate Newsletter, 9:13, 1970. (Brown Univ.)

Scott, P. P., Greaves, J. P., and Scott, M. G.: Nutrition of the cat. IV. Calcium and iodine deficiency on a meat diet. Br. J. Nutr., 15:35–51, 1961.

Swarts, J. L., and Thompson, R. L.: Accessory thyroid

tissue within the pericardium of the dog. J. Med. Res., 24:299–308, 1911.

Woods, J. W., Wayt, H. J., and Backer, H. J.: Cyclic fluctuations in I-131 content of thyroid glands of cats and monkeys. Proc. Soc. Exp. Biol. Med., 122:211–214, 1966.

Hypothyroidism

In the thyroid, as in the other endocrine glands, we are principally concerned with diseases that lead to insufficient or excessive production of thyroxine—hypothyroidism or hyperthyroidism, respectively.

The essential feature of hypothyroidism is an abnormally low basal metabolic rate. This can be measured by appropriate clinical techniques, but the disorder is commonly recognizable by a characteristic symptomatology. There is a disinclination to vigorous movement and a tendency to obesity, accompanied, in humans and doubtless in animals also, by an attitude of mental complacency. In cases of much severity, there is, in the young, retardation of growth as regards total stature, sexual development, and (in the human) mental acuity. The condition is called **cretinism,** and affected persons, even after they reach the stunted maturity which is their lot, are called cretins (Fr. *cretin,* an idiot). When the thyroid deficiency arises in an adult human, myxedema is the outstanding symptom. This is the accumulation in the subcutaneous and other connective tissues of a mucoid, or myxomatous, semifluid substance, essentially mucoid degeneration, which gives the face and other body surfaces a puffy and edematous appearance.

Aplasia or hypoplasia of the thyroid in the dog results in signs of hypothyroidism, including obesity, intolerance to cold, lethargy, muscular weakness, and bilaterally symmetrical alopecia. The lesions in the skin are equally characteristic, with atrophy of epidermis, sebaceous glands, and erector pili muscles, plus hyperkeratosis and distention of hair follicles with keratin (pilar hyperkeratosis). Serum cholesterol usually becomes elevated above 450 mg/100 ml serum; protein-bound iodine (PBI) is deficient, usually about 1.0 μg/100 ml. Thyroxine (T_4) is usually less than 0.6

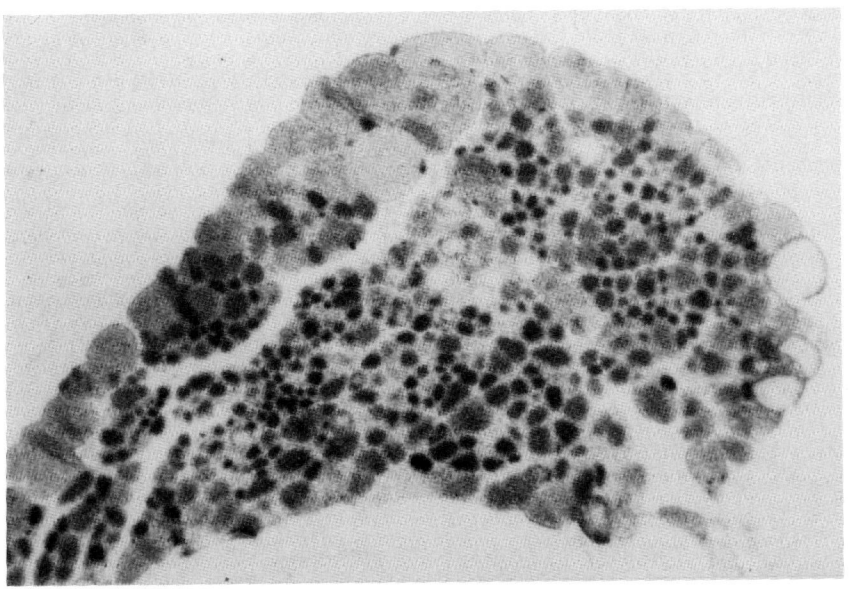

Fig. 26–2. Autoradiograph of normal rat thyroid gland prepared 12 hours following injection of [131]I. The radioactive iodine has been concentrated in the thyroid follicles; the radioactive emissions interacted with the photographic emulsion to produce the dark, roughly spherical masses.

μg/100 ml. Thyroidal radioactive iodine (^{131}I) uptake is less than 5% (Anderson and Capen, 1978).

Goiter

Goiter, or enlargement of the thyroid gland as a whole, may be accompanied by either hypo- or hyperthyroidism. The enlargement may be due to an increase of thyroid tissue, which is hyperplasia, or to an increased amount of colloid, distending the lumens of the acini, or much less commonly, to inflammatory proliferation. Hyperplasia of the thyroid is manifested, as in other glandular organs, (1) by an increase in the height of each individual columnar epithelial cell and (2) by an increase in the number of these epithelial cells. As explained in the study of hyperplasia in general, this results in the formation of complicated folds in the epithelial lining of the acini. Hyperplasia of the glandular epithelium does not mean hyperthyroidism, but quite the opposite. Neither does a large amount of colloid in distended acini have this significance. These facts are better understood if we consider the accepted explanations of thyroid function. The morphologic and functional activity of the thyroid is induced and sustained by a thyrotropic hormone which the circulating blood brings from the pituitary. The thyroid then releases into the blood its own secretion, thyroxine or a derivative thereof. The thyrotropic hormone from the pituitary stimulates the production of thyroxine; the presence of thyroxine inhibits the production of more thyrotropic hormone. Normally the two are in balance and thyroid effect is held at the proper level. But if something, like an absence of the essential ingredient, iodine, arises to prevent successful achievement of the thyroxine-making process, there is no thyroxine to inhibit the generation of pituitary thyrotropic hormone. The result is a continued, and even greater, stimulation of the thyroid cells, which react in the strongest way open to them, by prolifera-

tion. Thus develops the hyperplastic thyroid, a reaction to the organ's own impotency.

Certain other adverse influences besides lack of iodine can prevent the proper culmination of thyroxine synthesis and lead similarly to hyperplasia. Developmental anomalies of morphologic or functional nature doubtless occur rarely in the thyroid mechanism, as elsewhere, and may account for occasional cases of cretinism that appear unrelated to deficiency of iodine. We are principally concerned, however, with a number of substances that have this effect when ingested and are known as **goitrogenic substances.** Among these are thiouracil, which is used therapeutically to reduce hyperthyroidism, thiourea, cyanides, sulfocyanates, or thiocyanates, and even, to a lesser degree, sulfonamides. Certain plants are known to be goitrogenic when eaten in sufficient amount by man or animal. Soybeans are notable in this respect; cabbage and its near relatives, rape and kale, as well as turnips, are less potent goitrogens. Goitrogenic substances from weeds of these and related families have been transmitted through milk, at least in the ovine species. Cooking or heating (and the usual processing of soybean meal) destroys the goitrogenic substance in these plants. Most, and probably all, of these goitrogenic substances are neutralized by unusually liberal supplies of iodine in the diet. Evidence indicates that they act by interfering with the elaboration of the thyroid hormone. The resulting low level of the hormone not only causes the symptoms characterized as hypothyroidism, but also permits unrestrained stimulation by the pituitary thyrotropic hormone to institute hyperplastic enlargement of the gland.

Goiter, a clinical term applicable to any nonmalignant gross enlargement, is by far the most frequent disease of the thyroid gland. While there is still obscurity in respect to the cause of some forms, it will be helpful to classify goiters under the follow-

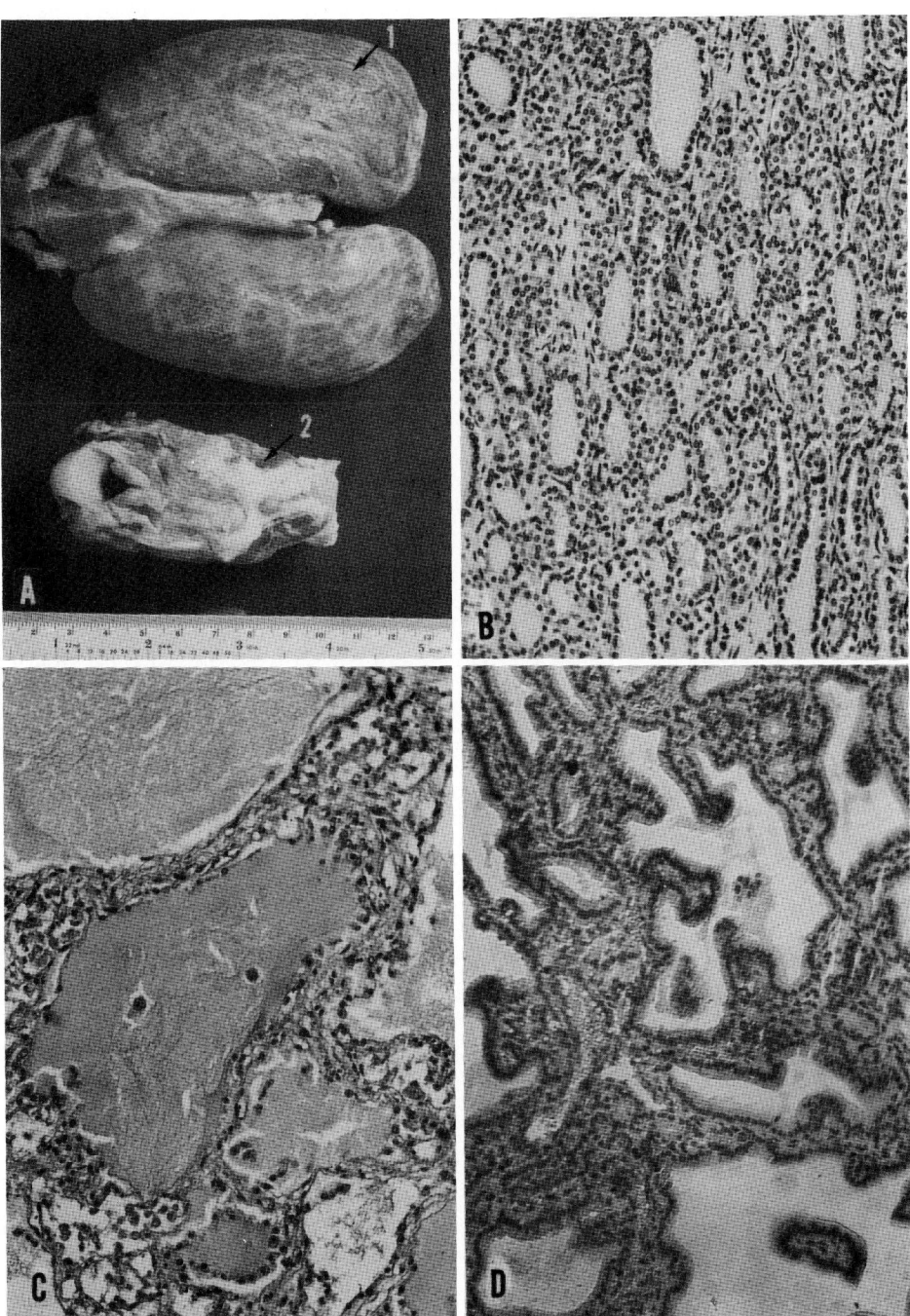

Fig. 26–3. *A,* Goiter in a newborn lamb. The enlarged thyroid glands *(1)* can be compared with those of a normal lamb *(2). B,* Normal thyroid (× 195) of the newborn lamb. Same specimen as a *A (2). C,* Goitrous thyroid of lamb (× 195), same specimen as *(1)* in *A.* Note large acini of irregular size. *D,* Thyroid of cretinism in a young calf (× 195). Tall cells line large, irregularly shaped acini. *(A-C,* Courtesy of Armed Forces Institute of Pathology.) Contributor: Dr. C. L. Davis.

ing four types: hyperplastic, colloid, adenomatous, and exophthalmic.

Hyperplastic Goiter. Hyperplasia is the first morphologic response to iodine deficiency. With reduced thyroxine production, the pituitary releases increased levels of thyrotropic hormone, which is the stimulus for hyperplasia leading to goiter. The hyperplastic gland may and usually does compensate for the reduced availability of iodine; thus goiter is not synonymous with hypothyroidism. Microscopically the follicles are lined with tall columnar epithelium which forms papillary projections into the lumens. Colloid is scant and often absent. In the adult Beagle deprived of sufficient iodine for many months, the follicular cells become tall columnar with abundant cytoplasm. Hyperplasia of these cells causes them to fold inward, into a papillary arrangement, eventually obliterating most or all of the colloid (Belshaw et al., 1973, 1975; Leav et al., 1976).

Hyperplastic goiter is not common; the usual goiter of animals is a colloid goiter. An exception is seen in congenital goiter or the **goiter of cretinism.** Cretinism has already been described as a severe hypothyroidism of the young. Actually, the disorder begins in prenatal life. The classic cretins were children of the Swiss Alps, a region where the soil and water are highly deficient in iodine, but the same effects of unrelieved iodine deficiency occur in other parts of the world. This is the type of goiter that has been common in newborn colts, calves, lambs, and pigs in iodine-deficient territories, which in the the United States are the regions of the Great Lakes and the Pacific Northwest. As the disease is readily prevented by supplying minute amounts of iodine to the pregnant mother, it is no longer common in the United States but is still reported from other parts of the world.

The thyroid is always enlarged, and in these newly born animals the massive lobes may protrude prominently on each side of the neck. Microscopically, there is typically an extreme degree of hyperplasia. The epithelium is tall and the acini, devoid of colloid, are perhaps almost filled with the papillary infoldings characteristic of hyperplasia of glands in general. Such extreme degrees of hyperplastic changes are differentiated from papillary carcinoma by the fact that the individual cells are not anaplastic, the basement membrane is not violated, and the epithelial layer can, perhaps with difficulty, be followed back to the wall of the acinus. In some species, particularly sheep, the goitrous change is more inclined to manifest itself by a "piling up" of more than one layer of epithelial cells without so much change in the architecture of the acini. In severe cases, there is an accompanying lack of hair, especially in pigs, and of wool in lambs. Subcutaneous edema, possibly akin to myxedema, has been described in the neck region. If only mildly affected, the young animal may be helped to a normal existence and eventual resolution of the goiter, but many are born dead or die soon after birth. There is said to be a certain dwarfing of animals that survive, but if this is true, the condition is not to be confused with the too-frequent occurrence of hereditary dwarfs in certain strains of beef cattle.

Familial goiter is a form of hyperplastic goiter that is not related to dietary deficiency of iodine, but rather to inborn errors of the enzyme systems involved in thyroxine synthesis. In man, five types of familial goiter have been recognized, each with a distinct metabolic basis. In animals, congenital goiter is occasionally seen that cannot be traced to iodine deficiency, and it seems most probable that certain of these goiters are analogous to familial goiter. Evidence of the existence of inherited goiter in swine, cattle, goats, and sheep has been reviewed by Rac and colleagues (1968). In their studies with sheep, the disorder appeared to be inherited as a recessive factor.

Colloid Goiter (Simple Goiter). This form of goiter is characterized by enlargement and distention of the acini, which are filled with colloid. The walls are stretched and the epithelium flattened. Although the colloid is abundant, it may stain weakly and unevenly. It contains little iodine and little thyroxine, and any symptoms are those of hypothyroidism. Frequently, there are no symptoms beyond the increased size of the gland. The cause is ordinarily a mild deficiency of iodine. The milder goitrogenic agents, such as soybeans, are likely to produce this type of goiter. The pathogenesis of colloid goiter has long been a mystery. As indicated, the response of the thyroid to iodine deficiency is hyperplasia mediated by thyrotropic hormone. How then does iodine deficiency result in colloid goiter? Experimental evidence (Follis, 1959) indicates that colloid goiter represents an involutional stage of hyperplastic goiter that results when iodine is returned to the diet, or when iodine deficiency is periodic, or when iodine deficiency is marginal. Severe deficiency of iodine in man and animals leads to hyperplastic goiter.

Adenomatous Goiter (Nodular Goiter). This form is characterized by nodules of thyroid tissue, more or less spherical, highly variable in size, and usually several in number, dispersed through the original tissue of the gland. As a rule, no two nodules show the same histologic appearance, there being all gradations between the colloid goiter with large, colloid-filled acini and low, inactive epithelium on the one hand, and the hyperplastic, cretinic type on the other. The picture within a given nodule, however, is usually rather constant. The nodules are often regarded as adenomas. It is idle to speculate on the accuracy of this conception until we have a precise definition of what constitutes an adenoma. The other view is that these forms represent merely a lobular distribution of what is essentially one of the other types of goiter. The nodules frequently resemble Graves' disease in being accompanied by unexplained lymphoid tissue. But at least it may be said that, like adenomas in other organs, they grow expansively at the expense of the surrounding tissue, which is easily seen, under the microscope, to be compressed.

Some of the nodules or adenomas are inert functionally; others actively secrete thyroid hormone, producing the usual symptoms of hyperthyroidism. The latter constitute the "toxic adenomas" of clinical terminology. Those adenomas seen in animals, chiefly horses and dogs, have seldom caused noticeable signs of toxicity (hyperthyroidism).

Exophthalmic Goiter (Goiter of Hyperthyroidism; Toxic Goiter). This disorder of humans is also known as Graves' disease or Basedow's disease. It may well be that this condition does not occur in animals, the occasional case of exophthalmos having a nervous or other cause. (Retrobulbar neoplasms produce exophthalmos, usually unilateral, and are not rare.) In man, exophthalmic goiter is the most formidable type. It produces hyperthyroidism which may be alleviated temporarily by iodine, only to be made worse in the course of a few weeks.

The thyroid may or may not be much enlarged; the enlargement may extend around to the dorsal side of the trachea, constituting the so called "inward goiter." Microscopically, there is hyperplasia, but not the extreme degree seen in the thyroid of cretinism. The epithelium is tall, but infolding papillae are absent or few. The colloid is usually present but thin and pale-staining. There is often a row of rounded vacuoles in the colloid where it adjoins the epithelial cells. This has been interpreted as resorption of colloid into the epithelial cells. New acini of small size may be formed. In company with the changes in the thyroid acini, there are almost always to be found areas of lymphoid tissue somewhere in the gland. Active germinal centers are usually present. The superabundance of lymphoid tissue extends to other organs, including the thymus. A tendency toward degenerative changes is described in various locations. Exophthalmos, or protrusion of the eyeballs with a white ring of sclera showing around the cornea, constitutes a startling aspect of the disease, but as stated previously, is thought to be due to some other derangement than the excess of thyroid hormone.

The cause of the condition is unknown, although an excess of pituitary thyrotropic hormone is presumed to be part of the mechanism. Surgical removal of part of the gland or "internal irradiation" by the administration of radioactive iodine usually relieves the condition. Untreated, the disease may lead to death from degenerative changes in an overstimulated heart, or rarely, to practically complete destruction of the exhausted thyroid and consequent myxedema.

Equine Goiter Due to Iodine Toxicity. This type of thyroid enlargement, described in Thoroughbred mares and foals by Baker and Lindsey (1968), has some unusual features. In the first place, it was closely associated with excessive dietary levels of iodine resulting from the addition of dried seaweed (kelp) to the prepared feed. The iodide level in the diet of each mare was measured and found to be from 48 to 432 mg/day/mare. This is, at a minimum, ten times the normal requirement for pregnant animals of this species.

The problem was seen in three farms over the course of two years; the disease disappeared on two farms following removal of the iodide from the diet. It continued on one farm where the diet was not corrected. The disease was manifest principally in newborn foals, which were born weak or dead or died soon after birth. The thyroids were extremely enlarged and visible grossly. A few mares also had obvious goiters. The microscopic appearance of the enlarged thyroids of the foals was characteristic, with the acini strikingly varied in size and most with an irregular, somewhat angular shape. The lining epithelium was low, flattened, and in some acini formed interfollicular tufts of hyperplastic cells. The colloid content was pale-staining and contained many vacuoles adjacent to the epithelium.

Anderson, M. P., and Capen, C. C.: The endocrine system. *In* Pathology of Laboratory Animals, edited by K. Benirschke, F. M. Garner, and T. C. Jones. New York, Springer-Verlag, 1978. pp. 423–508.

Baker, H. J., and Lindsey, J. R.: Equine goiter due to excess dietary iodide. J. Am. Vet. Med. Assoc., 153:1618–1630, 1968.

Belshaw, B. E., and Becker, D. V.: Necrosis of follicular cells and discharge of thyroidal iodine induced by administering iodine to iodine-deficient dogs. J. Clin. Endocrinol. Metab., 36:466–474, 1973.

Belshaw, B. E., Cooper, T. B., and Becker, D. V.: The iodine requirement and influence of iodine intake on iodine metabolism and thyroid function in the adult Beagle. Endocrinology, 96:1280–1291, 1975.

Care, A. D.: Goitrogenic properties of linseed. Nature, 173:172–173, 1954.

————: Goitrogenic activity in linseed. NZ J. Sci. Tech. (Sec. A.), 36:321–327, 1955.

Clements, F.: A goitrogenic factor in milk. Med. J. Aust., 2:645–646, 1957.

Coffin, D. L., and Munson, T. O.: Endocrine diseases of the dog associated with hair loss. Sertoli-cell tumor of testis, hypothyroidism, canine Cushing's syndrome. J. Am. Vet. Med. Assoc., 123:403–408, 1953.

Falconer, I. R.: Effect of thyroid deficiency in the ewe on lamb viability. Nature, 205:703, 1965.

Falconer, I. R., Roitt, I. M., Seamark, R. F., and Torrigiani, G.: Studies of the congenitally goitrous sheep. Iodoproteins of the goitre. Biochem. J., 117:417–424, 1970.

Follis, R. H.: Experimental colloid goitre produced by thiouracil. Nature, 183:1817–1818, 1959.

Follis, R. H.: Studies on the pathogenesis of colloid goiter. Trans. Assoc. Am. Physicians, 72:265–274, 1959.

Hemken, R. W., Vandershall, J. H., Sass, B. A., and Hibbs, J. W.: Goitrogenic effects of a corn silage-soybean meal supplemented ration. J. Dairy Sci., 52:85–88, 1971.

Holt, A. G., Cheek, D. B., and Kerr, G. R.: Prenatal hypothyroidism and brain composition in a primate. Nature, 243:413–415, 1973.

Jaarsveld, P. van, Theron, C. B. van der, and Zyl, A. van: Congenital goitre in South African Boer goats. J. S. Afr. Vet. Med. Assoc., 42:295–303, 1971.

Jamieson, S., and Harbour, H. E.: Congenital goitre in lambs. Vet. Rec., 59:102, 1947.

Kalkus, J. W.: Goitre and associated conditions in domestic animals. Exp. Sta. Bull. 156, State College of Washington, Pullman, 1920.

Leav, I., et al.: Adenomas and carcinomas of the canine and feline thyroid. Am. J. Pathol., 83:61–122, 1976.

McCauley, E. H., Linn, J. G., and Goodrich, R. D.: Experimentally induced iodide toxicosis in lambs. Am. J. Vet. Res., 34:65–70, 1973.

Norfeldt, S., Gellerstedt, N. and Falkmer, S.: Studies on rape-seed meal and its goitrogenic effects on pigs. Acta Pathol. Microbiol. Scand., 35:217–236, 1954.

Obel, A. L., Sjoberg, K., and Sandstedt, H.: (Congenital goitre in calves in Sweden.) Nord. Vet. Med., 2:491–507, 1950.

Ostertag, H. G.: Schilddrüsen befunde bei totgeborenen und verendeten Kälbern. Berl. Münch. Tierarztl. Wochenschr., 76:253–255, 1962.

Peltola, P.: Goitrogenic effects of cow's milk from the goitre district of Finland. Acta Endocrinol. Copenhagen , 34:121–128, 1960.

Rac, R., et al.: Congenital goitre in Merino sheep due to an inherited defect in the biosynthesis of thyroid hormone. Res. Vet. Sci., 9:209–223, 1968.

Scaccini, A.: I muscoli della ghiandola tiroide negli equini. Nuova Vet., 30:211–217, 1954.

Schlotthauer, C. F., McKenney, F. D., and Caylor, H. D.: The incidence of goiter and other lesions of the thyroid gland in dogs of southern Minnesota. J. Am. Vet. Med. Assoc., 76:811–819, 1930.

Schlumberger, H. G.: Spontaneous goiter and cancer of the thyroid in animals. Ohio J. Sci., 55:24–43, 1955.

Sinclair, D. P., and Andrews, E. D.: Goitre in newborn lambs (fed kale). NZ Vet. J., 2:72–79, 1954.

Sreekumaran, T., and Rajan, A.: Clinocopathological studies in experimental hypothyroidism in goats. Vet. Pathol., 15:549–555, 1978.

Statham, M., and Bray, A. C.: Congenital goitre in sheep in southern Tasmania. Aust. J. Agri. Res., 26:751–768, 1975.

Steyn, D. G., and Sunkel, W.: Goitre in animals in the Union of South Africa. J. S. Afr. Vet. Med. Assoc., 25:9–18, 1954.

Wilson, J. G.: Hypothyroidism in ruminants with special reference to foetal goitre. Vet. Rec., 97:161–164, 1975.

Wright, E., and Sinclair, D. P.: The goitrogenic effect of thousand-headed kale (Brassica oleracea, var. acephala) on adult sheep and rabbits. NZ J. Agri. Res., 1:477–485, 1958.

Zwart, D.: (Goiter in goats in Dutch New Guinea). Tijdschr. Diergeneeskd., 84:550–559, 1959.

Myxedema

The subcutaneous accumulation of mucoid material in this hypothyroid state has been described in the general discussion of hypothyroidism. The reason for the severe shortage of hormone is the result of goiter with hypothyroidism, or destruction of the gland by any inflammatory or neoplastic processes. In one form of hypothyroidism the thyroid is all but nonexistent. Compressed islets of thyroid parenchyma, buried in fibrous tissue, are the rule, perhaps with lymphocytes or other inflammatory cells still present. The term Riedel's struma is sometimes used to describe thyroid changes of this nature. The cause of this fibrous atrophy of the thyroid may or may not be readily apparent, but is usually the end result of some destructive inflammatory process of infectious origin, centered in either a neighboring or a distant area of the body. Accidents to the blood supply or damage from excessive use of goitrogenic drugs (thiocyanates) are other possibilities. Some cases are the terminal exhaustive phase of exophthalmic goiter. Myxedema, now rare because of therapy with artificial thyroid products, is principally a disease of human beings, but it would be a mistake to say that it cannot occur in animals. The same susceptibility to thyroid deficiency exists and tissue reactions paralleling those of humans are not unknown in domestic animals.

Hyperthyroidism

Hyperthyroidism is a syndrome quite opposite to hypothyroidism. The individual is unusually active and alert, does not store fat in spite of a vigorous appetite, and is often of an irritable or excitable disposition. The heart rate is unusually rapid (tachycardia), and there may be palpitation. The basal metabolic rate, a measure of oxidative process, is above normal. In the young, growth may be somewhat accelerated and maturity comes early. The bulging of the eyeballs known as exophthalmos appears to be only an indirect effect of the hyperthyroid state.

Hyperthyroidism in dogs is now well recognized as a clinical entity. The studies of Rijnberk (1971) are of particular merit and are briefly summarized. In his studies on iodine metabolism and thyroid disease, Rijnberk identified 59 dogs with thyroid tumors and subjected them to intensive clinical and laboratory study. In 13 of the 59 dogs studied, a hyperthyroid state was recognized as a result of excessive production of thyroxine. Each hyperthyroid dog had a small circumscribed tumor in one thyroid. In one case the tumor was located in an ectopic thyroid found ventral to the cranial aspect of the larynx. Each tumor was considered a carcinoma, although none had metastasized. The histologic features of these tumors are considered further in the section on thyroid neoplasms.

Clinical Signs. The clinical signs of this hyperthyroid state were described as follows: The signs appeared abruptly or gradually. Polydipsia and polyuria in the absence of primary renal lesions were the most consistent signs. The dogs lost weight although their food intake increased. Weakness and fatigue were noted in 8 of 13 dogs. An intolerance to slightly elevated ambient temperature was indicated by the dogs' tendency to seek cool places. Restlessness indicated by continuous pacing was often evident. The heart rate was generally high—up to 133 beats per minute. In three dogs, the electrocardiogram displayed high voltage in all leads. After treatment with radioiodine or surgical ablation of the thyroid, in all 13 cases the clinical signs disappeared and laboratory values returned to normal.

Laboratory and Clinical Objective Measurements. The **scintiscan** of the thyroid region of the neck following a diagnostic dose of radioiodine gave an outline of the radioactivity concentrated in the thyroid or thyroid tumors by the affinity of thyroid cells for iodine. This gave one indication of the thyroxine-producing activity of the thyroid tumor and provided a good indication of the depressed activity of the ipsilateral thyroid not involved by the tumor. A diagnostic dose of thyroid-stimulating hormone (TSH) from the pituitary restored the ipsilateral lobe to a functional state, stimulating the binding of radioactive iodine.

The **radioactive iodine uptake** (RIU) gave a clear differentiation between normal and hypersecreting thyroids. In the hyperthyroid animals, the RIU increased from a higher base level to a peak within four hours and gradually returned to baseline in 72 hours. In normal dogs the curve was quite different; starting from a lower point, the uptake curve climbed moderately during the first 24 hours and continued to rise more slowly, reaching a plateau above normal at 72 hours.

The **thyroidal iodine turnover index,** consisting of the ratio between the iodine uptake value at 24 hours and the same value at 72 hours, was also useful in detecting dogs with hypersecretion of thyroxine. **Protein-bound iodine (PBI)** in serum was generally elevated in dogs with hyperthyroidism. The **total hormone iodine (HI)** was also elevated. **Iodinated amino acids (IAA)** were also measured and a discrepancy between the PBI and the total hormone iodine (HI) plus iodinated amino acids (IAA) often indicated the probability of circulating iodoproteins.

Auclair, R. F., Bonofiglio, R. A., and Rosenkrantz, H.: Determination of serum thyroid hormone in laboratory animals. Am. J. Vet. Res., *31:*1655–1660, 1970.

Bohn, F. K.: Der Fall eines abnormen Herzbefundes in Verbindung mit Hyperthyrose beim Hund. Kleint. Prax. *8:*228–233, 1967.

Bustad, L. K., and Fuller, J. M.: Thyroid function in domestic animals. Lab. Anim. Care, *20:*561–581, 1970.

Decker, J. P.: I¹³¹ triiodothyronine red cell uptake as a test of thyroid function. Bull. Ayer Clin. Lab. Penn. Hosp., *4:*47–56, 1962.

Kallfelz, F. A., and Erali, R. P.: Thyroid function tests in domesticated animals: free thyroxine index. Am. J. Vet. Res., *34:*1449–1452, 1973.

Kodama, A. M.: Radioisotopic T-3 and T-4 thyroid function tests in the pig-tailed monkeys (*Macaca nemestrina*). Lab. Anim. Sci., *22:*68–71, 1972.

Leav, I., et al.: Adenomas and carcinomas of the canine and feline thyroid. Am. J. Pathol., *83:*61–122, 1976.

Marine, D.: On the occurrence and physiological nature of glandular hyperplasia of the thyroid (dog and sheep): together with remarks on important clinical (human) problems. Johns Hopkins Hosp. Bull., *18:*359–364, 1907.

Reid, C. F., Pensinger, R. R., Ferrigan, L. W., and Parkes, L.: Functioning adenocarcinoma of the thyroid gland in a dog with mitral insufficiency. J. Am. Vet. Radiol. Soc., *4:*36–40, 1963.

Rijnberk, A.: Hyperthyroidism in the dog and its treatment with radioactive iodide. Tijdschr. Diergeneeskd., *91*:789–794, 1966.

Rijnberk, A.: Iodine Metabolism and Thyroid Disease in the Dog. Drukkerij Elinkwijk, Utrecht, 1971.

Rijnberk, A., and Horst, C. J. G. van der: Investigations on iodine metabolism of normal and goitrous dogs. Zentralbl. Veterinaermed., (A), *16*:495–508, 1969.

Rijnberk, A., and Kinderen, P. J. der: Toxic thyroid carcinoma in the dog. Acta Endocrinol. (Suppl) (Kbh), *138*:177, 1969. (Abstr.)

Other Disorders

Other changes that occasionally affect the thyroid include hemorrhage, necrosis, amyloidosis, and metastatic infections, all of which are rare. A tendency to form abnormally small acini with little or no colloid has been reported as occurring in dogs with various infections, including experimental Chagas' disease. There were free cells in the acini, suspected of being phagocytes, but there was no inflammatory change. Toxins from the infections were presumed to be causative.

Lymphocytic Thyroiditis

In dogs of the Beagle breed, lymphocytic thyroiditis remarkably similar to Hashimoto's disease of man is frequently encountered, though only in a few advanced cases is it associated with clinical disease. The microscopic features consist of diffuse or nodular infiltration of the gland by lymphocytes and lesser numbers of plasma cells and macrophages. Lymphocytic nodules may have prominent germinal centers. Displacement and destruction of the follicles may be prominent, with colloid gaining entrance to the interstitium where it is engulfed by macrophages and occasionally giant cells. Nodules of hyperplastic interstitial or parafollicular cells often accompany the lesion. In addition to its similarity to Hashimoto's disease, the thyroiditis is also indistinguishable from experimental autoimmune thyroiditis in dogs and other experimental animals. Evidence now clearly supports the idea that in the laboratory Beagle this disease has a hereditary basis. Further studies are necessary to elucidate the pathogenesis of the spontaneous disease in dogs, but it would appear to represent an example of an autoimmune disease. Lymphocytic thyroiditis is occasionally seen in old dogs of any breed, but the relationship to the disease in Beagles has not been established.

Hajdu and Rona (1969) have reported spontaneous lymphocytic thyroiditis in laboratory rats which is also similar to Hashimoto's disease.

Beierwaltes, W. H., and Nishiyama, R. H.: Dog thyroiditis: Occurrence and similarity to Hashimoto's struma. Endocrinology, *83*:501–508, 1968.

Bigazzi, P. E., and Rose, N. R.: Spontaneous autoimmune thyroiditis in animals as a model of human disease. Prog. Allergy, *19*:245–274, 1975.

Cole, W. H., and Womack, N. A.: The thyroid in infections and toxemias. Proc. Soc. Exp. Biol. Med., *25*:188–191, 1927–1928.

Cole, R. K.: Hereditary hypothyroidism in the domestic fowl. Genetics, *53*:1021–1033, 1966.

Fritz, T. E., Zeman, R. C., and Zeele, M. R.: Pathology and familial incidence of thyroiditis in a closed Beagle colony. Exp. Mol. Pathol., *12*:14–30, 1970.

Goble, F. C.: Thyroid changes in acute experimental Chagas' disease in dogs. Am. J. Pathol., *30*:599–611, 1954.

Hajdu, A., and Rona, G.: Spontaneous thyroiditis in laboratory rats. Experientia, *25*:1325–1327, 1969.

Jones, H. E. H., and Roitt, I. M.: Experimental autoimmune thyroiditis in the rat. Br. J. Exp. Pathol., *42*:546–557, 1961.

Kite, J. H., Jr., and Witebsky, E.: Hereditary autoimmune thyroiditis in the fowl. Science, *160*:1357–1358, 1968.

Levy, B. M., Hampton, S., Dreizen, S., and Hampton, J. K.: Thyroiditis in the marmoset (*Callithrix spp.* and *Saquinus spp.*). J. Comp. Pathol., *82*:99–102, 1972.

Lucke, V. M.: An histological study of thyroid abnormalities in the domestic cat. J. Small Anim. Pract., *5*:351–358, 1964.

Manning, P. J., Corwin, L. A., Jr., and Middleton, C. C.: Familial hyperlipoproteinemia and thyroid dysfunction of Beagles. Exp. Mol. Pathol., *19*:378–388, 1973.

Mawdesley-Thomas, L. E., and Jolly, D. W.: Autoimmune disease in the Beagle. Vet. Rec., *80*:553–554, 1967.

Mizejewski, G. J., Baron, J., and Poissant, G.: Immunologic investigations of naturally occurring canine thyroiditis. J. Immunol., *10F*:1152–1160, 1971.

Musser, E., and Graham, W. R.: Familial occurrence of thyroiditis in purebred Beagles. Lab. Anim. Care, *18*:58–68, 1968.

Rajan, A., and Mohiyuddeen, S.: Pathology of the thyroid gland in canines (*Canis familiaris*). Indian J. Anim. Sci., *43*:760–765, 1974.

Reuber, M. D., and Glover, E. L.: Role of age and sex in chronic thyroiditis in rats fed 3'-methyl-4-dimethylaminoazobenzene. Vet. Pathol., *13*:295–302, 1976.

Schlotthauer, C. F.: Diseases of the thyroid gland of adult horses. J. Am. Vet. Med. Assoc., *78*:211–218, 1931.

Terplan, K. L., et al.: Experimental thyroiditis in rabbits, guinea pigs and dogs, following immunization with thyroid extracts of their own and of heterologous species. Am. J. Pathol., *36*:213–239, 1960.

Tucker, W. E., Jr.: Thyroiditis in a group of laboratory dogs. Am. J. Clin. Nutr., *38*:70–74, 1962.

Wick, G., and Graf, J.: Electron microscopic studies in chickens of the obese strain with spontaneous hereditary autoimmune thyroiditis. Lab. Invest., *27*:400–411, 1972.

Thyrocalcitonin (Calcitonin)

This is the latest hormone to have its functions identified, its cell of origin established, its composition unraveled, and its synthesis accomplished, all in about half a decade. Copp and associates (1962) were first to postulate that a second (after parathyroid hormone) serum calcium regulating hormone existed; they named it "calcitonin," and believed that it originated from the parathyroid. Hirsch et al. (1963, 1964) demonstrated a new hormone with the property of lowering blood calcium that arose in the thyroid, and they named it "thyrocalcitonin." Hirsch et al. (1964) demonstrated thyrocalcitonin activity in the thyroids of the rat, dog, rabbit, hog, ox, and monkey.

The cell of origin of thyrocalcitonin was postulated to be the "parafollicular" cell, to which no function had been ascribed up to that time. Nonidez (1932) described the parafollicular cell of the dog as a distinctive cell, somewhat larger than follicular cells, usually located near the basement membrane of the thyroid follicle but separated from the colloid by the follicle cells. In some species these cells are found outside of the basement membrane of the follicles. The cytoplasm of these cells contains numerous secretory granules of varying size and density, numerous mitochondria, and arrays of fine tubules, as seen by the electron microscope. The cytoplasm was faintly stained—"light"—in PAS preparations, hence the name "light cells." The term "C cell" was coined to distinguish it from A and B cells, and later used to indicate "C" for "calcitonin" (Pearse, 1966, 1968). Considerable evidence accumulated to indicate that this cell produced or, at least, stored thyrocalcitonin, culminating in the demonstration by immunofluorescent localization technique that C cells did contain thyrocalcitonin (Bussolati and Pearse, 1967). The parafollicular or C cells are believed to be possibly of neural crest origin, become part of the ultimobranchial body, and eventually are distributed to their ultimate sites in the thyroid. Each species has a characteristic distribution pattern for C cells. In cattle, the ultimobranchial body becomes incorporated into the vasculature and stroma at the hilus of the thyroid. This is a common site of origin for tumors of C cells in cattle.

The amino-acid sequences of porcine and human thyrocalcitonin were worked out (Potts et al., 1968), and in an amazingly short time, both of these hormones were synthesized (Rittel et al., 1968). Thyrocalcitonin is currently viewed as a polypeptide hormone from parafollicular cells of the thyroid, having the function of inhibiting bone resorption or stimulating its accretion, and thereby lowering the blood calcium.

Increased calcium in the blood stimulates both the parathyroids and the C cells to secrete their respective hormones. Parathyroid hormone tends to inhibit bone calcification and elevate blood calcium levels; thyrocalcitonin tends to promote bone growth and decrease the blood level of calcium.

Abnormally increased secretion of thyrocalcitonin may be stimulated by high levels of calcium in the diet or by the presence of a tumor of C cells (medullary adenoma or carcinoma of the thyroid—see

Neoplasms of the Thyroid). Medullary carcinoma with hypocalcemia and elevated serum thyrocalcitonin has been described in man, dog, cattle (bulls), and rats. In each species, morphologic characteristics of the tumors are similar and evidence of hypersecretion of thyrocalcitonin may be developed. Thyrocalcitonin also has the effect of increasing renal excretion of inorganic phosphorus, sodium, potassium, and calcium in sheep. Urinary excretion of magnesium by sheep is inhibited by physiologic doses of porcine or salmon calcitonin (Bartlet, 1972).

In cows with parturient hypocalcemia, the release of thyrocalcitonin may have an effect on the blood calcium levels seen in the disease (Capen and Young, 1967).

Aliapoulios, M. A., Bernstein, D. S., and Balodimos, M. C.: Thyrocalcitonin. Its role in calcium homeostasis. Arch. Intern. Med., 123:88–94, 1969.

Bartlet, J. P.: Effect of porcine, salmon and human calcitonin on urinary excretion of some electrolytes in sheep. J. Endocrinol., 55:153–161, 1972.

Berger, A. J.: Thyrocalcitonin: A review. Bull. Hosp. Joint Dis., 32:40–49, 1971.

Bussolati, G., and Pearse, A. G. E.: Immunofluorescent localization of calcitonin "C" cells of pig and dog thyroid. J. Endocrinol., 37:205, 1967.

Capen, C. C., and Young, D. M.: Thyrocalcitonin: evidence for release in a spontaneous hypocalcemic disorder. Science, 157:205–206, 1967.

———: The ultrastructure of the parathyroid glands and thyroid parafollicular cells of cows with parturient paresis and hypocalcemia. Lab. Invest., 17:717–737, 1967.

Chan, A. S., and Conen, P. E.: Ultrastructural observations on cytodifferentiation of parafollicular cells in the human fetal thyroid. Lab. Invest., 25:249–259, 1971.

Copp, D. H., et al.: Evidence for calcitonin—a new hormone from the parathyroid that lowers blood calcium. Endocrinology, 70:638–644, 1962.

Das, V. K., and Das, S.: Distribution of calcitonin cells in thyroid glands of normal adult rhesus monkey Macaca mulatta. Experientia, 34:541–542, 1978.

DeLellis, R. A., Nunnemacher, G., and Wolfe, H. J.: C cell hyperplasia: an ultrastructural analysis. Lab. Invest., 36:237–248, 1977.

Foster, G. V., MacIntyre, I., and Pearse, A. G. E.: Calcitonin and the mitochondrion-rich cells of the dog thyroid. Nature, 203:1029–1030, 1964.

Hargis, G. K., et al.: Radioimmunoassay of calcitonin in the plasma of rhesus monkey and man. Clin. Chem., 24:595–601, 1978.

Hirsch, P. F., Gauthier, G. T., and Munson, P. L.: Thyroid hypocalcemic principle and recurrent laryngeal nerve injury as factors affecting the response to parathyroidectomy in rats. Endocrinology, 73:244–249, 1963.

Hirsch, P. F., Voekel, E. F., and Munson, P. L.: Thyrocalcitonin: hypocalcemic principle of the thyroid gland. Science, 146: 412, 1964.

Mazzuli, G. F., Coen, G., and Bashievi, L.: Thyrocalcitonin excess syndrome. Lancet, 2:1192, 1966.

Meyer, J. S., and Abdel-Bari, W.: The syndrome of excessive calcitonin produced by medullary carcinoma of the thyroid gland. N. Engl. J. Med., 278:523, 1968.

Machardo, C. R. S.: Monoamines in C cells of thyroid gland of callithricid primates. Histochemistry, 48:187–190, 1976.

Nonidez, J. F.: The origin of the "parafollicular" cell, a second epithelial component of the thyroid gland of the dog. Am. J. Anat., 49:479–505, 1932.

Nunez, E. A., et al.: Ultrastructure of the parafollicular "C" cells and the parathyroid cell in growing dogs on a high calcium diet. Lab. Invest., 31:96–108, 1974.

Pearse, A. G. E.: The cytochemistry of the thyroid "C" cells and their relationship to calcitonin. Proc. R. Soc. Lond. (Biol), 164:478–480, 1966.

———: Common cytochemical and ultrastructural characteristics of cells producing polypeptide hormones (APUD series) and their relevance to thyroid and ultimobranchial C cells and calcitonin. Proc. R. Soc. Lond. (Biol), 170:71–76, 1968.

Potts, J. T., et al.: The amino acid sequence of porcine thyrocalcitonin. Proc. Natl. Acad. Sci. USA, 59:1321, 1968.

Rasmussen, H., and Pechet, M. M.: Calcitonin. Sci. Am., 223:42–50, 1970.

Reynolds, W. A., et al.: Calcitonin secretion in response to hypercalcemia in the fetal monkey. Gynec. Invest., 8:79–80, 1977.

Rittel, W., et al.: Thyrocalcitonin. III. Die Synthese der alpha Thyrocalcitonins. Helv. Chim. Acta, 51:924, 1968.

Roth, S. I., Feinblatt, J. D. and Roisz, L. G.: Effect of calcium on embryonic rat thyroid C cells in vitro. Am. J. Pathol., 75:27–44, 1974.

Tashjian, A. H., Jr., and Melvin, K. E. W.: Medullary carcinoma of the thyroid gland (studies of thyrocalcitonin in plasma and tumor extracts). N. Engl. J. Med., 279:279, 1968.

Tashjian, A. H., Jr.: Soft bones, hard facts and calcitonin therapy. N. Engl. J. Med., 283:588–594, 1970.

Weisbrode, S. E., and Capen, C. C.: Ultrastructural evaluation of the effects of calcitonin on bone in thyroparathyroidectomized rats administered vitamin D. Am. J. Pathol., 77:455–464, 1974.

Young, D. M., Capen, C. C., and Black, H. E.: Calcitonin activity in ultimobranchial neoplasms of bulls. Vet. Pathol., 8:19–27, 1971.

Neoplasms of the Thyroid

Neoplasms may originate, in approximate order of frequency, from any of the following: (1) follicular cells, (2) parafollicular or C cells, and (3) mesenchymal cells.

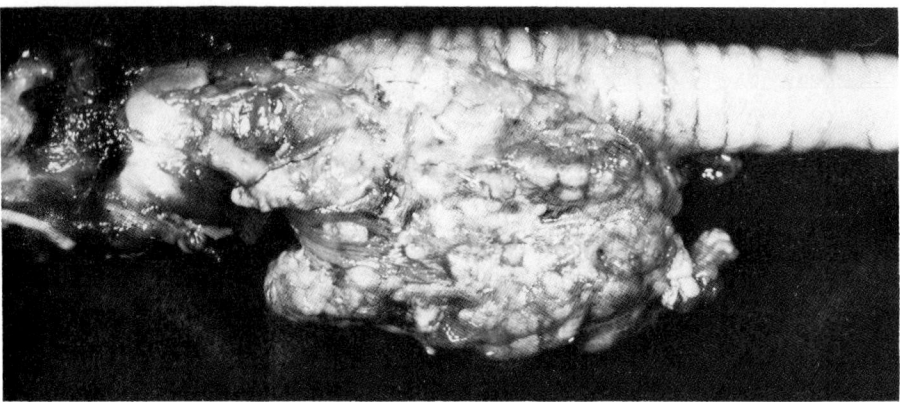

Fig. 26–4. Adenocarcinoma of the left thyroid of a 12-year-old male Cocker Spaniel. Note the relation of the tumor mass to the larynx and trachea. (Courtesy of Angell Memorial Animal Hospital.)

Follicular and C cells are cells of internal secretion, and neoplasms that arise from them may be associated with increased secretion. Thyroid tumors have been reported from all domestic animals and from many laboratory and wild mammals and birds. The WHO *International Histological Classification of Tumors of Domestic Animals* (von Sandersleben and Hänichen, 1974) provides classifications for epithelial, mesenchymal, and epithelial/mesenchymal tumors, and this classification is used in the discussion that follows.

Follicular adenoma is encountered as single or multiple nodules in one or both lobes of the thyroid. These nodules are circumscribed masses encapsulated by thin connective tissue, and they grow by expansion, compressing adjacent thyroid. The epithelial cells usually form follicles that are smaller than normal thyroid follicles ("microfollicular"), but may also form solid cords several cells in thickness. The resemblance to normal thyroid follicles is usually unmistakable and their presence within the thyroid is characteristic. The cells are usually low-cuboidal and quite uniform. In some cases, these cells form a papillary pattern and are called "papillary adenoma." The significance of this difference in growth pattern is not presently un-

derstood. Nodular hyperplasia of the thyroid may be difficult, if not impossible, to differentiate from adenoma.

Out of a series of 44 adenomas of the canine thyroid (Leav, et al., 1976), 43 were follicular adenomas and one was a papillary adenoma. Of these tumors, 13 contained a centrally placed cyst filled with mineralized necrotic debris and red blood cells. From the inner surface of the dense, fibrous capsule projected many fronds of epithelial cells forming follicles or a compact cellular pattern.

Follicular carcinoma constitutes one histologic type that is well recognized in animals. The cells are cuboidal or columnar and form follicles containing variable amounts of colloid. The follicles are usually microfollicular, but often contain both large and small follicles of various shapes. The follicular pattern is often mixed with papillary zones and the amount of stroma also is varied. This appears to be the least malignant histologic type, but local invasion into capsule and blood vessels and metastases to lungs and lymph nodes have been reported, particularly in the dog (Fig. 4–16).

Follicular carcinoma is the usual histologic type in which the cells produce thyroxine, which results in clinical signs of thyrotoxicosis or hyperthyroidism. In a

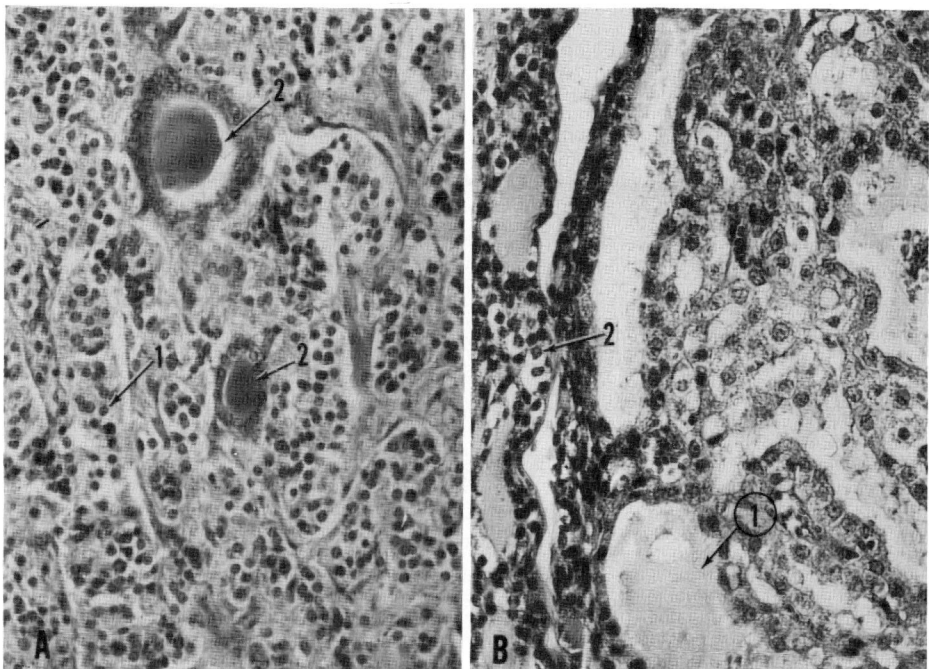

Fig. 26-5. *A*, Adenocarcinoma of the thyroid of an eight-year-old cow. Solid nests of cells *(1)* and acini containing colloid *(2)* are present. Contributor: Dr. C. L. Davis. *B*, Adenoma of the thyroid of a ten-year-old male cat. The tumor (× 335) is forming large acini *(1)* and compresses the adjacent normal thyroid tissue *(2)*. Contributor: Dr. Leo L. Lieberman. (Courtesy of Armed Forces Institute of Pathology.)

study of 58 canine thyroid tumors, Rijnberk (1971) identified 13 which produced clinical signs of hyperthyroidism.

The ultrastructure of the cells of follicular thyroid carcinomas has been described by Leav et al. (1976) as columnar cells with numerous microvilli projecting from their apical surfaces. Dense accumulations of free ribosomes give the cytoplasm of some cells a darker appearance than that of others. Mitochondria, varying in shape, are found throughout the cells, as are dense bodies. Colloid droplets are seen along the apices of most cells. The rough endoplasmic reticulum is dilated and filled with light-staining granular material. Golgi complexes are dispersed in small dense cysternal aggregates. Microvesicles are numerous.

Compact cellular or solid carcinomas of the thyroid have a gross appearance of firm masses with a smooth external surface and a uniform creamy, cut surface. The microscopic appearance is one of solid sheets of closely packed cells, with a fine stroma dividing the tumor into lobules. The cells are uniform in appearance, with a centrally placed nucleus and granular, lightly eosinophilic cytoplasm. Pleomorphic and large nuclei are not seen often and mitoses are rare. Clusters of cells with somewhat more abundant and dense granular cytoplasm (Hurthle cells) are occasionally evident. The cells often invade the capsule, adjacent thyroid, and blood or lymph vessels. This tumor must be differentiated from medullary carcinoma.

Compact cellular and follicular carcinoma (solid carcinoma and follicular carcinoma) are terms used to indicate a mixture of these two histologic types.

Papillary carcinoma of the thyroid is recognized by the tendency of the epithelial cells to be arranged in fronds of intermixed projections supported by a fine stroma. Nuclei are occasionally pleomorphic and sometimes vesicular; others may have a "ground-glass" appearance. Capsular and vascular invasions are often found. In most cases, the papillary structure is mixed with a follicular pattern in the same tumor. The papillary type is more often seen in the cat than in the dog.

Squamous cell carcinoma of the thyroid is an infrequent tumor in animals, but may occasionally be encountered. The cells are similar to those seen in squamous cell carcinoma arising at other sites. The epithelial cells are large, polyhedral, may form keratin, and are often connected by intercellular bridges. These tumors may arise from remnants of the thyroglossal duct or by metaplasia from thyroid epithelium. Squamous cell carcinomas originating in the tonsillar crypt in the dog may reach the thyroid, but are more apt to be found in the nearby lymph nodes.

Anaplastic (undifferentiated) carcinomas of the thyroid are so classified on the basis of their cellular pleomorphism and lack of differentiation. The pattern of growth is usually solid but cells may be individualized and the stroma desmoplastic. Some are made up of small, elongated epithelial cells and are called "spindle cell carcinoma." Others contain many large multinucleated giant cells—"giant-cell carcinoma"—or diffuse small cells— "diffuse small-cell carcinoma."

Medullary carcinoma of the thyroid is a distinctive neoplasm that develops from the parafollicular "light" or C cell of the thyroid. They are sometimes referred to as "C-cell carcinomas," although their morphologic uniqueness was recognized long before the functional nature of the cells was known. These tumors are encountered most frequently in the dog, man, bull, and rat, but other species may be affected. The functional effects of tumors whose cells produce thyrocalcitonin are described in the section on thyrocalcitonin.

The gross description of medullary carcinoma usually includes the fact that the tumors most often involve only one lobe of the thyroid; the cut surface is yellow or cream-colored, and may be divided into lobules by indistinct septa. In the bull, the tumors appear to arise most often in the hilus of one thyroid lobe. The tumor cells in the dog consist of two types: large polygonal cells (15 to 20 μ) with foamy or finely granular cytoplasm, or fusiform cells (5 to 15 μ) with bright eosinophilic, granular cytoplasm and hyperchromatic, irregular nuclei. Silver stains reveal the presence of argyrophilic granules in the tumor cells, and immunoperoxidase stain reveals the presence of thyrocalcitonin.

Histologically identifiable lobules may have characteristic rows of tall columnar cells with the nuclei in rows adjacent to the thin fibrous stroma. The granular cytoplasm of the tumor cells extends toward the center of the lobule in a palisaded array.

The ultrastructure of these neoplastic C cells reveals large (2500 Å), membrane-bound secretory granules with a central electron-dense core. Enlarged saccules of a Golgi system are often seen, and well-developed rough endoplasmic reticulum is present. Many cells contain large numbers of cytoplasmic vacuoles.

Hypocalcemia has been described in the dog, bull, and rat in association with elevated levels of thyrocalcitonin. Hyperplasia of C cells and probably neoplasia has been considered likely the result of long-term feeding of a diet high in calcium. This evidence is most convincing in the situation in cattle. Bulls receiving diets high in calcium are prone to develop medullary carcinomas ("ultimobranchial thyroid tumors"), but none of these tumors appear in cows, presumably because the requirements of pregnancy and lactation utilize the increased supply of calcium.

Histologically benign tumors of parafollicular cells **(medullary adenomas)** have been described in male cattle. The potential of these tumors to eventually become malignant has not yet been documented.

Mesenchymal tumors, such as fibrosarcomas, osteosarcomas and chondrosarcomas, may occasionally be encountered in the thyroid. Their features are described elsewhere.

Epithelial-mesenchymal tumors have been described in the canine thyroid. These tumors may contain both elements of follicular carcinoma and undifferentiated sarcoma in the same primary tumor or in its metastases. When these epithelial and mesenchymal elements are found adjacent to one another, they have been described as *coexistent*. On the other hand, should these cells be mixed together, the term carcinosarcoma has been applied. Whether this condition involves similar problems and controversies to those surrounding the canine mixed mammary tumor is not clear at this moment.

Secondary neoplasms, metastatic to the thyroid, may be observed in animals. Squamous cell carcinoma arising in the tonsillar crypt of the dog may occasionally involve the thyroid as well as the anterior cervical lymph nodes. Lymphosarcoma may also occur as a secondary tumor in the thyroid.

Allam, M. W., Lombard, L. S., Stubbs, E. L., and Shiver, J. F.: Transplant of a thyroid CA within the canine species. Cancer Res., 14:734–737, 1954.

Black, H. E., Capen, C. C., and Young, D. M.: Ultimobranchial thyroid neoplasms in bulls. A syndrome resembling medullary thyroid carcinoma in man. Cancer, 32:865–878, 1973.

Boorman, G. A., van Noord, M. J., and Hollander, C. F.: Naturally occurring medullary thyroid carcinoma in the rat. Arch. Pathol., 94:35–41, 1972.

Boorman, G. A., Heersche, J. N. M., and Hollander, C. F.: Transplantable calcitonin-secreting medullary carcinomas of the thyroid of the WAG/Rij rat. J. Natl. Cancer. Inst., 53:1011–1015, 1974.

Boorman, G. A., and Hollander, C. F.: Animal model of human disease: Medullary carcinoma of the thyroid. Model No. 102. In Handbook, Animal Models of Human Disease, Fasc. 6, edited by T. C. Jones, D. B. Hackel, and G. Migaki. Washington, D.C., Registry of Comparative Pathology, AFIP, 1977.

Capen, C. C., and Black, H. E.: Animal model of human disease: Medullary thyroid carcinoma, multiple endocrine neoplasia, Sipple's syndrome. Animal model: Ultimobranchial thyroid neoplasm in the bull. Am. J. Pathol., 74:377–380, 1974.

Cheville, N. F.: Ultrastructure of canine carotid body and aortic body tumors: Comparison with tissues of thyroid and parathyroid origin. Vet. Pathol., 9:166–189, 1972.

Cohrs, P.: Beitrag zur Kenntnis der intraperikardialen akzessorischen Schilddruesen und Epithelkoerperchen beim Hund (Canis familiaris). Berl. Tieraerztl. Wochenschr., 46:683–699, 1930.

Davis, D. J.: Goiter and malignant growth of the thyroid in the dog. Arch. Pathol., 26:339–347, 1938.

Eickhoff, W.: Zur Histologie und Pathologie der Wildschilddrüse. Arch. Exp. Vet. Med., 16:211–228, 1963.

Griesbach, W. E., Kennedy, T. H., and Purves, H. D.: Thyroid adenomata in rats on brassica seed diet. Br. J. Exp. Pathol., 26:18–24, 1945.

Hackel, D. B., Kinney, T. D., and Wendt, W.: Pathologic lesions in captive wild animals. II. Adenocarcinoma of thyroid in a bear. Lab. Invest., 2:154–163, 1952.

Holzworth, J., Husted, P., and Wind, A.: Arterial thrombosis and thyroid carcinoma in a cat. Cornell Vet., 45:487–496, 1955.

Johnson, K. H., and Osborne, C. A.: Adenocarcinoma of the thyroid gland in a cat. J. Am. Vet. Med. Assoc., 156:906–912, 1970.

Jones, E. E., Barker, J., and Dietrich, S.: Spontaneous tumors of the thyroid gland in mice. J. Natl. Cancer Inst., 36:1–14, 1966.

Joyce, J. R., Thompson, R. B., Kyzar, J. R., and Hightower, D.: Thyroid carcinoma in a horse. J. Am. Vet. Med. Assoc., 168:610–612, 1976.

Jubb, K. V., and McEntee, K.: The relationship of ultimobranchial remnants and derivatives to tumor of the thyroid gland in cattle. Cornell Vet., 44:41–69, 1958.

Krook, L., Olsson, S., and Rooney, J. R.: Thyroid carcinoma in the dog. A case of bone-metastasizing carcinoma simulating secondary hyperparathyroidism. Cornell Vet., 50:106–114, 1960.

Leav, I., et al.: Adenomas and carcinomas of the canine and feline thyroid. Am. J. Pathol., 83:61–122, 1976.

McClelland, R. B.: Carcinoma of the thyroid: a report of five cases in dogs. J. Am. Vet. Med. Assoc., 98:38–40, 1941.

Patnaik, A. K., et al.: Canine medullary carcinoma of the thyroid. Vet. Pathol., 15:590–599, 1978.

Rijnberk, A.: Iodine Metabolism and Thyroid Disease in the Dog. Utrecht, Drukkerij Elinksijk, 1971.

Schlumberger, H. G.: Spontaneous goiter and cancer of the thyroid in animals. Ohio J. Sci., 55:23–43, 1955.

Thake, D. C., Cheville, N. F., and Sharp, R. K.: Ectopic thyroid adenomas at the base of the heart of the dog: ultrastructural identification of dense tubular structures in endoplasmic reticulum. Vet. Pathol., 8:421–432, 1971.

Vitovec, J.: Epithelial thyroid tumors in cows. Vet. Pathol., 13:401–408, 1976.

von Sandersleben, J., and Hänichen, T.: III. Tumours of the thyroid gland. In International Histological

Classification of Tumours of Domestic Animals. Bull. WHO, *50*:35–42, 1974.

Wilkie, B. N., and Krook, L.: Ultimobranchial tumour of the thyroid and pheochromocytoma in the bull. Pathol. Vet., *7*:126–134, 1970.

Zarrin, K.: Naturally occurring parafollicular cell carcinoma of the thyroid in dogs. A histological and ultrastructural study. Vet. Pathol., *14*:556–566, 1977.

PARATHYROID GLANDS

The parathyroid glands, usually consisting of four glands, two on either side of the midline, occur in the upper cervical region and are often in contact or embedded within the thyroid. The parathyroids arise embryologically from the III and IV pharyngeal pouches. All air-breathing vertebrates have parathyroids. The functioning cells are called chief cells, which are concerned with the secretion of parathyroid hormone. This hormone is a straight-chain polypeptide, consisting of 84 amino-acid residues, with a molecular weight of 9500. A "proparathyroid hormone" is believed to be synthesized first on ribosomes of the chief cells, from which active parathyroid hormone is then cleaved enzymatically before it is released from the chief cells.

In concert with two other hormones, thyrocalcitonin and vitamin D, parathyroid hormone exercises precise control of the level of calcium ions in the blood. Calcium is involved in key roles in several biologic processes (blood coagulation, muscle contraction, neural excitability, enzyme activity, hormone release, and membrane permeability) and is an essential component of bone structure. The health of humans and animals therefore depends upon the precise control of calcium in circulating blood and body fluids. Although the hormones produced by parathyroids, thyroid C cells, and renal tubular cells (parathyroid hormone, thyrocalcitonin, and active vitamin D—1,25-dihydroxy-cholecalciferol) are central to the regulation of calcium homeostasis, other hormones may also be involved under some circum-stances. These include adrenal corticosteroids, somatotropin, thyroxine, estrogens, and glucagon.

Important diseases of the parathyroid glands, as with all endocrines, are those that either decrease or increase the secretion of parathyroid hormone (hypoparathyroidism and hyperparathyroidism, respectively). Parathyroid hormone exerts its effect upon calcium homeostasis by increasing the rate of resorption of bone. Intestinal absorption of calcium, renal tubular reabsorption of calcium, and urinary excretion of phosphorus appear to be influenced by parathyroid hormone. The normal secretion of parathyroid hormone is regulated by a negative feedback system in which increased blood levels of calcium cause decreased production of parathyroid hormone. Increased production of thyrocalcitonin, stimulated by high levels of blood calcium, acts to decrease blood levels of calcium.

Altenahr, E.: Ultrastructural pathology of parathyroid glands. Curr. Top. Pathol., *56*:1–54, 1972.

Bergdahl, L., and Boquist, L.: Parathyroid morphology in normal dogs. Pathol. Eur., *8*:95–103, 1973.

Boquist, L., and Lundgren, E.: Effects of variations in calcium concentration on parathyroid morphology in vitro. Lab. Invest., *33*:638–647, 1975.

Capen, C. C., Koestner, A., and Cole, C. R.: The ultrastructure and histochemistry of normal parathyroid glands of pregnant and non-pregnant cows. Lab. Invest., *14*:1673–1690, 1965.

Capen, C. C., and Rowland, G. N.: The ultrastructure of the parathyroid glands of young cats. Anat. Rec., *162*:327–331, 1968.

Capen, C. C.: Functional and fine structural relationships of parathyroid glands. Adv. Vet. Sci. Comp. Med. *19*:249–286, 1975.

Fetter, A. W., and Capen, C. C.: The ultrastructure of the parathyroid glands of young pigs. Acta Anat., *75*:359–372, 1970.

Fleischman, A. R., et al.: Perinatal primate parathyroid hormone metabolism. Biol. Neonate, *27*:40–49, 1975.

Jowsey, J., Reiss, E., and Canterbury, J. M.: Long-term effects of high phosphate intake on parathyroid hormone levels and bone metabolism. Acta Orthop. Scand., *45*: 801–808, 1974.

Mayer, G. P., Habener, J. F., and Potts, J. T., Jr.: Parathyroid hormone secretion *in vivo:* Demonstration of a calcium-independent nonsuppressible component of secretion (in calf). J. Clin. Invest., *57*:678–683, 1976.

Persson, J., and Luthman, J.: Some acute metabolic effects of parathyroid hormone in sheep. Acta Vet. Scand., 15:381–397, 1974.

Potts, J. T., Ambach, G. D., Sherwood, L. M., and Sandovel, A.: Structural basis of biological and immunological activity of parathyroid hormone. Proc. Natl. Acad. Sci., 54:1743–1751, 1965.

Raisz, L. G., and O'Brien, J. E.: Effect of calcium on uptake of alpha-aminoisobutyric acid by parathyroid glands. Am. J. Physiol., 205:816–820, 1963.

Raisz, L. G., O'Brien, J. E., and Au, W. Y. W.: Parathyroid size and uptake of alpha-aminoisobutyric acid in intact and hypophysectomized rats. Proc. Soc. Exp. Biol. Med., 119:1048–1053, 1965.

Roth, S. I., and Capen, C. C.: Ultrastructural and functional correlations of the parathyroid gland. Int. Rev. Exp. Pathol., 13:161–221, 1974.

Sherwood, L. M.: Magnesium ion and parathyroid function. N. Engl. J. Med., 282:752, 1970.

Smith, F. G., Jr., et al.: Parathyroid hormone in foetal and adult sheep: The effect of hypocalcaemia. J. Endocrinol., 53:339–348, 1972.

Waterhouse, C., and Heinig, R. E.: Parathormone levels vs. parathormone function. N. Engl. J. Med., 294:545–546, 1976.

Weisbrode, S. E., Capen, C. C., and Nagode, L. A.: Effects of parathyroid hormone on bone of thyroparathyroidectomized rats. An ultrastructural and enzymatic study. Am. J. Pathol., 75:529–542, 1974.

Williams, G. A., Henderson, W. J., and Bowser, E. N.: Amino acid transport by rat parathyroid glands *in vivo*: Effect of low calcium diet. Proc. Soc. Exp. Biol. Med., 116:651–653, 1964.

Wilson, J. W., Harris, S. G., Moore, W. D., and Leipold, H. W.: Primary hyperparathyroidism in a dog. J. Am. Vet. Med. Assoc., 164:942–946, 1974.

Hypoparathyroidism

A severely depressed level of parathyroid hormone results in a low concentration of blood calcium and tonic (or tetanic) spasms of muscle known as **parathyroid tetany.** These signs appear within two days following surgical extirpation of all parathyroid glands.

Several other natural and experimental conditions may destroy the parathyroids and result in hypoparathyroidism. Infection has been reported to have this effect in dogs. Replacement of the parathyroid by malignant thyroid or other tumors should have the same effect, although this seems not to have been reported.

Diets high in calcium fed to cows have caused atrophy of the chief cells and concomitant failure of secretion. Increased calcium dietary intake by growing dogs appears to cause accumulation of secretory granules and lipid bodies in chief cells, thus inhibiting secretion (Nunez, 1974; Black et al., 1973; Capen, 1975). Experimental administration of dietary levels of vitamin D to cattle increases the rate and amount of calcium absorbed from the intestine. The parathyroid glands, in this situation, have ultrastructural changes that suggest suppression of parathyroid synthesis and secretion (Capen et al., 1965).

Hypersecretion of thyrocalcitonin by medullary or C-cell adenomas or adenocarcinomas of bulls, rats, and dogs has an inhibiting effect upon parathyroid secretion. Experimental administration of L-asparaginase to rabbits is reported to result in severe hypoparathyroidism with tetany. Experimentally induced hypoparathyroidism is also reported as a result of production of isoimmune parathyroiditis in dogs (Capen, 1975).

Black, H. E., Capen, C. C., and Arnaud, C. D.: Ultrastructure of parathyroid glands and plasma immunoreactive parathyroid hormone in pregnant cows fed normal and high calcium diets. Lab. Invest., 29:173–185, 1973.

Capen, C. C., Koestner, A., and Cole, C. R.: The ultrastructure, histopathology, and histochemistry of the parathyroid glands of pregnant and non-pregnant cows fed a high level of vitamin D. Lab. Invest., 14:1809–1825, 1965.

Capen, C. C., and Young, D. M.: The ultrastructure of the parathyroid glands and thyroid parafollicular cells of cows with parturient paresis and hypocalcemia. Lab. Invest., 17:717–737, 1967.

Capen, C. C., Cole, C. R., and Hibbs, J. W.: Influence of vitamin D on calcium metabolism and the parathyroid glands of cattle. Fed. Proc., 27:141–152, 1968.

Capen, C. C.: Functional and fine structural relationships of parathyroid glands. Adv. Vet. Sci. Comp. Med., 19:249–286, 1975.

Hedhammer, A., et al.: Overnutrition and skeletal disease: An experimental study in growing Great Dane dogs. Cornell Vet., 64(Suppl. 5):1–160, 1974.

Meyer, D. J., and Terrell, T. G.: Idiopathic hypoparathyroidism in a dog. J. Am. Vet. Med. Assoc., 168:858–860, 1976.

Nunez, E. A., et al.: Ultrastructure of the parafollicular (C) cells and the parathyroid in growing dogs on high calcium diet. Lab. Invest., 31:96–108, 1974.

Tettenborn, D., Hobik, H. P., and Luckhaus, G.: Hypoparathyreoidismus beim Kaninchen nach Varabreichung von L-asparaginase. Arzneim. Forsch., 20:1753–1755, 1970.

Hyperparathyroidism

Increased synthesis and secretion of parathyroid hormone may result from any of several causes (to be described later). The clinical signs include weakness, polydipsia, and polyuria associated with hypercalcemia; serum phosphate is reduced; urinary excretion of inorganic phosphorus is increased; urinary calculi may be associated with nephrocalcinosis. Generalized demineralization of the skeleton may lead to bone pain and pathologic fractures. The cortex of long bones becomes thinner and the bones of skull, mandible, and maxilla less radiopaque. When the bones are involved, serum levels of alkaline phosphatase are elevated and increased secretion of urinary hydroxyproline occurs.

The effect on the skeleton is one of intensified resorption leading to fibrous osteodystrophy. Calcium is also deposited in soft tissues, especially in the elastica of aorta and arteries, pulmonary arteries, cardiac atria, and coronary arteries. Calcifica-

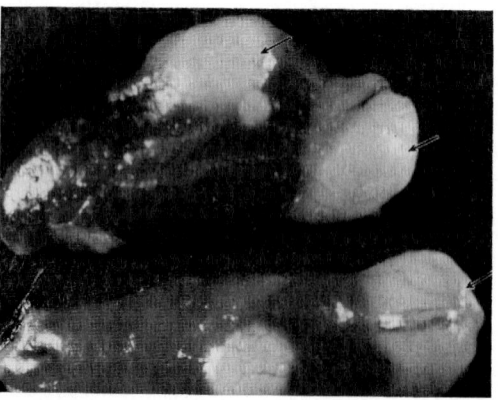

Fig. 26–6. Secondary hyperplasia of parathyroids in a seven-year-old male Airedale with chronic interstitial nephritis. The enlarged gray parathyroids (arrows) stand out against the dark-brown thyroids. (Courtesy of Angell Memorial Animal Hospital.)

tion in the kidneys and walls of bronchi and bronchioles may also be conspicuous (see metastatic calcification).

Primary Hyperparathyroidism. Primary hyperparathyroidism is a term used to identify hyperparathyroidism in humans due to (1) a functioning parathyroid adenoma or adenocarcinoma, or (2) hypersecretion of parathyroids from an unknown cause. Primary hyperparathyroidism due to functional parathyroid tumors has been described in dogs (see Neoplasms of the Parathyroid).

Secondary Hyperparathyroidism. Secondary hyperparathyroidism results from parathyroid hyperplasia and increased secretion of parathyroid hormone due to renal or nutritional causes. **Renal hyperparathyroidism** (renal osteodystrophy, renal rickets, osteorenal syndrome) is associated with chronic renal insufficiency in human beings, rats, and dogs. The secondary hyperparathyroidism associated with renal disease is ascribed to chronic hypocalcemia leading to excessive production of parathyroid hormone. In the progressive renal disease, reduction in glomerular filtration leads to retention of phosphorus and progressive hyperphosphatemia. This decreases the blood calcium. The relatively recent finding that the most active hormone of vitamin D (1,25-dihydrocholecalciferol) is synthesized in the kidney introduces another possible factor. Reduced synthesis of 1,25–dihydrocholecalciferol in a diseased kidney could diminish intestinal transport of calcium and its mobilization from the skeleton. A role for thyrocalcitonin has also been postulated in this process.

The skeletal lesions of secondary renal hypoparathyroidism are described in Chapter 19.

Nutritional secondary hyperparathyroidism has been described in man, horses, cats, dogs, cows, nonhuman primates, domestic and wild birds, and reptiles. The essential deficiency in the causal diets is either (1) inadequate amount of

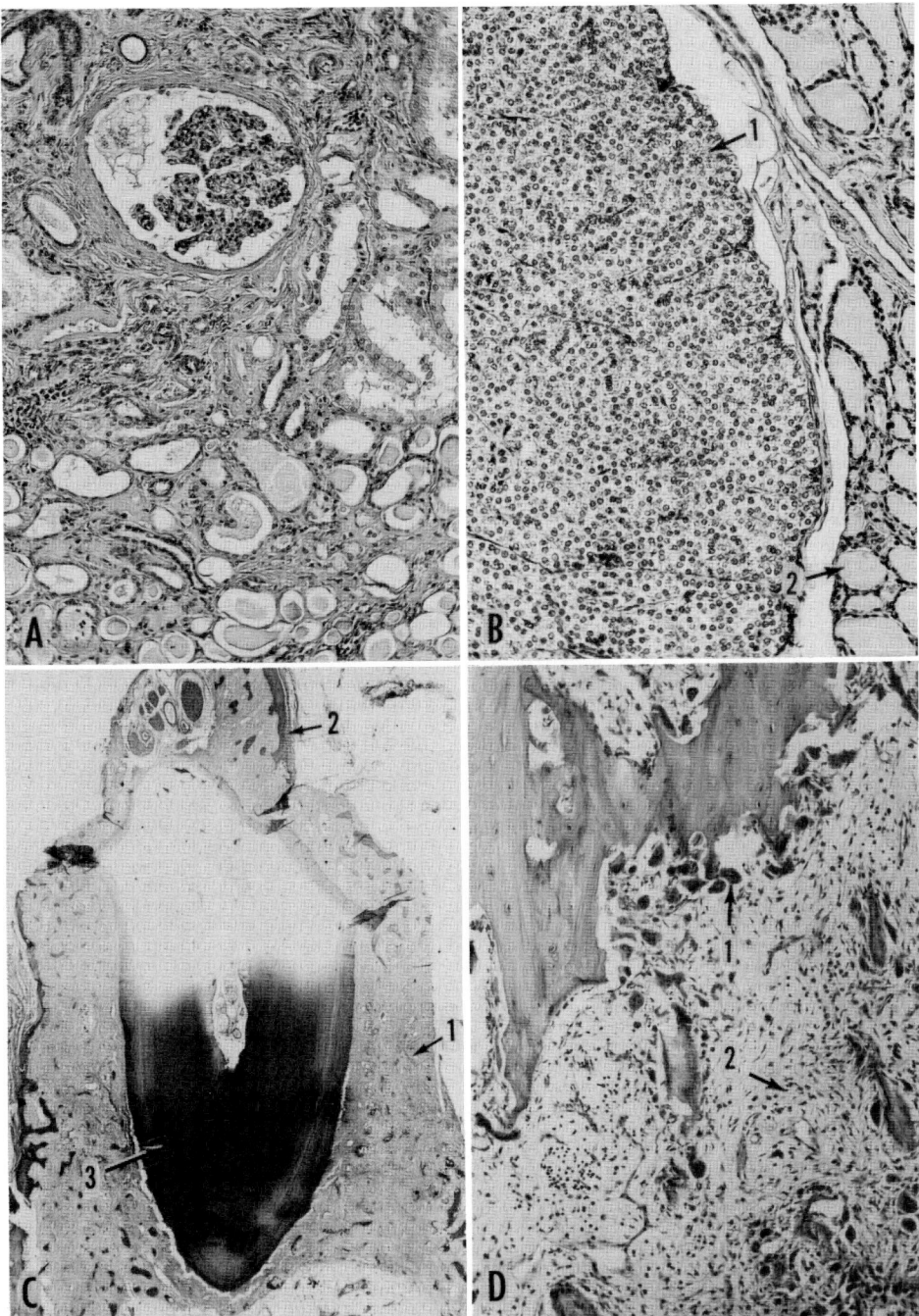

Fig. 26–7. Renal hyperparathyroidism in a dog. *A*, The kidney (× 110). *B*, The enlarged parathyroid *(1)* compressing adjacent thyroid *(2)*. *C*, A tooth (× 11) poorly supported by soft spongy bone. Note absence of bone trabeculae *(1)*. Gingival epithelium *(2)*, dentine of the root of the tooth *(3)*. *D*, The mandible (× 145). Note many osteoblasts *(1)*, fibrous marrow *(2)*, and irregular spicules of bone. (Courtesy of Armed Forces Institute of Pathology.) Contributor: Dr. Joseph M. Stoyak.

calcium, (2) inadequate or inappropriate vitamin D (vitamin D_3 is required by many species), (3) relatively high amounts of phosphorus in the presence of an otherwise adequate amount of calcium, or (4) some combination of the first three factors. Historical examples include all-bran diets fed to miller's horses, the all-meat diets (heart and kidneys) fed to kittens and wild felidae in zoos, and the all-meat diets fed to dogs. The lesions in all these situations are described in Chapter 19.

Anderson, M. P., and Capen, C. C.: Fine structural changes of bone cells in experimental nutritional osteodystrophy of green iguanas. Virchow's Arch. B (Cell Pathol.), 20:169–184, 1976.

Capen, C. C., and Young, D. M.: The ultrastructure of the parathyroid glands and thyroid parafollicular cells of cows with parturient paresis and hypocalcemia. Lab. Invest., 17:717–737, 1967.

Deluca, H. F.: The kidney as an endocrine organ involved in the function of vitamin D. Am. J. Med., 58:39–47, 1975.

Hunt, R. D., Garcia, F. G., and Hegsted, D. M.: A comparison of vitamin D_2 and D_3 in New World primates. I. Production and regression of osteodystrophy fibrosa. Lab. Anim. Care, 17:222–234, 1967.

Ichido, S.: Pathological studies on the osteorenal syndrome in the dog. Jpn. J. Vet. Sci., 28:217–228, 1966.

Ingelfinger, F. J.: Editorial: Pathogenesis of renal osteodystrophy—a role for calcitonin? N. Engl. J. Med., 296:1112–1114, 1977.

Itakura, C., Iida, M., and Goto, M.: Renal secondary hyperparathyroidism in aged Sprague-Dawley rats. Vet. Pathol., 14:463–469, 1977.

Jackson, C. E., Talbert, P. C., and Caylor, H. D.: Hereditary hyperparathyroidism. J. Indiana State Med. Assoc., 53:1313–1316, 1960.

Platt, H.: The parathyroid glands with particular reference to the "rubber jaw" syndrome. The skeletal system in "rubber jaw." J. Comp. Pathol. Therap., 61:188–196, 197–214, 1951.

Rowland, G. N., Capen, C. C., and Nagode, L. A.: Experimental hyperparathyroidism in young cats. Pathol. Vet., 5:504–509, 1968.

Scott, P. P.: Special features of nutrition of cats, with observations on wild felidae nutrition in the London Zoo. Symp. Zool. Soc. London, 21:21–36, 1968.

Pseudohyperparathyroidism. Pseudohyperparathyroidism is a term applied to a disease that closely resembles hyperparathyroidism but occurs in the presence of normal parathyroids. The source of the excessive parathyroid hormone is a tumor not of parathyroid origin. This phenomenon is known in man and dog. The secreting tumor may be a lymphosarcoma (malignant lymphoma) or hepatoma.

Knill-Jones, R. P., et al.: Hypercalcemia and increased parathyroid-hormone activity in a primary hepatoma. N. Engl. J. Med., 282:704–708, 1970.

Osborne, C. A., and Stevens, J. B.: Pseudohyperparathyroidism in the dog. J. Am. Vet. Med. Assoc., 162:125–135, 1973.

Rijnberk, A.: Pseudohyperparathyroidism in the dog. Tijdschr. Diergeneeskd., 95:515, 1970.

Neoplasms of the Parathyroid

Neoplasms of the parathyroid are rarely reported. Of the few reported in animals, most were recognized because of their functional effect (hyperparathyroidism). In nine cases from the literature, one was a nonfunctional tumor from a rat, and seven, all of which were functional, were from dogs (Krook, 1957; Stavrou, 1968; Legendre et al., 1976; Patnaik et al., 1978). One of the seven canine tumors was a large adenocarcinoma in the mediastinum with associated hypercalcemia. It is possible that this tumor arose from ectopic parathyroid in the mediastinum. It is equally possible that this tumor was not of parathyroid origin and represents another case of pseudoparathyroidism.

The clinical signs are usually abated following surgical removal of the parathyroid tumor, but several animals have been reported to have died following a stormy postsurgical course. Because the condition is so infrequent, limited experience has been obtained with the disease.

The tumors, localized in one parathyroid gland and associated with hyperparathyroidism, were small (2 to 3 cm in diameter), circumscribed, encapsulated nodules made up of cells closely resembling the chief cells of the normal parathyroid, or in some cases consisting of a mixture of chief and oxyphil cells. The chief cells had a central, dark-staining nucleus and light, essentially clear cytoplasm. The oxyphil cells had more abundant cytoplasm with a faint eosinophilic tint. In these few cases, the

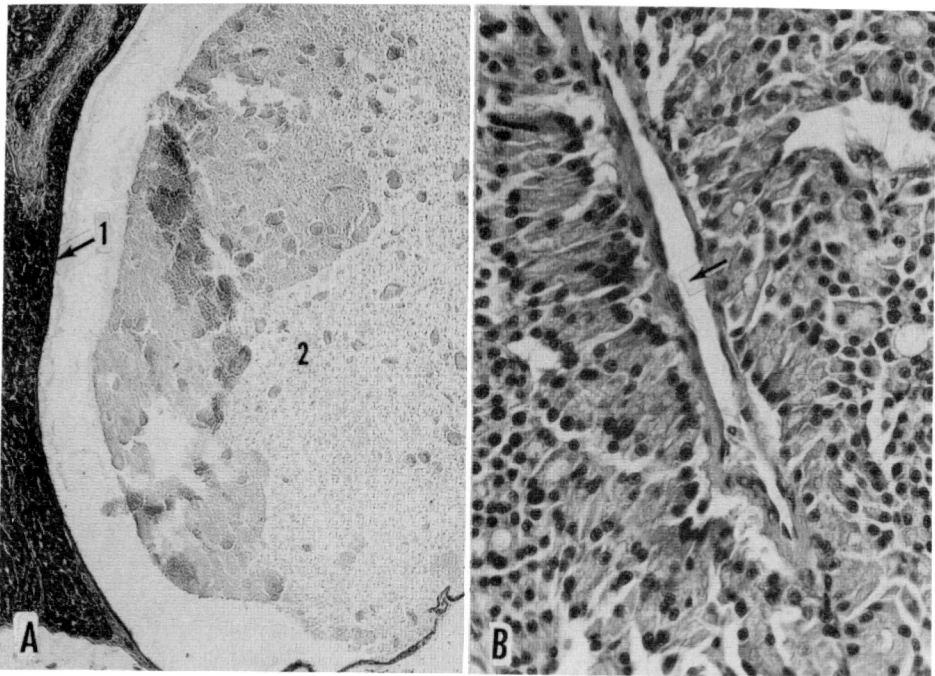

Fig. 26–8. *A*, Cyst of the parathyroid of a dog (× 60). This cyst, found iincidentally, was lined by columnar epithelium *(1)* and contains eosinophilic material *(2)*. Contributor: Dr. Elihu Bond. *B*, Adenocarcinoma of parathyroid of a dog (× 305). Intinate relationship of cells to blood vessels (arrow) is a feature of neoplasms of endocrine organs. (*A* and *B*, Courtesy of Armed Forces Institute of Pathology.) Contributor: Dr. M. M. Mason.

neoplasm was completely encapsulated, with no evidence of extension through the capsule. In human cases, some evidence indicated a familial or possibly inherited tendency to develop similar tumors. Genetic data on the canine tumors have not yet been generated.

Krook, L.: Spontaneous hyperparathyroidism in the dog. A pathologic-anatomic study. Acta Pathol. Microbiol. Scand., 41(Suppl. 122): 1–88, 1957.

Legendre, A. M., Merkley, D. F., Carrig, C. B., and Krehbiel, J. D.: Primary hyperparathyroidism in a dog. J. Am. Vet. Med. Assoc., 168:694–696, 1976.

Patnaik, A. K., et al.: Mediastinal parathyroid adeno-carcinoma in a dog. Vet. Pathol., 15:55–63, 1978.

Pearson, P. T., et al.: Primary hyperparathyroidism in a Beagle. J. Am. Vet. Med. Assoc., 147:1201–1206, 1965.

Stavrou, D.: Beitrag zum Hyperparathyreoidismus des Hundes. Dtsch. Tierarztl. Wochenschr., 75:117–121, 1968.

Warren, S., and Chute, R.: Parathyroid carcinoma in parabiont rats. Science, 135:927–928, 1962.

Wilson, J. W., Harris, S. G., Moore, W. D., and Leipold, H. W.: Primary hyperparathyroidism in a dog. J. Am. Vet. Med. Assoc., 164:942–946, 1974.

ADRENAL GLANDS

The adrenal glands may share, either through direct extension or blood-borne metastases, in degenerative, inflammatory, and neoplastic processes that affect other parts of the animal body. Hemorrhages, usually petechial, infarctions and similar disturbances may appear in the adrenals from the same causes as elsewhere. If one adrenal deteriorates for any one of a variety of reasons, its fellow is prone to undergo compensatory hypertrophy. Hence, except in the case of primary neoplasms or altered control by the pituitary, functional disease is likely to develop only if involvement is bilateral.

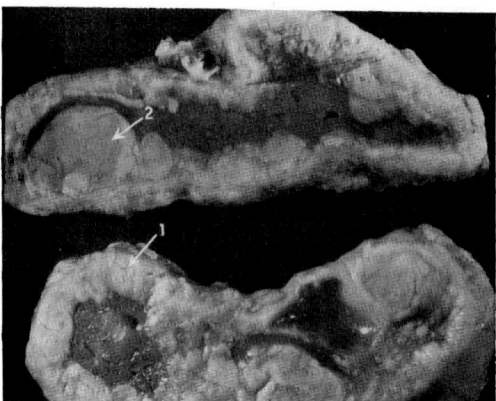

Fig. 26–9. Hyperplasia (1) and adenoma (2) of adrenal cortex of a 12-year-old male English Setter. (Courtesy of Angell Memorial Animal Hospital.)

Adrenal Cortex. Each adrenal gland consists of two parts, cortex and medulla, which embryologically as well as functionally are separate organs. As in some other structures such as the combined openings of the urinary and genital tracts, one wonders whether the arrangement of the adrenal medullary tissue inside the cortex does not represent an anatomic makeshift; indeed, in some lower animal species, the two tissues are anatomically separate.

The adrenal cortex arises from the urogenital ridge, in common with the several urinary and genital organs; thus it is of mesodermal origin. This tissue, under the stimulus and control of hormones from the pituitary gland (adrenocorticotropic hormone, ACTH) and juxtaglomerular apparatus of the kidney (renin-angiotensin), secretes a number of hormones of its own which control a variety of body functions. Because of the essential nature of these hormones, complete loss of adrenocortical tissue is fatal. Chemically the hormones are sterols (having a steroid nucleus), which relates them to cholesterol, ergosterol, and other forms of vitamin D, the sex hormones, certain carcinogenic compounds, and the drug, digitalis.

In general, the hormones produced by the adrenal cortex favor retention and inhibit renal excretion of sodium (but not potassium) and chlorides, thereby maintaining an osmotic pressure sufficient to retain appropriate amounts of water in the blood and tissues. Hormones of this group are under the control of renin-angiotensin from the juxtaglomerular apparatus and are believed to come from the zona glomerulosa and are designated, on the basis of chemical structure, as mineralocorticoids. They include aldosterone (natural) and desoxycorticosterone (synthetic).

Other hormones favor gluconeogenesis, raising the level of blood sugar and increasing the glycogen in the liver. They also tend to reduce the numbers of eosinophils in the blood and of lymphocytes in either the blood or lymphoid tissues. These hormones are called glucocorticoids; cortisone (17-hydroxy-11-dehydroxycorticosterone) and hydrocortisone (17-hydroxycorticosterone) are the outstanding examples. They come from the zona fasciculata and are under control of ACTH.

The adrenal sex hormones are androgenic and masculinizing, an effect that will be mentioned in connection with adrenocortical tumors. These hormones are characterized by a ketone group on the seventeenth carbon atom and, therefore, are known as the 17-ketosteroids. They are believed to come from the zona reticularis. Some effects of the hormones are more or less antagonistic to those of others, a proper balance being essential to health. Many of them are concerned, along with epinephrine from the medulla, in maintaining many bodily functions in their normal state of activity (homeostasis) against the "stress" of unfavorable environmental situations. Other effects attributable to cortical hormones include stimulating delivery of erythrocytes and neutrophils into the circulating blood, but inhibiting the same process for lymphocytes and eosinophils. There is, in fact, a general depression of the lymphoid tissues. Deposition of body fat is favored, although it is likely to be peculiarly localized. Sweating is increased. This, probably with other factors, assists in toleration of high ambient temperatures. Production of melanin in the skin is augmented. Blood pressure tends to be raised. Excretion of calcium is somewhat increased. Proliferation of cells of the reticuloendothelial and fibroblastic groups is inhibited. It is to this latter action that the drug cortisone (and indirectly ACTH) owes its value; chronic proliferative inflammations are inhibited, as are also certain immunologic processes. Where these inflammations are excessive, such inhibition is desirable, bringing symptomatic and often morphologic relief. In the case of active infections (such as the granulomas), the same action is harmful and may be lethal.

Adrenal Medulla. Cells that make up the adrenal medulla are derived embryologically from the neural crest and part of the chromaffin system. The hormones produced by these cells are epinephrine (adrenalin) and norepinephrine. Cells that produce each of these hormones may be distinguished by special stains. Both of these hormones have effects on maintaining or increasing blood pressure. In excessive amounts (as in a functional pheochromocytoma), these hormones produce paroxysmal hypertension.

Anderson, A. C.: The Beagle as an Experimental Dog. Ames, Iowa State Univ. Press, 1972.

Benirschke, K., and Richart, R.: Observations on the fetal adrenals of Marmoset monkeys. Endocrinology, 74:382–387, 1964.

Dellman, H. D.: Veterinary Histology. Philadelphia, Lea & Febiger, 1971.

King, M. P., and Angelakos, E. T.: Differentiation of noradrenaline and adrenaline containing cells in the adrenal medulla by the trihydroxyindole histochemical reaction. Acta Histochem. (Jena), 45:61–70, 1973.

McConnell, E. E., and Talley, F. A.: Intracytoplasmic hyaline globules in the adrenal medulla of laboratory animals. Vet. Pathol., 14:435–440, 1977.

Moser, H. G., and Benirschke, K.: Fetal zone of the adrenal gland in the nine-banded armadillo, Dasypus novemcinctus. Anat. Rec., 143:47–59, 1962.

Pauly, J. E.: The comparative anatomy of the adrenals. Anim. Care Panel, 9:143–154, 1959.

Hypoadrenocorticism

Atrophy, necrosis, or malfunction leads to a deficiency of the hormones produced by the adrenal cortex. The best known adrenal insufficiency is classically represented by Addison's disease, a syndrome affecting humans. Known since 1855, this disease was invariably fatal until the discovery and therapeutic use of adrenocortical hormones.

In Addison's disease, there is a gradually developing weakness with feeble heart action, accompanied by low blood pressure, decrease in blood volume (due to excessive excretion of sodium and chlorides and consequent loss of fluid), frequently hypoglycemia (due to failure of gluconeogenesis), and shock. Severe gastrointestinal malfunctions, including vomition, are the rule. A spectacular symptom regularly present is a marked increase in the pigmentation of the skin. This is believed to be due to an excess of pituitary melanocyte-stimulating hormone which develops reciprocally to a fall in an inhibitory adrenocortical hormone. Lesions of Addison's disease in other organs are of interest in showing the effects of adrenal insufficiency upon other structures and functions. The pituitary gland shows a decrease of basophils and an increase of chromophobes. Both the thyroid and the heart are often small and atrophic, with areas of atrophic or dying fibers in the myocardium. Lymphoid tissue is often greatly increased in the thyroid and in the lymphoid organs.

The cause of Addison's disease is the destruction of both adrenal glands. Frequently, this is the result of tuberculous involvement, but histoplasmosis, amyloidosis, bilateral metastatic tumors, and possibly the direct toxic effects of some drugs and chemicals in hypersensitive individuals are also causes of the same destructive lesions.

Canine Hypoadrenocorticism. This disorder is now recognized as a spontaneously occurring clinical and pathologic entity in dogs. The lesions were first identified as involving atrophy of the adrenal cortex (Hadlow, 1953; Nelson and Woodward, 1949); the clinical changes resulting from these lesions were described a few years thereafter (Freudiger and Lindt, 1958; Marshak et al., 1960). The clinical features included quickly induced fatigue or muscle weakness (asthenia), depression, anorexia, frequent vomiting, repeated diarrhea, tendency to hypothermia, disturbances of circulation, terminal dehydration, eosinophilia, anuria, azotemia, hyponatremia, and hyperkalemia. Thyroid and gonadal functions were normal, and administration of adrenocorticotropic hormone (ACTH) produced no significant change. Administration of cortisone and 9-α-fluorohydrocortisone produced dramatic relief of all signs.

The **lesions** in the adrenal are limited to the cortex; the medulla is unaffected. In later stages, the cortex is completely atrophied; all secreting cells are absent, giving the entire adrenal a much reduced size. In less advanced cases, one may see remnants of adrenal cortical cells with necrosis and some leukocytic response.

The **causes** of adrenal cortical atrophy are often not determined in individual spontaneous cases. Generalized infections may damage the adrenal cortex, although documentation is presently sparse. Experimental toxoplasmosis, histoplasmosis, and besnoitiosis in hamsters have produced specific necrotizing effects on the adrenal cortex (Frenkel, 1977). This localized affinity of these organisms is believed to be related to the anti-inflammatory effects of glucocorticoid hormones present at the site in the adrenal cortex.

A few specific toxins have a severe deleterious effect on the adrenal cortex. The first to be identified as a natural poison and its cytotoxicity demonstrated experimentally is a metabolite of DDT known as DDD or TDE (2,2-bis(parachlorophenyl) 1,1-Dichloroethane). This is an insecticide with such specific toxicity for cells of the adrenal cortex (in dogs and rats) that it is also useful in destroying the hyperplastic cells of the adrenal in hyperadrenocorticism.

Acryonitrile also has a severe cytotoxic effect on the adrenal cortex and has been used to develop a model for "adrenal apoplexy." A functional adrenal cortical tumor in one adrenal gland will cause severe atrophy in the cortex of the contralateral gland. Because of the excess production of cortical hormones by the tumor, the overall effect on the host is one of hyperadrenocorticism. Replacement of both adrenals by malignant metastatic tumor is a possibility, but has rarely been reported in animals.

Bovine Hypoadrenocorticism. A congenital hypoplasia of the adrenal cortex, inherited as a recessive trait, is believed to be the underlying lesion in cases of prolonged gestation that occur in Holstein and Ayrshire cattle.

Adlersberg, C., Schaefer, L. E., and Want, Chun-I: Adrenal cortex, lipid metabolism and atherosclerosis: Experimental studies in the rabbit. Science, 120:319–320, 1954.

Anderson, M. P., and Capen, C. C.: The endocrine system. *In* Pathology of Laboratory Animals, edited by K. Benirschke, F. M. Garner, and T. C. Jones. New York, Springer-Verlag, 1978.

Atkins, G., Marotta, S. F., and Hirai, K.: In vitro studies on distribution of cortisol in dog's blood. Proc. Soc. Exp. Biol. Med., 122:347–351, 1966.

Bowman, R. E., and Wolf, R. C.: Plasma 17-hydroxycorticosteroid response to ACTH in *M. mulatta*: Dose, age, weight, sex. Proc. Soc. Exp. Biol. Med., 130:61–64, 1969.

Cameron, E. H. D., and Grant, J. K.: Biochemistry of histologically defined zones in the adrenal cortex: Cortisol synthesis in the horse. J. Endocrinol., 37:413–420, 1967.

Frenkel, J. K.: Animal model of human disease: Adrenal infection, necrosis, and hypocorticism. Am. J. Pathol., 86:749–752, 1977.

Freudiger, U., and Lindt, S.: Beitrage zur Klinik der Nebennierenrinden-Funktions-störungen des

Hundes. Schweiz. Arch. Tierheilkd., *100*:362–378, 1958.

Hadlow, W. J.: Adrenal cortical atrophy in the dog. Am. J. Pathol., *29*:353–361, 1953.

Marshak, R. R., Webster, G. D., and Shelley, J. F.: Observations on a case of primary adrenocortical insufficiency in a dog. J. Am. Vet. Med. Assoc., *136*:274–280, 1960.

Nelson, A. A., and Woodward, G.: Severe adrenal cortical atrophy (cytotoxic) and hepatic damage produced in dogs by feeding 2,2-bis (parachlorophenyl) 1,1-dichloroethane (DDD or TDE). Archiv. Pathol., *48*:387–394, 1949.

Powers, J. M., Hennigar, G. R., Grooms, G., and Nichols, J.: Adrenal cortical degeneration and regeneration following administration of DDD. Am. J. Pathol., *75*:181–194, 1974.

Price, P. J., Greef, J., and Weber, H. W.: Pathological findings in the adrenal gland of Chacma baboons—160 consecutive cases. J. S. Afr. Vet. Med. Assoc., *42*:39–43, 1971.

Szabo, S., Reynolds, E. S., and Kovacs, K.: Animal model: Waterhouse-Fredricksen syndrome. Animal Model No. 101. *In* Handbook: Animal Models of Human Disease, Fasc. 6, edited by T. C. Jones, D. B. Hackel and G. Migaki. Washington, D.C., Registry of Comparative Pathology, AFIP, 1977.

Vilar, O., and Tullner, W. W.: Effects of o,p'-DDD on histology and 17 hydroxycorticosteroid output of the dog adrenal cortex. Endocrinology, *65*:80–86, 1959.

Wassermann, D., and Wassermann, M.: Adrenocortical zona fasciculata in rats receiving p,p',-DDT. Environ. Physiol. Biochem., *3*:274–280, 1973.

Hyperadrenocorticism

Excessive production of hormones by cells of the adrenal cortex, concomitant with hyperplasia or neoplasia, results in clinical manifestations called hyperadrenocorticism. The clinical signs produced by this excessive amount of adrenal cortical hormones may be listed as follows: bilaterally symmetric loss of hair (alopecia), weakness of muscles, enlarged pendulous abdomen, trembling, obesity, polyuria, and polydipsia. Lymphopenia, eosinophilia, and neutrophilia are rather consistent hematologic features. These signs are accompanied by elevated levels of cortisol in the serum and by excessive secretion of 17-ketogenic steroids. An exaggerated response to administration of adrenocorticotropic hormone (ACTH) results in at least a two-fold elevation in urinary 17-ketogenic steroids. Some effects may be due to ac-

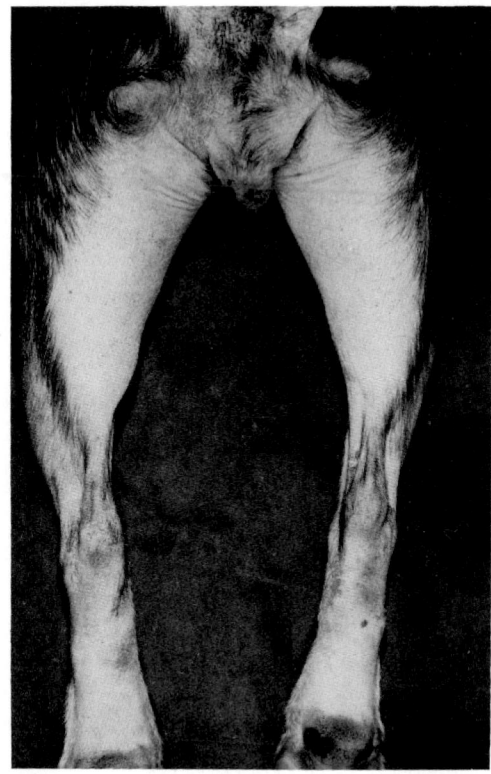

Fig. 26–10. Symmetrical alopecia of the thighs of a ten-year-old spayed female Boston Terrier with hyperadrenocorticism. (Courtesy of Angell Memorial Animal Hospital.)

companying destruction of hypothalamus by pituitary tumor (e.g., diabetes insipidus, behavioral changes, blindness). Other less constant changes, such as mineralization of the skin, lungs, and other tissues, hyperesthesia, hyperglycemia, and hypercholesterolemia are probably due to the excessive adrenal cortical hormones.

Three types of hyperadrenocorticism are recognized in dogs: canine Cushing's disease, canine Cushing's syndrome, and functional adrenal cortical neoplasms.

Canine Cushing's Disease. This disease of canines was so named because of its similarity to a human disease named in recognition of Harvey Cushing, a Boston physician who first described the disease. The hyperadrenocorticism in this type results

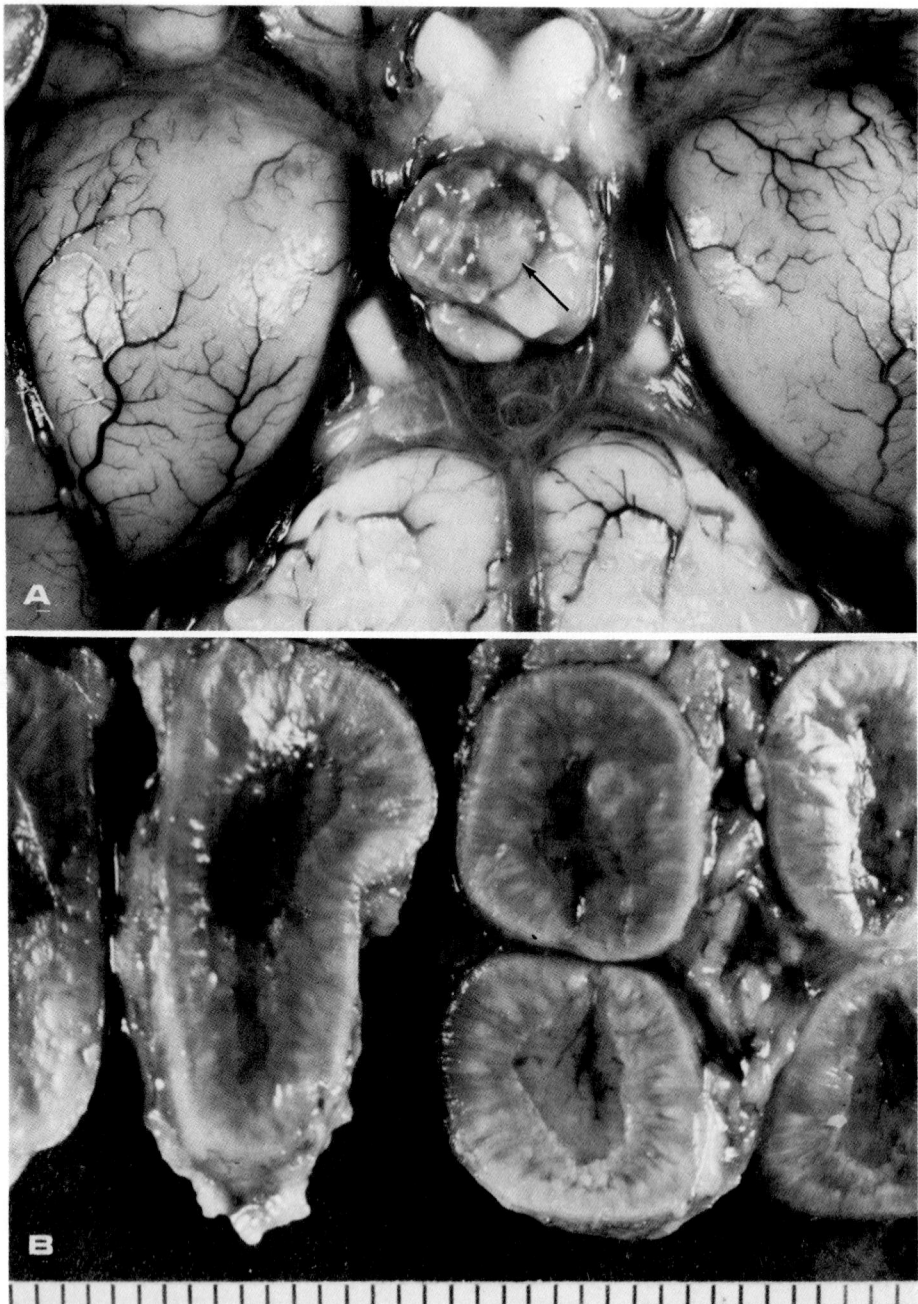

Fig. 26–11. *A,* Adenoma of the pituitary of a ten-year-old spayed female Boston Terrier with canine "Cushing's" disease. *B,* Hyperplasia of adrenal cortices, same dog. (Courtesy of Angell Memorial Animal Hospital.)

from hyperplasia and hypertrophy of the adrenal cortex, stimulated by adrenocorticotropic hormone (ACTH) secreted by a functional tumor of the pituitary. In one study (Capen et al., 1976), about 62% of the chromophobe adenomas (or adenomas of the intermediate lobe) of the pituitary were functionally active in secreting ACTH.

Among cases of diffuse hyperplasia of the adrenal cortex in another study, about 20% were associated with secreting pituitary adenomas (Siegal et al., 1970); 80% were not associated with any pituitary tumor or other lesion. These cases, similar to the human syndrome, have come to be called "canine Cushing's syndrome."

Canine Cushing's Syndrome. This phrase is used to distinguish those cases of hyperadrenocorticism stemming from adrenal cortical hyperfunction and hyperplasia in the absence of any pituitary lesion. These cases of idiopathic hyperadrenocorticism are distinguished by their long-term recovery following adrenalectomy and maintenance on cortisone and mineralocorticoid therapy.

The adrenal cortical hyperplasia in these cases may be diffuse or nodular, but is consistently bilateral. Extracapsular hyperplastic nodules of adrenal cortical cells are not uncommon in normal dogs and usually are not associated with hypersecretion. The zona reticularis and zona fasciculata are usually most involved. The zona glomerulosa may be essentially intact. No lesions are seen in other endocrine glands.

Adrenal Cortical Adenoma and Carcinoma. These tumors are considered the causative factors in the third type of canine hyperadrenocorticism. The underlying cause is essentially unknown. In one study, these neoplasms were responsible for 3 cases of 27 in dogs with hyperadrenocorticism (Kelley et al., 1971). The tumors usually involve only one adrenal gland; the cortex of the contralateral gland is severely atrophied. Excision of the adenomas, as a part of adrenalectomy, usually results in clinical recovery. One

carcinoma was recognized as malignant by its invasion of the vena cava and metastases to the lung. These tumors are described further under Neoplasms of the Adrenal.

Adrenogenital Syndrome. Excessive secretion of sex hormones, especially androgens, may occur in the adrenal cortex as a result of hyperadrenocorticism from any cause. In human patients, deficiency of an enzyme, 21-hydroxylase or 11-β-hydroxylase, leads to excessive production of androgens. Such an excess of androgens in dogs, horses, and cattle as well as humans results in precocious masculine sexual development and premature closure of epiphyses of the long bones. In the female, virilization occurs including hypertrophy of the clitoris, hirsutism, hypertrophy of the laryngeal muscles, anestrus, and in the mare, masculine development of the neck. The mammary glands and uterus undergo atrophy. The 17-ketosteroid metabolites of androgens may be demonstrable in the urine. This syndrome has been reported in several species, but needs further documentation (Anderson and Capen, 1978).

Anderson, M. P., and Capen, C. C.: The endocrine system. *In* Pathology of Laboratory Animals, edited by K. Benirschke, F. M. Garner, and T. C. Jones. New York, Springer-Verlag, 1978.

Bush, I. E., and Ferguson, K. A.: The secretion of the adrenal cortex of sheep. J. Endocrinol., 10:1–8, 1953.

Capen, C. C., and Martin, S. L.: Cushing's syndrome, hypercortisolism, Cushing's disease, Nelson's syndrome. Model No. 89. *In* Handbook: Animal Models of Human Disease, Fasc. 5, edited by T. C. Jones, D. B. Hackel, and G. Migaki. Washington, D.C., Registry of Comparative Pathology, AFIP, 1976.

Christian, J. J.: The relation of adrenal weight to body weight in mammals. Science, 117:78–80, 1952.

Coffin, D. L., and Munson, T. O.: Endocrine diseases of the dog associated with hair loss. Sertoli-cell tumor of testis, hypothyroidism, canine Cushing's syndrome. J. Am. Vet. Med. Assoc., 123:403–408, 1953.

Cohen, R. B., Chapman, W. B., and Castleman, B.: Hyperadrenocorticism (Cushing's disease). A study of surgically resected adrenal glands. Am. J. Pathol., 35:537–561, 1959.

Dahme, E., and Schlemmer, W.: Endokrin aktive Nebennierenmarktumoren des Hundes und ihre

Auswirkungen auf die arterielle Blutstromahn. Zentralbl. Veterinaermed. (A), 6:249–259, 1959.

Dämmrich, K.: Die Beeinflussung des Skeletts durch die Hormone der Nebennierenrinde unter besonderer Berücksichtigung des "Morbus Cushing" beim Hund. Berl. Münch. Tierarztl. Wochenschr. 75:331–337, 1962.

Dunn, T. G.: Normal and pathologic anatomy of the adrenal gland of the mouse, including neoplasms. J. Natl. Cancer Inst., 44:1323–1389, 1970.

Elias, H.: Growth of the adrenal cortex in domesticated ungulata. Am. J. Vet. Res., 9:173–189, 1948.

Fox, R. R., and Crary, D. D.: A lethal recessive gene for adrenal hyperplasia in the rabbit. Teratology, 5:255, 1972.

Fujii, K., and Sato, H.: Spontaneous endocrine tumors in mastomys. Gan, 63:135–137, 1972.

Gilman, J., Gilbert, C., and Spence, I.: Phaeochromocytoma in the rat. Pathogenesis and collateral reactions and its relation to comparable tumors in man. Cancer, 6:494–511, 1953.

Hamburger, F., and Russfield, A. B.: An inbred line of Syrian hamsters with frequent spontaneous adrenal tumors. Cancer Res., 30:305–308, 1970.

Kelley, D. F., Siegel, E. T., and Berg, P.: The adrenal gland in dogs with hyperadrenalcorticalism. A pathologic study. Vet. Pathol., 8:385–400, 1971.

Lindt, S.: Über die Pathologie der Nebenniere des Hundes. Dtsch. Tierarztl. Wochenschr., 69:586–588, 1962.

Lubberink, A.A.M.E., Rijnberk, A., Kinderen, P.J. der, and Thijssen, J.H.H.: Hyperfunction of the adrenal cortex: A review. Aust. Vet. J., 47:504–509, 1971.

Luke, D.: The effect of adrenocorticotrophic hormone and adrenal cortical extract on the differential white count in the pig. Br. Vet. J., 109:434–436, 1953.

Rijnberk, A., Kinderen, P.J. der, and Thijssen, J.H.H.: Spontaneous hyperadrenocorticism in the dog. J. Endocrinol., 41:397–406, 1968.

Rijnberk, A., Kinderen, P.J. der, and Thijssen, J.H.H.: Canine Cushing's syndrome. Zentralbl. Veterinaermed. [A], 16:13–28, 1969.

Ross, M.A., Gainer, J.H., and Innes, J.R.M.: Dystrophic calcification in the adrenal glands of monkeys, cats and dogs. Arch. Pathol., 60: 655–662, 1955.

Siegel, E.T.: Determination of 17-hydroxycorticosteroids in canine urine. Am. J. Vet. Res., 26:1152–1156, 1965.

Siegel, E.T., O'Brien, J. B., Pyle, L., and Schryver, H. F.: Functional adrenocortical carcinoma in a dog. J. Am. Vet. Med. Assoc., 150:760–766, 1967.

Siegel, E. T.: Assessment of pituitary-adrenal gland function in the dog. Am. J. Vet. Res., 29:173–180, 1968.

Siegel, E. T., Kelly, D.F., and Berg, P.: Cushing's syndrome in the dog. J. Am. Vet. Med. Assoc., 157:2081–2090, 1970.

Spaar, F.W., and Wille, H.: Zur vergleichenden Pathologie der Hypophosenadenom der Tiere. Zentralbl. Veterinaermed., 6:925–944, 1959.

Verstraete, A., and Thoonern, J.: Zwee nieuwe geval-

len van hypophysaire stoormissen bij de Hond. Vlaams Diergeneeskd. Tijdschr. 8:304–314, 1939.

Wilson, R. B., et al.: Response of dogs to corticotropin measured by 17-hydroxycorticosteroid excretion. Am. J. Vet. Res., 28:313–322, 1967.

Neoplasms of the Adrenal

The primary tumors of the adrenal originate either in the cortex or medulla. The cortical tumors are classified as adenomas or carcinomas of the adrenal cortex. The medullary tumors in animals include: pheochromocytoma, ganglioneuroma, ganglioneuroblastoma, and neuroblastoma. Each of these primary tumors is described briefly. Secondary neoplasms are infrequent in all species with the possible exception of lymphosarcoma. Tumors of the supporting tissues, such as fibrocarcinoma and hemangioma, may occur in the adrenal, but are also uncommon.

Adenoma of the adrenal cortex (adrenocortical adenoma) is encountered in about every species of mammal and is often functional, producing cortical steroid hormones. These tumors are usually unilateral and arise within the cortex, but may take origin from invaginations of cortical cells into the medulla. They are usually circumscribed and grow by expansion, but are usually incompletely encapsulated. The cells are usually well-differentiated and resemble the cells of one or more zones of the cortex. Most common are those made up of polyhedral cells in cords or sheets, with or without cytoplasmic lipid, and resembling the cells of the zona fasciculata or zona reticularis. Tumors of the zona glomerulosa are less frequent.

Small nodules of hyperplastic cells are often seen within and outside the adrenal capsule. These nodules may be numerous and some are clearly visible with the naked eye. Most of these nodules are believed to be nonfunctional and not neoplastic. The differentiation of such hyperplastic nodules from adenomas is often a problem for the pathologist. Most decisions involving the small lesions are arbitrary and

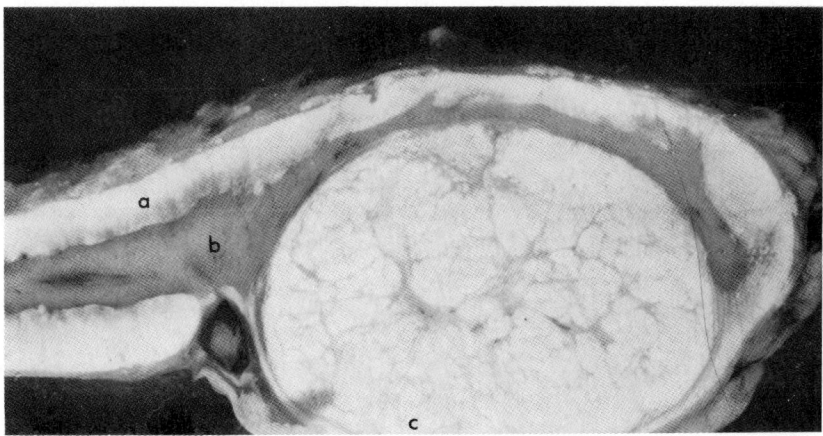

Fig. 26–12.   Adenoma of the adrenal cortex of an eight-year-old male hound. Adrenal cortex *(a)*, medulla *(b)*, tumor *(c)*.

perhaps incorrect. The clearly functional adenomas usually are larger, however, and contain many large cells with foamy cytoplasm and lipid vacuoles.

Reliable statistical data are not available concerning the frequency of these adenomas, but they are encountered and reported more frequently in the dog. They are of particular interest because they may secrete enough adrenocortical hormones to cause hyperadrenocorticism, a frequent problem in dogs.

Carcinoma of the adrenal cortex (adrenocortical carcinoma) is a neoplasm whose cells resemble those of the cortical adenoma, but differ in some respects. Mitoses and less well differentiated cells are more frequent, necrosis of tumor cells is more apt to be seen, and the neoplastic cells invade adjacent adrenal cortex, blood and lymph vessels, and metastasize. Extension into the vena cava and along its intima may occur and metastatic tumors may be found in lungs or other organs.

Carcinomas may also produce enough corticosteroid hormone to cause hyperadrenocorticism, as discussed elsewhere.

Pheochromocytoma is the most frequent tumor of the adrenal medulla in all species in which it has been reported. Cattle, dogs and horses are the domestic animals most often affected. Adrenal pheochromocytomas are more common in the rat than in other laboratory species; however the frequency of this tumor varies greatly with the strain of animal. In one study of "Holzman-source" random-bred rats (Schardein et al., 1968), involving 5086 animals of all ages, spontaneous adrenal cortical adenomas appeared in 91 rats (slightly more than half in females), pheochromocytomas were found in 7, and a myelolipoma in 1. In aged "Wistar" rats, one report gives frequencies up to 86%, with more tumors occurring in males than in females (Gillman et al., 1953). In Sprague-Dawley rats with an average age of 22 months, pheochromocytomas were found in 8% of the animals (Thompson and Hunt, 1963). The frequency of this tumor clearly varies with species, strain, age, and sex.

The pheochromocytoma arises in the adrenal medulla from the chromaffin cells and usually keeps a resemblance to them. The tumor cells are large with abundant cytoplasm, in which granules can be demonstrated with appropriate technique (Müller's, Zenker's, Orth's, or other fixative containing dichromate will usually help in demonstrating the granules). The tumor cells may be arranged in irregular cords or

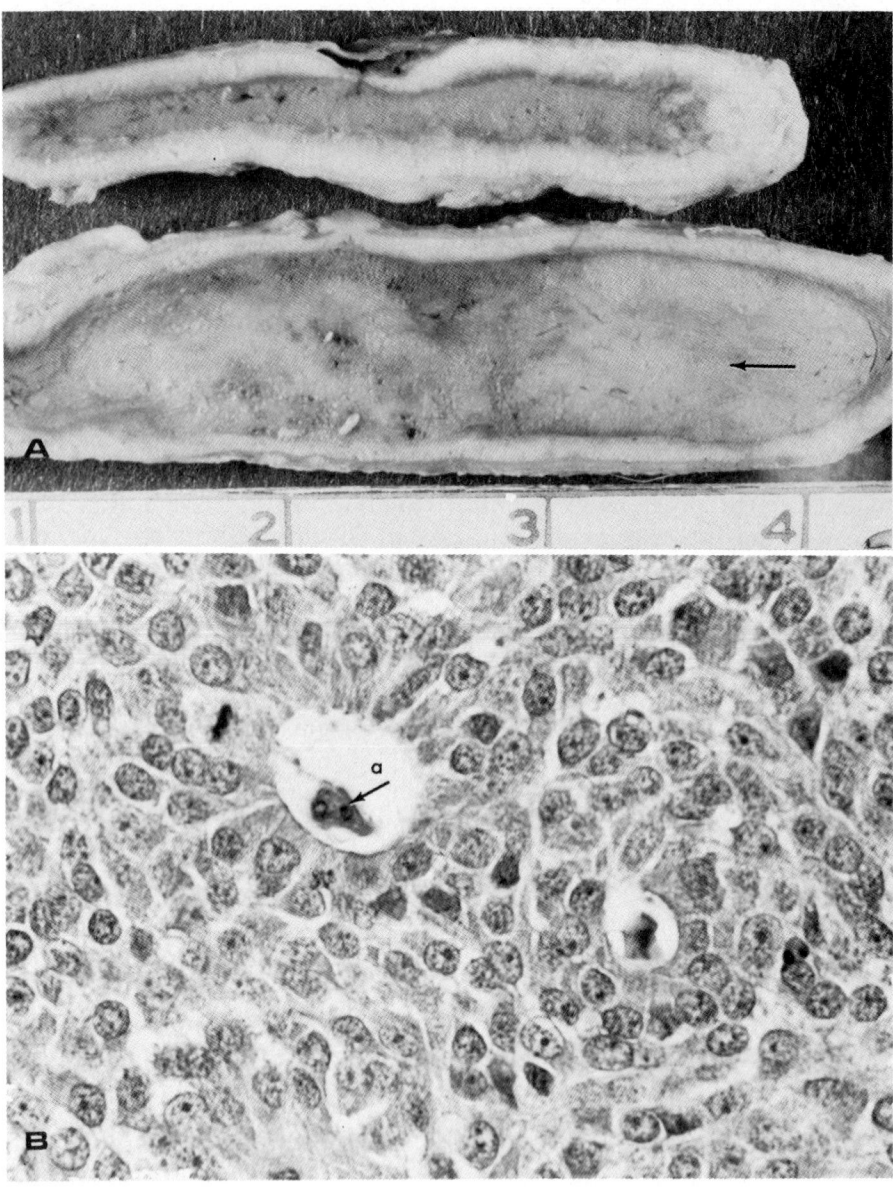

Fig. 26–13. *A,* Pheochromocytoma (arrow), medulla of the adrenal of an eight-year-old male Dalmatian dog. *B,* Same tumor. (H & E stain, × 1000.) Note intimate relationship of tumor cells to small capillaries *(a),* forming "pseudo rosettes" around them. The empty space around the capillary is due to shrinkage artifact. (Courtesy of Angell Memorial Animal Hospital.)

arcuate arrays, separated by a rich vascular system. The cells are usually elongated, but bovine tumors may also be spherical, giving the impression that two types of cells may be involved.

The pheochromocytoma grossly is dark reddish brown and may be single or multiple, involving one or both adrenals. The surrounding adrenal medulla and cortex may be compressed by the larger tumors. Encapsulation is usually incomplete at best, but some trabeculation may occur in the tumor. Brown pigment (lipofuscin) may be seen at the periphery of the tumor. Poorly differentiated tumor cells may invade the adjacent tissues and grow into the vena cava. Metastasis can be expected in this type.

Some pheochromocytomas have functional effects upon their host as a result of secreting either epinephrine, norepinephrine, or both. These effects have been described previously under "Adrenal Medulla."

Neurofibromas are infrequently recognized in animals, perhaps more so in cattle than other species. These tumors arise in the adrenal medulla, presumably from precursor cells that come from the neural crest. Histologically they are similar to neurofibromas of other sites, consisting of parallel arrays of spindle-shaped cells occasionally arranged in palisades and bizarre patterns.

Ganglioneuroma is a rare tumor, sharing its origin in neural crest with the chromaffin cells of the medulla. It is made up of nerve fibers and ganglion cells and may replace the adrenal medulla but does not metastasize. Although rare, at least three cases have been seen in rats (Todd et al., 1970).

Glanglioneuroblastoma resembles the neuroblastoma, but also contains pleomorphic ganglion cell neurons.

Neuroblastoma is a tumor of the adrenal medulla which is most often encountered in young animals. This tumor contains many fine fibrils in which small cells with hyperchromatic nuclei are entangled. The fibrils are more evident in the few places where cell nuclei are sparse. Rosettes and peculiar fan-shaped or windblown patterns may be seen. This tumor has been reported in the dog, but its natural history and significance are as yet unknown.

"Myelolipoma" is not clearly a tumor but consists of collections of myeloid cells in fat, sometimes accompanied by bone. It is a benign lesion, probably not neoplastic. It is seen occasionally as an incidental finding in the adrenal of rats and dogs.

Anderson, M. P., and Capen, C. C.: The endocrine system. *In* Pathology of Laboratory Animals, edited by K. Benirschke, F. M. Garner, and T. C. Jones. New York, Springer-Verlag, 1978.

Appleby, E. C.: XVII. Tumours of the adrenal gland and paraganglia. International Histological Classification of Tumours of Domestic Animals. Bull. WHO, *53*:227–235, 1976.

Dahme, E., and Schlemmer, W.: Endokin aktiv Nebennierenmarktumoren des Hundes und ihre Auswirkungen auf die arterielle Blutstrombahn. Zentralbl. Veterinaermed. (A), *6*:249–259, 1959.

Dunn, T. G.: Normal and pathologic anatomy of the adrenal gland of the mouse, including neoplasms. J. Natl. Cancer Inst., *44*:1323–1389, 1970.

Gillman, J., Gilbert, C., and Spense, I.: Phaeochromocytoma in the rat. Pathogenesis and collateral reactions and its relation to comparable tumours in man. Cancer, *6*:494–511, 1953.

Howard, E. B., and Nielsen, S. W.: Phaeochromocytomas associated with hypertensive lesions in dogs. J. Am. Vet. Med. Assoc., *147*:245–252, 1965.

Kelley, D. F., Siegel, E. T., and Berg, P.: The adrenal gland in dogs with hyperadrenalcorticalism. A pathologic study. Vet. Pathol., *8*:385–400, 1971.

McClure, H. M.: Tumors in non-human primates: Observations during a six year period in the Yerkes Primate Research Center. Am. J. Phys. Anthropol., *38*:425–450, 1973.

Richter, W. R.: Tubular adenomata of the adrenal of the goat. Cornell Vet., *47*:558–577, 1957.

Richter, W. R.: Adrenal cortical adenomata in the goat. Am. J. Vet. Res., *19*:895–901, 1958.

Seibold, H. R., and Wolf, R. H.: Neoplasms and proliferative lesions in 1065 non-human primate necropsies. Lab. Anim. Sci., *23*:533–539, 1973.

Schardein, J. L., Fitzgerald, J. E., and Kaump, D. H.: Spontaneous tumors in Holzman-source rats of various ages. Pathol. Vet., *5*:238–252, 1968.

Siegel, E. T., O'Brien, J. B., Pyle, L., and Schryver, H. F.: Functional adrenocortical carcinoma in a dog. J. Am. Vet. Med. Assoc., *150*:760–766, 1967.

Siegel, E. T., Kelley, D. R., and Berg, P.: Cushing's syndrome in the dog. J. Am. Vet. Med. Assoc., *157*:2081–2090, 1970.

Squire, R. A., et al.: Tumors. *In* Pathology of Laboratory Animals, edited by K. Benirschke, F. M.

Garner, and T. C. Jones. New York, Springer-
    Verlag, 1978. pp. 1051–1283.
Thompson, S. W., and Hunt, R. D.: Spontaneous
    tumors in the Sprague-Dawley rat: Incidence
    rates of some types of neoplasms as determined
    by serial section versus single section technics.
    Ann. NY Acad. Sci., 108:832–845, 1963.
Todd, G. C., Pierce, E. C., and Clevinger, W. G.:
    Ganglioneuroma of the adrenal medulla in rats. A
    report of three cases. Pathol. Vet., 7:139–144,
    1970.
West, J. L.: Bovine pheochromocytoma: Case report
    and review of literature. Am. J. Vet. Res.,
    36:1371–1374, 1975.

PANCREATIC ISLETS

The pancreatic islets (islets of Langerhans) develop embryonically as tiny buds of epithelial cells arising from the ultimate radicles of the pancreatic ducts. These solid masses of cells become detached from the pancreatic ducts and acquire vasculature by sprouting of capillaries. These primary islets contain specific granules of β and δ cells and insulin may be demonstrated. Later in embryonic life, the primary cells degenerate and a second generation of endocrine cells is produced from ductal cells.

The islets in humans and animals are made up of several endocrine types of cells. The β cells are the most numerous (60 to 70%) of the islet cells; they are distinctively stained by aldehyde fuchsin, which intensely stains their granules and demonstrates that they are concentrated in the central part of the normal islet. Ultrastructurally, these β cells contain many characteristic secretory granules, usually surrounded by a clear halo and enclosed by a membrane. The immunohistochemical peroxidase-antiperoxidase technique (PAP) may be used to identify insulin in these cells and glucagon in the α cells. The α cells are much less numerous than the β cells and are seen, in aldehyde-fuchsin preparations, as unstained cells around the periphery of the islet. These cells are known to be the source of glucagon.

A third cell, the δ cell, has been identified in the human pancreas and described as producing somatostatin, which mediates between glucagon and insulin.

Gastrin has been demonstrated in human islets, but its cell of origin has not yet been identified.

An "E" cell has been described in the opossum pancreas and an "F" cell in that of the dog. Their functions are as yet unknown. Several hormonal substances identified in the islets have been described, but not localized to a particular cell. These include somatostatin, avian pancreatic polypeptide, and human pancreatic polypeptide. These and other hormones represent part of the challenge for the future.

Lacy, P. E., and Kissane, J. M.: Pancreas and diabetes
    mellitus. In Pathology, 7th ed., edited by W.A.D.
    Anderson and J. M. Kissane. St. Louis, C. V.
    Mosby, 1977. pp. 1457–1482.
Like, A. A., and Chick, W. L.: β-cell replication in
    subhuman primates. Am. J. Pathol., 62:77a–78a,
    1971.
Like, A. A., and Chick, W. L.: Pancreatic beta cell
    replication induced by glucocorticoids in subhuman primates. Am. J. Pathol., 75:329–348,
    1974.
Pictet, R. L., Rall, L. B., Phelps, P., and Rutter, W. J.:
    The neural crest and the origin of the insulin-producing and other gastrointestinal hormone-producing cells. Science, 191:191–192, 1975.

Diabetes Mellitus

Under this name is collected a syndrome complex affecting man and animals, in which the unifying phenomenon is abnormal or inappropriate metabolism of glucose. Hyperglycemia is therefore one of the most consistent clinical signs. Studies over the years have increased the data available on the human disease and to a lesser extent, that on the animal disease, but the fundamental factors underlying this phenomenon are still unknown. The complexities of the human disease and the variations found in spontaneous disease in laboratory animals suggest that this is not just one disease of single cause, but a complex syndrome due to many yet undetermined factors. The literature presently abounds on this subject and limitations of space prevent little more than a brief review in this text. Excellent reviews are listed in the references to follow.

Diabetes means "to flow through" and mellitus refers to honey. Thus the original concept of an increased flow of urine (polyuria) that was sweet enough to attract bees emphasizes the clinical signs. The polyuria is considered due to the inability of the renal tubular epithelium to concentrate the urine against the osmotic attraction and possibly other effects of the sugar contained therein. Polydipsia follows as a result of polyuria. Sugar, in the form of glucose absorbed from digested food, reaches an abnormally high concentration in the blood. This is **hyperglycemia.** The normal concentration of glucose is about 80 to 100 mg/100 ml of blood in most species. When this level is increased above the "renal threshold" of 150 to 170 mg/100 ml, the kidneys begin to excrete the excess glucose in the urine (glycosuria).

Glucose in the blood is normally the animal's principal source of energy, but in this disease its utilization is prevented by two fundamental defects of metabolism: (1) the liver cannot convert glucose to glycogen for storage, and (2) the tissues cannot oxidize it or use it for energy. Therefore, glucose continues to accumulate in the blood until it can be excreted by the kidneys. Insulin, a hormone produced by the β cells of the pancreatic islets, facilitates the conversion of glucose to glycogen in the liver and its oxidation and utilization by all cells for energy. This essential function of the pancreatic islets was demonstrated by the now famous work of Banting and Best in Toronto in 1921, who established the diabetogenic effect of pancreatectomy in dogs and developed a pancreatic extract that controlled the diabetes mellitus. The role of the pancreatic islets and the specific secretion of insulin by the β cells has been amply confirmed, but the underlying mechanisms that prevent the β cells from secreting adequate amounts of effective insulin are still unknown.

Clinical Signs. The signs of diabetes mellitus may be summarized briefly as follows: Hyperglycemia and abnormal glucose tolerance curves are constant. Glycosuria follows, with increased secretion of urine (polyuria) of high specific gravity. Polydipsia results as a consequence of polyuria. In dogs, a voracious appetite appears in the early stages. Obesity is observed in some species (C57BL/6J-*ob/ob,* obese murine; KK mouse; C3Hf XI F$_1$ Hybrid mouse; Chinese hamster; *Psammomys obesus* and *Acomys cahirinus*). These laboratory animals are among those species that do not usually die in ketoacidosis, having the "nonlethal" type of diabetes mellitus (Like, 1977). In contrast, some species develop severe ketoacidosis and die in ketoacidotic or diabetic coma. These species include the dog; C57BLK/sJ *db/db, diabetic* mouse; Chinese hamster (those with severe syndrome); sand rats, *Psammomys obesus* (when first adapted to the laboratory); spiny "mice," *Acomys catarinus* (occasionally); and the B10 Breeding Lab (BBL) rat. Dogs and guinea pigs usually have pancreatic exocrine disease accompanying diabetes mellitus; hence they may exhibit signs of pancreatic exocrine deficiency as well.

The glucose-tolerance test is useful in detecting incipient diabetes. Circulating immunoreactive insulin (IRI) is elevated in the nonlethal types of the disease. In the lethal types, the IRI is transiently elevated, then becomes inappropriately low.

Lesions. The lesions of diabetes mellitus first involve the β cells of the pancreatic islets, particularly in the lethal types. The secretory granules are lost (degranulation) and the cells accumulate glycogen, then undergo necrosis and disappear from the islet. In some types, amyloid may accumulate around the capillaries within the islet. In the dog and guinea pig, the islets are lost as a result of the intense inflammation of exocrine pancreatitis. Generalized arteriosclerosis may be accentuated, and microangiopathic changes occur in the capillaries of the retina, renal glomeruli, and muscles. This is manifest by thickening of the basement membrane of afferent arterioles. The mesangial cells of the glomeruli undergo proliferation and accumulate PAS-positive material, which is continuous with the thickened afferent arteriole. Only rarely are thickenings encountered in the peripheral part of the glomerular capillaries, to produce changes resembling diffuse or focal nodular glomerulosclerosis (Kimmelstiel-Wilson nodules) of human diabetes. In the retina, whole mounts with trypsin digestion reveal degeneration of capillary pericytes and occasional typical microaneurysms.

Spontaneous diabetes mellitus has been encountered in all domestic animals and in several species of laboratory animals. The laboratory animals are undergoing continued study because of the interest in gaining information which might be applicable to the human disease.

Baker, J. R., and Ritchie, H. E.: Diabetes mellitus in the horse: A case report and review of the literature. Equine Vet. J., 6:7–11, 1974.

Balk, M. W., Lang, C. M., White, W. J., and Munger, B. L.: Exocrine pancreatic dysfunction in guinea pigs with diabetes mellitus. Lab. Invest., 32:28–32, 1975.

Bloodworth, J.M.B., Jr., and Engerman, R. L.: Spontaneous and induced diabetic microangiopathy. Acta Diabetol. Lat., 8:263–301, 1971.

Boquist, L.: Pancreatic islet morphology in diabetic Chinese hamsters. A light and electron microscopic study. Acta Pathol. Microbiol. Scand., 75:399, 1969.

Craighead, J. E.: Animal model of human disease diabetes mellitus (juvenile and maturity-onset types). Am. J. Pathol., 78:537, 1975.

DiGiacomo, R. F., Myers, R. E., and Baez, L. R.: Diabetes mellitus in a rhesus monkey (Macaca mulatta): A case report and literature review. Lab. Anim. Sci., 21:572–574, 1971.

Dixon, J. B., and Sanford, J.: Pathological features of spontaneous canine diabetes mellitus. J. Comp. Pathol., 72:153–164, 1962.

Goeken, J. A., Packer, J. T., Rose, S. D., and Stuhlman, R. A.: Structure of the islets of Langerhans. Pathological studies in normal and diabetic Mystromys albicaudatus. Arch. Pathol., 93:123–129, 1972.

Howard, C. F., Jr.: Diabetes in Macaca nigra: Metabolic and histologic changes. Diabetologia, 10:671–677, 1974.

Howard, C. F., Jr., and Palotay, J. L.: Spontaneous diabetes mellitus in Macaca cyclopis and Mandrillus leucophaeus: Case reports. Lab. Anim. Sci., 25:191–196, 1975.

Howard, C. F.: Basement membrane thickness in muscle capillaries of normal and spontaneously diabetic Macaca nigra. Diabetes, 24:201–206, 1975.

Howard, C. R., Jr., and Palotay, J. L.: Diabetes mellitus: Diabetic syndrome in Macaca nigra. Comp. Pathol. Bull., 8:3–4, 1976.

Howard, C. F., Jr.: Diabetes and lipid metabolism in nonhuman primates. Adv. Lipid Res., 13:91–134, 1976.

———: Insular amyloidosis and diabetes mellitus in Macaca nigra. Diabetes, 27:357–364, 1978.

———: Diabetes and atherosclerosis in Macaca nigra. Diabetes, 27(Suppl. 2):447, 1978.

Kaneko, J. J., and Rhode, E. A.: Diabetes mellitus in a cow. J. Am. Vet. Med. Assoc., 144:367–373, 1964.

Kuwabara, T., and Cogan, D. G.: Retinal vascular patterns. I. Normal architecture. Arch. Ophthalmol., 64:904–911, 1960.

Lang, C. M., and Munger, B. L.: Diabetes mellitus in guinea pig. Diabetes, 25:434–443, 1976.

Lang, C. M., Munger, B. L., and Rapp, F.: The guinea pig as an animal model of diabetes mellitus. Lab. Anim. Sci., 27:789–805, 1977.

Like, A. A.: Spontaneous diabetes in animals. In The Diabetic Pancreas, edited by B. W. Volk, and K. F. Wellmann. New York, Plenum, 1977.

Like, A. A., Lavine, R. L., Poffenbarger, P. L., and Chick, W. L.: Studies in the diabetic mutant mouse. VI. Evolution of glomerular lesions and associated proteinuria. Am. J. Pathol., 66:193–203, 1972.

Loppnow, H., and Gembardt, C.: Pathogenesis of spontaneous diabetes mellitus in cats. I. Diabetes mellitus due to primary lesions of the islets in ten cats. Berl. Münch. Tierärztl. Wochenschr. 89:79–83, 1976.

Mauer, S. M., Steffes, M. W., Michael, A. F., and Brown, D. M.: Studies of diabetic nephropathy in animals and man. Diabetes, 25:(2 Suppl.):850–857, 1976.

Meyer, J., Bates, M. W., and Dickie, M. M.: Hereditary diabetes in genetically obese mice. Science, 113:746–747, 1951.

Munger, B. L., and Lang, C. M.: Spontaneous diabetes mellitus in guinea pigs: The acute cytopathology of the islets of Langerhans. Lab. Invest., 29:685–702, 1973.

Nakamura, M., and Yamada, K.: Studies on a diabetic (KK) strain of the mouse. Diabetologia, 3:212–215, 1967.

Patz, A., et al.: Studies on diabetic retinopathy. II. Retinopathy and nephropathy in spontaneous canine diabetes. Diabetes, 14:700–708, 1965.

Renold, A. E.: Spontaneous diabetes and/or obesity in laboratory rodents. In Advances in Metabolic Disorders, Vol. 3, edited by R. Levine, and R. Luft. New York, Academic Press, 1968.

Renold, A. E., Burr, I. M., and Stauffacher, W.: Experimental and spontaneous diabetes in animals: What is their relevance to human diabetes mellitus? Proc. R. Soc. Med., 64:613–617, 1971.

Ricketts, H. T., et al.: Spontaneous diabetes mellitus in the dog. An account of 8 cases. Diabetes, 4:288–294, 1953.

Sheldon, W. G., and Gleiser, C. A.: Amyloidosis of the islets of Langerhans in a crab-eating monkey *(Macaca fascicularis).* Vet. Pathol., *8*:16–18, 1971.

Siegel, E. T.: Endocrine Diseases of the Dog. Philadelphia, Lea & Febiger, 1977.

Tasker, J. B., Whiteman, C. E., and Martin, B. R.: Diabetes mellitus in the horse. J. Am. Vet. Med. Assoc., *149*:393–399, 1966.

Wehner, H., et al.: Glomerular changes in mice with spontaneous hereditary diabetes. Lab. Invest., *27*:331–340, 1972.

Wilkinson, J. S.: Spontaneous diabetes mellitus. Vet. Rec., *72*:548–555, 1960.

Neoplasms of the Pancreatic Islets

Primary tumors of the pancreatic islet cells (islet cell tumors) identified so far in animals consist of adenoma and adenocarcinoma. These tumors are brought to the attention of the clinical veterinarian because they often secrete insulin, causing hyperinsulinism. The dog is most often recognized to be affected, but other species are susceptible. Data collected by 11 veterinary colleges in the United States (Priester, 1974) indicate the rarity of islet cell tumors in domestic animals. The frequency per 100,000 animal years in this study was estimated for domestic species as follows: canine, 11.4; feline, 2.8; bovine, less than 1.9; equine, less than 1.6; porcine, less than 13.2; and ovine, less than 30.2. The estimates for the last four species were based on an assumption of less than one islet cell tumor per species, although none were recognized in the populations studied.

Adenomas are recognized as circumscribed nodules in the pancreas with no evidence of invasion of adjacent pancreas or spread to lymphatics, lymph nodes, or other organs. The tumor cells are usually polyhedral with a centrally placed nucleus in abundant cytoplasm that is faintly granular in hematoxylin and eosin stains (Fig. 26–14). Special stains are useful in identifying the granules and the origin of the cells. Rows of cells may form a so-called ribbon pattern in some cases. Hyperplastic islets are difficult to distinguish from adenomas and in fact may rep-

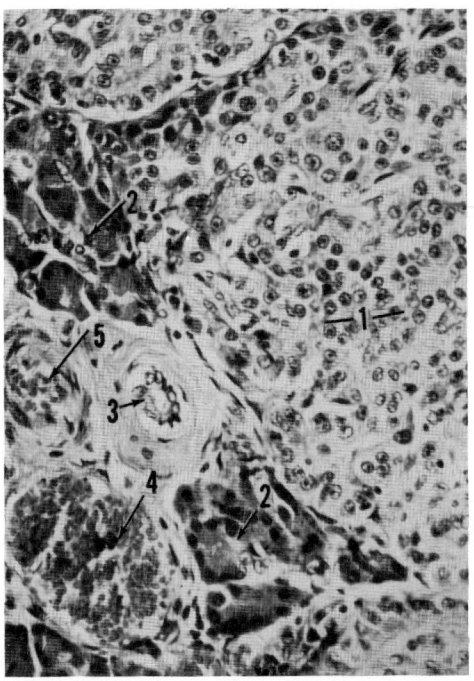

Fig. 26–14. Adenoma of islet cells, pancreas of a ten-year-old female Persian cat (× 575). Tumor *(1)* is compressing normal pancreatic acini *(2).* Pancreatic duct *(3),* vein *(4),* and artery *(5).* (Courtesy of Armed Forces Institute of Pathology.) Contributor: Dr. M. A. Troy.

resent a continuum which includes carcinomas. These are distinguished by their tendency to be multiple, to invade the adjacent pancreas, and to metastasize to the pancreatic lymph nodes and liver. In a limited survey of 43 cases reported in the literature, about twice as many carcinomas as adenomas were found, and more than half of both types were functional. So far, all reported functional islet tumors secreted insulin. Identification of tumors of α cells and others should be possible if suitable techniques are used.

The signs of hyperinsulinism are rather dramatic. The effects are principally due to hypoglycemia. The blood glucose level in affected dogs is usually below 50 mg/100 ml blood. The affected dog suddenly collapses and goes into convulsions or coma. Feeding of sugar or milk will produce slow re-

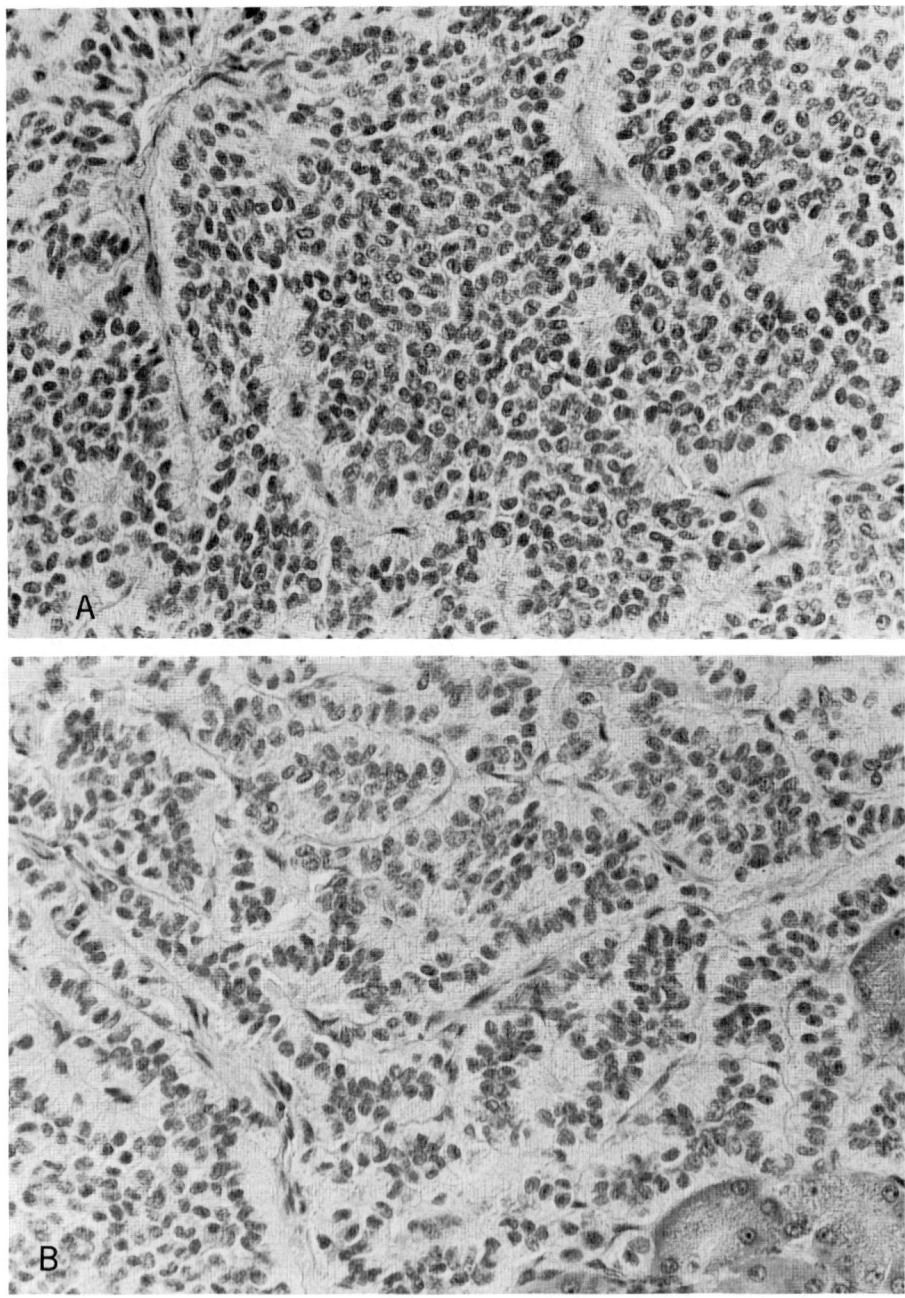

Fig. 26–15. Non-beta islet cell tumors (Zollinger-Ellison syndrome) in the dog. *A*, Solid masses of cells with ribbon pattern and pseudorosette formation. *B*, Ribbon pattern. (Courtesy of Dr. R. P. Happé and Veterinary Pathology.)

covery, but subcutaneous or intravenous administration of glucose is followed by prompt recovery. Surgical removal of the tumor when possible, as in the case of small, localized tumors, will result in prolonged alleviation of the disease.

Adenomas and adenocarcinomas of nonbeta islet cells have been reported in dogs (Jones et al., 1976; Straus et al., 1977; Happé et al., 1980). The tumor cells secrete gastrin, which may be detected in elevated levels in the plasma and is believed to be the cause of the associated ulcers in the jejunum. The clinical disease has been called **canine Zollinger-Ellison syndrome,** after the human disease which it closely resembles (Zollinger and Ellison, 1955). Happé et al. (1980) described three histologic patterns to these tumors: solid; ribbon or trabecular; and acinar (Fig. 26–15).

Cello, R. M., and Kennedy, P. C.: Hyperinsulinism in dogs due to pancreatic islet cell carcinoma. Cornell Vet., 47:538–557, 1957.

Grant, C. A.: Pancreatic insuloma with clinical manifestations in a dog. J. Comp. Pathol., 70:450–456, 1960.

Hansen, H. J.: Insulom hos hund. Nord. Vet. Med., 1:363–376, 1949.

Happé, R. P., et al.: Zollinger-Ellison syndrome in three dogs. Vet. Pathol., 17:177–186, 1980.

Hueper, W. C.: Islet adenoma in the pancreas of a mouse. Arch. Pathol., 22:220–221, 1936.

Jones, B. R., Nicholls, M. R., and Badman, R.: Peptic ulceration in a dog associated with an islet cell carcinoma of the pancreas and an elevated plasma gastrin level. J. Small Anim. Pract., 17:593–598, 1976.

Justus, A. A.: Pancreatic insuloma in a dog. J. Am. Vet. Med. Assoc., 142:1413–1414, 1963.

Kircher, C. H., and Nielsen, S. W.: XIV. Tumours of the pancreas. International Histological Classification of Tumours of Domestic Animals. Bull. WHO, 53:195–202, 1976.

Kovacs, K., Horvath, E., Ilse, R. G., and Ilse, D.: Spontaneous pancreatic beta cell tumor in the rat. A light and electron microscopic study. Vet. Pathol., 13:286–294, 1976.

Krook, L., and Kenney, R. M.: Central nervous system lesions in dogs with metastasizing islet cell carcinoma. Cornell Vet., 52:385–415, 1962.

Larsson, L. I., et al.: Mixed endocrine pancreatic tumors producing several peptide hormones. Am. J. Pathol., 79:271–284, 1975.

Marcus, L. C., Bucci, T. J., and Kraner, K. L.: Pancreatic islet cell tumor in a dog. J. Am. Vet. Med. Assoc., 145:1198–1203, 1964.

Priester, W. A.: Pancreatic islet cell tumors in domestic animals. Data from 11 colleges of veterinary medicine in the United States and Canada. J. Natl. Cancer Inst., 53:227–229, 1974.

Rouse, B. T., and Wilson, M. R.: A case of hypoglycaemia in a dog associated with neoplasia of the pancreas. Vet. Rec., 79:454–456, 1966.

Slye, M., and Wells, H.G.: Tumors of islet tissue with hyperinsulinism in a dog. Arch. Pathol., 19:537–542, 1935.

Strafuss, A. C., Njoku, C. O., Blauch, B., and Anderson, N. V.: Islet cell neoplasm in four dogs. J. Am. Vet. Med. Assoc., 159:1008–1011, 1971.

Straus, E., Johnson, G. F., and Yalow, R. S.: Canine Zollinger-Ellison syndrome. Gastroenterology, 72:380–381, 1977.

Takarnia, C. H.: Islet cell tumor of the bovine pancreas. J. Am. Vet. Med. Assoc., 138:541–547, 1961.

Teunissen, G. H. B., Verwer, M. A. J., and Van den Akker, S.: Spontaneous hypoglycemia caused by multiple insulomas in a dog. Tijdschr. Diergeneeskd., 86:1115–1128, 1961.

Zollinger, R. M., and Ellison, E. H.: Primary peptic ulceration of the jejunum associated with islet cell tumors of the pancreas. Ann. Surg., 142:709–728, 1955.

PINEAL GLAND

Although the pineal gland (pineal body or epiphysis cerebri) has long been thought to have an endocrine function, only recently has evidence been gathered which warrants placing it with the endocrine organs in mammals. Embryologically, the organ is thought to be a vestige of a "third eye" which exists in certain reptiles and amphibians. It has been demonstrated that the amphibian and mammalian pineal secretes a hormone-like compound known as **melatonin.** In amphibians, melatonin synthesis is controlled by photoreceptors within the pineal and the hormone causes skin lightening. In mammals, photoreceptor cells are not present and the pineal does not respond directly to light. Instead the pineal responds to light received by the retina; increased light depresses melatonin synthesis and decreased light stimulates melatonin synthesis. In mammals, melatonin inhibits gonadotropic hormone synthesis or release by the pituitary, and is believed to play a major role in the seasonal reproductive activity exhibited by many species.

Although knowledge of the ultrastructure and functions of the pineal has increased in recent years, information concerning the pathologic lesions of this interesting organ still remains limited. Necrosis, calcification, cystic degeneration, hyaline degeneration, deposition of hemosiderin, hyperemia and petechiae have been described in the equine pineal body but were asymptomatic. Hyperplastic enlargement to four times the normal, with consequent pressure on surrounding nervous structures, has been reported as causing a circling syndrome in a mule.

Pinealoma

This tumor, also known as pineal adenoma, is a rare neoplasm derived from the pineal gland. Its histologic appearance is distinctive in that it consists of an indiscriminate mingling of groups of large epithelioid cells with groups of small (neuroglial) cells with small round nuclei suggestive of lymphocytes. Sexual or other forms of precocity have accompanied some pinealomas in children, but these are suspected of being due to disturbance of nearby structures rather than to the direct effect of the tumors. A pinealoma has been reported in a silver fox, a horse and a rat.

Binkley, S., MacBride, S. E., Klein, D. C., and Ralph, C. L.: Pineal enzymes: regulation of avian melatonin synthesis. Science, 181:273–275, 1973.

Binkley, S., Riebman, J. B., and Reilly, K. B.: Timekeeping by the pineal gland. Science, 197:1181–1183, 1977.

Kerenyi, N. A., and von Westarp, C.: Post-natal transformation of the pineal gland: Effect of constant darkness. Endocrinology, 88:1077–1079, 1971.

Kitay, J. I., and Altschule, M. D.: The Pineal Gland: A Review of the Physiologic Literature. Cambridge, Harvard Univ. Press, 1954.

Lászlo, F.: Beiträge zur pathologischen Anatomie und Histologie der Zirbel. Dtsch. Tierarztl. Wochenschr., 42:685–689, 1934.

———: Weitere Beiträge zur vergleichenden pathologischen Anatomie der Zirbel. Dtsch. Tierärztl. Wochenschr., 43:245–247, 1935.

Louis, C. J., Kenny, G. C., and Anderson, R. M.: Autoradiographic localization of 5-hydroxytryptamine in monkey pineal gland. Experientia, 26:756–757, 1970.

Nobel, T. A.: Circling syndrome in a mule due to hyperplasia of the pineal gland. Cornell Vet., 45:570–575, 1955.

Reiter, F. J., and Sorrentino, S., Jr.: Reproductive effects of the mammalian pineal. Am. Zoologist, 10:247–258, 1970.

Roche, J. F., et al.: Effect of pinealectomy on estrus, ovulation and luteinizing hormone in ewes. Biol. Reprod., 2:251–254, 1970.

Santamarina, E., and Venzke, W. G.: Physiological changes in the mammalian pineal gland correlated with the reproductive system. Am. J. Vet. Res., 14:555–562, 1953.

Schlotthauer, C. F., and Kernohan, J. W.: Glioma in a dog and pinealoma in a silver fox (Vulpes fulvis). Am. J. Cancer, 24:350–356, 1935.

Symington, R. B., Knight, B., and Hayes M.: Microstructure of the pineal gland in man and baboon (Papio ursinus). J. Anat., 114:291, 1973.

Welser, J. R., Hinsman, E. J., and Stromberg, M. W.: Fine structure of the canine pinealocyte. Am. J. Vet. Res., 29:587–599, 1968.

Wurtman, R. J., and Moskowitz, M. A.: The pineal organ (two parts). N. Engl. J. Med., 296:1329–1333; 1383–1386, 1977.

CHAPTER 27

The Nervous System

While the general laws of pathology are by no means abrogated in the nervous system, certain peculiar characteristics of the nervous tissues have led to a number of names and concepts which, whether necessary or not, have to be added to the list of those encountered in the study of other bodily systems. Before concerning ourselves with these, we should like to examine briefly the functional aspects of some nervous disorders.

Certain anatomic, histologic, and biochemical features cause reactions in the central nervous system to differ somewhat from lesions of corresponding etiologic basis in other locations. Enclosed in unyielding bony cavities, the brain and spinal cord are encompassed by the thin but dense and fibrous dura mater, which in most places forms a tough white sheet, suspended, with few attachments, between the bony wall and the organ itself. The brain and cord proper are bound by a thin limiting membrane, the pia-arachnoid, whose few cell layers are intimately joined with the underlying soft parenchyma, following the convolutions of its surface into the depths of the sulci and over the summits of the gyri. In the sulci especially, the pia-arachnoid thickens slightly to form a matrix through which pass most of the blood and lymph vessels. Between the dura and the pia-arachnoid is the subdural space; its surfaces are lined with flat mesenchymal or endothelial cells, according to the terminology used.

With the exception of these membranes, known collectively as the meninges, and of a limited number of adventitial and perivascular fibroblasts accompanying the vessels which ramify into the parenchyma, there is no fibrous connective tissue in the brain and spinal cord. Instead, a soft but densely homogeneous supporting tissue called neuroglia (glia, a glue-like substance) constitutes the bulk of these organs and forms a matrix in which lie embedded the nerve cell bodies and their dendritic and axonal fibers. In this mass two varieties of tissue are grossly recognizable: the **white matter,** which forms the bulk of the inner substance, and the **gray matter,** which constitutes the cortical layer of the cerebrum and cerebellum and also composes certain islands of gray matter within the white, called "nuclei," including the basal ganglia. The white matter is composed principally of nerve fibers (axons and dendrites) with their myelin sheaths and a minimum of supporting tissue comprised of oligodendroglia and astrocytes. The gray matter is composed of neuroglia (principally astrocytes), with numerous nerve cell bodies (neurons) embedded in it. With light microscopy the

1637

neurons and glia are embedded in a background of fine, criss-crossing fibrils which stain pink with hematoxylin and eosin. When stained with special methods, such as silver impregnation, the fibrils are seen much better and more completely, and predominantly represent cytoplasmic processes of astrocytes and neurons.

The **neuron,** the functional unit of the nervous system, consists of a nucleus with a large nucleolus surrounded by a relatively abundant amount of cytoplasm, from which projects one or more dendrites and a single axon. Neurons vary in size from no larger than astrocytes (about 5 μ) to the large neurons in the cerebellum (Purkinje cells) and cerebral cortex (Betz cells), which exceed 75 μ in diameter. The cytoplasm contains basophilic granules or ribosomes called **Nissl substance,** which is uniformly distributed except at the base of the axon (axon hiloc). In older animals, the cytoplasm often contains lipofuscin pigment.

Three kinds of neuroglial cells can be distinguished. None of their nuclei have visible nucleoli with light microscopy, a fact that distinguishes them from nearly all the nerve cells. Of these, the **astrocytes** comprise the bulk of the neuroglia in most regions. Their nuclei are usually elliptical, somewhat pale and vesicular in tinctorial properties, and of a size somewhat smaller than the nucleus of a monocyte. Special preparations show that each nucleus has a star-like (*astro,* star) network of branching cytoplasmic processes around it, with at least one of these connected to a "footpad" at the wall of a nearby blood vessel, and others often extending to the pia mater. Astrocytes with long, thin processes are called *fibrous astrocytes,* and those with shorter, wider, and usually more highly branched processes are called *protoplasmic astrocytes.* In sections stained by ordinary methods, they are usually distinguishable from the smaller nerve cells by their less spherical and more vesicular nuclei (pale, without internal structure but with a dis-

tinct nuclear wall), and from the other neuroglial nuclei by the fact that the latter are still smaller, darker, and of denser appearance. The **oligodendroglial** cells (*oligo,* few; *dendro,* branches) have, as just implied, regularly round, darkly staining nuclei, comparable in size to the nuclei of lymphocytes. Their short and scanty fibrils are revealed only by special techniques, but the fact that a majority of these cells occur in the fiber tracts of the white matter and appear in straight rows between the fibers facilitates their recognition. Oligodendroglial cells are the source of myelin, a proteolipid formed from extensions of the cell's plasma membrane. In contrast to most plasma membranes, the lipid content is higher than the protein content. In peripheral nerves myelin is derived from Schwann cells.

The **microglial** cells have very small, round and dark nuclei; many of them are found in the vicinity of a nerve cell. Their fibrils are minimal in both number and length and, as usual, require special techniques for their demonstration. They are of mesodermal rather than neuroectodermal origin, as is the case with the other components of the neuroglia, and they are phagocytic.

Ependymal cells are cuboidal or columnar cells that line ventricles, the choroid plexus, and spinal canal. They may be ciliated and each contains a blepharoplast.

The white matter consists exclusively of nerve fibers separated from each other by myelin and a small amount of neuroglia. The fibers have a tendency to lie evenly spaced and parallel to each other as a number of them follow the same intercommunicating path from one area of gray matter to another. Such parallel groups are called fiber tracts; their particular functions are ascertainable and usually well known in human neurology.

The blood vessels within the central nervous parenchyma have the peculiarity of being surrounded by a zone of appreciable width in which the cells and fibers are so scanty as to be limited to a bare supporting framework. This encircling zone constitutes what is known as the Virchow-Robin space or, since it serves for the drainage of lymph, as the perivascular lymph space. In infectious inflammations lymphocytes commonly accumulate in it, constituting perivascular lymphocytic infiltrations ("cuffing").

Bernstein, J., and Landing, B.H.: Extraneural lesions associated with neonatal hyperbilirubinemia and kernicterus. Am. J. Pathol., 40:371–392, 1962.

Blackwood, W., et al.: Greenfield's Neuropathology. 2nd ed., London, Edward Arnold, 1963.

Croft, P.G.: Fits in dogs: A survey of 260 cases. Vet. Rec., 77:438–445, 1965.

Eager, R.P., and Eager, P.R.: Glial responses to degenerating cerebellar corticonuclear pathways in the cat. Science, 153:553–554, 1966.

Fankhauser, R.: Zur Frage des Hirnoedems beim Rind. Schweiz. Arch. Tierheilk., 104:261–274, 1962.

Fischer, K.: Herdförmige symetrische Hirngewebsnekrosen bei Hunden mit epileptiformen Krampfen. Path. Vet., 1:133–160, 1964.

Fox, M.W.: Gross structure and development of the canine brain. Am. J. Vet. Res., 24:1240–1247, 1963.

Fransen, J.M., and Andrews, F.N.: Cerebrospinal fluid pressure in dwarf and normal cattle. Am. J. Vet. Res., 19:336–337, 1958.

Frauchiger, E., and Fankhauser, R.: Die Nervenkrankheiten unserer Hunde. Bern, Hans Huber, 1949.

——: Vergleichende Neuropathologie. Berlin, J. Springer, 1957.

Innes, J.R.M., and Saunders, L.Z.: Diseases of the central nervous system of domesticated animals and comparisons with human neuropathology. In Advances in Veterinary Science. Vol. III. New York, Academic Press, Inc., 1957, pp. 33–196. (Extensive Bibliography).

——: Comparative Neuropathology. New York, Academic Press, 1962.

Kappers, C.U.A., Huber, G.C., and Crosby, E.C.: The Comparative Anatomy of the Nervous System of Vertebrates, Including Man. New York, The Macmillan Co., 1936.

Lim, R.K.S., Liu, C.N., and Moffitt, R.L.: A Stereotaxic Atlas of the Dog's Brain. Springfield, Charles C Thomas, 1960.

Luginbühl, H.: (Angiopathies of the CNS in Animals.) Schweiz. Arch. Tierheilk., 104:694–700, 1962.

——: Comparative aspects of tumors of the nervous system. Ann. NY Acad. Sci., 108:702–721, 1963.

McGrath, J.T.: Neurological Examination of the Dog. 2nd ed., Philadelphia, Lea & Febiger, 1960.

O'Daly, J.A., and Imaeda, T.: Electron microscopic study of wallerian degeneration in cutaneous nerves caused by mechanical injury. Lab. Invest., 17:744–766, 1967.

Penfield, W.: Cytology and Cellular Pathology of the Nervous System. New York, Paul B. Hoeber, Inc., 1932.

Saunders, L.Z.: A check list of hereditary and familial diseases of the central nervous system in domestic animals. Cornell Vet., 42:592–600, 1952.

——: Cerebrovascular siderosis in horses. A.M.A. Arch. Pathol., 56:637–642, 1953.

Scherer, H.J.: Vergleichende Pathologie des Nervensystems der Säugetiere. Leipzig, Georg Thieme, 1944.

Schoene, W.C.: The nervous system. In Pathologic Basis of Disease, 2nd ed., edited by S.L. Robbins and R.S. Cotran. Philadelphia, W.B. Saunders, 1979. pp. 1530–1598.

Sykes, J.F., and Moore, L.A.: The normal cerebrospinal fluid pressure and a method for its determination in cattle. Am. J. Vet. Res., 3:364–367, 1942.

TISSUE CHANGES

Postmortem autolysis becomes evident early in the central nervous system and, like necrosis, soon leads to liquefaction. It is not unusual for brains to be almost completely liquefied in three or four days at mild summer temperatures (70 to 90°F, 21 to 32°C). The differentiation between the two forms of death is made according to the principles already outlined in Chapter 1.

Necrosis ranges from slow death of an occasional neuron to softening and liquefaction of considerable volumes of central nervous tissue, the former occurring soonest and from milder causes. The usual causes of necrosis in the brain or cord are anoxia, chemical and plant poisons, mycotoxins, metabolic disorders, and infectious diseases. Among the poisons are cyanides in repeated small doses, mercury (chronic ingestion), lead (chronic), manganese, carbon monoxide, and alcohol, as well as various other organic and inorganic substances.

Anoxia is a frequent cause of death of nerve cells, usually in a limited area. The disorder results from interference with the blood supply, even though transient, the neurons being highly susceptible. It is probable that many of the poisons really act through an anoxic mechanism. Massive deprivation of blood through cerebral embolism and infarction, arteriosclerotic changes, or hemorrhage, however, is rare in domestic animals.

Necrosis involves some forms of change that are peculiar to nervous tissue and have not been discussed previously. This is particularly true with respect to necrosis of individual neurons, which occurs upon slight provocation of certain sorts. It is difficult to determine in these cells the exact point where various peculiar degenerative (and reversible) changes become (irreversible) necrosis. Since the former regularly lead to the latter, the several consecutive stages will be considered together.

Necrosis of Neurons (Nerve Cell Bodies). Changes in the neurons themselves that indicate their death or approaching death take several forms. Acute injury is characterized by cellular swelling, as is the case with other cells. The dendritic processes of multipolar cells tend to disappear, leaving the outline of the cell unduly smooth and rounded. The **Nissl substance** in a normal and perfectly preserved neuron should appear as a sharply granular, basophilic substance in the cytoplasm, giving the latter an appearance like the markings of a tiger, whence the synonym, **tigroid substance.** In a pathogenic environment, such as anoxia, these Nissl granules lose their sharpness and, in just a few hours, disappear first centrally (central chromatolysis) and then completely, often by fading, occasionally by a general blackening of the cytoplasm (known by some neurologists in their own exclusive dialect as "pyknosis"), but more usually by increased cytoplasmic eosinophilia. Concomitantly with the cytoplasmic loss of Nissl granules and loss of the normal cell outline, the nucleus tends to swell and the nucleolus within the nucleus enlarges even more. The more or less swollen nucleus is commonly displaced from its central to an eccentric position, even to lie against the cell membrane. Then the nucleus undergoes karyorrhexis or karyolysis and disappears from view.

The whole neuron tends to swell at first, then shrinks into some angular and unrecognizable form and likewise disappears. Incidental to this swelling and shrinking, the axon, if it chances to be visible, swells, loses its Nissl substance, and is distorted into a writhing, twisting form, and then passes from the scene. All this transpires in the course of a day or two. Exceptionally, as in the viral disease called "scrapie," slow dissolution and liquefaction of the neuron involve the formation of one or two large, clear vacuoles which eventually displace practically all of the cytoplasm.

Commonly, neurons are observed to be shrunken and angular, with either increased cytoplasmic basophilia or eosinophilia and distorted dendrites. Such shrunken cells are often encountered in the absence of observable cellular swelling. Although this change may represent a true degenerative process, such cells may be encountered in normal brains, in which case it has been suggested that they are "inactive" neurons. Shrinking of neurons is also a feature of improper fixation. The absence of other reactions in the nervous system or clinical signs of dysfunction must be used to differentiate between artifact and cell death.

Meantime, even while the hapless cell is dying, arrangements are already being made for disposal of its remains. Microglia cells gather about the dying neuron, as a magpie sits upon the back of a moribund horse in order to be present at the moment the animal's flesh becomes available to him. While vulture cells might be a better name, these clustering cells are politely called satellite cells and the process is called **satellitosis.** As the neuron dies, they not only surround but enter the cell, engulfing bits of its cystoplasm, and their true phagocytic nature becomes evident.

They are then known as neuronophages and the process is designated as **neuronophagia.** The small collection of microglia is known as a glial nodule. Satellitosis and neuronophagia are then indirect but no less reliable signs of necrosis of a neuron. Satellitosis is reported as developing within a matter of minutes after anoxic injury; neuronophagia within a few hours. Satellitosis is a reversible change; in other words, the neuron is injured but not dead. These two processes, unlike the intracellular regressive changes, do not occur in postmortem autolysis, but only in necrosis.

Astrocytes also respond to nerve cell injury. They may increase in number, a condition known as astrocytosis, with many cells containing two and four nuclei, and/or they may increase in size due to an increased amount of eosinophilic cytoplasm (which is ordinarily not visible except as background substance). Such swollen astrocytes are called gemistocytic astrocytes or gemistocytes.

Necrosis in the neuroglia is also a process of liquefaction, but it develops more slowly, and in the case of some of the milder injurious agents, it may not occur at all, even though the nerve cells of the area have been killed. Close observation and a precise knowledge of the normal histology of the area are necessary to detect accurately the absence of a few neurons under such circumstances. If an area of neuroglia (and the contained nerve cells and fibers) undergoes necrosis, it is at first (two to five days) softened grossly, a condition known as **encephalomalacia** (or myelomalacia), and in one to two weeks, disappears through a process of liquefaction, leaving an empty space of no characteristic shape, size, or type excepting its frayed and indefinite borders. Such an area may be difficult to distinguish from an artifact caused by imperfect cutting of the section, but the distinctions mentioned in Chapter 1 in connection with liquefactive necrosis apply. Where appreciable areas of central nervous tissue are destroyed (undergo necrosis), there may be after two or three weeks an increase of neuroglial tissue surrounding the vacant space, called gliosis, and an accumulation of macrophagic cells. These are discussed further in connection with proliferative inflammation in the nervous system.

Necrosis of nerve fibers, whether in the peripheral nerves or in the fiber tracts of the brain or cord, first becomes discernible through degeneration of the myelin sheaths of the affected fibers and swelling of the axons. Especially within the brain and cord, the change is usually called **demyelination.** The axons or nerve fibers eventually disappear, as well as, perhaps, much of the interstitial tissue (neuroglia), but loss of the myelin sheaths alone is sufficient to render the nerves nonfunctional (although regeneration may be possible).

Microglia assume their phagocytic role engulfing axonal fragments and myelin sheaths, converting the myelin to neutral fat. These lipid-containing microglia are known as **gitter cells,** and their presence is indicative of myelin damage which may otherwise be difficult to discern in ordinary hematoxylin-eosin tissue sections. In addition to microglia, phagocytes derived from blood monocytes participate in removing necrotic material. There is also evidence that oligodendrocytes participate as phagocytes in removing degenerated axoplasmic organelles. The presence of an excessive number and size of holes in an area of white matter is also a morphologic sign of myelin damage. The axon may still be visible in some of them, but there may be difficulty in deciding whether one is dealing with demyelination or spaces due to edema or to excessive shrinkage in the preparation of the tissue.

Since the lipid of the myelin goes through stages involving the presence of free neutral fats, it is possible to demonstrate demyelination by the usual stains for fats, or more particularly by Marchi's method, to be described shortly. However, since, in the central nervous system, whole fiber tracts usually share the same fate, it is often preferable to demonstrate the disorder by staining methods (myelin-sheath stains) that directly color normal myelin. Demyelination is then detected by a blank area, usually viewed under low magnification, in the midst of the more darkly staining healthy tissue. Such areas are usually only relatively colorless, for the remaining neuroglial cells and fibers absorb a minimal amount of stain. Damage to either an individual or group of axons results in these same changes. When isolated axons are affected, they may be recognizable as eosinophilic, spherical masses called **spheroids** (in cross section), composed of the swollen axon and altered myelin.

In the peripheral nerves, destruction of myelin (and of the functioning fiber) may be detected by similar means, but Marchi's method is often used, in spite of a certain reputed inconstancy of action. This involves the use of the oxidizing agent osmic acid (osmium peroxide) to stain the fat separated from the myelin a deep black. Since osmic acid would have the same effect on the lipids of myelin, the tissue is first exposed to a milder oxidizing agent, potassium dichromate, which oxidizes normal myelin without coloring it but leaves the fatty, injured myelin still susceptible to the osmic acid. Theoretically, at least, a delicate differentiation is obtainable. About two weeks must elapse between the injury to a peripheral nerve and the stainability of injured nerves by this method. Unless the injury is very close to the nerve-cell body, the cell body does not die, so this process is not usually necrosis but, rather, a degeneration. It is known as **wallerian degeneration.** The part of the neuron distal to the point of injury (which may well be mechanical severance) dies, undergoing wallerian degeneration throughout its length, and is

associated with an influx of macrophages and proliferation of Schwann cells. Macrophages derived from blood monocytes are the principal phagocytic cell, but some believe that Schwann cells may also become phagocytic. The nerve fiber is commonly regenerated by growth from the surviving proximal portion of the neuron, a process requiring a few months. While, as stated, the cell body seldom dies because of injury to its axon, it may suffer transiently a certain degree of degeneration, particularly a rounding of the cell, displacement of the nucleus, and fading of the Nissl granules. This is known as Nissl's degeneration. Recovery usually occurs. Demyelination of nerve fibers results from a variety of types of injury including mechanical pressure, brief or prolonged, and deficiency of thiamine and the vitamin-B complex.

Calcification and, less frequently, some of the other degenerative changes described in Chapter 2 may occur in the central nervous system, but usually in relation to the vessels or meninges.

Circulatory Lesions. **Passive congestion** of these tissues, most prominent in the pia-arachnoid, accompanies severe passive congestion of the rest of the body. It is readily recognized by virtue of the dark, distended veins that cover the meningeal surfaces and is usually acute and terminal. **Hyperemia** is part of the picture of inflammation. **Hemorrhages** of petechial size are frequent in those numerous acute infections and toxemias that injure capillaries in other parts of the body. However, pinpoint spots of blood seen on the cut surface when the brain is freshly sliced often mark, not hemorrhages, but the cut ends of congested capillaries.

Severe blows to the head may result in fracture of the skull, rupture of one or more branches of the meningeal arteries, and hemorrhage into the space between the dura and bone. This **epidural hemorrhage** is uncommon in the young or old due to close adherence between the dura and bone. When it does occur, the dura is compressed over the brain and may lead rapidly to hemiplegia, convulsions and death unless relieved surgically. **Subdural hemorrhage** on the other hand usually results from rupture of veins, and the blood is mixed with cerebrospinal fluid. The signs may be delayed as bleeding continues. It is possible for large areas of the cerebrum to be compressed by the resulting hematoma which also could become organized, leading to increasing pressure on the brain. The location of the hemorrhage is not necessarily at the site of the blow; it may be at the opposite side owing to the inertia of the brain within the cranium and its elasticity, propensity to rebound strongly, and rupture of vessels on the opposite side (*contrecoup*). If the animal survives the immediate injury of the blow, the effects are those of pressure and depend upon the size of the clot. Death from such a blow may then follow the accident by hours or days.

In man, a massive hemorrhage into the brain substance is an all-too-frequent complication of arteriosclerotic and hypertensive disease. The sudden unconsciousness is known as apoplexy; the result, if the patient lives, is paralysis of parts innervated from the portion of the brain that undergoes pressure necrosis. Commonly this is one side of the body, the condition being known popularly as a "paralytic stroke." (Infarction from embolism or occlusion also causes such "strokes.") Hemorrhages of this nature and strokes in general are infrequent in animals, doubtless because arteriosclerotic disease is rare, except in aged swine. (See also the discussion on concussion, later in this section.)

Edema of the brain occurs as a diffuse accumulation of fluid in the tissue, especially in the perivascular (Virchow-Robin) spaces, in the subarachnoid spaces, and in spaces that form around the neurons (Fig. 9–50). Grossly, the gyri are swollen and flattened and the sulci partly obliterated. The cut surface is moist and shiny; the parenchyma is softened. The causes are the same as the causes of edema elsewhere, either general or local.

Edema is also used in neuropathologic terminology to describe intracellular accumulation of fluid. Cytotoxic damage of neurons and glia results in membrane dysfunction with an influx of sodium and water leading to acute cellular swelling, as it does in other tissues.

Infarcts are not as frequent in animals as they are in human beings, where they are associated with the higher incidence of atherosclerosis. Infarcts may arise from lodged emboli and are seen in association with some of the infectious diseases of animals that lead to vasculitis. Focal necrosis of the brain unassociated with vascular disease may result from many infectious and noninfectious diseases and are sometimes incorrectly termed infarcts.

Anoxic (Hypoxic) Encephalopathy. The central nervous system is particularly susceptible to deprivation of oxygen. The lesions are comparable regardless of cause, e.g., anemia, heart failure, or cyanide or carbon monoxide poisoning. If death results from acute cerebral anoxia within minutes or up to eight hours, lesions will not be evident. Lesions become evident if survival is prolonged beyond eight hours. The morphologic features, which are not distinctive, are those of either poliomalacia or leukomalacia. The distribution of the lesions, however, is relatively distinctive. There is necrosis of the cerebral cortex, which is usually patchy but may involve the entire cortex. All layers may be affected or only the deeper lamina, a situation called *laminar necrosis.* The depths of sulci suffer greater damage than the crowns of gyri. Laminar necrosis may also be seen in other conditions, such as polioencephalomalacia of cattle or salt poisoning in swine. There is also selective necrosis of nuclei, with relatively consistent involvement of the globis pallidus, substantia nigra, and thalamus. There is focal malacia of cerebral white matter, especially the corpus callosum and anterior commissure (see porencephaly). The lesions in the gray and white matter are bilaterally symmetrical. Similar neuropathologic changes develop in the fetus from compression of the umbilical cord and other mechanisms.

Concussion and Compression. **Concussion** of the brain results from a nonfatal blow on the head, the cranial bones being fractured or not. It produces instant, though transient, unconsciousness. The concussion causes a sudden, violent displacement of the subarachnoid and other fluid in the brain and the unconsciousness is believed to be due to transient anemia as a certain amount of blood is jarred prematurely from the capillaries into larger vessels. The same sudden movement of intravascular blood and perivascular lymph (cerebrospinal fluid) may cause numerous hemorrhages of petechial size or lacerations of superficially placed tissues with

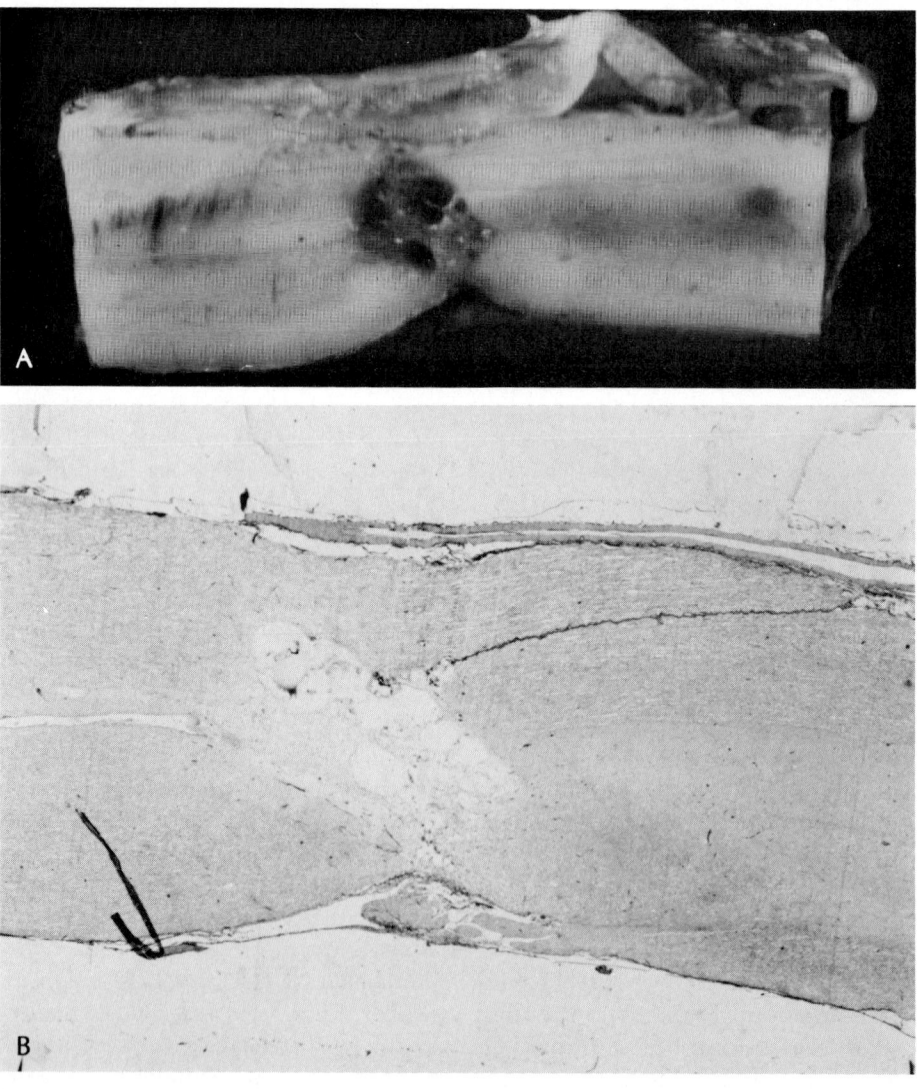

Fig. 27–1. Compression of spinal cord of an eight-month-old female Dachshund as result of dislocation of the first and second cervical vertebrae. *A,* The gross specimen incised after formalin fixation. *B,* Low power of a histologic section. (H & E, × 4.) (Courtesy of Angell Memorial Animal Hospital.)

more extensive hemorrhage into the subarachnoid spaces. These lesions are often on the side opposite to that of the blow, the injury then being caused as the somewhat movable brain, suspended in the cranial cavity, comes to a sudden stop against the opposite wall. It becomes apparent from these considerations that the interpretation of cephalic hemorrhages must be guarded in necropsy of an animal killed by a blow on the head. The fact remains, however, that this factor has seldom, if ever, been a significant cause of diagnostic error.

Diffuse compression of the brain or cord results from the pressure of extensive hemorrhages, tumors, abscesses, or edema. The symptoms may at first be manifested as hyperirritability, perhaps with convulsions, but as the pressure grows, mental depression, somnolence, and coma supervene. There may be paralysis as the effect of compression of motor centers. Headache is severe in humans and the same is doubtless true in animals. This is one, and possibly the principal, reason for the tendency of horses and cattle to press the forehead against objects (in various illnesses). It is difficult to evaluate this sign precisely. Vomiting in the absence of any digestive disorder is prominent in those species which vomit. The lesions are obviously those that belong to the individual causative disorder. Edematous swelling has been described. In a localized area of compression, softening and liquefaction necrosis develop if the patient survives a few days.

Pressure upon the cord leads to paralysis of the parts supplied from segments below the point of compression (for instance, a fractured vertebra), perhaps initiated with local hyperirritability. It is of the upper-motor-neuron type, that is, spastic. Flaccid paralysis involves parts that happen to be innervated directly from the injured segment. Sensation ceases from the parts below the lesion. As in the brain, softening and liquefaction necrosis result from local pressure. Myelin stains show demyelinization and loss of fibers in the motor tracts

below and the sensory tracts above the injured segment; however the development of this change requires several days.

Adamsons, K., and Myers, R.E.: Perinatal asphyxia: Causes, detection and neurologic sequelae. Pediatr. Clin. North Am., 20:465–480, 1973.

Brann, A.W., Jr., and Myers, R.E.: Central nervous system findings in newborn monkey following severe in utero partial asphyxia. Neurology, 25:327–338, 1975.

Fishman, R.A.: Brain edema. N. Engl. J. Med., 293:706–711, 1975.

Ginsberg, M.D., and Myers, R.E.: Experimental carbon monoxide encephalopathy in the primate. I. Physiologic and metabolic aspects. Arch. Neurol., 30:202–208, 1974.

Ginsberg, M.D., Myers, R.E., and McDonagh, B.F.: Experimental carbon monoxide encephalopathy in the primate. II. Clinical aspects, neuropathology, and physiologic correlation. Arch. Neurol., 30:209–216, 1974.

Innes, J.R.M., and Saunders, L.Z.: Comparative Neuropathology. New York, Academic Press, 1962.

Liu, H.M.: Schwann cell properties. II. The identity of phagocytes in the degenerating nerve. Am. J. Pathol., 75:395–416, 1974.

Myers, R.E.: Brain damage induced by umbilical cord compression at different gestational ages in monkeys. *In* Medical Primatology, edited by E.I. Goldsmith and J. Moor-Jankowski. Basel, Karger, 1971, pp. 394–425.

———: Two patterns of perinatal brain damage and their conditions of occurrence. Am. J. Obstet. Gynecol., 112:246–276, 1972.

———: Fetal asphyxia due to umbilical cord compression. Metabolic and brain pathologic consequences. Biol. Neonate, 26:21–43, 1975.

Myers, R.E., Valerio, M.G., Martin, D.P., and Nelson, K.B.: Perinatal brain damage: Porencephaly in a cynomolgous monkey. Biol. Neonate, 22:253–273, 1973.

Newberne, J.W., et al.: Granular structures in brains of apparently normal dogs. Am. J. Vet. Res., 21:782–786, 1960.

Sigurdsson, B., and Palsson, P.A.: Visna of sheep. A slow, demyelinating infection. Br. J. Exp. Pathol., 39:519–528, 1958.

Smith, A.D.M., Duckett, S., and Waters, A.H.: Neuropathological changes in chronic cyanide intoxication. Nature (Lond.), 200:179–181, 1963.

Spencer, P.S., and Thomas, P.K.: Ultrastructural studies of the dying-back process. II. The sequestration and removal of Schwann cells and oligodendrocytes of organelles from normal and diseased axons. J. Neurocytol., 3:763–783, 1974.

ENCEPHALITIS AND ENCEPHALOMALACIA

Inflammation and Inflammatory Disease. The same general laws of inflammation apply in the brain and spinal cord as elsewhere, but the manifestations of an inflammatory process are restricted in accordance with the kinds of cells and tissues present and anatomic limitations: (1) Since there are no mucous membranes, catarrhal inflammation does not occur. (2) Serous inflammatory reactions probably do not occur; if they do, they are not differentiated from edema. (3) Hemorrhagic exudates are seldom, if ever, encountered, although hemorrhages, by themselves, are frequent. (4) Fibrinous inflammation is limited practically to the meninges and to penetrating wounds. (5) Purulent, lymphocytic and proliferative inflammations are the types regularly encountered in the central nervous system.

Many infectious diseases are characterized by encephalitis as either their primary manifestation or as part of more generalized diseases. These include viruses, mycoplasma, chlamydia, bacteria, fungi, protozoa, and metazoan parasites, all of which have been discussed in earlier chapters. In many of these inflammatory diseases, malacia is an important feature of the lesion. Similarly, in most conditions primarily characterized by malacia, there is invariably an inflammatory reaction.

Purulent inflammation occurs as the result of infection by pyogenic microorganisms, to the usual list of which must be added *Listeria (Listerella) monocytogenes.* Listerellosis is the most frequent cause of a purulent reaction in the brains of farm animals. The accumulations of pus involve both the pia-arachnoid and the parenchymal tissue but are microscopic in amount. While diffuse in a given area, the distribution of the areas of neutrophilic infiltration is limited and variable. Lymphocytic infiltration is also prominent. If other pus-formers reach the brain, as they do occasionally as blood-borne metastases, the infection is usually confined, one or more abscesses being the result. The *Pasteurella* organism has been known to cause formation of intracranial abscesses in the bovine.

Infectious thromboembolic menin-goencephalitis of cattle caused by a *Haemophilus* organism is characterized by purulent inflammation of the brain and meninges, principally within and surrounding vascular walls. A limited amount of purulent exudation accompanies some forms (Eastern strain) of equine encephalomyelitis, although the reaction in this disease is fundamentally lymphocytic. Diffuse suppurative or fibrinopurulent meningitis occurs as a wound infection in the rare event of trauma which pierces the bony covering without being immediately fatal. It does not appear that animals have a copiously suppurative meningitis comparable to that caused by the meningococcus of man.

Subacute lymphocytic inflammation is a characteristic type in the central nervous tissues, the cells being trapped in the Virchow-Robin spaces as they leave the vessels and progress further only with difficulty. The cause is usually, but not invariably, one of the neurotropic viruses. Infiltrations of lymphocytes, which may be only perivascular, constitute the most conspicuous lesions in the viral infections. They may or may not be accompanied by petechial hemorrhages and notable hyperemia. The primary lesion in most types of viral encephalitis, however, is necrosis of neurons, the morphologic features of which have already been described. In the earlier stages of some of the viral diseases, such as rabies, practically no visible lesions may exist. Such infections as toxoplasmosis and even torulosis (cryptococcosis) also result in limited infiltrations of lymphocytes, usually perivascular, when they involve the nervous tissues. Lymphocytic cuffing is also seen adjacent to areas of necrosis (see malacia), cerebral abscesses, and neoplasms in the brain. Practically speaking, however, without the presence of other exudates, and without other apparent explanation, lymphocytic infiltrations may be considered indicative of an infectious disease, quite likely a viral disease. The localization of lesions and other

Table 27–1. Disorders Associated with Encephalomalacia

Deficiency Diseases
  Copper deficiency
  Thiamine deficiency
  Vitamin E deficiency in birds
  Polioencephalomalacia of sheep
    and cattle
Poisons
  Bracken fern
  Equisetum
  Yellow Star thistle
  Lead
  Mercury
  Cycads
  Clostridial enterotoxemia
  Mycotoxins
  Salt poisoning
Uncertain Cause
  Focal spinal poliomalacia of sheep
  Mulberry heart disease

---

features of viral diseases are discussed in Chapter 9.

Malacia. As stated earlier, necrosis in the central nervous system is called malacia: **encephalomalacia** in the brain and **myelomalacia** in the spinal cord. If the gray matter is affected, it is termed **poliomalacia,** and if white matter, **leukomalacia.** While malacia may be a feature of many of the infectious forms of encephalitis, necrosis in the brain or cord also accompanies many toxic and metabolic disorders. Certain of the latter conditions in which encephalomalacia is a prominent finding are listed in Table 27–1. Diseases characterized by destruction of myelin are also characterized by malacia, and are described as a group elsewhere.

The toxic degenerative and necrotic changes described earlier in this chapter may or may not be accompanied by any of the usual signs of inflammation. A reaction that is both striking and unique, however, does accompany softening and necrosis of appreciable amounts of central nervous tissue. This is the appearance, at the necrotic site, of what are called **scavenger cells,** also known as **compound granular corpuscles,**

Hortega cells or **gitter cells** (German, *gitterzellen*). These are large, lipid-filled phagocytes which, in the course of a few days, infiltrate the injured area in large numbers. Evidence indicates that they arise by proliferation and differentiation of the microglial cells, and probably also of the scanty connective-tissue cells which accompany the vascular network. At any rate, they are entirely comparable to the reticuloendothelial cells found in many inflammations elsewhere. The gitter cells phagocytize and assist in the removal of the large amount of lipid which is characteristic of central nervous tissue, slowly disappearing when this task has been completed. They thus represent a form of proliferative inflammation. Concurrently, the oligodendroglial cells swell and remain swollen throughout the period of active reaction.

Within two to three weeks, another proliferative change develops that is comparable to the formation of fibrous granulation tissue. It differs in that the proliferating cells are the fibrillary astrocytes of the neuroglia, hence the name, **gliosis.** Unlikely to be detected grossly, gliosis has the appearance microscopically of an area of neuroglia that is denser than the surrounding normal areas, with which it gradually blends. There occurs early an increase in the number of glial nuclei, but the increased density is due to the larger number of fibrils per unit of area and also to a somewhat greater diameter of some of the individual fibrils. The increase of glial tissue is mainly around the perimeter of the defect when there has been a complete loss of substance (liquefaction necrosis); the new glial tissue does not fill the empty space as would be done by proliferating fibrous granulation tissue. The glia-encircled empty space sometimes remains filled with clear fluid, constituting a cyst.

Proliferation of numerous small capillaries often accompanies proliferation of the glial cells, or the former may occur without the latter in an area that otherwise shows little change. This constitutes another form of proliferative inflammatory reaction. It first becomes conspicuous about a week after an anoxic or toxic injury.

Sometimes accompanying these several reactive phenomena is a change in the microglia consisting of the formation of **"rod cells."** These are microglial nuclei that elongate until their length is three or four times their diameter. They stain darkly.

Proliferation of fibrous connective tissue is limited to the immediate vicinity of blood vessels and to the meninges, where a parent fibrous tissue of mesodermal origin exists. Granulation tissue of this kind is rarely extensive except in the case of traumatic injury to the perivascular and meningeal fibroblastic tissues. Scars, be they glial or fibroblastic, tend to contract as they grow older and, in doing so, place unnatural strains and pressures on the neighboring tissue. In human beings, who are more likely than animals to live on after an anoxic, toxic or traumatic injury of the brain, malfunction of the distorted brain tissue sometimes leads to periodic convulsive seizures or lapses of consciousness known as traumatic epilepsy. However, animals seldom experience, and still more rarely survive, injuries of these kinds.

INCIDENTAL FINDINGS

A few incidental findings in the central nervous system deserve mention. Deposits of iron pigment are common in the cerebral blood vessels of the horse and less frequent in the cow. This "cerebrovascular siderosis" has been described by Saunders (1953). It is apparently a normal process and the amount of iron pigment increases with age.

Irregular plaques of melanin-laden cells are often seen grossly and microscopically in the meninges of cattle and sheep. These are considered incidental.

In the brains of senile dogs Braunmühl (1956) has described "Kongophile Angiopathie," characterized by the accumula-

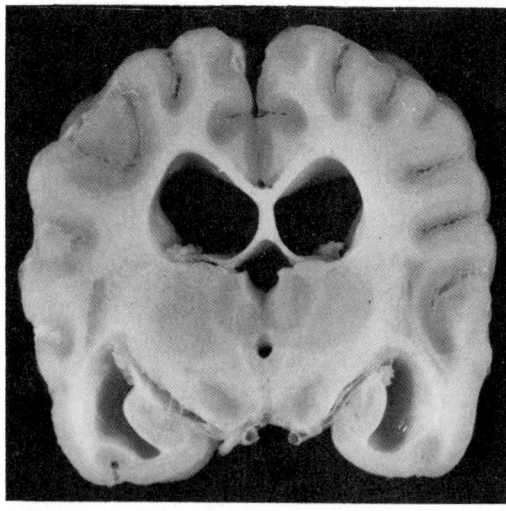

Fig. 27–2. Brain of an 18-year-old dog. Ventricles are enlarged, gyri narrowed, and blood vessels fibrotic. (Courtesy of Dr. H. Wisniewski and *Laboratory Investigation*.)

tion of lipid material in the walls of small arteries and veins. This writer also described focal glial scars designated as "senile plaques" in the cerebral cortex of aged dogs.

Wisniewski et al. (1970) have studied these **senile plaques** and **cerebral amyloidosis** in aged dogs with light and electron microscopy. These changes are of interest in comparison with the lesions in Alzheimer's presenile dementia and in aged human patients. The plaques were recognized in histologic preparations stained with acid phosphatase-Congo red preparations as small groups of rounded clusters of acid-phosphatase reactive elements resembling distended axons. Small foci of Congo-red positive, green birefringent materials were also mixed with linear and globular acid-phosphatase reaction products. A third type consisted of a rounded mass containing congophilic and green birefringent materials. Large macrophages containing acid-phosphatase reactive materials were often seen near small blood vessels. The ultrastructural fea-

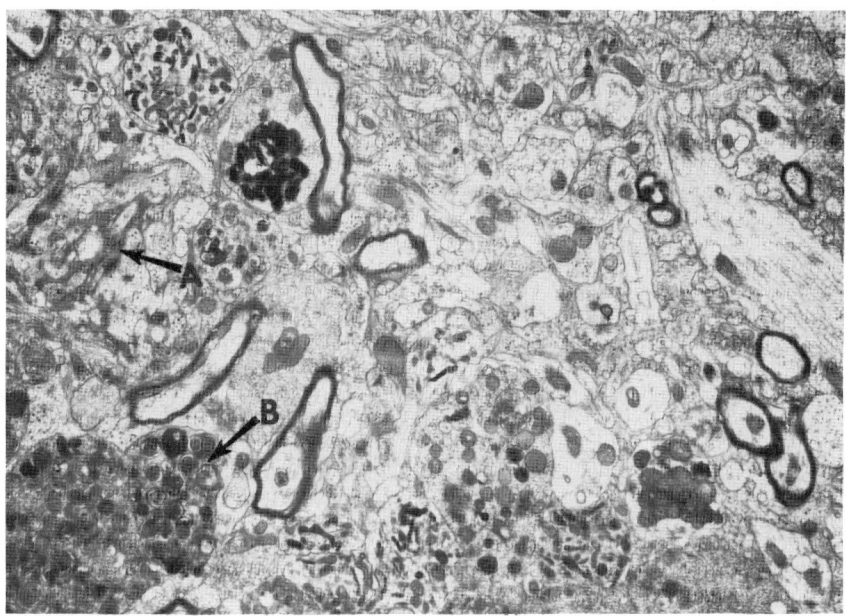

Fig. 27–3.   Senile plaque, brain of aged dog (× 4,800). Aggregates of degenerating neurites (*B*) and small amounts of amyloid (*A*). (Courtesy of Dr. H. Wisniewski and *Laboratory Investigation*.)

tures described by Wisniewski et al. consisted of aggregations of abnormal axons, amyloid, and reactive cells. The enlarged axons contained normal and degenerating mitochondria, laminated electron-dense bodies, vesicles, profiles of smooth membranes, and clusters of 100-Å filaments and 240-Å tubules. Amyloid was generally scattered as small wisps among the processes of the plaques (Figs. 27–3 to 27–5).

Organized hemorrhages in the choroid plexus are common in horses. These may

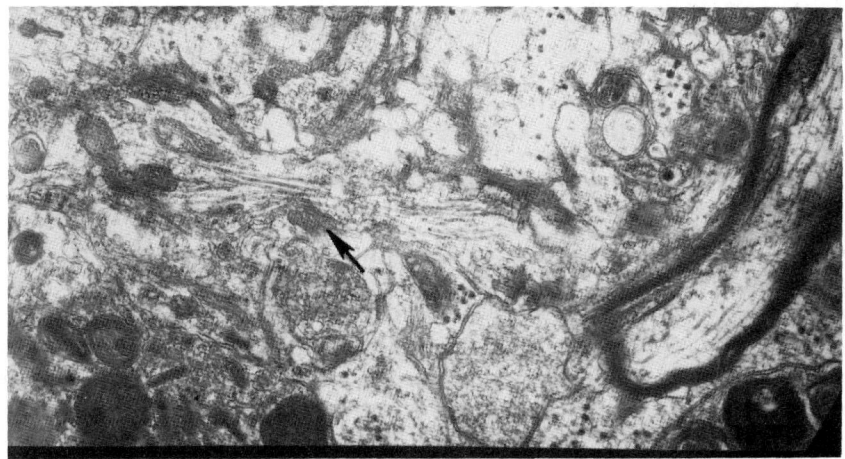

Fig. 27–4.   Senile plaque, brain of aged dog. Higher magnification of Fig. 27–3. (× 25,000). Note normal neurotubules, above amyloid (arrow). (Courtesy of Dr. H. Wisniewski and *Laboratory Investigation*.)

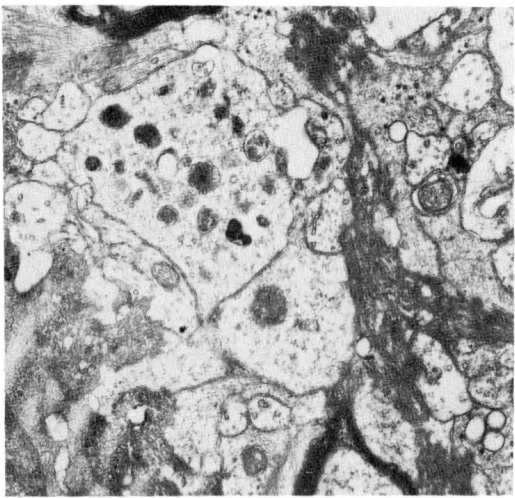

Fig. 27–5. Senile plaque, brain of an aged dog, × 16,000. Perimeter of amyloid (left) from a large plaque. (Courtesy of Dr. H. Wisniewski and *Laboratory Investigation*.)

reach rather large size (sometimes resulting in nervous signs), and because of their cholesterol content are called **cholesteatomas,** but preferably should be known as cholesterinic granulomas.

Braunmühl, A. von: "Kongophile Angiopathie" und "senile Plaques" beim greisen Hunden. Arch. f. Psychiat., *194*:396–414, 1956.
Saunders, L.Z.: Cerebrovascular siderosis in horses. Arch. Pathol., *56*:637–642, 1953.
Wisniewski, H., et al.: Senile plaques and cerebral amyloidosis in aged dogs. Lab. Invest., *23*:287–296, 1970.

DISEASES OF UNCERTAIN ETIOLOGY

The general neurophysiologic aspects of diseases of the nervous system have been discussed in the first part of this chapter and changes that constitute the reactions of nervous tissue to injury have been described. Important viral diseases affecting the nervous system specifically, such as rabies, equine, avian, ovine, and porcine encephalomyelitis, Aujeszky's disease, Borna disease, scrapie, mouse polioencephalitis and others are discussed in Chapter 9; bacterial diseases affecting the

nervous system, in Chapters 11 and 12. Cerebrospinal nematodiasis, a parasitic disease of the nervous system, is included in Chapter 14. Neoplasms of the brain and spinal cord appear at the end of this chapter. The neurologic aspects of certain poisonings are presented in Chapter 16, under the headings of the poison concerned. The bracken fern, mercury, cyanides, and especially the yellow star thistle are prominent in this category. Still requiring attention are diseases of the nervous system which, although of uncertain etiology, have distinguishing clinical or pathologic features. Certain diseases of animals that fulfill these criteria are described briefly. Since a number of the nervous disorders are at least suspected of being due to dietary deficiencies, further data on these are found under the appropriate titles in Chapter 17. In this section we include:

Congenital anomalies
Congenital lesions of cerebellum
Disorders of myelin
Neuroaxonal degeneration-dystrophy
Conditions characterized by vacuolation
Equine incoordination
Focal symmetrical poliomalacia of sheep
Poliomalacia of cattle and sheep

The classification is somewhat arbitrary, as there is considerable overlap within these groups.

Congenital Anomalies

The nervous system of animals and man is subject to many anomalies that originate during embryonic life. Some of these have already been described separately. Certain of these conditions are hereditary; others, of suspected nutritional deficiency. For many, the cause is unknown, and some are due to in-utero viral infection. Several congenital diseases of suspected hereditary origin have been shown to result from viral infections of the fetal central nervous system. These are listed in Table 27–2 and discussed further in Chapter 9.

Table 27–2. Some Virus-Induced CNS Malformations*

Virus	Malformation
Feline panleukopenia	Cerebellar hypoplasia in cats and ferrets
Bovine virus diarrhea	Cerebellar hypoplasia in cattle and sheep
Hog cholera	Cerebellar hypoplasia, microcephaly, hypomyelinogenesis in swine
Border disease	Hypomyelinogenesis in sheep
Bluetongue	Hydranencephaly, porencephaly in sheep
Influenza A (Newcastle disease)	Microcephaly and myeloschisis in chick embryos
Rat virus	Cerebellar hypoplasia in rats, hamsters, cats, and ferrets
Minute virus of mice	Cerebellar hypoplasia in mice
Lymphocytic choriomeningitis	Cerebellar hypoplasia in rats
Mumps, Parainfluenza II, Reovirus Type I, Ross River virus	Aqueductal stenosis and hydrocephalus in hamsters, mice, rats, and ferrets

* After Johnson, R.T.: Effects of viral infection on the developing nervous system. N. Engl. J. Med., 287:599–604, 1972.

The numbers and complexities of these anomalies make it impossible to cover the subject adequately in the space available. Mention is made of a few entities reported in animals. The reader is referred to the literature cited for further information in a complex field.

Anencephaly or agenesis of most of the brain or **microencephaly,** an abnormally small brain, occurs in most animal species. The cause is unknown, although in-utero infections or toxicities have been sug-

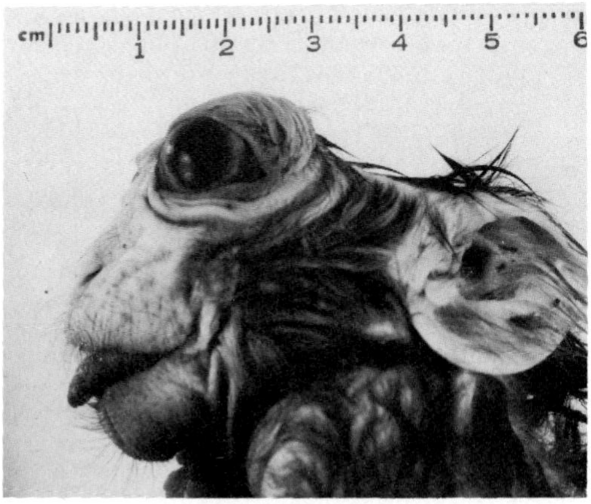

Fig. 27–6. Anencephaly, *Macaca fascicularis.* (Courtesy of New England Regional Primate Research Center, Harvard Medical School.)

gested when it occurs in small outbreaks. Anencephaly is usually associated with failure of closure of the skull. **Cranioschisis** or failure of cranial fusion is reported particularly in swine. It results in herniation of meninges known as **meningocele,** or meninges and brain called **meningoencephalocele,** which in swine appears to be inherited (Trautwein and Meyer, 1966; Wijeratne, et al., 1974).

Spina bifida or failure of closure of the vertebral arches is more frequent than the analogous cranial defect. Herniation results in formation of subcutaneous (cystic) blebs of meninges (meningocele) or meninges and cord called meningomyelocele. Various types and their postulated means of development are summarized by Padget (1968). They are common in Manx cats.

Hydromyelia is the term used to describe dilation of the central spinal canal. It is rarely seen.

Syringomyelia is a condition characterized by cavitation of the spinal cord. The cavity or syrinx is filled with watery fluid and lined by neuropil. Although rare, Weimaraner dogs appear more susceptible than other species. **Porencephaly** is a somewhat analogous situation in the brain, characterized by cystic cavities within the brain. Both result from failure of a part to develop or degeneration of preformed tissue. The cause of degeneration is usually unknown. Porencephaly is seen in lambs infected in-utero with bluetongue virus, as is hydranencephaly. **Hydranencephaly** results from destruction of most of the cerebral hemispheres, leaving a thin walled membranous sac composed of meninges and a thin rim of cortex lacking an ependymal lining. It is not to be confused with hydrocephalus. Occasional epizootics occur in cattle which are thought to result from an infectious or toxic disease.

Spinal dysraphism in the dog is believed to have an inherited basis (McGrath, 1965). This entity, which is principally a disease of Weimaraners, is manifest by numerous anomalies involving the dorsal septum of the spinal canal (hydromelia, syringomelia), central gray matter, dorsal or ventral horns, or the median fissure.

Caudal displacement of the medulla and all or part of the cerebellum below the foramen magnum into the spinal canal is another anomaly of the nervous system. In man it is often associated with hydrocephalus and other defects and is known as the Arnold-Chiari malformation. **Lissencephaly** or absence of cerebrocortical convolution has been reported in two Lhasa Apso dogs (Greene, et al., 1976).

Epidermoid cysts represent a rare anomaly produced by ectopic sequestration of epithelial tissue during closure of the neural tube. Microscopically they resemble those seen in the skin.

Hydrocephalus is most often seen as a congenital anomaly. It is discussed in the following section.

Bardens, J.W.: Congenital malformation of the foramen magnum in dogs. Swest. Vet., *18*:295–298, 1965.

Christie, R.J.: An occurrence of monozygotic twinning and anencephaly in *Macaca arctoides*. Lab. Anim. Care, *19*:531–532, 1969.

Dennis, S.M.: Congenital defects of the nervous system of lambs. Aust. Vet. J., *51*:385–388, 1975.

Epstein, H.: Phylogenetic significance of spina bifida in Zebu cattle. Indian J. Vet., *25*:313–315, 1955.

Field, B., and Wanner, R.A.: Cerebral malformation in Manx cat. Vet. Rec., *96*:42–43, 1975.

Geib, L.W., and Bistner, S.I.: Spinal cord dysraphism in a dog. J. Am. Vet. Med. Assoc., *150*:618–620, 1967.

Gitter, M., and Bowen, P.D.G.: Unusual cerebellar conditions in pigs. Cerebellar herniation associated with vitamin A deficiency; cerebellar hypoplasia. Vet. Rec., *74*:1150–1154, 1962.

Goss, L.J., and Hull, F.E.: Spina bifida in a calf. Cornell Vet., *29*:239–242, 1939.

Greene, C.E., Vandevelde, M., and Braund, K.: Lissencephaly in two Lhasa Apso dogs. J. Am. Vet. Med. Assoc., *169*:405–410, 1976.

Gunberg, D.L.: Spina bifida and the Arnold-Chiari malformation in the progeny of trypan-blue-injected rats. Anat. Rec., *126*:343–347, 1956.

Harding, J.D.J.: A cerebrospinal angiopathy in pigs. Pathol. Vet., *3*:83–88, 1966.

Hartley, W.J., and Haughey, K.G.: Attempted transmission of micrencephaly in newborn lambs. Aust. Vet. J., *50*:323–324, 1974.

Hartley, W.J., and Haughey, K.G.: An outbreak of micrencephaly in lambs in New South Wales. Aust. Vet. J., *50*:55–58, 1974.

James, C.C.M., Lassman, L.P., and Tomlinson, B.E.: Congenital anomalies of the lower spine and spinal cord in Manx cats. J. Pathol., *97*:269–276, 1969.

Johnson, R.T.: Effects of viral infection on the developing nervous system. N. Engl. J. Med., *287*:599–604, 1972.

Kelly, D.F., and Watson, W.J.B.: Epidermoid cyst of the brain in the horse. Equine Vet. J., *8*:110–112, 1976.

Kitchen, H., Murray, R.E., and Cockrell, B.Y.: Animal model for human disease: spina bifida, sacral dysgenesis and myelocele. Animal model: Manx cats. Am. J. Pathol., *68*:203–206, 1972.

Koens, H.: (A case of spina bifida in a lamb.) Tijdschr. Diergeneesk., *70*:307–309, 1945.

Levine, S.: Epidermoid cysts of the spinal cord: a spontaneous disease of rats. J. Neuropathol. Exp. Neurol., *25*:498–504, 1966.

McFarland, L.Z.: Spina bifida with myelomeningocele in a calf. J. Am. Vet. Med. Assoc., *132*:32–34, 1959.

McGrath, J.T.: Spinal dysraphism in the dog with comments on syringomyelia. Pathol. Vet., *2*(Suppl.):1–27, 1965.

McGrath, J.T.: Animal models of human disease: spinal dysraphism. Comp. Pathol. Bull., *8*:2, 4, 1976.

Nielsen, S.L., and Baringer, J.R.: Reovirus-induced aqueductal stenosis in hamsters: phase contrast and electron microscopic studies. Lab. Invest., *27*:531–537, 1972.

O'Hara, P.J., and Shortridge, E.H.: (I.) Some diseases of the porcine central nervous system. (II.) Congenital anomalies of the porcine nervous system. N. Z. Vet. J., *14*:1–12, 13–18, 1966.

Padget, D.H.: Spina bifida and neuroschisis—a

causal relationship. Definition of the postnatal conformations involving a bifid spine. Johns Hopkins Med. J., *123*:233–252, 1968.

Parker, A.J., and Byerly, C.S.: Meningomyelocele in a dog. Vet. Pathol., *10*:266–273, 1973.

Price, R.A., and Gilles, F.H.: Telencephalic remnants in simian and human anencephaly. Arch. Pathol., *91*:529–536, 1971.

Trautwein, G., and Meyer, H.: Experimental studies on hereditary meningocele cerebralis in pigs. II. Pathology. Pathol. Vet., *3*:543–555, 1966.

Wanner, R.A., and Gray, S.J.: Hydromyelia in a Weimaraner. Aust. Vet. J., *50*:282–283, 1974.

Wanner, R.A., and Husband, A.J.: Immunoglobulins in bovine congenital hydranencephaly. Aust. Vet. J., *50*:560–562, 1974.

Wijeratne, W.V.S., Beaton, D., and Cuthbertson, J.C.: A field occurrence of congenital meningo-encephalocele in pigs. Vet. Rec., *95*:81–84, 1974.

Hydrocephalus. Hydrocephalus is the slow accumulation of excessive cerebrospinal fluid in the lateral and other ventricles and sometimes in the subarachnoid spaces due to obstruction of normal drainage. When confined to the ventricles it is termed **internal hydrocephalus,** and when in the subarachnoid space, **external hydrocephalus.**

Normally there is a continual secretion of fluid from the choroid plexus of vessels located principally in the lateral ventricles. This drains through the aqueduct of Sylvius into the fourth ventricle. Thence it passes through some minute openings in the roof of that ventricle, known as the foramina of Luschka, into rather indefinite compartments called the basal cisterns in the subarachnoid space. Some of the fluid finds its way into the spinal canal as cerebrospinal fluid. The overflow continues from the basal cisterns anteriorly through the intercommunicating subarachnoid spaces, whence it is reabsorbed into the venous circulation, especially through the arachnoid villi, which project into the venous sinuses to afford increased absorptive surface.

The possibility of some obscure derangement of the resorptive process in the subarachnoid villi or elsewhere cannot be entirely excluded, but the causes of hydrocephalus are considered to lie ordinarily in some mechanical obstruction to the outflow of lymph. There are several obvious sites where such obstruction could easily occur and a variety of local disorders which could initiate the stoppage. The slender aqueduct of Sylvius is easily closed by external pressure, and the foramina of Luschka, which lead from the fourth ven-

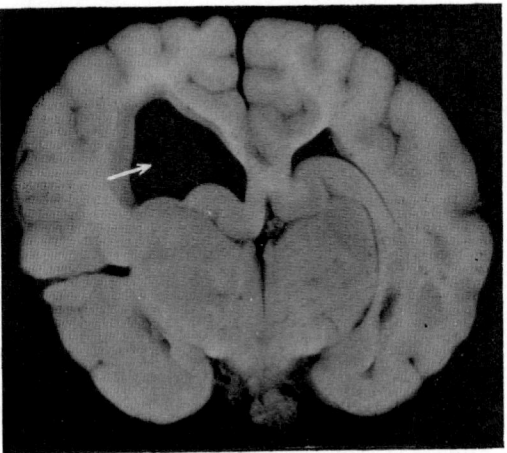

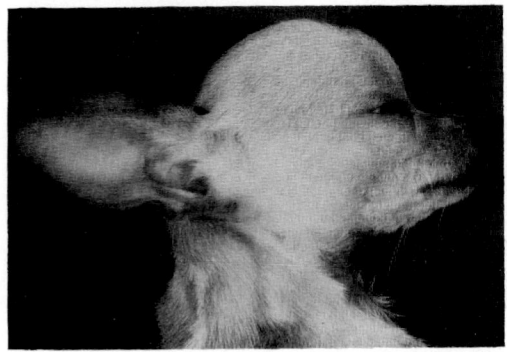

Fig. 27–7. Hydrocephalus in a three-year-old male Chihuahua. (Courtesy of Angell Memorial Animal Hospital.)

Fig. 27–8. Hydrocephalus involving left lateral ventricle (arrow) of a 15-year-old female Boston Terrier. An incidental finding at necropsy. (Courtesy of Angell Memorial Animal Hospital.)

tricle, are still more vulnerable. Inflammatory exudates, tumors, parasitic cysts (*Coenurus cerebralis*), and similar structures are ready sources of pressure in this region. Another potential barrier is the tentorium cerebelli; not only is the cranial cavity sharply narrowed here, facilitating obstruction of the subarachnoid passageways, but the same interference with flow is also achieved by slight displacement of the brain either forward or backward, its soft mass acting as a plug in the narrow incisura tentorii as a stopper plugs a bottle. Such displacement of the brain can be pro-

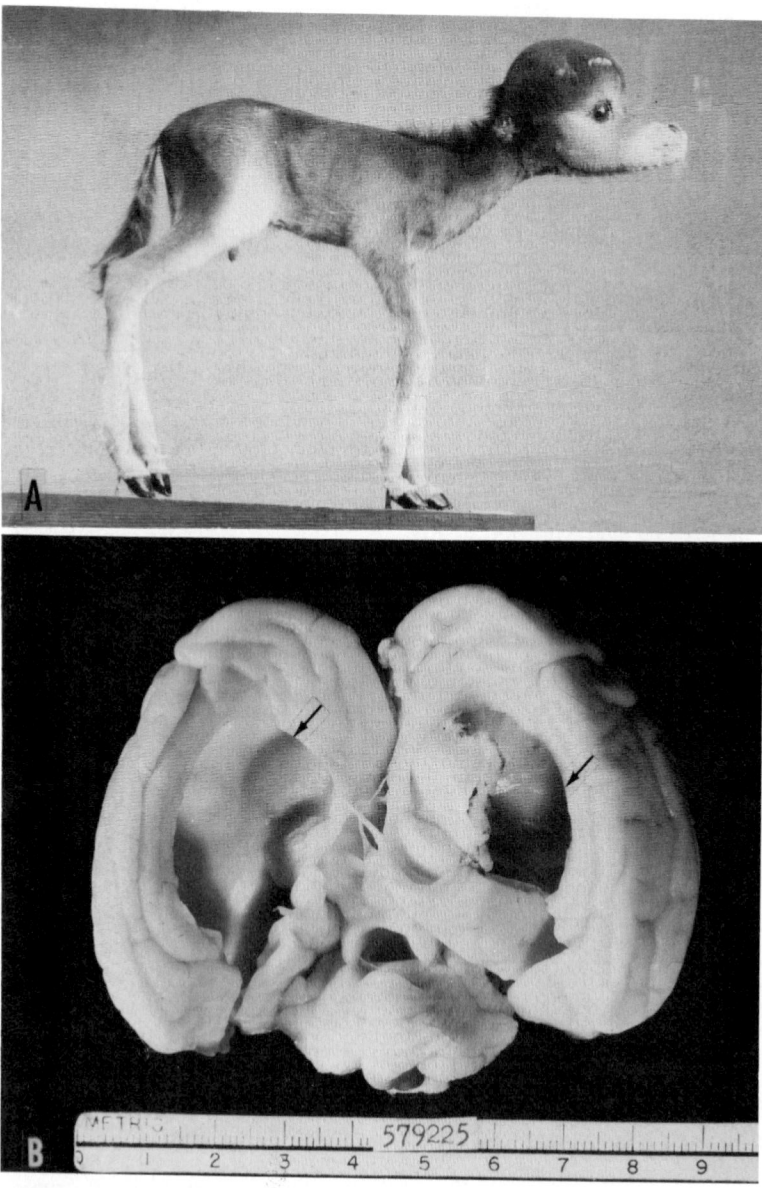

Fig. 27–9. Hydrocephalus. *A,* A mounted specimen of a newborn colt. (Mark Francis Collection, Texas School of Veterinary Medicine.) *B,* The brain of a newborn puppy with hydrocephalus. Arrows indicate the dilated lateral ventricle. (*B,* Courtesy of Armed Forces Institute of Pathology.) Contributor: Dr. Russell B. Oppenheimer.

duced by inflammatory or other swelling in either compartment of the cranial cavity. The brain is also occasionally forced backward into the foramen magnum until escape of fluid into the spinal canal is cut off.

While the preceding statements on causative mechanisms appear to be perfectly valid and are widely accepted, it must be admitted that there are many cases of hydrocephalus in humans and animals in which the exact etiology and manner of development have been impossible to demonstrate. In spite of the occasional development of hydrocephalus in connection with tumors and the circumstances just outlined, the usual occurrence of hydrocephalus is as a disease of the newborn and the cause is to be attributed to maldevelopment of the brain or cranium. As a general rule, **congenital hydrocephalus** is more severe than hydrocephalus acquired later in life.

Margolis and Kilham (1969) have shown that Reovirus type I inoculated into suckling ferrets, hamsters, mice, and rats regularly results in hydrocephalus. The virus specifically attacks ependymal cells, leading to destruction of those cells, ulceration, and healing by gliovascular proliferation, which results in obstructive hydrocephalus. Parainfluenza II, influenza A, and Ross River virus have also been shown to produce an analogous aqueductal stenosis and hydrocephalus in laboratory animals. It seems plausible that this viral mechanism may also account for natural cases of hydrocephalus. Other examples of congenital hydrocephalus appear to result from inherited defects. In Herefords and Shorthorns, several syndromes have been described and reviewed by Greene et al. (1974) which are thought to be passed as autosomal recessive traits. In what they termed "Hereford syndrome 1," calves were stillborn or died in the first few days of life, and in addition to hydrocephalus with doming of the forehead resulting from aqueductal stenosis, there was cerebellar hypoplasia, microphthalmia, and retinal

dysplasia. In "Hereford syndrome 2," which was not characterized by marked doming of the forehead, calves were stillborn or died in one or two days, and there was dorsal kinking of the midbrain. In the "Shorthorn syndrome," the hydrocephalus resulted from aqueductal stenosis and was also associated with microphthalmia and retinal dysplasia.

Hydrocephalus (and other anomalies) has been associated with several experimentally induced nutritional deficiencies in pregnant laboratory rodents to include vitamin A, folic acid, vitamin B_{12}, niacin, and zinc. Hypervitaminosis A during pregnancy may also lead to hydrocephalus.

The effect of the obstructed drainage—indeed, the essence of the disease, morphologically speaking—is pressure atrophy of the cerebral parenchyma. In the usual type of internal hydrocephalus due to obstruction in the flow of the fluid, the ventricles enlarge gradually at the expense of the parenchyma until the cerebral hemispheres are reduced to mere hollow rims around the lateral ventricles. In external hydrocephalus in which the interference with return flow lies somewhere in the subarachnoid course of drainage, pressure atrophy proceeds from the exterior of the brain. The eventual outcome of hydrocephalus is death, although, since the primitive vital centers are located in the less accessible midbrain and hindbrain, it is surprising how long a young animal can survive with almost no cerebrum.

Adeloye, A., and Warkany, J.: Experimental congenital hydrocephalus. A review with special consideration of hydrocephalus produced by zinc deficiency. Childs Brain, 2:325–360, 1976.

Greene, H.J., Leipold, H.W., and Hibbs, C.M.: Bovine congenital defects. Variations of internal hydrocephalus. Cornell Vet., 64:596–616, 1974.

Greene, H.J., Leipold, H.W., and Vestweber, J.E.: Experimentally induced hydrocephalus in calves. Am. J. Vet. Res., 35:945–951, 1974.

Halstead, J.R., and Kiel, F.W.: Hydrocephalus in a bear. J. Am. Vet. Med. Assoc., 141:367–368, 1962.

Higgins, R.J., Vandevelde, M., and Braund, K.B.: Internal hydrocephalus and associated periventricular encephalitis in young dogs. Vet. Pathol., 14:236–246, 1977.

Hyde, R.R.: An epidemic of hydrocephalus in a group of experimental rabbits. Am. J. Hyg., 31:1–8, 1940.

Johnson, R.T., Johnson, K.P., and Edmonds, C.J.: Virus-induced hydrocephalus: development of aqueductal stenosis in hamsters after mumps infection. Science, 157:1066–1067, 1967.

Kilham, L., and Margolis, G.: Hydrocephalus in hamsters, ferrets, rats, and mice following inoculations with Reovirus type I. I. Virologic studies. Lab. Invest., 21:183–188, 1969.

Krous, H.F., et al.: Congenital hydrocephalus produced by attenuated influenza A virus vaccine in Rhesus monkeys. Am. J. Pathol., 92:317–320, 1978.

Margolis, G., and Kilham, L.: Hydrocephalus in hamsters, ferrets, rats, and mice following inoculations with Reovirus type I. II. Pathologic studies. Lab. Invest., 21:189–198, 1969.

————: Experimental virus-induced hydrocephalus. Relation to pathogenesis of the Arnold-Chiari malformation. J. Neurosurg., 31:1–9, 1969.

Milhorat, T.H., Clark, R.G., and Hammock, M.K.: Experimental hydrocephalus II. Gross pathological findings in acute and subacute obstructive hydrocephalus in the dog and monkey. J. Neurosurg., 32:390–399, 1970.

Schlotthauer, C.F.: Internal hydrocephalus in a dog. J. Am. Vet. Med. Assoc., 85:788–794, 1934.

Selby, L.A., Hayes, H.M., and Becker, S.V.: Epizootiologic features of canine hydrocephalus. Am. J. Vet. Res., 40:411–413, 1979.

Weller, R.O., Wisniewski, H., Shulman, K., and Terry, R.D.: Experimental hydrocephalus in young dogs. Histological and ultrastructural study of the brain tissue damage. J. Neuropathol. Exp. Neurol., 30:613–626, 1971.

Williams, W.L., and Frost, J.N.: Subdural hydrocephalus in a calf. Cornell Vet., 28:340–345, 1938.

Wolinsky, J.S.: Mumps virus-induced hydrocephalus in hamsters: Ultrastructure of the chronic infection. Lab. Invest., 37:229–236, 1977.

Congenital Lesions of the Cerebellum

Severe destructive lesions of the cerebellum cause marked incoordination of gait, frequently referred to as "cerebellar ataxia." The signs referable to the lesions in the cerebellum are characteristic of involvement of this structure but may be the result of any one of several anatomically distinct entities. Their cause is often unknown. Some examples appear to be inherited, but others represent destructive lesions from viral infections in utero, as in cerebellar hypoplasia in cats caused by feline panleukopenia virus, in calves caused by bovine virus diarrhea, and in swine by hog cholera virus (which has also been associated with hypomyelinogenesis). Some of those that have been recognized in animals are described below.

Olivopontocerebellar Hypoplasia. Occurring in cats, olivopontocerebellar hypoplasia has been reported by numerous writers (Brouwer, 1934; Schut, 1946). The signs are not detectable in newborn kittens until the normal neonatal ataxia disappears, usually one month after birth. Lesions may be easily recognized in affected animals sacrificed at this time and occasionally will be detected in adult animals which have exhibited no abnormal signs. The anomaly results in a decided decrease in gross size of the cerebellum with corresponding hypoplasia of the olivary nuclei and pons. In a few cases the cerebellum is more severely involved on one side than the other, and then aplasia in the olive and pons is limited to the contralateral side. The cerebrum may also be reduced in size although not as obviously as the cerebellum.

In the cat, this hypoplasia or agenesis of the cerebellum in most cases is caused by the virus of feline panleukopenia (Kilham and Margolis, 1964). Cerebellar hypoplasia has been reported in kittens by Fatzer (1975) in association with dysmyelinogenesis or hypomyelinogenesis. The condition may represent a leukodystrophy.

Blood, D.C.: Cerebellar hypoplasia and degeneration in the kitten. Aust. Vet. J., 22:120–121, 1946.

Brouwer, B.: Familial olivo-ponto-cerebellar hypoplasia in cats. Folia Psychiat. Neurol. Neerl., 38:352–367, 1934.

Campbell, A.M.G.: Feline and human ataxia. Lancet, 2:265–266, 1967.

Fatzer, R. von: (Leucodystrophic lesions in the brain of young cats.) Schweiz. Arch. Tierheilkd., 117:641–648, 1975.

Harding, J.D.J., Done, J.T., and Darbyshire, J.H.: Congenital tremors in piglets and their relation to swine fever. Vet. Rec., 79:388–390, 1966.

Kilham, L., and Margolis, G.: Cerebellar ataxia in hamsters inoculated with rat virus. Science, 143:1047–1048, 1964.

Komar, G., and Meszaros, J.: (Congenital Cerebellar Ataxia in Cats.) Magy. Allatorv. Lap., 21:38–41, 1966. V.B. 36:4904, 1966.

Scheidy, S.F.: Familial cerebellar hypoplasia in cats. North Am. Vet., 34:118–119, 1953.

Schut, J.W.: Olivopontocerebellar atrophy in a cat. J. Neuropathol. Exp. Neurol., 5:77–81, 1946.

Feline Neuroaxonal Dystrophy. This condition, described by Woodard et al. (1974), is characterized by swelling and ballooning of axons and loss of neurons. Axonal swelling is most marked in the olivary nucleus and the lateral cuneate nucleus, with less extensive axonal degeneration in the brain stem, thalamus, and cerebellar vermis. There is loss of Purkinje cells and reduction in the granular cell layer as well as neuronal loss in the olivary nucleus and thalamus. The cerebellum in young animals is normal in size and only slightly smaller than normal in animals surviving longer periods. Woodard et al. presented evidence that it is inherited as an autosomal recessive trait in association with diluted coat color similar to the "lilac" Siamese. Kittens were affected at birth with incoordination which progressed with age.

Woodard, J.C., Collins, G.H., and Hessler, J.R.: Feline hereditary neuroaxonal dystrophy. Am. J. Pathol., 74:551–566, 1974.

Hereditary Cerebellar Ataxia of Calves. A specific cerebellar disease in Jersey calves has been described by Saunders et al. (1952), who presented evidence to indicate that it is inherited as a simple recessive character. Similar cases of ataxia have been reported in breeds of cattle (Hereford, Shorthorn) other than the Jersey, but the typical anatomic features have not been described in all instances.

The lesions in this disease are detectable only upon microscopic examination, for the brains are grossly well formed, of normal size and architecture. The microscopic changes are centered in the white matter of the cerebellum, but may involve cerebellar nuclei and extend into the medulla and midbrain. The outstanding feature is diffuse, nonsymmetric demyelination of large areas of central white matter, extending into the medullary portion of the cerebellar

folia. Affected areas assume a spongy appearance due to the replacement of myelinated fibers by vacuoles of irregular size, some of which contain albuminous fluid. The lesion is not confined within the boundaries of individual tracts, nor is this disorganization of myelinated fibers accompanied by leukocytic infiltration or glial proliferation. Neurons contiguous with affected white matter, as those in the reticular formation, dentate, and roof nuclei, are particularly susceptible to damage, most of them being absent, and the few that remain being misshapen. The molecular layer of the cerebellum in some instances is edematous, but the Purkinje cells are essentially unaffected.

Whether these changes are the consequence of developmental failure or degeneration has not been settled. It is possible that they are the result of demyelination during fetal life. The cerebellar lesions of this disease are somewhat reminiscent of the subcortical changes seen in the cerebrum and cerebellum of sheep affected with "swayback."

Inherited Cortical Cerebellar Atrophy. A disease of newborn lambs (called "daft lambs" in Britain, North Wales, and Scotland) has been characterized by Innes et al. (1949) as an inherited atrophy of cerebellar cortex which produces severe symptoms of cerebellar ataxia. The disease occurs not only in the British Isles, but also in Canada. The lesions do not result in recognizable gross atrophy of the central nervous system, hence are detected only upon microscopic examination. They are limited to the cerebellar cortex, where varying degrees of atrophy of individual folia are observed. The Purkinje cells are particularly affected, and in some folia almost all are lost. The changes in these cells consist of swelling and chromatolysis of varying degrees, or conversely, pyknosis of nuclei and basophilism of cytoplasm. Cytoplasmic vacuoles in affected Purkinje cells often push the nucleus to one side or altogether displace it from the cell. Loss of

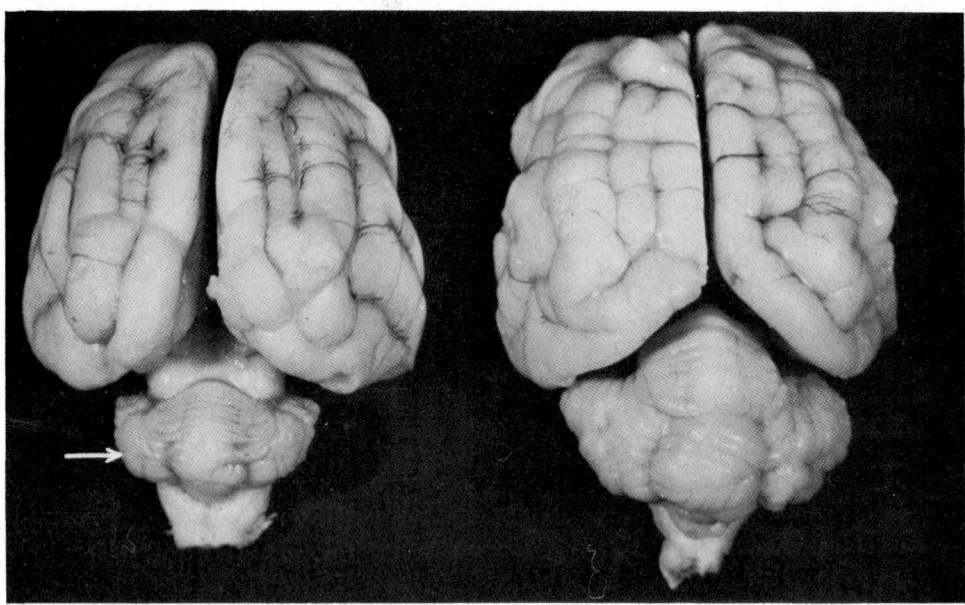

Fig. 27–10.   Hypoplasia of the cerebellum (arrow) in a two-month-old female kitten. The brain of a normal kitten of the same age is on the right for comparison. (Courtesy of Angell Memorial Animal Hospital.)

Purkinje cells is evidenced by the demonstration of empty "basket cells" with silver impregnation. These cells form a basket of dendrites that surround each Purkinje cell. If the Purkinje cell is lost, the basket remains; absence of "basket cells" is evidence that the Purkinje cells have never developed. The cerebellar white matter is not visibly affected. The molecular and granular layers are reduced in volume, decreasing the over-all width of affected folia, but rarely enough to be obvious upon gross examination.

Similar cortical atrophy of the cerebellum has been reported in calves and foals (Innes et al., 1940).

Other Forms of Cerebellar Agenesia, Hypoplasia and Abiotrophy. A type of hypoplasia of the cerebellum that is grossly evident in newborn or young calves, swine, and dogs has been reported by numerous authors (Blood, 1946; Cordy and Snelbaker, 1952; Sholl, et al., 1939). In some instances, evidence of a familial tendency has been presented, but many reports are

of only a single case, with no indication of a familial factor. In cattle there is supporting evidence to indicate it is inherited as an autosomal recessive trait in Shorthorn, but no hereditary pattern has been identified in Hereford, a breed in which it is also frequently seen, except as part of a syndrome also characterized by hydrocephalus and microphthalmia. The clinical features are those of cerebellar ataxia indistinguishable from those of other morphologic entities described in this group. The pathologic-anatomic features are evidenced by gross reduction in size of all lobes of the cerebellum with almost total absence of cerebellum in some cases. Microgyria and over-all atrophy of the cerebrum are sometimes described but are relatively minor in comparison with the cerebellar changes. Microscopically, in most reported examples, there is a notable reduction in all layers of the cerebellar cortex.

In horses, a type of cerebellar hypoplasia is seen in which there is no gross reduction

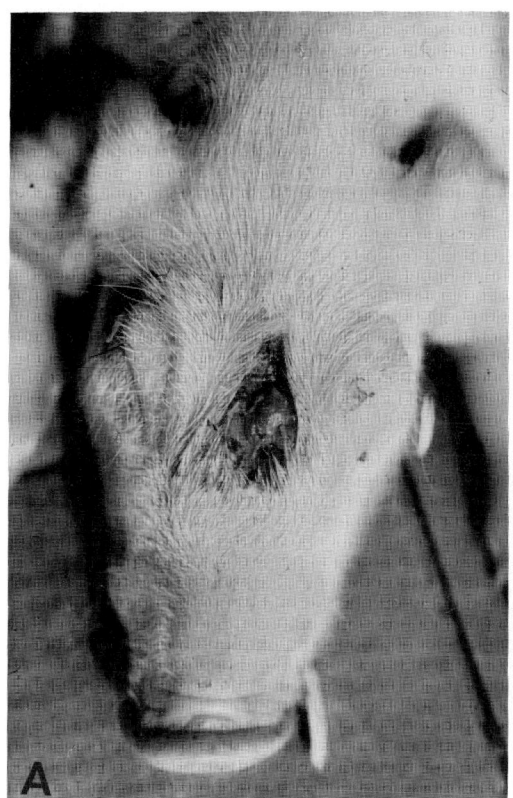 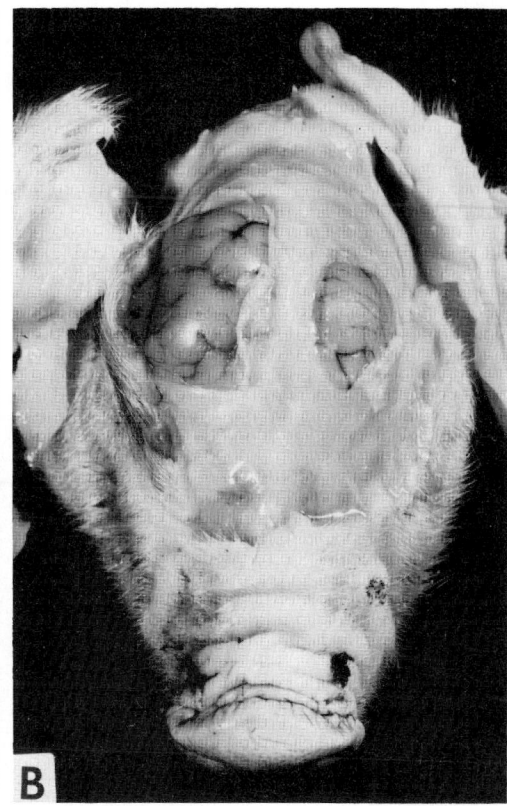

Fig. 27–11. Congenital meningoencephalocele. *A*, A small meningoencephalocele without a covering of skin, in a newborn piglet. *B*, Meningoencephalocele on each side of the frontal suture in a newborn piglet. The skin has been reflected. (Courtesy of Dr. W.S. Wijeratne. Reproduced with permission of *Veterinary Record* and the Controller of Her Britannic Majesty's Stationery Store.)

in the size of the cerebellum. Arabian or part-Arabian horses are affected, and develop incoordination within a few months of age. Microscopically, Purkinje cells and the granular layer are significantly reduced. A hereditary basis has been suggested but other mechanisms have not been eliminated. Cerebellar hypoplasia with gross reduction in size has been described in Gotland ponies (Bjorck et al., 1973).

In Kerry Blue Terriers, deLahunta and Averill (1976) have described a disease they termed **hereditary cerebellar cortical and extrapyramidal nuclear abiotrophy** which they report to have been seen in related dogs in California and New York as well as in Texas and England. The term abiotrophy is used to indicate degeneration after a period of normal development and implies premature degeneration due to an intrinsic abnormality. The condition became clinically apparent between 9 and 16 weeks of age. Early in the course, the cerebellum was normal in size, but grossly became progressively smaller with widened sulci between folia. Microscopically, there was degeneration of Purkinje cells followed by bilateral degeneration in the olivary nucleus, substantia nigra, and caudate nucleus.

What has also been termed **cerebellar abiotrophy** has been reported in Holstein heifers (White et al., 1975). Signs of incoordination developed between three to eight months, and progressed over several weeks. The cerebellum was normal in size, but microscopically there was degeneration of Purkinje cells and neurons of the cerebellar nuclei.

Anders, M.V.: The histopathology of a new type of hereditary loss of coordination in the domestic rabbit. Am. J. Anat., 76:183–199, 1945.

Anderson, W.A.D., and Davis, C.L.: Congenital cerebellar hypoplasia in a Holstein-Friesian calf. J. Am. Vet. Med. Assoc., 117:460–461, 1950.

Baird, J.D., and MacKenzie, C.D.: Cerebellar hypoplasia and degeneration in part-Arab horses. Aust. Vet. J., 50:25–28, 1974.

Barlow, R.M., Linklater, K.A., and Young, G.B.: Familial convulsions and ataxia in Angus calves. Vet. Rec., 83:60–65, 1968.

Bjork, G., Everz, K.E., Hansen, H.-J., and Henricson, B.: Congenital cerebellar ataxia in the Gotland pony breed. Zentralb. Vet. Med., 20A:341–354, 1973. Vet. Bull., 43:5102, 1973.

Blood, D.C.: Cerebellar hypoplasia and degeneration in the kitten. Aust. Vet. J., 22:120–121, 1946.

Cordy, D.R., and Snelbaker, H.A.: Cerebellar hypoplasia and degeneration in a family of Airedale dogs. J. Neuropathol. Exp. Neurol., 11:324–328, 1952.

D'Amato, C.J., and Hicks, S.P.: Neuropathologic alterations in the ataxic (paralytic) mouse. Arch. Pathol., 80:604–612, 1965.

deLahunta, A., and Averill, D.R., Jr.: Hereditary cerebellar cortical and extrapyramidal nuclear abiotrophy in Kerry Blue Terriers. J. Am. Vet. Med. Assoc., 168:1119–1124, 1976.

Dungworth, D.L., and Fowler, M.E.: Cerebellar hypoplasia and degeneration in a foal. Cornell Vet., 56:17–24, 1966.

Finnie, E.P., and Leaver, D.D.: Cerebellar hypoplasia in calves. Aust. Vet. J., 41:287–288, 1965.

Fraser, H.: Two dissimilar types of cerebellar disorder in the horse. Vet. Rec., 78:608–612, 1966.

Howell, J.McC., and Ritchie, H.E.: Cerebellar malformations in two Ayrshire calves. Pathol. Vet., 3:159–168, 1966.

Innes, J.R.M., Rowlands, W.T., and Parry, H.B.: An inherited form of cortical cerebellar atrophy in ("daft") lambs in Great Britain. Vet. Rec., 61:225–228, 1949.

Innes, J.R.M., Russell, D.S., and Wildson, A.J.: Familial cerebellar hypoplasia and degeneration in Hereford calves. J. Pathol. and Bacteriol., 50:455–461, 1940.

Kilham, L., and Margolis, G.: Cerebellar ataxia in hamsters inoculated with rat virus. Science, 143:1047–1048, 1964.

Kronevi, T., Hansen, H.-J., and Jonsson, O.J.: Cerebellar hypoplasia of unknown etiology in pigs. Vet. Rec., 96:403–404, 1975.

O'Leary, J.L., et al.: Hereditary ataxia of rabbits. Arch. Neurol., 6:123–137, 1962.

———: Ultrastructural lesions in rabbit hereditary ataxia. Arch. Neurol., 13:238–262, 1965.

O'Sullivan, B.M., and McPhee, C.P.: Cerebellar hypoplasia of genetic origin in calves. Aust. Vet. J., 51:469–471, 1975.

Palmer, A.C., et al.: Cerebellar hypoplasia and degeneration in the young Arab horse: Clinical and neuropathological features. Vet. Rec., 93:62–66, 1973.

Saunders, L.Z.: A check list of hereditary and familial diseases of the central nervous system in domestic animals. Cornell Vet., 42:592–600, 1952.

Saunders, L.Z., et al.: Herditary congenital ataxia in Jersey calves. Cornell Vet., 42:559–591, 1952.

Scheidy, S.F.: Familial cerebellar hypoplasia in cats. North Am. Vet., 34:118–119, 1953.

Sholl, L.B., Sales, E.K., and Langham, R.: Three cases of cerebellar agenesia. J. Am. Vet. Med. Assoc., 95:229–230, 1939.

Tuch, K., and Pohlenz, J.: Partielle Cerebellarhernie beim Lowen (Panthera leo L.) Vet. Pathol., 10:299–306, 1973.

Van Bogaert, L., and Innes, J.R.M.: Cerebellar disorders in lambs. A study in animal neuropathology with some comments on ovine neuroanatomy. Arch. Pathol., 50:36–62, 1950.

Ward, G.M.: Bovine cerebellar hypoplasia apparently caused by BVD-MD virus, a case report. Cornell Vet., 59:570–576, 1969.

White, M.E., Whitlock, R.H., and deLahunta, A.: A cerebellar abiotrophy of calves. Cornell Vet., 65:476–491, 1975.

Disorders of Myelin (Dysmyelinating Diseases, Demyelinating Diseases)

The integrity of the myelin sheath is disrupted in many disorders of the central nervous system that damage nerve fibers and oligodendroglial cells, including infarction, certain poisonings, and infectious encephalitis. Demyelination of this type, which is more of a form of necrosis, was discussed previously. There remain two groups of diseases in which the principal lesion focuses on myelin. They are classified as **dysmyelinating diseases** (hypomyelinogenesis), when there is a defect in myelin formation, and **demyelinating diseases,** when there is destruction of myelin. Distinction between the two mechanisms is, however, somewhat arbitrary especially in the case of fetal infections leading to destruction of myelin-forming cells. Dysmyelinating diseases include globoid cell leukodystrophy, metachromatic leukodystrophy, sudanophilic leukodystrophy, cerebellar ataxia of calves, feline neuroaxonal dystrophy, swayback, and several less-well-characterized hereditary forms of hypomyelinogenesis in calves, swine, dogs, cats, and other species which probably are specific leukodystrophies. The specific leukodystrophies are also discussed as a group with storage diseases, many others of which affect the brain with storage of material in neurons but do not cause dysmyelination.

Demyelinating diseases include allergic encephalomyelitis, multiple sclerosis in man, and certain viral infections that are discussed elsewhere, such as canine distemper (and old-dog encephalitis), measles, border disease, hog cholera, and visna. These are listed in Table 27–3.

Neuroaxonal dystrophies and degenerations also result in demyelination.

Congenital Hypo- or Dysmyelinogenesis. Congenital hypomyelinogenesis is occasionally seen in most species of animals. Certain of the better characterized forms are discussed elsewhere (leukodystrophies, cerebellar ataxia of calves). In swine, two hereditary forms of hypomyelinogenesis are recognized: a sex-linked recessive disease in Landrace pigs and an autosomal recessive trait in Saddleback pigs. Both are recognized clinically by congenital tremors and are included in what Done (1976) has called the *congenital tremor syndrome,* within which he also included viral-induced (hog cholera and possibly other viruses) cerebellar hypoplasia. In Landrace pigs and a similar disease in dogs (Greene et al., 1977), myelin formation in the central nervous system is almost totally absent, but in the peripheral nervous system, where myelin formation depends upon Schwann cells, it is normal. Saddleback pigs appear to have defective synthesis and degeneration of myelin. In Charolais cattle, a condition characterized by slowly progressive ataxia commencing after six months of age is characterized by loss of myelin apparently due to a defect in oligodendrocytes.

Table 27–3. Dysmyelinating and Demyelinating Diseases

Dysmyelinating
  Hereditary hypomyelinogenesis in swine
    (congenital tremor) and cattle
  Globoid cell leukodystrophy
  Metachromatic leukodystrophy
  Sudanophilic leukodystrophy in "quaking" and
    "jimpy" mice
  Hereditary cerebellar ataxia of calves
  Feline neuroaxonal dystrophy
  Swayback
Demyelinating
  Allergic encephalomyelitis
    Post-rabies vaccination
    Postinfectious
    Post-smallpox vaccination in man
  Polyradiculoneuritis (Coonhound paralysis)
  Viral encephalomyelitis
    Canine distemper
    Visna
    Mouse hepatitis
    Infectious leukoencephalomyelitis of goats
    Bluetongue (fetal)
    Border disease ("hairy shaker" disease) (fetal)
    Hog cholera (fetal)
  Suspected viral origin
    Subacute sclerosing panencephalitis in man
    Progressive multifocal leukoencephalopathy
      of man
    Multiple sclerosis of man
    Spinal demyelination in rats
  Poisonings
    Arsenilic acid
    Cycada
    Coyotillo
    Hexachlorophene
    Organic phosphates

Adams, J.M., et al.: Old dog encephalitis and demyelinating diseases in man. Vet. Pathol., 12:220–226, 1975.

Blakemore, W.F., and Harding, J.D.J.: Ultrastructural observations on the spinal cord of piglets affected with congenital tremor type AIV. Res. Vet. Sci., 17:248–255, 1974.

Blakemore, W.F., Harding, J.D.J., and Done, J.T.: Ultrastructural observations on the spinal cord of a Landrace pig with congenital tremor type AIII. Res. Vet. Sci., 17:174–178, 1974.

Blakemore, W.F., Palmer, A.C., and Barlow, R.M.: Progressive ataxia of Charolais cattle associated with disordered myelin. Acta Neuropathol., 29:127–139, 1974.

Cork, L.C., and Narayan, O.: The pathogenesis of viral leukoencephalomyelitis-arthritis of goats. I.

Persistent viral infection with progressive pathologic changes. Lab. Invest., 42:596–602, 1980.

Done, J.T.: The congenital tremor syndrome in pigs. Vet. Ann., 16:98–102, 1976.

Greene, C.E., Vandevelde, M., and Hoff, E.J.: Congenital cerebrospinal hypomyelinogenesis in a pup. J. Am. Vet. Med. Assoc., 171:534–536, 1977.

Hartley, W.J., and Palmer, A.C.: Ataxia in Jack Russell terriers. Acta Neuropathol., 26:71–74, 1973.

Herschkowitz, N., Vassella, F., and Bischoff, A.: Myelin differences in the central and peripheral nervous system in the "Jimpy" mouse. J. Neurochem., 18:1361–1363, 1971.

Kishimoto, Y.: Abnormality in sphingolipid fatty acids from sciatic nerve and brain of quaking mice. J. Neurochem., 18:1365–1368, 1971.

Palmer, A.C., Blakemore, W.F., Barlow, R.M., Fraser, J.A., and Ogden, A.L.: Progressive ataxia of Charolais cattle associated with a myelin disorder. Vet. Rec., 91:592–594, 1972.

Patterson, D.S.P., Done, J.T., Foulkes, J.A., and Sweasey, D.: Neurochemistry of the spinal cord in congenital tremor of piglets (type AII), a spinal dysmyelinogenesis of infectious origin. J. Neurochem., 26:481–485, 1976.

Patterson, D.S.P., et al.: Neurochemistry of the spinal cord in experimental border disease (hypomyelinogenesis congenita) of lambs. J. Neurochem., 18:883–894, 1971.

Patton, C.S.: Progressive ataxia in Charolais cattle. Vet. Pathol., 14:535–537, 1977.

Samorajski, T., Friede, R.L., and Reimer, P.R.: Hypomyelination in the quaking mouse. A model for the analysis of disturbed myelin formation. J. Neuropathol. Exp. Neurol., 29:507–523, 1971.

Weiner, L.P., Johnson, R.T., and Herndon, R.M.: Viral infections and demyelinating diseases. N. Engl. J. Med., 288:1103–1110, 1973.

Globoid-Cell Leukodystrophy.

This familial, apparently hereditary, disease in children was described by Krabbe (1916) as a type of diffuse sclerosis of the central nervous system. The principal lesion is disseminated failure of myelination with the accumulation of large "globoid" phagocytic cells around blood vessels in the vicinity of the altered myelin. A similar disease was originally reported by Fankhauser, et al. (1963) in dogs. Several other canine cases have subsequently appeared in the literature, most of which have concerned Cairn Terriers and West Highland White Terriers. It has also been described in Domestic Short-Hair cats. The disease is inherited as a simple autosomal recessive trait that results in a deficiency of β-galactocerebrosidase.

The signs appear usually about four to six months of age but may be recognized earlier. Impairment is usually evident first in the hind legs, with incoordination and slight diminution of placing reflexes. This progresses to motor incoordination, generalized tremor, twitching of head and neck, and eventually paraplegia. The lesions may be found in white matter throughout the central nervous system. They are usually bilaterally symmetrical, with loss of myelin and, in severe lesions, loss of axons. Associated with these lesions of altered myelin, and grouped around blood vessels, are many large globoid cells with cytoplasm filled with galactocerebroside which compresses the nucleus to one side of the cell. This material stains readily with periodic acid-Schiff (PAS) reagent, but is not metachromatic (with Giemsa's or toluidin blue stain), and stains gray with Sudan black B. Hypertrophied astrocytes are also numerous in the immediate vicinity.

Done, J.T.: The congenital tremor syndrome in pigs. Vet. Ann., 16:98–102, 1976.

Fankhauser, R., Luginbühl, H., and Hartley, W.J.: Leukodystrophie vom Typhus Krabbe beim Hund. Schweiz. Arch. Tierheilk., 105:198–207, 1963.

Fletcher, T.F., Kurtz, H.J., and Low, D.G.: Globoid cell leukodystrophy (Krabbe type) in the dog. J. Am. Vet. Med. Assoc., 149:165–172, 1966.

Greene, C.E., Vandevelde, M., and Hoff, E.J.: Congenital cerebrospinal hypomyelinogenesis in a pup. J. Am. Vet. Med. Assoc., 171:534–536, 1977.

Hirth, R.S., and Nielsen, S.W.: A familial canine globoid cell leukodystrophy ("Krabbe type"). J. Small Anim. Pract., 8:569–575, 1967.

Jortner, B.S., and Jonas, A.M.: The neuropathology of globoid-cell leucodystrophy in the dog. A report of two cases. Acta Neuropathol., 10:171–182, 1968.

Krabbe, K.: A new familial, infantile form of diffuse brain sclerosis. Brain, 39:74–114, 1916.

McGrath, J., et al.: A morphologic and biochemical study of canine globoid leukodystrophy. J. Neuropathol. Exp. Neurol., 28:171, 1969.

Wallace, B.J., Aronson, S.M., and Volk, B.W.: Histochemical and biochemical studies of globoid cell leucodystrophy (Krabbe's disease). J. Neurochem., 11:367–376, 1964.

Metachromatic Leukodystrophy. An- other metabolic defect in synthesis of lipids, known as a familial disease of in- fants, has also been recognized in mink (Brander and Palludan, 1965). The features shared by the human and mink disease are degeneration of myelin sheaths, disor- ganization of myelin, and the presence of metachromatic lipid material in macro- phages. In human beings, metachromatic leukodystrophy is recognized as due to a deficiency in the enzyme arylsulfatase A, which leads to accumulation of sulfatide in the brain as well as in other tissues such as the liver, kidney, and white blood cells. The evidence points toward an autosomal recessive mode of inheritance in the mink.

Anderson, H.A., and Palludan, B.: Leucodystrophy in mink. Acta Neuropathol., *11*:347–360, 1968.
Brander, N.R., and Palludan, B.: Leucoenceph- alopathy in mink. Acta Vet. Scand., *6*:41–51, 1965.
Christensen, E., and Palludan, B.: Late infantile famil- ial metachromatic leucodystrophy in mink. Acta Neuropathol., *4*:640–645, 1965.

Cerebellar Ataxia of Calves and Feline Neuroaxonal Dystrophy. These disorders are characterized by hypomyelinogenesis and have been previously discussed.

Congenital Demyelinating Disease of Lambs (Swayback, Enzootic Ataxia). New- born or young lambs are not infrequently affected with a specific demyelinating dis- ease known among shepherds in England, Scotland, and Wales as "swayback." The disease has also been reported from Aus- tralia as "enzootic ataxia" and is known colloquially in South Africa as "Lamkruis." It has also been reported in the United States. The disease is manifest in suckling or newborn lambs by severe ataxia; af- fected animals show incoordinated move- ments; they are unable to walk but able to nurse and they do not exhibit flaccid paralysis. Blindness is sometimes ob- served; fever is absent, and death usually results from starvation or exposure, fre- quently accompanied by bronchopneu- monia. Affected lambs, as a rule, are sac- rificed by the owner.

The disease is most prevalent among lambs born of ewes that have been main- tained on a diet low in copper. Many but not all such ewes manifest anemia, some have "stringy" wool, and most have low- ered copper levels in blood and liver. It is believed therefore that the disease is re- lated to copper deficiency, but the mecha- nism of its action is not known.

The lesions are limited to the central nervous system and are characterized by diffuse symmetric destruction of subcorti- cal white matter in the cerebrum accom- panied by descending destruction of cer- tain myelinated tracts in the spinal cord. In severe, acute cases the destruction of cere- bral white matter leads to grossly visible gelatinous softening in the subcortical white matter with formation of large sym- metric cavities. This cavitation may be fol- lowed by secondary internal hydro- cephalus. Chromatolysis in neurons of the red nucleus has been observed. The af- fected myelinated tracts appear spongy mi- croscopically, and in early cases may be bordered by areas containing globules of myelin and collections of gitter cells. All evidence of tissue reaction usually disap- pears shortly and inflammatory cells are rare in the adjacent viable parenchyma.

Allcroft, R., Clegg, F.G., and Uvarov, O.: Prevention of swayback in lambs. Vet. Rec., *71*:884–889, 1959.
Barlow, R.M.: Recent advances in swayback. Proc. Roy. Soc. Med., *51*:748–752, 1958.
Barlow, R.M., et al.: Swayback in Southeast Scotland. Field, clinical, pathological and biochemical as- pects. J. Comp. Pathol., *70*:396–428, 1960.
Barlow, R.M.: Further observations on swayback. I. Transitional pathology. II. Histochemical lo- calization of cytochrome oxidase activity in the central nervous system. J. Comp. Pathol., *73*:51– 60, 61–67, 1963.
Barlow, R.M., and Cancilla, P.A.: Structural changes of the central nervous system in swayback (en- zootic ataxia) of lambs. Acta Neuropathol., *6*:175–180, 1966.
Bennetts, H.W., and Beck, A.B.: Enzootic ataxia and copper deficiency of sheep in Western Australia. Aust. Council Sci. Indust. Res. Bull., *147*:55, 1942.
Bennetts, H.W., and Chapman, F.E.: Copper defi- ciency in sheep in Western Australia: A prelimi- nary account of the aetiology of enzootic ataxia of

lambs and anaemia of ewes. Aust. Vet. J., 13:138–149, 1937.

Butler, E.J., Barlow, R.M., and Smith, B.S.W.: Copper deficiency in relation to swayback in sheep. II. Effect of dosing young lambs with molybdate and sulphate. J. Comp. Pathol., 74:419–426, 1964.

Cancilla, P.A., and Barlow, R.M.: Structural changes of the central nervous system in swayback (enzootic ataxia) of lambs. IV. Electron microscopy of the white matter of the spinal cord. Acta Neuropathol., 11:294–300, 1968.

————: Structural changes of the central nervous system in swayback (enzootic ataxia) of lambs. V. Electron microscopic observations of the corpus callosum. Acta Neuropathol., 12:307–313, 1969.

Howell, J.McC.: Observation on the histology and possible pathogenesis of lesions in the central nervous system of sheep with swayback. Proc. Nutr. Soc., 27:85–88, 1968.

Innes, J.R.M., and Shearer, G.D.: I. "Swayback": A demyelinating disease of lambs with affinities to Schilder's encephalitis in man. J. Comp. Pathol. Therap., 53:1–41, 1940.

Jensen, R., Maag, D.D., and Flint, J.C.: Enzootic ataxia from copper deficiency in sheep in Colorado. J. Am. Vet. Med. Assoc., 133:336–340, 1958.

Roberts, H.E., Williams, B.M., and Harvard, A.: Cerebral oedema in lambs associated with hypocuprosis and its relationship to swayback. I. Field, clinical, gross anatomical and biochemical observations. II. Histopathological findings. J. Comp. Pathol., 76:279–290, 1966.

Schulz, K.C.A., van der Merwe, P.K., van Rensburg, P.J.J., and Swart, J.S.: Studies in demyelinating diseases of sheep associated with copper deficiency. Onderstepoort J. Vet. Res., 25:35–78, 1951.

"Allergic" Encephalitis (Postvaccination Encephalitis, Disseminated Encephalomyelitis).

It was observed many years ago that a few persons or animals suddenly exhibited paralytic symptoms several days after the administration of suspensions of nervous tissue (e.g., rabies vaccine). This "postvaccinal encephalitis" has since been reproduced experimentally by repeated parenteral injections of suspensions of normal brain tissue or by single injections of such tissue mixed with certain "adjuvants" that delay absorption. The causal relationship between injection of suspensions of brain tissue and the paralytic symptoms is evident, although the exact mechanism involved in the phenomenon is not clearly understood. It does appear that the process represents a type of induced autoimmune disease, and the experimental disease fits into the category of delayed (cellular) hypersensitivity. It can be passively transferred to isologous animals with mononuclear cells but not with serum. The antigen is the basic myelin protein.

Other forms of postvaccination encephalitis with demyelination as a prominent feature are recognized in human beings following smallpox vaccination, which does not contain nervous tissue. This reaction, and certain forms of postinfectious encephalitis in man such as measles, mumps, and influenza, are believed to represent a virus-induced immunologic reaction against myelin.

The signs in this disease usually start with motor paralysis of one or more limbs, which gradually extends to involve most of the body. Death is the usual outcome in animals with a severe form of the disease. Dogs are most commonly affected, presumably because antirabies vaccination is most frequent in this species, but many other species are susceptible.

The lesions are most evident upon microscopic examination of the brain and spinal cord. In the brain, the lesions are rather sharply limited to the white matter, destruction of myelinated tracts being the dominant feature. Tracts of all levels may be involved, although the largest lesions are usually seen in the cerebellar peduncles, internal capsule, and pyramids. Subcortical white matter is often affected and occasionally the corpus callosum is involved. The lesions appear as irregular, nonsymmetric areas of malacia with destruction of myelin followed by the usual glial and leukocytic response. Perivascular accumulation of lymphocytes is often intense in regions adjacent to foci of malacia. In the spinal cord, tracts in the myelinated white columns are similarly affected, but accumulation of lymphocytes around blood vessels is a more striking feature. There may also be considerable demyelination in peripheral nerves.

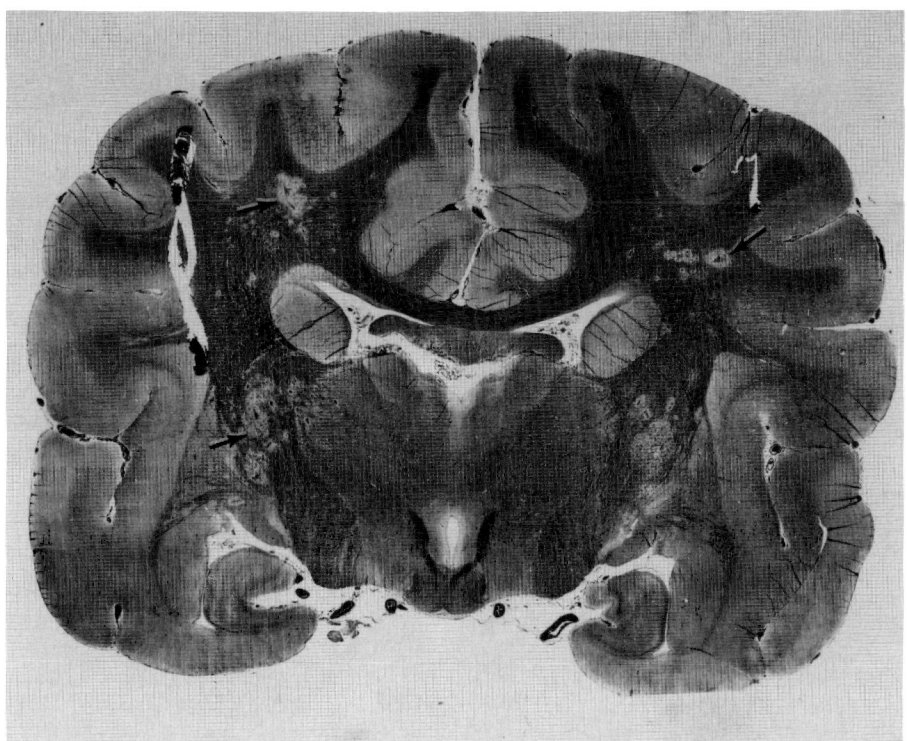

Fig. 27–12. Demyelinization in allergic encephalitis in a dog. Transverse section of brain. Weil's stain. Arrows indicate pale areas of demyelination in white matter. (Courtesy of Armed Forces Institute of Pathology.) Contributor: Dr. C.P. Zepp, Jr.

The diagnosis of "allergic encephalitis" can usually be based upon the history and on the demonstration of characteristic microscopic lesions in brain and cord.

Behan, P.O., et al.: Immunologic mechanisms in experimental encephalomyelitis in nonhuman primates. Arch. Neurol., 29:3–9, 1973.

Innes, J.R.M.: Experimental "allergic" encephalitis: Attempts to produce the disease in sheep and goats. J. Comp. Pathol. Therap., 61:241–251, 1951.

Jervis, G.A., Burkhart, R.L., and Koprowski, H.: Demyelinating encephalomyelitis in the dog associated with antirabies vaccination. Am. J. Hyg., 50:14–26, 1949.

Jervis, G.A., and Koprowski, H.: Encephalomyelitis of possible allergic etiology in mice injected with rabies vaccine. Can. J. Comp. Med., 13:116–121, 1949.

Levine, S., and Sowinski, R.: Reduction of allergic encephalomyelitis incubation period to five days. Am. J. Pathol., 56:97–110, 1969.

Oldstone, M.B.A., and Dixon, F.J.: Immunohis-tochemical study of allergic encephalomyelitis. Am. J. Pathol., 52:251–263, 1968.

Purdy, C.W., and Loan, R.W.: Induction of experimental allergic encephalomyelitis in the goat. Am. J. Vet. Res., 30:85–89, 1969.

Raine, C.S., Wisniewski, H., Dowling, P.C., and Cook, S.D.: An ultrastructural study of experimental demyelination and remyelination. IV. Recurrent episodes and peripheral nervous system plaque formation in experimental allergic encephalomyelitis. Lab. Invest., 25:28–34, 1971.

Rowe, M.J., III: Experimental allergic encephalomyelitis. A review. Bull. Los Angeles Neurol. Soc., 34:55–56, 1969.

Sherwin, A.L., et al.: Myelin-binding antibodies in experimental "allergic" encephalomyelitis. Science, 134:1370–1372, 1961.

Waksman, B.H., and Adams, R.D.: A histologic study of the early lesion in experimental allergic encephalomyelitis in the guinea pig and rabbit. Am. J. Pathol., 41:135–162, 1962.

Polyradiculoneuritis. An interesting syndrome in dogs, known colloquially as "Coonhound paralysis," has been associated for years with a prior bite or scratch by a raccoon. Coonhounds are most often affected, but other breeds are also susceptible. Cummings and Haas (1967) have demonstrated that the lesions consist of inflammation and segmental demyelination of ventral roots and spinal nerves and resemble the Landry-Guillain-Barré syndrome of man. The clinical features involve acute ascending flaccid paralysis starting 7 to 14 days following the bite of a raccoon. A viral etiology is suspected, perhaps operating on an allergic basis (Waksman and Adams, 1955, 1956). Attempts to isolate an infectious agent have been unsuccessful; however, an essentially identical condition has been experimentally induced in dogs by inoculation of canine ischiatic nerve and Freund's complete adjuvant, supporting its allergic basis (Holmes and de-Lahunta, 1975).

Axonal degeneration in the nerve roots and spinal nerves is accompanied by perivascular infiltration of leukocytes, mostly lymphocytes. Plasma cells may predominate in some sections. The peripheral nerves (sciatic) may be affected, but lesions are most consistent in the ventral nerve roots.

Cummings, J.F., and Haas, D.C.: Coonhound paralysis. An acute idiopathic polyradiculoneuritis in dogs resembling the Landry-Guillain-Barré syndrome. J. Neurol. Sci., 4:51–81, 1967.
————: Idiopathic polyneuritis, Guillain-Barré syndrome. Animal model: Coonhound paralysis, idiopathic polyradiculoneuritis of Coonhounds. Am. J. Pathol., 66:189–192, 1972.
Cummings, J.F., and deLahunta, A.: Chronic relapsing polyradiculoneuritis in a dog: A clinical, light- and electron-microscopic study. Acta Neuropathol., 18:191–204, 1974.
Holmes, D.F., and deLahunta, A.: Experimental allergic neuritis in the dog and its comparison with the naturally occurring disease: Coonhound paralysis. Acta Neuropathol., 30:329–337, 1974.
Kingma, F.J., and Catcott, E.J.: A paralytic syndrome in Coonhounds. North Am. Vet., 35:115–117, 1954.
Trayser, C.V., and Marshall, A.E.: A mild form of polyradiculoneuritis in a dog. J. Am. Vet. Med. Assoc., 164:150–151, 1974.
Waksman, B.H., and Adams, R.D.: Allergic neuritis:

An experimental disease of rabbits induced by injection of peripheral nervous tissue and adjuvants. J. Exp. Med., 102:213–236, 1955.
————: A comparative study of experimental allergic neuritis in the rabbit, guinea pig and mouse. J. Neuropathol. Exp. Neurol., 15:293–314, 1956.

Viral Demyelinating Diseases. Certain viral infections are associated with demyelinating encephalitis and some demyelinating diseases are suspected to be of viral cause. These are listed in Table 27–3. The mechanism of viral demyelination is generally unknown, but two basic processes are potentially operable. Destruction of oligodendrogliocytes and hence myelin by direct viral invasion and necrosis is believed to be the mechanism in neurotropic mouse hepatitis-encephalitis and possibly in canine distemper encephalitis. The alternate mechanism is analogous to allergic encephalomyelitis just discussed. In this case, it is believed the virus alters the membrane of oligodendrogliocytes or incorporates their membranes in the viral envelope, making myelin proteins antigenic and eliciting a cell-mediated immune response. This mechanism is believed to contribute to demyelination in canine distemper and subacute sclerosing panencephalitis in human beings, which is associated with measles virus. The mechanism in bluetongue infection in fetal lambs is direct necrosis, as is probably the case in border disease. In visna, the mechanism is unknown. Progressive multifocal leukoencephalopathy in man is believed to be caused by a papovavirus directly destroying oligodendrogliocytes. Multiple sclerosis is suspected of being caused by a virus, possibly a myxovirus, but is still under investigation. Postinfectious encephalitis in man may follow mumps, varicella, or influenza, and post-smallpox vaccination encephalitis is believed to result from virus-induced immunologic reactions. Cork et al. (1974) have described a demyelinating disease of young (one- to four-month-old) dairy goats, termed **infectious leukoencephalomyelitis,** which is caused by a virus serologically related to visna virus. Demyelination associated with astrocytosis and perivascular lymphocytic cuffing was most severe from the mesencephalon caudally including the spinal cord. The virus also causes interstitial pneumonia and arthritis.

Spinal Demyelination of Rats. Pappenheimer (1952) has described a spontaneous demyelinating disease in adult rats exhibiting progressive flaccid paralysis. The lesions are limited to the spinal cord, where ventral and lateral white columns undergo severe demyelination. The lesions are bilaterally symmetric and appear as sharply demarcated, spongy areas replacing most of the white matter. Dorsal columns are generally less severely affected. The cause remains unknown and attempts to transmit the disease and to demonstrate any relation to a viral disease of mice have been unsuccessful. The significance of this disease is not clear, although if it were reproducible or occurred spontaneously with more frequency it might be useful as a tool for investigation of demyelinating diseases.

Cork, L.C., et al.: Infectious leukoencephalomyelitis of young goats. J. Infect. Dis., *129*:134–141, 1974.
Pappenheimer, A.M.: Spontaneous demyelinating disease of adult rats. Am. J. Pathol., *28*:247–255, 1952.

Neuroaxonal Degeneration-Dystrophy

Several other disorders characterized by degeneration of neurons or their processes have been described in animals. Most are not common. Certain appear to be hereditary, but infectious agents have not been ruled out for most. Those included in this section are not readily classified with other degenerative diseases, such as leukodystrophies, cerebellar hypoplasias, or disorders of myelin, which are also degenerative diseases. The pathogenesis of these disorders is not understood, but each is characterized by degeneration of neurons or processes which is called *neuroaxonal degeneration or dystrophy*. Morphologic features of degenerating neurons and axons have been discussed earlier. Often, especially in dogs, isolated swollen axons (called spheroids) are encountered as an incidental finding without clinical correlation and of unknown pathogenesis.

Hereditary Neuronal Abiotrophy in Dogs. A previously unrecognized disease has been described by Sandefeldt et al. (1973) in Swedish Lapland dogs as due to a simple autosomal recessive trait. At five to seven weeks of age, there is a sudden onset of thoracic or pelvic limb weakening which progresses rapidly to paralysis of all four limbs (tetraparesis). Muscle atrophy and joint fixation follow and then further progression abates. Movement of the head, tail, and axial musculature is not affected.

Microscopically, neuronal degeneration (or abiotrophy) characterized by central chromatolysis and ultimately neuronophagia is widespread in spinal lower motor neurons, medullary rays of the cerebellum, Purkinje cells, spinal ganglia, and various nuclei. Wallerian degeneration is present in peripheral nerves in the limbs, especially motor nerves. Sandefeldt et al. (1976) suggested that the nerve cell body degeneration represents a retrograde response to axonal degeneration. The condition is similar to spinal muscular atrophy in man (Werdnig-Hoffmann disease).

Degenerative Myelopathy of German Shepherd Dogs. This has been described by Averill (1973); it results in a slowly progressive spastic paralysis of the pelvic limbs in older animals (mean age 8.2 years). Pathologically, there is degeneration of spinal cord myelin and axons in all fasciculi associated with astrocytosis. Lesions are most extensive in the midthoracic spinal cord. The pathogenesis has not been determined, although intervertebral disc protrusion, spondylosis deformans, or osseous metaplasia of the dura have been excluded.

Myelomalacia affecting the ventromedial spinal cord has been described in Afghan hounds by Cockrell et al. (1973). The dogs, which ranged from 3 to 13 months of age, developed ataxia and progressive paralysis leading to death or euthanasia. The cause is unknown.

Canine Spinal Muscular Atrophy. This disease, which has similarities to human juvenile spinal muscular atrophy and amyotropic lateral sclerosis, has been described in Brittany Spaniels by Cork et al. (1979). The condition, which is thought to be inherited as an autosomal recessive, is characterized by progressive muscular weakness and atrophy. Histopathologically, there is loss of motor neurons in the ventral horn of the spinal cord brain stem associated with astrogliosis and segmental swelling of axons.

Averill, D.R., Jr.: Degenerative myelopathy in the aging German Shepherd dog: Clinical and pathologic findings. J. Am. Vet. Med. Assoc., 162:1045–1051, 1973.

Cockrell, B.Y., Herigstad, R.R., Flo, G.L., and Legendre, A.M.: Myelomalacia in Afghan hounds. J. Am. Vet. Med. Assoc., 162:362–365, 1973.

Cork, L.C., et al.: Hereditary canine spinal muscular atrophy. J. Neuropathol. Exp. Neurol., 38:209–221, 1979.

Sandefeldt, E., et al.: Hereditary neuronal abiotrophy in the Swedish Lapland dog. Cornell Vet., 63(Suppl):71 pp, 1973.

————: Animal model of human disease. Infantile spinal muscular atrophy, Werdnig-Hoffmann disease. Animal model: Hereditary neuronal abiotrophy in Swedish Lapland dogs. Am. J. Pathol., 82:649–652, 1976.

Conditions Characterized by Vacuolation (Spongy Degeneration)

Several etiologically distinct disorders of the central nervous system are characterized by vacuolation of the gray and/or white matter. The vacuoles are usually within neurons, glial cells, or myelin, and in some disorders there is a defect in myelin formation. The terms "status spongiosis," "spongy degeneration," and "brain edema" have been loosely applied to these disorders; however, the occurrence of vacuoles is not a specific change and caution must be used in interpreting their presence. Care must also be exercised in discriminating these diseases from purely demyelinating diseases, although the two groups overlap.

Neuraxial Edema in Polled Herefords (Congenital Brain Edema). A congenital disorder of polled Herefords believed to be inherited as an autosomal recessive trait has been reported in the United States (Cordy et al., 1969), Australia (Blood and Gay, 1972), New Zealand (Davis et al., 1971; Jolly, 1974) and Europe (Weaver, 1974). Calves, which are affected at birth, are unable to stand and have tetanic spasms especially when touched or stimulated by noise. Most do not survive more than a week or two.

The lesions are confined to the central nervous system, which may appear wet on gross inspection and exhibit a slight internal hydrocephalus. Microscopically there is widespread spongy vacuolation (status spongiosus) in both gray and white matter, being most extensive in the medulla, pons, and midbrain. In the gray matter it results from hydropic swelling of astrocytes and their processes. Neurons are essentially normal. In the white matter the sponginess results from edema around axons and within myelin and hypomyelinogenesis. The lesion has been described as similar to "spongy degeneration" of children or Canavan's disease. It has been seen in polled Hereford/Friesian crosses but not in other breeds. (See Fig. 27–13.)

Spongy Degeneration in Kittens. A disorder similar to that just described has been reported in kittens by Kelly and Gaskell (1976). The principal neurologic signs are ataxia and dysmetria, and pathologically there is extensive intramyelinic vacuolation in the brain and spinal cord. Neurons and glial cells are unaffected. These authors also called attention to the similarity to Canavan's disease of human beings.

Subacute Spongiform Viral Encephalopathies. Entirely unrelated to the foregoing disorders is a group of slow virus diseases characterized by vacuolation of the gray and white matter. These include mink

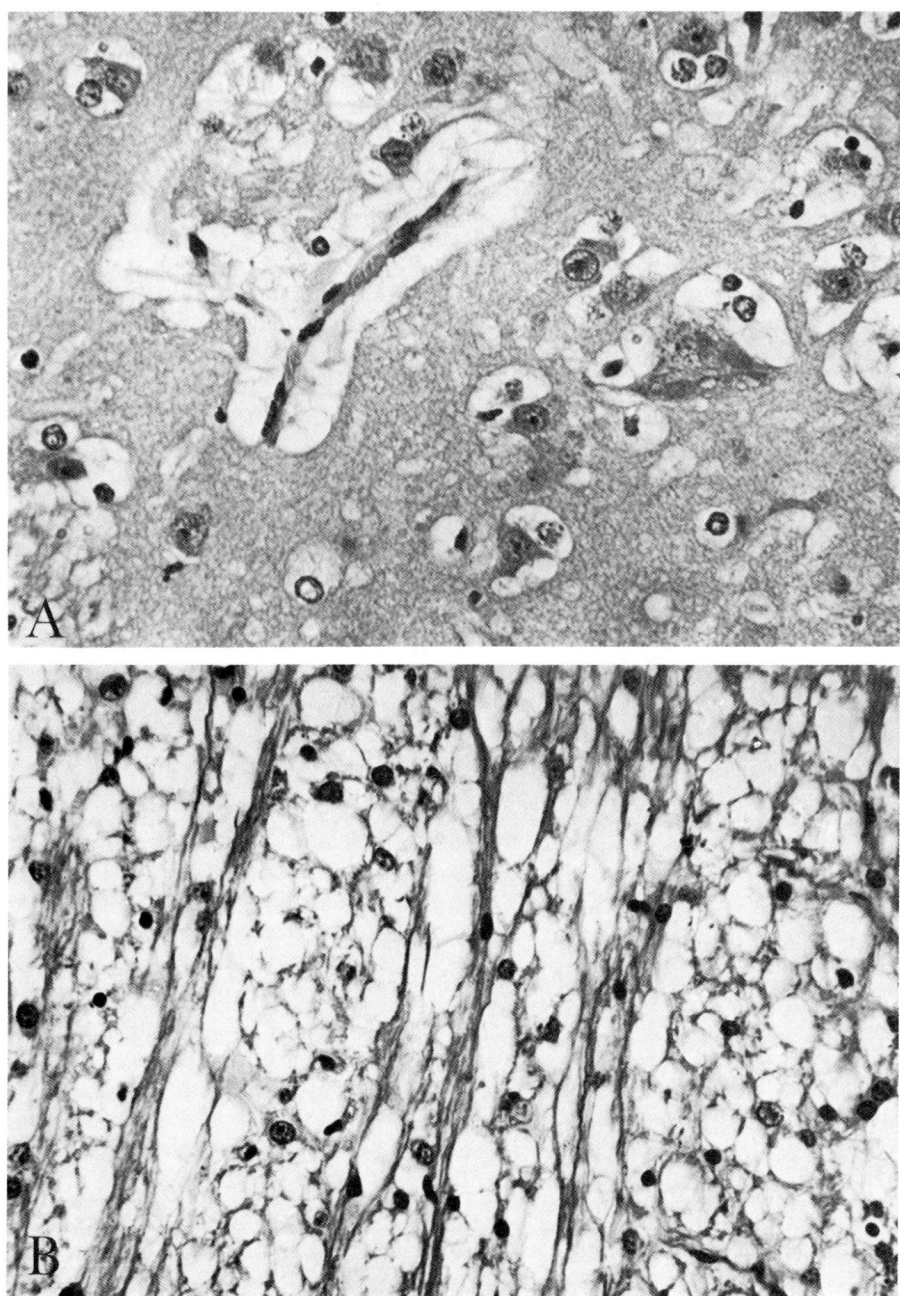

Fig. 27-13. Congenital brain edema of Hereford calves. *A,* Swollen hydropic astrocytes including foot processes around capillaries. *B,* Vacuolation of white matter. (Courtesy of Dr. R.D. Jolly.)

encephalopathy, scrapie in sheep, and kuru and Creutzfeldt-Jacob disease in human beings.

Hepatic Disease and Spongy Degeneration. Other examples of vacuolation of the central nervous system are occasionally encountered in most species of animals but the cause usually is not determined. Hooper (1975) believes that many of these represent a distinct entity as part of a hepatocerebral syndrome. He demonstrated underlying hepatic disease in examples of spongy degeneration of the brain in cattle, sheep, goats, swine, horses, dogs, and rabbits. He has presented evidence to indicate that it results from hyperammonemia. Pyrrolizidine alkaloids were the principal cause of the hepatic disease, but other hepatotoxins, parasites, hepatic viral infection, and congestive heart failure are also associated with spongy degeneration in the central nervous system.

Alpers, M., and Rail, L.: Kuru and Creutzfeldt-Jakob disease: Clinical and aetiological aspects. Proc. Aust. Assoc. Neurol., 8:7–15, 1971.

Blood, D.C., and Gay, C.C.: Hereditary neuraxial oedema of calves. Aust. Vet. J., 47:520, 1971. Vet. Bull., 42:1988, 1972.

Cordy, D.R., Richards, W.P.C., and Stormont, C.: Hereditary neuraxial edema in Hereford calves. Pathol. Vet., 6:487–501, 1969.

Davis, G.B., Thompson, E.J., and Kyle, R.J.: Hereditary neuraxial oedema of calves. NZ Vet. J., 23:520, 1971.

Gibbs, C.J., Jr., and Gajdusek, D.C.: Experimental subacute spongiform virus encephalopathies in primates and other laboratory animals. Science, 182:67–68, 1973.

Hooper, P.T.: Spongy degeneration in the central nervous system of domestic animals. I. Morphology. II. Chemical analysis and vascular permeability studies. III. Occurrence and pathogenesis—hepatocerebral disease caused by hyperammonaemia. Acta Neuropathol., 31:325–334, 335–341, 343–351, 1975.

Jolly, R.D.: Congenital brain oedema of Hereford calves. J. Pathol., 114:199–204, 1974.

Kelly, D.F., and Gaskell, C.J.: Spongy degeneration of the central nervous system in kittens. Acta Neuropathol., 35:151–158, 1976.

Weaver, A.D.: (Hereditary neuraxial oedema in polled Hereford calves.) DTW, 81:572–573, 1974.

Equine Incoordination (Ataxia of Foals)

A disease of young horses and mules, in which nonparalytic disturbances of gait are significant features, is referred to as equine incoordination, ataxia of foals, or "wobbles." The colloquial name is derived from the horseman's description of the incoordinated or wobbling gait of affected animals. Horses characteristically display the signs of this disorder during the first four years of life. The etiology is unknown.

The usual history indicates that severe symptoms become evident suddenly, usually after an accident such as a fall, but careful clinical observers report that the onset is, in reality, insidious. In the opinion of Jones, the accident accentuates the incoordination, bringing it to the owner's attention, but the usual sequence of events is that the animal's inability to coordinate muscle groups precedes and brings about the fall. There is no measurable loss of strength in the muscles, but rather a failure to synchronize their action, causing the animal to weave from side to side as it walks. The rear quarters are usually affected first, the incoordination later spreading to the forelimbs. The animal walks with its hind feet spread apart, has difficulty in turning and particularly in backing. The rear quarters sway from side to side during the walk or trot. After falls, which may be frequent, the animal has difficulty in regaining its feet. In early cases pressure on the neck in the anterior cervical region, or turning the head to one side will accentuate the "wobbling" and may cause the horse to fall. Slight excess mobility in the cervical region may be detected in early cases. The course is unpredictable. Affected animals may survive, with care, for years, or without warning, be found dead in pasture—apparently as the result of a fall. Paralysis is not a manifestation except in those singular cases in which subdural hemorrhage occurs in the cervical region. Affected animals are usually sacrificed as useless.

Lesions. The lesions in equine incoordination are confined to the spinal column and spinal cord. Distortion of the spinal canal may be seen in most cases at necropsy. Apparent relaxation of the intervertebral ligaments, particularly between the second and third, third and fourth, or fifth and sixth cervical vertebrae, allows them to become misaligned, giving the spinal canal a tortuous course. This kyphoscoliosis in some cases produces obvious constriction of the spinal canal and hence focal pressure upon the spinal cord. Osteoarthritis involving the vertebral joints

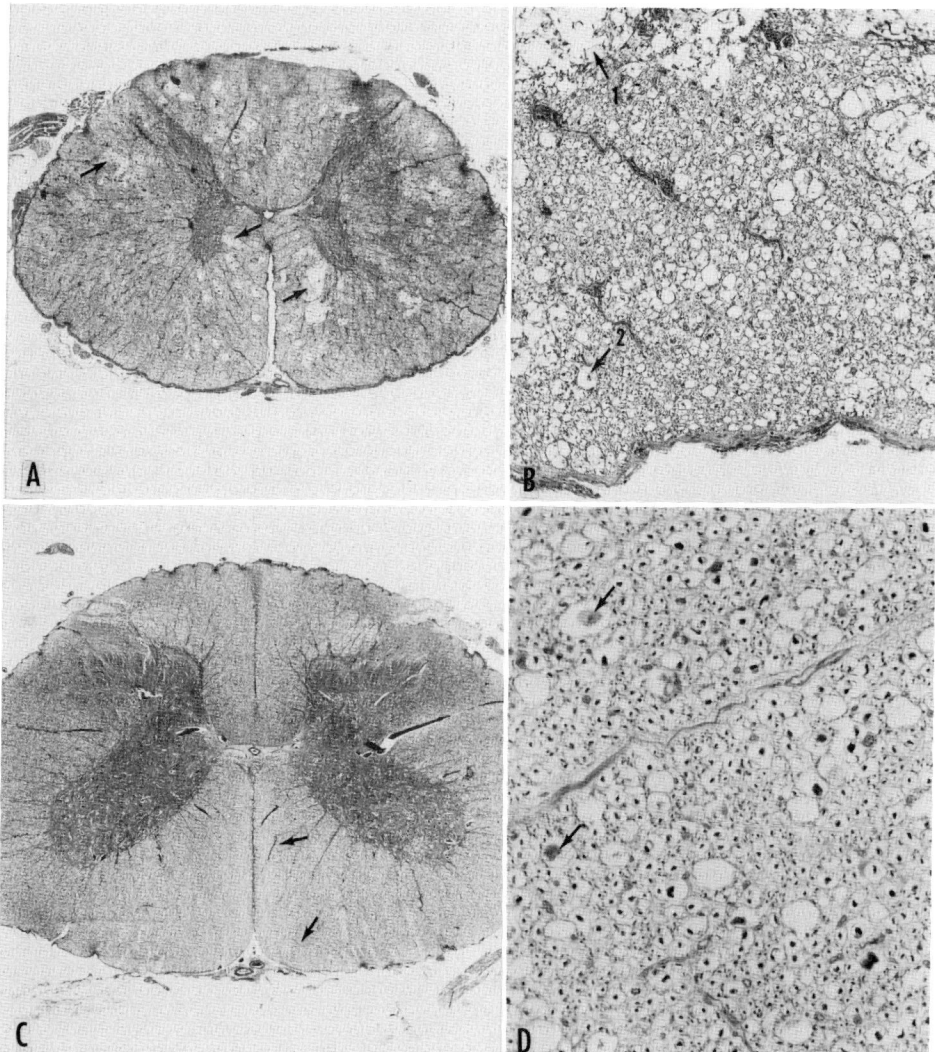

Fig. 27–14. Ataxia of foals (equine incoordination). *A,* Spinal cord (× 8) at level of junction of third and fourth cervical vertebrae. Areas of malacia (arrows) in several parts of white matter. The primary lesion. *B,* Same section as *A* (× 100). Large irregular spaces (*1*) and swollen axis sheaths (*2*). *C,* Spinal cord of same animal at level of the fifth cervical vertebra (× 8). Secondary (wallerian) degeneration is limited to certain fasciculi (arrows) adjacent to the ventral median fissure. *D,* Higher magnification (× 205) of secondary degeneration in *C*. Arrows indicate some swollen axons surrounded by a dilated axis sheath. (*D,* Courtesy of Armed Forces Institute of Pathology.) Contributor: Dr. E.R. Doll.

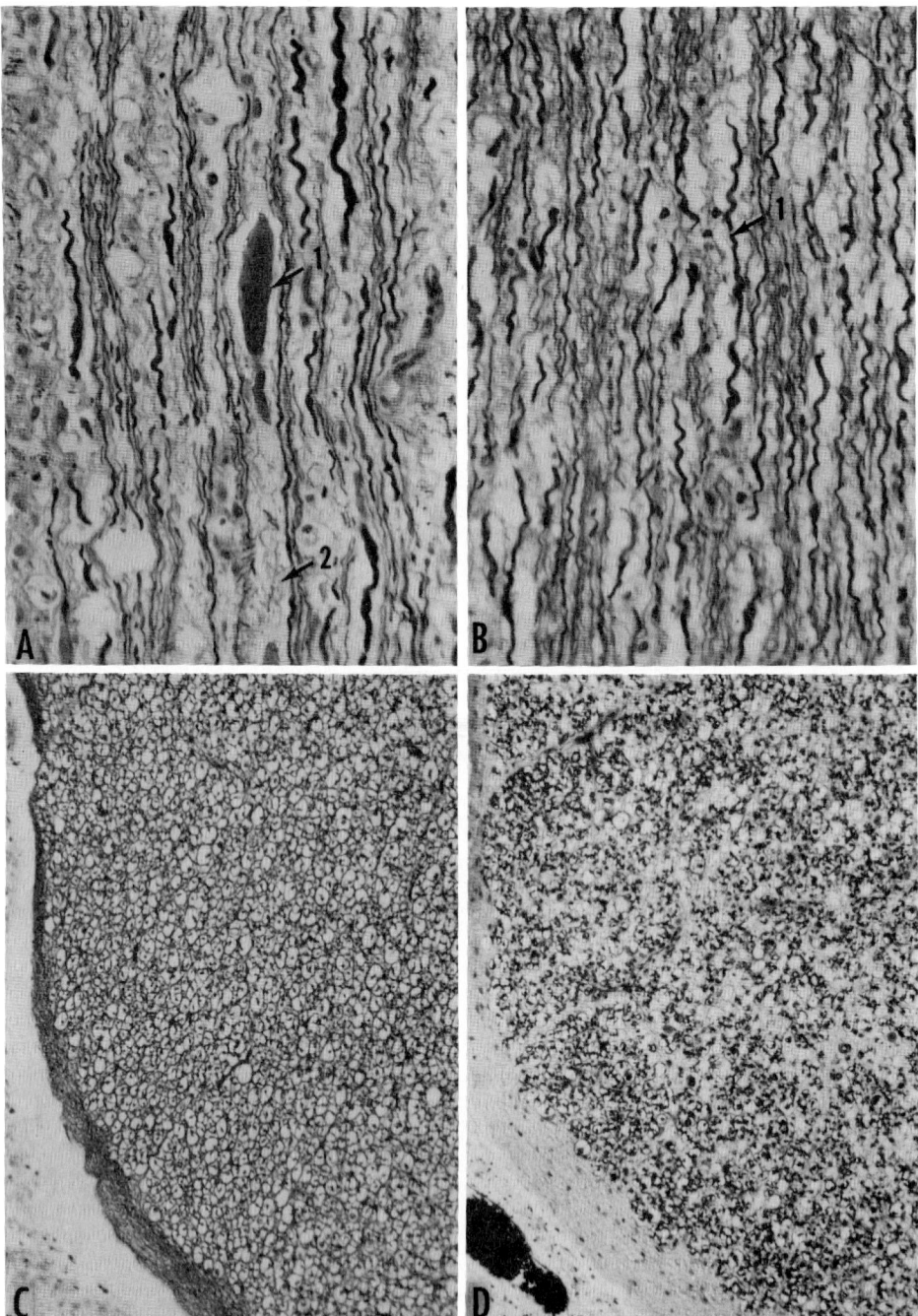

Fig. 27–15. Wallerian degeneration in equine incoordination. *A,* Longitudinal section (× 205) of an affected fasciculus in the cervical cord. Weil's stain. Enlarged, fragmented axon (*1*) and glial fibers (*2*). *B,* Normal spinal cord. Weil's stain. Axons (*1*) are of uniform width and surrounded by an intact myelin sheath. *C,* Normal spinal cord (× 100). Weil's stain. Note uniform size of myelin sheaths. Axons appear as dots within each myelin sheath. *D,* Cross section of an affected spinal cord (× 100). Weil's stain. Note irregular size of axons, disorganization and pale areas of glial scarring. (Courtesy of Armed Forces Institute of Pathology.) All contributed by Dr. E.R. Doll.

may be present, as evidenced by erosion of the joint cartilage and eburnation of the underlying bone. These articular lesions have been explained on the basis of excessive movement of the vertebrae; however, this is not firmly established.

In the spinal cord, gross lesions are not evident in most cases, although subdural hemorrhage may be present in the upper cervical region of a few animals dying after a fall or found dead in pasture. The microscopic lesions are characteristic but may be overlooked in casual or hurried examinations. Careful examination of many sections will usually disclose a primary zone of malacia in the cervical region, usually in relation to a constricted segment of the spinal canal. This primary malacic area in the cord usually is seen as several ragged cavities scattered through various white columns, although sometimes there is only one cavity. Loss of neurons in the gray columns may occur at this site but is not conspicuous, the white matter exhibiting the most severe changes. In these foci of malacia, the large, irregular, empty cavities are presumably the result of pooling of myelin and liquefaction necrosis. Swollen axons may be detected in cross section. Increased numbers of glial cells are present and gitter cells may be evident.

This "primary" focus of malacia in the upper cervical region is sharply delimited, only a few centimeters in length, but more than one such focus can occur. In cases with only one primary focus, its limits may be clearly defined by microscopic examination of transverse sections of the spinal cord on either side of the lesion. Above (cephalad to) the lesion, wallerian degeneration is seen in ascending nerve fibers, which for the most part are located in the dorsal funiculi. Caudal to this cervical lesion, wallerian degeneration will be seen in descending fibers. While such affected fibers may be found in lateral funiculi, they are more constant in ventral funiculi. In the lower cervical region the affected fibers are concentrated in the ventral funiculi on

either side of the ventral median fissure. Lesions in these columns may extend well into the thoracic and lumbar cord.

The lesions in ventral funiculi are bilaterally symmetric and typical of wallerian degeneration of any nerve tract, i.e., resulting from injury to the axon at a point nearer the nerve cell body. In early cases, swollen axon sheaths give this tissue a vacuolated, spongy appearance in contrast to the normal white column, in which the myelin sheaths are uniform in diameter. The axons are distorted, enlarged to many times their normal dimensions in some segments and broken off at other points along their course. In transverse sections these affected axons may appear as spherical, dark staining structures or may be absent. In sections cut parallel to the length of the tract, the axons appear thickened at some points, absent at others. Glial cells are increased in number and eventually replace the destroyed nerve fibers, giving the affected column a scarred appearance (gliosis). This change is best demonstrated microscopically by means of Weil's stain.

The diagnosis of equine incoordination may be established at necropsy by demonstration of characteristic gross and microscopic lesions in the spinal column and spinal cord.

Fraser, H., and Palmer, A.C.: Equine incoordination and wobbler disease of young horses. Vet. Rec., 80:338–355, 1967.

Jones, T.C., Doll, E.R., and Brown, R.G.: The pathology of equine incoordination (ataxia or "wobbles" of foals). Proc. 91st Ann. Meeting Am. Vet. Med. Assoc., 1954, pp. 139–149.

Matthias, D., Dietz, O., and Rechenberg, R.: (Clinical features and pathology of spinal ataxia in foals.) Arch. Exp. Veterinaermed. (Suppl.), 19:43–72, 1965. V.B. 36:1528, 1966.

Mayhew, I.G., deLahunta, A., Whitlock, R.H., and Geary, J.C.: Equine degenerative myeloencephalopathy. J. Am. Vet. Med. Assoc., 170:195–201, 1977.

Rooney, J.R.: Equine incoordination. I. Gross morphology. Cornell Vet., 53:411–422, 1963.

Rooney, J.R., Prickett, M.E., Delaney, F.M., and Drowe, M.W.: Focal myelitis-encephalitis in horses. Cornell Vet., 50:494–501, 1970.

Focal Symmetric Poliomalacia of Sheep

A singular paralytic disease of sheep seen on a farm located in the Rift Valley of Kenya, Africa, was described by Innes and Plowright (1955). The disease was first noticed between February and April 1952, in 10 of 40 lambs two to four months of age. The following year, 60 of 240 animals in the flock died from the disease and this outbreak also involved older animals. The disease apparently did not spread to other farms, but the unusual clinical and pathologic features it displayed justify its inclusion in this chapter.

The disease was sudden in onset, only a few sheep exhibiting premonitory signs such as motor weakness or incoordination of the forelimbs. Flaccid paralysis usually developed rapidly in all limbs, but in some instances spasticity was a feature. Only the forelimbs of some sheep were involved and animals thus affected hopped about on their hind legs like kangaroos during the days or weeks they survived. The muscles of the fixed, adducted front limbs usually underwent atrophy if the animal survived for some time, but most of them died within three weeks. The disease was afebrile and apparently not transmissible from one sheep to another. Cattle in the same pasture did not contract the disease.

Lesions. The lesions were limited to the spinal cord and could be recognized only upon microscopic examination. Symmetric malacic lesions in the ventral gray columns—never in the dorsal columns—were limited to certain segments in the cervical enlargement, except for a few cases in which the lesions were confined to segments of the lumbar enlargement. In a typical case the lesions in the gray columns started at the level of the fourth cervical vertebra (C4), disappeared at C6 and appeared again at the level of C7 and the first thoracic vertebra (T1). In another case lesions were found between C4 and C6 as well as in the lumbar enlargement.

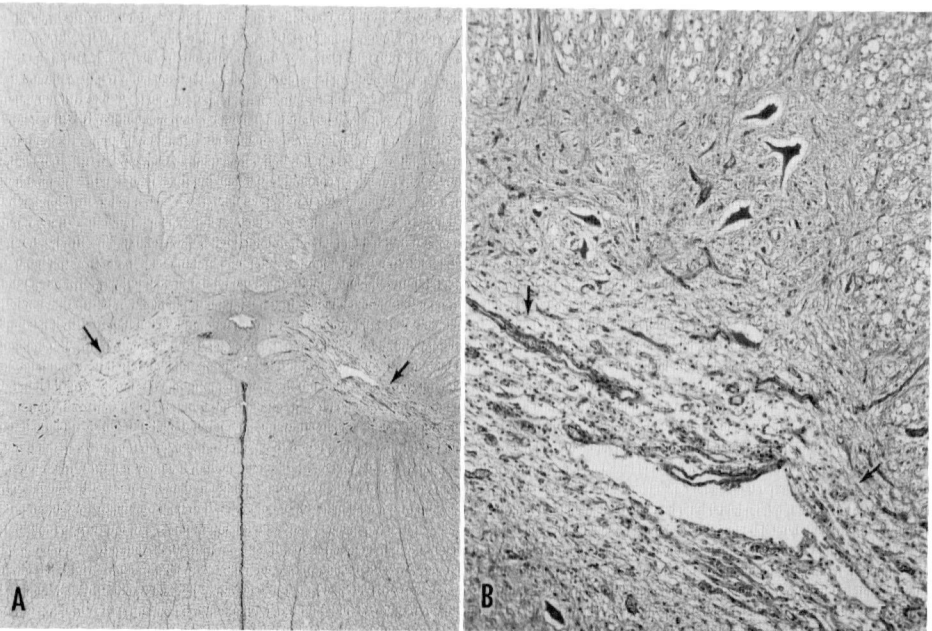

Fig. 27–16. Symmetrical poliomalacia of sheep. *A,* Spinal cord (× 16). Note symmetry of lesions in each of the ventral horns of gray matter (arrows). *B,* Higher magnification (× 110) of the malacic lesion in the gray matter (arrows). (*B,* Courtesy of Armed Forces Institute of Pathology.) Contributor: Dr. J.R.M. Innes.

Bilateral symmetry was particularly striking, the lesions in one ventral column being a mirror image of those in its opposite. These sharply delimited foci of malacia did not evoke a significant surrounding inflammatory reaction, but a rim of well-preserved gray matter containing neurons, was often evident around them and the commissural gray matter was intact. The involved areas of ventral gray matter were sharply demarcated, pale staining, with the neurons replaced by a ragged, spongy appearing lesion in which capillaries and glial fibers were predominant. In early lesions gitter cells were numerous, while in later stages astrocytes and newly proliferated capillaries filled the area of softening. Neither vascular lesions nor demyelination were observed in white columns.

The significance of this disease is not clear at this time, but it is an interesting addition to the growing list of pathologic entities that result in neurologic disturbances in sheep.

The diagnosis was made upon demonstration of the bilaterally symmetrical malacic lesions in the spinal cord of sheep which exhibited characteristic symptoms.

Innes, J.R.M., and Plowright, W.: Focal symmetrical poliomalacia of sheep in Kenya. J. Neuropathol. Exp. Neurol., *14*:185–197, 1955.
Pienaar, J.G., and Thornton, D.J.: Focal symmetrical encephalomalacia in sheep in South Africa. J. S. Afr. Vet. Med. Assoc., *35*:351–358, 1964. V.B. *35*:1051, 1965.

Polioencephalomalacia of Cattle and Sheep

The lesions of a noninfectious nervous disease of cattle, sheep, and goats known in certain western states as "forage poisoning" or "blind staggers," have been characterized by Jensen, Griner and Adams (1956) as necrotizing destruction of cortical gray matter, therefore the disease was named "polioencephalomalacia." These authors estimated that the incidence of this disease in cattle reached 100 per thousand animals in some regions of Colorado. The disorder was more frequently observed in cattle from 12 to 18 months of age; sheep of all ages were less often affected. The incidence increased during January among cattle in feedlots, while the incidence among those in pasture was highest in July. The disease has been recognized in cattle and sheep in Great Britain, where it is usually referred to as "cerebrocortical necrosis." The disease is also reported in ruminants in Australia and is apparently of worldwide distribution.

The dramatic response of certain clinical cases, diagnosed as polioencephalomalacia, to the administration of thiamine first suggested that this vitamin might be involved in some way in the etiology. Additional evidence pointing toward thiamine deficiency soon followed. Affected animals have increased levels of blood pyruvate, lactate, creatinine, phosphokinase, and pyruvate kinase, and low levels of thiamine in the brain and liver. Thiaminase has been identified in the rumen, a thiaminase-producing bacterium has been recovered from the rumen, and the disease has been reproduced by thiamine antagonists. Thiaminase can also cause depletion of nicotinic acid (a cosubstrate), but the possible role of the additional deficiency of this nutrient to the pathogenesis of the disease is uncertain. What appears to be the same entity has been described in Cuba in feedlot cattle fed a molasses-urea-based diet. Pyruvate oxidation was blocked, but brain and liver thiamine concentrations were normal. Thus the pathogenesis and definite etiologic role of thiamine remains to be incontrovertibly established. Thiamine deficiency diseases are further discussed in Chapter 17 (see also Bracken fern and *Equisetum* poisoning).

Clinical Manifestations. As originally described, the clinical manifestations in severely affected animals start with muscular tremors, twitching of the ears, eyelids, and facial muscles, followed in some in-

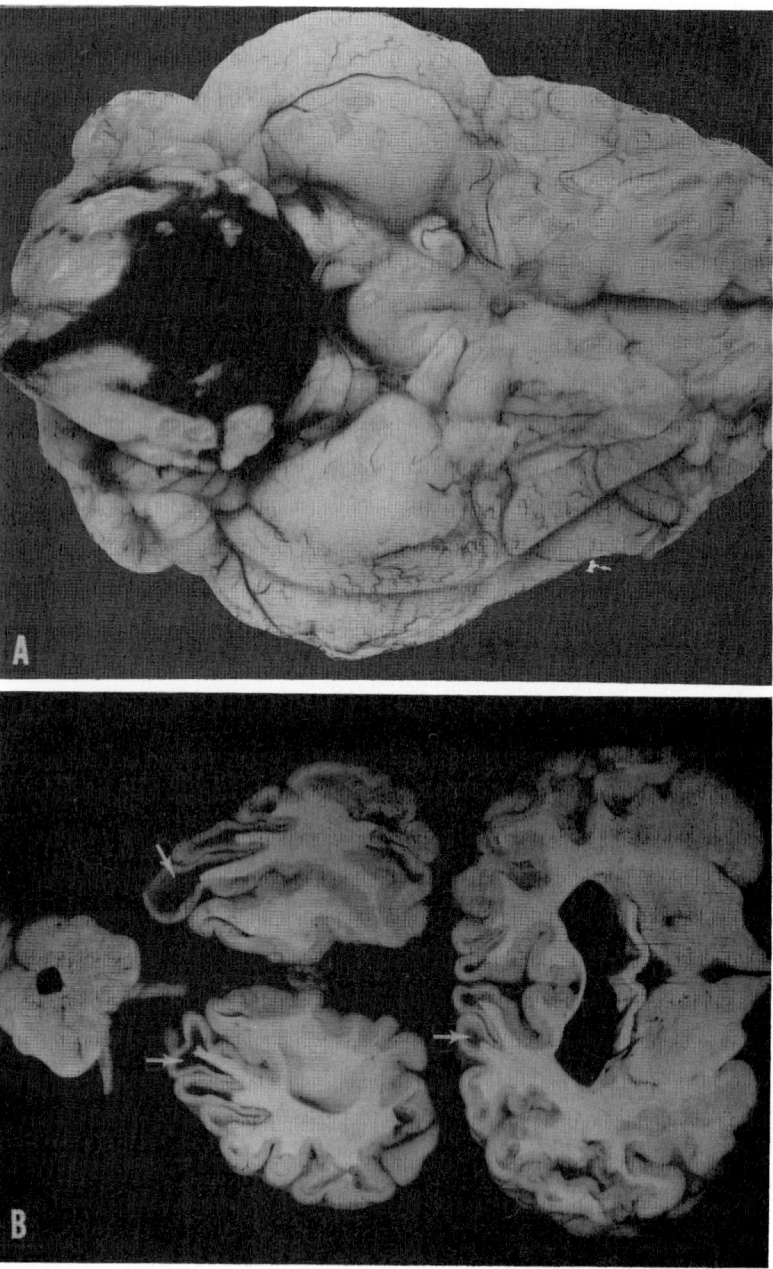

Fig. 27–17. *A,* Hemorrhage from the basilar artery, brain of a pig that was struck a blow on the forehead. *B,* Polioencephalomalacia in a young calf. Note cavities (arrows) in subcortical zones in the cerebrum.

stances by convulsions. Affected animals are unable to see, although no lesions can be detected in the eyes. Visible mucous membranes become injected; respiration and pulse rates accelerated, and temperature sometimes elevated. Mildly affected animals, seen more frequently during the summer months among those in pastures, separate themselves from the herd and occasionally push their heads against solid objects. They are unable to see, apathetic, and often exhibit purposeless masticatory movements accompanied by excessive salivation and, occasionally, twitching of facial or ear muscles. Death occurs in 50 to 90% of affected animals, depending upon the severity of the disorder.

The specific **lesions** are limited to the central nervous system, the changes in the cerebrum being most striking in the cortex, where focal, later diffuse, liquefaction necrosis destroys most of the gray matter. The adjacent white matter is spared. The cerebral convolutions thus collapse and give the appearance in cross section of having been sculptured away, appearing in bas relief against the underlying white matter. This gives the impression that the brain has decreased in size. Internal hydrocephalus is often recognized in severely affected brains.

This selective malacia is seen microscopically to affect only the gray matter, subcortical white matter showing only vascularization, a few gitter cells and occasional perivascular lymphocytic aggregations in regions adjacent to affected gray cortex. In light microscopy neurons appear to become necrotic first, but all cells are eventually involved in the areas of necrosis. Ultrastructural studies (Morgan, 1973) have, however, demonstrated that the earliest lesion is an increase in fluid in the cytoplasm of astrocytes and a perineuronal sponginess or vacuolation (edema) resulting from dilated astrocytic processes. In the cerebellum, necrosis of the granular layer precedes loss of Purkinje cells. Occasional

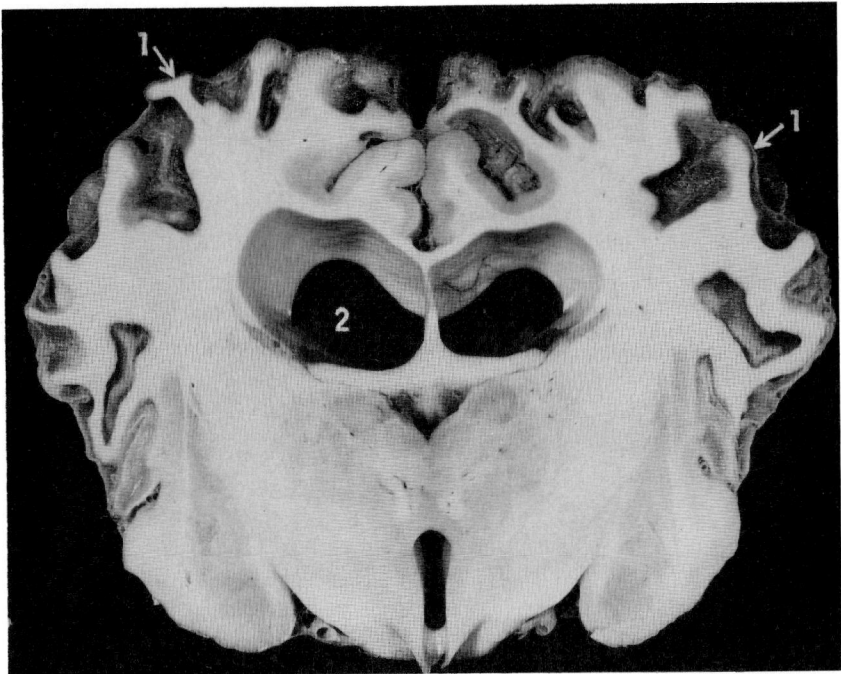

Fig. 27–18. Polioencephalomalacia, brain of a cow. Note loss of cortical gray matter (*1*) and hydrocephalus (*2*). (Courtesy of Drs. Jean C. Flint and Rue Jensen, Colorado State University.)

cystic cavities are observed, but in most cases debris is removed promptly by "gitter cells." Gliosis, with gemistocytic astrocytes predominating, is the usual change adjacent to cortical areas from which all viable tissue has been removed by liquefaction necrosis.

Anonymous: Thiamine deficiency in ruminants? Nutr. Rev., 27:176–178, 1968.

Deutsch, K.: An electron microscopical study of the cerebral cortex of the calf. II. The calf with amprolium-induced cerebrocortical necrosis. Zentralbl. Veterinaermed. (A), 20:692–698, 1973.

Edwin, E.E., and Jackman, R.: Thiaminase 1 in the development of cerebrocortical necrosis in sheep and cattle. Nature, 228:772–774, 1970.

Edwin, E.E., Lewis, G., and Allcroft, R.: Cerebrocortical necrosis: A hypothesis for the possible role of thiaminases in its pathogenesis. Vet. Rec., 83:176–177, 1968.

Evans, W.C., et al.: Induction of thiamine deficiency in sheep, with lesions similar to those of cerebrocortical necrosis. J. Comp. Pathol., 85:253–267, 1975.

Fenwick, D.C.: Polioencephalomalacia of sheep. Response to thiamine in a single case. Aust. Vet. J., 43:484, 1967.

Jarrett, J.: Thiaminase-induced encephalopathy (a review). Vet. Med. Small Anim. Clin., 65:704–708, 1970.

Jensen, R., Griner, L.A., and Adams, O.R.: Polioencephalomalacia of cattle and sheep. J. Am. Vet. Med. Assoc., 129:311–321, 1956.

Lilja, C.-G.: Cerebro-cortical necrosis (C.C.N.) in calf. An experimental reproduction of the disease. Acta Vet. Scand., 14:464–473, 1973.

———: Pyrimidinyl nicotinic acid and cerebrocortical necrosis. Acta Vet. Scand., 16:24–30, 1975.

Little, P.B.: Biochemical and pathologic studies of thiamin deficiency and polioencephalomalacia of cattle. Diss. Abstr. Int., 30B:4449–4450, 1970.

Markson, L.M., et al.:The aetiology of cerebrocortical necrosis: The effects of administering antimetabolites of thiamine to preruminant calves. Br. Vet. J., 128:488–499, 1972.

Markson, L.M., Terlecki, S., and Lewis, G.: Cerebrocortical necrosis in calves. Vet. Rec., 79:578–579, 1966.

Markson, L.M., and Terlecki, S.: The aetiology of cerebrocortical necrosis. Br. Vet. J., 124:309–315, 1968.

Mella, C.M., Margolles, E., and Loew, F.M.: Epinephrine-induced hyperglycemia in bulls and its relationship to polioencephalomalacia. Can. J. Comp. Med., 39:321–323, 1975.

Mella, C.M., Perez-Oliva, O., and Loew, F.M.: Induction of bovine polioencephalomalacia with a feeding system based on molasses and urea. Can. J. Comp. Med., 40:104–110, 1976.

Morgan, K.T.: An ultrastructural study of ovine polio-encephalomalacia. J. Pathol., 110:123–130, 1973.

Morgan, K.T., Coop, R.L., and Doxey, D.L.: Amprolium poisoning of preruminant lambs: An investigation of the encephalopathy and the haemorrhagic and diarrhoeic syndromes. J. Pathol., 116:73–81, 1975.

Morgan, K.T., and Lawson, G.H.K.: Thiaminase type 1-producing bacilli and ovine polioencephalomalacia. Vet. Rec., 95:361–363, 1974.

Peirson, R.E., and Jensen, R.: Polioencephalomalacia in feedlot lambs. J. Am. Vet. Med. Assoc., 166:257–259, 1975.

Pill, A.H.: Evidence of thiamine deficiency in calves affected with cerebrocortical necrosis. Vet. Rec., 81:178–181, 1967.

Roberts, G.W., and Boyd, J.W.: Cerebrocortical necrosis in ruminants. Occurrence of thiaminase in the gut of normal and affected animals and its effect on thiamine status. J. Comp. Pathol., 84:365–374, 1974.

Smith, M.C.: Polioencephalomalacia in goats. J. Am. Vet. Med. Assoc., 174:1328–1332, 1979.

LEUKODYSTROPHIES AND LIPIDODYSTROPHIES OF THE CENTRAL NERVOUS SYSTEM (NEURONAL STORAGE DISEASES)

Several inherited disorders of myelin, lipid, and glycoprotein metabolism lead to demyelination or dysmyelination and the accumulation of various metabolites within neurons or macrophages in the brain and often other tissues. In each, the basic defect is a specific enzyme deficiency. These disorders are discussed as a group in Chapter 2. Those that affect the central nervous system include Tay-Sachs disease (GM_2 gangliosidosis), globoid cell leukodystrophy (Krabbe's disease), metachromatic leukodystrophy, Niemann-Pick disease, Gaucher's disease, LaFora's disease, and sudanophilic leukodystrophy.

RETICULOSIS OF THE CENTRAL NERVOUS SYSTEM OF DOGS

In the course of study of more than a thousand neoplasms of the central nervous system of dogs, Fankhauser et al. (1972) distinguished 50 cases which they classified under the term "reticulosis of the central nervous system." This term was proposed earlier (Luginbühl, 1964; Luginbühl et al. 1968; Fankhauser et al., 1968) and based on a reasoned study of the evidence for the occurrence in man and animals of tumors and inflammatory lesions arising from the reticulohistiocytic elements of the brain. The cells of origin were believed to be the microglia, which are histiocytes existing on the neuropil side of the vascular limiting membrane. The existence of the "reticuloendothelial" system has been questioned and the exact origin of the cells has not yet been determined. Use of the term "reticulosis" presents a convenient and not unwieldy designation for the lesions described by Fankhauser et al. (1972) until more precise diagnosis, based on etiology, may be possible. They described lesions under three subheadings of granulomatous reticulosis, neoplastic reticulosis, and microgliomatosis.

The characteristic histologic features depend upon the association of the lesions with the vasculature. The proliferating cells accumulate around the vessels, forming concentric laminations in this perivascular location. Some are in isolated aggregations, separated from each other by intact nervous parenchyma; others form large, solid, tumor-like nodules. They are most extensive in the white matter of the cerebral hemispheres and in the brain stem. Rarely do the cells extend into the cerebral cortex. The leptomeninges are occasionally moderately involved, but in only a few cases are extensive meningeal infiltrations found. The spinal cord was involved in seven cases, but was not examined in all cases, so the extent of involvement cannot be stated.

Granulomatous reticulosis is used to designate those cases in which the proliferating cells are cellular elements of granulomatous proliferation, namely lymphocytes, monocytes, plasma cells, and reticulohistiocytes, with varying mixtures of granulocytes and multinucleated giant cells. Epithelioid (histiocytic) cells are also observed in syncytial nodules. These cells are large with ill-defined cytoplasm and small round or oval eccentric nuclei. In all but four of the ten cases of this type, no glial nodules were evident, but in these

four, disseminated encephalitis was present in addition to the granulomatous parts.

Neoplastic reticulosis is the term used to describe cases in which the typical cell is a large reticulohistiocyte with abundant cytoplasm and a round vesicular nucleus. In addition to these cells, which are often in mitosis, an admixture of lymphocytes, plasma cells, and eosinophil granulocytes are present. Giant cells with single or multiple nuclei are often present. Reticulum stains reveal a concentric pattern around many blood vessels and an intimate relationship of reticulum fibers with many of the tumor cells.

Microgliomatosis is the word used to describe diffuse and perivascular infiltrations of the neuropil by cells with large hyperchromatic nuclei and little visible cytoplasm. Mitotic figures are present in these areas also. The appearance of these cells and the lack of reticulin fibers suggested the use of the term microgliomatosis.

The clinical manifestations recorded in the literature include many neurologic signs, as would be expected with lesions involving large areas of the central nervous system. These include changes in behavior, depression, apathy or excitement and restlessness, ataxia, paresis of varying extent, epileptiform convulsions, other seizures, circling and other unmotivated movements, abnormal reflexes, impaired vision, neurovegetative disorders (anorexia, vomiting, allotriophagia), and salivation. No breed, age, or sex predisposition has been found.

Similar but not identical cases in dogs have been described under the term "canine granulomatous meningoencephalomyelitis" (Cordy, 1979). Until etiologic factors can be determined, it does not appear that exact comparisons can be made among the cases described in the literature.

Braund, K.D., Vandevelde, M., Walker, T.L., and Redding, R.W.: Granulomatous meningoencephalomyelitis in six dogs. J. Am. Vet. Med. Assoc., 172:1195–1200, 1978.

Cordy, D.R.: Canine granulomatous meningoencephalomyelitis. Vet. Pathol., *16*:325–333, 1979.

Fankhauser, R., and Luginbühl, H.: Zentrales Nervensystem. *In* Handbook der speziellen
pathologischen Anatomie der Haustiere, edited
by E. Joest. Vol. 3. Berlin, Parey, 1968, pp. 191–
436.

Fankhauser, R., Fatzer, R., Luginbühl, H., and
McGrath, J.T.: Reticulosis of the central nervous
system (CNS) in dogs. Adv. Vet. Sci. Comp.
Med., *16*:35–71, 1972.

Luginbühl, H.: A comparative study of neoplasms of
the central nervous system in animals. Acta
Neurochir. [Suppl.], *10*:30–42, 1964.

Luginbühl, H., Fankhauser, R., and McGrath, J.T.:
Spontaneous tumors of the nervous system in
animals. Prog. Neurol. Surg., *2*:85–164, 1968.

Koestner, A., and Zeman, W.: Primary reticulosis of
the central nervous system in dogs. Am. J. Vet.
Res., *23*:381–393, 1962.

NEOPLASMS OF NERVOUS TISSUE

Neoplasms arising in nervous tissue, ordinarily in the brain, come chiefly from the
neuroglia, and those having this source are
known as **gliomas.**

Gliomas. Gliomas can be subdivided
into a great many groups or varieties, but
the classes commonly recognized are (1)
astrocytoma; (2) *glioblastoma multiforme;* (3)
medulloblastoma, all varieties of which arise
from astrocytes or early, undifferentiated
forms of neuroglial tissue; (4) *ependymoma,*
which arises from the ependymal lining
cells; and (5) *oligodendroglioma.* These represent the recognized types of neuroglial
tissue except the microglia, which does not
form tumors. These classes are not sharply
demarcated and some gliomas partake of
the characteristics of two different classes.
The several classes of gliomas are characterized by different rates of growth, so that
the terms benign and malignant are used to
refer to them, but no glioma metastasizes
to locations outside the cranial cavity (or
spinal canal). Infiltration to adjoining areas
of the brain, however, is marked in the case
of the more malignant types, so that grossly
and even microscopically it may be difficult to discern the limits of the tumor.

In man, the usual location, biologic history, operability, and outcome are well

known with respect to each class of tumor.
Judging by the comparatively few cases of
glioma reported in animals, it appears that
this information has only a limited application to veterinary surgical problems. As
more case-records accumulate, our knowledge of these aspects of the gliomas found
in animals can be expected to increase. If
diagnosable, it would seem that surgical
treatment of such tumors need not be more
forbidding than it is in humans.

The **astrocytoma** varies considerably in
histologic appearance. Several different
types are recognized, whose description
would be beyond the scope of this work. In
general, the cells have round or somewhat
elongated nuclei which are relatively pale,
although chromatin granules can be seen.
The nuclei, which are rather sparsely distributed, may or may not be accompanied
by a poorly outlined cytoplasm, but the
bulk of the internuclear space is occupied
by pink-staining fibrils which crisscross in
various directions. This tumor occurs in
almost any part of the brain and is among
those of lesser malignancy. Astrocytomas
are most frequently seen in dogs of the
brachycephalic breeds. They are rare in
other species.

The **glioblastoma multiforme** differs histologically from the astrocytoma in that its
nuclei are more deeply stained, highly irregular, and pleomorphic in size, shape,
and position. Tumor giant cells and multinucleated cells are frequent. In man, this
tumor is the most frequent of the gliomas,
as well as the most malignant, and is usually located in the cerebral hemispheres.
These are also most frequently encountered in brachycephalic breeds of dogs.

The **medulloblastoma,** arising from
embryonal glial tissue, consists of masses
of round cells with deeply staining, round
nuclei. It thus resembles a malignant lymphoma in its microscopic appearance. At
times there is formed a kind of "rosette"
consisting of a flower-like circle or radially
arranged nuclei around a tiny pale central

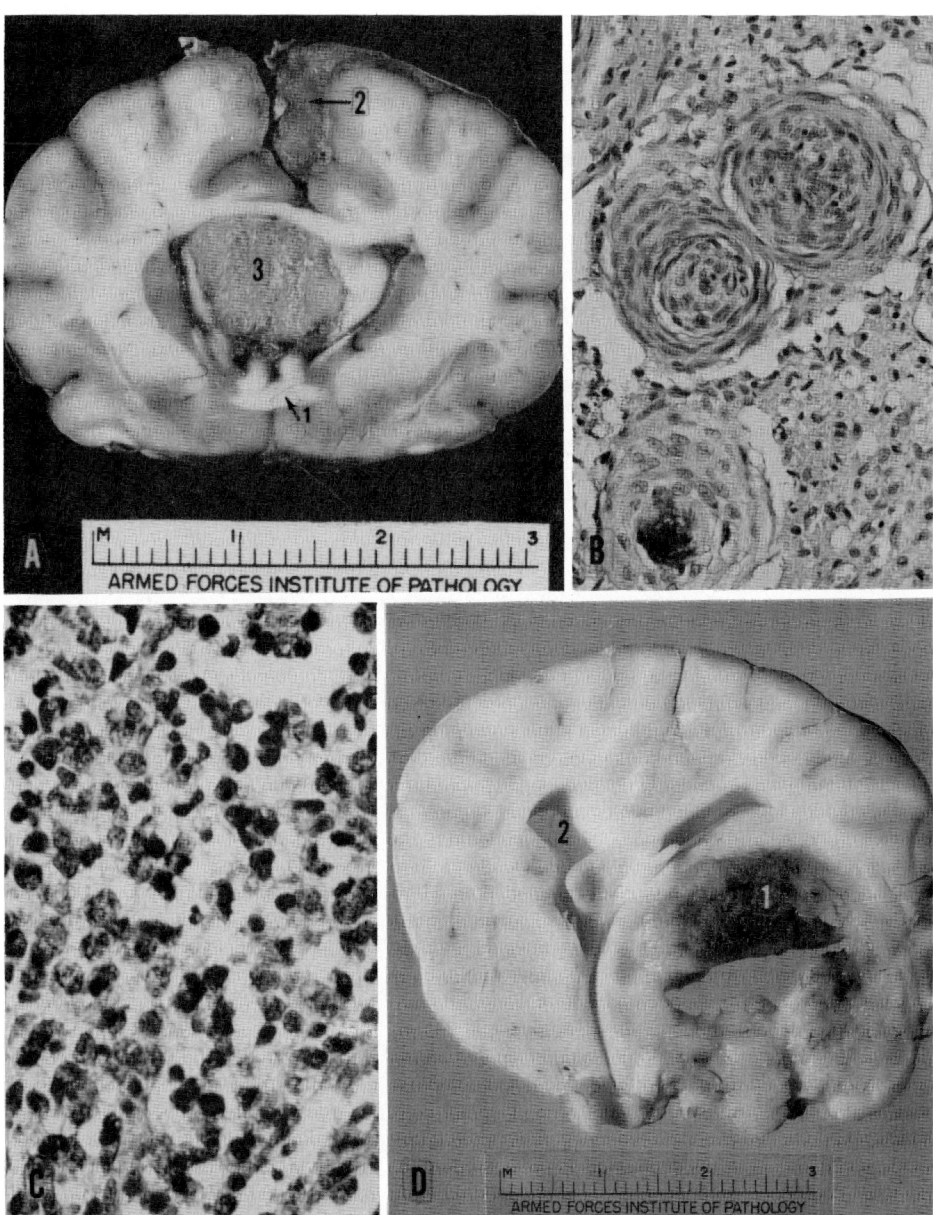

Fig. 27–19. *A*, Meningioma, brain of a 14-year-old castrated male cat. Section of brain through the anterior commissure (*1*), with tumor in pia (*2*) and in midline (*3*). *B*, Same tumor as *A* (× 210); note concentrically laminated structures. Contributor: Dr. J. Holzworth. *C*, Oligodendroglioma, brain of an eight-year-old female boxer. *D*, Gross specimen of same tumor. The tumor (*1*) displaces the midline. Slight hydrocephalus, lateral ventricle (*2*). (Courtesy of Armed Forces Institute of Pathology.) Contributor: Dr. L.N. Loomis.

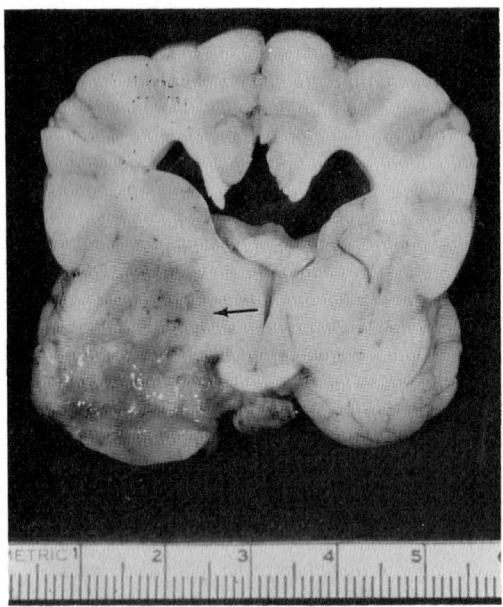

Fig. 27–20. Astrocytoma, right pyriform lobe of cerebrum of a nine-year-old castrated male Boxer. (Courtesy of Angell Memorial Animal Hospital.)

spot which may contain a capillary. Mitotic figures are numerous. This tumor occurs in young individuals and is located ordinarily just dorsal to the fourth ventricle, where it appears as a more or less spherical, discrete reddish-gray mass. Medulloblastomas are rare neoplasms. They occur most frequently in dogs and cattle, and have been reported in cats, swine, and mice.

The **ependymoma** consists of cells of medium size with irregularly rounded or polyhedral nuclei, which are centrally placed. The nuclei are moderately deep-staining; the cytoplasm, pink. The cells are put together in solid masses, broken here and there by a thin trabecula. Occasionally they reveal their innate tendency to line cavities by forming a tiny open space around which a single zone of cells is radially arranged. Such a structure is called a "rosette." Ependymomas form well-demarcated masses in the region of the fourth or the third ventricles, from whose lining they conceivably arise. They may

also arise from the lining of a choroid plexus and mimic its architecture with a papillary pattern of growth (*plexus papilloma*). Ependymomas are rare in all species, though most often seen in dogs, cats, and cattle.

The **oligodendroglioma,** not altogether rare in the dog, consists of polyhedral cells separated into compartments by thin trabeculae. The cytoplasm of the cells takes practically no stain by ordinary methods. This gives the tumor the appearance of rather small, round nuclei arranged alongside of, but separated from the trabeculae. The tumors infiltrate and destroy adjacent tissue. Mitotic figures are usually not frequent. Calcified granules equal to the size of several cells are often scattered through the tissue. Brachycephalic breeds are most prone to these tumors. There are a few reported examples in cats and cattle.

Pinealoma. This tumor, also known as pineal adenoma, is a rare neoplasm derived from the pineal body, or epiphysis cerebri. Its histologic appearance is distinctive in that it consists of an indiscriminate mingling of groups of large epithelioid cells with groups of small (neuroglial) cells with small round nuclei suggestive of lymphocytes. Sexual or other forms of precocity have accompanied some pinealomas in children, but these are suspected of being due to disturbance of nearby structures rather than to the direct effect of the tumors. A pinealoma has been reported in a silver fox, a horse, and a rat.

Cholesteatoma. This term relates to a tumor-like formation consisting of layers of epithelial-appearing cells containing so much cholesterol and other lipids that the gross tumor resembles a cluster of pearls. Some are in the brain tissue. In the horse, this term has been applied to a lesion in the choroid plexus which more appropriately should be called cholesterinic granuloma (Fig. 27–22). These are considered a result of degenerative processes and have been related to the granulomas. Those in the

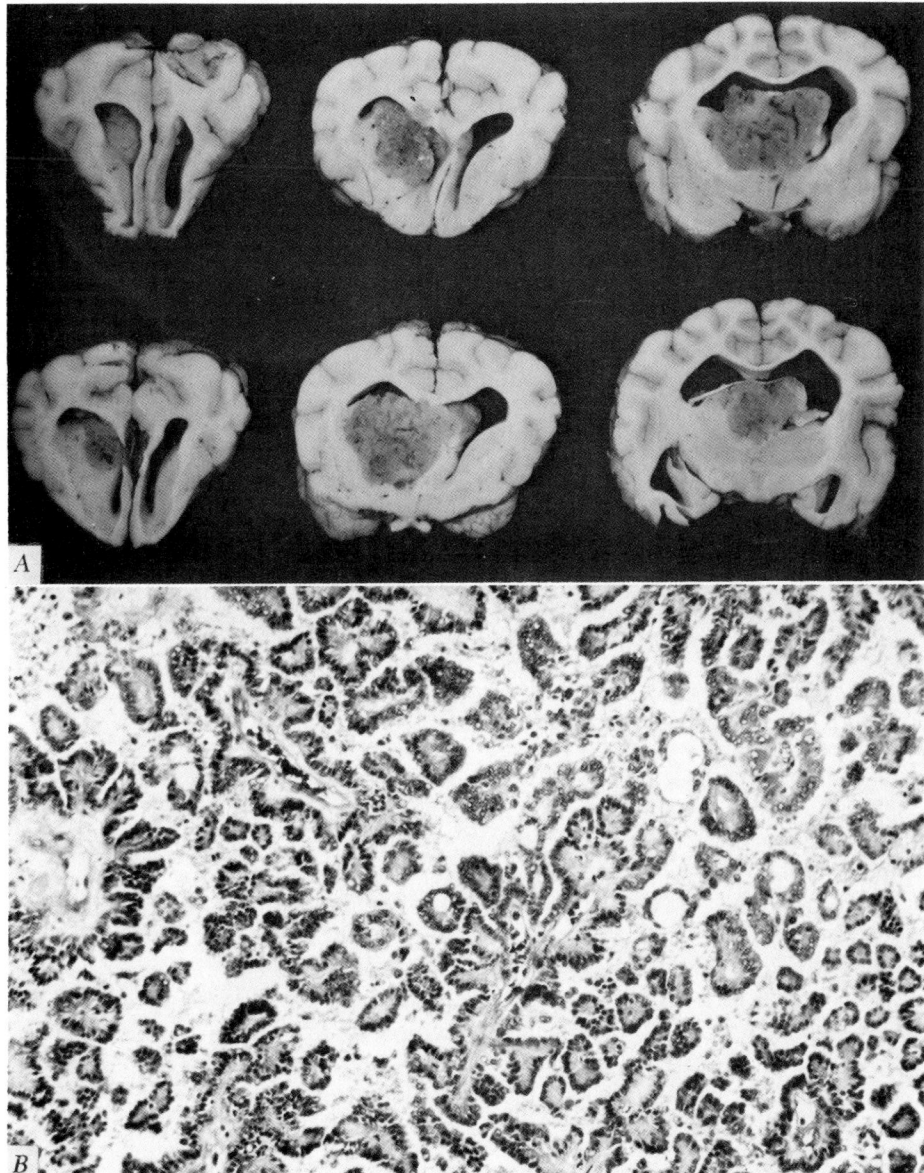

Fig. 27–21. Ependymoma, arising in third ventricle of an eight-year-old spayed female English Bulldog. *A*, The gross brain cut at 1-cm intervals. Note the deviation of the midline and the hydrocephalus of the lateral ventricles. *B*, Section of the tumor. (H & E, × 200.) (Courtesy of Angell Memorial Animal Hospital.)

brain tissue of man are said to be the result of epidermal or even dermal (dermoid cyst) remnants left there during embryonal development.

Psammoma. This is an old term used to designate intracranial tumors containing numerous calcified granules. Most of these were meningiomas, but some may have been overgrowths related to the cholesteatomas.

Neuroblastoma. These tumors consist of small, round cells of undifferentiated embryonal aspect. The microscopic appearance is similar to that of the medulloblastoma, to

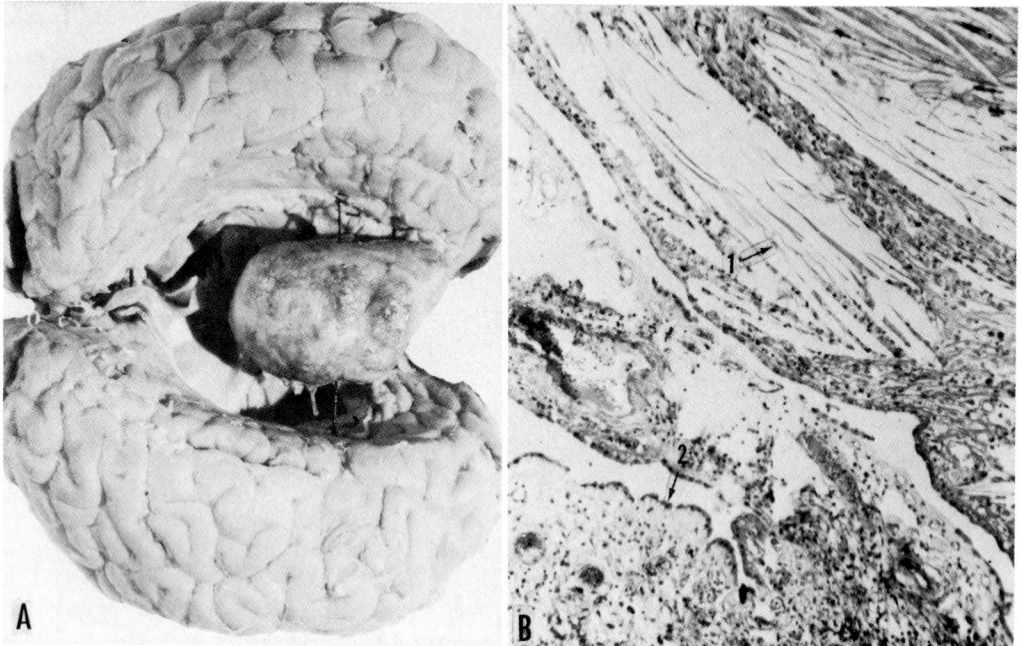

Fig. 27–22. Cholesterinic granulomas in the choroid plexus of lateral ventricle of a horse. *A,* The gross specimen. Note mass, which has been moved from the left lateral ventricle. Contributor: Lt. Col. T.C. Jones. *B,* Cholesterol clefts *(1)* and granulomatous tissue are prominent features in the choroid plexus. Ependyma *(2)*. (Courtesy of Armed Forces Institute of Pathology.) Contributor: Army Veterinary Research Laboratory.

which the neuroblastoma is embryologically related, since both arise from nervous tissue at an early stage of embryonal development. Like the medulloblastoma, this tumor also typically forms "rosettes," which are a prime aid in the microscopic diagnosis. In the case of the neuroblastoma, the cells of the rosette are arranged around a small tuft of fibrils of nervous origin.

The neuroblastoma can originate in the central nervous system, but the majority occur in the adrenal medulla; a few arise from sympathetic nervous tissue elsewhere in the abdominal cavity. In the adrenal medulla the tumor sometimes receives the name of **sympathoblastoma.** Wherever located, it occurs in the young and is highly malignant.

Retinoblastoma, or Neuroepithelioma. This tumor arises in the eye from the precursors of the neuroepithelial receptor cells of the retina. Like the medulloblastoma and the neuroblastoma, it consists of small cells with nuclei suggestive of lymphocytes. It also tends to form rosettes. It is malignant, metastasizing to the regional lymph nodes. It occurs in the very young and has a startlingly high incidence in some human families. These tumors appear to be rare in animals.

Ganglioneuroma. Arising from nervous tissue capable of forming neurons, this tumor is related to the neuroblastoma. But where the neuroblastoma is undifferentiated or anaplastic, the ganglioma is well differentiated into "ganglion cells" looking much like multipolar and other nerve cells with a supporting tissue suggestive of normal neuroglia. These rare tumors may occur in the brain but, like the neuroblastomas, are more likely to arise in the adrenal medulla or occasionally in sympathetic ganglia.

Chordoma. In humans, a rare neoplasm arises at the upper (spheno-occipital) or lower (sacrococcygeal) extremities of the vertebral column from "ecchordoses," which are remnants persisting from the fetal notochord. With a variable histologic appearance and frequently a superficial resemblance to cartilage, the chordoma consists of large rounded cells with central nuclei and clear, mucoid-appearing cytoplasm. These cells are seen in areas or clumps which are ordinarily connected to fibroblastic tissue but which sometimes appear surrounded by a noncellular mucinous matrix, probably a disintegration product of other similar cells. Both the cytoplasmic and the extracellular material usually contain numerous vacuoles. As one might guess, the chordoma consists grossly of a gelatinous, semitransparent tissue. The tumor infiltrates surrounding tissues and may reach considerable size.

There are but few reports of chordomas in animals.

Schwannoma, Neurilemmoma. Either of these terms describes a neoplasm, usually benign, which is believed to arise from Schwann cells (neurolemmal cells) surrounding the axons of the peripheral nerves. There is considerable difference of opinion about whether this tumor is distinguishable from the neurofibroma, which also arises from Schwann cells. Histologically, however, the tumors are distinct from one another. Studies on biologic behavior are needed to determine whether the continued recognition and separation of these two entities are justified.

The schwannoma is composed of elongated spindle-shaped cells arranged in a distinctive pattern. The cells, which are similar to those of a neurofibroma, and plumper than those of a fibroma, form interlacing fascicles, with clumps of cells

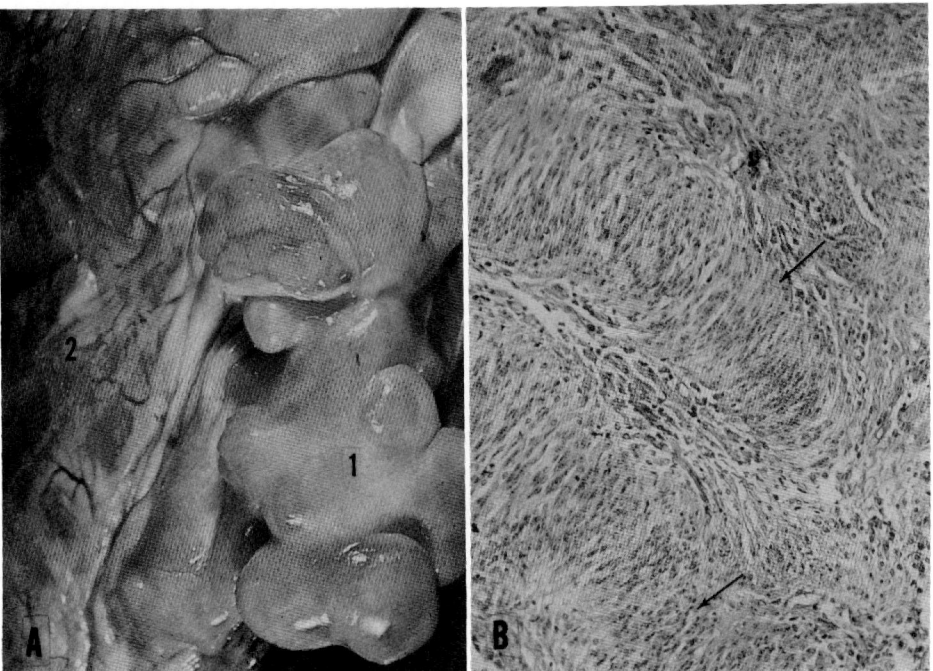

Fig. 27–23. *A*, Schwannoma (*1*) of the epicardium (*2*) in a steer. Photograph courtesy of Dr. C.L. Davis. *B*, Neurofibromatosis involving brachial plexus, myocardium, and intercostal nerves of an eight-year-old cow. Section (× 150) is from the tumor in the brachial plexus. (Courtesy of Armed Forces Institute of Pathology.) Contributor: Dr. C.L. Davis.

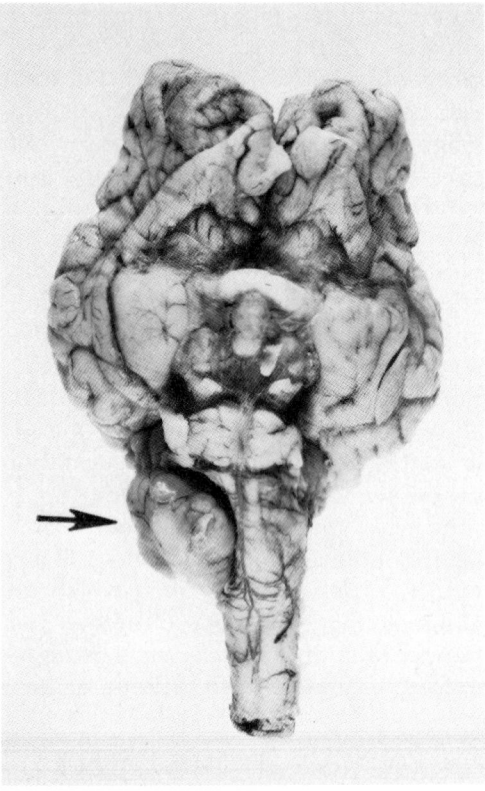

Fig. 27–24. Schwannoma of the eighth cranial nerve in a 14-year-old cow. (Courtesy of Dr. W.J. Hadlow.)

lying in windrows. This feature, referred to as palisading of nuclei, is the principal distinctive characteristic of the tumor. Often there are nodules or lobules of cells which are arranged in palisades at either end of a bundle of cytoplasmic processes or parallel fibers. Such a structure is termed a Verocay body. Fasciculi of cells run in wavy or undulating patterns and may also form tight whorls.

As would be expected, the growths are located along the course of a nerve or at a plexus or ganglion. They occur in most species, although infrequently. They are most common in cattle (in which many have been termed neurofibromas). The term acoustic neuroma has been applied to schwannomas of the eighth cranial nerve in humans. Schwannomas may also arise

from other cranial nerves (excluding the olfactory and optic nerves, which do not have Schwann cells). Cranial nerve schwannomas have been reported in dogs.

Neurofibroma; Neurofibrosarcoma; Neurosarcoma. These tumors arise from Schwann cells and therefore represent a histologic variant of schwannomas. Some hold that these tumors arise from "fibroblasts" in the perineurium and are variants of fibromas, but since Schwann cells cannot be differentiated from perineural cells except by position, this distinction is probably not valid. The neurofibroma is distinct from the ordinary fibroma and lacks the unique architecture of the schwannoma. Microscopically, the neurofibroma is composed of spindle-shaped cells arranged in circular whorls or wavy fasciculi.

Malignant tumors of this class occur rarely and are termed neurofibrosarcomas or neurogenic sarcomas. Microscopically, neurofibrosarcoma may closely resemble a fibrosarcoma, but the cells tend to have the form of plump spindles and retain a whorled or curly arrangement. Neurofibrosarcomas occur in most species but are seen most commonly in cattle, in which they are fairly frequent in the myocardium, sometimes with more than one occurring in a single heart. The tendency to form whorls is sometimes recognizable grossly in the moist, slightly bulging cut surface. In humans, large numbers of cutaneous neurofibromas occur in the same patient in what is known as von Recklinghausen's neurofibromatosis. A tumorous condition having similar characteristics has been reported in the dog (Antin, 1957), and neurofibromas are often multiple in cattle.

Meningioma. These tumors arise from the cranial or spinal meninges, presumably from their mesothelial (older histologists called them endothelial) cells which form the surface of these membranes. (Some say they arise from "arachnoid cells.") In most meningiomas, the cells are more plump and the nuclei more rounded than in the

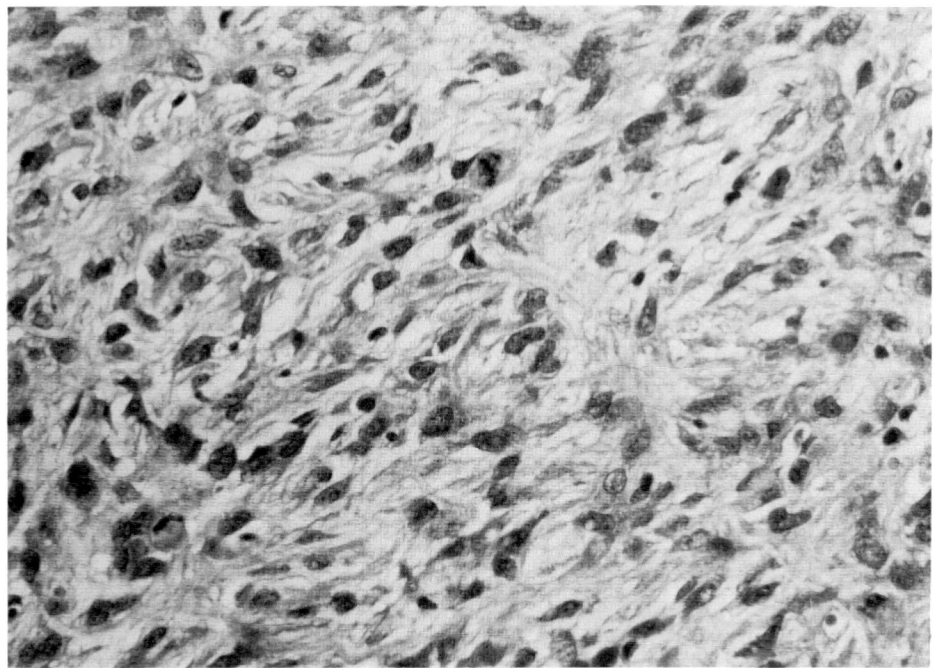

Fig. 27–25. Neurofibrosarcoma from the subcutis of the elbow of a dog. This neoplasm lacks the unique architecture of the Schwannoma (Fig. 27–23), more closely resembling a fibrosarcoma. (Courtesy of Dr. N.W. King, Jr.)

neurofibroma, but there is the same tendency toward a whorled arrangement. Occasionally meningiomas form areas of bone. Rather commonly at the center of many of the whorls, there is a compressed hyaline or calcified body suggestive grossly of a grain of sand. This form of meningioma is sometimes called a **psammoma** (from *psammos,* meaning sand), and the little granules are known as brain sand.

Grossly the meningioma forms a more or less spherical subdural mass. It compresses the underlying brain or cord and may extend deep into sulci. Meningiomas have been found somewhat frequently in dogs, cattle, and horses, and are the most common intracranial neoplasm in the cat (Fig. 27–19), where they are sometimes multiple.

Secondary Tumors. **Metastatic neoplasms** and direct invasion of neoplasms from adjacent tissues are not uncommon. Malignant lymphoma is the most frequent of the secondary tumors. It most often is located in the spinal canal and is especially frequent in cats and cattle. Melanomas and hemangioendotheliomas are also among the more frequent metastatic neoplasms.

Andrews, E.J.: Clinicopathologic characteristics of meningiomas in dogs. J. Am. Vet. Med. Assoc., *163*:151–157, 1973.

Antin, I.P.: Neurofibromatosis or von Recklinghausen's disease in a dog. J. Am. Vet. Med. Assoc., *130*:352, 1957.

Baronti, A.C., and Rhodes, D.A.: Meningioma in a dog. J. Am. Vet. Med. Assoc., *130*:520, 1957.

Beezley, D.N.: A trigeminal ganglioneuroma in a dog. Cornell Vet., *59*:585–594, 1969.

Bots, G.T.L.A.M., Kroes, R., and Feron, V.J.: Spontaneous tumors of the brain in rats. Pathol. Vet., *5*:290–296, 1968.

Buykmihci, N.: Orbital meningioma with intraocular invasion in a dog. Histology and ultrastructure. Vet. Pathol., *14*:521–523, 1977.

Canfield, P.: A light microscopic study of bovine peripheral nerve sheath tumours. Vet. Pathol., *15*:283–291, 1978.

Canfield, P.: The ultrastructure of bovine peripheral nerve sheath tumours. Vet. Pathol., *15*:292–300, 1978.

Cimprich, R., and Ardington, P.: Spinal ganglio-neuroma in a steer. Vet. Pathol., 12:59–60, 1975.

Cusick, P.K., and Parker, A.J.: Brain stem gliomas in cats. Vet. Pathol., 12:460–461, 1975.

Davies, H.W.: Tumors of the brain in the dog. Vet. Rec., 10:717–719, 1930.

Drew, R.A., and Greatorex, J.C.: Vertebral plasma cell myeloma causing posterior paralysis in a horse. Equine Vet. J., 6:131–134, 1974.

Duncan, T.E., and Harkin, J.C.: Electron microscopic studies of goldfish tumors previously termed neurofibromas and schwannomas. Am. J. Pathol., 55:191–202, 1969.

Ferrell, J.F., Hunt, R.D., and Nims, R.M.: Cervical ganglioneuroma in a dog. J. Am. Vet. Med. Assoc., 144:508–512, 1964.

Ferri, A.G., and Matera, E.A.: Glomus tumor in a dog. J. Comp. Pathol., 70:373–379, 1960.

Geib, L.W.: Ossifying meningioma with extracranial metastasis in a dog. Pathol. Vet., 3:247–254, 1966.

Hayes, K.C., and Schiefer, B.: Primary tumors in the CNS of carnivores. Pathol. Vet., 6:94–116, 1969.

Jacob, K.: Grosshirnmeningom beim Hund. Berl. Münch. Tierarztl. Wochenschr., 72:226–228, 1959.

Johnson, D.F., and Brown, D.G.: Intradural spinal lipoma in an experimental swine. Pathol. Vet., 6:342–347, 1969.

Jolly, R.D., and Alley, M.R.: Medulloblastoma in calves. A report of three cases. Pathol. Vet., 6:463–468, 1969.

Joshua, J.O., and Ottaway, C.W.: A case of cranial nerve tumor with acquired hydrocephalus in the dog. Vet. Rec., 59:649, 1947.

Kelly, D.F.: Neuroblastoma in the dog. J. Pathol., 116:209–212, 1975.

Koestner, A., and Zeman, W.: Primary reticuloses of the central nervous system in dogs. Am. J. Vet. Res., 23:381–393, 1962.

Kurtz, H.J., and Hanlon, G.F.: Choroid plexus papilloma in a dog. Vet. Pathol., 8:91–95, 1971.

Luginbühl, H.: Comparative aspects of tumors of the nervous system. Ann. NY Acad. Sci., 108:702–721, 1963.

———: Studies on meningiomas in cats. Review of the literature and report of eight cases. Am. J. Vet. Res., 22:1030–1040, 1961.

———: Zur vergleichenden pathologie der tumoren des nervensystems. I. Teil. Schweiz. Arch. Tierheilk., 104:305–322, 1962. V.B. 32:3853, 1962.

———: Spontaneous neoplasms of the nervous system in animals. Prog. Neurol. Surg., 2:85–164, 1968.

Milks, H.J., and Olafson, P.: Primary brain tumors in small animals. Cornell Vet., 26:159–170, 1936.

Misdorp, W., and Nauta-van Gelder, H.L.: "Granular cell myoblastoma" in the horse. A report of four cases. Pathol. Vet., 5:385–394, 1968.

Monlux, A.W., and Davis, C.L.: Multiple schwannomas of cattle. Am. J. Vet. Res., 14:499–509, 1953.

Nafe, L.A.: Meningiomas in cats: A retrospective clinical study of 36 cases. J. Am. Vet. Med. Assoc., 174:1224–1227, 1979.

Newman, A.J., and Mawdesley-Thomas, L.E.: Spontaneous tumours of the central nervous system of laboratory rats. J. Comp. Pathol., 84:39–50, 1974.

Pilleri, G.: Hirnlipom beim Buckelwal, Megaptera novaeangliae. Pathol. Vet., 3:341–349, 1966.

———: Cerebrale neurofibrome beim Finwal, Balaenoptera physalus. Pathol. Vet., 5:35–40, 1968.

Saliba, A.M., et al.: (Chordoma in two dogs.) Arq. Inst. Biol. (Sao Paulo), 34:45–50, 1967.

Savage, A., Isa, J.M., and Fischer, W.: Malignant ependymoma in a dog. Cornell Vet., 52:68–70, 1962.

Schlotthauer, C.F., and Kernohan, J.W.: Glioma in a dog and pinealoma in a Silver fox (Vulpes fulvus). Am. J. Cancer, 24:350–356, 1935.

Simon, J., and Brewer, R.L.: Multiple neurofibromatosis in cow and calf. J. Am. Vet. Med. Assoc., 142:1102–1104, 1963.

Strafuss, A.C., Martin, C.E., Blauch, B., and Guffy, M.: Schwannoma in a dog. J. Am. Vet. Med. Assoc., 163:245–247, 1973.

Teternik, D.M., et al.: (Neurogenous neoplasms in cattle.) Veterinariya, Moscow, 37:56–60, 1960.

Traver, D.S., et al.: Epidural melanoma causing posterior paresis in a horse. J. Am. Vet. Med. Assoc., 170:1400–1403, 1977.

Troy, M.A.: Granular-cell myoblastoma in a dog. J. Am. Vet. Med. Assoc., 126:397, 1955.

Vandevelde, M., Braund, K.G., and Hoff, E.J.: Central neurofibromas in two dogs. Vet. Pathol., 14:470–478, 1977.

Vandevelde, M., Higgins, R.J., and Greene, C.E.: Neoplasms of mesenchymal origin in the spinal cord and nerve roots of three dogs. Vet. Pathol., 13:47–58, 1976.

Zaki, F.A., and Hurvitz, A.I.: Spontaneous neoplasms of the central nervous system of the cat. J. Small Anim. Pract., 17:773–782, 1976.

Zaki, F.A., and Kay, W.J.: Carcinoma of the choroid plexus in a dog. J. Am. Vet. Med. Assoc., 164:1195–1197, 1974.

CHAPTER 28

Organs of Special Sense

EYE

The eye is a wondrously complex structure whose parts perform a function which even the most blasé must consider miraculous. The eyes of each animal or bird are remarkably adapted to its environment and habits. The hawk can spot his tiny prey from fantastic heights and the cat can see his victim on the darkest night. Such functional adaptations depend upon specific structural developments which are different in each species. This alone makes the study of diseased ocular structures in animals both difficult and fascinating.

Not only is the eye the organ of sight, but it also serves as a window through which some disease processes can be observed. With slit-lamp illumination and the corneal microscope, leukocytes or erythrocytes can be seen escaping from the iris, floating in the aqueous, and settling to the bottom of the anterior chamber. Capillaries in the retina can be studied with the ophthalmoscope, and sometimes they yield clues about the condition of capillaries in the rest of the body. It is unfortunate that the general pathologist often avoids the study of the eye, because this organ follows the general laws of biology in its response to injury and can teach much to the observant. This is not to disclaim the necessity for the special knowledge and interest of ophthalmic pathologists, whose contributions are vital, but rather to encourage veterinary pathologists to cultivate a deeper interest in this important organ in their animal patients.

The eye must be studied carefully in the living animal, the gross specimen approached systematically, and properly fixed for microscopic examination if the best evaluation is to be made. Some things are best detected in the living animal, including: the luster of the cornea; the size, shape, and response of the pupil to light; opacities in the media-cornea, aqueous, lens and vitreous; intraocular tension; and intraocular masses. The importance of systematic clinical evaluation and recording of findings is especially important to the pathologist in examining this system.

Adnexa

The **eyelids,** having cutaneous and conjunctival surfaces and containing both tear and sebaceous glands (i.e., meibomian glands), may be subject to lesions of any of these structures. Any lesion of the skin (Chapter 18) may involve the cutaneous part of the eyelid. The **conjunctiva** is frequently subject to nonspecific inflammation, which may at times result in hypertrophy and hyperplasia of subepithelial lymphocytic nodules. This may give the conjunctiva a grossly evident roughened, cobblestone appearance. Congenital inward turning of the eyelids, known as **entropion,** may lead to conjunctivitis and keratitis. It is frequent in sheep and dogs. A double row of eyelashes or **distichiasis,** may also cause conjunctivitis. It is reported in dogs. Inflammation or abscesses of sebaceous glands (stye) or meibomian glands (chalazion) are occasionally encountered. Meibomian glands are modified sebaceous glands on the inner surface of the eye.

Neoplasms of sebaceous and meibomian glands are most often encountered in dogs, where they resemble sebaceous gland tumors of the skin. Neoplasms of the conjunctiva are not infrequent, the most common being the squamous cell carcinoma of the bovine eye. This neoplasm most frequently originates in the conjunctiva but may arise from the skin of the eyelid. Basal cell carcinomas, cutaneous horns, and papillomas may also arise from the conjunctival or cutaneous portions of the eyelids.

The **membrana nictitans,** or nictitating membrane, is particularly well developed in most domestic animals, although vestigial in man. This membrane invests the nasal aspect of the globe and is usually barely visible at the medial canthus. It can be protruded like a "third eyelid" by voluntary or involuntary action to cover most, if not all, of the corneal surface. This is presumed to give the eye additional protection and may have a cleansing function. The membrane is covered by conjunctiva and is richly supplied with simple and compound tubular lacrimal glands. Rigidity is given the structure by a central core of cartilage which is concave to fit the eyeball. Eversion of the membrana nictitans has been reported to be an inherited anomaly in German Shorthaired Pointers (Martin and Leach, 1970).

Inflammation of the lacrimal glands (dacryoadenitis), may come to the attention of the veterinary pathologist. The superficial and deep glands of the membrana nictitans of the dog are most commonly involved. This inflammation results in congestion and enlargement of the gland, which, in turn, causes the third eyelid to protrude, usually necessitating its ablation. The microscopic findings in surgical specimens of the third eyelid are usually limited to inflammatory changes in the stroma and the connective tissue surrounding the tubular glands of the eyelid. The ducts of the glands are often dilated, occasionally filled with leukocytes, and the acinar elements are hypertrophic. Cysts of lacrimal ducts and glands are occasionally seen. They may be congenital or acquired. Frank neoplastic changes in the glands are rare, but adenomas may occur.

In most species, but not the dog, there is an accessory lacrimal gland, called the harderian gland, at the base of the third eyelid which may become inflamed or subject to neoplastic disease. In rats, a viral disease of this gland along with other lacrimal glands and the salivary glands (sialodacryoadenitis) is a relatively frequent disease (Jonas et al., 1969; Jacoby et al., 1975; Hunt, 1963); a similar disease is also seen in mice (Maronpot and Chavannes, 1977).

Anderson, D.R.: Ultrastructure of human and monkey lamina cribrosa and optic nerve head. Arch. Ophthal., *82*:800–814, 1969.

Cogan, M.J., and Zimmerman, L.E.: Ophthalmic Pathology. 2nd ed., Philadelphia, W.B. Saunders Co., 1962.

Cohrs, P.: Studien zur normalen und pathologischen Anatomie und Histologie des inneren Gehörorganes vom Pferde (*Equus caballus*). Leipzig, F.C.W. Vogel, 1928.

Duke-Elder, W.S.: Textbook of Ophthalmology, Vols. I–VI. St. Louis, C.V. Mosby Co., 1938–1954.

Gelatt, K.N.: Textbook of Veterinary Ophthalmology. Philadelphia, Lea & Febiger, 1981.

Gelatt, K.N.: Recent advances in veterinary and comparative ophthalmology. Adv. Vet. Sci. Comp. Med., *16*:1–33, 1972.

Hunt, R.D.: Dacryoadenitis in the Sprague-Dawley rat. Am. J. Vet. Res., *24*:638–641, 1963.

Jacoby, R.O., Blatt, P.N., and Jonas, A.M.: Pathogenesis of sialodacryoadenitis in gnotobiotic rats. Vet. Pathol., *12*:196–209, 1975.

Jonas, A.M., et al.: Sialodacryoadenitis in the rat, a light- and electron-microscopic study. Arch. Pathol., *88*:613–622, 1969.

Lawson, D.D.: Canine distichiasis. J. Small Anim. Pract., 14:469–478, 1973.

Magrane, W.G.: Canine Ophthalmology, 3rd ed. Philadelphia, Lea & Febiger, 1977.

Mann, I.C.: The Development of the Human Eye. 2nd ed. New York, Grune and Stratton, 1950.

Maronpot, R.R., and Chavannes, J.-M.: Dacryoadenitis, conjunctivitis, and facial dermatitis of the mouse. Lab. Anim. Sci., 27:277–278, 1977.

Martin, C.L., and Leach, R.: Everted membrana nictitans in German Shorthaired Pointers. J. Am. Vet. Med. Assoc., 157:1229–1232, 1970.

Miller, M.E., and Habel, R.E.: Harder's gland in the dog. J. Am. Vet. Med. Assoc., 118:155–156, 1951.

Playter, R.F., and Adams, L.G.: Lacrimal cyst (dacryops) in two dogs. J. Am. Vet. Med. Assoc., 171:736–737, 1977.

Prince, J.H., Diesem, C.D., Eglitis, I., and Ruskell, G.L.: Anatomy and Histology of the Eye and Orbit in Domestic Animals. Springfield, Ill., Charles C Thomas, 1960.

Saunders, L.Z.: Pathology of the Eye of Domestic Animals. Berlin, Paul Parey, 1968.

Shively, J.N., and Epling, G.P.: Fine structure of the canine eye: Iris. Am. J. Vet. Res., 30:13–26, 1969.

Shively, J.N., Epling, G.P., and Jensen, R.: Fine structure of the canine eye. Am. J. Vet. Res., 31:1339–1359, 1970.

Wolff, E.: The Anatomy of the Eye and Orbit. 3rd ed. Philadelphia, Blakiston, 1951.

Wyman, M., and Donovan, E.F.: The ocular fundus of the normal dog. J. Am. Vet. Med. Assoc., 147:7–26, 1965.

Cornea and Sclera

Some of the important anatomic differences between species will be mentioned as the specific anatomic structure is considered. The sclera is the relatively avascular tunic which gives the globe the structural rigidity to maintain its shape. In birds it normally contains cartilage, which may ossify to bone.

The cornea of animals of most species is subjected to a wide variety of deleterious influences but has a good capacity for recovery. Unfortunately, healing of lesions in the cornea may result in scarring, which is not objectionable in other structures, but may destroy sight by making all or part of the cornea opaque. Wounds, particularly when accompanied by penetrating foreign bodies, are a common cause of inflammation which may leave opacities in the cornea. Injuries that perforate the cornea are of serious import, often leading to loss of sight in the involved eye. Perforation of Descemet's membrane permits escape of aqueous humor followed by collapse of the cornea, with prolapse of the iris and dislocation of the lens further possibilities. Secondary infection often causes inflammation of the entire globe (panophthalmitis) which may cause permanent loss of sight.

Infectious Keratitis, Keratoconjunctivitis. So-called pink eye, this disease in sheep, goats, and cattle, may result in diffuse inflammation of the cornea, producing temporary blindness. Diffuse scarring with loss of transparency is a common sequel of this infection, which often occurs as an outbreak with a relatively high incidence (up to 50%). The cause is often not firmly established, although many organisms have been recovered from infected conjunctival sacs and in some cases specific organisms have proved to be pathogenic. In cattle, however, *Moraxella bovis* is the principal causative organism. It is recovered from many outbreaks, and instillation of the organism into the conjunctival sac of normal animals is followed by severe keratitis. Solar irradiation augments the disease, with most outbreaks occurring during the summer months. *Mycoplasma* have also been recovered from infected sheep and cattle. The herpesvirus of bovine rhinotracheitis also causes keratoconjunctivitis and is responsible for some outbreaks of pink-eye. In sheep, *Rickettsia conjunctivae* is a principal cause of keratoconjunctivitis. Although *Moraxella bovis* has been recovered from affected sheep as well as from horses, its role is uncertain. *Chlamydia* have also been associated with ocular infection in cattle and sheep. The problem of etiologies is still quite confused—apparently many organisms may cause this clinical disease.

Keratitis and keratoconjunctivitis in other species is usually sporadic with no single cause. Herpesviruses have a propensity to infect the conjunctiva and should be suspected in any species. Corneal edema and other ocular manifestations of infectious canine hepatitis are discussed elsewhere. In addition to cattle and sheep, *Chlamydia* have also been described as causes of keratitis in swine, guinea pigs, dogs, cats, and human beings. Nematodes of the genus *Thelazia* cause conjunctivitis in many different animal species. Other causes include vitamin A deficiency, exposure to ultraviolet light, chemical irritants, dust, and trauma. Allergic keratoconjunctivitis is well documented in human beings and may account for many examples in animals. Reduction in lacrimal secretion will also lead to keratitis (*keratoconjunctivitis sicca*). It is common in dogs, although the cause is usually unknown. Phenazopyridine hydrochloride has been shown to reduce tear flow in dogs.

Corneal opacity may also occur in the absence of keratitis as a congenital defect. It has been described in British Friesian cattle (Deas, 1959) as a hereditary disease. It results from edema, but the pathogenesis is uncertain.

Pigmentary Keratitis. In some instances, for reasons poorly understood, keratitis in dogs not only is accompanied by deep and superficial vascularization of the cornea, but also is followed by deposition of melanin pigment in the corneal epithelium and the underlying stroma. This may involve much of the cornea, giving it a brown or black color and rendering it opaque. Pigmentary keratitis is difficult to treat and often destroys sight in the affected eye.

Vascularization. Corneal vascularization may follow trauma to the cornea, especially any injury resulting in ulceration of the corneal epithelium, or may be a manifestation of dietary deficiency of certain vitamins (riboflavin) or amino acids (tryptophane). Capillaries that extend into the cornea toward an ulcer usually arise from the vessels in a small zone at the point in the limbus nearest the lesion. **Superficial vascularization,** i.e., formation of new capillaries in the stroma adjacent to the epithelium, usually is first to occur. Proliferation of blood vessels deeper in the stroma, **deep vascularization,** usually fol-

lows more prolonged effects on the cornea. Vascularization based upon nutritional deficiency is characterized by proliferation of new capillaries from the corneoscleral junction (limbus) all around the circumference of the cornea. These extend certripetally toward the centrum of the cornea, may occur in the absence of significant corneal opacity, and do not radiate toward or terminate in an ulcer or opacity of the cornea. Grossly, newly formed vessels in the cornea may appear as vascular arborizations, but microscopic study reveals that each blood vessel does not terminate blindly but forms a capillary loop through which the blood can return to the venules at the limbus (Fig. 28–2).

Pannus (pannus degenerativus). This term is applied to a lesion of the cornea in which vascular granulation tissue extends from the limbus over the cornea. This tissue, often containing leukocytes, lies between the corneal epithelium and Bowman's membrane, which at times may become duplicated. The granulation tissue may remain as scar tissue, may undergo calcification, and the overlying corneal epithelium is often disorganized and thickened. This condition is frequently associated with glaucoma. Pannus is especially common in German Shepherd dogs. A proliferative inflammatory lesion called **ophthalmic nodular fasciitis** has been described in dogs by Gwin et al. (1977). It was characterized by subconjunctival proliferation of fibroblasts and mononuclear inflammatory cells resembling a neoplasm. It did not affect the cornea.

Corneal Dermoid. A congenital lesion observed in newborn animals may involve one or both eyes. The affected cornea appears to be covered over part of its surface with haired, usually pigmented skin. Microscopically, the affected part of corneal epithelium is replaced with dermal epithelium having skin adnexa in its underlying stroma. Hair follicles, sebaceous glands, and cysts lined with epithelium and filled with keratin are common. The

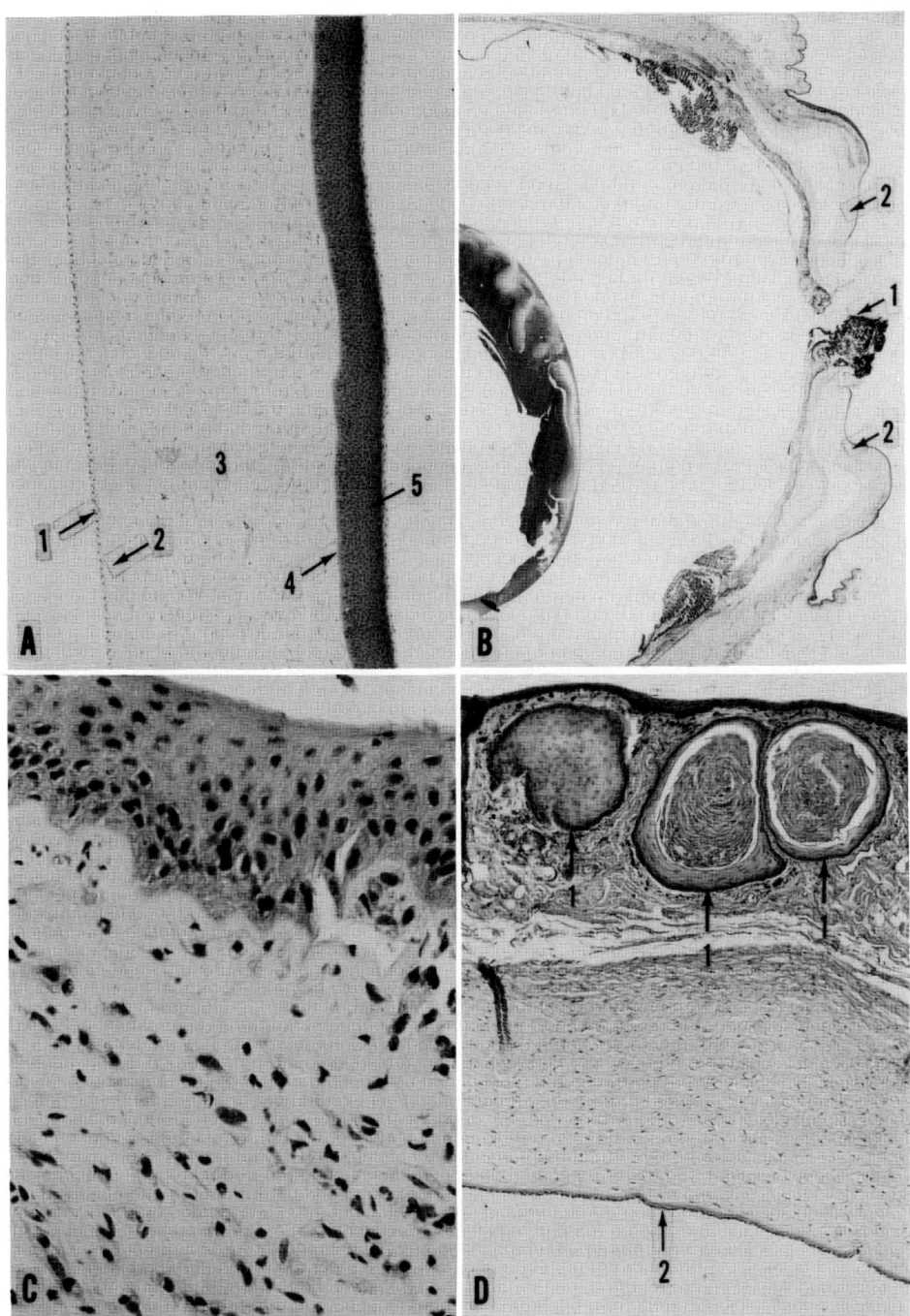

Fig. 28–1. *A,* Normal equine cornea (× 55). Corneal endothelium (*1*); Descemet's membrane (*2*); corneal stroma (substantia propria) (*3*); Bowman's membrane (*4*); corneal epithelium (*5*). Contributor: Army Veterinary Research Laboratory. *B,* Rupture of the equine cornea following trauma (× 2½). The iris (*1*) has prolapsed through the opening in the cornea (*2*). Contributor: Army Veterinary Research Laboratory. *C,* Keratitis, bovine eye (× 330). Note leukocytes in substantia propria of the cornea. Contributor: Dr. C.L. Davis. *D,* Corneal dermoid, eye of a lamb (× 70). Islands of pigmented epithelium (*1*), between the corneal epithelium and stroma. Corneal endothelium (*2*). (*A–D,* Courtesy of Armed Forces Institute of Pathology.) Contributor: Dr. Robert D. Courter.

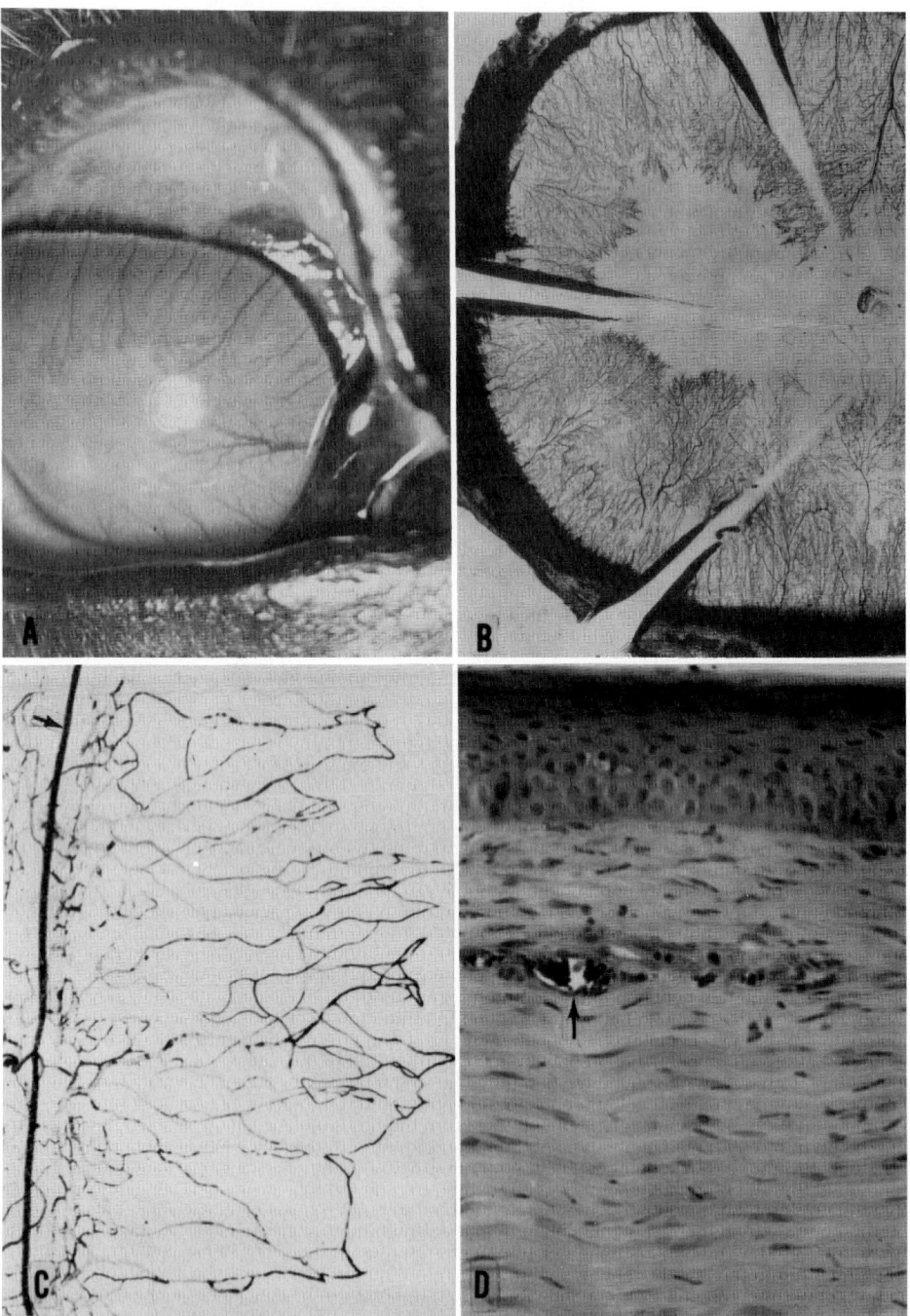

Fig. 28–2. Corneal vascularization. *A,* Eye of a horse during an acute recrudescence of periodic ophthal-mia. *B,* Cornea of a horse with periodic ophthalmia. The fixed cornea was mounted flat on a slide. The limbus is black because of its pigment. *C,* Cornea of a rat with riboflavin deficiency (× 36). Loops of capillaries extend into the cornea from the vessels at the limbus (*arrow*). *D,* New blood vessel (*arrow*) in the lamina propria of the cornea of a horse with periodic ophthalmia (× 300).

corneal stroma may be thickened and vascularized but is otherwise unaffected. Epithelial inclusion cysts may also affect the cornea. They resemble the lesions seen in the skin.

Aguirre, G.D., Rubin, L.F., and Harvey, C.E.: Keratoconjunctivitis sicca in dogs. J. Am. Vet. Med. Assoc., *158*:1566–1569, 1971.

Arora, A.K., Killinger, A.H., and Myers, W.L.: Detection of *Moraxella bovis* antibodies in infectious bovine keratoconjunctivitis by a passive hemagglutination test. Am. J. Vet. Res., *37*:1489–1492, 1976.

Baker, J.R., Faull, W.B., and Ward, W.R.: Conjunctivitis and keratitis in sheep associated with *Moraxella (Haemophilus)* organisms. Vet. Rec., *77*:402–406, 1965.

Bernis, W.O.: Partial penetrating keratoplasty in dogs. Southwest. Vet., *15*:30–44, 1961.

Bessey, O.A., and Wolbach, S.B.: Vascularization of the cornea of the rat in riboflavin deficiency, with a note on corneal vascularization in vitamin A deficiency. J. Exp. Med., *69*:1–12, 1939.

Bryan, H.S., et al.: Some bacteriologic and ophthalmologic observations on bovine infectious keratoconjunctivitis in an Illinois beef herd. J. Am. Vet. Med. Assoc., *163*:739–741, 1973.

Bryan, G.M., and Slatter, D.: Keratoconjunctivitis sicca induced by phenazopyridine in dogs. Arch. Ophthalmol., *90*:310–311, 1973.

Campbell, L.H., Okuda, H.K., Lipton, D.E., and Reed, C.: Chronic superficial keratitis in dogs: Detection of cellular hypersensitivity. Am. J. Vet. Res., *36*:669–671, 1975.

Campbell, L.H., and Snyder, S.B.: Chronic superficial keratitis in dogs: Negative results of isolation procedures for chlamydia. Am. J. Vet. Res., *34*:579–580, 1973.

Cooper, B.S.: Contagious conjunctivokeratitis (C.C.K.) of sheep in New Zealand. NZ Vet. J., *15*:79–84, 1967.

Davis, C.L.: An unusual occurrence of corneal dermatoma in newborn lambs. J. Am. Vet. Med. Assoc., *85*:679–682, 1934.

Deas, D.W.: A note on hereditary opacity of the cornea in British Friesian cattle. Vet. Rec., *71*:619–620, 1959.

Fairlee, G.: The isolation of a haemolytic neisseria from cattle and sheep in the North of Scotland. Vet. Rec., *78*:649–650, 1966.

Formston, C., Bedford, P.G.C., Staton, J.F., and Tripathi, R.C.: Corneal necrosis in the cat. J. Small Anim. Pract., *15*:19–25, 1974.

Gleeson, L.N., and Griffin, R.M.: A study of infectious kerato-conjunctivitis (I.K.C.). Irish Vet. J., *19*:163–182, 1965. V.B. *36*:1397, 1966.

Gwin, R.M., Gelatt, K.N., and Peiffer, R.L., Jr.: Ophthalmic nodular fasciitis in the dog. J. Am. Vet. Med. Assoc., *170*:611–614, 1977.

Hubbert, W.T., and Hermann, G.J.: A winter epizootic of infectious bovine keratoconjunctivitis. J. Am. Vet. Med. Assoc., *157*:452–454, 1970.

Hughes, D.E., and Pugh, G.W., Jr.: A five year study of infectious bovine keratoconjunctivitis in a beef herd. J. Am. Vet. Med. Assoc., *157*:443–451, 1970.

Hughes, D.E., Pugh, G.W., Jr., and McDonald, T.J.: Ultraviolet radiation and *Moraxella bovis* in the etiology of bovine infectious keratoconjunctivitis. Am. J. Vet. Res., *26*:1331–1338, 1965.

———: Experimental bovine infectious keratoconjunctivitis caused by sunlamp irradiation and *Moraxella bovis* infection: Determination of optimal irradiation. Am. J. Vet. Res., *29*:821–827, 1968.

———: Experimental bovine infectious keratoconjunctivitis caused by sunlamp irradiation and *Moraxella bovis* infection: Resistance to reexposure with homologous and heterologous *Moraxella bovis*. Am. J. Vet. Res., *29*:829–833, 1968.

Hughes, D.E., and Pugh, G.W., Jr.: Isolation and description of a *Moraxella* from horses with conjunctivitis. Am. J. Vet. Res., *31*:457–462, 1970.

Jones, F.S., and Little, R.B.: An infectious ophthalmia of cattle. J. Exp. Med., *38*:139–148, 1923.

Koch, S.A., Langloss, J.M., and Schmidt, G.: Corneal epithelial inclusion cysts in four dogs. J. Am. Vet. Med. Assoc., *164*:1190–1191, 1974.

Langford, E.V., and Dorward, W.J.: A mycoplasma isolated from cattle with infectious bovine keratoconjunctivitis. Can. J. Comp. Med., *33*:275–279, 1969.

Livingston, C.W., Moore, R.W., and Hardy, W.T.: Isolation of an agent producing ovine infectious keratoconjunctivitis (pink eye). Am. J. Vet. Res., *26*:295–302, 1965.

Mohanty, S.B., and Lillie, M.G.: Relationship of infectious bovine keratoconjunctivitis virus to the virus of infectious bovine rhinotracheitis. Cornell Vet., *60*:3–9, 1970.

Monlux, A.W., Anderson, W.A., and Davis, C.L.: The diagnosis of squamous cell carcinoma of the eye (cancer eye) in cattle. Am. J. Vet. Res., *18*:5–34, 1957.

Moreno, G., et al.: (Infectious keratoconjunctivitis of cattle caused by *Neisseria* [*Neisseria ovis* n. sp. Lindqvist, 1960]). Arqs. Inst. Biol. (Sao Paulo), *35*:173–179, 1968. V.B. *39*:2363, 1969.

Nichols, C.W., and Yanoff, M.: Dermoid of a rat cornea. Pathol. Vet., *6*:214–216, 1969.

Pavlov, P., Milanov, M., and Tschulew, D.: Studies on rickettsial keratoconjunctivitis in sheep. Zentralbl. Bakteriol. [Orig.], *194*:439–442, 1964. V.B. *35*:1788, 1965.

Pugh, G.W., Jr., and Hughes, D.E.: Experimental bovine infectious keratoconjunctivitis caused by sunlamp irradiation and *Moraxella bovis* infection: Correlation of hemolytic ability and pathogenicity. Am. J. Vet. Res., *27*:835–839, 1968.

Pugh, G.W., Jr., and Hughes, D.E.: Infectious bovine keratoconjunctivitis induced by different experimental methods. Cornell Vet., *61*:23–45, 1971.

———: Bovine infectious keratoconjunctivitis. *Moraxella bovis* as the sole etiologic agent in a winter epizootic. J. Am. Vet. Med. Assoc., *161*:481–486, 1972.

Pugh, G.W., Jr., Hughes, D.E., and McDonald, T.J.: Keratoconjunctivitis produced by *Moraxella bovis* in laboratory animals. Am. J. Vet. Res., *29*:2057–2061, 1968.

Pugh, G.W., Jr., Hughes, D.E., and Packer, R.A.: Bovine infectious keratoconjunctivitis: interactions of *Moraxella bovis* and infectious bovine rhinotracheitis virus. Am. J. Vet. Res., *31*:653–662, 1970.

Pugh, G.W., Jr., Hughes, D.E., and Schulz, V.D.: Infectious bovine keratoconjunctivitis: Experimental induction of infection in calves with mycoplasmas and *Moraxella bovis*. Am. J. Vet. Res., *37*:493–495, 1976.

Roberts, S.R.: The nature of corneal pigmentation in the dog. J. Am. Vet. Med. Assoc., *124*:208–211, 1944.

Roberts, S.R., Dawson, C.R., Coleman, V., and Togni, B.: Dendritic keratitis in a cat. J. Am. Vet. Med. Assoc., *161*:285–289, 1972.

Russell, W.O., Wynne, E.S., and Loquvam, G.S.: Studies on bovine ocular squamous carcinoma ("cancer eye"). Cancer, *9*:1–52, 1956.

Smith, J.S., Bistner, S., and Riis, R.: Infiltrative corneal lesions resembling fibrous histiocytoma: Clinical and pathologic findings in six dogs and one cat. J. Am. Vet. Med. Assoc., *169*:722–726, 1976.

Surman, P.G.: Cytology of "pink-eye" of sheep, including a reference to trachoma of man, by employing acridine orange and iodine stains, and isolation of mycoplasma agents from infected sheep eyes. Aust. J. Biol. Sci., *21*:447–467, 1968.

Sykes, J.A., et al.: Experimental induction of infectious bovine keratoconjunctivitis. Tex. Rep. Biol. Med., *22*:741–755, 1964.

Wagner, J.E., et al.: Spontaneous conjunctivitis and dacryoadenitis of mice. J. Am. Vet. Med. Assoc., *155*:1211–1217, 1969.

Wilcox, G.E.: Infectious bovine kerato-conjunctivitis: A review. Vet. Bull., *38*:349–360, 1968.

———: Isolation of adenoviruses from cattle with conjunctivitis and keratoconjunctivitis. Aust. Vet. J., *45*:265–270, 1969.

Iris and Ciliary Apparatus

Each species has its own peculiar pupillary outline. The contracted pupil of the cat is vertically slit-shaped; in the horse this slit is horizontal. In both these species the dilated pupil is smoothly circular. In the horse, along the dorsal margins of the pupil the iris bears one or more black nodules which may attain a diameter of nearly a centimeter. These structures, the **corpora nigra,** or **granula iridis,** are made up of pigmented cells from the epithelium of the iris and have been mistaken for neoplasms.

Similar but smaller structures occur in the bovine eye. The amount and distribution of pigment in the iris are highly variable between different species as well as individuals. True albinos, of course, do not have any pigment in the iris.

Iridal heterochromia and albinism are occasionally seen in cattle, dogs, and cats. In Hereford cattle it has been associated with incomplete albinism and coloboma (Gelatt et al., 1969).

The iris and ciliary apparatus (ciliary body and ciliary processes) are intimately associated in structure and function and thus are frequently involved simultaneously in disease. It is pertinent therefore to consider these structures together. The anterior segment of the vascular tunic, the **uvea,** is formed by the iris and ciliary apparatus, hence **anterior uvea** is often used as a collective term for these structures. The posterior segment of the uvea consists of the choroid.

Persistent Pupillary Membrane. Failure of the pupillary membrane to degenerate results in an absence of the pupil or strands of tissue bridging the pupil. It is seen most often in dogs, cats, cattle, and horses. In the Basenji dog, it may be inherited and associated with other anomalies (Roberts and Bistner, 1968). Remnants may adhere to the lens causing what have been called capsular cataracts. Persistent pupillary membrane of course leads to glaucoma.

Synechia. **Anterior synechia** is the term used to designate adhesion between the anterior surface of the iris and the posterior corneal surface, i.e., the corneal endothelium. This lesion may affect the movement of the iris profoundly, and when the iris is completely adherent all around the perimeter of the cornea (peripheral anterior synechia), an increase in intraocular pressure will be the sequel of occlusion of the filtration angle (see Glaucoma). Anterior synechia will result from iritis when the anterior chamber is collapsed, or in other situations in which the inflamed iris is forced forward to lie in contact with the

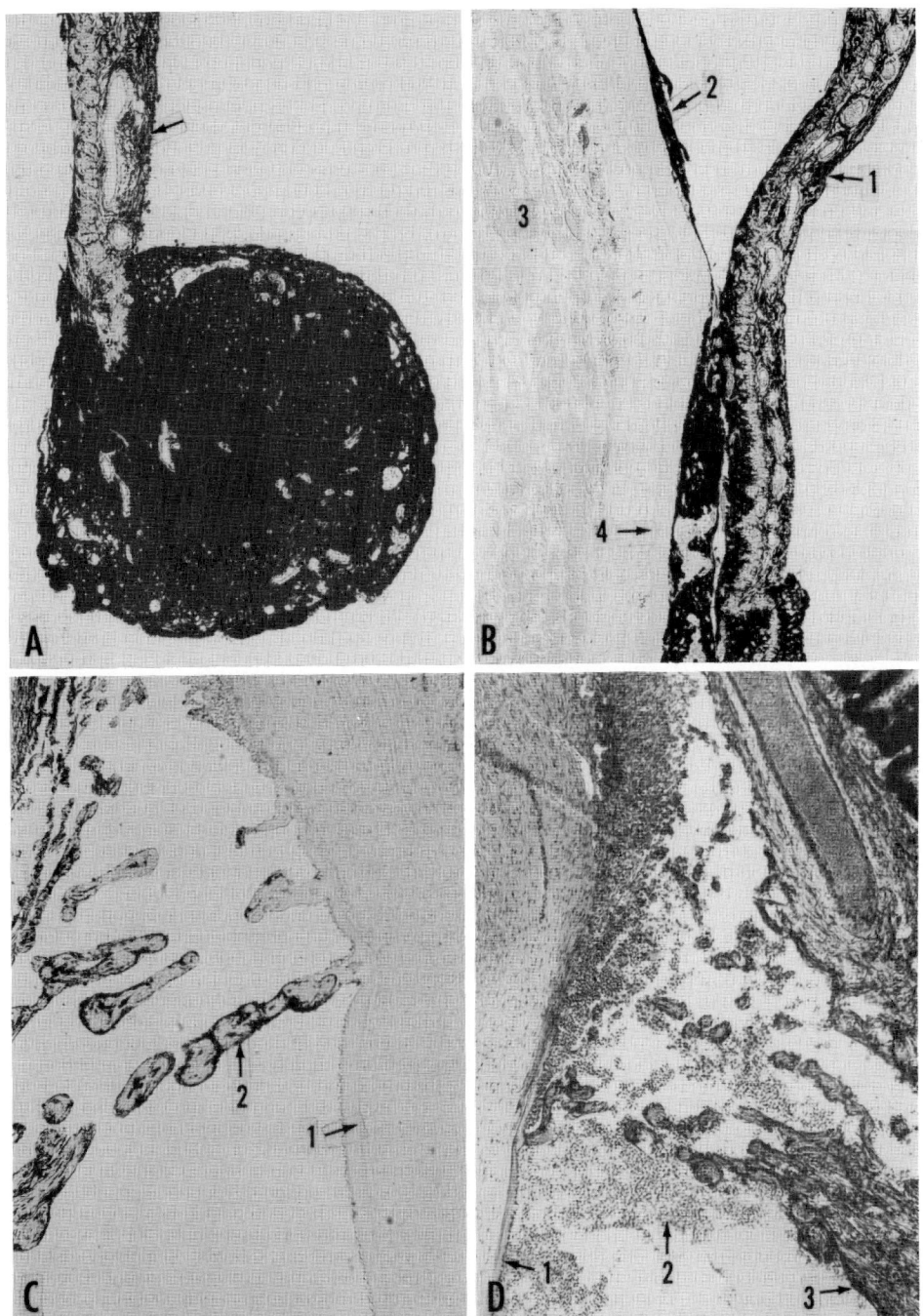

Fig. 28–3.   *A*, Normal iris of the horse (× 35) with the large corpora nigra on the dorsal pupillary margin. *B*, Posterior synechia, a sequel of periodic ophthalmia in the horse. The iris (*1*) is torn away from the lens but leaves pigment upon it at one point (*2*). The cortical lens fibers are disorganized (*3*) (cataract) and the anterior lens capsule (*4*) is firmly adherent to the iris in one zone. *C*, Normal filtration angle, eye of a horse (× 55). Descemet's membrane (*1*) and pectinate ligament (*2*) may be used as landmarks. *D*, The filtration angle in acute equine periodic ophthalmia (× 55). Descemet's membrane (*1*), leukocytes and plasma in anterior chamber (*2*), root of the iris (*3*). (*D*, Courtesy of Armed Forces Institute of Pathology.) Contributor: Army Veterinary Research Laboratory.

posterior corneal surface. In some instances the causative factors are obscure.

Posterior synechia means adhesion between the posterior surface of the iris and the anterior lens capsule. This is an even more frequent sequel of iritis than anterior synechia, because the iris normally lies in contact with the anterior lens capsule, at least when the pupil is partially or completely closed; thus it has a greater opportunity to adhere. Tenacious posterior synechiae may cause permanent closure of the pupil, or if the adhesions are forcibly torn loose by contraction of the iris, bits of iris pigment may be left clinging to the lens and cause the pupil to appear torn or ragged. Posterior synechia firmly fixed to the lens around the margin of the pupil (so-called ring synechia) and closing the pupillary orifice blocks the flow of aqueous from the posterior chamber. As a result, aqueous fluid accumulates behind the iris, causing it to bulge forward (*iris bombé*).

Posterior synechia may be indicated grossly by failure of the pupil to dilate with mydriatics, or, if it does dilate, by the ragged pupil or by iris pigment clinging to the anterior lens capsule. Microscopically, the iris is adherent to the lens and some fibrinous or, less often, leukocytic exudate is seen in the zone of adhesion. Usually the anterior lens capsule in this area is thickened or bits of iris pigment may be tightly fixed to its surface.

Iridocyclitis. Inflammation of the iris and ciliary apparatus, or **anterior uveitis,** is not unusual in animals and may have numerous different causes, not all of which are known. The classic example of iridocyclitis in animals is found in recurrent iridocyclitis or periodic ophthalmia of Equidae. The following description of this disease covers all the manifestations of iridocyclitis in any species and from any cause.

Equine Periodic Ophthalmia (Recurrent Iridocyclitis, Recurrent Uveitis). A specific disease of Equidae, periodic ophthalmia is the most common cause of blindness in horses and mules. It is characterized clinically by the sudden onset in one or both eyes of severe acute iridocyclitis which gradually abates in a week or more, to become quiescent for a period varying from a few days to many months. Acute exacerbations then follow at irregular intervals, each attack augmenting the damage to the eye. Repeated bouts of acute iridocyclitis usually end in complete loss of vision in the affected eye.

Clinical Signs. The significant clinical signs in the acute stage of the disease include: a tightly contracted pupil (myosis) which fails to dilate in darkness and only slowly after instillation of mydriatics; an iris that is yellowish instead of the normal brown; filling of the anterior chamber with finely particulate opacities (leukocytes) which usually settle to the ventral half of the chamber; severe congestion of the sclera and conjunctiva with tiny capillaries entering the cornea from the limbus (corneal vascularization). This is particularly evident (Fig. 28–2) in acute exacerbations. Photophobia is severe, lacrimation excessive, and intraocular tension diminished.

The acute signs abate quickly, usually within a week or so, leaving the disease in a quiescent stage, which, however, can be identified by the careful observer. Evidences of the disease during this period are posterior synechiae, indicated by iris pigment clinging to the anterior lens capsule, and tiny opacities in the vitreous humor on ophthalmoscopic examination. The fluorescein test (Jones et al., 1946) performed at this time reveals increased intraocular vascular permeability.

Repeated acute attacks result in posterior synechiae, subcapsular and diffuse cataracts, extensive corneal vascularization, opacities in the vitreous, detached retina, and decrease in the size of the globe **(phthisis bulbi).**

The etiology of periodic ophthalmia has been a matter of speculation over the years since the fourth century A.D. when the disease was first described by Vegetius. Ancients ascribed the periodic recrudescences of the disease to the lunar cycle, hence the term "moon blindness."

Studies done over the years have produced some reliable data relative to the etiology, but many facets remain to be elucidated. Good evidence has been obtained to show that affected horses frequently have a high serum titer of agglutinin-lysis antibodies to *Leptospira pomona*, but recovery of this organism from affected horses and reproduction of the disease have not been convincingly demonstrated. An allergic basis for the disease, comparable to that seen in canine infectious hepatitis, has been postulated. It has been shown that under certain circumstances addition of riboflavin to the ration of normal horses will prevent the appearance of new cases of the disease. Infection with *Onchocerca* has also been associated with the condition. More evidence is needed before it can be stated unequivocally that the causative factors are known.

Lesions. The microscopic lesions can be readily correlated with the gross changes, most of which can be seen in the living animal. During the acute stage, the changes are referable largely to the anterior uvea. The iris and ciliary body are severely congested and intensely infiltrated with leukocytes, among which neutrophils predominate at first but are soon replaced by lymphocytes. These cells, along with plasma, escape from the iris and ciliary processes into both the anterior and posterior chambers. A few leukocytes may gain access to the vitreous from the ciliary processes. The anterior choroid and sclera are congested and corneal vascularization is a constant feature. These new vessels start as tiny capillary loops extending from the scleral vessels at the limbus into the lamina propria adjacent to the epithelium, but in later stages well-developed vessels may be demonstrable deeper in the lamina propria of the cornea.

Affected eyes in the quiescent stage ex-hibit characteristic although subtle microscopic lesions even after only one acute attack. Nodules of lymphocytes in the ciliary body and iris are the most constant finding. It may be possible to detect some collections of lymphocytes and bits of fibrin on the surface of the ciliary processes, iris, or lens capsules. Similar exudates may sometimes be found in the vitreous humor.

Repeated acute attacks of periodic ophthalmia usually leave the eye partially or completely blind. Posterior synechiae commonly interfere seriously with vision, either by occlusion of the pupil or by leaving iris pigment and exudates on the anterior lens capsule. Exudates on both the anterior and posterior lens capsule produce capsular opacities which may eventuate in cataracts. The inflammatory changes in the anterior uvea eventually interfere with the nutrition of the lens, and it becomes opaque with a fused-quartz appearance. Occasionally the lens may be luxated. Exudates accumulate in the choroid and retina, and after a time cause their separation. The pigment layer of the retina usually remains attached to the choroid, while exudate accumulating between it and the layer of rods and cones detaches the retina and forces it into the vitreous. Often the atrophic retina comes to lie in contact with the posterior lens capsule, but it remains attached at the optic papilla and the ora ciliaris retinae. The entire globe becomes smaller in size (phthisis bulbi) and the sclera, thickened. Secondary degeneration may occur in the optic nerve as a consequence of destruction of the neurons in the retina.

Ectropion Uveae. A specialized term of ophthalmic pathology, ectropion uveae, applies to the extension of the pigmented layer of epithelium from the posterior surface of the iris, around the margin of the pupil, to the anterior surface of the iris. This results from scarring of the iris with eversion of the pupillary margin by contraction of the scars. It is seen following iritis, in glaucoma, and occasionally as a congenital anomaly. Contraction of the iris

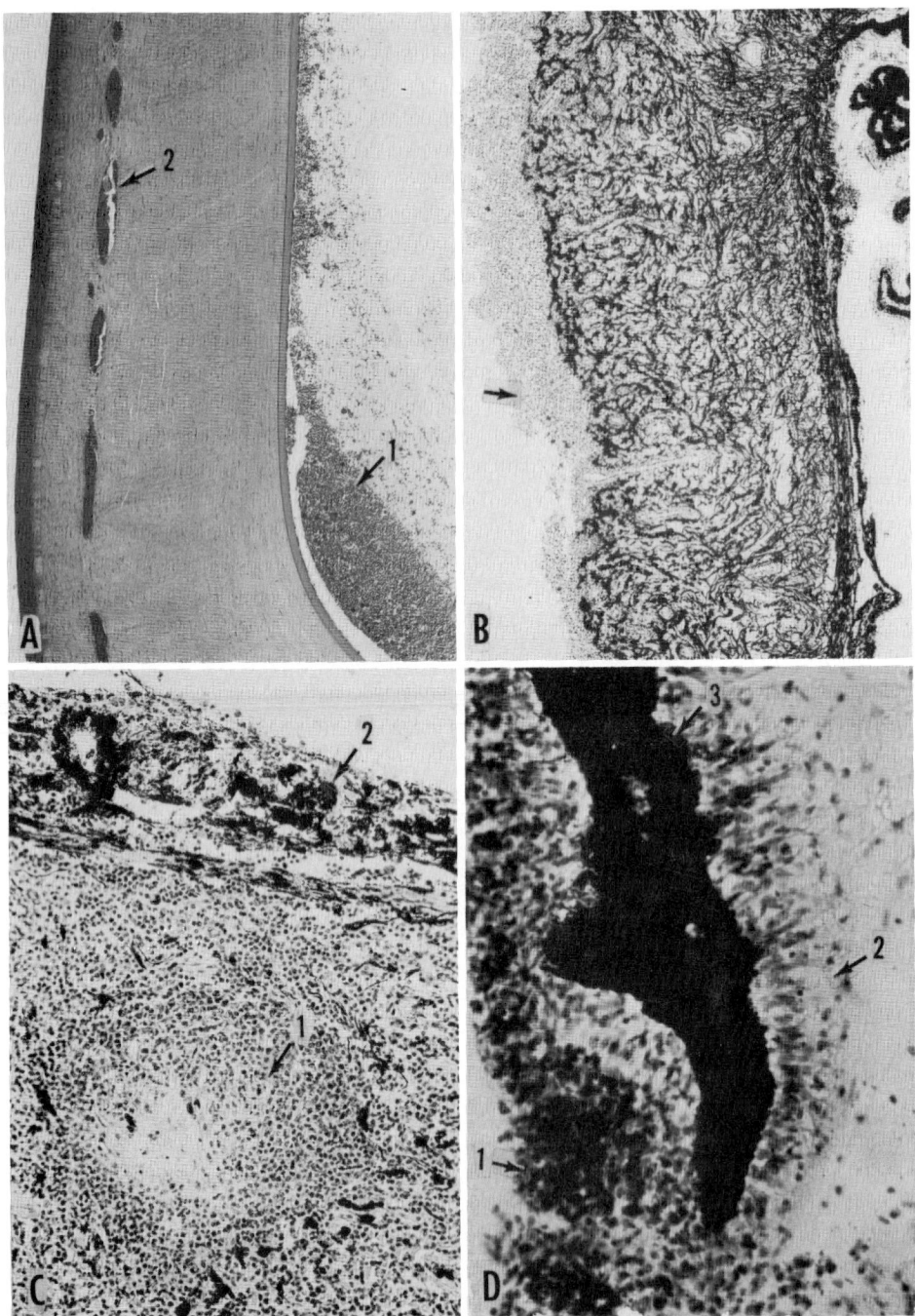

Fig. 28–4. Equine periodic ophthalmia (recurrent iridocyclitis). *A,* The acute stage. Leukocytes (*1*) in anterior chamber, corneal vascularization (*2*) (× 45). *B,* Leukocytes in anterior chamber (arrow) and iris in the acute stage (× 50). *C,* The iris in the acute stage (× 150). Circumscribed (*1*) and diffuse (*2*) collections of leukocytes in the iris. *D,* Ciliary process in the acute stage (× 240). Collections of leukocytes (*1*), disorganized ciliary epithelium (*2*) and pigment (*3*). (*D,* Courtesy of Armed Forces Institute of Pathology.) Contributor: Army Veterinary Research Laboratory.

which inverts the pupillary margin is known as **entropion uveae.**

Neoplasms. Primary neoplasms of the iris and ciliary apparatus are seldom recorded although their incidence is probably higher than published reports indicate. Malignant melanomas may arise from the iris or ciliary body, and hemangiomas have been observed in the iris. Adenomatous new growths (adenomas of ciliary epithelium) apparently arise from the non-pigmented ciliary epithelium and sometimes displace most of the internal structures of the eyeball (Saunders and Barron, 1958). Metastatic neoplasms may occur in the anterior uvea but are rare with the exception of malignant lymphoma. Ocular neoplasms are discussed more fully later in this chapter.

Ball, R.F.: A histopathological study of depigmented irises from single comb white Leghorns. Cornell Vet., 36:31–40, 1946.

Bryans, J.T.: Studies on equine leptospirosis. Cornell Vet., 45:16–50, 1955.

Gelatt, K.N.: Traumatic hyphema and iridocyclitis in the horse. Mod. Vet. Pract., 56:475–479, 1975.

Gelatt, K.N., Huston, K., and Leipold, H.W.: Ocular anomalies of incomplete albino cattle. Ophthalmoscopic examination. Am. J. Vet. Res., 30:1313–1316, 1969.

Heusser, H., et al.: Die periodische Augenentzundung der Pferde als Leptospirenerkrankung. Schweiz. Med. Wochenschr., 78:756–758, 1948.

Jones, T.C.: Equine periodic ophthalmia. Am. J. Vet. Res., 3:45–71, 1942.

Jones, T.C., Maurer, F.D., and Roby, T.O.: The role of nutrition in equine periodic ophthalmia. Am. J. Vet. Res., 6:67–80, 1945.

Jones, T.C., Roby, T.O., and Maurer, F.D.: The relation of riboflavin to equine periodic ophthalmia. Am. J. Vet. Res., 7:403–416, 1946.

Reese, A.B.: Tumors of the Eye. New York, Paul B. Hoeber, Inc., 1951.

Roberts, S.R.: Fundus lesions in equine periodic ophthalmia. J. Am. Vet. Med. Assoc., 141:229–239, 1962.

Roberts, S.R.: Etiology of equine periodic ophthalmia. Am. J. Ophthalmol., 55:1049–1055, 1963.

Roberts, S.R., and Bistner, S.I.: Persistent pupillary membrane in Basenji dogs. J. Am. Vet. Med. Assoc., 153:533–542, 1968.

Roby, T.O., and Jones, T.C.: The blood of equine periodic ophthalmia. Am. J. Vet. Res., 8:145–152, 1947.

Saunders, L.Z., and Barron, C.N.: Primary pigmented intraocular tumors in animals. Cancer Res., 18:234–245, 1958.

Trevino, G.S.: Canine blastomycosis with ocular involvement. Pathol. Vet., 3:652–658, 1966.

Wilder, H.C., and Paul, E.V.: Malignant melanoma of the choroid and ciliary body. A study of 2535 cases. Milit. Surg., 109:370–378, 1951.

Yager, R.H., Gochenour, W.S., Jr., and Wetmore, P.W.: Recurrent iridocyclitis (periodic ophthalmia) of horses. I. Agglutination and lysis of leptospiras by serums deriving from horses affected with recurrent iridocyclitis. J. Am. Vet. Med. Assoc., 117:207–209, 1950.

Vitreous

The vitreous body is that part of the transparent media that occupies the largest chamber of the eye. It may become distorted by luxation of the lens, persistence of the hyaloid artery, or detachment of the retina. Cells, pigment, and tissue debris may become suspended in the vitreous as opacities as a result of iridocyclitis or retinitis. During embryologic development of the lens, the primary vitreous is well vascularized. This vasculature and the hyaloid artery eventually atrophy under normal circumstances but may rarely persist, leaving the artery which terminates in a mass of fibrous, vascular tissue on the posterior capsule of the lens. Congenital cataract may accompany this anomaly.

Grimes, T.D., and Mullaney, J.: Persistent hyperplastic primary vitreous in a Greyhound. Vet. Rec., 85:607–611, 1969.

Rebhun, W.C.: Persistent hyperplastic primary vitreous in a dog. J. Am. Vet. Med. Assoc., 169:620–622, 1976.

Lens

The adult lens is composed entirely of epithelium without stroma or vasculature. It receives nourishment from the aqueous humor in which it is bathed. Its simple composition and structure sharply limit the range of morphologic changes which it can undergo, regardless of the type of injury to which it may be subjected. It is surrounded by a tough capsule within which is found the growing layer of epithelium (at the poles and on the anterior surface), whose inner layer of cells mature to become the lens fibers. These fibers are laid down in a concentric manner, the oldest being at the center, or nucleus, of the lens.

The morphologic changes that the lens itself can exhibit are limited to (1) abnormal growth changes in the epithelium, (2) deterioration of the lens protein with coagulation and disorganization of the lens fibers, and (3) rupture of the capsule, which exposes the lens substance to external forces which may lead to liquefaction, organization, or dissolution. The lens may be dislocated from its normal position (see Luxation), but if still in contact with normal aqueous humor may not be significantly altered.

The lens may be damaged by exposure to various toxic substances (naphthalein, ergot) or by nutritive or metabolic disturbances, especially in young animals (riboflavin deficiency, diabetes mellitus). The exact mode of action of substances harmful to the lens is not always clear, although it seems likely that changes in the aqueous probably precede any effect upon the lens.

Luxation. The lens is held in place by its ligaments which are attached to the ciliary body. A severe blow to the eyeball or a less severe one following damage to the suspensory ligaments may dislocate the lens from its normal position. The luxated lens may be displaced into the anterior chamber, into the ventral part of the posterior chamber, or into the vitreous (Fig. 28–6). The pathologist is sometimes faced with the problem of deciding whether a displaced lens in a specimen is actually luxated or is an artifact in sectioning the eye. This can usually be determined with certainty by careful gross and microscopic study to determine the status of the ocular tissue adjacent to the lens in its new site. Exudates around the lens, particularly if organized, are indications of luxation.

The luxated lens may be resorbed (*phacolysis*) if its capsule is ruptured, may

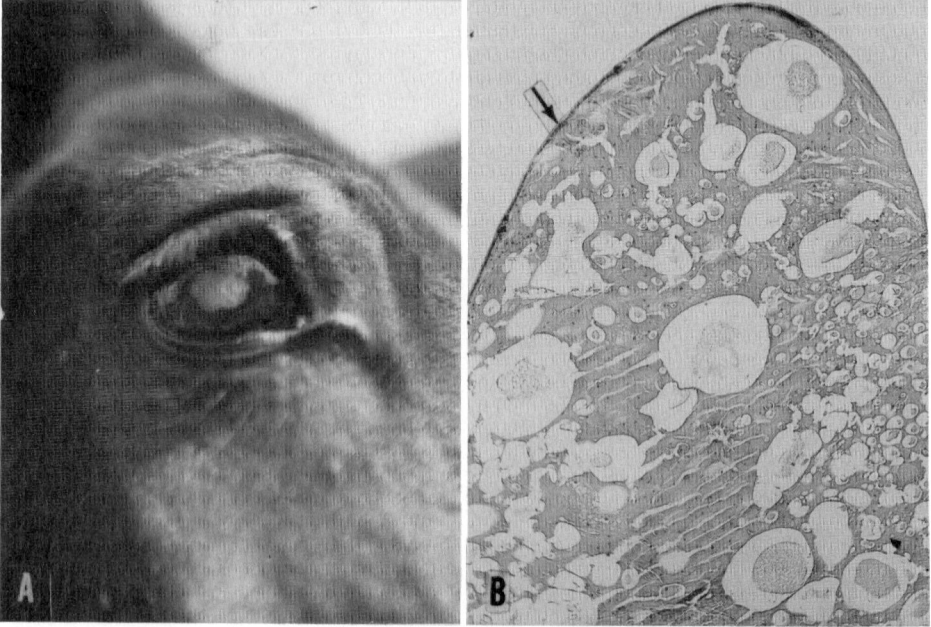

Fig. 28–5. *A*, Mature cataract in the eye of a horse following several attacks of periodic ophthalmia. *B*, Congenital cataract (× 40) in the eye of a newborn puppy. Anterior lens epithelium is indicated by the arrow. Note large vacuoles, disorganization of lens protein and retention of nuclei. (*B*, Courtesy of Armed Forces Institute of Pathology.) Contributor: Dr. Leo L. Lieberman.

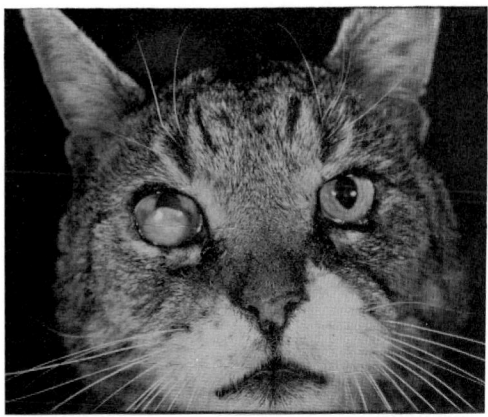

Fig. 28–6. Luxation of the lens into the anterior chamber of a 15-year-old castrated male cat. (Courtesy of Angell Memorial Animal Hospital.)

remain intact in its new site, or may become opaque and partially surrounded by leukocytic and fibrinous exudates which may become organized.

Cataract. A cataract is an opacity of the lens. It may be classified on the basis of its morphologic appearance, its etiology, or both. Opacities on the anterior or posterior lens capsule, usually resulting from iridocyclitis, may interfere with transparency of the lens but are not considered cataracts, nor are they believed to lead, per se, to cataracts.

The principal locations of cataracts are (1) the subcapsular epithelium, (2) the cortex, and (3) the nucleus of the lens. **Subcapsular cataracts** occurring under the anterior capsule (i.e., **anterior polar cataract**) are the result of abnormal proliferation of the lens epithelium at this site. The epithelial cells become redundant, disorganized, or laminated to form an opacity. This lesion may follow prolonged injury to the anterior segment of the lens as the result of a persistent posterior synechia. **Posterior polar cataract,** located under the capsule at the posterior face of the lens, also results from abnormal growth of lens epithelium. However, the absence of epithelium on the posterior surface in the normal adult eye means that epithelial cells must grow into

this area from the equator in order to form a cataract.

Cortical cataracts result from disorganization of the lens fibers, presumably following altered metabolism of the lens epithelium. The lens fibers lose their normal concentrically laminated structure to become disorganized and aggregated into irregularly spherical masses of material (*morgagnian globules*).

Nuclear cataracts are the result of changes in the transparency of the oldest lens fibers—those at the nucleus. These central fibers apparently become more dense and appear gray or (more often) yellowish in the center of the lens. This type appears most often in, but is not limited to, senile animals. The **morgagnian cataract** is characterized by complete liquefaction of cortical substance within which the sclerotic nucleus floats. To our knowledge, this type has not been described in animals.

Congenital cataracts are observed occasionally in newborn animals (Fig. 28–5). This defect is often attributable to failure of closure of the primary lens vesicle, hence such lesions are most likely to be found near the lens periphery toward the posterior lens surface, at the point where evidence of the lens vesicle is last demonstrable in the normal eye. Genetic factors may be the underlying cause in some congenital cataracts, but other factors may also be important. Many examples of congenital cataracts do, however, represent **hereditary cataracts.** Hereditary cataracts may not be evident at birth, and may be posterior or anterior. Examples of inherited or familial cataracts have been described in many different species. In some they appear to be inherited as an autosomal dominant trait (German Shepherd, Pointer, Beagle, Golden Retriever, Chesapeake Bay Retrievers) and in others as an autosomal recessive trait (Miniature Schnauzer, Standard Poodle, Holstein-Friesian, and Jersey cattle, certain strains of rats and mice), but in most the mode of inheritance is not clearly established. Congenital cataracts are seen in cats affected with the Chédiak-Higashi syndrome, but the relationship between the two is unclear, as cataracts are not associated with this disease in cattle, mink, or mice.

Viral infection in utero or early in life has been associated with cataracts in several species (rubella in man; *Herpesvirus canis* in dogs).

Cataracts can also be induced by a variety of experimental manipulations or exposure to certain drugs. Disophenol, an anthelmintic, has been shown to cause cataracts in dogs, as has dimethyl sulfoxide. The association of dinitrophenols and cataracts was first made in the 1930s in human beings when these drugs were used in weight control. Oxygen toxicity may lead to cataracts in mice and a variety of other ocular disorders in other species.

Congenital Anomalies. **Aphakia** (absence of the lens) and **microphakia** (small lens) are rare congenital anomalies of the lens usually associated with other ocular defects. Globular or cone-like protrusions of the posterior lens surface is a congenital defect of the lens known as posterior **lenticonus** and has been reported in dogs, calves, swine, mice, rabbits, and man. It is often associated with cataract within the protrusion or other areas of the lens. The lesion is believed to result from an overgrowth of lens fibers.

In dogs, capsular cataracts in the center of the lens may result from remnants of the pupillary membrane (Hirth et al., 1974).

Aguirre, G., and Bistner, S.I.: Posterior lenticonus in the dog. Cornell Vet., *63*:455–461, 1973.
Albanese, A.A., and Buschke, W.: On cataract and certain other manifestations of tryptophane deficiency in rats. Science, *95*:584–586, 1942.
Anderson, A.C.: Inherited (congenital) cataracts in the dog. Am. J. Pathol., *34*:965–975, 1958.
Clark, H.F.: Suckling mouse cataract agent. J. Infect. Dis., *114*:476–487, 1964.
Collier, L.L., Bryan, G.M., and Prieur, D.J.: Ocular manifestations of the Chédiak-Higashi syndrome in four species of animals. J. Am. Vet. Med. Assoc., *175*:587–590, 1979.
Farmston, C.: Observations on subluxations and luxations of the crystalline lens in the dog. J. Comp. Pathol. Therap., *55*:168–184, 1945.

Gelatt, K.N.: Cataracts in cattle. J. Am. Vet. Med. Assoc., *159*: 195–200, 1971.
———: Cataracts in the Golden Retriever dog. Vet. Med. Small Anim. Clin., *67*:113–115, 1972.
———: Congenital cataracts in a litter of rabbits. J. Am. Vet. Med. Assoc., *167*:598–599, 1975.
Gelatt, K.N., et al.: Cataracts in Chesapeake Bay Retrievers. J. Am. Vet. Med. Assoc., *175*:1176–1178, 1979.
Geyer, H., von, Morel, J., Lauvergne, J.J., and Winzernried, H.U.: Augenveranderungen bei blind geborenen Braunviehkalbern. Schweiz. Arch. Tierheilkd., *116*:147–153, 1974.
Gorthy, W.C., and Abdelbaki, Y.Z.: Morphology of a hereditary cataract in the rat. Exp. Eye Res., *19*:147–156, 1974.
Heywood, R.: Drug-induced lenticular lesions in the dog. Br. Vet. J., *127*:301–303, 1971.
———: Juvenile cataracts in the Beagle dog. J. Small Anim. Pract., *12*:171–177, 1971.
Hirth, R.S., Greenstein, E.T., and Peer, R.L.: Anterior capsular opacities (spurious cataracts) in Beagle dogs. Vet. Pathol., *11*:181–194, 1974.
Kirk, J.H.: Persistent pupillary membrane: Developmental review and an occurrence in *Macaca mulatta*. Lab. Anim. Sci., *22*:122–125, 1972.
Koch, S.A., and Rubin, L.F.: Probable nonhereditary congenital cataracts in dogs. J. Am. Vet. Med. Assoc., *150*:1374–1376, 1967.
Lapolla, L., and Mastronardi, M.: Cataract in young dogs. Acta Med. Vet. Napoli, *8*:311–321, 1962.
Martin, C.L.: The formation of cataracts in dogs with disophenol: Age susceptibility and production with chemical grade 2,6-diiodo-4-nitrophenol. Can. Vet. J., *16*:228–232, 1975.
Martin, C.L., Christmas, R., and Leipold, H.W.: Formation of temporary cataracts in dogs given a disophenol preparation. J. Am. Vet. Med. Assoc., *161*:294–302, 1972.
Martin, C.L., and Leipold, H.W.: Aphakia and multiple ocular defects in Saint Bernard puppies. Vet. Med. Small Anim. Clin., *69*:448–453, 1974.
Oleson, H.P., Jensen, O.A., and Norn, M.S.: Congenital hereditary cataract in Cocker Spaniels. J. Small Anim. Pract., *15*:741–750, 1974.
Peiffer, R.L., and Gelatt, K.N.: Cataracts in the cat. Feline Pract., *4*:34–38, 1974.
Prince, J.H., Diesem, C.D., Eglitis, I., and Ruskell, G.L.: Anatomy and Histology of the Eye and Orbit in Domestic Animals. Springfield, Ill., Charles C Thomas, 1960.
Ribelin, W.E., et al.: Development of cataracts in dogs and rats from prolonged feeding of sulfaethoxypyridazine. Toxicol. Appl. Pharmacol., *10*:557–564, 1967.
Roberts, S.R., and Helper, L.C.: Cataracts in Afghan hounds. J. Am. Vet. Med. Assoc., *160*:427–432, 1972.
Rubin, L.F.: Cataract in Golden Retrievers. J. Am. Vet. Med. Assoc., *165*:457–458, 1974.
Rubin, L.F., and Flowers, R.D.: Inherited cataract in a family of Standard Poodles. J. Am. Vet. Med. Assoc., *161*:207–208, 1972.
Rubin, L.F., Koch, S.A., and Huber, R.J.: Hereditary cataracts in Miniature Schnauzers. J. Am. Vet. Med. Assoc., *154*:1456–1458, 1969.

Schocket, S.S., et al.: Induction of cataracts in mice by exposure to oxygen. Israel J. Med. Sci., 8:1596–1601, 1972.

Smith, R.S., Hoffman, H., and Cisar, C.: Congenital cataract in the cat. Arch. Ophthalmol., 81:259–263, 1969.

Tissot, R.G., and Cohen, C.: A new congenital cataract in the mouse. J. Hered., 63:197–201, 1972.

Totter, J.R., and Day, P.L.: Cataract and other ocular changes resulting from tryptophane deficiency. J. Nutr., 24:159–166, 1942.

Warkany, J., and Schraffenberger, E.: Congenital malformations of the eyes induced in rats by maternal vitamin A deficiency. Proc. Soc. Exp. Biol. Med., 57:49–52, 1944.

Weisse, I., Niggeschulze, A., and Stotzer, H.: (Spontaneous congenital cataracts in rats, mice, and rabbits.) Arch. Toxicol., 32:199–207, 1974.

Williams, R.D.: Equine uveitis: A model system for study of immunologically mediated tissue injury. Diss. Abstr. Internat., 33B:4578–4579, 1973.

Worgul, B.V., and Rothstein, H.: Congenital cataracts associated with disorganized meridional rows in a new laboratory animal: The degu (Octodon degus). Biomedicine [Express], 23:1–4, 1975.

Retina

The retina is the light-sensitive inner coat that lines the posterior segment of the eyeball. Its inner surface is in contact with the vitreous and its outer surface with the choroid. The retina terminates anteriorly near the ciliary body to form a border which, though serrated in man (ora serrata), is usually smooth in most animals (ora ciliaris retinae). The retina is firmly attached at this anterior border as well as around the margin of the optic disc, but is more likely to be separated from its pigment epithelium, which coheres closely to the adjacent choroid.

In many animals a specific laminated structure, the **tapetum,** lies between the retina and choroid; in some species it is partially pigmented and then is called the **tapetum nigrum;** if unpigmented, the **tapetum lucidum.** In the horse, for example, a horizontal line in the globe just below the level of the optic disc separates the greenish iridescent tapetum lucidum above from the dark brown, nearly black, tapetum nigrum below. In some species, as the dog, the tapetum can be detected microscopically or with the ophthalmoscope and the overlying regions of the retina are designated as "tapetal" or "nontapetal." These two areas of the retina sometimes respond differently in disease.

The retinal vessels of each species have distinctive anatomic features which must be understood in order to interpret deviations from normal. In Equidae, for instance, the arteries and veins cannot be distinguished from one another with the ophthalmoscope and they emerge from the margins of the optic disc in a uniform radial manner which gives the disc the appearance of a conventionalized rising sun. In the dog and cat, as in many other species, veins and arteries are readily differentiated as they emerge from the center of the optic disc and follow a tortuous, branching course into the retina. The embryonic hyaloid artery, which extends from the optic disc to the posterior lens capsule, may still be present at birth in vestigial form. This persistence of the hyaloid may be normal in some species (dog, ox), abnormal in others.

The retina may be considered as having two components, the pigment epithelium (which develops from the outer layer of the embryonic cup) and the sensory retina (from the inner layer of the optic cup). The sensory retina has a complex structure consisting of nine layers which, from the innermost toward the outermost, are: (1) the inner limiting membrane; (2) layer of optic nerve fibers; (3) layer of ganglion cells; (4) inner plexiform layer; (5) inner nuclear layer; (6) outer plexiform layer; (7) outer nuclear layer; (8) outer limiting membrane; and (9) layer of rods and cones (bacillary layer). These layers vary in thickness in different regions in the retina and between species, but further consideration of these differences lies outside the scope of this book. It is important to recall that the layer of optic nerve fibers contains the axons of the neurons of the layer of ganglion cells; these axons assemble at the optic papilla and continue as the fibers within the optic nerve. Thus it is apparent that lesions in

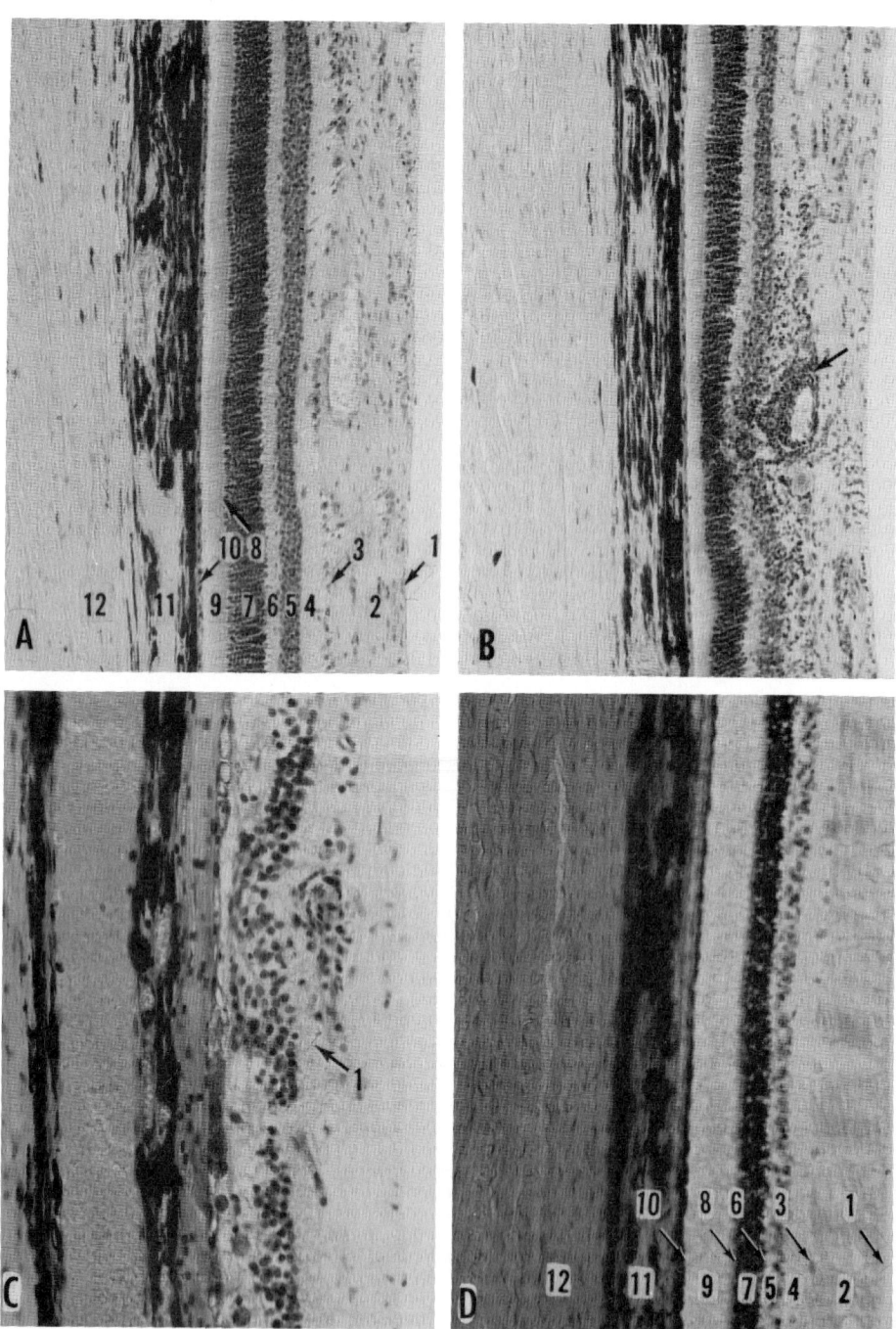

Fig. 28–7. *A,* Normal canine retina (× 130). Section from non-tapetal zone. Inner limiting membrane (*1*); layer of optic nerve fibers (*2*); layer of ganglion cells (*3*); inner plexiform layer (*4*); inner nuclear layer (*5*); outer plexiform layer (*6*); outer nuclear layer (*7*); outer limiting membrane (*8*); layer of rods and cones (*9*); pigment epithelium (*10*); choroid (*11*); and sclera (*12*). Contributor: Dr. Claude S. Perry. *B,* Early retinitis in a dog with toxoplasmosis (× 130). Leukocytes around blood vessels (arrow); layers of retina distorted. Contributor: Dr. Claude S. Perry. *C,* Retinal atrophy, tapetal zone of retina of a dog. Note atrophy of inner and outer nuclear layers (arrow) as well as layer of rods and cones. Note especially swollen cells of pigment epithelium adjacent to the tapetum. *D,* Normal equine retina (× 165). Numbers indicate same structures as *A.* (*A* and *B,* Courtesy of Armed Forces Institute of Pathology.)

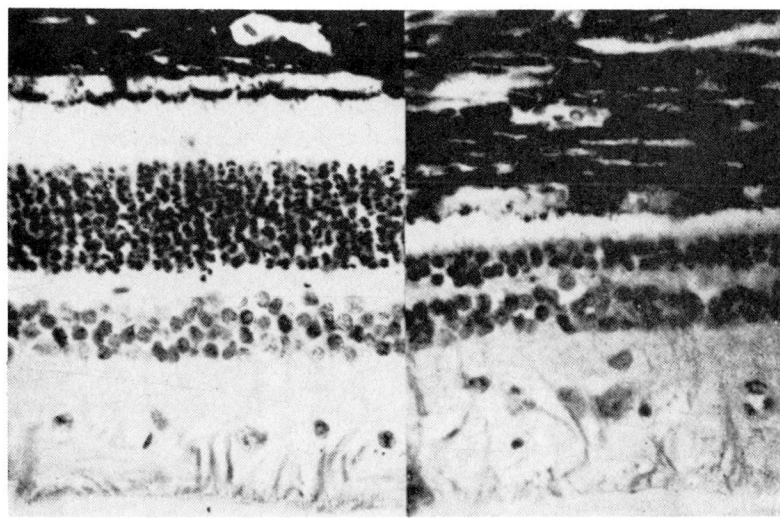

Fig. 28–8. Hereditary progressive retinal atrophy. Retina of two 3½-month-old dogs, normal on the left (× 270). Note reduction in width of outer nuclear and bacillary layers in the affected retina. The rod nuclei are almost completely lost, leaving only cone nuclei. The inner layers are not affected. (Courtesy of Dr. H.B. Parry and *British Journal of Ophthalmology.*)

the layer of ganglion cells or of nerve fibers could easily result in changes in the optic nerve.

The blood supply of the retina comes from two sources: (1) the choriocapillaris, which nourishes the pigment epithelium, the layer of rods and cones, and the outer nuclear layer, and (2) the retinal artery which emerges within or adjacent to the optic papilla and continues in the retina within the nerve-fiber layer, dividing dichotomously as it spreads out toward the ora ciliaris retinae. The capillaries from this arterial system anastomose only with each other and join only the retinal venous system. The retinal artery supplies the inner layers of the retina (nerve fiber, ganglion cell, inner plexiform, and inner nuclear layers).

The retinal artery grows out from the papilla into the retina toward the ora ciliaris retinae during embryonic life. In the human fetus, these vessels start growing from the papilla during the fourth month and reach the ora serrata during the eighth month in utero. In some animals

(dog, cat, rat), this development is slower; newborn kittens, puppies, or four-day-old rats have retinal vessels which reach about halfway to the ora ciliaris retinae, a stage of development reached by the human fetus during the seventh month of gestation.

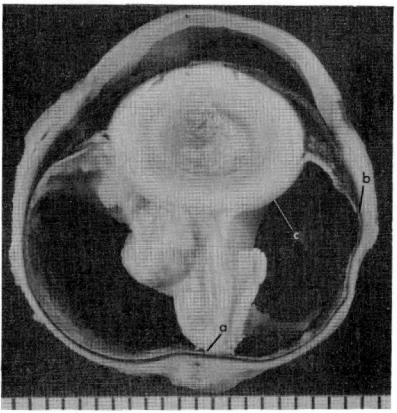

Fig. 28–9. Detachment of the retina, eye of a spayed female Beagle, five years old. Note that the retina remains attached around the margins of the optic disc (*a*) and at the *ora ciliaris retinae* (*b*), and is collapsed over the posterior surface of the lens (*c*). (Courtesy of Angell Memorial Animal Hospital.)

This species difference has been used in the experimental reproduction of retrolental fibroplasia or retinopathy of prematurity, a disease of premature infants. In an atmosphere high in oxygen (as in an incubator or oxygen tent), the immature retinal vessels of the newborn fail to grow normally, the endothelial cells forming nonfunctional nodules resembling glomerular tufts; this leads to retinal detachment, retinal edema and hemorrhages, and vitreous disorganization—features that closely simulate the lesions of retrolental fibroplasia of infants.

The retina may be affected by a large variety of injurious factors, not all of which are known. It is commonly involved in severe cases of iritis, iridocyclitis, and choroiditis—in fact, it is so intimately related to the choroid that inflammation of one usually involves the other. **Chorioretinitis** is therefore not an uncommon pathologic finding. Exudates that accumulate in the retina as a consequence of inflammation, especially in recurrent iridocyclitis, are usually found adjacent to the pigment epithelium. The presence of such exudates results in **detachment of the retina.** The accumulation of edema in the retina may dislodge it from its normal position and in extreme cases force it into the vitreous, sometimes to lie in contact with the posterior lens capsule where it becomes incorporated in an organized **cyclitic membrane.** The recognition of the presence of exudate is essential in order to differentiate between true retinal detachment and detachment as an artifact produced in preparation of the specimen. In either event, the retina remains attached at the optic papilla and ora ciliaris retinae.

The secondary changes in the retina resulting from glaucoma are described under "Glaucoma." In some specific diseases,

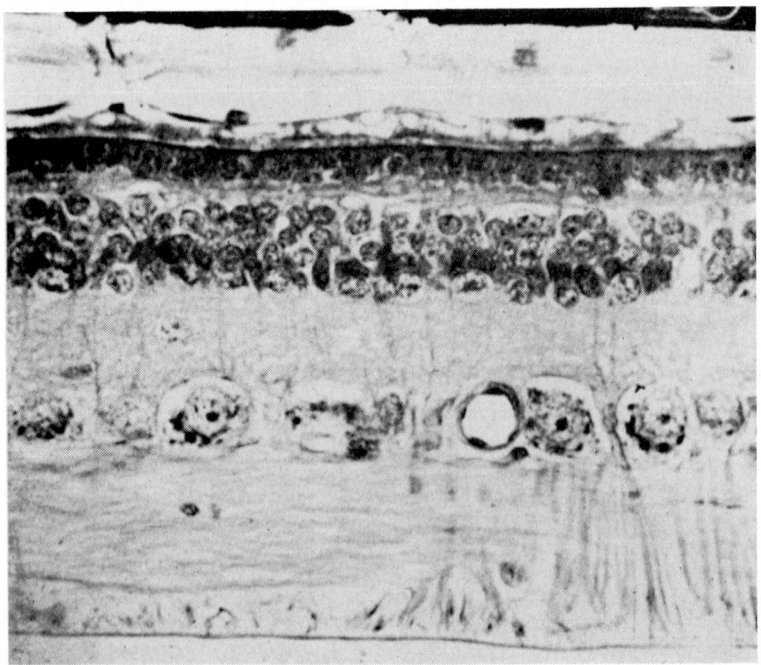

Fig. 28–10. Hereditary progressive retinal atrophy. Section of retina (× 450) of a six-month-old dog with a later stage of atrophy than shown in Fig. 28–8. Note complete loss of rod nuclei. Remnants of the cones form a thin layer between the atrophic pigment epithelium and the thickened external limiting membrane. (Courtesy of Dr. H.B. Parry and the *British Journal of Ophthalmology*.)

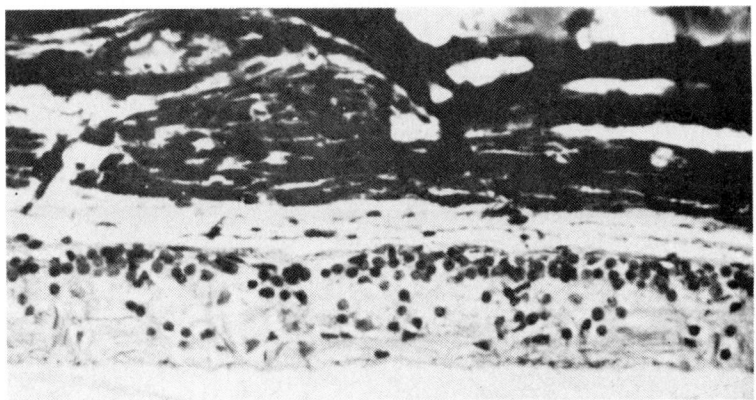

Fig. 28–11. Hereditary progressive retinal atrophy. Late stage in a six-year-old dog which had been blind for four years (× 240). The retina is completely disorganized, most nuclei have disappeared, and the pigment epithelium is missing. The remains of the atrophic retina are in direct contact with the tapetum. (Courtesy of Dr. H.B. Parry and the *British Journal of Ophthalmology*.)

i.e., canine distemper, feline panleukopenia, toxoplasmosis, and coccidioidomycosis, lesions may occur in the retina. Deficiencies of certain nutrients such as vitamin A or taurine may also lead to retinal degeneration, as can irradiation, severe anemia, and various poisons such as bracken fern.

Hereditary or suspected hereditary atrophy and degeneration of the retina occurs in several breeds of dogs as well as in cats, mice, and rats. The pathogenesis in different breeds and species is not entirely understood and therefore the conditions discussed under the single headings that follow should be viewed as categories of disease and not necessarily as specific syndromes.

Hereditary Progressive Retinal Atrophy in Dogs. Retinal atrophy in families of Red Irish Setter dogs was described by Parry (1953). Parry (1954) described a similar disease in Afghan dogs and a yellow Labrador Retriever under the designation *familial progressive retinal atrophy*. Similar retinal degenerations have since been described in many other breeds, including Norwegian Elkhounds, Poodles, Samoyed, Cocker Spaniel, Collie, as well as mixed breeds. All breeds are probably affected.

The condition has also been termed *rod dysplasia*. In Irish Setters, Norwegian Elkhounds, and Poodles, the disorder is inherited as a simple autosomal recessive trait. The mode of inheritance in other breeds has not been established.

Night blindness is the first indication of the disease, which may be apparent as early as six weeks of age in Irish Setters or as late as five years in Poodles. This progresses to complete blindness over a period of months to years. The lesions are similar in most examples, beginning in the outer layers of the retina with loss of rods, cones, and their nuclei, followed by disappearance of the inner layers. The disease terminates in total sclerosis of the retina, although the ganglion cell layer may be relatively spared. The rods in affected Norwegian Elkhounds and both the rods and cones in Irish Setters are never fully developed. In some breeds, especially Poodles, cataracts accompany the disease.

Three stages of the disease have been recognized and are of value in studying the lesions. During the first stage, 2 to 9 months in duration, there is uniform, bilaterally symmetric loss of rods and their nuclei, resulting in night blindness without detectable effect upon day vision. Al-

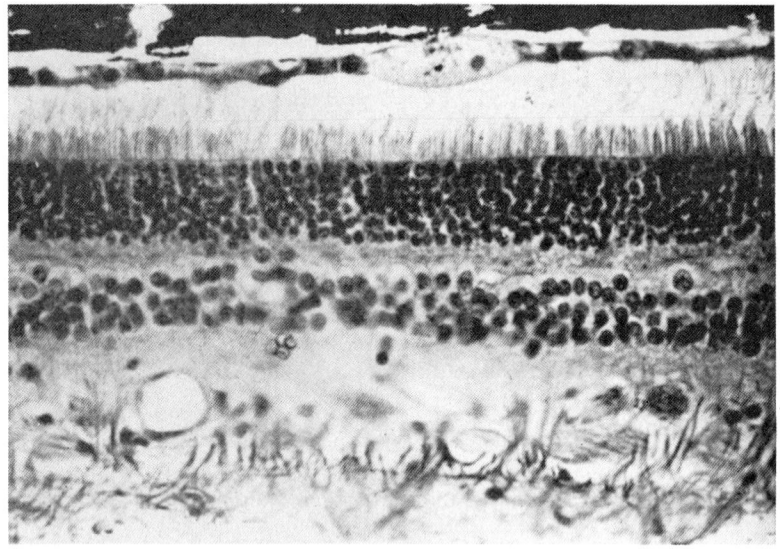

Fig. 28–12. Progressive central retinal atrophy with pigment epithelial dystrophy. Retina of a two-year-old red Irish Setter dog (× 330). Section near ventral edge of tapetal fundus near papilla. Giant cell in pigment epithelium and gliosis of optic nerve fiber layer. (Courtesy of Dr. H.B. Parry and the *British Journal of Ophthalmology*.)

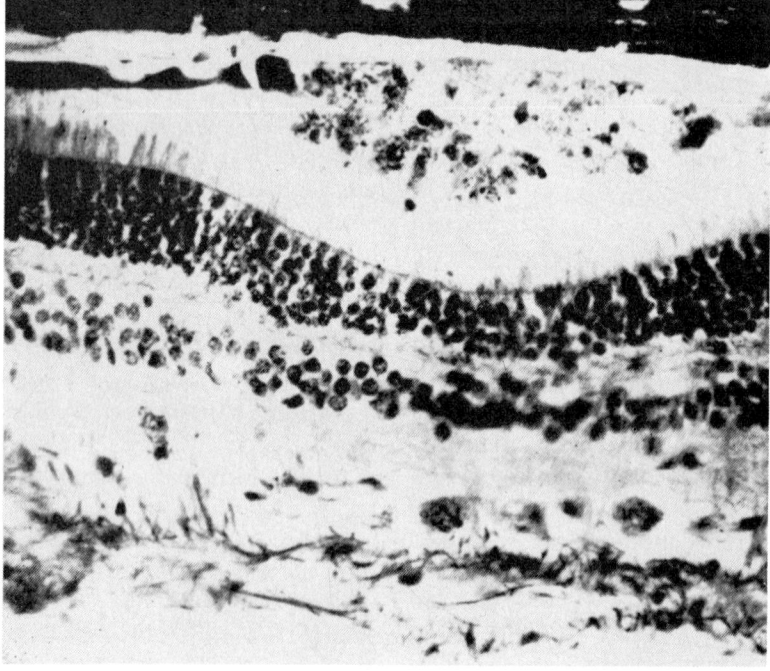

Fig. 28–13. Progressive central retinal atrophy. Same case as Fig. 28–12, section from midtapetal fundus near papilla. Note hypertrophied pigment epithelium, which displaces the adjacent layer of rods and cones. There is gliosis in the nerve fiber layer and atrophy of ganglion cells. (Courtesy of Dr. H.B. Parry and *British Journal of Ophthalmology*.)

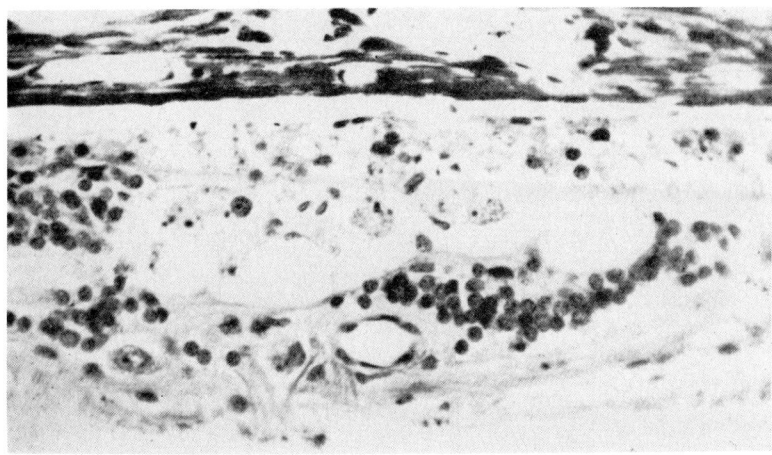

Fig. 28–14. Progressive central retinal atrophy. Retina of a three-year-old Border Collie dog (× 330). Note giant multicellular nest in pigment epithelium, cavities where rods and cones should be, atrophy and sclerosis of most of the retina. (Courtesy of Dr. H.B. Parry and the *British Journal of Ophthalmology*.)

though the entire retina is affected, the lesions are usually most severe at the periphery. In the second stage, lasting 3 to 24 months, retinal cones and cone nuclei are lost, causing progressive failure of day vision. The other layers of the retina remain normal. When the third stage is reached, both day and night blindness are complete as a result of the disorganization of all layers of the retina, glial proliferation and diffuse sclerosis of the retina. The pigment layer of the retina is atrophied and a few pigment-laden cells are dispersed in the sclerotic retina. Accumulations of pigment cells are not seen, as they are in human retinitis pigmentosa.

Progressive Central Retinal Atrophy in Dogs. Progressive atrophic changes in the central portion of the retina are distinguished by Parry (1954) from hereditary progressive retinal atrophy by the central distribution of the lesions and the occurrence of pigment aggregates which can be detected with the ophthalmoscope. The disease has been recognized in the Golden Retriever, Labrador, Shetland Sheepdog, Border Collie, and mixed breeds. It is thought to be inherited but the mode is not established.

The syndrome is recognized clinically by the appearance of small irregular foci of pigmentation in the tapetal fundus of middle-aged or old dogs, with bilateral impairment of central vision but with normal peripheral day and night vision. The lesions apparently start in the central part of the retina with swelling and proliferation of pigment epithelial cells, loss of adjacent rods and cones, and gliosis of the ganglion cell layer. As it progresses, nodular proliferation of the pigment epithelium increases, with displacement and sclerosis of all retinal layers. The final result is complete sclerosis of the retina around the papilla even though peripheral zones are unaffected.

Central Ganglion Cell Degeneration of Retina. An ocular syndrome has been described by Parry (1955) in a strain of Cocker Spaniels in which a central scotoma results from an anomaly of ganglion cells and optic nerve fibers of the central retina. These nonprogressive changes arise in puppyhood and are often associated with congenital cataracts, suggesting that the lesions develop in late intrauterine or early postnatal life. The cause is unknown.

The lesions are limited to the central part

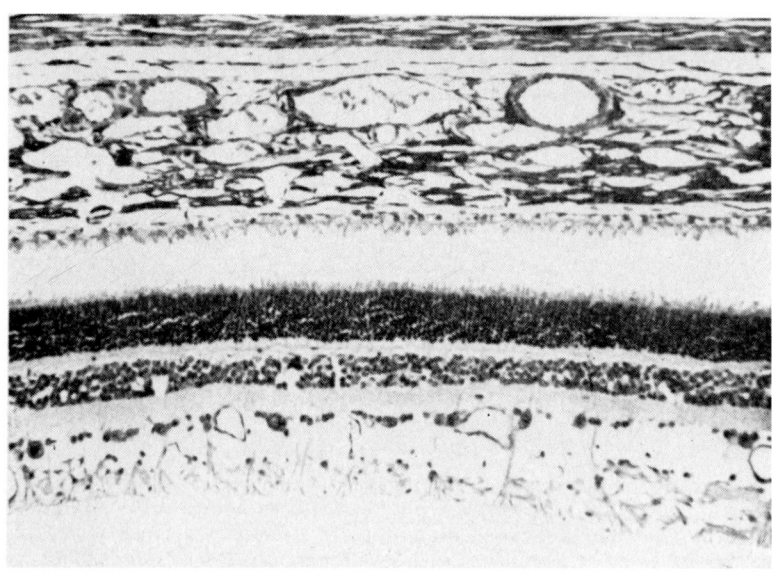

Fig. 28–15. Central ganglion cell degeneration of the retina. Retina of an eight-week-old Cocker Spaniel (× 120). Cavitation of optic nerve fiber and ganglion cell layers. Separation of the rod and cone layers from the pigment epithelium is an artifact. (Courtesy of Dr. H.B. Parry and *British Journal of Ophthalmology*.)

of the retina, usually extending a short distance from the papilla to involve the middle of the nontapetal zone ventrally and, to a smaller extent, the tapetal fundus dorsally. The outer layers of the neuroepithelium are normal and the choroid, sclera, and tapetum are unaffected. In the diseased central zone of the retina, the optic nerve fiber layer is seen microscopically to be much thickened and to contain many large vacuoles. Across these cavities run heavy strands of Müller's fibers, which fan out and terminate in the internal limiting membrane. The ganglion cells probably are fewer and the Nissl substance of those remaining is agglomerated into large clumps and stains deeply with basic dyes. The retinal vessels are not affected except that many are located rather deep in the thickened ganglion cell layer, and this may explain the apparent disappearance of central subsidiary vessels upon ophthalmoscopic examination.

Retinal Cone Atrophy in Dogs. A degenerative disease of the retina that affects only cones has been described in Alaskan Malamute dogs by Koch and Rubin (1971) and Aguirre and Rubin (1974). Loss of cones leads to day blindness or **hemeralopia**. The disease is inherited as a simple autosomal trait. Ultrastructural changes are evident as early as seven weeks of age and progress to lesions visible with light microscopy by six months of age and almost total absence of cones by two years of age.

Central Retinal Degeneration in Cats. Bellhorn and Fischer (1970) have described a central retinal degeneration in cats that occurs randomly and apparently is not inherited. The disease, also described by others (Bellhorn et al., 1974; Fischer, 1974), is characterized by degeneration and thinning of the outer layers of the central retina and macula, and has also been termed *macular retinal degeneration*. As the disease progresses, there is loss of all layers of the central retina with glial cell proliferation. Hayes and co-workers (1975) have shown experimentally that taurine deficiency leads to an essentially identical central ret-

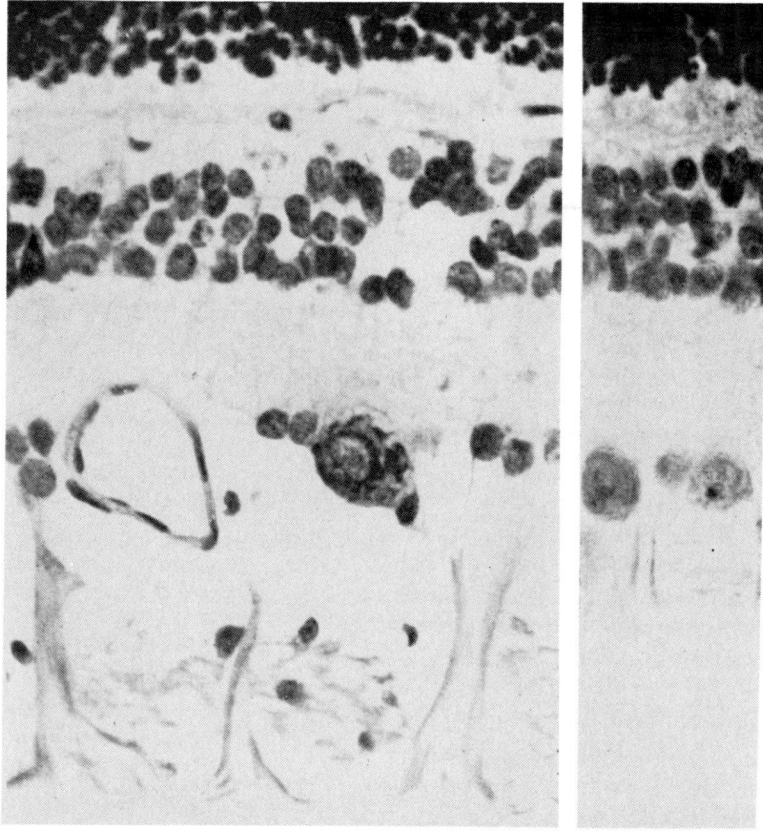

Fig. 28–16.   Central ganglion cell degeneration of the retina. Same case as Fig. 28–15 (× 590) with normal retina on the right for comparison. Note large vacuoles in the outer portion of the optic nerve fiber layer, with only a few fibers near the internal limiting membrane. The conspicuous strands transcending the cavities are Müller's fibers. (Courtesy of Dr. H.B. Parry and *British Journal of Ophthalmology*.)

inal degeneration in cats. The role of taurine in the spontaneous disease remains to be examined.

Diffuse Retinal Atrophy in Cats. This retinopathy is histologically similar to central degeneration in cats, except that the entire retina is affected. Rods and cones are affected first, and the disease progresses to affect all layers. The condition is considered an inherited disease (Rubin and Lipton, 1973).

Inherited Retinopathies in Mice and Rats. Several authors have described these retinopathies (Keeler, 1970; Sidman and Green, 1965; Sorsby et al., 1954; Tansley, 1951; Herron et al., 1974; Yates et al., 1974). In both species, lesions which begin in the outer layers and progress to the inner layers are evident as early as two to three weeks of age. In rats the degeneration commences centrally and spreads peripherally.

Retinopathy Associated With Canine Distemper. Blindness has often been described during or following outbreaks of distemper in dogs. It is difficult to obtain critical proof of the effect of the virus of Carré upon ocular structures, but much indirect evidence points toward such an effect, particularly in animals with involvement of the central nervous system. Parry (1954) and others have described changes in the choroid and retina of dogs which appear to be the direct result of distemper virus. This retinopathy occurs in peracute, subacute, and chronic forms, but all are characterized by generalized destruction of all layers of the retina with foci of more intense damage. These changes first involve the outer and inner layers, progressing toward the middle retinal layers. The damage is more severe over the peripheral than in the central fundus.

Early lesions consist of disorganization of the ganglion cell layer with loss of neurons and distortion of the layer of rods and cones. At first the intervening layers of the retina are not affected, but later they are also destroyed, the inner nuclear layer being the last to disappear. In some cases, intranuclear and cytoplasmic inclusion bodies have been observed in the ganglion cell layer. At the end stage, the retina is completely sclerotic, the choroid is thinned and has lost some pigment. The retinal pigment epithelium can no longer be distinguished, but numerous large cells laden with melanin may remain in the sclerosed retina. More study is needed on the possible effect of the distemper virus upon ocular and nervous structures.

Retinal degeneration is seen in sheep poisoned by bracken fern, and the various storage diseases discussed in Chapter 2 may involve the retina.

Aguirre, G.: Inherited retinal degenerations in the dog. Trans. Am. Acad. Ophthalmol. Otolaryngol., 81:667–676, 1976.

Aguirre, G.D., and Rubin, L.F.: Progressive retinal atrophy (rod dysplasia) in the Norwegian Elkhound. J. Am. Vet. Med. Assoc., 158:208–218, 1971.

———: The early diagnosis of rod dysplasia in the Norwegian Elkhound. J. Am. Vet. Med. Assoc., 159:429–433, 1971.

———: Pathology of hemeralopia in the Alaskan Malamute dog. Invest. Ophthalmol., 13:231–235, 1974.

———: Rod-cone dysplasia (progressive retinal atrophy) in Irish Setters. J. Am. Vet Med. Assoc., 166:157–164, 1975.

Barnett, K.C.: Canine retinopathies. I. History and review of the literature. II. The Miniature and Toy Poodle. III. The other breeds. IV. Causes of retinal atrophy. J. Small Anim. Pract., 6:41–55, 1965. II.

6:93–109, 1965. III. 6:185–196, 1965. IV. 6:229–242, 1965.

———: Retinal atrophy. Vet. Rec., 77:1543–1552, 1965.

Bellhorn, R.W.: Feline central retinal degeneration. Trans. Am. Acad. Ophthalmol. Otolaryngol., 81:683–686, 1976.

Bellhorn, R.W., Aguirre, G.D., and Bellhorn, M.B.: Feline central retinal degeneration. Invest. Ophthalmol., 13:608–616, 1974.

Bellhorn, R.W., and Fischer, C.A.: Feline central retinal degeneration. J. Am. Vet. Med. Assoc., 157:842–849, 1970.

Bourne, M.C., Campbell, D.A., and Tansley, K.: Hereditary degeneration of rat retina. Br. J. Ophthalmol., 22:613–623, 1938.

Cogan, D.G., and Kuwabara, T.: Photoreceptive abiotrophy of the retina in the Elkhound. Pathol. Vet., 2:101–128, 1965.

Fischer, C.A.: Retinopathy in anemic cats. J. Am. Vet. Med. Assoc., 156:1415–1427, 1970.

———: Retinal and retinochoroidal lesions in early neuropathic canine distemper. J. Am. Vet. Med. Assoc., 158:740–752, 1971.

———: Feline central retinal degeneration. Comp. Pathol. Bull., 5:3–4, 1974.

Hayes, K.C., Carey, R.E., and Schmidt, S.Y.: Retinal degeneration associated with taurine deficiency in the cat. Science, 188:949–951, 1975.

Hayes, K.C., Rabin, A.R., and Berson, E.L.: An ultrastructural study of nutritionally induced and reversed retinal degeneration in cats. Am. J. Pathol., 78:505–524, 1975.

Herron, W.L., Riegel, B.W., Brennan, E., and Rubin, M.L.: Retinal dystrophy in the pigmented rat. Invest. Ophthalmol., 13:87–94, 1974.

Heywood, R.: An anomaly of the ocular fundus of the Beagle dog. J. Small Anim. Pract., 13:213–215, 1972.

Keeler, C.: A new hereditary degeneration of the mouse retina. J. Hered., 61:62–63, 1970.

Koch, S.A., and Rubin, L.F.: Distribution of cones in the hemeralopic dog. J. Am. Vet. Med. Assoc., 159:1257–1259, 1971.

———: Distribution of cones in retina of the normal dog. Am. J. Vet. Res., 33:361–363, 1972.

Krahenmann, A.: (Progressive retinal atrophy in Swiss dog breeds. I. Peripheral retinal atrophy.) Schweiz. Arch. Tierheilkd., 116:645–652, 1974.

LaVail, M.M., Sidman, R.L., and Gerhardt, C.O.: Congenic strains of RCS rats with inherited retinal dystrophy. J. Hered., 66:242–244, 1975.

Mullen, R.J., and LaVail, M.M.: Inherited retinal dystrophy: Primary defect in pigment epithelium determined with experimental rat chimeras. Science, 193:799–801, 1976.

Parry, H.B.: Degenerations of the dog retina. I. Structure and development of the retina of the normal dog. Br. J. Ophthalmol., 37:385–404, 1953. (Abstr.) Vet. Rec., 68:77, 1956.

———: Degenerations of the dog retina. II. Generalized progressive atrophy of hereditary origin. Br. J. Ophthalmol., 37:487–502, 1953. (Abstr.) Vet. Rec., 68:77, 1956.

———: Degenerations of the dog retina. III. Retinopathy secondary to glaucoma. Br. J. Ophthalmol., *37*:670–679, 1953. (Abstr.) Vet. Rec., *68*:77, 1956.

———: Degenerations of the dog retina. IV. Retinopathies associated with dog distemper-complex virus infections. Br. J. Ophthalmol., *38*:295–309, 1954. (Abstr.) Vet. Rec., *68*:78, 1956.

———: Degenerations of the dog retina. V. Generalized progressive atrophy of uncertain aetiology. Br. J. Ophthalmol., *38*:545–552, 1954. (Abstr.) Vet. Rec., *68*:78, 1956.

———: Degenerations of the dog retina. VI. Central progressive atrophy with pigment epithelial dystrophy. Br. J. Ophthalmol., *38*:653–668, 1954.

———: Degeneration of the dog retina. VII. Central nonprogressive degeneration due to an anomaly of ganglion cells and their axons. Br. J. Ophthalmol., *39*:29–36, 1955. (Abstr.) Vet Rec., *68*:78, 1956.

———: Degeneration and pigment cell dystrophies of the dog retina. Excerpta Medica, Sect. VII, Neurology and Psychiatry, *8*:866–868, 1955.

Parry, H.B., Tansley, K., and Thomson, L.C.: Electroretinogram during development of the hereditary retinal degeneration in the dog. Br. J. Ophthalmol., *39*:349–352, 1955.

Priester, W.A.: Canine progressive retinal atrophy: Occurrence by age, breed and sex. Am. J. Vet. Res., *35*:571–574, 1974.

Rubin, L.F.: Atrophy of rods and cones in the cat retina. J. Am. Vet. Med. Assoc., *142*:1415–1420, 1963.

Rubin, L.F., and Lipton, D.E.: Retinal degeneration in kittens. J. Am. Vet. Med. Assoc., *162*:467–469, 1973.

Schardein, J.L., Lucas, J.A., and Fitzgerald, J.E.: Retinal dystrophy in Sprague-Dawley rats. Lab. Anim. Sci., *25*:323–326, 1975.

Shively, J.N., Epling, G.P., and Jensen, R.: Fine structure of the canine eye: Retina. Am. J. Vet. Res., *31*:1339–1359, 1970.

Shively, J.N., Phemister, R.D., Epling, G.P., and Jensen, R.: Dose relationships of pathologic alterations in the developing retina of irradiated dogs. Am. J. Vet. Res., *33*:2121–2134, 1972.

Sidman, R.L., and Green, M.C.: Retinal degeneration in the mouse. J. Hered., *56*:23–29, 1965.

Sorsby, A., et al.: Retinal dystrophy in the mouse: Histological and genetic aspects. J. Exp. Zool., *125*:171–197, 1954.

Steinberg, R.H., Reid, M., and Lacy, P.L.: The distribution of rods and cones in the retina of the cat (*Felis domesticus*). J. Comp. Neurol., *148*:229–248, 1973.

Tansley, K.: Hereditary degeneration of the mouse retina. Br. J. Ophthalmol., *35*:573–582, 1951.

von Sallman, L., and Grimes, P.: Retinal degeneration in mature rats. Comparison of the disease in an Osborne-Mendel and a spontaneously hypertensive Wistar strain. Invest. Ophthalmol., *13*:1010–1015, 1974.

Yates, C.M., et al.: Histological and biochemical studies on the retina of a new strain of dystrophic rat. Exp. Eye Res., *18*:119–133, 1974.

Retinal Dysplasia. Retinal dysplasia has been reported in young children, dogs, cattle, and rats as a congenital lesion, apparently present at birth. In children it may be associated with multiple anomalies; in puppies and rats it may be associated with microophthalmia. In dogs it has been reported in Sealyham Terriers, Bedlington Terriers, Beagles, Labrador Retrievers, Cocker Spaniels and English Springer Spaniels as an autosomal recessive inherited trait. Blindness is usually evident as soon as the behavior of the animal reaches a stage where detection is possible. In microscopic sections the retina is detached and thrown into disorganized folds and small rosettes. Differentiation of the retina may be incomplete, resulting in lack of definition of its multiple layers. In Herefords and Shorthorn cattle, retinal dysplasia and other ocular anomalies occur in association with hereditary congenital hydrocephalus.

Retinal dysplasia and necrosis have been produced in lambs with attenuated bluetongue virus vaccine as a component of the neurologic sequelae.

Ashton, N., Barnett, K.C., and Sachs, D.D.: Retinal dysplasia in the Sealyham Terrier. J. Pathol. Bacteriol., *96*:269–272, 1968.

Barnett, K.C., Bjorck, G.R., and Kock, E.: Hereditary retinal dysplasia in the Labrador Retriever in England and Sweden. J. Small Anim. Pract., *10*:755–759, 1970.

Carrig, C.B., et al.: Retinal dysplasia associated with skeletal abnormalities in Labrador Retrievers. J. Am. Vet. Med. Assoc., *170*:49–57, 1977.

Heywood, R., and Wells, G.A.H.: A retinal dysplasia in the Beagle dog. Vet. Rec., *87*:178–180, 1970.

Leipold, H.W., Gelatt, K.N., and Huston, K.: Multiple ocular anomalies and hydrocephalus in grade beef Shorthorn cattle. Am. J. Vet. Res., *32*:1019–1026, 1971.

Rubin, L.F.: Heredity of retinal dysplasia in Bedlington Terriers. J. Am. Vet. Med. Assoc., *152*:260–262, 1968.

Schmidt, G.M., et al.: Inheritance of retinal dysplasia in the English Springer Spaniel. J. Am. Vet. Med. Assoc., *174*:1089–1090, 1979.

Weisse, I., Stotzer, H., and Seitz, R.: (Neuroepithelial invagination, a form of retinal dysplasia in the Beagle.) Zentralbl. Veterinaermed., *20A*:89–99, 1973.

Choroid

The choroid is the posterior part of the middle, vascular tunic of the eye. It occupies the entire posterior part of the globe lying behind the ora ciliaris retinae except for the space containing the optic papilla. The retina lies on its inner surface, except in those areas where the two are separated by the tapetum. The sclera surrounds the choroid and gives it support and the entire globe its relative rigidity. The blood vessels of the choroid penetrate the sclera at various points, the locations depending upon the species.

The vascular nature of the choroid de-termines the kind of lesions to which it is subject. Metastatic neoplasms and bacterial emboli often lodge in the choroid, and leukocytes may readily escape the blood vessels to invade the choroidal stroma. The retina is commonly involved in inflammatory processes of the choroid, and to these the name **chorioretinitis** may be applied. The causes of chorioretinitis in animals are incompletely understood, but some of the infectious agents that have been demonstrated in chorioretinal lesions are *Toxoplasma gondii*, *Coccidioides immitis*, and *Mycobacterium tuberculosis*. Too few eyes of animals have been studied following or during the course of generalized infections

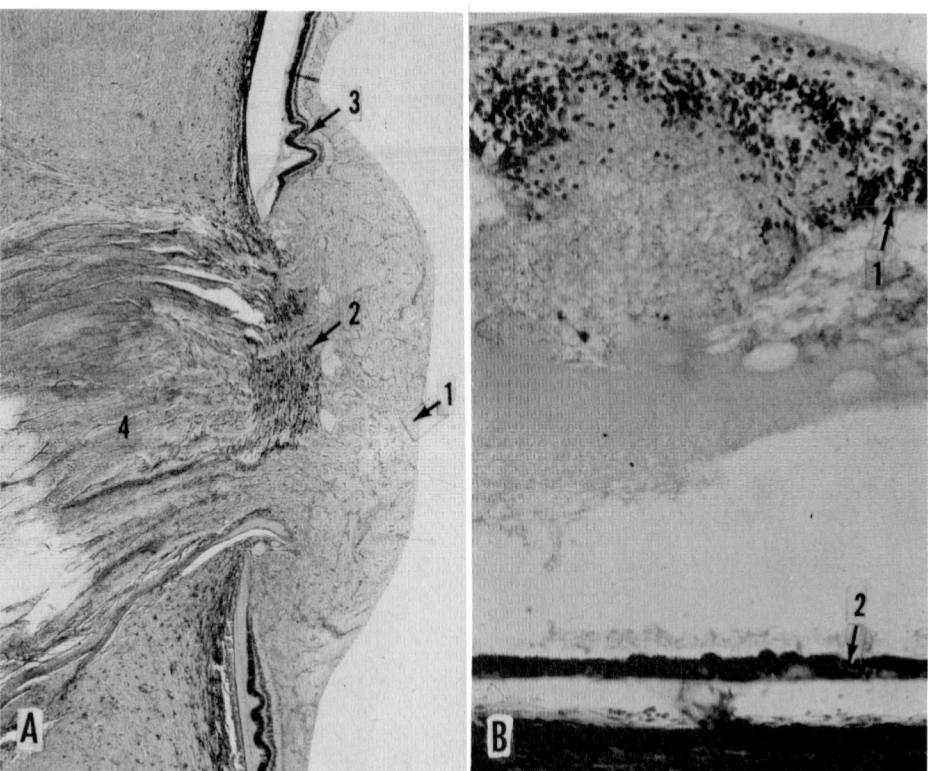

Fig. 28–17. *A*, Papilledema (× 17), eye of a ten-month-old Holstein calf which had been fed a ration low in vitamin A since birth. The optic papilla is elevated (*1*); the pigmented cribriform plate (2) is deflected inward; the retina folded (3); and the optic nerve edematous (4). Contributor: Dr. Louis L. Madsen. *B*, Detachment of the retina in equine periodic ophthalmia (× 165). Serous exudate in the layer of rods and cones and outer nuclear layer separates the latter (*1*) from the pigment epithelium (2). (*A*, Courtesy of Armed Forces Institute of Pathology.)

to determine how often the choroid is involved, but it probably is more frequent than the literature indicates.

Optic Nerve

Atrophy of the optic nerve has been reported in animals, usually secondary to retinopathy involving the ganglion cell layer. **Congenital hypoplasia** of the optic nerve has been reported by Saunders (1952) in purebred Merle Blue Collie puppies. In his cases, one or both of the optic nerves were grossly atrophic or absent and the optic nerve layer and ganglion cell layer of the retina were also atrophied. These changes were interpreted as resulting from degeneration in the retina, and no proof was found that they were inherited. Hypoplasia of the optic nerve has also been reported in cattle, cats, horses, and laboratory rodents. Complete agenesis of the optic nerve has been observed in rats and in swine with congenital anophthalmos; obviously the optic nerve would not develop in the absence of ganglion cells of the retina.

A proliferative optic neuropathy has been described in horses (Saunders et al., 1972). It was characterized by an accumulation of large foamy cells in the nerve and disc. It was thought to represent a storage disease.

Papilledema, or choked disc, is the term that denotes edema of the optic papilla and the adjacent retina. This lesion is sometimes associated with internal hydrocephalus but cannot always be explained on this basis. It has been observed in cattle maintained on diets deficient in vitamin A, but its pathogenesis in animals is by no means fully explained.

Ernest, J.T.: Bilateral optic nerve hypoplasia in a pup. J. Am. Vet. Med. Assoc., 168:125–128, 1976.

Gelatt, K.N., and Leipold, H.W.: Bilateral optic nerve hypoplasia in two dogs. Can. Vet. J., 12:91–96, 1971.

Gelatt, K.N., Leipold, H.W., and Coffman, J.R.: Bilateral optic nerve hypoplasia in a colt. J. Am. Vet. Med. Assoc., 155:627–631, 1969.

Moore, L.A., Huffman, C.F., and Duncan, C.W.: Blindness in cattle associated with constriction of optic nerve and probably of nutritional origin. J. Nutr., 9:533–551, 1935.

Saunders, L.Z.: Congenital optic nerve hypoplasia in Collie dogs. Cornell Vet., 42:67–80, 1952.

Saunders, L.Z., Bistner, S.I., and Rubin, L.F.: Proliferative optic neuropathy in horses. Vet. Pathol., 9:368–378, 1972.

Stubbs, E.L.: Blindness with papilledema in calves. J. Am. Vet. Med. Assoc., 105:209–211, 1944.

Other Hereditary and Congenital Anomalies

A variety of hereditary and congenital defects in addition to those already discussed may be encountered in the eye either singly or more often as multiple anomalies. They are observed in all species.

Coloboma, as it pertains to the eye, is defined as a congenital defect in the continuity of one of the tunics of the eye, usually the iris. The defect is seen as a cleft in the iris, and is believed to be the result of incomplete fusion of primordial parts in the optic vesicle during embryonic life.

Congenital anophthalmos, absence of the eye, has been observed in some animals, including swine, foals, dogs, cats, rats, and guinea pigs. This defect has been associated with maternal vitamin A deficiency in swine and is inherited in guinea pigs. Not only are the eyes absent, but also, as should be expected, the optic nerve and optic tract. Microscopically, however, remnants of the eye are usually present.

Congenital microphthalmos, decreased size of the eyes, has also been observed in dogs, rats, cattle, cats, and swine and is possibly related to the same factors that result in anophthalmos.

Congenital opacity of the cornea is most often encountered in cattle and dogs. The opacity results from edema but the pathogenesis is unknown. In Holstein-Friesian cattle in Germany and England, it is believed to be inherited as a recessive trait. It has also been described in Aberdeen Angus.

Hemeralopia (day-blindness) has been reported in two breeds of dogs, Alaskan Malamute and Poodles. Test crosses with clinically identified dogs indicate that this characteristic is inherited under the control of a single autosomal recessive gene. The lesions have not been reported.

Retinal lesions related to apparent hereditary or congenital factors have been discussed previously. Although such lesions as aplasia of optic nerves, albinism, and other defects have been reported in different species, it is not often that both the anatomic basis for the ocular defect and the evidence for their genetic background are entirely unequivocal. Much is still to be done by pathologists and geneticists to develop sound knowledge of this subject.

Barnett, K.C., and Grimes, T.D.: Verticillate corneal dystrophy in a dog. J. Small Anim. Pract., 12:297–299, 1971.

Barnett, K.C., and Ogden, A.L.: Ocular colobomata in Charolais cattle. Vet. Rec., 91:592, 1972.

Gelatt, K.N., Huston, K., and Leipold, H.S.: Ocular anomalies of incomplete albino cattle: Ophthalmoscopic examination. Am. J. Vet. Res., 30:1313–1316, 1969.

Gelatt, K.N., Leipold, H.H., and Huston, K.: Congenital ophthalmic anomalies in cattle. Mod. Vet. Pract., 57:105–109, 1976.

Gelatt, K.N., and McGill, L.D.: Clinical characteristics of microphthalmia with colobomas of the Australian Shepherd dog. J. Am. Vet. Med. Assoc., 162:393–396, 1973.

Herron, W.L., et al.: Retinal dystrophy in the rat—a pigment epithelial disease. Invest. Ophthal., 8:595–604, 1969.

Komich, R.J.: Anophthalmos: An inherited trait in a new stock of guinea pigs. Am. J. Vet. Res., 32:2099–2105, 1971.

Leipold, H.W., Gelatt, K.N., and Huston, K.: Multiple ocular anomalies and hydrocephalus in grade beef Shorthorn cattle. Am. J. Vet. Res., 32:1019–1026, 1971.

Leipold, H.W., and Huston, K.: Congenital syndrome of anophthalmia microphthalmia with associated defects in cattle. Pathol. Vet., 5:407–418, 1968.

McCormack, J., Powers, R.D., and Albert, R.A.: Typical colobomas in Charolais cattle. Vet. Med. Small Anim. Clin., 70:182–183, 185, 1975.

Priester, W.A.: Congenital ocular defects in cattle, horses, cats and dogs. J. Am. Vet. Med. Assoc., 160:1504–1511, 1972.

Roberts, S.R., and Bistner, S.I.: Persistent pupillary

membrane in Basenji dogs. J. Am. Vet. Med. Assoc., 153:533–542, 1968.

Rubin, L.F., Bourns, T.K.R., and Lord, L.H.: Hemeralopia in dogs: Heredity of hemeralopia in Alaskan Malamutes. Am. J. Vet. Res., 28:355–357, 1967.

Schmidt, R.E.: Colobomas in non-human primates. Folia Primatol., 14:256–268, 1971.

Überreiter, O.: (Retinochorioiditis maculosa disseminata in the dog.) Wien. Tierarztl. Mschr., 55:707–725, 1968. V.B. 39:2182, 1969.

Wikstrom, B., and Koch, E.: (Eye defects in Doberman puppies.) Svensk Veterinartidning, 26:37–38, 1974.

The Collie eye anomaly, first reported by Magrane (1953), has been referred to by many names which have resulted from the diverse clinical manifestations of the syndrome. Some of the names which have been applied are: Collie ectasia syndrome, congenital anomaly of optic nerve, congenital posterior ectasia of the sclera, ocular fundus anomaly, chorioretinal dysplasia, juxtapapillary staphyloma, retinal detachment, coloboma of optic disc, and excavated optic disc. This syndrome is now recognized as widespread in Collies, less frequent in other breeds. Evidence indicates that it is controlled by a single autosomal recessive gene with some variation in its expression (Yakely et al., 1968).

The lesions vary but may include any one or all of the following: Staphyloma or ectasia of the sclera near the optic disc (a defect in the sclera which allows the choroid and retina to dip into it), dysplasia of retina and choroid, detached retina, and intraocular hemorrhage. Some degree of microphthalmos may be present and pigmentary defects in the retina may be associated.

Barnett, K.C.: The collie eye anomaly. Vet. Rec., 84:431–434, 1969.

Latshaw, W.K., Wyman, M., and Venzke, W.G.: Embryologic development of an anomaly of ocular fundus in the Collie dog. Am. J. Vet. Res., 30:211–217, 1969.

Magrane, W.G.: Congenital anomaly of the optic nerve in Collies. North Am. Vet., 34:646, 1953.

Roberts, S.R.: The Collie eye anomaly. J. Am. Vet. Med. Assoc., 155:859–865, 1969.

Wyman, M., and Donovan, E.F.: Eye anomaly of the Collie. J. Am. Vet. Med. Assoc., *155*:866–870, 1969.

Yakely, W.L., et al.: Genetic transmission of an ocular fundus anomaly in Collies. J. Am. Vet. Med. Assoc., *152*:457–461, 1968.

Glaucoma

The term *glaucoma* appeared in the writings of Hippocrates but its present meaning has evolved over many centuries, and is broader than indicated by its derivation. Glaucoma is not a specific disease entity but a composite of the clinical and pathologic manifestations that result from persistent increase in intraocular pressure. Although the disease in the human subject has been studied for many centuries, many aspects of its causation and pathogenesis remain unknown. For example, the changes that initiate the intraocular hypertension often cannot be demonstrated. Although occlusion of the filtration angle is believed to be the basis for the hypertension, even this is uncertain in some instances. Because most glaucomatous eyes become available for pathologic study only after prolonged involvement, little is known of the early changes. The advantages of careful study of spontaneous glaucoma in animals would appear to be obvious, but little has been done to attack the problem from this approach.

Certain classifying terms concerning glaucoma in the human eye are well entrenched in the literature. For example, if the apparent underlying cause is demonstrable (anterior synechia following iridocyclitis or trauma to the eyeball, deformities of the lens, detachment of the retina, intraocular hemorrhage, intraocular neoplasms, or circulatory stasis), the condition is called **secondary glaucoma.** If a possible underlying pathologic process is not demonstrated, the term **primary glaucoma** is used. **Absolute glaucoma** is used to describe the distended, turgid, hopelessly blind eye that is the conse-

quence of prolonged intraocular hypertension.

Both primary and secondary glaucoma occur in animals. Primary glaucoma has been best studied in the dog; it is particularly frequent in Spaniels, Basset Hounds, and Beagles. Bedford (1975) has associated primary glaucoma in the dog with inherent structural defects of the iridocorneal angle, which for poorly understood reasons undergoes acute closure. A hereditary primary glaucoma occurs in certain strains of rabbits as an autosomal recessive trait.

Glaucoma may be unilateral or, more often, bilateral, and is recognized in early stages by increased intraocular tension which eventually enlarges the globe (buphthalmos), sometimes with apparent exophthalmos. Initially the cornea is edematous and opaque, and in later stages this opacity is accentuated by a degenerative pannus.

The underlying feature usually considered basic to the development of glaucoma is interference with the circulation of the intraocular fluid (aqueous). Aqueous is secreted into the posterior chamber by the ciliary epithelium. From the posterior chamber, this fluid moves through the pupil into the anterior chamber. The aqueous humor drains from the anterior chamber at the filtration angle near the limbus, where it passes through the spaces of Fontana and eventually reaches the veins at the limbus through the canals of Schlemm. If the filtration angle is occluded—for example, by peripheral anterior synechiae—and aqueous continues to enter the posterior chamber, the fluid pressure must increase. If the pupil is occluded for any reason, aqueous will accumulate behind the iris and force it to bulge forward into the anterior chamber (see iris bombé).

Lesions. The findings on pathologic study of the affected eye can be correlated with those of the clinical examination. The globe is enlarged, increasingly spherical,

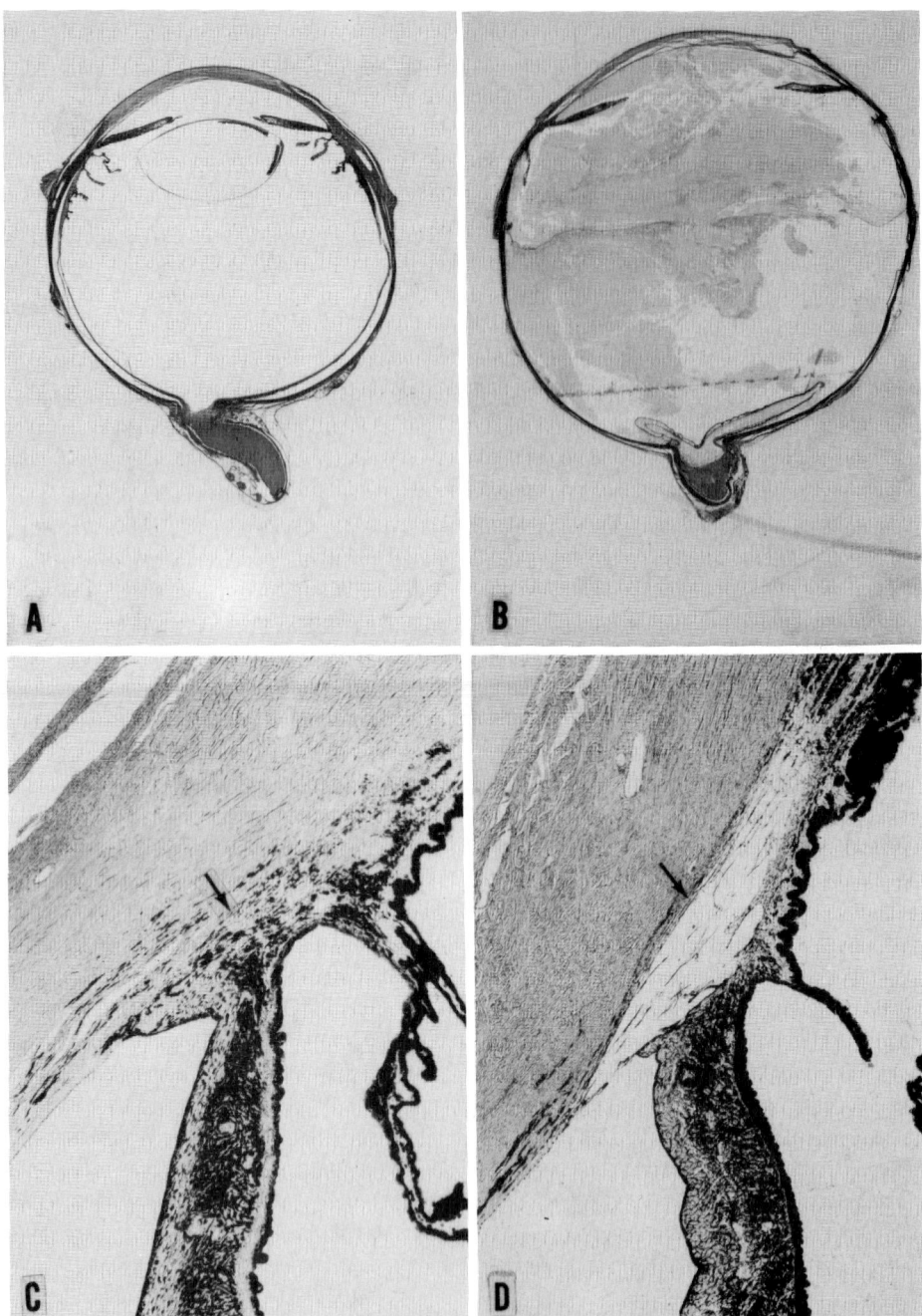

Fig. 28–18. Canine glaucoma. *A,* Section (× 2) of the left eye of a dog with moderately severe glaucoma. Note spherical outline of the eye, occlusion of the filtration angle, and cupping of the optic disc. *B,* Absolute glaucoma in the right eye of the same dog as *A* (× 2). Buphthalmos, severe cupping of the optic disc, disorganization of contents of globe. *C,* Filtration angle (× 35) of same eye as in *A.* Note occlusion (arrow). Contributor: Dr. Leon Z. Saunders. *D,* Normal filtration angle, eye of a dog (× 35). Compare with *C.* (*C,* Courtesy of Armed Forces Institute of Pathology.)

and turgid. The cornea is opaque, as also may be the lens and vitreous. Microscopically evident changes may be found in most of the ocular structures, depending upon the stage in which the eye is studied. In two human cases examined in the early stages, obliteration of one or more of the vortex veins by thrombosis, endophlebitis or periphlebitis has been reported, but this undoubtedly important feature has not been noted in animals. Edema in the corneal epithelium is usually seen in the form of small vacuoles which may coalesce to produce small bullae. It is thought that increased pressure in the anterior chamber forces this fluid through the corneal stroma and into the epithelium.

Significant changes are usually found at the filtration angle. Peripheral anterior synechiae may occlude the filtration angle (Fig. 28–18). The iris is usually thin and atrophic and its blood vessels sometimes are sclerotic. The ciliary processes are thin, compressed, and atrophic. The choroid may be similarly compressed and atrophied, eventually appearing only as a thin pigmented membrane containing some thick-walled hyaline vessels. The retina undergoes degenerative changes after prolonged intraocular hypertension, an effect believed to be due to retinal ischemia.

In the dog, Parry (1953) has described glaucomatous retinopathy, which results in complete blindness and is characterized histologically by atrophy, which is more severe in the inner than the outer layers of the retina. Ganglion cells are lost early, followed by disappearance of optic nerve fibers. The bipolar cells of the inner nuclear layer are next to disappear, but the outer nuclear layer and the layer of rods and cones are only slightly damaged. This degeneration is usually more advanced in the nontapetal areas of the retina; the tapetal fundus and central fundus are relatively spared. In the peripheral fundus the retina usually exhibits the most advanced sclerosis. There is little or no disturbance of the retinal pigment.

The optic nerve undergoes pathologic changes that are typical for glaucoma. In the advanced stages, the intraocular hypertension causes depression of the optic disc into the characteristic cup shape (cupping of the disc). This change starts with atrophy of the nerve fibers in the area where they go through the lamina cribrosa. The fibers of the lamina cribrosa are also deflected outward to form the cup-shaped space which is usually filled with vitreous. It must be remembered that in some animals (e.g., the elephant) the disc is normally cupped, hence the normal histologic features must be considered in interpreting this change. Cupping of the disc is usually considered to be the direct result of pressure upon the nerve fibers, but a divergent view holds that the pressure first affects the blood supply to the disc, the neuritic atrophy following secondarily.

Diagnosis. Diagnosis of glaucoma may be based upon the clinical and pathologic evidences of increased intraocular tension that have been described.

Beckh, W.: A case of spontaneous glaucoma in a rabbit. Am. J. Ophthalmol., 18:1144–1145, 1935.

Bedford, P.G.C.: The aetiology of primary glaucoma in the dog. J. Small Anim. Pract., 16:217–239, 1975.

Gelatt, K.N., Peiffer, R.L., Jr., Gwin, R.M., and Sauk, J.J., Jr.: Glaucoma in the Beagle. Trans. Am. Acad. Ophthalmol. Otolaryngol., 81:636–644, 1976.

Jourdan, R.J.: Pathogenesis of canine glaucoma. J. Am. Vet. Med. Assoc., 117:419–422, 1950.

Lovekin, L.G., and Bellhorn, R.W.: Clinicopathologic changes in primary glaucoma in the Cocker Spaniel. Am. J. Vet. Res., 29:379–385, 1968.

Parry, H.B.: Degenerations of the dog retina. III. Retinopathy secondary to glaucoma. Br. J. Ophthalmol., 37:670–679, 1953.

Podos, S.M.: Animal models of human glaucoma. Trans. Am. Acad. Ophthalmol. Otolaryngol., 81:632–635, 1976.

Wyman, M., and Ketring, K.: Congenital glaucoma in the Basset Hound: A biologic model. Trans. Am. Acad. Ophthalmol. Otolaryngol., 81:645–652, 1976.

Young, C., Festing, M.F.W., and Barnett, K.C.: Buphthalmos (congenital glaucoma) in the rat. Lab. Anim., 8:21–31, 1974.

Neoplasms

Extraocular Neoplasms. Neoplasms may arise from any of the specialized or sup-

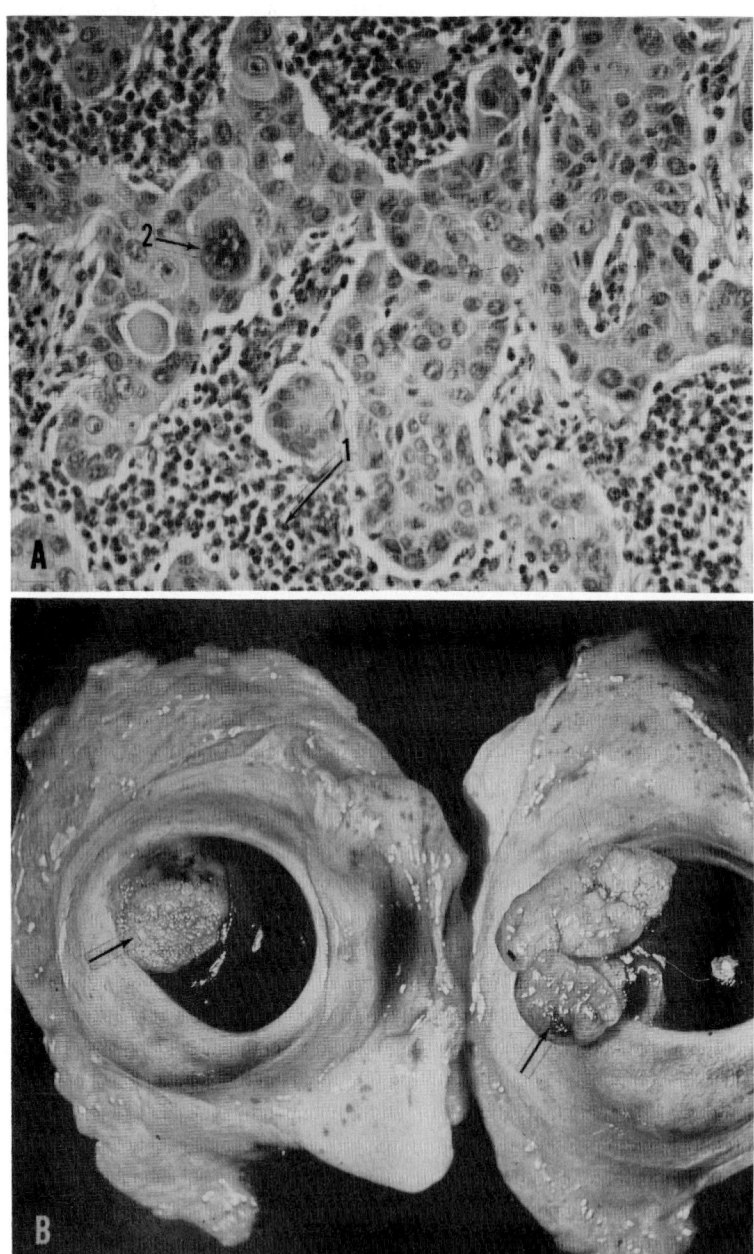

Fig. 28–19.   Squamous cell carcinoma ($\times$ 224) arising in corneal epithelium of an 11-year-old Hereford cow. The infiltrating tumor cells are surrounded by leukocytes (*1*) and have bizarre giant nuclei (*2*). (Courtesy of Armed Forces Institute of Pathology.) Contributor: Drs. C.N. Barron and G.T. Easley. *B*, Squamous cell carcinomas in both eyes of a Jersey cow. Note that each is attached at the limbus but extends over the cornea. Photograph courtesy of Dr. C.L. Davis.

porting tissues of the eyelids, conjunctiva, or orbit. Squamous cell carcinoma of the skin of the eyelid or conjunctiva is especially frequent in cattle, less so in horses and dogs, and infrequent in other species. In cattle this tumor most frequently arises from the corneal epithelium at the limbus and may invade and destroy the entire orbital contents. Papillomas may arise from the same structures. They are common in dogs but most frequent in cattle and are believed to be precursors of squamous cell carcinoma.

Basal cell tumors are less frequent than squamous cell carcinoma. Sebaceous gland (or meibomian gland) tumors of the eyelids are most common in dogs but reported in other species. Reference has already been made to dermoids and epidermal inclusion cysts. In dogs the eyelid is a frequent site for malignant melanomas. Mast cell tumors may also arise in the eyelid. Fibromas, leiomyomas, neurofibromas, lipomas, hemangiomas, and their malignant counterparts may arise in the orbit but are not common. Equine sarcoid occurs on the eyelid. Retrobulbar meningiomas are rarely seen, as are optic nerve gliomas.

Intraocular Neoplasms. Saunders and Barron (1958) reviewed intraocular tumors of animals and described 15 additional cases in dogs. They stated intraocular tumors have been observed in horses, cattle, sheep, cats, dogs, fish, a rabbit, and a hen.

Tumors arising within the orbit, however, are rare in animals. They are most frequent in dogs. They include malignant melanomas, adenomas and adenocarcinomas of the ciliary epithelium, retinoblastoma, and medulloepithelioma.

Malignant melanoma is the most frequent intraocular tumor. These tumors are most common in dogs, but are reported in cats, horses, cattle, and rats. They usually arise from the iris or ciliary body and less often from the choroid, which is the usual site in human beings. They may be heavily pigmented or amelanotic and take the many varied histologic patterns of malignant melanomas at other sites.

Adenomas and adenocarcinomas arising from pigmented or nonpigmented epithelium of the iris or ciliary body are most common in dogs and rarely reported in other species. Adenomas are comprised of cuboidal or columnar epithelial cells which form acinar, tubular, or papillary structures and less often, solid masses. They usually but not invariably contain melanin. The cells of adenocarcinomas tend to be more varied in shape and appear in more solid sheets. There is local invasion but rarely metastasis.

Retinoblastoma, or neuroepithelioma, arises in the eye from the precursors of the neuroepithelial receptor cells of the retina. Like the medulloblastoma and neuroblastoma, it consists of small cells with nuclei suggestive of lymphocytes. It also tends to form rosettes. Retinoblastoma is malignant, metastasizing to the regional lymph nodes. It occurs in the very young and has a startlingly high incidence in some human families. These tumors appear to be rare in animals. Saunders and Rubin (1975) state that there is no authentic case of retinoblastoma reported in a domestic animal.

Medulloepithelioma in the eye has been reported in a horse (Ramsey and Blodi, 1967), and a dog (Lahav et al., 1976). This neoplasm is composed of small round or oval cells that predominantly grow in solid masses, with collections of cells forming rosettes or tubular structures. The example reported in the dog included cartilage and ganglion cells, a feature seen in similar tumors of human beings and termed teratoid medulloepithelioma.

A single example of **ganglioglioma** has been described in a dog by Saunders et al. (1969). The tumor contained a mixture of large neurons, neoplastic glial cells, and ependyma-like cells.

Metastatic neoplasms in the orbit or eye are rare except for malignant lymphoma. In cattle it usually surrounds the orbit, whereas in dogs and cats there is frequent intraocular spread.

Barron, C.N., et al.: Intraocular tumors in animals. V. Transmissible venereal tumor of dogs. Am. J. Vet. Res., 24:1263–1269, 1963.

Bellhorn, R.W., and Henkind, P.: Adenocarcinoma of the ciliary body. A report of 2 cases in dogs. Pathol. Vet., 5:122–126, 1968.

Bistner, S.I.: Medullo-epithelioma of the iris and ciliary body in a horse. Cornell Vet., 64:588–595, 1974.

Blodi, F.C., and Ramsey, F.K.: Ocular tumors in domestic animals. Am. J. Ophthalmol., 64:627–633, 1967.

Gelatt, K.N., Leipold, H.W., Finocchio, E.J., and Coffman, J.R.: Optic disc astrocytoma in a horse. Can. Vet. J., 12:53–55, 1971.

Gelatt, K.N., Myers, V.S., Jr., Perman, V., and Jessen, C.: Conjunctival squamous cell carcinoma in the horse. J. Am. Vet. Med. Assoc., 165:617–620, 1974.

Krehbiel, J.D., and Langham, R.F.: Eyelid neoplasms of dogs. Am. J. Vet. Res., 36:115–119, 1975.

Lahav, M., Albert, D.M., Kircher, C.H., and Percy, D.H.: Malignant teratoid medulloepithelioma in a dog. Vet. Pathol., 13:11–16, 1976.

Lavach, J.D., and Severin, G.A.: Neoplasia of the equine eye, adnexa, and orbit: A review of 68 cases. J. Am. Vet. Med. Assoc., 170:202–208, 1977.

Ramsey, F.K., and Blodi, F.C.: Ocular tumors in domestic animals. Am. J. Ophthalmol., 64:627–633, 1967.

Saunders, L.Z., and Barron, C.N.: Primary intraocular tumors. Cancer Res., 18:234–245, 1958.

Saunders, L.Z., Geil, L.W., and Barron, C.N.: Intraocular ganglioglioma in a dog. Pathol. Vet., 6:525–533, 1969.

Saunders, L.Z., and Rubin, L.F.: Ophthalmic Pathology of Animals. An Atlas and Reference Book. Basel, S. Karger, 1975.

Simu, G., Ivascu, I., Muresan, E., and Papay, Z.: Histological and histoenzymochemical aspects of ocular tumours in cattle. Zentralbl. Veterinaermed., 20A:763–774, 1973.

Szymanski, C.M.: Bilateral metastatic intraocular hemangiosarcoma in a dog. J. Am. Vet. Med. Assoc., 161:803–805, 1972.

Williams, J.O., Garlick, E.C., and Beard, D.C.: Glioma of the optic nerve of a dog. J. Am. Vet. Med. Assoc., 138:377–378, 1961.

EAR

The ears of animals do not often come to the pathologist's attention as separate organs but are usually studied in connection with generalized lesions or because of some incidental finding. It seems desirable to describe the few specific lesions that have been recognized in ears of animals, and to recapitulate briefly some of the systemic diseases in which the ear may become involved. These lesions may be conveniently described in connection with the anatomic divisions of the ear, i.e., the external, middle, and inner ear.

External Ear

The external ear consists of the external auricular appendage (auricula) with its cartilage covered by skin, its muscles, and the external auditory meatus which is supported by the cartilage and surrounded by epidermis richly supplied with sebaceous glands, and specialized apocrine glands (ceruminous glands). The external ear is limited in its deepest aspect by the tympanic membrane (*tympanum*). The anatomic details (such as size and position of the auricular appendage, depth and course of the external auditory meatus) in each species are different, hence must be considered individually, but only those features that influence the nature of lesions are discussed here.

Inflammation of the external ear, **otitis externa,** is not uncommon in animals and may result from a variety of causes. Among the specific infectious agents is *Actinomyces bovis,* which may produce a specific granulomatous inflammation of the external ear of swine. This infection usually involves the auricular appendage only, giving it a thick, indurated appearance. Histologically, a granulomatous tissue reaction, characteristic of actinomycosis, is found in the subcutis around the cartilage and sometimes involving the cartilage. In other species, specific infections are uncommon, but nonspecific infections may result from wounds (usually caused by bites) of the external ear.

Parasitic infestations of the external ear are common in most animals and are usually due to parasites that have a specific affinity for the ear. The ear mites of rabbits, sheep, cattle, and horses, *Psoroptes communis* (var. *cuniculi, ovis,* etc.); cats

(*Notoedres cati*), and dogs (*Otodectes cynotis*) have an obligate affinity for the external ear. These acarid (mite) parasites are specific for each species; the variety that infests the rabbit is particularly common. These mites burrow into the epidermis lining the external auditory meatus and cause profuse exudation with accumulation of tenacious, brown, waxy material in the meatus and, in severe cases, over the inner surface of the external ear. Parasitic otitis externa may in some cases cause rupture of the tympanum and involve the middle ear.

Ticks may also attack the external ear, the most common being the spinose ear tick, *Otobius megnini*, of cattle.

Dermatomycosis is often particularly severe in, or limited to, the external ear. The lesions are not significantly different from those in the skin elsewhere in the body, but the term **otomycosis** may be used to designate infection of this type when limited chiefly to the ear.

Yeasts are often associated with chronic otitis externa in the dog but it is not known whether these organisms are actually the cause of the inflammation.

Otitis externa is extremely common in dogs. Anatomic peculiarities of the ear, mites, and various other organisms have been incriminated as the cause, but no single theory is universally accepted.

Of particular interest among the causes of severe otitis are the awns of certain grasses (particularly foxtail grass) which may lodge in the external ear. Otitis of this etiology is especially frequent in dogs in certain western states. When these bearded grasses penetrate deep into the external meatus, it is difficult to withdraw them. Severe otitis externa develops and the awns may even break through the tympanum to set up severe inflammation in the middle and internal ear.

Of interest is the occurrence, in cats and sometimes dogs, of **inflammatory polyps** which are attached by a thin pedicle to, or in the region of, the tympanum. These polyps may become relatively large, filling the external auditory meatus, and in some cases may be connected through the eustachian tube with a similar polyp which lies in the nasopharynx (Fig. 20–1). These polyps histologically consist of richly cellular connective tissue, liberally supplied with blood vessels and usually infiltrated by leukocytes, particularly when the squamous epithelium covering the mass is eroded. The cause and exact nature of these polyps is unknown. Although they may recur after surgical excision, they do not appear to be neoplastic.

Neoplasms which are likely to be encountered in the external ear include any new growth of the skin, its adnexa, or the cartilage. **Adenomas and adenocarcinomas of the ceruminous glands** of the external ear are occasionally encountered in the dog and cat (Fig. 28–20). They are usually be-

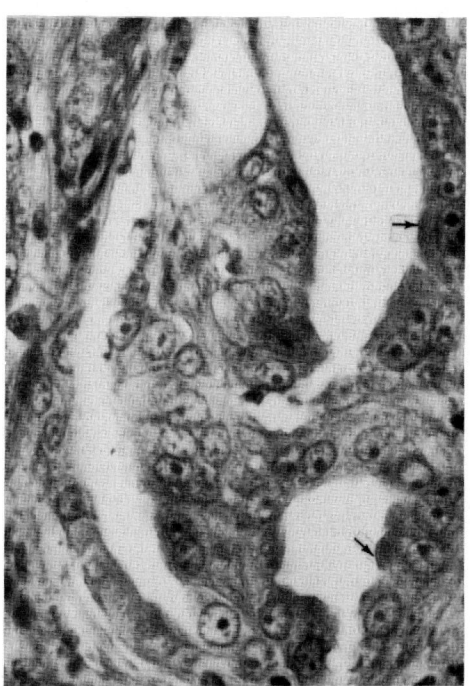

Fig. 28–20. Adenoma of ceruminous gland (× 545), ear of an eight-year-old mongrel dog. Tumor contains large columnar cells with granular cytoplasm (arrows). (Courtesy of Armed Forces Institute of Pathology.) Contributor: Dr. S.W. Stiles.

nign, nodular growths, 1 or 2 cm in diameter, which bulge into the auditory canal, but may become locally invasive or metastasize to the regional lymph nodes. Microscopically, they consist of rather ordinary glandular acini with lumens of generous size and linings of simple columnar or cuboidal epithelium (Black, 1949). These tumors are distinguished by a golden brown, crystalline pigment in the cytoplasm of the epithelial cells.

The specific neoplasm of horses and mules, **equine sarcoid,** appears at the base of the ear or even on the auricula. Chondromas and chondrosarcomas may arise from the auricular cartilage, but only a few have been reported.

Middle Ear

The middle ear includes the tympanic cavity with its contents and the auditive (eustachian) tubes. In the horse, two large diverticula of the eustachian tubes, the guttural pouches, are also part of the middle ear. The tympanic cavity is lined with epithelium which is continuous with that of the nasal mucosa through the eustachian tubes. The contents include the chain of auditory ossicles (malleus, incus, os lenticulare, and stapes) which communicate vibrations of the tympanum to the inner ear. This tympanic cavity is located within the tympanic and petrous parts of the temporal bone.

Infection of the middle ear **(otitis media)** may reach the tympanic cavity from the external ear by rupture of the tympanum, or may extend from the nasopharynx by way of the eustachian tubes. Extension of otitis externa to involve the middle ear is not infrequent in ear mite infestation and with penetrating foreign bodies (grass awns). The inflammation is usually purulent and tends to be chronic. Otitis media is especially frequent in laboratory rats with chronic murine pneumonia and rabbits with pasteurellosis. Occlusion of the eusta-

chian tube predisposes to otitis media. Spread of infection from the middle or internal ear sometimes leads to meningitis.

Non-neoplastic cholesteatomas are frequent in humans as sequelae to otitis media. Similar lesions have been described in rabbits and guinea pigs.

Inner Ear

The inner ear consists of two parts: (1) the membranous labyrinth in which are found the auditory cells and the peripheral ramifications of the auditory nerve, and (2) the osseous labyrinth, a series of cavities in the petrous temporal bone which enclose the membranous labyrinth. The osseous labyrinth is divided into three parts, the vestibule, the cochlea, and the semicircular canals. The membranous labyrinth, which occupies but does not completely fill the osseous labyrinth, is surrounded by the perilymphatic space. The labyrinth contains four divisions: the auricle, the saccule, the semicircular ducts, and the cochlear duct. The inner ear is concerned not only with hearing but also with the sense of equilibrium.

Involvement of the inner ear **(otitis interna; labyrinthitis),** in the presence of otitis media, is manifested clinically by disturbances in equilibrium. Examples are the otitis interna of rats and mice, presumably resulting from spread of otitis media caused by "pleuropneumonia-like organisms" (PPLO). One of the few studies on the pathologic anatomy of the inner ear of domesticated animals is by Cohrs (1928), who described the histologic features of the inner ear in the horse, and also atrophy of the cochlear apparatus of horses in which no clinical signs were recognized. Certain viruses in human beings may cause labyrinthitis and deafness (mumps, congenital rubella, measles).

Congenital deafness occurs in several species; cat, mink, dog, guinea pigs (waltzing), and mice (waltzing). In the mink and cat, deafness is the result of degenerative changes in the organ of Corti which are associated with white coat color. The deaf white cat was observed and commented upon by Darwin more than a hundred years ago and the histologic features of the affected organ of Corti have been known since the turn of the twentieth century. It appears to be established that the defect is associated with the white coat color (which is due to the dominant white gene [W] in the cat, not albino) and may occur in the presence of blue, yellow or "odd-eyed" (heterochromia iridis) iris color. The mode of inheritance of the deafness and eye color appears to be complex and is not completely understood. The deafness is more frequent, in our experience, in blue-eyed white cats, but may occur in dominant white cats of any iris color.

The lesions may be seen histologically in kittens after they reach four days of age. Starting with degeneration of the hair cells of the organ of Corti, the lesion progresses to collapse of the tunnel of Corti, contraction of the tectorial membrane, and complete sacculo-cochlear collapse by 21 days. There is loss of ganglion cells in the spiral ganglion, and the ventral cochlear nucleus and the superior olivary complex are reduced in size. The inner ear lesions may be bilateral or unilateral. Hereditary deafness in Dalmatian dogs and mink appears to follow the same process as in white cats.

Adams, E.W.: Hereditary deafness in a family of Foxhounds. J. Am. Vet. Med. Assoc., 128:302–303, 1956.

Alexander, G.: Zur vergleichenden, pathologischen Anatomie des Gehörorganes. I. Gehörorgan und Gehirn einer unvollkommen albino-tischen weissen Katze. Archiv. Ohrenheilkunde, 50:159–181, 1900.

Altman, F.: Histologic picture of inherited nerve deafness in man and animals. Arch. Otolaryngol., 51:852–890, 1950.

Anderson, H., et al.: Genetic hearing impairment in the Dalmatian dog. An audiometric, genetic and morphologic study in 53 dogs. Acta Otolaryngol. Suppl., 232:34 pp, 1967.

Bamber, R.C.: Correlation between white coat colour, blue eyes and deafness in cats. J. Genet., 27:407–413, 1927.

Black, M.B.: Adenoma of ceruminous gland in the dog. Arch. Pathol., 48:85–88, 1949.

Bosher, S.K., and Hallpike, C.S.: Observations on the histological features, development and pathogenesis of the inner ear degeneration of the deaf white cat. Proc. Roy. Soc. Lond. Ser. B, 162:147–170, 1965.

Brown, K.S., Bergsma, D.R., and Barrow, M.V.: Animal models of pigment and hearing abnormalities in man. Birth Defects, 7:102–109, 1971.

Cohrs, P.: Studien zur normalen und pathologischen Anatomie und Histologie des inneren Gehörorganes vom Pferde (Equus caballus). Leipzig, F.C.W. Vogel, 1928.

Davis, L.E., and Johnson, R.T.: Experimental viral infections of the inner ear. I. Acute infections of the newborn hamster labyrinth. Lab. Invest., 34:349–356, 1976.

Fernando, S.D.A.: Certain histopathologic features of the external auditory meatus of the cat and dog with otitis externa. Am. J. Vet. Res., 28:278–282, 1967.

Flatt, R.E., DeYoung, D.W., and Hogle, R.M.: Suppurative otitis media in the rabbit: Prevalence, pathology, and microbiology. Lab. Anim. Sci., 27:343–347, 1977.

Fraser, G.: Aetiology of otitis externa in the dog. J. Small Anim. Pract., 6:445–452, 1965.

Fraser, G., Withers, A.R., and Spreull, J.S.A.: Otitis externa in the dog. J. Small Anim. Pract., 2:32–47, 1961.

Fraser, G., et al.: Canine ear disease. J. Small Anim. Pract., 10:725–754, 1970.

Getty, R., Foust, H.L., Presley, E.T., and Miller, M.E.: Microscopic anatomy of the ear of the dog. Am. J. Vet. Res., 17:364–375, 1956.

Hilding, D.A., Sugiura, A., and Nakai, Y.: Deaf white mink: Electron microscopic study of the inner ear. Ann. Otol. Rhinol. Laryngol., 76:647–663, 1967.

Hudson, W.R., and Ruben, R.J.: Hereditary deafness in Dalmatians. Arch. Otolaryngol., 75:213–216, 1962.

Karmody, C.S.: Viral labyrinthitis—an experimental study. Ann. Otol. Rhinol. Laryngol., 84:179–181, 1975.

Krogh, H.V., Linnet, A., and Knudsen, P.B.: Otitis externa in the dog—clinical and microbiological study. Nord. Vet. Med., 27:285–295, 1975.

Mair, I.W.S.: Hereditary deafness in the Dalmatian dog. Arch. Otol. Rhinol. Laryngol., 212:1–14, 1976.

Olson, L.D., and McCune, E.L.: Histopathology of chronic otitis media in the rat. Lab. Anim. Care, 18:478–485, 1968.

Rankin, J.D., and Karmody, C.S.: Serous otitis media. An experimental model. Arch. Otolaryngol., 92:14–23, 1970.

Saunders, L.Z.: The histopathology of hereditary congenital deafness in white mink. Pathol. Vet., 2:256–263, 1965.

Sharma, V.D., and Rhoades, H.E.: The occurrence and microbiology of otitis externa in the dog. J. Small Anim. Pract., 16:241–247, 1975.

Smith, J.M.B.: The association of yeasts with chronic otitis externa in the dog. Aust. Vet. J., *44*:413–415, 1968. V.B. *39*:1518, 1968.

Strickland, J.H., and Calhoun, M.L.: The microscopic anatomy of the external ear of *Felis domesticus*. Am. J. Vet. Res., *21*:845–850, 1960.

Thoonen, J., and Hoorens, J.: Infection of the bulla tympanica and adjacent parts of the ear in pigs. Vlaams Diergeneesk. Tijdschr., *31*:237–243, 1962.

West, C.D., and Harrison, J.M.: Transneuronal cell atrophy in the congenitally deaf white cat. J. Comp. Neurol., *151*:377–398, 1973.

Index

Page numbers in **boldface** indicate principal discussion; numbers in *italics* indicate figures; numbers followed by t indicate tables.